KU-530-380

2006 Oncology Nursing Drug Handbook

Gail M. Wilkes, MSN, RNC, AOCN
Oncology Nurse Practitioner and
Clinical Instructor
Boston Medical Center
Boston, Massachusetts

Margaret Barton-Burke, PhD, RN
Assistant Professor
University of Massachusetts
Amherst, Massachusetts

JONES AND BARTLETT PUBLISHERS
Sudbury, Massachusetts
BOSTON TORONTO LONDON SINGAPORE

World Headquarters
Jones and Bartlett Publishers
40 Tall Pine Drive
Sudbury, MA 01776
978-443-5000
info@jbpub.com
www.jbpub.com

Jones and Bartlett Publishers Canada
6339 Ormindale Way
Mississauga, Ontario L5V 1J2
CANADA

Jones and Bartlett Publishers International
Barb House, Barb Mews
London W6 7PA
UK

Jones and Bartlett's books and products are available through most bookstores and online booksellers. To contact Jones and Bartlett Publishers directly, call 800-832-0034, fax 978-443-8000, or visit our website at www.jbpub.com.

Substantial discounts on bulk quantities of Jones and Bartlett's publications are available to corporations, professional associations, and other qualified organizations. For details and specific discount information, contact the special sales department at Jones and Bartlett via the above contact information or send an email to specialsales@jbpub.com.

Copyright © 2006, 2005, 2004, 2003, 2002, 2001, 2000, 1999, 1997, 1994 by Jones and Bartlett Publishers, Inc.

All rights reserved. No part of the material protected by this copyright notice may be reproduced or utilized in any form, electronic or mechanical, including photocopying, recording, or any information storage or retrieval system, without written permission from the copyright owner.

ISBN: 0-7637-3923-5
ISSN: 1536-0024
6048

Production Credits
Executive Publisher: Chris Davis
Associate Editor: Kathy Richardson
Production Director: Amy Rose
Production Editor: Renée Sekerak
Production Assistant: Rachel Rossi
Marketing Manager: Emily Ekle
Manufacturing and Inventory Coordinator: Amy Bacus
Cover Design: Kristin E. Ohlin
Composition: ATLIS Systems
Printing and Binding: Malloy, Inc.
Cover Printing: Malloy, Inc.

The drug information presented in the 2006 Oncology Nursing Drug Handbook has been derived from standard reference sources, recently published data, and respected pharmaceutical texts. The writers and publishers of this book have made every effort to ensure that the information and dosage regimens presented are accurate and in accord with current labeling at the time of publication. However, in view of the constant and rapid flow of information resulting from ongoing research and clinical experience, as well as changes in government regulations, readers are urged to check the package insert and consult with a pharmacist, if necessary, for each drug they plan to administer to be certain that changes have not been made in its indications or contraindications, or in the recommended dosage for each use. While the drugs included in this publication were chosen on the basis of frequency of use and appropriate indications, the publisher and authors do not necessarily advocate, and take no responsibility for, the use of products described herein.

Printed in the United States of America
09 08 07 06 05 10 9 8 7 6 5 4 3 2 1

Jones and Bartlett Series in Oncology
Recently Published

The Cancer Journal
Journal of the National Comprehensive Cancer Network
American Cancer Society Patient Education Guide to Oncology Drugs, Second Edition, Wilkes/Ades
American Cancer Society Consumer's Guide to Cancer Drugs, Second Edition, Wilkes/Ades/Krakoff
Biotherapy: A Comprehensive Overview, Second Edition, Reiger
Blood and Marrow Stem Cell Transplantation, Second Edition, Whedon
Cancer and HIV Clinical Nutrition Pocket Guide, Second Edition, Wilkes
Cancer Chemotherapy: A Nursing Process Approach, Third Edition, Barton-Burke/Wilkes/Ingwerson
Cancer Nursing: Principles and Practice, Sixth Edition, Yarbro/Frogge/Goodman/Groenwald
A Cancer Source Book for Nurses, Eighth Edition, American Cancer Society
Cancer Symptom Management, Third Edition, Yarbro/Frogge/Goodman
Cancer Symptom Management, Patient Self-Care Guides, Second Edition, Yarbro/Frogge/Goodman
Chemotherapy Care Plans Handbook, Third Edition, Barton-Burke/Wilkes/Ingwersen
A Clinical Guide to Cancer Nursing, Fifth Edition, Yarbro/Frogge/Goodman
A Clinical Guide to Stem Cell and Bone Marrow Transplantation, Shapiro et al.
Clinical Handbook for Biotherapy, Rieger
Contemporary Issues in Breast Cancer: A Nursing Perspective, Second Edition, Hassey Dow
Contemporary Issues in Colorectal Cancer: A Nursing Perspective, Berg
Contemporary Contemporary Issues in Lung Cancer: A Nursing Perspective, Haas
Contemorary Issues in Lymphoma, Poniatowski et al.
Contemporary Issues in Prostate Cancer: A Nursing Perspective, Held Warmkessel
Dx/Rx: Upper Gastrointestinal Malignancies: Cancers of the Stomach and Esophagus, Shah, Series Editor
Dx/Rx: Lung Cancer, Azzoli
Dx/Rx: Leukemia, Burke
Fatigue in Cancer: A Multidimensional Approach, Winningham/Barton-Burke
Glioblastoma Multiforme, Markert et al.
Handbook of Breast Cancer Risk-Assessment: Evidence-Based Guidelines for Evaluation, Prevention, Counseling, and Treatment, Vogel/Bevers
Handbook of Cancer Risk Assessment, Colditz/Stein
Handbook of Oncology Nursing, Third Edition, Johnson/Gross
Healthcare Instruments for Clinical Research, Third Edition, Frank-Stromborg
Homecare Management of the Bone Marrow Transplant Patient, Third Edition, Kelley/McBride/Randolph/Leum/Lonergan
How Cancer Works, Sompayrac
Human Embryonic Stem Cells, Kiessling/Anderson
Making the Decision: A Cancer Patient's Guide to Clinical Trials, Mulay
Malignant Liver Tumors, Second Edition, Clavien et al.
Management of Nausea and Vomiting in Cancer and Cancer Treatment, Hesketh

***Jones and Bartlett Series in Oncology** (continued)*

Memory Bank for Chemotherapy, Third Edition, Preston/Wilfinger
Molecular Oncology of Breast Cancer, Ross/Hortobagyi
Oncology Nursing in the Ambulatory Setting, Second Edition, Buchsel/Yarbro
Oncology Nursing Review, Second Edition, Yarbro/Frogge/Goodman
Outcomes in Radiation Therapy: Multidisciplinary Management, Watkins-Bruner/Moore-Higgs/Haas
Pancreatic Cancer, Von Hoff et al.
Pediatric Stem Cell Transplantation, Metha
Pocket Guide to Breast Cancer, Third Edition, Hassey Dow
Pocket Guide to Breast Cancer Drugs, Wilkes
Pocket Guide to Cancer Chemotherapy Protocols, Second Edition, Chu/DeVita
Pocket Guide to Colorectal Cancer, Berg
Pocket Guide To Colorectal Cancer Drugs and Treatment, Wilkes
Pocket Guide to Managing Cancer Fatigue, Schwartz
Pocket Guide to Prostate Cancer, Held-Warmkessel
Pocket Guide for Women and Cancer, Moore-Higgs/Almadrones/Colvin-Huff/Gossfield/Eriksson
Progress in Oncology 2004, DeVita/Hellman/Rosenberg
Quality of Life: From Nursing and Patient Perspectives, Second Edition, King/Hinds
2005–2006 Oncology Nursing Drug Handbook, Wilkes/Barton-Burke
Women and Cancer: A Gynecologic Oncology Nursing Perspective, Second Edition, Moore-Higgs/Almadrones/Colvin-Huff/Gossfield/Eriksson

Contents

Key to Abbreviations

ABV	doxorubicin (doxorubicin HCl Adriamycin) bleomycin vincristine
ac	"ante cibum;" before meals
ADH	antidiuretic hormone
Afib	atrial fibrillation
AIDS	acquired immunodeficiency syndrome
alkphos	alkaline phosphatase
ALL	acute lymphocytic leukemia
ALT	alanine aminotransferase (formerly SGPT)
AML	acute myelocytic leukemia
ANC	absolute neutrophil count
ANLL	acute nonlymphocytic leukemia
APL	acute promyelocytic leukemia
aPTT	activated partial thromboplastin time
ARDS	adult respiratory distress syndrome
ASA	acetylsalicylic acid
AST	aspartate aminotransferase (formerly SGOT)
AUC	area under curve
bili	bilirubin
BMT	bone marrow transplant
BP	blood pressure
BRM	biologic response modifier
BTP	break through pain
BUN	blood urea nitrogen
Ca	calcium
CAPD	continuous ambulatory periotoneal dialysis
CBC	complete blood count
CFU-GEM	colony forming unit-granulocyte, erythrocyte, megakaryocyte, and macrophage
CHF	congestive heart failure
CLL	chronic lymphocytic leukemia
CPK	creatinine phosphokinase

CR	complete response, e.g., disappearance of *all* detectable tumor cells
creat	creatinine
CSF	colony-stimulating factor
CTZ	chemoreceptor trigger zone
CVA	cerebrovascular accident
CXR	chest X-ray
D5W	5% dextrose in water
DEHP	diethylhexlphthalate
DHFR	difolate reductase
DLCO	diffusion capacity of the lung for carbon monoxide, which reflects rate of gas transfer across the alveolar-capillary membrane
DMSO	dimethyl sulfoxide
DTIC	dacarbazine
DVT	deep vein thrombosis
EDTA	edetic acid, one of several salts of edetic acid used as a chelating agent
EBV	Epstein-Barr virus
EPS	extra pyramidal side-effects
FAC	fluorouracil-adriamycin-cytoxan combination chemotherapy
FSH	follicle-stimulating hormone
FUDR-MP	5-fluoro-23-deoxyuridine-53-monophosphate
FVC	forced vital capacity
GABA	gamma-aminobutyric acid
GBPS	gated blood pool scan
GFR	glomerular filtration rate
GGT (SGGT)	gamma-glutamine transferase
G6PD	glucose-6-phosphate dehydrogenase
GU	genitourinary
HACA	human anti-chimeric antibody
HAMA	human anti-murine antibody
HCl	hydrochloride
hgb	hemoglobin
5-HIAA	5-hydroxyindoleacetic acid
HIV	human immunodeficiency virus
HCT	hematocrit
hs	"hora somni;" at bedtime
HSV	herpes simplex virus
5-HT2	5-hydroxytryptamine 2
5-HT3	5-hydroxytryptamine 3
HUS	hemolytic uremic syndrome

I/O	intake/output
ICP	intracranial pressure
ICU	intensive care unit
IFN	interferon
IL	interleukin
IOP	intraocular pressure
IT	intrathecal
IVB	intravenous bolus
IVP	intravenous push; intravenous pyelogram
LAK	lymphocyte activated killer cells
LDH	lactate dehydrogenase
LFTs	liver function tests
LH	luteinizing hormone
LHRH	luteinizing hormone-releasing hormone
LVEF	left ventricular ejection fraction
lytes	electrolytes
MAC	*mycobacterium avium* complex
MAO	monoamine oxidase
MAOI	monoamine oxidase inhibitor
MCV	mean corpuscular volume
MI	myocardial infarction
MIU	milli international units
MoAbs	monoclonal antibodies
MOPP	mustard-oncovin-prednisone-procarbazine combination chemotherpy for Hodgkin's disease
MTX	methotrexate
MU	milli units
NCI	National Cancer Institute
NHL	non-Hodgkin's lymphoma
NK	natural killer cells
NK_1	Neurokinin 1 receptor for Substance P
NMDA	N-methyl-D-aspartate pain receptor
NS	normal saline
NSAIDs	nonsteroidal antiinflammatory drugs
n/v	nausea/vomiting
OTC	over-the-counter
PACs	premature atrial contractions
PBPCs	packed red blood cells for transfusion
PCA	patient controlled analgesia
PCP	pneumocystis carinii pneumonia
PFTs	pulmonary function tests
phos	phosphorus
plts	platelets

	polymorphonuclear leukocyte
	partial response, e.g., reduction in tumor mass by 50% lasting for 3 months or longer
RN	"pro re na'ta;" as needed
PSA	prostate-specific antigen
PT	prothrombin time
PTH	parathyroid hormone
PTT	partial thromboplastin time
PVCs	premature ventricular contractions
QID	four times a day
RFTs	renal function tests
RUQ	right upper quadrant
SBP	systolic blood pressure
sed rate	sedimentation rate
SGPT	serum glutamic-pyruvic transferase
SIADH	syndrome of inappropriate antidiuretic hormone
SPF	skin protection factor
SQ	subcutaneous
SSRI	selective serotonin reuptake inhibitor
Sx	symptom
T	temperature
T4	thyroxine
TCA	tricyclic antidepressants
TFT	thyroid function tests
THC	tetrahydrocannabinol
TIL	tumor infiltrating lymphocytes
TLS	tumor lysis syndrome
TMP-SMX	trimethoprim-sulfamethoxazole
TNF	tumor necrosis factor
TTP/HUS	thrombotic thrombocytopenic purpura/hemolytic anemia syndrome
UA	urinalysis
US	ultrasound
UTI	urinary tract infection
VC	vomiting center
Vfib	ventricular fibrillation
VOD	veno-occlusive disease
VS	vital signs
VSCC	voltage-sensitive calcium channel
VZV	varicella zoster virus
WHO	World Health Organization
XRT	radiation therapy

Preface

Oncology nurses provide expert nursing care to patients with cancer and their families, as the patient moves along the disease trajectory from diagnosis to primary treatment and cure, or to remission, then relapse, and death. The nurse uses the nursing process to assess patient and family needs in the 14 high incidence problem areas identified in the Oncology Nursing Society (ONS) standards: prevention and early detection, information, coping, comfort, nutrition, protective mechanisms, mobility, elimination, sexuality, ventilation, oxygenation, complementary and alternative therapies, palliative and end-of-life care, and survivorship.

In 2003, Andrew von Eschenbach, MD, set the elimination of suffering and death due to cancer as the NCI challenge goal. He identified seven major initiatives to accomplish this goal, including developing more effective strategies for prevention and screening; early detection as well as improving our understanding of the molecular processes of carcinogenesis; and refinement of molecular targeted therapy (Miller, 2003). In this view, cancer becomes a chronic disease characterized by periods of exacerbations and remissions. As has been demonstrated in work on angiogenesis, malignant tumors must establish a blood supply when they reach a size of 1–2 mm in order to obtain oxygen and glucose, and to remove cellular waste products. Mortality is caused by metastasis in most people with cancer, and if a malignancy was confined to 1–2 mm with a combination of chemotherapy and anti-angiogenesis drug(s), then indeed, people can "live with cancer." Together, the nurse and patient, along with other members of the healthcare team, develop a plan of care. Since cancer, for many, is a chronic illness with periods of remission and relapse, nursing goals center around self-care and empowering the patient and family to live a high-quality, meaningful life outside the hospital. Nurses are involved in the pharmacologic management of disease (e.g., chemotherapy) and of symptoms that arise during the course of illness (e.g., pain, anxiety, constipation). In addition, as patients receive more aggressive treatment, nurses are deeply involved in the management of complications of disease or treatment, such as infection. As new technologies emerge, such as molecular targeted therapy, nurses need to stay abreast of newly approved agents, their mechanisms of action, and potential side effects. Finally, oncology nurses have long said that much of symptom management is in the domain of nursing practice, and they continue to advocate for effective management and symptom resolution. Knowledge of the drugs used in cancer care is critical for today's practicing nurse. In the past, rmacists wrote drug books for nurses that did not address the application of : nursing process to potential drug toxicities. Today, as the science of cancer eatment is rapidly exploding, it is imperative to keep current with new, emerging therapies.

This book is divided into sections addressing broad areas of nursing practice. There are individual chapters within each section presenting an introductory overview. For 2006, we have also added four antineoplastic agents (clofarabine, histrelin implant, paclitaxel protein bound particles for injection, TLK 286), four antimicrobial agents (micafungin, rifaximin, gemifloxacin, tigecycline), two immunotherapy/biotherapy symptom management agents (Imiquimod 5% cream, palifermin), and eight molecularly targeted drugs (lapatanib, panitumumab, pertuzumab, sorafenib (BAY 43-9006), sunitinib malate (sutent, SU11246), temsirolimus, tipifarnib, vatalanib), and two symptom management drugs (hydromorphone extended release tablets, ziconotide intrathecal infusion). In addition, indications and additional toxicity data have been updated for individual drugs, such as bevacizumab, cetuximab, and gefitinib. Specific drugs are described in terms of their mechanism of action, metabolism, drug interactions, laboratory effects/interference, and special considerations. The most important and common drug side effects are discussed. Chapter 5, Molecularly Targeted Therapies, discusses basic cell biology, carcinogenesis, malignant flaws resulting in abnormal cell division and cell death, invasiveness, and metastases. This is intended to provide a framework for understanding the new agents that target molecular flaws. Many of these agents inhibit steps in the processes of carcinogenesis and metastases in the areas of signal transduction (growth receptor over expression, ras, tyrosine kinases), cell cycle movement (cyclin-dependent kinases, apoptosis), angiogenesis, invasion, and metastases. In addition, the processes of apoptosis and ubiquitination are further explored. Standards may change as new scientific knowledge becomes available and as dictated by governmental regulations that affect practice. This book will be updated regularly with new drugs and nursing management strategies to reflect those changes. Every effort has been made to be accurate in describing drug doses and toxicities. However, errors may occur, so the nurse is referred to original documents and manufacturer's prescribing data. Software containing indications, dosaging, adverse reactions, and toxicity for chemotherapy drugs for use with your handheld device is available.

DRUG INFORMATION sections reflect current prescribing practices in the United States, which may differ from clinical practices in Europe and the United Kingdom. (Please see disclaimer, p. iv.)

References

American Nurses' Association (2004) ANA and ONS: *Standards of Oncology Nursing Practice*. Kansas City; ANA.

Miller M (2003) 2015: A target date for eliminating suffering and death due to cancer. Available at http://cancer.gov/newscenter/benchmarks-vol3-issue2. Accessed June 10, 2004.

Contributors

Deborah Berg, BSN, RN
Genentech Oncology
North Londonderry, NH

Catherine K. Bean, BSN, RN, BA
Bone Marrow Transplant Unit
H. Lee Moffitt Center
Tampa, FL

Karen Ingwersen MS, RN
Belmont, MA

Reginald King, Pharm D
Clinical Specialist
Oncology/BMT Hahnemann
University Hospital
Philadelphia, PA

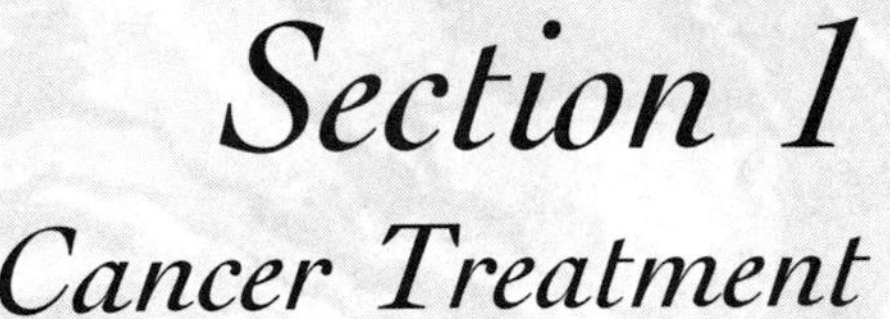

Section 1

Cancer Treatment

Chapter 1

Introduction to Chemotherapy Drugs

Chemotherapy drugs interfere with cell division, leading to cell kill, called *cytocidal effects*, or failure to replicate, called *cytostatic effects* (see Figure 1.1, Cell Cycle.) Unfortunately, drugs cannot discriminate between frequently dividing cells that are normal and those that are malignant. Consequently, normal cells as well as malignant cells are injured. Thus, anticipated acute side effects are found also in normal cell populations that divide frequently, i.e., bone marrow, gastrointestinal (GI) mucosa, gonads, and hair follicles. Since normal cells are better able to repair themselves, these side effects are usually reversible. Depending on drug properties, delayed, longer-term toxicities may occur, which may be irreversible. Properties to be aware of include route of administration, dose, excretion, and predilection for uptake by specific organ cells. Examples of toxicities are

- Lung toxicity from bleomycin, busulfan, and the nitrosureas (BCNU, CCNU)
- Cardiomyopathy from doxorubicin, daunorubicin, mitoxantrone, trastuzumab, and paclitaxel
- Renal dysfunction from cisplatin and high-dose methotrexate
- Hemorrhagic cystitis (bladder) from ifosfamide and cyclophosphamide
- Neurotoxicity from the platins, taxanes, and vinca alkaloids
- Development of second malignancies from melphalan, cyclophosphamide, and other drugs when combined with radiotherapy

Nurses play a critical role in patient education, drug administration, and minimization of toxicities. See Table 1.1 for prechemotherapy nursing assessment guidelines. Table 1.2 describes classifications of chemotherapeutic agents.

This ninth edition has been updated to include newly approved drugs as well as important investigational agents that should be approved in the near future. This section examines antineoplastic agents and classifies them by their mechanism(s) of action. As knowledge of cancer and its treatment emerges, drugs may be reclassified, such as the anthracycline antitumor antibiotics, which now appear to work by inhibiting topoisomerase II.

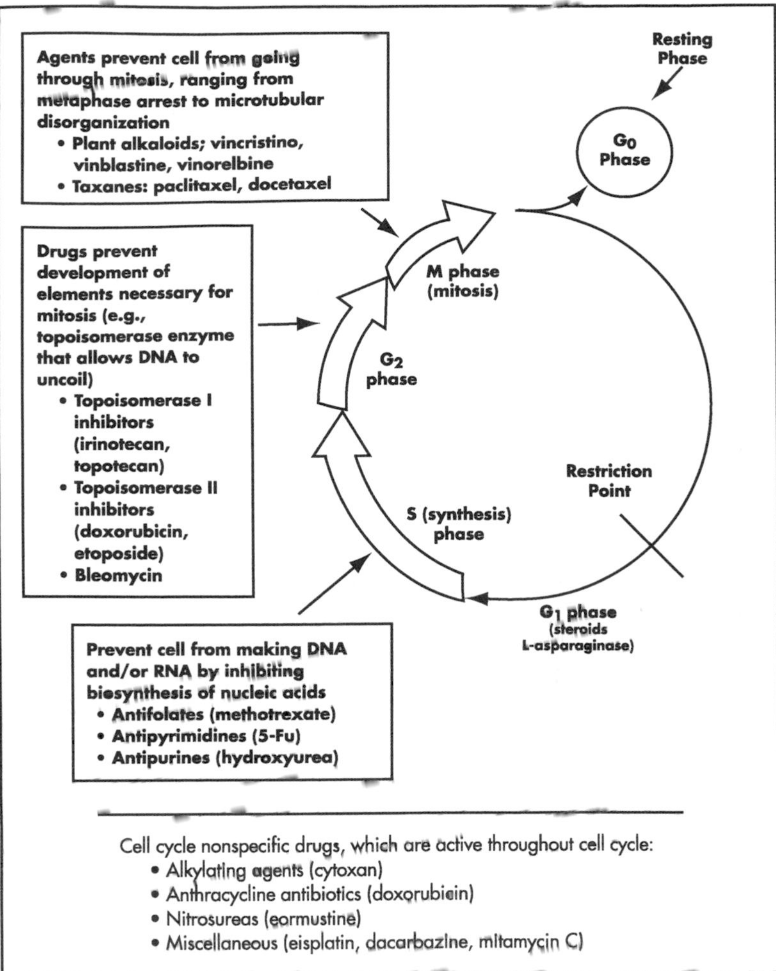

Figure 1.1 Mechanism of Action of Major Chemotherapy Drugs

As an example, the topoisomerase I inhibitors cause protein-linked DNA single-strand breaks and block DNA and RNA synthesis in dividing cells, thus preventing cells from entering mitosis. To better understand the topoisomerase inhibitors, it is important to go back to the DNA helix. The entire DNA genome consists of two strands wound into a double helix, which measures more

Table 1.1 Prechemotherapy Nursing Assessment Guidelines

Potential Problems/Nursing Diagnoses	Physical Status: Assessment Parameters/Signs and Symptoms	Drug and Dose-Limiting Factors/ Nursing Implications
Hematopoietic System		
1. Impaired tissue perfusion related to chemotherapy-induced anemia, leading to activity intolerance, changes in cardiopulmonary status due to compensatory changes	• Hgb g (norms 12–14; 14–16) • HCT% (norms 32–36; 36–40) • Vital signs (↓ BP, ↑ pulse, ↑ respiration) • Pallor (face, palms, conjunctiva) • Fatigue or weakness • Vertigo	Hgb < 8 g HCT < 20% and blood transfusions not initiated • Consider erythropoietin growth factor support when hgb < 10 g/dL (ASCO, 2002) or < 12 g/dL (Thomas, 2002) when receiving concomitant radiotherapy for cervical or head and neck cancers; also if patient is receiving anemia-causing chemotherapy, e.g. crisplatin.
2. Impaired immunocompetence and potential for infection related to chemotherapy-induced neutropenia	• WBC (norm 4500–9000/mm³); ANC > 2000/mm³ • Pyrexia/rigor, erythema, swelling, pain any site • Abnormal discharges, draining wounds, skin/mucous membrane lesions • Productive cough, SOB, rectal pain, urinary frequency	WBC ≤ 3,000/mm³; ANC < 1000/mm³ Fever > 38.3°C or 101°F • Hold all myelosuppressive agents (exceptions may include leukemia, lymphoma, and/or situations in which there is neoplastic marrow infiltration). • Consider growth factor support to prevent febrile neutropenia • Febrile neutropenia is a medical emergency

(continued)

Table 1.1 *(continued)*

Potential Problems/Nursing Diagnoses	Physical Status: Assessment Parameters/Signs and Symptoms	Drug and Dose-Limiting Factors/ Nursing Implications
		• Severe risk of infection ANC < 500 cells/ mm^3 • Protective precautions ANC < 500 cells/ mm^3
3. Potential for injury (bleeding) related to chemotherapy-induced thrombocytopenia	• Platelet count (150,000–400,000/ mm^3) • Spontaneous gingival bleeding or epistaxis • Presence of petechiae or easy bruisability • Hematuria, melena, hematemesis, hemoptysis • Hypermenorrhea • Signs and sx intracranial bleed (irritability, sensory loss, unequal pupils, headache, ataxia)	Platelet count ≤ 100,000/mm^3 • Hold all myelosuppressive agents (exceptions may include leukemia, lymphoma, and/or situations in which there is neoplastic marrow infiltration). • Platelet transfusion if bleeding • Platelet precaution: platelet count < 50,000 cells/mm^3

(continued)

Table 1.1 *(continued)*

Potential Problems/Nursing Diagnoses	Physical Status: Assessment Parameters/Signs and Symptoms	Drug and Dose-Limiting Factors/ Nursing Implications
Integumentary System		
Alteration in mucous membrane of mouth, nasopharynx, esophagus, rectum, anus, or ostomy stoma related to chemotherapy-induced tissue changes	Mucositis Scale 0 = pink, moist, intact mucosa; absence of pain or burning +1 = generalized erythema with or without pain or burning +2 = isolated small ulcerations and/or white patches +3 = confluent ulcerations with white patches on ≥ 25% mucosa +4 = hemorrhagic ulcerations	+2 mucositis • Hold antimetabolites (esp. methotrexate, 5-FU) • Hold antitumor antibiotics (esp. doxorubicin, dactinomycin) • Hold Irinotecan • In transplant settings, may require opioid analgesia, agressive antiemesis • Consider Kepivance™ before transplant chemotherapy
Gastrointestinal System		
Discomfort, nutritional deficiency, and/or fluid and electrolyte disturbances related to chemotherapy-induced:		
1. Anorexia	• Lab values: Albumin and total protein • Normal weight/present weight and % of body weight loss • Normal diet pattern/changes in diet pattern • Alterations in taste sensation • Early satiety	• Manage nutrition impact symptoms • Dietary teaching • Appetite stimulants as needed

(continued)

Table 1.1 *(continued)*

Potential Problems/Nursing Diagnoses	Physical Status: Assessment Parameters/Signs and Symptoms	Drug and Dose-Limiting Factors/ Nursing Implications
2. Nausea and vomiting	• Lab values: Electrolytes • Pattern of n/v (incidence, duration, severity) • Antiemetic plan: Drug(s), dosage(s), schedule, efficacy: Other (dietary adjustments, relaxation techniques, environmental manipulation)	Intractable n/v × 24 h if IV hydration not initiated • Consider aggressive combination antiemesis (serotonin antagonist and dexamethasone; or addition of aprepitant to serotonin-antagonist if delayed nausea and vomiting)
3. Bowel disturbances A. Diarrhea	• Normal pattern of bowel elimination • Consistency (loose, watery/bloody stools) • Frequency and duration (no./day and no. of days) • Antidiarrheal drug(s), dosage(s), efficacy	Diarrheal stools × 3/24 h above baseline • Hold antimetabolites (esp. methotrexate, 5-FU); irinotecan • Teach patient self-administration of antidiarrheal medicine • Antibiotic therapy for unresolved diarrhea per MD

(continued)

Table 1.1 *(continued)*

Potential Problems/Nursing Diagnoses	Physical Status: Assessment Parameters/Signs and Symptoms	Drug and Dose-Limiting Factors/ Nursing Implications
B. Constipation	• Normal pattern of bowel elimination • Consistency (hard, dry, small stools) • Frequency (hours or days beyond normal pattern) • Stool softener(s), laxative(s), efficacy	No BM × 48 h past normal bowel patterns • Hold vinca alkaloids (vinblastine, vincristine) • Teach patient to take stool softener with ondansetron antiemetic
4. Hepatotoxicity	• Lab values: LDH, ALT, AST, alk phos, bili • Pain/tenderness over liver, feeling of fullness • Increase in n/v or anorexia • Changes in mental status • Jaundice • High-risk factors: Hepatic metastasis Concurrent hepatotoxic drugs Viral hepatitis graft-vs.-host disease Abdominal XRT Blood transfusions	Evidence of chemical hepatitis • Hold hepatotoxic agents (esp. methotrexate, 6-MP) until differential dx established • Hold imatinib mesylate if lab thresholds exceeded • Hold oxaliplatin if venous acclusive disease suspected • Dose reduce drugs metabolized by liver if severe liver dysfunction

(continued)

Table 1.1 *(continued)*

Potential Problems/Nursing Diagnoses	Physical Status: Assessment Parameters/Signs and Symptoms	Drug and Dose-Limiting Factors/ Nursing Implications
Respiratory System		
Impaired gas exchange or ineffective breathing pattern related to chemotherapy-induced pulmonary fibrosis	• Lab values: PFTs CXR • Respirations (rate, rhythm, depth) • Chest pain • Nonproductive cough • Progressive dyspnea • Wheezing/stridor • High-risk factors: Total cumulative dose of bleomycin Age > 60 yr Preexisting lung disease Concomitant use of other pulmonary toxic drugs Prior/concomitant XRT Smoking hx	• Acute unexplained onset respiratory symptoms • Hold all antineoplastic agents until differential dx established (e.g., bleomycin, busulfan, oxaliplatin, gemcitabine) • Interstitial Lung Disease (ILD) is a class effect of EGFR antagonist (rare), eg., gefitinib, cetuximab, erlotinib. If pulmonary symptoms develop, hold drug until ILD can be ruled out.

(continued)

Table 1.1 *(continued)*

Potential Problems/Nursing Diagnoses	Physical Status: Assessment Parameters/Signs and Symptoms	Drug and Dose-Limiting Factors/ Nursing Implications
Cardiovascular System		
Decreased cardiac output related to chemotherapy-induced: 1. Cardiac arrhythmias 2. Cardiomyopathy 3. Hypertension	• Lab values: cardiac enzymes, electrolytes, ECG, ECHO, MUGA • Vital signs • Presence of arrhythmia (irregular radial/apical pulse) • Signs sx CHF (dyspnea, ankle edema, PND, decrease in LVEF, S_3 gallop, nonproductive cough, rales, cyanosis) • High-risk factors: Total cumulative dose anthracyclines Preexisting cardiac disease Prior/concurrent mediastinal XRT • Combined anthracycline, cyclophosphamide, and trastuzumab, and paclitaxel	Acute sx CHF and/or cardiac arrhythmia • Hypertension: bevacizumab • Hold all antineoplastic agents until differential dx established Total dose doxorubicin or daunorubicin > 550 mg/m^2 • Hold anthracyclines, trastuzumab, paclitaxel • Monitor baseline and serial ejection fractions (LVEF) while receiving treatment with potentially cardiotoxic drugs; evaluate any significant ↓ in LVEF. • Severe hypertension: hold bevacizumab until hypertension controlled

(continued)

Table 1.1 *(continued)*

Potential Problems/Nursing Diagnoses	Physical Status: Assessment Parameters/Signs and Symptoms	Drug and Dose-Limiting Factors/ Nursing Implications
Genitourinary System		
1. Alteration in fluid volume (excess) related to chemotherapy-induced: A. Glomerular or renal tubule damage B. Hyperuricemic nephropathy 2. Alteration in comfort related to chemotherapy-induced hemorrhagic cystitis	• Lab values: BUN, creatinine clearance, serum creatinine, uric acid, electrolytes, urinalysis, magnesium, calcium, phosphate • Color, odor, clarity of urine • 24-h fluid intake and output (estimate/actual) • Hematuria; proteinuria • Development of oliguria or anuria • High-risk factors: Preexisting renal disease Concurrent treatment with nephrotoxic drugs (esp. aminoglycoside antibiotics) • Bevacizumad: rare nephritic syndrome	• Hold cyclophosphamide, ifosfamide Serum creatinine > 2.0 and/or Creatinine clearance < 70 mL/min Hematuria • Hold cisplatin, streptozotocin Anuria × 24 h • Hold all antineoplastic agents Nephrotic syndrome (bevacizumab) • Check BUN/creatinine before treatment • 24 hour urine for protein if spilling protein • Drug dose reduction/hold if protein > 2g (e.g. Bevacizumab)

(continued)

Table 1.1 *(continued)*

Potential Problems/Nursing Diagnoses	Physical Status: Assessment Parameters/Signs and Symptoms	Drug and Dose-Limiting Factors/ Nursing Implications
Nervous System		
1. Impaired sensory/motor function related to chemotherapy-induced A. Peripheral neuropathy B. Cranial nerve neuropathy C. Acute oxliplatin neurotoxicity	• Paresthesias (numbness, tingling in feet, fingertips) • Trigeminal nerve toxicity (severe jaw pain) • Jaw or muscle spasm • Diminished or absent deep tendon reflexes (ankle and knee jerks) • Motor weakness/slapping gait/ataxia • Visual and auditory disturbances • Cold induced paresthesias and dysesthesias lasting < 14 days	Presence of any neurologic signs and symptoms or worsening: • Perform brief nursing neuro exam before each treatment focusing on symptom analysis and functional impairment; consult MD for full neuro exam if signs/symptoms or worsening of existing signs/ symptoms • Hold vinca alkaloids, cisplatin, hexamethyl melamine, oxaliplatin, procarbazine until differential dx established • Acute oxaliplation neurotoxicity: increase length of infusion time to 6 h (decreases peak serum level by 32%); teach patient to avoid cold exposure to hands/feet oral mucosa for 3–5 days after oxaliplatin drug administration.

(continued)

Table 1.1 *(continued)*

Potential Problems/Nursing Diagnoses	Physical Status: Assessment Parameters/Signs and Symptoms	Drug and Dose-Limiting Factors/ Nursing Implications
		• Assess for motor/sensory changes impact on function and ability to do ADLS prior to oxaliplatin, taxane or cisplatin administration; hold for grades 3 and 4 toxicity (see Appendix 2) • Teach avoidance of cold for 3–5 days after oxaliplatin administration
2. Impaired bowel and bladder elimination related to chemotherapy-induced autonomic nerve dysfunction	• Urinary retention • Constipation/abdominal cramping and distension • High-risk factors: Changes in diet or mobility Frequent use of opioid analgesics Obstructive disease process	Presence of any neurologic signs and symptoms • Hold vinca alkaloids until differential dx established

ALT = alanine aminotransferase; AST = aspartate aminotransferase; bili = bilirubin; BM = bowel movement; CHF = congestive heart failure; CXR = chest X-ray; dx = diagnosis; ECG = electrocardiogram; ECHO = echocardiogram; 5-FU = 5-fluorouracil; hx = history; LDH = lactate dehydrogenase; LVEF = left ventricular ejection fraction; MUGA = multigated acquisition (MUGA heart scan); n/v = nausea and vomiting; PFT = pulmonary function test; 6-MP = 6-mercaptopurine; SOB = shortness of breath; sx = symptoms; XRT = radiation therapy *Modified from:* Engleking C 1988 Prechemotherapy Nursing Assessment in Outpatient Settings. *Outpatient Chemotherapy* 3(1):10–11.

Table 1.2 Classifications of Antineoplastic Drugs

Classification	Mechanism of Action	Examples
	Cell Cycle Specific Agents	
Antimetabolites	Interfere with DNA and RNA synthesis by acting as false metabolites, which are incorporated into the DNA strand, or block essential enzymes, so that DNA synthesis is prevented.	Pemetraxate (slinta) Cytosine arabinoside (ara-C, Cytosar-U) Eniluracil 5-Fluorouracil (5-FU) Floxuridine (FUDR, 5-FUDR) Hydroxyurea (Hydrea) 6-Mercaptopurine (6-MP, Purinethol) Methotrexate (Amethopterin, Mexate, Folex) 6-Thioguanine (6-TG) Gemcitabine (Gemzar®) Fludarabine (Fludara®) Capecitabine (Xeloda®) Deoxycoformycin (Pentostatin)
Vinca Alkaloids	Crystallize microtubules of mitotic spindle causing metaphase arrest (vincristine, vinblastine, vindesine), role in blocking DNA and preventing cell division in M phase (vinorelbine).	Vincristine (VCR, Oncovin) Vinblastine (VLB, Velban) Vinorelbine (Navelbine®)
Epipodophyllotoxins	Damage the cell prior to mitosis, late S and G_2 phase; inhibit topoisomerase II.	Etoposide (VP-16, Vepesid) Teniposide (VM-26, Vumon)

(continued)

Table 1.2 *(continued)*

Classification	Mechanism of Action	Examples
	Cell Cycle Specific Agents	
Taxanes	Promotes early microtubule assembly. Prevents depolymerization, causing cell death (paclitaxel); enhances microtubule assembly and inhibits tubulin depolymerization, thus arresting cell division in metaphase (docetaxel).	Paclitaxel (Taxol®) Docetaxel (Taxotere®) Paclitaxe) protein bound
Camptothecins	Act in S phase to inhibit topoisomerase I and cause cell death.	Topotecan (HyCamptin®) Irinotecan (CPT-11, Camptosar®)
Miscellaneous		G_1 phase: L-asparaginase (ELSPAR), Prednisone G_2 phase: Bleomycin (Bleo, Blenoxane)
	Cell Cycle Non-Specific Agents	
Alkylating Agents	Substitute alkyl group for H+ ion causing single- and double-strand breaks in DNA, as well as cross-linkages; thus DNA strands are unable to separate during DNA replication.	Busulfan (Myleran®, oral; Busulfex®, IV) Carboplatin (Paraplatin) *Carmustine (BiCNU, BCNU) Chlorambucil (Leukeran) Cisplatin (*Cis*-Platinum, CDDP, Platinol) Cyclophosphamide (Cytoxan, CTX, Neosar) Dacarbazine (DTIC-Dome, Imidazole) Estramustine phosphate (Estracyte, Emcyt) Oxaliplatin (Eloxatin®)

(continued)

Table 1.2 *(continued)*

Classification	Mechanism of Action	Examples
	Cell Cycle Non-Specific Agents	
		Ifosfamide (IFEX) *Lomustine (CCNU) Mechlorethamine hydrochloride (nitrogen mustard, mustargen, HN_2) Melphalan (Alkeran, 1-PAM, Phenylalanine Mustard) Oxaliplatin (Eloxatin) *Streptozocin (Streptozotocin, Zanosar) Thiotepa (Triethylene Thiophosphoramide, TSPA)
Antibiotics	Use a variety of mechanisms to prevent cell division and death (DNA strand breakage, intercalation of base pairs, inhibition of RNA and DNA synthesis).	Dactinomycin (Actinomycin D, Cosmegan) Daunorubicin hydrochloride (Daunomycin, Cerubidine) Doxorubicin hydrochloride (Adria, Adriamycin) Epirubicin HCl (Ellenee) Indarubicin (Idamycin) Mithramycin (Mithramycin, Plicamycin) Mitomycin C (Mito, Mutamycin) Mitoxantrone (Novantrone)

*Nitrosoureas (cross blood-brain barrier)

Table 1.3 Common Agents Used in Dose-Intensive/High-Dose Chemothe[illegible] Associated Toxicities

Drug	Toxicity
Doxorubicin	1. Cardiotoxicity leading to degenerative cardiomyopa[illegible] over time Standard dose: 60–75 mg/m² Current lifetime dose: 450–550 mg/m² Current protocol dose ranges: 430–650 mg/m² (lifetime) When given over 96 hours in a dilute solution or at low weekly doses, cardiotoxicity appears to decrease. Prior radiation therapy to the chest or prior anthracycline therapy may predispose patient to or enhance cardiotoxicity. 2. Severe mucositis 3. Acute myelosuppression; late onset in children, even at low cumulative doses
Cyclophosphamide	1. Standard dose: 400–1600 mg/m² IV; high dose: up to 200 mg/kg 2. High dose: Cardiotoxicity, acute cardiomyopathy Diminished QRS complex on ECG Pulmonary congestion and pleural effusions Cardiomegaly Prior radiation therapy to the chest or prior anthracycline therapy may predispose patient to or enhance cardiotoxicity. Ejection fraction of > 50% not predictive of reduced risk for cardiotoxicity. 3. Hemorrhagic cystitis (occasionally chronic, severe) 5. Acral erythema and sloughing of skin on palms of hands and soles of feet 6. Diffuse hyperpigmentation 7. Gonadal dysfunction Delayed pubertal development Diminished testicular volume in adult males
Cisplatin	1. Standard dose: 15–120 mg/m²; high dose: 160–200 mg/m² 2. Renal and hepatic toxicity 3. Eighth cranial nerve damage and ototoxicity 4. Myelosuppression 5. Peripheral neuropathy 6. Intense nausea and vomiting

(continued)

(continued)

	Toxicity
ɔoplatin	1. Standard dose: 400–500 mg/m²; high dose: 800–1600 mg/m² 2. Myelosuppression (dose-limiting); pronounced thrombocytopenia 3. Severe nausea and vomiting 4. Hepatotoxicity 5. Auditory toxicity 6. Mild renal toxicity
Cytosine arabinoside	1. Standard dose: 100–200 mg/m²; high dose: 2–3 g/m² 2. Acute neurotoxicity: cerebellar toxicity Those over 50 at highest risk for minimal recovery from symptoms. Assess prior to each dose for ataxia, nystagmus, and slurred speech; hold dose if any indication of symptomatology (over baseline assessment). 3. Acral erythema and possible sloughing of skin on palms of hands and soles of feet 4. Conjunctivitis, Steroid eye drops may prevent or alleviate 5. Intense diarrhea, up to 2–3 liters/24 hours
Busulfan	1. Standard dose: 1–4 mg/m²; high dose: 16 mg/kg 2. Myelosuppression 3. Severe nausea and vomiting 4. Severe mucositis 5. Pneumonitis, pulmonary fibrosis; "busulfan lung" 6. Hepatic dysfunction leading to veno-occlusive disease 7. Diffuse hyperpigmentation; rare: development of bullae 8. Chronic alopecia
Etoposide	1. Standard dose: 60 mg/m²; high dose: 60 mg/kg or 80–250 mg/m² 2. Severe mucositis 3. Acral erythema and sloughing of skin or palms of hands and soles of feet 4. Myelosuppression 5. Severe blood pressure fluctuations 6. Fever and chills during infusion
Methotrexate	1. Standard dose: 10–500 mg/m²; high dose: 500 mg/m² and greater 2. Photosensitivity 3. Diffuse hyperpigmentation

(continued)

Table 1.3 *(continued)*

Drug	Toxicity
	4. Neurotoxicity: seizures, aphasia, cerebellar toxicity (rare; see cytosine arabinoside) 5. Severe diarrhea 6. Renal toxicity 7. Hepatotoxicity and coagulopathies 8. Thrombocytopenia 9. Pulmonary toxicities
Melphalan	1. Standard dose: 6–8 mg/m^2; high dose: 80–140 mg/m^2 2. Severe mucositis 3. Diarrhea 4. Severe nausea, especially in combination with another emetogenic drug 5. Renal toxicity 6. Profound myelosuppression 7. Severe liver toxicity
Carmustine	1. Standard dose: 200–240 mg/m^2; high dose: 600–1200 mg/m^2 2. Hepatic dysfunction leading to veno-occlusive disease 3. Central nervous system changes, including diffuse encephalopathy 4. Mild alopecia
5-Fluorouracil	1. Standard dose: 7–15 mg/kg for five days; high dose: 255–300 mg/m^2 continuous infusion weekly 2. Cardiotoxicity mimicking acute myocardial infarction, angina, cardiogenic shock 3. Photosensitivity and hyperpigmentation 4. Severe diarrhea 5. Cerebellar toxicity

Source: Brown KA, Esper P, Kelleher LO, et al (2001) *Chemotherapy and Biotherapy Guidelines and Recommendations for Practice*. Pittsburgh, Oncology Nursing Soc, pp 60–63. Reproduced with permission from Oncology Nursing Society Publishing.

than 3 feet and is condensed into chromosomes by torsion of the helix. During cell replication, the DNA strands that are coiled in the double helix need to unwind so that they can separate and be copied. This is made possible by the topoisomerase I and II enzymes (Chen and Liu, 1994).

Topoisomerase I relaxes tension in the DNA helix torsion by causing a transient single-strand break or nick in the DNA when it covalently bonds to the end of one of the DNA strands. The other, intact strand then passes through the break, and relaxation of the DNA helix occurs as the strands swivel at the strand break. The topoisomerase I enzyme then reseals the cleaved strand (religation step), and the enzyme is released from the DNA strand. Transcription (copying of the strands) is then initiated. Interestingly, topoisomerase I is found in greater concentrations in patients with cancers of the colon, non-Hodgkin's lymphoma, and some leukemias (Husain et al, 1994). Drugs developed within this decade, such as topotecan and irinotecan, work by inhibiting the religation or repair of the single-strand break by binding to topoisomerase I, and cells are arrested in G_2 phase.

Topoisomerase II is also involved in the relaxation of the helix torsion, but it causes a double-strand break to allow crossing of two double-stranded DNA segments. It then causes the closing of the two DNA strand breaks. This permits assembly of chromatin, as well as condensation and decondensation of the chromosomes, and separation of the DNA in the daughter cells during mitosis (Lui et al, 1980). Drugs that are well known to interfere with topoisomerase II are etoposide (nonintercalator, and cell cycle specific for M phase) and doxorubicin (intercalator of base pairs and cell cycle nonspecific) (Eber, 1996).

Descriptions of the drugs in the chapter have been updated to reflect new indications. Agents that have now been approved by the Food and Drug Administration (FDA) for use in cancer treatment have been updated, and investigational agents that are nearing FDA application or appear very promising, are included.

With the promise of increased survival in patients with solid tumors, standard chemotherapy agents are being combined at higher doses for marrow ablation, with subsequent stem cell rescue. However, more severe toxicity is seen (see Table 1.3). In addition, there have been advances in the approval of agents that provide organ protection from drug toxicity (cytoprotectants) which is discussed in Chapter 4.

New technology has permitted a reduction in toxicity from a number of drugs. For instance, the use of nanotechnology to manufacture liposomal delivery vehicles for doxorubicin, daunorubicin, cytarabine, amphotericin, paclitaxel and camptothecins are currently available or being studied. The liposomal "wrapping" of water-soluble or insoluble drugs permits the drug to be preferentially delivered to sites of infection, inflammation, or tumor. Liposomes may pass through gaps in the endothelial lining of blood capillaries within the tumor, where the drug may be unpackaged and released within the tumor. Healthy tissues, on the other hand, have capillary walls that prevent the leakage of liposomes into the tissues, so that toxicity is reduced. The targeting of liposomes for specific tissues or disease sites is accomplished by variation in the number of lipid layers, and the size, charge, and permeability of the layers (Bangham, 1992). In addition, oral formulations of intravenous drugs are being studied, such as topotecan, and the investigational camptothecins rubitecan and liposomal karenitecin. Efforts are being made to try to find agents offering equal efficacy but that can improve quality of life, such as new oral antineoplastic agents, by minimizing trips to the hospital or intrusive administration techniques.

Within the last few years, interest and clinical testing of new approaches to old drugs has occurred. 5-fluorouracil (5-FU) is an old drug that has good efficacy in colorectal cancer and other gastrointestinal cancers. However, it is limited, and increased doses are not necessarily more effective. Also, given by continuous infusion, 5-FU is often more effective because, being cell cycle specific for the S phase, more malignant cells are likely to be exposed to continuous infusion of chemotherapy than if the drug is given by bolus injection.

In an effort to improve the efficacy, new oral fluoropyrimidines have been developed, along with other agents that decrease the breakdown of 5-FU, so that serum drug levels are higher and more sustained, mimicking a continuous infusion. An example of a prodrug is tegafur, and an inhibitor of DPD is uracil, and also eniluracil. In an effort to reduce the toxicity of bolus 5FU/LV deGramont et al (1997) showed that infusional 5FU/LV was equivalent in efficacy but significantly less toxic. This has become the standard way to administer 5FU/LV in the United States at this time.

Capecitabine (Xeloda), a 5-FU prodrug that is preferentially taken up by tumor cells. The drug has been approved for both the adjuvant treatment of patients with colon cancer as well as patients with advanced metastatic breast and colon cancers. Capecitabine has been shown to be equivalent to 5FU/LV and is being studied as a replacement in combination with oxaliplatin, irinotecan, or alone during radiotherapy. It simulates a continuous infusion of 5-FU, and has been shown equivalent to 5FU/LV in both adjuvant and metastatic settings (Cassidy et al, 2004). Ideally, these oral agents could be used to provide radiosensitization for patients with gastrointestinal tumors undergoing external beam radiotherapy.

Antineoplastic agents are classified by mechanism of action (see Table 1.2). Cell cycle specific agents are most active during specific phases of the cell cycle and include antimetabolites (synthesis phase), vinca alkaloids (mitotic phase), and miscellaneous drugs. Examples of these include L-asparaginase and prednisone (G_1 phase) and bleomycin and etoposide (G_2 phase). In addition, effective drugs such as the taxanes, that have a clear mechanism of action at therapeutic doses, may in fact, have an antiangiogenic effect at lower, more frequent dosing. Endothelial cells appear to be very sensitive to the taxanes. Seidman et al (2004) demonstrated that paclitaxel given weekly at a lower dose (dose density) was superior to an increased dose given every 3 weeks.

Cell cycle nonspecific agents can damage cells in all phases of the cell cycle and include alkylating agents (cyclophosphamide, cisplatin), antitumor/antibiotics (doxorubicin, mitomycin-C), the nitrosureas (carmustine, lomustine), and others (dacarbazine, procarbazine) (see Table 1.2).

Antineoplastic agents are effective because they interfere with cellular metabolism and replication, resulting in cell death. When malignant cells evade programmed cell death, the tumor cells no longer are controlled by apoptosis, and resistance emerges. However, it is critical that nurses protect themselves when handling these drugs so that they are not exposed to the potential drug hazards. These drugs can be:

- *Mutagenic*: capable of causing a change in the genetic material within a cell that can be passed on to future cell generations;
- *Teratogenic*: capable of causing damage to a developing fetus exposed to the drug; the greatest risk is during the first trimester of pregnancy when the fetal organ systems are developing;
- *Carcinogenic*: capable of causing malignant change in a cell.

In 1985, the Occupational Safety and Health Administration (OSHA) developed guidelines for the safe handling of antineoplastic agents. These guidelines were revised in 1995 and then in 2004 to include all hazardous drugs (see Appendix I). NIOSH has updated recommendations as of March 2004.

Hormones are used in the management of hormonally sensitive cancers, such as breast and prostate cancers. The hormone changes the hormonal environment, probably affecting growth factors, so that the stimulus for tumor growth is suppressed or removed (see Table 1.4). New SERMs and aromatase inhibitors are being developed to improve on the demonstrated success of tamoxifen.

COMPLICATIONS OF DRUG ADMINISTRATION

All drugs can cause hypersensitivity reactions including anaphylaxis, but only a few drugs cause severe problems. These include:

- L-asparaginase
- Paclitaxel (related to carrier vehicle solution CR cremefor)
- Docetaxel (related to delivery vehicle solution Tween)
- Cisplatin
- Teniposide (Vumon, VM-26)
- Bleomycin (less common; 2% incidence in lymphoma patients)
- Cetuximab (Erbitux, discussed in Chapter 5), rare but may be fatal.
- Rituximab (Rituxan, discussed in Chapter 5)

In addition, certain drugs can cause delayed hypersensitivity, such as carboplatin and oxaliplatin, where the patient develops a range of signs and symptoms of hypersensitivity after receiving a number of cycles of the drug, such as 7 cycles of carboplatin (Markman et al. 2003). For nursing management of patients

Table 1.4 Common Hormonal Agents

Classification	Examples
Adrenocorticoids	cortisone hydrocortisone dexamethasone methylprednisone methylprednisolone prednisone prednisolone
Androgens	testosterone propionate (Neo-hombreol, Oreton) fluoxymesterone (Halotestin, Ora-Testryl) testolactone
Estrogens	chlorotrianisene (TACE) diethylstilbestrol (DES) diethylstilbestrol diphosphate (Stilphostrol) ethinyl estradiol (Estinyl) conjugated estrogen (Premarin) Stradiol
Selective Estrogen Receptor Modulators (SERM)	tamoxifen citrate (Nolvadex) toremifene citrate (Fareston) raloxifene (Evista)
Selective aromatase inhibitors	
• Reversible	Anastrozole (Arimidex) Letrozole (Femara)
• Irreversible	Exemestane (Aromasin)
Progesterones	medroxyprogesterone acetate (Provera, Depo-Provera) megestrol acetate (Megace, Pallace)
Antitestosterone	leuprolide acetate (Lupron) bicalutamide (Casodex) flutamide (Eulexin) nilutamide (Nilandron)

experiencing hypersensitivity or anaphylaxis, as recommended by the Oncology Nursing Society Practice Committee, see Table 1.5.

Table 1.5 Management of Hypersensitivity and Anaphylactic Reactions

1. Review the patient's allergy history.
2. Consider prophylactic medications with hydrocortisone or an antihistamine in atopic/allergic individuals. (This requires a physician's order.)
3. *Patient and family education:* Assess the patient's readiness to learn. Inform patient of the potential for an allergic reaction and instruct to report any unusual symptoms such as:
   A. Uneasiness or agitation
   B. Abdominal cramping
   C. Itching
   D. Chest tightness
   E. Light-headedness or dizziness
   F. Chills
4. Ensure that emergency equipment and medications are readily available.
5. Obtain baseline vital signs and note patient's mental status.
6. As appropriate, perform a scratch test, intradermal skin test, or test dose before administering the full dosage (this requires a physician's order). If there is no reaction, the remaining dose can be administered. If an allergic response is suspected, discontinue the test dose (unless it has been completed), maintain the intravenous line, and notify the physician.
7. For a *localized allergic response:*
   A. Evaluate symptoms; observe for urticaria, wheals, localized erythema.
   B. Administer diphenhydramine or hydrocortisone as per physician's order.
   C. Monitor vital signs every 15 minutes for 1 hour.
   D. Continue subsequent dosing or desensitization program according to a physician's order.
   E. If a "flare" reaction appears along the vein with doxorubicin (Adriamycin) or daunorubicin, flush the line with saline.
      a. Insure that extravasation has not occurred.
      b. Administer hydrocortisone 25–50 mg intravenously with a physician's order, followed by a 0.9% NS flush. This may be adequate to resolve the "flare" reaction.
      c. Once the "flare" reaction has resolved, continue slow infusion of the drug.
      d. Monitor for repeated "flare" episodes. It is preferable to change the intravenous site if possible.
8. For a generalized allergic response, *anaphylaxis* may be suspected if the following signs or symptoms occur (usually within the first 15 minutes of the start of the infusion or injection):
   A. Subjective signs and symptoms
      a. Generalized itching
      b. Chest tightness
      c. Agitation
      d. Uneasiness
      e. Dizziness
      f. Nausea
      g. Crampy abdominal pain
      h. Anxiety

Table 1.5 *(continued)*

i. Sense of impending doom
j. Desire to urinate or defecate
k.Chills

B. Objective signs
a. Flushed appearance (edema of face, hands, or feet)
b. Localized or generalized urticaria
c. Respiratory distress with or without wheezing
d. Hypotension
e. Cyanosis
f. Difficulty speaking

9. For a *generalized allergic response:*
A. Stop the infusion immediately and notify the physician.
B. Maintain the intravenous line with appropriate solution to expand the vascular space, e.g., NS.
C. If not contraindicated, ensure maximum rate of infusion if the patient is hypotensive.
D. Position the patient to promote perfusion of the vital organs; the supine position is preferred.
E. Monitor vital signs every 2 minutes until stable, then every 5 minutes for 30 minutes, then every 15 minutes as ordered.
F. Reassure the patient and the family.
G. Maintain the airway and anticipate the need for cardiopulmonary resuscitation.
H. All medications must be administered with a physician's order.
I. Anticipate administering the following medications for the following effects:
a) Vasoconstriction to increase cardiac output and blood pressure:
1) epinephrine (1:1000, 0.3–0.5 mL or 0.3–0.5 mg IM or SQ q 10–15 min; or if hypotensive, 1:10,000 concentration giving 0.5–1.0 mL (0.1 mg) IVP in Adults; in pediatrics, 1:1000 IM 0.01 mL/kg (up to 0.3 mL)
2) dopamine 2–20 micrograms/kg/min (adults)
b) Antihistamines to stop allergic release of histamines:
1) H1: diphenhydramine: 25–50 mg IVP (adults), 1 mg/kg (max 50 mg, pediatrics)
2) H2: ranitidine 50 mg IV or famotidine 20 mg IV (adults)
c) Bronchodilation: aminophylline 5 mg/kg IV over 30 min (adults)
d) Anti-inflammation/Bronchodilation: steroids. Methylprednisolone 30–50 mg IV (peds 0.3–0.5 mg/kg); or dexamethasone 10–20 mg IVP (peds 1–2 mg/kg); or hydrocortisone 100–500 mg IV (peds 1–2 mg/kg)

10. Document the incident in the medical record according to institution policy and procedures.
11. Physician-guided desensitization may be necessary for subsequent dosing.

References: Polovich M, White JM, Kelleher LC, (eds), *Chemotherapy and Biotherapy Guidelines and Recommendations for Practice.* 2nd ed. Pittsburgh, PA: ONS; 2005;86. Barton-Burke, M, Wilkes GM, Ingwersen K. *Cancer Chemotherapy: A Nursing process Approach,* 3rd ed. Sudbury, MA: Jones and Bartlett Publishers Inc.; 2001. Ellis AK and Day JH. Diagnosis and Management of Anaphylaxis. *Canadian Medical Association Journal* 2003;169(4): 307—312. Sheperd GM. Hypersensitivity Reactions to Chemotherapeutic Drugs. *Allergy and Immunology* 2003;24:253–262.

Table 1.6 Vesicants and Irritants

Vesicants				
Chemotherapeutic Agents	**Antidote**	**Antidote Preparation**	**Local Care**	**Comments**
Alkylating agents				
Mechlorethamine (nitrogen mustard)	Isotonic sodium (NA) thiosulfate	Prepare 1/6 molar solution: 1. If 10% Na thiosulfate solution, mix 4 mL with 6 ml sterile water for injection. 2. If 25% Na thiosufate solution, mix 1.6 mL with 8.4 ml sterile water.	1. Immediately inject Na thiosulfate through IV cannula, 2 mL for every mg extravasated. 2. Remove needle. 3. Inject antidote into subcutaneous (SC) tissue.	1. Na thiosulfate neutralizes nitrogen mustard, which then is excreted via the kidneys. 2. Time is essential in treating extravasation. 3. Heat and cold not proven effective. 4. Although clinically accepted, reports of the benefits are scant.
Cisplatin (Platinol®[a])	Same as above	Same as above	1. Use 2 ml of the 10% Na thiosulfate for each 100 mg of cisplatin. 2. Remove needle. 3. Inject SC.	1. Vesicant potential seen with a concentration of more than 20 cc of 0.5 mg/ml extravasates. If less than this, drug is an irritant; no treatment recommended.

(continued)

Table 1.6 *(continued)*

Vesicants				
Chemotherapeutic Agents	Antidote	Antidote Preparation	Local Care	Comments
Antitumor antibiotics				
Doxorubicin (Adriamycin®[b])	None		1. Apply cold pad with circulating ice water, ice pack, or cryogel pack for 15–20 minutes at least four times per day for the first 24–48 hours. Elevate site for 48 hrs, then resume normal activity	1. Extravasations of less than 1–2 cc often will heal spontaneously. If greater than 3 cc, ulceration often results. 2. Protect area from sunlight and heat. 3. Studies suggest benefit of 99% dimethyl sulfoxide (DMSO) 1–2 mL applied to site every 6 hours. Other studies show delayed healing with DMSO.
Daunorubicin (Cerubidine®[c])	None			1. Little information known. 2. In mouse experiments, some benefit from topical DMSO.
Mitomycin-C (mitamycin)	None			1. Protect from sunlight. 2. Delayed skin reactions have occurred in areas far from original IV site.

(continued)

Table 1.6 *(continued)*

Chemotherapeutic Agents	Antidote	Antidote Preparation	Local Care	Comments
Vesicants				
Taxanes				
Paclitaxel (Taxol®[a]) (concentrated solution)	Ice		Apply ice pack for 15–20 minutes at least four times per day for the first 24 hours.	1. Paclitaxel may have rare vesicant potential (probably due to dilution in 500 cc diluent. 2. Ice and hyaluronidase have been effective in decreasing local tissue damage in a mouse model.
Irritants				
Alkylating agents				
Dacarbazine (DTIC)				1. May cause phlebitis. 2. Protect drug from sunlight.
Ifosfamide Carboplatin				1. May cause phlebitis. 2. Antidote or local care measures unknown.

(continued)

Table 1.6 *(continued)*

Chemotherapeutic Agents	Antidote	Antidote Preparation	Local Care	Comments
		Irritants *(continued)*		
Oxaliplatin (however, has vesicant potential)				1. Oxaliplatin has vesicant potential so is best given via CL. If oxaliplatin given via peripheral line, drug can be diluted in 500 mL D5W (Sanofi Synthelabo, 2004) and infused over 6 hours to decrease discomfort. 2. High dose dexamethasone should be considered as a therapeutic intervention (Kretzschman et al., 2003)
Antitumor Antibiotics Daunorubicin citrace (DaunoXone®				
Nitrosoureas Carmustine (BCNU)				1. May cause phlebitis Local care measures are unknown. 2. Antidote or local care measures unknown.
Antitumor antibiotics Doxorubicin liposome (Doxil)®)				1. May produce redness and tissue edema. 2. Low ulceration potential. 3. If ulceration begins or pain, redness, or swelling persist, treat like doxorubicin.
Bleomycin (Blenoxan®)				1. May cause irritation to tissue. 2. Little information known.

(continued)

Table 1.6 *(continued)*

Irritants *(continued)*				
Chemotherapeutic Agents	**Antidote**	**Antidote Preparation**	**Local Care**	**Comments**
Epipodophyl-lotoxin				
Etoposide (VP-16)			1. Apply warm pack.	1. Treatment necessary only if large amount of a concentrated solution extravasates. In this case, treat like vincristine or vinblastine. 2. May cause phlebitis, urticaria, and redness.
Teniposide (VM-26)				Same as above.

[a]*Bristol-Myers-Squibb Oncology, Princeton, NJ;*
[b]*Pharmacia & Upjohn Co, Kalamazoo, MI;*
[c]*Chiron Therapeutics, Emeryville, CA;*
[d]*Andria Laboratories, Dublin, OH;*
[e]*Eli Lilly and Co., Indianapolis, IN;*
[f]*Glaxo Wellcome Oncology/HIV, Research Triangle Park, NC*

Note: Based on information from Bertelli, G., Gozzo, A., Forno, G.B., Vidili, M.G., Silvestro, S., Venturini, M., DelMastro, L., Garrone, O., Rosso, R., and Dini, D., 1995. Topical Dimethylsulfoxide for the Prevention of Soft Tissue Injury after Extravasation of Vesicant Cytotoxic Drugs: A Prospective Clinical Study. *Journal of Clinical Oncology,* 13(11):2851–2855; Lebredo, L., Barrie, R., and Woltering, E.A., 1992. DMSO Protection Against Adriamycin-induced Tissue Necrosis. *Journal of Surgery Research,* 53(1):62–65; Rospond, E.M., and Engel, L.M., 1993. Dimethyl Sulfoxide for Treating Anthracycline Extravesation. *Clinical Pharmatherapeutics* 12(8):560–561. *Source:* Brown KA, Esper P, Kellher LO, et al (2001) *Cancer Chemotherapy Guidelines and Recommendations for Practice,* pp 46–47. Reproduced with permission from Oncology Nursing Society Publishing.

Modified from Polovich M, White Jim, Kellner LO (Eds) (2005) *Chemotherapy and Biotherapy Guidelines and Recommendations for Practice*, 2nd Ed, pp. 79-81. Reproduced with permission from Oncology Nursing Society.

Table 1.7 Standardized Nursing Care Plan for Management of the Patient Experiencing Extravasation (Based on Oncology Nursing Press Cancer Chemotherapy Guidelines)

Nursing Diagnosis	Defining Characteristics	Expected Outcomes	Nursing Interventions
I. Potential alteration in skin integrity related to extravasation.	I. Vesicant drugs may cause erythema, burning, tissue necrosis, tissue sloughing.	I. Extravasation, if it occurs, is detected early with early intervention.	I. Careful technique is used during venipuncture. A. Select venipuncture site away from underlying tendons and blood vessels. B. Secure IV so that catheter/needle site is visible at all times. C. Administer vesicant through freely flowing IV, constantly monitoring IV site and patient response. Nurse should be thoroughly familiar with institutional policy and procedure for administration of a vesicant agent. D. If vesicant drug is administered as a continuous infusion, drug must be given through a patent central line and monitored closely.
II. Potential pain at site of extravasation.	II. Vesicant drugs include: A. Commercial agents 1. dactinomycin 2. daunorubicin 3. doxorubicin 4. mitomycin C	II. Skin and underlying tissue damage is minimized.	II. If extravasation is suspected: A. Stop drug administration. B. Aspirate any residual drug and blood from IV tubing, IV catheter/needle IV site if possible.

(continued)

Table 1.7 *(continued)*

Nursing Diagnosis	Defining Characteristics	Expected Outcomes	Nursing Interventions
	5. estramustine 6. mechlorethamine 7. vinblastine 8. vincristine 9. vinorelbine 10. idarubicin 11. vindesine 12. epirubicin 13. esorubicin 14. cisplatin (concentrated) 15. mitoxantrone 16. paclitaxel (concentrated) 17. fluorouracil (concentrated) B. Investigational agents 1. amsacrine 2. maytansine 3. bisantrene 4. pyrazofurin 5. adozelesin 6. anti-B4-blocked ricin		C. Instill antidote, if one exists, through needle if able to remove remaining drug in previous step. If standing orders are not available, notify MD and obtain order. D. Remove needle. E. Inject antidote into area of apparent infiltration, if antidote is recommended, using 25-gauge needle into subcutaneous tissue. F. Apply topical cream if recommended. G. Cover lightly with occlusive sterile dressing. H. Apply warm or cold applications as prescribed. I. Elevate arm. J. Assess site regularly for pain, progression of erythema, induration, and for evidence of necrosis: 1. If outpatient, arrange to assess site or teach patient to and to notify provider if condition worsens. Arrange next visit for assessment of site depending on drug, amount infiltrated, extent of potential injury, and patient variables.

(continued)

Table 1.7 *(continued)*

Nursing Diagnosis	Defining Characteristics	Expected Outcomes	Nursing Interventions
			2. Discuss with MD the need for plastic-surgical consult if erythema, induration, pain, tissue breakdown occurs. K. When in doubt about whether drug is infiltrating, treat as an infiltration. L. Document precise, concise information in patient's medical record: 1. Date, time 2. Insertion site, needle size and type 3. Drug administration technique, drug sequence, and approximate amount of drug extravasated 4. Appearance of site, patient's subjective response 5. Nursing interventions performed to manage extravasation, and notification of MD 6. Photo documentation if possible 7. Follow-up plan 8. Nurse's signature 9. Institutional policy and procedure for documentation should be adhered to
III. Potential loss of function of extremity related to extravasation			
IV. Potential infection related to skin breakdown			

Source: Barton-Burke M et al (2001) *Cancer Chemotherapy: A Nursing Process Approach,* pp 628–629. Reprinted with permission from Jones and Bartlett Publishers, Inc.

RAVASATION

ecific chemotherapeutic drugs called *vesicants* may cause severe tissue ne-osis if extravasated. Some of these drugs have antidotes that will minimize or prevent local tissue damage. These are shown in Table 1.6. For a Standardized Nursing Care Plan for management of patients experiencing extravasation, see Table 1.7.

When vesicants are administered as a continuous infusion, a central line is required. In addition, it is imperative that the IV insertion site be checked for signs/symptoms of extravasation at least hourly, and that the patient be instructed to tell the nurse immediately if stinging or burning is felt. As many continuous infusions of vesicant chemotherapy occur when the patient is at home, it is again imperative to instruct the patient to pay attention to any changes in sensation at the site, and to call the nurse if any discomfort, stinging, or burning is felt. A number of patients have had extravasation of drug from a needle dislodged from an implanted port onto the surrounding skin, which then caused a necrotic ulcer and necessitated explantation of the subcutaneous port.

Within the last decade, oncology nurses have been humbled by the reports of significant and lethal errors that have occurred during the chemotherapy prescription, admixing, and administration processes. It is clear that institutional and physician office practices must have systematic review of the entire linked process and steps taken to prevent the occurrence of these errors and tragic consequences through competent checks and balances (Fisher et al, 1996). Fortunately, the series of well-publicized errors have been a "wake-up" call, and oncology nurses, pharmacists, and physicians have worked together to develop safe environments for clinical practice. The Oncology Nursing Society position paper, "Regarding the Preparation of the Professional Registered Nurse Who Administers and Cares for the Individual Receiving Chemotherapy", states that the nurse administering chemotherapy and caring for patients receiving chemotherapy should complete a chemotherapy course and clinical practicum to safely and competently deliver chemotherapy. The course topics should include history of cancer chemotherapy; drug development; principles of cancer chemotherapy; chemotherapy preparation, storage, and transport; nursing assessment; chemotherapy administration; safety precautions during chemotherapy administration; disposal/accidental exposure and spills; and, finally, institutional considerations (ONS Position Paper, revised 6/99: ONS Safe Handeling of Hazardous Drugs, 2003; NISOH Safe Handeling of Hazardous Drugs, June 2004).

References

Ajani JA, Dodd LS, Daughtery K, et al. Taxol-Induced Soft-Tissue Injury Secondary Extravasation: Characterization by Histo-Pathology and Clinical Course. *JN* 1994;86:51–53

Alberts DS, Dorr RT. Case Report: Topical DMSO for Mitomycin-C-Induced Skin Ulceration. *Oncol Nurs Forum* 1991;18:693–695

Andre T, Boni C, Mounedji-Boudiaf L, et al. Oxaliplatin, fluorouracil and leucovorin as adjuvant treatment for colon cancer. *N Engl J Med* 2004;350(23):2342–2351

Anttila M, Laakso S, Nylanden P, Sotaniemi EA. Pharmacokinetics of the Novel Antiestrogenic Agent Toremifene in Subjects with Altered Liver and Kidney Function. *Clin Pharmacol Ther* 1995;57(6):628–635

AstraZeneca Pharmaceuticals LP. Prescribing Package Insert: Faslodex. Wilmington, DE:, AstraZeneca Pharmaceuticals LP; 2002

Aventis. Nilandron (Nilutamide) Product Information Center for Prostate Cancer. 2001; available at http://www.aventis-us.com/pls/nilandron_TXT.html. Accessed June 2004

Ayash LJ, Hunt M, Antman K. Hepatic Occlusive Disease in Autologous Bone Marrow Transplantition of Solid Tumor and Lymphomas. *J Clin Oncol* 1990;8:1699–1706

Bangham AC. Liposomes: Realizing Their Promise. *Hosp Pract* 1992;27(12):51–62

Barton-Burke M, Wilkes G, Berg D, et al. *Cancer Chemotherapy: A Nursing Process Approach,* 3rd ed Sudbury, MA: Jones and Bartlett; 2001

Baylin SB, Herman JG, Graff JR, et al. Alterations in DNA Methylation—A Fundamental Aspect of Neoplasia. *Adv Cancer Res* 1998;72:141–196

Berenson JR, et al. Efficacy of Pamidronate in Reducing Skeletal Events in Patients with Advanced Multiple Myeloma. *N Engl J Med* 1996;334:488–493

Bower M, Newlands ES, Bleehan NM, et al. Multicenter CRC Phase II Trial of Temozolomide in Recurrent or Progressive High Grade Glioma. *Cancer Chemother Pharmacol* 1997;40:484–488

Bristol-Myers Squibb Pharmaceutical Research Institute. Investigator Brochure for UFT (Uracil:Ftorafur in a molar ratio of 4:1); 1996

Brogden JM, Nevidjon B. Vinorelbine Tartare (Navelbine®): Drug Profile and Nursing Implications of a New Vinca Alkaloid. *Oncol Nurs Forum* 1995;22(4):635–646

Burris HA, Edelman MJ, Stewart F, et al. Phase II dose-ranging study of TLK286 (Telcyta), a novel glutathione analog prodrug, in combination with cisplatin as first-line treatment in locally advanced or metastatic non-small cell lung cancer (NSCLC). *Proc Am Soc Clin Oncol* 2005; abstract 7126, 41st Am Soc Clin Oncol Meeting, Orlando, FL

Camp-Sorrell D. Chemotherapy-Toxicity Management. Groenwald SL, Frogge MH, Goodman M, Yarbro CH, (eds), *Cancer Nursing: Principles and Practice.* Sudbury, MA: Jones and Bartlett; 1993

Cassidy J, Scheithauer W, McKendrick J, et al. *Capecitabine (X) vs bolus 5-FU/leucovorin (LV) as adjuvant therapy for colon cancer (the X-ACT study): efficacy results of a phase III trial J Clin Oncol 2004 ASCO Meeting Proceedings,* (Post-Meeting edition) 2004;22(14S):3509

Chabner BA, Longo DL. *Cancer Chemotherapy and Biotherapy: Principles and Practice,* 3rd ed. Philadelphia, Lippincott-Raven; 2001 g AY, Kuebler JP, Pandya KJ, et al. Pulmonary Toxicity Induced by Mitomycin C s Highly Responsive to Glucocorticoids. *Cancer* 1986;57:2285–2290

en AY, Liu LF. Topoisomerases: Essential Enzymes and Lethal Targets. *Annu Rev Pharmacol Toxicol* 1994;34:191–218

Cheson BD, Vena DA, Foss FM, Sorenson JM. Neurotoxicity of Purine Analogs: A Review. *J Clin Oncol* 1994;12(10):2216–2228

Chew T, Jacobs M. Pharmacology of Liposomal Daunorubicin and Its Use in Kaposi's Sarcoma. *Oncology* 1996;10(6):28–34

Chiron Therapeutics. Depocyt Package Insert. *Emeryville, CA, Chiron Therapeutics* 1999

Clinical Trials. *Colorectal Cancer Trials involving Irinotecan and the Saltz Regimen are Temporarily Suspended.* 2001; http://www.cancer.gov/clinicaltrials

Coombes RC, Haynes BP, Dowsett M, et al. Idoxifene: Report of a Phase I Study in Patients with Metastatic Breast Cancer. *Cancer Res* 1995;55:1070–1074

de Gramont A, Bossett JF, Milan C, et al. Randomized trial comparing monthly low-dose leucovorin and fluorouracil bolus with bimonthly high-dose leucovorin and fluorouracil bolus plus continuous infusion for advanced colorectal cancer: A French Intergroup study. *J Clin Oncol* 1997;15:808–815

de Gramont A, Banzi M, Navarro M, et al. Oxaliplatin/5-FU/LV in Adjuvant Colon Cancer: Results of the International Randomized Mosaic Trial. *Proc Am Society Clin Oncol* 2003; abstract 101,522:253

de Gramont A, Boni C, Navarro M, et al. Oxaliplatin/5FU/LV in the adjuvant treatment of stage II and stage III colon cancer: Efficacy results with a median follow-up of 4 years. Oral abstract presented at: ASCO 2005 Gastrointestinal Cancers Symposium; January 27–29, 2005; Hollywood, FL

Dorr R. Personal Communication, 8/22/95. 1995

Dorr RT. Antidotes to Vesicant Chemotherapy. *Blood Reviews* 1990;4(1):41–60

Dorr RT, Von Hoff DD. *Cancer Chemotherapy Handbook,* 2nd ed. Norwalk, CT: Appleton & Lange; 1994

Dowlati, et al. Phase 1 Clinical and Pharmacokinetic Study of Rebeccamycin Analog NSC 655649 Given Daily for Five Consecutive Days. *J Clin Oncol* 2001;19(8): 2309–2318

Eber JP. Camptothecins: New Traditionalists. *Adv Oncol* 1996;12(2):11–16

Ellis AK, Day JH. Diagnosis and Management of Anaphylaxis. *Canadian Medical Association Journal* 2003169(4):307–312

Fabian CJ, Molina R, Slavik M, et al. Pyridoxine Therapy for Palmar-Plantar Erythrodysesthesia Associated with Continuous 5-Fluorouracil Infusion. *Invest New Drugs* 1990;8(1):57–63

Fischer DS, Alfano S, Knof MT, et al. Improving the Cancer Chemotherapy Use Process. *J Clin Oncol* 1996;14(12):3148–3155

Fischer DS, Knobf MT, Durivage HJ, Beaulieu NJ. *The Cancer Chemotherapy Handbook,* 6th ed. St. Louis: Mosby Year-Book; 2003

Fishman M, Mrozek-Orlowski M. *Cancer Chemotherapy Guidelines and Recommendations for Practice,* 2nd ed. Pittsburgh, PA: Oncology Nursing Press; 1999

Franks AL, Steinberg KK. Encouraging News from the SERM Frontier: Selective Estrogen Receptor Modulators. *JAMA* 1999;281(23):2243–2244

Gianni L, Dombernowsky P, Sledge G, et al. Cardiac Function Following Combination Therapy with Taxol (T) and Doxorubicin (D) for Advanced Breast Cancer (ABC). *Proc Am SocClin Oncol* 1998;17:115a

Goodman M, Ladd LA, Pune S. Integumentary and Mucous Membrane Alterations. In Groenwald SL, Frogge M, Goodman M, Yarbro CH, (eds), *Cancer Nursing: Principles and Practice,* 3rd ed. Sudbury, MA: Jones and Bartlett; 1993;734–800

Harwood KV, Govin K. Short-Term vs Long-Term Local Cooling after Doxorubicin Extravasations: An Eastern Cooperative Oncology Group (ECOG) Study [abstract]. *Proceedings of the American Society of Clinical Oncology* 1994;13:447

Hortobagyi GM, et al. New Cytotoxic Agents for the Treatment of Breast Cancer. *Oncology* 1996;10(Suppl):21–29

Hortobagyi GM, et al. Reduction of Skeletal Related Complications in Breast Cancer Patients with Osteolytic Bone Metastases Receiving Chemotherapy by Monthly Pamidronate Sodium Infusion. Proceedings of 32nd Annual ASCO Meeting, Philadelphia, ASCO 1996; abstract 99

Hossan E, Logothetis CJ. The Medical Managment of Progressive Prostate Cancer. *Oncology Special Edition* 1999;2:13–16

Husain I, Mohler JL, Seigler HF, et al. Elevation of Topoisomerase I Messenger RNA, Protein, and Catalytic Activity in Human Tumors: Demonstration of Tumor-Type Specificity and Implications for Cancer Chemotherapy. *Cancer Res* 1994;54: 539–546

Ibrahim NK, Desai N, Legha S, et al. Phase I and pharmacokinetic study of ABI-007, a cremaphor-free protein-stabilized, nanoparticle formulation of paclitaxel. *Clin Cancer Res* 2002;8:1038–1044

Kaisery AV. Current Clinical Studies with a New Nonsteroidal Antiandrogen, CasodeX. *Prostate Suppl* 1994;5:27–33

Kaufmann M, Bajetta E, Dirix LY, et al. Exemestane Is Superior to Megestrol Acetate after Tamoxifen Failure in Postmenopausal Women with Advanced Breast Cancer: Results of a Phase III Randomized Double-blind Trial. The Exemestance Study Group. *J Clin Oncol* 2000;18(7):1399–1411

Kelland LR, Jarman M. Idoxifene. *Drugs of the Future* 1995;20(7):666–669

Larson DK. What Is the Appropriate Treatment for Tissue Extravasation by Antitumor Agents?. *Plastic and Reconstructive Surgery* 1985;75:397–405

Lathia C, Fleming G, Meyer M, Whitfield L. Pentostatin Pharmacokinetics and Dosing Guidelines in Patients with Renal Impairment. *PharmSci* 1998;1(1):Abstract 3360 American Association of Pharmaceutical Scientists Supplement, 1998 AAPS Annual Meeting, San Francisco, CA, November 1998

Laurie SW, Wilson KL, Keinahan DA, et al. Intravenous Extravasation Injuries: The Effectiveness of Hyaluronidase in Their Treatment. *Annals of Plastic Surgery* 1984; 13(3):191–194

Ligand Pharmaceuticals. Panretin Package Insert. San Diego, Ligand Pharmaceuticals 1999

Loprinzi CL, Pisansky TM, Fonseca R, et al. Pilot Evaluation of Venlafaxine Hydrochloride for the Therapy of Hot Flashes in Cancer Survivors. *J Clin Oncol* 1998;16: 2377–2381

Loprinzi CL, Sloane JA, Perez EA, et al. Phase III Evaluation of Fluoxetine for Treatment of Hot Flashes. *J Clin Oncol* 2002;20(6):1578–1583

Lui LF, Lui CC, Alberts BM. Type 2 DNA Topoisomerases: Enzymes That Can Unknot a Topologically Knotted DNA Molecule via a Reversible Double-Strand Break. *Cell* 1980;19:697–707

Mandelli F. Introduction to the Workshop on DNA Methyltransferase Inhibitors. *Leukemia* 1993;7(Suppl 1):1–2

Markman M. Prevention of paclitaxel-associated arthralgias and myalgias. *J Support Oncol* 2003;1:233–234

Markman M, Zanotti L, Peterson G, et al. Expanded experience with an intradermal skin test to predict for the presence or absence of carboplatin sensitivity. *J Clin Oncol* 2003;21:4611–4614

Matsuura T, Fukuda Y, Fujitaka T, et al. Preoperative Treatment with Tegafur Suppositories Enhances Apoptosis and Reduces the Intratumoral Microvessel Density of Human Colorectal Carcinoma. *Cancer* 2000;88(5):1007–1015

McEvoy GK, (ed). *AHFS 96 Drug Information.* Bethesda, MD: American Society of Health-System Pharmacists, Inc.; 1996

McFarland HM. Guide for the Administration and Use of Cancer Chemotherapeutic Agents. *Oncology Special Edition* 1999;2:82–87

Mouridsen H, Gershanovich M, Sun Y, et al. Superior Efficacy of Letrozole Versus Tamoxifen as First-line Therapy for Postmenopausal Women with Advanced Breast Cancer: Results of a Phase III Study of the International Letrozole Breast Cancer Group. *J Clin Oncol* 2001;19(10):2596–2606

Natelson EA, Giovanella BC, Verschraegen CF, et al. Phase I Clinical and Pharmacological Studies of 20-(S)-Camptothecin and 20-(S)-9-Nitrocamptothecin as Anticancer Agents. *Ann New York Acad Sci* 1996;803:224–230

Newlands ES, Stevens MFG, Wedge SR, et al. Temozolomide: A Review of Its Discovery, Chemical Properties, Pre-clinical Development and Clinical Trials. *Cancer Treat Rev* 1997;23:35–61

Niitsu N, Yamaguchi Y, Umeda M, Honma Y. Human Monocytoid Leukemia Cells Are Highly Sensitive to Apoptosis Induced by 2′-Deoxycoformycin and 2′-Deoxyadenosine: Association with dATP-dependent Activation of Caspase-3. *Blood* 1998;92(9): 3368–3375

Ninomoto J. Personal communication re rubitecan, decitabine, and pentostatin. San Ramon, CA: SuperGen; 2000

Novartis Pharmaceuticals. Aredia Package Insert. East Hanover, NJ: Novartis; 1998

Novotny WF, Holmgren E, Nelson B, et al. Bevacizumab (a monocolonal antibody to vascular endothelial growth factor) does not increase the incidence of venous thromboembolism when added to first-line chemotherapy to treat metastatic colorectal cancer. *Proc Am Soc Clin Oncol* 2004;23:252, abstract 3529

Occupational Safety and Health Administration. *Controlling Occupational Exposure to Hazardous Drugs.* 1995; Washington (OSHA Instruction CPL 2-2.20B)

Oktay, et al. JCO 2005

Oncology Nursing Society Board of Directors. *ONS Position Paper: Regarding t. Preparation of the Professional Registered Nurse who Administers and Cares fo the Individual Receiving Chemotherapy.* Pittsburgh, PA: Oncology Nursing Society; 1999

Orphan Medical. Busulfex (Busulfan) for Injection: Prescribing Information, 1999; available at http://www.orphan.com. Accessed June 2004

Perry MC, (ed). *The Chemotherapy Source Book,* 2nd ed. Baltimore: Williams & Wilkins; 1997

Pharmacia and Upjohn Company. *Patient Instructions for Management of Diarrhea Resulting from Camptosar®.* Kalamazoo, MI, Pharmacia and Upjohn Company 1996

Praecis Pharmaceuticals Incorporated. Plenaxis Package Insert. Waltham, MA: Praecis Pharmaceuticals Inc.; 2001

Polovich M, White JM, Kelleher LO, (eds), *Chemotherapy and Biotherapy Guidelines and Recommendations for Practice* 2nd ed. Pittsburgh, PA: Oncology Nursing Society; 2005

Rhone-Poulenc Rorer Pharmaceutical. Gliadel Package Insert. Collegeville, PA: Rhone-Poulenc Rorer 1997

Rittenberg CN, Gralla RJ, Rehmeyer TA. Assessing and Managing Venous Irritation Associated with Vinorelbine Tartare (Navelbine®). *Oncol Nurs Forum* 1995;22(4): 707–710

Sacchi S, Kantarjian HM, O'Brien S, et al. Chronic Myelogenous Leukemia in Nonlymphoid Blastic Phase: Analysis of the Results of First Salvage Therapy with Three Different Treatment Approaches for 162 Patients. *Cancer* 1999;86(12):2632–2641

Sanofi Synthelabo. Eloxatin Package Insert. New York: Sanofi Synthelabo, Inc.; 2004

Seidman AD, Berry D, Cirrincione L, et al. CALGB 9840: Phase III study of weekly (W) paclitaxel (P) via 1-hour (h) infusion versus standard (S) 3 h infusion every third week in the treatment of metastatic breast cancer (MBC), with trastuzumab (T) for HER2 positive MBC and randomized for T in HER2 normal MBC. *Proc Am Soc Clin Oncol* 2004;23:6, abstract 512

Sheperd GM. Hypersensitivity Reactions to Chemotherapeutic Drugs. *Allergy and Immunology* 2003;24:253–262

Shifflett SL, Harvey RD, Pfeiffer D, et al. Cancer Chemotherapeutic Regimens. *Oncology Special Edition* 1999;2:59–66

Slichenmyer WJ, Rowinsky EK, Donehower RC, Kaufmann SH. The Current Status of Camptothecin Analogues as Antitumor Agents. *J Natl Cancer Instit* 1993;85(4): 271–291

Smith IE, Johnston SRD, O'Brien MER, et al. Low-Dose Oral Fluorouracil with Eniluracil as First-Line Chemotherapy Against Advanced Breast Cancer: A Phase I Study. *J Clin Oncol* 2000;18(12):2378–2384

Solimando DA, Bressler L, Kintzel PE, Geraci MC. *Drug Information Handbook for Oncology,* 2nd ed. Cleveland, Ohio: Lexi-Comp, Inc.; 2000

Suwanawiboon B, Sumida KN. 5-azacitidine: An alternative treatment of myeloplastic syndromes in patient with refractory response to hematopoietic growth factor, a case report and review of the literature. *Hawaii Med J* 2004;63(1):14–16, 25

Taylor SCM. Raltitrexed for Advanced Colorectal Cancer: The Story So Far. *Cancer Practice* 2000;8(1):51–54

Thomas GM. Raising Hemoglobin: An Opportunity for Increasing Survival. *Oncology* 2002;63 Suppl 2:19–28

Trissel LA, Saenz CA, Ingram DS, Ogundele AB. Compatibility Screening of Oxaliplatin during Simulated Y-site Administration with Other Drugs. *J Oncol Pharm Practice* 2002;8(1):33–37

Venook AP, Egorin MJ, Rosner GL, et al. Phase I and Pharmacokinetic Trial of Paclitaxel in Patients with Hepatic Dysfunction: Cancer and Leukemia Group B 9264. *J Clin Oncol* 1998;16:1811–1819

Verschraegen CF, Hupta E, Loyer E, et al. A Phase II Clinical and Pharmacological Study of Oral 9-Nitrocamptothecin in Patients with Refractory Epithelial Ovarian, Tubal or Peritoneal Cancer. *Anti-Cancer Drugs* 1999;10:373–383

Verschraegen CF, Nateson E, Giovanella BC, et al. A Phase I Clinical and Pharmacological Study of Oral 9-Nitrocamptothecin, a Novel Water-Insoluble Topoisomerase I Inhibitor. *Anti Cancer Drugs* 1998;9:36–44

Vukelja SJ, Lombardo FA, James WD, Weiss RB. Pyridoxine for the Palmar-Plantar Erythrodysesthesia Syndrome [letter]. *Ann Intern Med* 1989;111:688–689

Wijermans P, Lubbert M, Verhoef G, et al. Low Dose 5-aza-2′-Deoxycytidine, a DNA Hypomethylating Agent, for the Treatment of High-Risk Myelodysplastic Syndrome: A Multicenter Phase II Study in Elderly Patients. *J Clin Oncol* 2000;18(5):956–967

Wilkes GM. New Therapeutic Options in Colon Cancer: Focus on Oxaliplatin. *Clinical Journal of Oncology Nursing* 2002;3:131–137

Wilkes GM. Therapeutic Options in the Management of Colon Cancer: 2005 Update. *Clinical Journal of Oncology Nursing* 2005;9(1):31–44

Drug: abarelix for injectable suspension (Plenaxis)

Class: Gonadotropin releasing-hormone (GnRH) antagonist.

Mechanism of Action: Directly and competitively blocks GnRH receptors in the pituitary: suppresses luteinizing hormone (LH) and follicle stimulating hormone (FSH) secretion, and thereby reduces the secretion of testosterone by the testes. There is no initial increase in serum testosterone concentrations.

Metabolism: Following IM administration, drug is slowly absorbed with a mean peak concentration 3 days after injection, and distributes extensively within the body. Drug is highly protein bound (96–99%), and is excreted in the urine, with 13% of drug unchanged.

Dosage/Range:

- 100 mg IM in the buttock days 1, 15, 29 (week 4), and every 4 weeks thereafter
- Assess efficacy by monitoring serum testosterone levels baseline, day 29, and then every 8 weeks thereafter

Drug Preparation/Administration:

- Reconstitute drug following manufacturer's recommendations to yield 50 mg/mL
- Administer in the buttock, and rotate sites

Drug Interactions:

Lab Effects/Interference:

- LFTs: transaminases may become elevated
- Serum testosterone levels should decrease to < 50 ng/dL. Slight decrease in hemoglobin
- Increase in serum triglycerides by 10%

Special Considerations:

- Drug is indicated for the palliative treatment of men with advanced symptomatic prostate cancer, in whom LHRH agonist therapy is not appropriate and who refuse surgical castration, and have one or more of the following:
    1) risk of neurological compromise due to metastases,
    2) ureteral or bladder outlet obstruction due to local encroachment of metastatic disease, or
    3) severe bone pain from skeletal metastases persisting on opioid analgesia
- Drug achieves castration levels of testosterone 24 hours after IM injection
- The effectiveness of abarelix in suppressing serum testosterone to castration levels decreases with continued dosing in patients weighing > 225 lbs, and effectiveness beyond 12 months has not been established. Assess total serum testosterone levels just prior to drug administration on day 29, and every 8 weeks thereafter to assure continued response in all patients. Periodic measurement of serum PSA will assist in assessing response.
- Immediate-onset systemic allergic reactions, with hypotension and syncope, may occur; risk increases with increased cumulative dose so patients should be observed for at least 30 minutes following the injection.
- Drug may cause QT interval prolongation in 20% of patients (changes from baseline of > 30 msec, or end-of-treatment QTc values > 450 msec; use cautiously if at all in patients taking class IA (quinidine, procainamide) or class III (amiodarone, sotalol) antiarrhythmic medications.
- Drug is not indicated for women or children; drug may cause fetal harm if administered to a pregnant woman.
- Transaminase levels became clinically significantly elevated in some patients, so levels should be assessed baseline, and periodically during treatment.
- Bone mineral density may decrease with extended treatment with GnRH antagonists and LHRH agonists.

Potential Toxicities/Side Effects and the Nursing Process

I. POTENTIAL FOR INJURY related to HYPERSENSITIVITY REACTION

Defining Characteristics: Allergic reactions can occur immediately after injection, and may result in hypotension and syncope, starting with the initial dose, or occurring later in the course of treatment. Risk increases with the duration of treatment.

Nursing Implications: Assess baseline VS and mental status prior to drug administration, and observe patient for 30 minutes following injection. Recall signs/symptoms of anaphylaxis, and if these occur, notify physician, and assess patient's vital signs. Subjective symptoms are generalized itching, nausea, chest tightness, crampy abdominal pain, difficulty speaking, anxiety, agitation, sense of impending doom, uneasiness, desire to urinate/defecate, dizziness, and chills. Objective signs are flushed appearance; angioedema of face, neck, eyelids, hands, and feet; localized or generalized urticaria; respiratory distress with or without wheezing; hypotension; and cyanosis. Review standing orders or nursing procedures for patient management of anaphylaxis, and be prepared to administer ordered medications, which may include epinephrine 1:1000, hydrocortisone sodium succinate, and diphenhydramine. Teach patient to report any unusual symptoms.

II. ALTERATION IN COMFORT related to HOT FLUSHES, SLEEP DISTURBANCES, PAIN, BREAST ENLARGEMENT/TENDERNESS, HEADACHE, EDEMA, AND DIZZINESS

Defining Characteristics: Signs and symptoms of androgen deprivation are: Hot flushes (79%), sleep deprivation (44%), breast enlargement (30%), breast pain/nipple tenderness (20%). Pain in general occurs in about 31% of patients, as well as back pain (17%).

Nursing Implications: Teach patient that symptoms may occur. Encourage patient to report symptoms early. Develop symptom management plan with patient and physician.

III. ALTERATION IN BOWEL AND BLADDER ELIMINATION related to HORMONAL CHANGES

Defining Characteristics: Diarrhea occurs in about 11% of patients, while constipation occurs in 15%. 10% of patients develop dysuria, micturition frequency, urinary retention, or urinary tract infection.

Nursing Implications: Assess baseline bowel and bladder elimination pattern, and teach patient to report any changes. Teach patient to modify diet to minimize either diarrhea or constipation. Discuss need for referral to urologist if dysuria, urinary retention, or urinary tract infections persist.

Drug: adrenocorticoids (Cortisone, Dexamethasone, Hydrocortisone, Methylprednisolone, Prednisolone, Prednisone)

Class: Hormones.

Mechanism of Action: Cause lysis of lymphoid cells, which leads to their use against lymphatic leukemia, myeloma, malignant lymphoma. May also recruit malignant cells out of G_0 phase, making them vulnerable to damage caused by cell-cycle-phase-specific agents.

Metabolism: Metabolized by the liver, excreted in urine. Prednisone is activated by the liver in its active form, prednisolone.

Dosage/Range:

- Varies according to which preparation is used. Dexamethasone is 25 times the potency of hydrocortisone.
- Cortisone 25 mg.
- Dexamethasone 0.75 mg.
- Hydrocortisone 20 mg.
- Methylprednisolone 4 mg.
- Prednisone, Prednisolone 5 mg.

Drug Preparation:

- None.

Drug Administration:

- Oral.

Drug Interactions:

- May increase K+ loss and hypokalemia when combined with amphotericin B or potassium-depleting diuretics.
- Warfarin (Coumadin) dose may need to be increased.
- Insulin or oral hypoglycemia dose may need to be increased.
- Oral contraceptives may inhibit steroid metabolism.

Lab Effects/Interference:

- Increased Na, decreased K with hypokalemic alkalosis.
- Decreased I^{131} uptake and protein-bound iodine concentration. May cause difficulty monitoring therapeutic response of patients treated for thyroid conditions.
- False-negative results in nitroblue tetrazolium test for systemic bacterial infections.
- May suppress reactions to skin tests.

Special Considerations:

- Chronic steroid use is associated with numerous side effects. Intermittent therapy is safer and in some conditions just as effective as daily therapy.

Potential Toxicities/Side Effects and the Nursing Process

I. ALTERATION IN NUTRITION, LESS THAN BODY REQUIREMENTS, related to GASTRIC IRRITATION, DECREASED CARBOHYDRATE METABOLISM, AND HYPERGLYCEMIA

Defining Characteristics: Steroids can cause increased secretion of hydrochloric acid and decreased secretion of protective gastric mucus, which can exacerbate an existing gastric ulcer. They are insulin antagonists and may cause gluconeogenesis. In addition, steroids may increase appetite and cause weight gain.

Nursing Implications: Administer drugs with meals or an antacid. Instruct patient to report evidence of gastric distress immediately; teach patient to take steroids prior to a meal or with milk or food. Obtain baseline glucose levels and monitor periodic blood sugars throughout therapy. Teach patient to recognize signs/symptoms of hyperglycemia (polyuria, polydipsia, polyphagia), and to report these to the doctor or nurse.

II. POTENTIAL FOR INJURY related to SODIUM AND WATER RETENTION, ALTERATIONS IN FLUID AND ELECTROLYTE BALANCE, AND STEROIDINDUCED IMMUNOSUPPRESSION

Defining Characteristics: Sodium and water retention may occur and lead to CHF, hypertension, and edema in susceptible individuals; hypokalemia and hypocalcemia may occur due to increased excretion of potassium and calcium. Osteoporosis may occur with long-term therapy. Steroids increase susceptibility to infections and tuberculosis, may mask or aggravate infection, and may prolong or delay healing of injuries.

Nursing Implications: Identify patients at risk for complications associated with fluid/sodium retention (i.e., patients with preexisting cardiac, renal, hepatic dysfunction); monitor fluid and electrolyte balance and assess for imbalance. Document baseline cardiac status and monitor through therapy. Instruct patient to report signs/symptoms of hypokalemia (anorexia, muscle twitching, tetany, polyuria, polydipsia) and of hypocalcemia (leg cramps, tingling in fingertips, muscle twitching); monitor electrolytes regularly and discuss abnormal values with physician. Encourage high-potassium, high-calcium diet, and instruct patient in safety measures as needed. Teach patient to report slow healing of wounds, signs/symptoms of infection (erythema, warmth, purulence) of skin areas, as well as sore throat and burning on urination. Reinforce/teach patient hygiene measures for mouth, perineum, and skin.

III. POTENTIAL FOR INJURY related to RAPID WITHDRAWAL OF THERAPY

Defining Characteristics: Long-term therapy leads to suppression of normal adrenal function. Rapid cessation of therapy will lead to adrenal insufficiency, characterized by anorexia, nausea, orthostatic hypotension, dizziness, depression, dyspnea, hypoglycemia, and rebound inflammation (fever, myalgias, arthralgia, malaise). It can be fatal.

Nursing Implications: Discuss with physician the taper of steroids and instruct patient/family carefully. Teach patient to report symptoms of rapid withdrawal to nurse or physician.

IV. POTENTIAL FOR BODY IMAGE DISTURBANCE related to CUSHINGOID CHANGES

Defining Characteristics: Cushingoid state may occur with prolonged use and may be diminished by every-other-day dosing. Changes include moonface, striae, purpura, acne, hirsutism. In addition, increased appetite from steroids may lead to weight gain.

Nursing Implications: Teach patient about potential changes and provide reassurance that they will resolve once therapy ceases; encourage patient to verbalize feelings and provide emotional support.

V. POTENTIAL FOR SENSORY/PERCEPTUAL ALTERATIONS related to CATARACTS OR GLAUCOMA, AND OCULAR INFECTIONS (increased risk)

Defining Characteristics: Cataracts or glaucoma may develop with prolonged steroid use; risk of ocular infections from virus or fungi is increased.

Nursing Implications: Teach patient to report signs/symptoms of eye infection, such as discharge, erythema, or visual changes; ophthalmologic exams are recommended every two to three months.

VI. INEFFECTIVE COPING related to AFFECTIVE/BEHAVIORAL CHANGES

Defining Characteristics: Emotional lability, insomnia, mood swings, euphoria, and psychosis may occur, causing ineffective coping and role-relationship problems if unprepared.

Nursing Implications: Teach patient and family that affective/behavioral changes may occur and that they will resolve once therapy is discontinued. Encourage patient and family to report these changes, especially if troublesome.

VII. IMPAIRED PHYSICAL MOBILITY related to MUSCULOSKELETAL CHANGES

Defining Characteristics: With chronic, high-dose usage, loss of muscle mass, muscle weakness (steroid myopathy), tendon rupture, osteoporosis, pathologic fractures, and aseptic necrosis of the heads of the humerus and femur can occur.

Nursing Implications: Teach patient that muscle weakness and other effects can occur with therapy and that muscle cramping may occur with discontinuation of therapy. Teach patient to report weakness, cramping, and any musculoskeletal changes. If weakness occurs, therapy may be discontinued.

Drug: altretamine (Hexalen, Hexamethylmelamine)

Class: Alkylating agent.

Mechanism of Action: The exact mechanism of action is unknown. May inhibit incorporation of thymidine and uridine into DNA and RNA, respectively. Altretamine is believed not to act as an alkylating agent in vitro, but it may be activated to an alkylating agent in vivo. Also may act as an antimetabolite with activity in S phase.

Metabolism: Well absorbed orally although bioavailability is variable. Peak plasma concentration in 1 hour. Metabolized extensively in the liver, with majority excreted in the urine. Some of the drug is excreted as respiratory CO_2. Half-life of the parent compound is 4.7–10.2 hours.

Dosage/Range:
- 4–12 mg/kg/day (divided in 3 or 4 doses) × 21–90 days, or
- 240 mg/m^2 (6 mg/kg)–320 mg/m^2 (8 mg/kg) daily × 21 days, repeated every 6 weeks.

Drug Preparation:
- Available in 50-mg and 100-mg capsules.

Drug Administration:
- Oral.

Drug Interactions:
- Concurrent administration of drug with monoamine oxidase inhibitor (MAO) antidepressants may cause severe orthostatic hypotension.

Lab Effects/Interference:
- Decreased CBC.
- Increased BUN, creatinine.

Special Considerations:

- Nausea and vomiting can be minimized if patient takes dose two hours after meals and at bedtime.
- Nadir three to four weeks after treatment.

Potential Toxicities/Side Effects and the Nursing Process

I. INFECTION AND BLEEDING related to BONE MARROW DEPRESSION

Defining Characteristics: Causes mild to moderate bone marrow suppression, with nadir occurring 21–28 days after beginning treatment, and rapid recovery within one week of cessation of drug. Anemia occurs in 33% of patients and is moderate to severe in 9% of patients.

Nursing Implications: Assess CBC, WBC, differential, and platelet count prior to drug administration, as well as for signs/symptoms of infection or bleeding. Teach patient signs/symptoms of infection and bleeding, and instruct to report them immediately. Teach self-care measures to minimize risk of infection and bleeding, including avoidance of OTC aspirin-containing medications. Assess energy and activity tolerance; discuss blood transfusion with physician as appropriate. Discuss with physician dose interruption and reduction if WBC $< 2000/mm^3$, ANC $< 1000/mm^3$, or platelet count $< 75{,}000/mm^3$.

II. SENSORY/PERCEPTUAL ALTERATIONS related to PERIPHERAL NEUROPATHY AND CNS EFFECTS

Defining Characteristics: Peripheral sensory neuropathy occurs in 31% of patients and is moderate to severe in 9% of patients. Paresthesia, hyperesthesia, hyperreflexia, and numbness may occur and are reversible. CNS effects of agitation, confusion, hallucinations, depression, mood disorders, and Parkinson-like symptoms may occur, and usually are reversible. Neurologic effects are more common with continuous dosing > 3 months, rather than pulse dosing.

Nursing Implications: Assess baseline neurologic status. Teach patient that possible side effects may occur, and instruct to report them. If neurologic toxicity is severe, drug should be dose reduced, then discontinued if symptoms do not improve.

III. ALTERATION IN NUTRITION, LESS THAN BODY REQUIREMENTS, related to NAUSEA AND VOMITING, DIARRHEA, ABDOMINAL CRAMPS, ANOREXIA

Defining Characteristics: Nausea occurs in 33% of patients and is dose related. Tolerance may develop after three weeks of drug administration. Diarrhea and cramps may be dose-limiting. Anorexia may occur.

Nursing Implications: Premedicate with antiemetics (phenothiazines are usually effective) at least initially, then as needed. Divide dose into four doses, and give 1–2 hours after meals and at bedtime. Instruct patient to report nausea/vomiting, diarrhea, abdominal cramping. Teach self-administration of prescribed antidiarrheals and self-care techniques to manage cramps, e.g., heat pads or position change. If GI side effects are refractory to symptom management, discuss interrupting dose and then dose reduction with physician.

IV. ALTERATION IN SKIN INTEGRITY related to SKIN RASHES

Defining Characteristics: Skin rashes, pruritus, eczematous skin lesions may occur but are rare.

Nursing Implications: Assess for changes in skin color, texture, and integrity. Teach patient to report any changes in skin, and discuss measures to minimize discomfort.

V. ALTERATION IN ELIMINATION related to RENAL DYSFUNCTION

Defining Characteristics: Elevations in BUN (9% of patients) or creatinine (7%) can occur.

Nursing Implications: Assess baseline renal status and monitor renal function studies throughout treatment.

VI. POTENTIAL SEXUAL DYSFUNCTION related to DRUG EFFECTS

Defining Characteristics: Drug is mutagenic, carcinogenic, and teratogenic. Drug causes testicular atrophy and decreased spermatogenesis. It is unknown whether drug is excreted in human milk.

Nursing Implications: Discuss with patient and partner normal sexual patterns and anticipated dysfunction resulting from drug or disease. Provide information, emotional support, and referral for counseling as appropriate.

Drug: 9-aminocamptothecin (9-AC) (investigational)

Class: Topoisomerase inhibitor.

Mechanism of Action: Induces protein-linked DNA single-strand breaks and blocks DNA and RNA synthesis in dividing cells, preventing cells from entering mitosis. Cell cycle specific.

Metabolism: 32% of the drug is excreted in the urine as unchanged drug at 96 hours.

Dosage/Range:
- 35 μg/m²/h every 2 weeks or 45 μg/m²/h every 3 weeks (Phase II trials) as 72-hour infusion.
- Prolonged infusion studies under way.

Drug Preparation:
- Per protocol.

Drug Administration:
- IV infusion over 72 hours.

Drug Interactions:
- Unknown.

Lab Effects/Interference:
- Decreased CBC.

Special Considerations:
- Neutropenia is dose-limiting toxicity.

Potential Toxicities/Side Effects and the Nursing Process

I. INFECTION AND BLEEDING related to BONE MARROW DEPRESSION

Defining Characteristics: Causes neutropenia (dose-limiting), thrombocytopenia, and anemia.

Nursing Implications: Assess CBC, WBC, differential, and platelet count prior to drug administration, as well as signs/symptoms of infection or bleeding. Teach patient signs/symptoms of infection and bleeding, and instruct to report them immediately. Teach self-care measures to minimize risk of infection and bleeding, including avoidance of OTC aspirin-containing medications. Assess energy and activity tolerance; discuss blood transfusion with physician as appropriate. Discuss with physician dose interruption and reduction if WBC $< 2000/mm^3$ or absolute neutrophil count $< 1000/mm^3$, platelet count $< 75{,}000/mm^3$.

II. ALTERATION IN NUTRITION, LESS THAN BODY REQUIREMENTS, related to NAUSEA AND VOMITING, DIARRHEA

Defining Characteristics: Nausea, vomiting, diarrhea, mucositis may occur.

Nursing Implications: Premedicate with antiemetics. Teach patient to report nausea/vomiting, diarrhea, and changes in oral mucosa. Teach self-administration of prescribed antidiarrheals, and self-care techniques for discomfort and mucosal integrity. Teach oral hygiene self-care measures, including self-assessment, and systematic oral cleansing. Refer to clinical protocol.

III. ALTERATION IN SKIN INTEGRITY related to ALOPECIA

Defining Characteristics: Alopecia may occur.

Nursing Implications: Teach patient about possible side effects and self-care measures, including obtaining a wig or cap as appropriate prior to hair loss. Encourage patient to verbalize feelings and provide patient emotional support.

IV. POTENTIAL FOR ACTIVITY INTOLERANCE related to FATIGUE

Defining Characteristics: Fatigue and anemia are common.

Nursing Implications: Teach patient to report increasing fatigue, signs of severe anemia (shortness of breath, chest pain/angina, headaches). Monitor hemoglobin/hematocrit; discuss transfusion with physician if signs/symptoms develop or hematocrit falls (refer to protocol).

Drug: aminoglutethimide (Cytadren, Elipten)

Class: Adrenal steroid inhibitor.

Mechanism of Action: Causes "chemical adrenalectomy." Blocks adrenal production of steroids, reducing levels of glucocorticoids, mineralocorticoids, and estrogens. Also inhibits peripheral aromatization of androgens to estrogens.

Metabolism: Well-absorbed orally. Hydroxylated in liver; undergoes enterohepatic circulation. Most of drug is excreted in urine.

Dosage/Range:
- 750–2000 mg PO daily in divided doses.
- 40 mg hydrocortisone daily given to replace glucocorticoid deficiencies.

Drug Preparation:
- None.

Drug Administration:
- Oral.

Drug Interactions:
- Drug enhances dexamethasone metabolism, so hydrocortisone should be used for glucocorticoid replacement.
- Warfarin (Coumadin) dose may need to be increased.
- Alcohol potentiates drug side effects.
- May need to increase doses of theophylline, digitoxin, or medroxyprogesterone.

Lab Effects/Interference:
- Hypothyroidism: monitor TFT.
- Elevated LFTs, especially SGOT, alk phos, bili.

Special Considerations:

- Skin rash may develop within 5–7 days, lasting 8 days, often with malaise and fever (37.7–39°C [100–102°F]). If not resolved in 7–14 days, drug should be discontinued.
- Adjuvant corticosteroids need to be administered.

Potential Toxicities/Side Effects and the Nursing Process

I. ALTERATION IN ENDOCRINE FUNCTION related to ADRENAL INSUFFICIENCY

Defining Characteristics: Drug causes reversible chemical adrenalectomy by blockade of steroid hormone production. Patient will experience signs/symptoms of adrenal insufficiency if enough replacement glucocorticoid steroids are not received. Signs/symptoms of adrenal insufficiency include hyponatremia, hypoglycemia, dizziness, and postural hypotension. In addition, possible ovarian blockade may result in virilization.

Nursing Implications: Teach patient about self-administration of hydrocortisone replacement therapy (i.e., administer in A.M. with breakfast), potential side effects, and tapering schedule; refer to section on adrenocorticoids. Teach patient side effects of hormone replacement and self-assessment techniques, including weekly weights and signs/symptoms of infection. Monitor electrolytes, especially Na+, K+, and Ca++. Assess for signs/symptoms of adrenal insufficiency (fatigue, anorexia, nausea, vomiting, diarrhea, weight loss, weakness, dizziness, and low blood sugar). As appropriate, explore with patient/significant other reproductive and sexuality patterns and impact chemotherapy may have. Recognize that patient may need increased hydrocortisone and mineralocorticoid support if surgery is needed (increased stress requirement).

II. IMPAIRED SKIN INTEGRITY related to DRUG RASH

Defining Characteristics: Area of erythema, pruritus, and unexplained dermatitis may appear within one week of treatment and disappear in 5–8 days. May be accompanied by malaise and low-grade fever.

Nursing Implications: Teach patient to report symptoms and to avoid scratching involved areas if rash develops. Assess skin for any changes and rash development. Consider use of Sarna cream, and use of OTC diphenhydramine.

III. SENSORY/PERCEPTUAL ALTERATIONS related to TRANSIENT SYMPTOMS

Defining Characteristics: Transient symptoms such as drowsiness, lethargy, somnolence, visual blurring, vertigo, and ataxia may occur, as may nystagmus. Lethargy may be severe in elderly patients.

Nursing Implications: Document baseline neurological function and general health assessment. Teach patient possible side effects, self-assessment, and to report symptoms. Discuss with physician possible dose reduction for significant symptoms.

IV. ALTERATION IN NUTRITION related to NAUSEA/VOMITING AND ANOREXIA

Defining Characteristics: Nausea/vomiting and anorexia occur in approximately 10–13% of patients and are mild.

Nursing Implications: Initially, premedicate (and teach patient to) with antiemetics prior to drug administration. Usually symptoms subside within two weeks. Encourage small, frequent feedings.

V. ALTERATION IN OXYGENATION/PERFUSION related to HYPOTENSION

Defining Characteristics: Drug may block aldosterone production leading to orthostatic or persistent hypotension. This is not usually a problem when hydrocortisone replacement is given.

Nursing Implications: Monitor BP regularly. Instruct patient to change position slowly and to report dizziness.

Drug: anastrozole (Arimidex)

Class: Nonsteroidal aromatase inhibitor.

Mechanism of Action: Inhibits the enzyme aromatase. Aromatase is one of the P-450 enzymes and is involved in estrogen biosynthesis. Circulating estrogen in postmenopausal women (mainly estradiol) arises from the aromatase-mediated conversion of androstenedione (made by the adrenals) to estrone, then estrone to estradiol, in the peripheral tissues, such as adipose tissue. Anastrozole is highly selective for this enzyme and does not affect steroid synthesis, so that estradiol synthesis is potently suppressed (to undetectable levels) while cortisol and aldosterone levels are unchanged.

Metabolism: Extensively metabolized, with 85% of the drug metabolized by the liver. About 10% of the unchanged drug and 60% of the drug as metabolites are excreted in the urine within 72 hours of drug administration.

Dosage/Range:
- 1 mg PO qd. No dosage adjustment required for mild to moderate hepatic impairment.

Drug Preparation:

- None. Available as 1-mg tablet.

Drug Administration:

- Take orally with or without food, at approximately the same time daily.

Lab Effects/Interference:

- Elevated GGT, especially in patients with liver metastases.

Special Considerations:

- Indicated for the adjuvant treatment of postmenopausal women with hormone receptor positive early breast cancer; as first-line therapy for postmenopausal women with hormone receptor-positive or hormone receptor-unknown locally advanced or metastatic breast cancer; and for treatment of advanced breast cancer in postmenopausal women with disease progression following tamoxifen therapy.
- In the large Arimidex Tamoxifen Alone or in Combination (ATAC) clinical trial, anastrozole was shown to reduce the relative risk of breast cancer recurrence by 17% over tamoxifen in hormone receptor-positive patients in the adjuvant setting.
- Well-tolerated with low toxicity profile.
- Coadministration of corticosteroids is not necessary.
- Absolutely contraindicated during pregnancy.

Potential Toxicities/Side Effects and the Nursing Process

I. SEXUAL DYSFUNCTION related to DECREASED ESTROGEN LEVELS

Defining Characteristics: Hot flashes (12%), asthenia or loss of energy (16%), and vaginal dryness may occur.

Nursing Implications: As appropriate, explore with patient and partner patterns of sexuality and impact therapy may have. Discuss strategies to preserve sexual health. Teach patient that the vaginal dryness may be from menopause, not the drug, and that the patient SHOULD NOT use estrogen creams. Teach patient to use lubricants.

II. POTENTIAL ALTERATION IN CARDIAC OUTPUT related to THROMBOPHLEBITIS

Defining Characteristics: Thrombophlebitis may occur, but is uncommon.

Nursing Implications: Identify patients at risk. Teach patients to report/come to emergency room for pain, redness, or marked swelling in arms or legs, or if shortness of breath or dizziness occur.

…TERATION IN COMFORT related to HEADACHES, …VEAKNESS

…ining Characteristics: Headaches are mild and occur in about 13% of pa-…nts. Decreased energy and weakness is common. Mild swelling of arms/legs …nay occur and is mild.

Nursing Implications: Teach patient that headache is usually relieved by nonprescription analgesics, and to report headaches that are unrelieved. Teach patient to elevate extremities when at rest, as needed.

IV. POTENTIAL ALTERATION IN NUTRITION, LESS THAN BODY REQUIREMENTS, related to NAUSEA

Defining Characteristics: Nausea is mild, with a 15% incidence.

Nursing Implications: Determine baseline weight, and monitor at each visit. Teach patient that nausea may occur, and to report this. Discuss strategies to minimize nausea, including diet and dosing time.

V. POTENTIAL ALTERATION IN BOWEL ELIMINATION related to DIARRHEA

Defining Characteristics: Diarrhea is uncommon (9% incidence) and mild.

Nursing Implications: Assess for change in bowel patterns and teach patient to report diarrhea. If diarrhea occurs, teach patient that diarrhea is usually relieved by nonprescription medications, such as loperamide HCl and kaopectate, and to report unrelieved diarrhea.

Drug: androgens: testosterone propionate (Testex), obfluoxymesterone (Halotestin), obtestolactone (Teslac)

Class: Hormones.

Mechanism of Action: Has stimulatory effect on red blood cells that results in an increased HCT. Other mechanism of action unknown.

Metabolism: Metabolized by the liver; excreted in the urine and feces.

Dosage/Range:
- Fluoxymesterone: 10–30 mg PO daily (3–4 divided doses).
- Testolactone: 100 mg IM 3 × weekly or 250 mg PO 4 × daily.
- Testosterone Propionate: 50–100 mg IM 3 × weekly.

Drug Preparation:
- Drug comes in ready-to-use vials or tablets.

Drug Administration:

- Before IM administration, shake vial vigorously and give injection immediately to avoid solution settling.

Drug Interactions:

- Pharmacological effects of oral anticoagulants may be enhanced; monitor patient and adjust dose.

Lab Effects/Interference:

- LFTs: possible hepatic dysfunction with long-term use.
- Increased serum Ca.
- May cause decreased total serum thyroxine (T_4) concentrations and increased T_3 and T_4.

Special Considerations:

- Fluoxymesterone may increase sensitivity to oral anticoagulants. Should be administered in divided doses because of its short action.

Potential Toxicities/Side Effects and the Nursing Process

I. POTENTIAL FOR INJURY related to SODIUM AND WATER RETENTION, HYPERCALCEMIA, AND OBSTRUCTIVE JAUNDICE

Defining Characteristics: Sodium and water retention may occur, necessitating dose reduction or diuretic use; hypercalcemia may occur initially in patients with bony metastases and needs to be distinguished from disease progression. Obstructive jaundice has occurred with methyltesterone, fluoxymesterone, and oxymethalone.

Nursing Implications: Identify patients most at risk for injury related to sodium and water retention: patients with cardiac, renal, or hepatic dysfunction, as well as patients with low serum albumin. Teach patient about potential side effects and instruct to report any changes to physician or nurse; assess patient at each visit for signs/symptoms of fluid and electrolyte imbalance. Identify patients at risk for hypercalcemia (those with bony metastases) and monitor serum calcium during first few weeks of therapy; hyperoalcemia is an indlcation to discontinue therapy. Teach patient/family signs/symptoms of hypercalcemia (drowsiness, increased thirst, constipation, polyuria) and to notify physician. Monitor LFTs and instruct patient/family to report signs/symptoms of GI distress, diarrhea, jaundice.

II. POTENTIAL FOR SEXUAL DYSFUNCTION related to MASCULINIZATION

Defining Characteristics: Commonly occurs in women receiving drug for > 3 months; with prolonged use masculinization may be irreversible. Symptoms include increased libido, deepening of voice, excessive growth of body (face) hair, acne, and clitoral hypertrophy. In men, priapism (sustained and often painful erections) and reduced ejaculatory volume may occur.

Nursing Implications: Instruct patient to report symptoms of changes in sexual health. Discuss strategies to preserve sexual health; if unacceptable, discuss alternative medications with physician.

III. ALTERATION IN NUTRITION, LESS THAN BODY REQUIREMENTS, related to NAUSEA AND VOMITING

Defining Characteristics: Nausea may occur.

Nursing Implications: Teach patient about possible side effects and administer antiemetics as ordered. Encourage small, frequent feedings and dietary modifications as appropriate.

Drug: arsenic trioxide (Trisenox)

Class: Miscellaneous antineoplastic agent.

Mechanism of Action: Not completely understood, but drug appears to cause changes in DNA with fragmentation typical of apoptosis or programmed cell death. Drug also damages and causes degradation of the fusion protein PMLRAR alpha characteristic of acute promyelocytic leukemia. The gene responsible for the fusion protein is corrected in many cases (cytogenetic complete response), so that immature malignant myelocytic cells mature into normal white blood cells.

Metabolism: Pharmacokinetics continue to be characterized. Drug is metabolized by methylation, primarily in the liver. Arsenic is stored primarily in the liver, kidney, heart, lung, hair, and nails. Drug appears to be excreted in the urine.

Dosage/Range:

Adult:

- Induction dose of 0.15 mg/kg/d IV until bone marrow remission, not to exceed 60 doses.
- Consolidation begins 3–6 weeks after induction therapy is completed, at a dose of 0.15 mg/kg/d IV for 25 doses over a period of up to 5 weeks.

Drug Preparation/Administration:

- Drug is available in 10 mL, single-use ampules containing 10 mg of arsenic trioxide, with a concentration of 1 mg/mL.
- Further dilute prescribed dose immediately in 100–250 ml 5% dextrose injection, USP or 0.9% Sodium Chloride Injection, USP.

- Administer IV over 1–2 hours, or up to 4 hours if acute vasomotor reactions occur (does not require a central line).
- Drug is chemically and physically stable for 24 hours at room temperature and 48 hours when refrigerated.
- Drug does not contain any preservatives, so unused portions should be discarded.
- Overdosage: If symptoms of serious acute arsenic toxicity appear (seizures, muscle weakness, confusion), discontinue drug immediately and chelation therapy should be considered: dimercaprol 3 mg/kg IMq 4 hours until immediate life-threatening toxicity has subsided, then give penicillamine 250 mg PO up to qid (1 Gm per day).

Drug Interactions:
- Unknown; do not mix with any other medications.
- Drugs that can prolong the QT interval (e.g., certain antiarrhythmics or thioridazine) or lead to electrolyte abnormalities (e.g., diuretics or amphotericin B) should be avoided if possible; otherwise, scrupulous monitoring and correction of abnormalities is critical.

Lab Effects/Interference:
- Hyperkalemia or hypokalemia.
- Hypomagnesemia.
- Hyperglycemia or hypoglycemia.
- Hypocalcemia.
- Increased hepatic transaminases ALT and AST.
- Leukocytosis (50% of patients).
- Anemia (14% of patients).
- Thrombocytopenia (19% of patients).
- Neutropenia (10% of patients).
- Disseminated intravascular coagulation (DIC) (8% of patients).

Special Considerations:
- Drug is indicated for induction of remission and consolidation in paients with acute promyelocytic leukemia (APL) who are refraotory to, or have relapsed from, retinoid and anthracycline chemotherapy, and whose APL is characterized by the presence of the t(15;17) translocation or PML/RAR-alpha gene expression.
- Arsenic has been used in medical care for the last 2000 years, and 100 years ago it was used to treat leukemia and infections. However, it was replaced with current chemotherapy and antibiotics. Certain traditional Chinese medicines were found to be anti-leukemic, and the active ingredient was shown to be arsenic trioxide.
- Preliminary studies showed high hematologic complete response rate (55–82%) and cytogenetic conversion to no detection of APL chromosome

rearrangement (29–100%) depending on response criteria. This led to a fast track status and early FDA approval. Additional post-approval toxicity reports will help clarify full toxicity profile of this drug.

- Drug may cause APL Differentiation Syndrome similar to the retinoicacidacute Promyelocytic Leukemia (RA-APL), which is characterized by fever, dyspnea, weight gain, pulmonary infiltrates, and pleural or pericardial effusions, with or without leukocytosis. This syndrome can be fatal, and, at the first suggestion, high-dose steroids should be instituted (dexamethasone 10 mg IV bid) for at least 3 days or longer until signs and symptoms abate. The drug manufacturer states that the majority of patients do not require termination of arsenic trioxide therapy during treatment of the syndrome (Cell Therapeutics, Inc., Trisenox package insert, 9/2000).
- Drug can cause QT interval prolongation and complete atrioventricular block. Prolonged QT interval can progress to a torsade de pointes-type fatal ventricular arrythmia. Risk factors for development of torsade de pointes are: significant QT prolongation; concomitant administraton of drugs that prolong the QT interval; history of torsades de pointes; preexisting QT prolongation; CHF; administration of potassium-wasting diuretics; conditions resulting in hypokalemia or hypomagnesemia, such as concurrent administration of amphotericin B.
- The manufacturer recommends the following: Prior to treatment with arsenic trioxide, the patient should have a baseline 12-lead EKG as well as serum electrolytes and renal function tests. Electrolyte abnormalities should be corrected. Any drugs that prolong the QT interval should be discontinued. If the QT interval prolongation is > 500 msec, this should be corrected prior to drug administration. During arsenic trioxide therapy, serum potassium should be kept > 4.0 mEq/dL and serum magnesium > 1.8 mg/dL. If the QT interval exceeds 500 msec, reassessment and correction of risk factors should occur. The patient should be hospitalized for monitoring if syncope, or rapid or irregular heart rate occurs, and serum electrolytes assessed and any abnormalities corrected. Drug should be stopped until QT interval falls below 460 msec, electrolyte abnormalities corrected, and symptoms resolve.
- Drug is a human carcinogen. Drug should not be used by pregnant or breast-feeding women.
- Standard monitoring: At least 2 times a week, the patient should have electrolyte, hematologic, and coagulation assessed; more frequently if abnormal during the induction phase, and at least weekly during the consolidation phase. EKGs should be done weekly; more frequently if abnormal.
- Most common side effects are manageable, are reversible, and include: leukocytosis, nausea, vomiting, diarrhea, abdominal pain, fatigue, edema, hyperglycemia, dyspnea, cough, rash, itching, headaches, and dizziness.

Potential Toxicities/Side Effects and the Nursing Process

I. ALTERATION IN OXYGENATION, POTENTIAL, related to APL DIFFERENTIATION SYNDROME

Defining Characteristics: Drug may cause APL Differentiation Syndrome similar to the retinoic-acid-acute Promyelocytic Leukemia (RA-APL), which is characterized by fever, dyspnea, weight gain, pulmonary infiltrates, and pleural or pericardial effusions, with or without leukocytosis. This syndrome develops in response to the differentiation of immature malignant cells into mature normal white blood cells and the increased white blood cell count. The body's response is an inflammatory reaction with fluid retention in the lining of the lungs and heart.) This syndrome can be fatal, and at the first suggestion, high-dose steroids should be instituted (dexamethasone 10 mg IV bid) for at least 3 days or longer until signs and symptoms abate. The drug manufacturer states that the majority of patients do not require termination of arsenic trioxide therapy during treatment of the syndrome. The reported incidence is 20%. Leucocytosis, if it occurs, at levels $> 10 \times 10^3/\mu L$ is unrelated to baseline or peak white blood cell counts. Leukocytosis was not treated with chemotherapy, and levels were lower during consolidation than during induction.

Nursing Implications: Assess temperature and VS, oxygen saturation, cardiopulmonary status baseline and at each visit. Assess weight daily, and teach patient to report any SOB, fever, or weight gain immediately. If signs or symptoms develop, notify physician immediately and discuss obtaining CXR, cardiac echo, and focused exam. Discuss CXR, ECHO, and laboratory findings with physician. Be prepared to administer high-dose steroids (e.g., dexamethasone 10 mg IV bid × 3 days or longer depending on symptom resolution). Provide pulmonary and hemodynamic support as necessary. Assess CBC, with focus on white blood cell count and presence of leukocytosis.

II. POTENTIAL ALTERATION IN CARDIAC FUNCTION related to QT PROLONGATION AND ARRYTHMIA

Defining Characteristics: Drug can cause QT interval prolongation and complete atrioventricular block. Prolonged QT interval can progress to a torsade de pointes-type fatal ventricular arrythmia. Risk factors for development of torsade de pointes are significant QT prolongation, concomitant administraton of drugs that prolong the QT interval, history of torsades de pointes, preexisting QT prolongation, CHF, administration of potassium-wasting diuretics, and conditions resulting in hypokalemia or hypomagnesemia such as concurrent administration of amphotericin B.

Nursing Implications: Assess baseline risk, cardiovascular status, EKG determined QT interval, electrolyte and renal blood studies, and medications the patient is taking that may prolong QT interval, such as serotonin antagonist antiemetics. At least 2 times a week, the patient should have electrolyte, hematologic and coagulation assessed; more frequently if abnormal during the induction phase, and at least weekly during the consolidation phase. EKGs should be done weekly, and more frequently if abnormal. Discuss correction of any electrolyte abnormalities, as well as other risk factors, with physician. Any drugs that prolong the QT interval should be discontinued. If the QT interval prolongation is > 500 msec, this should be corrected prior to drug administration. During arsenic trioxide therapy, serum potassium should be kept > 4.0 mEq/dL and serum magnesium > 1.8 mg/dL. If the QT interval exceeds 500 msec, reassessment and correction of risk factors should occur. The patient should be hospitalized for monitoring if syncope or rapid or irregular heart rate occurs, and serum electrolytes assessed and any abnormalities corrected. Drug should be stopped until QT interval falls below 460 msec, electrolyte abnormalities corrected, and symptoms resolve.

III. ALTERATION IN NUTRITION, LESS THAN BODY REQUIREMENTS related to GI DYSFUNCTION

Defining Characteristics: Nausea is most common (incidence 75%), followed by vomiting (58%), abdominal pain (58%), diarrhea (53%), constipation (28%), anorexia (23%), dyspepsia (10%), abdominal tenderness or distention (8%), and dry mouth (8%).

Nursing Implications: Assess GI and nutrition status and presence of GI dysfunction baseline, and with each visit. Administer antiemetics, and teach patient self-administration. Discuss risk of serotonin antagonists to prolong QT interval, and contraindication with physician. Teach patient to report signs and symptoms, and evaluate symptom management plan based on effectiveness of symptom control. Assess presence of pain, and discuss pharmacologic and nonpharmacologic analgesic plan with physician.

IV. ALTERATION IN PROTECTIVE MECHANISMS, related to FEVER, ANEMIA, DIC, BLEEDING

Defining Characteristics: Fever affects 63% of patients (13% febrile neutropenia), with 38% of patients having rigors. In clinical studies, 8% of patients had hemorrhage, 14% anemia, 19% thrombocytopenia, 10% neutropenia, and 8% DIC. Patients may develop infections, and in clinical studies, most commonly these were: sinusitis 20%, herpes simplex 13%, upper respiratory tract infection 13%, nonspecific bacterial 8%, herpes zoster 8%, oral candidiasis 5%, and (rarely) sepsis 5%.

Nursing Implications: At least 2 times a week, the patient should have electrolyte, hematologic and coagulation assessed; more frequently if abnormal during the induction phase, and at least weekly during the consolidation phase.

Monitor laboratory results, and discuss abnormalities with physician. Assess patient for fever, signs and symptoms of infection, rigors, and bleeding, and implement management plan to assure patient safety. Transfuse patient as ordered, and monitor closely.

V. ALTERATION IN COMFORT related to HEADACHE, CHEST PAIN, AND INJECTION SITE CHANGES

Defining Characteristics: Headache occurred in approximately 60% of patients while chest pain occurred in 25%. Injection site reactions of pain, erythema, and edema occurred in 20%, 13%, and 10% of patients, respectively.

Nursing Implications: Assess level of comfort, and develop plan for comfort, including pharmacologic, and non-pharmacologic measures. Assess effectiveness, and revise plan as needed. Assess patency of IV site and need for IV catheter change. Assess need for central line. Although not necessary for drug delivery, if patient venous access is limited this may provide enhanced patient comfort.

VI. ALTERATION IN ACTIVITY TOLERANCE related to FATIGUE, MUSCULOSKELETAL PROBLEMS

Defining Characteristics: 63% of patients reported fatigue. In clinical studies, musculoskeletal events were: arthralgias (33%), myalgias (25%), bone pain (23%), back pain (18%), neck pain, and pain in limbs (13%).

Nursing Implications: Assess baseline energy and activity level, and level of comfort. Assess need for assistance with ADLs and home assistance. Assess need for analgesics or local measures to relieve pain and discomfort. Teach patient self-care strategies to minimize exertion and maximize activity, such as clustering activity during shopping, alternating rest and activity periods, diet, gentle exercise. Evaluate success of plan and need for revisions.

VII. ALTERATION IN FLUID AND ELECTROLYTE BALANCE related to HYPOKALEMIA, HYPOMAGNESEMIA, HYPERGLYCEMIA, EDEMA

Defining Characteristics: Hypokalemia occurs in about 50% of patients, hypomagnesemia (45%), hyperglycemia (45%), and edema (40%). Other electrolyte abnormalities are hyperkalemia (18%), hypocalcemia (10%), hypoglycemia (8%), acidosis (5%), and increased transaminases (13–20%).

Nursing Implications: At least 2 times a week, the patient should have electrolyte, hematologic and coagulation assessed; more frequently if abnormal during the induction phase, and at least weekly during the consolidation phase. EKGs should be done weekly, and more frequently if abnormal. Teach patient that edema may occur, and to report it. Assess patient baseline and before each treatment for weight and presence of edema. Discuss abnormalities with physician, correct as ordered, and monitor closely for signs and symptoms of imbalance.

VIII. SENSORY/PERCEPTUAL ALTERATIONS, POTENTIAL related to PARESTHESIA, DIZZINESS, TREMOR, INSOMNIA

Defining Characteristics: Insomnia occurs in 43% of patients, paresthesia (33%), dizziness (23%), tremor (13%), seizures (8%), somnolence (8%), and (rarely) coma (5%).

Nursing Implications: Assess baseline mental and neurological status, and monitor frequently during therapy. Assess sensory function, and teach patient to report numbness, tingling, dizziness, tremor, seizure, decrease in alertness, and changes in sleep. Assess presence of paresthesias, and motor and sensory function prior to each treatment; discuss presence or worsening with physician. Teach patient self-care strategies, including maintaining safety when walking, getting up, taking a bath, or washing dishes if unable to feel temperature changes. Teach self-care measures to manage sleep problems, and discuss possible need for sleeping medication.

IX. ALTERATION IN GAS EXCHANGE, POTENTIAL, related to COUGH, DYSPNEA, HYPOXIA, PLEURAL EFFUSION

Defining Characteristics: Cough is common, affecting 65% of patients, followed by dyspnea (53%), epistaxis (25%), hypoxia (23%), pleural effusion (20%), postnasal drip (13%), wheezing (13%), decreased breath sounds (10%), crepitations (10%), rales (crackles) (10%), hemoptysis (8%), tachypnea (8%), and rhonchi (8%).

Nursing Implications: Assess baseline pulmonary status, including breath sounds and oxygen saturation, and monitor at least daily during treatment. Teach patient that symptoms may occur and to report them. Discuss management of patients experiencing cough, dyspnea, and other symptoms with physician, and develop individualized management plan.

X. ALTERATION IN SKIN INTEGRITY, POTENTIAL, related to SKIN IRRITATION

Defining Characteristics: Dermatitis affects about 43% of patients, pruritis (33%), ecchymosis (20%), dry skin (13%), erythema (10%), hyperpigmentation (8%), and urticaria (8%).

Nursing Implications: Assess baseline skin integrity and monitor at each visit. Teach patient to report any skin changes or itching. Teach patient symptomatic local measures to manage dermatitis, itch, or other changes. If plan ineffective, discuss other measures with physician.

Drug: asparaginase (Elspar)

Class: Miscellaneous agents (enzyme).

Mechanism of Action: Hydrolyzes serum asparagine, which deprives leukemia cells of the required amino acid. Normal cells are spared because they generally have the ability to synthesize their own asparagine. Cell cycle specific for G1 postmitotic phase. Some leukemic cells are unable to synthesize asparagine. These cells must obtain asparagine from an exogenous source, the patient's serum. Administration of the enzyme L-asparaginase causes hydrolysis of asparagine to aspartate, resulting in rapid depletion of the asparagine concentration in the patient's serum.

Metabolism: Metabolism of L-asparaginase is independent of renal and hepatic function. The drug is not recovered in the urine and does not appear to cross the blood-brain barrier.

Dosage/Range:

- IM or IV varies with protocol. Typical dosing is 200 IU/kg IV qd × 28 days (ALL).

Drug Preparation:

- IV injection: reconstitute with sterile water for injection or 0.9% Sodium Chloride injection (without preservative) and use within 8 hours of restoration.
- IV infusion: dilute with 0.9% Sodium Chloride injection or 5% Dextrose injection and use within 8 hours, only if clear; if gelatinous particles develop, filter through a 5.0-μm filter.
- The lyophilized powder must be stored under refrigeration. The reconstituted solution must also be stored under refrigeration if it is not used immediately. The solution must be discarded 8 hours after preparation.

Drug Administration:

- Use in a hospital setting. Make preparations to treat anaphylaxis at each administration of the drug.

Drug Interactions:

- Prednisone: potential additive hyperglycemic effect; monitor blood glucose levels.
- Cyclophosphamide, vincristine, 6-mercaptopurine: may increase or decrease drug's effect (CTX, VCR, 6-MP).
- 6-mercaptopurine: Enhanced hepatotoxicity; monitor LFTs closely.

- Methotrexate: Antagonism if administered immediately prior to methotrexate; when administered some time after methotrexate, may enhance methotrexate activity.
- Synergy with cytosine arabinoside.
- Increased hyperglycemia when given together with prednisone.
- Reduced hypersensitivity when given with 6-mercaptopurine or prednisone.
- Additive neurotoxicity when given with vincristine.

Lab Effects/Interference:
- Increased LFTs.
- Decreased hepatically derived clotting factors.
- Interferes with thyroid function tests after first two days of therapy: effect lasts four weeks.

Special Considerations:
- Potential reduction in antineoplastic effect of methotrexate when given in combination.
- Anaphylaxis is associated with the administration of this drug.
- Intravenous administration of L-asparaginase concurrently with or immediately before prednisone and vincristine administration may be associated with increased toxicity.

Potential Toxicities/Side Effects and the Nursing Process

I. POTENTIAL FOR INJURY related to HYPERSENSITIVITY OR ANAPHYLACTIC REACTIONS

Defining Characteristics: Occurs in 20–30% of patients. Increased incidence after several doses administered, but may occur with first dose. Occurs less often with IM route of administration. May be life-threatening reaction, but is usually mild.

Nursing Implications: Discuss with physician use of test dose prior to drug administration. Assess baseline vital signs and mental status prior to drug administration. Review standing orders or nursing procedure for management of anaphylaxis and be prepared to stop drug immediately if signs/symptoms occur; keep IV line open with 0.9% Sodium Chloride, notify physician, monitor vital signs, and administer ordered medications, which may include epinephrine 1:1000, hydrocortisone sodium succinate, and diphenhydramine. Teach patient the potential of a hypersensitivity or anaphylactic reaction and to immediately report any unusual symptoms. *Escherichia coli* preparation of L-asparaginase and *Erwinia carotovora* preparation are non-cross-resistant, so if an anaphylactic reaction occurs with one, the other preparation may be used.

II. POTENTIAL FOR INJURY related to HEPATIC DYSFUNCTION OR THROMBOEMBOLISM

Defining Characteristics: Two-thirds of patients have elevated LFTs starting within the first two weeks of treatment: e.g., SGOT, bili, and alk phos. Hepatically derived clotting factors may be depressed, resulting in excessive bleeding or blood clotting. Relatively uncommon.

Nursing Implications: Monitor SGOT, bili, alk phos, albumin, and clotting factors CPT, PTT, fibrinogen. Teach patient of the potential of excessive bleeding or blood clotting, and instruct to report any unusual symptoms. Assess patient for signs/symptoms of bleeding.

III. ALTERED NUTRITION, LESS THAN BODY REQUIREMENTS related to NAUSEA/VOMITING, ANOREXIA, HYPERGLYCEMIA

Defining Characteristics: 50–60% of patients experience mild to severe nausea and vomiting starting within 4–6 hours after treatment. Anorexia commonly occurs. Hyperglycemia is a transient reaction caused by effects on the pancreas with decreased insulin synthesis. Pancreatitis occurs in 5% of patients.

Nursing Implications: Premedicate with antiemetics and continue prophylactically for 24 hours to prevent nausea and vomiting. Encourage small, frequent meals of cool, bland foods and liquids, as well as favorite foods, especially high-calorie, high-protein foods. Encourage use of spices and do weekly weights. Teach patient about the potential of hyperglycemia and pancreatitis, and instruct to report any unusual symptoms, e.g., increased thirst, urination, and appetite. Monitor serum glucose, amylase, and lipase levels periodically during treatment. Report any laboratory elevations to physician. Treat hyperglycemia issues with diet or insulin as ordered by physician. Treat pancreatitis per physician orders.

IV. SENSORY/PERCEPTUAL ALTERATIONS related to CHANGES IN MENTAL STATUS

Defining Characteristics: 25% of patients experience some changes in mental status—commonly, lethargy, drowsiness, and somnolence; rarely coma. Predominantly seen in adults. Malaise (feeling "blah") occurs in most patients, and generally gets worse with subsequent doses. Drug does not cross BBB.

Nursing Implications: Teach patient about the potential of CNS toxicity, and instruct to report any unusual symptoms. Obtain baseline neurologic and mental function. Assess patient for any neurologic abnormalities and report changes to physician. Discuss with patient the impact of malaise on his/her general sense of well-being and strategies to minimize the distress.

V. POTENTIAL FOR SEXUAL DYSFUNCTION related to REPRODUCTION HAZARD

Defining Characteristics: Drug is teratogenic.

Nursing Implications: As appropriate, explore with patient and partner issues of reproductive and sexual patterns and impact chemotherapy will have. Discuss strategies to preserve sexuality and reproductive health (e.g., sperm banking, contraception).

VI. INFECTION, BLEEDING, AND FATIGUE related to BONE MARROW DEPRESSION

Defining Characteristics: Bone marrow depression is not common. Mild anemia may occur. Serious leukopenia and thrombocytopenia are rare.

Nursing Implications: Monitor CBC, platelet count prior to drug administration, as well as signs/symptoms of infection, bleeding, or anemia. Instruct patient in self-assessment of signs/symptoms of infection, bleeding, or anemia and to report immediately.

Drug: 5-azacytidine (Vidaza)

Class: Antimetabolite.

Mechanism of Action: Azacytidine causes hypomethylation of DNA, which may restore normal gene function to genes responsible for cell division and differentiation of the bone marrow. At higher doses, it also interferes with nucleic acid metabolism by acting as a false metabolite when incorporated into DNA and RNA; cell cycle phase specific for S phase.

Metabolism: Rapidly absorbed following subcutaneous administration, with peak plasma level in 30 minutes. Bioavailability of subcutaneously administered drug is 89% of IV dose. 85% of the total administered dose is excreted in the urine, and $<1\%$ in feces. Mean elimination half-life is about 4 hours in both subcutaneous and IV administered drug.

Dosage/Range:

- 75 mg/m^2 Subcutaneous injection qd $\times$ 7 days, repeated q 4 weeks for at least 4 cycles
- Dose may be increased to 100 mg/m^2 after 2 cycles if initial dose ineffective and toxicity manageable (no toxicity except nausea and vomiting)
- Decrease or hold dose if significant bone marrow depression
- If baseline WBC $>3000/mm^3$, ANC $>1500/mm^3$, and platelets $>75{,}000/mm^3$, modify dose based on nadir counts:
- ANC $<500/mm^3$, platelets $<25{,}000/mm^3$ = 50% dose next course

- ANC 500–1500/mm^3, platelets 25,000–50,000/mm^3 = 67% of dose next course
- ANC > 1500/mm^3, platelets > 50,000/mm^3 = 100% dose
- If baseline WBC < 3000/mm^3, ANC < 1500/mm^3, or platelets < 75,000/mm^3, dose modifications and bone marrow biopsy cellularity at time of nadir used, unless there is clear improvement in differentiation (% mature granulocytes is higher with ANC higher than at onset of treatment)- see package insert.
- Dose modification based on renal function and serum electrolytes
- If unexplained decreases in serum bicarbonate < 20 mEq/L, dose reduce 50% in next cycle
- If elevations of BUN or serum creatinine occur, delay next dose until values return to normal or baseline, and reduce dose by 50% in next cycle.

Drug Preparation:

- Drug is a lyophilized powder in 100 mg single-use vials
- Reconstitute asceptically with 4 mL sterile water for injection, adding diluent slowly into the vial
- Invert vial 2–3 times and gently rotate, yielding a cloudy suspension containing 25 mg/mL
- Divide doses greater than 4 mL into 2 syringes and administer within 1 hour of reconstitution at room temperature
- Reconstituted solution may be kept in the vial or drawn in a syringe(s) and refrigerated immediately for later use for up to 8 hours. After removal from the refrigerator, the suspension may be allowed to equilibrate to room temperature for up to 30 minutes prior to administration

Drug Administration:

- Invert syringe(s) 2–3 times and gently roll syringe(s) between palms for 30 seconds immediately prior to administration to provide a homogenous suspension.
- Rotate sites for each subcutaneous injection (thigh, abdomen, or upper arm), and give new injection at least 1 inch from old site, and never into areas where site is tender, bruised, red or hard.

Drug Interactions:

- None significant.

Lab Effects/Interference:

- Decreased ANC, platelets, red blood cell counts.
- Renal tubular acidosis
- Increased BUN and creatinine
- Hypokalemia

Special Considerations:

- Azacytidine is indicated for treatment of patients with all five Myelodysplastic subtypes: refractory anemia (RA) or refractory anemia with ringed sideroblasts (RARS) (if accompanied by neutropenia or thrombocytopenia or requiring transfusions), refractory anemia with excess blasts (RAEB), refractory anemia with excess blasts in transformation (RAEB-T), and chronic myelomonocytic leukemia (CMMoL).
- Overall response rate of patients with all patients except those with AML was 15.7% (Complete and partial responders).
- Drug is contraindicated in patients with hypersensitivity to mannitol, and in patients with advanced malignant hepatic tumors.
- Drug is fetotoxic and embryotoxic. Women of child-bearing age must use effective contraception methods; men should be advised not to father a child while receiving treatment with azacitidine. Women who are receiving azacitidine should not breast feed their infant as drug causes tumors in animals, and has the potential for severe toxicity.
- Monitor renal function closely in elderly patients.
- Use cautiously in patients with pre-existing hepatic disease as patients with extensive liver metastases have rarely been reported to develop coma and death.

Potential Toxicities/Side Effects and the Nursing Process

I. INFECTION AND BLEEDING related to BONE MARROW DEPRESSION

Defining Characteristics: Leukopenia is dose-limiting, with nadir occurring from days 14–17; lasts two weeks, with recovery in 14 days. Thrombocytopenia and anemia also occur. Bone marrow depression lessens once patient has a response to therapy.

Nursing Implications: Monitor CBC, neutrophil, and platelet count prior to drug administration and postchemotherapy; assess for signs/symptoms of infection, bleeding, and anemia. Teach patient/family signs/symptoms of infection, bleeding, and anemia, and instruct to report them to nurse or physician immediately. Teach patient to avoid aspirin-containing OTC medications.

II. ALTERATION IN NUTRITION, LESS THAN BODY REQUIREMENTS, related to NAUSEA AND VOMITING, ANOREXIA, STOMATITIS, CONSTIPATION and DIARRHEA

Defining Characteristics: Nausea/vomiting is dose-related, and occurs in about 70.5%/54.1% of patients, respectively, beginning 1–3 hours postchemotherapy. This tends to be worse in the first 1–2 cycles, and increases in incidence with increasing doses. Diarrhea develops in 36.4% of patients, with incidence increasing as dose increases. Constipation occurs in about 33% of patients and is worse during the first 2 cycles of therapy. Anorexia affects 20% of patients, and stomatitis occurs in 7% of patients.

Nursing Implications: Assess baseline nutritional status, and periodically at visits. Premedicate with antiemetics before injection, and teach patient self-administration of antiemetics at home; encourage small, frequent feedings as tolerated; if severe vomiting occurs, treat with alternative antiemetics and assess for signs/symptoms of fluid and electrolyte imbalance. Monitor serum potassium, as hypokalemia may be a side effect of treatment. Assess baseline bowel elimination stastus. Instruct patient to report onset of diarrhea and administer antidiarrheals as ordered. If diarrhea is protracted, ensure adequate hydration, monitor total body fluid balance, and teach/reinforce perineal hygiene. Instruct patient to monitor for constipation, and to use measures to prevent constipation if that is a problem. If patient has anorexia, teach patient to identify nutrient-dense foods and to eat small frequent meals, including a bedtime snack. Teach patient strategies to increase appetite, depending upon an individualized assessment. Teach patient to self-assess oral mucosa, and to use a systematic cleansing of teeth/mouth after meals and at bedtime. Monitor LFTs periodically during therapy and discuss abnormalities with physician.

III. ALTERATION IN COMFORT related to FEVER, FATIGUE, ARTHRALGIAS, and INJECTION SITE IRRITATION

Defining Characteristics: Fever occurs in 54% of patients, with rigors affecting about 25%; fatigue in 36% of patients; arthralgias in 22%; and injection site erythema (35%), injection site pain (23%), injection site bruising (14%), injection site reaction (14%). Injection site discomfort was more pronounced during the 1st and 2nd cycles of therapy.

Nursing Implications: Monitor temperature and teach patient to self-assess temperature. Teach patient that pyrexia may occur, and how to self-administer antipyretics. Teach patient to notify nurse/MD if rigors occur and are severe. Teach measures to reduce discomfort related to myalgias if they occur, such as application of heat and NSAIDs. Teach patient strategies to conserve energy, such as alternating activity with reset. Teach patient to rotate sites used for injection, and local measures to increase comfort.

Drug: bicalutamide (Casodex)

Class: Nonsteroidal antiandrogen.

Mechanism of Action: Binds to androgen receptors in the prostate; affinity is four times greater than that of flutamide.

Metabolism: Extensively metabolized in the liver. Decreased drug excretion in patients with moderate to severe hepatic dysfunction.

Dosage/Range:
- 50 mg PO qd.

Drug Preparation:
- None.

Drug Administration:
- Orally.

Drug Interactions:
- None known.

Lab Effects/Interference:
- Increased LFTs.

Special Considerations:
- Use cautiously in patients with moderate to severe hepatic dysfunction. Observe closely for toxicity, as dosage adjustment may be required.
- No dose modification needed for renal dysfunction.

Potential Toxicities/Side Effects and the Nursing Process

I. ALTERATION IN COMFORT, POTENTIAL related to GYNECOMASTIA AND HOT FLASHES

Defining Characteristics: Gynecomastia occurs in 23% of patients, breast tenderness in 26%, and hot flashes in 9.3%.

Nursing Implications: Teach patient that these side effects may occur, and discuss measures that may offer symptomatic relief.

II. ALTERATION IN NUTRITION, LESS THAN BODY REQUIREMENTS, related to NAUSEA, POTENTIAL

Defining Characteristics: Nausea may occur in 6% of patients.

Nursing Implications: Teach patient that nausea may occur, and instruct to report nausea. Determine baseline weight, and monitor at each visit. Discuss strategies to minimize nausea, including diet modification and time of dosing.

III. ALTERATION IN ELIMINATION, POTENTIAL, related to CONSTIPATION OR DIARRHEA

Defining Characteristics: Incidence of constipation is 6%, while that of diarrhea is 2.5%.

Nursing Implications: Assess baseline elimination pattern. Teach patient that alterations may occur, and instruct to report them if changes do not respond to usual nonprescription management strategies (OTC medications, dietary modifications).

Drug: bleomycin sulfate (Blenoxane)

Class: Antitumor action of bleomycin; isolated from fungus *Streptomyces verticullus*. Possesses both antitumor and antimicrobial actions.

Mechanism of Action: Induces single-strand and double-strand breaks in DNA. DNA synthesis is inhibited.

Metabolism: Excreted via the renal system. About 70% is excreted unchanged in urine; 30–60 minutes after IV infusion, urine levels are 10 times the serum level.

Dosage/Range:
- 5–20 U/m^2 once a week.
- 10–20 U/m^2 twice a week.
- Frequency and schedule may vary according to protocol and age.

Drug Preparation:
- Dilute powder in 0.9% Sodium Chloride or sterile water.

Drug Administration:
- IV, IM, or SQ doses may be administered. Some clinical trial protocols may use 24-hour infusions. There is a risk for anaphylaxis in lymphoma patients and hypotension with higher doses of drug. It may be recommended that a test dose be given before the first dose to detect hypersensitivity.

Drug Interactions:
- Digoxin dose may need to be increased.
- Phenytoin dose may need to be increased.

Lab Effects/Interference:
- None.

Special Considerations:
- Because of pulmonary toxicities with increasing dose, pulmonary function tests (PFTs) and CXR should be obtained before each course or as outlined by protocol.
- Maximum cumulative lifetime dose: 400 U.
- Oxygen (FIO2) increases risk of pulmonary toxicity.
- Reduce dose for impaired renal function (urinary creatinine clearance < 40–60 mL/min).
- Risk of pulmonary toxicity increased in elderly (> 70 years old); renal impairment; pulmonary disease or prior chest XRT; exposure to high oxygen concentration (i.e., surgery); cumulative doses > 400 U lifetime.

- May cause chemical fevers up to 39.4–40.5°C (103–105°F) in up to 60% of patients. May need to administer premedications such as acetaminophen, antihistamines, or in some cases steroids.
- Watch for signs/symptoms of hypotension and anaphylaxis with high drug doses; physician may order test dose in patients with lymphoma.
- May cause irritation at site of injection (is considered an irritant, not a vesicant).
- Decreases the oral bioavailability of digoxin when given together.
- Decreases the pharmacologic effects of phenytoin when given in combination.

Potential Toxicities/Side Effects and the Nursing Process

I. POTENTIAL FOR IMPAIRED GAS EXCHANGE related to PULMONARY TOXICITY

Defining Characteristics: Pneumonitis occurs in 10% of patients and is characterized by rales, dyspnea, infiltrate on CXR; in 1% may progress to irreversible pulmonary fibrosis. Risk factors include age > 70, dose > 400 U (but may occur at much lower doses), and concurrent or prior radiotherapy to the chest. Slower, continuous infusion may lower the risk.

Nursing Implications: Discuss with physician the need for PFTs and CXR prior to initiating therapy and monthly during therapy. Assess pulmonary status prior to each treatment (early symptom is dyspnea, and earliest sign is fine crackles). Instruct patient to report cough, dyspnea, shortness of breath. If patient needs surgery, discuss with physician the need to use low FIO2 during surgery since the lung tissue has been sensitized to bleomycin, and high concentrations of oxygen will cause further lung damage.

II. POTENTIAL FOR INJURY related to ANAPHYLAXIS

Defining Characteristics: Anaphylactoid reaction may occur in 1% of lymphoma patients, characterized by hypotension, confusion, tachycardia, wheezing, and facial edema. Reaction may be immediate or delayed for several hours and may occur after the first or second drug administration.

Nursing Implications: Discuss with physician the use of test dose prior to drug administration in lymphoma patients. Assess baseline vital signs (VS) and mental status prior to drug administration. Review standing orders or nursing procedure for patient management of anaphylaxis, and be prepared to stop drug immediately if signs/symptoms occur. Keep IV line open with 0.9% Sodium Chloride; notify physician, monitor VS, and administer ordered medications, which may include epinephrine 1:1000, hydrocortisone sodium succinate, and diphenhydramine.

III. POTENTIAL ALTERATION IN COMFORT related to FEVER AND CHILLS AND PAIN AT TUMOR SITE

Defining Characteristics: Fever (up to 39.4°–40.5°C [103°–105°F]) and chills, occurring in up to 60% of patients, begin 4–10 hours after drug administration and may last 24 hours. There appears to be tolerance with successive doses of bleomycin. Pain may occur at tumor site due to chemotherapy-induced cellular damage.

Nursing Implications: Teach patient that these side effects may occur, and assess patient during and postadministration. If fever occurs, notify physician and administer ordered acetaminophen, antihistamine, or steroid. If tumor pain occurs, reassure patient and discuss with physician the use of acetaminophen as analgesic.

IV. POTENTIAL FOR IMPAIRED SKIN INTEGRITY related to ALOPECIA, SKIN CHANGES, AND NAIL CHANGES

Defining Characteristics: Dose-related alopecia begins 3–4 weeks after first dose and is reversible. Skin changes occur in 50% of patients and include erythema, rash, striae, hyperpigmentation, skin peeling of fingertips, and hyperkeratosis; these are dose-related and begin after 150–200 U have been administered. Skin eruptions include a macular rash over hands and elbows, urticaria, and vesiculations. Pruritus may occur. Nail changes and possible nail loss may occur. Phlebitis at the IV site may occur.

Nursing Implications: Teach patient about possible side effects and self-care measures, including obtaining a wig or cap as appropriate prior to hair loss. Encourage patient to verbalize feelings and provide patient emotional support. Discuss with physician symptomatic treatment of skin changes. Assess IV site for phlebitis and restart IV at alternate site if phlebitis develops.

V. POTENTIAL ALTERATION IN NUTRITION, LESS THAN BODY REQUIREMENTS, related to NAUSEA AND VOMITING, ANOREXIA AND WEIGHT LOSS, AND STOMATITIS

Defining Characteristics: Nausea with or without vomiting may occur; anorexia and weight loss may occur and may continue after treatment is completed; stomatitis may occur and decrease ability and desire to eat.

Nursing Implications: Administer antiemetic prior to initial treatment and revise plan for successive treatments if no nausea/vomiting. Teach patient about possible anorexia and encourage patient to eat high-calorie, high-protein foods. Assess oral mucosa prior to drug administration; teach patient self-assessment and instruct to notify nurse or physician if stomatitis develops. Teach patient oral care prior to drug administration.

VI. POTENTIAL FOR SEXUAL DYSFUNCTION related to REPRODUCTIVE HAZARDS

Defining Characteristics: Drug is mutagenic and probably teratogenic.

Nursing Implications: Discuss with patient and partner both sexuality and reproductive goals, as well as possible impact of chemotherapy. Discuss contraception and sperm banking if appropriate.

Drug: busulfan (Myleran)

Class: Alkylating agent.

Mechanism of Action: Forms carbonium ions through the release of a methane sulfonate group, resulting in the alkylation of DNA. Acts primarily on granulocyte precursors in the bone marrow and is cell cycle phase nonspecific.

Metabolism: Well absorbed orally; almost all metabolites are excreted in the urine. Has a very short half-life.

Dosage/Range:

Chronic myelogenous leukemia:

- 4–8 mg/day PO for 2–3 weeks initially, then maintenance dose of 1–3 mg/m^2 PO qd or 0.05 mg/kg orally qd. Dose titrated based on leukocyte counts. Drug witheld when leukocyte count reaches 15,000/μL; resume when total leukocyte count is 50,000/μL; maintenance dose of 1–3 mg qd used if remission lasts < 3 months.

High doses with bone marrow transplantation:

- See Busulfan for Injection.

Drug Preparation:

- None.

Drug Administration:

- Available in 2-mg scored tablets given orally.

Drug Interactions:

- Combination treatment with thioguanine may cause hepatic dysfunction and the development of esophageal varices in a small number of patients.

Lab Effects/Interference:

- Decreased CBC.
- Increased LFTs.

Special Considerations:

Regular dose:

- If WBC is high, patient is at risk for hyperuricemia. Allopurinol and hydration may be indicated.

- Follow weekly CBC and platelet count initially, then monthly. Dose is decreased to maintenance level when leukocyte count falls below 50,000 mm^3.
- Hyperpigmentation of skin creases may occur due to increased melanin production.
- If given according to accepted guidelines, patients should have minimal side effects.

High dose:

- See Busulfan for Injection.

Potential Toxicities/Side Effects and the Nursing Process

I. POTENTIAL FOR INFECTION, BLEEDING, AND FATIGUE related to BONE MARROW DEPRESSION

Defining Characteristics: The nadir is at 11–30 days following initial drug administration, with recovery in 24–54 days; however, delayed, refractory pancytopenia has occurred.

Nursing Implications: Monitor CBC, WBC differential, and platelets, initially weekly, then at least monthly. Expect drug will be interrupted if counts fall rapidly or steeply. Teach patient to self-assess for signs/symptoms of infection, bleeding, or severe fatigue, and to notify nurse or physician immediately. Teach patient to avoid aspirin-containing OTC medications.

II. POTENTIAL FOR IMPAIRED GAS EXCHANGE related to INTERSTITIAL PULMONARY FIBROSIS

Defining Characteristics: Rarely, bronchopulmonary dysplasia progressing to pulmonary fibrosis can occur, beginning one to many years posttherapy. Symptoms are usually delayed (occurring after four years) and include anorexia, cough, dyspnea, and fever. High-dose corticosteroids may be helpful, but condition may be fatal due to rapid, diffuse fibrosis.

Nursing Implications: Assess pulmonary status routinely in all patients receiving long-term therapy. Discuss plan for regular pulmonary function studies with physician.

III. POTENTIAL FOR SEXUAL AND REPRODUCTIVE DYSFUNCTION related to REPRODUCTIVE HAZARDS

Defining Characteristics: Premenopausal female patients commonly experience ovarian suppression and amenorrhea with menopausal symptoms; men experience sterility, azoospermia, and testicular atrophy. Although successful pregnancies have occurred following busulfan therapy, the drug is potentially teratogenic.

Nursing Implications: Assess patient's/partner's sexual patterns and reproductive goals. Provide information, supportive counseling, and referral as needed. Teach importance of birth control measures as appropriate.

Drug: busulfan for injection (Busulfex)

Class: Alkylating agent.

Mechanism of Action: Forms carbonium ions through the release of a methane sulfonate group, resulting in the alkylation of DNA. Acts primarily on granulocyte precursors in the bone marrow, and is cell cycle, phase nonspecific.

Metabolism: After IV administration, drug achieves equal concentrations in the plasma and CSF. Drug is 32% protein-bound. Metabolized in the liver, and excreted in the urine (30%). Appears metabolites may be long-lived.

Dosage/Range:

Conditioning regimen:

- Indicated in combination with cyclophosphamide prior to allogeneic hematopoietic progenitor cell transplantation for chronic myelogenous leukemia.
- 0.8 mg/kg (IBW or actual weight, whichever is lower, or adjusted IBW) IV q6h × 4 days (total of 16 doses).
- Cyclophosphamide dose is given on each of 2 days as a 1-hour infusion at a dose of 60 mg/kg beginning on BMT day −3, 6 hours following the 16th dose of IV busulfan.

Drug Preparation:

- Asceptically open ampule, and using the 25-mm, 5-micron nylon membrane syringe filter provided, remove the ordered, calculated drug dose.
- Remove the syringe/filter, replace with a new needle, and dispense the syringe contents into a bag or syringe containing 10 times the volume of the drug, either 0.9% NS Injection or 5% Dextrose Injection. The final concentration of drug should be ≥ 0.5 mg/mL. For example, a 70-kg patient at a dose of 0.8 mg/kg given a concentration of 6 mg/mL would require 9.3 mL (56 mg) busulfan total dose. 9.3 mL of drug × 10 = 93 mL. As the further diluent needed is 0.9% NS Inj or D%W Inj, the total volume is 9.3 mL + 93 mL = 102.3 mL.
- Mix contents thoroughly.
- Ensure that this meets the recommended drug concentration, e.g., (9.3 mL × 6 mg/mL)/102.3 mL = 0.54 mg/mL.
- Unopened ampules must be refrigerated at 2–8°C (36–46°F).
- Diluted drug is stable at room temperature (25°C) for up to 8 hours, but infusion must be completed within this time. Drug diluted in 0.9% NS Inj,

USP, is stable refrigerated (2–8°C) for up to 12 hours, but the infusion must be completed within that time.

Drug Administration:

- Available in a 10-mL, single-use ampule containing 60 mg (6 mg/mL).
- Dilute in 0.9% NS Injection or 5% Dextrose Injection to 10 times volume of drug (see example in Preparation) prior to IV infusion.
- Infuse dose over 2 hours via infusion pump.
- Drug should be administered through a central line.
- All patients should be premedicated with phenytoin, as drug crosses BBB and causes seizures (see Drug Interactions).

Drug Interactions:

- Phenytoin decreases busulfan AUC by 15%, resulting in the target dose. If phenytoin is not used concomitantly, AUC and drug exposure may be greater.
- Other anticonvulsants may increase busulfan AUC, increasing the risk of veno-occlusive disease or seizures. Monitor busulfan exposure and toxicity closely.
- Itraconazole decreases busulfan clearance by up to 25% with potential significant increases in serum busulfan levels.
- Acetaminophen prior to (< 72 hours) or concurrent with busulfan may result in decreased drug clearance and increased serum busulfan levels.

Lab Effects/Interference:

- Profound myelosuppression/aplasia with decreased WBC, neutrophils, Hgb/HCT, and platelet counts.
- If liver veno-occlusive disease develops, increased serum transaminases, alk phos, and bili.
- Creatinine is elevated in 21% of patients.

Special Considerations:

- Drug clearance is best predicted when the busulfan dose is based on adjusted ideal body weight (AIBW).
- Ideal body weight (IBW in kg): men = 50 + 0.91 × (height in cm − 152); Women = 45 + 0.91 × (height in cm − 152).
- AIBW = IBW + 0.25 × (actual weight − IBW).
- No known antidote if overdose occurs; one report says that drug is dialyzable.

Drug is metabolized by conjugation with glutathione, so consider administration of same. Drug should only be given in combination with hematopoietic progenitor cell transplantation, as expected toxicity is profound myelosuppression.

CNS effects including seizures, hepatic veno-occlusive disease (VOD), cardiac tamponade, bronchopulmonary dysplasia with pulmonary fibrosis four months to ten years after therapy.

- Contraindicated in patients with a history of hypersensitivity to drug or its components.
- Women of childbearing age should use effective birth control measures; nursing mothers should interrupt breast-feeding during therapy.
- Drug is for adult use, and has not been studied in patients with hepatic insufficiency.
- Drug may cause cellular dysplasia in many organs (characterized by giant, hyperchromatic nuclei in lymph nodes, pancreas, thyroid, adrenal glands, liver, lungs, and bone marrow), which may cause difficult interpretation of subsequent cytologic examinations in lungs, bladder, and uterine cervix.
- Factors that may increase risk of veno-occlusive disease are history of XRT, more than three cycles of chemotherapy, prior progenitor cell transplantation, or busulfex dose AUC concentrations of > 1500 μm/min.

Potential Toxicities/Side Effects and the Nursing Process

I. POTENTIAL FOR INFECTION, BLEEDING, AND ANEMIA related to BONE MARROW DEPRESSION

Defining Characteristics: Myelosuppression is profound in 100% of patients. ANC < 500/mm^3 occurred a median of four days posttransplant in 100% of patients. Following progenitor cell infusion, the median recovery of neutrophil count to ≥ 500 cells/mm^3 was day 13 when prophylactic G-CSF was given. 51% of patients experienced 1+ episodes of infection; fever occurred in 80% of patients, with chills in 33%. Thrombocytopenia (< 25,000/mm^3 or requiring platelet transfusion) occurred in 5–6 days in 98% of patients. There was a median of six platelet transfusions per patient in clinical trials. Anemia affected 50% of patients, and the median number of red blood cell transfusions on clinical trials was 4 per patient.

Nursing Implications: Assess WBC, with differential, Hgb/HCT, and platelet count prior to drug administration, and at least daily during treatment. Discuss any abnormalities with physician. Monitor continuously for signs/symptoms of infection or bleeding. Teach patient signs/symptoms of infection and bleeding, self-assessment, and to report signs/symptoms immediately. Teach self-care measures to minimize infection and bleeding, including avoidance of OTC aspirin-containing medications. Discuss with physician use of granulocyte-colony stimulating factor (G-CSF) to prevent febrile neutropenia. Transfuse platelets and red blood cells per physician order.

II. ALTERATION IN CARDIAC OUTPUT, POTENTIAL related to TACHYCARDIA, THROMBOSIS, HYPERTENSION, VASODILATION

Defining Characteristics: Mild-to-moderate tachycardia has been noted in 44% of patients (11% during drug infusion), and, less commonly, other rhythm disturbances such as arrhythmia (5%), atrial fibrillation (2%), ventricular extrasystoles (2%), and third-degree heart block (2%). Mild-to-moderate thrombosis may occur in 33% of patients, usually associated with a central venous catheter. Hypertension has been seen in 36% of patients and grade ¾ in 3%. Mild vasodilation (flushing and hot flashes) occurs in 25% of patients. In clinical trials, most commonly in the postcyclophosphamide phase, other less common events were cardiomegaly (5%), mild EKG changes (2%), grades 3 and 4 CHF (2%), and moderate pericardial effusion (2%).

Nursing Implications: Assess baseline cardiac status and frequently during shift/care depending upon patient condition, including HR, BP, EKG, and total body fluid balance. Monitor patient for changes in cardiac function throughout treatment course, and report changes immediately. Monitor central venous lines for patency, and use scrupulous care in maintaining catheters; assess for signs/symptoms of venous thrombosis, and discuss management with physician as soon as it is discovered.

III. ALTERATION IN FLUID AND ELECTROLYTE BALANCE, POTENTIAL related to TREATMENT, CARDIAC RESPONSE

Defining Characteristics: 79% of patients develop edema, hypervolemia, or weight increase, mild or moderate.

Nursing Implications: Assess baseline fluid volume status, weight, orthostatic vital signs, and presence/absence of edema, and assess at least daily, especially after fluid or blood product infusion. Closely monitor I/O and daily total body balance, and discuss abnormalities with physician. Assess renal status, as BUN and creatinine can become elevated in 21% of patients. Assess patient for signs/symptoms of dysuria, oliguria, and hematuria, as hemorrhagic cystis may occur with cyclophosphamide.

IV. POTENTIAL FOR IMPAIRED GAS EXCHANGE related to DYSPNEA AND INTERSTITIAL PULMONARY FIBROSIS

Defining Characteristics: Mild or moderate dyspnea was seen in 25% of study patients, and was severe in 2% (severe hyperventilation). 5% of patients in the study developed alveolar hemorrhage and died. One patient developed nonspecific interstitial fibrosis and died from respiratory failure on BMT day +98. Other reported pulmonary events were mild or moderate, including pharyngitis (18%), hiccup (18%), asthma (8%), atelectasis (2%), pleural effusion

(3%), hypoxia (2%), hemoptysis (3%), and sinusitis (3%). As with oral busulfan, pulmonary fibrosis can occur one to many years post-therapy, with the average onset of symptoms four years after therapy (range 4 months to 10 years).

Nursing Implications: Assess pulmonary status, including breath sounds, rate, oxygen saturation, at baseline, and regularly during care. Assess for any underlying problems, such as infection, effusions, and leukemic infiltrates. Teach patient to report any dyspnea, SOB, or other change, and monitor closely. Provide oxygen and support and discuss management plan with physician and implement promptly. After therapy is completed, remind patient that pulmonary fibrosis may develop as a late effect. The patient should have long-term follow-up, and report any dyspnea or SOB, especially in the cold.

V. POTENTIAL FOR ALTERATION IN NUTRITION, LESS THAN BODY REQUIREMENTS, related to NAUSEA/VOMITING, ANOREXIA, STOMATITIS, DIARRHEA, AND ELECTROLYTE ABNORMALITIES

Defining Characteristics: The incidence of GI toxicities is high, but manageable: nausea 98%, vomiting 95%, stomatitis 97%, diarrhea 84%, anorexia 85%, dyspepsia 44%, and mild-to-moderate constipation 38%. Grade ¾ stomatitis occurred in 26% of patients, severe anorexia in 21%, and grade ¾ diarrhea in 5%. Additionally, hyperglycemia was seen in 67% of patients, with grade 3/4 in 15%. Hypomagnesemia was mild/moderate in 62%, and severe in 2%; hypokalemia was mild/moderate in 62% and severe in 2%; hypocalcemia was mild/moderate in 46%, and severe in 3%; hypophosphatemia was mild/moderate in 17%, and hyponatremia occurred in 2%.

Nursing Implications: Assess baseline weight, usual weight, and any changes. Assess appetite, and favorite foods. Assess baseline glucose, electrolytes, and minerals, and monitor throughout therapy. Premedicate with aggressive antiemetics (serotonin antagonist) and continue protection throughout treatment. Assess efficacy and modify regimen as needed. Assess oral mucosa and teach patient self-care strategies, including assessment, what to report, oral hygiene regimen. Encourage dietary modifications as needed. Assess bowel elimination pattern baseline and daily during therapy. Teach patient to report diarrhea, and discuss management with physician. Provide comfort measures, and teach patient scrupulous hygiene to prevent infection. Discuss abnormal lab values with physician, correct hyperglycemia, and replete magnesium, potassium, phosphate, calcium, and sodium as ordered.

VI. POTENTIAL FOR SENSORY/PERCEPTUAL ALTERATIONS related to NEUROLOGICAL TOXICITY

Defining Characteristics: Drug crosses BBB, achieving levels equivalent to plasma concentration. Neurologic changes observed in clinical testing were insomnia (84%), anxiety (75%), headaches (65%), dizziness (30%), depression (23%), confusion (11%), lethargy (7%), and hallucinations (5%). Less commonly, delirium occurred in 2%, agitation in 2%, encephalopathy in 2%, and somnolence in 2%. Despite prophylaxis with phenytoin, one patient developed seizures while receiving cyclophosphamide. Especial caution should be used when patients with a history of seizure disorder or head trauma receive the drug.

Nursing Implications: Assess baseline neurologic status and continue to monitor status throughout. Closely monitor patients who have a history of seizure disorder, or head trauma for the development of seizures (seizure precautions). Teach patient to report any changes in usual patterns. Discuss any abnormalities with physician, and develop collaborative symptom-management strategies, including medications. Assess patient interest in relaxation exercises or imagery, or other techniques, and teach self-care strategies. Be prepared to manage seizures as needed.

VII. ALTERATION IN HEPATIC FUNCTION, POTENTIAL related to VENOOCCLUSIVE DISEASE (VOD) AND GRAFT-VERSUS-HOST DISEASE (GVHD)

Defining Characteristics: Increased bilirubin occurred in 49% of patients, and grade ¾ hyperbilirubinemia occurred in 30% within 28 days of transplantation. This was associated with graft-versus-host disease in 6 patients in clinical studies, and with VOD in 8% of patients (5). Severe increases in SGPT occurred in 7%, while mild increases in alkaline phosphatase occurred in 15% of patients. Jaundice occurred in 12%, while hepatomegaly developed in 6%. VOD is a complication of conditioning therapy prior to transplant and occurred in 8% of patients (fatal in 2 of the 5 patients). Factors that may increase risk of venoocclusive disease are history of XRT, more than three cycles of chemotherapy, prior progenitor cell transplantation, or busulfex dose AUC concentrations of > 1500 μm/min. Use Jones' criteria to diagnose VOD hyperbilirubinemia, and two of the following: painful hepatomegaly, weight gain > 5%, or ascites. GVHD developed in 18% of patients (severe 3%, mild/moderate 15%, fatal in 3 patients).

Nursing Implications: Assess hepatic function baseline and daily during treatment. Discuss any abnormalities with physician. Teach the patient to report RUQ pain, weight gain, increasing girth, or yellowing of eyes or skin.

VIII. ALTERATION INCOMFORT, POTENTIAL, related to ASTHENIA, PAIN, INJECTION SITE INFLAMMATION, ARTHRALGIAS

Defining Characteristics: Symptoms leading to discomfort include: abdominal pain (mild/moderate 69%, severe 3%), asthenia (mild/moderate 49%, severe 2%), general pain (45%), injection site inflammation or pain (25%), chest or back pain (23–26%), and arthralgia (13%).

Nursing Implications: Assess baseline comfort, and usual strategies to promote comfort. Teach patient to report any pain, weakness, listlessness, injection site discomfort, or any other changes. Discuss strategies to promote comfort, such as use of heat or cold. If discomfort persists, discuss pharmacologic management to reduce symptom distress.

IX. POTENTIAL SEXUAL DYSFUNCTION related to DRUG EFFECTS

Defining Characteristics: Similar to oral busulfan: premenopausal female patients commonly experience ovarian suppression and amenorrhea with menopausal symptoms; men experience sterility, azoospermia, and testicular atrophy. The drug is potentially teratogenic.

Nursing Implications: Assess patient's signs/symptoms and partner's patterns of sexuality and reproductive goals. Teach patient/partner about need for effective contraception and provide other information as appropriate. Provide emotional support, supportive counseling, and referral as needed.

X. ALTERATION IN SKIN INTEGRITY, POTENTIAL related to SKIN RASH, ALOPECIA

Defining Characteristics: Rash is common (57%) and pruritus less so (28%). Alopecia occurred in 15% of patients. Character of rash ranged from mild vesicular rash (10%), mild/moderate maculopapular rash (8%), vesiculo-bullous rash (10%), and exfoliative dermatitis (5%). Other skin abnormalities described were erythema nodosum (2%).

Nursing Implications: Assess baseline skin integrity, presence of rashes, itching, and repeat qd. Teach patient skin changes may occur, and to report them. Discuss use of topical agents and antipruritic medications with physician.

Drug: capecitabine (Xeloda, N4-Pentoxycarbonyl-5-deoxy-5-fluorocytidine)

Class: Fluoropyrimidine carbamate.

Mechanism of Action: Metabolites bind to thymidylate synthetase, inhibiting the formation of uracil from thymidylate, and reducing the cell's ability to produce DNA. It also prevents cell division by hindering the formation of RNA, by causing nuclear transcription enzymes to mistakenly incorporate its metabolites in the process of RNA transcription.

Metabolism: Absorbed from the intestinal mucosa as an intact molecule, metabolized in the liver to intermediary metabolite, and then in the liver and tumor tissue to 5-FU precursor. It is then converted through catalytic activation to 5-FU at the tumor site. Metabolites are cleared in the urine.

Dosage/Range:

- 2500 mg/m^2/d PO in two divided doses with food for two weeks, although some patients require starting at 75% of the recommended dose.
- Two-week treatment followed by a one-week rest period and repeated every three weeks.
- Interrupt for grade 2 nausea, vomiting, diarrhea, stomatitis, or hand-foot syndrome.
- Dose reduce for renal dysfunction.
- Adjuvant colon regimen: 1250 mg/m2 po bid d1-14 repeated q 21 days × 8 cycles (24 weeks).
- In combination with docetaxel: 1250 mg/m^2 po bid × 14 days, followed by a 7 day rest period, repeated q 3 weeks, with docetaxel 75 mg/m^2 IV over 1 hr day 1, repeated q 3 weeks.

Drug Preparation/Administration:

- Oral.
- Administer within 30 min of a meal with plenty of water.
- Divide daily dose in half; take 12 hours apart.

Drug Interactions:

- Warfarin: ↑ INR, monitor closely and adjust warfarin dose as needed.
- Phenytoin: monitor phenytoin serum level closely and adjust dose as needed.
- Docetaxel: synergy due to up regulation of 5-FU enzyme.
- Leucovorin: synergy and ↑ toxicity; monitor closely.

Lab Effects/Interference:

- Increased bili, alk phos.

Special Considerations:

- Indications:

Adjuvant Colon Cancer: In patients who have undergone complete resection of the primary tumor when fluoropyrimidine therapy alone is preferred.

Metastatic Colorectal Cancer: First line treatment when treatment with fluropyrimidine therapy alone preferred.

Breast Cancer (metastatic): In patients who are resistant to both paclitaxel and an anthracycline-containing regimen, or resistant to paclitaxel in women who cannot receive anthracycline therapy.

Breast Cancer (metastatic): In combination with docetaxel, capecitabine is indicated for the treatment of patients after failure of prior anthracycline-containing chemotherapy.

- Many oncologists begin dosing at 1500 mg/m²–1875 mg/m²/d × 14 days.
- Monitor bili baseline and before each cycle, as dose modifications are necessary with hyperbilirubinemia.
- Folic acid should be avoided while taking drug.
- Contraindicated in patients hypersensitive to 5-fluorouracil or patients with creatinine clearance < 30 mL/mm.

Potential Toxicities/Side Effects and the Nursing Process

I. POTENTIAL FOR INFECTION AND BLEEDING related to BONE MARROW DEPRESSION

Defining Characteristics: Commonly causes anemia, neutropenia, and thrombocytopenia.

Nursing Implications: Assess baseline CBC, WBC with differential, and platelet count prior to chemotherapy, as well as for signs/symptoms of infection or bleeding. Teach patient signs/symptoms of infection and bleeding and instruct to report these immediately; teach patient self-care measures to minimize risk of infection and bleeding. This includes avoidance of crowds, proximity to people with infections, and avoidance of OTC aspirin-containing medications.

II. ALTERED NUTRITION, LESS THAN BODY REQUIREMENTS, related to NAUSEA AND VOMITING, STOMATITIS, AND DIARRHEA

Defining Characteristics: Nausea and vomiting occur in 30–50% of patients. Stomatitis and diarrhea also occur in about 50% of patients. Less common with reduced doses. Abdominal pain (35%), constipation (14%), anorexia (26%), dehydration (7%) also occur. Side effects are increased in the old elderly (≥ 80 yrs old).

Nursing Implications: Premedicate patient with antiemetics (phenothiazines usually effective), and continue for 24 hours, at least for first cycle. Encourage small, frequent meals of cool, bland foods. Assess oral mucosa prior to drug administration and teach patient to report changes. Teach patient oral hygiene measures and self-assessment. Instruct patient to report diarrhea, to self-administer prescribed antidiarrheal medications, and to drink adequate fluids. Moderate to severe stomatitis, diarrhea, or nausea and vomiting is an indication to interrupt therapy.

III. ALTERATION IN SKIN INTEGRITY/COMFORT related to HAND/FOOT SYNDROME

Defining Characteristics: Hand and foot syndrome occurs in more than half of patients and is characterized by tingling, numbness, pain, erythema, dryness, rash, swelling, and/or pruritus of hands and feet. Less common with reduced doses.

Nursing Implications: Teach patient about the possibility of this side effect and instruct to inform physician immediately should it occur. If patient has pain, expect dose interruption, with dose reduction if this is 2nd or subsequent episode at current dose. Teach patient self-assessment of soles of feet and palms of hands daily for erythema, pain, dry desquamation, and to report pain right away. Teach patients to avoid hot showers, whirlpools, paraffin treatments of nails, vigorous repetitive movements of hands, feet, as well as other body areas; avoid tight fitting shoes and clothes. Teach patients to take cool showers, keep skin surfaces intact and soft with skin emollients. Studies ongoing establishing evidence base for prophylaxis or treatment: vitamin B_6, urea moisturizers, nicotine patch.

IV. ALTERATION IN COMFORT related to FATIGUE, WEAKNESS, DIZZINESS, HEADACHE, FEVER, MYALGIAS, INSOMNIA, AND TASTE PROBLEMS

Defining Characteristics: Fatigue affects approximately 43% of patients, while 42% of patients complained of weakness. Fever was reported in 18% of patients, headache 10%, dizziness 8%, insomnia 7%, and taste problems 6%. Eye irritation was reported by 13% of patients and is related to the drug's excretion via tears.

Nursing Implications: Assess baseline comfort, and teach patient that these symptoms may occur. Teach patient strategies to manage fatigue, such as alternating rest and activity periods, and consolidating tasks. Teach patient to report fever, headache, and eye irritation, and discuss management plan with physician.

Drug: carboplatin (Paraplatin)

Class: Alkylating agent (heavy metal complex).

Mechanism of Action: A second-generation platinum analog. The cytotoxicity is identical to that of the parent, cisplatin, and it is cell cycle phase nonspecific. It reacts with nucleophilic sites on DNA, causing predominantly intrastrand and interstrand crosslinks rather than DNA-protein crosslinks. These crosslinks are similar to those formed with cisplatin but are formed later.

Metabolism: At 24 hours postadministration, approximately 70% of carboplatin is excreted in the urine. The mean half-life is roughly 100 minutes.

Dosage/Range:
- Dose usually given as a function of Area Under the Curve (AUC). Since carboplatin has predictable pharmokinetics based on the drug's excretion by the kidneys, area under the curve (AUC) dosing is recommended for this drug. This allows tailoring the drug dose precisely to the individual patient's excretion of the drug (renal function). The Calvert formula is used where the total dose (mg) = target AUC × GFR or glomerular filtration rate + 25. The GFR is approximated by the urine creatinine clearance, either estimated or actual, and can be calculated by hand. The target AUC is determined by the treatment plan depending upon the type of malignancy, such as an AUC of 6 for cancer of unknown primary. Then the dose calculation can be done by hand. Additionally, the manufacturer (Bristol-Myers-Squibb Oncology) distributes a calculator to determine dose.
- As a single agent, 360 mg/m^2 every 4 weeks, or 300 mg/m^2 when combined with cyclophosphamide for advanced ovarian cancer. Delay drug for neutrophil count $< 2000/mm^2$ or platelets $< 100{,}000/mm^2$.
- Drug dose reduction for urine creatinine clearance < 60 mL/minute.

Drug Preparation:
- Available as a white powder in amber vial.
- Reconstitute with sterile water for injection, 5% Dextrose, or 0.9% Sodium Chloride solution.
- Dilute further in 5% Dextrose or 0.9% Sodium Chloride.
- The solution is chemically stable for 24 hours; discard solution after 8 hours because of the lack of bacteriostatic preservative.

Drug Administration:
- Administered by IV bolus over 15 minutes to 1 hour.
- May also be given as a continuous infusion over 24 hours.
- May be administered intraperitoneally in patients with advanced ovarian cancer.

Drug Interactions:
- Increases in renal toxicity when combined with cisplatin.
- Increases in bone marrow depression when combined with myelosuppressive drugs.
- Avoid aluminum needles in drug handling.
- Taxol: administer following taxol to maximize cell kill.

Lab Effects/Interference:
- Increased LFTs, RFTs.

Special Considerations:

- Does not have the renal toxicity seen with cisplatin.
- Thrombocytopenia is dose-limiting toxicity, and correlates with GFR.
- Monitor urine creatinine clearance.
- Calculators that facilitate AUC dosing are available from Bristol-Myers-Squibb (Princeton, NJ) along with a helpful booklet entitled, *Individualized Dosing of Paraplatin Using Area Under the Curve (AUC)*.

Potential Toxicities/Side Effects and the Nursing Process

I. POTENTIAL FOR INFECTION AND BLEEDING related to BONE MARROW DEPRESSION

Defining Characteristics: Myelosuppression is dose-limiting toxicity; platelet nadir is 14–21 days, with usual recovery by day 28; WBC nadir follows 1 week later, but recovery may take 5–6 weeks. The risk of thrombocytopenia is severe, especially when the drug is combined with other myelosuppressive drugs, or if the patient has renal compromise. Anemia may occur with prolonged treatment.

Nursing Implications: Assess CBC, WBC, with differential, and platelet count prior to drug administration. Monitor for signs/symptoms of infection or bleeding. Drug dosage should be reduced if urine creatinine clearance is < 60 mL/min. Drug should be held or dose reduced if absolute neutrophil count (ANC) and/or platelet count is low. Teach the patient signs/symptoms of infection and bleeding, and instruct to report them immediately if they occur. Teach self-care measures to minimize infection and bleeding. Discuss with physician use of granulocyte-colony stimulating factor (G-CSF) to prevent neutropenia in heavily pretreated patients.

II. POTENTIAL FOR ALTERED URINARY ELIMINATION related to NEPHROTOXICITY

Defining Characteristics: The drug does not have the renal toxicity seen with cisplatin (Platinol), so that only minimal hydration is needed. However, the drug is excreted by the kidneys, and concomitant treatment with drugs causing nephrotoxicity (i.e., aminoglycoside antibiotics) can alter renal function studies. Nephrotoxicity does occur at high doses, and patients with renal dysfunction are at risk. In addition, serum electrolyte loss can occur (K+, Mg++, rarely Ca++). Monitor serum electrolytes prior to treatment and periodically after treatment. Replete electrolytes as ordered.

Nursing Implications: Assess renal function studies, (i.e., urine creatinine clearance, serum blood urea nitrogen [BUN], and creatinine) prior to drug administration. Discuss drug dose modification if creatinine clearance < 60 cc/min, or if other values are abnormal.

III. POTENTIAL FOR ALTERATION IN NUTRITION, LESS THAN BODY REQUIREMENTS, related to NAUSEA/VOMITING, ANOREXIA, STOMATITIS, DIARRHEA, AND HEPATIC DYSFUNCTION

Defining Characteristics: Nausea and vomiting begin 6+ hours after administration and last for <24 hours, but may be easily prevented by available antiemetics. Anorexia occurs in 10% of patients but is usually mild, lasting 1–2 days. Diarrhea occurs in 10% of patients and is mild. Reversible hepatic dysfunction is mild to moderate, as evidenced by changes in alk phos and SGOT and, rarely, serum glutamic pyruvic transaminase (SGPT) and bili.

Nursing Implications: Premedicate with antiemetics and continue protection for 24 hours, at least for the first cycle. Encourage dietary modifications as needed. Monitor LFTs prior to and periodically during treatment.

IV. POTENTIAL FOR SENSORY/PERCEPTUAL ALTERATIONS related to NEUROLOGICAL CHANGES

Defining Characteristics: Neurologic dysfunction is infrequent, but there is increased risk in patients >65 years old, or if previously treated with cisplatin and receiving prolonged carboplatin treatment.

Nursing Implications: Assess baseline neurologic status and continue to monitor status throughout treatment, looking for dizziness, confusion, peripheral neuropathy, ototoxicity, visual changes, and changes in taste. Teach patient the potential for side effects, and to report any changes.

V. POTENTIAL SEXUAL DYSFUNCTION related to DRUG EFFECTS

Defining Characteristics: Drug is mutagenic and probably teratogenic. It is unknown whether drug is excreted in breast milk.

Nursing Implications: Assess patient's signs/symptoms and partner's patterns of sexuality and reproductive goals. Teach patient/partner about need for contraception and provide other information as appropriate. Provide emotional support.

VI. POTENTIAL FOR INJURY related to HYPERSENSITIVITY REACTIONS

Defining Characteristics: Drug may cause allergic reactions, ranging from rash, urticaria, erythema, and pruritus to anaphylaxis; they can occur within minutes of drug administration.

Nursing Implications: Assess baseline VS. During drug administration, observe for signs/symptoms of hypersensitivity reaction. If signs/symptoms of anaphylaxis (tachycardia, wheezing, hypotension, facial edema) occur, stop drug immediately. Keep IV patent with 0.9% Sodium Chloride, notify physician, monitor VS, and be prepared to administer ordered drugs (i.e., steroid, epinephrine, or antihistamines).

Drug: carmustine (BCNU, BiCNU)

Class: Nitrosourea.

Mechanism of Action: Alkylates DNA by causing crosslinks and strand breaks in the same manner as classic mustard agents; it also carbamoylates cellular proteins, thus inhibiting DNA repair. Cell cycle phase nonspecific.

Metabolism: Rapidly distributed and metabolized with a plasma half-life of 1 hour; 70% of IV dose is excreted in urine within 96 hours. Significant concentrations of drug remain in cerebrospinal fluid for 9 hours due to lipid solubility of drug.

Dosage/Range:

Usual:

- 75–100 mg/m^2 IV/day × 2 days, OR
- 200–225 mg/m^2 every 6 weeks, OR
- 40 mg/m^2/day on 5 successive days, repeating cycle every 6–8 weeks.

High dose with autologous BMT (*investigational*):

- 450–600 mg/m^2 IV; however, doses of 900 mg/m^2 (in combination with cyclophosphamide) or 1200 mg/m^2 as single agent have been reported.
- These doses are fatal and require AUTOLOGOUS BMT after drug administration.
- Refer to protocol for exact dosages.

Drug Preparation/Administration:

- Add sterile alcohol (provided with drug) to vial, then add sterile water for injection.
- May be further diluted with 100–250 mL 5% Dextrose or 0.9% Sodium Chloride.

High dose (*investigational*):

- IV bolus in at least 500 mL of 5% Dextrose over 2 hours; can also divide dose into two equal fractions administered 12 hours apart. Refer to protocol for exact information.
- When given for gliomas as a single agent, administer with dexamethasone or mannitol infusion to reduce cerebral edema.
- Usually given in combination with other cytotoxic agents in BMT protocols.

Mycosis fungoides:

- Carmustine topical solution 0.5–3.0 mg/mL may be painted on body after showering, qd × 14 days (investigational).

Drug Interactions:

- Cimetidine may increase myelosuppression when given concurrently. AVOID IF POSSIBLE.
- Possible increased cellular uptake of drug when administered in combination with amphotericin B.
- Carmustine may decrease the pharmacologic effects of phenytoin.

Lab Effects/Interference:

- Pulmonary, hepatic, and renal function tests.

Special Considerations:

- Drug is an irritant; avoid extravasation.
- Pain at the injection site or along the vein is common. Treat by applying ice pack above the injection site and decreasing the infusion flow rate.
- Patient may act inebriated related to the alcohol diluent and may experience flushing.

High dose:

- Pulmonary toxicity related to higher systemic levels (higher AUC).

Potential Toxicities/Side Effects and the Nursing Process

I. POTENTIAL FOR INFECTION AND BLEEDING related to BONE MARROW DEPRESSION

Defining Characteristics: Delayed myelosuppression is dose-limiting toxicity and is cumulative. WBC nadir 3–5 weeks after dose and persists 1–2 weeks; platelet nadir at 4 weeks, persisting 1–2 weeks. Drug should not be dosed more frequently than once every 6 weeks.

Nursing Implications: Assess baseline CBC, WBC with differential, and platelet count prior to chemotherapy and at least weekly postchemotherapy for the first cycle. Discuss dose reductions with physician for subsequent cycles if counts are lower than normal since bone marrow depression is cumulative. Teach patient and family self-assessment for signs/symptoms of infection and bleeding, and instruct to report them immediately. Teach self-care measures to minimize risk of infection and bleeding, including avoidance of aspirin-containing medicines.

II. POTENTIAL FOR IMPAIRED GAS EXCHANGE related to PULMONARY FIBROSIS

Defining Characteristics: Pulmonary toxicity appears to be dose-related, with risk greatest in patients receiving total doses > 1400 mg (although it can occur at lower doses). Other risk factors include patients with abnormal PFTs prior to drug administration; i.e., baseline forced vital capacity (FVC) < 70% of predicted; carbon monoxide diffusion capacity (DLCO) < 70% of predicted; or if patient is receiving concurrent cyclophosphamide or thoracic radiation. Presents as insidious cough and dyspnea, or may be the sudden onset of respiratory failure. CXR shows interstitial infiltrates. Incidence is 20–30% of patients, with a mortality of 24–80%.

Nursing Implications: Assess patient's risk and baseline pulmonary function prior to chemotherapy, as well as the results of pulmonary function testing periodically during treatment, for evidence of pulmonary dysfunction. Teach patient to report any changes in respiratory pattern.

III. ALTERATION IN NUTRITION, LESS THAN BODY REQUIREMENTS, related to NAUSEA/VOMITING AND LIVER DYSFUNCTION

Defining Characteristics: Severe nausea and vomiting may occur 2 hours after administration and last 4–6 hours. Reversible liver dysfunction, although rare, is related to subacute hepatitis and is characterized by abnormal LFTs, painless jaundice, and (rarely) coma.

Nursing Implications: Premedicate with antiemetics and continue antiemetic protection for 24 hours, at least for the first treatment. Encourage small, frequent feedings of cool, bland foods, and liquids. Infuse drug over 60–120 minutes. Monitor LFTs (SGOT, SGPT, lactic dehydrogenase [LDH], alk phos, bili) during treatment and discuss any abnormalities with physician.

IV. ALTERATION IN COMFORT related to DRUG ADMINISTRATION

Defining Characteristics: Drug diluent is absolute alcohol, so irritation may result in pain along the vein path. Thrombosis is rare, but venospasms and flushing of skin or burning of the eyes can occur with rapid drug infusion.

Nursing Implications: Administer drug only through patent IV and dilute drug in 250 mL of 5% Dextrose or 0.9% Sodium Chloride and infuse over 1–2 hours. If pain along vein occurs, use ice packs above injection site, decrease infusion rate, or further dilute drug. If patient will receive ongoing therapy, consider venous access device.

V. ALTERED URINARY ELIMINATION related to NEPHROTOXICITY

Defining Characteristics: Increase in BUN occurs in 10% of patients and is usually reversible. However, decreased kidney size, progressive azotemia, and renal failure have occurred in patients receiving large cumulative doses over long periods.

Nursing Implications: Assess baseline renal function and monitor BUN and creatinine prior to each successive cycle. Since drug is excreted by the kidneys, drug dosage should be reduced if renal dysfunction exists. If abnormalities occur and persist, discuss discontinuing drug with physician.

VI. POTENTIAL SEXUAL DYSFUNCTION related to DRUG EFFECTS

Defining Characteristics: Drug is mutagenic and teratogenic.

Nursing Implications: Assess patient's and partner's pattern of sexuality and reproductive goals. Teach patient and partner the need for contraception as appropriate. Provide emotional support and counseling, or referral as appropriate.

VII. SENSORY/PERCEPTUAL ALTERATIONS related to OCULAR TOXICITY

Defining Characteristics: Infarcts of optic nerve fiber, retinal hemorrhage, and neuroretinitis have been associated with high-dose therapy.

Nursing Implications: Assess baseline vision and appearance of eyes. Instruct patient to report any visual changes to physician or nurse.

Drug: chlorambucil (Leukeran)

Class: Alkylating agent.

Mechanism of Action: Alkylates DNA by causing strand breaks and cross-links in the DNA. The drug is a derivative of a nitrogen mustard.

Metabolism: Pharmacokinetics are poorly understood. It is well absorbed orally, with a plasma half-life of 1.5 hours. Degradation is slow; it appears to be eliminated by metabolic transformation, with 60% excreted in urine in 24 hours.

Dosage/Range:
- 0.1–0.2 mg/kg/day (equals 4–8 $mg/m^2/day$) to initiate treatment, OR
- 14 $mg/m^2/day$ × 5 days with a repeat every 21–28 days, depending on platelet count and WBC.

Drug Preparation:
- 2-mg tablets.

Drug Administration:
- Oral.

Drug Interactions:
- None significant.
- Simultaneous administration of barbiturates may increase toxicity of chlorambucil due to hepatic drug activation.

Lab Effects/Interference:
- BUN, uric acid.
- LFTs, especially alk phos and AST (SGOT).
- CBC, especially WBC with differential.

Special Considerations:
- None.

Potential Toxicities/Side Effects and the Nursing Process

I. POTENTIAL FOR INFECTION related to BONE MARROW DEPRESSION

Defining Characteristics: Neutropenia after third week of treatment lasting for 10 days after the last dose. Neutropenia and thrombocytopenia occur with prolonged use and may be irreversible occasionally (especially if high total doses are given; i.e., > 6.5 mg/kg). Increased toxicity may occur with prior barbiturate use.

Nursing Implications: Assess baseline CBC, including WBC with differential, and platelet count prior to dosing, as well as weekly for the first cycle of therapy. Discuss dose reduction with physician if blood values are abnormal. Teach patient self-assessment of signs/symptoms of infection and bleeding and instruct to report them immediately. Teach self-care measures to minimize risk of infection and bleeding, including avoidance of OTC aspirin-containing medications.

II. POTENTIAL FOR SEXUAL DYSFUNCTION related to REPRODUCTIVE HAZARD

Defining Characteristics: Drug is mutagenic, teratogenic, and suppresses gonadal function with consequent temporary or permanent sterility. Amenorrhea occurs in females, and oligospermia/azoospermia occur in males.

Nursing Implications: Assess patient's and partner's sexual patterns and reproductive goals. Provide teaching and emotional support; encourage birth control measures as appropriate.

III. POTENTIAL FOR ALTERATION IN NUTRITION, LESS THAN BODY REQUIREMENTS, related to NAUSEA/VOMITING, ANOREXIA/ WEIGHT LOSS, AND HEPATIC DYSFUNCTION

Defining Characteristics: Nausea and vomiting are rare. Anorexia and weight loss may occur and be prolonged. Hepatotoxicity with jaundice is rare, but abnormal LFTs may occur.

Nursing Implications: Administer antiemetics as needed and instruct patient in self-administration. Suggest weekly weights and dietary instruction if patient develops anorexia and weight loss. Monitor LFTs baseline and periodically during treatment. Discuss any abnormalities with physician and consider dose modification.

IV. POTENTIAL FOR IMPAIRED GAS EXCHANGE related to PULMONARY FIBROSIS

Defining Characteristics: Bronchopulmonary dysplasia and pulmonary fibrosis may occur rarely with long-term use.

Nursing Implications: Assess patients at risk: increased risk with cumulative dose > 1 g/m^2, preexisting lung disease, concurrent treatment with cyclophosphamide or thoracic radiation. Assess pulmonary status prior to chemotherapy and at each visit, notifying physician of dyspnea. Monitor PFTs periodically for evidence of pulmonary dysfunction. Teach patient to report any changes in pulmonary pattern, such as dyspnea.

V. POTENTIAL FOR SENSORY/PERCEPTUAL ALTERATIONS related to OCULAR DISTURBANCES, CNS ABNORMALITIES

Defining Characteristics: Ocular disturbances may occur, e.g., diplopia, papilledema, retinal hemorrhage. Tremors, muscular twitching, confusion, agitation, ataxia, flaccid paresis, and hallucinations have been described. Seizures, although uncommon, have occurred in adults and children during normal dosing, as well as with overdosing.

Nursing Implications: Assess baseline neurologic status prior to treatment and at each visit. Instruct patient to report any abnormalities.

Drug: cisplatin (Platinol)

Class: Heavy metal that acts like alkylating agent.

Mechanism of Action: Inhibits DNA synthesis by forming inter- and intrastrand crosslinks and by denaturing the double helix, preventing cell replication. Cell cycle phase nonspecific; the chemical properties are similar to those of bifunctional alkylating agents.

Metabolism: Rapidly distributed to tissues (predominately the liver and kidneys) with less than 10% in the plasma 1 hour after infusion. Clearance from plasma proceeds slowly after the first 2 hours due to platinum's covalent bonding with serum proteins; 20–74% of administered drug is excreted in the urine within 24 hours.

Dosage/Range:
- 50–120 mg/m^2 every 3–4 weeks, OR

- 15–20 mg/m² × 5 repeated every 3–4 weeks.
- Radiosensitizing effect: Administer 1–3 times per week at doses of 15–50 mg/m² (total weekly dose 50 mg/m²) with concomitant radiotherapy.

High dose (investigational):

- 200 mg/m² given in 250 mL of 3% Sodium Chloride (hypertonic).

Drug Preparation:

- 10-mg and 50-mg vials. Add sterile water to develop a concentration of 1 mg/mL.
- Further dilute solution with 250 mL or more of 0.9% Sodium Chloride (recommended) or 5% Dextrose (D_5 ½ NS) Sodium Chloride.
- Never mix with 5% Dextrose, as a precipitate will form. Drug stability increased in 0.9% Sodium Chloride.
- Available as an aqueous solution.
- Do not refrigerate.

Drug Administration:

- Avoid aluminum needles when administering, as precipitate will form.

Drug Interactions:

- Decreases pharmacologic effect of phenytoin, so dose may need to be increased.
- Possible increase in ototoxicity when combined with loop diuretics.
- Increased renal toxicity with concurrent use of aminoglycosides, amphotericin B.
- Cisplatin reduces drug clearance of high-dose methotrexate (MTX) and standard-dose bleomycin by increasing the drugs' half-life; enhances toxicity of ifosfamide (myelosuppression) and etoposide.
- Synergy when cisplatin is combined with etoposide.
- Radiosensitizing effect.
- Sodium thiosulfate and mesna: Each directly inactivates cisplatin.
- Taxol: Administer cisplatin *after* taxol to prevent delayed taxol excretion with subsequent increased bone marrow depression.

Lab Effects/Interference:

- Decreased Mg, K, Ca, Na, phos.
- Increased creatinine, uric acid.

Special Considerations:

- Administer cautiously, if at all, to patients with renal dysfunction, hearing impairment, peripheral neuropathy, or prior allergic reaction to cisplatin.
- Hydrate vigorously before and after administering drug. Urine output should be at least 100–150 mL/hour. Mannitol or furosemide diuresis may be needed to ensure this output.

- Hypersensitivity reactions have occurred, manifested by wheezing, flushing, hypotension, tachycardia. Usually occurs within minutes of starting infusion. Treat with epinephrine, corticosteroids, antihistamines.
- Drug causes potassium and magnesium wasting. Some ideas to help increase magnesium follow.
- To help increase absorption, it is recommended that excessive milk, cheese, or other high-calcium products be limited when eating foods high in magnesium.

Calcium and magnesium compete to gain entrance to the body in the intestines, so a high-calcium diet increases requirements for dietary magnesium. Foods high in magnesium are those with 100 mg or greater per 100 grams, including

Nuts:
Almonds
Brazil nuts
Cashews
Peanut butter
Peanuts
Pecans
Walnuts

Peas and beans:
Red beans
Split peas
White beans

Other good sources:
Blackstrap molasses
Brewer's yeast
Chocolate (bitter)
Cocoa (dry breakfast)
Cornmeal
Instant coffee and tea
Oatmeal
Shredded wheat
Wheat germ
Whole wheat breads and cereals

- Phase I studies are ongoing, evaluating an oral platinum (JM-216) agent in small-cell lung cancer.
- Amifostine has been shown to be renally protective in patients at risk for renal toxicity from cisplatin; in addition, drug offers protection from neurotoxicity. Other agents being studied, e.g., BNP7787.

Potential Toxicities/Side Effects and the Nursing Process

I. POTENTIAL ALTERATION IN URINARY ELIMINATION related to DRUG-INDUCED RENAL DAMAGE

Defining Characteristics: Dose-limiting toxicity, which may be cumulative. The drug accumulates in the kidneys, causing necrosis of proximal and distal renal tubules. Damage to renal tubules prevents reabsorption of Mg++, Ca++, and K+, with resultant decreased serum levels. Renal damage becomes most obvious 10–20 days after treatment, is reversible, and can be prevented by adequate hydration and diuresis, as well as slower infusion time. Hyperuricemia may occur due to impaired tubular transport of uric acid, but it is responsive to allopurinol. Concurrent administration of nephrotoxic agents is not recommended.

Nursing Implications: Assess renal function studies prior to administration (BUN, creatinine, 24-hour creatinine clearance) and discuss any abnormalities with physician. Assess cardiac and pulmonary status in terms of tolerance of aggressive hydration. Anticipate vigorous hydration regimen with or without forced diuresis (i.e., mannitol, lasix). The typical hydration schedule is 0.9% Sodium Chloride or D_5 ½ NS at 250 mL/hr × 3–5 hours prechemotherapy and 3–5 hours postchemotherapy (total hydration 3 L). Outpatient hydration of 1–2 L over 1–2 hours prechemotherapy and 1 L postchemotherapy, is typical. Strictly monitor I/O and total body fluid balance. Assess for signs/symptoms of fluid overload and notify physician for supplemental furosemide or other diuretic as needed. Monitor serum electrolytes (Na+, K+, Mg++, Ca++, PO_4) and replete as ordered by physician. Teach patient and family the need for increased oral fluids on discharge—up to 3 L or more for 5 days posttherapy.

II. ALTERATION IN NUTRITION, LESS THAN BODY REQUIREMENTS, related to SEVERE NAUSEA AND VOMITING, TASTE ALTERATIONS

Defining Characteristics: Nausea and vomiting may be severe and will occur in 100% of patients if antiemetics are not given. They begin 1 or more hours postchemotherapy and last 8–24 hours. Since the drug is slowly excreted over five days, delayed nausea and vomiting may occur 24–72 hours after dose. Taste alterations and anorexia occur with long-term use.

Nursing Implications: Premedicate with combination antiemetics (i.e., serotonin antagonist plus dexamethasone), especially for high-dose cisplatin, and continue antiemetics for up to five days with dopamine antagonist. Encourage small, frequent intake of cool, bland foods as tolerated. Infuse cisplatin over at least 1 hour to minimize emesis, since slower infusion rates decrease emesis. Taste alterations may be improved with the use of spices and zinc dietary supplementation. Refer the patient for dietary consultation as needed.

III. POTENTIAL FOR INJURY related to ANAPHYLAXIS

Defining Characteristics: Anaphylaxis has occurred, characterized by wheezing, bronchoconstriction, tachycardia, hypotension, and facial edema, in patients who have previously received the drug.

Nursing Implications: Assess baseline VS and continue to assess patient during infusion. Prior to drug administration, review standing orders or protocols for nursing management of anaphylaxis: stop infusion; keep line open with 0.9% Sodium Chloride; notify physician; monitor VS; be prepared to administer epinephrine, antihistamines, corticosteroids.

IV. POTENTIAL FOR SENSORY/PERCEPTUAL ALTERATIONS related to NEUROLOGIC TOXICITY

Defining Characteristics: Severe neuropathy may occur in patients receiving high doses or prolonged treatment and may be irreversible and is seen in stocking-and-glove distribution, with numbness, tingling, and sensory loss in arms and legs. Areflexia, loss of proprioception and vibratory sense, and loss of motor function can occur. Ototoxicity, beginning with loss of high-frequency hearing, affects > 30% of patients. It may be preceded by tinnitus, is doserelated, and can be unilateral or bilateral. The damage results from destruction of hair cells lining the organ of Corti and is cumulative and may be permanent. Rarely, ocular toxicity has occurred, but it is reversible (optic neuritis, papilledema, cerebral blindness).

Nursing Implications: Assess baseline neurologic, motor, and sensory functions prior to drug administration. Discuss use of neuroprotector in high-risk patients. Discuss baseline audiogram with physician as appropriate. Instruct patient to report changes in function or sensation, as well as diminished hearing. Discuss with physician risks vs benefits of continuing therapy if/when symptoms develop. If severe neuropathies develop, provide teaching related to activity, emotional support, and referral to physical/occupational therapy as appropriate. Discuss use of neuroprotector in high-risk patients.

V. POTENTIAL FOR ACTIVITY INTOLERANCE related to ANEMIA

Defining Characteristics: Drug may interfere with renal erythropoietin production, resulting in late development of anemia.

Nursing Implications: Teach patient to report increasing fatigue, signs of severe anemia (shortness of breath, chest pain/angina, headaches). Monitor hemoglobin/hematocrit; discuss transfusion with physician if signs/symptoms develop or hematocrit falls < 25 mg/dL. Teach patient about diet high in iron. Exogenous erythropoietin (epoetin alpha) may be helpful.

VI. INFECTION AND BLEEDING related to BONE MARROW DEPRESSION

Defining Characteristics: Bone marrow depression is mild with low to moderate doses, but may be significant when high doses are used, or when drug is given in combination with radiation as a radiation-sensitizer. Nadir is in 2–3 weeks, with recovery in 4–5 weeks.

Nursing Implications: Assess CBC, WBC, differential, and platelet count, as well as any signs/symptoms of infection or bleeding, prior to drug administration. Teach patient to self-assess for signs/symptoms of infection and bleeding. Teach self-care measures to minimize infection and bleeding, including avoidance of aspirin-containing medications.

VII. POTENTIAL SEXUAL DYSFUNCTION related to DRUG EFFECTS

Defining Characteristics: Drug is mutagenic and probably teratogenic.

Nursing Implications: Assess patient's and partner's sexual patterns and reproductive goals. Provide emotional support and discuss strategies to preserve sexual and reproductive health (i.e., contraception and sperm banking).

VIII. POTENTIAL FOR ALTERATIONS IN CARDIOVASCULAR FUNCTION related to CISPLATIN-CONTAINING COMBINATION CHEMOTHERAPY

Defining Characteristics: Angina, myocardial infarction, cerebrovascular accident, thrombotic microangiopathy, cerebral arteritis, and Raynaud's phenomenon have occurred, although they are uncommon. Combination drugs include bleomycin, vinblastine, vincristine, and etoposide.

Nursing Implications: Assess cardiopulmonary status, especially if patient has preexisting cardiac disease, both prior to and throughout treatment.

Drug: cladribine (Leustatin, 2-CdA)

Class: Antimetabolite.

Mechanism of Action: Selectively damages normal and malignant lymphocytes and monocytes that have large amounts of deoxycytidine kinase but small amounts of deoxynucleotidase. The drug, a chlorinated purine nucleoside, enters passively through the cell membrane, is phosphorylated into the active metabolite 2-CdATP, and accumulates in the cell. 2-CdATP interferes with DNA synthesis and prevents repair of DNA strand breaks in both actively dividing and normal cells. The process may also involve programmed cell death (apoptosis).

Metabolism: Drug is 20% protein-bound and is cleared from the plasma within 1–3 days after cessation of treatment.

Dosage/Range:
- 0.09 mg/kg/day IV as a continuous infusion for 7 days for one course of therapy of hairy-cell leukemia.

Drug Preparation:
- Available in 10 mg/10 mL preservative-free, single-use vials (1 mg/mL), which must be further diluted in 0.9% Sodium Chloride injection. Diluted drug stable at room temperature for at least 24 hours in normal light. Once prepared, the solution may be refrigerated up to 8 hours prior to use.
- Single daily dose: add calculated drug dose to 500 mL of 0.9% Sodium Chloride injection, and administer over 24 hours; repeat daily for a total of 7 days.
- 7-day continuous infusion by ambulatory infusion pump: add calculated drug dose for 7 days to infusion reservoir using a sterile 0.22-μm hydrophilic syringe filter. Then add, again using 0.22-μm filter, sufficient sterile bacteriostatic 0.9% Sodium Chloride injection containing 0.9% benzyl alcohol to produce 100 mL in the infusion reservoir.
- Do not use 5% Dextrose, as it accelerates degradation of drug.

Drug Administration:
- Dilute in minimum of 100 mL.
- Administer as continuous infusion over 24 hours for 7 days.

Drug Interactions:
- None known.

Lab Effects/Interference:
- Decreased CBC, platelets.
- Increased LFTs, RFTs.

Special Considerations:
- Indicated for the treatment of active hairy-cell leukemia.
- Unstable in 5% Dextrose; should not be used as diluent or infusion fluid.
- Store unopened vials in refrigerator and protect from light.
- Drug may precipitate when exposed to low temperatures. Allow solution to warm to room temperature and shake vigorously. DO NOT HEAT OR MICROWAVE.
- Drug is structurally similar to pentostatin and fludarabine.
- Contraindicated in patients who are hypersensitive to the drug.
- Administer with caution in patients with renal or hepatic insufficiency.
- Embryotoxic; women of childbearing age should use contraception.

Potential Toxicities/Side Effects and the Nursing Process

I. INFECTION AND BLEEDING related to BONE MARROW DEPRESSION

Defining Characteristics: Neutropenia occurs in 70% of patients with nadir 1–2 weeks after infusion, recovery by weeks 4–5. Incidence of infection 28%, with 40% caused by bacterial infection of lungs and venous access sites. Prolonged hypocellularity of bone marrow occurs in 34% of patients, and may last for at least four months. Infections most common in patients with pancytopenia and lymphopenia due to hairy-cell leukemia. Lymphopenia is common with decreased CD4 (helper T cells) and CD8 (suppressor T cells), with recovery by weeks 26–34. Common infectious agents are viral (20%) and fungal (20%). Thrombocytopenia occurs commonly, along with purpura (10%), petechiae (8%), and epistaxis (5%). Platelet recovery occurs by day 12, but 14% of patients require platelet support.

Nursing Implications: Monitor CBC, platelet count prior to therapy, and periodically posttherapy at expected time of nadir. Monitor for, and teach patient self-assessment of signs/symptoms of infection, bleeding. Instruct patient to call physician or nurse or go to emergency room if temperature (T) is greater than 101°F (38.3°C) or bleeding. Transfuse platelets per physician order.

II. ALTERATION IN COMFORT related to FEVER, HEADACHES

Defining Characteristics: Fever (> 100°F [37.5°C]) occurs in 66% of patients during the month following treatment due either to infection (47%) or the release of endogenous pyrogen from lysed lymphocytes. Other symptoms include chills (9%), diaphoresis (9%), malaise (7%), dizziness (9%), insomnia (7%), myalgia (7%), arthralgias (5%). Headaches occur in 22% of patients.

Nursing Implications: Assess patient for fever, chills, diaphoresis during visits; assess signs/symptoms of infection. Teach patient self-assessment, how to report this, and measures to reduce fever. Anticipate laboratory and X-ray tests to rule out infection and perform according to physician order.

III. POTENTIAL IMPAIRMENT OF SKIN INTEGRITY related to RASH

Defining Characteristics: Rash occurs in 27–50% of patients. Other symptoms include pruritus (6%), erythema (6%), injection site reactions (erythema, swelling, pain, phlebitis).

Nursing Implications: Assess skin for any cutaneous changes, such as rash or changes at injection site, and any associated symptoms such as pruritus; discuss with physician. Instruct patient in self-care measures, including avoiding abrasive skin products and clothing; avoiding tight-fitting clothing; use of skin emolients appropriate to specific skin alteration; measures to avoid scratching involved areas. Consider venous access device if skin is at risk for reaction.

IV. FATIGUE related to ANEMIA

Defining Characteristics: Fatigue occurs in 45% of patients. Red cell recovery is by week 8, but 40% of patients require red cell transfusion.

Nursing Implications: Monitor Hgb and HCT and transfuse per physician order. Administer erythropoietin per physician order and teach patient selfadministration. Teach patient about diet and instruct to alternate rest and activity; stress reduction/relaxation techniques may improve energy level.

V. ALTERATION IN ELIMINATION related to DIARRHEA, CONSTIPATION

Defining Characteristics: Diarrhea occurs in 10% of patients while constipation occurs in 9%. Abdominal pain affects 6% of patients.

Nursing Implications: Encourage patient to report onset of change in bowel habits (diarrhea or constipation) and assess factors contributing to changes. Administer or teach patient self-administration of antidiarrheal medication or cathartic as ordered. Teach patient diet modification regarding foods that minimize diarrhea or constipation.

VI. POTENTIAL FOR IMPAIRED GAS EXCHANGE related to COUGH

Defining Characteristics: Cough affects 10%, while abnormal breath sounds occur in 11% and shortness of breath in 7%.

Nursing Implications: Assess baseline pulmonary status, including breath sounds, presence of cough, shortness of breath. Instruct patient to report symptoms of cough, shortness of breath, other abnormalities.

VII. ALTERATION IN NUTRITION, LESS THAN BODY REQUIREMENTS, related to NAUSEA, VOMITING

Defining Characteristics: Nausea is mild and occurs in 28% of patients, while vomiting may occur in 13%. If antiemetics are required, nausea/vomiting is easily controlled by phenothiazines. Renal and hepatic function studies are rarely affected.

Nursing Implications: Premedicate with antiemetics. If nausea and/or vomiting occur, teach patient to self-administer antiemetics per physician order. Encourage small, frequent feedings of cool, bland foods and liquids. Teach patient to record diet history for 2–3 days and weekly weights. If patient has decreased appetite, assess food preferences (encourage or discourage) and suggest use of spices.

VIII. POTENTIAL ALTERATION IN CARDIAC OUTPUT related to TACHYCARDIA

Defining Characteristics: Occurs rarely, with edema and tachycardia each affecting 6% of patients.

Nursing Implications: Assess baseline cardiac status, including apical heart rate, presence of peripheral edema. Instruct patient to report rapid heartbeat or swelling of ankles.

Drug: clofarabine

Class: Purine nucleoside anti-metabolite.

Mechanism of Action: Drug inhibits DNA and DNA repair, causing cell death of both cycling and quiescent cancer cells. In addition, it breaks down the mitochondrial membranes, releasing cytochrome C and apoptosis-inducing factor, leading to programmed cell death.

Metabolism: Drug is 47% protein bound (mostly to albumin), with a terminal half-life of 5.2 hours. 49–60% of the dose is excreted unchanged in the urine. Other non-renal excretion is unknown.

Dosage/Range:
52 mg/m2 IV over 2 hr qd × 5, to be repeated after recovery of all baseline organ function, about q 2–6 weeks. IV hydration should be continued during the 5 days of treatment.

Drug Preparation: Drug is supplied as a 20 mg in 20 mL vial. Withdraw drug using a sterile 0.2 μm syringe filter and then further diluted with 5% dextrose injection USP or 0.9% sodium chloride injection USP prior to IV infusion. This admixture may be stored at room temperature but must be used within 24 hr of preparation.

Drug Administration: Administer IV over 2 hours; if hyperuricemia (tumor lysis syndrome), patient should receive allopurinol, and may need urine alkalinization and aggressive hydration as well.

Drug Interactions: Concurrent administration with other renally cleared drugs may alter drug levels so should be avoided during the 5 days of treatment; avoid other hepatotoxic drugs, as well as those affecting blood pressure or cardiac function if possible during drug administration.

Lab Effects/Interference: Severe bone marrow depression with decreased white blood cells, neutrophils, red blood cells and platelets. Drug may cause tumor lysis syndrome with increased levels of potassium, phosphate, uric acid, creatinine, and changes in other electrolyte values. Renal and hepatic function studies should be monitored during the 5 days of drug treatment.

Special Considerations:

- Drug is indicated for the treatment of pediatric patients aged 1–21 years old with relapsed or refractory acute lymphoblastic leukemia after at least 2 prior regimens.
- Treatment results in the rapid lysis of peripheral leukemia cells.
- Drug is fetotoxic so all patients should be taught to use effective contraceptive measures to prevent pregnancy; female patients shold be taught not to breast feed during treatment.
- Drug may cause dehydration, hypotension, capillary leak syndrome.

Potential Toxicities/Side Effects and the Nursing Process

I. INFECTION AND BLEEDING related to BONE MARROW DEPRESSION

Defining Characteristics: Bone marrow depression is dose limiting. Febrile neutropenia occurs in 57% of patients. Pyrexia affects 41% of patients, while 38% experience rigors. Infections include bacteremia, cellulites, herpes simplex, oral candidiasis, pneumonia, sepsis, and staphylococcal infections.

Nursing Implications: Assess WBC, neutrophil, and platelet count, and discuss any abnormalities with physician prior to drug administration; assess for signs/symptoms of skin infections (all mucosal surfaces, body orifices) and bleeding; instruct patient in signs/symptoms of infection and bleeding, as well as to report them or come to emergency room. Teach patient self-care measures to minimize risk of infection and bleeding, including avoidance of OTC aspirin-containing medications. Assess patient's Hgb/HCT and signs/symptoms of fatigue; teach patient self-assessment and to alternate rest and activity as needed.

II. ALTERED NUTRITION, LESS THAN BODY REQUIREMENTS, related to NAUSEA AND VOMITING, ANOREXIA, DIARRHEA, and HEPATOTOXICITY

Defining Characteristics: Nausea and vomiting occur in 75% and 83% of patients respectively. Can be successfully prevented with combination antiemetics. Anorexia occurs in about 1/3 of patients. Diarrhea is frequent, affecting about 50% of patients. Constipation affects 21% of patients. Hepatotoxicity and jaundice occur in 15% of patients.

Nursing Implications: Premedicate with antiemetics depending on dose, using aggressive, combination antiemetics, and continue throughout chemotherapy. If patient develops nausea/vomiting, assess fluid and electrolyte balance and the need for replacements. Assess oral mucosa prior to chemotherapy and teach patient oral hygiene regimen and self-assessment; encourage patient to report diarrhea, discuss use of antidiarrheals with physician, and teach self-care PRN. Since patients become neutropenic, all mucosal surfaces need to be assessed for infection, and patients must be taught scrupulous perineal hygiene. Monitor LFTs prior to, during, and posttherapy.

III. IMPAIRED SKIN/MUCOSAL INTEGRITY related to RASH, ANAL INFLAMMATION/ULCERATION, ALOPECIA

Defining Characteristics: Maculopapular rash, with or without fever, myalgia, bone pain, occasional chest pain, conjunctivitis, and malaise (cytarabine syndrome) may occur. Syndrome is not common, but occurs 6–12 hours after drug administration; corticosteroids have been helpful in treating/preventing syndrome. Mucosal inflammation and ulceration of anus/rectum may occur, especially in patients with prior hemorrhoids or history of abscesses. Alopecia occurs less frequently.

Nursing Implications: Assess baseline skin and mucous membranes prior to chemotherapy and identify patients at risk for problems. Consider including corticosteroid in antiemetic regimen, especially for high-dose therapy, and discuss with physician prophylactic use of dexamethasone eye drops to prevent conjunctivitis. Teach patient scrupulous perineal hygiene, instruct to report any rectal discomfort, and assess rectal mucosa daily with high-dose therapy. Discuss with patient potential coping strategies if alopecia occurs (i.e., wig, scarves).

IV. ALTERATION IN COMFORT, POTENTIAL, related to EDEMA, FATIGUE, LETHARGY, PAIN

Defining Characteristics: In clinical studies, the frequency of occurrence of these symptoms was: edema 20%, fatigue 36%, injection site pain 14%, pain 19%, arthralgia 11%, back pain 13%, myalgia 14%, pain in limb 29%, dermatitis 41%, erythema 18%, pruritis 47%, palmar plantar erythrodyesthesia syndrome (PPE) 13%, and flushing 18%.

Nursing Implications: Teach patient that these symptoms may occur and to report them. Teach patient self-care measures to reduce discomfort, such as application of heat or cold for pain, arthralgias and myalgias. Teach patient to report redness and pain on palms of hands or soles of feet as this may be PPE, and would require close monitoring and follow-up to prevent moist desquamation. Instruct patient to report any symptoms that do not resolve or improve with self-care measures.

Drug: cyclophosphamide (Cytoxan)

Class: Alkylating agent.

Mechanism of Action: Causes crosslinkage in DNA strands, thus preventing DNA synthesis and cell division. Cell cycle phase nonspecific.

Metabolism: Inactive until converted by microsomes in liver and serum enzymes (phosphamidases). Both cyclophosphamide and its metabolites are excreted by the kidneys. Plasma half-life: 6–12 hours, with 25% of drug excreted after 8 hours. Prolonged plasma half-life in patients with renal failure results in increased myelosuppression.

Dosage/Range:
- 400 mg/m^2 IV × 5 days.
- 100 mg/m^2 PO × 14 days.
- 500–1500 mg/m^2 IV q3–4 weeks.

High dose with BMT (*investigational*):
- 1.8–7 gm/m^2 in combination with other cytotoxic agents.

Drug Preparation:
- Dilute vials with sterile water. Shake well. Allow solution to clear if lyophilized preparation is not used. Do not use solution unless crystals are fully dissolved. Available in 25- and 50-mg tablets.

Drug Administration:
- Oral use: Administer in morning or early afternoon to allow adequate excretion time. Should be taken with meals.
- IV use: For doses > 500 mg, pre- and posthydration to total 500–3000 mL is needed to ensure adequate urine output and to avoid hemorrhagic cystitis. Administer drug over at least 20 minutes for doses > 500 mg.
- Mesna given with high-dose cyclophosphamide to prevent hemorrhagic cystitis.
- Solution is stable for 24 hours at room temperature, 6 days if refrigerated.
- Rapid infusion may result in dizziness, nasal stuffiness, rhinorrhea, sinus congestion during or soon after infusion.

Drug Interactions:
- Increases chloramphenicol half-life.
- Increases duration of leukopenia when given in combination with thiazide diuretics.
- Increases effect of anticoagulant drugs.

- Decreases digoxin level, so dose may need to be increased.
- Potentiation of doxorubicin-induced cardiomyopathy.
- Increased succinylcholine action with prolonged neuromuscular blockage.
- Increased drug action of barbiturates; induction of hepatic microsomes.

Lab Effects/Interference:

- Increased K, uric acid secondary to tumor lysis.
- Monitor electrolytes for symptoms of SIADH.
- Decreased CBC, platelets.

Special Considerations:

- Metabolic and leukopenic toxicity is increased by simultaneous administration of barbiturates, corticosteroids, phenytoin, and sulfonamides.
- Activity and toxicity of both cyclophosphamide and the specific drug may be altered by allopurinol, chloroquine, phenothiazides, potassium iodide, chloramphenicol, imipramine, vitamin A, warfarin, succinylcholine, digoxin, thiazide diuretics.
- Test urine for occult blood.
- High-dose cyclophosphamide therapy may require catheterization and constant bladder irrigation. Mesna should be given, either as a continuous infusion or in bolus doses, around drug administration. Consult protocol. See Chapter 4.

Potential Toxicities/Side Effects and the Nursing Process

I. INFECTION AND BLEEDING related to BONE MARROW DEPRESSION

Defining Characteristics: Leukopenia nadir occurs days 7–14, with recovery in 1–2 weeks; thrombocytopenia is less frequent and anemia is mild. Drug is a potent immunosuppressant.

Nursing Implications: Assess CBC, WBC with differential, platelet count, and signs/symptoms of infection and bleeding prior to treatment. Teach patient signs/symptoms of infection and instruct to report them if they occur. Teach patient self-care measures to minimize infection and bleeding. Increased risk of bone marrow depression in patients with prior radiation or chemotherapy.

II. ALTERED URINARY ELIMINATION related to HEMORRHAGIC CYSTITIS

Defining Characteristics: Metabolites of drug, if allowed to accumulate in the bladder, irritate bladder wall capillaries, causing hemorrhagic cystitis. This occurs in 7–40% of patients, is evidenced by microscopic or gross hematuria, is common with high doses, and is preventable. Long-term drug exposure may lead to bladder fibrosis.

Nursing Implications: Monitor BUN and creatinine prior to drug dose and as drug is excreted by the kidneys. Assess for signs/symptoms of hematuria, urinary frequency, or dysuria; instruct patient to report these if they occur. Instruct patient to take in at least 3 L of fluid per day and to empty bladder every 2–3 hours, as well as at bedtime. If patient is receiving a high dose, ensure vigorous hydration prior to drug administration. Bladder irrigation per protocol. Instruct patient to take oral cyclophosphamide early in the day to prevent drug accumulation in bladder during the night.

III. ALTERATION IN NUTRITION, LESS THAN BODY REQUIREMENTS, related to NAUSEA AND VOMITING, ANOREXIA, STOMATITIS, DIARRHEA, AND HEPATOTOXICITY

Defining Characteristics: Nausea and vomiting are dose-related and begin 2–4 hours after dose, peak in 12 hours, and may last 24 hours. Anorexia is common; stomatitis, if it occurs, is mild; and diarrhea is mild and infrequent. Hepatotoxicity is rare.

Nursing Implications: Premedicate with antiemetics prior to drug administration and continue prophylactically for 24 hours, at least for the first cycle. Encourage small feedings of bland foods and liquids. Encourage favorite foods and consult dietitian regarding anorexia if needed. Assess oral mucosa prior to drug administration; teach patient self-assessment techniques and oral care. Monitor LFTs before, during, and after therapy.

IV. ALTERED BODY IMAGE related to ALOPECIA, CHANGES IN NAILS AND SKIN

Defining Characteristics: Alopecia occurs in 30–50% of patients, especially with IV dosing, but some degree of hair loss occurs in all patients. Hair loss begins after 3+ weeks; hair may grow back while on therapy, but will grow back after therapy is discontinued (may be softer in texture). Hyperpigmentation of nails and skin, as well as transverse ridging of nails (banding), may occur.

Nursing Implications: Teach patient about potential hair loss and other changes. Discuss impact of hair loss on patient and strategies to minimize it (i.e., wig, scarf, cap) prior to drug administration. Assess ongoing coping during treatment. If nail changes are distressing, discuss the use of nail polish or other measures.

V. POTENTIAL SEXUAL DYSFUNCTION related to DRUG EFFECTS

Defining Characteristics: Drug is mutagenic and teratogenic. Amenorrhea often occurs in females, and testicular atrophy, possibly with reversible oligospermia/azoospermia, occurs in males. Drug is excreted in breast milk.

Nursing Implications: Assess patient's/partner's sexual patterns and reproductive goals. Discuss strategies to preserve sexual and reproductive health, including contraception and sperm banking, as appropriate. Mothers receiving cyclophosphamide should not breast-feed.

VI. POTENTIAL FOR INJURY related to ACUTE WATER INTOXICATION (SIADH) AND SECOND MALIGNANCY

Defining Characteristics: SIADH may occur with high-dose administration (> 50 mg/kg). Prolonged therapy may cause bladder cancer and acute leukemia.

Nursing Implications: Assess patients receiving high-dose cyclophosphamide: monitor serum Na+, osmolality, and urine osmolality and electrolytes; strictly monitor I/O, total body fluid balance, and daily weight. Screen patients who are receiving prolonged cyclophosphamide therapy for secondary malignancies.

VII. ALTERATION IN CARDIAC OUTPUT related to HIGH-DOSE CYCLOPHOSPHAMIDE

Defining Characteristics: Cardiomyopathy may occur with high doses as well as hemorrhagic cardiac necrosis, transmural hemorrhage, and coronary artery vasculitis at doses of 120–240 mg/kg. The mechanism is endothelial injury with subsequent hemorrhagic necrosis. The incidence is 22%, with 11% mortality, which may be decreased by dividing the dose into two split daily infusions. The risk at standard doses is increased by coadministration of doxorubicin (Adriamycin).

Nursing Implications: Assess cardiac status, especially if patient is receiving a high dose. Discuss baseline cardiac function test (GBPS) and assess for signs/symptoms of cardiomyopathy as treatment continues. Instruct patient to report dyspnea, shortness of breath, or other changes.

VIII. POTENTIAL FOR IMPAIRED GAS EXCHANGE related to PULMONARY TOXICITY

Defining Characteristics: Rare, but may occur with prolonged, high-dose therapy or continuous, low-dose therapy. Onset is insidious and appears as interstitial pneumonitis, which may progress to fibrosis. May respond to steroids.

Nursing Implications: Assess patients receiving high-dose or continuous low-dose cyclophosphamide for signs/symptoms of pulmonary dysfunction. Discuss pulmonary function studies with physician. Assess lung sounds prior to drug administration and periodically during treatment. Teach patient to report dyspnea, cough, or any abnormalities.

Drug: cytarabine, cytosine arabinoside (Ara-C, Cytosar-U)

Class: Antimetabolite.

Mechanism of Action: Incorporated into DNA, slowing its synthesis and causing defects in the linkages to new DNA fragments. Also, cells exposed to cytarabine in the S phase reinitiate DNA synthesis when the drug, a pyrimidine analogue, is removed, resulting in erroneous duplication of the early portions of the DNA strands. Most effective when cells are undergoing rapid DNA synthesis.

Metabolism: Inactivated by liver enzymes in biphasic manner: half-lives 10–15 minutes and 2–3 hours. Crosses the BBB with cerebrospinal fluid concentration of 50% that of plasma; 70% of dose excreted in urine as Ara-U; 4–10% excreted 12–24 hours after administration.

Dosage/Range:
- Varies depending on disease.
- Leukemia: 100 mg/m^2/day IV continuous infusion × 5–10 days; 100 mg/m^2 q12h × 1–3 weeks IV or SQ.
- Head and neck: 1 mg/kg q12h × 5–7 days IV or SQ.
- High dose: 2–3 g/m^2 IV q12h × 4–12 doses to treat refractory acute leukemia.
- Differentiation: 10 mg/m^2 SQ q12h × 15–21 days.
- Intrathecal: 20–30 mg/m^2.

Drug Preparation:
- 100-mg vials: add water with benzyl alcohol then dilute with 0.9% Sodium Chloride or 5% Dextrose.
- 500-mg vials: add water with benzyl alcohol then dilute with 0.9% Sodium Chloride or 5% Dextrose.
- For intrathecal use and high dose: use preservative-free diluent.
- Reconstituted drug is stable 48 hours at room temperature and 7 days refrigerated.

Drug Administration:
- Doses of 100–200 mg can be given SQ.
- Doses less than 1 g: Administer via pump over 10–20 minutes.
- Doses over 1 g: Administer over 2 hours.

Drug Interactions:
- May be a decreased bioavailability of digoxin when given in combination.

Lab Effects/Interference:
- Decreased CBC.
- Increased LFTs, RFTs.
- Increased uric acid due to tumor lysis.

Special Considerations:

- Thrombophlebitis, pain at the injection site, should be treated with warm compresses.
- Dizziness has occurred with too rapid IV infusions.
- Use with caution if hepatic dysfunction exists.
- Drug is excreted in tears requiring protection of eye conjunctiva with high-dose therapy.

Potential Toxicities/Side Effects and the Nursing Process

I. INFECTION AND BLEEDING related to BONE MARROW DEPRESSION

Defining Characteristics: Bone marrow depression is related to dose and duration of therapy. WBC depression is biphasic. After a 5-day continuous infusion at doses of 50–600 mg/m^2, WBC begins to fall within 24 hours, reaching nadir in 7–9 days, briefly rises around day 12, and begins to fall again, reaching nadir at days 15–24, with recovery within 10 days. Platelet drop begins day 5, reaching nadir at days 12–15, with recovery within 10 days. Anemia is seen frequently, with megaloblastic changes common in the bone marrow. Potent but transient suppression of primary and secondary antibody responses occur.

Nursing Implications: Assess WBC, neutrophil, and platelet count, and discuss any abnormalities with physician prior to drug administration; assess for signs/symptoms of skin infections (all mucosal surfaces, body orifices) and bleeding; instruct patient in signs/symptoms of infection and bleeding, as well as to report them or come to emergency room. Teach patient self-care measures to minimize risk of infection and bleeding, including avoidance of OTC aspirin-containing medications. Assess patient's Hgb/HCT and signs/symptoms of fatigue; teach patient self-assessment and to alternate rest and activity as needed.

II. ALTERED NUTRITION, LESS THAN BODY REQUIREMENTS, related to NAUSEA AND VOMITING, ANOREXIA, STOMATITIS, DIARRHEA, HEPATOTOXICITY

Defining Characteristics: Nausea and vomiting occurs in 50% of patients, is dose related, and lasts for several hours. Can be successfully prevented with combination antiemetics. Anorexia commonly occurs. Stomatitis occurs 7–10 days after therapy is initiated, occurs in 15% of patients, and is dose related. May be preceded by angular stomatitis (reddened area at juncture of lips). Diarrhea is infrequent and mild. Hepatotoxicity is usually mild and reversible, but drug should be used cautiously in patients with impaired hepatic function.

Nursing Implications: Premedicate with antiemetics depending on dose, using aggressive, combination antiemetics for high-dose therapy, and continue throughout chemotherapy. If patient develops nausea/vomiting, assess fluid and electrolyte balance and the need for replacements. Assess oral mucosa prior to chemotherapy and teach patient oral hygiene regimen and self-assessment; encourage patient to report diarrhea, discuss use of antidiarrheals with physician, and teach self-care PRN. Since patients become neutropenic, all mucosal surfaces need to be assessed for infection, and patients must be taught scrupulous perineal hygiene. Monitor LFTs prior to, during, and posttherapy.

III. IMPAIRED SKIN/MUCOSAL INTEGRITY related to RASH, ANAL INFLAMMATION/ULCERATION, ALOPECIA

Defining Characteristics: Maculopapular rash, with or without fever, myalgia, bone pain, occasional chest pain, conjunctivitis, and malaise (cytarabine syndrome) may occur. Syndrome is not common, but occurs 6–12 hours after drug administration; corticosteroids have been helpful in treating/preventing syndrome. Mucosal inflammation and ulceration of anus/rectum may occur, especially in patients with prior hemorrhoids or history of abscesses. Alopecia occurs less frequently.

Nursing Implications: Assess baseline skin and mucous membranes prior to chemotherapy and identify patients at risk for problems. Consider including corticosteroid in antiemetic regimen, especially for high-dose therapy, and discuss with physician prophylactic use of dexamethasone eye drops to prevent conjunctivitis. Teach patient scrupulous perineal hygiene, instruct to report any rectal discomfort, and assess rectal mucosa daily with high-dose therapy. Discuss with patient potential coping strategies if alopecia occurs (i.e., wig, scarves).

IV. POTENTIAL FOR INJURY related to NEUROTOXICITY

Defining Characteristics: Neurotoxicity can occur at high doses. If cerebellar toxicity (characterized by nystagmus, dysarthria, ataxia, slurred speech, and/or disdiadochokinesia or inability to make fine, coordinated movements) develops, it is an indication to terminate therapy. Onset usually 6–8 days after first dose, lasts 3–7 days. Lethargy and somnolence have resulted from rapid infusion of the drug. Incidence of CNS toxicity is 10% and may be related to total cumulative drug dose, impaired renal function, and/or age > 50 years old. Ocular toxicity may occur, characterized by injection of conjunctive, corneal opacities, decreased visual acuity. This may be a result of inhibition of DNA synthesis of corneal epithelium. Conjunctivitis occurs due to excretion of drug in lacrimal tearing and can be prevented by corticosteroid eye drops. Other visual symptoms that may occur are increased lacrimation, blurred vision, photophobia, eye pain.

Nursing Implications: Assess baseline neurologic status and cerebellar function (coordinated movements such as handwriting and gait) prior to and during therapy. Teach patient to self-assess and report changes in coordination, control of eye movement, handwriting. Monitor patient for somnolence and lethargy during infusion, and infuse drug according to established guidelines. With high-dose therapy, discuss with physician use of prophylactic corticosteroid eye drops. Assess and teach patient self-assessment of eyes and instruct to report increased lacrimation, blurred vision, photophobia, eye pain.

V. POTENTIAL FOR INJURY related to TUMOR LYSIS SYNDROME (TLS)

Defining Characteristics: May develop with initial therapy if patient has a large tumor burden; results from rapid lysis of tumor cells. This usually begins 1–5 days after initiation of therapy and causes elevations in serum uric acid, potassium, phosphorus, BUN, creatinine.

Nursing Implications: If this is induction therapy for a patient with acute leukemia or high tumor burden, expect medical orders to include IV hydration at 150 mL/hour with or without alkalinization, oral allopurinol, strict monitoring of I/O, daily weight, and total body fluid balance determination. Monitor baseline and daily BUN, creatinine, K+, phosphorus, uric acid, and calcium. Monitor for renal, cardiac, neuromuscular signs/symptoms of TLS.

VI. POTENTIAL SEXUAL DYSFUNCTION related to DRUG EFFECTS

Defining Characteristics: Drug is mutagenic and probably teratogenic. Although normal babies have been delivered by mothers receiving drug in first trimester, other babies have had congenital defects. It is unknown whether the drug is excreted in breast milk.

Nursing Implications: Discuss with patient and partner sexuality and reproductive goals and possible impact of chemotherapy. Discuss contraception and sperm banking if appropriate. Discourage breast-feeding if the mother is receiving chemotherapy.

Drug: cytarabine, liposome injection (DepoCyt)

Class: Antimetabolite.

Mechanism of Action: Drug is converted to the metabolite ara-CTP intracellularly. Ara-CTP is thought to inhibit DNA polymerase, thereby affecting DNA synthesis. Incorporation into DNA and RNA may also contribute to cytarabine cellular toxicity.

Metabolism: With systemically administered cytarabine, the drug is metabolized to an inactive compound, ara-U, and is then renally excreted. In the CSF, however, conversion to the ara-U is negligible, because CNS tissue and CSF lack the enzyme necessary for the conversion to occur. Liposomal formulation gives sustained effect over 2 weeks.

Dosage/Range:

Indicated for the intrathecal treatment of lymphomatous meningitis only. To be given as follows:

- Induction therapy: DepoCyt, 50 mg, administered intrathecally (intraventricular or lumbar puncture) every 14 days for 2 doses (weeks 1 and 3).
- Consolidation therapy: DepoCyt, 50 mg, administered intrathecally (intraventricular or lumbar puncture) every 14 days for 3 doses (weeks 5, 7, and 9) followed by 1 additional dose at week 13.
- Maintenance therapy: DepoCyt, 50 mg, administered intrathecally (intraventricular or lumbar puncture) every 28 days for 4 doses (weeks 17, 21, 25, and 29).
- If drug-related neurotoxicty develops, the dose should be reduced to 25 mg. If toxicity persists, treatment with DepoCyt should be terminated.

Drug Preparation/Administration:

- Drug is supplied in single-use vials and comes as a white to off-white suspension in 5 mL of fluid.
- Drug is to be withdrawn immediately before use and should not be used later than 4 hours from the time of withdrawal from vial.
- DepoCyt should be administered directly into the CSF over 1–5 minutes. Patients should lie flat for 1 hour after administration.
- Patients should be started on dexamethasone 4 mg bid either PO or IV for 5 days beginning on the day of DepoCyt injection.

Drug Interactions:

- No formal drug interaction studies of DepoCyt and other drugs have been done.
- Expect increased neurotoxicity if drug is administered at same time as other intrathecal, cytotoxic agents.

Lab Effects/Interference:

- DepoCyt particles are similar in size and appearance to white blood cells, so care must be taken when interpreting CSF samples.

Special Considerations:

- Do not use inline filters with DepoCyt; administer directly into CSF.
- Must be administered with concurrent dexamethasone as described above.
- FDA indication based on controlled clinical trial showing superior CR rate (41%) compared to standard intrathecal cytarabine.

Potential Toxicities/Side Effects and the Nursing Process

I. ALTERATION IN NUTRITION, LESS THAN BODY REQUIREMENTS, related to NAUSEA AND VOMITING

Defining Characteristics: Nausea, vomiting, and headache are common, and are physical manifestations of chemical arachnoiditis.

Nursing Implications: Administer dexamethasone throughout treatment course as described above. Observe patient for at least 1 hour after administration for toxicity. Administer antiemetics as ordered. Encourage small, frequent feedings of cool, bland foods. Instruct patient to report nausea and vomiting and to self-administer antiemetics as ordered.

II. ALTERATION IN COMFORT related to HEADACHE, NECK AND/ OR BACK PAIN, FEVER, NAUSEA, AND VOMITING

Defining Characteristics: Some degree of chemical arachnoiditis is expected in about one-third of patients: incidence approaches 100% of patients when dexamethasone is NOT given with DepoCyt. Causes headache, neck pain, and/ or rigidity, back pain, fever, nausea, and vomiting, which are reversible.

Nursing Implications: Instruct patient in dexamethasone self-administration and to report to physician if oral doses are not tolerated. Patients should lie flat for one hour after lumbar puncture and should be observed for immediate toxic reactions. Administer medications to treat pain.

Drug: dacarbazine (DTIC-Dome, Dimethyl-triazeno-imidazolecarboximide)

Class: Alkylating agent.

Mechanism of Action: Appears to methylate nucleic acids (particularly DNA) causing crosslinkage and breaks in DNA strands, which inhibits RNA and DNA synthesis. Also interacts with sulfhydral groups in proteins. Generally, cell cycle phase nonspecific.

Metabolism: Thought to be activated by liver microsomes. Excreted renally, with a plasma half-life of 0.65 hour, and terminal half-life of 5 hours.

Dosage/Range:
- 375 mg/m^2 every 3–4 weeks, OR
- 150–250 mg/m^2/day × 5 days, repeat every 3–4 weeks, OR
- 800–900 mg/m^2 as a single dose every 3–4 weeks.

High dose (investigational):
- 350 mg/m^2–2.5 g/m^2 IV as 24-hour infusion with hemibody radiotherapy.

Drug Preparation:

- Add sterile water or 0.9% Sodium Chloride to vial.

Drug Administration:

- Administer via pump over 20 minutes or give via IV push over 2–3 minutes.
- Stable for 8 hours at room temperature, for 72 hours if refrigerated. Store lyophilized drug in refrigerator and protect from light. Drug decomposition is denoted by a change in color from yellow to pink.

Drug Interactions:

- Increased drug metabolism with concurrent administration of dilantin, phenobarbital; potential increased toxicity with (Imuran) and 6-MP.

Lab Effects/Interference:

- Decreased CBC.
- Increased LFTs.

Special Considerations:

- Irritant—avoid extravasation.
- Pain may occur above site: Usually unrelieved by slowing IV, but may be relieved by applying ice to painful area. May cause venospasm; slow rate if this occurs.
- Anaphylaxis has occurred with infusion of dacarbazine.

Potential Toxicities/Side Effects and the Nursing Process

I. INFECTION AND BLEEDING related to BONE MARROW DEPRESSION

Defining Characteristics: Nadir occurs days 14–28 following drug administration; anemia may occur with long-term treatment.

Nursing Implications: Evaluate WBC, neutrophil, and platelet count and discuss any abnormalities with physician prior to drug administration; assess for signs/symptoms of infection or bleeding; instruct patient in identifying signs/symptoms of infection and bleeding, and to report them. Teach patient selfcare measures to minimize risk of infection and bleeding, including avoidance of OTC aspirin-containing medications. Assess patient's Hgb/HCT and signs/symptoms of fatigue; teach patient self-assessment and instruct to alternate rest and activity as needed.

II. ALTERATION IN NUTRITION, LESS THAN BODY REQUIREMENTS, related to NAUSEA AND VOMITING, DIARRHEA, ANOREXIA, HEPATOTOXICITY

Defining Characteristics: Nausea/vomiting occurs in 90% of patients and is moderate to severe, beginning 1–3 hours after dose. Nausea and vomiting decrease with each consecutive day the drug is given. Preventable by aggressive combination antiemetics. Diarrhea is uncommon. Anorexia is common, occurring in 90% of patients; drug may also cause a metallic taste. Hepatotoxicity is rare, but hepatic venoocclusive disease has been described (hepatic vein thrombosis and hepatocellular necrosis).

Nursing Implications: Premedicate with combination antiemetics and continue protection during infusions. Administer drug over at least one hour. Use relaxation exercises, imagery, or other techniques; teach patient exercises prior to drug treatment. Teach patient to report diarrhea and administer antidiarrheal medication as ordered, or teach patient self-administration as appropriate. Encourage small, frequent feedings of favorite foods; teach patient/caregiver to make foods ahead of time so patient will have them ready for snacks when hungry; encourage use of spices if food tastes bland; encourage patient to weigh self weekly. Monitor LFTs and discuss abnormalities with physician.

III. ALTERATION IN COMFORT related to FLULIKE SYNDROME, PAIN AT INJECTION SITE

Defining Characteristics: Flulike syndrome may occur, characterized by malaise, headache, myalgia, hypotension; may occur up to 7 days after first dose, lasting 7–21 days, and may recur with subsequent doses of drug. Drug is an irritant and may cause phlebitis of vein.

Nursing Implications: Teach patient flulike symptoms may occur; suggest symptom management using acetaminophen as needed; encourage fluid intake of > 3 L/day and rest, as determined by healthcare team. Assess patient vein selection prior to drug administration and suggest venous access device early on if patient is to receive ongoing treatment with dacarbazine (DTIC). Administer drug in 100–250-mL IV fluid and infuse slowly over 1 hour. Consider premedications when drug is given peripherally and discuss with physician: hydrocortisone IVP (DTIC forms precipitate with hydrocortisone sodium succinate [Solucortef] but not with hydrocortisone), lidocaine 1–2% IVP, or heparin IVP to minimize vein trauma prior to DTIC infusion. Apply heat or ice above injection site to reduce venous burning.

IV. IMPAIRED SKIN INTEGRITY related to ALOPECIA, FACIAL FLUSHING, ERYTHEMA, URTICARIA

Defining Characteristics: Alopecia occurs in 90% of patients. Facial flushing occurs rarely and is self-limiting; erythema and urticaria may occur around injection site. High dose-related photosensitization may occur, with resulting severe reaction to sunlight, e.g., burning, pain.

Nursing Implications: Teach patient about expected hair loss; encourage patient to verbalize feelings regarding anticipated/actual hair loss and discuss strategies to minimize impact of alopecia. Encourage female patients to obtain wig prior to hair loss; ask male patients to identify how they will manage hair loss. Provide emotional support. In cold climates, encourage patient to wear cap at night to prevent loss of body heat. Teach patient receiving high-dose therapy to cover body, head, and hands when exposed to sunlight, or to avoid direct sunlight. Patient should also use sunblock.

V. POTENTIAL FOR SENSORY/PERCEPTUAL ALTERATIONS related to FACIAL PARESTHESIA, PHOTOSENSITIVITY

Defining Characteristics: Photosensitivity may occur in bright sunlight or ultraviolet light. Facial paresthesias may occur.

Nursing Implications: Instruct patient to report facial paresthesias and in self-care measures if sensory changes occur: wear sunglasses in strong sunlight; wear sunscreens when out in the sun; as well as protective clothing, including a hat, avoid UV or strong sunlight exposure if possible.

VI. POTENTIAL SEXUAL DYSFUNCTION related to DRUG EFFECTS

Defining Characteristics: Drug is teratogenic. It is unknown whether drug is excreted in breast milk. Drug is probably carcinogenic.

Nursing Implications: Assess patient's and partner's patterns of sexuality and reproductive goals. Teach need for contraception and provide information and referral as appropriate. Encourage verbalization of feelings and provide emotional support. Discourage breast-feeding if patient is a lactating mother.

Drug: dactinomycin (Actinomycin D, Cosmegen)

Class: Antitumor antibiotic isolated from *Streptomyces* fungus.

Mechanism of Action: Binds to guanine portion of DNA and blocks the ability of DNA to act as a template for both DNA and RNA. At lower drug doses, the predominant action inhibits RNA, whereas at higher doses both RNA and DNA are inhibited. Cell cycle specific for G1 and S phases.

Metabolism: Most of drug is excreted unchanged in bile and urine. There is a rapid clearance of drug from plasma (approximately 36 hours). Dose reduction in the presence of liver or renal failure may be needed.

Dosage/Range:
- 10–15 μg/kg/day × 5 days q3–4 weeks.
- 15–30 μg/kg/week, 400–600 μg/m^2 day for 5 days IV.
- Frequency and schedule may vary according to protocol and age.

Drug Preparation:

- Add sterile water for a concentration of 500 μg/mL. Use preservative-free water, as precipitate may develop otherwise.

Drug Administration:

- IV: Drug is a vesicant and should be given through a running IV to avoid extravasation, which can lead to ulceration, pain, and necrosis. Be sure to check the nursing policy and procedure for administration of vesicants.

Drug Interactions:

- None significant.

Lab Effects/Interference:

- Decreased CBC.
- Increased LFTs.
- Decreased calcium.

Special Considerations:

- Drug is a vesicant. Give through a running IV to avoid extravasation, which may develop into ulceration, necrosis, and pain.
- Nausea and vomiting are moderate to severe. Usually occurs 2–5 hours after administration; may persist up to 24 hours.
- Potent myelosuppressive agent: Severity of nadir is dose-limiting toxicity.
- GI toxicity: Mucositis, diarrhea, and abdominal pain.
- Skin changes: Radiation recall phenomenon. Skin discoloration along vein used for injection.
- Alopecia.
- Malaise, fatigue, mental depression.
- Contraindicated in patients with chickenpox or herpes zoster, as life-threatening systemic disease may develop.

Potential Toxicities/Side Effects and the Nursing Process

I. POTENTIAL FOR INFECTION AND BLEEDING related to BONE MARROW DEPRESSION

Defining Characteristics: Myelosuppression often dose-limiting toxicity. Onset of decreasing WBC and platelets in 7–10 days, with nadir 14–21 days after dose and recovery in 21–28 days. Delayed anemia.

Nursing Implications: Assess CBC, WBC, differential, and platelet count prior to drug administration, as well as for signs/symptoms of infection and bleeding, and discuss any abnormalities with physician prior to drug administration. Instruct patient in signs/symptoms of infection and bleeding and instruct to report this; teach patient self-care measures to minimize risk of infection and bleeding, including avoidance of OTC aspirin-containing medications. Assess patient's Hgb/HCT and signs/symptoms of fatigue; teach patient self-assessment and instruct to alternate rest and activity as needed.

II. ALTERATION IN NUTRITION, LESS THAN BODY REQUIREMENTS, related to NAUSEA/VOMITING, DIARRHEA, ANOREXIA

Defining Characteristics: Nausea/vomiting may be severe and begins 2–5 hours after dose, lasting 24 hours. Diarrhea with/without cramps occurs in 30% of patients. Anorexia occurs frequently.

Nursing Implications: Use combination antiemetics to prevent nausea and vomiting. Nausea/vomiting may be prevented by aggressive, combination antiemetics, such as serotonin antagonist plus dexamethasone. Encourage small, frequent feedings of bland foods. Encourage patient to eat favorite foods and use seasonings on foods if anorexia persists; refer to dietitian as needed.

III. ALTERATION IN MUCOUS MEMBRANES related to STOMATITIS, ESOPHAGITIS, AND PROCTITIS

Defining Characteristics: Irritation and ulceration may occur along the entire GI mucosa.

Nursing Implications: Assess baseline oral mucosa and presence of irritation along GI tract. Instruct patient in self-assessment and teach patient to report irritation; instruct regarding oral hygiene regimen.

IV. POTENTIAL IMPAIRED SKIN INTEGRITY related to RADIATION RECALL, RASH, ALOPECIA, AND DRUG EXTRAVASATION

Defining Characteristics: Recalls damage to skin from previous radiation, resulting in erythema or increased pigmentation at the radiation site. Acnelike rash and alopecia can occur in 47% of patients. Drug is a potent vesicant.

Nursing Implications: Conduct baseline skin, hair assessment. Discuss with patient impact of potential changes on body image, as well as possible coping/adaptive strategies (e.g., obtain wig prior to hair loss). When administering the drug, ensure use of a patent vein to avoid extravasation; consider the use of venous access device early. Be familiar with institution's policy and procedure for administration of a vesicant and management of extravasation.

V. ALTERATION IN COMFORT related to FLULIKE SYMPTOMS

Defining Characteristics: Flulike symptoms can occur, including symptoms of malaise, myalgia, fever, depression.

Nursing Implications: Inform patient this may occur. Assess for occurrence during and after treatment. Discuss with physician symptomatic management.

VI. POTENTIAL FOR ALTERATION IN METABOLISM related to HEPATOTOXICITY AND RENAL TOXICITY

Defining Characteristics: Hepatotoxicity is related to drug metabolism in liver; renal toxicity is related to drug excretion by kidneys.

Nursing Implications: Monitor LFTs, BUN, and creatinine. Discuss abnormalities with physician, as drug doses may need to be reduced.

VII. POTENTIAL FOR SEXUAL DYSFUNCTION

Defining Characteristics: Drug is carcinogenic, mutagenic, and teratogenic. It is unknown if drug is excreted in breast milk.

Nursing Implications: Assess patient's/partner's sexual patterns and reproductive goals. Provide information, supportive counseling, and referral as needed. Teach importance of birth control measures as appropriate. Discourage breast-feeding if patient is a lactating mother.

Drug: daunorubicin citrate liposome injection (DaunoXome)

Class: Anthracycline antibiotic that is isolated from streptomycin products, in particular the rhodomycin products, and encapsulated in a liposome.

Mechanism of Action: No clearly defined mechanism. Intercalates DNA, therefore blocking DNA, RNA, and protein synthesis. Binds to DNA and inhibits DNA replication and DNA-dependent RNA synthesis. Drug is encapsulated within liposomes (lipid vesicles) and is preferentially delivered to solid tumor sites. The liposomal encapsulated drug is protected from chemical and enzymatic degradation, protein binding, and uptake by normal tissues while circulating in the blood. The exact mechanism for selective targeting of tumor sites is unknown but is believed to be related to increased permeability of the tumor neovasculature. Once delivered to the tumor, the drug is slowly released and exerts its antineoplastic action.

Metabolism: Cleared from the plasma at 17 mL/min with a small steady-state volume of distribution. As compared to standard IV daunorubicin, the liposomal encapsulated daunorubicin has higher daunorubicin exposure (plasma area under the curve, ARC). The elimination half-life (4.4 hours) is shorter than standard daunorubicin.

Dosage/Range:

- 40 mg/m^2/day IV bolus over 60 minutes every 2 weeks.

Drug Preparation:

- Drug is available as 50 mg of daunorubicin base in a total volume of 25 mL (2 mg/mL).

- Visually inspect for particulate matter and discoloration (drug appears as a translucent dispersion of liposomes that scatters light, but should not be opaque or have precipitate or foreign matter present).
- Withdraw the calculated volume of drug and add to an equal volume of 5% Dextrose to deliver a 1:1, or 1 mg/mL solution.
- Administer immediately, or may be stored in the refrigerator at 2–8°C (36–46°F) for 6 hours.
- Use ONLY 5% Dextrose, NOT 0.9% Sodium Chloride or any other solution.
- Drug contains no preservatives.
- Unopened drug vials should be stored in the refrigerator at 2–8°C (36–46°F), but should not be frozen. Protect from light.

Drug Administration:
- IV bolus over 60 minutes, repeated every 2 weeks.
- Do not use an inline filter.
- Drug is an irritant, not a vesicant.
- Dose should be reduced in patients with renal or hepatic dysfunction.
- Hold dose if absolute granulocyte count is < 750 cells/mm^3.

Drug Interactions:
- Unknown at this time, so do not mix with any other drugs.

Lab Effects/Interference:
- Increased LFTs, RFTs (especially if elevated prior to administration).
- Increased uric acid secondary to tumor lysis.

Special Considerations:
- Drug is embryotoxic, so female patients should use contraceptive measures as appropriate.
- Back pain, flushing, and chest tightness may occur during the first 5 minutes of drug administration and resolve with cessation of the infusion. Most patients do not experience recurrence when the infusion is restarted at a slower rate.
- Drug indicated in the treatment of Kaposi's sarcoma. Activity reported to be equivalent to treatment with ABV (doxorubicin, vincristine, bleomycin) but with less alopecia, cardiotoxicity, and neurotoxicity.

Potential Toxicities/Side Effects and the Nursing Process

I. POTENTIAL FOR INFECTION AND BLEEDING related to BONE MARROW DEPRESSION

Defining Characteristics: Myelosuppression can be severe and affects the granulocytes primarily. Incidence of neutropenia of 36% is similar to that of patients receiving ABV (doxorubicin, vincristine, bleomycin), which is 35%.

Neutropenia with < 500 cells/mm³ occurs in 15% of patients (vs 5% in patients receiving ABV). Fever incidence is 47%. Concurrent antiretroviral and antiviral agents received for HIV infection may enhance this. Patients are immunocompromised; therefore, monitoring for opportunistic infection is essential. Platelets and RBCs are less affected.

Nursing Implications: Monitor CBC, WBC, differential, and platelet count prior to drug administration, and discuss any abnormalities with physician. Drug should not be given if ANC is < 750 cells/mm³. Assess for signs/symptoms of infection or bleeding, and instruct patient in self-assessment and to report signs/symptoms immediately. Teach patient self-care measures to minimize risk of infection and bleeding, including avoidance of OTC aspirin-containing medications. Drug dosage must be reduced if patient has hepatic dysfunction: 75% of drug dose if serum bili 1.2–3.0 mg/dL, 50% reduction if bili is > 3.0 mg/dL. Drug dosage must be reduced if patient has renal impairment: creatinine > 3 mg/dL, give 50% of normal dose.

II. ALTERATION IN COMFORT related to TRIAD OF BACK PAIN, FLUSHING, CHEST TIGHTNESS

Defining Characteristics: This occurs in 13.8% of patients and is mild to moderate. The syndrome resolves with cessation of the infusion, and does not usually recur when the infusion is resumed at a slower infusion rate.

Nursing Implications: Infuse drug at prescribed rate over 60 minutes. Assess for, and teach patient to report, back pain, flushing, and chest tightness. Stop infusion if this occurs, and once symptoms subside, resume infusion at a slower rate.

III. POTENTIAL FOR ALTERATION IN SKIN INTEGRITY related to ALOPECIA, CHANGES IN SKIN

Defining Characteristics: Mild alopecia occurs in 6% of patients and moderate alopecia in 2% of patients, as compared to 36% of patients receiving ABV chemotherapy. The drug is considered an irritant, NOT a vesicant. Folliculitis, seborrhea, and dry skin occur in < 5% of patients.

Nursing Implications: Teach patient that hair loss is unlikely, and to report this or any skin changes.

IV. POTENTIAL FOR ALTERATION IN NUTRITION, LESS THAN BODY REQUIREMENTS, related to NAUSEA AND VOMITING, ANOREXIA, DIARRHEA

Defining Characteristics: Mild nausea occurs in 35% of patients, moderate nausea in 16% of patients, and severe nausea in 3% of patients. Vomiting is less common, with 10% experiencing mild, 10% experiencing moderate, and 3% experiencing severe vomiting. Anorexia may occur (21%) or increased appetite may occur in < 5% of patients. Diarrhea may occur in 38% of patients. Other GI problems, occurring < 5% of the time, are dysphagia, gastritis, hemorrhoids, hepatomegaly, dry mouth, and tooth caries.

Nursing Implications: Premedicate with antiemetics. Encourage small, frequent feedings of bland foods. If patient has anorexia, teach patient or caregiver to make foods ahead of time, use spices, and encourage weekly weights. Instruct patient to report diarrhea, and to use self-management strategies (medications as ordered, diet modification). Instruct patient to report other GI problems.

V. POTENTIAL FOR ALTERATION IN CARDIAC OUTPUT related to CARDIAC CHANGES

Defining Characteristics: Daunorubicin may cause cardiotoxicity and CHF, but studies with liposomal daunorubicin show rare clinical cardiotoxicity at cumulative doses > 600 mg/m². However, especially in patients with preexisting cardiac disease or prior anthracycline treatment, assessment of cardiac function (history and physical) should be performed prior to each dose. In addition, testing of cardiac ejection fraction and echocardiogram should be performed at cumulative doses of 320 mg/m², 480 mg/m², and every 160 mg/m² thereafter.

Nursing Implications: Assess cardiac status prior to chemotherapy administration: signs/symptoms of CHF, quality/regularity and rate of heartbeat, results of prior tests of left ventricular ejection fraction (LVEF) or echocardiogram, if performed. Instruct patient to report dyspnea, palpitations, swelling in extremities. Maintain accurate records of total dose, and expect GBPS to be repeated periodically during treatment and the drug to be discontinued if there is a significant drop in heart function.

VI. POTENTIAL FOR ACTIVITY INTOLERANCE related to FATIGUE

Defining Characteristics: Fatigue occurs in 49% of patients.

Nursing Implications: Assess baseline activity level. Instruct patient to report fatigue and activity intolerance. Teach self-management strategies, including alternating rest and activity periods, and stress reduction.

Drug: daunorubicin hydrochloride (Cerubidine, Daunomycin HCl, Rubidomycin)

Class: Anthracycline antibiotic isolated from streptomycin products, in particular the rhodomycin products.

Mechanism of Action: No clearly defined mechanism. Intercalates DNA, therefore blocking DNA, RNA, and protein synthesis. Binds to DNA and inhibits DNA replication and DNA-dependent RNA synthesis.

Metabolism: Site of significant metabolism is in the liver. Doses need to be modified in presence of abnormal liver function. Excreted in urine and bile.

Dosage/Range:
- 30–60 mg/m^2/day IV for 3 consecutive days.

Drug Preparation:
- Add sterile water to produce liquid. Drug will form a precipitate when mixed with heparin and is incompatible with dexamethasone.

Drug Administration:
- IV: This drug is a potent vesicant. Give through a running IV to avoid extravasation, which can lead to ulceration, pain, and necrosis. Check individual hospital policy and procedure on administration of a vesicant.

Drug Interactions:
- Incompatible with heparin (forms a precipitate).

Lab Effects/Interference:
- Increased bili, AST, alk phos.
- Increased uric acid secondary to tumor lysis.

Special Considerations:
- Drug is a potent vesicant. Give through running IV to avoid/minimize effects of extravasation.
- Moderate to severe nausea and vomiting occur in 50% of patients within first 24 hours.
- Causes discoloration of urine (pink to red for up to 48 hours after administration).
- Potent myelosuppressive agent. Nadir occurs within 10–14 days.
- Alopecia.
- Cardiac toxicity: Dose limit at 550 mg/m^2. Patients may exhibit irreversible CHF. Acute toxicity may be seen within hours after administration. This is unrelated to cumulative dose and may manifest symptoms of pump or conduction dysfunction. Rarely, transient EKG abnormalities, CHF; pericardial effusion (whole syndrome referred to as myocarditis-pericarditis syndrome) may occur, which may lead to death.
- Dose reduction necessary in patients with impaired liver function.

- Available in liposomal encapsulated vehicle (Daunoxome) that has less myelosuppression and cardiotoxicity. Drug is currently approved for therapy of Kaposi's sarcoma.

Potential Toxicities/Side Effects and the Nursing Process

I. POTENTIAL FOR INFECTION AND BLEEDING related to BONE MARROW DEPRESSION

Defining Characteristics: WBC and platelet counts begin to decrease in 7 days, with nadir 10–14 days after drug dose; recovery in 21–28 days. Dose reduction indicated with renal or hepatic dysfunction as drug is excreted by these routes.

Nursing Implications: Evaluate WBC, neutrophil, and platelet count and discuss any abnormalities with physician prior to drug administration; assess for signs/symptoms of infection and bleeding; instruct patient in signs/symptoms of infection and bleeding and to report these immediately. Teach patient self-care measures to minimize risk of infection and bleeding, including avoidance of OTC aspirin-containing medications.

II. POTENTIAL FOR ALTERATION IN CARDIAC OUTPUT related to ACUTE AND CHRONIC CARDIAC CHANGES

Defining Characteristics: Acute effects (i.e., EKG changes, atrial arrhythmias) occur in 6–30% of patients 1–3 days after dose and are not life-threatening. Chronic myofibril damage resulting in irreversible cardiomyopathy is life-threatening and dose-related. Cumulative dose should not exceed 550 mg/m^2 or 450 mg/m^2 if patient is receiving/has received radiation to chest or with concurrent administration of cyclophosphamide or other cardiotoxic agent. CHF may develop 1–16 months after therapy ceases if cumulative dose is exceeded.

Nursing Implications: Assess baseline cardiac status, quality and regularity of heartbeat, and baseline EKG. Patient should have baseline GBPS or other measure of left ventricular ejection fraction at baseline, and periodically during treatment. If there is a significant drop in ejection fraction, then drug should be stopped. Maintain accurate documentation of doses administered so that cumulative dose is known. Instruct patient to report dyspnea, shortness of breath, edema, orthopnea.

III. ALTERATION IN NUTRITION, LESS THAN BODY REQUIREMENTS, related to NAUSEA AND VOMITING, STOMATITIS

Defining Characteristics: Mild nausea and vomiting on the day of therapy occur in 50% of patients and can be prevented with antiemetics. Stomatitis is infrequent but may occur 3–7 days after dose.

Nursing Implications: Premedicate with antiemetics, and continue for 24 hours for protection. Assess oral mucosa prior to chemotherapy, teach patient oral hygiene regimen and self-assessment; encourage patient to report burning or oral irritation. Assess pain in mouth, and administer analgesics as needed and ordered.

IV. POTENTIAL FOR IMPAIRED SKIN INTEGRITY related to ALOPECIA, HYPERPIGMENTATION OF FINGERNAILS AND TOENAILS, RADIATION RECALL, AND DRUG EXTRAVASATION

Defining Characteristics: Reversible total alopecia occurs 3–4 weeks after treatment begins; nail beds become hyperpigmented. Drug is a potent vesicant and will result in severe soft tissue damage if extravasated. Damage to skin from prior irradiation may be reactivated (radiation recall). Rash may occur, as may onycholysis (nail loosening from nail bed).

Nursing Implications: Teach patient that alopecia will occur and discuss impact hair loss will have on body image. Discuss coping strategies, including obtaining wig or cap prior to hair loss. Encourage patient to verbalize feelings and provide patient with emotional support. Drug dose may be decreased with prior irradiation; assess for skin changes from radiation recall. Hyperpigmentation of nail beds may cause body image problem; discuss with patient and identify measures to minimize distress. Ensure that drug is administered only through a patent IV and that nurse is familiar with institution's policy for vesicant administration and management of extravasation. Manufacturer recommends aspiration of any remaining drug from IV tubing, discontinuing IV, and applying ice. Assess need for venous access device early.

V. POTENTIAL SEXUAL DYSFUNCTION related to DRUG EFFECTS

Defining Characteristics: Drug is mutagenic and teratogenic. Drug may cause testicular atrophy and azoospermia. It is unknown whether drug is excreted in breast milk.

Nursing Implications: Assess patient's and partner's sexual patterns and reproductive goals. Provide information, supportive counseling, and referral as needed. Male patients may wish to try sperm banking. Teach importance of birth control measures as appropriate. Women receiving the drug should not breast-feed.

VI. POTENTIAL FOR ALTERATION IN COMFORT related to ABDOMINAL PAIN, FEVER, CHILLS

Defining Characteristics: Abdominal pain may occur but is uncommon. Fever and chills, with or without rash, occur rarely.

Nursing Implications: Assess patient for occurrence and provide symptomatic management.

Drug: decitabine (5-Aza-2-deoxycytidine) (investigational)

Class: Antimetabolite, molecular/genetic modulator.

Mechanism of Action: Drug is a pyrimidine analogue, and prevents DNA synthesis in the S phase, leading to cell death. In addition, and more important, drug inhibits methyltransferase, an enzyme necessary for the expression of cellular genes. The cells in tumors that have progressed or that are resistant to therapy, characteristically have DNA *hyper*methylation. Decitabine "traps" DNA methyltranferase, thus greatly reducing its activity, which results in the synthesis of DNA that is *hypo*methylated. DNA hypomethylation results in activating genes that have been silent, causing the cell to differentiate, and then to die (cell death through disorganized gene expression or extinction of clones of cells that were terminally differentiated). Research has shown that the drug modulates Tumor Suppressor Genes (TSG), the expression of tumor antigens, other genes, and overall cell differentiation. (Mandelli, 1993; Wijermans et al, 2000; Ninomoto, 2000; Baylin et al, 1998).

Metabolism: Unknown.

Dosage/Range:
- Per protocol.
- Myelodysplastic syndrome: 15 mg/m^2 IV q4h q8h × 3 days (total dose 45 mg/m^2/d), repeated q6 weeks.
- Chronic myelogenous leukemia: 25–50 mg/m^2 IV over 6 h q12h × 5 days (reduce dose 25–50% to permit drug delivery q4–5 weeks).

Drug Preparation:
- Per protocol.

Drug Administration:
- Intravenously, per protocol.

Drug Interactions:

- Appears to be synergistic with biological agents such as interferons and reinoids (retinoic acid).
- Synergistic cytotoxic effects when given together with each of the following: cisplatin, 4-hydroperoxycyclophosphamide, 3-deazauridine, cyclopentenyl cytosine, cytosine arabinoside, topotecan, and thymidine.

Lab Effects/Interference:

- Unknown.

Special Considerations:

- Contraindicated in patients with a history of hypersensitivity reactions to the drug or any of its components.
- Current clinical trials (phase): Myelodysplastic syndrome (II), CML (II), relapse postautoBMT (I/II), alloBMT for acute myelogenous leukemia and CML (I/II), metastatic breast cancer (II), lung cancer (I), stage III/IV melanoma (I), advanced solid malignancies (I).

Potential Toxicities/Side Effects and the Nursing Process

I. POTENTIAL FOR INFECTION AND BLEEDING related to BONE MARROW DEPRESSION

Defining Characteristics: Dose-limiting factor is bone marrow suppression. In one study of patients with CML blast crisis, the incidence of neutropenia was 85% with most patients experiencing fever. Nadir is delayed, occurring on day 21, with recovery on day 35. Thrombocytopenia occurs, with nadir platelet count on day 15, and recovery by day 21.

Nursing Implications: Assess baseline CBC and differential, and platelet count prior to chemotherapy, as well as for signs/symptoms of infection or bleeding. Teach patient signs/symptoms of infection or bleeding, to report these immediately, and to come to the emergency room or clinic if febrile, and teach patient self-care measures to minimize risk of infection and bleeding. This includes avoidance of crowds and proximity to people with infections, and avoidance of OTC aspirin-containing medications.

II. ALTERED NUTRITION, LESS THAN BODY REQUIREMENTS, RELATED TO NAUSEA AND VOMITING, STOMATITIS

Defining Characteristics: Nausea and vomiting occur commonly, are mild to moderate, and preventable by antiemetic medicines.

Nursing Implications: Premedicate patient with antiemetic. If patient develops nausea and/or vomiting, encourage small, frequent intake of cool, bland foods. Instruct patient to report nausea, and teach self-administration of antiemetic medications. If nausea/vomiting occur and are severe, assess for signs/

symptoms of fluid/electrolyte imbalance. Teach patient to self-administer antidiarrheal medications if needed. Assess baseline oral mucous membranes. Teach patient oral assessment, hygiene measures, and to report any alterations.

Drug: docetaxel (Taxotere)

Class: Taxoid, mitotic spindle poison.

Mechanism of Action: Enhances microtubule assembly and inhibits disassembly. Disrupts microtubule network that is essential for mitotic and interphase cellular function. Stabilization of microtubules inhibits mitosis.

Metabolism: Drug is extensively protein-bound (94–97%). Triphasic elimination. Metabolism involves P-450 3A (CYP3A4) isoenzyme system (in vitro testing). Fecal elimination is main route, accounting for excretion of 75% of the drug and its metabolites within seven days; 80% of the fecal excretion occurs during the first 48 hours. Mild to moderate liver impairment (SGOT and/or SGPT > 1.5 times normal and alk phos > 2.5 times normal) results in decreased clearance of drug by an average of 27%, resulting in a 38% increase in systemic exposure (AUC).

Dosage/Range:

- Adjuvant breast cancer: docetaxel 75 mg/m^2 IV 1-hour after doxorubicin 50 mg/m^2 IVP and cyclophamide 500 mg/m^2 IV q3 weeks × 6 courses, with G-CSF support PRN.
- Breast cancer: 60–100 mg/m^2 IV as a 1-hour infusion every 3 weeks.
- Non-small-cell lung cancer: 1) 75 mg/m^2 as a 1-hour infusion as a single agent, 2) 75 mg/m^2 as a 1-hour infusion, followed by cisplatin over 30–60 minutes every 3 weeks.
- Prostate cancer: docetaxel 75 mg/m^2 day 1 repeated q 21 days, in combination with prednisone 5 mg PO bid continuously, to be repeated for 10 cycles.
- Dose reductions for nadir ANC < 500 cells/mm^3 for > 1 week, or severe and cumulative cutaneous reactions, or moderate neurosensory signs and/or symptoms, should have a dose reduction when symptoms resolve (see package insert).
- Premedication regimen with corticosteroids: e.g., dexamethasone 8 mg bid × 3 days, starting 1 day prior to docetaxel to reduce the incidence and severity of fluid retention and hypersensitivity reactions. For patients with prostate cancer receiving prednisone, the doses of oral dexamethasone are: 8 mg at 12 hours, 3 hours, and 1 hour prior to docetaxel dose.

Drug Preparation: (requires 2 dilutions prior to administration):

- Vials available as 80-mg and 20-mg concentrate as single-dose blister packs with diluent. Do not reuse single-dose vials. Drug contains polysorbate 80.
- Unopened vials require protection from bright light. May be stored at room temperature or in refrigerator (36–77°F). Allow to stand at room temperature for at least 5 minutes prior to reconstitution.
- Reconstitute 20-mg and 80-mg vials with the entire contents of accompanying diluent vial (13% Ethanol in water for injection). Reconstituted vials contain 10 mg/mL docetaxel (initial diluted solution).
- Gently invert repeatedly, but do not shake the initial diluted solution for approximately 45 seconds.
- Reconstituted vials (10 mg/mL initial diluted solution) are stable for 8 hours at either room temperature or under refrigeration.
- Use only glass or polypropylene or polyolefin plastic (bag) IV containers.
- Withdraw ordered dose, and further dilute in 250 mL volume of 5% Dextrose or 0.9% Sodium Chloride to a final concentration of 0.3–0.74 mg/mL. Thoroughly mix by manual rotation.
- Inspect for any particulate matter or discoloration, and if found, discard.
- Use infusion solution immediately or within 4 hrs.

Drug Administration:

- Assess patient's ANC and liver function studies, and if abnormal, discuss with physician. See Special Considerations.
- Use only glass or polypropylene bottles, or polypropylene or polyolefin plastic bags for drug infusion, and administer infusion ONLY through polyethylenelined administration sets.
- Patient should receive corticosteroid premedication (e.g., dexamethasone 8 mg bid) for 3 days beginning 1 day before drug administration to reduce the incidence and severity of fluid retention and hypersensitivity reactions.
- Infuse drug over 1 hour.

Drug Interactions:

- Radiosensitizing effect.
- Theoretically, CYP3A4 inhibitors, such as ketoconazole, erythromycin, troleandomycin, cyclosporine, terfenadine, and nifedipine, can inhibit docetaxel metabolism and result in elevated serum levels of docetaxel; use together with caution or not at all.
- Theoretically, CYP3A4 inducers, such as anticonvulsants and St. John's Wort, may increase metabolism, and decrease serum levels of docetaxel.
- Capecitabine.

Lab Effects/Interference:

- Decreased CBC.

Special Considerations:

- Indicated for the treatment of (1) adjuvant treatment of operable node-positive breast cancer; (2) locally advanced or metastatic breast cancer after failure of prior chemotherapy; (3) as a single agent in locally advanced or metastatic non-small-cell lung cancer (NSCLC) after failure of prior platinum-based chemotherapy; (4) in combination with cisplatin, in patients with unresectable locally advanced or metastatic NSCLC who have not received prior chemotherapy; and (5) in combination with prednisone for the treatment of androgen-independent (hormone-refractory) metastatic prostate.
- Contraindicated in patients with history of severe hypersensitivity reactions to docetaxel or to other drugs formulated with polysorbate 80; drug should not be used in patients with neutrophil counts of < 1500 cells/mm^3. Drug should not be used in pregnant or breast-feeding women; women of child-bearing age should use effective birth control measures.
- Docetaxel generally should not be administered to patients with bilirubin > upper limit of normal (ULN) or to patients with SGOT and/or SGPT > 1.5 × ULN concomitant with alkaline phosphatase > 2.5 × ULN. Patients treated with elevated bilirubin or abnormal transaminases plus alkaline phosphatase have an increased risk of grade 4 neutropenia, febrile neutropenia, severe stomatitis, infections, severe thrombocytopenia, severe skin toxicity, and toxic death. Serum bilirubin, SGOT or SGPT, and alkaline phosphatase should be obtained and reviewed by the treating physician before each cycle of docetaxel treatment.
- Dose modifications during treatment: (1) Patients with breast cancer dosed initially at 100 mg/m^2 who experience either febrile neutropenia, ANC < 500/mm^3 for > 1 week, or severe or cumulative cutaneous reactions, or other grade ¾ non-hematologic toxicity, should have dose reduced to 75 mg/m^2. If reactions continue at the reduced dose, further reduce to 55 mg/m^2 or discontinue drug. Patients dosed initially at 60 mg/m^2 who do not experience febrile neutropenia, ANC < 500/mm^3 for > 1 week, nadir platelets < 25,000 cells/mm^3, or severe cutaneous reactions, or severe peripheral neuropathy during drug therapy may tolerate higher drug doses and may be dose-escalated. Patients who develop ≥ grade 3 peripheral neuropathy should have drug discontinued. (2) Patients with NSCLC dosed initially at 75 mg/m^2 who experience febrile neutropenia, ANC < 500 mg/m^2 for > 1 week, nadir platelets < 25,000 cells/mm^3, or severe or cumulative cutaneous reactions, or other nonhematologic toxicity grades 3 or 4 should have treatment withheld until toxicity resolves and then have dose reduced to 55 mg/m^2; patients who developμgrade 3 peripheral neuropathy should discontinue docetaxel chemotherapy. (3) Patients with Prostate cancer who experience febrile neutropenia, ANC < 500/mm^3 for > 1 week, or severe or

cumulative cutaneous reactions, or moderate neuro-sensory signs and/or symptoms during docetaxel therapy should have dose reduced from 75mg/m² to 60 mg/m². If the same symptoms arise at the reduced dosage, the drug should be discontinued.

- Patients should receive dexamethasone premedication (such as 8 mg bid × 3 days starting 1 day prior to taxotere).
- Administration of docetaxel in Europe is not subject to United States Federal Drug Administration recommendations—non-PVC containers and tubing are not required.
- Incomplete cross-resistance between paclitaxel and docetaxel in many tumor types.
- Studies are ongoing to determine the effectiveness of docetaxel 25–40 mg/m² weekly in breast cancer, lung cancer, prostate cancer, and other cancers as drug given in this "dose-dense" fashion may act as an antiangiogenesis agent, and may provide less opportunity for malignant cells to develop resistant clones. Weekly dose schedules being studied include 3 weeks of treatment followed by 1 week of rest every 4 weeks, and 6 weekly treatments followed by 2 weeks off every 8 weeks. Docetaxel is administered as a 15–30-minute infusion. Hematologic side effects are uncommon with these schedules. Nonhematologic side effects of weekly therapy include asthenia, fluid retention, nail changes, and tearing. Corticosteroid premedication is often dexamethasone 4 or 8 mg PO q12h × 3 doses beginning the day before treatment.

Potential Toxicities/Side Effects and the Nursing Process

I. POTENTIAL FOR INJURY related to HYPERSENSITIVITY OR ANAPHYLAXIS REACTIONS

Defining Characteristics: Severe hypersensitivity reactions characterized by hypotension, dyspnea and/or bronchospasm, or generalized rash/erythema occurred in 2.2% (2/92) patients who received 3-day dexamethasone premedication. If patient experiences a severe hypersensitivity reaction, patient should not be rechallenged with docetaxel (e.g., patients with bronchospasm, angioedema, systolic BP < 80 mmHg, generalized urticaria). Minor allergic reactions are characterized by flushing, chest tightness, or low back pain.

Nursing Implications: Ensure that patient has taken premedication (e.g., dexamethasone 8 mg bid starting 1 day prior to chemotherapy). Assess baseline VS and mental status prior to drug administration, especially first and second doses of the drug. Monitor VS every 15 minutes, and remain with patient during first 15 minutes of drug infusion, as most reactions occur during the first 10 minutes. Stop drug if cardiac arrhythmia (irregular apical pulse) or hypo- or hypertension occur and discuss continuance of infusion with physician. Recall signs/symptoms of anaphylaxis, and if these occur, stop drug immediately and notify physician. Subjective symptoms are generalized itching, nausea, chest tightness, crampy abdominal pain, difficulty speaking, anxiety, agitation, sense of impending doom, uneasiness, desire to urinate/defecate, dizziness, chills. Objective signs are flushed appearance; angioedema of face, neck, eyelids, hands, feet; localized or generalized urticaria; respiratory distress with or without wheezing, hypotension, cyanosis. Review standing orders or nursing procedure for patient management of anaphylaxis, and be prepared to stop drug immediately if signs/symptoms occur, keep IV line open with 0.9% Sodium Chloride, notify physician, monitor VS, and administer ordered medications, which may include epinephrine 1:1000, hydrocortisone sodium succinate, and diphenhydramine. Teach patient the potential of a hypersensitivity or anaphylactic reaction and to immediately report any unusual symptoms. Depending upon severity of reaction, when planning subsequent treatment discuss with physician administration of antihistamine prior to docetaxel and also gradual increase in infusion rate, e.g., starting at 8-hour rate × 5 minutes, then increasing to 4-hour rate × 5 minutes, then 2-hour rate × 5 minutes, and finally 1-hour infusion rate.

II. POTENTIAL FOR INFECTION AND BLEEDING related to BONE MARROW DEPRESSION

Defining Characteristics: Neutropenia may be severe, is dose-related, is the dose-limiting toxicity, and is noncumulative. Nadir is day 7, with recovery by day 15. Incidence of grade 4 neutropenia (ANC < 500 mm^3) in 2045 patients (any tumor type) with normal hepatic function was 75% at a dose of 100 mg/m^2. Incidence of febrile neutropenia requiring IV antibiotics and/or hospitalization in these patients was 11% and the incidence of septic deaths was 1.6%. Severe thrombocytopenia was less common (8%). However, fatal GI bleeding has been reported in patients with severe hepatic impairment who received docetaxel.

Nursing Implications: Assess LFTs, as dose generally should not be given if SGOT, SGPT, alk phos, or bili suggest moderate to severe hepatic dysfunction (see Special Considerations section). Assess baseline CBC and differential to ensure that ANC is > 1500/mm^3, and platelet count is > 100,000/mm^3 prior to chemotherapy, as well as for signs/symptoms of infection or bleeding. Teach patient signs/symptoms of infection or bleeding and to report these immediately, and teach patient self-care measures to minimize risk of infection and bleeding. This includes avoidance of crowds and proximity to people with infections, and avoidance of OTC aspirin-containing medications. Teach patient self-administration of G-CSF as ordered to prevent severe neutropenia, and EPO as ordered to prevent severe anemia/transfusion requirements. Instruct patient to alternate rest and activity periods, and to report increased fatigue, shortness of breath, or chest pain that might herald severe anemia.

III. POTENTIAL ALTERATION IN ACTIVITY TOLERANCE related to ASTHENIA, FATIGUE

Defining Characteristics: Fatigue, weakness, and malaise may last from a few days to several weeks, but is rarely severe enough to be dose-limiting. Incidence of asthenia (all grades) is 50–66%. Incidence of anemia is 90%, with grades of 3 and 4 occurring in 8% at doses of 100 mg/m^2 and in 9% at doses of 75 mg/m^2.

Nursing Implications: Assess Hgb/HCT prior to each treatment and at nadir counts. Assess patient activity tolerance and ability to do ADLs. Teach patient self-care strategies to minimize exertion, and maximize activity, such as clustering activity during shopping, alternating rest and activity periods, diet, gentle exercise. Teach self-administration of EPO, if ordered, to prevent severe anemia/transfusion requirements. Instruct patient to alternate rest and activity periods, and to report increased fatigue, shortness of breath, or chest pain that might herald severe anemia.

IV. POTENTIAL ALTERATION IN FLUID BALANCE related to FLUID RETENTION

Defining Characteristics: Fluid retention is a cumulative toxicity that may occur in docetaxel treated patients. Peripheral edema usually begins in the lower extremities and may become generalized with weight gain (2kg avg). Fluid retention is not associated with cardiac, renal, or hepatic impairment and may be minimized by use of dexamethasone 8 mg bid for 3 days beginning the day prior to therapy. Severe fluid retention may occur in up to 6.5% of patients despite premedication, and is characterized by generalized edema, poorly tolerated peripheral edema, pleural effusion requiring drainage, dyspnea at rest, cardiac tamponade, or abdominal distention (due to ascites). Fluid retention usually resolves completely within 16 weeks of last docetaxel dose (range, 0–42+ weeks).

Nursing Implications: Ensure that patient takes corticosteroids as ordered to minimize risk of developing fluid retention. Assess baseline weight and skin turgor, especially in the extremities. Assess respiratory status, including breath sounds. Instruct patient to report any alterations in breathing patterns, swelling in the extremities, and weight gain. If patient has preexisting effusion, monitor effusion closely during treatment. If fluid retention occurs, instruct patient to elevate extremities while at rest. Teach patient not to use added salt when eating or cooking. Discuss with physician use of diuretics for new-onset edema, progression of edema, and weight gain, e.g., >2 lb.

V. POTENTIAL IMPAIRMENT OF SKIN INTEGRITY related to RASH, ALOPECIA, NAIL CHANGES

Defining Characteristics: Maculopapular, violaceous/erythematous, and pruritic rash may occur, usually on the feet and/or hands, but may also occur on arms, face, or thorax. These localized eruptions usually occur within one week of last docetaxel treatment, and are reversible and usually resolve prior to next treatment. Overall, about 50% of patients experience skin problems. Palmar-plantar erythrodysesthia (hand-foot syndrome) may occur but can be minimized by adherence to three-day corticosteroid premedication. Drug extravasation may cause skin discoloration, but no necrosis. Most patients on every-3-week schedules experience alopecia (75% at dose of 100 mg/m^2 and 56% at dose of 75%). Changes in nails may occur in 11–40% of patients, and be severe in 1–2% of patients (hypo- or hyperpigmentation, onycholysis [loss of nail]).

Nursing Implications: Assess skin for any cutaneous changes, such as rash, and any associated symptoms, such as pruritus, and discuss management with physician. If patient develops severe or cumulative skin toxicity, docetaxel dose should be reduced (see Special Considerations). Instruct patient in self-care measures such as avoidance of abrasive skin products and clothing, avoidance of tight-fitting clothes, use of skin emollients appropriate for skin problem, and measures to prevent itching. Discuss potential impact of hair loss prior to drug administration, coping strategies, and plan to minimize body image distortion (e.g., wig, scarf, cap). Assess patient for signs/symptoms of hair loss. Assess patient's response and use of coping strategies; help patient to build on effective strategies. Teach patient self-care measures to preserve hair, such as washing hair with warm water, use of a gentle shampoo and conditioner, use of a softbristle brush, cutting hair short to reduce pressure on hair shaft, and use of a satin pillowcase to minimize friction on hair shaft. Teach patient to wear a wide-brimmed hat and sunglasses when outside, and to use sunscreen (at least SPF 15) on scalp when outdoors without a hat. Assess nails baseline, and teach patient to report changes. Teach patient to keep nails clean and trimmed, not to wear nail polish or imitation nails, and to wear protective gloves when doing house cleaning, and gardening. Teach patient to use a nail hardener if nails appear soft, and to use Lotrimin cream if ordered.

VI. SENSORY/PERCEPTUAL ALTERATIONS related to SENSORY NEUROPATHY

Defining Characteristics: Grade 1–4 Peripheral neuropathy may affect up to 49% of patients (severe 5.5%). Sensory alterations are paresthesias in a glove and stocking distribution, and numbness. There may be loss of sensation symmetrically, of vibration, and of proprioception. Risk is increased in patients receiving both docetaxel and cisplatin, or in patients with prior neuropathy from diabetes mellitus or alcohol. Extremity weakness or transient myalgia may also occur. Patients described spontaneous reversal of symptoms in a median of 9 weeks from onset (range 0–106).

Nursing Implications: Assess baseline neurologic status. Instruct patient to report signs/symptoms of pins and needle sensation, numbness, pain, increased discomfort with certain sensations, especially in the extremities, or motor weakness. Identify patients at risk: prior cisplatin, or having preexisting neuropathies (ethanol- and diabetes mellitus-related). Assess sensory and motor function prior to each treatment, and if abnormality found, assess impact on patient function, safety, independence, and quality of life. Test patient's ability to button a shirt, or pick up a dime from a flat surface. If severely impacting safety or quality of life, discuss with patient and physician drug discontinuance or use of cytoprotective agent. Teach self-care strategies, including maintaining safety when walking, getting up, taking bath, or washing dishes and unable to sense temperature, and the need to keep extremities warm in cold weather. Docetaxel should be discontinued if patient develops grades 3 or 4 peripheral neuropathy (see NCI Common Toxicity Criteria, Appendix II). Grade 3 motor = objective weakness, interfering with ADLs; grade 3 sensory = sensory loss or paresthesia interfering with ADLs; grade 4 motor = paralysis; grade 4 sensory = permanent sensory loss that interferes with function.

VII. ALTERED NUTRITION, LESS THAN BODY REQUIREMENTS, related to NAUSEA AND VOMITING, DIARRHEA, STOMATITIS

Defining Characteristics: Nausea and vomiting may occur, but are mild and preventable with antiemetics. Diarrhea occurs and is mild; incidence of any grade of nausea is 33–42%, vomiting 22%, and diarrhea 22–42%. Incidence of stomatitis is 26–51% (severe 5.5%). Only 1.1% of breast cancer patients who received three-day corticosteroid treatment developed severe mucositis.

Nursing Implications: Premedicate patient with antiemetic. If patient develops nausea and/or vomiting, encourage small, frequent intake of cool, bland foods. Instruct patient to report nausea, and teach self-administration of antiemetic medications. If nausea/vomiting occur and are severe, assess for signs/symptoms of fluid/electrolyte imbalance. Encourage patient to report onset of diarrhea. Teach patient to self-administer antidiarrheal medications if needed. Assess baseline oral mucous membranes. Ensure that patient takes three-day corticosteroid regimen. Teach patient oral assessment, hygiene measures, and to report any alterations.

VIII. ALTERATION IN VISION, POTENTIAL, related to HYPERLACRIMATION

Defining Characteristics: Epiphora or hyperlacrimation occurs as a result of lacrimal duct stenosis. There is inflammation of the conjunctiva and ductal epithelium, which occurs chronically, especially with weekly docetaxel therapy. This appears related to cumulative dose, usually about 300 mg/m^2 and resolves after treatment is stopped. Stenosis of tear ducts is reversible.

Nursing Implications: Assess baseline vision and function of tear ducts. Teach patient that this may occur, and to report it. If this occurs, teach patient to use "Artificial Tears" frequently throughout day, or saline eyewash. Discuss with physician use of prophylactic steroid ophthalmic solution, such as prednisolone acetate 2 gtt bid × 3 days, beginning the day before docetaxel treatment, if patient does not have a history of herpetic eye infection. If the patient is on weekly therapy, discuss with physician treatment break × 2 weeks for symptoms to resolve, and resumption of therapy on a three-week-on, one-week-off schedule.

Drug: doxorubicin hydrochloride (Adriamycin)

Class: Anthracycline antibiotic isolated from streptomycin products, in particular from the rhodomycin products.

Mechanism of Action: Topoisomerase-inhibitor; antitumor antibiotic binds directly to DNA base pairs (intercalates) and inhibits DNA and DNA-dependent RNA synthesis, as well as protein synthesis. Cell cycle specific for S phase.

Metabolism: Excretion of drug predominates in the liver; renal clearance is minor. Alteration in liver function requires modification of doses, whereas with renal failure there is no need to alter doses. Drug is excreted through urine and may discolor urine from 1–48 hours after administration.

Dosage/Range:
- 30–75 mg/m^2 every 3–4 weeks.
- 20–45 mg/m^2/IV for 3 consecutive days.
- For bladder instillation: 3–60 mg/m^2.
- For interperitoneal instillation: 40 mg in 2 L dialysate (no heparin).
- Continuous infusion: Varies with individual protocol.

Drug Preparation:
- Drug will form a precipitate if mixed with heparin or 5-FU. Dilute with 0.9% Sodium Chloride (preservative-free) to produce 2-mg/mL concentration.

Drug Administration:

- This drug is a potent vesicant. Give through a running IV to avoid extravasation, which may lead to ulceration, pain, and necrosis. Be sure to check nursing procedure for administration of a vesicant.

Drug Interactions:

- When given with barbituates there is increased plasma clearance of doxorubicin.
- When given with cyclophosphamide there is risk of hemorrhage and cardiotoxicity.
- When given with mitomycin there is increased risk of cardiotoxicity.
- There is decreased oral bioavailability (decreased serum levels) of digoxin when given together.
- When given with mercaptopurine there is increased risk of hepatotoxicity.
- Incompatible with heparin, forming a precipitate.

Lab Effects/Interference:

- Decreased CBC.
- Increased LFTs.
- Increased uric acid secondary to tumor lysis.

Special Considerations:

- Drug is a potent vesicant. Give through running IV to avoid extravasation and tissue necrosis.
- Give through central line if drug is to be given by continuous infusion.
- Nausea and vomiting are dose-related. Occur in 50% of patients and begin 1–3 hours after administration.
- Causes discoloration of urine (from pink to red for up to 48 hours).
- Skin changes: May cause radiation recall phenomenon—recalls reaction in previously irradiated tissue.
- Potent myelosuppressive agent causes GI toxicities: mucositis, esophagitis, and diarrhea.
- Cardiac toxicity: Dose limit at 550 mg/m^2. Patients may exhibit irreversible CHF. Acute toxicity may be seen within hours after administration. This is unrelated to cumulative dose and may manifest symptoms of pump or conduction dysfunction. Rarely, transient EKG abnormalities, CHF, pericardial effusion (whole syndrome referred to as *myocarditis-pericarditis syndrome*) may occur, which may lead to death of patient.
- Vein discoloration.
- Increased pigmentation in black patients.
- Drug dosage reductions necessary for hepatic dysfunction: 50% dose given for serum bili 1.2–2.9 mg/dL, 25% dose given for serum bili 3 mg/dL.
- Prior chest radiation therapy (XRT): reduce total lifetime dose to 300–350 mg/m^2.

- Concomitant cyclophosphamide administration: may limit to 450 mg/m^2.
- Obesity: use ideal body weight table found in nutrition books to calculate dose.
- Dexrazoxane available for patients at risk for cardiotoxicity but for whom doxorubicin continues to be effective. See Chapter 4.

Potential Toxicities/Side Effects and the Nursing Process

I. POTENTIAL FOR INFECTION AND BLEEDING related to BONE MARROW DEPRESSION

Defining Characteristics: WBC and platelet nadir 10–14 days after drug dose, with recovery from days 15–21. Myelosuppression may be severe but is less severe with weekly dosing.

Nursing Implications: Monitor CBC, WBC, differential, and platelet count prior to drug administration; discuss any abnormalities with physician. Assess for signs/symptoms of infection or bleeding; instruct patient in self-assessment and to report signs/symptoms immediately. Teach patient self-care measures to minimize risk of infection and bleeding, including avoidance of OTC aspirin-containing medications. Drug dosage must be reduced if patient has hepatic dysfunction: 50% reduction of drug dose if bili is 1.2–3.0 mg/dL; 75% reduction if bili is > 3.0 mg/dL.

II. POTENTIAL FOR ALTERATION IN CARDIAC OUTPUT related to ACUTE AND CHRONIC CARDIAC CHANGES

Defining Characteristics: Acutely, pericarditis-myocarditis syndrome may occur during infusion or immediately after (non–life-threatening EKG changes of flat T waves, ST segment, PVCs). With high cumulative doses > 550 mg/m^2 (450 mg/m^2 if concurrent treatment with cardiotoxic drugs or radiation to the chest), cardiomyopathy may occur. Risk is decreased if drug given as continuous infusion.

Nursing Implications: Assess cardiac status prior to chemotherapy administration: signs/symptoms of CHF, quality/regularity and rate of heartbeat, results of prior GBPS or other test of LVEF. Instruct patient to report dyspnea, palpitations, swelling in extremities. Maintain accurate records of total dose; expect GBPS to be repeated periodically during treatment and the drug to be discontinued if there is a significant drop in heart function.

III. POTENTIAL FOR ALTERATION IN NUTRITION, LESS THAN BODY REQUIREMENTS, related to NAUSEA AND VOMITING, ANOREXIA, STOMATITIS

Defining Characteristics: Nausea/vomiting occurs in 50% of patients, is moderate to severe, and is preventable with combination antiemetics. Onset 1–3 hours after drug dose and lasts 24 hours. Anorexia occurs frequently, and stomatitis occurs in 10% of patients.

Nursing Implications: Premedicate with combination antiemetics and continue protection for 24 hours. If patient has a central line, slower infusion of drug over 1 hour decreases nausea/vomiting. Encourage small, frequent feedings of bland foods. Anorexia occurs frequently: teach patient or caregiver to make foods ahead of time and use spices; encourage taking weekly weight. Stomatitis occurs in 10% of patients, and esophagitis may occur in patients who have received prior radiation to the chest. Perform oral assessment prior to drug administration and during posttreatment visits. Teach patient oral hygiene and self-assessment techniques.

IV. POTENTIAL ALTERATION IN SKIN INTEGRITY related to ALOPECIA, RADIATION RECALL, NAIL AND SKIN CHANGES, AND DRUG EXTRAVASATION

Defining Characteristics: Complete alopecia occurs with doses > 50 mg/m^2, occurring after therapy begins. Regrowth usually begins a few months after drug is stopped. Hyperpigmentation of nail beds and dermal creases of hands is greatest in dark-skinned individuals. Skin damage from prior radiation may be reactivated. Adriamycin "flare" may occur during peripheral drug administration, often with urticaria and pruritus, and is due to local allergic reaction. Drug is a potent vesicant and causes SEVERE tissue destruction if drug extravasates.

Nursing Implications: Discuss with patient hair loss, anticipated impact, and strategies to decrease distress, e.g., obtaining wig prior to hair loss. Assess body disturbance from hyperpigmentation and discuss strategies to minimize this, e.g., nail polish for dark nail beds. Drug must be administered via patent IV. If flare occurs, this must be distinguished from extravasation, where there is leakage of drug into the perivascular tissue. Stop or slow drug injection and flush with plain IV solution. Wait to see whether reaction will resolve. If confirmed flare, consider diphenhydramine 25 mg IVP to resolve pruritus and/or urticaria, and then resume administration of drug slowly into freely flowing IV. Assess need for venous access device early. If drug administered as a continuous infusion, IT MUST BE GIVEN VIA A CENTRAL LINE.

V. POTENTIAL SEXUAL DYSFUNCTION related to DRUG EFFECT

Defining Characteristics: Drug is teratogenic, mutagenic, and carcinogenic.

Nursing Implications: Assess patient's/partner's sexual patterns and reproductive goals. Provide information, supportive counseling, and referral as needed. Teach importance of birth control measures as appropriate. Male patients may wish to use a sperm bank prior to therapy.

Drug: doxorubicin hydrochloride liposome injection (Doxil)

Class: Anthracycline antibiotic isolated from streptomycin products.

Mechanism of Action: Topoisomerase-inhibitor; antitumor antibiotic binds directly to DNA base pairs (intercalates) and inhibits DNA and DNA-dependent RNA synthesis, as well as protein synthesis. Cytotoxic in all phases of cell cycle but maximally in S phase. Cell cycle nonspecific. Drug is encapsulated in STEALTH liposomes, which have surface-bound methoxypolyethylene glycol to protect the liposome from detection by blood phagocytes, and thus prolong circulation time. It is believed that the liposomal-encapsulated drug is able to penetrate the tumor through abnormal capillaries (tumor neovasculature) and then, once inside the tumor, accumulates and the drug is released.

Metabolism: Slower clearance from the body than doxorubicin (0.041 L/h/m^2 vs 24–35 L/h/m^2) with resulting larger AUC than a similar dose of doxorubicin. Half-life is approximately 55 hours. Has preferential uptake in Kaposi's sarcoma tumors.

Dosage/Range:
- Treatment of metastic carcinoma of the ovary refractory to both paclitaxel and platinum-based chemotherapy: 50 mg/m^2 every 4 weeks × at least 4 cycles (in clinical trials, median time to response was 4 months).
- AIDS/Kaposi's sarcoma: 20 mg/m^2 IV over 30 minutes once every 3 weeks.
- Dose-reduce for palmar-plantar erythrodysesthesia, hematologic toxicity, or stomatitis.

Drug Preparation:
- Drug is available as 20-mg doxorubicin HCl in a 2-mg/mL concentration.
- Inspect drug for any particulate matter or discoloration; drug is translucent, with red liposomal dispersion.
- Further dilute drug (dose up to 90 mg) in 250 mL 5% Dextrose USP ONLY; use 500 mL 5% Dextrose USP for doses > 90 mg.
- Administer at once or store diluted drug for 24 hours refrigerated at 2–8°C (36–46°F).

Drug Administration:

- Ovarian cancer: Administer IV at an initial rate of 1 mg/min to minimize risk of infusion reaction; if no reaction, increase rate to complete administration over 1 hour.
- AIDS/Kaposi's sarcoma: Administer IV over 30 minutes through patent IV.
- Dose-reduce for hepatic dysfunction: 50% dose reduction for bilirubin 1.2–3.0 mg/dL; 75% dose reduction if bilirubin > 3.0 mg/dL.
- Do not use inline filter.
- Monitor for infusion reactions if drug is infused too rapidly.
- DO NOT ADMINISTER IM OR SQ.

Drug Interactions:

- Doxorubicin may potentiate the toxicity of (1) cyclophosphamide-induced hemorrhagic cystitis; (2) hepatotoxicity of 6-mercaptopurine; (3) radiation toxicity to heart, mucous membranes, skin, liver.

Lab Effects/Interference:

- Decreased CBC.

Special Considerations:

- Drug is an irritant, not a vesicant.
- Acute, infusion-associated reactions may occur (7% incidence) during drug infusion, characterized by flushing, shortness of breath, facial swelling, headache, chills, back pain, chest or throat tightness, and/or hypotension. Infusion should be stopped. If symptoms are minor, infusion may be resumed at a slower rate, but discontinue if symptoms resume.
- Assessment for cardiac toxicity similar to that for doxorubicin should be done since limited information is available as to cardiotoxicity of liposomal doxorubicin at high cumulative doses.
- Drug dosage reductions.
- FDA-approved at this time for treatment of progressive AIDS-related Kaposi's sarcoma after treatment with combination chemotherapy or in patients unable to tolerate combination chemotherapy, and FDA indicated for the treatment of refractory ovarian cancer.
- Drug has been used for the treatment of breast cancer.

Potential Toxicities/Side Effects and the Nursing Process

I. POTENTIAL FOR INFECTION AND BLEEDING related to BONE MARROW DEPRESSION

Defining Characteristics: Dose-limiting toxicity in the treatment of HIV-infected patients, possibly due to HIV disease and/or concomitant medications. Leukopenia occurs in 91% of patients, with anemia and thrombocytopenia (< 150,000/mm^3) less common (55% and 60%, respectively). Neutropenia (< 2000/mm^3) occurred in 85% and ANC (< 500/mm^3) occurred in 13% of patients. In ovarian cancer patients, incidence of neutropenia (< 2000cells/mm^3) was 51%, but ANC < 500 cells/mm^3 was only 8.3%. Thrombocytopenia (< 150,000/mm^3) occurred in 24%, while severe (< 25,000/mm^3) occurred in 1.1% of patients with ovarian cancer.

Nursing Implications: Monitor CBC, WBC, differential, and platelet count prior to drug administration, and discuss any abnormalities with physician. Assess for signs/symptoms of infection or bleeding, and instruct patient in self-assessment and to report signs/symptoms immediately. Teach patient self-care measures to minimize risk of infection and bleeding, including avoidance of OTC aspirin-containing medications. See drug dosage reductions in Special Considerations section.

II. POTENTIAL FOR ALTERATION IN CARDIAC OUTPUT related to ACUTE AND CHRONIC CARDIAC CHANGES

Defining Characteristics: Experience and data is limited in the cardiotoxicity of liposomal doxorubicin at high cumulative doses. Therefore, the manufacturer recommends the adoption of cardiotoxicity warnings made for doxorubicin HCl. With high cumulative doses > 550 mg/m^2 (400 mg/m^2 if concurrent treatment with cardiotoxic drugs such as cyclophosphamide, or radiation to the chest), cardiomyopathy may occur. In clinical trials, the incidence of "possibly or probably related" cardiac-related adverse events, including cardiomyopathy, arrhythmia, heart failure, pericardial effusion, and tachycardia, was 1–5% in patients with AIDS/Kaposi's sarcoma and < 1% in ovarian cancer patients.

Nursing Implications: Assess patient risk (history of prior anthracycline chemotherapy, history of cardiovascular disease). Assess cardiac status prior to chemotherapy administration: signs/symptoms of CHF, quality/regularity and rate of heart beat, results of prior GBPS or other test of LVEF. Instruct patient to report dyspnea, palpitations, swelling in extremities. Maintain accurate records of total dose. Expect GBPS to be repeated periodically during treatment and the drug to be discontinued if there is a significant drop in heart function.

III. POTENTIAL FOR INJURY related to ALLERGIC INFUSION REACTION TO LIPOSOMAL COMPONENT(S)

Defining Characteristics: During the initial infusion, patients may experience an acute reaction characterized by flushing, shortness of breath, facial swelling, headache, chills, back pain, chest or throat tightness, and/or hypotension. Incidence is 5–6%. Reactions generally resolve after the immediate termination of the infusion in several hours to a day, or in some patients, after slowing of the infusion rate. Of those patients who experienced reactions, many were able to tolerate subsequent treatment without problem; however, some patients terminated therapy with liposomal doxorubicin because of the reaction.

Nursing Implications: Assess baseline comfort, vital signs, general condition. Infuse liposomal doxorubicin at 1 mg/min to minimize risk of acute reaction. Teach patient to report signs/symptoms of reaction immediately during infusion, and assess patient frequently during initial infusion. If signs/symptoms occur, stop infusion immediately. Discuss with the physician, but anticipate that if signs/symptoms are mild, infusion will resume at slower rate, and if signs/symptoms are severe, patient may not receive additional liposomal doxorubicin.

IV. POTENTIAL ALTERATIONS IN COMFORT AND ACTIVITY related to PALMAR-PLANTAR ERYTHRODYSESTHESIA (HAND-FOOT SYNDROME)

Defining Characteristics: Incidence is approximately 3.4% in patients receiving a dose of 20 mg/m^2 and 37% in patients with ovarian cancer (16% grades 3 and 4). Toxicity becomes dose-limiting in clinical studies at doses of 60 mg/m^2, or when treatment is administered more frequently than every three weeks. signs/symptoms are swelling, pain, erythema, possibly progressing to desquamation of the skin on hands and feet, and usually occur after six weeks of treatment. Reaction is generally mild, not requiring treatment delays. However, in some patients, reaction can be severe and debilitating, necessitating discontinuance of treatment.

Nursing Implications: Assess baseline skin of patients' hands and feet, and in women with ovarian cancer, skin under areas of pressure, such as under the breasts of women with large breasts or skin folds, before each treatment. Teach patient to report signs/symptoms of reaction (e.g., tingling or burning, redness, flaking of skin in areas of pressure such as soles of feet, under breasts in large-breasted women, small blisters, or small sores on the palms of hands or soles of feet). If signs/symptoms occur, discuss treatment, treatment delays, or discontinuance. Do not use hydrocortisone cream as this will cause greater desquamation of skin.

V. POTENTIAL FOR ALTERATION IN NUTRITION, LESS THAN BODY REQUIREMENTS, related to NAUSEA AND VOMITING, STOMATITIS, DIARRHEA, ANOREXIA

Defining Characteristics: Nausea and/or vomiting occur in 17% and 8% of patients, respectively, are mild to moderate, and are preventable with antiemetics. Stomatitis occurs in 7% of patients. Incidence of diarrhea is 8%. Anorexia may affect 1–5% of patients.

Nursing Implications: Premedicate with antiemetic (dopamine antagonist or serotonin antagonist). Encourage small, frequent feeding of bland foods. Stomatitis occurs in 7% of patients. Perform oral assessment prior to drug administration, and during posttreatment visits. Dose reductions or delay necessary for grades 2–4 stomatitis. Teach patient oral hygiene, and self-assessment techniques. Instruct patient to report diarrhea, and teach self-management strategies for diarrhea.

VI. POTENTIAL FOR ALTERATION IN SKIN INTEGRITY related to ALOPECIA, RASH, PRURITUS, AND RADIATION RECALL

Defining Characteristics: Incidence of alopecia significantly less with liposomal delivery of doxorubicin, and is about 9% in AIDS/Kaposi's sarcoma patients and 15% in women with ovarian cancer. Skin damage from prior radiation may be reactivated. Rash and itching occur in 1–5% of the patients. Rarely, significant skin reactions may occur, such as exfoliative dermatitis. Drug is an irritant, but extravasation should be avoided.

Nursing Implications: Discuss with patient low incidence of hair loss, and to report hair thinning if it occurs. At that time, discuss impact and strategies to decrease distress. Instruct patient to report skin rash or itching, and discuss significance and management with physician. Teach patient to assess for skin changes in prior radiated sites, including mucous membranes, and to report this immediately. Assess and develop management strategies depending on site and extent. Use caution to avoid drug extravasation; if infiltration occurs, stop infusion, apply ice for 30 minutes, and restart a new IV elsewhere.

VII. POTENTIAL ALTERATION IN NUTRITION related to NAUSEA AND/OR VOMITING, STOMATITIS

Defining Characteristics: Nausea occurs in 37% (severe, grade ¾ in 8%) of ovarian cancer patients and 17% of AIDS/Kaposi's sarcoma patients. Vomiting occurs in 22% of ovarian cancer patients and 7.8% of patients with AIDS/Kaposi's sarcoma. Stomatitis occurs in 37% of women with ovarian cancer and is severe in 7.7%; overall incidence in AIDS/Kaposi's sarcoma patients is 6.8%.

Nursing Implications: Assess baseline nutritional status. Teach patient that these side effects may occur and teach self-care measures, including self-assessment, oral hygiene regimen, and to report occurrence of symptoms. Administer antiemetic prior to chemotherapy, especially in ovarian cancer patients, and assess efficacy after treatment. Revise antiemetic regimen as needed to provide complete protection from nausea and/or vomiting. Assess oral mucosa prior to each treatment. If stomatitis develops, dose reduction be considered.

VIII. POTENTIAL SEXUAL DYSFUNCTION related to DRUG EFFECTS

Defining Characteristics: Drug is embryotoxic. Doxorubicin has been shown to be carcinogenic and mutagenic.

Nursing Implications: Assess patient's/partner's sexual pattern and reproductive goals. Provide information, supportive counseling, and referral as needed. Teach importance of birth control measures for female patients of childbearing age. Mothers who are nursing should discontinue nursing during treatment.

IX. ACTIVITY INTOLERANCE related to ASTHENIA AND FATIGUE

Defining Characteristics: Anemia is the most common hematologic event, affecting 52.6% of women with ovarian cancer, but only 25% experienced severe anemia (Hgb < 8 gm/dL). Incidence for patients with AIDS/Kaposi's syndrome overall is 55%, with 4% experiencing severe anemia. Asthenia is more common in women with ovarian cancer, affecting 33%, while patients with AIDS/Kaposi's syndrome had an incidence of 9.9%.

Nursing Implications: Assess activity tolerance, and HCT/Hgb baseline, and prior to each treatment. Teach patients to report any changes in energy and activity level. Teach patients self-care strategies to maximize energy use and conservation. Evaluate efficacy of strategies at each visit, and if ineffective, assist patient to problem solve other alternative solutions, such as friends, volunteers, to help with activities such as shopping, food preparation.

Drug: eniluracil (776C85) (investigational)

Class: Dihydropyrimidine dehydrogenase inhibitor. When used with 5-fluorouracil (5-FU), together they become dihydropyrimidine dehydrogenase inhibitory fluoropyrimidines.

Mechanism of Action: Dihydropyrimidine dehydrogenase (DPD) is the ratelimiting enzyme in the degradation of 5-FU. By inhibiting DPD, eniluracil permits higher and longer sustained serum levels of 5-FU. In early studies, a single dose of eniluracil increased plasma half-life of oral 5-FU 6 times, and produced 100% bioavailability (Smith et al, 2000).

Metabolism: Unclear.

Dosage/Range:
- Per protocol.
- Advanced breast cancer: 10 mg/m^2 bid qd × 28 days, with oral 5-FU 1.0 mg/m^2 bid qd × 28 days, then rest × 7 days, cycle repeated q35 days.
- Dose reduce for hematologic or gastrointestinal toxicity.

Drug Preparation:
- None, oral, available as 2.5-mg and 10-mg tablets.

Drug Administration:

- Take with large amount of water (e.g., 180 mL) at least 1 hour before or after eating.

Drug Interactions:

- Significantly increases 5-FU serum level and half-life, mimicking continuous 5-FU infusions.

Lab Effects/Interference:

- Unknown.

Special Considerations:

- Eniluracil dose is in 10:1 ratio with 5-FU.
- In study of patients with advanced breast cancer, using oral 5-FU concurrently with eniluracil, incidence of grade 1 hand-foot syndrome was 15% and neuropathy 9%, grade 1 only.
- Concurrent oral eniluracil and oral 5-FU well tolerated with low toxicity profile.

Potential Toxicities/Side Effects and the Nursing Process (when used together with oral 5-FU in study on advanced breast cancer)

I. POTENTIAL FOR INFECTION AND BLEEDING related to BONE MARROW DEPRESSION

Defining Characteristics: Neutropenia and thrombocytopenia are dose-related and occur rarely. In the advanced breast cancer trial of oral eniluracil and 5-FU, 30% of patients had granulocytopenia (6% grade 3, 1 patient had neutropenic sepsis), and 42% had thrombocytopenia (3% grade 3). 36% of patients had anemia. Toxicity is enhanced when combined with leucovorin calcium.

Nursing Implications: Assess baseline CBC, WBC, differential, and platelet count prior to chemotherapy, as well as for signs/symptoms of infection or bleeding. Teach patient signs/symptoms of infection or bleeding, and instruct to report these immediately. Teach patient self-care measures to minimize risk of infection and bleeding, including avoidance of crowds, proximity to people with infections, and OTC aspirin-containing medications.

II. ACTIVITY INTOLERANCE, POTENTIAL, related to ASTHENIA, FATIGUE, MALAISE

Defining Characteristics: Malaise and fatigue were reported in 45% of patients, grades 1–2. Anemia occurred in 36% of patients, all grades 1–2.

Nursing Implications: Assess baseline activity level, tolerance, and self-care ability. Teach patients that these side effects are common, but manageable. Assess need for home care assistance and arrange if possible. If not, and needed, involve social worker to assist in coordinating care. Teach patient to alternate rest and activity periods, and strategies to conserve energy.

III. ALTERED NUTRITION, LESS THAN BODY REQUIREMENTS, related to NAUSEA AND VOMITING, STOMATITIS, AND DIARRHEA

Defining Characteristics: Nausea occurred in 27% and vomiting in 12% of patients but was mild. Mucositis was uncommon, affecting 6% of patients, all grades 1–2. Diarrhea can be severe, and in prolonged courses is the dose-limiting toxicity.

Nursing Implications: Premedicate patient with antiemetics (phenothiazines are usually effective), and continue for 24 hours, at least for the first cycle. Encourage small, frequent meals of cool, bland foods. Assess oral mucosa prior to drug administration and instruct patient to report changes. Teach patient oral hygiene measures and self-assessment. Instruct patient to report diarrhea, to self-administer prescribed antidiarrheal medications, and to drink adequate fluids.

Drug: epirubicin HCl (Ellence, Farmorubicin(e), Farmorubicina, Pharmorubicin)

Class: Anthracycline antitumor antibiotic analogue.

Mechanism of Action: Drug complexes with DNA by intercalation of planar rings between DNA base pairs; this inhibits nucleic acid (DNA and RNA) and protein synthesis. This also causes cleavage of DNA by topoisomerase II, causing cell death. Drug also prevents enzymatic separation of DNA, interfering with replication and transcription. Drug also causes the production of cytotoxic free radicals.

Metabolism: Following IV administration, drug rapidly disperses into body tissues and into red blood cells; drug is 77% bound to plasma proteins. Drug is rapidly and extensively metabolized in the liver, excreted primarily through the biliary system, and to a lesser extent in the urine. Drug clearance is reduced in elderly women (35% lower in women aged ≥ 70 years old). Drug clearance is reduced 30% in mild hepatic dysfunction, and 50% in moderate hepatic dysfunction. Drug clearance is reduced (50%) in patients with severe renal impairment (serum creatinine ≥ 5 mg/dL). Dose reductions should be made for patients with hepatic dysfunction and patients with severe renal dysfunction.

Dosage/Range:
FDA indication:

Starting dose as part of adjuvant therapy in patients with axillary node positive breast cancer: 100 mg/m² to 120 mg/m² IV every 3–4 weeks.

- Drug dose may be given in one day, or divided equally and given on day 1 and day 8.
- Other dosing schedules that have been studied: 60–90 mg/m² IV as a single dose q3weeks (dose divided over 2–3 days; 45 mg/m² IV qd × 3 repeated q3weeks; 20 mg IV qweek; intravesicular dose of 50 mg weekly as a 0.1% solution × 8 weeks, with dose reduction for chemical cystitis.

Dose modifications:

- Bone marrow dysfunction: Consider dose of 75–90 mg/m² if patient heavily pretreated (e.g., with existing BMD or bone marrow infiltration by tumor).
- Hepatic dysfunction: Bilirubin 1.2–3 mg/dL or AST 2–4 × Upper Limit of Normal (ULN) = 50% of recommended starting dose; bilirubin > 3 mg/dL or AST > 4 × ULN = 25% of recommended starting dose.
- Renal dysfunction: Consider lower doses if serum creatinine > 5 mg/dL.
- Dosage adjustment after first treatment cycle: Platelet count < 50,000/mm³, ANC < 250/mm³, neutropenic fever, or grades ¾ nonhematologic toxicity: day 1 dose should be 75% of prior day 1 dose. Delay day 1 chemo until platelet count ≥ 100,000/mm³, ANC ≥ 1500/mm³, and nonhematologic toxicities have recovered to ≤ grade 1. If patient is receiving dose divided into day 1 and 8, day 8 dose should be 75% of day 1 dose if platelet counts are 75,000/mm³–100,000/mm³ and ANC is 1000–1499/mm³. If day 8 platelet counts are < 75,000/mm³, ANC < 1000, or grade ¾ nonhematologic toxicity has occurred, omit the day 8 dose.
- Patients receiving dose of 120 mg/m² regimen should also receive prophylactic antibiotic therapy with trimethoprim-sulfamethoxazole or a fluoroquinolone.

Drug Preparation:

- Drug is provided as a preservative-free, ready-to-use solution (50-mg/25-mL and 200-mg/100-mL single-use vials).
- Use within 24 hours of penetration of rubber stopper; discard any unused drug.
- Store unopened vials in refrigerator between 36–46°F (2–8°C).

Drug Administration:

- Drug is a vesicant, so vesicant precautions should be used (check nursing procedure for administration of a vesicant).
- Administer via slow IVP into the tubing of a freely flowing IV infusion of 0.9% NS or 5% Glucose solution over 3–5 minutes, checking blood return every few ml of drug.

Drug Interactions:

- Cytotoxic drugs: Additive toxicity (hematologic and gastrointestinal).

- Cardioactive drugs (e.g., calcium channel blockers): May increase risk of congestive heart failure; use together cautiously, and monitor cardiac function closely during treatment.
- Radiation therapy: Tissue sensitization to cytotoxic effects of radiation therapy; when drug is given after prior radiation therapy, a radiation recall inflammatory reaction may occur at site of prior radiation.
- Cimetidine: Increases drug AUC by 50%, DO NOT use together. Hold cimetidine during treatment with epirubicin.
- Other drugs extensively metabolized by the liver: Changes in hepatic function caused by concomitant therapies may affect clearance of epirubicin; use together with caution, if at all, and monitor for hematologic and gastrointestinal toxicity closely during treatment.

Lab Effects/Interference:

- Decreased white blood and neutrophil cell counts, platelet counts.

Special Considerations:

- Drug is a vesicant, and severe local tissue necrosis will occur if drug infiltrates; avoid IV sites over joints, into small veins, or in veins on arms that have compromised venous or lymphatic drainage.
- Drug should never be given intramuscularly.
- Myocardial toxicity (e.g., CHF) may occur during therapy or months to years after cessation of therapy, and risk increases according to dose. Cumulative doses >900 mg/m^2 should generally not be exceeded. Risk increases with prior anthracycline or anthracenedione therapy, past or concurrent radiation therapy to mediastinal/pericardial area, active or history of cardiovascular disease, or concomitant use of other cardiotoxic drugs.
- Rarely, secondary cancers (e.g., acute myelogenous leukemia) have been reported, and risk is increased when given in combination with other cytotoxic drugs or when doses of anthracycline chemotherapy have been escalated. The estimated risk is 0.2% at three years, and 0.8% at five years.
- Myelosuppression is the dose-limiting toxicity, and severe myelosuppression may occur.
- Doses must be reduced in patients with hepatic dysfunction.
- Drug is mutagenic, carcinogenic, and genotoxic. Men and women of childbearing age should use effective birth control measures.
- Nursing mothers should not breast-feed during chemotherapy treatment.
- Teach patients that urine will be pink-red for the first 1–2 days following drug administration.

Potential Toxicities/Side Effects and the Nursing Process

I. POTENTIAL FOR INFECTION, BLEEDING, FATIGUE related to BONE MARROW DEPRESSION

Defining Characteristics: WBC and platelet nadir 10–14 days after drug dose, with recovery by day 21. Leukopenia and neutropenia may be severe, especially when given with other myelosuppressive chemotherapy. Thrombocytopenia may be severe, and anemia may occur.

Nursing Implications: Monitor CBC, WBC, differential, and platelet count prior to drug administration; discuss any abnormalities with physician. Assess for signs/symptoms of infection or bleeding; instruct patient in self-assessment and to report signs/symptoms immediately. Teach patient self-care measures to minimize risk of infection and bleeding, including avoidance of company of people with colds and OTC aspirin-containing medications. Dose reduction necessary in patients with hepatic dysfunction, as decreased metabolism of drug results in increased serum levels of drug and hematologic toxicity. Patients receiving 120 mg/m^2 dose should also receive prophylactic antibiotic therapy with trimethoprim-sulfamethoxazole or a fluoroquinolone antibiotic.

II. POTENTIAL FOR ALTERATION IN CARDIAC OUTPUT related to ACUTE AND CHRONIC CARDIAC CHANGES

Defining Characteristics: Cardiotoxicity is dose-related, cumulative, and may occur during or months to years after cessation of therapy. The estimated probability of developing clinically evident CHF is 0.9% at a cumulative dose of 500 mg/m^2, 1.6% at 700 mg/m^2, and 3.3% at a cumulative dose of 900 mg/m^2. The risk of CHF increases rapidly with cumulative doses in excess of 900 mg/m^2. Risk of developing cardiotoxicity is increased by history of cardiovascular disease, prior anthracycline or anthrocenedione therapy, prior or concomitant radiation therapy to mediastinum and/or pericardial area, and concomitant use of other cardiotoxic drugs. Cardiotoxicity may be acute (early) or delayed (late). signs/symptoms of early toxicity are not usually of clinical significance, do not predict late cardiotoxicity, and usually do not require change in epirubicin therapy. These include: sinus tachycardia and EKG abnormalities (nonspecific ST–T wave changes, and, rarely, PVCs, VT, bradycardia, atrioventricular and bundle branch block). Delayed cardiotoxocity is related to cardiomyopathy, characterized by decreased left ventricular ejection fraction (LVEF) and classic signs/symptoms of CHF (tachycardia, dyspnea, pulmonary edema, dependent edema, hepatomegaly, ascites, pleural effusion, gallop rhythm). If late cardiotoxicity occurs, it is in the late stages of treatment or within months following treatment, and is cumulative dose-related.

Nursing Implications: Assess cardiac status prior to chemotherapy administration: risk factors and signs/symptoms of CHF, quality/regularity and rate of heartbeat, results of baseline and periodic prior gated blood pool scan (GBPS), multigated radionuclide angiography (MUGA), echocardiogram (ECHO), or other test of LVEF. Instruct patient to report dyspnea, palpitations, and swelling in extremities. Maintain accurate records of total dose; expect GBPS or measure of LVEF to be repeated periodically during treatment and the drug to be discontinued if there is a significant drop in heart function as evidenced by LVEF falling below normal range.

III. POTENTIAL FOR ALTERATION IN NUTRITION, LESS THAN BODY REQUIREMENTS, related to NAUSEA AND VOMITING, DIARRHEA, STOMATITIS

Defining Characteristics: Nausea/vomiting occurs in > 90% of patients, can moderate to severe especially when drug is given together with other emetogenic chemotherapy, and is preventable with combination antiemetics. Onset 1–3 hours after drug dose and lasts 24 hours. Mucositis may occur; stomatitis is most common. Esophagitis is less common but may occur, especially if patient has had prior radiotherapy to the chest. Drug dose must be reduced in patients with hepatic dysfunction; otherwise, increased gastrointestinal toxicity will occur.

Nursing Implications: Assess baseline LFTs, and discuss with physician dose reduction if abnormal. Premedicate with combination antiemetics and continue protection for 24 hours. If patient has a central line, slower infusion of drug over 1 hour decreases nausea/vomiting. Encourage small, frequent feedings of bland foods. Perform oral assessment prior to drug administration and during posttreatment visits. Teach patient oral hygiene and self-assessment techniques. Teach patient to report pain, burning sensation, erythema, erosions, ulcerations, bleeding, or oral infections.

IV. POTENTIAL ALTERATION IN SKIN INTEGRITY related to ALOPECIA, RADIATION RECALL, FACIAL FLUSHING, FLARE REACTION, NAIL/SKIN/ORAL MUCOUS MEMBRANE HYPERPIGMENTATION, AND DRUG EXTRAVASATION

Defining Characteristics: Alopecia is universal, but is reversible, with hair regrowth in two to three months following cessation of therapy. Skin damage and inflammation from prior radiation may be reactivated when drug is given. Drug may cause "flare" reaction or streaking along vein during peripheral drug administration, often with facial flushing, and may be related to excessively rapid drug administration. If it occurs, slow drug administration time, flush line with plain IV solution, and slowly complete therapy. This must be distinguished from extravasation, where there is leakage of drug into the perivascular tissue. Skin and nail hyperpigmentation may occur.

Nursing Implications: Discuss with patient hair loss, anticipated impact, and strategies to decrease distress, e.g., obtaining wig prior to hair loss. Assess body disturbance from hyperpigmentation and discuss strategies to minimize this, e.g., nail polish for dark nail beds. Drug must be administered via patent IV. Local phlebitis or thrombophlebitis may follow a flare reaction, so assess vein path closely, and teach patient to report any pain, erythema, or swelling following drug administration. Drug is a potent vesicant and causes SEVERE tissue destruction if drug extravasates. Teach patient to report any stinging or burning during drug administration, and stop administration if there is any question at all. Assess need for venous access device early.

V. POTENTIAL FOR SEXUAL DYSFUNCTION related to REPRODUCTIVE HAZARD

Defining Characteristics: Drug is genotoxic, mutagenic, and carcinogenic. In laboratory animals receiving very high doses of the drug, testicular atrophy occurred. Drug may cause irreversible amenorrhea in premenopausal women (premature menopause).

Nursing Implications: Assess patient's/partner's sexual patterns and reproductive goals. Provide information, supportive counseling, and referral as needed. Teach importance of birth control measures as appropriate. Male patients may wish to use a sperm bank, and women may wish to investigate cryopreservation of oocytes prior to therapy.

Drug: estramustine (Estracyte, Emcyt)

Class: Alkylating agent.

Mechanism of Action: Acts as a weak alkylator at usual therapeutic concentrations. A chemical combination of mechlorethamine and estradiol phosphate, estramustine is believed to selectively enter cells with estrogen receptors, where the drug acts as an alkylating agent due to bischlorethyl side-chain and liberated estrogens. Believed to have antimicrotubule activity. Cell cycle nonspecific.

Metabolism: Well-absorbed orally, metabolized in liver, partly excreted in urine. Induces a marked decline in serum calcium and phosphate levels.

Dosage/Range:
- 600 mg/m^2 (15 mg/kg) orally daily in three divided doses (range, 10–16 mg/kg/day in most studies with evaluation after 30–90 days).
- IV: Available for investigational use; 150 mg IV initially, then may increase to 300 mg/day per protocol.

Drug Preparation:

- Available in 140-mg capsules.
- Store in refrigerator (2–8°C [36–46°F]); may be stored at room temperature for 24–48 hours.
- IV: Dissolve in at least 10 mL sterile water.

Drug Administration:

- Oral with water, at least 1 hour before or 2 hours after meals.
- IV (investigational): Slow IVP via IV containing 5% Dextrose.

Drug Interactions:

- Drug/food: milk, milk products, and Ca++ rich foods may decrease drug absorption.
- Synergy with vinblastine.

Lab Effects/Interference:

- Changes in Ca.
- Increased LFTs, RFTs.
- May affect certain endocrine and LFTs because it contains estrogen.

Special Considerations:

- Avoid taking drug with milk, milk products, and calcium-rich foods (i.e., antacids), as this will delay or impair drug absorption.
- Contraindicated or to be used with great caution in patients who are children or who have thrombophlebitis or thromboembolic disorders, peptic ulcers, severe hepatic dysfunction, cardiac disease, hypertension, or diabetes.
- IV preparation is a vesicant; avoid extravasation.
- Transient perineal itching and pain after IV administration.

Potential Toxicities/Side Effects and the Nursing Process

I. POTENTIAL ALTERATION IN TISSUE PERFUSION related to THROMBOPHLEBITIS, THROMBOSIS

Defining Characteristics: Increased risk of clot formation, with risk for development of thrombophlebitis, pulmonary emboli, myocardial infarction, and cerebrovascular accident.

Nursing Implications: Assess patient risk; drug is contraindicated in patients with thrombophlebitis or thromboembolic disorders, unless caused by the malignancy. Should be used cautiously in these patients, and in those patients with coronary artery disease. Drug may worsen CHF. Assess baseline cardiac and peripheral vascular status, including signs/symptoms of CHF. Monitor blood pressure and glucose tolerance during therapy. Instruct patient to report immediately any signs/symptoms, e.g., dyspnea, edema, pain, and erythema in legs.

II. BODY IMAGE DISTURBANCE related to GYNECOMASTIA

Defining Characteristics: Mild to moderate breast enlargement may occur, with nipple tenderness initially.

Nursing Implications: Teach patient about potential side effects; discuss potential impact on body image and comfort. Encourage patient to verbalize feelings; provide information and emotional support.

III. POTENTIAL ALTERATION IN COMFORT related to PERINEAL SYMPTOMS, HEADACHE, RASH, URTICARIA, TRANSIENT PARESTHESIAS (IV)

Defining Characteristics: Perineal itching and pain, as well as transient paresthesias of the mouth, may occur after IV administration (investigational). Other symptoms that may accompany oral dosing are rash, pruritus, dry skin, peeling skin of fingertips, thinning hair, night sweats, lethargy, pain in eyes, and breast tenderness.

Nursing Implications: Assess patient for occurrence of symptoms and discuss measures for symptomatic relief.

IV. POTENTIAL FOR ALTERATION IN NUTRITION, LESS THAN BODY REQUIREMENTS, related to NAUSEA AND VOMITING, DIARRHEA, HEPATIC DYSFUNCTION

Defining Characteristics: Nausea and vomiting occur at higher dosing; tolerance may develop, but dose may need to be reduced. Nausea and vomiting may be delayed but become intractable and necessitate discontinuance of the drug. Diarrhea occurs occasionally. Mild elevations in liver function tests may occur (LDH, SGOT, bili) with or without jaundice, but are usually self-limiting. Abnormal Ca++ and P levels may occur.

Nursing Implications: Assess baseline nutritional fluid and electrolyte status. Premedicate with antiemetics prior to drug administration and continue through treatment. Assess baseline LFTs and Ca++ and P levels; monitor during therapy and discuss any abnormalities with physician. Monitor daily or weekly weights.

Drug: estrogens: diethylstilbestrol (DES), ethinyl estradiol (Estinyl), conjugated estrogen (Premarin), chlorotrianisene (Tace)

Class: Hormones.

Mechanism of Action: Unknown; estrogens change the hormonal milieu of the body.

Metabolism: Metabolized mainly in the liver. Undergoes enterohepatic recirculation. DES is metabolized more slowly than natural estrogens.

Dosage/Range:
- DES: Prostate cancer: 1–3 mg PO daily; breast cancer: 5 mg PO tid.
- Diethylstilbestrol diphosphate: Prostate cancer: 50–200 mg PO tid, 0.5–1.0 g IV daily × 5 days, then 250–1000 mg each week.
- Chlorotrianisene: 1–10 mg PO tid.
- Ethinyl estradiol: 0.5–1.0 mg PO tid.

Drug Preparation:
- None.

Drug Administration:
- Oral.

Drug Interactions:
- None significant.

Lab Effects/Interference:
- Increased Ca.
- Increased T_4 levels.
- Increased clotting factors.
- Decreased serum folate.

Special Considerations:
- Long-term dosage of DES in men has been associated with cardiovascular deaths. Maximum dose should be 1 mg tid for prostate cancer.
- Can cause inaccurate laboratory results (liver, adrenal, thyroid).
- Causes rapid rise in serum calcium in patients with bony metastases; watch for symptoms of hypercalcemia.

Potential Toxicities/Side Effects and the Nursing Process

I. POTENTIAL FOR INJURY related to THROMBOEMBOLIC COMPLICATIONS, HYPERCALCEMIA, SODIUM AND WATER RETENTION, AND CARDIOTOXICITY

Defining Characteristics: Thromboembolic complications are infrequent but serious, and increased risk occurs with long-term use and higher doses. Hypercalcemia occurs in 5–10% of women with breast cancer metastatic to bone, appears in first two weeks of therapy, and is aggravated by preexisting renal disease. There is an increased risk of cardiovascular-related deaths, especially in men on high-dose estrogens for prostate cancer. Drug should be used cautiously, if at all, in patients with underlying cardiac, renal, or hepatic disease.

Nursing Implications: Assess risk (preexisting cardiac, hepatic, and renal disease), baseline cardiac, and vascular status; discuss abnormalities with physician. Monitor status during therapy. Teach patient to report signs/symptoms of edema, dyspnea, localized swelling, pain, tenderness, erythema, and CNS changes. Teach female patient signs/symptoms of hypercalcemia (drowsiness, increased thirst, constipation, increased urine output) and to report this. Monitor Ca++ level in women with metastatic breast cancer closely during first few weeks of therapy.

II. ALTERATION IN NUTRITION, LESS THAN BODY REQUIREMENTS, related to NAUSEA AND VOMITING

Defining Characteristics: Occurs in 25% of patients; intensity is related to specific drug and dose. Tolerance occurs after a few weeks of therapy.

Nursing Implications: Inform patient that this may occur; teach self-administration of antiemetics prior to drug administration per physician order, and to take drug at bedtime to decrease nausea. Discuss with physician starting patient at low dose, with increase as tolerated.

III. ALTERATION IN MALE SEXUAL FUNCTION related to GYNECOMASTIA, LOSS OF LIBIDO, IMPOTENCE, AND VOICE CHANGE

Defining Characteristics: Gynecomastia may be prevented by pretreatment of breast with low dose of radiotherapy. Feminine characteristics disappear when therapy is stopped.

Nursing Implications: Explore with patient and partner reproductive and sexual patterns and impact that chemotherapy may have. Provide information, supportive counseling, and referral as indicated. Since alternative, superior hormonal manipulative drugs are available, discuss these with physician.

IV. POTENTIAL FOR FEMALE SEXUAL DYSFUNCTION related to BREAST TENDERNESS/ENGORGEMENT, UTERINE PROLAPSE, AND URINARY INCONTINENCE

Defining Characteristics: Breast engorgement may occur in postmenopausal women; uterine prolapse and exacerbation of preexisting uterine fibroids with possible uterine bleeding may occur, as may urinary incontinence.

Nursing Implications: Explore with patient sexual and reproductive patterns, and any impact the drug may have. Provide information, supportive counseling, and referral as needed. Discuss with physician alternative hormonal manipulative drugs as needed.

Drug: etoposide (VP-16, VePesid, Etopophos)

Class: Plant alkaloid, a derivative of the mandrake plant (mayapple plant).

Mechanism of Action: Inhibits DNA synthesis in S and G_2 so that cells do not enter mitosis. Causes single-strand breaks in DNA. Cell cycle specific for S and G_2 phases.

Metabolism: VP-16 is rapidly excreted in the urine and, to a lesser extent, in the bile. About 30% of drug is excreted unchanged. Binds to serum albumin (94%) and then becomes extensively tissue-bound.

Dosage/Range:

- 50–100 mg/m² IV qd × 5 days (testicular cancer) q3–4 weeks.
- 75–200 mg/m² IV qd × 3 days (small-cell lung cancer) q3–4 weeks.
- Many other doses based on tumor type being treated (e.g., lymphomas, ANLL, bladder, prostate, uterus, Kaposi's sarcoma).
- Oral dose is twice the intravenous dose, rounded to the nearest 50 mg.
- High dose (bone marrow transplantation): 750–2400 mg/m² IV, or 10–60 mg/kg over 1–4 hours to 24 hours, usually combined with other cytotoxic agents or total body irradiation.
- Dose modification if renal or hepatic dysfunction (see Special Considerations section).

Drug Preparation:

- Available in 5-cc (100-mg) vial as VePesid; the 100-mg Etopophos vial is reconstituted with 5 mL or 10 mL Normal Saline, D5W, sterile water, bacteriostatic sterile water, or bacteriostatic Normal Saline with benzyl alcohol to 20 mg/mL or 10 mg/mL, respectively. May be further diluted with NS or D5W to 0.1 mg/mL final concentration.
- Oral capsules are available in 50-mg and 100-mg capsules, and should be stored in the refrigerator.

Drug Administration:

- IV infusion: VePesid over 30–60 minutes to minimize risk of hypotension and bronchospasm (wheezing). In some instances, a test dose may be infused slowly (0.5 mL in 50 0.9% Sodium Chloride) and the remaining drug infused if no untoward reaction after 5 minutes. Etopophos: IVB over 5 minutes as drug is significantly less likely to cause hypotension.
- Stability: Drug must be diluted with either 5% Dextrose Injection USP or 0.9% Sodium Chloride solution and is stable 96 hours in glass and 48 hours in plastic containers at room temperature (25°C [77°F]) under normal fluorescent light at a concentration of 0.2 mg/mL.
- Inspect for clarity of solution prior to administration.
- Oral administration: may give as a single dose up to 400 mg; otherwise, divide dose into 2–4 doses.

Drug Interactions:

- Enhances warfarin action by increasing prothrombin time (PT); need to monitor closely.
- Increased toxicity of methotrexate when given concurrently.
- Cyclosporin: additive cytotoxicity when given concurrently.

Lab Effects/Interference:

- Increased PT with patients on warfarin.
- Increased LFTs, metabolic acidosis with higher doses.

Special Considerations:

- Nadir 7–14 days after treatment.
- Dose modifications: reduce drug dose by 50% if bili > 1.5 mg/dL, by 75% if bili > 3.0 mg/dL. Reduce drug 25% if creatinine clearance 10–50 mL/min; reduce by 50% if creatinine clearance < 10 mL/min.
- Synergistic drug effect in combination with cisplatin.
- Radiation recall may occur when combined therapies are used.
- Patients receiving high-dose therapy are at risk for the development of second malignancy or ethanol intoxication (injection contains polyethylene glycol with absolute alcohol).
- VePesid: drug stability is concentration-dependent, while Etopophos is prepared as a phosphate esther, which negates the need for concentration-dependent stability (equally stable for 24 hours at concentrations of 20 mg/mL to 0.1 mg/mL).

Table 1.9

Etoposide concentration (mg/mL)	5% Dextrose	0.9% Sodium Chloride
2	0.5 hour*	0.5 hour*
1	2 hours	2 hours
0.6	8 hours	8 hours
0.4	48 hours	48 hours
0.2	96 hours	96 hours

* Check for fine precipitate.
Source: Data from Dorr RT, Von Hoff DD (1994) *Cancer Chemotherapy Handbook* (2nd ed). Norwalk, CT: Appleton & Lange, p 462.

Potential Toxicities/Side Effects and the Nursing Process

I. POTENTIAL FOR INJURY related to ALLERGIC REACTION, HYPOTENSION, ANAPHYLAXIS DURING DRUG INFUSION

Defining Characteristics: Bronchospasm (wheezing) may occur, with or without fever, chills; hypotension may occur during rapid infusion. Anaphylaxis may occur, but is rare.

Nursing Implications: Infuse drug over at least 30–60 minutes in correct amount of IV solution (stability related to volume). Monitor temperature, vital signs prior to drug administration, and periodically during treatment. Remain with patient during first 15 minutes of infusion and assess for signs/symptoms of bronchospasm. Discontinue drug and notify physician if bronchospasm or signs/symptoms of anaphylacticlike reaction occur. Maintain patent IV, monitor VS, and have ready epinephrine, diphenhydramine, and hydrocortisone, as well as emergency equipment. Be familiar with institution's practice guidelines for management of anaphylaxis.

II. POTENTIAL FOR INFECTION AND BLEEDING related to BONE MARROW DEPRESSION

Defining Characteristics: Nadir 10–14 days after drug dose, with recovery on days 21–22. Neutropenia may be severe. Profound bone marrow suppression when given in high doses for bone marrow/stem cell rescue.

Nursing Implications: Monitor CBC, WBC, differential, and platelet count prior to chemotherapy and at expected nadir. Assess for signs/symptoms of infection or bleeding prior to drug administration; instruct patient in self-assessment and to report signs/symptoms immediately. Teach patient self-care measures to minimize risk of infection and bleeding, including avoidance of OTC aspirin-containing medications.

III. ALTERED NUTRITION, LESS THAN BODY REQUIREMENTS, related to NAUSEA AND VOMITING, ANOREXIA

Defining Characteristics: Nausea and vomiting are usually mild, occurring soon after infusion. Oral dosing has higher incidence of nausea/vomiting. Anorexia is mild but may be severe with oral dosing. Severe nausea and vomiting when given in high doses, requiring aggressive, maximal antiemesis. In addition, hepatitis, stomatitis, and metabolic acidosis may occur with high-dose therapy.

Nursing Implications: Premedicate with antiemetics and continue prophylactically for at least 4–6 hours after drug administration. Encourage small feedings of bland, cool foods and liquids; encourage spices as desired. Consult dietitian if anorexia is severe. Patients receiving high-dose therapy should have baseline and periodic assessment of laboratory parameters (e.g., LFTs and chemistries), as well as assessment of oral mucosa. Teach patients self-care, including oral assessment, use of oral hygiene regimen, and to report pain, burning, oral lesions.

IV. BODY IMAGE DISTURBANCE related to ALOPECIA

Defining Characteristics: Incidence is 20–90% and is dose-dependent; regrowth may occur between drug cycles.

Nursing Implications: Discuss with patient possible hair loss and potential coping strategies, including obtaining wig or cap. If hair loss is complete, instruct patient to wear cap or scarf at night to prevent loss of body heat in cold climates.

V. POTENTIAL SEXUAL DYSFUNCTION related to DRUG EFFECTS

Defining Characteristics: Drug is mutagenic and teratogenic.

Nursing Implications: Explore with patient and partner sexual patterns and reproductive goals. Teach about need for contraception as appropriate. Provide information, emotional support, and referral as needed.

VI. ALTERED SKIN INTEGRITY related to RADIATION RECALL, PERIVASCULAR IRRITATION IF DRUG INFILTRATES, AND SKIN LESIONS WITH HIGH DOSE THERAPY

Defining Characteristics: Drug is a radiosensitizer and an irritant. Patients receiving high-dose therapy may develop bullae on the skin (similar to Steven's Johnson syndrome).

Nursing Implications: Assess skin in area of prior radiation when combined therapies are given as well as mucous membranes. Drug may need to be withheld until skin healing occurs if radiation recall results in skin breakdown. Teach patient wound-management techniques. Use careful venipuncture and infuse drug through patent IV over 30–60 minutes, diluted according to manufacturer's specifications. Teach patients receiving high-dose therapy to report any skin changes.

VII. ALTERATION IN CARDIAC OUTPUT related to RARE MYOCARDIAL INFARCTION, ARRHYTHMIAS

Defining Characteristics: Rare myocardial infarction has been reported after prior mediastinal XRT in patients receiving etoposide-containing regimens. Arrhythmias are uncommon but may occur, especially in patients with preexisting coronary artery disease.

Nursing Implications: Monitor patient during infusion and instruct patient to report any unusual sensations. Discuss any abnormalities with physician.

VIII. SENSORY/PERCEPTUAL ALTERATION related to NEUROTOXICITY

Defining Characteristics: Peripheral neuropathies may occur but are uncommon and mild.

Nursing Implications: Assess motor and sensory function prior to drug administration. Instruct patient to report any changes in sensation or function. Discuss any abnormalities with physician. Encourage patient to verbalize feelings about discomfort and sensory loss, and discuss alternative coping strategies.

Drug: exemestane (Aromasin)

Class: Steroidal aromatase inactivator.

Mechanism of Action: Aromatase converts adrenal and ovarian androgens into estrogen, peripherally, in postmenopausal women. Exemestane acts as a false substrate (looks like androstenedione) and binds irreversibly to the aromatase enzyme, making it inactive ("suicide inhibition"). This results in a significant decrease (up to 95%) in circulating estrogen levels in postmenopausal women without affecting other adrenal enzymes. In the absence of estrogen, the stimulus for breast cancer growth is removed.

Metabolism: Oral drug is rapidly absorbed from the GI tract, with plasma levels increased by about 40% if taken after a high-fat breakfast. Drug is extensively distributed into the tissues, and is highly protein-bound (90%). Drug is extensively metabolized in the liver by the P450 3A4 (CYP 3A4) isoenzyme system, and excreted equally in urine and feces. After a single dose of 25 mg, maximal suppression of circulating estrogen occurs 2–3 days after the dose, and lasts for 4–5 days. In patients with either hepatic or renal insufficiency, the dose of exemestane was three times higher than in patients with normal liver or renal function. This does not require dosage adjustment, but studies looking at the safety of chronic dosing in these groups of patients have not been done.

Dosage/Range:
- 25 mg tab PO daily.

Drug Preparation:
- None. Store tablets at 77°F (25°C).

Drug Administration:
- Oral, once daily, after a meal.

Drug Interactions:
- Although metabolized by the P450 3A4 (CYP 3A4) isoenzyme system, it is unlikely that inhibitors of this system will significantly increase exemestane

serum levels; however, manufacturer cautions that known inducers of the enzyme system may decrease serum levels, and should be used together cautiously (see Chapter 15).

Lab Effects/Interference:

- Lymphopenia (20% incidence).
- Elevated LFTs (AST, ALT, alk phos, GGT) rarely.

Special Considerations:

- Drug is indicated for the 1) adjuvant treatment of post-menopausal women with ER positive early breast cancer who received 2–3 years of tamoxifen and who are switched to exemestane for completion of a total of five consecutive years of adjuvant hormonal therapy and 2) treatment of advanced breast cancer in postmenopausal women ONLY, whose disease has progressed following tamoxifen therapy. Drug should not be used for premenopausal women as the presence of estrogen may interfere with exemestane action.
- Drug should not be given to pregnant women.
- Drug is well tolerated, with mild to moderate side effects.
- Differs from other selective aromatase inhibitors in that drug irreversibly binds to aromatase, and androgens cannot displace drug from this enzyme. Body must synthesize new aromatase to start estrogen production again.
- Drug similar to or superior to megestrol acetate after tamoxifen failure in metastatic breast cancer (Kaufmann et al, 2000).

Potential Toxicities/Side Effects and the Nursing Process

I. ALTERATION IN ACTIVITY related to FATIGUE

Defining Characteristics: Overall incidence in studies is 22%, while incidence considered drug-related or of indeterminate cause is 8%.

Nursing Implications: Assess baseline activity tolerance, and self-care ability. Teach patient that fatigue may occur, but is usually mild to moderate. Teach patient to alternate rest and activity. Teach patient to manage activities of daily living using energy-saving strategies, e.g., shopping, cooking. Teach patient to accept assistance from friends and family as needed.

II. ALTERATION IN COMFORT related to HOT FLASHES, INCREASED SWEATING, PAIN

Defining Characteristics: Incidence of events attributable to exemestane were hot flashes, 13%, and increased sweating, 4%. In total evaluation of all adverse events, all patients, pain was reported in 13%.

Nursing Implications: Assess patient baseline comfort, and incidence and tolerance of hot flashes and increased sweating. Assess whether patient has any pain, and effectiveness of current pain-management regimen. Teach patient self-care strategies to maximize comfort, to keep cool (e.g., light, loose clothing, fans, cool drinks) and dry (e.g., use of corn starch after bathing, fan), and to minimize any painful discomfort (e.g., depending upon type and location of pain, OTC analgesics, application of heat, cold, Tiger Balm).

III. ALTERATION IN NUTRITION, POTENTIAL related to NAUSEA, INCREASED APPETITE

Defining Characteristics: Nausea appeared drug-related or of indeterminate cause in 9% of patients, and 3% of patients noted an increased appetite. 8% of patients receiving drug complained of weight gain (greater than 10% of baseline). These side effects are mild to moderate if they occur.

Nursing Implications: Assess baseline nutritional status, optimal and desired weight, and any changes. Teach patient to report nausea or weight gain. Teach patient strategies to minimize nausea (e.g., dietary modification, taking drug after meals) if it occurs, and discuss with physician antiemetic medication if dietary modification not effective. If patient experiences weight gain, discuss patient interest in gentle exercising, such as progressive muscle resistance, which would encourage weight gain as lean body mass rather than fat.

IV. SENSORY/PERCEPTION ALTERATIONS, POTENTIAL, related to DEPRESSION, INSOMNIA

Defining Characteristics: While not reported as side effects considered drugrelated or of indeterminate cause, depression and insomnia occurred in 13% and 11%, respectively, of patients participating in the clinical trials.

Nursing Implications: Assess baseline affect, use of effective coping strategies in dealing with disease and treatment, and usual sleep patterns. Teach patient to report changes in mood, such as depression, and difficulty falling asleep, or early awakening. If this occurs, further assess symptom, and suggest self-care strategies to minimize symptom. If nonpharmacologic measures are ineffective, discuss use of antidepressant or sleeping medication with physician, depending upon assessment.

Drug: floxuridine (FUDR, 2′-Deoxy-5-fluorouridine)

Class: Antimetabolite.

Mechanism of Action: Antimetabolite (fluorinated pyrimidine) that is metabolized to 5-FU when given by IV bolus, or metabolized to 5-FUDR-MP 5-fluoro-2′-deoxyuridine-5′-monophosphate when smaller doses are given, by continuous infusion intraarterially. FUDR-MP is four times more effective in inhibiting the enzyme thymidine synthetase than 5-FU. The inhibition prevents the synthesis of thymidine, an essential component of DNA, resulting in interruption of DNA synthesis and cell death. Other FUDR metabolites inhibit RNA synthesis. Drug is cell cycle specific, with activity during the S phase.

Metabolism: When given IV, drug is transformed to 5-FU; 70–90% of drug is extracted by liver on first pass. Metabolites are excreted by kidneys and lungs. Continuous infusion decreases metabolism of drug with more of the drug being converted to the active metabolite FUDR-MP.

Dosage/Range:

- Intraarterially by slow infusion pump: 0.3 mg/kg/day (range, 0.1–0.6 mg/kg/day), OR
- 5–20 mg/m^2/day every day × 14–21 days.
- IV: Investigational.

Drug Preparation:

- Reconstitute 500-mg vial of lyophilized powder with sterile water, then dilute with 0.9% Sodium Chloride.

Drug Administration:

- Usually administered by slow intraarterial infusion using a surgically placed catheter or percutaneous catheter in a major artery.
- H_2 antagonist antihistamine (i.e., ranitidine 150 mg PO bid) administered concurrently during intraarterial infusion to prevent development of peptic ulcer disease.

Drug Interactions:

- None significant.

Lab Effects/Interference:

- Decreased WBC, platelets.
- PT, total protein, sedimentation rate (abnormal values).
- Increased LFTs.

Special Considerations:

- Drug usually given for 14 days, then heparinized saline for 14 days to maintain line patency.
- Dose reductions or infusion breaks may be necessary depending on toxicity.
- FDA-approved for intrahepatic arterial infusion only.

Potential Toxicities/Side Effects and the Nursing Process

I. ALTERED NUTRITION, LESS THAN BODY REQUIREMENTS, related to NAUSEA/VOMITING, ANOREXIA, STOMATITIS/ ESOPHOPHARYNGITIS, DIARRHEA, GASTRITIS, HEPATIC DYSFUNCTION

Defining Characteristics: Nausea and vomiting occur infrequently and are mild; anorexia is common. Mucositis is milder than 5-FU when administered intrahepatically, but more severe when given via carotid artery. Diarrhea is mild to moderately severe. Gastritis may occur, with abdominal cramping and pain. Incidence is greater in patients receiving hepatic artery infusion. Duodenal ulcers may occur in 10% of patients, be painless, and lead to gastric outlet obstruction and vomiting. Chemical hepatitis may be severe, with increased alk phos in patients receiving drug via hepatic artery infusions.

Nursing Implications: Premedicate with antiemetics as ordered and teach patient in self-administration of prescribed antiemetics. Encourage small, frequent feedings of cool, bland foods. If intractable nausea and vomiting, severe diarrhea, or severe cramping occur, notify physician, stop drug, and infuse heparinized saline. Teach patient oral assessment and oral hygiene regimen, and instruct to report any signs/symptoms of stomatitis, esophopharyngitis. Instruct patient to report diarrhea. Teach self-care measures, including diet modification and self-administration of prescribed antidiarrheal medication. Assess for signs/symptoms of abdominal stress, cramping prior to and during infusion. Discuss with physician use of antacids and antisecretory medications. Catheter placement should be verified prior to each infusion cycle, and inadvertent drug infusion into gastric/duodenal-supplying arteries should be investigated. Monitor LFTs prior to drug initiation, during treatment, and at end of 14-day cycle. Discuss abnormalities and dose reductions with physician. Assess patient for signs/symptoms of liver dysfunction: lethargy, weakness, malaise, anorexia, fever, jaundice, icterus.

II. POTENTIAL FOR INJURY related to INTRAARTERIAL CATHETER PROBLEMS

Defining Characteristics: Catheter problems that may occur include leakage, arterial ischemia or aneurysm, bleeding at catheter site, catheter occlusion, thrombosis or embolism of artery, vessel perforation or dislodged catheter, infection, and biliary sclerosis.

Nursing Implications: Assess catheter carefully prior to each cycle of therapy for patency, signs/symptoms of infection. Ensure that catheter position and patency are determined prior to each cycle of therapy; do not force flushing solution—reaccess and try again. If still unsuccessful, notify physician.

III. SENSORY/PERCEPTUAL ALTERATIONS related to HAND-AND-FOOT SYNDROME AND OTHER CNS SYMPTOMS

Defining Characteristics: Hand-and-foot syndrome occurs in 30–40% of patients (numbness, sensory changes in hands and feet). Uncommonly, cerebellar ataxia, vertigo, nystagmus, seizures, depression, hemiplegia, hiccups, lethargy, and blurred vision may occur.

Nursing Implications: Assess baseline neurologic status prior to and during therapy. Teach patient that hand/foot syndrome may occur and instruct to report signs/symptoms. Discuss with physician use of pyridoxine 50 mg tid to prevent hand/foot syndrome. Assess ability to do activities of daily living and level of comfort.

IV. ALTERATION IN SKIN INTEGRITY related to LOCALIZED ERYTHEMA, DERMATITIS, NONSPECIFIC SKIN TOXICITY, OR RASH

Defining Characteristics: Erythema, dermatitis, pruritus, or rash may occur.

Nursing Implications: Assess for skin changes. Assess impact on comfort and body image. Teach patient self-care.

V. POTENTIAL FOR INFECTION AND BLEEDING related to BONE MARROW DEPRESSION

Defining Characteristics: Occurs rarely when FUDR is given as a single agent via continuous intraarterial infusion.

Nursing Implications: Assess baseline WBC, neutrophil count, and platelets, during treatment and at completion of 14-day infusion. Discontinue drug infusion if WBC $< 3500/mm^3$ or if platelet count $< 100{,}000/mm^3$, or per established physician orders; refill pump with heparinized saline.

Drug: fludarabine phosphate (Fludara)

Class: Antimetabolite.

Mechanism of Action: Inhibits DNA synthesis, probably by inhibiting DNA-polymerase-alpha, ribonucleotide reductase, and DNA primase.

Metabolism: Drug is rapidly converted to the active metabolite 2-fluoroara-A when given intravenously. The drug's half-life is about 10 hours. The major route of elimination is via the kidneys, and approximately 23% of the active drug is excreted unchanged in the urine.

Dosage/Range:

- 25 mg/m^2 IV over 30 minutes daily × 5 days, repeated every 28 days.

Drug Preparation:

- Aseptically add 2 mL sterile water for injection USP to the vial, resulting in a final concentration of 25 mg/mL. The drug may then be diluted further in 100 mL of 5% Dextrose or 0.9% Sodium Chloride. Once reconstituted, the drug should be used within 8 hours.

Drug Administration:

- IV infusion over 30 minutes.

Lab Effects/Interference:

- Decreased CBC.
- Tumor lysis syndrome.

Special Considerations:

- Indicated for the treatment of patients with B-cell chronic lymphocytic leukemia (CLL) who have not responded to treatment with at least one standard alkylating agent-containing regimen, or who have progressed on treatment.
- Dose-dependent toxicity: overdosage (four times recommended dose) has been associated with delayed blindness, coma, and death.
- Do not administer in combination with pentostatin, as fatal pulmonary toxicity can occur.
- Administer cautiously in patients with renal insufficiency.
- Drug is teratogenic.
- Drug may cause severe bone marrow depression.

Potential Toxicities/Side Effects and the Nursing Process

I. INFECTION AND BLEEDING related to BONE MARROW DEPRESSION

Defining Characteristics: Severe and cumulative bone marrow depression may occur; nadir, 13 days (range, 3–25 days).

Nursing Implications: Monitor CBC, platelet count prior to drug administration, as well as signs/symptoms of infection and bleeding. Instruct patient in self-assessment of signs/symptoms of infection and bleeding as well as self-care measures, including avoidance of OTC aspirin-containing medication.

II. POTENTIAL FOR ACTIVITY INTOLERANCE related to ANEMIA-INDUCED FATIGUE

Defining Characteristics: Bone marrow depression often includes red cell line.

Nursing Implications: Monitor Hgb, HCT; discuss transfusion with physician if HCT doesn't recover postchemotherapy. Teach patient high-iron diet as appropriate.

III. SENSORY/PERCEPTUAL ALTERATIONS related to CNS EFFECTS, PERIPHERAL NEUROPATHIES

Defining Characteristics: Agitation, confusion, visual disturbances, and coma have occurred. Objective weakness has been reported (9–65%), as have paresthesias (4–12%).

Nursing Implications: Assess baseline neurologic status; monitor neurologic vital signs. Teach patient signs/symptoms and instruct to report them if they occur. Evaluate these changes with physician and discuss continuation of therapy.

IV. POTENTIAL FOR IMPAIRED GAS EXCHANGE related to PULMONARY TOXICITY

Defining Characteristics: Pneumonia occurs in 16–22% of patients. Pulmonary hypersensitivity reaction characterized by dyspnea, cough, interstitial pulmonary infiltrate has been observed. Fatal pulmonary toxicity has occurred when drug is given in combination with pentostatin (Deoxycofomycin).

Nursing Implications: Instruct patient in possible side effects and to report dyspnea, cough, signs of breathlessness following exertion. Assess lung sounds prior to chemotherapy administration. DO NOT administer drug in combination with pentostatin.

V. POTENTIAL FOR SEXUAL DYSFUNCTION, related to TERATOGENICITY

Defining Characteristics: Drug is teratogenic; may cause testicular atrophy. It is unknown whether drug is excreted in breast milk.

Nursing Implications: As appropriate, explore with patient and partner issues of reproduction and sexuality patterns, and impact chemotherapy may have. Discuss strategies to preserve sexual and reproductive health (sperm banking, contraception). Mothers receiving drug should not breast-feed.

VI. ALTERED NUTRITION, LESS THAN BODY REQUIREMENTS, related to NAUSEA/VOMITING, DIARRHEA

Defining Characteristics: Nausea/vomiting occurs in about 30% of patients and can be prevented with standard antiemetics; diarrhea occurs in 15% of patients.

Nursing Implications: Premedicate with antiemetics; evaluate response to emetic protection. Encourage small, frequent meals of cool, bland foods and liquids. If vomiting occurs, assess for signs/symptoms of fluid/electrolyte imbalance; monitor I/O and daily weights, lab results. Encourage patient to report onset of diarrhea; teach patient to administer antidiarrheal medication as ordered.

Drug: 5-fluorouracil (Fluorouracil, Adrucil, 5-FU, Efudex [topical])

Class: Pyrimidine antimetabolite.

Mechanism of Action: Acts as a "false" pyrimidine, inhibiting the formation of an enzyme (thymidine synthetase) necessary for the synthesis of DNA. Also incorporates into RNA, causing abnormal synthesis. Methotrexate given prior to 5-FU results in synergism and enhanced efficacy.

Metabolism: Metabolized by the liver; most is excreted as respiratory CO_2, remainder is excreted by the kidneys. Plasma half-life is 20 minutes.

Dosage/Range:

- 12–15 mg/kg IV once per week, OR
- 12 mg/kg IV every day × 5 days every 4 weeks, OR
- 500 mg/m^2 every week or every week × 5 weeks.
- Hepatic infusion: 22 mg/kg in 100 mL 5% Dextrose infused into hepatic artery over 8 hours for 5–21 consecutive days.
- Head and neck: 1000 mg/m^2 day × 4–5 days as continuous infusion.
- Colon cancer: A variety of regimens, such as 500 mg/m^2 IVB 1 hour after start of leucovorin (500 mg/m^2 in a 2-hour IV infusion) every week × 6 weeks, or together with irinotecan and leucovorin as first line for metastatic colon cancer.

Drug Preparation:

- No dilution required. Can be added to 0.9% Sodium Chloride or 5% Dextrose.
- Store at room temperature; protect from light. Solution should be clear: if crystals do not disappear after holding vial under hot water, discard vial.

Drug Administration:

- Given via IV push or bolus (slow drip), or as continuous infusion.
- Topical: As cream.

Drug Interactions:

- When given with cimetidine, there are increased pharmacologic effects of fluorouracil.

- When given with thiazide diuretics, there is increased risk of myelosuppression.
- Leucovorin causes increased 5-fluorouracil cytotoxicity.

Lab Effects/Interference:
- Decreased CBC.

Special Considerations:
- Cutaneous side effects occur, e.g., skin sensitivity to sun, splitting of fingernails, dry flaky skin, and hyperpigmentation on face, palms of hands.
- Patients who have had adrenalectomy may need higher doses of prednisone while receiving 5-FU, or dose of 5-FU may be reduced in postadrenalectomy patients.
- Reduce dose in patients with compromised hepatic, renal, or bone marrow function and malnutrition.
- Inspect solution for precipitate prior to continuous infusion.

Potential Toxicities/Side Effects and the Nursing Process

I. POTENTIAL FOR INFECTION AND BLEEDING related to BONE MARROW DEPRESSION

Defining Characteristics: Nadir 10–14 days after drug dose; neutropenia, thrombocytopenia are dose-related. Toxicity is enhanced when combined with leucovorin calcium.

Nursing Implications: Assess baseline CBC, WBC, differential, and platelet count prior to chemotherapy, as well as for signs/symptoms of infection or bleeding. Teach patient signs/symptoms of infection or bleeding, and instruct to report these immediately; teach patient self-care measures to minimize risk of infection and bleeding. This includes avoidance of crowds, proximity to people with infections, and avoidance of OTC aspirin-containing medications.

II. ALTERED NUTRITION, LESS THAN BODY REQUIREMENTS, related to NAUSEA AND VOMITING, STOMATITIS, AND DIARRHEA

Defining Characteristics: Nausea and vomiting occur in 30–50% of patients and severity is dose-dependent. Stomatitis can be severe, with onset in 5–8 days; and may herald severe bone marrow depression. Diarrhea can be severe, and in combination with leucovorin calcium is the dose-limiting toxicity.

Nursing Implications: Premedicate patient with antiemetics (phenothiazines are usually effective), and continue for 24 hours, at least for the first cycle. Encourage small, frequent meals of cool, bland foods. Assess oral mucosa prior to drug administration and instruct patient to report changes. Teach patient oral hygiene measures and self-assessment. Instruct patient to report diarrhea, to self-administer prescribed antidiarrheal medications, and to drink adequate fluids. Moderate to severe stomatitis or diarrhea is an indication to interrupt therapy.

III. ALTERATION IN SKIN INTEGRITY related to ALOPECIA, CHANGES IN NAILS AND SKIN

Defining Characteristics: Alopecia is more common with five-day course and involves diffuse thinning of scalp hair, eyelashes, and eyebrows. Brittle nail cracking and loss may occur. Photosensitivity occurs. Chemical phlebitis may occur during continuous infusion with higher doses (pH > 8.0).

Nursing Implications: Teach patient about possible hair loss and skin changes; discuss possible impact on body image. Assess patient's risk for hair loss and skin changes during the therapy and discuss with patient strategies to minimize distress (wig, scarf, nail polish). Instruct patient to use sunblock when outdoors. Suggest implanted venous access device for continuous infusion of 5-FU, especially if patient will receive ongoing therapy.

IV. SENSORY/PERCEPTUAL ALTERATIONS related to PHOTOPHOBIA, CEREBELLAR ATAXIA, OCULAR CHANGES

Defining Characteristics: Photophobia may occur. Occasional cerebellar ataxia may occur and will disappear once drug is stopped. Drug is excreted in tears. Ocular changes that may occur are conjunctivitis, increased lacrimation, photophobia, oculomotor dysfunction, and blurred vision.

Nursing Implications: Assess baseline neurologic status, including vision. Instruct patient to report any changes. Teach patient safety precautions as needed.

Drug: flutamide (Eulexin)

Class: Antiandrogen.

Mechanism of Action: Inhibits androgen uptake or inhibits nuclear binding of androgen in target tissues or both.

Metabolism: Rapidly and completely absorbed. Excreted mainly via urine. Biologically active metabolite reaches maximum plasma levels in approximately 2 hours. Plasma half-life is 6 hours. Largely plasma-bound.

Dosage/Range:
- 250 mg every 8 hours.

Drug Preparation:
- None (provided in 125-mg tablets).

Drug Administration:
- Oral.

Drug Interactions:
- None reported.

Lab Effects/Interference:
- Increased LFTs.
- Increased BUN, creatinine.
- Monitor PSA for changes.

Special Considerations:
- None.

Potential Toxicities/Side Effects and the Nursing Process

I. POTENTIAL SEXUAL DYSFUNCTION related to DRUG EFFECTS

Defining Characteristics: Decreased libido and impotence can occur in 33% of patients; gynecomastia occurs in 10% of patients.

Nursing Implications: Assess patient's sexual pattern, any alterations, and patient response. Encourage patient to verbalize feelings; provide information, emotional support, and referral for counseling as available and appropriate.

II. ALTERATION IN COMFORT related to HOT FLASHES

Defining Characteristics: Hot flashes occur commonly.

Nursing Implications: Teach patient that this may occur, and encourage patient to report symptoms. Provide symptomatic support.

III. ALTERED NUTRITION, LESS THAN BODY REQUIREMENTS, related to DIARRHEA, NAUSEA AND VOMITING

Defining Characteristics: Diarrhea and nausea/vomiting occur in 10% of patients.

Nursing Implications: Teach patient that these may occur, and instruct to report them. Assess for occurrence; teach patient self-administration of prescribed antidiarrheal or antiemetic medications.

Agent: fulvestrant injection (Faslodex)

Class: Estrogen Downregulator.

Mechanism of Action: Fulvestrant is an estrogen receptor antagonist that binds to the estrogen receptor of cells that are dependent upon estrogen for growth, including breast cancer cells that are hormone positive. There is no agonist effect as with other antiestrogens, such as tamoxifen. In addition, the estrogen receptor is also degraded so that it is lost from the cell. Because of this, there is no chance that the hormone receptor can be stimulated by low concentrations of estrogen, as with other antiestrogens, and this theoretically reduces the development of resistance.

Metabolism: When given IM, it takes 7 days for the drug to reach maximal plasma levels, which are maintained for at least one month. Half-life is about 40 days, and after 3-6 monthly doses, steady-state plasma area under the curve levels are reached at 2.5 times that of a single-dose injection. Drug undergoes biotransformation similar to endogenous steroids (oxidation, aromatic hydroxylation, conjugation), and oxidative pathway is via cytochrome P-450 (CYP 3A4). Drug is metabolized by the liver and rapidly cleared from the plasma via the hepatobiliary route. 90% is excreted via the feces; renal excretion is < 1%. There were no pharmacokinetic differences found in the elderly and younger adults, men and women, different races, patients with renal impairment, and patients with mild hepatic impairment. However, patients with moderate to severe liver dysfunction have not been studied.

Dosage/Range:

- 250 mg given IM into the buttock monthly as either one 5 mL slow injection or 2 separate 2.5-mL slow injections into each buttock.

Drug Preparation:

- Drug available in refrigerated 5 ml/250 mg, and 2.5 ml/125 mg prefilled syringes; concentration is 50 mg/mL.
- Unopened vials should be stored in the refrigerator at 2°–8°C (36°–46°F), but do not freeze. Drug can be left at room temperature for a short period of time prior to injection to increase patient comfort.
- Remove glass syringe barrel from tray and ensure it is undamaged.
- Unopen Safety Glide needle and attach to luer lock end of the syringe.
- Expel any air.

Drug Administration:

- Administer slow IM in one buttock 5 mL (250 mg) or 2.5 mL (125 mg) into each buttock as solution is viscous.
- Z-track administration is recommended to prevent drug leakage into subcutaneous tissue.
- Following drug injection, activate needle protectin device when withdrawing needle from patient by pushing lever arm completely forward until needle tip is fully covered.
- If unable to activate, drop into sharps disposal container.

Drug Interactions:

- None significant as drug does not significantly inhibit the major CYP isoenzymes, including rifampin.

Lab Effects/Interference: None.

Special Considerations:

- Indicated for the treatment of hormone receptor positive metastatic breast cancer in postmenopausal women with disease progression following antiestrogen therapy.
- Contraindicated in pregnancy or in patients hypersensitive to the drug or its components.
- Drug should not be used by breastfeeding mothers.
- Injection site reactions more common when drug is given in two divided doses.

Potential Toxicities/Side Effects and the Nursing Process

I. ALTERATION IN COMFORT related to INJECTION SITE REACTION, ABDOMINAL PAIN, BACK PAIN

Defining Characteristics: Injection site reactions (pain and inflammation) occurred in 7% of patients receiving a single 5-mL injection (European Trial) as compared to 27% of patients (North American Trial) receiving two 2.5-mL injections, one in each buttock. Back and bone pain occurred in 15.8% of patients, while abdominal pain occurred in 11.8% of patients and often was associated with other gastrointestinal symptoms.

Nursing Implications: Teach patient this may occur and to report it. Consider using Z-track method, and if using 2 separate injection of 2.5 mL, try a single-dose injection to see if discomfort is reduced. Teach patient to report bone and/or back pain. Teach patient to use over-the-counter analgesics such as acetaminophen or nonsteroidal anti-inflammatory drugs as appropriate to bleeding history or risk factors. Discuss alternatives with physician if ineffective in symptom management.

II. ALTERATION IN NUTRITION, POTENTIAL related to NAUSEA, VOMITING, CONSTIPATION, DIARRHEA

Defining Characteristics: Nausea occurs in 26%, vomiting 13%, constipation 12.5%, diarrhea 12.3%, and anorexia 9%.

Nursing Implications: Assess baseline appetite, presence of nausea and/or vomiting, and bowel elimination pattern. Teach patient that these side effects may occur, self-care measures to minimize nausea and vomiting such as dietary modification, and to report these side effects. Discuss antiemetics with physician if dietary modification is ineffective. Teach patient to use dietary modification to relieve constipation or diarrhea and, if ineffective, to use over-the-counter laxatives or anti-diarrheal medicine. If ineffective, discuss pharmacologic management with physician.

III. ALTERATION IN SKIN INTEGRITY, POTENTIAL, related to HOT FLASHES AND PERIPHERAL EDEMA

Defining Characteristics: Vasodilation or hot flashes occurred in 17.7% of patients, and peripheral edema in 9% of patients.

Nursing Implications: Assess baseline skin integrity, history of hot flashes in post-menopausal patients, and presence of peripheral edema. Teach patient these side effects may occur and to report them. If hot flashes are severe, review common hot flash management including wearing loose, layered clothing that can be removed when the woman becomes hot, sipping cold beverages throughout the day, sleeping with light nightgown and window open, avoiding triggers such as caffeine or alcohol, and if ineffective, discuss use of venlaxafine (Effexor) or fluoxetine (Paxil) to reduce intensity and frequency of hot flashes (Loprinski et al, 2000). Teach patient self-assessment of peripheral edema, to wear loose stockings and shoes, to keep skin moisturized to prevent cracking, and comfort measures. Teach patient to report increasing edema or related problems.

Drug: gemcitabine (Gemzar, Difluorodeoxycitidine)

Class: Antimetabolite.

Mechanism of Action: Inhibits DNA synthesis by inhibiting DNA polymerase activity through a process called *masked chain termination*. It is a prodrug, structurally similar to ara-C, needing intracellular phosphorylation. It then inhibits DNA synthesis. Cell cycle specific for S phase, causing cells to accumulate at the G-S boundary.

Metabolism: Pharmacokinetics vary by age, gender, and infusion time. Half-life for short infusions ranges from 32–94 minutes, while that of long infusions ranges from 245–638 minutes. Following short infusions (< 70 minutes), the drug is not extensively tissue-bound; following long infusions (70–285 minutes), the drug slowly equilibrates within tissues. The terminal half-life of the parent drug, gemcitabine, is 17 minutes. There is negligible binding to serum proteins. Drug and metabolites are excreted in the urine, with 92–98% of the drug dose recovered in the urine within one week. Mean systemic clearance is 90 L/h/m^2. Clearance is about 30% lower in women than in men, and also reduced in the elderly, but this does not necessarily require a dose reduction.

Dosage/Range:

Adults:

- Breast cancer: 1250 mg/m^2 IV over 30 minutes d 1, 8 q 21 days, in combination with paclitaxel 175mg/m^2 IV over 3 hr administered prior to gemcitabine, day 1 repeated q 21 days.
- Pancreatic cancer: 1000 mg/m^2 IV infusion over 30 min every week for up to 7 weeks (or until toxicity necessitates dose reduction or delay), then followed by 1-week break. Treatment then continues weekly for 3 weeks, followed by 1 week off (i.e., treatment 3 weeks out of 4). See dose modifications for hematologic toxicity in Special Considerations. For patients who complete the initial 7 weeks, or a subsequent 3-week cycle at a dose of 1000 mg/m^2, the dose may be increased by 25% to 1250 mg/m^2 if the following conditions are met: the ANC NADIR is > 1500 × 10/L, platelet count NADIR is > 100,000 × 10/L, and nonhematologic toxicity has not been greater than WHO grade 1. If patient tolerates this course well, the dose for the next cycle can be increased an additional 20% if the above three criteria are met. (Source: Eli Lilly Co., Gemzar package insert.)
- Non-small-cell lung cancer (inoperable, locally advanced Stage IIIA and IIIB or metastatic) in combination with cisplatin: 4-week cycle: 1000 mg/m^2 IV over 30 minutes on day 1, 8, 15, repeat q28 days, with cisplatin 100 mg/m^2 IV on day 1 after the gemcitabine infusion; or as a 3-week cycle, with gemcitabine 1250 mg/m^2 IV over 30 minutes on day 1, 8; cisplatin 100 mg/m^2 IV is given following gemcitabine infusion on day 1, repeated q3 weeks.

Drug Preparation:

- Drug available in single-use vials of 200 mg/10 mL and 1 g/50 mL. Use 0.9% Sodium Chloride USP and reconstitute the 200-mg vial with 5 mL, and the 1-g vial with 25 mL. Shake to dissolve the powder. This results in a concentration of 38 mg/mL. Withdraw recommended dose and further dilute in 0.9% Sodium Chloride injection. Discard unused portion. Inspect solution for particulate matter or discoloration and do not use if these occur. Stable 24 hours at room temperature (20–25°C [68–77°F]). DO NOT refrigerate, as drug crystallization may occur.

Drug Administration:

- Administer IV over 30 minutes.

Drug Interactions:

- Administer cisplatin after gemcitabine to enhance renal drug clearance; paclitaxel should be administered before gemcitabine.

Lab Effects/Interference:

- Decreased CBC.
- Increased LFTs, RFTs.

Special Considerations:

- FDA-approved for first-line treatment of patients with unresectable non-small-cell lung cancer, in combination with cisplatin.
- FDA-approved for first-line treatment of patients with locally advanced (nonresectable Stage II or III), or metastatic (Stage IV) adenocarcinoma of the pancreas, in combination with paclitaxel, as first-line therapy for treatment of women with metastatic breast cancer who have failed prior anthracycline adjuvant chemotherapy, unless anthracyclines are contraindicated. Drug is also indicated for patients with pancreatic cancer previously treated with 5-FU.
- FDA-approved in combination with paclitaxel, as first-line therapy for treatment of patients with metastatic breast cancer who have failed prior anthracycline adjuvant chemotherapy, unless anthracyclines are contraindicated.
- Monitor liver and renal function at baseline and throughout therapy.
- Dose reduction or delay required for hematologic toxicity.

Table 1.10

ANC (× 10^6/L)		Platelet Count (× 10^6/L)	% of full dose
≥ 1000	and	≥ 100,000	100
500–999	or	50,000–99,000	75
< 500	or	< 50,000	hold

Source: Gemzar package insert (1998). Eli Lilly Company, Indianapolis, IN.

- Use with caution in patients with impaired renal function or hepatic dysfunction. (Studies have not been done to identify risks in this population.)
- Rarely, HUS (hemolytic uremic syndrome) has occurred. Discontinue drug if signs/symptoms occur (rapid decrease in hemoglobin and thrombocytopenia, together with elevated BUN/creatinine). Observe for elevation of serum bili or LDH.
- Drug can rarely cause severe pulmonary toxicity (interstitial pneumonitis, pulmonary fibrosis, pulmonary edema, adult respiratory distress syndrome), occurring up to 2 weeks following the last gemcitabine infusion. If patients develop dyspnea, with or without bronchospasm, stop gemcitabine until further pulmonary evaluation can proceed; discontinue drug if related to gemcitabine.
- Drug may cause sedation in 10% of patients; caution patient not to drive or operate heavy machinery until it is determined whether patient develops this side effect.
- Drug is embryotoxic; women of childbearing age should avoid pregnancy while receiving the drug.
- Drug may be irritating to the vein, requiring local heat; may require a central line for (long-term) administration.

Potential Toxicities/Side Effects and the Nursing Process

I. POTENTIAL FOR INFECTION AND BLEEDING related to BONE MARROW DEPRESSION

Defining Characteristics: Myelosuppression is dose-limiting toxicity. Incidence of leukopenia is 63%, thrombocytopenia 36%, and anemia 73%. Dose reductions required are shown in the Special Considerations section. Grades 3–4 thrombocytopenia are more common in the elderly, and grades 3–4 neutropenia and thrombocytopenia are more common in women (especially older women). Older women were less able to complete subsequent courses of therapy. Myelosuppression is usually short-lived with recovery within one week. Approximately 19% of patients require RBC transfusions.

Nursing Implications: Assess baseline CBC, WBC, differential, and platelet count prior to chemotherapy, as well as for signs/symptoms of infection or bleeding. Discuss dose reductions or delay based on neutrophil and platelet counts. Teach patient signs/symptoms of infection or bleeding, and instruct to report these immediately. Teach patient self-care measures to minimize risk of infection and bleeding. This includes avoidance of crowds, proximity to people with infections, and OTC aspirin-containing medications. Transfuse red blood cells and platelets as needed per physician order.

II. POTENTIAL ALTERATION IN NUTRITION, LESS THAN BODY REQUIREMENTS, related to NAUSEA AND VOMITING, DIARRHEA, STOMATITIS, AND ALTERATIONS IN LFTS

Defining Characteristics: Nausea and vomiting occur in 69% of patients, and of these, < 15% are severe. Nausea and vomiting are usually mild to moderate and are easily prevented or controlled by antiemetics. Diarrhea may occur (19% incidence), as may stomatitis (11% incidence). Abnormalities in liver transaminases occur in two-thirds of patients; rarely does this require drug discontinuance.

Nursing Implications: Premedicate patient with antiemetics (phenothiazides are usually effective). Encourage small, frequent meals of cool, bland foods. Teach patient self-administration of prescribed antiemetic medications, and to drink adequate fluids. Assess oral mucosa prior to drug administration, and instruct patient to report changes. Teach patient oral hygiene measures and self-assessment. Instruct patient to report diarrhea, to self-administer prescribed antidiarrheal medications, and to drink adequate fluids. Monitor LFTs baseline and periodically during therapy. Notify physician of any abnormalities and discuss implications. Drug should be used cautiously in any patient with hepatic dysfunction.

III. POTENTIAL ALTERATION IN COMFORT related to FLULIKE SYMPTOMS

Defining Characteristics: Flulike symptoms occur in 20% of patients with first treatment dose. Transient febrile episodes occur in 41% of patients.

Nursing Implications: Encourage patient to report flulike symptoms. Treat fevers with acetaminophen per physician. Assess for alterations in comfort, and discuss symptomatic measures. If severe, discuss drug discontinuance with physician.

IV. IMPAIRED SKIN INTEGRITY related to ALOPECIA, RASH, PRURITUS, EDEMA

Defining Characteristics: Skin rash occurs in about 30% of patients, often within 2–3 days of starting drug. The rash is erythematous, pruritic, and/or maculopapular, and may occur on the neck and extremities. Edema occurs in about 30% of patients, and is primarily peripheral but can rarely be facial or pulmonary. Edema is reversible after drug is discontinued, and appears unrelated to cardiac, renal, or hepatic impairment. Edema is usually mild to moderate. Minimal hair loss occurs in 15% of patients, and is reversible.

Nursing Implications: Assess skin integrity and presence of rash, pruritus, alopecia, and edema prior to dosing. Assess impact of these alterations on patient, and develop plan to manage symptom distress and promote skin integrity. Instruct patient to report rash, itching; discuss treatment of rash with topical corticosteroids. Teach patient self-assessment of signs/symptoms of edema, and instruct to notify health care provider if swelling occurs. If severe, discuss drug discontinuance with physician.

Drug: goserelin acetate (Zoladex)

Class: Synthetic analogue of luteinizing hormone-releasing hormone (LHRH).

Mechanism of Action: Inhibits pituitary gonadotropin, achieving a chemical orchiectomy in 2–4 weeks. Sustained-release medication provides continuous drug diffusion from the depot into subcutaneous tissue. This permits monthly injection instead of daily.

Metabolism: Absorbed slowly for first 8 days, then more rapid and constant absorption for remaining 28 days.

Dosage/Range:

Adults:

- Subcutaneous: 3.6-mg dose into upper abdominal wall, q28 days 10.8 mg q 3 months.

Drug Preparation/Administration:

- Inspect package for damage. Open package and inspect drug in translucent chamber.
- Select site on upper abdomen.
- Prepare site with alcohol swab, cleansing from center outward.
- Administer local anesthetic as ordered.
- Aseptically, stretch skin at site with nondominant hand, and insert needle into subcutaneous tissue with dominant hand at 45-degree angle.
- Redirect needle so it is parallel to the abdominal wall. Advance needle forward until hub touches skin. Withdraw needle 1 cm (approximately ½ inch).
- Depress plunger fully, expelling depot into prepared site.
- Withdraw needle carefully. Apply gentle pressure bandage to site. Confirm that tip of plunger is visible within needle tip.
- Document in chart.

Drug Interactions:

- None.

Lab Effects/Interference:

- Hypercalcemia in patients with bone metastases.
- Tests of pituitary/gonadal function may be inaccurate while on therapy due to suppression of pituitary/gonadal system.

Special Considerations:

- Compliance to 28-day injection schedule is important.
- Indicated for palliative treatment of advanced prostate cancer; treatment of Stage B2 (locally advanced) prostate cancer in combination with flutamide; palliative treatment of advanced breast cancer in pre- or peri-menopausal women; and for the treatment of endometriosis.
- Initially, there is transient increase in serum testosterone levels, with flare of symptoms.
- Well-tolerated treatment.

Potential Toxicities/Side Effects and the Nursing Process

I. SEXUAL DYSFUNCTION related to DECREASED TESTOSTERONE LEVELS

Defining Characteristics: Hot flashes, sexual dysfunction, and decreased erections can occur.

Nursing Implications: Assess normal sexual pattern. Refer as needed for sexual counseling.

II. POTENTIAL ALTERATION IN CARDIAC OUTPUT related to ARRYTHMIA, CARDIOVASCULAR DYSFUNCTION

Defining Characteristics: Arrhythmia, cerebrovascular accident (CVA), hypertension, myocardial infarction, peripheral vascular disease, chest pain may occur in 1–5% of patients.

Nursing Implications: Assess heart rate, blood pressure, peripheral pulses. Teach patient to report palpitations, shortness of breath, chest pain, or leg pain immediately. Evaluate abnormalities with physician.

III. SENSORY/PERCEPTUAL ALTERATION related to ANXIETY, DEPRESSION, HEADACHE

Defining Characteristics: Anxiety, depression, headache may occur (< 5%).

Nursing Implications: Assess baseline affect, comfort. Instruct patient to report mood disorder. Encourage patient to verbalize feelings, provide patient with emotional support. Assess efficacy of supportive care, and if needed, discuss pharmacologic management of symptoms with physician.

IV. ALTERATION IN NUTRITION, LESS THAN BODY REQUIREMENTS, related to VOMITING, HYPERGLYCEMIA

Defining Characteristics: Vomiting may occur (< 5%); also increased weight, ulcer, hyperglycemia.

Nursing Implications: Teach patient to report GI disturbances. Assess severity and discuss management with physician. Assess serum glucose, and if abnormal, discuss dietary or pharmacologic management, depending upon severity, with physician.

V. ALTERATION IN BOWEL ELIMINATION related to CONSTIPATION OR DIARRHEA

Defining Characteristics: Constipation or diarrhea may occur (< 5%).

Nursing Implications: Instruct patient to report problems in elimination. Teach symptomatic management.

VI. ALTERATION IN URINARY ELIMINATION related to OBSTRUCTION OR INFECTION

Defining Characteristics: Urinary obstruction, urinary tract infection, renal insufficiency may occur.

Nursing Implications: Monitor baseline urinary elimination pattern, baseline kidney function tests, and continue to monitor through therapy. Instruct patient to report signs/symptoms of urinary tract infection (UTI).

VII. ALTERATION IN COMFORT related to FEVER, CHILLS, TENDERNESS

Defining Characteristics: Chills, fever, breast swelling, and tenderness. Also, discomfort may result from injection, as a 16-gauge needle is used to inject depot.

Nursing Implications: Instruct patient to report discomfort. Discuss strategies to increase comfort. Administer local anesthetic prior to injection of medication (per physician's order).

Drug: histrelin implant (Vantas)

Class: Synthetic analogue of gonadotropin releasing factor (GnRH) or luteinizing hormone-releasing hormone (LHRH).

Mechanism of Action: Histrelin inhibits pituitary gonadotropin, achieving a chemical orchiectomy.

Metabolism: Implant delivers histrelin continuously for 12 months at 50–60 micrograms per day. Drug serum concentration 50% higher in patients with severe renal dysfunction, but this is not considered clinically significant.

Dosage/Range:
Adults:
- Histrelin implant (50 mg) is asceptically inserted subcutaneously under skin on upper, inner arm using implant tool; at 12 months, implant must be removed before new one is implanted.

Drug Preparation:
- Keep implant refrigerated until implant.
- Select site on upper inner arm, and follow guidelines in package insert using asceptic technique and implant tool.
- Implant is NOT radio-opaque so care must be given to carefully secure the implant as directed.

Drug Interactions:
- Unknown.

Lab Effects/Interference:
- Hypercalcemia in patients with bone metastases.
- Tests of pituitary/gonadal function may be inaccurate while on therapy due to suppression of pituitary/gonadal system.
- Decreased serum testosterone to below castrate levels (< ng/dL)

Special Considerations:
- Indicated for palliative treatment of advanced prostate cancer.

- Initially (1st week of treatment), there is transient increase in serum testosterone levels, with flare of symptoms or onset of new symptoms such as bone pain, neuropathy, hematuria, or ureteral/bladder outlet obstruction. If severe (rarely spinal cord compression, ureteral obstruction), these should be managed immediately.
- Patients with metastatic vertebral and/or urinary tract obstruction should be monitored very closely during the first few weeks of treatment.
- Generally well-tolerated treatment.
- Contraindicated in children and women.

Potential Toxicities/Side Effects and the Nursing Process

I. SEXUAL DYSFUNCTION related to DECREASED TESTOSTERONE LEVELS

Defining Characteristics: Hot flashes (66% with 2.3% severe), testicular atrophy (5.3%), gynecomastica (4.1%), decreased libido (2.3%) and erectile dysfunction (3.5%) can occur.

Nursing Implications: Assess normal sexual pattern. Encourage patient to verbalize feelings to assess impact of symptoms on sexual function; refer as needed for sexual counseling. Teach patient self-care strategies to reduce distress of hot flashes.

II. ALTERATION IN BOWEL ELIMINATION related to CONSTIPATION

Defining Characteristics: Constipation may occur (< 5%).

Nursing Implications: Instruct patient to report problems in elimination. Teach symptomatic management.

III. ALTERATION IN URINARY ELIMINATION related to OBSTRUCTION OR INFECTION

Defining Characteristics: Urinary obstruction, urinary tract infection, renal insufficiency may occur. Renal impairment occurs in 4.7% of patients.

Nursing Implications: Monitor baseline urinary elimination pattern, baseline kidney function tests, and continue to monitor through therapy. Instruct patient to report signs/symptoms of urinary tract infection (UTI).

IV. ALTERATION IN COMFORT related to IMPLANT SITE IRRITATION, ASTHENIA, AND INSOMNIA

Defining Characteristics: Implantation site reactions occur in at least 5.8% of patients: these include bruising, pain/soreness/tenderness after insertion or removal; rarely, erythema, and swelling may occur. Asthenia occurs in about 10% of patients, and insomnia 2.9% of patients.

Nursing Implications: Instruct patient to report discomfort. Discuss strategies to increase comfort. Teach patient to self-assess and reassure local effects will resolve. Teach patient to report any signs/symptoms of infection.

Drug: hydroxyurea (Hydrea, Droxia)

Class: Miscellaneous/antimetabolite.

Mechanism of Action: Prevents conversion of ribonucleotides to deoxyribonucleotides by inhibiting the converting enzyme ribonucleoside diphosphate reductase. DNA synthesis is thus inhibited. Cell cycle phase specific for S phase. May also sensitize cells to the effects of radiation therapy, although the process is not clearly understood.

Metabolism: Rapidly absorbed from GI tract. Peak plasma level reached in 2 hours, with plasma half-life of 3–4 hours. About half the drug is metabolized in the liver and half is excreted in urine as urea and unchanged drug. Some of the drug is eliminated as respiratory CO_2. Crosses BBB.

Dosage/Range:

- 500–3000 mg PO daily (dose reduced in renal dysfunction).
- 20–30 mg/kg/day PO as a continuous dose.
- 100 mg/kg IV daily × 3 days.
- Radiation sensitization: 80 mg/kg as a single dose every 3rd day starting at least 7 days before initiation of radiation.
- Sickle cell disease: To prevent painful crises, initial 15 mg/kg/day, increased by 5 mg/kg every 12 weeks to a maximum dose of 35 mg/kg/day as tolerated.

Drug Preparation:

- None. Hydrea available in 500-mg capsules or Droxia in 200-mg, 300-mg, and 400-mg tablets.

Drug Administration:

- Oral.
- High-dose IV continuous infusions are being studied with doses of 0.5–1 $g/m^2/day$ × 5–12 weeks (investigational).

Drug Interactions:

- None significant.

Lab Effects/Interference:

- Decreased CBC.
- Increased BUN, creatinine, uric acid.

- Increased hepatic enzymes.

Special Considerations:

- Hydroxyurea has a side effect of dramatically lowering the WBC in a relatively short period of time (24–48 hours). In leukemia patients endangered by the potential complication of leukostasis, this is the desired effect.
- May need to pretreat with allopurinol to protect patient from tumor lysis syndrome.
- Dermatologic radiation recall phenomena may occur.
- In combination with radiation therapy, mucosal reactions in the radiation field may be severe.
- Drug used in the treatment of chronic myelogenous leukemia (CML) in chronic phase, as a radiosensitizer (primary brain tumors, head and neck cancer, cancer of the cervix or uterus, non-small-cell lung cancer), and in sickle cell anemia.
- Drug should not be used during pregnancy, or by breast-feeding mothers as drug is excreted in breast milk.
- Dose modification in renal dysfunction: Reduce dose by 50% if creatinine clearance 10–50 mL/min; reduce dose 80% (give only 20% of dose) if creatinine clearance < 10 mL/min.

Potential Toxicities/Side Effects and the Nursing Process

I. INFECTION AND BLEEDING related to BONE MARROW DEPRESSION

Defining Characteristics: WBC begins to decrease 24–48 hours after beginning therapy, with nadir in 10 days and recovery within 10–30 days. Leukopenia more common than thrombocytopenia and anemia, and is dose-related.

Nursing Implications: Assess CBC, WBC with differential, and platelet count prior to drug administration, as well as for signs/symptoms of infection or bleeding. Doses may need to be reduced if patient has undergone prior radiotherapy or chemotherapy. Dose must be reduced if patient has renal dysfunction. Discuss any abnormalities with physician prior to drug administration. Teach patient signs/symptoms of infection and bleeding, and instruct to report them immediately. Teach self-care measures to minimize risk of infection and bleeding, including avoidance of OTC aspirin-containing medications.

II. ALTERED NUTRITION, LESS THAN BODY REQUIREMENTS, related to NAUSEA AND VOMITING, DIARRHEA, STOMATITIS, ANOREXIA, HEPATIC DYSFUNCTION

Defining Characteristics: Nausea and vomiting are uncommon, anorexia is mild to moderate, stomatitis is uncommon, diarrhea is uncommon, and hepatic dysfunction is rare, although abnormal LFTs may occur.

Nursing Implications: Premedicate with antiemetics as needed. Teach self-administration of prescribed medications. Instruct patient to report nausea/vomiting, diarrhea, anorexia, and stomatitis. Teach patient oral hygiene regimen and assess baseline oral mucosa. Monitor baseline LFTs, and monitor them periodically during therapy.

III. POTENTIAL ALTERATION IN FLUID/ELECTROLYTES/RENAL ELIMINATION STATUS related to TUMOR LYSIS SYNDROME

Defining Characteristics: When drug is first started in patients with high tumor burden, e.g., CML with high WBC, this often results in rapid death of a large number of malignant cells. The lysis or breakdown of these cells results in the release of intracellular contents into the systemic circulation. The resulting metabolic abnormalities are hyperkalemia, hyperphosphatemia, hypocalcemia, and hyperuricemia. If these persist, renal failure with oliguria can result.

Nursing Implications: Assess baseline chemistries, including metabolic panel, renal function. Expect that if the patient is at risk for the development of tumor lysis syndrome, the patient will begin allopurinol 200–300 mg/m^2/day prior to therapy, and receive hydration with alkalination (e.g., 50–100 mEq bicarbonate added per liter) to deliver 3 liters/m^2/day. Assess serum potassium, phosphate, calcium, uric acid, and BUN and creatinine at least daily, and discuss any abnormalities with physician to revise current regimen. Monitor I/O, weights, and total body balance carefully, and at least daily.

IV. SENSORY/PERCEPTUAL ALTERATIONS related to DROWSINESS, HALLUCINATIONS, OTHER CNS EFFECTS

Defining Characteristics: Drug crosses the BBB, so CNS effects may occur, such as drowsiness, confusion, disorientation, headache, vertigo; symptoms last $<$ 24 hours.

Nursing Implications: Assess baseline mental status and neurologic functioning. Instruct patient to report signs/symptoms, and reassure that they will resolve. If symptoms persist, discuss interrupting drug with physician.

V. POTENTIAL SEXUAL/REPRODUCTIVE DYSFUNCTION related to DRUG EFFECTS

Defining Characteristics: Drug is mutagenic and teratogenic. Drug is excreted in breast milk.

Nursing Implications: Assess patient's sexual patterns and reproductive goals. Discuss with patient and partner potential toxicity and impact on sexuality. Provide information, emotional support, and referral as needed. Patient should use contraceptive measures; a mother receiving the drug should not breast-feed.

Drug: idarubicin (Idamycin, 4-Demethoxydaunorubicin)

Class: Antitumor antibiotic.

Mechanism of Action: Cell cycle phase specific for S phase. Analogue of daunorubicin. Has a marked inhibitory effect on RNA synthesis.

Metabolism: Excreted primarily in the bile and urine, with approximately 25% of the intravenous dose accounted for over 5 days. The half-life is 6–9.4 hours.

Dosage/Range:

- 12 mg/m^2 qd × 3 days in combination with ara-C 100 mg/m^2 continuous infusion × 7 days, OR
- In combination with ara-C, 25 mg/m^2 IVP followed by ara-C 200 mg/m^2 continuous infusion daily × 5 days.
- 8–15 mg/m^2 IV every 3 weeks has been studied.

Drug Preparation:

- Available as a red powder.
- The drug is reconstituted with 0.9% Sodium Chloride injection to give a final concentration of 1 mg/1 mL.

Drug Administration:

- Drug is a vesicant. Administer IV over 10 to 15 minutes into the sidearm of a freely running IV.

Drug Interactions:

- Other myelosuppressive drugs: additive bone marrow suppression; monitor patient closely.
- Incompatible with heparin—causes precipitant.

Lab Effects/Interference:

- Decreased CBC.
- Increased LFTs, RFTs.

Special Considerations:

- Vesicant.
- Discolored urine (pink to red) may occur up to 48 hours after administration.
- Cardiomyopathy is less common and less severe than with doxorubicin and daunorubicin.
- Drug is light-sensitive.
- Dose-reduce for renal dysfunction.

- Dose-reduce for hepatic dysfunction: give 50% of dose if serum bili is 2.5 mg/dL; do not give dose if serum bili is > 5 mg/dL.

Potential Toxicities/Side Effects and the Nursing Process

I. INFECTION AND BLEEDING related to BONE MARROW DEPRESSION

Defining Characteristics: Hematologic toxicity is dose limiting. Leukopenia nadir 10–20 days with recovery in 1–2 weeks. Thrombocytopenia usually follows leukopenia and is mild. Bone marrow toxicity is not cumulative.

Nursing Implications: Evaluate WBC, neutrophil, and platelet count and discuss any abnormalities with physician prior to drug administration. Assess for signs/symptoms of infection or bleeding and instruct patient in signs/symptoms of infection and bleeding and to report them immediately. Suggest strategies to minimize risk of infection and bleeding, including avoidance of OTC aspirin-containing medications.

II. ALTERATION IN CARDIAC OUTPUT related to CUMULATIVE DOSES OF IDARUBICIN

Defining Characteristics: Cardiac toxicity is similar characteristically but less severe than that seen with daunorubicin and doxorubicin; CHF due to cardiomyopathy seen after large cumulative doses.

Nursing Implications: Assess cardiac status prior to chemotherapy administration: signs/symptoms of CHF, quality/regularity and rate of heartbeat, results of prior GBPS or other test of LVEF. Teach patient to report dyspnea, palpitations, swelling in extremities. Maintain accurate records of total dose; expect GBPS to be repeated periodically during treatment and the drug to be discontinued if there is a significant drop in heart function.

III. ALTERED NUTRITION, LESS THAN BODY REQUIREMENTS, related to NAUSEA/VOMITING, ANOREXIA, STOMATITIS, DIARRHEA, AND HEPATIC DYSFUNCTION

Defining Characteristics: Nausea/vomiting is usually mild to moderate, although it is seen to some degree in most patients; anorexia commonly occurs; stomatitis is mild; diarrhea is infrequent and mild; hepatitis is rare but may occur, and there are also disturbances in LFTs.

Nursing Implications: Premedicate with combination antiemetics and continue protection for 24 hours. If patient has a central line, slower infusion of drug over 1 hour decreases nausea/vomiting. Encourage small, frequent meals of bland foods. Anorexia occurs frequently: teach patient or caregiver to make foods ahead of time and use spices; encourage weekly weights. Stomatitis and esophagitis may occur in patients who have received prior radiation and during posttreatment visits. Teach patient oral hygiene regimen and self-assessment techniques. Encourage patient to report onset of diarrhea; administer or teach patient to self-administer antidiarrheal medications. Monitor SGOT, SGPT, LDH, alk phos, and bili periodically during treatment. Notify physician of any elevations.

IV. ALTERATION IN SKIN INTEGRITY related to ALOPECIA, SKIN CHANGES

Defining Characteristics: Alopecia occurs in about 30% of patients after oral drug and can be partial after IV drug; begins after 3+ weeks and hair may grow back while on therapy; may be slight to diffuse thinning. Skin changes include darkening of nail beds, skin ulcer/necrosis, sensitivity to sunlight, skin itching at irradiated areas, radiation recall, and potential necrosis with extravasation.

Nursing Implications: Discuss with patient hair loss, anticipated impact, and strategies to decrease distress, e.g., obtaining wig prior to hair loss. Assess disturbance of body image from hyperpigmentation and discuss strategies to minimize this, e.g., nail polish. Drug must be administered via patent IV. Assess need for venous access device early. If drug administered as continuous infusion, IT MUST BE GIVEN VIA A CENTRAL LINE.

V. POTENTIAL SEXUAL/REPRODUCTIVE DYSFUNCTION related to DRUG EFFECTS

Defining Characteristics: Gonadal function and fertility may be affected (may be permanent or transient). Reported to be excreted in breast milk.

Nursing Implications: As appropriate, explore with patient and partner issues of reproductive and sexuality patterns and impact chemotherapy will have; discuss strategies to preserve sexuality and reproductive health (e.g., contraception, sperm banking).

Drug: idoxifene (investigational)

Class: Synthetic tamoxifen analogue, nonsteroidal antiestrogen.

Mechanism of Action: Overcomes tamoxifen limitations, such as the estrogenic effects that tamoxifen possesses, and maximizes antiestrogen activity. (Only about 50% of estrogen-positive women with breast cancer respond to tamoxifen, acquired resistance to tamoxifen eventually develops, and it is probable that the estrogen agonist activity of tamoxifen accounts for the increased risk of developing endometrial cancer after tamoxifen therapy.) Drug has 2.5–5-fold higher affinity for estrogen receptors than tamoxifen. It is 1.5-fold more effective in inhibiting estrogen-induced growth in tumor cells, and potently inhibits calmodulin activity (important in breast cancer cell growth) (Coombes et al, 1995).

Metabolism: Peak plasma levels at 2–8 hours after a single dose, achieving steady-state levels with daily dosing in 6–12 weeks, as compared to tamoxifen's 2–6 weeks, and possessing a very long elimination phase (terminal half-life is 23.3 ± 5 days, about three times longer than tamoxifen).

Dosage/Range:

- Doses studied include 10- to 60-mg daily dosing for 2 weeks, and then 20-mg maintenance doses.
- Refer to study protocol.

Drug Preparation:

- None.

Drug Administration:

- Oral.

Drug Interactions:

- Unknown, but probably similar to tamoxifen.

Lab Effects/Interference:

- None known.

Special Considerations:

- Possesses ability to reverse multi-anticancer drug resistance mediated by P-glycoprotein (at least as effective as tamoxifen and verapamil).
- Probably has partial cross-resistance with tamoxifen, so may be effective in tamoxifen-resistant patients.

Potential Toxicities/Side Effects and the Nursing Process

I. ALTERATION IN NUTRITION, LESS THAN BODY REQUIREMENTS, related to NAUSEA AND VOMITING

Defining Characteristics: Nausea and vomiting may occur and are transient.

Nursing Implications: Inform patient of possibility of nausea, vomiting, and anorexia. Encourage small, frequent feedings of high-calorie, high-protein foods. Assess need for antiemetic medications, and discuss with physician. Teach patient self-administration as needed.

II. ACTIVITY INTOLERANCE related to TIREDNESS, LETHARGY, WEAKNESS

Defining Characteristics: Tiredness, lethargy, weakness may occur, but do not appear to be dose-related.

Nursing Implications: Assess baseline activity level and changes that occur with drug. Discuss with patient impact of activity intolerance or symptoms on quality of life.

Drug: ifosfamide (Ifex)

Class: Alkylating agent.

Mechanism of Action: Destroys DNA throughout the cell cycle by binding to protein and by DNA crosslinking and causing chain scission as well as inhibition of DNA synthesis. Analogue of cyclophosphamide and is cell cycle phase nonspecific. Ifosfamide has been shown to be effective in tumors previously resistant to cyclophosphamide. Activated by microsomes in the liver.

Metabolism: Only about 50% of the drug is metabolized, with much of the drug excreted in the urine almost completely unchanged. Half-life is 13.8 hours for high dose vs 3–10 hours for lower doses.

Dosage/Range:
- IV bolus/push: 50 mg/kg/day, OR.
- 700 mg–2 grams/m²/day × 5 days, OR.
- 2400 mg/m²/day × 3 days.
- Continuous infusion: 1200 mg/m²/day × 5 days.
- Single dose: 5000 mg/m² q3–4 weeks.
- Dose-reduce by 25–50% if serum creatinine is 2.1–3.0 mg/dL and hold if creatinine > 3.0 mg/dL.
- High dose (bone marrow transplant/stem cell rescue): 7.5–16 grams/m² IV in divided doses over several days.

Drug Preparation:
- Available as a powder and should be reconstituted with sterile water for injection.
- Solution is chemically stable for 7 days, but discard after 8 hours due to lack of bacteriostatic preservative in the solution.
- May be diluted further in either 5% Dextrose or 0.9% Sodium Chloride.

Drug Administration:
- IV bolus: Administer over 30 minutes. Mesna (20% of ifosfamide dose) should be administered with ifosfamide: mesna is begun 15 minutes prior to ifosfamide and repeated at 4 and 8 hours after the ifosfamide (see drug sheet on mesna). Mesna, ascorbic acid, and mucomycin have been used to protect the bladder. Pre- and posthydration (1500–2000 mL/day) or continuous bladder irrigations are recommended to prevent hemorrhagic cystitis.
- Continuous infusion: Administer intravenously for 5 days. Mesna is mixed with ifosfamide in equal amounts (1:1 mix). Prior to initiating continuous

infusion, mesna is given IVB (10% of total ifosfamide dose). Following completion of the infusion, mesna alone should be infused for 12–24 hours to protect from delayed drug excretion activity against the bladder.

Drug Interactions:

- Activity/toxicity affected by allopurinol, chloroquine, phenothiazides, potassium iodide, chloramphenicol, imipramine, vitamin A, corticosteroids, succinylcholine.
- Mesna binds to and inactivates ifosfamide metabolite, thus preventing bladder toxicity.

Lab Effects/Interference:

- Decreased CBC.
- Increased RFTs.

Special Considerations:

- Metabolic toxicity is increased by simultaneous administration of barbiturates.
- Renal function: BUN, serum creatinine, and creatinine clearance must be determined prior to treatment.
- Therapy requires the concomitant administration of a uroprotector such as mesna and pre- and posthydration; may also require catheterization and constant bladder irrigation, and/or ascorbic acid.
- Test urine for occult blood.
- Dose-limiting toxicity has been renal and bladder dysfunction.
- Increased risk for toxicity in patients who have received prior or concurrent radiotherapy or other antineoplastic agents.
- Drug active in cancers of lung, breast, ovary, pancreas, and stomach; Hodgkin's and NHL, acute and chronic lymphocytic leukemias.

Potential Toxicities/Side Effects and the Nursing Process

I. ALTERED URINARY ELIMINATION related to HEMORRHAGIC CYSTITIS AND RENAL TOXICITY

Defining Characteristics: Symptoms of bladder irritation; hemorrhagic cystitis with hematuria, dysuria, urinary frequency; preventable with uroprotection and hydration. Symptoms of renal toxicity; increased BUN and serum creatinine, decreased urine creatinine clearance (usually reversible); acute tubular necrosis, pyelonephritis, glomerular dysfunction; metabolic acidosis.

Nursing Implications: Assess presence of RBC in urine prior to successive doses, especially if symptoms are present, as well as BUN and creatinine. Administer drug with concomitant uroprotector (e.g., mesna). Encourage prehydration: oral intake of 2–3 L/day prior to chemotherapy; posthydration: increase oral fluids to 2–3 L for 2 days after chemotherapy. If possible, administer drug in morning to minimize drug accumulation in bladder during sleep. Instruct patient to empty bladder every 2–3 hours, before bedtime, and during night when awake. Monitor urinary output and total body balance. Assess urinary elimination pattern prior to each drug dose. If rigorous regimen is adhered to, minimal renal toxicity will result. Monitor BUN and creatinine.

II. ALTERED NUTRITION, LESS THAN BODY REQUIREMENTS, related to NAUSEA AND VOMITING, HEPATOTOXICITY

Defining Characteristics: Nausea and vomiting occur in 58% of patients; dose and schedule-dependent, with increased severity with higher dose and rapid injection. Occurs within a few hours of drug administration and may last 3 days. Elevations of serum transaminase and alk phos may occur; usually transient and resolve spontaneously without apparent sequelae.

Nursing Implications: Premedicate with antiemetics and continue prophylactically to prevent nausea and vomiting for 24 hours at least for the first treatment. Encourage small, frequent feedings of cool, bland foods and liquids. Refer to section on nausea and vomiting. Monitor LFTs during treatment.

III. INFECTION AND BLEEDING related to BONE MARROW DEPRESSION

Defining Characteristics: Leukopenia is mild to moderate. Thrombocytopenia and anemia are rare. Dosage adjustment may be necessary when ifosfamide is combined with other chemotherapy agents. Patients at risk for bone marrow depression include patients with impaired renal function and decreased bone marrow reserve (bone marrow metastases, prior XRT).

Nursing Implications: Evaluate WBC, with neutrophil, and platelet count and discuss any abnormalities with physician prior to drug administration. Assess for signs/symptoms of infection or bleeding and instruct patient in signs/symptoms of infection and bleeding, and to report them immediately; discuss strategies to minimize risk of infection and bleeding, including avoidance of OTC aspirin-containing medications. Assess patient's Hgb/HCT and signs/symptoms of fatigue; teach patient self-assessment and to alternate rest and activity as needed.

IV. ALTERATION IN SKIN INTEGRITY related to ALOPECIA, STERILE PHLEBITIS, SKIN CHANGES

Defining Characteristics: The incidence of alopecia is 83%, with 50% experiencing severe hair loss in 2–4 weeks. Sterile phlebitis may occur at injection site; irritation occurs with extravasation. Hyperpigmentation, dermatitis, and nail ridging may occur.

Nursing Implications: Discuss with patient anticipated impact of hair loss; suggest wig, as appropriate, prior to actual hair loss. Explore with patient response to hair loss and alternative strategies to minimize distress. Carefully monitor injection site during drug administration for signs/symptoms of phlebitis, irritation, vein patency. Assess skin integrity. Assess impact of skin changes on body image. Discuss strategies to minimize distress.

V. POTENTIAL SEXUAL/REPRODUCTIVE DYSFUNCTION related to DRUG EFFECTS

Defining Characteristics: Drug is carcinogenic, mutagenic, and teratogenic. Drug is excreted in breast milk.

Nursing Implications: As appropriate, explore with patient and partner issues of reproductive and sexual patterns, and impact chemotherapy will have. Discuss strategies to preserve sexuality and reproductive health (e.g., sperm banking, contraception).

VI. SENSORY/PERCEPTUAL ALTERATIONS related to CONFUSION, ACTIVITY INTOLERANCE, FATIGUE

Defining Characteristics: Intact drug passes easily into CNS; however, active metabolites do not. Lethargy and confusion may be seen with high doses, lasting 1–8 hours, usually spontaneously reversible. CNS side effects occur in about 12% of patients treated, including somnolence, confusion, depressive psychosis, hallucinations. Less frequent side effects: dizziness, disorientation, cranial nerve dysfunction, seizures. Incidence of CNS side effects may be higher in patients with compromised renal function, as well as in patients receiving high doses.

Nursing Implications: Identify patients at risk (decreased renal function) and observe closely. Assess neurologic and mental status prior to and during drug administration and on follow-up. Instruct patient to report any alterations in behavior, sensation, perception. Develop a plan of care with patient and family if side effects develop to manage distress and promote safety.

Drug: irinotecan (Camptosar, Camptothecan-11, CPT-11)

Class: Topoisomerase I inhibitor.

Mechanism of Action: Induces protein-linked DNA single-strand breaks and blocks DNA and RNA synthesis in dividing cells, thus preventing cells from entering mitosis. The active metabolite, SN-38, prevents repair (religation) of previous, reversible single-strand breaks in DNA by binding to topoisomerase I. Topoisomerase I is an enzyme that relaxes tension in the DNA helix torsion by initially causing this single-strand break in DNA so that DNA replication can occur. Topoisomerases I and II then work together to bring about replication, transcription, and recombination of DNA material. Topoisomerase I is found in higher-than-normal concentrations in certain malignant cells, such as colon adenocarcinoma cells and non-Hodgkin's lymphoma cells.

Metabolism: Metabolized to its active metabolite SN-38 in the liver; 11–20% of the drug is excreted in the urine, and 5–39% in the bile over a 48-hour period. Mean terminal half-life is 6 hours, while that of SN-38 is 10 hours. Drug is moderately protein-bound (30–68%), while SN-38 is highly protein-bound (95%).

Dosage/Range:
IFL (Saltz) regimen:
- Metastatic colorectal cancer (in combination with 5-FU and leukovorin): Irinotecan 125 mg/m^2 IV over 90 minutes (day 1, 8, 15, 22); leukovorin 20 mg/m^2 IVB immediately after irinotecan (day 1, 8, 15, 22); 5-FU 500 mg/m^2 IVB immediately after leukovorin (day 1, 8, 15, 22), followed by 2-week rest period (total, 6-week cycle). Requires *very* close monitoring and supportive care.
- Colon and rectal cancers that have recurred following 5-FU-based therapy: Starting dose is 125 mg/m^2 IV over 90 minutes weekly × 4 weeks, followed by a 2-week rest period. This 6-week cycle is then repeated.
- Dose increase up to 150 mg/m^2 as tolerated.
- 350 mg/m^2 IV day 1 repeated every 21 days (300 mg/m^2 for patients > 70 years old, those who have received prior pelvic/abdominal radiotherapy, or those with a performance status of 2).
- Dose modifications based on tolerance of prior cycle of therapy (see Tables 1.9a–d).

Douillard
- Metastatic colorectal cancers: Day 1: Irinotecan 180 mg/m^2 IV over 90 min, at the same time as Leucovorin 200 mg/m^2 IV over 2hr through separate arms of a Y-tubing, followed by 5-FU 400 mg/m^2 IVB, then 22 hr 5-FU 600 mg/m^2 IV continuous infusion (CI). Day 2: leucovorin 200 mg/m^2 IV over 2 hr, then 5-FU 400 mg/m^2 IVB, then 22 hr 5-FU 600 mg/m^2 IV continuous infusion (CI). Repeat q 2 weeks.

Drug Preparation:
- Store unopened vials at room temperature and protect from light.
- Dilute and mix drug in 5% Dextrose (preferred) or 0.9% Sodium Chloride to a final concentration of 0.12–1.1 mg/mL. Commonly, the drug is diluted in 500 mL 5% Dextrose.

- Diluted drug is stable 24 hours at room temperature. If diluted in 5% Dextrose, the drug is stable for 48 hours if refrigerated (2–8°C [36–46°F]) and protected from light.

Drug Administration:

- Administer IV bolus over 90 minutes.

Lab Effects/Interference:

- Decreased CBC.

Special Considerations:

- IFL (Saltz) regimen may result in increased deaths. Use cautiously and monitor patients closely, especially patients with ↓ Performance Status (2), elderly, or patients with prior pelvic/abdominal radiation, or with hepatic dysfunction. Assess for s/s dehydration, febrile neutropenia, diarrhea. Modify dose per manufacturer's guidelines.
- Independent expert panel reviewed clinical trial data and did not recommend changes in starting doses; potential life-threatening toxicity was highlighted, especially severe myelosuppression, and both *early* and late diarrhea.
- Patient must have weekly assessment for toxicity.
- Patient must have dose reduction as recommended; drug should not be administered if the patient is neutropenic or has diarrhea.
- Patient must be taught to notify provider if toxicity develops, and how to manage diarrhea, nausea, vomiting, potential infection. (www.asco.org/people/nr/html/jco-early.htm.)
- Drug is indicated for first-line treatment of metastatic colon or rectal cancer in combination with 5-FU and leukovorin, and as a single agent for colorectal cancer recurring or progressing after treatment with 5-FU.
- Dose-limiting toxicities are diarrhea and severe myelosuppression.
- Drug is teratogenic and thus contraindicated in pregnant women; women of childbearing age should be taught and encouraged to use birth control.
- Drug is an irritant. If extravasation occurs, the manufacturer recommends flushing the IV site with sterile water, and then applying ice.
- All patients should receive self-care instructions on management of diarrhea, self-administration of loperamide for delayed diarrhea, and assessment of the patient's ability to purchase loperamide, and ability to comply with instructions.
- Patient response to treatment is usually apparent within two courses of therapy (12 weeks).
- Flushing (vasodilation) may occur during drug infusion, and usually does not require intervention.
- Patient educational material is available from Pharmacia/Upjohn Co.

- Rarely, patients may lack an enzyme necessary for drug metabolism, resulting in increased toxicity (Gilbert's syndrome, abnormal gucouronidation of bilirubin).
- Dose reductions must be made for neutropenia and severe diarrhea, and are different for combination therapy (irinotecan/5-FU/leukovorin) and irinotecan as a single agent.
- Contraindications: serum BR > 2.0 mg/dL although no studies done, grades ¾.neutropenia occurred in patients with BR 1–2 mg/dL.

Potential Toxicities/Side Effects and the Nursing Process

I. ALTERATION IN ELIMINATION related to DIARRHEA

Defining Characteristics: Diarrhea may be early or late. Early diarrhea is characterized by onset within 24 hours of drug dose and is mediated by cholinergic pathway(s), as the metabolite SN-38 inhibits acetylcholinesterase; diaphoresis and abdominal cramping may precede diarrhea, and may be prevented by atropine. Other cholinergic effects that may appear are salivation, lacrimation, visual disturbances, piloerection, and bradycardia. This can be managed effectively with atropine 0.25–1.0 mg IV or scopalomine. Late diarrhea occurs > 24 hours after the drug dose, can be severe, prolonged, and lead to dehydration and electrolyte imbalance; the etiology appears related to changes in intestinal mucosal epithelium that prevent the reabsorption of water and electrolytes, which are then lost during diarrhea. 88% of patients may experience late diarrhea, and 31% have severe, or grade ¾ diarrhea. Loperamide is effective in halting late diarrhea. Irinotecan should be held for grade 3 diarrhea (7–9 stools/day, incontinence, or severe cramping) and grade 4 (> 10 stools/day, grossly bloody stool, or need for parenteral support). Once recovered, decrease drug dose at next treatment per manufacturer's guidelines and per physician order.

Nursing Implications: Acute diarrhea: teach patient to report diarrhea, sweating, and abdominal cramping during or after drug administration. Administer atropine 0.25–1 mg IVP per physician order, unless contraindicated, to prevent diarrhea. Delayed diarrhea: teach patient self-management of diarrhea (diet, fluids, avoidance of laxatives), and to notify nurse or physician of vomiting, fever, or if signs/symptoms of dehydration occur (fainting, light-headedness, dizziness). Teaching about diet should include drinking 8–10 large glasses of fluid/day, including soup/broth, soda, Gatorade; avoiding dairy products; eating small meals often; using BRAT diet (bananas, rice, applesauce, toast); and adding other foods as tolerated, such as bland, low-fiber foods, white chicken meat without skin, scrambled eggs, crackers, or pasta without sauce. Also teach patient to avoid foods that worsen diarrhea (fatty, fried, or greasy foods, high-fiber foods with bran, raw fruits and vegetables, popcorn, beans, nuts, chocolate). Review patient's medication profile, including over-the-counter medicines, and teach patient to stop taking any laxatives. Teach patient to avoid cigarette smoking to promote comfort. Instruct patient to record stools, and to take loperamide, not as indicated on the medication package, but as instructed: At the first episode of late-onset diarrhea, take 4 mg (2 [2-mg] capsules) of loperamide, then 2 mg (1 capsule) every 2 hours until free of diarrhea for at least 12 hours. Take a 4-mg dose (2 [2-mg] capsules) at bedtime (Camptosar recommendations). Patient should notify doctor or nurse if diarrhea is unrelieved by loperamide taken as instructed. Assess patient's ability to purchase loperamide if impoverished, and identify other sources that can provide the medication prior to patient's discharge from clinic after drug therapy. Review patient's medication profile to ensure that the patient is not taking any cathartics. Diarrhea must be monitored closely and managed aggressively to prevent morbidity and mortality.

II. POTENTIAL FOR INFECTION, ANEMIA related to BONE MARROW DEPRESSION

Defining Characteristics: Leukopenia has been noted in 63% of patients on single-dose schedules, with an overall neutropenia incidence of 54%, and grade ¾ neutropenia occurring in 26% of patients. Thrombocytopenia is uncommon, occurring in about 3% of patients. Anemia is common (61%). Nadir is commonly on day 6–9.

Nursing Implications: Evaluate WBC, with neutrophil, and platelet count, and discuss any abnormalities with physician prior to drug administration. Refer to Special Considerations section for dosage modifications based on hematologic toxicity. Assess patient tolerance of chemotherapy and nadir blood counts, especially Cycle 1. Assess for signs/symptoms of infection or bleeding; instruct patient in signs/symptoms of infection and bleeding, and to report them immediately. If febrile neutropenia develops, assess and begin antibiotic therapy ASAP. Instruct in measures to minimize risk of infection and bleeding, including avoidance of OTC aspirin-containing medications. Assess patient's Hgb/HCT and signs/symptoms of fatigue; teach patient self-assessment and to alternate rest and activity as needed.

III. POTENTIAL ALTERATION IN NUTRITION, LESS THAN BODY REQUIREMENTS, related to NAUSEA AND VOMITING, DEHYDRATION

Defining Characteristics: Moderate to severe nausea and vomiting occur in 35–60% of patients, with 17% experiencing NCI grade ¾ nausea and 13% experiencing NCI grade ¾ vomiting. Aggressive combination antiemetics are effective in preventing nausea/vomiting.

Nursing Implications: Premedicate with aggressive combination antiemetics such as serotonin antagonist (dolestron, granisetron, or ondansetron) plus dexamethasone 10 mg IV 30 minutes prior to chemotherapy to prevent nausea and vomiting. Encourage small, frequent meals of cool, bland foods and liquids. Teach patients to monitor their fluid intake, and take daily weights if nausea/vomiting occurs. Assess for signs/symptoms of fluid and electrolyte imbalance. Teach patients self-assessment, and instruct to notify doctor or nurse if these occur. Late-onset nausea and vomiting may occur, and dopamine antagonists such as prochlorperazine are then recommended. If dehydration develops, replace fluid and electrolytes to prevent worsening dehydration and cardiovascular complications.

IV. POTENTIAL FOR IMPAIRED GAS EXCHANGE, POTENTIAL related to DYSPNEA, PULMONARY INFILTRATES, FEVER

Defining Characteristics: Pulmonary effects may occur in up to 22% of patients, ranging from transient dyspnea to pulmonary infiltrates, fever, increased cough, and decreased DLCO in a small number of patients.

Nursing Implications: Assess baseline pulmonary status, and teach patient to report any changes. Assess pulmonary status prior to each treatment and at visits between treatment. If patient develops dyspnea, discuss patient having PFTs with physician, and evaluating whether related to drug. Teach patient to manage dyspnea if it occurs, including alternating activity and rest periods.

Drug: ketoconazole (investigational as an anticancer agent)

Class: Azole antifungal, antiadrenal.

Mechanism of Action: High-dose therapy interferes with conversion of lanosterol to cholesterol, a major precursor of several hormones. Drug has inhibitory effect on gonadal and adrenal steroid synthesis, thus lowering serum testosterone concentrations and suppressing corticosteroid secretion. Both hormones return to baseline levels when ketoconazole therapy is discontinued.

Metabolism: Rapidly absorbed from GI tract in acid environment. Decreased absorption in patients with gastric hypochlorhydria (25% of all AIDS patients) or in patients taking medications that raise pH (antacids, H_2 antagonists). Distributed widely but cerebrospinal penetration is unpredictable. Drug is ~90% protein-bound. Partially metabolized in liver, and mostly excreted in the feces via bile.

Dosage/Range:

- For lymphoma: 200 mg/day PO.

- For metastatic prostate cancer: 400 mg PO 3 times per day with hydrocortisone 20 mg PO q A.M. and 10 mg PO q P.M.

Drug Preparation:

- Store in tightly closed container at < 40°C (104°F).

Drug Administration:

- Orally in single dose.
- May take with meals to decrease GI side effects (unclear whether food increases absorption).
- In patients with gastric achlorhydria, patient may be instructed to dissolve ketoconazole in 4 mL aqueous solution of 0.2 N hydrochloric acid and drink through a straw; follow with 4 oz (120 mL) water.

Drug Interactions:

- Drugs that increase gastric pH: Antacids, cimetidine, rantidine, famotidine, sucralfate decrease ketoconazole absorption; give these drugs at least 2 hours after ketoconazole.
- Other hepatotoxic drugs: Use cautiously, and monitor liver function studies closely.
- Rifampin or rifampin plus isoniazid: Decreased ketoconazole levels, especially if isoniazid is taken as well. Increase ketoconazole dose.
- Acyclovir: Synergism and increased antiviral action against herpes simplex virus.
- Norfloxacin: Theoretically increases antifungal action of ketoconazole, but studies are inconsistent.
- Coumarin anticoagulants: Increased PT; monitor patient closely and decrease anticoagulant dose accordingly.
- Cyclosporine: Increased cyclosporine serum level; monitor serum level and decrease cyclosporine dose accordingly.
- Phenytoin: May have altered serum levels of phenytoin or ketoconazole; monitor serum levels of each and adjust dosages accordingly.
- Theophylline: May decrease theophylline serum concentrations; monitor serum levels and increase dosage accordingly.
- Terfenadine (Seldane): May increase terfenadine serum level with possible prolongation of QT interval on EKG, and/or ventricular tachycardia. Do not administer concomitantly.
- Corticosteroids: May increase corticosteroid serum level; may need to decrease dosage.

Lab Effects/Interference:

Major clinical significance:

- ALT, alk phos, AST, serum bili values may be elevated.
- ACTH-induced serum corticosteroid concentrations and serum testosterone concentrations may be decreased by doses of 800 mg/day of ketoconazole;

serum testosterone concentrations are abolished by values of 1.6 g/day of ketoconzole but return to baseline values when ketoconazole is discontinued.

Special Considerations:

- Monitor liver function studies.
- High failure rate in HIV-infected patients due to achlorhydria.
- Addisonian crisis may occur if ketoconazole not given with hydrocortisone.

Potential Toxicities/Side Effects and the Nursing Process

I. ALTERATION IN MALE SEXUAL FUNCTION related to GYNECOMASTIA, BREAST TENDERNESS, OLIGOSPERMIA, DECREASED LIBIDO, AND IMPOTENCE

Defining Characteristics: Breast enlargement and tenderness may occur in some men, lasting weeks to duration of therapy. Oligospermia, azoospermia, decreased libido, and impotence may also occur.

Nursing Implications: Inform patient that these side effects may occur. Explore with patient and partner reproductive and sexual patterns, and impact that therapy may have. Provide information and supportive counseling, and referral as appropriate. Assess for presence of side effects on follow-up, as well as comfort level, breast tenderness, and impact on body image and sexual relationships.

II. ALTERATION IN NUTRITION, LESS THAN BODY REQUIREMENTS, related to GI SIDE EFFECTS

Defining Characteristics: Nausea, vomiting is seen in 3–10% of patients; anorexia affects about 10% as well. Diarrhea, abdominal pain, flatulence, constipation may occur less frequently. Increased LFTs may occur: AST, ALT, alk phos. Hepatotoxicity is less common, is usually reversible, and is rarely fatal.

Nursing Implications: Assess baseline nutritional and elimination status. Instruct patient to report GI disturbances. Administer and teach patient to self-administer antiemetics and antidiarrheals as needed and as ordered. Although an acidic environment enhances absorption, taking ketoconazole with milk or food reduces nausea. Alternatively, starting patient at lower dose and gradually increasing dose will also reduce nausea. Teach patient importance of nutritious diet, and suggest small, frequent, high-calorie, high-protein meals as appropriate. Assess baseline LFTs and monitor periodically during treatment. Discuss abnormalities and drug interruption with physician. Assess whether taking other hepatotoxic drugs (see Special Considerations section). Assess for increased fatigue, jaundice, dark urine, pale stools (signs of hepatotoxicity) and discuss drug discontinuance immediately with physician.

III. ALTERATION IN COMFORT related to GYNECOMASTIA AND BREAST TENDERNESS

Defining Characteristics: Breast enlargement and tenderness may occur in some men, lasting weeks to duration of therapy.

Nursing Implications: Assess for occurrence in male patients. Assess comfort level, degree of tenderness, and self-care measures used to increase comfort. Assess impact on body image.

IV. ALTERATION IN SKIN INTEGRITY related to ALLERGIC REACTION

Defining Characteristics: Rash, dermatitis, purpura, urticaria occur in 1% of patients; rarely, anaphylaxis may occur.

Nursing Implications: Assess baseline skin condition and integrity. Teach patient to report itch, rash, other skin changes. Teach patient skin care and symptomatic measures. If rash or dermatitis progresses, discuss drug discontinuance with physician. Assess for signs/symptoms of anaphylaxis.

V. ALTERATIONS IN SENSORY/PERCEPTUAL PATTERNS related to CNS EFFECTS

Defining Characteristics: Dizziness, headache, nervousness, insomnia, lethargy, somnolence, and paresthesia have occurred in ~1% of patients.

Nursing Implications: Assess baseline neurologic function and comfort, and monitor during treatment. Instruct patient to report any changes. Discuss any abnormalities with physician.

Drug: letrozole (Femara)

Class: Nonsteroidal aromatase inhibitor.

Mechanism of Action: Highly selective, potent agent that significantly suppresses (90%) serum estradiol levels within 14 days, without interfering with other steroid hormone synthesis. Binds to the heme group of aromatase, a cytochrome P-450 enzyme necessary for the conversion of androgens to estrogens. Aromatase is thus inhibited, leading to a significant reduction in plasma estradiol, estrone, and estrone sulfate. After six weeks of therapy, there is 97% suppression of estradiol.

Metabolism: Rapidly and completely absorbed after oral administration, with a terminal half-life of 2 days. Metabolized in the liver and excreted in the urine.

Dosage/Range:
- 2.5 mg PO qd.

Drug Preparation/Administration:
- Oral.

Drug Interactions:
- None known.

Lab Effects/Interference:
- Liver transaminases may be transiently elevated.

Special Considerations:
- Indicated for the first-line treatment of post-menopausal women with hormone receptor positive or unknown, locally advanced or metastatic breast cancer; the extended adjuvant treatment of early breast cancer in postmenopausal women who have received 5 years of adjuvant tamoxifen therapy; and treatment of advanced breast cancer in postmenopausal women with disease progression following antiestrogen therapy.
- Indicated for the first-line treatment of postmenopausal women with hormone receptor positive or unknown locally advanced or metastatic breast cancer. Also indicated for the treatment of postmenopausal women with disease progression on antiestrogen therapy.
- Letrozole was compared to tamoxifen in postmenopausal women and found to be superior in terms of response (30% vs 20%), time to disease progression (41 weeks vs 25 weeks), and rate of clinical benefit (49% vs 38%) (Mouridsen et al, 2001).
- Potent aromatase inhibitor with response rate of 20%.
- Drug has not been evaluated in premenopausal women.
- Glucocorticoid replacement is not necessary.
- About 200 times more potent than aminoglutethamide.
- Letrozole is being studied as an adjunct to in vitro fertilization (IVF) for women with breast cancer who wish to have a child, given with FSH. The addition of either tamoxifen or letrozole with FSH increased the number of ovarian follicles, more mature eggs, and more embryos. At 1.5 years, there is no increased risk of recurrence compared to controls (Oktay et al, 2005).

Potential Toxicities/Side Effects and the Nursing Process

I. ALTERATION IN COMFORT related to PAIN, FATIGUE, AND HOT FLASHES

Defining Characteristics: Most common side effects were musculoskeletal pain (21%: muscle, skeletal, back, arm, leg), arthralgia (8%), headache (9%), fatigue (8%), and chest pain (6%). Hot flashes occur in approximately 6% of patients.

Nursing Considerations: Assess baseline comfort levels, and teach patient that this discomfort may occur. Teach patient symptomatic measures, and instruct to report if symptoms are unrelieved.

II. ALTERATION IN NUTRITION, LESS THAN BODY REQUIREMENTS, related to NAUSEA/VOMITING, ANOREXIA

Defining Characteristics: Nausea occurs in 13% of patients, with less frequent vomiting and anorexia.

Nursing Implications: Determine baseline weight, and monitor at each visit. Teach patient that these side effects may occur, and instruct to report this. Discuss strategies to minimize nausea, including diet and dosing time.

III. ALTERATION IN BOWEL ELIMINATION related to DIARRHEA AND CONSTIPATION

Defining Characteristics: Diarrhea or constipation occurs in about 6% of patients.

Nursing Implications: Assess for change in bowel patterns, and instruct patient to report diarrhea or constipation. Teach patient that diarrhea or constipation are usually relieved by nonprescription medications such as Kaolin pectate combinations (Kaopectate) for diarrhea, and stool softeners or Psyllium for constipation. Instruct patient to report unrelieved diarrhea or constipation.

Drug: leuprolide acetate (Lupron, Viadur)

Class: Antihormone.

Mechanism of Action: It is a luteinizing hormone-releasing hormone (LHRH) analogue that suppresses the secretion of follicle-stimulating hormone (FSH) and luteinizing hormone (LH) from the pituitary gland. The decrease in LH causes the Leydig cells to reduce testosterone production to castrate levels.

Metabolism: 95% of the drug is absorbed after SQ injection, and 85–100% of the drug is absorbed after IM or SQ injection. Drug is slightly protein bound (7–15%).

Dosage/Range:
- For palliative treatment of prostate cancer: Depot suspension 7.5 mg IM q month, OR 22.5 mg IM q 3 months, OR 30 mg IM q 4 months, OR Viadur implant 65 mg q 12 months, OR 1 mg/day SQ injection.

Drug Preparation:
- Use syringes, diluent, kit provided by manufacturer.
- Injection: 5 mg/mL; kit 5 mg/mL for 7.5-mg, 22.5-mg doses.

- Powder for injection: 7.5 mg.
- Viadur implant kit contains implant, implanter, and sterile field/supplies. Sterile gloves must be added. Procedure is sterile, and uses a special implant technology.

Drug Administration:
- Depot is administered IM or SQ.
- Daily solution is given SQ.
- Viadur: Kit contains specific directions for insertion of implant, removal, and reinsertion of subsequent dose after 1 year.

Drug Interactions:
- None reported.

Lab Effects/Interference:
- Decreased PSA, testosterone levels; increased calcium, decreased WBC, decreased serum total protein.
- Injection: Increased BUN and creatinine.
- Depot: Increased LDH, alk phos, AST, uric acid, cholesterol, LDL, triglycerides, glucose, WBC, phosphate; decreased potassium, platelets.

Special Considerations:
- Patient should be instructed in proper administration techniques, and in signs/symptoms of infection at site. Sites should be rotated. For Viadur, patient has implant inserted by MD/RN once yearly.
- Initially, drug causes increased LH secretion, resulting in increased testosterone secretion and tumor flare. Usually disappears after 2 weeks.
- Drug has been studied in the treatment of breast and islet cell cancers.
- Studies on Viadur show that implant delivers 120 micrograms of leuprolide acetate per day over 12 months, reducing testosterone levels to castration levels within 2–4 weeks after insertion.

Potential Toxicities/Side Effects and the Nursing Process

I. ALTERATION IN COMFORT related to HOT FLASHES, TUMOR FLARE, EDEMA

Defining Characteristics: Headache, dizziness, and hot flashes may occur. Vasodilation most common, with 67.9% incidence. Sweating may affect 5% of patients. Tumor flare may also occur initially (bone and tumor pain, transient increase in tumor size due to transient increase in testosterone levels). Breast tenderness has been reported. Peripheral edema may occur in 8% of patients.

Nursing Implications: Inform patient that symptoms may occur, that flare reaction will subside after the initial two weeks of therapy. Encourage patient to report symptoms early. Develop symptom management plan with patient and physician.

II. POTENTIAL SEXUAL DYSFUNCTION related to LIBIDO, IMPOTENCE

Defining Characteristics: Frequently causes decreased libido and erectile impotence in men. Gynecomastia occurs in 3–6.9% of patients. In women, amenorrhea occurs after ten weeks of therapy.

Nursing Implications: As appropriate, explore with patient and significant other issues of reproductive and sexual patterns and the impact chemotherapy may have on them. Discuss strategies to preserve sexuality and reproductive health.

III. DEPRESSION, POTENTIAL related to DRUG EFFECT

Defining Characteristics: Depression may affect up to 5.3% of patients, and less commonly, patients may develop emotional lability, insomnia, nervousness, anxiety.

Nursing Implications: Assess baseline affect and usual coping strategies. Teach patient to report change in affect. Assess effectiveness of coping strategies, encourage patient to verbalize feelings, and provide emotional support. Assess need for referral to psychiatric nurse specialist or social worker if supportive efforts ineffective.

IV. ALTERED NUTRITION, LESS THAN BODY REQUIREMENTS, related to GI SIDE EFFECTS

Defining Characteristics: Anorexia, nausea, and vomiting may occur rarely, with an incidence of < 5%.

Nursing Implications: If patients experience symptoms, encourage small, frequent feedings of favorite foods, especially high-calorie, high-protein foods. Monitor weight weekly. Assess incidence and pattern of nausea, vomiting, or anorexia if they occur. Discuss need for antiemetic with physician and patient.

V. ALTERATION IN SKIN INTEGRITY, POTENTIAL related to INSERTION, REMOVAL OF 12-MONTH IMPLANT

Defining Characteristics: Insertion and removal of implant caused local site bruising (34.8%) and burning (5.6%). In general, the reactions lasted two weeks, and then resolved completely. In about 10% of patients, reactions lasted longer than two weeks, or reactions didn't develop until after two weeks.

Nursing Implications: Assess baseline skin integrity after implant insertion, or removal. Teach patient that these reactions may occur, and will resolve, usually within two weeks. Teach patients to use local measures to minimize feeling of burning.

Drug: lomustine (CCNU, CeeNU)

Class: Alkylating agent (nitrosourea).

Mechanism of Action: Nitrosourea alkylates DNA with a reactive chloroethyl carbonium ion, producing strand breaks and crosslinks that inhibit RNA and DNA synthesis. Interferes with enzymes and histadine utilization. Is cell cycle phase nonspecific.

Metabolism: Completely absorbed from GI tract. Metabolized rapidly, partly protein-bound. Undergoes hepatic recirculation. Lipid soluble: crosses BBB; 75% excreted in urine within 4 days.

Dosage/Range:
- 130 mg/m^2 PO every 6 weeks.
- 100 mg/m^2 if given with other myelosuppressive drugs.

Drug Preparation:
- Oral: Available in 10-mg, 30-mg, and 100-mg capsules.

Drug Administration:
- Administer on an empty stomach at bedtime.

Drug Interactions:
- Myelosuppressive drugs increase hematologic toxicity; reduce dose.

Lab Effects/Interference:
- Decreased CBC.
- Increased LFTs, RFTs.

Special Considerations:
- Give orally on an empty stomach.
- Consumption of alcohol should be avoided for a short period after taking CCNU.
- Absorbed 30–60 minutes after administration; consequently, vomiting does not usually affect efficacy.

Potential Toxicities/Side Effects and the Nursing Process

I. INFECTION AND BLEEDING related to MYELOSUPPRESSION

Defining Characteristics: Nadir of platelets: 26–34 days, lasting 6–10 days; nadir of WBC: 41–46 days, lasting 9–14 days. Delayed and cumulative bone marrow depression with successive dosing: recovery takes 6–8 weeks. Bone marrow depression is dose-limiting toxicity.

Nursing Implications: Drug should be administered every 6–8 weeks due to delayed nadir and recovery. Monitor CBC, platelets prior to drug administration (WBC > 4000/mm^3 and platelets > 100,000/mm^3). Dispense only one dose at a time.

II. ALTERATION IN NUTRITION, LESS THAN BODY REQUIREMENTS related to NAUSEA/VOMITING, ANOREXIA, DIARRHEA

Defining Characteristics: Onset of nausea/vomiting occurs 2–6 hours after taking dose; may be severe. Anorexia may last for several days. Diarrhea is uncommon.

Nursing Implications: Administer drug on an empty stomach at bedtime. Premedicate with antiemetic and sedative or hypnotic to promote sleep. Discourage food or fluid intake for two hours after drug administration. Encourage small, frequent feedings of favorite foods. Encourage high-calorie, high-protein foods; monitor weekly weights. Encourage patient to report onset of diarrhea. Administer or teach patient to self-administer antidiarrheal medication.

III. ALTERATION IN URINARY ELIMINATION related to RENAL COMPROMISE

Defining Characteristics: After prolonged therapy with high cumulative doses, tubular atrophy, glomerular sclerosis, and interstitial nephritis have occurred, leading to renal failure.

Nursing Implications: Monitor BUN, creatinine prior to dosing, especially in patients receiving prolonged or high cumulative dose therapy. If abnormalities are noted, a creatinine clearance should be determined.

IV. POTENTIAL FOR SEXUAL DYSFUNCTION related to MUTAGENIC AND TERATOGENIC QUALITIES OF CCNU

Defining Characteristics: Drug is teratogenic, mutagenic, and carcinogenic.

Nursing Implications: As appropriate, discuss birth control measures.

V. ACTIVITY INTOLERANCE related to LETHARGY, CONFUSION

Defining Characteristics: Neurologic dysfunction may occur rarely: confusion, lethargy, disorientation, ataxia.

Nursing Implications: Perform neurologic assessment as part of prechemotherapy assessment. Assess orientation and level of consciousness, gait, activity tolerance.

VI. POTENTIAL SENSORY/PERCEPTUAL ALTERATIONS (VISUAL) related to OCULAR DAMAGE

Defining Characteristics: Ocular damage may occur rarely: optic neuritis, retinopathy, blurred vision.

Nursing Implications: Assess vision during prechemotherapy assessment. Encourage patient to report any visual changes.

Drug: mechlorethamine hydrochloride (Mustargen, Nitrogen Mustard, HN_2)

Class: Alkylating agent.

Mechanism of Action: Produces interstrand and intrastrand cross-linkages in DNA, causing miscoding, breakage, and failures of replication. Cell cycle phase nonspecific.

Metabolism: Undergoes chemical transformation after injection with less than 0.01% excreted unchanged in urine. Drug is rapidly inactivated by body fluids. 50% of the inactive metabolites are excreted in the urine within 24 hours.

Dosage/Range:

- IV: 0.4 mg/kg, or 12–16 mg/m² IV as single agent; 6 mg/m² IV days 1 and 8 of 28-day cycle with MOPP regimen.
- Topical: Dilute 10 mg in 60 mL sterile water; apply with rubber gloves.
- Intracavitary: Pleural, peritoneal, pericardial: 0.2–0.4 mg/kg.

Drug Preparation:

- Add sterile water or 0.9% Sodium Chloride to each vial. Wear eye and hand protection when mixing.
- Administer via sidearm or rapidly running IV.
- Drug must be used within 15 minutes of reconstitution.

Drug Administration:

- Intravenous: This drug is a potent vesicant. Give through a freely running IV to avoid extravasation, which can lead to ulceration, pain, and necrosis. Check hospital's policy and procedure for administration of a vesicant.

Drug Interactions:

- Myelosuppressive drugs: Additive hematologic toxicity; dose reduce or monitor patient closely.

Lab Effects/Interference:

- Decreased CBC.
- Increased uric acid, RFTs.

Special Considerations:

- Drug is a vesicant. Give through a running IV to avoid extravasation. Antidote is sodium thiosulfate: dilute 4 mL sodium thiosulfate injection USP (10%) with 6 mL sterile water for injection, USP and inject SQ in area of infiltration.
- Nadir is 6–8 days after treatment.
- Side effects occur in the reproductive system, such as amenorrhea and azoospermia.
- Severe nausea and vomiting.
- Systemic toxic effects may occur with intracavitary drug administration.

Potential Toxicities/Side Effects and the Nursing Process

I. ALTERATION IN NUTRITION, LESS THAN BODY REQUIREMENTS related to NAUSEA AND VOMITING, ANOREXIA, DIARRHEA

Defining Characteristics: Nausea and vomiting occur in ~100% of patients, within 30 minutes to 2 hours of drug administration, and up to 8 hours afterward. Nausea and vomiting can be severe, but can be prevented by the use of combination antiemetics such as serotonin antagonist (granisetron or ondansetron) and dexamethasone. Anorexia and taste distortion (metallic taste) occur commonly. Diarrhea may occur up to several days after drug administration.

Nursing Implications: Premedicate with combination antiemetics such as serotonin antagonist (granisetron or ondansetron) and dexamethasone. Continue prophylactically. Antiemetic and sedative may need to be started the evening before if patient develops anticipatory nausea and vomiting. Encourage small, frequent feedings of cool, bland foods, dry toast, crackers. Monitor I/O to detect fluid volume deficit. Notify physician of the need for more aggressive antiemetic if vomitus >750 mL. Encourage small, frequent feedings of high-calorie, high-protein foods. Encourage use of spices for anorexia, weekly weights. Encourage patient to report onset of diarrhea. Administer or teach patient to self-administer antidiarrheal medication and teach diet modifications (low residue) as appropriate.

II. INFECTION AND BLEEDING related to BONE MARROW DEPRESSION

Defining Characteristics: Potent myelosuppressant with nadir 6–8 days, recovery in 4 weeks. Patients at risk for profound bone marrow depression are those with previous extensive XRT, previous chemotherapy, or compromised bone marrow function. Lymphocyte depression occurs within 24 hours of drug dose.

Nursing Implications: Evaluate WBC, with neutrophil, and platelet count, and discuss any abnormalities with physician prior to drug administration. Assess for signs/symptoms of infection or bleeding; instruct patient in signs/symptoms of infection and bleeding, and to notify nurse or physician if they arise. Teach patient self-care measures to minimize risk of infection and bleeding, including avoidance of OTC aspirin-containing medications. Assess patient's Hgb/HCT and signs/symptoms of fatigue; teach patient self-assessment and to alternate rest and activity as needed. Transfuse red blood cells and platelets per physician order.

III. IMPAIRED SKIN INTEGRITY related to ALOPECIA, DRUG EXTRAVASATION

Defining Characteristics: Alopecia usually occurs as diffuse thinning. Drug is a potent vesicant, causing tissue necrosis and sloughing if extravasation occurs. Thrombosis or thrombophlebitis may occur despite all precautions, and venous access device may be required. Delayed cutaneous hypersensitivity is seen with topical application.

Nursing Implications: Discuss with patient hair loss, anticipated impact, and strategies to decrease distress, e.g., obtaining wig prior to hair loss. Assess body disturbance from hyperpigmentation and discuss strategies to minimize this, e.g., nail polish. Drug must be administered via patent IV. Assess need for venous access device early. Delayed cutaneous hypersensitivity (topical application) is not an indication to stop the drug. Discuss symptomatic management with physician. If extravasation is suspected, stop drug; aspirate any residual drug and blood from IV tubing, IV catheter/needle, and IV site if possible; instill antidote, sodium thiosulfate (1–6 molar), into area of apparent infiltration as per physician orders and institutional policy and procedure; apply cold or topical medication as per physician orders and institutional policy and procedure. Assess site regularly for pain, progression of erythema, induration, and for evidence of necrosis. When in doubt about whether drug is infiltrating, TREAT AS AN INFILTRATION. Teach patient to assess site, and instruct to notify physician if condition worsens. Arrange next clinic visit for assessment of site depending on drug, amount infiltrated, extent of potential injury, and patient variables. Document in patient's record as per institutional policy. Warm packs may decrease discomfort of phlebitis. Have standing orders and sodium thiosulfate injection USP (10%) close by in the event of actual infiltration of drug; dilute sodium thiosulfate with sterile water for injection and inject SQ in area of infiltration.

IV. ALTERATION IN COMFORT related to CHILLS, FEVER, DIARRHEA

Defining Characteristics: Chills, fever, diarrhea may occur after drug administration. Also weakness, drowsiness, headache may occur.

Nursing Implications: Assess patient for these symptoms during hour following treatment. Instruct patient to report these symptoms and teach self-management at home if outpatient. Provide symptomatic management per physician with acetaminophen, antidiarrheal medication.

V. POTENTIAL SEXUAL DYSFUNCTION related to DRUG EFFECTS

Defining Characteristics: Drug is teratogenic, carcinogenic. Amenorrhea occurs in females. Impaired spermatogenesis occurs in males. If administered to pregnant patients, spontaneous abortion or fetal abnormalities may occur.

Nursing Implications: As appropriate, explore with patient and partner issues of reproductive and sexual patterns, and anticipated impact chemotherapy will have. Discuss strategies to preserve sexuality and reproductive health (sperm banking, contraception).

VI. POTENTIAL FOR SENSORY/PERCEPTUAL ALTERATIONS related to CRANIAL NERVE INJURY

Defining Characteristics: Tinnitus, deafness, and other signs of eighth cranial nerve damage occur rarely, with high drug doses or regional perfusion techniques. Temporary aphasia and paresis occurs very rarely.

Nursing Implications: Assess hearing ability, presence of tinnitus prior to drug doses. If high doses of drug are given, or regional perfusion used, schedule patient for periodic audiometry. Instruct patient to report signs/symptoms of hearing loss.

Drug: melphalan hydrochloride (Alkeran, L-Phenylalanine Mustard, L-PAM, L-Sarcolysin)

Class: Alkylating agent.

Mechanism of Action: Prevents cell replication by causing breaks and cross-linkages in DNA strands with subsequent miscoding and breakage. Cell cycle phase nonspecific. Drug is derivative of nitrogen mustard.

Metabolism: Variable bioavailability after oral administration, especially if taken with food. Therefore, dose is titrated to WBC count; 20–50% of drug is excreted in feces over 6 days, 50% excreted in urine within 24 hours. After IV administration, parent compound disappears from plasma, with a half-life of about 2 hours.

Dosage/Range:
- Multiple myeloma: Several regimens, including 0.25 mg/kg/day × 4 days, in combination with prednisone 2 mg/kg/day, repeated every 6 weeks; OR 6 mg/m^2 orally daily × 5 days every 6 weeks for myeloma; OR 0.1 mg/kg PO × 2–3 weeks, then maintenance of 2–4 mg daily when bone marrow has recovered.
- 8 mg/m^2 IV daily × 5 days (investigational).
- Bone marrow transplantation: 50–60 mg/m^2 IV, but may be as high as 140–200 mg/m^2 (investigational).

Drug Preparation:
- Oral: Available in 2-mg tablets. Take on empty stomach.

- IV: Reconstitute 50-mg vial with 10 mL of provided diluent resulting in concentration of 5 mg/mL. Further dilute in 100–150 mL to produce a final concentration ≤ 2 mg/mL in 0.9% Sodium Chloride. Use provided 0.45-μm filter. Administer over 30–45 minutes. Stable for 1 hour at room temperature.

Drug Administration:
- Serious hypersensitivity reactions reported with IV administration.
- IV drug can cause anaphylaxis.
- IV drug is an irritant—avoid extravasation.

Drug Interactions:
- Myelosuppressive chemotherapy: Increases hematologic toxicity; dose-reduce or monitor patient very carefully.
- Cyclosporine: Increases nephrotoxicity.
- Drug activity is enhanced with concurrent administration of misonidazol (investigational).

Lab Effects/Interference:
- Decreased CBC.

Special Considerations:
- Nadir is 14–21 days after treatment.
- Increased risk of nephrotoxicity when given with cyclosporine.
- Drug dose reductions are recommended in patients with renal compromise.
- Drug is used in regional perfusion.

Potential Toxicities/Side Effects and the Nursing Process

I. INFECTION AND BLEEDING related to BONE MARROW DEPRESSION

Defining Characteristics: Bone marrow depression may be pronounced; leukopenia and thrombocytopenia occur 14–21 days after intermittent dosing schedules. May be delayed in onset, and cumulative with nadir extended to 5–6 weeks. Combined immunosuppression from disease (e.g., multiple myeloma) and drug may prolong vulnerability to infection. Thrombocytopenia may be persistent.

Nursing Implications: Evaluate WBC, with neutrophil, and platelet count and discuss any abnormalities with physician prior to drug administration. Assess for signs/symptoms of infection or bleeding; instruct patient in signs/symptoms of infection and bleeding, and to notify nurse or physician if they arise. Teach patient self-care measures to minimize risk of infection and bleeding, including avoidance of OTC aspirin-containing medications. Assess patient for Hgb/HCT and signs/symptoms of fatigue; teach patient self-assessment and to alternate rest and activity as needed. Transfuse packed red blood cells and platelets per physician order.

II. ALTERATION IN NUTRITION, LESS THAN BODY REQUIREMENTS, related to NAUSEA AND VOMITING, ANOREXIA

Defining Characteristics: Nausea and vomiting are mild at low, continuous dosing; severe following high doses. Anorexia occurs rarely.

Nursing Implications: Administer drug (oral) on empty stomach. Premedicate with antiemetic (oral) one hour before oral dose. Use aggressive antiemetic regimen for IV Alkeran. Encourage small, frequent feedings of favorite foods, especially high-calorie, high-protein foods. Encourage use of spices; weekly weights.

III. ALTERATION IN CARDIAC OUTPUT, PERFUSION related to ANAPHYLAXIS

Defining Characteristics: Severe hypersensitivity reactions can occur with IV administration, including diaphoresis, hypotension, and cardiac arrest.

Nursing Implications: Review standing orders for management of patient in anaphylaxis and identify location of anaphylaxis kit containing epinephrine 1:1000, hydrocortisone sodium succinate (Solucortef), diphenhydramine HCl (Benadryl), aminophylline, and others. Prior to drug administration, obtain baseline vital signs and record mental status. Administer drug slowly, diluted as per physician's order. Observe for following signs/symptoms, usually occurring within first 15 minutes of infusion. Subjective signs are generalized itching, nausea, chest tightness, crampy abdominal pain, difficulty speaking, anxiety, agitation, sense of impending doom, uneasiness, desire to urinate/defecate, dizziness, chills. Objective signs are flushed appearance (angioedema of face, neck, eyelids, hands, feet), localized or generalized urticaria, respiratory distress ± wheezing, hypotension, cyanosis. For generalized allergic reaction, stop infusion and notify physician. Place patient in supine position to promote perfusion of visceral organs. Monitor VS. Provide emotional reassurance to patient and family. Maintain patent airway and have CPR equipment ready if needed. Document incident. Discuss with physician desensitization for further dosing vs drug discontinuance.

IV. POTENTIAL SEXUAL DYSFUNCTION related to DRUG EFFECTS

Defining Characteristics: Potentially mutagenic and teratogenic.

Nursing Implications: Encourage patient to verbalize goals about family; discuss options, such as sperm banking. As appropriate, discuss or refer for counseling about birth control measures during therapy.

V. POTENTIAL FOR INJURY related to SECOND MALIGNANCY

Defining Characteristics: Acute myelogenous and myelomonocytic leukemias may occur after continuous long-term dosing, especially in patients with ovarian cancer and multiple myeloma. Heralded by preleukemic pancytopenia of several weeks' duration. Chromosomal abnormalities characteristic of acute leukemia.

Nursing Implications: Patients receiving prolonged continuous therapy should be closely followed during and after treatment.

VI. POTENTIAL FOR IMPAIRED GAS EXCHANGE related to PULMONARY TOXICITY

Defining Characteristics: Rare, but may occur, especially with continued chronic dosing. Bronchopulmonary dysplasia and pulmonary fibrosis.

Nursing Implications: Assess pulmonary status for signs/symptoms of pulmonary dysfunction. Assess lung sounds prior to dosing. Instruct patient to report cough or dyspnea. Discuss PFTs to be performed periodically with physician. Long-term follow-up is important.

VII. IMPAIRED SKIN INTEGRITY related to ALOPECIA, MACULOPAPULAR RASH, URTICARIA

Defining Characteristics: Alopecia is minimal if it occurs at all. Maculopapular rash and urticaria are infrequent.

Nursing Implications: Assess skin integrity and presence of rash, urticaria, alopecia prior to dosing. Assess impact of these alterations on patient and develop plan to manage symptom distress.

Drug: menogaril (Menogarol) (investigational)

Class: Antitumor (anthracycline) antibiotic.

Mechanism of Action: Appears to have a mechanism different from other anthracyclines in that the drug does not appear to bind too strongly to DNA for its cytotoxicity; drug also appears to act in the cytoplasm of the cell rather than in the cell nucleus.

Metabolism: Metabolized in the liver to its metabolite(s) following IV administration. Limited oral bioavailability; 5% elimination via either the bile or kidneys. Drug elimination half-life of 30 hours, and of its metabolite 58 hours.

Dosage/Range:
- 140–200 mg/m^2 IV over 2 hours every 3–4 weeks (investigational).
- 50 mg/m^2/day × 5 days every 3–4 weeks (investigational).

Drug Preparation:
- Vial is kept refrigerated and protected from light.
- Reconstitute 50-mg vial with 10 mL sterile water and shake well for 2 minutes; solution is stable for 14 days at room temperature and 6 weeks refrigerated.
- Withdraw dose and further dilute in 5% Dextrose ONLY to a final concentration of 0.1 mg/mL. Commonly, drug is mixed in 500 mL of 5% Dextrose.

Drug Administration:
- Administer by slow IV infusion over 1–2 hours by central line if possible to avoid phlebitis.
- Oral administration has been studied: drug is mixed in grape juice.

Drug Interactions:
- Drug becomes a gel when mixed in sodium-containing solutions.
- Incompatible with heparin and sodium bicarbonate.

Lab Effects/Interference:
- Decreased CBC.
- Increased LFTs.

Special Considerations:
- Drug is being studied in a number of malignancies.

Potential Toxicities/Side Effects and the Nursing Process

I. POTENTIAL FOR INFECTION AND BLEEDING related to BONE MARROW DEPRESSION

Defining Characteristics: Neutropenia is dose-limiting toxicity, with nadir occurring 2–3 weeks after treatment, and recovery by week 4. Thrombocytopenia and anemia are less common, with 10–12% incidence.

Nursing Implications: Evaluate WBC, ANC, and platelet count, and discuss any abnormalities with physician prior to drug administration. Assess for signs/symptoms of infection or bleeding, and teach patient to notify nurse or physician if they arise. Teach patient self-care measures to minimize risk of infection and bleeding, including avoidance of OTC aspirin-containing medications. Assess patient for Hgb/HCT and signs/symptoms of fatigue; teach patient self-assessment and to alternate rest and activity as needed. HIGH DOSE: Bone marrow aplasia expected; refer to investigational protocol.

II. ALTERATION IN NUTRITION, LESS THAN BODY REQUIREMENTS, related to NAUSEA, DIARRHEA, STOMATITIS, ANOREXIA, HEPATIC ENZYME ELEVATIONS

Defining Characteristics: Nausea/vomiting is mild if it occurs. Stomatitis is dose-limiting in leukemic patients. Anorexia has an incidence of 25%, and diarrhea has been reported. SGOT and SGPT may become mildly elevated.

Nursing Implications: Teach patient to report GI side effects, and teach self-care measures as appropriate. Monitor SGOT, SGPT, LDH, alk phos, and bili baseline and monitor SGPT and SGOT periodically during treatment. Notify physician of any elevations.

III. POTENTIAL FOR IMPAIRED SKIN INTEGRITY related to ALOPECIA, PHLEBITIS, URTICARIA

Defining Characteristics: Drug is irritating to vein. Phlebitis, inflammation, and pain at the IV injection site are common. Erythema may occur along the vein path during administration in 10% of patients. Urticaria may be severe, is dose-related, and may result in blister formation. Alopecia occurs and is mild.

Nursing Implications: Consider central line, especially if higher dose is given. Assess patient for signs/symptoms of hair loss. Discuss with patient impact of hair loss, and strategies to minimize distress. Teach patient that skin reactions may occur, and instruct to report them. Develop management strategies to maintain skin integrity and comfort.

IV. POTENTIAL ALTERATION IN OXYGENATION related to CARDIOTOXICITY

Defining Characteristics: Drug is less cardiotoxic than doxorubicin. However, atrial fibrillation, sinus bradycardia, myocardial infarction, ventricular arrythmias, and decreased LVEF may occur. Incidence of the last abnormality is 10%.

Nursing Implications: Assess patient risk (history of prior anthracycline chemotherapy, history of cardiovascular disease). Assess cardiac status prior to chemotherapy administration: signs/symptoms of CHF, quality/regularity and rate of heart beat, results of prior GBPS or other test of LVEF. Instruct patient to report dyspnea, palpitations, swelling in extremities. Maintain accurate records of total dose, and expect GBPS to be repeated periodically during treatment, and the drug to be discontinued if there is a significant drop in heart function.

Drug: mercaptopurine (Purinethol, 6-MP)

Class: Antimetabolite.

Mechanism of Action: One of two thiopurine antimetabolites (with 6-TG) that are converted to monophosphate nucleotides and inhibit de novo purine synthesis. The nucleotides are also incorporated into DNA. Cell cycle phase specific for S phase.

Metabolism: Metabolized by the enzyme xanthine oxidase in the kidney and liver; 50% of the drug is excreted in the urine. Plasma half-life is 20–40 minutes.

Dosage/Range:
- 100 mg/m^2 PO daily × 5 days.
- Children: 70 mg/m^2 daily for induction, then 40 mg/m^2 daily for maintenance.
- IV: 500–1000 mg/m^2/day × 2–3 days (investigational).

Drug Preparation:
- Oral: none; available in 50-mg tablets.
- IV: reconstitute 500-mg vial with sterile water for concentration of 10 mg/mL; store IV solution at room temperature; discard after 8 hours.
- Further dilute to a final concentration of 1–2 mg/mL in 5% Dextrose or 0.9% Sodium Chloride. Stable 3 days either refrigerated or at room temperature.

Drug Administration:
- Oral.
- IV: Infuse over 1 hour or longer per protocol.

Drug Interactions:
- Allopurinol: increased mercaptopurine levels; reduce dose to 25–35% of normal.
- Hepatotoxic drugs: additive hepatotoxicity; monitor LFTs closely.
- Warfarin: decreases or increases PT; monitor PT closely.
- Nonpolarizing muscle relaxants: decreased neuromuscular blockage; use together cautiously.

Lab Effects/Interference:
- Decreased CBC.
- Increased LFTs.
- Increased RFTs: tumor lysis.

Special Considerations:
- Elevated serum glucose levels and elevated serum uric acid levels could be related to the effects of medication.
- Reduce dose in cases of hepatic or renal dysfunction.

- Because xanthine oxidase is inhibited by allopurinol, concurrent use of the latter necessitates a dose reduction of 6-MP to ¼ the normal dose.

Potential Toxicities/Side Effects and the Nursing Process

I. POTENTIAL FOR INFECTION AND BLEEDING related to BONE MARROW DEPRESSION

Defining Characteristics: Nadir varies from 5 days to 6 weeks after treatment. Leukopenia more prominent than thrombocytopenia. Blood counts may continue to fall after therapy is stopped.

Nursing Implications: Evaluate WBC, with neutrophil, and platelet count, and discuss any abnormalities with physician prior to drug administration. Assess for signs/symptoms of infection or bleeding; instruct patient to notify nurse or physician if they arise. Teach patient self-care measures to minimize risk of infection and bleeding, including avoidance of OTC aspirin-containing medications. Assess patient's Hgb/HCT and signs/symptoms of fatigue; teach patient self-assessment and to alternate rest and activity as needed.

II. ALTERATION IN NUTRITION, LESS THAN BODY REQUIREMENTS related to HEPATOTOXICITY, GI SYMPTOMS

Defining Characteristics: Reversible cholestatic jaundice may develop after 2–5 months of treatment. Hepatic necrosis may develop. Nausea, vomiting, anorexia, diarrhea are infrequent. Stomatitis uncommon, but appears as white patchy areas similar to thrush.

Nursing Implications: Monitor SGOT, SGPT, LDH, alk phos, and bili periodically during treatment. Notify physician of any elevations. Hepatic toxicity may be an indication for discontinuing treatment. Instruct patient to report GI side effects and to perform self-care measures as appropriate.

III. POTENTIAL FOR IMPAIRED SKIN INTEGRITY related to RASH

Defining Characteristics: Skin eruptions; rash may occur.

Nursing Implications: Advise patient these changes may occur. Instruct patient in symptomatic care if distress related to skin reactions occurs.

Drug: methotrexate (Amethopterin, Mexate, Folex)

Class: Antimetabolite, folic acid antagonist.

Mechanism of Action: Blocks the enzyme dihydrofolate reductase (DHFR), which inhibits the conversion of folic acid to tetrahydrofolic acid, resulting in an inhibition of the key precursors of DNA, RNA, and cellular proteins. May synchronize malignant cells in the S phase: at high plasma levels, passive entry of the drug into tumor cells can potentially overcome drug resistance.

Metabolism: Bound to serum albumin; concurrent use of drugs that displace methotrexate from serum albumin should be avoided. Salicylates, sulfonamides, dilantin, some antibacterials—including tetracycline, chloramphenicol, paraminobenzoic acid—and alcohol should be avoided, as they will delay excretion. Drug is absorbed from GI tract and peaks in 1 hour. Plasma half-life is 2 hours; 50–100% of dose is excreted into the systemic circulation, with peak concentration 3–12 hours after administration.

Dosage/Range:

- IV: Low: 10–50 mg/m^2; med: 100–500 mg/m^2; high: 500 mg/m^2 and above with leucovorin rescue.
- IT: 10–15 mg/m^2.
- IM: 25 mg/m^2.

Drug Preparation:

- 5-, 50-, 100-, and 200-mg vials are available already reconstituted.
- Powder is available in vials without preservative for IT and high-dose administration (reconstitute with preservative-free 0.9% Sodium Chloride).

Drug Administration:

- 5–149 mg: slow IVP.
- 150–499 mg: IV drip over 20 minutes.
- 500–1500 mg: infusion, per protocol, with leucovorin rescue.

Drug Interactions:

- Protein-bound drugs (aspirin, sulfonamides, sulfonylureas, phenytoin, tetracycline, chloramphenicol) increase toxicity; give together cautiously and monitor patient closely.
- NSAIDs (nonsteroidal anti-inflammatory drugs, e.g., indomethacin, ketoprofen) increased and prolonged methotrexate levels; DO NOT administer concurrently with high doses of methotrexate; monitor patients closely who are receiving moderate or low-dose methotrexate.
- Cotrimoxazole increased methotrexate serum level; DO NOT use concurrently.
- Pyrimethamine increased methotrexate serum level; DO NOT use concurrently.

Lab Effects/Interference:

- Decreased CBC.
- Increased LFTs, RFTs.

Special Considerations:

- High doses cross the BBB; reconstitute with preservative-free 0.9% Sodium Chloride.
- With high doses (1–7.5 gm/m^2), urine should be alkalinized both before and after administration, as the drug is a weak acid and can crystallize in the kidneys at an acid pH. Alkalinize with bicarbonate; add to pre- and posthydration. High doses should only be given under the direction of a qualified oncologist at an institution that can provide rapid serum methotrexate level readings.
- Leucovorin rescue must be given on time per orders to prevent excessive toxicity and to achieve maximum therapeutic response (see Leucovorin Calcium).
- Avoid folic acid and its derivatives during methotrexate therapy. Kidney function must be adequate to excrete drug and avoid excessive toxicity. Check BUN and creatinine before each dose.

Potential Toxicities/Side Effects and the Nursing Process

I. ALTERATION IN NUTRITION, LESS THAN BODY REQUIREMENTS, related to GI SIDE EFFECTS

Defining Characteristics: Nausea and vomiting are uncommon with low dose; more common (39%) with high dose; may occur during drug administration and last 24–72 hours. Anorexia is mild. Stomatitis is a common indication for interruption of therapy: occurs in 3–5 days with high dose, 3–4 weeks with low dose; appears initially at corners of mouth. Diarrhea is common and is an indication for interruption of therapy, as enteritis and intestinal perforation may occur; melena, hematemesis may occur. Hepatotoxicity is usually subclinical and reversible, but can lead to cirrhosis; increased risk of hepatotoxicity when given with other agents, like alcohol; transient increase in LFTs with high dose 1–10 days after treatment—may cause jaundice.

Nursing Implications: Premedicate with antiemetics if giving high-dose methotrexate; continue prophylactically for 24 hours (at least) to prevent nausea and vomiting. Encourage small, frequent feedings of cool, bland foods and liquids. Assess for symptoms of fluid and electrolyte imbalance: monitor I/O, daily weights if administered to inpatient. Assess oral cavity every day. Teach patient oral assessment and mouth care regimens. Encourage patient to report early stomatitis. Provide pain relief measures, if indicated. Explore patient compliance to rescue; discuss increase in rescue dose if moderate GI toxicity. Assess patient for diarrhea: guaiac all stools; encourage patient to report onset of diarrhea. Administer or teach patient to self-administer antidiarrheal medications. Monitor LFTs prior to drug dose, especially with high-dose methotrexate. Assess patient prior to and during treatment for signs/symptoms of hepatotoxicity.

II. POTENTIAL FOR INFECTION AND BLEEDING related to BONE MARROW DEPRESSION

Defining Characteristics: Nadir is seen 7–9 days after drug administration. Bone marrow depression occurs in about 10% of patients.

Nursing Implications: Monitor CBC and platelet count prior to drug administration, as well as signs/symptoms of infection or bleeding. Instruct patient in self-assessment of signs/symptoms of infection or bleeding measures to decrease risk. Administer leucovorin calcium as ordered.

III. POTENTIAL FOR ALTERATION IN URINARY ELIMINATION related to RENAL TOXICITY

Defining Characteristics: As an organic acid, methotrexate is insoluble in acid urine. At doses greater than 1 gm/m^2 (i.e., high dose), drug may precipitate in renal tubules, causing acute renal tubular necrosis (ATN).

Nursing Implications: Prehydrate patient with alkaline solution for several hours prior to drug administration. Maintain high urine output with a urine pH greater than 7.0 (hydration fluid may need further alkalinization); dipstick each void. Record I/O. Monitor BUN and serum creatinine before, during, and after drug administration. Increases in these values may require methotrexate dose reductions or leucovorin dose increases.

IV. POTENTIAL FOR IMPAIRED GAS EXCHANGE related to PULMONARY TOXICITY

Defining Characteristics: Pneumothorax (high dose): rare, occurs within first 48 hours after drug administration in patients with pulmonary metastasis. Allergic pneumonitis (high dose): rare but accompanied by eosinophilia, patchy pulmonary infiltrates, fever, cough, shortness of breath. Occurs 1–5 months after initiation of treatment. Pneumonitis (low dose) symptoms usually disappear within a week, with or without use of steroids; interstitial pneumonitis may be a fatal complication.

Nursing Implications: Assess for signs/symptoms of pulmonary dysfunction before each dose and between doses (see Defining Characteristics section). Discuss PFTs to be performed periodically with physician. Assess lung sounds prior to drug administration. Instruct patient to report cough or dyspnea.

V. POTENTIAL FOR ALTERATION IN SKIN INTEGRITY related to ALOPECIA, DERMATITIS

Defining Characteristics: Alopecia and dermatitis are uncommon. Pruritus, urticaria may occur. Photosensitivity, sunburnlike rash 1–5 days after treatment; also, patient can develop radiation recall reaction.

Nursing Implications: Assess patient for signs/symptoms of hair loss. Discuss with patient impact of hair loss and strategies to minimize distress. Instruct patient to avoid sun if possible and to stay covered or wear sunblock if sun exposure is unavoidable.

VI. POTENTIAL FOR SENSORY AND PERCEPTUAL ALTERATIONS related to CNS CHANGES

Defining Characteristics: CNS effects: dizziness, malaise, blurred vision. IT administration may increase CSF pressure. Brain XRT followed by IV methotrexate may also cause neurologic changes.

Nursing Implications: Monitor for CNS effects of drug: dizziness, blurred vision, malaise. Monitor for symptoms of increased CSF pressure: seizures, paresis, headache, nausea and vomiting, brain atrophy, fever. If IV methotrexate follows brain XRT, monitor for symptoms of increased CSF pressure.

VII. POTENTIAL FOR ALTERATIONS IN COMFORT related to PAIN

Defining Characteristics: Sometimes causes back pain during administration.

Nursing Implications: Monitor patient for back and flank pain. Slow down infusion rate if it occurs. Administer analgesics if pain occurs (must avoid aspirin-containing products, as they displace methotrexate from serum albumin).

Drug: methyl-CCNU (Semustine, MeCCNU) (investigational)

Class: Alkylating agent (nitrosourea); investigational agent.

Mechanism of Action: Alkylation and carbamoylation by semustine metabolites interfere with the synthesis and function of DNA, RNA, and proteins. Also inhibits DNA repair. Semustine is lipid-soluble and easily enters the brain. Cell cycle phase nonspecific.

Metabolism: 10–20% of the drug is excreted in the urine.

Dosage/Range:

- 150–200 mg/m^2 PO once every 6–12 weeks.

Drug Preparation:

- Oral: Available in 10-, 50-, and 100-mg capsules.

Drug Administration:

- Administer at bedtime on an empty stomach or 3–4 hours after a meal to minimize nausea and vomiting.

Drug Interactions:

- Myelosuppressive drugs: Additive toxicity if similar nadir; use cautiously at decreased dose.

Lab Effects/Interference:

- Decreased WBC and platelets.
- Increased BUN, creatinine.
- Increased SGOT, alk phos, bili.

Special Considerations:

- Dose reduction necessary if patient has liver impairment.
- Dispense one dose of semustine at a time.
- Bone marrow recovery should occur prior to administration: WBC > 4000/ mm^3 and platelets > 100,000/mm^3.

Potential Toxicities/Side Effects and the Nursing Process

I. POTENTIAL FOR INFECTION AND BLEEDING related to MYELOSUPPRESSION

Defining Characteristics: Nadir of platelets: 4 weeks, but may be delayed to 8 weeks, with recovery 4–10 weeks later; nadir of WBC: occurs later than platelets. Cumulative bone marrow suppression with subsequent dosing may occur: Second or third drug dose may need to be reduced 25–50%. Persistent thrombocytopenia may occur.

Nursing Implications: Monitor WBC and platelets prior to drug administration (see Special Considerations section). WBC should be > 4000/mm^3 and platelets > 100,000/mm^3. Dispense only one drug dose at a time. Do not administer more often than once every 6 weeks. Dose-reduce with bone marrow or liver impairment.

II. ALTERED NUTRITION, LESS THAN BODY REQUIREMENTS, related to GI SIDE EFFECTS

Defining Characteristics: Onset of nausea and vomiting occurs 4–6 hours after drug dosing and may be severe. Stomatitis, hepatic dysfunction are rare.

Nursing Implications: Premedicate with antiemetic and sedative or hypnotic. Administer at night on empty stomach. Discourage food or fluid for 6 hours after drug dose. Encourage favorite foods, especially those that are high-calorie, high-protein. Encourage small, frequent meals. Inspect oral mucosa prior to dosing. Teach patient oral exam, mouth care after meals and at bedtime. Monitor SGOT, LDH, alk phos, bili. Notify physician of elevations and discuss prior to administering subsequent dose.

III. ALTERATION IN URINARY ELIMINATION related to RENAL DYSFUNCTION

Defining Characteristics: Renal dysfunction infrequent but may occur late in treatment. Tubular atrophy and glomerular sclerosis; ultimately, renal failure.

Nursing Implications: Monitor BUN, creatinine prior to dosing, especially in patients receiving prolonged or high cumulative doses. If abnormalities are noted, determine renal creatinine clearance.

IV. POTENTIAL SEXUAL DYSFUNCTION related to DRUG EFFECT

Defining Characteristics: Drug is teratogenic and mutagenic.

Nursing Implications: Assess patient's risk of becoming pregnant. Give information about adverse effects on fetus. As appropriate, discuss birth control measures.

V. ACTIVITY INTOLERANCE related to NEUROLOGIC DYSFUNCTION

Defining Characteristics: Neurologic dysfunction may occur rarely, including disorientation, lethargy, ataxia.

Nursing Implications: Perform neurologic assessment as part of prechemotherapy assessment. Assess orientation and level of consciousness, gait, activity tolerance.

VI. SENSORY/PERCEPTUAL ALTERATIONS (VISUAL) related to OCULAR DAMAGE

Defining Characteristics: Ocular damage may occur rarely, including optic neuritis, retinopathy, blurred vision.

Nursing Implications: Assess vision during prechemotherapy assessment. Encourage patient to report any visual changes.

VII. IMPAIRED GAS EXCHANGE related to PULMONARY FIBROSIS

Defining Characteristics: Pulmonary fibrosis occurs rarely.

Nursing Implications: Assess patients at risk, particularly those with (1) preexisting lung disease and (2) high cumulative doses. Monitor PFTs periodically for pulmonary dysfunction.

Drug: mitomycin (Mitomycin C, Mutamycin, 3 Mitozytrex)

Class: Antitumor antibiotic.

Mechanism of Action: Drug acts as alkylating agent and inhibits DNA synthesis by crosslinking of DNA. Alkylating and crosslinking mitomycin metabolites interfere with structure and function of DNA.

Metabolism: Drug is rapidly cleared by the liver. May need to modify dose in presence of liver abnormalities; 10% of drug is excreted unchanged.

Dosage/Range:
- 2 mg/m^2 IV every day × 5 days.
- 5–20 mg/m^2 IV every 6–8 weeks.
- Bladder instillations 20–60 mg (1 mg/mL).
- May be used at different dosages for autologous bone marrow transplant.

Drug Preparation:
- Depending on vial size, dilute with sterile water to obtain concentration of 0.5 mg/mL.

Drug Administration:
- IV: Drug is potent vesicant.
- Give through the sidearm of a running IV to avoid extravasation, which can lead to ulceration, pain, and necrosis. Check individual hospital policy for administration of a vesicant.

Drug Interactions:
- Myelosuppressive agents: Additive toxicity if overlapping nadirs; use cautiously.

Lab Effects/Interference:
- Decreased CBC, especially WBC and platelets.
- Hemolytic uremic syndrome (rare): Decreased hemoglobin, platelets, and increased creatinine.

Special Considerations:
- Indicated for treatment of disseminated adenocarcinoma of the stomach or pancreas in proven combinations with other approved chemotherapeutic agents and as palliative treatment when other modalities have failed.
- May cause interstitial pneumonitis.
- Rarely, hemolytic uremic syndrome can occur (characterized by rapid fall in hemoglobin, renal failure, severe thrombocytopenia) and progress to pulmonary edema and hypotension.
- Drug may be given intraarterially.
- Manufacturer's recommendations on dosage modification based on hematologic toxicity (NADIR AFTER PRIOR DOSE).

Potential Toxicities/Side Effects and the Nursing Process

I. POTENTIAL FOR INFECTION related to MYELOSUPPRESSION

Defining Characteristics: Myelosuppression is the dose-limiting toxicity. Toxicity is delayed and cumulative. Initial nadir occurs at approximately 4–6 weeks. Usually by the third course, 50% drug modifications are necessary.

Nursing Implications: Monitor WBC, HCT, platelets prior to drug administration. Monitor patients for signs/symptoms of infection. Teach patient self-assessment. Drug dosage should be reduced or held for lower-than-normal blood values.

II. ALTERATION IN NUTRITION, LESS THAN BODY REQUIREMENTS, related to NAUSEA, VOMITING, ANOREXIA, STOMATITIS

Defining Characteristics: Mild-to-moderate nausea and vomiting occur within 1–2 hours, lasting up to 3 days, but may be prevented by adequate premedication. Anorexia occurs commonly, and stomatitis may occur.

Nursing Implications: Premedicate with aggressive antiemetics, i.e., serotonin antagonist to prevent nausea and vomiting at least for the first treatment. Encourage small, frequent feedings of cool, bland foods and liquids. Teach patient and family member preparation of meals in advance, and encourage the use of spices when patient has little appetite. Teach patient oral assessment and oral hygiene regimen, and encourage patient to report early stomatitis.

III. POTENTIAL FOR ACTIVITY INTOLERANCE related to FATIGUE

Defining Characteristics: Fatigue is common.

Nursing Implications: Assess baseline activity level. Teach patient to report fatigue and activity intolerance. Teach self-management strategies, including alternating rest and activity periods, as well as stress reduction.

IV. POTENTIAL FOR IMPAIRED SKIN INTEGRITY related to DRUG EXTRAVASATION, ALOPECIA

Defining Characteristics: Extravasation of drug can cause severe tissue necrosis, erythema, burning, tissue sloughing. Delayed erythema or ulceration has been reported weeks to months after drug dose, at the injection site or distant from it, and despite the fact that there was no evidence of extravasation. Alopecia occurs frequently.

Nursing Implications: Use scrupulous IV technique to prevent extravasation of the drug. If there is doubt as to whether drug has infiltrated, treat as an infiltration, aspirate any drug in the tubing, and discontinue IV. IV line must be patent. Assess for need of venous access device early. Refer to hospital policy for management of extravasation. (If unclear what best strategy is, application of 1–2 mL 99% DMSO to the site every 6 hours × 14 days may offer some benefit [Alberts and Dorr, 1991].) Assess site regularly for pain, progression of erythema, induration, and evidence of necrosis. Discuss with patient hair loss, anticipated impact, and strategies to decrease distress, e.g., obtaining wig prior to hair loss.

V. POTENTIAL FOR INJURY related to HEMOLYTIC UREMIC SYNDROME

Defining Characteristics: 2% of patients may experience significant increase in creatinine unrelated to total dose or duration of therapy. Hold drug if creatinine is > 1.7 mg/dL. Thrombotic microangiopathy may occur with anemia, thrombocytopenia. Blood transfusions may exacerbate condition. Can often be fatal.

Nursing Implications: Monitor renal function, HCT, and platelets prior to each drug dose; hold dose if serum creatinine is > 1.7 mg/dL. If renal failure occurs, hemofiltration or dialysis may be necessary. Discuss risks and benefits with physician and patient if renal insufficiency is present and blood transfusion(s) is required.

VI. POTENTIAL ALTERATION IN OXYGENATION related to INTERSTITIAL PNEUMONITIS

Defining Characteristics: Rarely, interstitial pneumonitis occurs and can be quite severe (ARDS). signs/symptoms include nonproductive cough, dyspnea, hemoptysis, pneumonia, pulmonary infiltrates on X-ray. Incidence may be reduced by dexamethasone 20 mg IV prior to dose (Chang et al, 1986).

Nursing Implications: Assess baseline pulmonary status, and monitor prior to each drug dose. Teach patient to report dyspnea, new onset cough, or any respiratory symptoms. Discuss abnormalities with physician, and plan for further diagnostic workup.

VII. POTENTIAL FOR INJURY related to VENO-OCCLUSIVE DISEASE OF THE LIVER AFTER BONE MARROW TRANSPLANT

Defining Characteristics: Hepatic veno-occlusive disease has been reported in patients who have received mitomycin C and autologous bone marrow transplant. signs/symptoms are abdominal pain, hepatomegaly, and liver failure.

Nursing Implications: Assess baseline LFTs, and monitor periodically during therapy. Notify physician of any abnormalities, and discuss further diagnostic workup and management. Refer to autologous bone marrow transplant protocol.

Drug: mitotane (o, p′-DDD, Lysodren)

Class: Antihormone.

Mechanism of Action: Adrenocortical suppressant with direct cytotoxic effect on mitochondria of adrenal cortical cells. Forces a drop in steroid secretion and alters the peripheral metabolism of steroids.

Metabolism: 34–45% of oral dose is absorbed from the GI tract. Metabolized partly in the liver and kidneys to a water-soluble metabolite that is then excreted in the bile and urine. Small amount of drug passes into the CSF.

Dosage/Range:
- Dose ranges from 2–16 g/day PO.
- Usual doses 2–10 g/day.
- Treatment usually begins with low doses (2 g/day) and gradually increases.
- Daily dose is divided into 3–4 doses.

Drug Preparation:
- None.

Drug Administration:
- Oral.

Drug Interactions:
- Neurotoxic drugs may have additive toxicity; use cautiously.

Lab Effects/Interference:
- None.

Special Considerations:
- Hypersensitivity reactions are rare but have occurred.

Potential Toxicities/Side Effects and the Nursing Process

I. ALTERATION IN NUTRITION, LESS THAN BODY REQUIREMENTS, related to GI SIDE EFFECTS

Defining Characteristics: Nausea and vomiting occur in 75% of patients and may be dose-limiting toxicity. Anorexia may also occur. Diarrhea occurs in 20% of patients.

Nursing Implications: Nausea and vomiting may be reduced by beginning therapy with a low dose and increasing it as tolerated. Premedicate with antiemetics to prevent nausea and vomiting; continue as needed. Encourage small, frequent meals of cool, bland foods and liquids. Inform patient that nausea and vomiting can occur; encourage patient to report onset. Encourage patient to report onset of diarrhea. Administer or teach administration of antidiarrheal medication. If diarrhea is protracted, ensure adequate hydration, monitor I/O and electrolytes, teach perineal hygiene.

II. POTENTIAL FOR INJURY related to NEUROLOGIC TOXICITY

Defining Characteristics: Lethargy and somnolence are most common; resolve with discontinuation of therapy. Dizziness, vertigo occur in about 15% of patients. Other CNS manifestations are depression, muscle tremors, confusion, headache.

Nursing Implications: Teach the patient and family about possible neurologic toxicity; assess safety of planned activities (e.g., patient should avoid activities that require alertness). Encourage patient and family to report onset of symptoms, as they may necessitate discontinuing therapy.

III. POTENTIAL FOR IMPAIRED SKIN INTEGRITY related to RASH

Defining Characteristics: Skin irritation or rash occurs in about 15% of patients. Sometimes resolves during treatment.

Nursing Implications: Inform patient that rash is expected and will resolve when treatment is finished. Assess skin for integrity; recommend measures to decrease irritation, if indicated.

Drug: mitoxantrone (Novantrone)

Class: New class of antineoplastics—anthracenediones. Antitumor antibiotic.

Mechanism of Action: Inhibits both DNA and RNA synthesis regardless of the phase of cell division. Intercalates between base pairs, thus distorting DNA structure. DNA-dependent RNA synthesis and protein synthesis are also inhibited.

Metabolism: Excreted in both the bile and urine for 24–36 hours as virtually unchanged drug. Mean half-life is 5.8 hours. Peak levels achieved immediately. FDA-approved for acute nonlymphocytic leukemia in adults.

Dosage/Range:

- 12 mg/m^2 IV daily for 3 days, in combination with cytosine arabinoside 100 mg/m^2/day × 7 days continuous infusion for induction therapy of ANLL.
- 10–14 mg/m^2 IV every 3–4 weeks (refer to protocol).

Drug Preparation:

- Available as dark blue solution.

- May be diluted in 5% Dextrose, 0.9% Sodium Chloride, or 5% Dextrose in 0.9% Sodium Chloride.
- Solution is chemically stable at room temperature for at least 48 hours.
- Intact vials should be stored at room temperature. If refrigerated, a precipitate may form. This precipitate can be redissolved when vial is warmed to room temperature.

Drug Administration:

- IV push over 3 minutes through the sidearm of a freely running infusion.
- IV bolus over 5–30 minutes.

Drug Interactions:

- Myelosuppressive agents: Increased hematologic toxicity if nadir overlaps; use together cautiously.

Lab Effects/Interference:

- Decreased CBC.
- Decreased electrolytes.
- Increased LFTs, uric acid.

Special Considerations:

- Nonvesicant. There have been rare reports of tissue necrosis after drug infiltration.
- Incompatible with admixtures containing heparin.
- Patient may experience blue-green urine for 24 hours after drug administration.
- Cardiotoxicity is less than that of doxorubicin or daunorubicin.

Potential Toxicities/Side Effects and the Nursing Process

I. POTENTIAL FOR INJURY related to BONE MARROW DEPRESSION

Defining Characteristics: Potent bone marrow depression; nadir 9–10 days. Granulocytopenia is usually the dose-limiting toxicity, and toxicity may be cumulative. Thrombocytopenia uncommon, but can be severe when it occurs. Hypersensitivity has been reported occasionally with hypotension, urticaria, dyspnea, rashes.

Nursing Implications: Monitor WBC, HCT, platelets prior to drug administration. Instruct patient in self-assessment for signs/symptoms of infection. Drug dosage should be reduced or held for lower-than-normal blood values. Instruct patient in self-assessment of signs/symptoms of bleeding. Prior to drug administration, obtain baseline vital signs. Observe for signs/symptoms of allergic reaction. Subjective signs/symptoms: generalized itching, dizziness. Objective signs/symptoms: flushed appearance (angioedema of face, neck, eyelids, hands, feet), localized or generalized urticaria. Document incident. Discuss with physician desensitization for future dose vs drug discontinuance.

II. POTENTIAL FOR ALTERATION IN CARDIAC OUTPUT related to CARDIOTOXICITY

Defining Characteristics: CHF with decreased LVEF occurs in about 3% of patients. Increased cardiotoxicity with cumulative dose greater than 180 mg/m^2; cumulative lifetime dose must be reduced if patient has had previous anthracycline therapy.

Nursing Implications: Assess for signs/symptoms of cardiomyopathy. Assess quality and regularity of heartbeat. Baseline EKG. Instruct patient to report dyspnea, shortness of breath, swelling of extremities, orthopnea. Discuss frequency of GBPS with physician.

III. ALTERATION IN NUTRITION, LESS THAN BODY REQUIREMENTS, related to NAUSEA/VOMITING AND MUCOSITIS

Defining Characteristics: Nausea and vomiting are typically not severe and occur in 30% of patients. Mucositis is more common with prolonged dosing; occurs in 5% of patients, usually within one week of therapy.

Nursing Implications: Premedicate with antiemetic and continue prophylactically for 24 hours to prevent nausea and vomiting, at least for the first treatment. Encourage small, frequent feedings of cool, bland foods and liquids. Teach patient oral assessment and oral hygiene regimen. Encourage patient to report early stomatitis.

IV. POTENTIAL FOR IMPAIRED SKIN INTEGRITY related to ALOPECIA AND EXTRAVASATION

Defining Characteristics: Alopecia is mild to moderate; occurs in 20% of patients. Drug is not a vesicant. Stains skin blue without ulcers. There have been rare reports of tissue necrosis following extravasation.

Nursing Implications: Discuss with patient impact of hair loss. Suggest wig as appropriate prior to actual hair loss. Explore with patient response to actual hair loss and plan strategies to minimize distress, e.g., wig, scarf, cap. Use careful technique during venipuncture and IV administration. Administer drug through freely flowing IV, constantly monitoring IV site and patient response.

V. POTENTIAL FOR ANXIETY related to ABNORMAL COLOR OF URINE SCLERA

Defining Characteristics: Urine will be green-blue for 24 hours. Sclera may become discolored blue.

Nursing Implications: Explain to patient changes that may occur with therapy and that they are only temporary.

VI. POTENTIAL SEXUAL DYSFUNCTION related to DRUG EFFECT

Defining Characteristics: Drug is mutagenic and teratogenic.

Nursing Implications: As appropriate, explore with patient and partner issues of reproductive and sexuality patterns and impact chemotherapy may have. Discuss strategies to preserve sexual and reproductive health (e.g., sperm banking, contraception).

Drug: nilutamide (Nilandron)

Class: Antiandrogen.

Mechanism of Action: Irreversibly binds to androgen receptors and inhibits androgen binding. Unlike steroidal antiandrogens, nilutamide binds specifically to adrenal androgen receptor and does not interact with progestin or glucocorticoid receptors.

Metabolism: Following oral administration, nilutamide is rapidly and completely absorbed. Steady-state levels are achieved after about two weeks. Though the drug is extensively metabolized, it appears that the parent drug is the active compound. The drug is excreted in the urine as metabolite. Renal impairment does not alter the properties of the drug.

Dosage/Range:
- 300 mg/day for 30 days, then 150 mg/day.

Drug Preparation/Administration:
- Oral.

Drug Interactions:
- Has been shown to inhibit the liver cytochrome P-450 isoenzymes and may decrease the metabolism of compounds requiring these systems.
- Drugs with a low therapeutic margin, such as vitamin K antagonists, phenytoin, and theophylline, could delay elimination. Dose reduction of these drugs may be necessary.

Contraindications:
- In patients with severe hepatic impairment (baseline hepatic enzymes should be evaluated prior to treatment).
- In patients with severe respiratory insufficiency.
- In patients with hypersensitivity to nilutamide or any component of this preparation.

Lab Effects/Interference:
- Causes increased liver enzymes (see below); may cause increased serum glucose.

Special Considerations:

- Treatment should begin the day of or the day after surgical castration.
- If transaminases rise to greater than 2–3 times the upper limit of normal, therapy should be discontinued.

Potential Toxicities/Side Effects and the Nursing Process

I. ALTERATION IN NUTRITION, LESS THAN BODY REQUIREMENTS, related to NAUSEA, ANOREXIA

Defining Characteristics: Nausea, anorexia occur infrequently.

Nursing Implications: Teach patient to report occurrence of loss of appetite or nausea. Encourage small, frequent feedings and consider antiemetic if necessary.

II. ALTERATION IN CARDIAC OUTPUT related to HYPERTENSION, ANGINA

Defining Characteristics: Angina occurs in 2% of patients; unclear whether increased incidence of hypertension (9%) due to drug alone.

Nursing Implications: Instruct patient in signs and symptoms of angina, and to report to physician if they occur. Monitor BP on follow-up visits.

III. ALTERATION IN COMFORT related to DIZZINESS, HOT FLASHES, DYSPNEA, VISUAL CHANGES

Defining Characteristics: Hot flashes occur in 28% of patients and are the most common side effect. Dyspnea is rare but is related to interstitial pneumonitis, a serious side effect of the drug. Many patients experience impaired adaptation to light.

Nursing Implications: Inform patient that side effects may occur and to report dyspnea immediately to physician, as therapy must be discontinued if it occurs. Baseline chest X-ray should be done prior to treatment. Patients should be discouraged from driving at night because of visual changes and may find it helpful to wear tinted glasses during the day.

Drug: oxaliplatin (Eloxatin)

Class: Alkylating agent (3rd-generation platinum analogue).

Mechanism of Action: Blocks DNA replication and transcription into RNA by causing intrastrand and interstrand crosslinks in DNA strands.

Metabolism: Heavily bound (90%) to plasma proteins; following 2-hour drug infusion, 15% of drug is found in plasma and 85% in tissue or excreted in the urine. Binds irreversibly in red blood cells. The drug concentrates in the kidney and spleen, and is excreted as platinum-containing metabolites.

Dosage/Range:

- FOLFOX 4: *Day 1*: Oxaliplatin 85 mg/m² IV infusion in 250–500 ml 5% Dextrose in water and leucovorin 200 mg IV infusion in 5% dextrose in water, each over 2 hours simultaneously in different bags connected by a Y-line, followed by 5-FU 400 mg/m² IVB over 2–4 minutes, followed by 5-FU 600 mg/m² in 250–500 mL D5W as a 22-hour continuous infusion. *Day 2*: Leucovorin 200 mg/m² IVB over 2 hours, followed by 5-FU 400 mg/m² IVB over 2–4 minutes, followed by 5-FU 600 mg/m² in 250–500 mL D5W as a 22-hour continuous infusion.

Dose Reductions:

- Persistent grade 2 neurotoxicity: Reduce oxaliplatin to 65 mg/m².
- Grade 3 neurotoxicity: Discontinue oxaliplatin.
- Grades 3–4 gastrointestinal toxicity: Decrease oxaliplatin dose to 65 mg/m² and 5-FU by 20% (300mg/m² IVB and 500 mg/m² CI).
- Grades 3–4 hematological toxicity (ANC < 1500/l, platelets < 100,000/l): Decrease oxaliplatin dose to 65 mg/m² and 5-FU by 20% (300 mg/m² IVB and 500 mg/m² CI).
- Nausea, vomiting or other acute symptoms: Infuse oxaliplatin over a period of up to 6 hours as this lowers peak serum levels by 32%, revise antiemetic regime.

Drug Preparation:

- Add 10 mL bacteriostatic water for injection or 5% dextrose injection to the 50-mg vial of lyophilized powder and 20 mL to the 100-mg vial. Further dilute in 250–500 mL of 5% dextrose injection.
- DO NOT use chloride-containing solutions.
- DO NOT use aluminum needles or infusion sets containing aluminum.

Drug Administration:

- Administer IV infusion over 2 or more hours through central line, preferably.
- Drug classified as an irritant, but extravasations have resulted in induration and formation of nodule lasting 9 months or more.
- If given peripherally, it may cause infusion site pain; relieve this by further diluting the drug in 500 mL 5% Dextrose in water.

Drug Interactions:

- Incompatible with 5-FU and other highly alkaline solutions.
- Incompatible with chloride-containing solutions (forms precipitate).
- Physically incompatible with diazepam (forms precipitate).

- Nephrotoxic drugs: renal excretion of oxaliplatin could be reduced with increased serum levels of oxaliplatin.
- At high doses (130 mg/m^2), increases plasma levels of 5-FU by 20%.

Lab Effects/Interference:
- Decreased CBC, especially WBC and platelets.

Special Considerations:
- Indicated for the (1) adjuvant treatment of patients with Stage III colon cancer, and (2) first-line treatment of metastatic colon and rectal cancers in combination with infusional 5-fluorouracil (5-FU) and leucovorin (LV) for the treatment of patients with metastatic carcinoma of the colon or rectum. In the MOSAIC study of 2246 patients receiving adjuvant chemotherapy for colon cancer, Stage III patients receiving FOLFOX 4 had a superior survival compared to patients receiving 5FU/LV alone (24% risk reduction for recurrence) 4 years out (de Gramont, 2005). In addition, 99% of patients with grade 3 neurotoxicity had resolved or decreased by 1-year post treatment (deGramont et al, 2003).
- Peripheral neuropathy (sensory) is dose-limiting toxicity. Two distinct neurotoxicity syndromes: acute, lasting less than 14 days, and chronic persistent peripheral neuropathy (PN) similar to cisplatin.
- Rare pulmonary fibrosis and veno-occlusive disease of the liver.

Potential Toxicities/Side Effects and the Nursing Process

I. SENSORY/PERCEPTUAL ALTERATIONS related to ACUTE SENSORY NEUROPATHY

Defining Characteristics: Acute neurotoxicity appears related to ion channelopathy. It is common, affecting up to 56% of patients. It is temporary, and occurs during, within hours of, or up to 14 days following oxaliplatin administration. Often precipitated by exposure to cold and characterized by dysesthesias, transient paresthesias, or hypothesias of the hands, feet, perioral area, and throat. Acute events can be minimized by slower infusion of oxaliplatin, increasing the infusion time from 2 to 6 hours, as this lowers peak serum levels. Studies are ongoing to determine whether glutamine can prevent these, and also studies exploring 1 gm calcium/1 gm magnesium IVB prior to and after the oxaliplatin infusion. Most frightening for patients is pharyngolaryngeal dysesthesia characterized by a sensation of discomfort or tightness in the back of the throat and inability to breathe. It may be accompanied by jaw pain, and is often precipitated by exposure to cold. Cramping of muscles, such as fisted hand, occurs due to prolonged action potential. Rarely, dysarthria (difficulty articulating words), eye pain, and a feeling of chest pressure can occur.

Nursing Implications: Teach patient that acute neurotoxicity can occur but is not dangerous. Teach patient to minimize occurrence by avoiding exposure to cold during and for 3–5 days after drug administration, such as wearing scarves over the face in the winter, warm gloves if going outside or reaching into the refrigerator or freezer. Teach patient to avoid exposure to cold and cold liquids, if lip paresthesias present. Teach patient to use straw if drinking cool liquids. Teach patient to avoid cold air conditioning in the car or home during the summer. Teach patient how to reassure themselves they are breathing if pharyngolaryngeal dysesthesia occurs (cup hands in front of mouth or hold mirror so that breath can be felt or seen on the mirror). Teach patient to warm area, such as fingers or toes, if they become cold, such as running warm water over affected area, as this may help resolve the feeling.

II. SENSORY/PERCEPTUAL ALTERATIONS related to PERSISTENT, CHRONIC SENSORY NEUROPATHY

Defining Characteristics: Peripheral neurotoxicity affects about 48% of patients, and usually occurs when a cumulative dose of 800 mg/m^2 is reached. Symptoms include paresthesias, dysesthesias, hypoesthesias, in a stocking and glove distribution, and altered proprioception (knowing where body parts are in relation to the whole). This can become manifest in difficulty writing, walking, swallowing, and buttoning buttons. IF allowed to progress, motor pathways will become involved. When drug is stopped, symptoms resolve in 4–6 months in many patients. Ongoing studies are looking at temporarily stopping the drug when grade 2 or 3 neurotoxicity occurs, and resuming when the patient has grade 0 or 1 toxicity (OPTIMOX trial). In the MOSAIC trial, an adjuvant trial, although 23% of patients developed grade 3 neurotoxicity after 6 months, all patients except 1% had complete resolution of toxicity (de Gramont, 2003).

Nursing Implications: Assess baseline neurologic status (sensory and motor); instruct patient to report signs/symptoms. Identify patients at risk: those with preexisting neuropathies (e.g., ethanol- and diabetes mellitus-related). Assess motor function, and monitor over time prior to each treatment, such as picking up a dime from a smooth/flat surface, buttoning shirt, and writing name. Specifically, assess whether function impaired, as this necessitates a dose reduction, or if ability to perform activities of daily living impaired, as this necessitates drug cessation. In either case, discuss with physician as complete neurological exam should be performed prior to treatment decision. Assess impact on patient and quality of life. Drug holiday or discontinuance based on grade of neurotoxicity.

III. POTENTIAL FOR INFECTION, BLEEDING, and FATIGUE related to BONE MARROW DEPRESSION

Defining Characteristics: Mild leukopenia, and mild to moderate thrombocytopenia occur. Anemia common.

Nursing Implications: Assess baseline CBC, WBC, differential, and platelet count prior to chemotherapy as well as signs/symptoms of infection, bleeding, or fatigue. Teach patient signs/symptoms of infection or bleeding, and to report these immediately. Teach patient self-care measures to minimize risk of infection and bleeding. This includes avoidance of crowds, proximity to people with infections, and OTC aspirin-containing medications. Teach energy-conserving techniques and ways to minimize fatigue, such as gentle exercise as tolerated.

IV. ALTERATION IN NUTRITION, LESS THAN BODY REQUIREMENTS, related to NAUSEA AND VOMITING

Defining Characteristics: Nausea and vomiting occur commonly and are severe if patient does not receive aggressive antiemesis.

Nursing Implications: Premedicate patient with aggressive combination antiemetics: serotonin antagonist (granisetron or ondansetron) and dexamethasone. Encourage small, frequent feedings of cool, bland foods. Instruct patient to report nausea, and teach self-administration of antiemetics if patient is receiving drug as an outpatient.

V. POTENTIAL FOR INJURY related to DELAYED HYPERSENSITIVITY OR ANAPHYLAXIS REACTIONS (often after 10–12 cycles of therapy)

Defining Characteristics: Delayed hypersensitivity may occur after 10–12 cycles of therapy with symptoms ranging from local rash or vague symptoms such as new onset of vomiting, to anaphylaxis and severe hypersensitivity (characterized by dyspnea, hypotension requiring treatment, angioedema, and generalized urticaria). Anecdotal reports show successful desensitization using carboplatin desensitization regimens.

Nursing Implications: Assess baseline VS and mental status prior to drug administration. If patient has symptoms, discuss premedication using corticosteroid, antihistamine, and H2 antagonist as ordered. Monitor VS every 15 minutes, and remain with patient during first 15 minutes of drug infusion. Stop drug if signs/symptoms of hypersensitivity or anaphylaxis occur, and notify physician. *Subjective symptoms*: generalized itching, nausea, chest tightness, crampy abdominal pain, difficulty speaking, anxiety, agitation, sense of impending doom, uneasiness, desire to urinate/defecate, dizziness, chills. *Objective signs*: flushed appearance; angioedema of face, neck, eyelids, hands, feet; localized or generalized urticaria; respiratory distress with or without wheezing; hypotension; cyanosis. Provide fluid resuscitation for hypotension per MD order, and maintain a patent airway.

Drug: paclitaxel (Taxol)

Class: Taxoid, mitotic inhibitor.

Mechanism of Action: Promotes early microtubule assembly and prevents depolymerization, resulting in cell death.

Metabolism: Extensively protein-bound, resulting in an initial sharp decline in serum level. Metabolized primarily by hepatic hydroxylation using the P-450 enzyme system. Metabolites are excreted in the bile. Less than 10% of the intact drug is excreted in the urine.

Dosage/Range:

- Previously untreated ovarian cancer: 135 mg/m^2 IV over 24 hours, followed by cisplatin 75 mg/m^2 every 3 weeks or paclitaxel 175 mg IV over 3 hours followed by cisplatin 75 mg/m^2 q 3 weeks.
- Previously treated ovarian cancer: 135mg or 175 mg/m^2 IV over 3 hours every 3 weeks.
- Adjuvant node positive breast cancer: 175 mg/m^2 IV over 3 hours, every 3 weeks, for 4 courses, administered sequentially to doxorubicin-containing combination chemotherapy.
- Metastatic breast cancer, after failure of initial therapy or relapse within 6 months of adjuvant therapy: 175 mg/m^2 IV over 3 hours every 3 weeks.
- Metastatic breast cancer, weekly paclitaxel 80 mg/m^2 IV over 1 hour q wk.
- Non-small-cell lung cancer (NSCLC): 135 mg/m^2 IV over 24 hours, followed by cisplatin 75 mg/m^2 repeated every 3 weeks.
- AIDS-related Kaposi's sarcoma: 135 mg/m^2 IV over 3 hours, repeated every 3 weeks, or 100 mg/m^2 IV over 3 hours, repeated every 2 weeks (dose intensity of 45–50 mg/m^2 per week.
- Less myelosuppression with 3-hour vs 24-hour infusion.

Other regimens used/being studied/reported:

- Metastatic breast cancer overexpressing *HER*-2 protein: 175 mg/m^2 IV over 3 hours, every 3 weeks in combination with trastuzumab.
- Advanced or metastatic NSCLC; Weekly paclitaxel 50 mg/m^2 IV over 1 hour in combination with carboplatin AUC 2 with concurrent XRT, and after completion of XRT, paclitaxel 200 mg/m^2 and carboplatin AUC 6 q3 weeks × 2 cycles.
- Activity in other tumor types (bladder, small-cell lung, head and neck cancers).

Drug Preparation:

- Drug is poorly soluble in water, so is formulated using polyoxyethylated castor oil (Cremaphor EL) and dehydrated alcohol.
- Further dilute in 5% Dextrose or 0.9% Sodium Chloride.

Drug Administration:

- Glass or polyolefin containers MUST BE USED, and polyethylene-lined administration sets must be used. DO NOT USE polyvinylchloride containers or tubing since the polyoxyethlated caster oil (Cremaphor EL) causes leaching of plasticizer diethylhexlphthalate (DEHP) from polyvinylchloride plastic into the infusion fluid. Do not use Chemo Dispensing Pin device or similar devices since the device may cause the stopper to collapse, sacrificing sterility of the paclitaxel solution.
- Inline filter of < 0.22 microns MUST be used.
- Assess vital signs baseline, and remain with patient during first 15 minutes of infusion. Monitor vital signs every 15 minutes or per hospital policy.
- Assess CBC: Patients with solid tumors: absolute neutrophil count (ANC) must be at least 1500 cells/mm^3 and platelet count at least 100,000/mm^3; patients with AIDS-related Kaposi's sarcoma: ANC at least 1,000 cells/mm^3.

Premedication with corticosteroids:

- Solid Tumors: Dexamethasone 20 mg PO 12 and 6 hours prior to treatment. Administer diphenydramine 50 mg and H2 antagonist (cimetidine 300 mg, famotidine 20 mg, or ranitidine 50 mg) IV 30–60 minutes prior to treatment.
- AIDS-related Kaposi's sarcoma: Dexamethasone 10 mg PO 12 and 6 hours prior to treatment; administer diphenydramine 50 mg and H2 antagonist (cimetidine 300 mg, famotidine 20 mg, or ranitidine 50 mg) IV 30–60 minutes prior to treatment.
- Administer paclitaxel IV over 3 hours via infusion controller.
- DO NOT give drug as a bolus, as this may cause bronchospasm and hypotension.
- Assess for hypersensitivity reaction (most often occurs during first 10 minutes of infusion) and for cardiovascular effects (arrhythmia, hypotension).
- Keep resuscitation equipment nearby.
- Administer paclitaxel first when given in combination with cisplatin or carboplatin. There is increased cytotoxic activity when given in this sequence.
- Paclitaxel is being studied as a radiosensitizer, given weekly doses 80–100 mg/m^2 as a 1-hour infusion.
- Intraperitoneal infusion (investigational): Dilute dose into 1–2 liters of 0.9% NS, or as ordered; warm to 37°C and infuse as rapidly as tolerated into peritoneal cavity; assist patient to change position every 15 minutes per protocol × 2 hours to maximize distribution in peritoneal cavity.

Drug Interactions:

- Cisplatin: Myelosuppression is more severe when cisplatin is administered prior to paclitaxel (due to 33% reduction in paclitaxel clearance from the plasma). Therefore, paclitaxel must be given prior to cisplatin when drugs are administered sequentially.

- Ketoconazole, other azole antifungal agents: May inhibit metabolism of paclitaxel. Use together cautiously, and closely monitor for paclitaxel toxicity.
- Carboplatin: Possible increased cytotoxicity when given *after* taxol. Also, combination of paclitaxel and carboplatin results in less thrombocytopenia than would be expected from dose of carboplatin alone (etiology of plateletsparing effect unknown).
- Paclitaxel is metabolized by P450 cytochrome isoenzymes CYP2C8 and CYP3A4. Potential interactions may occur, including antiretroviral protease inhibitors. Use together cautiously with other drugs metabolized by this system (substrates or inhibitors).
- Doxorubicin and liposomal doxorubicin: Increased incidence of neutropenia and stomatitis when paclitaxel is administered prior to doxorubicin (due to significant decrease in doxorubicin clearance, possibly due to competition for biliary excretion of both agents). Therefore, doxorubicin should be given prior to paclitaxel.
- Doxorubicin: Increased risk of cardiotoxicity when given in combination with paclitaxel, with sharp increase in risk of congestive heart failure once cumulative dose of doxorubicin is > 380 mg/m^2. Consider stopping combination therapy when cumulative doxorubicin dose is 340–380 mg/m^2 and continuing paclitaxel as a single agent, as this does not increase risk of CHF (Gianni et al, 1998).
- Beta-blockers, calcium-channel blockers, digoxin: Additive bradycardia may occur; assess/monitor patients closely.
- Immunosuppressive agents, other antineoplastic agents: Additive immunosuppression may occur; assess toxicity and patient response closely.

Lab Effects/Interference:

- Decreased CBC.
- Increased LFTs.

Special Considerations:

- Reversal of multidrug resistance has been studied with quinidine, cyclosporine, quinine, verapamil.
- Drug has radiosensitizing effects.
- Drug is embryotoxic; avoid use in pregnancy. Women of childbearing age should use effective contraception.
- Drug may be excreted in breast milk, so breast-feeding should be avoided during drug therapy.
- ANC should be ≥ 1500/mm^3 prior to initial or subsequent doses of paclitaxel.
- Dose reductions: 20% dose reduction if severe neuropathy or severe neutropenia (ANC < 500/mm^3 for 7+ days) develop and/or consider addition of colony-stimulating factor support with next cycle; 25–50% dose reduction if hepatic dysfunction (hepatic metastasis > 2 cm) occurs (Chabner and Lon-

go, 2001); 50% or more dose reduction for moderate or severe hyperbilirubinemia or significantly increased serum transferase levels, with dose of paclitaxel not exceeding 50–75 mg/m² IV over 24 hours, or 75–100 mg/m² IV over 3 hours; if AST > 2 times upper limit of normal, patient dose should not exceed 50 mg/m² IV over 24 hours (Venook et al, 1998).

- One-hour infusion of paclitaxel as well as weekly dosing regimens are being studied/used. Lower doses, e.g., 80–100 mg/m² IV over 1 hour weekly × 3 with 1 week off per cycle, weekly × 6 with 2 weeks off per cycle, or weekly > 12 weeks, appear to inhibit angiogenesis, and allow for increased dose density.

Potential Toxicities/Side Effects and the Nursing Process

I. POTENTIAL FOR INJURY related to HYPERSENSITIVITY OR ANAPHYLAXIS REACTIONS

Defining Characteristics: Hypersensitivity occurs in 10% of patients, with anaphylaxis and severe hypersensitivity reactions in 2–4% (characterized by dyspnea, hypotension requiring treatment, angioedema, and generalized urticaria). Reaction is to cremaphor in paclitaxel preparation. Signs/symptoms include tachycardia, wheezing, hypotension, facial edema; incidence of supraventricular tachycardia with hypotension and chest pain occurs in 1–2%. Patients who have severe hypersensitivity reaction should not be rechallenged with drug. Those who have less severe reactions have received 24 hours of corticosteroid prophylaxis, and have been successfully rechallenged with drug infused at a slower rate.

Nursing Implications: Assess baseline VS and mental status prior to drug administration. Ensure that patient has taken dexamethasone premedication, and administer diphenhydramine and H2 antagonist as ordered. Monitor VS every 15 minutes, and remain with patient during first 15 minutes of drug infusion as most reactions occur during the first 10 minutes. Stop drug if cardiac arrhythmia (irregular apical pulse), hypotension, or hypertension occur, and discuss continuance of infusion with physician. Recall signs/symptoms of anaphylaxis, and if these occur, stop drug immediately and notify physician. *Subjective symptoms*: generalized itching, nausea, chest tightness, crampy abdominal pain, difficulty speaking, anxiety, agitation, sense of impending doom, uneasiness, desire to urinate/defecate, dizziness, chills. *Objective signs*: flushed appearance; angioedema of face, neck, eyelids, hands, feet; localized or generalized urticaria; respiratory distress with or without wheezing; hypotension; cyanosis. Review standing orders or nursing procedure for patient management of anaphylaxis, and be prepared to stop drug immediately if signs/symptoms occur, keep IV line open with 0.9% Sodium Chloride, notify physician, monitor VS, and administer ordered medications, which may include epinephrine 1:1000, hydrocortisone sodium succinate, and diphenhydramine. Teach patient the potential of a hypersensitivity or anaphylactic reaction and to immediately report any unusual symptoms.

II. POTENTIAL FOR INFECTION AND BLEEDING related to BONE MARROW DEPRESSION

Defining Characteristics: Neutropenia may be severe, especially when drug is administered via 24-hour infusion. Neutropenia is also more severe when cisplatin precedes paclitaxel in sequential administration, as it reduces paclitaxel clearance by 33%. Neutropenia is also more pronounced in patients who have received prior radiotherapy. Nadir is 7–10 days after dose with recovery in one week. Neutropenia is dose-dependent, with severe neutropenia (ANC $< 500/mm^3$) occurring in 47–67% of patients. Anemia occurs frequently, but thrombocytopenia is uncommon.

Nursing Implications: Assess baseline CBC, WBC, differential, and platelet count prior to chemotherapy, as well as signs/symptoms of infection or bleeding. Teach patient the signs/symptoms of infection or bleeding, and to report these immediately, and teach patient self-care measures to minimize risk of infection and bleeding. This includes avoidance of crowds, proximity to people with infections, and OTC aspirin-containing medications. Administer paclitaxel PRIOR to cisplatin or carboplatin when either is given in combination with paclitaxel. Teach patient self-administration of G-CSF as ordered to prevent severe neutropenia. Transfuse red blood cells and platelets per physician order.

III. SENSORY/PERCEPTUAL ALTERATIONS related to SENSORY NEUROPATHY

Defining Characteristics: Frequency and incidence is dose-dependent but appears not to be influenced by infusion duration. Overall incidence is 60%, with 3% severe neuropathy in women with breast or ovarian cancer treated with single-agent paclitaxel, but severe neuropathy occurred in 8–13% of patients with NSCLC who also received cisplatin. Onset related to cumulative dose, with incidence after first course 27% and remainder occurring after 2–10 courses. Sensory symptoms usually resolve after two or more months following paclitaxel discontinuance. Sensory alterations are paresthesias in a glove-and-stocking distribution, and numbness. There may be a loss of sensation, symmetrically, vibration, proprioception, temperature, and pinprick. Sensory and motor neuropathy may occur in patients receiving both paclitaxel and cisplatin. There is an increased risk for motor and autonomic dysfunction in patients with neuropathy from diabetes mellitus or alcohol ingestion prior to treatment with paclitaxel. Arthralgias and myalgias affect 60% of patients, begin 2–3 days after treatment, then resolve in a few days; may be ameliorated by low-dose dexamethasone.

Nursing Implications: Assess baseline neurologic status. Instruct patient to report signs/symptoms of pins and needle sensation, numbness, pain, increased discomfort with certain sensations, especially in the extremities, or motor weakness. Identify patients at risk: prior cisplatin, or having preexisting neuropathies (ethanol- and diabetes mellitus-related). Assess sensory and motor function prior to each treatment, and if abnormality found, assess impact on patient function, safety, independence, and quality of life. Test patient's ability to button a shirt, or pick up a dime from a flat surface. If severely impacting safety or quality of life, discuss with patient and physician drug reduction (20%) or discontinuance or use of cytoprotective agent. Teach self-care strategies, including maintaining safety when walking, getting up, taking bath or washing dishes and unable to sense temperature, and the need to keep extremities warm in cold weather. See NCI Common Toxicity Criteria, Appendix II: grade 3 motor = objective weakness, interfering with ADLs; grade 3 sensory = sensory loss or paresthesia interfering with ADLs; grade 4 motor = paralysis; grade 4 sensory = permanent sensory loss that interferes with function.

IV. ALTERATION IN SKIN INTEGRITY related to ALOPECIA

Defining Characteristics: Complete alopecia occurs in most patients and is reversible.

Nursing Implications: Discuss potential impact of hair loss prior to drug administration. Discuss coping strategies and plan to minimize body image distortion (e.g., wig, scarf, cap). Assess patient for signs/symptoms of hair loss. Assess patient's response and use of coping strategies, and help patient to build on effective strategies.

V. ALTERATION IN NUTRITION, LESS THAN BODY REQUIREMENTS, related to NAUSEA AND VOMITING, DIARRHEA, STOMATITIS, HEPATOTOXICITY

Defining Characteristics: Nausea and vomiting occur commonly in 52% of patients and are mild and preventable with antiemetics. Diarrhea occurs in 38% of patients and is mild. Stomatitis occurs in 31% and is mild, appears to be dose- and schedule-dependent, and is more common with 24-hour infusions than 3-hour infusions. Mild increase in LFTs may occur (7% bilirubin, 22% alk phos, 19% AST). Rarely, hepatic necrosis and hepatic encephalopathy leading to death have been reported. If severe hepatic dysfunction occurs, paclitaxel dose should be reduced (see Special Considerations section).

Nursing Implications: Premedicate patient with antiemetic (either serotonin antagonist or dopamine antagonist). Encourage small, frequent meals of cool, bland foods. Instruct patient to report nausea, and teach self-administration of antiemetics if receiving drug as an outpatient. If nausea/vomiting occur and is severe, assess for signs/symptoms of fluid/electrolyte imbalance. Encourage patient to report onset of diarrhea and to self-administer antidiarrheal medications. Assess baseline oral mucous membranes. Teach patient oral assessment and to report any alterations. Assess LFTs prior to drug administration and periodically during treatment.

VI. POTENTIAL ALTERATION IN CIRCULATION related to HYPOTENSION, ARRYTHMIA

Defining Characteristics: Hypotension during first three hours of infusion in 12% of patients, and bradycardia in 3% of patients have been reported; most often patients were asymptomatic, and patients did not require intervention. Significant cardiovascular events (syncope, rhythm abnormalities, hypertension, and venous thrombosis) occurred in 1% of patients receiving single-agent paclitaxel, but the incidence was 12–13% in patients with NSCLC receiving cisplatin as well. Of those patients with normal baseline EKGs at the beginning of paclitaxel therapy, 14% of patients developed an abnormal EKG tracing (nonspecific repolarization abnormalities, sinus bradycardia, sinus tachycardia, premature beats). Whether or not the patient received prior anthracycline therapy did not influence these events. Prior anthracycline therapy did influence the rare incidence of CHF. Rarely, patients developed myocardial infarction, atrial fibrillation, and supraventricular tachycardia. For patients receiving doxorubicin in combination with paclitaxel, there is increased risk of CHF once the cumulative dose of doxorubicin is >380 mg/m^2. (Gianni et al, 1998). Severe conduction abnormalities have been described in $<1\%$ of patients, and required pacemaker insertion in some patients.

Nursing Implications: Assess baseline cardiac status, history, and risk for development of CHF. Closely monitor patient during paclitaxel infusion, especially if patient has history of hypertension, or is on cardiac medications (see Drug Interactions section). Teach patient to report any dyspnea, SOB, chest pain, or heart palpitations, or any unusual feeling. If any abnormalities occur, stop infusion as appropriate and discuss further management with physician. If patient is receiving doxorubicin and paclitaxel, discuss with physician stopping combination therapy when cumulative doxorubicin dose is 340–380 mg/m^2, and continuing paclitaxel as a single agent, as this does not increase risk of CHF (Gianni et al, 1998). If the patient develops significant conduction abnormalities, discuss medical management with physician, and expect that patient will have cardiac monitoring during subsequent paclitaxel therapy.

VII. ALTERATION IN COMFORT related to FATIGUE, ARTHRALGIAS AND MYALGIAS

Defining Characteristics: Fatigue occurs commonly, and arthalgias and myalgias affect about 44% of all patients, with 8% experiencing severe symptoms.

Arthralgias and myalgias commonly occurred 2–3 days after the drug was given, and resolved within a few days.

Nursing Implications: Teach patient that fatigue may occur, and ways to minimize exertion and energy expenditure by alternating rest and activity, and organizing chores so that they are done as efficiently as possible. Arthalgias and myalgias may be troublesome, and can be managed with NSAIDs, application of warmth, and other comfort measures. Some patients report that swimming is helpful in minimizing discomfort. Studies of gabapentin, glutamine, and steroids have been disappointing. Opioids may be needed if severe.

Drug: paclitaxel protein bound particles for injectable suspension, albumin-bound (Abraxane, nab paclitaxel)

Class: Taxane, Nanoparticle albumin-bound paclitaxel, mitotic inhibitor.

Mechanism of Action: Promotes early microtubule assembly and prevents depolymerization, resulting in cell death; drug is combined with human albumin in a nanoparticle state, resulting in increased intra-tumoral concentrations of paclitaxel, lower drug concentrations in normal tissue, and potentially greater anti-tumor activity as higher doses can be given compared to cremaphor-dissolved paclitaxel.

Metabolism: Lower AUC, slower metabolism of paclitaxel nanoparticles, more rapid and extensive distribution into tissues; and longer half-life than paclitaxel.

Dosage/Range:

- 260 mg/m^2 q 21 day cycle, IV over 30 min; ANC must be > 1500 cells/mm^3;
- Dose reduce to 220 mg/m^2 if nadir ANC < 500/mm^3 for 1+ weeks or severe neuropathy; further reduce to 180 mg/m^2 if severe neutropenia or neuropathy recur; resume chemotherapy only when neuropathy resolves to grades 1–2, and ANC > 1500 cells/mm^3.
- Also being studied: 100 g/m^2 IV weekly.

Drug Preparation/Administration:

- Available in single use 100 mg vials. Gently dilute in Normal Saline, place in IV bag, and administer IV over 30 minutes. If not used immediately after mixing, may be stored in refrigerator for 8 hours. See package insert.

Drug Interactions:

- Metabolism of paclitaxel is catalyzed by the P450 micro-enzyme system: CYP2C8 and CYP3A4, but studies have not been done to determine extent of interaction; use together cautiously with protease inhibitors, e.g., retonivir.

- Cisplatin: Myelosuppression is more severe when cisplatin is administered prior to paclitaxel (due to 33% reduction in paclitaxel clearance from the plasma). Therefore, paclitaxel must be given prior to cisplatin when drugs are administered sequentially.
- Ketoconazole, other azole antifungal agents: May inhibit metabolism of paclitaxel. Use together cautiously, and closely monitor for paclitaxel toxicity.
- Carboplatin: Possible increased cytotoxicity when given *after* paclitaxel. Also, combination of paclitaxel and carboplatin results in less thrombocytopenia than would be expected from dose of carboplatin alone (etiology of plateletsparing effect unknown).
- Doxorubicin and liposomal doxorubicin: Increased incidence of neutropenia and stomatitis when paclitaxel is administered prior to doxorubicin (due to significant decrease in doxorubicin clearance, possibly due to competition for biliary excretion of both agents). Therefore, doxorubicin should be given prior to paclitaxel.
- Doxorubicin: Increased risk of cardiotoxicity when given in combination with paclitaxel, with sharp increase in risk of congestive heart failure once cumulative dose of doxorubicin is > 380 mg/m^2. Consider stopping combination therapy when cumulative doxorubicin dose is 340–380 mg/m^2 and continuing paclitaxel as a single agent, as this does not increase risk of CHF (Gianni et al, 1998).
- Beta-blockers, calcium-channel blockers, digoxin: Additive bradycardia may occur; assess/monitor patients closely.

Lab Effects/Interference:

- Decreased white blood cell count, neutrophil count, platelet count, decreased red blood cell count; 1/3 of patients had elevated alkaline phosphatase, AST.

Special Considerations:

- Indicated for the treatment of breast cancer after failure of combination chemotherapy for metastatic disease or relapse within six months of adjuvant chemotherapy. Prior therapy should have included an anthracycline unless clinically contraindicated.
- Drug is a Cremaphor-free, protein-engineered nanotransporter of paclitaxel. No pre-medication for hypersensitivity is required.
- Drug needs no special tubing, filter.
- Rarely, pneumothorax, interstitial pneumonia, lung fibrosis, pulmonary embolism have been reported.

Potential Toxicities/Side Effects and the Nursing Process

I. POTENTIAL FOR INJURY related to HYPERSENSITIVITY OR ANAPHYLAXIS REACTIONS

Defining Characteristics: Neutropenia is dose dependent and reversible, with grade 4 reported as 9% at doses of 260mg/m^2, without growth factor support. Febrile neutropenia occurred in 2% of patients, compared to 1% in the paclitaxel arm. Neutropenia may be more pronounced in patients who have received prior radiotherapy. Infectious complications occurred in 24% of patients, with oral candidiasis, respiratory tract infection, and pneumonia the mose commonly reported. Thrombocytopenia is uncommon, with bleeding reported in 2% of patients. Anemia occurred in 33% of patients, and was severe in 1% of patients (hgb < 8 g/dL).

Nursing Implications: Assess baseline CBC, WBC, differential, and platelet count prior to chemotherapy, as well as signs/symptoms of infection or bleeding. Teach patient the signs/symptoms of infection or bleeding, and to report these immediately, and teach patient self-care measures to minimize risk of infection and bleeding. This includes avoidance of crowds, proximity to people with infections, and OTC aspirin-containing medications. Administer paclitaxel PRIOR to cisplatin or carboplatin when either is given in combination with paclitaxel.

II. SENSORY/PERCEPTUAL ALTERATIONS related to SENSORY NEUROPATHY

Defining Characteristics: Sensory neuropathy is dose related, and common, occurring in 71% of patients in clinical studies (10% severe), compared to 56% in patients receiving paclitaxel. Grade 3 neuropathy reversible in many patients, within a mean 22 days. No grade 4 severity have been reported in clinical trials. Rare motor or autonomic neuropathy (e.g., ileus). Ocular/visual disturbances may occur rarely, especially at higher doses, and in the literature, persistent optic nerve damage related to paclitaxel has been reported.

Nursing Implications: Assess baseline neurologic status. Instruct patient to report signs/symptoms of pins and needle sensation, numbness, pain, increased discomfort with certain sensations, especially in the extremities, or motor weakness. Identify patients at risk: prior cisplatin, or having pre-existing neuropathies (ethanol- and diabetes mellitus-related). Assess sensory and motor function prior to each treatment, and if abnormality found, assess impact on patient function, safety, independence, and quality of life. Test patient's ability to button a shirt, or pick up a dime from a flat surface. Teach self-care strategies as needed, including maintaining safety when walking, getting up, taking bath or washing dishes and unable to sense temperature, and the need to keep extremities warm in cold weather (see NCI Common Toxicity Criteria, Appendix).

III. POTENTIAL ALTERATION IN CIRCULATION related to HYPOTENSION, ARRYTHMIA

Defining Characteristics: Hypotension during first three hours of infusion in 5% of patients, and bradycardia in < 1% of patients have been reported; most often patients were asymptomatic, and patients did not require intervention. Significant cardiovascular events (chest pain, cardiac arrest, supraventricular tachycardia, edema, thombosis, pulmonary embolism, hypertension, cerebral vascular accident) occurred in 3% of patients receiving single-agent paclitaxel albumin-bound particles for injection. Of those patients with normal baseline EKGs at the beginning of single-agent paclitaxel albumin-bound particles for injection therapy, 35% of patients developed an abnormal EKG tracing (non-specific repolarization abnormalities, sinus bradycardia, sinus tachycardia).

Nursing Implications: Assess baseline cardiac status, history, and risk for development of CHF. Closely monitor patient during paclitaxel infusion, especially if patient has history of hypertension, or is on cardiac medications (see Drug Interactions section). Teach patient to report any dyspnea, SOB, chest pain, or heart palpitations, or any unusual feeling. If any abnormalities occur, stop infusion as appropriate and discuss further management with physician.

IV. ALTERATION IN SKIN INTEGRITY related to ALOPECIA

Defining Characteristics: Alopecia occurs commonly (90% of patients studied).

Nursing Implications: Discuss potential impact of hair loss prior to drug administration. Discuss coping strategies and plan to minimize body image distortion (e.g., wig, scarf, cap). Assess patient for signs/symptoms of hair loss. Assess patient's response and use of coping strategies, and help patient to build on effective strategies.

V. ALTERATION IN NUTRITION, LESS THAN BODY REQUIREMENTS, related to NAUSEAVOMITING, DIARRHEA, MUCOSITIS, AND HEPATOTOXICITY

Defining Characteristics: Nausea, vomiting, diarrhea and mucositis were reported in 30%, 18%, 26%, and 7% of patients respectively. Rarely, hepatic necrosis, hepatic encephalopathy, intestinal obstruction, intestinal perforation, pancreatitis, and ischemic colitis have been reported in patients receiving paclitaxel albumin-bound injection.

Nursing Implications: Premedicate patient with antiemetic (either serotonin antagonist or dopamine antagonist). Encourage small, frequent meals of cool, bland foods. Instruct patient to report nausea, and teach self-administration of antiemetics. If nausea/vomiting occur and is severe, assess for signs/symptoms of fluid/electrolyte imbalance. Assess bowel elimination pattern and oral mucosa baseline and prior to each treatment. Teach patient to report diarrhea unrelieved with self-administered anti-diarrheal medications and adequate fluid replacement. Teach patient to assess oral mucosa and to use systematic oral cleansing after meals and at bedtime. Teach patient to report difficulty drinking fluids or ingesting food.

VI. ALTERATION IN COMFORT related to FATIGUE, ARTHRALGIAS AND MYALGIAS

Defining Characteristics: Fatigue occurs commonly, and arthalgias and myalgias affect about 44% of all patients, with 8% experiencing severe symptoms. Arthralgias and myalgias commonly occurred 2–3 days after the drug was given, and resolved within a few days.

Nursing Implications: Teach patient that fatigue may occur, and ways to minimize exertion and energy expenditure by alternating rest and activity, and organizing chores so that they are done as efficiently as possible.

Drug: pamidronate disodium (Aredia)

Class: Biphosphonate; hypocalcemic agent.

Mechanism of Action: Probably inhibits osteoclast activity in bone (which causes bone breakdown and lytic bone lesions) and may also block dissolution of minerals (hydroxyapatite) in bone, thus preventing calcium release from bone. Indicated for skeletal metastasis of breast cancer and multiple myeloma.

Metabolism: Not metabolized, renally excreted.

Dosage/Range:
- For bone metastases from breast cancer: 90 mg in 250 mL NS or D5W IV over 2 hours every 3–4 weeks.
- For bone metastases from multiple myeloma: 90 mg in 500 mL NS or D5W IV over 4 hours every 4 weeks.

Drug Preparation/Administration:
- Reconstitute by adding 10 mL sterile water for injection to 30-mg vial. Further dilute in 1 L 0.95 Sodium Chloride or 5% Dextrose Injection as per manufacturer's directions.
- Infuse over 2–24 hours via infusion pump or rate controller.

Drug Interactions:
- None.

Lab Effects/Interference:
- Decreased Ca.
- Decreased K+, decreased Mg, decreased P (phosphate).

Special Considerations:
- Saline hydration to maintain urinary output of 2 L/day should be maintained during treatment.
- Clinical studies show 64% of patients have corrected serum calcium levels by 24 hours after beginning therapy, and after 7 days 100% of the 90-mg group had normal corrected levels. For some (33–53%), normal or partially corrected calciums in the 60-mg and 90-mg groups persisted × 14 days.
- Has been shown to reduce bony metastasis in patients with multiple myeloma and to reduce pain.
- Patients with preexisting anemia, leukopenia, or thrombocytopenia should be monitored closely for 2 weeks after pamidronate disodium treatment.

Potential Toxicities/Side Effects and the Nursing Process

I. ALTERATIONS IN NUTRITION, LESS THAN BODY REQUIREMENTS, related to GI SIDE EFFECTS

Defining Characteristics: Rarely, nausea, vomiting, abdominal discomfort, constipation, and anorexia may occur.

Nursing Implications: Assess baseline nutritional and elimination status and monitor during treatment. Ensure adequate hydration and urinary output of 2 L/day. Administer ordered antiemetics. Administer oral phosphates as cathartics if ordered. Assess food differences and offer small, frequent feedings.

II. ALTERATION IN ELECTROLYTES related to HYPOCALCEMIA, HYPERCALCEMIA

Defining Characteristics: Rarely, if drug is very effective, hypocalcemia may occur; conversely, if drug is ineffective, hypercalcemia may occur. Hypokalemia, hypomagnesemia, hypophosphatemia may occur.

Nursing Implications: Monitor serum Ca+ closely. Assess for signs/symptoms of hypocalcemia (muscle twitching, spasm tetany, seizures) and hypercalcemia (bone pain, nausea, vomiting, polyuria, polydipsia, constipation, bradycardia, lethargy, muscle weakness, psychosis). Notify physician, recheck serum calcium immediately, and institute corrective measures as ordered. Monitor serum potassium, magnesium, phosphate levels, and notify physician of abnormalities.

III. ALTERATIONS IN COMFORT related to LOCAL VEIN IRRITATION

Defining Characteristics: Transient fever (1°C or 3°F elevation) may occur 24–48 hours after drug administration (27% of patients); local reactions (pain, irritation, phlebitis) are common with 90-mg dose.

Nursing Implications: Assess baseline temperature, and monitor during and after infusion. Administer antipyretics as ordered. Assess IV site and restart new IV as needed for 90-mg dose in large vein where drug can be rapidly diluted. Apply warm packs as needed to site.

IV. ALTERATIONS IN FLUID BALANCE related to AGGRESSIVE HYDRATION

Defining Characteristics: Patients receive aggressive saline hydration to ensure urinary output of 2 L/day. Hypertension may occur. Patients with history of heart disease or renal insufficiency are at risk for fluid overload.

Nursing Implications: Assess baseline hydration status, total body fluid balance; monitor q4h. Discuss with physician need for diuretics once hydrated to keep body fluid balance equal (I = O). Monitor VS q4h during hydration, and notify physician of changes.

Drug: pegasparaginase

Class: Miscellaneous agent (enzyme).

Mechanism of Action: Pegasparaginase is a modified form of L-asparaginase, wherein units of monomethoxypolethylene glycol (PEG) are covalently conjugated to L-asparaginase, forming the active ingredient PEG-L-asparaginase. The enzyme hydrolyzes serum asparagine, a nonessential amino acid for both normal and leukemic cells. Unlike normal cells, leukemic cells are unable to synthesize their own asparagine, resulting in cell death.

Metabolism: Unclear.

Dosage/Range:
- Adults under 21 and adolescents: 2500 IU/m^2 every 14 days.
- Children with BSA $\geq$ 0.6 m^2: 2500 IU/m^2 every 14 days.
- Children with BSA $\leq$ 0.6 m^2: 82.5 IU/kg body weight every 14 days.
- NOTE: Safety and efficacy have been established only in patients from 1–21 years of age.

Drug Preparation/Administration:
- For intravenous use, reconstitute with sterile water for injection, and dilute further in 100 cc NS or D5W. If giving IM, reconstitute in no more than 2

cc NS for injection. If more than 2 cc of NS is used, more than one injection site must be used.

- IM is the preferred route of administration, because of the lower incidence of hepatotoxicity, coagulopathy, and gastrointestinal and renal disorders as compared with the intravenous route.

Drug Interactions:

- Nonsteroidal anti-inflammatory drugs (NSAIDs), aspirin, dipyridamole, heparin, warfarin, and blood-dyscrasia-causing medications: Pegasparaginase causes imbalances in coagulation factors, predisposing patients to bleeding and/or thrombosis.
- Hepatotoxic medications (increased risk of toxicity).
- Methotrexate: Drug antagonizes antifolate effects of MTX if given before MTX administration. If given 24 hours after MTX, its antifolate activity will be terminated at that point.
- Vaccines, both live and killed virus: Patient's antibody response to the killed vaccine may be reduced for up to one year by the immunosuppression brought on by pegasparaginase. Such immunosuppression may also potentiate the replication of live-virus vaccines, increase the side effects of the vaccine virus, and/or may decrease the patient's antibody response to the vaccine.

Lab Effects/Interference:

- Increased LFTs, serum glucose, BUN, and uric acid.
- Prolonged PT.

Special Considerations:

- Drug should NOT be given in patients with:
  - —Pegasparaginase allergy
  - —Bleeding disorders associated with prior asparaginase therapy
  - —Pancreatitis, or history of
- Hypersensitivity reactions occur more frequently with pegasparaginase than with the vast majority of chemotherapeutic agents. Patients must be closely monitored for signs of allergic/anaphylactic reactions. Ensure immediate access to adverse-reaction kit.

Potential Toxicities/Side Effects and the Nursing Process

I. POTENTIAL FOR INJURY related to HYPERSENSITIVITY OR ANAPHYLACTIC REACTIONS

Defining Characteristics: Occurs less often with IM route of administration. May be life-threatening reaction, but is usually mild.

Nursing Implications: Discuss with physician use of test dose prior to drug administration. Assess baseline VS and mental status prior to drug administration. Review standing orders or nursing procedure for management of anaphylaxis and be prepared to stop drug immediately if signs/symptoms occur; keep IV line open with 0.9% Sodium Chloride, notify physician, monitor vital signs, and administer ordered medications, which may include epinephrine 1:1000, hydrocortisone sodium succinate, and diphenhydramine. Teach patient the potential of a hypersensitivity or anaphylactic reaction and to immediately report any unusual symptoms. *Escherichia coli* preparation of L-asparaginase and *Erwinia carotovora* preparation are non-cross-resistant, so if an anaphylactic reaction occurs with one, the other preparation may be used.

II. POTENTIAL FOR INJURY related to HEPATIC DYSFUNCTION OR THROMBOEMBOLISM

Defining Characteristics: Most patients have elevated LFTs starting within first two weeks of treatment, e.g., SGOT, bili, and alk phos. Hepatically derived clotting factors may be depressed, resulting in excessive bleeding or blood clotting. Relatively uncommon.

Nursing Implications: Monitor SGOT, bili, alk phos, albumin, and clotting factors CPT, PTT, fibrinogen. Teach patient of the potential for excessive bleeding or blood clotting, and instruct to report any unusual symptoms. Assess patient for signs/symptoms of bleeding.

III. ALTERED NUTRITION, LESS THAN BODY REQUIREMENTS, related to NAUSEA/VOMITING, ANOREXIA, HYPERGLYCEMIA

Defining Characteristics: Many patients experience mild-to-moderate nausea and vomiting. Anorexia commonly occurs. Hyperglycemia is a transient reaction caused by effects on the pancreas with decreased insulin synthesis. Pancreatitis occurs in some patients.

Nursing Implications: Premedicate with antiemetics and continue prophylactically for 24 hours to prevent nausea and vomiting. Encourage small, frequent meals of cool, bland foods and liquids, as well as favorite foods, especially high-calorie, high-protein foods. Encourage use of spices and do weekly weights. Teach patient about the potential of hyperglycemia and pancreatitis, and instruct to report any unusual symptoms: e.g., increased thirst, urination, and appetite (hyperglycemia) and abdominal or stomach pain, constipation, or nausea and vomiting (pancreatitis). Monitor serum glucose, amylase, and lipase levels periodically during treatment. Report any laboratory elevations to physician. Treat hyperglycemia issues with diet or insulin as ordered by physician. Treat pancreatitis per physician orders.

IV. SENSORY/PERCEPTUAL ALTERATIONS related to NEUROTOXICITY

Defining Characteristics: Neurotoxicity may occur in some patients—commonly, lethargy, drowsiness, and somnolence; rarely coma. Seen more frequently in adults.

Nursing Implications: Teach patient about the potential of CNS toxicity, and instruct to report any unusual symptoms. Obtain baseline neurologic and mental function. Assess patient for any neurologic abnormalities and report changes to physician. Discuss with patient the impact of malaise on his/her general sense of well-being and strategies to minimize the distress.

V. INFECTION, BLEEDING, AND FATIGUE related to BONE MARROW DEPRESSION

Defining Characteristics: Bone marrow depression is not common. Mild anemia may occur. Serious leukopenia and thrombocytopenia are rare.

Nursing Implications: Monitor CBC, platelet count prior to drug administration, as well as signs/symptoms of infection, bleeding, or anemia. Instruct patient in self-assessment of signs/symptoms of infection, bleeding, or anemia and to report immediately.

Drug: pemetrexed (Alimta)

Class: Multi-targeted antifolate (antimetabolite).

Mechanism of Action: Inhibits key metabolic enzymatic steps (Thymidylate synthase [TS], dihydrofolate reductase [DHFR], and glycinamide ribonucleotide formyl-transferase [GARFT]) critical to pyrimidine and purine synthesis, thus preventing DNA synthesis and cell division. Drug is carried into tumor cells via reduced folate carriers, metabolized intracellularly to polyglutamated form of pemetrexed that potently inhibits purine and pyrimidine synthesis. Antitumor effect dependent upon size of cellular folate pools, so folic acid must be co-administered to increase drug efficacy and minimize toxicity. Polyglutamates accumulate in the cell, with a long cellular half-life, and increased cytotoxicity.

Metabolism: Following IV administration, peak plasma levels are achieved within 30 minutes. Drug is widely distributed in body tissues, especially liver, kidneys, small intestines and colon. Excreted by kidneys (glomerular and tubular) into the urine, with up to 90% of the drug excreted unchanged during the first 24 hours after administration. Plasma half-life is about 3 hours, with prolonged terminal half-life of 20 hours.

Dosage/Range:

- Malignant-pleural mesothelioma: 500 mg/m^2 IV over 10 minutes q 21 days together with cisplatin 75 mg/m^2 IV over 2 hours, beginning 30 minutes after the end of the pemetrexed dose.
- Non-Small Cell Lung Cancer: 500 mg/m^2 IV over 10 minutes q 21 days

Drug Preparation/Administration:

- Reconstitute pemetrexed 500 mg vial by adding 20 mL 0.9% sodium chloride for injection, resulting in a concentration of 25 mg/mL.
- Asceptically remove dose and add to 100 mL 0.9% sodium chloride for injection.
- Administer as a 10-minute IV infusion.
- Patient should take dexamethasone 4 mg PO twice daily on the day before, day of, and day after treatment to help prevent skin rash.
- Patient must take daily folic acid supplement (350 to 1000 μg) po beginning 1 week prior to treatment, and continuing throughout treatment and post-treatment.
- Patient must receive vitamin B_{12} (1000 μg) IM injections every 3 cycles, beginning 1 week prior to treatment, and continuing throughout treatment every 3 cycles thereafter
- Full dose if ANC > 1500 cells/mm^3, platelets > 100,000 cells/mm^3, AND creatinine clearance > 45 mL/min.

Dose Reductions:

- Hematologic: Nadir ANC < 500 cells/mm^3 and platelet count > 50,000 cells/mm^3 DOSE REDUCE both drugs to 75% of previous doses.
- Hematologic: Nadir platelets < 50,000 cells/mm^3 regardless of ANC nadir DOSE REDUCE both drugs to 50% of previous doses.
- Pemetrexed should be discontinued for any grade 3 or 4 hematologic or non-hematologic toxicity after 2 dose reductions, or immediately if grade 3 or 4 neurologic toxicity.
- If grade 1 neurotoxicity, no dose modifications of either drug. If grade 2 neurotoxicity, 100% pemetrexed dose, but cisplatin is 50% of previous dose.

Drug Interactions:

- Nephrotoxic drugs: Potentially delayed pemetrexed excretion.
- Drugs secreted by renal tubules (e.g., probenecid): potential delayed pemetrexed excretion.
- Ibuprofen in people with normal renal function: 20% increase in AUC of pemetrexed, due to 20% reduction in pemetrexed clearance.
- NSAIDs (short half-lives, e.g., ibuprofen): AVOID if renal compromise (creatinine clearance < 80 mL/min), stop NSAIDs 2 days prior to peme-

trexed administration, the day of administration, and for 2 days following pemetrexed administration.

- NSAIDs (long half-lives): stop NSAID 5 days before, the day of, and for 2 days following pemetrexed administration.

Lab Effects/Interference: None known.

Special Considerations:

- FDA indicated in combination with cisplatin for the treatment of patients with malignant pleural mesothelioma whose disease is unresectable or who are otherwise not candidates for curative surgery.
- FDA indicated as a single agent for the treatment of patients with locally advanced or metastatic nonsmall cell lung cancer after prior chemotherapy.
- Do not administer drug if creatinine clearance is <45 mL/min using Cockcroft and Gault formula (estimated creatinine clearance).
  [140 − age in years] × actual body weight (kg)
  Males = 72 × Serum creatinine (mg/dL) = mL/min
  Females = Estimated creatinine clearance for males × 0.85
- Pemetrexed is fetotoxic and teratogenic. Women of child-bearing age should use effective birth control measures. Women should not breast feed an infant while receiving pemetrexed.

Potential Toxicities/Side Effects and the Nursing Process

I. POTENTIAL INFECTION, BLEEDING, AND FATIGUE related to BONE MARROW DEPRESSION

Defining Characteristics: Bone marrow depression is dose-limiting toxicity. Nadir is day 8 with recovery by day 15 of each cycle. Neutropenia occurred in 58% of patients, with grade 3 (19%), and grade 4 (5%). For grades 3 and 4 neutropenia, the incidence in between patients who were fully supplemented was 24%, in contrast to patients who were never supplemented (38%). The overall incidence of thrombocytopenia is 27%, with grades 3 and 4 (4%/1%, respectively). Anemia occurred in 33% of patients overall.

Nursing Implications: Assess baseline CBC, WBC, differential and ANC, and platelet count prior to chemotherapy as well as for signs and symptoms of infection, bleeding, or anemia. Ensure labs ANC >1500 cells/mm^3, platelets $>100{,}000$ cells/mm^3, AND creatinine clearance >45 mL/min prior to drug administration. Ensure that patient has taken vitamin supplements prior to drug administration: low dose oral folic acid or multivitamin with folic acid q d (at least 5 daily doses of folic acid must be taken during the 7-day period prior to the first dose of pemetrexed, and dosing should continue during the full course of therapy, and for 21 days after the last drug dose; Vitamin B_{12} 100 μg IM during the week prior to cycle 1, then every 3 cycles. Subsequent doses can be given on same day as pemetrexed treatment). Discuss dose reductions based on nadir counts with physician as needed. Teach patient signs/symptoms of infection, and bleeding, and instruct to report them right away. Teach measures to minimize infection and bleeding, such as avoidance of crowds, proximity to people with infection, and to avoid aspirin or NSAID-containing medications. Teach patient strategies to minimize fatigue, such as alternating rest with activity, and ways to organize shopping to minimize energy expenditure.

II. POTENTIAL ALTERATION IN NUTRITION, LESS THAN BODY REQUIREMENTS, related to NAUSEA, CONSTIPATION, ANOREXIA, DIARRHEA, STOMATITIS

Defining Characteristics: Nausea occurs in 84% of patients, vomiting 58%, constipation 44%, anorexia 35%, stomatitis/pharyngitis 28%, and diarrhea 26%, in combination with cisplatin.

Nursing Implications: Premedicate with antiemetics, and ensure patient has antiemetics to take to prevent delayed emesis from cisplatin. Teach patient and family delayed emesis regime. Encourage small, frequent meals of cool, bland foods, and to increase fluid intake. Assess oral mucosa prior to drug administration and instruct patient to report changes. Teach patient oral hygiene measures and self-assessment. Instruct patient to report diarrhea, to self-administer prescribed antidiarrheal medications and to drink adequate fluids. Monitor LFTs baseline and periodically during therapy. Notify physician of any abnormalities and discuss implications as drug studied only in patients with elevated LFTs related to liver metastases.

III. ALTERATION IN SKIN INTEGRITY related to RASH

Defining Characteristics: Incidence of rash with or without desquamation was 22%.

Nursing Implications: Assess baseline skin integrity. Teach patient that this may occur, and to take recommended dexamethasone premedication 4 mg po bid the day before, the day of, and the day after pemetrexed administration. Teach patient potential side effects of corticosteroid administration, including difficulty sleeping, mood alterations, and depression.

IV. POTENTIAL FOR IMPAIRED GAS EXCHANGE related to DYSPNEA

Defining Characteristics: Dyspnea was reported in 66% of patients receiving pemetrexed and cisplatin therapy; 10% had grade 3 dyspnea, and 1% had grade 4 toxicity.

Nursing Implications: Teach patient that this may occur, and to report it right away if severe or worsening. Assess baseline pulmonary status, at rest, and with activity. Assess oxygen saturation with vital signs. Discuss severe or worsening dyspnea with physician.

Drug: plicamycin (Mithramycin, Mithracin)

Class: Antibiotic isolated from *Streptomyces plicatus*.

Mechanism of Action: In the presence of magnesium ions the drug binds with guanine bases of DNA and inhibits DNA-directed RNA synthesis. Cell cycle specific for S phase.

Metabolism: Metabolism is not clearly understood. About half of the drug is excreted within 18–24 hours. Crosses BBB. Concentrations of drug in CSF equal blood concentration 4–6 hours after elimination.

Dosage/Range:

- Dose for testicular cancer: 25–30 μg/kg IV, alternating days until toxicity occurs.
- Hypercalcemia: 25 μg/kg IV for one dose.

Drug Preparation:

- For each 2.5-mg vial, add sterile water to obtain concentration of 500 μg/mL.

Drug Administration:

- IV drug is an irritant; avoid extravasation. Administer over 4–6 hours to minimize nausea and vomiting.

Drug Interactions:

- Myelosuppressive agents: Increased hematologic toxicity if overlapping nadirs; use cautiously and monitor patient closely or reduce drug dose.

Lab Effects/Interference:

- Decreased CBC (especially platelets).
- Decreased electrolytes, especially Ca, K, P.
- Increased LFTs, RFTs.
- Increased PT, bleeding time.

Special Considerations:

- Alternate-day therapy greatly reduces the incidence and severity of stomatitis, hemorrhage, and facial flushing and swelling.
- Do not administer to patient with a coagulation disorder or impaired bone marrow function because of the risk of hemorrhagic diathesis.
- Crosses the BBB.
- Metallic taste with administration.

Potential Toxicities/Side Effects and the Nursing Process

I. ALTERATION IN NUTRITION, LESS THAN BODY REQUIREMENTS, related to NAUSEA/VOMITING, ANOREXIA, AND STOMATITIS

Defining Characteristics: Severe nausea and vomiting begin 6+ hours after dose and may last 24 hours (at therapeutic doses); anorexia commonly occurs; alternate-day therapy greatly reduces the incidence and severity of stomatitis; taste alterations can occur.

Nursing Implications: Premedicate with antiemetics and continue prophylactically to prevent nausea and vomiting, at least for the first treatment. Encourage small, frequent meals of cool, bland foods and liquids. Encourage small, frequent feedings of favorite foods, especially high-calorie, high-protein foods. Encourage use of spices; weekly weights. Teach patient oral assessment and oral hygiene regimens. Encourage patient to report early stomatitis. Administer pain relief measures, e.g., diclone, viscous xylocaine oral gargles if needed. Suggest increased use of spices as tolerated. Help patient and partner develop menu based on past favorite foods. Dietary consultation as needed. Discuss dietary supplements of zinc and selenium.

II. POTENTIAL FOR IMPAIRED SKIN INTEGRITY related to ALOPECIA

Defining Characteristics: Occurs in 30–50% of patients, especially with IV dosing. Some degree of hair loss is expected in all patients. Begins after 3+ weeks, and hair may grow back in therapy. May be slight to diffuse thinning.

Nursing Implications: Assess patient for signs/symptoms of hair loss. Discuss with patient impact of hair loss and strategies to minimize distress (e.g., wig, scarf, cap); begin before therapy initiated. Assess patient for changes in skin, nails. Discuss with patient impact of changes and strategies to minimize distress; e.g., wearing nail polish, long-sleeved tops. Hyperpigmentation of nails and skin, transverse ridging of nails ("banding") may occur.

III. POTENTIAL FOR INFECTION AND BLEEDING related to BONE MARROW DEPRESSION

Defining Characteristics: Leukopenia nadir 7–14 days with recovery by 1–2 weeks. Less frequent thrombocytopenia, but one-third of patients develop a coagulopathy. Alternate-day instead of daily dosing reduces bleeding complications. Mild anemia. Potent immunosuppressant.

Nursing Implications: Monitor CBC, platelet count prior to drug administration, as well as signs/symptoms of infection or bleeding. Instruct patient in self-assessment of signs/symptoms of infection or bleeding and risk reduction. Dose reduction often necessary (35–50%) if there is compromised bone marrow function.

IV. POTENTIAL SEXUAL DYSFUNCTION related to DRUG EFFECTS

Defining Characteristics: Drug is mutagenic and teratogenic. Testicular atrophy sometimes occurs with reversible oligo- and azoospermia. Amenorrhea often occurs in females. Drug is excreted in breast milk.

Nursing Implications: As appropriate, explore with patient and partner issues of reproductive and sexuality patterns and the impact chemotherapy will have. Discuss strategies to preserve sexual and reproductive health (e.g., sperm banking, contraception).

V. ALTERATION IN METABOLISM related to HYPOCALCEMIA

Defining Characteristics: Drug may decrease calcium and lead to hypocalcemia. Monitor for muscle stiffness, twitching. In some cases when calcium is abnormally high (as in hypercalcemia from breast cancer), this drug may be used to decrease calcium level.

Nursing Implications: Monitor blood calcium levels. Instruct patient about signs/symptoms of neuromuscular involvement such as muscle stiffness, weakness, or twitching. Instruct patient about CNS manifestations of hypocalcemia: weakness, drowsiness, lethargy, irritability, headache, confusion, depression.

Drug: polifeprosan 20 with carmustine (BCNU) implant (Gliadel®)

Class: Alkylating agent.

Mechanism of Action: Wafer (copolymer) containing carmustine is implanted in the surgical cavity created when brain tumor is resected. In water, the anhydride bonds of the wafer are hydrolyzed, releasing the carmustine into the surgical cavity. The carmustine diffuses into the surrounding brain tissue, reaching any residual tumor cells, and causing cell death by alkyating DNA and RNA.

Metabolism: Unknown. Dime-sized wafer is biodegradable in brain tissue, with a variable rate. More than 70% of the copolymer degrades by three weeks, slowly releasing 7.7 mg of carmustine in concentrations. In some patients, wafer fragments remained up to 232 days after implantation, with almost all drug gone.

Dosage/Range:

- Each wafer contains 7.7 mg of carmustine, and the recommended dose is 8 wafers, or a total dose of 61.6 mg of carmustine.

Drug Preparation:

- Drug must be stored at or below 20°C (−4°F) until time of use.

- Unopened foil packages can stay at room temperature for a maximum of 6 hours at a time. The manufacturer recommends that the treatment box be removed from the freezer and taken to the operating room just prior to surgery.
- The box and pouches should be opened just before the surgeon is ready to implant the wafers. Open the sealed treatment box and remove double foil packages, handling the unsterile outer foil packet by the crimped edge VERY CAREFULLY to prevent damage to the wafers. See product information for opening the inner foil pouch and removing the wafer with sterile technique.
- Chemotherapy precautions should be used to limit exposure to the chemotherapy: surgical instruments used to remove and implant the wafers should be kept separate from other instruments and sterile fields, and should be cleaned after the procedure according to hospital chemotherapy procedure; all personnel handling the wafers of the inner foil pouches containing the wafers should wear double gloves, which, along with unused wafers or fragments, inner foil packages, and opened outer foil package, should be disposed of as chemotherapeutic waste.

Drug Administration:

- Neurosurgeon places 8 wafers into surgical resection cavity if size and shape appropriate; wafers are placed contiguously or with slight overlapping.
- Wafer may be broken into 2 pieces *only* if needed.

Drug Interactions:

- Unknown but unlikely as drug is probably not systemically absorbed.

Lab Effects/Interference:

- Unknown, but unlikely.

Special Considerations:

- Indicated for the treatment of newly diagnosed patients with high-grade malignant glioma as an adjunct to surgery and radiation.
- Indicated for use as an adjunct to surgery to prolong survival in patients with recurrent glioblastoma multiforme for whom surgical resection is indicated.
- Manufacturer reports that in a study of 222 patients with recurrent glioma who failed initial surgery and radiotherapy, the six-month survival rate after surgery increased from 47% (placebo) to 60%, and in patients with glioblastoma multiforme, the six-month survival for patients receiving placebo was 36% vs 56% for patients receiving polifeprosan 20 with camustine implant.
- Patients require close monitoring for complications of craniotomy, as intracerebral mass effect has occurred that does not respond to corticosteroid treatment; in one case, this resulted in brain herniation.

- Studies have not been conducted during pregnancy or in nursing mothers. Carmustine is a known teratogen, and is embryotoxic. Use during pregnancy should be avoided, and mothers should stop nursing during use of the drug.

Potential Toxicities/Side Effects and the Nursing Process

I. POTENTIAL SENSORY/PERCEPTUAL ALTERATIONS related to SEIZURES, BRAIN EDEMA, MENTAL STATUS CHANGES

Defining Characteristics: In clinical testing, the incidence of new or worsened seizures was 19% in both the group receiving the implant and those receiving the placebo. Seizures were mild to moderate in severity. In patients with new or worsened seizures postoperatively, the group receiving the implant had a 56% incidence, with median time to first new or worsened seizure of 3.5 days, versus placebo incidence of 9%, and median time to first new or worsened seizure of 61 days. Incidence of brain edema was 4%, and there were cases of intracerebral mass effect that did not respond to corticosteroids. Other nervous system effects were hydrocephalus (3%), depression (3%), abnormal thinking (2%), ataxia (2%), dizziness (2%), insomnia (2%), visual field defect (2%), monoplegia (2%), eye pain (1%), coma (1%), amnesia (1%), diplopia (1%), and paranoid reaction (1%). Rarely (< 1%), cerebral infarct or hemorrhage may occur.

Nursing Implications: Monitor neurovital signs closely postoperatively, and notify physician of any abnormalities. If intracranial pressure increases, a mass effect is suspected, and if it is nonresponsive to corticosteroids, expect the patient to be taken to surgery, with possible removal of wafer or remnants. Assess baseline mental status and regularly during postoperative care. Validate changes with family members. Discuss abnormalities with physician immediately and continue to monitor closely.

II. POTENTIAL FOR INFECTION related to HEALING ABNORMALITIES

Defining Characteristics: Most abnormalities were mild to moderate, occurred in 14% of patients, and included cerebrospinal leaks, subdural fluid collections, subgaleal or wound effusions, and breakdown. The incidence of intracranial infection (e.g., meningitis or abscess) was 4%. Incidence of deep wound infection was 6% (same as placebo) and included infection of subgaleal space, bone, meninges, and brain tissue.

Nursing Implications: Using aseptic technique, assess postoperative wound/dressing immediately postoperatively, and regularly thereafter. Assess systematically for signs/symptoms of infection or wound breakdown. Notify physician immediately and discuss antimicrobial therapy.

III. ALTERATION IN NUTRITION, LESS THAN BODY REQUIREMENTS, related to GI SIDE EFFECTS, ELECTROLYTE ABNORMALITIES

Defining Characteristics: Rarely, GI disturbances occurred: diarrhea (2%), constipation (2%), dysphagia (1%), gastrointestinal hemorrhage (1%), fecal incontinence (1%). Hyponatremia (3%), hyperglycemia (3%), and hypokalemia (1%) also occurred.

Nursing Implications: Assess baseline nutritional status, including electrolytes. Assess bowel elimination status and monitor nutritional and bowel elimination status closely during postoperative time. Discuss interventions for abnormalities with physician.

IV. ALTERATION IN CIRCULATION, POTENTIAL, related to CHANGES IN BLOOD PRESSURE

Defining Characteristics: Hypertension occurred in 3% of patients, and hypotension in 1%.

Nursing Implications: Assess baseline VS and monitor closely during postoperative phase. Discuss abnormalities with physician.

V. ALTERATION IN COMFORT related to EDEMA, PAIN, ASTHENIA

Defining Characteristics: The following occur rarely: peripheral edema (2%), neck pain (2%), rash (2%), back pain (1%), asthenia (1%), chest pain (1%).

Nursing Implications: Assess baseline comfort level and monitor closely during postoperative phase. Provide comfort measures. If ineffective, discuss symptom-management strategies with physician.

Drug: procarbazine hydrochloride (Matulane)

Class: Miscellaneous agent.

Mechanism of Action: Uncertain but appears to affect preformed DNA, RNA, and protein. It is a methylhydrazine derivative.

Metabolism: Most of the drug is excreted in the urine. Procarbazine crosses the BBB. Rapidly absorbed from the GI tract; metabolized by the liver.

Dosage/Range:
- 100 mg/m^2 PO daily from 7–14 days every 4 weeks.
- Given in combination with other drugs.

Drug Preparation:
- None.

Drug Administration:

- Oral.
- Available in 50-mg capsules.

Drug Interactions:

- Procarbazine is synergistic with CNS depressants. Barbiturate, antihistamine, narcotic, and hypotensive agents or phenothiazine antiemetics should be used with caution.
- Disulfirim (Antabuse)-like reaction may result if the patient consumes alcohol. Symptoms include headache, respiratory difficulties, nausea and vomiting, chest pain, hypotension, and mental status changes.
- Exhibits weak MAO(monoamine oxidase) inhibitor activity. Foods containing high amounts of tyramine should be avoided: substances such as beer, wine, cheese, brewer's yeast, chicken livers, and bananas. Consumption of foods high in tyramine in combination with procarbazine may lead to intracranial hemorrhage or hypertensive crisis.
- When taken in combination with digoxin, there is a decreased bioavailability of digoxin.

Lab Effects/Interference:

- Decreased CBC.
- Increased LFTs, RFTs.

Special Considerations:

- Discontinue if CNS signs/symptoms (paresthesia, neuropathy, confusion), stomatitis, diarrhea, or hypersensitivity reaction occur.

Potential Toxicities/Side Effects and the Nursing Process

I. POTENTIAL FOR INFECTION AND BLEEDING related to BONE MARROW DEPRESSION

Defining Characteristics: Major dose-limiting toxicity. Thrombocytopenia occurs in 50% of patients, evidenced by a delayed onset (28 days after treatment) and lasting 2–3 weeks. Leukopenia seen in two-thirds of patients, with nadirs occurring after initial thrombocytopenia. Anemias may be due to bone marrow depression or hemolysis.

Nursing Implications: Monitor CBC, platelet count prior to drug administration, as well as signs/symptoms of infection, bleeding, and anemia. Instruct patient in self-assessment of signs/symptoms of infection, bleeding, and anemia and to report this immediately. Dose reduction often necessary (35–50%) if compromised bone marrow function. Platelet and red cell transfusions per physician order.

II. ALTERATION IN NUTRITION, LESS THAN BODY REQUIREMENTS, related to GI SIDE EFFECTS

Defining Characteristics: Nausea and vomiting occur in 70% of patients and may be a dose-limiting toxicity. Diarrhea is uncommon, but rarely may be protracted and thus would be an indication for dose reduction.

Nursing Implications: Premedicate with antiemetics and continue prophylactically for 24 hours to prevent nausea and vomiting. Encourage small, frequent meals of cool, bland foods and liquids. Minimize nausea and vomiting by dividing the total daily dosage into 3–4 doses. Also, taking the pills at bedtime may decrease the sense of nausea. May administer nonphenothiazine antiemetics. Encourage patients to report onset of diarrhea. Administer, or teach patient to self-administer, antidiarrheal medications.

III. POTENTIAL FOR SENSORY/PERCEPTUAL ALTERATIONS

Defining Characteristics: Symptoms occur in 10–30% of patients and are seen as lethargy, depression, frequent nightmares, insomnia, nervousness, or hallucinations. Tremors, coma, convulsions are less common. Symptoms usually disappear when drug is discontinued. Crosses into CSF.

Nursing Implications: Teach patient the potential for neurotoxicity and provide early counseling about these effects. Assess patients for any symptoms of neurotoxicity. Discuss strategies with patient to preserve general sense of well-being. Obtain baseline neurologic and motor function. CNS toxicity may be manifested as reactions to other drugs, e.g., barbiturates, narcotics, and phenothiazine antiemetics.

IV. ACTIVITY INTOLERANCE related to PERIPHERAL NEUROPATHY

Defining Characteristics: 10% of patients exhibit paresthesias, decrease in deep tendon reflexes. Foot drop and ataxia occasionally reported. Reversible when drug is discontinued.

Nursing Implications: Obtain baseline neurologic and motor function. Assess patient for any changes in motor function, e.g., ability to pick up pencil, button buttons.

V. ALTERATION IN COMFORT related to FLULIKE SYNDROME

Defining Characteristics: Fever, chills, sweating, lethargy, myalgias, and arthralgias commonly occur.

Nursing Implications: Teach patient the potential for flulike syndromes and how to distinguish from actual infection. Instruct patient to report any changes in condition.

VI. POTENTIAL FOR IMPAIRED SKIN INTEGRITY related to RARE DERMATITIS REACTIONS

Defining Characteristics: Rarely occurs as alopecia, pruritus, rash, hyperpigmentation.

Nursing Implications: Assess patient for changes in skin, nails, and hair loss. Discuss with patient impact of changes and strategies to minimize distress, e.g., wearing nail polish, long-sleeved tops, wigs, scarfs, caps.

VII. POTENTIAL SEXUAL DYSFUNCTION related to DRUG EFFECTS

Defining Characteristics: Drug is teratogenic. Causes azoospermia. Causes cessation of menses, although may be reversible.

Nursing Implications: As appropriate, explore with patient and partner issues of reproductive and sexuality patterns and the impact chemotherapy may have. Discuss strategies to preserve sexual and reproductive health (e.g., sperm banking, contraception).

Drug: progestational agents: medroxyprogesterone acetate (Provera, Depo-Provera), megestrol acetate (Megace)

Class: Hormone.

Mechanism of Action: Unclear, but progestational agents compete for androgen and progestational receptor sites on the cell. Has potent antiestrogenic properties that disturb estrogen receptor cycle. Also increases synthesis of RNA by interacting with DNA.

Metabolism: Rapidly absorbed from GI tract. Metabolized in the liver. Excreted in the urine. Peak plasma levels reached in 1–3 hours; biological half-life, 3.5 days.

Dosage/Range:

Medroxyprogesterone acetate:

- Provera: 20–80 mg PO daily.

Depo-Provera:

- —400–800 mg IM every month
- —100 mg IM three times weekly
- —1000–1500 mg daily (high dose)

Megestrol acetate:

- Megace, mg PO qid (breast cancer): 80 mg PO qid (endometrial cancer).

Drug Preparation:

- IM preparation is ready to use; shake vial well before drawing up medication.

Drug Administration:
- Give via deep IM injection.

Drug Interactions:
- None.

Lab Effects/Interference:
- Increased LFTs.
- Changes in TFTs.

Special Considerations:
- Patients may become sensitive to oil carrier (oil in which drug is mixed).
- Small risk of hypersensitivity reaction.

Potential Toxicities/Side Effects and the Nursing Process

I. POTENTIAL FOR INJURY related to FLUID RETENTION, THROMBOEMBOLISM

Defining Characteristics: Fluid retention. Thromboembolic complications may occur. Sterile abscess may occur with IM injection.

Nursing Implications: Inform patient of potential for fluid retention and of signs/symptoms to watch for and to report to nurse or physician. Assess for signs/symptoms of fluid overload. Teach patient and family signs/symptoms of thromboembolic events: positive Homan's sign, localized pain, tenderness, erythema, sudden CNS changes, shortness of breath. Instruct patient to notify nurse or physician if any of the above occur. Give drug via deep IM injection: apply pressure to injection site after administering. Inspect used sites; rotate sites systematically.

II. ALTERED NUTRITION, LESS THAN BODY REQUIREMENTS, related to NAUSEA

Defining Characteristics: Nausea is rare.

Nursing Implications: Inform patient that nausea can occur; encourage patient to report nausea. Encourage small, frequent meals of cool, bland foods and liquids.

Drug: raloxifene hydrochloride (Evista®)

Class: Selective estrogen receptor modulator (SERM).

Mechanism of Action: Selectively modulates estrogen receptors by binding to estrogen receptors. This binding causes expression of multiple estrogen-regulated genes in different tissues. Acts as antagonist by inhibiting breast epithelial and uterine/endometrial proliferation; acts as an agonist (like estrogen) in bone to preserve bone mineral density, and on lipid metabolism to lower low-density lipids and total cholesterol, while not affecting high-density lipids or triglycerides.

Metabolism: Primarily metabolized in the liver, with rapid systemic clearance.

Dosage/Range:

- 60 mg PO qd.

Drug Preparation:

- Oral, available in 60-mg tablets.

Drug Administration:

- Take orally without regard to food or meals.

Drug Interactions:

- Cholestyramine: Causes 60% reduction in absorption of raloxifene. DO NOT GIVE CONCURRENTLY.
- Warfarin: 10% decrease in PT has been noted; monitor prothrombin closely if drugs are given concurrently.
- Highly protein-bound drugs: Raloxifene is >95% protein-bound. Use together with the following drugs cautiously, and monitor for underdosing or toxicity: clofibrate, indomethacin, naproxen, ibuprofen, diazepam, diazoxide.

Lab Effects/Interference:

- Unknown.

Special Considerations:

- Indicated for the prevention of osteoporosis in postmenopausal women, at doses of 30 mg–150 mg/day, together with calcium replacement.
- Recent evidence shows that raloxifene used to treat osteoporosis in postmenopausal women reduces risk of invasive breast cancer by 76% (*Multiple Outcomes of Raloxifene Evaluation*, 1999). Raloxifene decreased estrogen receptor-positive breast cancer by 90% but did not decrease estrogen receptor-negative breast cancer risk; benefit seems to be for postmenopausal women who commonly have receptor-positive receptor status.
- As compared to tamoxifen, raloxifene has 3 times the risk of causing thromboembolic disease but does significantly increase the risk of endometrial cancer (tamoxifen increases the risk 4 times).
- Currently being tested against tamoxifen in preventing breast cancer [National Surgical Adjuvant Breast and Bowel Project—PT (Prevention Trial) 2, sometimes referred to as the STAR (Study of Tamoxifen and Raloxifene)].

- Contraindicated in individuals who are hypersensitive to the drug, have or have had thromboembolic disorders, pregnant women, women who may become pregnant.
- Use cautiously in patients with cardiovascular disease, uterine cancer, or renal or hepatic dysfunction.
- When used to preserve bone density in postmenopausal women, drug should be combined with supplemental calcium and vitamin D, weight-bearing exercises, lifestyle changes such as cessation of smoking and reduced alcohol consumption.

Potential Toxicities/Side Effects and the Nursing Process

I. ALTERATION IN CIRCULATION, POTENTIAL, related to THROMBOEMBOLIC EVENT

Defining Characteristics: Drug can cause thromboembolic events, including deep vein thrombosis, pulmonary embolism, and retinal vein thrombosis. Greatest risk is during first four months of treatment. Rarely, patients may experience chest pain. Drug is contraindicated for individuals who have had or currently have thromboembolic events.

Nursing Implications: Assess baseline risk (e.g., history of CHF, malignancy). Teach patient to report pain in the legs, especially the calves, any redness or swelling of the legs, sudden-onset shortness of breath with chest pain. If leg pain, assess Homan's sign, and if positive, discuss with physician and anticipate sending patient to radiology for a duplex ultrasound to rule out thromboembolism or thrombophlebitis. If pulmonary embolism suspected, assess pulmonary status, discuss VQ scan with physician. Drug should be discontinued at least 72 hours prior to and during prolonged bed rest (e.g., postoperative care) resumed when the patient is fully ambulatory. Teach patient to move around while traveling to avoid prolonged time in one position.

II. ALTERATION IN NUTRITION related to GASTROINTESTINAL SYMPTOMS

Defining Characteristics: Nausea, vomiting, dyspepsia, flatulence, gastroenteritis, and weight gain have all been reported as occurring > 2% of the time.

Nursing Implications: Assess baseline nutritional status. Teach patient that these symptoms may occur and to report them. Teach patient symptomatic management. If problems persist or are severe, discuss pharmacologic symptom management and possible drug discontinuance.

III. SENSORY/PERCEPTUAL ALTERATIONS related to CNS CHANGES

Defining Characteristics: Migraine headaches, depression, insomnia, and fever have all been reported as occurring in > 2% of patients.

Nursing Implications: Assess baseline neurological status, including affect and sleeping pattern. Teach patient that these symptoms may occur and to report them. Teach symptomatic management. If symptoms do not resolve or become severe, discuss with physician pharmacologic symptom management and possible discontinuance of drug.

IV. ALTERATION IN COMFORT related to HOT FLASHES, ARTHRALGIAS, MYALGIAS, COUGH, RASH

Defining Characteristics: Hot flashes (25%), arthralgias (11%), myalgias (8%), leg cramps (6%), arthritis (4%), rash (6%), and flulike syndrome (15%) have all been described. Hot flashes usually occur during first six months of treatment.

Nursing Implications: Assess baseline comfort level and history of muscle and joint aches or pains. Assess skin integrity and respiratory status. Teach patient that these symptoms may occur and to report them, especially rash. Teach symptomatic management. If symptoms persist or become severe, discuss drug discontinuance with physician.

V. ALTERATION IN SEXUALITY related to VAGINITIS, LEUKORRHEA

Defining Characteristics: Vaginitis, urinary tract infections (UTIs), cystitis, and leukorrhea have been reported to occur in at least 2% of patients.

Nursing Implications: Assess baseline gynecologic status and history of UTIs and cystitis. Teach patient that these problems may occur and to report them. Teach patient symptomatic management and, if these are ineffective, discuss other strategies with physician.

Drug: raltitrexed (Tomudex, NSC-639186, ZD 1694, ICI-D1694) (investigational)

Class: Antimetabolite folate antagonist.

Mechanism of Action: Quinazoline-based folic acid analogue that acts as a folic acid antagonist; by selectively inhibiting the enzyme thymidylate synthase, it blocks purine synthesis. This causes breaks in DNA strands, and thus, DNA, RNA, and protein synthesis cannot proceed and the cell dies.

Metabolism: Drug has triphasic kinetics when administered intravenously over 15 minutes. The drug is rapidly distributed into tissue, with peak plasma levels occurring during or immediately after drug infusion. Cells actively take up drug, which is metabolized intracellularly into polyglutamates (more potent inhibitors of thymidylate synthase than parent drug). Polyglutamates have a long half-life in the cell, simulating continuous infusion therapy, with a terminal elimination half-life 8.2–105+ hours. Except for cellular metabolism, drug is excreted unchanged in the urine and is actively excreted by the renal tubules.

Dosage/Range:
- Per protocol.
- Colorectal cancer: 3 mg/m^2 IV q3 weeks.

Drug Preparation:
- Available in 2-mg vials, which should be protected from light, and refrigerated at 2–8°C (36–46°F).
- Reconstitute with 4 mL sterile water for injection, producing a concentration of 0.5 mg/mL.
- Withdraw dose, and further dilute in 50–250 mL 0.9% Normal Saline or 5% Dextrose.
- Reconstituted and diluted solutions are stable refrigerated for 24 hours.

Drug Administration:
- IV infusion over 15 minutes.
- Hold if urine creatinine clearance is < 25 mL/min.
- Contraindicated in patients with uncontrolled diarrhea, or hypersensitivity.

Drug Interactions:
- Potential interaction with other drugs that compete for excretion in the renal tubules: penicillin, indomethacin, methotrexate (Taylor, 2000).
- Folate, folic acid: Interferes, decreases cytotoxicity.

Lab Effects/Interference:
- Decreased WBC, neutrophil count, platelet count, Hgb/HCT.
- Increased bili and/or alk phos, liver transaminases (ALT, AST).

Special Considerations:
- Has been used for a long time in Europe; is being studied in the United States in the following tumor types: colorectal, with and without 5-FU/leucovorin and/or irinotecan, oxaliplatin; breast; NSCLC; ovary; pancreas.
- Some U.S. clinical studies in colorectal cancer have shown conflicting results and higher mortality, possibly because dose was not adjusted in renal dysfunction.
- Use cautiously, and monitor closely patients who have previously been heavily pretreated with chemotherapy or radiotherapy, especially if persistent stomatitis, bone marrow depression, hepatic or renal dysfunction; pa-

tients with history of gastrointestinal problems (e.g., diarrhea); and patients with hepatic or renal dysfunction.

- Patients should NOT take folate or folate-containing vitamins during therapy, as this interferes with cytotoxicity of drug.
- Drug should not be used during pregnancy or by breast-feeding mothers.
- Dose reduce for myelosuppression, gastrointestinal toxicity, renal dysfunction per protocol; reduced dose should be given only when toxicity resolved.
- Allergic responses (e.g., stridor and wheezing) following first dose are rare, but have been reported.

Potential Toxicities/Side Effects and the Nursing Process

I. POTENTIAL FOR INFECTION, BLEEDING, AND FATIGUE related to BONE MARROW DEPRESSION

Defining Characteristics: Bone marrow depression is one of dose-limiting toxicity. 60% incidence of leukopenia, and severe in 10–22% of patients. Nadir is day 8, but may be delayed to day 21; recovery begins day 10. Thrombocytopenia is less common, occurring in 25% of patients, and is severe in 2%.

Nursing Implications: Assess baseline WBC, differential, platelet and Hgb/HCT prior to chemotherapy, as well as for signs/symptoms of infection or bleeding. Teach patient signs/symptoms of infection and bleeding and to report these immediately; teach patient self-care measures to minimize risk of infection and bleeding. This includes avoidance of crowds, proximity to people with infections, and OTC aspirin-containing medications. Teach patient to report fatigue and teach measures to conserve energy, such as alternating rest and activity periods. Discuss transfusion of red blood cells as needed. Consult protocol for dose reductions if patient has severe bone marrow suppression, renal dysfunction, or severe hepatic dysfunction.

II. ALTERATION IN NUTRITION, LESS THAN BODY REQUIREMENTS, related to DIARRHEA, NAUSEA, VOMITING, STOMATITIS

Defining Characteristics: Diarrhea may be dose-limiting in some studies. Incidence is 11–26%, and drug is contraindicated in patients with uncontrollable diarrhea. Nausea and vomiting are mild to moderate if they occur, with an incidence of 11–19%, and are preventable with antiemetics. Stomatitis may occur, and in some studies had an incidence of 48%. Rarely, patients may experience anorexia or constipation (1–10% incidence).

Nursing Implications: Teach patient that these side-effects may occur and to report them. Assess baseline weight and nutritional status, bowel elimination pattern, and oral mucosal integrity, and monitor before each treatment and throughout treatment. Administer premedication to prevent nausea/vomiting. Teach patient to self-administer antiemetics at home, and to report unrelieved or persistent nausea/vomiting. Teach patient to notify provider if diarrhea occurs, to take OTC antidiarrheal medications if diarrhea develops, and to call nurse/physician if diarrhea persists or recurs. Teach patient self-care of oral mucosa, including assessment, when to notify provider, and oral hygiene regimen. Refer to protocol for dose reductions for gastrointestinal toxicity.

III. ALTERATION IN ACTIVITY related to ASTHENIA, FATIGUE

Defining Characteristics: Asthenia is very common, and may be severe. Appears to be dose-related. Anemia is very common, affecting up to 70% of patients.

Nursing Implications: Assess baseline activity tolerance, and level of fatigue. Teach patient that these side-effects may occur and to report them. Teach patient to alternate rest and activity periods. Teach fatigue self-care measures, such as strategies to maximize energy use and conservation while shopping, interacting with friends, and other activities.

IV. POTENTIAL FOR ALTERATION IN COMFORT related to FEVER, RASH, PAIN

Defining Characteristics: Fever occurs in 20% of patients, usually 1–3 days after drug administration. Rash may occur (35% incidence), is papular and pruritic, and commonly affects head and upper trunk. Alopecia and cellulitis have been reported rarely (1–10%). Pain may occur.

Nursing Implications: Assess baseline skin texture, presence of rashes, general comfort level, and also, whether patient commonly has fevers. Teach patient to report fever, pain, or rash. Teach patient to take acetaminophen or other agent to relieve fever or pain. Teach patient to use skin emollient or cream if rash appears to reduce itching. If itching and/or rash persist or are severe, discuss further management with physician.

Drug: rebeccamycin analogue (NSC 655649) (investigational)

Class: Antitumor antibiotic.

Mechanism of Action: Rebeccamycin is isolated from an actinomycete strain, but is not water soluble. It causes breaks in DNA. Its analogue, NSC 655649, has a tartrate salt (glycosyl-dichloro-indolecarbazole) that is water soluble and that appears to bind to or intercalate into the base pairs of DNA. It causes unwinding of the supercoiled DNA double helix. It also inhibits topoisomerase II.

Metabolism: Long terminal half-life of drug, and large volume of distribution, leading to marked bone marrow suppression. Appears to be exclusively metabolized in the liver and excreted in the bile. Five-day treatment provides therapeutic plasma concentrations for 7–8 days versus 2–3 days with one-day treatment q 21 days.

Dosage/Range:
- Per protocol, in studies, given as a 30–60 minute IV infusion q 21 days at MTD of 500 mg/m^2 (heavily pretreated patients) or 572 mg/m^2 (minimal pretreatment), or IV qd × 5, repeated q 21 days at 141 mg/m^2/d (heavily pretreated) or 165 mg/m^2/d (minimal pretreatment).

Drug Preparation/Administration:
- Drug available from NCI in 20 mL vials containing 10 mg/mL with one equivalent (2.24 mg/mL) of l-tartaric acid in sterile water for injection. Desired drug dose is further diluted in 0.9% Normal Saline and infused over 1 hour via a central line.

Drug Interactions:
- Unknown.

Lab Effects/Interference:
- Transient elevation of hepatic transaminases peaking on day 8 or 15 of each cycle.

Special Considerations:
- Bone marrow suppression is dose-limiting toxicity (Dowlati et al, 2001).
- Phlebitis related to dose necessitates use of central venous catheter for MTD infusions.
- One patient developed acute myeloid leukemia 13 months after completing therapy (described with topoisomerase II inhibitor therapy).
- Appears marked activity in hepatobiliary cancers in chemotherapy-naïve patients (2 PRs, 2 minor responses, and 6 prolonged (> 6 month); stable disease in 3 patients with gallbladder cancer and 1 patient cholangiocarcinoma.

Potential Toxicities/Side Effects and the Nursing Process

I. POTENTIAL FOR INFECTION, BLEEDING, FATIGUE related to NEUTROPENIA, THROMBOCYTOPENIA, ANEMIA

Defining Characteristics: Neutropenia and thrombocytopenia may occur at MTD. Anemia is uncommon but may occur at highest dose level. Many patients required dose delays due to neutropenia, but neutropenic fever is rare.

Nursing Implications: Evaluate WBC, ANC, platelet count, hemoglobin/hematocrit baseline and monitor regularly during therapy per protocol. Discuss abnormalities with physician prior to drug administration. Assess for signs/symptoms of infection or bleeding, and teach patient to notify nurse or physician if they arise. Teach patient self-care measures to minimize risk of infection and bleeding, including avoidance of OTC aspirin-containing medications. Assess patient Hgb/Hct and signs/symptoms of fatigue. Teach patient self-assessment and energy conservation strategies, such as alternating rest and activity periods.

II. ALTERATION IN NUTRITION, LESS THAN BODY REQUIREMENTS related to NAUSEA, VOMITING, MUCOSITIS, AND TRANSIENT INCREASED TRANSAMINASES

Defining Characteristics: Nausea and vomiting is mild and easily prevented by serotonin antagonists. Mild stomatitis may occur. Hepatic transaminases often increase, usually between days 8–15 of each cycle.

Nursing Implications: Assess nutritional status and weight baseline and monitor regularly at each visit. Premedicate with antiemetic prior to each treatment. Assess efficacy of plan, and revise as needed. Assess oral mucosa and dentition baseline and prior to each treatment. Teach patient systematic oral hygiene, self-assessment, and to report development of stomatitis. Teach patient dietary modifications if following symptoms develop: nausea, vomiting, stomatitis, and weight loss. Assess LFTs baseline and prior to each treatment per protocol. Discuss elevated transaminases with physician.

Drug: rubitecan (9-Nitro-20(S)-Camptothecin, 9NC, RFS 2000) (investigational)

Class: Topoisomerase I inhibitor.

Mechanism of Action: Induces protein-linked DNA single-strand breaks and blocks DNA and RNA synthesis in dividing cells, thus preventing cells from entering mitosis. Prevents repair (religation) of previous, reversible single-strand breaks in DNA by binding to topoisomerase I. Topoisomerase I is an enzyme that relaxes tension in the DNA helix torsion by initially causing this single-strand break in DNA so that DNA replication can occur. Topoisomerases I and II then work together to bring about replication, transcription, and recombination of DNA material. Topoisomerase I is found in higher-than-normal concentrations in certain malignant cells, such as colon adenocarcinoma cells and non-Hodgkin's lymphoma cells.

Metabolism: Drug is well absorbed after oral administration, with maximal serum levels in 2–4 hours after the first dose, and is converted to 9-aminocamptothecin and other metabolites. Drug is water insoluble, unlike other topoisomerase inhibitors (e.g., irinotecan, topotecan), which are water soluble.

Drug is metabolized in the liver, and slowly excreted in the urine, with a terminal half-life of 10.6 hours.

Dosage/Range:

- Studies in solid tumors: 1.5 mg/m²/d PO on days 1–5, with no therapy on days 6–7, repeated q week.
- Studies in hematologic malignancies: 2 mg/m²/d on days 1–5, with no therapy on days 6–7, repeated q week.

Drug Preparation:

- Per protocol.

Drug Administration:

- Oral, available in 1.25-mg and 0.5-mg capsules.

Drug Interactions:

- Unknown.

Lab Effects/Interference:

- Unknown.

Special Considerations:

- Drug is a radiosensitizer.
- Being studied in the following cancers: pancreatic (phase III), myelodysplastic syndrome (phase II), refractory ovarian (phase II), advanced colorectal (phase II), metastatic melanoma (phase II), previously treated NSCLC (phase II), sarcoma (phase II), relapsed metastatic breast cancer (phase II), refractory prostate cancer (phase II), recurrent glioma (phase II), chronic phase CML (phase II), refractory/relapsed AML (phase II), refractory lymphoma (phase II).
- Patients should drink 3 L of fluid daily to prevent hemorrhagic cystitis.
- Drug is contraindicated in patients with hypersensitivity to the drug, or to 9-amino-camptothecin.

Potential Toxicities/Side Effects and the Nursing Process

I. POTENTIAL FOR INFECTION, BLEEDING, AND FATIGUE related to BONE MARROW DEPRESSION

Defining Characteristics: Bone marrow depression is the dose-limiting toxicity. 30% of patients in pancreatic clinical trials experienced neutropenia, 11% severe (grades 3/4). Thrombocytopenia in these studies affected 35%, with 21% graded severe (grades 3/4). Finally, anemia was common, with an incidence of 53%, with 16% severe (grades 3/4).

Nursing Implications: Assess baseline WBC, differential, platelet, and Hgb/HCT prior to chemotherapy as well as for signs/symptoms of infection or bleeding. Teach patient signs/symptoms of infection and bleeding and to report these immediately; teach patient self-care measures to minimize risk of infection and bleeding. This includes avoidance of crowds, proximity to people with infections, and OTC aspirin-containing medications. Teach patient to report fatigue and teach measures to conserve energy, such as alternating rest and activity periods. Discuss transfusion of red blood cells as needed.

II. ALTERATION IN NUTRITION, LESS THAN BODY REQUIREMENTS, related to NAUSEA, VOMITING, AND DIARRHEA

Defining Characteristics: Nausea and vomiting are common, but preventable with antiemetics. Incidence in pancreatic studies was 50%, with only 5% having severe (grades 3/4). The incidence of diarrhea in these studies was 28%, with 5% severe (grades 3/4).

Nursing Implications: Teach patient that these side-effects may occur and to report them. Teach patients to take ordered antiemetic medications one hour prior to their dose, and to notify provider right away if nausea and/or vomiting persist, or if unable to drink/keep down fluids. Teach patient to take antidiarrheal medications if diarrhea develops, and to notify provider if diarrhea persists or recurs.

III. POTENTIAL FOR ALTERATION IN COMFORT related to FEVER

Defining Characteristics: In the pancreatic studies, 13% of patients reported fever.

Nursing Implications: Teach patient to report fever. Teach patient to take acetaminophen or other agent to relieve fever if it occurs.

IV. ALTERATION IN URINE ELIMINATION, related to CYSTITIS

Defining Characteristics: Interstitial cystitis may occur and be hemorrhagic; in clinical studies, cystoscopy revealed punctate mucosal ulcerations. Histopathologic exam revealed interstitial cystitis, coagulative mucosal necrosis, and little inflammatory infiltrate (Natelson et al, 1996). This is preventable by maintaining hydration. Incidence in patients described in pancreatic studies was 3%.

Nursing Implications: Teach patient that it is imperative to drink 3 L of fluid a day, and to avoid alcoholic beverages, as they may cause diuresis. Teach patient that if nausea and/or vomiting develop, and unable to drink this amount, to notify provider immediately.

Drug: streptozocin (Zanosar)

Class: Alkylating agent (nitrosourea).

Mechanism of Action: A weak alkylating agent (nitrosourea) that causes interstrand cross-linking in DNA and is cell cycle phase nonspecific. Appears to have some specificity for neoplastic pancreatic endocrine cells. Glucose attached to nitrosourea appears to diminish myelotoxicity.

Metabolism: 60–70% of total dose and 10–20% of parent drug appear in urine. Drug is rapidly eliminated from serum in 4 hours, with major concentrations occurring in liver and kidneys.

Dosage/Range:
- 500 mg/m^2 IV qd × 5 days. Repeat every 3–4 weeks; OR
- 1500 mg/m^2 IV every week.

Drug Preparation:
- Add sterile water or 0.9% Sodium Chloride to vial.
- If powder or solution contacts skin, wash immediately with soap and water.
- Solution is stable 48 hours at room temperature, 96 hours if refrigerated.

Drug Administration:
- Administer via pump over 1 hour.
- Has also been given as continuous infusion or continuous arterial infusion into the hepatic artery.
- If local pain or burning occurs, slow infusion and apply cool packs above injection site.
- Irritant; avoid extravasation.
- Administer with 1–2 L of hydration to prevent nephrotoxicity.

Drug Interactions:
- Nephrotoxic drugs: additive nephrotoxicity; avoid concurrent use.

Lab Effects/Interference:
- Decreased CBC.
- Increased RFTs (especially BUN).
- Increased LFTs.
- Changes in glucose, phosphorus.

Special Considerations:
- Renal function must be monitored closely.
- Drug is an irritant; give through the sidearm of a running IV over 15 minutes to 6 hours.

Metabolism: Well absorbed from GI tract and metabolized by liver. Undergoes enterohepatic circulation, prolonging blood levels. Excreted in feces. Elimination half-life is 7 days.

Dosage/Range:
- 20–80 mg PO daily (most often, 10 mg bid).

Drug Preparation:
- Available in 10-mg tablets.

Drug Administration:
- Oral.

Drug Interactions:
- Anticoagulants: increased PT; monitor PT closely and reduce anticoagulant dose.

Lab Effects/Interference:
- Decreased CBC.
- Increased LFTs.
- Increased Ca.
- Interference in lab tests such as TFTs and hyperlipidemia.

Special Considerations:
- Measurement of estrogen receptors in tumor may be important in predicting tumor response and should be performed at same time as biopsy and before antiestrogen treatment is started.
- Avoid antacids within 2 hours of taking enteric-coated tablets.
- A flare reaction with bony pain and hypercalcemia may occur. Such reactions are short-lived and usually result in a tumor response if therapy is continued.
- No evidence exists that doses > 20 mg/day are more efficacious.
- FDA-approved to reduce the incidence of breast cancer in high-risk women.
- FDA-indicated also for reducing the risk of contralateral breast cancer.
- FDA-approved for use to reduce the risk of invasive breast cancer in women with ductal carcinoma.
- Tamoxifen resulted in a significant decrease in development of invasive breast cancer in woman with atypical hyperplasia (88%).
- Rare side effects include uterine sarcoma, stroke, uterine cancer, blood clot formation.
- Tamoxifen is being studied as an adjunct to in vitro fertilization (IVF) for women with breast cancer who wish to have a child, given with FSH. The addition of either tamoxifen or letrozole with FSH increased the number of ovarian follicles, more mature eggs, and more embryos (Oktay et al, 2005).

Potential Toxicities/Side Effects and the Nursing Process

I. POTENTIAL FOR SEXUAL DYSFUNCTION related to CHANGES IN MENSES, HOT FLASHES

Defining Characteristics: May cause menstrual irregularity, hot flashes, milk production in breasts, vaginal discharge, and bleeding. Symptoms occur in about 10% of patients and are usually not severe enough to discontinue therapy.

Nursing Implications: As appropriate, explore with patient and partner issues of reproductive and sexuality patterns and the impact drug may have on them. Discuss strategies to preserve sexual and reproductive health.

II. POTENTIAL FOR ALTERATION IN COMFORT related to FLARE REACTION

Defining Characteristics: May cause flare reaction initially (bone and tumor pain, transient increase in tumor size). Nausea, vomiting, and anorexia may occur.

Nursing Implications: Inform patient of possibility of flare reaction, signs/symptoms to be aware of, and encourage patient to report any signs/symptoms. Inform patient of possibility of nausea, vomiting, and anorexia. Encourage small, frequent meals of high-calorie, high-protein foods.

III. POTENTIAL FOR SENSORY/PERCEPTUAL ALTERATION related to VISUAL CHANGES

Defining Characteristics: Retinopathy has been reported with high doses. Corneal changes (infrequent), decreased visual acuity, and blurred vision have occurred. Headache, dizziness, and light-headedness are rare.

Nursing Implications: Obtain visual assessment prior to starting therapy. Encourage patient to report any visual changes. Instruct patient to report headache, dizziness, light-headedness.

IV. POTENTIAL FOR INFECTION AND BLEEDING related to BONE MARROW DEPRESSION

Defining Characteristics: Mild, transient leukopenia and thrombocytopenia occur rarely.

Nursing Implications: Monitor CBC, platelets prior to drug administration and after therapy has begun. Instruct patient in self-assessment of signs/symptoms of infection or bleeding.

V. POTENTIAL FOR SKIN INTEGRITY IMPAIRMENT related to RASH, ALOPECIA

Defining Characteristics: Skin rash, alopecia, peripheral edema are rare.

Nursing Implications: Assess patient for signs/symptoms of hair loss, edema, and skin rash. Instruct patient to report any of these symptoms. Discuss with patient the impact of skin changes.

VI. POTENTIAL FOR INJURY related to HYPERCALCEMIA

Defining Characteristics: Hypercalcemia uncommon.

Nursing Implications: Obtain serum calcium levels prior to therapy and at regular intervals during therapy. Instruct patient in signs/symptoms of hypercalcemia: nausea, vomiting, weakness, constipation, loss of muscle tone, malaise, decreased urine output.

Drug: temozolamide (Temodar®)

Class: Alkylating agent.

Mechanism of Action: Drug is a member of the imidazotetrazine class and related to dacarbazine. Drug is a pro-drug, forming the metabolite monomethyl triazenoimidazole carboxamide (MTIC) when chemically degraded, and is further metabolized to 5-aminoimidazole-4-carboxamide (AIC), the active cytotoxic metabolite. Drug can pass through the BBB, where it has been shown to be effective against some brain tumors, possibly because of the alkyline pH. MTIC causes alkylation of DNA and RNA strands.

Metabolism: Well absorbed from the GI tract following oral dose (100% bioavailability), with peak concentrations in 1 hour when taken on empty stomach. The elimination half-life is 1.8 hours. The drug is degraded into MTIC in plasma and tissues. 15% of drug is excreted unchanged in the urine. Differs from dacarbazine in that formation of MTIC does not require liver metabolism. Food decreases the rate and extent of drug absorption.

Dosage/Range:

Refractory anaplastic astrocytoma that has failed prior chemotherapy:

- 150 mg/m^2/day × 5 days if patient has received prior chemotherapy, repeated q28 days.
- Dose should be adjusted to keep ANC 1000–1500/mm^3 and platelet count 50,000–100,000/mm^3.

Newly diagnosed glioblastoma multiforme (GBM) concomitantly with (at the same time as) radiotherapy and then as maintenance treatment.

- 75 mg/m^2 qd starting the first day of RT through the last day of RT, for 42 days (maximum 49 days) as long as ANC > 1500 cells/mm^3, platelet count > 100,000 cells/mm^3, and other toxicity (except alopecia, nausea, vomiting) are less than grade 1 (CTC),
- Prophylaxis for Pneumocystis carinii pneumonia while receiving concomitant RT and temozolamide, then 4 weeks after completion of RT.
- Maintenance dose (temozolamide PO qd × 5, then 23 days without treatment, repeated × 6):
- Cycle 1: Temozolamide 150 mg/m^2 PO qd × 5, then 23 days without treatment (as long as ANC > 1500 cells/mm^3, platelet count >100,000 cells/mm^3, and other toxicity (except alopecia, nausea, vomiting) are less than grade 1 (CTC),
- Cycle 2-6: Temozolamide 200 mg/m^2 PO qd × 5 then 23 days without treatment, repeated for 5 more cycles (as long as ANC > 1500 cells/mm^3, platelet count > 100,000 cells/mm^3, and other toxicity (except alopecia, nausea, vomiting) are <, grade 1 (CTC),
- Monitor CDC on day 22 then weekly until ANC > 1500 cells/mm^3, and platelets > 100,000 cells/mm^3; see package insert for dose reductions based on nadir counts and worst CTC toxicity.

Drug Preparation:
- None.
- Available in 250-mg, 100-mg, 20-mg, and 5-mg strengths.
- Drug is stored at room temperature, protected from light and moisture.

Drug Administration:
- Give orally with full glass of water on an empty stomach. Patient should take medicine at around the same time of day each day, e.g., bedtime.
- Do not crush or dissolve capsule.

Drug Interactions:
- Valproic acid: reduces temozolomide clearance by 5% but may not be clinically significant; monitor drug effect closely if used together.

Lab Effects/Interference:
- Elevated liver function tests (e.g., ALT, AST; occur in up to 40% of patients), increase in alk phos; decreased WBC, Hgb and platelet count; hyperglycemia; elevated renal function tests.

Special Considerations:
- Drug is indicated for the treatment of adults with 1) refractory anaplastic astrocytoma who have experienced disease progression on a nitrosurea and procarbazine (after first relapse), and 2) with newly diagnosed glioblastoma multiforme (GBM) concomitantly with (at the same time as) radiotherapy and then as maintenance treatment.

- Drug has also been used for treatment of glioma after first relapse and advanced metastatic malignant melanoma, and is being studied in a variety of solid tumors.
- Drug causes severe myelosuppression, and thrombocytopenia is the dose-limiting factor.
- Active in high-grade malignant glioma (gioblalstoma multiforme, anaplastic astrocytoma) and metastatic melanoma.
- Use with caution, if at all, in the following patients: hypersensitive to dacarbazine; myelosuppressed; have bacterial or viral infection; have renal dysfunction; have received prior chemotherapy or radiation; and women who are pregnant or who are breast-feeding.
- Rarely (1% of patients), hypercalcemia may occur with the 5-day regimen.
- PET (positive emission tomography) scanning showed reduced uptake of fluorodeoxyglucose (FDG) in patients who responded, in 7–14 days following a 5-day course of treatment, as opposed to those patients who did not respond, and who showed increased FDG uptake (Newlands et al, 1997).
- Overall response rate in some studies of patients with malignant glioma that had recurred or progressed after surgery and radiation therapy was 15–25% and 30% in newly diagnosed patients prior to XRT (Bower et al, 1997).

Potential Toxicities/Side Effects and the Nursing Process

I. POTENTIAL FOR INFECTION, BLEEDING, AND FATIGUE related to BONE MARROW DEPRESSION

Defining Characteristics: Thrombocytopenia and leukopenia are dose-limiting factors and occur in grade 2 or higher 40% of the time. This does not usually require administration of G-CSF. Nadir at 21–22 days, unless using 5-day treatment schedule, where nadir is day 28–29. Recovery for platelets is 7–42 days and in shorter time for WBC. Anemia may also occur, but is infrequent and less severe. Severity of bone marrow depression depends on dose and schedule, as well as disease process. In one trial, patients with malignant glioma had severe lymphopenia (41% grade 3 and 15% grade 4).

Nursing Implications: Assess baseline WBC, differential, platelet and Hgb/HCT prior to chemotherapy, as well as for signs/symptoms of infection or bleeding. Teach patient signs/symptoms of infection and bleeding and to report these immediately; teach patient self-care measures to minimize risk of infection and bleeding. This includes avoidance of crowds, proximity to people with infections, and OTC aspirin-containing medications. Teach patient to report fatigue and teach measures to conserve energy, such as alternating rest and activity periods. Discuss transfusion of red blood cells as needed.

II. ALTERED NUTRITION, LESS THAN BODY REQUIREMENTS, related to NAUSEA AND VOMITING, STOMATITIS, AND DIARRHEA

Defining Characteristics: Nausea and vomiting occur in 75% of patients, usually grade 1 or 2, and usually occurring on day 1. In one trial, using a 5-day treatment regimen, 21% had grade 3 nausea, and 23% had grade 4. Stomatitis may occur in up to 20% of patients. Diarrhea, constipation, and/or anorexia may affect up to 40% of patients.

Nursing Implications: Teach patient to self-medicate with antiemetics (serotonin antagonist effective) one hour prior to dose and suggest evening dosing to minimize nausea/vomiting. Encourage small, frequent feedings of cool, bland foods. Teach patient to notify provider right away if nausea/vomiting persists. Assess oral mucosa prior to drug administration and teach patient to report changes. Teach patient oral hygiene measures and self-assessment. Teach patient to report diarrhea, to self-administer prescribed antidiarrheal medications, and to drink adequate fluids. Teach patient to report constipation, and manage with stool softeners or laxatives. If patient has anorexia, teach patient to select acceptable foods and to eat small portions q2 hours and at bedtime.

III. ALTERATION IN SKIN INTEGRITY/COMFORT related to RASH, PRURITUS, ALOPECIA

Defining Characteristics: Skin rash, itching, and mild alopecia may occur, and are mild.

Nursing Implications: Teach patient about the possibility of these side effects and to notify the nurse if any develop. Discuss rash with physician if moderate or severe. Teach patient local symptom-management strategies for itch. Reassure patient that hair loss is usually thinning with mild hair loss and will grow back.

IV. ACTIVITY INTOLERANCE POTENTIAL, related to CENTRAL NERVOUS SYSTEM EFFECTS

Defining Characteristics: Lethargy (up to 40% in patients with malignant glioma), fatigue, headache, ataxia, and dizziness may occur, and in clinical testing, it was unclear whether this was due to neurological disease (i.e., malignant glioma), concurrent other drug therapy, or temozolomide.

Nursing Implications: Assess baseline energy and activity level. Teach patients that these side effects may occur, especially if the primary diagnosis is malignant glioma. Teach patient to report them. Teach patient to alternate rest and activity periods, to use supportive device such as a cane if ataxia or dizziness occurs, and other measures to maximize activity tolerance and to prevent injury.

Drug: teniposide (Vumon, VM-26)

Class: Plant alkaloid, a derivative of the mandrake plant (*Mandragora officinarum*).

Mechanism of Action: Cell cycle specific in late S phase, early G_2 phase, causing arrest of cell division in mitosis. Inhibits uptake of thymidine into DNA so DNA synthesis is impaired.

Metabolism: Drug binds extensively to serum protein. Metabolized by the liver and excreted in bile and urine.

Dosage/Range:
- 100 mg/m^2 weekly for 6–8 weeks.
- 50 mg/m^2 twice weekly × 4 weeks.

Drug Preparation:
- Available in 50-mg/5-mL glass ampules.
- Add desired 0.9% Sodium Chloride for injection or 5% Dextrose in water to reach final concentration of 0.1 mg/mL–0.4 mg/mL (stable 24 hours) or 1.0 mg/mL (stable 4 hours).
- USE ONLY non-DEHP containers such as glass or polyolefin plastic bags or containers.
- DO NOT USE polyvinylchloride IV bags, as the plasticizer DEHP will leach into the solution.

Drug Administration:
- Assess for presence of precipitate and do not administer solution if precipitate is seen.
- Administer over at least 30–60 minutes.

Drug Interactions:
- Doses of tolbutamide, sodium salicylate, and sulfamethizole will need to be reduced.
- Heparin causes a precipitate.

Lab Effects/Interference:
- Increased LFTs, RFTs.
- Decreased CBC.

Special Considerations:
- Rapid infusion may cause hypotension and sudden death.
- Chemical phlebitis may occur if drug is not properly diluted, or infused too rapidly.

- Severe myelosuppression may occur.
- Hypersensitivity reactions, including anaphylaxis-like symptoms, may occur with initial or repeated doses.

Potential Toxicities/Side Effects and the Nursing Process

I. POTENTIAL FOR INJURY DURING DRUG ADMINISTRATION related to HYPOTENSION AND HYPERSENSITIVITY REACTION

Defining Characteristics: Hypotension may occur during rapid IV infusion. Hypersensitivity reactions occur in 5% of patients, characterized by fever, chills, tachycardia, dyspnea, flushing, lumbar pain, bronchospasm, and progressive hypotension or hypertension. It is thought that hypersensitivity may be to the drug suspension of castor oil and denatured alcohol, which is used because the drug is poorly water-soluble.

Nursing Implications: Assess baseline temperature (T), VS prior to drug administration, and periodically during infusion. Ensure that drug is properly diluted, and infuse over at least 30–60 minutes. Instruct patient to report untoward signs/symptoms immediately. Have emergency equipment and medications, including epinephrine, diphenhydramine, hydrocortisone nearby. If signs/symptoms develop, stop infusion, keep IV line open, notify physician, monitor VS, and support patient. Be familiar with institution's standing orders or practice guidelines on management of anaphylaxis.

II. POTENTIAL FOR INFECTION AND BLEEDING related to BONE MARROW DEPRESSION

Defining Characteristics: Leukopenia is dose-limiting toxicity but thrombocytopenia may occur; nadir day 7 (3–14 days). Dose reductions need to be made if patient previously received chemotherapy or radiotherapy.

Nursing Implications: Assess CBC, WBC, differential, and platelet count prior to drug administration, as well as for signs/symptoms of infection and bleeding. Teach patient signs/symptoms of infection and bleeding, and instruct to report them immediately. Teach patient self-care measures to minimize infection and bleeding, including avoidance of OTC aspirin-containing medications.

III. ALTERATION IN NUTRITION, LESS THAN BODY REQUIREMENTS, related to NAUSEA AND VOMITING, HEPATIC DYSFUNCTION, MUCOSITIS

Defining Characteristics: Nausea and vomiting occur in 29% of patients but are usually mild; mucositis occurs at high drug doses. Mild elevation of LFTs may occur.

Nursing Implications: Premedicate with antiemetics prior to drug administration, and continue prophylactically for 24 hours, at least for the first cycle. Assess oral mucosa at baseline prior to drug administration; teach patient self-assessment and self-care measures. Monitor LFTs prior to drug administration; discuss dose reduction with physician if results abnormal.

IV. POTENTIAL FOR IMPAIRED SKIN INTEGRITY related to ALOPECIA AND PHLEBITIS

Defining Characteristics: Alopecia is uncommon (9–30% of patients) and is reversible. Phlebitis can occur if drug is improperly diluted or administered too rapidly.

Nursing Implications: If patient develops hair loss, discuss impact of loss and suggest coping strategies, such as wig or cap. Encourage patient to verbalize feelings and provide emotional support. Administer drug only through patent IV, properly diluted, and over at least 30–60 minutes.

V. POTENTIAL FOR SENSORY/PERCEPTUAL ALTERATIONS related to NEUROLOGIC TOXICITY

Defining Characteristics: Peripheral neuropathies may occur and are mild.

Nursing Implications: Assess baseline neurologic status. Teach patient to report any changes in motor or sensory functioning. Encourage patient to verbalize feelings regarding discomfort and sensory loss if these occur.

VI. POTENTIAL FOR ALTERATION IN CARDIAC OUTPUT related to HYPOTENSION AND PALPITATIONS

Defining Characteristics: Hypotension is related to rapid infusion of drug. Palpitations may occur during drug infusion.

Nursing Implications: Assess baseline cardiac status, noting heart rate, rhythm, and monitor heart rate and BP periodically during infusion. Infuse drug over at least 30–60 minutes.

VII. POTENTIAL SEXUAL DYSFUNCTION related to DRUG EFFECT

Defining Characteristics: Drug is carcinogenic, mutagenic, and teratogenic. It is not known if drug is excreted in breast milk.

Nursing Implications: Assess patient's and partner's sexual patterns and reproductive goals. Provide information, supportive counseling, and referral as needed and appropriate. Teach importance of contraception and discuss coping strategies for alterations in fertility (e.g., sperm banking). Mothers receiving drug should not breastfeed.

Drug: thioguanine (Tabloid, 6-Thioguanine, 6-TG)

Class: Thiopurine antimetabolite.

Mechanism of Action: Converts to monophosphate nucleotides and inhibits *de novo* purine synthesis. The nucleotides are also incorporated into DNA. Cell cycle phase specific for S phase. Thioguanine interferes with nucleic acid biosynthesis, resulting in sequential blockage of the synthesis and utilization of the purine nucleotides.

Metabolism: Absorption is incomplete and variable orally. Is metabolized in the liver by deamination and methylation. Metabolites are excreted in the urine and feces. Plasma half-life is 80–90 minutes.

Dosage/Range:

- Children and adults: 100 mg/m^2 PO q12h for 5–10 days, usually in combination with cytarabine.
- 100 mg/m^2 IV daily × 5 days (investigational).
- 1–3 mg/kg PO daily.

Drug Preparation:

- Available in 40-mg tablets.
- Dilute 75-mg vial with 5 mL 0.9% Sodium Chloride USP (15 mg/mL).
- Further dilute drug in 5% Dextrose or 0.9% Sodium Chloride (stable for 24 hours at room temperature or under refrigeration).

Drug Administration:

- Given orally between meals; can be given as a single dose.
- Given via IV bolus over 5–30 minutes (investigational).

Drug Interactions:

- Busulfan: increased hepatotoxicity; use caution when used together; monitor patient closely during long-term therapy.

Lab Effects/Interference:

- Decreased CBC.
- Increased LFTs.
- Increased uric acid.

Special Considerations:

- Oral dose is to be given on empty stomach to facilitate complete absorption.
- Dose is titrated to avoid excessive stomatitis and diarrhea.
- Thioguanine can be used in full doses with allopurinol.

Potential Toxicities/Side Effects and the Nursing Process

I. ALTERATION IN NUTRITION, LESS THAN BODY REQUIREMENTS, related to GI SIDE EFFECTS

Defining Characteristics: Nausea and vomiting occur commonly, especially in children, but are dose-related; anorexia is rare; stomatitis is rare, but most common with high doses; hepatotoxicity is rare, but may be associated with hepatic veno-occlusive disease or jaundice.

Nursing Implications: Treat symptomatically with antiemetics. Encourage small, frequent feedings of cool, bland foods and liquids. If vomiting occurs, assess for fluid and electrolyte imbalance. Monitor I/O and daily weights if patient is hospitalized. Encourage small, frequent meals of favorite foods, especially high-calorie, high-protein foods. Encourage use of spices; weekly weights. Teach oral assessment and oral hygiene regimen. Encourage patient to report early stomatitis. Provide pain relief measures, if indicated. Monitor LFTs prior to drug dose. Assess patient prior to and during treatment for signs/symptoms of hepatotoxicity.

II. POTENTIAL FOR INFECTION AND BLEEDING related to BONE MARROW DEPRESSION

Defining Characteristics: Bone marrow depression occurs 1–4 weeks after treatment. Leukopenia and thrombocytopenia are most common. Drug may have prolonged or delayed nadir.

Nursing Implications: Monitor CBC, platelet count prior to drug administration as well as for signs/symptoms of infection or bleeding. Instruct patient in self-assessment of signs/symptoms of infection or bleeding. Administer platelet, red cell transfusions per physician's order.

III. POTENTIAL FOR SENSORY/PERCEPTUAL ALTERATION related to LOSS OF VIBRATORY SENSE

Defining Characteristics: Loss of vibratory sensation; unsteady gait may occur.

Nursing Implications: Assess vibratory sensation, gait before each dose and between treatments. Report changes to physician. Encourage patient to report any changes.

Drug: thiotepa (Thioplex, Triethylenethiophosphoramide)

Class: Alkylating agent.

Mechanism of Action: Selectively reacts with DNA phosphate groups to produce chromosome cross-linkage with blocking of nucleoprotein synthesis. Acts as a polyfunctional alkylating agent. Cell cycle phase nonspecific agent. Mimics radiation-induced injury.

Metabolism: Rapidly cleared following IV administration; 60% of dose is eliminated in urine within 24–72 hours. Slow onset of action, slowly bound to tissues, extensively metabolized.

Dosage/Range:

Intravenous:

- 8 mg/m^2 (0.2 mg/kg) IV every day × 5 days, repeated every 3–4 weeks, OR
- 0.3–0.4 mg/kg IV, q 1–4 weeks.

Intracavitary:

- Bladder: 60 mg in 60 mL sterile water once a week for 3–4 weeks.

Drug Preparation:

- Add sterile water to vial of lyophilized powder.
- Further dilute with 0.9% Sodium Chloride or 5% Dextrose.
- Do not use solution unless it is clear.
- Refrigerate vial until use (reconstituted solution is stable for 5 days).

Drug Administration:

- IV, IM; intracavitary, intratumor, intraarterial.

Drug Interactions:

- Myelosuppressive drugs: additive hematologic toxicity.

Lab Effects/Interference:

- Decreased CBC (especially WBC and platelets).
- Increased LFTs and RFTs.

Special Considerations:

- Hypersensitivity reactions have occurred with this drug.
- Is an irritant; should be given IVP via a sidearm of a running IV.
- Increased neuromuscular blockage when given with nondepolarizing muscle relaxants.

Potential Toxicities/Side Effects and the Nursing Process

I. POTENTIAL FOR INFECTION AND BLEEDING related to BONE MARROW DEPRESSION

Defining Characteristics: Nadir is 5–30 days after drug administration. Thrombocytopenia and leukopenia may occur. Anemia may occur with prolonged use. May be cumulative toxicity with recovery of bone marrow in 40–50 days. Thrombocytopenia is dose-limiting.

Nursing Implications: Monitor CBC, platelet count prior to drug administration; monitor for signs/symptoms of infection or bleeding. Instruct patient in self-assessment of signs/symptoms of infection or bleeding and to report them immediately. Administer red cells and platelet transfusions per physician's orders.

II. ALTERATION IN NUTRITION, LESS THAN BODY REQUIREMENTS, related to GI SIDE EFFECTS

Defining Characteristics: Nausea and vomiting occur in 10–15% of patients; dose-dependent; occurs 6–12 hours after drug dose; anorexia occurs occasionally.

Nursing Implications: Premedicate with antiemetics especially with parenteral dosing of high dose. Continue antiemetics at least 12 hours after drug is given. Encourage small, frequent meals of cool, bland, dry foods, and favorite foods, especially high-calorie, high-protein foods. Encourage use of spices; assess weight weekly.

III. POTENTIAL SEXUAL DYSFUNCTION related to DRUG EFFECT

Defining Characteristics: Drug is mutagenic. Sterility may be reversible and incomplete. Amenorrhea often reverses in 6–8 months.

Nursing Implications: As appropriate, explore with patient and partner issues of reproductive and sexuality patterns and the anticipated impact chemotherapy may have. Discuss strategies to preserve sexuality and reproductive health (e.g., sperm banking).

IV. POTENTIAL FOR INJURY related to ALLERGIC REACTION

Defining Characteristics: Allergic responses occur rarely: hives, bronchospasm, skin rash (dermatitis). Secondary malignancies may occur with prolonged therapy.

Nursing Implications: Assess for signs/symptoms of allergic response during drug administration. Stop drug if bronchospasm occurs and notify physician. Discuss symptomatic treatment with physician. Instruct patient receiving prolonged therapy about importance of regular health maintenance examinations during and after therapy by primary care provider and oncologist.

V. ALTERATION IN COMFORT related to DIZZINESS, FEVER, PAIN

Defining Characteristics: Dizziness, headache, fever, and local pain may occur.

Nursing Implications: Assess for alterations in comfort. Treat symptomatically.

Drug: TLK 286 (Telcyta, investigational)

Class: Cell activated chemotherapeutic agent.

Mechanism of Action: Drug is a prodrug, and is activated when split into its two component parts—glutathione analogue and cytotoxic fragment, by the enzyme glutathione S-transferase P1-1(GST P1-1). This enzyme is overexpressed in many cancers, and confers a poor prognosis, and resistance to many chemo agents. The cytotoxic fragment then interacts with DNA, RNA and proteins to bring about cell death. The glutathione fragment may bind to GST P1-1 and reduce its ability to inactivate other chemotherapeutic agents, thus reducing drug resistance.

Metabolism: Unknown.

Dosage/Range:
Per protocol, phase II study 75 mg/m^2.

Drug Interactions: Unknown.

Lab Effects/Interference: Decreased neutrophil and platelet counts.

Special Considerations:

- Drug appears synergistic with platinums, taxanes, and anthracyclines.
- Drug is being studied in breast, ovarian, NSCLC, colorectal cancers.
- Drug has activity in patients with NSCLC resistant to cisplatin.

Potential Toxicities/Side Effects and the Nursing Process

I. INFECTION AND BLEEDING, POTENTIAL, related to BONE MARROW DEPRESSION

Defining Characteristics: Neutropenia is the dose-limiting toxicity. Grade 3 neutropenia occurred in 28% of NSCLC study patients, and grade 3 thrombocytopenia in 5%.

Nursing Implications: Monitor CBC and platelet count prior to drug administration as well as signs/symptoms of infection or bleeding. Instruct patient in self-assessment of signs/symptoms of infection or bleeding.

II. ALTERATION IN NUTRITION, LESS THAN BODY REQUIREMENTS, related to NAUSEA AND VOMITING,

Defining Characteristics: Nausea and vomiting in patients with NSCLC who received drug with cisplatin.

Nursing Implications: Premedicate with anti-emetics per protocol, and teach patient self-administration of anti-emetics at home if needed. Encourage small, frequent feedings of cool, bland, dry foods. Assess for symptoms of fluid and electrolyte imbalance: monitor I/O and daily weights if administered to an inpatient.. Ensure adequate hydration, nutrition, and monitor I/O.

Drug: topotecan hydrochloride for injection (Hycamptin)

Class: Topoisomerase I inhibitor.

Mechanism of Action: Causes single-strand breaks in DNA to permit relaxation of DNA helix prior to DNA replication. Topotecan binds to the topoisomerase I-DNA complex thus preventing repair (religation) of the strand breaks. This leads to double-strand DNA breaks that cannot be repaired; thus, drug prevents DNA synthesis and replication and leads to cell death.

Metabolism: 30% of dose is excreted in the urine. Patients with moderate renal impairment have a 34% decrease in plasma clearance and require a dosage adjustment. Minor metabolism by the liver, so patients with liver dysfunction do not require dose modification.

Dosage/Range:

- Metastatic carcinoma of the ovary after failure of initial or subsequent chemo: 1.5 mg/m^2 IV infusion over 30 minutes for 5 consecutive days every 21 days, but many oncologists use dose of 1.25 mg/m^2, which the manufacturer says has equal efficacy.
- Small-cell lung cancer after failure of first-line chemotherapy: same.

Drug Preparation:

- Available as a 4 mg vial.
- Reconstitute vial with 4 mL sterile water for injection.
- Further dilute in 0.9% Sodium Chloride or 5% Dextrose.
- Use immediately.

Drug Administration:

- Administer IV over 30 minutes × 5 days.
- Baseline ANC for initial course must be ≥ 1500/mm^3 and platelets ≥ 100,000/mm^3, and for subsequent courses, ANC ≥ 1000/mm^3, platelets ≥ 100,000/mm^3, and hemogloblin ≥ 9mg/dL.
- G-CSF may be required if neutropenia develops.

Drug Interactions:

- None known.

Lab Effects/Interference:

- Decreased CBC.
- Increased LFTs, RFTs.

Special Considerations:

Dosage Modifications:

- Renal impairment: MILD (creatinine clearance 40–60 mL/minute): use reduced dose of 0.75 mg/m²; MODERATE (creatinine clearance 29–39 mL/minute): manufacturer makes no recommendation, but physician may discontinue drug.
- Hematologic toxicity: SEVERE NEUTROPENIA: reduce dose by 0.25 mg/m² for subsequent doses, or may use G-CSF instead to prevent neutropenia beginning on day 6 of the course (24 hours after last day of topotecan infusion).
- Minimum of 4 courses needed, as clinical responses occur 9–12 weeks after beginning of therapy.
- Indicated for the treatment of relapsed or refractory metastatic ovarian cancer and small-cell lung cancer sensitive disease after first relapse.
- Currently, an oral formulation of the drug is being studied in clinical trials.
- Drug appears to cross BBB.

Potential Toxicities/Side Effects and the Nursing Process

I. INFECTION AND BLEEDING related to BONE MARROW DEPRESSION

Defining Characteristics: Myelosuppression is the dose-limiting toxicity. Severe grade 4 neutropenia is seen during the first course of therapy in 60% of patients. Febrile neutropenia or sepsis may occur in up to 26% of patients. Nadir occurs on day 11. Prophylactic G-CSF is needed in 27% of courses after the first cycle. Thrombocytopenia (grade 4 with platelet count $< 25{,}000/mm^3$) occurs in 26% of patients. Platelet nadir occurs on day 15. Severe anemia (Hgb < 8 gm/dL) occurs in 40% of patients, and transfusions were needed for 56% of patients.

Nursing Implications: Monitor CBC and platelet count prior to drug administration as well as signs/symptoms of infection or bleeding. Assess renal function baseline and prior to each treatment. Discuss dose reductions with physician (see Special Considerations section). Instruct patient in self-assessment of signs/symptoms of infection or bleeding. Administer RBCs and platelet transfusions per physician's orders. Teach patient self-administration of G-CSF as ordered.

II. ALTERATION IN NUTRITION, LESS THAN BODY REQUIREMENTS, related to NAUSEA AND VOMITING, DIARRHEA, ELEVATED LFTS

Defining Characteristics: Nausea occurs in 77% of patients, and vomiting in 58% without premedication with antiemetics. Diarrhea occurs in 42% of patients, while constipation occurs in 39%. Abdominal pain may occur in 33% of patients. Asparate aminotransferase (AST, previously SGOT) and alanine aminotransferase (ALT, previously SGPT) elevations occur in 5% of patients.

Nursing Implications: Premedicate with a serotonin antagonist or dopamine antagonist antiemetic, and continue prophylactically for 24 hours to prevent nausea and vomiting, at least for the first treatment. Encourage small, frequent feedings of cool, bland, dry foods. Assess for symptoms of fluid and electrolyte imbalance: monitor I/O and daily weights if administered to an inpatient. Teach patient oral assessment and oral hygiene regimen. Encourage patient to report early stomatitis. Provide pain relief measures if indicated (e.g., topical anesthetics). Encourage patient to report onset of diarrhea. Administer or teach patient to self-administer antidiarrheal medication. Ensure adequate hydration, monitor I/O. Monitor LFTs baseline and periodically during treatment.

III. POTENTIAL FOR HEPATOTOXICITY related to HYPOALBUMINEMIA, PREEXISTING HEPATIC INSUFFICIENCY

Defining Characteristics: Evidence of increased drug toxicity in patients with low protein and hepatic dysfunction. Dose reductions may be necessary.

Nursing Implications: Monitor LFTs prior to drug dose. Assess patient prior to administering drug and during treatment for signs/symptoms of hepatotoxicity.

Drug: toremifene citrate (Fareston)

Class: Synthetic tamoxifen analogue.

Mechanism of Action: Estrogen antagonist.

Metabolism: Extensively metabolized in the liver by the P-450 enzyme system. Peak serum level after single dose is 3 hours, with terminal half-life of 6.2 days. Increased terminal half-life (decreased clearance) in patients with hepatic dysfunction to 10.9 days and 21 days for the principal metabolite. Only slightly protein-bound (0.3%). Clearance not significantly changed with renal impairment.

Dosage/Range:
- 60 mg PO qd.

Drug Preparation:

- None.

Drug Administration:

- Oral.

Drug Interactions:

- Metabolism is inhibited by testosterone and cyclosporin.
- Appears to enhance inhibition of multidrug-resistant cell lines by vinblastine.
- Appears to be cross-resistant with tamoxifen.

Lab Effects/Interference:

- Decreased WBC and platelets (mild).

Special Considerations:

- Activity, side effects, toxicity in postmenopausal women or women with unknown receptor status appear similar.

Potential Toxicities/Side Effects and the Nursing Process

I. POTENTIAL FOR SEXUAL DYSFUNCTION related to MENSTRUAL IRREGULARITIES, HOT FLASHES

Defining Characteristics: Similar to tamoxifen toxicity profile. May cause menstrual irregularity, hot flashes (most common), milk production in breasts, and vaginal discharge and bleeding.

Nursing Implications: As appropriate, explore with patient and partner issues of reproductive and sexuality patterns and the impact drug may have on them. Discuss strategies to preserve sexual and reproductive health.

II. POTENTIAL FOR ALTERATION IN COMFORT related to FLARE REACTION

Defining Characteristics: May cause flare reaction initially (bone and tumor pain, transient increase in tumor size). Nausea, vomiting, and anorexia may occur. Tremor may occur and be significant in some patients.

Nursing Implications: Inform patient of flare reaction, signs/symptoms to be aware of, and encourage patient to report any signs/symptoms. Inform patient of possibility of nausea, vomiting, and anorexia. Encourage small, frequent feedings of high-calorie, high-protein foods. Teach patients to report tremor, and discuss impact on self-care ability and comfort.

III. POTENTIAL FOR INFECTION AND BLEEDING related to BONE MARROW DEPRESSION

Defining Characteristics: Mild, transient leukopenia and thrombocytopenia occur rarely. Lowest WBC count in clinical trials was 2500/mm^3.

Nursing Implications: Monitor CBC and platelet count prior to drug administration and after therapy has begun. Instruct patient in self-assessment of signs/symptoms of infection or bleeding.

IV. POTENTIAL FOR SKIN INTEGRITY IMPAIRMENT related to RASH, ALOPECIA

Defining Characteristics: Skin rash, alopecia, and peripheral edema are rare.

Nursing Implications: Assess patient for signs/symptoms of hair loss, edema, and skin rash. Instruct patient to report any of these symptoms. Discuss with patient the impact of skin changes.

Drug: trimetrexate (Neutrexin)

Class: Antimetabolite.

Mechanism of Action: Nonclassical folate antagonist; potent inhibitor of dihydrofolate reductase. May be able to overcome mechanism(s) of methotrexate resistance as drug reaches higher concentration within tumor cells. Also, inhibits growth of parasitic infective agents (causing *Pneumocystis carinii* pneumonia [PCP], toxoplasmosis) in patients with immunodeficiency or myelodysplastic disorders.

Metabolism: Significant percentage of drug is protein-bound. Metabolized by liver; 10–20% of dose is excreted by kidneys in 24 hours.

Dosage/Range:

For PCP indication:

- 45 mg/m^2 qd IV infusion over 60–90 minutes × 21 days.
- Leucovorin 20 mg/m^2 IV over 5–10 minutes q6 hours (80 mg/m^2 24-hour total dose), or 20 mg/m^2 PO qid for days of trimetrexate treatment, extending 72 hours past the last dose of trimetrexate, for a total of 24 days.

Drug Preparation:

- Reconstitute with 2 mL 5% Dextrose USP or sterile water for injection (12.5 mg of trimetrexate/mL).
- Filter with 0.22-μm filter prior to further dilution; observe for cloudiness or precipitate.
- Further dilute in 5% Dextrose to a final concentration of 0.25–2.00 mg/mL.
- Stable 24 hours at room temperature or refrigerated.

Drug Administration:

- IV infusion over 60 minutes.
- Incompatible with chloride solutions, as precipitate forms immediately, and leucovorin.
- Leucovorin can be started either before or after first trimetrexate dose, but ensure that IV line is flushed with at least 10 mL of 5% Dextrose between drugs.

Drug Interactions:

- Drug is metabolized by P-450 enzyme system, so interactions are possible with erythromycin, fluconazole, ketoconazole, rifabutin, rifampin, protease inhibitors.

Lab Effects/Interference:

- Decreased CBC.
- Increased LFTs, RFTs (especially creatinine).
- Decreased Ca, Na.

Special Considerations:

- Indicated for alternative treatment of moderate-to-severe PCP in patients with immunodeficiency, including AIDS patients who are intolerant or refractory to trimethoprim-sulfamethoxazole (TMP-SMX), or for whom TMP-SMX is contraindicated.
- Increased toxicity is seen in patients with low protein (drug is highly proteinbound) and hepatic dysfunction. Dose reduction is indicated.
- Leukopenia is dose-limiting toxicity.
- Other side effects are nausea and vomiting, rash, mucositis, AST elevations, thrombocytopenia.
- Drug is fetotoxic and embryotoxic. Women of childbearing age should use contraceptive measures to prevent pregnancy while receiving the drug.
- Zidovudine (AZT) therapy should be interrupted while receiving trimetrexate.
- Use cautiously in patients with renal, hepatic, or hematologic impairment.
- Transaminase levels or alk phos > 5 times upper limit of normal: HOLD DOSE.
- Serum creatinine ≥ 2.5 mg/dL due to trimetrexate: HOLD DOSE.
- Severe mucosal toxicity (unable to eat): HOLD DOSE, and continue leucovorin.
- Temperature ≥ 40.5°C (105°F) uncontrolled by antipyretics: HOLD DOSE.
- Hematologic toxicity: HOLD DOSE and consult package insert.

Potential Toxicities/Side Effects and the Nursing Process

I. INFECTION AND BLEEDING related to BONE MARROW DEPRESSION

Defining Characteristics: Leukopenia is a dose-limiting toxicity. Thrombocytopenia also occurs commonly.

Nursing Implications: Monitor CBC, platelet count prior to drug administration, as well as for signs/symptoms of infection or bleeding. Instruct patient in self-assessment of signs/symptoms of infection or bleeding. Administer red cells and platelet transfusions per physician's orders.

II. ALTERATION IN NUTRITION, LESS THAN BODY REQUIREMENTS, related to GI SIDE EFFECTS

Defining Characteristics: Nausea and vomiting have been reported in clinical trials; drug has been reported to cause stomatitis; diarrhea may occur also.

Nursing Implications: Premedicate with antiemetics and continue prophylactically for 24 hours to prevent nausea and vomiting, at least for the first treatment. Encourage small, frequent feedings of cool, bland, dry foods. Assess for symptoms of fluid and electrolyte imbalance: monitor I/O, daily weights if administered to an inpatient. Teach patient oral assessment and oral hygiene regimen. Encourage patient to report early stomatitis. Provide pain relief measures if indicated (e.g., topical anesthetics). Encourage patient to report onset of diarrhea. Administer or teach patient to self-administer antidiarrheal medication. Guaiac all stools. Ensure adequate hydration; monitor I/O.

III. POTENTIAL FOR IMPAIRED SKIN INTEGRITY related to ALOPECIA

Defining Characteristics: Alopecia is total in 42% of patients.

Nursing Implications: Discuss with patient the impact of hair loss. As appropriate, suggest wig prior to actual hair loss. Explore patient's response to actual hair loss and plan strategies to minimize distress (e.g., wig, scarf, cap).

IV. ALTERATION IN COMFORT related to HEADACHE

Defining Characteristics: Headache occurs in 21% of patients. Paresthesias may affect 9% of patients.

Nursing Implications: Teach patient that headache may occur and is usually relieved by acetaminophen. Instruct patient to report headache that is not relieved by usual methods.

V. ALTERATION IN OXYGEN POTENTIAL related to DYSPNEA

Defining Characteristics: Dyspnea may occur in 20% of patients, and is severe in 4% of patients.

Nursing Implications: Assess baseline pulmonary status, including presence of dyspnea, and history since last treatment prior to successive drug administrations. Instruct patient to report new onset or worsening of dyspnea. Discuss occurrences with physician to determine further diagnostic evaluation.

Drug: UFT (Ftorafur [Tegafur] and Uracil) (investigational)

Class: Dihydropyrimidine dehydrogenase inhibitory fluoropyrimidines.

Mechanism of Action: Tegafur is a fluorouracil pro-drug, which then acts as a "false" pyrimidine, inhibiting the formation of an enzyme (thymidine synthetase) necessary for the synthesis of DNA. Also incorporates into RNA, causing abnormal synthesis and resultant suppression of tumor cell multiplication. Uracil competitively inhibits the degradation of 5-FU (see Metabolism section). Tegafur appears to directly increase apoptosis in cancer cells, but may also decrease intratumoral angiogenesis.

Metabolism: Quickly absorbed by the GI tract. Tegafur is metabolized by the liver into 5-FU; most is excreted as respiratory CO_2 and a small amount is excreted by the kidneys. Uracil is rapidly metabolized and excreted but enhances the cytotoxic effect of 5-FU by increasing its concentration in tumors and inhibiting its degradation.

Dosage/Range:

Check protocol, but these are examples:

- 200 mg/m^2/day and may be combined with with 5 or 50 mg leucovorin × 28 days per cycle.
- 300–350 mg/m^2/day in three divided doses (8 h apart) × 28 days.

Drug Preparation:

- Oral.

Drug Administration:

- Oral.

Drug Interactions:

- Unknown.

Lab Effects/Interference:

- Decreased CBC.
- Decreased K, Mg.
- Increased or decreased Ca.

- Increased PT.
- Increased LFTs.

Special Considerations:

- Cutaneous side effects occur, e.g., pigmentation changes.
- Can cause asthenia, paresthesias, and headaches.
- Uracil may increase 5-FU concentrations within tumor more than within normal tissues.

Potential Toxicities/Side Effects and the Nursing Process

I. POTENTIAL FOR INFECTION AND BLEEDING related to BONE MARROW DEPRESSION

Defining Characteristics: Usually mild, reversible.

Nursing Implications: Assess baseline CBC, WBC, differential, and platelet count prior to chemotherapy, as well as for signs/symptoms of infection or bleeding. Teach patient signs/symptoms of infection or bleeding, and instruct to report these immediately. Teach patient self-care measures to minimize risk of infection and bleeding, including avoidance of crowds, proximity to people with infections, and OTC aspirin-containing medications.

II. ALTERATION IN NUTRITION, LESS THAN BODY REQUIREMENTS, related to NAUSEA AND VOMITING, STOMATITIS, AND DIARRHEA

Defining Characteristics: Nausea and vomiting, anorexia, and diarrhea can be severe, and are the dose-limiting toxicities. Dehydration may result. Mucositis and stomatitis also occur.

Nursing Implications: Premedicate patient with antiemetics, and continue for 24 hours, at least for the first cycle. Encourage small, frequent meals of cool, bland foods. Assess oral mucosa prior to drug administration and instruct patient to report changes. Teach patient oral hygiene measures and self-assessment. Instruct patient to report diarrhea, to self-administer prescribed antidiarrheal medications, and to drink adequate fluids.

Drug: UFT (Ftorafur [Tegafur] and Uracil) plus leucovorin (Orzel) (investigational)

Class: Dihydropyrimidine dehydrogenase inhibitory fluoropyrimidines.

Mechanism of Action: Tegafur is a fluorouracil pro-drug, which then acts as a “false” pyrimidine, inhibiting the formation of an enzyme (thymidine synthetase) necessary for the synthesis of DNA. Also incorporates into RNA, causing abnormal synthesis and resultant suppression of tumor cell multiplication. Uracil competitively inhibits the dihydropyrimidine dehydrogenase (DPD), which is the primary enzyme degrading 5-FU into its metabolites. This results in sustained levels of 5-FU in plasma and tumor (see Metabolism section). Leucovorin potentiates the activity of 5-fluorouracil (5-FU). Tegafur appears to directly increase apoptosis in cancer cells, but may also decrease intratumoral angiogenesis.

Metabolism: Quickly absorbed by the GI tract. Tegafur is metabolized by the liver into 5-FU (via hepatic microsomal cytochrome P-450 system as well as by thymidine phosphorylase, which exists in tumor and body tissues); most is excreted as respiratory CO_2; small amount is excreted by the kidneys. Uracil is rapidly metabolized and excreted but enhances the cytotoxic effect of 5-FU by increasing its concentration in tumors and inhibiting its degradation.

Dosage/Range:
- Metastatic colorectal cancer: UFT 300 mg/m^2/day PO in 3 divided doses × 28 days with 1-week rest period. Leucovorin 75–90 mg/da PO in 3 divided doses.

Drug Preparation:
- Oral. Capsules contain uracil (224 mg) and tegafur (100 mg) in a 4:1 molar ratio.

Drug Administration:
- Oral.

Drug Interactions:
- Unknown.

Lab Effects/Interference:
- Decreased CBC.
- Decreased K, Mg.
- Increased or decreased Ca.
- Increased PT.
- Increased bili.

Special Considerations:
- Combination gives double modulation of 5-FU.
- Cutaneous side effects occur, e.g., pigmentation changes.
- Can cause asthenia, paresthesias, and headaches.
- Single daily dose causes more myelosuppression and diarrhea than if drug dose is given in three divided doses.
- Does NOT cause hand-foot syndrome seen with 5-FU or 5-FU analogues.
- Drug may have usefulness in breast, head and neck, and other gastrointestinal cancers.

- Appears to have efficacy comparable to IV fluorouracil and leucovorin with less toxicity.
- 5-FU is excreted in human tears, so increased lacrimation, conjunctivitis may occur.

Potential Toxicities/Side Effects and the Nursing Process

I. POTENTIAL FOR INFECTION AND BLEEDING related to BONE MARROW DEPRESSION

Defining Characteristics: Usually mild, reversible.

Nursing Implications: Assess baseline CBC, WBC, differential, and platelet count prior to chemotherapy, as well as for signs/symptoms of infection or bleeding. Teach patient signs/symptoms of infection or bleeding, and instruct to report these immediately; teach patient self-care measures to minimize risk of infection and bleeding, including avoidance of crowds, proximity to people with infections, and OTC aspirin-containing medications.

II. ALTERATION IN NUTRITION, LESS THAN BODY REQUIREMENTS, related to NAUSEA AND VOMITING, STOMATITIS, AND DIARRHEA

Defining Characteristics: Nausea and vomiting, and diarrhea may occur; diarrhea is the dose-limiting toxicity. Dehydration may result. Mucositis and stomatitis also occur.

Nursing Implications: Premedicate patient with antiemetics, and continue for 24 hours, at least for the first cycle. Teach patient to report nausea and/or vomiting so that antiemetic regimen can be revised, and patient can be compliant with oral regimen. If nausea, vomiting occur, encourage small, frequent meals of cool, bland foods. Assess oral mucosa prior to drug administration, and instruct patient to report changes. Teach patient oral hygiene measures and self-assessment. Instruct patient to report diarrhea, to self-administer prescribed antidiarrheal medications, to drink adequate fluids, and to call provider right away if diarrhea does not resolve. Consult protocol re dose modifications for diarrhea and other gastrointestinal toxicity.

Drug: valrubicin (Valstar)

Class: Anthracycline antitumor antibiotic.

Mechanism of Action: Semisynthetic analogue of doxorubicin; drug is highly lipophilic and is made soluble in Cremophor EL. Apparently, the drug does not interact with negatively charged molecules, and thus is less irritating to bladder mucosa. Drug metabolites appear to inhibit topoisomerase II so that cellular DNA cannot replicate, thus inhibiting DNA synthesis and causing chromosomal damage and cell death.

Metabolism: Drug is well absorbed by bladder mucosa with little if any systemic absorption unless bladder is injured/perforated. Used for bladder instillation, and excreted unchanged in the urine (98.6%).

Dosage/Range:

- Intravesicular therapy of BCG-refractory carcinoma in situ of the urinary bladder: 800 mg q week × 6 weeks.
- High incidence of metastases in patients receiving drug in clinical trials, probably due to delayed cystectomy. Therefore, therapy should be discontinued in patients not responding to treatment after three months.

Drug Preparation:

- Available as injection form, 200 mg in 5-mL vial, which should be stored in the refrigerator 2–8°C (36–46°F).
- Remove vials from refrigerator and allow to warm to room temperature without heating; dilute by adding 800 mg (20 mL) to 55 mL of 0.9% Normal Saline Injection, USP.

Drug Administration:

- Bladder lavage by intravesicular administration of drug (total volume of 75 mL when diluted as above), allowed to dwell for 2 hours, and then voided out.
- Non-PVC tubing and non-DEHP containers and administration sets should be used to prevent leaching of PVC into drug volume (due to Cremophor EL).

Drug Interactions:

- None known due to limited, if any, systemic absorption.

Lab Effects/Interference:

- Hyperglycemia.

Special Considerations:

- Contraindicated in patients with hypersensitivity to anthracycline antibiotics, Cremophor EL, or any drug components, during pregnancy, in breastfeeding mothers, or in patients with urinary tract infection at time treatment is planned or with small bladder unable to hold 75 mL.
- Drug should NOT be given if bladder is injured, inflamed, or perforated, as systemic absorption will occur via loss of mucosal integrity.
- Use with caution in patients with severe irritable bladder symptoms, as drug may cause symptoms of irritable bladder (during instillation and dwell time).
- Teach patients that urine will be red- or pink-tinged for 24 hours.

- Patients with diabetes need to check blood glucose levels, as hyperglycemia may occur with treatment (1% incidence).

Potential Toxicities/Side Effects and the Nursing Process

I. ALTERATION IN URINE ELIMINATION related to DRUG EFFECTS

Defining Characteristics: Intravesicular administration of drug is associated with signs/symptoms of bladder irritation: frequency (61% of patients), dysuria (56%), urgency (57%), bladder spasm (31%), hematuria (29%), pain in bladder (28%), incontinence (22%), cystitis (15%), and urinary tract infection (15%). Less commonly, nocturia (7%), burning on urination (5%), urinary retention (4%), pain in the urethra (3%), pelvic pain (1%).

Nursing Implications: Assess baseline urinary elimination pattern, history of signs/symptoms of bladder irritation. Teach patient that these side effects may occur and to report them. Teach patient to drink 3 L of fluid for at least 2–3 days beginning day of treatment to flush bladder. Reassure patient that signs/symptoms will resolve and to report any persistent symptoms.

II. ALTERATION IN OXYGENATION, POTENTIAL, related to RARE CARDIAC EFFECTS

Defining Characteristics: Rarely, chest pain may occur (2%) as may vasodilation (2%) or peripheral edema (1%).

Nursing Implications: Assess patient's baseline cardiac status, and history of chest pain, peripheral edema. Teach patient to report any pain, or swelling in hands or feet. If this occurs, discuss management with physician. If possible, do EKG while patient is having chest pain to see if ischemia exists. Systemic absorption is possible only if bladder mucosal surfaces are injured, so this should be considered.

III. ALTERATION IN COMFORT, POTENTIAL, related to PAIN, RASH, WEAKNESS, MYALGIA

Defining Characteristics: The following discomfort may occur: headache (4%), malaise (4%), dizziness (3%), fever (2%), rash (3%), abdominal pain (5%), weakness (4%), back pain (3%), myalgia (1%).

Nursing Implications: Assess baseline comfort level, and any pain and the usual pain relief plan. Teach patient that these problems may occur rarely and to report them if they do. Teach patient these symptoms should resolve, and to use local measures to minimize discomfort. Teach patient to report any symptoms that do not resolve or that become worse.

IV. ALTERATION IN NUTRITION, POTENTIAL, related to NAUSEA, DIARRHEA, VOMITING

Defining Characteristics: Rarely, gastrointestinal symptoms may occur: nausea affects approximately 5% of patients, diarrhea 3% of patients, and vomiting 2% of patients.

Nursing Implications: Assess baseline nutritional status, history of nausea, vomiting, or diarrhea. Teach patient that these may occur rarely and to report them if they do. If patient does develop symptoms, teach patient to take antiemetic medication as ordered, and OTC antidiarrheal medicine. Teach patient to call right away if symptoms do not resolve.

Drug: vinblastine (Velban)

Class: Plant alkaloid extracted from the periwinkle plant (*Vinca rosea*).

Mechanism of Action: Drug binds to microtubular proteins, thus arresting mitosis during metaphase; may inhibit RNA, DNA, and protein synthesis. Cell cycle phase specific for M phase and active in S phase.

Metabolism: About 10% of drug is excreted in feces. Vinblastine is partially metabolized by the liver. Minimal amount of the drug is excreted in urine and bile. Dose modification may be necessary in the presence of hepatic failure.

Dosage/Range:

- 0.1 mg/kg; 6 mg/m^2 IV weekly: continuous infusion 1.5–2.0 mg/m^2/d in 1L D_5W or NS × 5 days.

Drug Preparation:

- Available in 10-mg vials. Store in refrigerator until use.

Drug Administration:

- IV: This drug is a vesicant. Give slow IVP over 1–2 min through the sidearm of a running IV so as to avoid extravasation, which can lead to ulceration, pain, and necrosis. Refer to individual hospital policy and procedure for administration of a vesicant.

Drug Interactions:

- Decreased pharmacologic effects of phenytoin when given with this drug.
- Increases cellular uptake of methotrexate by certain malignant cells when administered sequentially, but less so than vincristine.

Lab Effects/Interference:

- Decreased WBC.

Special Considerations:

- Drug is a vesicant; give through a running IV to avoid extravasation.

- Dose modification may be necessary in the presence of hepatic failure.

Potential Toxicities/Side Effects and the Nursing Process

I. POTENTIAL FOR INFECTION AND BLEEDING related to BONE MARROW DEPRESSION

Defining Characteristics: May cause severe bone marrow depression; nadir 4–10 days. Neutrophils greatly affected. In patients with prior XRT or chemotherapy, thrombocytopenia may be severe.

Nursing Implications: Monitor CBC, platelet count prior to drug administration. Assess for signs/symptoms of infection or bleeding. Instruct patient in self-assessment of signs/symptoms of infection or bleeding. Dose reduction if hepatic dysfunction: 50% if bili > 1.5 mg/dL; 75% if bili > 3.0 mg/dL. Administer red blood cell and platelet transfusions per physician's orders.

II. POTENTIAL FOR SENSORY/PERCEPTUAL ALTERATIONS related to PERIPHERAL OR CENTRAL NEUROPATHY

Defining Characteristics: Occur less frequently than with vincristine. Occur in patients receiving prolonged or high-dose therapy. Symptoms: paresthesias, peripheral neuropathy, depression, headache, malaise, jaw pain, urinary retention, tachycardia, orthostatic hypotension, seizures. Rare ocular changes: diplopia, ptosis, photophobia, oculomotor dysfunction, optic neuropathy.

Nursing Implications: Assess sensory/perceptual changes prior to each drug dose, especially if dose is high (> 10 mg) or patient is receiving prolonged therapy. Notify physician of alterations. Discuss with patient the impact changes have had, as well as strategies to minimize dysfunction and decrease distress.

III. ALTERATION IN BOWEL ELIMINATION related to CONSTIPATION

Defining Characteristics: Constipation results from neurotoxicity (central) and is less common than with vincristine. Risk factor: high dose (> 20 mg). May lead to adynamic ileus, abdominal pain.

Nursing Implications: Assess bowel elimination pattern with each drug dose, especially if dose > 20 mg. Teach patient to promote bowel elimination with fluids (3 L/day), high-fiber, bulky foods, exercise, stool softeners. Suggest laxative if unable to move bowels at least once a day. Instruct patient to report abdominal pain.

IV. ALTERATION IN NUTRITION, LESS THAN BODY REQUIREMENTS, related to GI SIDE EFFECTS

Defining Characteristics: Nausea and vomiting rarely occur. Stomatitis is uncommon but can be severe.

Nursing Implications: Premedicate with antiemetics and continue prophylactically for 24 hours to prevent nausea and vomiting, at least for the first treatment. Encourage small, frequent feedings of cool, bland foods and liquids. Assess for symptoms of fluid and electrolyte imbalance: monitor I/O, daily weights if administered to an inpatient. Teach patient oral assessment. Teach, reinforce teaching, regarding oral hygiene regimen. Encourage patient to report early stomatitis. Provide pain relief measures if indicated (e.g., topical anesthetics).

V. POTENTIAL FOR IMPAIRED SKIN INTEGRITY related to ALOPECIA

Defining Characteristics: Alopecia is reversible and mild and occurs in 45–50% of patients receiving drug. Drug is a potent vesicant and can cause irritation and necrosis if infiltrated.

Nursing Implications: Discuss with patient the impact of hair loss. Suggest wig as appropriate prior to actual hair loss. Explore with patient response to actual hair loss and plan strategies to minimize distress (e.g., wig, scarf, cap). Careful technique is used during venipuncture and intravenous administration. Administer vesicant through freely flowing IV, constantly monitoring IV site and patient response. Nurse should be THOROUGHLY familiar with institutional policy and procedure for administration of a vesicant agent. If vesicant drug is administered as a continuous infusion, drug must be given through a PATENT CENTRAL LINE. If extravasation is suspected, stop drug administration and aspirate any residual drug and blood from IV tubing, IV catheter/needle, and IV site if possible. If drug infiltration is suspected, manufacturer suggests the following after withdrawing any remaining drug from IV: local installation of hyaluronidase; application of moderate heat. Assess site regularly for pain, progression of erythema, induration, and for evidence of necrosis. When in doubt about whether drug is infiltrating, TREAT AS AN INFILTRATION. Teach patient to assess site, and instruct to notify physician if condition worsens. Arrange next clinic visit for assessment of site depending on drug, amount infiltrated, extent of potential injury, and patient variables. Document in patient's record as per institutional policy and procedure.

VI. POTENTIAL FOR SEXUAL DYSFUNCTION related to REPRODUCTIVE HAZARD

Defining Characteristics: Drug is possibly teratogenic. Likely to cause azoospermia in men.

Nursing Implications: As appropriate, explore with patient and partner issues of reproductive and sexuality patterns and the anticipated impact chemotherapy may have. Discuss strategies to preserve sexual health (e.g., sperm banking).

Drug: vincristine (Oncovin)

Class: Plant alkaloid extracted from the periwinkle plant (*Vinca rosea*).

Mechanism of Action: Drug binds to microtubular proteins, thus arresting mitosis during metaphase. Cell cycle phase specific for M phase and active in S phase.

Metabolism: The primary route for excretion is via the liver with about 70% of the drug being excreted in feces and bile. These metabolites are a result of hepatic metabolism and biliary excretion. A small amount is excreted in the urine. Dose modification may be necessary in the presence of hepatic failure.

Dosage/Range:
- 0.4–1.4 mg/m^2 weekly (initially limited to 2 mg per dose).

Drug Preparation:
- Supplied in 1-mg, 2-mg, and 5-mg vials. Refrigerate vials until use.

Drug Administration:
- IV: This drug is a vesicant. Give IVP through sidearm of a running IV to avoid extravasation, which can lead to ulceration, pain, and necrosis. Refer to hospital's policy and procedure for administration of a vesicant.

Drug Interactions:
- Neurotoxic drugs: additive neurotoxicity can occur; use cautiously.
- Decreased bioavailability of digoxin when given with this drug.
- Increased cellular uptake of methotrexate by some malignant cells when given sequentially.

Lab Effects/Interference:
- Decreased WBC, platelets.
- Increased uric acid.

Special Considerations:
- Dose is a vesicant; give through a running IV to avoid extravasation.
- Dose modifications may be necessary in the presence of hepatic failure.

Potential Toxicities/Side Effects and the Nursing Process

I. POTENTIAL FOR SENSORY/PERCEPTUAL ALTERATIONS related to PERIPHERAL CENTRAL NEUROPATHY

Defining Characteristics: Peripheral neuropathies occur as a result of toxicity to nerve fibers: absent deep tendon reflexes, numbness, weakness, myalgias, cramping, and late severe motor difficulties. Reversal or discontinuance of therapy is necessary. Increased risk exists in elderly. Cranial nerve dysfunction may occur (rare), as well as jaw pain (trigeminal neuralgia), diplopia, vocal cord paresis, mental depression, and metallic taste.

Nursing Implications: Assess sensory/perceptual changes prior to each drug dose, e.g., presence of numbness or tingling of fingertips or toes. Assess for loss of tendon reflexes: foot drop, slapping gait. Assess for motor difficulties: clumsiness of hands, difficulty climbing stairs, buttoning shirt, walking on heels. Notify physician of alterations; discuss holding drug if loss of deep tendon reflexes occurs. Discuss with patient the impact alterations have had, and strategies to minimize dysfunction and decrease distress. Discuss with patient type of alteration: memory and sensory/perceptual changes are temporary and reversible when drug is stopped. Assess patient for signs/symptoms of nerve dysfunction before each dose. Notify physician of any changes.

II. ALTERATION IN BOWEL ELIMINATION related to CONSTIPATION

Defining Characteristics: Autonomic neuropathy may lead to constipation and paralytic ileus. A concurrent use of vincristine, narcotic analgesics, or cholinergic medication may increase risk of constipation.

Nursing Implications: Assess bowel elimination pattern prior to each chemotherapy administration. Teach patient to include bulky and high-fiber foods in diet, increase fluids to 3 L/day, and exercise moderately to promote elimination. Suggest stool softeners if needed. Teach patient to use laxative if unable to move bowels at least once every two days. Instruct patient to report abdominal pain.

III. POTENTIAL FOR IMPAIRED SKIN INTEGRITY related to ALOPECIA

Defining Characteristics: Complete hair loss occurs in 12–45% of patients. Both men and women are at risk for body image disturbance. Hair will grow back. Dermatitis is uncommon. Drug is potent vesicant causing irritation and necrosis if infiltrated.

Nursing Implications: Discuss with patient anticipated impact of hair loss. Suggest wig or toupee as appropriate prior to actual hair loss. Explore with patient response to actual hair loss and plan strategies to minimize distress (e.g., wig, scarf, cap). Assess impact on patient: body image, comfort. Careful technique is used during venipuncture and intravenous administration. Administer vesicant through freely flowing IV, constantly monitoring IV site and patient response. Nurse should be THOROUGHLY familiar with institutional policy and procedure for administration of a vesicant agent. If vesicant drug is administered as a continuous infusion, drug must be given THROUGH A PATENT CENTRAL LINE. If extravasation is suspected, stop drug administration and aspirate any residual drug and blood from IV tubing, IV catheter/needle, and IV site if possible. If drug infiltration is suspected, manufacturer suggests the following after withdrawing any remaining drug from IV: local installation of hyaluronidase, application of moderate heat. Assess site regularly for pain, progression of erythema, induration, and evidence of necrosis. When in doubt about whether drug is infiltrating, TREAT AS AN INFILTRATION. Teach patient to assess site and notify physician if condition worsens. Arrange next clinic visit for assessment of site depending on drug, amount infiltrated, extent of potential injury, and patient variables. Document in patient's record as per institutional policy and procedure.

IV. POTENTIAL FOR INFECTION AND BLEEDING related to BONE MARROW DEPRESSION

Defining Characteristics: Rare myelosuppression, mild when it occurs. Nadir 10–14 days after treatment begins.

Nursing Implications: Monitor CBC, HCT, platelet count prior to drug administration. Dose reduction if hepatic dysfunction: 50% reduction if bili > 1.5 mg/dL; 75% reduction if bili > 3.0 mg/dL.

V. POTENTIAL SEXUAL DYSFUNCTION related to IMPOTENCE

Defining Characteristics: Impotence may occur related to neurotoxicity.

Nursing Implications: As appropriate, explore with patient and partner issues of reproductive and sexuality patterns, and impact chemotherapy may have. Discuss strategies to preserve sexual health, e.g., alternative expressions of sexuality. Reassure patient that impotency, if it occurs, is usually temporary, and reversible after drug discontinuance.

Drug: vindesine (Eldisine, Desacetylvinblastine) (investigational)

Class: Synthetic derivative of vinblastine; synthetic vinca alkyloid.

Mechanism of Action: Inhibits microtubule formation, causing metaphase arrest during M phase. Causes some cell death during S phase. Cell cycle phase specific.

Metabolism: Short plasma half-life (probably binds to tissue). Prolonged elimination suggesting drug may accumulate with repeated dosing. Excreted primarily by bile.

Dosage/Range:
- 3–4 mg/m^2 every 1–2 weeks.
- 1.0–1.3 mg/m^2/day × 5–7 days, repeated every 3 weeks.
- 1.5–2.0 mg/m^2 twice weekly.

Drug Preparation:
- 10-mg vial of lyophilized powder, reconstituted with provided diluent or 0.9% Sodium Chloride. Solution is stable for two weeks if refrigerated.

Drug Administration:
- Vesicant precautions: administer slowly as intravenous push through side-arm of freely running IV; also may be given as continuous infusion.

Drug Interactions:
- Do not give with other vinca alkaloids, such as vincristine or vinblastine, as there is potential for cumulative neurotoxicity.

Lab Effects/Interference:
- Decreased CBC, especially WBC.

Special Considerations:
- Dose reduction may be necessary in patients with abnormal liver function or if patient has received maximal doses of other vinca alkaloids.

Potential Toxicities/Side Effects and the Nursing Process

I. POTENTIAL FOR INFECTION AND BLEEDING related to BONE MARROW DEPRESSION

Defining Characteristics: Dose-limiting side effect. Nadir 5–10 days. Neutropenia is mild to moderate. Thrombocytopenia is mild, rare (may increase on treatment).

Nursing Implications: Monitor CBC, HCT, platelet count prior to drug administration as well as for signs/symptoms of infection or bleeding. Instruct patient in self-assessment of signs/symptoms of infection or bleeding. Dose reduction is often necessary (35–50%) if compromised bone marrow function exists.

II. POTENTIAL FOR SENSORY/PERCEPTUAL ALTERATIONS related to PERIPHERAL, CENTRAL NEUROPATHIES

Defining Characteristics: Neurotoxicity is similar to vincristine. Cumulative toxicity, mild. Begins with distal paresthesias, proximal muscle weakness, loss of deep tendon reflexes. Abdominal cramping is common; constipation and paralytic ileus are less common. Hoarseness, jaw pain (severe and transient) may occur.

Nursing Implications: Obtain visual assessment prior to starting therapy. Encourage patient to report any visual changes. Instruct patient to report headache, dizziness, light-headedness.

III. POTENTIAL FOR IMPAIRED SKIN INTEGRITY related to ALOPECIA

Defining Characteristics: Alopecia affects 80–90%, with 25–50% experiencing complete hair loss. Alopecia may be progressive. Both men and women are at risk for body image disturbance. Hair will grow back. Drug is a vesicant. Inapparent or obvious infiltrations can occur. Presentation is delayed; pain, phlebitis, blister formation occur; may progress to ulceration and necrosis. Management similar to vincristine extravasation.

Nursing Implications: Discuss with patient anticipated impact of hair loss. Suggest wig or toupee as appropriate prior to actual hair loss. Explore with patient response to actual hair loss and plan strategies to minimize distress (e.g., wig, scarf, cap). Assess impact on patient: body image, comfort. Careful technique is used during venipuncture and intravenous administration. Administer vesicant through freely flowing IV, constantly monitoring IV site and patient response. Nurse should be THOROUGHLY familiar with institutional policy and procedure for administration of a vesicant agent. If vesicant drug is administered as a continuous infusion, drug must be given THROUGH A PATENT CENTRAL LINE. If extravasation is suspected, stop drug administration and aspirate any residual drug and blood from IV tubing, IV catheter/needle, and IV site if possible. If drug infiltration is suspected, manufacturer suggests the following after withdrawing any remaining drug from IV: local installation of hyaluronidase, application of moderate heat. Assess site regularly for pain, progression of erythema, induration, and for evidence of necrosis. When in doubt about whether drug is infiltrating, TREAT AS AN INFILTRATION. Teach patient to assess site and instruct to notify physician if condition worsens. Arrange next clinic visit for assessment of site depending on drug, amount infiltrated, extent of potential injury, and patient variables. Document in patient's record as per institutional policy and procedure.

IV. ALTERATION IN BOWEL ELIMINATION related to CONSTIPATION

Defining Characteristics: Autonomic neuropathy may lead to constipation and paralytic ileus.

Nursing Implications: Assess bowel elimination pattern prior to each chemotherapy administration. Teach patient to include bulky and high-fiber foods in diet, increase fluids to 3 L/day, and exercise moderately to promote elimination. Suggest stool softeners if needed. Teach patient to use laxative if unable to move bowels at least once every two days. Instruct patient to report abdominal pain.

V. ALTERATION IN NUTRITION, LESS THAN BODY REQUIREMENTS, related to GI SIDE EFFECTS

Defining Characteristics: Nausea and vomiting typically not severe; occur in 30% of patients. Diarrhea is uncommon but rarely may be protracted and thus would be an indication for dose reduction.

Nursing Implications: Premedicate with antiemetic and continue prophylactically for 24 hours to prevent nausea and vomiting, at least for the first treatment. Encourage small, frequent feedings of cool, bland food and liquids. Encourage patient to report onset of diarrhea. Administer, or teach patient to self-administer, antidiarrheal medications.

Drug: vinorelbine tartrate (Navelbine)

Class: Semisynthetic vinca alkaloid derived from vinblastine.

Mechanism of Action: Inhibits mitosis at metaphase by interfering with microtubule assembly. Also appears to interfere with some aspects of cellular metabolism, including cellular respiration and nucleic acid biosynthesis. Cell cycle specific.

Metabolism: Slow elimination; extensive tissue binding (80% bound to plasma proteins); metabolized by the liver. Terminal half-life is 27–43 hours. Excreted in feces (46%) and urine (18%).

Dosage/Range:
- 30 mg/m² IV weekly or in combination with cisplatin.

Drug Preparation:
- Drug is available as 10 mg/mL in 1- or 5-mL vials.
- Further dilute drug in syringe or IV bag in 0.9% Sodium Chloride or 5% Dextrose to a final concentration of 1.5–3.0 mg/mL in a syringe, or 0.5–2.0 mg/mL in an IV bag.
- Stable for 24 hours if refrigerated.
- Also available as a 40-mg gelatin capsule.

Drug Administration:
- Infuse diluted drug IV over 6–10 minutes into sidearm port of freely flowing IV infusion, either peripherally or via central line. Use port CLOSEST TO THE IV BAG, not the patient.

- Flush vein with at least 75–125 mL of IV fluid after drug infusion.
- Use vesicant precautions.
- Oral capsule should be taken on an empty stomach at bedtime.

Drug Interactions:
- Increased granulocytopenia occurs when given in combination with cisplatin.
- Possible pulmonary reactions occur when given in combination with mitomycin C, characterized by dyspnea and severe bronchospasm. May require management with bronchodilators, corticosteroids, and/or supplemental oxygen.

Lab Effects/Interference:
- Decreased CBC (especially WBC).
- Increased LFTs.

Special Considerations:
- Drug indicated as single agent or in combination with cisplatin for the first-line treatment of advanced, unresectable, non-small-cell lung cancer (Stage III, combination therapy; Stage IV, single agent, or in combination with cisplatin).
- Increased nausea, vomiting, and diarrhea with oral administration.
- Drug is embryotoxic and mutagenic, so female patients of childbearing age should use contraception.
- Administer cautiously to patients with hepatic insufficiency. Contraindicated in patients with ANC < $1000/mm^3$.

Dosage modifications:
- Hematologic toxicity: if ANC on day of treatment is $1000–1499/mm^3$, use 50% dose (i.e., 15 mg/m^2); drug should be held if ANC < $1000/mm^3$. If drug is held for 3 consecutive weeks due to ANC < $1000/mm^3$, discontinue drug. If patient develops neutropenic fever or sepsis, or drug is held for neutropenia for 2 consecutive doses, dose should be reduced 25% (i.e., 22.5 mg/m^2) if ANC < $1500/mm^3$; if ANC is $1000–1499/mm^3$, drug should be decreased to 11.25 mg/m^2 as per package insert.
- Hepatic dysfunction: if total bili is 2.1–3.0 mg/dL, use 50% dose reduction (i.e., 15 mg/m^2); if total bili is > 3.0 mg/dL, use 75% dose reduction (i.e., 7.5 mg/m^2).

Potential Toxicities/Side Effects and the Nursing Process

I. INFECTION AND BLEEDING related to BONE MARROW DEPRESSION

Defining Characteristics: Leukopenia is dose-limiting toxicity; bone marrow depression noncumulative and short-lived (< 7 days), with nadir at 7–10 days.

Use with caution in patients with history of prior radiotherapy or chemotherapy. Severe thrombocytopenia and anemia are uncommon.

Nursing Implications: Monitor CBC, ANC, HCT, and platelet count prior to drug administration, as well as for signs/symptoms of infection or bleeding. Instruct patient in self-assessment of signs/symptoms of infection or bleeding. Teach patient self-care measures, including avoidance of OTC aspirin-containing medications. Dose reduction necessary for hematologic toxicity (see Special Considerations section).

II. POTENTIAL FOR SENSORY/PERCEPTUAL ALTERATIONS related to NEUROLOGIC TOXICITY

Defining Characteristics: Incidence of mild-to-moderate neuropathy is 25%. Paresthesias occur in 2–10% of patients, but incidence is increased if patient has received prior chemotherapy with vinca alkaloids or abdominal XRT. Decreased deep tendon reflexes occur in 6–29% of patients. Constipation may occur in 29% of patients. Neuropathy is reversible.

Nursing Implications: Assess baseline neuromuscular function, and reassess prior to drug infusion, especially in the presence of paresthesias; risk is increased if drug is given concurrently with cisplatin. Teach patient to report any changes in sensation or function. Identify strategies to promote comfort and safety.

III. ALTERATION IN NUTRITION, LESS THAN BODY REQUIREMENTS, related to NAUSEA/VOMITING, DIARRHEA, STOMATITIS, HEPATOTOXICITY

Defining Characteristics: Incidence of nausea/vomiting increases with oral dosing; mild in IV dosing, with an incidence of 44%. Vomiting occurs in 20% of patients. Diarrhea increases with oral dosing (17% incidence). Stomatitis is mild to moderate with < 20% incidence. Transient increases in LFTs (AST) occur in 67% of patients, and are without clinical significance.

Nursing Implications: Premedicate with antiemetic, such as a serotonin antagonist, prior to drug administration. Encourage small, frequent meals of cool, bland foods and liquids. Assess for symptoms of fluid/electrolyte imbalance if patient has severe nausea and vomiting. Monitor I/O, daily weights, and lab electrolyte values. Encourage patient to report onset of diarrhea. Administer, or teach patient to self-administer, antidiarrheal medications. Teach patient oral assessment. Teach and reinforce teaching of systemic oral hygiene regimen. Instruct patient to report early stomatitis, and provide pain relief measures as needed. Assess LFTs prior to drug administration baseline and periodically during treatment. Dose modifications may be necessary for hepatic dysfunction (see Special Considerations section).

IV. POTENTIAL FOR ALTERATION IN SKIN INTEGRITY related to ALOPECIA, EXTRAVASATION

Defining Characteristics: Gradual alopecia occurs in 10% of patients, rarely progressing to complete hair loss or requiring a wig. Severity is related to treatment duration. Drug is a moderate vesicant, primarily causing venous irritation and phlebitis; 30% of patients experience injection-site reactions commonly characterized by erythema, vein discoloration, tenderness; rarely, pain and venous irritation at sites proximal to injection site.

Nursing Implications: Discuss potential impact of hair loss prior to drug administration, coping strategies, and plans to minimize body-image distortion (e.g., wig, scarf, cap). Assess patient for signs/symptoms of hair loss. Assess patient's response and use of coping strategies. Scrupulous venipuncture technique is used during venipuncture. Administer vesicant through freely flowing IV via IV port closest to IV fluid bag, not patient, and administer maximally diluted drug over 6–10 minutes (not longer). If extravasation is suspected, TREAT AS AN INFILTRATION and aspirate any remaining drug from IV tubing, locally instill hyaluronidase in area of suspected infiltration, and apply moderate heat. Assess site regularly for pain, progression of erythema, and evidence of necrosis. Document in patient's record. Schedule next clinic visit for assessment of site depending on drug, amount infiltrated, extent of potential injury, and other patient variables.

V. POTENTIAL FOR SEXUAL/REPRODUCTIVE DYSFUNCTION related to TERATOGENICITY

Defining Characteristics: Drug is teratogenic and fetotoxic.

Nursing Implications: As appropriate, explore with patient and partner issues of reproductive and sexuality patterns and the anticipated impact chemotherapy may have. Counsel female patients of childbearing age in contraceptive options.

Chapter 2

Biologic Response Modifier Therapy

Surgery, chemotherapy, and radiation therapy are the three most commonly used treatments against cancer. Biotherapy, or the use of biologic response modifiers (BRMs), comprises the fourth traditional treatment modality for cancer management. BRMs work in a variety of ways to modify the immune response so that cancer cells are injured or killed. This category includes antibodies, cytokines, and other substances that stimulate the immune system. It has recently been greatly expanded to include gene therapy and immunomodulating agents, such as vaccines. In this book, Chapter 5 addresses new agents that target specific abnormal molecular events that promote malignant transformation, such as over-expression of cell surface growth factors like Epidermal Growth Factor receptor. Inhibitors that target abnormal signal transduction and transcription factors are also included. Monoclonal antibodies are classically targeted against molecular flaws, such as the angiogenesis inhibitor, bevaacizumab (Avastin) and epidermal growth factor receptor inhibitor cetuximab (Erbitux). Even though they are technically biological agents, for this edition, they appear in Chapter 5, Molecular Targeted Therapies. Biological response modifiers can

- Have direct antitumor activity or help cancer cells become recognizable as foreign so that the host immune system can kill the cancer cells.
- Restore, augment, or modulate the host's immune system, such as inhibiting viral infection, and activating natural killer (NK) and lymphocyte-activated killer (LAK) cells.
- Help the host's normal ability to repair or replace damaged cells (e.g., damaged by chemotherapy or radiotherapy).
- Interfere with tumor cell differentiation, transformation, or metastasis.

Cytokines are substances released from activated lymphocytes and include the interferons (IFNs), interleukins (ILs), tumor necrosis factor (TNF), and colony stimulating factors (CSFs). Other BRMs are the monoclonal antibodies (MoAbs or MAbs), and vaccine.

Interferons occur naturally in the body and were the first cytokine to be studied. IFN-alfa (α) is stimulated by viruses and tumor cells; its antiviral activity is greater than its antiproliferative activity, which is greater than its immunomodulatory effects. There are twenty subtypes of IFN-α. IFN-beta (β) is also stimulated by viruses; it has equal antiviral, antiproliferative, and immunomodulatory effects. There are two subtypes of IFN-β. IFN-gamma (γ) is stimulated by cell-mediated immune response and IL-2; it is released by activated T lymphocytes and natural killer cells. Its immunomodulatory action is greater than its antiproliferative effect, which is greater than its antiviral effect. There is only one type of this interferon. IFN-alfa 2a is used in the treatment of hairy-cell leukemia, acquired immunodeficiency syndrome (AIDS)-related Kaposi's sarcoma, chronic myelogenous leukemia (CML), chronic hepatitis C, and adjuvant therapy of malignant melanoma. IFN-alpha 2b is used for condyloma acuminata, hepatitis B and C, hairy-cell leukemia, high-risk malignant melanoma, and AIDS-related Kaposi's sarcoma. IFN-beta 1a is being studied as to its usefulness in treating AIDS-related Kaposi's sarcoma, metastatic renal cell cancer, malignant melanoma, and cutaneous T-cell lymphoma. IFN-gamma is used for B-cell malignancies, chronic myelogenous leukemia, renal cell cancer, and is being studied in ovarian cancer. Common side effects of interferons include flulike symptoms, anorexia, and fatigue.

Colony stimulating factors include hematopoietic growth factors. They too occur naturally in the body and help immature blood cell elements develop into mature, effective white blood cells, red blood cells, and platelets. Recombinant DNA techniques have permitted the manufacture of large quantities of these substances. An "r" prefix (e.g., r-IL-2) indicates that it was produced using recombinant technology. The use of these cytokines has permitted increased doses of chemotherapy to be safely given. Filgrastim, or granulocyte-colony stimulating factor (G-CSF), is approved to prevent febrile neutropenia following bone marrow suppressive chemotherapy, as well as for other uses, and a sustained-duration pegylated formulation requiring less frequent dosing is available (pegfilgrastim or Neulasta). Sargramostim, or granulocyte-macrophage colony stimulating factor (GM-CSF), is approved for myeloid reconstitution after autologous bone marrow transplantation and for other uses. It is now being studied in use with dendritic cell vaccines. Both G-CSF and GM-CSF can be used to mobilize stem cells that will be used to rescue the bone marrow after high-dose chemotherapy. EPO or rHuEPO (erythropoietin) has become standard therapy in many situations, especially in radiation therapy, as it has become clear that cytotoxic damage from radiation is enhanced if the hemoglobin is > 12–14g/dL (hypoxic cells require almost three times the dose of radiation therapy to kill the cell than normally oxygenated cells [Kumar, 1999]). In addition, EPO helps prevent the need for red blood cell transfusions during chemotherapy and helps to minimize the fatigue associated with anemia. Efforts to produce an erythropoietin growth factor requiring less frequent dosing has resulted in the drug darbapoietin, now available.

Platelet growth factor, oprelvekin (Neumega), or interleukin-11 can be used to prevent and treat thrombocytopenia following myelosuppressive chemotherapy, and results in a modest increase in platelets. Research continues on thrombopoietin (TPO), which has a peak effect in twelve days, which often is when the nadir effect of chemotherapy occurs. In addition, new technology permits fused growth factors, such as GM-CSF fused together with interleukin-3 (IL-3) in the molecule PIXY-321. Common side effects of colony stimulating factors may include bone pain, fatigue, anorexia, and fever. In order to provide guidance and recommendations for evidence-based practice, the American Society of Clinical Oncology (ASCO) published guidelines for the use of colony stimulating factors. Together with American Society of Hematology colleagues, both organizations said there is strong evidence to use epoetin as a treatment option for patients with chemotherapy-associated anemia with a hemoglobin concentration below 10g/dL (Rizzo et al, 2002).

IL-2 is another naturally occurring cytokine that is made using recombinant technology. It is indicated for the treatment of adults with metastatic renal cell carcinoma and adults with metastatic malignant melanoma; recently, an inhaled high-dose form given together with dacarbazine has been shown to reduce lung metastases from malignant melanoma (Enk et al, 2000). IL-12 is gaining much attention due to its ability to stimulate natural killer (NK) activity and antitumor potential, as well as its synergistic action with IL-2, GM-CSF, and calcium ionophore to enhance dendritic cell function (Bedrosian et al, 2000). IL-12 is being studied in gene therapy (Divino et al, 2000). Side effects of interleukins include flulike symptoms, fatigue, and anorexia, as well as substance-specific side effects; for example, IL-2 can cause serious side effects, depending upon dose, such as capillary leak syndrome.

While many BRMs are still investigational (i.e., being studied in clinical research trials to determine their effectiveness, optimal dose, and method of administration), many are quickly being approved for use. Expected side effects vary according to agent, dose, and patient characteristics. In general, flulike symptoms (fever, chills, rigor, malaise, arthralgias, headache, myalgias, and anorexia) may occur. Routes of administration include intravenous (IV), intramuscular (IM), intraperitoneal (IP), subcutaneous (SQ), intralesional, inhaled and topical.

Currently, palifermin or recombinant human keratinocyte growth factor has shown remarkable success in decreasing the oral mueositis associated with bone marrow transplant, and is being considered for approval by the FDA.

Monoclonal antibodies are produced to target a single foreign antigen, and are designed to attach to specific cancer antigens. Monoclonal antibodies can become targeted therapies and have demonstrated an active role in molecularly targeted therapies. Therefore, further discussion of monoclonal antibodies and specific agents can be found in Chapter 5, Molecular Targeted Therapies.

References

Amgen. Prescribing Package Insert: Neulasta. Thousand Oaks, CA: Amgen, Inc. 2002

Bedrosian I, Roras JG, Xu S, et al. Granulocyte-Macrophage Colony-Stimulating Factor, Interleukin-2a and Interleukin-12 Synergize with Calcium Ionophore to Enhance Dendritic Cell Function. *J Immunother* 2000;23(3):311–320

Benstein K. Future of Basic/Clinical Hematopoiesis: Research in the Era of Hematopoietic Growth Factor Availability. *Semin Oncol* 1992;19(4):441–448

Bronchud MH, Scarffe JH, Thatcher N, et al. Phase I/II Study of Recombinant Human Granulocyte Colony-Stimulating Factor in Patients Receiving Intensive Chemotherapy for SCLC. *Br J Cancer* 1987;56:809–813

Chabner BA, Longo DL. *Cancer Chemotherapy and Biotherapy,* 2nd ed. Philadelphia: Lippincott-Raven; 1996

Clark JW, Longo DL. Biologic Response Modifiers. *Mediguide Oncology* 1986;6:1–10

Dorr RT, Von Hoff DD. *Cancer Chemotherapy Handbook,* 2nd ed. Norwalk, CT: Appleton & Lange; 1994

Egrie JC, Dwyer E, Lykos M, et al. Novel Erythropoiesis Stimulating Protein (NESP) Has a Longer Serum Half-life and Greater in vivo Biological Activity than Recombinant Human Erythropoietin (rHuEPO). *Blood* 1997;90(10): abstract 243 (Suppl 1)

Enk AH, Nashan D, Rubben A, Knop J. High Dose Inhalation Interleukin-2 Therapy for Lung Metastases in Patients with Malignant Melanoma. *Cancer* 2000;88(9): 2042–2046

Farese AM, Roskos L, Cheung E, et al. A Single Administration of r-met-HuGCSF-SD/01 (SD/01) Significantly Improves Neutrophil Recovery Following Autologous Bone Marrow Transplantation. *Blood* 1998;92 (suppl):112A (abstract 455)

Gabrilove JL, Cleeland CS, Livingston RB. Clinical Evaluation of Once Weekly Dosing of Epoetin Alfa in Chemotherapy Patients: Improvements in Hemoglobin and Quality of Life are Similar to Three Times Weekly Dosing. *J Clin Oncol* 2001;19 (11):2875–2882

Genentech. Herceptin Package Insert S. San Francisco,, Genentech BioOncology 1998

Glaspy JA, Glode DW. Clinical Applications of the Myeloid Growth Factors. *Semin Hematol* 1989;26 (Suppl 2):14–17

Hahn MB, Jassak PF. Nursing Management of Patients Receiving Interferon. *Semin Oncol Nurs* 1988;4:120–125

Irwin MM. Patients Receiving Biologic Response Modifiers: Overview of Nursing Care. *Oncol Nurs Forum* 1987;14 (Suppl):32–37

Jassak PF. Biotherapy. In Groenwald SL, Frogge MH, Goodman M, Yarbro CH, (eds), *Cancer Nursing Principles and Practice,* 2nd ed. Sudbury, MA: Jones and Bartlett;1990;284–306

Kammula US, White D, Rosenberg SA. Trends in the Safety of High Dose Bolus Interleukin-2 Administration in Patients with Metastatic Cancer. *Cancer* 1998;83(4): 797–805

Kumar P. Tumor Hypoxia and Anemia: Impact upon the Efficacy of Radiation Therapy. *Anemia YK Symposium* New Orleans, LA 3 December 1999

MacDougall IC, Gray SJ, Orlaith E, et al. Pharmacokinetics of Novel Erythropoiesis Stimulating Protein Compared with Epoetin Alfa in Dialysis Patients. *J Am Soc of Nephrology* 1999;10(11):2411–2419

Moldawer NP, Figlin RA. Tumor Necrosis Factor: Current Clinical Status and Implications for Nursing Management. *Semin Oncol Nurs* 1988;4:95–101

Neumega Prescribing Information. Cambridge, MA: Genetics Institute, Inc.; 1998

Rizzo JD, Lichtin AE, Woolf SH, et al. Use of Epoetin in patients with Cancer: Evidence-based Clinical Practice Guidelines of the American Society of Clinical Oncology and the American Society of Hematology. *Blood* 2002;100(7):2303–2320

Simpson C, Seipp CA, Rosenbery SA. The Current Status and Future Applications of Interleukin-2 and Adoptive Immunotherapy in Cancer Treatment. *Semin Oncol Nurs* 1988;4:132–141

Solimando DA, Bressler LR, Kintzel PE, Geraci MC. *Drug Information Handbook for Oncology,* 2nd ed. Cleveland, OH: Lexi-Comp Inc.; 2000

Spielberger R, Emmanouilides C, Stiff P, et al. Use of recombinant human keratinocyte growth factor (rHuKGF) can reduce severe oral mucositis in patients with hematologic malignancies undergoing autologous peripheral blood progenitor cell transplantation (auto-PBPCT) after radiation-based conditioning—results of a phase 3 trial. *Proc Am Soc Clin Oncol* 2003;22:122, abstract 3642

Swanson G, Bergstrom K, Stump E, et al. Growth Factor Usage Patterns and Outcomes in the Community Setting: Collection through a Practice-based Computerized Clinical Information System. *J Clin Oncol* 2000;18(8):1764–1770

Yasko JM, Dudjak LA, eds. *Biological Response Modifier Therapy: Symptom Management.* New York: Park Row Publishers; 1990

Agent: darbepoetin alfa (Aranesp)

Class: Cytokine, CSF.

Mechanism of Action: Recombinant DNA protein that is an erythropoiesis-stimulating protein, closely resembling erythropoietin. Drug is produced in the Chinese hamster ovary. Drug stimulates erythropoiesis in the same way that endogenous erythropoietin does in response to hypoxia. Darbepoetin alfa interacts with progenitor stem cells to stimulate red blood cell production.

Metabolism: Drug is slowly absorbed after subcutaneous injection, with bioavailabilty of 37%, a peak serum level 34 hours after administration (24–72 hour range), and half-life of 49 hours (27–89 hour range) in patients with Chronic Renal Failure. In patients with cancer, the peak serum concentration occurs at 90 hours with a range of 71–123 hours. When given IV, the drug has a biphasic profile, with a distribution half-life of 1.4 hours, and terminal half-life of 21 hours, which is about 3 times longer than Epoetin alfa.

Dosage/Range:

- Cancer Patients Receiving Chemotherapy: 2.25 mcg/kg SQ q week as starting dose
  - —If less than 1.0 g/dL increase in hgb after 6 weeks of therapy, increase dose to 4.5 mcg/kg.

  - —If hgb increases by > 1.0 g/dL in 2-week period or exceeds 12 g/dL, reduce dose by 25%.
  - —If hgb > 13 g/dL, hold dose until hgb falls to 12g/dL and restart at 75% of prior dose.
- Chronic Renal Failure Patients: 0.45 mcg/kg IV or SC q week as starting dose
  - —Titrate to achieve/maintain hemoglobin at 12 g/dL, increasing dose q month.
  - —If increase in hgb is < 1.0 g/dL over 4 weeks and iron stores are adequate, increase dose by 25% of the previous dose; dose may be increased at 4-week intervals until target hemoglobin reached.
  - —If hgb increases by > 1 g/dL in 2-week period, decrease dose by 25%.
  - —Convert from Epoetin alfa to darbepoetin alfa (Special Considerations).
  - —May be able to give drug every 2 weeks.

Drug Preparation:

- Drug available in single-dose vials containing 25, 40, 60, 100, 150, 200, 300, or 500 mcg of darbepoetin alfa; contains no preservative so should not be pooled.
- Do not shake drug as it may denature it; do not dilute; visually inspect drug for discoloration or particulate matter prior to parenteral administration, and discard if found.
- Drug available with either polysorbate or albumin solution.
- Store at 2° to 8°C (36° to 46°F). Do not freeze or shake, and protect from light.

Drug Administration:

- Administer SQ or IV weekly to start, and may be able to give every 2 weeks depending upon response to drug.

Drug Interactions:

- No studies have been performed.

Lab Effects/Interference:

- Increased hemoglobin and hematocrit.

Special Considerations:

- Contraindicated in patients with uncontrolled hypertension, or known hypersensitivity to any of the active substance or excipients (albumin or polysorbate).
- Drug may increase the risk of cardiovascular events in patients with Chronic Renal Failure (CRF) due to high hemoglobin and risk increased in patients who had a rise of 1 g/dL or more in a 2-week period.
- Once starting drug, weekly hemoglobin should be monitored until stabilized and maintenance dose has been established; once dose has been adjusted, the hemoglobin should be monitored weekly for at least 4 weeks until stabi-

lization occurs; once maintenance established, hemoglobin should be monitored at regular intervals.

- Rarely, patients may develop antibodies that neutralize the effect, and rarely can lead to red cell aplasia. If a patient loses response to darbepoetin alfa, evaluation should be done to find cause, including presence of binding and neutralizing antibodies to darbepoetin alfa, native erythropoietin, and any other recombinant erythropoietin administered to the patient.
- Overall incidence of thrombotic events 6.2% compared to 4.1% for placebo, characterized by pulmonary embolism, thromboembolism, thrombosis, and thrombophlebitis (deep and/or superficial).
- Edema occurred in 21% of patients as compared to 10% with placebo.
- The possibility that darbepoetin alfa can stimulate tumor growth, especially as a growth factor of myeloid malignancies, has not been studied.
- Iron status should be assessed before and during treatment to ensure effective erythropoiesis; supplemental iron is recommended for patients with serum ferritin < 100 mcg/L or whose serum transferring saturation is < 20%. If patient does not respond to darbepoetin alfa, folic acid and vitamin B_{12} levels should also be assessed and deficiencies corrected.
- No studies have been performed on use of the drug in pregnant women. Drug should be used only if potential benefit outweighs risk to the fetus; it is unknown if the drug is excreted in human milk, so caution should be used if used in a nursing mother.
- Rarely, allergic reactions can be severe, including skin rash and urticaria. Drug should be discontinued if serious allergic or anaphylactic reactions occur.
- Patients who have controlled hypertension should have regular assessment of blood pressure. Patients should be encouraged to be compliant with their anti-hypertensive medication regime.
- Dosing in Chronic Renal Faillure: Estimated Darbepoetin alfa starting doses (mcg/week) based on Prior Epoetin alfa dose (units/week):

Previous Weekly Epoetin alfa dose (units/wk)	Weekly Darbepoetin alfa dose (mcg/week)
< 2500	6.25
2500–4999	12.5
5000–10,999	25

Previous Weekly Epoetin alfa dose (units/wk)	Weekly Darbepoetin alfa dose (mcg/week)
11,000–17,999	40
18,000–33,999	60
34,000–89,999	100
≥ 90,000	200

Potential Toxicities/Side Effects and the Nursing Process

I. ACTIVITY INTOLERANCE related to FATIGUE

Defining Characteristics: 33% of cancer patients reported fatigue compared to 30% in the placebo group. Patients had advanced disease, which may explain the high incidence.

Nursing Implications: Assess baseline activity and energy levels. Assess baseline fluid.

II. ALTERATION IN SKIN INTEGRITY, POTENTIAL related to PERIPHERAL EDEMA, RASH

Defining Characteristics: Peripheral edema occurred in 21% of cancer patients in clinical trials as compared to 10% in the placebo group; rash occurred in 7% of patients receiving darbepoietin alfa compared to 3% in the placebo group.

Nursing Implications: Perform baseline skin assessment, assess baseline weight and presence of edema. Teach patient to report development of peripheral edema. Teach patient self-assessment of skin, weight, and peripheral edema, and to report rash right away. Assess degree of peripheral edema if it develops, and discuss significant edema with physician to determine etiology and management. Teach patient local skin care, including avoidance of tight clothing and shoes, keeping skin moisturized to prevent cracking, and local comfort measures. If rash develops, assess extent, presence of urticaria, and implications regarding allergic reaction and drug discontinuance.

III. ALTERATION IN COMFORT related to HEADACHE, DIZZINESS, FEVER, MYALGIA, ARTHRALGIA

Defining Characteristics: Headache occurred in 12% of cancer patients in the clinical trials compared to 8% in the placebo group; dizziness 14% compared to 8% in placebo group; fever 19% compared to 16% in placebo group; myalgias 13% compared to 6% in placebo group, and myalgias 8% compared to 5% in the placebo group, probably due to bone marrow expansion.

Nursing Implications: Teach patient bone pain may occur and discuss use of nonsteroidal anti-inflammatory drugs with patient and physician for symptom management. Teach patient to remain seated or lying down if feeling dizzy, and when dizziness has resolved, to change position gradually. Monitor hemoglobin weekly during dose determination period, and weekly for at least 4 weeks after each dose adjustment. Teach patient headache, fever, dizziness, myalgia, and arthralgia may occur and to report them if they do not respond to usual management strategies.

IV. ALTERATION IN ELIMINATION related to DIARRHEA

Defining Characteristics: Diarrhea occurred in 22% of cancer patients receiving the drug in clinical trials compared to 12% of placebo group; 18% experienced constipation compared to 17% in the placebo group.

Nursing Implications: Assess baseline patient bowel elimination pattern. Teach patient to report these side effects so that they can be evaluated. Teach patient self-care measures, including dietary modification, local comfort measures, and over-the-counter anti-diarrheal medication. Teach patient to report symptoms that persist, and discuss with physician possible other etiologies and management plan.

V. KNOWLEDGE DEFICIT related to SELF-ADMINISTRATION TECHNIQUE

Defining Characteristics: Drug is administered once weekly or if response is adequate, may be given once every 2 weeks.

Nursing Implications: Assess baseline psychomotor ability, knowledge, and willingness to learn technique of self-injection. Teach how to refrigerate drug, self-administer using pre-filled syringes, how to activate needle guard, and safely collect used syringes for proper disposal. Drug insert has "Information for Patients and Caregivers." Use written and video supplements to teaching process and have patient correctly demonstrate technique prior to performing at home. Make referral to visiting-nurse agency to reinforce teaching if needed. Teach patient telephone number and who to call if questions or problems arise, and ensure patient can correctly repeat information.

Agent: epoetin alfa (Epogen, Erythropoietin, Procrit)

Class: Cytokine, colony stimulating factor (CSF).

Mechanism of Action: Stimulates the division and differentiation of erythrocyte stem cells in the bone marrow and is a hormone produced by recombinant DNA techniques. Has a naturally occurring counterpart, erythropoietin. Results in the release of reticulocytes into the bloodstream in 7–10 days, where they mature into erythrocytes, taking 2–6 weeks to increase hemoglobin.

Metabolism: Following SC injection, 21–31% of drug is bioavailable, with rapid distribution to tissues. Drug is taken up in the liver, kidneys, and bone marrow. Onset of action in a few days to 2 weeks; peak effect in 2–3 weeks. Half-life is 4–13 h. Eliminated via the liver and urine (10% unchanged drug).

Dosage/Range:

I. 50–150 units/kg TIW; if no increase in HCT within 8 weeks, increase dose by 25–50 units/kg/dose up to 300 units/kg TIW.

II. 40,000 U as a single dose once a week SQ; if HCT does not rise 5–6% in 8 weeks, increase dose to 60,000 units/week; if no response, increase dose to 80,000 units/week (maximum).

- Interrupt therapy if HCT > 40%, and resume at 75% of dose when HCT is 36%.
- Usual target range 30–36% HCT.
- IV doses must be 40–50% higher than subcutaneous doses to achieve same effect.

Drug Preparation:

- DO NOT SHAKE vial as it may denature the glycoprotein.
- Available as preservative-free injection in 2000-U/mL, 3000-U/mL, 4000-U/mL, 10,000-U/mL, and 40,000-U/mL vials. These must be refrigerated and unused portions should be discarded.
- Injection, preserved with benzyl alcohol: available as 10,000–U/mL (2 mL multidose) and 20,000-U/mL vials.

Drug Administration:

- SQ or IV injection.

Drug Interactions:

- None reported.

Lab Effects/Interference:

- Expect increase in Hgb/HCT in 2–6 weeks.

Special Considerations:

- Drug is contraindicated in patients with uncontrolled hypertension.
- Iron stores need to be checked, and replaced to maximize response to therapy.
- Used for management of chemotherapy-related anemia and anemia of chronic disease.

Potential Toxicities/Side Effects (Dose- and Schedule-Dependent) and the Nursing Process

I. ALTERATION IN COMFORT related to PYREXIA, FATIGUE, HEADACHE

Defining Characteristics: May be due to HIV disease, rather than drug, and occurs in 20–25% of patients. Allergic reactions including urticaria may occur. Anaphylaxis has not been reported.

Nursing Implications: Assess baseline temperature (T) and energy level. Instruct patient to report signs/symptoms, and discuss measures to increase comfort.

II. POTENTIAL ALTERATION IN OXYGENATION related to POLYCYTHEMIA

Defining Characteristics: Polycythemia may result if target range is exceeded (HCT of 40%).

Nursing Implications: Monitor weekly HCT: dose should be interrupted if HCT > 40%, then resumed at 75% dose once HCT is 36%. When HCT is stabilized, discuss monitoring HCT with physician (e.g., testing).

III. KNOWLEDGE DEFICIT related to SELF-ADMINISTRATION TECHNIQUE

Defining Characteristics: Most often drug is administered SQ three times per week.

Nursing Implications: Assess baseline psychomotor ability, knowledge, and willingness to learn technique of self-injection. Teach how to prepare drug, self-administer, and safely collect used syringes for proper disposal. Use written and video materials as supplements to teaching process and have patient correctly demonstrate technique prior to performing at home. Make referral to visiting-nurse agency to reinforce teaching.

Agent: filgrastim (Neupogen, G-CSF)

Class: Cytokine, CSF.

Mechanism of Action: Recombinant DNA protein (G-CSF) that regulates the production of neutrophils in the bone marrow (proliferation, differentiation, activation of mature neutrophils). Drug is produced by the insertion of the human G-CSF gene into *Escherichia coli* bacteria.

Metabolism: Elimination half-life is 3.5 hours.

Dosage/Range:

- Starting dose 5 μg/kg/day SQ or IV; dose increase by 5 μg/kg for each chemotherapy cycle, based on duration and severity of neutropenia at nadir.
- BMT: After BMT, 10 μg/kg/day as IV infusion of 4 or 24 hours, or as a continuous subcutaneous, 24-hour infusion, and then titrated based on ANC.
- Mobilization of peripheral blood progenitor cells (PBPC) is 10 mcg/kg/day SQ × at least 4 days until the first leukapheresis procedure, and continued until the last leukapheresis. Modify dose if WBC > 100,000/mm^3.
- Patients with acute myeloid leukemia receiving induction or consolidation: 5 mcg/kg/da SQ beginning 24 hrs after last dose of chemotherapy until ANC > 1000/mm^3 for 3 consecutive days.

Drug Preparation:

- Drug available in refrigerated vials of 300 μg/mL; discard unused portions.
- Unopened vials should be stored in the refrigerator at 2–8°C (36–46°F).
- Avoid shaking.
- Remove from refrigerator 30 minutes prior to injection. Discard if left out > 6 hours.

Drug Administration:

- SQ or IV, daily, beginning at least 24 hr postadministration of chemotherapy, continuing up to 2 weeks or until ANC > 10,000/mm^3.

Drug Interactions:

- None significant.

Lab Effects/Interference:

- Increased WBC and neutrophil counts.

Special Considerations:

- PEGylated form of filgrastim (sustained duration) is available and is given once a treatment cycle; it is equivalent to daily injections of filgrastim (see p.364, pegfilgrastim).
- Indicated for accelerating the recovery of neutrophil counts after myelosuppressive chemotherapy, including BMT and prevention of febrile neutropenia.
- Indicated for the mobilization of hematopoietic progenitor cells into the periphery for collection by leukopheresis, and reinfusion for stem cell rescue.
- Studies showed no statistical difference between Neupogen or placebo group in complete remission rate, disease-free survival, time to disease progression, or overall survival when used in patients with acute myeloid leukemia after induction or consolidation therapy.

Potential Toxicities/Side Effects (Dose- and Schedule-Dependent) and the Nursing Process

I. ALTERATION IN COMFORT related to SKELETAL PAIN

Defining Characteristics: Patients (22%) may report transient skeletal pain, believed due to the expansion of cells in the bone marrow in response to G-CSF.

Nursing Implications: Teach patient this may occur and discuss use of nonsteroidal anti-inflammatory drugs (NSAIDs) with patient and physician for symptom management. Monitor WBC and ANC twice weekly during therapy; dose should be discontinued when ANC > $10{,}000/mm^3$.

II. KNOWLEDGE DEFICIT related to SELF-ADMINISTRATION TECHNIQUE

Defining Characteristics: Drug is administered daily for up to two weeks by SQ injection (outpatients).

Nursing Implications: Assess baseline psychomotor ability, knowledge, and willingness to learn technique of self-injection. Teach how to prepare drug, self-administer, and safely collect used syringes for proper disposal. Use written and video supplements to teaching process and have patient correctly demonstrate technique prior to performing at home. Make referral to visiting-nurse agency to reinforce teaching. Patient instructions in English are on package insert. Video and more detailed patient education are available from Amgen (Thousand Oaks, CA) representative.

Agent: Imiquimod 5% topical cream (Aldara®)

Class: Immune response modifier.

Mechanism of Action: Stimulates the immune system to release cytokines, including interferon, which stimulate Langerhans cells to kill skin cancer cells. Has been shown to reduce the expression of Bcl-2 (a protein that causes the cell to avoid apoptosis, or programmed cell death, by preventing the activation of the proapoptotic proteins called capases) and increase apoptosis of basal skin cancer cells.

Metabolism: Unknown.

Dosage/Range:
Imiquimod 5% topical cream is applied to the superficial basal cell carcinoma (sBCC) lesion (must be 2 cm or less in diameter), including a 1cm margin around the lesion as shown in the table below.

Target tumor diameter	Size of cream droplet to be used (diameter)	Amount of Imiquimod cream used
0.5cm—< 1.0 cm	4 mm	10 mg
> 1.0 cm—< 1.5 cm	5 mm	25 mg
> 1.5 cm—2.0cm	7 mm	40 mg

Available in single use packets, supplied 12 per box.

Drug Preparation/Administration: Wash hands before and after application of cream, and wear gloves. Wash skin area(s) with mild soap and water, then dry thoroughly before application, and again, after 8 hours application. Apply cream to lesion with an additional 1 cm surrounding the lesion(s), at bedtime leaving the cream on at least 8 hours, 5 nights a week, × 6 weeks.

Drug Interactions: Unknown.

Lab Effects/Interference: None known.

Special Considerations:

- Indicated for the treatment of sBCC on the body, neck, arms or legs (not the face, hands or feet) when surgical removal is not an option.
- Drug is also used for the treatment of external genital and non-genital warts, molluscum contagiosum, solar keratoses.

Potential Toxicities/Side Effects (More Severe with Higher Dosing) and the Nursing Process

I. POTENTIAL ALTERATION IN SKIN INTEGRITY AND COMFORT related to SKIN IRRITATION

Defining Characteristics: Redness, swelling, development of a sore or blister, peeling, itching, and burning are common application site reactions. Response to therapy cannot be determined until the skin reaction resolves, sometimes up to 12 weeks.

Nursing Implications: Explain to the patient that these side effects may occur. Teach patient to wash skin prior to application, and again after 8 hours. Teach patient to assess skin reactions, and to report any symptoms that interfere with activities of daily living as a rest period of a few days may be necessary if symptoms are severe. In addition, instruct patient to stop cream and report infection in the application area right away.

II. KNOWLEDGE DEFICIT related to SELF-ADMINISTRATION OF CREAM

Defining Characteristics: Treatment is for 6 weeks and must be applied properly for adequate tumor exposure.

Nursing Implcations: Teach patient self-administration of the cream, and to keep a diary to keep track of the application schedule. Teach patient to wash hands before and after application. Teach patient verbally and through demonstration to wash treatment area with mild soap and water, then to dry prior to application. Cream should be applied to extend 1 cm beyond the lesion borders, and rubbed into the treatment area until no longer visible. Keep cream away from eyes. Cream should be on for at least 8 hours, and then removed using mild soap and water.

Agent: interferon alfa (α) (Alpha interferon, IFN, Interferon alpha-2a, rIFN-A, Roferon A)

Class: Cytokine.

Mechanism of Action: Antiviral, antiproliferative, and immunomodulatory effects. Activates prenatural killer cells, increases cytotoxicity of NK cells, and enhances immune response.

Metabolism: Well absorbed following SQ or IM injection with 90% bioavailability after SQ injection. Drug peaks at 6–8 hours, and has an elimination half-life of 2 hours (IM/IV) and 3 hours (SQ). Renal filtration and tubular reabsorption as catabolites; minor hepatic metabolism and biliary excretion.

Dosage/Range:

- Hairy-cell leukemia: IFN-α_{2a}: Induction 3 mIU qd for 16–24 weeks (IM, SQ); maintenance 3 mIU three times per week for 6–24 months.
- CML: 9mIU qd SQ × up to 18 months.
- AIDS-related Kaposi's sarcoma: IFN-α_{2a}: Induction 3 mIU qd for 10–12 weeks (IM, SQ); can escalate dose from 3 mIU → 9 mIU → 18 mIU over 3 days to 36 mIU; maintenance 36 mIU three times per week.
- Malignant melanoma: 3mIU qd × 8–48 weeks.

Drug Preparation:

- IFN-α_{2a} available as injection solution (3–mIU vial or 18–mIU multidose vial) or powder for injection (3 mIU/0.5 mL in 18–mIU vial). Do not shake or freeze. Store in refrigerator and use reconstituted solution within 30 days.

Drug Administration:

- IM, SQ, or IV.

Drug Interactions:

- May decrease elimination of aminophylline by 33–81% via inhibition of cytochrome P-450 enzyme system.
- Increased effects of CNS depressants.
- Increased bone marrow suppressant effects with zidovudine (AZT).

- Cimetidine may increase antitumor effect in melanoma.
- Vinblastine: may increase incidence of peripheral neuropathy.

Lab Effects/Interference:

- Dose-dependent; leukopenia; elevated liver serum transaminases.

Potential Toxicities/Side Effects (More Severe with Higher Dosing) and the Nursing Process

I. ALTERATION IN COMFORT related to FLULIKE SYNDROME

Defining Characteristics: Chills 3–6 hours after dose in 40–60% of patients; fever (74–98% of patients) with onset 30–90 minutes after chill, lasting up to 24 hours. Temperature 39–40°C (102–104°F), tachyphylaxis (decrease in severity/occurrence after successive treatments) common. Fatigue (89–95% of patients) and malaise are cumulative and dose-limiting. Headache, myalgias occur in 60–70% of patients, as well as arthralgias (5–24% of patients).

Nursing Implications: Assess baseline T, vital signs (VS), neurologic status, and comfort level; monitor every 4–6 hours if patient is in hospital. Discuss with physician premedication and regular dosing of antipyretic (e.g., acetaminophen ± diphenhydramine, NSAID). Teach patient self-care measures, including monitoring T, comfort level, self-administration of prescribed medications prior to dose and regularly postdose, as well as the use of heat or cold for myalgias, arthralgias. Encourage patient to increase oral fluids and alternate rest and activity periods. If patient is in hospital and experiences rigor, discuss with physician IV meperidine (25 mg IVq15min to maximum 100 mg in 1 hour) and monitor BP for hypotension. Teach patient to alternate rest and activity periods.

II. POTENTIAL FOR INFECTION AND BLEEDING related to NEUTROPENIA AND THROMBOCYTOPENIA

Defining Characteristics: Although uncommon, increased risk with increased dose; dose-limiting thrombocytopenia; reversible. Onset usually in 7–10 days, nadir at day 14, but may be delayed in hairy-cell leukemia (20–40 days); recovery in 21 days.

Nursing Implications: Assess baseline CBC, WBC, differential, and platelet count, and signs/symptoms of infection or bleeding. Discuss any abnormalities with physician before drug administration. Teach patient signs/symptoms of infection and bleeding, and to report them immediately. Teach patient self-care measures to minimize infection and bleeding, including avoidance of OTC aspirin-containing medications, and oral hygiene regimen.

III. ALTERATION IN NUTRITION, LESS THAN BODY REQUIREMENTS, related to NAUSEA, DIARRHEA, ANOREXIA

Defining Characteristics: Anorexia occurs (46–65% of patients) and is cumulative and dose-limiting. Nausea (32–51% of patients) is mild with tachyphylaxis after one week. Diarrhea (29–42% of patients) is mild, and vomiting is rare (10–17% of patients). Taste alterations and xerostomia may occur.

Nursing Implications: Assess baseline nutritional status. Teach patient potential side effects and self-care measures, including oral hygiene. Encourage patient to prepare favorite high-calorie, high-protein foods ahead of time so can snack when hungry. Teach self-administration of prescribed antiemetics and antidiarrheals as needed. Refer to dietitian as appropriate.

IV. SENSORY/PERCEPTUAL ALTERATION related to CNS EFFECTS

Defining Characteristics: Dizziness (21–41% of patients), confusion (8–10% of patients), decreased mental status (17% of patients), and depression (16% of patients). Somnolence, irritability, poor concentration, seizures, paranoia, hallucinations, psychoses may occur in 70% of patients but are reversible. Use drug cautiously in patients with history of seizures or CNS dysfunction.

Nursing Implications: Assess baseline mental status and neurologic status prior to drug administration. Assess patient for changes (impaired memory/attention, disorientation, slow/vague responses to questions, increased lethargy) during treatment. Instruct patient to report signs/symptoms; provide information and emotional support, as well as interventions to ensure safety if signs/symptoms occur.

V. POTENTIAL ALTERATION IN CARDIAC OUTPUT related to TACHYCARDIA, CHEST PAIN, DYSRHYTHMIAS

Defining Characteristics: Uncommon but dose-related with increased risk in elderly and patients with preexisting cardiac dysfunction: tachycardia, pallor, cyanosis, chest pain, orthostatic hypotension or hypertension arrhythmias, CHF, syncope.

Nursing Implications: Assess baseline cardiopulmonary status and risk (elderly, preexisting cardiac dysfunction). EKG testing is done baseline and during treatment for high-risk individuals. Monitor VS and I/O, every four hours while receiving drug in hospital. Teach patient to report signs/symptoms of dyspnea, chest pain, edema, or other abnormalities immediately.

VI. POTENTIAL ALTERATION IN ELIMINATION related to RENAL AND HEPATIC DYSFUNCTION

Defining Characteristics: Dose-related increased BUN, creatinine, LFTs (increased AST 42–46%) may occur, as well as proteinuria. Patient may develop interstitial nephritis.

Nursing Implications: Assess baseline renal and hepatic function studies and urinalysis prior to drug initiation, and periodically during therapy. Discuss abnormalities with physician.

VII. POTENTIAL FOR SEXUAL DYSFUNCTION related to IMPOTENCE, MENSTRUAL IRREGULARITIES

Defining Characteristics: Impotence and decreased libido, menstrual irregularities, and increased spontaneous abortions have occurred. Drug is excreted in breast milk.

Nursing Implications: Assess patient's baseline sexual patterns and discuss potential alterations. Provide information, emotional support, and referral as appropriate and needed. Encourage patient to use contraceptive measures; mothers receiving the drug should not breast feed.

VIII. POTENTIAL ALTERATION IN SKIN INTEGRITY related to RASH, PARTIAL ALOPECIA, DRYNESS

Defining Characteristics: Partial alopecia (8–22% of patients), rash (11–18% of patients), throat dryness (15% of patients), as well as skin dryness, flushing, pruritus, and irritation at injection site may occur.

Nursing Implications: Assess baseline skin integrity. Instruct patient to report signs/symptoms. Discuss/teach symptomatic management, including the use of mild soaps and rinsing skin thoroughly after bathing. Encourage patient to use alcohol-free, oil-based moisturizers on skin.

IX. KNOWLEDGE DEFICIT related to SELF-ADMINISTRATION TECHNIQUE

Defining Characteristics: Often patients must receive daily dosing or thrice weekly dosing in the home setting by SQ injection, and they are unfamiliar with technique.

Nursing Implications: Assess baseline psychomotor ability, knowledge, and willingness to learn technique of self-injection. Teach how to prepare drug, self-administer, and safely collect used syringes for proper disposal. Use written and video materials as supplements to teaching process and have patient correctly demonstrate technique prior to performing at home. Make referral to visiting-nurse agency to reinforce teaching.

Agent: interferon alfa-2b (Intron A, IFN-alpha-2b Recombinant, α-2–Interferon, rIFN-α-2)

Class: Cytokine.

Mechanism of Action: Antiviral, antiproliferative, and immunomodulatory effects. Activates prenatural killer cells, increases cytotoxicity of NK cells, and enhances immune response.

Metabolism: Well absorbed following SQ or IM injection with 90% bioavailability after SQ injection. Drug peaks at 6–8 hours, and has an elimination half-life of 2 hours (IM/IV) and 3 hours (SQ). Renal filtration and tubular reabsorption as catabolites; minor hepatic metabolism and biliary excretion.

Dosage/Range:

- Hairy-cell leukemia: IFN-α_{2b}: 2 mIU/m^2 IM or SQ three times per week × 2–6 months.
- AIDS-related Kaposi's sarcoma: IFN-α_{2b}: 30 mIU/m^2 SQ or IM three times per week.
- Malignant melanoma: Induction: 20 mIU/m^2 IV days 1–5/week for 4 weeks; maintenance: 10 mIU/m^2 SQ three times per week for 48 weeks.
- NHL: 5 mIU TIW.

Drug Preparation:

- IFN-α_{2b} (Intron A): Available in powder for injection (3-, 5-, 10-, 25-, 50-mIU vials).
- Albumin free: in 3-, 5-, 10-, 18-, and 25-mIU vials.
- Powder for injection (lyophilized): 3-, 5-, 10-, 18-, 25-, and 50-mIU vials.
- Multidose pens with 6 doses of 3 mIU (18 mIU) or 5 mIU (30 mIU) or 10 mIU (60 mIU).

Drug Administration:

- IM, SQ, or IV (IVB, intermittent or continuous infusion).

Drug Interactions:

- May decrease elimination of aminophylline by 33–81% via inhibition of cytochrome P-450 enzyme system.
- Increased effects of CNS depressants.
- Increased bone marrow suppressant effects with zidovudine (AZT).
- Increased risk of peripheral neuropathy when combined with vinblastine.

Lab Effects/Interference:

- Dose-dependent; leukopenia; elevated liver serum transaminases.

Potential Toxicities/Side Effects (More Severe with Higher Dosing) and the Nursing Process

I. ALTERATION IN COMFORT related to FLULIKE SYNDROME

Defining Characteristics: Chills 3–6 hours after dose in 40–60% of patients; fever (74–98% of patients) with onset 30–90 minutes after chill, lasting up to 24 hours. Temperature 39–40°C (102–104°F); tachyphylaxis (decrease in severity/occurrence after successive treatments) common. Fatigue (89–95% of patients) and malaise are cumulative and dose-limiting. Headache, myalgias occur in 60–70% of patients, as well as arthralgias (5–24% of patients).

Nursing Implications: Assess baseline T, vital signs (VS), neurologic status, and comfort level; monitor every 4–6 hours if patient is in hospital. Discuss with physician premedication and regular dosing of antipyretic (e.g., acetaminophen ± diphenhydramine, NSAID). Teach patient self-care measures, including monitoring T, comfort level, self-administration of prescribed medications prior to dose and regularly postdose, as well as the use of heat or cold for myalgias, arthralgias. Encourage patient to increase oral fluids and alternate rest and activity periods. If patient is in hospital and experiences rigor, discuss with physician IV meperidine (25 mg IV q15min to maximum 100 mg in 1 hour) and monitor BP for hypotension. Teach patient to alternate rest and activity.

II. POTENTIAL FOR INFECTION AND BLEEDING related to NEUTROPENIA AND THROMBOCYTOPENIA

Defining Characteristics: Although uncommon, increased risk with increased dose; dose-limiting thrombocytopenia, reversible. Onset in 7–10 days, nadir in 14 days (may be delayed 20–40 days in patients with hairy-cell leukemia), and recovery at day 21.

Nursing Implications: Assess baseline CBC, WBC, differential, and platelet count, and signs/symptoms of infection or bleeding. Discuss any abnormalities with physician before drug administration. Teach patient signs/symptoms of infection and bleeding, and to report them immediately. Teach patient self-care measures to minimize infection and bleeding, including avoidance of OTC aspirin-containing medications, and oral hygiene regimen.

III. ALTERATION IN NUTRITION, LESS THAN BODY REQUIREMENTS, related to NAUSEA, DIARRHEA, ANOREXIA

Defining Characteristics: Anorexia occurs (46–65% of patients) and is cumulative and dose-limiting. Nausea (32–51% of patients) is mild with tachyphylaxis after one week. Diarrhea (29–42% of patients) is mild, and vomiting is rare (10–17% of patients). Taste alterations and xerostomia may occur.

Nursing Implications: Assess baseline nutritional status. Teach patient potential side effects and self-care measures including oral hygiene. Encourage patient to prepare favorite high-calorie, high-protein foods ahead of time so can snack when hungry. Teach self-administration of prescribed antiemetics and antidiarrheals as needed. Refer to dietitian as appropriate.

IV. SENSORY/PERCEPTUAL ALTERATION related to CNS EFFECTS

Defining Characteristics: Dizziness (21–41% of patients), confusion (8–10% of patients), decreased mental status (17% of patients), and depression (16% of patients). Somnolence, irritability, poor concentration, seizures, paranoia, hallucinations, psychoses may occur in 70% of patients but are reversible. Use drug cautiously in patients with history of seizures or CNS dysfunction.

Nursing Implications: Assess baseline mental status and neurologic status prior to drug administration. Assess patient for changes (impaired memory/attention, disorientation, slow/vague responses to questions, increased lethargy) during treatment. Instruct patient to report signs/symptoms; provide information and emotional support, as well as interventions to ensure safety if signs/symptoms occur.

V. POTENTIAL ALTERATION IN CARDIAC OUTPUT related to TACHYCARDIA, CHEST PAIN, DYSRHYTHMIAS

Defining Characteristics: Uncommon but dose-related with increased risk in elderly and patients with preexisting cardiac dysfunction: tachycardia, pallor, cyanosis, chest pain, orthostatic hypotension or hypertension arrhythmias, CHF, syncope.

Nursing Implications: Assess baseline cardiopulmonary status and risk (elderly, preexisting cardiac dysfunction). EKG testing is done baseline and during treatment for high-risk individuals. Monitor VS and I/O, every four hours while receiving drug in hospital. Teach patient to report signs/symptoms of dyspnea, chest pain, edema, or other abnormalities immediately.

VI. POTENTIAL ALTERATION IN ELIMINATION related to RENAL AND HEPATIC DYSFUNCTION

Defining Characteristics: Dose-related increased BUN, creatinine, LFTs (increased AST in 42–46%) may occur, as well as proteinuria. Patient may develop interstitial nephritis.

Nursing Implications: Assess baseline renal and hepatic function studies and urinalysis prior to drug initiation, and periodically during therapy. Discuss abnormalities with physician.

VII. POTENTIAL FOR SEXUAL DYSFUNCTION related to IMPOTENCE, MENSTRUAL IRREGULARITIES

Defining Characteristics: Impotence and decreased libido, menstrual irregularities, and increased spontaneous abortions have occurred. Drug is excreted in breast milk.

Nursing Implications: Assess patient's baseline sexual patterns and discuss potential alterations. Provide information, emotional support, and referral as appropriate and needed. Encourage patient to use contraceptive measures; mothers receiving the drug should not breast feed.

VIII. POTENTIAL ALTERATION IN SKIN INTEGRITY related to RASH, PARTIAL ALOPECIA, DRYNESS

Defining Characteristics: Partial alopecia (8–22% of patients), rash (11–18% of patients), throat dryness (15% of patients), as well as skin dryness, flushing, pruritus, and irritation at injection site may occur.

Nursing Implications: Assess baseline skin integrity. Instruct patient to report signs/symptoms. Discuss/teach symptomatic management, including the use of mild soaps and rinsing skin thoroughly after bathing. Encourage patient to use alcohol-free, oil-based moisturizers on skin.

IX. KNOWLEDGE DEFICIT related to SELF-ADMINISTRATION TECHNIQUE

Defining Characteristics: Often patients must receive daily dosing or thrice weekly dosing in the home setting by SQ injection, and they are unfamiliar with technique.

Nursing Implications: Assess baseline psychomotor ability, knowledge, and willingness to learn technique of self-injection. Teach how to prepare drug, self-administer, and safely collect used syringes for proper disposal. Use written and video materials as supplements to teaching process and have patient correctly demonstrate technique prior to performing at home. Make referral to visiting-nurse agency to reinforce teaching.

Agent: interferon gamma (Actimmune, IFN-gamma (γ), rIFN-gamma)

Class: Cytokine.

Mechanism of Action: Antiviral, antiproliferative, and immunomodulatory effects. Activates phagocytes and appears to generate toxic oxidative metabolites in phagocytes; interacts with interleukins to orchestrate immune effect, and enhances antibody-dependent cellular cytotoxicity, NK activity, and mounting of antigen on monocytes (Fc expression).

Metabolism: Slowly absorbed following SQ or IM injection, with 89% bioavailability. Peaks in 4–13 hours following IM injection, and 6–7 hours after SQ injection. Elimination half-lives for IV injection is 30–60 minutes, and 2–8 hours for IM or SC injection. Renal filtration and tubular reabsorption as catabolites; minor hepatic metabolism and biliary excretion.

Dosage/Range:
- Per protocol.
- CML: 0.5–1.5 mg/m² IV TIW OR 0.75–1.5 mg/m² IV 5 times/week OR 1.5 mg/m² IV qd.
- Renal cell carcinoma: 100 micrograms SQ q week OR 0.25 mg IM qd × 8 days q21–28 days.

Drug Preparation:
- Available in 100-μg (3 million units) vials, which should be refrigerated at 2–8°C (36–46°F); do not freeze. Vials stable at room temperature for up to 12 hours.

Drug Administration:
- IM, SQ, or IV.

Drug Interactions:
- May decrease elimination of aminophylline by 33–81% via inhibition of cytochrome P-450 enzyme system.
- Increased effects of CNS depressants.
- Increased bone marrow suppressant effects with zidovudine (AZT).

Lab Effects/Interference:
- Dose-dependent, leukopenia; clevated liver serum transaminases.
- Increased serum creatinine, BUN, proteinuria.

Potential Toxicities/Side Effects (More Severe with Higher Dosing) and the Nursing Process

I. ALTERATION IN COMFORT related to FLULIKE SYNDROME

Defining Characteristics: Chills 3–6 hours after dose in 20% of patients; fever (80% of patients), with onset 30–90 minutes after chill. Tachyphylaxis (decrease in severity/occurrence after successive treatments) common. Fatigue (20% of patients) and myalgia (10%) can occur. Headache occurs in 50% of patients.

Nursing Implications: Assess baseline T, vital signs (VS), neurologic status, and comfort level; monitor every 4–6 hours if patient is in hospital. Discuss with physician premedication and regular dosing of antipyretic (e.g., acetaminophen ± diphenhydramine, NSAID). Teach patient self-care measures, including monitoring T, comfort level, self-administration of prescribed medications prior to dose and regularly postdose, as well as the use of heat or cold for myalgias, arthralgias. Encourage patient to increase oral fluids and alternate rest and activity periods. If patient is in hospital and experiences rigor, discuss with physician IV meperidine (25 mg IV q15min to maximum 100 mg in 1 hour) and monitor BP for hypotension. Teach patient to alternate rest and activity.

II. POTENTIAL FOR INFECTION AND BLEEDING related to NEUTROPENIA AND THROMBOCYTOPENIA

Defining Characteristics: Although uncommon, increased risk with increased dose; dose-limiting thrombocytopenia; reversible.

Nursing Implications: Assess baseline CBC, WBC, differential, and platelet count, and signs/symptoms of infection or bleeding. Discuss any abnormalities with physician before drug administration. Teach patient signs/symptoms of infection and bleeding, and to report them immediately. Teach patient self-care measures to minimize infection and bleeding, including avoidance of OTC aspirin-containing medications, and oral hygiene regimen.

III. ALTERATION IN NUTRITION, LESS THAN BODY REQUIREMENTS, related to NAUSEA, DIARRHEA, ANOREXIA

Defining Characteristics: Anorexia occurs (46–65% of patients) and is cumulative and dose-limiting. Nausea (32–51% of patients) is mild with tachyphylaxis after one week. Diarrhea (29–42% of patients) is mild, and vomiting is rare (10–17% of patients). Taste alterations and xerostomia may occur.

Nursing Implications: Assess baseline nutritional status. Teach patient potential side effects and self-care measures, including oral hygiene. Encourage patient to prepare favorite high-calorie, high-protein foods ahead of time so can snack when hungry. Teach self-administration of prescribed antiemetics and antidiarrheals as needed. Refer to dietitian as appropriate.

IV. SENSORY/PERCEPTUAL ALTERATION related to CNS EFFECTS

Defining Characteristics: Incidence 1–10%: dizziness, confusion, seizures, gait instability, and depression (3% of patients). Use drug cautiously in patients with history of seizures or CNS dysfunction.

Nursing Implications: Assess baseline mental status and neurologic status prior to drug administration. Assess patient for changes (impaired memory/attention, disorientation, slow/vague responses to questions, increased lethargy) during treatment. Instruct patient to report signs/symptoms; provide information and emotional support, as well as interventions to ensure safety if signs/symptoms occur.

V. POTENTIAL ALTERATION IN CARDIAC OUTPUT related to TACHYCARDIA, CHEST PAIN, DYSRHYTHMIAS

Defining Characteristics: Uncommon but dose-related with increased risk in elderly and patients with preexisting cardiac dysfunction: tachycardia, pallor, cyanosis, chest pain, orthostatic hypotension or hypertension arrhythmias, CHF, syncope.

Nursing Implications: Assess baseline cardiopulmonary status and risk (elderly, preexisting cardiac dysfunction). EKG testing is done baseline and during treatment for high-risk individuals. Monitor VS and I/O, every four hours while receiving drug in hospital. Teach patient to report signs/symptoms of dyspnea, chest pain, edema, or other abnormalities immediately.

VI. POTENTIAL ALTERATION IN ELIMINATION related to RENAL AND HEPATIC DYSFUNCTION

Defining Characteristics: Dose-related increased BUN, creatinine, LFTs (increased AST in 42–46%) may occur, as well as proteinuria. Patient may develop interstitial nephritis.

Nursing Implications: Assess baseline renal and hepatic function studies and urinalysis prior to drug initiation, and periodically during therapy. Discuss abnormalities with physician.

VII. POTENTIAL FOR SEXUAL DYSFUNCTION related to IMPOTENCE, MENSTRUAL IRREGULARITIES

Defining Characteristics: Impotence and decreased libido, menstrual irregularities, and increased spontaneous abortions have occurred. It is unknown whether drug is excreted in breast milk.

Nursing Implications: Assess patient's baseline sexual patterns and discuss potential alterations. Provide information, emotional support, and referral as appropriate and needed. Encourage patient to use contraceptive measures; mothers receiving the drug should not breast feed.

VIII. KNOWLEDGE DEFICIT related to SELF-ADMINISTRATION TECHNIQUE

Defining Characteristics: Often patients must receive daily dosing or thrice weekly dosing in the home setting by SQ injection, and they are unfamiliar with technique.

Nursing Implications: Assess baseline psychomotor ability, knowledge, and willingness to learn technique of self-injection. Teach how to prepare drug, self-administer, and safely collect used syringes for proper disposal. Use written and video materials as supplements to teaching process and have patient correctly demonstrate technique prior to performing at home. Make referral to visiting-nurse agency to reinforce teaching.

Agent: interleukin-2 (Aldesleuken, Proleukin)

Class: Cytokine.

Mechanism of Action: IL-2, previously called T-cell growth factor, is produced by helper T cells following antibody-antigen reaction (processed antigen is mounted on macrophage) and IL-1. IL-2 amplifies the immune response to an antigen by immunomodulation and immunorestoration. IL-2 stimulates T-lymphocyte proliferation, enhances killer T-cell activity, increases antibody production (secondary to increased B-cell proliferation), helps to increase synthesis of other cytokines (IFNs, IL-1, -3, -4, -5, -6, CSFs), and stimulates production and activation of natural killer (NK) cells and other cytotoxic cells (LAK and TIL).

Metabolism: Half-life is 3–10 minutes when given by IV bolus, but 30–120 minutes when given by continuous infusion.

Dosage/Range:
Metastic renal cell carcinoma and metastatic malignant melanoma:
- 600,000 IU/kg (0.037 mg/kg) IVB over 15 minutes every 8 hours for a maximum of 14 doses over 5 days, then a 9-day rest, followed by 14 additional doses every 8 hours, for a maximum of 28 doses per course as tolerated. Evaluate for response 4 weeks after completion of a course and prior to next treatment course. Tumor shrinkage should be seen before retreatment. 7-week rest period should separate discharge from the hospital and retreatment. Delay and drug holiday should be used rather than drug dose reduction to manage toxicity.

Contraindications (based on toxicity) to retreatment:
- Sustained ventricular tachycardia (5 beats), uncontrolled cardiac rhythm disturbances, ECG changes showing angina or MI, cardiac tamponade.
- Intubation > 72 hours.
- Renal failure requiring dialysis > 72 hrs.
- Coma or toxic psychosis lasting > 48 hrs; difficult to control seizures.
- Bowel ischemia or perforation, GI bleeding requiring surgery.

Delay with resumption of dose after resolution of symptoms and condition resolved or ruled out.

- Persistent atrial fibrillation, supraventricular tachycardia or bradycardia.
- Hypotension (SBP < 90 mmHg with need for pressors).
- ECG change showing MI, ischemia, myocarditis.
- O2 sat < 90%.
- Mental status changes (confusion, agitation).
- Sepsis.
- Serum creatinine > 4.5 mg/dL or ≥ with severe volume overload, acidosis, or hyperkalemia; persistent oliguria, urine output < 10 mL/hr for 16–24 hours with increasing serum creatinine.
- Signs of hepatic failure (encephalopathy, increasing ascites, liver pain, hypoglycemia): stop this course of treatment, and reinitiate new course after at least 7 weeks of rest.
- Stool guaiac repeatedly > 3–4+.
- Bullous dermatitis or marked worsening of pre-existing skin condition (don't use topical steroid therapy).

Drug Preparation:

- Vial containing 22 mIU (1.3 mg) should be reconstituted with 1.2 mL of sterile water for injection, USP so each mL contains 18 IU of drug. DO NOT SHAKE. Further dilute in 50 mL of 5% Dextrose injection, USP. If patient weight < 40 kg, use smaller volume. Refrigerate and use within 48 hrs of preparation. Bring to room temperature prior to administration.

Drug Administration:

- IV (IVB or 24–hour continuous infusion); SQ; intraperitoneal (IP).
- Administer IV over 15 minutes.

Drug Interactions:

- Potentiation of CNS effects when given in combination with psychotropic drugs.
- Combination with nephrotoxic, myelotoxic, cardiotoxic, or hepatotoxic will increase toxicity of aldesleukin in these organ systems.
- Increased risk of hypersensitivity reactions when sequential high dose aldesleukin combined with dacarbazine, cisplatin, tamoxifen, and interferon-alpha.
- Interferon alpha and aldesleukin concurrently: increased risk of myocardial injury (MI, myocarditis, severe rhabdomyolysis).
- Glucocorticoid steroids: decreased antitumor effectiveness, do not use together.
- Beta-blockers, antihypertensives: potentiate hypotension of aldesleukin.
- Iodinated contrast medium: increased risk of atypical adverse reaction (12.6% incidence) characterized by fever, chills, nausea, vomiting, pruritus, rash, diarrhea, hypotension, edema, and oliguria, and can happen when contrast is given within 4 weeks of aldesleukin dosing.

Lab Effects/Interference:
- Anemia, leukopenia, thrombocytopenia.
- Elevated LFTs.

Special Considerations:
- FDA-indicated for treatment patients with metastatic renal cell cancer or metastatic malignant melanoma.
- Patient must have NORMAL cardiac, pulmonary, hepatic, renal (serum creatinine ≤ 1.5 mg/dL) and CNS function prior to treatment, and be free of any known infection.
- Drug may worsen symptoms of patients with unknown/untreated CNS metastases. Thorough evaluation and treatment of CNS metastases should precede treatment so patient has a negative scan before starting aldesleukin.
- Use caution when patient receiving other drugs that are hepatic or renally toxic.
- Drug may increase rejection in allogeneic transplant patients, exacerbation of autoimmune disease and inflammatory disorders.
- Contraindicated in male or female patients of child-bearing age/intention not using effective contraception; nursing mothers should not nurse while taking the drug unless benefit outweighs unknown risk.
- Pegylated interleukin-2 with a longer drug half-life is being studied but still has the same cardiopulmonary toxicity; inhaled interleukin-2 for patients with pulmonary metastases continues to be studied, and offers few systemic side effects.

Potential Toxicities/Side Effects (Dose-1 and Schedule-Dependent) and the Nursing Process

I. ALTERATION IN COMFORT related to FLULIKE SYNDROME

Defining Characteristics: Chills may occur 2–4 hours after dose; rigors are possible; fever to 39–40°C (102–104°F); and headache. Myalgia and arthralgias may occur at high doses due to accumulation of cytokine deposits/lymphocytes in joint spaces. Incidence of chills 52%, fever 29%, malaise 27%, asthenia 23%, anorexia 20%.

Nursing Implications: Assess baseline T, VS, neurologic status, and comfort level, and monitor every 4–6 hours if patient in hospital. Discuss with physician premedication and regular dosing of antipyretic (e.g., acetaminophen ± diphenhydramine, NSAID). Teach patient self-care measures, including monitoring T, comfort level, self-administration of prescribed medications prior to dose and regularly postdose, as well as the use of heat or cold for myalgias, arthralgias. Encourage patient to increase oral fluids and alternate rest and activity periods. If patient is in hospital and experiences rigor, discuss with physician IV meperidine (25 mg IV every 15 minutes to maximum 100 mg in 1 hour), and monitor BP for hypotension.

II. SENSORY/PERCEPTUAL ALTERATION related to CNS EFFECTS

Defining Characteristics: Confusion, irritability, disorientation, impaired memory, expressive aphasia, sleep disturbances, depression, hallucinations, and psychoses may occur, resolving within 24–48 hours after last drug dose. Mental status abnormalities exaggerated by anxiety and sleep deprivation.

Nursing Implications: Assess baseline mental status and neurologic status prior to drug administration. Assess patient for changes (impaired memory/attention, disorientation, slow/vague responses to questions, increased lethargy) during treatment. Teach patient to report signs/symptoms. Provide information, emotional support, and interventions to ensure safety if signs/symptoms occur.

III. ALTERATION IN CARDIAC OUTPUT related to HYPOTENSION (HIGH-DOSE THERAPY)

Defining Characteristics: Increased risk with doses > 100,000 IU/kg. Capillary leak syndrome (peripheral edema, CHF, pleural effusions, and pericardial effusions) may occur and is reversible once treatment is stopped. Atrial arrhythmias may occur; occasionally, supraventricular tachycardia, myocarditis, chest pain; and rarely, myocardial infarction. IL-2 causes peripheral vasodilation, decreased systemic vascular resistance, and hypotension that may lead to decreased renal perfusion. A decrease in SBP occurs 2–12 hours after start of therapy, and typically will progress to significant hypotension (SBP < 90 mmHg or a 20 mmHg drop from baseline SBP) with hypoperfusion. In addition, protein and fluids will extravasate into the extravascular space forming edema and new effusions.

Nursing Implications: Assess baseline cardiopulmonary status and patients at risk (the elderly, those with preexisting cardiac dysfunction). Monitor VS and pulse oximetry frequently, at least q 4 hour (if hypotensive, q 1 hr), noting rate, rhythm of heartbeat, blood pressure, urinary output, fluid status, I/O q 4 hours or more frequent, and daily weights during therapy. Discuss any abnormalities with physician and revise plan as needed (e.g., diuretics, plasma expanders, ICU transfer). Instruct patient to report signs/symptoms of dyspnea, chest pain, edema, or other abnormalities immediately. Hypotension requires fluid replacement, and patient should be monitored with continuous cardiac monitoring if SBP < 90 mmHg. Any ectopy should be documented on EKG. Manufacturer states that early administration of dopamine (1–5 μg/kg/min) to patients with capillary leak syndrome before the onset of hypotension can improve organ perfusion and preserve urinary output. Increased dopamine doses (6–10 μg/kg/min) or the addition of phenylephrine hydrochloride (1–5 μg/kg/min) to low dose dopamine have been described. Once blood pressure stabilized, use of diuretics often effective in relieving edema and pulmonary congestion.

IV. POTENTIAL ALTERATION IN OXYGENATION

Defining Characteristics: Pulmonary symptoms are dose-related, such as dyspnea and tachypnea. Pulmonary edema may occur with hypoxia, due to fluid shifts.

Nursing Implications: Assess baseline cardiopulmonary status every four hours during therapy, noting rate, rhythm, depth of respirations, presence of dyspnea, and breath sounds (presence of wheezes, crackles, rhonchi). Identify patients at risk: those with preexisting cardiac or pulmonary disease, prior treatment with cardio- or pulmonary-toxic drugs or radiation, and smoking history. Instruct patient to report cough, dyspnea, or change in respiratory status. Strictly monitor I/O, total fluid balance, and daily weight. Discuss abnormalities with physician, as well as the need for oxygen, diuretics, or transfer to ICU.

V. POTENTIAL ALTERATION IN NUTRITION, LESS THAN BODY REQUIREMENTS, related to NAUSEA/VOMITING, DIARRHEA, MUCOSITIS, ANOREXIA

Defining Characteristics: Nausea and vomiting are mild and are effectively controlled by antiemetics. Diarrhea is common, can be severe, and may require bicarbonate replacement. Stomatitis is common but mild.

Nursing Implications: Assess patient's baseline nutritional status. Administer antiemetics as ordered. Teach patient potential side effects and self-care measures, including oral hygiene, and encourage patient to eat favorite high-calorie, high-protein foods. Teach self-administration of prescribed antiemetics and antidiarrheals as needed. Refer to dietitian as appropriate.

VI. POTENTIAL ALTERATION IN ELIMINATION related to RENAL DYSFUNCTION, HEPATOTOXICITY

Defining Characteristics: IL-2 causes direct tubular cell injury and decreased renal blood flow with cumulative doses. Oliguria, proteinuria, increased serum creatinine and BUN, increased LFTs (bili, AST, ALT, LDH, alk phos). Anuria (i.e., 10 mL of urine/hour for 8 hours) occurs in 38% of patients; renal dysfunction is reversible after drug discontinuance. Hepatomegaly and hypoalbuminemia may occur.

Nursing Implications: Assess baseline renal and hepatic functions and monitor during treatment. Assess fluid and electrolyte balance, urine output hourly, and total body balance. Dipstick urine for protein. Discuss abnormalities with physician and revise plan.

VII. POTENTIAL FOR FATIGUE AND BLEEDING related to ANEMIA, THROMBOCYTOPENIA

Defining Characteristics: Severe anemia occurs in 70% of patients, requiring RBC transfusion. Thrombocytopenia occurs commonly but rarely requires transfusion.

Nursing Implications: Assess baseline CBC and platelet count, and signs/symptoms of fatigue, severe anemia, bleeding. Instruct patient to report signs/symptoms immediately and to manage self-care (alternate rest/activity, minimize bleeding by avoidance of OTC aspirin-containing medicines). Transfuse red cells and platelets as ordered.

VIII. POTENTIAL ALTERATION IN SKIN INTEGRITY related to DIFFUSE RASH

Defining Characteristics: All patients develop diffuse erythematous rash, which may desquamate (soles of feet, palms of hands, between fingers). Pruritus may occur with or without rash.

Nursing Implications: Assess baseline skin integrity. Teach patient to report signs/symptoms. Discuss/teach symptomatic management, including the use of mild soaps and rinsing skin thoroughly after bathing. Encourage the use of alcohol-free, oil-based moisturizers on skin and the protection of desquamated areas.

Agent: interleukin-3 (investigational)

Class: Cytokine.

Mechanism of Action: Binds to early progenitor cells. Species-specific stimulator of bone marrow progenitor cells (CFU-GEMM [colony forming unit-granulocyte, erythrocyte, megakaryocyte, and macrophage]). Production of immature neutrophils is enhanced when drug is administered after GM-CSF.

Metabolism: IL-3 is produced by activated T lymphocytes. Other cytokines released after administration of IL-3 include IL-6 (B-lymphocyte growth factor). Short half-life of 4–8 minutes.

Dosage/Range:

- Per investigational protocol, but effective doses have been found to be 60 $\mu g/m^2$/day to 500 $\mu g/m^2$/day for 15 days.

Drug Preparation:

- Per protocol.

Drug Administration:

- SQ qd for 15 days (no difference between IV or SQ injection, and less toxicity; best delivery may be via depot injection or prolonged infusions).

Drug Interactions:

- None reported, but data is being accumulated in clinical trials.

Lab Effects/Interference:

- Expect increase in neutrophils, platelets.

Special Considerations:

- Bone marrow depression/bone marrow failure after chemotherapy: dose-dependent increases in neutrophils in 15 days, and in platelets.
- Myelodysplastic syndrome: respond more slowly, with neutrophil production peak at 19 days, and peak platelet count at 15–25 days.

Potential Toxicities/Side Effects (Dose-1 and Schedule-Dependent) and the Nursing Process

I. ALTERATION IN COMFORT related to FLULIKE SYNDROME

Defining Characteristics: Fever occurs, especially on first day of therapy, and lasts 2–16 hours after administration. Headache and stiff neck also affect comfort but are not severe. Facial flushing, erythema at the injection site, mild bone pain, and edema may occur. When given IV, flulike symptoms, hypotension, rash, headache, and purpura occur (Dorr and Von Hoff, 1994).

Nursing Implications: Assess baseline T, VS, neurologic status, and comfort level, and monitor every 2–16 hours if patient is in hospital. Discuss with physician premedication and regular dosing of antipyretic (e.g., acetaminophen ± diphenhydramine, NSAID). Teach patient self-care measures, including monitoring T, comfort level, self-administration of prescribed medications prior to dose and regularly postdose, and use of heat or cold for myalgias and arthralgias. Encourage patient to increase oral fluids and alternate periods of rest and activity.

Agent: interleukin-6 (investigational)

Class: Cytokine.

Mechanism of Action: Acts primarily as a cofactor in the differentiation and proliferation of cytotoxic T cells (Dorr and Von Hoff, 1994) but has some antitumor activity. Also stimulates differentiation of megakaryocytes, resulting in increased peripheral platelets (thrombopoiesis). Mediates increased osteoclast activity and bone absorption. Probably augments IL-3 activity. IL-6 is produced by T lymphocytes, monocytes, endothelial cells, and fibroblasts.

Metabolism: Probably triphasic elimination, with peak serum levels five hours after administration.

Dosage/Range:
- Per investigational protocol, but effective doses have been found to be 2.5 μg/kg/day administered by SQ injection.

Drug Preparation:
- Per protocol.

Drug Administration:
- SQ.

Drug Interactions:
- None reported, but data is being accumulated in clinical trials.

Lab Effects/Interference:
- Anemia.
- Increased LFTs.

Special Considerations:
- Not recommended therapy for patients with history of cardiac disease, as atrial fibrillation has occurred.
- Contraindicated in patients with diabetes, T- or B-cell malignancy, and multiple myeloma.
- Clinical studies in patients with melanoma, ovarian cancer, and post-BMT in Hodgkin's disease.

Potential Toxicities/Side Effects (Dose- and Schedule-Dependent) and the Nursing Process

I. ALTERATION IN COMFORT related to FLULIKE SYNDROME

Defining Characteristics: Fever and chills commonly occur, along with headaches, which can be severe. These occur 1–4 hours after drug administration. Anorexia and arthralgias can occur. Symptoms can be ameliorated or prevented by prophylactic antipyretics and anti-inflammatory agents.

Nursing Implications: Assess baseline T, VS, neurologic status, and comfort level, and monitor if patient is in hospital. Discuss with physician premedication and regular dosing of antipyretic (e.g., acetaminophen ± diphenhydramine, NSAID). Teach patient self-care measures, including monitoring T, comfort level, self-administration of prescribed medications prior to dose and regularly postdose, and use of heat or cold for myalgias and arthralgias. Encourage patient to increase oral fluids and alternate rest and activity periods.

II. POTENTIAL ALTERATION IN NUTRITION, LESS THAN BODY REQUIREMENTS, related to ALTERATIONS IN HEPATIC FUNCTION STUDIES AND GLUCOSE

Defining Characteristics: Transient alterations in serum alk phos, transaminases, and fasting blood glucose can occur. Development of significant alteration in alk phos in one patient who developed hepatic necrosis has been reported at higher doses (30 μg/kg/day).

Nursing Implications: Assess patient's baseline LFTs and blood glucose. Monitor during therapy. Discuss any alterations with physician.

III. POTENTIAL FOR ACTIVITY INTOLERANCE related to ANEMIA

Defining Characteristics: Anemia appears a few days after beginning therapy. Recovery occurs within one week of cessation of IL-2. Platelet counts rise and neutrophil counts are unchanged.

Nursing Implications: Assess baseline WBC, Hgb/HCT hematocrit, and platelet counts, and monitor during therapy. Assess impact of anemia on patient, and reassure that Hgb/HCT will rise once treatment has stopped.

Agent: interleukin-12 (investigational)

Class: Cytokine.

Mechanism of Action: Stimulates strong natural-killer (NK) cell-mediated antitumor response and enhances cytotoxic lymphocytes (called *cytotoxic lymphocyte maturation factor* and *NK stimulatory factor*). Synergistic with GMCSF, IL-2, and calcium ionophore to enhance maturation of dendritic cell function (Bedrosian et al, 2000); being studied in gene therapy.

Metabolism: Unknown.

Dosage/Range:
- Per investigational protocol.

Drug Preparation:
- Per protocol.

Drug Administration:
- Per protocol.

Drug Interactions:
- Unknown.

Lab Effects/Interference:
- Increased triglycerides and LFTs.
- Hyperglycemia.

- Decreased white and red blood cell counts, platelet count.

Special Considerations:

- Interleukin-12 gene therapy being studied in patients with unresectable/recurrent or refractory squamous cell cancer of the head and neck, and AIDS-related Kaposi's sarcoma.

Potential Toxicities/Side Effects (Dose- and Schedule-Dependent) and the Nursing Process

I. ALTERATION IN COMFORT related to FLULIKE SYNDROME

Defining Characteristics: Flulike symptoms and delayed fever commonly occur.

Nursing Implications: Assess baseline T, VS, neurologic status, and comfort level, and monitor if patient is in hospital. Discuss with physician pre-medication and regular dosing of antipyretic (e.g., acetaminophen ± diphenhydramine, NSAID) and per protocol. Teach patient self-care measures, including monitoring T, comfort level, self-administration of prescribed medications prior to dose and regularly post-dose, and use of heat or cold for myalgias and arthralgias. Encourage patient to increase oral fluids and alternate rest and activity periods.

II. POTENTIAL ALTERATION IN NUTRITION, LESS THAN BODY REQUIREMENTS, related to STOMATITIS, ALTERATIONS IN HEPATIC FUNCTION STUDIES AND GLUCOSE

Defining Characteristics: Stomatitis occurs, as do transient alterations in LFTs, triglycerides, and fasting blood glucose. Hyperglycemia, elevated triglycerides, and LFTs common.

Nursing Implications: Assess oral mucosa baseline and regularly during therapy. Teach patient self-care strategies, including self-assessment, self-administration of oral hygiene regimen, and to report alterations. Assess patient's baseline LFTs, triglycerides, and blood glucose. Monitor during therapy. Discuss any alterations with physician.

III. POTENTIAL FOR INFECTION, BLEEDING, FATIGUE related to BONE MARROW SUPPRESSION

Defining Characteristics: Bone marrow suppression can occur.

Nursing Implications: Assess baseline CBC, WBC, differential, and platelet count, and signs/symptoms of infection or bleeding. Discuss any abnormalities with physician before drug administration. Teach patient signs/symptoms of infection and bleeding, and to report them immediately. Teach patient self-care measures to minimize infection and bleeding, including avoidance of OTC aspirin-containing medications. Teach patient to alternate rest and activity periods and strategies to conserve energy.

Nursing Implications: Assess baseline WBC, Hgb/HCT, and platelet counts, and monitor during therapy. Assess impact of anemia on patient, and reassure that Hgb/HCT will rise once treatment has stopped.

Agent: levamisole hydrochloride (Ergamisol)

Class: Anthelmintic.

Mechanism of Action: Stimulate immunorestoration in deficient host. Nonspecific immunomodulating agent has antiproliferating action against tumor metastases (with small tumor burdens) rather than primary tumor. Thus, drug is combined with chemotherapy (e.g., 5-FU) and/or surgery (e.g., colon resection).

Metabolism: Rapidly absorbed from GI tract, with elimination half-life of 3–4 hours. Extensively metabolized by liver, and metabolites excreted by kidneys (70% over three days). Unchanged drug is excreted in urine (< 5%) and feces (< 0.2%).

Dosage/Range:

Adjuvant chemotherapy with 5-FU for Duke's Stage C colon cancer:

- Initial therapy: 50 mg PO q8h × 3 days (starting day 7–30 postsurgery); 5-FU 450 mg/m²/day IV × 5 days (concomitant with levamisole, starting 21–34 days postsurgery).
- Maintenance: 50 mg PO q8h × 3 days every 2 weeks for 1 year; 5-FU 450 mg/m²/day every week beginning 28 days after initiation of 5-day course.
- See package insert for 5-FU dose reductions for stomatitis, diarrhea, leukopenia.

Drug Preparation:

- Available as 50-mg tablets in 36-tablet blister pack.

Drug Administration:

- Oral.

Drug Interactions:

- Alcohol may produce disulfiram-like effect (flushing, throbbing in head and neck, throbbing headaches, respiratory difficulty, nausea and vomiting, sweating, chest pain, dyspnea, hypotension, weakness, blurred vision, confusion, coma, and death).
- Increased phenytoin levels occur when coadministered with levamisole and 5-FU: phenytoin dose may need to be decreased.

Lab Effects/Interference:

- Leukopenia, increased bili when given together with 5-FU.

Special Considerations:

- Indicated for adjuvant treatment in combination with 5-FU after surgical resection of Duke's Stage C colon cancer.
- May be used investigationally with other protocols.

Potential Toxicities/Side Effects (in Combination with 5-fluorouracil) and the Nursing Process

I. ALTERATION IN NUTRITION, LESS THAN BODY REQUIREMENTS, related to NAUSEA/VOMITING, DIARRHEA, STOMATITIS, ANOREXIA

Defining Characteristics: Stomatitis or diarrhea (i.e., 5 stools/day) is an indication to interrupt 5-day course and weekly 5-FU injection; if stomatitis or diarrhea develops during weekly 5-FU, dose-reduce subsequent 5-FU doses. Nausea may occur more commonly than vomiting.

Nursing Implications: Assess baseline oral mucosa, elimination pattern. Inform patient of potential side effects and need to report them if they develop. Premedicate with antiemetic, at least for the first cycle. Assess oral mucosa; ask about incidence of diarrhea during and prior to each course of therapy. Teach patient self-care measures, including diet modifications, self-medication with prescribed antiemetic, and oral hygiene regimen. If stomatitis or diarrhea develops, discuss modification of therapy with physician.

II. POTENTIAL FOR INFECTION AND BLEEDING related to BONE MARROW DEPRESSION

Defining Characteristics: Agranulocytosis may occur and may be preceded by flulike syndrome (fever, chills). Neutropenia is usually reversible on discontinuance of therapy.

Nursing Implications: Monitor CBC, WBC, differential, platelet count prior to initial drug treatment and then weekly prior to each 5-FU dose. Discuss with physician if abnormalities occur. Manufacturer recommends holding 5-FU dose until WBC > 3500/mm^3, and holding both 5-FU and levamisole if platelets < 100,000/mm^3. If 5-FU nadir < 2500/mm^3, next 5-FU dose should be reduced by 20%. Teach patient signs/symptoms of infection and bleeding, and instruct to report these immediately. Teach patient self-care measures to minimize infection and bleeding, including avoidance of OTC aspirin-containing medications.

III. POTENTIAL ALTERATION IN SKIN INTEGRITY related to DERMATITIS, SKIN CHANGES

Defining Characteristics: Dermatitis (23% of patients), alopecia (22% of patients), and pruritus may occur.

Nursing Implications: Assess skin and teach patient about potential side effects. Discuss potential impact hair loss will have, as well as coping strategies (e.g., wig, scarf). Discuss/teach symptom management depending on character of dermatitis.

IV. SENSORY/PERCEPTUAL ALTERATIONS related to NEUROLOGIC CHANGES

Defining Characteristics: Dizziness, headaches, paresthesia, ataxia, taste perversion, and altered sense of smell may occur (4–8% of patients). Less commonly, somnolence, depression, nervousness, insomnia, and anxiety may occur (2% of patients).

Nursing Implications: Assess baseline mental status and neurologic status. Instruct patient to report any abnormalities. Notify physician of any abnormalities and discuss therapy modification depending on severity of side effects.

V. ALTERATION IN COMFORT related to FLULIKE SYMPTOMS

Defining Characteristics: Fever, chills, fatigue, chest pain may occur, although they are rare. Fever and chills may precede agranulocytosis.

Nursing Implications: Teach patient that these may occur, and instruct to report fever and chills. Assess CBC, WBC, differential if fever and chills occur. Discuss symptom management with patient, self-administration of prescribed NSAIDs or acetaminophen, and alternation of rest/activity periods.

Agent: megakaryocyte growth and development factor (MGDF) (investigational)

Class: Cytokine.

Mechanism of Action: Growth-factor-specific for megakaryocyte precursor lineage.

Metabolism: Unknown.

Dosage/Range:
- Per protocol.

Drug Preparation/Administration:
- SQ daily for 5 days, or per protocol.

Drug Interactions:
- None known.

Lab Effects/Interference:
- Expect increase in platelet count.

Special Considerations:
- Minimal toxicity.
- Current studies are exploring platelet recovery after induction therapy for acute myelogenous leukemia (AML), and activity of MGDF as a mobilizing agent for peripheral blood stem cells.
- For further information, contact Amgen (Thousand Oaks, CA).

Potential Toxicities/Side Effects and the Nursing Process

I. POTENTIAL FOR KNOWLEDGE DEFICIT related to INVESTIGATIONAL AGENT

Nursing Diagnosis: Knowledge deficit related to drug's status as an investigational agent.

Defining Characteristics: Clinical studies are defining a toxicity profile, but no toxicity has been reported as yet.

Nursing Interventions: Reinforce teaching about cytokine, including indication, expected benefit, and administration. Instruct patient to report any side effects or unusual occurrences.

Drug: novel erythropoiesis stimulating protein (darbepoietin, NESP) (investigational)

Class: Cytokine, colony simulating factor (CSF).

Mechanism of Action: NESP is a hyperglycosylated analogue of recombinant human erythropoietin (EPO, r-HuEPO), which has a terminal half-life 3 times longer than EPO (r-HuEPO). Stimulates the division and differentiation of erythrocyte stem cells in the bone marrow and is a hormone produced by recombinant DNA techniques. Has a naturally occurring counterpart, erythropoietin. When administered once weekly, drug is 20 times more efficacious than rHuEPO (Egrie et al, 1997). NESP has five N-linked carbohydrate chains as compared to endogenous hormone and rHuEPO, which each have only three.

Metabolism: When given IV, terminal half-life is 25.3 hours (compared to 8.5 for rHuEPO), with significantly increased serum concentration-time curve and lower clearance as compared to rHuEPO. When given SQ, mean terminal half-life was 48.8 hours, with peak concentration 10% of the level achieved when given IV, with 37% bioavailability.

Dosage/Range:

- Per protocol; in renal failure patients, optimal dose appeared to be 0.45 μg/kg SQ or IV once weekly, although in some studies every-2-week dosing showed effectiveness.

Drug Preparation:

- Per protocol.

Drug Administration:

- SQ or IV.

Special Considerations:

- Studies have shown NESP to be equally effective when given weekly as compared to rHuEPO given TIW in patients with renal dysfunction (MacDougall et al, 1999).

Potential Toxicities/Side Effects and the Nursing Process

I. POTENTIAL ALTERATION IN OXYGENATION related to POLYCYTHEMIA

Defining Characteristics: Polycythemia may result if target range is exceeded (HCT of 40%).

Nursing Implications: Monitor weekly HCT: dose should be interrupted if HCT > 40%, then resumed at 75% dose once hematocrit is 36%. When HCT is stabilized, discuss monitoring HCT with physician (e.g., testing).

II. KNOWLEDGE DEFICIT related to SELF-ADMINISTRATION TECHNIQUE

Defining Characteristics: Drug is administered IV or SQ once a week to once every two weeks. If the drug is to be given SQ, patient must be instructed in self-injection technique.

Nursing Implications: Assess baseline psychomotor ability, knowledge, and willingness to learn technique of self-injection. Teach how to prepare drug, self-administer, and safely collect used syringes for proper disposal. Use written and video materials as supplements to teaching process and have patient correctly demonstrate technique prior to performing at home. Make referral to visiting-nurse agency to reinforce teaching.

Drug: oprelvekin (Neumega)

Class: Biological (interleukin).

Mechanism of Action: IL-11 is a thrombopoietin growth factor that stimulates directly the bone marrow stem cells and megakaryocyte progenitor cells so that the production of platelets is increased. Produced by recombinant DNA technology. Results in higher platelet nadir and accelerates time to platelet recovery postchemotherapy.

Metabolism: Peak serum concentrations reached in approximately 3 ± 2 hours, with a terminal half-life of approximately 7 ± 1 hours. Bioavailability is < 80%. Clearance decreases with age, and drug is rapidly cleared from the serum, is distributed to organs with high perfusion, metabolized, and excreted by the kidneys. Little intact drug is found in the urine.

Dosage/Range:

- Adults: 50 μg/kg SQ qd.

Drug Preparation/Administration:

- Available as single-use vial containing 5 mg of oprelvekin as a lyophilized, preservative-free powder. This is reconstituted with 1 mL sterile water for injection, USP, gently swirled to mix, and results in a concentration of 5 mg/1 mL in a single-use vial. NOTE: 5 mL of diluent is supplied, but only 1 mL should be withdrawn to reconstitute drug. Drug should be used within 3 hours of reconstitution. If not used immediately, store reconstitued solution in refrigerator or at room temperature, but DO NOT FREEZE OR SHAKE.
- The drug should be administered SQ every day (abdomen, thigh or hip, or upper arm). Begin daily administration 6–24 hours after the completion of chemotherapy, and continue until the postnadir platelet count is equal to or greater than 50,000 cells/mL. Do not give for more than 21 days, and stop at least 2 days before starting the next planned cycle of chemotherapy. Drug has *not* been evaluated in patients receiving chemotherapy regimens longer than 5 days, nor has it been shown to cause delayed myelosuppression (e.g., Mitomycin C, nitrosoureas).

Drug Interactions:

- Unknown.

Lab Effects/Interference:

- Increase in platelet count.
- Anemia associated with increased circulating plasma volume.

Special Considerations:

- Indicated for the prevention of severe thrombocytopenia and to decrease the need for platelet transfusion in patients with nonmyeloid malignancies receiving myelosuppressive chemotherapy.

- Causes fluid retention, so must be used with caution in patients with CHF or in patients receiving chronic diuretic therapy (sudden deaths reported in patients receiving ifosfamide and chronic diuretic therapy due to severe hypokalemia).
- Monitor platelet count frequently during oprelvekin therapy, and at the time of the expected nadir to identify when recovery will begin.
- Contraindicated in pregnant females and nursing mothers.

Potential Toxicities/Side Effects and the Nursing Process

I. ALTERATIONS IN FLUID AND ELECTROLYTE BALANCE related to FLUID RETENTION

Defining Characteristics: Most patients develop mild to moderate fluid retention (peripheral edema, dyspnea on exertion) but without weight gain. Fluid retention is reversible in a few days after drug is stopped. Patients with preexisting pleural effusions, pericardial effusions, or ascites may develop increased fluid, and may require drainage. Patients receiving chronic administration of potassium-excreting diuretics should be monitored extremely closely, as there are reports of sudden death due to severe hypokalemia in patients receiving ifosfamide and chronic diuretic therapy. Capillary leak syndrome has *not* been reported.

Nursing Implications: Assess baseline fluid and electrolyte balance, and weight prior to beginning drug. Assess presence of history of cardiac problems, or CHF, and risk of developing fluid volume overload. If diuretic therapy is ordered, monitor fluid and electrolyte balance very carefully, and replete electrolytes as indicated and ordered. Teach patients that mild-to-moderate peripheral edema and shortness of breath on exertion are likely to occur during the first week of treatment and will disappear after treatment ends. If the patient has CHF or pleural effusions, instruct to report worsening dyspnea to their nurse or physician.

II. ALTERATION IN CIRCULATION related to ATRIAL FIBRILLATION

Defining Characteristics: 10% of patients experience transient arrhythmias, including atrial fibrillation or flutter, after treatment with oprelvekin; it is believed to be due to increased plasma volume rather than the drug itself. Arrhythmias may be symptomatic, are usually brief in duration, and are not clinically significant. Some patients have spontaneous conversion to a normal sinus rhythm, while others require rate-controlling drug therapy. Most patients can receive drug without recurrence of the atrial arrhythmia. Risk factors for developing atrial arrhythmias are: (1) advancing age, (2) use of cardiac medications, (3) history of doxorubicin exposure, (4) history of atrial arrhythmia.

Other cardiovascular events include tachycardia, vasodilatation, palpitations, and syncope.

Nursing Implications: Assess baseline risk. If patient has history or presence of atrial arrhythmias, discuss with the physician potential benefit versus risk, and monitor very closely. Monitor baseline heart rate and other VS at each visit. Instruct patient to report immediately palpitations, lightheadedness, dizziness, or any other change in condition, especially if patient has any risk factors.

III. ALTERATION IN SENSORY PERCEPTION related to VISUAL BLURRING

Defining Characteristics: Transient, mild visual blurring has been reported, as has papilledema in 1.5% of patients. Dizziness (38%), insomnia (33%), and injection of conjunctiva (19%) may also occur.

Nursing Implications: Assess risk for papilledema (existing papilledema, CNS tumors); assess for changes in pupillary response in these patients. Teach patients that dizziness and insomnia may occur, and to change positions slowly and to hold onto supportive structures.. If insomnia is severe, discuss sleep medications with physician.

IV. ALTERATION IN NUTRITION, LESS THAN FULL BODY REQUIREMENTS, related to GI SYMPTOMS

Defining Characteristics: Nausea, vomiting, mucositis, and diarrhea may occur, although percentage was not significantly greater than placebo control. Oral candidiasis occurred in 14% of patients, and this was significantly greater than control.

Nursing Implications: Instruct patient to report changes, and assess impact on nutrition. Inspect oral mucosa and teach patient to as well. Since patient is receiving myelosuppressive chemotherapy, teaching should include oral hygiene regimen, and frequent self-assessment by patient.

V. ALTERATIONS IN BREATHING PATTERN, INEFFECTIVE, POTENTIAL, related to DYSPNEA, COUGH

Defining Characteristics: Dyspnea (48% of patients), rhinitis (42%), increased cough (29%), pharyngitis (25%), and pleural effusions (10%) may occur.

Nursing Implications: Assess baseline pulmonary status and presence of pleural effusions. Instruct patient to report dyspnea and any other changes. Discuss significant changes with physician.

Drug: palifermin (Kepivance)

Class: Keratinocyte Growth Factor.

Mechanism of Action: Palifermin is a keratinocyte growth factor (KGF) produced by recombinant DNA technology, similar to the naturally occurring, endogenous KGF. Once EGF binds to its receptor found on epithelial cells including those of the tongue, buccal mucosa, mammary gland, skin (hair follicles and sebaceous gland), lung, liver, and the lens of the eye, it stimulates proliferation, differentiation, and migration of epithelial cells. KGF decreases the incidence and duration of severe stomatitis in patients with hematologic malignancies who undergo high dose chemotherapy and radiation therapy with stem cell rescue.

Metabolism: Palifermin has an elimination half-life of 4.5 hour (average).

Dosage/Range:

- 60 mcg/kg/day IV bolus for 3 consecutive days before and 3 consecutive days after myelotoxic therapy for a total of 6 doses.

Drug Preparation:

- Reconstitute Kepivance lyophilized powder with Sterile Water for Injection USP, asceptically, by slowly injecting 1.2 mL Sterile Water for Injection USP to yield final volume of 5 mg/mL. Do not shake or agitate the vial.
- Protect from light.
- Reconstituted solution may be refrigerated in its carton for up to 24 hours at 2°–8° C (36°–46° F); prior to injection, may leave at room temperature for up to 1 hour protected from light. Inspect for discoloration or particulates, and if found, do not use.
- Do not filter drug during reconstitution or administration.

Drug Administration:

- Pre-myelotoxic therapy: the 3rd dose should be 24–48 hours before myelotoxic chemotherapy is administered.
- Post-myelotoxic therapy: the first of the 3 doses should be given after, but on the same day of the hematopoietic stem cell infusion, and at least 4 days after the most recent administration of palifermin.

Drug Interactions:

- Heparin: palifermin binds to heparin, so drugs should not be used concomitantly; flush central line well with saline prior to administration of palifermin.
- Myelotoxic chemotherapy: if given with chemotherapy, KGF increases the severity and duration of oral mucositis. Palifermin should NOT be administered within 24 hours before, during infusion of, or after the administration of myelotoxic chemotherapy.

Lab Effects/Interference:

- Increase in serum amylase and lipase.

Special Considerations:

- Palifermin is FDA-approved to decrease the incidence and duration of severe oral mucositis in patients with hematologic malignancies receiving myelotoxic therapy requiring hermatopoietic stem cell support.
- Drug is being studied in the treatment of patients with solid tumors, but the safety and efficacy has not been established at this time. KFG in laboratory studies can enhance malignant cell growth in tissues with KFG receptors.
- Drug is contraindicated in patients with known hypersensitivity to *E. coli* derived proteins.
- Drug is embryotoxic to lab animals when given in higher doses; drug should be used in pregnant women only when the potential benefit to the mother exceeds the risk to the fetus.

Potential Toxicities/Side Effects and the Nursing Process

I. POTENTIAL ALTERATION IN SKIN INTEGRITY related to SKIN RASH

Defining Characteristics: Skin rash was the most common serious adverse reaction, and occurred in 62% of patients in clinical studies. Skin toxicity was manifested by rash, erythema (32%), edema (28%), pruritis (35%). Median time to onset was 6 days after the first of 3 doses, and lasted a median of 5 days.

Nursing Implications: Teach patient that skin changes may occur and to report them. Teach patient self-care strategies to promote comfort and reduce the risk of infection.

II. ALTERATION IN NUTRITION AND COMFORT, related to ORAL TOXICITIES

Defining Characteristics: Dysesthesia, tongue discoloration, tongue thickening, alterations in taste occur related to the increased keratin layer on the lining of the oral cavity.

Nursing Implications: Inform patient that these side effects may occur. Teach patient systematic oral cleansing after meals and at hs. Inform patient to report discomfort or inability to chew or swallow, and develop plan with measures to promote comfort and nutrition. Many patients are already receiving TPN. If taste alterations are bothersome, suggest dietitian referral for measures to stimulate taste.

III. ALTERATION IN COMFORT related to PAIN, ARTHRALGIAS, AND DYSESTHESIAS

Defining Characteristics: Dysesthesia, pain, and arthralgias may occur and affect about 12% of patients.

Nursing Implications: Assess baseline comfort, as well as existing arthralgias and dysesthesias. Perform a basic neurologic assessment. Inform patient these side effects may occur and to report them if they occur. Develop a plan of care that includes self-care activities to promote comfort, such as the use of heat or cold for arthralgias. If pain related to stomatitis is severe, then patient-controlled analgesia may be necessary. Teach patient to report any dysesthesias, hyperesthesias, hypoesthesia, or paresthesias that occur. Develop a plan to minimize discomfort, such as keeping sheets off feet if patient has hyperesthesias.

Agent: pegfilgrastim (Neulasta)

Class: Cytokine, CSF.

Mechanism of Action: Recombinant DNA protein (G-CSF) that regulates the production of neutrophils in the bone marrow (proliferation, differentiation, activation of mature neutrophils). Drug is produced by the insertion of the human G-CSF gene into Escherichia coli bacteria. Drug has longer half-life and different excretion pattern as compared to the parent drug, filgrastim.

Metabolism: Clearance of drug decreases with increased dose, body weight, and is directly related to the number of neutrophils so that as neutrophil recovery begins after myelosuppressive chemotherapy, serum concentration of pegfilgrastim declines rapidly. In patients with increased body weight, systemic exposure to the drug was higher despite dose normalized for body weight. Pharmacokinetics variable, with a half-life of 15–80 hours after SQ injection. Pharmacokinetics did not vary with age (elderly) or gender.

Dosage/Range:

- 6 mg SQ once per chemotherapy cycle.

Drug Preparation:

- Drug available in refrigerated 6 mg (0.6mL) prefilled syringes with UltraSafe needle guards.
- Unopened vials should be stored in the refrigerator at 2–8°C (36–46°F) in the original carton to protect from light.
- Avoid shaking. Screen for visible particulate matter or discoloration and do not use if found.

- Remove from refrigerator 30 minutes prior to injection, but drug may be left at room temperature for up to 48 hours.
- If drug accidently freezes, allow to thaw in the refrigerator prior to administration; if frozen a second time, discard.

Drug Administration:

- SQ × 1 *at least 14 days prior to or more than 24 hours after* chemotherapy administration.
- Following injection, activate UltraSafe Needle Guard holding hands behind the needle, and sliding the guard forward until the needle is completely covered and guard clicks into place. If no click is heard, drop entire syringe/needle into sharps disposal container.

Drug Interactions:

- Lithium: may potentiate the release of neutrophils from the bone marrow: monitor neutrophil count more frequently.

Lab Effects/Interference:

- Increased white blood cell count and neutrophil count.
- Elevated LDH, alkaline phosphatase, uric acid may occur but is reversible and less frequent than with filgrastim.

Special Considerations:

- Indicated to decrease the incidence of infection (febrile neutropenia) in patients with non-myeloid malignancies receiving myelosuppressive anti-cancer therapy associated with a significant incidence of febrile neutropenia.
- Contraindicated in patients with known hypersensitivity to *E. coli* derived proteins, pegfilgrastim, filgrastim, or any product component; contraindicated in peripheral blood progenitor cell (PBPC) mobilization as the drug has not been studied in this population.
- Splenic rupture has been reported in patients receiving the parent drug, filgrastim, for PBPC. If a patient receiving pegfilgrastim complains of left upper abdominal or shoulder tip pain, s/he should be evaluated immediately for an enlarged spleen or splenic rupture.
- Adult Respiratory Distress Syndrome (ARDS) has been reported in neutropenic patients with sepsis receiving the parent drug filgrastim, probably related to the influx of neutrophils to inflammed pulmonary sites. Neutropenic patient receiving pegfilgrastim who develop fever, lung infiltrates, or respiratory distress should be immediately evaluated for ARDS. If ARDS is suspected, pegfilgrastim should be stopped until ARDS resolves with appropriate medical care.
- Severe sickle cell crisis, rarely fatal, has been reported in patients with sickle cell disease (homozygous sickle cell anemia, sickle/hemoglobin C disease, sickle/α-thalassemia) who received filgrastim, the parent drug. Pegfilgrastim should be used in this population only when the potential ben-

efit outweighs the risk, and patients should be well hydrated and closely monitored for sickle cell crisis, with immediate intervention.

- Pegfilgrastim should not be administered within *14 days prior to* and *for 24 hours after chemotherapy administration* as this will increase the sensitivity of rapidly dividing myeloid cells to the chemotherapy.
- G-CSF receptor to which drug binds is also found in tumor cell lines (some myeloid, T-lymphoid, lung, head and neck, and bladder cancer) and the potential for the drug to be a tumor growth factor exists.
- Drug should be used in pregnant women only when the potential benefit outweighs risk of fetal harm as there are no adequate controlled studies in pregnant women, and laboratory animals had increased number of abortions and wavy ribs in fetuses.
- Do not use in infants, children, and smaller adolescents whose weight is <45 kg.

Potential Toxicities/Side Effects (dose and schedule-dependent) and the Nursing Process

I. ALTERATION IN COMFORT related to SKELETAL PAIN, HEADACHE, MYALGIA, ABDOMINAL PAIN, ARTHRALGIA

Defining Characteristics: Patients (26%) may report transient mild to moderate skeletal pain believed due to the expansion of cells in the bone marrow in response to G-CSF. About 12% used non-opioid analgesics and less than 6% required opioid analgesics. Leukocytosis of more than 100–109/L occurred in <1% of patients. Other pain related to headache, myalgia and arthralgia, and abdominal pain may occur less commonly, but is easily managed.

Nursing Implications: Teach patient bone pain may occur and discuss use of nonsteroidal anti-inflammatory drugs with patient and physician for symptom management. Monitor white blood cell count (WBC), hematocrit and platelet count as appropriate prior to each cycle of chemotherapy. Teach patient headache, myalgia, arthralgia, abdominal pain may occur and to report them if they do not respond to usual management strategies.

II. ALTERATION IN NUTRITION, POTENTIAL, related to NAUSEA, VOMITING, CONSTIPATION, DIARRHEA, ANOREXIA, STOMATITIS, MUCOSITIS

Defining Characteristics: Nutritional symptoms are rarely reported and may be related to the underlying malignancy.

Nursing Implications: Perform baseline patient nutritional assessment, history of nausea and vomiting, bowel elimination pattern, oral assessment, and usual appetite. Teach patient to report these sideeffects so that they can be evaluated. Teach patient self-care measures, including dietary modification, local comfort measures as well as pharmacologic management as determined by the nurse/physician team. Teach patient to report symptoms that persist and do not respond to the planned therapy.

III. ALTERATION IN SKIN INTEGRITY, POTENTIAL related to PERIPHERAL EDEMA, ALOPECIA

Defining Characteristics: Peripheral edema and alopecia are rarely reported, and may be related to other factors, such as the chemotherapy agents administered.

Nursing Implications: Perform baseline skin and scalp assessment. Teach patient to report development of peripheral edema, hair loss. Discuss with patient acceptable management strategies depending upon impact of hair loss, if it occurs. Assess degree of peripheral edema if it develops, and discuss significant edema with physician to determine etiology and management. Teach patient local skin care, including avoidance of tight clothing and shoes, keeping skin moisturized to prevent cracking, and local comfort measures.

IV. KNOWLEDGE DEFICIT related to SELF-ADMINISTRATION TECHNIQUE

Defining Characteristics: Drug is administered once per chemotherapy cycle, more than 14 days prior to chemotherapy administration or more than 24 hours after chemotherapy is given.

Nursing Implications: Assess baseline psychomotor ability, knowledge, and willingness to learn technique of self-injection. Teach how to refrigerate drug, self-administer using pre-filled syringes, how to activate needle guard, and safely collect used syringes for proper disposal. Drug insert has "Information for Patients and Caregivers." Use written and video supplements in teaching process and have patient correctly demonstrate technique prior to performing at home. Make referral to visiting-nurse agency to reinforce teaching if needed. Teach patient telephone number and whom to call if questions or problems arise, and ensure that patient can correctly repeat information.

Drug: PIXY-321 (GM-CSF/IL-3 fusion protein)

Class: Fusion protein.

Mechanism of Action: Synergism of IL-3 together with GM-CSF causes a rapid rise in neutrophils due to GM-CSF and a slower rise in platelets due to IL-3.

Metabolism: Unknown in humans.

Dosage/Range:

- 750–1000 μg/m² SQ or IV 24 hours after chemotherapy per protocol.

Drug Preparation/Administration:

- SQ or IV (per protocol).

Drug Interactions:

- Under investigation.

Lab Effects/Interference:

- Increase in neutrophils, with slower increase in platelets.

Special Considerations:

- Has been studied in patients with breast or ovarian cancers, and patients undergoing BMT. In patients with breast cancer receiving PIXY-321, there was decreased incidence and duration of severe (grades 3 and 4) neutropenia, with more rapid recovery of neutrophils than those patients not receiving it; however, patients had more pronounced systemic toxicity and thrombocytopenia in later cycles of therapy.
- Limited data as to toxicity profile in humans, but it is expected that toxicity from each component (i.e., flulike symptoms), did not occur at doses > 500 μg/m².

Potential Toxicities/Side Effects (Dose- and Schedule-Dependent) and the Nursing Process

I. POTENTIAL ALTERATION IN SKIN INTEGRITY related to ERYTHEMA AT INJECTION SITE

Defining Characteristics: This is the most common toxicity at doses up to 500 μg/m². More toxicity may be seen with higher doses.

Nursing Implications: Select and rotate sites, assess and monitor skin for reaction and skin integrity. Implement strategies to maintain intact skin.

II. ALTERATION IN COMFORT related to FEVER

Defining Characteristics: Fever is mild if it occurs. Flulike symptoms do not occur at doses < 500 μg/m², but toxicity may be more pronounced at higher doses. Toxicity is being studied in humans at higher doses.

Nursing Implications: Monitor T at baseline and during therapy. Teach patient to take own T and to report elevations. If severe, discuss premedication with physician.

Drug: recombinant human keratinocyte growth factor (Palifermin, rHuKGF) (investigational)

Class: Cytokine.

Mechanism of Action: Selectively stimuates the growth and differentiation of epithelial cells. Reduces duration and incidence of severe oral mucositis in patients undergoing high-dose chemotherapy, radiotherapy, and total body irradiation (TBI) followed by stem cell support, such as peripheral blood progenitor cell transplantation (PBPCT).

Metabolism: Unknown.

Dosage/Range:
Per protocol, but in one study 60 μg/kg/day for 3 consecutive days before TBI and 3 consecutive days after PBPCT.

Drug Preparation/Administration: Per protocol.

Drug Interactions: Unknown.

Lab Effects/Interference: Transient, asymptomatic increases in serum amylase and lipase.

Special Considerations:
- Preliminary studies show drug significantly reduces duration and incidence of severe oral mucositis of patients with hematologic malignancies undergoing PBPCT after TBI and chemotherapy conditioning (Spielberger et al, 2003).
- Keratinocytes stimulate the growth and development of epithelial cells, such as those lining the oral mucosa; keratinocyte growth factor occurs naturally, and stimulates the growth of keratinocytes.

Potential Toxicities/Side Effects and the Nursing Process

I. POTENTIAL ALTERATION IN SKIN INTEGRITY related to SKIN AND ORAL ERYTHEMA

Defining Characteristics: Mild to moderate skin and oral erythema may occur, with or without edema.

Nursing Implications: Assess oral mucosa and skin baseline, and during treatment. Teach patient to self-assess, and use systematic cleansing pc and hs.

Agent: sargramostim (Leukine, GM-CSF) (investigational)

Class: Cytokine.

Mechanism of Action: Granulocyte-macrophage colony-stimulating factor that regulates growth of all levels of granulocytes and stimulates production of monocytes and macrophages; GM-CSF induces synthesis of other cytokines and enhances cytotoxic action. Manufactured using recombinant DNA technology.

Metabolism: Peak serum levels 2–3 hours after injection. Initial half-life 12–17 min, with a terminal half-life of 1.6–2.6 hours.

Dosage/Range:

- 250 $\mu g/m^2$/day as a 2–hour infusion for 21 days, beginning 2–4 hours after autologous marrow infusion, > 24 hours after last chemotherapy dose, and > 12 hours after last radiation treatment; administer for 14 days when used for BMT failure.
- Neutrophil recovery after chemotherapy for AML: 250 $\mu g/m^2$/day IV over 4 hours beginning on day 11 (4 days after completion of induction chemotherapy if day 10 bone marrow biopsy shows hypoplasia with < 5% blasts).
- Mobilization of peripheral blood progenitor cells (PBPCs): 250 $\mu g/m^2$/day IV over 24 hours or SQ daily; continue through PBPC collection.

Drug Preparation:

- Reconstitute per manufacturer's directions. Do *not* filter.
- Further dilute in 0.9% Sodium Chloride.
- If final concentration is < 10 $\mu g/mL$, human albumin (dilute to final concentration of 0.1% human albumin in 0.9% Sodium Chloride) should be added before adding GM-CSF to prevent absorption of drug in IV container and tubing.

Drug Administration:

- Administer IV over 2 hours, or according to research protocol.

Drug Interactions:

- Corticosteroids, lithium: may ↑ myeloproliferation.
- Sargramostim effect may be ↓ in patients who have received chemotherapy containing alkylating agents, anthracyclines, antibiotics, antimetabolites.

Lab Effects/Interference:

- Increased stem cell, granulocyte, macrophage production.
- Serum glucose, BUN, cholesterol, bili, creatinine, ALT, alk phos; ↓ serum albumin, Ca.
- Leukocytosis, eosinophilia.

Special Considerations:

- Indicated for acceleration of bone marrow recovery (myeloid cells) after autologous or allogeneic BMT; following induction chemotherapy in acute myelogenous leukemia; mobilization and following transplant of autologous PBPCs; and in BMT failure or engraftment delay.
- Produces fever more commonly than G-CSF, and fluid retention.
- Stop drug when WBC > 50,000 cells/mm³, or ANC > 20,000 cells/mm³.
- Administer > 24 hours after last chemotherapy, or > 12 hours after radiotherapy.

Potential Toxicities/Side Effects (Dose- and Schedule-Dependent) and the Nursing Process

I. ALTERATION IN COMFORT related to FLULIKE SYNDROME

Defining Characteristics: Fever, myalgias, chills, rigors, fatigue, and headache may occur.

Nursing Implications: Assess baseline T, VS, neurologic status, and comfort level, and monitor q4–6h if patient in hospital. Discuss with physician premedication and regular dosing of antipyretic (e.g., acetaminophen ± diphenhydramine, NSAID). Teach patient self-care measures, including monitoring T, comfort level, self-administration of prescribed medications prior to dose and regularly postdose, as well as the use of heat or cold for myalgias, arthralgias. Encourage patient to increase oral fluids and alternate rest and activity periods. If patient is in hospital and experiences rigor, discuss with physician IV meperidine (25 mg IV every 15 minutes to maximum 100 mg in 1 hour) and monitor BP for hypotension.

II. ALTERATION IN COMFORT related to SKELETAL PAIN

Defining Characteristics: Transient skeletal pain may occur and is believed to be due to bone marrow expansion in response to GM-CSF.

Nursing Implications: Teach patient this may occur and discuss use of NSAIDS with patient and physician for symptom management. Monitor WBC, ANC twice weekly during therapy; dose reduction or discontinuation depends on purpose of drug.

III. POTENTIAL ALTERATION IN SKIN INTEGRITY related to RASH, FLUSHING, INJECTION SITE REACTION

Defining Characteristics: Facial flushing, generalized rash, and inflammation at injection site may occur.

Nursing Implications: Teach patient that these may occur, and instruct to report rash, inflammation. Teach patient to rotate injection sites. Assess rash, and teach symptomatic management.

IV. POTENTIAL ALTERATION IN OXYGENATION related to DYSPNEA AND FLUID RETENTION

Defining Characteristics: Some patients developed dyspnea during initial 2–6 hours of continuous infusion GM-CSF, thought to be due to migration of neutrophils in the lung. Fluid retention may also occur.

Nursing Implications: Assess baseline pulmonary and fluid status. Teach patient to weigh self daily and instruct to report any changes in weight, breathing (e.g., dyspnea).

Agent: tumor necrosis factor (TNF) (investigational)

Class: Cytokine.

Mechanism of Action: Binds to target cell membranes. TNF (cachectin) is produced by activated macrophages. It appears to halt cell growth in G_2 phase of cell cycle (cytostatic), is cytotoxic, and may cause vascular endothelial injury in tumor capillaries, leading to hemorrhage and necrosis of tumor cells. It also activates immune elements: increased NK cytotoxic activity, increased production of NK cells, B cells, and neutrophils.

Metabolism: Half-life is 20 minutes when given as IV bolus but varies with dose and route of administration.

Dosage/Range:

- Per individual protocol.

Drug Preparation:

- Per individual protocol.

Drug Administration:

- IVB or continuous infusion SQ and IM. Refer to protocol for guidelines. When given IV, agent must be administered using a solution of 0.9% Sodium Chloride containing human serum albumin at a concentration of 2 mg/mL. This albumin prevents TNF from adhering to bag or tubing; prime tubing with solution before adding TNF to bag.

Drug Interactions:

- None reported, but data is being accumulated in clinical trials.

Lab Effects/Interference:

- Granulocytopenia, thrombocytopenia.

Potential Toxicities/Side Effects (Dose- and Schedule-Dependent) and the Nursing Process

I. ALTERATION IN COMFORT related to FLULIKE SYMPTOMS

Defining Characteristics: Fever to 39–40°C (102–104°F) and chills occur within 1–6 hours of dose, dependent on administration route; rigor, fatigue, myalgia, arthralgia, headache (dull, aching), and back pain may occur. Gradual disappearance of symptoms with repeated dosing (tachyphylaxis).

Nursing Implications: Assess baseline T, VS, neurologic status, and comfort level, and monitor every 4–6 hours if patient in hospital. Discuss with physician premedication and regular dosing of antipyretic (e.g., acetaminophen ± diphenhydramine, NSAID). Teach patient self-care measures, including monitoring T, comfort level, self-administration of prescribed medications prior to dose and regularly postdose, as well as the use of heat or cold for myalgias, arthralgias. Encourage patient to increase oral fluids and alternate rest and activity periods. If patient is in hospital and experiences rigor, discuss with physician IV meperidine (25 mg IV every 15 minutes to maximum 100 mg in 1 hour) and monitor BP for hypotension.

II. POTENTIAL ALTERATION IN NUTRITION, LESS THAN BODY REQUIREMENTS, related to ANOREXIA, NAUSEA, VOMITING, DIARRHEA

Defining Characteristics: Do not appear dose-dependent. Weight loss is not significant, and nausea/vomiting can be effectively managed.

Nursing Implications: Assess baseline nutritional status. Teach patient potential side effects, and self-care measures, including oral hygiene and preparing favorite high-calorie, high-protein foods ahead of time so patient can snack when hungry. Teach self-administration of prescribed antiemetics and antidiarrheals as needed. Refer to dietitian as appropriate.

III. ALTERATION IN CARDIAC OUTPUT related to ORTHOSTATIC HYPOTENSION

Defining Characteristics: Transient orthostatic hypotension (SBP $<$ 90 mm Hg) may occur after IV or SQ injection and resolve with IV saline infusion. Hypertension may occur secondary to rigors.

Nursing Implications: Assess baseline cardiovascular status and orthostatic BP. Teach patient to change position slowly, to report light-headedness, and to increase oral fluids to 3 L/day.

IV. POTENTIAL FOR INFECTION AND BLEEDING related to GRANULOCYTOPENIA, THROMBOCYTOPENIA

Defining Characteristics: Dose-related, especially if > 100 mg/m^2 day, with normalization when treatment terminated.

Nursing Implications: Assess baseline CBC, WBC, differential, and platelet count, and signs/symptoms of infection or bleeding. Discuss any abnormalities with physician before drug administration. Teach patient signs/symptoms of infection, bleeding, and instruct to report them immediately. Teach patient self-care measures to minimize infection and bleeding, including avoidance of OTC aspirin-containing medications, and oral hygiene regimen.

V. POTENTIAL SENSORY/PERCEPTUAL ALTERATIONS related to NEUROLOGIC TOXICITY

Defining Characteristics: Seizures, confusion, aphasia may occur transiently and rarely.

Nursing Implications: Assess baseline mental status and history of seizures. Instruct patient to report any changes and ensure patient safety.

VI. POTENTIAL ALTERATION IN OXYGENATION related to DYSPNEA

Defining Characteristics: Dyspnea may occur, possibly related to alveolar endothelial damage.

Nursing Implications: Assess patient's risk (preexisting pulmonary dysfunction) and baseline pulmonary status. Instruct patient to report any changes.

Chapter 3

Antineoplastic Treatment Agonists: Radiosensitizers, Chemosensitizers, and Chemical Adjuncts

Radiation is the third major cancer treatment modality. Ionizing radiation causes cell damage and death to frequently dividing cells within the radiation port (site being radiated). Damage to DNA in malignant cells depends on the oxygenation of the tumor—cells that are well supplied with oxygen are sensitive to radiation effects, while those that are hypoxic (i.e., large, necrotic tumors) are radioresistant. Oxygen appears to be necessary at the time of radiation because it promotes formation of free radicals, causing DNA damage and preventing DNA repair (Noll, 1992).

Certain drugs called *radiosensitizers* may be administered concurrently with radiation therapy to increase the radiation damage to sensitive cells, thus increasing the tumor response (i.e., tumor reduction) to radiation therapy. Radiosensitizers are classified into three broad groups based on ability to sensitize hypoxic tumor cells and mechanism of action (Noll, 1992).

Hypoxic cell sensitizers mimic oxygen in chemical reactions that occur after ionizing radiotherapy, thus making the hypoxic cells sensitive to radiation damage. Examples are etanidazole, Fluosol DA with 100% oxygen breathing, and buthionine, which depletes sulfhydryl-containing compounds from damaged cells so they are unable to repair their DNA.

Nonhypoxic cell sensitizers include the halogenated pyrimidines, which, because they are analogues of the DNA pyrimidine thymidine, are actively taken up by dividing cells and incorporated into DNA. This enhances radiosensitivity of the tumor cells and theoretically increases tumor response to radiotherapy. Drugs undergoing clinical testing include bromodeoxyuridine (BUdR) and iododeoxyuridine (IUdR).

A third group is composed of *chemotherapy agents* that are capable of radiosensitization. They are administered either prior to radiotherapy as part of combined modality therapy or concurrently in low doses to enhance radiosensitivity of tumor cells. These drugs include cisplatin, 5-fluorouracil, gemcitabine, carboplatin, paclitaxel, gemcitabine, bleomycin, and mitomycin. Recent research on gemcitabine showed that the radiosensitization mechanism of action is different than when the drug is used as a chemotherapy agent (cytotoxic): When the cancer cells start to move through the Synthesis phase of the cell cycle and the DNA strands are damaged by radiation, the cell undergoes programmed cell death (apoptosis) (Symon Z et al, 2002).

Finally, a fourth group called *molecular targeted agents* can also produce radiosensitization, thus increasing the therapeutic index (so cancer cells are killed rather than normal cells). These include epidermal growth factor receptor (EGFR) tyrosine kinase inhibitors cetuximab (Erbitux), the EGFR tyrosine kinase inhibitor gefitinib (Iressa), and farnesyl transferase inhibitors (Lawrence TS and Nyati MK, 2002).

This is a promising frontier in cancer treatment, and the next decade will bring greater understanding and options in radiotherapy, chemosensitization, and new adjuncts.

References

Brown JM. Therapeutic Targets In Radiotherapy. *Int J Radiat Oncol Biol Phys* 2001; 49(2):319–326

Bunn PA. Triplet Combination Chemotherapy and Targeted Therapy Regimens. *Oncology* 2001;15(3 Suppl 6):26–32

Coleman CN. Radiation and Chemotherapy Sensitizers and Protectors. In Chabner BA, Longo DL, (eds), *Cancer Chemotherapy and Biotherapy,* 2nd ed. Philadelphia: Lippincott Raven;1996;553–584

Coleman CN, Bump EA, Kramer RA. Chemical Modifiers of Cancer Treatment. *J Clin Oncol* 1989;6:709–733

Craighead PS, Pearcey R, Stuart G. A Phase I/II Evaluation of Tirapazamine Administered Intravenously Concurrent with Cisplatin and Radiotherapy in Women with Locally Advanced Cervical Cancer. *Int J Radiat Oncol Biol Phys* 2000;48(3):791–795

Denny WA, Wilson WR. Tirapazamine: A Bioreductive Anticancer Drug that Exploits Tumour Hypoxia. *Expert Opin Investig Drugs* 2000;9(12):2889–2901

Dische S. Chemical Sensitizers for Hypoxic Cells: A Decade of Experience in Clinical Radiotherapy. *Radiother Oncol* 1985;3:97–111

Fowler JF. Chemical Modifiers of Radiosensitivity: Theory and Reality: A Review. *Int J Radiat Oncol Biol Phys* 1985;11:665–674

Goldberg Z, Evans J, Birrell G, Brown JM. An Investigation of the Molecular Basis for the Synergistic Interaction of Tirapazamine and Cisplatin. *Int J Radiat Oncol Biol Phys* 2001;49(1):175–182

Kinsella TJ, Mitchell JB, Russo A, et al. The Use of Halogenated Thymidine Analogues as Clinical Radiosensitizers: Rationale, Current Status, and Future Prospects. *Int J of Radiat Oncol Biol Phys* 1984;10:1399–1406

Lawrence TS, Nyati MK. Small-molecule Tyrosine Kinase Inhibitors as Radiosensitizers. *Semin Radiat Oncol* 2002;12 (suppl 2):33–36

Mallinkckrodt Phosphocol P32 Package Insert. St. Louis: Mallinkckrodt Inc.; 1997

Noll L. Chemical Modifiers of Radiation Therapy. In Hassey-Dow K, Hilderly LJ, (eds), *Nursing Care in Radiation Oncology* Philadelphia: WB Saunders; 1992

Rischin D, Peters L, Hicks R, et al. Phase I Trial of Concurrent Tirapazamine, Cisplatin, and Radiotherapy in Patients with Advanced Head and Neck Cancer. *J Clin Oncol* 2000;19(2):535–545

Symon Z, Davis M, McGinn CJ, et al. Concurrent Chemoradiotherapy with Gemcitabine and Cisplatin for Pancreatic Cancer: From Laboratory to the Clinic. *Int J Radiat Oncol Biol Phys* 2002;53:140–145

Drug: chromic phosphate P32 suspension (Phosphocol™ P32)

Class: Radiopharmaceutical agent.

Mechanism of Action: Provides local irradiation by beta emission and is administered into cavities for the treatment of peritoneal or pleural effusions due to metastatic cancer; it may also be given interstitially to treat cancer.

Metabolism: Phosphorus P32 decays by beta emission with a physical half-life of 14.3 days, with a residence time of 495 hours. The mean energy of the beta particle is 695 keV. Distribution in the pleural or peritoneal space is non-uniform, with extremes of local dosage.

Dosage/Range:

- Intraperitoneal: 370–740 megabecquerels (10–20 millicuries).
- Intrapleural: 222–444 megabecquerels (6–12 millicuries).
- Interstitial (e.g., prostate): based on estimated gram weight of tumor, about 3.7–18.5 megabecquerels/gm (0.2–0.5 millicuries/gm).
- 37 kilobecquerels = 1 millicurie (mCi) = 7.3 grays = 730 rads.

Drug Preparation:

- None.
- Available as chromic phosphate P32 suspension in 10–mL vials containing 555 megabecquerels (15 mCi) with a concentration of up to 185 megabecquerels (5 mCi)/mL.

Drug Administration:

- Always given into pleural or peritoneal cavity, or may be given interstitially (e.g., prostate), but NEVER intravenously.
- For pleural effusions:

Interventional radiologist visualizes pleural space with ultrasound to ensure that it is open without adhesions.

Interventional radiologist places a thoracentesis catheter in the pleural space, having a three-way stopcock, and verifies position by ultrasound; removes pleural fluid by opening ports 1 and 2.

Port 2 is closed and port 3 is opened for a qualified M.D. to administer chromic phosphate P32 suspension (injecting 6–12 mCi into the port, then rinses with 10 mL 0.9% NS).
Close ports and ensure that they are closed to prevent leakage of radionucleotide and radiation contamination. The catheter is then removed. If there is leakage or contamination, refer to institutional policy/procedure for radiation spill.
Reposition patient from supine to prone, onto the right side, and onto the left side, and lastly, have the patient stand and bend over.
CXR is done to make certain there is no pneumothorax.
Patient is given one-month follow-up appointment for a CXR, and is asked to return if shortness of breath occurs, as this may signify reaccumulation of effusion.

Drug Interactions:
- Unknown.

Lab Effects/Interference:
- Unknown.

Special Considerations:
Eligible candidates for treatment of pleural effusion:
- History of prior pleurodesis with talc.
- Evidence of pleural plaques.
- Prior treatment using a chest tube.
- Emphysema.
- History of pleural asbestos exposure.

Contraindications:
- Presence of ulcerative tumors.
- Pregnant or nursing mothers, unless benefit outweighs risks.
- Presence of large tumor masses.
- Risk of improper placement: intestinal fibrosis or necrosis, and chronic fibrosis of body wall have been described.
- Radiation damage may occur if injected interstitially or into a loculation.
- Treatment may be less effective if effusion bloody.

Potential Toxicities/Side Effects and the Nursing Process

I. POTENTIAL FOR INFECTION, BLEEDING, AND FATIGUE related to BONE MARROW DEPRESSION

Defining Characteristics: Bone marrow suppression, if it occurs, is transitory.

Nursing Implications: Assess baseline WBC, differential, platelet and Hgb/HCT prior to treatment, as well as for signs/symptoms of infection or bleeding. Teach patient signs/symptoms of infection and bleeding and to report these immediately; teach patient self-care measures to minimize risk of infection and bleeding. This includes avoidance of crowds, proximity to people with infections, and avoidance of OTC aspirin-containing medications. Teach patient to report fatigue, and teach measures to conserve energy, such as alternating rest and activity periods. Discuss transfusion of red blood cells as needed.

II. PAIN related to PLEURITIS, PERITONITIS, AND ABDOMINAL CRAMPING

Defining Characteristics: Symptoms depend upon area treated, with pleuritis arising from treatment of pleural effusion, and peritonitis, abdominal cramping, and nausea arising from treatment of peritoneal effusion.

Nursing Implications: Assess baseline pain level. Teach patient of potential side effects and to report them. Teach patient symptom-management techniques and discuss with physician medications for analgesia and nausea. Teach patient to report if symptoms do not subside or improve.

III. ALTERATION IN COMFORT related to RADIATION SICKNESS

Defining Characteristics: Exposure to ionizing radiation causes symptoms, the severity of which are dependent upon the volume of radiation, the length of time of exposure, and the area of the body affected. Moderate symptoms may occur from treatment with chromic phosphate P32 suspension, and these include headache, nausea, vomiting, anorexia, and diarrhea. Long-term exposure may result in sterility, malformation of the fetus in a pregnant woman, and cancer.

Nursing Implications: Assess baseline comfort level. Teach patient that moderate symptoms may arise. Teach patient to report symptoms as soon as possible, and discuss management strategies. Discuss pharmacologic management of nausea/vomiting and diarrhea with physician and give patient prescriptions for antiemetic and antidiarrheal medications for PRN use.

Drug: etanidazole (investigational)

Class: Nitrolmidazole, hypoxic radiosensitizer.

Mechanism of Action: Sensitizes hypoxic tumor cells to the effects of ionizing radiotherapy by mimicking oxygen. This enhances formation of free radicals, which damage cellular DNA and prevent DNA repair so that tumor cell kill is enhanced.

Metabolism: Metabolized by liver.

Dosage/Range:
- Per protocol.

Drug Preparation/Administration:

- Per protocol, but may be administered as a rapid intravenous infusion three times per week, immediately prior to radiotherapy.

Drug Interactions:

- Unknown.

Special Considerations:

- Peripheral neuropathy is dose-limiting toxicity.
- Less toxic than nitrolmidazole, with less nerve tissue penetration.

Potential Toxicities/Side Effects and the Nursing Process

I. SENSORY PERCEPTUAL ALTERATION related to PERIPHERAL NEUROPATHY

Defining Characteristics: Peripheral neuropathy occurs, with sensory loss and paresthesias of feet, toes, hands. May have decreased sensitivity to pinprick, decreased vibratory sense. May resolve over days, while severe neuropathies may be permanent. Related to cumulative drug exposure.

Nursing Implications: Assess baseline neurologic status. Assess for numbness, tingling, burning, loss of temperature sensation, and ache at each visit. Instruct patient to report these or other changes immediately. Discuss drug discontinuance with physician as appropriate to prevent permanent severe neuropathy.

II. ALTERATION IN NUTRITION, LESS THAN BODY REQUIREMENTS, related to GI SIDE EFFECTS

Defining Characteristics: Nausea and vomiting may occur.

Nursing Implications: Assess baseline nutritional status and signs/symptoms of nausea, vomiting. Instruct patient to report occurrence of nausea, vomiting. Discuss premedication with physician and administer prescribed antiemetic prior to drug. Teach patient to self-administer prescribed antiemetic at home.

III. ALTERATION IN COMFORT related to RASH, ARTHRALGIAS

Defining Characteristics: Rash, transient arthralgias may occur.

Nursing Implications: Assess baseline comfort level. Assess for rash, arthralgias, and instruct patient to report these side effects. If they occur, provide and teach patient symptomatic measures to reduce discomfort.

Drug: fluosol DA (20%) (investigational)

Class: Perfluorocarbon emulsion, hypoxic radiosensitizer.

Mechanism of Action: Hydrocarbon with hydrogen atom replaced by fluorine, so acts as artifical oxygen carrier. Thus, it decreases cell hypoxia and enhances formation of free radicals, which damage tumor cell DNA and prevent DNA repair.

Metabolism: By liver.

Dosage/Range:
- Per protocol.

Drug Preparation/Administration:
- Per protocol.

Drug Interactions:
- None known.

Special Considerations:
- Administer prior to radiation with patient breathing 100% oxygen before and during radiation.
- Increases solid tumor response to radiotherapy without increased damage to normal cells.
- Mild myelosuppression may be due to radiotherapy rather than drug.

Potential Toxicities/Side Effects and the Nursing Process

I. ALTERATION IN COMFORT related to DRUG ALLERGY

Defining Characteristics: Allergic-type reaction may occur with first dose, characterized by facial flushing, chest pressure, and/or chills and fever. Premedication with antihistamines and corticosteroids prevents further episodes.

Nursing Implications: Assess baseline drug allergies, temperature, VS. Teach patient to report sensation of warmth, chest pressure, chllls, facial flushing. Discuss with physician premedication with antihistamines and corticosteroids.

II. ALTERATION IN NUTRITION, LESS THAN BODY REQUIREMENTS, related to HEPATOTOXICITY

Defining Characteristics: Transient, self-limited increases in LFTs may occur (AST, ALT, alk phos).

Nursing Implications: Assess baseline LFTs and monitor throughout treatment. Discuss abnormalities with physician.

Drug: leucovorin calcium (Folinic Acid, Citrovorum Factor)

Class: Water-soluble vitamin in the folate group (folinic acid).

Mechanism of Action: Potentiates antitumor activity of 5-FU when given prior to or concurrently with 5-FU, ± XRT. Acts as an antidote for methotrexate and other folic acid antagonists. Circumvents the biochemical block of the enzyme inhibitors (e.g., dihydrofolate reductase [DHFR]) to permit DNA and RNA synthesis.

Metabolism: Leucovorin is metabolized to polyglutamates that are more effective in potentiating 5-FU tumor cell kill. Metabolized primarily in the liver; 50% of the single dose is excreted in 6 hours in the urine (80–90% of the dose) and stool (8% of the dose).

Dosage/Range:

Antidote for methotrexate:

- Dose of drug and duration of rescue is dependent on serum methotrexate levels:

Methotrexate Level	Leucovorin
$< 5.0\ (10)^{-7}$M	10 mg/m^2 q6h
$5\ (10)^{-7}$M$(10)^{-6}$M	30–40 mg/m^2 q6h
$> 5\ (10)^{-6}$M	100 mg/m^2 q3–6h

- Potentiation of 5-FU ± XRT: dose varies leucovorin 20 mg/m^2/d–2.5 g/m^2 CI.

Drug Preparation:

- Drug is supplied in ampules or vials.
- Reconstitute vials with sterile water for injection.
- Dilute reconstituted vials or ampules further with 5% Dextrose or 0.9% Sodium Chloride.

Drug Administration:

- With 5-FU, in a variety of combinations; e.g., leucovorin: 500 mg/m^2/week for 6 weeks as a 2-hour infusion; 5-FU: 500–600 mg/m^2/week for 6 weeks, IVB midway through leucovorin infusion, then 2-week rest, then repeat 6-week cycle.
- Administered 24 hours after first methotrexate dose is begun. Dose every 6 hours for up to 12 doses.
- First dose is given IV; others can be given IM or PO when given as methotrexate "rescue."
- IV doses are given via bolus over 15 minutes unless otherwise specified.
- When given as a rescue dose, must be given exactly on time in order to rescue normal cells from methotrexate toxicity.

Drug Interactions:
- 5-FU: potentiation.
- Folic acid: provides folinic acid so cells can make DNA (antagonizes drug effect).
- Phenobarbital, phenytoin, primidone: decreases anticonvulsant action (when leucovorin given in large doses); monitor patient closely and increase anticonvulsant as needed.

Lab Effects/Interference:
- None.

Special Considerations:
- It is imperative that the patient receive the leucovorin on schedule to avoid fatal methotrexate toxicity. Notify the physician if the patient is unable to take the dose orally, as it must then be given IV.
- Usually free of side effects, but allergic reaction and local pain may occur.

Potential Toxicities/Side Effects and the Nursing Process

I. POTENTIAL FOR INJURY related to HYPERSENSITIVITY, DRUG INTERACTIONS

Defining Characteristics: Allergic sensitization has been reported: facial flushing, itching. Leucovorin in large amounts may counteract the antiepileptic effects of phenobarbital, phenytoin, and primidone.

Nursing Implications: Monitor patient for signs/symptoms of allergic reaction. Diphenhydramine is effective for relieving symptoms of allergic reaction. Monitor patient for symptoms of increased seizure activity (if on antiepileptic drugs); monitor antiepileptic drug levels.

II. ALTERED NUTRITION, LESS THAN BODY REQUIREMENTS, related to NAUSEA, VOMITING

Defining Characteristics: Oral leucovorin rarely causes nausea or vomiting.

Nursing Implications: Administer oral leucovorin with antacids, milk, or juice.

Drug: porfirmer (Photofrin)

Class: Photosensitizing agent.

Mechanism of Action: Porfirmer is selectively distributed and maintained in tumor tissue. When exposed to 630 nanometer laser light, porfirmer is activated and a chain reaction ensues, resulting in damage to tumor cell mitochondria and intracellular membranes. The therapy also causes the release of thromboxane A, resulting in vasoconstriction, activation and aggregation of platelets, and increased clotting. Ischemic necrosis ensues, causing tissue and tumor death.

Metabolism: Distributed through a variety of tissues, but is selectively retained by tumors, skin, and organs of the reticuloendothelial system (liver, spleen). Drug is not dialysable.

Dosage/Range:
- 2 mg/kg body weight, injected over 3–5 minutes.
- May be given for a total of 3 courses of therapy, each separated by at least 30 days.

Drug Preparation/Administration:
- Add 31.8 mL D5W or NS to the 75-mg vial, producing a concentration of 2.5 mg/ml.
- Protect reconstituted solution from bright light and use immediately.

Drug Interactions:
- The following drugs may decrease the effectiveness of profirmer therapy: allopurinol, corticosteroids (glucocorticoid), calcium channel blockers, prostaglandin synthesis inhibitors, Thromboxane A inhibitors, beta carotene, DMSO, ethanol, formate, and mannitol.
- Some drugs may increase photosensitivity, including griseofulvin, phenothiazines, sulfonamides, sulfonylurea hypoglycemia agents, tetracyclines, and thiazide diuretics.

Lab Effects/Interference:
- None.

Special Considerations:
- Drug is for use in esophageal and non-small-cell lung carcinoma (NSCLC).
- Photodynamic therapy should NOT be used in patients with:
  porphyria
  tumor erosion into a major blood vessel
  bronchoesophageal fistula
  tracheoesophageal fistula
  tumor erosion into the trachea or bronchial tree
- Extreme caution should be exercised when deciding candidacy for therapy, as it can cause an initial inflammation at the site and can cause fistulas as tumors shrink.
- When photodynamic therapy is preceded or followed by local radiation therapy, sufficient time should be allowed between treatments for inflammation to subside (e.g., radiation therapy should not be given to the site until at least 2–4 weeks after photodynamic therapy).

- If extravasation occurs during IV administration, the area should be protected from light for 30 days.

Potential Toxicities/Side Effects and the Nursing Process

I. POTENTIAL FOR INJURY related to ANEMIA, INFLAMMATION AT SITE OF THERAPY

Defining Characteristics: Photodynamic therapy can cause significant tumor bleeding at the site of treatment, sometimes resulting in anemia. Inflammation at the site can cause narrowing and/or obstruction of vital structures and pulmonary and cardiovascular changes (pleural effusion or edema, atrial fibrillation and angina), particularly since much of this therapy occurs in the mediastinal area.

Nursing Implications: Monitor respiratory, cardiovascular systems during treatment. Instruct patient to contact physician immediately for dyspnea, excessive coughing, abdominal pain, fever, dysphagia, bleeding/hemoptysis, chest pain, etc. Substernal chest pain in esophageal cancer patients can be treated with opioids.

II. POTENTIAL FOR INJURY related to PHOTOSENSITIVITY

Defining Characteristics: May cause photosensitivity reactions for 30 days after administration, both to sunlight and bright indoor light. Skin around the eyes may be particularly sensitive. Sunscreens are not protective, as phototherapy causes sensitivity to visible light. Porfirmer is slowly inactivated by ambient light.

Nursing Implications: Patients should test skin (do not use facial skin) by exposing a small area to sunlight for 10 minutes. If area is free of erythema, blistering, and edema 24 hours later, patient may gradually increase exposure. Patients should wear dark glasses that transmit less than 4% of white light for 30 days after treatment.

Drug: tirapazamine (investigational)

Class: Hypoxic cell cytoxin (benzotriazine bioreductive compound).

Mechanism of Action: When given concurrently with radiotherapy, increases damage to aerobic malignant cells throughout different oxygen levels, probably due to the fact that in hypoxic conditions, tirapazamine is reduced to a free radical form, which produces DNA strand breaks. Drug also shows marked potentiation of cisplatin, probably by preventing repair of cisplatin-induced DNA cross-linkages in hypoxic cells. Additive effect when given with cisplatin, and synergy when given before cisplatin. It is possible that under hypoxic conditions, tirapazamine may act as a topoisomerase II inhibitor.

Metabolism: Is metabolized by reductases to form a transient oxidizing radical, which is scavenged by molecular oxygen. In hypoxic conditions, the oxidizing radical removes a proton from DNA to form DNA radicals (at the C4' position on the ribose ring). The radicals are then oxidized, forming DNA strand breaks, preventing cell division, and causing cell death.

Dosage/Range:
Maximum tolerated dose is 290 mg/m^2 IV on days 1, 15, and 29, and 220 mg/m^2 on days 8, 10, 12, 22, 24, and 26 concurrent with cisplatin and radiotherapy (Craighead PS et al, 2000).

Drug Preparation/Administration: Administer IV over 2 hours followed 1 hour later by cisplatin IV given over 1 hour, followed immediately by radiotherapy. When given without cisplatin, radiotherapy follows 30–120 minutes after tirapazamine infusion.

Drug Interactions:
- Additive cytotoxicity when given concurrently with cisplatin.
- Synergy with increased cell kill when given prior to cisplatin.

Lab Effects/Interference:
- Unknown.

Special Considerations:
- Administer prior to cisplatin chemotherapy.
- Is being studied in treatment of head and neck, advanced cervical and ovarian cancers.

Potential Toxicities/Side Effects and the Nursing Process

I. ALTERATION IN NUTRITION, LESS THAN BODY REQUIREMENTS, related to NAUSEA, VOMITING, DIARRHEA

Defining Characteristics: Nausea and vomiting can be severe, especially when drug is given in combination with cisplatin. Diarrhea can also occur, but is usually mild.

Nursing Implications: Ensure aggressive antiemesis, with serotonin antagonists and dexamethasone recommended to prevent nausea and vomiting. Assess efficacy of regime, and modify as needed. Explain to patient that this may occur, and teach dietary modifications, including the avoidance of greasy, spicy foods.

II. POTENTIAL FOR INFECTION AND BLEEDING related to NEUTROPENIA AND THROMBOCYTOPENIA

Defining Characteristics: In one study, febrile neutropenia necessitated decreasing the dose and frequency of tirapazamine. Thrombocytopenia was uncommon.

Nursing Implications: Assess baseline CBC and differential prior to therapy, and at least weekly during therapy. Teach patient to report signs and symptoms of infection and bleeding right away. Teach patient to check temperature during treatment, and to report T > 100.5°F. If infection occurs, discuss antibiotic treatment, and teach patient self-care strategies.

III. ALTERATION IN COMFORT related to MUSCLE CRAMPS

Defining Characteristics: Muscle cramps can occur, especially during the first 2 weeks of treatment, generally resolving by the 3rd week of treatment.

Nursing Implications: Teach patient that muscle cramps may occur, and to report them. Teach patient self-care measures to minimize discomfort. Discuss alternative approaches with physician if plan is ineffective. Refer to protocol for other management strategies.

IV. POTENTIAL ALTERATION IN SKIN INTEGRITY related to RASH

Defining Characteristics: Rash that is transient may occur.

Nursing Implications: Teach patient that rash may occur, and to report it. Discuss local management with physician.

Chapter 4

Cytoprotective Agents

Advances in the development of effective, new chemotherapeutic agents have been slow, although a number of excellent agents have recently been approved for use. All traditional chemotherapeutic agents work by interfering with DNA and RNA replication, and protein synthesis, causing cell death or stasis. Unfortunately, the chemotherapy, unless attached to a targeted vehicle, such as a monoclonal antibody, is nonselective, and normal cells are damaged by the chemotherapy. Often, the dose-limiting toxicity is myelosuppression, but organ toxicity specific to the chemotherapy agent may limit the drug's usefulness. Specific organ toxicity that can occur includes neurotoxicity (e.g., cisplatin, oxaliplatin, the taxanes), cardiotoxicity (e.g., anthracyclines, alone or together with trastuzumab), bladder toxicity (e.g., high-dose cyclophosphamide, ifosfamide), and nephrotoxicity (e.g., cisplatin). Thus, both doses and duration of therapy of treatment are often limited by these organ toxicities. This can compromise optimal treatment, as well as compromise quality of life. Similarly, radiation therapy causes cell damage (e.g., ionization causes the formation of free radicals, which, in the presence of oxygen, cause damage to DNA, leading to cell death when the cell tries to replicate). Again, normal tissue in the radiation port also are damaged, such as the bone marrow in the skull, sternum, and heads of long bones, and can lead to side effects such as bone marrow depression, which results in the need for treatment breaks and less-than-optimal radiotherapy.

In an effort to protect normal cells from treatment toxicity and to limit organ toxicities, a number of agents have been developed that offer cyto (cell) or organ protection, and even more are being studied (investigational agents). Agents that are currently approved for use are amifostine (Ethyol), Mesna, and dexrazoxane (Zinecard, a chelating agent). Amifostine has shown "broad spectrum" activity in protecting multiple organ systems, such as the kidneys, bone marrow, and nerves. In addition, it protects the parotid glands from radiation damage. Amifostine is indicated for the reduction of cumulative nephrotoxicity from cisplatin in patients with advanced ovarian and NSCLC, as well as for reducing the incidence of moderate-to-severe xerostomia in patients with head and neck cancer whose radiation port covers the parotid glands. Mesna is included in this chapter because it provides bladder protection from the toxic effects of high-dose cyclophosphamide and ifosfamide. Leucovorin is also a classic cytoprotectant in that it "rescues" normal cells from methotrexate toxicity (bone marrow and mucosal cells). This drug appears in Chapter 3. In an effort to help establish a practice standard for the use of currently available cytoprotectants in patients not enrolled on clinical trials, the American Society of Clinical Oncology (ASCO) has developed guidelines (ASCO, 1999).

One organ toxicity that is receiving increased attention is neurotoxicity. Many highly effective agents are limited in both dose and duration of treatment by the development of peripheral neuropathy, such as the taxanes (paclitaxel causes axonal degeneration and demyelination), oxaliplatin, and cisplatin (segmental demyelination). This side effect can be one of the most clinically challenging problems for oncology nurses. See Table 4.1 for a list of antitumor agents that cause neurotoxicity. Peripheral neuropathy is defined as the injury, inflammation, or degeneration of any nerve outside the central nervous system. Chemotherapy may cause damage to the sensory and motor axons. Symptoms of sensory damage include tingling, pricking or numbness of the extremities, a sensation of wearing an invisible glove or sock and thus the term *glove and stocking distribution*; burning or freezing pain; sharp, stabbing, or electric shock-like pain; and extreme sensitivity to touch. Patients, in some cases, will be reluctant to admit to these symptoms because they believe that if they do, their chemotherapy drug will be stopped. If the motor neurons are affected, then symptoms include muscle weakness and loss of balance or coordination. If myelinated nerves are injured, then there is a reduction in conduction velocity of the nerve impulse, and on examination, the patient has depressed or absent deep tendon reflexes (Wilkes, 2004). Although in many instances, peripheral neuropathy may be reversible, it may take many months for this to occur. Unfortunately, damage to peripheral nerves can have long-term effects on quality of life, and cause much discomfort, injury, and distress. In addition, while the exact percentage of patients with cancer who experience peripheral neuropathy is unknown, the economic impact is considerable. It has been estimated that it costs $5,507 per patient to treat neuropathy (both medical and indirect costs) (Calhoun et al, 1999). Nurses have been pivotal in performing assessments of sensory and motor function, and assessing the impact of peripheral neuropathy on the patient's safety and quality of life, making them strong advocates for patients. Nurses monitor patients' neurological status prior to each treatment and between treatment cycles. A simple six-step neurosensory exam should be performed throughout the course of chemotherapy to identify any potential deficits. The exam should include a history, such as the questionnaire developed by Berghorn and shown in Figure 4.1, as well as a physicial exam of gait, motor and sensory systems, and testing of reflexes. Grading of neurotoxicity is based on a neurosensory exam that includes assessment of gait, motor and sensory system, functional ability, and reflexes, and is scored from 0–4 according to the National Cancer Institute (NCI) Common Toxicity Criteria (see Appendix II). In obtaining the history, since it is imperative to involve patients in the assessment of function and ability to perform activities of daily living, an excellent patient neurotoxicity questionnaire has been developed by Berghorn et al (2000) and incorporated in one clinical trial evaluating neuroprotectants. (see Figure 4.1.) Patients are asked if they have difficulties in performing their normal activities of daily living, such as buttoning a shirt or holding a fork to eat (fine motor movement), mobility in terms of difficulty going up or down stairs, and communicating. Currently, in clinical practice, the offending drug is usually stopped if the patient develops grade 3 or 4 toxicity. Fortunately, clinical studies are being conducted to find effective neuroprotectants that have little or no toxicity. Agents being studied include amifostine, BNP7787, and glutamine. These agents are included in this chapter.

Table 4.1 Chemotherapy Agents Likely to Cause Neurotoxicity

High Incidence (very common > 80% incidence)	
Cisplatin	Interferon (especially at HD)
Interleukin-2 (if patient develops capillary leak syndrome)	
Moderate Incidence (common, 20–80% incidence)	
Arsenic trioxide	Methotrexate (IT, HD)
Carmustine (intra-arterial)	Oxaliplatin, ormaplatin
Cytosine arabinoside (HD)	Paclitaxel
Docetaxel	Procarbazine
Hexamethylmelamine	Suramin
Ifosfamide	Tretinoin
l-asparaginase	Vincristine, vinblastine, vinorelbine
Uncommon (< 20% incidence)	
Busulfan	Fludarabine
Capecitabine	5-fluorouracil
Cladrabine	Pentostatin
Etoposide	Teniposide

IT = intrathecal; HD = high dose

Data from: Armstrong T, Rust D, and Kohtz JR (1997); Cheson BD, Vena DA, Foss FM, and Sorensen JM (1994); Furlong TG (1993); Weiss RB (2001).

References

Armstrong T, Rust D, Kohtz JR. Neurologic, Pulmonary, and Cutaneous Toxicities of High-Dose Chemotherapy. *Oncology Nursing Forum* 1997;24(Suppl 1):23–33

Berghorn E, Hausheer F. Bionumerik Patient Neurotoxicity Questionnaire. San Antonio, TX: Bionumerick Pharmaceuticals, Inc.; 2000

For each of the following 2 items, please indicate by placing a check in the box that best describes how you have felt over the past 4 weeks.

1. ☐ I have no numbness, pain, or tingling in my hands or feet.
   ☐ I have mild tingling, pain, or numbness in my hands or feet. This does not interfere with my activities.
   ☐ I have moderate tingling, pain, or numbness in my hands or feet. This interferes with some of my activities.
   ☐ I have moderate to severe tingling, pain, or numbness in my hands or feet. This interferes with my activities of daily living.
   ☐ I have severe tingling or numbness in my hands or feet. It completely prevents me from doing most activities.
2. ☐ I have no weakness in my arms or legs.
   ☐ I have a mild weakness in my arms or legs. This does not interfere with my activities.
   ☐ I have moderate weakness in my arms or legs. This interferes with some of my actities.
   ☐ I have moderate to severe weakness in my arms or legs. This interferes with my activities of daily living.
   ☐ I have severe weakness in my arms or legs. It completely prevents me from doing most activities.

To help you complete this form, listed below are some examples of activities of daily living:

Dressing:	ability to button blouse/shirt, put on earrings, tying shoes, put in contact lenses
Eating:	ability to use knife, fork, and spoon or chopsticks
Mobility:	ability to walk, climb stairs
Communication:	writing, typing on a keyboard
Other:	interference with sleep, driving, operation of remote controls

Figure 4.1 Patient Neurotoxicity Questionnaire
Source: Berghorn E and Hausheer F (2000) Bionumerik Patient Neurotoxicity Questionnaire. San Antonio, TX, Bionumerik Pharmaceuticals, Inc.

Boyle FM, Wheeler HR, Shenfield GM. Glutamine Ameliorates Experimental Vincristine Neuropathy. *J Pharmacol Exp Ther* 1996;279(1):410–415

Boyle FM, Wheeler HR, Shenfield GM. Amelioration of Experimental Cisplatin and Paclitaxel Neuropathy with Glutamate. *J Neuro-Oncol* 1999;41:107–116

Calhoun EA, Fishman DA, Roland PY, Lurain JR, Bennett CL. Total Cost of Chemotherapy-induced Hematologic and Neurologic Toxicity. *Proc Am Soc Clin Oncol* 1999;18A:1606

Cheson BD, Vena DA, Foss FM, Sorensen JM. Neurotoxicity of Purine Analogues: A Review. *J Clin Oncology* 1994;12(10):2216–2228

Furlong TG. Neurologic Complications of Immunosuppressive Cancer Therapy. *Oncology Nursing Forum* 1993;20(9):1337–1352

Hensley ML, Schuchter LM, Lindley C, et al. American Society of Clinical Oncology Clinical Practice Guidelines for the Use of Chemotherapy and Radiotherapy Protectants. *J Clin Oncol* 1999;17(10):3333–3355

Liu T, Liu Y, He S, et al. Use of Radiation with or without WR-2721 in Advanced Rectal Cancer. *Cancer* 1992;69(11):2820–2825

Savarese D, Boucher J, Corey B. Glutamine Treatment of Paclitaxel-induced Myalgias and Arthralgias [letter]. *J Clin Oncol* 1998;16(12):3918–3939

Schuchter LM, Luginbuhl WE, Meropol NJ. The Current Status of Toxicity Protectants in Cancer Therapy. *Semin Oncol* 1992;19(6):742–751

Viele CS, Holmes BC. Amifostine: Drug Profile and Nursing Implications of the First Pancytoprotectant. *Oncol Nurs Forum* 1998;25(3):515–523

Weiss RB. Miscellaneous Toxicities. In DeVita VT Jr, Hellman S, Rosenberg SA, (eds), *Principles and Practice of Oncology,* 5th ed. New York, NY: Lippincott-Raven Publishers;1997;2802

Weiss RB. Miscellaneous Toxicities, Adverse Effects of Treatment. DeVita VT Jr, Hellman S, Rosenberg SA, (eds), *Principles and Practice of Oncology,* 6th ed. New York, NY: Lippincott-Raven Publishers; 2001: Chapter 55

Wilkes GM. Peripheral Neuropathy. In Yarbro CH, Frogge MH, Goodman M, (eds), *Cancer Symptom Management,* 3rd ed. Sudbury, MA: Jones and Bartlett Publishers;2004;362–367

Drug: allopurinol sodium (Aloprim, Zyloprim, Zurinol)

Class: Xanthine oxidase inhibitor.

Mechanism of Action: Drug inhibits xanthine oxidase, the enzyme necessary for conversion of hypoxanthine (natural purine base) to xanthine, and then xanthine to uric acid, without affecting biosynthesis of purines. This lowers serum and urinary uric acid levels.

Metabolism: Well absorbed orally and IV with comparable oxypurinol (major pharmacologic component) serum levels with the relative bioavailability of oxypurinol 100%. Time to peak serum concentration is 30–120 minutes, with half-life of allopurinol 1–3 hours, and of oxypurinol 18–30 hours. Drug metabolized in liver to active metabolite oxypurinol, and excreted by kidneys and enterohepatic circulation.

Dosage/Range:

- Oral: 600 mg–800 mg/day for 2–3 days with hydration (dose-reduce if creatinine clearance is < 60 mg/mL.
- IV: in management of patients with leukemia, lymphoma, and solid tumors receiving cancer therapy expected to cause elevated serum and urinary uric acid levels and who cannot tolerate oral therapy:

Adults: 200–400 mg/m²/day, maximum 600 mg/day as a single dose or in divided doses every 6, 8, or 12 hours; optimally begin allopurinol 24–48 hours prior to chemotherapy.
Dose-reduce for renal dysfunction based on creatinine clearance (10–20 mL/min = 200 mg/day; 3–10 mL/min = 100 mg/day).

Drug Preparation:

- Oral: available in 100-mg and 300-mg tablets.
- IV: available as 30-mL vial containing 500 mg allopurinol lyophilized powder, which is stable at room temperature (25°C, 77°F).
- Reconstitute by adding 25 mL Sterile Water for Injection.
- The ordered dose should be withdrawn, and further diluted in 0.9% NS Injection or 5% Dextrose for Injection to achieve a final concentration of no greater than 6 mg/mL.
- Store at 20–25°C (68–77°F) for up to 10 hours after reconstitution.
- Do not refrigerate reconstituted or diluted product.

Drug Administration:

- Oral: give with food or immediately after meals to decrease gastric irritation.
- IV: administer over appropriate period of time given volume of diluted drug.

Drug Interactions:

- Dicoumarol: PT may be prolonged due to prolonged half-life; monitor PT closely and adjust dose as needed.
- Mercaptopurine/azathioprine: allopurinol decreased drug metabolism so dose of mercaptopurine or azathioprine must be reduced to 1/3 or 1/4 the usual dose, and then subsequent dose adjusted based on clinical response.
- Uricosuric agents: decreases the inhibition of xanthine oxidase by oxypurinol and increases the urinary excretion of uric acid. Avoid concomitant use.
- Ampicillin/amoxicillin: increased frequency of skin rash; use together cautiously.
- Chlorpropamide: allopurinol may prolong half-life of drug as both drugs compete for excretion in renal tubule; monitor closely for hypoglycemia if drugs used concomitantly in a patient with renal dysfunction.
- Cyclosporin: cyclosporine levels may be increased, so drug levels should be monitored closely, and dose of cyclosporine adjusted accordingly.
- Theophylline: prolonged half-life when used together; monitor theophylline levels closely and adjust dose accordingly.

Physical incompatibilities with IV allopurinol:

- Amikacin sulfate, amphotericin B, carmustine, cefotaxime sodium, chlorpromazine HCl, cimetidine HCl, clindamycin phosphate, cyarabine, dacarbazine, daunorubicin HCl, diphenhydramine HCl, doxorubicin HCl, doxycycline hyclate, droperidol, floxuridine, gentamycin sulfate, haloperidol lactate, hydroxyzine HCl, idarubicin HCl, imipenem-cilastin sodium, mechlorethamine HCl, meperidine HCl, metoclopramide HCl, methylprednisolone sodium succinate, minocycline HCl, nalbuphine HCl, netimicin sulfate, ondansetron HCl, prochlor perazine edisylate, promethazine HCl, sodium bicarbonate, streptozocin, tobramycin sulfate, vinorelbine tartrate.

Lab Effects/Interference:
- Increased alk phos, AST, ALT, bili.

Special Considerations:
- Dose reduction necessary in renal dysfunction.
- Contraindicated in patients hypersensitive to drug (even mild allergic reaction).
- Discontinue at first sign of a rash.
- Use cautiously with patients on diuretics, as may decrease renal function and increase serum levels of allopurinol.
- Allopurinol hypersensitivity syndrome may occur rarely and is characterized by fever, chills, leukopenia or leukocytosis, eosinophilia, arthralgias, rash, pruritus, nausea, vomiting, renal and hepatic compromise.
- Drug MUST be discontinued immediately if rash develops.
- To prevent tumor lysis syndrome, patient should receive aggressive IV hydration and alkalinization of urine, together with allopurinol.

Potential Toxicities/Side Effects and the Nursing Process

I. POTENTIAL SENSORY/PERCEPTUAL ALTERATIONS related to CNS EFFECTS

Defining Characteristics: Drowsiness, chills, and fever have been reported in > 10% of patients. Headaches, and somnolence occur in 1–10% of patients. Rarely, seizure, myoclonus, twitching, agitation, mental status changes, cerebral infarction, coma, paralysis, and tremor can occur. If fever and chills are associated with rash, eosinophilia, nausea, vomiting, they are most likely related to rare allopurinol hypersensitivity reaction.

Nursing Implications: Assess baseline neurological status, including mental status, and periodically during treatment. If any abnormalities, discuss with physician right away. Teach patient to report chills, fever, drowsiness, or any changes, if they occur. If they do, teach patient self-management strategies, and to report if they are ineffective. If so, discuss management strategies with physician. If fever and chills are associated with rash, eosinophilia, nausea, vomiting, they are most likely related to rare allopurinol hypersensitivity reaction and should be discussed with the physician immediately, and drug discontinued.

II. ALTERATION IN SKIN INTEGRITY, POTENTIAL, related to RASH, STEVENS-JOHNSON SYNDROME

Defining Characteristics: More than 10% of patients develop maculopapular rash, often associated with urticaria and pruritus; may be exfoliative. Less common but more severe, 1–10% of patients develop Stevens-Johnson syndrome or toxic epidermal necrolysis, which may be fatal. For IV administration, local injection site reactions may occur. Alopecia has been reported in 1–10% of patients.

Nursing Implications: Assess baseline skin integrity and intactness of scalp hair. Teach patient that rash may occur, and to report it right away, as drug must be discontinued. Teach patient self-care strategies, including skin cream to moisturize the skin and to prevent itching. Discuss drug discontinuance and management with physician. Teach patient to report any hair loss. If it occurs, discuss impact on patient, self-care strategies, and if severe, discuss drug discontinuance with physician.

Drug: amifostine for injection (Ethyol, WR-2721)

Class: Cytoprotectant; free-radical scavenger, metabolized to a free thiol.

Mechanism of Action: Drug is phosphorylated by alkaline phosphatase bound in tissue membranes, producing free thiol. Inside the cell, free thiol binds to and detoxifies reactive metabolites of cisplatin and other chemotherapeutic agents, thus neutralizing the chemotherapy drug in normal tissues so that cellular DNA and RNA are not damaged. Normal cells are protected because of differences in cell physiology (higher alkaline phosphatase concentrations and tissue pH, as well as more effective vascularity in normal cells as compared to malignant cells) and transport mechanisms that promote the preferential uptake of free thiol into normal tissues. Free thiol may also scavenge reactive free-radical reactive oxygen molecules resulting from chemotherapy or radiotherapy. Free thiol may also upregulate p53 expression, so that cells accumulate in the G_1-S cell cyle phase, enabling DNA repair.

Metabolism: Drug is rapidly metabolized to an active free-thiol metabolite and cleared from the plasma, so the drug should be administered 30 minutes prior to drug dose.

Dosage/Range:

- Chemoprotectant: 740 mg/m^2 in 50 mL 0.9% NS administered intravenously (IV) over 5 minutes, 30 minutes prior to beginning chemotherapy.
- Radioprotectant: 200 mg/m^2/day IVP over 3 minutes, 15–30 minutes prior to standard fraction radiation therapy (1.8–2.0 Gy).

- Clinical studies: myelodysplastic syndrome: 200 mg/m² IV 3d/week × 3 weeks, then 2 weeks off, q5 weeks; evaluate response after 2 cycles (10 weeks).
- Clinical studies: reversal of neurotoxicity: 500 mg/m² IV qd × 5q 21 days × 3 cycles (evaluate response after 2 cycles).

Drug Preparation:

- Available in 10-mL vials containing 500 mg of drug; store at room temperature.
- Use only 0.9% Sodium Chloride.
- Reconstitute vial with 9.7 mL of sterile 0.9% Sodium Chloride.
- Further dilute with sterile 0.9% Sodium Chloride to total 50 mL.
- Stable at 5 mg/mL to 40 mg/mL for 5 hours at room temperature, and for 24 hours if refrigerated.

Drug Administration:

- Hypertension medicines should be stopped 24 hours prior to drug administration.
- Place patient in supine position.
- Administer combination antiemetics.
- Infuse amifostine IV over 15 minutes, beginning 30 minutes prior to chemotherapy or IVP 15–30 minutes prior to radiotherapy.
- Administer IV antiemetic medication 1 hour prior, and oral antiemetic 2 hours prior to amifostine administration.
- Generally, patients should be hydrated with 1 L 0.9% NS prior to amifostine when used as a chemoprotectant.
- Monitor BP baseline, immediately after amifostine infusion and as needed until BP returns to baseline.
- Resume diuretic(s) and/or antihypertensive medications 30 minutes after amifostine infusion is complete as long as patient is normotensive.

Drug Interactions:

- Antihypertensive and diuretic medications may potentiate hypotension.

Lab Effects/Interference:

- May cause hypocalcemia.

Special Considerations:

- Patients unable to tolerate cessation of antihypertensive medications are not candidates for the drug.
- Drug is indicated to reduce the cumulative renal toxicity from cisplatin in patients with advanced ovarian cancer or non-small-cell lung cancer.
- Studies have shown no decrease in drug efficacy when given with first-line therapy in ovarian cancer.
- No evidence exists that drug interferes with tumor response from chemotherapy in other cancers, but research is ongoing.

- Offers significant protection of kidneys.
- Offers protection of bone marrow and nerves.
- Drug has been shown to protect skin, mucous membranes, and bladder and pelvic structures against late moderate-to-severe radiation reactions.

Potential Toxicities/Side Effects and the Nursing Process

I. ALTERATION IN NUTRITION, LESS THAN BODY REQUIREMENTS, related to NAUSEA AND VOMITING, HYPOCALCEMIA

Defining Characteristics: Incidence is frequent, and nausea and vomiting may be severe. These are preventable by using serotonin antagonist and dexamethasone. Hypocalcemia noted in trials using higher doses.

Nursing Implications: Administer serotonin antagonist (e.g., granisetron, ondansetron, or dolasetron) and dexamethasone 20 mg IV prior to amifostine. Encourage small, frequent meals of cool, bland foods and liquids. Teach patient self-management tips and to avoid greasy or heavy foods. Instruct patient to report nausea and/or vomiting that is not resolved by antiemetics. Teach patient to maintain oral hydration as tolerated. Identify patients at risk for hypocalcemia, i.e., nephrotic syndrome and depletion from many courses of cisplatin. Check baseline calcium and albumin, and monitor during therapy. Assess for signs/symptoms of hypocalcemia. Patients may receive calcium supplements as needed.

II. ALTERATION IN OXYGENATION related to HYPOTENSION, POTENTIAL

Defining Characteristics: Drug causes transient, reversible hypotension in 62% of patients at a dose of 910 mg/m^2. Hypotension is usually manifested by a 5- to 15-minute transient decrease in systolic BP of ≥ 20 mm Hg. Incidence is less when dose is 740 mg/m^2, and infused over 5 minutes.

Nursing Implications: Assess patient's medication profile. Antihypertensives should be stopped 24 hours prior to drug administration. Assess baseline BP, heart rate, and hydration status. Ensure that patient is well hydrated, and per physician, administer 1 L of 0.9% NS IV prior to amifostine if needed to assure euhydration; if dehydrated, patient may require 2 L. Place patient in supine position during administration of drug, and monitor BP q5min during administration, immediately after administration, and as needed postinfusion. If the BP falls below threshold (see tabulation below), interrupt infusion and give an IVB of 0.9% NS per physician order. If BP comes back above threshold (returns to threshold within 5 minutes and patient is asymptomatic), then resume infusion and give full dose. If BP does not return to threshold within 5 minutes, infusion should be terminated and IV hydration fluids administered per physician, and patient placed in Trendelenburg position, if symptomatic. If

BP does not return to normal in 5 minutes, dose should be reduced in next cycle. Manufacturer recommends the following thresholds for supine BP:

Systolic BP (SBP)	Threshold SBP in mm Hg
< 100	< 80
100–119	75–94
120–139	90–109
140–179	100–139
≥180	≥130

III. ALTERATION IN COMFORT related to FLUSHING, CHILLS, DIZZINESS, SOMNOLENCE, HICCUPS, AND SNEEZING

Defining Characteristics: These effects may occur during or after drug infusion and are mild. Allergic reactions are rare, ranging from skin rash to rigors, but anaphylaxis has not been reported.

Nursing Implications: Assess comfort level, and ask patient to report these symptoms. Discuss with patient comfort measures.

Drug: dexrazoxane for injection (Zinecard)

Class: Cardioprotector.

Mechanism of Action: Enters easily through cell membranes, but the exact mechanism of cardiac cell protection is unclear. A possible mechanism is that the drug becomes a chelating agent within the cell and interferes with ironmediated free-radical formation that otherwise would cause cardiotoxicity from anthracyclines. Drug is a derivative of edetic acid (EDTA).

Metabolism: 42% of the dose is excreted in the urine. No plasma protein binding of drug.

Dosage/Range:
- 10:1 ratio of dexrazoxane to doxorubicin (i.e., 500 mg/m^2 of dexrazoxane to 50 mg/m^2 of doxorubicin).

Drug Preparation:
- Available in 250- or 500-mg vials.
- Reconstitute drug with provided diluent.
- Drug may be further diluted in 0.9% Sodium Choride or 5% Dextrose to a concentration of 1.3–5 mg/mL.
- Stable 6 hours at room temperature or refrigerated.
- USE SAFE CHEMOTHERAPEUTIC AGENT HANDLING PRECAUTIONS!

Drug Administration:
- Give slow IV push or IVB < 30 minutes prior to beginning doxorubicin.

Drug Interactions:
- None known.

Lab Effects/Interference:
- May increase myelosuppression of concomitant doxorubicin, with leukopenia, neutropenia, and thrombocytopenia.

Special Considerations:
- Drug is indicated for reduction of the incidence and severity of cardiomyopathy associated with doxorubicin in women with metastatic breast cancer who have received a cumulative doxorubicin dose of 300 mg/m^2 and who would benefit from continuing doxorubicin.
- Drug may reduce the response from 5–FU, doxorubicin, and cyclophosphamide (FAC) chemotherapy when given concurrently on the first cycle of therapy (48% response rate vs. 63% without the drug, and shorter time to disease progression).
- Drug requires SAFE CHEMOTHERAPEUTIC AGENT HANDLING PRECAUTIONS!

Potential Toxicities/Side Effects and the Nursing Process

I. POTENTIAL FOR INJURY related to ENHANCED BONE MARROW DEPRESSION

Defining Characteristics: Drug may increase doxorubicin-induced bone marrow depression.

Nursing Implications: Monitor WBC, HCT/Hgb, and platelets bascline and prior to each dose. Instruct patient in self-assessment for signs/symptoms of infection and bleeding, and how to report them. Teach patient self-care measures to minimize risk.

II. POTENTIAL ALTERATION IN METABOLISM related to HEPATIC AND RENAL ALTERATIONS

Defining Characteristics: Possible elevations in liver and renal function studies may occur. Incidence did not differ from patients who received same chemotherapy (FAC) without the protector.

Nursing Implications: Assess hepatic and renal function tests (bili, BUN, creatinine, and alk phos), baseline and prior to each treatment. Notify physician of any abnormalities.

III. ALTERATION IN COMFORT related to PAIN AT INJECTION SITE

Defining Characteristics: Pain at the injection site may occur.

Nursing Implications: Assess site during and after infusion. Instruct patient to notify nurse if discomfort arises. Apply local measures to reduce discomfort.

Drug: glutamine (investigational)

Class: Nutrient (amino acid).

Mechanism of Action: Glutamine is the most abundant amino acid in blood and human tissues. It is a precursor of neurotransmitters and necessary in nucleic acid and nucleotide synthesis. Deficiency can occur during metabolic stress or catabolic periods. It is unclear how glutamine may protect or reduce neurotoxicity related to taxanes, or how it may reduce the arthralgias and myalgias related to paclitaxel administration.

Metabolism: Unknown.

Dosage/Range:
- Per research protocol.
- Neuroprotectant: glutamine 10 g PO tid beginning 24 hours after HD paclitaxel × 3–4 days prior to autologous BM.
- Prevention of arthralgias and myalgias: paclitaxel dose > 135 mg/m^2: glutamine 10 g tid starting on day 2 × 4 days; paclitaxel plus radiotherapy: glutamine 10 g tid 24 hours after paclitaxel × 3 days.

Drug Preparation:
- Oral, available in packets of 10 g per envelope; mix powder with water or preferred beverage.

Drug Administration:
- Per research protocol; drink immediately after mixing tid.

Drug Interactions:
- None known.

Lab Effects/Interference:
- None known.

Special Considerations:
- In laboratory animals, glutamine was shown to improve neuropathy associated with vincristine, cisplatin and paclitaxel.
- Anecdotal reports have shown prevention of arthralgias and myalgias in patients receiving paclitaxel who were their own controls.
- Numerous clinical research studies are ongoing to determine effectiveness, mechanism of action, pharmacokinetics.

- Glutamine available from health food stores.

Potential Toxicities/Side Effects and the Nursing Process

I. LACK OF KNOWLEDGE RE DRUG, SELF-ADMINISTRATION related to NEW PRODUCT

Defining Characteristics: Unclear how nutrient may work, but there are published reports suggesting its effectiveness. Randomized clinical trials are being undertaken to determine effectiveness, pharmacokinetics, and mechanism of action. There are no known side effects.

Nursing Implications: Assess baseline knowledge of nutrient, and its use. Teach patient dosing and self-administration per protocol.

Drug: mesna for injection (Mesnex)

Class: Sulfhydryl.

Mechanism of Action: Used to prevent ifosfamide-induced hemorrhagic cystitis. Drug is rapidly metabolized to the metabolite dimesna. In the kidney, dimesna is reduced to mesna, which binds to the urotoxic ifosfamide and cyclophosphamide metabolites acrolein and 4-hydroxyfosfamide, resulting in their detoxification.

Metabolism: Rapidly metabolized, remains in the intravascular compartment, and is rapidly eliminated by the kidneys. The drug is eliminated in 24 hours as mesna (32%) and dimesna (33%). Majority of the dose is eliminated within 4 hours. Oral mesna has 50% bioavailability of IV dose.

Dosage/Range: Initial dose should be given IV; subsequent doses can be given PO or IV

- Recommended IV-IV-IV: clinical dose 20% of the Mesna dose IV bolus 15 minutes before (or at the same time as the Ifosfamide), 4 hours and 8 hours after ifosfamide or cyclophosphamide dose. Mesna dose is 20% of ifosfamide or cyclophosphamide dose, with total daily dose 60% of the ifosphamide or cyclophosphamide dose.
- IV-oral-oral: Mesna is given as an IV bolus injection in a dosage equal to 20% of the ifosfamide dosage at the time of ifosfamide administration. Mesna tablets are given orally in a dosage equal to 40% of the ifosfamide dose at 2 and 6 hours after each dose of ifosfamide. The total daily dose of mesna is 100% of the ifosfamide dose.
- Patients who vomit within two hours of taking oral mesna should repeat the dose or receive IV mesna. The efficacy and safety of this ratio of IV-oral-

oral mesna has not been established as being effective for daily doses of ifosfamide higher than 2.0 gm/m² for 3–5 days.

- For continuous ifosfamide infusions, mesna is mixed with ifosfamide in equal amounts (1:1 mix). Prior to initiating continuous infusion, mesna is given IVB (10% of total ifosfamide dose). Following completion of the infusion, mesna alone should be infused for 12–24 hours to protect against delayed drug excretion activity against the bladder.
- Oral mesna: dose is 40% of ifosfamide or cyclophosphamide dose (not recommended for initial dose if the patient experiences nausea and vomiting).

Drug Preparation:

- Dilute mesna with 5% Dextrose, 5% Dextrose/0.9% Sodium Chloride, or 0.9% Sodium Chloride to create a designated fluid concentration.
- For continuous ifosfamide infusion, mesna should be mixed together with the ifosfamide.

Drug Administration:

- Diluted solution is stable for 24 hours at room temperature.
- Refrigerate and use reconstituted solution within 6 hours.
- Oral preparation can be diluted from 1:1–1:10 in cola, chilled fruit juice, or plain or chocolate milk (if patient vomits within 1 hour, patient should receive repeated IV dose).

Drug Interactions:

- Ifosfamide: mesna binds to drug metabolites; is given concurrently for bladder protection.

Lab Effects/Interference:

- None.

Special Considerations:

- At clinical doses, mild nausea, vomiting, and diarrhea are the only side effects expected.
- Can cause false-positive result on urinalysis for ketones.

Potential Toxicities/Side Effects and the Nursing Process

I. POTENTIAL FOR INJURY related to MAINTENANCE OF BLADDER MUCOSAL INTEGRITY

Defining Characteristics: Mesna uniquely concentrates in the bladder and has a very low degree of toxicity, making it the uroprotector of choice against ifosfamide-related urotoxicity.

Nursing Implications: Assess daily urinalysis. Assess for hematuria per hospital policy and procedure. Hydrate vigorously.

II. ALTERATION IN NUTRITION, LESS THAN BODY REQUIREMENTS, related to NAUSEA/VOMITING, DIARRHEA

Defining Characteristics: Nausea and vomiting are minor in incidence and severity. Diarrhea is mild if it occurs.

Nursing Implications: Assess baseline nutritional status. Usual antiemetics for ifosfamide or cyclophosphamide-induced nausea/vomiting protect against mesna contribution. Encourage small, frequent meals and liquids. Teach patient to avoid greasy, fried, or fatty foods. Encourage patient to report onset of nausea/vomiting or diarrhea.

Chapter 5
Molecularly Targeted Therapies

The new millennium has brought exciting promise to patients with cancer and to their nurses. As a better understanding of the process of carcinogenesis and metastases has emerged, with it has come identified molecular flaws that can be therapeutically targeted. For the past decades, systemic and local therapies have provided cure, disease stabilization, and palliation for many patients with cancer. However, the physical cost of these benefits was often significant, and included bone marrow depression with increased risk of infection and bleeding, nausea, and vomiting. The "magic bullet" was always sought so that benefit could be achieved with minimal toxicity. Today, a number of molecularly targeted agents have been FDA approved and thousands more are undergoing clinical testing. This chapter lays the groundwork for a sound understanding of the molecular basis of cancer, the identified and potential molecular flaws and targets, and the agents that target them. The presentation is simplified, and if the reader wishes more in-depth discussion of the material covered, please consult the references for more advanced readings.

Dr. Andrew von Eschenbach MD, NCI Director, describes our knowledge of the process of cancer (http://cancer.gov/BenchMarks/archives/2003_04/feature_article.html#q3):

"Today we understand cancer as both a genetic disease and a cell signaling failure. Genes that control orderly replication become damaged, allowing the cells to reproduce without restraint. A single cell's progress from normal, to malignant, to metastatic, appears to involve a series of interactive processes, each controlled by a different gene or set of genes. These altered genes produce defective protein signals, which are, in turn, mishandled by the cell. This understanding of the biology of cancer is enabling us to design interventions to preempt the cancer's progression to uncontrolled growth."

In order to better understand the molecular basis of cancer, it is important to recall early courses in biology and genetics. The following will be reviewed: basic cell biology, genetic mutations, malignant transformation, communication within the cell (signal transduction), over-expression of growth factor genes and their receptors, cell cycle regulation, loss of apoptosis, loss of telomerase activity, invasion, angiogenesis, and metastases.

BASIC CELL BIOLOGY

Cancer is a disease of the cell. The nucleus of the cell is where the genetic material, or Deoxyribonucleic Acid (DNA), is located. DNA is the building block of life, an incredibly simple yet complex double helix in which each strand is made up of millions of chemical bases, and each chemical base attaches to its complementary pair in a specific way (cytosine with guanine, thymine with adenosine). See Figure 5.1.

Genes are a subunit of DNA, and each gene contains a code for a specific product, such as a protein or enzyme. Scientists have now identified all the 35,000 or so genes in the human genome. Genes carry the blueprint of who we are. All cells have the genetic blueprint, but only the genes we need are "turned on," such as blue eyes. The genes we don't need at the moment are turned off. In early fetal growth, many genes are turned on, and then when the embryo develops into a baby, the unnecessary genes are "turned off." Genes code for specific proteins and are contained in a chromosome. Humans have 46 chromosomes: 22 autosomal pairs and 1 pair of sex chromosomes. When the body needs to make a specific protein or enzyme, or to make more cells, this requirement message comes to the cell, attaches to a receptor, such as a growth receptor, on the outside of the cell membrane. Once complexed at the growth factor receptor site, there is dimerization or pairing of receptors, or the receptor can be autostimulated; this begins the message, which is now sent through the membrane to tyrosine kinase molecules, which exchange the currency of a phosphate (phosphorylation) to send the message from one molecule to another (signal transduction). The information goes to the cell nucleus, the DNA strands separate exposing the gene that codes for that enzyme or protein, and information from the gene is copied.

The sequence of chemical bases in the gene are copied base by base onto a new strand of messenger ribonucleic acid (m-RNA) so that the complementary base is shown on the m-RNA. This piece of m-RNA then travels out of the nucleus into the cytoplasm of the cell to the ribosomes, which are the cell's "protein factory." Here the gene copy is transferred by transfer RNA (t-RNA) to the ribosome, and the copy is now identical to the original gene, telling the ribosome to make the specific protein or enzyme. Amino acids are then assembled into a completed protein molecule. See Figure 5.2

When a cell needs to divide, such as a cell lining the gastrointestinal tract, the cell's nucleus receives a message from a growth factor to divide. Recall the process of cell division in terms of the cell cycle, as discussed in Chapter 1. When each cell prepares to divide, the DNA is copied during the Synthesis (S) Phase to make a duplicate set of DNA for the daughter cell. Millions of coded genes are copied during cell division, or when the necessary proteins or enzymes are being made. Occasionally a mistake is made, such as when one

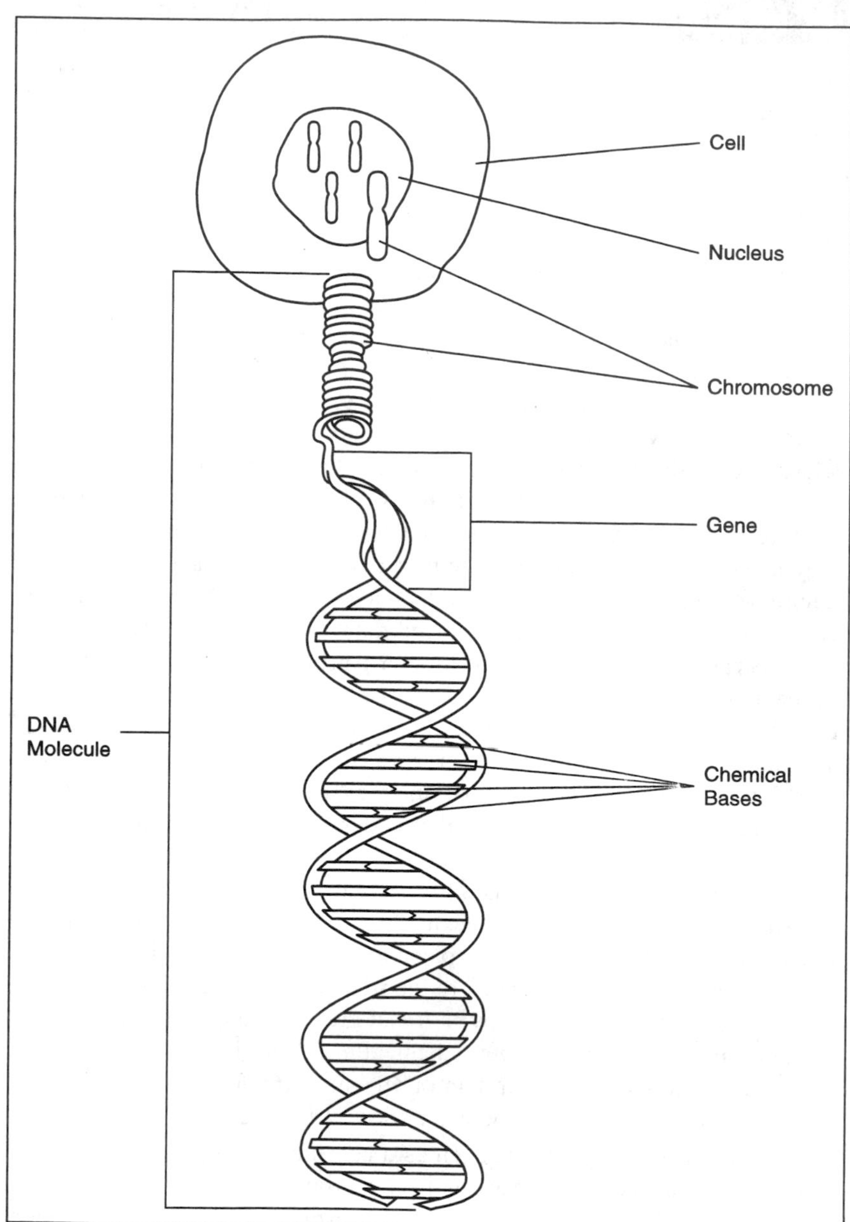

Figure 5.1 DNA: base pairs and double helix (NCI, Understanding Gene Testing, p ii, 1997)

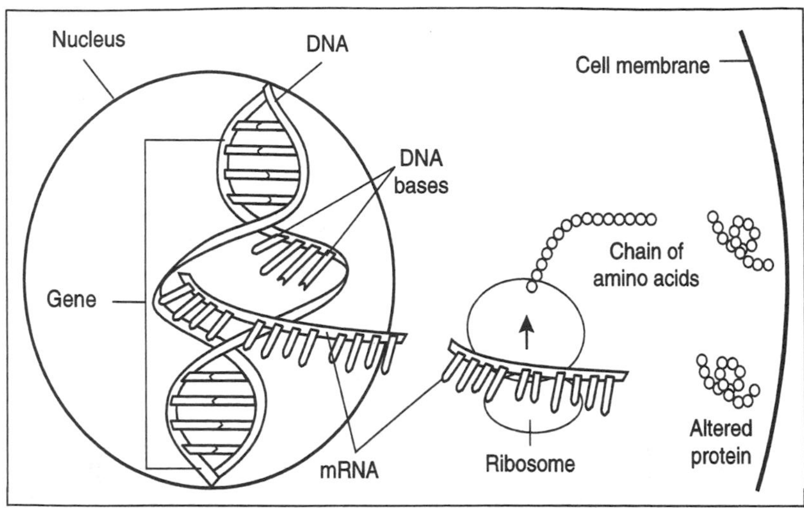

Figure 5.2 Protein synthesis (NCI, Understanding Gene Testing p 2, 1995)

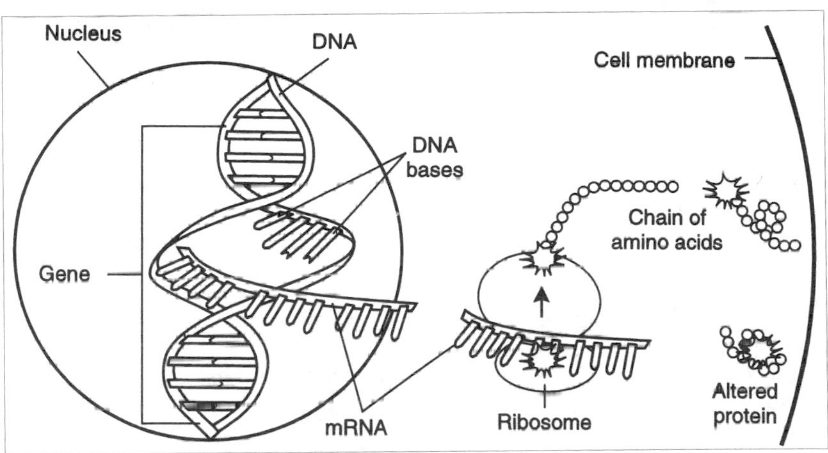

Figure 5.3 Mutation Leading to Abnormal Protein Production (NCI, Understanding Gene Testing p 4, 1995)

chemical base is not correctly copied. Often this is quickly fixed, but sometimes a mutation can result in the production of an abnormal protein, enzyme, or product. Figure 5.3 shows how a mutation can lead to the production of an abnormal protein. Different types of mutations are shown in Figure 5.4.

One example of a serious mutation is the reciprocal translocation between chromosome 9 and 22, forming an extra-long chromosome 9. The other chro-

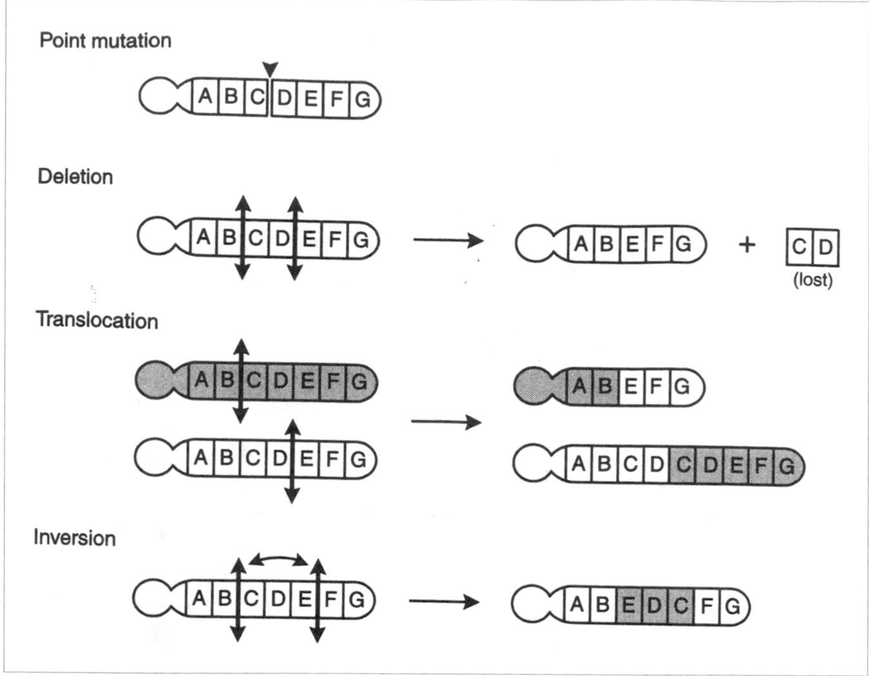

Figure 5.4 Types of Chromosomal Mutations

mosome is short, called the Philadelphia chromosome (Ph[1]) which contains the fused ABL-BCR gene, and is shown in Figure 5.5. This genetic abnormality occurs in 90% of patients with Chronic Myelogenous Leukemia (CML), and results in the formation of an abnormal receptor tyrosine kinase. Imatinib mesylate (Gleevec), a receptor tyrosine kinase inhibitor that selectively targets this flaw, has been FDA approved due to its extraordinary ability to block this mutation.

It appears that all malignancies are caused by mutations in cellular DNA. However, it usually takes at least four mutations to cause malignant transformation. This is shown in Figure 5.6.

Approximately 10% of these mutations are inherited or carried in the DNA of reproductive cells in individuals with parents carrying the gene, while 90% of mutations are acquired and considered sporadic. These develop during the course of one's life, due to exposure to carcinogens and are related to relationships among and between genes and the environment. Most cancers are not inherited, although two examples of inherited vulnerability to cancer are:

- Women who carry the BRCA-1 gene, who represent 5% or so of women who develop breast cancer, and

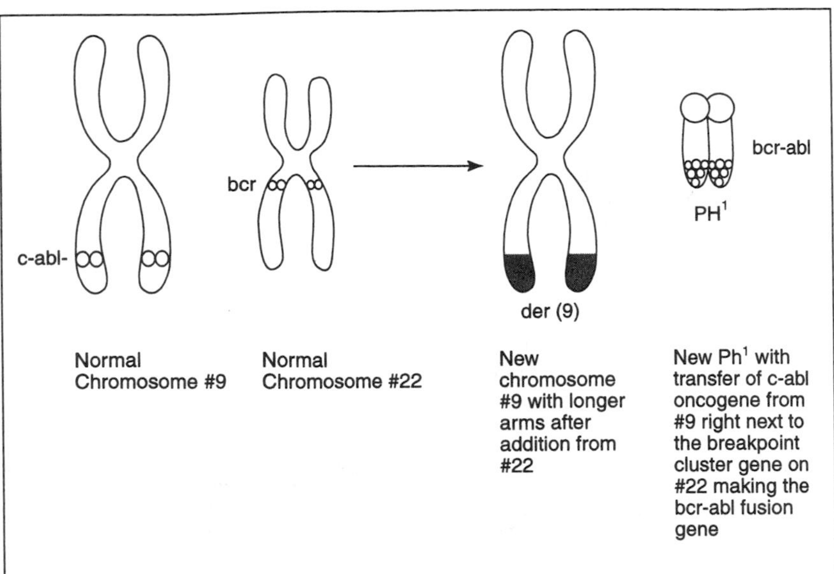

Figure 5.5 Philadelphia Chromosome

- Individuals with hereditary polyposis in which one allele of the APC tumor suppressor gene is silenced. This gene is located in the intraepithelial cells of the intestines. When the second allele becomes mutated, the gene no longer functions as a tumor suppressor gene. Thousands of polyps are formed, and many can progress to malignancy. Fortunately, COX-2 inhibitors appear to prevent many polyps from forming. This also suggests that cyclo-oxygenase 2 (COX-2) is an important mediator of not only inflammation, but also of malignant transformation. COX-2 is overexpressed in many premalignant and malignant tumors, in addition to colorectal adenomas and cancer, such as pancreatic cancer, oral leucoplakia and head and neck cancer, prostate intraepithelial neoplasia and prostate cancer, ductal carcinoma in situ, and breast cancer. Specifically, it appears that COX-2 plays a role in angiogenesis, apoptosis, inflammation, immunosuppression, and invasiveness (Dannenberg AJ et al, 2001).

Thus, people who have a genetic mutation start with one mutation. Most cancers, however, are related to acquired mutations, occurring when the genes become damaged during one's lifetime by factors in the environment or chemicals made in the cells. Genetic errors may be added during cell division when enzymes are copying DNA so that the mutation is copied into permanent DNA. Usually the body's DNA repair mechanism catches the mistake, and if unable to repair it, causes the cell to die (programmed cell death or apoptosis).

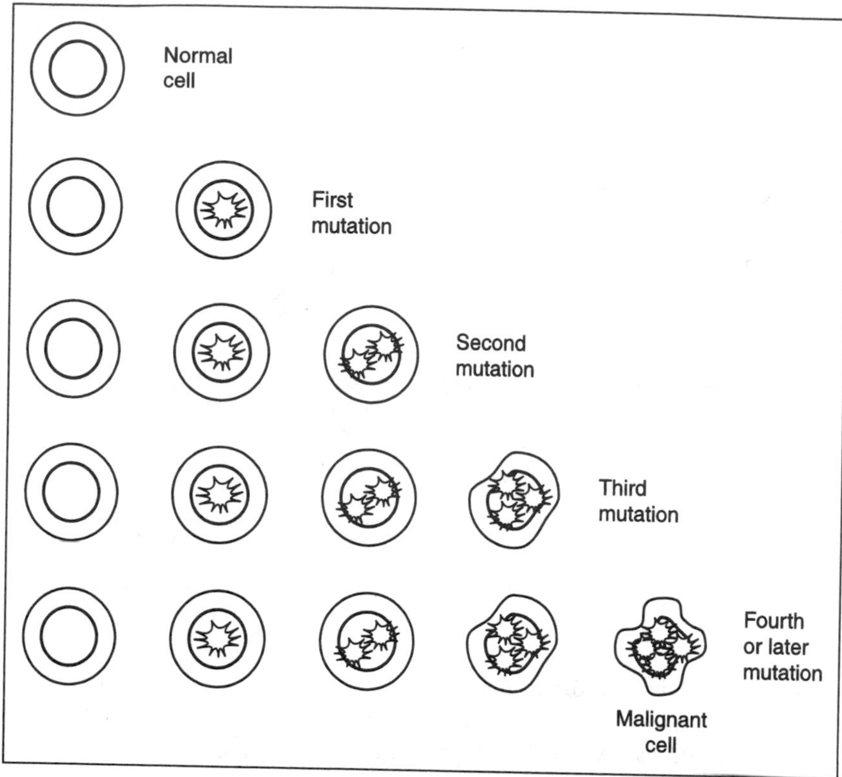

Figure 5.6 Mutations and Malignant Transformation (NCI, Understanding Gene Testing, p 13, 1995)

Sometimes, the system fails, and the error becomes permanent, and are passed on to successive generations of cells.

According to Lippman (2000) mutations in DNA can result from:

- **Gain of function:** The mutation activates one or more genes that lead to malignant transformation, such as with the *Ras, Myc, Epidermal Growth Factor Receptor* family. This results in the speeding up of cell growth and division, which makes more cells than the body needs.
- **Loss of function:** The mutation(s) inactivate genes that control cell growth, such as the tumor suppressor gene p53. In this case, the genetic mutation is not caught, the DNA is not repaired or destroyed, and the genetic flaw is perpetuated with each further cell division.

CELL COMMUNICATION (SIGNAL TRANSDUCTION)

How does a cell know when it needs to divide or make proteins or other cellular products? Signal transduction is the communication link between and among cells. It depends on signals that often originate on the cell surface, such as the growth factors or hormones that attach to cell surface receptors. These are called *ligands*. Once the growth factor attaches to the receptor, the receptor dimerizes with another receptor, and a message is generated. The receptor has three domains: one that sticks outside the cell (external), one that is transmembrane, and one that is internal. The message from a growth factor telling the cell to divide starts when it attaches to the receptor's external domain or "docking station." The message passes through the transmembrane domain into the internal domain, which changes in shape to allow it to interact with the receptor tyrosine kinases or "information-relaying molecules" in the cytoplasm (Scott and Pawson, 2000). Receptor tyrosine kinases pick the message up from the internal end of the receptor and pass it along from one molecule to another until it gets to the cell nucleus. The name *kinase* means enzyme, and this group adds a specific phosphate group to the amino acid tyrosine, called phosphorylation. This transfer of chemical energy activates the tyrosine kinase and it passes the message along from one molecule to another, like a "bucket brigade" or "signal cascade" (Weinberg, 1996). This way, the message is relayed "downstream" to the cell nucleus or down specific signaling pathways to get the desired effect, such as normal cell growth, cell division, differentiation (specialization), or cell death (apoptosis). It is a precise system and has many redundant parallel pathways. As the understanding of the complexity of cell signal transduction has grown, the many potential targets for anticancer therapy have skyrocketed! Figures 5.7 and 5.8 show schemas of cell signals resulting in important cell functions.

Important growth factors are the epidermal growth factor family (EGF or erb-1, erb-2 or HER-2-neu, erb-3, and erb-4), platelet derived growth factor (PDGF), vascular endothelial growth factor (VEGF), transforming growth factor α (TGF-α), and fibroblast growth factor (FGF). The EGF receptor family is very important for cell growth, differentiation, and survival. Many cancers overexpress this receptor resulting in a more aggressive tumor with increased tendency for invasion and metastases and shorter survival. HER-2-neu has become well known because it is overexpressed in about 20% of breast cancer cases, again conferring a poor prognosis. A number of monoclonal antibodies have been developed to block the external domain of the EGF-1 receptor (cetuximab or Erbitux), and the EGF-2 receptor (trastuzumab or Herceptin), and the internal domain [receptor tyrosine kinase inhibitors such as imatinib mesylate (Gleevec).

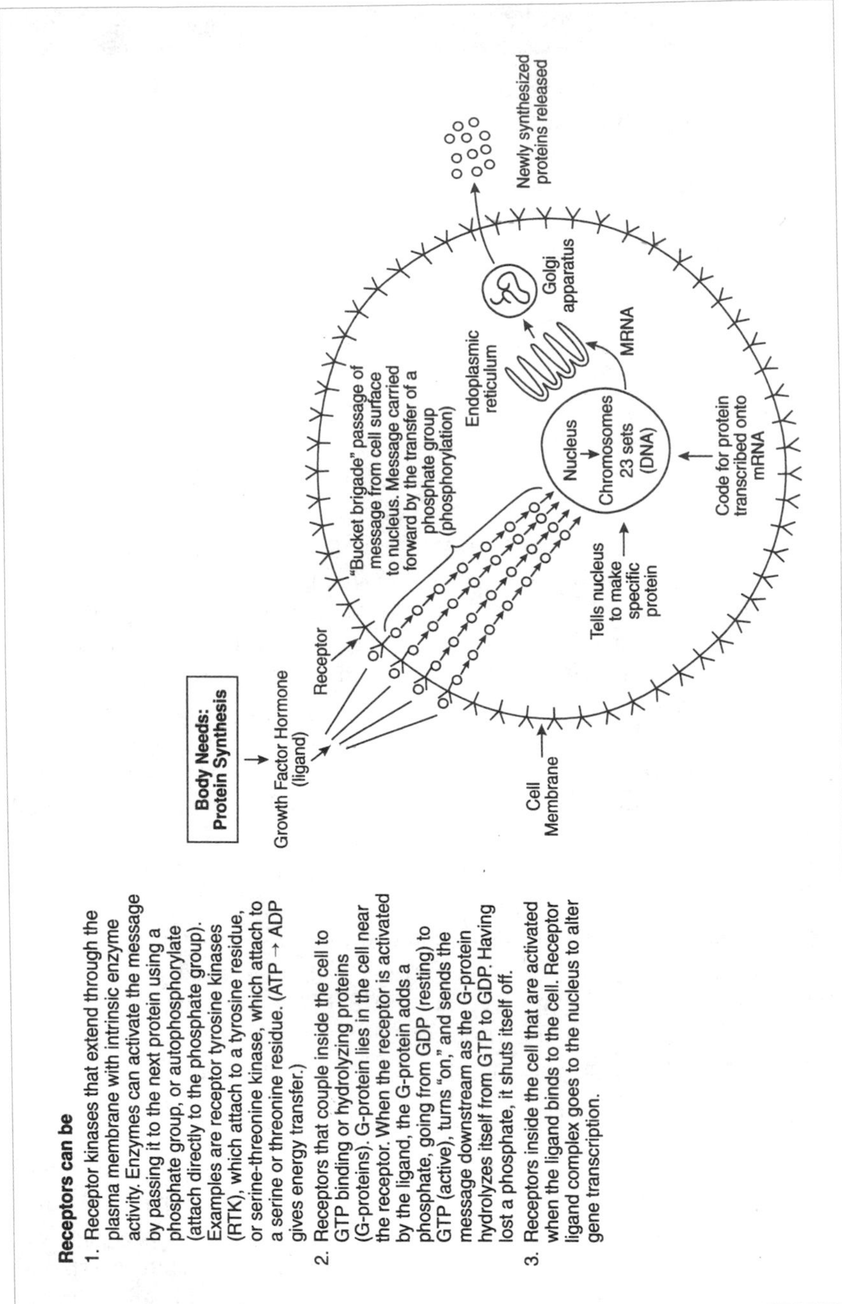

Figure 5.7 Cell Communication: The Inside Story (Scott JD and Pawson T. Scientific American, June 2000)

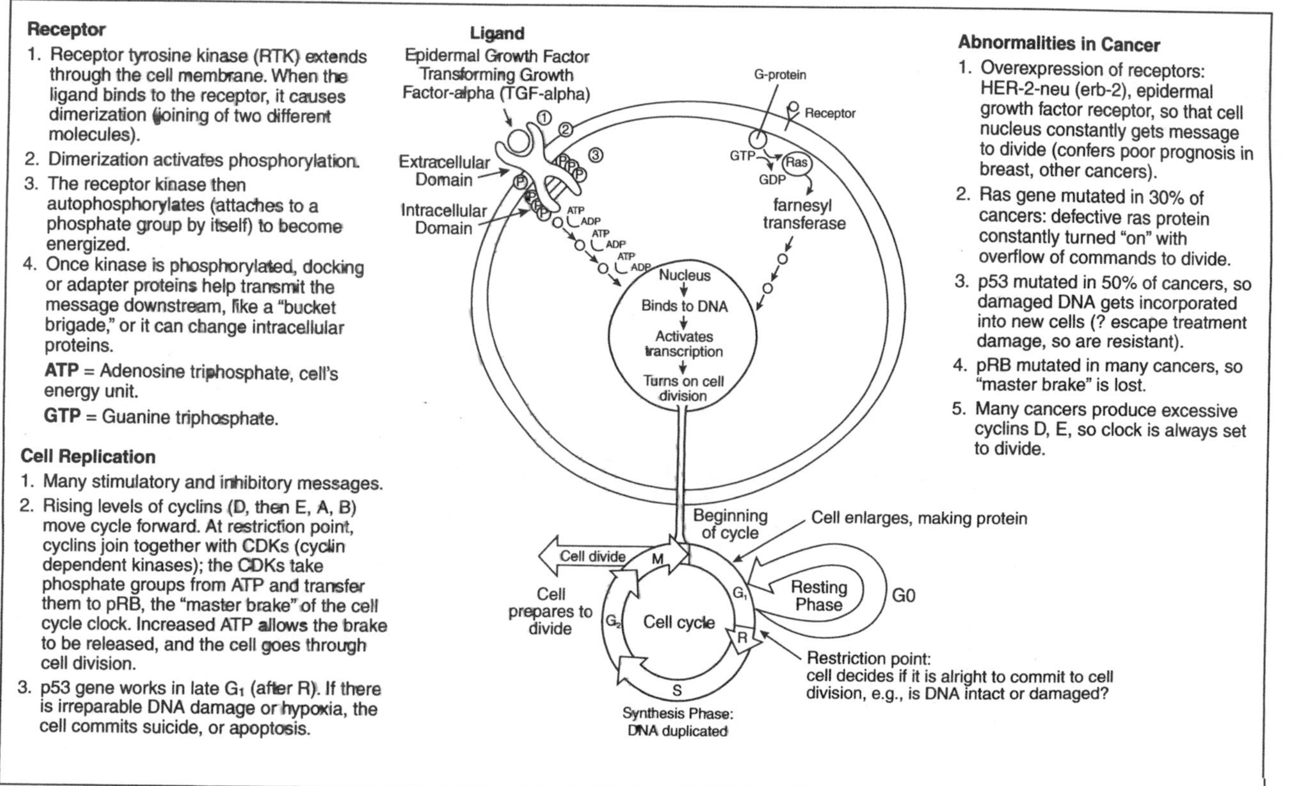

Figure 5.8 Epidermal Growth Factor Receptor and Its Role in Signal Transduction and Tumor Progression (Harari and Huang, 2000)

MALIGNANT TRANSFORMATION

How exactly does the malignant transformation occur? Normally, cell division occurs only when the tissue needs to replace lost or dead cells. Proto-oncogenes are normal cells that encourage cell growth. They are balanced by tumor suppressor genes that not only tell the cell nucleus not to divide if cells are not needed, but they also prevent injured or mutated cells from going through cell division and passing on genetic errors. Mutations must occur in both oncogenes and suppressor genes to get malignant transformation.

For example, a mutation in a proto-oncogene can start the process. This is because proto-oncogenes often produce the protein molecules in the bucket brigade. As a result, the mutates oncogene keeps sending the message to the nucleus for the cell to divide over and over again, leading to uncontrolled cell division. Other mutated oncogenes can also lead to the overproduction of growth factors. PDGF or TGF-α can repeatedly tell the cell to divide, while HER-2-neu overexpression causes proliferation of cell surface receptors that flood the cell with signals to divide, again leading to uncontrolled cell division.

Other proto-oncogenes code for other molecules in the signal cascade, such as the *ras* family of proto-oncogenes which are the H-ras gene, the K-ras-gene, and the N-ras gene (Weinberg, 1996). Normally, the *ras* gene, a proto-oncogene, codes for proteins that bring the message from the cell surface growth factor receptors to other protein messengers further down the signal cascade as part of the bucket brigade, activating downstream effectors such as the Raf-1/mitogen-activating protein kinase (MAPK) pathway, and the Rac/Rho pathway (Rowinsky et al, 1999). Once the message is sent to the nucleus, the ras protein is turned ''off,'' and remains off until recruited again to the cell membrane to bring another message from the extracellular growth factor to inside the cell, and down to the cell nucleus. If the ras proto-oncogene is mutated and then activated, it becomes locked in an ''on'' position, and keeps sending the message to divide even when there is no growth factor binding to the surface receptor, and no message was actually generated. In order to become activated and to attach to the inner surface of the cell membrane, ras has a molecule added called farnesyl isoprenoid; it depends upon an enzyme called farnesytansferase (FTase) to catalyze this addition. If the enzyme is inhibited, then the ras protein is blocked, and in many tumors, causes cells to undergo dysregulation of the cell cycle and programmed cell death (apoptosis). Tipifarnib (R115777, Zarnestra) is a farnesyltransferase inhibitor (FTI) that has shown exciting results in phase III clinical trials. If farnesylation is not blocked, and the ras protein goes to the cell membrane, then Raf-1 kinase is activated and phosphorylates two MAPK kinases (MEK_1 and MEK_2 that are also known as extracellular signal-regulated kinases 1 and 2). Once activated, (phosphorylated), the MAPKs move to the nucleus, where they start a chain reaction leading to cell proliferation (Rowinsky et al, 1999). Sorafenib (BAY 43-9006) is a multi-targeted protein kinase inhibitor that inhibits Raf-kinase, as well as two kinases involved in angiogenesis (VEGF-2, PDGF-β, which is being studied in Phase III trials. It is estimated that 33% of all cancers have a mutated *ras* oncogene, especially cancers Sorof the colon, pancreas, and lungs (Weinberg, 1996). These oncogenes, or their products, are therapeutic targets being studied in clinical trials to block their function so that, for example, the abnormal *ras* proteins are not produced.

Another key pathway that appears to play an important role in cancer is the STAT (Signal Transducers and Activators of Transcription) pathway. This pathway is made up of proteins in the cytoplasm of the cell that join together (dimerize) when activated by tyrosine phosphorylation (Haura et al, 2005). This causes the activated STAT proteins to move into the cell nucleus, then into the DNA where they bind to gene promoters and regulate the expression of certain genes involved in malignancy. The STAT proteins that are activated by themselves without normal growth regulation (constitutive) during malignant transformation regulate pathways such as cell-cycle progression, programmed cell death (apoptosis), angiogenesis, invasion, metastases, and evasion of the immune system by tumor (Haura et al, 2005). Many tumors have dysregulation of Stat 3, Stat 4, and loss of Stat 1 function. Agents are being studied to target the flaws in the STAT signaling pathway.

Via an analogous bucket brigade of inhibitory signals from the cell surface to the nucleus, the normal cell nucleus also receives messages from tumor suppressor genes telling it not to divide unless the body tissues need more cells. This normally prevents the mutated oncogene from causing uncontrolled cell growth, and can be thought of as "putting brakes on" the cell division process. However, tumor suppressor genes also become mutated, and this must occur in order for the malignant transformation to happen. The most famous of these tumor suppressor genes is p53; it appears to be mutated in over 50% of human cancers.

Once there are mutations in both the proto-oncogene and tumor suppressor genes, then there is no longer balance between cell growth and division. Instead, there is uncontrolled cell growth. How does this happen? Again, recall the cell cycle as shown in Figures 5.8 and 5.9. Normally, the nucleus activates the cell cycle by putting the cell into cell division mode only when the stimulatory signals are greater than the inhibitory signals. When this happens, levels of cyclins rise (cyclin D, followed by E, A, and B) as the cell moves through the phases of the cell cycle. This starts the cell to cycle, initiating in the G_1 phase. During this phase, the cell produces new proteins that make RNA in preparation for cell division. The cell enlarges, and the time spent in this phase is highly variable. If division is not needed, then the cell goes into a resting phase called G_0. Near the end of G_1, the cell decides whether to proceed into cell division that is called the *Restriction point.* Weinberg (1996) describes this as a time when the molecular switch needs to be moved from the "off" mode to "on mode," as follows: Cyclins D then E combine/activate cyclin-dependent kinases, enzymes which then transfer phosphate groups from adenosine triphosphate (ATP), the energy molecule, to the retinoblastoma protein (pRB) which is the "master brake" of the cell cycle. If no phosphate groups are added to pRB, the brake stays in the "off" position; however, the brake is lifted when sufficient phosphate groups are added. When the brake is lifted, transcription factors are released which interact with genes so that proteins are actively synthesized for progression through the cell cycle. Mutations can also occur in important inhibitory proteins that would otherwise stop the cell cycle from progressing forward, specifically p53, pRB, p16, and p15. This is important because the cell's DNA is examined to see whether there are any mutations or mistakes, and, if so, the cell tries to repair them. If the DNA cannot be repaired, p53 causes the cell to go into "programmed cell death," or apoptosis. This normally eliminates any abnormal cells from the body. Unfortunately, in over 50% of cancers this protein is inactive. In some cancers, such as cervical cancer, both p53 and pRB are both inactivated (Weinberg, 1996), and in small cell lung cancer and retinoblastoma, pRB is lost. Other proteins such as the cyclins or cyclin-dependent kinases (CDK), which can be synthesized in greater number, or loss of CDK inhibitors, can move the cell through the cell cycle relentlessly. Unfortunately, most cancers have some abnormalities in the cell cycle machinery, and each of these becomes a molecular flaw that can be targeted.

The genes for p53 and pRB are also active in regulating normal cell senescence, leading to programmed cell death. All somatic cells have a finite life of 50–60 doublings after which the cell dies. At the end of the chromosomes, caps called *telomeres* count each of the cell divisions, and snip off a piece of the chromosome with each division. After 50–60 divisions, the chromosome is too short to divide again. In a developing embryo, where there is rapid cell division, the chromosome is protected from being snipped off with each division by the enzyme telomerase, which replaces each snipped piece. This enzyme is not found in normal cells after the embryo develops into a fetus but is found in all tumor cells. If there is a mutation that inactivates either of these genes, the cells can use telomerase to replace each of the snipped off pieces of chromosome, to become immortal. Again, telomerase becomes a molecular target.

2003 saw the arrival of a unique class of antineoplastic targeted therapy: proteasome inhibitors. Bortezomib (Velcade) is the first of this class that is FDA approved for cancer therapy, specifically multiple myeloma as it interferes with the interaction of the myeloma cells with the bone marrow microenvironment. Proteasomes are enzyme complexes that are the housekeeping enzymes which degrade or breakdown proteins in the cell nucleus so that the

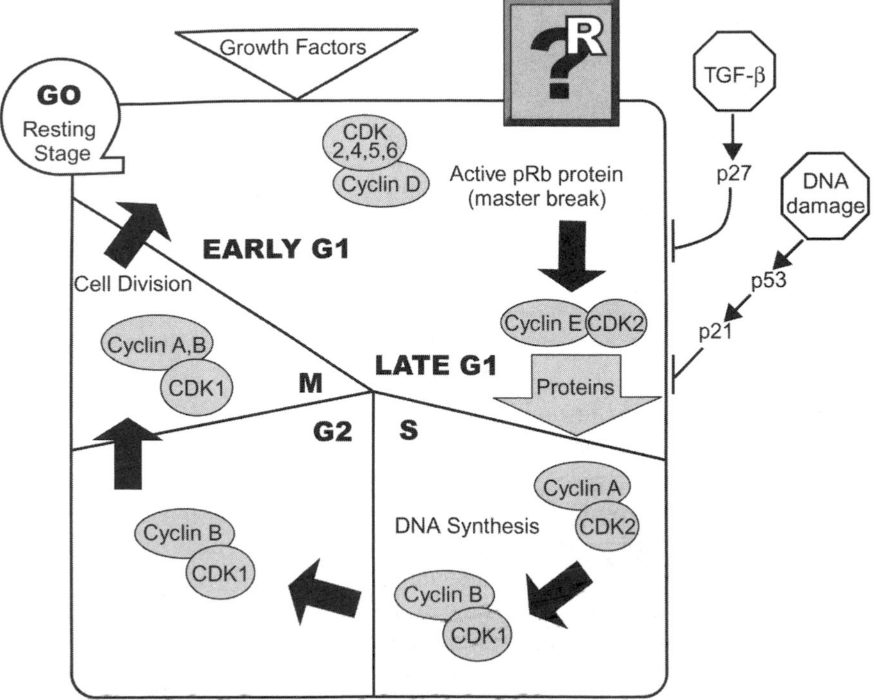

Figure 5.9 The Cell Cycle (Merkle CJ, Loescher LJ. The Biology of Cancer. In Yarbro CH, Frogge MH and Goodman M, (eds). *Cancer Nursing: Principles and Practice*, 6th ed. Sudbury, MA: Jones and Bartlett Inc; 2005;15)

proteins can be recycled and used again. They are found in every cell of the body. The proteasomes know which proteins to degrade because they are tagged with ubiquitin. The ubiquitin-proteasome pathway regulates protein homeostasis within the cell (Kemple, 2003). Proteasome inhibitors block this process from occurring, so the cell gets conflicting signals about cell regulation. The high volume of the conflicting messages the cell nucleus receives causes malignant cells to go into apoptosis or programmed cell death, while normal cells are less sensitive to this overload and can recover. Specifically, 3 pathways are affected by proteasome inhibition: the cell cycle (proteins active in the cell cycle such as cyclins, cyclin-dependent kinase inhibitors, tumor suppressor p53), apoptosis (proteins which inhibit apoptosis like XIAP, cIAP, and Bcl-2 proteins), and Nuclear Factor-kappa B dependent signaling (inhibitor of this pathway is I kappa B-alpha) [Glickman and Ciechanover, 2002]. Nuclear Factor (NF)-kappa B is a transcription factor that has been found to regulate a number of genes that control malignant transformation and metastases. Inactive proteins p50, p65, I kappa B- alpha, and NF-kappa B are found in the cytoplasm of the cell (outside the nucleus). When NF-kappa B is activated by carcinogens, tumor promoter factors, inflammatory cytokines, and some chemotherapy agents, I kappa B-alpha is broken down and the other two proteins move into the nucleus. They attach to DNA in the nucleus at a promoter region and activate the gene. Once NF-kappa B is activated, it can stop apoptosis, which leads to tumor formation and resistance to chemotherapy. There is much excitement about using chemoprevention strategies to block activation of the NF-kappa B by inhibiting its signaling pathway, such as the proteasome does. In addition, it theoretically increases tumor sensitivity to chemotherapy (Bharti and Aggarwal, 2002).

A number of agents are being investigated that target Bcl-2 or other proteins that may suppress apoptosis. Since Bcl-2 protein inhibits apoptosis and makes the cells resistant to treatment with standard chemotherapy, drugs such as anti-sense oligonucleotides theoretically can disable Bcl-2 and restore responsiveness to chemotherapy. Oblimersen sodium is an anti-sense oligonucleotide that binds to Bcl-2 messenger RNA (mRNA), leading to the degradation of Bcl-2 mRNA, which then results in decreased Bcl-2 protein translation or downregulation of Bcl-2 (Klaska et al, 2002).

Another exciting group of agents being explored is the histone deacetylase (HDAC) inhibitors. HDACs complex with cell regulatory proteins to regulate gene transcription, and are key components of cell proliferation, angiogenesis, apoptosis, and cell differentiation. HDAC inhibitors are intended to help malignant cells become normal again, since they target and accumulate in malignant cells. An example of one such agent is suberoylanilide hydroxamic acid (SAHA), which has demonstrated activity in cutaneous T-cell lymphoma, diffuse large B-cell lymphoma, and mesothelioma. SAHA is synergistic with radiation, tyrosine kinase inhibitors, and cytotoxic agents (NCI, 2004).

INVASION AND METASTASES

Once a mutation of an epithelial cell occurs, for example, further development and transformation into malignancy occurs in stages. In this case, the first mutation causes hyperplasia or increased proliferation of normal-appearing cells, and the second leads to dysplasia. The cells now appear abnormal. A third mutation may cause a change to carcinoma in situ, in which the cells remain within normal tissue boundaries. If allowed to continue, the cells may again mutate and develop invasiveness, allowing them to invade underlying tissue and enter blood and lymphatic vessels. As cells are shed, they travel via the blood or lymph system to distant sites. This is called *metastases*. It initially seemed that metastasis begins after the development of a detectable tumor, but it is now clear that, in some tumors, metastases can begin even before the primary tumor is detectable. In general, a tumor cannot grow beyond a size of 2 mm (the head of a pin) unless it forms new blood vessels (angiogenesis).

However, not all cancers are invasive or metastasize. The explosion of scientific discovery about cell function and the molecular processes of metastases has led to the clinical trials of numerous molecularly targeted therapies, including agents that interrupt different steps in the metastases process. Fortunately, it appears that the metastatic process is highly inefficient, especially in late disease, and, in addition, each of the steps is "rate limiting," so that if one step is not achieved, the process can't move forward (Stetler-Stevenson and Kleiner, 2001).

Stetler-Stevenson and Kleiner (2001) identify eight steps in the "metastatic cascade," each controlled by a number of gene products in the malignant cell. Some aggressively permit invasion and others subvert the normal body's defenses against metastases. These steps include the detachment of cells from the primary tumor, invasion of the underlying basement membrane and extracellular tissue, movement of cells into blood vessels, and survival in the venous or lymphatic circulation until reaching a capillary bed. There the malignant cell must attach to the basement membrane of the blood vessel, enter the tissue of the organ fed by the capillary bed, respond to local growth factors, begin cell division to form a small tumor, and begin the formation of local blood vessels to support growth beyond 2 mm.

1. As seen, a cell undergoes multiple mutations during malignant transformation. A single cell (clone) that goes through multiple mutations usually results in cells that are not all alike (heterogenous). Some of the cells are more likely to metastasize than others. Activation of the *ras* oncogene turns a malignant cell into one that invades and metastasizes, and there appears to be a survival advantage for more aggressive cells that respond to local growth factors. The new, tiny tumor gets nourishment by simple diffusion. However, once the tumor reaches 2 mm, it can grow no bigger until it gets its own blood supply to increase the delivery of nutrients.
2. As the tumor grows, the cells on the outside get nourishment (e.g., oxygen), but the cells in the inside (core) become hypoxic. This causes the activation of an "angiogenic switch," involving secretion of angiogenic growth factors (e.g., Vascular Endothelial Growth Factor, VEGF) and suppressing normal inhibitors of angiogenesis (e.g., angiostatin). The blood vessels that form are leaky but have an invasiveness not seen in normal new blood vessels. If the tumor grows near an existing vessel, it may invade and use existing vessels before making its own. Unfortunately, studies have shown that turning on the angiogenic switch is associated with increased frequency of metastases, disease recurrence, and shorter survival (Weidner, 1998).

3. Cells continue to mutate in the primary tumor, and a clone of cells emerges that is superior in growth and is highly invasive. This clone of cells turns down (down regulates) the activity of substances that keep normal cells sticking to their neighboring cells (cell-cell adhesion molecules called *cadherins*, and in epithelial cells, *E-cadherin*) and to the extracellular matrix (integrins). Thus, the tumor cells become mobile and can separate from the rest of the primary tumor. Stromolysin-1 is a matrix metalloproteinase (MMP) that can degrade E-cadherin, and is associated with tumor progression. The tumor cell then uses enzymes (e.g., MMPs) to destroy the integrity of the basement membrane that the tumor lies on, as well as the extracellular matrix. Imagine it like a tank destroying the area ahead so that the invading army can move forward. Now the malignant cells can invade neighboring normal tissue and the newly made leaky blood vessels or nearby thin-walled lymph vessels. Normal cells must remain attached to the extracellular matrix or they die. It is unclear how malignant cells can overcome this. Integrins are critical molecules in the extracellular matrix and also have a role in cell signal transduction and cell growth. Changes in integrin-mediated signaling allow the malignant cell to become invasive and to migrate. Integrin attached to the extracellular matrix gives the malignant cell adhesive traction. As the actin filaments in the cell's cytoskeleton contract, the cell body is propelled forward. Proportionate to the age and size of the primary tumor, huge numbers and clumps of malignant cells can be shed into the bloodstream. The clinical effect depends on whether the embolized cells reach a favorable environment and can achieve the steps in metastases.
4. Individual cells or clumps of cells are carried in the blood or lymph circulation, and many do not survive. The cells need to survive the turbulence of blood flow as well as the circulating cell-mediated and humoral immune cell elements (e.g., cytotoxic and killer lymphocytes). Most die.
5. Cells that survive the ride to distant organs or lymph nodes either get stuck in the microcirculation or attach to specific endothelial cells in capillaries or lymph vessels. In addition, they may attach to an exposed basement membrane of the organ or lymph node.
6. The cells "extravasate" from the blood or lymph vessel into the extracellular tissue and either grow in response to growth factors or stay dormant in this secondary site. Malignant cells migrate to find a "favorable" site. Many die.
7. If successful in finding an hospitable local environment, after some growth to 2 mm, the tumor cells release angiogenic growth factors to build blood vessels in this secondary site. This increases the ability of the metastastic cells to metastasize again.

8. How the metastatic cells evade the body's host immune responses is not well known.

ANGIOGENESIS

Many similarities exist between angiogenesis and tumor invasion and, as a result, they may have similar molecular targets. The body normally needs the ability to make new blood vessels for processes such as wound healing, female menstruation, rebuilding the endometrial lining, or making the placenta during pregnancy. The body maintains a fine balance between turning angiogenesis on and turning it off. When there are more factors favoring angiogenesis than opposing it (inhibitors), angiogenesis occurs. Factors that are angiogenic growth factors are shown in Table 5.1. When cells are hypoxic or lacking oxygen, they release vascular endothelial growth factor (VEGF), also known as vascular permeability factor. VEGF initiates new blood vessel growth and casuses the release of nitric oxide (NO) from the endothelial cells lining the blood vessel, which causes them to dilate. There are a number of VEGF receptors on the endothelial cells, and the most important appears to be VEGF-R2. Others are VEGF-R1, VEGF-R3 (Flt-4), which when stimulated send the message for proliferation and migration of endothelial cells via a tyrosine kinase system, and neuropilin, which is a non-tyrosine kinase receptor. Neuropilin is hypothesized to be a survival factor for tumors (Parikh et al, 2004). Bevacizumab prevents VEGF (the ligand) from binding to VEGF-R2. Numerous agents are being developed and tested to block the VEGF-R2 receptor (monoclonal anti-

Table 5.1 Natural Factors that Stimulate or Inhibit Angiogenesis

Factors Stimulating Angiogenesis	Factors Inhibiting Angiogenesis
• Angiopoietin-1	• Cartilage derived inhibitor (CDI)
• Fibroblast growth factor	• Herparinases
• Interleukin-8	• Human chorionic gonadotropin (hCG)
• Tumor Necrosis Factor (TNF) alpha	• Interferon (alpha, beta, gamma)
• Transforming Growth Factor (TGF) alpha and beta	• Interleukin-12
• Plasminogen activator inhibitor retinoids	• Plasminogen activator inhibitor retinoids
• Platelet derived growth factor (PDGF) BB	• Tissue inhibitors of metaloproteinases called TIMPs
• Granulocyte-Colony Stimulating Factor (G-CSF)	• Thrombospondin-1
• VEGF, also known as vascular permeability factor (VPF)	• Vasculostatin
	• Platelet factor-4

bodies with longer half-lives), and tyrosine kinases (TKIs, which are given orally and have short-half-lives). Of interest, clinical trials with bevacizumab showed not only the cessation of tumor angiogenesis and growth, but also tumor regression suggesting that when combined with chemotherapy, anti-angiogenesis agents alter the tumor blood flow so that the chemotherapy is more effective in killing tumor cells. In addition, it is now believed that there are VEGF- receptors are on tumor cells which are involved in tumor cell migration and invasion; thus, anti-angiogenesis agents appear to directly affect tumor cells (Fan et al, 2005). New agents with ability to target multiple receptors are being developed.

Platelet derived growth factor is necessary for the pericytes outside the newly formed blood vessel to give it stability. Sorafenib (BAY 43-9006), a multiple targeted protein tyrosine kinase inhibitor as well as an anti-angiogenesis agent, appears to block the Raf kinase step in the ras pathway, as well as VEGF-2 and PDGF-β.

Drugs such as bevacizumab (Avastin) neutralize Vascular Endothelial Growth Factor (VEGF), which is released by tumors to start the process of angiogenesis. This drug has shown a significant delay in disease recurrence and increased overall survival in patients with metastatic colon and rectal cancers when combined with chemotherapy. The drug is being studied in the adjuvant setting and it is hoped that it may prevent metatases in patients with Stage III colon cancer. It has also been shown to increase overall survival when combined with carboplatin and paclitaxel in patients with non-squamous NSCLC.

Some substances in the extracellular matrix components undergo proteolysis and release angiogenesis inhibitors such as endostatin and others (Stetler-Stevenson and Kleiner, 2001). On their Web site, http://www.angio.org/providers/oncology/oncology.html, the Angiogenesis Foundation describes the process of angiogenesis (see also Figure 5.10) as follows:

- Angiogenic growth factors are released, normally by injured tissue, and in the case of malignancy, by tumor cells that require blood vessels to grow beyond their current size. The growth factors diffuse into the neighboring tissue.
- The growth factors bind to receptors on the endothelial cells of a nearby blood vessel, activating the endothelial cells.
- Once activated, the endothelial cells send a signal from the cell membrane into the cell nucleus telling the nucleus (genes) to make new molecules, including enzymes.
- The enzymes dissolve tiny holes in the basement membrane of the blood vessels in the area.
- The endothelial cells are stimulated to divide, making more endothelial cells that migrate through the holes in the basement membrane and move toward

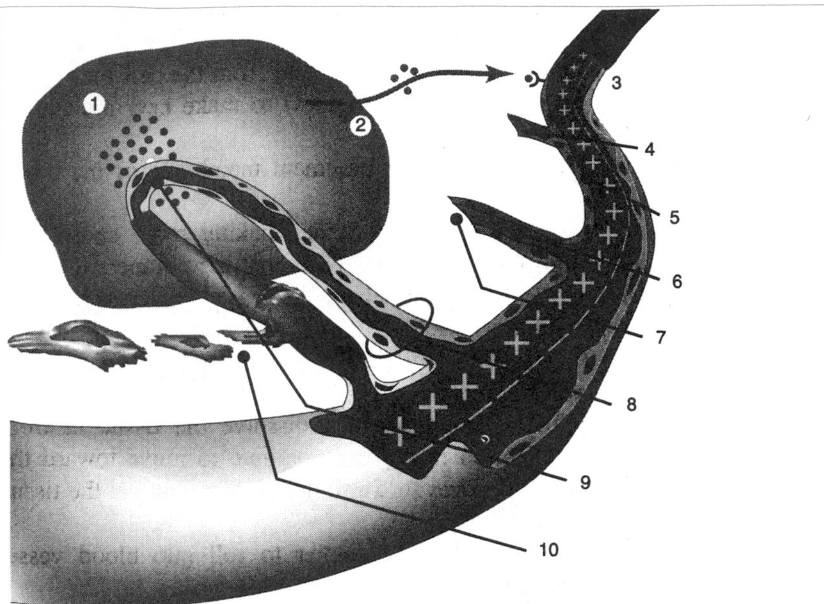

1. Hypoxic or injured tissues produce and release angiogenic growth factors (proteins) that diffuse into the nearby tissues.
2. The angiogenic growth factors bind to endothelial receptors located on the endothelial cells (EC) of nearby preexisting blood vessels.
3. Once growth factors bind to their receptors, the endothelial cells become activated. Signals are sent from the cell's surface to the nucleus. The endothelial cell's machinery begins to produce new molecules, including enzymes
4. Enzymes dissolve tiny holes in the sheath-like covering (basement membrane) surrounding all existing blood vessels.
5. The endothelial cells begin to divide (proliferate), and they migrate out through the dissolved holes of the existing vessels towards the diseased tissue (tumor),
6. Specialized molecules called adhesion molecules, or integrins (avb3, avb5), serve as grappling hooks to help pull the sprouting new blood vessel forward.
7. Additional enzymes (matrix metalloproteinases, or MMP) are produced to dissolve the tissue in front of the sprouting vessel tip in order to accommodate it. As the vessel extends, the tissue is remolded around the vessel.
8. Sprouting endothelial cells roll up to form a blood vessel tube.
9. Individual blood vessel tubes connect to form blood vessel loops that can circulate blood.
10. Finally, newly formed blood vessel tubes are stabilized by specialized muscle cells (smooth muscle cells, pericytes) that provide structural support. Blood flow then begins.

Figure 5.10 The Angiogenesis Cascade (Modified from the Angiogenesis Foundation, 2000, Angiogenesis Cascade)

the injured tissue or malignant cells that released the growth factor, like tiny sprouting new blood vessels.

- Adhesion molecules (integrins) act like little grappling hooks and pull the sprouting new blood vessels forward toward the tumor.
- Additional enzymes (MMPs) are made and dissolve the tissue in front of the sprouting blood vessel so that it can continue to move toward the tumor. After the blood vessel moves forward, the MMPs remodel the tissue to anchor the blood vessel.
- The sprouting endothelial cells come together to roll into blood vessel tubes.
- The individual blood vessel tubes connect to form blood vessel loops.
- Smooth muscle cells stabilize the blood vessels, and blood begins to flow from the parent blood vessel to the new blood vessel loops.

Table 5.2 lists agents currently being tested to inhibit angiogenesis. These are only some of the many agents undergoing clinical testing. In addition, altering the dose and administration schedule of some standard chemotherapy agents appears to change the mechanism of action. As illustrated in the complex steps of metatastases, there are innumerable opportunities for interruption, causing the arrest of the metastatic cascade.

FINDING AND ESTABLISHING A METASTATIC SITE

Ruoslahti (1996) describes the "area code" hyposthesis first developed by Dreyer and Sperry in the late 1960s. The theory helps to explain how certain malignancies develop metastases in preferential areas given that, as we have seen, metastatic cells are blindly embolized into the bloodstream.

First, in order to be embolized, malignant epithelial cells must overcome two types of adhesion, which keep normal cells adhering to one another and attached to the protein meshwork (extracellular matrix), especially in epithelial tissue. This is important because most cancers are epithelial, arising from the epithelial covering of the outer layer of skin and outer layer and lining of many organs, such as the gut and lungs.

Cell-to-cell adhesion molecules keep normal cells orderly. One molecule is especially important, E-cadherin, which ensures intercellular adhesion. Early studies show that when this molecule is manipulated in cancer cells, it changes a cell from a non-invasive cell to an invasive cell capable of forming tumors. When functional E-cadherin is restored, this tendency can be reversed. Malignant cells are able to inactivate E-cadherin and are released from this requirement of cell-to-cell adhesion.

Table 5.2 Agents Currently Being Tested to Inhibit Angiogenesis

MMP Inhibitors	Growth Factor Inhibitors	Small Molecule Inhibitors
• COL-3 (synthetic, tetracycline derivative) • BMS-275291 (synthetic) • Marimastat (synthetic) • AG3340 (synthetic) • Neovastat (natural)	• SU 6668 (blocks vascular endothelial growth factor (VEGF), fibroblast growth factor (FGF), and epidermal growth factor (EGF) signaling from the receptor to the cell nucleus) • Anti-VEGF Ab (monoclonal antibody to VEGF) • Interferon alfa (inhibits bFGF) • Thalidomide (recently found to inhibit VEGF, others) • SU5416 (blocks VEGF signaling from the receptor to cell nucleus)	• Angiostatin (inhibits proliferation of endothelial cells) • Endostatin (inhibits proliferation of endothelial cells) • EMD 121974 (blocks endothelial integrin) • TNP-470 (inhibits proliferation of endothelial cells) • Combretastatin (causes programmed cell death of proliferating endothelial cells) • IM862 (inhibits endothelial cells)

Source: From Folkman (2001), others

In addition, for cell survival and reproduction, normal cells must adhere to the extracellular matrix. In laboratory tests, cells in culture cannot grow unless they attach to a surface, or achieve *anchorage dependence* (Ruoslahti and Reed, 1994). The molecules on the cell surface that actually do the attachment are *integrins.* Integrins must be intact for cell growth and cell division. It appears that integrins influence a protein in the cell nucleus called cyclin E-CDK2 complex (cyclin dependent kinase [CDK]), which is necessary for the cell cycle (division) clock to move toward cell growth and division. When cells do not adhere to the extracellular matrix, the lack of integrin adherence causes inhibition of cyclin E-CDK2 in the cell nucleus; the cell cycle clock stops; and the cell commits suicide (programmed cell death, or apoptosis). Unfortunately, cancer cells are able to circumvent this process, to become *anchorage independent* so cyclin E-CDK2 stays active whether or not the cell is attached, and cells keep growing and dividing, thus avoiding programmed death. In addition, with only a few exceptions (e.g., neutrophils), normal cells cannot penetrate through the underlying basement membrane on which they rest, or through basement membranes of blood vessels (endothelial lining). Like neutrophils, malignant cells release the enzymes called *matrix metalloproteinases (MMPs)* that dissolve parts of the basement membrane as well as the extracellular matrix, like a military tank, so that the cells can migrate away from the primary tumor and into the blood vessels for the process of metastases.

Once in the blood vessel, it is estimated that only one cell in 10,000 is successful in setting up a new metastatic site distant from the primary tumor. As stated, it must attach to the inner lining of capillaries and dissolve holes in the blood vessel basement membrane to escape into the extravascular tissue. It appears that most cells get trapped in the nearest capillary bed they encounter after leaving the primary tumor. Metastatic cells tend to be large and easily trapped, and many secrete clotting factors that cause platelets to aggregate around them. The primary destination for venous blood from most organs is the lungs, thus this is the most common metastatic site. Venous blood leaves the gut and goes to the liver first; the liver is the most common metastatic site for intestinal tumors. While this is true, it appears that, in addition, the cell surface adhesion molecules are directed to specific organ locations, via a code much like telephone area codes, so that malignant cells migrate to specific areas, such as prostate cancer to bone. This was further defined by Muller et al (2001). It also appears that there is "metastatic inefficiency"; some cells go to places without "area codes," or cells from a primary tumor that lacks metastatic qualities undergo apoptosis (Wong et al, 2001).

By studying neutrophils, normal cells that migrate where needed to fight infection, Muller et al (2001) were able to demonstrate that chemokines, soluble substances that carry messages between cells, are responsible for directing breast cancer cells to the primary organs where breast cancer metastasizes: lymph nodes, bone marrow, lung, and liver. Chemokines are small molecules that resemble cytokines and that connect with specific receptors on the cell surface causing rearrangement of the cell's cytoskeleton. This allows cells to adhere firmly to endothelial cells (lining blood vessels) and migrate in a specific direction. Chemokines work with integrins and other proteins on the surface of the cell to direct the breast cancer cells to specific organs. The authors found that breast cancer cells have functionally active chemokine receptors. When these receptors are activated by binding with a ligand (a substance that binds to a receptor on the cell surface and that turns on signal transduction within a cell), the cell starts active actin (which gives structure to a cell) polymerization and formation of pseudopods (fake feet) that allow the cell to migrate and invade tissue. The tissues in which these ligands are overexpressed are the primary metastatic sites in breast cancer. Further, by neutralyzing interactions between the chemokines and their receptors, there is a significant inhibition of metastases to lymph nodes and lung. As more is learned about the process of metastases, new agents can be developed to inhibit each of the critical steps, thus preventing the process.

Thus, as the twenty-first century moves forward, there is tremendous momentum in transforming cancer care. The human genome project and other molecular research have given great insight into the process of carcinogenesis, metastases, and molecular flaws that can be targeted to provide cytostatic and cytocidal effects. This chapter presents investigational as well as FDA approved agents in which the mechanism of action is taking advantage of the molecular flaw, and interrupting the malignant process. As targets are identified, often they can be directly attacked, as with the fusion protein denileukin diftitox (Ontak) which carries the diphtheria toxin directly to high-affinity IL-2 receptors containing a CD25 component, such as activated T- and B-cell lymphocytes. The drug is indicated in the treatment of persistent or recurrent cutaneous T-cell lymphoma (CTCL or mycoses fungoides). The uses of monoclonal antibodies include:

- blocking a receptor, such as the Erb-B1 (EGFR) or Erb-B2 (HER-2-neu) which prevents over-expressed growth factor receptors from sending the signal for cell division
- targeting the internal ptotein receptor kinases, such as gefitinib (Iressa) or erlotinib (OSI-774, Tarceva) which are tyrosine kinase inhibitors.
- carrying chemotherapy or radioisotopes which, when internalized into the cell, cause cell death, such as gemtuzumab ozogamicin (Mylotarg) and ^{90}Y ibritumomab (Zevalin).

Figure 5.11 shows mechanisms of monoclonal antibody therapy.

Tables 5.3 and 5.4 show current agents in clinical trials that target molecular flaws.

Matrix metalloproteases (*MMPs*) have been shown to be overexpressed in breast, lung, and prostate cancers, and it appears that certain MMPs are necessary for the formation of new capillaries (angiogenesis), movement of the cancer cells into neighboring tissue (invasion), and metastases. Normally, the extracellular matrix provides structure between cells, with basement membranes that separate subdivisions within tissues. This matrix prevents aberrant cells from invading other tissues or moving into the bloodstream to go elsewhere in the body. MMPs are zinc-dependent enzymes that maintain the extracellular matrix of tissues by breaking down different parts of the matrix as needed for ongoing remodeling (synthesis and breakdown of these proteins) over time. There are five main subcategories, based on their site of action: collagenases (MMP-1, MMP-8, MMP-13); gelatinases (MMP-2, MMP-9); stromelysins (MMP-3, MMP-7, MMP-10); membrane-type MMPs or MT-MMPs (MMP-14, MMP-15, MMP-16, MMP-17); and others (MMP-11, MMP-12, MMP-18) (Agouron Pharmaceuticals, 1999; Chambers and Matrisian, 1997). The principal MMPs that appear to be involved in tumor angiogenesis, invasion, and metastases are gelatinase A (MMP-2), gelatinase B (MMP-9), and MT-MMP-1 (MMP-14). It is known that tumors larger than 2 mm require new blood vessels to nourish the tumor cells and support tumor growth. As the tu-

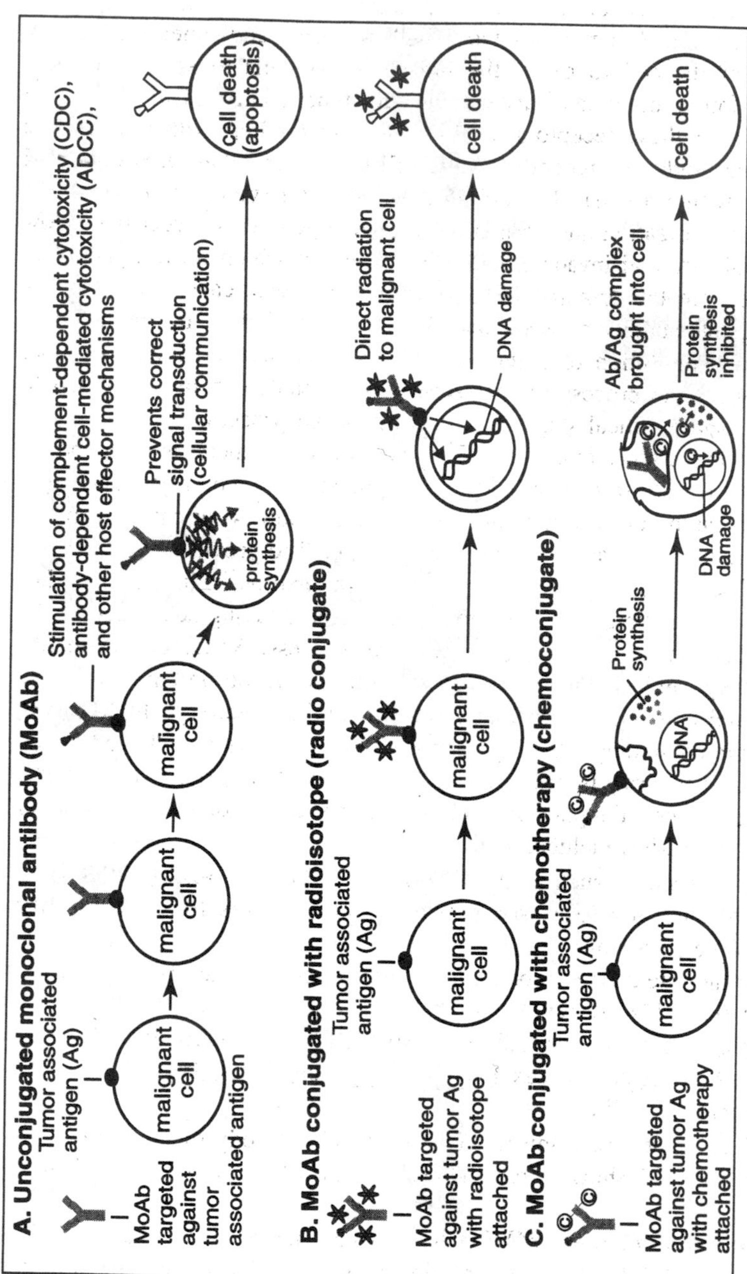

Figure 5.11 Mechanisms of Monoclonal Antibody Therapy

Source: Modified from Wyeth-Ayerest Laboratories (1999) *Antibody-Targeted Chemotherapy.* Philadelphia, PA: Wyeth-Ayerest Laboratories, p. 3

Table 5.3 Molecular Targeted Therapy: Selected Agents Undergoing Clinical Testing

Agent	Mechanism of Action
Cetuximab (Erbitux)	Monoclonal Antibody (MoAb) against EGF receptor
Erlotinib	Small molecule directed against EGF receptor tyrosine kinase
(Tarceva)	MoAb against VEGF Oral immunomodulatory analogue of thalidomide which as
Bevacizumab (Avastin)	
Lenalidomide (Revimid)	Oral iMID (immunomodulatory) analogue of thalidomide which has VEGF antagonist activity
Arasentan (ABT-627)	Endothelin-A receptor antagonist
SCH 44342, BMS-186511, others	Farnesyl Transferase Inhibitors

Table 5.4 Quick Tips on Understanding Monoclonal Antibody Names

1st syllable	Name unique to the product	Tras
2nd syllable	Target, tumor = tu	Tu
3rd syllable	Identifies the source, where 0 = mouse u = human I = chimeric (mouse and human)	U
4th syllable	mab = monoclonal antibody	Mab
X and z	Consonants to link syllables	Tras tu z u mab

mor grows, it releases MMPs to enable cells to break from the tumor and attach to pieces of the extracellular matrix, then to break down the extracellular matrix so the cells can move through the tissue compartments, and, finally, to move through the created openings to invade blood and lymphatic vessels and travel to distant sites. It is hoped that through inhibiting the MMPs, new blood vessel growth (angiogenesis), invasion, and metastases can be prevented. Currently, MMP inhibitors (MMPIs) can be specific, such as inhibiting MMP-2 and MMP-9, or broad spectrum, and are being clinically tested either alone as a single agent, or together with chemotherapy, and then continued as a maintenance agent. Clinical studies with MMPIs have been disappointing, and this book will be updated as more promising agents appear.

Retinoids appear to function by interfering with tumor differentiation. They are believed to have a role in cancer prevention as well as therapy. There are receptors in the cell nucleus that are retinoid-dependent and function in the transcription of proteins. When retinoids bind to the receptors, it is believed that they dimerize nuclear proteins, the complex then binds to DNA, and then there is transcription of a number of target genes. Thus, these activated retinoid receptors regulate the expression of genes responsible for differentiation and replication of cells. Retinoids have been effective in treating superficial Kaposi's sarcoma lesions (alitretinoin) and acute promyelocytic leukemia (tretinoin). In acute promyelocytic leukemia (APL), there is a translocation of a gene called retinoic-receptor alpha (RAR-alpha) on chromosome 17 that is switched with a gene called PML on chromosome 15. It appears that this translocation of RAR-alpha is part of the etiology of APL. Treatment with all-trans retinoic acid induces the primitive leukemic blast cells to differentiate, with replacement by normal myelocyte cells. This drug is now indicated for induction remission in patients with APL with subtype 3, including the M3 variant of AML. Other cancers that appear sensitive to 13-*cis* retinoic acid in combination with interferon alpha are squamous cell cancers of the skin and cervix. Alitretinoin (9-*cis*-retinoic acid) occurs naturally in the body and is able to bind and activate intracellular retinoid receptors. It has been shown to inhibit the growth of Kaposi's sarcoma when used topically and is now indicated for topical treatment of cutaneous lesions in patients with AIDS-related Kaposi's sarcoma who do not require systemic therapy.

It is an exciting time in cancer care. Genetic arrays are being perfected, thus improving diagnosis and treatment and promising to pave the way for individualized multidimensional therapy. It may be possible in the near future to prevent tumors from enlarging beyond 2 mm, and to prevent metastases. Given world politics and individual lifestyle choices, it is probably not possible to eliminate environmental carcinogens. However, the future looks promising that cancer, if not cured, will soon be a chronic, not terminal, disease.

References

Agus DB, Gordon MS, Taylor C, et al. Phase I clinical study of pertuzumab, a novel HER dimerization inhibitor, in patients with advanced cancer. *J Clin Oncol* 2005; 23(11):2534–2543

Agus DB, Sweeny CJ, Morris M, et al. Efficacy and safety of single agent pertuzumab (rhuMAb 2C4), a HER dimerization inhibitor, in hormone refractory prostate cancer after failure of taxane-based therapy. *J Clin Oncol* 2005;23(16s):408s, abstact 4624

Bartlett JB, Dredge K, Dalgleish AG. The evolution of thalidomide and its IMiD derivatives as anticancer agents *Nat Rev Cancer* 2004;4(4):314–322

Bharti AC, Aggarwal BB. Nuclear Factor-kappa B and Cancer:Its Role in Prevention and Therapy. *Biochem Pharmacol* Sept 2002;64(5-6):883–888

Blankenberg F, Chang JT, Tidmarsh G, et al. Independent Review of Response to Iodine-131 Anti-B1 Antibodies in Low Grade or Transformed Low Grade NHL. *Proc Am Soc Clin Oncol* 1998;17:20, abstract 77

Browder T, Butterfield CE, Kraling BM, et al. Antiangiogenic Scheduling of Chemotherapy Improves Efficacy Against Experimental Drug-Resistant Cancer. *Cancer Res* 2000;60:1878–1886

Carducci MA, Nelson JB, Padley RJ, et al. The Endothelin-A Receptor Antagonist Atrasentan (ABT-627) Delays Clinical Progression in Hormone Refractory Prostate Cancer: A Multinational, Randomized Double-Blind, Placebo-Controlled Trial. *Proc Am Soc Clin Oncol* 2001;20(Part 1):174a Abstract 694. 37th Annual Meeting: San Francisco, CA

Chan S, Scheulen ME, Johnston S. et al. Phase II study of temsirolimus (CCI-779), a novel inhibitor of mTOR, in heavily pretreated patients with locally advanced or metastatic breast cancer. *J Clin Oncol* 2005;23:1–9

Connor KM. Understanding Vaccine Therapy. 1998; www.oncolink.upenn.edu/specialty/med onc/vaccine therapy.html

Cortes J, Baselga J, Kellokumpu-Lehtinen P, et al. Open label, randomized phase II study of pertuzumab (P) in patients (pat) with metastatic breast cancer with low expression of HER-2. *Proc Am Soc Clin Oncol* 2005; abstract 3068

Cunningham D, Humblet Y, Siena S, et al. Cetuximab (C225) alone or in combination with irinotecan (CPT-11) in patients with epidermal growth factor receptor (EGFR)-positive, irinotecan refractory metastatic colorectal cancer (MCRC). *Proc Am Soc Clin Oncol* 2003;22:252, abstract 1012

Dannenberg AJ, Altorki NK, Boyle JO, et al. Cyclo-oxygenase 2: A pharmacological target for the Prevention of Cancer. *Lancet Oncology* 2001;2(9):544–551

Demetri GD, Desai J, Fletcher JA, et al. SU11248: a multi-targeted tyrosine kinase inhibitor, can overcome imatinib (IM) resistance caused by diverse genomic mechanisms in patients with metastatic gastrointestinal stromal tumor (GIST). *Proc Am Soc Clin Oncol* 2004;23:195, abstract 3001

Dimopoulous M, Weber D, Chen C, et al. Evaluating oral lenalidomide (revlimid) and dexamethasone versus placebo and dexamethasone in patients with relapsed or refractory multiple myeloma. *European Hematology Assoc 10th Conference* June 2–5 2005, Stockholm, Sweden, abstract 0402

Divino CM, Chen SH, Yang W, et al. Anti-tumor Immunity Induced by Interleukin-12 Gene Therapy in a Metastatic Model of Breast Cancer Is Mediated by Natural Killer Cells. *Breast Cancer Res Treat* 2000;60(2):129–134

Fan F, Wey JS, McCarty MF, et al. Expression and function of vascular endothelial growth factor receptor 1 on human colorectal cancer cancer cells. *Oncogene* 2005; 24:2647–2653

Ferrara N, Alitalo K. Clinical Applications of Angiogenic Growth Factors and Their Inhibitors. *Nature Medicine* 1999;5:1359–1364

Folkman J. Pharmacology of Cancer Biotherapeutics: Antiangiogenesis Agents. In DeVita VT, Hellman S, Rosenberg SA, (eds), *Principles and Practice of Oncology,* 6th ed. Philadelphia, PA: Lippincott, Williams and Wilkins 2001;509–521

Fonseca R, Anderson KC, Weber D. Scientific Symposium: IMiDs: Results of Phase III Studies in Relapsed/Refractory Myeloma (SS10). Program of the 41st Annual Meeting of the American Society of Clinical Oncology. May 13–17, 2005; Orlando, FL

Francois B, Jourdes P, Benabid A. AE-941 (Neovastat) Induces the Expression of Angiostatin in Experimental Glioma. *Proc Am Soc Clin Oncol* 2001;20(Part 1):100a. Abstract 395. 37th Annual Meeting: San Francisco

Galanis E, Buckner JC, Maurer MJ, et al. N997B: Phase II trial of CCI-779 in recurrent glioblastoma multiforme (GBM): Updated results and correlative laboratory analysis. *Proc Am Soc Clin Oncol* 2005;Abstract 1505. 41st Annual Meeting: Orlando, FL

Gasparini G. Prognostic Value of Vascular Endothelial Growth Factor in Breast Cancer. *The Oncologist* 2000;5(suppl 1):37–44

Genentech, Avastin package insert. South San Francisco, CA: Genetech, Inc. 2004

Glickman MH, Ciechanover A. The Ubiquitin-Proteasome Proteolytic Pathway: Destruction for the Sake of Construction. *Physiology Review* 2002;82:373–428

Gorre ME, Mohammed M, Ellwood K, et al. Clinical Resistance to STI-571 Cancer Therapy Caused by Bcr-Abl Gene Mutation or Amplification. *Science* 2001; 293(5531):876–880

Hanahan D, Folkman J. Patterns and Emerging Mechanisms of the Angiogenic Switch During Tumorigenesis. *Cell* 1996;86:353–358

Harari PM, Huang SM. Modulation of Molecular Targets to Enhance Radiation. *Clin Cancer Res* 2000;6:323–325

Harris AL, Zhang H, Moghaddam A, et al. Breast Cancer Angiogenesis. New Approaches to Therapy Via Antiangiogenesis, Hypoxic Activated Drugs, and Vascular Targeting. *Breast Cancer Research Treatment* 1996;38:97–108

Haura EB, Turkson J, Jove R. Mechanisms of Disease: Insights into the Emerging Role of Signal Transducers and Activators of Transcription in Cancer. *Nature Clinical Practice Oncology* 2(6):315–324

Hidalgo M, Siu LL, Neumanitis J, et al. Phase I and Pharmacologic Study of OSI-774, an Epidermal Growth Factor Receptor Tyrosine Kinase Inhibitor, in Patients with Advanced Solid Malignancies. *J Clin Oncol* 2001;19(13):3267–3279

Hurwitz H, Fehrenbacher L, Novotny W, et al. Bevacizumab plus irinotecan, fluorouracil, and leucovorin for metastatic colorectal cancer. *N Engl J Med* 2004;350(23): 2335–2342

Imclone Systems, Erbitux package insert. NY.Imclone Systems, Inc. 2004

Keating M, Byrd J, Rai K, et al. Multicenter Study of Campath-1H in Patients with CLL Refractory to Fludarabine. *Blood* 1999;94:3118 (abstract)

Keefe DL. Trasuzumab-associated Cardiotoxicity. *Cancer* 2002;95(7):1592–1600

Kemple SN. *The proteasome: A novel target in multiple myeloma.* Cambridge, MA: Millennium Pharma 2003

Kern FG, Lippman ME. The Role of Angiogenic Growth Factors in Breast Cancer Progression. *Cancer Metastatasis Rev* 1996;15:213–219

Lancet JE, Gotlib J, Gojo I, et al. Tipifarnib (ZARNESTRA™ in Previously Untreated Poor-Risk AML of the Elderly: Updated Results of a Multicenter Phase 2 Trial. *Blood* (ASH Annual Meeting Abstracts), November 2004;104:874

Li F. Angiogenesis. The Angiogenesis Foundation. 2000; (http://www.angio.org)

Liekens S, DeClercq E, Neyts J. Angiogenesis: Regulators and Clinical Applications. *Biochem Pharmacol* 2001;61(3):253–270

Linderholm B, Grankvist K, Wilking N, et al. Correlation of Vascular Endothelial Growth Factor Content with Recurrences, Survival, and First Relapse Site in Primary Node-postiive Breast Carcinoma after Adjuvant Treatment. *J Clin Oncology* 2000;18:1423–1431

List A, Kurtin S, Roe DJ, et al. Efficacy of lenalidomide in myelodysplastic syndromes. *N Eng J Med* 2005;352:549–557

Lippman ME. New Approaches to the Treatment of Breast Cancer in the Next Century. *Clinical Dialogues in Oncology,* Kingston, NJ: Medicom; 2000

Liu ET. Tumor Suppressor Genes: Changing Concepts. ASCO Educational Book. 35th Annual Meeting, Atlanta, GA: 1999

Maloney DG, Grillo-Lopez AJ, White CA, et al. IDEC-C2B8 (Rituximab) Anti-CD_{20} Monoclonal Antibody Therapy in Patients with Relapsed Low-Grade Non-Hodgkin's Lymphoma. *Blood* 1997;90(6):2188–2195

Lynch TJ, Bell DW, Sordella R, et al. Activating Mutations in the Epidermal Growth Factor Receptor Underlying Responsiveness of Non-Small-Cell Lung Cancer to Gefitinib. *N Eng J Med* 2004;350(21):2129–2139

Malik I, Hecht J, Patnaik A, et al. Safety and efficacy of panitumumab monotherapy in patients with metastatic colorectal cancer (mCRC). Poster presented at the 41st Annual American Society of Clinical Oncologists (ASCO). Orlando, FL;May 2005, abstract K4, 3520

McMahon G. VEGF Receptor Signaling in Tumor Angiogenesis. *The Oncologist* 2000; 5(suppl 1):3–10

Merkle CJ , Loescher LJ. The Biology of Cancer. In Yarbro CH, Frogge MH, Goodman M, (eds), *Cancer Nursing: Principles and Practice,* 6th ed. Sudbury, MA:Jones and Bartlett Publishers, Inc.;2005;15

Meyerson M. Role of Telomerase in Normal and Cancer Cells. *J Clin Oncol* 2000; 18(13):2626–2634

Muller A, Homey B, Soto H, et al. Involvement of Chemokine Receptors in Breast Cancer Metastases. *Nature* 2001;410:50–56

Motzer RJ, Rini BL, Michaelson MD, et al. SU 11248, a novel tyrosine kinase inhibitor, shows antitumor activity in second-line therapy for patients with metastatic renal cell carcinoma. Results of a Phase II trial. *Proc Am Soc Clin Oncol* 2004;23:381, abstract 4500

Murray JL, Witzig TE, Wiseman GA, et al. Zevalin Therapy Can Convert Peripheral Blood bcl-2 Status from Positive to Negative in Patients with Low-grade, Follicular or Transformed Non-Hodgkin's Lymphoma (NHL). *Proc ASCO* 2000;19:22a (77) New Orleans, LA: May 20–23, 2000

National Cancer Institute, *Histone Deacetylase Inhibitors.* 2004; Available at http://cancer.gov/clinicaltrials. Accessed June 13, 2004

Nelson JB, Carducci MA. The Role of Endothelin-1 and Endothelin Receptor Antagonists in Prostate Cancer. *BJU Int* 2000;85(Suppl 2):45–48

Nelson JB, Carducci MA, Padley RJ, et al. The Endothelial-A Receptor Antagonist Atrasentan (ABT-627) Reduces Skeletal Remodeling Activity in Men with Advanced, Hormone Refractory Prostate Cancer. *Proc Am Soc Clin Oncol* 2001; 20(Part 1):4a. Abstract 12. 37th Annual Meeting: San Francisco, CA

Novartis. Gleevec Package Insert. New Jersey: Novartis Pharma AG; May 2001

Onyx Pharmaceuticals . Sorafenib. http://www.onyx-pharma.com/wt/page/bay 43 9006. Accessed June 22, 2005

Parikh AA, Fan F, Liu WB, et al. Neuropilin-1 in human colon cancer: Expression, regulation, and role in induction of angiogenesis. *Am J Pathology* 2004;164(6): 2139–2151

Perez EA, et al. Interim cardiac safety analysis of NCCTG N9831. *Proc Am Soc Clin Oncol* 2005; Scientific Session presented May 16, 2005, 41st Am Soc Clin Oncol Meeting, Orlando, FL

Piccart-Gebhart MJ. First results of the HERA trial. *Proc Am Soc Clin Oncol* 2005; Scientific Session presented May 16, 2005, 41st Am Soc Clin Oncol Meeting, Orlando, FL

Punt CJ, Nagy A, Douillard JY, et al. Edrecolomab alone or in combination with fluorouracil and folinic acid in the adjuvant treatment of Stage III colon cancer: A randomized study. *Lancet* 2002;360:671–677

Raponi M, Lowenberg R, Lancet JE, et al. Identification of Molecular Predictors of Response to ZARNESTRA™ (Tipifarnib, R115777) in Relapsed and Refractory Acute Myeloid Leukemia. *Blood* (ASH Annual Meeting Abstracts) November, 2004;104: 861

Riethmuller G, Schneider-Gadicke E, Schlimok G, et al. Randomised trial of monoclonal antibody for adjuvant therapy of resected Dukes' C colorectal carcinoma. *Lancet* 1994;343:1177–1183

Rituximab Prescribing Information. San Francisco/San Diego,, IDEC Pharmaceuticals and Genentech, Inc 1997

Robert F, Ezekiel MP, Spencer SA, et al. Phase I Study of Anti-epidermal Growth Factor Receptor Antibody Cetuximab in Combination with Radiation Therapy in Patients with Advanced Head and Neck Cancer. *J Clin Oncol* 2001;19(13):3234–3243

Romond EH, et al. Doxorubicin and cyclophosphamide followed by paclitaxel with or without trastuzumab as adjuvant therapy for patients with HER-2 positive operable breast cancer: Combined analysis of NSABP-B31/NCCTG-N9831. *Proc Am Soc Clin Oncol* 2005; Scientific Session presented May 16, 2005, 41st Am Soc Clin Oncol Meeting, Orlando, FL

Rosenberg SA. Molecular Targets and Early Clinical Trials of New Therapeutics and Prevention. ASCO 2000 Educational Book 36th Annual Meeting, New Orleans. 2000

Rowinsky EK, Schwartz GH, Gollob JA, et al. Safety, pharmakinetics, and activity of ABX-EGF, a fully human anti-epidermal growth factor receptor monoclonal antibody in patients with metastatic renal cell cancer. *J Clin Onco* 2004;22(15): 3003–3015

Rowinsky EK, Windle JJ, Von Hoff DD. Ras protein farnesyltransferase: A strategic target for anticancer therapeutic development. *J Clin Oncol* 1999;17(11):3631–3652

Ruoslahti E. How Cancer Spreads. Scientific American (Sept 1996). 1996; http://www.sciam.com/0996issue/0996ruoslahti.html

Ruoslahti E, Reed JC. Anchorage Dependence, Integrins, and Apoptosis. *Cell* 1994; 77(4):477–478

Sandler AB, Blumenschein GR, Henderson T, et al. Phase I/II trial evaluating the anti-VEGF MAb bevacizumab in combination with erlotinib, a HER1/EGFR-TK inhibitor, for patients with recurrent non-small cell lung cancer. 2004 ASCO Annual Meeting Proceedings, Post Meeting Edition. *J Clin Oncol* 2004;22(14S):2000

Sandler AB, Gray R, Bhramer J, et al. Randomized phase II/III trial of paclitaxel (P) plus carboplatin © with or without bevacizumab (NSC 704865) in patients with advanced non-squamous non-small cell lung cancer: An Eastern Cooperative Oncology Group (ECOG) trial-E4599. *Proc Am Soc Clin Oncol* 2005; abstract LBA4

Sausville EA. Cyclin Dependent Kinases: Novel Targets for Cancer Development. ASCO 1999 Educational Book 35th Annual Meeting, Atlanta: 1999

Shi N, Pardridge WM. Noninvasive Gene Targeting to the Brain. *Proc Natl Acad Sci USA* 2000;97(13):7567–7572

Siegel JA. Revised Nuclear Regulatory Commission Regulation for Release of Patients Administered Radioactive Materials: Outpatient Iodine-131 Anti-B1 Therapy. *J Nucl Med* 1998;39(8):285–335

Siemeister G, Martiny-Baron G, Marme D. The Pivotal Role of VEGF in Tumor Angiogenesis: Molecular Facts and Therapeutic Opportunities. *Cancer Metastases Rev* 1998;17:241–245

Singh A, Padley RJ, Ashraf T. The Selective Endothelin-A Receptor Antagonist Atrasentan Improves Quality of Life Adjusted Time to Progression (QATTP) in Hormone Refractory Prostate Cancer Patients. *Proc Am Soc Clin Oncol* 2001;20(Part 2): 393a. Abstract 1567. 37th Annual Meeting: San Francisco

Sledge G, Milelr K, Novotny W, et al. A Phase II Trial of Single-Agent rhuMAb VEGF (Recombinant Humanized Monoclonal Antibody to Vascular Endothelial Cell Growth Factor) in Patients with Relapsed Metastatic Breast Cancer. *Proc Am Soc Oncol* 2000;19:3a, abstract 5C

Stetler-Stevenson WG, Kleiner DE. Molecular Biology of Cancer: Invasion and Metastases. In DeVita VT, Hellman S, Rosenberg SA, (eds), *Principles and Practice of Oncology,* 6th ed. Philadelphia, PA: Lippincott Williams and Wilkins;2001:123–137

U.S. Department of Health and Human Services. Understanding Gene Testing. Washington, DC, National Cancer Institute, NIH Publication,1995;96–3905

Vose J, Saleh M, Lister A, et al. Iodine-131 Anti-B1 Antibody for Non-Hodgkin's Lymphoma (NHL): Overall Clinical Trial Experience. *Proc Am Soc Clin Oncol* 1998;17:38, abstract 38

Wahl RL, Tidmarsh G, Krolls , et al. Successful Retreatment of Non-Hodgkin's Lymphoma (NHL) with Iodine-131 Anti-B1 Antibody. *Proc Am Soc Clin Oncol* 1998; 17:40, abstract 156

Weidner N. Tumoural Vascularity as a Prognostic Factor in Cancer Patients: The Evidence Continues to Grow. *J Pathol* 1998;184:119–120

Weinberg RA. Fundamental Understandings: How Cancer Arises. Scientific American. Sept 1996; http://www.sciam.com/0996

Weiner LM. Phase 1 Open-Label Dose Escalation Trial, poster presented at the 41st Annual American Society of Clinical Oncologists (ASCO), Orlando, FL, May 2005, abstract K4, 3509

Wilkes GM, Ingwersen K, Barton-Burke M. Oncology Nursing Drug Reference. Sudbury, MA: Jones and Bartlett; 2001

Wiseman GA, Leigh BR, Gordon LI, et al. Zevalin Radioimmunotherapy (RIT) for B-Cell Non-Hodgkin's Lymphoma (NHL): Biodistribution and Dosimetry Result. *Proc ASCO* 2000;19:10a (29) New Orleans, LA: May 20–23, 2000

Witzig TE, White CA, Wiseman GA, et al. Phase I/II trial of IDEC-Y2B8 Radioimmunotherapy for Treatment of Relapsed or Refractory CD_{20} + B-Cell Non-Hodgkin's Lymphoma. *J Clin Oncol* 1999;17:3793–3803

Wong CW, Lee A, Shientag L, et al. Apoptosis: An Early Event in Metastatic Inefficiency. *Cancer Res* 2001;61(1):333–338

Wyeth-Ayerst Laboratories. Antibody-Targeted Chemotherapy: Coming of Age. Philadelphia, PA: Wyeth-Ayerest Laboratories; 1999

Drug: alemtuzumab (campath-1H anti-CD52 Monoclonal Antibody, Humanized IgG1 MoAb)

Class: Monoclonal antibody.

Mechanism of Action: Humanized monoclonal antibody, which targets the CD52 antigen present on the surface of most normal human lymphocyte cells, as well as malignant T cell and B-cell malignant lymphocytes (lymphomas). Once the monoclonal antibody binds with the CD52 antigen, it initiates antibodydependent cellular toxicity and complement binding, which then lead to apoptosis, or programmed cell death, and activation of normal T-cell cytotoxicity against the malignant cells.

Metabolism: When given subcutaneously or intravenously, bioavailability appears similar. Host antibodies may develop 14–21 days after the first dose and theoretically can decrease lymphocyte killing. Drug half-life 12 days.

Drug Preparation:

- Available in single use vials containing 30 mg alemtuzumab in 1 mL of diluent. Draw up ordered dose, and dilute in 100 mL sterile 0.9% sodium chloride USP or 5% dextrose in water. Gently invert IV bag to mix. Use within 8 hours. Store at room temperature or refrigerated.

Drug Administration:

- TIW dose initially is 3 mg, then dose escalated to 10 mg, then 30 mg if well tolerated during the first week (tolerance usually achieved within 3–7 days) as IV infusion over 2 hours.
- Stop drug if reaction during infusion.
- Premedicate with acetaminophen 650 mg and diphenhydramine 50 mg 30 min prior to beginning infusion. Severe reactions may require hydrocortisone 200 mg.
- Subsequent dosing: 30 mg IV over 2 h 3-times-a-week, for a minimum of 4 weeks, but may continue up to 12 weeks. Give on Mon, Wed, Fri.
- If dose held more than 7 days, reinstitute gradually with dose escalation.

- Anti-infective prophylaxis recommended, starting on day 8 and continuing for 2 months after treatment completed or stopped, or CD4 count ≥ 200 cells/μL, e.g., with trimethoprim and sulfamethoxazole (Bactrim) DS/bid.
- Dose Reduce ANC < 250/μL and/or platelet count ≤ 25,000/μL. See package insert.

Drug Interactions:
- Unknown.

Lab Effects/Interference:
- An immune e response to the drug may interfere with subsequent serum laboratory tests using antibodies.

Special Considerations:
- Indicated for the treatment of B-cell chronic lymphocytic leukemia (B-CLL) in patients who have received alkylating agents and failed fludarabine.
- Patients who have received multiple courses of chemotherapy prior to campath-1H are at increased risk for bacterial, viral, and other opportunistic infections.
- Immunosuppression related to drug may reactivate herpes simplex infections, septicemia.
- Subcutaneous and intravenous have similar efficacy and effect.
- Following 3-times-a-week therapy, destruction of CLL cells takes about 14 days before being removed from the blood, with no cells detectable at 5 weeks (Solimandro et al, 2000).
- Is being studied in the treatment of chronic lymphocytic leukemia, lowgrade lymphoma, graft-versus-host disease, multiple sclerosis, and rheumatoid arthritis.

Potential Toxicities/Side Effects (Dose- and Schedule-Dependent) and the Nursing Process

I. POTENTIAL FOR INJURY related to HYPERSENSITIVITY REACTION DURING INFUSION

Defining Characteristics: Infusion reactions are common and require premedication to prevent them. Hypotension occurs in 16%, rash in 50%, nausea in 62% of patients, and fever and rigors in 80% of patients. Infusion reactions usually resolve after one week of therapy.

Nursing Implications: Assess vital signs baseline and frequently during infusion, especially during dose escalation. Teach patient that reactions may occur and to tell nurse or physician immediately. Administer premedication as ordered, usually acetaminophen and diphenhydramine. Dose is begun low at 3 mg, then gradually increased based on patient tolerance to 10-mg dose, then to a 30-mg dose. If the patient has a treatment break of seven days or more, then it is necessary to reintroduce drug at the lower dose and gradually escalate dose. If reaction happens, stop infusion but keep main IV line open, notify physician, and, if rigors, give meperidine and any other medications ordered by physician. Expect reaction to resolve in 20 minutes or so, and gradually resume infusion per physician order. Assess skin for integrity and presence of rash. Teach patient to report this, and discuss management with physician. Teach patient that nausea may develop, and to report it right away. Discuss antiemetic agent with physician, and administer as ordered.

II. POTENTIAL FOR INFECTION AND BLEEDING related to BONE MARROW DEPRESSION

Defining Characteristics: All patients develop leukopenia, with approximately 28% of patients developing neutropenia. There is a dramatic fall in WBC during the first week. As both T and B cell lymphocytes are injured, patients are at an increased risk for bacterial, viral, and other opportunistic infections. Most patients require prophylactic antibiotic with/without antiviral therapy, especially heavily pretreated patients. Most common pulmonary infections are opportunistic: *Pneumocystis carinii* pneumonia, cytomegalus virus (CMV) pneumonia, and pulmonary aspergillosis. Commonly, there is reactivation of herpes simplex infections and development of oral candidiasis. Thrombocytopenia affects 22%, with platelet recovery weeks 7 to 12. Incidence of anemia is 36%.

Nursing Implications: Assess baseline leukocyte, platelet, and Hgb/HCT and monitor before each treatment, during therapy, and more often as needed. Hold drug for ANC $< 250/\mu L$ or platelets $\leq 25{,}000/\mu L$. See package insert for dose modifications. Assess risk for infection and integrity of skin and mucous membranes, pulmonary status, and ability to clear secretions, as well as history of past infections, baseline and prior to each treatment. Teach patient to self-administer prophylactic antibiotics and antiviral agents as ordered by physician. Teach patient to self-administer oral antifungal agent if oral candidiasis develops. Teach patient to self-assess for signs/symptoms of infection, and to call provider immediately or come to the emergency room if temperature $> 100.5°F$, shaking chills, or rash, productive cough, burning on urination, or any signs/symptoms of infection or bleeding. Teach self-care strategies to minimize risk of infection and bleeding, including avoidance of OTC aspirin-containing medications.

III. ALTERATION IN COMFORT related to PAIN, ASTHENIA, PERIPHERAL EDEMA, HEADACHE, DYSTHESIAS, DIZZINESS

Defining Characteristics: Pain is common, and in clinical studies 24% of patients experienced skeletal pain, 13% asthenia, 13% peripheral edema, 10%

back or chest pain, 9% malaise, 24% headache, 15% dysthesias, and 12% dizziness.

Nursing Implications: Assess comfort and presence of peripheral edema, baseline and prior to each treatment. Teach patient that these side effects may occur and to report them. Teach patient local comfort measures, and discuss management plan with physician if ineffective.

IV. ALTERATION IN OXYGENATION, POTENTIAL, related to HYPOTENSION, HYPERTENSION, TACHYCARDIA

Defining Characteristics: Hypotension is common, affecting 32% of patients in clinical studies, while 11% had hypertension. 11% of patients also had sinus or supraventricular tachycardia.

Nursing Implications: Assess baseline cardiac status, including blood pressure and heart rate, noting rhythm and rate. Assess past medical history for arrhythmia, hypertension. If heart rate irregular, document rhythm on EKG, monitor blood pressure for evidence of decompensation, and discuss management with physician. If hypertension noted, discuss management with physician. If hypotension noted, assess patient tolerance and need for intervention; discuss management with physician.

Drug: alitretinoin gel 0.1% (Panretin®)

Class: Retinoid.

Mechanism of Action: A9-*cis*-retinoic acid, alitretinoin is a naturally occurring, endogenous retinoid necessary for regulation of gene expression responsible for cell differentiation and replication. 9-*cis*-retinoic acid binds to and activates intracellular retinoid receptors that enable transcription of these genes. Alitretinoin has been found to inhibit the growth of Kaposi's sarcoma (KS) cells directly.

Metabolism: Drug is used topically, without any detectable plasma concentrations or metabolites.

Dosage/Range:
- Sufficient gel applied to cover the lesion with "generous" coating.
- Available in 60-gram tube.

Drug Preparation:
- None.
- Gel tube should be stored at room temperature.

Drug Administration:
- Use glove to apply generous coating of gel to lesions bid, avoiding surrounding skin.
- DO NOT APPLY on or near mucosal surfaces.
- Allow to dry for 3–5 minutes before covering with clothing.
- Gradually increase applications to 3–4 per day.
- If severe skin irritation develops, stop application for a few days until irritation resolves.
- DO NOT USE an occlusive dressing over gel.

Drug Interactions:
- DEET (*N*, *N*-diethyl-*m*-toluamide) insect repellent or products containing DEET, as gel increases DEET toxicity.
- No testing has been done to assess possible interactions between systemic antiretroviral agents, or other agents used in the systemic management of HIV infection.

Lab Effects/Interference:
- None known.

Special Considerations:
- Responses may be seen in 2 weeks, but most often take longer, rarely 14 weeks. Gel should be used as long as there is clinical benefit.
- Indicated for TOPICAL treatment of cutaneous KS lesions in patients with AIDS. It should not be used when systemic therapy for KS is necessary (> 10 KS lesions in prior month, or symptomatic lymphedema, pulmonary KS, or visceral involvement).
- Contraindicated in patients having hypersensitivity to retinoids.
- Women of childbearing age should use contraception to prevent pregnancy, as it is unknown whether topical gel can modulate endogenous 9-*cis*-retinoic levels. 9-*Cis*-retinoic acid is teratogenic.
- Drug SHOULD NOT BE USED by nursing mothers; mothers must discontinue nursing prior to using the drug.
- Drug may increase photosensitivity, so patients should be taught to AVOID sunlamps and to minimize sunlight exposure.
- Safety testing has not been done in pediatric or geriatric (> 65 yr) populations.
- Toxicity almost exclusively related to skin reactions at the application site.

Potential Toxicities/Side Effects and the Nursing Process

I. ALTERATION IN COMFORT AND SKIN INTEGRITY, POTENTIAL, related to APPLICATION SITE REACTIONS

Defining Characteristics: Toxicity begins as erythema. This may increase, and edema may develop with continued application. Most of reactions are mild to moderate, but in some patients (10%), severe reactions may occur with intense erythema, edema, and formation of vesicles. Other skin reactions occurring in >5% of patients are rash, pain, pruritus, exfoliative dermatitis, cracking, crusting, drainage, oozing, stinging, or tingling.

Nursing Implications: Assess baseline skin integrity and condition of KS cutaneous lesions. Teach patient to apply gel only to lesions and AVOID surrounding skin, as irritation will occur. Teach patient to assess and report any changes in the lesions, such as erythema, and edema. Teach patient to reduce frequency of application if skin reaction occurs, to stop use of the gel if severe reactions occur, and to report this as soon as possible.

Drug: arasentan (ABT-627) (investigational)

Class: Endothelin-A receptor antagonist.

Mechanism of Action: Cytostatic. Blocks the endothelin-A (ET-A) receptor, which, when stimulated, would inhibit apoptosis (programmed cell death) resulting in malignant cell proliferation (prostate cancer cells and osteoblasts). Endothelin-1 is important in inducing osteoblastic changes (G-protein couples with RT-A receptor).

Dosage/Range:
- Per protocol. Doses studied are 2.5-mg and 10-mg tablets.

Drug Preparation/Administration:
- Administer orally, once daily.

Drug Interactions:
- Unknown.

Lab Effects/Interference:
- Unknown.

Special Considerations:
- Drug showed improved quality of life (37% higher) in patients using 10 mg dose (Singh et al, 2001).
- Drug appears to inhibit progression of skeletal metastases in hormone-refractory prostate cancer (Nelson et al, 2001).
- Significant increase in median time to clinical progression for men with hormone-refractory prostate cancer (196 days at 10 mg dose) compared to placebo (129 days) and time to PSA progression (155 days at 10 mg dose) compared to placebo (71 days) (Carducci et al, 2001).
- Toxicity profile mild and drug is well tolerated.

Potential Toxicities/Side Effects and the Nursing Process

I. ALTERATION IN COMFORT related to PERIPHERAL EDEMA, RHINITIS, AND HEADACHE

Defining Characteristics: Peripheral edema developed in 35% of patients receiving the drug as compared to 14% receiving placebo. Edema was mild and easily managed. Rhinitis affected 28% in the treatment group and 13% receiving placebo, while 20% receiving the drug had headache as compared to 10% in the placebo group.

Nursing Implications: Assess comfort and presence of edema baseline and at each visit, and teach patient these side effects may occur and to report them. Assess degree of peripheral edema if it develops, and discuss need for diuretics if permitted by protocol with physician. Discuss symptomatic treatment of rhinitis if it develops with physician based on protocol.

Drug: bevacizumab (Avastin)

Class: Recombinant humanized Monoclonal Antibody targeted against Vascular Endothelial Growth Factor (VEGF); Angiogenesis inhibitor.

Mechanism of Action: VEGF binds to receptors on endothelial cells, turning on the cell surface receptors KDR and Flt-1, which then function as tyrosine kinases sending the message to the cells to proliferate and migrate. This leads to the establishment of new blood vessels (neovascularization) in tumors. Studies show that tumors that express VEGF tend to be more aggressive, more invasive, and more likely to metastasize. Bevacizumab binds to all human forms of VEGF, thus preventing it from binding to its receptors on the endothelial cells. This theoretically prevents one step in the process of angiogenesis from occurring.

Metabolism: Humanized via recombinant technologies resulting in a 93% human monoclonal antibody. It is widely distributed throughout the body and has a terminal half-life of approximately 20 days (range 11–50 days). It appears to reach steady state in 100 days. Drug clearance varies by body weight, gender, and tumor burden: men and patients with a large tumor burden have higher clearances than females, but this does not appear to decrease drug efficiency. Drug clearance has not been studied in patients with either renal or hepatic impairment. Concurrent administration of 5-fluourouracil, carboplatin, doxorubicin, cisplatin, or paclitaxel does not affect pharmacokinetics of the drug.

Dosage/Range:
5 mg/kg IV q 2 weeks

Drug Preparation/Administration:

- Single use vials contain 4 mL to deliver 100 mg, and 16 mL to deliver 400 mg per vial. Use within 8 hours of opening. Store at 2–8°C (36–46°F). Protect from light. Do not freeze or shake.
- Further dilute in 100 mL 0.9% Normal Saline for injection.
- Administer IV over 90 minutes as an infusion. If tolerated well without fever and/or chills, may give second dose over 60 minutes; if this is well tolerated, administer all subsequent doses as a 30 minute infusion.

Drug Interactions:

- SN-38 (the active metabolite of irinotecan) concentration is 33% higher when bevacuzimab is given concurrently
- Incompatible with dextrose solutions

Lab Effects/Interference:

- Thrombocytopenia
- Proteinuria
- Leukopenia
- Hypokalemia
- Bilirubinemia

Special Considerations:

- FDA approved for first-line treatment of patients with metastatic colon or rectal cancer in combination with a fluorouracil-based regimen. Is being studied in adjuvant treatment of patients with Stage III colon cancer. Bevacuzimab has been shown to increase the overall survival of patients with metastatic colorectal cancer when given with IFL (irinotecan, 5-fluorouracil or 5-FU, leucovorin or LV) chemotherapy by 4.7 months as compared to IFL alone, and by 4.1 months in combination with 5-FU/LV as compared to 5-FU/LV alone (Hurwitz et al, 2004).
- Interim analysis of a phase III study showed that patients receiving bevacizumab together with paclitaxel and carboplatin had a 30% improvement in overall survival compared to patients receiving paclitaxel and carboplatin alone (Sandler et al, 2005).
- Black box warnings include risk of 1) gastrointestinal perforations/complications of wound healing, and 2) hemorrhage (fatal hemoptysis occurred in 5 patients with NSCLC- squamous cell and adenocarcinoma histologies); Postmarketing: UP to 5% incidence of arterial thrombi with risk of stroke, myocardial infarction, transient ischemic attacks, angina. Risk factors for development of arterial thromboembolic events: history of arterial thromboembolism and age > 65.
- Discontinue drug in patients who develop gastrointestinal perforation, wound dehiscence requiring medical intervention, serious bleeding, nephrotic syndrome, hypertensive crisis.

- Temporarily suspend drug in patients with moderate to severe hypertension uncontrolled with medical management, and for patients who require elective surgery, at least several weeks prior to surgery.
- Bevacuzimab may increase the incidence and severity of hypertension, and severe hypertensive crisis may rarely occur.
- Proteinuria may occur, and rarely, nephrotic syndrome.
- Contraindicated in patients with hemoptysis.
- Drug may impair fertility, and is teratogenic. Women of child bearing age taking drug should use contraceptive measures during treatment, and for the expected time of drug elimination from the body (half-life is 20 days, with a range of 11–50 days) after the drug is stopped. Nursing mothers should discontinue nursing during treatment with bevacuzimab and for the expected time of drug elimination after the drug is stopped.
- Drug toxicities that occur more commonly in the elderly (> 2%) were asthenia, sepsis, deep thrombophlebitis, hypertension, hypotension, myocardial infarction, congestive heart failure, diarrhea, constipation, anorexia, leukopenia, anemia, dehydration, hypokalemia, and hyponatremia. In those aged 75 or older, in addition, dyspepsia, gastrointestinal hemorrhage, edema, epistaxis, increased cough, and voice alteration occurred more commonly than those under age 65.

Potential Toxicities/Side Effects and the Nursing Process

I. ALTERATION IN INTESTINAL AND SKIN INTEGRITY related to GASTROINTESTINAL PERFORMATION AND WOUND DEHISCENCE

Defining Characteristics: Rarely, patients may develop gastrointestinal perforation, sometimes fatal. It may be associated with intra-abdominal abcesses, and occur at variable times during the treatment. Incidence in pre-approval studies was 2–4%, as compared to 0.3% in the bolus IFL-only arm. Presenting symptoms were abdominal pain associated with nausea and constipation. Colonoscopy has a similar risk of GI perforation, so drug should be stopped 28 days before a planned colonoscopy. Also in clinical testing, 1% of patients receiving bevacuzimab plus either IFL or 5-FU/LV developed wound dehiscence, compared to 0.5% in the IFL arm alone. It is unknown how long the interval between surgery and treatment with bevacuzimab should be, but it may be greater than 2 months; similarly, it is not known how long the interval should be between treatment with bevacuzimab and elective surgery, but it certainly should be longer than the elimination time of the drug (half life 20 days). In one small clinical study, 15% of patients who had surgery following bevacuzimab treatment had wound healing or bleeding complications (Genentech, 2004). Exfoliative dermatitis occurred in 19% of patients receiving 5-FU/LV plus bevacuzimab.

Nursing Implications: Assess baseline bowel, skin integrity, and healing of any wounds or incisions; assess for dehiscence, and presence of rash at each visit. Teach patient that very rarely GI perforation or wound dehiscence may occur, to report abdominal pain associated with nausea, constipation, or other symptoms; or problems with wound healing right away for immediate evaluation. Bevacuzimab should be discontinued if perforation or wound dehiscence occur. Bevacuzimab should not be started until at least 28 days before or after major surgery, and the surgical incision is fully healed. Drug should be stopped at least 28 days (drug half-life is 20 days, with a range of 10–50 days) before elective surgery. Teach patient to self-assess skin for rash, and to report it right away.

II. ALTERATION IN HEMOSTASIS related to BLEEDING and THROMBOSIS

Defining Characteristics: Two patterns of bleeding may rarely occur: minor hemorrhage such as mild epistaxis, and serious hemorrhage. Of note, hemorrhage (pulmonary) occurred when drug was being studied in patients with lung cancer, with a higher incidence (31% in a small study) in patients with squamous cell histology. Many of these patients bled from a cavitation or area of necrosis in the pulmonary tumor. CNS bleeding has not been evaluated at this time, as patients with brain metastases were excluded from clinical trials following CNS hemorrhage in a patient with brain metastases. Rarely, the following other events were described in clinical trials: gastrointestinal hemorrhage (24% compared to 6% In IFL alone patients), subarachnoid hemorrhage, hemorrhagic stroke, thrombosis (grade 3/4 incidence 3% compared to 1% in IFL only group), embolism, epistaxis, hematemesis, hemoptysis, and bleeding at tumor sites. Epistaxis occurred in 35% of patients rcceiving bevacizumab + IFL, compared to 10% in IFL-alone arm. Epistaxis is easily controlled with pressure application.Thrombocytopenia may occur in 5% of patients. Deep vein thrombosis may occur in 6–9%, and epistaxis in 32–35% of patients. Patients on low-dose coumadin for implanted port patency had no increased risk of bleeding. There was no increased venous thromboembolism in a review of clinical studies when bevacizumab was added to chemotherapy, although there may be a small increase in arterial thromboembolic events (Novotny et al, 2004).

Nursing Implications: Assess baseline hematologic parameters and monitor during therapy. Teach patient that bleeding may occur and is most commonly epistaxis; but may also rarely occur as bleeding in the gastrointestinal tract, vagina in women, or elsewhere, and to report signs/symptoms of bleeding, changes in mental status, mobility, vision, weakness, or any new sign or symptom right away. Teach patient to assess for and report right away signs/symptoms of thrombosis: new swelling, pain, skin warmth and/or change in color (e.g., erythema, mottling) on the legs or thighs; new onset pain in the abdomen; dysnpnea or shortness of breath, rapid heartbeat, chest pain, or pressure that may signal a pulmonary embolism; and any changes in vision, new onset of severe headache, lightheadedness, or dizziness. Assess baseline mental status and neurological signs and monitor during therapy, especially in patients with brain metastases. Teach patients to apply pressure if epistaxis occurs. Discuss any abnormalities with physician. Bevacuzimab should be discontinued if the patient develops serious hemorrhage, and is contraindicated in patients with recent hemoptysis.

III. POTENTIAL ALTERATION IN CIRCULATION related to HYPERTENSION and CONGESTIVE HEART FAILURE

Defining Characteristics: Bevacuzimab may increase the incidence and severity of hypertension. Incidence of hypertension (> 150/100 mm Hg) was 60% in the clinical study arm IFL+ bevacuzimab and 67% in the arm 5-FU/LV + bevacuzimab arm, compared to 43% in the IFL arm. Severe hypertension defined as > 200/110 mm Hg occurred in 7% of patients in the clinical study arm IFL+ bevacuzimab and 10% in the arm 5-FU/LV+bevacuzimab arm, compared to 2% in the IFL-only arm. Hypertension may persist following drug cessation, as shown in clinical studies: 69% in patients receiving IFL+bevacuzimab, and 80% in the IFL-only arm. Grade 3/4 hypertension occurred in 12% of patients in clinical trials, compared to 2% in the IFL group. Severe hypertension necessitated hospitalization or drug discontinuation, and was complicated by hypertensive encepthalopathy or subarachnoid hemorrhage in some patients. Overall incidence of hypertension is 23–34%, with 12% grade 3/4. Rarely, 2% of patients may develop grade 2–4 congestive heart failure (CHF). Incidence is higher in combination with, or if a past history of, receiving anthracycline chemotherapy with or without left chest wall irradiation.

Nursing Implications: Assess baseline BP prior to and during treatment, at least for the first treatment, then prior to each drug administration. If the patient has a history of hypertension, monitor BP more closely, although hypertension develops over time rather than during the drug infusion. Blood pressure should continue to be monitored after patient has stopped the drug. Teach patient drug administration, potential side-effects, and self care measures if prescribed antihypertensive medication, such as angiotensin-converting enzyme inhibitors, beta blockers, diuretics, and calcium channel blockers. Drug should be permanently discontinued if the patient develops hypertensive crisis (diastolic blood pressure > 120 mm Hg). Drug can be temporarily suspended in patients with severe hypertension until BP can be controlled with medical management.

IV. POTENTIAL FOR INJURY related to HYPERSENSITIVITY REACTION DURING INFUSION

Defining Characteristics: Although the recombinant DNA product is 93% humanized, allergic reactions are still possible. Incidence is < 3%, and slower infusion time greatly reduces the incidence. Infusion syndrome is characterized by fever, rigors, chills, or myalgias. Premedication is not necessary unless the patient experiences an infusion reaction in prior treatments. However, stridor and wheezing may occur. Rash with desquamation may also occur.

Nursing Implications: Assess vital signs baseline and as needed. Teach patient that reactions may occur and to tell nurse or physician immediately. First dose is MENT administered over 90 minutes, 2nd infusion over 60 minutes if previously well tolerated, and then subsequent infusions can be given over 30 minutes if tolerated well. If a reaction occurs, stop infusion but keep main IV line open, notify physician, and if rigors, give meperidine and any other medications ordered by physician. Expect reaction to resolve over 20 minutes or so, and gradually resume infusion per physician order. Monitor blood pressure, and implement ordered medical management plan. Stop drug if severe infusion reactions occur, such as stridor or wheezing, and be prepared to administer oxygen, fluids, and/or antihistamines. Monitor baseline skin integrity, and teach patient to report rash or skin changes. Develop local management plan, and discuss plan revision with physician if ineffective. Fever is treated symptomatically.

V. ALTERATION IN RENAL FUNCTION related to NEPHROTIC SYNDROME

Defining Characteristics: Nephrotic syndrome and proteinuria may occur. 17–28% of patients receiving bevacuzimab in combination with IFL or 5-FU/LV had 2+ proteinuria compared to 14% of patients on IFL alone. 2–4% had grade 3 proteinuria (> 3.5 g protein/24 h), as compared to 0% in the IFL arm. Nephrotic syndrome is rare, occuring in 0.5% of patients, but 1 of the 5 affected patients required dialysis and 1 patient died. Although there may be an improvement in renal function, no patient had normalization following drug discontinuation.

Nursing Implications: Assess baseline renal function and presence of protein in urine (1+ or greater by dipstick), and monitor prior to and between treatments. Discuss any abnormalities with the physician. Patients with 2+ or higher proteinuria by urine dipstick should be asked to collect a 24 hour urine sample for protein. Drug should be held for proteinuria > 2 g/24 h, and resume when proteinuria < 2 g/24 h. Monitor patients closely if moderate to severe proteinuria until improved or resolved.

VI. ALTERATION IN NUTRITION, LESS THAN BODY REQUIREMENTS related to DIARRHEA, STOMATITIS, VOMITING, CONSTIPATION, and TASTE DISORDER

Defining Characteristics: Patients on clinical studies developed the following symptoms compared to patients receiving IFL-only: stomatitis (30–32% vs 18%), dyspepsia (17–24% vs 15%), flatulence (11–19% vs 10%), and vomiting (47–52% vs 47%). Grade 3/4 diarrhea occurred in 34% of patients, compared to 25% receiving IFL-only. Grade 3/4 constipation occurred in 4% of patients, compared to 2% receiving IFL-only. GI hemorrhage occurred in 19–24% vs 6% in the IFL group. Taste disorder occurred in 14–21% of patients compared to 9% in the IFL-alone arm.

Nursing Implications: Assess baseline weight, nutritional status, taste distortion and monitor prior to each treatment. Teach patient that these side effects may occur and to report them. Develop symptom management plan with physician. Make referral to dietitian as appropriate.

VII. ALTERATION IN COMFORT related to ARTHRALGIA, ASTHENIA, PAIN, HEADACHE, COUGH, DYSPNEA, EXCESS LACRIMATION

Defining Characteristics: Discomfort may occur, with symptoms occuring with the following frequency: arthralgias, asthenia (73–74%), myalgia (8–15%), pain (61–62%), headache (26%), cough, or dyspnea (25–26%). Pain and asthenia were common grade 3/4 toxicities in clinical studies. Voice alterations occurred in 6–9% of patients. Underlying disease process may account for many of these symptoms rather than drug, but it was unclear in clinical studies. Excess lacrimation occurred in 18% of patients receiving 5-FU/LV+bevacuzimab, compared to 2–6% in IFL alone or with bevacuzimab arm.

Nursing Implications: Assess baseline comfort, pulmonary status, and eye tearing, and teach patient to report any changes. Discuss further evaluation of symptoms with physician. Develop symptom management plan with physician and implement. Revise plan as appropriate.

VIII. POTENTIAL FOR INFECTION related to LEUKOPENIA

Defining Characteristics: Infection may occur without neutropenia. The incidence of Grade 3/4 leukopenia was 37% in patients receiving the combination, compared to 31% in patients receiving IFL alone. Grade 3/4 neutropenia was 21% in the combination arm, compared to 14% in the IFL arm. Thrombocytopenia occurs in 5% of patients.

Nursing Implications: Assess baseline white blood cell count, differential, and absolute neutrophil count, and monitor closely prior to each treatment when given in combination with irinotecan. Teach patient to avoid opportunities for infection (crowds, people with colds), and to report signs/symptoms of infection right away. Ensure that patient has a thermometer and knows how to use it; alternatively, a family member can monitor patient's temperature at home. Teach patient to monitor temperature, and report temperature > 100.5°F. If patient develops febrile neutropenia, discuss immediate antibiotics and hospitalization as needed.

Drug: bexarotene (Targretin oral capsules and topical gel)

Class: Retinoid

Mechanism of Action: Retinoid that selectively binds to and activates retinoid × receptors, which have biologic activity distinct from retinoic acid receptors. The activated receptors can partner with receptor partners (e.g., retinoic acid receptors), and then function as transcription factors that regulate the expression of genes which control cellular differentiation and proliferation. The exact mechanism of action in cutaneous T-cell lymphoma is unknown.

Metabolism: Drug is well absorbed after oral administration, especially after a fat-containing meal, with a terminal half-life of seven hours. Drug is highly protein-bound (> 99%). Drug appears to be metabolized by the cytochrome P4503A4 isoenzyme system in the liver, forming glucuronidated oxidative metabolites. Four metabolites are formed and are active, but it is unclear which metabolites or whether the parent drug are responsible for the efficacy of the drug. Probably excreted via the hepatobiliary system.

Dosage/Range:

Oral capsules:

- Indicated for the treatment of cutaneous manifestations of cutaneous T-cell lymphoma in patients who are refractory to at least one prior systemic therapy.
- Initial dose of 300 mg/m^2 PO per day for up to 97 weeks (maximum in clinical trials).
- Dose-reduce for toxicity to 200 mg/m^2 PO qd, then down to 100 mg/m^2 PO qd, or stop temporarily until toxicity resolves. After resolution, gradually titrate dose upward.
- Evaluate treatment efficacy at 8 weeks, and if no tumor response but the drug is well tolerated, increase dose to 400 mg/m^2 PO qd and monitor closely.

Topical gel:

- 1% gel indicated for the topical treatment of skin lesions in patients with early stage cutaneous T-cell lymphoma who have failed other therapies.

Drug Preparation:
- Available as 75-mg gelatin capsules in bottles of 100 capsules. The contents of the bottle should be protected from light, high temperatures, and humidity once opened.
- Store at 2–25°C (36–77°F).
- 1% gel available in tube.

Drug Administration:
- Oral: single daily oral dose with a meal.
- Topical gel: apply to affected areas only (NOT entire body) as needed.

Drug Interactions: *Oral capsules:*
- Presumed to be related to P4503A4 isoenzyme system metabolism.
- Inhibitors of cytochrome P4503A4 enzyme system (e.g., ketoconazole, itraconazole, erythromycin, gemfibrozil, grapefruit juice) theoretically can increase serum levels of bexarotene; DO NOT GIVE GEMFIBROZIL concomitantly with bexarotene.
- Inducers of cytochrome P4503A4 enzyme system (e.g., rifampin, phenytoin, Phenobarbital) may cause a decrease in serum bexarotene concentrations. If used concomitantly, assess response, and increase bexarotene accordingly.
- Theoretically, as drug is highly protein bound, it is possible that baxarotene can displace drugs or be displaced by drugs which bind to plasma proteins; use together cautiously.
- Insulin, sulfonylureas, or insulin-sensitizers: may increase action with resultant hypoglycemia; use together cautiously.

Lab Effects/Interference: *Oral capsules:*
- CA 125 assay values in patients with ovarian cancer may be increased.
- Significantly increased serum triglycerides, total cholesterol, and decreased HDL.
- Increased LFTs.
- Decreased TSH and total T4.
- Leukopenia and neutropenia.
- Increased LDH.

Special Considerations:
Oral capsules:
- Baseline serum lipid levels must be assessed prior to initiation of therapy, and any abnormalities treated so that fasting triglycerides are normal before starting therapy.
- Drug is contraindicated during pregnancy as it is teratogenic. Women of childbearing age should use effective contraception — optimally, two forms

unless abstinence is chosen. This should continue during therapy and for one month after the completion of therapy. A pregnancy test should be done one week prior to beginning therapy, and repeated monthly during therapy. If pregnancy occurs, the drug must be stopped immediately and the woman counseled.

- Male patients with sexual partners who are pregnant, possibly pregnant, or who could become pregnant, should use condoms during therapy, and for one month after therapy is ended.
- Most patients have major lipid abnormalities, and one patient died of pancreatitis. In general, patients with risk factors for pancreatitis should not take the drug (e.g., history of pancreatitis, uncontrolled hyperlipidemia, uncontrolled diabetes mellitus, biliary tract disease, or medications known to increase triglyceride levels or to be associated with pancreatic toxicity).
- Drug is contraindicated in nursing mothers.
- Drug should be used cautiously in patients who have hypersensitivity to other retinoids.
- Drug may cause cataracts; patients who experience visual difficulties should have an opthamologic exam.
- Baseline laboratory assessment prior to starting drug should include WBC with differential, thyroid function tests, fasting blood lipid profile, and liver function tests.
- Patients should limit vitamin A intake to ≤ 15,000 IU/day to avoid possible additive toxicity.
- Patients should avoid direct sunlight and artificial ultraviolet light while taking bexarotene as severe sunburn and skin sensitivity reactions may occur due to photosensitization.
- No studies have been done with patients having hepatic dysfunction, but theoretically, hepatic dysfunction would greatly reduce metabolism/excretion and increase serum drug levels. Use cautiously if at all in this setting.
- Response rate in patients with cutaneous T-cell lymphoma who were refractory to one prior systemic therapy was 32%.
- Drug being studied in clinical trials of patients with advanced breast cancer or moderate/severe psoriasis.

1% gel:

- Main side effects are rash, itching, and pain at application site.

Potential Toxicities/Side Effects and the Nursing Process

I. ALTERATION IN NUTRITION, POTENTIAL, related to ABNORMAL LIPID LEVELS, PANCREATITIS, ELEVATED LFTs, AND NAUSEA (oral capsules)

Defining Characteristics: Almost all patients experience major lipid abnormalities, including elevated fasting triglycerides (70% receiving doses of ≥ 300 mg/m²/day had elevations of more than 2.5 times upper limits of normal (ULN), and 55% had values over 800 mg/dL with a median of 1200 mg/dL), elevated cholesterol (60% of patients receiving 300 mg/m²/day, and 75% of patients receiving doses of ≥ 300 mg/m²/day), and decreased levels of the protective high-density lipoproteins (HDL) to < 25 mg/dL (55% of patients receiving a dose of 300 mg/m²/day, and 90% of patients receiving a dose of > 300 mg/m²/day). These values normalize after bexarotene is stopped. In most patients, either antilipemic medication or dose reduction of bexarotene allowed contol over elevated levels. Rarely, patients with markedly elevated triglycerides (lowest level 770 mg/dL) can develop pancreatitis, which can be fatal. Patients with risk factors for pancreatitis should not receive the drug (e.g., history of pancreatitis, uncontrolled hyperlipidemia, uncontrolled diabetes mellitus, biliary tract disease, or medications known to increase triglyceride levels or to be associated with pancreatic toxicity). Uncommonly, patients may have elevated LFTs (5% of patients receiving an initial dose of 300 mg/m²/day and 7% when doses of > 300 mg/m²/day were used), but one patient developed cholestasis and died of liver failure in clinical trials. Nausea/vomiting occurs in 15%/3% of patients receiving a dose of 300 mg/m²/day and 7%/13% of patients receiving doses of > 300 mg/m²/day. Anorexia affects 2% of patients receiving a dose of 300 mg/m²/day, and 22% of patients receiving higher doses.

Nursing Implications: Assess baseline triglyceride, cholesterol, and HDL levels. If abnormal, discuss pharmacological management plan, e.g., atorvastatin, as fasting triglyceride level should be normal before patient begins therapy. Gemfibrozzil should NOT be used. Fasting triglyceride level should then be monitored weekly until the lipid response to bexarotene is known (2–4 weeks), then at 8-week intervals. Goal is to keep fasting triglyceride level < 400 mg/dL to prevent pancreatitis. If fasting triglyceride level becomes elevated during treatment, discuss with physician antilipemic medication, e.g., atorvastatin, and if no response, discuss with physician bexarotene dose reduction or drug holiday. Teach patient about importance of testing fasting triglycerides, and monitoring level throughout treatment. LFTs should be assessed baseline, and after 1, 2, and 4 weeks of starting treatment; if stable, then assess every 8 weeks during treatment. Monitor serum LFTs, HDL, and discuss any abnormalitites with physician (manufacturer recommends suspension or discontinuance of bexarotene if LFTs (SGOT/AST, SGPT/ALT, and bilirubin) > 3x ULN). Assess baseline nutritional status, teach patient that nausea, vomiting, and anorexia may occur and to report them. If these occur, teach strategies to minimize occurrence, and if ineffective or symptoms are severe, discuss pharmacologic management with physician.

II. ALTERATION IN ACTIVITY, POTENTIAL, related to HYPOTHYROIDISM (oral capsules)

Defining Characteristics: Bexarotene binds and activates retinoid × receptors, and can partner with thyroid receptor; once activated, the receptor functions as a transcription factor that regulates gene expression controlling cellular differentiation and proliferation. Drug induces reversible clinical hypothyroidism in about 50% of patients (decrease in TSH in 60% of patients, and total T4 in 45% of patients at a dose of 300 mg/m^2/day), and hypothyroidism was reported in 29% of patients. Asthenia occurs in 29.8% of patients at a dose of 300 mg/m^2/day and in 45% of patients at higher doses.

Nursing Implications: Assess baseline thyroid function tests (TFTs), and discuss pharmacologic replacement of thyroid hormone with physician if values indicate hypothyroidism. Monitor TFTs during treatment. Teach patient that this may occur, importance of laboratory testing, fact that hypothyroidism induced by drug is reversible following discontinuance of drug, and to report signs/symptoms of hypothyroidism (e.g., weight gain, lethargy, slowed thinking, skin dryness, constipation, joint pain/stiffness). Teach patient to alternate rest and activity periods, and other measures to conserve energy.

III. POTENTIAL FOR INFECTION related to LEUKOPENIA (oral capsules)

Defining Characteristics: Reversible leukopenia (WBC/mm^3 1000–3000) occurred in 18% of patients receiving dose of 300 mg/m^2/day, and in 43% of patients receiving higher doses. Patients receiving 300 mg/m^2/day had grade 3 (12%) and grade 4 (4%) neutropenia. Incidence of bacterial infection was 1.2% in patients receiving dose of 300 mg/m^2/day (overall body infection was 13%), and bacterial infection was 13% (overall infections 22%) in patients receiving higher doses. Onset of leukopenia was 4–8 weeks. Resolution of leukopenia/neutropenia occurred in 30 days with drug dose reduction or discontinuance in most patients (82–93%). There were rare serious adverse events associated with leukopenia/neutropenia.

Nursing Implications: Assess baseline WBC, ANC and periodically during therapy. Teach patient that leukopenia may occur, and teach self-care measures, including self-assessment for infection, minimizing risk of infection, and when to notify provider. Teach patient/family signs/symptoms of infection, and how to take temperature if this is not known.

IV. ALTERATION IN BOWEL ELIMINATION related to DIARRHEA (oral capsules)

Defining Characteristics: Diarrhea is uncommon in patients receiving dose of 300 mg/m^2/day, but is more common (41%) when dose is increased.

Teach self-care strategies to minimize risk of infection and bleeding, including avoidance of OTC aspirin-containing medications.

III. ALTERATION IN NUTRITION, LESS THAN BODY REQUIREMENTS, related to NAUSEA, DIARRHEA, DECREASED APPETITE, CONSTIPATION, VOMITING, AND DEHYDRATION

Defining Characteristics: Patients on clinical studies developed these symptoms with the following incidence: nausea (64%), diarrhea (51%), decreased appetite (43%), constipation (43%), vomiting (36%), dehydration (18%). Diarrhea, nausea, and vomiting occur 6–24 hours after infusion. Diarrhea and constipation may occur during cycles 1 and 2, and then disappear.

Nursing Implications: Assess baseline weight and nutritional status, and monitor prior to each treatment. Assess electrolytes prior to each treatment to weekly, especially serum sodium and potassium; replete as necessary and teach diet high in sodium and potassium. Teach patient that serum electrolytes may be decreased and to assess for s/s: hyponatremia (confusion, weakness, seizures), hypokalemia (muscle weakness, confusion, irregular heart beats), hypercalcemia (constipation, thirst, confusion, muscle cramps, sleepiness), and hypomagnesemia (muscle cramps, headache, weakness). Teach patient that side effects may occur, self-care strategies, and to report them if symptoms do not resolve. Use aggressive antiemetics to prevent nausea and vomiting: serotonin antagonist IV prior to bortezomib dose, and for 36 hours after each drug dose. If diarrhea develops after 1st treatment, teach patient to take loperamide prior to next dose of bortezomib and after every loose stool × 36 hours (not to exceed 8 tablets a day), as well as to use the BRAT diet (bananas, rice, applesauce, toast). If patient develops constipation, teach preventative self-care (stool softener, flax seed oil, MOM, prunes or prune juice q am to ensure BM at least q o day). Teach patient to drink 2 quarts of fluid daily, drinking 1 glass an hour while awake to prevent dehydration. Teach patient to report dizziness, lightheadedness, or fainting spells, and to avoid operating heavy machinery or driving a car if these occur. Develop symptom management plan with physician. Make referral to dietitian as appropriate.

IV. ALTERATION IN OXYGENATION, POTENTIAL, related to HYPOTENSION

Defining Characteristics: Orthostatic hypotension/postural hypotension can affect up to 12% of patients throughout therapy.

Nursing Implications: Identify patients at risk: patients with history of syncope, dehydration, or taking medications associated with hypotension. Assess baseline cardiac status, including blood pressure and heart rate, noting rhythm and rate. Teach patient to prevent injury by gradual change in position, and to report any dizziness. Teach patients to avoid dehydration, especially in warm climates. If hypotension noted, assess patient tolerance and need for intervention; discuss management with physician.

V. ALTERATION IN COMFORT related to ASTHENIA, PYREXIA, HEADACHE, INSOMNIA, EDEMA, DIZZINESS, RASH, MYALGIA, MUSCLE CRAMPS, BLURRED VISION

Defining Characteristics: Asthenia (characterized by fatigue, malaise, and weakness) was most common, affecting 65% of patients in clinical trials. Other symptoms included pyrexia (36%), headache (28%), insomnia (27%), arthralgias (26%), edema (26%), dyspnea (22%), dizziness (21%), myalgia (14%), pruritus (11%) and blurred vision (11%).

Nursing Implications: Assess comfort and presence of discomfort, fatigue, peripheral edema, baseline and prior to each treatment. Teach patient that these side effects may occur and to report them. Teach patient local comfort measures as well as energy conservation, and discuss management plan with physician if ineffective.

Drug: cetuximab (Erbitux)

Class: Chimeric (mouse/human) monoclonal antibody targeted against epidermal growth factor receptor (EGFR).

Mechanism of Action: Blocks growth factor (ligand, such as epidermal growth factor and transforming growth factor-alpha) from binding to EGFR, thus preventing dimerization and initiation of cell signaling via receptor tyrosine kinase phosphorylation; thus, the message telling the cell to divide does not occur. In addition to cell growth inhibition, there is induction of apoptosis, and decreased matrix metalloproteinase and vascular endothelial growth factor production. Drug is synergistic with chemotherapy and radiotherapy as it appears to prevent the malignant cell from repairing DNA damage.

Metabolism: Drug is an IgG_1 chimerized antibody, and it is postulated that clearance is via binding of the antibody to EGFR of hepatocytes with internalization of the cetuximab-EGFR complex. Mean elimination half-life is approximately 97 hours (range, 41–213 h). Steady state reached by 3rd weekly infusion. Mean half-life is 114 hours (range 75–188 h). Females have a 25% lower clearance of drug than males, but there was no difference in efficacy. No differences were found related to race, age, and hepatic and renal functional impairment.

- Responses have been shown in irinotecan refractory colorectal cancer when adding cetuximab to irinotecan, cisplatin refractory squamous cell cancer of the head and neck when adding cetuximab to cisplatin, and when added to radiotherapy in the treatment of patients with unresectable squamous cell cancer of the head and neck.
- Early testing in patients with pancreatic, nonsmall cell lung cancer or ovarian cancers is underway.
- Drug is antigenically similar to humanized monoclonal antibodies.
- Very rarely (< 0.5%), interstitial lung disease may occur, which may be complicated with non cardiogenicpulmonary edema and death. Onset is between 4–11th cycle of cetuximab, and is more likely in patients with pre-existing fibrotic lung disease. Hold drug and evaluate patients who develop acute or worsening pulmonary symptoms. Discontinue the drug if interstitial lung disease is found.
- Skin toxicity (acneform rash) is major toxicity; patients should be taught to wear sunscreen and hats, as well as to limit sun exposure. Rash is not acne.
- EGFR overexpression determination should be done by a laboratory with demonstrated proficiency.
- Women of childbearing age should use effective contraception, and for 60 days from the last dose of cetuximab; nursing mothers should not nurse during cetuximab and for 60 days from the last dose of the drug.

Potential Toxicities/Side Effects and the Nursing Process

I. POTENTIAL FOR INJURY related to HYPERSENSITIVITY/ ANAPHYLAXIS and INFUSION REACTION

Defining Characteristics: 19–25% of patients experience an infusion reaction. Rarely it is severe (3% of patients receiving drug in combination with Irinotecan, and 2% In patients receiving monotherapy), characterized by rapid onset of airway obstruction (bronchospams, stridor, hoarseness), urticaria, and/or hypotension. In some cases this may be fatal. Most (90%) occur during the 1st infusion. Mild-to-moderate infusion reactions characterized by chills, fever, dyspnea usually occur during the 1st infusion in 16% of patients receiving combination therapy, and 23% of patients receiving monotherapy. In addition, 73% of patients who received the combination reported asthenia vs 49% who received monotherapy; 33% fever, 9% chills, 7% headache, and 7% mucous membrane disorder (MMD).

Nursing Implications: Ensure patient receives premedication with diphenhydramine as ordered. Assess baseline VS and mental status prior to drug administration, at 15 minutes, and periodically during infusion, as needed. Remain with patient during first 15 minutes of first infusions. Recall signs/symptoms of anaphylaxis, and if these occur, stop drug immediately, notify physician, and assess patient's vital signs. Subjective symptoms are generalized itching, nausea, chest tightness, crampy abdominal pain, difficulty speaking, anxiety, agitation, sense of impending doom, uneasiness, desire to urinate/defecate, dizziness, and chills. Objective signs are flushed appearance; angioedema of face, neck, eyelids, hands, and feet; localized or generalized urticaria; respiratory distress with or without wheezing; hypotension; and cyanosis. Review standing orders or nursing procedures for patient management of anaphylaxis, and be prepared to stop drug immediately, notify physician, monitor VS, and administer ordered medications, which may include epinephrine 1:1000, hydrocortisone sodium succinate, and diphenhydramine. Teach patient to report any unusual symptoms. For mild-to-moderate infusion reactions (grade 1–2), decrease infusion rate permanently by 50%. Drug should be discontinued in patients who experience severe infusion reactions (grade 3/4).

II. POTENTIAL ALTERATION IN BODY IMAGE, SKIN INTEGRITY, COMFORT related to SKIN RASH

Defining Characteristics: Drug inhibits epidermal growth factor receptor, so major toxicity is manifested in the skin. Most patients (88%–90%) develop a mild-to-moderate acne-like rash that is self-limiting. 14% report a grade 3 rash, and in clinical studies 1.6% of patients discontinued treatment due to skin rash. Rash is a sterile, suppurative rash with multiple follicular or pustular lesions that appear during the first 2 weeks of therapy on the face, upper chest and back, but in some cases, extended to the arms. Rash resolves when treatment is stopped, without scar formation. However, in 50% of patients, it takes longer than 28 days to resolve. 7% of patients reported dry skin, which may be associated with fissures and in some cases, inflammation and infection such as blepharitis and cellulitis. Infection can be treated with topical clindamycin, or oral antibiotics. Do not use topical corticosteroid cream. It appears that patients who have significant rash, also have a tumor response.

Nursing Implications: Teach patient that rash most likely will occur due to mechanism of drug action. Assess baseline skin integrity on areas of face, neck, and trunk; assess baseline comfort and satisfaction with body image, and monitor at each treatment. Teach patient to report any distress and assess extent of rash. Drug is held for 1–2 weeks for severe rash, and if it resolves, dose is reduced on and after the 2nd occurrence. If rash does not resolve, drug is stopped. If skin appears to be infected, discuss with physician, the prescription of clindamycin gel (Cleocin T) or oral cephalexin (Keflex) 250 mg PO bid × 3 days, then 250 mg qd × 7 days, for a total of 10 days for skin infection. Rash is not acne, and so usual anti-acne treatment will not be effective.

III. ALTERATION IN NUTRITION, LESS THAN BODY REQUIREMENTS, related to NAUSEA, VOMITING, DIARRHEA, STOMATITIS/ MUCOUS MEMBRANE DISORDER, CONSTIPATION, WEIGHT LOSS

Defining Characteristics: Incidence of mild-to-moderate digestive symptoms include nausea (55% for combination patients, and 29% for monotherapy), diarrhea (72% vs 28%), vomiting (41% vs 25%), stomatitits/mucous membrane disorder (26% vs 11%), weight loss (21% vs 9%), anorexia (36% vs 25%), and constipation (30%).

Nursing Implications: Assess baseline weight and nutritional status. Teach patient that these symptoms may occur, and to report them. Administer antiemetic and other symptom management medications as ordered. Teach patient self-administration of these medications at home. Teach patient dietary modifications to address symptoms such as anorexia (small, frequent high-calorie, high-protein foods, stimulants as permitted by protocol); constipation (high-fiber, high-fluid, high-roughage foods, stool softeners); diarrhea (bananas, rice, applesauce, and toast); nausea (avoid food preparation odors by cooking in zipped plastic bag, or having someone else cook; choose cool, soft, non-spicy, or fatty foods). Assess efficacy of intervention, and revise plan as needed.

IV. POTENTIAL FOR INFECTION AND FATIGUE related to LEUKOPENIA AND ANEMIA

Defining Characteristics: Leukopenia occurs in about 25% of patients (combination vs 1% monotherapy) with 17% grade 3–4 (combination) and anemia in 16% (combination vs 10% monotherapy (4–5% grade 3–4).

Nursing Implications: Assess baseline wbc, hematocrit and hemoglobin, and monitor prior to each treatment, especially if drug is given in combination with irinotecan Teach patient to monitor temperature, and report temperature > 100.5°F. Assess level of fatigue and teach energy baseline and prior to each treatment. Teach patient that fatigue may occur due to anemia, and teach energy conserving strategies such as alternating rest and activity periods.

Drug: denileukin diftitox (ONTAK®)

Class: Fusion protein.

Mechanism of Action: Agent is recombinant DNA-derived cytotoxic protein containing diphtheria toxin fragments, and IL-2. It targets cells with high affinity for IL-2 receptors containing a CD25 component, such as activated T and B lymphocytes, and activated macrophages. The IL-2 portion of the fusion protein binds to the IL-2 receptor on malignant cells, which contain a CD25 component. The diphtheria toxin fragments are brought into the cell through the receptor (receptor-mediated endocytosis) and into the endosomal vesicles. Acidification cleaves the active fragment of diphtheria toxin, which is then actively transported into the cytoplasm. There, it catalyzes a reaction that inhibits protein synthesis and causes cell death within hours.

Metabolism: Distribution phase has half-life of 2–5 minutes, and terminal phase half-life of 70–80 minutes; the development of antibodies to denileukin diftitox significantly increases clearance 2–3 times, with a consequent decrease in mean systemic exposure of about 75%. Metabolized by proteolytic degradation and primarily excreted via the liver and kidneys; excreted material is < 25% of total dose.

Dosage/Range:

- 9 or 18 mcg/kg/day IV daily × 5 days, repeated every 3 weeks × at least 3 cycles.

Drug Preparation:

- Bring ONTAK vial to room temperature (25°C, or 77°F); may thaw in refrigerator at 2–8°C (36–46°F) over less than 24 hours, or at room temperature for 1–2 hours. DO NOT HEAT.
- Mix by gentle swirling. DO NOT SHAKE VIGOROUSLY.
- DO NOT REFREEZE DRUG.
- Inspect solution for clarity and discard if it remains hazy (will be hazy after thawing, but becomes clear when at room temperature).
- Withdraw ordered dose from vial and inject into an empty IV infusion bag; add up to 9 mL of sterile saline without preservative for each 1 mL of ONTAK to the IV bag, for a final concentration of at least 15 mcg/mL.
- Discard any unused portion of the drug.

Drug Administration:

- Give by IV infusion over at least 15 minutes, but less than 80 minutes.
- Slow or stop infusion if infusion reaction occurs, depending upon severity of symptoms.
- DO NOT administer with other drugs, or give through an inline filter.
- Administer prepared IV solution within 6 hours, using a syringe pump or infusion bag.

Drug Interactions:

- Unknown.

Lab Effects/Interference:

- Hypoalbuminemia may occur in up to 83% of patients, with nadir 1–2 weeks after drug administration.

Nursing Implications: Teach patient that flulike symptoms may occur commonly following treatment, and teach symptom management with antipyretics (e.g., acetaminophen) and dietary modification if nausea experienced. Discuss with physician giving patient prescription for antiemetic agent in case nausea is severe or vomiting develops. Discuss use of meperidine, diphenhydramine if patient develops rigors. Teach patient to call nurse or physician if symptoms do not respond, become worse, if unable to take at least 1 qt of fluid orally per day, or new symptoms develop.

V. ALTERATION IN NUTRITION related to DIARRHEA, ANOREXIA, NAUSEA/VOMITING, HYPOALBUMINEMIA

Defining Characteristics: Nausea/vomiting occurs in 64% of patients as part of flulike syndrome, anorexia occurs in 36% of patients, and diarrhea occurs in 29%. Hypoalbuminemia occurs in 83%, weight loss in 14%, and elevated transaminases 61%. Elevation of serum transaminases occurred during first cycle of therapy, and resolved within two weeks. Hypocalcemia (17%) and hypokalemia (6%) have also been reported. Constipation occurred in 9%, dyspepsia 7%, and dysphagia 6%. Rarely, pancreatitis, hyperthyroidism, and hypothyroidism may occur.

Nursing Implications: Assess baseline nutritional status, as well as baseline LFTs and serum albumin, and monitor weekly during therapy. Teach patient to eat high-calorie, high-protein foods. Assess for occurrence of symptoms of nausea, vomiting, diarrhea, anorexia, other problems, and teach patient to report them. Teach patient self-administration of prescribed medications to manage symptoms.

VI. ALTERATION IN COMFORT related to SKIN RASHES, PAIN AT TUMOR SITES

Defining Characteristics: During clinical trials, rash occurred in 34%, pruritus 20%, and sweating 10%. Rashes occurred during/after treatment or were delayed. They were varied, as generalized maculopapular, petechial, vesicular bullous, urticarial, or as eczema.

Nursing Implications: Assess baseline skin integrity and presence of rashes. Assess daily during treatment and weekly thereafter; teach patient to report any skin changes. Assess need for diphenhydramine or other antihistamines for pruritus, and use of topical and/or oral corticosteroids for moderate to severe rashes and discomfort.

VII. POTENTIAL ALTERATION IN CARDIAC OUTPUT related to HYPOTENSION, TACHYCARDIA, THROMBOTIC EVENTS

Defining Characteristics: The following cardiovascular side effects occurred in clinical testing: hypotension (36%), vasodilation (22%), tachycardia (12%), thrombotic events (7%), hypertension (6%), and arrythmia (6%). Two patients with preexisting coronary artery disease developed myocardial infarctions while receiving the drug. Thrombotic events included deep vein thrombosis, pulmonary embolus, arterial thrombosis, and superficial thrombophlebitis.

Nursing Implications: Assess baseline cardiovascular status and presence of risk factor of coronary artery disease. Teach patient to report any chest pain or discomfort, palpitations, pain in calf, heat/redness of calf immediately, or to come to the emergency room if at home. Discuss onset of hypotension, tachycardia with physician, relationship to drug administration, and management strategies. If symptoms severe, stop drug infusion and discuss use of saline hydration to raise BP and decrease HR.

VIII. POTENTIAL FOR FATIGUE AND BLEEDING related to BONE MARROW SUPPRESSION

Defining Characteristics: Anemia occurs in about 18% (6% grades 3 or 4), thrombocytopenia in 8% (2% grades 3 or 4), and leukopenia in 6% (3% grades 3 or 4).

Nursing Implications: Monitor CBC/differential, HCT, and platelet count and assess for signs/symptoms of infection, fatigue, and bleeding baseline prior to treatment, and weekly during treatment. Instruct patient in self-assessment of signs/symptoms of infection, fatigue, bleeding. Transfuse platelet, red cell transfusions per physician's order.

IX. POTENTIAL ALTERATION IN OXYGENATION related to DYSPNEA, COUGH

Defining Characteristics: In clinical trials, 29% of patients reported dyspnea, 26% increased cough, 17% pharyngitis, 13% rhinitis, and 8% "lung disorder."

Nursing Implications: Assess VS, pulmonary exam, and weight prior to each treatment, and at each weekly visit. Teach patient to do daily weights, and to report any SOB, weight gain, increased cough, or other problems. If this occurs, notify physician and discuss obtaining CXR and focused exam. Discuss chest X-ray findings with physician.

X. POTENTIAL SENSORY/PERCEPTUAL ALTERATIONS related to NERVOUSNESS, CONFUSION, INSOMNIA

Defining Characteristics: Nervousness may affect 11%, confusion 8%, and insomnia 9%.

Nursing Implications: Teach patient that these symptoms may occur and to report them. Assess baseline mental status, affect, and sleep pattern prior to each treatment cycle, and weekly during treatment. Discuss need for pharmacologic symptom management if symptoms are severe.

XI. POTENTIAL ALTERATION IN URINE ELIMINATION related to HEMATURIA, ALBUMINURIA, PYURIA

Defining Characteristics: Patients in clinical trials experienced hematuria (10%), albuminuria (10%), and pyuria (10%). 7% had increases in serum creatinine. Rarely, acute renal insufficiency occurs.

Nursing Implications: Assess baseline urinary elimination status, urinalysis, as well as serum renal function studies. Teach patient to report blood in urine, and dysuria, or any problems in voiding. Discuss abnormalities with physician.

Drug: edrecolomab (moAb 17–1A) (investigational)

Class: Monoclonal antibody.

Mechanism of Action: Murine monoclonal antibody that recognizes the human tumor-associated antigen glycoprotein 17–1A or Ep-CAM, that is expressed on epithelial tissues, and in many colon and rectal cancers.

Metabolism: Unknown.

Dosage/Range:
Per protocol in combination with 5-FU/LV.

Drug Preparation/Administration: Per protocol.

Drug Interactions: Unknown.

Lab Effects/Interference: Unknown.

Special Considerations:

- An initial study of 189 patients showed survival benefit of 32% in patients with resected Stage III colon cancer when given in the adjuvant setting (Riethmuller et al, 1994), compared to surgery alone, but these data were not replicated in a later international study of 2761 patients (Punt et al, 2002), which showed that edrecolomab alone is inferior to 5-FU/LV adjuvant chemotherapy and that, when given in combination with 5-FU/LV adjuvant chemotherapy, it did not increase overall survival.

- Drug is well tolerated and did not increase the incidence of neutropenia, diarrhea, or mucositis when combined with 5-FU/LV.

Potential Toxicities/Side Effects and the Nursing Process

I. POTENTIAL FOR INJURY related to HYPERSENSITIVITY/ ANAPHYLAXIS and INFUSION REACTION

Defining Characteristics: 25% of patients experienced a hypersensitivity reaction, causing discontinuation in 4% of patients. Drug is a murine monoclonal antibody, largely made up of mouse antibody. Allergic reactions may be mild characterized by chills, fever, dyspnea, or severe, characterized by rapid onset of airway obstruction (bronchospams, stridor, hoarseness), urticaria, and/or hypotension.

Nursing Implications: Ensure patient receives premedication with diphenhydramine per protocol. Assess baseline VS and mental status prior to drug administration, at 15 minutes, and periodically during infusion, as needed. Remain with patient during first 15 minutes of first infusions. Recall signs/ symptoms of anaphylaxis, and if these occur, stop drug immediately, notify physician, and assess patient's vital signs. Subjective symptoms are generalized itching, nausea, chest tightness, crampy abdominal pain, difficulty speaking, anxiety, agitation, sense of impending doom, uneasiness, desire to urinate/ defecate, dizziness, and chills. Objective signs are flushed appearance; angioedema of face, neck, eyelids, hands, and feet; localized or generalized urticaria; respiratory distress with or without wheezing; hypotension; and cyanosis. Review standing orders or nursing procedures for patient management of anaphylaxis, and be prepared to stop drug immediately, notify physician, monitor VS, and administer ordered medications, which may include epinephrine 1:1000, hydrocortisone sodium succinate, and diphenhydramine. Teach patient to report any unusual symptoms.

Drug: erlotinib (OSI-774, Tarceva™)

Class: Epidermal Growth Factor Receptor (HER1/EGFR) tyrosine kinase inhibitor (quinazoline type).

Mechanism of Action: Mechanism of anti-tumor activity not fully characterized. Inhibits the cytoplasmic protein (tyrosine kinase) domain of the EGFR.

Metabolism: Drug bioavailability is about 60% after oral administration with peak plasma concentration ocurring 4 hours after ingestion. Drug is highly protein-bound (90–95%). It is primarily metabolized by the cytochrome P450 hepatic microsomal enzyme system (CYP3A4). Food can increase drug bioavailability by 100%.

Dosage/Range:
- 150 mg PO q day.

Drug Preparation/Administration:
- Oral, available in 150-, 100-, and 25-mg tablets.
- Dose should be taken on an empty stomach, either 1 hour before meals or 2 hours after meals.

Drug Interactions:
- *Inducers of the CYP3A4* (may increase metabolism of erlotinib and decrease its plasma concentration): rifampin, phenytoin, phenobarbitol, St. John's Wort, carbamazepine, rifapentin, rifabuten. May need to increase dose of erlotinib.
- *Inhibitors of the CYP3A4* (may increase metabolism of erlotinib and increase its plasma concentration): ketoconazole, itraconazole, grapefruit (fruit or juice), clarithromycin, ritonavir, indinavir, atanazavir, nelfinavir, saquinavir, metronidazole, isoniazid, telithromycin, troleandomycin, voriconazole. May need to decrease dose of erlotinib.
- *Warfarin* increases INR and bleeding possible; monitor INR, patient bleeding, and decrease warfarin dose as needed.

Lab Effects/Interference:
- May increase liver function tests (serum transaminases).

Special Considerations:
- Drug is FDA approved for the treatment of patients with locally advanced or metastatic Non-Small Cell lung cancer after failure of at least one prior chemotherapy regimen.
- Infrequently, drug can cause interstitial lung disease (ILD) (< 1% of patients), which can be serious. This is a class effect, and similar to that of gelfitinib. Drug should be stopped immediately in patients who develop worsening or unexplained pulmonary symptoms, and appropriate diagnostic work-up begun to establish the cause. If ILD is diagnosed, erlotinib should be discontinued.
- Drug can cause conjunctivitis and drying of eyes, ameliorated by artificial tears.
- Patients may require temporary interruption or dose reduction for severe diarrhea that does not resolve with anti-diarrheals, or for severe and intolerable rash; dose modification if refractory or intolerable. Also, consider if patient has severe liver dysfunction.

Potential Toxicities/Side Effects and the Nursing Process

I. ALTERATION IN SKIN INTEGRITY related to RASH

Defining Characteristics: As expected, because EGFR is important in skin function, this is the area of major toxicity. Rash ranges from maculopapular to pustular on the face, neck, chest, back, and arms, affecting up to 75% of patients. Most rashes are mild to moderate (Sandler et al, 2004). Typically, rash begins on days 8–10 of therapy, maximizing in intensity by week 2, and resolving gradually on therapy (often by week 4). Use of skin treatments (corticosteroids, topical clindamycin, or minocycline) have been used with varying results.

Nursing Implications: Assess skin integrity of face, neck, arms, and upper trunk baseline, and regularly during treatment. Teach patient that rash may occur, its usual course, and self-care measures for comfort. Emphasize the need to keep skin with rash clean to prevent infection, and to continue taking erlotinib until told to stop by nurse or physician. Teach patient that skin may become dry, and to use skin emollients or moisturizers. Assess body image intactness, and if rash develops, its threat to body image. Encourage patient to verbalize feelings; provide emotional support, and individualize care plan to patient response.

II. ALTERATION IN ELIMINATION PATTERN related to DIARRHEA

Defining Characteristics: Affects approximately 54% of patients, and is mild to moderate with only 6% of patients experiencing grade 3 diarrhea. Diarrhea usually beginning weeks 3–4. Symptoms may be self-limited or require an anti-diarrheal agent, such as loperamide. Severe diarrhea not responsive to anti-diarrheal medication may require temporary dose-interruption or adjustment if refractory.

Nursing Implications: Assess bowel elimination pattern baseline, and regularly during therapy. Teach patient to report diarrhea; teach patient self-care strategies to manage diarrhea such as dietary modification and self-administration of loperamide; teach patient to minimize potential complications such as dehydration and electrolye depletion. If diarrhea does not resolve or is severe, discuss with physician dose interruption, as well as fluid and electrolyte replacement.

III. SENSORY/PERCEPTUAL ALTERATION, POTENTIAL related to CONJUNCTIVITIS AND EYE DRYNESS

Defining Characteristics: Conjunctivits and eye dryness may occur, and are generally mild to moderate (grades 1–2).

Nursing Implications: Teach patient to report any eye irritation or change in visual acuity. Teach patient to use artificial tears to keep eyes lubricated.

IV. POTENTIONAL ALTERATION IN NUTRITION, LESS THAN BODY REQUIREMENTS related to MUCOSITIS and ANOREXIA

Defining Characteristics: Stomatitis is uncommon, occurring in 17% of patients receiving erlotinib, compared to 3% receiving placebo. Grade 3/4 occurs in <1% of patients. It is usually mild to moderate and is generally self-limited. Anorexia affects about 52% of patients with 8% experiencing grade 3.

Nursing Implications: Assess oral hygiene practices, and status of oral mucosa, gums, and teeth baseline, and regularly throughout therapy. Teach patient to report stomatitis, and to use a systematic cleansing regime as determined by institutional policy.

Drug: gefitinib (Iressa)

Class: Tyrosine kinase inhibitor.

Mechanism of Action: Drug inhibits the intracellular phosphorylation of a number of tyrosine kinases associated with transmembrane cell surface receptors, including the epidermal growth factor receptor (EGFR-TK). This prevents the message for cell division from being sent to the nucleus. Thus cell division, growth, and angiogenesis do not occur.

Metabolism: Absorbed slowly from the gastrointestinal tract following oral administration with peak plasma levels occurring 3–7 hours after dosing. Bioavailability 60%, and unaffected by food. Drug is 90% protein bound (serum albumin). Drug is metabolized via the P450 microenzyme system, primarily the CYP 3A4 subsystem, and excreted in the feces (86%). Elimination half-life 48 hours with steady state plasma level achieved within 10 days.

Dosage/Range:

250 mg po qd. As of 9/15/05, the manufacturer, Astra Zeneca, is limiting availability of the drug to patients who have previously taken the drug and are benefiting, or who have benefited. The drug will be available through the IRESSA access program only. In clinical trials, the drug will be available to patients who are enrolled. If new study data shows an improvement in survival, then the labeling will change.

Drug Preparation: Available as 250 mg tablets in a bottle of 30 tablets.

Drug Administration: Administer with or without food at about the same time each day

- If severe diarrhea or skin reaction, briefly interrupt therapy for up to 14 days, and then resume at same dose.
- If new onset or worsening of pulmonary symptoms (dyspnea, cough, fever), interrupt therapy until pulmonary evaluation can rule out interstitial lung disease. IF interstitial lung disease confirmed, STOP gefitinib and treat pulmonary toxicity.
- If new onset eye pain or other eye symptoms, interrupt therapy and evaluate cause.
- If patient receiving concomitant potent CYP3A4 inducer (e.g., rifampicin or phenytoin), consider increasing dose to 500 mg q d in the absence of severe drug reaction.

Drug Interactions:

- Inducers of CYP3A4 (increase metabolism of gefitinib and decrease its plasma concentrations or AUC by 85%): rifamicin, phenytoin; consider increasing gefitinib dose to 500 mg/da.
- Inhibitors of CYP 3A4 (decrease metabolism of gefitinib and increase its plasma concentration or AUC by 88%): Itraconazole; consider another antifungal or decrease gefitinib if increased toxicity.
- High gastric pH > 5.0 (e.g., ranitidine with sodium bicarbonate: decrease gefitinib AUC by 44%).
- Warfarin: increased INR and bleeding; monitor INR frequently and patient for s/s bleeding and decrease warfarin dose accordingly.

Lab Effects/Interference:

- Asymptomatic elevations in liver function tests (transaminases, bilirubin and alkaline phosphatase).

Special Considerations:

- Indicated as monotherapy for the treatment of patients with locally advanced or metastatic non-small cell lung cancer (NSCLC) after failure of both platinum-based and docetaxel chemotherapies. Given the response rate of 10%, and the fact that there was no survival advantage together with the fact that erlotinib (Tarceva) has since been FDA approved, based on clinical evidence of a survival advantage, gelfitinib is now restricted. Effective 9/15/05, drug is only available to 1) patients who are currently or who have previously taken the drug and are benefiting, or who have benefited and 2) previously enrolled patients or new patients in non-Investigational New Drug (IND) clinical trials approved by an IRB prior to 6/17/05. The drug will be available through the IRESSA access program only.

Nursing Implications: Assess baseline comfort, energy/activity level, and ability to do self-care. Teach patient that these side effects may occur, and energy conservation strategies to manage them. If patient unable to do ADLs, assess need for home support from outside agency.

VI. SENSORY/PERCEPTUAL ALTERATIONS, POTENTIAL related to VISUAL AND OCULAR CHANGES

Defining Characteristics: Amblyopia occurred in 2% of patients, and conjunctivitis 1%. There are reports of patients with eye pain and corneal erosion/ulceration, sometimes associated with abnormal eyelash growth. In addition, rarely, corneal membrane sloughing and ocular ischemia/hemorrhage occurred.

Nursing Implications: Teach patient to stop drug and report any eye discomfort or visual changes immediately. Discuss referral of patient to ophthalmologist for evaluation and advice. Discuss drug continuance with physician depending upon cause of problem.

Drug: gemtuzumab ozogamicin for injection (Mylotarg)

Class: Monoclonal antibody conjugated to a cytotoxic antibiotic.

Mechanism of Action: Drug is composed of a recombinant hymanized Ig4 kappa antibody conjugated with a cytotoxic antitumor antibiotic, calicheamicin. The antibody portion of the drug binds to the CD33 antigen found on the cell surface of leukemic blast and immature normal cells in the myeloid cell line but not the pleuripotent stem cell. The CD33 antigen is expressed on more than 80% of patients with acute myeloid leukemia. 98.3% of the amino acids used are of human origin, while the remainder are derived from murine antibody. Once the MoAb binds to the CD33 antibody, the complex is brought inside the cell, calicheamicin is released inside lysosomes within the myeloid cell and then binds to DNA, resulting in DNA double-strand breaks and cell death.

Metabolism: Following first dose, terminal half-lives of total and unconjugated calicheamicin were 45 and 100 hours, while after the second dose 14 days later, the terminal half-life of total calicheamicin was 60 hours, and the area under the concentration-time curve was double that following the first treatment. The cytotoxic drug calicheamicin derivative is hydrolyzed to release it from the monoclonal antibody and forms many metabolites.

Dosage/Range:
9 mg/m^2 given as a 2-hour IV infusion q14 days × 2.

- Premedicate 1 hour before the drug is given with diphenhydramine 50 mg PO and acetaminophen 650–1000 mg PO, with acetaminophen repeated q4h × 2 PRN.

Drug Preparation:
- Protect from direct and indirect sunlight and unshielded fluorescent light during preparation and administration of drug (fluorescent light must be turned off in biological safety cabinet during preparation).
- Allow refrigerated vials to come to room temperature.
- Reconstitute 5 mg vial with 5 mL sterile water for injection, USP, using sterile syringes. Gently swirl the vial to dissolve. Final concentration is 1 mg/mL. While in the amber vial, the reconstituted solution can be refrigerated (2–8°C, 36–36°F) and protected from light for up to 8 hrs.
- Withdraw ordered dose and inject into 100 mL bag of 0.9% Normal Saline Injection, and then place the bag inside an UV-protectant bag. Use the medication immediately.

Drug Administration:
- Premedicate 1 hour before the drug is given with diphenhydramine 50 mg PO and acetaminophen 650–1000 mg PO, with acetaminophen repeated q4h × 2 PRN.
- Administer in light-protected bag IV over 2 hours via separate IV tubing containing a 1.2 micron terminal filter.
- Can be given via peripheral or central IV line.
- DO NOT administer by IVP or bolus.

Drug Interactions:
- Unknown.

Lab Effects/Interference:
- Increased LFTs.
- Hyperglycemia (part of post-infusion syndrome).
- Significant decrease in WBC, Hgb/HCT, platelet count.
- Increased LDH.
- Decreased serum K, Mg.

Special Considerations:
- Drug is indicated for the treatment of patients with CD33 positive acute myeloid leukemia in first relapse who are 60 years or older, and who are not considered candidates for cytotoxic chemotherapy.
- Drug is contraindicated in patients with known hypersensitivity to gemtuzumab ozogamicin or its components (anti-CD33 antibody), calicheamicin derivatives, or inactive ingredients and in pregnant or nursing women.
- Give premedication to prevent post-infusion symptom complex.
- Severe myelosuppression will occur in all patients, and systemic infections must be treated.

- Use cautiously in patients with renal or hepatic dysfunction.
- Women of childbearing age should use effective contraception measures.
- Rarely, patient may develop antibodies to calicheamicin/calicheamicin-linker portion of gemtuzumab ozogamicin (2 patients, after 3 doses of drug, characterized by transient fever, hypotension, dyspnea in 1 patient), but in clinical trials no patient developed antibody responses to the antibody portion of Mylotarg.
- Tumor lysis syndrome may occur commonly in leukemic patients, so patients should be well hydrated, receive allopurinol, and receive alkalinization if at risk (high tumor burden).

Potential Toxicities/Side Effects and the Nursing Process

I. POTENTIAL FOR INJURY related to ACUTE INFUSION-RELATED EVENTS

Defining Characteristics: Patients often experience a post-infusion syndrome characterized by chills (62%), fever (61%), nausea (38%), vomiting (32%), headache (12%), hypotension (11%), hypertension (6%), hypoxia (6%), dyspnea (4%), and hyperglycemia (2%). Syndrome may occur any time within 24 hours after administration, and resolves about 2–4 hours later with supportive therapy of acetaminophen, diphenhydramine, and IV fluids. Patients are less likely to experience this syndrome when receiving the second treatment.

Nursing Implications: Premedicate patient as ordered with acetaminophen and diphenhydramine one hour before drug therapy. Ensure that medications necessary for the management of hypersensitivity/anaphylaxis are readily available (e.g., epinephrine, antihistamines, corticosteroids). Assess baseline VS and monitor frequently during the infusion, and for 4 hours post infusion; keep IV line patent. Monitor VS, and notify physician of abnormalities. Be prepared to provide emergency support as necessary (including IV saline, epinephrine, antihistamines, bronchodilators).

II. POTENTIAL FOR INFECTION, BLEEDING, AND FATIGUE related to BONE MARROW DEPRESSION

Defining Characteristics: Severe (grade 3 or 4) neutropenia occurs in 98% of patients, with recovery of an ANC of 500 cells/micro liter by day 40 (after first dose) in those patients who respond. During treatment phase, 28% developed grades 3 and 4 infections, with 16% experiencing sepsis and 7% pneumonia. 22% of patients developed herpes simplex infection. Thrombocytopenia is common, with 99% of patients developing grades 3 and 4. For those responding to treatment, platelet recovery (25,000/microliter) occurs by day 39 after first day of drug. 23% of patients required platelet transfusions. During treatment phase, bleeding occurred in 15% of patients (grades 3 and 4). These episodes included epistaxis (3%), cerebral hemorrhage (2%), disseminated intravasuclar coagulation (2%), intracranial hemorrhage (2%) and hematuria (1%). Anemia also was common, with 47% of patients developing grades 3 and 4 anemia, and 26% of patients requiring transfusions.

Nursing Implications: Monitor CBC, platelets baseline and regularly during treatment. Assess for signs/symptoms of infection, bleeding, and fatigue baseline, between treatment, and prior to each treatment. Teach patient to self-assess for these, including taking temperature, and instruct to report them immediately. Teach patient measures to minimize infection, bleeding, and fatigue, including avoidance of crowds, and not taking OTC medications containing aspirin. Transfuse red blood cells and platelets as ordered. Teach patient strategies to conserve energy and minimize fatigue.

III. ALTERATION IN NUTRITION, POTENTIAL, related to NAUSEA, MUCOSITIS, VOMITING, HEPATOTOXICITY

Defining Characteristics: Nausea is common, affecting 70% of patients, with 63% developing vomiting. Stomatitis affected 35% of patients, with 4% having grades 3 or 4 toxicity. Transient increases in LFTs occurred, and were usually reversible. In clinical studies, 23% of patients developed grades 3 or 4 hyperbilirubinemia, 9% in levels of ALT, and 17% in levels of AST. In clinical studies, there were deaths reported: one patient died with liver failure as part of multisystem failure related to tumor lysis syndrome, another patient died of persistent jaundice and hepatosplenomegaly five months after treatment, and finally, 4 (of 27) patients died of veno-occlusive disease following stem cell transplantation after Mylotarg administration.

Nursing Implications: Assess baseline nutritional status, integrity of oral mucosa, and liver function studies and regularly after treatment. Administer antiemetic medications prior to chemotherapy to prevent nausea/vomiting, and teach patient self-administration of antiemetics after discharge if drug is given on an outpatient basis. Teach patient to report persistent or continued nausea and/or vomiting. Assess efficacy and discuss change in antiemetic drug with physician if regimen ineffective. Teach patient to assess oral mucosa regularly, use oral hygiene regimen, and report signs/symptoms of stomatitis. If patient develops stomatitis, teach patient self-administration of oral analgesics, antifungals, as ordered and appropriate. Monitor liver function tests, and discuss any abnormalities with physician.

IV. ALTERATION IN BOWEL ELIMINATION related to CONSTIPATION OR DIARRHEA

Defining Characteristics: Diarrhea affects 38% of patients, and constipation 25%.

tered biodistribution of Indium-111 Zevalin, patients with ≥ 25% lymphoma marrow involvement or impaired bone marrow reserve.

- 2% incidence of development of secondary malignancy (acute myeloid leukemia, myelodysplastic syndrome). Radiation is a potent carcinogen and mutagen.

Potential Toxicities/Side Effects and the Nursing Process

I. POTENTIAL FOR INJURY related to ANAPHYLAXIS

Defining Characteristics: Rare but potentially life-threatening reaction may occur. Mouse antibodies are used that are foreign and may stimulate anaphylaxis. Rare, fatal anaphylactic reactions have occurred within 24 hours of rituximab dose. Of the reactions, 80% occur during the first rituximab infusion, and within 30–120 minutes of the infusion. Severe infusion reactions include pulmonary infiltrates, acute respiratory distress syndrome, myocardial infarction, ventricular fibrillation, and cardiogenic shock.

Nursing Implications: Assess baseline T, VS. Administer premedications prior to rituximab as ordered, usually acetaminophen and diphenhydramine. Initiate infusion at 50 mg/hr, and increase in 50mg/hr increments q 30 min to a maximum of 400 mg/hr. If patient develops discomfort, slow infusion; stop infusion if reaction is severe. Once symptoms have improved, resume rate at 50% of previous rate. Have emergency equipment and medications nearby, including epinephrine and corticosteroids. Assess patient for signs/symptoms, including generalized flushing andurticaria leading to pallor, cyanosis, bronchospasm, hypotension, unconsciousness. Teach patient to report signs/symptoms, including sense of doom, tickle in throat. If signs/symptoms occur, stop infusion immediately, assess VS, notify physician. Physician may prescribe epinephrine 0.3 mL (1:1000) SQ if hypotensive. Oxygen, antihistamines, corticosteroids may also be used.

II. POTENTIAL FOR INFECTION, BLEEDING, AND FATIGUE related to BONE MARROW SUPPRESSION

Defining Characteristics: Neutropenia common, with 77% incidence, and 25–32% of patients experiencing grade 4 neutropenia, with a median nadir of $900/mm^3$–$1100/mm^3$; Thrombocytopenia incidence 95% with median platelet nadir of $49{,}500/mm^3$; Anemia incidence 61% with median nadir for red blood cells 9.9 g/dL hemoglobin. Nadir occurred around 7–9 weeks after treatment, and duration of cytopenias was 22–35d. Chills and fever were common, affecting 27.5% and 21.6% of patients in one study. There appears to be increased hematologic toxicity in patients with bone marrow involvement by tumor, as expected. Rare fatal cerebral hemorrhage, severe infections.

Nursing Implications: Drug contraindicated in patients with > 25% bone marrow hypocellular bone marrow, or history of failed stem cell collection. Assess baseline CBC, platelet count, and monitor closely during and after therapy at least weekly for the first 12 weeks after treatment. Assess risk for increased hematological toxicity, e.g., whether bone marrow involvement by tumor. Teach patient that blood counts will fall and potential signs/symptoms of infection, bleeding, and fatigue. Teach patient self-care measures including self-assessment for signs/symptoms of infection, bleeding, and anemia; self-care strategies to minimize risk for infection (e.g., avoiding crowds, proximity to people with colds), bleeding (e.g., avoid aspirin-containing OTC medicines), and fatigue (e.g., alternating rest and activity periods), and what/where to report fever, bleeding, signs/symptoms of infection. Most studies show that few patients developed severe infections, and there were few if any deaths from treatment-related infections. Transfuse red blood cells and platelets as ordered.

III. ALTERATION IN COMFORT related to ASTHENIA, NAUSEA, ABDOMINAL PAIN, HEADACHE

Defining Characteristics: Asthenia commonly affects 21.6%, nausea (grades 1 or 2) 21.6%, and abdominal pain and headache 9.8%. Nausea, vomiting, diarrhea, increased cough, dizziness, arthralgia, anxiety may occur.

Nursing Implications: Assess baseline comfort and energy level. Teach patient that these side effects may occur, and strategies to manage them. If the symptom persists or is unresolved, teach patient to report it, and discuss with physician other management strategies.

IV. POTENTIAL FOR INJURY related to RADIATION EXPOSURE

Defining Characteristics: Y-90 Zevalin is a beta-emitter so that patients should protect others from exposure to their body secretions (saliva, stool, blood, urine).

Nursing Implications: Teach patient importance of specific radiation precautions, beginning at the start of treatment, and continuing for 1 week after treatment is completed: use condom during sexual intercourse, refrain from deep kissing; avoid transfer of body fluids; wash hands thoroughly after using the toilet, and continue effective contraception for 12 months following completion of treatment.

Drug: imatinib mesylate (Gleevec, STI 571)

Class: Protein tyrosine kinase inhibitor.

Mechanism of Action: Inhibits sending of message for cell division from abnormal tyrosine kinase encoded by the Philadelphia chromosome (BCR-ABL) in Chronic Myelocytic Leukemia (CML), thus preventing cell proliferation. Drug also inhibits receptor tyrosine kinases for platelet-derived growth factor (PDGF) and stem cell factor (SCF) and thus prevents their respective cell cycle stimulation. Inhibits c-Kit receptor tyrosine kinases as well, which has resulted in marked responses in GIST (gastrointestinal stromal tumors). 15–85% of GISTs have kit mutations; imatinib mesylate selectively inhibits this tyrosine kinase.

Metabolism: Well absorbed after oral administration with 98% bioavailability and Cmax in 2–4 hours after dosing. Elimination half-life of imatinib is 18 hours, and 40 hours for primary active metabolite N-desmethyl derivative. Drug is 95% protein bound. It is metabolized via CYP3A4 hepatic cytochrome P450 enzyme system, with 81% of the dose eliminated in 7 days, primarily via fecal route (68%) and, to a lesser degree, urinary (13%). 25% of drug dose is excreted unchanged in feces and urine.

Dosage/Range:

- 400 mg/da PO (single dose) for patients in chronic phase of CML.
- 600 mg/da PO (single dose) for patients in accelerated phase or blast crisis.
- Treatment continued as long as patient derives benefit from drug.
- If disease progression, failure of hematologic response after 3 months of treatment, or loss of a hematologic remission: increase dose to 600 mg/da (chronic CML), or to 800 mg/da given as 400 mg bid qd (accelerated or blast crisis) if no severe adverse drug reactions occur.
- GIST dosing: 400–600 mg/day.
- Peidatric dosing: 260 mg/m^2/day; if disease progression or no response in 3 months or no cytogenetic response in 6–12 months, or relapse: may increase to 340 mg/m^2/day if no severe drug reaction or treatment complication.

Drug Preparation/Administration:

- Available in hard gelatin 100-mg capsules or scored 100 mg tablets, in bottles of 120.
- Administer dose orally, once daily (unless the total dose is 800 mg, which is given as 400 mg bid), with a meal and a large glass of water.

Drug Interactions:

- CYP3A4 inhibitors (ketoconazole, itraconazole, erythropmycin, clarithromycin) may increase imatinib plasma concentrations; do not coadminister with ketoconazole.

- CYP3A4 substrates (simvastatin): imatinib decreases simvastatin metabolism with simvastatin serum levels increased 2–3.5 times. Use together cautiously, if at all.
- CYP3A4 inducers (dexamethasone, phenytoin, carbamazepine, rifampicin, Phenobarbital, St. John's Wort) may increase metabolism of imatinib so imatinib serum levels are reduced. Use together cautiously, if at all.
- Other CYP3A4 substrates (Cyclosporine, pimozide) increased plasma concentrations if co-administered with imatinib. Do not administer together because drug has a narrow therapeutic window.
- Other CYP3A4 substrates (Triazolo-benzadiazepines, dihydropyridine calcium channel blockers, HMG-CoA reductase inhibitors) may have increased serum levels when given together with imatinib. Use together cautiously, and monitor patient closely.
- Warfarin: Do not give together with imatinib because imatinib inhibits warfarin metabolism by CYP2C9 enzymes. Use low molecular heparin or standard heparin instead.

Lab Effects/Interference:

- Neutropenia, thrombocytopenia.
- Elevated hepatic transaminases (SGOT/AST, SGPT/ALT) and bilirubin.

Special Considerations:

- Imatinib mesylate is indicated for the treatment of patients with CML: 1) initial treatment of newly diagnosed patients with Ph+ chromosome CML, 2) patients in blast crisis, in accelerated phase, or in chronic phase after failure of interferon alpha therapy, 3) patients with metastatic and/or unresectable malignant gastrointestinal stromal tumor (GIST), 4) pediatric patients with chronic phase Ph+ CML recurring after stem cell transplant or resistant to interferon alpha.
- Clinical trials results were remarkable: Chronic phase (n > 500 patients): hematologic complete response (88%), complete cytogenic response (genetic correction) (30%); Accelerated phase (n = 235): hematologic (28%), complete cytogenic response (14%); Blast crisis: hematologic complete response (4%), cytogenic complete response (5%).
- Emerging evidence indicates that resistance can develop with reactivation of the BCR-ABL signal transduction, and, in some patients, an inverted duplicate Philadelphia chromosome with amplification of the BCR-ABL fusion gene occurs (Gorre et al, 2001).
- Drug is teratogeneic. Women should avoid pregnancy or breast-feeding while taking the drug.
- Drug often causes edema that may be serious in some patients. There is increased risk in patients at higher drug doses and in the elderly (> 65 years).
- Drug is associated with neutropenia and thrombocytopenia. Blood counts should be checked weekly for the first month, biweekly for the second

month, and then every 2–3 months as clinically indicated. Patients with accelerated phase CML or blast crisis require closer monitoring.
- Liver function tests (LFTs) should be monitored baseline and monthly or as clinically indicated. Drug should be stopped if bilirubin is increased to 3 times institutional upper limit of normal (IULN), or if liver transaminases is > 5 times IULN and held until these tests have returned to bilirubin < 1.5 times IULN or transaminase levels to < 2.5 times IULN. Drug should then be resumed at a reduced dose (400 mg dose reduced to 300 mg qd, and 600 mg dose reduced to 400 mg qd).
- Use cautiously in patients with liver impairment, and monitor liver function tests closely prior to and throughout treatment.
- Drug modifications for hematologic toxicity: *Chronic phase CML at initial dose of 400 mg/da or GIST at initial dose of 400–600 mg/da:* ANC < 1000/mm^3 and/or platelets < 50,000/mm^3: stop drug until ANC ≥ 1500/mm^3 and/or platelets > 75,000/mm^3 and then resume at usual dose; if recurrence of ANC < 1000/mm^3, and/or platelets < 50,000/mm^3, hold until recovered, and reduce dose to 300 mg qd if initial dose 400 mg/da, and 400 mg/da if initial dose was 600 mg/da.
- *Accelerated phase and Blast Crisis:* ANC < 500/mm^3 and/or platelets < 10,000/mm^3: determine if related to leukemia by bone marrow aspirate/biopsy; if unrelated to leukemia, reduce dose to 400 mg qd; if cytopenia persists 2 weeks, reduce again to 300 mg qd; if cytopenia persists 4 weeks and is still unrelated to leukemia, stop imatinib until ANC ≥ 1000/mm^3 and platelets ≥ 20/mm^3, and then resume at 300 mg/da.

Potential Toxicities/Side Effects and the Nursing Process

I. POTENTIAL FOR INFECTION AND BLEEDING related to BONE MARROW DEPRESSION

Defining Characteristics: Neutropenia and thrombocytopenia were common, especially in patients who received higher doses, and in patients with advanced stages of disease (blast crisis and accelerated phase). Median duration of neutropenia was 2–3 weeks, and thrombocytopenia from 3–4 weeks. Dose needs to be held and reduced as noted in *Special Considerations.* Fever affected 14% (chronic phase) to 38% (accelerated phase) of patients. Hemorrhage (CNS and GI) was treated in 13% (chronic phase) to 48% (accelerated phase) of patients.

Nursing Implications: Assess baseline cbc, including wbc and differential and platelet count prior to dosing, as well as at least weekly during first month of treatment, at least every other week for the second month of treatment, and then as clinically indicated and ordered. Discuss dose interruption and reduction as above for neutropenia and thombocytopenia. Teach patient self-assessment of signs/symptoms of infection and bleeding (including epistaxis and development of petechiae), and instruct patient to report them right away. Teach patient self-care measures to minimize risk of infection and bleeding, including avoidance of OTC aspirin-containing medications.

II. ALTERATION IN FLUID AND ELECTROLYTE BALANCE related to FLUID RETENTION, EDEMA, AND HYPOKALEMIA

Defining Characteristics: Fluid retention is common (52% chronic phase and 67% accelerated phase patients), especially in the elderly, and primarily reflects periorbital and lower extremity edema. However, pleural effusions, ascites, rapid weight gain, and pulmonary edema may develop, and in some cases, be life-threatening (pleural effusion, congestive heart failure, renal failure, pericardial effusion, anasarca). Hypokalemia was reported to occur in 2–12% of patients.

Nursing Implications: Assess baseline parameters of weight, presence of edema, pulmonary function, and monitor closely during therapy. Teach patient to monitor weight daily at home, and to report weight gain of 2 pounds in one week, development of edema, or dyspnea. With physician, discuss drug interruption if fluid retention occurs, and the prescription of diuretics.

III. ALTERATION IN NUTRITION, POTENTIAL, LESS THAN BODY REQUIREMENTS, related to NAUSEA, VOMITING, DIARRHEA, HEPATOTOXICITY

Defining Characteristics: Nausea affected 68% of patients with accelerated phase, and 55% with chronic phase; vomiting affected 54% and 28%, respectively. Diarrhea affected 54%, while constipation affected 13%. Dyspepsia affected about 19%.

Nursing Implications: Teach patient to self-administer antiemetics one hour prior to each dose, and to call if nausea/vomiting develop. Discuss with physician more effective antiemetic regime if nausea/vomiting develop. Encourage small, frequent intake of cool, bland foods as tolerated if nausea develops. Refer to dietitian as needed for meal planning.

IV. ALTERATION IN COMFORT related to MUSCLE CRAMPS, MUSCULOSKELETAL PAIN, HEADACHE, FATIGUE, ARTHRALGIA, AND ABDOMINAL PAIN

Defining Characteristics: Muscle cramps are common, affecting 25–46% of patients. Musculoskeletal pain affects 27–37% of patients, headache 24–29% of patients, fatigue 33% of patients, and arthralgias 26% of patients. In clinical studies, abdominal pain affected 20% of patients with chronic phase, and 26% of patients in blast crisis.

Nursing Implications: Teach patient that these events may occur and to report them. Assess baseline comfort, and monitor closely during treatment. Develop plan to assure comfort depending on symptoms reported. Discuss ineffective strategies with physician, and revise plan as needed.

V. ALTERATION IN SKIN INTEGRITY, POTENTIAL, related to RASH

Defining Characteristics: Rash may occur. In clinical studies, 32% of patients with accelerated phase, and 36% of patients in chronic phase CML reported rash. 10% of patients complained of pruritis.

Nursing Implications: Teach patient that rash may occur and to report it. Assess patient skin integrity baseline and regularly during treatment. Teach patient local comfort measures. Discuss rash and management plan with physician, especially if severe.

Drug: lapatinib ditosylate (investigational)

Class: Tyrosine kinase inhibitor.

Mechanism of Action: Drug inhibits tyrosine kinases of both Human Epidermal growth factor Receptor (HER)-1 and HER-2-neu, leading to arrest of cell growth and/or apoptosis in tumor cells that depend upon ErbB1 and ErbB2 cell signaling. Normally, HER-2 dimerizes with other members of the HER family, including HER-1. The message is then sent repeatedly via the tyrosine kinases to the cell nucleus telling the cell to divide. In 20% of patients with breast cancer, HER-2-neu is overexpressed, leading to increased cell proliferation, invasiveness, and conferring a poor prognosis associated with reduced survival. By blockading the tyrosine kinases, the message for repeated cell division is halted.

Dosage/Range:
Per protocol. For example, 1500 mg PO qd.

Drug Preparation/Administration: Oral.

Drug Interactions: Unknown.

Lab Effects/Interference: Unknown.

Special Considerations:

- Drug is being studied in women with metastatic breast cancer who overexpress HER-2-neu, as well as patients with solid tumors, such as NSCLC and colorectal cancers.

Potential Toxicities/Side Effects and the Nursing Process

I. ALTERATION IN COMFORT related to RASH, FATIGUE

Defining Characteristics: Rash is usually mild to moderate. Rash and fatigue are common, with 5% of patients with advanced metastatic breast cancer reporting severe (grade 3) rash and fatigue.

Nursing Implications: Assess patient's baseline comfort, and teach that these symptoms may occur. Assess skin integrity baseline, and during therapy. Teach symptom management strategies to minimize discomfort. Teach patient to notify nurse or physician if fatigue or rash is severe, or does not resolve with local management. Interrupt or delay dose based on protocol.

II. ALTERATION IN NUTRITION, LESS THAN BODY REQUIREMENTS related to DIARRHEA, NAUSEA, VOMITING, ANOREXIA

Defining Characteristics: In patients with metatastic breast cancer studied, diarrhea occurred commonly and was severe (grade 3) in 10% of patients.

Nursing Implications: Assess baseline nutritional status, bowel elimination pattern, and appetite. Inform patient these side effects may occur. Teach self-administration of anti-nausea and anti-diarrheal medications according to protocol, and to notify provider if symptoms persists so dose can be interrupted per protocol. Teach patient dietary modification if nausea and vomiting or diarrhea occur, (e.g., for diarrhea, bananas, rice, applesauce, and toast) and to increase oral fluids to prevent dehydration. Consult dietitian to see patient for dietary counseling for anorexia.

Drug: lenalidomide (Revlimid, CC-5013, investigational)

Class: Immunomodulator with anti-angiogenesis properties.

Mechanism of Action: Drug induces G0/G1 growth arrest and apoptosis, increases expression of genes found on 5q locus including genes involved in cell adhesion. Inhibits COX-2 expression, stimulates T-cell proliferation, as well as the anti-inflammatory cytokines Interleukin-2, Interleukin-10, and Interferon-gamma. Decreases the secretion of proinflammatory cytokines that mediate cell growth and survival (TNF-α, Interleukin-1β, and Interleukin-6); stimulates host natural killer cell immunity (Bartlett et al, 2004).

Metabolism: Unknown.

Dosage/Range:
Per protocol.

Drug Preparation/Administration: Oral, per protocol; for example in multiple myeloma, 25 mg PO qd × 21 days, repeated q 28 days in combination with dexamethasone.

Drug Interactions:

- Bone marrow suppressive agents: additive bone marrow suppression.
- Additive anti-tumor effect when combined with dexamethasone in the treatment of multiple myeloma.

Lab Effects/Interference:

Special Considerations:

- Selectively designed to be more potent (10,000 times) and to have a different adverse event profile than thalidomide; drug is not teratogenic at similar doses, but has been found embryotoxic in animal studies.
- Drug has shown efficacy in treating patients with MDS who are have refractory anemia (5q31–33 chromosomal mutation), so that they achieved transfusion independence.
- Drug does not cause sleepiness, constipation, or peripheral neuropathy like thalidomide.
- Drug may cause tumor lysis syndrome in newly diagnosed multiple myeloma patients with large tumor burdens that lyse quickly when lenalidomide is given.
- Drug is being studied in the treatment of type-1 Complex Regional Pain Syndrome.
- In the treatment of patients with relapsed or refractory multiple myeloma, patients receiving lenalidomide plus dexamethasone had significantly longer TTP (40 to > 60 weeks vs about 20 weeks) and ORR (51.3% vs 22.9%) [Dimopoulous et al, 2004]; and more mature results reported by Fonseca et al (2005) showed a 61% RR compared to 24% with dexamethasone alone, and a 26% CR.
- Drug has hematologic activity in patients with low risk myelodysplastic syndromes who have no response to erythropoietin (List et al, 2005).

Potential Toxicities/Side Effects and the Nursing Process

I. POTENTIAL FOR INFECTION AND BLEEDING related to BONE MARROW SUPPRESSION

Defining Characteristics: Neutropenia occurs in 57% of patients, and thrombocytopenia in 58% of patients studied in multiple myeloma trials.

Nursing Implications: Assess baseline CBC, WBC, differential, and platelet count prior to chemotherapy, as well as signs/symptoms of infection or bleeding. Teach patient the signs/symptoms of infection or bleeding, and to report these immediately, and teach patient self-care measures to minimize risk of infection and bleeding. This includes avoidance of crowds, proximity to people with infections, and OTC aspirin-containing medications. Drug should be used in combination with another agent that does not cause bone marrow suppression, like bortezomib (Velcade) rather than chemotherapy.

II. ALTERATION IN COMFORT related to RASH, FATIGUE, LIGHT-HEADEDNESS AND LEG CRAMPS

Defining Characteristics: Mild rash, light-headedness have been reported, as have fatigue and leg cramps. Pruritis may be limited to the scalp and occur within 1 week of treatment.

Nursing Implications: Assess patient's baseline comfort, and teach patient that these symptoms may occur. Assess skin integrity baseline and during therapy. Teach symptom management strategies to minimize discomfort. Teach patient to notify nurse or physician if fatigue, rash, itching, or leg cramps are severe, or do not resolve with local management.

III. ALTERATION IN NUTRITION, LESS THAN BODY REQUIREMENTS, related to DIARRHEA

Defining Characteristics: In patients with MDS studied, diarrhea occurred in 21% of patients receiving prolonged treatment.

Nursing Implications: Assess baseline bowel elimination pattern, and inform patient diarrhea may occur. Teach self-administration of anti-diarrheals according to protocol, and to notify provider if diarrhea persists for dose interruption. Teach patient dietary modification if diarrhea occurs, (e.g., bananas, rice, applesauce, and toast) and to increase oral fluids to prcvent dehydration.

Drug: neovastat (investigational)

Class: Angiogenesis inhibitor made from cartilaginous spine of dogfish shark.

Mechanism of Action: Appears to inhibit Vascular Endothelial Growth Factor (VEGD) signaling, to inhibit matrix metalloproteinases (MMPs), and to induce apoptosis (programmed cell death).

Dosage/Range:

- Per protocol.

Drug Preparation/Administration:

- Available orally in liquid form, taken bid, per protocol.

Drug Interactions:

- Unknown.

Lab Effects/Interference:
- Unknown.

Special Considerations:
- Differs from OTC shark cartilage, which is made primarily from shark fins.
- In a small study of patients with renal cell cancer, patients receiving a higher dose of neovastat survived 16.3 months compared to those receiving a lower dose whose survival was 7.1 months (Bukowski, 2001).
- Well tolerated without reported side effects.
- Clinical trials in patients with lung or ovarian cancer, multiple myeloma, with or without chemotherapy, are ongoing (NCI, others).

Potential Toxicities/Side Effects and Nursing Implications

I. KNOWLEDGE DEFICIT relating to LACK OF KNOWLEDGE, MEDIA MISINFORMATION

Defining Characteristics: Media about shark cartilage has been rife with misinformation, because there is no distinction between the cartilage-derived drug and that sold as an OTC miracle drug. Neovastat is made from shark spine cartilage, and the active substance is found in all animal cartilage. Shark is used because there is a high percentage of cartilage per body weight, and it is abundantly available. OTC shark cartilage is made from shark fins.

Nursing Implications: Assess basic understanding of drug and its mechanism of action, and explain how it differs from OTC shark cartilage. Teach the patient self-administration of the drug. Provide information, and answer questions. Ensure patient makes an informed consent prior to entering the study.

Drug: oblimersen sodium (Gentasense, G3139) (investigational)

Class: Antisense oligonucleotide.

Mechanism of Action: Downregulates Bcl-2 protein, which suppresses apoptosis, thus increasing sensitivity to programmed cell death. Increased levels of Bcl-2 protein are associated with resistance to chemotherapy and radiation, so Bcl-2 is also known as a multidrug-resistance protein. Oblimersen sodium, an antisense oligonucleotide, binds to the first 6 codons of the human Bcl-2 mRNA sequence, causing the degradation of Bcl-2 mRNA, and a reduction in Bcl-2 protein translation. This helps to re-establish apoptosis, or programmed cell death of the cell, and theoretically, sensitivity to chemotherapy or radiotherapy.

Metabolism: Rapidly metabolized in plasma and tissues. Steady state plasma concentratons of oblimersen achieved in 24–48 hours when given as a continuous infusion × 5 (IV)-14 (SQ) days. Plasma concentration directly related to dose. Plasma half-life is 2 hours and is dose independent. Drug excreted essentially unchanged by kidneys into urine.

Dosage/Range:
Per protocol. One study used 7 mg/kg IV continuous infusion daily × 5 days, with chemotherapy given on day 5.

Drug Preparation/Administration: Intravenous or subcutaneous continuous infusion for 5–14 days, given prior to or together with chemotherapy. Half-life of Bcl-2 protein is long. Maximal Bcl-2 protein downregulation reached at 5 days.

Drug Interactions: Synergy with chemotherapy.

Lab Effects/Interference: Unknown.

Special Considerations:
- Being studied in malignant melanoma, 1 chronic lymphocytic leukemia, multiple myeloma, colorectal cancer, small cell lung cancer.
- Toxicity related to Oblimersen sodium: fatigue, thrombocytopenia, pyrexia.
- Patients in study had toxicity from chemotherapy included in treatment as well as infectious complications of venous access devices (VADs).

Potential Toxicities/Side Effects and the Nursing Process

I. POTENTIAL FOR INFECTION AND BLEEDING related to NEUTROPENIA AND THROMBOCYTOPENIA

Defining Characteristics: Risk of neutropenia and thrombocytopenia is increased in combination with bone marrow suppressive chemotherapy.

Nursing Implications: Assess baseline blood counts and platelets. Teach patient to report fever, and signs/symptoms of infection or bleeding right away. Assess medication profile and OTC medications taken. Teach patient to avoid OTC medications containing NSAIDs or aspirin. Teach patient to talk to nurse or physician before beginning any OTC medications.

II. POTENTIAL ALTERATION IN COMFORT related to FATIGUE, PYREXIA

Defining Characteristics: Fatigue and pyrexia appeared to be increased in studies. However, there were also infectious complications of VADs.

Nursing Implications: Teach patient that fatigue and pyrexia may occur and to report pyrexia right away. Teach patient to alternate rest and activity periods, to plan shopping and chores so that it minimizes energy expenditure, and to explore whether family members can help with necessary chores. Teach patient measures to manage pyrexia: acetaminophen, tepid baths, increase oral fluids.

Drug: panitumumab (ABX-EGF) (investigational)

Class: Human monoclonal antibody targeted against epidermal growth factor receptor (EGFR).

Mechanism of Action: Blocks growth factor (ligand, such as epidermal growth factor and transforming growth factor-alpha) from binding to EGFR, thus preventing dimerization and initiation of cell signaling via receptor tyrosine kinase phosphorylation; thus, the message telling the cell to divide does not occur. In addition to cell growth inhibition, there is induction of apoptosis, and decreased matrix metalloproteinase and vascular endothelial growth factor production.

Metabolism: Unknown.

Dosage/Range:
Per protocol; 0.01–5.0 mg/kg IV q wk, 6.0 mg/kg q 2 weeks, and 9.0 mg/kg q 3 weeks are some dosages and frequencies being studied.

Drug Preparation/Administration: Per protocol; administered as IV infusion per protocol. Does not require premedication to prevent hypersensitivity reactions as drug is a human monoclonal antibody.

Drug Interactions: Unknown.

Lab Effects/Interference: Unknown.

Special Considerations:

- Tumors over-expressing epidermal growth factor receptors are colorectal, lung, breast, bladder, pancreas, kidney, head and neck cancers. Principal study is in patients with metasatic colorectal cancer.
- Drug exposure and tolerability similar between weekly, every-other-week, and every-three-week dosing schedules (Weiner LM, 2005).
- Rarely, a patient may develop an infusion reaction. During clinical trials, at least 1 patient developed rigors, dyspnea, wheezing on the day of the 2nd cycle of panitumumab infusion, effectively treated with meperidine, lorazepam, and diphenhydramine. The patient successfully received subsequent treatment with the same premedication (Malik et al, 2005).
- In patients studied, no patient developed HAHA formation (Malik et al, 2005).
- Theoretically, interstitial lung disease, a class effect, may occur; however, this was not seen in clinical trials.

Potential Toxicities/Side Effects and the Nursing Process

I. POTENTIAL ALTERATION IN BODY IMAGE, SKIN INTEGRITY, COMFORT related to SKIN RASH

Defining Characteristics: Drug inhibits epidermal growth factor receptor, so major toxicity is manifested in the skin with 95% of patients experiencing some type of skin toxicity. Most patients (80%, 3% of these grade 3) develop a mild-to-moderate acne-like rash that is self-limiting. 14% report a grade 3 rash, and in clinical studies 1% of patients discontinued treatment due to skin rash. Rash is a sterile, suppurative rash with multiple follicular or pustular lesions that appear during the first 2 weeks of therapy on the face, upper chest and back, but in some cases, extended to the arms. Rash resolves when treatment is stopped, without scar formation. Pruritis affects 34%, dry-skin 26%, acneiform dermatitis 16%, skin desqumation 13%, erythema 11%, paronychia 11%, macular rash 10%, skin fissures 6%, maculopapular rash 7%, popular rash 7%, exfoliative dermatitis 6%. Fissures can become infected; infection can be treated with topical clindamycin, or oral antibiotics. Do not use topical corticosteroid cream. Median time to first skin toxicity was 7 days, and median time to most severe skin toxicity was 12 days in clinical studies.

Nursing Implications: Teach patient that rash most likely will occur due to mechanism of drug action. Assess baseline skin integrity on areas of face, neck, and trunk; assess baseline comfort and satisfaction with body image, and monitor at each treatment. Teach patient to report any distress and assess extent of rash. Consult protocol for drug holiday (e.g., drug may be held for 1–2 weeks for severe rash, and if it resolves, dose reduced on and after the 2nd occurrence. If rash does not resolve, drug may be stopped). If skin appears to be infected, discuss with physician, the prescription of clindamycin gel (Cleocin T) or oral cephalexin (Keflex) 250 mg PO bid × 3 days, then 250 mg qd × 7 days, for a total of 10 days for skin infection. Rash is not acne, and so usual anti-acne treatment will not be effective.

II. ALTERATION IN NUTRITION, LESS THAN BODY REQUIREMENTS, related to NAUSEA, VOMITING, DIARRHEA, STOMATITIS, CONSTIPATION, ANOREXIA, ABDOMINAL PAIN

Defining Characteristics: Incidence of mild-to-moderate digestive symptoms include nausea (39%), diarrhea (36%), abdominal pain (30%), anorexia (27%), vomiting (27%), constipation (25%), stomatitits (18%) in patients on clinical trials.

Nursing Implications: Assess baseline weight and nutritional status. Inform patient that these symptoms may occur, and to report them. Administer antiemetic and other symptom management medications as ordered. Teach patient self-administration of these medications at home. Teach patient dietary modifications to address symptoms such as anorexia (small, frequent high-calorie, high-protein foods, stimulants as permitted by protocol); constipation (high-fiber, high-fluid, high-roughage foods, stool softeners); diarrhea (bananas, rice, applesauce, and toast); nausea (avoid food preparation odors by cooking in zipped plastic bag, or having someone else cook; choose cool, soft, non-spicy, or fatty foods). Teach patient to report any symptoms that do not resolve or improve on the plan. Assess efficacy of intervention, and revise plan as needed.

III. POTENTIAL FOR ALTERATION IN COMFORT related to FATIGUE, DYSPNEA, PERIPHERAL EDEMA, PYREXIA, ARTHRALGIA

Defining Characteristics: In clinical trials, the following symptoms were reported in patients with advanced colorectal cancer: fatigue (51%), cough (18%), dyspnea (14%), peripheral edema (14%), pyrexia (14%), arthralgia (14%), back pain (12%), headache (12%), dizziness (11%), insomnia (11%).

Nursing Implications: Assess patient comfort level, self-care measures baseline and periodically during therapy. Teach patient that these symptoms may arise, either from the drug and/or the treatment. Develop a plan for symptom management, assess efficacy and revise as needed. Assess level of fatigue and teach energy baseline and prior to each treatment. Inform patient that fatigue may occur due to anemia, and teach energy conserving strategies such as alternating restand activity periods.

Drug: pertuzumab (Omnitarg, rhuMab 2C4) (investigational)

Class: First of a new class called Human Epidermal (Growth Factor) Receptor dimerization inhibitors (HDI). Multiple targeted Tyrosine kinase inhibitor, anti-angiogenesis agent.

Mechanism of Action: In order for a growth signal to be sent to the cell nucleus, a growth factor (ligand) attaches to the Human Epidermal Growth Factor Receptor, or HER. The growth factor receptor now needs to dimerize or pair with another growth factor receptor, e.g., HER-2 receptor needs to dimerize or pair with another HER receptor, such as HER-1. Pertuzumab binds to the dimerization domain of HER so the binding of the antibody directly inhibits the ability of HER-2 to dimerize with other HER (EGFR) proteins. This disrupts the activation of downstream effectors so that the growth signal is not sent, notably the AKT pathway (cell survival). Drug is a recombinant, humanized monoclonal antibody.

Metabolism: Unknown.

Dosage/Range:
Per protocol; studies have included doses 0.5–15mg/kg q 3 wk.

Drug Preparation/Administration: Per protocol; IV infusion.

Drug Interactions: Unknown.

Lab Effects/Interference: Unknown.

Special Considerations:

- Drug is being investigated in prostate, NSCLC, metastatc breast, ovarian cancers, but may need to be given with chemotherapy to improve response.
- Drug is targeted against tumors that do not over-express HER-2.
- Side effects varied according to patient population with diarrhea and rash most common in prostate cancer patients studied, and diarrhea, fatigue, nausea, vomiting, and uncommon drop in LVEF in patients with metastatic breast cancer who previously had received anthracyclines (Cortes et al, 2005).

Potential Toxicities/Side Effects and the Nursing Process

I. POTENTIAL ALTERATION IN NUTRITION related to DIARRHEA, NAUSEA, VOMITING

Defining Characteristics: Diarrhea was most common affecting about 50–59% of patients, and ranging in severity from grade 1–3; nausea and vomiting affected patients with metasttic breast cancer, affecting 32% and 23% of women respectively.

Nursing Implications: Assess bowel elimination patterns and nutritional status baseline prior to each treatment. Teach patient to take anti-diarrheal medication per protocol. Administer anti-emetics prior to drug administration per protocol, and teach patient to self-administer anti-emetics as permitted on protocol. Teach patient to report any symptoms that do not resolve or improve with the established plan

II. ACTIVITY INTOLERANCE, POTENTIAL, related to FATIGUE

Defining Characteristics: Fatigue occurs commonly in patients with advanced cancer who were studied.

Nursing Implications: Assess baseline activity and energy level, and teach patient that this symptom may occur. Assess patient's activity patterns, and suggest ways to conserve energy.

Drug: rituximab (Rituxan)

Class: Monoclonal antibody (anti-CD_{20} antibody).

Mechanism of Action: Anti-CD_{20} antibody that is genetically engineered (chimeric monoclonal antibody, or part mouse part human) directed against the CD_{20} antigen found on the surface of normal and malignant B-cell lymphocytes. The CD_{20} antigen is also present (expressed) on more than 90% of B-cell non-Hodgkin's lymphoma (NHL) cells, but fortunately is not found on normal bone marrow stem cells, pre-B cells, or other normal tissues. A section of the rituximab (Fab domain) CD_{20} binds to the CD_{20} antigen on B lymphocytes; another section of the rituximab (Fc domain) calls together other immune effectors, resulting in lysis of the B lymphocyte.

Metabolism: Serum and half-life of drug varies with dose and sequence, and at 375 mg/m^2, the median serum half-life was 76.3 hours after the first infusion, as compared to 205 hours after the fourth infusion. Drug was detected in patient serum up to 3–6 months after completion of treatment.

Dosage/Range:
- 375 mg/m^2 given as IV infusion weekly for × 4 weeks or 8 doses.

Drug Preparation/Administration:
- Do not mix with or dilute with other drugs.
- Store at 2–8°C (36–46°F) and protect vials from direct sunlight.
- Available as 100-mg (10-mL) and 500-mg (50-mL) single-use vials.
- Add ordered dose to 0.9% Sodium Chloride USP or 5% Dextrose, resulting in a final concentration of 1–4 mg/mL; gently invert to mix, and inspect for presence of any particulate matter or discoloration.
- Drug is stable in infusion solution at 2–8°C (36–46°F) for 24 hours, and at room temperature for another 24 hours.
- Must not be given IVB due to risk of hypersensitivity or infusion reactions.
- First infusion: initial infusion rate should be 50 mg/hr; if no hypersensitivity or infusion-related problems occur, increase the infusion rate in 50 mg/hr increments every 30 minutes to a maximum of 400 mg/hr. If infusion or hypersensitivity problems occur, slow or stop the infusion depending on severity. May continue the infusion at half the previous rate once symptoms resolve.
- Second, third, fourth infusions: administer at initial rate of 100 mg/hr, and increase by 100 mg/hr increments every 30 minutes, to a maximum of 400 mg/hr as tolerated.

Drug Interactions:
- None known.

Lab Effects/Interference:

- Decreased lymphocyte count (B cells); decreased IgM and IgG serum levels.

Special Considerations:

- Drug is indicated for the treatment of patients with low-grade or follicular, CD_{20}-positive, B-cell non-Hodgkin's lymphoma who have relapsed or who are refractory to standard therapy, and as initial therapy for patients with bulky disease.
- Severe mucocutaneous reactions may occur, resulting in death. Drug should be stopped if a reaction develops and a skin biopsy performed.
- Contraindicated in patients with known Type 1 hypersensitivity or anaphylactic reactions to murine proteins or product components.
- Infusion reactions common (fever, chills) during the first infusion. Hypotension, bronchospasm, and angioedema may occur. STOP infusion for severe reactions, and manage symptoms with diphenhydramine and acetaminophen, and additional treatment with bronchodilators, epinephrine, or IV saline as indicated. Infusion may be resumed at 50% of the previous rate once symptoms have resolved.
- Emergency medications should be readily available: epinephrine, antihistamines, and corticosteroids.
- STOP infusion if serious cardiac arrhythmias develop; patient should receive cardiac monitoring during and after subsequent infusions of the drug. Patients with a history of arrhythmias and angina should be cardiac monitored during infusion and immediately post-infusion for evidence of recurrence of these problems.
- Monitor CBC, platelet count regularly during therapy.
- Possibility of developing antibodies to the human antimurine (HAMA) and human antichimeric (HACA) exists, and may be as low as 1% incidence; these individuals are at risk for developing allergic/hypersensitivity reactions when treated with rituximab or other MoAbs (murine or chimeric).
- Birth control practices during and for 12 months following therapy should be used by individuals of childbearing potential.
- Women should not breast-feed infants while drug is detectable in the serum.

Potential Toxicities/Side Effects and the Nursing Process

I. POTENTIAL FOR INJURY related to INFUSION-RELATED REACTIONS AND HYPERSENSITIVITY

Defining Characteristics: Infusion-related reactions occurred within 30 minutes to 2 hours of the beginning of the first infusion, and occurred in 80% of patients receiving a first infusion (7% severe), as opposed to 40% of patients (5–10% severe) receiving subsequent infusions. Fever and chills/rigors affect

Nursing Implications: Assess baseline comfort prior to each infusion, and tolerance of past infusion. Discuss strategies to manage symptoms. If symptoms are severe, discuss management with physician.

Drug: Sorafenib (BAY 43-9006) (investigational)

Class: Multiple targeted Tyrosine kinase inhibitor, anti-angiogenesis agent.

Mechanism of Action: Drug inhibits a number of tyrosine kinases, including Raf kinase, an enzyme in the RAS pathway (RAS is mutated in about 20–30% of solid tumors), as well as receptor tyrosine kinases VEGFR-2 and PDGFR-β, thus preventing cell proliferation and angiogenesis. First, sorafenib inhibits the signaling cascade in the RAS pathway, blocking uncontrolled cell growth from either excessive stimulation of the RAS pathway, or through mutations of RAS and RAF proteins. In addition, sorafenib inhibits angiogenesis by preventing the message from Vascular Endothelial Growth Factor (VEGF), telling endothelial cells to proliferate and migrate, from reaching the cell nucleus (signal transduction) and angiogenesis is prevented. It also inhibits the message that would be sent to the cell nucleus when the ligand Platelet Derived Growth Factor (PDGF) attaches to it's receptor PDGFR-β; PDGF is necessary for pericytes around the blood vessels to provide external structure during angiogenesis, and when they are not available, angiogenesis is stopped (Onyx, 2005).

Metabolism: Unknown.

Dosage/Range:
Per protocol, varies with other chemotherapy agents administered in combination.

Drug Preparation/Administration: None, oral.

Drug Interactions: Unknown.

Lab Effects/Interference: Unknown.

Special Considerations:
- Drug is being studied in Phase III clinical trials of patients with clear cell metastatic renal cell cancer, as well as patients with malignant melanoma in combination with chemotherapy.
- Drug is well tolerated with principal side effects being hypertension (11% vs 1% placebo), rash (34% vs 13%), hand-foot syndrome (27% vs 5%) and diarrhea (33% vs 10%).
- In patients with malignant melanoma, a specific RAS kinase. BRAF, is mutated in 66% of patients and some patients with colorectal cancer (Onyx Pharmaceuticals, 2005).

Potential Toxicities/Side Effects and the Nursing Process

I. POTENTIAL ALTERATION IN CIRCULATION related to HYPERTENSION

Defining Characteristics: Hypertension occurred in 11% of renal cell cancer patients being studied, compared to 1% receiving placebo.

Nursing Implications: Assess baseline blood pressure, and monitor prior to each treatment cycle. Discuss persistent elevations with physician, and consult protocol.

II. ALTERATION IN SKIN INTEGRITY AND COMFORT related to HAND-FOOT SYNDROME, RASH, POTENTIAL

Defining Characteristics: In renal cell cancer patients being studied, rash occurred in 34% of patients, and hand-foot syndrome in 27% of patients compared to 13% and 5% of patients, respectively, receiving placebo.

Nursing Implications: Assess baseline skin integrity, including soles of feet and palms of hands, and teach patient that these symptoms may occur. Teach patient to self assess all skin areas, and to report rash, as well as redness, swelling, and/or pain anywhere, particularly the soles of feet and palms of hands. Teach patient to avoid activities that increase blood flow in the hands and feet, such as hot showers and baths, and to take tepid showers to reduce likelihood and severity of hand-foot syndrome. Teach patient to avoid constrictive clothing and repetitive movements that can irritate the opposing skin. Teach patient to use skin emollients to prevent skin from drying and cracking.

Drug: sunitinib malate (Sutent, U-11248) (investigational)

Class: Multi-targeted tyrosine kinase inhibitor.

Mechanism of Action: Drug has both anti-tumor and anti-angiogenesis activity. When a growth factor or ligand binds to the receptor on the outside of the cell, it sends a message to the cell nucleus telling the cell to proliferate, make new blood vessels (angiogenesis, by releasing VEGF) and to ignore programmed cell death signals (apoptosis). Protein tyrosine kinases are inside the cell membrane, and then receive the message from outside the cell and send it down through a process called phosphorylation, to the nucleus via multiple signaling pathways, called signal transduction. Sunitinib malate blocks multiple tyrosine kinases, thus preventing the message from getting to the nucleus of the cell via blockage of multiple signaling pathways, and preventing cell division, the formation of new blood vessels, and permitting programmed cell death. The receptor tyrosine kinases blocked are platelet derived growth factor receptor (PDGFR α and β), Vascular endothelial growth factor receptor (VEGFR 1,2,3), c-KIT, and Flt-3 in GastroIntestinal Stomal Tumor (GIST) and VEGF and PDGF pathways in renal cell cancer.

Metabolism: Unknown.

Dosage/Range:
50mg PO qd in 6 week cycles per protocol. Dose reduced for grade 3 and 4 toxicities.

Drug Preparation/Administration: None, oral tablet.

Drug Interactions: Unknown at this time.

Lab Effects/Interference:
- Decreased lymphocyte, neutrophil, red blood cell, and platelet counts; elevated serum lipase and amylase.

Special Considerations:
- Most active in the treatment of Gastrointestinal stromal tumors (GIST) that were refractory to imatinib (Gleevec) and renal cell cancer.
- Hypertension affected 5–14% of patients on clinical trials.

Potential Toxicities/Side Effects and the Nursing Process

I. POTENTIAL FOR INFECTION AND BLEEDING related to NEUTROPENIA AND THROMBOCYTOPENIA

Defining Characteristics: Neutropenia occurred in 39–45% of patients, anemia 25-37% of patients, and thrombocytopenia 18–19% of patients in clinical trials.

Nursing Implications: Assess baseline blood counts and platelets. Teach patient to report fever, and signs/symptoms of infection or bleeding right away. Assess medication profile and OTC medications taken. Teach patient to avoid OTC medications containing NSAIDs or aspirin. Teach patient to talk to nurse or physician before beginning any OTC medications.

II. POTENTIAL ACTIVITY INTOLERANCE related to FATIGUE, DIZZINESS

Defining Characteristics: Fatigue occurred in 22–38% of patients in clinical trials.

Nursing Implications: Teach patient that fatigue may occur and self-care measures. Teach patient to alternate rest and activity periods, to plan shopping and chores to minimize energy expenditure, and to explore whether family members can help with necessary chores.

III. ALTERATION IN NUTRITION, LESS THAN BODY REQUIREMENTS, related to NAUSEA, STOMATITIS, DIARRHEA, ELEVATED AMYLASE AND LIPASE LEVELS

Defining Characteristics: Diarrhea occurred in 16–24% of patients, nausea in 13–19% of patients, and stomatitis in 14–19%, hyperamylasemia in 8-10% (renal cell cancer), and hyperlipasemia in 24–28% (renal cell cancer) of patients in clinical studies.

Nursing Implications: Assess baseline nutritional status, bowel elimination patterns, integrity of oral mucosa, and lipase and amylase function studies regularly during treatment. Teach patient self-administration of anti-diarrheal medications and to report if ineffective. Teach patient self-administration of antiemetics prior to administration of drug. Teach patient to report persistent or continued nausea and/or vomiting. Assess efficacy and discuss change in antiemetic drug with physician if regimen ineffective. Teach patient to assess oral mucosa regularly, use oral hygiene regimen, and report signs/symptoms of stomatitis. If patient develops stomatitis, teach patient self-administration of oral analgesics, antifungals, as ordered and appropriate. Monitor amylase and lipase tests in patients with renal cell cancer, and discuss any abnormalities with physician.

IV. ALTERATION IN SKIN INTEGRITY, POTENTIAL, related to DERMATITIS

Defining Characteristics: In clinical studies, 5–11% of patients complained of dermatologic problems, including skin discoloration and hand-foot syndrome in patients with GIST.

Nursing Implications: Assess patient skin integrity baseline and regularly during treatment. Teach patient local comfort measures. Teach patient to report skin changes and if self-care ineffective, discuss plan with physician, especially if severe.

Drug: suberoylanilide hydroxamic acid (SAHA)

Class: Histone deacetylase (HDAC) inhibitor.

Mechanism of Action: Histone deacetylases work with other regulatory proteins to modulate gene expression (transcriptional activity). By inhibiting selected gene expression of genes involved in cancer, histone deacetylase inhibitors are able to block angiogenesis and cell cycling, and promote apoptosis and differentiation. Drug is cytostatic.

Metabolism: Excellent bioavailability; metabolism unknown.

Dosage/Range:
Per protocol.

Drug Preparation/Administration: Per protocol, administered orally (breast, lung cancers) and intravenously (prostate, breast, colon cancers).

Drug Interactions: Unknown.

Lab Effects/Interference: Unknown.

Special Considerations:
- In Phase I and II clinical trials, SAHA causes accumulation of acetylated histones in peripheral blood mononuclear cells as well as tumor cells, so is being studied in hematologic and solid tumors.
- Synergistic with radiation, tyrosine kinase inhibitors (imatinib), chemotherapy (5-FU), differentiating agents (ATRA).
- As a single agent, demonstrated antitumor activity in cutaneous T-cell lymphoma, diffuse B-cell lymphoma, laryngeal cancer, and mesothelioma.
- Side effects occur after several weeks or months of therapy, and following a drug holiday, drug can be resumed.

Potential Toxicities/Side Effects and the Nursing Process

I. POTENTIAL FOR BLEEDING AND FATIGUE related to BONE MARROW DEPRESSION

Defining Characteristics: In clinical trials, fatigue, anemia and thrombocytopenia were reversible.

Nursing Implications: Monitor CBC, platelet count baseline and periodically during therapy per protocol. Assess for signs and symptoms of bleeding, fatigue, and anemia. Teach patient to self-assess for signs and symptoms of bleeding, anemia, and to call if they occur. Assess patient medication profile, and any OTC medications such as contain aspirin or NSAIDs that would increase risk of bleeding. Teach patient to avoid these drugs, and not to begin any OTC medications without first discussing with nurse or physician. Teach patient to alternate rest and activity periods if feeling fatigued; to organize shopping and chores in a way to minimize energy expenditures.

II. ALTERATION IN NUTRITION, LESS THAN BODY REQUIREMENTS related to DEHYDRATION AND ANOREXIA

Defining Characteristics: In clinical trials, anorexia and dehydration occurred, and were reversible following drug holiday.

Nursing Implications: Assess weight, and baseline nutritional status. Teach patient that anorexia and dehydration can occur, and ways to minimize this effect. Teach patient to identify nutritionally-dense (high calories and protein in the smallest amount) foods and to keep them handy in the refrigerator. Teach patient to eat small, frequent meals and to have a bedtime snack. Teach patient to drink a glass of fluid every hour while awake if patient is at risk for developing dehydration (elderly, forgetful).

Drug: temsirolimus (CCI-779) (investigational)

Class: Protein Kinase Inhibitor.

Mechanism of Action: Drug binds to the immunophilin FKBP and inhibits mTOR (mammalian Target of Rapamycin or FKBP 12) kinase. mTOR is responsible for sensing the nutrients in the cell's environment, and also for organizing actin, trafficking of the membrane, insulin secretion, protein degradation, protein kinase C signaling, and tRNA synthesis. Inhibition of the kinase makes the cell think it is starving and it stops growing (arrests cell growth in G1 phase of the cell cycle). As more is learned about the function of this pathway, it appears that rapamycin and mTOR inhibitors affect only some of mTOR functioning.

Metabolism: Unknown.

Dosage/Range:
Per protocol, but have ranged from 25–250 mg IV weekly; dose reduction for neutropenia, thrombocytopenia, and mucositis.

Drug Preparation/Administration: IV infusion over 30 minutes; premedication with diphenhydraminde 25–50 mg 30 minutes before drug administration. If hypersensitivity occurs, an H2-receptor antagonist is given 30 minutes prior to resuming drug administration.

Drug Interactions: Unknown.

Lab Effects/Interference: Hyperglycemia, hypertriglyceridemia, hypophospatemia; elevated GGT levels; rare neutropenia, thrombocytopenia, anemia.

Special Considerations:

- Drug is well tolerated with most common toxicities: maculopapular rash (76%), mucositis (70%), asthenia (50%) and nausea (43%) when studied in patients with advanced refractory renal cell carcinoma (Atkins et al, 2004); depression is a significant toxicity when the dose of 250 mg IV is used (Chen et al, 2005).
- Drug has shown anti-tumor activity in patients with advanced renal cell and advanced breast cancer. In the treatment of gliobolastoma multiforme, the drug is called a ''smart drug,'' because it targets molecular changes in the malignant cell related to its unfortunate aggressiveness (Galanis et al, 2005).

Potential Toxicities/Side Effects and the Nursing Process

I. POTENTIAL FOR INJURY related to INFUSION-RELATED REACTIONS AND HYPERSENSITIVITY

Defining Characteristics: The incidence of hypersensitivity was uncommon, as most patients received premedicaton with diphenhydramine (Chan et al, 2005).

Nursing Implications: Consult protocol. Discuss with physician the use of premedications such as diphenhydramine before drug therapy. In one study, patients who developed hypersensitivity despite diphenhudramine, the addition of an H2 antagonist 30 minutes prior to resuming the infusion prevented further hypersensitivity. Ensure that medications necessary for the management of hypersensitivity/anaphylaxis are readily available (e.g., epinephrine, antihistamines, corticosteroids). Assess baseline VS and monitor frequently during the infusion, as specified by the infusion. Be prepared to provide emergency support as necessary (including IV saline, epinephrine, antihistamines, bronchodilators). If/when symptoms resolve, resume the infusion at 50% of the rate of the previous infusion, as directed by the physician.

II. POTENTIAL FOR INFECTION AND BLEEDING related to NEUTROPENIA AND THROMBOCYTOPENIA

Defining Characteristics: Although rare, Grade 3 or 4 neutropenia occurred in 7% of patients, thrombocytopenia in 5%, and anemia in 9% of patients in clinical trials comparing doses 75–250 mg weekly.

Nursing Implications: Assess baseline blood counts and platelets. Teach patient to report fever, and signs/symptoms of infection or bleeding right away. Assess medication profile and OTC medications taken. Teach patient to avoid OTC medications containing NSAIDs or aspirin. Teach patient to talk to nurse or physician before beginning any OTC medications.

III. ALTERATION IN SKIN INTEGRITY, POTENTIAL, related to RASH

Defining Characteristics: Maculopapular rash is the most common toxicity, affecting between 51–76%; 33% had acne, 31% had a nail disorder, 19% had dry skin.

Nursing Implications: Assess patient skin integrity, including nails baseline and regularly during treatment. Teach patient self-assessment and local comfort measures. Teach patient to report skin changes and if self-care ineffective, discuss plan with physician, especially if severe.

IV. POTENTIAL ALTERATION IN NUTRITION, LESS THAN BODY REQUIREMENTS, related to MUCOSITIS, NAUSEA, ANOREXIA, DIARRHEA, HYPERGLYCEMIA, HYPERTRIGLYCERIDEMIA

Defining Characteristics: In clinical studies, mucositis affected 70% of patients, nausea 43%, diarrhea 27%, and anorexia 40% of patients; in terms of grade 3 and 4 toxicities, hyperglycemia occurred in 17% of patients, hypophosphatemia 13%, and hypertriglyceridemia in 6% of patients. mTOR is involved in insulin signaling, which possibly explains the hypertriglyceridemia and hypoglycemia.

Nursing Implications: Premedicate with antiemetics per protocol. Encourage small, frequent meals of cool, bland foods, and increase fluid intake. Assess oral mucosa prior to drug administration and instruct patient to report changes. Teach patient oral hygiene measures and self-assessment. Monitor glucose, triglyceride and phosphate serum levels baseline and during therapy per protocol. Notify physician of any abnormalities and discuss implications and management per protocol.

V. ALTERATION IN COMFORT AND ACTIVITY TOLERANCE, POTENTIAL, related to ASTHENIA, SOMNOLENCE AND DEPRESSION

Defining Characteristics: Asthenia affects 50% of patients in clinical studies, depression 17%, but at the higher dose of 250 mg q week, 5% had grade 3 and 4 depression; somnolence 30%, with 6% grade 3 and 4.

Nursing Implications: Assess baseline comfort, mental status, and activity tolerance, and reassess during treatment, asking patient to identify what activities now unable to do, sleep habits, and also feeling state. Discuss alternating rest and activity periods, and also possibility of other family members or friends assisting with energy consuming responsibilities to increase energy reserve. Assess baseline alertness, sleep patterns. Assess other drugs taken, especially those with sedating qualities, and alcohol ingestion. Instruct patient to avoid alcohol and to take drug at bedtime. Assess degree of drowsiness and dizziness for safety of patient. If significant, teach measures to ensure safety.

Drug: thalidomide (investigational)

Class: Inhibitor of TNF-alpha, antiangiogenesis agent.

Mechanism of Action: Drug exerts its immunomodulatory action in an unknown way. Hypothesized that drug may modulate VEGF (vascular epithelial growth factor) by inhibiting neovasculature and thus have an antiangiogenesis effect in malignant tumors.

Metabolism: Well absorbed after oral administration. Mean peak serum level reached at 4–5 hours. Elimination half-life is 4–12 hours, with drug found in the plasma after 24 hours. NOT metabolized using P450 hepatic enzyme system, and has low renal excretion.

Dosage/Range:
- Per protocol.
- Advanced multiple myeloma after relapse (after high-dose chemotherapy): begin dose of 200 mg PO qd, increase dose by 200 mg every 2 weeks up to 800 mg PO qd.

Drug Preparation/Administration:
- Oral, give at bedtime.
- Available for investigational or compassionate use in 50–mg capsules.

Drug Interactions:
- Barbiturates, alcohol, chlorpromazine, reserpine: increased sedation.

Lab Effects/Interference:
- Rare neutropenia.

Special Considerations:
- ABSOLUTE CONTRAINDICATION IS PREGNANCY. Pregnancy tests must be routinely negative prior to beginning therapy in women of childbearing age. Contraception is mandatory in men and women.
- Women taking hormonal contraception as well as any of the following drugs — barbiturates, glucocorticoids, phenytoin, carbamazepine—have decreased efficacy of the hormonal contraception and must use barrier contraception as well.
- Most common side effects are dry skin, occasional tingling of extremities, somnolence, fatigue, constipation, and neutropenia, followed by rash, peripheral neuropathy, lightheadedness, dizziness and edema. Uncommonly, severe rash, DVT, PE, URI and pneumonia, renal insufficiency, severe neutropenia and bradycardia may occur.

Potential Toxicities/Side Effects and the Nursing Process

I. ALTERATION IN SEXUALITY/REPRODUCTION related to POTENTIAL TERATOGENICITY

Defining Characteristics: Drug is teratogenic and a single dose can cause birth defects. Unclear if drug is excreted in semen.

Nursing Implications: Assess reproductive status, sexual activity, and birth control measures used for both men and women. Instruct male patients to use barrier contraception, and women to use both barrier and hormonal contraception. Women of childbearing age must have a negative pregnancy test baseline to begin the drug, and pregnancy test should be repeated every two weeks for two months, then every month. Instruct patient to continue contraception one month after drug is discontinued. Physicians, patients, and pharmacists must participate in drug manufacturer (Celgene, Warren, NJ) STEPS program (System for Thalidomide Education and Prescription Safety).

II. ALTERATION IN SENSORY/PERCEPTUAL PATTERNS related to PERIPHERAL NEUROPATHY

Defining Characteristics: Peripheral neuropathy occurs in about 25% of patients (range, 10–50%). If drug is discontinued at the first sign of neuropathy, symptoms are reversible. Neuropathy is a distal axonal degeneration affecting long and large-diameter motor and sensory axons in hands and feet. Initially, there is numbness of toes/feet, described often as a "tightness around the feet." There may be decreased sensitivity to light touch, pinprick (sensory loss) in hands and feet, muscle cramps, symmetrical sensorimotor neuropathy, painful paresthesias in hands and feet, distal hypoesthesia, proximal weakness in lower limbs, slight postural tremor, leg cramps, absent ankle jerks. If treatment is continued, there is permanent paresthesias of feet and hands, which progresses proximally. Increased risk of occurrence with increased age (> 70 years old) and high total doses > 14 g (40–50 g).

Nursing Implications: Assess baseline neurologic status, especially presence of peripheral neuropathy. Teach patient to stop drug and report immediately dysesthesias, numbness, and/or muscle cramps. Perform assessment for peripheral neuropathy at every visit.

III. ALTERATION IN SENSORY/PERCEPTUAL PATTERNS related to DROWSINESS

Defining Characteristics: Drug has nonbarbiturate sedative qualities, and drowsiness is the most frequent side effect. Tolerance to daytime drowsiness occurs over several weeks of use. Drowsiness and dizziness are more frequent at doses of 20–400 mg/day than at lower doses. HIV-infected patient studies reported drowsiness, dizziness, and mood changes 33–100% of the time.

Nursing Implications: Assess baseline alertness, sleep patterns. Assess other drugs taken, especially those with sedating qualities, and alcohol ingestion. Instruct patient to avoid alcohol and to take drug at bedtime. Assess degree of drowsiness and dizziness and safety of patient. If significant, teach measures to ensure safety. Tell patient that tolerance develops over 2–3 weeks.

IV. ALTERATION IN SKIN INTEGRITY, POTENTIAL, related to RASH

Defining Characteristics: Pruritic, erythematous macular rash may appear over trunk and back 2–13 days after initiation of therapy. Increased incidence in patients with HIV infection with low CD4 counts. Drug rechallenge often

either infusion: reduce infusion rate by 50% for mild to moderate infusional reactions; stop if reactions severe. After complete resolution of severe symptoms, resume infusion at 50% slower rate.

- Dosing: patients with platelet count $\geq$ 150,000/mm^3: dose is activity of I-131 calculated to deliver 75 cGy total body irradiation and 35 mg tositumomab; patients with platelet count 100,000/mm^3 but $<$ 150,000/mm^3: dose is activity of I-131 that will deliver 65 cGy total body irradiation and 35 mg tositumomab.

Drug Interactions:

- Unknown.

Lab Effects/Interference:

- Bone marrow suppressive agents: further depression of red blood cells, white blood cells, and platelets.
- If human anti-murine antibodies (HAMA) develop: interference with accuracy and results of diagnostic tests relying on murine antibody technology may occur.

Special Considerations:

- Indicated for the treatment of patients with CD_{20} positive, follicular, non-Hodgkin's lymphoma, whose disease is refractory to rituximab and has relapsed following chemotherapy.
- In rituximab-resistant patients, 63% responded with a median duration of 25 months.
- Therapeutic regimen should be prescribed by a physician certified or in the process of being certified by Corixa Corporation in dose calculation and administration of BEXXAR.
- Bexxar should be administered only once.
- Contraindicated in patients with known hypersensitivity to murine (mouse) proteins, patients with $>$25% lymphoma marrow involvement and/or impaired bone marrow reserve.
- Drug causes fetal harm so avoid use in pregnant women; women who are breast-feeding should discontinue nursing.
- Delayed adverse reactions that can develop are hypothyroidism, HAMA, myelodysplasia/leukemia, and secondary malignancies.
- Oral iodine supplements are given one day prior to dosimetric dose, and continued for 2 weeks after the therapeutic dose (to block the thyroid uptake of I-131).
- Overall summary of responses in 116 patients with low-grade or transformed low-grade NHL showed 78% responses (11.7-month median duration of response), with 46% complete responses (36.5-month median duration of response). 24 patients with no prior chemotherapy had a 100% response, with 71% having a complete response (Vose, 1998).

- The development of human antimouse antibodies (HAMA) was related to extent of prior chemotherapy: in chemonaïve patients, 38% developed HAMA, while only 4% did who received more than one prior chemotherapy regimen.
- Response rate and duration of response were lower in patients aged 65 and older, and duration of severe hematologic toxicity was longer.

Potential Toxicities/Side Effects and the Nursing Process

I. POTENTIAL FOR INJURY related to ANAPHYLAXIS

Defining Characteristics: Rare but potentially life-threatening reaction may occur. Mouse antibodies are used that are foreign and may stimulate anaphylaxis. No grade 4 adverse experiences have been reported. Approximately 8% of patients in clinical trials require slowing of the infusion to manage symptoms.

Nursing Implications: Assess baseline T, VS. If patient develops discomfort, slow infusion per protocol. Have emergency equipment and medications nearby. Assess patient for signs/symptoms, including generalized flushing and urticaria leading to pallor, cyanosis, bronchospasm, hypotension, unconsciousness. Teach patient to report signs/symptoms, including sense of doom, tickle in throat. If signs/symptoms occur, stop infusion immediately, assess VS, notify physician. Physician may prescribe epinephrine 0.3 mL (1:1000) SQ if hypotensive. Oxygen, antihistamines, corticosteroids may also be used.

II. POTENTIAL FOR INFECTION, BLEEDING, AND FATIGUE related to NEUTROPENIA, THROMBOCYTOPENIA, AND ANEMIA

Defining Characteristics: Prolonged Bone marrow suppression is the dose-limiting toxicity. Patients at risk are patients who have been heavily pretreated with minimal bone marrow reserve, who have lower nadir counts with longer times to recovery. The maximum tolerated total body dose is 75 cGy to avoid severe myelosuppression. Nadir counts occur approximately six weeks post-therapy. Median nadirs were ANC 1,000 cells/m^3, platelets 62,000 cells/m^3, and hemoglobin 11.1 gm/dL. Grade 4 toxicity occurred in < 5% of patients: absolute neutropenia < 100 cells/mm^3 (3%), platelet count < 10,000 cells/mm^3 (5%), and Hgb < 6.5% (4%). Supportive use of growth factors and transfusions was 18%, especially in patients heavily pretreated.

Nursing Implications: Assess prior bone marrow suppressive therapy and risk for toxicity. Assess baseline WBC, differential, Hgb/HCT and platelet count, and signs/symptoms of infection, bleeding, or fatigue. Discuss any abnormalities with physician before drug administration. Teach patient signs/symptoms of infection and bleeding, and to report them immediately. Teach patient self-care measures to minimize infection and bleeding, including avoidance of aspirin-containing OTC medication, and oral hygiene regimen. Teach patient signs/symptoms of fatigue, and self-care measures to maximize energy, and to minimize fatigue (e.g., alternate rest and activity periods, organize activities).

III. ALTERATION IN COMFORT related to INFUSION REACTION

Defining Characteristics: Approximately 29% of patients have infusion-related reactions, despite premedication with acetaminophen and diphenhydramine. Symptoms include fever, rigots or chills, sweating, hypotension, dyspnea, bronchospasm and nausea either during or up to 48 hours after the infusion.

Nursing Implications: Assess baseline T, VS, neurological status, and comfort level; monitor q4–6h if patient is in hospital. Assure patient receives premedication and regular dosing of antipyretic (e.g., acetaminophen ± diphenhydramine, nonsteroidal anti-inflammatory drug [NSAID]), and antiemetic as ordered by physician. Teach patient self-care measures, including monitoring T, comfort level, self-administration of prescribed medications prior to dose and regularly postdose, as well as the use of heat or cold for myalgias, anthralgias. Encourage patient to increase oral fluids and alternate rest and activity periods. If patient is in hospital and experiences rigor, discuss with physician IV meperidine (25 mg IV q15 min to maximum 100 mg in 1 hour) and monitor BP for hypotension.

IV. KNOWLEDGE DEFICIT, POTENTIAL, related to RADIATION PRECAUTIONS

Defining Characteristics: The Nuclear Regulatory Commission recommends that patients receiving outpatient I-131 anti-B1 therapy follow measures to prevent radiation contamination of others. Patients may receive outpatient treatment as long as total dose to an individual at 1 meter is < 500 millirem.

Nursing Implications: Teach patient rules of time and distance, and review protocol patient discharge instructions. If in doubt, discuss with radiotherapist or radiation physicist. Patients are advised to sleep alone for at least the first night. Discuss need for longer separation based on dose received. Other teaching is based on dose and should include (1) remain at distances of > 3 feet from other people, except for brief periods as necessary, for at least two days; (2) infants, young children, and pregnant women should not visit the patient; if necessary, visits should be brief, and a distance of at least 9 feet from the patients should be maintained; (3) do not travel by commercial transportation or go on a prolonged automobile trip with others for at least the first two days; (4) have sole use of the bathroom for at least two days; and (5) drink "plenty" of fluids for at least the first two days, e.g., 3+ quarts per day.

Drug: trastuzumab (Humanized anti-*Her*-2 Antibody, rhuMAbHER2, Herceptin)

Mechanism of Action: Recombinant humanized monoclonal antibody targeted against the human epidermal growth factor receptor (*Her*-2). *Her*-2 is overexpressed in a number of cancers, including 25–30% of breast cancers. This monoclonal antibody is believed to act through three different mechanisms: (1) the antagonizing function of the growth-signaling properties of *Her*-2, (2) signaling immune cells to attack and kill malignant cells with this receptor, and (3) synergistic and/or additive effects seen with many chemotherapeutic agents.

Metabolism: Initial studies using a loading dose of 4 mg/kg followed by a weekly maintenance dose of 2 mg/kg, a mean half-life of 5.8 days, with a range of 1–32 days was seen. More recent studies with trastuzumab suggest the half-life may be longer in the 21–28 day range.

Dosage/Range: (in HER-2 positive patients)

- Loading dose: 4 mg/kg IV infusion (never IV push) week 1.
- Maintenance dose: 2 mg/kg IV infusion weekly beginning at week 2 until at least disease progression.

Alternative dosing:

- Loading dose 8 mg/kg IV infusion.
- Maintenance dose: 6 mg/kg IV infusion q 3 weeks.

Drug Preparation:

- Drug is available as a lyophilized sterile powder of 440 mg per vial for parenteral administration. Requires refrigeration at 2–8°C (36–46°F). DO NOT FREEZE.
- Reconstitute with 20 mL of Bacteriostatic Water for Injection, USP, containing 1.1% benzyl alcohol, which is supplied with each vial. DO NOT SHAKE.
- Reconstituted solution contains 22 mg/mL. Further dilute desired dose in 250 mL of 0.9% Sodium Chloride Injection, USP.
- Vial is designed for multiple use, and is stable for 28 days following reconstitution at 2–8°C (36–46°F).

Drug Administration:

- Administered IV infusion; initial loading dose is administered over 90 minutes, and initial maintenance dose (week or dose 2) is administered over 90 minutes. Never give as IV push or bolus.
- Observe patient for 1 hour following completion of initial loading dose, and if well tolerated, observe patient for 30 minutes following completion of initial maintenance dose (week 2). If well tolerated, no further post-infusion observation is needed in subsequent weekly infusions.

- Subsequent maintenance doses are administered over 30 minutes if prior administration was well tolerated without fever, chills.
- Continue to administer over 90 minutes if fever, chills experienced in prior administrations.

Drug Interactions:

- Paclitaxel: 2 fold decrease in trastuzumab clearance in animals and a 1.5 fold increase in trastuzumab serum level in human clinical studies.
- No suggested interactions when combined with cisplatin, doxorubicin, epirubicin plus cyclophosphamide.
- No formal drug interaction studies done.

Lab Effects/Interference:

- None known.

Special Considerations:

- Trastuzumab is indicated in combination with paclitaxel for treatment of patients with metastatic breast cancer whose tumors overexpress the HER2 protein and have not received chemotherapy for their metastatic disease. It may also be given as a single agent in patients who overexpress HER2 protein and who have received one or more chemotherapy regimens for metastatic disease.
- Phase III clinical trials studied co-administration together with doxorubicin/cyclophosphamide and/or paclitaxel, and an increased risk of cardiomyopathy was seen. Left ventricular function should be evaluated prior to and during treatment with trastuzumab therapy.
- FISH appears more accurate in identifying HER2 overexpression.
- Trastuzumab is very well tolerated; given that it is a humanized antibody, no pre-medication is recommended.
- Rarely, trastuzumab may cause hypersensitivity/allergic reactions, so emergency equipment should be available during infusions.
- Trastuzumab at a dose of 6–8 mg/kg q 3 weeks × 1 year in the adjuvant setting was shown to reduce the risk of breast cancer recurrence significantly. Interim analysis of the HERA study (2005) showed that the group receiving trastuzumab for 1–2 yrs after adjuvant chemotherapy in HER-2 positive women had an estimated 2-year survival of 86% compared to 77% for the observation group. $P < 0.01$. Cardiac toxicity was higher in the trastuzumab arm, with CHF occurring 3–4% more commonly in high risk patients in the trastuzumab arm so cardiac function must be monitored (Piccan-Gebart et al, 2005).
- Romond et al (2005) summarized the NSABP B-31 and NCCTG N0931 trials showing that the addition of trastuzumab to paclitaxel (concurrent not sequential) following AC in the adjuvant setting, at 2 years, there was increased disease free and overall survival. Perez (2005) showed that after 4

years on study, 15% of the women treated with trastuzumab plus paclitaxel concurrently had recurrence, compared to 33% of women receiving paclitaxel alone. At this point, there was a 49% improvement in survival (Perez, 2005). While there was increased cardiotoxicity, it was within the 4% acceptable range.

Potential Toxicities/Side Effects and the Nursing Process

I. ALTERATION IN CIRCULATION related to CARDIOMYOPATHY

Defining Characteristics: Trastuzumab administration may result in ventricular dysfunction and congestive heart failure. A significant decrease in left ventricular function was found in patients who received concurrent anthracycline and cyclophosphamide chemotherapy. Incidence in one study with trastuzumab alone was 7%; in combination with paclitaxel it was 11%; paclitaxel alone, 1%; and in combination with doxorubicin (A) and cyclophosphamide (C) it was 28% compared to AC alone (7%). If allowed to progress, failure may be severe, and the following have been reported: severe cardiac failure, death, and mural thrombosis leading to stroke. Rare events described following treatment with trastuzumab were vascular thrombosis, pericardial effusion, heart arrest, hypotension, syncope, hemorrhage, shock, and arrythmia.

Nursing Implications: Assess baseline cardiac function, including apical pulse, BP. Review history, and identify patients at risk who have CHF, hypertension, coronary artery disease, or who are receiving trastuzumab in combination with either paclitaxel or AC. Patients should have baseline ECHO or gated blood pool scan to determine left ventricular ejection fraction, and this should be monitored periodically, especially in patients at risk. Assess for signs and symptoms at each visit: dyspnea, increased cough, paroxysmal nocturnal dyspnea, peripheral edema, S_3 gallop, and decrease in left ventricular function when tested. Teach patient to report cough, weight gain, edema of ankles, difficulty breathing, or need to use more pillows at night. Drug should be discontinued in patients who develop clinically significant congestive heart failure.

II. POTENTIAL FOR INJURY related to HYPERSENSITIVITY

Defining Characteristics: Infusion-related reactions (e.g., fever and/or chills) were reported in about 40% of paients with their first treatment, and > 10% with subsequent infusions. Severe hypersensitivity reactions are rare but have been seen.

Nursing Implications: Assess VS baseline and frequently during infusion, especially during initial loading and maintenance infusions. Observe patient for one hour following completion of loading dose, and 30 minutes after initial maintenance dose if loading dose was well tolerated. If not well tolerated, continue to monitor for 60 minutes until well tolerated. Notify physician if fever, chills develop and assess need for acetaminophen, and slowing of infusion. Although severe allergic reactions are uncommon, have emergency equipment available and nearby, and be prepared to provide emergency support if necessary.

III. ALTERATION IN COMFORT related to PAIN, ASTHENIA, DYSPNEA

Defining Characteristics: Generalized pain may affect 11% of patients, dyspnea 6%, and asthenia 5%. Abdominal pain may specifically affect 3% of patients.

Nursing Implications: Teach patients to report alterations in comfort, especially pain and dyspnea. Distinguish new onset of symptoms versus those experienced prior to treatment due to malignancy. Discuss intensity of symptoms and need for pharmacologic and nonpharmacologic interventions. Monitor response to intervention between weekly treatments, and need for alternative strategies.

Drug: tretinoin (Vesanoid®, ATRA, All-Trans-Retinoic Acid)

Class: Retinoid.

Mechanism of Action: Induces maturation of acute promyelocytic leukemia (APL) cells, thus decreasing proliferation. In patients who achieve a complete response to this therapy, there is an initial maturation of primitive leukemic cells, and then cells in both the bone marrow and peripheral blood are normal, polyclonal blood cells. The exact mechanism is unknown.

Metabolism: This drug is well absorbed orally into the systemic circulation, with peak concentrations in 1–2 hours. Drug is > 95% protein-bound, primarily to albumin. Oxidative metabolism occurs via the cytochrome P450 enzyme system in the liver. Drug is excreted in the urine (63% in 72 hours) and feces (31% in 6 days).

Dosage/Range:
- 45 mg/m^2 per day.

Drug Preparation:
- None: oral.
- Available as 10–mg capsules.
- Protect from light.

Drug Administration:
- Drug is to be used for induction remission only.

- Administer in evenly divided doses until complete remission (CR) is achieved, then for an additional 30 days, or after 90 days of treatment, whichever comes first.

Drug Interactions:
- Drugs that either inhibit or induce the cytochrome P450 hepatic enzyme system potentially will interact with this drug, but there is no data to suggest that these drugs either increase or decrease tretinoin activity.
- Drugs that induce the enzyme system: rifampin, glucocorticoids, phenobarbitol, pentobarbitol; drugs that inhibit the enzyme system: ketoconazole, cimetidine, erythromycin, verapamil, diltiazem, cyclosporin.

Lab Effects/Interference:
- Increased cholesterol and triglyceride levels (60% of patients) and elevated LFTs (50–60% of patients).

Special Considerations:
- Indicated for the induction remission of patients with APL (FAB-M3), characterized by the presence of the t(15:17) translocation and/or presence of the PML/RARα (alpha) gene.
- Absorption is enhanced when taken with food.
- Monitor CBC, platelets, coagulation studies, liver function tests, and triglyceride and cholesterol levels frequently during therapy.

Potential Toxicities/Side Effects and the Nursing Process

I. ALTERATION IN OXYGENATION, POTENTIAL, related to RETINOIC ACID-APL SYNDROME

Defining Characteristics: Syndrome occurs in approximately 25% of patients and varies in severity, but has resulted in death. Syndrome is characterized by fever, dyspnea, weight gain, pulmonary infiltrates on X-ray, and pleural and/or pericardial effusions. May also be accompanied by impaired myocardial contractility, hypotension, ± leukocytosis, and because of progressive hypoxemia and multisystem organ failure, some patients have died. Usually occurs during first month of treatment, but may follow initial drug dose.

Nursing Implications: Assess VS, pulmonary exam, and weight at each visit. Teach patient to do daily weights, and to report any SOB, fever, weight gain. If this occurs, notify physician and discuss obtaining CXR and focused exam. Discuss chest X-ray findings with physician. Be prepared to give high-dose steroids at the first sign of the syndrome, e.g., dexamethasone 10 mg IV q12h × 3 days or until symptom resolution (necessary in 60% of patients). Provide pulmonary and hemodynamic support as necessary. Discuss whether drug should be discontinued based on severity and patient's response to high-dose steroids.

II. ALTERATION IN COMFORT related to VITAMIN A TOXICITY

Defining Characteristics: Almost all patients experience some toxicity, but they do not usually have to discontinue the drug. Toxicity of high-dose vitamin A includes headache (86%) starting the first week of treatment, but fading after that; fever (83%); skin/mucous membrane dryness (77%); bone pain (77%); nausea/vomiting (57%); rash (54%); mucositis (26%); pruritus (20%); increased sweating (20%); visual disturbances (17%); ocular disorders (17%); skin changes (17%); alopecia (14%); changed visual acuity (6%); visual field defects (3%).

Nursing Implications: Teach patient about possible side effects of high-dose vitamin A as above and to report them if they occur. Teach patient symptom management. Assess severity of symptom(s) and discuss with physician symptom management of fever, headache unresponsive to acetaminophen, nausea/vomiting. If headache is severe in a child, have child evaluated for pseudotumor cerebri.

III. POTENTIAL FOR INJURY related to PSEUDOTUMOR CEREBRI

Defining Characteristics: Benign intracranial hypertension has occurred in children treated with retinoids. Early signs and symptoms are papilledema, headache, nausea and vomiting, and visual disturbances.

Nursing Implications: Teach patient/parents to report symptoms. Assess patient for symptomatology on regular basis. If headache is severe, discuss with physician analgesics and therapeutic lumbar puncture.

IV. POTENTIAL DISTURBANCE IN CIRCULATION

Defining Characteristics: The following disturbances may occur: arrythmia (23%), flushing (23%), hypotension (14%), hypertension (11%), phlebitis (11%), cardiac failure (6%); 3% of patients studied developed cardiac arrest, myocardial infarction, enlarged heart, heart murmur, ischemia, stroke, and other serious disturbances.

Nursing Implications: Assess cardiac status baseline and presence of risk factors (e.g., hypertension). Assess VS at each visit and teach patient in a manner not to induce anxiety to report any symptoms such as chest pain, SOB, heart palpitations, or any changes that occur.

V. ALTERATION IN NUTRITION, LESS THAN BODY REQUIREMENTS, related to GI DYSFUNCTION

Defining Characteristics: Some problems are related to APL, and together with drug may emerge, such as GI bleeding/hemorrhage, which may occur in up to 34% of patients. Other GI problems include abdominal pain (31%), diarrhea (23%), constipation (17%), dyspepsia (14%), abdominal distention (11%), hepatosplenomegaly (9%), hepatitis (3%), and ulcer (3%).

Nursing Implications: Assess GI status and presence of GI dysfunction baseline. Teach patient to report any GI disturbances or changes in bowel status. If these occur, assess severity and need for symptom management, or discussion/intervention with physician. Monitor liver function studies frequently during therapy.

VI. SENSORY/PERCEPTUAL ALTERATIONS related to CHANGES IN EAR SENSATION/HEARING

Defining Characteristics: 23% of patients report earache or fullness in ears. Other ear problems that may occur are reversible hearing loss (5%) and irreversible hearing loss (1%).

Nursing Interventions: Teach patient that this may occur and to report it if it occurs. Assess severity and need for intervention.

VII. POTENTIAL FOR INJURY related to CNS, PERIPHERAL NERVOUS SYSTEM CHANGES, AND AFFECT CHANGES

Defining Characteristics: Changes that may occur include dizziness (20%), paresthesias (17%), anxiety (17%), insomnia (14%), depression (14%), confusion (11%), cerebral hemorrhage (9%), agitation (9%), and hallucinations (6%). Rarely, the following may occur: forgetfulness, gait disturbances, convulsions, coma, facial paralysis, tremor, leg weakness, somnolence, slow speech, aphasia, and other CNS changes.

Nursing Implications: Teach patient in a manner that does not cause anxiety to report any changes in affect, sensorium, or functional ability (e.g., to walk, speak). Assess severity of symptom(s) if they arise and potential for injury. If severe, modify patient's environment to minimize risk of injury and discuss medical intervention with physician.

VIII. ALTERED URINARY ELIMINATION, POTENTIAL, related to RENAL CHANGES

Defining Characteristics: Uncommonly, renal insufficiency may occur (11%), dysuria (9%), acute renal failure (3%), urinary frequency (3%), renal tubular necrosis (3%), and enlarged prostate (3%).

Nursing Implications: Assess baseline urinary elimination pattern. Teach patient to report any changes. Monitor BUN/creatinine periodically during therapy and discuss any abnormalities with physician.

Drug: liposomal tretinoin (Atragen®, All-Trans-Retinoic Acid Liposomal, AR-623. LipoATRA, Tretinoin Liposomal) (investigational)

Class: Retinoid.

Mechanism of Action: Induces maturation of acute promyelocytic leukemia (APL) cells, thus decreasing proliferation. In patients who achieve a complete response to this therapy, there is an initial maturation of primitive leukemic cells, and then cells in both the bone marrow and peripheral blood are normal, polyclonal blood cells. The exact mechanism is unknown. Liposomal drug permits IV administration, with less toxicity, as it is believed the liposome overcomes resistance seen with continued oral therapy (possibly due to declining serum levels during oral administration since IV administration of liposome gives higher and more sustained plasma levels of drug (Estey et al, 1999).

Metabolism: IV administration of liposome gives higher and more sustained plasma levels of drug as compared to oral administration. Probably has oxidative metabolism via the cytochrome P450 enzyme system in the liver. Drug is probably excreted in the urine and feces.

Dosage/Range:

- Per research protocol.
- Newly diagnosed acute promyelocytic leukemia (APL) 90 mg/m^2 IV every other day for induction, followed by maintenance with the same dose 3 times a week × 9 months.
- AIDS-related Kaposi's sarcoma: 120 mg/m^2 three times a week × 4 weeks (Bernstein et al, 1998).

Drug Preparation:

- Per research protocol.

Drug Administration:

- IV, per research protocol.

Drug Interactions:

- Drugs that either inhibit or induce the cytochrome P450 hepatic enzyme system potentially will interact with this drug, but there is no data to suggest that these drugs either increase or decrease tretinoin activity.
- Drugs that induce the enzyme system: rifampin, glucocorticoids, phenobarbitol, pentobarbitol; drugs that inhibit the enzyme system: ketoconazole, cimetidine, erythromycin, verapamil, diltiazem, cyclosporin.

Lab Effects/Interference:

- Increased cholesterol and triglyceride levels.
- Elevated LFTs.
- Elevated renal function test.

Special Considerations:

- Has shown effectiveness in the induction remission of patients with APL (FAB-M3) characterized by the presence of the t(15:17) translocation and/or presence of the PML/RARα (alpha) gene. It should be considered in patients relapsing after oral tretinoin, refractory to oral tretinoin and chemotherapy, or unable to take oral tretinoin.
- In one clinical trial, for newly diagnosed patients with APL, time to hematologic complete remission (CR) was a median of 34 days (range, 22–64 days), but at this time only 10% had a molecular CR. However, after an additional three months of therapy, all patients with a hematologic CR achieved a molecular CR (Estey et al, 1999). Complete hematologic remission is defined as $< 5\%$ blasts and $< 8\%$ promyelocytes in bone marrow (with normal appearing myelocytes), ANC $\geq 1000/mm^3$, and platelet count of $\geq 100{,}000/mm^3$; molecular remission means the PML-RAR-alpha gene rearrangement has disappeared, as shown by PCR (polymerase chain reaction) at a sensitivity of 10(-4).
- In newly diagnosed APL, high response rates were seen in patients with low white counts, e.g., $< 10{,}000/mm^3$, and were minimal in patients with high white counts (Estey et al, 1999).
- Drug appears to slow progression of lesions in AIDS-related Kaposi's sarcoma.
- Drug is being studied in cancer of the prostate, bladder (superficial), and non-Hodgkin's lymphoma.
- Toxicity profile is less than with oral tretinoin.
- Monitor CBC, platelets, coagulation studies, liver function tests, and triglyceride and cholesterol levels, renal function tests baseline, and frequently during therapy.
- Drug is contraindicated during pregnancy as drug is teratogenic, and women should not breast-feed while taking the drug; drug is contraindicated in patients hypersensitive to tretinoin or any of the liposomal components.
- Drug, as with oral version, can cause retinoic acid-acute promyelocytic leukemia syndrome (RA-APL): fever, dyspnea, joint pain.
- Drug should be used cautiously in patients with renal dysfunction, patients with prior sensitivity to acitretin, etretinate, isotretinoin, or other vitamin A derivatives; and patients with pretherapy leukocytosis, as the risk for developing RA-APL syndrome is increased.

Potential Toxicities/Side Effects and the Nursing Process

I. ALTERATION IN OXYGENATION, POTENTIAL, related to RETINOIC ACID-APL SYNDROME

Defining Characteristics: Syndrome occurs in approximately 25% of patients and varies in severity, but has resulted in death in studies of the oral drug. Syndrome is characterized by fever, dyspnea, weight gain, pulmonary infiltrates on X-ray, and pleural and/or pericardial effusions, and joint pain. May also be accompanied by impaired myocardial contractility, hypotension, ± leukocytosis, and because of progressive hypoxemia and multisystem organ failure, some patients have died in studies using the oral drug. Usually occurs during first month of treatment, but may follow initial drug dose. With liposomal drug, when dose was reduced and it was given with steroids, patients successfully continued/completed liposomal tretinoin treatment.

Nursing Implications: Assess VS, pulmonary exam, and weight at each visit. Teach patient to do daily weights, and to report any SOB, fever, weight gain. If this occurs, notify physician and discuss obtaining CXR and focused exam. Discuss chest X-ray findings with physician. Be prepared to give high-dose steroids at the first sign of the syndrome, e.g., dexamethasone 10 mg IV q12h × 3 days or until symptom resolution (necessary in 60% of patients). Provide pulmonary and hemodynamic support as necessary. Discuss whether drug should be discontinued based on severity and patient's response to high-dose steroids.

II. ALTERATION IN COMFORT related to VITAMIN A TOXICITY

Defining Characteristics: Toxicity is less with liposomal IV drug than when given orally. Almost all patients experience some toxicity, but they do not usually have to discontinue the drug. Toxicity of high-dose vitamin A includes headache starting the first week of treatment (87% incidence in one study), but fading after that; fever; skin/mucous membrane dryness; bone pain; nausea/vomiting; rash; mucositis; pruritus; increased sweating; visual disturbances (ocular disorders); skin changes; alopecia; changed visual acuity; visual field defects.

Nursing Implications: Teach patient about possible side effects of high-dose vitamin A as above and to report them if they occur. Teach patient symptom management. Assess severity of symptom(s) and discuss with physician symptom management of fever, headache unresponsive to acetaminophen, nausea/vomiting. Teach patient to avoid other administration of vitamin A preparations, e.g., beta carotene. If headache is severe in a child, have child evaluated for pseudotumor cerebri.

III. POTENTIAL FOR INJURY related to PSEUDOTUMOR CEREBRI

Defining Characteristics: Benign intracranial hypertension has occurred in children treated with retinoids. Early signs and symptoms are papilledema, headache, nausea and vomiting, and visual disturbances.

Nursing Implications: Teach patient/parents to report symptoms. Assess patient for symptomatology on regular basis. If headache is severe, discuss with physician analgesics and therapeutic lumbar puncture.

IV. POTENTIAL DISTURBANCE IN CIRCULATION

Defining Characteristics: Toxicity is less than in incidence of patients receiving oral tretinoin. The following disturbances may occur: arrythmia, flushing, hypotension, hypertension, phlebitis, cardiac failure; one patient studied developed fatal acute heart failure myocardial infarction occurring day after starting therapy, with death the following day in a patient with a history of coronary artery disease and hypertension, and in whom ACE inhibitor was discontinued day prior to starting liposomal tretinoin. In oral studies, enlarged heart, heart murmur, ischemia, stroke, and other serious disturbances occurred.

Nursing Implications: Assess cardiac status baseline and presence of risk factors (e.g., hypertension). Assess VS at each visit and teach patient, in a manner not to induce anxiety, to report any symptoms such as chest pain, SOB, heart palpitations, or any changes that occur.

V. ALTERATION IN NUTRITION, LESS THAN BODY REQUIREMENTS, related to GI DYSFUNCTION

Defining Characteristics: Toxicity with liposomal tretinoin is less severe or frequent than with oral drug. Some problems are related to APL, and together with drug, may emerge, such as GI bleeding/hemorrhage, abdominal pain, diarrhea, constipation, dyspepsia, abdominal distention, hepatosplenomegaly, hepatitis, and ulcer.

Nursing Implications: Assess GI status and presence of GI dysfunction baseline. Teach patient to report any GI disturbances or changes in bowel status. If these occur, assess severity and need for symptom management, or discuss intervention with physician. Monitor liver function studies frequently during therapy.

VI. SENSORY/PERCEPTUAL ALTERATIONS related to CHANGES IN EAR SENSATION/HEARING

Defining Characteristics: Toxicity with liposomal tretinoin is less severe or frequent than with oral drug. Patients may report earache or fullness in ears, and hearing loss.

Nursing Interventions: Teach patient that this may occur and to report it if it occurs. Assess severity and need for intervention.

VII. POTENTIAL FOR INJURY related to CNS, PERIPHERAL NERVOUS SYSTEM CHANGES, AND AFFECT CHANGES

Defining Characteristics: Toxicity with liposomal tretinoin is less severe or frequent than with oral drug. Changes that may occur include dizziness, paresthesias, anxiety, insomnia, depression, confusion, cerebral hemorrhage, agitation, and hallucinations. Rarely, the following may occur: forgetfulness, gait disturbances, convulsions, coma, facial paralysis, tremor, leg weakness, somnolence, slow speech, aphasia, and other CNS changes.

Nursing Implications: Teach patient in a manner that does not cause anxiety to report any changes in affect, sensorium, or functional ability (e.g., to walk, speak). Assess severity of symptom(s) if they arise and potential for injury. If severe, modify patient's environment to minimize risk of injury and discuss medical intervention with physician.

VIII. ALTERED URINARY ELIMINATION, POTENTIAL, related to RENAL CHANGES

Defining Characteristics: Toxicity with liposomal tretinoin is less severe or frequent than with oral drug. Uncommonly, renal insufficiency may occur, dysuria, acute renal failure, urinary frequency, renal tubular necrosis, and enlarged prostate.

Nursing Implications: Assess baseline urinary elimination pattern. Teach patient to report any changes. Monitor BUN/creatinine periodically during therapy and discuss any abnormalities with physician.

Drug: vatalanib (PTK787/ZK222584)

Class: Angiogenesis inhibitor; protein tyrosine kinase inhibitor.

Mechanism of Action: Drug is a potent inhibitor of all known vascular endothelial growth factor (VEGF) tyrosine kinases (VEGFR-1, 2, 3) that are expressed on endothelial cells; also inhibits c-KIT and platelet-derived growth factor receptor (PDGFR).

Metabolism: Rapidly absorbed in 1–2 hours following oral ingestion; half-life of 4–5 hrs.

Dosage/Range:

Per protocol, eg, 50–1500 mg/day; probably requires multiple dosing per day given half-life of q 4–5 hrs

Drug Preparation: Oral.

Drug Interactions: Unknown

Lab Effects/Interference: Unknown

Special Considerations:

- Drug is being studied in patients with colorectal cancer, and glioblastoma multiforme.
- CONFIRM-1 (Colrectal Oral Novel Therapy for the Inhibition of Angiogenesis and Retarding of Metastases) trial: phase III trial comparing patients with advanced colorectal cancer receiving FOLFOX ± vetalinib. Although there appeared to be a significant difference favoring patients receiving the combination (17% reduction in risk of disease progression) this was not significant when reviewed by central reviewers. Survival data is being accrued. It is questioned that perhaps drug was not given frequently enough (qd instead of bid or more frequent) since the half-life of the drug is only 4–5 hrs.
- CONFIRM 2: Phase III trial comparing patients with metastatic colorectal cancer who have progressed after 1st line irinotecan containing chemotherapy. Overall survival data are expected in mid-2006.
- Grade 3 thrombopenia and Grade 4 neutropenia higher in the patients receiving vatalinib and FOLFOX compared to patients receiving FOLFOX alone.

Potential Toxicities/Side Effects and the Nursing Process

I. ALTERATION IN HEMOSTASIS related to BLEEDING and THROMBOSIS

Defining Characteristics: In the CONFIRM trials, Grade 3 venous thrombosis occurred in 7% of patients compared to 4% in the FOLFOX alone arm, and Grade 4 pulmonary embolism occurred in 6% versus 1% in the FOLFOX only arm.

Nursing Implications: Assess baseline hematologic parameters and monitor during therapy. Teach patient to assess for and report right away signs/symptoms of thrombosis: new swelling, pain, skin warmth and/or change in color (e.g., erythema, mottling) on the legs or thighs; new onset pain in the abdomen; dysnpnea or shortness of breath, rapid heartbeat, chest pain, or pressure that may signal a pulmonary embolism; and any changes in vision, new onset of severe headache, lightheadedness, or dizziness. Assess baseline mental status and neurological signs and monitor during therapy.

II. POTENTIAL ALTERATION IN CIRCULATION related to HYPERTENSION

Defining Characteristics: Grade 3 hypertension occurred in 21% of patients receiving the combination in the CONFIRM trial compared to 6% receiving FOLFOX alone.

Nursing Implications: Assess baseline BP prior to and during treatment, at least for the first treatment, then prior to each drug administration. If the patient has a history of hypertension, monitor BP more closely, although hypertension develops over time rather than during the drug infusion. Blood pressure should continue to be monitored after patient has stopped the drug. Teach patient drug administration, potential side-effects, and self care measures if prescribed antihypertensive medication, such as angiotensin-converting enzyme inhibitors, beta blockers, diuretics, and calcium channel blockers, consult protocol and expect that drug should be permanently discontinued if the patient develops hypertensive crisis (diastolic blood pressure > 120 mm Hg). Drug can be temporarily suspended in patients with severe hypertension until BP can be controlled with medical management per protocol.

III. POTENTIAL FOR ACTIVITY INTOLERANCE related to FATIGUE,

Defining Characteristics: Fatigue occurs commonly in patients with advanced colorectal cancer treated with vatalinib and FOLFOX; dizziness was more common in the patiens receiving the combination, and 7% of patients receiving the combination had grade 3 dizziness compared to 2% receiving FOLFOX alone.

Nursing Implications: Teach patient that fatigue and dizziness may occur and self-care measures. Teach patient to alternate rest and activity periods, to plan shopping and chores to minimize energy expenditure, and to explore whether family members can assist with necessary chores. Teach patient to slowly change position to minimize feeling dizzy, and to hold onto secure objects such as the wall and not a small table, when arising and moving from a sitting to a standing position. Teach patient to report increasing or severe dizziness.

Section 2
Symptom Management

Chapter 6
Pain

Pain in the patient with cancer may result from a variety of stimuli. A careful assessment is critical in order to identify the physical causes and psychosocial factors that modulate pain intensity and perception. Pain can be acute or chronic. Acute pain results from stimuli such as surgical procedures, pathological fractures, and obstruction of a hollow viscus, while chronic pain reflects the more common cancer pain resulting from tissue inflammation caused by tumor, but patients often have both acute and chronic components of pain. Acute pain lasts from minutes to months and ceases when the cause of pain is removed (e.g., pain caused by spinal cord compression is removed when the patient undergoes laminectomy or radiotherapy to relieve the compression). This type of pain is often associated with anxiety, and as well one sees symptoms of sympathetic nervous system arousal (increased heart rate, increased/decreased BP). In contrast, chronic pain lasts from months to years; the cause cannot be removed, and this type of pain is often associated with depression. The long duration of chronic pain dampens sympathetic response, so the patient does not manifest changes in heart rate or BP.

Symptoms often accompanying unrelieved pain are sleeplessness, anorexia (loss of appetite), fatigue, irritability, and fear. Nurses play a critical role in advocating for effective cancer pain management and alleviation of other accompanying symptoms. Fortunately, there are a variety of available analgesic medications, including non-opioid and opioid, adjuvant agents such as antidepressants, as well as nonpharmacologic techniques such as relaxation exercises.

In addition, opioid agents are available in immediate-onset formulations for acute pain, and long-duration agents that allow superior control for chronic pain as long-acting preparations avoid the peaks and valleys of serum levels and relief associated with immediate preparations. While analgesics do not remove the source or stimulus for the pain, they decrease or modulate the impulse so that the pain impulse perceived by the patient is reduced or absent, thus decreasing the distress and discomfort perceived by the patient. *Non-opioid* medications are helpful for mild to moderate pain. Most non-opioid analgesics work peripherally to decrease prostaglandin synthesis (NSAIDs), but some agents may have a central action as well, possibly at the level of the hypothalamus (McEvoy, Litvak, and Welsh, 1992). Pain receptors appear to be sensitized to mechanical and chemical stimulation by prostaglandins, so interruption of prostaglandin synthesis diminishes the painful impulse. For example, bone destruction and pain from metastasis appear to be mediated by prostaglandins, so NSAIDs that inhibit prostaglandin synthesis are first-line analgesics (Foley 2000). In addition, the anti-inflammatory action of NSAIDs contributes to analgesia. Principal side effects of this class are alteration in hemostasis (aspirin inhibits platelet aggregation, while other salicylates may alter hepatic synthesis of blood coagulation factors); alteration in GI mucosal integrity (aspirin and other NSAIDs can erode GI mucosal surface, causing bleeding or ulceration); and altered renal elimination due to inhibition of renal prostaglandins responsible for renal blood flow and function.

Recently, COX-2 inhibitors came upon the health care scene, in relation to the treatment of rheumatoid and osteoarthritis. Their role in the management of cancer-related bony pain is unclear, but the selective inhibition of prostaglandins responsible for inflammation is an achievement that will undoubtedly find a niche. In addition, these agents at slightly higher dosing may have anti-tumor effects as well as they decrease angiogenesis and increase apoptosis ability on the cellular level. NSAIDs achieve their anti-inflammatory effect by inhibiting the enzyme cyclooxygenase (COX), which is necessary for synthesis of prostaglandins and thromboxanes. There are two isoforms of the enzyme, COX-1, which appears to protect the gastric mucosa and is found in most tissues including platelets, and COX-2, which is found in brain and kidney tissue, as well as other body tissues at the site of inflammation. NSAIDs traditionally inhibit both COX-1 and COX-2 isoforms, resulting in a high risk of gastric ulceration and perforation. The risk of gastrointestinal bleeding is significantly less with the selective COX-2 inhibitors but still may occur. In addition, the selective COX-2 inhibitors do not affect bleeding time. The effect of the new COX-2 inhibitors on acute pain remains to be seen. In one study, 50 mg of refecoxib was equally effective as 550 mg of naproxen sodium or 400 mg of ibuprofen. Two other selective COX-2 inhibitors are celecoxib (Celebrex®) and rofecoxib (Vioxx®). Of interest as the applications of these new agents are explored is their possible role in prevention or treatment of colon cancer. An American Cancer Society study (Thun et al, 1991) showed that the regular ingestion of aspirin diminished colon cancer mortality 40% in men and 42% in women over six years. In addition, it appears that prostaglandin E2 may have a role in colon cancer development, and it appears that a COX-2–derived prostanoid promotes survival of colonic adenomas (Lipsky 1999). Currently, research is underway to better define the role of COX-2 inhibitors in the prevention and/or management of colon cancer.

Adjuvant analgesics play a vital role in cancer pain management. These drugs are indicated for purposes other than analgesia but can be combined with primary analgesics to increase analgesia and/or manage symptoms related to pain or the adverse effects of the opioids. There may be wide variations in patient responses. The major classes used as adjuvant drugs are antidepressant (Chapter 9), corticosteroid (Chapter 1), anticonvulsant (Chapter 7), and specialty drugs for bony metastasis (Chapter 10).

The *antidepressants* enhance pain-modulating pathways that are mediated by serotonin and norepinephrine, and, interestingly, clomipramine and amitriptyline have been shown to increase morphine levels (Wilkie, 1995). Not only can these agents help reduce the depression associated with chronic pain, but they can also relieve sleep problems, and often offer significant benefit in the management of neuropathic pain. Most commonly, the tricyclic antidepressants are used, such as amitriptyline and desipramine. The drug selection should be individualized to the patient and the risk for developing side effects. The advent of serotonin-reuptake inhibitors (SSRI) brought great hope to oncology nurses. However, there have been conflicting resports of the efficacy of these SSRIs in managing chronic pain syndromes (Belcheva et al, 1995; Tokunaga et al, 1998). Of the non-tricyclic antidepressants, paroxetine (Paxil) has shown benefit in reducing the painful symptoms of peripheral neuropathy in diabetic patients (Sindrup et al, 1990) and itching in patients with advanced cancer (Zycliz, 1996). In dosing antidepressants, the starting dosage should be low (i.e., 10 mg amitriptyline for the elderly patient, or 25 mg for the young adult) and given at bedtime. The dose should be titrated up slowly to the usually effective range of 50–150 mg. It is important to allow one week between dose titrations to evaluate the benefit of a given dose. Side effects include: sedation, orthostatic hypotension, constipation, dry mouth, dizziness and, less commonly, precipitation of acute angle-closure glaucoma, urinary retention, and arrhythmia.

Corticosteroids are useful in both acute and chronic pain management, such as that associated with metastatic bone pain, neuropathic pain, lymphedema, hepatic capsular distension, and brain metastasis. The dosing is individualized to the etiology of the pain and patient requirements, from low doses to high doses for patients with brain metastasis. It is important to identify patients at risk for peptic ulceration, and then to use corticosteroids cautiously if at all. In addition, patients need to be cautioned not to take concomitant aspirin.

Anticonvulsants may provide analgesia for lancinating, neuropathic pain. Drugs such as gabapentin, carbamazepine, phenytoin, clonazepam, and valproate are often used, and the dosing is the same as that used for seizure prevention.

Specialty drugs for the management of bony metastasis are biphosphonate pamidronate disodium (Aredia) and zolendronate (Zometa), indicated for use in managing pain related to bony metastases. Pamidronate and zolendronate have been shown to inhibit osteoclast activity and reduce pain from bony metastasis. Treatment is given IV every four weeks. Radiopharmaceuticals such as Strontium-89 is taken up in bone mineral preferentially, in sites of metastasis. However, the subsequent development of acute leukemia has limited interest in radiopharmaceutical management of pain.

Opioid analgesics are the cornerstone of management of moderate to severe cancer pain. These drugs, opiate agonists, attach to specific opiate receptors in the limbic system, thalamus, hypothalamus, spinal cord, and organs such as intestines. This leads to altered pain perception at the spinal cord and higher CNS levels. Because of this action, side effects that may occur include suppressed cough reflex; alterations in consciousness and mood (drowsiness, sedation, euphoria, dysphoria, mental clouding); respiratory depression; nausea/vomiting; and constipation. Opiate agonists may cause physical dependence (causing physical signs and symptoms of withdrawal if drug is stopped abruptly after chronic usage) and addiction (psychological dependence). However, addiction is VERY RARE in cancer patients, occurring in less than 0.1% of patients.

Unfortunately, some patients with cancer pain suffer needlessly because health care providers (physicians) underprescribe and (nurses) undermedicate (Marks and Sacher 1973). Chronic cancer pain requires the patient to self-administer opioids "around-the-clock" rather than "as needed (PRN)" to prevent moderate-to-severe pain. Tolerance is the ability to receive larger amounts of a drug without ill effect and to show decreased effect (i.e., pain relief) with continued use of the same drug dose. Tolerance occurs over time, depending on the drug and the route of administration. In addition, tolerance to the respiratory depressant effects of opiates develops over time with chronic usage for prevention of cancer pain. For instance, a patient with severe cancer pain who has been receiving escalating doses over a period of time may require very high doses to finally eliminate or reduce the pain to acceptable levels, as in the case of a patient with head and neck cancer who required 1200 mg/hour of morphine yet was still ambulatory and able to interact with family and friends. According to McCaffery (1982), pain is "whatever the patient says it is, occurring where the patient says it is." Use of quantifiable measurement tools is helpful to identify pain intensity (see Figure 6.1) and pain *relief* in response to intervention. The World Health Organization recommends a two-step approach to cancer pain management, beginning with non-opioids for slight-to-mild pain and adding a opioid as the pain intensity increases. Opioids have different potencies, and when a patient is changed from one opioid to another, it is imperative that equianalgesic dosages be used. Equianalgesic dose tables are based on comparative potencies to morphine (see Table 6.1). Opioids and non-opioids can be combined for additive analgesia. Opioid agonist-antagonists, such as pentazocine (e.g., Talwin), should be used with caution, if at all, since they may cause withdrawal syndrome. NSAIDs and opioid analgesics are available

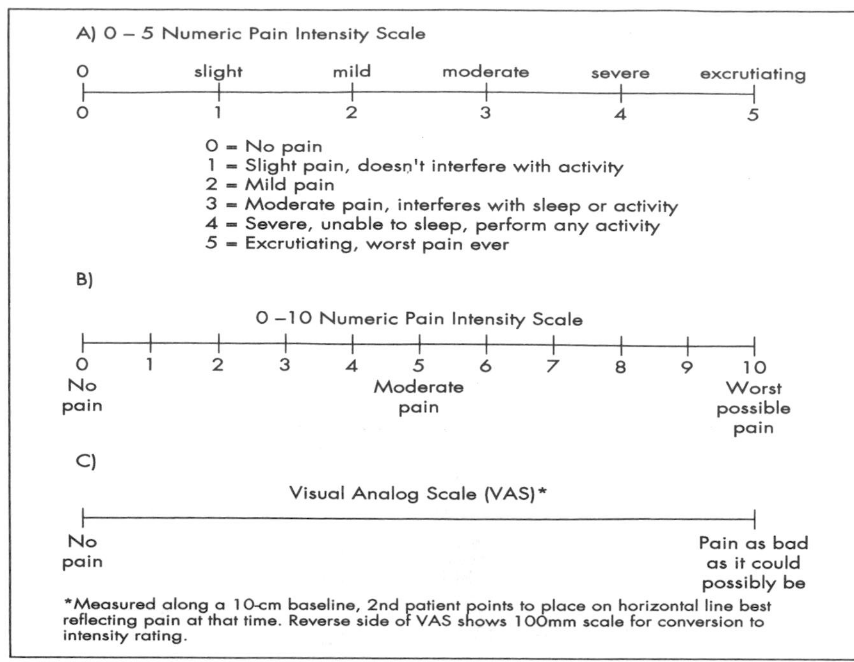

Figure 6.1 Examples of Measurement Tools of Pain Intensity

for oral, parenteral, and rectal administration. The United States Food and Drug Administration (FDA) approved ketorolac in 1996, and it is the only available *parenteral* NSAID. Also, transdermal patch delivery of fentanyl (20 times more potent than morphine) has been available for some time, and an immediate-release oral with mucosal absorption system is available (Actiq). Finally, awareness of the benefits of patient-controlled analgesia (PCA) has made this method of drug delivery for IV analgesics more widely available.

When trying to evaluation an opioid intervention, it is important to again recall that this is the century of genomics. It is now clear that there is considerable genetic polymorphism in the cytochrome P-450 family of enzymes (Bernard & Bruera, 2000), and that this can influence analgesic effect. For example, Payne (1998) states that 15% of Caucasians lack the enzyme CYPD211 that is required to metabolize codeine to morphine, so this group will require higher doses to achieve the same effect. As genotyping becomes more a part of designing a plan of care, it is important to remember this. In addition, as nurses have always done, when one opioid is ineffective, care planning with physician colleagues is to make sure that another opioid from a different class are tried.

Table 6.1 Equianalgesic Dose Table

Drug	Approximate Equianalgesic Oral Dose	Approximate Equianalgesic Parenteral Dose	Recommended Starting Dose Adults > 50 kg Body Weight)	
Opioid Agonist			**Oral**	**Parenteral**
Morphine	30 mg q3–4h (around-the-clock dosing) 60 mg q3–4h (single dose or intermittent dosing)	10 mg q3–4h	30 mg q3–4h	10 mg q3–4h
Codeine	130 mg q3–4h	75 mg q3–4h	60 mg q3–4h	60 mg q2h (IM, SQ)
Hydromorphone (Dilaudid)	7.5 mg q3–4h	1.5 mg q3–4h	6 mg q3–4h	1.5 mg q3–4h
Hydrocodone (in Lorcet, Lortab, Vicodin, others)	30 mg q3–4h	Not available	10 mg q3–4h	Not applicable
Levorphanol (Levo-Dromoran)	4 mg q6–8 h	2 mg q6–8 h	4 mg q6–8 h	2 mg q6–8 h
Meperldine (Demerol)	300 mg q2-3h	100 mg q3h	Not recommended	100 mg q3h
Methadone (Dolophine, others)	20 mg q6-8h	10 mg q6-8h	20 mg q6-8h	10 mg q6-8h
Oxycodone (Roxicodone, also in Percocet, Percodan, Tylox, others)	30 mg q3–4h	Not available	10 mg q3–4h	Not applicable
Oxymorphone (Numorphan)	Not available	1 mg q3–4h	Not available	1 mg q3–4h

Source: From AHCPR, Public Health Service, US Department of Health and Human Services. Rockville, MD. AHCPR Publication No. 92-0032.

MANAGEMENT

Numerous practice guidelines are available, and most recently the National Comprehensive Cancer Network (NCCN). Practice emphasize the need for rapid titration of short-acting opioids to manage severe pain, before then determining the optimal analgesic regime to control the patient's pain (Grossman et al, 1999). The recommended guidelines (2002) are available on the Internet at http://www.nccn.org/physician_gls/f_guidelines.html.

New horizons are being explored, and new medications that act directly at the spinal cord level are being studied. Recently, research has identifed alpha-adrenergic receptors for epinephrine at presynaptic and postjunctional sites in the dorsal horn of the spinal cord, located near the opioid receptors. Stimulation of these alpha-2 adrenergic receptors by agonists such as clonidine appears to block the transmission of the pain signal up the spinal cord to the brain, thus blocking pain perception, and this does not compete with opioids at opioid binding sites. One such agent that has been approved is clonidine hydrochloride (Duraclon), which is given along with opioids. Other agents being studied are *N*-methyl-D-aspartate (NMDA) antagonists (such as ketamine and dextromethorphan), which decrease pain due to inflammation and ischemia, and are effective in reducing neuropathic pain. NMDA receptors are found in the brain, spinal cord, and periphery, and are responsible for recognizing neuropathic pain. Unfortunately, side effects such as hallucinations and disassociation may be problematic.

Drugs intended to limit the development of tolerance are ongoing. Mu agonists (e.g., morphine) activate the mu-opioid receptor to inhibit the neuron from passing along incoming pain impulses, thus effecting analgesia. When morphine binds to the mu receptor, it increases the sensitization of the *N*-methyl-D-aspartate receptor, or NMDA receptor, and leads to an overactivation of protein-kinase C. This in turn leads to a desensitization of the mu-opioid receptor so that the effect of morphine is less, and tolerance may develop. By combining morphine with a NMDA antagonist, this stimulates the mu-opioid receptor and at the same time prevents activation of the protein-kinase C, thus preventing desensitization of the mu-opioid receptor, and theoretically increasing analgesia and preventing tolerance.

A second group that is being studied are the calcium channel blockers, which may also offer analgesia. By antagonizing the voltage-sensitive calcium channels in the synaptic membranes of neurons, these *N*-type voltage-sensitive calcium channel (VSCC) antagonists have shown some success in relieving neuropathic pain. Intrathecal administration of selective neuronal channel are being studied and offer promise of relief of chronic intractable pain.

As a nurse negotiating with patients with cancer-related pain around goals, often patients choose a 2–3 on a scale of 0–10 as the goal because they would rather have some pain in exchange for not being too sleepy. One possible intervention that is being studied is the use of modafinil (Provigil) to help treat fatigue and help patients stay awake (NCI, accessed July 2002; Breitbart et al, 1998). This agent could also be useful to help patients try to achieve a goal of pain intensity of 0–1 and not be afraid of becoming too sleepy with a lower quality of life.

References

Algos Pharmaceutical Corporation; *Understanding NMDA-Enhanced Analgesia.* Neptune, NJ: Algos Pharmaceutical Corporation; 1999

Belcheva S, Petkov VD, Konstantinova E, et al. Effects on Nociception of the Calcium and 5-HT Antagonist Dotarizine and Other 5-HT Receptor Agonists and Antagonists. *Acta Physiol Pharmacol Bulg* 1995;21:93–98

Bernard SA, Bruera E. Drug Interactions in Palliative Care. *J Clin Oncol* 2000;18(8): 1780–1799

Breitbart W, Passik S, Payne D. Psychological and Psychiatric Interventions In Pain Control. Doyle D, Hanks GW, MacDonald N, (eds), *Oxford Textbook of Palliative Medicine,* 2nd ed. New York: Oxford University Press;1998;437–454

Eliot L, Geiser R, Loewen G. Steady State Pharmacokinetic Comparison of a New Once-daily, Extended Release Morphine Formulation (Morphelan) and OxyContin Twice Daily. *J Oncol Pharm Pract* 2001;7:1–8

Fan G-H, Zhao J, Wu Y-L, et al. *N*-methyl-D-aspartate Attenuates Opioid Receptor-Mediated G Protein Activation and This Process Involves Protein Kinase C. *Mol Pharmacol* 1998;53:684–690

Ferrell BR, Rivera LM. Cancer Pain Education for Patients. *Semin Oncol Nurs* 1997;13: 42–48

Foley KM. The Treatment of Cancer Pain. *N Engl J Med* 1995;313:84–95

Foley KM. Controlling Cancer Pain. *Hospital Practice* 2000; http://www.hosppract.com/issues/2000/04/foley.htm. Accessed June 26, 2003

Grossman SA, Benedetti C, Payne R, Syrjala K, et al. NCCN Practice Guidelines for Cancer Pain. *Oncology* 1999;13(11A):1–20

Jacox A, Carr DB, Payne R, et al. Management of Cancer Pain. *Clinical Practice Guideline No 9 (AHCPR Pub No 94–0592).* Rockville, MD:Agency for Health Care Policy & Research USDHHS; 1994

Kaiko RF, Wallenstein SL, Rogers AG, et al. Opioids in the Elderly. *Med Clin North Am* 1982;66:1079–1089

Lipsky PE. COX-2 Specific Inhibitors: Basic Science and Clinical Implications. *Am J Med* 1999;106(5B):1–515 (proceeding of a symposium)

Lipsky PE. The Clinical Potential of Cyclooxygenase 2-Specific Inhibitors. *Am J Med* 1999;106(5B):515–575

Marks RM, Sacher EJ. Undertreatment of Medical Inpatients with Opioid Analgesics. *Ann Intern Med* 1973;78:173–181

McCaffery M. Nursing. *Management of the Patient with Pain.* Philadelphia, PA: JB Lippincott Co.; 1982

McEvoy GK, Litvak K, Welsh OH, et al. (eds.) *AHFS Drug Information.* Bethesda, MD: American Society of Health-System Pharmacists; 1992

Merck & Co. Vioxx Package Insert. West Point, NY: Merck & Co; 1992

Miaskowski C. Innovations in Pharmacologic Therapies. *Semin Oncol Nurs* 1997;13: 30–35

National Cancer Institute. Fatigue PDQ: Intervention, Pschostimulants. July 2002; Available at http://www.nci.org. Accessed August 2002

Paice J. Pain, Yarbro CH, Frogge MH, Goodman M, (eds), *Cancer Symptom Management,* 3rd ed. Sudbury, MA: Jones and Bartlett Publishers; 2003

Payne R. Pharmacologic Management of Pain, Section IA3. Berger A, Portenoy RK, Weissman DE, (eds), *Principles and Practice of Supportive Oncology,* Philadelphia, PA: Lippincott-Raven Publishers; 1998

Searle. Celebrex Package Insert. Skokie, IL: Searle Co.; 1999

Syndrup SH, Gram LF, Brosenk EO Jr, et al. The Selective Serotonin Reuptake Inhibitor Paroxetine is Effective in the Treatment of Diabetic Neuropathy Symptoms. *Pain* 1990;42:135–144

Thun MJ, Namboodri MM, Heath CW Jr. Aspirin Use and Reduced Risk of Fatal Colon Cancer. *N Engl J Med* 1991;325:1593–1596

Tokunaga A, Saika M, Senba E. 5-HT2A Receptor Subtype is Involved in the Thermal Hyperalgesic Mechanism of Serotonin in the Periphery. *Pain* 1998;76:349–355

Wilkie D. Neural Mechanisms of Pain: A Foundation for Cancer Pain Assessment and Management. Maguire DB, Yarbro CH, Ferrell BR, (eds), *Cancer Pain Management,* 2nd ed. Sudbury, MA: Jones and Bartlett Publishers;1995;61–87

Zycliz Z, Smits C, Krajnik M. Paroxetine for Pruritis in Advanced Cancer. *J Pain Symptom Management* 1996;16:121–124

NON-OPIOD ANALEGICS

Drug: acetaminophen (Acephen, Actamin, Anacin-3, Apacet, Anesin, Dapa, Datril, Genapap, Genebs, Gentabs, Halenol, Liquiprin, Meda Cap, Panadol, Panex, Suppap, Tempra, Tenol, Ty Caps, Tylenol)

Class: Miscellaneous analgesic/antipyretic.

Mechanism of Action: Appears to inhibit prostaglandin synthesis centrally, thus preventing sensitization of pain receptors to chemical or mechanical stimulation. Mechanism is similar to salicylates but is not uricosuric. May have weak anti-inflammatory effects in nonrheumatoid conditions (e.g., after oral surgery). Reduces fever by direct effect on hypothalamus; heat is lost through vasodilation and increased peripheral blood flow. Analgesic and antipyretic action similar to aspirin.

Metabolism: Rapidly absorbed from GI tract; 25% serum protein-binding. Elimination half-life is 1–3 hours. Metabolized by the liver and excreted in the urine.

Dosage/Range:
325–650 mg every 4–6 hours PRN for pain, discomfort, not to exceed 4 g/24 hours. Some individuals may need increased single doses of 1 g.

Drug Preparation:
- Ensure seals on tamper-resistant package are intact when opening new package.

Drug Administration:
- Oral, rectal, elixir.

Drug Interactions:
- Hepatotoxicity of acetaminophen may be increased by chronic use of high doses of drugs using hepatic microsomal enzyme system: barbiturates, carbamazepine, rifampin, phenytoin, sulfinpyrazone.
- Alcohol: increased risk of hepatic damage with chronic, excessive use.
- Diflunisal: increased acetaminophen serum level; avoid concurrent use.
- Phenothiazines: possible severe hypothermia may occur when used concomitantly.

Lab Effects/Interference:
- None known.

Special Considerations:
- Elixirs contain alcohol (Tylenol, Valadol).
- Contraindicated in patients with known hypersensitivity; use cautiously, if at all, in patients with hepatic or renal dysfunction.
- Chronic ingestion of large doses of acetaminophen may slightly potentiate effects of coumarin and other anticoagulants.

Potential Toxicities/Side Effects and the Nursing Process

I. KNOWLEDGE DEFICIT related to SELF-ADMINISTRATION

Defining Characteristics: Fever curve or excessive fever can be masked by self-dosing with acetaminophen.

Nursing Implications: Instruct patient to report temperature over 38.3°C (101°F) or persistent or recurrent fever. Assess other over-the-counter (OTC) medicines the patient may be taking.

II. POTENTIAL INJURY related to HEPATOTOXICITY

Defining Characteristics: Excessive alcoholic intake and other drugs can increase risk for hepatotoxicity.

Nursing Implications: Assess total acetaminophen dosage/24 hours, taking into account OTC medications. Assess baseline LFTs, especially if the patient has primary hepatoma or liver metastasis. Teach patient to avoid excessive alcohol intake and/or excessive acetaminophen intake.

Drug: aspirin, acetylsalicylic acid (ASA, Aspergum, Bayer Aspirin, Easprin, Ecotrin, Empirin)

Class: Salicylate.

Mechanism of Action: Inhibits prostaglandin synthesis peripherally preventing sensitization of pain receptors by mechanical and chemical stimuli. Also, has anti-inflammatory effect, producing analgesic and antipyretic effects. Central action via hypothalamus unclear.

Metabolism: Rapidly and well absorbed from GI tract, and distributed throughout the body with high concentrations in liver and kidney. Drug is bound to serum proteins, especially albumin. Metabolized by liver and excreted in urine.

Dosage/Range:

- 325–650 mg PO or PR every 4 hours PRN for pain or fever (maximum 3.9 g/day).

Drug Preparation:

- Keep in closed container, away from heat, to prevent drug decomposition.
- Do not use if strong, vinegar-like odor is present. Do not crush enteric-coated aspirin.

Drug Administration:

- Oral or rectal suppositories. Give oral dose with 240 mL water or milk to decrease gastric irritation. Oral solution may be made from effervescent aspirin powders (e.g., Alka-Seltzer); Alka-Seltzer chewable aspirin tablets available.

Drug Interactions:

- Ammonium chloride, ascorbic acid, or methionine (urine acidifiers): Decrease ASA excretion, so increase risk of ASA toxicity.
- Antacids, urinary alkalizers: may increase ASA excretion, so may decrease the ASA effect. Alcohol increases the risk of GI ulceration, bleeding.
- Decreased effect of angiotensin-converting enzyme (ACE) inhibitors. When used together, the effect of anticoagulants may be enhanced (additive hypothrombinemic effect), leading to prolonged bleeding time. DO NOT USE TOGETHER.
- Beta-adrenergic blockers (e.g., propranolol): Possible decrease in antihypertensive effect.
- Corticosteroids: increase in aspirin excretion with decrease in aspirin effect.

- Methotrexate: increase in methotrexate serum levels with increased toxicity. DO NOT USE CONCURRENTLY.
- NSAIDs: decrease in NSAID serum concentration; may have increased incidence of GI side effects. Not recommended to be used together.
- Probenecid, sulfinpyrazone: aspirin (doses ≥ 3 g/day) antagonizes uricosuric drug effect.
- Spirolactone: aspirin may inhibit diuretic effect.
- Sulfonylureas, exogenous insulin: Aspirin may have hypoglycemic effect and may potentiate these drug actions. Monitor for hypoglycemia.
- Valproic acid: aspirin displaces drug and decreases its excretion, resulting in increased serum levels and possible valproic acid toxicity.

Lab Effects/Interference:

- Prolonged bleeding time, leukopenia, thrombocytopenia.

Special Considerations:

- Patients receiving myelosuppressive chemotherapy should be cautioned not to take aspirin due to increased risk of bleeding.
- Patients should be instructed to take drug with food or milk.
- Use cautiously in patients with asthma, rhinitis, or nasal polyps (can cause severe bronchospasm).
- Drug is contraindicated in patients with GI ulcer, GI bleeding, hypersensitivity to aspirin, increased bleeding tendencies.
- Use cautiously in patients with liver damage, hypoprothrombinemia, or with vitamin K deficiency.

Potential Toxicities/Side Effects and the Nursing Process

I. ALTERATION IN NUTRITION, LESS THAN BODY REQUIREMENTS, related to GI TOXICITY

Defining Characteristics: Nausea, dyspepsia (5–25% of patients), heartburn, epigastric discomfort, anorexia, and acute, reversible hepatotoxicity may occur. Risk increases with dose. May potentiate peptic ulcer disease.

Nursing Implications: Teach patient self-administration with 8 oz (240 mL) water or milk. If GI distress develops, discuss use of enteric-coated aspirin (e.g., Ecotrin). If patient receiving high doses of aspirin, monitor LFTs. Drug contraindicated in patients with peptic ulcer disease.

II. POTENTIAL FOR BLEEDING related to INHIBITION OF PLATELET AGGREGATION

Defining Characteristics: Aspirin may cause prolongation of bleeding time, leukopenia, thrombocytopenia, purpura, shortened erythrocyte survival time.

Nursing Implications: Teach patient to avoid aspirin and aspirin-containing drugs if receiving myelosuppressive chemotherapy. Review concurrent medications to identify risk for drug interactions. Monitor Hgb, HCT over time; teach patient signs/symptoms of anemia, and instruct to report them (headache, fatigue, chest pain, irritability). Monitor stool guaiacs.

III. INJURY related to MILD SALICYLISM

Defining Characteristics: Administration of large doses of salicylates may cause salicylism, characterized by dizziness, tinnitus, diminished hearing, nausea, vomiting, diarrhea, mental confusion, CNS depression, headache, sweating, and hyperventilation at serum salicylate concentration 150–300 μg/mL (use in cancer patients usually 100 μg/mL).

Nursing Implications: Teach patient to reduce dose, interrupt dose if signs/symptoms occur. Assess concurrent medications for possible drug interactions.

Drug: celecoxib (Celebrex®)

Class: Nonsteroidal anti-inflammatory drug.

Mechanism of Action: Drug has anti-inflammatory and antipyretic properties effected by inhibition of prostaglandin synthesis via selective inhibition of cyclooxygenase-2 (COX-2) pathway. It does not inhibit the cyclooxygenase-1 (COX-1) isoenzyme.

Metabolism: Following an oral dose, peak serum levels are reached at 3 hours, with a terminal half-life of 11 hours, and with multiple doses, steady-state is reached on or before 5 days. Drug is highly protein-bound (97%) and extensively distributed into tissue. Drug is metabolized in the liver via the cytochrome P450 2C9 system, with little unchanged drug recoverable in the urine or feces. Higher area under the curve (AUC) concentrations are found in the elderly (women > men), in African Americans, and in patients with moderate hepatic dysfunction.

Dosage/Range:
- Adults: 200 mg PO qd, or 100–200 mg PO.
- Patients with moderate hepatic dysfunction or weighing < 50 kg should get lowest dose.

Drug Preparation:
- Oral, available in 100-mg and 200-mg capsules.

Drug Administration:
- Administer orally in morning or evening, without regard to food.

Drug Interactions:

- Celecoxib inhibits cytochrome P450 2D6 system, so when given concurrently with drugs metabolized by this system, may result in increased doses of the second drug; also, celecoxib is metabolized primarily by P450 2C9 system, so if given concomitantly with drugs that inhibit this system, increased serum levels of celecoxib may result (e.g., fluconazole results in 2 × serum levels of celecoxib; use lowest dose possible of celecoxib, if at all).
- Angiotensin converting enzyme (ACE) inhibitors, e.g., lisinopril: may have decreased antihypertensive effect when used together.
- Furosemide, thiazide diuretics: reduced natriuretic effect due to inhibition of renal prostaglandin synthesis; assess diuretic effect and adjust dose as necessary.
- Lithium: use together cautiously, and monitor serum lithium levels if used together.
- Warfarin: monitor INR, PT closely, especially the first few days following initiation of celecoxib therapy or after changing the dose.
- Aspirin: low dose well tolerated, but higher doses may result in GI ulceration or other complications; use only together with low-dose aspirin.
- Methotrexate: no significant interaction.

Lab Effects/Interference:

- Increase in serum chloride, decrease in serum phosphate, and increased BUN; if there is GI bleeding, HCT and Hgb will be reduced. Also, rarely, borderline elevations of liver function tests (e.g., ALT, AST) may occur.

Special Considerations:

- Lowest doses should be used for individuals weighing < 50 kg or those with moderate hepatic impairment. DO NOT ADMINISTER to patients with severe hepatic impairment.
- DO NOT GIVE to pregnant women or nursing mothers unless benefits outweigh risk; DO NOT GIVE to women in last trimester of pregnancy.
- Celecoxib does not affect platelet aggregation or bleeding time. Studies showed significantly fewer GI ulcers in patients receiving celecoxib as compared to naproxen or ibuprofen.
- Indicated for the relief of signs and symptoms of osteoarthritis or rheumatoid arthritis in adults.
- Celecoxib is contraindicated in patients hypersensitive to celecoxib or allergic to sulfonamides, patients with severe hepatic disease, advanced renal disease, or patients who have or have had asthma, urticaria, or allergic-type reactions after taking aspirin or other NSAIDs, as anaphylaxis may occur.
- Use cautiously, if at all, in patients with preexisting asthma, preexisting kidney disease, fluid retention, cardiac failure, hypertension, prior history of ulcer disease or bleeding.

Drug: choline magnesium trisalicylate (Trilisate)

Class: Choline and magnesium salicylate combination.

Mechanism of Action: Analgesic effect through peripheral and central pathways, decreasing pain perception. Prostaglandin inhibition probably involved in peripheral mechanism. Antipyretic effect via hypothalamic heat regulation center. Does not interfere with platelet aggregation.

Metabolism: Rapidly absorbed from GI tract. Metabolized by the liver and excreted in the urine.

Dosage/Range:
- Trilisate 750 mg bid or dose-increase to maximum 3200 mg/day.

Drug Preparation:
- Trilisate liquid 5 mL or Trilisate 500-mg tablet contains ASA equivalent of 650 mg.
- Trilisate 750-mg tablet contains 975 mg ASA.
- Trilisate 1000-mg tablet contains 1300 mg ASA.

Drug Administration:
- Oral.

Drug Interactions:
- Antacids, urine alkylinizers: increase salicylate excretion and decrease drug effect. Do not administer with antacids.
- Ammonium chloride, ascorbic acid, methionine (urine acidifiers): decrease salicylate excretion so increase risk of salicylate toxicity.
- Concomitant administration with alcohol, steroids, other NSAIDs may increase GI side effects.
- Corticosteroids: may increase salicylate excretion and decrease Trilisate effect.
- Warfarin: may have increased warfarin levels and increased PT; monitor patient closely, and reduce warfarin dosage as needed.

Lab Effects/Interference:
- Free T4 may be increased with a concurrent decrease in total plasma T4 (does not affect thyroid function).

Special Considerations:
- Drug does not interfere with platelet aggregation.
- Use cautiously in patients with chronic renal failure, gastritis.
- Contraindicated if known hypersensitivity to salicylates.
- Drug contains magnesium, so periodic evaluation of serum magnesium should be performed.

Potential Toxicities/Side Effects and the Nursing Process

I. ALTERATION IN NUTRITION, LESS THAN BODY REQUIREMENTS, related to GI TOXICITY

Defining Characteristics: Fewer GI side-effects than aspirin. Nausea, dyspepsia (5–25% of patients), heartburn, epigastric discomfort, anorexia, and acute reversible hepatotoxicity may occur. Risk increases with dose. May potentiate peptic ulcer disease.

Nursing Implications: Teach patient self-administration with food, or 8 oz (240 mL) water or milk. If patient is receiving antacid, administer antacid two hours after meals and Trilisate before meals. Assess baseline liver and renal function and monitor if patient receiving high doses on ongoing basis. Guaiac stool to assess occult blood, as gastric ulceration may occur.

II. INJURY related to MILD SALICYLISM

Defining Characteristics: Administration of large doses of salicylates may cause salicylism, characterized by dizziness, tinnitus, diminished hearing, nausea, vomiting, diarrhea, mental confusion, CNS depression, headache, sweating, and hyperventilation at serum salicylate concentration 150–300 μg/mL (use in cancer patients usually 100 μg/mL).

Nursing Implications: Teach patient to reduce dose, interrupt dose if signs/symptoms occur. Assess concurrent medications for possible drug interactions.

III. POTENTIAL ALTERATION IN URINARY ELIMINATION related to RENAL PROSTAGLANDIN INHIBITION

Defining Characteristics: Rarely, elevated serum BUN and creatinine may occur.

Nursing Implications: Assess baseline serum BUN, creatinine, and monitor during therapy.

Drug: clonidine hydrochloride (Duraclon)

Class: Antiadrenergic agent.

Mechanism of Action: Acts centrally to stimulate alpha-2-adrenergic receptors in the CNS, thus inhibiting sympathetic vasomotor centers. When given epidurally, the drug is believed to mimic norepinephrine activity at presynaptic and postjunctional alpha-2-adrenoceptors in the dorsal horn of the spinal cord. Is administered together with opioids for severe cancer pain to maximize analgesia. Clonidine HCl shows best efficacy against neuropathic pain.

Metabolism: Drug is highly lipid-soluble and rapidly distributes into extravascular sites and into the CNS; enters the plasma via the epidural veins, leading to hypotensive effect. Drug is metabolized and excreted in the urine (72% of the administered dose in 96 hours, and 40–50% of that is unchanged drug).

Dosage/Range:

To be administered in combination with opioids via epidural route:

- Initial: starting dose is 30 μg/hr.
- May be titrated up to 40 μg/hr or down, based on degree of pain relief and extent of side effects.

Drug Preparation/Administration:

- Preservative-free preparation.
- Given epidurally in combination with opioid via continuous epidural infusion device.

Drug Interactions:

- CNS depressants (e.g., alcohol, barbiturates): potentiation of CNS depression.
- Opioid analgesics: may potentiate hypotension due to clonidine.
- Tricyclic antidepressants: may antagonize hypotensive effect of clonidine.
- Beta-blockers: may exacerbate hypertensive symptoms of clonidine withdrawal.
- Epidural local anesthetics: clonidine may prolong pharmacologic effects of local anesthetic; both motor and sensory blockade.

Lab Effects/Interference:

- None known.

Special Considerations:

- Contraindicated in patients sensitive or allergic to clonidine HCl; epidural administration contraindicated if (1) injection site infection occurs, (2) patient is receiving anticoagulation, (3) patient has bleeding diathesis, (4) administered above the C4 dermatome, (5) patient has severe cardiac disease or is hemodynamically unstable, or (6) used in obstetrical or postoperative analgesia.
- Use cautiously in patients receiving digitalis, calcium channel blockers, and beta-blockers, as there may be additive effects of bradycardia and AV block.
- Severe hypotension may occur during first 2 days of clonidine therapy, especially when drug is infused into the upper thoracic spinal segments—monitor vital signs frequently.
- Do not suddenly withdraw drug, as this may result in nervousness, agitation, headache, tremor, rapid increase in blood pressure; scrupulously maintain drug administration equipment to prevent accidental interruption of drug. Drug dose should be gradually decreased over 2–4 days. If patient is

receiving a beta-blocker, the beta-blocker should be discontinued several days before the gradual discontinuaton of epidural clonidine. Teach patient NOT to discontinue drug on own.

Potential Toxicities/Side Effects and the Nursing Process

I. ALTERED TISSUE PERFUSION related to HYPOTENSION

Defining Characteristics: Hypotension usually occurs within the first four days after beginning epidural clonidine but may also occur throughout treatment. Increased risk in patients receiving infusion into upper-thoracic spinal segments, in women, and in patients who have low body weight. Hypotension may be accentuated by concurrent opiate administration. Clonidine decreases sympathetic CNS outflow, decreasing peripheral resistance, decreasing renal vascular resistance, and decreasing heart rate and BP.

Nursing Implications: Monitor T, BP, HR frequently, especially during first few days of therapy. Notify physician of significant changes. Expect IV fluids to be given to correct hypotension, and if needed, IV ephedrine. Symptomatic bradycardia can be treated with atropine.

II. ALTERED TISSUE PERFUSION related to REBOUND HYPERTENSION

Defining Characteristics: Withdrawal symptoms can occur if drug is interrupted or stopped abruptly; characterized by nervousness, agitation, headache, tremor, rapid increase in BP. Increased risk in patients receiving high drug doses, patients receiving beta-blockers, or patients with a history of hypertension. Rarely, this may result in CVA, hypertensive encephalopathy, or death.

Nursing Implications: Scrupulously manage/maintain catheter and pump to prevent interruption in flow; teach patient catheter and pump care and use; instruct patient never to abruptly discontinue medicine; anticipate physician will discontinue beta-blockers prior to gradual taper of drug over 2–4 days when drug is being discontinued.

III. POTENTIAL FOR INFECTION related to IMPLANTED DEVICE

Defining Characteristics: Implanted epidural catheter may become infected, leading to epidural abcess or meningitis.

Nursing Implications: Scrupulously maintain catheter, using sterile technique; teach patient catheter care and management; monitor for signs/symptoms of infection and teach patient this assessment. If in the hospital, monitor for fever and pain and notify the physician immediately if either is found. Instruct patient to report fever, pain to the physician immediately if at home.

Drug: gabapentin (Neurontin)

Class: Anticonvulsant.

Mechanism of Action: Not clearly understood. Drug is stucturally related to neurotransmitter GABA (gamma-amino-butyric acid), but drug does not bind to GABA receptor sites. It is unclear whether drug has activity at NMDA receptor sites. Drug has been shown to bind to receptor sites in neocortex and hippocampus.

Metabolism: Bioavailability of drug decreases as dose increases, and drug absorption unaffected by food. Drug half-life is 5–7 hours, and drug excreted unchanged in the urine. Plasma clearance may be reduced in elderly and is reduced in renal insufficiency.

Dosage/Range:
- Initial titration: 300 mg on day 1, 300 mg bid on day 2, and 300 mg tid on day 3.
- As needed, dose may be titrated up to 400 mg tid, in increments, to a maximum dose of 600 mg tid (1800 mg total dose per day).
- Dose-reduce in renal insufficiency:

Creatinine Clearance	Drug Dose
30–60 mL/min	300 mg bid
15–30 mL/min	300 mg/day
< 15 mL/min	300 mg every other day

Drug Preparation/Administration:
- Oral, take without regard to food intake.
- Take 1 hour before, or 2 hours after, antacid.
- Take initial dose at bedtime to enhance somnolence and minimize dizziness, fatigue and ataxia.
- Doses should not be separated by > 12 hours (must be tid, e.g., every 8 hours).
- If drug is discontinued or changed to another anticonvulsant, gradually discontinue drug over 1 week.

Drug Interactions:
- Antacids: decrease bioavailability of drug.
- Cimetidine: decreases renal excretion of drug with potential for excess toxicity; monitor patient closely and dose reduce if both drugs must be given concommitantly.

Lab Effects/Interference:
- Urinary protein test using Ames N-Multistix may be falsely positive.
- Drug may cause leukopenia, anemia, thrombocytopenia.

Special Considerations:

- Dose-reduce in patients with renal insufficiency, and consider dose reduction in the elderly.
- Drug helpful in the management of painful peripheral neuropathies.
- Drug may cause dizziness, fatigue, drowsiness, ataxia, so patient should be taught to avoid activities requiring mental acuity, such as driving, until after full effect of drug is known.

Potential Toxicities/Side Effects and the Nursing Process

I. SENSORY/PERCEPTUAL ALTERATIONS related to CNS CHANGES

Defining Characteristics: The most common side effects are somnolence, ataxia, dizziness, and fatigue. Less commonly, nystagmus, tremor, nervousness, dysarthria, amnesia, depression, abnormal thought processes, incoordination, headache, confusion, emotional lability, paresthesia, areflexia, anxiety, hostility, syncope, hypesthesia may occur. Seizures have been reported, as have suicidal tendencies. Other sensory side effects that rarely occur are diplopia, abnormal vision, dry eyes, photophobia, ptosis, and hearing loss.

Nursing Implications: Assess baseline neurological status and document. Instruct patient of general side effects that may occur, and to report them. Assess for suicidal ideation. If significant CNS changes occur, discuss dose reduction or change to an alternative drug with physician. Instruct patient not to drive a car or to do activities that require mental acuity until full effect of drug is known.

II. ALTERATION IN NUTRITION related to GI TOXICITY

Defining Characteristics: Nausea and vomiting may occur. Less commonly, dyspepsia, dry mouth, constipation, increased or decreased appetite, thirst, stomatitis, taste changes, increased salivation, fecal incontinence may occur.

Nursing Implications: Assess patient tolerance of GI side effects. Instruct patient to report side effects. If nausea and vomiting occur, discuss changing to another medication or adding antiemetic agent to regimen if relief of peripheral neuropathy is achieved.

III. ALTERATION IN SKIN INTEGRITY related to RASH

Defining Characteristics: Rash may occur, as may pruritus, acne, alopecia, hirsutism, herpes simplex, dry skin, and increased sweating.

Nursing Implications: Perform baseline skin assessment, and note any areas that are not intact. Teach patient to self-assess for rash, other changes, and to report them. If rash develops, instruct patient to notify provider immediately. If itch occurs, discuss symptomatic management.

IV. ALTERATION IN RESPIRATORY PATTERN related to RHINITIS, COUGH

Defining Characteristics: Rhinitis, pharyngitis, coughing, pneumonia, dyspnea may occur. Rarely, epistaxis and apnea have been reported.

Nursing Implications: Assess baseline respiratory pattern, and instruct patient to report any changes. Discuss any significant changes with physician, and discuss management versus change of drug.

V. ALTERATION IN URINARY ELIMINATION related to URINARY CHANGES

Defining Characteristics: Hematuria, dysuria, frequency, urinary incontinence, cystitis, urinary retention may occur.

Nursing Implications: Assess baseline urinary elimination pattern, and instruct patient of possible side effects and to report them. Discuss symptomatic management, or discuss drug change with physician if changes are significant.

VI. POTENTIAL FOR SEXUAL DYSFUNCTION related to VAGINAL CHANGES AND IMPOTENCE

Defining Characteristics: Vaginal hemorrhage, amenorrhea, dysmenorrhea, menorrhagia, inability to climax, abnormal ejaculation, and impotence have been reported.

Nursing Implications: Assess baseline sexuality, and instruct patient to report any changes. If changes occur, discuss impact and distress caused, and together with physician and patient, discuss drug alternatives.

VII. POTENTIAL ALTERATION IN OXYGENATION related to TACHYCARDIA, HYPOTENSION

Defining Characteristics: Rarely, hypertension, vasodilatation, hypotension, angina pectoris, peripheral vascular disease, palpitation, tachycardia, and appearance of a murmur may occur.

Nursing Implications: Assess baseline cardiovascular status, and instruct patient to notify provider if any changes occur. Instruct patient to report palpitations, fast heart beat, dizziness, or chest pain immediately. If significant changes occur, discuss alternative drug therapy with physician.

Drug: ibuprofen (Advil, Genpril, Haltran, Ibuprin, Midol 200, Nuprin, Rufen)

Class: NSAID.

Mechanism of Action: Peripherally acting analgesic, anti-inflammatory, and antipyretic agent; anti-inflammatory action probably due to prostaglandin inhibition and/or release.

Metabolism: 80% of dose absorbed from GI tract, and absorption rate is slowed by administration with food. Peak serum concentrations with tablet occur in 2 hours; suspension in 1 hour. Highly protein bound (90–99%) and has a plasma half-life of 2–4 hours. Excreted in urine.

Dosage/Range:

200–800 mg every 4–8 hours PRN to maximum of 3200 mg/24 hours.

Drug Preparation:

- Tablets: 200 mg, 300 mg, 400 mg, 600 mg, 800 mg.
- Caplets: 200 mg.
- Oral suspension: 100 mg/5 mL.

Drug Administration:

- Oral.

Drug Interactions:

- Oral anticoagulants, thrombolytic agents: possible increase in PT with increased bleeding; use with caution and monitor patient closely.
- Other NSAIDs: possible increase in GI toxicity; do not administer concomitantly.
- Furosemide, thiazide diuretics: decreased diuretic effect when administered concomitantly.

Lab Effects/Interference:

- Slight decrease in Hgb not exceeding 1 g/dL without signs of bleeding; decrease in Hgb > 1 g/dL may be associated with signs of bleeding.

Special Considerations:

- Contraindicated in patients with known hypersensitivity, asthmatic patients with nasal polyps and other patients who develop bronchospasm or angioedema with aspirin or other NSAIDs, patients with peptic or duodenal ulcer.
- Use cautiously in patients with cardiac or renal dysfunction.

Potential Toxicities/Side Effects and the Nursing Process

I. ALTERATION IN NUTRITION, LESS THAN BODY REQUIREMENTS, related to GI SIDE EFFECTS

Defining Characteristics: Dyspepsia, heartburn, nausea, vomiting, anorexia, diarrhea, constipation, stomatitis, bloating, epigastric and abdominal pain may occur.

Nursing Implications: Assess history of GI symptoms and history of ulcer disease. Teach patient to take NSAID with meals or milk. Teach patient potential side effects, and instruct to report them. If symptoms are severe, discuss alternative NSAIDs with physician.

II. POTENTIAL FOR BLEEDING related to INHIBITION OF PLATELET AGGREGATION

Defining Characteristics: Drug can prolong bleeding time and inhibit platelet aggregation. Peptic ulceration and occult GI bleeding can occur and be life-threatening. Increased risk factors: smoking, alcoholism.

Nursing Implications: Assess risk, history of peptic ulcer disease or GI bleeding. Assess baseline Hgb, HCT, and presence/absence of occult bleeding by guaiac of stools. Instruct patient to report signs/symptoms of abdominal pain, black stools, blood per rectum, epistaxis, menorrhagia. If patient is at risk for bleeding, discuss with physician use of misoprostol to protect GI mucosa. Teach patient to avoid concurrent use of aspirin, other NSAIDs.

III. POTENTIAL SENSORY/PERCEPTUAL ALTERATIONS related to CNS CHANGES

Defining Characteristics: Dizziness, headache, nervousness, fatigue, drowsiness, malaise/light-headedness, anxiety, confusion, mental depression, and emotional lability may occur. Decreased hearing, visual acuity, changes in color vision, conjunctivitis, diplopia, and cataracts have been reported. In addition, though rare, aseptic meningitis has occurred.

Nursing Implications: Assess baseline neurologic and mental status. Instruct patient to report changes in sensory/perceptual pattern, especially VISUAL CHANGES. If visual changes occur, discuss with physician referral to ophthalmologist as soon as possible. Assess for rare occurrence of aseptic meningitis (fever, coma). Discuss drug continuance with physician for significant symptoms.

IV. ALTERATION IN NUTRITION, LESS THAN BODY REQUIREMENTS, related to HEPATIC TOXICITY

Defining Characteristics: Severe and sometimes fatal hepatotoxicity has occurred. Jaundice, hepatitis occur rarely. Borderline increase in LFTs occurs in 15% of patients, while values increase by three times in 1%.

Nursing Implications: Assess baseline LFTs and monitor periodically during long-term therapy. Instruct patient to report jaundice, abdominal pain. Discuss discontinuance of drug with physician for significant toxicity.

V. ALTERATION IN RENAL ELIMINATION related to INHIBITION OF RENAL PROSTAGLANDINS

Defining Characteristics: Acute renal failure may occur rarely within first few days of treatment in patients with preexisting renal dysfunction. Other signs/symptoms of renal dysfunction that may occur rarely are azotemia, cystitis, hematuria, increased serum BUN and creatinine, and decreased creatinine clearance. Peripheral edema has also been described.

Nursing Implications: Assess baseline renal function. Instruct patient to report any changes in urinary function. Monitor periodic serum BUN, creatinine during chronic therapy.

VI. ALTERATION IN SKIN INTEGRITY related to RASH

Defining Characteristics: Rash (urticaria, vesicles, or erythematous macular) may occur, as may Stevens-Johnson syndrome, flushes, alopecia, rectal itching, and acne.

Nursing Implications: Assess baseline skin integrity and presence of lesions. Teach patient to report abnormalities. Provide symptomatic relief for rashes, pruritus.

VII. POTENTIAL FOR FATIGUE AND INFECTION related to BONE MARROW INJURY

Defining Characteristics: Neutropenia, agranulocytosis, aplastic anemia, hemolytic anemia, and THROMBOCYTOPENIA may occur *rarely*.

Nursing Implications: Assess baseline CBC, WBC, differential, and platelet count. Discuss abnormalities with physician. Instruct patient to report severe fatigue, infection, bleeding. Monitor lab values periodically during treatment.

Drug: indomethacin (Indocin, Indocin SR, Indotech)

Class: NSAID, structurally related to sulindac.

Mechanism of Action: Actions similar to other NSAIDs: anti-inflammatory action, probably by inhibition of prostaglandin synthesis, as well as by inhibiting migration of leukocytes to infection site and stabilization of neutrophils so lysosomal enzymes cannot be released; may also interfere with the production of autoantibodies (mediated by prostaglandins). Analgesic and antipyretic effects appear to result from inhibition of prostaglandin synthesis. Probably reduces tumor-associated fever by inhibition of synthesis of prostaglandin (PGE_1) in hypothalamus. However, drug has serious side effects, so should not be used routinely as an antipyretic.

Metabolism: Rapidly and completely absorbed from GI tract. When administered with food or antacid (aluminum and magnesium hydroxide), peak plasma drug concentrations may be slightly decreased or delayed. Drug is 99% bound to plasma proteins. Crosses BBB slightly, and placenta freely. Metabolized by liver, undergoes enterohepatic circulation, and is excreted in urine.

Dosage/Range:
- Capsules: 10 mg, 25 mg, 50 mg, 75 mg, given in 2–4 divided doses.
- Sustained release: 75 mg, given once or bid.
- Oral suspension: 25 mg/5 mL, given in 2–4 divided doses.
- Suppositories: 50 mg, given in 2–4 divided doses.

Drug Preparation:
- Drug is sensitive to light. Store capsules in well-closed containers at temperatures < 40°C (104°F).
- Oral suspension should be stored in tight, light-resistant containers at 30°C (86°F).
- Suppositories should be stored at temperatures < 30°C (86°F).

Drug Administration:
- Give with food or antacid to protect GI mucosa.
- Rectal suppository must remain in rectum for at least 1 hour for maximum absorption.
- Consider reduced dose in patients with renal dysfunction.
- Indocin suspension contains 1% alcohol.

Drug Interactions:
- Indomethacin can displace or be displaced by other protein-bound drugs: oral anticoagulants, hydantoins (e.g., phenytoin), salicylates, sulfonamides, sulfonylureas. Therefore, if taking any of these medications with indomethacin, the patient must be assessed for increased toxicity of each drug.

- Antihypertensive effect of hydralazine, captopril, furosemide, beta-adrenergic blockers, or thiazide diuretics may be decreased.
- NSAIDs: concurrent administration with salicylates does not improve drug effects but increases toxicity (GI, aplastic anemia) so should NOT be given concurrently. Diflunisal may decrease renal excretion of indomethacin and increase risk of GI hemorrhage; AVOID concurrent use.
- Triamterene: may precipitate renal failure. DO NOT USE CONCURRENTLY.
- Digoxin: serum levels may be increased and prolonged, so digoxin levels should be monitored closely.
- Methotrexate, especially HIGH DOSE: increased, prolonged serum methotrexate levels can be fatal; AVOID concurrent use.
- Potassium (K+) supplements, K+ sparing diuretics: indomethacin may increase serum K+ concentrations, especially in the elderly or patients with renal dysfunction. Use with caution and monitor K+ serum levels.
- Lithium: may increase plasma lithium levels; assess patient for lithium toxicity.
- Cyclosporine: possible increased nephrotoxicity; use with caution and monitor renal function.
- Probenecid: increased plasma level and therapeutic effects of indomethacin; decrease indomethacin dose.

Lab Effects/Interference:

- May prolong bleeding time.
- Rarely, hemolytic anemia, leukopenia, thrombocytopenia.

Special Considerations:

- Avoid use or use cautiously in the elderly or in patients with epilepsy, Parkinson's disease, renal dysfunction, mental illness.

Potential Toxicities/Side Effects and the Nursing Process

I. POTENTIAL SENSORY/PERCEPTUAL ALTERATIONS

Defining Characteristics: Dose-related headache occurs in 25–50% of patients (more severe in morning); may be associated with frontal throbbing, vomiting, tinnitus, ataxia, tremor, vertigo, and insomnia. Dizziness, depression, fatigue, and peripheral neuropathy may occur in 3–9% of patients; 1% of patients may have confusion, psychic disturbances, hallucinations, and nightmares. May accentuate epilepsy and Parkinson's disease symptomatology. Blurred vision, corneal and retinal damage, and hearing loss may occur with long-term use.

Nursing Implications: Assess baseline mental and neurologic status. Teach patient to report headache, changes in sensation or perception, and sleep problems. Discuss drug discontinuance with physician if neurologic side effects occur. Patients with visual disturbances or pain, or changes from baseline, should be seen by an ophthalmologist.

II. ALTERATION IN NUTRITION, LESS THAN BODY REQUIREMENTS, related to GI TOXICITY

Defining Characteristics: Nausea, with or without vomiting and indigestion, heartburn, and epigastric pain occur in ~10% of patients. Diarrhea, abdominal pain/distress, and constipation may occur in ~ 3%. Other effects occurring in ~ 1% are anorexia, distension, flatulence, gastroenteritis, rectal bleeding, stomatitis. Severe GI bleeding may occur in 1% of patients, as drug decreases platelet aggregation.

Nursing Implications: Teach patient potential side effects and to self-administer drug with food or antacid. Teach patient to avoid OTC aspirin-containing drugs, alcohol, or steroids, all of which can increase GI toxicity and risk for GI bleeding. Instruct patient to report any signs/symptoms of GI bleeding, abdominal pain immediately, and to stop taking the drug. Guaiac stool for occult blood periodically. If drug must be used, and risk of GI ulceration is high, discuss with physician use of misoprostol to protect the GI mucosa.

III. POTENTIAL FOR INFECTION, FATIGUE, BLEEDING related to BONE MARROW INJURY

Defining Characteristics: Although rare (1%), potential toxicities include hemolytic anemia, bone marrow depression (leukopenia, thrombocytopenia), aplastic anemia, thrombocytopenic purpura. Drug inhibits platelet aggregation but this will reverse to normal within 24 hours of drug discontinuance. May prolong bleeding time, especially in patients with underlying bleeding problems.

Nursing Implications: Assess all medicines the patient is taking and teach patient to avoid OTC aspirin-containing drugs. Teach patient to self-assess and instruct to report signs/symptoms of bleeding, fatigue, and infection.

IV. POTENTIAL FOR ALTERATION IN ELIMINATION PATTERN related to RENAL DYSFUNCTION

Defining Characteristics: Acute interstitial nephritis with hematuria, proteinuria, nephrotic syndrome may occur in 1% of patients. Patients with renal dysfunction may have worsening of renal function. Increased K+ levels may occur in the elderly or in patients with renal dysfunction. Risk increases with long-term therapy.

Nursing Implications: Assess baseline renal status. Discuss alternate drugs if renal dysfunction. Monitor serum K+, sodium (Na+), especially if receiving other drugs that affect serum K+ level (e.g., amphotericin, diuretics), or in the elderly.

V. POTENTIAL FOR ALTERATION IN CARDIAC OUTPUT related to CARDIAC EFFECTS

Defining Characteristics: CHF, tachycardia, chest pain, arrhythmias, palpitations, hypertension, and edema may occur in < 1% of patients.

Nursing Implications: Assess baseline cardiovascular status and monitor periodically while receiving the drug. Assess efficacy of antihypertensive medication due to possible drug interaction.

VI. POTENTIAL FOR INJURY related to DERMATOLOGIC AND SENSITIVITY REACTIONS

Defining Characteristics: Dermatologic effects occur in < 1% of patients and include pruritus, urticaria, rash, exfoliative dermatitis, and Stevens-Johnson syndrome. Allergic reactions occur in < 1%, characterized by asthma in aspirin-sensitive individuals, dyspnea, fever, acute anaphylaxis.

Nursing Implications: Assess baseline dermatologic, pulmonary status, and continue during drug use. Instruct patient to report any adverse reactions immediately.

Drug: ketorolac tromethamine (Toradol)

Class: NSAID.

Mechanism of Action: Inhibits prostaglandin synthesis peripherally to exert analgesic, antiinflammatory, and antipyretic activity.

Metabolism: Drug completely absorbed following PO or IM administration of the drug, with peak serum levels in 44 minutes and 50 minutes, respectively. Drug is extensively bound to serum protein (99%). Terminal half-life is 2.4–9.2 hours. Excreted by the kidney.

Dosage/Range:

- Single dose: IM, 60 mg; IV, 30 mg.
- Multiple dose: IM/IV, 30 mg q6h (maximum daily dose is 120 mg).
- 50% dose reduction for patients aged ≥ 65 years, renally impaired, or weight < 50 kg.
- Oral: for continuation therapy.

- Patients < 65 years old: 20 mg × 1, then 10 mg q4–6h (max 40 mg/24 hours).
- Patients ≥ 65: 10 mg q4–6h (max 40 mg/24 hrs).
- MAXIMUM USE OF KETOROLAC IS 5 DAYS.

Drug Preparation:
- Store at controlled room temperature of 15–30°C (59–86°F) and protect from light.

Drug Administration:
- PO, IM, or IV.

Drug Interactions:
- Other salicylates: displace ketorolac from protein binding. DO NOT USE together or dose-reduce ketorolac.
- Anticoagulants: possible increase in bleeding time; use with caution and monitor closely.
- Furosemide: decreased diuretic response; need to increase diuretic dose.
- Probenecid: causes prolonged, increased serum ketorolac levels; use cautiously, and reduce dose.
- Lithium, methotrexate: theoretically increased serum levels, so should be dose-reduced if given with ketorolac.

Lab Effects/Interference:
- None known.

Special Considerations:
- Drug indicated for the treatment of ACUTE, short-term pain, not chronic pain.
- Concurrent use with other NSAIDs NOT recommended due to risk of additive toxicity.
- Contraindicated in persons with hypersensitivity to ketorolac, or patients with asthma, nasal polyps, angioedema, and bronchospastic reaction to aspirin or other NSAIDs; also in patients with active peptic ulcer disease or GI bleeding, and patients with advanced renal insufficiency.

Equianalgesic Dosing:

Ketorolac	Meperidine		Morphine
IM			
30 or 90 mg	100 mg		12 mg
10 mg	50 mg		6 mg
Ketorolac	**Ibuprofen**	**Aspirin**	**Acetaminophen**
PO			
10 mg	400 mg	650 mg	600 mg

Potential Toxicities/Side Effects and the Nursing Process

I. ALTERATION IN NUTRITION, LESS THAN BODY REQUIREMENTS, related to GI SIDE EFFECTS

Defining Characteristics: Dyspepsia, heartburn, nausea, vomiting, anorexia, diarrhea, constipation, stomatitis, bloating, epigastric and abdominal pain may occur.

Nursing Implications: Assess history of GI symptoms and history of ulcer disease. Teach patient to take NSAID with meals or milk. Teach patient potential side effects and instruct to report them. If symptoms are severe, discuss alternative NSAIDs with physician.

II. POTENTIAL FOR BLEEDING related to INHIBITION OF PLATELET AGGREGATION

Defining Characteristics: Drug can prolong bleeding time and inhibit platelet aggregation. Peptic ulceration and occult GI bleeding can occur and be life-threatening. Increased risk factors: smoking, alcoholism.

Nursing Implications: Assess risk, history of peptic ulcer disease or GI bleeding. Assess baseline Hgb, HCT and presence/absence of occult bleeding by guaiac of stools. Instruct patient to report signs/symptoms of abdominal pain, black stools, blood per rectum, epistaxis, menorrhagia. If patient at risk for bleeding, discuss with physician use of misoprostol to protect GI mucosa. Teach patient to avoid concurrent use of aspirin, other NSAIDs.

III. POTENTIAL SENSORY/PERCEPTUAL ALTERATIONS related to CNS CHANGES

Defining Characteristics: Dizziness, headache, nervousness, fatigue, drowsiness, malaise/light-headedness, anxiety, confusion, mental depression, and emotional lability may occur. Decreased hearing, visual acuity, changes in color vision, conjunctivitis, diplopia, and cataracts have been reported. In addition, though rare, aseptic meningitis has occurred.

Nursing Implications: Assess baseline neurologic and mental status. Instruct patient to report changes in sensory/perceptual pattern, especially VISUAL CHANGES. If visual changes occur, discuss with physician referral to ophthalmologist as soon as possible. Assess for rare occurrence of aseptic meningitis (fever, coma). Discuss drug continuance with physician for significant symptoms.

IV. ALTERATION IN NUTRITION, LESS THAN BODY REQUIREMENTS, related to HEPATIC TOXICITY

Defining Characteristics: Severe and sometimes fatal hepatotoxicity has occurred. Jaundice, hepatitis occur rarely. Borderline increase in LFTs occurs in 15% of patients, while values increase by three times in 1%.

Nursing Implications: Assess baseline LFTs and monitor periodically during long-term therapy. Instruct patient to report jaundice, abdominal pain. Discuss discontinuance of drug with physician for significant toxicity.

V. ALTERATION IN RENAL ELIMINATION related to INHIBITION OF RENAL PROSTAGLANDINS

Defining Characteristics: Acute renal failure may occur rarely within first few days of treatment in patients with preexisting renal dysfunction. Other signs/symptoms of renal dysfunction that may occur rarely are azotemia, cystitis, hematuria, increased serum BUN and creatinine, and decreased creatinine clearance. Peripheral edema has also been described.

Nursing Implications: Assess baseline renal function. Teach patient to report any changes in urinary function. Monitor periodic serum BUN, creatinine during chronic therapy.

VI. ALTERATION IN SKIN INTEGRITY related to RASH

Defining Characteristics: Rash (urticaria, vesicles, or erythematous macular) may occur, as may Stevens-Johnson syndrome, flushes, alopecia, rectal itching, and acne.

Nursing Implications: Assess baseline skin integrity and presence of lesions. Instruct patient to report abnormalities. Provide symptomatic relief for rashes, pruritus.

VII. POTENTIAL FOR FATIGUE AND INFECTION related to BONE MARROW INJURY

Defining Characteristics: Neutropenia, agranulocytosis, aplastic anemia, hemolytic anemia, and thrombocytopenia may occur rarely.

Nursing Implications: Assess baseline CBC, WBC, differential, and platelet count. Discuss abnormalities with physician. Instruct patient to report severe fatigue, infection, bleeding. Monitor lab values periodically during treatment.

Drug: salsalate (Disalcid, Salsalate, Salflex)

Class: Salicylic acid derivative, NSAID.

Mechanism of Action: Hydrolyzed into two molecules of salicylic acid. Has central and peripheral action that decreases pain perception, probably through inhibition of prostaglandin synthesis. Anti-inflammatory action via prostaglandin inhibition.

Metabolism: Absorbed completely from small intestines and widely distributed into body tissues and fluids. Elimination half-life is 1 hour. Metabolized by liver and excreted in urine. Drug DOES NOT accumulate in plasma after multiple doses, unlike salicylates.

Dosage/Range:

- 500 mg q4h or 750 mg q6h, to maximum 3 g/24 hours.

Drug Preparation:

- Not significant.

Drug Administration:

- Oral: Administer with food or 8 oz (240 mL) of water or milk.

Drug Interactions:

- Antacids, urine alkylinizers: increase salicylate excretion and decrease drug effect. Do not administer with antacids.
- Ammonium chloride, ascorbic acid, methionine (urine acidifiers): decrease salicylate excretion, so increase risk of salicylate toxicity.
- Concomitant administration with alcohol, steroids, other NSAIDs may increase GI side effects.
- Corticosteroids may increase salicylate excretion and decrease drug effect.

Lab Effects/Interference:

- Competes with thyroid hormone for protein binding, so plasma T4 may be decreased but thyroid function is unaffected.

Special Considerations:

- Use cautiously if patient has history of GI bleeding, hepatic dysfunction, renal dysfunction, hypoprothrombinemia, vitamin K deficiency, bleeding hypersensitivity.
- Contraindicated if known Salsalate hypersensitivity.

Potential Toxicities/Side Effects and the Nursing Process

I. ALTERATION IN NUTRITION, LESS THAN BODY REQUIREMENTS, related to GI TOXICITY

Defining Characteristics: Fewer GI side effects than aspirin. Nausea, dyspepsia (5–25% of patients), heartburn, epigastric discomfort, anorexia, and acute reversible hepatotoxicity may occur. Risk increases with dose. May potentiate peptic ulcer disease.

Nursing Implications: Teach patient self-administration with food or 8 oz (240 mL) water or milk. If patient is receiving antacid, administer antacid two hours after meal and Salsalate before meal. Assess baseline liver and renal function, and monitor if patient is receiving high doses on ongoing basis.

II. INJURY related to MILD SALICYLISM

Defining Characteristics: Administration of large doses of salicylates may cause salicylism, characterized by dizziness, tinnitus, diminished hearing, nausea, vomiting, diarrhea, mental confusion, CNS depression, headache, sweating, and hyperventilation at serum salicylate concentration 150–300 μg/mL (use in cancer patients usually 100 μg/mL).

Nursing Implications: Teach patient to reduce dose, interrupt dose if signs/symptoms occur. Assess concurrent medications for possible drug interactions.

III. POTENTIAL FOR BLEEDING related to INHIBITION OF PLATELET AGGREGATION, OCCULT BLEEDING, BRUISING

Defining Characteristics: Salsalate may cause prolongation of bleeding time, leukopenia, thrombocytopenia, purpura, shortened erythrocyte survival time.

Nursing Implications: Teach patient to avoid aspirin and Salsalate-containing drugs if receiving myelosuppressive chemotherapy. Review concurrent medications to identify risk for drug interactions. Monitor Hgb, HCT over time; teach patient signs/symptoms of anemia, and instruct to report them (headache, fatigue, chest pain, irritability). Monitor stool guaiacs.

IV. POTENTIAL FOR INJURY related to ALLERGIC REACTION

Defining Characteristics: Rash; hypersensitivity characterized by asthma and anaphylaxis has occurred rarely.

Nursing Implications: Assess for reactions to prior salicylate-containing medications or salsalates. Teach patient to report rash, asthmalike symptoms. If these occur, discuss alternative non-opioid analgesics. Provide systemic support if anaphylaxis occurs.

Drug: ziconotide intrathecal infusion (Prialt)

Class: Selective blocker of neuronal N-type calcium channels in the nerves which normally conduct pain signals from the periphery to the spinal cord.

Mechanism of Action: Synthetic equivalent to a naturally occurring conopeptide found in a marine snail (*Conus magus*), which binds to N-type calcium channels on the primary afferent nerves (A-δ and C) of the dorsal horn of the spinal cord. Voltage sensitive calcium channels (VSCC) permit the cell to regulate the amount of calcium entering and leaving the cell; this directly inflences membrane excitability, among other cellular processes. Ziconotide appears to block these channels so that pain messages from the periphery do not get passed through to the spinal cord and up the spinal cord where pain perception occurs.

Metabolism: Following 1 hour IT administration of 1–10 micrograms of drug, total and peak exposure were variable but dose proportional; as a continuous IT infusion, once a quantifiable serum level of drug is identified, the serum level remains constant at least up to 9 months. Drug is 50% bound to human plasma proteins, and CSF volume of distribution is the same as the total CSF volume of 140 mL. Terminal half-life in the CSF is 4.6 hours, and is cleared from the CSF at approximately the human CSF turnover rate of 0.3–0.4 mL/min. Drug passes across the blood brain barrier into systemic circulation with a serum half-life of 1.3 hrs; Drug is cleaved at multiple sites of the peptide; it is degraded via the ubiquitin-protease system in many organs (kidney, liver, lung) into component amino acids. < 1% of intact ziconotide is recovered in the urine.

Dosage/Range:

- Initial dose no more than 2.4 micrograms (mcg)/day (0.1 mcg/hr) and titrated to patient response.
- Increase dose by up to 2.4 mcg/day (0.1 mcg/hr) at intervals of no more than 2–3 times/week based on patient response, up to recommended MAXIMUM of 19.2 mcg/da (0.8 mcg/hr) by day 21.
- May use dose increases in increments of less than 2.4 mg/da less frequently than 2–3 times a week.
- With each dosage titration ensure that the pump infusion rate is adjusted correctly (either implanted microinfusion device or external microinfusion device and catheter).
- Available in 1, 2, 5 mL vials (100 micrograms/mL) for diluted use; and 20 mL vial (25 micrograms/mL) for undiluted use.
- Diluted ziconotide: use 0.9% Sodium Chloride Injection USP (preservative free) using aseptic procedures to achieve pump manufacturer's recommended concentration.

- Once the appropriate dose has been established, the 100mcg/mL formulation may be used undiluted.
- Store unopened vials at 2°C–8°C (36°F–46°F) but do not freeze; Refrigerate (2°C–8°C) after preparation, protect from light, and use within 24 hours.
- **Initial (naïve) pump priming:** use 2 mL of undiluted 25 mcg/mL formulation to rinse the internal surfaces of the pump; repeat 2× more for a total of 3 rinses.
- **Initial pump fill:** Use undiluted 25 mcg/mL ONLY to fill the naïve pump after priming; begin dosing NO HIGHER than 2.4 mcg/da (0.1mcg/hr). Initial pump fill loses drug through adsorption on internal device surfaces and by dilution in the residual space in the device—this does not occur with subsequent pump filling. Refill the pump reservoir within 14 days of the initial fill to ensure accurate drug administration.
- **Pump Refills:** Fill the pump at least every 40 days if used diluted; if undiluted drug, fill the pump at least every 60 days. Use the Medtronic refill kit to empty the pump contents prior to refill with new drug. If an implanted pump must be surgically replaced while the patient is receiving the drug, the replacement pump should be primed, and the initial drug replaced in 14 days as above.

Drug Preparation:

Ziconotide IT infusion	Initial Fill (expiration)	Refill (expiration)
25 mcg/mL undiluted	14 days	60 days
100 mcg/mL undiluted	N/A	60 days
100 mcg/mL, diluted	N/A	40 days

- Refer to manufacturer's pump manual for specific instructions. When using an external microinfusion device, and filling it the first time, use a concentration of 5 mcg/mL; dilute drug with 0.9% Sodium Chloride USP (preservative free); the flow rate for the external microinfusor usually starts at 0.02 mL/hr to deliver the initial dose rate of 2.4 mcg/day (0.1 mcg/hr).

Drug Administration:

- Continuous IT infusion via Medronic SynchroMed® EL (Medtronic Inc), SynchroMed® II Infusion System (Medtronic Inc), Simms Deltec Cadd Micro® (Ardus Medical, Inc.) External Microinfusion Device and Catheter pumps.
- Most patients continue to receive opioids.
- There is no known antidote for the drug; if overdosage, most patients recover within 24 hours after drug withdrawal; if inadvertent IV or epidural injection of drug, support blood pressure by recumbent positioning, and BP support as needed.

Drug Interactions:

- Additive effect when given with opioid medications as drug does not bind to opiate receptors.
- CNS depressant drugs: increased incidence of CNS adverse events (e.g., dizziness, confusion).

Lab Effects/Interference:

- Increased serum creatine kinase levels (40% of patients) which may be associated with muscle weakness; rare renal failure related to rhabdomyolysis and very high CK elevations.

Special Considerations:

- Severe psychiatric symptoms and neurological impairment may occur during ziconotide IT infusion; patients with a history of psychosis should NOT receive the drug; monitor patients frequently for signs/symptoms of cognitive impairment, hallucinations, or changes in mood or level of consciousness; interrupt or discontinue drug for severe psychiatric or neurological symptoms/signs.
- Drug can be interrupted or discontinued abruptly without risk of withdrawal syndrome.
- Drug is embryotoxic in animals.
- Use cautiously in elderly patients as incidence of confusion is higher; start at lower dose and titrate more slowly.
- Patients should be taught not to engage in hazardous activity, such as operation of heavy machinery.
- Patients should notify provider IMMEDIATELY for any of the following:
  - Change in mental status such as lethargy, confusion, disorientation, decreased alertness.
  - Change in mood or perception, such as hallucinations (e.g., unusual tactile sensations in oral cavity).
  - Symptoms of depression or suicidal ideation.
  - Nausea, vomiting, seizures, fever, headache, and/or stiff neck as these may herald developing meningitis.

Potential Toxicities/Side Effects and the Nursing Process

I. SENSORY/PERCEPTUAL ALTERATIONS related to CNS CHANGES

Defining Characteristics: CNS depression and changes in mental status may occur, including psychiatric symptoms, cognitive impairment and decreased alertness/unresponsiveness. These are characterized by confusion (33%, with a higher incidence in the elderly), memory impairment (22%), speech disorder (14%), aphasia (12%), abnormal thinking (8%), and amnesia (1%). Psychiatric symptoms are more likely to occur in patients with pretreatment psychiatric disorders, and include hallucinations (12%), paranoid ideation (2%), hostility

(2%), delirium (2%), psychosis (1%), and manic reactions (0.4%). Cognitive impairment may be gradual a few weeks after starting therapy. Once dose is interrupted or discontinued, symptoms usually resolve in 2 weeks. Patients may become depressed with suicidal ideation. Other sensory/perceptual alterations include: dizziness (47%), somnolence (22%), abnormal vision (22%), ataxia (16%), abnormal gait (15%), hypertonia (11%), nystagmus (8%), dysesthesia (7%), paresthesia (7%), and vertigo (7%).

Nursing Implications: Assess past medical history for psychiatric and neurological problems. Assess baseline gait, movement, mental, affective, and neurologic status. Assess medication profile to identify other contributions, i.e., CNS depressants, antiepileptics, neuroleptics, sedatives, diuretics. Teach patient and family that these side effects may occur, and instruct patient/family to report any changes. Teach patient/family to notify provider IMMEDIATELY for any of the following:

- Change in mental status such as lethargy, confusion, disorientation, decreased alertness.
- Change in mood or perception, such as hallucinations (e.g., unusual tactile sensations in oral cavity).
- Symptoms of depression or suicidal ideation.

Assess patient safety, and measures to ensure safety. Discuss any significant changes with physician, and need to interrupt/discontinue drug based on severity of symptoms.

OPIOID ANALGESICS

Drug: codeine (as Sulfate or Phosphate); may be combined with acetaminophen (Phenaphen with Codeine, Tylenol with Codeine, Capital and Codeine, Codaphen (Odalan), or with aspirin (Empirin with Codeine, Soma Compound with Codeine, Fiorinal with Codeine)

Class: Opioid analgesic (opioid agonist).

Mechanism of Action: Resembles morphine but has milder action; binds to opiate receptors in CNS (limbic system, thalamus, striatum, hypothalamus, midbrain, spinal cord), altering pain perception at level of spinal cord and higher centers, as well as the emotional response to pain. Also suppresses cough reflex.

Metabolism: Well absorbed after oral or parenteral administration. Metabolized by liver; excreted in urine, and small amount in feces.

Dosage/Range:

- Mild pain: 30 mg q4h (range 15–60 mg), PO, SQ, or IM.

Drug Preparation:
- Store tablets in tight, light-resistant containers at 15–30°C (59–86°F).
- Injection should be protected from light and stored at 15–40°C (59–104°F).
- At home, teach patient to store oral doses in a safe place away from children and pets.

Drug Administration:
- PO, SQ, IM.

Drug Interactions:
- Injection is incompatible with solutions containing aminophylline, ammonium chloride, amobarbital sodium, chlorothiazide sodium, heparin sodium, methicillin sodium, nitrofurantoin, phenobarbital sodium, sodium bicarbonate.
- Alcohol, CNS depressants: additive effects.

Lab Effects/Interference:
- None known.

Special Considerations:
- Parenteral dose is 2/3 oral dose for equianalgesic effect.
- Onset of action after PO or SQ dose is 15–30 minutes, with duration of analgesia 4–6 hours.
- Indicated for relief of mild-to-moderate pain unrelieved by nonopiate analgesia.
- Addition of acetaminophen or aspirin gives additive analgesia.
- Give smallest effective dose to prevent development of tolerance, physical dependency.
- Reduce dose in debilitated patients, or patients receiving other CNS depressants.
- Use with caution in patients with hepatic or renal dysfunction, hypothyroidism, Addison's disease, severe CNS depression, respiratory depression, head injury, elevated intracranial pressure.
- If required, naloxone HCl (Narcan) will reverse opiate toxicity (e.g., respiratory depression). However, it is important that acute withdrawal symptoms be prevented by giving only enough naloxone to reverse respiratory depression and that this be continued for opioid drug half-life.

Potential Toxicities/Side Effects and the Nursing Process

I. SENSORY/PERCEPTUAL ALTERATIONS related to CNS DEPRESSION

Defining Characteristics: Drowsiness, sedation, mood changes, euphoria, dysphoria, dizziness, mental clouding may occur. At high doses, may cause seizures. Miosis (papillary constriction) may occur.

Nursing Implications: Assess baseline neurologic status. Use cautiously, if at all, in patients with head injury, increased intracranial pressure, severe CNS depression, acute alcoholism, or who are elderly or debilitated. Assess other concurrent medications. Use with caution in patients receiving other opioids, tranquilizers, hypnotics, monoamine oxidase (MAO) inhibitors, since increasing CNS depressant effects can occur. Monitor neurologic status closely. Teach patient to avoid driving and operating machinery while taking the medicine, and to AVOID concurrent alcohol.

II. ALTERATION IN OXYGENATION related to RESPIRATORY DEPRESSION

Defining Characteristics: Opiate agonists directly depress respiratory center in brain stem, causing decreased sensitivity and responsiveness to increased pCO2 (CO2 tension in serum). Also may depress deep breathing and reflex to sigh. Tolerance to respiratory depressant effects occurs with chronic use.

Nursing Implications: Assess baseline pulmonary status, and monitor periodically during drug use. Use cautiously in patients with bronchial asthma, chronic obstructive pulmonary disease (COPD), respiratory depression, and monitor closely.

III. ALTERATION IN ELIMINATION related to CONSTIPATION, ILEUS

Defining Characteristics: Opium agonists bind to opiate receptors in bowel, slowing peristalsis, leading to constipation. Untreated constipation may result in bowel perforation.

Nursing Implications: Assess baseline elimination, fluid intake, diet, and exercise patterns. Teach patient about prevention of constipation: goal is to move bowels at least every two days by increasing fluid intake to 3 L/day, following a diet high in fiber (beans, vegetables, fruit), and taking moderate exercise. Assess need for bowel softeners, bulk-forming laxatives, and osmotic cathartics, and discuss prescription with physician. Teach patient self-administration of medications.

IV. ALTERATION IN NUTRITION, LESS THAN BODY REQUIREMENTS, related to GI TOXICITY

Defining Characteristics: Nausea, vomiting, dry mouth may occur. Gastric, biliary, and pancreatic secretions are decreased by opiate agonists; digestion is delayed. Biliary tract muscle tone is increased, and spasm of Oddi's sphincter may occur (morphine > meperidine > codeine).

Nursing Implications: Assess patient tolerance of GI side effects. Teach patient to report side effects. If nausea/vomiting occur, change to another opioid, or premedicate with antiemetic to prevent nausea/vomiting. Assess GI pain, biliary spasm, and consider alternative opioid.

V. ALTERATION IN CARDIAC OUTPUT related to HYPOTENSION, BRADYCARDIA

Defining Characteristics: Orthostatic hypotension, bradycardia due to cholinergic effect, and peripheral vasodilation may occur with rapid IV dosing. There may be histamine-related flushing, pruritus, diaphoresis with chronic drug usage; tolerance develops to this effect.

Nursing Implications: Assess baseline cardiovascular status. Teach patient to change position slowly and to hold onto stable, nearby structure for support as needed. Be careful when giving IV push opioids, and caution patient to remain in supine position for 15–20 minutes after injection. Monitor cardiovascular status after injection.

VI. ALTERATION IN URINE ELIMINATION related to URINARY RETENTION

Defining Characteristics: Increased smooth muscle tone in urinary tract and spasm may occur. Bladder tone is increased, with may cause urgency. Vesical sphincter tone may be increased, leading to difficulty urinating. Increased risk of urinary retention in patients with prostatic hypertrophy or urethral stricture.

Nursing Implications: Assess baseline urinary elimination pattern. Teach patient to increase fluids to 3 L/day, and encourage voiding every 2–3 hours. Instruct patient to report problems with urination.

VII. KNOWLEDGE DEFICIT related to DRUG ADMINISTRATION, POTENTIAL FOR TOLERANCE, AND DEPENDENCY

Defining Characteristics: Psychological dependence (addiction) occurs rarely in patients taking opioid agonists for cancer pain (< 1%). Physical dependence (precipitation of withdrawal symptoms) occurs with chronic use of the drug for the relief of chronic cancer pain. In addition, tolerance, or less analgesic effect over time with the same drug dose, occurs and requires increased dosage of drug.

Nursing Implications: Assess baseline knowledge of opioid analgesics, and attitude about their use for cancer pain management. Teach patient about proper self-administration, possible side effects, and self-care measures. Suggest patient maintain diary of pain intensity, precipitating and alleviating factors, drug dose and time taken, and relief. Teach patient to self-administer opioid agonists for relief of chronic cancer pain around-the-clock, not PRN, to prevent pain. Explain use of prescribed short-acting opioid for rescue or to manage breakthrough pain. Discuss with physician dose increase or change in frequency of administration if tolerance develops. Teach patient that withdrawal symptoms may occur if chronic, around-the-clock dosing is interrupted. Withdrawal (abstinence) symptoms that may be seen are restlessness, lacrimation, rhinorrhea, yawning, perspiration, gooseflesh, restless sleep, mydriasis in first 24 hours. These are followed by twitching and leg spasm; severe aching of the back, abdomen, and legs; cramping in abdomen and legs; hot/cold flashes; insomnia; nausea/vomiting, diarrhea; severe sneezing; and increased heart rate, BP, and temperature (T), which peak at 36–72 hours. Withdrawal syndrome can be prevented by administration of at least 1/4 of previous opioid dose.

VIII. SEXUAL DYSFUNCTION related to IMPOTENCE, ↓ LIBIDO

Defining Characteristics: Opiate agonists may suppress gonadotropin, causing impotence and decreased libido.

Nursing Implications: Assess baseline sexual pattern. Discuss potential toxicity and impact on sexuality. Provide information, emotional support, and referral as needed.

Drug: fentanyl citrate (Oral Transmucosal Fentanyl, Actiq)

Class: Opioid analgesic (opioid agonist).

Mechanism of Action: Fentanyl is a pure opioid agonist that binds to opioid μ-receptors located in the brain, spinal cord, and smooth muscle. The oral transmucosal preparation of the drug is a solid formulation of fentanyl citrate placed on a handle so the drug is sucked. Sucking, the drug dose coats the oral mucosa, through which the drug is rapidly absorbed, reportedly as fast as IV morphine. Onset of analgesia is approximately 5 minutes from onset of administration, with maximum effect in 20–30 minutes.

Metabolism: Initial rapid absorption of about 25% of total dose across buccal mucosa, into systemic circulation, and longer prolonged absorption of swallowed fentanyl (75% of dose) from GI tract. One-third of drug escapes first-pass elimination and enters the systemic circulation for a total of 50% of the total dose that is bioavailable. Following absorption, drug is rapidly distributed to brain, heart, lungs, kidneys, spleen. Plasma binding is 80–85%. The drug is primarily metabolized in the liver, and less than 7% of the dose is excreted in the urine. The terminal elimination half-life is approximately 219 minutes.

Dosage/Range:

Adult:

- Titrate to patient's individual needs: available in six strengths that are color-coded: 200-, 400-, 600-, 800-, 1200-, and 1600-μg fentanyl base.

- Drug CANNOT be used in opioid-naïve patients, and is indicated for the management of chronic pain, especially breakthrough pain in patients who are ALREADY RECEIVING AND WHO ARE TOLERANT to opioid therapy (e.g., taking at least 60 mg of morphine/day, 50 μg/hr of transdermal fentanyl, or an equianalgesic dose of another opioid for a week or longer).
- Patient begins using 200 μg unit for breakthrough pain (BTP) and sucks the medicine for 15 minutes. If the pain is unrelieved, the patient waits an additional 15 minutes then administers a second 200-μg unit. If the pain is unrelieved, the patient waits another 15 minutes and administers a third 200-μg unit. Three units of any dosage is the maximum drug per BTP episode.
- If the patient required two units of 200-μg dosage, then the patient would give 400-μg dose for the next episode of BTP. If using two 200-μg units, the patient would wait 15 minutes between taking units.
- If the patient needed three units of 200-μg dose, the patient would take the 600-μg strength the next dose for BTP.
- The patient should notify the physician if drug is required more than four times per day, so that the long-acting opioid can be increased.

Drug Preparation/Administration:

- Drug is on a handle, sealed in a child-resistant foil pouch that requires scissors to open. The drug dose is color-coded.
- Open foil pack immediately before use. Patient should place drug dose unit in the mouth between cheek and lower gum. Patient should suck, NOT CHEW, the medication over 15 minutes.
- If the patient achieves adequate analgesia or develops excessive side effects, the drug should be removed from the mouth and discarded immediately. The remaining drug is very dangerous if a child or pet ingests it, so maximum precautions must be taken.
- To discard the remaining drug, twist drug off handle using tissue paper, and flush medicine down the toilet. Destroy any medication remaining on the handle by dissolving it under hot water.
- Keep medication away from patient's eyes, skin, or mucous membranes when not sucking the medication, and the patient should wash hands after discarding unused medication portion.
- At home, teach patient to store oral doses in a safe place away from children and pets.

Drug Interactions:

- CNS depressants (e.g., other opioids, alcohol, sedatives, hypnotics, general anesthetics, phenothiazines, tranquilizers, skeletal muscle relaxants, sedating antihistamines) may increase CNS depression (hypoventilation, hypotension, profound sedation, especially in opioid nontolerant patients).

Lab Effects/Interference:

- None known.

Special Considerations:

- CONTRAINDICATED in opioid-nontolerant patients, as life-threatening hypoventilation may occur; in children < 10 kg for management of acute postoperative pain; in patients with hypersensitivity to fentanyl; in patients with head injury and increased intracranial pressure (ICP); and in nursing mothers.
- Administer cautiously to patients with hepatic or renal dysfunction.
- Teach patient drug must be kept out of reach of children as dose can be LETHAL to children.
- Use cautiously in patients with chronic pulmonary disease (degree of hypoventilation), cardiac conduction disease (bradycardia), and the elderly.
- Respiratory depression may be associated with opioids, and patients should be monitored for this. This was not reported in the clinical trials with Actiq.
- Patients should be taught to call nurse or physician if taking four of the same strength units within 60 minutes without relief or if taking drug more than four times per day.
- Once effective dose determined, drug provides rapid relief of BTP.
- Some reported toxicities may be due to advanced malignancy rather than the drug.

Potential Toxicities/Side Effects and the Nursing Process

I. ALTERATION IN OXYGENATION related to HYPOVENTILATION

Defining Characteristics: Dyspnea (10%), increased cough and pharyngitis (3–10%).

Nursing Implications: Assess baseline pulmonary status. Use with caution in patients with COPD, bradycardia, renal or hepatic dysfunction, and in the elderly. Teach patient to report any pulmonary difficulties immediately. Ensure patient knows that if respiratory difficulty develops, the drug must be removed from mouth and discarded immediately; also, to suck and not chew drug. Ensure that patient understands how to handle drug safely to prevent additional absorption of unused drug.

II. SENSORY/PERCEPTUAL ALTERATIONS related to CNS CHANGES

Defining Characteristics: CNS depression and changes in mental status may occur, characterized by somnolence or dizziness (10%); abnormal gait, anxiety, confusion, depression, insomnia, hypesthesia, vasodilation, abnormal vision (3–10% incidence).

Nursing Implications: Assess baseline gait, mental, affective, and neurologic status. Assess medication profile to identify other contributions, i.e., CNS depressants. Instruct patient to report any changes. Assess patient safety, and measures to ensure safety. Discuss any significant changes with physician.

III. ALTERATION IN COMFORT related to HEADACHE, FEVER

Defining Characteristics: Headache, fever, asthenia are reported in ~10% of patients; less commonly, myalgia, pruritus, rash, sweating occur in 3–10% of patients.

Nursing Implications: Assess baseline comfort. Teach patient to report symptoms and manage based on severity. Assess impact on patient's quality of life. If severe, discuss alternative strategies with physician.

IV. ALTERATION IN NUTRITION, LESS THAN BODY REQUIREMENTS, related to NAUSEA/VOMITING

Defining Characteristics: Nausea, vomiting are reported in ~10% of patients; less commonly, anorexia, dehydration, edema, and dyspepsia occur in 3–10% of patients.

Nursing Implications: Assess baseline nutritional status. Teach patient to report nausea, vomiting, anorexia, dyspepsia. Manage symptomatically. Assess severity and impact on quality of life. Discuss severe or unmanaged symptoms with physician.

V. ALTERATION IN ELIMINATION related to CONSTIPATION OR DIARRHEA

Defining Characteristics: Opium agonists bind to opiate receptors in bowel, slowing peristalsis, leading to constipation. Untreated constipation may result in bowel perforation. Opiate receptors in bowel decrease peristalsis. Constipation and diarrhea were each reported in < 10% of patients.

Nursing Implications: Assess baseline elimination, fluid intake, diet, and exercise patterns. Instruct patient regarding prevention of constipation: goal is to move bowels at least every two days by increasing fluids to 3 L/day, following a diet high in fiber (beans, vegetables, fruit), and taking moderate exercise. Assess need for bowel softeners, bulk-forming laxatives, and osmotic cathartics, and discuss prescription with physician. Teach patient self-administration of medications. MUST be started on bowel regimen.

Drug: fentanyl transdermal system (Duragesic)

Class: Opioid analgesic (opioid agonist).

Mechanism of Action: Strong opioid analgesic; 20–30 times more potent than parenteral morphine when given transdermally to opioid-naïve patients. Drug interacts primarily with opioid μ-receptors, found in the brain, spinal cord, and other tissues, causing analgesia and sedation. Duragesic patches provide continuous-released fentanyl from a transdermal reservoir system at a constant amount per unit time. The drug moves from areas of higher concentration (patch) to areas of lower concentration (skin). Initially, the skin under the patch absorbs the fentanyl, and the drug is concentrated in the upper skin layers. The drug gradually enters the systemic circulation, leveling off 2–24 hours later, and remaining fairly constant for the 72-hour application period.

Metabolism: Primarily metabolized by the liver; 75% of IV dose excreted in urine, 9% in feces, and < 10% as unchanged drug. Peak levels occur 24–72 hours after a single application. Half-life is approximately 17 hours (after system removal, serum fentanyl concentrations fall to 50% in approximately 17 hours; range, 13–22 hours).

Dosage/Range:

25 μg/hour is initial dosage for non-opioid-tolerant patients.

Doses for patients currently receiving opioid analgesics who are tolerant can be calculated from the following table:

Duragesic Dose Prescription Based on Daily Morphine Equivalence Dose

Oral 24-hour Morphine (mg/day)	IM 24-hour Morphine (mg/day)	DURAGESIC Dose (μg/hr)
45–134	8–22	25
135–224	23–37	50
225–314	38–52	75
315–404	53–67	100
405–494	68–82	125
495–584	83–97	150
585–674	98–112	175
675–764	113–127	200
765–854	128–142	225
855–944	143–157	250
945–1034	158–172	275
1035–1124	173–187	300

Drug Preparation:

- None.

Drug Administration:

- Apply to nonirritated and nonirradiated skin; clip hair (not shave) as needed. May cleanse with water only and dry completely if necessary. Apply patch immediately after removal from package. Press firmly into place with palm of hand for 10–20 seconds, making sure contact is complete, especially around edges. Patient wears for 72 hours, then changes patch. Some patients may need to reapply new patches every 48 hours. Short-acting opioids must be continued for 24 hours until serum fentanyl level achieved.
- Disposal: at home, patient must fold so adhesive side of system adheres to itself, then flush down toilet. In hospital, used patches must be returned to pharmacy for proper disposal.
- At home, teach patient to store oral doses in a safe place away from children and pets.

Drug Interactions:

- Potentiation of CNS depressant effects, when administered concurrently with other opioids, benzodiazepines, or other CNS depressants.

Lab Effects/Interference:

- None known.

Special Considerations:

- Indications: patients with chronic pain requiring opioid analgesia.
- Contraindicated in patients with known hypersensitivity to fentanyl or adhesives. Use with caution in the following patients: patients with COPD predisposed to hypoventilation; patients with head injuries, brain tumor (very sensitive to effects of CO_2 retention); patients with cardiac disease (may cause bradyarrhythmias); patients with hepatic dysfunction.
- Availability: Dosages: 25 μg/h, 50 μg/h, 75 μg/h, and 100 μg/h. Supplied in one carton containing five individually wrapped patches.

Potential Toxicities/Side Effects and the Nursing Process

I. ALTERATION IN OXYGENATION related to HYPOVENTILATION

Defining Characteristics: Dyspnea, hypoventilation, apnea (3–10% of patients); hemoptysis, pharyngitis, hiccups rare; stertorous breathing, asthma, respiratory dysfunction.

Nursing Implications: Assess baseline pulmonary status. Use with caution in patients with COPD, brain tumors, increased intracranial pressure (ICP), hepatic failure. NEVER exceed 25 μg/h if patient not tolerant to opioids. Must continue to observe patient for 17 hours after dose removed for signs/symptoms of toxicity—same is true if naloxone HCl (Narcan) required to reverse opioid. Theoretically, a temperature of 39°C (102°F) will increase serum fentanyl by 33% due to drug delivery and skin absorption. If patient develops fever, observe for signs/symptoms of overdosage. Elderly patients (> 60–65 years old) may have reduced ability to clear drug, so start at 25 μg/hr unless already tolerant of > 135 mg morphine sulfate/24 hours.

II. SENSORY/PERCEPTUAL ALTERATIONS related to CNS CHANGES

Defining Characteristics: CNS depression and changes in mental status may occur, characterized by somnolence, confusion, depression, asthenia (> 10%), dizziness, nervousness, hallucinations, anxiety, depression, euphoria (3–10%), tremors, abnormal coordination, speech disorder, abnormal thinking, dreams. Rare: aphasia, vertigo, stupor, hypotonia, hypertonia, hostility.

Nursing Implications: Assess baseline mental, neurologic status. Dose of other opioids and benzodiazepines should be 50%. Use cautiously in substance abusers.

III. ALTERATION IN CARDIAC OUTPUT related to ARRYTHMIA, ANGINA

Defining Characteristics: Arrhythmia, chest pain may occur; IV fentanyl has caused bradyarrhythmias.

Nursing Implications: Assess baseline cardiac status, and monitor during drug use. Instruct patient to report palpitations, chest pain.

IV. ALTERATION IN NUTRITION, LESS THAN BODY REQUIREMENTS, related to NAUSEA, VOMITING

Defining Characteristics: Nausea, vomiting, anorexia, dyspepsia, rare abdominal distension.

Nursing Implications: Assess baseline nutritional status. Instruct patient to report nausea, vomiting, anorexia, dyspepsia.

V. ALTERATION IN ELIMINATION related to CONSTIPATION, ILEUS

Defining Characteristics: Opium agonists bind to opiate receptors in bowel, slowing peristalsis, leading to constipation. Untreated constipation may result in bowel perforation. Opiate receptors in bowel decrease peristalsis.

Nursing Implications: Assess baseline elimination, fluid intake, diet, and exercise patterns. Instruct patient regarding prevention of constipation: goal is to move bowels at least every two days, by increasing fluids to 3 L/day, following a diet high in fiber (beans, vegetables, fruit), and taking moderate exercise. Assess need for bowel softeners, bulk-forming laxatives, and osmotic cathartics, and discuss prescription with physician. Teach patient self-administration of medications. MUST be started on bowel regimen.

VI. ALTERATION IN CARDIAC OUTPUT related to HYPOTENSION, BRADYCARDIA

Defining Characteristics: Orthostatic hypotension, bradycardia due to cholinergic effect, and peripheral vasodilation may occur with rapid IV dosing. There may be histamine-related flushing, pruritus, diaphoresis with chronic drug usage; tolerance develops to this effect.

Nursing Implications: Assess baseline cardiovascular status. Teach patient to change position slowly and to hold onto stable, nearby structure for support as needed. Be careful when giving IV push opioids, and caution patient to remain in supine position for 15–20 minutes after injection. Monitor cardiovascular status after injection.

VII. ALTERATION IN URINE ELIMINATION related to URINARY RETENTION

Defining Characteristics: Increased smooth muscle tone in urinary tract and spasm may occur. Bladder tone is increased, which may cause urgency. Vesical sphincter tone may be increased, leading to difficulty urinating. Increased risk of urinary retention in patients with prostatic hypertrophy or urethral stricture. Rare bladder pain, oliguria, urinary frequency.

Nursing Implications: Assess baseline urinary elimination pattern. Teach patient to increase fluids to 3 L/day, and encourage voiding every 2–3 hours. Instruct patient to report problems with urination.

VIII. ALTERATION IN SKIN INTEGRITY/COMFORT related to RASH, PRURITUS

Defining Characteristics: Sweating, pruritus, rash; erythema, papules, itching, edema, exfoliative dermatitis, pustules at application site; headache rare.

Nursing Implications: Teach patient proper drug application and to rotate sites.

Drug: hydromorphone (Dilaudid)

Class: Opioid analgesic (opioid agonist).

Mechanism of Action: Resembles morphine but has milder action; binds to opiate receptors in CNS (limbic system, thalamus, striatum, hypothalamus, midbrain, spinal cord), altering pain perception at level of spinal cord and higher centers as well as the emotional response to pain. Also suppresses cough reflex.

Metabolism: Well absorbed after oral, rectal, and parenteral administration. Onset of action is 15–30 minutes (more rapid than morphine), with a duration of action of 4–5 hours. Metabolized by liver and excreted in urine.

Dosage/Range:
- Use caution in patients who have not received opiates before and have not developed tolerance.
- Moderate pain: oral: 1–6 mg q4–6h; SQ or IM: 2–4 mg q4–6h, 3 mg rectal suppository.
- Severe pain: oral: 4 mg or more q4h; SQ or IM: 4 mg or more, then titrate based on patient response and tolerance.

Drug Preparation:
- Store tablets in tight, light-resistant containers at 15–30°C (59–86°F).
- Injection should be protected from light and stored at 15–40°C (59–104°F).

Drug Administration:
- PO, SQ, IM. Use highly concentrated injectable solution for patients who are tolerant to opiate agonists.
- At home, teach patient to store oral doses in a safe place away from children and pets.

Drug Interactions:
- Alcohol, CNS depressants: Additive effects.

Lab Effects/Interference:
- None known.

Special Considerations:
- Parenteral dose is 1/5 oral dose for equianalgesic effect.
- Indicated for relief of moderate-to-severe pain.
- Additive benefit when combined with acetaminophen or aspirin.
- Give smallest effective dose to prevent development of tolerance, physical dependency.
- Reduce dose in debilitated patients or patients receiving other CNS depressants.
- Use with caution in patients with hepatic or renal dysfunction, hypothyroidism, Addison's disease, severe CNS depression, respiratory depression, head injury, elevated ICP.
- If required, naloxone HCl will reverse opiate toxicity (e.g., respiratory depression). However, it is important that acute withdrawal symptoms be prevented by giving only enough naloxone to reverse respiratory depression and that this be continued for opioid drug half-life.

Potential Toxicities/Side Effects and the Nursing Process

I. SENSORY/PERCEPTUAL ALTERATIONS related to CNS DEPRESSION

Defining Characteristics: Drowsiness, sedation, mood changes, euphoria, dysphoria, dizziness, mental clouding may occur. At high doses, may cause seizures. Miosis (papillary constriction) may occur.

Nursing Implications: Assess baseline neurologic status. Use cautiously, if at all, in patients with head injury, increased ICP, severe CNS depression, acute alcoholism, the elderly, and the debilitated. Assess other concurrent medications. Use with caution in patients receiving other opioids, tranquilizers, hypnotics, MAO inhibitors, since increasing CNS depressant effects can occur. Monitor neurologic status closely. Teach patient to avoid driving and operating machinery while taking the medicine, and to AVOID concurrent alcohol.

II. ALTERATION IN OXYGENATION related to RESPIRATORY DEPRESSION

Defining Characteristics: Opiate agonists directly depress respiratory center in brain stem, causing decreased sensitivity and responsiveness to increased pCO_2. Also may depress deep breathing and reflex to sigh. Tolerance to respiratory depressant effects occurs with chronic use.

Nursing Implications: Assess baseline pulmonary status, and monitor periodically during drug use. Use cautiously in patients with bronchial asthma, COPD, respiratory depression, and monitor closely.

III. ALTERATION IN ELIMINATION related to CONSTIPATION, ILEUS

Defining Characteristics: Opium agonists bind to opiate receptors in bowel, slowing peristalsis, leading to constipation. Untreated constipation may result in bowel perforation.

Nursing Implications: Assess baseline elimination, fluid intake, diet, and exercise patterns. Instruct patient about prevention of constipation: goal is to move bowels at least every two days by increasing fluids to 3 L/day, following a diet high in fiber (beans, vegetables, fruit), and taking moderate exercise. Assess need for bowel softeners, bulk-forming laxatives, and osmotic cathartics, and discuss prescription with physician. Teach patient self-administration of medications.

IV. ALTERATION IN NUTRITION related to GI TOXICITY

Defining Characteristics: Nausea, vomiting, and dry mouth may occur. Gastric, biliary, and pancreatic secretions are decreased by opiate agonists; digestion is delayed. Biliary tract muscle tone is increased, and spasm of Oddi's sphincter may occur (morphine > meperidine > codeine).

Nursing Implications: Assess patient tolerance of GI side effects. Teach patient to report side effects. If nausea/vomiting occur, change to another opioid, or premedicate with antiemetic to prevent nausea/vomiting. Assess GI pain, biliary spasm, and consider alternative opioid.

V. ALTERATION IN CARDIAC OUTPUT related to HYPOTENSION, BRADYCARDIA

Defining Characteristics: Orthostatic hypotension, bradycardia due to cholinergic effect, and peripheral vasodilation may occur with rapid IV dosing. There may be histamine-related flushing, pruritus, diaphoresis with chronic drug usage; tolerance develops to this effect.

Nursing Implications: Assess baseline cardiovascular status. Teach patient to change position slowly and to hold onto stable, nearby structure for support as needed. Be careful when giving IV push opioids, and caution patient to remain in supine position for 15–20 minutes after injection. Monitor cardiovascular status after injection.

VI. ALTERATION IN URINE ELIMINATION related to URINARY RETENTION

Defining Characteristics: Increased smooth muscle tone in urinary tract and spasm may occur. Bladder tone is increased, which may cause urgency. Vesical sphincter tone may be increased, leading to difficulty urinating. Increased risk of urinary retention in patients with prostatic hypertrophy or urethral stricture.

Nursing Implications: Assess baseline urinary elimination pattern. Teach patient to increase fluids to 3 L/day, and encourage voiding every 2–3 hours. Instruct patient to report problems with urination.

VII. KNOWLEDGE DEFICIT related to DRUG ADMINISTRATION, POTENTIAL FOR TOLERANCE, AND DEPENDENCY

Defining Characteristics: Psychological dependence (addiction) occurs rarely in patients taking opioid agonists for cancer pain (< 1%). Physical dependence (precipitation of withdrawal symptoms) occurs with chronic use of the drug for the relief of chronic cancer pain. In addition, tolerance, or less analgesic effect over time with the same drug dose, occurs and requires increased dosage of drug.

Nursing Implications: Assess baseline knowledge of opioid analgesics and attitude about their use for cancer pain management. Teach patient about proper self-administration, possible side effects, and self-care measures. Suggest patient maintain diary of pain intensity, precipitating and alleviating factors, drug dose and time taken, and relief. Teach patient to self-administer opioid agonists for relief of chronic cancer pain around-the-clock, not PRN, to prevent pain. Explain use of prescribed short-acting opioid for rescue or to manage BTP. Discuss with physician dose increase or change in frequency of administration if tolerance develops. Teach patient that withdrawal symptoms may occur if chronic, around-the-clock dosing is interrupted. Withdrawal (abstinence) symptoms that may be seen are restlessness, lacrimation, rhinorrhea, yawning, perspiration, gooseflesh, restless sleep, mydriasis in first 24 hours. These are followed by twitching and leg spasm; severe aching of the back, abdomen, and legs; cramping in abdomen and legs; hot/cold flashes; insomnia; nausea/vomiting, diarrhea; severe sneezing; and increased heart rate, BP, T, which peak at 36–72 hours. Withdrawal syndrome can be prevented by administration of at least 1/4 of previous opioid dose.

VIII. SEXUAL DYSFUNCTION related to IMPOTENCE, ↓ LIBIDO

Defining Characteristics: Opiate agonists may suppress gonadotropin, causing impotence and decreased libido.

Nursing Implications: Assess baseline sexual pattern. Discuss potential toxicity and impact on sexuality. Provide information, emotional support, and referral as needed.

Drug: hydromorphone extended release capsules (Palladone)

Class: Opioid analgesic (opioid agonist, extended release).

Mechanism of Action: Resembles morphine but has milder action; binds to opiate receptors in CNS (limbic system, thalamus, striatum, hypothalamus, midbrain, spinal cord), altering pain perception at level of spinal cord and higher centers as well as the emotional response to pain. Also suppresses cough reflex.

Metabolism: Well absorbed after oral administration, with biphasic absorption: initial, rapid peak with second, braoder peak characterized by therapeutic serum concentration maintained over 24 hours. Two- to three-fold reduction in serum concentration fluctuations compared to immediate release hydromorphone. Terminal half-life of 18 hours, and steady state plasma concentration reached in 2–3 days so dose titration should be every 2–3 days. Metabolized by liver and excreted in urine.

Dosage/Range:

- For use in patients who have received opiates before and who are opioid tolerant; DO NOT USE in patients for whom this is the first opioid product prescribed, or in patients who require opioid analgesia for a short period of time.
- Available in 12, 16, 24, and 32 mg dosage strengths.
- To determine dosage,
  - Use standard equianalgesic dosing table, or conversion table below, to determine equivalent total daily dose of oral hydromorphone in a 24-hour period—these tables provide a ''reasonable starting point'' but have not been verified in well-controlled, multiple-dose trials.
  - Adjust dose as needed based on patient variables.
  - Round off dose to nearest capsule strength.
  - Discontinue all other around-the-clock opioid analgesics when extended release hydromorphone is initiated.
  - Titrate dose based on patient response, recognizing the steady state serum levels require 2–3 days until it is possible to assess full drug effect.
- Dose conversion from other opioids to hydromorphone from manufacturer Purdue Pharma; multiplication factors for converting the daily dose of prior opioids to the daily dose of oral hydromorphone* (mg/day prior opioid X factor = mg/day oral hydromorphone):

Prior Opioid	ORAL	PARENTERAL
Codeine	0.04	—
Hydrocodone	0.22	–
Hydromorphone	1.00	5.00
Levorphanol	1.88	3.75
Meperidine	0.02	0.10
Methadone	0.38	0.75
Morphine	0.12	0.75
Oxycodone	0.25	–

***To be used only for conversion TO oral hydromorphone. For patients receiving high-dose parenteral opioids, a more conservative conversion is warranted. For example, for high dose parenteral morphine, use 0.38 instead of 0.75 as a multiplication factor, i.e., halve the multiplication factor** (http://www.fda.gov/cder/foi/label/2004/021044lbl.pdf, accessed July 5, 2005.)

Drug Preparation:

- Store capsules at 25°C (77°F), with excursions permitted from 15–30°C (59–86°F). Teach patient to store in a safe place away from children and pets.

Drug Administration:

- Oral; DO NOT crush, open, dissolve or break the capsules–must be swallowed whole as otherwise a potentially lethal rapid release and absorption of hydromorphone will occur.

Drug Interactions:

- Alcohol, CNS depressants: Additive effects.

Lab Effects/Interference:

- None known.

Special Considerations:

- Parenteral dose is 1/5 oral dose for equianalgesic effect.
- Indicated for relief of persistent moderate-to-severe pain in patients requiring continuous, around-the-clock analgesia with a high potency opioid for an extended period of time.
    - Patients MUST be opioid tolerant, and pain must require at least an equivalent opioid dose of 12 mg of hydromorphone a day (24-hour period).
    - For example, the patient must be taking at least 60 mg of oral morphine/day or at least 30 mg of oxycodone/day or at least 8 mg of hydromorphone/day or an equianalgesic dose of another opioid, *for a week or longer.*
- Additive benefit when combined with acetaminophen or aspirin.
- Give smallest effective dose to prevent development of physical dependency. *Adequate dose* is defined as providing effective pain control so the patient requires *2 or less break-through opioid immediate release doses per 24-hour period.*
- Reduce dose in debilitated patients or patients receiving other CNS depressants.
- Use with caution in patients with hepatic or renal dysfunction, hypotension, severe CNS depression, respiratory depression or pulmonary diseases such as Chronic Obstructive Pulmonary Disease, head injury, elevated ICP.
- Contraindicated in patients: requiring opioids on an as needed basis (e.g., PRN); in situations of significant respiratory depression (especially in unmonitored settings); acute or severe bronchial asthma; who have or are suspected of having paralytic ileus; who have known hypersensitivity to hydromorphone or any of the ingredients.

- If required, naloxone HCl will reverse opiate toxicity (e.g., respiratory depression). However, it is important that acute withdrawal symptoms be prevented by giving only enough naloxone to reverse respiratory depression and that this be continued for opioid drug half-life of 18 hours.

Potential Toxicities/Side Effects and the Nursing Process

I. SENSORY/PERCEPTUAL ALTERATIONS related to CNS DEPRESSION

Defining Characteristics: Drowsiness, sedation, mood changes, euphoria, dysphoria, dizziness, mental clouding may occur. At high doses, may cause seizures. Miosis (papillary constriction) may occur.

Nursing Implications: Assess baseline neurologic status. Use cautiously, if at all, in patients with head injury, increased ICP, severe CNS depression, acute alcoholism, the elderly, and the debilitated. Assess other concurrent medications. Use with caution in patients receiving other opioids, tranquilizers, hypnotics, MAO inhibitors, since increasing CNS depressant effects can occur. Monitor neurologic status closely. Teach patient to avoid driving and operating machinery while taking the medicine, and to AVOID concurrent alcohol.

II. ALTERATION IN OXYGENATION related to RESPIRATORY DEPRESSION

Defining Characteristics: Opiate agonists directly depress respiratory center in brain stem, causing decreased sensitivity and responsiveness to increased pCO_2. Also may depress deep breathing and reflex to sigh. Tolerance to respiratory depressant effects occurs with chronic use.

Nursing Implications: Assess baseline pulmonary status, and monitor periodically during drug use. Use cautiously in patients with bronchial asthma, COPD, respiratory depression, and monitor closely.

III. ALTERATION IN ELIMINATION related to CONSTIPATION, ILEUS

Defining Characteristics: Opium agonists bind to opiate receptors in bowel, slowing peristalsis, leading to constipation. Untreated constipation may result in bowel perforation.

Nursing Implications: Assess baseline elimination, fluid intake, diet, and exercise patterns. Instruct patient about prevention of constipation: goal is to move bowels at least every two days by increasing fluids to 3 L/day, following a diet high in fiber (beans, vegetables, fruit), and taking moderate exercise. Assess need for bowel softeners, bulk-forming laxatives, and osmotic cathartics, and discuss prescription with physician. Teach patient self-administration of medications.

IV. ALTERATION IN NUTRITION related to GI TOXICITY

Defining Characteristics: Nausea, vomiting, and dry mouth may occur. Gastric, biliary, and pancreatic secretions are decreased by opiate agonists; digestion is delayed. Biliary tract muscle tone is increased, and spasm of Oddi's sphincter may occur

Nursing Implications: Assess patient tolerance of GI side effects. Teach patient to report side effects. If nausea/vomiting occur, change to another opioid, or premedicate with antiemetic to prevent nausea/vomiting. Assess GI pain, biliary spasm, and consider alternative opioid.

V. ALTERATION IN CARDIAC OUTPUT related to HYPOTENSION, BRADYCARDIA

Defining Characteristics: Orthostatic hypotension, bradycardia due to cholinergic effect, and peripheral vasodilation may occur. There may be histamine-related flushing, pruritus, diaphoresis with chronic drug usage; tolerance develops to this effect.

Nursing Implications: Assess baseline cardiovascular status. Teach patient to change position slowly and to hold onto stable, nearby structure for support as needed. Caution patient to remain in supine position for 15–20 minutes after dose if dizziness occurs. Monitor status closely if patient has other factors contributing to hypotension.

VI. ALTERATION IN URINE ELIMINATION related to URINARY RETENTION

Defining Characteristics: Increased smooth muscle tone in urinary tract and spasm may occur. Bladder tone is increased, which may cause urgency. Vesical sphincter tone may be increased, leading to difficulty urinating. Increased risk of urinary retention in patients with prostatic hypertrophy or urethral stricture.

Nursing Implications: Assess baseline urinary elimination pattern. Teach patient to increase fluids to 3 L/day, and encourage voiding every 2–3 hours. Instruct patient to report problems with urination.

VII. KNOWLEDGE DEFICIT related to DRUG ADMINISTRATION, POTENTIAL FOR TOLERANCE, AND DEPENDENCY

Defining Characteristics: Psychological dependence (addiction) occurs rarely in patients taking opioid agonists for cancer pain (< 1%). Physical dependence (precipitation of withdrawal symptoms) occurs with chronic use of the drug for the relief of chronic cancer pain. In addition, tolerance, or less analgesic effect over time with the same drug dose, occurs and requires increased dosage of drug.

Nursing Implications: Assess baseline knowledge of opioid analgesics and attitude about their use for cancer pain management. Teach patient about proper self-administration, possible side effects, and self-care measures. Suggest patient maintain diary of pain intensity, precipitating and alleviating factors, drug dose and time taken, and relief. Teach patient to self-administer opioid agonists for relief of chronic cancer pain around-the-clock, not PRN, to prevent pain. Explain use of prescribed short-acting opioid for rescue or to manage BTP. Discuss with physician dose increase or change in frequency of administration if tolerance develops. Teach patient that withdrawal symptoms may occur if chronic, around-the-clock dosing is interrupted. Withdrawal (abstinence) symptoms that may be seen are restlessness, lacrimation, rhinorrhea, yawning, perspiration, gooseflesh, restless sleep, mydriasis in first 24 hours. These are followed by twitching and leg spasm; severe aching of the back, abdomen, and legs; cramping in abdomen and legs; hot/cold flashes; insomnia; nausea/vomiting, diarrhea; severe sneezing; and increased heart rate, BP, T, which peak at 36–72 hours. Withdrawal syndrome can be prevented by administration of at least 1/4 of previous opioid dose.

VIII. SEXUAL DYSFUNCTION related to IMPOTENCE, ↓ LIBIDO

Defining Characteristics: Opiate agonists may suppress gonadotropin, causing impotence and decreased libido.

Nursing Implications: Assess baseline sexual pattern. Discuss potential toxicity and impact on sexuality. Provide information, emotional support, and referral as needed.

Drug: levorphanol tartrate opioid (Levo-Dromoran)

Class: Opioid analgesic (opioid agonist).

Mechanism of Action: A synthetic opioid agonist, levorphanol resembles morphine but has milder action; binds to opiate receptors in CNS (limbic system, thalamus, striatum, hypothalamus, midbrain, spinal cord), altering pain perception at level of spinal cord and higher centers, as well as the emotional response to pain. Also suppresses cough reflex.

Metabolism: Well absorbed after oral (peak analgesia 60–90 minutes) or SQ (peak analgesia 20 minutes) administration. Metabolized by liver and excreted in urine.

Dosage/Range:

For moderate to severe pain:

- PO: 2–3 mg PO q6–8h.
- SQ: 2–3 mg SQ q6–8h.

Drug Preparation:

- Store tablets in tight, light-resistant containers at 15–30°C (59–86°F).
- Injectable preparation should be stored at 15–40°C (59–104°F).
- At home, teach patient to store oral doses in a safe place away from children and pets.

Drug Administration:

- PO, SQ, IV.

Drug Interactions:

- Injection incompatible with solutions containing aminophylline, ammonium chloride, amobarbital sodium, chlorothiazide sodium, heparin sodium, methicillin sodium, nitrofurantoin, phenobarbital sodium, sodium bicarbonate.
- Alcohol, CNS depressants: additive effects.

Lab Effects/Interference:

- None known.

Special Considerations:

- Oral dose is twice parenteral dose.
- Produces less nausea, vomiting, constipation than morphine, but more sedation and smooth muscle stimulation.
- Additive benefit when combined with acetaminophen or aspirin.
- Give smallest effective dose to prevent development of tolerance, physical dependency.
- Reduce dose in debilitated patients, or patients receiving other CNS depressants.
- Use with caution in patients with hepatic or renal dysfunction, hypothyroidism, Addison's disease, severe CNS depression, respiratory depression, head injury, elevated ICP.
- If required, naloxone HCl will reverse opiate toxicity (e.g., respiratory depression). However, it is important that acute withdrawal symptoms be prevented by giving only enough naloxone to reverse respiratory depression and that this be continued for opioid drug half-life.

Potential Toxicities/Side Effects and the Nursing Process

I. SENSORY/PERCEPTUAL ALTERATIONS related to CNS DEPRESSION

Defining Characteristics: Drowsiness, sedation, mood changes, euphoria, dysphoria, dizziness, mental clouding may occur. At high doses, may cause seizures. Miosis (papillary constriction) may occur.

Nursing Implications: Assess baseline neurologic status. Use cautiously, if at all, in patients who are elderly, debilitated, have a head injury, increased ICP, severe CNS depression, acute alcoholism. Assess other concurrent medications. Use with caution in patients receiving other opioids, tranquilizers, hypnotics, MAO inhibitors, since increasing CNS depressant effects can occur. Monitor neurologic status closely. Instruct patient to avoid driving and operating machinery while taking the medicine, and to AVOID concurrent alcohol.

II. ALTERATION IN OXYGENATION related to RESPIRATORY DEPRESSION

Defining Characteristics: Opiate agonists directly depress respiratory center in brain stem, causing decreased sensitivity and responsiveness to increased pCO_2. Also may depress deep breathing and reflex to sigh. Tolerance to respiratory depressant effects occurs with chronic use.

Nursing Implications: Assess baseline pulmonary status, and monitor periodically during drug use. Use cautiously in patients with bronchial asthma, COPD, respiratory depression, and monitor closely.

III. ALTERATION IN ELIMINATION related to CONSTIPATION, ILEUS

Defining Characteristics: Opium agonists bind to opiate receptors in bowel, slowing peristalsis, leading to constipation. Untreated constipation may result in bowel perforation.

Nursing Implications: Assess baseline elimination, fluid intake, diet, and exercise patterns. Instruct patient regarding prevention of constipation: goal is to move bowels at least every two days by increasing fluids to 3 L/day, following a diet high in fiber (beans, vegetables, fruit), and taking moderate exercise. Assess need for bowel softeners, bulk-forming laxatives, and osmotic cathartics, and discuss prescription with physician. Teach patient self-administration of medications.

IV. ALTERATION IN NUTRITION, LESS THAN BODY REQUIREMENTS, related to GI TOXICITY

Defining Characteristics: Nausea, vomiting, dry mouth may occur. Gastric, biliary, and pancreatic secretions are decreased by opiate agonists; digestion is delayed. Biliary tract muscle tone is increased, and spasm of Oddi's sphincter may occur (morphine > meperidine > codeine).

Nursing Implications: Assess patient tolerance of GI side effects. Teach patient to report side effects. If nausea/vomiting occur, change to another opioid, or premedicate with antiemetic to prevent nausea/vomiting. Assess GI pain, biliary spasm, and consider alternative opioid.

V. ALTERATION IN CARDIAC OUTPUT related to HYPOTENSION, BRADYCARDIA

Defining Characteristics: Orthostatic hypotension, bradycardia due to cholinergic effect, and peripheral vasodilation may occur with rapid IV dosing. There may be histamine-related flushing, pruritus, and diaphoresis with chronic drug usage; tolerance develops to this effect.

Nursing Implications: Assess baseline cardiovascular status. Teach patient to change position slowly and to hold onto stable, nearby structure for support as needed. Be careful when giving IV push opioids, and caution patient to remain in supine position for 15–20 minutes after injection. Monitor cardiovascular status after injection.

VI. ALTERATION IN URINE ELIMINATION related to URINARY RETENTION

Defining Characteristics: Increased smooth muscle tone in urinary tract and spasm may occur. Bladder tone is increased, which may cause urgency. Vesical sphincter tone may be increased, leading to difficulty urinating. Increased risk of urinary retention in patients with prostatic hypertrophy or urethral stricture.

Nursing Implications: Assess baseline urinary elimination pattern. Teach patient to increase fluids to 3 L/day, and encourage voiding every 2–3 hours. Instruct patient to report problems with urination.

VII. KNOWLEDGE DEFICIT related to DRUG ADMINISTRATION, POTENTIAL FOR TOLERANCE, AND DEPENDENCY

Defining Characteristics: Psychological dependence (addiction) occurs rarely in patients taking opioid agonists for cancer pain (< 1%). Physical dependence (precipitation of withdrawal symptoms) occurs with chronic use of the drug for the relief of chronic cancer pain. In addition, tolerance, or less analgesic effect over time with the same drug dose, occurs and requires increased dosage of drug.

Nursing Implications: Assess baseline knowledge of opioid analgesics, and attitude about their use for cancer pain management. Teach patient about proper self-administration, possible side effects, and self-care measures. Suggest patient maintain diary of pain intensity, precipitating and alleviating factors, drug dose and time taken, and relief. Teach patient to self-administer opioid agonists for relief of chronic cancer pain around-the-clock, not PRN, to prevent pain. Explain use of prescribed short-acting opioid for rescue or to manage BTP. Discuss with physician dose increase or change in frequency of administration if tolerance develops. Teach patient that withdrawal symptoms may occur if chronic, around-the-clock dosing is interrupted. Withdrawal (abstinence) symptoms that may be seen are restlessness, lacrimation, rhinorrhea, yawning, perspiration, gooseflesh, restless sleep, mydriasis in first 24 hours. These are followed by twitching and leg spasm; severe aching of the back, abdomen, and legs; cramping in abdomen and legs; hot/cold flashes; insomnia; nausea/vomiting, diarrhea; severe sneezing; and increased heart rate, BP, and T, which peak at 36–72 hours. Withdrawal syndrome can be prevented by administration of at least 1/4 of previous opioid dose.

VIII. SEXUAL DYSFUNCTION related to IMPOTENCE, ↓ LIBIDO

Defining Characteristics: Opiate agonists may suppress gonadotropin, causing impotence and decreased libido.

Nursing Implications: Assess baseline sexual pattern. Discuss potential toxicity and impact on sexuality. Provide information, emotional support, and referral as needed.

Drug: meperidine hydrochloride (Demerol, Mepergan Fortis)

Class: Opioid analgesic (opioid agonist).

Mechanism of Action: A synthetic opioid agonist, meperidine resembles morphine but has milder action; binds to opiate receptors in CNS (limbic system, thalamus, striatum, hypothalamus, midbrain, spinal cord), altering pain perception at level of spinal cord and higher centers, as well as the emotional response to pain. Also suppresses cough reflex.

Metabolism: After oral administration, metabolized by liver (first pass) with 50–60% reaching systemic circulation; thus oral administration is < 50% as effective as IM dose. After IM dose, 80–85% of drug is absorbed. Peak analgesia is ~ 1 hour after oral administration, 40–60 minutes after SQ, and 30–50 minutes after IM. Duration is 2–4 hours. Drug is 60–80% bound to plasma proteins. Metabolism is by the liver, into metabolites such as normeperidine, and excreted in the urine. Normeperidine has a longer half-life and accumulates in patients with decreased renal function. It is a potent CNS stimulant, producing seizures, agitation, irritability, nervousness, tremors, twitches, and myoclonus.

Dosage/Range:

For moderate to severe pain:

- PO: 50–150 mg q3–4h.
- IM: 50–150 mg q3–4h.
- SQ: 50–150 mg q3–4h.
- IV: 15–35 mg/hr by continuous IV infusion.

Drug Preparation:

- Store tablets in tight, light-resistant containers at 15–30°C (59–86°F).
- Injectable preparation should be stored at 15–40°C (59–104°F).

Drug Administration:

- PO, IM, SQ, IV.
- At home, teach patient to store oral doses in a safe place away from children and pets.

Drug Interactions:

- May increase isoniazid side effects; use concurrently with caution.
- Enhanced toxicity with MAO inhibitors (coma, severe respiratory depression, hypotension), so drug is contraindicated for patients who have received MAO inhibitors in previous 14 days.
- Injection incompatible with solutions containing aminophylline, barbiturates, ephedrine sulfate, heparin sodium, hydrocortisone sodium succinate, methicillin sodium, methylprednisolone sodium succinate, morphine sulfate, tetracycline.
- Alcohol, CNS depressants: additive effects.

Lab Effects/Interference:

- None known.

Special Considerations:

- Drug has many side effects, unfavorable oral to parenteral ratio, so is not recommended in the treatment of cancer-related pain. Drug is NOT used to treat or prevent chronic cancer pain because of short duration of action, bioavailability, and severe risk of neurotoxicity related to metabollte normeperidine.
- Oral meperidine, 50 mg, is equivalent in analgesia (equianalgesic) to acetaminophen 650 mg or aspirin 650 mg.
- Sedative and euphoric effect greater than morphine (equianalgesic dose).
- Oral dose is three times parenteral dose for equianalgesic effect.
- Use with caution in patients with atrial flutter or other supraventricular tachycardias (drug can increase ventricular response rate via vagolytic action).
- Formulation may contain sodium metabisulfite, which may cause anaphylactic or other allergic reactions.
- Additive benefit when combined with acetaminophen or aspirin.

- Give smallest effective dose to prevent development of tolerance, physical dependency.
- Reduce dose in debilitated patients or patients receiving other CNS depressants.
- Use with caution in patients with hepatic or renal dysfunction, hypothyroidism, Addison's disease, severe CNS depression, respiratory depression, head injury, elevated ICP.
- If required, naloxone HCl will reverse opiate toxicity (e.g., respiratory depression). However, it is important that acute withdrawal symptoms be prevented by giving only enough naloxone to reverse respiratory depression and that this be continued for opioid drug half-life.

Potential Toxicities/Side Effects and the Nursing Process

I. SENSORY/PERCEPTUAL ALTERATIONS related to CNS DEPRESSION

Defining Characteristics: Drowsiness, sedation, mood changes, euphoria, dysphoria, dizziness, mental clouding may occur. At high doses, may cause seizures. Miosis (papillary constriction) may occur.

Nursing Implications: Assess baseline neurologic status. Use cautiously, if at all, in the elderly, the debilitated, and patients with head injury, increased ICP, severe CNS depression, acute alcoholism. Assess other concurrent medications. Use with caution in patients receiving other opioids, tranquilizers, hypnotics, MAO inhibitors, since increasing CNS depressant effects can occur. Monitor neurologic status closely. Instruct patient to avoid driving and operating machinery while taking the medicine, and to AVOID concurrent alcohol.

II. ALTERATION IN OXYGENATION related to RESPIRATORY DEPRESSION

Defining Characteristics: Opiate agonists directly depress respiratory center in brain stem, causing decreased sensitivity and responsiveness to increased pCO_2. Also may depress deep breathing and reflex to sigh. Tolerance to respiratory depressant effects occurs with chronic use.

Nursing Implications: Assess baseline pulmonary status, and periodically during drug use. Use cautiously in patients with bronchial asthma, COPD, respiratory depression, and monitor closely.

III. ALTERATION IN ELIMINATION related to CONSTIPATION, ILEUS

Defining Characteristics: Opium agonists bind to opiate receptors in bowel, slowing peristalsis, leading to constipation. Untreated constipation may result in bowel perforation.

Nursing Implications: Assess baseline elimination, fluid intake, diet, and exercise patterns. Instruct patient regarding prevention of constipation: goal is to move bowels at least every two days by increasing fluids to 3 L/day, following a diet high in fiber (beans, vegetables, fruit), and taking moderate exercise. Assess need for bowel softeners, bulk-forming laxatives, and osmotic cathartics, and discuss prescription with physician. Teach patient self-administration of medications.

IV. ALTERATION IN NUTRITION related to GI TOXICITY

Defining Characteristics: Nausea, vomiting, and dry mouth may occur. Gastric, biliary, and pancreatic secretions are decreased by opiate agonists; digestion is delayed. Biliary tract muscle tone is increased, and spasm of Oddi's sphincter may occur (morphine > meperidine > codeine).

Nursing Implications: Assess patient tolerance of GI side effects. Teach patient to report side effects. If nausea/vomiting occur, change to another opioid, or premedicate with antiemetic to prevent nausea/vomiting. Assess GI pain, biliary spasm, and consider alternative opioid.

V. ALTERATION IN CARDIAC OUTPUT related to HYPOTENSION, BRADYCARDIA

Defining Characteristics: Orthostatic hypotension, bradycardia due to cholinergic effect, and peripheral vasodilation may occur with rapid IV dosing. There may be histamine-related flushing, pruritus, diaphoresis with chronic drug usage; tolerance develops to this effect.

Nursing Implications: Assess baseline cardiovascular status. Teach patient to change position slowly and to hold onto stable, nearby structure for support as needed. Be careful when giving IV push opioids, and caution patient to remain in supine position for 15–20 minutes after injection. Monitor cardiovascular status after injection.

VI. ALTERATION IN URINE ELIMINATION related to URINARY RETENTION

Defining Characteristics: Increased smooth muscle tone in urinary tract and spasm may occur. Bladder tone is increased, which may cause urgency. Vesical sphincter tone may be increased, leading to difficulty urinating. Increased risk of urinary retention in patients with prostatic hypertrophy or urethral stricture.

Nursing Implications: Assess baseline urinary elimination pattern. Teach patient to increase fluids to 3 L/day, and encourage voiding every 2–3 hours. Instruct patient to report problems with urination.

VII. KNOWLEDGE DEFICIT related to DRUG ADMINISTRATION, POTENTIAL FOR TOLERANCE, AND DEPENDENCY

Defining Characteristics: Psychological dependence (addiction) occurs rarely in patients taking opioid agonists for cancer pain (< 1%). Physical dependence (precipitation of withdrawal symptoms) occurs with chronic use of the drug for the relief of chronic cancer pain. In addition, tolerance, or less analgesic effect over time with the same drug dose, occurs and requires increased dosage of drug.

Nursing Implications: Assess baseline knowledge of opioid analgesics and attitude about their use for cancer pain management. Teach patient about proper self-administration, possible side effects, and self-care measures. Suggest patient maintain diary of pain intensity, precipitating and alleviating factors, drug dose and time taken, and relief. Teach patient to self-administer opioid agonists for relief of chronic cancer pain around-the-clock, not PRN, to prevent pain. Explain use of prescribed short-acting opioid for rescue or to manage breakthrough pain. Discuss with physician dose increase or change in frequency of administration if tolerance develops. Teach patient that withdrawal symptoms may occur if chronic, around-the-clock dosing is interrupted. Withdrawal (abstinence) symptoms that may be seen are restlessness, lacrimation, rhinorrhea, yawning, perspiration, gooseflesh, restless sleep, mydriasis in first 24 hours. These are followed by twitching and leg spasm; severe aching of the back, abdomen, and legs; cramping in abdomen and legs; hot/cold flashes; insomnia; nausea/vomiting, diarrhea; severe sneezing; and increased heart rate, BP, T, which peak at 36–72 hours. Withdrawal syndrome can be prevented by administration of at least 1/4 of previous opioid dose.

VIII. SEXUAL DYSFUNCTION related to IMPOTENCE, ↓ LIBIDO

Defining Characteristics: Opiate agonists may suppress gonadotropin, causing impotence and decreased libido.

Nursing Implications: Assess baseline sexual pattern. Discuss potential toxicity and impact on sexuality. Provide information, emotional support, and referral as needed.

Drug: methadone (Dolophine, Methadose)

Class: Opioid analgesic (opioid agonist).

Mechanism of Action: A synthetic opioid agonist, methadone resembles morphine but has milder action; binds to opiate receptors in CNS (limbic system, thalamus, striatum, hypothalamus, midbrain, spinal cord), altering pain perception at level of spinal cord and higher centers, as well as the emotional response to pain. Also suppresses cough reflex.

Metabolism: Well absorbed from GI tract; onset and duration of single dose similar to morphine. With chronic administration (physical dependency) half-life is 22–48 hours. Highly tissue-bound; metabolized by liver, excreted by renal filtration, then is reabsorbed (pH dependent).

Dosage/Range:

For moderate to severe pain:

- PO: 5–20 mg q6–8h, or more for severe cancer pain.
- SQ, IM: 2.5–10 mg q3–4h.

Drug Preparation:

- Store tablets in tight, light-resistant containers at 15–30°C (59–86°F).
- Injection should be protected from light and stored at 15–40°C (59–104°F).
- At home, teach patient to store oral doses in a safe place away from children and pets.

Drug Administration:

- PO, IM, SQ.

Drug Interactions:

- Injection incompatible with solutions containing aminophylline, ammonium chloride, amobarbital sodium, chlorothiazide sodium, heparin sodium, methicillin sodium, nitrofurantoin, phenobarbital sodium, sodium bicarbonate.
- Alcohol, CNS depressants: additive effects.

Lab Effects/Interference:

- None known.

Special Considerations:

- Oral dose is twice parenteral dose (equianalgesic effect).
- May produce similar or slightly greater respiratory depression than equivalent doses of morphine.
- Additive benefit when combined with acetaminophen or aspirin.
- Give smallest effective dose to prevent development of tolerance, physical dependency.
- Reduce dose in debilitated patients or patients receiving other CNS depressants.
- Use with caution in patients with hepatic or renal dysfunction, hypothyroidism, Addison's disease, severe CNS depression, respiratory depression, head injury, elevated ICP.
- If required, naloxone HCl will reverse opiate toxicity (e.g., respiratory depression). However, it is important that acute withdrawal symptoms be pre-

vented by giving only enough naloxone to reverse respiratory depression and that this be continued for opioid drug half-life.

Potential Toxicities/Side Effects and the Nursing Process

I. SENSORY/PERCEPTUAL ALTERATIONS related to CNS DEPRESSION

Defining Characteristics: Drowsiness, sedation, mood changes, euphoria, dysphoria, dizziness, mental clouding may occur. At high doses, may cause seizures. Miosis (papillary constriction) may occur.

Nursing Implications: Assess baseline neurologic status. Use cautiously, if at all, in the elderly, the debilitated, and patients with head injury, increased ICP, severe CNS depression, acute alcoholism. Assess other concurrent medications. Use with caution in patients receiving other opioids, tranquilizers, hypnotics, MAO inhibitors, since increasing CNS depressant effects can occur. Monitor neurologic status closely. Instruct patient to avoid driving and operating machinery while taking the medicine, and to AVOID concurrent alcohol.

II. ALTERATION IN OXYGENATION related to RESPIRATORY DEPRESSION

Defining Characteristics: Opiate agonists directly depress respiratory center in brain stem, causing decreased sensitivity and responsiveness to increased pCO2. Also may depress deep breathing and reflex to sigh. Tolerance to respiratory depressant effects occurs with chronic use.

Nursing Implications: Assess baseline pulmonary status, and periodically during drug use. Use cautiously in patients with bronchial asthma, COPD, respiratory depression, and monitor closely.

III. ALTERATION IN ELIMINATION related to CONSTIPATION, ILEUS

Defining Characteristics: Opium agonists bind to opiate receptors in bowel, slowing peristalsis, leading to constipation. Untreated constipation may result in bowel perforation.

Nursing Implications: Assess baseline elimination, fluid intake, diet, and exercise patterns. Instruct patient regarding prevention of constipation: goal is to move bowels at least every two days by increasing fluids to 3 L/day, following a diet high in fiber (beans, vegetables, fruit), and taking moderate exercise. Assess need for bowel softeners, bulk-forming laxatives, and osmotic cathartics, and discuss prescription with physician. Teach patient self-administration of medications.

IV. ALTERATION IN NUTRITION, LESS THAN BODY REQUIREMENTS, related to GI TOXICITY

Defining Characteristics: Nausea, vomiting, and dry mouth may occur. Gastric, biliary, and pancreatic secretions are decreased by opiate agonists; digestion is delayed. Biliary tract muscle tone is increased, and spasm of Oddi's sphincter may occur (morphine > meperidine > codeine).

Nursing Implications: Assess patient tolerance of GI side effects. Instruct patient to report side effects. If nausea/vomiting occur, change to another opioid, or premedicate with antiemetic to prevent nausea/vomiting. Assess GI pain, biliary spasm, and consider alternative opioid.

V. ALTERATION IN CARDIAC OUTPUT related to HYPOTENSION, BRADYCARDIA

Defining Characteristics: Orthostatic hypotension, bradycardia due to cholinergic effect, and peripheral vasodilation may occur with rapid IV dosing. There may be histamine-related flushing, pruritus, diaphoresis with chronic drug usage; tolerance develops to this effect.

Nursing Implications: Assess baseline cardiovascular status. Teach patient to change position slowly and to hold onto stable, nearby structure for support as needed. Be careful when giving IV push opioids, and caution patient to remain in supine position for 15–20 minutes after injection. Monitor cardiovascular status after injection.

VI. ALTERATION IN URINE ELIMINATION related to URINARY RETENTION

Defining Characteristics: Increased smooth muscle tone in urinary tract and spasm may occur. Bladder tone is increased, which may cause urgency. Vesical sphincter tone may be increased leading to difficulty urinating. Increased risk of urinary retention in patients with prostatic hypertrophy or urethral stricture.

Nursing Implications: Assess baseline urinary elimination pattern. Teach patient to increase fluids to 3 L/day, and encourage voiding every 2–3 hours. Instruct patient to report problems with urination.

VII. KNOWLEDGE DEFICIT related to DRUG ADMINISTRATION, POTENTIAL FOR TOLERANCE, AND DEPENDENCY

Defining Characteristics: Psychological dependence (addiction) occurs rarely in patients taking opioid agonists for cancer pain (< 1%). Physical dependence (precipitation of withdrawal symptoms) occurs with chronic use of the drug for the relief of chronic cancer pain. In addition, tolerance, or less analgesic effect over time with the same drug dose, occurs and requires increased dosage of drug.

Nursing Implications: Assess baseline knowledge of opioid analgesics, and attitude about their use for cancer pain management. Teach patient about proper self-administration, possible side effects, and self-care measures. Suggest patient maintain diary of pain intensity, precipitating and alleviating factors, drug dose and time taken, and relief. Teach patient to self-administer opioid agonists for relief of chronic cancer pain around-the-clock, not PRN, to prevent pain. Explain use of prescribed short-acting opioid for rescue or to manage BTP. Discuss with physician dose increase or change in frequency of administration if tolerance develops. Teach patient that withdrawal symptoms may occur if chronic, around the-clock dosing is interrupted. Withdrawal (abstinence) symptoms that may be seen are restlessness, lacrimation, rhinorrhea, yawning, perspiration, gooseflesh, restless sleep, mydriasis in first 24 hours. These are followed by twitching and leg spasm; severe aching of the back, abdomen, and legs; cramping in abdomen and legs; hot/cold flashes; insomnia; nausea/vomiting, diarrhea; severe sneezing; and increased heart rate, BP, T, which peak at 36–72 hours. Withdrawal syndrome can be prevented by administration of at least 1/4 of previous opioid dose.

VIII. SEXUAL DYSFUNCTION related to IMPOTENCE, ↓ LIBIDO

Defining Characteristics: Opiate agonists may suppress gonadotropin, causing impotence and decreased libido.

Nursing Implications: Assess baseline sexual pattern. Discuss potential toxicity and impact on sexuality. Provide information, emotional support, and referral as needed.

Drug: morphine (Astramorph, Avinza, Duramorph, Infumorph, Kadian Morphine Sulfate Sustained Release, MS Contin, MSIR, Morphelan, Oramorph, Roxanol)

Class: Opioid analgesic (opioid agonist).

Mechanism of Action: Binds to opiate receptors in CNS (limbic system, thalamus, striatum, hypothalamus, midbrain, spinal cord). This opioid agonist alters pain perception at level of spinal cord and higher centers, as well as the emotional response to pain. Also suppresses cough reflex.

Metabolism: Variable absorption from GI tract; increased absorption when taken with food. Peak analgesia 60 minutes (oral), 20–60 minutes (rectal), 50–90 minutes (SQ), 30–60 minutes (IM), 20 minutes (IV). Duration is 4–7 hours. Maximum respiratory depression is 30 minutes (IM), 7 minutes (IV), 90 minutes (SQ). Drug is slowly absorbed into systemic circulation after intrathecal (IT) administration. Peak CSF concentrations occur 60–90 minutes after epidural dose. Metabolized by liver and excreted in urine and, to a small degree, feces.

Dosage/Range:

For moderate to severe pain:

- Oral: 10–60 mg PO q3–4h titrated to pain; 10–240 mg sustained release q8–12h, titrated to pain.
- Rectal: 10–60 mg q4h.
- SQ, IM: 4–15 mg q3–4h.
- IV: 1–100 mg/h, and higher, titrated to need in physically dependent patients.
- Intrathecal: dose is 1/10 the epidural dose.
- Epidural: 5 mg q24h.
- At home, teach patient to store oral doses in a safe place away from children and pets.

Drug Preparation:

- Store tablets in tight, light-resistant containers at 15–30°C (59–86°F).
- Injection should be protected from light, and stored at 15–40°C (59–104°F).

Drug Administration:

- Begin morphine therapy using immediate-release oral preparations and increase dose to control pain; once optimal dose identified, convert to sustained-release formulation by dividing 24-hour total morphine dose by 2, giving two (q12h) doses.
- Intrathecal or epidural: use preservative-free morphine only, e.g., Astramorph PF, Duramorph PF, Infumorph; consult individual policies/procedures for administration.

Drug Interactions:

- Injection incompatible with solutions containing aminophylline, ammonium chloride, amobarbital sodium, chlorothiazide sodium, heparin sodium, methicillin sodium, nitrofurantoin, phenobarbital sodium, sodium bicarbonate.
- Alcohol, CNS depressants: additive effects.

Lab Effects/Interference:

- None known.

Special Considerations:

- Oral to parenteral dose is 3–6 to 1 (equianalgesic dose).
- Highly concentrated formulations are available and are for use in continuous infusion pumps.

- Do not crush sustained-release formulations (e.g., MS Contin, Oramorph).
- When epidural or intrathecal route is used, refer to institutional policy/procedure for administration and patient monitoring.
- Additive benefit when combined with acetaminophen or aspirin.
- Give smallest effective dose to prevent development of tolerance, physical dependency.
- Reduce dose in debilitated patients, or patients receiving other CNS depressants.
- Use with caution in patients with hepatic or renal dysfunction, hypothyroidism, Addison's disease, severe CNS depression, respiratory depression, head injury, elevated intracranial pressure.
- If required, naloxone HCl will reverse opiate toxicity (e.g., respiratory depression). However, it is important that acute withdrawal symptoms be prevented by giving only enough naloxone to reverse respiratory depression and that this be continued for opioid drug half-life.
- Kadian as well as Avinza are sustained-release morphine formulated for once-a-day dosing; available in 20-, 50-, and 100-mg tablets (Kadian) and 30-, 60-, 90-, and 120 mg capsules (Avinza).

Potential Toxicities/Side Effects and the Nursing Process

I. SENSORY/PERCEPTUAL ALTERATIONS related to CNS DEPRESSION

Defining Characteristics: Drowsiness, sedation, mood changes, euphoria, dysphoria, dizziness, mental clouding may occur. At high doses, may cause seizures. Miosis (papillary constriction) may occur.

Nursing Implications: Assess baseline neurologic status. Use cautiously, if at all, in the elderly, the debilitated, and patients with head injury, increased intracranial pressure, severe CNS depression, acute alcoholism. Assess other concurrent medications. Use with caution in patients receiving other opioids, tranquilizers, hypnotics, MAO inhibitors, since increasing CNS depressant effects can occur. Monitor neurologic status closely. Instruct patient to avoid driving and operating machinery while taking the medicine, and to AVOID concurrent alcohol.

II. ALTERATION IN OXYGENATION related to RESPIRATORY DEPRESSION

Defining Characteristics: Opiate agonists directly depress respiratory center in brain stem, causing decreased sensitivity and responsiveness to increased pCO2. Also may depress deep breathing and reflex to sigh. Tolerance to respiratory depressant effects occurs with chronic use.

Nursing Implications: Assess baseline pulmonary status, and periodically during drug use. Use cautiously in patients with bronchial asthma, COPD, respiratory depression, and monitor closely.

III. ALTERATION IN ELIMINATION related to CONSTIPATION, ILEUS

Defining Characteristics: Opium agonists bind to opiate receptors in bowel, slowing peristalsis, leading to constipation. Untreated constipation may result in bowel perforation.

Nursing Implications: Assess baseline elimination, fluid intake, diet, and exercise patterns. Instruct patient regarding prevention of constipation: goal is to move bowels at least every two days by increasing fluids to 3 L/day, following a diet high in fiber (beans, vegetables, fruit), and taking moderate exercise. Assess need for bowel softeners, bulk-forming laxatives, and osmotic cathartics, and discuss prescription with physician. Teach patient self-administration of medications.

IV. ALTERATION IN NUTRITION, LESS THAN BODY REQUIREMENTS, related to GI TOXICITY

Defining Characteristics: Nausea, vomiting, and dry mouth may occur. Gastric, biliary, and pancreatic secretions are decreased by opiate agonists; digestion is delayed. Biliary tract muscle tone is increased, and spasm of Oddi's sphincter may occur (morphine > meperidine > codeine).

Nursing Implications: Assess patient tolerance of GI side effects. Teach patient to report side effects. If nausea/vomiting occur, change to another opioid, or premedicate with antiemetic to prevent nausea/vomiting. Assess GI pain, biliary spasm, and consider alternative opioid.

V. ALTERATION IN CARDIAC OUTPUT related to HYPOTENSION, BRADYCARDIA

Defining Characteristics: Orthostatic hypotension, bradycardia due to cholinergic effect, and peripheral vasodilation may occur with rapid IV dosing. There may be histamine-related flushing, pruritus, diaphoresis with chronic drug usage; tolerance develops to this effect.

Nursing Implications: Assess baseline cardiovascular status. Teach patient to change position slowly and to hold onto stable, nearby structure for support as needed. Be careful when giving IV push opioids, and caution patient to remain in supine position for 15–20 minutes after injection. Monitor cardiovascular status after injection.

VI. ALTERATION IN URINE ELIMINATION related to URINARY RETENTION

Defining Characteristics: Increased smooth muscle tone in urinary tract and spasm may occur. Bladder tone is increased, which may cause urgency. Vesical sphincter tone may be increased, leading to difficulty urinating. Increased risk of urinary retention in patients with prostatic hypertrophy or urethral stricture.

Nursing Implications: Assess baseline urinary elimination pattern. Teach patient to increase fluids to 3 L/day, and encourage voiding every 2–3 hours. Instruct patient to report problems with urination.

VII. KNOWLEDGE DEFICIT related to DRUG ADMINISTRATION, POTENTIAL FOR TOLERANCE, AND DEPENDENCY

Defining Characteristics: Psychological dependence (addiction) occurs rarely in patients taking opioid agonists for cancer pain (< 1%). Physical dependence (precipitation of withdrawal symptoms) occurs with chronic use of the drug for the relief of chronic cancer pain. In addition, tolerance, or less analgesic effect over time with the same drug dose, occurs and requires increased dosage of drug.

Nursing Implications: Assess baseline knowledge of opioid analgesics, and attitude about their use for cancer pain management. Teach patient about proper self-administration, possible side effects, and self-care measures. Suggest patient maintain diary of pain intensity, precipitating and alleviating factors, drug dose and time taken, and relief. Teach patient to self-administer opioid agonists for relief of chronic cancer pain around-the-clock, not PRN, to prevent pain. Explain use of prescribed short-acting opioid for rescue or to manage breakthrough pain. Discuss with physician dose increase or change in frequency of administration if tolerance develops. Teach patient that withdrawal symptoms may occur if chronic, around-the-clock dosing is interrupted. Withdrawal (abstinence) symptoms that may be seen are restlessness, lacrimation, rhinorrhea, yawning, perspiration, gooseflesh, restless sleep, mydriasis in first 24 hours. These are followed by twitching and leg spasm; severe aching of the back, abdomen, and legs; cramping in abdomen and legs; hot/cold flashes; insomnia; nausea/vomiting, diarrhea; severe sneezing; and increased heart rate, BP, T, which peak at 36–72 hours. Withdrawal syndrome can be prevented by administration of at least 1/4 of previous opioid dose.

VIII. SEXUAL DYSFUNCTION related to IMPOTENCE, ↓ LIBIDO

Defining Characteristics: Opiate agonists may suppress gonadotropin, causing impotence and decreased libido.

Nursing Implications: Assess baseline sexual pattern. Discuss potential toxicity and impact on sexuality. Provide information, emotional support, and referral as needed.

Drug: oxycodone (Percodan, Endodan, Roxiprin)

Class: Opioid analgesic (opioid agonist).

Mechanism of Action: A synthetic opioid agonist, oxycodone resembles morphine but has milder action; binds to opiate receptors in CNS (limbic system, thalamus, striatum, hypothalamus, midbrain, spinal cord), altering pain perception at level of spinal cord and higher centers, as well as the emotional response to pain. Also suppresses cough reflex.

Metabolism: Onset of analgesia in 10–15 minutes, peaks 30–60 minutes, duration 3–6 hours. Metabolized by liver and kidney; excreted in urine.

Dosage/Range:

For moderate to moderately severe pain:

- 5 mg q6h (Roxicodone).
- 5 mg q6h, combined with acetaminophen: 300 mg (e.g., Oxycet, Percocet, Roxicet caplets), OR 500 mg (e.g., Roxicet caplets, Tylox); OR combined with aspirin: 325 mg (e.g., Percodan, Codoxy, Roxiprin); OR combined with ibuprofen 5 mg/400 mg (e.g., Combunox).
- Oral solution: 5 mg/5 mL (Roxicodone); 20 mg/mL (Roxicodone, Intensol).
- Oxycontin 10-mg, 20-mg, 40-mg (sustained-release) tablets q12h.

Drug Preparation:

- Store tablets in tight, light-resistant containers at 15–30°C (59–86°F) and protect from light.
- At home, teach patient to store oral doses in a safe place away from children and pets.

Drug Administration:

- Oral.

Drug Interactions:

- Alcohol, CNS depressants: additive CNS depressant effects.
- Anticoagulants, chemotherapy: aspirin-oxycodone combination may increase bleeding risk; AVOID concurrent use.

Lab Effects/Interference:

- None known.

Special Considerations:

- Adverse effects are milder than morphine.

- Preparations may contain sodium metabisulfite and may cause allergic reactions, including anaphylaxis and severe asthma-like reactions.
- Additive benefit when combined with acetaminophen or aspirin.
- Give smallest effective dose to prevent development of tolerance, physical dependency.
- Reduce dose in debilitated patients or patients receiving other CNS depressants.
- Use with caution in patients with hepatic or renal dysfunction, hypothyroidism, Addison's disease, severe CNS depression, respiratory depression, head injury, elevated ICP.
- If required, naloxone HCl will reverse opiate toxicity (e.g., respiratory depression). However, it is important that acute withdrawal symptoms be prevented by giving only enough naloxone to reverse respiratory depression and that this be continued for opioid drug half-life.
- Oxycontin is a sustained-release oxycodone preparation that is taken q12h; available in 10-mg, 20-mg, and 40-mg tablets.

Potential Toxicities/Side Effects and the Nursing Process

I. SENSORY/PERCEPTUAL ALTERATIONS related to CNS DEPRESSION

Defining Characteristics: Drowsiness, sedation, mood changes, euphoria, dysphoria, dizziness, mental clouding may occur. At high doses, may cause seizures. Miosis (papillary constriction) may occur.

Nursing Implications: Assess baseline neurologic status. Use cautiously, if at all, in the elderly, the debilitated, and patients with head injury, increased ICP, severe CNS depression, acute alcoholism. Assess other concurrent medications. Use with caution in patients receiving other opioids, tranquilizers, hypnotics, MAO inhibitors, since increasing CNS depressant effects can occur. Monitor neurologic status closely. Instruct patient to avoid driving and operating machinery while taking the medicine, and to AVOID concurrent alcohol.

II. ALTERATION IN OXYGENATION related to RESPIRATORY DEPRESSION

Defining Characteristics: Opiate agonists directly depress respiratory center in brain stem, causing decreased sensitivity and responsiveness to increased pCO_2. Also may depress deep breathing and reflex to sigh. Tolerance to respiratory depressant effects occurs with chronic use.

Nursing Implications: Assess baseline pulmonary status, and periodically during drug use. Use cautiously in patients with bronchial asthma, COPD, respiratory depression, and monitor closely.

III. ALTERATION IN ELIMINATION related to CONSTIPATION, ILEUS

Defining Characteristics: Opium agonists bind to opiate receptors in bowel, slowing peristalsis, leading to constipation. Untreated constipation may result in bowel perforation.

Nursing Implications: Assess baseline elimination, fluid intake, diet, and exercise patterns. Instruct patient regarding prevention of constipation: goal is to move bowels at least every two days by increasing fluids to 3 L/day, following a diet high in fiber (beans, vegetables, fruit), and taking moderate exercise. Assess need for bowel softeners, bulk-forming laxatives, and osmotic cathartics, and discuss preparation with physician. Teach patient self-administration of medications.

IV. ALTERATION IN NUTRITION, LESS THAN BODY REQUIREMENTS, related to GI TOXICITY

Defining Characteristics: Nausea, vomiting, dry mouth may occur. Gastric, biliary, and pancreatic secretions are decreased by opiate agonists; digestion is delayed. Biliary tract muscle tone is increased, and spasm of Oddi's sphincter may occur (morphine > meperidine > codeine).

Nursing Implications: Assess patient tolerance of GI side effects. Teach patient to report side effects. If nausea/vomiting occur, change to another opioid, or premedicate with antiemetic to prevent nausea/vomiting. Assess GI pain, biliary spasm, and consider alternative opioid.

V. ALTERATION IN CARDIAC OUTPUT related to HYPOTENSION, BRADYCARDIA

Defining Characteristics: Orthostatic hypotension, bradycardia due to cholinergic effect, and peripheral vasodilation may occur with rapid IV dosing. There may be histamine-related flushing, pruritus, diaphoresis with chronic drug usage; tolerance develops to this effect.

Nursing Implications: Assess baseline cardiovascular status. Teach patient to change position slowly and to hold onto stable, nearby structure for support as needed. Be careful when giving IV push opioids, and caution patient to remain in supine position for 15–20 minutes after injection. Monitor cardiovascular status after injection.

VI. ALTERATION IN URINE ELIMINATION related to URINARY RETENTION

Defining Characteristics: Increased smooth muscle tone in urinary tract and spasm may occur. Bladder tone is increased, which may cause urgency. Vesical sphincter tone may be increased, leading to difficulty urinating. Increased

Chapter 7

Nausea and Vomiting

Nausea and/or vomiting can occur commonly during the course of the cancer experience, related to disease, such as liver metastases, or to treatment, such as with chemotherapy or radiation to the abdomen. In addition, if acute nausea and vomiting were not prevented following cancer chemotherapy, delayed nausea and vomiting often followed. This problem continues. Nausea is often underreported and under-assessed (Wickham, 2003). A replication of the Coates et al (1983) study by de Boer-Dennert et al (1997) showed that patients rated nausea as more distressing than vomiting since much has been done to prevent and control chemotherapy-induced nausea and vomiting (CINV). Complete control of CINV has improved greatly with the advent of serotonin 5-hydroxytryptamine type 3 (5-HT_3) receptor antagonists used in combination with dexamethasone, bringing complete control to about 70% for patients receiving high-dose cisplatin. This new century of genomics has led to the understanding that the effectiveness of many drugs, and in particular, 5-HT_3 receptor antagonists, is influenced by the recipient's genotype. This is because the liver's microenzyme system, Cytochrome P450, and subtypes are determined by an individual's genotype. If the genotype is a ultrarapid metabolizer, the drug is rapidly cleared and eliminated from the body with decreased effect and undertreatment, while slow or poor metabolizers slowly clear the drug from the body with the risk of overtreatment. A study by Kaiser et al (2002) evaluated whether patients who vomited after receiving their first cycle of emetogenic chemotherapy with 5-HT_3 receptor antagonist protection by either ondansetron or tropisetron were either ultrarapid or slow metabolizers of the P450 subsystem CYP 2D6. They found that 30% had nausea and vomiting. The ultrarapid metabolizers had a higher incidence of nausea and vomiting, which was more marked for tropisetron- than ondansetron-receiving patients, and the poor metabolizers had higher serum concentrations and were protected. As we look to the future, not only do we see patients having genotypic evaluation of their tumors for an individualized prescription of anti-cancer treatment, but it will also include individual prescription of antiemetic dose based on genotype.

CHEMOTHERAPY INDUCED NAUSEA AND VOMITING

CINV appears mediated by multiple pathways. Nausea usually precedes vomiting, and is controlled by cerebral and autonomic input, with common accompanying signs and symptoms of tachycardia, pallor, and diaphoresis. Vomiting involves the ejection of stomach contents, and is a critical protection mechanism which helps the body excrete poisons. Most commonly, receptors in the gut enterochromaffin cells are stimulated, and release serotonin. Serotonin binds to 5-HT_3 receptors which stimulate the vagus nerve. This leads to stimulaton of the chemotherapy trigger zone (CTZ) in the area postrema on the floor of the 4th ventricle, leading to activation of the vomiting center (VC) in the medulla, or to stimulation of the vomiting center directly. The 5-HT_3 receptor antagonists, such as dolasetron, granisetron, and ondansetron, block the emetic impulses from reaching the CTZ and VC. In addition, other neuroreceptors in the CTZ can transmit impulses to the VC, such as dopamine, endorphin, and Substance P. Dopamine antagonists include phenothiazines and butyrophenones, and Substance P/Neurokinin1 receptor antagonist antiemetics include aprepitant, which has been newly FDA approved as Emend. Emotional and cognitive factors can influence the occurrence and severity of CINV through a descending pathway from the cerebral cortex to the vomiting center, such as with anticipatory nausea and vomiting. Here a conditioned response is set up based on 3–4 past episodes of severe nausea and/or vomiting. The benzodiazepine lorazepam has been effective in preventing or lessening this effect through the drug's amnesiac qualities.

Dexamethasone has long been known to reduce the incidence of CINV, through a probable anti-inflammatory effect, leading to a closing of spaces in the gut wall that would permit leakage of emetogens into the bloodstream (Wickham, 2003). However, the exact mechanism is unknown.

Delayed nausea and vomiting is difficult to control, but appears to be influenced by slowed gastric emptying. Thus, delayed antiemetic regimes usually include metoclopramide to speed gastric emptying, along with dexamethasone, and a phenothiazine or serotonin antagonist. Recently, it became clear that Substance P and its receptor Neurokinin-1 (NK_1), in the gut and brainstem, were important mediators in delayed CINV. The NK_1 receptors are located near the vomiting center, the "final common pathway" for emesis, so it is expected the NK_1 receptor antagonists will have broader application (Wickham, 2003). Although great strides have been made in the prevention and control of CINV, even with maximal pharmacologic blockade of known pathways, 100% protection is not obtained, so it is clear other pathways await discovery. See Figure 7.1 for a review of pathophysiology of CINV. See Table 7.1 for the emetogenicity of cancer chemotherapy agents, and Table 7.2 for a schematic for antiemetic drugs and doses for CINV.

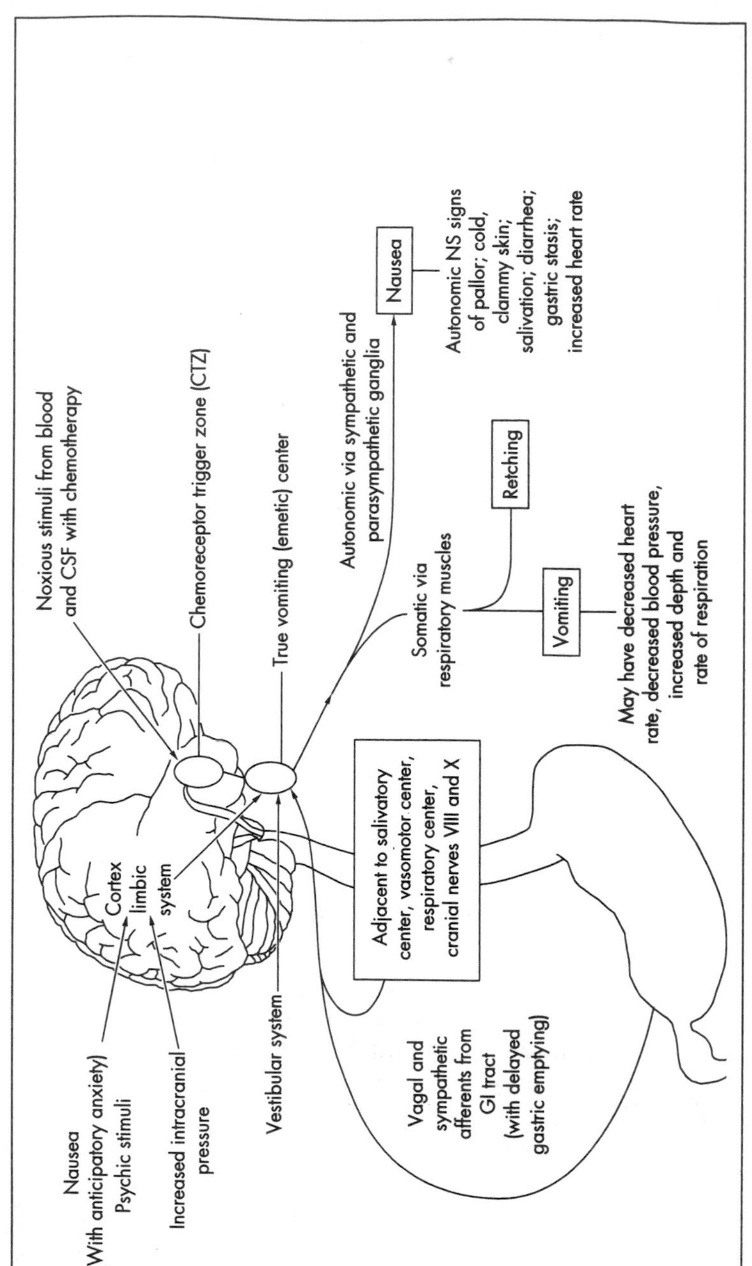

Figure 7.1 The Physiology of Nausea and Vomiting.

Source: Reproduced from Burke MM, Wilkes GM, Ingwersen K et al (1996) *Chemotherapy and the Nursing Process,* Sudbury, MA, Jones and Bartlett Publishers. *Drawing adapted from original by Gail Wilkes.*

Table 7.1 Emetogenic Risk by Antineoplast Agent

High Risk > 90%	Moderate Risk 0–90%	Low Risk 10-30%	Minimal Risk < 10%
Carmustine > 250 mg/m²	Carmustine < 250 mg/m²	Aldesleukin (IL=2)	Bleomycin
Cisplatin > 50 mg/m²	Carboplatin < 250 mg/m²	Asparaginase	Capecitabine
Cyclophosphamide > 1000 mg/m²	Cyclophosphamide < 1000 mg/m²	Docetaxel	Etoposide IV
Dacarbazine > 500 mg/m²	Cyclophosphamide PO	Doxorubicin < 20 mg/m²	Fludarabine
Dactinomycin	Cytarabine > 1 g/m²	Etoposide PO	Methotrexate < 100 mg/m²
Lomustine > 60 mg/m²	Doxorubicin	Fluorouracil	Rituximab
Mechlorethamine	Epirubicin	Gemcitabine	Tenoposide IV
Pentostatin	Hexamethylmelamine	Methotrexate > 100mg/m²	Traztuzumab
Streptozocin	Idarubicin	Mitomycin C	Vinblastine
	Ifosfamide	Mitoxantrone < 12 mg/m²	Vinorelbine IV
	Irinotecan	Paclitaxel	
	Melphalan	Temozolomide	
	Mitoxantrone > 12 mg/m²	Thiotepa	
	Procarbazine	Topotecan	
	Oxaliplatin		

Source: From Wickham R (2003) Nausea and Vomiting, Chapter 11. In Yarbro CH, Goodman M, and Frogge MH *Cancer Symptom Mangement*, 3rd ed. Sudbury, MA, Jones and Bartlett Publishers.

MANAGEMENT

CINV can occur *acutely*, during the first 24 hours following chemotherapy administration, *delayed*, occurring after the first 24 hours, or in anticipation (*anticipatory*).

Factors which influence the occurrence and severity of CINV include sex (female has higher risk than male), age (younger have higher risk than older), drug dose and emetogenic potential, combination of drugs versus single agent, history of alcohol intake (increased alcohol intake confers protection), and past experience with nausea and vomiting, such as air sickness, which increase risk.

Delayed nausea and vomiting are influenced by the effectiveness of control/prevention of the acute phase of CINV (Roila, 2000; Koeller et al, 2002), as well as the half-life of the antineoplastic agent. For example, the metabolites of cisplatin continue to be excreted for 3–5 days after drug administration, so protection must be provided for that period of time; and for cyclophosphamide, the half-life is at least 12 hours, so only half the drug is excreted by that time,

Table 7.2 Antiemetic Agents used in CINV

Antiemetic Agent	IV Doses (Acute)	Oral Doses (Acute)	Oral (Delayed)
Serotonin Receptor Antagonists			
• Dolasetron	100 mg or 1.8 mg/kg IV	100 mg (acute)	100 mg qd delayed
• Granisetron	0.01 mg/kg or 1 mg IV	1–2 mg oral (acute)	1 mg bid delayed
• Ondansetron	0.15 mg/kg or 8mg IV	24 mg oral (acute)	8 mg bid delayed
Corticosteroids			
• Dexamethasone	20 mg	20 mg	8 mg bid days 2–4 highly emetogenic 4–8 mg bid days 2–3 moderately emetogenic
Substance P/NK1 Receptor Antagonist			
• Aprepitant		125 mg po day 1 with dexamethasone 12 mg po with serotonin receptor antagonist	80 mg day 2,3 with dexamethasone 8 mg po
Dopamine Receptor Antagonists			
• Metoclopramine			20–40 mg bid-qid
• Prochlorperazine			15–30mg LA spansules bid PRN
Benzodiazepines			
• Lorazepam	0.5–1 mg	1–2 mg	

Source: Modified from Wickham R (2003) Nausea and Vomiting, Chapter 11. In Yarbro CH, Goodman M, and Frogge MH *Cancer Symptom Mangement*, 3rd ed. Sudbury, MA, Jones and Bartlett Publishers.

and full antiemetic protection must continue for at least 24 hours to prevent delayed nausea and vomiting.

Insofar as CINV involves multiple pathways, multiple antiemetics to block these pathways are needed, especially for aggressive antiemesis. Antiemetics must be administered to prevent nausea and vomiting, so the drug(s) should be administered prior to chemotherapy administration in order to block stimulation of the pathways. Oral antiemetics should be administered 30–40 minutes before treatment; rectal (PR) preparations 60 minutes before; intramuscular (IM) injections 20–30 minutes before; and intravenous bolus (IVB) 10–30 minutes prior to chemotherapy (Barton Burke et al, 1997).

In order to better identify treatment approaches for CINV, American Society for Clinical Oncology (ASCO) published "Recommendations for the Use of Antiemetics: Evidence-Based Clinical Practice Guidelines" and stated that "at equivalent doses, serotonin receptor antagonists have equivalent safety and efficacy and can be used intrchangeably based on convenience, availability, and cost" (Gralla et al, 1999). They listed four agents in this class, three of which are commercially available in the United States: dolasetron, granisetron, and ondansetron. In addition, the National Community Network (NCCN) has developed supportive care guidelines for antiemesis, which can be found at http://www.nccn.org/physician_gls/f_guidelines.html. Finally, key members of the Supportive Care in Cancer organization have developed consensus guidelines for the study and prescription of antiemetic care (Koeller et al, 2002).

2003 has seen the advent of a new class of antiemetics for the control of chemotherapy-induced nauseas and vomiting. Aprepitant (Emend) is the first substance P/Neurokinin 1 receptor antagonist indicated for the prevention of acute and delayed nausea and vomiting related to highly emetogenic chemotherapy, in combination with other antiemetic agents. First identified in 1931, and reaching notoriety in 1950 when linked with pain transmission, substance P has continued to be prominent in the symptom management field. Substance P is a member of the tachykinin family of peptides and, together with NK1 receptors, is found in high concentrations in the chemotherapy trigger zone (CTZ, in the medulla oblongata) and the dorsal horn of the spinal cord (posterior column of gray matter), as well as the gut. Substance P is released from peripheral sensory as well as central sensory nerve endings and plays a key role in transmitting noxious sensory information to the brain. Substance P initiates its activity by binding to the Neurokinin 1 (NK_1) receptor, a site distinctly different from the serotonin-mediated $5HT_3$ site (Hesketh, 2001).

In an effort to design a serotonin-antagonist with a long half-life, and activity against delayed chemotherapy-induced nausea and vomiting, palonestron (Aloxi) was created. Recently approved for the prevention of chemotherapy-induced nausea and vomiting, palonestron is the only serotonin-antagonist with an indication for delayed nausea and vomiting.

RADIATION INDUCED NAUSEA AND VOMITING

Radiation therapy to the gastrointestinal tract usually causes nausea and vomiting. Highest risk (90%) is when Total Body Irradiation (TBI) or external beam radiation is administered to the upper or total abdomen or upper hemithorax, with emesis occurring within 10–15 minutes with TBI or hemithorax treatment, and within 1–2 hours when external beam therapy is administered to the upper abdomen (Wickham, 2003). Antiemesis is effective using serotonin-antagonists or phenothiazines.

DISEASE INDUCED NAUSEA AND VOMITING

Site of advanced disease is a strong predictor of the risk for nausea and vomiting. Metastases to the liver is often associated with difficult to control nausea and vomiting. Pressure from ascites or obstruction of a hollow viscus, as with advanced ovarian cancer, can also lead to intractable nausea and vomiting. A factor here, along with advanced pancreatic cancer, may be delayed gastric emptying, or gastric outlet syndrome. Increased intracranial pressure (ICP) from a malignant brain tumor often causes nausea and vomiting. Other conditions related to disease that cause nausea and vomiting include hypercalcemia, hyperglycemia, electrolyte imbalance, and severe constipation. Strategies to relieve nausea and vomiting in these circumstances vary with the cause, and range from aggressive antiemesis to correction of delayed gastric emptying (metoclopramide) or the obstruction (stent if possible, or if not, release of gastric contents via a gastrostomy tube), to correction of electrolyte abnormalities.

In summary then, nausea and/or vomiting can arise from treatment or complications of disease. There are a variety of agents useful for blocking a number of neurotransmitter pathways to prevent or control nausea and vomiting in cancer. Specifically, it is known that chemotherapy stimulates nausea and vomiting via multiple pathways and often, therefore, multiple drugs are necessary for the prevention of nausea and vomiting associated with aggressive chemotherapy. These include a $5HT_3$ receptor (serotonin) antagonist, a corticosteroid (Gralla et al, 1999), and a Substance P/NK 1 receptor antagonist if there is a delayed component anticipated (Koeller et al, 2002).

References

Barnhart ER. *Physicians' Desk Reference.* Oradell, NJ, Medical Economics Data 1998

Barton Burke M, Wilkes G, Berg D, et al. *Cancer Chemotherapy: A Nursing Process Approach,* 2nd ed. Sudbury, MA, Jones and Bartlett Publishers 1997

Barton Burke M, Wilkes G, Ingwersen K. *Chemotherapy Care Plans: Designs for Nursing Care.* Sudbury, MA, Jones and Bartlett Publishers 1997

Coates A, Abraham S, Kaye SB, et al. On the Receivin End–Patient Perception of the Side-Effects of Cancer Chemotherapy. *Eur J Cancer Clin Oncol* 1983;19:203–208

Cotanch PM, Stum S. Progressive Muscle Relaxation as Antiemetic Therapy for Cancer Patients. *Oncol Nurs Forum* 1987;14(1):33–37 de Boer-Dennert M, de Wit R, Schmitz PIM, et al. Patient Perceptions of the Side-effects of Chemotherapy: The Influence of 5HT3 Antagonists. *Br J Cancer* 1997;76: 1055–1061

Gralla RJ, Osoba D, Kris MG, et al. ASCO Special Article: Recommendations for the Use of Antiemetics: Evidence-Based Clinical Practice Guidelines. *J Clin Oncol* 1999;17(9):2971–2994

Hesketh PJ. Potential Role of the NK1 Receptor Antagonists in Chemotherapy-induced Nausea and Vomiting. *Supportive Care in Cancer* 2001;9:350–354

Hesketh PJ, Beck TM, Uhlenhopp M, et al. Adjusting the Dose of Intravenous Ondansetron plus Dexamethasone to the Emetogenic Potential of the Chemotherapy Regimen. *J Clin Oncol* 1995;13(8):2117–2122

Hesketh PJ, Kris MG, Grunberg SM, et al. Proposal for Classifying the Acute Emetogenicity of Cancer Chemotherapy. *J Clin Oncol* 1997;15(1):103–109

Hesketh PJ, Murphy WK, Khojasten A, et al. GR-C507175 (GR38032F): A Novel Compound Effective in the Treatment of Cisplatin-Induced Nausea and Vomiting. *Proc American Society of Clinical Oncologists* 1988;7:280

Hui YF, Ignoffo RJ. Dolasetron: A New 5-Hydroxytryptamine3 Receptor Antagonist. *Cancer Practice* 1997;(Sept/Oct) 5(5):324–327

Kaiser R, Sezer O, Papies A, et al. Patient-tailored Antiemetic Treatment with 5-hydroxytryptamine Type 3 Receptor Antagonists according to Cytochrome P-450 Genotypes. *J Clin Oncol* 2002;20(12):2805–2811

Koeller JM, Aapro MS, Gralla RJ, et al. Antiemetic Guidelines: Creating a More Practical Treatment Approach. *Supportive Care in Cancer* 2002;10:519–522

Nolte MJ, Berkery R, Pizzo B, et al. Assuring the Optimal Use of Serotonin Antagonist Antiemetics: The Process for Development and Implementation of Institutional Antiemetic Guidelines at Memorial Sloan-Kettering Cancer Center. *J Clin Oncol* 1998; 16:771–778

Roila F, Ballatori E, Ruggeri B, et al. Dexamethasone Alone or in Combination with Ondansetron for the Prevention of Delayed Nausea and Vomiting Induced by Chemotherapy. *New Engl J Med* 2000;342(21):1554–1559

Roxane Laboratories. Marinol (Dronabinol) Manufacturer's Information Sheet. Columbus, Ohio: Roxane Laboratories 1986

Rubenstein EB, Gralla RJ, Hainsworth JD, et al. Randomized, Double Blind, Dose-Response Trial across Four Oral Doses of Dolasetron for the Prevention of Acute Emesis after Moderately Emetogenic Chemotherapy. *Cancer* 1997;79(6): 1216–1224

Sylvester RK, Etzell R, Levitt R, et al. Comparison of 16-mg vs 32-mg Ondansetron and Dexamethasone in Patients Receiving Cisplatin. *Proc Am Soc Clin Oncol* 1996; 15:547 (abstract 1781)

Van Belles, Cocquyt V, DeSmet M, et al. Comparison of a Neurokinin-1 Antagonist L-758, 298 to Ondansetron in the Prevention of Cisplatin-induced Emesis. *Proc American Society of Clinical Oncologists* 1998;17:51a (abstract 198)

Wickham R. Nausea and Vomiting, chapter 11. Yarbro CH, Frogge MH, Goodman M, (eds), *Cancer Symptom Management,* 3rd ed. Sudbury, MA: Jones and Bartlett Publishers 2003

Drug: aprepitant (Emend®)

Mechanism of Action: Selective Substance P/Neurokinin 1 (NK_1) receptor antagonist (high affinitiy). Drug has no affinity for $5HT_3$, dopamine, or corticosteroid receptors. Drug crosses the blood brain barrier to saturate brain NK_1 receptors. Drug increases the activity of serotonin receptor antagonists and corticosteroids in preventing acute nausea and vomiting, and inhibits both acute and delayed nausea and vomiting related to cisplatin chemotherapy.

Class: Substance P/Neurokinin 1 Receptor Antagonist.

Dosage/Range:
Day 1, 125 mg po 1 hour before chemotherapy, together with a serotonin (HT3) receptor antagonist and dexamethasone (dose reduced to 12 mg day 1, 8 mg days 2&3); days 2 and 3, 80 mg po each morning.

Drug Preparation/Administration: Oral drug supplied as 1) 80 mg capsules in bottle of 30 capsules or in unit dose packs of 5 capsules, 2) 125 mg tablets in bottle of 30 capsules or in unit dose packs of 5 capsules, and 3) tri-fold pack containing 1–125 mg capsule, and 2–80 mg capsules. Capsules should be stored at room temperature. Day 1, give 125 mg capsule po 1 hour before chemotherapy, and then the 80 mg capsule in the morning on days 2 and 3. Give with or without food.

Drug Interactions:
- Drugs that inhibit the CYP3A4 isoenzyme system can increase the serum level of aprepitant: ketoconazole, itraconazole, nefazodone, troleandomycin, claritromycin, ritonavir, nelfinavir; diltiazem (2-fold increase in aprepitant plasma concentration), so coadminister cautiously and monitor for aprepitant toxicity or dose reduce aprepitant.
- Drugs that strongly induce CYP3A4 isoenzyme system can lower aprepitant serum levels: rifampin, carbamazepine, phenytoin; assess for efficacy of aprepitant and need for drug dose increase.
- Drug is a moderate inhibitor of P450 hepatic isoenzyme system CYP3A4, so the plasma concentrations of the following drugs can theoretically be increased if coadministered:
  - Chemotherapy agents docetaxel, paclitaxel, etoposide, irinotecan, ifosfamide, imatinib, vinorelbine, vinblastine, vincristine.
  - dexamethasone (dose-reduce dexamethasone by 50%).
  - methylprednisolone (dose-reduce 25% if IV, 50% if po).
  - benzodiazepines: midazolam, lorazepam, alprazolam, triazolam.
- Drug is an inducer of CYP2C9, and the plasma concentrations of the following drugs can theoretically be decreased if coadministered:

- Warfarin (34% decrease with 14% decrease in INR; closely monitor INR 7–10 days after 3-day antiemetic regime, and modify warfarin dose as needed.
- Phenytoin, tolbutamide, oral contraceptives.

Lab Effects/Interference: Lab Effects/Interactions: Decreased INR if patient taking warfarin.

Special Considerations:

- Contraindications: do not give concomitantly with pimozide, terfenadine, astemizole, or cisapride; do not give if hypersensitive to aprepitant or any of its components; use cautiously if at all during pregnancy or breast-feeding; no studies have been done in patients with severe liver failure.
- Indications: in combination, with other antiemetic agents, for the prevention of acute and delayed nausea and vomiting associated with initial and repeat courses of highly emetogenic chemotherapy, including high-dose cisplatin.
- Significant drug interactions (see above).
- Drug is well tolerated with few side effects.

Potential Toxicities/Side Effects and the Nursing Process

I. ALTERATION IN NUTRITION, LESS THAN BODY REQUIREMENTS related to CONSTIPATION, DIARRHEA, NAUSEA, ANOREXIA, HICCUPS

Defining Characteristics: Gastrointestinal side effects may occur but are infrequent with the following incidences: constipation (10.3%), diarrhea (10.3%), nausea (12.7%), vomiting (7.5%), hiccups (10.8%), and anorexia (10.1%).

Nursing Implications: Teach patient that these side effects may occur, and to report them if unrelieved by symptom-management measures. Teach patient self-care measures to manage and prevent symptoms.

II. ALTERATION IN COMFORT related to ASTHENIA/FATIGUE, ABDOMINAL PAIN, HEADACHE

Defining Characteristics: Asthenia/fatigue occurred in 17.8% of patients; abdominal pain 4.6%; headache 8.5%.

Nursing Implications: Teach patient that these side effects may occur and measures to minimize their occurrence. Teach energy-conserving measures, management of abdominal pain and headache. Teach patient to report signs and symptoms which worsen or are unrelieved.

Drug: dexamethasone (Decadron)

Class: Glucocorticoid steroid.

Mechanism of Action: May inhibit prostaglandin release by stabilizing lysosomal membranes, thereby interrupting hypothalamic prostaglandin release and subsequent stimulation of nausea and vomiting. Causes demargination of marginated WBCs, with leukocytosis. Decreases inflammation by suppression of migration of polymorphonuclear leukocytes.

Metabolism: Half-life is 3–4 hours; oral dose peaks in 1–2 hours, with duration of two days; IM peaks in 8 hours, with duration of six days.

Dosage/Range:

Adult (as antiemetic):

- Oral: 4 mg q4h × four doses beginning 1–8 hours before chemotherapy.
- IV: 10–20 mg prior to chemotherapy, then q4–6h.

Drug Preparation/Administration:

- Oral: administer with food or milk.
- IV: may be given with H_2-antagonist (e.g., ranitidine) to prevent gastric irritation.

Drug Interactions:

- Indomethacin, aspirin: increased GI irritation and bleeding; avoid concurrent administration.
- Barbiturates, phenytoin, rifampin: decreased dexamethasone effect; increase dose as needed.

Lab Effects/Interference: Lab Effects/Interactions:

- Increased WBC may occur due to demargination.
- Increased serum glucose level.
- May cause decreased K.

Special Considerations:

- Contraindicated in patients with psychosis, hypersensitivity, idiopathic thrombocytopenia, acute glomerulonephritis, amebiasis, fungal infections, and nonasthmatic bronchial disease.
- Indicated in the management of inflammation, allergies, neoplasms, cerebral edema, and in combination antiemetic therapy.
- If patient received dexamethasone chronically, drug must be tapered to prevent withdrawal (i.e., signs/symptoms of adrenal insufficiency, rebound weakness, arthralgia, fever, dizziness, orthostatic hypotension, dyspnea, hypoglycemia).

Potential Toxicities/Side Effects and the Nursing Process

I. ALTERATION IN NUTRITION, LESS THAN BODY REQUIREMENTS, related to GI TOXICITY

Defining Characteristics: Increased appetite, abdominal distension, pancreatitis, GI hemorrhage; diarrhea may occur.

Nursing Implications: Assess baseline nutritional status and monitor throughout therapy. Discuss symptomatic management of diarrhea, abdominal distension, and increased appetite with patient. Assess stool for occult blood and notify physician if positive. Monitor Hgb and HCT values.

II. ALTERATIONS IN SENSORY/PERCEPTUAL PATTERNS related to CHANGES IN MOOD, VASODILATION, CATARACTS

Defining Characteristics: Euphoria, insomnia, depression, flushing, sweating, headache, mood changes, and cataracts may occur.

Nursing Implications: Assess baseline mental status and monitor during therapy. Discuss symptomatic management or drug discontinuance, based on severity, with physician.

III. ALTERATION IN CARDIAC OUTPUT related to CHF

Defining Characteristics: Congestive heart failure (CHF), hypertension, fluid retention, and edema may occur.

Nursing Implications: Assess baseline vital signs (VS), and monitor during therapy. Discuss hypertension with physician, monitor daily weights, and assess for edema.

IV. ALTERATION IN CARBOHYDRATE METABOLISM related to CARBOHYDRATE INTOLERANCE

Defining Characteristics: May cause hyperglycemia, hypokalemia, and carbohydrate intolerance.

Nursing Implications: Assess baseline blood glucose, K, and monitor during therapy. Teach patient signs/symptoms of hyperglycemia (polyuria, polydipsia), especially if receiving drug for extended period.

Drug: diphenhydramine hydrochloride (Benadryl)

Class: Antihistamine.

Mechanism of Action: Inhibits histamine, and has slight, if any, antiemetic activity by blocking the CTZ and decreasing vestibular stimulation. Acts on blood vessels, GI, respiratory systems by competing with histamine for H1-receptor site; decreases allergic response by blocking histamine.

Metabolism: Biologically transformed in the liver; half-life is 2.4–9.3 hours; 80–85% protein-bound; excreted by the kidney. Metabolized in the liver, crosses placenta, and is excreted in breast milk.

Dosage/Range:

Adult:

- Oral: 25–50 mg q4h.
- IM: 25–50 mg q4h.
- IV: 50 mg prior to chemotherapy or 25 mg q4h × 4 doses, beginning prior to antiemetic.

Drug Preparation/Administration:

- Available forms include 25-, 50-mg capsules; elixir 12.5 mg/mL; syrup 12.5 mg/mL; injection available as 10 mg/mL and 50 mg/mL. Administer IM deep in large muscle mass.

Drug Interactions:

- CNS depressants: increased sedation; monitor patient closely.

Lab Effects/Interference: Lab Effects/Interactions:

- None known.

Special Considerations:

- Useful in treatment or prevention of extrapyramidal side effects (EPS) related to antiemetics (dopamine antagonists).
- Contraindicated in patients with prior hypersensitivity to H1-receptor antagonist, acute asthma attack, or lower respiratory tract disease.

Potential Toxicities/Side Effects and the Nursing Process

I. ALTERATIONS IN SENSORY/PERCEPTUAL PATTERNS related to CNS CHANGES

Defining Characteristics: Sedation/drowsiness, dizziness, confusion (especially in the elderly), hyperexcitability, blurred vision/diplopia, tinnitus, dry mouth/nose/throat may all occur.

Nursing Implications: Assess patient's level of consciousness and risk for increased sedation (i.e., elderly, concomitant CNS depressant drugs). Monitor neurologic VS closely if sedated. Instruct patient to avoid alcohol ingestion, operation of equipment, or driving a car while drowsy. Teach strategies to protect safety.

II. ALTERED URINARY ELIMINATION related to URINARY RETENTION, DYSURIA

Defining Characteristics: Urinary retention, dysuria, frequency may occur.

Nursing Implications: Assess baseline urinary elimination pattern. Teach patient potential side effects and instruct to report them. Use drug cautiously in men with prostatic hypertrophy; if side effect occurs, instruct patient not to take drug and discuss with physician.

III. ALTERATION IN COMFORT related to RASH

Defining Characteristics: Rash, urticaria, photosensitivity, hypotension, palpitations may occur.

Nursing Implications: Assess baseline drug allergy history. Instruct patient to report rash, itching, and to avoid sunlight while taking the drug. Assess VS and monitor patient closely for hypotension, especially if patient is elderly or sedated, or taking other sedating drugs.

IV. POTENTIAL FOR INJURY related to BONE MARROW DEPRESSION

Defining Characteristics: Thrombocytopenia, agranulocytosis, hemolytic anemia may occur rarely.

Nursing Implications: Assess baseline CBC, platelet count. Discuss abnormalities with physician.

Drug: dolasetron mesylate (Anzemet)

Class: Serotonin antagonist.

Mechanism of Action: Together with the active metabolite hydrodolasetron, drug is a selective serotonin 5-HT_3 receptor antagonist, blocking transmission of impulses via the vagus nerve peripherally and centrally in the chemotherapy receptor trigger zone (CTZ). Blocks chemotherapy-induced nausea and vomiting produced by the release of serotonin from the enterochromaffin cells of the small intestines, which otherwise would stimulate the 5-HT_3 receptors on the vagus efferents that begin the vomiting reflex.

Metabolism: IV: Parent drug is rapidly eliminated from the plasma and completely metabolized into the major metabolite hydrodolasetron, as is the oral drug. Hydrodolasetron is metabolized by the cytochrome P-450 enzyme system in the liver, with an approximate half-life of 7.3 hours. Oral and orally administered IV solution are bioequivalent, and apparent absolute bioavailability of oral dolasetron is 75%, determined by the active metabolite; 66% of drug is excreted in the urine unchanged, and 33% in the feces. Metabolite is 77% protein-bound.

Dosage/Range:

For the prevention of cancer chemotherapy-induced nausea and vomiting:

Adult:

- IV: 1.8 mg/kg IV, 30 minutes prior to chemotherapy, diluted in 50 mL and infused over a period of up to 15 min, or 100-mg IV fixed dose for most adults given IV over 30 sec.
- Oral: 100 mg given within 1 hour prior to chemotherapy.

Pedi (2–16 years of age):

- IV: the recommended intravenous dosage is 1.8 mg/kg given as a single dose approximately 30 minutes before chemotherapy, up to a maximum of 100 mg. Safety and effectiveness in pediatric patients under 2 years of age have not been established.
- Oral: Anzemet injection mixed in apple or apple-grape juice may be used for oral dosing of pediatric patients. When Anzemet injection is administered orally, the recommended dosage in pediatric patients 2–16 years of age is 1.8 mg/kg, up to a maximum 100-mg dose given within 1 hour before chemotherapy.

For the prevention or treatment of postoperative nausea and/or vomiting:

Adult:

- IV: 12.5 mg given as a single dose 15 minutes before the cessation of anesthesia for prevention, or as soon as nausea or vomiting presents (treatment).
- Oral: 100 mg given within 2 hours before surgery.

Pedi (2–16 years of age):

- IV: 0.35 mg/kg, with a maximum dose of 12.5 mg, given as a single dose 15 minutes prior to the cessation of anesthesia (prevention), or as soon as nausea or vomiting presents (treatment).
- Oral: Anzemet injection mixed in apple or apple-grape juice may be used for oral dosing of pediatric patients. When Anzemet injection is administered orally, the recommended dose is 1.2 mg/kg, up to a maximum 100-mg dose given within 2 hours before surgery.
- Safety and efficacy have not been established for children under 2 years of age.
- Diluted product can be up to 2 hours at room temperature before use. The recommended dose of Anzemet should not be exceeded.

Drug Preparation/Administration:

- Injectable drug available in 100-mg/5-mL single-use vials, and 12.5-mg/0.625 mL single-use vials.
- Tablets available in 50-mg and 100-mg doses, each in a 5-count bottle or blister pack, or in a 10-count unit dose.

- IV dose given IVP over 30 sec or further diluted in 50 mL of 0.9% NS, 5% D_5W, D_5 1/2 NS, D_5LR, LR, or 10% mannitol injection and infused over a period of up to 15 minutes. Diluted drug stable 24 hours at room temperature, or 48 hours refrigerated.
- Oral: administer within 1 hour before chemotherapy, or within 2 hours prior to surgery.

Drug Interactions:

- Anzemet injection has been safely coadministered with other drugs used in chemotherapy and surgery. As with other agents that prolong ECG intervals, caution should be exercised in patients taking other drugs that prolong ECG intervals, particularly QT_c. See Special Considerations section.
- Increased hydrodolasetron serum levels (24%) when given with cimetidine (nonselective inhibitor of cytochrome P-450 enzyme system).
- Decreased hydrodolasetron serum levels (28%) when combined with rifampin (potent inducer of P-450 enzyme system).

Lab Effects/Interference:

- Transient increased liver transaminases (AST, ALT) in $< 1\%$ of patients; rare increase in bili, GGT, alk phos.

Special Considerations:

- Administer with caution in patients who have or may develop cardiac conduction defects, especially prolongation of QT interval (e.g., patients with hypokalemia, hypomagnesemia, receiving diuretics, congenital QT syndrome, receiving antiarrhythmic drugs or other drugs causing QT segment prolongation, and with high cumulative doses of anthracycline chemotherapy). Prolongation of PR, QRS, and QT_c intervals was observed in some patients. These changes are mild, transient, asymptomatic, and do not require medical treatment. Of note, other 5-HT_3 antagonists were also associated with similiar electrocardiographic changes.
- Rare anaphylaxis, facial edema, urticaria.
- No dosage modifications necessary in elderly or patients with hepatic or renal impairment.
- IV preparation indicated for highly emetogenic chemotherapy, including high-dose cisplatin; oral dose indicated for prevention of chemotherapy-induced nausea and vomiting due to moderately emetogenic chemotherapy.

Potential Toxicities/Side Effects and Nursing Process

I. ALTERATION IN COMFORT related to HEADACHE

Defining Characteristics: Headache (24%), fever (4%), fatigue (4%), and, rarely, arthralgia, myalgia occur.

Nursing Implications: Assess baseline comfort. Teach patient to report any unusual occurrence. Provide symptomatic management.

II. ALTERATION IN NUTRITION, LESS THAN BODY REQUIREMENTS, related to CONSTIPATION, DYSPEPSIA

Defining Characteristics: Constipation, dyspepsia, anorexia, and, rarely, pancreatitis may occur. In less than 1% of patients, there is an increase in LFTs.

Nursing Implications: Assess baseline weight, nutritional pattern. Instruct patient to report alterations, and manage symptomatically. Discuss alterations in LFTs and/or abdominal pain suggestive of pancreatitis with physician.

III. POTENTIAL ALTERATIONS IN SENSORY/PERCEPTUAL PATTERNS related to VERTIGO, PARESTHESIA

Defining Characteristics: Rarely, flushing, vertigo, paresthesia, agitation, sleep disorder, depersonalization may occur, as may ataxia, twitching, confusion, anxiety, abnormal dreams.

Nursing Implications: Teach patient to report any changes, and assess patient safety. Discuss any significant alterations with physician and consider alternative antiemetics.

Drug: dronabinol (Marinol)

Class: Cannabinoid.

Mechanism of Action: Active ingredient is δ-9-tetrahydrocannabinol (THC). Probably depresses CNS and may disrupt higher cortical input, inhibit prostaglandin synthesis, or bind to opiate receptors in the brain to indirectly block the VC.

Metabolism: Metabolized by the liver.

Dosage/Range:

Adult:

- Oral: 5 mg/m^2–7.5 mg/m^2 1–3 hours prior to chemotherapy, then 2–4 hours postchemotherapy for 4–6 doses per day.

Drug Preparation/Administration:

- If ineffective at above dose and no toxicity, may be increased by 2.5 mg/m^2 to a maximum of 15 mg/m^2/day.

Drug Interactions:

- CNS depressants: increased sedation; avoid concurrent use.

Lab Effects/Interference: Lab Effects/Interactions:
- None known.

Special Considerations:
- More effective than placebo and in some instances may be better than prochlorperazine.
- Indicated in the management of chemotherapy-induced nausea and vomiting refractory to usual antiemetics.
- Can produce physical and psychological dependency.
- May increase appetite.
- May produce dry mouth.

Potential Toxicities/Side Effects and the Nursing Process

I. ALTERATIONS IN SENSORY/PERCEPTUAL PATTERNS related to CNS CHANGES

Defining Characteristics: Mood changes, disorientation, drowsiness, muddled thinking, dizziness, and brief impairment of perception, coordination, and sensory functions may occur. Increased toxicity in elderly (up to 35%).

Nursing Implications: Explain to patient these changes may occur to decrease anxiety, fear. Assess baseline mental status, and monitor during therapy. Assess patient safety and implement measures to ensure this. Avoid use in the elderly.

II. ALTERATION IN CARDIAC OUTPUT related to TACHYCARDIA

Defining Characteristics: Tachycardia, orthostatic hypotension may occur.

Nursing Implications: Assess baseline VS, and monitor during therapy. If hypotension occurs, notify physician and anticipate increasing rate of IV fluids to increase BP.

Drug: droperidol (Inapsine)

Class: Butyrophenone.

Mechanism of Action: Neuroleptic compound that produces a state of quiescence with reduced motor activity, reduced anxiety, and indifference to surroundings. Dopamine antagonist that suppresses CTZ and VC; more potent than phenothiazines. Decreases stimulation of the VC along vestibular pathway.

Metabolism: When given IM/IV, has onset of action in 3–10 minutes, peak 30 minutes, duration 3–6 hours; metabolized in liver, excreted in urine as metabolites; crosses placenta.

Dosage/Range:
Adults:
- IM/IV: 0.5–2.5 mg q4–6h or drip, but reports suggest large loading dose, then intermittent IVB or continuous infusion for 6–10 hours.

Drug Preparation/Administration:
- IM: 2.5 mg/mL.
- IV: 2.5 mg/mL initial reconstitution then further dilute in at least 25 mL 0.9% Sodium Chloride or 5% Dextrose.

Drug Interactions:
- Epinephrine: reversal of vasopressor effects; avoid concurrent use.
- CNS depressants: increased sedation; monitor patient closely.

Lab Effects/Interference:
- None known.

Special Considerations:
- Contraindicated in patients with hypersensitivity or who are pregnant.
- Indicated for premedication prior to surgery; induction and maintenance of general anesthesia; also useful as an antiemetic prior to chemotherapy for some patients.

Potential Toxicities/Side Effects and the Nursing Process

I. ALTERATIONS IN SENSORY/PERCEPTUAL PATTERNS related to SEDATION, RESTLESSNESS

Defining Characteristics: Sedation, restlessness, and EPS may occur, although are less severe than with phenothiazines. Tardive dyskinesia may occur in older patients.

Nursing Implications: Assess baseline level of consciousness and monitor during therapy. Assess for signs/symptoms of EPS (dystonia, tongue protrusion, trismus, opisthotonus), and administer diphenhydramine as ordered.

II. ALTERATION IN OXYGENATION/PERFUSION related to RESPIRATORY DEPRESSION

Defining Characteristics: Can induce respiratory depression when used with narcotic analgesics; rarely, laryngospasm or bronchospasm may occur.

Nursing Implications: Assess baseline pulmonary status and monitor during therapy. Identify risk factors (concomitant narcotics, CNS depressants), notify physician, and hold drug if respiratory depression occurs or is suspected. Be prepared to institute respiratory support if necessary, and to reverse opiate.

III. ALTERATION IN CARDIAC OUTPUT related to TACHYCARDIA

Defining Characteristics: Tachycardia and hypotension may occur.

Nursing Implications: Assess baseline VS, and monitor during therapy. If hypotension occurs, notify physician and anticipate increasing rate of IV fluids to increase BP. Epinephrine should not be used since drug reverses vasopressor effect; rather, metaraminol or norepinephrine should be used.

IV. ALTERATION IN COMFORT related to CHILLS, FACIAL SWEATING

Defining Characteristics: Rarely, chills, facial sweating, and shivering occur.

Nursing Implications: Assess baseline comfort. Teach patient to report any unusual occurrence. Provide symptomatic management.

Drug: granisetron hydrochloride (Kytril)

Class: Serotonin antagonist.

Mechanism of Action: Binds to vagal afferents (serotonin receptors) adjacent to the enterochromaffin cells in the GI mucosa, thus preventing the stimulation of afferent fibers that would otherwise stimulate the VC and CTZ. In addition, granisetron inhibits a positive feedback loop located on the enterochromaffin cells that normally responds to high levels of serotonin released from chemotherapy injury to the gut mucosa by releasing a surge of additional serotonin. Thus, granisetron blocks two pathways of serotonin release to prevent chemotherapy-induced nausea and vomiting.

Metabolism: Rapidly and extensively metabolized by the liver using the P-450 cytochrome enzymes; 12% of unchanged drug is eliminated in the urine at 48 hours. The half-life of IV granisetron in cancer patients is 9 hours.

Dosage/Range:
- IV: 10 μg/kg IV over 5 minutes, beginning within 30 minutes prior to chemotherapy.
- Oral: 1 mg bid (q12h).

Drug Preparation:
- Dilute in 20–50 mL 0.9% Sodium Chloride or 5% Dextrose.

Drug Administration:
- IV infusion over 5 minutes.

- Drug can also be given IV push over 5 minutes.

Drug Interactions:
- None known, but, because the drug is metabolized by the P-450 cytochrome enzymes, drugs that induce or inhibit this may theoretically change the drug serum levels and half-life.

Lab Effects/Interference:
- Rarely, increased AST, ALT.

Special Considerations:
- Useful in the management of high-dose cisplatin, in combination with dexamethasone, either with oral tablets or IV preparation.
- Preliminary study data showed little difference in efficacy between oral dosing of 1 mg bid versus a single dose of 2 mg.
- Both IV and tablet formulation are indicated for the prevention of nausea and vomiting associated with initial and repeat courses of emetogenic chemotherapy, including cisplatin.

Potential Toxicities/Side Effects and the Nursing Process

I. ALTERATION IN COMFORT related to HEADACHE, ASTHENIA, SOMNOLENCE

Defining Characteristics: Side effects are uncommon but may include headache, asthenia, and somnolence.

Nursing Implications: Teach patient that side effects may occur. Headache is usually relieved by OTC analgesics such as acetaminophen.

II. ALTERATION IN ELIMINATION related to CONSTIPATION OR DIARRHEA

Defining Characteristics: A small percentage of patients may experience constipation or diarrhea.

Nursing Implications: Assess baseline elimination pattern. Instruct patient to report alterations. Identify patients at risk, such as those receiving narcotic analgesics for cancer pain, who may develop constipation. Assist patient in modifying bowel regimen.

Drug: haloperidol (Haldol)

Class: Butyrophenone.

Mechanism of Action: Tranquilizer that depresses cerebral cortex, hypothalamus, limbic system (controls activity and aggression); appears to block dopamine receptors in CTZ, giving antiemetic activity.

Metabolism: Metabolized by the liver, excreted in the urine, bile, and crosses placenta. Enters breast milk. Half-life is 21 hours.

Dosage/Range:

Adult:

- Oral: 3–5 mg q2h × 3–4 doses, beginning 30 minutes before chemotherapy.
- IM: 0.5–2 mg (dose-reduce in elderly patients).

Drug Preparation/Administration:

- Available as 0.5-, 1-, 2-, 5-, 10-, 20-mg tablets; injection: 5 mg/mL.

Drug Interactions:

- Epinephrine: reversal of vasopressor effects; avoid concurrent use.
- CNS depressants: increased sedation; monitor patient closely.

Lab Effects/Interference:

- Rarely, increased alk phos, bili, serum transaminases (AST, ALT).
- Rarely, decreased PT (if patient on warfarin).
- Rarely, decreased serum cholesterol.

Special Considerations:

- Indicated for the management of psychotic disorders, short-term treatment of hyperactive children showing excessive motor activity, schizophrenia; may be used in the management of nausea and vomiting.
- Contraindicated in severe toxic CNS depression or comatose states; individuals with hypersensitivity; patients with Parkinson's disease, blood dyscrasias, brain damage, bone marrow depression, and alcohol or barbiturate withdrawal states.
- Shown to be equivalent to THC and superior to phenothiazines when tested as an antiemetic.

Potential Toxicities/Side Effects and the Nursing Process

I. ALTERATIONS IN SENSORY/PERCEPTUAL PATTERNS related to TARDIVE DYSKINESIA

Defining Characteristics: With chronic use, tardive dyskinesia syndrome occurs, characterized by involuntary, dyskinetic movements; sedation, EPS may occur when used as an antiemetic.

MANAGEMENT

Nursing Implications: Assess baseline level of consciousness and monitor during therapy. Assess for signs/symptoms of EPS (dystonia, tongue protrusion, trismus, opisthotonus), and administer diphenhydramine as ordered.

II. ALTERATION IN OXYGENATION related to LARYNGOSPASM

Defining Characteristics: Laryngospasm, respiratory depression occur rarely.

Nursing Implications: Assess baseline pulmonary status and monitor during therapy. Identify risk factors (concomitant narcotics, CNS depressants), notify physician, and hold drug if respiratory depression occurs or is suspected. Be prepared to institute respiratory support if necessary, and to reverse opiate.

III. ALTERATION IN CARDIAC OUTPUT/PERFUSION related to ORTHOSTATIC HYPOTENSION

Defining Characteristics: Orthostatic hypotension may occur and may precipitate angina; also, tachycardia, EKG changes, and rare cardiac arrest may occur.

Nursing Implications: Assess VS baseline, and monitor during therapy. If hypotension occurs, notify physician and anticipate increasing rate of IV fluids to increase BP. Epinephrine should NOT be used since drug reverses vasopressor effect; rather, metaraminol or norepinephrine should be used.

Drug: metoclopramide hydrochloride (Reglan)

Class: Substituted benzamide.

Mechanism of Action: Procainamide derivative without cardiac effects. Acts both centrally and peripherally. Acts peripherally to enhance the action of acetylcholine at muscarinic synapses and in the CNS to antagonize dopamine. Is primarily a dopamine antagonist blocking the CTZ; also stimulates upper GI tract motility, thus increasing gastric emptying, and opposes retrograde peristalsis of retching.

Metabolism: Metabolized by the liver, excreted in the urine, with a half-life of 4 hours.

Dosage/Range:

Adult:

- Oral: 10 mg qid (gastroparesis).
- IV: 2 mg/kg q2h × 3–5 doses OR 3 mg/kg q2h × 2 doses, beginning 30 minutes prior to chemotherapy. Dose-reduce if renal insufficiency.

Drug Preparation/Administration:

- IV: further dilute in 50 mL 0.9% Sodium Chloride or 5% Dextrose and administer over 15 minutes.

Drug Interactions:

- Digoxin: may decrease absorption; monitor digoxin effectiveness and modify dose as needed.
- Aspirin, acetaminophen, tetracycline, ethanol, levodopa, diazepam: may increase absorption; monitor for drug toxicity.
- CNS depressants: increased depressant effects; monitor patient closely.

Lab Effects/Interference:

- None known.

Special Considerations:

- Indicated as an antiemetic to prevent nausea and vomiting from chemotherapy, delayed gastric emptying, gastroesophageal reflux.
- There is an increased incidence of dystonic reactions in men under 35 years old. Consider diphenhydramine q4h or lorazepam and decadron to minimize dystonic reactions.
- Efficacy as an antiemetic: 60% complete protection against high-dose cisplatin, and increased to 66% with the addition of steroids and lorazepam.
- Contraindicated in patients with prior hypersensitivity to this drug, procaine, or procainamide; patients with seizure disorder, pheochromocytoma, GI obstruction.
- Use cautiously in patients with breast cancer, as may increase prolactin levels, and in patients with renal insufficiency.

Potential Toxicities/Side Effects and the Nursing Process

I. ALTERATIONS IN SENSORY/PERCEPTUAL PATTERNS related to SEDATION, EPS

Defining Characteristics: Sedation, akathisia (restlessness), adverse dystonic or extrapyramidal effects may occur; increased risk in patients < 30 years old.

Nursing Implications: Assess baseline neurologic status, and monitor during therapy. Protect patient safety, and keep all necessary patient equipment at the bedside, e.g., commode. Assess for extrapyramidal side effects, and administer diphenhydramine as ordered. In addition, lorazepam administered as part of combination antiemetics helps to decrease akathisia.

II. POTENTIAL FOR ALTERED BOWEL ELIMINATION related to DIARRHEA

Defining Characteristics: Increase in both esophageal sphincter pressure and gastric emptying, leading to diarrhea with high doses. Action antagonized by narcotics.

Nursing Implications: Assess baseline bowel elimination status. Teach patient to report diarrhea, and administer kaolin/pectin as ordered, or other antidiarrheals. Arrange for commode at the bedside if bathroom far from bed. Also, diarrhea may be prevented by administration of dexamethasone as part of antiemetic regimen.

III. ALTERATION IN COMFORT related to DRY/MOUTH, RASH

Defining Characteristics: Dry mouth, rash, urticaria, hypotension may occur.

Nursing Implications: Assess baseline comfort. Teach patient to report rash, urticaria, and treat symptomatically. Monitor VS, and slow infusion rate if hypotensive, as well as replace IV fluids per physician's order.

Drug: ondansetron hydrochloride (Zofran)

Class: Serotonin antagonist.

Mechanism of Action: Selective 5-HT_3 (serotonin) receptor antagonist and may block 5-HT_3 receptors found peripherally on the vagus nerve terminals and centrally in the CTZ, thus preventing chemotherapy-induced vomiting.

Metabolism: Extensively metabolized, with only 5% of parent compound found in urine.

Dosage/Range:

Adults:

- IV: 0.15 mg/kg q4h × 3 doses OR as a single 32-mg dose, beginning 30 minutes prior to chemotherapy.
- Highly emetogenic chemo: 24 mg po 30 minutes before chemotherapy.
- Moderately emetogenic chemotherapy.
- Oral: 8 mg PO bid, beginning 30 minutes before chemotherapy, and continuing for 1–2 days after chemotherapy.

Drug Preparation/Administration:

- IV available as 2 mg/mL or 32 mg/50 mL; mix in 50 mL 5% Dextrose or 0.9% Sodium Chloride and infuse over 15 minutes.
- Note: single-dose ondansetron (> 22 mg) needs to be given over at least 30 minutes to minimize risk of headache/hypotension.

- Tablets available as either regular tablet or ODT (oral disintegrating tablet), which is freeze-dried and dissolves instantly on the tongue, available in 4-mg and 8-mg strengths.
- Available as an oral solution, 4 mg/5 mL.

Drug Interactions:
- None significant.

Lab Effects/Interference:
- Rarely, increased LFTs.

Special Considerations:
- Contraindicated in patients hypersensitive to the drug.
- Does not affect the dopamine system, so does not cause EPS.
- Approved for use to prevent nausea/vomiting related to chemotherapy, radiation therapy to the abdomen or total body, and following surgery (postoperative).

Potential Toxicities/Side Effects and the Nursing Process

I. ALTERATION IN ELIMINATION related to DIARRHEA or CONSTIPATION

Defining Characteristics: Patients may experience diarrhea (22%) or constipation (11%).

Nursing Implications: Assess baseline elimination status. Teach patient to report alterations, and treat symptomatically.

II. ALTERATION IN COMFORT related to HEADACHE

Defining Characteristics: Headache may occur (16%).

Nursing Implications: Assess comfort level. Teach patient to report headache. Administer acetaminophen as ordered.

III. ALTERATION IN NUTRITION, LESS THAN BODY REQUIREMENTS, related to ↑ LFTs

Defining Characteristics: Transient increases in LFTs may occur (5%).

Nursing Implications: Assess LFTs baseline, and monitor during therapy.

Drug: palonosetron (Aloxi)

Class: Serotonin antagonist antiemetic

Mechanism of Action: Selective serotonin antagonist with strong binding affinity to receptor.

Metabolism: Drug is excreted via renal and metabolic pathways

Dosage/Range:

- Single 0.25 mg IV over 30 seconds 30 minutes before the start of chemotherapy
- Give once every 7 days

Drug Preparation/Administration: Draw up in a syringe to administer IVP over 30 seconds; flush line with Normal Saline prior to and after drug administration.

Drug Interactions: None known.

Lab Effects/Interference: Rare prolongation of QTc interval on ECG (> 500 msec, changes > 60 msec from baseline).

Special Considerations:

- Drug is indicated for:
  - Prevention of acute nausea and vomiting associated with initial and repeat courses of moderately and highly emetogenic cancer chemotherapy.
  - Prevention of delayed nausea and vomiting associated with initial and repeat courses of moderately emetogenic cancer chemotherapy.
- Palonosetron has greater potency, higher binding affinity to the 5-HT3 receptor, and has a longer half life (40 hours) than any of the 1st generation serotonin antagonists.
- Drug should be administered with caution to patients with prolonged conduction intervals (QTc), such as patients who have hypokalemia, hypomagnesemia, are taking diuretics, have congenital QT syndrome, taking anti-arrhythmic drugs or other drugs leading to QTc prolongation such as arsenic, and cumulative high dose anthracycline therapy.

Potential Toxicities/Side Effects and the Nursing Process

I. ALTERATION IN COMFORT related to HEADACHE

Defining Characteristics: Headache occurs in 9% of patients.

Nursing Implications: Teach patients that this may occur, and to take acetaminophen to relieve headache if it occurs.

II. ALTERATION IN BOWEL ELIMINATION related to CONSTIPATION

Defining Characteristics: Constipation occurs in about 5% of patients

Nursing Implications: Assess baseline bowel elimination status. Teach patients that constipation may occur, and to use usual strategies to prevent constipation. If constipation occurs, teach patient to use bowel softeners, laxatives as needed, and to increase oral fluids, fiber, and exercise to promote peristalsis.

Drug: perphenazine

Class: Phenothiazine.

Mechanism of Action: Antipsychotic agent. Blocks dopamine receptors in CTZ; also decreases vagal stimulation of VC by peripheral afferents.

Metabolism: Metabolized by the liver, excreted in the urine, crosses placenta, enters breast milk.

Dosage/Range:

Adult:

- Oral: 4 mg q4–6h.
- IM/IV: 5 mg IVB q4–6h OR 5 mg IVB then infusion at 1 mg/hour for 10 hours.
- Maximum: 30 mg in 24 hours (inpatient), or 15 mg in 24 hours (outpatient).

Drug Preparation/Administration:

- Further dilute IV drug in 50 mL 0.9% Sodium Chloride, and infuse over 20 minutes.

Drug Interactions:

- Antacids: decreased perphenazine absorption; take 2 hours before or after antacid.
- Antidepressants: increased Parkinsonian symptoms; avoid concomitant use or use cautiously.
- Barbiturates: increased CNS depressant effect; use together cautiously, if at all.

Lab Effects/Interference:

- Rarely, increased LFTs.

Special Considerations:

- Effective in management of nausea and vomiting related to moderately emetogenic drugs.
- Contraindicated in patients hypersensitive to the drug, or who have blood dyscrasias, coma.

IV. ALTERATION IN URINARY ELIMINATION related to URINARY RETENTION

Defining Characteristics: Urinary retention may occur.

Nursing Implications: Instruct patient to report this symptom; discuss alternative drug with physician for control of emesis.

Drug: scopolamine

Class: Antimuscarinic; used as an antiemetic.

Mechanism of Action: Appears to prevent nausea/vomiting associated with motion sickness by blocking cholinergic impulses, thus preventing stimulation of the VC.

Dosage/Range:
Adult:
- Patch: transdermal patch 1.5 mg q72h.

Drug Preparation/Administration:
- Apply 4 hours prior to time protection is needed.
- Apply to clean and dry hairless area behind ear; remove clear plastic cover, exposing adhesive layer; apply directly to skin behind ear and press firmly; wash hands.

Drug Interactions:
- None significant.

Lab Effects/Interference:
- None known.

Special Considerations:
- Use cautiously in patients with glaucoma, urinary bladder-neck obstruction.
- Wash hands after handling patch to prevent exposure to scopolamine.
- If patch falls off, wash area, then reapply new patch in another location.

Potential Toxicities/Side Effects and the Nursing Process

I. ALTERATION IN MUCOUS MEMBRANE INTEGRITY related to DRY MOUTH

Defining Characteristics: Dry mouth occurs in 67% of patients.

Nursing Implications: Teach patient this may occur. Suggest patient suck ice chips, sugar-free candy, or practice usual oral hygiene regimen more frequently.

II. ALTERATIONS IN SENSORY/PERCEPTUAL PATTERNS related to DROWSINESS, BLURRED VISION

Defining Characteristics: Drowsiness, blurred vision, mydriasis may occur; rarely, disorientation, restlessness, confusion may occur.

Nursing Implications: Assess baseline mental status. Instruct patient to report changes in vision or feeling state. Assess patient safety needs, and provide safe environment.

Drug: thiethylperazine (Torecan)

Class: Phenothiazine derivative; antiemetic.

Mechanism of Action: Blocks stimulation of CTZ and VC.

Metabolism: Metabolized by liver, excreted by kidneys, crosses placenta, and may be excreted in breast milk.

Dosage/Range:
Adult:
- Oral/PR/IM: 10 mg qd-tid.

Drug Preparation/Administration:
- IM: give deep IM into large muscle mass.
- Do not give IV (causes hypotension).

Drug Interactions:
- Barbiturates: may decrease antiemetic effect; increase dose as needed.
- Antacids: may decrease absorption of thiethylperazine; administer 2 hours before or after antacid.
- Epinephrine: may reverse vasopressor effect of epinephrine; avoid concurrent use.

Lab Effects/Interference:
- Rarely, increased LFTs.

Special Considerations:
- Contraindicated in patients with severe CNS depression, coma, prior sensitivity reaction.
- Contraindicated in patients allergic to dye tartazine (FD + C yellow No 5) as it may cause bronchial asthma.
- Torecan injection contains sodium metabisulfite; contraindicated in patients allergic to sulfites.
- Increased risk of dystonic reactions in men under 35 years old. Consider diphenhydramine or lorazepam and decadron every 4 hours to minimize dystonia.

Potential Toxicities/Side Effects and the Nursing Process

I. ALTERATIONS IN SENSORY/PERCEPTUAL PATTERNS related to DROWSINESS, EPS

Defining Characteristics: Drowsiness may occur after IM injection. Rarely, extrapyramidal side effects may occur (i.e., dystonia, torticollis, akathisia, gait disturbances), as may blurred vision and tinnitus.

Nursing Implications: Assess baseline level of consciousness, and monitor during therapy. Assess for signs/symptoms of EPS (dystonia, tongue protrusion, trismus, opisthotonus), and administer diphenhydramine as ordered.

II. ALTERATION IN CARDIAC OUTPUT related to HYPOTENSION

Defining Characteristics: Hypotension may occur after IM dosing; rarely, tachycardia, EKG changes occur.

Nursing Implications: Assess baseline VS, and monitor during IV administration. Administer drug slowly, and notify physician if hypotension occurs. Anticipate increasing IV fluids.

Chapter 8
Anorexia and Cachexia

Anorexia and weight loss may be presenting symptoms of cancer, or symptoms of advanced disease. No other symptoms may cause more powerful distress to a patient than being confronted with weight loss and inability to eat due to anorexia. Consequences of severe anorexia include nutritional depletion and further weight loss, which result in decreased functional status, diminished treatment responses to chemotherapy, and apparent decreased quality of life. Primary cachexia, or wasting syndrome, occurs in at least two-thirds of patients with advanced cancer or human immunodeficiency virus (HIV) disease. The associated extreme weakness and fatigue lead to incapacity, dependency, social isolation, and again, apparent diminished quality of life.

In addition, anorexia and cachexia can be terrifying and frustrating to family members. The patient's spouse may be used to nurturing the patient and preparing meals, and feel rejected and frightened by a loved one's inability to eat. This may symbolize personal failure on the part of the spouse, as well as failure of current treatment to reverse the disease process and a poor prognosis.

Metabolically, cachexia appears to result from chronic, systemic inflammation with the release of acute-phase proteins and orchestration by cytokines such as tumor necrosis factor, IL-1 and IL-6 (Laviano et al, 2002). This leads to the preferential breakdown of skeletal muscle protein and body fat, resulting in the profound wasting syndrome characterized by anorexia, early satiety, weight loss, decreased function, and death (Inui, 2002). Secondary cachexia is simple starvation from decreased food intake or defective nutrient absorption, and results from situations such as nausea, vomiting, and anorexia due to chemotherapy. As expected, patients responding to chemotherapy will show a weight gain.

Pharmacologic agents used to stimulate appetite are varied in mechanism of action, efficacy, and strength of evidence. Corticosteroids have been tried for many years, with usual effect within 1-3 weeks (Ottery et al, 1998; Loprinzi et al, 1999). However, side effects have limited their usefulness, such as insomnia, muscle catabolism, hyperglycemia. Of the studies of pharmacologic agents in the treatment of anorexia and cachexia in cancer, megestrol acetate has shown statistical improvement in nonfluid weight gain (Ottery, 1998). Mantovani et al (1998) suggest that megestrol acetate, in fact, downregulates cytokine production, resulting in increased appetite and anabolism. There appears to be a dose-response effect, and Loprinzi et al (1992) showed optimal weight gain at a dose of 800 mg/day. Patients showed increased appetite, increased food intake, weight gain, and less nausea and vomiting. The incidence of thrombophlebitis was 6%. Loprinzi et al also demonstrated that the weight gain resulting from megestrol acetate is increased fat and lean body mass, not water gain (i.e., edema, ascites).

Thalidomide, an agent originally developed as a nonbarbiturate sedative but which was never marketed as such due to its teratogenicity, has been shown to increase weight gain and lean body mass in HIV-infected individuals with cachexia (Ottery, 1998).

Metoclopramide, at low doses for stimulation of GI motility, has been shown to decrease early satiety and postprandial fullness, and may be helpful for some patients (Kris et al, 1985). Cannabinoid derivatives, such as δ-9-tetrahydrocannabinol (THC) and dronabinol, appear to stimulate appetite and possible weight gain in some patients (Beal et al, 1997; Klausner et al, 1996; Kaplan et al, 1998). Other agents that are being studied are eicosapentaenoic (EPA) acid (fish oil, stabilize acute phase proteins) and melatonin (regulation of circadian rhythm) [Cunningham, 2003].

References

Beal JE, et al. Long-term Efficacy and Safety of Dronabinol for Acquired Immunodeficiency Syndrome-associated Anorexia. *J Pain Symptom Manage.* 1997;14(1):7–14

Brown JK. A Systematic Review of the Evidence on Symptom Management of Cancer-related Anorexia and Cachexia. *Oncol Nurs Forum* 2002;29:517–530

Bruera E, Macmillan K, Kuehn N, et al. A Controlled Trial of Megestrol Acetate on Appetite, Caloric Intake, Nutritional Status, and Other Symptoms in Patients with Advanced Cancer. *Cancer* 1990;66:1279–1282

Chlebowski RT, Bulcavage L, Grosvenor M, et al. Hydrazine Sulfate Influence on Nutritional Status and Survival in NSCLC. *J Clin Oncol* 1990;8:9–15

Cunningham RS. The Anorexia-Cachexia Syndrome, chapter 9. Yarbro CH, Frogge MH, Goodman M, (eds), *Cancer Symptom Management,* 3rd ed. Sudbury, MA: Jones and Bartlett Publishers 2003;137–155

Dreizen S, McCredie KB, Keating MJ, et al. Nutritional Deficiencies in Patients Receiving Cancer Chemotherapy. *Postgrad Med J* 1990;87:163–170

Enck RE. Anorexia and Cachexia: An Update. *Am J Hospice Palliative Care* 1990;7(5):13–15

Inui A. Cancer Anorexia-Cachexia Syndrome: Current issues in Research and Management. *CACancer J Clin* 2002;52:72–91

Kaplan G, Schambelan M, Gottleib C, et al. Thalidomide Reverses Cachexia in HIV-Wasting Syndrome. *5th International Conf on Retroviruses and Opportunistic Infections, Abstract 476. February 1-5, 1998, Chicago, IL* 1998

Klausner JD, Makonkawkeyoon S, Akarasewi P, et al. The Effect of Thalidomide on the Pathogenesis of Human Immunodeficiency Virus Type 1 and M. tuberculosis Infection. *J Acquir Immune Defic Syndr and Hum Retrovirology* 1996;11:247–257

Kornblith AB, Hollis D, Phillips CA, et al. Effect of Megestrol Acetate upon Quality of Life in Advanced Breast Cancer Patients in a Dose Response Trial. . *Proc American Society of Clinical Oncologists* 1992;11:377

Kris MG, Yeh SDJ, Gralla RJ, et al. Symptomatic Gastroparesis in Cancer Patients: Possible Cause of Anorexia That Can Be Improved with Oral Metoclopramide. *Proc American Society of Clinical Oncologists* 1985;4:267

Laviano A, Russo M, Freda F, et al. Neurochemical Mechanisms for Cancer Cachexia. *Nutrition* 2002;18:100–105

Loprinzi CL, Ellison NM, Schard OJ, et al. Controlled Trial of Megestrol Acetate for the Treatment of Cancer Anorexia and Cachexia. *J Natl Cancer Inst* 1990;82: 1127–1132

Loprinzi CL, Jensen M, Burnham N, et al. Body Composition Changes in Cancer Patients Who GainWeight from Megestrol Acetate. *Proc American Society of Clinical Oncologists* 1992;11:378

Loprinzi CL, Kugler JW, Sloan JA, et al. Randomized Comparison of Megestrol Acetate versus Dexamethasone versus Fluoxymesterone for the Treatment of Cancer Anorexia/Cachexia. *J Clin Oncol* 1999;17:3299–3306

Loprinzi CL, Mailliard J, Schaid D, et al. Dose/Response Evaluation of Megestrol Acetate for the Treatment of Cancer Anorexia/Cachexia: A Mayo Clinic and North Central Cancer Treatment Group Trial. *Proc American Society of Clinical Oncologists* 1992;11:378

Mantovani G, Maccio A, Paola L, et al. Cytokine Activity in Cancer-related Anorexia/Cachexia: Role of megestrol Acetate and Medroxyprogesterone Acetate. *Semin Oncol* 1998;25 (suppl):45–52

Ottery FD, Walsh D, Strawford A. Pharmacologic Management of Anorexia/Cachexia. *Semin Oncol* 1998;25 (suppl):35–44

Drug: dronabinol (Marinol)

Class: Cannabinoid.

Mechanism of Action: Stimulates appetite in acquired immunodeficiency syndrome (AIDS) patients, leading to trends toward improved body weight and mood.

Metabolism: 90–95% absorption after oral dose, but because of first-pass effect of the liver and high lipid solubility, only about 20% of the dose reaches the systemic circulation. Large area of distribution so that drug continues to be excreted for a long period of time. The appetite stimulation effect may persist for 24 hours from a single dose.

Dosage/Range:
- 2.5 mg bid before lunch and supper, or if patient is intolerant, a single 2.5-mg dose may be taken at bedtime.

Drug Preparation:
- Available in 2.5-, 5-, or 10-mg gel capsules that harden under refrigeration.

Drug Administration:
- Oral.

Drug Interactions:
- Amphetamines, cocaine: additive hypertension, tachycardia.
- Atropine, scopolamine: tachycardia, drowsiness.
- Amitriptyline, tricyclic antidepressants: additive tachycardia, hypertension.
- Barbiturates, CNS depressants, buspirone: drowsiness and additive CNS depression.
- Theophylline: increased metabolism.

Lab Effects/Interference:
- None known.

Special Considerations:
- Drug has antiemetic qualities.

Potential Toxicities/Side Effects and the Nursing Process

I. ALTERATIONS IN SENSORY/PERCEPTUAL PATTERNS related to CNS CHANGES

Defining Characteristics: Drug can cause changes in mood, cognition, memory, and perception. In addition, nervousness, anxiety, confusion, dizziness, depersonalization, euphoria, paranoid reaction, somnolence, and thinking abnormalities can occur. Drug has abuse potential.

Nursing Implications: Assess appropriateness of drug for patient, as this would not be the drug of choice for a substance abuser, either one who is actively using or who has withdrawn and is abstaining because of abuse potential. Teach patient of possible side effects, and self-care strategies to avoid heightened fear or anxiety.

II. POTENTIAL FOR ALTERATION IN OXYGENATION related to SYMPATHOMIMETIC EFFECTS

Defining Characteristics: Tachycardia and conjunctival injection may occur. Drug interactions may cause hypertension.

Nursing Implications: Review patient medication profile to identify any possible drug interactions. Monitor appetite stimulation effects, and weigh these against any sympathomimetic changes.

Drug: megestrol acetate (Megace)

Class: Synthetic progestin.

Mechanism of Action: Alters malignant cell environment in hormonally sensitive tumors, discouraging tumor cell proliferation; appears to stimulate appetite and weight gain in cancer cachexia directly or indirectly through antagonism of TNF. Designated as orphan drug by FDA for management of anorexia, cachexia, or weight loss > 10% of baseline. Approved for AIDS-related cachexia.

Metabolism: Well absorbed from GI tract. Metabolized in liver and excreted by kidneys.

Dosage/Range:
- Optimal dose for management of cachexia is 800 mg/day in a single dose.

Drug Preparation/Administration:
- Store in tight container at temperature < 40°C (104°F).
- Oral administration.

Drug Interactions:
- None.

Lab Effects/Interference:
- Rarely, may increase glucose, lactic dehydrogenase (LDH).

Special Considerations:
- Drug is expensive.
- One-third of patients with metastatic cancer gain weight.
- Weight gain appears to be from increased fat stores rather than water gain (Loprinzi, et al 1992).

Potential Toxicities/Side Effects and the Nursing Process

I. ALTERATIONS IN PERFUSION related to DEEP VEIN THROMBOSIS

Defining Characteristics: Rarely, 6% of patients may experience deep vein thrombosis (DVT) or pulmonary emboli.

Nursing Implications: Assess baseline peripheral vascular status and monitor during therapy. Teach patient to report pain in calf, erythema, shortness of breath, chest pain immediately.

II. ALTERATION IN COMFORT related to CARPAL TUNNEL SYNDROME NIV, TUMOR FLARE

Defining Characteristics: Carpal tunnel syndrome, nausea, vomiting, tumor flare may occur rarely.

MANAGEMENT

limbs, slight postural tremor, leg cramps, absent ankle jerks. IF treatment is continued, there is permanent paresthesias of feet and hands, which progresses proximally. Increased risk of occurrence with increased age (> 70 years old) and high total doses > 14 g (40–50 g).

Nursing Implications: Assess baseline neurologic status, especially presence of peripheral neuropathy. Teach patient to stop drug and report immediately dysesthesias, numbness, and/or muscle cramps. Perform assessment for peripheral neuropathy at every visit.

III. ALTERATION IN SENSORY/PERCEPTUAL PATTERNS related to DROWSINESS

Defining Characteristics: Drug has nonbarbiturate sedative qualities, and drowsiness is the most frequent side effect. Tolerance to daytime drowsiness occurs over several weeks of use. Drowsiness and dizziness are more frequent at doses of 20–400 mg/day than at lower doses. HIV-infected patient studies reported drowsiness, dizziness, and mood changes 33–100% of the time.

Nursing Implications: Assess baseline alertness, sleep patterns. Assess other drugs taken, especially those with sedating qualities, and alcohol ingestion. Instruct patient to avoid alcohol and to take drug at bedtime. Assess degree of drowsiness and dizziness and safety of patient. If significant, teach measures to ensure safety. Tell patient that tolerance develops over 2–3 weeks.

IV. ALTERATION IN SKIN INTEGRITY, POTENTIAL, related to RASH

Defining Characteristics: Pruritic, erythematous macular rash may appear over trunk and back 2–13 days after initiation of therapy. Increased incidence in patients with HIV infection with low CD4 counts. Drug rechallenge often results in immediate reaction of rash, tachycardia, and fever. Rash resolves with drug discontinuation.

Nursing Implications: Teach patient to self-assess for rash, and instruct to discontinue drug and report rash to nurse or physician immediately. If necessary, manage symptomatic itching with antihistamines.

V. ALTERATION IN ELIMINATION related to CONSTIPATION

Defining Characteristics: Mild constipation occurs in 3–30% of patients.

Nursing Implications: Instruct patient to prevent constipation by using stool softeners, mild laxatives if needed (e.g., milk of magnesia), and to use bulk (e.g., psyllium). In addition, teach dietary interventions (e.g., increased fiber, fluids of 3 qt/day), and mild exercise. Instruct patient to report constipation unresponsive to these interventions.

VI. POTENTIAL FOR INFECTION related to NEUTROPENIA

Defining Characteristics: Rare (< 1%) in most patients, but increased incidence of 2–20% in HIV-infected patients. Average onset 6–7 weeks after initiation of treatment (range, 3–12 weeks).

Nursing Implications: Determine baseline WBC and absolute neutrophil count (ANC). Do not initiate therapy if ANC < 750/mm^3. If on treatment, ANC < 750/ mm^3, consider drug discontinuance, but definitely drug should be discontinued if ANC < 500/mm^3. Drug may be reinstituted after neutrophil recovery (e.g., G-CSF). WBC and ANC should be monitored closely in HIV-infected patients (e.g., every other week for three months), and then at least every month. In non-HIV-infected patients, monitor baseline and monthly.

Chapter 9

Anxiety and Depression

Anxiety and depression in response to uncertainty and hopelessness are frequently associated with the cancer experience. Studies have shown that anxiety increases with the cancer diagnosis and remains elevated to some degree throughout treatment, regardless of modality or setting (Clark, 1990). Nursing efforts are aimed at anxiety-reducing strategies such as helping the patient explore the anxiety and find anxiety-reducing activities (e.g., relaxation exercises, verbalization of feelings). Nurses can also refer patients for specialized support if necessary, and, as appropriate, teach patients and their families about prescribed anxiolytic medications. Depression is an often expected response to the cancer experience, to an actual or perceived loss of health, role, and life. It also may be associated with chronic cancer pain and can clearly adversely affect quality of life. Prominent features may be perceived loss of self-esteem, worthlessness, hopelessness, guilt, and sadness. Symptoms include a change in appetite, sleeplessness, lethargy, and social withdrawal. Nurses use caring and compassion to help patients who are depressed acknowledge and explore their feelings. Through patient teaching and supportive counseling, short-term realistic and achievable goals can often be negotiated by patient and nurse. Now, nurses are helping patients to make the "mountain" more "manageable."

It is generally accepted that depression results from a deficiency in key neurotransmitters, resulting in either an over- or underexpression of neurotransmitters that control the release or breakdown of the neurotransmitters (Barsevick and Much, 2003).

The tricyclic antidepressant (TCA) medications have long been the cornerstone of managing cancer-related depression, partially because of their ability to improve sleeplessness and to enhance analgesia. However, these drugs also have undesirable side effects, such as dry mouth, constipation, and blurred vision. Newer antidepressant medications are now available and have found a firm niche in oncology care. The selective serotonin reuptake inhibitors (SSRIs) are quite effective for many patients and have few side effects, together with a short half-life. More recently, serotonin-norepinephrine reuptake inhibitors (SNRIs) have been developed. An example included in this chapter is venlafaxine, which has shown equal efficacy to fluoxetine (Prozac) without the significant side effects (Silverstone, 1999; Costa SJ, 1998).

Massie and Popkin (1998) suggest principles to guide antidepressant therapy in patients with cancer: start with a lower dose, slowly increase the dose as the therapeutic dose may be lower than that in non-cancer patients, and monitor very carefully for side effects as there may be overlapping toxicity in organ systems (with chemotherapy, the malignancy).

In addition, it is important to do a thorough assessment of herbs used in the management of anxiety and depression, as these may be interact with pharmacologic agents. For example, Mathijssen et al (2002) found that St. John's wort induces the metabolism of SN-38 via the cytochrome P450 CYP3A4 subsystem, lowering serum levels by up 42% with an effect lasting up to 3 weeks. Table 9.1 depicts anti-anxiety and antidepressant agents commonly prescribed.

Table 9.1 Agents Commonly Used in the Management of Anxiety and Depression in Patients with Cancer

Drug	Dose Range (oral)	Half-Life or Onset of Therapeutic Effect	Common Side Effects	Comments
Anti-anxiety				
Alprazolam (Xanax)	0.5–0.6 mg/day (max 2 mg/day)	10–15 hrs half-life	Sedation, confusion, motor incoordination, somnolence	Short half-life
Diazepam (Valium, valrelease)	2–40 mg/day (usual max dose 20 mg/day)	20–70 hrs half-life	Drowsiness, fatigue, lethargy, weakness, rash, vivid dreams, feeling "hung over"	Long half-life, so accumulation of active metabolites; fast absorption
Lorazepam (Ativan)	2–6 mg/day (usual max dose 3 g/day)	10–20 hr half-life	Drowsiness, fatigue, lethargy, weakness, rash, vivid dreams	Short half-life with intermediate absorption
Oxazepam (Serax)	30–120 mg/day (usual max dose 60 mg/day)	5–15 hrs	Drowsiness, fatigue, lethargy, weakness, rash, vivid dreams	Short half life
Antidepressants				
SSRIs				
Paroxetine (Paxil)	10–50 mg	Onset 3–10 days	Nausea, dry mouth, rash, headache, drowsiness, loss of libido, postural hypotension	Caution in elderly, patients with renal or hepatic dysfunction, suicidal ideation

Table 9.1 *(continued)*

Drug	Dose Range (oral)	Half-Life or Onset of Therapeutic Effect	Common Side Effects	Comments
Sertraline (Zoloft)	50–200 mg	Onset 7 days	Same as paroxetine	Same
Fluoxetine (Prozac)	20 mg	Onset 2–4 weeks	Same as paroxetine	Same
TCAs				
Amitriptyline (Elavil)	25–250 mg	Onset 4–6 weeks	Anticholinergic (urinary retention, dry mouth, thirst, blurred vision, sedation) and antihistaminic (sedation); tachycardia, orthostatic hypotension, arrythmia; withdrawal reaction	Caution in patients with suicidal ideation, cardiac/renal or hepatic dysfunction; don't stop drug abruptly; do baseline EKG and assess toxicity
Desipramine (Norpramin)	25–150 mg	4–6 weeks	Same as amitriptyline	Same as amitriptyline; serum level correlates with therapeutic effect
Doxepin (Sinequan)	50–150 mg	4–6 weeks	Same amitriptyline	Same as amitriptyline
Imipramine (Tofranil)	25–150 mg	4–6 weeks	Same amitriptyline	Same as amitriptyline; serum level correlates with therapeutic effect
Nortriptyline (Pamelor)	50–150 mg	4–6 weeks	Same as amitriptyline	Same as amitriptyline; serum level correlates with therapeutic effect
Trazodone (Dyseril)	50–250 mg	1–4 weeks	Same as amitriptyline	Same as amitriptyline

Table 9.1 *(continued)*

Drug	Dose Range (oral)	Half-Life or Onset of Therapeutic Effect	Common Side Effects	Comments
SNRI				
Venlafaxine HCl (Effexor)	75–225 mg/da	1–4 weeks	Emotional lability, vertigo, trismus, nausea	Use cautiously in elderly, patients with cardiac/renal or hepatic dysfunction
Nefazodone HCl (Serzone)	200–600 mg/da	1–4 weeks	Dizziness, drowsiness, dry mouth, headache	Use cautiously in elderly, patients with cardiac/renal or hepatic dysfunction

Modified from: Barsevick AM and Much JK (2003) Depression, chapter 34 in *Cancer Symptom Management,* 3rd ed, Yarbro CH, Frogge MH, Goodman M (eds). Sudbury, MA, Jones and Bartlett Publishers, pp. 668–692; Goebel BH (2003) Anxiety, chapter 33 in *Cancer Symptom Management,* 3rd ed, Yarbro CH, Frogge MH, Goodman M (eds). Sudbury, MA, Jones and Bartlett Publishers, pp. 651–668

MANAGEMENT

References

Barsevick AM, Much JK. Depression, chapter 34. Yarbro CH, Frogge MH, Goodman M, (eds), *Cancer Symptom Management,* 3rd ed. Sudbury, MA: Jones and Bartlett Publishers 2003;668–692

Clark J. Psychosocial Dimensions: The Patient. Groenwald S, Frogge MH, Goodman M, Yarbro CH, (eds), *Cancer Nursing Principles and Practice,* 2nd ed. Sudbury, MA: Jones and Bartlett Publishers 1990

Costa E Silva J. Randomized, Double-blind Comparison of Venlafaxine and Fluoxetine in Outpatients with Major Depression. *J Clin Psychiatry* 1998;59:352–353

Forest Pharmaceuticals. Celexa® package Insert. St. Louis, Forest Pharmaceuticals, Inc 1998

Gerchufsky M. The Art and Science of Prescribing Psychiatric Medications. *ADVANCE for Nurse Practitioners* 1997;4(3):33–36

Goebel BH. Anxiety, chapter 33. Yarbro CH, Frogge MH, Goodman M, (eds), *Cancer Symptom Management,* 3rd ed. Sudbury, MA: Jones and Bartlett Publishers 2003; 651–668

Massie MJ, Popkin MK. Depressive disorders, chapter 10. Holland JC, (eds), *Psycho-Oncology.* New York NY: Oxford University Press 1998;518–540

Mathijssen RH, Verweij J, de Bruijn P, et al. Effects of St. John's Wort on Irinotecan Metabolism. *J Natl Cancer Instit* 2002;94(16):1247–9

..rstone PH, Ravindran A. Once Daily Venlafaxine Extended Release (XR) Compared with Fluoxetine in Outpatients with Depression and Anxiety. *J Clin Psychiatry* 1999;60:22–24

Drug: alprazolam (Xanax)

Class: Benzodiazepine (anxiolytic).

Mechanism of Action: Binds to benzodiazepine receptors in the CNS (limbic and cortical areas, cerebellum, brain stem, and spinal cord), resulting in the following effects: anxiolytic, ataxia, anticonvulsant, muscle relaxation. Appears to potentiate the effects of γ-aminobutyric acid (GABA).

Metabolism: Well absorbed from GI tract. Widely distributed in body tissues and fluids, including CSF. Crosses placenta and is excreted in breast milk. Highly bound to plasma proteins. Metabolized in liver and excreted in urine. Short elimination time; half-life of 12–15 hours. May produce psychological and physical dependence. Indicated for management of anxiety, the short-term relief of anxiety associated with depression, and panic disorder.

Dosage/Range:

Adult:

- Anxiety: 0.25–0.5 mg PO tid (may gradually increase dose q3–4 days over time to maximum 4 mg/day in divided doses).
- Elderly/debilitated: 0.25 mg PO bid.
- Discontinue drug by decreasing dose by 0.25–0.5 mg q3–7 days.
- Drug should be used for short-term use only (< 4 months).
- Panic: optimal dosage not determined; titrate dose and increase slowly.

Drug Preparation:

- Store in tight, light-resistant containers at 15–30°C (59–86°F).

Drug Administration:

- Orally, in divided doses.
- May take with food if stomach upset occurs.

Drug Interactions:

- CNS depressants (alcohol, anticonvulsants, phenothiazines, opiates): additive CNS depression; avoid concurrent use or use cautiously and monitor carefully.
- Oral contraceptives, isoniazid, ketoconazole, or cimetidine: decrease plasma clearance of alprazolam so may increase effect (e.g., sedation); monitor patient closely.
- Tricyclic antidepressants: increased serum levels of antidepressant possible; use together cautiously.

- Digoxin: may decrease renal excretion of digoxin; monitor for overdosage; may need to decrease digoxin.

Lab Effects/Interference:

- No consistent pattern of interaction between benzodiazepines and laboratory tests.

Special Considerations:

- Wide margin of safety between therapeutic and toxic doses.
- May impair ability to perform activities requiring mental alertness (e.g., driving a car, operating machinery).
- May produce psychological and physical dependence.
- Administer cautiously in patients with liver or renal impairment.
- Use cautiously in patients with chronic pulmonary disease or sleep apnea.
- Contraindicated in patients with depressive neuroses, psychotic reactions (without prominent anxiety), acute alcoholic intoxication (with depressed VS), known hypersensitivity to the drug, or acute angle-closure glaucoma.
- May cause fetal damage so should not be used during pregnancy or if the mother is breast-feeding.
- Withdrawal symptoms (including seizure, delirium) can occur with rapid drug discontinuance in patients taking high or chronic doses.
- If manic episodes or hyperactivity occur soon after drug started, drug should be discontinued.
- Drug should not be used to manage "everyday stress."

Potential Toxicities/Side Effects and the Nursing Process

I. ALTERATIONS IN SENSORY/PERCEPTUAL PATTERNS related to CNS DEPRESSION

Defining Characteristics: CNS depressant effects include drowsiness, fatigue, lethargy, confusion, weakness, headache, which may occur initially and resolve with continued therapy or dose reduction. Vivid dreams, suicidal ideation, and bizarre behavior also may occur. Patient risk factors: elderly, debilitated, liver dysfunction, low serum albumin.

Nursing Implications: Assess baseline neurologic status and risk factors, and monitor during treatment. Instruct patient to report signs/symptoms and discuss drug modification with physician. Evaluate patient satisfaction with drug efficacy. If patient expresses suicidal ideation (more common in panic disorders), refer patient for psychiatric evaluation and drug modification. Instruct patient to avoid alcohol while taking drug. Teach patient prescribed schedule for discontinuing drug when used chronically: assess for signs/symptoms of withdrawal (increased anxiety, rebound insomnia; may also include agitation, dysphoria, nausea/vomiting, irritability, muscle cramps, hallucinations, seizures).

II. ALTERATION IN NUTRITION, LESS THAN BODY REQUIREMENTS, related to GI SIDE EFFECTS

Defining Characteristics: Nausea, vomiting, weight increase or decrease, dry mouth, constipation may occur; also, elevated serum LFTs.

Nursing Implications: Assess baseline nutrition and elimination patterns and LFTs, and monitor during therapy. Discuss abnormalities and drug modification with physician. Teach patient to self-administer prescribed antiemetics as appropriate.

III. POTENTIAL FOR INJURY related to DECREASE IN MENTAL ALERTNESS, PHYSICAL COORDINATION

Defining Characteristics: Drug may cause drowsiness, dizziness, and impair physical coordination, mental alertness.

Nursing Implications: Assess other medications that may increase risk (e.g., opiates, phenothiazenes) and response to drug. Instruct patient to avoid potentially hazardous activities, including driving a car, operating machinery.

IV. ALTERATIONS IN CARDIAC OUTPUT related to RHYTHM DISTURBANCES, VASODILATION

Defining Characteristics: Drug may cause bradycardia, tachycardia, hyper- or hypotension, palpitations, edema.

Nursing Implications: Assess baseline VS, and monitor during therapy. Discuss abnormalities with physician. Instruct patient to report dizziness on standing or other changes.

V. ALTERATIONS IN SKIN INTEGRITY related to RASH

Defining Characteristics: Urticaria, pruritus, rash (morbilliform, urticarial, or maculopapular) may occur.

Nursing Implications: Assess baseline skin integrity, and instruct patient to report changes. Teach symptomatic skin management, and discuss drug discontinuance with physician if severe.

Drug: amitriptyline hydrochloride (Elavil)

Class: Tricyclic antidepressant.

Mechanism of Action: Blocks reuptake of neurotransmitters at neuronal membrane, thus increasing available serotonin, norepinephrine in CNS, and potentiating their effects. Appears to have analgesic effect separate from antidepressant action. May increase bioavailability of morphine. Indicated in the treatment of depressive (affective) mood disorders. Also used as an adjuvant analgesic in cancer pain management.

Metabolism: Well absorbed from GI tract. Distributed to lungs, heart, brain, liver; highly bound to plasma, proteins. Plasma half-life of 10–50 hours. Metabolized in liver, excreted in urine and, to a lesser degree, in bile and feces.

Dosage/Range:

Adult:

- Oral: 25–100 mg PO hs divided or single dose; may increase to 200–300 mg/day (300 mg maximum).
- Cancer pain: 25 mg/day hs; may increase by 25 mg of 1–2 days to 75–150 mg, when desired relief level is reached; may start at 10 mg in elderly.
- Elderly: 30 mg/day in divided doses.
- Intramuscular (IM): 20–30 mg qid or as single dose at bedtime.

Drug Preparation/Administration:

- Oral: store in well-closed containers at 15–30°C (59–86°F); store Elavil 10-mg capsules away from light. Administer as a single bedtime dose.
- IM: administer IM in large muscle mass; change to oral as soon as possible.

Drug Interactions:

- Monamine oxidase inhibitors (MAOIs): increased excitation, hyperpyrexia, seizures; use together cautiously (especially if high dose is used).
- CNS depressants (alcohol, sedatives, hypnotics): increase CNS depression; use together cautiously.
- Sympathomimetic (epinephrine, amphetamines): increased hypertension; AVOID concurrent use.
- Cimetidine methylphenidate: increased amitriptyline levels, increased toxicity; use cautiously and monitor for increased toxicity.
- Warfarin: may increase PT; monitor closely and decrease dose of warfarin as needed.

Lab Effects/Interference:

- None known; bone marrow depression uncommon.

Special Considerations:

- Antidepressant effect may take two weeks or longer.
- Adjuvant analgesic useful in cancer pain management.
- May also decrease depression associated with chronic cancer pain and promote improved sleep.
- Contraindicated in patients with myocardial infarction, seizure disorder, or benign prostatic hypertrophy.
- Use cautiously in patients with urine retention, narrow-angle glaucoma, hyperthyroidism, hepatic dysfunction, or suicidal ideation.

- Drug should be gradually discontinued rather than abruptly withdrawn to prevent anxiety, malaise, dizziness, nausea/vomiting.
- May be helpful in treating hiccups.
- Increased anticholinergic side effects in elderly.

Potential Toxicities/Side Effects and the Nursing Process

I. ALTERATIONS IN SENSORY/PERCEPTUAL PATTERNS related to DROWSINESS, FATIGUE, EPS

Defining Characteristics: Drowsiness, dizziness, weakness, lethargy, and fatigue are common; confusion, disorientation, hallucinations may occur in the elderly. Extrapyramidal symptoms may occur (fine tremor, rigidity, dystonia, dysarthria, dysphagia), as may peripheral neuropathy and blurred vision.

Nursing Implications: Assess baseline gait, neurologic and mental status, and monitor during therapy. Instruct patient to report signs/symptoms; discuss benefit/risk ratio with physician. Assess for signs/symptoms of suicidal ideation; if they occur, refer for psychiatric evaluation. Inform patient that drowsiness, dizziness will resolve after 1–2 weeks; instruct to avoid hazardous activities while drowsy (e.g., driving a car, operating machinery).

II. ALTERATION IN CARDIAC OUTPUT related to POSTURAL HYPOTENSION, TACHYCARDIA

Defining Characteristics: Postural hypotension, EKG changes, tachycardia, hypertension may occur.

Nursing Implications: Assess baseline orthostatic BP, heart rate, and monitor during therapy. Instruct patient to report abnormalities, including postural dizziness, palpitations. Drug should be stopped several days before surgery to prevent hypertensive crisis, especially if high dose.

III. ALTERATION IN NUTRITION, LESS THAN BODY REQUIREMENTS, related to GI SIDE EFFECTS

Defining Characteristics: Dry mouth, anorexia, nausea, vomiting, diarrhea, abdominal cramping may occur; also, elevated LFTs.

Nursing Implications: Assess baseline nutrition and elimination patterns and LFTs, and monitor during therapy. Discuss abnormalities with physician, and discuss drug modification. Teach patient to self-administer prescribed antiemetics as appropriate. LFTs should be repeated, and if still elevated, the drug should be discontinued. Teach patient to take full dose at bedtime. Suggest patient use sugar-free hard candy, frequent ice chips, or artificial saliva for dry mouth.

IV. ALTERATION IN URINARY ELIMINATION related to URINARY RETENTION

Defining Characteristics: Urinary retention may occur. Increased risk if patient has history of urinary retention.

Nursing Implications: Assess baseline urinary elimination pattern and risk. Assess for urinary retention, and instruct patient to report signs/symptoms. Discuss alternative drug with physician if this occurs.

V. ALTERATIONS IN SKIN INTEGRITY related to ALLERGY

Defining Characteristics: Urticaria, erythema, rash, and photosensitivity may occur.

Nursing Implications: Assess baseline drug allergy history and skin integrity. Instruct patient to report skin changes. If angioedema of face, tongue develops, discuss drug discontinuance with physician. Instruct patient to avoid sunlight or to use sunblock protection.

Drug: bupropion hydrochloride (Wellbutrin)

Class: Aminoketone antidepressant.

Mechanism of Action: Unknown. Does block reuptake of serotonin, norepinephrine, and dopamine weakly; does not inhibit MAO; has CNS stimulant effects.

Metabolism: Peak plasma level 2 hours after oral administration, and it appears that only a small percentage of the dose reaches the systemic circulation. Half-life about 14 hours (8–24 hours average). Four major metabolites, with significantly longer elimination half-lives. Primarily excreted in the urine (87%) and to a lesser extent in the feces (10%).

Dosage/Range:

Adult:

- Initial dose: 100 mg bid for at least 3 days.
- Based on response, may increase to usual dose of 100 mg tid (300 mg total dose/day).
- If after 4 weeks of treatment there is no clinical response, may increase to a maximum of 450 mg/day (150 mg tid).

Drug Preparation/Administration:

- Available in 75-mg and 100-mg tablets.
- Protect tablets from light and moisture.
- Ensure at least 4 hours between doses (optimally, give in morning and evening).

Drug Interactions:

- Because of extensive drug metabolism by liver, when given with other drugs that have hepatic metabolism may have decreased effect of that drug (e.g., carbamazepine, cimetidine, phenobarbital, phenytoin).
- MAOIs may increase drug toxicity.
- Use cautiously in patients receiving L-dopa, starting with small initial dose, and slowly increasing dose.
- Use cautiously in patients receiving other seizure-threshold-lowering drugs, starting with small initial dose, and slowly and gradually increasing dose.
- Bupropion, (Zyban; smoking cessation aid): DO NOT USE TOGETHER, as will increase risk of seizures.

Lab Effects/Interference:

- Rarely, anemia and pancytopenia.

Special Considerations:

- Contraindicated in patients with seizure disorder, present/past history of bulimia, or anorexia nervosa.
- Contraindicated in patients receiving MAOI; if MAOI is discontinued, wait at least 14 days before starting bupropion HCl.
- Risk of seizures for patients receiving drug at a dose of 450 mg is 0.4% and appears related to dose and predisposing factors, such as prior seizure, head trauma, CNS tumor, and concomitant medications that lower seizure threshold (e.g., antipsychotics, other antidepressants, abrupt cessation of a benzodiazepine medication, use or abrupt cessation of alcohol).
- Avoid alcohol when taking drug.
- Can precipitate manic episodes in patients with bipolar manic depression or can activate latent psychoses.
- Use cautiously, if at all, in individuals who are underweight, as drug may cause weight loss of at least 2.25 kg (5 lb) (28% of patients), and most patients do not gain weight (only 9% of patients gain weight).
- Drug contains same ingredient found in burpropion, which is used in smoking cessation. DO NOT USE TOGETHER.
- Use cautiously in patients with a recent history of myocardial infarction or unstable heart disease.

Potential Toxicities/Side Effects and the Nursing Process

I. ALTERATIONS IN SENSORY/PERCEPTUAL PATTERNS related to RESTLESSNESS, AGITATION, INSOMNIA

Defining Characteristics: Many patients experience increased restlessness, agitation, anxiety, and insomnia, especially after initiation of therapy. This may be severe enough to require treatment with sedative/hypnotic or drug discontinuation. Restlessness, agitation, hostility, decreased concentration, ataxia, incoordination, confusion, paranoia, anxiety, manic episodes in bipolar manic depressives, migraine, insomnia, euphoria, and psychoses may occur. Akathesia, dyskinesia, dystonia, muscle spasms, bradykinesia, and sensory disturbances may occur.

Nursing Implications: Assess baseline gait, neurologic and mental status, and monitor during therapy. Teach patient to report signs/symptoms; discuss benefit/risk ratio with physician. Assess for signs/symptoms of suicidal ideation; if they occur, refer for psychiatric evaluation. Inform patient that drowsiness, dizziness will resolve after 1–2 weeks; instruct to avoid hazardous activities while drowsy (e.g., driving a car, operating machinery). Instruct patient to avoid alcohol ingestion, as this may precipitate seizures.

II. ALTERATION IN CARDIAC OUTPUT related to CHANGES IN BP, HR

Defining Characteristics: Dizziness, tachycardia, hypertension or hypotension, palpitations, edema, syncope, and cardiac arrhythmias may occur.

Nursing Implications: Assess baseline orthostatic BP, heart rate, presence of peripheral edema, and monitor during therapy. Patient should have a baseline EKG. Instruct patient to report abnormalities including postural dizziness, palpitations. Discuss any significant changes with physician, and discuss interventions. If the patient has had a recent myocardial infarction, expect that dose of drug may be reduced.

III. ALTERATION IN NUTRITION, LESS THAN BODY REQUIREMENTS, related to GI SIDE EFFECTS

Defining Characteristics: Dry mouth, anorexia, nausea, vomiting, diarrhea, constipation, weight loss of up to 2.25 kg (5 lb), dyspepsia, weight gain and increased appetite, increased salivation, taste changes, stomatitis may occur rarely.

Nursing Implications: Assess baseline nutrition and elimination patterns, weight, and monitor during therapy. Discuss abnormalities with physician, and discuss drug modification. Teach patient to self-administer prescribed antiemetics as appropriate. Suggest patient use sugar-free hard candy, frequent ice chips, or artificial saliva for dry mouth.

IV. ALTERATION IN URINARY ELIMINATION related to URINARY RETENTION

Defining Characteristics: Urinary retention, frequency, and nocturia may occur. Increased risk in patients with history of urinary retention.

Nursing Implications: Assess baseline urinary elimination pattern and risk. Assess for urinary retention, and instruct patient to report signs/symptoms. Discuss alternative drug with physician if this occurs.

V. ALTERATIONS IN SKIN INTEGRITY related to ALLERGY

Defining Characteristics: Urticaria, erythema, rash, pruritus may occur.

Nursing Implications: Assess baseline drug allergy history and skin integrity. Instruct patient to report skin changes. If angioedema of face or tongue develops, tell patient to stop drug and discuss drug discontinuance with physician.

VI. POTENTIAL SEXUAL DYSFUNCTION related to IMPOTENCE, IRREGULAR MENSES

Defining Characteristics: Impotence in men and irregular menses in women may occur.

Nursing Considerations: Assess baseline sexual functioning. Inform patient that alterations may occur, and instruct to report them. If severe, discuss dysfunction with physician, and whether another antidepressant would provide equal benefit with less dysfunction.

Drug: buspirone hydrochloride (BuSpar)

Class: Antianxiety agent.

Mechanism of Action: Unclear; drug is considered a midbrain modulator and affects many neurotransmitters (serotonin, dopamine, and cholinergic and noradrenergic systems).

Metabolism: Rapid and complete GI absorption. Food may delay absorption but does not affect total serum drug level. Distributed to body tissues and fluids, especially brain. Metabolized in liver and excreted in urine.

Dosage/Range:

Adult:

- Oral: 10–15 mg in 2–3 divided doses.
- May be increased in 5-mg increments every 2–4 days to achieve goal (maximum 60 mg/day).
- Maintenance: usual is 5–10 mg tid.

Drug Preparation/Administration:

- Store tablets in tight, light-resistant containers at < 30°C (86°F).
- Administer with food.

Drug Interactions:

- MAOIs: increased BP; AVOID CONCURRENT USE.
- Haloperidol: increased haloperidol serum levels; AVOID CONCURRENT USE or reduce haloperidol dose.
- Alcohol: may increase fatigue, drowsiness, dizziness; AVOID CONCURRENT USE.
- Other CNS depressants (analgesics, sedatives): may increase fatigue, drowsiness, dizziness; AVOID CONCURRENT USE.

Lab Effects/Interference:

- None known.

Special Considerations:

- Selective anxiolytic; causes little sedation or psychomotor dysfunction.
- Anxiolytic effect comparable to oral diazepam.
- Onset slower, so patients should be told to expect full anxiolytic effect in 3–4 weeks.
- Use with caution if renal insufficiency; dose-reduce in anuric patients.

Potential Toxicities/Side Effects and the Nursing Process

I. ALTERATIONS IN SENSORY/PERCEPTUAL PATTERNS related to DIZZINESS, DROWSINESS

Defining Characteristics: Far less sedation than with other anxiolytics. May cause dizziness, drowsiness, headache in 10% of patients; fatigue, nightmares, weakness, paresthesia occur less frequently.

Nursing Implications: Assess baseline neurologic status, and monitor during therapy. Instruct patient to report signs/symptoms, and discuss drug modification with physician. Instruct patient to avoid alcohol while taking drug.

II. ALTERATION IN NUTRITION, LESS THAN BODY REQUIREMENTS, related to GI SIDE EFFECTS

Defining Characteristics: Nausea occurs in 8% of patients; less common is dry mouth, vomiting, diarrhea, or constipation.

Nursing Implications: Assess baseline nutrition and elimination patterns, and monitor during therapy. Instruct patient to report signs/symptoms.

Drug: citalopram hydrobromide (Celexa®)

Class: Antidepressant.

Mechanism of Action: Selective serotonin reuptake inhibitor (SSRI) with unique structure unlike other antidepressants (racemic bicyclic phthalane derivative).

Drug inhibits the reuptake of neurotransmitter serotonin in the CNS, thus potentiating serotonin activity in the CNS and relieving depressive symptoms.

Metabolism: Steady-state plasma level reached in one week. Bioavailability is 80% following single daily dose, unaffected by food intake, and peak plasma level is reached in 4 hours. Metabolism is primarily hepatic, with a terminal half-life of 25 hours. Renal excretion accounts for 20% of drug excretion. In the elderly, drug is more slowly cleared, with increases in area under the curve (AUC) by 23% and half-life by 30%. Patients with hepatic dysfunction have reduced drug clearance (37%), with half-life of drug extended to 8 hours.

Dosage/Range:
- Adult: 20 mg qd, increased 40 mg qd after at least 1 week.
- Patients with hepatic dysfunction or elderly: 20 mg qd.
- If changing to or from monamine oxidase inhibitor therapy, wait at least 14 days between drugs.

Drug Preparation:
- Oral: available in 20-mg (pink) and 40-mg (white) oval, scored tablets.

Drug Administration:
- Administer orally in morning or evening, without regard to food.

Drug Interactions:
- Monamine oxidase inhibitors: potential for serious, sometimes fatal interactions (hyperthermia, rigidity, myoclonus, autonomic instability, mental status changes, including coma). DO NOT USE TOGETHER, and if changing to/from citaloprom HBr, drugs MUST be separated by at least 14 days.
- Alcohol: possible potentiation of depression of cognitive and motor function; DO NOT USE TOGETHER.
- Cimetidine: increases AUC of citaloprom HBr by 43%. Use together with caution, if at all; assess for toxicity and reduce dose as needed if must use together.
- Lithium: use together cautiously, and monitor serum lithium levels if used together.
- Warfarin: monitor INR, PT closely.
- Carbamazepine, ketoconazole, itraconazole, fluconazole, erythromycin: possible increase in clearance of citaloprom HBr, monitor drug effectiveness and increase dose as needed.

- Metoprolol: may increase metoprolol levels; monitor BP and HR.
- Tricyclic antidepressants, e.g., imipramine: possible increases in plasma tricyclic antidepressant level; use together cautiously, if at all.

Lab Effects/Interference:
- Infrequently, increased liver function tests, alk phos, and abnormal glucose tolerance test.
- Rarely, bilirubinemia, hypokalemia, and hypoglycemia.

Special Considerations:
- At high doses in animals, drug is teratogenic, and, in some tests, mutagenic and carcinogenic (> 20 times the human maximum dose). DO NOT give to pregnant women or nursing mothers.
- Most responses occur within 1–4 weeks of therapy, but if no benefit has yet occurred, patients should be taught to continue taking medicine as prescribed.
- Use cautiously in patients with a seizure disorder, and monitor closely during therapy.

Potential Toxicities/Side Effects and the Nursing Process

I. ALTERATION IN NUTRITION related to GI SIDE EFFECTS

Defining Characteristics: Nausea (21%) and dry mouth (20%) are common. Less common are diarrhea (8%), dyspepsia (5%), vomiting (4%), and abdominal pain (3%). Infrequent are gastritis, stomatitis, eructation, dysphagia, teeth grinding, change in weight, and gingivitis. The following were rare: colitis, cholecystitis, gastroesophageal reflux, diverticulitis, and hiccups.

Nursing Implications: Assess baseline nutrition and elimination patterns, and monitor during therapy. Discuss abnormalities with physician, and discuss drug modification. Teach patient to self-administer prescribed antiemetics as appropriate. Suggest patient use sugar-free hard candy, frequent ice chips, or artificial saliva for dry mouth.

II. ALTERATION IN CARDIAC OUTPUT, POTENTIAL, related to CHANGES IN BLOOD PRESSURE

Defining Characteristics: Tachycardia, postural hypotension, and hypotension are common. The following are infrequent: hypertension, bradycardia, peripheral edema, angina, arrythmias, flushing, and cardiac failure. Rarely, transient ischemic attacks, phlebitis, changes in cardiac conduction (atrial fibrillation, bundle branch block), and cardiac arrest.

Nursing Implications: Assess baseline orthostatic BP, heart rate, and monitor during therapy. Teach patient to report abnormalities, including postural dizziness, palpitations. Discuss significant changes with physician. If patient has orthostatic hypotension, teach patient to change position slowly and to hold on to support.

III. SENSORY/PERCEPTUAL ALTERATIONS related to CHANGES IN MENTAL STATUS

Defining Characteristics: The following may occur: somnolence (18%), insomnia (15%), agitation (3%), impaired concentration, amnesia, apathy, confusion, taste perversion, abnormal ocular accommodation, and possibly worsening depression and suicide attempt. Infrequently, increased libido, aggressive reaction, depersonalization, hallucination, euphoria, paranoia, emotional lability, and panic reaction may occur.

Nursing Implications: Assess baseline gait, neurologic, affective, and mental status, and monitor during therapy. Teach patient to report signs and symptoms; discuss benefit/risk ratio with physician. Assess for signs and symptoms of suicidal ideation; if they occur, refer for psychiatric evaluation. Teach patient that drowsiness may occur, and teach to avoid hazardous activities while drowsy (e.g., driving a car, operating machinery).

IV. POTENTIAL FOR INJURY related to DRUG OVERDOSE

Defining Characteristics: Although rare, drug overdoses have resulted in fatalities (total drug 3920 mg and 2800 mg in two cases resulting from this drug only) while other total doses of 6000 mg have not resulted in death. Symptoms resulting from overdose include: dizziness, sweating, nausea, vomiting, tremor, somnolence, sinus tachycardia, amnesia, confusion, coma, convulsions, hyperventilation, cyanosis, rhabdomyolysis, and EKG changes (QT interval prolongation, nodal rhythm, and ventricular arrythmias).

Nursing Implications: Teach patient self-administration schedule and to keep drug in tightly closed container out of reach of children and pets. Teach patient not to double doses if a dose is missed. Give prescriptions in smallest number of pills possible (e.g., one month's worth at a time). In the event of an overdosage, teach patient to come to nearest emergency department where focus is on maintaining a patent airway and oxygenation, gastric evacuation by lavage and use of activated charcoal, and close monitoring of cardiac and overall status. Because of large area of drug distribution, dialysis is unlikely to be beneficial.

V. ALTERATIONS IN SKIN INTEGRITY related to RASH, SKIN CHANGES

Defining Characteristics: Rash and pruritus may occur. Less commonly, photosensitivity, urticaria, eczema, acne, dermatitis, alopecia, and dry skin may occur. Rarely, angioedema, epidermal necrolysis, erythema multiforme have been reported.

Nursing Implications: Assess baseline skin integrity. Teach patient to report skin changes. If angioedema of face, tongue develops, discuss drug discontinuance with physician. Assess impact of changes on patient and discuss strategies to minimize distress and preserve skin integrity and comfort.

VI. SEXUAL DYSFUNCTION, POTENTIAL, related to ↓ LIBIDO, IMPOTENCE, ANORGASMIA

Defining Characteristics: While difficult to separate from sexual dysfunction related to depression, the following have been reported in men: decreased ejaculation disorder (6.1%), libido (3.8%), and impotence (2.8%), and in women: decreased libido (1.3%) and anorgasmia (1.1%). Dysmenorrhea and amenorrhea may occur in female patients.

Nursing Implications: Assess baseline sexual functioning. Teach patient that alterations may occur and to report them. If severe, discuss dysfunction with physician and whether an antidepressant other than a SSRI would provide equal benefit with less dysfunction.

VII. ALTERATION IN URINE ELIMINATION related to CHANGES IN PATTERNS

Defining Characteristics: Polyuria is common. Less commonly, the following may occur: urinary frequency, incontinence, retention, and dysuria. Rarely, hematuria, liguria, pyelonephritis, renal calculus, and renal pain have been reported.

Nursing Implications: Assess baseline urinary elimination pattern and risk for alterations. Assess for changes in urinary elimination and teach patient to report signs and symptoms. Discuss alternative drug with physician if severe or bothersome symptoms occur.

Drug: clonazepam (Klonopin)

Class: Benzodiazepine.

Mechanism of Action: Appears to enhance the activity of γ-aminobutyric acid (GABA), which inhibits neurotransmitter activity in the CNS. Drug is able to suppress absence seizures (petit mal) and decrease the frequency, amplitude, and duration of minor motor seizures. Unclear mechanism in relieving panic episodes.

Metabolism: Completely absorbed after oral administration, with peak plasma levels of 1–2 hours. Drug half-life is 18–60 hours (typically 30–40 hours), and therapeutic serum level is 20–80 ng/mL; 80% protein-bound, metabolized by the liver via the P-450 cytochrome enzyme system, and inactive metabolites are excreted in the urine.

Dosage/Range:

Adult (panic attacks):

- Initial: 0.25 mg bid.
- May increase as needed to target dose of 1 mg/day after at least 3 days on the previous dose. Some individuals may require doses of up to 4 mg/day in divided doses, and dose is titrated up to that dose in increments of 0.125–0.25 mg bid every 3 days until panic disorder is controlled or as limited by side effects.
- Withdrawal of treatment must be gradual, with a decrease of 0.125 mg bid every 3 days until drug is completely withdrawn.

Adult (seizure disorders):

- Initial dose: 1.5 mg/day in 3 divided doses.
- Dosage may be increased in increments of 0.5–1 mg every 3 days until seizures are controlled or as limited by side effects.
- Maximum recommended daily dose is 20 mg/day.

Drug Preparation/Administration:

- Oral.
- Available in 0.5-, 1-, and 2-mg tablets.
- Discontinuance of drug when used for panic attacks: gradually discontinue, by 0.125 mg bid every 3 days, until drug is completely withdrawn.

Drug Interactions:

- CNS depressants (narcotics, barbiturates, hypnotics, anxiolytics, phenothiazines): potentiation of CNS depressive effects; use together cautiously, if at all, and monitor patient closely.
- Alcohol: potentiates CNS depressant effects; DO NOT use together.
- Phenobarbital: increases hepatic metabolism of clonazepam so that decreased serum levels lead to decreased clonazepam effect; assess patient for drug efficacy and need for increased drug dose.
- Phenytoin: increased hepatic metabolism of clonazepam so that decreased serum levels lead to decreased clonazepam effect; assess patient for drug efficacy and need for increased drug dose.
- Valproic acid: increased risk of absence seizure activity.

Lab Effects/Interference:

- Rarely, anemia, leukopenia, thrombocytopenia, eosinophilia.
- Transient elevation of liver function studies (serum transaminases and alk phos).

Special Considerations:

- Contraindicated during pregnancy, for breast-feeding mothers, and patients with severe liver dysfunction or acute narrow-angle glaucoma.

- May cause psychological and physical dependency.

I. ALTERATIONS IN SENSORY/PERCEPTUAL PATTERNS related to CNS DEPRESSION

Defining Characteristics: CNS depressant effects include drowsiness (37%), and, less commonly, dizziness (8%); abnormal coordination (6%); ataxia (5%); dysarthria (2%); depression (7%); memory disturbance (4%); nervousness (3%); decreased intellectual ability (2%); emotional lability; confusion; paresthesia; feeling of drunkenness; paresis; tremor; head fullness; hyperactivity, or hypoactivity. Rarely, suicidal ideation.

Nursing Implications: Assess baseline gait, neurologic status, affects, and monitor during treatment. Instruct patient to report signs/symptoms, and discuss drug modification with physician. Evaluate patient satisfaction with drug efficacy. Instruct patient to avoid alcohol while taking drug. Instruct patient prescribed schedule for discontinuing drug when used chronically: assess for signs/symptoms of withdrawal. Assess patient risk for suicide, and if at risk, refer to psychiatry for supportive counseling.

II. ALTERATION IN NUTRITION, LESS THAN BODY REQUIREMENTS, related to GI SIDE EFFECTS

Defining Characteristics: Constipation (1%), decreased appetite (1%), and less commonly, abdominal pain, flatulence, increased salivation, dyspepsia, decreased appetite; also elevated serum transaminases and alk phos.

Nursing Implications: Assess baseline nutrition and elimination patterns and serum transaminases, alk phos, and monitor during therapy. Assess degree of discomfort and interference with nutrition. Discuss significant abnormalities with physician and discuss drug modification.

III. INJURY related to DECREASE IN MENTAL ALERTNESS, PHYSICAL COORDINATION

Defining Characteristics: Drug may cause drowsiness, dizziness, and impair physical coordination, mental alertness.

Nursing Implications: Assess other medications that may increase risk (e.g., opiates, phenothiazenes) and response to drug. Instruct patient to avoid potentially hazardous activities, including driving a car, operating machinery. Instruct patient to avoid alcohol.

IV. ALTERATIONS IN CARDIAC OUTPUT related to POSTURAL HYPOTENSION

Defining Characteristics: Drug may cause postural hypotension, palpitations, chest pain, edema.

Nursing Implications: Assess baseline VS, and monitor during therapy. Discuss abnormalities with physician. Instruct patient to report dizziness on standing or other changes, and to change position slowly and hold on to support if this occurs.

V. ALTERATIONS IN SKIN INTEGRITY related to SKIN DISORDERS

Defining Characteristics: Acne flare, xeroderma, contact dermatitis, pruritus, skin disorders may occur.

Nursing Implications: Assess baseline skin integrity, and instruct patient to report changes. Teach symptomatic skin management, and discuss drug discontinuance with physician if severe.

VI. SEXUAL DYSFUNCTION related to CHANGES IN LIBIDO, MENSTRUAL IRREGULARITIES

Defining Characteristics: Loss or increase in libido, menstrual irregularities in women; decreased ejaculation in men.

Nursing Implications: Assess baseline sexual functioning. Inform patient that alterations may occur, and instruct to report them. If severe, discuss dysfunction with physician, and whether another antidepressant would provide equal benefit with less dysfunction.

VII. ALTERATION IN ELIMINATION, URINARY, related to DYSURIA, BLADDER DYSFUNCTION

Defining Characteristics: Dysuria, polyuria, cystitis, urinary incontinence, bladder dysfunction, urinary retention, urine discoloration, and urinary bleeding may occur uncommonly.

Nursing Implications: Assess baseline urinary elimination pattern. Instruct patient to report any changes. Discuss impact on patient, and severity, and discuss significant problems with physician.

Drug: desipramine hydrochloride (Norpramin, Pertofrane)

Class: Tricyclic antidepressant.

Mechanism of Action: Blocks reuptake of neurotransmitters at neuronal membrane, thus increasing available serotonin, norepinephrine in CNS, and potentiating their effects. Appears to have analgesic effect separate from antidepressant action. May increase bioavailability of morphine. Indicated in the treatment of depressive (affective) mood disorders. Also used as an adjuvant analgesic in cancer pain management.

Metabolism: Well absorbed from GI tract. Highly protein-bound. Plasma half-life of 7–60 hours. Metabolized in liver, and primarily excreted in urine.

Dosage/Range:

Adult:

- Oral: 75–150 mg hs, or in divided doses.
- May be gradually increased to 300 mg/day if needed.
- Elderly: 25–50 mg/day, maximum 150 mg/day.

Drug Preparation/Administration:

- Store in tight containers at < 40°C (104°F).
- Administer as a single bedtime dose.

Drug Interactions:

- MAOIs: increased excitation, hyperpyrexia, seizures; use together cautiously (especially if high dose used).
- Sympathomimetic (epinephrine, amphetamines): increased hypertension; AVOID concurrent use.
- Cimetidine methylphenidate: increased amitriptyline levels, increased toxicity; use cautiously and monitor for increased toxicity.
- Warfarin: may increase PT; monitor closely and decrease dose of warfarin as needed.
- Barbiturates: may decrease desipramine serum level; monitor for decreased antidepressant effect; may need increased dose.
- Alcohol: may antagonize antidepressant effects; AVOID CONCURRENT USE.

Lab Effects/Interference:

- Rarely, altered liver function studies.
- Rarely, increased or decreased serum glucose levels.
- Rarely, increased pancreatic enzymes.
- Rarely, bone marrow depression with agranulocytosis, eosinophilia, purpura, thrombocytopenia.

Special Considerations:

- Antidepressant effect may take two weeks or longer.

- Adjuvant analgesic useful in cancer pain management.
- May also decrease depression associated with chronic cancer pain and promote improved sleep.
- Contraindicated in patients with myocardial infarction, seizure disorder, or benign prostatic hypertrophy.
- Use cautiously in patients with urine retention, narrow-angle glaucoma, hyperthyroidism, hepatic dysfunction, or suicidal ideation.
- Drug should be gradually discontinued rather than abruptly withdrawn to prevent anxiety, malaise, dizziness, nausea/vomiting.
- May be helpful in treating hiccups.
- Increased anticholinergic side effects in elderly.

Potential Toxicities/Side Effects and the Nursing Process

I. ALTERATIONS IN SENSORY/PERCEPTUAL PATTERNS related to DROWSINESS, EPS

Defining Characteristics: Drowsiness, dizziness, weakness, lethargy, fatigue are common; confusion, disorientation, hallucinations may occur in the elderly. Extrapyramidal symptoms may occur (fine tremor, rigidity, dystonia, dysarthria, dysphagia), as may peripheral neuropathy and blurred vision. Less sedation than amitriptyline.

Nursing Implications: Assess baseline gait, neurologic and mental status, and monitor during therapy. Instruct patient to report signs/symptoms; discuss benefit/risk ratio with physician. Assess for signs/symptoms of suicidal ideation; if they occur, refer for psychiatric evaluation. Inform patient that drowsiness, dizziness will resolve after 1–2 weeks; instruct to avoid hazardous activities while drowsy (e.g., driving a car, operating machinery).

II. ALTERATION IN CARDIAC OUTPUT related to POSTURAL HYPOTENSION, TACHYCARDIA

Defining Characteristics: Postural hypotension, EKG changes, tachycardia, hypertension may occur. Less severe than with other tricyclics.

Nursing Implications: Assess baseline orthostatic BP, heart rate, and monitor during therapy. Instruct patient to report abnormalities, including postural dizziness, palpitations. Drug should be stopped several days before surgery to prevent hypertensive crisis, especially if high dose is used.

III. ALTERATION IN NUTRITION, LESS THAN BODY REQUIREMENTS, related to GI SIDE EFFECTS

Defining Characteristics: Dry mouth, anorexia, nausea, vomiting, diarrhea, abdominal cramping may occur; also, elevated LFTs.

Nursing Implications: Assess baseline nutrition and elimination patterns and LFTs, and monitor during therapy. Discuss abnormalities with physician, and discuss drug modification. Teach patient to self-administer prescribed antiemetics as appropriate. LFTs should be repeated, and if still elevated, the drug should be discontinued. Instruct patient to take full dose at bedtime. Suggest patient use sugar-free hard candy, frequent ice chips, or artificial saliva for dry mouth.

IV. ALTERATION IN URINARY ELIMINATION related to URINARY RETENTION

Defining Characteristics: Urinary retention may occur. Increased risk in patients with history of urinary retention.

Nursing Implications: Assess baseline urinary elimination pattern and risk. Assess for urinary retention, and instruct patient to report signs/symptoms. Discuss alternative drug with physician if this occurs.

V. ALTERATIONS IN SKIN INTEGRITY related to ALLERGY

Defining Characteristics: Urticaria, erythema, rash, and photosensitivity may occur.

Nursing Implications: Assess baseline drug allergy history and skin integrity. Instruct patient to report skin changes. If angioedema of face or tongue develops, discuss drug discontinuance with physician. Instruct patient to avoid sunlight or to use sunblock protection.

Drug: diazepam (Valium)

Class: Benzodiazepine (anxiolytic).

Mechanism of Action: Binds to benzodiazepine receptors in the CNS (limbic and cortical areas, cerebellum, brain stem, and spinal cord), resulting in the following effects: anxiolytic, ataxia, anticonvulsant, muscle relaxation. Appears to potentiate the effects of GABA.

Metabolism: Well absorbed from GI tract. Widely distributed in body tissues and fluids, including CSF. Crosses placenta and is excreted in breast milk. Highly bound to plasma proteins. Metabolized in liver and excreted in urine. Half-life of 20–80 hours. May produce psychological and physical dependence. Indicated for management of anxiety, the relief of reflex spasm or spasticity, and as an anticonvulsant for termination of status epilepticus.

Dosage/Range:
Adult:

- Oral: 2–10 mg tid-qid or 15–30 mg/day extended-release preparation.
- Intravenous (IV) (tension): 5–10 mg IV, maximum 30 mg/8 h.
- IV (seizures): 5–10 mg IV, maximum 30 mg; may repeat in 2–4 hours if needed.
- IV (status epilepticus): 5–20 mg slow IV push (IVP) (2–5 mg/min), q5–10 min, maximum 60 mg.
- IV (elderly, debilitated): 2–5 mg slow IVP.

Drug Preparation/Administration:

- Oral: protect tablets from light and store at 15–30°C (59–86°F).
- IV: do not administer with other drugs; drug may absorb to sides of plastic syringe or to plastic IV bag and tubing if added to IV infusion bag; consult hospital pharmacist for IV infusion protocol; administer IVP slowly 2–5 mg/min; have emergency equipment available.

Drug Interactions:

- CNS depressants (alcohol, anticonvulsants, phenothiazines, opiates): additive CNS depression; avoid concurrent use or use cautiously and monitor carefully.
- Oral contraceptives, isoniazid, ketoconazole, or cimetidine: decrease plasma clearance of diazepam so may increase effect (e.g., sedation); monitor patient closely.
- Tricyclic antidepressants: increased serum levels of antidepressant possible; use together cautiously.
- Digoxin: may decrease renal excretion of digoxin; monitor for overdosage; may need to decrease digoxin.
- Levodopa: may decrease levodopa effect; monitor patient response; may have to increase levodopa dose.

Lab Effects/Interference:

- Rarely, altered liver function studies.
- Rarely, neutropenia.

Special Considerations:

- Wide margin of safety between therapeutic and toxic doses.
- May impair ability to perform activities requiring mental alertness (e.g., driving a car, operating machinery).
- May produce psychological and physical dependence.
- Administer cautiously in patients with liver or renal impairment.
- Use cautiously in patients with chronic pulmonary disease or sleep apnea.
- Contraindicated in patients with depressive neuroses, psychotic reactions (without prominent anxiety), acute alcoholic intoxication (with depressed VS), known hypersensitivity to the drug, or acute angle-closure glaucoma.
- May cause fetal damage, so should not be used during pregnancy or if the mother is breast-feeding.

- Withdrawal symptoms (including seizure, delirium) can occur with rapid drug discontinuance in patients taking high or chronic doses.

Potential Toxicities/Side Effects and the Nursing Process

I. ALTERATIONS IN SENSORY/PERCEPTUAL PATTERNS relating to CNS DEPRESSION

Defining Characteristics: CNS depressant effects include drowsiness, fatigue, lethargy, confusion, weakness, headache, which may occur initially and resolve with continued therapy or dose reduction. Vivid dreams, visual disturbances, slurred speech, "hangover," and bizarre behavior may also occur. Patient risk factors: elderly, debilitated, liver dysfunction, low serum albumin.

Nursing Implications: Assess baseline neurologic status and risk factors, and monitor during treatment. Instruct patient to report signs/symptoms and discuss drug modification with physician. Evaluate patient satisfaction with drug efficacy. Instruct patient to avoid alcohol while taking drug. Teach patient prescribed schedule for discontinuing drug when used chronically: assess for signs/symptoms of withdrawal (increased anxiety, rebound insomnia; may also include agitation, dysphoria, nausea/vomiting, irritability, muscle cramps, hallucinations, seizures).

II. ALTERATION IN NUTRITION, LESS THAN BODY REQUIREMENTS, related to GI SIDE EFFECTS

Defining Characteristics: Nausea, vomiting, abdominal discomfort may occur; also, elevated LFTs.

Nursing Implications: Assess baseline nutrition and elimination patterns and LFTs, and monitor during therapy. Discuss abnormalities with physician and discuss drug modification. Teach patient to self-administer prescribed antiemetics as appropriate.

III. INJURY related to DECREASE IN MENTAL ALERTNESS, PHYSICAL COORDINATION

Defining Characteristics: Drug may cause drowsiness, dizziness, and impair physical coordination, mental alertness.

Nursing Implications: Assess other medications that may increase risk (e.g., opiates, phenothiazines) and response to drug. Instruct patient to avoid potentially hazardous activities, including driving a car, operating machinery.

IV. ALTERATIONS IN PERFUSION related to CARDIOPULMONARY COMPROMISE

Defining Characteristics: Drug may cause transient hypotension, bradycardia, cardiovascular collapse, respiratory depression.

Nursing Implications: Assess baseline VS; have resuscitation equipment nearby. Monitor q5–15 min and before IV dose of drug. Discuss abnormalities with physician.

V. ALTERATIONS IN SKIN INTEGRITY related to RASH

Defining Characteristics: Urticaria, rash may occur; also phlebitis, pain at injection site.

Nursing Implications: Assess baseline skin integrity, and instruct patient to report changes. Teach symptomatic skin management, and discuss drug discontinuance with physician if severe. Assess IV site for evidence of pain, phlebitis, and change site; apply heat as needed.

Drug: doxepin hydrochloride (Sinequan)

Class: Antidepressant of the dibenzoxepine tricyclic class.

Mechanism of Action: Appears to exert adrenergic effect at the synapses, preventing deactivation of norepinephrine by reuptake into the nerve terminals.

Metabolism: Metabolized in the liver by the P-450 enzyme system, into active metabolite. Effective serum level of doxepin and metabolite is 100–200 ng/mL. Takes 2–8 days to reach steady-state.

Dosage/Range:

Adult:

- Initial dose of 75 mg/day is recommended; in elderly, dose should start at 25–50 mg/day.
- Dose may be titrated up or down based on response. Usual dose is 75 mg/day to 150 mg/day.
- Patients with mild symptoms may require only 25 mg/day to 50 mg/day.
- Patients with severe symptoms may require gradual titration up to 300 mg/day.

Drug Preparation/Administration:

- Oral, taken in a single dose (maximum 150-mg dose) or in divided doses. Single dose given at bedtime enhances sleep.
- Available in 10-, 25-, 50-, 75-, 100-, and 150-mg capsules.
- If changing a patient from MAOI to doxepin HCl, wait at least 14 days before the careful initiation of doxepin.

Drug Interactions:
- Alcohol: do not use concomitantly, as increases drug toxicity.
- MAOI: severe reaction, including death may occur; DO NOT USE TOGETHER.
- Cimetidine: increased serum levels of drug and anticholinergic side effects (severe dry mouth, urinary retention, blurred vision); avoid concurrent use.
- Tolazamide: may cause severe hypoglycemia; monitor patient's serum glucose carefully.

Lab Effects/Interference:
- Rarely, eosinophilia, bone marrow depression (e.g., agranulocytosis, leukopenia, thrombocytopenia, purpura).
- Increased or decreased blood glucose levels.

Special Considerations:
- Contraindicated in patients with glaucoma or urinary retention.
- Antianxiety effect appears before the antidepressant effect, which takes 2–3 weeks.
- Most sedating of antidepressants, so useful in enhancing sleep, and single dose (up to 150 mg) should be taken at bedtime.
- Recommended for the treatment of depression accompanied by anxiety and insomnia, depression associated with organic illness or alcohol, psychotic depressive disorders with associated anxiety.

Potential Toxicities/Side Effects and the Nursing Process

I. ALTERATIONS IN SENSORY/PERCEPTUAL related to DROWSINESS, EPS

Defining Characteristics: Drowsiness, which may disappear as therapy continues. Rarely, dizziness, confusion, disorientation, hallucinations, numbness, paresthesia, ataxia, extrapyramidal symptoms, seizures, blurred vision, tardive dyskinesia, tremor may occur.

Nursing Implications: Assess baseline gait, neurologic, affective and mental status, and monitor during therapy. Instruct patient to report signs/symptoms; discuss benefit/risk ratio with physician and measures to reduce extrapyramidal side effects if they occur. Assess for signs/symptoms of suicidal ideation; if they occur, refer for psychiatric evaluation. Inform patient that drowsiness will decrease after 1–2 weeks, and instruct to avoid hazardous activities while drowsy (e.g., driving a car, operating machinery). Instruct patient to avoid alcohol while taking drug.

II. ALTERATION IN CARDIAC OUTPUT related to BLOOD PRESSURE CHANGES

Defining Characteristics: Hypotension or hypertension, tachycardia may occur.

Nursing Implications: Assess baseline orthostatic BP, heart rate, and monitor during therapy. Instruct patient to report abnormalities, including postural dizziness, palpitations.

III. ALTERATION IN NUTRITION, LESS THAN BODY REQUIREMENTS, related to GI SIDE EFFECTS

Defining Characteristics: Dry mouth, anorexia, nausea, vomiting, diarrhea, indigestion, taste changes, aphthous stomatitis may occur rarely.

Nursing Implications: Assess baseline nutrition and elimination patterns. Discuss abnormalities with physician, and discuss drug modification. Teach patient to self-administer prescribed antiemetics as appropriate. Instruct patient to take full dose at bedtime (if 150 mg or less). Suggest patient use sugar-free hard candy, frequent ice chips, or artificial saliva for dry mouth.

IV. ALTERATION IN URINARY ELIMINATION related to URINARY RETENTION

Defining Characteristics: Urinary retention may occur. Increased risk in patients with history of urinary retention.

Nursing Implications: Assess baseline urinary elimination pattern and risk. Assess for urinary retention, and instruct patient to report signs/symptoms. Discuss alternative drug with physician if this occurs.

V. ALTERATIONS IN SKIN INTEGRITY related to ALLERGY

Defining Characteristics: Urticaria, erythema, rash, and photosensitivity may occur.

Nursing Implications: Assess baseline drug allergy history and skin integrity. Instruct patient to report skin changes. If severe changes occur, discuss drug discontinuance with physician. Instruct patient to avoid sunlight or to use sunblock protection.

VI. SEXUAL DYSFUNCTION related to CHANGES IN LIBIDO

Defining Characteristics: Increased or decreased libido, testicular swelling, gynecomastia in males; enlargement of breasts and galactorrhea in women.

Nursing Implications: Assess baseline sexual functioning. Inform patient that alterations may occur, and instruct to report them. If severe, discuss dysfunction with physician and whether another antidepressant would provide equal benefit with less dysfunction.

Drug: fluoxetine hydrochloride (Prozac)

Class: Antidepressant.

Mechanism of Action: Inhibits CNS neuronal uptake of serotonin.

Metabolism: Well absorbed after oral administration, and peak serum levels occur in 6–8 hours. Peak plasma concentrations are 15–55 ng/mL. Time to steady-state in serum level is 2–4 weeks; 94.5% protein-bound. Drug is extensively metabolized in the liver to norfluoxetine and other metabolites using P-450 enzyme pathway; inactive metabolites are excreted in the urine. Elimination half-life is 1–3 days when administered acutely, and 4–6 days with chronic administration.

Dosage/Range:

Adult (for depression):

- 20 mg/day initially.
- After several weeks of therapy, if no response, may increase dose gradually to a maximum dose of 80 mg/day.
- Patients with hepatic dysfunction, elderly, or patients with concurrent diseases: start at lower dose or give less frequently.
- Weekly 90 mg tablets: begin 7 days after last 20-mg daily dose.

Drug Preparation/Administration:

- Give orally with or without food in the morning; with higher doses, e.g., 80 mg/day, may give two doses, one in the morning and one at noon.
- Available in pulvules of 10 mg and 20 mg; liquid/oral solution available as 20 mg/5 mL; weekly 90-mg tablets.
- Allow at least 14 days between stopping an MAOI and beginning fluoxetine; when stopping fluoxetine to begin an MAOI, wait at least five weeks before beginning the MAOI.

Drug Interactions:

- Alcohol: DO NOT USE CONCOMITANTLY, as increases impaired judgment, thinking, and motor skills.
- Tricyclic antidepressants (TCA): decreased metabolism and increased serum levels of TCA; monitor for increased toxicity and dose-reduce TCA as necessary when drug is given concomitantly with fluoxetine.
- MAOIs: when drug is given concomitantly or within a short time period, severe, potentially life-threatening interactions may occur, including symptoms resembling neuroleptic malignant syndrome. DO NOT GIVE

TOGETHER, AND END SEPARATELY, as stated in Administration section.

- Buspirone: reduced effects of buspirone; assess need to increase dose.
- Carbamazepine: increased serum levels of carbamazepine, with potential increased toxicity; monitor closely and dose-reduce as necessary.
- Cyproheptadine: decreased fluoxetine serum levels, so that effect was reduced or reversed; avoid concomitant administration if possible.
- Dextromethorphan: increased risk of hallucinations.
- Diazepam: increased diazepam half-life with increased circulating serum levels, leading to increased toxicity (e.g., excessive sedation or impaired psychomotor skills); dose-reduce diazepam or avoid concurrent administration.
- Digoxin: displaces fluoxetine from plasma protein binding, leading to increased fluoxetine serum levels and effect; monitor for toxicity and dosereduce as necessary.
- Lithium: increased lithium serum levels leading to possible increased neurotoxicity; monitor patient closely, and reduce lithium dose as needed.
- Phenytoin: increased phenytoin serum levels; monitor effect and serum levels, and modify dose accordingly.
- Thioridazine: DO NOT administer together. Discontinue fluoxetine at least 5 weeks before starting thioridazine.
- Tryptophan: increased risk of CNS toxicity (e.g., headache, sweating, dizziness, agitation, aggressiveness) and peripheral toxicity (e.g., nausea, vomiting); use together cautiously if at all; avoid if possible.
- Warfarin: displaces fluoxetine from plasma protein binding sites, leading to increased fluoxetine serum levels, and effect; monitor for toxicity and dosereduce as necessary.

Lab Effects/Interference:

- None known.

Special Considerations:

- Weekly dosing is for patients whose depression is stable on daily dosing. Diarrhea and cognitive changes are more common with weekly dosing.
- May take up to four weeks of therapy before benefit is seen.
- Possibility of suicide attempt may exist in depression and persist until depression managed by drug; monitor high-risk patients closely and give smallest prescription of tablets possible to ensure frequent follow-up and reduce the risk of overdosage.
- Has slight-to-no anticholinergic, sedative, or orthostatic hypotensive side effects.
- Avoid use in women who are pregnant or breast-feeding.
- Drug is also indicated for treatment of obsessive-compulsive disorder and bulimia disorder.

Potential Toxicities/Side Effects and the Nursing Process

I. ALTERATIONS IN SKIN INTEGRITY related to RASH

Defining Characteristics: Urticaria, rash may occur (7%). In initial trials, in one-third of patients developing rash, rash was associated with fever, leukocytosis, arthralgias, edema, carpal tunnel syndrome, respiratory distress, lymphadenopathy, proteinuria, and/or mildly elevated liver transaminase levels that required drug discontinuation, which largely resolved symptoms.

Nursing Implications: Assess baseline skin integrity, and instruct patient to report rash immediately. Discuss drug discontinuance with physician if severe or associated with other symptoms as above. Teach symptomatic skin management.

II. ALTERATIONS IN SENSORY/PERCEPTUAL PATTERNS related to CNS EFFECTS

Defining Characteristics: CNS effects include headache and, less commonly, activation of mania or hypomania, insomnia, anxiety, decreased ability to concentrate, tremor, sensory disturbances, abnormal dreams, nervousness, dizziness, fatigue, sedation, lightheadedness, blurred vision. Rarely, seizures may occur. Patients at risk for suicide may commit suicide during initial period of treatment.

Nursing Implications: Assess baseline neurologic status and risk factors, and monitor during treatment. Instruct patient to report signs/symptoms, and discuss drug modification with physician. Evaluate patient satisfaction with drug efficacy. Instruct patient to avoid alcohol while taking drug. Assess suicide risk, and if at high risk, monitor closely, provide supportive counseling, and prescribe only small numbers of pills to prevent overdosage. May take up to four weeks for therapeutic effect to be seen.

III. ALTERATION IN NUTRITION, LESS THAN BODY REQUIREMENTS, related to GI SIDE EFFECTS

Defining Characteristics: Nausea and, less commonly, vomiting, diarrhea, constipation, dry mouth, dyspepsia, anorexia, abdominal discomfort, flatulence, taste changes, gastroenteritis, and increased hunger may occur. Significant weight loss can occur in underweight, depressed patients.

Nursing Implications: Assess baseline nutrition and elimination patterns. Discuss abnormalities with physician and discuss drug modification. Teach patient to self-administer prescribed antiemetics as appropriate. If patient is losing weight, instruct patient to report this immediately, and discuss benefit of continuation of drug with physician.

IV. INJURY related to DECREASE IN MENTAL ALERTNESS, PHYSICAL COORDINATION

Defining Characteristics: Drug may cause drowsiness, dizziness, and impair physical coordination, mental alertness.

Nursing Implications: Assess other medications that may increase risk (e.g., opiates, phenothiazines) and response to drug. Instruct patient to avoid potentially hazardous activities, including driving a car, operating machinery.

V. SEXUAL DYSFUNCTION, POTENTIAL, related to IMPOTENCE

Defining Characteristics: Sexual dysfunction, impotence, anorgasmia may occur.

Nursing Implications: Assess baseline sexual functioning. Inform patient that alterations may occur, and instruct to report them. If severe, discuss dysfunction with physician, and whether another antidepressant would provide equal benefit with less dysfunction.

VI. ALTERATION IN OXYGENATION, POTENTIAL, related to ALTERED BREATHING PATTERNS

Defining Characteristics: Bronchitis, upper respiratory infections, pharyngitis, cough, dyspnea, rhinitis, nasal congestion, and sinusitis may occur infrequently.

Nursing Implications: Assess baseline respiratory status, and instruct patient to report any changes. Discuss serious changes with physician, and interventions necessary.

VII. ALTERATION IN COMFORT, POTENTIAL, related to PAIN

Defining Characteristics: Pain in muscles, joints, or back may occur; flulike symptoms are infrequent, as are asthenia, chest pain, and limb pain.

Nursing Implications: Assess baseline comfort level; instruct patient to report any changes. Discuss symptom management strategies, unless severe, and then discuss benefit of changing to another antidepressant medicine.

Drug: imipramine pamoate (Tofranil-PM)

Class: Tricyclic antidepressant.

Mechanism of Action: Blocks reuptake of neurotransmitters at neuronal membrane, thus increasing available serotonin, norepinephrine in CNS, and potentiating their effects. Appears to have analgesic effect separate from antidepressant action. May increase bioavailability of morphine. Indicated in the treatment of depressive (affective) mood disorders. Also used as an adjuvant analgesic in cancer pain management.

Metabolism: Completely absorbed from GI tract; highly protein bound. Plasma half-life is 8–16 hours. Metabolized in liver; excreted in urine and, to lesser degree, in bile and feces.

Dosage/Range:

Adult:

- Oral: 75–100 mg/day (may increase on patient response, to maximum 300 mg; reduce dose in elderly, 30–40 mg/day, to maximum 100 mg).
- IM: used only when oral route cannot be used.

Drug Preparation/Administration:

- Oral: store in well-closed containers at 15–30°C (59–86°F). Administer as a single bedtime dose.
- IM: administer IM in large muscle mass; change to oral as soon as possible.

Drug Interactions:

- MAOIs: increased excitation, hyperpyrexia, seizures; use together cautiously (especially if high dose is used).
- CNS depressants (alcohol, sedatives, hypnotics): increase CNS depression; use together cautiously.
- Sympathomimetic (epinephrine, amphetamines): increased hypertension; AVOID concurrent use.
- Cimetidine methylphenidate: increased imipramine levels, increased toxicity; use cautiously and monitor for increased toxicity.
- Warfarin: may increase PT; monitor closely and decrease dose of warfarin as needed.
- Barbiturates; may decrease imipramine level; monitor patient response; may need to increase dose.

Lab Effects/Interference:

- Increased metanephrine (Pisano test).
- Decreased urinary 5-HIAA.

Special Considerations:

- Antidepressant effect may take two weeks or longer.
- Adjuvant analgesic useful in cancer pain management.
- May also decrease depression associated with chronic cancer pain and promote improved sleep.
- Contraindicated in patients with myocardial infarction, seizure disorder, or benign prostatic hypertrophy.
- Use cautiously in patients with urine retention, narrow-angle glaucoma, hyperthyroidism, hepatic dysfunction, or suicidal ideation.

- Drug should be gradually discontinued rather than abruptly withdrawn to prevent anxiety, malaise, dizziness, nausea/vomiting.
- May be helpful in treating hiccups.
- Increased anticholinergic side effects in elderly.
- Some preparations may contain sodium bisulfite, which can cause allergic reactions, including anaphylaxis, in hypersensitive individuals. Check ingredients. Assess allergy history.

Potential Toxicities/Side Effects and the Nursing Process

I. ALTERATIONS IN SENSORY/PERCEPTUAL PATTERNS related to DROWSINESS, CNS EFFECT

Defining Characteristics: Drowsiness, dizziness, weakness, lethargy, fatigue are common; confusion, disorientation, hallucinations may occur in the elderly. Extrapyramidal symptoms may occur (fine tremor, rigidity, dystonia, dysarthria, dysphagia), as may peripheral neuropathy and blurred vision.

Nursing Implications: Assess baseline gait, neurologic and mental status, and monitor during therapy. Instruct patient to report signs/symptoms; discuss benefit/risk ratio with physician. Assess for signs/symptoms of suicidal ideation; if they occur, refer for psychiatric evaluation. Inform patient that drowsiness, dizziness will resolve after 1–2 weeks; instruct to avoid hazardous activities while drowsy (e.g., driving a car, operating machinery).

II. ALTERATION IN CARDIAC OUTPUT related to POSTURAL HYPOTENSION, TACHYCARDIA

Defining Characteristics: Postural hypotension, EKG changes, tachycardia, hypertension may occur.

Nursing Implications: Assess baseline orthostatic BP, heart rate, and monitor during therapy. Instruct patient to report abnormalities, including postural dizziness, palpitations. Drug should be stopped several days before surgery to prevent hypertensive crisis (especially if high dose is used).

III. ALTERATION IN NUTRITION related to GI SIDE EFFECTS

Defining Characteristics: Dry mouth, anorexia, nausea, vomiting, diarrhea, and abdominal cramping may occur; also, elevated LFTs.

Nursing Implications: Assess baseline nutrition and elimination patterns and LFTs, and monitor during therapy. Discuss abnormalities with physician, and discuss drug modification. Teach patient to self-administer prescribed antiemetics as appropriate. LFTs should be repeated, and if still elevated, the drug should be discontinued. Instruct patient to take full dose at bedtime. Suggest patient use sugar-free hard candy, frequent ice chips, or artificial saliva for dry mouth.

IV. ALTERATION IN URINARY ELIMINATION related to URINARY RETENTION

Defining Characteristics: Urinary retention may occur. Increased risk in patients with history of urinary retention.

Nursing Implications: Assess baseline urinary elimination pattern and risk. Assess for urinary retention, and instruct patient to report signs/symptoms. Discuss alternative drug with physician if this occurs.

V. ALTERATIONS IN SKIN INTEGRITY related to ALLERGY

Defining Characteristics: Urticaria, erythema, rash, photosensitivity may occur.

Nursing Implications: Assess baseline drug allergy history and skin integrity. Instruct patient to report skin changes. If angioedema of face, tongue develops, discuss drug discontinuance with physician. Instruct patient to avoid sunlight or to use sunblock protection.

Drug: lorazepam (Ativan)

Class: Benzodiazepine (anxiolytic).

Mechanism of Action: Binds to benzodiazepine receptors in the CNS (limbic and cortical areas, cerebellum, brain stem, and spinal cord), resulting in the following effects: anxiolytic, ataxia, anticonvulsant, muscle relaxation. Appears to potentiate the effects of GABA.

Metabolism: Well absorbed from GI tract. Widely distributed in body tissues and fluids, including CSF. Crosses placenta and is excreted in breast milk. Highly bound to plasma proteins. Metabolized in liver and excreted in urine. Short half-life of 10–20 hours. May produce psychological and physical dependence. Indicated for management of anxiety and short-term relief of anxiety associated with depression.

Dosage/Range:

Adult:

- Oral: 1–6 mg/day in divided doses (maximum 10 mg/day).
- IM: 0.044 mg/kg or 2 mg, whichever is smaller (initial dose).
- IV: 0.044 mg/kg (up to 2 mg) given 15–20 minutes prior to surgery; 1.4 mg/m^2 given 30 minutes prior to chemotherapy; or 0.05 mg/kg (maximum 4 mg) if perioperative amnesia is desired.

- Use maximum dose (2 mg) in patients > 50 years old.

Drug Preparation/Administration:

- Oral: may administer with food to decrease stomach upset; has been given sublingually for more rapid onset (investigational).
- IM and IV: store drug in refrigerator until use.
- IM: administer undiluted, deep IM in large muscle mass (e.g., gluteus maximus).
- IV: dilute in equal volume of 0.9% Sodium Chloride or 5% Dextrose for IVP administration (administer slowly; not > than 2 mg/min) OR dilute in 50 mL 0.9% Sodium Chloride or 5% Dextrose immediately prior to administering IVB over 15 minutes.

Drug Interactions:

- CNS depressants (alcohol, anticonvulsants, phenothiazines, opiates): additive CNS depression; avoid concurrent use or use cautiously and monitor carefully.
- Oral contraceptives, isoniazid, ketoconazole: decrease plasma clearance of lorazepam so may increase effect (e.g., sedation); monitor patient closely.
- Tricyclic antidepressants: increased serum levels of antidepressant possible; use together cautiously.
- Digoxin: may decrease renal excretion of digoxin; monitor for overdosage; may need to decrease digoxin.

Lab Effects/Interference:

- Rarely, leukopenia, elevated LDH.
- Less frequently, elevated liver function studies.

Special Considerations:

- Wide margin of safety between therapeutic and toxic doses.
- May impair ability to perform activities requiring mental alertness (e.g., driving a car, operating machinery).
- May produce psychological and physical dependence.
- Administer cautiously in patients with liver or renal impairment.
- Use cautiously in patients with chronic pulmonary disease or sleep apnea.
- Contraindicated in patients with depressive neuroses, psychotic reactions (without prominent anxiety), acute alcoholic intoxication (with depressed VS), known hypersensitivity to the drug, or acute angle-closure glaucoma.
- May cause fetal damage, so should not be used during pregnancy or if the mother is breast-feeding.
- Withdrawal symptoms (including seizure, delirium) can occur with rapid drug discontinuance in patients taking high or chronic doses.
- If manic episodes or hyperactivity occur soon after drug started, drug should be discontinued.
- Drug should not be used to manage “everyday stress.”

Berenson JR, Lichtenstein A, Porter L, et al. Efficacy of Pamidronate in Reducing Skeletal Events in Patients with Advanced Multiple Myeloma. *N Engl J Med* 1996; 334:488–493

Berenson JR, Rosen LS, Howell A. Zoledronic Acid Reduces Skeletal-related Events in Patients with Osteolytic Metastases. A Double-blind, Randomized Dose-response Study. *Cancer* 2001;91:144–154

Bilezikian JP. Management of Acute Hypercalcemia. *N Engl J Med* 1992;326(18): 1196–1203

Fitton A, McTavish D. Pamidronate: A Review of its Pharmacological Properties and Therapeutic Efficacy in Resorptive Bone Disease. *Drugs* 1991;41(2):289–318

Major P, Lortholary A, Hon J. Zoledronic Acid is Superior to Pamidronate in the Treatment of Hypercalcemia of Malignancy: A Pooled Analysis of Two Randomized, Controlled Clinical Trials. *J Clin Oncol* 2001;19:558–567

Novartis. Zometa Package Insert. East Hanover, NJ: Novartis; 2003

Solimandro DA, Bressler LR, Kintzel PE, Geraci MC. *Drug Information Handbook for Oncology*. Cleveland, OH: Lexi-Comp Inc.; 2000

Drug: calcitonin-salmon (Calcimar, Miacalcin)

Class: Thyroid hormone.

Mechanism of Action: Inhibits bone absorption (breakdown) by inhibiting bone osteoclasts and blocking osteolysis. Decreases high serum calcium concentrations in hypercalcemia of malignancy, beginning 2 hours after dose and lasting 6–8 hours. Promotes renal excretion of calcium, phosphate; also, acts on GI tract to decrease volume, acidity of gastric fluid, and enzyme content in pancreatic fluid.

Metabolism: Rapidly converted to smaller fragments by kidneys; excreted in urine.

Dosage/Range:

Adult (hypercalcemia):

- Subcutaneous (SQ) or intramuscular (IM): 4 IU/kg q12h × 2 days; if no effect, increase dose to 8 IU/kg q12h × 2 days, then to 8 IU q6h (maximum).

Drug Preparation/Administration:

- Refrigerate for 2–6 hours (36–43°F, 2–6°C).
- Reconstitute according to manufacturer's recommendations.
- If allergy suspected, perform skin test first: withdraw 0.05 mL of the 200 IU/mL solution in tuberculin syringe, then fill syringe with 1 mL 0.9% Sodium Chloride. After mixing, discard 0.9 mL; inject 0.1 mL intradermally on forearm and inspect for urticaria, wheal at 15 minutes.

Drug Interactions:

- None.

Lab Effects/Interference:

- Decreased alk phos.
- Decreased 24-hour urinary excretion of hydroxyproline.
- Casts in urine (indicate kidney damage).
- Decreased Ca++.

Special Considerations:

- Calcitonin-salmon consists of a foreign protein, so allergic reactions may occur. Perform skin test first if sensitivity is suspected. Do not use drug if wheal forms.
- It is unknown whether drug crosses placenta or is excreted in breast milk; use cautiously in pregnancy or breast-feeding.
- Patient should receive adequate saline hydration to keep urinary output at ~2 L/day throughout treatment.
- 80% of patients have reduction in calcium in 24 hours.
- Antibodies to drug may develop with long-term use.
- Rapid onset of action and mild side effects.
- Short duration of response.

Potential Toxicities/Side Effects and the Nursing Process

I. INJURY related to HYPERSENSITIVITY

Defining Characteristics: Rare hypersensitivity may occur.

Nursing Implications: Perform skin testing as ordered when sensitivity suspected; if positive, suggest use of human calcitonin or other hypocalcemic agent. Assess for signs/symptoms of hypersensitivity (generalized itching, agitation, dizziness, nausea, sense of impending doom, urticaria, angioedema, respiratory distress, hypotension). If this develops, stop drug immediately, notify physician, maintain IV access, and be prepared to administer epinephrine, hydrocortisone, diphenhydramine.

II. ALTERATION IN NUTRITION, LESS THAN BODY REQUIREMENTS, related to GI SIDE EFFECTS

Defining Characteristics: Transient nausea/vomiting is mild and tolerance develops; anorexia, diarrhea, epigastric discomfort, and abdominal pain may occur as well.

Nursing Implications: Assess baseline nutrition and elimination patterns. Since nausea/vomiting may occur within 30 minutes after injection, administer at bedtime to decrease distress.

III. ALTERATION IN COMFORT related to DRUG EFFECTS

Defining Characteristics: Flushing of face, hands, feet may occur soon after injection, as well as tingling of palms and soles. Rarely, rash (maculopapular), erythema, urticaria, headache, chills have developed. Inflammation may occur at IM or SQ injection site.

Nursing Implications: Assess comfort level. Administer drug at bedtime if possible. If symptoms are uncomfortable, consider symptomatic relief measures (e.g., heat, cold). Reassure patient that flushing lasts ~1 hour and is transient. Assess rash if severe; discuss with physician drug discontinuance.

IV. ALTERATIONS IN ELECTROLYTES related to HYPOCALCEMIA, HYPERCALCEMIA

Defining Characteristics: Rarely, if drug is very effective, hypocalcemia may occur; conversely, if drug is ineffective, hypercalcemia may occur.

Nursing Implications: Monitor serum Ca+ closely. Assess for signs/symptoms of hypocalcemia (muscle twitching, spasm tetany, seizures) and hypercalcemia (bone pain, nausea, vomiting, polyuria, polydipsia, constipation, bradycardia, lethargy, muscle weakness, psychosis). Notify physician, recheck serum calcium immediately, and institute corrective measures as ordered.

Drug: cinacalcet HCl (Sensipar)

Class: Hypocalcemic agent

Mechanism of Action: The calcium-sensing receptor on the surface of the chief cell of the parathyroid gland regulates PTH secretion. PTH is responsible for telling the bones to break down bone (osteoclastic) and release calcium into the blood when it is needed. Cinacalcet HCl directly decreases PTH levels by increasing the sensitivity of calcium-sensing receptors to activation by extracellular calcium. As PTH levels decrease, the level of calcium in the blood decreases.

Metabolism: Oral drug is well absorbed, and maximum plasma levels are achieved in 2–6 hours. Drug AUC levels are increased 82% when ingested with a high fat meal. Drug is metabolized by CYP3A4, CYP2D6, and CYP1A2 enzymes of the P450 microenzyme system. Drug is excreted in the urine (80%) primarily, and to a lesser degree in the feces (15%). Drug is poorly excreted in patients with moderate-to-severe hepatic impairment, with a half-life prolonged 33% and 70% respectively. Drug is highly protein bound so hemodialysis does not treat over dosage.

Dosage/Range:
30 mg PO bid, titrated every 2–4 weeks through sequential doses of 30 mg PO bid, then 60 mg PO bid, then 90 mg PO bid, and 90 mg tid or quid as necessary to normalize serum calcium levels.

- Monitor patients with moderate or severe hepatic impairment closely.
- Do not administer if serum calcium is < 8.4 mg/dL.
- Monitor calcium levels frequently during dose titration.

Drug Preparation/Administration:

- Drug available in 30, 60, and 90 mg tablets.
- Administer with food or shortly after a meal.

Drug Interactions:

- Drug is a potent inhibitor of CYP2D6: Dosage adjustment may be needed for flecainide, vinblastine, thioridazine, tricyclic antidepressants.
- Ketoconazole: increased AUC by 2.3 times of cinacalcet HCl.
- Amitriptyline: increased amitriptyline and nortriptyline by 20% in CYP2D6 extensive metabolizers.
- Warfarin: no effect.

Lab Effects/Interference:

- Hypocalcemia
- Hyperphosphatemia

Special Considerations:

- Drug is indicated for treatment of hypercalcemia in patients with parathyroid carcinoma.
- Patients should be monitored for signs and symptoms of hypocalcemia.
- Drug should not be used by pregnant or breast-feeding mothers, unless benefit outweighs risk.

Potential Toxicities/Side Effects and the Nursing Process

I. POTENTIAL FOR INJURY related to HYPOCALCEMIA

Defining Characteristics: Drug lowers serum calcium. Signs and symptoms of hypocalcemia are paresthesia, myalgias, cramping, tetany, and seizures.

Nursing Implications: Assess baseline serum calcium, phosphate, magnesium levels, as well as PTH level. Develop a plan for titration with the patient, and frequency of laboratory monitoring. Teach patient symptoms of hypocalcemia, and to report them right away if they occur. Serum calcium should be assessed within 1 week after initiation or dose adjustment. Once dose has been established, serum calcium should be assessed q month. If serum calcium > 7.5 mg/dL but < 8.4 mg/dL, or if symptoms of hypocalcemia occur, discuss with physician the addition of calcium-containing phosphate binders and/or vitamin D sterols to raise the serum calcium. If the serum calcium falls to < 7.5 mg/dL or if symptoms of hypocalcemia persist, stop drug until serum calcium level reaches 8.0 mg/dL and/or symptoms resolve. Resume dose per physician, at next lowest dose of drug.

II. ALTERATION IN NUTRITION, LESS THAN BODY REQUIREMENTS, related to GI SIDE EFFECTS

Defining Characteristics: Nausea (31%), vomiting (27%) are most common adverse effects, but diarrhea may also occur (21%).

Nursing Implications: Assess baseline nutritional and elimination status, and monitor during treatment. Ensure adequate hydration and urinary output of 2 L/day. Teach patient to administer oral antiemetics prior to taking drug, and as needed between drug doses. Assess food preferences, and suggest small, frequent feedings. Teach patient to report symptoms that worsen or do not resolve with supportive care.

III. ALTERATION IN COMFORT related to MYALGIA AND DIZZINESS

Defining Characteristics: Myalgia affects about 15% of patients and dizziness 10% of patients.

Nursing Implications: Assess baseline hydration, comfort status, and teach patient that these side effects may occur. Teach patient to change position slowly if dizziness occurs, and to notify nurse or physician if dizziness worsens or does not resolve. Teach patient symptom management strategies such as local application of heat for myalgias, and to notify provider if myalgias worsen.

Drug: etidronate disodium (Didronel)

Class: Biphosphonate; hypocalcemic agent.

Mechanism of Action: Inhibits osteoclastic bone resorption (bone breakdown), thereby decreasing calcium release, and serum calcium levels. Indicated in the management of hypercalcemia of malignancy.

Metabolism: Oral absorption is variable and decreased by food. Following IV injection, drug is distributed into bone, then excreted unchanged in the urine.

Dosage/Range:

Adult (hypercalcemia of malignancy):

- IV (induction): 7.5* mg/kg/day × 3 days (may increase to 7 days; if hypercalcemia recurs, wait at least 7 days before treatment using same induction regimen).
- Oral (maintenance): 20 mg/kg/day beginning on day after last IV dose, for up to 90 days if effective.

Drug Preparation/Administration:

- Oral: give as single oral dose (may be advised if GI distress); give at least 2 hours before or after a meal.
- IV: dilute drug in at least 250 mL 0.9% Sodium Chloride and infuse over at least 2 hours.

Drug Interactions:

- Nephrotoxic drugs: additive nephrotoxicity; AVOID concurrent use.

Lab Effects/Interference:

- Decreased P, decreased Mg.
- Abnormal renal function tests.
- Decreased Ca.

Special Considerations:

- Saline hydration should be maintained during treatment to keep urinary output at 2 L/day.
- Use with caution.
- It is unknown whether drug crosses placenta or is excreted in breast milk; use with caution, if at all, in pregnant or breast-feeding women.
- 60–70% response rate when given with hydration and diuresis, and one-half of this when based on corrected calcium value.

Potential Toxicities/Side Effects and the Nursing Process

I. ALTERATIONS IN NUTRITION, LESS THAN BODY REQUIREMENTS, related to GI SIDE EFFECTS

Defining Characteristics: Diarrhea, nausea, vomiting, abdominal discomfort, and guaiac-positive stools may occur rarely.

Nursing Implications: Assess baseline nutritional and elimination status and monitor during treatment. Instruct patient to report nausea and vomiting, and consider dividing dose (if oral) or slowing infusion rate >2 hours. Guaiac stools and notify physician if positive.

*Dose reduction necessary in patients with renal insufficiency.

II. ALTERATION IN URINE ELIMINATION related to NEPHROTOXICITY

Defining Characteristics: Drug is nephrotoxic and may cause rises in serum BUN and creatinine. Increased risk when concurrent nephrotoxic drugs administered.

Nursing Implications: Assess baseline hydration status and total body fluid balance to ensure adequate urinary output (> 2 L/day). Assess baseline serum BUN and creatinine, and monitor throughout treatment. Dose reduction necessitated by renal insufficiency.

III. ALTERATIONS IN ELECTROLYTES related to HYPOCALCEMIA, HYPERCALCEMIA

Defining Characteristics: Rarely, if drug is very effective, hypocalcemia may occur; conversely, if drug is ineffective, hypercalcemia may occur. Increased sodium phosphate levels may occur during oral therapy but are less frequent with IV dosing (serum phosphate levels are inversely proportional to serum calcium).

Nursing Implications: Monitor serum calcium closely. Assess for signs/symptoms of hypocalcemia (muscle twitching, spasm tetany, seizures) and hypercalcemia (bone pain, nausea, vomiting, polyuria, polydipsia, constipation, bradycardia, lethargy, muscle weakness, psychosis). Notify physician, recheck serum calcium immediately, and institute corrective measures as ordered.

Drug: furosemide (Lasix)

Class: Loop diuretic.

Mechanism of Action: Inhibits renal reabsorption of sodium and chloride in proximal loop of Henle. Useful in management of edema, hypertension related to CHF or renal disease, and with 0.9% Sodium Chloride IV hydration/diuresis to increase renal excretion of calcium in patients with hypercalcemia of malignancy.

Metabolism: Variable GI absorption of oral drug. Diuretic effect of oral dose occurs within 30–60 minutes, lasting 6–8 hours; with IV dose, occurs within 5 minutes, maximal 20–60 minutes, and lasts 2 hours. Highly protein-bound. Slight hepatic metabolism and is excreted in urine.

Dosage/Range:

- Edema: 20–80 mg PO in morning; if no response, dose-increase in 20–40 mg increments q6–8h.

- Hypertension: 10–20 mg PO bid, increasing to 40 mg bid based on BP response.
- Hypercalcemia: 80–100 mg IV q1–2h.

Drug Preparation/Administration:

- Oral: store in tight, light-resistant containers.
- IV: slow IVP over 1–2 minutes (use multidose vial or draw up drug from ampule through filtered needles).

Drug Interactions:

- Ascorbic acid, tetracycline, epinephrine form a precipitate; DO NOT give together with IV.
- Diuretics: enhanced diuretic effect; dose-reduce furosemide.
- Digoxin: toxicity enhanced by furosemide-induced hypokalemia; keep potassium level 4.5–5.0 mEq/dL.
- Drugs causing potassium loss (corticosteroids, amphotericin B): enhanced hypokalemia; monitor potassium level closely.
- Antidiabetic agents: decreases effect of insulin or oral hypoglycemics; monitor blood glucose and adjust antidiabetic drug as needed.
- Indocin: may decrease diuretic effect; monitor patient response and increase furosemide dose as needed.
- Aminoglycosides: increased ototoxicity; use cautiously.
- High doses of salicylates: increase salicylate toxicity at lower doses; monitor carefully and decrease salicylate dose.

Lab Effects/Interference:

- Decreased potassium, decreased chloride, decreased sodium, increased uric acid.
- Rarely, anemia, thrombocytopenia, neutropenia, leukopenia.

Special Considerations:

- Contraindicated in anuric patients and patients hypersensitive to the drug.
- May produce profound diuresis and electrolyte depletion.
- Should not be used by pregnant women, and breast-feeding should be interrupted during drug therapy.
- Use with caution in patients with liver cirrhosis.

Potential Toxicities/Side Effects and the Nursing Process

I. ALTERATIONS IN FLUID AND ELECTROLYTE BALANCE related to HYDRATION/DIURESIS

Defining Characteristics: Aggressive hydration with 0.9% Sodium Chloride and IV furosemide is used to promote calcium excretion. Hypokalemia, hypochloremia, hyperuricemia, hypomagnesemia may occur.

Nursing Implications: Assess baseline electrolyte (K+, Mg++, Cl−, Ca++), renal BUN, creatinine, and fluid balance, and monitor during therapy. Strictly monitor intake/output (I/O), assess daily weights, and maintain total body fluid balance (I = O). Administer prescribed replacement electrolytes. Assess for signs/symptoms of hypokalemia. Assess orthostatic BP, heart rate, and monitor during therapy.

II. ALTERATION IN SENSORY/PERCEPTUAL PATTERNS related to OTOTOXICITY, CNS EFFECTS

Defining Characteristics: Tinnitus and reversible or permanent hearing impairment may occur, often related to high doses of drug given IVP (high serum drug concentrations). Headache, vertigo, paresthesias can occur.

Nursing Implications: Assess baseline hearing (ability to hear spoken voice) and neurologic status. Teach patient to report tinnitus, decreased hearing, and any other symptoms. Discuss administration of high doses as IV infusion (4 mg/min).

III. ALTERATIONS IN SKIN INTEGRITY related to RASH, SENSITIVITY

Defining Characteristics: Purpura, photosensitivity, rash, urticaria, pruritus, exfoliative dermatitis, erythema multiforme may occur. Anaphylaxis has occurred in patients allergic to sulfonamides.

Nursing Implications: Assess drug allergies, especially to furosemide and sulfonamides. Assess baseline skin integrity, and instruct patient to report changes. Discuss drug discontinuance if severe reaction occurs.

Drug: gallium nitrate (Ganite)

Class: Hypocalcemic agent.

Mechanism of Action: Inhibits calcium release from bone by inhibiting bone resorption and turnover. Indicated for the treatment of hypercalcemia of malignancy refractory to hydration.

Metabolism: Excreted by kidneys.

Dosage/Range:

Adult:

- IV: Severe hypercalcemia: 200 mg/m^2 as continuous 24-hour infusion × 5 days (or when serum calcium normalizes if before 5 days). Moderate hypercalcemia: 100 mg/m^2 as continuous 24-hour infusion × 5 days (or less if patient achieves normal serum calcium).

Drug Preparation/Administration:

- Dilute daily dose in 1 L 0.9% Sodium Chloride or 5% Dextrose injection and infuse over 24 hours (42 mL/hour) via infusion pump.

Drug Interactions:

- Nephrotoxic drugs (amphotericin B, aminoglycosides, cisplatin): additive nephrotoxicity; avoid concurrent use.

Lab Effects/Interference:

- Increased BUN, creatinine.
- Decreased calcium; transient decrease in phosphorus, decrease bicarbonate.
- Rarely, anemia, leukopenia.

Special Considerations:

- Contraindicated in patients with severe renal dysfunction (serum creatinine > 2.5 mg/dL).
- Unknown if drug crosses placenta or is excreted in breast milk; use cautiously in pregnancy, and suggest mother interrupt breast-feeding while taking drug.
- 92% patient response (reduction in serum calcium corrected for albumin), lasting for 7.5 days.
- Saline hydration to maintain urinary output of 2 L/day should be maintained during treatment.

Potential Toxicities/Side Effects and the Nursing Process

I. ALTERATION IN URINE ELIMINATION related to NEPHROTOXICITY

Defining Characteristics: Increased serum BUN, creatinine in 13% of patients. Decreased risk if concurrent administration of other nephrotoxic drugs.

Nursing Implications: Assess baseline hydration status and total body fluid balance to ensure adequate urinary output (> 2 L/day). Assess baseline serum BUN and creatinine, and monitor throughout treatment. Dose reduction necessitated by renal insufficiency. Drug should NOT be given if serum creatinine > 2.5 mg/dL.

II. ALTERATIONS IN ELECTROLYTES related to HYPOCALCEMIA, HYPERCALCEMIA

Defining Characteristics: Rarely, if drug is very effective, hypocalcemia may occur; conversely, if drug is ineffective, hypercalcemia may occur. Transient hypophosphatemia occurs in up to 79% of hypercalcemic patients after treatment with drug. Also, decreased serum bicarbonate occurs in 40–50% of patients.

Nursing Implications: Monitor serum calcium closely. Assess for signs/symptoms of hypocalcemia (muscle twitching, spasm tetany, seizures) and hypercalcemia (bone pain, nausea, vomiting, polyuria, polydipsia, constipation, bradycardia, lethargy, muscle weakness, psychosis). Notify physician, recheck serum calcium immediately, and institute corrective measures as ordered. Monitor serum phosphate levels, and administer replacement oral phosphates as ordered.

III. ALTERATIONS IN NUTRITION, LESS THAN BODY REQUIREMENTS, related to GI SIDE EFFECTS

Defining Characteristics: Diarrhea, nausea, vomiting, constipation may occur.

Nursing Implications: Assess baseline nutritional and elimination status, and monitor during treatment. Instruct patient to report nausea and vomiting. Administer ordered antiemetics. Ensure adequate hydration with urinary output > 2 L/day.

Drug: pamidronate disodium (Aredia)

Class: Biphosphonate; hypocalcemic agent.

Mechanism of Action: Probably inhibits osteoclast activity in bone (bone breakdown) and may also block dissolution of minerals (hydroxyapatite) in bone, thus preventing calcium release from bone. Does not inhibit bone formation or bone mineralization. Indicated for the treatment of hypercalcemia of malignancy, in conjunction with adequate hydration.

Metabolism: Excreted by kidneys.

Dosage/Range:

Adult (hypercalcemia of malignancy):

- IV(moderate hypercalcemia, 12–13.5 mg/dL corrected): 60–90 mg as continuous infusion over 24 hours.
- IV (severe hypercalcemia > 13.5 mg/dL): 90 mg as continuous infusion over 24 hours.

Osteolytic bone metastases of breast cancer:

- 90 mg in 250 mL of IV fluid via 2-hour infusion q3–4 weeks.

Osteolytic lesions of multiple myeloma:

- 90 mg in 500 mL IV fluid via 4-hour infusion every month.

Drug Preparation/Administration:
- Reconstitute by adding 10 mL sterile water for injection to 30-mg vial. Further dilute in 1 L 0.9% Sodium Chloride or 5% Dextrose injection as per manufacturer's directions.
- Infuse over 2–24 hours via infusion pump or rate controller.

Drug Interactions:
- None.

Lab Effects/Interference:
- Decreased calcium.
- Decreased K+, decreased Mg, decreased P (phosphate).

Special Considerations:
- Saline hydration to maintain urinary output of 2 L/day should be maintained during treatment.
- Clinical studies show 64% of patients have corrected serum calcium levels by 24 hours after beginning therapy, and after 7 days 100% of the 90-mg group had normal corrected levels. For some (33–53%), normal or partially corrected calciums in 60-mg and 90-mg groups persisted × 14 days.
- Has been shown to reduce bony metastasis in patients with multiple myeloma and to reduce pain.
- Patients with preexisting anemia, leukopenia, or thrombocytopenia should be monitored closely for 2 weeks after pamidronate disodium treatment.

Potential Toxicities/Side Effects and the Nursing Process

I. ALTERATIONS IN NUTRITION, LESS THAN BODY REQUIREMENTS, related to GI SIDE EFFECTS

Defining Characteristics: Nausea, vomiting, abdominal discomfort, constipation, and anorexia may occur rarely.

Nursing Implications: Assess baseline nutritional and elimination status and monitor during treatment. Ensure adequate hydration and urinary output of 2 L/day. Administer ordered antiemetics. Administer oral phosphates as cathartics if ordered. Assess food differences and offer small, frequent feedings.

II. ALTERATION IN ELECTROLYTES related to HYPOCALCEMIA, HYPERCALCEMIA

Defining Characteristics: Rarely, if drug is very effective, hypocalcemia may occur; conversely, if drug is ineffective, hypercalcemia may occur. Hypokalemia, hypomagnesemia, hypophosphatemia may occur.

Nursing Implications: Monitor serum calcium closely. Assess for signs/symptoms of hypocalcemia (muscle twitching, spasm tetany, seizures) and hypercalcemia (bone pain, nausea, vomiting, polyuria, polydipsia, constipation, bradycardia, lethargy, muscle weakness, psychosis). Notify physician, recheck serum calcium immediately, and institute corrective measures as ordered. Monitor serum potassium, magnesium, phosphate levels and notify physician of abnormalities.

III. ALTERATIONS IN COMFORT related to LOCAL VEIN IRRITATION

Defining Characteristics: Transient fever (1°C or 3°F elevation) may occur 24–48 hours after drug administration (27% of patients), local reactions (pain, irritation, phlebitis) are common with 90-mg dose.

Nursing Implications: Assess baseline temperature, and monitor during and after infusion. Administer antipyretics as ordered. Assess IV site and restart new IV as needed for 90-mg dose in large vein where drug can be rapidly diluted. Apply warm packs as needed to site.

IV. ALTERATIONS IN FLUID BALANCE related to AGGRESSIVE HYDRATION

Defining Characteristics: Patients receive aggressive saline hydration to ensure urinary output of 2 L/day. Hypertension may occur. Patients with history of heart disease or renal insufficiency are at risk for fluid overload.

Nursing Implications: Assess baseline hydration status, total body fluid balance; monitor q4h. Discuss with physician need for diuretics once hydrated to keep body fluid balance equal (I = O). Monitor vital signs q4h during hydration, and notify physician of changes.

Drug: zoledronic acid (Zometa)

Class: Third-generation bisphosphonate.

Mechanism of Action: Inhibits bone resorption. Inhibits tumor related osteoclast activity in bone (bone breakdown) and may also block dissolution of minerals (hydroxyapatite) in bone, thus preventing calcium release from bone. Does not inhibit bone formation or bone mineralization. Drug is very rapidly taken up in the bone, but very slowly released. Drug appears to inhibit endothelial cell proliferation and to inhibit the beta fibroblast growth factor (βFGF)-mediated angiogenesis.

Metabolism: Drug is primarily eliminated intact via the kidney. Long terminal half life in plasma of 167 hours. Rapid injection results in 30% increase in serum drug concentration and renal damage.

Dosage/Range:
4 mg (maximum dose)

Drug Preparation/Administration:

- Drug is available in 4-mg vials. Reconstitute drug by adding 5 mL sterile water for injection, USP.
- Further dilute in 100 ml 5% dextrose injection, USP or 0.9% Sodium Chloride Injection, USP.
- Administer IV over *at least* 15 minutes.
- Assure that patient has been adequately rehydrated prior to drug administration, and the BUN and creatinine are WNL.
- Patients who require retreatment and who have had altered renal status after receiving the drug (manufacturer's recommendations):
- Normal serum creatinine prior to receiving drug, but have an increase of 0.5 mg/dL within 2 weeks of their next dose: hold drug until serum creatinine is at least within 10% of their baseline value.
- Abnormal serum creatinine prior to receiving drug: but have an increase of 1.0 mg/dL within 2 weeks of next dose, drug should be held until serum creatinine is at least within 10% of their baseline value.

Drug Interactions:

- Incompatible with calcium-containing fluids, such as Lactated Ringer's.
- Use cautiously together with aminoglycoside antibiotics, as there may be an additive effect resulting in hypocalcemia for prolonged periods.
- Use cautiously together with loop diuretics as the risk of hypocalcemia may be increased.

Lab Effects/Interference:

- Hypocalcemia.
- Hypophosphatemia.
- Hypomagnesemia.
- Increased BUN and serum creatinine.

Special Considerations:

- Indicated for the treatment of hypercalcemia of malignancy. Indicated for the treatment of patients with multiple myeloma and patients with documented bone metastases from solid tumors, in conjunction with standard antineoplastic therapy. Indicated for patients with prostate cancer who have progressed after treatment with at least one hormonal therapy.
- Serum creatinine must be monitored prior to each treatment, and abnormal values discussed with physician, as risk must be weighed against benefit.
- As compared to pamidronate in the management of hypercalcemia of malignancy, Zometa had a 45.3% response rate by day 4, and an 82.6% response rate by day 7, as compared to a 33.3% response rate and a 63.6% response rate, respectively, when pamidronate was given. Time to relapse was 30 days with Zometa, and 17 days with pamidronate (package insert for Zometa, Novartis, 2001).

- Use drug cautiously in patients who have aspirin-sensitive asthma, as well as in elder patients.
- Use drug in pregnant or nursing women only if benefit outweighs risk.

Potential Toxicities/Skin Effects and the Nursing Process

I. ALTERATION IN COMFORT, related to FEVER, NAUSEA AND VOMITING, INSOMNIA, AND FLU-LIKE SYMPTOMS

Defining Characteristics: Fever occurred in 44% of patients during clinical trials. Flu-like symptoms of chills, bone pain, and/or arthralgias and myalgias may occur less commonly. Nausea occurred in 29% of patients, and vomiting 14%. Insomnia affects 15%.

Nursing Implications: Assess baseline comfort and temperature. Teach patient that these side effects may occur and to report them. Administer or teach patient self-administration of acetaminophen or over-the-counter NSAIDs as appropriate to manage fever, arthralgias myalgias, if they occur. Teach patient to report if symptoms do not resolve. Administer antiemetics as ordered to minimize nausea and vomiting.

II. ALTERATION IN BOWEL ELIMINATION PATTERN related to CONSTIPATION, DIARRHEA, ABDOMINAL PAIN, AND ANOREXIA

Defining Characteristics: Diarrhea affected 17% of patients in clinical trials, while 27% developed constipation. 16% of patients developed abdominal pain, and 9% anorexia.

Nursing Implications: Assess baseline bowel elimination status, and teach patient to report alterations. Teach patient to use diet modifications depending upon changes, and over-the-counter antidiarrheals or laxatives as necessary. Teach patient to report persistent diarrhea or constipation (lasting more than 24 hours), presence of blood, abdominal cramping, or pain.

III. ALTERATION IN ACTIVITY TOLERANCE related to ANEMIA, FATIGUE

Defining Characteristics: Anemia occurred in 22% of patients during clinical trials.

Nursing Implications: Assess baseline hemoglobin and hematocrit. Teach patient to report fatigue, and discuss strategies to conserve energy, such as alternating rest and activity. Discuss with physician transfusion if symptoms are severe.

IV. ALTERATION IN FLUID AND ELECTROLYTE BALANCE related to CHANGES IN RENAL EXCRETION

Defining Characteristics: Drug will cause renal dysfunction with rise in serum creatinine if drug is given rapidly or in less than 15 minutes. Hypophosphatemia occurred in 13% of patients during clinical trials, hypokalemia in 12%, and hypomagnesemia in 10%.

Nursing Implications: Assess baseline renal function and electrolytes prior to initial therapy, post therapy, and prior to any additional therapy as needed. Hold drug if renal abnormalities do not correct, as indicated in administration section.

Chapter 11
Infection

Patients with cancer are susceptible to infection because chemotherapy, radiation therapy, or the malignancy itself results in immunosuppression. Risk for infection results from damage to the bone marrow stem cells that form blood cell elements. Leukocytes, or white blood cells (WBCs), are composed of five different cell types; they are further divided into cells that contain granules in their cytoplasm (granulocytes) and those that do not. Granulocytes include the neutrophils, basophils, and eosinophils. Neutrophils fight infection against invading micro-organisms by migrating to the site of infection. See Figure 11.1 for maturation of the formed blood cell elements. The absolute neutrophil count [ANC], the number of neutrophils in the body, determines the risk for infection. This calculation is shown in Table 11.1.

The risk of infection increases as the number of neutrophils decreases, as shown in Table 11.2. The longer the duration of neutropenia, the greater the risk for infection. Infection and fever in a neutropenic patient represent a medical emergency, and, if untreated, can result in sepsis and death within 48 hours. Initial therapy with third-generation cephalosporins containing a β-lactam ring (i.e., ceftazidime) or combination therapy with broadspectrum antibiotics should be instituted immediately. Fortunately, the use of colony stimulating factor (CSFs), such as granulocyte-colony stimulating factor (G-CSF) and granulocyte-macrophage colony stimulating factor (GM-CSF), has helped to reduce the incidence of febrile neutropenia.

Gram-negative bacilli are responsible for a high incidence of life-threatening infections (*Escherichia coli*, *Klebsiella* spp., *Proteus* spp., and *Pseudomonas aeruginosa*). However, gram-positive organisms such as *Staphylococcus epidermidis* and streptococci have become more prominent, probably due to a decrease in gram-negative sepsis resulting from prompt empiric antimicrobial therapy against gram-negative organisms, as well as the wide use of central venous access lines that become infected by gram-positive organisms.

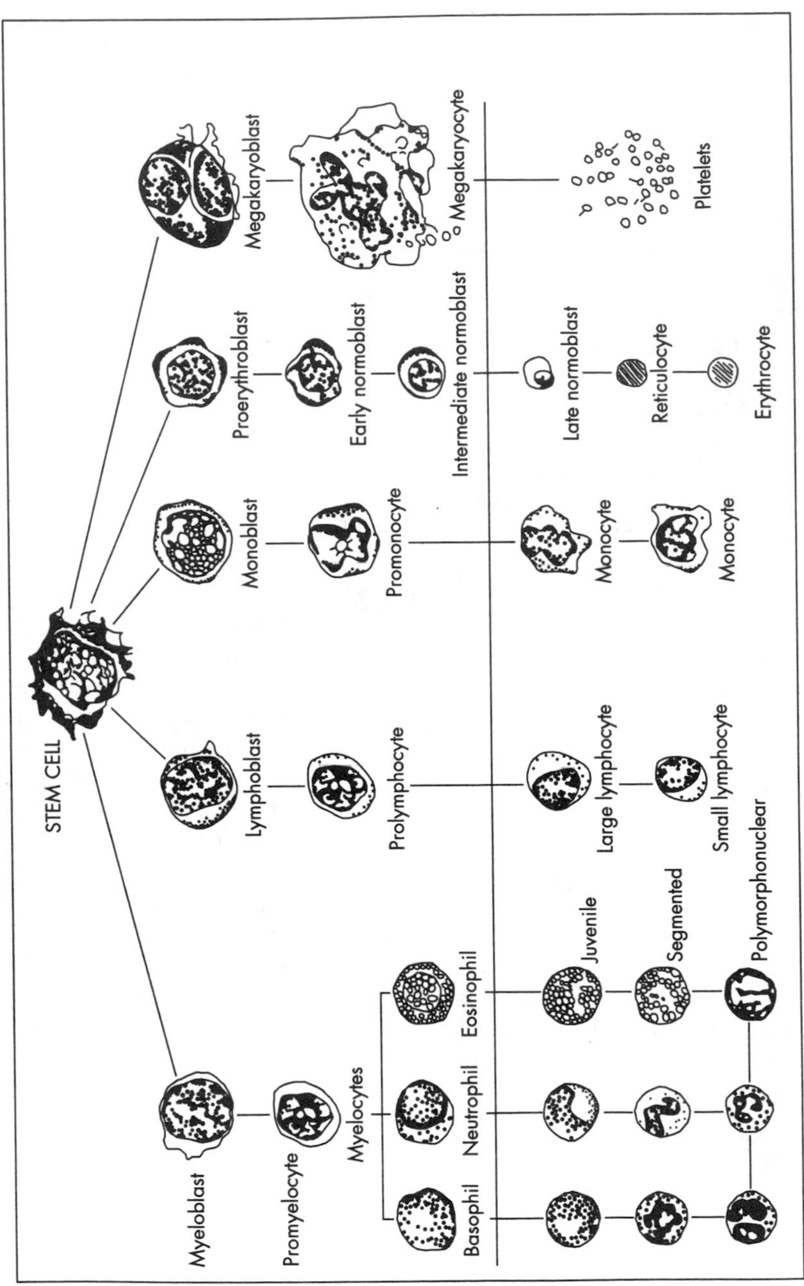

Figure 11.1 The development of formed blood cell elements

Table 11.1 Calculation of Absolute Neutrophil Count (ANC)

Patient Example	Normal Values
1. Lab results: total white blood count (WBC) = 4000/mm^3	5000–10,000/mm^3
neutrophils = 40	50–70%
lymphocytes = 50	20–40%
monocytes = 6	2–6%
eosinophils = 1	0.5–1%
bands = 2	
2. Total WBC × % (neutrophils + bands)	2500–7000/mm^3
4000 × % (40 + 2) =	
4000 × 42/100 =	
4000 × 0.42 = 1680/mm^3	
3. Assessment: low but no significant risk	

Table 11.2 Relative Risk of Infection

Risk	Number/Neutrophils
No significant risk	> 1500–2000/mm^3
Minimal risk	1000–1500/mm^3
Moderate risk	500–1000/mm^3
Severe risk	< 500/mm^3

Disease-related immunosuppression is related to defects in the cell-mediated immunity (thymus-dependent lymphocytes), such as with certain lymphomas. This leads to an increased risk for bacterial infections (*Mycobacterium, Nocardia asteroides, Legionella, Salmonella*), as well as infections caused by fungi (*Cryptococcus, Histoplasma, Candida, Aspergillus*), parasites (*Pneumocystis carinii* pneumonia, *Toxoplasma gondii*), and viruses (varicella zoster, cytomegalovirus). Other malignancies may have defects in the humoral immune system (B lymphocytes), as in multiple myeloma and chronic lymphocytic leukemia (CLL). Patients with these malignancies are at risk for infection from bacteria (*Streptococcus pneumoniae, Haemophilus influenzae, Neisseria meningitidis, Klebsiella pneumoniae, Staphylococcus aureus*) and certain enteroviruses.

Another antibiotic-related concern is the emergence of antibiotic resistance, such as vancomycin-resistant enterococci (VRE) and methacillin-resistant *Staphylococcus aureus* (MRSA). Since 1989, US hospitals report a rapid increase in the incidence of infection and colonization with vancomycin-resistant enterococci (VRE). This increase poses important problems, including (a) the lack of available antimicrobial therapy for VRE infections, since most VRE infections are also resistant to drugs previously used to treat these infections (e.g., aminoglycosides and ampicillin), and (b) the possibility that the vancomycin-resistant genes present in VRE can be transferred to other gram-positive microorganisms (e.g., *Staphylococcus aureus*).

The increased risk for VRE infection and colonization is associated with previous vancomycin and/or multiantimicrobial therapy, severe underlying disease or immunosuppression, and intraabdominal surgery. Because enterococci are found in the normal gastrointestinal and female genital tracts, most enterococcal infections are attributed to endogenous sources within the patient. Whenever possible, empiric antimicrobial therapy should be modified based on culture and sensitivity results so that the most specific therapy is administered.

The Food and Drug Administration (FDA) has approved tigecycline, the first of a new class of agents called glycylcyclines. The drug is indicated for the treatment of complicated intra-abdominal infections and complicated skin and skin structure infections in adults. Approval of this first-in-class agent is opportune as the need for new antimicrobial options is increasing.

Antimicrobial medications are intended to kill or to inhibit the growth of the organism without harming the patient. Antimicrobial agents may be bacteriostatic (inhibit growth of organisms) or bactericidal (kill microorganisms). Drug activity varies, so that at low concentrations a drug may be bacteriostatic, but bactericidal at higher concentrations. Usually antimicrobial drugs target some difference between the microorganism and the host. Overall, antibiotics are prescribed based on patient factors—the condition of the renal and hepatic systems, as well as drug allergies, the spectrum of antibiotic activity, and the site of infection.

This section focuses on antimicrobial medications used to treat infections in patients with cancer: antibacterial, antiviral, and antifungal. These drugs target specific cellular mechanisms of the infectious agent. For example, sulfonamide antibiotics inhibit para-aminobenzoic acid, an essential requirement for nucleic acid synthesis in many bacteria but not in humans. Penicillins and the cephalosporins contain a β-lactam ring that disrupts the synthesis of peptidoglycan. Peptidoglycan gives shape and strength to the bacterial cell wall. Table 11.3 provides an overview of one of the oldest (penicillins/cephalosporins) as well as the newest groups of antibacterials (streptogramins/oxazolidinones).

Table 11.3 Comparison of Antibiotic Categories

Antibacterial Category	Examples	Mechanism of Action, Including Differences Among or Between Categories or Unique Characteristics
Penicillins		Penicillins are derived from the fungus *Penicillium* and contain a β-lactam ring.
Natural penicillins	• penicillin V • penicillin G	The first group comprises natural penicillins, which are active against many aerobic Gram-positive cocci (*S. aureus, Streptococcus*), Gram-negative aerobic cocci (*N. meningitidis,* some *H. influenzae*), and some spirochetes. However, they are resistant to *Pseudomonas,* most *Enterobacter,* and to bacteria that produce the enzyme penicillinase, which inactivates the penicillin molecule.
Penicillinase-resistant penicillins	• cloxacillin • dicloxacillin • nafcillin • oxacillin	The second group contains the penicillinase-resistant penicillins. These are semisynthetic drugs that can withstand the action of the enzyme penicillinase and continue to exert their antibiotic action. They are primarily used to treat *S. aureus* and *S. epidermidis* strains that secrete penicillinase; they also have some activity against Gram-negative bacteria and spirochetes.
Aminopenicillins	• amoxicillin • ampicillin • bacampicillin	The third group includes the aminopenicillins; this group has heightened activity against Gram-negative bacteria as compared to the first two groups. These drugs are resistant to penicillinase-producing bacteria.
Extended-spectrum penicillins	• carbenicillin • mezlocillin • piperacillin • ticarcillin	The fourth group is composed of the extended-spectrum penicillins; drugs in this group have enhanced activity against gram-negative bacilli, both aerobic and nonaerobic.

(continued)

Table 11.3 *(continued)*

Antibacterial Category	Examples	Mechanism of Action, Including Differences Among or Between Categories or Unique Characteristics
Cephalosporins		The cephalosporins are derived from cephalosporin C (produced by a fungus) and have broad bactericidal activity. They contain a β-lactam ring and may also be referred to as β-lactam antibiotics. Bacterial resistance can develop, and a major mechanism is the development by the bacteria of an enzyme, β-lactamase, which inactivates the cephalosporin antibiotic by destroying the β-lactam ring.
First generation	• cefadroxil • cefalothin • cefazolin • cephalexin • cephapirin • cephradine	First-generation cephalosporins are active against Gram-positive cocci (*Staphylococcus* and *Streptococcus*) and have only limited activity against Gram-negative bacteria (e.g., *E. coli*); they have no activity against enterococci.
Second generation	• cefaclor • cefamandole • cefmetazole • cefonicid • ceforanide • cefotetan • cefoxitin • cefprozil • cefuroxime • cefuroxime • axetil	Second-generation cephalosporins are active against the same organisms as the first-generation drugs but are slightly more active against Gram-negative bacteria. In addition, they are active against *H. influenzae*

(continued).

Table 11.3 *(continued)*

Antibacterial Category	Examples	Mechanism of Action, Including Differences Among or Between Categories or Unique Characteristics
Third generation	• cefdinir • cefixime • cefoperazone • cefotaxime • cefpodoxime • ceftazidime • ceftibuten • ceftizoxime • ceftriaxone • loracarbef	Third-generation cephalosporins are less active against gram-positive organisms but have broader activity against Gram-negative organisms than either first- or second-generation drugs.
Fourth generation	• cefepime	Fourth-generation cephalosporins are projected to have many attributes including: • Extended spectrum of activity for Gram-negative and Gram-positive organisms (different from third-generation cephalosporins) • Minimal β-lactamase activity due to rapid periplasmic penetration and high penicillin-binding protein (PBP) access • Spectrum of activity to include Gram-negative organisms with multiple drug resistance patterns (*Enterobacter* and *Klebsiella*)

(continued)

Table 11.3 *(continued)*

Antibacterial Category	Examples	Mechanism of Action, Including Differences Among or Between Categories or Unique Characteristics
Streptogramins	• quinupristin/ dalfopristin	This new class of antibiotics, the streptogramin group, is a separate family of antimicrobials. Synercid is an intravenous combination of two semisynthetic, water-soluble derivatives of naturally occurring pristinamycin. The two distinct compounds are quinupristin and dalfopristin, derived from pristinamycin I and pristinamycin II. These two compounds work synergistically to kill susceptible bacteria through a two-pronged attack on protein synthesis in bacterial cells. Each component of the drug binds irreversibly to different sites on the bacterial cell's ribosomal subunit to form a stable quinupristin-ribosome-dalfopristin complex, which disables the cell's ability to make cellular protein. Without the ability to manufacture new proteins, the bacterial cell dies.
Oxazolidinones	• linezolid	Inhibits initiation of protein synthesis by binding to a site on bacterial 23S ribosomal RNA of the 50S subunit. This mechanism of inhibiting protein synthesis is not shared by other antibacterials. Cross-resistance is unlikely.
Macrolides	• azithromycin • clarithromycin • erythromycin	Binds to 50S ribosomal subunit resulting in inhibition of protein synthesis. In some cases the drug metabolite is twice as active as the parent compound.
Lipopeptides	• daptomycin	Derived from the fermentation of *Streptomyces roseosporus*. The mechanism of action is not fully understood. Binds to bacterial membranes and causes a rapid depolarization of membrane potential. This loss of membrane potential leads to inhibition of protein, DNA, and RNA synthesis resulting in bacterial cell death.
Ketolide	telithromycin	Similar to that of macrolides and is related to the 50S-ribosomal subunit binding with inhibition of bacterial protein synthesis. Telithromycin appears to have greater affinity for the ribosomal binding site than macrolides. It concentrates in phagocytes where it exhibits activity against intracellular respiratory pathogens.

Within the past few years, the FDA approved daptomycin and telithromycin. These new antibiotics have largely been developed by making minor modifications to an existing class of drugs. Daptomycin is the first drug in a new structural class, the cyclic lipopeptides. Its mode of action is to rapidly kill gram-positive bacteria by disrupting multiple aspects of bacterial membrane function. Telithromycin, a first-in-class antibiotic group called the ketolides, is structurally related to the macrolide antibiotics and specifically designed to offer optimal spectrum activity for the first-line treatment of upper and lower respiratory tract infections. The latest antibiotic group, the glycylcyclines, is structurally similar to the tetracyclines and tigecycline is the first agent in this class to be FDA-approved for the treatment of MRSA.

Another class of antimicrobial agents, the echinocandins or glucan synthesis inhibitors, has recently been added to the options available for treating opportunistic fungal infections. Caspofungin, the first-in-class, inhibits the synthesis of a key component of the fungal cell wall. Caspofungin demonstrates fungicidal activity against *Candida* species; it is indicated for the treatment of invasive *Aspergillus* in patients who are refractory to, or intolerant of, other therapies. Ideal candidates for this drug are patients with amphotericin B–induced nephrotoxicity. Caspofungin appears to be well tolerated.

The latest FDA-approved anti-fungal agent is micafungin. This drug inhibits the synthesis of 1,3-β-D-glucan, an essential component of fungal cell walls, which is not present in mammalian cells. It is indicated for the treatment of patients with esophageal candidiasis and as prophylaxis of *Candida* infections in patients undergoing hematopoietic stem cell transplantation.

COMPLICATIONS

References

American Thoracic Society. Guidelines for the management of adults with hospital-acquired, ventilatory-associated and health care-associated pneumonia. *Am J of Respiratory Critical Care* 2005;171:388–416171:388–416

Ampicillin sodium/sulbactam sodium. Available at http://hcunviweb05/mdxcgi/quiklocn.exe?CTL=E:/Mdx/mdxcgi/MEGAT.SYS&SET=1C573 June 2005

Antman KD, Griffin JD, Elias A, et al. Effect of Recombinant Human Granulocyte-Macrophage Colony Stimulating Factor on Chemotherapy-Induced Myelosuppression. *N Engl J Med* 1998;319(19):593–598

Aumercier M, Bouhallab S, Capmau M, et al. RP 59500: A Proposed Mechanism for Its Bactericidal Activity. *J Antimicrob Chemother* 1992;30 (Suppl A):9–14

Bodey G, Buckley M, Sathe YS, et al. Quantitative Relationship between Circulating Leukocytes and Infections in Patients with Acute Leukemia. *Ann Intern Med* 1966; 64(2):328–340

Brandt B. A Nursing Protocol for the Client with Neutropenia. *Oncol Nurs Forum* 1984;11(2):24–28

Carlson AC. Infection Prophylaxis in the Patient with Cancer. *Oncol Nurs Forum* 1985; 12(3):60

Cubicin. Product Information. Cubist Pharmaceutical Inc. September 2003

Cunningham R. Infection Prophylaxis for the Patient with Cancer. *Oncol Nurs Forum* 1990;17(1) (Suppl 1):16–19

Declomycin. Product Information. Lederle Pharmaceutical Division, American Cynamid Co. Pearl River, NY: 2003

Declomycin, Available at http://www.rxmed.com/b.main/b2.pharmaceutical/b2.1monographs/CPS-%20Monographs. Accessed June 2004

Drugs.com. Drug Information Online. Daptomycin. Available at http://www.drugs.com/MTM/daptomycin.html. Accessed June 2004

Gemifloxacin mesylate [package insert]. http://hcunviweb05/mdxcgi/quiklocn.exe?CTL=E:/Mdx/mdxcgi/MEGAT.SYS&SET=1C573. June 2005

Goh K.P., Management of hyponatremia. *AM Fam Physician* 2004;69(10):2387–2394

Hughes WT, Armstrong D, Bodey GP, et al. Guidelines for the Use of Antimicrobial Agents in Neutropenic Patients with Unexplained Fever. *J Infect Dis* 1989;161: 381–396

Ketek. Product Information.Aventis Pharmaceutical Inc. March 2004

Kucers A, Bennett N. *The Use of Antibiotics: A Comprehensive Review with Clinical Analysis,* 4th ed. Philadelphia, PA: JB Lippincott Co.; 1987

Medline. Drug Information: Daptomycin. Available at http://www.nlm.nih.gov/medline. Accessed June 2004

Meropenem [package insert]. http://hcunviweb05/mdxcgi/quiklocn.exe?CTL=E:/Mdx/mdxcgi/MEGAT.SYS&SET=1C573. June 2005

Mycamine [Package Insert]. Osaka Japan: Fujisawa Pharmaceutical Company LTD; 2005

Morstyn G, Campbell L, Souza LM, et al. Effect of Granulocyte Colony Stimulating Factor on Neutropenia Induced by CytotoxicChemotherapy. *Lancet* 1988;1:667–671

Pizzo PA, Hathorn MD, Hiemenz J, et al. A Randomized TrialComparing Ceftazidime Alone with Combination Antibiotic Therapy in Cancer Patients with Fever and Neutropenia. *N Engl J Med* 1986;315:552–558

Recommendations for Preventing the Spread of Vancomycin Resistance (Sept 22, 1994). *Recommendations of the Hospital Infection Control Practices Advisory Committee (HICPAC) MMWR (Morbidity and Mortality Weekly Report)* 44 (RR-12):1–712

Rifaximin [package insert]. http://hcunviweb05/mdxcgi/quiklocn.exe?CTL=E:/Mdx/mdxcgi/MEGAT.SYS&SET=1C573. June 2005

Rostad ME. Current Strategies for Managing Myelosuppression in Patients with Cancer. *Oncol Nurs Forum* 1991;18(2):7–15

Telithromycin. Thompson Center Watch. Clinical Trials Listing Service. Drugs approved by the FDA. Available at http://www.mcromedex.com/products/updates/drugdex_updates/de/tilithromycinfull.html. Accessed June 2004

Telithromycin. Available at http://www.centerwatch.com/patient/drugs/dru853.html. Accessed June 2004

Tygacil [package insert]. Philadelphia, PA: Wyeth Pharmaceuticals, Inc.; 2005.

United States Pharmacopoeia Drug Information for Health Care Professionals. Rockville, MD: 18th ed.

The United States Pharmacopoeia Convention, Inc.; 1998

VHA Pharmacy Benefits Management Strategic Healthcare Group and Medical Advisor Panel. Daptomycin.

Warner-Lambert Co. Omnicef Package Insert. Morris Plains, NJ: Parke-Davis; 1998

Wujik D. Infection. Groenwald SL, Frogge MH, Goodman M, Yarbro CH, (eds), *Cancer Symptom Management.* Sudbury, MA: Jones and Bartlett; 1996;289–308

ANTIBIOTICS

Drug: amikacin sulfate (Amikin)

Class: Aminoglycoside antibacterial antibiotic.

Mechanism of Action: Synthetic antibiotic derived from kanamycin; bactericidal, most probably by inhibition of protein synthesis. Active against aerobic microorganisms: many sensitive gram-negative organisms (including *Acinetobacter, Citrobacter, Enterobacter, E. coli, Klebsiella, Proteus, Pseudomonas, Salmonella, Serratia,* and *Shigella*), and some sensitive gram-positive organisms (*S. aureus* and *S. epidermidis*). Over time, bacterial resistance may develop, either naturally or acquired.

Metabolism: Well absorbed following parenteral administration, but variability in absorption after IM injection (peak serum level 0.5–2 hours, duration 8–12 hours). Widely distributed into body fluids. Minimally protein-bound. Readily crosses placenta and into breast milk. Drug excreted unchanged in the urine.

Dosage/Range:

- 15 mg/kg/day given in 8-hour or 12-hour doses IV or IM.
- Desired peak serum concentration is 15–30 μg/mL, and trough serum concentration is 5–10 μg/mL. DOSE-REDUCE IF RENAL IMPAIRMENT.

Drug Preparation:

- Store injectable at < 40°C (104°F).
- Potency not affected by pale yellow color that may develop.
- Stable for 24 hours at concentrations of 0.25 and 5 mg/mL in 0.9% Sodium Chloride, 5% Dextrose.

Drug Administration:

- IV: in 100–200 mL IV fluid (e.g., 0.9% Sodium Chloride or 5% Dextrose injection), infused over 30–60 minutes.

Drug Interactions:

- Increased risk of toxicity with other ototoxic drugs: acyclovir, other aminoglycosides, amphotericin B, bacitracin, cephalosporins, colistin, cisplatin, ethacrynic acid, furosemide, vancomycin.
- Potentiation of neuromuscular blockade when given concurrently with general anesthetics (succinylcholine, tubocurarine) — use cautiously; observe for signs/symptoms of respiratory depression.
- Synergism with extended-spectrum penicillins, but must be administered separately.

Lab Effects/Interference:

- Serum ALT, serum alk phos, serum AST, serum bili, and serum LDH values all may be increased.
- BUN and serum creatinine values may be increased.
- Serum Ca+, serum Mg+, serum K+, and serum Na+ concentrations may be decreased.

Special Considerations:

- Used as first-line treatment in short-term treatment of serious gram-negative infections (e.g., septicemia, respiratory tract infections).
- Use against gram-positive organisms only as second-line treatment.
- Use in pregnancy only if infection is life-threatening and no safer drug exists; drug crosses placenta and may cause fetal toxicity.

Potential Toxicities/Side Effects and the Nursing Process

I. ALTERATIONS IN SENSORY/PERCEPTUAL PATTERNS related to OTOTOXICITY

Defining Characteristics: Damage to eighth cranial nerve (auditory) may result in dizziness, nystagmus, vertigo, ataxia (vestibular damage) and less commonly, tinnitus, roaring sound in ears, and impaired hearing (auditory damage). Hearing loss usually begins with high-frequency loss, followed by clinical hearing loss, then permanent hearing loss if damage continues. Increased risk in elderly or renally impaired patients.

Nursing Implications: Assess baseline hearing (ability to hear spoken voice) and continue during therapy. Teach patient potential side effects, and instruct patient to report any hearing/perceptual problems (e.g., tinnitus, vertigo, decreased hearing). Discuss drug discontinuance and audiogram with physician to confirm hearing dysfunction if symptoms arise. Assess for increased risk if given concurrently with other ototoxic medications (e.g., cisplatin, furosemide).

II. ALTERATION IN URINARY ELIMINATION related to NEPHROTOXICITY

Defining Characteristics: Renal damage characterized by tubular necrosis with increased serum BUN, creatinine; decreased urine creatinine clearance and specific gravity; proteinuria and casts in urine. Azotemia usually not associated with oliguria. Rarely, electrolyte wasting with hypomagnesemia, hypocalcemia, and hypokalemia may occur. Renal dysfunction usually reversible after drug discontinuance. Increased risk in elderly and in patients with preexisting renal dysfunction. Risk is low in well-hydrated patients with normal renal function when normal doses given.

Nursing Implications: Assess baseline renal function and electrolytes, and monitor periodically during therapy. Discuss any abnormalities with physician, as drug should be dose-reduced or discontinued if renal dysfunction develops. Assess baseline total body fluid balance, weight, and monitor periodically during antibiotic therapy. Monitor hydration status to keep patient well hydrated. Assess drug peak and trough levels as ordered so that drug dosage is correctly titrated. Increased risk of toxicity if peak serum concentration > 30–35 μg/mL. Draw blood for peak drug concentration 30 minutes after end of 30-minute infusion or at the end of a 60-minute infusion; draw trough immediately before next dose.

III. ALTERATIONS IN SENSORY/PERCEPTUAL PATTERNS related to CNS EFFECTS, NEUROMUSCULAR BLOCKADE

Defining Characteristics: Headache, tremor, lethargy may occur. Peripheral neuropathy or encephalopathy (numbness, skin tingling, muscle twitching) may occur rarely. Neuromuscular blockade is dose related, self-limiting, and uncommon: risk is greater with topical application or when drug is administered to patient with neuromuscular disease (myasthenia gravis) or hypocalcemia.

Nursing Implications: Assess baseline neurologic status. Assess coexisting risk factors, neuroblockade medications. Teach patient about side effects, and instruct to report headache, tremor, lethargy. Observe for respiratory depression. If signs/symptoms arise, discuss drug discontinuance with physician.

IV. POTENTIAL FOR INJURY related to HYPERSENSITIVITY

Defining Characteristics: Rash, urticaria, pruritus, fever, and eosinophilia have occurred rarely. CROSS-SENSITIVITY between AMINOGLYCOSIDES exists!

Nursing Implications: Assess for drug allergies to any aminoglycoside—amikacin, gentamycin, kanamycin, neomycin, netilmicin, streptomycin, tobramycin—prior to drug administration. Instruct patient to report any allergic reactions. Assess for signs/symptoms of allergic reaction after drug dose.

V. ALTERATION IN NUTRITION, LESS THAN BODY REQUIREMENTS, related to GI SIDE EFFECTS

Defining Characteristics: Nausea, vomiting, anorexia have occurred rarely. Also, transient hepatomegaly with elevated LFTs—AST, ALT, LDH, alk phos—has occurred.

Nursing Implications: Assess baseline nutritional status, preexisting nausea/ vomiting, anorexia. Assess baseline LFTs and monitor periodically during treatment. Instruct patient to report side effects. Provide symptomatic interventions if side effects occur; discuss with physician use of alternative drug(s).

VI. POTENTIAL FOR FATIGUE, INFECTION, AND BLEEDING related to BONE MARROW INJURY

Defining Characteristics: Anemia, leukopenia, granulocytopenia, and thrombocytopenia may occur. Also, patients receiving antibiotics are at risk for overgrowth of nonsusceptible microorganisms, such as fungi (superinfection). Rare.

Nursing Implications: Assess baseline CBC, differential, and monitor periodically during treatment. Instruct patient to report signs/symptoms of fatigue, infection, or bleeding immediately. Assess for signs/symptoms of superinfection. Discuss any adverse effects with physician.

Drug: amoxicillin (Amoxil, Polymox, Trimox, Wymox; amoxicillin plus potassium clavulanate is Augmentin)

Class: Penicillin (aminopenicillin antibiotic); β-lactam.

Mechanism of Action: Semisynthetic antibiotic prepared from fungus *Penicillium.* Contains β-lactam ring and is bactericidal by inhibiting cell wall synthesis. Aminopenicillins have increased activity against gram-negative bacilli (*H. influenzae, E. coli*), as well as some activity against gram-positive bacilli (*Streptococci* and *Staphylococci*). Used for treatment of infections of upper and lower respiratory tract, genitourinary (GU) tract, and skin by sensitive organisms.

Metabolism: Well absorbed from GI tract; rate of absorption slowed by food but total amount of drug absorbed remains unchanged. Widely distributed in body tissues and fluids. Crosses placenta and is found in breast milk. Excreted in urine and bile.

Dosage/Range:

Adult:

- 125–500 mg PO q8h 48–72 hours after infection eradicated; for uncomplicated urinary tract infection, may use single dose of 3 gm PO.
- Drug dose should be reduced if severe renal failure occurs.
- Augmentin dose: mild to moderate infection: 500 mg PO 2 × /day; severe infection: 875 mg PO 2 × /day

Drug Preparation/Administration:

- Store capsules in tight container at 15–30°C (59–86°F).
- Administer on empty stomach.

Drug Interactions:

- Aminoglycosides: synergism.
- Aminoglycosides (e.g., gentamicin): incompatible when mixed together; administer at separate sites at different times. Also, penicillinase-resistant penicillins can inactivate aminoglycoside serum samples from patients receiving both drugs.
- Rifampin: possible antagonism, only at high doses of penicillin.
- Probenecid: increased serum level of penicillin; may be co-administered to exert this effect.
- Allopurinol: increased incidence of rash; avoid concurrent administration if possible.
- Clavulanic acid (β-lactamase inhibitor): synergistic bactericidal effect. Amoxicillin plus potassium clavulanate = Augmentin.

Lab Effects/Interference:

Major clinical significance:

- Urine glucose: high urinary concentrations of a penicillin may produce false-positive or falsely elevated test results with copper-reduction tests (Benedict's, Clinitest, or Fehling's); glucose enzymatic tests (Clinistix or Testape) are not affected.

Clinical significance:

- Coombs' tests: false-positive result may occur during therapy with any penicillin.
- ALT, alk phos, AST, serum bili, and serum LDH values may be increased.
- Estradiol, total conjugated estriol, estriol-glucuronide, or conjugated estrone concentrations may be transiently decreased in pregnant women following administration of amoxicillin.
- WBC: leukopenia or neutropenia is associated with the use of all penicillins; the effect is more likely to occur with prolonged and severe hepatic function impairment.

Special Considerations:

- Contraindicated in patients with prior hypersensitivity to penicillins. Use with caution in patients sensitive to other β-lactams (e.g., cephalosporins) since partial cross-allergenicity exists.
- Obtain ordered specimen and send for culture and sensitivity prior to first antibiotic dose.
- Consider alternative antibiotic therapy if eosinophilia, drug fever or rash, arthralgia, hematuria, or unexplained rise in BUN and serum creatinine occur.
- Monitor electrolytes and renal, hepatic, and hematologic laboratory parameters during extended treatment periods.
- Use with caution in pregnancy or with nursing women.
- Amoxicillin rash may occur that is distinct from drug-allergic rash; increased risk if concurrent use of allopurinol.
- Less diarrhea as a GI side effect than ampicillin.
- May cause false-positive with Clinitest glucose testing.

Potential Toxicities/Side Effects and the Nursing Process

I. POTENTIAL FOR INJURY related to HYPERSENSITIVITY REACTION

Defining Characteristics: Urticaria, pruritus, rash (maculopapular or erythematous), fever and chills, eosinophilia, myalgia, edema, erythema, angioedema, Stevens-Johnson syndrome, and exfoliative skin reactions occur in 5% of patients. Increased risk in individuals allergic to cephalosporin antibiotics. A nonimmunologic rash may occur 3–14 days after drug started, characterized as a generalized erythematous/maculopapular rash, and worse over pressure areas of elbows and knees. Rash usually subsides in 6–14 days, even if drug is continued. If drug is stopped, resolves in 1–7 days.

Nursing Implications: Assess allergy to cephalosporin antibiotics and penicillin: if patient states "yes," determine actual response, e.g., "swollen lips = angioedema." If angioedema, patient SHOULD NOT receive drug. Discuss other patient responses with physician to determine whether drug should be given. Assess baseline skin condition, including integrity and allergy history to drugs. Instruct patient to report rash, itching, other skin changes. Teach patient skin care and symptomatic measures as appropriate. If skin rash develops, discuss drug discontinuance with physician. If rash progresses, drug should be discontinued, as fatal Stevens-Johnson syndrome may develop. Be prepared to treat severe acute hypersensitivity reactions with airway management, oxygen, epinephrine, corticosteroids, antihistamines as ordered.

II. ALTERATION IN NUTRITION, LESS THAN BODY REQUIREMENTS, related to GI SIDE EFFECTS

Defining Characteristics: Nausea, vomiting, diarrhea, anorexia may occur; rarely, pseudomembranous colitis caused by *Clostridium difficile* resistant to the antibiotic occurs. Rarely, transient increases in LFTs—AST, ALT, alk phos, bili—may occur.

Nursing Implications: Assess baseline nutritional status. Instruct patient to report GI disturbances. Administer and instruct patient to self-administer antiemetics as needed and as ordered. Teach patient importance of nutritious diet, and suggest small, frequent, high-calorie, high-protein meals as appropriate. Assess baseline LFTs and monitor periodically during treatment. Discuss abnormalities and drug interruption with physician.

III. FUNGAL SUPERINFECTION related to OVERGROWTH of ENDOGENOUS MICROORGANISMS

Defining Characteristics: Vaginal candidiasis, vaginitis may occur as endogenous bacteria are eliminated, and normal fungal population expands.

Nursing Implications: Teach female patient to report vaginal itching or discharge. Discuss appropriate antifungal treatment with physician. Teach perineal hygiene and symptomatic management.

IV. ALTERATIONS IN PROTECTIVE MECHANISMS (RARE) related to TRANSIENT LEUKOPENIA

Defining Characteristics: Rarely, transient leukopenia, lymphocytosis, anemia, eosinophilia may occur. Prolonged PT, prolonged activated partial thromboplastin time (APTT), and hypoprothrombinemia have occurred rarely, especially in elderly or debilitated patients, or in individuals with vitamin K deficiency.

Nursing Implications: Assess baseline laboratory parameters, and monitor periodically during treatment. Assess patient for response to antibiotics. Discuss abnormalities with physician.

V. KNOWLEDGE DEFICIT related to SELF-ADMINISTRATION OF MEDICATION

Defining Characteristics: Increased compliance when patient is instructed in self-care activities.

Nursing Implications: Assess knowledge regarding infection and planned treatment. Teach drug action, potential side effects, and when and how to take drug (take medication as directed, 1 hour before or 2 hours after food). Instruct patient to report any possible drug side effects that occur.

Drug: ampicillin sodium/sulbactam sodium (UNASYN)

Class: Penicillin (aminopenicillin antibiotic).

Mechanism of Action: Semisynthetic antibiotic prepared from fungus *Penicillium.* Contains β-lactam ring and is bactericidal by inhibiting cell wall synthesis. Aminopenicillins have increased activity against gram-negative bacilli *(H. influenzae, E. coli),* as well as some activity against gram-positive bacilli *(Streptococci* and *Staphylococci).* Although sulbactam alone possesses little useful antibacterial activity, whole organism studies have shown that sulbactam restores ampicillin activity against beta-lactamase producing strains of bacteria. Used for treatment of infections of the skin, intra-abdominal infections, and gynecologic infections by sensitive organisms. In combination with sulbactam there is irreversible inhibition of beta lactamases, thus making ampicillin effective against beta lactamase bacteria that would otherwise be resistant to it.

Metabolism: Metabolism: Well absorbed from GI tract, but rate and amount of drug absorbed is decreased with food. Widely distributed in body tissues and fluids. Crosses placenta and is found in breast milk. Excreted in urine and bile.

Dosage/Range:

Adult:

- Dose modification necessary if renal impairment occurs. See manufacturer's package insert.
- UNASYN: 1.5–3 grams ampicillin and 0.5–1 gram sulbactam IV/IM every 6 hours (dose not to exceed 4 g sulbactam a day).

Drug Preparation/Administration:

- IV dilute with Normal Saline only, give over 10–30 minutes.
- IM: reconstitute per manufacturer's directions and use within 1 hour after reconstitution.

Drug Interactions:

- Aminoglycosides: synergism.
- Aminoglycosides (e.g., gentamicin): incompatible when mixed together; administer at separate sites at different times. Also, penicillinase-resistant penicillins can inactivate aminoglycoside serum samples from patients receiving both drugs.
- Rifampin: possible antagonism, only at high doses of ampicillin.
- Probenecid: decreases renal tubular secretion of ampicillin and sulbactam.
- Oral contraceptives: may decrease efficacy of contraceptive and increase incidence of breakthrough bleeding. Suggest additional use of barrier contraception.

- Sulbactam: broadens antibacterial coverage of ampicillin against resistant beta lactamase-producing microorganisms.
- Concurrent administration of allopurinal and ampicillin increases the incidence of rashes.

Lab Effects/Interference:

- Urine glucose: high urinary concentrations of a penicillin may produce false-positive or falsely elevated test results with copper-reduction tests (Benedict's Clinitest, or Fehling's); glucose enzymatic tests (Clinistix or Testape) are not affected
- Estradiol, total conjugated estriol, estriol-glucuronide or conjugated estrone concentrations may be transiently decreased in pregnant women following administration of ampicillin.
- Increased AST (SGOT), ALT (SGPT), alkaline phosphatase, and LDH.
- Decreased serum albumin and total protein.
- WBC: leukopenia or neutropenia is associated with the use of all penicillins; the effect is more likely to occur with prolonged and severe hepatic function impairment.
- BUN and serum creatinine: increased concentrations have been associated with ampicillin.

Special Considerations:

- Contraindicated in patients with prior hypersensitivity to penicillins. Use with caution in patients sensitive to other β-lactams (e.g., cephalosporins) since partial cross-allergenicity exists.
- Obtain ordered specimen and send for culture and sensitivity prior to first antibiotic dose.
- Consider alternative antibiotic therapy if eosinophilia, drug fever or rash, arthralgia, hematuria, or unexplained rise in BUN and serum creatinine occur.
- Monitor electrolytes and renal, hepatic, and hematologic laboratory parameters during extended treatment periods.
- Use with caution in pregnancy or with nursing women.
- Renal dysfunction: Unasyn dose must be reduced.

Potential Toxicities/Side Effects and the Nursing Process

I. POTENTIAL FOR INJURY related to HYPERSENSITIVITY REACTION and LOCAL REACTIONS (pain at injection site & thrombophlebitis)

Defining Characteristics: Urticaria, pruritus, rash (maculopapular or erythematous), fever and chills, eosinophilia, myalgia, edema, erythema, angioedema, Stevens-Johnson syndrome, and exfoliative skin reactions occur in 5% of patients. Increased risk in individuals allergic to cephalosporin antibiotics.

Nursing Implications: Assess allergy to cephalosporin antibiotics and penicillin: if patient states "yes," determine actual response, e.g., "swollen lips = angioedema." If angioedema, patient SHOULD NOT receive drug. Discuss other patient responses with physician to determine whether drug should be given. Assess baseline skin condition, including integrity and allergy history to drugs. Instruct patient to report rash, itching, other skin changes. Teach patient skin care and symptomatic measures as appropriate. If skin rash develops, discuss drug discontinuance with physician. If rash progresses, drug should be discontinued, as fatal Stevens-Johnson syndrome may develop. Be prepared to treat severe acute hypersensitivity reactions with airway management, oxygen, epinephrine, corticosteroids, antihistamines as ordered.

II. ALTERATION IN NUTRITION, LESS THAN BODY REQUIREMENTS, related to GI SIDE EFFECTS

Defining Characteristics: Nausea, vomiting, diarrhea may occur; rarely, pseudomembranous colitis caused by *C. difficile* resistant to the antibiotic occurs. Rarely, transient increases in LFTs—AST, ALT, alk phos, bili—may occur.

Nursing Implications: Assess baseline nutritional status. Instruct patient to report GI disturbances. Administer and teach patient to self-administer antiemetics as needed and as ordered. Teach patient importance of nutritious diet, and suggest small, frequent, high-calorie, high-protein meals as appropriate. Assess baseline LFTs, and monitor periodically during treatment. Discuss abnormalities and drug interruption with physician.

III. FUNGAL SUPERINFECTION related to REDISTRIBUTION OF ENDOGENOUS MICROORGANISMS

Defining Characteristics: Vaginal candidiasis, vaginitis may occur as endogenous bacteria are eliminated, and normal fungal population expands.

Nursing Implications: Instruct female patient to report vaginal itching or discharge. Discuss appropriate antifungal treatment with physician. Teach perineal hygiene and symptomatic management.

IV. KNOWLEDGE DEFICIT related to SELF-ADMINISTRATION OF MEDICATION

Defining Characteristics: Increased compliance when patient is instructed in self-care activities.

Nursing Implications: Assess knowledge regarding infection and planned treatment. Teach about drug action, potential side effects, and when and how to take drug. (Take medication as directed, 1 hour before or 2 hours after food.) Instruct patient to report any possible drug side effects.

Drug: azithromycin (Zithromax)

Class: Antibacterial (macrolide).

Mechanism of Action: Azithromycin binds to the 50S ribosomal subunit of the 70S ribosome of susceptible organisms, thereby inhibiting RNA-dependent protein synthesis. Bactericidal for *S. pyogenes, S. pneumoniae,* and *H. influenzae.* It is bacteriostatic for staphylococci and most aerobic gram-negative species.

Metabolism: Rapidly and widely distributed throughout the body; concentrates intracellulary, resulting in tissue concentrations 10 to 100 times those in plasma and serum. Rapidly absorbed with decreased absorption when given with food. Concentrates intracellularly, resulting in tissue concentration 10 to 100 times those in plasma or serum. Azithromycin is highly concentrated in phagocytes and fibroblasts. Over 50% of the dose is eliminated through biliary excretion as unchanged drug; approximately 4.5% of the dose is excreted unchanged in the urine within 72 hours.

Dosage/Range:

- Oral: loading dose of 500 mg as a single dose on day 1, then 250 mg once a day on days 2–5.
- No adjustment in dose is required in patients with mild renal function impairment. No data available for patients with more severe renal function impairment.
- IV: if indicated, 500 mg may be given daily × 1–2 days, then followed by oral therapy 250 mg to complete course.

Drug Preparation:

- Reconstitute 500-mg vial with 4.8 mL sterile water for concentration of 100 mg/mL.
- Further dilute with 250 or 500 mL of compatible IV solution.

Drug Administration:

- Oral: give at least 1 hour before and 2 hours after meals.
  Give at least 1 hour before and 2 hours after aluminum- and magnesium-containing antacids.
- IV: infuse 500 mg/500 mL over 3 hours and 500 mg/250 mL over 1 hour.

Drug Interactions:

- Concurrent use with antacids has decreased the peak serum concentration by approximately 24%.

Lab Effects/Interference:

- Serum SGPT, serum SGOT values may be increased.
- Creatinine clearance ≥ 40 mL per minute is desired.

Special Considerations:

- Do not use when there is a known hypersensitivity to erythromycins or other macrolides.
- Use with caution in patients with severe, impaired hepatic function.

Potential Toxicities/Side Effects and the Nursing Process

I. POTENTIAL FOR INJURY related to HYPERSENSITIVITY

Defining Characteristics: Rarely, serious allergic reactions such as anaphylaxis and angioedema have been known to occur. Fever, joint pain, skin rash, urticaria, pruritus, difficulty breathing, swelling of face, mouth, neck, hands, and feet have occurred rarely.

Nursing Implications: Assess for drug allergies to erythromycin or macrolide antibiotic prior to drug administration. Teach patient to report any allergic reactions. Assess for signs/symptoms of allergic reaction after drug dose.

II. ALTERATION IN NUTRITION related to GI SIDE EFFECTS

Defining Characteristics: Abdominal pain, diarrhea, nausea, and vomiting have occurred rarely.

Nursing Implications: Assess baseline nutritional status, preexisting nausea/vomiting, anorexia. Assess baseline LFTs and monitor periodically during treatment. Teach patient to report side effects. Provide symptomatic interventions if side effects occur; discuss with physician use of alternative drug(s).

III. ALTERATION IN URINARY ELIMINATION related to ACUTE INTERSTITIAL NEPHRITIS

Defining Characteristics: Risk is low, but patient may manifest symptoms of acute interstitial nephritis—fever, joint pain, skin rash.

Nursing Implications: Assess baseline renal function and electrolytes, and monitor periodically during therapy. Monitor hydration status to keep patient well hydrated.

IV. SENSORY/PERCEPTUAL ALTERATIONS related to CNS EFFECTS OF DIZZINESS AND HEADACHE

Defining Characteristics: Dizziness and headache may occur.

Nursing Implications: Assess baseline neurological status. Teach patient about side effects and to report dizziness or headache. If signs/symptoms arise, discuss drug discontinuance with physician.

Drug: aztreonam (Azactam)

Class: Antibacterial (systemic).

Mechanism of Action: Bactericidal by inhibition of cell wall synthesis, which results in cell wall disintegration, lysis, and cell death. Narrow-spectrum of activity against aerobic, gram-negative microorganisms (*Enterobacteriaceae* and *P. aeruginosa*). Used to treat gram-negative infections of urinary and lower respiratory tract, septicemia, and gynecologic and intraabdominal infections.

Metabolism: Poorly absorbed from GI tract. Widely distributed in body tissue and fluids, including CSF and peritoneal fluid. Crosses placenta and is excreted in breast milk. Partially metabolized, and excreted primarily in urine.

Dosage/Range:

- Given IV or IM (IV preferred for doses > 1 g, and for serious infections).
- Adults: 500 mg–2 g IV/IM q6–12h (maximum 8 g/day).
- Dose modification needed for renal dysfunction (creatinine clearance < 30 mL/min); may need to modify dosage in hepatic impairment.

Drug Preparation/Administration:

- IV: reconstitute by adding 10 mL sterile water for injection or compatible IV fluid. Further dilute by adding to a volume of IV fluid (50 mL for each gram of drug) so final concentration is < 20 mg/mL. Administer over 20–60 minutes. Flush line with plain IV fluid before and after drug infusion to prevent incompatibilities.
- IM: reconstitute drug with 3 mL for each gram of drug using sterile or bacteriostatic water for injection, or 0.9% Sodium Chloride. Do not mix with local anesthetics. Administer deep IM in large muscle mass (e.g., gluteus maximus).

Drug Interactions:

- Probenecid: increased serum concentrations of antibiotic; monitor and decrease dose if needed.
- Aminoglycosides, penicillins: may have synergistic antibacterial effect against some organisms.
- Nephrotoxic drugs (aminoglycosides, colistin, vancomycin): may increase risk of renal dysfunction; avoid if possible.
- Magnesium, calcium: incompatible in IV fluid.
- Oral anticoagulants, ASPIRIN: may increase risk of bleeding.
- Alcohol: disulfiramlike reaction (flushing, throbbing headache, dyspnea, nausea, vomiting, diaphoresis, chest pain, palpitation, hyperventilation, tachycardia, hypertension, syncope, weakness, blurred vision) when alcohol is ingested within 48–72 hours of aztreonam; does not occur if alcohol is ingested prior to first antibiotic dose. If no alcohol prior to first dose, avoid alcohol for 72 hours after last dose.

Lab Effects/Interference:
- Coombs' (antiglobulin) tests may become positive during therapy.
- Serum ALT, serum alk phos, serum AST, and serum LDH values may be transiently increased during therapy.
- Serum creatinine concentrations may be transiently increased during therapy.
- PTT and PT may be prolonged during therapy.

Special Considerations:
- Obtain and send specimen for culture and sensitivity prior to first drug dose.
- May cause false-positive Clinitest glucose result.
- Use with caution in patients with renal or hepatic dysfunction.
- Drug crosses placenta and is excreted in breast milk. Use with caution if patient is pregnant; weigh potential risks and benefits carefully if lactating; suggest interruption of breast-feeding during antibiotic therapy.
- Use cautiously if prior immediate hypersensitivity reaction to penicillins or cephalosporins; little risk of cross-allergenicity, but monitor patient closely.
- Comparable antiinfective effectiveness to aminoglycosides against gram-negative organisms without ototoxicity or nephrotoxicity.

Potential Toxicities/Side Effects and the Nursing Process

I. ALTERATIONS IN SKIN INTEGRITY related to ALLERGY HYPERSENSITIVITY REACTION

Defining Characteristics: 1–2% incidence of rash that is mild, transient, pruritic, and/or erythematous. Less than 1% of patients develop purpura, erythema multiforme, urticaria, or exfoliative dermatitis. Less than 1% incidence occurs of immediate hypersensitivity reaction characterized by angioedema, bronchospasm, severe shock. Little cross-allergenicity with penicillins, cephalosporins (less than 1%).

Nursing Implications: Assess baseline skin integrity and presence of drug allergies; if anaphylactic reaction to penicillins or cephalosporins, monitor patient closely during drug infusions. Instruct patient to report immediately signs/symptoms of rash, pruritus, shortness of breath, and adverse sensation. Teach patient skin care and symptomatic measures as appropriate. If skin rash develops, discuss drug discontinuance with physician. If rash progresses, especially in HIV-infected patients, drug should be discontinued, as fatal Stevens-Johnson syndrome may develop. Be prepared to treat severe acute hypersensitivity reactions with airway management, oxygen, epinephrine, corticosteroids, antihistamines as ordered.

II. ALTERATION IN NUTRITION, LESS THAN BODY REQUIREMENTS, related to GI SIDE EFFECTS

Defining Characteristics: Nausea, vomiting, diarrhea, anorexia may occur; rarely, pseudomembranous colitis caused by *C. difficile* resistant to the antibiotic occurs. Rarely, transient increases in LFTs—AST, ALT, alk phos—may occur. May develop taste alteration and halitosis.

Nursing Implications: Assess baseline nutritional status. Instruct patient to report GI disturbances. Administer and teach patient to self-administer antiemetics as needed and as ordered. Teach patient importance of nutritious diet, and suggest small, frequent, high-calorie, high-protein meals as appropriate. Assess baseline LFTs, and monitor periodically during treatment. Discuss abnormalities and drug interruption with physician. Encourage oral hygiene after meals and at bedtime.

III. FUNGAL SUPERINFECTION related to REDISTRIBUTION OF ENDOGENOUS MICROORGANISMS

Defining Characteristics: Vaginal candidiasis, vaginitis may occur as endogenous bacteria are eliminated, and normal fungal population expands.

Nursing Implications: Instruct female patient to report vaginal itching or discharge. Discuss appropriate antifungal treatment with physician. Teach perineal hygiene and symptomatic management.

IV. ALTERATIONS IN PROTECTIVE MECHANISMS (RARE) related to PANCYTOPENIA

Defining Characteristics: Pancytopenia, neutropenia, thrombocytopenia, anemia, leukocytosis, thrombocytosis may occur rarely. Eosinophilia occurs in 11% of patients. May have slight prolongation of bleeding time with high doses (e.g., 2-gm IV q6h).

Nursing Implications: Assess baseline laboratory parameters, and monitor periodically during treatment. Assess patient for response to antibiotics. Discuss abnormalities with physician. Assess for signs/symptoms of bleeding. If taking anticoagulants, assess for increased PT, signs/symptoms of bleeding.

V. ALTERATIONS IN SENSORY/PERCEPTUAL PATTERNS related to DIZZINESS, SOMNOLENCE

Defining Characteristics: Dizziness, headache, somnolence, seizures occur rarely.

Nursing Implications: Assess baseline neurologic function and comfort, and monitor during treatment. Instruct patient to report any changes. Discuss any abnormalities with physician.

VI. ALTERATIONS IN COMFORT related to LOCAL INJECTION IRRITATION

Defining Characteristics: 2–3% incidence of phlebitis and thrombophlebitis when administering IV; 3% incidence of pain and swelling at injection site when given IM.

Nursing Implications: Rotate IM injection sites, and administer drug deep IM in large muscle mass (e.g., gluteus maximus). Use IM injection when IV administration is not possible. Change IV sites q48h, and assess for signs/symptoms of phlebitis prior to each administration. Administer drug slowly. Apply warm packs to increase comfort.

VII. ALTERATIONS IN CARDIAC OUTPUT related to CARDIOVASCULAR CHANGES

Defining Characteristics: Rare, ~1% incidence of hypotension, transient EKG changes (e.g., premature ventricular contractions), bradycardia, flushing, and chest pain.

Nursing Implications: Assess baseline heart rate and BP; monitor during therapy, at least with initial dose.

Drug: carbenicillin indanyl sodium (Geocillin, Geopen)

Class: Extended-spectrum penicillin antibacterial.

Mechanism of Action: Semisynthetic penicillin prepared from fungus *Penicillium*. Contains β-lactam ring and is bactericidal by inhibiting cell wall synthesis. Active against gram-positive and gram-negative organisms, but most active against *Pseudomonas* and *Proteus,* except those that have developed resistance to carbenicillin.

Metabolism: After oral administration, rapidly converted to carbenicillin by hydrolysis. Widely distributed in body tissues and fluids. Crosses placenta and is excreted in breast milk. Excreted via urine and bile.

Dosage/Range:

Adult:

- 1 tablet (382 mg).

Urinary tract infections:

- *Escherichia coli Proteus* species *Enterobacter:* 1–2 tabs QID (QID = 4 times a day).
- *Pseudomonas, Enterococcus:* 2 tabs QID.
- *Prostatitis* due to *Escherichia coli, Proteus mirabilis, Enterobacter, Enterococcus:* 2 tabs QID.

Drug Preparation/Administration:

- Oral, none.

Drug Interactions:

- Probenecid: increased serum level of penicillin; may be coadministered to exert this effect.

Lab Effects/Interference:

Major clinical significance:

- Urine glucose: high urinary concentrations of a penicillin may produce falsepositive or falsely elevated test results with copper sulfate tests (Benedict's, Clinitest, or Fehling's); glucose enzymatic tests (Clinistix or Testape) are not affected.
- PTT and PT: an increase has been associated with intravenous carbenicillin.

Clinical significance:

- Coombs' (direct antiglobulin) tests: false-positive result may occur during therapy with any penicillin.
- ALT, alk phos, AST, and serum LDH values may be decreased.
- WBC: leukopenia or neutropenia is associated with the use of all penicillins; the effect is more likely to occur with prolonged therapy and severe hepatic function impairment.

Special Considerations:

- Contraindicated in patients with prior hypersensitivity to penicillins. Use with caution in patients sensitive to other β-lactams (e.g., cephalosporins) since partial cross-allergenicity exists.
- Obtain ordered specimen and send for culture and sensitivity prior to first antibiotic dose.
- Consider alternative antibiotic therapy if eosinophilia, drug fever or rash, arthralgia, hematuria, or unexplained rise in BUN and serum creatinine occur.
- Use with caution in pregnancy or with nursing women.

Potential Toxicities/Side Effects and the Nursing Process

I. POTENTIAL FOR INJURY related to HYPERSENSITIVITY REACTION

Defining Characteristics: Urticaria, pruritus, rash (maculopapular or erythematous), fever and chills, eosinophilia, myalgia, edema, erythema, angioedema, Stevens-Johnson syndrome, and exfoliative skin reactions occur in 5% of patients. Increased risk in individuals allergic to cephalosporin antibiotics.

Nursing Implications: Assess allergy to cephalosporin antibiotics and penicillin: if patient states "yes," determine actual response, e.g., "swollen lips = angioedema." If angioedema, patient SHOULD NOT receive drug. Discuss other patient responses with physician to determine whether drug should be given.

Assess baseline skin condition, including integrity and allergy history to drugs. Instruct patient to report rash, itching, other skin changes. Teach patient skin care and symptomatic measures as appropriate. If skin rash develops, discuss drug discontinuance with physician. If rash progresses, drug should be discontinued, as fatal Stevens-Johnson syndrome may develop.

II. ALTERATION IN NUTRITION, LESS THAN BODY REQUIREMENTS, related to GI SIDE EFFECTS

Defining Characteristics: Nausea, vomiting, diarrhea may occur; rarely, "furry" tongue, abdominal cramps, transient increases in LFTs—AST, ALT, alk phos, bili—may occur.

Nursing Implications: Assess baseline nutritional status. Instruct patient to report GI disturbances. Administer and teach patient to self-administer antiemetics as needed and as ordered. Teach patient importance of nutritious diet, and suggest small, frequent, high-calorie, high-protein meals as appropriate. Assess baseline LFTs and monitor periodically during treatment. Discuss abnormalities and drug interruption with physician.

III. FUNGAL SUPERINFECTION related to REDISTRIBUTION OF ENDOGENOUS MICROORGANISMS

Defining Characteristics: Vaginal candidiasis, vaginitis may occur as endogenous bacteria are eliminated, and normal fungal population expands.

Nursing Implications: Instruct female patient to report vaginal itching or discharge. Discuss appropriate antifungal treatment with physician. Teach perineal hygiene and symptomatic management.

IV. ALTERATIONS IN PROTECTIVE MECHANISMS (RARE) related to LEUKOPENIA

Defining Characteristics: Rarely, transient leukopenia, lymphocytosis, anemia, eosinophilia may occur. Prolonged PT, prolonged APTT, and hypoprothrombinemia have occurred rarely, especially in elderly or debilitated patients, or in individuals with vitamin K deficiency.

Nursing Implications: Assess baseline laboratory parameters, and monitor periodically during treatment. Assess patient for response to antibiotics. Discuss abnormalities with physician. Assess for signs/symptoms of bleeding.

Drug: cefaclor (Ceclor)

Class: Second-generation cephalosporin antibiotic.

Mechanism of Action: Semisynthetic derivative of cephalosporin C (produced by fungus); contains β-lactam ring and is related to penicillins and cephamycins (e.g., cefoxitin). Bactericidal through inhibition of cell wall synthesis, with resulting cell wall instability and cell lysis. Active against organisms causing lower respiratory tract infections (*H. influenzae, Klebsiella, Proteus, S. aureus, Streptococcus pneumoniae*); urinary tract infections (*Enterobacter, E. coli*); skin and soft tissue infections (*S. aureus, E. coli*); septicemia; and biliary infections. (Active against *H. influenzae, S. pneumoniae, Streptococcus pyogenes, E. coli, Proteus mirabilis, Klebsiella,* and staphylococci.)

Metabolism: Well absorbed from GI tract; delayed GI absorption if taken with food, but total amount of drug absorption is the same. Widely distributed in body tissues, fluids except CSF; readily crosses placenta and is excreted in breast milk. Unchanged drug rapidly excreted by the kidneys.

Dosage/Range:

- Oral: 250–500 mg q8h (maximum total 4 gm/day).

Drug Preparation/Administration:

- Store in tight container at 15–30°C (59–86°F).

Drug Interactions:

- Probenecid: increased serum concentrations of cefaclor, but does not usually require dose reduction of antibiotic.

Lab Effects/Interference:

Major clinical significance:

- Coombs' (antiglobulin) tests: a positive reaction frequently appears in patients who receive large doses of cephalosporins; hemolysis rarely occurs, but it has been reported; test may be positive in neonates whose mothers received cephalosporins before delivery.
- Urine glucose: cefaclor may produce false-positive or falsely elevated test results with copper sulfate tests (Benedicts, Clinitest, or Fehling's); glucose enzymatic tests (Clonistix or Testape) are not affected.
- PT: may be prolonged; cephalosporins may inhibit vitamin K synthesis by suppressing gut flora.

Clinical significance:

- Serum ALT, serum alk phos, serum AST, serum bili, or serum LDH values may be increased.
- BUN and serum creatinine concentrations may be increased.

- CBC or platelet count: transient leukopenia, neutropenia, agranulocytosis, thrombocytopenia, eosinophilia, lymphocytosis, and thrombocytosis have been seen on rare occasions.

Special Considerations:
- Use cautiously if renal impairment is present.
- Contraindicated if hypersensitive to other cephalosporins, or if has had angioedema response to penicillin.
- Urine glucose testing with Clinitest may result in false-positive.

Potential Toxicities/Side Effects and the Nursing Process

I. POTENTIAL FOR INJURY related to HYPERSENSITIVITY REACTION

Defining Characteristics: Urticaria, pruritus, rash (maculopapular or erythematous), fever and chills, eosinophilia, myalgia, edema, erythema, angioedema, Stevens-Johnson syndrome, and exfoliative skin reactions occur in 5% of patients. Increased risk in individuals allergic to penicillin.

Nursing Implications: Assess allergy to cephalosporin antibiotics and penicillin: if patient states "yes," determine actual response, e.g., "swollen lips = angioedema." If angioedema, patient SHOULD NOT receive drug. Discuss other patient responses with physician to determine whether drug should be given. Assess baseline skin condition, including integrity and allergy history to drugs. Instruct patient to report rash, itching, and other skin changes. Teach patient skin care and symptomatic measures as appropriate. If skin rash develops, discuss drug discontinuance with physician. If rash progresses, drug should be discontinued, as fatal Stevens-Johnson syndrome may develop. Be prepared to treat severe acute hypersensitivity reactions with airway management, oxygen, epinephrine, corticosteroids, antihistamines as ordered.

II. ALTERATION IN NUTRITION, LESS THAN BODY REQUIREMENTS, related to GI SIDE EFFECTS

Defining Characteristics: Nausea, vomiting, diarrhea, and anorexia may occur; rarely, pseudomembranous colitis caused by *C. difficile* resistant to the antibiotic occurs. May cause transient increases in LFTs.

Nursing Implications: Assess baseline nutritional status. Instruct patient to report GI disturbances. Administer and teach patient to self-administer antiemetics as needed and as ordered. Teach patient importance of nutritious diet, and suggest small, frequent, high-calorie, high-protein meals as appropriate. Assess baseline LFTs and monitor periodically during treatment. Discuss abnormalities and drug interruption with physician.

III. FUNGAL SUPERINFECTION related to REDISTRIBUTION OF ENDOGENOUS MICROORGANISMS

Defining Characteristics: Vaginal candidiasis, vaginitis may occur as endogenous bacteria are eliminated, and normal fungal population expands.

Nursing Implications: Instruct female patient to report vaginal itching or discharge. Discuss appropriate antifungal treatment with physician. Teach perineal hygiene and symptomatic management.

IV. ALTERATIONS IN PROTECTIVE MECHANISMS (RARE) related to CHANGES IN BLOOD CELL ELEMENTS, CLOTTING FACTOR

Defining Characteristics: Rarely, transient leukopenia, lymphocytosis, anemia, eosinophilia may occur. Prolonged PT, prolonged APTT, and hypoprothrombinemia have occurred rarely, especially in elderly or debilitated patients, or in individuals with vitamin K deficiency.

Nursing Implications: Assess baseline laboratory parameters, and monitor periodically during treatment. Assess patient for response to antibiotics. Discuss abnormalities with physician.

V. ALTERATIONS IN SENSORY/PERCEPTUAL PATTERNS related to DIZZINESS, SOMNOLENCE

Defining Characteristics: Dizziness, headache, somnolence occur rarely.

Nursing Implications: Assess baseline neurologic function and comfort, and monitor during treatment. Instruct patient to report any changes. Discuss any abnormalities with physician.

VI. KNOWLEDGE DEFICIT related to SELF-ADMINISTRATION OF MEDICATION

Defining Characteristics: Increased compliance when patient is instructed in self-care activities.

Nursing Implications: Assess knowledge regarding infection and planned treatment. Teach about drug action, potential side effects, and when and how to take drug. Instruct patient to report any possible side effects that occur.

Drug: cefadroxil (Duracef)

Class: First-generation cephalosporin antibacterial.

Mechanism of Action: Semisynthetic derivative of cephalosporin C, contains beta-lactam ring, and is related to penicillins and cephamycins. Bactericidal through inhibition of cell wall synthesis by binding to one or more of the penicillin-binding proteins (PBPs) that in turn inhibit the final transpeptidation step of peptidoglycan synthesis in bacterial cell walls, thus inhibiting cell wall biosynthesis. Bacteria eventually lyse due to ongoing activity of cell wall autolytic enzymes (autolysins and murein hydrolases) while cell wall assembly is arrested.

Metabolism: Well absorbed from GI tract; delayed GI absorption if taken with food, but total amount of drug absorption is the same. Widely distributed in body tissues, fluids except cerebrospinal fluid; readily crosses placenta and is excreted in breast milk. Unchanged drug rapidly excreted by the kidneys.

Dosage/Range:
- Adults: 1–2 g/day every 12 hours.
- Dose reduce if creatinine clearance is reduced per manufacturer's recommendations.

Drug Preparation/Administration:
- Store suspension in refrigerator, discard after 14 days.
- Oral administration.

Drug Interactions:
- Furosemide and aminoglycosides increase nephrotic potential and increase toxicity.
- Probenecid may decrease cephalosporin elimination and increase effect.

Lab Effects/Interference:
- Serum SGPT, serum Alk Phos, serum SGOT, serum bilirubin, or serum LDH—values may be increased
- BUN and serum creatinine—concentrations may be increased

Special Considerations:
- Use with caution in patients with renal dysfunction—dose reduction required if severe impairment exists.
- Contraindicated in patients hypersensitive to other cephalosporin antibiotics
- Use cautiously if sensitive to penicillin; contraindicated if angioedema reaction to penicillin.
- Obtain ordered specimen and send for culture and sensitivity prior to first drug dose.

Potential Toxicities/Side Effects and the Nursing Process

I. POTENTIAL FOR INJURY related to HYPERSENSITIVITY REACTION

Defining Characteristics: Urticaria, pruritis, rash (maculopapular or erythematous), fever and chills, eosinophilia, myalgia, edema, erythema, angioedema. Increased risk in individuals allergic to penicillin.

Nursing Implications: Assess allergy to cephalosporin antibiotics and penicillin: if patient states "yes," determine actual response, e.g., "swollen lips = angioedema." If angioedema, patient SHOULD NOT receive drug. Discuss other patient responses with physician to determine whether drug should be given. Assess baseline skin condition, including integrity and allergy history to drugs. Teach patient to report rash, itching, other skin changes. Teach patient skin care and symptomatic measures as appropriate. If skin rash develops, discuss drug discontinuance with physician.

II. ALTERATION IN NUTRITION, LESS THAN BODY REQUIREMENTS related to GI SIDE EFFECTS

Defining Characteristics: Nausea and vomiting and diarrhea and anorexia may occur. Rarely, transient increases in LFTs—AST (SGOT), ALT (SGPT), ALKPHOS, BR—may occur.

Nursing Implications: Assess baseline nutritional status. Teach patient to report GI disturbances. Administer and teach patient to self-administer medication as needed and as ordered. Teach patient importance of nutritious diet, and suggest small, frequent, high-calorie, high-protein meals as appropriate. Assess baseline LFTs and monitor periodically during treatment. Discuss abnormalities and drug interruption with physician.

III. FUNGAL SUPERINFECTION related to REDISTRIBUTION OF ENDOGENOUS MICROORGANISMS

Defining Characteristics: Vaginal moniliasis, vaginitis may occur as endogenous bacteria are eliminated and normal fungal population expands.

Nursing Implications: Teach female patient to report vaginal itching or discharge. Discuss appropriate antifungal treatment with physician. Teach perineal hygiene and symptomatic management.

Drug: cefamandole nafate (Mandol)

Class: Second-generation cephalosporin antibacterial.

Mechanism of Action: Semisynthetic derivative of cephalosporin C (produced by fungus); contains β-lactam ring and is related to penicillins and cephamycins (e.g., cefoxitin). Bactericidal through inhibition of cell wall synthesis, with resulting cell wall instability and cell lysis. Active against organisms causing lower respiratory tract infections (*H. influenzae, Klebsiella, Proteus, S. aureus, S. pneumoniae*); urinary tract infections (*Enterobacter, E. coli*); skin and soft tissue infections (*S. aureus, E. coli*); septicemia; and biliary infections.

Metabolism: Not absorbed from GI tract, so must be given IV or IM. Rapidly hydrolyzed to active metabolite. Widely distributed to body tissues and fluids except CSF; 65–75% bound to serum proteins. Readily crosses placenta and is excreted in breast milk. Rapidly excreted by kidneys in urine.

Dosage/Range:

Adult:

- 500 mg–1 g q4–8h; severe infections: 1–2 g q4–6h.
- Dose modification if renal impairment, based on creatinine clearance: refer to manufacturer's package insert.

Drug Preparation/Administration:

- Store powder for injection at T < 40°C (104°F). Reconstituted solution stable for 24 hours at room temperature, or 96 hours refrigerated.
- IV or deep IM injection. IV: reconstitute with 10 mL sterile water for injection, 5% Dextrose or 0.9% Sodium Chloride injection, then further dilute in 100-mL piggyback set and infuse over 30 minutes. IM: reconstitute 1-g vial with 3 mL sterile or bacteriostatic water for injection, 0.9% Sodium Chloride. Administer deep IM into large muscle mass (e.g., gluteus maximus).

Drug Interactions:

- Probenecid: increased serum concentrations of antibiotic; monitor and decrease dose if needed.
- Aminoglycosides, penicillins: may have synergistic antibacterial effect against some organisms.
- Nephrotoxic drugs (aminoglycosides, colistin, vancomycin): may increase risk of renal dysfunction; avoid if possible.
- Magnesium, calcium: incompatible in IV fluid.
- Oral anticoagulants, ASPIRIN: may increase risk of bleeding.
- Alcohol: disulfiramlike reaction (flushing, throbbing headache, dyspnea, nausea, vomiting, diaphoresis, chest pain, palpitations, hyperventilation, tachycardia, hypertension, syncope, weakness, blurred vision) when alcohol ingested within 48–72 hours of cefamandole; does not occur if alcohol ingested prior to first antibiotic dose. If no alcohol prior to first dose, avoid alcohol for 72 hours after last dose.

Lab Effects/Interference:

Major clinical significance:

- Coombs' (antiglobulin) tests: a positive reaction frequently appears in patients who receive large doses of cephalosporins; hemolysis rarely occurs, but it has been reported; test may be positive in neonates whose mothers received cephalosporins before delivery.
- Urine glucose: cefamandole may produce false-positive or falsely elevated test results with copper sulfate tests (Benedicts, Clinitest, or Fehling's); glucose enzymatic tests (Clonistix or Testape) are not affected.

- PT: may be prolonged; cephalosporins may inhibit vitamin K synthesis by suppressing gut flora; also, cephalosporins with the NMTT side chain (cefamandole) have been associated with an increased incidence of hypoprothrombinemia; patients who are critically ill, malnourished, or have liver function impairment may be at the highest risk of bleeding.

Clinical significance:

- Urine protein may produce false-positive tests for proteinuria with acid and denaturization-precipation tests.
- Serum ALT, serum alk phos, serum AST, serum bili, or serum LDH values may be increased.
- BUN and serum creatinine concentrations may be increased.
- CBC or platelet count: transient leukopenia, neutropenia, agranulocytosis, thrombocytopenia, eosinophilia, lymphocytosis, and thrombocytosis have been seen on rare occasions.

Special Considerations:

- Use cautiously if renal impairment is present.
- Contraindicated if hypersensitive to other cephalosporins, or if has had angioedema response to penicillin.
- Urine glucose testing with Clinitest may result in false-positive.

Special Considerations:

- Use with caution in patients with renal dysfunction—dose reduction required if severe impairment exists.
- Use cautiously if history of colitis exists.
- Contraindicated in patients hypersensitive to other cephalosporin antibiotics.
- Use cautiously if sensitive to penicillin; contraindicated if angioedema reaction to penicillin.
- Obtain ordered specimen and send for culture and sensitivity prior to first drug dose.
- May cause false-positive direct Coombs' test.
- May cause false-positive Clinitest glucose result.

Potential Toxicities/Side Effects and the Nursing Process

I. POTENTIAL FOR INJURY related to HYPERSENSITIVITY REACTION

Defining Characteristics: Urticaria, pruritus, rash (maculopapular or erythematous), fever and chills, eosinophilia, myalgia, edema, erythema, angioedema, Stevens-Johnson syndrome, and exfoliative skin reactions occur in 5% of patients. Increased risk in individuals allergic to penicillin.

Nursing Implications: Assess allergy to cephalosporin antibiotics and penicillin: if patient states "yes," determine actual response, e.g., "swollen lips = angioedema." If angioedema, patient SHOULD NOT receive drug. Discuss other patient responses with physician to determine whether drug should be given. Assess baseline skin condition, including integrity and allergy history to drugs. Instruct patient to report rash, itching, other skin changes. Teach patient skin care and symptomatic measures as appropriate. If skin rash develops, discuss drug discontinuance with physician. If rash progresses, drug should be discontinued, as fatal Stevens-Johnson syndrome may develop. Be prepared to treat severe acute hypersensitivity reactions with airway management, oxygen, epinephrine, corticosteroids, antihistamines as ordered.

II. ALTERATION IN NUTRITION, LESS THAN BODY REQUIREMENTS, related to GI SIDE EFFECTS

Defining Characteristics: Nausea, vomiting, diarrhea, anorexia may occur; rarely, pseudomembranous colitis caused by *C. difficile* resistant to the antibiotic occurs. Rarely, transient increases in LFTs—AST, ALT, alk phos, bili—may occur.

Nursing Implications: Assess baseline nutritional status. Instruct patient to report GI disturbances. Administer and teach patient to self-administer antiemetics as needed and as ordered. Teach patient importance of nutritious diet, and suggest small, frequent, high-calorie, high-protein meals as appropriate. Assess baseline LFTs, and monitor periodically during treatment. Discuss abnormalities and drug interruption with physician.

III. FUNGAL SUPERINFECTION related to REDISTRIBUTION OF ENDOGENOUS MICROORGANISMS

Defining Characteristics: Vaginal candidiasis, vaginitis may occur as endogenous bacteria are eliminated and normal fungal population expands.

Nursing Implications: Teach female patient to report vaginal itching or discharge. Discuss appropriate antifungal treatment with physician. Teach perineal hygiene and symptomatic management.

IV. ALTERATIONS IN PROTECTIVE MECHANISMS (RARE) related to TRANSIENT LEUKOPENIA

Defining Characteristics: Rarely, transient leukopenia, lymphocytosis, anemia, eosinophilia may occur. Prolonged PT, prolonged APTT, and hypoprothrombinemia have occurred rarely, especially in elderly or debilitated patients, or in individuals with vitamin K deficiency.

Nursing Implications: Assess baseline laboratory parameters, and monitor periodically during treatment. Assess patient for response to antibiotics. Discuss abnormalities with physician. Assess for signs/symptoms of bleeding. If they occur, especially in elderly or debilitated patients, discuss vitamin K administration with physician. Instruct patient to avoid aspirin. If taking oral anticoagulants, assess for increased PT, signs/symptoms of bleeding.

V. ALTERATIONS IN SENSORY/PERCEPTUAL PATTERNS related to DIZZINESS, HEADACHE, SOMNOLENCE

Defining Characteristics: Dizziness, headache, somnolence occur rarely.

Nursing Implications: Assess baseline neurologic function and comfort, and monitor during treatment. Instruct patient to report any changes. Discuss any abnormalities with physician.

VI. ALTERATIONS IN COMFORT related to LOCAL INJECTION IRRITATION

Defining Characteristics: Pain, induration, sterile abscesses may form in IM injection sites; phlebitis may develop in IV sites.

Nursing Implications: Rotate IM injection sites, and administer drug deep IM in large muscle mass (e.g., gluteus maximus). Use IM injection when IV administration is not possible. Change IV sites q48h, and assess for signs/symptoms of phlebitis prior to each administration. Administer drug slowly. Apply warm packs to increase comfort.

Drug: cefazolin sodium (Ancef)

Class: First-generation cephalosporin antibacterial.

Mechanism of Action: Semisynthetic derivative of cephalosporin C (produced by fungus); contains β-lactam ring and is related to penicillins and cephamycins (e.g., cefoxitin). Bactericidal through inhibition of cell wall synthesis, with resulting cell wall instability and cell lysis. Active against many gram-positive aerobic cocci (*S. aureus*, groups A and B streptococci); some susceptible gramnegative organisms (*E. coli, H. influenzae, Klebsiella, Proteus*); and gramnegative organisms causing intraabdominal and biliary infections.

Metabolism: Not absorbed from GI tract so must be given IV or IM. Widely distributed to body tissues and fluids, including bile; 74–86% bound to serum proteins. Excreted unchanged in urine. Crosses placenta and is excreted in breast milk.

Dosage/Range:

- IV is same as IM.
- Adults: 250 mg–1.5 g q6–8h (maximum 12 g/day in life-threatening infections).

- May give loading dose of 500 mg.
- Dose-reduce if serum creatinine = 1.5 mg/dL according to manufacturer's package insert.

Drug Preparation/Administration:

- Store powder at < 40°C (104°F) and protect from light. Is available as frozen solution that should be stored at T < −20°C (−4°F).
- Reconstitute powder with sterile water for injection, bacteriostatic water for injection, or 0.9% Sodium Chloride; solution stable for 24 hours at room temperature or 96 hours at 5°C (41°F).
- Further dilute in 50–100 mL 0.9% Sodium Chloride or 5% Dextrose for IV administration.
- For IM administration, reconstitute with 2–2.5 mL sterile or bacteriostatic water for injection or 0.9% Sodium Chloride injection. Administer deep IM in large muscle mass (e.g., gluteus maximus).

Drug Interactions:

- Probenecid: increased serum concentrations of antibiotic; monitor and decrease dose if needed.
- Aminoglycosides, penicillins: may have synergistic antibacterial effect against some organisms.
- Nephrotoxic drugs (aminoglycosides, colistin, vancomycin): may increase risk of renal dysfunction; avoid if possible.

Lab Effects/Interference:

Major clinical significance:

- Coombs' (antiglobulin) tests: a positive reaction frequently appears in patients who receive large doses of cephalosporins; hemolysis rarely occurs, but it has been reported; test may be positive in neonates whose mothers received cephalosporins before delivery.
- Urine glucose: cefazolin may produce false-positive or falsely elevated test results with copper sulfate tests (Benedicts, Clinitest, or Fehling's); glucose enzymatic tests (Clonistix or Testape) are not affected.
- PT may be prolonged; cephalosporins may inhibit vitamin K synthesis by suppressing gut flora.

Clinical significance:

- Serum ALT, serum alk phos, serum AST, serum bili, or serum LDH values may be increased.
- BUN and serum creatinine concentrations may be increased.
- CBC or platelet count: transient leukopenia, neutropenia, agranulocytosis, thrombocytopenia, eosinophilia, lymphocytosis, and thrombocytosis have been seen on rare occasions.

Special Considerations:

- Used in treatment of serious infections of respiratory tract, urinary tract, skin and soft tissues, and biliary tree.
- Use with caution in patients with renal dysfunction—dose reduction required if severe impairment exists.
- Use cautiously if history of colitis exists.
- Contraindicated in patients hypersensitive to other cephalosporin antibiotics.
- Use cautiously if sensitive to penicillin; contraindicated if angioedema reaction to penicillin.
- Obtain ordered specimen and send for culture and sensitivity prior to first drug dose.
- May cause false-positive direct Coombs' test.
- May cause false-positive Clinitest glucose result.

Potential Toxicities/Side Effects and the Nursing Process

I. POTENTIAL FOR INJURY related to HYPERSENSITIVITY REACTION

Defining Characteristics: Urticaria, pruritus, rash (maculopapular or erythematous), fever and chills, eosinophilia, myalgia, edema, erythema, angioedema, Stevens-Johnson syndrome, and exfoliative skin reactions occur in 5% of patients. Increased risk in individuals allergic to penicillin.

Nursing Implications: Assess allergy to cephalosporin antibiotics and penicillin: if patient states "yes," determine actual response, e.g., "swollen lips = angioedema." If angioedema, patient SHOULD NOT receive drug. Discuss other patient responses with physician to determine whether drug should be given. Assess baseline skin condition, including integrity and allergy history to drugs. Instruct patient to report rash, itching, other skin changes. Teach patient skin care and symptomatic measures as appropriate. If skin rash develops, discuss drug discontinuance with physician. If rash progresses, drug should be discontinued, as fatal Stevens-Johnson syndrome may develop. Be prepared to treat severe acute hypersensitivity reactions with airway management, oxygen, epinephrine, corticosteroids, antihistamines as ordered.

II. ALTERATION IN NUTRITION, LESS THAN BODY REQUIREMENTS, related to GI SIDE EFFECTS

Defining Characteristics: Nausea, vomiting, diarrhea, anorexia may occur; rarely, pseudomembranous colitis caused by *C. difficile* resistant to the antibiotic occurs. Rarely, transient increases in LFTs—AST, ALT, alk phos, bili—may occur.

Nursing Implications: Assess baseline nutritional status. Instruct patient to report GI disturbances. Administer and teach patient to self-administer antiemetics as needed and as ordered. Teach patient importance of nutritious diet, and suggest small, frequent, high-calorie, high-protein meals as appropriate. Assess baseline LFTs, and monitor periodically during treatment. Discuss abnormalities and drug interruption with physician.

III. FUNGAL SUPERINFECTION related to REDISTRIBUTION OF ENDOGENOUS MICROORGANISMS

Defining Characteristics: Vaginal candidiasis, vaginitis may occur as endogenous bacteria are eliminated and normal fungal population expands.

Nursing Implications: Teach female patient to report vaginal itching or discharge. Discuss appropriate antifungal treatment with physician. Teach perineal hygiene and symptomatic management.

IV. ALTERATIONS IN PROTECTIVE MECHANISMS (RARE) related to CHANGES IN FORMED BLOOD CELL ELEMENTS

Defining Characteristics: Rarely, transient leukopenia, lymphocytosis, anemia, eosinophilia may occur. Prolonged PT, prolonged APTT, and hypoprothrombinemia have occurred rarely, especially in elderly or debilitated patients, or in individuals with vitamin K deficiency.

Nursing Implications: Assess baseline laboratory parameters, and monitor periodically during treatment. Assess patient for response to antibiotics. Discuss abnormalities with physician. Assess for signs/symptoms of bleeding. If they occur, especially in elderly or debilitated patients, discuss vitamin K administration with physician. Instruct patient to avoid aspirin. If taking oral anticoagulants, assess for increased PT, signs/symptoms of bleeding.

V. ALTERATIONS IN SENSORY/PERCEPTUAL PATTERNS related to DIZZINESS, SOMNOLENCE

Defining Characteristics: Dizziness, headache, somnolence occur rarely.

Nursing Implications: Assess baseline neurologic function and comfort, and monitor during treatment. Teach patient to report any changes. Discuss any abnormalities with physician.

VI. ALTERATIONS IN COMFORT related to LOCAL INJECTION IRRITATION

Defining Characteristics: Pain, induration, sterile abscesses may form in IM injection sites; phlebitis may develop in IV sites.

Nursing Implications: Rotate IM injection sites, and administer drug deep IM in large muscle mass (e.g., gluteus maximus). Use IM injection when IV administration is not possible. Change IV sites q48h, and assess for signs/symptoms of phlebitis prior to each administration. Administer drug slowly. Apply warm packs to increase comfort.

Drug: cefdinir (Omnicef)

Class: Cephalosporin broad-spectrum antibiotic.

Mechanism of Action: Inhibits cell wall synthesis, thus destroying microorganisms. Stable in presence of some β-lactamase enzymes, so active against many microorganisms that are resistant to the penicillins and other cephalosporin antibiotics.

Metabolism: Well absorbed from the GI tract following oral dosing, with maximal plasma concentration in 2–4 hrs. Drug largely unmetabolized and eliminated by the kidneys. Mean plasma half-life is 1.7 hours. Dose must be adjusted in patients with severe renal dysfunction or who receive hemodialysis.

Dosage/Range:

Adults with:

- Community-acquired pneumonia: 300 mg PO q12h × 10 days.
- Acute exacerbation of chronic bronchitis: 300 mg PO q12h or 600 mg PO q24h × 10 days.
- Acute maxillary sinusitis: 300 mg PO q12h or 600 mg PO q24h × 10 days.
- Pharyngitis/tonsilitis: 300 mg PO q12h × 5–10 days or 600 mg PO q24h × 10 days.
- Uncomplicated skin/skin structures: 300 mg PO q12h × 10 days.
- Patients with renal insufficiency (creatinine clearance < 30 mL/min) is 300 mg PO q24h.
- Patients on hemodialysis: 300 mg PO every other day with 300 mg given at the end of each dialysis.

Drug Preparation:

- Oral, available as 300-mg tablets or oral suspension that, when reconstituted as directed, results in 125 mg/5 mL in 60- or 100-mL bottles.

Drug Administration:

- Take orally without regard to meals or food intake.

Drug Interactions:

- Antacids containing magnesium or aluminum decrease absorption of cefdinir; take cefdinir at least 2 hours before or after the antacid.

- Iron or iron supplements decrease absorption by up to 80%; separate drugs by at least 2 hours.
- Probenecid inhibits the renal excretion of cefdinir, increasing peak plasma levels by 54% and prolonging half-life by 50%; decrease cefdinir dose if must use together.

Lab Effects/Interference:

- False-positive reaction for ketones in testing using nitroprusside.
- False-positive test for glucose in the urine using Clinitest, Benedict's solution, or Fehling's solution (suggest using Clinistix or Testape).
- False-positive Coombs' test (rare).
- Increased gamma glutamyltransferase (1%); rarely other liver function tests.

Special Considerations:

Indicated for the treatment of adults with mild-tomoderate infections:

- Community-acquired pneumonia caused by *Haemophilus influenzae* (including β-lactamase–producing strains), penicillin-susceptible strains of *Streptococcus pneumoniae, Moraxella catarrhalis* (including β-lactamase–producing strains).
- Acute exacerbation of chronic bronchitis cased by *Haemophilus influenzae,* (including β-lactamase–producing strains), penicillin-susceptible strains of *Streptococcus pneumoniae, Moraxella catarrhalis* (including β-lactamase–producing strains).
- Acute maxillary sinusitis caused by *Haemophilus influenzae* (including β-lactamase–producing strains), penicillin-susceptible strains of *Streptococcus pneumoniae, Moraxella catarrhalis* (including β-lactamase–producing strains).
- Pharyngitis/tonsillitis caused by *Streptococcus pyogenes.*
- Uncomplicated skin and skin structure infections caused by *Staphylococcus aureus* (including β-lactamase–producing strains) and *Streptococcus pyogenes.*
- Contraindicated in patients with an allergy to the cephalosporin class of antibiotics as well as penicillin (cross-sensitivity in 10% of patients).
- Use cautiously, if at all, in patients with a history of colitis.
- Use in pregnancy only when benefits outweigh risks.
- If patient has severe renal dysfunction as evidenced by creatinine clearance < 30 mL/min, the dose should be reduced to 300 mg q day.
- Diabetic patients should know that the oral suspension has 2.86 g of sucrose per teaspoon.

Potential Toxicities/Side Effects and the Nursing Process

I. ALTERATION IN NUTRITION related to GI SIDE EFFECTS

Defining Characteristics: Diarrhea occurs in approximately 16% of patients, and nausea in 3%. Less common are abdominal discomfort (1%), vomiting < 1%, anorexia (< 1%). The following rarely occur: dyspepsia, flatulence, constipation, abnormal stools (red-colored in patients taking iron). As with all antibiotics, psuedomembranous colitis may occur, ranging in severity from mild to life-threatening. Treatment with antibiotics changes the intestinal microflora, so *Clostridiaum difficile* bacteria may overgrow. Once diagnosis is made, mild diarrhea may stop with cessation of drug; if moderate to severe, it will require, in addition, hydration, electrolyte replacement, nutritional support, and antibacterial coverage against *C. difficile.*

Nursing Implications: Assess baseline nutritional and elimination status. Teach patient to report GI disturbances. Teach patient to report diarrhea immediately, consider whether this is pseudomembranous colitis, and send stool specimen for *C. difficile;* if positive, discuss drug discontinuance with physician. Administer and teach patient to self-administer antiemetics, antidiarrheals as needed and as ordered. Teach patient importance of nutritious diet, and suggest small, frequent, high-calorie, high-protein meals as appropriate. Assess baseline LFTs and monitor periodically during treatment. Discuss abnormalities and drug interruption with physician.

II. SENSORY/PERCEPTUAL ALTERATIONS related to CNS EFFECTS

Defining Characteristics: Headaches occur in 2% of patients, and less common (< 1%) are dizziness, asthenia, insomnia, somnolence.

Nursing Implications: Assess baseline neurological function and comfort, and monitor during treatment. Teach patient to report any changes. Teach patient how to manage symptoms. If unrelieved or persistent, discuss any abnormalities with physician.

III. ALTERATION IN SKIN INTEGRITY related to ALLERGY/HYPERSENSITIVITY

Defining Characteristics: Uncommonly (< 1%) rash and pruritus may occur; other manifestations include eosinophilia, urticaria, flushing, fever, chills, photosensitivity, angioedema. Rarely, Stevens-Johnson reaction, toxic epidermal necrolysis, and exfoliative dermatitis have occurred. Anaphylactic reactions have occurred rarely.

Nursing Implications: Assess baseline skin condition, including integrity and drug allergy history. Teach patient to report rash, itching, other skin changes. Teach patient skin care and symptomatic measures as appropriate. If skin rash develops, discuss drug discontinuance with physician. If rash progresses, drug should be discontinued, as fatal Stevens-Johnson syndrome may develop. Be prepared to treat severe acute hypersensitivity reactions with airway management, oxygen, epinephrine, corticosteroids, antihistamines as ordered.

IV. FUNGAL SUPERINFECTION related to REDISTRIBUTION OF ENDOGENOUS MICROORGANISMS

Defining Characteristics: Vaginal moniliasis, vaginitis may occur as endogenous bacteria are eliminated and normal fungal population expands.

Nursing Implications: Teach female patient to report vaginal itching or discharge. Discuss appropriate antifungal treatment with physician. Teach perineal hygiene and symptomatic management.

Drug: cefditoren pivoxil (Spectracef)

Class: Cephalosporin antibacterial

Mechanism of Action: Semisynthetic derivative of cephalosporin C, contains beta-lactam ring, and is related to penicillins and cephamycins. Bactericidal through inhibition of cell wall synthesis, with resulting cell wall instability and cell lysis.

Metabolism: Well absorbed from GI tract.

Dosage/Range:
- Oral (adult 12 years and older): 200–400 mg q 12 hours
- Dose modification if renal impairment, based on creatinine clearance—refer to manufacturer's recommendations.
- Dose modification if hepatic impairment, based on LFTs—refer to manufacturer's recommendations.

Drug Preparation/Administration:
- Take with food.

Drug Interactions:
- Probenecid: increased serum concentrations of antibiotic; monitor and decrease dose if needed.
- Histamine H_2 antagonists: Famotidine decreases oral absorption; concomitant use should be avoided.
- Nephrotoxic drugs: may increase risk of renal dysfunction; avoid if possible.
- Magnesium- and aluminum-containing antacids decrease oral absorption; concomitant use should be avoided.

Lab Effects/Interference:
- Serum ALT (SGPT), serum Alk Phos, serum AST (SGOT), and serum bilirubin—values may be increased.
- BUN and serum creatinine—concentrations may be increased.

Special Considerations:
- Use cautiously if renal impairment is present.
- Contraindicated if hypersensitive to other cephalosporins, or if has had angioedema response to penicillin.

Potential Toxicities/Side Effects and the Nursing Process

I. POTENTIAL FOR INJURY related to HYPERSENSITIVITY REACTION

Defining Characteristics: Urticaria, pruritis, rash (maculopapular or erythematous), fever and chills, eosinophilia, myalgia, edema, erythema, angioedema. Increased risk in individuals allergic to penicillin.

Nursing Implications: Assess allergy to cephalosporin antibiotics and penicillin: if patient states "yes," determine actual response, e.g., "swollen lips = angioedema." If angioedema, patient SHOULD NOT receive drug. Discuss other patient responses with physician to determine whether drug should be given. Assess baseline skin condition, including integrity and allergy history to drugs. Teach patient to report rash, itching, other skin changes. Teach patient skin care and symptomatic measures as appropriate. If skin rash develops, discuss drug discontinuance with physician.

II. ALTERATION IN NUTRITION, LESS THAN BODY REQUIREMENTS, related to GI SIDE EFFECTS

Defining Characteristics: Nausea, vomiting, diarrhea, and anorexia may occur.

Nursing Implications: Assess baseline nutritional status. Teach patient to report GI disturbances. Administer and teach patient to self-administer antiemetics as needed and as ordered. Teach patient importance of nutritious diet, and suggest small, frequent, high-calorie, high-protein meals as appropriate. Discuss abnormalities and drug interruption with physician.

III. FUNGAL SUPERINFECTION related to REDISTRIBUTION OF ENDOGENOUS MICROORGANISMS

Defining Characteristics: Vaginal moniliasis, vaginitis may occur as endogenous bacteria are eliminated and normal fungal population expands.

Nursing Implications: Teach female patient to report vaginal itching or discharge. Discuss appropriate antifungal treatment with physician. Teach perineal hygiene and symptomatic management.

Drug: cefepime (Maxipime)

Class: Fourth-generation cephalosporin antibacterial.

Mechanism of Action: Exerts bactericidal action by inhibiting cell wall synthesis. Highly resistant to hydrolysis by β-lactamases, and exhibits rapid penetration into gram-negative bacterial cells. Active against gram-negative and grampositive organisms. Spectrum of activity includes gram-negative organisms with multiple drug resistance patterns (*Enterobacter* and *Klebsiella*.) Drug is used for treatment of infections in lower respiratory tract, skin, abdomen, and urinary tract.

Metabolism: Given intramuscularly and parenterally. Widely distributed into body tissues and fluids. Serum protein binding is less than 19% and is independent of its concentration in the serum. Excreted in urine. The average elimination half-life is approximately 2 hours.

Dosage/Range:

Adult:

- IV and IM are similar.
- Mild–mod UTI: 0.5–1 g IV or IM q12h × 7–10 days.
- Severe UTI, Klebsiella pneumonia: 2 g IV q12h × 10 days.
- Mod–severe pneumonia: 1–2 g IV q12h × 10 days.
- Febrile neutropenia: 2 g IV q8h × 7 days or neutrophil recovery.

Drug Preparation/Administration:

- IV or IM: add diluent recommended by manufacturer into vial.

Drug Interactions:

- Solutions of cefepime should not be added to solutions of metronidazole, vancomycin hydrochloride, gentamicin sulfate, tobramycin sulfate, or netilmicin sulfate and aminophylline because of potential side effects. If necessary, administer each drug separately.

Lab Effects/Interference:

Major clinical significance:

- Coombs' (antiglobulin) tests: a positive reaction has appeared in clinical trials without evidence of hemolysis.
- PT or PTT: may be prolonged; cephalosporins may inhibit vitamin K synthesis by suppressing gut flora.

Clinical significance:

- Serum SGPT, serum alk phos, serum SGOT, serum bilirubin, or serum LDH: values may be increased.
- BUN and serum creatinine: concentrations may be increased.
- CBC or platelet count: transient leukopenia, neutropenia, agranulocytosis, thrombocytopenia, eosinophilia, lymphocytosis, and thrombocytosis have been seen on rare occasions.

Special Considerations:

- Contraindicated in patients hypersensitive to other cephalosporin antibiotics.
- Use cautiously if sensitive to penicillin; contraindicated if angioedema reaction to penicillin.
- Obtain specimen and send for culture and sensitivity prior to first drug dose.
- May cause false-positive Clinitest glucose result.

Potential Toxicities/Side Effects and the Nursing Process

I. POTENTIAL FOR INJURY related to HYPERSENSITIVITY REACTION

Defining Characteristics: Urticaria, pruritus, rash (maculopapular or erythematous), fever and chills, eosinophilia, myalgia, edema, erythema, angioedema, Stevens-Johnson syndrome, and exfoliative skin reactions occur in 5% of patients. Increased risk in individuals allergic to penicillin.

Nursing Implications: Assess allergy to cephalosporin antibiotics and penicillin: if patient states "yes," determine actual response, e.g., "swollen lips = angioedema." If angioedema, patient SHOULD NOT receive drug. Discuss other patient responses with physician to determine whether drug should be given. Assess baseline skin condition, including integrity and allergy history to drugs. Teach patient to report rash, itching, other skin changes. Teach patient skin care and symptomatic measures as appropriate. If skin rash develops, discuss drug discontinuance with physician. If rash progresses, drug should be discontinued, as fatal Stevens-Johnson syndrome may develop. Be prepared to treat severe acute hypersensitivity reactions with airway management, oxygen, epinephrine, corticosteroids, antihistamines as ordered.

II. ALTERATION IN NUTRITION, LESS THAN BODY REQUIREMENTS, related to GI SIDE EFFECTS

Defining Characteristics: Nausea, vomiting, diarrhea, constipation, abdominal pain, and dyspepsia may occur; rarely, pseudomembranous colitis caused by *C. difficile* resistant to the antibiotic occurs. Rarely, transient increases in LFTs—AST (SGOT), ALT (SGPT), alk phos, BR—may occur.

Nursing Implications: Assess baseline nutritional status. Teach patient to report GI disturbances. Administer and teach patient to self-administer antiemetics, antidiarrheals as needed and as ordered. Teach patient importance of nutritious diet, and suggest small, frequent, high-calorie, high-protein meals as appropriate. Assess baseline LFTs and monitor periodically during treatment. Discuss abnormalities and drug interruption with physician.

III. FUNGAL SUPERINFECTION related to REDISTRIBUTION OF ENDOGENOUS MICROORGANISMS

Defining Characteristics: Vaginal moniliasis, vaginitis may occur as endogenous bacteria are eliminated and normal fungal population expands.

Nursing Implications: Teach female patient to report vaginal itching or discharge. Discuss appropriate antifungal treatment with physician. Teach perineal hygiene and symptomatic management.

IV. ALTERATIONS IN PROTECTIVE MECHANISMS (RARE) related to CHANGES IN FORMED BLOOD CELL ELEMENTS

Defining Characteristics: Rarely, transient leukopenia, lymphocytosis, anemia, eosinophilia may occur. Prolonged PT, prolonged APTT, and hypoprothrombinemia have occurred rarely, especially in elderly or debilitated patients, or in individuals with vitamin K deficiency.

Nursing Implications: Assess baseline laboratory parameters and monitor periodically during treatment. Assess patient for response to antibiotics. Discuss abnormalities with physician. Assess for signs and symptoms of bleeding. If they occur, especially in elderly or debilitated patients, discuss vitamin K administration with physician. Teach patient to avoid aspirin. If taking oral anticoagulants, assess for increased PT, signs and symptoms of bleeding.

V. SENSORY/PERCEPTUAL ALTERATIONS related to DIZZINESS, SOMNOLENCE

Defining Characteristics: Dizziness, headache, somnolence occur rarely.

Nursing Implications: Assess baseline neurological function and comfort, and monitor during treatment. Teach patient to report any changes. Discuss any abnormalities with physician.

Drug: cefixime (Suprax)

Class: Third-generation cephalosporin antibacterial.

Mechanism of Action: Semisynthetic derivative of cephalosporin C (produced by fungus); contains β-lactam ring and is related to penicillins and cephamycins (e.g., cefoxitin). Bactericidal through inhibition of cell wall synthesis, with resulting cell wall instability and cell lysis. Active against sensitive gramnegative bacteria (e.g., urinary tract infections caused by *E. coli, Proteus, H. influenzae*), as well as *S. pneumoniae* and *H. influenzae* related to acute bronchitis and acute exacerbations of chronic bronchitis.

Metabolism: 30–50% absorbed from GI tract; rate of absorption slowed by food but does not affect total dose absorbed; 65–70% protein-bound. Eliminated unchanged in urine, and to a lesser degree in bile and feces.

Dosage/Range:

- Adult: 400 mg/day PO (single, or two divided doses q12h).
- Duration: 5–10 days for uncomplicated urinary tract infection or upper respiratory infection; 10–14 days for lower respiratory tract infections.
- Dose-reduce if creatinine clearance < 60 mL/min per manufacturer's package insert.

Drug Preparation/Administration:

- Store tablets in tight container at 15–30°C (59–86°F).
- Oral administration.

Drug Interactions:

- Probenecid: increased serum concentrations of antibiotic; monitor and decrease dose if needed.

Lab Effects/Interference:

Major clinical significance:

- Coombs' (antiglobulin) tests: a positive reaction frequently appears in patients who receive large doses of cephalosporins; hemolysis rarely occurs, but it has been reported; test may be positive in neonates whose mothers received cephalosporins before delivery.
- PT: may be prolonged; cephalosporins may inhibit vitamin K synthesis by suppressing gut flora.

Clinical significance:

- Serum ALT, serum alk phos, serum AST, serum bili, or serum LDH values may be increased.
- BUN and serum creatinine concentrations may be increased.
- CBC or platelet count: transient leukopenia, neutropenia, agranulocytosis, thrombocytopenia, eosinophilia, lymphocytosis, and thrombocytosis have been seen on rare occasions.

Special Considerations:

- Use with caution in patients with renal dysfunction; dose reduction required if severe impairment exists.
- Use cautiously if history of colitis exists.
- Contraindicated in patients hypersensitive to other cephalosporin antibiotics.

- Use cautiously if sensitive to penicillin; contraindicated if angioedema reaction to penicillin.
- Obtain ordered specimen and send for culture and sensitivity prior to first drug dose.
- May cause false-positive direct Coombs' test.
- May cause false-positive Clinitest glucose result.

Potential Toxicities/Side Effects and the Nursing Process

I. POTENTIAL FOR INJURY related to HYPERSENSITIVITY REACTION

Defining Characteristics: Urticaria, pruritus, rash (maculopapular or erythematous), fever and chills, eosinophilia, myalgia, edema, erythema, angioedema, Stevens-Johnson syndrome, and exfoliative skin reactions occur in 5% of patients. Increased risk in individuals allergic to penicillin.

Nursing Implications: Assess allergy to cephalosporin antibiotics and penicillin: if patient states "yes," determine actual response, e.g., "swollen lips = angioedema." If angioedema, patient SHOULD NOT receive drug. Discuss other patient responses with physician to determine whether drug should be given. Assess baseline skin condition, including integrity and allergy history to drugs. Instruct patient to report rash, itching, other skin changes. Teach patient skin care and symptomatic measures as appropriate. If skin rash develops, discuss drug discontinuance with physician. If rash progresses, drug should be discontinued, as fatal Stevens-Johnson syndrome may develop. Be prepared to treat severe acute hypersensitivity reactions with airway management, oxygen, epinephrine, corticosteroids, antihistamines as ordered.

II. ALTERATION IN NUTRITION, LESS THAN BODY REQUIREMENTS, related to GI SIDE EFFECTS

Defining Characteristics: Nausea, vomiting, diarrhea, anorexia may occur; rarely, pseudomembranous colitis caused by *C. difficile* resistant to the antibiotic occurs. Rarely, transient increases in LFTs—AST, ALT, alk phos, bili—may occur.

Nursing Implications: Assess baseline nutritional status. Instruct patient to report GI disturbances. Administer and teach patient to self-administer antiemetics as needed and as ordered. Teach patient importance of nutritious diet, and suggest small, frequent, high-calorie, high-protein meals as appropriate. Assess baseline LFTs and monitor periodically during treatment. Discuss abnormalities and drug interruption with physician.

III. FUNGAL SUPERINFECTION related to REDISTRIBUTION OF ENDOGENOUS MICROORGANISMS

Defining Characteristics: Vaginal candidiasis, vaginitis may occur as endogenous bacteria are eliminated, and normal fungal population expands.

Nursing Implications: Teach female patient to report vaginal itching or discharge. Discuss appropriate antifungal treatment with physician. Teach perineal hygiene and symptomatic management.

IV. ALTERATIONS IN PROTECTIVE MECHANISMS (RARE) related to TRANSIENT LEUKOPENIA

Defining Characteristics: Rarely, transient leukopenia, lymphocytosis, anemia, eosinophilia may occur. Prolonged PT, prolonged APTT, and hypoprothrombinemia have occurred rarely, especially in elderly or debilitated patients, or in individuals with vitamin K deficiency.

Nursing Implications: Assess baseline laboratory parameters, and monitor periodically during treatment. Assess patient for response to antibiotics. Discuss abnormalities with physician. Assess for signs/symptoms of bleeding. If they occur, especially in elderly or debilitated patients, discuss vitamin K administration with physician. Instruct patient to avoid aspirin. If taking oral anticoagulants, assess for increased PT, signs/symptoms of bleeding.

V. ALTERATIONS IN SENSORY/PERCEPTUAL PATTERNS related to DIZZINESS, SOMNOLENCE

Defining Characteristics: Dizziness, headache, somnolence occur rarely.

Nursing Implications: Assess baseline neurologic function and comfort, and monitor during treatment. Instruct patient to report any changes. Discuss any abnormalities with physician.

Drug: cefoperazone sodium (Cefobid)

Class: Third-generation cephalosporin antibacterial.

Mechanism of Action: Semisynthetic derivative of cephalosporin C, contains beta-lactam ring, and is related to penicillins and cephamycins. Bactericidal through inhibition of cell wall synthesis, with resulting cell wall instability and cell lysis.

Metabolism: Not absorbed from GI tract so must be given IV or IM. Widely distributed in body fluids, including bile and cerebrospinal fluid at high doses, and body tissues. Metabolized by liver and excreted by kidneys into urine.

Dosage/Range:

- IV route when possible, but IV and IM doses are the same.
- Adults: 2–12 gm q 6–12 hours IM/IV; MAX 16 gm/day.
- Pediatrics: 100–150 mg/kg/day q 8–12 hours IV; MAX 6 gm/day.

Drug Preparation/Administration:

- Store vial containing powder at < 30°C (86°F).
- IV: Reconstitute with sterile water for injection, and further dilute in 50–100 mL of 0.9% Sodium Chloride or 5% Dextrose injection and infuse over 15–30 minutes at maximum concentration of 50 mg/ml.
- IM: Reconstitute by adding sterile or bacteriostatic water for injection. Depending on dose, divide dose and give in separate IM sites; may need to administer large doses to avoid discomfort. Administer IM injections deeply into large muscle (e.g., gluteus maximus).

Drug Interactions:

- Probenecid: increased serum concentrations of antibiotic; monitor and decrease dose if needed.
- Aminoglycosides, penicillins: may have synergistic antibacterial effect against some organisms.
- Nephrotoxic drugs (aminoglycosides, colistin, vancomycin): may increase risk of renal dysfunction; avoid if possible.
- Heparin and warfarin-cephalosporins may inhibit vitamin K synthesis by suppressing gut flora.
- Typhoid vaccine.

Lab Effects/Interference:

- PT: may be prolonged; cephalosporins may inhibit vitamin K synthesis by suppressing gut flora.
- Serum SGPT, serum Alk Phos, serum SGOT, serum bilirubin, or serum LDH: values may be increased.
- BUN and serum creatinine: concentrations may be increased.

Special Considerations:

- Use with caution in patients with renal dysfunction; dose reduction required if severe impairment exists.
- Contraindicated in patients hypersensitive to other cephalosporin antibiotics.
- Use cautiously if sensitive to penicillin; contraindicated if angioedema reaction to penicillin.
- Obtain ordered specimen and send for culture and sensitivity prior to first drug dose.

Potential Toxicities/Side Effects and the Nursing Process

I. POTENTIAL FOR INJURY related to HYPERSENSITIVITY REACTION

Defining Characteristics: Urticaria, pruritis, rash (maculopapular or erythematous), fever and chills, eosinophilia, myalgia, edema, erythema, and angioedema. Increased risk in individuals allergic to penicillin.

Nursing Implications: Assess allergy to cephalosporin antibiotics and penicillin: if patient states "yes," determine actual response, e.g., "swollen lips = angioedema." If angioedema, patient SHOULD NOT receive drug. Discuss other patient responses with physician to determine whether drug should be given. Assess baseline skin condition, including integrity and allergy history to drugs. Teach patient to report rash, itching, or other skin changes. Teach patient skin care and symptomatic measures as appropriate. If skin rash develops, discuss drug discontinuance with physician.

II. ALTERATION IN NUTRITION, LESS THAN BODY REQUIREMENTS, related to GI SIDE EFFECTS

Defining Characteristics: Diarrhea or anorexia may occur.

Nursing Implications: Assess baseline nutritional status. Teach patient to report GI disturbances. Administer and teach patient to self-administer antidiarrheal agent as needed and as ordered.

III. FUNGAL SUPERINFECTION related to REDISTRIBUTION OF ENDOGENOUS MICROORGANISMS

Defining Characteristics: Vaginal moniliasis, vaginitis may occur as endogenous bacteria are eliminated and normal fungal population expands.

Nursing Implications: Teach female patient to report vaginal itching or discharge. Discuss appropriate antifungal treatment with physician. Teach perineal hygiene and symptomatic management.

IV. ALTERATIONS IN PROTECTIVE MECHANISMS (RARE)

Defining Characteristics: Prolonged PT, prolonged APTT, and hypoprothrombinemia have occurred rarely, especially in elderly or debilitated patients, or in individuals with vitamin K deficiency.

Nursing Implications: Assess baseline laboratory parameters, and monitor periodically during treatment. Assess patient for response to antibiotics. Discuss abnormalities with physician. Assess for signs/symptoms of bleeding. If they occur, especially in elderly or debilitated patients, discuss vitamin K administration with physician. Teach patient to avoid aspirin. If taking oral anticoagulants, assess for increased PT, signs/symptoms of bleeding.

V. ALTERATIONS IN COMFORT related to LOCAL INJECTION IRRITATION

Defining Characteristics: Pain, induration, and sterile abscesses may form in IM injection sites; phlebitis may develop in IV sites.

Nursing Implications: Rotate IM injection sites, and administer drug deep IM in large muscle mass (e.g., gluteus maximus). Use IM injection when IV administration is not possible. Change IV sites q 48 hours, and assess for signs/symptoms of phlebitis prior to each administration. Administer drug slowly. Apply warm packs to increase comfort.

Drug: cefotaxime sodium (Claforan)

Class: Third-generation cephalosporin antibacterial.

Mechanism of Action: Semisynthetic derivative of cephalosporin C (produced by fungus); contains β-lactam ring and is related to penicillins and cephamycins (e.g., cefoxitin). Bactericidal through inhibition of cell wall synthesis, with resulting cell wall instability and cell lysis. Active against gramnegative cocci (*Enterobacter,* some strains of *Pseudomonas, E. coli, Klebsiella, Serratia*), as well as gram-positive *S. aureus* and *Staphylococcus epidermidis*, and *S. pneumoniae.* Used to treat serious lower respiratory tract, urinary tract, gynecologic, CNS, blood, and skin infections caused by sensitive bacteria.

Metabolism: Not absorbed from GI tract, so must be given IV or IM. Widely distributed in body fluids, including bile and CSF at high doses, and body tissues. Crosses placenta and is excreted in breast milk. Metabolized by liver and excreted by kidneys into urine.

Dosage/Range:

- IV route when possible, but IV and IM doses are the same.
- Adults: 1–2 g q6–8h (severe, 2 g q4h) × 48–72 hours after infection eradicated.

Drug Preparation/Administration:

- Store vial containing powder at < 30°C (86°F).
- Frozen injection should be stored at < −20°C (−4°F).
- IV: reconstitute with 10 mL sterile water for injection, and further dilute in 50–100 mL of 0.9% Sodium Chloride or 5% Dextrose injection and infuse over 20–30 minutes.
- IM: reconstitute by adding 2–5 mL sterile or bacteriostatic water for injection. Depending on dose, divide dose and give in separate IM sites; may need to administer large doses (2 g) IV to avoid discomfort. Administer IM injections deeply into large muscle (e.g., gluteus maximus).

Drug Interactions:

- Probenecid: increased serum concentrations of antibiotic; monitor and decrease dose if needed.
- Aminoglycosides, penicillins: may have synergistic antibacterial effect against some organisms.
- Nephrotoxic drugs (aminoglycosides, colistin, vancomycin): may increase risk of renal dysfunction; avoid if possible.

Lab Effects/Interference:

Major clinical significance:

- Coombs' (antiglobulin) tests: a positive reaction frequently appears in patients who receive large doses of cephalosporins; hemolysis rarely occurs, but it has been reported, test may be positive in neonates whose mothers received cephalosporins before delivery.
- PT: may be prolonged; cephalosporins may inhibit vitamin K synthesis by suppressing gut flora.

Clinical significance:

- Serum ALT, serum alk phos, serum AST, serum bili, or serum LDH values may be increased.
- BUN and serum creatinine concentrations may be increased.
- CBC or platelet count: transient leukopenia, neutropenia, agranulocytosis, thrombocytopenia, eosinophilia, lymphocytosis, and thrombocytosis have been seen on rare occasions.

Special Considerations:

- Use with caution in patients with renal dysfunction; dose reduction required if severe impairment exists.
- Use cautiously if history of colitis exists.
- Contraindicated in patients hypersensitive to other cephalosporin antibiotics.
- Use cautiously if sensitive to penicillin; contraindicated if angioedema reaction to penicillin.
- Obtain ordered specimen and send for culture and sensitivity prior to first drug dose.
- May cause false-positive direct Coombs' test.

Potential Toxicities/Side Effects and the Nursing Process

I. POTENTIAL FOR INJURY related to HYPERSENSITIVITY REACTION

Defining Characteristics: Urticaria, pruritus, rash (maculopapular or erythematous), fever and chills, eosinophilia, myalgia, edema, erythema, angioedema, Stevens-Johnson syndrome, and exfoliative skin reactions occur in 5% of patients. Increased risk in individuals allergic to penicillin.

Nursing Implications: Assess allergy to cephalosporin antibiotics and penicillin: if patient states "yes," determine actual response, e.g., "swollen lips = angioedema." If angioedema, patient SHOULD NOT receive drug. Discuss other patient responses with physician to determine whether drug should be given. Assess baseline skin condition, including integrity and allergy history to drugs. Instruct patient to report rash, itching, other skin changes. Teach patient skin care and symptomatic measures as appropriate. If skin rash develops, discuss drug discontinuance with physician. If rash progresses, drug should be discontinued, as fatal Stevens-Johnson syndrome may develop. Be prepared to treat severe acute hypersensitivity reactions with airway management, oxygen, epinephrine, corticosteroids, antihistamines as ordered.

II. ALTERATION IN NUTRITION, LESS THAN BODY REQUIREMENTS, related to GI SIDE EFFECTS

Defining Characteristics: Nausea, vomiting, diarrhea, anorexia may occur; rarely, pseudomembranous colitis caused by *C. difficile* resistant to the antibiotic occurs. Rarely, transient increases in LFTs—AST, ALT, alk phos, bili—may occur.

Nursing Implications: Assess baseline nutritional status. Instruct patient to report GI disturbances. Administer and teach patient to self-administer antiemetics as needed and as ordered. Teach patient importance of nutritious diet, and suggest small, frequent, high-calorie, high-protein meals as appropriate. Assess baseline LFTs, and monitor periodically during treatment. Discuss abnormalities and drug interruption with physician.

III. FUNGAL SUPERINFECTION related to REDISTRIBUTION OF ENDOGENOUS MICROORGANISMS

Defining Characteristics: Vaginal candidiasis, vaginitis may occur as endogenous bacteria are eliminated and normal fungal population expands.

Nursing Implications: Instruct female patient to report vaginal itching or discharge. Discuss appropriate antifungal treatment with physician. Teach perineal hygiene and symptomatic management.

IV. ALTERATIONS IN PROTECTIVE MECHANISMS (RARE) related to TRANSIENT LEUKOPENIA

Defining Characteristics: Rarely, transient leukopenia, lymphocytosis, anemia, eosinophilia may occur. Prolonged PT, prolonged APTT, and hypoprothrombinemia have occurred rarely, especially in elderly or debilitated patients, or in individuals with vitamin K deficiency.

Nursing Implications: Assess baseline laboratory parameters, and monitor periodically during treatment. Assess patient for response to antibiotics. Discuss abnormalities with physician. Assess for signs/symptoms of bleeding. If they occur, especially in elderly or debilitated patients, discuss vitamin K administration with physician. Instruct patient to avoid aspirin. If taking oral anticoagulants, assess for increased PT, signs/symptoms of bleeding.

V. ALTERATIONS IN SENSORY/PERCEPTUAL PATTERNS related to DIZZINESS, SOMNOLENCE

Defining Characteristics: Dizziness, headache, somnolence occur rarely.

Nursing Implications: Assess baseline neurologic function and comfort, and monitor during treatment. Instruct patient to report any changes. Discuss any abnormalities with physician.

VI. ALTERATIONS IN COMFORT related to LOCAL INJECTION IRRITATION

Defining Characteristics: Pain, induration, and sterile abscesses may form in IM injection sites; phlebitis may develop in IV sites.

Nursing Implications: Rotate IM injection sites, and administer drug deep IM in large muscle mass (e.g., gluteus maximus). Use IM injection when IV administration is not possible. Change IV sites q48h, and assess for signs/symptoms of phlebitis prior to each administration. Administer drug slowly. Apply warm packs to increase comfort.

Drug: cefotetan (Cefotan)

Class: Second-generation cephalosporin antibiotic.

Mechanism of Action: Semisynthetic derivative of cephalosporin C; contains beta-lactam ring, and is related to penicillins and cephamycins. Bactericidal through inhibition of cell wall synthesis by binding to one or more of the penicillin-binding proteins (PSPs) that in turn inhibit the final transpeptidation step of peptidoglycan synthesis in bacterial cell walls, thus inhibiting cell wall biosynthesis. Bacteria eventually lyse due to ongoing activity of cell wall autolytic enzymes (autolysins and murein hydrolases) while cell wall assembly is arrested.

Metabolism: Widely distributed in body tissues, fluids except cerebrospinal fluid; readily crosses placenta and is excreted in breast milk. Unchanged drug rapidly excreted by the kidneys.

Dosage/Range:

- Oral (adult): 1–6 g/day in divided doses every 12 hours, usual dose: 1–2 g every 12 hours for 5–10 days; 1–2 g may be given every 24 hours for urinary tract infection.
- Oral (child): 20–40 mg/kg/dose q 12 hours.

Drug Preparation/Administration:

- Refrigerate suspension.

Drug Interactions:

- Probenecid: increased serum concentrations of cefotetan but does not usually require dose reduction of antibiotic.
- Aminoglycosides and furosemide can increase nephrotoxicity.
- Disulfiram-like reaction has been reported when taken within 72 hours of ethanol consumption.

Lab Effects/Interference:

- Serum ALT (SGPT), serum Alk Phos, serum AST (SGOT), and serum bilirubin—values may be increased.
- BUN and serum creatinine—concentrations may be increased.

Special Considerations:

- Use cautiously if renal impairment is present.
- Contraindicated if hypersensitive to other cephalosporins, or if has had angioedema response to penicillin.

Potential Toxicities/Side Effects and the Nursing Process

I. POTENTIAL FOR INJURY related to HYPERSENSITIVITY REACTION

Defining Characteristics: Urticaria, pruritis, rash (maculopapular or erythematous), fever and chills, eosinophilia, myalgia, edema, erythema, angioedema. Increased risk in individuals allergic to penicillin.

Nursing Implications: Assess allergy to cephalosporin antibiotics and penicillin: if patient states "yes," determine actual response, e.g., "swollen lips = angioedema." If angioedema, patient SHOULD NOT receive drug. Discuss other patient responses with physician to determine whether drug should be given. Assess baseline skin condition, including integrity and allergy history to drugs. Teach patient to report rash, itching, and other skin changes. Teach patient skin care and symptomatic measures as appropriate. If skin rash develops, discuss drug discontinuance with physician.

II. ALTERATION IN NUTRITION, LESS THAN BODY REQUIREMENTS related to GI SIDE EFFECTS

Defining Characteristics: Nausea, vomiting, diarrhea, and anorexia may occur. May cause transient increases in LFTs.

Nursing Implications: Assess baseline nutritional status. Teach patient to report GI disturbances. Administer and teach patient to self-administer antiemetics as needed and as ordered. Teach patient importance of nutritious diet, and suggest small, frequent, high-calorie, high-protein meals as appropriate. Assess baseline LFTs and monitor periodically during treatment. Discuss abnormalities and drug interruption with physician.

III. FUNGAL SUPERINFECTION related to REDISTRIBUTION OF ENDOGENOUS MICROORGANISMS

Defining Characteristics: Vaginal moniliasis, vaginitis may occur as endogenous bacteria are eliminated, and normal fungal population expands.

Nursing Implications: Teach female patient to report vaginal itching or discharge. Discuss appropriate antifungal treatment with physician. Teach perineal hygiene and symptomatic management.

IV. KNOWLEDGE DEFICIT related to SELF-ADMINISTRATION OF MEDICATION

Defining Characteristics: Increased compliance when patient is instructed in self-care activities.

Nursing Implications: Assess knowledge re: infection and planned treatment. Teach about drug action, potential side effects, and when and how to take drug. Teach patient to report any possible side effects that occur.

Drug: cefoxitin sodium (Mefoxin)

Class: Considered second-generation cephalosporin based on activity spectrum; technically, a cephamycin antibacterial.

Mechanism of Action: β-lactam antibiotic that inhibits bacterial cell wall synthesis, leading to cell lysis. Active against sensitive gram-negative bacteria causing lower respiratory infections (*H. influenzae, E. coli, Klebsiella*); GU infections (*E. coli, Klebsiella, Proteus*); septicemia; pelvic infections (*E. coli, Neisseria gonorrheae*); or skin infections (*E. coli, Klebsiella*). Also, some grampositive infections, including lower respiratory tract infections (*S. aureus, S. pneumoniae,* streptococci).

Metabolism: Not absorbed from GI tract, so must be administered IV or IM.

Dosage/Range:
- IV route preferred; IV and IM dosages the same.
- Adult: 1–2 g q6–8h (maximum 12 g/day in divided doses).

- Dose-reduce for renal compromise (based on manufacturer's package insert).

Drug Preparation/Administration:

- Store sterile powder at < 30°C (86°F); frozen injection should be stored at < −20°C (−4°F).
- IV: reconstitute drug by adding 10 mL sterile water for injection. Further dilute in 50–100 mL 0.9% Sodium Chloride or 5% Dextrose injection and infuse over 30–60 minutes.
- IM: reconstitute drug by adding 2 mL sterile water for injection or 0.5% or 1% lidocaine HCl injection without epinephrine to 1 g of cefoxitin. Administer IM deeply into large muscle mass (e.g., gluteus maximus). Using proper technique, ensure that injection is not into blood vessel. (Make certain patient is NOT ALLERGIC to lidocaine.)

Drug Interactions:

- Probenecid: increased serum concentrations of antibiotic; monitor and decrease dose if needed.
- Aminoglycosides, penicillins: may have synergistic antibacterial effect against some organisms.
- Nephrotoxic drugs (aminoglycosides, colistin, vancomycin): may increase risk of renal dysfunction; avoid if possible.
- Magnesium, calcium: incompatible in IV fluid.
- Oral anticoagulants, ASPIRIN: may increase risk of bleeding.
- Alcohol: disulfiramlike reaction (flushing, throbbing headache, dyspnea, nausea, vomiting, diaphoresis, chest pain, palpitation, hyperventilation, tachycardia, hypertension, syncope, weakness, blurred vision) when alcohol ingested within 48–72 hours of cefoxitin; does not occur if alcohol ingested prior to first antibiotic dose. If no alcohol prior to first dose, avoid alcohol for 72 hours after last dose.

Lab Effects/Interference:

Major clinical significance:

- Coombs' (antiglobulin) tests: a positive reaction frequently appears in patients who receive large doses of cephalosporins; hemolysis rarely occurs, but it has been reported; test may be positive in neonates whose mothers received cephalosporins before delivery.
- Urine glucose: some cephalosporins (cefoxitin) may produce false-positive or falsely elevated test results with copper sulfate tests (Benedict's, Fehling's, or Clinitest); glucose enzymatic tests (Clinistix and Testape) are not affected.
- PT: may be prolonged; cephalosporins may inhibit vitamin K synthesis by suppressing gut flora.

Clinical significance:

- Serum and urine creatinine may falsely elevate test values when the Jaffe reaction is used; serum samples should not be obtained within 2 hours of administration.
- Serum ALT, serum alk phos, serum AST, serum bili, or serum LDH values may be increased.
- BUN and serum creatinine concentrations may be increased.
- CBC or platelet count: transient leukopenia, neutropenia, agranulocytosis, thrombocytopenia, eosinophilia, lymphocytosis, and thrombocytosis have been seen on rare occasions.

Special Considerations:

- Use with caution in patients with renal dysfunction; dose reduction required if severe impairment exists.
- Use cautiously if history of colitis exists.
- Contraindicated in patients hypersensitive to other cephalosporin antibiotics.
- Use cautiously if sensitive to penicillin; contraindicated if angioedema reaction to penicillin.
- Obtain ordered specimen and send for culture and sensitivity prior to first drug dose.
- May cause false-positive direct Coombs' test.
- May cause false-positive Clinitest glucose result.

Potential Toxicities/Side Effects and the Nursing Process

I. POTENTIAL FOR INJURY related to HYPERSENSITIVITY REACTION

Defining Characteristics: Urticaria, pruritus, rash (maculopapular or erythematous), fever and chills, eosinophilia, myalgia, edema, erythema, angioedema, Stevens-Johnson syndrome, and exfoliative skin reactions occur in 5% of patients. Increased risk in individuals allergic to penicillin.

Nursing Implications: Assess allergy to cephalosporin antibiotics and penicillin: if patient states "yes," determine actual response, e.g., "swollen lips = angioedema." If angioedema, patient SHOULD NOT receive drug. Discuss other patient responses with physician to determine whether drug should be given. Assess baseline skin condition, including integrity and allergy history to drugs. Instruct patient to report rash, itching, and other skin changes. Teach patient skin care and symptomatic measures as appropriate. If skin rash develops, discuss drug discontinuance with physician. If rash progresses, drug should be discontinued, as fatal Stevens-Johnson syndrome may develop. Be prepared to treat severe acute hypersensitivity reactions with airway management, oxygen, epinephrine, corticosteroids, antihistamines as ordered.

II. ALTERATION IN NUTRITION, LESS THAN BODY REQUIREMENTS, related to GI SIDE EFFECTS

Defining Characteristic: Nausea, vomiting, diarrhea, anorexia may occur; rarely, pseudomembranous colitis caused by *C. difficile* resistant to the antibiotic occurs. Rarely, transient increases in LFTs—AST, ALT, alk phos, bili—may occur.

Nursing Implications: Assess baseline nutritional status. Instruct patient to report GI disturbances. Administer and teach patient to self-administer antiemetics as needed and as ordered. Teach patient importance of nutritious diet, and suggest small, frequent, high-calorie, high-protein meals as appropriate. Assess baseline LFTs and monitor periodically during treatment. Discuss abnormalities and drug interruption with physician.

III. FUNGAL SUPERINFECTION related to REDISTRIBUTION OF ENDOGENOUS MICROORGANISMS

Defining Characteristics: Vaginal candidiasis, vaginitis may occur as endogenous bacteria are eliminated and normal fungal population expands.

Nursing Implications: Instruct female patient to report vaginal itching or discharge. Discuss appropriate antifungal treatment with physician. Teach perineal hygiene and symptomatic management.

IV. ALTERATIONS IN PROTECTIVE MECHANISMS (RARE) related to TRANSIENT LEUKOPENIA

Defining Characteristics: Rarely, transient leukopenia, lymphocytosis, anemia, eosinophilia may occur. Prolonged PT, prolonged APTT, and hypoprothrombinemia have occurred rarely, especially in elderly or debilitated patients, or in individuals with vitamin K deficiency.

Nursing Implications: Assess baseline laboratory parameters, and monitor periodically during treatment. Assess patient for response to antibiotics. Discuss abnormalities with physician. Assess for signs/symptoms of bleeding. If they occur, especially in elderly or debilitated patients, discuss vitamin K administration with physician. Instruct patient to avoid aspirin. If taking oral anticoagulants, assess for increased PT, signs/symptoms of bleeding.

V. ALTERATIONS IN SENSORY/PERCEPTUAL PATTERNS related to DIZZINESS, SOMNOLENCE

Defining Characteristics: Dizziness, headache, somnolence occur rarely.

Nursing Implications: Assess baseline neurologic function and comfort, and monitor during treatment. Instruct patient to report any changes. Discuss any abnormalities with physician.

VI. ALTERATIONS IN COMFORT related to LOCAL INJECTION IRRITATION

Defining Characteristics: Pain, induration, sterile abscesses may form in IM injection sites; phlebitis may develop in IV sites.

Nursing Implications: Rotate IM injection sites, and administer drug deep IM in large muscle mass (e.g., gluteus maximus). Use IM injection when IV administration is not possible. Change IV sites q48h, and assess for signs/symptoms of phlebitis prior to each administration. Administer drug slowly. Apply warm packs to increase comfort.

Drug: cefpodoxime proxetil (Vantin)

Class: Cephalosporin antibacterial.

Mechanism of Action: Semisynthetic derivative of cephalosporin C, contains beta-lactam ring, and is related to penicillins and cephamycins. Bactericidal through inhibition of cell wall synthesis, with resulting cell wall instability and cell lysis.

Metabolism: Well absorbed from GI tract.

Dosage/Range:
- Oral (adult 13 years and older): 100–400 mg q 12 hours.
- Oral (gonorrhea indication): 200-mg single dose.
- Oral (child 6 months–12 years): 10 mg/kg/daily (divided QD-BID), (MAX 400 mg/day).
- Dose modification if renal impairment, based on creatinine clearance: refer to manufacturer's recommendations.

Drug Preparation/Administration:
- Take with food.

Drug Interactions:
- Probenecid: increased serum concentrations of antibiotic; monitor and decrease dose if needed.
- Aminoglycosides, penicillins: may have synergistic antibacterial effect against some organisms.
- Nephrotoxic drugs: may increase risk of renal dysfunction; avoid if possible.
- Magnesium and aluminum.

Lab Effects/Interference:
- Serum ALT (SGPT), serum Alk Phos, serum AST (SGOT), and serum bilirubin: values may be increased.
- BUN and serum creatinine: concentrations may be increased.

Special Considerations:

- Use cautiously if renal impairment is present.
- Contraindicated if hypersensitive to other cephalosporins, or if has had angioedema response to penicillin.

Potential Toxicities/Side Effects and the Nursing Process

I. POTENTIAL FOR INJURY related to HYPERSENSITIVITY REACTION

Defining Characteristics: Urticaria, pruritis, rash (maculopapular or erythematous), fever and chills, eosinophilia, myalgia, edema, erythema, angioedema. Increased risk in individuals allergic to penicillin.

Nursing Implications: Assess allergy to cephalosporin antibiotics and penicillin: if patient states "yes," determine actual response, e.g., "swollen lips = angioedema." If angioedema, patient SHOULD NOT receive drug. Discuss other patient responses with physician to determine whether drug should be given. Assess baseline skin condition, including integrity and allergy history to drugs. Teach patient to report rash, itching, other skin changes. Teach patient skin care and symptomatic measures as appropriate. If skin rash develops, discuss drug discontinuance with physician.

II. ALTERATION IN NUTRITION, LESS THAN BODY REQUIREMENTS, related to GI SIDE EFFECTS

Defining Characteristics: Nausea, vomiting, diarrhea, and anorexia may occur.

Nursing Implications: Assess baseline nutritional status. Teach patient to report GI disturbances. Administer and teach patient to self-administer antiemetics as needed and as ordered. Teach patient importance of nutritious diet, and suggest small, frequent, high-calorie, high-protein meals as appropriate. Discuss abnormalities and drug interruption with physician.

III. FUNGAL SUPERINFECTION related to REDISTRIBUTION OF ENDOGENOUS MICROORGANISMS

Defining Characteristics: Vaginal moniliasis, vaginitis may occur as endogenous bacteria are eliminated and normal fungal population expands.

Nursing Implications: Teach female patient to report vaginal itching or discharge. Discuss appropriate antifungal treatment with physician. Teach perineal hygiene and symptomatic management.

Drug: cefprozil (Cefzil)

Class: Second-generation cephalosporin antibiotic.

Mechanism of Action: Semisynthetic derivative of cephalosporin C; contains beta-lactam ring, and is related to penicillins and cephamycins. Bactericidal through inhibition of cell wall synthesis, with resulting cell wall instability and cell lysis.

Metabolism: Well absorbed from GI tract; delayed GI absorption if taken with food, but total amount of drug absorption is the same. Widely distributed in body tissues and fluids, except cerebrospinal fluid; readily crosses placenta and is excreted in breast milk. Unchanged drug rapidly excreted by the kidneys.

Dosage/Range:

- Oral (adult 13 years and older): 250–500 mg q 12–24 hours.
- Oral (child 7 months–12 years): 7.5–15 mg/kg q 12 hours (MAX 1 gm/day).

Drug Preparation/Administration:

- Refrigerate suspension.
- Discard after 14 days.

Drug Interactions:

- Probenecid: increased serum concentrations of cefprozil but does not usually require dose reduction of antibiotic.
- Aminoglycosides, penicillins: may have synergistic antibacterial effect against some organisms.
- Typhoid vaccine.

Lab Effects/Interference:

- Serum ALT (SGPT), serum Alk Phos, serum AST (SGOT), and serum bilirubin: values may be increased.
- BUN and serum creatinine: concentrations may be increased.

Special Considerations:

- Use cautiously if renal impairment is present.
- Contraindicated if hypersensitive to other cephalosporins, or if has had angioedema response to penicillin.

Potential Toxicities/Side Effects and the Nursing Process

I. POTENTIAL FOR INJURY related to HYPERSENSITIVITY REACTION

Defining Characteristics: Urticaria, pruritis, rash (maculopapular or erythematous), fever and chills, eosinophilia, myalgia, edema, erythema, angioedema. Increased risk in individuals allergic to penicillin.

Nursing Implications: Assess allergy to cephalosporin antibiotics and penicillin: if patient states "yes," determine actual response, e.g., "swollen lips = angioedema." If angioedema, patient SHOULD NOT receive drug. Discuss other patient responses with physician to determine whether drug should be given. Assess baseline skin condition, including integrity and allergy history to drugs. Teach patient to report rash, itching, and other skin changes. Teach patient skin care and symptomatic measures as appropriate. If skin rash develops, discuss drug discontinuance with physician.

II. ALTERATION IN NUTRITION, LESS THAN BODY REQUIREMENTS, related to GI SIDE EFFECTS

Defining Characteristics: Nausea, vomiting, diarrhea, and anorexia may occur. May cause transient increases in LFTs.

Nursing Implications: Assess baseline nutritional status. Teach patient to report GI disturbances. Administer and teach patient to self-administer antiemetics as needed and as ordered. Teach patient importance of nutritious diet, and suggest small, frequent, high-calorie, high-protein meals as appropriate. Assess baseline LFTs and monitor periodically during treatment. Discuss abnormalities and drug interruption with physician.

III. FUNGAL SUPERINFECTION related to REDISTRIBUTION OF ENDOGENOUS MICROORGANISMS

Defining Characteristics: Vaginal moniliasis, vaginitis may occur as endogenous bacteria are eliminated and normal fungal population expands.

Nursing Implications: Teach female patient to report vaginal itching or discharge. Discuss appropriate antifungal treatment with physician. Teach perineal hygiene and symptomatic management.

IV. KNOWLEDGE DEFICIT related to SELF-ADMINISTRATION OF MEDICATION

Defining Characteristics: Increased compliance when patient is instructed in self-care activities.

Nursing Implications: Assess knowledge regarding infection and planned treatment. Teach about drug action, potential side effects, and when and how to take drug. Teach patient to report any possible side effects that occur.

Drug: ceftazidime (Fortaz, Tazicef, Tazidime)

Class: Third-generation cephalosporin antibacterial.

Mechanism of Action: Semisynthetic derivative of cephalosporin C (produced by fungus); contains β-lactam ring and is related to penicillins and cephamycins (e.g., cefoxitin). Bactericidal through inhibition of cell wall synthesis, with resulting cell wall instability and cell lysis. Active against sensitive microorganisms causing lower respiratory tract, urinary tract, skin, bone and joint, gynecologic, intraabdominal infections. These include primarily gram-negative bacteria (*Enterobacter, E. coli, Klebsiella, Proteus, Serratia,* and *Pseudomonas*) and, to a lesser degree, some gram-positive bacteria (*S. aureus, S. epidermidis,* streptococci).

Metabolism: Not absorbed from GI tract so must be administered parenterally. Small degree of protein binding (5–24%). Widely distributed in body fluids (including CSF and bile) and body tissues. Crosses placenta and is excreted unchanged in urine.

Dosage/Range:

- IV and IM doses are the same.
- Adult: maximum 6 g/d.
- Uncomplicated pneumonia, skin/structure infections: 0.5–1 g IV q8h.
- Bone, joint infection: 2 g q12h.
- Severe GYN, abdominal infections or febrile neutropenia: 2 g IV q8h.
- Lung infection by pseudomonas in patients with cystic fibrosis: 30–50 mg/kg q8h.
- Dose should be reduced in renal insufficiency according to manufacturer's package insert.

Drug Preparation/Administration:

- Store sterile powder vials at 15–30°C (59–86°F) and protect from light; frozen injection containers should be stored at < −20°C (−4°F).
- IV: reconstitute according to manufacturer's package insert, as some preparations contain sodium carbonate. Further dilute in 100 mL of 0.9% Sodium Chloride or 5% Dextrose and infuse over 30–60 minutes.
- IM: reconstitute according to manufacturer's package insert, which may suggest the addition of 0.5–1% lidocaine HCl to decrease discomfort. Make certain patient is NOT ALLERGIC to lidocaine. Administer deep IM in large muscle mass (e.g., gluteus maximus).

Drug Interactions:

- Probenecid: increased serum concentrations of antibiotic; monitor and decrease dose if needed.
- Aminoglycosides, penicillins: may have synergistic antibacterial effect against some organisms.
- Nephrotoxic drugs (aminoglycosides, colistin, vancomycin): may increase risk of renal dysfunction; avoid if possible.
- Sodium bicarbonate: incompatible; DO NOT administer concurrently through same IV site.

Lab Effects/Interference:
Major clinical significance:
- Coombs' (antiglobulin) tests: a positive reaction frequently appears in patients who receive large doses of cephalosporins; hemolysis rarely occurs, but it has been reported; test may be positive in neonates whose mothers received cephalosporins before delivery.
- PT: may be prolonged; cephalosporins may inhibit vitamin K synthesis by suppressing gut flora.

Clinical significance:
- Serum ALT, serum alk phos, serum AST, serum bili, or serum LDH values may be increased.
- BUN and serum creatinine concentrations may be increased.
- CBC or platelet count: transient leukopenia, neutropenia, agranulocytosis, thrombocytopenia, eosinophilia, lymphocytosis, and thrombocytosis have been seen on rare occasions.

Special Considerations:
- Empiric use in management of febrile neutropenic patient appears to be as effective as combination antibiotic regimens; vancomycin may need to be added to ceftazidime to better cover gram-positive bacteria (e.g., *S. epidermidis*).
- Has excellent coverage against *P. aeruginosa.*
- Use with caution in patients with renal dysfunction; dose reduction required if severe impairment exists.
- Use cautiously if history of colitis exists.
- Contraindicated in patients hypersensitive to other cephalosporin antibiotics.
- Use cautiously if sensitive to penicillin; contraindicated if angioedema reaction to penicillin.
- Obtain specimen and send for culture and sensitivity prior to first drug dose.
- May cause false-positive direct Coombs' test.
- May cause false-positive Clinitest glucose result.

Potential Toxicities/Side Effects and the Nursing Process

I. POTENTIAL FOR INJURY related to HYPERSENSITIVITY REACTION

Defining Characteristics: Urticaria, pruritus, rash (maculopapular or erythematous), fever and chills, eosinophilia, myalgia, edema, erythema, angioedema, Stevens-Johnson syndrome, and exfoliative skin reactions occur in 5% of patients. Increased risk in individuals allergic to penicillin.

Nursing Implications: Assess allergy to cephalosporin antibiotics and penicillin: if patient states "yes," determine actual response, e.g., "swollen lips = angioedema." If angioedema, patient SHOULD NOT receive drug. Discuss other patient responses with physician to determine whether drug should be given. Assess baseline skin condition, including integrity and allergy history to drugs. Instruct patient to report rash, itching, other skin changes. Teach patient skin care and symptomatic measures as appropriate. If skin rash develops, discuss drug discontinuance with physician. If rash progresses, drug should be discontinued, as fatal Stevens-Johnson syndrome may develop. Be prepared to treat severe acute hypersensitivity reactions with airway management, oxygen, epinephrine, corticosteroids, antihistamines as ordered.

II. ALTERATION IN NUTRITION, LESS THAN BODY REQUIREMENTS, related to GI SIDE EFFECTS

Defining Characteristics: Nausea, vomiting, diarrhea, anorexia may occur; rarely, pseudomembranous colitis caused by *C. difficile* resistant to the antibiotic occurs. Rarely, transient increases in LFTs—AST, ALT, alk phos, bili—may occur.

Nursing Implications: Assess baseline nutritional status. Instruct patient to report GI disturbances. Administer and teach patient to self-administer antiemetics as needed and as ordered. Teach patient importance of nutritious diet, and suggest small, frequent, high-calorie, high-protein meals as appropriate. Assess baseline LFTs, and monitor periodically during treatment. Discuss abnormalities and drug interruption with physician.

III. FUNGAL SUPERINFECTION related to REDISTRIBUTION OF ENDOGENOUS MICROORGANISMS

Defining Characteristics: Vaginal candidiasis, vaginitis may occur as endogenous bacteria are eliminated, and normal fungal population expands.

Nursing Implications: Instruct female patient to report vaginal itching or discharge. Discuss appropriate antifungal treatment with physician. Teach perineal hygiene and symptomatic management.

IV. ALTERATIONS IN PROTECTIVE MECHANISMS (RARE) related to TRANSIENT LEUKOPENIA

Defining Characteristics: Rarely, transient leukopenia, lymphocytosis, anemia, eosinophilia may occur. Prolonged PT, prolonged APTT, and hypoprothrombinemia have occurred rarely, especially in elderly or debilitated patients, or in individuals with vitamin K deficiency.

Nursing Implications: Assess baseline laboratory parameters, and monitor periodically during treatment. Assess patient for response to antibiotics. Discuss abnormalities with physician.

V. ALTERATIONS IN SENSORY/PERCEPTUAL PATTERNS related to DIZZINESS, SOMNOLENCE

Defining Characteristics: Dizziness, headache, somnolence occur rarely.

Nursing Implications: Assess baseline neurologic function and comfort, and monitor during treatment. Instruct patient to report any changes. Discuss any abnormalities with physician.

VI. ALTERATIONS IN COMFORT related to LOCAL INJECTION IRRITATION

Defining Characteristics: Pain, induration, sterile abscesses may form in IM injection sites; phlebitis may develop in IV sites.

Nursing Implications: Rotate IM injection sites, and administer drug deep IM in large muscle mass (e.g., gluteus maximus). Use IM injection when IV administration is not possible. Change IV sites q48h, and assess for signs/symptoms of phlebitis prior to each administration. Administer drug slowly. Apply warm packs to increase comfort.

Drug: ceftibuten (Cedax)

Class: Third-generation cephalosporin antibacterial.

Mechanism of Action: Semisynthetic derivative of cephalosporin C, contains beta-lactam ring, and is related to penicillins and cephamycins. Bactericidal through inhibition of cell wall synthesis, with resulting cell wall instability and cell lysis.

Metabolism: Well absorbed from GI tract; delayed GI absorption if taken with food, but total amount of drug absorption is the same. Widely distributed in body tissues and fluids, except cerebrospinal fluid; readily crosses placenta and is excreted in breast milk. Unchanged drug rapidly excreted by the kidneys.

Dosage/Range:

- Adults: 400 mg orally QD × 10 days.
- Dose reduce if creatinine clearance is reduced per manufacturer's recommendations.

Drug Preparation/Administration:

- Store suspension in refrigerator; discard after 14 days.
- Oral administration.

Drug Interactions:

- Aminoglycosides, penicillins: may have synergistic antibacterial effect against some organisms.

- Typhoid vaccine.

Lab Effects/Interference:

- Serum SGPT, serum Alk Phos, serum SGOT, serum bilirubin, or serum LDH: values may be increased.
- BUN and serum creatinine: concentrations may be increased.

Special Considerations:

- Use with caution in patients with renal dysfunction; dose reduction required if severe impairment exists.
- Contraindicated in patients hypersensitive to other cephalosporin antibiotics.
- Use cautiously if sensitive to penicillin; contraindicated if angioedema reaction to penicillin.
- Obtain ordered specimen and send for culture and sensitivity prior to first drug dose.

Potential Toxicities/Side Effects and the Nursing Process

I. POTENTIAL FOR INJURY related to HYPERSENSITIVITY REACTION

Defining Characteristics: Urticaria, pruritis, rash (maculopapular or erythematous), fever and chills, eosinophilia, myalgia, edema, erythema, angioedema. Increased risk in individuals allergic to penicillin.

Nursing Implications: Assess allergy to cephalosporin antibiotics and penicillin: if patient states "yes," determine actual response, e.g., "swollen lips = angioedema." If angioedema, patient SHOULD NOT receive drug. Discuss other patient responses with physician to determine whether drug should be given. Assess baseline skin condition, including integrity and allergy history to drugs. Teach patient to report rash, itching, other skin changes. Teach patient skin care and symptomatic measures as appropriate. If skin rash develops, discuss drug discontinuance with physician.

II. ALTERATION IN NUTRITION, LESS THAN BODY REQUIREMENTS, related to GI SIDE EFFECTS

Defining Characteristics: Nausea, vomiting, diarrhea, and anorexia may occur. Rarely, transient increases in LFTs—AST (SGOT), ALT (SGPT), ALK-PHOS, BR—may occur.

Nursing Implications: Assess baseline nutritional status. Teach patient to report GI disturbances. Administer and teach patient to self-administer medication as needed and as ordered. Teach patient importance of nutritious diet, and suggest small, frequent, high-calorie, high-protein meals as appropriate. Assess baseline LFTs and monitor periodically during treatment. Discuss abnormalities and drug interruption with physician.

III. FUNGAL SUPERINFECTION related to REDISTRIBUTION OF ENDOGENOUS MICROORGANISMS

Defining Characteristics: Vaginal moniliasis, vaginitis may occur as endogenous bacteria are eliminated and normal fungal population expands.

Nursing Implications: Teach female patient to report vaginal itching or discharge. Discuss appropriate antifungal treatment with physician. Teach perineal hygiene and symptomatic management.

Drug: ceftriaxone sodium (Rocephin)

Class: Third-generation cephalosporin antibacterial.

Mechanism of Action: Semisynthetic derivative of cephalosporin C (produced by fungus); contains β-lactam ring and is related to penicillins and cephamycins (e.g., cefoxitin). Bactericidal through inhibition of cell wall synthesis, with resulting cell wall instability and cell lysis. Active primarily against gram-negative cocci (*H. influenzae, Enterobacter, E. coli, Klebsiella, Proteus, Pseudomonas*) and, to a lesser degree, gram-positive cocci (*S. aureus* and streptococci). Drug is used for treatment of infections in lower respiratory tract, skin, bone and joint, abdomen, urinary tract, and pelvis (gonorrhea), as well as for treatment of meningitis and sepsis.

Metabolism: Not absorbed from GI tract and must be given parenterally. Widely distributed into body tissues and fluids, including bile and CSF. Crosses placenta and excreted in breast milk. Protein binding depends on drug concentration, and varies from 58–96%. Excreted in urine and feces to a lesser extent. Has long half-life.

Dosage/Range:

- IV and IM doses same.
- 1–2 g/day, or in equally divided doses q12h.
- CNS infections may require maximum recommended of 4 g/day in divided doses.

Drug Preparation/Administration:

- Store vial of sterile drug powder at ≤ 25°C (77°F) and protect from light. Frozen injection containers should be stored at ≤ −20°C (−4°F).
- IV: Add diluent recommended by manufacturer into vial, then further dilute in 100 mL 0.9% Sodium Chloride or 5% Dextrose. Infuse over 30–60 minutes.
- IM: Add 0.9–7.2 mL of sterile or bacteriostatic water for injection, or 1% lidocaine HCl without epinephrine to appropriate vial, resulting in 250

mg/mL. Administer deep IM into large muscle mass (e.g., gluteus maximus). Make certain patient is NOT ALLERGIC to lidocaine.

Drug Interactions:
- Probenecid: increased serum concentrations of antibiotic; monitor and decrease dose if needed.
- Aminoglycosides, penicillins: may have synergistic antibacterial effect against some organisms.
- Nephrotoxic drugs (aminoglycosides, colistin, vancomycin): may increase risk of renal dysfunction; avoid if possible.

Lab Effects/Interference:

Major clinical significance:
- Coombs' (antiglobulin) tests: a positive reaction frequently appears in patients who receive large doses of cephalosporins; hemolysis rarely occurs, but it has been reported; test may be positive in neonates whose mothers received cephalosporins before delivery.
- PT: may be prolonged; cephalosporins may inhibit vitamin K synthesis by suppressing gut flora.

Clinical significance:
- Serum ALT, serum alk phos, serum AST, serum bili, or serum LDH values may be increased.
- BUN and serum creatinine concentrations may be increased.
- CBC or platelet count: transient leukopenia, neutropenia, agranulocytosis, thrombocytopenia, eosinophilia, lymphocytosis, and thrombocytosis have been seen on rare occasions.

Special Considerations:
- Use cautiously if history of colitis exists.
- Contraindicated in patients hypersensitive to other cephalosporin antibiotics.
- Use cautiously if sensitive to penicillin; contraindicated if angioedema reaction to penicillin.
- Obtain specimen and send for culture and sensitivity prior to first drug dose.
- May cause false-positive direct Coombs' test.
- May cause false-positive Clinitest glucose result.

Potential Toxicities/Side Effects and the Nursing Process

I. POTENTIAL FOR INJURY related to HYPERSENSITIVITY REACTION

Defining Characteristics: Urticaria, pruritus, rash (maculopapular or erythematous), fever and chills, eosinophilia, myalgia, edema, erythema, angioedema, Stevens-Johnson syndrome, and exfoliative skin reactions occur in 5% of patients. Increased risk in individuals allergic to penicillin.

Nursing Implications: Assess allergy to cephalosporin antibiotics and penicillin: if patient states "yes," determine actual response, e.g., "swollen lips = angioedema." If angioedema, patient SHOULD NOT receive drug. Discuss other patient responses with physician to determine whether drug should be given. Assess baseline skin condition, including integrity and allergy history to drugs. Instruct patient to report rash, itching, other skin changes. Teach patient skin care and symptomatic measures as appropriate. If skin rash develops, discuss drug discontinuance with physician. If rash progresses, drug should be discontinued, as fatal Stevens-Johnson syndrome may develop. Be prepared to treat severe acute hypersensitivity reactions with airway management, oxygen, epinephrine, corticosteroids, antihistamines as ordered.

II. ALTERATION IN NUTRITION, LESS THAN BODY REQUIREMENTS, related to GI SIDE EFFECTS

Defining Characteristics: Nausea, vomiting, diarrhea, anorexia may occur; rarely, pseudomembranous colitis caused by *C. difficile* resistant to the antibiotic occurs. Rarely, transient increases in LFTs—AST, ALT, alk phos, bili—may occur.

Nursing Implications: Assess baseline nutritional status. Instruct patient to report GI disturbances. Administer and teach patient to self-administer antiemetics, antidiarrheals as needed and as ordered. Teach patient importance of nutritious diet, and suggest small, frequent, high-calorie, high-protein meals as appropriate. Assess baseline LFTs and monitor periodically during treatment. Discuss abnormalities and drug interruption with physician.

III. FUNGAL SUPERINFECTION related to REDISTRIBUTION OF ENDOGENOUS MICROORGANISMS

Defining Characteristics: Vaginal candidiasis, vaginitis may occur as endogenous bacteria are eliminated and normal fungal population expands.

Nursing Implications: Instruct female patient to report vaginal itching or discharge. Discuss appropriate antifungal treatment with physician. Teach perineal hygiene and symptomatic management.

IV. ALTERATIONS IN PROTECTIVE MECHANISMS (RARE) related to TRANSIENT LEUKOPENIA

Defining Characteristics: Rarely, transient leukopenia, lymphocytosis, anemia, eosinophilia may occur. Prolonged PT, prolonged APTT, and hypoprothrombinemia have occurred rarely, especially in elderly or debilitated patients, or in individuals with vitamin K deficiency.

Nursing Implications: Assess baseline laboratory parameters, and monitor periodically during treatment. Assess patient for response to antibiotics. Discuss abnormalities with physician. Assess for signs/symptoms of bleeding. If they occur, especially in elderly or debilitated patients, discuss vitamin K administration with physician. Instruct patient to avoid aspirin. If taking oral anticoagulants, assess for increased PT, signs/symptoms of bleeding.

V. ALTERATIONS IN SENSORY/PERCEPTUAL PATTERNS related to DIZZINESS, SOMNOLENCE

Defining Characteristics: Dizziness, headache, somnolence occur rarely.

Nursing Implications: Assess baseline neurologic function and comfort, and monitor during treatment. Instruct patient to report any changes. Discuss any abnormalities with physician.

VI. ALTERATIONS IN COMFORT related to LOCAL INJECTION IRRITATION

Defining Characteristics: Pain, induration, and sterile abscesses may form in IM injection sites; phlebitis may develop in IV sites.

Nursing Implications: Rotate IM injection sites, and administer drug deep IM in large muscle mass (e.g., gluteus maximus). Use IM injection when IV administration is not possible. Change IV sites q48h, and assess for signs/symptoms of phlebitis prior to each administration. Administer drug slowly. Apply warm packs to increase comfort.

Drug: cefuroxime (Ceftin; Kefurox; Zinacef)

Class: Second-generation cephalosporin antibiotic.

Mechanism of Action: Semisynthetic derivative of cephalosporin C; contains beta-lactam ring, and is related to penicillins and cephamycins. Bactericidal through inhibition of cell wall synthesis by binding to one or more of the penicillin-binding proteins (PSPs) that in turn inhibit the final transpeptidation step of peptidoglycan synthesis in bacterial cell walls, thus inhibiting cell wall biosynthesis. Bacteria eventually lyse due to ongoing activity of cell wall autolytic enzymes (autolysins and murein hydrolases) while cell wall assembly is arrested.

Metabolism: Widely distributed in body tissues, fluids; crosses blood-brain barrier, therapeutic concentrations achieved in cerebrospinal fluid even when meninges are not inflamed; readily crosses placenta and is excreted in breast milk. Unchanged drug rapidly excreted by the kidneys.

Dosage/Range:

- Oral (adult): 250–500 mg twice daily for 10 days.
- IM & IV (adult): 750 mg to 1.5 g/dose every 8 hours or 100–150 mg/kg/day in divided doses every 6–8 hours; maximum dose—6 g/24 hours.

Drug Preparation/Administration:

- Refrigerate suspension; solution stable for 48 hours.
- IV infusion in NS or D5W solution stable for 7 days when refrigerated.

Drug Interactions:

- Probenecid: increased serum concentrations of cefotetan, but does not usually require dose reduction of antibiotic.
- Aminoglycosides: can increase nephrotoxicity.

Lab Effects/Interference:

- Serum ALT (SGPT), serum Alk Phos, serum AST (SGOT), and serum bilirubin—values may be increased.
- BUN and serum creatinine—concentrations may be increased.

Special Considerations:

- Use cautiously if renal impairment is present.
- Contraindicated if hypersensitive to other cephalosporins, or if has had angioedema response to penicillin.

Potential Toxicities/Side Effects and the Nursing Process

I. POTENTIAL FOR INJURY related to HYPERSENSITIVITY REACTION

Defining Characteristics: Urticaria, pruritis, rash (maculopapular or erythematous), fever and chills, eosinophilia, myalgia, edema, erythema, angioedema. Increased risk in individuals allergic to penicillin.

Nursing Implications: Assess allergy to cephalosporin antibiotics and penicillin: if patient states "yes," determine actual response, e.g., "swollen lips = angioedema." If angioedema, patient SHOULD NOT receive drug. Discuss other patient responses with physician to determine whether drug should be given. Assess baseline skin condition, including integrity and allergy history to drugs. Teach patient to report rash, itching, and other skin changes. Teach patient skin care and symptomatic measures as appropriate. If skin rash develops, discuss drug discontinuance with physician.

II. ALTERATION IN NUTRITION, LESS THAN BODY REQUIREMENTS, related to GI SIDE EFFECTS

Defining Characteristics: Nausea, vomiting, diarrhea, and anorexia may occur. May cause transient increases in LFTs.

Nursing Implications: Assess baseline nutritional status. Teach patient to report GI disturbances. Administer and teach patient to self-administer antiemetics as needed and as ordered. Teach patient importance of nutritious diet, and suggest small, frequent, high-calorie, high-protein meals as appropriate. Assess baseline LFTs and monitor periodically during treatment. Discuss abnormalities and drug interruption with physician.

III. FUNGAL SUPERINFECTION related to REDISTRIBUTION OF ENDOGENOUS MICROORGANISMS

Defining Characteristics: Vaginal moniliasis, vaginitis may occur as endogenous bacteria are eliminated and normal fungal population expands.

Nursing Implications: Teach female patient to report vaginal itching or discharge. Discuss appropriate antifungal treatment with physician. Teach perineal hygiene and symptomatic management.

IV. KNOWLEDGE DEFICIT related to SELF-ADMINISTRATION OF MEDICATION

Defining Characteristics: Increased compliance when patient is instructed in self-care activities.

Nursing Implications: Assess knowledge re: infection and planned treatment. Teach about drug action, potential side effects, and when and how to take drug. Teach patient to report any possible side effects that occur.

Drug: cephalexin (Biocef; Keflex; Keftab)

Class: First-generation cephalosporin antibacterial.

Mechanism of Action: Semisynthetic derivative of cephalosporin C, contains beta-lactam ring, and is related to penicillins and cephamycins. Bactericidal through inhibition of cell wall synthesis by binding to one or more of the penicillin-binding proteins (PBPs) that in turn inhibits the final transpeptidation step of peptidoglycan synthesis in bacterial cell walls, thus inhibiting cell wall biosynthesis. Bacteria eventually lyse due to ongoing activity of cell wall autolytic enzymes (autolysins and murein hydrolases) while cell wall assembly is arrested.

Metabolism: Well absorbed from GI tract; delayed GI absorption if taken with food, but total amount of drug absorption is the same. Widely distributed in body tissues, fluids except cerebrospinal fluid; readily crosses placenta and is excreted in breast milk. Unchanged drug rapidly excreted by the kidneys.

Dosage/Range:
- Adults: 250–1000 mg every 6 hours, maximum—4 g/day.
- Dose reduce if creatinine clearance is reduced per manufacturer's recommendations.

Drug Preparation/Administration:
- Store suspension in refrigerator, discard after 14 days.
- Oral administration.

Drug Interactions:
- Aminoglycosides increase nephrotic potential and increase toxicity.
- Probenecid may decrease cephalosporin elimination and increase effect.

Lab Effects/Interference:
- Serum SGPT, serum Alk Phos, serum SGOT, serum bilirubin, or serum LDH—values may be increased.
- BUN and serum creatinine—concentrations may be increased.

Special Considerations:
- Use with caution in patients with renal dysfunction—dose reduction required if severe impairment exists.
- Contraindicated in patients hypersensitive to other cephalosporin antibiotics.
- Use cautiously if sensitive to penicillin; contraindicated if angioedema reaction to penicillin.
- Obtain ordered specimen and send for culture and sensitivity prior to first drug dose.

Potential Toxicities/Side Effects and the Nursing Process

I. POTENTIAL FOR INJURY related to HYPERSENSITIVITY REACTION

Defining Characteristics: Urticaria, pruritis, rash (maculopapular or erythematous), fever and chills, eosinophilia, myalgia, edema, erythema, angioedema. Increased risk in individuals allergic to penicillin.

Nursing Implications: Assess allergy to cephalosporin antibiotics and penicillin: if patient states "yes," determine actual response, e.g., "swollen lips = angioedema." If angioedema, patient SHOULD NOT receive drug. Discuss other patient responses with physician to determine whether drug should be given. Assess baseline skin condition, including integrity and allergy history to drugs. Teach patient to report rash, itching, other skin changes. Teach patient skin care and symptomatic measures as appropriate. If skin rash develops, discuss drug discontinuance with physician.

II. ALTERATION IN NUTRITION, LESS THAN BODY REQUIREMENTS, related to GI SIDE EFFECTS

Defining Characteristics: Nausea and vomiting and diarrhea and anorexia may occur. Rarely, transient increases in LFTs—AST (SGOT), ALT (SGPT), ALKPHOS, BR—may occur.

Nursing Implications: Assess baseline nutritional status. Teach patient to report GI disturbances. Administer and teach patient to self-administer medication as needed and as ordered. Teach patient importance of nutritious diet, and suggest small, frequent, high-calorie, high-protein meals as appropriate. Assess baseline LFTs and monitor periodically during treatment. Discuss abnormalities and drug interruption with physician.

III. FUNGAL SUPERINFECTION related to REDISTRIBUTION OF ENDOGENOUS MICROORGANISMS

Defining Characteristics: Vaginal moniliasis, vaginitis may occur as endogenous bacteria are eliminated and normal fungal population expands.

Nursing Implications: Teach female patient to report vaginal itching or discharge. Discuss appropriate antifungal treatment with physician. Teach perineal hygiene and symptomatic management.

Drug: cephapirin (Cefadyl; Cephapirin Sodium)

Class: First-generation cephalosporin antibacterial.

Mechanism of Action: Semisynthetic derivative of cephalosporin C, contains beta-lactam ring, and is related to penicillins and cephamycins. Bactericidal through inhibition of cell wall synthesis by binding to one or more of the penicillin-binding proteins (PBPs) that in turn inhibit the final transpeptidation step of peptidoglycan synthesis in bacterial cell walls, thus inhibiting cell wall biosynthesis. Bacteria eventually lyse due to ongoing activity of cell wall autolytic enzymes (autolysins and murein hydrolases) while cell wall assembly is arrested.

Metabolism: Well absorbed from GI tract; delayed GI absorption if taken with food, but total amount of drug absorption is the same. Widely distributed in body tissues, fluids except cerebrospinal fluid; readily crosses placenta and is excreted in breast milk. Unchanged drug rapidly excreted by the kidneys.

Dosage/Range:
- Adults: 500–1000 mg every 6 hours, maximum—4 g/day
- Dose reduce if creatinine clearance is reduced per manufacturer's recommendations.

Drug Preparation/Administration:

- Reconstituted solution is stable for 10 days when refrigerated.
- IV infusion in NS or D5W solution stable for 10 days when refrigerated.

Drug Interactions:

- Aminoglycosides increase nephrotic potential and increase toxicity.
- Probenecid may decrease cephalosporin elimination and increase effect.

Lab Effects/Interference:

- Serum SGPT, serum Alk Phos, serum SGOT, serum bilirubin, or serum LDH—values may be increased.
- BUN and serum creatinine—concentrations may be increased.

Special Considerations:

- Use with caution in patients with renal dysfunction—dose reduction required if severe impairment exists.
- Contraindicated in patients hypersensitive to other cephalosporin antibiotics.
- Use cautiously if sensitive to penicillin; contraindicated if angioedema reaction to penicillin.
- Obtain ordered specimen and send for culture and sensitivity prior to first drug dose.

Potential Toxicities/Side Effects and the Nursing Process

I. POTENTIAL FOR INJURY related to HYPERSENSITIVITY REACTION

Defining Characteristics: Urticaria, pruritis, rash (maculopapular or erythematous), fever and chills, eosinophilia, myalgia, edema, erythema, angioedema. Increased risk in individuals allergic to penicillin.

Nursing Implications: Assess allergy to cephalosporin antibiotics and penicillin: if patient states "yes," determine actual response, e.g., "swollen lips = angioedema." If angioedema, patient SHOULD NOT receive drug. Discuss other patient responses with physician to determine whether drug should be given. Assess baseline skin condition, including integrity and allergy history to drugs. Teach patient to report rash, itching, other skin changes. Teach patient skin care and symptomatic measures as appropriate. If skin rash develops, discuss drug discontinuance with physician.

II. ALTERATION IN NUTRITION, LESS THAN BODY REQUIREMENTS, related to GI SIDE EFFECTS

Defining Characteristics: Nausea and vomiting and diarrhea and anorexia may occur. Rarely, transient increases in LFTs—AST (SGOT), ALT (SGPT), ALKPHOS, BR—may occur.

Nursing Implications: Assess baseline nutritional status. Teach patient to report GI disturbances. Administer and teach patient to self-administer medication as needed and as ordered. Teach patient importance of nutritious diet, and suggest small, frequent, high-calorie, high-protein meals as appropriate. Assess baseline LFTs and monitor periodically during treatment. Discuss abnormalities and drug interruption with physician.

III. FUNGAL SUPERINFECTION related to REDISTRIBUTION OF ENDOGENOUS MICROORGANISMS

Defining Characteristics: Vaginal moniliasis, vaginitis may occur as endogenous bacteria are eliminated and normal fungal population expands.

Nursing Implications: Teach female patient to report vaginal itching or discharge. Discuss appropriate antifungal treatment with physician. Teach perineal hygiene and symptomatic management.

Drug: cephradine (Anspor, Velosef)

Class: First-generation cephalosporin antibacterial.

Mechanism of Action: Semisynthetic derivative of cephalosporin C (produced by fungus); contains β-lactam ring and is related to penicillins and cephamycins (e.g., cefoxitin). Bactericidal through inhibition of cell wall synthesis, with resulting cell wall instability and cell lysis. Active against many gram-positive aerobic cocci (streptococci, staphylococci) and has limited gram-negative activity (*Klebsiella, H. influenzae, E. coli, Proteus*). Used in treatment of infections of respiratory tract, GU tract, skin, bone and joint, and in meningitis, sepsis.

Metabolism: Poorly absorbed from GI tract so must be given parenterally. Widely distributed throughout body tissues and fluids, including CSF; 65–79% protein-bound. Crosses placenta and is excreted in breast milk. Metabolized in liver and kidneys and is excreted in the urine.

Dosage/Range:
- Adult: 500 mg–1 g IM or IV q4–6h; and in life-threatening infections, 2 g q4h.
- Dose reduction in renal insufficiency according to manufacturer's package insert.

Drug Preparation/Administration:
- Store vial of powder for injection at < 40°C (< 104°F), and frozen injection containers at ≤ −20° (−4°F).

COMPLICATIONS

- IV: Reconstitute with at least 10 mL sterile water for injection according to manufacturer's package insert. Further dilute in 100 mL 0.9% Sodium Chloride or 5% Dextrose injection and administer over 30–60 minutes.
- IM: Reconstitute each gram of drug with 4 mL sterile water for injection. Administer deep IM in large muscle mass (e.g., gluteus maximus).

Drug Interactions:
- Probenecid: increased serum concentrations of antibiotic; monitor and decrease dose if needed.
- Aminoglycosides, penicillins: may have synergistic antibacterial effect against some organisms.
- Nephrotoxic drugs (aminoglycosides, colistin, vancomycin): may increase risk of renal dysfunction; avoid if possible.

Lab Effects/Interference:
Major clinical significance:
- Coombs' (antiglobulin) tests: a positive reaction frequently appears in patients who receive large doses of cephalosporins; hemolysis rarely occurs, but it has been reported; test may be positive in neonates whose mothers received cephalosporins before delivery.
- Urine glucose: some cephalosporins (cephradine) may produce a false-positive or falsely elevated test results with copper sulfate tests (Benedict's, Fehling's, or Clinitest); glucose enzymatic tests (Clinistix and Testape) are not affected.
- PT: may be prolonged; cephalosporins may inhibit vitamin K synthesis by suppressing gut flora.

Clinical significance:
- Serum ALT, serum alk phos, serum AST, serum bili, or serum LDH values may be increased.
- BUN and serum creatinine concentrations may be increased.
- CBC or platelet count: transient leukopenia, neutropenia, agranulocytosis, thrombocytopenia, eosinophilia, lymphocytosis, and thrombocytosis have been seen on rare occasions.

Special Considerations:
- Use with caution in patients with renal dysfunction; dose reduction required if severe impairment exists.
- Use cautiously if history of colitis exists.
- Contraindicated in patients hypersensitive to other cephalosporin antibiotics.
- Use cautiously if sensitive to penicillin; contraindicated if angioedema reaction to penicillin.
- Obtain specimen and send for culture and sensitivity prior to first drug dose.
- May cause false-positive direct Coombs' test.

- May cause false-positive Clinitest glucose result.

Potential Toxicities/Side Effects and the Nursing Process

I. POTENTIAL FOR INJURY related to HYPERSENSITIVITY REACTION

Defining Characteristics: Urticaria, pruritus, rash (maculopapular or erythematous), fever and chills, eosinophilia, myalgia, edema, erythema, angioedema, Stevens-Johnson syndrome, and exfoliative skin reactions occur in 5% of patients. Increased risk in individuals allergic to penicillin.

Nursing Implications: Assess allergy to cephalosporin antibiotics and penicillin: if patient states "yes," determine actual response, e.g., "swollen lips = angioedema." If angioedema, patient SHOULD NOT receive drug. Discuss other patient responses with physician to determine whether drug should be given. Assess baseline skin condition, including integrity and allergy history to drugs. Instruct patient to report rash, itching, other skin changes. Teach patient skin care and symptomatic measures as appropriate. If skin rash develops, discuss drug discontinuance with physician. If rash progresses, drug should be discontinued, as fatal Stevens-Johnson syndrome may develop. Be prepared to treat severe acute hypersensitivity reactions with airway management, oxygen, epinephrine, corticosteroids, antihistamines as ordered.

II. ALTERATION IN NUTRITION, LESS THAN BODY REQUIREMENTS, related to GI SIDE EFFECTS

Defining Characteristics: Nausea, vomiting, diarrhea, anorexia may occur; rarely, pseudomembranous colitis caused by *C. difficile* resistant to the antibiotic occurs. Rarely, transient increases in LFTs—AST, ALT, alk phos, bili—may occur.

Nursing Implications: Assess baseline nutritional status. Instruct patient to report GI disturbances. Administer and teach patient to self-administer antiemetics as needed and as ordered. Teach patient importance of nutritious diet, and suggest small, frequent, high-calorie, high-protein meals as appropriate. Assess baseline LFTs and monitor periodically during treatment. Discuss abnormalities and drug interruption with physician.

III. FUNGAL SUPERINFECTION related to REDISTRIBUTION OF ENDOGENOUS MICROORGANISMS

Defining Characteristics: Vaginal candidiasis, vaginitis may occur as endogenous bacteria are eliminated and normal fungal population expands.

Nursing Implications: Instruct female patient to report vaginal itching or discharge. Discuss appropriate antifungal treatment with physician. Teach perineal hygiene and symptomatic management.

IV. ALTERATIONS IN PROTECTIVE MECHANISMS (RARE) related to TRANSIENT LEUKOPENIA

Defining Characteristics: Rarely, transient leukopenia, lymphocytosis, anemia, eosinophilia may occur. Prolonged PT, prolonged APTT, and hypoprothrombinemia have occurred rarely, especially in elderly or debilitated patients, or in individuals with vitamin K deficiency.

Nursing Implications: Assess baseline laboratory parameters, and monitor periodically during treatment. Assess patient for response to antibiotics. Discuss abnormalities with physician.

V. ALTERATIONS IN SENSORY/PERCEPTUAL PATTERNS related to DIZZINESS, SOMNOLENCE

Defining Characteristics: Dizziness, headache, somnolence occur rarely.

Nursing Implications: Assess baseline neurologic function and comfort, and monitor during treatment. Instruct patient to report any changes. Discuss any abnormalities with physician.

VI. ALTERATIONS IN COMFORT related to LOCAL INJECTION IRRITATION

Defining Characteristics: Pain, induration, sterile abscesses may form in IM injection sites; phlebitis may develop in IV sites.

Nursing Implications: Rotate IM injection sites, and administer drug deep IM in large muscle mass (e.g., gluteus maximus). Use IM injection when IV administration is not possible. Change IV sites q48h, and assess for signs/symptoms of phlebitis prior to each administration. Administer drug slowly. Apply warm packs to increase comfort.

VII. KNOWLEDGE DEFICIT related to SELF-ADMINISTRATION OF MEDICATION

Defining Characteristics: Increased compliance when patient is instructed in self-care activities.

Nursing Implications: Assess knowledge about infection and planned treatment. Teach about drug action, potential side effects, and when and how to take drug. Teach patient to report any side effects that occur.

Drug: ciprofloxacin (Cipro)

Class: Fluoroquinolone.

Mechanism of Action: Antiinfective; appears to inhibit DNA replication in susceptible bacteria. Has a broad spectrum, and is active against most gramnegative bacteria (e.g., *Enterobacter, Pseudomonas*), some gram-positive organisms (e.g., methicillin-resistant staphylococci), and some mycobacteria.

Metabolism: Well absorbed from GI tract; rate decreased by food but not extent of absorption. Widely distributed in body tissues and fluids with highest concentrations in organs, such as liver, kidneys, and lungs. Partially metabolized in liver; excreted in urine and feces. Crosses placenta and is excreted in breast milk.

Dosage/Range:
- 250–750 mg q12h × 1–2 weeks.
- IV: 200–400 mg q12h × 1–2 weeks (IV used if patient unable to take oral formulation).
- Dose modification necessary if renal impairment exists.

Drug Preparation/Administration:
- Oral: Take drug with 1 large glass of fluid, preferably 2 hours after meal/ food. Encourage oral fluids of 2–3 qt(liters)/day.
- IV: Further dilute drug in 0.9% Sodium Chloride or 5% Dextrose in water to final concentration of < 2 mg/mL. Administer over 60 minutes.

Drug Interactions:
- Antacids (containing magnesium, aluminum, or calcium): decrease oral ciprofloxacin serum level; do not administer concurrently. If must administer antacids, administer at least 2 hours apart.
- Other antiinfectives: potential synergism with clindamycin, aminoglycosides, β-lactam antibiotics against certain organisms.
- Probenecid: 50% increase in ciprofloxacin serum levels; decrease ciprofloxacin dose if given concurrently.
- Theophylline: increases theophylline serum level; avoid if possible since fatal reactions have occurred. Otherwise, monitor theophylline level very closely and decrease theophylline dose as needed.
- Caffeine: delays caffeine clearance from body. Instruct patient to limit coffee, tea, soft drinks, especially if CNS side effects.

Lab Effects/Interference:
- Serum ALT, serum alk phos, serum AST, and serum LDH values may be increased.

Special Considerations:

- Used in the treatment of infections of urinary and lower respiratory tract, skin, bone and joint, and GI tract, as well as gonorrhea.
- Contraindicated in pregnancy and in women who are breast-feeding.
- Obtain ordered specimen for culture and sensitivity prior to first drug dose.
- Use cautiously in patients with seizure disorders.
- Use cautiously in patients receiving concurrent theophylline, as cardiopulmonary arrest has occurred.

Potential Toxicities/Side Effects and the Nursing Process

I. ALTERATION IN NUTRITION, LESS THAN BODY REQUIREMENTS, related to GI SIDE EFFECTS

Defining Characteristics: 2–10% incidence of nausea, vomiting, abdominal discomfort, diarrhea, anorexia.

Nursing Implications: Assess baseline nutritional and elimination status. Instruct patient to report GI disturbances. Administer and teach patient to selfadminister antiemetics, antidiarrheals as needed and as ordered. Teach patient importance of nutritious diet, and suggest small, frequent, high-calorie, high-protein meals as appropriate. Assess baseline LFTs and monitor periodically during treatment. Discuss abnormalities and drug interruption with physician. Assess whether taking other hepatotoxic drugs. (See Special Considerations section.)

II. ALTERATIONS IN SENSORY/PERCEPTUAL PATTERNS related to CNS EFFECTS

Defining Characteristics: 1–2% incidence of headache, restlessness. Dizziness, hallucinations, and seizures may also occur. Exacerbated by caffeine, as ciprofloxacin delays caffeine excretion.

Nursing Implications: Assess baseline neurologic function and comfort, and monitor during treatment. Instruct patient to report any changes. Discuss any abnormalities with physician. Teach patient to limit or restrict all caffeinecontaining fluids, medications, e.g., tea, coffee, soft drinks containing caffeine.

III. ALTERATION IN SKIN INTEGRITY related to ALLERGY/HYPERSENSITIVITY

Defining Characteristics: 1–4% incidence of rash; other manifestations include eosinophilia, urticaria, flushing, fever, chills, photosensitivity, angioedema. Fatal hypersensitivity reactions have occurred rarely. Direct exposure to sunlight can cause sunburn (moderate to severe phototoxicity).

Nursing Implications: Assess baseline skin condition, including integrity and drug allergy history. Instruct patient to report rash, itching, other skin changes. Teach patient skin care and symptomatic measures as appropriate. If skin rash develops, discuss drug discontinuance with physician. If rash progresses, especially in HIV-infected patients, drug should be discontinued as fatal Stevens-Johnson syndrome may develop. Be prepared to treat severe acute hypersensitivity reactions with airway management, oxygen, epinephrine, corticosteroids, antihistamines as ordered. Instruct patient to avoid excessive sun exposure and to use skin protection factor (SPF) 15 or higher.

IV. ALTERATION IN URINARY ELIMINATION related to RENAL TOXICITY

Defining Characteristics: Increased BUN and creatinine, crystal and stone formation in urine, interstitial nephritis, and renal failure may occur.

Nursing Implications: Assess baseline renal function; expect that drug dose will be decreased in presence of renal dysfunction. Instruct patient to take drug with at least 8 oz (240 mL) of water, and to increase oral fluids to 2–3 qt/day.

V. ALTERATION IN COMFORT related to IV ADMINISTRATION

Defining Characteristics: Drug may cause pain, inflammation, and rare thrombophlebitis at IV site.

Nursing Implications: Change IV site q48h. Assess for phlebitis, discomfort, and IV patency prior to each administration. Administer drug slowly over 60–90 minutes in large volume of 5% Dextrose (see Drug Preparation/Administration). Apply heat to promote comfort.

VI. FUNGAL SUPERINFECTION related to REDISTRIBUTION OF ENDOGENOUS MICROORGANISMS

Defining Characteristics: Vaginal candidiasis, vaginitis may occur as endogenous bacteria are eliminated and normal fungal population expands.

Nursing Implications: Instruct female patient to report vaginal itching or discharge. Discuss appropriate antifungal treatment with physician. Teach perineal hygiene and symptomatic management.

Drug: clarithromycin (Biaxin; Biaxin XL)

Class: Antibacterial (macrolide).

Mechanism of Action: Clarithromycin exerts its antibacterial action by binding to 50S ribosomal subunit resulting in inhibition of protein synthesis. The

14-OH metabolite of clarithromycin is twice as active as the parent compound against certain organisms.

Metabolism: Rapidly and widely distributed throughout the body. Highly stable in presence of gastric acid (unlike erythromycin); food delays but does not affect extent of absorption. Widely distributed in body tissues but does not cross blood brain barrier into CSF. Metabolized by liver and excreted by kidneys into urine.

Dosage/Range:

- Adults: Usual dosage 250–500 mg every 12 hours or 1000 mg (two 500 mg extended release tablets) once daily for 7–14 days.
- Children ≥ 6 months: 15 mg/kg/day divided every 12 hours for 10 days.

Drug Preparation/Administration:

- Store tablets and granules for oral suspension at controlled room temperature.
- Reconstituted oral suspension should not be refrigerated because it might gel.
- Microencapsulated particles of clarithromycin in suspension are stable for 14 days when stored at room temperature.

Drug Interactions:

- Alfentanil (and possible other narcotic analgesics): Serum levels may be increased by clarithromycin—monitor for increased effect.
- Astemizole: Concomitant use is contraindicated—may lead to QT prolongation or torsade de pointes.
- Benzodiazepines (those metabolized CYP3A4, including alprazolam and triazolam): Serum levels may be increased by clarithromycin—somnolence and confusion have been reported.
- Bromocriptine: Serum levels may be increased by clarithromycin—monitor for increased effect.
- Buspirone: Serum levels may be increased by clarithromycin—monitor.
- Calcium channel blockers (felodipine, verapamil, and potentially others metabolized by CYP3A4): Serum levels may be increased by clarithromycin—monitor.
- Carbamazepine: Serum levels may be increased by clarithromycin—monitor.
- Cisapride: Serum levels may be increased by clarithromycin—monitor.
- Cilostazol: Serum levels may be increased by clarithromycin—monitor.
- Clozapine: Serum levels may be increased by clarithromycin—monitor.
- Cyclosporine: Serum levels may be increased by clarithromycin—monitor serum levels.
- Delavirdine: Serum levels may be increased by clarithromycin.

- Digoxin: Serum levels may be increased by clarithromycin; digoxin toxicity and potentially fatal arrhythmias have been reported; monitor digoxin levels.
- Dispyramide: Serum levels may be increased by clarithromycin—monitor.
- Ergot alkaloids: Concurrent use may lead to acute ergot toxicity (severe peripheral vasospasm and dysesthesia).
- Fluconazole: Increases clarithromycin levels and AUC by ~25%.
- Indinavir: Serum levels may be increased by clarithromycin—monitor.
- Loratadine: Serum levels may be increased by clarithromycin—monitor.
- Neuromuscular-blocking agents: May be potentate by clarithromycin (case reports)
- Oral contraceptives: Serum levels may be increased by clarithromycin—monitor.
- Phenytoin: Serum levels may be increased by clarithromycin; other evidence suggests phenytoin levels may be decreased in some patients—monitor.
- Pimozide: Serum levels may be increased, leading to malignant arrhythmias; concomitant use is contraindicated.
- Quinolone antibiotics (sparfloxacin, gatifloxacin, or moxifloxacin): Concomitant use may increase the risk of malignant arrhythmias—avoid concomitant use.
- Rifabutin: Serum levels may be increased by clarithromycin—monitor.
- Ritonavir: Concurrent use results in a 77% increase in clarithromycin levels (100% increase in metabolite levels); may be given together without dosage adjustment in patients with normal renal function; dosage of clarithromycin must be decreased in renal impairment.
- Sildenafil: Serum levels may be increased by clarithromycin—monitor.
- Tacrolimus: Serum levels may be increased by clarithromycin—monitor serum concentrations.
- Terfenadine: Serum levels may be increased by clarithromycin; may lead to QT prolongation, ventricular tachycardia, ventricular fibrillation or torsade de pointes; concomitant use is contraindicated.
- Theophylline: Serum levels may be increased by clarithromycin (by as much as 20%)—monitor.
- Valproic acid (and derivatives): Serum levels may be increased by clarithromycin—monitor.
- Warfarin: Effects may be potentiated—monitor INR closely and adjust warfarin dose as needed or choose another antibiotic.
- Zidovudine: Peak levels (but not AUC) of zidovudine may be increased—other studies suggest levels may be decreased.
- St. John's Wort: May decrease clarithromycin levels.
- CYP3A3/4 enzyme substrate—CYP1A2 and 3A3/4 enzyme inhibitor.

Lab Effects/Interference:
- PT/INR—may be prolonged.
- Serum SGPT, serum Alk Phos, serum SGOT, serum bilirubin, or serum LDH—values may be increased.
- BUN and serum creatinine—concentrations may be increased.

Special Considerations:
- Use with caution in patients with renal dysfunction—dose reduction required if severe impairment exists.
- Do not use when there is known hypersensitivity to erythromycins or other macrolides.
- Obtain ordered specimen and send for culture and sensitivity prior to first drug dose.

Potential Toxicities/Side Effects and the Nursing Process

I. POTENTIAL FOR INJURY related to HYPERSENSITIVITY REACTION

Defining Characteristics: Urticaria, pruritis, rash (maculopapular or erythematous), fever and chills, eosinophilia, myalgia, edema, erythema, angioedema.

Nursing Implications: Assess allergy to erythromycin: if patient states "yes," determine actual response, e.g., "swollen lips = angioedema." If angioedema, patient SHOULD NOT receive drug. Discuss other patient responses with physician to determine whether drug should be given. Assess baseline skin condition, including integrity and allergy history to drugs. Teach patient to report rash, itching, other skin changes. Teach patient skin care and symptomatic measures as appropriate. If skin rash develops, discuss drug discontinuance with physician.

II. ALTERATION IN NUTRITION, LESS THAN BODY REQUIREMENTS, related to GI SIDE EFFECTS

Defining Characteristics: Abdominal pain, diarrhea, nausea, and vomiting may occur.

Nursing Implications: Assess baseline nutritional status, preexisting nausea/vomiting, anorexia. Assess baseline LFTs and monitor periodically during treatment. Teach patient to report GI disturbances. Administer and teach patient to self-administer symptomatic interventions if side effects occur; discuss with physician use of alternative drug(s).

III. FUNGAL SUPERINFECTION related to REDISTRIBUTION OF ENDOGENOUS MICROORGANISMS

Defining Characteristics: Vaginal moniliasis, vaginitis may occur as endogenous bacteria are eliminated and normal fungal population expands.

Nursing Implications: Teach female patient to report vaginal itching or discharge. Discuss appropriate antifungal treatment with physician. Teach perineal hygiene and symptomatic management.

IV. ALTERATIONS IN PROTECTIVE MECHANISMS (RARE)

Defining Characteristics: Prolonged PT, prolonged INR, and hypoprothrombinemia have occurred rarely, especially in elderly or debilitated patients, or in individuals with vitamin K deficiency.

Nursing Implications: Assess baseline laboratory parameters, and monitor periodically during treatment. Assess patient for response to antibiotics. Discuss abnormalities with physician. Assess for signs/symptoms of bleeding. If they occur, especially in elderly or debilitated patients, discuss vitamin K administration with physician. Teach patient to avoid aspirin. If taking oral anticoagulants, assess for increased PT, signs/symptoms of bleeding.

Drug: clindamycin phosphate (Cleocin)

Class: Antibacterial (systemic); antiprotozoal.

Mechanism of Action: Bacteriostatic or bactericidal depending on drug concentration or when used against highly susceptible organisms; binds to bacterial ribosomes and prevent peptide bond formation, thus inhibiting protein synthesis. Active against gram-positive cocci (e.g., staphylococci, streptococci) and some anaerobic gram-positive and gram-negative bacilli (e.g., clostridia, mycobacteria).

Metabolism: Well absorbed (90% of dose) from GI tract. Food may delay absorption but does not affect amount absorbed. Widely distributed in body tissues and fluids, including bile. Crosses placenta and is excreted in breast milk. Excreted in urine, bile, and feces.

Dosage/Range:

Adult:

- Oral: 150–450 mg PO q6h; IM/IV: 300 mg q6–12h (maximum 2.7 g/day).

Drug Preparation/Administration:

- Oral: Administer with 8 oz (240 mL) of water to prevent esophageal irritation.
- IM: Single dose should not exceed 600 mg.

- Further dilute in 0.9% Sodium Chloride or 5% Dextrose in water to final concentration < 12 mg/mL, and infuse over 20 minutes (600-mg dose) or 30–40 minutes (1.2-g dose). Maximum 1.2 gm in single 1-hour period. May be given as continuous infusion.

Drug Interactions:
- Neuromuscular blocking agents (tubocurarine, ether, pancuronium): may increase neuromuscular blockade; use concurrently with caution.
- Erythromycin: decreases bactericidal activity of clindamycin.
- Kaolin: decreases GI absorption of clindamycin. Avoid concurrent administration, or administer at least 2 hours apart.

Lab Effects/Interference:
- Serum ALT, serum alk phos, and serum AST concentrations may be increased.

Special Considerations:
- Contraindicated in patients with hypersensitivity to clindamycin or lincomycin; contraindicated in patients with history of colitis.
- Can cause severe, sometimes fatal colitis. Stop drug if diarrhea develops, or if necessary, continue only under close monitoring and endoscopy.
- Used in the treatment of serious infections of respiratory tract, skin/soft tissues, female pelvic/genital tract. May be used investigationally with other drugs in treatment of *Mycobacterium avium* complex (MAC); also may be used to treat *P. carinii* pneumonia, cryptosporidiosis, and toxoplasmosis in AIDS patients.
- Also used for prophylaxis of bacterial endocarditis in penicillin-allergic, erythromycin-intolerant patients.
- DO NOT GIVE rapid IVB: cardiopulmonary arrest has occurred.
- Avoid use in pregnant or breast-feeding women.

Potential Toxicities/Side Effects and the Nursing Process

I. ALTERATION IN NUTRITION, LESS THAN BODY REQUIREMENTS, related to GI SIDE EFFECTS

Defining Characteristics: Nausea, vomiting, diarrhea, abdominal pain, and tenesmus may occur. Flatulence, bloating, anorexia, and esophagitis may occur as well. Fatal pseudomembranous colitis has occurred, characterized by severe diarrhea, abdominal cramping, and melena. Usually begins 2–9 days after drug is initiated.

Nursing Implications: Assess elimination and nutrition pattern, baseline and during therapy. Instruct patient to report diarrhea and/or abdominal pain immediately. Discuss drug discontinuance with physician if diarrhea occurs. Guaiac stool for occult blood, and notify physician if positive. If severe diarrhea develops, discuss management plan including endoscopy, fluid and electrolyte replacement. Do not administer antiperistaltic agents such as opiates and diphenoxylate with atropine (Lomotil), since it may worsen condition. Assess for nausea/vomiting, and administer prescribed antiemetic medications. Encourage small, frequent feedings as tolerated. Instruct patient to take oral dose with a full glass of water.

II. ALTERATION IN SKIN INTEGRITY related to HYPERSENSITIVITY

Defining Characteristics: Maculopapular rash, urticaria may occur. Rarely, erythema multiforme may occur. Increased risk of allergic reaction in asthma patients. Anaphylaxis may rarely occur.

Nursing Implications: Assess baseline allergy history. Assess baseline skin integrity. Instruct patient to report rash, pruritus. Teach patient symptomatic management of rash, pruritus. Assess for hypersensitivity reaction: if it occurs, monitor vital signs (VS), discontinue drug, notify physician, and institute supportive measures.

III. ALTERATION IN COMFORT related to LOCAL ADMINISTRATION EFFECTS

Defining Characteristics: IM administration may cause pain, induration, sterile abscesses, and transient increase in creatine phosphokinase (CPK) due to muscle injury. IV administration may cause erythema, pain, swelling, and thrombophlebitis.

Nursing Implications: Administer maximum 600-mg dose IM deeply in large muscle mass (e.g., gluteus maximus). Rotate sites. Assess IV site prior to each dose for phlebitis or swelling, and change site at least q48h. Administer dose slowly: 300–600 mg in 50 mL over 20–30 minutes, and 900–1200-mg dose in 100 mL IV over 40–60 minutes. Apply heat to painful IV sites as ordered.

IV. ALTERATION IN HEPATIC FUNCTION related to TRANSIENT INCREASE LFTs

Defining Characteristics: Transient increases in serum bili, AST, alk phos have occurred.

Nursing Implications: Assess baseline LFTs, and monitor during therapy.

V. FUNGAL SUPERINFECTION related to REDISTRIBUTION OF ENDOGENOUS MICROORGANISMS

Defining Characteristics: Vaginal candidiasis, vaginitis may occur as endogenous bacteria are eliminated, and normal fungal population expands.

Nursing Implications: Instruct female patient to report vaginal itching or discharge. Discuss appropriate antifungal treatment with physician. Teach perineal hygiene and symptomatic management.

Drug: co-trimoxazole; trimethoprim and sulfamethoxazole (Bactrim, Bactrim DS, Cotrim, Septra)

Class: Sulfonamide antibacterial (systemic); antiprotozoal.

Mechanism of Action: Bactericidal by preventing folic acid synthesis so microorganism cannot undergo cell division (sequential inhibition of folic acid synthesis, first by sulfamethoxazole, then by trimethoprim). Active against gram-positive bacteria (streptococci, *S. aureus, Nocardia*), gram-negative bacteria (*Enterobacter, E. coli, Proteus, Klebsiella, Shigella*), and protozoa (*P. carinii*).

Metabolism: Rapidly absorbed from GI tract. Widely distributed into body tissues and fluids; crosses the placenta and is excreted in breast milk. Highly protein-bound. Metabolized by the liver and excreted in the urine.

Dosage/Range:

Adult:

- Oral: Trimethoprim 160 mg and sulfamethoxazole 800 mg (double-strength tablet DS) q12h × 7–14 days (depending on infection).
- Oral: *P. carinii* pneumonia prophylaxis: 1 DS tablet twice daily 2 days per week (typically consecutive) or 1 DS tablet every other day.
- IV: 10–20 mg/kg in two to four divided doses q6–8h (usually 21 days for *P. carinii* pneumonia in AIDS patients).
- Dose modification if renal impairment exists.

Drug Preparation:

- Oral tablets should be stored in tight, light-resistant containers; vials of powder for injection and suspension should be stored at 15–30°C (59–86°F).

Drug Administration:

- Oral: Administer with full (8 oz or 240 mL) glass of water.
- IV: Add each 5 mL of drug to 125 mL of 5% Dextrose in water ONLY. Stable for 6 hours. If patient is fluid restricted, can mix each 5 mL in 75 mL of 5% Dextrose immediately prior to administration and give within 2 hours. DO NOT REFRIGERATE. Administer over 60–90 minutes.

Drug Interactions:

- Warfarin: increases PT. Monitor PT closely and decrease dose of warfarin as needed.

- Sulfonylureas: increases hypoglycemic effect. Monitor blood glucose closely and reduce sulfonylurea dose as needed.
- Phenytoin: increases and prolongs serum levels. Monitor serum phenytoin level closely and reduce dose as needed.
- Thiazide diuretics (in elderly): increases toxicity (thrombocytopenia with purpura). AVOID CONCURRENT USE.
- Cyclosporine: decreases cyclosporine effect; increases risk of nephrotoxicity. AVOID CONCURRENT USE when possible.
- Methotrexate: increases methotrexate level and potential toxicity (e.g., bone marrow depression). Monitor levels or decrease methotrexate dose as needed.
- Oral contraceptives: decreases contraceptive effect. Monitor for breakthrough bleeding and counsel patient to use barrier contraceptive in addition during antibiotic therapy.
- Ammonium chloride or ascorbic acid: causes antibiotic drug precipitation in kidneys. AVOID CONCURRENT USE.

Lab Effects/Interference:

- Jaffe alkaline picrate reaction overestimation of creatinine by 10%.

Special Considerations:

- Drug is teratogenic, so should not be used in pregnant women if avoidable.
- Drug is excreted in breast milk and can cause kernicterus in infants. Alternative drug should be used or mother should interrupt breast-feeding during drug use.
- Contraindicated if patient has porphyria.
- Contraindicated in patients with hypersensitivity to sulfites, sulfonamides, or to trimethoprim.
- Contraindicated if severe renal failure (creatinine clearance < 15 mL/minute).
- Use with caution at reduced dosage in patients with glucose-6-phosphate dehydrogenase deficiency (G6PD); hemolysis may occur. Also, use with caution in patients with impaired renal or hepatic function, severe allergy, bronchial asthma, and blood dyscrasias.
- Use cautiously in patients with known hypersensitivity to sulfonamide-derivative drugs such as thiazides, acetazolamide, tolbutamide.
- Increased incidence of adverse side effects in AIDS patients, especially allergic, hematologic reactions. Monitor closely for toxicity.
- Drug is first line treatment for *P. carinii* pneumonia; it is at least as effective as pentamidine, with a cure rate of 70–80%.
- Send specimen for culture and sensitivity prior to initial drug dose, as appropriate.

Potential Toxicities/Side Effects and the Nursing Process

I. ALTERATION IN SKIN INTEGRITY related to HYPERSENSITIVITY REACTION

Defining Characteristics: Skin reactions ranging from mild maculopapular rash with urticaria, pruritus to erythema multiforme, exfoliative dermatitis, and Stevens-Johnson syndrome. Risk for rash is increased in AIDS patients; usually occurs 7–14 days after beginning drug. Other allergic manifestations include fever, chills, photosensitivity, angioedema, and anaphylaxis.

Nursing Implications: Assess for prior hypersensitivity to drug. Assess for signs/symptoms of drug allergy. Instruct patient to report rash, allergic reaction immediately. Discuss any drug continuance with physician if rash appears. Teach patient symptomatic management of discomfort and skin irritation. Be prepared to treat severe acute hypersensitivity reactions with airway management, oxygen, epinephrine, corticosteroids, antihistamines as ordered.

II. POTENTIAL FOR INFECTION, BLEEDING, AND FATIGUE related to HEMATOLOGIC TOXICITY

Defining Characteristics: Leukopenia, neutropenia, and thrombocytopenia are common in AIDS patients. Agranulocytosis, aplastic and megaloblastic anemia, thrombocytopenia, hemolytic anemia, neutropenia, hypoprothrombinemia, and eosinophilia may occur less commonly. Increased risk exists in folate-deficient patients: elderly, alcoholic, malnourished; also, patients receiving folate antimetabolites, e.g., phenytoin, methotrexate, or thiazide diuretics; or in patients with renal dysfunction.

Nursing Implications: Assess baseline risk, CBC, and monitor CBC periodically during treatment. Assess for and teach patient to monitor signs/symptoms of infection, bleeding, fatigue, and to report these. If side effects occur, discuss with physician use of folinic acid (leucovorin).

III. ALTERATIONS IN NUTRITION, LESS THAN BODY REQUIREMENTS, related to GI TOXICITY

Defining Characteristics: Nausea, vomiting, and anorexia are most common; pseudomembranous colitis, glossitis, stomatitis, abdominal pain, diarrhea may occur.

Nursing Implications: Assess GI function. Teach patient to assess for and instruct to report GI side effects, and to administer prescribed antiemetics or antidiarrheals as needed. Assess oral mucosa, and if stomatitis develops, discuss with physician use of leucovorin (folinic acid). Teach patient oral hygiene. Take drug with 8 oz (240 mL) water to prevent esophageal ulcerations. Discuss food preferences, use of spices, and suggest small, frequent meals if anorexia develops.

IV. SENSORY/PERCEPTUAL DYSFUNCTION related to FATIGUE, WEAKNESS

Defining Characteristics: Headache, vertigo, insomnia, fatigue, weakness, mental depression, seizures, and hallucinations may occur.

Nursing Implications: Assess baseline neurologic function and comfort, and monitor during treatment. Instruct patient to report any changes. Discuss any abnormalities with physician.

V. ALTERATION IN URINARY ELIMINATION related to RENAL TOXICITY

Defining Characteristics: Increased BUN and creatinine, crystal and stone formation in urine, interstitial nephritis, and renal failure may occur.

Nursing Implications: Assess baseline renal function; expect that drug dose will be decreased in presence of renal dysfunction. Instruct patient to take drug with at least 8 oz water and to increase oral fluids to 2–3 qt (liters)/day.

VI. ALTERATION IN COMFORT related to IV ADMINISTRATION

Defining Characteristics: Drug may cause pain, inflammation, and rare thrombophlebitis at IV site.

Nursing Implications: Change IV site q48h. Assess for phlebitis, discomfort, and IV patency prior to each administration. Administer drug slowly over 60–90 minutes in large volume of 5% Dextrose (see Drug Administration). Apply heat to promote comfort.

VII. FUNGAL SUPERINFECTION related to REDISTRIBUTION OF ENDOGENOUS MICROORGANISMS

Defining Characteristics: Vaginal candidiasis, vaginitis may occur as endogenous bacteria are eliminated and normal fungal population expands.

Nursing Implications: Instruct female patient to report vaginal itching or discharge. Discuss appropriate antifungal treatment with physician. Teach perineal hygiene and symptomatic management.

Drug: daptomycin (Cubicin)

Class: Cyclic lipopeptide antibiotic

Mechanism of Action: This antibiotic is the first in a new structural class. It is derived from the fermentation of *Streptomyces roseosporus*. The mechanism of action is not fully understood. Daptomycin binds to bacterial membranes and causes a rapid depolarization of membrane potential. This loss of membrane potential leads to inhibition of protein, DNA, and RNA synthesis resulting in bacterial cell death. It acts against Gram-positive bacteria, and retains in vitro potency against isolates resistant to methicillin, vancomycin, and linezolid.

Metabolism: Excreted by the kidney. Renal excretion is primary route of elimination.

Dosage/Range:
Adult: 4 mg/kg by IV infusion q d for 7–14 days
Drug dose should be reduced or adjusted in patients with severe renal insufficiency.

Drug Preparation/Administration:
- 0.9% sodium chloride injection
- Administer over 30 minutes

Drug Interactions:
- Tobramycin: interaction between daptomycin and tobramycin is unknown. Caution is warranted when daptomycin is co-administered with tobramycin.
- Warfarin: anticoagulant activity in patients receiving daptomycin and warfarin should be monitored for the first several days.

Lab Effects/Interference:
- There are no reported drug-laboratory test interactions.

Special Considerations:
- Contraindicated in patients with known hypersensitivity to daptomycin.
- Obtain ordered specimen and send for culture and sensitivity prior to first antibiotic dose.
- Consider alternative antibiotic therapy if anemia, drug rash or fever, arthralgia, or unexplained rise in BUN and serum creatinine occur.

Potential Toxicities/Side Effects and the Nursing Process

I. ALTERATION IN NUTRITION, LESS THAN BODY REQUIREMENTS, related to GI SIDE EFFECTS

Defining Characteristics: Constipation, nausea, diarrhea, vomiting, dyspepsia

Nursing Implications: Assess baseline nutritional status, preexisiting nausea/ vomiting, anorexia. Assess baseline bowel pattern. Administer symptomatic interventions if side effects occur; discuss with physician use of alternative drug(s).

II. POTENTIAL FOR INJURY related to HYPERSENSITIVITY REACTION

Defining Characteristics: Rash, urticaria, pruritis, and fever can occur in individuals with hypersensitivity to daptomycin.

Nursing Implications: Assess for drug allergies prior to drug administration. Instruct patient to report any allergic reactions. Assess for signs/symptoms of allergic reaction after drug dose.

III. SENSORY/PERCEPTUAL ALTERATIONS related to CNS EFFECTS OF DIZZINESS AND HEADACHE

Defining Characteristics: Dizziness, headache and insomnia may occur.

Nursing Implications: Assess baseline neurological status. Teach patient about side effects and to report dizziness or headache. If signs/symptoms arise, discuss drug discontinuance with physican.

Drug: demeclocycline hydrochloride (Declomycin)

Class: Antibacterial (systemic); tetracycline; antiprotozoal

Mechanism of Action: Bacteriostatic but may be bactericidal at high concentrations. Binds to bacterial ribosomes and prevents protein synthesis. Active against broad range of Gram-negative and Gram-positive organisms. Demeclocycline hydrochloride may also be used in special cases of fluid retention (SIADH). A syndrome of polyuria, polydipesia, and weakness has been shown to be nephrogenic, dose-dependent, and reversible on discontinuation of therapy.

Metabolism: Absorbed from the GI tract. Widely distributed into body tissues and fluids. Crosses placenta and is excreted in breast milk. Concentrated in the liver, excreted into the bile. The rate of demeclocycline hydrochloride clearance is less than half that of tetracycline.

Dosage/Range:
Adult: Oral: 150 mg q 6 hours or 300 mg q 12 hours

- Duration of therapy depends on indication
- As treatment for hyponatremia: 600–1200 mg daily.
- Drug dose should be reduced or adjusted in patients with hepatic or renal insufficiency.

Drug Preparation/Administration:

- Oral: Take 1 hour before meals or 2 hours after meals. Dose reduce in patients with renal and liver impairment.

Drug Interactions:

- Oral anticoagulants: increase PT. Monitor patient closely and decrease anticoagulant dose as needed.
- Concurrent use of tetracyclines with oral contraceptives may render oral contraceptives less effective. Advise patient to use barrier contraceptive as well during a course of tetracycline therapy.
- Methoxyflurane: fatal renal toxicity has been reported with concurrent use.
- Iron preparations: decreases oral absorption. Administer iron preparations 3 hours after or 2 hours before any tetracycline.
- Antacids & antidiarrheals: may decrease absorption of tetracyclines. Avoid concurrent use.

Lab Effects/Interference:

- There are no reported drug-laboratory test interactions.
- SGPT, alk phos, Amylase, SGOT, and bilirubin: serum concentrations may be increased.

Special Considerations:

- Avoid use in pregnant or lactating women.
- Contraindicated in patients with known hypersensitivity to tetracyclines.
- Obtain ordered specimen and send for culture and sensitivity prior to first antibiotic dose.

Potential Toxicities/Side Effects and the Nursing Process

I. ALTERATION IN NUTRITION related to GI SIDE EFFECTS

Defining Characteristics: Anorexia, nausea, vomiting, diarrhea, glossitis, dysphagia, enterocolitis, pancreatitis.

Nursing Implications: Assess baseline nutritional status. Assess for and teach patient to report any symptoms. Administer and teach patient self-administration of prescribed antiemetic or antidiarrheal medication as appropriate. Administer and teach to self-administer oral dose with at least 8 oz of water at least 1 hour before or 2 hours after a meal or sleep.

II. ALTERATION IN SKIN INTEGRITY related to RASH, PHOTOSENSITIVITY

Defining Characteristics: Maculopapular and erythematous rash may occur. Photosensitivity risk (exaggerated sunburn) persists 1–2 days after completion of drug therapy.

Nursing Implications: Teach patient about potential side effects, to avoid sunlight during drug therapy, and to report rash, and other abnormalities. Teach symptomatic skin care as appropriate.

III. INJURY related to HYPERSENSITIVITY

Defining Characteristics: Urticaria, angioneurotic edema, anaphylaxis may occur; also fever, arthralgias, eosinophilia, and pericarditis.

Nursing Implications: Assess drug allergy history. Assess baseline allergy history. Assess baseline skin integrity. Teach patient to report rash, pruritis, Teach patient symptomatic management of rash, pruritis. Assess for hypersensitivity reacton: if it occurs, monitor VS, discontinues drug, notify physician, and institute supportive measures.

IV. FUNGAL SUPERINFECTION related to REDISTRIBUTION OF ENDOGENOUS MICROORGANISMS

Defining Characteristics: Vaginal moniliasis, vaginitis may occur as endogenous bacteria are eliminated and normal fungal population expands.

Nursing Implications: Teach female patient to report vaginal itching or discharge. Discuss appropriate antifungal treatment with physician. Teach perineal hygiene and symptom management.

Drug: dicloxacillin sodium (Dycill, Dynapen, Pathocil)

Class: Penicillin antibacterial.

Mechanism of Action: Semisynthetic antibiotic prepared from fungus *Penicillium.* Contains β-lactam ring and is bactericidal by inhibiting cell wall synthesis. Penicillinase-resistant and active against penicillin-resistant staphylococci, which produce the enzyme penicillinase. Used to treat upper and lower respiratory tract and skin infections.

Metabolism: Well absorbed from GI tract, but food decreases rate and extent of absorption. Widely distributed through body tissues and fluids; crosses placenta and is excreted in breast milk; 95–99% bound to serum proteins. Excreted in urine and bile.

Dosage/Range:

- Adult: 125 mg–500 mg PO q6h × 14 days (but depends on severity of infection).

Drug Preparation:

- Store in tight containers at <40°C (104°F).

Drug Administration:

- Oral: administer at least 1 hour before or 2 hours after meals.

Drug Interactions:

- Aminoglycosides: synergism.
- Rifampin: possible antagonism, only at high doses of penicillin.
- Probenecid: increased serum level of penicillin; may be coadministered to exert this effect.

Lab Effects/Interference:

Major clinical significance:

- Urine glucose: high urinary concentrations of a penicillin may produce false-positive or falsely elevated test results with copper sulfate tests (Benedict's, Clinitest, or Fehling's); glucose enzymatic tests (Clinistix or Tes-tape) are not affected

Clinical significance:

- Coombs' (direct antiglobulin) test: false-positive result may occur during therapy with any penicillin.
- ALT, alk phos, AST, serum LDH values may be increased.
- WBC: leukopenia or neutropenia is associated with the use of all penicillins; the effect is more likely to occur with prolonged therapy and severe hepatic function impairment.

Special Considerations:

- Contraindicated in patients with prior hypersensitivity to penicillins. Use with caution in patients sensitive to other β-lactams (e.g., cephalosporins) since partial cross-allergenicity exists.
- Obtain ordered specimen and send for culture and sensitivity prior to first antibiotic dose.
- Consider alternative antibiotic therapy if eosinophilia, drug fever or rash, arthralgia, hematuria, or unexplained rise in BUN and serum creatinine occur.
- Monitor electrolytes and renal, hepatic, and hematologic laboratory parameters during extended treatment periods.
- Use with caution in pregnancy or with nursing women.

Potential Toxicities/Side Effects and the Nursing Process

I. POTENTIAL FOR INJURY related to HYPERSENSITIVITY REACTION

Defining Characteristics: Urticaria, pruritus, rash (maculopapular or erythematous), fever and chills, eosinophilia, myalgia, edema, erythema, angioedema, Stevens-Johnson syndrome, and exfoliative skin reactions occur in 5% of patients. Increased risk exists in individuals allergic to cephalosporin antibiotics.

Nursing Implications: Assess allergy to cephalosporin antibiotics and penicillin: if patient states "yes," determine actual response, e.g., "swollen lips = angioedema." If angioedema, patient SHOULD NOT receive drug. Discuss other patient responses with physician to determine whether drug should be given. Assess baseline skin condition, including integrity and allergy history to drugs. Instruct patient to report rash, itching, and other skin changes. Teach patient skin care and symptomatic measures as appropriate. If skin rash develops, discuss drug discontinuance with physician. If rash progresses, drug should be discontinued as fatal Stevens-Johnson syndrome may develop. Be prepared to treat severe acute hypersensitivity reactions with airway management, oxygen, epinephrine, corticosteroids, antihistamines as ordered.

II. ALTERATION IN NUTRITION, LESS THAN BODY REQUIREMENTS, related to GI SIDE EFFECTS

Defining Characteristics: Nausea, vomiting, diarrhea may occur; rarely, pseudomembranous colitis caused by *C. difficile* resistant to the antibiotic occurs. Rarely, transient increases in LFTs—AST, ALT, alk phos, bili—may occur.

Nursing Implications: Assess baseline nutritional status. Instruct patient to report GI disturbances. Administer and teach patient to self-administer antiemetics as needed and as ordered. Teach patient importance of nutritious diet, and suggest small, frequent, high-calorie, high-protein meals as appropriate. Assess baseline LFTs, and monitor periodically during treatment. Discuss abnormalities and drug interruption with physician.

III. FUNGAL SUPERINFECTION related to REDISTRIBUTION OF ENDOGENOUS MICROORGANISMS

Defining Characteristics: Vaginal candidiasis, vaginitis may occur as endogenous bacteria are eliminated and normal fungal population expands.

Nursing Implications: Instruct female patient to report vaginal itching or discharge. Discuss appropriate antifungal treatment with physician. Teach perineal hygiene and symptomatic management.

IV. ALTERATIONS IN PROTECTIVE MECHANISMS (RARE) related to TRANSIENT LEUKOPENIA

Defining Characteristics: Rarely, transient leukopenia, lymphocytosis, anemia, eosinophilia may occur. Prolonged PT, prolonged APTT, and hypoprothrombinemia have occurred rarely, especially in elderly or debilitated patients, or in individuals with vitamin K deficiency.

Nursing Implications: Assess baseline laboratory parameters, and monitor periodically during treatment. Assess patient for response to antibiotics. Discuss abnormalities with physician.

V. KNOWLEDGE DEFICIT related to SELF-ADMINISTRATION OF MEDICATION

Defining Characteristics: Increased compliance when patient is instructed in self-care activities.

Nursing Implications: Assess knowledge about infection and planned treatment. Teach about drug action, potential side effects, and when and how to take drug (take medication as directed, 1 hour before or 2 hours after food). Instruct patient to report any possible drug side effects that occur.

Drug: doxycycline hyclate (Vibramycin, Doryx, MonoDox)

Class: Antibacterial (systemic); antiprotozoal.

Mechanism of Action: Bacteriostatic but may be bactericidal at high concentrations. Binds to bacterial ribosomes and prevents protein synthesis. Active against broad range of gram-positive and gram-negative bacteria, Chlamydia, and Mycoplasma.

Metabolism: Absorbed (60%–80%) from GI tract. Widely distributed into body tissues and fluids. Crosses placenta and is excreted in breast milk. Excreted unchanged in urine.

Dosage/Range:
Adult:
- Oral: 100 mg q12 hours for the first day, then 100–200 mg once daily, or 50–100 mg q12 hours. Duration of therapy depends on indication.
- IV: 200 mg QD or 100 mg q12 hours for the first day, then 100–200 mg QD or 50–100 mg q12 hours. Duration of therapy depends on indication.

Drug Preparation/Administration:
- Oral: may be taken with food, water, milk, or carbonated beverages.
- IV: add 10 mL sterile water for injection to 100-mg vial or 20 mL to each 200-mg vial. Further dilute in 100 to 1000 mL or in 200 to 2000 ml, respectively, of lactated Ringer's injection or 5% dextrose and lactated Ringer's injection. Infuse over 1 to 4 hours.
- CONCENTRATIONS LESS THAN 100 MCG PER ML OR GREATER THAN 1 MG PER ML ARE NOT RECOMMENDED.
- AVOID RAPID ADMINISTRATION.

- Solution stable for 6 hours, so use after mixing. Avoid exposure to heat or sunlight. Convert to oral preparation as soon as possible as there is risk of thrombophlebitis.
- DO NOT ADMINISTER INTRAMUSCULARLY OR SUBCUTANEOUSLY.

Drug Interactions:

- Hepatotoxic drugs: may increase hepatotoxicity if given concurrently. Assess baseline and periodically during treatment.
- Iron preparations: decrease oral and possibly IV absorption. Administer iron preparations 3 hours after or 2 hours before any tetracycline.
- Oral anticoagulants: increase PT. Monitor patient closely and decrease anticoagulant dose as needed.
- Antidiarrheals (containing kaolin, pectate, or bismuth): may decrease absorption of tetracyclines. Avoid concurrent use.
- Oral contraceptives: decreased effectiveness of contraceptive and increased incidence of breakthrough bleeding. Advise patient to use barrier contraceptive as well during a course of tetracycline therapy.
- Lithium: may decrease lithium levels. Monitor serum levels and increase dose as needed.

Lab Effects/Interference:

- Urine catecholamine determinations: may produce false elevations of urinary catecholamines because of interfering fluorescence in the Hingerty method.
- SGPT, alk phos, Amylase, SGOT, and bilirubin: serum concentrations may be increased.

Special Considerations:

- Use cautiously in patients with myasthenia gravis: may increase muscle weakness.
- Avoid use in pregnant or lactating women.
- Obtain ordered specimen for culture and sensitivity prior to first dose.
- IV preparation contains ascorbic acid and may cause false-positive result using Clinitest, or false-negative result when using Clinistix and Testape.
- Drug has affinity for ischemic, necrotic tissue, and may localize in tumors.

Potential Toxicities/Side Effects and the Nursing Process

I. ALTERATION IN NUTRITION related to GI SIDE EFFECTS

Defining Characteristics: Nausea, vomiting, diarrhea, anorexia, abdominal discomfort, epigastric burning and distress, glossitis, black hairy tongue may occur.

Nursing Implications: Assess baseline nutritional status. Assess for and teach patient to report any symptoms. Administer and teach patient self-administration of prescribed antiemetic or antidiarrheal medication as appropriate. Administer and teach patient to self-administer oral dose with at least 8 oz of water taken at least 1 hour before lying down for sleep.

II. ALTERATION IN SKIN INTEGRITY related to RASH, PHOTOSENSITIVITY

Defining Characteristics: Maculopapular and erythematous rashes may occur. Rarely, exfoliative dermatitis, onycholyis, and nail discoloration. Photosensitivity risk (exaggerated sunburn) persists 1–2 days after completion of drug therapy.

Nursing Implications: Each patient about potential side effects, to avoid sunlight during drug therapy, and to report rash, other abnormalities. Teach symptomatic skin care as appropriate.

III. INJURY related to HYPERSENSITIVITY

Defining Characteristics: Urticaria, angioneurotic edema, anaphylaxis may occur; also, fever, rash, arthralgias, eosinophilia, and pericarditis.

Nursing Implications: Assess drug allergy history. Assess baseline allergy history. Assess baseline skin integrity. Teach patient to report rash, pruritus. Teach patient symptomatic management of rash, pruritus. Assess for hypersensitivity reaction: if it occurs, monitor VS, discontinue drug, notify physician, and institute supportive measures.

IV. FUNGAL SUPERINFECTION related to REDISTRIBUTION OF ENDOGENOUS MICROORGANISMS

Defining Characteristics: Vaginal moniliasis, vaginitis may occur as endogenous bacteria are eliminated, and normal fungal population expands.

Nursing Implications: Teach female patient to report vaginal itching or discharge. Discuss appropriate antifungal treatment with physician. Teach perineal hygiene and symptomatic management.

V. ALTERATION IN HEPATIC FUNCTION

Defining Characteristics: Associated with high IV doses (> 2 gm/day): hepatotoxicity and cholestasis may occur.

Nursing Implications: Assess baseline LFTs and monitor during therapy.

VI. INFECTION AND BLEEDING related to NEUTROPENIA, THROMBOCYTOPENIA

Defining Characteristics: Neutropenia, leukocytosis, leukopenia, atypical lymphocytes, thrombocytopenia, thrombocytopenic purpura, hemolytic anemia occur rarely with long-term therapy.

Nursing Implications: Assess baseline WBC, hematocrit, and platelets, and monitor periodically during long-term therapy.

VII. ALTERATION IN COMFORT related to LOCAL ADMINISTRATION EFFECTS

Defining Characteristics: IM administration may cause pain, induration due to muscle injury. IV administration may cause erythema, pain, swelling, and thrombophlebitis.

Nursing Implications: Rotate sites. Apply ice as ordered to painful buttock. Assess IV site prior to each dose for phlebitis or swelling and change site at least q 48 hours. Apply heat to painful IV sites as ordered.

VIII. SENSORY/PERCEPTUAL ALTERATION

Defining Characteristics: Light-headedness, dizziness, headache may occur.

Nursing Implications: Assess baseline neurological status. Teach patient to report any changes and discuss them with physician.

Drug: ertapenem sodium (Invanz)

Class: antibiotic, carbapenem.

Mechanism of Action: The bactericidal activity results from the inhibition of cell wall synthesis. Penetrates the cell wall of most gram-positive and gram-negative bacteria to reach penicillin-binding protein (PBP) targets.

Metabolism: Widely distributed in body tissues and fluids, excreted in urine.

Dosage/Range:

Adult:

- Acute Pelvic Infection: 1 gram IV/IM once a day for 3–10 days
- Community Acquired Pneumonia: 1 gram IV/IM once a day for 10–14 days
- Intrabdominal infection: 1 gram IV/IM once a day for 5–14 days
- Skin/Skin Structure Infections: 1 gram IV/IM once a day for 7–14 days
- Urinary Tract Infections: 1 gram IV/IM once a day for 10–14 days
- Adjust dose in patients with renal impairment and on hemodialysis

Drug Preparation/Administration:

- IV infusion for up to 14 days.
- IV infusion for up to 14 days.
- IM injection for up to 7 days.
- DO NOT DILUTE WITH Diluents containing dextrose.

Drug Interactions:

- Probenecid competes with ertapenem for active tubular secretion; increasing AUC by 25% and reducing the plasma and renal clearances by 20% and 35% respectively.

Lab Effects/Interference:

- Ertapenem posses the characteristic low toxicity of the beta-lactam group of antibiotics.
- Periodically assess organ system function: renal, hepatic & hematopoietic.

Potential Toxicities/Side Effects and the Nursing Process

I. POTENTIAL FOR INJURY related to HYPERSENSITIVITY REACTION and LOCAL REACTIONS (pain at injection site)

Defining Characteristics: Urticaria, pruritus, rash (maculopapular or erythematous), fever and chills, eosinophilia, myalgia, edema, erythema, angioedema.

Nursing Implications: Assess allergy to cephalosporin antibiotics and penicillin; if patient states "yes," determine actual response, e.g., "swollen lips = angioedema." If angioedema, patient SHOULD NOT receive drug. Discuss other patient responses with physician to determine whether drug should be given. Assess baseline skin condition, including integrity and allergy history to drugs. Instruct patient to report rash, itching, and other skin changes. Teach patient skin care and symptomatic measures as appropriate. If skin rash develops, discuss drug discontinuance with physician. Be prepared to treat severe acute hypersensitivity reactions with airway management, oxygen, epinephrine, corticosteroids, antihistamines as ordered.

II. ALTERATION IN NUTRITION, LESS THAN BODY REQUIREMENTS, related to GI SIDE EFFECTS

Defining Characteristics: Nausea, vomiting, diarrhea may occur; rarely, pseudomembranous colitis caused by antibiotic resistance occurs.

Nursing Implications: Assess baseline nutritional status. Instruct patient to report GI disturbances. Administer and teach patient to self-administer antiemetics as needed and as ordered. Teach patient importance of nutritious diet, and suggest small, frequent, high-calorie, high-protein meals as appropriate. Assess baseline LFTs, and monitor periodically during treatment. Discuss abnormalities and drug interruption with physician.

III. FUNGAL SUPERINFECTION related to REDISTRIBUTION OF ENDOGENOUS MICROORGANISMS

Defining Characteristics: Vaginal candidiasis, vaginitis may occur as endogenous bacteria are eliminated, and normal fungal population expands.

Nursing Implications: Instruct female patient to report vaginal itching or discharge. Discuss appropriate antifungal treatment with physician. Teach perineal hygiene and symptomatic management.

Drug: erythromycin (ERYC, E-Mycin, Illotycin, Erythrocin)

Class: Antibacterial (macrolide).

Mechanism of Action: Erythromycin is a broad spectrum antibiotic with activity against gram-positive and gram-negative bacteria, and other infectious agents, including *Chlamydia trachomatis,* mycoplasmas (*Mycoplasma pneumoniae* and *Ureaplasma urealyticum*), and spirochetes (*Treponema pallidum* and *Borrelia* species). Erythromycin has good activity against *S. pyogenes, Streptococcus pneumoniae (group A beta-hemolytic streptococci)*, and *Straphylococcus aureus*.

Erythromycin is a bacteriostatic macrolide antibiotic. It may be bactericidal in high concentrations or when used against highly susceptible organisms. It is thought to penetrate the bacterial cell membrane and to reversibly bind to the 50 S ribosomal subunit. It does not directly inhibit peptide formation rather, it inhibits the translocation of peptides from the acceptor site on the ribosome to the donor site, inhibiting subsequent protein synthesis. Effective against actively dividing organisms.

Metabolism: 90% of the drug is metabolized by the liver; may accumulate in patients with severe hepatic disease. Primarily excreted into the bile. Between 2 to 5% is excreted unchanged by the kidneys following oral administration; 12 to 15% excreted unchanged following IV administration. Erythromycins cross the placental barrier in pregnancy; can be found in breast milk.

Dosage/Range:

- Oral: 250 mg once q6h for 10 days; or 500 mg q6h for 10 days; or 333 mg q8h
- IV: 500 mg q6h; up to 1000 mg q6h (Legionnaires' Disease).

Drug Preparation:

- Further dilute in 0.9% Sodium Chloride to a concentration of 1–5 mg/mL (500 mg/100 mL, 1000 mg/250 mL).
- Reconstitute 500 mg or 1 g vials with 10 or 20 mL, respectively, of sterile water for injection only (no preservatives).

Drug Administration:

- Must not be given IV push.
- Intermittent IV infusion over 1 hour is appropriate.

Drug Interactions:

- Use of alcohol concurrently with IV erythromycin increases peak blood alcohol concentrations by 40%; this is thought to be related to rapid gastric emptying, less exposure to alcohol dehydrogenase in the gastric mucosa, and slower small intestine transit time.
- Concurrent use of astemizole or terfenadine with erythromycins is contraindicated and may increase risk of cardiotoxicity, such as *torsades de points*, ventricular tachycardia, and death.
- Erythromycins may inhibit carbamazepine and valproic acid metabolism, resulting in increased anticonvulsant plasma concentration and toxicity.
- Concurrent use of chloramphenicol, lincomycins, and erythromycins is not recommended due to their antagonizing effects. It is best to avoid concurrent use of bactericidal and bacteriostatic drugs until culture and sensitivity results are determined.
- Erythromycin can increased cyclosporin plasma concentrations and may increase the risk of nephrotoxicity.
- Erythromycins inhibit the metabolism of ergotamine and increase the vasospasm associated with ergotamines.
- Simultaneous administration of erythromycin and lovastatin should be used with caution since concurrent use may increase the risk of rhabdomyolysis.
- Concurrent use of midazolam and triazolam with erythromycins can increase the pharmacological effect of these drugs.
- Erythromycins may cause prolonged prothrombin time and increased risk of hemorrhage, especially in the elderly.
- Use of erythromycins and xanthines (i.e., Aminophylline, caffeine, Oxtriphylline, and Theophylline) may lead to increased serum levels of xanthines and toxicity.

Lab Effects/Interference:

- Serum SGPT, serum SGOT serum bilirubin, and alkaline phosphatase—values may be increased by all erythromycins.
- Urinary catecholamines may produce false positive results when patient is on erythromycin.

Special Considerations:

- Do not use when there is a known hypersensitivity to erythromycins.
- Use with caution in patients with impaired hepatic function.
- Patients with a history of hearing loss, may be at risk of further hearing loss especially if hepatic or renal function is present or if on high dose erythromycins, or if patient is elderly.

Potential Toxicities/Side Effects and the Nursing Process

I. ALTERATION IN NUTRITION related to GI SIDE EFFECTS

Defining Characteristics: Nausea, vomiting, anorexia have occurred frequently. Also, transient increase LFTs—AST (SGOT), ALT (SGPT), LDH, ALK-PHOS, BR—has occurred. Hepatotoxicity (fever, nausea, skin rash, stomach pain, severe and unusual tiredness or weakness, yellow eyes or skin, and vomiting) has occurred less frequently. Pancreatitis (severe abdominal pain, nausea and vomiting) has occurred but is rare.

Nursing Implications: Assess baseline nutritional status, preexisting nausea/vomiting, anorexia. Assess baseline LFTs and monitor periodically during treatment. Teach patient to report side effects. Provide symptomatic interventions if side effects occur; discuss with physician use of alternative drug(s).

II. POTENTIAL FOR INJURY related to HYPERSENSITIVITY REACTION

Defining Characteristics: Urticaria, pruritus, rash (maculopapular or erythematous), fever and chills, eosinophilia, myalgia, edema, erythema, angioedema.

Nursing Implications: Assess for drug allergies to erythromycin or macrolide antibiotic prior to drug administration. Teach patient to report any allergic reactions. Assess for signs/symptoms of allergic reaction after drug dose. Assess baseline skin integrity and presence of drug allergies; monitor patient closely during drug infusions. Teach patient to report immediately signs/symptoms of rash, pruritus, shortness of breath, any adverse sensation. Teach patient skin care and symptomatic measures as appropriate. If skin rash develops, discuss drug discontinuance with physician. If rash progresses, especially in human immunodeficiency virus (HIV)-infected patients, drug should be discontinued as fatal Stevens-Johnson syndrome may develop. Be prepared to treat severe acute hypersensitivity reactions with airway management, oxygen, epinephrine, corticosteroids, antihistamines as ordered.

III. ALTERATIONS IN COMFORT related to LOCAL INJECTION IRRITATION

Defining Characteristics: Incidence of phlebitis, thrombophlebitis, and pain when administering IV.

Nursing Implications: Change IV sites q 48 hours, and assess for signs/symptoms of phlebitis prior to each administration. Administer drug slowly. Apply warm packs to increase comfort.

IV. ALTERATIONS IN CARDIAC OUTPUT related to CARDIOVASCULAR CHANGES

Defining Characteristics: Rare incidence of cardiac arrhythmias, electrocardiogram (EKG) changes (e.g., QT prolongation), torsades de points (irregular or slow heart rate: recurrent fainting, sudden death).

Nursing Implications: Assess baseline heart rate and blood pressure (BP); monitor during therapy, at least with initial dose.

V. SENSORY/PERCEPTUAL ALTERATIONS related to OTOTOXICITY

Defining Characteristics: Damage to eighth cranial nerve (auditory) may result in dizziness, nystagmus, vertigo, ataxia (vestibular damage), and more commonly tinnitus, roaring sound in ears, and impaired hearing (auditory damage). Hearing loss usually begins with high-frequency loss, followed by clinical hearing loss, then permanent hearing loss if damage continues. Increased risk in elderly, renally, hepatically impaired patients.

Nursing Implications: Assess baseline hearing (ability to hear spoken voice) and continue to assess during therapy. Teach patient potential side effects, and instruct patient to report any hearing/perceptual problems (e.g., tinnitus, vertigo, decreased hearing). Discuss drug discontinuance and audiogram with physician to confirm hearing dysfunction if symptoms arise. Assess for increased risk if given concurrently with other ototoxic medications (e.g., cisplatin, furosemide).

VI. FUNGAL SUPERINFECTION related to REDISTRIBUTION OF ENDOGENOUS MICROORGANISMS

Defining Characteristics: Vaginal candidiasis (sore mouth or tongue; white patches in mouth and/or tongue); vaginitis (vaginal candidiasis); vaginal itching and discharge may occur as endogenous bacteria are eliminated and normal fungal population expands.

Nursing Implications: Teach female patient to report vaginal itching or discharge. Discuss appropriate antifungal treatment with physician. Teach perineal hygiene and symptomatic management.

Drug: gatifloxacin (Tequin)

Class: Quinolone.

Mechanism of Action: Gatifloxacin is a broad-spectrum anti-infective, active against a wide range of aerobic gram-positive and gram-negative organisms. Acts intracellularly by inhibiting DNA gyrase (bacterial topoisomerase IV).

Metabolism: Widely distributed to most body fluids and tissues with highest concentrations in organs such as kidneys, gallbladder, lungs, liver, gynecological tissue, prostatic tissue, phagocytic cells, urine, sputum, and bile. Well absorbed from GI tract. Metabolized in liver; excreted in urine and feces. Crosses placenta and is excreted in breast milk.

Dosage/Range:

- 400 mg PO or IV QD.

Drug Preparation/Administration:

- Oral: Take drug with large glass of water; preferably 2 hours after meal/food. Encourage oral fluids of 2–3 qt (liters)/day.
- IV: Further dilute drug in 0.9% Sodium Chloride or 5% Dextrose in water to final concentration of 2 mg/mL.

Drug Interactions:

- Antacids (containing magnesium, aluminum, or calcium) and iron decrease absorption of serum level of gatifloxacin; do not administer concurrently. If must administer antacids or iron, administer at least 4 hours apart. The administration of antacids containing aluminum, magnesium, calcium, sucralfate, zinc, or iron may substantially reduce the absorption of gatofloxacin; do not administer concurrently.
- Serum digoxin concentrations should be monitored; gatifloxacin may raise serum levels in some patients.
- Probenecid: decreases the renal tubular secretion of gatifloxacin resulting in a prolonged elimination half-life and increased risk of toxicity.
- Gatifloxacin may have the potential to prolong the Q-T interval of the EKG in some patients. Gatifloxacin should not be used in patients with prolonged Q-T interval; patients with uncorrected hypokalemia; and patients taking quinidine, procanamide, amiodrone, and sotalol (antiarrhythmic agents).
- Increased intracranial pressure and psychosis have been reported along with CNS stimulation.
- Hypersensitivity reactions have been reported.

Lab Effects/Interference:

- Serum SGPT, serum Alk Phos, serum SGOT, and serum LDH: values may be increased.

Special Considerations:

- Used in treatment of infections of urinary and lower respiratory tracts, skin, bone and joint, and GI tract, as well as gonorrhea.
- Contraindicated in pregnancy or in women who are breast-feeding.
- Obtain ordered specimen for culture and sensitivity prior to first drug dose.
- Use cautiously in patients with seizure disorders.
- Used in the treatment of infections or most bacterial infections.

Potential Toxicities/Side Effects and the Nursing Process

I. ALTERATION IN NUTRITION related to GI SIDE EFFECTS

Defining Characteristics: Incidence of nausea, vomiting, abdominal discomfort, diarrhea, anorexia.

Nursing Implications: Assess baseline nutritional and elimination status. Teach patient to report GI disturbances. Administer and teach patient to self-administer antiemetics and antidiarrheals as needed and as ordered. Teach patient importance of nutritious diet, and suggest small, frequent, high-calorie, high-protein meals as appropriate. Assess baseline LFTs and monitor periodically during treatment. Discuss abnormalities and drug interruption with physician. Assess taking other hepatotoxic drugs (see Special Considerations).

II. SENSORY/PERCEPTUAL ALTERATIONS related to CNS EFFECTS

Defining Characteristics: Incidence of headache, restlessness. Dizziness, hallucinations, and seizures may also occur. Exacerbated by caffeine as quinolones delay caffeine excretion.

Nursing Implications: Assess baseline neurological function and comfort, and monitor during treatment. Teach patient to report any changes. Discuss any abnormalities with physician. Teach patient to limit or restrict all medications and caffeine-containing fluids (e.g., tea, coffee, caffeinated soft drinks).

III. ALTERATION IN SKIN INTEGRITY related to ALLERGY/HYPERSENSITIVITY

Defining Characteristics: Incidence of rash; other manifestations include eosinophilia, urticaria, flushing, fever, chills, photosensitivity, angioedema. Fatal hypersensitivity reactions have occurred rarely. Direct exposure to sunlight can cause sunburn (moderate to severe phototoxicity).

Nursing Implications: Assess baseline skin condition, including integrity and drug allergy history. Teach patient to report rash, itching, other skin changes. Teach patient skin care and symptomatic measures as appropriate. If skin rash develops, discuss drug discontinuance with physician. Be prepared to treat severe acute hypersensitivity reactions with airway management, oxygen, epinephrine, corticosteroids, antihistamines as ordered. Teach patient to avoid excessive sun exposure and to use skin protection factor (SPF) 15 or higher. If rash progresses, especially in HIV-infected patients, drug should be discontinued as fatal Stevens-Johnson syndrome may develop.

IV. FUNGAL SUPERINFECTION related to REDISTRIBUTION OF ENDOGENOUS MICROORGANISMS

Defining Characteristics: Vaginal moniliasis, vaginitis may occur as endogenous bacteria are eliminated and normal fungal population expands.

Nursing Implications: Teach female patient to report vaginal itching or discharge. Discuss appropriate antifungal treatment with physician. Teach perineal hygiene and symptomatic management.

V. ALTERATION IN URINARY ELIMINATION related to RENAL TOXICITY

Defining Characteristics: Increased BUN and creatinine, crystal and stone formation in urine, interstitial nephritis, and renal failure may occur.

Nursing Implications: Assess baseline renal function; expect that drug dose will be decreased in presence of renal dysfunction. Teach patient to take drug with at least 8 oz of water, and to increase oral fluids to 2–3 qt/day.

VI. ALTERATION IN COMFORT related to IV ADMINISTRATION

Defining Characteristics: Drug may cause pain, inflammation, and rare thrombophlebitis at IV site.

Nursing Implications: Change IV site q 48 hours. Assess for phlebitis, discomfort, and IV patency prior to each administration. Administer drug slowly over 60–90 minutes in large volume of 5% Dextrose (see Drug Preparation/Administration). Apply heat to promote comfort.

Drug: gemifloxacin mesylate (Factive)

Class: Quinolone.

Mechanism of Action: Gemifloxacin is a broad-spectrum anti-infective, active against a wide range of aerobic gram-positive and gram-negative organisms. Acts inhibiting DNA synthesis through the inhibition of DNA gyrase and topoisomerase IV, which are essential for bacterial growth.

Metabolism: Widely distributed to most body fluids and tissues after oral administration. Gemifloxacin penetrates well into lung tissues and fluids. Well absorbed from GI tract. Metabolized to a limited extent in the liver; excreted in urine and feces. The safety in pregnant women has not been established. The drug is excreted in breast milk in animal studies.

Dosage/Range:

- 320 mg orally once a day for 5–7 days.

Drug Preparation/Administration:

- Oral: Take drug with or without food. Take with large glass of water; encourage oral fluids of 2–3 qt (liters)/day.

Drug Interactions:

- Antacids (containing magnesium, aluminum, or calcium) and iron decrease absorption of serum level of gemifloxacin; do not administer concurrently. If must administer antacids or iron, administer at least 3 hours before or 2 hours after. The administration of antacids containing aluminum, magnesium, calcium, sucralfate, zinc, or iron may substantially reduce the absorption of gemifloxacin; do not administer concurrently.
- Probenecid: decreases the renal tubular secretion of gemifloxacin resulting in a prolonged elimination half-life and increased risk of toxicity.
- Gemifloxacin may have the potential to prolong the Q-T interval of the EKG in some patients. Gemifloxacin should not be used in patients with prolonged Q-T interval; patients with uncorrected hypokalemia or hypomagnesemia; and patients taking quinidine, procanamide, amiodrone, and sotalol (Class 1A antiarrhythmic agents).
- Increased intracranial pressure and psychosis have been reported along with CNS stimulation.
- Hypersensitivity reactions have been reported.
- Fluroquinolones have been shown to cause arthropathy and osteochondrosis in animal studies. Discontinue if patient experiences pain, inflammation, or rupture of a tendon. Elderly patients, athletes, and patients taking corticosteroids are more prone to tendonitis.
- Pseudomembranous colitis has been reported and may range from mild to life-threatening.

Lab Effects/Interference:

- Serum SGPT, serum Alk Phos, serum SGOT, and serum LDH: values may be increased.

Special Considerations:

- Used in treatment of infections of lower respiratory tracts.
- Contraindicated in pregnancy or in women who are breast-feeding.
- Obtain ordered specimen for culture and sensitivity prior to first drug dose.
- Use cautiously in patients with seizure disorders.
- Used in the treatment of infections or most bacterial infections.

Potential Toxicities/Side Effects and the Nursing Process

I. ALTERATION IN NUTRITION related to GI SIDE EFFECTS

Defining Characteristics: Incidence of nausea, vomiting, abdominal discomfort, diarrhea, anorexia.

Nursing Implications: Assess baseline nutritional and elimination status. Teach patient to report GI disturbances. Administer and teach patient to self-administer antiemetics and antidiarrheals as needed and as ordered. Teach patient importance of nutritious diet, and suggest small, frequent, high-calorie, high-protein meals as appropriate. Assess baseline LFTs and monitor periodically during treatment. Discuss abnormalities and drug interruption with physician. Assess taking other hepatotoxic drugs.

II. SENSORY/PERCEPTUAL ALTERATIONS related to CNS EFFECTS

Defining Characteristics: Incidence of headache, restlessness. Dizziness, hallucinations, and seizures may also occur. Exacerbated by caffeine as quinolones delay caffeine excretion.

Nursing Implications: Assess baseline neurological function and comfort, and monitor during treatment. Teach patient to report any changes. Discuss any abnormalities with physician. Teach patient to limit or restrict all medications and caffeine-containing fluids (e.g., tea, coffee, caffeinated soft drinks).

III. ALTERATION IN SKIN INTEGRITY related to ALLERGY/ HYPERSENSITIVITY

Defining Characteristics: Incidence of rash; other manifestations include eosinophilia, urticaria, flushing, fever, chills, photosensitivity, angioedema. Fatal hypersensitivity reactions have occurred rarely. Direct exposure to sunlight can cause sunburn (moderate to severe phototoxicity).

Nursing Implications: Assess baseline skin condition, including integrity and drug allergy history. Teach patient to report rash, itching, and other skin changes. Teach patient skin care and symptomatic measures as appropriate. If skin rash develops, discuss drug discontinuance with physician. Be prepared to treat severe acute hypersensitivity reactions with airway management, oxygen, epinephrine, corticosteroids, antihistamines as ordered. Teach patient to avoid excessive sun exposure and to use skin protection factor (SPF) 15 or higher. If rash progresses, especially in HIV-infected patients, drug should be discontinued as fatal Stevens-Johnson syndrome may develop.

IV. FUNGAL SUPERINFECTION related to REDISTRIBUTION OF ENDOGENOUS MICROORGANISMS

Defining Characteristics: Vaginal moniliasis, vaginitis may occur as endogenous bacteria are eliminated and normal fungal population expands.

Nursing Implications: Teach female patient to report vaginal itching or discharge. Discuss appropriate antifungal treatment with physician. Teach perineal hygiene and symptomatic management.

V. ALTERATION IN URINARY ELIMINATION related to RENAL TOXICITY

Defining Characteristics: Increased BUN and creatinine, crystal and stone formation in urine, interstitial nephritis, and renal failure may occur.

Nursing Implications: Assess baseline renal function; expect that drug dose will be decreased in presence of renal dysfunction. Teach patient to take drug with at least 8 oz of water, and to increase oral fluids to 2–3 qt/day.

Drug: gentamicin sulfate (Garamycin, Gentamicin)

Class: Aminoglycoside antibacterial.

Mechanism of Action: Derived from *Micromonospora*; bactericidal, most probably by inhibition of protein synthesis. Active against aerobic microorganisms: many sensitive gram-negative organisms (including *Acinetobacter, Brucella, Citrobacter, Enterobacter, E. coli, Klebsiella, Proteus, Pseudomonas, Salmonella, Serratia,* and *Shigella*) and some sensitive gram-positive organisms (*S. aureus* and *S. epidermidis*). Over time, bacterial resistance may develop, either naturally or acquired.

Metabolism: Well absorbed following IV administration, but variability in absorption after IM injection (peak serum level 0.5–2 hours, duration 8–12 hours). Widely distributed into body fluids. Minimally protein-bound. Readily crosses placenta and into breast milk. Drug excreted unchanged in the urine.

Dosage/Range:
- IM, IV: Loading dose, 2 mg/Kg, then 3–6 mg/Kg/day in one daily dose, 2 equal doses in split 8-hour dosing.
- IT: 4–8 mg (preservative-free).
- Desired peak serum concentration 4–10 μg/mL, and trough serum concentration is 1–2 μg/mL.
- DOSE REDUCTION IF RENAL DYSFUNCTION.

Drug Preparation:
- Store injectable at < 40°C (104°F). Stable for 24 hours at room temperature in 0.9% Sodium Chloride or 5% Dextrose.

Drug Administration:
- Do not mix with other drugs.
- IV: Mix in 50–200 mL 0.9% Sodium Chloride or 5% Dextrose injection and infuse over 30 minutes to 2 hours. Can also be given IM.

Drug Administration:

- Increased risk of toxicity with other ototoxic drugs: acyclovir, other aminoglycosides, amphotericin B, bacitracin, cephalosporins, colistin, cisplatin, ethacrynic acid, furosemide, vancomycin.
- Potentiation of neuromuscular blockade when given concurrently with general anesthetics (succinylcholine, tubocurarine); use cautiously, observe for signs/symptoms of respiratory depression.
- Synergism with extended-spectrum penicillins, but must be administered separately.

Lab Effects/Interference:

- Serum ALT, serum alk phos, serum AST, serum bili, and serum LDH values may be increased.
- BUN and serum creatinine concentrations may be increased.
- Serum Ca++, serum Mg++, serum K+, and serum Na+ concentrations may be decreased.

Special Considerations:

- Used as first-line treatment in short-term treatment of serious gram-negative infections (e.g., septicemia, respiratory tract infections).
- Use against gram-positive organisms only as second-line treatment.
- Use in pregnancy only if infection is life-threatening and no safer drug exists; drug crosses placenta and may cause fetal toxicity.

Potential Toxicities/Side Effects and the Nursing Process

I. ALTERATIONS IN SENSORY/PERCEPTUAL PATTERNS related to OTOTOXICITY

Defining Characteristics: Damage to eighth cranial nerve (auditory) may result in dizziness, nystagmus, vertigo, ataxia (vestibular damage), and more commonly tinnitus, roaring sound in ears, and impaired hearing (auditory damage). Hearing loss usually begins with high-frequency loss, followed by clinical hearing loss, then permanent hearing loss if damage continues. Increased risk in elderly or renally impaired patients.

Nursing Implications: Assess baseline hearing (ability to hear spoken voice) and continue to access during therapy. Teach patient potential side effects and instruct patient to report any hearing/perceptual problems (e.g., tinnitus, vertigo, decreased hearing). Discuss drug discontinuance and audiogram with physician to confirm hearing dysfunction if symptoms arise. Assess for increased risk if given concurrently with other ototoxic medications (e.g., cisplatin, furosemide).

II. ALTERATION IN URINARY ELIMINATION related to NEPHROTOXICITY

Defining Characteristics: Renal damage characterized by tubular necrosis with increased serum BUN, creatinine; decreased urine creatinine clearance and specific gravity; proteinuria and casts in urine. Azotemia usually not associated with oliguria. Rarely, electrolyte wasting with hypomagnesemia, hypocalcemia, and hypokalemia may occur. Renal dysfunction is usually reversible after drug discontinuance. Increased risk exists in elderly and if preexisting renal dysfunction. Risk low in well-hydrated patients with normal renal function when normal doses given.

Nursing Implications: Assess baseline renal function and electrolytes, and monitor periodically during therapy. Discuss any abnormalities with physician, as drug should be dose-reduced or discontinued if renal dysfunction develops. Assess baseline total body fluid balance, weight, and monitor periodically during antibiotic therapy. Monitor hydration status to keep patient well hydrated. Assess drug peak and trough levels as ordered so that drug dosage is correctly titrated. Increased risk of toxicity if peak serum concentration > 10–12 μg/mL. Draw blood for peak drug concentration 30 minutes after end of 30-minute infusion or at the end of a 60-minute infusion; draw trough immediately before next dose.

III. ALTERATIONS IN SENSORY/PERCEPTUAL PATTERNS related to CNS EFFECTS, NEUROMUSCULAR BLOCKADE

Defining Characteristics: Headache, tremor, lethargy may occur. Peripheral neuropathy or encephalopathy (numbness, skin tingling, muscle twitching) may occur rarely. Neuromuscular blockade is dose-related, self-limiting, and uncommon; risk is greater with topical application or when drug is administered to patient with neuromuscular disease (myasthenia gravis) or hypocalcemia.

Nursing Implications: Assess baseline neurologic status. Assess coexisting risk factors, neuromuscular blockade medications. Teach patient about side effects and to report headache, tremor, lethargy. Observe for respiratory depression. If signs/symptoms arise, discuss drug discontinuance with physician.

IV. POTENTIAL FOR INJURY related to HYPERSENSITIVITY

Defining Characteristics: Rash, urticaria, pruritus, fever, eosinophilia have occurred rarely. CROSS-SENSITIVITY between AMINOGLYCOSIDES exists!

Nursing Implications: Assess for drug allergies to any aminoglycoside—amikacin, gentamicin, kanamycin, neomycin, netilmicin, streptomycin, tobramycin—prior to drug administration. Instruct patient to report any allergic reactions. Assess for signs/symptoms of allergic reaction after drug dose.

V. ALTERATION IN NUTRITION, LESS THAN BODY REQUIREMENTS, related to GI SIDE EFFECTS

Defining Characteristics: Nausea, vomiting, anorexia have occurred rarely. Also, transient hepatomegaly with increased LFTs—AST, ALT, LDH, alk phos, bili—has occurred.

Nursing Implications: Assess baseline nutritional status, preexisting nausea/vomiting, anorexia. Assess baseline LFTs and monitor periodically during treatment. Instruct patient to report side effects. Provide symptomatic interventions if side effects occur; discuss with physician use of alternative drug(s).

VI. POTENTIAL FOR FATIGUE, INFECTION, AND BLEEDING related to BONE MARROW INJURY

Defining Characteristics: Anemia, leukopenia, granulocytopenia, and thrombocytopenia may occur. Also, patients receiving antibiotics are at risk for overgrowth of nonsusceptible microorganisms, such as fungi (superinfection). Rare.

Nursing Implications: Assess baseline CBC, differential, and monitor periodically during treatment. Instruct patient to report signs/symptoms of fatigue, infection, or bleeding immediately. Assess for signs/symptoms of superinfection. Discuss any adverse effects with physician.

Drug: imipenem/cilastatin sodium (Primaxin)

Class: Antibacterial. Imipenem is a β-lactam antibiotic, carbapenem type; cilastatin inhibits an enzyme in the kidneys that breaks down imipenem, increasing drug potency and protecting kidneys.

Mechanism of Action: Semisynthetic derivative of cephalosporin C (produced by fungus); contains β-lactam ring and is related to penicillins and cephamycins (e.g., cefoxitin). Bactericidal through inhibition of cell wall synthesis, with resulting cell wall instability and cell lysis. Active against most anaerobic and aerobic gram-positive and gram-negative organisms. These include *Staphylococcus, Streptococcus, E. coli, P. aeruginosa, Proteus, Klebsiella, Enterobacter.* Some activity against *Mycobacterium.* Resists hydrolysis by β-lactamase enzymes produced by microorganisms, so resistance to these organisms is much less than other β-lactam antibiotics (e.g., cephalosporins, penicillins). Used in treatment of serious infections of lower respiratory tract, urinary tract, abdomen, female pelvis, skin, bone, and joint, as well as polymicrobial infections and infections resistant to other antibiotics.

Metabolism: Not well absorbed from GI tract, so must be given IV. Incompletely absorbed after IM injection. Widely distributed in body tissues and fluids, including bile; does not result in significant CSF drug levels. Crosses placenta and is excreted in breast milk. Cilastatin decreases renal metabolism of imipenem; both drugs are excreted in urine, and to a lesser degree in feces.

Dosage/Range:

Adult:

- IV: 250 mg–1 g q6–8h (maximum 50 mg/kg or 4 g/day, whichever is less).
- IM (if unable to give IV): 500–750 mg q12h (maximum 1.5 g/day). Reduce dose if renal insufficiency, according to manufacturer's package insert.

Drug Preparation/Administration:

- Store vial of sterile powder at < 30°C (86°F).
- IV: Reconstitute according to manufacturer's package insert and further dilute in 100 mL 0.9% Sodium Chloride or 5% Dextrose injection. Infuse over 60 minutes for each gram of drug administered. Slow infusion if nausea/vomiting develop.
- IM: Reconstitute drug with lidocaine HCl 1% injection (without epinephrine) as directed by package insert. Administer deep IM in large muscle mass (e.g., gluteus maximus). Assess allergy to lidocaine. IM preparation SHOULD NOT BE USED FOR IV ADMINISTRATION.

Drug Interactions:

- Probenecid: increases serum concentrations of imipenem. DO NOT USE CONCURRENTLY.
- Aminoglycosides: may have synergistic antimicrobial effect.
- β-lactam antibiotics (cephalosporins, extended-spectrum penicillins): Antagonism. Imipenem stimulates production of β-lactamase enzymes by the bacteria that inactivate the cephalosporins and penicillins. DO NOT USE CONCURRENTLY.
- Ganciclovir: may decrease seizure threshold. Do not use concurrently unless critical for life-saving treatment.
- Co-trimoxazole: possible synergy against *Nocardia asteroides.*
- Chloramphenicol: possible antagonism. Consider chloramphenicol administration 2+ hours after imipenem (requires clinical study).

Lab Effects/Interference:

- Serum ALT, serum alk phos, and serum AST values may be transiently increased.

Clinical significance:

- Coombs' (direct antiglobulin) tests: may occur during therapy.
- Serum LDH values may be transiently increased.

- Serum bili, BUN concentrations, and serum creatinine concentrations may be transiently increased.
- HCT and Hgb concentrations may be decreased.

Special Considerations:

- Contraindicated in patients hypersensitive to imipenem or cilastatin. Use cautiously in patients sensitive to penicillin or other β-lactams, as partial cross-allergenicity exists.
- Do not give IM preparation reconstituted with 1% lidocaine if hypersensitive to lidocaine.
- Drug may cause false-positive glucose determination when using Clinitest.
- Ensure specimen sent for culture and sensitivity prior to first antibiotic dose.
- Drug has significantly broad antibacterial properties.
- Drug dosage needs to be reduced if severe renal insufficiency.
- Slow IV infusion if nausea/vomiting develops.

Potential Toxicities/Side Effects and the Nursing Process

I. POTENTIAL FOR INJURY related to HYPERSENSITIVITY REACTION

Defining Characteristics: Urticaria, pruritus, rash (maculopapular or erythematous), fever and chills, eosinophilia, myalgia, edema, erythema, angioedema, Stevens-Johnson syndrome, and exfoliative skin reactions occur in 5% of patients. Increased risk in individuals allergic to penicillin.

Nursing Implications: Assess allergy to cephalosporin antibiotics and penicillin: if patient states "yes," determine actual response, e.g., "swollen lips = angioedema." If angioedema, discuss with physician RISK versus benefit prior to drug administration, as there is partial cross-allergenicity. Discuss other patient responses with physician to determine whether drug should be given. Assess baseline skin condition, including integrity and allergy history to drugs. Instruct patient to report rash, itching, other skin changes. Teach patient skin care and symptomatic measures as appropriate. If skin rash develops, discuss drug discontinuance with physician. If rash progresses, drug should be discontinued, as fatal Stevens-Johnson syndrome may develop. Be prepared to treat severe acute hypersensitivity reactions with airway management, oxygen, epinephrine, corticosteroids, antihistamines as ordered.

II. ALTERATION IN NUTRITION, LESS THAN BODY REQUIREMENTS, related to GI SIDE EFFECTS

Defining Characteristics: Nausea, vomiting occurs more frequently than diarrhea, anorexia; rarely, pseudomembranous colitis caused by *C. difficile* resistant to the antibiotic occurs. Rarely, transient increases in LFTs—AST, ALT, alk phos, bili—may occur.

Nursing Implications: Assess baseline nutritional status. Instruct patient to report GI disturbances. Administer and teach patient to self-administer antiemetics as needed and as ordered. Teach patient importance of nutritious diet and suggest small, frequent, high-calorie, high-protein meals as appropriate. Assess baseline LFTs and monitor periodically during treatment. Discuss abnormalities and drug interruption with physician.

III. FUNGAL SUPERINFECTION related to REDISTRIBUTION OF ENDOGENOUS MICROORGANISMS

Defining Characteristics: Vaginal candidiasis, vaginitis may occur as endogenous bacteria are eliminated and normal fungal population expands.

Nursing Implications: Instruct female patient to report vaginal itching or discharge. Discuss appropriate antifungal treatment with physician. Teach perineal hygiene and symptomatic management.

IV. ALTERATIONS IN PROTECTIVE MECHANISMS (RARE) related to TRANSIENT LEUKOPENIA

Defining Characteristics: Rarely, transient leukopenia, lymphocytosis, anemia, eosinophilia may occur. Prolonged PT, prolonged APTT, and hypoprothrombinemia have occurred rarely, especially in elderly or debilitated patients, or in individuals with vitamin K deficiency.

Nursing Implications: Assess baseline laboratory parameters, and monitor periodically during treatment. Assess patient for response to antibiotics. Discuss abnormalities with physician.

V. ALTERATIONS IN SENSORY/PERCEPTUAL PATTERNS related to DIZZINESS, SOMNOLENCE

Defining Characteristics: Dizziness, headache, somnolence, seizures occur rarely. Most seizures have occurred in patients with preexisting CNS problems, those who had received higher-than-recommended IV doses, the elderly, and patients with impaired renal function.

Nursing Implications: Assess baseline neurologic function and comfort, and monitor during treatment. Instruct patient to report any changes. Discuss any abnormalities with physician. Institute seizure precautions. If seizures occur, discuss with physician anticonvulsant therapy or discontinuance of antibiotic.

VI. ALTERATIONS IN COMFORT related to LOCAL INJECTION IRRITATION

Defining Characteristics: Pain, induration, sterile abscesses may form in IM injection sites; phlebitis may develop in IV sites.

Nursing Implications: Rotate IM injection sites, and administer drug deep IM in large muscle mass (e.g., gluteus maximus). Use IM injection when IV administration is not possible. Change IV sites q48h, and assess for signs/symptoms of phlebitis prior to each administration. Administer drug slowly. Apply warm packs to increase comfort.

Drug: kanamycin sulfate (Kantrex)

Class: Aminoglycoside antibacterial.

Mechanism of Action: Synthetic antibiotic derived from *Streptomyces;* bactericidal, most probably by inhibition of protein synthesis. Active against aerobic microorganisms: many sensitive gram-negative organisms (including *Acinetobacter, Citrobacter, Enterobacter, E. coli, Klebsiella, Proteus, Salmonella, Serratia, and Shigella)* and some sensitive gram-positive organisms (*S. aureus* and *S. epidermidis).* Over time, bacterial resistance may develop, either naturally or acquired.

Metabolism: Well absorbed following parenteral administration, but variable absorption after IM injection (peak serum level 0.5–2 hours, duration 8–12 hours). Widely distributed into body fluids. Minimally protein-bound. Readily crosses placenta and into breast milk. Drug excreted unchanged in the urine.

Dosage/Range:

- IM, IV: 15 mg/kg/day in equally divided doses at 8- or 12-hour intervals.
- Desired peak serum concentration 15–30 μg/mL, and trough serum concentration is 5–10 μg/mL.
- DOSE REDUCTION IF RENAL IMPAIRMENT.

Drug Preparation:

- Store capsules in tight containers at temperature < 40°C (104°F).
- Injection should be stored at < 40°C (104°F), preferably 15–30°C (59–86°F).
- Mix 500 mg in 100–200 mL of IV infusion solution. Stable for 24 hours at room temperature in 0.9% Sodium Chloride or 5% Dextrose. DO NOT MIX WITH OTHER MEDICATIONS.

Drug Administration:

- Deep IM: upper outer quadrant of buttock.
- IV: Infuse over 30–60 minutes.
- Orally (pre-op bowel sterilization): 1 g PO qh × four doses, then q4h × four doses.
- Wound irrigation: 2–2.5 mg/mL in 0.9% Sodium Chloride irrigant.

Drug Interactions:

- Increased risk of toxicity with other ototoxic drugs: acyclovir, other aminoglycosides, amphotericin B, bacitracin, cephalosporins, colistin, cisplatin, ethacrynic acid, furosemide, vancomycin.
- Potentiation of neuromuscular blockade when given concurrently with general anesthetics (succinylcholine, tubocurarine); use cautiously, observe for signs/symptoms of respiratory depression.
- Synergism with extended-spectrum penicillins, but must be administered separately.

Lab Effects/Interference:

- Serum ALT, serum alk phos, serum AST, serum bili, and serum LDH values may be increased.
- BUN and serum creatinine concentrations may be increased.
- Serum Ca++, serum Mg++, serum K+, and serum Na+ concentrations may be decreased.

Special Considerations:

- Used as first-line treatment in short-term treatment of serious gram-negative infections (e.g., septicemia, respiratory tract infections).
- Use against gram-positive organisms only as second-line treatment.
- Use in pregnancy only if infection is life-threatening and no safer drug exists; drug crosses placenta and may cause fetal toxicity.

Potential Toxicities/Side Effects and the Nursing Process

I. ALTERATIONS IN SENSORY/PERCEPTUAL PATTERNS related to OTOTOXICITY

Defining Characteristics: Damage to eighth cranial nerve (auditory) may result in dizziness, nystagmus, vertigo, ataxia (vestibular damage), and less commonly tinnitus, roaring sound in ears, and impaired hearing (auditory damage). Hearing loss usually begins with high-frequency loss, followed by clinical hearing loss, then permanent hearing loss if damage continues. Increased risk in elderly or renally impaired patients.

Nursing Implications: Assess baseline hearing (ability to hear spoken voice) and continue during therapy. Teach patient potential side effects, and instruct patient to report any hearing/perceptual problems (e.g., tinnitus, vertigo, decreased hearing). Discuss drug discontinuance and audiogram with physician to confirm hearing dysfunction if symptoms arise. Assess for increased risk if given concurrently with other ototoxic medications (e.g., cisplatin, furosemide).

II. ALTERATION IN URINARY ELIMINATION related to NEPHROTOXICITY

Defining Characteristics: Renal damage characterized by tubular necrosis with increased serum BUN, creatinine; decreased urine creatinine clearance and specific gravity; proteinuria and casts in urine. Azotemia usually not associated with oliguria. Rarely, electrolyte wasting with hypomagnesemia, hypocalcemia, and hypokalemia may occur. Renal dysfunction usually reversible after drug discontinuance. Increased risk exists in elderly and if there is preexisting renal dysfunction. Risk is low in well-hydrated patients with normal renal function when normal doses given.

Nursing Implications: Assess baseline renal function and electrolytes, and monitor periodically during therapy. Discuss any abnormalities with physician, as drug should be dose-reduced or discontinued if renal dysfunction develops. Assess baseline total body fluid balance, weight, and monitor periodically during antibiotic therapy. Monitor hydration status to keep patient well hydrated. Assess drug peak and trough levels as ordered so that drug dosage is correctly titrated. Increased risk of toxicity if peak serum concentration > 30–35 μg/mL. Draw blood for peak drug concentration 30 minutes after end of 30-minute infusion or at the end of a 60-minute infusion; draw trough immediately before next dose.

III. ALTERATIONS IN SENSORY/PERCEPTUAL PATTERNS related to CNS EFFECTS, NEUROMUSCULAR BLOCKADE

Defining Characteristics: Headache, tremor, lethargy may occur. Peripheral neuropathy or encephalopathy (numbness, skin tingling, muscle twitching) may occur rarely. Neuromuscular blockade is dose-related, self-limiting, and uncommon; risk is greater with topical application or when drug is administered to patient with neuromuscular disease (myasthenia gravis) or hypocalcemia.

Nursing Implications: Assess baseline neurologic status. Assess coexisting risk factors, neuromuscular blockade medications. Teach patient about side effects, and instruct to report headache, tremor, lethargy. Observe for respiratory depression. If signs/symptoms arise, discuss drug discontinuance with physician.

IV. POTENTIAL FOR INJURY related to HYPERSENSITIVITY

Defining Characteristics: Rash, urticaria, pruritus, fever, eosinophilia have occurred rarely. CROSS-SENSITIVITY between AMINOGLYCOSIDES exists!

Nursing Implications: Assess for drug allergies to any aminoglycoside—amikacin, gentamicin, kanamycin, neomycin, netilmicin, streptomycin, tobramycin—prior to drug administration. Instruct patient to report any allergic reactions. Assess for signs/symptoms of allergic reaction after drug dose.

V. ALTERATION IN NUTRITION, LESS THAN BODY REQUIREMENTS, related to GI SIDE EFFECTS

Defining Characteristics: Nausea, vomiting, anorexia have occurred rarely. Also, transient hepatomegaly with increased LFTs—AST, ALT, alk phos—has occurred.

Nursing Implications: Assess baseline nutritional status, preexisting nausea/vomiting, anorexia. Assess baseline LFTs and monitor periodically during treatment. Instruct patient to report side effects. Provide symptomatic interventions if side effects occur; discuss with physician use of alternative drug(s).

VI. POTENTIAL FOR FATIGUE, INFECTION, AND BLEEDING related to BONE MARROW INJURY

Defining Characteristics: Anemia, leukopenia, granulocytopenia, and thrombocytopenia may occur. Also, patients receiving antibiotics are at risk for overgrowth of nonsusceptible microorganisms, such as fungi (superinfection). Rare.

Nursing Implications: Assess baseline CBC, differential, and monitor periodically during treatment. Instruct patient to report signs/symptoms of fatigue, infection, or bleeding immediately. Assess for signs/symptoms of superinfection. Discuss any adverse effects with physician.

Drug: levofloxacin (Levaquin)

Class: Fluoroquinolone antibiotic.

Mechanism of Action: Drug is a synthetic, broad-spectrum antibacterial agent. Inhibits DNA gyrase (bacterial topoisomerase II), which is necessary for DNA replication, transcription, and repair. Has activity against a wide range of gramnegative and gram-positive bacteria, as well as against some bacteria resistant to β-lactam antibiotics.

Metabolism: Drug is well absorbed from the GI tract without regard to food, with 99% bioavailability; peak serum levels occur in 1–2 hours. Steady-state is reached in 48 hours. Drug is not extensively metabolized, with 87% of drug excreted largely unchanged in the urine at 48 hours. Terminal half-life is 6–8 hours.

Dosage/Range:

- 500 mg qd × 7 days (acute bacterial exacerbation of chronic bronchitis), × 7–14 days (community-acquired pneumonia), × 7–10 days (uncomplicated skin and skin structure infection), × 10–14 days (acute maxillary sinusitis), × 10 days (uncomplicated UTI, acute pyelonephritis).

Drug Preparation:

- Oral, available in 250-mg and 500-mg tablets.
- IV: Administer over 60 min to prevent hypotension; IV available in premixed 250-mg or 500-mg bags, or 20-mL vial containing 500 mg that is further diluted in 5% Dextrose, 0.9% Sodium Chloride.

Drug Administration:

- Administer without regard to food.
- Dose-reduce if renal compromise (see Special Considerations section).
- Administer oral doses at least 2 hours before or 2 hours after antacids containing magnesium or aluminum, as well as sucralfate, metal cations such as iron, and multivitamins containing zinc.

Drug Interactions:

- Antacids containing magnesium or aluminum, sucralfate, iron, multivitamins containing zinc: may decrease serum levels of levofloxacin; take any of these agents at least 2 hours before or 2 hours after levofloxacin.
- Theophylline: possible increase in theophylline serum levels; monitor levels and change dose accordingly.
- Warfarin: theoretically could enhance effects of oral anticoagulants; monitor INR closely and modify dose accordingly.
- NSAIDs: possible increase in the risk of CNS stimulation and seizures; assess patient risk for seizures, and use cautiously if at all in patients at risk.
- Antidiabetic agents: changes in glucose (hyper- or hypoglycemia); monitor blood sugar closely, and modify dose accordingly.

Lab Effects/Interference:

- Decreased glucose, decreased lymphocytes.

Special Considerations:

- Indicated for the treatment of acute maxillary sinusitis due to *Streptococcus pneumoniae, Haemophilus influenzae, Moraxella catarrhalis;* acute bacterial exacerbation of chronic bronchitis due to *Staphylococcus aureus, Streptococcus pneumoniae, Haemophilus influenzae, Haemophilus parainfluenzae,* or *Moraxella catarrhalis;* community-acquired pneumonia due to *Staphylococcus aureus, Streptococcus pneumoniae, Haemophilus influenzae, Haemophilus parainfluenzae, Klebsiella pneumoniae, Moraxella catarrhalis, Chlamydia pneumoniae, Legionella pneumonophila,* or *Mycoplasma pneumoniae.*

- Active against the above as well as aerobic gram-positive *Enterococcus faecalis* and *Streptococcus pyogenes* and aerobic gram-negative microorganisms *Enterobacter cloacae, Escherichia coli, Proteus mirabilis,* and *Pseudomonas aeruginosa.*
- Dose modifications for renal dysfuncion:

Acute Bacterial Exacerbation of:	**Chronic Bronchitis, Community-Acquired**	**Pneumonia, Acute Maxillary Sinusitis, Uncomplicated Skin Infections**
Renal status	Initial dose	Subsequent dose
Cr cl 20–49 mL/min	500 mg	250 mg q24h
Cr cl 10–19 mL/min	500 mg	250 mg q48h
Hemodialysis	500 mg	250 mg q48h
CAPD	500 mg q48h	250 mg q48h
Uncomplicated UTI/Acute Pyelonephritis		
Cr cl 10–19 mL/min	250 mg	250 mg q48h

- Use drug cautiously, if at all, in the following patients: (1) known or suspected CNS or seizure disorder (e.g., severe cerebral arteriosclerosis or epilepsy); (2) possess factors lowering seizure threshold (e.g., renal dysfunction, other drug therapy); (3) pregnant or nursing mothers; (4) children < 18 years old.
- Obtain ordered specimen for culture and sensitivity prior to first drug dose.

Potential Toxicities/Side Effects and the Nursing Process

I. ALTERATION IN NUTRITION related to GI SIDE EFFECTS

Defining Characteristics: 0.1–3.0% incidence of nausea, vomiting, abdominal discomfort, diarrhea, anorexia. As with all antibiotics, pseudomembranous colitis may occur, ranging in severity from mild to life-threatening. Treatment with antibiotics changes the intestinal microflora, so *C. difficile* bacteria may overgrow. Once diagnosis is made, mild diarrhea may stop with cessation of drug; if moderate to severe, it will require hydration, electrolyte replacement, nutritional support, and antibacterial coverage against *C. difficile.*

Nursing Implications: Assess baseline nutritional and elimination status. Teach patient to report GI disturbances. Teach patient to report diarrhea immediately, and consider whether this is pseudomembranous colitis and send stool specimen for *C. difficile;* if positive, discuss drug discontinuance with physician. Administer and teach patient to self-administer antiemetics, antidiarrheals as needed and as ordered. Teach patient importance of nutritious diet, and suggest small, frequent, high-calorie, high-protein meals as appropriate. Assess baseline LFTs and monitor periodically during treatment. Discuss abnormalities and drug interruption with physician.

II. SENSORY/PERCEPTUAL ALTERATIONS related to CNS EFFECTS

Defining Characteristics: 1–2% incidence of insomnia, dizziness, taste perversion, headache, nervousness, anxiety, tremors, and seizures may also occur.

Nursing Implications: Assess baseline neurological function and comfort, and monitor during treatment. Teach patient to report any changes. Discuss any abnormalities with physician. Teach patient to avoid caffeine-containing fluids, medications, e.g., tea, coffee, soft drinks.

III. ALTERATION IN SKIN INTEGRITY related to ALLERGY/HYPERSENSITIVITY

Defining Characteristics: 1–4% incidence of rash; other manifestations include eosinophilia, urticaria, flushing, fever, chills, photosensitivity, angioedema. Fatal hypersensitivity reactions have occurred rarely. Direct exposure to sunlight can cause sunburn (moderate-to-severe phototoxicity).

Nursing Implications: Assess baseline skin condition, including integrity and drug allergy history. Teach patient to report rash, itching, other skin changes. Teach patient skin care and symtomatic measures as appropriate. If skin rash develops, discuss drug discontinuance with physician. If rash progresses, especially in HIV-infected patients, drug should be discontinued, as fatal Stevens-Johnson syndrome may develop. Be prepared to treat severe acute hypersensitivity reactions with airway management, oxygen, epinephrine, corticosteroids, antihistamines as ordered. Teach patient to avoid excessive sun exposure and to use skin protection factor (SPF) 15 or higher.

IV. FUNGAL SUPERINFECTION related to REDISTRIBUTION OF ENDOGENOUS MICROORGANISMS

Defining Characteristics: Vaginal moniliasis, vaginitis may occur as endogenous bacteris are eliminated and normal fungal population expands.

Nursing Implications: Teach female patient to report vaginal itching or discharge. Discuss appropriate antifungal treatment with physician. Teach perineal hygiene and symptomatic management.

Drug: linezolid (Zyvox)

Class: Oxazolidinone class of antibiotic.

Mechanism of Action: Linezolid inhibits initiation of protein synthesis by preventing the formation of the fmet-tRNA:mRNA:30S subunit ternary complex. Oxazolidinones bind to the 50S subunit in a region shared with the peptidyl transferase inhibitor chloramphenicol. Oxazolidinones are not peptidyl transferase inhibitors, and it is not known which specific ribosome reaction is inhibited by 50S subunit binding. Linezolid has a specific mechanism of action against bacteria resistant to other antibiotics, including methicillin-resistant *Staphylococcus aureus* (MRSA), multi-resistant strains of *Streptococcus pneumoniae,* and vancomycin-resistant (VRE) *enterococcus faecium.*

Metabolism: Primarily metabolized by oxidation of the morpholine ring, resulting in two inactive carboxylic acid metabolites. Only about 30% of a dose is excreted unchanged in the urine.

Dosage/Range:
- Oral: 400–600 mg q12h for 10 to 14 days; up to 28 days for VRE.
- IV: 600 mg q12h for 10–14 days; up to 28 days for VRE.

Drug Preparation:
- Available in single-use, ready-to-use infusion bags.

Drug Administration:
- IV infusion over 30–120 minutes.

Drug Administration:
- Linezolid has the potential to interact with adrenergic (phenylpropanolamine, pseudoephedrine) and serotonergic agents since it is a reversible, nonselective monoamine oxidase inhibitor.
- Large quantities of foods or beverages with high tyramine content should be avoided.

Lab Effects/Interference:
- Thrombocytopenia has been seen when this drug is administered long-term (up to 28 days).

Special Considerations:
- IV and PO doses are the same.

Potential Toxicities/Side Effects and the Nursing Process

I. ALTERATION IN NUTRITION related to GI SIDE EFFECTS

Defining Characteristics: Nausea, vomiting, anorexia have occurred frequently.

Nursing Implications: Assess baseline nutritional status, preexisting nausea/vomiting, anorexia. Teach patient to report side effects. Provide symptomatic interventions if side effects occur; discuss with physician use of alternative drug(s).

II. POTENTIAL FOR INJURY related to HYPERSENSITIVITY REACTION

Defining Characteristics: Urticaria, pruritus, rash (maculopapular or erythematous), fever and chills, eosinophilia, myalgia, edema, erythema, angioedema.

Nursing Implications: Assess for drug allergies to erythromycin or macrolide antibiotic prior to drug administration. Teach patient to report any allergic reactions. Assess for signs/symptoms of allergic reaction after drug dose. Assess baseline skin integrity and presence of drug allergies; monitor patient closely during drug infusions. Teach patient to report immediately signs/symptoms of rash, pruritus, shortness of breath, any adverse sensation. Teach patient skin care and symptomatic measures as appropriate. If skin rash develops, discuss drug discontinuance with physician. If rash progresses, especially in human immunodeficiency virus (HIV)-infected patients, drug should be discontinued, as fatal Stevens-Johnson syndrome may develop. Be prepared to treat severe acute hypersensitivity reactions with airway management, oxygen, epinephrine, corticosteroids, antihistamines as ordered.

III. ALTERATION IN COMFORT related to HEADACHE

Defining Characteristics: Headache has occurred in some patients.

Nursing Implications: Assess baseline hearing (ability to hear spoken voice) and continue to assess during therapy. Teach patient potential side effects, and instruct patient to report any hearing/perceptual problems (e.g., tinnitus, vertigo, decreased hearing). Discuss drug discontinuance and audiogram with physician to confirm hearing dysfunction if symptoms arise. Assess for increased risk if given concurrently with other ototoxic medications (e.g., cisplatin, furosemide).

IV. FUNGAL SUPERINFECTION related to REDISTRIBUTION OF ENDOGENOUS MICROORGANISMS

Defining Characteristics: Vaginal or oral candidiasis (sore mouth or tongue; white patches in mouth and/or tongue); vaginitis (vaginal candidiasis); vaginal itching and discharge may occur as endogenous bacteria are eliminated and normal fungal population expands.

Nursing Implications: Teach female patient to report vaginal itching or discharge. Discuss appropriate antifungal treatment with physician. Teach perineal hygiene and symptomatic management.

Drug: meropenem (Merrem)

Class: antibiotic, carbapenem.

Mechanism of Action: The bactericidal activity results from the inhibition of cell wall synthesis. Penetrates the cell wall of most gram-positive and gram-negative bacteria to reach penicillin-binding protein (PBP) targets.

Metabolism: Widely distributed in body tissues and fluids, excreted in urine.

Dosage/Range:

Adult:

- Intrabdominal infection: 1 gram IV every 8 hours.
- Meningitis: bacterial 2 grams IV every 8 hours.

Drug Preparation/Administration:

- IV bolus, dilute with 5–20 ml. Sterile Water for Injection and give over 3–5 minutes,
- IV infusion dilute with D5W or normal saline, infuse over 15–30 minutes, maximum concentration 50 mg/ml

Drug Interactions:

- Probenecid competes with meropenem for active tubular secretion and thus inhibits the renal excretion of meropenem.
- Meropenem may reduce serum levels of valproic acid to subtherapeutic levels.

Lab Effects/Interference:

- Meropenem posses the characteristic low toxicity of the beta-lactam group of antibiotics.
- Periodically assess organ system function; renal, hepatic & hematopoietic.

Potential Toxicities/Side Effects and the Nursing Process

I. POTENTIAL FOR INJURY related to HYPERSENSITIVITY REACTION and LOCAL REACTIONS (pain at injection site)

Defining Characteristics: Urticaria, pruritus, rash (maculopapular or erythematous), fever and chills, eosinophilia, myalgia, edema, erythema, angioedema.

Nursing Implications: Assess allergy to cephalosporin antibiotics and penicillin: if patient states ''yes,'' determine actual response, e.g., ''swollen lips = angioedema.'' If angioedema, patient SHOULD NOT receive drug. Discuss other patient responses with physician to determine whether drug should be given. Assess baseline skin condition, including integrity and allergy history to drugs. Instruct patient to report rash, itching, and other skin changes. Teach patient skin care and symptomatic measures as appropriate. If skin rash develops, discuss drug discontinuance with physician. Be prepared to treat severe acute hypersensitivity reactions with airway management, oxygen, epinephrine, corticosteroids, antihistamines as ordered.

II. ALTERATION IN NUTRITION, LESS THAN BODY REQUIREMENTS, related to GI SIDE EFFECTS

Defining Characteristics: Nausea, vomiting, diarrhea may occur; rarely, pseudomembranous colitis caused by antibiotic resistance occurs.

Nursing Implications: Assess baseline nutritional status. Instruct patient to report GI disturbances. Administer and teach patient to self-administer antiemetics as needed and as ordered. Teach patient importance of nutritious diet, and suggest small, frequent, high-calorie, high-protein meals as appropriate. Assess baseline LFTs, and monitor periodically during treatment. Discuss abnormalities and drug interruption with physician.

III. FUNGAL SUPERINFECTION related to REDISTRIBUTION OF ENDOGENOUS MICROORGANISMS

Defining Characteristics: Vaginal candidiasis, vaginitis may occur as endogenous bacteria are eliminated, and normal fungal population expands.

Nursing Implications: Instruct female patient to report vaginal itching or discharge. Discuss appropriate antifungal treatment with physician. Teach perineal hygiene and symptomatic management.

Drug: metronidazole hydrochloride (Flagyl)

Class: Antibacterial (systemic); antiprotozoal.

Mechanism of Action: Disrupts DNA, inhibits nucleic acid synthesis in susceptible organisms. Active against anaerobic gram-negative (*Bacteroides*) and gram-positive bacilli (*Clostridium*), and protozoa (*Trichomonas, Giardia*).

Metabolism: Well absorbed after oral administration; rate affected by food, but not amount absorbed. Oral and IV serum levels are similar. Widely distributed in body tissues and fluids, including CSF, placenta, breast milk. Excreted in urine (60–80%) and feces.

Dosage/Range:

Adult:

- Oral: 250–750 mg PO tid × 7–10 days or single dose of 2 g PO (trichomoniasis).
- Pseudomembranous colitis: 250 mg PO qid × 7–14 days or 500 mg PO tid × 7–14 days.

- IV: Loading dose of 15 mg/kg IV over 1 hour (1 g); then maintenance dose of 7.5 mg/kg IV (500 mg) q8h (maximum 4 g/day).

Drug Preparation/Administration:
- Oral: Store in light-resistant container at < 30°C (86°F).
- IV: Protect from light and freezing. Reconstitute according to manufacturer's package insert. Further dilute with 0.9% Sodium Chloride or 5% Dextrose to concentration of ≤ 8 mg/mL. Do not use aluminum needles. Administer over 30–60 minutes. May be given as continuous or intermittent infusion.

Drug Interactions:
- Coumarin anticoagulants: increase anticoagulant effect. Avoid concurrent use if possible; otherwise, monitor PT closely and decrease anticoagulant drug dose as needed.
- Alcohol: inhibits alcohol metabolism, causing a disulfiram-like reaction (flushing, headache, nausea, vomiting, abdominal cramps, diaphoresis). Avoid alcohol and alcohol-containing medications for 48 hours after last metronidazole dose.
- Disulfiram: causes acute psychoses and confusion. Avoid concurrent use and separate use by 2 weeks.
- Phenobarbital/phenytoin: decrease metronidazole activity. Monitor effectiveness and increase metronidazole dose as needed.
- Cimetidine: increases metronidazole levels with potential for increased toxicity. Avoid concurrent administration.

Lab Effects/Interference:
- Serum ALT, serum AST, and LDH: metronidazole has a high absorbance at the wavelength at which NADH is determined; therefore, elevated liver enzyme concentrations may appear to be suppressed by metronidazole when measured by continuous-flow methods based on endpoint decrease.

Special Considerations:
- Carcinogenic in rodents, so drug is used only when necessary.
- Contraindicated in first trimester of pregnancy and administered only as salvage therapy in second and third trimesters when other agents have failed; lactating mothers should interrupt breast-feeding during treatment with drug.
- Use with caution in patients with a history of blood dyscrasias, CNS disorders/dysfunction, hepatic dysfunction, or alcoholism.
- May interfere with laboratory determinations of LFTs (AST, ALT, LDH).

Potential Toxicities/Side Effects and the Nursing Process

I. ALTERATION IN NUTRITION, LESS THAN BODY REQUIREMENTS, related to GI SIDE EFFECTS

Defining Characteristics: Nausea (with/without headache), anorexia, dry mouth, metallic taste in mouth have occurred; less frequently, vomiting, diarrhea, epigastric distress, or constipation. Rare pseudomembranous colitis.

Nursing Implications: Assess baseline nutritional and elimination status. Instruct patient to report GI disturbances. Administer and teach patient to self-administer antiemetics, antidiarrheals as needed and as ordered. Teach patient importance of nutritious diet, and suggest small, frequent, high-calorie, high-protein meals as appropriate. Assess baseline LFTs and monitor periodically during treatment. Discuss abnormalities and drug interruption with physician. Assess whether taking other hepatotoxic drugs (see Special Considerations section). Instruct patient to avoid alcohol and alcohol-containing medications for 48 hours after last drug dose.

II. ALTERATIONS IN SENSORY/PERCEPTUAL PATTERNS related to PERIPHERAL NEUROPATHY

Defining Characteristics: Peripheral neuropathy (numbness, tingling, paresthesia) is reversible with drug discontinuance. Headache, dizziness, ataxia, confusion, mood changes have also occurred.

Nursing Implications: Assess baseline neurologic function and comfort, and monitor during treatment. Instruct patient to report any changes. Discuss abnormalities and drug discontinuance with physician.

III. ALTERATIONS IN SKIN INTEGRITY related to SENSITIVITY REACTIONS

Defining Characteristics: Urticaria, erythematous rash, pruritus, flushing, transient joint pain may occur.

Nursing Implications: Assess drug allergy history. Assess baseline skin integrity. Instruct patient to report rash, pruritus. Teach patient symptomatic management of rash, pruritus.

IV. ALTERATIONS IN URINARY ELIMINATION related to DYSURIA

Defining Characteristics: Urethral burning, dysuria, cystitis, polyuria, incontinence, sensation of pelvic pressure may occur with oral dose. Urine may be dark or reddish-brown.

Nursing Implications: Assess baseline elimination status. Instruct patient to report side effects, and to increase oral fluids to 2–3 qt (liters)/day. Reassure patient urine color change is related to drug and will disappear when drug therapy is completed.

V. ALTERATIONS IN SEXUALITY related to DECREASED LIBIDO, DYSPAREUNIA

Defining Characteristics: Decreased libido, dyspareunia, dryness of vagina and vulva may occur.

Nursing Implications: Assess pattern of sexuality. Inform patient and partner that these effects, if they occur, are temporary. Suggest frequent perineal hygiene as needed to relieve dryness and use of lubricants during intercourse.

VI. FUNGAL SUPERINFECTION related to REDISTRIBUTION OF ENDOGENOUS MICROORGANISMS

Defining Characteristics: Vaginal candidiasis, vaginitis may occur as endogenous bacteria are eliminated and normal fungal population expands.

Nursing Implications: Instruct female patient to report vaginal itching or discharge. Discuss appropriate antifungal treatment with physician. Teach perineal hygiene and symptomatic management.

VII. ALTERATIONS IN COMFORT related to PHLEBITIS

Defining Characteristics: Phlebitis and thrombophlebitis may occur with IV administration.

Nursing Implications: Assess IV site prior to each dose for phlebitis, erythema, swelling, and change site at least q48h. Apply heat to painful IV site as ordered.

Drug: mezlocillin sodium (Mezlin)

Class: Antibacterial (extended spectrum penicillin).

Mechanism of Action: Semisynthetic antibiotic prepared from fungus *Penicillium.* Contains β-lactam ring and is bactericidal by inhibiting cell wall synthesis. Active against most gram-positive (except penicillinase-producing strains) and most gram-negative bacilli. Used in the treatment of serious gram-negative infections, especially *P. aeruginosa*–related infections of lower respiratory tract, urinary tract, and skin.

Metabolism: Poorly absorbed from GI tract, so must be given parenterally. Widely distributed in body tissues and fluids. Crosses placenta and is excreted in breast milk. Excreted via urine and bile.

Dosage/Range:

Adult:

- IV: 200–300 mg/kg/day in four to six divided doses (usual dose 3 g q4–6h).
- Dose modification if severe renal insufficiency; refer to manufacturer's package insert.

Drug Preparation/Administration:

- IV: Reconstitute each gram with at least 10 mL sterile water for injection. Further dilute in 50–100 mL 0.9% Sodium Chloride or 5% Dextrose injection. Administer over 30 minutes.
- IM: Reconstitute each gram with 3–4 mL sterile water for injection or 0.5–1% lidocaine HCl (without epinephrine). Maximum dose is 2 g. Divide dose into two injections, as needed, and administer deep IM in large muscle mass. Administer slowly. Make certain patient is NOT ALLERGIC to lidocaine.

Drug Interactions:

- Aminoglycosides: synergism.
- Aminoglycosides (e.g., gentamicin): incompatible when mixed together; administer at separate sites at different times. Also, penicillinase-resistant penicillins can inactivate aminoglycoside serum samples from patients receiving both drugs.
- Clavulanic acid (inhibits β-lactamase): increases antibacterial action.
- Probenecid: increased serum level of mezlocillin; may be coadministered to exert this effect.

Lab Effects/Interference:

Major clinical significance:

- Urine glucose: high urinary concentrations of a penicillin may produce false-positive or falsely elevated test results with copper sulfate tests (Benedict's, Clinitest, or Fehling's); glucose enzymatic tests (Clinistix or Tes-tape) are not affected.

Clinical significance:

- Coombs' (direct antiglobulin) test: false-positive result may occur during therapy with any penicillin.
- Urine protein: high urinary concentrations of mezlocillin may produce false-positive protein reactions (pseudoproteinuria) with the sulfosalicylic acid and boiling test, the acetic acid test, the biuret reaction, and the nitric acid test; bromophenol blue reagent test strips (Multistix) are reportedly unaffected.
- ALT, alk phos, AST, serum LDH values may be increased.
- Serum bili: an increase has been associated with mezlocillin.
- BUN and serum creatinine: an increase has been associated with mezlocillin.

- Serum K+: hypokalemia may occur following the administration of parenteral mezlocillin, which may act as a non-reabsorbable anion in the distal renal tubules; this may cause an increase in pH and result in increased urinary K+ loss. The risk of hypokalemia increases with the use of larger doses.
- Serum Na+: hypernatremia may occur following administration of large doses of parenteral mezlocillin because of the high Na+ content of these medications.
- WBC: leukopenia or neutropenia is associated with the use of all penicillins; the effect is more likely to occur with prolonged therapy and severe hepatic function impairment.

Special Considerations:

- Contraindicated in patients with prior hypersensitivity to penicillins. Use with caution in patients sensitive to other β-lactams (e.g., cephalosporins) since partial cross-allergenicity exists.
- Obtain ordered specimen, and send for culture and sensitivity test prior to first antibiotic dose.
- Consider alternative antibiotic therapy if eosinophilia, drug fever or rash, arthralgia, hematuria, or unexplained rise in BUN and serum creatinine occur.
- Monitor electrolytes and renal, hepatic, and hematologic laboratory parameters during extended treatment periods.
- Use with caution in pregnancy or with nursing women.
- Na content is 1.85 mEq/g of drug.

Potential Toxicities/Side Effects and the Nursing Process

I. POTENTIAL FOR INJURY related to HYPERSENSITIVITY REACTION

Defining Characteristics: Urticaria, pruritus, rash (maculopapular or erythematous), fever and chills, eosinophilia, myalgia, edema, erythema, angioedema, Stevens-Johnson syndrome, and exfoliative skin reactions occur in 5% of patients. Increased risk in individuals allergic to cephalosporin antibiotics.

Nursing Implications: Assess allergy to cephalosporin antibiotics and penicillin: if patient states "yes," determine actual response, e.g., "swollen lips = angioedema." If angioedema, patient SHOULD NOT receive drug. Discuss other patient responses with physician to determine whether drug should be given. Assess baseline skin condition, including integrity and allergy history to drugs. Instruct patient to report rash, itching, and other skin changes. Teach patient skin care and symptomatic measures as appropriate. If skin rash develops, discuss drug discontinuance with physician. If rash progresses, drug should be discontinued, as fatal Stevens-Johnson syndrome may develop. Be prepared to treat severe acute hypersensitivity reactions with airway management, oxygen, epinephrine, corticosteroids, antihistamines as ordered.

II. ALTERATION IN NUTRITION, LESS THAN BODY REQUIREMENTS, related to GI SIDE EFFECTS

Defining Characteristics: Nausea, vomiting, diarrhea may occur; rarely, pseudomembranous colitis caused by *C. difficile* resistant to the antibiotic occurs. Rarely, transient increases in LFTs—AST, ALT, alk phos, bili—may occur.

Nursing Implications: Assess baseline nutritional status. Instruct patient to report GI disturbances. Administer and teach patient to self-administer antiemetics as needed and as ordered. Teach patient importance of nutritious diet, and suggest small, frequent, high-calorie, high-protein meals as appropriate. Assess baseline LFTs, and monitor periodically during treatment. Discuss abnormalities and drug interruption with physician.

III. FUNGAL SUPERINFECTION related to REDISTRIBUTION OF ENDOGENOUS MICROORGANISMS

Defining Characteristics: Vaginal candidiasis, vaginitis may occur as endogenous bacteria are eliminated and normal fungal population expands.

Nursing Implications: Instruct female patient to report vaginal itching or discharge. Discuss appropriate antifungal treatment with physician. Teach perineal hygiene and symptomatic management.

IV. ALTERATIONS IN PROTECTIVE MECHANISMS (RARE) related to TRANSIENT LEUKOPENIA

Defining Characteristics: Rarely, transient leukopenia, lymphocytosis, anemia, eosinophilia may occur. Prolonged PT, prolonged APTT, and hypoprothrombinemia have occurred rarely, especially in elderly or debilitated patients, or in individuals with vitamin K deficiency.

Nursing Implications: Assess baseline laboratory parameters, and monitor periodically during treatment. Assess patient for response to antibiotics. Discuss abnormalities with physician. Assess for signs/symptoms of bleeding.

V. ALTERATIONS IN SENSORY/PERCEPTUAL PATTERNS related to DIZZINESS, SOMNOLENCE

Defining Characteristics: Dizziness, headache, somnolence occur rarely. Neuromuscular irritability and seizures may occur with high drug serum levels.

Nursing Implications: Assess baseline neurologic function and comfort, and monitor during treatment. Instruct patient to report any changes. Discuss any abnormalities with physician. Institute seizure precautions.

VI. ALTERATIONS IN COMFORT related to LOCAL INJECTION IRRITATION

Defining Characteristics: Vein irritation (pain, erythema), phlebitis, and thrombophlebitis may occur at IV administration site.

Nursing Implications: Change IV sites q48h, and assess for signs/symptoms of phlebitis prior to each administration. Administer drug slowly. Apply warm packs to increase comfort. Discuss central line with patient and physician to facilitate administration.

VII. ALTERATION IN FLUID AND ELECTROLYTE BALANCE related to HYPOKALEMIA AND INCREASED SODIUM INTAKE

Defining Characteristics: Prolonged therapy may cause hypokalemia; also, drug is prepared as sodium salt. Frequent IV infusions increase fluid intake.

Nursing Implications: Assess baseline electrolytes, fluid balance, weight, and monitor throughout therapy. Monitor renal function studies, especially if patient has preexisting renal dysfunction.

Drug: minocycline hydrochloride (Minocin, Vectrin, Dynacin)

Class: Antibacterial (systemic); antiprotozoal.

Mechanism of Action: Bacteriostatic, but may be bactericidal at high concentrations. Binds to bacterial ribosomes and prevents protein synthesis. Active against broad range of gram-positive and gram-negative bacteria, Chlamydia, and Mycoplasma.

Metabolism: Absorbed (60%–80%) from GI tract. Widely distributed into body tissues and fluids. Crosses placenta and is excreted in breast milk. Excreted unchanged in urine.

Dosage/Range:

Adult:

- Oral: 200 mg initially, then 100 mg q12h for 5–15 days; or 100–200 mg initially, then 50 mg q6h for 5–15 days.
- IV: 200 mg initially, then 100 mg q12h for 5–15 days (depends on indication).
- Dose modification necessary if renal dysfunction exists.

Drug Preparation/Administration:

- Oral: may be taken with food, water, or milk.
- IV: add 5–10 mL sterile water for injection to 100-mg vial. Further dilute in 500 to 1000 mL of 0.9% Sodium Chloride injection, Dextrose injection, Dextrose and Sodium Chloride injections, Ringer's injection, or lactated

Ringer's injection. Do not use other calcium-containing solutions, since precipitate may form.

- AVOID RAPID ADMINISTRATION.
- Solution stable for 24 hours at room temperature. Avoid exposure to heat or sunlight. Convert to oral preparation as soon as possible, as there is risk of thrombophlebitis.
- DO NOT ADMINISTER INTRAMUSCULARLY or SUBCUTANEOUSLY.

Drug Interactions:

- Hepatotoxic drugs: may increase hepatotoxicity if given concurrently. Assess baseline and periodically during treatment.
- Iron preparations: decrease oral and possibly IV absorption. Administer iron preparations 3 hours after or 2 hours before any tetracycline.
- Oral anticoagulants: increase PT. Monitor patient closely and decrease anticoagulant dose as needed.
- Antidiarrheals (containing kaolin, pectate, or bismuth): may decrease absorption of tetracyclines. Avoid concurrent use.
- Oral contraceptives: decreased effectiveness of contraceptive and increased incidence of breakthrough bleeding. Advise patient to use barrier contraceptive as well during a course of tetracycline therapy.
- Lithium: may decrease lithium levels. Monitor serum levels and increase dose as needed.

Lab Effects/Interference:

- Urine catecholamine determinations: may produce false elevations of urinary catecholamines because of interfering fluorescence in the Hingerty method.
- SGPT, alk phos, amylase, SGOT, and bilirubin: serum concentrations may be increased.

Special Considerations:

- May cause dizziness, lightheadedness, or unsteadiness (CNS toxicity).
- Pigmentation of skin and mucous membranes may occur.
- Use cautiously in patients with myasthenia gravis: may increase muscle weakness.
- Avoid use in pregnant or lactating women.
- Obtain ordered specimen for culture and sensitivity prior to first dose.
- IV preparation contains ascorbic acid and may cause false-positive result using Clinitest, or false-negative when using Clinistix and Testape.
- Drug has affinity for ischemic, necrotic tissue, and may localize in tumors.

Potential Toxicities/Side Effects and the Nursing Process

I. ALTERATION IN NUTRITION related to GI SIDE EFFECTS

Defining Characteristics: Nausea, vomiting, diarrhea, anorexia, abdominal discomfort, epigastric burning and distress, glossitis, black hairy tongue may occur.

Nursing Implications: Assess baseline nutritional status. Assess for and teach patient to report any symptoms. Administer and teach patient self-administration of prescribed antiemetic or antidiarrheal medication as appropriate. Administer and teach patient to self-administer oral dose with at least 8 oz of water taken at least 1 hour before lying down for sleep.

II. ALTERATION IN SKIN INTEGRITY related to RASH, PHOTOSENSITIVITY

Defining Characteristics: Maculopapular and erythematous rashes may occur. Rarely, exfoliative dermatitis, onycholysis, and nail discoloration. Photosensitivity risk (exaggerated sunburn) persists 1–2 days after completion of drug therapy.

Nursing Implications: Teach patient about potential side effects, to avoid sunlight during drug therapy, and to report rash, other abnormalities. Teach symptomatic skin care as appropriate.

III. INJURY related to HYPERSENSITIVITY

Defining Characteristics: Urticaria, angioneurotic edema, anaphylaxis may occur; also, fever, rash, arthralgias, eosinophilia, and pericarditis.

Nursing Implications: Assess drug allergy history. Assess baseline allergy history. Assess baseline skin integrity. Teach patient to report rash, pruritus. Teach patent symptomatic management of rash, pruritus. Assess for hypersensitivity reaction; if it occurs, monitor VS, discontinue drug, notify physician, and institute supportive measures.

IV. FUNGAL SUPERINFECTION related to REDISTRIBUTION OF ENDOGENOUS MICROORGANISMS

Defining Characteristics: Vaginal moniliasis, vaginitis may occur as endogenous bacteria are eliminated and normal fungal population expands.

Nursing Implications: Teach female patient to report vaginal itching or discharge. Discuss appropriate antifungal treatment with physician. Teach perineal hygiene and symptomatic management.

V. ALTERATION IN HEPATIC FUNCTION

Defining Characteristics: Associated with high IV doses (> 2 g/day): hepatotoxicity and cholestasis may occur.

Nursing Implications: Assess baseline LFTs and monitor during therapy.

VI. INFECTION AND BLEEDING related to NEUTROPENIA, THROMBOCYTOPENIA

Defining Characteristics: Neutropenia, leukocytosis, leukopenia, atypical lymphocytes, thrombocytopenia, thrombocytopenic purpura, hemolytic anemia occur rarely with long-term therapy.

Nursing Implications: Assess baseline WBC, HCT, and platelets, and monitor periodically during long-term therapy.

VII. ALTERATION IN COMFORT related to LOCAL ADMINISTRATION EFFECTS

Defining Characteristics: IM administration may cause pain, induration due to muscle injury. IV administration may cause erythema, pain, swelling, and thrombophlebitis.

Nursing Implications: Rotate sites. Apply ice as ordered to painful buttock. Assess IV site prior to each dose for phlebitis or swelling, and change site at least q48h. Apply heat to painful IV sites as ordered.

VIII. SENSORY/PERCEPTUAL ALTERATION

Defining Characteristics: Light-headedness, dizziness, headache may occur.

Nursing Implications: Assess baseline neurological status. Teach patient to report any changes and discuss them with physician.

Drug: moxifloxacin (ABC Pack; Avelox)

Class: Antibiotic; Quinolone.

Mechanism of Action: Moxifloxacin is a broad-spectrum anti-infective, active against a wide range of aerobic gram-positive and gram-negative organisms. Acts intracellularly by inhibiting DNA gyrase and bacterial topoisomerase IV. DNA gyrase is required for DNA replication and transcription, DNA repair, recombination, and transposition; inhibition is bactericidal.

Metabolism: Widely distributed to most body fluids and tissues with highest concentrations in organs, such as kidneys, gallbladder, lungs, liver, gynecological tissue, prostatic tissue, phagocytic cells, urine, sputum, and bile. Well absorbed from GI tract. Metabolized in liver; excreted in urine and feces. Crosses placenta and is excreted in breast milk.

Dosage/Range:

- 400 mg PO or IV QD.

Drug Preparation/Administration:

- Oral: Take drug with large glass of water, preferably 2 hours after meal/ food. Encourage oral fluids of 2–3 qt (liters)/day.
- IV: Further dilute drug in 0.9% Sodium Chloride or 5% Dextrose in water to final concentration of 2 mg/mL. Administer over 60 minutes, do not infuse by rapid or bolus intravenous infusion.
- Do not refrigerate.

Drug Interactions:

- Antacids (containing magnesium, aluminum, or calcium) and iron decrease absorption of serum level of moxifloxacin; do not administer concurrently. If must administer antacids or iron, administer at least 4 hours apart. The administration of antacids containing aluminum, magnesium, calcium, sucralfate, zinc, or iron may substantially reduce the absorption of moxifloxacin; do not administer concurrently.
- Serum digoxin concentrations should be monitored; moxifloxacin may raise serum levels in some patients.
- Probenecid: decreases the renal tubular secretion of moxifloxacin, resulting in a prolonged elimination half-life and increased risk of toxicity.
- Moxifloxacin may have the potential to prolong the Q-T interval of the EKG in some patients. Moxifloxacin should not be used in patients with prolonged Q-T interval; patients with uncorrected hypokalemia; and patients on quinidine, procanamide, amiodrone, and sotalol (antiarrhythmic agents).
- Increased intracranial pressure and psychosis has been reported along with CNS stimulation.
- Hypersensitivity reactions have been reported.

Lab Effects/Interference:

- Serum SGPT, serum Alk Phos, serum SGOT, and serum LDH—values may be increased.

Special Considerations:

- Used in the treatment of respiratory tract infections (acute bacterial exacerbation of chronic bronchitis, acute bacterial sinusitis, and commonly acquired pneumonia).
- Used in the treatment of uncomplicated infections of the skin and skin structures.
- Contraindicated in pregnancy or women who are breast-feeding.
- Obtain ordered specimen for culture and sensitivity prior to first drug dose.

- Use cautiously in patients with seizure disorders.

Potential Toxicities/Side Effects and the Nursing Process

I. ALTERATION IN NUTRITION related to GI SIDE EFFECTS

Defining Characteristics: Incidence of nausea, vomiting, abdominal discomfort, diarrhea, anorexia.

Nursing Implications: Assess baseline nutritional and elimination status. Teach patient to report GI disturbances. Administer and teach patient to self-administer antiemetics, antidiarrheals as needed and as ordered. Teach patient importance of nutritious diet, and suggest small, frequent, high-calorie, high-protein meals as appropriate. Assess baseline LFTs and monitor periodically during treatment. Discuss abnormalities and drug interruption with physician.

II. SENSORY/PERCEPTUAL ALTERATIONS related to CNS EFFECTS

Defining Characteristics: Incidence of headache, restlessness. Dizziness, hallucinations, and seizures may also occur. Exacerbated by caffeine as quinolones delay caffeine excretion.

Nursing Implications: Assess baseline neurological function and comfort, and monitor during treatment. Teach patient to report any changes. Discuss any abnormalities with physician. Teach patient to limit or restrict all caffeine-containing fluids, medications, e.g., tea, coffee, soft drinks.

III. ALTERATION IN SKIN INTEGRITY related to ALLERGY/HYPERSENSITIVITY

Defining Characteristics: Incidence of rash; other manifestations include eosinophilia, urticaria, flushing, fever, chills, photosensitivity, angioedema. Fatal hypersensitivity reactions have occurred rarely. Direct exposure to sunlight can cause sunburn (moderate to severe phototoxicity).

Nursing Implications: Assess baseline skin condition, including integrity and drug allergy history. Teach patient to report rash, itching, and other skin changes. Teach patient skin care and symptomatic measures as appropriate. If skin rash develops, discuss drug discontinuance with physician. Be prepared to treat severe acute hypersensitivity reactions with airway management, oxygen, epinephrine, corticosteroids, antihistamines as ordered. Teach patient to avoid excessive sun exposure and to use skin protection factor (SPF) 15 or higher. If rash progresses, especially in HIV-infected patients, drug should be discontinued as fatal Stevens-Johnson syndrome may develop.

IV. FUNGAL SUPERINFECTION related to REDISTRIBUTION OF ENDOGENOUS MICROORGANISMS

Defining Characteristics: Vaginal moniliasis, vaginitis may occur as endogenous bacteria are eliminated and normal fungal population expands.

Nursing Implications: Teach female patient to report vaginal itching or discharge. Discuss appropriate antifungal treatment with physician. Teach perineal hygiene and symptomatic management.

V. ALTERATION IN URINARY ELIMINATION related to RENAL TOXICITY

Defining Characteristics: Increased BUN and creatinine, crystal and stone formation in urine, interstitial nephritis, and renal failure may occur.

Nursing Implications: Assess baseline renal function; expect that drug dose will be decreased in presence of renal dysfunction. Teach patient to take drug with at least 8 oz of water, and to increase oral fluids to 2–3 qt/day.

VI. ALTERATION IN COMFORT related to IV ADMINISTRATION

Defining Characteristics: Drug may cause pain, inflammation, and rare thrombophlebitis at IV site.

Nursing Implications: Change IV site q 48 hours. Assess for phlebitis, discomfort, and IV patency prior to each administration. Administer drug slowly over 60–90 minutes in large volume of 5% Dextrose (see Drug Preparation/Administration). Apply heat to promote comfort.

Drug: nafcillin sodium (Unipen)

Class: Antibacterial (systemic).

Mechanism of Action: Semisynthetic antibiotic. Contains β-lactam ring and is bactericidal by inhibiting cell wall synthesis. Penicillinase-resistant penicillin; active against penicillin-resistant staphylococci that produce the enzyme penicillinase.

Metabolism: Incompletely absorbed from GI tract; rapidly absorbed when given IM or IV. Widely distributed in body tissues and fluid, including bile. Crosses placenta and is excreted in breast milk; 70–90% bound to serum proteins. Metabolized in liver, excreted in bile, and to a lesser degree in the urine.

Dosage/Range:

Adult:

- Oral: 500 mg–1 g PO q6h.

- IM/IV: 500 mg–2 g q4h.

Drug Preparation/Administration:

- Oral: Reconstitute per manufacturer's recommendation or by capsules or tablets. Administer 1 hour before meals or 2 hours after meals.
- IM: Reconstitute with sterile or bacteriostatic water for injection, and give deep IM in large muscle (e.g., gluteus maximus).
- IV: Reconstitute with sterile water for injection or 0.9% Sodium Chloride for injection according to manufacturer's package insert. Further dilute in 100 mL IV solution and infuse over 40–60 minutes.

Drug Interactions:

- Aminoglycosides: synergism.
- Aminoglycosides (e.g., gentamicin): incompatible when mixed together; administer at separate sites at different times. Also, penicillinase-resistant penicillins can inactivate aminoglycoside serum samples from patients receiving both drugs.
- Rifampin: possible antagonism, only at high doses of penicillin.
- Probenecid: increased serum level of nafcillin; may be coadministered to exert this effect.

Lab Effects/Interference:

Major clinical significance:

- Urine glucose: high urinary concentrations of a penicillin may produce false-positive or falsely elevated test results with copper sulfate tests (Benedict's, Clinitest, or Fehling's); glucose enzymatic tests (Clinistix or Tes-tape) are not affected.

Clinical significance:

- Coombs' (direct antiglobulin) test: false-positive result may occur during therapy with any penicillin.
- ALT, alk phos, AST, serum LDH: values may be increased.
- WBC: leukopenia or neutropenia is associated with the use of all penicillins; the effect is more likely to occur with prolonged therapy and severe hepatic function impairment.

Special Considerations:

- Contraindicated in patients with prior hypersensitivity to penicillins. Use with caution in patients sensitive to other β-lactams (e.g., cephalosporins) since partial cross-allergenicity exists.
- Obtain ordered specimen and send for culture and sensitivity prior to first antibiotic dose.
- Consider alternative antibiotic therapy if eosinophilia, drug fever or rash, arthralgia, hematuria, or unexplained rise in BUN and serum creatinine occur.

- Monitor electrolytes and renal, hepatic, and hematologic laboratory parameters during extended treatment periods.
- Use with caution in pregnancy or with nursing women.

Potential Toxicities/Side Effects and the Nursing Process

I. POTENTIAL FOR INJURY related to HYPERSENSITIVITY REACTION

Defining Characteristics: Urticaria, pruritus, rash (maculopapular or erythematous), fever and chills, eosinophilia, myalgia, edema, erythema, angioedema, Stevens-Johnson syndrome, and exfoliative skin reactions occur in 5% of patients. Increased risk in individuals allergic to cephalosporin antibiotics.

Nursing Implications: Assess allergy to cephalosporin antibiotics and penicillin: if patient states "yes," determine actual response, e.g., "swollen lips = angioedema." If angioedema, patient SHOULD NOT receive drug. Discuss other patient responses with physician to determine whether drug should be given. Assess baseline skin condition, including integrity and allergy history to drugs. Instruct patient to report rash, itching, other skin changes. Teach patient skin care and symptomatic measures as appropriate. If skin rash develops, discuss drug discontinuance with physician. If rash progresses, drug should be discontinued, as fatal Stevens-Johnson syndrome may develop. Be prepared to treat severe acute hypersensitivity reactions with airway management, oxygen, epinephrine, corticosteroids, antihistamines as ordered.

II. ALTERATION IN NUTRITION, LESS THAN BODY REQUIREMENTS, related to GI SIDE EFFECTS

Defining Characteristics: Nausea, vomiting, diarrhea may occur; rarely, pseudomembranous colitis caused by *C. difficile* resistant to the antibiotic occurs. Rarely, transient increases in LFTs—AST, ALT, alk phos, bili—may occur.

Nursing Implications: Assess baseline nutritional status. Instruct patient to report GI disturbances. Administer and teach patient to self-administer antiemetics, antidiarrheals as needed and as ordered. Teach patient importance of nutritious diet, and suggest small, frequent, high-calorie, high-protein meals as appropriate. Assess baseline LFTs and monitor periodically during treatment. Discuss abnormalities and drug interruption with physician.

III. FUNGAL SUPERINFECTION related to REDISTRIBUTION OF ENDOGENOUS MICROORGANISMS

Defining Characteristics: Vaginal candidiasis, vaginitis may occur as endogenous bacteria are eliminated and normal fungal population expands.

Nursing Implications: Instruct female patient to report vaginal itching or discharge. Discuss appropriate antifungal treatment with physician. Teach perineal hygiene and symptomatic management.

IV. ALTERATIONS IN PROTECTIVE MECHANISMS (RARE) related to TRANSIENT LEUKOPENIA

Defining Characteristics: Rarely, transient leukopenia, lymphocytosis, anemia, eosinophilia may occur. Prolonged PT, prolonged APTT, and hypoprothrombinemia have occurred rarely, especially in elderly or debilitated patients, or in individuals with vitamin K deficiency.

Nursing Implications: Assess baseline laboratory parameters, and monitor periodically during treatment. Assess patient for response to antibiotics. Discuss abnormalities with physician.

V. ALTERATIONS IN COMFORT related to PHLEBITIS

Defining Characteristics: Phlebitis and thrombophlebitis may occur with IV administration. Increased risk in elderly.

Nursing Implications: Assess IV site prior to each dose for phlebitis, erythema, swelling, and change site at least q48h. Apply heat to painful IV site as ordered.

Drug: oxacillin sodium (Bactocill, Prostaphlin)

Class: Antibacterial (systemic).

Mechanism of Action: Semisynthetic antibiotic. Contains β-lactam ring and is bactericidal by inhibiting cell wall synthesis. Penicillinase-resistant penicillin and active against penicillin-resistant staphylococci, which produce the enzyme penicillinase.

Metabolism: Incompletely absorbed from GI tract; rapidly absorbed when given IM or IV. Widely distributed in body tissues and fluid, including bile. Crosses placenta and is excreted in breast milk; 89–94% bound to serum proteins. Metabolized in liver, excreted in urine.

Dosage/Range:

Adult:

- Oral: 500 mg–1 g PO q6h.
- IM/IV: 500 mg–2 g q4h.

Drug Preparation/Administration:

- Oral: Reconstitute per manufacturer's package insert or by capsules or tablets. Administer 1 hour before meals or 2 hours after meals.

- IM: Reconstitute with sterile or bacteriostatic water for injection, and give deep IM in large muscle (e.g., gluteus maximus).
- IV: Reconstitute with sterile water for injection or 0.9% Sodium Chloride for injection according to manufacturer's package insert. Further dilute in 100 mL IV solution and infuse over 40–60 minutes.

Drug Interactions:
- Aminoglycosides: synergism.
- Aminoglycosides (e.g., gentamicin): incompatible when mixed together; administer at separate sites at different times. Also, penicillinase-resistant penicillins can inactivate aminoglycoside serum samples from patients receiving both drugs.
- Rifampin: possible antagonism, only at high doses of oxacillin.
- Probenecid: increased serum level of oxacillin; may be coadministered to exert this effect.

Lab Effects/Interference:
Major clinical significance:
- Urine glucose: high urinary concentrations of a penicillin may produce false-positive or falsely elevated test results with copper sulfate tests (Benedict's, Clinitest, or Fehling's); glucose enzymatic tests (Clinistix or Testape) are not affected.

Clinical significance:
- Coombs' (direct antiglobulin) test: false-positive result may occur during therapy with any penicillin.
- ALT, alk phos, AST, serum LDH values may be increased.
- WBC: leukopenia or neutropenia is associated with the use of all penicillins; the effect is more likely to occur with prolonged therapy and severe hepatic function impairment.

Special Considerations:
- Contraindicated in patients with prior hypersensitivity to penicillins. Use with caution in patients sensitive to other β-lactams (e.g., cephalosporins) since partial cross-allergenicity.
- Obtain ordered specimen and send for culture and sensitivity prior to first antibiotic dose.
- Consider alternative antibiotic therapy if eosinophilia, drug fever or rash, arthralgia, hematuria, or unexplained rise in BUN and serum creatinine occur.
- Monitor electrolytes and renal, hepatic, and hematologic laboratory parameters during extended treatment periods.
- Use with caution in pregnant or nursing women.

Potential Toxicities/Side Effects and the Nursing Process

I. POTENTIAL FOR INJURY related to HYPERSENSITIVITY REACTION

Defining Characteristics: Urticaria, pruritus, rash (maculopapular or erythematous), fever and chills, eosinophilia, myalgia, edema, erythema, angioedema, Stevens-Johnson syndrome, and exfoliative skin reactions occur in 5% of patients. Increased risk in individuals allergic to cephalosporin antibiotics.

Nursing Implications: Assess allergy to cephalosporin antibiotics and penicillin: if patient states "yes," determine actual response, e.g., "swollen lips = angioedema." If angioedema, patient SHOULD NOT receive drug. Discuss other patient responses with physician to determine whether drug should be given. Assess baseline skin condition, including integrity and allergy history to drugs. Instruct patient to report rash, itching, and other skin changes. Teach patient skin care and symptomatic measures as appropriate. If skin rash develops, discuss drug discontinuance with physician. If rash progresses, drug should be discontinued, as fatal Stevens-Johnson syndrome may develop. Be prepared to treat severe acute hypersensitivity reactions with airway management, oxygen, epinephrine, corticosteroids, antihistamines as ordered.

II. ALTERATION IN NUTRITION, LESS THAN BODY REQUIREMENTS, related to INCREASED LFTs

Defining Characteristics: Oral lesions may occur, as may hepatitis (rare) and increased LFTs.

Nursing Implications: Assess baseline oral mucosa, and LFTs—AST, ALT, alk phos, bili. Teach patient to practice oral hygiene after meals and at bedtime, and instruct to report any oral lesions. Monitor LFTs periodically during treatment, and discuss abnormalities with physician.

III. FUNGAL SUPERINFECTION related to REDISTRIBUTION OF ENDOGENOUS MICROORGANISMS

Defining Characteristics: Vaginal candidiasis, vaginitis may occur as endogenous bacteria are eliminated and normal fungal population expands.

Nursing Implications: Instruct female patient to report vaginal itching or discharge. Discuss appropriate antifungal treatment with physician. Teach perineal hygiene and symptomatic management.

IV. ALTERATIONS IN PROTECTIVE MECHANISMS (RARE) related to TRANSIENT LEUKOPENIA

Defining Characteristics: Rarely, transient leukopenia, lymphocytosis, anemia, eosinophilia may occur. Prolonged PT, prolonged APTT, and hypoprothrombinemia have occurred rarely, especially in elderly or debilitated patients, or in individuals with vitamin K deficiency.

Nursing Implications: Assess baseline laboratory parameters, and monitor periodically during treatment. Assess patient for response to antibiotics. Discuss abnormalities with physician.

V. ALTERATIONS IN COMFORT related to PHLEBITIS

Defining Characteristics: Phlebitis and thrombophlebitis may occur with IV administration. Increased risk in elderly.

Nursing Implications: Assess IV site prior to each dose for phlebitis, erythema, swelling, and change site at least q48h. Apply heat to painful IV site as ordered.

VI. ALTERATIONS IN URINARY ELIMINATION related to RENAL DAMAGE

Defining Characteristics: Interstitial nephritis, transient proteinuria, hematuria may occur.

Nursing Implications: Assess baseline liver, renal function tests (e.g., serum BUN, creatinine, and urinalysis), and monitor during therapy.

VII. ALTERATIONS IN SENSORY/PERCEPTUAL PATTERNS related to NEUROPATHY

Defining Characteristics: Neuropathy, seizures, neuromuscular irritability may occur rarely.

Nursing Implications: Assess baseline neurologic function and comfort, and monitor during treatment. Instruct patient to report any changes. Discuss any abnormalities with physician.

Drug: penicillin G (PenG Potassium, PenG Sodium, Intravenous; PenVK, Oral Preparation)

Class: Natural penicillin.

Mechanism of Action: Produced by fermentation of *Penicillium chrysogenum.* Active against many gram-positive bacteria (streptococci, staphylococci) but resistant to *S. aureus* and *S. epidermidis* strains that produce penicillinases. Also active against some gram-negative bacteria (*Neisseria, H. influenzae*), and spirochetes.

Metabolism: Decreased oral absorption, but IM or IV absorption is quite rapid and complete. Widely distributed in body tissues and fluids; 45–68% bound to proteins. Eliminated in urine and bile.

Dosage/Range:
- Oral: 250–500 mg qid.
- IV: 200,000–4 million U q4h.
- Dose modification may be necessary in patients with renal impairment.

Drug Preparation/Administration:
- Oral: Administer at least 1 hour before or 2 hours after meals.
- IM: Reconstitute drug as directed. Administration of greater than 100,000 U is likely to result in some discomfort. Give IM deep in large muscle mass.
- IV: Reconstitute drug as directed. Further dilute in 0.9% Sodium Chloride or 5% Dextrose in water, and administer over 1–2 hours.

Drug Interactions:
- Aminoglycosides: synergism.
- Aminoglycosides (e.g., gentamicin): incompatible when mixed together; administer at separate sites at different times. Also, penicillinase-resistant penicillins can inactivate aminoglycoside serum samples from patients receiving both drugs.
- Rifampin: possible antagonism, only at high doses of penicillin.
- Probenecid: increased serum level of penicillin; may be coadministered to exert this effect.

Lab Effects/Interference:
Major clinical significance:
- Urine glucose: high urinary concentrations of a penicillin may produce false-positive or falsely elevated test results with copper sulfate tests (Benedict's, Clinitest, or Fehling's); glucose enzymatic tests (Clinistix or Testape) are not affected.

Clinical significance:
- Coombs' (direct antiglobulin) test: false-positive result may occur during therapy with any penicillin.
- ALT, alk phos, AST, serum LDH values may be increased.
- Serum K+: hyperkalemia may occur following administration of parenteral penicillin G potassium because of the high potassium content.
- Serum Na+: hypernatremia may occur following administration of large doses of parenteral penicillin G sodium because of the high sodium content.
- WBC: leukopenia or neutropenia is associated with the use of all penicillins; the effect is more likely to occur with prolonged therapy and severe hepatic function impairment.

Special Considerations:

- Contraindicated in patients with prior hypersensitivity to penicillins. Use with caution in patients sensitive to other β-lactams (e.g., cephalosporins) since partial cross-allergenicity exists.
- Obtain ordered specimen and send for culture and sensitivity test prior to first antibiotic dose.
- Consider alternative antibiotic therapy if eosinophilia, drug fever or rash, arthralgia, hematuria, or unexplained rise in BUN and serum creatinine occur.
- Monitor electrolytes and renal, hepatic, and hematologic laboratory parameters during extended treatment periods.
- Hyperkalemia may occur with high dose therapy: monitor serum K+.
- Use with caution in pregnant or nursing women.
- Penicillin G benzathine should never be given IV (suspension); give IM only.

Potential Toxicities/Side Effects and the Nursing Process

I. POTENTIAL FOR INJURY related to HYPERSENSITIVITY REACTION

Defining Characteristics: Urticaria, pruritus, rash (maculopapular or erythematous), fever and chills, eosinophilia, myalgia, edema, erythema, angioedema, Stevens-Johnson syndrome, and exfoliative skin reactions occur in 5% of patients. Increased risk exists in individuals allergic to cephalosporin antibiotics.

Nursing Implications: Assess allergy to cephalosporin antibiotics and penicillin: if patient states "yes," determine actual response, e.g., "swollen lips = angioedema." If angioedema, patient SHOULD NOT receive drug. Discuss other patient responses with physician to determine whether drug should be given. Assess baseline skin condition, including integrity and allergy history to drugs. Instruct patient to report rash, itching, and other skin changes. Teach patient skin care and symptomatic measures as appropriate. If skin rash develops, discuss drug discontinuance with physician. If rash progresses, drug should be discontinued, as fatal Stevens-Johnson syndrome may develop. Be prepared to treat severe acute hypersensitivity reactions with airway management, oxygen, epinephrine, corticosteroids, antihistamines as ordered.

II. ALTERATION IN NUTRITION, LESS THAN BODY REQUIREMENTS, related to GI SIDE EFFECTS

Defining Characteristics: Rarely, nausea, vomiting, diarrhea, and pseudomembranous colitis caused by *C. difficile* resistant to the antibiotic may occur. Rarely, transient increases in LFTs—AST, ALT, alk phos, bili—may occur.

Nursing Implications: Assess baseline nutritional status. Instruct patient to report GI disturbances. Administer and teach patient to self-administer antiemetics as needed and as ordered. Teach patient importance of nutritious diet, and suggest small, frequent, high-calorie, high-protein meals as appropriate. Assess baseline LFTs and monitor periodically during treatment. Discuss abnormalities and drug interruption with physician.

III. FUNGAL SUPERINFECTION related to REDISTRIBUTION OF ENDOGENOUS MICROORGANISMS

Defining Characteristics: Vaginal candidiasis, vaginitis may occur as endogenous bacteria are eliminated and normal fungal population expands.

Nursing Implications: Instruct female patient to report vaginal itching or discharge. Discuss appropriate antifungal treatment with physician. Teach perineal hygiene and symptomatic management.

IV. ALTERATIONS IN PROTECTIVE MECHANISMS (RARE) related to RARE LEUKOPENIA

Defining Characteristics: Rarely, hemolytic anemia, leukopenia, thrombocytopenia may occur.

Nursing Implications: Assess baseline laboratory parameters, and monitor periodically during treatment. Assess patient for response to antibiotics. Discuss abnormalities with physician.

V. ALTERATIONS IN SENSORY/PERCEPTUAL PATTERNS related to NEUROPATHY

Defining Characteristics: Neuropathy, seizures may occur with high doses.

Nursing Implications: Assess baseline neurologic function and comfort, and monitor during treatment. Instruct patient to report any changes. Discuss any abnormalities with physician.

VI. ALTERATIONS IN COMFORT related to LOCAL INJECTION IRRITATION

Defining Characteristics: Pain, induration may form in IM injection sites; phlebitis may develop in IV sites.

Nursing Implications: Rotate IM injection sites, and administer drug deep IM in large muscle mass (e.g., gluteus maximus). Use IM injection when IV administration is not possible. Change IV sites q48h, and assess for signs/symptoms of phlebitis prior to each administration. Administer drug slowly. Apply warm packs to increase comfort.

Drug: piperacillin sodium (Pipracil); combined with tazobactam sodium (Zosyn)

Class: Antibacterial (systemic) (extended-spectrum penicillin).

Mechanism of Action: Semisynthetic antibiotic prepared from fungus *Penicillium.* Contains β-lactam ring and is bactericidal by inhibiting cell wall synthesis. Active against most gram-positive (except penicillinase-producing strains) and most gram-negative bacilli. Used in the treatment of serious gram-negative infections, especially *P. aeruginosa*–related infections of lower respiratory tract, urinary tract, and skin. When combined with tazobactam sodium, which inhibits β-lactamases, piperacillin sodium is effective against resistant bacteria.

Metabolism: Poorly absorbed from GI tract, so must be given parenterally. Widely distributed in body tissues and fluids. Crosses placenta and is excreted in breast milk. Excreted via urine and bile.

Dosage/Range:
- IV route preferred.

Adult:

piperacillin sodium:
- IV: 3–4 g q4–6h (maximum 24 g, but higher doses may be used in severe infection); IM: maximum 2 g/per dose.

Zosyn:
- 3 g piperacillin and 0.375 g tazobactam (3.375 g)–4 g piperacillin and 0.50 g tazobactam (4.50 g) q6h IV × 7–10 days.
- Moderate-to-severe pneumonia caused by piperacillin-resistant s. aureus that produces β-lactamase: 3.375 g IV q6h plus aminoglycoside × 7–10 days.
- Dose modification necessary if severe renal insufficiency exists.

Drug Preparation/Administration:
- IV: Reconstitute each gram of drug with at least 5 mL of sterile or bacteriostatic water. Further dilute in 50–100 mL 0.9% Sodium Chloride or 5% Dextrose injection and infuse over 30 minutes.
- IM: Reconstitute with 2 mL of sterile or bacteriostatic water, or 0.5–1.0% lidocaine HCl (without epinephrine), with final concentration 1 g/2.5 mL. Administer as deep IM injection in large muscle mass (e.g., gluteus maximus). Make certain patient is NOT ALLERGIC to lidocaine.

Drug Interactions:
- Aminoglycosides: synergism.
- Aminoglycosides (e.g., gentamicin): incompatible when mixed together; administer at separate sites at different times. Also, penicillinase-resistant penicillins can inactivate aminoglycoside serum samples from patients receiving both drugs.

- Clavulanic acid (inhibits β-lactamase): increases antibacterial action.
- Probenecid: increased serum level of piperacillin; may be coadministered to exert this effect.
- Tazobactam: inhibits β-lactamase, thus broadening drug's antimicrobial effectiveness.

Lab Effects/Interference:
Major clinical significance:
- Urine glucose: high urinary concentrations of a penicillin may produce false-positive or falsely elevated test results with copper sulfate tests (Benedict's, Clinitest, or Fehling's); glucose enzymatic tests (Clinistix or Testape) are not affected.
- PTT and PT: an increase has been associated with intravenous piperacillin.

Clinical significance:
- Coombs' (direct antiglobulin) test: false-positive result may occur during therapy with any penicillin.
- Urine protein: high urinary concentrations of piperacillin may produce false-positive protein reactions (pseudoproteinuria) with the sulfosalicyclic acid and boiling test; bromophenol blue reagent test strips (Multistix) are reportedly unaffected.
- ALT, alk phos, AST, serum LDH values may be increased.
- Serum bili: an increase has been associated with piperacillin.
- BUN and serum creatinine: increased concentrations have been associated with piperacillin.
- Serum K+: hypokalemia may occur following administration of parenteral piperacillin, which may act as a non-reabsorbable anion in the distal tubals; this may cause an increase in pH and result in increased urinary potassium loss: the risk of hypokalemia increases with use of larger doses.
- WBC: leukopenia or neutropenia is associated with the use of all penicillins; the effect is more likely to occur with prolonged therapy and severe hepatic function impairment.

Special Considerations:
- Contraindicated in patients with prior hypersensitivity to penicillins. Use with caution in patients sensitive to other β-lactams (e.g., cephalosporins), since partial cross-allergenicity exists.
- Obtain ordered specimen, and send for culture and sensitivity test prior to first antibiotic dose.
- Consider alternative antibiotic therapy if eosinophilia, drug fever or rash, arthralgia, hematuria, or unexplained rise in BUN and serum creatinine occur.
- Monitor electrolytes and renal, hepatic, and hematologic laboratory parameters during extended treatment periods.
- Use with caution in pregnant or nursing women.

- Low Na content: 1.98 mEq/g of drug.
- Increased activity against *P. aeruginosa*.

Potential Toxicities/Side Effects and the Nursing Process

I. POTENTIAL FOR INJURY related to HYPERSENSITIVITY REACTION

Defining Characteristics: Urticaria, pruritus, rash (maculopapular or erythematous), fever and chills, eosinophilia, myalgia, edema, erythema, angioedema, Stevens-Johnson syndrome, and exfoliative skin reactions occur in 5% of patients. Increased risk exists in individuals allergic to cephalosporin antibiotics.

Nursing Implications: Assess allergy to cephalosporin antibiotics and penicillin: if patient states "yes," determine actual response, e.g., "swollen lips = angioedema." If angioedema, patient SHOULD NOT receive drug. Discuss other patient responses with physician to determine whether drug should be given. Assess baseline skin condition, including integrity and allergy history to drugs. Instruct patient to report rash, itching, other skin changes. Teach patient skin care and symptomatic measures as appropriate. If skin rash develops, discuss drug discontinuance with physician. If rash progresses, drug should be discontinued, as fatal Stevens-Johnson syndrome may develop. Be prepared to treat severe acute hypersensitivity reactions with airway management, oxygen, epinephrine, corticosteroids, antihistamines as ordered.

II. ALTERATION IN NUTRITION, LESS THAN BODY REQUIREMENTS, related to GI SIDE EFFECTS

Defining Characteristics: Nausea, vomiting, diarrhea may occur; rarely, pseudomembranous colitis caused by *C. difficile* resistant to the antibiotic occurs. Rarely, transient increases in LFTs—AST, ALT, alk phos, bili—may occur.

Nursing Implications: Assess baseline nutritional status. Instruct patient to report GI disturbances. Administer and teach patient to self-administer antiemetics as needed and as ordered. Teach patient importance of nutritious diet, and suggest small, frequent, high-calorie, high-protein meals as appropriate. Assess baseline LFTs and monitor periodically during treatment. Discuss abnormalities and drug interruption with physician.

III. FUNGAL SUPERINFECTION related to REDISTRIBUTION OF ENDOGENOUS MICROORGANISMS

Defining Characteristics: Vaginal candidiasis, vaginitis may occur as endogenous bacteria are eliminated and normal fungal population expands.

Nursing Implications: Instruct female patient to report vaginal itching or discharge. Discuss appropriate antifungal treatment with physician. Teach perineal hygiene and symptomatic management.

IV. ALTERATIONS IN PROTECTIVE MECHANISMS (RARE) related to HEMATOLOGIC ABNORMALITIES

Defining Characteristics: Rarely, transient leukopenia, lymphocytosis, anemia, eosinophilia may occur. Prolonged PT, prolonged APTT, and hypoprothrombinemia have occurred rarely, especially in elderly or debilitated patients, or in individuals with vitamin K deficiency.

Nursing Implications: Assess baseline laboratory parameters, and monitor periodically during treatment. Assess patient for response to antibiotics. Discuss abnormalities with physician. Assess for signs/symptoms of bleeding.

V. ALTERATIONS IN SENSORY/PERCEPTUAL PATTERNS related to DIZZINESS, SOMNOLENCE

Defining Characteristics: Dizziness, headache, somnolence occur rarely. Neuromuscular irritability and seizures may occur with high drug serum levels.

Nursing Implications: Assess baseline neurologic function and comfort, and monitor during treatment. Instruct patient to report any changes. Discuss any abnormalities with physician. Institute seizure precautions.

VI. ALTERATIONS IN COMFORT related to LOCAL INJECTION IRRITATION

Defining Characteristics: Vein irritation (pain, erythema), phlebitis, and thrombophlebitis may occur at IV administration site.

Nursing Implications: Change IV sites q48h, and assess for signs/symptoms of phlebitis prior to each administration. Administer drug slowly. Apply warm packs to increase comfort. Discuss central line with patient and physician to facilitate administration.

VII. ALTERATION IN FLUID AND ELECTROLYTE BALANCE related to HYPOKALEMIA AND INCREASED SODIUM INTAKE

Defining Characteristics: Prolonged therapy may cause hypokalemia; also, drug is prepared as sodium salt. Frequent IV infusions increase fluid intake.

Nursing Implications: Assess baseline electrolytes, fluid balance, weight, and monitor throughout therapy. Monitor renal function studies, especially if patient has preexisting renal dysfunction.

Nursing Implications: Assess IV site prior to each dose for phlebitis or swelling, and change site at least q 48 hours. Administer dose slowly over 60 minutes. Apply heat to painful IV sites as ordered. Infuse via central line if possible.

IV. ALTERATION IN COMFORT

Defining Characteristics: Myalgias and arthralgias may occur.

Nursing Implications: Assess baseline T, VS, neurologic status, and comfort level and monitor q4–6 hours if patient in hospital. Teach patient self-care measures, including use of prescribed medications as well as use of heat or cold for myalgias and arthralgias.

V. ALTERATION IN HEPATIC FUNCTION

Defining Characteristics: Transient increases in serum BR, AST (SGOT), alk phos have occurred.

Nursing Implications: Assess baseline LFTs and monitor during therapy.

VI. FUNGAL SUPERINFECTION related to REDISTRIBUTION OF ENDOGENOUS MICROORGANISMS

Defining Characteristics: Vaginal moniliasis, vaginitis, and oral moniliasis may occur as endogenous bacteria are eliminated and normal fungal population expands.

Nursing Implications: Teach female patient to report vaginal itching or discharge. Discuss appropriate antifungal treatment with physician. Teach perineal hygiene and symptomatic management.

Drug: rifaximin (Xifaxan)

Class: anti-infective, antidiarrheals, gastrointestinal, rifamycin.

Mechanism of Action: Acts by binding to the beta-subunit of bacterial DNA-dependent RNA polymerase resulting in inhibition of bacterial RNA synthesis. Structural analog of rifampin. Active against Eschericha coli (enterotoxigenic and enteroaggregative strains).

Metabolism: Well absorbed following PO administration. Poorly absorbed from the gastrointestinal tract. Drug excreted unchanged in the feces.

Dosage/Range:

- Traveler's diarrhea: 200mg orally three times daily for 3 days.

Drug Preparation:

- Oral preparation.

Drug Administration:

- May be taken with or without food.

Drug Interactions:

- Rifaximin has not been shown to significantly affect intestinal or hepatic CYP3A4 activity.
- Rifaximin has not been shown to effect contraceptives containing ethinyl estradiol and norgestimate.

Lab Effects/Interference:

- None reported.

Special Considerations:

- Rifaximin was teratogenic in animal studies. There are no adequate and well-controlled studies in pregnant women.

Potential Toxicities/Side Effects and the Nursing Process

I. ALTERATION IN NUTRITION related to GI SIDE EFFECTS

Defining Characteristics: Gas, abdominal pain, nausea, vomiting, constipation, and pseudomembranous enterocolitis may occur.

Nursing Implications: Assess elimination and nutrition pattern, baseline and during therapy. Teach patient to report changes in diarrhea and/or abdominal pain immediately. Guaiac stool for occult blood, and notify physician if positive. Discuss management plan, including fluid and electrolyte replacement. Assess for nausea/vomiting, and administer prescribed antiemetic medications. Encourage small, frequent feedings as tolerated.

Drug: streptomycin sulfate

Class: Antibacterial; antimyobacterial (systemic).

Mechanism of Action: Synthetic antibiotic derived from *Streptomyces;* bactericidal, most probably by inhibition of protein synthesis; active against *Mycobacterium tuberculosis.* Active as second-line agent against sensitive microorganisms (including *Brucella, Nocardia, M. avium-intracellulare*).

Metabolism: Well absorbed following IM administration. Widely distributed into body fluids; 35% bound to plasma proteins. Readily crosses placenta and into breast milk. Drug excreted unchanged in the urine.

Dosage/Range:

- Antituberculosis regimen: Adults: 15 mg/kg/day or 1 g/day IM × 2–3 months, then 1 g 2–3 × per week. Elderly: dose may be limited to 10 mg/kg (or 750 mg). Desired serum peak is 5–25 μg/mL, and trough < 5 μg/mL.

Drug Preparation:

- Prepare a solution with concentration of ≤ 500 mg/mL, using sterile water for injection or 0.9% Sodium Chloride. Use within 2 days if kept at room temperature, or within 2 weeks if refrigerated at 2–8°C (36–46°F).

Drug Administration:

- Deep IM: into large muscle mass; rotate sites as sterile abscesses may form. DO NOT GIVE IV.

Drug Interactions:

- Increased risk of toxicity with other ototoxic drugs: acyclovir, other aminoglycosides, amphotericin B, bacitracin, cephalosporins, colistin, cisplatin, ethacrynic acid, furosemide, vancomycin.
- Potentiation of neuromuscular blockade when given concurrently with general anesthetics (succinylcholine, tubocurarine)—use cautiously, observe for signs/symptoms of respiratory depression.
- Synergism with extended-spectrum penicillins, but must be administered separately.

Lab Effects/Interference:

- Serum ALT, serum alk phos, serum AST, serum bili, and serum LDH values may be increased.
- BUN and serum creatinine concentrations may be increased.
- Serum Ca++, serum Mg++, serum K+, and serum Na+ concentrations may be decreased.

Special Considerations:

- Used parenterally with at least one other agent in treatment of tuberculosis.
- Use in pregnancy only if infection is life-threatening and no safer drug exists; drug crosses placenta and may cause fetal toxicity.

Potential Toxicities/Side Effects and the Nursing Process

I. ALTERATIONS IN SENSORY/PERCEPTUAL PATTERNS related to OTOTOXICITY

Defining Characteristics: Damage to eighth cranial nerve (auditory) may result in dizziness, nystagmus, vertigo, ataxia (vestibular damage), and more commonly, tinnitus, roaring sound in ears, and impaired hearing (auditory damage). Hearing loss usually begins with high-frequency loss, followed by clinical hearing loss, then permanent hearing loss if damage continues. Increased risk in elderly or renally impaired patients.

Nursing Implications: Assess baseline hearing (ability to hear spoken voice) and continue during therapy. Teach patient potential side effects, and instruct patient to report any hearing/perceptual problems (e.g., tinnitus, vertigo, decreased hearing). Discuss drug discontinuance and audiogram with physician to confirm hearing dysfunction if symptoms arise. Assess for increased risk if given concurrently with other ototoxic medications (e.g., cisplatin, furosemide).

II. ALTERATION IN URINARY ELIMINATION related to NEPHROTOXICITY

Defining Characteristics: Risk of nephrotoxicity is less than with other aminoglycosides. Renal damage characterized by tubular necrosis with increased serum BUN, creatinine; decreased urine creatinine clearance and specific gravity; proteinuria and casts in urine. Azotemia usually not associated with oliguria. Rarely, electrolyte wasting with hypomagnesemia, hypocalcemia, and hypokalemia may occur. Renal dysfunction is usually reversible after drug discontinuance. Increased risk exists in elderly and if there is preexisting renal dysfunction. Risk is low in well-hydrated patients with normal renal function when normal doses are given.

Nursing Implications: Assess baseline renal function and electrolytes, and monitor periodically during therapy. Discuss any abnormalities with physician, as drug should be dose-reduced or discontinued if renal dysfunction develops. Assess baseline total body fluid balance, weight, and monitor periodically during antibiotic therapy. Monitor hydration status to keep patient well hydrated. Assess drug peak and trough levels as ordered so that drug dosage is correctly titrated. Increased risk of toxicity if peak serum concentration >40 μg/mL. Draw blood for peak drug concentration 30 minutes after end of 30-minute infusion or at the end of a 60-minute infusion; draw trough immediately before next dose.

III. ALTERATIONS IN SENSORY/PERCEPTUAL PATTERNS related to CNS EFFECTS, NEUROMUSCULAR BLOCKADE

Defining Characteristics: Headache, tremor, lethargy may occur. Peripheral neuropathy or encephalopathy (numbness, skin tingling, muscle twitching) may occur rarely. Neuromuscular blockade is dose-related, self-limiting, and uncommon. Risk is greater with topical application or when drug is administered to patient with neuromuscular disease (myasthenia gravis) or hypocalcemia.

Nursing Implications: Assess baseline neurologic status. Assess coexisting risk factors, neuromuscular blockade medications. Teach patient about side effects and instruct to report headache, tremor, lethargy. Observe for respiratory depression. If signs/symptoms arise, discuss drug discontinuance with physician.

IV. POTENTIAL FOR INJURY related to HYPERSENSITIVITY

Defining Characteristics: Rash, urticaria, pruritus, fever, eosinophilia have occurred rarely. CROSS-SENSITIVITY between AMINOGLYCOSIDES existsHandling of drug can cause sensitization to the drug.

Nursing Implications: Assess for drug allergies to any aminoglycoside—amikacin, gentamicin, kanamycin, neomycin, netilmicin, streptomycin, tobramycin—prior to drug administration. Instruct patient to report any allergic reactions. Assess for signs/symptoms of allergic reaction after drug dose. Take special care in preparing drug or wear gloves.

V. ALTERATION IN NUTRITION, LESS THAN BODY REQUIREMENTS, related to GI SIDE EFFECTS

Defining Characteristics: Nausea, vomiting, anorexia have occurred rarely. Also, transient hepatomegaly with increased LFTs—AST, ALT, LDH, alk phos—has occurred.

Nursing Implications: Assess baseline nutritional status, preexisting nausea/vomiting, anorexia. Assess baseline LFTs and monitor periodically during treatment. Instruct patient to report side effects. Provide symptomatic interventions if side effects occur; discuss with physician use of alternative drug(s).

VI. POTENTIAL FOR FATIGUE, INFECTION, AND BLEEDING related to BONE MARROW INJURY

Defining Characteristics: Anemia, leukopenia, granulocytopenia, and thrombocytopenia may occur. Also, patients receiving antibiotics are at risk for overgrowth of nonsusceptible microorganisms, such as fungi (superinfection). Rare.

Nursing Implications: Assess baseline CBC, differential, and monitor periodically during treatment. Instruct patient to report signs/symptoms of fatigue, infection, or bleeding immediately. Assess for signs/symptoms of superinfection. Discuss any adverse effects with physician.

VII. ALTERATION IN SKIN INTEGRITY related to IRRITATION AT INJECTION SITE, EXFOLIATIVE DERMATITIS

Defining Characteristics: Exfoliative dermatitis rarely occurs; may develop pain, irritation, and sterile abscesses at injection site.

Nursing Implications: Assess skin integrity and presence of lesions. Monitor for changes during treatment, and instruct patient to report them. Rotate injection sites and give injection deeply into large muscle mass, e.g., upper outer quadrant of buttock. Administer solutions of ≤ 500 mg/mL.

Drug: telithromycin (Ketek)

Class: Antimicrobial agent. This antibiotic is a new structural class called ketolides.

Mechanism of Action: Similar to that of macrolides and is related to the 50S-ribosomal subunit binding with inhibition of bacterial protein synthesis. Telithromycin appears to have greater affinity for the ribosomal binding site than macrolides. Demonstrated efficacy against *Staphylococcus aureus, Streptococcus aureus, Streptococcus pheumoniae, Haemophilus influenzae, Moraxella catarrhalis, Chlamydia pneumoniae*, and *Mycoplasma pneumoniae.*

Metabolism: Absorbed from the GI tract. Eliminated by multiple pathways: 7% of the dose is excreted unchanged by biliary and/or intestinal secretion; 13% of the dose is excreted unchanged in urine; and 37% of the dose is metabolized by the liver. May accumulate in patients with severe hepatic disease.

Dosage/Range:

- Adult: Oral: 800 mg daily for 5–10 days. Duration of therapy depends on indication. Drug dose should be reduced or adjusted in patients with hepatic or renal insufficiency

Drug Preparation/Administration:

- Oral: Administration of telithromycin with food had no significant effect on extent or rate of oral absorption in healthy subjects.

Drug Interactions:

- Class I, IA, & III Anti-arrhythmic Agents: Concomitant use is contraindicated as it may lead to QT prolongation. Serum levels may be increased.
- CYP 3A4 inhibitors: Itraconazole and Ketoconazole: Increases telithromycin levels and AUC by ~54% and 95%, respectively.
- CYP3A4 substrates: Cisapride, Simvastin, and Midazolam: Increases serum concentration of cisapride by 95%; significantly increases serum concentration of simvastin and midazolam. These drugs SHOULD NOT be used when a patient is taking telithromycin.
- CYP 2D6 substrates: Metoprolol: Increases serum concentrations. Administer with caution. Rifampin: Decreases serum concentrations. Digoxin: Increases serum concentration. Theophylline: Increases serum concentrations. Take 1 hour apart to decrease the gastrointestinal side effects. Sotalol: Decreases serum concentrations.

Lab Effects/Interference:

- There are no reported drug-laboratory test interactions. SGPT, alk phos, Amylase, SGOT, and bilirubin: serum concentrations may be increased in patients with pre-existing hepatic disease.

Special Considerations:

- Avoid use in pregnant or lactating women.
- Contraindicated in patients with known hypersensitivity.
- Obtain ordered specimen and send for culture and sensitivity prior to first antibiotic dose.

Potential Toxicities/Side Effects and the Nursing Process

I. ALTERATION IN NUTRITION related to GI SIDE EFFECTS

Defining Characteristics: Anorexia, nausea, vomiting, diarrhea, glossitis, dysphagia, gastroenteritis, gastritis, constipation.

Nursing Implications: Assess baseline nutritional status. Assess for and teach patient to report any symptoms. Administer and teach patient self-administration of prescribed antiemetic or antidiarrheal medication as appropriate.

II. ALTERATION IN PROTECTIVE MECHANISMS

Defining Characteristics: Prolonged PT, prolonged INR, cardiac arrhythmias including atrial arrhythmias, bradycardia, and hypotension.

Nursing Implications: Monitor and teach patient about potential side effects and to report abnormalities such as fainting & dizziness.

III. POTENTIAL FOR INJURY related to VISUAL DISTURBANCES

Defining Characteristics: Blurred vision and difficulty focusing.

Nursing Implications: Assess baseline visual and neurologic status. Teach patient to report any changes in vision. If signs/symptoms arise, discuss discontinuance with physician, and institute supportive measures.

IV. FUNGAL SUPERINFECTION related to REDISTRIBUTION OF ENDOGENOUS MICROORGANISMS

Defining Characteristics: Vaginal moniliasis, vaginitis may occur as endogenous bacteria are eliminated and normal fungal population expands.

Nursing Implications: Teach female patient to report vaginal itching or discharge. Discuss appropriate antifungal treatment with physician. Teach perineal hygiene and symptom management.

Drug: ticarcillin disodium (Ticar); combined with clavulanate potassium (Timentin)

Class: Antibacterial (systemic) (extended spectrum penicillin).

Mechanism of Action: Semisynthetic antibiotic prepared from fungus *Penicillium*. Contains β-lactam ring and is bactericidal by inhibiting cell wall synthesis. Active against most gram-positive (except penicillinase-producing strains) and most gram-negative bacilli. Used in the treatment of serious gram-negative infections, especially *P. aeruginosa*–related infections of lower respiratory tract, urinary tract, and skin. When combined with clavulanate potassium, the drug is protected from breakdown by bacterial β-lactamase enzymes, thus keeping therapeutic antibiotic serum levels.

Metabolism: Poorly absorbed from GI tract, so must be given parenterally. Widely distributed in body tissues and fluids. Crosses placenta and is excreted in breast milk. Excreted via urine and bile.

Dosage/Range:

- IV dosing preferred but drug can be given IM or IV.

Adult:

Ticarcillin disodium:

- 3 g q4–6h (200–300 mg/kg/day in divided doses).
- Dosage modification required if renal insufficiency exists; refer to manufacturer's package insert.

Timentin:

- 3 g ticarcillin plus 0.1 g clavulanic acid (3.1 g) IV q4–6h × 10–14 days if weight < 60 kg: 200–300 mg ticarcillin/kg/d in divided doses q4–6h IV.

Drug Preparation/Administration:

- IV: reconstitute each gram with 4 mL 0.9% Sodium Chloride or 5% Dextrose injection. Further dilute in 50–100 mL IV solution and infuse over 30 minutes to 2 hours.
- IM: reconstitute each gram with 2 mL sterile water for injection or 1% lidocaine HCl (without epinephrine). Ensure patient is NOT ALLERGIC to lidocaine. Inject drug deep IM in large muscle mass (e.g., gluteus maximus). Maximum 2 g at one site.

Drug Interactions:

- Aminoglycosides: synergism.
- Aminoglycosides (e.g., gentamicin): incompatible when mixed together; administer at separate sites at different times. Also, penicillinase-resistant penicillins can inactivate aminoglycoside serum samples from patients receiving both drugs.
- Probenecid: increased serum level of penicillin; may be coadministered to exert this effect.

- Clavulanic acid (β-lactamase inhibitor): Synergistic bactericial effect.

Lab Effects/Interference:

Major clinical significance:

- Urine glucose: high urinary concentrations of a penicillin may produce false-positive or falsely elevated test results with copper sulfate tests (Benedict's, Clinitest, or Fehling's); glucose enzymatic tests (Clinistix or Testape) are not affected.
- PTT and PT: an increase has been associated with ticarcillin.

Clinical significance:

- Coombs' (direct antiglobulin) test: false-positive result may occur during therapy with any penicillin.
- Urine protein: high urinary concentrations of ticarcillin may produce false-positive protein reactions (pseudoproteinuria) with the sulfosalicylic acid and boiling test; bromophenol blue reagent test strips (Multistix) are reportedly unaffected.
- ALT, alk phos, AST, serum LDH values may be increased.
- Serum bili: an increase has been associated with ticarcillin.
- BUN and serum creatinine: increased concentrations have been associated with ticarcillin.
- Serum K+: hypokalemia may occur following administration of parenteral ticarcillin, which may act as a non-reabsorbable anion in the distal tubules; this may cause an increase in pH and result in increased urinary potassium loss. The risk of hypokalemia increases with use of larger doses.
- WBC: leukopenia or neutropenia is associated with the use of all penicillins; the effect is more likely to occur with prolonged therapy and severe hepatic function impairment

Special Considerations:

- Contraindicated in patients with prior hypersensitivity to penicillins. Use with caution in patients sensitive to other β-lactams (e.g., cephalosporins) since partial cross-allergenicity exists.
- Obtain ordered specimen, and send for culture and sensitivity test prior to first antibiotic dose.
- Consider alternative antibiotic therapy if eosinophilia, drug fever or rash, arthralgia, hematuria, or unexplained rise in BUN and serum creatinine occur.
- Monitor electrolytes and renal, hepatic, and hematologic laboratory parameters during extended treatment periods.
- Use with caution in pregnant or nursing women.
- Decreased incidence of hypokalemia, and less salt load, than other extended spectrum penicillins.

Potential Toxicities/Side Effects and the Nursing Process

I. POTENTIAL FOR INJURY related to HYPERSENSITIVITY REACTION

Defining Characteristics: Urticaria, pruritus, rash (maculopapular or erythematous), fever and chills, eosinophilia, myalgia, edema, erythema, angioedema, Stevens-Johnson syndrome, and exfoliative skin reactions occur in 5% of patients. Increased risk in individuals allergic to cephalosporin antibiotics.

Nursing Implications: Assess allergy to cephalosporin antibiotics and penicillin: if patient states "yes," determine actual response, e.g., "swollen lips = angioedema." If angioedema, patient SHOULD NOT receive drug. Discuss other patient responses with physician to determine whether drug should be given. Assess baseline skin condition, including integrity and allergy history to drugs. Instruct patient to report rash, itching, other skin changes. Teach patient skin care and symptomatic measures as appropriate. If skin rash develops, discuss drug discontinuance with physician. If rash progresses, drug should be discontinued, as fatal Stevens-Johnson syndrome may develop. Be prepared to treat severe acute hypersensitivity reactions with airway management, oxygen, epinephrine, corticosteroids, antihistamines as ordered.

II. ALTERATION IN NUTRITION, LESS THAN BODY REQUIREMENTS, related to GI SIDE EFFECTS

Defining Characteristics: Nausea, vomiting, diarrhea may occur; rarely, pseudomembranous colitis caused by *C. difficile* resistant to the antibiotic occurs. Rarely, transient increases in LFTs—AST, ALT, alk phos, bili—may occur.

Nursing Implications: Assess baseline nutritional status. Instruct patient to report GI disturbances. Administer and teach patient to self-administer antiemetics, antidiarrheals as needed and as ordered. Teach patient importance of nutritious diet, and suggest small, frequent, high-calorie, high-protein meals as appropriate. Assess baseline LFTs, and monitor periodically during treatment. Discuss abnormalities and drug interruption with physician.

III. FUNGAL SUPERINFECTION related to REDISTRIBUTION OF ENDOGENOUS MICROORGANISMS

Defining Characteristics: Vaginal candidiasis, vaginitis may occur as endogenous bacteria are eliminated, and normal fungal population expands.

Nursing Implications: Instruct female patient to report vaginal itching or discharge. Discuss appropriate antifungal treatment with physician. Teach perineal hygiene and symptomatic management.

IV. ALTERATIONS IN PROTECTIVE MECHANISMS (RARE) related to TRANSIENT LEUKOPENIA

Defining Characteristics: Rarely, transient leukopenia, lymphocytosis, anemia, eosinophilia may occur. Prolonged PT, prolonged APTT, and hypoprothrombinemia have occurred rarely, especially in elderly or debilitated patients, or in individuals with vitamin K deficiency.

Nursing Implications: Assess baseline laboratory parameters, and monitor periodically during treatment. Assess patient for response to antibiotics. Discuss abnormalities with physician. Assess for signs/symptoms of bleeding.

V. ALTERATIONS IN SENSORY/PERCEPTUAL PATTERNS related to DIZZINESS, SOMNOLENCE

Defining Characteristics: Dizziness, headache, somnolence occur rarely. Neuromuscular irritability and seizures may occur with high drug serum levels.

Nursing Implications: Assess baseline neurologic function and comfort, and monitor during treatment. Instruct patient to report any changes. Discuss any abnormalities with physician. Institute seizure precautions.

VI. ALTERATIONS IN COMFORT related to LOCAL INJECTION IRRITATION

Defining Characteristics: Vein irritation (pain, erythema), phlebitis, and thrombophlebitis may occur at IV administration site.

Nursing Implications: Change IV sites q48h, and assess for signs/symptoms of phlebitis prior to each administration. Administer drug slowly. Apply warm packs to increase comfort. Discuss central line with patient and physician to facilitate administration.

VII. ALTERATION IN FLUID AND ELECTROLYTE BALANCE related to HYPOKALEMIA AND INCREASED SODIUM INTAKE

Defining Characteristics: Prolonged therapy may cause hypokalemia; also, drug is prepared as sodium salt. Frequent IV infusions increase fluid intake.

Nursing Implications: Assess baseline electrolytes, fluid balance, weight, and monitor throughout therapy. Monitor renal function studies, especially if patient has preexisting renal dysfunction.

Drug: tigecycline (Tygacil)

Class: Antimicrobial agent. This antibiotic is the first in a new class called glycylcyclines. This novel IV antibiotic has a broad spectrum of antimicrobial activity, including activity against the drug-resistant bacteria methicillin-resistant Staphylococcus aureus (MRSA).

Mechanism of Action: Inhibits protein transplation in bacteria by binding to the 30Sribosomal subunit and blocking entry of amino-acyl tRNA molecules into the A site of the ribosome. Demonstrated efficacy against methicillin-susceptible and -resistant Staphylococcus aureus (MRSA), Escherichia coli, Enterococcus faecalis (vancomycin-resistant isolates), Streptococcus anginosus, Streptococcus intermedius, and Streptococcus constellatus, Bacteroides fragilis, Bacteroides thetaiotaomicron, Bacteroides uniformis, Bacteroides vulgatus, Clostridium perfringens, and Peptostreptococcus micros.

Metabolism: Is not extensively metabolized. Eliminated by multiple pathways: 7% of the dose is excreted unchanged by biliary and/or intestinal secretion; 59% of the dose is excreted unchanged in bile/feces and 33% of the dose is excreted in the urine. May accumulate in patients with severe hepatic disease.

Dosage/Range:

Adult:

Initial dose 100 mg IV, followed by 50 mg every 12 hours. Duration of therapy depends on indication. Drug dose should be reduced or adjusted in patients with severe hepatic insufficiency.

Drug Preparation/Administration:

- Intravenous injection should be administered over 30–60 minutes every 12 hours.

Drug Interactions:

- Monitor prothrombin time if administered with warfarin.
- Concurrent use of antibacterial drugs with oral contraceptives may render the oral contraceptives less effective.

Lab Effects/Interference:

- There are no reported drug-laboratory test interactions. SGPT, alk phos, Amylase, SGOT, and bilirubin: serum concentrations may be increased in patients with pre-existing hepatic disease.

Special Considerations:

- Avoid use in pregnant or lactating women.
- Contraindicated in patients with known hypersensitivity.
- Obtain ordered specimen and send for culture and sensitivity prior to first antibiotic dose.

Potential Toxicities/Side Effects and the Nursing Process

I. ALTERATION IN NUTRITION related to GI SIDE EFFECTS

Defining Characteristics: Anorexia, nausea, vomiting, diarrhea, glossitis, dysphagia, gastroenteritis, gastritis, constipation.

Nursing Implications: Assess baseline nutritional status. Assess for and teach patient to report any symptoms. Administer and teach patient self-administration of prescribed antiemetic or antidiarrheal medication as appropriate.

II. POTENTIAL FOR INJURY related to HYPERSENSITIVITY REACTION

Defining Characteristics: Urticaria, pruritus, rash (maculopapular or erythematous), fever and chills, eosinophilia, myalgia, edema, erythema, angioedema, Stevens-Johnson syndrome, and exfoliative skin reactions occur.

Nursing Implications: Assess allergy to antibiotics: if patient states "yes," determine actual response, e.g., "swollen lips = angioedema." If angioedema, patient SHOULD NOT receive drug. Discuss other patient responses with physician to determine whether drug should be given. Assess baseline skin condition, including integrity and allergy history to drugs. Instruct patient to report rash, itching, and other skin changes. Teach patient skin care and symptomatic measures as appropriate. If skin rash develops, discuss drug discontinuance with physician. If rash progresses, drug should be discontinued, as fatal Stevens-Johnson syndrome may develop. Be prepared to treat severe acute hypersensitivity reactions with airway management, oxygen, epinephrine, corticosteroids, and antihistamines as ordered.

III. ALTERATIONS IN COMFORT related to LOCAL INJECTION IRRITATION

Defining Characteristics: Vein irritation (pain, erythema), phlebitis, and thrombophlebitis may occur at IV administration site.

Nursing Implications: Change IV sites q48h, and assess for signs/symptoms of phlebitis prior to each administration. Administer drug slowly. Apply warm packs to increase comfort. Discuss central line with patient and physician to facilitate administration.

IV. FUNGAL SUPERINFECTION related to REDISTRIBUTION OF ENDOGENOUS MICROORGANISMS

Defining Characteristics: Vaginal moniliasis, vaginitis may occur as endogenous bacteria are eliminated and normal fungal population expands.

Nursing Implications: Teach female patient to report vaginal itching or discharge. Discuss appropriate antifungal treatment with physician. Teach perineal hygiene and symptom management.

Drug: tobramycin sulfate (Nebcin)

Class: Aminoglycoside antibacterial (systemic).

Mechanism of Action: Synthetic antibiotic derived from *Streptomyces;* bactericidal, most probably by inhibition of protein synthesis. Active against aerobic microorganisms: many sensitive gram-negative (including *Acinetobacter, Citrobacter, Enterobacter, E. coli, Klebsiella, Proteus, Pseudomonas, Salmonella, Serratia,* and *Shigella*) and some sensitive gram-positive organisms (*S. aureus* and *S. epidermidis*). Over time, bacterial resistance may develop, either naturally or acquired.

Metabolism: Well absorbed following parenteral administration, but variability in absorption after IM injection (peak serum level 0.5–2 hours, duration 8–12 hours). Widely distributed into body fluids. Minimally protein-bound. Readily crosses placenta and into breast milk. Drug excreted unchanged in the urine.

Dosage/Range:
- 3 mg/kg/day given in equally divided doses q8h.
- Desired peak serum concentration is 4–10 μg/mL, and trough serum concentration is 1–2 μg/mL.
- May use 5–6 mg/kg/day in three equally divided doses to treat life-threatening infections.
- If loading dose required, 2 mg/kg; usual dosing q8h, but q12 or q24 dosing may also be used.
- DOSE-REDUCE IF RENAL IMPAIRMENT.

Drug Preparation:
- Store unreconstituted vials at 15–30°C (59–86°F).
- Store injections at 25°C (77°F).
- Store reconstituted solution (using sterile water for injection, with final concentration 40 mg/mL) at room temperature (stable 24 hours) or in refrigerator at 2–8°C (36–46°F) (stable 96 hours).

Drug Administration:
- IV: further dilute by adding dose to 50–100 mL in 0.9% Sodium Chloride and administer over 30–60 minutes.

Drug Interactions:

- Increased risk of toxicity with other ototoxic drugs: acyclovir, other aminoglycosides, amphotericin B, bacitracin, cephalosporins, colistin, cisplatin, ethacrynic acid, furosemide, vancomycin.
- Potentiation of neuromuscular blockade when given concurrently with general anesthetics (succinylcholine, tubocurarine); use cautiously; observe for signs/symptoms of respiratory depression.
- Synergism with extended-spectrum penicillins, but must be administered separately.

Lab Effects/Interference:

- Serum ALT, serum alk phos, serum AST, serum bili, and serum LDH values may be increased.
- BUN and serum creatinine concentrations may be increased.
- Serum Ca++, serum Mg++, serum K+, and serum Na+ concentrations may be decreased.

Special Considerations:

- Used as first-line treatment in short-term treatment of serious gram-negative infections (e.g., septicemia, respiratory tract infections).
- Use against gram-positive organisms only as second-line treatment.
- Use in pregnancy only if infection is life-threatening and no safer drug exists; drug crosses placenta and may cause fetal toxicity.

Potential Toxicities/Side Effects and the Nursing Process

I. ALTERATIONS IN SENSORY/PERCEPTUAL PATTERNS related to OTOTOXICITY

Defining Characteristics: Damage to eighth cranial nerve (auditory) may result in dizziness, nystagmus, vertigo, ataxia (vestibular damage), and more commonly, tinnitus, roaring sound in ears, and impaired hearing (auditory damage). Hearing loss usually begins with high-frequency loss, followed by clinical hearing loss, then permanent hearing loss if damage continues. Increased risk in elderly or renally impaired patients.

Nursing Implications: Assess baseline hearing (ability to hear spoken voice) and continue during therapy. Teach patient potential side effects, and instruct patient to report any hearing/perceptual problems (e.g., tinnitus, vertigo, decreased hearing). Discuss drug discontinuance and audiogram with physician to confirm hearing dysfunction if symptoms arise. Assess for increased risk if given concurrently with other ototoxic medications (e.g., cisplatin, furosemide).

II. ALTERATION IN URINARY ELIMINATION related to NEPHROTOXICITY

Defining Characteristics: Risk of nephrotoxicity is less than with other aminoglycosides. Renal damage characterized by tubular necrosis with increased serum BUN, creatinine; decreased urine creatinine clearance and specific gravity; proteinuria and casts in urine. Azotemia usually not associated with oliguria. Rarely, electrolyte wasting with hypomagnesemia, hypocalcemia, and hypokalemia may occur. Renal dysfunction is usually reversible after drug discontinuance. Increased risk exists in elderly and if there is preexisting renal dysfunction. Risk is low in well-hydrated patients with normal renal function when normal doses given.

Nursing Implications: Assess baseline renal function and electrolytes, and monitor periodically during therapy. Discuss any abnormalities with physician, as drug should be dose-reduced or discontinued if renal dysfunction develops. Assess baseline total body fluid balance, weight, and monitor periodically during antibiotic therapy. Monitor hydration status to keep patient well hydrated. Assess drug peak and trough levels as ordered so that drug dosage is correctly titrated. Increased risk of toxicity if peak serum concentration > 10–12 μg/mL. Draw blood for peak drug concentration 30 minutes after end of 30-minute infusion or at the end of a 60-minute infusion; draw trough immediately before next dose.

III. ALTERATIONS IN SENSORY/PERCEPTUAL PATTERNS related to CNS EFFECTS, NEUROMUSCULAR BLOCKADE

Defining Characteristics: Headache, tremor, lethargy may occur. Peripheral neuropathy or encephalopathy (numbness, skin tingling, muscle twitching) may occur rarely. Neuromuscular blockade is dose-related, self-limiting, and uncommon. Risk is greater with topical application or when drug is administered to patient with neuromuscular disease (myasthenia gravis) or hypocalcemia.

Nursing Implications: Assess baseline neurologic status. Assess coexisting risk factors, neuromuscular blockade medications. Teach patient about side effects, and instruct to report headache, tremor, lethargy. Observe for respiratory depression. If signs/symptoms arise, discuss drug discontinuance with physician.

IV. POTENTIAL FOR INJURY related to HYPERSENSITIVITY

Defining Characteristics: Rash, urticaria, pruritus, fever, eosinophilia have occurred rarely. CROSS-SENSITIVITY between AMINOGLYCOSIDES exists!

Nursing Implications: Assess for drug allergies to any aminoglycoside—amikacin, gentamicin, kanamycin, neomycin, netilmicin, streptomycin, tobramycin—prior to drug administration. Instruct patient to report any allergic reactions. Assess for signs/symptoms of allergic reaction after drug dose.

V. ALTERATION IN NUTRITION, LESS THAN BODY REQUIREMENTS, related to GI SIDE EFFECTS

Defining Characteristics: Nausea, vomiting, anorexia have occurred rarely. Also, transient hepatomegaly with increased LFTs—AST, ALT, LDH, alk phos—has occurred.

Nursing Implications: Assess baseline nutritional status, preexisting nausea/vomiting, anorexia. Assess baseline LFTs and monitor periodically during treatment. Instruct patient to report side effects. Provide symptomatic interventions if side effects occur; discuss with physician use of alternative drug(s).

VI. POTENTIAL FOR FATIGUE, INFECTION, AND BLEEDING related to BONE MARROW INJURY

Defining Characteristics: Anemia, leukopenia, granulocytopenia, and thrombocytopenia may occur. Also, patients receiving antibiotics are at risk for overgrowth of nonsusceptible microorganisms, such as fungi (superinfection). Rare.

Nursing Implications: Assess baseline CBC, differential, and monitor periodically during treatment. Instruct patient to report signs/symptoms of fatigue, infection, or bleeding immediately. Assess for signs/symptoms of superinfection. Discuss any adverse effects with physician.

Drug: vancomycin hydrochloride (Vancocin)

Class: Antibacterial (systemic).

Mechanism of Action: Derived from cultures of *Streptomyces orientalis;* drug is bactericidal by binding to bacterial cell wall, thus blocking protein polymerization and cell wall synthesis. Also damages cell membrane and acts at a different site than the penicillins. Bacteriostatic for enterococci. Active against many gram-positive organisms (staphylococci, group A β-hemolytic streptococci, *S. pneumoniae, C. difficile,* enterococci, *Corynebacterium, Clostridium*).

Metabolism: Not well absorbed from the GI tract—except in those patients with colitis—especially if patient has renal compromise. Effective when administered IV and is widely distributed in body tissues and fluid, including bile. Crosses placenta; unknown whether drug is excreted in breast milk;

52–60% bound to plasma proteins. IV dose excreted primarily by kidneys and, to a small degree, in bile; oral dose excreted in feces.

Dosage/Range:

Adult:

- Oral (for use in pseudomembranous colitis): capsules or powder: 0.5–1 g/day in four divided doses × 7–10 days.
- IV: 500 mg or 1 g q12h.
- Desired peak serum concentration is 20 to 40 mg/mL; and trough serum concentration is 5–15 μg/ml.
- Dose reduction necessary if renal dysfunction; see manufacturer's package insert.

Drug Preparation/Administration:

- Oral dose for treatment of *C. difficile* pseudomembranous colitis. Oral dose not recommended for treating systemic infections.
- Reconstituted by adding 10 mL of sterile water to 500-mg vial (20 mL to 1-g vial). Further dilute in at least 100 mL 0.9% Sodium Chloride or 5% Dextrose in water, and infuse over 1 hour (central line).
- For peripheral lines, further dilution in 250 mL is recommended.
- Causes tissue necrosis if given IM; DO NOT ADMINISTER IM.

Drug Interactions:

- Nephrotoxic drugs (aminoglycoside antibiotics, amphotericin B, cisplatin, colistin): increased risk of nephrotoxicity; avoid concurrent use if possible.

Lab Effects/Interference:

- BUN concentrations may be increased.

Special Considerations:

- Use cautiously in patients with renal dysfunction.
- DO NOT USE in patients with hearing loss—or use at reduced doses if necessary in life-threatening infections.
- Contraindicated in patients with known hypersensitivity.
- Obtain ordered specimen for culture and sensitivity prior to first antibiotic dose.
- Use with caution in pregnancy, as fetal effects are unknown, and in lactating mothers, as drug may be excreted in breast milk.

Potential Toxicities/Side Effects and the Nursing Process

I. ALTERATIONS IN SENSORY PERCEPTUAL PATTERNS related to OTOTOXICITY

Defining Characteristics: IV drug appears to damage eighth cranial nerve (auditory). First symptom of ototoxicity is tinnitus and may progress to deafness; may also be associated with vertigo and dizziness (vestibular branch). High risk exists in patients with renal impairment who are receiving concurrent ototoxic drugs (e.g., cisplatin) or prolonged therapy, or those whose age > 60 years old.

Nursing Implications: Assess baseline hearing (ability to hear spoken voice) or audiogram if patient is at high risk—both at baseline and throughout therapy. Monitor serum drug concentrations during therapy if at high risk. Teach patient potential side effects, and instruct patient to report any hearing/perceptual problems (e.g., tinnitus, decreased hearing, vertigo). Discuss drug discontinuance with physician if symptoms arise.

II. ALTERATION IN URINARY ELIMINATION related to NEPHROTOXICITY

Defining Characteristics: Renal damage may occur, characterized by transient increases in serum BUN or creatinine, hyaline casts, and albuminuria. May cause acute interstitial nephritis. High risk in patients with renal impairment who are receiving concurrent nephrotoxic drugs (e.g., cisplatin) or prolonged therapy, or those whose age > 60 years.

Nursing Implications: Assess baseline renal function and electrolytes, and monitor periodically during therapy. Discuss any abnormalities with physician, as drug should be dose-reduced or discontinued if renal dysfunction develops. Assess baseline hydration status, including urinary output, total body balance, daily weights; keep patient well hydrated.

III. ALTERATION IN COMFORT related to LOCAL TISSUE EFFECTS

Defining Characteristics: Vesicant if given IM (causing tissue necrosis). Irritating to veins when given IV, causing pain and thrombophlebitis.

Nursing Implications: Administer drug IV *NOT* IM. Assess IV site prior to each dose and at completion of dose; instruct patient to report pain or burning; change IV site if irritation, phlebitis develop. Change site at least q48h and consider central line for prolonged therapy. AVOID EXTRAVASATION.

IV. ALTERATION IN CARDIAC OUTPUT related to RAPID IV INFUSION

Defining Characteristics: Rapid IV administration may cause histamine release and "red-neck" syndrome, characterized by rapid onset of hypotension, flushing, and erythematous or maculopapular rash of neck, face, chest. May be associated with wheezing, dyspnea, angioedema, urticaria, pruritus. Rarely, seizures and cardiac arrest may occur. Syndrome occurs minutes after beginning infusion, but may occur at end; usually resolves spontaneously over 2+

hours, but may require antihistamines, corticosteroids, or IV fluids. Rare when drug is administered over 1 hour.

Nursing Implications: Monitor temperature, VS at baseline, 5 minutes into IV administration, and at end of infusion, at least with the initial dose; infuse over at least 1 hour, using infusion controller if necessary. Observe patient during first 5 minutes, and instruct patient to report rash, wheezing, itching immediately. If reaction occurs, stop infusion, assess VS, and notify physician. Patient may be treated with antihistamine or IV fluids, or both. Completion of dose and subsequent doses may be ordered at very slow rate. Document episode in medical record and update care plan/medication sheet to reflect change in drug administration.

V. INJURY related to BONE MARROW SUPPRESSION

Defining Characteristics: Rarely, leukopenia, thrombocytopenia, agranulocytosis may occur, especially with cumulative doses > 25 g.

Nursing Implications: Monitor baseline and periodic WBC, differential, platelet count, especially if receiving other bone marrow-suppressive drugs. Discuss abnormalities with physician.

VI. INFECTION related to OVERGROWTH OF NONSUSCEPTIBLE MICROORGANISMS

Defining Characteristics: Normal microflora populations altered by drug, with possible overgrowth by nonsusceptible microorganisms, i.e., fungi, gram-negative bacteria.

Nursing Implications: Assess for signs/symptoms of other infections of skin, mucous membranes. Instruct patient to report signs/symptoms. Discuss further antimicrobial therapy with physician.

ANTIFUNGALS

Drug: amphotericin B (deoxycholate) (Fungizone); amphotericin B lipid complex (Abelcet); amphotericin B cholesteryl sulfate complex (Amphotec); liposomal amphotericin B (AmBisome)

Class: Antifungal (systemic); antiprotozoal.

Mechanism of Action: Produced by *Streptomyces;* binds to sterol molecule in fungal membrane, causing disruption and leakage of intracellular ions. Is fungistatic (prevents replication at normal doses) and fungicidal (kills fungi at high doses). Active against systemic fungal infections (*Aspergillus, Candida,*

II. ALTERATION IN URINARY ELIMINATION related to NEPHROTOXICITY

Defining Characteristics: 80% incidence; multiple toxic effects (vasoconstriction, lytic action on renal tubular cell membranes, calcium deposits in distal nephron); hypokalemia may precede azotemia with increased BUN and creatinine, decreased creatinine clearance, and increased excretion of K+, uric acid, and protein. Renal tubular acidosis may occur. Renal impairment usually diminishes after drug discontinuance, but some degree of impairment may be permanent.

Nursing Implications: Assess baseline renal function and electrolytes; monitor every other day during dosage escalation, then at least weekly. Discuss any abnormalities with physician. Drug should be dose-reduced if renal dysfunction develops. Slowly administer initial test dose, then gradually increase doses over first week. Assess fluid status and total body balance closely to keep patient well hydrated. Assess for signs/symptoms of hypokalemia: arthralgia, myalgia, muscle weakness. Administer potassium and magnesium replacements as ordered.

III. FATIGUE related to ANEMIA

Defining Characteristics: High incidence of reversible normocytic, normochromic anemia that rarely requires transfusion.

Nursing Implications: Assess baseline cbc, HCT; monitor Hgb and HCT during treatment. Instruct patient to report fatigue, shortness of breath, headache. Transfuse red blood cells as needed and ordered by physician.

IV. ALTERATION IN COMFORT, PAIN related to PAIN AT INJECTION SITE

Defining Characteristics: Drug may cause pain at injection site, phlebitis, thrombophlebitis; extravasation causes local irritation.

Nursing Implications: Select veins for IV administration distally and then more proximally, avoiding phlebitic veins or small veins. Apply heat to increase comfort. Administer drug slowly.

V. ALTERATION IN CARDIAC OUTPUT related to CARDIOPULMONARY DYSFUNCTION

Defining Characteristics: Rarely, hypertension, ventricular fibrillation, cardiac arrest, failure, pulmonary edema may occur. Pulmonary hypersensitivity may occur with bronchospasm, wheezing, or pulmonary pneumonitis.

Nursing Implications: Monitor VS closely, noting heart rate and rhythm, BP, breath sounds at baseline and during infusion. Instruct patient to report dyspnea, other changes in breathing pattern, or general feeling state ASAP. Discuss any changes, abnormalities with physician. Administer granulocyte transfusions as far apart from amphotericin administration as possible, and monitor pulmonary status closely. Be prepared to provide basic life support/resuscitation if needed.

VI. ALTERATIONS IN SENSORY/PERCEPTUAL PATTERNS related to PERIPHERAL AND CNS DYSFUNCTION

Defining Characteristics: Rarely, hearing loss, tinnitus, transient vertigo, blurred vision or diplopia, peripheral neuropathy, and seizures may occur. Following intrathecal drug administration, headache, lumbar nerves, arachnoiditis, and visual changes may occur.

Nursing Implications: Assess baseline neurologic function and monitor during drug administration and over time, especially when drug is given intrathecally. Notify physician if abnormalities occur. Discuss with physician coadministration of small doses of intrathecal corticosteroids to decrease CNS irritation.

VII. ALTERATION IN NUTRITION, LESS THAN BODY REQUIREMENTS, related to GI TOXICITY

Defining Characteristics: Anorexia, nausea, vomiting, dyspepsia, cramping, epigastric pain, and diarrhea may occur. Rarely, melena and hemorrhagic gastroenteritis may occur. Elevated LFTs may occur.

Nursing Implications: Assess baseline nutritional status, including weight and usual weight. Administer antiemetics as ordered and needed, then prophylactically prior to infusion if nausea and/or vomiting develop. Administer antidiarrheal medicine as ordered and needed. Instruct patient to report any symptoms; teach/reinforce importance of high-calorie, high-protein diet; suggest family/significant other bring in favorite foods from home as appropriate. Assess LFT results at baseline and periodically during treatment as elevated serum aminotransferase, bili, and alk phos may occur. Discuss abnormalities with physician. Encourage patient to eat favorite foods, especially those high in calories, protein, potassium, and magnesium. Monitor daily weight during treatment, and discuss weight loss with dietitian, patient, and physician to revise nutritional plan.

VIII. ALTERATION IN PROTECTIVE MECHANISMS related to BONE MARROW INJURY

Defining Characteristics: Rarely, thrombocytopenia, leukopenia, agranulocytosis, and coagulation defects may occur.

Nursing Implications: Assess baseline CBC, differential. Assess for any signs/symptoms of bleeding or infection, and discuss with physician if they occur. Teach patient general self-assessment guidelines, such as taking temperature and reporting any changes from baseline condition.

Drug: caspofungin (Cancidas)

Class: Echinocandin; glucan synthesis inhibitor.

Mechanism of Action: Caspofungin inhibits the synthesis of β (1, 3)-D-glucan, an integral component of the fungal cell wall of susceptible filamentous fungi. It has demonstrated activity in regions of active cell growth of *Aspergillus fumigatus*.

Metabolism: Caspofungin is slowly metabolized by hydrolysis and N-acetylation. Elimination route is via feces and urine.

Dosage/Range:
- The recommended dose of caspofungin is a 70-mg loading dose on the first day, followed by 50 mg/daily.
- No dosage adjustment is necessary for the elderly.
- No dosage adjustment is necessary for patients with renal insufficiency. Caspofungin is not dialyzable.
- No dosage adjustment is recommended for patients with mild hepatic insufficiency (Child-Pugh score 5 to 6). In those with moderate hepatic insufficiency (Child-Pugh score 7 to 9), a daily dose of 35 mg after the 70-mg loading dose is recommended.

Drug Administration:
- Caspofungin should be given as a slow IV infusion in 250 ml 0.9% Sodium Chloride over 1 hour.
- Caspofungin is not compatible with dextrose-containing solutions.

Drug Interactions:
- Transient increase in AST and ALT have been observed when caspofungin and cyclosporine are coadministered. Therefore, concomitant use of these two agents is not recommended unless the potential benefit outweighs the potential risk.

I. I. ALTERATIONS IN COMFORT related to LOCAL VEIN IRRITATION (IV ADMINISTRATION)

Defining Characteristics: Erythema, irritation, pain, swelling, phlebitis may occur at injection site. Consider use of central line.

Nursing Implications: Assess IV site for patency, irritation prior to each dose. Change IV site at least q 48 hours. Apply warmth/heat to painful area as needed.

II. POTENTIAL FOR INJURY related to HYPERSENSITIVITY REACTION

Defining Characteristics: Fever and erythema. Increased risk in allergic individuals.

Nursing Implications: Assess allergy/allergic potential to drug. Discuss other patient responses with physician to determine whether drug should be given. Assess baseline skin condition, including integrity and allergy history to drugs. Teach patient to report rash, itching, and other skin changes. Teach patient skin care and symptomatic measures as appropriate. If reaction occurs, discuss drug discontinuance with physician.

III. ALTERATION IN NUTRITION, LESS THAN BODY REQUIREMENTS, related to GI SIDE EFFECTS

Defining Characteristics: Nausea and vomiting may occur. Rarely, transient increases in LFTs—AST (SGOT), ALT (SGPT), ALKPHOS, bilirubin (BR)—may occur with coadministration of cyclosporine.

Nursing Implications: Assess baseline nutritional status. Teach patient to report GI disturbances. Administer and teach patient to self-administer antiemetics as needed and as ordered. Teach patient importance of nutritious diet, and suggest small, frequent, high-calorie, high-protein meals as appropriate. Assess baseline LFTs and monitor periodically during treatment. Discuss abnormalities and drug interruption with physician.

IV. SENSORY/PERCEPTUAL ALTERATIONS

Defining Characteristics: Headache.

Nursing Implications: Assess baseline neurological function and comfort, and monitor during treatment. Teach patient to report any changes. Discuss any abnormalities with physician.

Drug: fluconazole (Diflucan)

Class: Azole, antifungal (systemic).

Mechanism of Action: Fungistatic; causes increased permeability of fungal cell membrane, so intracellular nutrients leak out (potassium, amino acids) and cell is unable to take in nutrients to make DNA (precursors for purine, pyrimidines). Active against most fungi, including yeast.

Metabolism: Drug is rapidly and highly absorbed from GI tract, with > 90% of drug bioavailable. GI absorption is unaffected by food or gastric pH. Steady-state plasma levels achieved in 5–10 days, or by second day if loading dose given. Widely distributed in body tissues and fluids, including CSF. There is minimal protein binding. It is unknown whether drug crosses the placenta or is excreted in human milk; 60–80% of drug is excreted unchanged in the urine. Renal dysfunction results in higher circulating serum levels with prolonged drug effect and potential toxicity. Drug elimination in elderly clients may be decreased.

Dosage/Range:

- Oral and parenteral dosages are the same; IV dosage recommended for patients unable to take oral form. Dose is a single daily dose.
- Dosage depends on fungal infection. Candidiasis (oropharyngeal or esophageal): 200 mg day 1, followed by 100 mg/day (may titrate based on patient's response up to 400 mg/day) × 2 weeks (oropharyngeal); × 3 weeks or at least × 2 weeks after symptoms resolve (esophageal). Candidiasis (systemic): 400 mg day 1, followed by 200 mg/day × 4 weeks at least, then × 2 weeks after symptoms resolve (esophageal). Cryptococcal infections: Initial: 400 mg day 1, followed by 200–400 mg/day × 10–12 weeks after CSF cultures for *Cryptococcus* are negative. Maintenance (AIDS patients): 200 mg/day indefinitely.
- DOSE-REDUCE AFTER LOADING DOSE IF RENAL COMPROMISE based on creatinine clearance (e.g., 21–50 mL/min, dose-reduce 50%; if 11–20 mL/min, dose-reduce 75%).

Drug Preparation:

- Oral: store in tight containers at < 30°C (86°F).
- Parenteral: glass vials for injection should be stored at 5–30°C, (41–86°F); protect from freezing. Plastic containers should be stored at 5–25°C (41–77°F). Inspect for any discoloration, particulate matter, or leaks in plastic bags. If found, do not use.

Drug Administration:

- Oral: once daily without regard to food intake.
- IV: once daily at a rate ≤ 200 mg/hour. DO NOT ADD ADDITIVES. DO NOT ADMINISTER IV IN SERIES THAT COULD INTRODUCE AIR EMBOLISM.

Drug Interactions:

- Coumarin anticoagulants: increased PT; monitor PT closely.
- Cyclosporine: increased cyclosporine serum levels; monitor closely and adjust dose.
- Phenytoin: increased phenytoin serum level; monitor closely and reduce phenytoin dose as needed.

- Rifampin: decreased fluconazole serum level; increase fluconazole dose when given concurrently.
- Sulfonylurea antidiabetic agents (tolbutamide, glyburide, glipizide): increased drug serum levels; monitor blood glucose levels closely and decrease dose as needed.
- Thiazide diuretics: increased fluconazole serum level; do not appear to increase fluconazole toxicity so dose adjustment not necessary.
- Rifampin, isoniazid, phenytoin, valproic acid, oral sulfonylurea: increased risk of elevated hepatic transaminases exists.

Lab Effects/Interference:

Major clinical significance:

- ALT, alk phos, AST, and serum bili values may be elevated.

Special Considerations:

- Drug is being studied as a prophylactic antifungal agent in patients at risk for neutropenia and fungal infections (cancer patients receiving myelosuppressive chemotherapy, bone marrow transplant patients).
- Use cautiously in patients with renal dysfunction; dose reduction based on creatinine clearance (see Dosage/Range section).
- Absorption NOT affected by gastric pH or food intake.
- Risk of drug toxicity may be higher in patients with HIV infection.

Potential Toxicities/Side Effects and the Nursing Process

I. ALTERATION IN NUTRITION, LESS THAN BODY REQUIREMENTS, related to GI SIDE EFFECTS

Defining Characteristics: 2–8% incidence of mild-to-moderate nausea, vomiting, abdominal pain, diarrhea is seen; anorexia, dyspepsia, dry mouth, flatus, bloating occur rarely; 5–7% incidence of mild, transient increases in LFTs, which are reversible with drug discontinuance.

Nursing Implications: Assess baseline nutritional and elimination status. Instruct patient to report GI disturbances. Administer and teach patient to selfadminister antiemetics, antidiarrheals as needed and as ordered. Teach patient importance of nutritious diet, and suggest small, frequent, high-calorie, high-protein meals as appropriate. Assess baseline LFTs and monitor periodically during treatment. Discuss abnormalities and drug interruption with physician. Assess whether patient is taking other hepatotoxic drugs (see Special Considerations section).

II. ALTERATION IN SKIN INTEGRITY related to ALLERGY/HYPERSENSITIVITY

Defining Characteristics: 5% incidence is seen of rash, often diffuse, associated with eosinophilia and pruritus; rarely, exfoliative dermatitis and Stevens-Johnson syndrome may occur in patients receiving multiple drugs.

Nursing Implications: Assess baseline skin condition, including integrity and drug allergy history. Instruct patient to report rash, itching, and other skin changes. Teach patient skin care and symptomatic measures as appropriate. If skin rash develops, discuss drug discontinuance with physician. If rash progresses, especially in HIV-infected patients, drug should be discontinued, as fatal Stevens-Johnson syndrome may develop. Be prepared to treat severe acute hypersensitivity reactions with airway management, oxygen, epinephrine, corticosteroids, antihistamines as ordered.

III. ALTERATIONS IN SENSORY/PERCEPTUAL PATTERNS related to CNS EFFECTS

Defining Characteristics: Dizziness and headache occur in 2% of patients. Rarely, somnolence, delirium/coma, dysesthesia, malaise, fatigue, seizure, and psychiatric disturbance may occur.

Nursing Implications: Assess baseline neurologic function and comfort, and monitor during treatment. Instruct patient to report any changes. Discuss any abnormalities with physician.

Drug: flucytosine (Ancobon)

Class: Antifungal (systemic).

Mechanism of Action: Nonantibiotic antifungal; enters fungal cell and undergoes deamination to fluorouracil, which acts as an antimetabolite, preventing RNA and protein synthesis; may also inferfere with DNA synthesis. Active against *Candida* and *Cryptococcus.*

Metabolism: Oral preparation well absorbed from GI tract; decreased rate of absorption when taken with food. Widely distributed into body tissues and fluids, including CSF; 75–90% of dose excreted unchanged by kidneys, with increased serum levels and toxicity in patients with renal dysfunction.

Dosage/Range:

- Oral: 50–150 mg/kg/day in four equally divided doses given q6h × weeks or months until fungal studies are negative. Dose may be 150–250 mg/kg/day in *Cryptococcus* meningitis.
- Dose must be reduced in patients with renal dysfunction:

Dose must be determined by flucytosine levels (therapeutic range is 25–120 μg/mL).

Dose may be determined by creatinine clearance. Individual dose of 12.5–37.5 mg/kg given:

- q12h if creatinine clearance is 20–40 mL/min.
- q24h if creatinine clearance is 10–20 mL/min.
- q24–48h if creatinine clearance is < 10 mL/min.

Drug Preparation/Administration:

- Store in tight, light-resistant container at < 40°C (104°F).
- Oral.

Drug Interactions:

- Amphotericin B: theoretical synergism.
- Norfloxacin: theoretical synergism.

Lab Effects/Interference:

- Rare anemia, leukopenia, agranulocytosis, thrombocytopenia, pancytopenia, eosinophilia.

Special Considerations:

- Use only in severe infections, as drug is toxic.
- Theoretically synergistic with amphotericin, but some studies do not show significant benefit of combination.
- Therapeutic response (negative fungal cultures) may take weeks to months.
- Drug has no antineoplastic activity.
- Drug is teratogenic, capable of causing fetal malformations when given to pregnant women. Risks and benefits should be carefully considered before drug is used in a pregnant patient.

Potential Toxicities/Side Effects and the Nursing Process

I. POTENTIAL FOR INFECTION, BLEEDING, AND FATIGUE related to BONE MARROW DEPRESSION

Defining Characteristics: Anemia, leukopenia, thrombocytopenia may occur; agranulocytosis and aplastic anemia occur rarely. Increased risk exists with increased serum flucytosine levels (100 μg/mL), especially in patients with renal compromise or those receiving concurrent amphotericin B.

Nursing Implications: Assess baseline CBC, differential, BUN, and creatinine, and monitor closely during therapy, especially if receiving concurrent amphotericin B. Assess for signs/symptoms of bleeding, fatigue, infection during therapy. Teach patient to self-assess for signs/symptoms of infection, bleeding, and instruct to report them immediately. Discuss dose with physician; dose modification is needed if renal dysfunction occurs. Monitor flucytosine therapeutic levels (to maintain level of 25–100 μg/mL).

II. ALTERATION IN NUTRITION, LESS THAN BODY REQUIREMENTS, related to MUCOSITIS, NAUSEA, VOMITING

Defining Characteristics: Frequently dividing epithelial cells of GI mucosa are damaged, leading to diarrhea and possible bowel perforation (rare). Nausea, vomiting, anorexia, abdominal bloating may also occur. Elevated LFTs may occur, but are dose-related and reversible; liver enlargement may occur.

Nursing Implications: Assess elimination and nutritional status, baseline and throughout treatment. Assess baseline LFTs. Instruct patient to report diarrhea, nausea, vomiting immediately, and teach self-administration of prescribed antiemetics and antidiarrheal medication. Monitor weight, and teach patient importance of high-protein, high-calorie diet. Instruct patient to administer dose over 15 minutes to decrease nausea and vomiting. If weight loss occurs/persists, refer to dietitian/nutritionist. Monitor LFTs during treatment: AST, ALT, bili, and alk phos.

III. INJURY related to ANAPHYLAXIS

Defining Characteristics: Rare anaphylaxis has occurred in patients with AIDS, characterized by diffuse erythema, pruritus, injection of conjunctiva, fever, tachycardia, hypotension, edema, and abdominal pain.

Nursing Implications: Instruct AIDS patients to report any signs/symptoms of rash, pruritus, conjunctivitis, abdominal pain immediately. Use drug cautiously in AIDS patients. Monitor any adverse sensations over time. Assess for signs/symptoms.

IV. ALTERATION IN SENSORY/PERCEPTUAL PATTERNS related to CNS CHANGES

Defining Characteristics: Confusion, sedation, hallucinations, and headaches occur infrequently.

Nursing Implications: Assess baseline mental status. Instruct patient to report headaches, abnormal thoughts, mental status changes. Discuss alternative drug if mental status changes occur.

Drug: itraconazole (Sporanox)

Class: Azole; antifungal.

Mechanism of Action: Fungistatic; may be fungicidal, depending on concentration; azole antifungals interfere with cytochrome P-450 activity, which is necessary for the demethylation of 14-α-methylsterols to ergosterol. Ergosterol, the principal sterol in the fungal cell membrance, becomes depleted. This damages the cell membrane, producing alterations in membrane function and permeability. In *Candida albicans,* azole antifungals inhibit transformation of blastospores into invasive mycelial form.

Metabolism: Rapidly absorbed from GI tract in acid environment. Decreased absorption in patients with gastric hypochlorhydria or achlorhydria, or in patients taking medications that raise pH (antacids, H_2 antagonists).

Dosage/Range:

- Oral: 100–200 mg/day × 7–14 days (candidiasis); longer for other infections (400 mg/day in severe infections).
- Although studies did not provide a loading dose, in life-threatening situations a loading dose of 200 mg three times a day (600 mg/day) for the first 3 days is recommended, based on pharmacokinetic data.
- Doses above 200 mg/day should be given in two divided doses.
- IV: 200 mg bid × 4 doses followed by 200 mg qd; gave each dose over 1 hour—do not use for more than 14 days.

Drug Preparation:

- Store in tightly closed container at < 40°C (104°F).
- Itraconazole injection must be diluted prior to IV infusion. The entire 250 mg ampule should be diluted in the 50 mL bag of 0.9% Sodium Chloride provided by the manufacturer. The final concentration of the solution is 3.33 mg/mL (250 mg/75 mL).

Drug Administration:

- Orally in single or split dose, depending on total daily dose.
- Should take with meals to increase absorption of medication.
- Oral solution should be taken on an empty stomach to increase absorption of the medication.
- To administer a 200 mg dose of itraconazole, 60 mL should be given by IV infusion over 60 minutes. The infusion should be given using a controlled-infusion device, the manufacturer-provided infusion set, and a dedicated IV line. When the infusion is complete, the manufacturer recommends that the infusion set be flushed via the 2-way stopcock using 15–20 mL of 0.9% Sodium Chloride over 30 seconds to 15 minutes. The entire IV line should then be discarded.

Drug Interactions:

- Drugs that increase gastric pH: antacids, anticholinergics/antispasmodics, histamine H_2-receptor antagonists, or omeprazole will decrease the absorption of itraconazole.
- Didanosine contains a buffer to increase its absorption; this will decrease the absorption of itraconazole since itraconazole needs an acidic environment.

- Use with oral antidiabetic agents has increased the plasma concentration of these sulfonylurea agents, leading to hypoglycemia.
- Use with carbamazepine may decrease itraconazole plasma concentrations, leading to clinical failure or relapse.
- Itraconazole may increase digoxin concentrations, leading to digoxin toxicity.
- Use with lovastatin or simvastatin may increase the plasma concentrations of these cholesterol-lowering agents and may increase the risk of rhabdomyolysis.
- Use with midazolam or triazolam may potentiate the hyponotic and sedative effects of these benzodiazepines.

Lab Effects/Interference:

Major clinical significance:

- ALT, alk phos, AST, serum bili values may be elevated.
- Serum K+: hypokalemia has occurred in approximately 2–6% of patients treated with itraconazole and has resulted in ventricular fibrillation, especially in higher doses.

Special Considerations:

- High failure rate in HIV-infected patients due to achlorhydria.

Potential Toxicities/Side Effects and the Nursing Process

I. ALTERATION IN NUTRITION, LESS THAN BODY REQUIREMENTS, related to GI SIDE EFFECTS

Defining Characteristics: Increased LFTs may occur: AST, ALT, alk phos. Hepatotoxicity is less common, is usually reversible, and is rarely fatal.

Nursing Implications: Assess baseline nutritional and elimination status. Instruct patient to report GI disturbances. Administer and teach patient to selfadminister antiemetics, antidiarrheals as needed and as ordered. Teach patient importance of nutritious diet, and suggest small, frequent, high-calorie, high-protein meals as appropriate. Assess baseline LFTs and monitor periodically during treatment. Discuss abnormalities and drug interruption with physician. Assess whether taking other hepatotoxic drugs (see Special Considerations section). Assess for increased fatigue, jaundice, dark urine, pale stools (signs of hepatotoxicity), and discuss drug discontinuance immediately with physician.

II. ALTERATION IN SKIN INTEGRITY related to ALLERGIC REACTION

Defining Characteristics: Rash, dermatitis, purpura, urticaria occur; rarely, anaphylaxis may occur.

Nursing Implications: Assess baseline skin condition and integrity. Instruct patient to report itch, rash, other skin changes. Teach patient skin care and symptomatic measures. If rash or dermatitis progresses, discuss drug discontinuance with physician. Assess for signs/symptoms of anaphylaxis.

Drug: ketoconazole (Nizoral)

Class: Azole; antifungal (systemic).

Mechanism of Action: Fungistatic by damaging fungal cell membrane and increasing permeability, altering cell metabolism, and inhibiting cell growth. Fungicidal at high concentrations. Active against mucocutaneous candidiasis, histoplasmosis, coccidioidomycosis, and blastomycosis.

Metabolism: Rapidly absorbed from GI tract in acid environment. Decreased absorption in patients with gastric hypochlorhydria (25% of all AIDS patients) or in patients taking medications that raise pH (antacids, H_2 antagonists). Distributed widely but cerebrospinal penetration is unpredictable. Drug is ~90% protein-bound. Partially metabolized in liver, and mostly excreted in the feces via bile.

Dosage/Range:
- Oral: 200 mg/day × 7–14 days (candidiasis); longer for other infections (400 mg/day in severe infections).

Drug Preparation:
- Store in tightly closed container at < 40°C (104°F).

Drug Administration:
- Orally in single dose.
- May take with meals to decrease GI side effects (unclear if food increases absorption).
- In patients with gastric achlorhydria, patient may be instructed to dissolve ketoconazole in 4 mL aqueous solution of 0.2 N hydrochloric acid and drink through a straw; follow with 4 oz (120 mL) water.

Drug Interactions:
- Drugs that increase gastric pH: antacids, cimetidine, rantidine, famotidine, sucralfate decrease ketoconazole absorption; give these drugs at least 2 hours after ketoconazole.
- Other hepatotoxic drugs: use cautiously, and monitor liver function studies closely.
- Rifampin or rifampin plus isoniazid: decreased ketoconazole levels, especially if isoniazid is taken as well. Increase ketoconazole dose.
- Acyclovir: synergism and increased antiviral action against herpes simplex virus.

- Norfloxacin: theoretically increases antifungal action of ketoconazole, but studies are inconsistent.
- Coumarin anticoagulants: increased PT; monitor patient closely and decrease anticoagulant dose accordingly.
- Cyclosporine: increased cyclosporine serum level; monitor serum level and decrease cyclosporine dose accordingly.
- Phenytoin: may have altered serum levels of phenytoin or ketoconazole; monitor serum levels of each and adjust dosages accordingly.
- Theophylline: may decrease theophylline serum concentrations; monitor serum levels and increase dosage accordingly.
- Corticosteroids: may increase corticosteroid serum level; may need to decrease dosage.

Lab Effects/Interference:

Major clinical significance:

- ALT, alk phos, AST, serum bili values may be elevated.
- ACTH-induced serum corticosteroid concentrations and serum testosterone concentrations may be decreased by doses of 800 mg/day of ketoconazole; serum testosterone concentrations are abolished by values of 1.6 g/day of ketoconazole, but return to baseline values when ketoconazole is discontinued.

Special Considerations:

- Monitor liver function studies.
- High failure rate in HIV-infected patients due to achlorhydria.

Potential Toxicities/Side Effects and the Nursing Process

I. ALTERATION IN NUTRITION, LESS THAN BODY REQUIREMENTS, related to GI SIDE EFFECTS

Defining Characteristics: Nausea, vomiting is seen in 3–10% of patients. Diarrhea, abdominal pain, flatulence, constipation may occur less frequently. Increased LFTs may occur: AST, ALT, alk phos. Hepatotoxicity is less common, is usually reversible, and is rarely fatal.

Nursing Implications: Assess baseline nutritional and elimination status. Instruct patient to report GI disturbances. Administer and teach patient to self-administer antiemetics, antidiarrheals as needed and as ordered. Teach patient importance of nutritious diet, and suggest small, frequent, high-calorie, high-protein meals as appropriate. Assess baseline LFTs and monitor periodically during treatment. Discuss abnormalities and drug interruption with physician. Assess whether taking other hepatotoxic drugs (see Special Considerations section). Assess for increased fatigue, jaundice, dark urine, pale stools (signs of hepatotoxicity), and discuss drug discontinuance immediately with physician.

II. ALTERATION IN COMFORT related to GYNECOMASTIA AND BREAST TENDERNESS

Defining Characteristics: Breast enlargement and tenderness may occur in some men, lasting weeks to duration of therapy.

Nursing Implications: Assess for occurrence in male patients. Assess comfort level, degree of tenderness, and self-care measures used to increase comfort. Assess impact on body image.

III. ALTERATION IN SKIN INTEGRITY related to ALLERGIC REACTION

Defining Characteristics: Rash, dermatitis, purpura, urticaria occur in 1% of patients; rarely, anaphylaxis may occur.

Nursing Implications: Assess baseline skin condition and integrity. Teach patient to report itch, rash, and other skin changes. Teach patient skin care and symptomatic measures. If rash or dermatitis progresses, discuss drug discontinuance with physician. Assess for signs/symptoms of anaphylaxis.

IV. ALTERATIONS IN SENSORY/PERCEPTUAL PATTERNS related to CNS EFFECTS

Defining Characteristics: Dizziness, headache, nervousness, insomnia, lethargy, somnolence, and paresthesia have occurred in ~1% of patients.

Nursing Implications: Assess baseline neurologic function and comfort, and monitor during treatment. Instruct patient to report any changes. Discuss any abnormalities with physician.

Drug: micafungin sodium (Mycamine)

Class: antifungal.

Mechanism of Action: Fungistatic by damaging fungal cell membrane increasing permeability, altering cell metabolism, and inhibiting cell growth. Fungicidal at high concentrations. Inhibits the synthesis of 1,3-β-D-glucan, an integral component of the fungal cell wall.

Metabolism: Metabolized by liver and excreted in urine.

Dosage/Range:

- Esophageal Candidiasis: 150 mg/day × 15 days.
- Prophylaxis of Candida Infections in HSCT recipients 50 mg/day × 19 days.

Drug Preparation/Administration:
- Do not mix or co-infuse with other medications. Mycafungin has been shown to precipitate when mixed directly with a number of other commonly used medications.
- No dose adjustment is required with concomitant use of mycophenolate mofetil, cyclosporine, tacrolimus, prednisolone, Sirolimus, nifedipine, fluconazole, ritonavir, or rifampin.
- A loading dose is not required; typically, 85% of the steady-state is achieved after three daily doses.
- IV: Dilute in 0.9% Sodium Chloride, USP (without a bacteriostatic agent) or 5% Dextrose injection, USP.
- Infuse over 1 hour. Stable × 24 hours at room temperature.

Drug Interactions:
- Coumarin anticoagulants: increased PT. Monitor patient closely and decrease anticoagulant dose accordingly.
- Norfloxacin: may increase antifungal action.
- Cyclosporine: increased cyclosporine serum level. Monitor serum level and decrease cyclosporine dose accordingly.

Lab Effects/Interference: *Major clinical significance:*
- ALT, alk phos, AST, serum bili values may be elevated.

Special Considerations:
- Used in treatment of fungal infections.
- Monitor HCT, Hgb, serum electrolytes, and lipids, as changes may occur during treatment.

Potential Toxicities/Side Effects and the Nursing Process

I. POTENTIAL FOR INJURY related to ANAPHYLAXIS

Defining Characteristics: Anaphylaxis with tachycardia, arrhythmias, and cardiac arrest may occur.

Nursing Implications: Assess baseline VS and monitor throughout infusion. Instruct patient to report signs/symptoms immediately. Assess for signs/symptoms: nausea, generalized itching, crampy abdominal pain, chest tightness, anxiety, agitation, sense of impending doom, wheezing, and dizziness.

II. ALTERATION IN COMFORT related to PRURITUS, PHLEBITIS, SKIN ERUPTIONS, FEVER

Defining Characteristics: Phlebitis, pruritus with or without rash may occur.

Nursing Implications: Assess temperature, skin integrity, and comfort prior to drug administration, and monitor throughout treatment. Discuss with physician use of diphenhydramine to decrease itching. Change IV sites q48h to decrease phlebitis, or discuss with patient and physician use of central line. If rash and pruritus worsen, discuss with physician drug discontinuance.

III. ALTERATION IN NUTRITION, LESS THAN BODY REQUIREMENTS, related to GI SIDE EFFECTS

Defining Characteristics: Nausea, vomiting, diarrhea, and anorexia may occur.

Nursing Implications: Assess baseline nutritional and elimination status. Instruct patient to report GI disturbances. Administer and teach patient to self-administer antiemetics, antidiarrheals as needed and as ordered. Teach patient importance of nutritious diet, and suggest small, frequent, high-calorie, high-protein meals as appropriate.

IV. ALTERATIONS IN SENSORY/PERCEPTUAL PATTERNS related to CNS, ENDOCRINE EFFECTS

Defining Characteristics: Dizziness, headache, and somnolence may occur.

Nursing Implications: Assess baseline neurologic function and comfort, and monitor during treatment. Instruct patient to report any changes. Discuss any abnormalities with physician.

Drug: miconazole nitrate (Monistat)

Class: Azole; antifungal (systemic).

Mechanism of Action: Fungistatic by damaging fungal cell membrane and increasing permeability, altering cell metabolism, and inhibiting cell growth. Fungicidal at high concentrations. Active against most fungi, especially candidiasis, coccidioidomycosis, cryptococcosis.

Metabolism: Limited (50%) oral absorption so usually given parenterally; 91–93% protein-bound to plasma proteins. Unpredictable penetration into CSF, so must be given intrathecally to achieve therapeutic levels. Metabolized by liver and excreted in urine.

Dosage/Range:

IV:

- Coccidioidomycosis: 1.8–3.6 g/day × 3–20+ weeks.
- Cryptococcosis: 1.2–2.4 g/day × 3–12+ weeks.
- Candidiasis: 600 mg–1.8 g/day × 1–20+ weeks.
- Intrathecal: refer to protocol; usually 20 mg q1–2 days, or q3–7 days if given by lumbar puncture.

- Intravesical: 200 mg in dilute solution 2–4 × day or by continuous bladder irrigation.

Drug Preparation/Administration:
- IV: Dilute in 200 mL of 0.9% Sodium Chloride (preferred) or 5% Dextrose injection and infuse over 30–60 min; daily dosage usually given in three divided doses q8h. Stable × 24 hours at room temperature.
- Intrathecal: is administered undiluted.
- Intravesical: as above (dosage) in conjunction with IV drug as well.

Drug Interactions:
- Coumarin anticoagulants: increased PT. Monitor patient closely and decrease anticoagulant dose accordingly.
- Norfloxacin: may increase antifungal action.
- Oral sulfonylureas: increased hypoglycemia effect. Monitor blood glucose and decrease dose of oral sulfonylurea.
- Rifampin or rifampin plus isoniazid: decreased miconazole levels, especially if isoniazid taken as well. Increase miconazole dose.
- Phenytoin: may have altered serum levels of phenytoin or miconazole.
- Monitor serum levels of each and adjust dosages accordingly.
- Cyclosporine: increased cyclosporine serum level. Monitor serum level and decrease cyclosporine dose accordingly.

Lab Effects/Interference:

Major clinical significance:
- ALT, alk phos, AST, serum bili values may be elevated.

Clinical significance:
- Serum lipid profile: hyperlipidemia has occurred in patients receiving intravenous miconazole; this is reportedly due to the vehicle in the miconazole solution, PEG 40 castor oil (Cremophor EL).

Special Considerations:
- Used in treatment of severe fungal infections.
- Initial dose should be in hospital with resuscitation equipment available to determine hypersensitivity (cardiac arrest has occurred with initial dose). Drug is suspended in castor oil base, which stimulates allergic reaction. Subsequent dosing can be safely given to selected patients in ambulatory settings.
- IV push injection of drug may cause arrhythmias, so drug must be diluted (200+ mL) and administered over 30–60 minutes.
- Monitor HCT, Hgb, serum electrolytes, and lipids, as changes may occur during treatment.

Potential Toxicities/Side Effects and the Nursing Process

I. POTENTIAL FOR INJURY related to ANAPHYLAXIS

Defining Characteristics: Anaphylaxis with tachycardia, arrhythmias, and cardiac arrest may occur on first IV dose, probably related to suspension medium of drug (castor oil).

Nursing Implications: Ensure first dose is given in inpatient setting with resuscitation equipment and physician available. Assess baseline VS and monitor throughout infusion. Instruct patient to report signs/symptoms immediately. Assess for signs/symptoms: nausea, generalized itching, crampy abdominal pain, chest tightness, anxiety, agitation, sense of impending doom, wheezing, and dizziness.

II. ALTERATION IN COMFORT related to PRURITUS, PHLEBITIS, SKIN ERUPTIONS, FEVER

Defining Characteristics: Phlebitis, pruritus with or without rash may occur.

Nursing Implications: Assess temperature, skin integrity, and comfort prior to drug administration, and monitor throughout treatment. Discuss with physician use of diphenhydramine to decrease itching. Change IV sites q48h to decrease phlebitis, or discuss with patient and physician use of central line. If rash and pruritus worsen, discuss with physician drug discontinuance.

III. ALTERATION IN NUTRITION, LESS THAN BODY REQUIREMENTS, related to GI SIDE EFFECTS

Defining Characteristics: Nausea, vomiting, diarrhea, anorexia, and bitter taste may occur.

Nursing Implications: Assess baseline nutritional and elimination status. Instruct patient to report GI disturbances. Administer and teach patient to self-administer antiemetics, antidiarrheals as needed and as ordered. Teach patient importance of nutritious diet, and suggest small, frequent, high-calorie, high-protein meals as appropriate.

IV. ALTERATIONS IN SENSORY/PERCEPTUAL PATTERNS related to CNS, ENDOCRINE EFFECTS

Defining Characteristics: Dizziness, flushing, anxiety, increased libido, blurred vision, eye dryness, headache may occur.

Nursing Implications: Assess baseline neurologic function and comfort, and monitor during treatment. Instruct patient to report any changes. Discuss any abnormalities with physician.

Drug: nystatin (Mycostatin, Nilstat)

Class: Antifungal.

Mechanism of Action: Binds to sterol molecule in fungi cell membrane, increasing permeability so that potassium and other intracellular ions are lost. Active against yeast and fungi, especially *Candida.*

Metabolism: Drug is not absorbed from intact skin, mucous membranes, and is poorly absorbed from GI tract. Excreted as unchanged drug in the feces.

Dosage/Range:

- Oral (for treatment of oral or intestinal candidiasis): 500,000–1 million U tid; continue therapy for 48 hours after clinical remission to prevent recurrence.
- Powder: topical for candidal rash infections.
- Vaginal: 100,000 U as vaginal tablet, inserted into vagina qd or bid × 14 days.

Drug Preparation:

- Oral suspension and tablets should be stored in tight, light-resistant containers < 40°C (104°F).

Drug Administration:

- Oral suspension. Instruct patient to:
  - Rinse mouth with oral hygiene solution to clean food debris.
  - Hold suspension in mouth and swish for 1–2 minutes, then swallow or spit solution.
  - Do not rinse mouth or eat for 15–30 minutes.

Drug Interactions:

- None.

Lab Effects/Interference:

- None known.

Special Considerations:

- For patients with oral thrush who have difficulty taking oral suspension:
  - Oral suspension can be frozen in medicine cups so it is easier to administer if the patient has stomatitis.
  - Vaginal suppository may be sucked as this increases mucosal contact with drug.
  - Cannot be used to treat systemic infections.
  - Adverse effects are infrequent.

Potential Toxicities/Side Effects and the Nursing Process

I. ALTERATION IN NUTRITION, LESS THAN BODY REQUIREMENTS, related to GI SIDE EFFECTS

Defining Characteristics: High oral doses may cause nausea, vomiting, diarrhea.

Nursing Implications: Assess baseline nutritional status. Instruct patient to report GI disturbances. Administer and teach patient to self-administer antiemetics, antidiarrheals as needed and as ordered. Teach patient importance of nutritious diet, and suggest small, frequent, high-calorie, high-protein meals as appropriate.

II. KNOWLEDGE DEFICIT related to SELF-ADMINISTRATION OF MEDICATION

Defining Characteristics: Increased compliance when patient is instructed in self-care activities.

Nursing Implications: Assess knowledge about infection and planned treatment. Teach about drug action, potential side effects, and when and how to take drug. Instruct patient to rinse mouth with saline gargle (or other rinse) to remove food debris prior to taking nystatin suspension; solution should be swished in mouth 1–2 minutes, then swallowed or spit out. Patient should not eat or rinse mouth for 15–30 minutes.

Drug: voriconazole (VFEND)

Class: Triazole; antifungal (systemic).

Mechanism of Action: Fungistatic by damaging fungal cell membrane and increasing permeability, altering cell metabolism, and inhibiting cell growth. Fungicidal at high concentrations. Active against invasive aspergillosis fumigatus, Fusarium spp. infection, and Scedosporium apiospermum infection.

Metabolism: Rapidly absorbed from GI tract in acid environment. Partially metabolized in liver, and mostly excreted in the feces via bile.

Dosage/Range:

- Oral: 200 mg q 12 hours for 7–14 days; dose may be increased if there is an inadequate response to infections (300 mg q 12 hours).
- IV preparation is available. The final voriconazole preparation must be infused over 1–2 hours at a maximum rate of 3 mg/kg per hour.

Drug Preparation:

- Once reconstituted, drug should be used immediately, or it can be stored for no longer than 24 hours at 2–8°C (37–46°F).

Drug Administration:

- Orally. May take 1 hour before meals or 1 hour after meals.
- The final voriconazole preparation must be infused over 1–2 hours at a maximum rate of 3 mg/kg per hour.

Drug Interactions:

- Drugs that increase gastric pH: antacids, cimetidine, rantidine have minor or no significant effect on voriconazole.
- Hepatotoxic drugs: use cautiously, and monitor liver function studies closely.
- Rifampin decreases the steady state of voriconazole.
- Coumarin anticoagulants: increases PT; monitor patient closely and decrease anticoagulant dose accordingly.
- Cyclosporine: increases cyclosporine serum level; monitor serum level and decrease cyclosporine dose accordingly.
- Phenytoin: may have altered serum levels of phenytoin or ketoconazole; monitor serum levels of each and adjust dosages accordingly.
- Carbamazepine and long-acting barbiturates and macrolide antibiotics reduce the efficacy of voriconazole.

Lab Effects/Interference:

Major clinical significance:

- ALT, alk phos, AST, serum bili values may be elevated.

Special Considerations:

- Monitor liver function studies.

Potential Toxicities/Side Effects and the Nursing Process

I. ALTERATION IN NUTRITION, LESS THAN BODY REQUIREMENTS, related to GI SIDE EFFECTS

Defining Characteristics: Nausea, vomiting is seen in 3–10% of patients. Diarrhea, abdominal pain, flatulence, constipation may occur less frequently. Increased LFTs may occur: AST, ALT, alk phos. Hepatotoxicity is less common, is usually reversible, and is rarely fatal.

Nursing Implications: Assess baseline nutritional and elimination status. Instruct patient to report GI disturbances. Administer and teach patient to self-administer antiemetics, antidiarrheals as needed and as ordered. Teach patient importance of nutritious diet, and suggest small, frequent, high-calorie, high-protein meals as appropriate. Assess baseline LFTs and monitor periodically during treatment. Discuss abnormalities and drug interruption with physician. Assess whether taking other hepatotoxic drugs (see Special Considerations section). Assess for increased fatigue, jaundice, dark urine, pale stools (signs of hepatotoxicity), and discuss drug discontinuance immediately with physician.

II. ALTERATION IN SENSORY/PERCEPTUAL PATTERNS related to VISUAL DISTURBANCES

Defining Characteristics: Treatment-related visual disturbances are common (30%). Generally mild and rarely result in discontinuing treatment.

Nursing Implications: Assess for occurrence. Assess comfort level. Educate patient about this side effect. Assess impact on body image.

III. ALTERATION IN SKIN INTEGRITY related to ALLERGIC REACTION

Defining Characteristics: Rash, dermatitis, purpura, urticaria occur in 6% of patients.

Nursing Implications: Assess baseline skin condition and integrity. Teach patient to report itch, rash, and other skin changes. Teach patient skin care and symptomatic measures. If rash or dermatitis progresses, discuss drug discontinuance with physician. Assess for signs/symptoms of anaphylaxis.

ANTIVIRALS

Drug: acyclovir (Zovirax)

Class: Antiviral (systemic).

Mechanism of Action: Interferes with DNA synthesis so that viral replication cannot occur. Active against herpes simplex virus (HSV-1, HSV-2), varicella-zoster virus (VZV) (shingles), Epstein-Barr virus (EBV), and cytomegalovirus (CMV).

Metabolism: Variable GI absorption; unaffected by food. Widely distributed in body tissue and fluids, including CSF. Variable protein-binding (9–33%). Crosses placenta and is excreted in breast milk.

Dosage/Range:

Adult:

- Oral: 200 mg PO q4h (genital herpes) to 800 mg PO 5 × /day (acute herpes zoster).
- IV (initial/recurrent infections in immunocompromised patients): 5–10 mg/kg q8h × 7 days; 5 mg/kg q8h × 7–14 days (herpes simplex); 10 mg/kg q8h × 7–14 days (herpes zoster, herpes encephalitis).
- Use ideal body weight for dose calculation.

- Avoid doses greater than 1000 mg/dose.
- Dose modification is required if renal dysfunction is present.

Drug Preparation/Administration:
- Oral: store in tight, light-resistant containers at 15–25°C (59–77°F).
- IV: reconstitute with sterile water for injection per manufacturer's directions and further dilute in 50–100 mL IV fluid; a final concentration of 7 mg/mL or less is recommended to minimize the incidence of phlebitis; infuse over 1 hour.

Drug Interactions:
- Zidovudine: potentiates antiretroviral activity of zidovudine, but may cause increased neurotoxicity (drowsiness, lethargy) in AIDS patients. Monitor for increased neurotoxicity.
- Probenecid: may increase plasma half-life. Monitor for increased acyclovir toxicity.
- Antifungals: potential antiviral synergy.
- Interferon: potential synergistic antiviral effect, potential increased neurotoxicity. Use together with caution.
- Methotrexate (intrathecal): possible increased neurotoxicity. Use together with caution.

Lab Effects/Interference:

Major clinical significance:
- BUN and serum creatinine concentrations required prior to and during therapy, since intravenous acyclovir may be nephrotoxic; if acyclovir is given by rapid intravenous injection or its urine solubility is exceeded, precipitation of acyclovir crystals may occur in renal tubules; renal tubular damage may occur and may progress to acute renal failure.

Clinical significance:
- Pap test: although clear association has not been shown to date, patients with genital herpes may be at increased risk of developing cervical cancer. Pap test should be done at least once a year to detect early cervical changes.

Special Considerations:
- Use cautiously in patients with preexisting renal dysfunction or dehydration; underlying neurologic dysfunction or neurologic reactions to cytotoxic drugs, intrathecal methotrexate, or interferon and in patients with hepatic dysfunction.
- It is imperative that patients be well hydrated, with adequate urine output prior to and for up to 2 hours after IV dosing.
- Administer with caution if patient is receiving other nephrotoxic drugs.
- Contraindicated in patients hypersensitive to drug.
- Minimal injury to normal cells, so few adverse effects exist.

Potential Toxicities/Side Effects and the Nursing Process

I. ALTERATION IN URINARY ELIMINATION related to RENAL TOXICITY

Defining Characteristics: Transient increase is seen in renal function tests (serum BUN, creatinine) and decreased urine creatinine clearance, as drug may precipitate in renal tubules during dehydration or rapid IV drug administration. Increased risk exists if preexisting renal disease or concurrent administration of nephrotoxic drugs.

Nursing Implications: Assess baseline renal function, and monitor periodically during therapy. Notify physician of any abnormalities before administering next dose. Ensure adequate hydration and urine output prior to and for 2 hours after IV drug administration. Administer IV drug slowly over 1 hour.

II. ALTERATIONS IN SENSORY/PERCEPTUAL PATTERNS related to ENCEPHALOPATHY

Defining Characteristics: IV administration: encephalopathy (lethargy, tremors, confusion, agitation, seizures, dizziness) may occur rarely. Oral: headache occurs in 13% of patients receiving chronic suppressive treatment.

Nursing Implications: Assess baseline neurologic function and comfort, and monitor during treatment. Instruct patient to report any changes. Discuss any abnormalities with physician.

III. ALTERATIONS IN COMFORT related to LOCAL VEIN IRRITATION (IV ADMINISTRATION)

Defining Characteristics: Erythema, irritation, pain, swelling, phlebitis may occur at injection site.

Nursing Implications: Assess IV site for patency, irritation prior to each dose. Change IV site at least q48h. Apply warmth/heat to painful area as needed.

IV. ALTERATION IN NUTRITION, LESS THAN BODY REQUIREMENTS, related to GI SIDE EFFECTS (ORAL DOSAGE)

Defining Characteristics: Nausea, vomiting, and diarrhea occur in 2–5% of patients receiving chronic therapy.

Nursing Implications: Assess history of nausea/vomiting, diarrhea, and instruct patient to report any occurrence. Teach patient self-medication of prescribed antinausea or antidiarrheal medicines. Discuss drug discontinuance with physician if symptoms are severe.

V. ALTERATION IN SKIN INTEGRITY related to RASH

Defining Characteristics: Rash, urticaria, pruritus may occur.

Nursing Implications: Assess baseline history of drug allergy and skin integrity. Instruct patient to report any occurrence of rash, pruritus. Teach symptomatic management measures unless severe; if severe, discuss drug discontinuance with physician.

VI. KNOWLEDGE DEFICIT related to (ORAL) DRUG ADMINISTRATION

Defining Characteristics: Patient may not realize drug does not cure viral infection, nor does it prevent spread of virus to others. Prodrome of tingling, itching, or pain can herald mucocutaneous herpes.

Nursing Implications: Teach patient about herpetic infection and goal of therapy to suppress infection. When used to treat recurrent episodes of chronic infection, teach patient to recognize prodromal symptoms and to take prescribed drug then or within two days of onset of lesions. Teach patient about routes of viral spread, and instruct to avoid contacts with others that may lead to viral spread.

Drug: cidofovir (Vistide)

Class: Antiviral (systemic).

Mechanism of Action: Suppresses CMV replication by selective inhibition of viral DNA synthesis.

Metabolism: Less than 6% bound to plasma proteins. Renal clearance is reduced with the concomitant administration of probenecid.

Dosage/Range:
- Weekly induction regimen: 5 mg/kg infused every week × 2 weeks.
- Twice monthly maintenance regimen: 5 mg/kg infused every other week.

Drug Preparation:
- Requires chemotherapy safety handling (drug is mutagenic, tumorogenic, embryotoxic).
- Reconstitute drug (single use, nonpreserved); vial contains 75 mg/mL.
- Further dilute in 100 mL 0.9% Sodium Chloride.

Drug Administration:
- Administer 2 g probenecid (four 500-mg tabs) 3 hours prior to drug infusion.

- Infuse 1 L of 0.9% Sodium Chloride over 1–2 hours immediately prior to drug infusion.
- Infuse IV drug over 1 hour.
- As ordered by physician, may administer second liter of 0.9% Sodium Chloride at the start of the drug infusion, and continue for 1–3 hours.
- 2 hours after end of drug infusion, administer 1 g probenecid (two 500-mg tabs).
- 8 hours after end of the drug infusion, administer 1 g probenecid (two 500-mg tabs).

Drug Interactions:
- Probenecid: interacts with the metabolism or renal tubular excretion of acetaminophen, acyclovir, angiotensin-converting enzyme (ACE) inhibitors, barbiturates, NSAIDS, theophylline, zidovudine.
- Increased nephrotoxicity when combined with other nephrotoxic drugs.

Lab Effects/Interference:
- Serum creatinine levels may be elevated.

Special Considerations:
- Indicated for the treatment of AIDS patients who have newly diagnosed or relapsed CMV retinitis.
- Dose-limiting toxicity is nephrotoxicity evidenced by proteinuria and increased serum creatinine.
- Treatment requires prehydration and posthydration use of concomitant probenecid.
- Drug contraindicated in patients with baseline serum creatinine > 1.5 mg/dL, creatinine clearance ≤ 55 mL/min, proteinuria ≥ 3+, past severe hypersensitivity to probenecid or other sulfa-containing medications, hypersensitivity to cidofovir, and patients who are pregnant or breast-feeding.

DOSE REDUCTIONS:
- (a) Patients with baseline normal renal function:

Renal abnormality	Cidofovir dosage
Serum creatinine 0.3–0.4 mg/dL > baseline	3 mg/kg
Serum creatinine = 0.5 mg/dL above baseline	discontinue cidofovir
Proteinuria ≥ 3+	discontinue cidofovir

- (b) Patients with baseline renal impairment:

Creatinine clearance (mL/min)	Induction (once a week × 2 weeks)	Maintenance (once every 2 weeks)
41–55	2.0 mg/kg	2.0 mg/kg

COMPLICATIONS

Creatinine clearance (mL/min)	Induction (once a week × 2 weeks)	Maintenance (once every 2 weeks)
30–40	1.5 mg/kg	1.1 mg/kg
20–29	1.0 mg/kg	1.0 mg/kg
≤ 19	0.5 mg/kg	0.1 mg/kg

- Patient teaching:
  - Encourage increased oral intake of fluids to 1–3 L as tolerated.
  - Return to clinic for appointments (induction: weekly × 2 weeks, maintenance every other week).
  - Report side effects immediately.
  - Ophthalmologic appointments as scheduled for intraocular pressure (IOP), visual acuity monitoring.

Potential Toxicities/Side Effects and the Nursing Process

I. POTENTIAL FOR INJURY related to NEUTROPENIA

Defining Characteristics: Neutropenia ($< 750/mm^2$) may occur in 28% of patients, and $< 500/mm^3$ occurred in 20% of patients. Infections occurred in 25% of patients.

Nursing Implications: Monitor WBC and ANC prior to each drug dose, and hold treatment if neutropenic. Discuss with physician use of G-CSF. If the patient is receiving zidovudine, the zidovudine should be temporarily discontinued or dose decreased by 50% on days of probenecid therapy. Instruct patient to monitor temperature and to report fever > 101°F immediately. Discuss use of G-CSF with physician as needed (up to 34% required G-CSF in clinical trials).

II. ALTERATION IN NUTRITION, LESS THAN BODY REQUIREMENTS, related to NAUSEA/VOMITING

Defining Characteristics: Nausea/vomiting occurs in about 65% of patients.

Nursing Implications: Encourage patients to eat food prior to each dose of probenecid. Discuss antiemetic prior to the first dose of probenecid, and then during period of probenecid therapy.

III. ALTERATION IN COMFORT related to FEVER, CHILLS, RASH, HEADACHE FROM PROBENECID

Defining Characteristics: Fever occurs in up to 57% of patients, rash in 30%, headache in 27%, chills in 24%. Asthenia (46% incidence), diarrhea (27%), alopecia (25%), anorexia (22%), dyspnea (22%), abdominal pain (17%), and anemia (20%). In clinical trials, 25% of patients withdrew from treatment due to adverse events.

Nursing Implications: Assess baseline comfort, and instruct patient to report symptoms. Discuss symptom management with physician, such as antihistamine and/or antipyretic (acetaminophen) for fever, and then use prophylactically in subsequent doses.

IV. ALTERATION IN ELIMINATION related to RENAL TOXICITY

Defining Characteristics: Creatinine elevations to > 1.5 mg/dL occur in approximately 17% of patients, proteinuria in 80% of patients, and decreased serum bicarbonate in > 5% of patients.

Nursing Implications: Encourage patients to increase their daily oral fluid intake to 2–3 L. Closely monitor renal function; patients who have received foscarnet are at increased risk for nephrotoxicity. Ensure that patient receives prehydration and posthydration, and is able to take oral fluids. Discuss dose reductions based on alterations in renal function with physician. Check urine for protein. If positive, discuss additional hydration and rechecking of urine for blood with physician.

V. ALTERATIONS IN SENSORY/PERCEPTUAL PATTERNS related to OCULAR HYPOTONY

Defining Characteristics: OCULAR HYPOTONY occurs rarely, may be increased risk for patients with concomitant diabetes mellitus.

Nursing Implications: Patients should see ophthalmologist for IOP assessments and visual acuity periodically.

VI. METABOLIC ACIDOSIS related to DECREASED SERUM BICARBONATE

Defining Characteristics: Occurs rarely (2%).

Nursing Implications: Assess for decreases in serum bicarbonate < 16 mEq/L associated with evidence of renal tubular damage (incidence 9%). Serious metabolic acidosis in association with liver failure, mucormycosis, aspergillus, and disseminated MAC has occurred, with subsequent death in one patient. Monitor baseline chemistries, and review results prior to each treatment.

Drug: famciclovir (Famvir)

Class: Antiviral (systemic).

Mechanism of Action: Rapidly transformed into antiviral penciclovir, which inhibits herpes simplex types HSV-1, HSV-2, or VZV by inhibiting HSV-2 polymerase. Herpes viral DNA synthesis and viral replication are selectively inhibited.

Metabolism: Oral bioavailability is 77%, with peak plasma levels 30–90 minutes after dosing. Plasma half-life is 2.3 hours. In the virus, the active form of the drug has a long intracellular half-life. Low protein binding and rapid and complete elimination in the urine (73%) and feces (27%).

Dosage/Range:
- Herpes zoster: 500 mg q8h × 7 days.
- Genital herpes: 125 mg bid × 5 days.

Drug Preparation:
- Available in 125-, 250-, 500-mg tablets.

Drug Administration:
- Oral, without regard to meals.

Drug Interactions:
- None.

Lab Effects/Interference:
- None known.

Special Considerations:
- Treatment of herpes zoster: viral shedding stopped 50% faster than with placebo, with full crusting in < 1 week, and shorter time to relief from acute pain. In addition, drug significantly reduces the duration of postherpetic neuralgia by two months compared to placebo.
- Dose should be reduced in patients with renal impairment according to schedule below:

Condition	Creatinine clearance cc/min	Dose
Herpes zoster	40–59	500 mg q12h
	20–39	500 mg q24h
	< 20	250 mg q48h
Recurrent genital herpes	20–39	125 mg q24h
	< 20	125 mg q48h

Condition	Creatinine clearance cc/min	Dose

Potential Toxicities/Side Effects and the Nursing Process

I. ALTERATION IN COMFORT related to HEADACHE, NAUSEA

Defining Characteristics: Headache occurred in approximately 22% of patients. Nausea occurred in 12% of patients.

Nursing Implications: Teach patient that side effects may occur and are usually mild. Instruct patient to report headache that does not resolve with acetaminophen, or nausea that does not resolve with diet modification.

Drug: foscarnet sodium (Foscavir)

Class: Antiviral (systemic).

Mechanism of Action: Inhibits binding sites on virus-specific DNA polymerases and reverse transcriptases without affecting cellular DNA polymerases. Thus, prevents viral replication of all known herpes viruses: CMV, HSV-1, HSV-2, EBV, and VZV. Active against resistant herpes simplex viruses that are resistant via thymidine kinase deficiency. Indicated for treatment of CMV retinitis in AIDS patients.

Metabolism: 14–17% bound to plasma proteins, and excreted into urine 80–90% unchanged by kidneys. Variable penetration into CSF.

Dosage/Range:

Adult (normal renal function):

- IV induction: 60 mg/kg IV over 1 hour q8h × 2–3 weeks.
- Maintenance: 90–120 mg/kg/day IV over 2 hours.
- Dose modification is necessary if renal insufficiency. See manufacturer's package insert.

Drug Preparation/Administration:

- Add drug solution (24 mg/mL) to 0.9% Sodium Chloride or 5% Dextrose to achieve a final concentration ≤ 12 mg/mL.
- Administer via rate controller or infusion pump over 1 hour (induction) or 2 hours (maintenance) via peripheral or central vein.
- Do not administer or give concurrently with other drugs or solutions.

Drug Interactions:

- Incompatible with $D_{30}W$, amphotericin B, Ringer's lactate, total parenteral nutrition (TPN), acyclovir, ganciclovir, trimetrexate, pentamidine, vancomycin, trimethoprim/sulfamethoxazole, diazepam, digoxin, phenytoin, leucovorin, prochlorperazine.

- Pentamidine: potentially fatal HYPOCALCEMIA; seizures have occurred; AVOID CONCURRENT USE.
- Nephrotoxic drugs (amphotericin B, aminoglycosides): additive nephrotoxicity; AVOID CONCURRENT USE.
- Hypocalcemic agents: additive hypocalcemia; AVOID CONCURRENT USE.
- Zidovudine: increased anemia; monitor patient closely and transfuse with red blood cells as ordered.

Lab Effects/Interference: Lab Effects/Alterations:

Major clinical significance:

- Serum calcium (ionized), serum calcium (total), and serum phosphate: concentrations of phosphate may be increased or decreased; concentrations of total calcium may be decreased; although the total calcium concentration may also appear normal, the level of ionized calcium may be decreased and result in symptomatic hypocalcemia.
- Serum creatinine concentrations may be increased.
- Serum Mg++ concetrations may be decreased.

Clinical significance:

- ALT, alk phos, AST, and serum bili values may be increased.
- Serum K+ concentrations may be decreased.

Special Considerations:

- Contraindicated in patients hypersensitive to foscarnet.
- DO NOT administer concomitantly with IV pentamidine.
- Avoid use during pregnancy; lactating women should interrupt breast-feeding while receiving the drug.
- Regular monitoring of renal function IMPERATIVE; dose modifications must be made if renal insufficiency exists.
- Use measures for safe handling of cytotoxic drugs (see Appendix 1).

Potential Toxicities/Side Effects and the Nursing Process

I. ALTERATION IN URINARY ELIMINATION related to RENAL TOXICITY

Defining Characteristics: Abnormal renal function occurs commonly; increased serum creatinine, decreased creatinine clearance, acute renal failure may occur.

Nursing Implications: Assess baseline elimination pattern and renal function studies, and monitor closely throughout treatment. Manufacturer suggests creatinine clearance be calculated 2–3 × per week (induction) and q1–2 weeks (maintenance). Creatinine clearance can be calculated from modified Cockcroft and Gault equation:

For males: $$\frac{140 - \text{age}}{\text{serum creatinine} \times 72}$$

For females: $$\frac{140 - \text{age}}{\text{serum creatinine} \times 72} \times 0.085$$

Discuss dose modifications with physician if renal dysfunction occurs. Ensure adequate hydration and urinary output prior to and following dose; administer drug slowly over 1–2 hours, at no more than 1 mg/kg/min. Teach patient to increase oral fluids as tolerated to clear drug from kidneys.

II. ALTERATION IN ELECTROLYTE BALANCE related to METABOLIC ABNORMALITIES

Defining Characteristics: Hypocalcemia, hypophosphatemia, hyperphosphatemia, hypomagnesemia, and hypokalemia occur. Transient decreased ionized calcium may not appear in serum total calcium value. Tetany and seizures may occur, especially in patients receiving foscarnet and IV pentamidine. Increased risk exists if renal impairment or neurologic impairment.

Nursing Implications: Assess baseline calcium, phosphorus, magnesium, potassium, and concurrent drugs that might affect these values. Assess patient for signs/symptoms of hypocalcemia, such as perioral tingling, numbness, or paresthesias during or after infusion. Instruct patient to report these signs/symptoms immediately. If signs/symptoms occur, stop infusion, notify physician, and evaluate serum electrolyte, renal studies. Administer ordered electrolyte repletion.

III. ALTERATIONS IN SENSORY/PERCEPTUAL PATTERNS related to NEUROLOGIC CHANGES

Defining Characteristics: Headache, paresthesia, dizziness, involuntary muscle contractions, hypoesthesia, neuropathy, and seizures (including grand mal) have occurred. Increased risk exists of hypocalcemia (ionized Ca++) and renal insufficiency.

Nursing Implications: Assess baseline risk factors and neurologic status, and monitor during treatment. Assess for and instruct patient to report signs/symptoms. Discuss abnormalities with physician, and possible drug discontinuance.

IV. FATIGUE related to ANEMIA

Defining Characteristics: Anemia occurs in 33% of patients, and in 60% of patients receiving concomitant zidovudine.

Nursing Implications: Assess baseline HCT/Hgb, activity tolerance, cardiopulmonary status, and monitor during therapy. Instruct patient to report increasing fatigue, headache, irritability, shortness of breath, chest pain. Transfuse RBCs as ordered by physician. Discuss with clinic patient self-care ability; refer for home health assistance as needed.

V. ALTERATION IN NUTRITION, LESS THAN BODY REQUIREMENTS, related to GI SIDE EFFECTS

Defining Characteristics: Nausea, vomiting, diarrhea are common; anorexia, abdominal pain may also occur.

Nursing Implications: Assess baseline nutrition, liver function and monitor during therapy. Instruct patient to report GI side effects. Administer or teach patient to self-administer prescribed antiemetic or antidiarrheal medications. Encourage adequate oral or IV hydration. Notify physician of abnormal LFTs. If anorexia occurs, encourage favorite foods and small, frequent meals as tolerated.

VI. INFECTION related to NEUTROPENIA

Defining Characteristics: May occur in 17% of patients; increased risk when receiving concurrent zidovudine.

Nursing Implications: Assess baseline WBC, ANC, and temperature; monitor during therapy. Assess for signs/symptoms of infection and discuss these with physician. Instruct patient to report signs/symptoms of infection.

VII. ALTERATIONS IN COMFORT related to LOCAL VEIN IRRITATION (IV ADMINISTRATION)

Defining Characteristics: Erythema, irritation, pain, swelling, phlebitis may occur at injection site. Consider use of central line.

Nursing Implications: Assess IV site for patency, irritation prior to each dose. Change IV site at least q48h. Apply warmth/heat to painful area as needed.

VIII. ALTERATION IN SKIN INTEGRITY related to RASH

Defining Characteristics: Rash, sweating may occur. Also, rarely, local irritation and ulcerations of penile epithelium in males, and vulvovaginal mucosa in females has occurred—perhaps related to drug in urine.

Nursing Implications: Assess skin integrity baseline and during treatment. Instruct patient to report any irritation or lesions. Teach patient to perform frequent perineal hygiene.

Drug: ganciclovir (Cytovene)

Class: Antiviral (systemic).

Mechanism of Action: Interferes with DNA synthesis so that viral replication cannot occur. Active against HSV-1, HSV-2, VZV (shingles), EBV, and CMV.

Metabolism: Poorly absorbed from GI tract. Appears to be widely distributed, concentrates in kidneys, and is well distributed to the eyes. Crosses BBB. Drug crosses placenta and is excreted in breast milk in animals. Excreted unchanged in urine. Active against CMV infections, especially in the retina.

Dosage/Range:

Adult:

- IV induction: 5 mg/kg IV q12h × 14–21 days.
- Maintenance: 5 mg/kg IV 7 days/week or 6 mg/kg/day × 5 days/week.
- Intravitreous by ophthalmologist (investigational).
- DOSE MUST BE REDUCED IN RENAL IMPAIRMENT.

Drug Preparation/Administration:

- Drug is CARCINOGENIC and TERATOGENIC: use chemotherapy handling precautions (see Appendix 1) when preparing and administering ganciclovir.
- Administer only if ANC is > 500 cells/mm^3 and platelet count > 25,000/mm^3.
- Add 10 mL of sterile water for injection to 500-mg vial. Further dilute dose in 50–250 mL of IV fluid and infuse over at least 1 hour.

Drug Interactions:

- Zidovudine: increased hematologic toxicity (neutropenia, anemia); do not use together if possible. Consider didanosine (ddI) instead of zidovudine (AZT) or concomitant use of neutrophil growth factor (e.g., G-CSF or GM-CSF).
- Foscarnet: additive or synergistic antiviral activity.
- Probenecid: may increase ganciclovir serum levels. Monitor closely and decrease ganciclovir dose as needed.
- Immunosuppressant (corticosteroids, cyclosporine, azathioprine): increased bone marrow suppression; dose reduce or hold immunosuppressants during ganciclovir treatment.
- Interferon: potent synergism against herpes virus, VZV.
- Imipenem/cilastatin: increase neurotoxicity with seizures. AVOID CONCURRENT USE.
- Cytotoxic antineoplastic agents: additive toxicity in bone marrow, gonads, GI epithelium/mucosa.

- Other cytotoxic drugs (dapsone, pentamidine, flucytosine, amphotericin B, trimethoprim-sulfamethoxazole): increase toxicity. Use cautiously if unable to avoid concurrent use.

Lab Effects/Interference:

- Serum ALT, serum alk phos, serum AST, and serum bili values may be increased.
- BUN and serum creatinine values may be increased.

Special Considerations:

- Do not use in pregnancy.
- Patient should be well hydrated; use with caution at reduced doses if renal insufficiency exists.
- Drug is mutagenic; patient should use barrier contraceptive.
- For CMV retinitis patient, should see ophthalmologist at least every 6 weeks during ganciclovir therapy.
- Administer over at least 1 hour.
- Monitor blood counts frequently (3 × per week).

Potential Toxicities/Side Effects and the Nursing Process

I. INFECTION, BLEEDING related to BONE MARROW DEPRESSION

Defining Characteristics: Neutropenia (< 1000/mm^3) occurs in 25–50% of patients, especially in patients with AIDS or those undergoing bone marrow transplant. Thrombocytopenia (< 50,000/mm^3) occurs in 20% of patients. Anemia occurs in 1% of patients.

Nursing Implications: Assess baseline WBC, ANC, and platelet count; monitor throughout therapy (every other day initially, then 3 × per week). Hold ganciclovir if ANC < 500/mm^3, platelet count < 25,000/mm^3. Assess for signs/symptoms of infection or bleeding; instruct patient in signs/symptoms of infection and bleeding, and instruct to report these immediately. Teach patient self-care measures to minimize risk of infection, bleeding, including avoidance of OTC aspirin-containing medicines. Administer or teach patient to self-administer prescribed G-CSF or GM-CSF. Assess Hgb/HCT and signs/symptoms of fatigue. Instruct patient to alternate rest and activity periods.

II. ALTERATIONS IN SENSORY/PERCEPTUAL PATTERNS related to SENSORY CHANGES

Defining Characteristics: Retinal detachment may occur in 30% of patients treated for CMV retinitis. Local reactions (foreign body sensation, conjunctival or vitreal hemorrhage) may occur with intravitreal injection. CNS effects include headache, confusion, altered dreams, ataxia, dizziness, and affect 5–17% of patients.

Nursing Implications: Assess baseline neurologic status, including vision, and monitor during treatment. Patient should see ophthalmologist at least every six weeks. Instruct patient to report any abnormalities and discuss them with physician.

III. ALTERATION IN NUTRITION, LESS THAN BODY REQUIREMENTS, related to GI SIDE EFFECTS

Defining Characteristics: Nausea, vomiting, diarrhea, anorexia may occur in 2% of patients. Elevated LFTs may occur due to drug, but may be difficult to distinguish from CMV infection of liver or biliary tree.

Nursing Implications: Assess baseline nutrition, liver function, and monitor during therapy. Instruct patient to report GI side effects. Administer or teach patient to self-administer prescribed antiemetic or antidiarrheal medications. Encourage adequate oral or IV hydration. Notify physician of abnormal LFTs. If anorexia occurs, encourage favorite foods and small, frequent meals as tolerated.

IV. ALTERATION IN URINARY ELIMINATION related to RENAL TOXICITY

Defining Characteristics: 2% of patients have increased serum BUN, creatinine, hematuria. Increased risk exists in elderly or patients with renal insufficiency.

Nursing Implications: Ensure adequate hydration with urinary output prior to drug administration and infuse drug over at least 1 hour. Dose should be reduced in patients with decreased renal function.

V. ALTERATIONS IN COMFORT related to LOCAL VEIN IRRITATION (IV ADMINISTRATION)

Defining Characteristics: Inflammation, phlebitis, pain occur often at IV infusion site due to high pH of drug.

Nursing Implications: Assess IV site for patency, irritation, prior to each dose. Change IV site at least q48h. Apply warmth/heat to painful area as needed. Assess need for tunneled central line. Avoid drug extravasation.

VI. ALTERATION IN CARDIAC OUTPUT related to CHANGES IN BP

Defining Characteristics: Rarely, hypotension, or hypertension, arrhythmia, myocardial infarction, arrest occur.

Nursing Implications: Assess baseline VS and monitor throughout treatment. Notify physician of any changes from baseline.

VII. ALTERATION IN SEXUALITY/REPRODUCTIVE PATTERNS related to REPRODUCTIVE HAZARD

Defining Characteristics: Drug is carcinogenic, mutagenic, and teratogenic; may produce infertility in males. It is unknown whether drug crosses placenta and is excreted in breast milk.

Nursing Implications: Assess sexuality/reproductive patterns. Teach patient and partner about reproductive hazards; offer contraceptive counseling or refer for counseling, as barrier contraceptive should be used by patient.

Drug: valacyclovir hydrochloride (Valtrex)

Class: Antiviral (systemic).

Mechanism of Action: Drug is well absorbed and rapidly converted to acyclovir. Drug interferes with DNA synthesis so that viral replication cannot occur. Active against HSV-1, HSV-2, VZV (shingles), EBV, and CMV.

Metabolism: Widely distributed in body tissues and fluids including the CNS.

Dosage/Range:

- Herpes zoster: 1 g tid × 7 days.

Drug Preparation/Administration:

- Available in 500-mg caplets.
- Oral, without regard to meals.

Drug Interactions:

- Cimetidine and probenecid decrease renal clearance of valacyclovir.

Lab Effects/Interference:

- None known.

Special Considerations:

- Dose-reduce for renal impairment:

Creatinine Clearance (cc/min)	Dose
≥ 50	1 g q8h
30–49	1 g q12h
10–29	1 g q24h
< 10	500 mg q24h

- Treatment should be started within 48 hours of rash onset.
- AVOID DRUG IN IMMUNOCOMPROMISED PATIENTS, as patients with advanced HIV infection, and those undergoing bone marrow and renal transplants, have developed thrombotic thrombocytopenic purpura/hemolytic uremic syndrome (TTP/HUS).

Potential Toxicities/Side Effects and the Nursing Process

I. ALTERATION IN COMFORT related to HEADACHE, NAUSEA

Defining Characteristics: Headache occurred in approximately 22% of patients. Nausea occurred in 12% of patients.

Nursing Implications: Teach patient that side effects may occur and are usually mild. Patient 1/4 should report headache that does not resolve with acetaminophen or nausea that does not resolve by diet modification.

Chapter 12
Constipation

Constipation is a decreased frequency of defecation that is difficult or uncomfortable (Walsh 1989). Levy (1992) reports five causes of constipation in cancer patients. They include:

1. Disease itself: i.e., primary bowel cancers, paraneoplastic autonomic neuropathy.
2. Disease sequelae: i.e., dehydration, paralysis, immobility, alterations in bowel elimination patterns.
3. Prior history of laxative abuse, hemorrhoids/anal fissures, other diseases.
4. Cancer therapy: chemotherapy (vinca alkaloids, e.g., vincristine, vinblastine); bowel surgery.
5. Medications used to manage symptoms: opioids, antihistamines, tricyclic antidepressants, aluminum antacids.

Complications of constipation can be severe (i.e., bowel perforation), extremely painful, and compromise quality of life. Nurses play an enormous role in preventing morbidity from constipation in patients with cancer. Assessment of the patient's previous and current nutrition and elimination patterns, along with assessment of probable etiology of constipation, are critical, as is patient/ family teaching about constipation management and prevention. Teaching should include dietary modifications to include high-fiber intake (fruits, vegetables, or nutritional supplements high in fiber); fluid intake of 3 L/day; and moderate exercise as tolerated. Patients receiving drugs (i.e., opioids) that are likely to be constipating should also receive a bowel regimen to prevent constipation. Available laxatives include the following types:

- *Bulk-forming* laxatives cause the stool to retain water, and thus increase peristalsis (fiber, bran, psyllium, methylcellulose).
- *Lubricants* coat and soften the stool so it can move more smoothly through the intestines (mineral oil).
- *Saline laxatives* pull water into the gut and into the stool, increasing peristalsis (magnesium citrate, sodium biphosphate, magnesium hydroxide).
- *Osmotic laxatives* work through colonic bacteria that metabolize osmotic laxatives causing increased osmotic pressure gradient, pulling water into the

gut and then into the stool, thus increasing peristalsis (glycerin, lactulose, sorbitol).

- *Detergent laxatives* reduce surface tension of the colonic cells, so water and fats enter the stool; in addition, electrolyte and water absorption is decreased (docusate salts).
- *Stimulant laxatives* irritate the gut, increasing gut motility (senna, bisacodyl).

References

Levy MH. Constipation and Diarrhea in Cancer Patients, Part I. *Prim Care Cancer* 1992;12(4):11–18

Massey RL, Haylock PJ, Curtiss C. *Constipation,* Chapter 27. Yarbro CH, Frogge MH, Goodman M, (eds), *Cancer Symptom Management,* 3rd ed. Sudbury, MA: Jones and Bartlett, 2003

Twycross RG, Harcourt JMV. The Use of Laxatives at a Palliative Care Centre. *Pallia Med* 1991;5:27–33

Walsh TD. Constipation. Walsh TD, (eds), *Symptom Control.* Cambridge: Blackwell Scientific Publications Inc.,1989;331–381

Drug: bisacodyl (Dulcolax)

Class: Stimulant laxative.

Mechanism of Action: Stimulates/irritates smooth muscle of intestines, increasing peristalsis; increases fluid accumulation in colon and small intestines. Indicated for relief of constipation and bowel preparation prior to bowel surgery.

Metabolism: Minimal oral absorption. Evacuation occurs in 6–10 hours when taken orally, or within 15 minutes to 1 hour when administered rectally.

Dosage/Range:

Adult:

- Oral: 5–15 mg at bedtime or early morning. Bowel preparation may use up to 30 mg.
- Suppository: 10 mg PR.

Drug Preparation/Administration:

- Administer oral tablet > 1 hour after antacids or milk.
- Insert suppository as high as possible against wall of rectum.

Drug Interactions:

- None.

Lab Effects/Interference:

- None known.

Special Considerations:

- Contraindicated in patients with signs/symptoms of acute abdomen (nausea, vomiting, abdominal pain), intestinal obstruction, fecal impaction, or ulcerative bowel lesions.

Potential Toxicities/Side Effects and the Nursing Process

I. ALTERATIONS IN BOWEL ELIMINATION related to CHRONIC USE

Defining Characteristics: Removes defecation reflexes when used chronically (laxative dependence). Narcotic analgesics and vinca alkaloid chemotherapy may predispose to constipation.

Nursing Implications: Assess baseline elimination pattern. Teach patient how to self-administer laxative. Encourage patient to normalize bowel habits through adequate fluid intake (2–3 L/day), diet high in fiber and bulk (bran, cereals, fruits, and vegetables), and exercise as tolerated. Teach patient bowel regimen when on narcotics or vinca alkaloids to promote regular evacuation.

II. ALTERATION IN NUTRITION, LESS THAN BODY REQUIREMENTS, related to GI SIDE EFFECTS

Defining Characteristics: Constipation or drug may cause nausea, vomiting, abdominal pain; rectal suppository may cause burning in rectum as it is absorbed.

Nursing Implications: Assess comfort level and GI distress related to constipation. Encourage patient to drink cold fluids or ginger ale as tolerated. Encourage patient to try resting in different positions; warm packs may decrease abdominal pain. Teach patient to expect burning sensation with suppository use; reassure that it will resolve in 5–10 minutes.

III. ALTERATION IN FLUID AND ELECTROLYTE BALANCE related to LAXATIVE ABUSE

Defining Characteristics: Diarrhea resulting from laxative abuse can deplete fluid volume, nutrients, and electrolytes.

Nursing Implications: Teach patient regular bowel regimen when receiving constipating drugs (narcotics, vinca alkaloids). Teach patient to replace lost fluids and electrolytes (encourage chicken soup, sports drink).

Drug: docusate calcium, docusate potassium, docusate sodium (Dioctyl Calcium Sulfosuccinate, Dioctyl Potassium Sulfosuccinate, Dioctyl Sodium Sulfosuccinate, Colace, Diocto-K, Diosuccin, DOK-250, Doxinate, Duosol, Laxinate 100, Regulax SS, Stulex)

Class: Stool softener.

Mechanism of Action: The calcium, sodium, and potassium salts of docusate soften stool by decreasing surface tension, emulsification, and wetting action, thus increasing stool absorption of water in the bowel.

Metabolism: Appears to be absorbed somewhat in the duodenum and jejunum, and excreted in bile. Stool softening occurs in 1–3 days.

Dosage/Range:

Adult:

- Oral: 50–360 mg/day, in single or divided doses, depending on stool-softening response.

Drug Preparation/Administration:

- Oral: store gelatin capsule in tight container; store syrup in light-resistant containers.
- Rectal: according to manufacturer's package insert.

Drug Interactions:

- Mineral oil: increased mineral oil absorption; AVOID CONCURRENT USE.

Lab Effects/Interference:

- None known.

Special Considerations:

- Useful in prevention of straining-at-stool in patients receiving narcotics; when combined with other agents/laxatives, prevents constipation in these patients.
- Does not increase intestinal peristalsis; stop drug if severe abdominal cramping occurs.
- Is effective only in prevention of constipation, not in treating constipation.

Potential Toxicities/Side Effects and the Nursing Process

I. KNOWLEDGE DEFICIT related to BOWEL ELIMINATION

Defining Characteristics: Oncology patients who are receiving narcotic analgesics, vinca alkaloid chemotherapy (vincristine, vinblastine, vindesine), or who are dehydrated or hypercalcemic are at increased risk of constipation.

Nursing Implications: Assess baseline elimination pattern. Teach patient need for bowel movement at least every other day, depending on usual pattern.

Teach patient importance of adequate fluid intake (2–3 L/day), diet high in fiber and bulk (bran, cereals, fruits, vegetables, and supplements with fiber), and exercise as tolerated. Teach self-administration of stool softeners and prescribed laxatives.

Drug: glycerin suppository (Fleet Babylax, Sani-Supp)

Class: Hyperosmotic laxative.

Mechanism of Action: Local irritant, with hyperosmotic action, drawing water from tissues into feces and stimulating fecal evacuation within 15–30 minutes.

Metabolism: Poorly absorbed from rectum.

Dosage/Range:

Adult:

- Rectal suppository: 2–3 g PR.
- Enema: 5–15 mL PR.

Drug Preparation/Administration:

- Rectal administration must be retained for 15 minutes.

Drug Interactions:

- None.

Lab Effects/Interference:

- None known.

Special Considerations:

- Contraindicated in patients with undiagnosed abdominal pain, intestinal obstruction.

Potential Toxicities/Side Effects and the Nursing Process

I. ALTERATIONS IN BOWEL ELIMINATION related to CHRONIC USE

Defining Characteristics: Removes defecation reflexes when used chronically (laxative dependence). Narcotic analgesics and vinca alkaloid chemotherapy may predispose to constipation.

Nursing Implications: Assess baseline elimination pattern. Teach patient how to self-administer laxative. Encourage patient to normalize bowel habits through adequate fluid intake (2–3 L/day), diet high in fiber and bulk (bran, cereals, fruits, and vegetables), and exercise as tolerated. Teach patient bowel regimen when on narcotics or vinca alkaloids to promote regular evacuation.

II. ALTERATION IN FLUID AND ELECTROLYTE BALANCE related to LAXATIVE ABUSE

Defining Characteristics: Diarrhea resulting from laxative abuse can deplete fluid volume, nutrients, and electrolytes.

Nursing Implications: Teach patient regular bowel regimen when receiving constipating drugs (narcotics, vinca alkaloids). Teach patient to replace lost fluids and electrolytes (encourage chicken soup, sports drink).

III. ALTERATION IN COMFORT related to CRAMPING PAIN, RECTAL IRRITATION, OR DISCOMFORT

Defining Characteristics: Cramping pain, rectal irritation, and inflammation or discomfort may occur.

Nursing Implications: Teach patient this may occur. If discomfort is not self-limited, suggest sitz bath, warm or cold packs, and position changes.

Drug: lactulose (Cholac, Constilac, Constulose, Duphalac)

Class: Hyperosmolar sugar.

Mechanism of Action: Delivers osmotically active molecules to intestine, drawing fluid into colon and causing distension; this stimulates peristalsis and evacuation in 24–48 hours. Also used to lower blood ammonia in hepatic encephalopathy.

Metabolism: Less than 3% absorbed; metabolized by bacteria in colon into lactic acid.

Dosage/Range:

Adult:

- Oral: 10–20 g (15–30 mL)/day to 40 g (60 mL)/day.

Drug Preparation/Administration:

- Store solution at 15–30°C (59–86°F).
- Give with juice.

Drug Interactions:

- Antacids: may decrease lactulose effect; avoid administering together.

Special Considerations:

- Diarrhea indicates overdosage; dose should be reduced.

Potential Toxicities/Side Effects and the Nursing Process

I. ALTERATION IN COMFORT related to GI SIDE EFFECTS

Defining Characteristics: Gaseous distension, flatulence, abdominal pain may occur.

Nursing Implications: Encourage patient to find comfortable position; apply warmth to decrease abdominal pain; reassure that symptoms will resolve.

II. ALTERATION IN FLUID AND ELECTROLYTE BALANCE related to DIARRHEA

Defining Characteristics: Diarrhea resulting from laxative abuse can deplete fluid volume, nutrients, and electrolytes.

Nursing Implications: Teach patient regular bowel regimen when receiving constipating drugs (narcotics, vinca alkaloids). Teach patient to replace lost fluids and electrolytes (encourage chicken soup, sports drink).

Drug: magnesium citrate

Class: Saline laxative.

Mechanism of Action: Draws water into small intestinal lumen, stimulating peristalsis and evacuation in 3–6 hours.

Metabolism: 15–30% absorbed, excreted in urine.

Dosage/Range:

Adult:

- Oral: 11–25 g (5–10 oz or 150–300 mL)/day as single or divided dose at bedtime.

Drug Preparation/Administration:

- Refrigerate and serve with ice. Taste can be masked by adding small amount of juice.

Drug Interactions:

- None.

Lab Effects/Interference:

- None known.

Special Considerations:

- Contraindicated in patients with signs/symptoms of acute abdomen (nausea, vomiting, abdominal pain), intestinal obstruction, fecal impaction, or ulcerative bowel lesions.

- Contraindicated in patients with rectal fissures, myocardial infarction, renal disease.

Potential Toxicities/Side Effects and the Nursing Process

I. ALTERATIONS IN BOWEL ELIMINATION related to CHRONIC USE

Defining Characteristics: Removes defecation reflexes when used chronically (laxative dependence). Narcotic analgesics and vinca alkaloid chemotherapy may predispose to constipation.

Nursing Implications: Assess baseline elimination pattern. Teach patient how to self-administer laxative. Encourage patient to normalize bowel habits through adequate fluid intake (2–3 L/day), diet high in fiber and bulk (bran, cereals, fruits, and vegetables), and exercise as tolerated. Teach patient bowel regimen when on narcotics or vinca alkaloids to promote regular evacuation.

II. ALTERATION IN NUTRITION, LESS THAN BODY REQUIREMENTS, related to GI SIDE EFFECTS

Defining Characteristics: Constipation or drug may cause nausea and abdominal pain.

Nursing Implications: Assess comfort level and GI distress related to constipation. Encourage patient to drink cold fluids or ginger ale as tolerated. Encourage patient to try resting in different positions; warm packs may decrease abdominal pain.

III. ALTERATION IN FLUID AND ELECTROLYTE BALANCE related to LAXATIVE ABUSE

Defining Characteristics: Diarrhea resulting from laxative abuse can deplete fluid volume, nutrients, and electrolytes.

Nursing Implications: Teach patient regular bowel regimen when receiving constipating drugs (narcotics, vinca alkaloids). Teach patient to replace lost fluids and electrolytes (encourage chicken soup, sports drink).

COMPLICATIONS

Drug: methylcellulose (Citrucel)

Class: Bulk-producing laxative.

Mechanism of Action: Absorbs water; bulk expansion stimulates peristalsis and evacuation in 12–24 hours. May also be used to slow diarrhea.

Metabolism: Not absorbed by GI tract.

Dosage/Range:

Adult:

- Oral: up to 6 g/day PO in 2–3 divided doses.

Drug Preparation/Administration:

- Administer each dose with at least 250 mL of water or juice.

Drug Interactions:

- None.

Lab Effects/Interference:

- None known.

Special Considerations:

- Safest and most physiologically normal laxative.

Potential Toxicities/Side Effects and the Nursing Process

I. ALTERATIONS IN BOWEL ELIMINATION related to CHRONIC USE

Defining Characteristics: Removes defecation reflexes when used chronically (laxative dependence). Narcotic analgesics and vinca alkaloid chemotherapy may predispose to constipation.

Nursing Implications: Assess baseline elimination pattern. Teach patient how to self-administer laxative. Encourage patient to normalize bowel habits through adequate fluid intake (2–3 L/day), diet high in fiber and bulk (bran, cereals, fruits, and vegetables), and exercise as tolerated. Teach patient bowel regimen when on narcotics or vinca alkaloids to promote regular evacuation.

II. ALTERATION IN NUTRITION, LESS THAN BODY REQUIREMENTS, related to GI SIDE EFFECTS

Defining Characteristics: Constipation or drug may cause nausea, vomiting, cramps.

Nursing Implications: Assess comfort level and GI distress related to constipation. Encourage patient to drink cold fluids or ginger ale as tolerated. Encourage patient to try resting in different positions; warm packs may decrease abdominal pain. Teach patient laxative effect may take 12–24 hours, and assess need for other cathartic(s).

Drug: mineral oil (Fleet Mineral Oil)

Class: Lubricant laxative.

Mechanism of Action: Lubricates intestine, preventing fecal fluid from being absorbed in colon; water retention distends colon, stimulating peristalsis and evacuation in 6–8 hours.

Metabolism: Minimal GI absorption occurs following oral or rectal administration.

Dosage/Range:

Adult:

- Oral: 15–45 mL PO in single or divided doses.
- Rectal enemas: 120 mL PR as a single dose.

Drug Preparation/Administration:

- Administer plain mineral oil at bedtime on an empty stomach.
- Administer mineral oil emulsion with food if desired at bedtime.
- May mix with juice to mask taste.

Drug Interactions:

- Docusate salts: increase mineral oil absorption; DO NOT ADMINISTER concurrently.
- Fat-soluble vitamins: decrease absorption with chronic mineral oil administration.

Lab Effects/Interference:

- Decreased fat-soluble vitamins, e.g., vitamins A, D, E, K with chronic drug administration.

Special Considerations:

- Contraindicated in patients with signs/symptoms of acute abdomen (nausea, vomiting, abdominal pain), intestinal obstruction, fecal impaction, or ulcerative bowel lesions.
- Do not use for more than 1 week.

Potential Toxicities/Side Effects and the Nursing Process

I. ALTERATIONS IN BOWEL ELIMINATION related to CHRONIC USE

Defining Characteristics: Removes defecation reflexes when used chronically (laxative dependence). Narcotic analgesics and vinca alkaloid chemotherapy may predispose to constipation.

Nursing Implications: Assess baseline elimination pattern. Teach patient how to self-administer laxative. Encourage patient to normalize bowel habits through adequate fluid intake (2–3 L/day), diet high in fiber and bulk (bran, cereals, fruits, and vegetables), and exercise as tolerated. Teach patient bowel regimen when on narcotics or vinca alkaloids to promote regular evacuation.

II. ALTERATION IN NUTRITION, LESS THAN BODY REQUIREMENTS, related to GI SIDE EFFECTS

Defining Characteristics: Constipation or drug may cause nausea, vomiting, cramps.

Nursing Implications: Assess comfort level and GI distress related to constipation. Encourage patient to drink cold fluids or ginger ale as tolerated. Encourage patient to try resting in different positions; warm packs may decrease abdominal pain. Teach patient to expect burning sensation with suppository use; reassure that it will resolve in 5–10 minutes.

Drug: polyethylene glycol 3350, NF powder (Miralax®)

Class: Osmotic cathartic.

Mechanism of Action: Drug is an osmotic agent that pulls water into the intestines with the stool, softening the stool and causing peristalsis and evacuation in 2–4 days.

Metabolism: Is not fermented by colonic microflora and does not affect intestinal absorption or secretion of glucose or electrolytes.

Dosage/Range:
- 17 g (1 heaping T) (product comes with a measuring cup).

Drug Preparation:
- Mix in 8 oz of water and take orally once a day.

Drug Administration:
- Oral. Available in 14-oz and 26-oz containers.
- Store at room temperature.

Drug Interactions:
- None.

Lab Effects/Interference:
- None.

Special Considerations:
- Contraindicated in patients with bowel obstruction.
- Indicated for the treatment of occasional constipation for up to 2 weeks.
- Use during pregnancy only if clearly needed.
- Excessive or frequent use or use > 2 weeks may result in electrolyte imbalance and dependence on laxatives.

Potential Toxicities/Side Effects and the Nursing Process

I. ALTERATIONS IN BOWEL ELIMINATION related to CHRONIC USE

Defining Characteristics: Removes defecation reflexes when used chronically (laxative dependence). Narcotic analgesics and vinca alkaloid chemotherapy may predispose to constipation.

Nursing Implications: Assess baseline elimination pattern. Teach patient how to self-administer laxative. Encourage patient to normalize bowel habits through adequate fluid intake (2–3 L/day), diet high in fiber and bulk (bran, cereals, fruits, and vegetables), and exercise as tolerated. Teach patient bowel regimen when on narcotics or vinca alkaloids to promote regular evacuation.

II. ALTERATION IN NUTRITION related to GI SIDE EFFECTS

Defining Characteristics: Constipation or drug may cause nausea, cramps, abdominal bloating, flatulence. High doses may cause diarrhea, especially in the elderly. Continued use beyond 2 weeks may cause electrolyte imbalance.

Nursing Implications: Assess comfort level and GI distress related to constipation. Encourage patient to drink cold fluids or ginger ale as tolerated. Encourage patient to try resting in different positions; warm packs may decrease abdominal pain. Teach patient laxative effect may take 2–4 days and assess need for other cathartic(s).

Drug: senna (Senexon, Senokot)

Class: Irritant/stimulant laxative.

Mechanism of Action: Stimulates/irritates smooth muscle of intestines, increasing peristalsis; increases fluid accumulation in colon and small intestines. Indicated for relief of constipation or bowel preparation prior to bowel surgery.

Metabolism: Minimal oral absorption occurs. Evacuation occurs in 6–10 hours when taken orally.

Dosage/Range:
- Senexon: 2 tablets at bedtime (187 mg senna).
- Senokot: 2–4 tablets bid (187 mg senna); 1–2 tsp granules bid (326 mg senna); 1 suppository at bedtime, repeat PRN in 2 hours (652 mg senna).
- Black-Draught: 2 tablets (600 mg senna) or 1/4–1/2 level tsp granules (1.65 gm senna).

Drug Preparation/Administration:
- Store in a tightly closed bottle.

II. ALTERATION IN FLUID AND ELECTROLYTE BALANCE related to LAXATIVE ABUSE

Defining Characteristics: Diarrhea resulting from laxative abuse can deplete fluid volume, nutrients, and electrolytes.

Nursing Implications: Teach patient regular bowel regimen when receiving constipating drugs (narcotics, vinca alkaloids). Teach patient to replace lost fluids and electrolytes (encourage chicken soup, sports drink).

III. ALTERATION IN COMFORT related to CRAMPING PAIN, RECTAL IRRITATION OR DISCOMFORT

Defining Characteristics: Cramping pain, rectal irritation, and inflammation or discomfort may occur.

Nursing Implications: Teach patient this may occur. If discomfort is not self-limited, suggest sitz bath, warm or cold packs, and position changes.

Chapter 13

Diarrhea

Rutledge and Engleking (1998) define diarrhea as an abnormal increase in liquidity and frequency, and occurring as acute (within 24–48 hours of a stimulus, resolving in 7–14 days) or chronic (late onset, lasting > 2–3 weeks). Diarrhea occurring in patients with cancer is most often related to osmotic, malabsorptive, secretory, exudative, dysmotility-associated, or chemotherapy-induced (Levy, 1992; Engleking, 2003). Engleking (2003) gives examples of each.

- *Osmotic diarrhea* occurs as a result of hyperosmolar or non-absorbable substances, which draw large volumes of fluid into the intestines, producing watery stools that usually resolve with removal of the cause. Causative factors include high osmolality tube feedings, lactulose or sorbital, and gastrointestinal hemorrhage.
- *Malabsorptive diarrhea* results from changes in mucosal integrity causing changes in membrane permeability, or loss of absorptive surfaces, resulting in diarrhea that is large volume, frothy, and foul-smelling (steatorrhea). Causes include deficiency of an enzyme responsible for digestion of fats (lactose intolerance, pancreatic insufficiency) or surgical resection or removal of the intestines.
- *Secretory diarrhea* results from intestinal hypersecretion of large volumes (> 1 L/da) of watery stool with an osmolality equal to that in the plasma. Causes are endocrine tumors (VIPoma and carcinoid), enterotoxin-producing pathogens like c. difficile, acute graft-versus-host disease, and short gut syndrome.
- *Exudative diarrhea* is caused by inflammation or ulceration of the bowel mucosa, resulting in stools containing mucous, blood, and serum protein; the patient experiences frequent stooling, although the total volume is usually < 1 L/da. Unfortunately, this type of diarrhea is associated with hypoalbuminemia and anemia. Causes are radiation to the bowel (radiation enteritis) or opportunistic infection in the denuded bowel, such as with neutropenic typhlitis.
- *Dysmotility-associated diarrhea* is related to factors which increase or decrease normal peristalsis, such as with irritable bowel syndrome, the inges-

tion of food or medication that affects peristalsis, or psychological factors such as anxiety or fear that cause parasympathetic stimulation. Diarrhea of this type is usually semi-solid to liquid, small, and frequent.

- *Chemotherapy-induced diarrhea* occurs as a result of chemotherapy-induced cell death of the intestinal mucosa causing over-stimulation of intestinal water and electrolyte secretion. The patient experiences frequent watery to semi-solid stools within 24–96 hours of chemotherapy administration. With irinotecan chemotherapy, acute diarrhea occurs initially during or soon after administration related to cholinergic stimulation, and then delayed diarrhea occurs about 9–12 days later. In combination with 5-fluorouracil, the delayed diarrhea can lead to dehydration, and together with neutropenia, sepsis. Nurses play a very important role in teaching patients about the potential life-threatening diarrhea that may occur from this chemotherapy, self-adminsitration of anti-diarrheal medicines, increased fluid and diet modifications, and triage if these efforts are not effective.

Nurses are key in the management of diarrhea. Nurses play a significant role in patient assessment and patient/family teaching. Assessment of the patient's previous and current nutrition and elimination patterns, as well as assessment of probable etiology of diarrhea, are critical, as is patient/family teaching about the management and prevention of diarrhea.

Patient teaching includes (Wadler et al, 1998):

1. Diet modification: recommend low-residue foods high in protein and calories; high fluid intake of 3 L/day; avoidance of milk and milk products, foods high in potassium.
2. Care of irritated skin, mucosa in perirectal area; critical in neutropenic or immunocompromised patients.
3. Self-administration of prescribed antidiarrheal medication(s).
4. Need for blood tests to assess electrolyte imbalance and hydration if diarrhea is severe. Diarrhea can lead to severe fluid and electrolyte imbalance, as well as significant patient discomfort. Common electrolyte imbalances related to diarrhea include metabolic acidosis, hypokalemia, hyperchloremia, hypocalcemia, and hypomagnesemia.

Ippoliti (1998) describes antidiarrheal agents as:

- *Intraluminal agents*: decrease water in gut by absorption, increasing bulk of the stool, and protecting intestinal mucosa; includes absorbents such as activated charcoal and mucilloid preparations, and adsorbents such as psyllium, kaolin and pectate; less commonly used as more effective agents available without possible drug interactions or difficulty ingesting them.
- *Intestinal transit inhibitors*: Primarily anti-cholinergic (atropine sulfate and scopolamine) and opiate agonists (DTO and the synthetic opioids diphenox-

ylate and loperamide) which slow intestinal peristalsis and increasing fluid absorption.

- *Proabsorptive agents*: Intraluminal absorbent agents as above.
- *Antisecretory agents*: Octreotide (Sandostatin) is a synthetic somatostatin analogue that inhibits the secretion of gut hormones like serotonin and motilin, and thus slows transit time and improves regulation of water and electolyte movement in the gut. Bismuth subsalicylate (Pepto-Bismol) also works to decrease gut mucosal inflammation and hypermotility by binding to toxins and inhibition of prostaglandin synthesis.

References

Engleking C. Diarrhea, Chapter 28. Yarbro CH, Frogge MH, Goodman M, (eds), *Cancer Symptom Management,* 3rd ed. Sudbury, MA: Jones and Bartlett Publishers, 2003

Harris AG. Consensus Statement Recommendations: Octreotide Dose Titration in Secretory Diarrhea. *Dig Dis Sci* 1995;40(7):1464–1473

Ippoliti C. Antidiarrheal Agents for the Management of Treatment-related Diarrhea in Cancer Patients. *Am J Health Syst Pharm* 1998;55(15):1573–80

Levy MH. Constipation and Diarrhea, Part II. *Prim Care Cancer* 1992;12(5):53–58

Rutledge D, Engleking C. Cancer-related Diarrhea: Selected Findings of a National Survey of Oncology nurse experiences. *Oncol Nurs Forum* 1998;25:861–878

Wadler S, Benson AB, Engelking C, et al. Recommended Guidelines for the Treatment of Chemotherapy-Induced Diarrhea. *J Clin Oncol* 1998;16(9):3169–3178

Drug: deodorized tincture of opium (DTO, Laudanum)

Class: Opium antidiarrheal agent.

Mechanism of Action: Increases GI smooth muscle tone and inhibits GI motility, delaying movement of intestinal contents; water is absorbed from fecal contents, decreasing diarrhea.

Metabolism: Variable absorption from GI tract; metabolized by liver and excreted in urine.

Dosage/Range:

Adult:

- Oral: 0.3–1 mL qid (maximum 6 mL/day).

Drug Preparation/Administration:

- Store in tight, light-resistant bottle. Administer with water or juice.

Drug Interactions:

- None.

Lab Effects/Interference:
- None known.

Special Considerations:
- DTO contains 25 times more morphine than paregoric.
- Physical dependence may develop if drug is used chronically (e.g., colitis).
- Controlled substance.
- May be used in combination with kaolin and pectin mixtures.
- Do not use in diarrhea that results from poisoning until poison is removed (e.g., by lavage or cathartics).

Potential Toxicities/Side Effects and the Nursing Process

I. ALTERATION IN NUTRITION, LESS THAN BODY REQUIREMENTS, related to GI SIDE EFFECTS

Defining Characteristics: Nausea, vomiting may occur.

Nursing Implications: Assess baseline nutrition, GI status. If nausea/vomiting appears to follow dose administration, administer DTO with juice to disguise taste.

Drug: diphenoxylate hydrochloride and atropine (Lomotil)

Class: Antidiarrheal agent.

Mechanism of Action: Diphenoxylate is a synthetic opiate agonist that inhibits intestinal smooth muscle activity, thereby slowing peristalsis so that excess water is absorbed from feces. Atropine discourages deliberate overdosage.

Metabolism: Well absorbed from GI tract. Metabolized in liver. Excreted principally via feces in bile. Onset of action 45 minutes to 1 hour; duration 3–4 hours.

Dosage/Range:
Adult:
- Oral: 5 mg PO qid then titrate to response × 2 days (if no response in 48 hours, drug ineffective).

Drug Preparation/Administration:
- Oral: one tablet contains 2.5 mg diphenoxylate HCl and 0.025 mg atropine sulfate.

Drug Interactions:
- CNS depressants (alcohol, barbiturates): potentiate CNS depressant action; use together cautiously.

- MAOIs: may cause hypertensive crisis (similar structure to meperidine); use together cautiously.

Lab Effects/Interference:
- None known.

Special Considerations:
- May be habit-forming when used in high doses (40–60 mg); physical dependence.
- Use with extreme caution in patients with hepatic cirrhosis, as drug may precipitate hepatic coma, and in patients with acute ulcerative colitis.
- Contraindicated in patients with jaundice, diarrhea resulting from poisoning or pseudomembranous colitis caused by antibiotics.

Potential Toxicities/Side Effects and the Nursing Process

I. ALTERATION IN NUTRITION, LESS THAN BODY REQUIREMENTS, related to GI SIDE EFFECTS

Defining Characteristics: Nausea, vomiting, abdominal distension or discomfort, anorexia, mouth dryness, and (rarely) paralytic ileus may occur.

Nursing Implications: Assess baseline nutrition and elimination status. Instruct patient to report signs and symptoms. Discuss drug discontinuance with physician. Instruct patient that drug should be used for two days and physician notified if diarrhea persists.

II. ALTERATIONS IN SENSORY/PERCEPTUAL PATTERNS related to SEDATION

Defining Characteristics: Sedation, dizziness, lethargy, restlessness or insomnia, headache, paresthesia occur rarely with higher doses and prolonged therapy. Blurred vision may occur due to mydriasis.

Nursing Implications: Teach patient that drug is for short-term relief of diarrhea. Assess for and instruct patient to report signs/symptoms. Discuss drug discontinuance with physician if symptoms are severe.

III. ALTERATION IN SKIN INTEGRITY related to RASH, SENSITIVITY

Defining Characteristics: Pruritus, angioedema (swelling of lips, face, gums), giant urticaria may occur.

Nursing Implications: Assess for and instruct patient to report signs/symptoms immediately. Drug should be discontinued if angioedema or giant urticaria occur.

Drug: kaolin/pectin (Kaodene, K-P, Kaopectate, K-Pek)

Class: Antidiarrheal agent.

Mechanism of Action: Drug acts as absorbent and protectant; decreases stool fluidity but not total amount of fluid excreted.

Metabolism: Not absorbed from GI tract and excreted in stool.

Dosage/Range:

Adult:

- Oral: 60–120 mL regular or 45–90 mL concentrated suspension after each loose bowel movement < 48 hours.

Drug Preparation/Administration:

- Shake well prior to administration.

Drug Interactions:

- Oral lincomycin: decreases lincomycin absorption; administer kaolin/pectin at least 2 hours before or 3–4 hours after lincomycin dose.
- Oral digoxin: decreases digoxin absorption; administer kaolin/pectin 2 hours after digoxin dose.

Lab Effects/Interference:

- None known.

Special Considerations:

- Few adverse effects.
- Used for temporary relief of diarrhea.

Potential Toxicities/Side Effects and the Nursing Process

I. KNOWLEDGE DEFICIT related to SELF-ADMINISTRATION

Defining Characteristics: Transient constipation may occur.

Nursing Implications: Assess understanding of medication and self-administration schedule. Instruct patient in self-administration and to notify nurse/physician if diarrhea persists beyond 48 hours or fever develops. Reinforce need to drink fluids, especially in elderly or debilitated patients, to prevent constipation.

Drug: loperamide hydrochloride (Imodium)

Class: Antidiarrheal agent.

Mechanism of Action: Slows intestinal motility by inhibiting peristalsis (direct effect on circular and longitudinal intestinal muscles); increases stool bulk and viscosity.

Metabolism: Well absorbed from GI tract. Metabolized and small amounts are excreted in urine and feces as intact drug.

Dosage/Range:

Adult:

- Oral: 4 mg followed by 2 mg after each unformed stool (maximum 16 mg or higher if under direction of a physician; 8 mg per 24-hour period if self-medicating).

Drug Preparation/Administration:

- Oral.

Drug Interactions:

- None.

Lab Effects/Interference:

- None known.

Special Considerations:

- Reduces electrolyte and fluid loss from intestines; may be used to reduce volume of ileostomy drainage. 2–3 times more potent than diphenoxylate.
- Use cautiously in patients with acute ulcerative colitis; drug should be discontinued if abdominal distension occurs (risk of megacolon).
- Intended for self-medication × 48 hours; patients should be taught to notify nurse/physician if symptoms persist or fever occurs.
- Contraindicated in diarrhea due to pseudomembranous colitis (antibioticrelated), in acute diarrhea caused by mucosal-penetrating organisms (*Shigella, E. coli, Salmonella*), or if hypersensitivity to drug exists.
- Use cautiously in pregnant or nursing women.

Potential Toxicities/Side Effects and the Nursing Process

I. ALTERATION IN NUTRITION, LESS THAN BODY REQUIREMENTS, related to GI SIDE EFFECTS

Defining Characteristics: Less frequent adverse reactions occur than with diphenoxylate/atropine. Nausea, vomiting, abdominal pain, and distension may occur.

Nursing Implications: Assess baseline nutrition and elimination status. Instruct patient to report signs and symptoms. Discuss drug discontinuance with physician. Instruct patient that drug should be used for two days and physician notified if diarrhea persists.

II. ALTERATIONS IN SENSORY/PERCEPTUAL PATTERNS related to DROWSINESS

Defining Characteristics: Drowsiness, dizziness, fatigue may occur.

Nursing Implications: Teach patient that drug is for short-term relief of diarrhea. Assess for and instruct patient to report signs/symptoms. Discuss drug discontinuance with physician if symptoms are severe.

III. ALTERATION IN SKIN INTEGRITY related to RASH, SENSITIVITY

Defining Characteristics: Rarely, rash may develop.

Nursing Implications: Assess baseline skin integrity. Instruct patient to report rash. Discuss drug discontinuance with physician.

Drug: octreotide acetate (Sandostatin)

Class: Cyclic cotapeptide that mimics the pharmacologic actions of the natural hormone somatostatin and is long-acting.

Mechanism of Action: More potent inhibitor than somatostatin of growth hormone, glucagon, insulin; also suppresses LH (luteinizine hormone) response to GnRH (gonadotropin-releasing hormone); decreases splanchnic blood flow; and inhibits release of serotonin, gastrin, vasoactive intestinal peptide, secretin, motilin, and pancreatic polypeptide like somatostatin. Stimulates fluid and electrolyte absorption from GI tract, and lengthens transit time of intestinal contents. Controls symptoms associated with carcinoid syndrome (e.g., flushing, levels of serotonin metabolite 5-HIAA).

Metabolism: Absorbed rapidly and completely after injection, with peak concentrations after 24 minutes. Protein binding 65%, and eliminated from plasma with a half-life of 1.7 hours (natural hormone is 1–3 minutes). Duration of action approximately 12 hours depending upon tumor type. Excreted in urine, with decreased clearance by 26% in the elderly.

Dosage/Range:

Adult (immediate release injection):

- Carcinoid: Starting dose of 100–600 mcg/day (median 450 mcg/day) in 2–4 divided doses SQ.
- VIPoma: 200–300 mcg/day SQ in 2–4 divided doses during initial 2 weeks, then titrated to response with range of 150–750 mcg/day to control symptoms.

- Acromegaly: 50 mcg SQ tid, titrated to need every 2 weeks based on IGF (somatomedin C) levels.
- AIDS-related diarrhea: 500 mcg SQ q8h.
- Chemotherapy-induced diarrhea (high dose): 300 mcg/day continuous infusion.
- Radiation-induced diarrhea: 50 mcg SQ q8h.
- Graft-versus-host disease (GVHD): 100 mcg IV q8h.
- Short bowel syndrome: 50 mcg SQ q8h.
- Chronic idiopathic secretory diarrhea: 100 mcg SQ q8h.

Sandostatin LAR Depot:

- If patient not currently on octreotide acetate, begin therapy with immediate release dosing q8h at an initial dose of 50 mcg tid, and gradually increase as needed (based on growth hormone (GH) levels) as the goal is to normalize GH and IGF-1 (somatomedin C) levels. After 2 weeks, tolerance and response should be evident, so that patient can be changed to LAR Depot at a dose of 20 mg q4 weeks if tolerance and effectiveness positive.
- For patients currently on octreotide, they can be changed directly to LAR Depot q4 weeks, and at the end of three months, the LAR Depot dose should be titrated based on growth hormone level:
  - —GH ≤ 2.5 ng/mL, IGF-1 (somatomedin C) normal and controlled symptoms, 20 mg IM (intragluteally) q4 weeks.
  - —GH > 2.5 ng/mL, IGF-1 elevated and/or uncontrolled symptoms, increase dose to 30 mg IM q4 weeks.
  - —GH ≤ 1 ng/mL, IGF-1 normal and controlled symptoms, reduce dose to 10 mg IM q4 weeks.

Drug Preparation/Administration:

- Available in 1-mL ampules and 5-mL (5 mg) multidose vials or as LAR Depot 10–30 mg SQ q28 days.
- Immediate release injection: administer SQ, IV over 15–30 minutes, or IVP over 3 minutes.
- Stable in solution in 0.9% Sodium Chloride or 5% Dextrose in Water for 24 hours; dilute drug in 50–200 mL of 0.9% Sodium Chloride or 5% Dextrose for IV infusions over 15–30 minutes.
- Patient may develop pain, stinging, tingling, or burning sensation at injection site, with redness and swelling.

LAR Depot:

- Administer in gluteal muscle as other sites too painful (never give IV or SC).

Drug Interactions:

- May affect absorption of orally administered drugs.
- Cyclosporine: decreased serum levels of cyclosporine, resulting in transplant rejection.

- Insulin, oral hypoglycemic agents, beta-blockers, calcium channel blockers: assess patient response and need for dosage adjustment of these drugs.

Lab Effects/Interference:
- Hypoglycemia or hyperglycemia: suppression of TSH may result in hypothyroidism and decreased total/free T_4 (generally patients with acromegaly receiving long-term therapy).
- Decreased vitamin B_{12} levels (Shilling's test).

Special Considerations:
- Octreotide acetate is appropriate when other conventional antidiarrheal medications have failed, and other treatable causes of diarrhea have been excluded (e.g., obstruction, infection).
- Patient should be taught sterile SQ injection technique.
- Laboratory test monitoring (efficacy) based on treatment intent:
  - Carcinoid: 5-HIAA (urinary 5-hydroxyindoleacetic acid), plasma substance P and serotonin.
  - VIPoma: VIP (plasma vasoactive intestinal peptide).
  - Acromegaly: growth hormone, IGF-1 (somatomedin C).
- Adverse reactions of diabetes mellitus, hypothyroidism, and cardiovascular disease occur in patients treated for acromegaly.
- May change to long-acting depot if already controlled on immediate-release preparation, or in a new patient, after response is assessed after 2 weeks of immediate-release dosing.
- Drug inhibits gallbladder contraction and decreases bile secretion in 63% of patients with acromegaly or psoriasis when treated for long periods of time.

Potential Toxicities/Side Effects and the Nursing Process

I. ALTERATION IN NUTRITION, LESS THAN BODY REQUIREMENTS, related to CARBOHYDRATE METABOLISM

Defining Characteristics: Rarely, transient hypoglycemia or hyperglycemia due to altered balance between hormones regulating serum glucose (insulin, glucagon, growth hormone). Rarely, diarrhea, nausea and vomiting, abdominal pain or discomfort. Incidence 3–10%.

Nursing Implications: Assess baseline nutritional balance. Instruct patient to report any changes, and assess for hyperglycemia (drowsiness, dry mouth, flushing, dry skin, fruity breath, polyuria, polydipsia, polyphagia, weight loss, stomach ache, nausea/vomiting, fatigue), hypoglycemia (anxiety, chills, cool/pale skin, difficulty concentrating, headache, hunger, shakiness, diaphoresis, fatigue, weakness, nausea). If patient is hypoglycemic, teach patient to carry candy. Monitor serum glucose, and discuss alterations with physician. Treat nausea and vomiting symptomatically, and discuss need for antiemetic if significant.

II. ALTERATION IN COMFORT related to HEADACHE, FLUSHING

Defining Characteristics: Rarely (1–3%) patient may experience lightheadedness, dizziness, fatigue, pedal edema, headache, flushing of the face, weakness.

Nursing Implications: Assess baseline comfort, and instruct patient to report any changes. Assess safety, and manage symptoms symptomatically. If unrelieved or significant, discuss with physician.

Appendix 1

Controlling Occupational Exposure to Hazardous Drugs

A. Introduction

In response to numerous inquiries,[1] OSHA published guidelines for the management of cytotoxic (antineoplastic) drugs in the workplace in 1986.[106] At that time, surveys indicated little standardization in the use of engineering controls and personal protective equipment (PPE).[56,73] Although practices have improved in subsequent years, problems still exist.[111] In addition, the occupational management of these chemicals has been further clarified. These trends, in conjunction with many information requests, have prompted OSHA to revise its recommendations for hazardous drug handling. In addition, some of these agents are covered under the Hazard Communication Standard (HCS) [29 CFR 1910.1200].[107] In order to provide recommendations consistent with current scientific knowledge, this informational guidance document has been expanded to cover hazardous drugs (HD), in addition to the cytotoxic drugs (CD) that were covered in the 1986 guidelines. The recommendations apply to all settings where employees are occupationally exposed to HDs, such as hospitals, physicians' offices, and home health care agencies. This review will:

- provide criteria for classifying drugs as hazardous,
- summarize the evidence supporting the management of HDs as an occupational hazard,
- discuss the equipment and worker education recommended as well as the legal requirements of standards for the protection of workers exposed and potentially exposed to HDs,
- update the important aspects of medical surveillance and,
- list some common HDs currently in use.

Anesthetic agents have not been considered in this review. However, exposure to some of these agents is a recognized health hazard,[104] and they have been considered in a separate Technical Manual Chapter.

B. Categorization of Drugs as Hazardous

The purpose of this section is to describe the biological effects of those pharmaceuticals that are considered hazardous. A number of pharmaceuticals in the health care setting may pose occupational risk to employees through acute and chronic workplace exposure. Past attention focused on drugs used to treat cancer. However, it is clear that many other agents also have toxicity profiles of concern. This recognition prompted the American Society of Hospital Pharmacists (ASHP) to define a class of agents as "hazardous drugs."[3] That report specified concerns about antineoplastic and nonantineoplastic hazardous drugs in use in most institutions throughout the country. OSHA shares this concern. The ASHP Technical Assistance

Bulletin (TAB) described four drug characteristics, each of which could be considered hazardous:

- genotoxicity,
- carcinogenicity,
- teratogenicity or fertility impairment, and
- serious organ or other toxic manifestation at low doses in experimental animals or treated patients.

Table A.1 of this review lists some common drugs that are considered hazardous by the above criteria. There is no standardized reference for this information nor is there complete consensus on all agents listed. Professional judgment by personnel trained in pharmacology/toxicology is essential in designating drugs as hazardous, and reference 65 provides information regarding the development of such a list at one institution. Some drugs, which have a long history of safe use in humans despite *in vitro* or animal evidence to toxicity, may be excluded by the institution's experts by considerations such as those used to formulate GRAS *(Generally Regarded as Safe)* lists by the FDA under the Food, Drug, and Cosmetics Act.

Table A.1 is not all inclusive, should not be construed as complete, and represents an assessment of some, but not all, marketed drugs at a fixed point in time. Table A.1 was developed through consultation with institutions that have assembled teams of pharmacists and other health care personnel to determine which drugs should be used with caution. These teams reviewed product literature and drug information when considering each product.

Sources for this appendix are the *Physicians' Desk Reference,* Section 10:00 in the American Hospital Formulary Service Drug Information,[68] IARC publications (particularly volume 50),[43] the Johns Hopkins Hospital, and the National Institutes of Health, Clinical Center Nursing Department. No attempt to include investigational drugs was made, but they should be prudently handled as hazardous drugs until adequate information becomes available to exclude them. Any determination of the hazard status of drug should be periodically reviewed and updated as new information becomes available. Importantly, new drugs should routinely undergo a hazard assessment.

Table A.1 Some Common Drugs Considered Hazardous

Chemical/Generic Name	Source*
ALTRETAMINE	C
AMINOGLUTETHIMIDE	A
AZATHIOPRINE	ACE
L-ASPARAGINASE	ABC
BLEOMYCIN	ABC
BUSULFAN	ABC
CARBOPLATIN	ABC
CARMUSTINE	ABC
CHLORAMBUCIL	ABCE
CHLORAMPHENICOL	E
CHLOROTRIANISENE	B
CHLOROZOTOCIN	E
CYCLOSPORIN	E
CISPLATIN	ABCE

Table A.1 *(continued)*

Chemical/Generic Name	Source*
CYCLOPHOSPHAMIDE	ABCE
CYTARABINE	ABC
DACARBAZINE	ABC
DACTINOMYCIN	ABC
DAUNORUBICIN	ABC
DIETHYLSTILBESTROL	BE
DOXORUBICIN	ABCE
ESTRADIOL	B
ESTRAMUSTINE	AB
ETHINYL ESTRADIOL	B
ETOPOSIDE	ABC
FLOXURIDINE	AC
FLUOROURACIL	ABC
FLUTAMIDE	BC
GANCICLOVIR	AD
HYDROXYUREA	ABC
IDARUBICIN	AC
IFOSFAMIDE	ABC
INTERFERON-α	BC
ISOTRETINOIN	D
LEUPROLIDE	BC
LEVAMISOLE	C
LOMUSTINE	ABCE
MECHLORETHAMINE	BC
MEDROXYPROGESTERONE	B
MEGESTROL	BC
MELPHALAN	ABCE
MERCAPTOPURINE	ABC
METHOTREXATE	ABC
MITOMYCIN	ABC
MITOTANE	ABC
MITOXANTRONE	ABC
NAFARELIN	C
PIPOBROMAN	C
PLICAMYCIN	BC
PROCARBAZINE	ABCE
RIBAVIRIN	D
STREPTOZOCIN	AC
TAMOXIFEN	BC
TESTOLACTONE	BC
THIOGUANINE	ABC
THIOTEPA	ABC
URACIL MUSTARD	ACE

Table A.1 *(continued)*

Chemical/Generic Name	Source*
VIDARABINE	D
VINBLASTINE	ABC
VINCRISTINE	ABC
ZIDOVUDINE	D

*Sources:
A The National Institutes of Health, Clinical Center Nursing Department
B Antineoplastic drugs in the *Physicians' Desk Reference*
C American Hospital Formulary, Antineoplastics
D Johns Hopkins Hospital E International Agency for Research on Cancer

List of Abbreviations

ANSI	American National Standards Institute
ASHP	American Society of Hospital Pharmacists
BSC	Biological Safety Cabinet
CD	Cytotoxic Drug
EPA	Environmental Protection Agency
HD	Hazardous Drug
HCS	Hazard Communication Standard
HEPA	High Efficiency Particulate Air
IARC	International Agency for Research on Cancer
MSDS	Material Safety Data Sheet
NIOSH	National Institute for Occupational Safety and Health
NTP	National Toxicology Program
OSHA	Occupational Safety and Health Administration
PPE	Personal Protective Equipment

In contrast, investigational drugs are new chemicals for which there is often little information on potential toxicity. Structure or activity relationships with similar chemicals and in vitro data can be considered in determining potential toxic effects. Investigational drugs should be prudently handled as HDs unless adequate information becomes available to exclude them.

Some major considerations by professionals trained in pharmacology/toxicology[65] in designating a drug as hazardous are:

- Is the drug designated as Therapeutic Category 10:00 (Antineoplastic Agent) in the American Hospital Formulary Service Drug Information?[68]
- Does the manufacturer suggest the use of special isolation techniques in its handing, administration, or disposal?
- Is the drug known to be a human mutagen, carcinogen, teratogen, or reproductive toxicant?
- Is the drug known to be carcinogenic or teratogenic in animals (drugs known to be mutagenic in multiple bacterial systems or animals should also be considered hazardous)?
- And, is the drug known to be acutely toxic to an organ system?

C. Background: Hazardous Drugs as Occupational Risk

Preparation, administration, and disposal of HDs may expose pharmacists, nurses, physicians, and other health care workers to potentially significant workplace levels of these chemicals. The literature establishing these agents as occupational hazards deals primarily with CDs; however, documentation of adverse exposure effects from other HDs is rapidly accumulating.[15,40,41,42,43,59] The degree of absorption that takes place during work and the significance of secondary early biological effects on each individual encounter are difficult to assess and may vary depending on the HD. As a result, it is difficult to set safe levels of exposure on the basis of current scientific information.

However, there are several lines of evidence supporting the toxic potential of these drugs if handled improperly. Therefore, it is essential to minimize exposure to all HDs. Summary tables of much of the data presented below can be found in Sorsa[95] and Rogers.[84]

1. Mechanism of Action

Most HDs either bind directly to genetic material in the cell nucleus or affect cellular protein synthesis. Cytotoxic drugs may not distinguish between normal and cancerous cells. The growth and reproduction of the normal cells are often affected during treatment of cancerous cells.

2. Animal Data

Numerous studies document the carcinogenic, mutagenic, and teratogenic effects of HD exposure in animals. They are well summarized in the pertinent IARC publications.[37–43] Alkylating agents present the strongest evidence of carcinogenicity (e.g., *cyclophosphamide, mechlorethamine hydrochloride [nitrogen mustard]*). However, other classes, such as some antibiotics, have been implicated as well. Extensive evidence for mutagenic and reproductive effects can be found in all antineoplastic classes. The antiviral agent *ribavirin* has additionally been shown to be teratogenic in all rodent species tested.[31,49] The ASHP recommends that all pharmaceutical agents that are animal carcinogens be handled as if human carcinogens.

3. Human Data at Therapeutic Levels

Many HDs are known human carcinogens, for which there is no safe level of exposure. The development of secondary malignancies is a well-documented side effect of chemotherapy treatment.[52,86,90,115] Leukemia has been most frequently observed. However, other secondary malignancies, such as bladder cancer and lymphoma, have been documented in patients treated for other, usually solid, primary malignancies.[52,114] Chromosomal aberrations can result from chemotherapy treatment as well. One study, on *chlorambucil,* reveals chromosomal damage in recipients to be cumulative and related to both dose and duration of therapy.[77]

Numerous case reports have linked chemotherapeutic treatment to adverse reproductive outcomes.[7,88,91,98] Testicular and ovarian dysfunction, including permanent sterility, have occurred in male and female patients who have received CDs either singly or in combination.[14] In addition, some antineoplastic agents are known or suspected to be transmitted to infants through breast milk.[79]

The literature also documents the effects of these drugs on other organ systems. Extravasation of some agents can cause severe soft-tissue injury, consisting of necrosis and sloughing of exposed areas.[23,78,87] Other HDs, such as *pentamidine* and *zidovudine* (formerly AZT), are known to have significant side effects (i.e., hematologic abnormalities), in treated patients.[4,33] Serum transaminase elevation has also been reported in treated patients.[4,33]

4. Occupational Exposure—Airborne Levels

Monitoring efforts for cytotoxic drugs have detected measurable air levels when exhaust biological safety cabinets (BSC) were not used for preparation or when monitoring was performed inside the BSC.[50,73]

Concentrations of *fluorouracil* ranging from 0.12 to 82.26 ng/m^3 have been found during monitoring of drug preparation without a BSC implying an opportunity for respiratory exposure.[73] Elevated concentrations of *cyclophosphamide* were found by these authors as well. *Cyclophosphamide* has also been detected on the HEPAfilters of flow hoods used in HDpreparation, demonstrating aerosolization of the drug and an exposure opportunity mitigated by effective engineering controls.[81]

A recent study has reported wipe samples of *cyclophosphamide,* one of the Class I IARC carcinogens, on surfaces of work stations in an oncology pharmacy and outpatient treatment areas (sinks and countertops). Concentrations ranged from 0.005 to 0.03 μg/cm^2, documenting opportunity for dermal exposure.[60]

Administration of drugs via aerosolization can lead to measurable air concentrations in the breathing zone of workers providing treatment. Concentrations up to 18 μg/m^3 have been found by personal air sampling of workers administering *pentamidine.*[67] Similar monitoring for *ribavirin* has found concentrations as high as 316 μg/m[331]

5. Occupational Exposure—Biological Evidence of Absorption

Urinary Mutagenicity

Falk et al. were the first to note evidence of mutagenicity in the urine of nurses who handled cytotoxic drugs.[26] The extent of this effect increased over the course of the work week. With improved handling practices, a decrease in mutagenic activity was seen.[27] Researchers have also studied pharmacy personnel who reconstitute antineoplastic drugs. These employees showed increasingly mutagenic urine over the period of exposure; when they stopped handling the drugs, activity fell within 2 days to the level of unexposed controls.[5,76] They also found mutagenicity in workers using horizontal laminar flow BSCs that decreased to control levels with the use of vertical flow containment BSCs.[76] Other studies have failed to find a relationship between exposure and urine mutagenicity.[25] Sorsa[95] summarizes this information and discusses the factors, such as differences in urine collection timing and variations in the use of PPE, which could lead to disparate results. Differences may also be related to smoking status; smokers exposed to CDs exhibit greater urine mutagenicity than exposed non-smokers or control smokers, suggesting contamination of the work area by CDs and some contribution of smoking to their mutagenic profile.[9]

Urinary Thioethers

Urinary thioethers are glutathione conjugated metabolites of alkylating agents that have been evaluated as an indirect means of measuring exposure. Workers who handle cytotoxic drugs have been reported to have increased levels compared to controls and also have increasing thioether levels over a five-day work week.[44,48] Other studies of nurses who handle CDs and of treated patients have yielded variable results that could be due to confounding by smoking, PPE, and glutathione-S-transferase activity.[11]

Urinary Metabolites

Venitt[112] assayed the urine of pharmacy and nursing personnel handling cisplatin and found platinum concentrations at or below the limit of detection for both workers and controls.

Hirst[35] found *cyclophosphamide* in the urine of two nurses who handled the drug, documenting worker absorption. (Hirst also documented skin absorption in human volunteers by using gas chromatography after topical application of the drug.) Urinary *pentamidine* recovery has also been reported in exposed health care workers.[94]

6. Occupational Exposure—Human Effects

Cytogenetic Effects

A number of studies have examined the relationship of exposure to CDs in the workplace to chromosomal aberrations. These studies have looked at a variety of markers for damage, including sister chromatid exchanges (SCE), structural aberrations (e.g., gaps, breaks, translocations), and micronuclei in peripheral blood lymphocytes. The results have been somewhat conflicting. Several authors found increases in one or more markers.[74,75,88,113] Increased mutilation frequency has been reported as well.[17] Other studies have failed to find a significant difference between workers and controls.[99,101] Some researchers have found higher individual elevations[28] or a relationship between number of drugs handled and SCEs.[8] These disparate results are not unexpected. The difficulties in quantitating exposure have resulted in different exposure magnitudes between studies; workers in several negative studies appear to have a lower overall exposure.[10] In addition, differences in the use of PPE and work technique will alter absorption of CDs and resultant biologic effects.

Finally, techniques for SCE measurement may not be optimal. A recent study that looked at correlation of phosphoramide-induced SCE levels with duration of anticancer drug handling found a statistically significant correlation coefficient of 0.[63,66]

Taken together, the evidence indicates an excess of markers of mutagenic exposure in unprotected workers.

Reproductive Effects

Reproductive effects associated with occupational exposure to CDs have been well documented. Hemminki et al.[32] found no difference in exposure between nurses who had spontaneous abortions and those who had normal pregnancies. However, the study group consisted of nurses who were employed in surgical or medical floors of a general hospital. When the relationship between CD exposure and congenital malformations was explored, the study group was expanded to include oncology nurses, among others, and an odds ratio of 4:7 was found for exposures of more than once per week. This observed odds ratio is statistically significant. Selevan et al.[39] found a relationship between CD exposure and spontaneous abortion in a case-control study of Finnish nurses. This well-designed study reviewed the reproductive histories of 568 women (167 cases) and found a statistically significant odds ratio of 2:3. Similar results were obtained in another large casecontrol study of French nurses,[102] and a study of Baltimore area nurses found a significantly higher proportion of adverse pregnancy outcomes when exposure to antineoplastic agents occurred during the pregnancy.[85] The nurses involved in these studies usually prepared and administered the drugs. Therefore, workplace exposure of these groups of professionals to such products has been associated with adverse reproductive outcomes in several investigations.

Other Effects

Hepatocellular damage has been reported in nurses working in an oncology ward; the injury appeared to be related to intensity and duration of work exposure to CDs.[96] Symptoms such as light-headedness, dizziness, nausea, headache, and allergic reactions have also been described in employees after the preparation and administration of antineoplastic drugs in unventilated areas.[22,96] In occupational settings, these agents are known to be toxic to the skin and mucous membranes, including the cornea.[69,82]

Pentamidine has been associated with respiratory damage in one worker who administered the aerosol. The injury consisted of a decrease in diffusing capacity that improved after exposure ceased.[29] The onset of bronchospasm in a pentamidine-exposed worker has also been reported.[22] Employees involved in the aerosol administration of *ribavirin* have noted symptoms of respiratory tract irritation.[55] A number of medications including *psyllium* and various antibiotics are known respiratory and dermal sensitizers. Exposure in susceptible individuals can lead to asthma or allergic contact dermatitis.

D. Work Areas

Risks to personnel working with HDs are a function of the drugs' inherent toxicity and the extent of exposure. The main routes of exposure are: inhalation of dusts or aerosols, dermal absorption, and ingestion. Contact with contaminated food or cigarettes represents the primary means of ingestion. Opportunity for exposure to HDs may occur at many points in the handling of these drugs.

1. Pharmacy or Other Preparation Areas

In large oncology centers, HDs are usually prepared in the pharmacy. However, in small hospitals, outpatient treatments areas, and physicians' offices they have been prepared by physicians or nurses without appropriate engineering controls and protective apparel.[16,20] Many HDs must be reconstituted, transferred from one container to another, or manipulated before administration to patients. Even if care is taken, opportunity for absorption through inhalation or direct skin contact can occur.[35,36,73,116] Examples of manipulations that can cause splattering, spraying, and aerosolization include:

- withdrawal of needles from drug vials,
- drug transfer using syringes and needles or filter straws,
- breaking open of ampules, and
- expulsion of air from a drug-filled syringe.

Evaluation of these preparation techniques, using fluorescent dye solutions, has shown contamination of gloves and the sleeves and chest of gowns.[97]

Horizontal airflow work benches provide an aseptic environment for the preparation of injectable drugs. However, these units provide a flow of filtered air originating at the back of the workspace and exiting toward the employee using the unit. Thus, they increase the likelihood of drug exposure for both the preparer and other personnel in the room. As a result, the use of horizontal BSCs is contraindicated in the preparation of HDs. Smoking, drinking, applying cosmetics, and eating where these drugs are prepared, stored, or used also increase the chance of exposure.

2. Administration of Drugs to Patients

Administration of drugs to patients is generally performed by nurses or physicians. Drug injection into the IV line, clearing of air from the syringe or infusion line, and leakage at the tubing, syringe, or stopcock connection present opportunities for skin contact and aerosol generation. Clipping used needles and crushing used syringes can produce considerable aerosolization as well.

practice is the sharing of a cabinet (e.g., several medical offices share a cabinet) or sending the patient to a center where HDs can be prepared in a BSC. Alternatively, preparation can be performed in a facility with a BSC and the drugs transported to the area of administration. Use of a dedicated BSC, where only HDs are prepared, is prudent medical practice.

Types of BSCs

Four main types of Class II BSCs are available. They all have downward airflow and HEPA filters. They are differentiated by the amount of air recirculated within the cabinet, whether this air is vented to the room or the outside, and whether contaminated ducts are under positive or negative pressure. These four types are:

- Type A cabinets recirculate approximately 70% of cabinet air through HEPA filters back into the cabinet; the rest is discharged through a HEPA filter into the preparation room. Contaminated ducts are under positive pressure.
- Type B1 cabinets have higher velocity air inflow, recirculate 30% of the cabinet air, and exhaust the rest to the outside through HEPA filters. They have negative pressure contaminated ducts and plenums.
- Type B2 systems are similar to Type B1 except that no air is recirculated.
- Type B3 cabinets are similar to Type A in that they recirculate approximately 70% of cabinet air. However, the other 30% is vented to the outside and the ducts are under negative pressure.

Class III cabinets are totally enclosed with gas-tight construction. The entire cabinet is under negative pressure, and operations are performed through attached gloves. All air is HEPA filtered.

Class II, type B, or Class III BSCs are recommended since they vent to the outside.[3] Those without air recirculation are the most protective. If the BSC has an outside exhaust, it should be vented away from air intake units.

The blower on the vertical airflow hood should be on at all times. If the BSC is turned off, it should be decontaminated and covered in plastic until airflow is resumed.[3,72] Each BSC should be equipped with a continuous monitoring device to allow confirmation of adequate air flow and cabinet performance. The cabinet should be in an area with minimal air turbulence; this will reduce leakage to the environment.[6,70] Additional information on design and performance testing of BSCs can be found in papers by Avis and Levchuck,[6] Bryan and Marback,[10] and the National Sanitation Foundation.[70] Practical information regarding space needs and conversion possibilities is contained in the ASHP's 1990 technical assistance bulletins.[3]

Ventilation and biosafety cabinets installed should be maintained and evaluated for proper performance in accordance with the manufacturer's instructions.

Decontamination

The cabinet should be cleaned according to the manufacturer's instructions. Some manufacturers have recommended weekly decontamination as well as whenever spills occur or when the cabinet requires moving, service, or certification.

Decontamination should consist of surface cleaning with water and detergent, followed by thorough rinsing. The use of detergent is recommended because there is no single accepted method of chemical deactivation for all agents involved.[13,45] Quaternary ammonium cleaners should be avoided due to the possibility of vapor build-up in recirculated air.[3] Ethyl alcohol or 70% isopropyl alcohol may be used with the cleaner if the contamination is soluble only in alcohol.[3] Alcohol vapor build-up has also been a concern, so the use of alcohol should be avoided in BSCs where air is recirculated.[3] Spray cleaners should also be avoided due to the risk of spraying the HEPA filter. Ordinary decontamination procedures, which include fumigation with a germicidal agent, are inappropriate in a BSC used for HDs because such procedures do not remove or deactivate the drugs.

Removable work trays, if present, should be lifted in the BSC, so the back and the sump below can be cleaned. During cleaning, the worker should wear PPE similar to that used for spills. *Ideally, the sash should remain down during cleaning; however, a NIOSH-approved respirator appropriate for the hazard must be worn by the worker if the sash will be lifted during the process.* The exhaust fan/blower should be left on. Cleaning should proceed from least to most contaminated areas. The drain spillage trough area should be cleaned twice since it can be heavily contaminated. All materials from the decontamination process should be handled as HDs and disposed of in accordance with federal, state, and local laws.

Service and Certification

The ASHP recommends that BSCs be serviced and certified by a qualified technician every 6 months or any time the cabinet is moved or repaired.[3,71] Technicians servicing these cabinets or changing the HEPA filters should be aware of HD risk through hazard communication training from their employers and should use the same personal protective equipment as recommended for large spills. Certification of the BSC includes performance testing as outlined in the procedures of the National Sanitation Foundation's Standard Number 49.[70] Helpful information on such testing can be found in the ASHP 1990 technical assistance bulletins,[3] the BSC manufacturer's equipment manuals, and Bryan and Marback's paper.[10] HEPA filters should be changed when they restrict air flow or if they are contaminated by an accidental spill. They should be bagged in plastic and disposed of as HDs. Any time the cabinet is turned off or transported, it should be sealed with plastic.

Personal Protective Equipment

1. Gloves

Research indicates that the thickness of gloves used in handling HDs is more important than the type of material, since all materials tested have been found to be permeable to some HDs.[3,19,53] The best results are seen with latex gloves. Therefore, latex gloves should be used for the preparation of HDs unless the drug-product manufacturer specifically stipulates that some other glove provides better protection.[19,53,72,93,100] Thicker, longer latex gloves that cover the gown cuff are recommended for the use with HDs. *Individuals with latex allergy should consider the use of vinyl or nitrile gloves or glove liners.* Gloves with minimal or no powder are preferred since the powder may absorb contamination.[3,104]

The above referenced sources have noted great variability in permeability within and between glove lots. Therefore, double gloving is recommended if it does not interfere with an individual's technique.[3] Because all gloves are permeable to some extent and their permeability increases with time, they should be changed regularly (hourly) or immediately if they are torn, punctured, or contaminated with a spill. Hands should always be washed before gloves are put on and after they are removed. Employees need thorough training in proper methods for contaminated glove removal.

2. Gowns

A protective disposable gown made of lint-free, low-permeability fabric with a closed front, long sleeves, and elastic or knit closed cuff should be worn. The cuffs should be tucked under the gloves. If double gloves are worn, the outer glove should be over the gown cuff and the inner glove should be under the gown cuff. When the gown is removed, the inner glove should be removed last. Gowns and gloves in use in the HD preparation area should not be used outside the HD preparation area.[3]

As with gloves, there is no ideal material. Research has found non-porous Tyvek and Kaycel to be more permeable than Saranex-laminated Tyvek and polyethylene-coated Tyvek after 4 hours of exposure to the CDs tested.[54] However, little airflow is allowed with the latter materials. As a result, manufacturers have produced gowns with Saranex or polyethylene reinforced sleeves and front in an effort to decrease permeability in the most exposure-prone areas, but little data exists on decreasing exposure.

3. Respiratory Protection

A BSC is essential for the preparation of HDs. Where a BSC is not currently available, a *NIOSH-approved respirator* appropriate for the hazard must be worn to afford protection until the BSC is installed.* The use of respirators must comply with OSHA's Respiratory Protection Standard,[105] which outlines the aspects of a respirator program, including selection, fit testing, and worker training. Surgical masks are *not appropriate* since they *do not prevent* aerosol inhalation. Permanent respirator use, in lieu of BSCs, is imprudent practice and should not be a substitute for engineering controls.

4. Eye and Face Protection

Whenever splashes, sprays, or aerosols of HDs may be generated, which can result in eye, nose, or mouth contamination, chemical barrier face and eye protection must be provided and used in accordance with 29 CFR 1910.133. Eye glasses with temporary side shields are inadequate protection.

When a respirator is used to provide temporary protection as described above, and splashes, sprays, or aerosols are possible, employee protection should be:

- a respirator with a full face piece, or
- a plastic face shield or splash goggles complying with ANSI standards[2] when using a respirator of less than full face piece design.

Eyewash facilities should also be made available.

5. PPE Disposal and Decontamination

All gowns, gloves, and disposable materials used in preparation should be disposed of according to the hospital's hazardous drug waste procedures and as described under this review's section on Waste Disposal. Goggles, face shields, and respirators may be cleaned with mild detergent and water for reuse.

Work Equipment

NIH has recommended the work with HDs be carried out in a BSC on a disposable, plastic-backed paper liner. The liner should be changed after preparation is completed for the day, or after a shift. whichever comes first. Liners should also be changed after a spill.[103]

*NIOSH recommendation at the time of this publication is for a respirator with a high-efficiency filter, preferably a powered air-purifying respirator.

Syringes and IV sets with Luer-Lok fittings should be used for HDs. Syringe size should be large enough so that they are not full when the entire drug dose is present.

A covered disposable container should be used to contain excess solution. A covered sharps container should be in the BSC.

The ASHP recommends that HD-labeled plastic bags be available for all contaminated materials (including gloves, gowns, and paper liners), so that contaminated material can be immediately placed in them and disposed of in accordance with ASHP recommendations.[3]

Work Practices

Correct work practices are essential to worker protection. *Aseptic technique* is assumed as a standard practice in drug preparation. The general principles of aseptic technique, therefore, will not be detailed here. It should be noted, however, that BSC benches differ from horizontal flow units in several ways that require special precautions. Manipulations should not be performed close to the work surface of a BSC. Unsterilized items, including liners and hands, should be kept downstream from the working area. Entry and exit of the cabinet should be perpendicular to the front. Rapid lateral hand movements should be avoided. Additional information can be found in the National Sanitation Foundation Standard 49 for Class II (Laminar Flow) Biohazard Cabinetry[70] and Avis and Levchuck's paper.[6] All operators should be trained in these containment-area protocols.

All PPE should be donned before work is started in the BSC. All items necessary for drug preparation should be placed within the BSC before work is begun. Extraneous items should be kept out of the work area.

1. Labeling

In addition to standard pharmacy labeling practices, all syringes and IV bags containing HDs should be labeled with a distinctive warning label such as

SPECIAL HANDLING/Disposal Precautions

In addition, those HDs covered under HCS must have labels in accordance with section (f) of the standard to warn employees handling the drug(s) of the hazards.

2. Needles

The ASHP recommends that all syringes and needles used in the course of preparation be placed in *"sharps"* containers for disposal without being crushed, clipped, or capped.[3,103]

3. Priming

Prudent practice dictates that drug administration sets be attached and primed within the BSC, prior to addition of the drug. This eliminates the need to prime the set in a less well-controlled environment and ensures that any fluid that escapes during priming contains no drug. If priming must occur at the site of administration, the intravenous line should be primed with non-drug containing fluid, or backflow closed system should be used.[3]

4. Handling Vials

Extremes of positive and negative pressure in medication vials should be avoided, e.g., attempting to withdraw 10 mL of fluid from a 10-mL vial or placing 10 mL of a fluid into an air filled 10-mL vial. The use of large-bore needles, #18 or #20, avoids *high-pressure syring-*

ing of solutions. However, some experienced personnel believe that large-bore needles are more likely to drip. Multi-use dispensing pins are recommended to avoid these problems.

Venting devices such as filter needles or dispensing pins permit outside air to replace the withdrawn liquid. Proper worker education is essential before using these devices.[3] Although venting devices are recommended, another technique is to add diluent slowly to the vial by alternately injecting small amounts and allowing displaced air to escape into the syringe. When all diluent has been added, a small amount of additional air may be withdrawn to create a slight negative pressure in the vial. This should not be expelled into room air because it may contain drug residue. It should either be injected into a vacuum vial or remain in the syringe to be discarded.

If any negative pressure must be applied to withdraw a dosage from a stoppered vial and handling safety is compromised, an air-filled syringe should be used to equalize pressure in the stoppered vial. The volume of drug to be withdrawn can be replaced by injecting small amounts of air into the vial and withdrawing equal amounts of liquid until the required volume is withdrawn. The drug should be cleared from the needle and hub (neck) of the syringe before separating to reduce spraying on separation.

5. Handling Ampules

Prudent practice requires that ampules with dry material should be "*gently tapped down*" before opening to move any material in the top of the ampule to the bottom quantity. A sterile gauze pad should be wrapped around the ampule neck before breaking the top.[3] This can protect against cuts and catch airborne powder or aerosol. If diluent is to be added, it should be injected slowly down the inside wall of the ampule. The ampule should be tilted gently to ensure that all the powder is wet before agitating it to dissolve the contents.

After the solution is withdrawn from the ampule with a syringe, the needle should be cleared of solution by holding it vertically with the point upwards; the syringe should be tapped to remove air bubbles. Any bubbles should be expelled into a closed container.

6. Packaging HDs for Transport

The outside of bags or bottles containing the prepared drug should be wiped with moist gauze.

Entry ports should be wiped with moist alcohol pads and capped. Transport should occur in sealed plastic bags and in containers designed to avoid breakage.

HDs that are shipped and which are subject to EPA regulation as hazardous waste are also subject to Department of Transportation (DOT) regulations as specified in 49 CFR part 172.101.

7. Non-liquid HDs

The handling of non-liquid forms of HDs requires special precautions as well. Tablets that may produce dust or potential exposure to the handler should be counted in a BSC. Capsules, i.e., gel caps or coated tablets, are unlikely to produce dust unless broken in handling.

These are counted in a BSC on equipment designated for HDs only, because even manual counting devices may be covered with dust from the drugs handled. Automated counting machines should not be used unless an enclosed process isolates the hazard from the employee(s).

Compounding should also occur in a BSC. A gown and gloves should be worn. *(If a BSC is unavailable, an appropriate NIOSH-approved respirator must be worn.)*

Drug Administration

1. Personal Protective Equipment

The National Study Commission on Cytotoxic Exposure has recommended that personnel administering HDs wear gowns, latex gloves, and chemical splash goggles or equivalent safety glasses as described under the PPE section, preparation.[71] *NIOSH-approved respirators should be worn when administering aerosolized drugs.*

2. Administration Kit

Protective and administration equipment may be packaged together and labeled as an HD administration kit. Such a kit should include:

- personal protective equipment,
- gauze (4 × 4) for cleanup,
- alcohol wipes,
- disposable plastic-backed absorbent liner,
- puncture-resistant container for needles and syringes,
- a thick sealable plastic bag (with warning label), and
- accessory warning labels.

3. Work Practices

Safe work practices when handling HDs should include:

- Hands should be washed before donning and after removing gloves. Gowns or gloves that become contaminated should be changed immediately. Employees should be trained in proper methods to remove contaminated gloves and gowns. After use, gloves and gowns should be disposed of in accordance with ASHP recommendations.
- Infusion sets and pumps, which should have Luer-Lok fittings, should be observed for leakage during use. A plastic-backed absorbent pad should be placed under the tubing during administration to catch any leakage. Sterile gauze should be placed around any push sites; IV tubing connection sites should be taped.
- Priming IV sets or expelling air from syringes should be carried out in a BSC. If done at the administration site, ASHP recommends that the line be primed with non-drug-containing solution or that a backflow closed system be used. IV containers with venting tubes should not be used.[3]
- Syringes, IV bottles and bags, and pumps should be wiped clean of any drug contamination with sterile gauze. Needles and syringes should not be crushed or clipped. They should be placed in a puncture-resistant container then into the HD disposal bag with all other HD contaminated materials. Administration sets should be disposed of intact. Disposal of the waste bag should follow HD disposal requirements. Unused drugs should be returned to the pharmacy.
- Protective goggles should be cleaned with detergent and properly rinsed. All protective equipment should be disposed of upon leaving the patient care area.
- Nursing stations where these drugs will be administered should have spill and emergency skin and eye decontamination kits available and relevant MSDSs for guidance. The HCS requires MSDSs to be readily available in the workplace to all employees working with hazardous chemicals.
- PPE should be used during the administration of oral HDs if splashing is possible.

A large number of investigational HDs are under clinical study in health care facilities. Personnel not directly involved in the investigation should not administer these drugs unless they have received adequate instructions regarding safe handling procedures. Literature regarding potential toxic effects of investigational drugs should be evaluated prior to the drug's introduction into the workplace.[65]

The increased use of HDs in the home environment necessitates special precautions. Employees involved in home care delivery should follow the above work practices, and employers should make administration and spill kits available. Home health care workers should have emergency protocols with them as well as phone numbers and addresses in the event emergency care becomes necessary.[3] Waste disposal for drugs delivered for home use and other home-contaminated material should also be considered by the employer and should follow applicable regulations.

4. Aerosolized Drugs

The administration of aerosolized HDs requires special engineering controls to prevent exposure to health care workers and others in the vicinity. In the case of *pentamidine,* these controls include treatment booths with local exhaust ventilation designed specifically for its administration. A variety of ventilation methods have also been used for the administration of *ribavirin.* These include isolation rooms with separate HEPA-filtered ventilation systems and administration via endotracheal tube.[30,47] Engineering controls used to manage employee exposure to anesthetic gases is a traditional example of occupational chemical management. Both isolation and ventilation are used for these volatile HDs.

Caring for Patients Receiving HDs

In accordance with the Bloodborne Pathogens Standard, universal precautions must be observed to prevent contact with blood or other potentially infectious materials. Under circumstances in which differentiation between body fluid types is difficult or impossible, all body fluids should be considered potentially infectious materials and must be managed as dictated in the Bloodborne Pathogens Standard.[109]

1. Personal Protective Equipment

Personnel dealing with excreta, primarily urine, from patients who have received HDs in the last 48 hours should be provided with and wear latex or other appropriate gloves and disposable gowns, to be discarded after each use or whenever contaminated, as detailed under Waste Disposal. Eye protection should be worn if splashing is possible. Such excreta contaminated with blood, or other potentially infectious materials as well, should be managed according to the Bloodborne Pathogen Standard. Hands should be washed after removal of gloves or after contact with the above substances.

2. Linen

Linen contaminated with HDs or excreta from patients who have received HDs in the past 48 hours is a potential source of exposure to employees. Linen soiled with blood or other potentially infectious materials as well as contaminated with excreta must also be managed according to the Bloodborne Pathogens Standard.[109] Linen contaminated with HDs should be placed in specially marked laundry bags and then placed in a labeled, impervious bag. The laundry bag and its contents should be prewashed, and then the linens added to other laundry for a second wash. Laundry personnel should wear latex gloves and gowns while handling prewashed material.

3. Reusable Items

Glassware or other contaminated reusable items should be washed twice with detergent by a trained employee wearing double latex gloves and a gown.

Waste Disposal

1. Equipment

Thick, leakproof plastic bags, colored differently from other hospital trash bags, should be used for routine accumulation and collection of used containers, discarded gloves, gowns, and any other disposable material. Bags containing hazardous chemicals (as defined by Section C of HCS), shall be labeled in accordance with Section F of the Hazard Communication Standard where appropriate. Where the Hazard Communication Standard does not apply, labels should indicate that bags contain HD-related wastes.

Needles, syringes, and breakable items not contaminated with blood or other potentially infectious materials should be placed in a *"sharps"* container before they are stored in the waste bag. Such items that are contaminated with blood or other potentially infectious material *must* be placed in a *"sharps"* container. Similarly, needles should not be clipped or capped nor syringes crushed. If contaminated by blood or other potentially infectious material, such needles/syringes *must not* be clipped, capped, or crushed (except as on a rare instance where a *medical* procedure requires recapping). The waste bag should be kept inside a covered waste container clearly labeled "HD Waste Only." At least one such receptacle should be located in every area where the drugs are prepared or administered. Waste should not be moved from one area to another. The bag should be sealed when filled and the covered waste container taped.

2. Handling

Prudent practice dictates that every precaution be taken to prevent contamination of the exterior of the container. Personnel disposing of HD waste should wear gowns and protective gloves when handling waste containers with contaminated exteriors. Prudent practice further dictates that such a container with a contaminated exterior be placed in a second container in a manner that eliminates contamination of the second container. HD waste handlers should also receive hazard communication training as discussed below in Section H.

3. Disposal

Hazardous drug-related wastes should be handled separately from other hospital trash and disposed of in accordance with applicable EPA, state, and local regulations for hazardous waste.[24,110] This disposal can occur at either an incinerator or a licensed sanitary landfill for toxic wastes, as appropriate. Commercial waste disposal is performed by a licensed company. While awaiting removal, the waste should be held in a secure area in covered, labeled drums with plastic liners.

Chemical inactivation traditionally has been a complicated process that requires specialized knowledge and training. The MSDS should be consulted regarding specific advice on cleanup. IARC13 and Lunn et al.[56] have validated inactivation procedures for specific agents that are effective. However, these procedures vary from drug to drug and may be impractical for small amounts. Care must be taken because of unique problems presented by the cleanup

3. Transport

HDs should be securely capped or sealed, placed in sealed clear plastic bags, and transported in containers designed to avoid breakage.

Personnel involved in transporting HDs should be trained in spill procedures, including sealing off the contaminated area and calling for appropriate assistance.

All HD containers should be labeled as noted in Drug Preparation Work Practices. If transport methods that produce stress on contents, such as pneumatic tubes are used, guidance from the OSHA clarification of 1910.1030 with respect to transport (M.4.b.(8)(c)) should be followed. This clarification provides for use of packaging material inside the tube to prevent breakage. These recommendations that pertain to the Bloodborne Pathogens Standard are prudent practice for HDs, e.g., padded inserts for carriers.

F. Medical Surveillance

Workers who are potentially exposed to chemical hazards should be monitored in a systematic program or medical surveillance intended to prevent occupational injury and disease.[3,7] The purpose of surveillance is to identify the earliest reversible biologic effects so that exposure can be reduced or eliminated before the employee sustains irreversible damage. The occurrence of exposure-related disease or other adverse health effects should prompt immediate re-evaluation of primary preventive measures (e.g., engineering controls, personal protective equipment). In this manner, medical surveillance acts as a check on the appropriateness of controls already in use.[62]

For detection and control of work-related health effects, *job-specific* medical evaluations should be performed:

- before job placement,
- periodically during employment,
- following acute exposures, and
- at the time of job termination or transfer (exit examination).

This information should be collected and analyzed in a systematic fashion to allow early detection of disease patterns in individual workers and groups of workers.

1. Pre-placement Medical Examinations

Sound medical practice dictates that employees who will be working with HDs in the workplace have an initial evaluation consisting of a history, physical exam, and laboratory studies.

Information made available, by the employer, to the examining physician should be:

- a description of the employee's duties as they relate to the employee's exposure,
- the employee's exposure levels or anticipated exposure levels,
- a description of any personal protective equipment used or to be used, and
- information from previous medical examinations of the employee, which is not readily available to the examining physician.

The history details the individual's medical and reproductive experience with emphasis on potential risk factors, such as past hematopoietic, malignant, or hepatic disorders. It also includes a complete occupational history with information on extent of past exposures (including environmental sampling data, if possible) and use of protective equipment. Surrogates for worker exposure, in the absence of environmental sampling data, include:

- records of drugs and quantities handled,

- hours spent handling these drugs per week,
- number of preparations/administrations per week.

The physical examination should be complete, but the skin, mucous membranes, cardiopulmonary, lymphatic system, and liver should be emphasized. An evaluation for respirator use must be performed in accordance with 29 CFR 1910.134, if the employee will wear a respirator. The laboratory assessment may include a complete blood count with differential, liver function tests, blood urea nitrogen, creatinine, and a urine dipstick. Other aspects of the physical and laboratory evaluation should be guided by known toxicities of the HD of exposure. Due to poor reproducibility, interindividual variability, and lack of prognostic value regarding disease development, no biological monitoring tests (e.g., genotoxic markers) are currently recommended for routine use in employee surveillance. Biological marker testing should be performed only within the context of a research protocol.

2. Periodic Medical Examinations

Recognized occupational medicine experts in the HD area recommend these exams to update the employee's medical, reproductive, and exposure histories. They are recommended on a yearly basis or every 2–3 years. The interval between exams is a function of the opportunity for exposure, duration of exposure, and possibly the age of the worker at the discretion of the occupational medicine physician, guided by the worker's history. Careful documentation of an individual's routine exposure and any acute accidental exposures are made. The physical examination and laboratory studies follow the format outlined in the pre-placement examination.[54]

3. Post-exposure Examinations

Post-exposure evaluation is tailored to the type of exposure (e.g., spills or needle sticks from syringes containing HDs). An assessment of the extent of exposure is made and included in the confidential database (discussed below) and in an incident report. The physical examination focuses on the involved area as well as other organ systems commonly affected (i.e., for CDs the skin and mucous membranes; for aerosolized HDs the pulmonary system). Treatment and laboratory studies follow as indicated and should be guided by emergency protocols.

4. Exit Examinations

The exit examination completes the information on the employee's medical, reproductive and exposure histories. Examination and laboratory evaluation should be guided by the individual's history of exposures and follow the outline of the periodic evaluation.

5. Exposure/Health Outcome Linkage

Exposure assessment of all employees who have worked with HDs is important, and the maintenance of records is required by 29 CFR 1910.20. The use of previously outlined exposure surrogates is acceptable, although actual environmental or employee monitoring data is preferable. An MSDS can serve as an exposure record. Details of the use of personal protective equipment and engineering controls present should be included. A confidential database should be maintained with information regarding the individual's medical and reproductive history, with linkage to exposure information to facilitate epidemiologic review.

6. Reproductive Issues

The examining physician should consider the reproductive status of employees and inform them regarding relevant reproductive issues. The reproductive toxicity of hazardous drugs should be carefully explained to all workers who will be exposed to these chemicals, and is required for those chemicals covered by the HCS. Unfortunately, no information is available regarding the reproductive risks of HD handling with the current use of BSCs and PPE. However, as discussed earlier, both spontaneous abortion and congenital malformation excesses have been documented among workers handling some of these drugs without currently recommended engineering controls and precautions. The facility should have a policy regarding reproductive toxicity of HDs and worker exposure in male and female employees and should follow that policy.

G. Hazard Communication

This section is for informational purposes only and is not a substitute for the requirements of the Hazard Communication Standard.

The Hazard Communication Standard (HCS),107 is applicable to some drugs. It defines a hazardous chemical as *any chemical that is a physical hazard or a health hazard.*

Physical hazard refers to characteristics such as combustibility or reactivity. A health hazard is defined as *a chemical for which there is statistically significant evidence based on at least one study conducted in accordance with established scientific principles that acute or chronic health effects may occur in exposed employees.* Appendixes A and B of the HCS outline the criteria used to determine whether an agent is hazardous.

According to HCS Appendix A, agents with any of the following characteristics would be considered hazardous:

- carcinogens,
- corrosives,
- toxic or highly toxic (defined on the basis of median lethal doses),
- irritants,
- sensitizers, or
- target organ effectors, including reproductive toxins, hepatotoxins, nephrotoxins, neurotoxins, agents that act on the hematopoietic system, and agents that damage the lungs, skin, eyes, or mucous membranes.

Both human and animal data are to be used in this determination. HCS Appendix C lists sources of toxicity information.

As a result of the February 21, 1990 Supreme Court decision,21 all provisions of the Hazard Communication Standard [29 CFR 1910.1200]107 are now in effect for all industrial segments. This includes the coverage of drugs and pharmaceuticals in the non-manufacturing sector. On February 9, 1994, OSHA issued a revised Hazard Communication Final Rule with technical clarification regarding drugs and pharmaceutical agents.

The Hazard Communication Standard (HCS) requires that drugs posing a health hazard (with the exception of those in solid, final form for direct administration to the patient, i.e., tablets or pills) be included on lists of hazardous chemicals to which employees are exposed.[107] Their storage and use locations can be confirmed by reviewing purchasing office records of currently used and past used agents such as those in Table I.1. Employee exposure records, including workplace monitoring, biological monitoring, and MSDSs, as well as employee medical records related to drugs posing a health hazard must be maintained and access to them provided to employees in accordance with 29 CFR 1910.20. Training required under the HCS should include all employees potentially exposed to these agents, not only health care professional staff, but also physical plant, maintenance, or support staff.

MSDSs are required to be prepared and transmitted with the initial shipment of all hazardous chemicals including covered drugs and pharmaceutical products. This excludes drugs defined by the Federal Food, Drug and Cosmetic Act, which are in solid, final form for direct administration to the patient (e.g., tablets, pills, or capsules) or which are packaged for sale to consumers in a retail establishment. Package inserts and the *Physicians' Desk Reference* are not acceptable in lieu of requirements of MSDSs under the Standard. Items mandated by the Standard will use the term *shall* instead of *should.*

1. Written Hazard Communication Program

Employers shall develop, implement, and maintain at the workplace, a written hazard communication program for employees handling or otherwise exposed to chemicals, including drugs that represent a health hazard to employees. The written program will describe how the criteria specified in the Standard concerning labels and other forms of warning, MSDSs, and employee information and training will be met. This also includes the following:

- a list of the covered hazardous drugs known to be present using an identity that is referenced on the appropriate MSDS,
- the methods the employer will use to inform employees of the hazards of non-routine tasks in their work areas, and
- the methods the employer will use to inform employees of other employers of hazards at the worksite.

The employer shall make the written hazard communication program available, upon request, to employees, their designated representatives, and the Assistant Secretary of OSHA in accordance with requirements of the HCS.

2. MSDSs

In accordance with requirements in the Hazard Communication Standard, the employer must maintain MSDSs accessible to employees for all covered HDs used in the hospital. Specifics regarding MSDS content are contained in the Standard. Essential information includes: health hazards, primary exposure routes, carcinogenic evaluations, acute exposure treatment, chemical inactivators, solubility, stability, volatility, PPE-required and spill procedures for each covered HD. MSDSs shall also be made readily available upon request to employees, their designated representatives, or the Assistant Secretary of OSHA.

H. Training and Information Dissemination

In compliance with the Hazard Communication Standard, all personnel involved in any aspect of the handling of covered HDs (physicians, nurses, pharmacists, housekeepers, employees involved in receiving, transport, or storage) must receive information and training to appraise them of the hazards of HDs present in the work area.[71] Such information should be provided at the time of an employee's initial assignment to a work area where HDs are present and prior to assignments involving new hazards. The employer should provide annual refresher information and training.

The National Study Commission on Cytotoxic Exposure has recommended that knowledge and competence of personnel be evaluated after the first orientation or training session, and then yearly, or more often if a need is perceived.[71] Evaluation may involve direct observation of an individual's performance on the job. In addition, non-HD solutions should be used for evaluation of preparation technique; quinine, which will fluoresce under ultraviolet light, provides an easy mechanism for evaluation of technique.

1. Employee Information

Employees must be informed of the requirements of the Hazard Communication Standard, 29 CFR 1910.1200

- any operation/procedure in their work area where drugs that present a hazard are present, and
- the location and availability of the written hazard communication program.

In addition, they should be informed regarding:

- any operations or procedure in their work area where other HDs are present, and
- the location and availability of any other plan regarding HDs.

2. Employee Training

Employee training must include at least:

- methods of observations that may be used to detect the presence or release of a HCS-covered hazardous drug in the work area (such as monitoring conducted by the employer, continuous monitoring devices, visual appearance, or odor of covered HDs being released, etc.),
- the physical and health hazards of the covered HDs in the area,
- the measures employees can take to protect themselves from these hazards. This includes specific procedures that the employer has implemented to protect the employees from exposure to such drugs, such as identification of covered drugs and those to be handled as hazardous, appropriate work practices, emergency procedures (for spills or employee exposure), and personal protective equipment, and
- the details of the hazard communication program developed by the employer, including an explanation of the labeling system and the MSDS, and how employees can obtain and use the appropriate hazard information.

It is essential that workers understand the carcinogenic potential and reproductive hazards of these drugs. Both females and males should understand the importance of avoiding exposure, especially early in pregnancy, so they can make informed decisions about the hazards involved. In addition, the facility's policy regarding reproductive toxicity of HDs should be explained to workers. Updated information should be provided to employees on a regular basis and whenever their jobs involve new hazards. Medical staff and other personnel who are not hospital employees should be informed of hospital policies and of the expectation that they will comply with these policies.

I. Record Keeping

Any workplace-exposure record created in connection with HD handling shall be kept, transferred, and made available for at least thirty years and medical records shall be kept for the duration of employment plus thirty years in accordance with the Access to Employee Exposure and Medical Records Standard (29 CFR 1910.20).[108] In addition, sound practice dictates that training records should include the following information:

- the dates of the training sessions,
- the contents or a summary of the training sessions,
- the names and qualifications of the persons conducting the training, and
- the names and job titles of all persons attending the training sessions.

Training records should be maintained for three years from the date on which the training occurred.

Position Statement

For the handling of cytotoxic agents by women who are pregnant, attempting to conceive, or breastfeeding. There are substantial data regarding the mutagenic, teratogenic, and abortifacient properties of certain cytotoxic agents both in animals and humans who have received therapeutic doses of these agents. Additionally, the scientific literature suggests a possible association of occupational exposure to certain cytotoxic agents during the first trimester of pregnancy with fetal loss or malformation. These data suggest the need for caution when women who are pregnant, or attempting to conceive, handle cytotoxic agents. Incidentally, there is no evidence relating male exposure to cytotoxic agents with adverse fetal outcome. There are no studies that address the possible risk associated with the occupational exposure to cytotoxic agents and the passage of these agents into breast milk. Nevertheless, it is prudent that women who are breast-feeding should exercise caution in handling cytotoxic agents.

If all procedures for safe handling, such as those recommended by the Commission, are complied with, the potential for exposure will be minimized. Personnel should be provided with information to make an individual decision. This information should be provided in written form, and it is advisable that a statement of understanding be signed. It is essential to refer to individual state right-to-know laws to ensure compliance.

Approved by the National Study Commission on Cytotoxic Exposure, September 1987.

References

1. American Medical Association Council on Scientific Affairs. Guidelines for handling parenteral antineoplastics. *JAMA* 1985;253:1590–2
2. American National Standards Institute. Occupational and Educational Eye and Face Protection. *ANSI* 1968;Z87:1
3. American Society of Hospital Pharmacists. ASHP Technical Assistance Bulletin on Handling Cytotoxic and Hazardous Drugs. *Am. J. Hosp. Pharm.* 1990;47:1033–49
4. Andersen R, Boedicker M, Ma M, Goldstein EJC. Adverse Reactions Associated with Pentamidine Isethionate in AIDS Patients: Recommendations for Monitoring Therapy. *Drug Intell. Clin. Pharm.* 1986;20:862–8
5. Anderson RW, Puckett WH, Dana WJ, et al. Risk of handling injectable antineoplastic agents. *Am. J. Hosp. Pharm.* 1982;39:1881–87
6. Avis KE, Levchuck JW. Special considerations in the use of vertical laminar flow workbenches. *Am. J. Hosp. Pharm.* 1984;41:81–7
7. Barber RK. Fetal and neonatal effects of cytotoxic agents. *Obstet. Gynecol.* 1981;51: 41S–47S

8. Benhamou S, Pot-Deprun J, Sancho-Garnier H, Chouroulinkov I. Sister chromatid exchanges and chromosomal aberrations in lymphocytes of nurses handling cytostatic drugs. *Int. J. Cancer* 1988;41:350–3
9. Bos RP, Leenars AO, Theuws JL, Henderson PT. Mutagenicity of urine from nurses handling cytostatic drugs, influence of smoking. *Int. Arch. Occ. Envir. Health* 1982; 50:359–69
10. Bryan D, Marback RC. Laminar-airflow equipment certification: What the pharmacist needs to know. *Am. J. Hosp. Pharm.* 1984;41:1343–9
11. Burgaz S, Ozdamar YN, Karakaya AE. A signal assay for the detection of toxic compounds: Application on the urines of cancer patients on chemotherapy and of nurses handling cytotoxic drugs. *Human Toxicol.* 1988;7:557–60
12. California Department of Health Services Occupational Health Surveillance and Evaluation Program. *Health care worker exposure to ribavirin aerosol: field investigation FI-86-009.* Berkeley: California Department of Health Services. 1986
13. Castegnaro M, Adams J, Armour MA, eds, et al. *Laboratory decontamination and destruction of carcinogens in laboratory wastes: Some antineoplastic agents.* International Agency for Research on Cancer. Scientific Publications No. 73. Lyons, France: IARC 1985
14. Chapman RM. Effect of cytotoxic therapy on sexuality and gonadal function. Perry MC, Yarbro JW, (eds), *Toxicity of Chemotherapy* Orlando: Grune & Stratton.1984; 343–363
15. Chen CH, Vazquez-Padua M, Cheng YC. Effect of antihuman immunodeficiency virus nucleoside analogs on mDNA and its implications for delayed toxicity. *Mol. Pharm.* 1990;39:625–628
16. Christensen CJ, Lemasters GK, Wakeman MA. Work practices and policies of hospital pharmacists preparing antineoplastic agents. *J. Occup. Med.* 1990;32:508–12
17. Chrysostomou A, Morley AA, Seshadri R. Mutation frequency in nurses and pharmacists working with cytotoxic drugs. *Aust. N. Z. J. Med.* 1984;14:831–4
18. Connor JD, Hintz M, Van Dyke R. Ribavirin pharmacokinetics in children and adults during therapeutic trials. Smith RA, Knight V, Smith JAD, (eds), *In Clinical Applications of Ribavirin* Orlando: Academic Press, 1984
19. Connor TH, Laidlaw JL, Theiss JC, et al. Permeability of latex and polyvinyl chloride gloves to carmustine. *Am. J. Hosp. Pharm.* 1984;41:676–9
20. Crudi CB. A compounding dilemma: I've kept the drug sterile but have I contaminated myself? *Nat. Intra. Therapy J.* 1980;3:77–80
21. Dole *v.* United Steelworkers. 1990;494 U.S.26.
22. Doll C. Aerosolised pentamidine. *Lancet* 1989;ii:1284–5
23. Duvall E, Baumann B. An unusual accident during the administration of chemotherapy. *Cancer Nurs.* 1980;3:305–6
24. Environmental Protection Agency. *Discarded commercial chemical products, off specification species, container residues, and spill residues thereof.* 40 CFR:1991; 261.33(f)
25. Everson RB, Ratcliffe JM, Flack PM, et al. Detection of low levels of urinary mutagen excretion by chemotherapy workers which was not related to occupational drug exposures. *Cancer Research* 1985;45:6487–97
26. Falck K, Grohn P, Sorsa M, et al. Mutagenicity in urine of nurses handling cytostatic drugs. *Lancet* 1979;i:1250–1
27. Falck K, Sorsa M, Vainio H. Use of the bacterial fluctuation test to detect mutagenicity in urine of nurses handling cytostatic drugs (abstract). *Mutation Res.* 1981;85: 236–7

28. Ferguson LR, Everts R, Robbie MA, et al. The use within New Zealand of cytogenetic approaches to monitoring of hospital pharmacists for exposure to cytotoxic drugs: Report of a pilot study in Auckland. *Aust J Hosp Pharm.* 1988;18:228–33
29. Gude JK. Selective delivery of pentamidine to the lung by aerosol. *Am. Rev. Resp. Dis.* 1989;139:1060
30. Guglielmo BJ, Jacobs RA, Locksley RM. The exposure of health care workers to ribavirin aerosol. *JAMA* 1989;261:1880–1
31. Harrison R, Bellows J, Rempel D, et al. Assessing exposures of health-care personnel to aerosols of ribavirin—California. *Morbidity and Mortality Weekly Report* 1988;37: 560–3
32. Hemminki K, Kyyronen P, Lindbohm ML. Spontaneous abortions and malformations in the offspring of nurses exposed to anaesthetic gases, cytostatic drugs, and other potential hazards in hospitals, based on registered information of outcome. *J. Epidem. Comm. Health* 1985;39:141–7
33. Henderson DK, Gerberding JL. Prophylactic zidovudine after occupational exposure to the human immunodeficiency virus: An interim analysis. *J. Infectious Diseases* 1989;160:321–7
34. Hillyard IW. The preclinical toxicology and safety of ribavirin. Smith RA, Kirkpatrick W, (eds), *In Ribavirin: a broad spectrum antiviral agent.* New York: Academic Press 1980
35. Hirst M, Tse S, Mills DG, et al. Occupational exposure to cyclophosphamide. *Lancet* 1984;i:186–8
36. Hoy RH, Stump LM. Effect of an air-venting filter device on aerosol production from vials. *Am. J. Hosp. Pharm.* 1984;41:324–6
37. International Agency for Research on Cancer. *IARC Monographs on the Evaluation of the Carcinogenic Risk of Chemicals to Man: Some Aziridines, N-, S-, and O-mustards and selenium. Lyons, France.* 1975;Vol. 9
38. International Agency for Research on Cancer. *IARC Monographs on the Evaluation of the Carcinogenic Risk of Chemicals to Man: Some naturally occurring substances.* Lyons, France: IARC. 1976;Vol. 10
39. International Agency for Research on Cancer. *IARC Monographs on the Evaluation of the Carcinogenic Risk of Chemicals to Humans: Some Antineoplastic and Immunosuppressive Agents.* Lyons, France: IARC. 1981;Vol. 26
40. International Agency for Research on Cancer. *IARC Monographs on the Evaluation of the Carcinogenic Risk of Chemicals to Humans: Chemicals, Industrial Processes and Industries Associated with Cancer in Humans.* Lyons, France: IARC. 1982;Vol. 1–29 (Suppl. 4)
41. International Agency for Research on Cancer. *IARC Monographs on the Evaluation of the Carcinogenic Risk of Chemicals to Humans: Genetic and related effects: An updating of selected IARC Monographs from Volumes 1–42.* Lyons, France: IARC. 1987;Vol. 1–42 (Suppl. 6)
42. International Agency for Research on Cancer. *IARC Monographs on the Evaluation of the Carcinogenic Risk of Chemicals to Humans; Overall evaluations of carcinogenicity: An updating of IARC Monographs Volumes 1 to 42.* Lyons, France: IARC. 1987;Vol. 1–42 (Suppl. 7)
43. International Agency for Research on Cancer. *IARC Monographs on the Evaluation of the Carcinogenic Risk of Chemicals to Humans: Pharmaceutical Drugs.* Lyons, France: IARC.
44. Jagun O, Ryan M, Waldron HA. Urinary thioether excretion in nurses handling cytotoxic drugs. *Lancet* 1982;i:443–4

45. Johnson EG, Janosik JE. Manufacturer's recommendations for handling spilled antineoplastic agents. *Am. J. Hosp. Pharm.* 1989;46:318–9
46. Juma FD, Rogers HJ, Trounce JR, Bradbrook ID. Pharmacokinetics of intravenous cyclophosphamide in man, estimated by gas-liquid chromatography. *Cancer Chemother. Pharmacol.* 1978;1:229–31
47. Kacmarek RM. Ribavirin and pentamidine aerosols: Caregiver beware! *Respiratory Care* 1990;35:1034–6
48. Karakaya AE, Burgaz S, Bayhan A. The significance of urinary thioethers as indicators of exposure to alkylating agents. *Arch. Toxicol.* 1989;13(suppl):117–9
49. Kilham L, Ferm VH. Congenital anomalies induced in hamster embryos with ribavirin. *Science* 1977;195:413–4
50. Kleinberg ML, Quinn MJ. Airborne drug levels in a laminar-flow hood. *Am. J. Hosp. Pharm.* 1981;38:1301–3
51. Kolmodin-Hedman B, Hartvig P, Sorsa M, Falck K. Occupational handling of cytostatic drugs. *Arch. Toxicol.* 1983;54:25–33
52. Kyle RA. Second malignancies associated with chemotherapy. Perry MC, Yarbro JW, (eds), *Toxicity of Chemotherapy.* Orlando: Grune & Stratton.1984;479–506
53. Laidlaw JL, Connor TH, Theiss JC, et al. Permeability of latex and polyvinyl chloride gloves to 20 antineoplastic drugs. *Am. J. Hosp. Pharm.* 1984;41:2618–23
54. Laidlaw JL, Connor TH, Theiss JC, et al. Permeability of four disposable protective clothing materials to seven antineoplastic drugs. *Am. J. Hosp. Pharm.* 1985;42: 2449–54
55. Lee SB. Ribavirin—Exposure to health care workers. *Am. Ind. Hyg. Assoc.* 1988;49: A13–A14
56. LeRoy ML, Roberts MJ, Theisen JA. Procedures for handling antineoplastic injections in comprehensive cancer centers. *Am. J. Hosp. Pharm.* 1983;40:601–3
57. Lunn G, Sansone EB. Validated methods for handling spilled antineoplastic agents. *Am. J. Hosp. Pharm.* 1989;46:1131
58. Lunn G, Sansone EB, Andrews AW, Hellwig LC. Degradation and disposal of some antineoplastic drugs. *J. Pharm. Sciences.* 1989;78:652–9
59. Matthews T, Boehme R. Antiviral activity and mechanism of action of ganciclovir. *Rev. Infect. Diseases* 1988;10 (suppl 3):S490–94
60. McDevitt JJ, Lees PSJ, McDiarmid MA. Exposure of hospital pharmacists and nurses to antineoplastic agents. *J. Occup. Med.* 1993;35:57–60
61. McDiarmid MA, Egan T, Furio M, et al. Sampling for airborne fluorouracil in a hospital drug preparation area. *Am. J. Hosp. Pharm.* 1988;43:1942–5
62. McDiarmid MA, Emmett EA. Biological monitoring and medical surveillance of workers exposed to antineoplastic agents. *Seminars in Occup. Med.* 1987;2:109–17
63. McDiarmid MA, Jacobson-Kram D. Aerosolized pentamidine and public health. *Lancet* 1989;ii:863
64. McDiarmid MA. Medical surveillance for antineoplastic-drug handlers. *Am. J. Hosp. Pharm.* 1990;47:1061–6
65. McDiarmid MA, Gurley HT, Arrington D. Pharmaceuticals as hospital hazards: Managing the risks. *J. Occup. Med.* 1991;33:155–8
66. McDiarmid MA, Kolodner K, Humphrey F, et al. Baseline and phosphoramide mustard-induced sister chromatid exchanges in pharmacists handling anti-cancer drugs. *Mutation Research* 1992;279:199–204
67. McDiarmid MA, Schaefer J, Richard CL, Chaisson RE, Tepper BS. Efficacy of engineering controls in reducing occupational exposure to aerosolized pentamidine. *Chest* 1992;102:1764–6

68. McEvoy GK, ed. *American Hospital Formulary Service Drug Information.* Bethesda: American Society of Hospital Pharmacists, 1993
69. McLendon BF, Bron AF. Corneal toxicity from vinblastine solution. *Br. J. Ophthalmol.* 1978;62:97–9
70. National Sanitation Foundation. *Standard No. 49 for Class II (Laminar Flow) Biohazard Cabinetry.* Ann Arbor: National Sanitation Foundation, 1990
71. National Study Commission on Cytotoxic Exposure. Louis P Jeffrey Sc.D Chairman, (eds), *Recommendations for Handling Cytotoxic Agents.* Providence, Rhode Island: Rhode Island Hospital, 1983
72. National Study Commission on Cytotoxic Exposure. Consensus Responses to Unresolved Questions Concerning Cytotoxic Agents. Louis P Jeffrey Sc. D, (eds), Providence, Rhode Island. Chairman, Rhode Island Hospital, 1984
73. Neal AD, Wadden RA, Chiou WL. Exposure of hospital workers to airborne antineoplastic agents. *Am. J. Hosp. Pharm.* 1983;40:597–601
74. Nikula E, Kiviniitty K, Leisti J, Taskinen P. Chromosome aberrations in lymphocytes of nurses handling cytostatic agents. *Scand. J. Work Environ. Health.* 1984;10:71–4
75. Norppa H, Sorsa M, Vainio H, et al. Increased sister chromatid exchange frequencies in lymphocytes of nurses handling cytostatic drugs. *Scand. J. Work Environ. Health* 1980;6:299–301
76. Nguyen TV, Theiss JC, Matney TS. Exposure of pharmacy personnel to mutagenic antineoplastic drugs. *Cancer Research* 42:4792–6
77. Palmer RG, Dore CJ, Denman AM. Chlorambucil-induced chromosome damage to human lymphocytes is dose-dependent and cumulative. *Lancet* 1984;i:246–9
78. Perry MC, Yarbro JW, eds. *Toxicity of Chemotherapy.* Orlando: Grune & Stratton. 1984
79. Physician's Desk Reference. Barnhart ER, (eds), *Physician's Desk Reference,* 45th ed. Oradell, New Jersey: Medical Economics Data.1991;730
80. Pohlova H, Cerna M, Rossner P. Chromosomal aberrations, SCE and urine mutagenicity in workers occupationally exposed to cytostatic drugs. *Mutation Res.* 1986;174: 213–7
81. Pyy L, Sorsa M, Hakala E. Ambient monitoring of cyclophosphamide in manufacture and hospitals. *Am. Ind. Hyg. Assoc. J.* 1988;49:314–7
82. Reich SD, Bachur NR. Contact dermatitis associated with adriamycin (NSC-123127) and daunorubicin (NSC-82151). *Cancer Chemotherap. Reports* 1975;59:677–8
83. Reynolds RD, Ignoffo R, Lawrence J, et al. Adverse reactions to AMSA in medical personnel. *Cancer Treat. Rep.* 1982;66:1885
84. Rogers B. Health hazards to personnel handling antineoplastic agents. *Occupational Medicine: State of the Art Reviews* 1987;2:513–24
85. Rogers B, Emmett EA. Handling antineoplastic agents: Urine mutagenicity in nurses. *IMAGE Journal of Nursing Scholarship.* 1987;19:108–113
86. Rosner F. Acute leukemia as a delayed consequence of cancer chemotherapy. *Cancer* 1976;37:1033–6
87. Rudolph R, Suzuki M, Luce JK. Experimental skin necrosis produced by adriamycin. *Cancer Treat. Reports* 1979;63:529–37
88. Schafer AI. Teratogenic effects of antileukemic therapy. *Arch. Int. Med.* 1981;141: 514–5
89. Selevan SG, Lindbolm ML, Homung RW, Hemminki K. A study of occupational exposure to antineoplastic drugs and fetal loss in nurses. *New Engl. J. Med.* 1985;313: 1173–8
90. Sieber SM. Cancer chemotherapeutic agents and carcinogenesis. *Cancer Chemotherap. Reports* 1975;59:915–8

91. Sieber SM, Adamson RH. Toxicity of antineoplastic agents in man: Chromosomal aberrations, antifertility effects, congenital malformations, and carcinogenic potential. *Adv. Cancer Res.* 1975;22:57–155
92. Siebert D, Simon U. Cyclophosphamide: Pilot study of genetically active metabolites in the urine of a treated human patient. *Mutat. Res.* 1973;19:65–72
93. Slevin ML, Ang LM, Johnston A, Turner P. The efficiency of protective gloves used in the handling of cytotoxic drugs. *Cancer Chemo. Pharmacol.* 1984;12:151–3
94. Smaldone GC, Vincicuerra C, Marchese J. Detection of inhaled pentamidine in health care workers. *New Engl. J. Med.* 1991;325:891–2
95. Sorsa M, Hemminki K, Vanio H. Occupational exposure to anticancer drugs—Potential and real hazards. *Mut. Res.* 1985;154:135–49
96. Sotaniemi EA, Sutinen S, Arranto AJ, et al. Liver damage in nurses handling cytostatic agents. *Acta Med. Scand.* 1983;214:181–9
97. Stellman JM. The spread of chemotherapeutic agents at work: Assessment through stimulation. *Cancer Investigation* 1987;5:75–81
98. Stephens JD, Golbus MS, Miller TR, et al. Multiple congenital abnormalities in a fetus exposed to 5-fluorouracil during the first trimester. *Am. J. Obstet. Gynecol.* 1980;137:747–9
99. Stiller A, Obe G, Bool I, Pribilla W. No elevation of the frequencies of chromosomal aberrations as a consequence of handling cytostatic drugs. *Mut. Res.* 1983;121:253–9
100. Stoikes ME, Carlson JD, Farris FF, Walker PR. Permeability of latex and polyvinyl chloride gloves to fluorouracil and methotrexate. *Am. J. Hosp. Pharm.* 1987;44: 1341–6
101. Stucker I, Hirsch A, Doloy T, et al. Urine mutagenicity, chromosomal abnormalities and sister chromatid exchanges in lymphocytes of nurses handling cytostatic drugs. *Int. Arch. Occup. Environ. Health* 1986;57:195–205
102. Stucker I, Caillard JF, Collin R, et al. Risk of spontaneous abortion among nurses handling antineoplastic drugs. *Scand. J. Work Environ. Health* 1990;16:102–7
103. U.S. Department of Health and Human Services. Public Health Service. National Institutes of Health. *Recommendations for the Safe Handling of Cytotoxic Drugs.* NIH Publication No. 92-2621. 1992
104. U.S. Department of Health and Human Services. Public Health Service. Centers for Disease Control. National Institute for Occupational Safety and Health. *Guidelines for Protecting the Safety and Health of Health Care Workers.* DHHS (NIOSH) Publication No. 88-119. 1988
105. U.S. Department of Labor, Occupational Safety and Health Administration. *Respiratory Protection Standard.* 1984;29 CFR 1910.134
106. U.S. Department of Labor, Occupational Safety and Health Administration. *Work practice guidelines for personnel dealing with cytotoxic (antineoplastic) drugs.* OSHA Publication #8-1.1. 1986
107. U.S. Department of Labor, Occupational Safety and Health Administration. *Hazard Communication Standard.* 1989;29 CFR 1910.1200, as amended February 9, 1994.
108. U.S. Department of Labor, Occupational Safety and Health Administration. *Access to Employee and Medical Records Standard.* 1990;29 CFR 1910.20
109. U.S. Department of Labor, Occupational Safety and Health Administration. *Occupational Exposure to Bloodborne Pathogens Standard.* 1991;29 CFR 1910.1030
110. Vaccari FL, Tonat K, DeChristoforo R, et al. Disposal of antineoplastic waste at the NIH. *Am. J. Hosp. Pharm.* 1984;41:87–92
111. Valanis B, Vollmer WM, Labuhn K, Glass A, Corelle C. Antineoplastic drug handling protection after OSHA guidelines: Comparison by profession, handling activity, and work site. *J. Occup. Med.* 1992;34:149–55

112. Venitt S, Crofton-Sleigh C, Hunt J, et al. Monitoring exposure of nursing and pharmacy personnel to cytotoxic drugs. Urinary mutation assays and urinary platinum as markers of absorption. *Lancet* 1984;i:74:6
113. Waksvik H, Klepp O, Brogger A. Chromosome analyses of nurses handling cytostatic agents. *Cancer Treat. Reports* 1981;65:607–10
114. Wall RL, Clausen KP. Carcinoma of the urinary bladder in patients receiving cyclophosphamide. *New Engl. J. Med.* 1975;293:271–3
115. Weisburger JH, Griswold DP, Prejean JD, et al. Tumor induction by cytostatics. The carcinogenic properties of some of the principal drugs used in clinical cancer chemotherapy. *Recent Results Cancer Res.* 1975;52:1–17
116. Zimmerman PF, Larsen RK, Barkley EW, Gallelli JF. Recommendations for the safe handling of injectable antineoplastic drug products. *Am. J. Hosp. Pharm.* 1981; 38:1693–5

Appendix 2

Common Toxicity Criteria for Adverse Events v. 3.0 (CTCAE)

Source: From *National Cancer Institute Common Toxicity Criteria, Version 2.0* [Online], revised March 23, 1998. Available: http://ctep.info.nih.gov/CTC3/ctc.htm

Appendix 2

ALLERGY/IMMUNOLOGY						
		Grade				
Adverse Event	**Short Name**	**1**	**2**	**3**	**4**	**5**
Allergic reaction/hypersensitivity (including drug fever)	Allergic reaction	Transient flushing or rash; drug fever <38°C (<100.4°F)	Rash; flushing; urticaria; dyspnea; drug fever ≥38°C (≥100.4°F)	Symptomatic bronchospasm, with or without urticaria; parenteral medication(s) indicated; allergy-related edema/angioedema; hypotension	Anaphylaxis	Death
REMARK: Urticaria with manifestations of allergic or hypersensitivity reaction is graded as Allergic reaction/hypersensitivity (including drug fever). ALSO CONSIDER: Cytokine release syndrome/acute infusion reaction.						
Allergic rhinitis (including sneezing, nasal stuffiness, postnasal drip)	Rhinitis	Mild, intervention not indicated	Moderate, intervention indicated	—	—	—
REMARK: Rhinitis associated with obstruction or stenosis is graded as Obstruction/stenosis of airway – *Select* in the PULMONARY/UPPER RESPIRATORY CATEGORY.						
Autoimmune reaction	Autoimmune reaction	Asymptomatic and serologic or other evidence of autoimmune reaction, with normal organ function and intervention not indicated	Evidence of autoimmune reaction involving a nonessential organ or function (e.g., hypothyroidism)	Reversible autoimmune reaction involving function of a major organ or other adverse event (e.g., transient colitis or anemia)	Autoimmune reaction with life-threatening consequences	Death
ALSO CONSIDER: Colitis; Hemoglobin; Hemolysis (e.g., immune hemolytic anemia, drug-related hemolysis); Thyroid function, low (hypothyroidism).						

(continued)

Appendix 2 *(continued)*

		Grade				
Adverse Event	**Short Name**	**1**	**2**	**3**	**4**	**5**
Serum sickness	Serum sickness	—	—	Present	—	Death
NAVIGATION NOTE: Splenic function is graded in the BLOOD/BONE MARROW CATEGORY.						
NAVIGATION NOTE: Urticaria as an isolated symptom is graded as Urticaria (hives, welts, wheals) in the DERMATOLOGY/SKIN CATEGORY.						
Vasculitis	Vasculitis	Mild, intervention not indicated	Symptomatic, nonsteroidal medical intervention indicated	Steroids indicated	Ischemic changes; amputation indicated	Death
Allergy/Immunology – Other (Specify, ______)	Allergy – Other (Specify)	Mild	Moderate	Severe	Life-threatening; disabling	Death
		AUDITORY/EAR				
		Grade				
Adverse Event	**Short Name**	**1**	**2**	**3**	**4**	**5**
NAVIGATION NOTE: Earache (otalgia) is graded as Pain – *Select* in the PAIN CATEGORY.						

(continued)

Appendix 2 *(continued)*

		Grade				
Adverse Event	**Short Name**	**1**	**2**	**3**	**4**	**5**
Hearing: patients with/without baseline audiogram and enrolled in a monitoring program [1]	Hearing (monitoring program)	Threshold shift or loss of 15 – 25 dB relative to baseline, averaged at 2 or more contiguous test frequencies in at least one ear; or subjective change in the absence of a Grade 1 threshold shift	Threshold shift or loss of >25 – 90 dB, averaged at 2 contiguous test frequencies in at least one ear	Adult only: Threshold shift of >25 – 90 dB, averaged at 3 contiguous test frequencies in at least one ear Pediatric: Hearing loss sufficient to indicate therapeutic intervention, including hearing aids (e.g., ≥20 dB bilateral HL in the speech frequencies; ≥30 dB unilateral HL; and requiring additional speech-language related services)	Adult only: Profound bilateral hearing loss (>90 dB) Pediatric: Audiologic indication for cochlear implant and requiring additional speech-language related services	—
REMARK: Pediatric recommendations are identical to those for adults, unless specified. For children and adolescents (≤18 years of age) without a baseline test, pre-exposure/pretreatment hearing should be considered to be <5 dB loss.						
Hearing: patients without baseline audiogram and not enrolled in a monitoring program[1]	Hearing (without monitoring program)	—	Hearing loss not requiring hearing aid or intervention (i.e., not interfering with ADL)	Hearing loss requiring hearing aid or intervention (i.e., interfering with ADL)	Profound bilateral hearing loss (>90 dB)	—

(continued)

Appendix 2 *(continued)*

		Grade				
Adverse Event	**Short Name**	**1**	**2**	**3**	**4**	**5**
REMARK: Pediatric recommendations are identical to those for adults, unless specified. For children and adolescents (≤18 years of age) without a baseline test, pre-exposure/pretreatment hearing should be considered to be <5 dB loss.						
Otitis, external ear (non-infectious)	Otitis, external	External otitis with erythema or dry desquamation	External otitis with moist desquamation, edema, enhanced cerumen or discharge; tympanic membrane perforation; tympanostomy	External otitis with mastoiditis; stenosis or osteomyelitis	Necrosis of soft tissue or bone	Death
ALSO CONSIDER: Hearing: patients with/without baseline audiogram and enrolled in a monitoring program[1]; Hearing: patients without baseline audiogram and not enrolled in a monitoring program[1].						
Otitis, middle ear (non-infectious)	Otitis, middle	Serous otitis	Serous otitis, medical intervention indicated	Otitis with discharge; mastoiditis	Necrosis of the canal soft tissue or bone	Death
Tinnitus	Tinnitus	—	Tinnitus not interfering with ADL	Tinnitus interfering with ADL	Disabling	—
ALSO CONSIDER: Hearing: patients with/without baseline audiogram and enrolled in a monitoring program[1]; Hearing: patients without baseline audiogram and not enrolled in a monitoring program[1].						
Auditory/Ear – Other (Specify, ______)	Auditory/Ear – Other (Specify)	Mild	Moderate	Severe	Life-threatening; disabling	Death

[1] Drug-induced ototoxicity should be distinguished from age-related threshold decrements or unrelated cochlear insult. When considering whether an adverse event has occurred, it is first necessary to classify the patient into one of two groups. (1) The patient is under standard treatment/enrolled in a clinical trial <2.5 years, and has a 15 dB or greater threshold shift averaged across two contiguous frequencies; or (2) The patient is under standard treatment/enrolled in a clinical trial >2.5 years, and the difference between the expected agerelated and the observed threshold shifts is 15 dB or greater averaged across two contiguous frequencies. Consult standard references for appropriate age- and gender-specific

(continued)

Appendix 2 *(continued)*

hearing norms, e.g., Morrell, et al. Age- and gender-specific reference ranges for hearing level and longitudinal changes in hearing level. Journal of the Acoustical Society of America 100:1949-1967, 1996; or Shotland, et al. Recommendations for cancer prevention trials using potentially ototoxic test agents. Journal of Clinical Oncology 19:1658-1663, 2001.

In the absence of a baseline prior to initial treatment, subsequent audiograms should be referenced to an appropriate database of normals. ANSI. (1996) American National Standard: Determination of occupational noise exposure and estimation of noise-induced hearing impairment, ANSI S 3.44-1996. (Standard S 3.44). New York: American National Standards Institute. The recommended ANSI S3.44 database is Annex B.

BLOOD/BONE MARROW

		Grade				
Adverse Event	**Short Name**	**1**	**2**	**3**	**4**	**5**
Bone marrow cellularity	Bone marrow cellularity	Mildly hypocellular or ≤25% reduction from normal cellularity for age	Moderately hypocellular or >25 – ≤50% reduction from normal cellularity for age	Severely hypocellular or >50 – ≤75% reduction cellularity from normal for age	—	Death
CD4 count	CD4 count	<LLN – 500/mm³ <LLN – 0.5 × 10^9/L	<500 – 200/mm³ <0.5 – 0.2 × 10^9/L	<200 – 50/mm³ <0.2 × 0.05 – 10^9/L	<50/mm³ <0.05 × 10^9/L	Death
Haptoglobin	Haptoglobin	<LLN	—	Absent	—	Death
Hemoglobin	Hemoglobin	<LLN – 10.0 g/dL <LLN – 6.2 mmol/L <LLN – 100 g/L	<10.0 – 8.0 g/dL <6.2 – 4.9 mmol/L <100 – 80g/L	<8.0 – 6.5 g/dL <4.9 – 4.0 mmol/L <80 – 65 g/L	<6.5 g/dL <4.0 mmol/L <65 g/L	Death
Hemolysis (e.g., immune hemolytic anemia, drugrelated hemolysis)	Hemolysis	Laboratory evidence of hemolysis only (e.g., direct antiglobulin test [DAT, Coombs'] schistocytes)	Evidence of red cell destruction and ≥2 gm decrease in hemoglobin, no transfusion	Transfusion or medical intervention (e.g., steroids) indicated	Catastrophic consequences of hemolysis (e.g., renalfailure, hypotension, bronchospasm, emergency splenectomy)	Death

ALSO CONSIDER: Haptoglobin; Hemoglobin.

(continued)

Appendix 2 *(continued)*

		Grade				
Adverse Event	**Short Name**	**1**	**2**	**3**	**4**	**5**
Iron overload	Iron overload	—	Asymptomatic iron overload, intervention not indicated	Iron overload, intervention indicated	Organ impairment (e.g., endocrinopathy, cardiopathy)	Death
Leukocytes (total WBC)	Leukocytes	<LLN – 3000/mm^3 <LLN – 3.0 × 10^9/L	<3000 – 2000/mm^3 <3.0 – 2.0 × 10^9/L	<2000 – 1000/mm^3 <2.0 – 1.0 × 10^9/L	<1000/mm^3 <1.0 × 10^9/L	Death
Lymphopenia	Lymphopenia	<LLN – 800/mm^3 <LLN × 0.8 – 10^9/L	<800 – 500/mm^3 <0.8 – 0.5 × 10^9/L	<500 – 200 mm^3 <0.5 – 0.2 × 10^9/L	<200/mm^3 <0.2 × 10^9/L	Death
Myelodysplasia	Myelodysplasia	—	—	Abnormal marrow cytogenetics (marrow blasts ≤5%)	RAEB or RAEB-T (marrow blasts >5%)	Death
Neutrophils/granulocytes (ANC/AGC)	Neutrophils	<LLN – 1500/mm^3 <LLN – 1.5 × 10^9/L	<1500 – 1000/mm^3 <1.5 – 1.0 × 10^9/L	<1000 – 500/mm^3 <1.0 – 0.5 × 10^9/L	<500/mm^3 <0.5 × 10^9/L	Death
Platelets	Platelets	<LLN – 75,000/mm^3 <LLN – 75.0 × 10^9/L	<75,000 – 50,000/mm^3 <75.0 – 50.0 × 10^9/L	<50,000 – 25,000/mm^3 <50.0 – 25.0 × 10^9/L	<25,000/mm^3 <25.0 × 10^9/L	Death
Splenic function	Splenic function	Incidental findings (e.g., Howell-Jolly bodies)	Prophylactic antibiotics indicated	—	Life-threatening consequences	Death
Blood/Bone Marrow–Other (Specify, ______)	Blood – Other (Specify)	Mild	Moderate	Severe	Life-threatening; disabling	Death

(continued)

Appendix 2 *(continued)*

CARDIAC ARRHYTHMIA

		Grade				
Adverse Event	**Short Name**	**1**	**2**	**3**	**4**	**5**
Conduction abnormality/atrioventricular heart block – *Select*: – Asystole – AV Block-First degree – AV Block-Second degree Mobitz Type I (Wenckebach) – AV Block-Second degree Mobitz Type II – AV Block-Third degree (Complete AV block) – Conduction abnormality NOS – Sick Sinus Syndrome – Stokes-Adams Syndrome – Wolff-Parkinson-White Syndrome	Conduction abnormalit – *Select*	Asymptomatic, intervention not indicated	Non-urgent medical intervention indicated	Incompletely controlled medically or controlled with device (e.g., pacemaker)	Life-threatening (e.g., arrhythmia associated with CHF, hypotension, syncope, shock)	Death
Palpitations	Palpitations	Present	Present with associated symptoms (e.g., lightheadedness, shortness of breath)	—	—	—

REMARK: Grade palpitations only in the absence of a documented arrhythmia.

(continued)

Appendix 2 *(continued)*

		Grade				
Adverse Event	**Short Name**	**1**	**2**	**3**	**4**	**5**
Prolonged QTc interval	Prolonged QTc	QTc >0.45 – 0.47 second	QTc >0.47 – 0.50 second; ≥0.06 second above baseline	QTc >0.50 second	QTc >0.50 second; lifethreatening signs or symptoms (e.g., arrhythmia, CHF, hypotension, shock syncope); Torsade de pointes	Death
Supraventricular and nodal arrhythmia – *Select*:	Supraventricular arrhythmia – *Select*	Asymptomatic, intervention not indicated	Non-urgent medical intervention indicated	Symptomatic and incompletely controlled medically, or controlled with device (e.g., pacemaker)	Life-threatening (e.g., arrhythmia associated with CHF, hypotension, syncope, shock)	Death
–Atrial fibrillation –Atrial flutter –Atrial tachycardia/Paroxysmal Atrial Tachycardia –Nodal/Junctional –Sinus arrhythmia –Sinus bradycardia –Sinus tachycardia –Supraventricular arrhythmia NOS –Supraventricular extrasystoles (Premature Atrial Contractions; Premature Nodal/Junctional Contractions) –Supraventricular tachycardia						
NAVIGATION NOTE: Syncope is graded as Syncope (fainting) in the NEUROLOGY CATEGORY.						
Vasovagal episode	Vasovagal episode	—	Present without loss of consciousness	Present with loss of consciousness	Life-threatening consequences	Death

(continued)

Appendix 2 *(continued)*

		Grade				
Adverse Event	**Short Name**	**1**	**2**	**3**	**4**	**5**
Ventricular arrhythmia – *Select:* – Bigeminy – Idioventricular rhythm – PVCs – Torsade de pointes – Trigeminy – Ventricular arrhythmia NOS – Ventricular fibrillation – Ventricular flutter – Ventricular tachycardia	Ventricular arrhythmia– Select	Asymptomatic, no intervention indicated	Non-urgent medical intervention indicated	Symptomatic and incompletely controlled medically or controlled with device (e.g., defibrillator)	Life-threatening (e.g., arrhythmia associated with CHF, hypotension, syncope, shock)	Death
Cardiac Arrhythmia – Other (Specify, ______)	Cardiac Arrhythmia – Other (Specify)	Mild	Moderate	Severe	Life-threatening; disabling	Death

CARDIAC GENERAL

		Grade				
Adverse Event	**Short Name**	**1**	**2**	**3**	**4**	**5**
NAVIGATION NOTE: Angina is graded as Cardiac ischemia/infarction in the CARDIAC GENERAL CATEGORY.						
Cardiac ischemia/ infarction	Cardiac ischemia/ infarction	Asymptomatic arterial narrowing without ischemia	Asymptomatic and testing suggesting ischemia; stable angina	Symptomatic and testing consistent with ischemia; unstable angina; intervention indicated	Acute myocardial infarction	Death

(continued)

Appendix 2 *(continued)*

		Grade				
Adverse Event	**Short Name**	**1**	**2**	**3**	**4**	**5**
Cardiac troponin I (cTnI)	cTnI	—	—	Levels consistent with unstable angina as defined by the manufacturer	Levels consistent with myocardial infarction as defined by the manufacturer	Death
Cardiac troponin T (cTnT)	cTnT	0.03 – <0.05 ng/mL	0.05 – <0.1 ng/mL	0.1 – <0.2 ng/mL	0.2 ng/mL	Death
Cardiopulmonary arrest, cause unknown (non-fatal)	Cardiopulmonary arrest	—	—	—	Life-threatening	—

REMARK: Grade 4 (non-fatal) is the only appropriate grade. CTCAE provides three alternatives for reporting Death:

1. A CTCAE term associated with Grade 5.
2. A CTCAE 'Other (Specify, ______)' within any CATEGORY.
3. Death not associated with CTCAE term – *Select* in the DEATH CATEGORY.

NAVIGATION NOTE: Chest pain (non-cardiac and non-pleuritic) is graded as Pain – *Select* in the PAIN CATEGORY.

NAVIGATION NOTE: CNS ischemia is graded as CNS cerebrovascular ischemia in the NEUROLOGY CATEGORY.

(continued)

Appendix 2 *(continued)*

		Grade				
Adverse Event	**Short Name**	**1**	**2**	**3**	**4**	**5**
Hypertension	Hypertension	Asymptomatic, transient (<24 hrs) increase by >20 mmHg (diastolic) or to >150/100 if previously WNL; intervention not indicated Pediatric: Asymptomatic, transient (<24 hrs) BP increase >ULN; intervention not indicated	Recurrent or persistent (≥24 hrs) or symptomatic increase by >20 mmHg (diastolic) or to >150/100 if previously WNL; monotherapy may be indicated Pediatric: Recurrent or persistent (≥24 hrs) BP >ULN; monotherapy may be indicated	Requiring more than one drug or more intensive therapy than previously Pediatric: Same as adult	Life-threatening consequences (e.g., hypertensive crisis) Pediatric: Same as adult	Death
REMARK: Use age and gender-appropriate normal values >95th percentile ULN for pediatric patients.						
Hypotension	Hypotension	Changes, intervention not indicated	Brief (<24 hrs) fluid replacement or other therapy; no physiologic consequences	Sustained (≥24 hrs) therapy, resolves without persisting physiologic consequences	Shock (e.g., acidemia; impairment of vital organ function)	Death
ALSO CONSIDER: Syncope (fainting).						

(continued)

Appendix 2 *(continued)*

		Grade				
Adverse Event	**Short Name**	**1**	**2**	**3**	**4**	**5**
Left ventricular diastolic dysfunction	Left ventricular diastolic dysfunction	Asymptomatic diagnostic finding; intervention not indicated	Asymptomatic, intervention indicated	Symptomatic CHF responsive to intervention	Refractory CHF, poorly controlled; intervention such as ventricular assist device or heart transplant indicated	Death
Left ventricular systolic dysfunction	Left ventricular systolic dysfunction	Asymptomatic, resting ejection fraction (EF) <60 – 50%; shortening fraction (SF) <30 – 24%	Asymptomatic, resting EF <50 – 40%; SF <24 – 15%	Symptomatic CHF responsive to intervention; EF <40 – 20% SF <15%	Refractory CHF or poorly controlled; EF <20%; intervention such as ventricular assist device, ventricular reduction surgery, or heart transplant indicated	Death
NAVIGATION NOTE: Myocardial infarction is graded as Cardiac ischemia/infarction in the CARDIAC GENERAL CATEGORY.						
Myocarditis	Myocarditis	—	—	CHF responsive to intervention	Severe or refractory CHF	Death
Pericardial effusion (non-malignant)	Pericardial effusion	Asymptomatic effusion	—	Effusion with physiologic consequences	Life-threatening consequences (e.g., tamponade); emergency intervention indicated	Death

(continued)

Appendix 2 *(continued)*

		Grade				
Adverse Event	**Short Name**	**1**	**2**	**3**	**4**	**5**
Pericarditis	Pericarditis	Asymptomatic, ECG or physical exam (rub) changes consistent with pericarditis	Symptomatic pericarditis (e.g., chest pain)	Pericarditis with physiologic consequences (e.g., pericardial constriction)	Life-threatening consequences; emergency intervention indicated	Death
NAVIGATION NOTE: Pleuritic pain is graded as Pain – *Select* in the PAIN CATEGORY.						
Pulmonary hypertension	Pulmonary hypertension	Asymptomatic without therapy	Asymptomatic, therapy indicated	Symptomatic hypertension, responsive to therapy	Symptomatic hypertension, poorly controlled	Death
Restrictive cardiomyopathy	Restrictive cardiomyopathy	Asymptomatic, therapy not indicated	Asymptomatic, therapy indicated	Symptomatic CHF responsive to intervention	Refractory CHF, poorly controlled; intervention such as ventricular assist device, or heart transplant indicated	Death
Right ventricular dysfunction (cor pulmonale)	Right ventricular dysfunction	Asymptomatic without therapy	Asymptomatic, therapy indicated	Symptomatic cor pulmonale, responsive to intervention	Symptomatic cor pulmonale poorly controlled; intervention such as ventricular assist device, or heart transplant indicated	Death

(continued)

Appendix 2 *(continued)*

		Grade				
Adverse Event	**Short Name**	**1**	**2**	**3**	**4**	**5**
Valvular heart disease	Valvular heart disease	Asymptomatic valvular thickening with or without mild valvular regurgitation or stenosis; treatment other than endocarditis prophylaxis not indicated	Asymptomatic; moderate regurgitation or stenosis by imaging	Symptomatic; severe regurgitation or stenosis; symptoms controlled with medical therapy	Life-threatening; disabling; intervention (e.g., valve replacement, valvuloplasty) indicated	Death
Cardiac General – Other (Specify, ______)	Cardiac General – Other (Specify)	Mild	Moderate	Severe	Life-threatening; disabling	Death

COAGULATION

		Grade				
Adverse Event	**Short Name**	**1**	**2**	**3**	**4**	**5**
DIC (disseminated intravascular coagulation)	DIC	—	Laboratory findings with no bleeding	Laboratory findings and bleeding	Laboratory findings, lifethreatening or disabling consequences (e.g., CNS hemorrhage, organ damage, or hemodynamically significant blood loss)	Death

REMARK: DIC (disseminated intravascular coagulation) must have increased fibrin split products or D-dimer.
ALSO CONSIDER: Platelets.

(continued)

Appendix 2 *(continued)*

		Grade				
Adverse Event	**Short Name**	**1**	**2**	**3**	**4**	**5**
Fibrinogen	Fibrinogen	<1.0 – 0.75 × LLN or <25% decrease from baseline	<0.75 – 0.5 × LLN or 25 – <50% decrease from baseline	<0.5 – 0.25 × LLN or 50 – <75% decrease from baseline	<0.25 × LLN or 75% decrease from baseline or absolute value <50 mg/dL	Death
REMARK: Use % decrease only when baseline is <LLN (local laboratory value).						
INR (International Normalized Ratio of prothrombin time)	INR	>1 – 1.5 × ULN	>1.5 – 2 × ULN	>2 × ULN	—	—
ALSO CONSIDER: Hemorrhage, CNS; Hemorrhage, GI – *Select*; Hemorrhage, GU – *Select*; Hemorrhage, pulmonary/upper respiratory – *Select.*						
PTT (Partial Thromboplastin Time)	PTT	>1 – 1.5 × ULN	>1.5 – 2 × ULN	>2 × ULN	—	—
ALSO CONSIDER: Hemorrhage, CNS; Hemorrhage, GI – *Select*; Hemorrhage, GU – *Select*; Hemorrhage, pulmonary/upper respiratory – Select.						
Thrombotic microangiopathy (e.g., thrombotic thrombocytopenic purpura [TTP] or hemolytic uremic syndrome [HUS])	Thrombotic microangiopathy	Evidence of RBC destruction (schistocytosis) without clinical consequences	—	Laboratory findings present with clinical consequences (e.g., renal insufficiency, petechiae)	Laboratory findings and life-threatening or disabling consequences, (e.g., CNS hemorrhage/ bleeding or thrombosis/ embolism or renal failure)	Death
REMARK: Must have microangiopathic changes on blood smear (e.g., schistocytes, helmet cells, red cell fragments). ALSO CONSIDER: Creatinine; Hemoglobin; Platelets.						
Coagulation – Other (Specify, ______)	Coagulation – Other (Specify)	Mild	Moderate	Severe	Life-threatening; disabling	Death

(continued)

Appendix 2 *(continued)*

CONSTITUTIONAL SYMPTOMS

		Grade				
Adverse Event	**Short Name**	**1**	**2**	**3**	**4**	**5**
Fatigue (asthenia, lethargy, malaise)	Fatigue	Mild fatigue over baseline	Moderate or causing difficulty performing some ADL	Severe fatigue interfering with ADL	Disabling	—
Fever (in the absence of neutropenia, where neutropenia is defined as ANC $<1.0 \times 10^9/L$)	Fever	38.0 – 39.0°C (100.4 – 102.2°F)	>39.0 – 40.0°C (102.3 – 104.0°F)	>40.0°C (>104.0°F) for ≤24 hrs	>40.0°C (>104.0°F) for >24 hrs	Death
REMARK: The temperature measurements listed are oral or tympanic.						
ALSO CONSIDER: Allergic reaction/hypersensitivity (including drug fever).						
NAVIGATION NOTE: Hot flashes are graded as Hot flashes/flushes in the ENDOCRINE CATEGORY.						
Hypothermia	Hypothermia	—	35 – >32°C 95 – >89.6°F	32 – >28°C 89.6 – >82.4° F	≤28 °C 82.4°F or life-threatening consequences (e.g., coma, hypotension, pulmonary edema, acidemia, ventricular fibrillation)	Death
Insomnia	Insomnia	Occasional difficulty sleeping, not interfering with function	Difficulty sleeping, interfering with function but not interfering with ADL	Frequent difficulty sleeping, interfering with ADL	Disabling	—
REMARK: If pain or other symptoms interfere with sleep, do NOT grade as insomnia. Grade primary event(s) causing insomnia.						

(continued)

Appendix 2 *(continued)*

		Grade				
Adverse Event	**Short Name**	**1**	**2**	**3**	**4**	**5**
Obesity[2]	Obesity	—	BMI 25 – 29.9 kg/m^2	BMI 30 – 39.99 kg/m^2	BMI ≥40 kg/m^2	—
REMARK: BMI = (weight [kg])/ (height [m])^2						
Odor (patient odor)	Patient odor	Mild odor	Pronounced odor	—	—	—
Rigors/chills	Rigors/chills	Mild	Moderate, narcotics indicated	Severe or prolonged, not responsive to narcotics	—	—
Sweating (diaphoresis)	Sweating	Mild and occasional	Frequent or drenching	—	—	—
ALSO CONSIDER: Hot flashes/flushes.						
Weight gain	Weightgain	5 – <10% of baseline	10 – <20% of baseline	≥20% of baseline	—	—
REMARK: Edema, depending on etiology, is graded in the CARDIAC GENERAL or LYMPHATICS CATEGORIES.						
ALSO CONSIDER: Ascites (non-malignant); Pleural effusion (non-malignant).						
Weight loss	Weight loss	5 to <10% from baseline; intervention not indicated	10 – <20% from baseline; nutritional support indicated	≥20% from baseline; tube feeding or TPN indicated	—	—
Constitutional Symptoms – Other (Specify, ______)	Constitutional Symptoms – Other (Specify)	Mild	Moderate	Severe	Life-threatening; disabling	Death

[2] NHLBI Obesity Task Force. Clinical Guidelines on the Identification, Evaluation, and Treatment of Overweight and Obesity in Adults, *The Evidence Report,* Obes Res 6:51S-209S, 1998.

(continued)

Appendix 2 *(continued)*

DEATH

		Grade				
Adverse Event	**Short Name**	**1**	**2**	**3**	**4**	**5**
Death not associated with CTCAE term – *Select*: – Death NOS – Disease progression NOS – Multi-organ failure – Sudden death	Death not associated with CTCAE term – Select	—	—	—	—	Death

REMARK: Grade 5 is the only appropriate grade. 'Death not associated with CTCAE term – *Select'* is to be used where a death:

1. Cannot be attributed to a CTCAE term associated with Grade 5.
2. Cannot be reported within any CATEGORY using a CTCAE 'Other (Specify, ______)'.

DERMATOLOGY/SKIN

		Grade				
Adverse Event	**Short Name**	**1**	**2**	**3**	**4**	**5**
Atrophy, skin	Atrophy, skin	Detectable	Marked	—	—	—
Atrophy, subcutaneous fat	Atrophy, subcutaneous fat	Detectable	Marked	—	—	—
ALSO CONSIDER: Induration/fibrosis (skin and subcutaneous tissue).						
Bruising (in absence of Grade 3 or 4 thrombocytopenia)	Bruising	Localized or in a dependent area	Generalized	—	—	—

(continued)

Appendix 2 *(continued)*

		Grade				
Adverse Event	**Short Name**	**1**	**2**	**3**	**4**	**5**
Burn	Burn	Minimal symptoms; intervention not indicated	Medical intervention; minimal debridement indicated	Moderate to major debridement or reconstruction indicated	Life-threatening consequences	Death
REMARK: Burn refers to all burns including radiation, chemical, etc.						
Cheilitis	Cheilitis	Asymptomatic	Symptomatic, not interfering with ADL	Symptomatic, interfering with ADL	—	—
Dry skin	Dry skin	Asymptomatic	Symptomatic, not interfering with ADL	Interfering with ADL	—	—
Flushing	Flushing	Asymptomatic	Symptomatic	—	—	—
Hair loss/alopecia (scalp or body)	Alopecia	Thinning or patchy	Complete	—	—	—
Hyperpigmentation	Hyperpigmentation	Slight or localized	Marked or generalized	—	—	—
Hypopigmentation	Hypopigmentation	Slight or localized	Marked or generalized	—	—	—

(continued)

Appendix 2 *(continued)*

		Grade				
Adverse Event	**Short Name**	**1**	**2**	**3**	**4**	**5**
Induration/fibrosis (skin and subcutaneous tissue)	Induration	Increased density on palpation	Moderate impairment of function not interfering with ADL; marked increase in density and firmness on palpation with or without minimal retraction	Dysfunction interfering with ADL; very marked density, retraction or fixation	—	—
ALSO CONSIDER: Fibrosis-cosmesis; Fibrosis-deep connective tissue.						
Injection site reaction/extravasation changes	Injection site reaction	Pain; itching; erythema	Pain or swelling, with inflammation or phlebitis	Ulceration or necrosis that is severe; operative intervention indicated	—	—
ALSO CONSIDER: Allergic reaction/hypersensitivity (including drug fever); Ulceration.						
Nail changes	Nail changes	Discoloration; ridging (koilonychias); pitting	Partial or complete loss of nail(s); pain in nailbed(s)	Interfering with ADL	—	—
NAVIGATION NOTE: Petechiae is graded as Petechiae/purpura (hemorrhage/bleeding into skin or mucosa) in the HEMORRHAGE/BLEEDING CATEGORY.						
Photosensitivity	Photosensitivity	Painless erythema	Painful erythema	Erythema with desquamation	Life-threatening; disabling	Death
Pruritus/itching	Pruritus	Mild or localized	Intense or widespread	Intense or widespread and interfering with ADL	—	—

(continued)

Appendix 2 *(continued)*

		Grade				
Adverse Event	**Short Name**	**1**	**2**	**3**	**4**	**5**
ALSO CONSIDER: Rash/desquamation.						
Rash/desquamation	Rash	Macular or papular eruption or erythema without associated symptoms	Macular or papular eruption or erythema with pruritus or other associated symptoms; localized desquamation or other lesions covering <50% of body surface area (BSA)	Severe, generalized erythroderma or macular, papular or vesicular eruption; desquamation covering ≥50% BSA	Generalized exfoliative, ulcerative, or bullous dermatitis	Death
REMARK: Rash/desquamation may be used for GVHD.						
Rash: acne/ acneiform	Acne	Intervention not indicated	Intervention indicated	Associated with pain, disfigurement, ulceration, or desquamation	—	Death
Rash: dermatitis associated with radiatio – *Select*: – Chemoradiation – Radiation	Dermatitis – *Select*	Faint erythema or dry desquamation	Moderate to brisk erythema; patchy moist desquamation, mostly confined to skin folds and creases; moderate edema	Moist desquamation other than skin folds and creases; bleeding induced by minor trauma or abrasion	Skin necrosis or ulceration of full thickness dermis; spontaneous bleeding from involved site	Death

(continued)

Appendix 2 *(continued)*

		Grade				
Adverse Event	**Short Name**	**1**	**2**	**3**	**4**	**5**
Rash: erythema multiforme (e.g., Stevens-Johnson syndrome, toxic epidermal necrolysis)	Erythema multiforme	—	Scattered, but not generalized eruption	Severe (e.g., generalized rash or painful stomatitis); IV fluids, tube feedings, or TPN indicated	Life-threatening; disabling	Death
Rash: hand-foot skin reaction	Hand-foot	Minimal skin changes or dermatitis (e.g., erythema) without pain	Skin changes (e.g., peeling, blisters, bleeding, edema) or pain, not interfering with function	Ulcerative dermatitis or skin changes with pain interfering with function	—	—
Skin breakdown/ decubitus ulcer	Decubitus	—	Local wound care; medical intervention indicated	Operative debridement or other invasive intervention indicated (e.g., hyperbaric oxygen)	Life-threatening consequences; major invasive intervention indicated (e.g., tissue reconstruction, flap, or grafting)	Death
REMARK: Skin breakdown/decubitus ulcer is to be used for loss of skin integrity or decubitus ulcer from pressure or as the result of operative or medical intervention.						
Striae	Striae	Mild	Cosmetically significant	—	—	—
Telangiectasia	Telangiectasia	Few	Moderate number	Many and confluent	—	—

(continued)

Appendix 2 *(continued)*

		Grade				
Adverse Event	**Short Name**	**1**	**2**	**3**	**4**	**5**
Ulceration	Ulceration	—	Superficial ulceration <2 cm size; local wound care; medical intervention indicated	Ulceration ≥2 cm size; operative debridement, primary closure or other invasive intervention indicated (e.g., hyperbaric oxygen)	Life-threatening consequences; major invasive intervention indicated (e.g., complete resection, tissue reconstruction, flap, or grafting)	Death
Urticaria (hives, welts, wheals)	Urticaria	Intervention not indicated	Intervention indicated for <24 hrs	Intervention indicated for ≥24 hrs	—	—
ALSO CONSIDER: Allergic reaction/hypersensitivity (including drug fever).						
Wound complication, non-infectious	Wound complication, non-infectious	Incisional separation of ≤25% of wound, no deeper than superficial fascia	Incisional separation >25% of wound with local care; asymptomatic hernia	Symptomatic hernia without evidence of strangulation; fascial disruption/dehiscence without evisceration; primary wound closure or revision by operative intervention indicated; hospitalization or hyperbaric oxygen indicated	Symptomatic hernia with evidence of strangulation; fascial disruption with evisceration; major reconstruction flap, grafting, resection, or amputation indicated	Death
REMARK: Wound complication, non-infectious is to be used for separation of incision, hernia, dehiscence, evisceration, or second surgery for wound revision.						

(continued)

Appendix 2 *(continued)*

		Grade				
Adverse Event	**Short Name**	**1**	**2**	**3**	**4**	**5**
Dermatology/Skin – Other (Specify, ______)	Dermatology – Other (Specify)	Mild	Moderate	Severe	Life-threatening; disabling	Death

ENDOCRINE

		Grade				
Adverse Event	**Short Name**	**1**	**2**	**3**	**4**	**5**
Adrenal insufficiency	Adrenal insufficiency	Asymptomatic, intervention not indicated	Symptomatic, intervention indicated	Hospitalization	Life-threatening; disabling	Death
REMARK: Adrenal insufficiency includes any of the following signs and symptoms: abdominal pain, anorexia, constipation, diarrhea, hypotension, pigmentation of mucous membranes, pigmentation of skin, salt craving, syncope (fainting), vitiligo, vomiting, weakness, weight loss. Adrenal insufficiency must be confirmed by laboratory studies (low cortisol frequently accompanied by low aldosterone). ALSO CONSIDER: Potassium, serum-high (hyperkalemia); Thyroid function, low (hypothyroidism).						
Cushingoid appearance (e.g., moon face, buffalo hump, centripetal obesity, cutaneous striae)	Cushingoid	—	Present	—	—	—
ALSO CONSIDER: Glucose, serum-high (hyperglycemia); Potassium, serum-low (hypokalemia).						
Feminization of male	Feminization of male	—	—	Present	—	—
NAVIGATION NOTE: Gynecomastia is graded in the SEXUAL/REPRODUCTIVE FUNCTION CATEGORY.						
Hot flashes/flushes[3]	Hot flashes	Mild	Moderate	Interfering with ADL	—	—

(continued)

Appendix 2 *(continued)*

		Grade				
Adverse Event	**Short Name**	**1**	**2**	**3**	**4**	**5**
Masculinization of female	Masculinization of female	—	—	Present	—	—
Neuroendocrine: ACTH deficiency	ACTH	Asymptomatic	Symptomatic, not interfering with ADL; intervention indicated	Symptoms interfering with ADL; hospitalization indicated	Life-threatening consequences (e.g., severe hypotension)	Death
Neuroendocrine: ADH secretion abnormality (e.g., SIADH or low ADH)	ADH	Asymptomatic	Symptomatic, not interfering with ADL; intervention indicated	Symptoms interfering with ADL	Life-threatening consequences	Death
Neuroendocrine: gonadotropin secretion abnormality	Gonadotropin	Asymptomatic	Symptomatic, not interfering with ADL; intervention indicated	Symptoms interfering with ADL; osteopenia; fracture; infertility	—	—
Neuroendocrine: growth hormone secretion abnormality	Growth hormone	Asymptomatic	Symptomatic, not interfering with ADL; intervention indicated	—	—	—
Neuroendocrine: prolactin hormone secretion abnormality	Prolactin	Asymptomatic	Symptomatic, not interfering with ADL; intervention indicated	Symptoms interfering with ADL; amenorrhea; galactorrhea	—	Death

(continued)

Appendix 2 *(continued)*

		Grade				
Adverse Event	**Short Name**	**1**	**2**	**3**	**4**	**5**
Pancreatic endocrine: glucose intolerance	Diabetes	Asymptomatic, intervention not indicated	Symptomatic; dietary modification or oral agent indicated	Symptoms interfering with ADL; insulin indicated	Life-threatening consequences (e.g., ketoacidosis, hyperosmolar nonketotic coma)	Death
Parathyroid function, low (hypoparathyroidism)	Hypoparathyroidism	Asymptomatic, intervention not indicated	Symptomatic; intervention indicated	—	—	—
Thyroid function, high (hyperthyroidism, thyrotoxicosis)	Hyperthyroidism	Asymptomatic, intervention not indicated	Symptomatic, not interfering with ADL; thyroid suppression therapy indicated	Symptoms interfering with ADL; hospitalization indicated	Life-threatening consequences (e.g., thyroid storm)	Death
Thyroid function, low (hypothyroidism)	Hypothyroidism	Asymptomatic, intervention not indicated	Symptomatic, not interfering with ADL; thyroid replacement indicated	Symptoms interfering with ADL; hospitalization indicated	Life-threatening myxedema coma	Death
Endocrine – Other (Specify, ______)	Endocrine – Other (Specify)	Mild	Moderate	Severe	Life-threatening; disabling	Death

[3] Sloan JA, Loprinzi CL, Novotny PJ, Barton DL, Lavasseur BI, Windschitl HJ. Methodologic Lessons Learned from Hot Flash Studies, *J Clin Oncol* 2001;19(23):4280-90

(continued)

Appendix 2 *(continued)*

GASTROINTESTINAL

		Grade				
Adverse Event	**Short Name**	**1**	**2**	**3**	**4**	**5**
NAVIGATION NOTE: Abdominal pain or cramping is graded as Pain – *Select* in the PAIN CATEGORY.						
Anorexia	Anorexia	Loss of appetite without alteration in eating habits	Oral intake altered without significant weight loss or malnutrition; oral nutritional supplements indicated	Associated with significant weight loss or malnutrition (e.g., inadequate oral caloric and/or fluid intake); IV fluids, tube feedings or TPN indicated	Life-threatening consequences	Death
ALSO CONSIDER: Weight loss.						
Ascites (non-malignant)	Ascites	Asymptomatic	Symptomatic, medical intervention indicated	Symptomatic, invasive procedure indicated	Life-threatening consequences	Death
REMARK: Ascites (non-malignant) refers to documented non-malignant ascites or unknown etiology, but unlikely malignant, and includes chylous ascites.						
Colitis	Colitis	Asymptomatic, pathologic or radiographic findings only	Abdominal pain; mucus or blood in stool	Abdominal pain, fever, change in bowel habits with ileus; peritoneal signs	Life-threatening consequences (e.g., perforation, bleeding, ischemia, necrosis, toxic megacolon)	Death
ALSO CONSIDER: Hemorrhage, GI – *Select*.						

(continued)

Appendix 2 *(continued)*

		Grade				
Adverse Event	**Short Name**	**1**	**2**	**3**	**4**	**5**
Constipation	Constipation	Occasional or intermittent symptoms; occasional use of stool softeners, laxatives, dietary modification, or enema	Persistent symptoms with regular use of laxatives or enemas indicated	Symptoms interfering with ADL; obstipation with manual evacuation indicated	Life-threatening consequences (e.g., obstruction, toxic megacolon)	Death
ALSO CONSIDER: Ileus, GI (functional obstruction of bowel, i.e., neuroconstipation); Obstruction, GI – *Select*.						
Dehydration	Dehydration	Increased oral fluids indicated; dry mucous membranes; diminished skin turgor	IV fluids indicated <24 hrs	IV fluids indicated ≥24 hrs	Life-threatening consequences (e.g., hemodynamic collapse)	Death
ALSO CONSIDER: Diarrhea; Hypotension; Vomiting.						
Dental: dentures or prosthesis	Dentures	Minimal discomfort, no restriction in activities	Discomfort preventing use in some activities (e.g., eating), but not others (e.g., speaking)	Unable to use dentures or prosthesis at any time	—	—
Dental: periodontal disease	Periodontal	Gingival recession or gingivitis; limited bleeding on probing; mild local bone loss	Moderate gingival recession or gingivitis; multiple sites of bleeding on probing; moderate bone loss	Spontaneous bleeding; severe bone loss with or without tooth loss; osteonecrosis of maxilla or mandible	—	—
REMARK: Severe periodontal disease leading to osteonecrosis is graded as Osteonecrosis (avascular necrosis) in the MUSCULOSKELETAL CATEGORY.						

(continued)

Appendix 2 *(continued)*

		Grade				
Adverse Event	**Short Name**	**1**	**2**	**3**	**4**	**5**
Dental: teeth	Teeth	Surface stains; dental caries; restorable, without extractions	Less than full mouth extractions; tooth fracture or crown amputation or repair indicated	Full mouth extractions indicated	—	—
Dental: teeth development	Teeth development	Hypoplasia of tooth or enamel not interfering with function	Functional impairment correctable with oral surgery	Maldevelopment with functional impairment not surgically correctable	—	—
Diarrhea	Diarrhea	Increase of <4 stools per day over baseline; mild increase in ostomy output compared to baseline	Increase of 4 – 6 stools per day over baseline; IV fluids indicated <24hrs; moderate increase in ostomy output compared to baseline; not interfering with ADL	Increase of ≥7 stools per day over baseline; incontinence; IV fluids ≥24 hrs; hospitalization; severe increase in ostomy output compared to baseline; interfering with ADL	Life-threatening consequences (e.g., hemodynamic collapse)	Death
REMARK: Diarrhea includes diarrhea of small bowel or colonic origin, and/or ostomy diarrhea. ALSO CONSIDER: Dehydration; Hypotension.						
Distension/bloating, abdominal	Distension	Asymptomatic	Symptomatic, but not interfering with GI function	Symptomatic, interfering with GI function	—	—
ALSO CONSIDER: Ascites (non-malignant); Ileus, GI (functional obstruction of bowel, i.e., neuroconstipation); Obstruction, GI – *Select*.						

(continued)

Appendix 2 *(continued)*

		Grade				
Adverse Event	**Short Name**	**1**	**2**	**3**	**4**	**5**
Dry mouth/salivary gland (xerostomia)	Dry mouth	Symptomatic (dry or thick saliva) without significant dietary alteration; unstimulated saliva flow >0.2 ml/min	Symptomatic and significant oral intake alteration (e.g., copious water, other lubricants, diet limited to purees and/or soft, moist foods); unstimulated saliva 0.1 to 0.2 ml/min	Symptoms leading to inability to adequately aliment orally; IV fluids, tube feedings, or TPN indicated; unstimulated saliva <0.1 ml/min	—	—
REMARK: Dry mouth/salivary gland (xerostomia) includes descriptions of grade using both subjective and objective assessment parameters. Record this event consistently throughout a patient's participation on study. If salivary flow measurements are used for initial assessment, subsequent assessments must use salivary flow. ALSO CONSIDER: Salivary gland changes/saliva.						
Dysphagia (difficulty swallowing)	Dysphagia	Symptomatic, able to eat regular diet	Symptomatic and altered eating/swallowing (e.g., altered dietary habits, oral supplements); IV fluids indicated <24 hrs	Symptomatic and severely altered eating/swallowing (e.g., inadequate oral caloric or fluid intake); IV fluids, tube feedings, or TPN indicated ≥24 hrs	Life-threatening consequences (e.g., obstruction, perforation)	Death
REMARK: Dysphagia (difficulty swallowing) is to be used for swallowing difficulty from oral, pharyngeal, esophageal, or neurologic origin. Dysphagia requiring dilation is graded as Stricture/stenosis (including anastomotic), GI – *Select*. ALSO CONSIDER: Dehydration; Esophagitis.						

(continued)

Appendix 2 *(continued)*

		Grade				
Adverse Event	**Short Name**	**1**	**2**	**3**	**4**	**5**
Enteritis (inflammation of the small bowel)	Enteritis	Asymptomatic, pathologic or radiographic findings only	Abdominal pain; mucus or blood in stool	Abdominal pain, fever, change in bowel habits with ileus; peritoneal signs	Life-threatening consequences (e.g., perforation, bleeding, ischemia, necrosis)	Death
ALSO CONSIDER: Hemorrhage, GI – *Select*; Typhlitis (cecal inflammation).						
Esophagitis	Esophagitis	Asymptomatic pathologic, radiographic, or endoscopic findings only	Symptomatic; altered eating/swallowing (e.g., altered dietary habits, oral supplements); IV fluids indicated <24 hrs	Symptomatic and severely altered eating/swallowing (e.g., inadequate oral caloric or fluid intake); IV fluids, tube feedings, or TPN indicated ≥24 hrs	Life-threatening consequences	Death
REMARK: Esophagitis includes reflux esophagitis. ALSO CONSIDER: Dysphagia (difficulty swallowing).						

(continued)

Appendix 2 *(continued)*

		Grade				
Adverse Event	**Short Name**	**1**	**2**	**3**	**4**	**5**
Fistula, GI – *Select*: – Abdomen NOS – Anus – Biliary tree – Colon/cecum/appendix – Duodenum – Esophagus – Gallbladder – Ileum – Jejunum – Oral cavity – Pancreas – Pharynx – Rectum – Salivary gland – Small bowel NOS – Stomach	Fistula, GI – *Select*	Asymptomatic, radiographic findings only	Symptomatic; altered GI function (e.g., altered dietary habits, diarrhea, or GI fluid loss); IV fluids indicated <24 hrs	Symptomatic and severely altered GI function (e.g., altered dietary habits, diarrhea, or GI fluid loss); IV fluids, tube feedings, or TPN indicated ≥24 hrs	Life-threatening consequences	Death
REMARK: A fistula is defined as an abnormal communication between two body cavities, potential spaces, and/or the skin. The site indicated for a fistula should be the site from which the abnormal process is believed to have originated. For example, a tracheo-esophageal fistula arising in the context of a resected or irradiated esophageal cancer is graded as Fistula, GI – esophagus.						
Flatulence	Flatulence	Mild	Moderate	—	—	—

(continued)

Appendix 2 *(continued)*

		Grade				
Adverse Event	**Short Name**	**1**	**2**	**3**	**4**	**5**
Gastritis (including bile reflux gastritis)	Gastritis	Asymptomatic radiographic or endoscopic findings only	Symptomatic; altered gastric function (e.g., inadequate oral caloric or fluid intake); IV fluids indicated <24 hrs	Symptomatic and severely altered gastric function (e.g., inadequate oral caloric or fluid intake); IV fluids, tube feedings, or TPN indicated ≥24 hrs	Life-threatening consequences; operative intervention requiring complete organ resection (e.g., gastrectomy)	Death
ALSO CONSIDER: Hemorrhage, GI – *Select*; Ulcer, GI – *Select*.						
NAVIGATION NOTE: Head and neck soft tissue necrosis is graded as Soft tissue necrosis – *Select* in the MUSCULOSKELETAL/SOFT TISSUE CATEGORY.						
Heartburn/dyspepsia	Heartburn	Mild	Moderate	Severe	—	—
Hemorrhoids	Hemorrhoids	Asymptomatic	Symptomatic; banding or medical intervention indicated	Interfering with ADL; interventional radiology, endoscopic, or operative intervention indicated	Life-threatening consequences	Death
Ileus, GI (functional obstruction of bowel, i.e., neuroconstipation)	Ileus	Asymptomatic, radiographic findings only	Symptomatic; altered GI function (e.g., altered dietary habits); IV fluids indicated <24 hrs	Symptomatic and severely altered GI function; IV fluids, tube feeding, or TPN indicated ≥24 hrs	Life-threatening consequences	Death
REMARK: Ileus, GI is to be used for altered upper or lower GI function (e.g., delayed gastric or colonic emptying). ALSO CONSIDER: Constipation; Nausea; Obstruction, GI – *Select*; Vomiting.						

(continued)

Appendix 2 *(continued)*

		Grade				
Adverse Event	**Short Name**	**1**	**2**	**3**	**4**	**5**
Incontinence, anal	Incontinence, anal	Occasional use of pads required	Daily use of pads required	Interfering with ADL; operative intervention indicated	Permanent bowel diversion indicated	Death
REMARK: Incontinence, anal is to be used for loss of sphincter control as sequelae of operative or therapeutic intervention.						
Leak (including anastomotic), GI – *Select*: – Biliary tree – Esophagus – Large bowel – Leak NOS – Pancreas – Pharynx – Rectum – Small bowel – Stoma – Stomach	Leak, GI – *Select*	Asymptomatic radiographic findings only	Symptomatic; medical intervention indicated	Symptomatic and interfering with GI function; invasive or endoscopic intervention indicated	Life-threatening consequences	Death
REMARK: Leak (including anasomotic), GI – *Select* is to be used for clinical signs/symptoms or radiographic confirmation of anastomotic or conduit leak (e.g., biliary, esophageal, intestinal, pancreatic, pharyngeal, rectal), but without development of fistula.						
Malabsorption	Malabsorption	—	Altered diet; oral therapies indicated (e.g., enzymes, medications, dietary supplements)	Inability to aliment adequately via GI tract (i.e., TPN indicated)	Life-threatening consequences	Death

(continued)

Appendix 2 *(continued)*

		Grade				
Adverse Event	**Short Name**	**1**	**2**	**3**	**4**	**5**
Mucositis/stomatitis (clinical exam) – *Select*: – Anus – Esophagus – Large bowel – Larynx – Oral cavity – Pharynx – Rectum – Small bowel – Stomach – Trachea	Mucositis (clinical exam) – *Select*	Erythema of the mucosa	Patchy ulcerations or pseudomembranes	Confluent ulcerations or pseudomembranes; bleeding with minor trauma	Tissue necrosis; significant spontaneous bleeding; life-threatening consequences	Death

REMARK: Mucositis/stomatitis (functional/symptomatic) may be used for mucositis of the upper aero-digestive tract caused by radiation, agents, or GVHD.

(continued)

Appendix 2 *(continued)*

		Grade				
Adverse Event	**Short Name**	**1**	**2**	**3**	**4**	**5**
Mucositis/stomatitis (functional/symptomatic) – *Select*: – Anus – Esophagus – Large bowel – Larynx – Oral cavity – Pharynx – Rectum – Small bowel – Stomach – Trachea	Mucositis (functional/symptomatic) – *Select*	*Upper aerodigestive tract sites:* Minimal symptoms, normal diet; minimal respiratory symptoms but not interfering with function *Lower GI sites:* Minimal discomfort, intervention not indicated	*Upper aerodigestive tract sites:* Symptomatic but can eat and swallow modified diet; respiratory symptoms interfering with function but not interfering with ADL *Lower GI sites:* Symptomatic, medical intervention indicated but not interfering with ADL	*Upper aerodigestive tract sites:* Symptomatic and unable to adequately aliment or hydrate orally; respiratory symptoms interfering with ADL *Lower GI sites:* Stool incontinence or other symptoms interfering with ADL	Symptoms associated with life-threatening consequences	Death
Nausea	Nausea	Loss of appetite without alteration in eating habits	Oral intake decreased without significant weight loss, dehydration or malnutrition; IV fluids indicated <24 hrs	Inadequate oral caloric or fluid intake; IV fluids, tube feedings, or TPN indicated ≥24 hrs	Life-threatening consequences	Death
ALSO CONSIDER: Anorexia; Vomiting.						

(continued)

Appendix 2 *(continued)*

		Grade				
Adverse Event	**Short Name**	**1**	**2**	**3**	**4**	**5**
Necrosis, GI – *Select*: – Anus – Colon/cecum/appendix – Duodenum – Esophagus – Gallbladder – Hepatic – Ileum – Jejunum – Oral – Pancreas – Peritoneal cavity – Pharynx – Rectum – Small bowel NOS – Stoma – Stomach	Necrosis, GI – *Select*	—	—	Inability to aliment adequately by GI tract (e.g., requiring enteral or parenteral nutrition); interventional radiology, endoscopic, or operative intervention indicated	Life-threatening consequences; operative intervention requiring complete organ resection (e.g., total colectomy)	Death
ALSO CONSIDER: Visceral arterial ischemia (non-myocardial).						

(continued)

Appendix 2 *(continued)*

		Grade				
Adverse Event	**Short Name**	**1**	**2**	**3**	**4**	**5**
Obstruction, GI – *Select*: – Cecum – Colon – Duodenum – Esophagus – Gallbladder – Ileum – Jejunum – Rectum – Small bowel NOS – Stoma – Stomach	Obstruction, GI – *Select*	Asymptomatic radiographic findings only	Symptomatic; altered GI function (e.g., altered dietary habits, vomiting, diarrhea, or GI fluid loss); IV fluids indicated <24 hrs	Symptomatic and severely altered GI function (e.g., altered dietary habits, vomiting, diarrhea, or GI fluid loss); IV fluids, tube feedings, or TPN indicated ≥24 hrs; operative intervention indicated	Life-threatening consequences; operative intervention requiring complete organ resection (e.g., total colectomy)	Death

NAVIGATION NOTE: Operative injury is graded as Intra-operative injury – *Select Organ or Structure* in the SURGERY/INTRA-OPERATIVE INJURY CATEGORY.

NAVIGATION NOTE: Pelvic pain is graded as Pain – *Select* in the PAIN CATEGORY.

(continued)

Appendix 2 *(continued)*

		Grade				
Adverse Event	**Short Name**	**1**	**2**	**3**	**4**	**5**
Perforation, GI – *Select*: – Appendix – Biliary tree – Cecum – Colon – Duodenum – Esophagus – Gallbladder – Ileum – Jejunum – Rectum – Small bowel NOS – Stomach	Perforation, GI – *Select*	Asymptomatic radiographic findings only	Medical intervention indicated; IV fluids indicated <24 hrs	IV fluids, tube feedings, or TPN indicated ≥24 hrs; operative intervention indicated	Life-threatening consequences	Death
Proctitis	Proctitis	Rectal discomfort, intervention not indicated	Symptoms not interfering with ADL; medical intervention indicated	Stool incontinence or other symptoms interfering with ADL; operative intervention indicated	Life-threatening consequences (e.g., perforation)	Death
Prolapse of stoma, GI	Prolapse of stoma, GI	Asymptomatic	Extraordinary local care or maintenance; minor revision indicated	Dysfunctional stoma; major revision indicated	Life-threatening consequences	Death
REMARK: Other stoma complications may be graded as Fistula, GI – *Select*; Leak (including anastomotic), GI – *Select*; Obstruction, GI – *Select;* Perforation, GI – *Select*; Stricture/stenosis (including anastomotic), GI – *Select.*						

(continued)

Appendix 2 *(continued)*

		Grade				
Adverse Event	**Short Name**	**1**	**2**	**3**	**4**	**5**
NAVIGATION NOTE: Rectal or perirectal pain (proctalgia) is graded as Pain – *Select* in the PAIN CATEGORY.						
Salivary gland changes/saliva	Salivary gland changes	Slightly thickened saliva; slightly altered taste (e.g., metallic)	Thick, ropy, sticky saliva; markedly altered taste; alteration in diet indicated; secretioninduced symptoms not interfering with ADL	Acute salivary gland necrosis; severe secretion-induced symptoms interfering with ADL	Disabling	—
ALSO CONSIDER: Dry mouth/salivary gland (xerostomia); Mucositis/stomatitis (clinical exam) – *Select*; Mucositis/stomatitis (functional/symptomatic) – *Select*; Taste alteration (dysgeusia).						
NAVIGATION NOTE: Splenic function is graded in the BLOOD/BONE MARROW CATEGORY.						

(continued)

Appendix 2 *(continued)*

Adverse Event	Short Name	Grade 1	Grade 2	Grade 3	Grade 4	Grade 5
Stricture/stenosis (including anastomotic), GI – *Select*: – Anus – Biliary tree – Cecum – Colon – Duodenum – Esophagus – Ileum – Jejunum – Pancreas/pancreatic duct – Pharynx – Rectum – Small bowel NOS – Stoma – Stomach	Stricture, GI – *Select*	Asymptomatic radiographic findings only	Symptomatic; altered GI function (e.g., altered dietary habits, vomiting, bleeding, diarrhea); IV fluids indicated <24 hrs	Symptomatic and severely altered GI function (e.g., altered dietary habits, diarrhea, or GI fluid loss); IV fluids, tube feedings, or TPN indicated ≥24 hrs; operative intervention indicated	Life-threatening consequences; operative intervention requiring complete organ resection (e.g., total colectomy)	Death
Taste alteration (dysgeusia)	Taste alteration	Altered taste but no change in diet	Altered taste with change in diet (e.g., oral supplements); noxious or unpleasant taste; loss of taste	—	—	—

(continued)

Appendix 2 *(continued)*

		Grade				
Adverse Event	**Short Name**	**1**	**2**	**3**	**4**	**5**
Typhlitis (cecal inflammation)	Typhlitis	Asymptomatic, pathologic or radiographic findings only	Abdominal pain; mucus or blood in stool	Abdominal pain, fever, change in bowel habits with ileus; peritoneal signs	Life-threatening consequences (e.g., perforation, bleeding, ischemia, necrosis); operative intervention indicated	Death
ALSO CONSIDER: Colitis; Hemorrhage, GI – *Select* ; Ileus, GI (functional obstruction of bowel, i.e., neuroconstipation).						
Ulcer, GI – *Select*: – Anus – Cecum – Colon – Duodenum – Esophagus – Ileum – Jejunum – Rectum – Small bowel NOS – Stoma – Stomach	Ulcer, GI – *Select*	Asymptomatic, radiographic or endoscopic findings only	Symptomatic; altered GI function (e.g., altered dietary habits, oral supplements); IV fluids indicated <24 hrs	Symptomatic and severely altered GI function (e.g., inadequate oral caloric or fluid intake); IV fluids, tube feedings, or TPN indicated ≥24 hrs	Life-threatening consequences	Death
ALSO CONSIDER: Hemorrhage, GI – *Select*.						
Vomiting	Vomiting	1 episode in 24 hrs	2 – 5 episodes in 24 hrs; IV fluids indicated <24 hrs	≥6 episodes in 24 hrs; IV fluids, or TPN indicated ≥24 hrs	Life-threatening consequences	Death

(continued)

Appendix 2 *(continued)*

		Grade				
Adverse Event	**Short Name**	**1**	**2**	**3**	**4**	**5**
ALSO CONSIDER: Dehydration.						
Gastrointestinal – Other (Specify, ______)	GI – Other (Specify)	Mild	Moderate	Severe	Life-threatening; disabling	Death

GROWTH AND DEVELOPMENT

		Grade				
Adverse Event	**Short Name**	**1**	**2**	**3**	**4**	**5**
Bone age (alteration in bone age)	Bone age	—	±2 SD (standard deviation) from normal	—	—	—
Bone growth: femoral head; slipped capital femoral epiphysis	Femoral head growth	Mild valgus/varus deformity	Moderate valgus/varus deformity, symptomatic, interfering with function but not interfering with ADL	Mild slipped capital femoral epiphysis; operative intervention (e.g., fixation) indicated; interfering with ADL	Disabling; severe slipped capital femoral epiphysis >60%; avascular necrosis	—
Bone growth: limb length discrepancy	Limb length	Mild length discrepancy <2 cm	Moderate length discrepancy 2 – 5 cm; shoe lift indicated	Severe length discrepancy >5 cm; operative intervention indicated; interfering with ADL	Disabling; epiphysiodesis	—

(continued)

Appendix 2 *(continued)*

		Grade				
Adverse Event	**Short Name**	**1**	**2**	**3**	**4**	**5**
Bone growth: spine kyphosis/lordosis	Kyphosis/lordosis	Mild radiographic changes	Moderate accentuation; interfering with function but not interfering with ADL	Severe accentuation; operative intervention indicated; interfering with ADL	Disabling (e.g., cannot lift head)	—
Growth velocity (reduction in growth velocity)	Reduction in growth velocity	10 – 29% reduction in growth from the baseline growth curve	30 – 49% reduction in growth from the baseline growth curve	≥50% reduction in growth from the baseline growth curve	—	—
Puberty (delayed)	Delayed puberty	—	No breast development by age 13 yrs for females; no Tanner Stage 2 development by age 14.5 yrs for males	No sexual development by age 14 yrs for girls, age 16 yrs for boys; hormone replacement indicated	—	—
REMARK: Do not use testicular size for Tanner Stage in male cancer survivors.						
Puberty (precocious)	Precocious puberty	—	Physical signs of puberty <7 years for females, <9 years for males	—	—	—
Short stature	Short stature	Beyond two standard deviations of age and gender mean height	Altered ADL	—	—	—
REMARK: Short stature is secondary to growth hormone deficiency.						

(continued)

Appendix 2 *(continued)*

		Grade				
Adverse Event	**Short Name**	**1**	**2**	**3**	**4**	**5**
ALSO CONSIDER: Neuroendocrine: growth hormone secretion abnormality.						
Growth and Development – Other (Specify, ______)	Growth and Development – Other (Specify)	Mild	Moderate	Severe	Life-threatening; disabling	Death

HEMORRHAGE/BLEEDING

		Grade				
Adverse Event	**Short Name**	**1**	**2**	**3**	**4**	**5**
Hematoma	Hematoma	Minimal symptoms, invasive intervention not indicated	Minimally invasive evacuation or aspiration indicated	Transfusion, interventional radiology, or operative intervention indicated	Life-threatening consequences; major urgent intervention indicated	Death
REMARK: Hematoma refers to extravasation at wound or operative site or secondary to other intervention. Transfusion implies pRBC. ALSO CONSIDER: Fibrinogen; INR (International Normalized Ratio of prothrombin time); Platelets; PTT (Partial Thromboplastin Time).						
Hemorrhage/bleeding associated with surgery, intra-operative or postoperative	Hemorrhage with surgery	—	—	Requiring transfusion of 2 units non-autologous (10 cc/kg for pediatrics) pRBCs beyond protocol specification; postoperative interventional radiology, endoscopic, or operative intervention indicated	Life-threatening consequences	Death

(continued)

Appendix 2 *(continued)*

		Grade				
Adverse Event	**Short Name**	**1**	**2**	**3**	**4**	**5**
Hemorrhage, GU – *Select*: – Bladder – Fallopian tube – Kidney – Ovary – Prostate – Retroperitoneum – Spermatic cord – Stoma – Testes – Ureter – Urethra – Urinary NOS – Uterus – Vagina – Vas deferens	Hemorrhage, GU – *Select*	Minimal or microscopic bleeding; intervention not indicated	Gross bleeding, medical intervention, or urinary tract irrigation indicated	Transfusion, interventional radiology, endoscopic, or operative intervention indicated; radiation therapy (i.e., hemostasis of bleeding site)	Life-threatening consequences; major urgent intervention indicated	Death

REMARK: Transfusion implies pRBC.

ALSO CONSIDER: Fibrinogen; INR (International Normalized Ratio of prothrombin time); Platelets; PTT (Partial Thromboplastin Time).

(continued)

Appendix 2 *(continued)*

		Grade				
Adverse Event	**Short Name**	**1**	**2**	**3**	**4**	**5**
Hemorrhage, pulmonary/upper respiratory – *Select*: – Bronchopulmonary NOS – Bronchus – Larynx – Lung – Mediastinum – Nose – Pharynx – Pleura – Respiratory tract NOS – Stoma – Trachea	Hemorrhage pulmonary – *Select*	Mild, intervention not indicated	Symptomatic and medical intervention indicated	Transfusion, interventional radiology, endoscopic, or operative intervention indicated; radiation therapy (i.e., hemostasis of bleeding site)	Life-threatening consequences; major urgent intervention indicated	Death
REMARK: Transfusion implies pRBC.						
ALSO CONSIDER: Fibrinogen; INR (International Normalized Ratio of prothrombin time); Platelets; PTT (Partial Thromboplastin Time).						
Petechiae/purpura (hemorrhage/bleeding into skin or mucosa)	Petechiae	Few petechiae	Moderate petechiae; purpura	Generalized petechiae or purpura	—	—
ALSO CONSIDER: Fibrinogen; INR (International Normalized Ratio of prothrombin time); Platelets; PTT (Partial Thromboplastin Time).						
NAVIGATION NOTE: Vitreous hemorrhage is graded in the OCULAR/VISUAL CATEGORY.						

(continued)

Appendix 2 *(continued)*

		Grade				
Adverse Event	**Short Name**	**1**	**2**	**3**	**4**	**5**
Hemorrhage/Bleeding – Other (Specify, ______)	Hemorrhage – Other (Specify)	Mild without transfusion	—	Transfusion indicated	Catastrophic bleeding, requiring major nonelective intervention	Death

HEPATOBILIARY/PANCREAS

		Grade				
Adverse Event	**Short Name**	**1**	**2**	**3**	**4**	**5**
NAVIGATION NOTE: Biliary tree damage is graded as Fistula, GI – *Select*; Leak (including anastomotic), GI – *Select*; Necrosis, GI – *Select*; Obstruction, GI – *Select*; Perforation, GI – *Select*; Stricture/stenosis (including anastomotic), GI – *Select* in the GASTROINTESTINAL CATEGORY.						
Cholecystitis	Cholecystitis	Asymptomatic, radiographic findings only	Symptomatic, medical intervention indicated	Interventional radiology, endoscopic, or operative intervention indicated	Life-threatening consequences (e.g., sepsis or perforation)	Death
ALSO CONSIDER: Infection (documented clinically or microbiologically) with Grade 3 or 4 neutrophils – *Select*; Infection with normal ANC or Grade 1 or 2 neutrophils – *Select*; Infection with unknown ANC – *Select*.						
Liver dysfunction/failure (clinical)	Liver dysfunction	—	Jaundice	Asterixis	Encephalopathy or coma	Death
REMARK: Jaundice is not an AE, but occurs when the liver is not working properly or when a bile duct is blocked. It is graded as a result of liver dysfunction/failure or elevated bilirubin. ALSO CONSIDER: Bilirubin (hyperbilirubinemia).						
Pancreas, exocrine enzyme deficiency	Pancreas, exocrine enzyme deficiency	—	Increase in stool frequency, bulk, or odor; steatorrhea	Sequelae of absorption deficiency (e.g., weight loss)	Life-threatening consequences	Death

(continued)

Appendix 2 *(continued)*

Adverse Event	Short Name	Grade 1	Grade 2	Grade 3	Grade 4	Grade 5
ALSO CONSIDER: Diarrhea.						
Pancreatitis	Pancreatitis	Asymptomatic, enzyme elevation and/or radiographic findings	Symptomatic, medical intervention indicated	Interventional radiology or operative intervention indicated	Life-threatening consequences (e.g., circulatory failure, hemorrhage, sepsis)	Death
ALSO CONSIDER: Amylase. NAVIGATION NOTE: Stricture (biliary tree, hepatic or pancreatic) is graded as Stricture/stenosis (including anastomotic), GI – *Select* in the GASTROINTESTINAL CATEGORY.						
Hepatobiliary/Pancreas – Other (Specify, ______)	Hepatobiliary – Other (Specify)	Mild	Moderate	Severe	Life-threatening; disabling	Death

INFECTION

Adverse Event	Short Name	Grade 1	Grade 2	Grade 3	Grade 4	Grade 5
Colitis, infectious (e.g., Clostridium difficile)	Colitis, infectious	Asymptomatic, pathologic or radiographic findings only	Abdominal pain with mucus and/or blood in stool	IV antibiotics or TPN indicated	Life-threatening consequences (e.g., perforation, bleeding, ischemia, necrosis or toxic megacolon); operative resection or diversion indicated	Death
ALSO CONSIDER: Hemorrhage, GI – *Select*; Typhlitis (cecal inflammation).						

(continued)

Appendix 2 *(continued)*

		Grade				
Adverse Event	**Short Name**	**1**	**2**	**3**	**4**	**5**
Febrile neutropenia (fever of unknown origin without clinically or microbiologically documented infection) (ANC $<1.0 \times 10^9$/L, fever ≥38.5°C)	Febrile neutropenia	—	—	Present	Life-threatening consequences (e.g., septic shock, hypotension, acidosis, necrosis)	Death
ALSO CONSIDER: Neutrophils/granulocytes (ANC/AGC).						
Infection (documented clinically or microbiologically) with Grade 3 or 4 neutrophils (ANC $<1.0 \times 10^9$/L) – *Select* '*Select*' AEs appear at the end of the CATEGORY.	Infection (documented clinically) – *Select*	—	Localized, local intervention indicated	IV antibiotic, antifungal, or antiviral intervention indicated; interventional radiology or operative intervention indicated	Life-threatening consequences (e.g., septic shock, hypotension, acidosis, necrosis)	Death
REMARK: Fever with Grade 3 or 4 neutrophils in the absence of documented infection is graded as Febrile neutropenia (fever of unknown origin without clinically or microbiologically documented infection). ALSO CONSIDER: Neutrophils/granulocytes (ANC/AGC).						

(continued)

Appendix 2 *(continued)*

		Grade				
Adverse Event	**Short Name**	**1**	**2**	**3**	**4**	**5**
Infection with normal ANC or Grade 1 or 2 neutrophils – *Select* '*Select*' AEs appear at the end of the CATEGORY.	Infection with normal ANC – *Select*	—	Localized, local intervention indicated	IV antibiotic, antifungal, or antiviral intervention indicated; interventional radiology or operative intervention indicated	Life-threatening consequences (e.g., septic shock, hypotension, acidosis, necrosis)	Death
Infection with unknown ANC – *Select* '*Select*' AEs appear at the end of the CATEGORY.	Infection with unknown ANC – *Select*	—	Localized, local intervention indicated	IV antibiotic, antifungal, or antiviral intervention indicated; interventional radiology or operative intervention indicated	Life-threatening consequences (e.g., septic shock, hypotension, acidosis, necrosis)	Death
REMARK: Infection with unknown ANC – *Select* is to be used in the rare case when ANC is unknown.						
Opportunistic infection associated with ≥Grade 2 Lymphopenia	Opportunistic infection	—	Localized, local intervention indicated	IV antibiotic, antifungal, or antiviral intervention indicated; interventional radiology or operative intervention indicated	Life-threatening consequences (e.g., septic shock, hypotension, acidosis, necrosis)	Death
ALSO CONSIDER: Lymphopenia.						

(continued)

Appendix 2 *(continued)*

		Grade				
Adverse Event	**Short Name**	**1**	**2**	**3**	**4**	**5**
Viral hepatitis	Viral hepatitis	Present; transaminases and liver function normal	Transaminases abnormal, liver function normal	Symptomatic liver dysfunction; fibrosis by biopsy; compensated cirrhosis	Decompensated liver function (e.g., ascites, coagulopathy, encephalopathy, coma)	Death
REMARK: Non-viral hepatitis is graded as Infection – *Select*.						
ALSO CONSIDER: Albumin, serum-low (hypoalbuminemia); ALT, SGPT (serum glutamic pyruvic transaminase); AST, SGOT (serum glutamic oxaloacetic transaminase); Bilirubin (hyperbilirubinemia); Encephalopathy.						
Infection – Other (Specify, ______)	Infection – Other (Specify)	Mild	Moderate	Severe	Life-threatening; disabling	Death

INFECTION – *SELECT*

AUDITORY/EAR
- External ear (otitis externa)
- Middle ear (otitis media)

CARDIOVASCULAR
- Artery
- Heart (endocarditis)
- Spleen
- Vein

DERMATOLOGY/SKIN
- Lip/perioral
- Peristomal
- Skin (cellulitis)
- Ungual (nails)

GENERAL
- Blood
- Catheter-related
- Foreign body (e.g., graft, implant, prosthesis, stent)
- Wound

HEPATOBILIARY/PANCREAS
- Biliary tree
- Gallbladder (cholecystitis)
- Liver
- Pancreas

LYMPHATIC
- Lymphatic

PULMONARY/UPPER RESPIRATORY
- Bronchus
- Larynx
- Lung (pneumonia)
- Mediastinum NOS
- Mucosa
- Neck NOS
- Nose
- Paranasal
- Pharynx
- Pleura (empyema)
- Sinus
- Trachea

(continued)

Appendix 2 *(continued)*

GASTROINTESTINAL
- Abdomen NOS
- Anal/perianal
- Appendix
- Cecum
- Colon
- Dental-tooth
- Duodenum
- Esophagus
- Ileum
- Jejunum
- Oral cavity-gums (gingivitis)
- Peritoneal cavity
- Rectum
- Salivary gland
- Small bowel NOS
- Stomach

MUSCULOSKELETAL
- Bone (osteomyelitis)
- Joint
- Muscle (infection myositis)
- Soft tissue NOS

NEUROLOGY
- Brain (encephalitis, infectious)
- Brain + Spinal cord (encephalomyelitis)
- Meninges (meningitis)
- Nerve-cranial
- Nerve-peripheral
- Spinal cord (myelitis)

OCULAR
- Conjunctiva
- Cornea
- Eye NOS
- Lens
- Upper aerodigestive NOS
- Upper airway NOS

RENAL/GENITOURINARY
- Bladder (urinary)
- Kidney
- Prostate
- Ureter
- Urethra
- Urinary tract NOS

SEXUAL/REPRODUCTIVE FUNCTION
- Cervix
- Fallopian tube
- Pelvis NOS
- Penis
- Scrotum
- Uterus
- Vagina
- Vulva

LYMPHATICS

		Grade				
Adverse Event	**Short Name**	**1**	**2**	**3**	**4**	**5**
Chyle or lymph leakage	Chyle or lymph leakage	Asymptomatic, clinical or radiographic findings	Symptomatic, medical intervention indicated	Interventional radiology or operative intervention indicated	Life-threatening complications	Death
ALSO CONSIDER: Chylothorax.						

(Continued)

Appendix 2 *(continued)*

		Grade				
Adverse Event	**Short Name**	**1**	**2**	**3**	**4**	**5**
Dermal change lymphedema, phlebolymphedema	Dermal change	Trace thickening or faint discoloration	Marked discoloration; leathery skin texture; papillary formation	—	—	—
REMARK: Dermal change lymphedema, phlebolymphedema refers to changes due to venous stasis. ALSO CONSIDER: Ulceration.						
Edema: head and neck	Edema: head and neck	Localized to dependent areas, no disability or functional impairment	Localized facial or neck edema with functional impairment	Generalized facial or neck edema with functional impairment (e.g., difficulty in turning neck or opening mouth compared to baseline)	Severe with ulceration or cerebral edema; tracheotomy or feeding tube indicated	Death

(Continued)

Appendix 2 *(continued)*

		Grade				
Adverse Event	**Short Name**	**1**	**2**	**3**	**4**	**5**
Edema: limb	Edema: limb	5 – 10% inter-limb discrepancy in volume or circumference at point of greatest visible difference; swelling or obscuration of anatomic architecture on close inspection; pitting edema	>10 – 30% inter-limb discrepancy in volume or circumference at point of greatest visible difference; readily apparent obscuration of anatomic architecture; obliteration of skin folds; readily apparent deviation from normal anatomic contour	>30% inter-limb discrepancy in volume; lymphorrhea; gross deviation from normal anatomic contour; interfering with ADL	Progression to malignancy (i.e., lymphangiosarcoma); amputation indicated; disabling	Death
Edema: trunk/genital	Edema: trunk/genital	Swelling or obscuration of anatomic architecture on close inspection; pitting edema	Readily apparent obscuration of anatomic architecture; obliteration of skin folds; readily apparent deviation from normal anatomic contour	Lymphorrhea; interfering with ADL; gross deviation from normal anatomic contour	Progression to malignancy (i.e., lymphangiosarcoma); disabling	Death

(Continued)

Appendix 2 *(continued)*

		Grade				
Adverse Event	**Short Name**	**1**	**2**	**3**	**4**	**5**
Edema:viscera	Edema: viscera	Asymptomatic; clinical or radiographic findings only	Symptomatic; medical intervention indicated	Symptomatic and unable to aliment adequately orally; interventional radiology or operative intervention indicated	Life-threatening consequences	Death
Lymphedema-related fibrosis	Lymphedema-related fibrosis	Minimal to moderate redundant soft tissue, unresponsive to elevation or compression, with moderately firm texture or spongy feel	Marked increase in density and firmness, with or without tethering	Very marked density and firmness with tethering affecting ≥40% of the edematous area	—	—
Lymphocele	Lymphocele	Asymptomatic, clinical or radiographic findings only	Symptomatic; medical intervention indicated	Symptomatic and interventional radiology or operative intervention indicated	—	—
Phlebolymphatic cording	Phlebolymphatic cording	Asymptomatic, clinical findings only	Symptomatic; medical intervention indicated	Symptomatic and leading to contracture or reduced range of motion	—	—
Lymphatics – Other (Specify, ______)	Lymphatics – Other (Specify)	Mild	Moderate	Severe	Life-threatening; disabling	Death

(Continued)

Appendix 2 *(continued)*

METABOLIC/LABORATORY

		Grade				
Adverse Event	**Short Name**	**1**	**2**	**3**	**4**	**5**
Acidosis (metabolic or respiratory)	Acidosis	pH <normal, but ≥7.3	—	pH <7.3	pH <7.3 with life-threatening consequences	Death
Albumin, serum-low (hypoalbuminemia)	Hypoalbuminemia	<LLN – 3 g/dL <LLN – 30 g/L	<3 – 2 g/dL <30 – 20 g/L	<2 g/dL <20 g/L	—	Death
Alkaline phosphatase	Alkaline phosphatase	>ULN – 2.5 × ULN	>2.5 – 5.0 × ULN	>5.0 – 20.0 × ULN	>20.0 × ULN	—
Alkalosis (metabolic or respiratory)	Alkalosis	pH >normal, but ≥7.5	—	pH >7.5	pH >7.5 with life-threatening consequences	Death
ALT, SGPT (serum glutamic pyruvic transaminase)	ALT	>ULN – 2.5 × ULN	>2.5 – 5.0 × ULN	>5.0 – 20.0 × ULN	>20.0 × ULN	—
Amylase	Amylase	>ULN – 1.5 × ULN	>1.5 – 2.0 × ULN	>2.0 – 5.0 × ULN	>5.0 × ULN	—
AST, SGOT (serum glutamic oxaloacetic transaminase)	AST	>ULN – 2.5 × ULN	>2.5 – 5.0 × ULN	>5.0 – 20.0 × ULN	>20.0 × ULN	—
Bicarbonate, serum-low	Bicarbonate, serum-low	<LLN – 16 mmol/L	<16 – 11 mmol/L	<11 – 8 mmol/L	<8 mmol/L	Death
Bilirubin (hyperbilirubinemia)	Bilirubin	>ULN – 1.5 × ULN	>1.5 – 3.0 × ULN	>3.0 – 10.0 × ULN	>10.0 × ULN	—

(Continued)

Appendix 2 *(continued)*

		Grade				
Adverse Event	**Short Name**	**1**	**2**	**3**	**4**	**5**
REMARK: Jaundice is not an AE, but may be a manifestation of liver dysfunction/failure or elevated bilirubin. If jaundice is associated with elevated bilirubin, grade bilirubin.						
Calcium, serum-low (hypocalcemia)	Hypocalcemia	<LLN – 8.0 mg/dL <LLN – 2.0 mmol/L Ionized calcium: <LLN – 1.0 mmol/L	<8.0 – 7.0 mg/dL <2.0 – 1.75 mmol/L Ionized calcium: <1.0 – 0.9 mmol/L	<7.0 – 6.0 mg/dL <1.75 – 1.5 mmol/L Ionized calcium: <0.9 – 0.8 mmol/L	<6.0 mg/dL <1.5 mmol/L Ionized calcium: <0.8 mmol/L	Death
REMARK: Calcium can be falsely low if hypoalbuminemia is present. Serum albumin is <4.0 g/dL, hypocalcemia is reported after the following corrective calculation has been performed: Corrected Calcium (mg/dL) = Total Calcium (mg/dL) – 0.8 [Albumin (g/dL) – 4][4]. Alternatively, direct measurement of ionized calcium is the definitive method to diagnose metabolically relevant alterations in serum calcium.						
Calcium, serum-high (hypercalcemia)	Hypercalcemia	>ULN – 11.5 mg/dL >ULN – 2.9 mmol/L Ionized calcium: >ULN – 1.5 mmol/L	>11.5 – 12.5 mg/dL >2.9 – 3.1 mmol/L Ionized calcium: >1.5 – 1.6 mmol/L	>12.5 – 13.5 mg/dL >3.1 – 3.4 mmol/L Ionized calcium: >1.6 – 1.8 mmol/L	>13.5 mg/dL >3.4 mmol/L Ionized calcium: >1.8 mmol/L	Death
Cholesterol, serum-high (hypercholesteremia)	Cholesterol	>ULN – 300 mg/dL >ULN – 7.75 mmol/L	>300 – 400 mg/dL >7.75 – 10.34 mmol/L	>400 – 500 mg/dL >10.34 – 12.92 mmol/L	>500 mg/dL >12.92 mmol/L	Death
CPK (creatine phosphokinase)	CPK	>ULN – 2.5 × ULN	>2.5 × ULN – 5 × ULN	>5 × ULN – 10 × ULN	>10 × ULN	Death
Creatinine	Creatinine	>ULN – 1.5 × ULN	>1.5 – 3.0 × ULN	>3.0 – 6.0 × ULN	>6.0 × ULN	Death
REMARK: Adjust to age-appropriate levels for pediatric patients. ALSO CONSIDER: Glomerular filtration rate.						
GGT (γ-Glutamyl transpeptidase)	GGT	>ULN – 2.5 × ULN	>2.5 – 5.0 × ULN	>5.0 – 20.0 × ULN	>20.0 × ULN	—

(Continued)

Appendix 2 *(continued)*

		Grade				
Adverse Event	**Short Name**	**1**	**2**	**3**	**4**	**5**
Glomerular filtration rate	GFR	<75 – 50% LLN	<50 – 25% LLN	<25% LLN, chronic dialysis not indicated	Chronic dialysis or renal transplant indicated	Death
ALSO CONSIDER: Creatinine.						
Glucose, serum-high (hyperglycemia)	Hyperglycemia	>ULN – 160 mg/dL >ULN – 8.9 mmol/L	>160 – 250 mg/dL >8.9 – 13.9 mmol/L	>250 – 500 mg/dL >13.9 – 27.8 mmol/L	>500 mg/dL >27.8 mmol/L or acidosis	Death
REMARK: Hyperglycemia, in general, is defined as fasting unless otherwise specified in protocol.						
Glucose, serum-low (hypoglycemia)	Hypoglycemia	<LLN – 55 mg/dL <LLN – 3.0 mmol/L	<55 – 40 mg/dL <3.0 – 2.2 mmol/L	<40 – 30 mg/dL <2.2 – 1.7 mmol/L	<30 mg/dL <1.7 mmol/L	Death
Hemoglobinuria	Hemoglobinuria	Present	—	—	—	Death
Lipase	Lipase	>ULN – 1.5 × ULN	>1.5 – 2.0 × ULN	>2.0 – 5.0 × ULN	>5.0 × ULN	—
Magnesium, serum-high (hypermagnesemia)	Hypermagnesemia	>ULN – 3.0 mg/dL >ULN – 1.23 mmol/L	—	>3.0 – 8.0 mg/dL >1.23 – 3.30 mmol/L	>8.0 mg/dL >3.30 mmol/L	Death
Magnesium, serum-low (hypomagnesemia)	Hypomagnesemia	<LLN – 1.2 mg/dL <LLN – 0.5 mmol/L	<1.2 – 0.9 mg/dL <0.5 – 0.4 mmol/L	<0.9 – 0.7 mg/dL <0.4 – 0.3 mmol/L	<0.7 mg/dL <0.3 mmol/L	Death
Phosphate, serum-low (hypophosphatemia)	Hypophosphatemia	<LLN – 2.5 mg/dL <LLN – 0.8 mmol/L	<2.5 – 2.0 mg/dL <0.8 – 0.6 mmol/L	<2.0 – 1.0 mg/dL <0.6 – 0.3 mmol/L	<1.0 mg/dL <0.3 mmol/L	Death
Potassium, serum-high (hyperkalemia)	Hyperkalemia	>ULN – 5.5 mmol/L	>5.5 – 6.0 mmol/L	>6.0 – 7.0 mmol/L	>7.0 mmol/L	Death

(Continued)

Appendix 2 *(continued)*

		Grade				
Adverse Event	**Short Name**	**1**	**2**	**3**	**4**	**5**
Potassium, serum-low (hypokalemia)	Hypokalemia	<LLN – 3.0 mmol/L	—	<3.0 – 2.5 mmol/L	<2.5 mmol/L	Death
Proteinuria	Proteinuria	1+ or 0.15 – 1.0 g/24 hrs	2+ to 3+ or >1.0 – 3.5 g/24 hrs	4+ or >3.5 g/24 hrs	Nephrotic syndrome	Death
Sodium, serum-high (hypernatremia)	Hypernatremia	>ULN – 150 mmol/L	>150 – 155 mmol/L	>155 – 160 mmol/L	>160 mmol/L	Death
Sodium, serum-low (hyponatremia)	Hyponatremia	<LLN – 130 mmol/L	—	<130 – 120 mmol/L	<120 mmol/L	Death
Triglyceride, serum-high (hypertriglyceridemia)	Hypertriglyceridemia	>ULN – 2.5 × ULN	>2.5 – 5.0 × ULN	>5.0 – 10 × ULN	>10 × ULN	Death
Uric acid, serum-high (hyperuricemia)	Hyperuricemia	>ULN – 10 mg/dL ≤0.59 mmol/L without physiologic consequences	—	>ULN – 10 mg/dL ≤0.59 mmol/L with physiologic consequences	>10 mg/dL >0.59 mmol/L	Death
ALSO CONSIDER: Creatinine; Potassium, serum-high (hyperkalemia); Renal failure; Tumor lysis syndrome.						
Metabolic/Laboratory – Other (Specify, ______)	Metabolic/Lab – Other (Specify)	Mild	Moderate	Severe	Life-threatening; disabling	Death

[4]Crit Rev Clin Lab Sci 1984;21(1):51-97

(Continued)

Appendix 2 *(continued)*

MUSCULOSKELETAL/SOFT TISSUE

		Grade				
Adverse Event	**Short Name**	**1**	**2**	**3**	**4**	**5**
Arthritis (non-septic)	Arthritis	Mild pain with inflammation, erythema, or joint swelling, but not interfering with function	Moderate pain with inflammation, erythema, or joint swelling interfering with function, but not interfering with ADL	Severe pain with inflammation, erythema, or joint swelling and interfering with ADL	Disabling	Death
REMARK: Report only when the diagnosis of arthritis (e.g., inflammation of a joint or a state characterized by inflammation of joints) is made. Arthralgia (sign or symptom of pain in a joint, especially non-inflammatory in character) is graded as Pain – *Select* in the PAIN CATEGORY.						
Bone: spine-scoliosis	Scoliosis	≤20 degrees; clinically undetectable	>20 – 45 degrees; visible by forward flexion; interfering with function but not interfering with ADL	>45 degrees; scapular prominence in forward flexion; operative intervention indicated; interfering with ADL	Disabling (e.g., interfering with cardiopulmonary function)	Death
Cervical spine-range of motion	Cervical spine ROM	Mild restriction of rotation or flexion between 60 – 70 degrees	Rotation <60 degrees to right or left; <60 degrees of flexion	Ankylosed/fused over multiple segments with no C-spine rotation	—	—
REMARK: 60 – 65 degrees of rotation is required for reversing a car; 60 – 65 degrees of flexion is required to tie shoes.						
Exostosis	Exostosis	Asymptomatic	Involving multiple sites; pain or interfering with function	Excision indicated	Progression to malignancy (i.e., chondrosarcoma)	Death

(Continued)

Appendix 2 *(continued)*

		Grade				
Adverse Event	**Short Name**	**1**	**2**	**3**	**4**	**5**
Extremity-lower (gait/walking)	Gait/walking	Limp evident only to trained observer and able to walk ≥1 kilometer; cane indicated for walking	Noticeable limp, or limitation of limb function, but able to walk ≥0.1 kilometer (1 city block); quad cane indicated for walking	Severe limp with stride modified to maintain balance (widened base of support, marked reduction in step length); ambulation limited to walker; crutches indicated	Unable to walk	—
ALSO CONSIDER: Ataxia (incoordination); Muscle weakness, generalized or specific area (not due to neuropathy) – *Select*.						
Extremity-upper (function)	Extremity-upper (function)	Able to perform most household or work activities with affected limb	Able to perform most household or work activities with compensation from unaffected limb	Interfering with ADL	Disabling; no function of affected limb	—
Fibrosis-cosmesis	Fibrosis-cosmesis	Visible only on close examination	Readily apparent but not disfiguring	Significant disfigurement; operative intervention indicated if patient chooses	—	—
Fibrosis-deep connective tissue	Fibrosis-deep connective tissue	Increased density, ''spongy'' feel	Increased density with firmness or tethering	Increased density with fixation of tissue; operative intervention indicated; interfering with ADL	Life-threatening; disabling; loss of limb; interfering with vital organ function	Death

(Continued)

Appendix 2 *(continued)*

		Grade				
Adverse Event	**Short Name**	**1**	**2**	**3**	**4**	**5**
ALSO CONSIDER: Induration/fibrosis (skin and subcutaneous tissue); Muscle weakness, generalized or specific area (not due to neuropathy) – *Select*; Neuropathy: motor; Neuropathy: sensory.						
Fracture	Fracture	Asymptomatic, radiographic findings only (e.g., asymptomatic rib fracture on plain x-ray, pelvic insufficiency fracture on MRI, etc.)	Symptomatic but nondisplaced; immobilization indicated	Symptomatic and displaced or open wound with bone exposure; operative intervention indicated	Disabling; amputation indicated	Death
Joint-effusion	Joint-effusion	Asymptomatic, clinical or radiographic findings only	Symptomatic; interfering with function but not interfering with ADL	Symptomatic and interfering with ADL	Disabling	Death
ALSO CONSIDER: Arthritis (non-septic).						
Joint-function[5]	Joint-function	Stiffness interfering with athletic activity; ≤25% loss of range of motion (ROM)	Stiffness interfering with function but not interfering with ADL; >25 – 50% decrease in ROM	Stiffness interfering with ADL; >50 – 75% decrease in ROM	Fixed or non-functional joint (arthrodesis); >75% decrease in ROM	—
ALSO CONSIDER: Arthritis (non-septic).						

(Continued)

Appendix 2 *(continued)*

		Grade				
Adverse Event	**Short Name**	**1**	**2**	**3**	**4**	**5**
Local complication – device/prosthesis-related	Device/prosthesis	Asymptomatic	Symptomatic, but not interfering with ADL; local wound care; medical intervention indicated	Symptomatic, interfering with ADL; operative intervention indicated (e.g., hardware/device replacement or removal, reconstruction)	Life-threatening; disabling; loss of limb or organ	Death
Lumbar spine-range of motion	Lumbar spine ROM	Stiffness and difficulty bending to the floor to pick up a very light object but able to do activity	Some lumbar spine flexion but requires a reaching aid to pick up a very light object from the floor	Ankylosed/fused over multiple segments with no L-spine flexion (i.e., unable to reach to floor to pick up a very light	—	—

(Continued)

Appendix 2 *(continued)*

		Grade				
Adverse Event	**Short Name**	**1**	**2**	**3**	**4**	**5**
Muscle weakness, generalized or specific area (not due to neuropathy) – *Select*: – Extraocular – Extremity-lower – Extremity-upper – Facial – Left-sided – Ocular – Pelvic – Right-sided – Trunk – Whole body/generalized	Muscle weakness – *Select*	Asymptomatic, weakness on physical exam	Symptomatic and interfering with function, but not interfering with ADL	Symptomatic and interfering with ADL	Life-threatening; disabling	Death
ALSO CONSIDER: Fatigue (asthenia, lethargy, malaise).						
Muscular/skeletal hypoplasia	Muscular/skeletal hypoplasia	Cosmetically and functionally insignificant hypoplasia	Deformity, hypoplasia, or asymmetry able to be remediated by prosthesis (e.g., shoe insert) or covered by clothing	Functionally significant deformity, hypoplasia, or asymmetry, unable to be remediated by prosthesis or covered by clothing	Disabling	—

(Continued)

Appendix 2 *(continued)*

		Grade				
Adverse Event	**Short Name**	**1**	**2**	**3**	**4**	**5**
Myositis (inflammation/damage of muscle)	Myositis	Mild pain, not interfering with function	Pain interfering with function, but not interfering with ADL	Pain interfering with ADL	Disabling	Death
REMARK: Myositis implies muscle damage (i.e., elevated CPK). ALSO CONSIDER: CPK (creatine phosphokinase); Pain – *Select*.						
Osteonecrosis (avascular necrosis)	Osteonecrosis	Asymptomatic, radiographic findings only	Symptomatic and interfering with function, but not interfering with ADL; minimal bone removal indicated (i.e., minor sequestrectomy)	Symptomatic and interfering with ADL; operative intervention or hyperbaric oxygen indicated	Disabling	Death
Osteoporosis[6]	Osteoporosis	Radiographic evidence of osteoporosis or Bone Mineral Density (BMD) t-score –1 to –2.5 (osteopenia) and no loss of height or therapy indicated	BMD t-score < –2.5; loss of height <2 cm; antiosteoporotic therapy indicated	Fractures; loss of height ≥2 cm	Disabling	Death
Seroma	Seroma	Asymptomatic	Symptomatic; medical intervention or simple aspiration indicated	Symptomatic, interventional radiology or operative intervention indicated	—	—

(Continued)

Appendix 2 *(continued)*

		Grade				
Adverse Event	**Short Name**	**1**	**2**	**3**	**4**	**5**
Soft tissue necrosis – *Select*: – Abdomen – Extremity-lower – Extremity-upper – Head – Neck – Pelvic – Thorax	Soft tissue necrosis – *Select*	—	Local wound care; medical intervention indicated	Operative debridement or other invasive intervention indicated (e.g., hyperbaric oxygen)	Life-threatening consequences; major invasive intervention indicated (e.g., tissue reconstruction, flap, or grafting)	Death
Trismus (difficulty, restriction or pain when opening mouth)	Trismus	Decreased range of motion without impaired eating	Decreased range of motion requiring small bites, soft foods or purees	Decreased range of motion with inability to adequately aliment or hydrate orally	—	—
NAVIGATION NOTE: Wound-infectious is graded as Infection – *Select* in the INFECTION CATEGORY.						
NAVIGATION NOTE: Wound non-infectious is graded as Wound complication, non-infectious in the DERMATOLOGY/SKIN CATEGORY.						
Musculoskeletal/Soft Tissue – Other (Specify, ______)	Musculoskeletal – Other (Specify)	Mild	Moderate	Severe	Life-threatening; disabling	Death

[5] Adapted from the *International SFTR Method of Measuring and Recording Joint Motion, International Standard Orthopedic Measurements (ISOM),* Jon J. Gerhardt and Otto A.
[6] Assessment of Fracture Risk and its Application to Screening for Postmenopausal Osteoporosis, Report of a *WHO Study Group Technical Report Series*, No. 843, 1994, v + 129

(Continued)

Appendix 2 *(continued)*

NEUROLOGY

		Grade				
Adverse Event	**Short Name**	**1**	**2**	**3**	**4**	**5**
NAVIGATION NOTE: ADD (Attention Deficit Disorder) is graded as Cognitive disturbance.						
NAVIGATION NOTE: Aphasia, receptive and/or expressive, is graded as Speech impairment (e.g., dysphasia or aphasia).						
Apnea	Apnea	—	—	Present	Intubation indicated	Death
Arachnoiditis/meningismus/radiculitis	Arachnoiditis	Symptomatic, not interfering with function; medical intervention indicated	Symptomatic (e.g., photophobia, nausea) interfering with function but not interfering with ADL	Symptomatic, interfering with ADL	Life-threatening; disabling (e.g., paraplegia)	Death
ALSO CONSIDER: Fever (in the absence of neutropenia, where neutropenia is defined as ANC <1.0 × 10^9/L); Infection (documented clinically or microbiologically) with Grade 3 or 4 neutrophils (ANC <1.0 × 10^9/L) – *Select*; Infection with normal ANC or Grade 1 or 2 neutrophils – *Select*; Infection with unknown ANC – *Select*; Pain – *Select*; Vomiting.						
Ataxia (incoordination)	Ataxia	Asymptomatic	Symptomatic, not interfering with ADL	Symptomatic, interfering with ADL; mechanical assistance indicated	Disabling	Death
REMARK: Ataxia (incoordination) refers to the consequence of medical or operative intervention.						
Brachial plexopathy	Brachial plexopathy	Asymptomatic	Symptomatic, not interfering with ADL	Symptomatic, interfering with ADL	Disabling	Death
CNS cerebrovascular ischemia	CNS ischemia	—	Asymptomatic, radiographic findings only	Transient ischemic event or attack (TIA) ≤24 hrs duration	Cerebral vascular accident (CVA, stroke), neurologic deficit >24 hrs	Death

(Continued)

Appendix 2 *(continued)*

		Grade				
Adverse Event	**Short Name**	**1**	**2**	**3**	**4**	**5**
NAVIGATION NOTE: CNS hemorrhage/bleeding is graded as Hemorrhage, CNS in the HEMORRHAGE/BLEEDING CATEGORY.						
CNS necrosis/cystic progression	CNS necrosis	Asymptomatic, radiographic findings only	Symptomatic, not interfering with ADL; medical intervention indicated	Symptomatic and interfering with ADL; hyperbaric oxygen indicated	Life-threatening; disabling; operative intervention indicated to prevent or treat CNS necrosis/cystic progression	Death
Cognitive disturbance	Cognitive disturbance	Mild cognitive disability; not interfering with work/school/life performance; specialized educational services/devices not indicated	Moderate cognitive disability; interfering with work/school/life performance but capable of independent living; specialized resources on part-time basis indicated	Severe cognitive disability; significant impairment of work/school/life performance	Unable to perform ADL; full-time specialized resources or institutionalization indicated	Death
REMARK: Cognitive disturbance may be used for Attention Deficit Disorder (ADD).						
Confusion	Confusion	Transient confusion, disorientation, or attention deficit	Confusion, disorientation, or attention deficit interfering with function, but not interfering withC ADL	Confusion or delirium interfering with ADL	Harmful to others or self; hospitalization indicated	Death
REMARK: Attention Deficit Disorder (ADD) is graded as Cognitive disturbance.						
NAVIGATION NOTE: Cranial neuropathy is graded as Neuropathy-cranial – *Select*.						

(Continued)

Appendix 2 *(continued)*

		Grade				
Adverse Event	**Short Name**	**1**	**2**	**3**	**4**	**5**
Dizziness	Dizziness	With head movements or nystagmus only; not interfering with function	Interfering with function, but not interfering with ADL	Interfering with ADL	Disabling	—
REMARK: Dizziness includes disequilibrium, lightheadedness, and vertigo. ALSO CONSIDER: Neuropathy: cranial – *Select*; Syncope (fainting).						
NAVIGATION NOTE: Dysphasia, receptive and/or expressive, is graded as Speech impairment (e.g., dysphasia or aphasia).						
Encephalopathy	Encephalopathy	—	Mild signs or symptoms; not interfering with ADL	Signs or symptoms interfering with ADL; hospitalization indicated	Life-threatening;disabling	Death
ALSO CONSIDER: Cognitive disturbance; Confusion; Dizziness; Memory impairment; Mental status; Mood alteration – *Select*; Psychosis (hallucinations/delusions); Somnolence/depressed level of consciousness.						
Extrapyramidal/involuntary movement/ restlessness	Involuntary movement	Mild involuntary movements not interfering with function	Moderate involuntary movements interfering with function, but not interfering with ADL	Severe involuntary movements or torticollis interfering with ADL	Disabling	Death
NAVIGATION NOTE: Headache/neuropathic pain (e.g., jaw pain, neurologic pain, phantom limb pain, post-infectious neuralgia, or painful neuropathies) is graded as Pain – *Select* in the PAIN CATEGORY.						
Hydrocephalus	Hydrocephalus	Asymptomatic, radiographic findings only	Mild to moderate symptoms not interfering with ADL	Severe symptoms or neurological deficit interfering with ADL	Disabling	Death

(Continued)

Appendix 2 *(continued)*

Adverse Event	Short Name	Grade 1	Grade 2	Grade 3	Grade 4	Grade 5
Irritability (children <3 years of age)	Irritability	Mild; easily consolable	Moderate; requiring increased attention	Severe; inconsolable	—	—
Laryngeal nerve dysfunction	Laryngeal nerve	Asymptomatic, weakness on clinical examination/testing only	Symptomatic, but not interfering with ADL; intervention not indicated	Symptomatic, interfering with ADL; intervention indicated (e.g., thyroplasty, vocal cord injection)	Life-threatening; tracheostomy indicated	Death
Leak, cerebrospinal fluid (CSF)	CSF leak	Transient headache; postural care indicated	Symptomatic, not interfering with ADL; blood patch indicated	Symptomatic, interfering with ADL; operative intervention indicated	Life-threatening; disabling	Death
REMARK: Leak, cerebrospinal fluid (CSF) may be used for CSF leak associated with operation and persisting >72 hours.						
Leukoencephalopathy (radiographic findings)	Leukoencephalopathy	Mild increase in subarachnoid space (SAS); mild ventriculomegaly; small (+/− multiple) focal T2 hyperintensities, involving periventricular white matter or <1/3 of susceptible areas of cerebrum	Moderate increase in SAS; moderate ventriculomegaly; focal T2 hyperintensities extending into centrum ovale or involving 1/3 to 2/3 of susceptible areas of cerebrum	Severe increase in SAS; severe ventriculomegaly; near total white matter T2 hyperintensities or diffuse low attenuation (CT)	—	—
REMARK: Leukoencephalopathy is a diffuse white matter process, specifically NOT associated with necrosis. Leukoencephalopathy (radiographic findings) does not include lacunas, which are areas that become void of neural tissue.						

(Continued)

Appendix 2 *(continued)*

		Grade				
Adverse Event	**Short Name**	**1**	**2**	**3**	**4**	**5**
Memory impairment	Memory impairment	Memory impairment not interfering with function	Memory impairment interfering with function, but not interfering with ADL	Memory impairment interfering with ADL	Amnesia	—
Mental status[7]	Mental status	—	1 – 3 point below age and educational norm in Folstein Mini-Mental Status Exam (MMSE)	>3 point below age and educational norm in Folstein MMSE	—	—
Mood alteration – *Select*: – Agitation – Anxiety – Depression – Euphoria	Mood alteration – *Select*	Mild mood alteration not interfering with function	Moderate mood alteration interfering with function, but not interfering with ADL; medication indicated	Severe mood alteration interfering with ADL	Suicidal ideation; danger to self or others	Death
Myelitis	Myelitis	Asymptomatic, mild signs (e.g., Babinski's or Lhermitte's sign)	Weakness or sensory loss not interfering with ADL	Weakness or sensory loss interfering with ADL	Disabling	Death

NAVIGATION NOTE: Neuropathic pain is graded as Pain – *Select* in the PAIN CATEGORY.

(Continued)

Appendix 2 *(continued)*

		Grade				
Adverse Event	**Short Name**	**1**	**2**	**3**	**4**	**5**
Neuropathy: cranial – *Select*: – CN I Smell – CN II Vision – CN III Pupil, upper eyelid, extra ocular movements – CN IV Downward, inward movement of eye – CN V Motor-jaw muscles; Sensory-facial – CN VI Lateral deviation of eye – CN VII Motor-face; Sensory-taste – CN VIII Hearing and balance – CN IX Motor-pharynx; Sensory-ear, pharynx, tongue – CN X Motor-palate; pharynx, larynx – CN XI Motor-sternomastoid and trapezius – CN XII Motor-tongue	Neuropathy: cranial – *Select*	Asymptomatic, detected on exam/testing only	Symptomatic, not interfering with ADL	Symptomatic, interfering with ADL	Life-threatening; disabling	Death
Neuropathy: motor	Neuropathy-motor	Asymptomatic, weakness on exam/testing only	Symptomatic weakness interfering with function, but not interfering with ADL	Weakness interfering with ADL; bracing or assistance to walk (e.g., cane or walker) indicated	Life-threatening; disabling (e.g., paralysis)	Death

REMARK: Cranial nerve *motor* neuropathy is graded as Neuropathy: cranial – *Select*.
ALSO CONSIDER: Laryngeal nerve dysfunction; Phrenic nerve dysfunction.

(Continued)

Appendix 2 *(continued)*

		Grade				
Adverse Event	**Short Name**	**1**	**2**	**3**	**4**	**5**
Neuropathy: sensory	Neuropathy-sensory	Asymptomatic; loss of deep tendon reflexes or paresthesia (including tingling) but not interfering with function	Sensory alteration or paresthesia (including tingling), interfering with function, but not interfering with ADL	Sensory alteration or paresthesia interfering with ADL	Disabling	Death
REMARK: Cranial nerve *sensory* neuropathy is graded as Neuropathy: cranial – *Select*.						
Personality/ behavioral	Personality	Change, but not adversely affecting patient or family	Change, adversely affecting patient or family	Mental health intervention indicated	Change harmful to others or self; hospitalization indicated	Death
Phrenic nerve dysfunction	Phrenic nerve	Asymptomatic weakness on exam/ testing only	Symptomatic but not interfering with ADL; intervention not indicated	Significant dysfunction; intervention indicated (e.g., diaphragmatic plication)	Life-threatening respiratory compromise; mechanical ventilation indicated	Death
Psychosis (hallucinations/delusions)	Psychosis	—	Transient episode	Interfering with ADL; medication, supervision or restraints indicated	Harmful to others or self; life-threatening consequences	Death
Pyramidal tract dysfunction (e.g., ↑ tone, hyperreflexia, positive Babinski, ↓ fine motor coordination)	Pyramidal tract dysfunction	Asymptomatic, abnormality on exam or testing only	Symptomatic; interfering with function but not interfering with ADL	Interfering with ADL	Disabling; paralysis	Death

(Continued)

Appendix 2 *(continued)*

		Grade				
Adverse Event	**Short Name**	**1**	**2**	**3**	**4**	**5**
Seizure	Seizure	—	One brief generalized seizure; seizure(s) well controlled by anticonvulsants or infrequent focal motor seizures not interfering with ADL	Seizures in which consciousness is altered; poorly controlled seizure disorder, with breakthrough generalized seizures despite medical intervention	Seizures of any kind which are prolonged, repetitive, or difficult to control (e.g., status epilepticus, intractable epilepsy)	Death
Somnolence/depressed level of consciousness	Somnolence	—	Somnolence or sedation interfering with function, but not interfering with ADL	Obtundation or stupor; difficult to arouse; interfering with ADL	Coma	Death
Speech impairment (e.g., dysphasia or aphasia)	Speech impairment	—	Awareness of receptive or expressive dysphasia, not impairing ability to communicate	Receptive or expressive dysphasia, impairing ability to communicate	Inability to communicate	—
REMARK: Speech impairment refers to a primary CNS process, not neuropathy or end organ dysfunction.						
ALSO CONSIDER: Laryngeal nerve dysfunction; Voice changes/dysarthria (e.g., hoarseness, loss, or alteration in voice, laryngitis).						
Syncope (fainting)	Syncope (fainting)	—	—	Present	Life-threatening consequences	Death
ALSO CONSIDER: CNS cerebrovascular ischemia; Conduction abnormality/atrioventricular heart block – *Select*; Dizziness; Supraventricular and nodal arrhythmia – *Select*; Vasovagal episode; Ventricular arrhythmia – *Select*.						
NAVIGATION NOTE: Taste alteration (CN VII, IX) is graded as Taste alteration (dysgeusia) in the GASTROINTESTINAL CATEGORY.						

(Continued)

Appendix 2 *(continued)*

		Grade				
Adverse Event	**Short Name**	**1**	**2**	**3**	**4**	**5**
Tremor	Tremor	Mild and brief or intermittent but not interfering with function	Moderate tremor interfering with function, but not interfering with ADL	Severe tremor interfering with ADL	Disabling	—
Neurology – Other (Specify, ______)	Neurology – Other (Specify)	Mild	Moderate	Severe	Life-threatening; disabling	Death

[7] Folstein MF, Folstein SE, and McHugh PR 1975; Mini-Mental State: A Practical Method for Grading the State of Patients for the Clinician, *Journal of Psychiatric Research*, 12:189-198.

OCULAR/VISUAL

		Grade				
Adverse Event	**Short Name**	**1**	**2**	**3**	**4**	**5**
Cataract	Cataract	Asymptomatic, detected on exam only	Symptomatic, with moderate decrease in visual acuity (20/40 or better); decreased visual function correctable with glasses	Symptomatic with marked decrease in visual acuity (worse than 20/40); operative intervention indicated (e.g., cataract surgery)	—	—

(Continued)

Appendix 2 *(continued)*

		Grade				
Adverse Event	**Short Name**	**1**	**2**	**3**	**4**	**5**
Dry eye syndrome	Dry eye	Mild, intervention not indicated	Symptomatic, interfering with function but not interfering with ADL; medical intervention indicated	Symptomatic or decrease in visual acuity interfering with ADL; operative intervention indicated	—	—
Eyelid dysfunction	Eyelid dysfunction	Asymptomatic	Symptomatic, interfering with function but not ADL; requiring topical agents or epilation	Symptomatic; interfering with ADL; surgical intervention indicated	—	—
REMARK: Eyelid dysfunction includes canalicular stenosis, ectropion, entropion, erythema, madarosis, symblepharon, telangiectasis, thickening, and trichiasis. ALSO CONSIDER: Neuropathy: cranial – *Select*.						
Glaucoma	Glaucoma	Elevated intraocular pressure (EIOP) with single topical agent for intervention; no visual field deficit	EIOP causing early visual field deficit (i.e., nasal step or arcuate deficit); multiple topical or oral agents indicated	EIOP causing marked visual field deficits (i.e., involving both superior and inferior visual fields); operative intervention indicated	EIOP resulting in blindness (20/200 or worse); enucleation indicated	—

(Continued)

Appendix 2 *(continued)*

		Grade				
Adverse Event	**Short Name**	**1**	**2**	**3**	**4**	**5**
Keratitis (corneal inflammation/corneal ulceration)	Keratitis	Abnormal ophthalmologic changes only; intervention not indicated	Symptomatic and interfering with function, but not interfering with ADL	Symptomatic and interfering with ADL; operative intervention indicated	Perforation or blindness (20/200 or worse)	—
NAVIGATION NOTE: Ocular muscle weakness is graded as Muscle weakness, generalized or specific area (not due to neuropathy) – *Select* in the MUSCULOSKELETAL/SOFT TISSUE CATEGORY.						
Night blindness (nyctalopia)	Nyctalopia	Symptomatic, not interfering with function	Symptomatic and interfering with function but not interfering with ADL	Symptomatic and interfering with ADL	Disabling	—
Nystagmus	Nystagmus	Asymptomatic	Symptomatic and interfering with function but not interfering with ADL	Symptomatic and interfering with ADL	Disabling	—
ALSO CONSIDER: Neuropathy: cranial – *Select*; Ophthalmoplegia/diplopia (double vision).						
Ocular surface disease	Ocular surface disease	Asymptomatic or minimally symptomatic but not interfering with function	Symptomatic, interfering with function but not interfering with ADL; topical antibiotics or other topical intervention indicated	Symptomatic, interfering with ADL; operative intervention indicated	—	—

(Continued)

Appendix 2 *(continued)*

		Grade				
Adverse Event	**Short Name**	**1**	**2**	**3**	**4**	**5**
REMARK: Ocular surface disease includes conjunctivitis, keratoconjunctivitis sicca, chemosis, keratinization, and palpebral conjunctival epithelial metaplasia.						
Ophthalmoplegia/ diplopia (double vision)	Diplopia	Intermittently symptomatic, intervention not indicated	Symptomatic and interfering with function but not interfering with ADL	Symptomatic and interfering with ADL; surgical intervention indicated	Disabling	—
ALSO CONSIDER: Neuropathy: cranial – *Select*.						
Optic disc edema	Optic disc edema	Asymptomatic	Decreased visual acuity (20/40 or better); visual field defect present	Decreased visual acuity (worse than 20/40); marked visual field defect but sparing the central 20 degrees	Blindness (20/200 or worse)	—
ALSO CONSIDER: Neuropathy: cranial – *Select*.						
Proptosis/ enophthalmos	Proptosis/ enophthalmos	Asymptomatic, intervention not indicated	Symptomatic and interfering with function, but not interfering with ADL	Symptomatic and interfering with ADL	—	—
Retinal detachment	Retinal detachment	Exudative; no central vision loss; intervention not indicated	Exudative and visual acuity 20/40 or better but intervention not indicated	Rhegmatogenous or exudative detachment; operative intervention indicated	Blindness (20/200 or worse)	—

(Continued)

Appendix 2 *(continued)*

		Grade				
Adverse Event	**Short Name**	**1**	**2**	**3**	**4**	**5**
Retinopathy	Retinopathy	Asymptomatic	Symptomatic with moderate decrease in visual acuity (20/40 or better)	Symptomatic with marked decrease in visual acuity (worse than 20/40)	Blindness (20/200 or worse)	—
Scleral necrosis/melt	Scleral necrosis	Asymptomatic or symptomatic but not interfering with function	Symptomatic, interfering with function but not interfering with ADL; moderate decrease in visual acuity (20/40 or better); medical intervention indicated	Symptomatic, interfering with ADL; marked decrease in visual acuity (worse than 20/40); operative intervention indicated	Blindness (20/200 or worse); painful eye with enucleation indicated	—
Uveitis	Uveitis	Asymptomatic	Anterior uveitis; medical intervention indicated	Posterior or pan-uveitis; operative intervention indicated	Blindness (20/200 or worse)	—
Vision-blurred vision	Blurred vision	Symptomatic not interfering with function	Symptomatic and interfering with function, but not interfering with ADL	Symptomatic and interfering with ADL	Disabling	—
Vision-flashing lights/floaters	Flashing lights	Symptomatic not interfering with function	Symptomatic and interfering with function, but not interfering with ADL	Symptomatic and interfering with ADL	Disabling	—

(Continued)

Appendix 2 *(continued)*

		Grade				
Adverse Event	**Short Name**	**1**	**2**	**3**	**4**	**5**
Vision-photophobia	Photophobia	Symptomatic not interfering with function	Symptomatic and interfering with function, but not interfering with ADL	Symptomatic and interfering with ADL	Disabling	—
Vitreous hemorrhage	Vitreous hemorrhage	Asymptomatic, clinical findings only	Symptomatic, interfering with function, but not interfering with ADL; intervention not indicated	Symptomatic, interfering with ADL; vitrectomy indicated	—	—
Watery eye (epiphora, tearing)	Watery eye	Symptomatic, intervention not indicated	Symptomatic, interfering with function but not interfering with ADL	Symptomatic, interfering with ADL	—	—
Ocular/Visual – Other (Specify, ______)	Ocular – Other (Specify)	Symptomatic not interfering with function	Symptomatic and interfering with function, but not interfering with ADL	Symptomatic and interfering with ADL	Blindness (20/200 or worse)	Death

(Continued)

Appendix 2 *(continued)*

PAIN

		Grade				
Adverse Event	**Short Name**	**1**	**2**	**3**	**4**	**5**
Pain – *Select*: '*Select*' AEs appear at the end of the CATEGORY.	Pain – *Select*	Mild pain not interfering with function	Moderate pain; pain or analgesics interfering with function, but not interfering with ADL	Severe pain; pain or analgesics severely interfering with ADL	Disabling	—
Pain – Other (Specify, ______)	Pain – Other (Specify)	Mild pain not interfering with function	Moderate pain; pain or analgesics interfering with function, but not interfering with ADL	Severe pain; pain or analgesics severely interfering with ADL	Disabling	—

PAIN – *SELECT*

AUDITORY/EAR
- External ear
- Middle ear

CARDIOVASCULAR
- Cardiac/heart
- Pericardium

DERMATOLOGY/SKIN
- Face
- Lip
- Oral-gums
- Scalp
- Skin

HEPATOBILIARY/PANCREAS
- Gallbladder
- Liver

LYMPHATIC
- Lymph node

MUSCULOSKELETAL
- Back
- Bone
- Buttock
- Extremity-limb
- Intestine
- Joint

PULMONARY/UPPER RESPIRATORY
- Chest wall
- Chest/thorax NOS
- Larynx
- Pleura
- Sinus
- Throat/pharynx/larynx

RENAL/GENITOURINARY
- Bladder
- Kidney

SEXUAL/REPRODUCTIVE FUNCTION
- Breast

(Continued)

Appendix 2 *(continued)*

GASTROINTESTINAL
- Abdomen NOS
- Anus
- Dental/teeth/peridontal
- Esophagus
- Oral cavity
- Peritoneum
- Rectum
- Stomach

GENERAL
- Pain NOS
- Tumor pain

- Muscle
- Neck
- Phantom (pain associated with missing limb)

NEUROLOGY
- Head/headache
- Neuralgia/peripheral nerve

OCULAR
- Eye

- Ovulatory
- Pelvis
- Penis
- Perineum
- Prostate
- Scrotum
- Testicle
- Urethra
- Uterus
- Vagina

PULMONARY/UPPER RESPIRATORY						
		Grade				
Adverse Event	**Short Name**	**1**	**2**	**3**	**4**	**5**
Adult Respiratory Distress Syndrome (ARDS)	ARDS	—	—	Present, intubation not indicated	Present, intubation indicated	Death
ALSO CONSIDER: Dyspnea (shortness of breath); Hypoxia; Pneumonitis/pulmonary infiltrates.						

(Continued)

Appendix 2 *(continued)*

		Grade				
Adverse Event	**Short Name**	**1**	**2**	**3**	**4**	**5**
Aspiration	Aspiration	Asymptomatic ("silent aspiration"); endoscopy or radiographic (e.g., barium swallow) findings	Symptomatic (e.g., altered eating habits, coughing or choking episodes consistent with aspiration); medical intervention indicated (e.g., antibiotics, suction or oxygen)	Clinical or radiographic signs of pneumonia or pneumonitis; unable to aliment orally	Life-threatening (e.g., aspiration pneumonia or pneumonitis)	Death
Also Consider: Infection (documented clinically or microbiologically) with Grade 3 or 4 neutrophils (ANC <1.0 × 10^9/L) – *Select;* Infection with normal ANC or Grade 1 or 2 neutrophils – *Select;* Infection with unknown ANC – *Select;* Laryngeal nerve dysfunction; Neuropathy: cranial – *Select*; Pneumonitis/pulmonary infiltrates.						
Atelectasis	Atelectasis	Asymptomatic	Symptomatic (e.g., dyspnea, cough), medical intervention indicated (e.g., bronchoscopic suctioning, chest physiotherapy, suctioning)	Operative (e.g., stent, laser) intervention indicated	Life-threatening respiratory compromise	Death
Also Consider: Adult Respiratory Distress Syndrome (ARDS); Cough; Dyspnea (shortness of breath); Hypoxia; Infection (documented clinically or microbiologically) with Grade 3 or 4 neutrophils (ANC <1.0 × 10^9/L) – *Select*; Infection with normal ANC or Grade 1 or 2 neutrophils – *Select*; Infection with unknown ANC – *Select*; Obstruction/stenosis of airway – *Select*; Pneumonitis/pulmonary infiltrates; Pulmonary fibrosis (radiographic changes).						

(Continued)

Appendix 2 *(continued)*

		Grade				
Adverse Event	**Short Name**	**1**	**2**	**3**	**4**	**5**
Bronchospasm, wheezing	Bronchospasm	Asymptomatic	Symptomatic not interfering with function	Symptomatic interfering with function	Life-threatening	Death
ALSO CONSIDER: Allergic reaction/hypersensitivity (including drug fever); Dyspnea (shortness of breath).						
Carbon monoxide diffusion capacity (DL_{CO})	DL_{CO}	90 – 75% of predicted value	<75 – 50% of predicted value	<50 – 25% of predicted value	<25% of predicted value	Death
ALSO CONSIDER: Hypoxia; Pneumonitis/pulmonary infiltrates; Pulmonary fibrosis (radiographic changes).						
Chylothorax	Chylothorax	Asymptomatic	Symptomatic; thoracentesis or tube drainage indicated	Operative intervention indicated	Life-threatening (e.g., hemodynamic instability or ventilatory support indicated)	Death
Cough	Cough	Symptomatic, non-narcotic medication only indicated	Symptomatic and narcotic medication indicated	Symptomatic and significantly interfering with sleep or ADL	—	—
Dyspnea (shortness of breath)	Dyspnea	Dyspnea on exertion, but can walk 1 flight of stairs without stopping	Dyspnea on exertion but unable to walk 1 flight of stairs or 1 city block (0.1km) without stopping	Dyspnea with ADL	Dyspnea at rest; intubation/ventilator indicated	Death
ALSO CONSIDER: Hypoxia; Neuropathy: motor; Pneumonitis/pulmonary infiltrates; Pulmonary fibrosis (radiographic changes).						

(Continued)

Appendix 2 *(continued)*

		Grade				
Adverse Event	**Short Name**	**1**	**2**	**3**	**4**	**5**
Edema, larynx	Edema, larynx	Asymptomatic edema by exam only	Symptomatic edema, no respiratory distress	Stridor; respiratory distress; interfering with ADL	Life-threatening airway compromise; tracheotomy, intubation, or laryngectomy indicated	Death
ALSO CONSIDER: Allergic reaction/hypersensitivity (including drug fever).						
FEV_1	FEV_1	90 – 75% of predicted value	<75 – 50% of predicted value	<50 – 25% of predicted value	<25% of predicted	Death
Fistula, pulmonary/ upper respiratory – *Select*: – Bronchus – Larynx – Lung – Oral cavity – Pharynx – Pleura – Trachea	Fistula, pulmonary – *Select*	Asymptomatic, radiographic findings only	Symptomatic, tube thoracostomy or medical management indicated; associated with altered respiratory function but not interfering with ADL	Symptomatic and associated with altered respiratory function interfering with ADL; or endoscopic (e.g., stent) or primary closure by operative intervention indicated	Life-threatening consequences; operative intervention with thoracoplasty, chronic open drainage or multiple thoracotomies indicated	Death
REMARK: A fistula is defined as an abnormal communication between two body cavities, potential spaces, and/or the skin. The site indicated for a fistula should be the site from which the abnormal process is believed to have arisen. For example, a tracheo-esophageal fistula arising in the context of a resected or irradiated esophageal cancer should be graded as Fistula, GI – esophagus in the GASTROINTESTINAL CATEGORY.						
NAVIGATION NOTE: Hemoptysis is graded as Hemorrhage, pulmonary/upper respiratory – *Select* in the HEMORRHAGE/BLEEDING CATEGORY.						
Hiccoughs (hiccups, singultus)	Hiccoughs	Symptomatic, intervention not indicated	Symptomatic, intervention indicated	Symptomatic, significantly interfering with sleep or ADL	—	—

(Continued)

Appendix 2 *(continued)*

		Grade				
Adverse Event	**Short Name**	**1**	**2**	**3**	**4**	**5**
Hypoxia	Hypoxia	—	Decreased O_2 saturation with exercise (e.g., pulse oximeter <88%); intermittent supplemental oxygen	Decreased O_2 saturation at rest; continuous oxygen indicated	Life-threatening; intubation or ventilation indicated	Death
Nasal cavity/paranasal sinus reactions	Nasal/paranasal reactions	Asymptomatic mucosal crusting, blood-tinged secretions	Symptomatic stenosis or edema/narrowing interfering with airflow	Stenosis with significant nasal obstruction; interfering with ADL	Necrosis of soft tissue or bone	Death
ALSO CONSIDER: Infection (documented clinically or microbiologically) with Grade 3 or 4 neutrophils (ANC <1.0 × 10^9/L) – *Select;* Infection with normal ANC or Grade 1 or 2 neutrophils – *Select;* Infection with unknown ANC – *Select.*						
Obstruction/stenosis of airway – *Select*: – Bronchus – Larynx – Pharynx – Trachea	Airway obstruction – *Select*	Asymptomatic obstruction or stenosis on exam, endoscopy, or radiograph	Symptomatic (e.g., noisy airway breathing), but causing no respiratory distress; medical management indicated (e.g., steroids)	Interfering with ADL; stridor or endoscopic intervention indicated (e.g., stent, laser)	Life-threatening airway compromise; tracheotomy or intubation indicated	Death
Pleural effusion (non-malignant)	Pleural effusion	Asymptomatic	Symptomatic, intervention such as diuretics or up to 2 therapeutic thoracenteses indicated	Symptomatic and supplemental oxygen, >2 therapeutic thoracenteses, tube drainage, or pleurodesis indicated	Life-threatening (e.g., causing hemodynamic instability or ventilatory support indicated)	Death

(Continued)

Appendix 2 *(continued)*

		Grade				
Adverse Event	**Short Name**	**1**	**2**	**3**	**4**	**5**
ALSO CONSIDER: Atelectasis; Cough; Dyspnea (shortness of breath); Hypoxia; Pneumonitis/pulmonary infiltrates; Pulmonary fibrosis (radiographic changes).						
NAVIGATION NOTE: Pleuritic pain is graded as Pain – *Select* in the PAIN CATEGORY.						
Pneumonitis/pulmonary infiltrates	Pneumonitis	Asymptomatic, radiographic findings only	Symptomatic, not interfering with ADL	Symptomatic, interfering with ADL; O_2 indicated	Life-threatening; ventilatory support indicated	Death
ALSO CONSIDER: Adult Respiratory Distress Syndrome (ARDS); Cough; Dyspnea (shortness of breath); Hypoxia; Infection (documented clinically or microbiologically) with Grade 3 or 4 neutrophils (ANC <1.0 × 10^9/L) – *Select;* Infection with normal ANC or Grade 1 or 2 neutrophils – *Select;* Infection with unknown ANC – *Select*; Pneumonitis/pulmonary infiltrates; Pulmonary fibrosis (radiographic changes).						
Pneumothorax	Pneumothorax	Asymptomatic, radiographic findings only	Symptomatic; intervention indicated (e.g., hospitalization for observation, tube placement without sclerosis)	Sclerosis and/or operative intervention indicated	Life-threatening, causing hemodynamic instability (e.g., tension pneumothorax); ventilatory support indicated	Death
Prolonged chest tube drainage or air leak after pulmonary resection	Chest tube drainage or leak	—	Sclerosis or additional tube thoracostomy indicated	Operative intervention indicated (e.g., thoracotomy with stapling or sealant application)	Life-threatening; debilitating; organ resection indicated	Death
Prolonged intubation after pulmonary resection (>24 hrs after surgery)	Prolonged intubation	—	Extubated within 24 – 72 hrs postoperatively	Extubated >72 hrs postoperatively, but before tracheostomy indicated	Tracheostomy indicated	Death

(Continued)

Appendix 2 *(continued)*

		Grade				
Adverse Event	**Short Name**	**1**	**2**	**3**	**4**	**5**
NAVIGATION NOTE: Pulmonary embolism is graded as Grade 4 either as Thrombosis/embolism (vascular access-related) or Thrombosis/thrombus/embolism in the VASCULAR CATEGORY.						
Pulmonary fibrosis (radiographic changes)	Pulmonary fibrosis	Minimal radiographic findings (CT patchy or bibasilar changes) with estimated radiographic proportion of total lung volume that is fibrotic of <25%	Patchy or bi-basilar changes with estimated radiographic proportion of total lung volume that is fibrotic of 25 – <50%	Dense or widespread infiltrates/consolidation with estimated radiographic proportion of total lung volume that is fibrotic of 50 – <75%	Estimated radiographic proportion of total lung volume that is fibrotic is ≥75%; honeycombing	Death
REMARK: Fibrosis is usually a ''late effect'' seen >3 months after radiation or combined modality therapy (including surgery). It is thought to represent scar/fibrotic lung tissue. It may be difficult to distinguish from pneumonitis that is generally seen within 3 months of radiation or combined modality therapy.						
ALSO CONSIDER: Adult Respiratory Distress Syndrome (ARDS); Cough; Dyspnea (shortness of breath); Hypoxia; Infection (documented clinically or microbiologically) with Grade 3 or 4 neutrophils (ANC <1.0 × 10^9/L) – *Select;* Infection with normal ANC or Grade 1 or 2 neutrophils – *Select;* Infection with unknown ANC – *Select.*						
NAVIGATION NOTE: Recurrent laryngeal nerve dysfunction is graded as Laryngeal nerve dysfunction in the NEUROLOGY CATEGORY.						
Vital capacity	Vital capacity	90 – 75% of predicted value	<75 – 50% of predicted value	<50 – 25% of predicted value	<25% of predicted value	Death

(Continued)

Appendix 2 *(continued)*

		Grade				
Adverse Event	**Short Name**	**1**	**2**	**3**	**4**	**5**
Voice changes/dysarthria (e.g., hoarseness, loss or alteration in voice, laryngitis)	Voice changes	Mild or intermittent hoarseness or voice change, but fully understandable	Moderate or persistent voice changes, may require occasional repetition but understandable on telephone	Severe voice changes including predominantly whispered speech; may require frequent repetition or face-to-face contact for understandability; requires voice aid (e.g., electrolarynx) for ≤50% of communication	Disabling; nonunderstandable voice or aphonic; requires voice aid (e.g., electrolarynx) for >50% of communication or requires >50% written communication	Death
ALSO CONSIDER: Laryngeal nerve dysfunction; Speech impairment (e.g., dysphasia or aphasia).						
Pulmonary/Upper Respiratory – Other (Specify, ________)	Pulmonary – Other (Specify)	Mild	Moderate	Severe	Life-threatening; disabling	Death

RENAL/GENITOURINARY

		Grade				
Adverse Event	**Short Name**	**1**	**2**	**3**	**4**	**5**
Bladder spasms	Bladder spasms	Symptomatic, intervention not indicated	Symptomatic, antispasmodics indicated	Narcotics indicated	Major surgical intervention indicated (e.g., cystectomy)	—

(Continued)

Appendix 2 *(continued)*

		Grade				
Adverse Event	**Short Name**	**1**	**2**	**3**	**4**	**5**
Cystitis	Cystitis	Asymptomatic	Frequency with dysuria; macroscopic hematuria	Transfusion; IV pain medications; bladder irrigation indicated	Catastrophic bleeding; major non-elective intervention indicated	Death
ALSO CONSIDER: Infection (documented clinically or microbiologically) with Grade 3 or 4 neutrophils (ANC <1.0 × 10^9/L) – *Select*; Infection with normal ANC or Grade 1 or 2 neutrophils – *Select*; Infection with unknown ANC – *Select*; Pain – *Select*.						
Fistula, GU – *Select*: – Bladder – Genital tract-female – Kidney – Ureter – Urethra – Uterus – Vagina	Fistula, GU – *Select*	Asymptomatic, radiographic findings only	Symptomatic; noninvasive intervention indicated	Symptomatic interfering with ADL; invasive intervention indicated	Life-threatening consequences; operative intervention requiring partial or full organ resection; permanent urinary diversion	Death
REMARK: A fistula is defined as an abnormal communication between two body cavities, potential spaces, and/or the skin. The site indicated for a fistula should be the site from which the abnormal process is believed to have originated.						
Incontinence, urinary	Incontinence, urinary	Occasional (e.g., with coughing, sneezing, etc.), pads not indicated	Spontaneous, pads indicated	Interfering with ADL; intervention indicated (e.g., clamp, collagen injections)	Operative intervention indicated (e.g., cystectomy or permanent urinary diversion)	—

(Continued)

Appendix 2 *(continued)*

		Grade				
Adverse Event	**Short Name**	**1**	**2**	**3**	**4**	**5**
Leak (including anastomotic), GU – *Select*: – Bladder – Fallopian tube – Kidney – Spermatic cord – Stoma – Ureter – Urethra – Uterus – Vagina – Vas deferens	Leak, GU – *Select*	Asymptomatic, radiographic findings only	Symptomatic; medical intervention indicated	Symptomatic, interfering with GU function; invasive or endoscopic intervention indicated	Life-threatening	Death

REMARK: Leak (including anastomotic), GU – *Select* refers to clinical signs and symptoms or radiographic confirmation of anastomotic leak but without development of fistula.

(Continued)

Appendix 2 *(continued)*

		Grade				
Adverse Event	**Short Name**	**1**	**2**	**3**	**4**	**5**
Obstruction, GU – *Select*: – Bladder – Fallopian tube – Prostate – Spermatic cord – Stoma – Testes – Ureter – Urethra – Uterus – Vagina – Vas deferens	Obstruction, GU – *Select*	Asymptomatic, radiographic or endoscopic findings only	Symptomatic but no hydronephrosis, sepsis or renal dysfunction; dilation or endoscopic repair or stent placement indicated	Symptomatic and altered organ function (e.g., sepsis or hydronephrosis, or renal dysfunction); operative intervention indicated	Life-threatening consequences; organ failure or operative intervention requiring complete organ resection indicated	Death

NAVIGATION NOTE: Operative injury is graded as Intra-operative injury – *Select Organ or Structure* in the SURGERY/INTRA-OPERATIVE INJURY CATEGORY.

(Continued)

Appendix 2 *(continued)*

		Grade				
Adverse Event	**Short Name**	**1**	**2**	**3**	**4**	**5**
Perforation, GU – *Select*: – Bladder – Fallopian tube – Kidney – Ovary – Prostate – Spermatic cord – Stoma – Testes – Ureter – Urethra – Uterus – Vagina – Vas deferens	Perforation, GU – *Select*	Asymptomatic radiographic findings only	Symptomatic, associated with altered renal/GU function	Symptomatic, operative intervention indicated	Life-threatening consequences or organ failure; operative intervention requiring organ resection indicated	Death
Prolapse of stoma, GU	Prolapse stoma, GU	Asymptomatic; special intervention, extraordinary care not indicated	Extraordinary local care or maintenance; minor revision under local anesthesia indicated	Dysfunctional stoma; operative intervention or major stomal revision indicated	Life-threatening consequences	Death
REMARK: Other stoma complications may be graded as Fistula, GU – *Select*; Leak (including anastomotic), GU – *Select*; Obstruction, GU – *Select;* Perforation, GU – *Select*; Stricture/stenosis (including anastomotic), GU – *Select.*						
Renal failure	Renal failure	—	—	Chronic dialysis not indicated	Chronic dialysis or renal transplant indicated	Death

(Continued)

Appendix 2 *(continued)*

		Grade				
Adverse Event	**Short Name**	**1**	**2**	**3**	**4**	**5**
ALSO CONSIDER: Glomerular filtration rate.						
Stricture/stenosis (including anastomotic), GU – *Select*: – Bladder – Fallopian tube – Prostate – Spermatic cord – Stoma – Testes – Ureter – Urethra – Uterus – Vagina – Vas deferens	Stricture, anastomotic, GU – *Select*	Asymptomatic, radiographic or endoscopic findings only	Symptomatic but no hydronephrosis, sepsis or renal dysfunction; dilation or endoscopic repair or stent placement indicated	Symptomatic and altered organ function (e.g., sepsis or hydronephrosis, or renal dysfunction); operative intervention indicated	Life-threatening consequences; organ failure or operative intervention requiring organ resection indicated	Death
ALSO CONSIDER: Obstruction, GU – *Select*.						
Urinary electrolyte wasting (e.g., Fanconi's syndrome, renal tubular acidosis)	Urinary electrolyte wasting	Asymptomatic, intervention not indicated	Mild, reversible and manageable with replacement	Irreversible, requiring continued replacement	—	—
ALSO CONSIDER: Acidosis (metabolic or respiratory); Bicarbonate, serum-low; Calcium, serum-low (hypocalcemia); Phosphate, serum-low (hypophosphatemia).						

(Continued)

Appendix 2 *(continued)*

		Grade				
Adverse Event	**Short Name**	**1**	**2**	**3**	**4**	**5**
Urinary frequency/ urgency	Urinary frequency	Increase in frequency or nocturia up to 2 × normal; enuresis	Increase >2 × normal but <hourly	≥1 x/hr; urgency; catheter indicated	—	—
Urinary retention (including neurogenic bladder)	Urinary retention	Hesitancy or dribbling, no significant residual urine; retention occurring during the immediate postoperative period	Hesitancy requiring medication; or operative bladder atony requiring indwelling catheter beyond immediate postoperative period but for <6 weeks	More than daily catheterization indicated; urological intervention indicated (e.g., TURP, suprapubic tube, urethrotomy)	Life-threatening consequences; organ failure (e.g., bladder rupture); operative intervention requiring organ resection indicated	Death
REMARK: The etiology of retention (if known) is graded as Obstruction, GU – *Select*; Stricture/stenosis (including anastomotic), GU – *Select*.						
ALSO CONSIDER: Obstruction, GU – *Select*; Stricture/stenosis (including anastomotic), GU – *Select*.						
Urine color change	Urine color change	Present	—	—	—	—
REMARK: Urine color refers to change that is not related to other dietary or physiologic cause (e.g., bilirubin, concentrated urine, and hematuria).						
Renal/Genitourinary – Other (Specify, ________)	Renal – Other (Specify)	Mild	Moderate	Severe	Life-threatening; disabling	Death

(Continued)

Appendix 2 *(continued)*

SECONDARY MALIGNANCY

		Grade				
Adverse Event	**Short Name**	**1**	**2**	**3**	**4**	**5**
Secondary Malignancy – possibly related to cancer treatment (Specify, ________)	Secondary Malignancy (possibly related to cancer treatment)	—	—	Non-life-threatening basal or squamous cell carcinoma of the skin	Solid tumor, leukemia or lymphoma	Death

REMARK: Secondary malignancy excludes metastasis from initial primary. Any malignancy possibly related to cancer treatment (including AML/MDS) should be reported via the routine reporting mechanisms outlined in each protocol. Important: Secondary Malignancy is an exception to NCI Expedited Adverse Event Reporting Guidelines. Secondary Malignancy is "Grade 4, present'' but NCI does not require AdEERS Expedited Reporting for any (related or unrelated to treatment) Secondary Malignancy. A diagnosis of AML/MDS following treatment with an NCI-sponsored investigational agent is to be reported using the form available from the CTEP Web site at http://ctep.cancer.gov. Cancers not suspected of being treatment-related are not to be reported here.

SEXUAL/REPRODUCTIVE FUNCTION

		Grade				
Adverse Event	**Short Name**	**1**	**2**	**3**	**4**	**5**
Breast function/lactation	Breast function	Mammary abnormality, not functionally significant	Mammary abnormality, functionally significant	—	—	—
Breast nipple/areolar deformity	Nipple/areolar	Limited areolar asymmetry with no change in nipple/areolar projection	Asymmetry of nipple areolar complex with slight deviation in nipple projection	Marked deviation of nipple projection	—	—

(Continued)

Appendix 2 *(continued)*

		Grade				
Adverse Event	**Short Name**	**1**	**2**	**3**	**4**	**5**
Breast volume/ hypoplasia	Breast	Minimal asymmetry; minimal hypoplasia	Asymmetry exists, ≤1/3 of the breast volume; moderate hypoplasia	Asymmetry exists, >1/3 of the breast volume; severe hypoplasia	—	—
REMARK: Breast volume is referenced with both arms straight overhead.						
NAVIGATION NOTE: Dysmenorrhea is graded as Pain – *Select* in the PAIN CATEGORY.						
NAVIGATION NOTE: Dyspareunia is graded as Pain – *Select* in the PAIN CATEGORY.						
NAVIGATION NOTE: Dysuria (painful urination) is graded as Pain – *Select* in the PAIN CATEGORY.						
Erectile dysfunction	Erectile dysfunction	Decrease in erectile function (frequency/ rigidity of erections) but erectile aids not indicated	Decrease in erectile function (frequency/ rigidity of erections), erectile aids indicated	Decrease in erectile function (frequency/ rigidity of erections) but erectile aids not helpful; penile prosthesis indicated	—	—
Ejaculatory dysfunction	Ejaculatory dysfunction	Diminished ejaculation	Anejaculation or retrograde ejaculation	—	—	—
NAVIGATION NOTE: Feminization of male is graded in the ENDOCRINE CATEGORY.						
Gynecomastia	Gynecomastia	—	Asymptomatic breast enlargement	Symptomatic breast enlargement; intervention indicated	—	—
ALSO CONSIDER: Pain – *Select*.						

(Continued)

Appendix 2 *(continued)*

		Grade				
Adverse Event	**Short Name**	**1**	**2**	**3**	**4**	**5**
Infertility/sterility	Infertility/sterility	—	Male: oligospermia/ low sperm count Female: diminished fertility/ovulation	Male: sterile/azoo- spermia Female: infertile/ anovulatory	—	—
Irregular menses (change from baseline)	Irregular menses	1 – 3 months with- out menses	>3 – 6 months with- out menses but con- tinuing menstrual cycles	Persistent amenor- rhea for >6 months	—	—
Libido	Libido	Decrease in interest but not affecting re- lationship; interven- tion not indicated	Decrease in interest and adversely affect- ing relationship; in- tervention indicated	—	—	—
NAVIGATION NOTE: Masculinization of female is graded in the ENDOCRINE CATEGORY.						
Orgasmic dysfunction	Orgasmic function	Transient decrease	Decrease in orgasm- ic response requiring intervention	Complete inability of orgasmic re- sponse; not respond- ing to intervention	—	—
NAVIGATION NOTE: Pelvic pain is graded as Pain – *Select* in the PAIN CATEGORY.						
NAVIGATION NOTE: Ulcers of the labia or perineum are graded as Ulceration in DERMATOLOGY/SKIN CATEGORY.						
Vaginal discharge (non-infectious)	Vaginal discharge	Mild	Moderate to heavy; pad use indicated	—	—	—

(Continued)

Appendix 2 *(continued)*

		Grade				
Adverse Event	**Short Name**	**1**	**2**	**3**	**4**	**5**
Vaginal dryness	Vaginal dryness	Mild	Interfering with sexual function; dyspareunia; intervention indicated	—	—	—
ALSO CONSIDER: Pain – *Select.*						
Vaginal mucositis	Vaginal mucositis	Erythema of the mucosa; minimal symptoms	Patchy ulcerations; moderate symptoms or dyspareunia	Confluent ulcerations; bleeding with trauma; unable to tolerate vaginal exam, sexual intercourse or tampon placement	Tissue necrosis; significant spontaneous bleeding; life-threatening consequences	—
Vaginal stenosis/ length	Vaginal stenosis	Vaginal narrowing and/or shortening not interfering with function	Vaginal narrowing and/or shortening interfering with function	Complete obliteration; not surgically correctable	—	—
Vaginitis (not due to infection)	Vaginitis	Mild, intervention not indicated	Moderate, intervention indicated	Severe, not relieved with treatment; ulceration, but operative intervention not indicated	Ulceration and operative intervention indicated	—
Sexual/Reproductive Function – Other (Specify, ________)	Sexual – Other (Specify)	Mild	Moderate	Severe	Disabling	Death

(Continued)

Appendix 2 *(continued)*

SURGERY/INTRA-OPERATIVE INJURY

		Grade				
Adverse Event	**Short Name**	**1**	**2**	**3**	**4**	**5**
NAVIGATION NOTE: Intra-operative hemorrhage is graded as Hemorrhage/bleeding associated with surgery, intra-operative or postoperative in the HEMORRHAGE/BLEEDING CATEGORY.						
Intra-operative injury – *Select Organ or Structure* *'Select'* AEs appear at the end of the CATEGORY.	Intraop injury – *Select*	Primary repair of injured organ/structure indicated	Partial resection of injured organ/structure indicated	Complete resection or reconstruction of injured organ/structure indicated	Life threatening consequences; disabling	—
REMARK: The *'Select'* AEs are defined as significant, unanticipated injuries that are recognized at the time of surgery. These AEs do not refer to additional surgical procedures that must be performed because of a change in the operative plan based on intra-operative findings. Any sequelae resulting from the intra-operative injury that result in an adverse outcome for the patient must also be recorded and graded under the relevant CTCAE Term.						
Intra-operative Injury – Other (Specify, _________)	Intraop Injury – Other (Specify)	Primary repair of injured organ/structure indicated	Partial resection of injured organ/structure indicated	Complete resection or reconstruction of injured organ/structure indicated	Life threatening consequences; disabling	—

REMARK: Intra-operative Injury – Other (Specify, ______)is to be used only to report an organ/structure not included in the *'Select'* AEs found at the end of the CATEGORY. Any sequelae resulting from the intra-operative injury that result in an adverse outcome for the patient must also be recorded and graded under the relevant CTCAE Term.

(Continued)

Appendix 2 *(continued)*

SYNDROMES

		Grade				
Adverse Event	**Short Name**	**1**	**2**	**3**	**4**	**5**
NAVIGATION NOTE: Acute vascular leak syndrome is graded in the VASCULAR CATEGORY.						
NAVIGATION NOTE: Adrenal insufficiency is graded in the ENDOCRINE CATEGORY.						
NAVIGATION NOTE: Adult Respiratory Distress Syndrome (ARDS) is graded in the PULMONARY/UPPER RESPIRATORY CATEGORY.						
Alcohol intolerance syndrome (antabuse-like syndrome)	Alcohol intolerance syndrome	—	—	Present	—	Death
REMARK: An antabuse-like syndrome occurs with some new anti-androgens (e.g., nilutamide) when patient also consumes alcohol.						
NAVIGATION NOTE: Autoimmune reaction is graded as Autoimmune reaction/hypersensitivity (including drug fever) in the ALLERGY/IMMUNOLOGY CATEGORY.						
Cytokine release syndrome/acute infusion reaction	Cytokine release syndrome	Mild reaction; infusion interruption not indicated; intervention not indicated	Requires therapy or infusion interruption but responds promptly to symptomatic treatment (e.g., antihistamines, NSAIDS, narcotics, IV fluids); prophylactic medications indicated for ≤24 hrs	Prolonged (i.e., not rapidly responsive to symptomatic medication and/or brief interruption of infusion); recurrence of symptoms following initial improvement; hospitalization indicated for other clinical sequelae (e.g., renal impairment, pulmonary infiltrates)	Life-threatening; pressor or ventilatory support indicated	Death

(Continued)

Appendix 2 *(continued)*

		Grade				
Adverse Event	**Short Name**	**1**	**2**	**3**	**4**	**5**
REMARK: Cytokine release syndromes/acute infusion reactions are different from Allergic/hypersensitive reactions, although some of the manifestations are common to both AEs. An acute infusion reaction may occur with an agent that causes cytokine release (e.g., monoclonal antibodies or other biological agents). Signs and symptoms usually develop during or shortly after drug infusion and generally resolve completely within 24 hrs of completion of infusion. Signs/symptoms may include: Allergic reaction/hypersensitivity (including drug fever); Arthralgia (joint pain); Bronchospasm; Cough; Dizziness; Dyspnea (shortness of breath); Fatigue (asthenia, lethargy, malaise); Headache; Hypertension; Hypotension; Myalgia (muscle pain); Nausea; Pruritis/itching; Rash/desquamation; Rigors/chills; Sweating (diaphoresis); Tachycardia; Tumor pain (onset or exacerbation of tumor pain due to treatment); Urticaria (hives, welts, wheals); Vomiting. ALSO CONSIDER: Allergic reaction/hypersensitivity (including drug fever); Bronchospasm, wheezing; Dyspnea (shortness of breath); Hypertension; Hypotension; Hypoxia; Prolonged QTc interval; Supraventricular and nodal arrhythmia – *Select*; Ventricular arrhythmia – *Select.*						
NAVIGATION NOTE: Disseminated intravascular coagulation (DIC) is graded in the COAGULATION CATEGORY.						
NAVIGATION NOTE: Fanconi's syndrome is graded as Urinary electrolyte wasting (e.g., Fanconi's syndrome, renal tubular acidosis) in the RENAL/GENITOURINARY CATEGORY.						
Flu-like syndrome	Flu-like syndrome	Symptoms present but not interfering with function	Moderate or causing difficulty performing some ADL	Severe symptoms interfering with ADL	Disabling	Death
REMARK: Flu-like syndrome represents a constellation of symptoms which may include cough with catarrhal symptoms, fever, headache, malaise, myalgia, prostration, and is to be used when the symptoms occur in a cluster consistent with one single pathophysiological process.						
NAVIGATION NOTE: Renal tubular acidosis is graded as Urinary electrolyte wasting (e.g., Fanconi's syndrome, renal tubular acidosis) in the RENAL/GENITOURINARY CATEGORY.						

(Continued)

Appendix 2 *(continued)*

		Grade				
Adverse Event	**Short Name**	**1**	**2**	**3**	**4**	**5**
Retinoic acid syndrome	Retinoic acid syndrome	Fluid retention; less than 3 kg of weight gain; intervention with fluid restriction and/or diuretics indicated	Mild to moderate signs/symptoms; steroids indicated	Severe signs/symptoms; hospitalization indicated	Life-threatening; ventilatory support indicated	Death
REMARK: Patients with acute promyelocytic leukemia may experience a syndrome similar to ''retinoic acid syndrome'' in association with other agents such as arsenic trioxide. The syndrome is usually manifested by otherwise unexplained fever, weight gain, respiratory distress, pulmonary infiltrates and/or pleural effusion, with or without leukocytosis. ALSO CONSIDER: Acute vascular leak syndrome; Pleural effusion (nonmalignant); Pneumonitis/pulmonary infiltrates.						
NAVIGATION NOTE: SIADH is graded as Neuroendocrine: ADH secretion abnormality (e.g., SIADH or low ADH) in the ENDOCRINE CATEGORY.						
NAVIGATION NOTE: Stevens-Johnson syndrome is graded as Rash: erythema multiforme (e.g., Stevens-Johnson syndrome, toxic epidermal necrolysis) in the DERMATOLOGY/SKIN CATEGORY.						
NAVIGATION NOTE: Thrombotic microangiopathy is graded as Thrombotic microangiopathy (e.g., thrombotic thrombocytopenic purpura [TTP] or hemolytic uremic syndrome [HUS]) in the COAGULATION CATEGORY.						
Tumor flare	Tumor flare	Mild pain not interfering with function	Moderate pain; pain or analgesics interfering with function, but not interfering with ADL	Severe pain; pain or analgesics interfering with function and interfering with ADL	Disabling	Death
REMARK: Tumor flare is characterized by a constellation of signs and symptoms in direct relation to initiation of therapy (e.g., anti-estrogens/androgens or additional hormones). The symptoms/signs include tumor pain, inflammation of visible tumor, hypercalcemia, diffuse bone pain, and other electrolyte disturbances. ALSO CONSIDER: Calcium, serum-high (hypercalcemia).						

(Continued)

Appendix 2 *(continued)*

		Grade				
Adverse Event	**Short Name**	**1**	**2**	**3**	**4**	**5**
Tumor lysis syndrome	Tumor lysis syndrome	—	—	Present	—	Death
ALSO CONSIDER: Creatinine; Potassium, serum-high (hyperkalemia).						
Syndromes – Other (Specify, ________)	Syndromes – Other (Specify)	Mild	Moderate	Severe	Life-threatening; disabling	Death

VASCULAR

		Grade				
Adverse Event	**Short Name**	**1**	**2**	**3**	**4**	**5**
Acute vascular leak syndrome	Acute vascular leak syndrome	—	Symptomatic, fluid support not indicated	Respiratory compromise or fluids indicated	Life-threatening; pressor support or ventilatory support indicated	Death
Peripheral arterial ischemia	Peripheral arterial ischemia	—	Brief (<24 hrs) episode of ischemia managed nonsurgically and without permanent deficit	Recurring or prolonged (≥24 hrs) and/or invasive intervention indicated	Life-threatening, disabling and/or associated with end organ damage (e.g., limb loss)	Death
Phlebitis (including superficial thrombosis)	Phlebitis	—	Present	—	—	—
ALSO CONSIDER: Injection site reaction/extravasation changes.						

(Continued)

Appendix 3

Cancer Chemotherapeutic Regimens (Adult)

The use of cancer chemotherapeutic agents in combination is well established. The knowledge of cell kinetics and the pharmacology of antitumor agents have allowed the clinician to use combination therapy to maximize tumor cell kill with minimal or acceptable toxicity to the patient. The basic principles of combination therapy are to use agents that are individually active against a given tumor, in a dosage as close as possible to that used in single-agent therapy; agents with different mechanisms of action; and agents with different or minimally overlapping toxicities.

This review lists some of the common combination regimens and doses used in the cancers noted. It also lists selected single-agent regimens. The included regimens and doses were selected based on the following criteria: regimens published in 2 tertiary references; regimens positively evaluated in Phase II or III trials published in major English language journals; or regimens/agents that have received approval by the Food and Drug Administration with or without published literature. The accuracy of all regimens in this review has been checked against and matched with findings in the scientific literature. Therefore, in each case, references are provided.

This review should serve as a general reference only, as variations of many of the combinations exist, and the dose and frequency of administration may be altered because of tumor response or patient toxicity. These regimens may vary from institution to institution and from physician to physician. *Source:* Modified from Adams VR, DeRemer D, Holdsworth MT. Guide to Cancer Chemotherapy Regimens 2005. *Oncology Special Edition,* volume 7. NY: McMahon Publishing 2005

Adenocarcinoma—Unknown Primary

Carbo-Tax

Carboplatin dose targeted by Calvert equation to AUC 6 mg/mL/min I.V.

FOLLOWED BY

Paclitaxel* 200 mg/m² I.V. over 3 hours, day 1

G-CSF 300 mcg/d SQ, days 5–12

Repeat cycle every 21 days

EP

Cisplatin 60–100 mg/m² I.V., day 1

	Etoposide 80–120 mg/m²/d I.V., days 4, 6, 8, or 3, 5, 7
	Repeat cycle every 21–28 days
Paclitaxel/Carboplatin/ Etoposide	**Paclitaxel*** 200 mg/m² I.V. over 1 hour, day 1
	FOLLOWED BY
	Carboplatin dose targeted by Calvert equation to AUC 6 mg/mL/min I.V.
	Etoposide 50 mg/d PO alternated with 100 mg/d PO, days 1–10
	Repeat cycle every 21 days

References

Carbo-Tax

Briasoulis E, Kalofonos H, Bafaloukos D, et al. Carboplatin plus paclitaxel in unknown primary carcinoma: a phase II Hellenic Cooperative Oncology Group Study. *J Clin Oncol.* 2000;18:3101–3107.

EP

Longeval E, Klastersky J. Combination chemotherapy with cisplatin and etoposide in bronchogenic squamous cell carcinoma and adenocarcinoma. *Cancer.* 1982;50: 2751–2756.

Shepherd FA Treatment of advanced non-small cell lung cancer. *Semin Oncol.* 1994; 21(Suppl 7):7–18.

Paclitaxel, Carboplatin, Etoposide

Hainsworth JD, Erland JB, Kalman LA, et al. Carcinoma of unknown primary site: treatment with 1-hour paclitaxel, carboplatin, and extended-schedule etoposide. *J Clin Oncol.* 1997;15:2385–2393.

AIDS-Related Kaposi's Sarcoma

Single-Agent Regimens

Alitretinoin	Apply generous coat to cutaneous Kaposi's sarcoma lesions bid initially, then gradually increase to tid or qid according to individual lesion tolerance.
Liposomal daunorubicin	**Liposomal daunorubicin** 40 mg/m² I.V. over 60 minutes
	Repeat cycle every 14 days
Pegylated liposomal doxorubicin	**Pegylated liposomal doxorubicin** 20 mg/m² I.V. over 30 minutes
	Repeat cycle every 21 days

Single-Agent Regimen (2nd Line)

Paclitaxel	**Paclitaxel*** 135 mg/m² I.V. over 3 hours
	Repeat cycle every 21 days

OR
Paclitaxel* 100 mg/m^2 I.V. over 3 hours
Repeat cycle every 14 days

References

Alitretinoin

Panretin Gel 0.1% (alitretinoin) (package insert). San Diego, CA: Ligand Pharmaceuticals Inc., 2001.

Liposomal daunorubicin

DaunoXome (package insert). San Dimas, CA: Gilead Sciences; 2002.

Pegylated liposomal doxorubicin

Doxil (package insert). Raritan, NJ: Ortho Biotech Products, LP; 2003.

Paclitaxel

Taxol (package insert). Princeton, NJ: Bristol-Myers Squibb Oncology; 2003.

AIDS-Related Lymphoma

CDE

Cyclophosphamide 200 mg/m^2/d I.V. Cl for 96 hours
Doxorubicin 12.5 mg/m^2/d I.V. CI for 96 hours
Etoposide 60 mg/m^2/d I.V. CI for 96 hours
Repeat cycle every 28 days

CHOP

Cyclophosphamide 750 mg/m^2 I.V., day 1
Doxorubicin 50 mg/m^2 I.V., day 1
Vincristine# 1.4 mg/m^2 I.V., day 1
Prednisone 100 mg/d PO, days 1–5
Doses of doxorubicin/cyclophosphamide may be reduced by up to 50% in high-risk patients
Repeat cycle every 21 days

m-BACOD

Methotrexate 200 mg/m^2 I.V., day 15
Bleomycin 4 units/m^2 I.V., day 1
Doxorubicin 25 mg/m^2 I.V., day 1
Cyclophosphamide 300 mg/m^2 I.V., day 1
Vincristine# 1.4 mg/m^2 I.V., day 1
Dexamethasone 3 mg/m^2/d PO, days 1–5
GM-CSF 5 mcg/kg/d SQ, days 4–13
Repeat cycle when ANC ≥1,000/mm^3 but not earlier than day 22

References

CDE

Sparano JA, Wiernik PH, Hu X, et al. Pilot trial of infusional cyclophosphamide, doxorubicin, and etoposide plus didanosine and filgrastim in patients with human immunodeficiency virus-associated non-Hodgkin's lymphoma. *J Clin Oncol.* 1996;14: 3026–3035.

CHOP

Ratner L, Lee J, Tang S, et al. Chemotherapy for human immunodeficiency virus-associated non-Hodgkin's lymphoma in combination with highly active antiretroviral therapy. *J Clin Oncol.* 2001;19:2171–2178.

Levine AM Acquired immunodeficiency syndrome–related lymphoma: clinical aspects. *Semin Oncol.* 2000;27:442–453.

m-BACOD

Kaplan LD, Straus DJ, Testa MA, et al. Low-dose compared with standard-dose m-BACOD chemotherapy for non-Hodgkin's lymphoma associated with human immunodeficiency virus infection. *N Engl J Med.* 1997;336:1641–1648.

Breast Cancer

Combination Regimens

AC	**Doxorubicin** 60 mg/m^2 I.V., day 1 **Cyclophosphamide** 600 mg/m^2 I.V., day 1 *Repeat cycle every 21 days*
AT	**Doxorubicin** 50 mg/m^2 I.V., day 1 **FOLLOWED 24 HOURS LATER BY** **Paclitaxel*** 220 mg/m^2 I.V. over 3 hours, day 2 *Repeat cycle every 21 days for up to 8 cycles*
A→T→C→ (dose dense)	**Doxorubicin** 60 mg/m^2 I.V. q 2 wk × 4 cycles (dose dense) **FOLLOWED BY** **Paclitaxel** 175 mg/m^2 I.V. q 2 wk × 4 cycles **FOLLOWED BY** **Cyclophosphamide** 600 mg/m^2 I.V. q 2 wk × 4 cycles *Administer filgrastim 5 mcg/kg SQ on days 3-10 of each 2 week cycle*
CAF	**Cyclophosphamide** 500 mg/m^2 I.V., day 1 **Doxorubicin** 50 mg/m^2 I.V., day 1 **Fluorouracil** 500 mg/m^2 I.V., day 1 *Repeat cycle every 21 days*
CEF (FEC)	**Cyclophosphamide** 75 mg/m^2/d PO, days 1–14 **Epirubicin** 60 mg/m^2/d I.V., days 1, 8 **Fluorouracil** 500 mg/m^2/d I.V., days 1, 8

	Repeat cycle every 28 days for 6 cycles
	OR
	Cyclophosphamide 500 mg/m^2 I.V., day 1
	Epirubicin 100 mg/m^2 I.V., day 1
	Fluorouracil 500 mg/m^2 I.V., day 1
	Repeat cycle every 21 days for 4 cycles
CFM (CNF, FNC)	**Cyclophosphamide** 600 mg/m^2 I.V., day 1
	Fluorouracil 600 mg/m^2 I.V., day 1
	Mitoxantrone 12 mg/m^2 I.V., day 1
	Repeat cycle every 21 days
CMF	**Cyclophosphamide** 100 mg/m^2/d PO, days 1–14 or 600 mg/m^2/d I.V., days 1, 8
	Methotrexate 40 mg/m^2/d I.V., days 1, 8 (for patients >60 years, 30 mg/m^2)
	Fluorouracil 600 mg/m^2/d I.V., days 1, 8 (for patients >60 years, 400 mg/m^2)
	Repeat cycle every 28 days
	OR
	Cyclophosphamide 600 mg/m^2 I.V., day 1
	Methotrexate 40 mg/m^2 I.V., day 1
	Fluorouracil 600 mg/m^2 I.V., day 1
	Repeat cycle every 21 days
Gem/Tax	**Gemcitabine** 1,250 mg/m^2 I.V. over 30 min. days 1,8
	Paclitaxel 175 mg/m^2 I.V. over 3 hr. before gemcitabine day 1
	Repeat cycle every 21 days
HEC	**Epirubicin** 100 mg/m^2 I.V., day 1
	Cyclophosphamide 830 mg/m^2 I.V., day 1
	Repeat cycle every 21 days for up to 8 cycles
NA	**Vinorelbine** 25 mg/m^2/d I.V., days 1, 8
	Doxorubicin 50 mg/m^2 I.V., day 1
	Repeat cycle every 21 days
NFL	**Mitoxantrone** 10 mg/m^2 I.V., day 1
	Fluorouracil 1,000 mg/m^2/d I.V. CI, days 1–3
	Leucovorin 100 mg/m^2/d I.V. over 15 minutes, days 1–3
	Repeat cycle every 21 days
	OR
	Mitoxantrone 12 mg/m^2 I.V., day 1
	Fluorouracil 350 mg/m^2/d I.V. bolus, days 1–3 after leucovorin
	Leucovorin 300 mg/d I.V. over 30–60 minutes, days 1–3
	Repeat cycle every 21 days

Paclitaxel/Virorelbine	**Paclitaxel*** 135 mg/m^2 I.V. CI over 3 hours, starting 1 hour after vinorelbine, day 1 **Vinorelbine** 30 mg/m^2/d I.V. over 20 minutes, days 1, 8 *Repeat cycle every 28 days*
Sequential AC/ Paclitaxel	**Doxorubicin** 60–90 mg/m^2 I.V., day 1 **Cyclophosphamide** 600 mg/m^2 I.V., day 1 *Repeat cycle every 21 days for 4 cycles,* **FOLLOWED BY** **Paclitaxel*** 175 mg/m^2 I.V. *Repeat cycle every 21 days for 4 cycles*
Sequential Dox-CMF	**Doxorubicin** 75 mg/m^2 I.V. every 21 days for 4 cycles, **FOLLOWED BY** 21- or 28-day CMF *(see previous page)* for 8 cycles
TAC	**Doxorubicin** 50 mg/m^2 as a 15-minute I.V. bolus, **FOLLOWED IMMEDIATELY BY** **Cyclosphosphamide** 500 mg/m^2 as 15-minute I.V. bolus, **FOLLOWED 1 HOUR AFTER COMPLETION OF THE DOXORUBICIN INFUSION BY** **Docetaxel** 75 mg/m^2 I.V. over 1 hour
Tamoxifen/Epirubicin Epirubicin	**Tamoxifen** 20 mg/d PO for 4 years **Epirubicin** 50 mg/m^2/d I.V., days 1, 8 *Repeat epirubicin cycle every 28 days for 6 cycles*
Trastuzumab/Paclitaxel	**Trastuzumab** 4 mg/kg I.V. loading dose over 90 minutes, **FOLLOWED BY** **Trastuzumab** 2 mg/kg I.V. over 30 minutes, weekly **Paclitaxel*** 175 mg/m^2 over 3 hours, every 21 days for at least 6 cycles
X + T	**Capecitabine** 1,250 mg/m^2 PO bid, days 1–14 **Docetaxel** 75 mg/m^2 as a 1-hour I.V. infusion, day 1 *Repeat cycle every 21 days*

Monoclonal Antibody Regimen

Trastuzumab	**Trastuzumab** 4 mg/kg I.V. loading dose over 90 minutes, **FOLLOWED BY** 2 mg/kg I.V. over 30 minutes, weekly

Single-Agent Regimens

Abraxane	**Paclitaxel** protein-bound particles for injectable suspension 260 mg/m^2 I.V. every 3 weeks

Anastrozole	**Anastrozole** 1 mg/d PO
Capecitabine	**Capecitabine** 1,250–1,255 mg/m^2 PO bid, days 1–14, followed by 7 days rest *Repeat cycle every 21 days*
Docetaxel	**Docetaxel** 60–100 mg/m^2 I.V., over 1 hour, every 21 days All patients should be premedicated with oral corticosteroids such as dexamethasone 16 mg/d (e.g., 8 mg bid) for 3 days starting 1 day prior to docetaxel administration. **Docetaxel** 40 mg/m^2 q wk × 6, repeated q 8 weeks
Exemestane	**Exemestane** 25 mg/d PO
Fulvestrant	**Fulvestrant** 250 mg IM into the buttock every month
Gemcitabine	**Gemcitabine** 725 mg/m^2/d I.V. over 30 minutes, days 1, 8, 15 *Repeat cycle every 28 days*
Letrozole	**Letrozole** 2.5 mg/d PO
Megestrol	**Megestrol** 40 mg PO qid
Paclitaxel	**Paclitaxel*** 250 mg/m^2 I.V. over 3 or 24 hours, every 21 days **OR** **Paclitaxel*** 175 mg/m^2 I.V. over 3 hours, every 21 days
Tamoxifen	**Tamoxifen** 20–40 mg/d, dosages >20 mg/d should be given in divided doses (morning and evening)
Toremifene	**Toremifene** 60 mg/d PO
Vinorelbine	**Vinorelbine** 30 mg/m^2 I.V. every 7 days

References

AC

Fisher B, Brown AM, Dimitrov NV, et al. Two months of doxorubicin–cyclophosphamide with and without interval reinduction therapy compared with 6 months of cyclophosphamide, methotrexate, and fluorouracil in positive-node breast cancer patients with tamoxifen-nonresponsive tumors: results from the National Surgical Adjuvant Breast and Bowel Project B-15. *J Clin Oncol.* 1990;8:1483–1496.

ATC

Citron ML, Berry DA, Cirrincione C, et al. Randomized trial of dose-dense versus conventionally scheduled and sequential versus concurrent combination chemotherapy as postoperative adjuvant treatment of node-positive primary breast cancer: First report of intergroup trial C9741/Cancer and Leukemia Group B Trial 9741 *Clin J Oncol* 2003;21:1431–1439.

AT

Jassem J, Pienkowski T, Pluzanska A, et al. Doxorubicin and paclitaxel versus fluorouracil, doxorubicin, and cyclophosphamide as first-line therapy for women with metastatic breast cancer: final results of a randomized phase III multicenter trial. *J Clin Oncol.* 2001;19:1707–1715.

CAF

Smalley RV, Lefante J, Bartolucci A, et al. A comparison of cyclophosphamide, adriamycin, and 5-fluorouracil (CAF) and cyclophosphamide, methotrexate, 5-fluorouracil, vincristine, and prednisone (CMFVP) in patients with advanced breast cancer. *Breast Cancer Res Treat.* 1983;3:209–220.

CEF (FEC)

Levine MN, Bramwell VH, Pritchard KI, et al. Randomized trial of intensive cyclophosphamide, epirubicin, and fluorouracil chemotherapy compared with cyclophosphamide, methotrexate, and fluorouracil in premenopausal women with node-positive breast cancer. *J Clin Oncol.* 1998;16:2651–2658.

French Epirubicin Study Group. Epirubicin-based chemotherapy in metastatic breast cancer patients: role of dose intensity and duration of treatment. *J Clin Oncol.* 2000;18: 3115–3124.

CFM (CNF, FNC)

Alonso MC, Tabernero JM, Ojeda B, et al. A phase III randomized trial of cyclophosphamide, mitoxantrone and 5-fluorouracil (CNF) versus cyclophosphamide, adriamycin, and 5-fluorouracil (CAF) in patients with metastatic breast cancer. *Breast Cancer Res Treat.* 1995;34:15–24.

CMF

Bonadonna G, Valagussa P, Moliterni A, Zambetti M, Brambilla C. Adjuvant cyclophosphamide, methotrexate, and fluorouracil in node-positive breast cancer: the results of 20 years of follow-up. *N Engl J Med.* 1995;332:901–906.

Bonadonna G, Zambetti M, Valagussa P. Sequential or alternating doxorubicin and CMF regimens in breast cancer with more than three positive nodes: ten year results. *JAMA.* 1995;273:542–547.

Gemcitabine/Paclitaxel

Gemzar [package insert]. Indianapolis, IN: Eli Lilly and Company; 2004

HEC

Piccart MJ, Di Leo A, et al. Phase III trial comparing two dose levels of epirubicin combined with cyclophosphamide with cyclophosphamide, methotrexate, and fluorouracil in node-positive breast cancer. *J Clin Oncol.* 2001;19:3103–3110.

NA

Blajman C, Balbiani L, Block J, et al. A prospective, randomized Phase III trial comparing combination chemotherapy with cyclophosphamide, doxorubicin, and 5-fluorouracil with vinorelbine plus doxorubicin in the treatment of advanced breast carcinoma. *Cancer.* 1999;85:1091–1097.

NFL

Jones SE, Mennel RG, Brooks B, et al. Phase II study of mitoxantrone, leucovorin, and infusional fluorouracil for treatment of metastatic breast cancer. *J Clin Oncol.* 1991;9: 1736–1739.

Hainsworth JD, Jolivet J, Birch R, et al. Mitoxantrone, 5-fluorouracil, and high-dose leucovorin (NFL) versus intravenous cyclophosphamide, methotrexate, and 5-fluorouracil (CMF) in first-line chemotherapy for patients with metastatic breast carcinoma: a randomized phase II trial. *Cancer.* 1997;79:740–748.

Paclitaxel/Vinorelbine

Acuña LR, Langhi M, Pérez J, et al. Vinorelbine and paclitaxel as first-line chemotherapy in metastatic breast cancer. *J Clin Oncol.* 1999;17:74–81.

Sequential AC/Paclitaxel

Henderson IC, Berry DA, Demetri GD, et al. Improved outcomes from adding sequential paclitaxel but not from escalating doxorubicin dose in an adjuvant chemotherapy regimen for patients with node-positive primary breast cancer. *J Clin Oncol.* 2003;21: 976–983.

Taxol (package insert). Princeton, NJ: Bristol-Myers Squibb Oncology; 2003.

Sequential Dox-CMF

Bonadonna G, Zambetti M, Valagussa P. Sequential or alternating doxorubicin and CMF regimens in breast cancer with more than three positive nodes: ten year results. *JAMA.* 1995;273:542–547.

TAC

Nabholtz JM, Pienkowski T, Mackey J, et al. Phase III trial comparing TAC (docetaxel, doxorubicin, cyclophosphamide) with FAC (5-fluorouracil, doxorubicin, cyclophosphamide) in the adjuvant treatment of node-positive breast cancer (BC) patients: interim analysis of the BCIRG 001 study (abstract). *Proc Am Soc Clin Oncol.* 2002;21: 36a. Abstract 141.

Tamoxifen/Epirubicin

Wils JA, Bliss JM, Marty M, et al. Epirubicin plus tamoxifen versus tamoxifen alone in node-positive postmenopausal patients with breast cancer: a randomized trial of the International Collaborative Cancer Group. *J Clin Oncol.* 1999;17:1988–1998.

Trastuzumab/Paclitaxel

Slamon D, Leyland-Jones B, Shak S, et al. Use of chemotherapy plus a monoclonal antibody against HER2 for metastatic breast cancer that overexpresses HER2. *N Engl J Med.* 2001;344:783–792.

Herceptin (package insert). South San Francisco, CA: Genentech, Inc; 2003.

X + T

Xeloda (package insert). Nutley, NJ: Roche Pharmaceuticals; 2003.

Trastuzumab

Herceptin (package insert). South San Francisco, CA: Genentech, Inc; 2003.

Abraxane

(package insert). South San Francisco, CA: Genentech, Inc; 2004.

Anastrozole

Arimidex (package insert). Wilmington, DE: AstraZeneca Pharmaceuticals; 2003.

Capecitabine

Blum JL, Jones SE, Buzdar AU, et al. Multicenter phase II study of capecitabine in paclitaxel-refractory metastatic breast cancer. *J Clin Oncol.* 1999;17:485–493.

Xeloda (package insert). Nutley, NJ: Roche Pharmaceuticals; 2003.

Docetaxel

Burstein HJ, Manol J, Younger J, et al. Docetaxel administered on a weekly basis for metastatic breast cancer. *J Clin Oncol.* 2001;18(6):1212–1219.

Chan S, Friedrichs K, Noel D, et al. Prospective randomized trial of docetaxel versus doxorubicin in patients with metastatic breast cancer. *J Clin Oncol.* 1999;17: 2341–2354.

Nabholtz JM, Senn HJ, Bezwoda WR, et al. Prospective randomized trial of docetaxel versus mitomycin plus vinblastine in patients with metastatic breast cancer progressing despite previous anthracycline-containing chemotherapy. *J Clin Oncol.* 1999;17: 1413–1424.

Taxotere (package insert). Bridgewater, NJ: Aventis Pharmaceuticals; 2003.

Exemestane

Lønning PE, Bajetta E, Murray R, et al. Activity of exemestane in metastatic breast cancer after failure of nonsteroidal aromatase inhibitors: a phase II trial. *J Clin Oncol.* 2000;18:2234–2244.

Kaufmann M, Bajetta E, Dirix LY, et al. Exemestane is superior to megestrol acetate after tamoxifen failure in postmenopausal women with advanced breast cancer: results of a phase III randomized double-blind trial. The Exemestane Study Group. *J Clin Oncol.* 2000;18:1399–1411.

Coombes RC, Hall E, Gibson LJ, et al. A randomized trial of exemestane after two to three years of tamoxifen therapy in postmenopausal women with primary breast cancer. *N Engl J Med.* 2004;350:1081–1092.

Aromasin (package insert). New York, NY: Pfizer; 2003.

Fulvestrant

Faslodex (package insert). Wilmington, DE: AstraZeneca Pharmaceuticals LP; 2003.

Gemcitabine

Carmichael J, Possinger K, Phillip P, et al. Advanced breast cancer: a phase II trial with gemcitabine. *J Clin Oncol.* 1995;13:2731–2736.

Letrozole

Dombernowsky P, Smith I, Falkson G, et al. Letrozole, a new oral aromatase inhibitor for advanced breast cancer: double-blind randomized trial showing a dose effect and improved efficacy and tolerability compared with megestrol acetate. *J Clin Oncol.* 1998; 16:453–461.

Ingle JN, et al. A randomized phase II trial of two dosage levels of letrozole as third-line hormonal therapy for women with metastatic breast cancer. *Cancer.* 1997;80: 218–224.

Goss PE, Ingle JN, Martino S, et al. A randomized trial of letrozole in postmenopausal women after five years of tamoxifen therapy for early-stage breast cancer. *N Engl J Med.* 2003;349:1793–1802.

Megestrol

Megace (package insert). Princeton, NJ: Bristol-Myers Squibb Oncology; 2002.

Paclitaxel

Seidman AD, Tiersten A, Hudis C, et al. Phase II trial of paclitaxel by 3-hour infusion as initial and salvage chemotherapy for metastatic breast cancer. *J Clin Oncol.* 1995;13: 2575–2581.

Smith RE, et al. Randomized trial of 3-hour versus 24-hour infusion of high-dose paclitaxel in patients with metastatic or locally advanced breast cancer: National Surgical Adjuvant Breast and Bowel Project Protocol B-26. *J Clin Oncol.* 1999;17:3403–3411.

Tamoxifen

Nolvadex (package insert). Wilmington, DE: AstraZeneca; 2003.

Toremifene

Hayes DF, Van Zyl JA, Hacking A, et al. Randomized comparison of tamoxifen and two separate doses of toremifene in postmenopausal patients with metastatic breast cancer. *J Clin Oncol.* 1995;13:2556–2566.

Fareston (package insert). Newport, KY: Shire Pharmaceuticals; 1999.

Vinorelbine

Weber BL, Vogel C, Jones S, et al. Intravenous vinorelbine as first-line and second-line therapy in advanced breast cancer. *J Clin Oncol.* 1995;13:2722–2730.

Colorectal Cancer

Combination Regimens

Cetuximab/Irinotecan	**Cetuximab** 400 mg/m² I.V. initial dose, then 250 mg/m² I.V. every 7 days **Irinotecan** 350 mg/m² I.V. every 21 days **OR** 180 mg/m² I.V. every 14 days **OR** 125 mg/m² I.V. every 7 days × 4 doses every 6 weeks
Fluorouracil/Leucovorin (Mayo regimen)	**Fluorouracil** 370 mg/m²/d I.V. bolus 1 hour after start of leucovorin, days 1–5 **Leucovorin** 200 mg/m²/d I.V. bolus, days 1–5 *Repeat cycle at 4 and 8 weeks, and every 5 weeks thereafter*
Fluorouracil/Leucovorin (Roswell Park regimen)	**Fluorouracil** 600 mg/m²/d I.V. bolus 1 hour after start of leucovorin, days 1, 8, 15, 22, 29, 35 **Leucovorin** 500 mg/m²/d I.V. over 2 hours, days 1, 8, 15, 22, 29, 35 *Repeat cycle every 8 weeks*
IFL (Saltz regimen)	**Irinotecan** 125 mg/m²/d I.V. over 90 minutes, days 1, 8, 15, 22 **Leucovorin** 20 mg/m²/d I.V. bolus, days 1, 8, 15, 22 **Fluorouracil** 500 mg/m²/d I.V. bolus, days 1, 8, 15, 22 *Repeat cycle every 6 weeks*

IFL/BV	**IFL** (see above) **Bevacizumab** 5 mg/kg I.V. every 14 days
Douillard regimen	**Irinotecan** 180 mg/m² I.V., day 1 **Leucovorin** 200 mg/m²/d I.V., days 1, 2 **Fluorouracil** 400 mg/m² I.V. bolus and **Fluorouracil** 600 mg/m² I.V. over 22 hours, day 1 *Repeat cycle every 14 days*
Oxaliplatin/ Fluorouracil/ Leucovorin (FOLFOX4)	**Oxaliplatin** 85 mg/m² I.V. and Leucovorin 200 mg/m² I.V. over 120 minutes at same time (separate bags, Y-line), day 1, **FOLLOWED BY** **Fluorouracil** 400 mg/m² I.V. bolus over 2–4 minutes, day 1, **FOLLOWED BY** **Fluorouracil** 600 mg/m² I.V. CI over 22 hours, day 1 **Leucovorin** 200 mg/m² I.V. over 120 minutes, day 2, **FOLLOWED BY** **Fluorouracil** 400 mg/m² I.V. bolus over 2–4 minutes, day 2, **FOLLOWED BY** **Fluorouracil** 600 mg/m² I.V. CI over 22 hours, day 2 *Repeat cycle every 14 days*
(FOLFOX6)	**Oxaliplatin** 85-100 mg/m² I.V. and Leucovorin 200 mg/m² I.V. over 120 minutes at same time (separate bags, Y-line), day 1, **FOLLOWED BY** **Fluorouracil** 400 mg/m² I.V. bolus day 1 **FOLLOWED BY** **Fluorouracil** 2,400-3,000 mg/m² I.V. CI over 46 hours *Repeat cycle every 14 days*
FOLFOX+BV	**FOLFOX regimen as above** **Bevacizumab** 5 mg/kg I.V. over 90 min then repeated q 2 wk; if well tolerated, next infusion is over 60 min; if this goes well; subsequent infusions are over 30 min
XELIRI	**Irinotecan** 250 mg/m² I.V. day 1 **Capecitabine** 1,000 mg/m² PO bid from the evening of day 1 to morning of day 15. *Repeat cycle every 21 days*
XELOX	**Oxaliplatin** 130 mg/m² I.V. day 1 **Capecitabine** 1,000 mg/m² PO bid from the evening of day 1 to morning of day 15. *Repeat cycle every 21 days*

Single-Agent Regimens

Capecitabine	**Capecitabine** 2,500 mg/m²/d PO in 2 divided doses, days 1–14, followed by 7 days rest *Repeat cycle every 21 days*
Cetuximab	**Cetuximab** 400 mg/m² I.V. initial dose, then 250 mg/m² I.V. every 7 days *For irinotecan-intolerant patients*
5-Fluorouracil	**5-Fluorouracil** 1,000 mg/m²/d I.V. CI, days 1–5 *Repeat cycle every 28 days*
Irinotecan	**Irinotecan** 125 mg/m²/d I.V. over 90 minutes, days 1, 8, 15, 22 *Repeat cycle every 6 weeks* **OR** **Irinotecan** 350 mg/m² I.V. over 90 minutes, day 1 *Repeat cycle every 21 days*

References

Cetuximab/Irinotecan

Erbitux (package insert). Branchburg, NJ and Princeton, NJ: ImClone Systems/Bristol-Myers Squibb; 2004.

Fluorouracil/Leucovorin (Mayo regimen)

Poon MA, O'Connell MJ, Moertel CG. Biochemical modulation of fluorouracil: evidence of significant improvement of survival and quality of life in patients with advanced colorectal carcinoma. *J Clin Oncol.* 1989;7:1407–1418.

Fluorouracil/Leucovorin (Roswell Park regimen)

Petrelli N, et al. The modulation of fluorouracil with leucovorin in metastatic colorectal carcinoma: a prospective randomized phase III trial. *J Clin Oncol.* 1989;7:1419–1426.

Petrelli N, Herrera L, Rustum Y, et al. A prospective randomized trial of 5-fluorouracil versus 5-fluorouracil and high-dose leucovorin versus 5-fluorouracil and methotrexate in previously untreated patients with advanced colorectal carcinoma. *J Clin Oncol.* 1987;5:1559–1565.

IFL (Saltz regimen)

Saltz LB, Cox JV, Blanke C, et al. Irinotecan plus fluorouracil and leucovorin for metastatic colorectal cancer. *N Engl J Med.* 2000;343:905–914.

IFL/BV and FOLFOX/BV

Avastin (package insert). South San Francisco, CA: Genentech, Inc; 2004.

Hurwitz H, Fehrenbacher L, Cartwright T, et al. Bevacizumab prolongs survival in first-line colorectal cancer: results of a phase III trial of bevacizumab in combination with bolus IFL as first-line therapy in subjects with metastatic CRC. Abstract presented at: The 39th Annual Meeting of the American Society of Clinical Oncology. May 31, June 3, 2003; Chicago, Ill. Abstract 3646.

Douillard

Douillard JY, Cunningham D, Roth AD, et al. Irinotecan combined with fluorouracil compared with fluorouracil alone as first-line treatment for metastatic colorectal cancer: a multicentre randomised trial. *Lancet.* 2000;355:1041–1047.

Oxaliplatin/Fluorouracil/Leucovorin (FOLFOX4)

Eloxatin (package insert). New York, NY: Sanofi Aventis; 2004.

FOLFOX6

Tournigand C, Andre T, Achille E, et al. FOLFIRI followed by FOLFOX6 on the reverse sequence in advanced colorectal cancer: a randomized GERCOR study. *J Clin Oncol.* 2004;22:229–237.

XELOX

Cassidy J, Tabernero J, Twelves C, et al. XELOX (capecitabine plus oxaliplatin): active first-line therapy for patients with metastatic colorectal cancer. *J Clin Oncol.* 2004;22: 2084–2091.

Capecitabine

Cox JV, Pazdur R, Thibault A, et al. A phase III trial of Xeloda (capecitabine) in previously untreated advanced/metastatic colorectal cancer (abstract). *Proc Am Soc Clin Oncol.* 1999;18:265a. Abstract 1016.

Patt YZ, Liebmann J, Diamandidis D, et al. Capecitabine (X) plus irinotecan (XELIRI) as first-line treatment for metastatic colorectal cancer (MCRC): Final safety findings from a phase II trial [Abstract 3602]. *Proc Am Soc Clin Oncol.* 23:271.

Van Cutsem E, Findlay M, Osterwalder B, et al. Capecitabine, an oral fluoropyrimidine carbamate with substantial activity in advanced colorectal cancer: results of a randomized phase II study. *J Clin Oncol.* 2000;18:1337–1345.

Cetuximab

Erbitux (package insert). Branchburg, NJ and Princeton NJ: ImClone Systems; Bristol-Myers Squibb; 2004.

5-Fluorouracil

Kemeny N, Israel K, Neidzweiki D, et al. Randomized study of continuous-infusion fluorouracil versus fluorouracil plus cisplatin in patients with metastatic colorectal cancer. *J Clin Oncol.* 1990;8:313–318.

Schmoll HJ. Development of treatment for advanced colorectal cancer: infusional 5-FU and the rôle of new agents. *Eur J Cancer.* 1996;32A(suppl 5):S18–S22.

Irinotecan

Rougier P, Bugat R, Douillard JY, et al. Phase II study of irinotecan in the treatment of advanced colorectal cancer in chemotherapy-naïve patients and patients pretreated with fluorouracil-based chemotherapy. *J Clin Oncol.* 1997;15:251–260.

Camptosar (package insert). New York, NY: Pfizer; 2002.

Conti JA, Kemeny NE, Saltz LB, et al. Irinotecan is an active agent in untreated patients with metastatic colorectal cancer. *J Clin Oncol.* 1996;14:709–715.

Cunningham D, Pyrhönen S, James RD, et al. Randomised trial of irinotecan plus supportive care versus supportive care alone after fluorouracil failure for patients with metastatic colorectal cancer. *Lancet.* 1998;352:1413–1418.

Gastric Cancer

Docetaxel/Cisplatin	**Docetaxel** 85 mg/m² I.V. over 1 hour, day 1, **FOLLOWED BY** **Cisplatin** 75 mg/m² I.V. over 1 hour, day 1 *Repeat cycle every 21 days for a maximum of 8 cycles*
ECF	**Epirubicin** 50 mg/m² I.V., day 1 **Cisplatin** 60 mg/m² I.V., day 1 *Repeat cycle every 21 days for a maximum of 8 cycles* **WITH** **Fluorouracil** 200 mg/m²/d I.V. CI, for up to 6 months
ELF	**Leucovorin** 150 mg/m²/d I.V. over 10 minutes, **FOLLOWED BY** **Etoposide** 120 mg/m²/d I.V. over 30 minutes, **FOLLOWED BY** **Fluorouracil** 500 mg/m²/d I.V. over 10 minutes *Give all agents on days 1–3; repeat cycle every 3 weeks* **OR** **Leucovorin** 300 mg/m²/d I.V. over 10 minutes, **FOLLOWED BY** **Etoposide** 120 mg/m²/d I.V. over 50 minutes, **FOLLOWED BY** **Fluorouracil** 500 mg/m²/d I.V. bolus *Give all agents on days 1–3; repeat cycle every 3 weeks*
FAMTX	**Methotrexate** 1,500 mg/m² I.V., day 1, **FOLLOWED 1 HOUR LATER BY** **Fluorouracil** 1,500 mg/m² I.V., day 1, FOLLOWED 24 HOURS AFTER METHOTREXATE DOSE BY **Leucovorin** 15 mg/m² PO every 6 hours for 48 hours **Doxorubicin** 30 mg/m² I.V., day 15 *Repeat cycle every 28 days*
5-FU/LV	**Fluorouracil** 425 mg/m²/d for 5 days **Leucovorin** 20 mg/m²/d for 5 days **FOLLOWED BY** **Radiation** 4,500 cGy (180 cGy/d), 5 days a week for 5 weeks **Fluorouracil** 400 mg/m²/d I.V., on the first 4 and last 3 days of radiation **Leucovorin** 20 mg/m²/d, on the first 4 and last 3 days of radiation **FOLLOWED 1 AND 2 MONTHS LATER BY** **Fluorouracil** 425 mg/m²/d for 5 days

	Leucovorin 20 mg/m²/d for 5 days
FUP	**Fluorouracil** 1,000 mg/m²/d I.V. CI, days 1–5
	Cisplatin 100 mg/m² I.V. over 1 hour, day 2
	Repeat cycle every 4 weeks

References

Docetaxel/Cisplatin

Roth AD, Maibach R, Martinelli G, et al. Docetaxel (Taxotere)-cisplatin (TC): an effective drug combination in gastric carcinoma. *Ann Oncol.* 2000;11:301–306.

ECF

Waters JS, Norman A, Cunningham D, et al. Long-term survival after epirubicin, cisplatin and fluorouracil for gastric cancer: results of a randomized trial. *Br J Cancer.* 1999;80:269–272.

ELF

di Bartolomeo M, Bajetta E, de Braud F, et al. Phase II study of the etoposide, leucovorin and fluorouracil combination for patients with advanced gastric cancer unsuitable for aggressive chemotherapy. *Oncology.* 1995;52:41–44.

Vanhoefer U, Rougier P, Wilke H, et al. Final results of a randomized phase III trial of sequential high-dose methotrexate, fluorouracil, and doxorubicin versus etoposide, leucovorin, and fluorouracil versus infusional fluorouracil and cisplatin in advanced gastric cancer: a trial of the European Organization for Research and Treatment of Cancer Gastrointestinal Tract Cancer Cooperative Group. *J Clin Oncol.* 2000;18: 2648–2657.

FAMTX

Wils J, Bleiberg H, Dalesio O, et al. An EORTC Gastrointestinal Group evaluation of the combination of sequential methotrexate and 5-fluorouracil, combined with adriamycin in advanced measurable gastric cancer. *J Clin Oncol.* 1986;4:1799–1803.

5-FU/LV

Macdonald JS, Smalley SR, Benedetti J, et al. Chemoradiotherapy after surgery compared with surgery alone for adenocarcinoma of the stomach or gastroesophageal junction. *N Engl J Med.* 2001;345:725–730.

FUP

Vanhoefer U, Rougier P, Wilke H, et al. Final results of a randomized phase III trial of sequential high-dose methotrexate, fluorouracil, and doxorubicin versus etoposide, leucovorin, and fluorouracil versus infusional fluorouracil and cisplatin in advanced gastric cancer: a trial of the European Organization for Research and Treatment of Cancer Gastrointestinal Tract Cancer Cooperative Group. *J Clin Oncol.* 2000;18: 2648–2657.

Genitourinary Malignancy—Bladder

Combination Regimens

CISCA	**Cyclophosphamide** 650 mg/m^2 I.V. over 15 minutes, day 1
	Doxorubicin 50 mg/m^2 I.V. over 15 minutes, day 1
	Cisplatin 100 mg/m^2 I.V. over 2 hours, day 2
	Repeat cycle every 21 days
Cisplatin/Docetaxel	**Cisplatin** 30 mg/m^2/d I.V. over 30 minutes, days 1, 8, 15, 22, 29, 36, 43, 50
	Docetaxel 40 mg/m^2/d I.V. over 1 hour, days 4, 11, 18, 25, 32, 39, 46, 53 with radiation
	OR
	Cisplatin 75 mg/m^2 I.V., day 1
	Docetaxel 75 mg/m^2 I.V. over 1 hour, day 1
	Repeat cycle every 21 days
CMV	**Cisplatin** 100 mg/m^2 I.V. over 4 hours, day 2 (12 hours after methotrexate and vinblastine)
	Methotrexate 30 mg/m^2/d I.V., days 1, 8
	Vinblastine 4 mg/m^2/d I.V., days 1, 8
	Repeat cycle every 21 days
Gemcitabine/Cisplatin	**Gemcitabine** 1,000 mg/m^2/d I.V. over 30–60 minutes, days 1, 8, 15
Cisplatin	**Cisplatin** 70 mg/m^2 I.V., day 2
	Repeat cycle every 28 days
MVAC	**Methotrexate** 30 mg/m^2/d I.V., days 1, 15, 22
	Vinblastine 3 mg/m^2/d I.V., days 2, 15, 22
	Doxorubicin 30 mg/m^2 I.V., day 2
	Cisplatin 70 mg/m^2 I.V., day 2
	Repeat cycle every 28 days
PC	**Paclitaxel*** 200 mg/m^2 or 150–225 mg/m^2 over 3 hours, day 1
	Carboplatin targeted by Calvert equation to AUC 5 or 6 mg/mL/min I.V., after paclitaxel, day 1
	Repeat cycle every 21 days

Single-Agent Regimens

Gemcitabine	**Gemcitabine** 1,200 mg/m^2/d I.V. over 30 minutes, days 1, 8, 15
	Repeat cycle every 28 days
Paclitaxel	**Paclitaxel*** 250 mg/m^2 I.V. over 24 hours, day 1
	Repeat cycle every 21 days

References

CISCA

Sternberg JJ, Bracken RB, Handel PB, Johnson DE. Combination chemotherapy (CISCA) for advanced urinary tract carcinoma: a preliminary report. *JAMA.* 1977;238: 2282–2287.

Cisplatin/Docetaxel

Varveris H, Delakas D, Anezinis P, et al. Concurrent platinum and docetaxel chemotherapy and external radical radiotherapy in patients with invasive transitional cell bladder carcinoma: a preliminary report of tolerance and local control. *Anticancer Res.* 1997; 17:4771–4780.

Sengelov L, Kamby C, Lund B, Engelholm SA. Docetaxel and cisplatin in metastatic urothelial cancer: a phase II study. *J Clin Oncol.* 1998;16:3392–3397.

CMV

Harker WG, Meyers FJ, Freiha FS, et al. Cisplatin, methotrexate, and vinblastine (CMV): an effective chemotherapy regimen for metastatic transitional cell carcinoma of the urinary tract: a Northern California Oncology Group study. *J Clin Oncol.* 1985;3: 1463–1470.

Gemcitabine/Cisplatin

von der Maase H, Hansen SW, Roberts JT, et al. Gemcitabine and cisplatin versus methotrexate, vinblastine, doxorubicin, and cisplatin in advanced or metastatic bladder cancer: results of a large, randomized, multinational, multicenter, phase III study. *J Clin Oncol.* 2000;17:3068–3077.

MVAC

von der Maase H, Hansen SW, Roberts JT, et al. Gemcitabine and cisplatin versus methotrexate, vinblastine, doxorubicin, and cisplatin in advanced or metastatic bladder cancer: results of a large, randomized, multinational, multicenter, phase III study. *J Clin Oncol.* 2000;17:3068–3077.

PC

Redman BG, Smith DC, Flaherty L, Du W, Hussain M. Phase II trial of paclitaxel and carboplatin in the treatment of advanced urothelial carcinoma. *J Clin Oncol.* 1998;16: 1844–1848.

Vaughn DJ, Malkowicz SB, Zoltick B, et al. Paclitaxel plus carboplatin in advanced carcinoma of the urothelium: an active and tolerable outpatient regimen. *J Clin Oncol.* 1998;16:255–260.

Gemcitabine

Moore MJ, Tannock IF, Ernst DS, Huan S, Murray N. Gemcitabine: a promising new agent in the treatment of advanced urothelial cancer. *J Clin Oncol.* 1997;15: 3441–3445.

Stadler WM, Kuzel T, Roth B, Roghavan D, Dorr FA. Phase II study of single-agent gemcitabine in previously untreated patients with metastatic urothelial cancer. *J Clin Oncol.* 1997;15:3394–3398.

Paclitaxel

Roth BJ, Dreicer R, Einhorn LH, et al. Significant activity of paclitaxel in advanced transitional cell carcinoma of the urothelium: a phase II trial of the Eastern Cooperative Oncology Group. *J Clin Oncol.* 1994;12:2264–2270.

Genitourinary Malignancy—Prostate

Combination Regimens

Regimen	Drugs
Docetaxel/Estramustine	**Docetaxel** 70 mg/m² I.V. over 1 hour, 12 hours after first dose of estramustine
	Estramustine 280 mg PO every 6 hours for 5 doses
	Repeat cycle every 21 days for maximum of 6 cycles
Docetaxel/prednisone	**Docetaxel** 75 mg/m² I.V. over 1 hr, day 1
	Prednisone 5 mg PO bid, days 1–21
	Repeat cycle every 21 days
Estramustine/ Vinblastine	**Estramustine** 600 mg/m²/d PO bid or tid, days 1–42
	Vinblastine 4 mg/m² I.V. weekly for 6 weeks, begin day 1
	Repeat cycle every 8 weeks
FL	**Flutamide** 250 mg PO tid
	WITH
	Leuprolide 1 mg/d SQ
	OR
	Leuprolide depot 7.5 mg IM every 28 days
FZ	**Flutamide** 250 mg PO tid
	WITH
	Goserelin implant 3.6 mg SQ every 28 days, beginning 8 weeks prior to radiotherapy for 4 cycles
	OR
	Goserelin implant 3.6 mg SQ 8 weeks prior to radiotherapy
	Goserelin implant 10.8 mg SQ 4 weeks prior to radiotherapy
Mitoxantrone/ Prednisone	**Mitoxantrone** 12 mg/m² I.V., day 1
	Prednisone 5 mg PO bid
	Repeat cycle every 21 days
No Known Acronym	**Bicalutamide** 50 mg/d PO
	WITH
	Leuprolide depot 7.5 mg IM every 28 days
	OR
	Goserelin implant 3.6 mg SQ every 28 days
PE	**Paclitaxel*** 120 mg/m² by 96-hour I.V. infusion, days 1–4
	Estramustine 600 mg/m²/d PO in 2 or 3 divided doses, starting 24 hours before paclitaxel
	Repeat cycle every 21 days

Single-Agent Regimens

Estramustine	**Estramustine** 14 mg/kg/d PO in 3 or 4 divided doses
Goserelin	**Goserelin implant** 3.6 mg SQ every 28 days or 10.8 mg SQ every 12 weeks
Leuprolide	**Leuprolide depot** 7.5 mg IM every 28 days, 22.5 mg IM every 3 months, or 30 mg IM every 4 months
Nilutamide	**Nilutamide** 300 mg/d PO, days 1–30, then 150 mg/d PO, in combination with surgical castration; begin on same day or day after castration
Prednisone	**Prednisone** 5 mg PO bid
Triptorelin	**Triptorelin** 3.75 mg IM every 28 days

References

Docetaxel/Estramustine

Sinibaldi VJ, Carducci MA, Moore-Cooper S, Laufer M, Zahurak M, Eisenberger MA. Phase II evaluation of docetaxel plus one-day oral estramustine phosphate in the treatment of patients with androgen independent prostate carcinoma. *Cancer*. 2002;94: 1457–1465.

Docetaxel/Predinisone

Tannock IF, de Wit R, Berry WR, et al. Docetaxel plus prednisone or mitoxantrone plus prednisone for advanced prostate cancer. *New Engl J Med.* 2004;351:1502–1512.

Estramustine/Vinblastine

Hudes G, Einhorn L, Ross E, et al. Vinblastine versus vinblastine plus oral estramustine phosphate for patients with hormone-refractory prostate cancer: a Hoosier Oncology Group and Fox Chase Network phase III trial. *J Clin Oncol.* 1999;17:3160–3166.

FL

Fischer DS, Knobf MT, Durivage HJ, eds. *The Cancer Chemotherapy Handbook*, 5th ed. St. Louis, MO: CV Mosby1997;369.

Sarosdy MF, Schellhammer PF, Johnson R, Carroll K, Kolvenbag GJCM. Does prolonged combined androgen blockade have survival benefits over short-term combined androgen blockade therapy? *Urology*. 2000;15:391–396.

FZ

Zoladex 3.6 mg, Zoladex 10.8 mg (package inserts). Wilmington, DE: AstraZeneca; 2003.

Jurincic CD, Horlbeck R, Klippel KF. Combined treatment (goserelin plus flutamide) versus monotherapy (goserelin alone) in advanced prostate cancer: a randomized study. *Semin Oncol.* 1991;18(suppl 6):21–25.

Mitoxantrone/Prednisone

Tannock IF, Osoba D, Stockler MR, et al. Chemotherapy with mitoxantrone plus prednisone or prednisone alone for symptomatic hormone-resistant prostate cancer: a Canadian randomized trial with palliative endpoints. *J Clin Oncol.* 1996;14:1756–1764.

No Known Acronym

Schellhammer P, Sharifi R, Block N, et al. A controlled trial of bicalutamide versus flutamide, each in combination with luteinizing hormone-releasing hormone analogue therapy, in patients with advanced prostate cancer. *Urology.* 1995;45:745–752.

PE

Hudes GR, Nathan F, Khater C, et al. Phase II trial of 96-hour paclitaxel plus oral estramustine phosphate in metastatic hormone-refractory prostate cancer. *J Clin Oncol.* 1997;15:3156–3163.

Estramustine

Emcyt (package insert). New York, NY: Pfizer; 2003.

Goserelin

Zoladex 3.6 mg, Zoladex 10.8 mg (package inserts). Wilmington, DE: AstraZeneca; 2003.

Leuprolide

Lupron Depot 7.5 mg, Lupron Depot 22.5 mg, Lupron Depot 30 mg (package inserts.) Lake Forest, IL: TAP Pharmaceuticals; 2003.

Nilutamide

Nilandron (package insert). New York, NY: Pfizer; 2004.

Prednisone

Tannock IF, Osoba D, Stockler MR, et al. Chemotherapy with mitoxantrone plus prednisone or prednisone alone for symptomatic hormone-resistant prostate cancer: a Canadian randomized trial with palliative endpoints. *J Clin Oncol.* 1996;14:1756–1764.

Triptorelin

Kuhn JM, Abourachid H, Brucher P, et al. A randomized comparison of the clinical and hormonal effects of two GnRH agonists in patients with prostate cancer. *Eur Urol.* 1997;32:397–403.

Genitourinary Malignancy—Renal

Combination Regimens

Interleukin-2/ Interferon alfa	**Interleukin-2** 18 million units/m²/d I.V. CI, days 1–5, × 2, separated by 6 days rest (induction) **THEN, AFTER 3 WEEKS** 18 million units/m²/d I.V. CI, days 1–5 (maintenance) *Repeat maintenance cycle for 4 cycles, with 3 weeks rest after each cycle* **WITH**

Interferon alfa-2a
6 million units SQ, 3 times per week during each interleukin-2 cycle (induction and maintenance)

Vinblastine/ Interferon alfa

Vinblastine 0.1 mg/kg I.V. every 3 weeks

Interferonalfa-2a 3 million units SQ, 3 times per week for the first week, then 18 million units 3 times per week for subsequent weeks (9 million units for those unable to tolerate higher dose)

Single-Agent Regimens

Interferon alfa

Interferon alfa-2b 10 million units SQ, 3 times per week for 12 weeks (first week: 5, 5, and 10 million units)

Interleukin-2

Interleukin-2
High Dose: 600,000–720,000 units/kg I.V. over 15 minutes, every 8 hours until toxicity or 14 doses; administer 2 courses separated by 5–9 days
Repeat 2-course cycle every 6–12 weeks
Low Dose: 18 million units/d SQ, days 1–5, week 1
THEN,
9 million units/d SQ, days 1, 2 and 18 million units/d, days 3–5, weeks 2–6
Cycle may be repeated after 3 weeks rest
OR
3 million units/m^2/d I.V. CI, days 1–5 and 12–17; *repeat cycle on day 35*
THEN,
3 million units/m^2/d I.V. CI, days 1–5
Repeat second cycle every 28 days for 4 cycles

References

Interleukin-2/Interferon alfa

Negrier S, Escudier B, Lasset C, et al. Recombinant human interleukin-2, recombinant human interferon alfa-2a, or both in a metastatic renal-cell carcinoma. *N Engl J Med.* 1998;338:1272–1278.

Vinblastine/Interferon alfa

Pyrhönen S, Salminen E, Ruutu M, et al. Prospective randomized trial of interferon alfa-2a plus vinblastine versus vinblastine alone in patients with advanced renal cell cancer. *J Clin Oncol.* 1999;17:2859–2867.

Interferon alfa

Medical Research Council Renal Cancer Collaborators.. Interferon-α and survival in metastatic renal carcinoma: early results of a randomised controlled trial. *Lancet.* 1999; 353:14–17.

Interleukin-2

Fyfe G, Fisher RI, Rosenberg SA, Sznol M, Parkinson DR, Louie AC. Results of treatment of 255 patients with metastatic renal cell carcinoma who received high-dose recombinant interleukin-2 therapy. *J Clin Oncol.* 1995;13:688–696.

Sleijfer DT, Janssen RAJ, Buter J, et al. Phase II study of subcutaneous interleukin-2 in unselected patients with advanced renal cell cancer on an outpatient basis. *J Clin Oncol.* 1992;10:1119–1123.

Stoter G, Fossa SD, Rugarli C, et al. Metastatic renal cell cancer treated with low-dose interleukin-2: a phase II multicentre study. *Cancer Treat Rev.* 1989;16(suppl A): 111–113.

Genitourinary Malignancy—Testicular

BEP	**Bleomycin** 30 units I.V. bolus, weekly for 12 weeks **Etoposide** 100 mg/m²/d I.V. over 30–60 minutes, days 1–5 **Cisplatin** 20 mg/m²/d I.V. over 30–60 minutes, days 1–5 *Repeat cycle every 21 days*
EP	**Etoposide** 100 mg/m²/d I.V., days 1–5 **Cisplatin** 20 mg/m²/d I.V., days 1–5 *Repeat cycle once after 21 days*
PVB	**Cisplatin** 20 mg/m²/d I.V. over 15–30 minutes, days 1–5 **Vinblastine** 0.15 mg/kg/d I.V. bolus, days 1, 2 **Bleomycin** 30 units/d I.V. bolus, days 2, 9, 16 *Repeat cycle every 21 days*
VIP	**Vinblastine** 0.11 mg/kg/d I.V., days 1, 2 **OR** **Etoposide** 75 mg/m²/d I.V., days 1–5 AND **Ifosfamide** 1,200 mg/m²/d I.V., days 1–5 **Cisplatin** 20 mg/m²/d I.V., days 1–5 **Mesna** 400 mg I.V. 15 minutes prior to ifosfamide, then 1,200 mg/d I.V. CI, days 1–5 *Repeat cycle every 21 days for 4 cycles*

References

BEP

Nichols CR, Catalano PJ, Crawford ED, et al. Randomized comparison of cisplatin and etoposide and either bleomycin or ifosfamide in treatment of advanced disseminated germ cell tumors: an Eastern Cooperative Oncology Group, Southwest Oncology Group, and Cancer and Leukemia Group B Study. *J Clin Oncol.* 1998;16:1287–1293.

EP

Motzer RJ, Sheinfeld J, Mazumdar M, et al. Etoposide and cisplatin adjuvant therapy for patients with pathologic stage II germ cell tumors. *J Clin Oncol.* 1995;13:2700–2704.

PVB

Williams SD, Birch R, Einhorn LH, et al. Treatment of disseminated germ cell tumors with cisplatin, bleomycin, and either vinblastine or etoposide. *N Engl J Med.* 1987; 316:1435–1440.

VIP

Loehrer PJ, Lauer R, Roth BJ, et al. Salvage therapy in recurrent germ cell cancer: ifosfamide and cisplatin plus either vinblastine or etoposide. *Ann Intern Med.* 1988;109: 540–546.

Gynecologic Malignancy—Cervical

Combination Regimens

Cisplatin/Fluorouracil	**Cisplatin** 75 mg/m² I.V. over 4 hours, day 1, given within 16 hours of the first dose of radiotherapy **Fluorouracil** 4,000 mg/m² I.V. CI over 96 hours, days 2–5 *Repeat cycle every 21 days for 3 cycles* **OR** **Cisplatin** 50 mg/m²/d I.V., days 1, 29, given 4 hours before the first dose of radiotherapy **Fluorouracil** 1,000 mg/m²/d I.V., days 2–5, 30–33
C-P	**Cisplatin** 50 mg/m² I.V. day 1, IMMEDIATELY AFTER **Paclitaxel** 135 mg/m² I.V. over 24 hours, day 1 *Repeat cycle every 21 days for 6 cycles*
Cisplatin/Vinorelbine	**Cisplatin** 80 mg/m² I.V., day 1 **Vinorelbine** 25 mg/m²/d, days 1, 8 *Repeat cycle every 21 days for 3 to 6 cycles*

Single-Agent Regimen

Cisplatin	**Cisplatin** 40 mg/m² I.V. once per week during radiation therapy for up to 6 doses, followed by hysterectomy 3–6 weeks later; do not exceed 70 mg per dose

References

Cisplatin/Fluorouracil

Morris M, Eifel PJ, Lu J, et al. Pelvic radiation with concurrent chemotherapy compared with pelvic and para-aortic radiation for high-risk cervical cancer. *N Engl J Med.* 1999;340:1137–1143.

Whitney CW, Sause W, Bundy BN, et al. Randomized comparison of fluorouracil plus cisplatin versus hydroxyurea as an adjunct to radiation therapy in stage IIB-IVA carcinoma of the cervix with negative para-aortic lymph nodes: a Gynecologic Oncology Group and Southwest Oncology Group study. *J Clin Oncol.* 1999;17:1339–1348.

Cisplatin/Paclitaxel

Moore DH, Blessing JA, McQuellon RP, et al. Phase III study of cisplatin with or without paclitaxel in stage IV, recurrent or persistent squamous cell carcinoma of the cervix: A Gynecologic Oncology Study Group study. *J Clin Oncol.* 2004;22:3113–3119.

Cisplatin/Vinorelbine

Pignata S, Silvestro G, Ferrari E, et al. Phase II study of cisplatin and vinorelbine as first-line chemotherapy in patients with carcinoma of the uterine cervix. *J Clin Oncol.* 1999;17:756–760.

Cisplatin

Keys HM, Bundy BN, Stehman FB, et al. Cisplatin, radiation, and adjuvant hysterectomy compared with radiation and adjuvant hysterectomy for bulky stage IB cervical carcinoma. *N Engl J Med.* 1999;340:1154–1161.

Gynecologic Malignancy—Endometrial

Combination Regimen

TAP

Doxorubicin 45 mg/m² I.V. day 1
Cisplatin 50 mg/m² I.V. day 1
Paclitaxel* 160 mg/m² I.V. over 3 hours, day 2
Filgrastim 5 mcg/kg SQ, days 3–21
Repeat cycle every 21 days for a maximum of 7 cycles

Single-Agent Regimens

Doxorubicin

Doxorubicin 60 mg/m² I.V. every 21 days (maximum cumulative dose, 500 mg/m²)

Medroxyprogesterone

Medroxyprogesterone acetate 200 mg/d PO

References

TAP

Fleming GF, Brunetto VL, Cella D, et al. Phase III trial of doxorubicin plus cisplatin with or without paclitaxel plus filgrastim in advanced endometrial carcinoma: a Gynecologic Oncology Study Group. *J Clin Oncol.* 2004;22:2159–2166.

Doxorubicin

Morrow CP, Bundy BN, Homesley HD, et al. Doxorubicin as an adjuvant following surgery and radiation therapy in patients with high-risk endometrial carcinoma, stage I and occult stage II: a Gynecologic Oncology Group study. *Gynecol Oncol.* 1990;36:166–171.

Medroxyprogesterone

Thigpen JT, Brady MF, Alvarez RD, et al. Oral medroxyprogesterone acetate in the treatment of advanced or recurrent endometrial carcinoma: a dose-response study by the Gynecological Oncology Group. *J Clin Oncol.* 1999;17:1736–1744.

Gynecologic Malignancy—Ovarian/Epithelial

Combination Regimens

Carbo-Docetaxel	**Docetaxel** 75 mg/m^2 I.V. over 1 hour, day 1 **FOLLOWED BY** **Carboplatin** AUC 5 I.V. over 1 hour, day 1 *Repeat cycle every 21 days*
Carbo-Tax	**Paclitaxel*** 175 mg/m^2 I.V. over 3 hours, day 1 **Carboplatin** dose targeted by Calvert equation to AUC 5 units, I.V., day 1 *Repeat cycle every 21 days*
CT**	**Paclitaxel*** 135 mg/m^2 I.V. over 24 hours, day 1 **Cisplatin** 75 mg/m^2 I.V., day 1 *Repeat cycle every 21 days* **OR** **Paclitaxel*** 175 mg/m^2 I.V. over 3 hours, day 1 **Cisplatin** 75 mg/m^2 I.V., day 1 *Repeat cycle every 21 days*

Single-Agent Regimens

Altretamine	**Altretamine** 260 mg/m^2/d PO in 4 divided doses after meals and at bedtime for 14 days *Repeat cycle every 28 days*
Gemcitabine	**Gemcitabine** 800 mg/m^2/d I.V., days 1, 8, 15 *Repeat cycle every 28 days*
Paclitaxel	**Paclitaxel*** 175 mg/m^2 I.V. over 3 hours, every 21 days
Pegylated liposomal doxorubicin	**Pegylated liposomal doxorubicin** 50 mg/m^2 I.V. every 28 days at an initial rate of 1 mg/min; if no infusion-related adverse events are observed, the infusion rate can be increased to complete administration over 1 hour
Topotecan	**Topotecan** 1.5 mg/m^2/d I.V. over 30 minutes, days 1–5 *Repeat cycle every 21 days*

References

Carbo-Docetaxel

Vasey PA, Jayson GC, Gordon A, et al. Phase III randomized trial of docetaxel-carboplatin versus paclitaxel-carboplatin as first-line chemotherapy for ovarian carcinoma. *J Natl Cancer Instit.* 2004;96:1682–1691.

Carbo-Tax

Neijt JP, Engelholm SA, Tuxen MK, et al. Exploratory phase III study of paclitaxel and cisplatin versus paclitaxel and carboplatin in advanced ovarian cancer. *J Clin Oncol.* 2000;18:3084–3092.

CT

McGuire WP, Hoskins WJ, Brady MF, et al. Cyclophosphamide and cisplatin compared with paclitaxel and cisplatin in patients with stage III and stage IV ovarian ancer. *N Engl J Med.* 1996;334:1–6.

Neijt JP, Engelholm SA, Tuxen MK, et al. Exploratory phase III study of paclitaxel and cisplatin versus paclitaxel and carboplatin in advanced ovarian cancer. *J Clin Oncol.* 2000;18:3084–3092.

Altretamine

Markman M, Blessing JA, Moore D, Ball H, Lentz SS. Altretamine (hexamethylmelamine) in platinum-resistant and platinum-refractory ovarian cancer: a Gynecologic Oncology Group phase II trial. *Gynecol Oncol.* 1998;69:226–229.

Gemcitabine

Lund B, Hansen OP, Theilade K, et al. Phase II study of gemcitabine (2',2' difluorodeoxycitidine) in previously treated ovarian cancer patients. *J Natl Cancer Instit.* 1994;86: 1530–1533.

Paclitaxel

ten Bokkel Huinink W, Gore M, Carmichael J, et al. Topotecan versus paclitaxel for the treatment of recurrent epithelial ovarian cancer. *J Clin Oncol.* 1997;15:2183–2193.

Pegylated liposomal doxorubicin

Gordon AN, Granal CO, Rose PG, et al. Phase II study of liposomal doxorubicin in platinum- and paclitaxel-refractory epithelial ovarian cancer. *J Clin Oncol.* 2000;18: 3093–3100.

Doxil (package insert). Bridgewater, NJ: Tibotec Therapeutics, Division of Ortho Biotech Products, LP; 2005.

Topotecan

ten Bokkel Huinink W, Gore M, Carmichael J, et al. Topotecan versus paclitaxel for the treatment of recurrent epithelial ovarian cancer. *J Clin Oncol.* 1997;15:2183–2193.

Head and Neck/Esophageal Malignancies

Carboplatin/ Fluorouracil

Carboplatin 400 mg/m^2 I.V. CI over 24 hours, day 1
Fluorouracil 5,000 mg/m^2 I.V. CI over 120 hours
Repeat cycle every 21 days

Cisplatin/Fluorouracil	**Cisplatin** 100 mg/m^2 I.V., day 1 **Fluorouracil** 5,000 mg/m^2 I.V. CI over 120 hours *Repeat cycle every 21 days*

References

Carboplatin/Fluorouracil

De Andrés L, Brunt J, López-Pousa A, et al. Randomized trial of neoadjuvant cisplatin and fluorouracil versus carboplatin and fluorouracil in patients with stage IV-M0 head and neck cancer. *J Clin Oncol.* 1995;13:1493–1500.

Cisplatin/Fluorouracil

De Andrés L, Brunt J, López-Pousa A, et al. Randomized trial of neoadjuvant cisplatin and fluorouracil versus carboplatin and fluorouracil in patients with stage IV-M0 head and neck cancer. *J Clin Oncol.* 1995;13:1493–1500.

Leukemia—AML

Combination Regimens (Induction)

Idarubicin/Cytarabine/ Etoposide	**Idarubicin** 5 mg/m^2/d slow I.V. push, days 1–5 **Cytarabine** 2 g/m^2 every 12 hours as 3-hour infusion, days 1–5 **Etoposide** 100 mg/m^2/d as 1-hour infusion, days 1–5 **OR** **Idarubicin** 6 mg/m^2/d I.V. bolus, days 1–5 **Cytarabine** 600 mg/m^2/d I.V. over 2 hours, days 1–5 **Etoposide** 150 mg/m^2/d over 2 hours, days 1–3
5 + 2	**Cytarabine** 100 mg/m^2/d I.V. CI, days 1–5 **WITH** **Daunorubicin** 45 mg/m^2/d I.V., days 1–2 **OR** **Mitoxantrone** 12 mg/m^2/d I.V., days 1–2 For reinduction or consolidation
7 + 3	**Cytarabine** 100 mg/m^2/d I.V. CI, days 1–7 **WITH** **Daunorubicin** 45 mg/m^2/d I.V., days 1–3 **OR** **Idarubicin** 12 mg/m^2/d I.V., days 1–3 **OR** **Mitoxantrone** 12 mg/m^2/d I.V., days 1–3
7 + 3 + 7	**Cytarabine** 100 mg/m^2/d I.V. CI, days 1–7 **Daunorubicin** 50 mg/m^2/d I.V., days 1–3 **Etoposide** 75 mg/m^2/d I.V. over 1 hour, days 1–7

Monoclonal Antibody Regimen

Gemtuzumab — **Gemtuzumab** 2 doses of 9 mg/m^2 I.V., each as a 2-hour infusion, separated by 14 days

Single-Agent Regimens (Induction)

Arsenic — **Arsenic trioxide** 0.15 mg/kg I.V. daily until remission, not to exceed 50 doses

ATRA — **All-*trans*-retinoic acid (ATRA)** 45 mg/m^2/d PO

Single-Agent Regimens (Post-Remission)

Arsenic — **Arsenic trioxide** 0.15 mg/kg/d I.V., days 1–5
Repeat cycle every week for 5 weeks (25 doses)

Cytarabine — **Cytarabine** 100 mg/m^2/d I.V. CI, days 1–5
For patients ≥ 60 years of age
Repeat cycle every 28 days

HiDAC — **Cytarabine** 3,000 mg/m^2 I.V. over 3 hours, every 12 hours, days 1, 3, 5
For patients <60 years of age
Repeat cycle every 28 days

References

Idarubicin/Cytarabine/Etoposide

Mehta J, Powles R, Singhai S, et al. Idarubicin, high-dose cytarabine, and etoposide for induction of remission in acute leukemia. *Semin Hematol.* 1996;33(suppl 3):18–23.

Carella AM, Carlier P, Pungolino E, et al. Idarubicin in combination with intermediate-dose cytarabine and VP-16 in the treatment of refractory or rapidly relapsed patients with acute myeloid leukemia. *Leukemia.* 1993;7:196–199.

5 + 2

Skeel RT, Lachant NA, eds. *Handbook of Cancer Chemotherapy*, 4th ed. Boston, MA: Little, Brown and Co;1995:400.

7 + 3

Preisler H, Davis RB, Kirshner J, et al. Comparison of three remission induction regimens and two post-induction strategies for the treatment of acute nonlymphocytic leukemia: a cancer and leukemia group B study. *Blood.* 1987;69:1441–1449.

Skeel RT, Lachant NA, eds. *Handbook of Cancer Chemotherapy*, 4th ed. Boston, MA: Little, Brown and Co; 1995:400.

7 + 3 + 7

Bishop JF, Lowenthal RM, Joshua D, et al. Etoposide in acute nonlymphocytic leukemia. *Blood.* 1990;75:27–32.

Gemtuzumab

Mylotarg (package insert). Philadelphia, PA: Wyeth-Ayerst Pharmaceuticals; 2004.

Arsenic

Trisenox (package insert). Seattle, WA: Cell Therapeutics, Inc; 2003.

ATRA

Degos L, Dombret H, Chomienne C, et al. All-*trans*-retinoic acid as a differentiating agent in the treatment of acute promyelocytic leukemia. *Blood.* 1995;85:2643–2653.

Single-Agent Regimens (Post-Remission)

Arsenic

Trisenox (package insert). Seattle, WA: Cell Therapeutics, Inc; 2003.

Cytarabine

Stone RM. Leukemia in the elderly. *Hematology.* Washington, DC: American Society of Hematology. 1999;510–516. Available at www.hematology.org/education/hema99/stone.pdf

HiDAC

Mayer RJ, Davis RB, Schiffer CA, et al. Intensive postremission chemotherapy in adults with acute myeloid leukemia. *N Engl J Med.* 1994;331:896–903.

Leukemia—Chronic Lymphocytic

Alemtuzumab	**Alemtuzumab** 3 mg/d I.V. over 2 hours initial dose, increasing to maintenance dose of 30 mg/d I.V. over 2 hours, 3 times per week on alternating days for up to 12 weeks. Do not exceed 30 mg per single dose or 90 mg per week.
Chlorambucil	**Chlorambucil** 0.1–0.2 mg/kg/d PO for 3–6 weeks as required **THEN** (as intermittent therapy) **Chlorambucil** 0.4 mg/kg PO *Repeat intermittent therapy every 14–28 days, increasing dose by 0.1 mg/kg until control of lymphocytosis or toxicity is observed*
Cyclophosphamide	**Cyclophosphamide** 2–3 mg/kg/d PO **OR** **Cyclophosphamide** 20 mg/kg I.V. every 2–3 weeks
Fludarabine	**Fludarabine** 25 mg/m^2/d I.V. over 30 minutes, days 1–5 *Repeat cycle every 28 days*
Prednisone	**Prednisone** 60–100 mg/m^2/d PO for 3–6 weeks *Use if patient symptomatic with autoimmune hemolytic anemia or immune thrombocytopenia*

References

Alemtuzumab

Campath (package insert). Richmond, CA: Berlex Laboratories; 2004.

Chlorambucil

Leukeran (package insert). Research Triangle Park, NC: GlaxoSmithKline; 2004.

Cyclophosphamide

Han T, Rai KR. Management of chronic lymphocytic leukemia. *Hematol Oncol Clin North Am.* 1990;4:431–445.

Fludarabine

The French Cooperative Group on CLL., Johnson S, Smith AG, Löffler H, et al. Multicentre prospective randomised trial of fludarabine versus cyclophosphamide, doxorubicin, and prednisone (CAP) for treatment of advanced-stage chronic lymphocytic leukemia. *Lancet.* 1996;347:1432–1438.

Prednisone

Skeel RT, Lachant NA, eds. *Handbook of Cancer Chemotherapy,* 4th ed. Boston, MA: Little, Brown and Co;1995;430–431.

Leukemia—Chronic Myelogenous

Combination Regimen (Induction)

Interferon alfa-2b/ Hydroxyurea/ Cytarabine	**Interferon alfa-2b** 5 million units/m^2/d SQ qd (dose dependent on granulocyte and platelet count)
	Hydroxyurea 50 mg/kg/d (dose dependent on WBC count)
	Cytarabine 20 mg/m^2/d SQ for 10 days starting 2 weeks after initiation of induction (interferon alfa-2b + hydroxyurea) therapy, repeating every month (dose dependent on WBC, granulocyte, and platelet count)

Single-Agent Regimens (Post-Remission)

Hydroxyurea	**Hydroxyurea** 20–30 mg/kg/d PO
Imatinib mesylate	**Imatinib mesylate** 400–800 mg/d PO
Interferon alfa-2a	**Interferon alfa-2a** 9 million units/d SQ or IM 120 Tolerance dose: 3 million units/d for 3 days, then 6 million units/d to a target dose of 9 million units/d for the duration of the treatment period

References

Interferon alfa-2b/Hydroxyurea/Cytarabine

Guilhot F, Chastang C, Michallet M, et al. Interferon alfa-2b combined with cytarabine versus interferon alone in chronic myelogenous leukemia. *N Engl J Med.* 1997;337: 223–229.

Hydroxyurea

Hydrea (package insert). Princeton, NJ: Bristol-Myers Squibb; 2001.

Imatinib mesylate

Gleevec (package insert). East Hanover, NJ: Novartis; 2004.

Interferon alfa-2a

Roferon-A (package insert). Nutley, NJ: Roche Pharmaceuticals; 2004.

Leukemia—Hairy Cell

Cladribine	**Cladribine** 0.09 mg/kg/d I.V. CI, days 1–7 *Administer 1 cycle only*
Interferon alfa-2a	**Interferon alfa-2a** 3 million units SQ 3 times per week for 6 months
Pentostatin	**Pentostatin** 4 mg/m² I.V. every 14 days

References

Cladribine

Leustatin (package insert). Raritan, NJ; Ortho Biotech Products, LP; 1996.

Interferon alfa-2a

Grever M, Kopecky K, Foucar MK, et al. Randomized comparison of pentostatin versus interferon alfa-2a in previously untreated patients with hairy cell leukemia: an intergroup study. *J Clin Oncol.* 1995;13:974–982.

Pentostatin

Grever M, Kopecky K, Foucar MK, et al. Randomized comparison of pentostatin versus interferon alfa-2a in previously untreated patients with hairy cell leukemia: an intergroup study. *J Clin Oncol.* 1995;13:974–982.

Lung Cancer-Small Cell

Combination Regimens

CAE	**Cyclophosphamide** 1,000 mg/m² I.V., day 1 **Doxorubicin** 45 mg/m² I.V., day 1 **Etoposide** 50 mg/m²/d I.V., days 1–5 *Repeat cycle every 21 days*

Carboplatin/Paclitaxel/ Etoposide	**Carboplatin** dose targeted by Calvert equation to AUC 6 units I.V., day 1 **Paclitaxel*** 200 mg/m^2 I.V. over 1 hour, day 1 **Etoposide** 50 mg alternating with 100 mg PO, days 1–10 *Repeat cycle every 21 days for 4 cycles*
CAV	**Cyclophosphamide** 800–1,000 mg/m^2 I.V., day 1 **Doxorubicin** 45–50 mg/m^2 I.V., day 1 **Vincristine#** 1.4–2.0 mg/m^2 I.V., day 1 *Repeat cycle every 21–28 days*
CAV/EP	**CAV:** **Cyclophosphamide** 1,000 mg/m^2 I.V., day 1 **Doxorubicin** 50 mg/m^2 I.V., day 1 **Vincristine#** 1.2 mg/m^2 I.V., day 1 **EP:** **Etoposide** 100 mg/m^2/d I.V., days 1–3 **Cisplatin** 25 mg/m^2/d I.V., days 1–3 *Alternate regimens every 21 days*
CDDP + CPT-11	**Cisplatin** 60 mg/m^2, day 1 **Irinotecan** 60 mg/m^2/d, days 1, 8, 15 *Repeat cycle every 28 days*
EC	**Etoposide** 100 mg/m^2/d I.V., days 1–3 **Carboplatin** 450 mg/m^2 I.V., day 1 *Repeat cycle every 28 days*
EP (PE)	**Etoposide** 80 mg/m^2/d I.V., days 1–3 **Cisplatin** 80 mg/m^2 I.V., day 1 (standard dose) *Repeat cycle every 21 days* **OR** **Etoposide** 80 mg/m^2/d I.V., days 1–5 **Cisplatin** 27 mg/m^2/d I.V., days 1–5 (high dose) *Repeat cycle every 21 days*
VIP	**Etoposide** 75 mg/m^2/d I.V., days 1–4 **Ifosfamide** 1,200 mg/m^2/d I.V., days 1–4 **Cisplatin** 20 mg/m^2/d I.V., days 1–4 **Mesna** 300 mg/m^2 I.V. bolus before the first dose of ifosfamide, then 1,200 mg/m^2/d I.V. CI, days 1–4 *Repeat cycle every 21 days for 4 cycles*

Single-Agent Regimens

Etoposide	**Etoposide** 160 mg/m^2/d PO, days 1–5 *Repeat cycle every 28 days* **OR** **Etoposide** 50 mg PO, bid for 14 days

	Repeat cycle every 21 days
Paclitaxel	**Paclitaxel*** 250 mg/m^2 I.V. over 24 hours, every 21 days
Topotecan	**Topotecan** 1.5 mg/m^2/d I.V. over 30 minutes, days 1–5
	Repeat cycle every 21 days

References

CAE

Bunn PA Jr, Greco FA, Einhorn L. *Cyclophosphamide, doxorubicin, and etoposide as first-line therapy in the treatment of small-cell lung cancer. Semin Oncol.* 1986;13(3 suppl 3):45–53.

Fischer DS, Knobf MT, Durivage HJ, eds. *The Cancer Chemotherapy Handbook,* 5th ed. St. Louis, MO: CV Mosby;1997;370–371.

Carboplatin/Paclitaxel/Etoposide

Hainsworth JD, Gray JR, Stroup SL, et al. Paclitaxel, carboplatin, and extended-schedule etoposide in the treatment of small cell lung cancer: comparison of sequential Phase II trials using different dose intensities. *J Clin Oncol.* 1997;15:3464–3470.

CAV

Fukuoka M, Furuse K, Saijo N, et al. Randomized trial of cyclophosphamide, doxorubicin, and vincristine versus cisplatin and etoposide versus alternation of these regimens in small cell lung cancer. *J Natl Cancer Inst.* 1991;83:855–861.

DeVita VT, Hellman S, Rosenberg SA, eds. *Cancer: Principles and Practice of Oncology,* 5th ed. Philadelphia, PA: JB Lippincott Co; 1997;911–949.

CAV/EP

Murray N, Livingston RB, Shepherd FA, et al. Randomized study of CODE versus alternating CAV/EP for extensive-stage small cell lung cancer: an intergroup study of the National Cancer Institute of Canada Clinical Trials Group and the Southwest Oncology Group. *J Clin Oncol.* 1999;17:2300–2308.

CDDP + CPT-11

Noda K, Nishiwaki Y, Kawahara M, et al. Irinotecan plus cisplatin compared with etoposide plus cisplatin for extensive small-cell lung cancer. *N Engl J Med.* 2002;346: 85–91.

EC

Viren M, Liippo K, Ojala A, et al. Carboplatin and etoposide in extensive small-cell-lung cancer. *Acta Oncol.* 1994;33:921–924.

EP (PE)

Ihde DC, Mulshine JL, Kramer BS, et al. Prospective randomized comparison of high-dose and standard-dose etoposide and cisplatin chemotherapy in patients with extensive-stage small-cell lung cancer. *J Clin Oncol.* 1994;12:2022–2034.

VIP

Loehrer PJ Sr, Rynard S, Ansari R, et al. Etoposide, ifosfamide, and cisplatin in extensive small-cell lung cancer. *Cancer.* 1992;69:669–673.

Etoposide

Johnson DH. Recent developments in chemotherapy treatment of small-cell lung cancer. *Semin Oncol.* 1993;20:315–325.

Paclitaxel

Ettinger DS, Finkelstein DM, Sarma RP, Johnson DH. Phase II study of paclitaxel in patients with extensive-disease small-cell lung cancer: an Eastern Cooperative Oncology Group study. *J Clin Oncol.* 1995;13:1430–1435.

Kirschling RJ, Grill JP, Marks RS, et al. Paclitaxel and G-CSF in previously untreated patients with extensive-stage small-cell lung cancer: a phase II study of the North Central Cancer Treatment Group. *Am J Clin Oncol.* 1999;22:517–522.

Topotecan

Adrizzoni A, Hansen H, Dombernowsky P, et al. Topotecan, a new active drug in the second-line treatment of small-cell lung cancer: a phase II study in patients with refractory and sensitive disease. *J Clin Oncol.* 1997;15:2090–2096.

von Pawel J, Schiller JH, Shepherd FA, et al. Topotecan versus cyclophosphamide, doxorubicin, and vincristine for the treatment of recurrent small-cell lung cancer. *J Clin Oncol.* 1999;17:658–667.

Lung Cancer—Non-Small Cell

Combination Regimens

Carbo-Tax	**Paclitaxel*** 225 mg/m² I.V. over 3 hours, day1
	Carboplatin dose targeted by Calvert equation to AUC 6 mg/mL/min, day 1
	Repeat cycle every 21 days
Docetaxel/Cisplatin**	**Docetaxel** 75 mg/m² I.V., day 1
	Cisplatin 75 mg/m² I.V., day 1
	Repeat cycle every 21 days
Gemcitabine/Cisplatin**	**Gemcitabine** 1,000 mg/m²/d I.V., days 1, 8, 15
	Cisplatin 100 mg/m² I.V., day 1
	Repeat cycle every 28 days
	OR
	Gemcitabine 1,250 mg/m²/d I.V., days 1, 8
	Cisplatin 100 mg/m² I.V., day 1
	Repeat cycle every 21 days
Gemcitabine/Docetaxel	**Gemcitabine** 1,100 mg/m²/d I.V., days 1, 8
	Docetaxel 100 mg/m² I.V., day 8
	Filgrastim 150 mcg/m²/d SQ, days 9-15
	Repeat cycle every 21 days
Gemcitabine/Paclitaxel	**Paclitaxel*** 200 mg/m² I.V. over 3 hours, day 1
	Repeat cycle every 21 days

Gemcitabine/ Vinorelbine	**Gemcitabine** 1,200 mg/m²/d I.V., days 1, 8 **Vinorelbine** 30 mg/m²/d I.V., days 1, 8 *Repeat cycle every 21 days* **OR** **Gemcitabine** 800–1,000 mg/m²/d I.V., days 1, 8, 15 **Vinorelbine** 20 mg/m²/d I.V., days 1, 8, 15 *Repeat cycle every 28 days*
PC**	**Paclitaxel*** 135 mg/m² over 24 hours, day 1 **Cisplatin** 75 mg/m² I.V., day 1 *Repeat cycle every 21 days* **OR** **Paclitaxel*** 175 mg/m² over 3 hours, day 1 **Cisplatin** 80 mg/m² I.V., day 1 *Repeat cycle every 21 days*
Vinorelbine/ Cisplatin**	**Vinorelbine** 30 mg/m² I.V. over 20 minutes, every 7 days **Cisplatin** 120 mg/m² I.V. over 1 hour, days 1, 29, then every 6 weeks

Single-Agent Regimens

Docetaxel	**Docetaxel** 75 mg/m² I.V. over 1 hour, every 21 days
Erlotinib	**Erlotinib** 150 mg PO qd at least 1 hour before or 2 hours after eating
Gefitinib	**Gefitinib** 250 mg PO daily
Gemcitabine	**Gemcitabine** 1,000 mg/m²/d I.V. over 30 minutes, days 1, 8, 15 *Repeat cycle every 28 days*
Vinorelbine	**Vinorelbine** 30 mg/m² I.V. over 20 minutes, every 7 days

References

Carbo-Tax

Schiller JH, Harrington D, Belani CP, et al. Comparision of four chemotherapy regimens for advanced non-small-cell lung cancer. *N Engl J Med.* 2002;346:92–98.

Docetaxel/Cisplatin**

Schiller JH, Harrington D, Belani CP, et al. Comparision of four chemotherapy regimens for advanced non-small-cell lung cancer. *N Engl J Med.* 2002;346:92–98.

Gemcitabine/Cisplatin**

Schiller JH, Harrington D, Belani CP, et al. Comparision of four chemotherapy regimens for advanced non-small-cell lung cancer. *N Engl J Med.* 2002;346:92–98.

Cardenal F, Ĺopez-Cabrerizo MP, Anton A, et al. Randomized phase III study of gemcitabinecisplatin versus etoposide-cisplatin in the treatment of locally advanced or metastatic non-small cell lung cancer. *J Clin Oncol.* 1999;17:12–18.

Gemcitabine/Docetaxel

Georgoulias V, Papadakis E, Alexopoulos A, et al. Platinum-based and non-platinum based chemotherapy in advanced non-small-cell-lung-cancer: A randomized multicentre trial. *Lancet.* 2001;357:1478–1484.

Gemcitabine/Paclitaxel

Kosmidis P, Mylonakis N, Nicolaides C, et al. Paclitaxel plus carboplatin versus gemcitabine plus paclitaxel in advanced non-small-cell-lung-cancer: A phase III randomized trial. *J Clin Oncol.* 2002;20:3578–3585.

Gemcitabine/Vinorelbine

Frasci G, Lorusso V, Panza N, et al. Gemcitabine plus vinorelbine versus vinorelbine alone in elderly patients with advanced non-small cell lung cancer. *J Clin Oncol.* 2000;18:2529–2536.

Chen YM, Perng RP, Young KY, et al. A multicenter phase II trial of vinorelbine plus gemcitabine in previously untreated inoperable (stage IIIB/IV) non-small-cell lung cancer. *Chest.* 2000;117:1583–1589.

Hainsworth JD, Burris HA 3rd, Litchy S, et al. Gemcitabine and vinorelbine in the secondline treatment of non-small cell lung carcinoma patients: a Minnie Pearl Cancer Research Network phase II trial. *Cancer.* 2000;88:1353–1358.

PC**

Schiller JH, Harrington D, Belani CP, et al. Comparision of four chemotherapy regimens for advanced non-small-cell lung cancer. *N Engl J Med.* 2002;346:92–98.

Smit EF, van Meerbeeck JP, Lianes P, et al. Three-arm randomized study of two cisplatin-based regimens and paclitaxel plus gemcitabine in advanced non-small-cell lung cancer: a phase III trial of the European Organization for Research and Treatment of Cancer Lung Cancer Group—EORTC 08975. *J Clin Oncol.* 2003;21:3909–3917.

Vinorelbine/Cisplatin**

Le Chevalier T, Brisgand D, Douillard JY, et al. Randomized study of vinorelbine and cisplatin versus vindesine and cisplatin versus vinorelbine alone in advanced non-small-cell lung cancer: results of a European multicenter trial including 612 patients. *J Clin Oncol.* 1994;12:360–367.

Docetaxel

Shepherd FA, Dancey J, Ramlau R, et al. Prospective randomized trial of docetaxel versus best supportive care in patients with non-small-cell lung cancer previously treated with platinum-based chemotherapy. *J Clin Oncol.* 2000;18:2095–2103.

Fossella FV, DeVore R, Kerr RN, et al. Randomized phase III trial of docetaxel versus vinorelbine or ifosfamide in patients with advanced non-small cell lung cancer previously treated with platinum-containing chemotherapy regimens. *J Clin Oncol.* 2000; 18:2354–2362.

Erlotinib

Tarceva (package insert). Melville NY and South San Francisco, CA: OSI Pharmaceuticals Inc and Genentech Inc; 2004

Gefitinib

Iressa (package insert). Wilmington, DE: AstraZeneca Pharmaceuticals LP; 2004.

Gemcitabine

Crinò L, Mosconi AM, Scagliotti G, et al. Gemcitabine as second-line treatment for advanced non-small-cell lung cancer: a phase II trial. *J Clin Oncol.* 1999;17:2081–2085.

Ricci S, Antonuzzo A, Galli L, et al. Gemcitabine monotherapy in elderly patients with advanced non-small-cell lung cancer: a multicenter phase II study. *Lung Cancer.* 2000;27:75–80.

Vinorelbine

Le Chevalier T, Brisgand D, Douillard JY, et al. Randomized study of vinorelbine and cisplatin versus vindesine and cisplatin versus vinorelbine alone in advanced non-small-cell lung cancer: results of a European multicenter trial including 612 patients. *J Clin Oncol.* 1994;12:360–367.

Lymphoma—Hodgkin's

ABVD	**Doxorubicin** 25 mg/m² I.V., days 1, 15
	Bleomycin 10 mg/m² I.V., days 1, 15
	Vinblastine 6 mg/m² I.V., days 1, 15
	Dacarbazine 375 mg/m² I.V., days 1, 15
	Repeat cycle every 28 days
ChlVPP	**Chlorambucil** 6 mg/m²/d PO (maximum, 10 mg/d), days 1–14
	Vinblastine mg/m²/d I.V. (maximum, 10 mg/single dose), days 1, 8
	Procarbazine mg/m²/d PO (maximum, 150 mg/d), days 1–14
	Prednisolone 40 mg/d PO, days 1–14
	Repeat cycle every 28 days
MOPP	**Mechlorethamine** 6 mg/m²/d I.V., days 1, 8
	Vincristine[#] 1.4 mg/m²/d I.V., days 1, 8
	Procarbazine 100 mg/m²/d PO, days 1–14
	Prednisone 40 mg/m²/d PO, days 1–14, cycles 1 and 4
	Repeat cycle every 28 days
MOPP/ABVD	Refer to MOPP and ABVD regimens
	Alternating months of MOPP and ABVD
Stanford V	**Doxorubicin** 25 mg/m²/d I.V., days 1 and 15
	Vinblastine[a] 6 mg/m²/d I.V., days 1 and 15
	Mechlorethamine 6 mg/m² I.V., day
	Vincristine[#] 1.4 mg/m²/d I.V., days 8 and 22
	Bleomycin 5 units/m²/d I.V., days 8 and 22
	Etoposide 60 mg/m²/d I.V., days 15 and 16
	Prednisone[b] 40 mg/m² PO qod;
	repeat regimen every 28 days for 3 cycles

[a]For patients >e;50 years old, decrease dose to 4 mg/m^2 and 1mg/m^2 for vinblastine and vincristine, respectively, during cycle 3

[b] Tapered by 10 mg qod starting at week 10

References

ABVD

Harker WG, Kushlan P, Rosenberg SA. Combination chemotherapy for advanced Hodgkin's disease after failure of MOPP: ABVD and B-CAVe. *Ann Intern Med.* 1984;101: 440–446.

Longo DL. The use of chemotherapy in the treatment of Hodgkin's disease. *Semin Oncol.* 1990;17:716–735.

ChlVPP

Selby P, Patel P, Milan S, et al. ChlVPP combination chemotherapy for Hodgkin's disease: long-term results. *Br J Cancer.* 1990;62:279–285.

MOPP

DeVita VT Jr, Serpick AA, Carbone PP. Combination chemotherapy in the treatment of advanced Hodgkin's disease. *Ann Intern Med.* 1970;73:881–895.

Longo D. The use of chemotherapy in the treatment of Hodgkin's disease. *Semin Oncol.* 1990;17:716–735.

MOPP/ABVD

DeVita VT Jr, Hellman S, Rosenberg SA, eds. *Cancer: Principles & Practices of Oncology,* 5th ed. Philadelphia, PA: JB Lippincott Co;1997:1839.

Longo DL. The use of chemotherapy in the treatment of Hodgkin's disease. *Semin Oncol.* 1990;17:716–735.

Stanford V

Bartlett NL, Rosenberg SA, Hoppe RT, Hancock SL, Hornig SJ. Brief chemotherapy, Stanford V, and adjuvant radiotherapy for bulky or advanced-stage Hodgkin's disease: a preliminary report. *J Clin Oncol.* 1995;13:1080–1088.

Lymphoma—Non-Hodgkin's

Combination Regimens

CHOP	**Cyclophosphamide** 750 mg/m^2 I.V., day 1
	Doxorubicin 50 mg/m^2 I.V., day 1
	Vincristine[#] 1.4 mg/m^2 I.V., day 1
	Prednisolone 50 mg/m^2/d PO, days 1–5
	Repeat cycle every 21 days
CHOP + Rituximab	**Cyclophosphamide** 750 mg/m^2 I.V., day 1
	Doxorubicin 50 mg/m^2 I.V., day 1
	Vincristine[#] 1.4 mg/m^2 I.V., day 1
	Prednisone 40 mg/m^2/d PO, days 1–5

Rituximab 375 mg/m² I.V., day 1
Repeat cycle every 21 days for 8 cycles (diffuse large B-cell lymphoma)
OR
Cyclophosphamide 750 mg/m² I.V., day 1
Doxorubicin 50 mg/m² I.V., day 1
Vincristine# 1.4 mg/m² I.V., day 1
Prednisone 100 mg/m²/d PO, days 1–5
Rituximab 375 mg/m² I.V., given 7 and 2 days before 1st CHOP cycle; then 2 days before 3rd and 5th CHOP cycles; then 134 and 141 days after 6th CHOP cycle
Repeat CHOP cycle every 21 days for 6 cycles (follicular or low-grade lymphoma)

CNOP
Cyclophosphamide 750 mg/m² I.V., day 1
Mitoxantrone 10 mg/m² I.V., day 1
Vincristine# 1.4 mg/m² I.V., day 1
Prednisolone 50 mg/m²/d PO, days 1–5
Repeat cycle every 21 days

COP
Cyclophosphamide 800 mg/m² I.V., day 1
Vincristine# 2 mg (total dose) I.V., day 1
Prednisone 60 mg/m²/d PO, days 1–5, then taper over 3 days
Repeat cycle every 14 days

CVP
Cyclophosphamide 300 mg/m²/d PO, days 1–5
Vincristine# 1.2 mg/m² (maximum, 2 mg) I.V., day 1
Prednisone 40 mg/m²/d PO, days 1–5
Repeat cycle every 21 days for 8 cycles

DHAP
Dexamethasone 40 mg/d PO or I.V. over 24 hours, days 1–4
Cisplatin 100 mg/m² I.V. CI, day 1
Cytarabine 2,000 mg/m² I.V. over 3 hours every 12 hours for 2 doses, day 2
Repeat cycle every 21–28 days for 6–10 cycles

ESHAP
Etoposide 40 mg/m²/d I.V., days 1–4
Methylprednisolone 500 mg/d I.V., days 1–5
Cytarabine 2,000 mg/m² I.V. over 2–3 hours, day 5
Cisplatin 25 mg/m²/d I.V. CI, days 1–4
OR
Etoposide 60 mg/m²/d I.V., days 1–4
Methylprednisolone 500 mg/d I.V., days 1–4
Cisplatin 25 mg/m²/d I.V. CI, days 1–4

	Cytarabine 2,000 mg/m^2 I.V. over 2 hours, day 5, immediately following completion of cisplatin *Repeat cycle every 21–28 days*
Hyper-CVAD/ MTX-Ara-C	*Course 1:* Cyclophosphamide 300 mg/m^2 over 3 hours every 12 hours × 6 doses, days 1–3 **Doxorubicin** 50 mg/m^2 over 48 hours after cyclophosphamide, days 4–5 **Vincristine**[#] 2 mg administered 12 hours after last cyclophosphamide dose, repeated on day 11 **Dexamethasone** 40 mg/d I.V. or PO, days 1–4 and days 11–14 **Filgrastim** 5 mcg/kg I.V. or SQ beginning 24 hours after doxorubicin is complete *Course 2 (begin after clinical and hermatologic recovery from Course 1):* **Methotrexate** 200 mg/m^2 I.V. bolus, day 1, **FOLLOWED BY** **Methotrexate** 800 mg/m^2 over 24 hours, day 1, **FOLLOWED BY** **Cytarabine** 3,000 mg/m^2 I.V. every 12 hours × 4 doses, days 2–3 (dose reduced to 1,000 mg/m2 in patients older than 60 years or with serum creatinine > 1.5 mg/dL) **Leucovorin** 50 mg PO 24 hours after end of MTX infusion, FOLLOWED 6 HOURS LATER BY **Leucovorin** 15 mg PO every 6 hours × 8 doses (dose adjusted for MTX concentration at 24 and 48 hours after completion of MTX infusion) **Filgrastim** 5 mcg/kg I.V. or SQ beginning 24 hours after cytarabine *Repeat courses every 21 days*
MINE-ESHAP	**Mesna** 1,330 mg/m^2/d I.V. over 1 hour, administered at same time as ifosfamide, then 500 mg/d PO 4 hours after ifosfamide, days 1–3 **Ifosfamide** 1,330 mg/m^2/d I.V. over 1 hour, days 1–3 **Mitoxantrone** 8 mg/m^2 I.V., day 1 **Etoposide** 65 mg/m^2/d I.V., days 1–3 *Repeat cycle every 21 days for 6 cycles, followed by 3–6 cycles of ESHAP*
ProMACE/cytaBOM	**Prednisone** 60 mg/m^2/d PO, days 1–14 **Doxorubicin** 25 mg/m^2 I.V., day 1 **Cyclophosphamide** 650 mg/m^2 I.V., day 1

Etoposide 120 mg/m^2 I.V., day 1
Cytarabine 300 mg/m^2 I.V., day 8
Bleomycin 5 units/m^2 I.V., day 8
Vincristine# 1.4 mg/m^2 I.V. (no cap at 2 mg total dose), day 8
Methotrexate 120 mg/m^2 I.V., day 8
Leucovorin 25 mg/m^2 PO every 6 hours for 4 doses, beginning 24 hours after methotrexate
Repeat cycle every 21 days

Monoclonal Antibody Regimens

Ibritumomab tiuxetan

Ibritumomab tiuxetan is administered in 2 steps:
Step 1: Rituximab 250 mg/m2 infusion followed within 4 hours by a fixed 5.0 mCi (1.6 mg total antibody dose) of **In-111 Ibritumomab tiuxetan** administered as a 10-minute I.V. push
Step 2 (7–9 days after step 1): Rituximab 250 mg/m^2 infusion followed within 4 hours by **Y-90 Ibritumomab tiuxetan** 0.4 mCi/kg (maximum 32 mCi) administered as a 10-minute I.V. push

Rituximab

Rituximab 375 mg/m^2/d I.V., days 1, 8, 15, 22
Infuse at 50 mg/h initially; increase rate if tolerated

Tositumomab

Dosimetric step: Tositumomab 450 mg infused over 60 minutes
Iodine I^{131} tositumomab (35 mg tositumomab containing 5.0 mCi I^{131}) infused over 20 minutes
Therapeutic step: Tositumomab 450 mg infused over 60 minutes
Iodine I^{131} tositumomab (dose individualized for each patient based on results of dosimetric step)

Single-Agent Regimens

Bexarotene

Bexarotene 300 mg/m^2/d PO with a meal until benefit is no longer derived

Denileukin diftitox

Denileukin diftitox 9 or 18 mcg/kg/d I.V. over 15–60 minutes, days 1–5
Repeat cycle every 21 days

Fludarabine

Fludarabine 25 mg/m^2/d I.V. over 10 minutes, days 1–5
Repeat cycle every 21–28 days

Lymphoma–Primary CNS

MTX

Methotrexate 2.5 g/m^2 I.V. over 2–3 hours every other wk × 5 doses (weeks 1, 3, 5, 7, 9)

Leucovorin 20 mg PO q 6 hours × 12 doses (weeks 1, 3, 5, 7, 9)

Methotrexate 12 mg IT via Ommaya reservoir (weeks 2, 4, 6, 8, 10)

FOLLOWED BY

Leucovorin 10 mg PO bid × 8 doses beginning the evening after Methotrexate administration

Vincristine 1.4 mg/m^2 I.V. (max 2.8 mg) every other wk × 5 doses (week 1, 3, 5, 7, 9)

Procarbazine 100 mg/m^2 PO × 7 days (weeks 1, 5, 9)

Dexamethasone 16 mg/d PO week 1, 12 mg/d week 2, 8 mg/d week 3, 6 mg/d week 4, 4 mg/d week 5, and 2 mg/d week 6.

Whole-brain RT 1.20 Gy fractions, bid × 15 days (if CR after week 10)

Cytarabine 3 mg/m ^{2}/d I.V. over 3 hr × 2 days × 2 cycles (begin after RT on weeks 16, 19)

References

CHOP

Bezwoda W, Ristogi RB, Erazo Valla A, et al. Long-term results of a multicentre randomised, comparative phase III trial of CHOP versus CNOP regimens in patients with intermediate and high-grade non-Hodgkin's lymphomas. *Eur J Cancer.* 1995;31A: 903–911.

CHOP+ Rituximab

Coiffier B, Lepage E, Brière J, et al. CHOP chemotherapy plus rituximab compared with CHOP alone in elderly patients with diffuse large B-cell lymphoma. *N Engl J Med.* 2002;346:235–242.

Czuczman MS, Grillo-López AJ, White CA, et al. Treatment of patients with low-grade B-cell lymphoma with the combination of chimeric anti-CD20 monoclonal antibody and CHOP chemotherapy. *J Clin Oncol.* 1999;17:268–276.

CNOP

Bezwoda W, Ristogi RB, Erazo Valla A, et al. Long-term results of a multicentre randomised, comparative phase III trial of CHOP versus CNOP regimens in patients with intermediate and high-grade non-Hodgkin's lymphomas. *Eur J Cancer.* 1995;31A: 903–911.

COP

Luce JK, Gamble JF, Wilson HE, et al. Combined cyclophosphamide, vincristine, and prednisone therapy of malignant lymphoma. *Cancer.* 1971;28:306–317.

CVP

Hagenbeek A, Carde P, Meerwaldt JH, et al. Maintenance of remission with human recombinant interferon alfa-2a in patients with stages III and IV low-grade malignant non-Hodgkin's lymphoma. *J Clin Oncol.* 1998;16:41–47.

DHAP

Velasquez WS, Cabanillas F, Salvador P, et al. Effective salvage therapy for lymphoma with cisplatin in combination with high-dose Ara-C and dexamethasone (DHAP). *Blood.* 1988;71:117–122.

ESHAP

Velasquez WS, McLaughlin P, Tucker S, et al. ESHAP—an effective chemotherapy regimen in refractory and relapsing lymphoma: a 4-year follow-up study. *J Clin Oncol.* 1994;12:1169–1176.

Rodriguez MA, Cabanillas FC, Velasquez W, et al. Results of a salvage treatment program for relapsing lymphoma: MINE consolidated with ESHAP. *J Clin Oncol.* 1995;13:1734–1741.

Fischer DS, Knobf MT, Durivage HJ, eds. *The Cancer Chemotherapy Handbook,* 5th ed. St. Louis, MO: CV Mosby;1997;397.

Casciato CA, Lowitz BB, eds. *Manual of Clinical Oncology*, 4th ed. Boston, MA: Little, Brown and Co; 2000;379.

Hyper-CVAD/MTX-Ara-C

Khouri IF, Romaguera J, Kantarjian H, et al. Hyper-CVAD and high-dose methotrexate/cytarabine followed by stem-cell transplantation: an active regimen for aggressive mantle-cell lymphoma. *J Clin Oncol.* 1998;16:3803–3809.

MINE-ESHAP

Velasquez WS, McLaughlin P, Tucker S, et al. ESHAP—an effective chemotherapy regimen in refractory and relapsing lymphoma: a 4-year follow-up study. *J Clin Oncol.* 1994;12:1169–1176.

Rodriguez MA, Cabanillas FC, Velasquez W, et al. Results of a salvage treatment program for relapsing lymphoma: MINE consolidated with ESHAP. *J Clin Oncol.* 1995;13:1734–1741.

Fischer DS, Knobf MT, Durivage HJ, eds. *The Cancer Chemotherapy Handbook,* 5th ed. St. Louis, MO: CV Mosby;1997;397.

Casciato CA, Lowitz BB, eds. *Manual of Clinical Oncology*, 4th ed. Boston, MA: Little, Brown and Co;2000;379.

ProMACE/cytaBOM

Longo DL, DeVita VT Jr, Duffey PL, et al. Superiority of ProMACE-CytaBOM over ProMACE-MOPP in the treatment of advanced diffuse aggressive lymphoma: results of a prospective randomized trial. *J Clin Oncol.* 1991;9:25–38.

Ibritumomab tiuxetan

Zevalin (package insert). San Diego, CA: IDEC Pharmaceutical Corporation; 2003.

Wiseman GA, White CA, Sparks RB, et al. Biodistribution and dosimetry results from a phase III prospectively randomized controlled trial of Zevalin radioimmunotherapy for low-grade, follicular, or transformed B-cell non-Hodgkin's lymphoma. *Crit Rev Oncol Hematol.* 2001;39:181–194.

Rituximab

McLaughlin P, Grillo-López AJ, Link BK, et al. Rituximab chimeric anti-CD20 monoclonal antibody therapy for relapsed indolent lymphoma: half of patients respond to a four-dose treatment program. *J Clin Oncol.* 1998;16:2825–2833.

Maloney DG, Grillo-López AJ, White CA, et al. IDEC-C2B8 (rituximab) anti-CD20 monoclonal antibody therapy in patients with relapsed low-grade non-Hodgkin's lymphoma. *Blood.* 1997;90:2188–2195.

Tositumomab

Bexxar (package insert). Seattle, WA, and Philadelphia, PA: Corixa Corp and GlaxoSmithKline; 2003.

Bexarotene

Targretin (package insert). San Diego, CA: Ligand Pharmaceuticals, Inc; 2001.

Denileukin diftitox

Olsen E, Duvic M, Frankel A, et al. Pivotal phase III trial of two dose levels of denileukin diftitox for the treatment of cutaneous T-cell lymphoma. *J Clin Oncol.* 2001;19: 376–388.

Fludarabine

Pigaditou A, Rohantiner AZS, Whelan JS, et al. Fludarabine in low-grade lymphoma. *Semin Oncol.* 1993;20(suppl 7):24–27.

MTX

DeAngelis LM, Seiferheld W, Schold SC, et al. Combination chemotherapy and radiotherapy for primary central nervous system lymphoma: Radiation Oncology Group Study 93-10. *J Clin Oncol.* 2002;20(suppl 7):2643–4648.

Melanoma

Combination Regimens

Cisplatin/Dacarbazine/ Carmustine/Tamoxifen	**Cisplatin** 25 mg/m²/d I.V., days 1–3
	Dacarbazine 220 mg/m²/d I.V., days 1–3
	Carmustine 150 mg/m² I.V., day 1 of every odd 21-day cycle
	Tamoxifen 10 mg PO bid
	Repeat cycle every 21 days
CVD	**Cisplatin** 20 mg/m²/d I.V., days 2–5
	Vinblastine 1.6 mg/m²/d I.V., days 1–5
	Dacarbazine 800 mg/m² I.V., day 1
	Repeat cycle every 21 days
CVD + IL-2	**Cisplatin** 20 mg/m²/d I.V., days 1–4
	Vinblastine 1.6 mg/m²/d I.V., days 1–4
	Dacarbazine 800 mg/m² I.V., day 1

Interleukin-2 9 million units/m^2/d I.V. CI, days 1–4
Interferon alfa 5 million units/m^2/d SQ, days 1–5, 7, 9, 11, 13
Repeat cycle every 21 days

Single-Agent Regimens

Aldesleukin	**Aldesleukin** 0.037 mg/kg I.V. over 15 minutes, every 8 hours (maximum, 14 doses) *Repeat cycle after 9 days; treatment course (28 doses) may be repeated following rest period of at least 7 weeks*
Dacarbazine	**Dacarbazine** 2.0–4.5 mg/kg/d I.V., days 1–10 *Repeat cycle every 28 days* **OR** **Dacarbazine** 250 mg/m^2/d I.V., days 1–5 *Repeat cycle every 21 days*
Interferon alfa-2a	**Interferon alfa-2a** 20 million units/m^2 IM 3 times a week for 12 weeks
Interferon alfa-2b	**Interferon alfa-2b** 20 million units/m^2/d I.V., days 1–5 for 4 weeks, then 10 million units/m^2 SQ 3 times a week for 48 weeks
Temozolomide	**Temozolomide** 200 mg/m^2/d PO under fasting conditions, days 1–5 *Repeat cycle every 28 days*

References

Cisplatin/Dacarbazine/Carmustine/Tamoxifen

Chapman PB, Einhorn LH, Meyers ML, et al. Phase III multicenter randomized trial of the Dartmouth regimen versus dacarbazine in patients with metastatic melanoma. *J Clin Oncol.* 1999;17:2745–2751.

CVD

Legha SS, Ring S, Papadopoulos N, et al. A prospective evaluation of a triple drug regimen containing cisplatin, vinblastine, and dacarbazine (CVD) for metastatic melanoma. *Cancer.* 1989;64:2024–2029.

CVD + IL-2

Legha SS, Ring S, Eton O, et al. Development of a biochemotherapy regimen with concurrent administration of cisplatin, vinblastine, dacarbazine, interferon alfa, and interleukin-2 for patients with metastatic melanoma. *J Clin Oncol.* 1998;16:1752–1759.

Aldesleukin

Proleukin (package insert). Emeryville, CA: Chiron Corporation; 2000.

Dacarbazine

Middleton MR, Grob JJ, Aaronson N, et al. Randomized phase III study of temozolomide versus dacarbazine in the treatment of patients with advanced metastatic malignant melanoma. *J Clin Oncol.* 2000;18:158–166.

DTIC-Dome (package insert). West Haven, CT: Bayer Corporation; 1998.

Interferon alfa-2a

Creagan ET, Dalton RJ, Ahmann DL, et al. Randomized, surgical adjuvant clinical trial of recombinant interferon alfa-2a in selected patients with malignant melanoma. *J Clin Oncol.* 1995;13:2776–2783.

Interferon alfa-2b

Kirkwood JM, Strawderman MH, Ernstoff MS, et al. Interferon alfa-2b adjuvant therapy of high-risk resected cutaneous melanoma: the Eastern Cooperative Oncology Trial EST 1684. *J Clin Oncol.* 1996;14:7–17.

Intron A (package insert). Kenilworth, NJ: Schering Corporation; 2002.

Temozolomide

Middleton MR, Grob JJ, Aaronson N, et al. Randomized phase III trial study of temozolomide versus dacarbazine in the treatment of patients with advanced metastatic malignant melanoma. *J Clin Oncol.* 2000;18:158–166.

Multiple Myeloma

Combination Regimens

M2	**Vincristine#** 0.03 mg/kg I.V., day 1
	Carmustine 0.5 mg/kg I.V., day 1
	Cyclophosphamide 10 mg/kg I.V., day 1
	Melphalan 0.25 mg/kg/d PO, days 1–4 OR 0.1 mg/kg/d PO, days 1–7 or 1–10
	Prednisone 1 mg/kg/d PO, days 1–7, then taper and discontinue on day 21, unless continued therapy is warranted
	Repeat cycle every 35 days
MP	**Melphalan** 10 mg/m²/d PO, days 1–4
	Prednisone 60 mg/m²/d PO, days 1–4
	Repeat cycle every 42 days
Thalidomide/ Dexamethasone	**Thalidomide** 200 mg/d PO
	Dexamethasone 40 mg/d PO d 1–4, 9–12, 17–20 during odd cycles, and 40 mg PO d 1–4 during even cycles
VAD	**Vincristine#** 0.4 mg/d I.V. CI, days 1–4
	Doxorubicin 9 mg/m²/d I.V. CI, days 1–4
	Dexamethasone 40 mg PO, days 1–4, 9–12, 17–20
	Repeat cycle every 25 days
VBMCP	**Vincristine#** 1.2 mg/m² I.V., day 1

Carmustine 20 mg/m^2 I.V., day 1
Melphalan 8 mg/m^2/d PO, days 1–4
Cyclophosphamide 400 mg/m^2 I.V., day 1
Prednisone 40 mg/m^2/d PO, days 1–7 (all cycles), and 20 mg/m^2/d PO, days 8–14 (first 3 cycles only)
Repeat cycle every 35 days for 10 cycles (induction), then every 42 days for 3 cycles, then every 56 days until relapse

Single-Agent Regimens

Bortezomib	**Bortezomib** 1.3 mg/m^2/d I.V. bolus, days 1, 4, 8, 11 *Repeat cycle every 21 days*
Dexamethasone	**Dexamethasone** 20 mg/m^2/d PO, days 1–4, 9–12, and 17–20 *Repeat cycle after 14–day rest period*
Interferon alfa-2b	**Interferon alfa-2b** 2 million units/m^2 SQ 3 times per week for maintenance therapy in selected patients with significant response to initial melphalan treatment. Continue until evidence of relapse.
Melphalan	**Melphalan** 90–200 mg/m^2 I.V. *Administer 1 cycle*
Thalidomide	**Thalidomide** 200 mg/d PO at hs with dose escalation q 2 weeks over 6 weeks to target dose of 800 mg/d

References

M2

Case DC Jr, Lee DJ 3rd, Clarkson BD. Improved survival times in multiple myeloma treated with melphalan, prednisone, cyclophosphamide, vincristine and BCNU: M-2 protocol. *Am J Med.* 1977;63:897–903.

MP

Southwest Oncology Group Study.. Remission maintenance therapy for multiple myeloma. *Arch Intern Med.* 1975;135:147–152.

Fischer DS, Knobf MT, Durivage HJ, eds. *The Cancer Chemotherapy Handbook,* 5th ed. St. Louis, MO: CV Mosby; 1997;408.

Thalidomide/Dexamethasone

Rajkumar SV, Hayman S, Gertz MA, et al. Combination therapy with thalidomide plus dexamethasone for newly diagnosed myeloma. *J Clin Oncol* 2002;20:4319–4323

VAD

Barlogie B, Smith L, Alexanian R. Effective treatment of advanced multiple myeloma refractory to alkylating agents. *N Engl J Med.* 1984;310:1353–1356.

VBMCP

Oken MM, Harrington DP, Abramson N, et al. Comparison of melphalan and prednisone with vincristine, carmustine, melphalan, cyclophosphamide, and prednisone in the treatment of multiple myeloma: results of Eastern Cooperative Oncology Group study E2479. *Cancer.* 1997;79:1561–1567.

Bortezomib

Richardson PG, Barlogie B, Berenson J, et al. A phase 2 study of bortezomib in relapsed, refractory myeloma. *N Engl J Med.* 2003;348:2609–2617.

Dexamethasone

Alexanian R, Dimopoulos MA, Delasalle K, Barlogie B. Primary dexamethasone treatment of multiple myeloma. *Blood.* 1992;80:887–890.

Interferon alfa-2b

Browman GP, Bergsagel D, Sicheri D, et al. Randomized trial of interferon maintenance in multiple myeloma: a study of the National Cancer Institute of Canada Clinical Trials Group. *J Clin Oncol.* 1995;13:2354–2360.

Melphalan

Cunningham D, Paz-Ares L, Gore ME, et al. High-dose melphalan for multiple myeloma: long-term follow-up data. *J Clin Oncol.* 1994;12:764–768.

Vesole DH, Barlogie B, Jagannath S, et al. High-dose therapy for refractory multiple myeloma: improved prognosis with better supportive care and double transplants. *Blood.* 1994;84:950–956. Thalidomide

Singhal S, Mehta J, Desikan R, et al. Antitumor activity of thalidomide in refractory multiple myeloma. *N Engl J Med.* 1999;341:1565–1571.

Pancreatic Cancer

Combination Regimens

GEMOX

Gemcitabine 1 g/m², day 1 as 100-minute infusion
Oxaliplatin 100 mg/m², day 2 as 2-hour infusion

SMF

Streptozocin 1,000 mg/m²/d I.V. over 10–20 minutes, days 1, 8, 29, 36
Mitomycin-C 10 mg/m² I.V., day 1
Fluorouracil 600 mg/m²/d I.V., days 1, 8, 29, 36
Repeat cycle every 56 days

Single-Agent Regimen

Gemcitabine

Gemcitabine 1,000 mg/m² I.V. over 30 minutes once weekly for 7 weeks, followed by a 1-week rest period
Subsequent cycles once weekly for 3 consecutive weeks out of every 4 weeks

References

GEMOX

Louvet C, Labianca R, Hammel P. Gemcitabine versus GEMOX (gemcitabine + oxaloplatin) in nonresectable pancreatic adenocarcinoma: interim results of GERCOR/GISCAD Intergroup Phase III. Abstract presented at: American Society for Clinical Oncology 39th Annual Meeting;. May 31–June 1, 2003; Chicago, Ill. Abstract 1004.

SMF

The Gastrointestinal Tumor Study Group,. Phase II studies of drug combinations in advanced pancreatic carcinoma: fluorouracil plus doxorubicin plus mitomycin C and two regimens of streptozotocin plus mitomycin C plus fluorouracil. *J Clin Oncol.* 1986;4:1794–1798.

Gemcitabine

Burris HA, Moore MJ, Andersen J, et al. Improvements in survival and clinical benefit with gemcitabine as first-line therapy for patients with advanced pancreas cancer: a randomized trial. *J Clin Oncol.* 1997;15:2403–2413.

Pleural Mesothelioma

Pemetrexed/Cisplatin
Cisplatin

Pemetrexed 500 mg/m² I.V. over 10 minutes, day 1
Cisplatin 75 mg/m² I.V. over 2 hours, 30 minutes after pemetrexed dose
Premedications:
Dexamethasone 4 mg PO day 0, day 1, day 2
Folic acid 400 µg; PO qd starting 7 days prior to pemetrexed dose (Cycle 1), continuing qd during treatment, then for 21 days following last cycle of pemetrexed
Vit B12 1000 µg; IM/SQ beginning week prior to cycle 1, and continuing q 3 cycles during pemetrexed therapy
Repeat cycle every 21 days

References

Pemetrexed/Cisplatin

Alimta (package insert). Indianapolis, IN: Eli Lilly and Company; 2004.

Sarcoma

Combination Regimens

AD — **Doxorubicin** 15 mg/m²/d I.V. CI, days 1–4

	Dacarbazine 250 mg/m²/d I.V. CI, days 1–4
	Repeat cycle every 21 days
DI	**Doxorubicin** 50 mg/m² I.V. bolus, day 1
	Ifosfamide 5,000 mg/m² I.V. CI following doxorubicin, day 1
	Mesna 600 mg/m² I.V. bolus before ifosfamide, followed by 2,500 mg/m² I.V. CI with ifosfamide, and 1,250 mg/m² I.V. over 12 hours following ifosfamide
	Repeat cycle every 21 days
MAID	**Mesna** 2,500 mg/m²/d I.V. CI, days 1–4
	Doxorubicin 15 mg/m²/d I.V. CI, days 1–4
	Ifosfamide 2,500 mg/m²/d I.V. CI, days 1–3
	Dacarbazine 250 mg/m²/d I.V. CI, days 1–4
	Repeat cycle every 21 days

Single-Agent Regimen

Doxorubicin	**Doxorubicin** 75 mg/m² I.V. every 21 days

References

AD

Antman K, Crowley J, Balcerzak SP, et al. An intergroup phase III randomized study of doxorubicin and dacarbazine with or without ifosfamide and mesna in advanced soft tissue and bone sarcomas. *J Clin Oncol.* 1993;11:1276–1285.

DI

Santoro A, Tursz T, Mouridsen H, et al. Doxorubicin versus CYVADIC versus doxorubicin plus ifosfamide in first-line treatment of advanced soft tissue sarcomas: a randomized study of the European Organization for Research and Treatment of Cancer Soft Tissue and Bone Sarcoma Group. *J Clin Oncol.* 1995;13:1537–1545.

MAID

Antman K, Crowley J, Balcerzak SP, et al. An intergroup phase III randomized study of doxorubicin and dacarbazine with or without ifosfamide and mesna in advanced soft tissue and bone sarcomas. *J Clin Oncol.* 1993;11:1276–1285.

Doxorubicin

Nielsen OS, Dombernowsky P, Mouridsen H, et al. High-dose epirubicin is not an alternative to standard-dose doxorubicin in the treatment of advanced soft tissue sarcomas: a study of the EORTC soft tissue and bone sarcoma group. *Br J Cancer.* 1998;78:1634–1639.

---

*All patients should be premedicated with dexmethasone, diphenhydramine, and either ranitidine or cimetidine prior to paclitaxel administration. See paclitaxel package insert for dosages.

#Maximum vincristine dose should never exceed 2 mg.

**Amifostine 910 mg/m²/d I.V. over 15 min can be administered 30 min prior to chemotherapy with cisplatin to reduce cumulative renal toxicity in patients with ovarian cancer or non-small-cell lung cancer.

Index

Note: Page numbers followed by f indicate figures; those followed by t indicate tables. Generic drug names are in bolface type.

WY 156 WIL £35.00

2006
Oncology Nursing Drug Handbook

THE STATESMAN'S YEAR-BOOK

STATISTICAL AND HISTORICAL ANNUAL
OF THE STATES OF THE WORLD
FOR THE YEAR

1991–1992

EDITED BY

BRIAN HUNTER

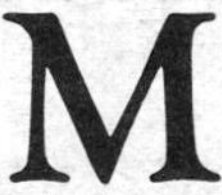

© The Macmillan Press Ltd, 1991

All rights reserved. No reproduction, copy or transmission of this publication may be made without written permission.

No paragraph of this publication may be reproduced, copied or transmitted save with written permission or in accordance with the provisions of the Copyright, Designs and Patents Act 1988, or under the terms of any licence permitting limited copying issued by the Copyright Licensing Agency, 33-4 Alfred Place, London WC1E 7DP (as amended).

Any person who does any unauthorised act in relation to this publication may be liable to criminal prosecution and civil claims for damages.

Published annually since 1864
128th edition first published 1991 by
THE MACMILLAN PRESS LTD
London and Basingstoke

Associated companies in Auckland, Delhi, Dublin, Gaborone, Hamburg, Harare, Hong Kong, Johannesburg, Kuala Lumpur, Lagos, Manzini, Melbourne, Mexico City, Nairobi, New York, Singapore, Tokyo.

British Library Cataloguing in Publication Data
Statesman's year-book.—1991-1992
1. Social conditions—Serials
909.82'8'05 HN1

ISSN 0081–4601
ISBN 0–333–39155–1

Typeset in Great Britain by
A. J. LATHAM LIMITED
Dunstable, Bedfordshire

Printed in Great Britain by
Richard Clay (The Chaucer Press) Ltd, Bungay, Suffolk

PREFACE

The year that has elapsed since THE STATESMAN'S YEAR-BOOK'S last account of the states of the world has again been marked by momentous events. The countries of the former communist bloc have continued to transform themselves in their various ways. East and West Germany have been re-unified, and the Warsaw Pact demilitarized. The Cold War's automatic confrontations are no longer a factor in global politics, and the world has seen how successful an international policing action can be when the United States and the Soviet Union acted in concert at the United Nations to compel Iraq to withdraw from Kuwait.

In different parts of the world several eras have ended. South Africa has abandoned apartheid; a number of single-party African states have held or announced democratic elections; and Britain has seen the departure from office of one of the few prime ministers to bestow an epithet upon the English language.

The editor would like to express his thanks to the correspondents and colleagues who contributed to this edition, and particularly to his predecessor, John Paxton, for the care and patience with which he handed on the task he loved so well.

Dr Paxton has thoroughly revised THE STATESMAN'S YEAR-BOOK WORLD GAZETTEER for its fourth edition, and this is now available for those who want more details about towns and regions.

THE STATESMAN'S YEAR-BOOK OFFICE,
THE MACMILLAN PRESS LTD,
LITTLE ESSEX STREET,
LONDON, WC2R 3LF

B.H.

WEIGHTS AND MEASURES

On 1 Jan. 1960 following an agreement between the standards laboratories of Great Britain, Canada, Australia, New Zealand, South Africa and the USA, an international yard and an international pound (avoirdupois) came into existence. 1 yard = 91·44 centimetres; 1 lb. = 453·59237 grammes.

The abbreviation 'm' signifies 'million(s)' and tonnes implies metric tons.

Length		Dry Measure	
Centimetre	0·394 inch	Litre	0·91 quart
Metre	1·094 yards	Hectolitre	2·75 bushels
Kilometre	0·621 mile		
		Weight—Avoirdupois	
Liquid Measure			
Litre	1·75 pints	Gramme	15·42 grains
Hectolitre	22 gallons	Kilogramme	2·205 pounds
		Quintal (= 100 kg)	220·46 pounds
		Tonne (= 1,000 kg)	0·984 long ton 1·102 short tons
Surface Measure			
		Weight—Troy	
Square metre	10·76 sq. feet	Gramme	15·43 grains
Hectare	2·47 acres	Kilogramme	32·15 ounces 2·68 pounds
Square kilometre	0·386 sq. mile		

BRITISH WEIGHTS AND MEASURES

Length		Weight	
1 foot	0·305 metre	1 ounce (= 437·2 grains)	28·350 grammes
1 yard	0·914 metre	1 lb. (= 7,000 grains)	453·6 grammes
1 mile (= 1,760 yds)	1·609 kilometres	1 cwt. (= 112 lb.)	50·802 kilogrammes
		1 long ton (= 2,240 lb.)	1·016 tonnes
		1 short ton (= 2,000 lb.)	0·907 tonne
Surface Measure		**Liquid Measure**	
1 sq. foot	9·290 sq. decimetres		
1 sq. yard	0·836 sq. metre	1 pint	0·568 litre
1 acre	0·405 hectare	1 gallon	4·546 litres
1 sq. mile	2·590 sq. kilometres	1 quarter	2·909 hectolitres

ABBREVIATIONS

Abbreviations of the names of organizations also appear in the index.

The three-letter groups in parentheses after the names of currencies are the codes of the International Standardization Organization (ISO).

ACP	African Caribbean Pacific
bbls.	barrels
CFA	Communauté Financière Africaine
CFP	Communauté Financière Pacifique
c.i.f.	cost, insurance, freight
C.-in-C.	Commander-in-Chief
cu.	cubic
CUP	Cambridge University Press
DWT	dead weight tonnes
ECOWAS	Economic Community of West African States
EEZ	Exclusive Economic Zone
ERM	Exchange Rate Mechanism
f.o.b.	free on board
GDP	gross domestic product
GNP	gross national product
GRT	gross registered tonnes
ha	hectare(s)
ind	independent(s)
kg	kilogramme(s)
kl	kilolitre(s)
km	kilometre(s)
kwh	kilowatt hours
m.	million
mw	megawatt
NRT	net registered tonnes
OUP	Oxford University Press
oz.	ounce(s)
SADCC	South African Development Co-ordination Council
SDR	Special Drawing Rights
sq.	square
TAFE	technical and further education
Univ.	University
vfd	value for duty

CONTENTS

Part I: International Organizations

Part II: Countries of the World A–Z

WHEAT[2]

Countries	Area (1,000 ha) Average 1979-81	1986	1987	1988	1989	Production (1,000 tonnes) Average 1979-81	1986	1987	1988	1989
Afghanistan	2,220	2,313	2,300	2,372	1,619	2,754	2,750	2,800	2,900	1,925
Argentina	5,245	4,893	4,875	4,617*	5,415*	8,060	8,700	9,000*	7,769*	10,000*
Australia [1]	11,440	11,135	9,005	9,301	8,827	14,468	16,119	12,287	14,102	14,200
Bulgaria [1]	986	1,127	1,085	1,181	1,138	3,881	4,327	4,149	4,713	5,402
Canada	11,386	14,239	13,474	12,921	13,638	20,430	31,378	25,950	15,655	24,382
Chile [1]	513	569	677	577	540	882	1,626	1,874	1,734	1,766
China [1]	28,930	29,617	28,799	29,001	29,801	59,196	90,044	87,775	87,505	91,002
Czechoslovakia	1,121	1,205	1,212	1,239	1,239	4,482	5,305	6,154	6,547	6,356
Egypt [1]	577	507	577	598	630*	1,844	1,928	2,721	2,839	3,148*
France	4,473	4,859	4,932	4,825	5,012	22,362	26,475	27,415	29,677	31,817
Germany, Fed. Rep. of	1,642	1,648	1,671	1,761	1,783	8,177	10,406	9,932	12,044	11,065
Greece	1,022	905	886	875	890	2,770	2,839	2,213	2,550	2,005
Hungary [1]	1,187	1,318	1,315*	1,281*	1,242	4,800	5,793	5,748	6,962	6,559
India	22,364	22,997	23,131	22,604	24,092	34,550	47,052	44,323	45,096	53,995
Iran	5,824	6,405	6,725	6,900	6,000	6,215	7,577	7,960	8,200	5,800
Iraq	1,215	1,240	859	1,300	500	854	1,036	722	1,200*	491*
Italy	3,373	3,136	3,087	2,895	2,951	8,989	9,102	9,381	7,945	7,408
Japan [1]	188	246	271	282*	284*	571	876	864	1,021*	985*
Mexico	723	1,201	988	900*	950*	2,754	4,770	4,415	3,700*	3,900*
Morocco	1,673	2,223	2,288	2,332	2,630	1,500	3,809	2,427	4,035	3,927
Pakistan [1]	6,865	7,403	7,706	7,307	7,730	10,760	13,923	12,016	12,675	14,419
Poland [1]	1,525	2,025	2,133	2,179	2,195	4,189	7,502	7,942	7,582	8,462
Romania [1]	2,154	2,360	2,400*	2,500*	2,600*	5,471	7,320	9,672	9,000	6,000*
S. Africa, Republic of	1,770	1,926	1,927	1,985*	1,830	1,965	2,321	3,135	3,400*	2,720
Spain	2,628	2,114	2,221	2,332	2,295	4,510	4,392	5,791	6,514	5,465
Turkey	9,208	9,356	9,331	9,341	9,300	17,058	19,032	18,932	20,500	15,729
USSR [1,3]	59,463	48,728	46,684	48,000*	47,635	89,859	92,306	83,312	84,500	90,500
UK	1,434	1,991	1,992	1,891	2,106	8,116	13,911	11,941	11,605	13,900
USA	28,898	24,574	22,646	21,519	25,150	66,229	56,926	57,357	49,295	55,407
Yugoslavia	1,475	1,346	1,498	1,506	1,479	4,624	4,776	5,345	6,303	5,599
World total	235,073	228,319	221,609	220,406	225,951	443,618	536,709	517,152	509,952	538,056

* Unofficial figures. [1] Sown area. [2] Includes spelt. [3] Does not include spelt.

RYE

Countries	Area (1,000 ha) Average 1979–81	1986	1987	1988	1989	Production (1,000 tonnes) Average 1979–81	1986	1987	1988	1989
Argentina	199	65	96	55	75	169	60	88	41	71
Austria	105	83	85	80*	91	327	284	309	280*	381
Belgium	12	5	5*	3*	2*	43	22	20	14*	12*
Bulgaria [1]	21	30	32	32	25	29	52	49	58	51
Canada	362	315	313	245	364	636	609	493	257	835
China	733	550	650	650	650	1,167	900	1,000	1,000	1,000
Czechoslovakia	192	155	142	143	175	534	547	496	534	708
Denmark	59	120	136*	80	101*	221	546	513	366	485*
Finland	44	27	38	26	69	88	71	74	49	202
France	121	81	82	79	74	368	229	299	276	262
German Demo. Rep.	671	680	655	606	624	1,848	2,406	2,283*	1,783	2,103
Germany, Fed. Rep. of	532	414	412	373	384	1,980	1,768	1,599	1,558	1,797
Hungary [1,2]	72	89	94	97*	97	117	172	186	245	261
Netherlands	10	4	6	7	7	39	19	25	27	33
Poland [1]	2,970	2,760	2,647	2,325	2,275	6,166	7,074	6,817	5,501	6,216
Portugal	166	124	128	124	122	128	100	108	73	97
Romania [1]	33	35	37*	37	37	38	66*	55	60*	63
Spain	219	221	222	222	227	239	220	318	357	337
Sweden	58	40	40	36	67	197	154	137	140	316
Turkey	439	221	240	222	165	558	350	380	293	183
USSR [1]	7,557	8,741	9,725	9,000	10,598	9,309	15,296	18,082	16,000*	18,800
USA	295	274	276	246	194	474	496	503	382	343
Yugoslavia	56	42	41	40	37	78	74	69	76	75
World total	15,076	15,283	16,272	14,903	16,655	24,980	31,794	34,145	29,617	34,893

* Unofficial figures. [1] Sown area. [2] Fields crops and other crops.

BARLEY

Countries	Area (1,000 ha) Average 1979–81	1986	1987	1988	1989	Production (1,000 tonnes) Average 1979–81	1986	1987	1988	1989
Australia [1]	2,539	2,274	2,346	2,272	2,190	3,278	3,548	3,417	3,270	3,242
Austria	370	333	291	277*	292	1,288	1,292	1,179	1,135	1,422
Belgium	173	146	139	131*	122	844	858	736	802*	693
Bulgaria [1]	425	318	295	345	360	1,439	1,144	1,091	1,306	1,568
Canada	4,631	4,829	5,005	4,132	4,701	11,199	14,569	13,957	10,125	11,672
China	1,295	1,100	990	990	1,295	3,133	2,520	2,800	3,000	3,200
Czechoslovakia	972	821	834	793	751	3,524	3,530	3,551	3,411	3,550
Denmark	1,580	1,078	943	1,154	1,001*	6,250	5,134	4,292	5.419	4,982*
Finland	579	589	583	682	517	1,421	1,714	1,306	1,612	1,614
France	2,670	2,090	1,992	1,916	1,830	10,997	10,063	10,489	10,086	9,810
German Demo. Rep.	959	895	891	874	895	3,592	4,293	4,198	3,798	4,683
Germany, Fed. Rep. of	2,011	1,947	1,850	1,841	1,753	8,566	9,377	8,571	9,609	9,757
Greece	344	266	241	261	225	838	681	573	695	496
Hungary [1,2]	265	253	208*	264*	282	848	857	794	1,161	1,339
India	1,802	1,369	1,225	1,148	1,093	2,020	1,962	1,669	1,593	1,721
Iran	1,336	2,200	2,200	2,200	2,500	1,397	2,500	2,500	2,500	2,600
Ireland	349	283	276	275	258	1,603	1,428	1,599	1,538	1,470
Italy	324	465	445	450	477	914	1,543	1,710	1,561	1,702
Japan [1]	120	107	105*	114*	113*	392	344	353	399*	371*
Korea, South [1]	386	190	204*	284	230*	1,059	453	516	733*	552*
Morocco	2,190	2,472	2,314	2,552	2,399	1,712	3,563	1,543	3,501	2,999
Poland [1]	1,362	1,335	1,286	1,250	1,175	3,563	4,412	4,335	3,804	3,909
Romania [1]	833	575*	560*	660	680	2,360	2,497	3,231	2,200*	1,800*
Spain	3,520	4,340	4,401	4,175	4,257	6,571	7,431	9,836	12,070	9,308
Sweden	678	638	545	2,323	480*	537	2,327	1,907	1,942	1,889*
Syria	1,220	1,548	1,570	1,844	859	1,129	1,116	576	2,836	271
Turkey	2,846	3,343	3,298	3,300	2,800	5,480	7,000	6,900	7,500	4,500
USSR [1]	33,456	29,964	30,654	30,000	27,611	46,540	53,889	58,409	47,000	52,000
UK	2,333	1,917	1,831	1,895	1,622	10,058	10,014	9,226	8,765	7,977
USA	3,214	4,859	4,070	3,049	3,360	8,838	13,292	11,529	6,325	8,784
World total	81,044	79,448	78,088	75,961	71,962	156,844	182,387	181,699	168,423	168,964

* Unofficial figures. [1] Sown area. [2] Field crops and other crops.

OATS

	Area (1,000 ha)					Production (1,000 tonnes)				
Countries	*Average 1979–81*	*1986*	*1987*	*1988*	*1989*	*Average 1979-81*	*1986*	*1987*	*1988*	*1989*
Argentina	353	312	476	446	445	431	495	718	620	668
Australia	1,201	1,140	1,275	1,439	1,309	1,386	1,584	1,698	1,815	1,838
Austria	93	73	69	70*	67	298	270	246	250*	249
Belgium	39	23	22	21*	20	171	98	65	95*	63*
Canada	1,501	1,287	1,263	1,418*	1,705	2,993	3,251	2,995	2,993	3,549
Chile	84	64	56	61	69	151	124	128	157	185
China	400	400	400	400	400	600	500	600	500	600
Czechoslovakia	132	115	108	102	103	418	419	406	366	330
Denmark	40	27	23	44	21*	166	111	95	202	110*
Finland	444	403	368	388*	446	1,183	1,175	813*	857	1,455
France	525	312	281	273	226	1,850	1,066	1,122	1,074	1,025
German Demo. Rep.	154	163	149	148	143	571	666	637	508	476
Germany, Fed.Rep.of	700	506	459	474	421	2,777	2,276	2,008	2,036	1,552
Ireland	25	21	20	22	19	95	102	106	117	103
Italy	223	184	177	171	168	433	397	361	383	293
Netherlands	20	7	9	13	8	106	40	47	63	32
Norway	108	126	115	128	128	424	401	466	480	500*
Poland [1]	1,082	924	856	850	803	2,387	2,486	2,429	2,222	2,186
Spain	453	393	353	335	345	527	433	502	537	494
Sweden	461	455	397	423	412*	1,635	1,486	1,440	1,402	1,466*
Turkey	199	158	178	158	150	350	300	325	276	215
USSR [1]	12,160	13,173	11,790	12,000	10,880	14,372	21,929	18,495	16,500	17,000
UK	142	97	99	121	121	587	503	451	557	600
USA	3,743	2,776	2,802	2,262	2,780	7,234	5,608	5,429	3,175	5,425
Yugoslavia	199	152	140	135	144	296	260	232	253	279
World total	25,691	24,847	23,489	23,549	23,167	42,582	47,417	43,223	38,848	42,197

* Unofficial figures. [1] Sown area.

MAIZE

Countries	Area (1,000 ha)					Production (1,000 tonnes)				
	Average 1979–81	1986	1987	1988	1989	Average 1979–81	1986	1987	1988	1989
Argentina	2,895	3,231	2,900	2,438	1,520	9,333	12,100	9,250	9,200	4,260
Austria	190	217	207	202*	194	1,338	1,740	1,685	1,640*	1,491
Brazil	11,430	12,466	13,499	13,142	12,859	19,265	20,531	26,787	24,709	26,508
Bulgaria	605	574	497	494	563	2,626	2,848	1,858	1,625	2,421
Canada	1,039	994	999	981	1,014	5,904	5,912	7,015	5,369	6,400
China	19,986	19,199	20,291	19,792*	20,385	60,720	71,128	80,127	73,820	75,840*
Egypt	800	623	761	900	644*	3,159	2,918	3,367	4,088*	3,748*
France	1,774	1,884	1,743	1,936	1,920	9,641	11,641	12,470	13,996	12,926
Greece	157	218	262	212	200	1,165	1,994	2,156	2,116	1,700
Hungary	1,270	1,146	1,170	1,122*	1,124	7,022	7,261	7,234	6,027	6,949
India	5,887	5,923	5,542	5,900*	5,800*	6,486	7,593	5,629	7,500*	7,800*
Indonesia	2,761	3,143	2,626	3,203	2,969	4,035	5,920	5,155	6,668	6,324
Italy	956	849	768	843	807	6,590	6,461	5,764	6,318	6,251*
Kenya	1,273	1,426	1,600*	1,800*	1,554	1,714	2,898	2,250*	2,685	2,925
Malawi	1,120	1,193	1,153	1,216*	1,271	1,268	1,295	1,225	1,445*	1,510
Mexico	6,836	6,417	6,788	6,800	5,900*	11,866	11,721	11,575	11,800	9,900*
Nigeria	443	600	700	700	1,500	591	1,336	1,202	1,500	1,600
Philippines	3,267	3,595	3,683	3,745	3,489	3,174	4,091	4,278	4,428	4,522
Portugal	333	258	262	230	271	486	628	655	663	674
Romania	3,309	2,976	2,894	3,200	3,100*	11,823	20,158	18,378	19,500	11,800
S. Africa, Republic of	4,900	4,044	4,014*	3,600*	3,778*	11,207	8,077	7,372	6,900*	11,700*
Spain	450	524	542	556	576	2,227	3,423	3,557	3,577	3,224
Tanzania	1,350	1,626	1,650*	1,720*	1,950*	1,762	2,787	2,359	2,339*	3,159
Thailand	1,408	1,815	1,357	1,950	1,793	3,103	4,309	2,781	5,166	4,456
Turkey	583	560	570	560	500	1,263	2,300	2,400	2,100	2,000
USSR [1]	3,063	4,223	4,573	4,200*	4,786	9,076	12,479	14,808	16,000	17,000
USA	29,661	27,988	23,960	23,538	27,223	192,084	209,555	179,638	125,003	191,197
Yugoslavia	2,250	2,369	2,218	2,269	2,279	9,736	12,526	8,863	7,697	9,415
Zimbabwe	1,097	1,314	1,211	1,300	1,198*	1,829	2,545	931	2,253	1,931*
World total	126,060	128,337	125,983	126,613	129,664	421,873	485,066	458,028	405,460	470,318

* Unofficial figures. [1] For dry grain only.

RICE (Paddy)

Countries	Area (1,000 ha) Average 1979–81	1986	1987	1988	1989	Production (1,000 tonnes) Average 1979–81	1986	1987	1988	1989
Bangladesh	10,310	10,610	10,322	10,000	10,630	20,125	23,110	23,120	21,900	26,600*
Brazil	5,932	5,585	6,000	5,961	5,273	8,533	10,374	10,425	11,804	11,107
Burma	4,684	4,666	4,641	4,715	4,760	12,637	14,126	13,722	14,000	13,581
Cambodia	1,186	1,700	1,546	1,600	2,100	1,160	2,000	1,855	2,000	1,800
China	34,323	32,798	32,694	32,500	32,400*	145,665	174,790	176,958	172,365	179,403*
Colombia	428	325	385	389	432	1,831	1,521	1,865	1,775	1,884
Egypt	416	423	412	330*	413*	2,376	2,445	2,279	1,900*	2,680*
India	40,091	41,167	38,319	41,000	41,500*	74,557	90,779	84,538	101,950	107,500*
Indonesia	9,063	9,988	9,923	10,090	10,304	29,570	39,727	40,078	41,769	43,566
Iran	433	489	510	482	400	1,448	1,828	1,920	1,757*	1,200
Italy	176	192	190	198	203	989	1,137	1,064	1,094	1,130*
Japan	2,384	2,303	2,146	2,132*	2,097*	13,320	14,559	13,284	12,419	12,934*
Korea, North	793	860	875	885	890	4,970	6,000	6,200	6,350	6,400
Korea, South	1,230	1,236	1,262	1,260	1,215*	6,780	7,872	7,596	8,400*	8,200*
Madagascar	1,182	1,188	1,214	1,200	1,200	2,055	2,230	2,296	2,100	2,290*
Malaysia	658	628	641	630	636*	2,053	1,745	1,697	1,669	1,697*
Mexico	153	158	155	120*	161*	528	545	591	420*	441*
Nepál	1,275	1,333	1,423	1,400	1,088	2,361	2,372	2,982	2,787	2,870
Nigeria	517	720*	730*	650	700	1,027	1,416	1,450*	1,400	1,400*
Pakistan	1,981	2,066	1,963	1,939	2,114	4,884	5,230	4,861	4,577	4,796
Philippines	3,513	3,464	3,256	3,293	3,497	7,893	9,247	8,540	8,971	9,459
Sri Lanka	819	836	679	811	730*	2,093	2,588	2,128	2,466	1,949*
Thailand	8,953	9,194	9,083	10,417	10,256*	16,967	18,868	18,042	20,813	21,300*
USSR	637	621	657	660	654	2,558	2,633	2,683	2,900	2,525
USA	1,345	955	944	1,172	1,087	6,968	6,049	5,879	7,237	7,007
Vietnam	5,558	5,689	5,594	5,600	5,860*	11,663	16,003	15,103	15,200*	18,100*
World total	145,602	145,157	141,497	145,602	146,455	396,290	472,482	464,514	483,466	506,291

* Unofficial figures.

MILLET

Countries	Area (1,000 ha) Average 1979–81	1986	1987	1988	1989	Production (1,000 tonnes) Average 1979–81	1986	1987	1988	1989
Argentina	203	94	59	45	45	245	107	80	50	50
Australia	26	31	42	39	26	26	32	39	45	21
Burkina Faso	803	1,054	1,168	1,277	1,278	390	687	632	817	649
Cameroon	503	500	465	470	110	402	450	400	410	100
Chad	774	1,078*	950	990*	400*	409	624*	518*	690*	257*
China	3,981	2,981	2,689	2,701*	2,651*	5,790	4,541	4,539	5,501	5,701
Egypt	172	156	133	155	...	641	606	551	578*	...
Ethiopia	226	230	230	230	200	203	188	180	200	180
Ghana	182	240	220	240	244	117	140	121*	140	180
India	17,845	16,645	13,886	16,000*	16,000*	9,189	8,383	6,775	8,500	10,000*
Kenya	80	60	60	60	96*	84	65	60	60	60*
Korea, North	418	440	445	448	450	447	545	560	575	600
Korea, South	3	3	2	2	2	4	3	3	3	2
Mali	1,077	1,634	1,540	1,624	980	801	1,301	1,207*	1,900*	862*
Nepal	122	151	165	169	175	121	138	150	160	170
Niger	3,011	3,239	3,000	3,482	3,385	1,311	1,383	1,020	1,783	1,293
Nigeria	2,882	3,900*	3,700	3,400	3,400	3,600*	4,111	3,905	4,000	3,500
Pakistan	509	509	293	270	558	255	233	135	125	220
Senegal	1,062	993	1,074	1,026	977*	603	634	801	634	671*
Sudan	1,094	1,543	1,091*	2,300*	1,550*	458	285	153*	550*	167*
Tanzania	450	308	290*	300	300	370	259	291*	280*	300
Togo	121	116	128	120*	120*	44	82	71	50*	78
Uganda	297	342	295	300*	270	473	350	471	414	380
USSR	2,794	2,485	2,763	2,800	2,736	1,759	2,368	3,926	2,700	4,000
Zimbabwe [1]	250	295*	310	374	296*	153	141*	81	278	142*
World total	40,101	40,419	36,284	40,641	37,464	27,784	28,711	27,679	31,536	30,512

* Unofficial figures. [1] On farms and estates.

SORGHUM

Countries	Area (1,000 ha)					Production (1,000 tonnes)				
	Average 1979–81	*1986*	*1987*	*1988*	*1989*	*Average 1979–81*	*1986*	*1987*	*1988*	*1989*
Argentina	1,866	1,322	1,005	956	597	5,641	4,061	3,040	3,200	1,360
Australia	548	734	818	745	625	1,084	1,416	1,419	1,633	1,244
Burkina Faso	1,051	1,210	1,176	1,295	1,362	620	1,012	848	1,009	991
China	2,828	1,896	1,884	1,902*	1,903*	7,034	5,481	5,531	6,115	6,125
Colombia	220	227	259	266	239	488	600	704	707	689
Ethiopia [1]	1,048	910	900	910	900	1,420	1,092	950	1,100	964
France	75	45	36	43	70	332	172	209	234	300
India	16,361	15,948	15,648	16,000*	15,500*	11,380	9,185	11,847	11,000	11,500*
Mexico	1,491	1,533	1,853	1,800	1,300*	4,991	4,833	6,296	5,500	3,800*
Niger	822	1,109	1,100	1,470	1,566	347	360	360	603	452
Nigeria	3,047	4,800	4,200	4,500	4,200	3,545	5,455	5,182	4,940	4,587
S. Africa, Republic of	377	307	314	313*	281	540	437	467	482*	466
Sudan	3,163	4,960	3,360	5,882*	3,682*	2,361	3,282	1,300	4,640*	1,924*
Thailand	220	184	160	184	184	237	211	192	215	229
Uganda	175	208	185	199*	180	312	280	286	289*	260
USA	5,273	5,609	4,291	3,663	4,513	19,157	23,829	18,778	14,670	15,694
Venezuela	227	381*	350*	350*	330*	365	756	777	600*	450*
Yemen Arab Republic	631	601	566	584	585	616	457	450	542	547
World total	44,143	46,200	42,684	45,590	44,441	64,522	67,265	62,843	61,787	57,976

* Unofficial figures. [1] Includes teff.

CENTRIFUGAL RAW SUGAR
(in 1,000 tonnes)

Countries	*Average 1979–81*	*1984*	*1985*	*1986*	*1987*	*1988*	*1989*
Argentina	1,584	1,545	1,174	1,120*	1,063	1,150*	915*
Australia [1]	3,243	3,548	3,379	3,371	3,440	3,580*	3,679
Barbados [2]	113	100	100	111	83	83*	66*
Brazil	7,991	9,332*	8,274*	8,649*	8,458*	8,500*	7,409*
Canada	118	113	54	122	147*	109*	135*
China	3,809	5,352*	6,347*	6,340*	5,219*	5,925*	5,634*
Colombia	1,192	1,178	1,367	1,297	1,390	1,415	1,425
Cuba	7,510	8,331*	8,101*	7,467	7,232	7,548*	8,188*
Czechoslovakia	808	844*	939*	862	818	614	755*
Dominican Rep.	1,142	1,156	921	895	866	800*	810*
Egypt	666	780	887*	959	1,007	1,029*	977*
France	4,720	4,305	4,324	3,734*	3,973*	4,424*	4,130*
Fiji [1]	446	480	341	502	401	420	385*
German Demo.Rep.	675	778*	798*	790*	760*	445*	668*
Germany, Fed.Rep.of	3,261	3,151	3,454	3,479	2,963*	3,130	3,109
Guyana	294	238	265	249	234*	168*	166*
India [3]	5,380	6,430	6,650	7,051	8,533	9,100	10,200*
Indonesia [4]	1,286	1,500	1,767	2,013	2,073	1,800*	1,817
Italy	1,956	1,385*	1,352*	1,868*	1,867*	1,607*	1,800*
Jamaica	238	193	225	206	189*	221*	192*
Mauritius	615	610	684	707	694	634	568
Mexico	2,796	3,297*	3,489*	4,031*	3,986*	3,822*	3,678*
Pakistan [3]	734	1,258	1,430	1,210	1,364	1,936	2,011*
Peru	571	620*	757*	599	560*	565*	580*
Philippines	2,289	2,335	1,718	1,447	1,337	1,369	1,590*
Poland	1,530	1,878	1,811	1,891	1,823	1,824*	1,850
Puerto Rico	156	87	98	87	87	93	83*
S. Africa, Rep.of	2,011	2,560	2,280	2,248*	2,235*	2,260*	2,276*
Spain	934	1,166	976	1,111	1,108	1,088*	1,038*
Sweden	350	392	346	386	275	396*	422*
Thailand	1,534	2,350*	2,572	2,586	2,637	2,705	4,052*
Trinidad	117	70	81	92	85	91*	97*
Turkey	1,178	1,655*	1,398*	1,414*	1,784*	1,595*	1,314*
USSR	7,017	8,685*	8,260*	8,700*	9,565*	9,240*	9,565*
UK	1,215	1,400	1,317	1,433	1,335*	1,413*	1,304
USA	5,345	5,363	5,473	6,075	6,651	6,260	6,464
World total	88,622	99,976	99,283	101,273	101,781	102,779	105,639

[1] 94° net titre.
[2] Includes the sugar equivalent of fancy molasses.
[3] Includes sugar (raw value) refined from gur.
[4] Tel quel.
* Unofficial figures.

WORLD ESTIMATED CRUDE OIL PRODUCTION[1]

(in 1,000 tonnes)

	1960	*1970*	*1989*	*1990*
Africa				
Algeria*	8,630	47,253	51,370	56,678
Angola	70	5,066	22,642	23,963
Congo	—	—	7,396	7,835
Côte d'Ivoire	—	—	350	215
Egypt	—	—	42,956	44,197
Gabon*	850	5,460	10,998	13,772
Libya*	—	159,201	53,694	65,784
Nigeria*	880	53,420	83,129	90,811
Tunisia	—	4,151	4,740	4,422
Zaïre	—	—	1,358	1,350
Caribbean Area				
Colombia	8,100	11,071	20,383	22,600
Cuba	—	—	718	736
Trinidad	6,075	7,225	7,881	7,333
Venezuela*	148,690	193,209	94,591	110,526
Far East				
Australia	—	8,292	22,783	27,340
Brunei	4,690	6,916	7,449	7,449
Burma	530	750	756	781
China	5,000	20,000	136,068	137,679
India	440	6,809	33,685	31,633
Indonesia*	20,560	42,102	68,034	69,777
Japan	510	750	542	518
Malaysia	—	—	26,545	28,584
New Zealand	—	—	1,702	1,657
Pakistan	360	486	2,530	3,042
Thailand	—	—	1,812	1,816
Vietnam	—	—	1,022	2,482
Middle East				
Abu Dhabi*	—	33,288	70,706	70,956
Bahrain	2,250	3,834	2,102	2,058
Dubai*	—	—	20,706	20,902
Iran*	52,065	191,663	144,347	156,078
Iraq*	47,480	76,600	139,185	100,262
Kuwait*	81,860	137,397 [2]	91,886 [2]	58,401 [2]
Oman	—	—	31,819	33,056
Qatar*	8,210	17,257	19,139	19,403
Saudi Arabia*	61,090	176,851 [2]	257,176 [2]	320,720 [2]
Sharjah*	—	—	1,681	1,802
Syria	—	4,350	16,998	20,292
Turkey	350	3,461	2,843	3,447
Yemen	—	—	9,410	9,931

[1] Excluding small scale production in Afghanistan, Bangladesh and Mongolia; including other small producers not specified here.

[2] Figures for Saudi Arabia and Kuwait include shares of production from the Neutral Zone, all counted as Saudi from Aug. 1990.

*Member of OPEC.

WORLD ESTIMATED CRUDE OIL PRODUCTION

(contd.)

(in 1,000 tonnes)

	1960	*1970*	*1989*	*1990*
North America				
Canada	27,480	69,954	92,404	91,024
USA	384,080	533,677	425,830	409,634
Latin America				
Argentina	9,160	19,969	23,596	24,168
Bolivia	990	1,128	930	903
Brazil	390	8,009	30,229	32,002
Chile		1,620	1,102	980
Ecuador*	2,680	191	14,604	14,484
Mexico	14,125	21,877	143,617	146,678
Peru	450	3,450	6,975	6,831
USSR and Eastern Europe				
Albania	600	1,199	2,135	1,986
Bulgaria	200	334	303	322
Czechoslovakia	140	203	144	113
Hungary	1,215	1,937	1,966	2,000
Poland	195	424	154	100
Romania	11,500	13,377	9,237	8,228
USSR	148,000	352,667	607,181	569,309
Yugoslavia	1,040	2,854	3,393	3,250
Western Europe				
Austria	2,440	2,798	1,158	1,222
Denmark	—	—	5,530	5,784
France	2,260	2,308	3,243	3,017
Germany, Fed. Rep. of	5,560	7,536	3,792	3,648
Italy	1,990	1,408	4,355	4,788
Netherlands	1,920	1,919	3,814	4,142
Norway	—	49,500	74,594	81,080
Spain	—	156	1,039	825
UK	90	84	91,749	93,471
World total	1,090,080	2,336,153	3,113,280	3,150,358

*Member of OPEC.

MARITIME LIMITS (IN MILES)

State	*Territorial Sea*	*Jurisdiction over fisheries (measured from the baseline of the territorial sea)*
Albania	15 (1976)	—
Algeria	12 (1963)	—
Angola	20 (1975)	200 (1975)
Antigua and Barbuda	12 (1982)	200 (1982) [1]
Argentina	200 (1967)	—
Australia	3 (1973)	200 (1979)
Bahamas	3 (1878)	200 (1977)
Bahrain	3	—
Bangladesh	12 (1974)	200 (1974) [1]
Barbados	12 (1977)	200 (1979) [1]
Belgium	3	up to median line (1978)
Belize	3 (1878)	—
Benin	200 (1976)	—
Brazil	200 (1970)	—
Brunei Darussalam	12 (1983)	200 (1983) (or median line)
Bulgaria	12 (1951)	200 (1987) [1]
Burma	12 (1968)	200 (1977) [1]
Cambodia	12(1969)	200 (1979) [1]
Cameroon	50 (1974)	—
Canada	12 (1970)	200 (1977)
Cape Verde	12 (1977)	200 (1977) [1]
Chile	12 (1986)	200 (1986) [1]
China	12 (1958)	—
Colombia	12 (1978)	200 (1978) [1]
Comoros	12 (1976)	200 (1982) [1]
Congo	200 (1977)	—
Costa Rica	12 (1982)	200 (1975) [1]
Côte d'Ivoire	12 (1977)	200 (1977) [1]
Cuba	12 (1977)	200 (1977) [1]
Cyprus	12 (1964)	—
Denmark (including Faroe Islands and Greenland)	3 (1966)	200 (1977)
Djibouti	12 (1979)	200 (1979) [1]
Dominica	12 (1981)	200 (1981) [1]
Dominican Republic	6 (1967)	200 (1977) [1]
Ecuador	200 (1966)	—
Egypt	12 (1958)	—
El Salvador	200 (1983)	—
Equatorial Guinea	12 (1984)	200 (1984) [1]
Ethiopia	12 (1953)	—
Fiji	12 (1978)	200 (1981) [1]
Finland	4 (1956)	12 (1975) (or agreed boundary)
France	12 (1971)	200 (1977) [1] (except Mediterranean)
Gabon	12 (1986)	200 (1986) [1]
Gambia	12 (1969)	200 (1978)
Germany	3 [2]	200 (1977)
Ghana	12 (1986)	200 (1986) [1]
Greece	6 (1936)	—
Grenada	12 (1978)	200 (1978) [1]
Guatemala	12 (1976)	200 (1976) [1]
Guinea	12 (1980)	200 (1980) [1]
Guinea-Bissau	12 (1978)	200 (1978) [1]

[1] Economic zone. [2] In the Baltic Sea; off the former GDR, 12 miles; in the German Bight, at least 12 miles; area defined by coordinates.

MARITIME LIMITS (IN MILES)—*contd.*

State	*Territorial Sea*	*Jurisdiction over fisheries (measured from the baseline of the territorial sea)*
Guyana	12 (1977)	200 (1977)
Haiti	12 (1972)	200 (1977) [1]
Honduras	12 (1965)	200 (1951) [1]
Iceland	12 (1979)	200 (1979) [1]
India	12 (1967)	200 (1977) [1]
Indonesia	12 (1957) [2]	200 (1980) [1,7]
Iran	12 (1959)	[8]
Iraq	12 (1958)	—
Ireland	12 (1988)	200 (1977)
Israel	6 (1956)	—
Italy	12 (1974)	—
Jamaica	12 (1971)	—
Japan	12 (1977)	200 (1977)
Jordan	3 (1943)	—
Kenya	12 (1971)	200 (1979) [1]
Kiribati	12 (1983)	200 (1983) [1]
Korea (North)	12 (1967)	200 (1977) [1]
Korea (South)	12 (1978)	12
Kuwait	12 (1967)	—
Lebanon	12 (1983)	—
Liberia	200 (1976)	—
Libya	12 (1959)	—
Madagascar	12 (1985)	200 (1985) [1]
Malaysia	12 (1969)	200 (1984) [1]
Maldive, Republic of	12 (1975)	(1976) [1,3]
Malta	12 (1978)	25 (1978)
Mauritania	12 (1988)	200 (1988) [1]
Mauritius	12 (1977)	200 (1977) [1]
Mexico	12 (1972)	200 (1976) [1]
Monaco	12 (1973)	(1985) [9]
Morocco	12 (1973) [4]	200 (1981) [1,4]
Mozambique	12 (1976)	200 (1976) [1]
Namibia	6 (1963)	12 (1963)
Nauru	12 (1971)	200 (1978)
Netherlands	12 (1985)	200 (1977)
New Zealand	12 (1977)	200 (1978) [1]
Nicaragua	(1979) [5]	200 (1979) [5]
Nigeria	30 (1971)	200 (1978) [1]
Norway	4 (1812)	200 (1977) [1]
Oman	12 (1977)	200 (1981) [1]
Pakistan	12 (1976)	200 (1976) [1]
Panama	200 (1967)	—
Papua New Guinea	12 (1978)	200 (1978) (offshore waters)
Peru	(1947) [5]	200 (1947) [5]
Philippines	[6]	200 (1978) [1]

[1] Economic zone.
[2] The territorial sea of Indonesia is measured by straight lines surrounding the archipelago.
[3] Territorial limits and economic zone defined by geographical co-ordinates.
[4] Limits with opposite or adjacent states to be fixed by agreement, failing which median line principle to apply.
[5] Sovereignty and jurisdiction over the sea, its soil and subsoil up to 200 miles.
[6] The territorial sea of the Philippines is determined by straight base-lines joining appropriate points of the outermost islands forming the Philippine archipelago in accordance with Treaties of 1898, 1900 and 1930 (1961).
[7] 200 mile exclusive fisheries zone established 1985.
[8] Outer limits of the superjacent waters of the continental shelf. 50-mile fishing zone in the Sea of Oman (1973).
[9] Half way to Corsica.

MARITIME LIMITS (IN MILES)—*contd.*

State	*Territorial Sea*	*Jurisdiction over fisheries (measured from the baseline of the territorial sea)*
Poland	12 (1978)	to be determined (1978)
Portugal	12 (1977)	200 (1977) [2]
Qatar	3	[1]
Romania	12 (1956)	200 (1986) [2]
St Christopher (St Kitts)–Nevis	12 (1984)	200 (1984) [2]
St Lucia	12 (1984)	200 (1984) [2]
St Vincent and the Grenadines	12 (1983)	200 (1983) [2]
São Tomé and Principe	12 (1978)	200 (1978) [2]
Saudi Arabia	12 (1958)	[6]
Senegal	12 (1985)	200 (1985) [2]
Seychelles	12 (1977)	200 (1977) [2]
Sierra Leone	200 (1971)	—
Singapore	3 (1878)	—
Solomon Islands	12 (1978)	200 (1986)
Somalia	200 (1972)	—
South Africa, Republic of	12 (1977)	200 (1977)
Spain	12 (1977)	200 (1978) [2] (except Mediterranean)
Sri Lanka	12 (1977)	200 (1977) [2]
Sudan	12 (1987)	—
Suriname	12 (1978)	200 (1978) [2]
Sweden	12 (1980)	200 (1978)
Syria	35 (1981)	—
Tanzania	12 (1989)	200 (1989) [1]
Thailand	12 (1966)	200 (1980) [2]
Togo	30 (1977)	200 (1977) [2]
Tonga	[3]	—
Trinidad and Tobago	12 (1969)	200 (1986) [2]
Tunisia	12 (1973)	—
Turkey	[7]	12 (1964) 200 (1986) [2] (Black Sea)
Tuvalu	12 (1984)	200 (1984) [2]
USSR	12 (1982)	200 (1984) [2]
United Arab Emirates	3 [4]	[5]
UK	12 (1987)	200 (1977)
USA	12 (1988)	200 (1983) [2]
Uruguay	200 (1969)	—
Vanuatu	12 (1978–82)	200 (1978–82) [2]
Venezuela	12 (1956)	200 (1978) [2]
Vietnam	12 (1977)	200 (1977) [2]
Western Samoa	12 (1971)	200 (1980) [2]
Yemen [8]	—	—
Yugoslavia	12 (1979)	—
Zaïre	12 (1974)	—

[1] Limited by agreement by the outer limits of the superjacent waters of the continental shelf or by a median line (1974).

[2] Economic zone.

[3] Territorial limits defined by geographical co-ordinates (173–177° W. and 15–23° 30' S.) (1887).

[4] Sharjah, 12 miles.

[5] Limits to be defined by agreement, failing which median line to apply (1980).

[6] Outer limits of the superjacent waters of the continental shelf.

[7] 6 Aegean (1964), 12 Black Sea and Mediterranean.

[8] Situation under review following the unification of the Republic and People's Democratic Republic.

The table above, reproduced from a survey prepared by the FAO of the UN shows: *(a)* the territorial sea limit, and *(b)* jurisdiction over fisheries.

Further Reading

Attard, D. J., *The Exclusive Economic Zone in International Law*. Oxford, 1987

Booth, K., *Law, Force and Diplomacy at Sea*. London, 1985

Buzan, B., *Seabed Politics*. New York, 1976

Churchill, R. R. and Lowe, A. V., *The Law of the Sea*. Manchester, 1988

Janis, M. W., *Sea Power and the Law of the Sea*. Lexington, 1977

Luard, E., *The Control of the Sea-Bed*. London, 1974

Moore, G., *Coastal State Requirements for Foreign Fishing. FAO Legislative Study No. 21*. Rev. 2. Rome, 1985

Sangar, C., *Ordering the Oceans: The Making of the Law of the Sea*. Univ. of Toronto Press, 1987

CHRONOLOGY

1990

April 4 Hong Kong. National People's Congress of China approves Basic Law, to be Hong Kong's constitution after 1997.

8 Greece. Konstantinos Mitsotakis's New Democracy wins election.
Hungary. Hungarian Democratic Forum wins general election.

19 Nepal. New reforming government led by Krishna Prasad Bhattarai.

May 2 South Africa. Meeting between representatives of the government and the African National Congress.

4 Afghanistan. President Najibullah lifts state of emergency.
Greece. Konstantinos Karamanlis elected president by parliament.

5 Germany. GDR and Federal German foreign ministers meet foreign ministers of France, USSR, UK and USA ('two-plus-four' talks) to discuss re-unification.

8 Israel. Formation of coalition government under Prime Minister Shamir of right-wing Likud party.
Czechoslovakia. First free general elections since 1946 won by Civic Forum and its Slovak cognate Public Against Violence.

10 Bulgaria. Socialist Party (formerly Communists) wins elections.

20 Romania. National Salvation Front wins general elections.
USA and PLO. US President Bush announces suspension of dialogue with Palestine Liberation Organization begun in Dec. 1988.

22 Yemen. Yemen Arab Republic and People's Democratic Republic of Yemen united as Republic of Yemen.

24 North Korea. Kim Il Sung re-elected president.

27 Colombia. César Gaviria Trujillo elected president.

29 EBRD. Founding charter of the European Bank for Reconstruction and Development signed.

June 1 USA and USSR. Presidents Bush and Gorbachev sign agreements banning the production of chemical weapons, normalizing commercial relations between their two countries, and a provisional treaty on nuclear weapons.

5 USA. Primary elections in 9 states.

7 South Africa. State of emergency lifted except in Natal.

8 Israel. Formation of new coalition government under Prime Minister Shamir of the right-wing Likud party.

10 Peru. Alberto Fujimori elected president.

July 5 Czechoslovakia. Václav Havel re-elected president for 2-year term.

8 Mozambique. First peace talks between Frelimo government and Mozambique National Resistance rebels.

25 Zimbabwe. State of emergency, first imposed in 1965, lifted.

28 Russia. Boris Yeltsin elected chairman of Supreme Soviet.

CHRONOLOGY—*contd.*

1990

Aug. 1 Bulgaria. Zhelyu Zhelev elected president by parliament.

2 Kuwait. Occupation by Iraq.

3 USA. Budget negotiations between President Bush and bipartisan Congressional panel adjourned in deadlock.

6 Pakistan. President Khan dismisses Prime Minister Benazir Bhutto.

UN. Security Council invokes sanctions against Iraq for its occupation of Kuwait.

7 South Africa. African National Congress suspends its 29-year armed insurrection.

USA. Decides to send ground, naval and air units to Saudi Arabia as part of a coalition force to end Iraq's occupation of Kuwait.

8 Kuwait. Iraq announces annexation.

15 Iraq and Iran. Iraq accepts Iranian peace terms.

28 Serbia. New constitution reduces autonomy of Kosovo and Vojvodina.

31 Germany. State treaty signed by GDR and Federal Germany outlining constitutional arrangements for unification.

Sept. 4 New Zealand. Mike Moore becomes prime minister.

Korea. North and South Korean prime ministers meet.

9 USA and USSR. Meeting of Presidents Bush and Gorbachev in Helsinki results in joint statement calling on Iraq to leave Kuwait.

10 Cambodia. Cambodian parties accept UN peace plan.

11 Liberia. President Doe killed in continuing civil war.

UK. Announcement that UK ground units would be deployed in Saudi Arabia as part of coalition force.

Russia. Unilateral adoption by Russian Supreme Soviet of Shatalin programme to establish market economy in 500 days.

12 Germany. Foreign ministers of GDR, Federal Germany, France, UK, USA and USSR sign Treaty on Final Settlement, covering external aspects of German re-unification.

24 USSR. President Gorbachev granted emergency powers.

25 Iraq. UN Security Council embargo on air traffic with Iraq.

27 Iran and UK. Resumption of diplomatic relations.

Oct. 3 Germany. GDR re-unified with Federal Germany.

5 UK. Chancellor of the Exchequer John Major announces that sterling will enter the European Exchange Rate Mechanism.

6 USA. House of Representatives approves stop-gap funding measure after the defeat of the budget agreement for fiscal year 1990–91.

7 Austria. Socialist Party wins general election.

15 Lebanon. Syrian and Lebanese troops expel Gen. Aoun.

18 South Africa. State of emergency lifted in Natal also.

CHRONOLOGY—*contd.*

1990

Oct. 24 Pakistan. Benazir Bhutto's Pakistan People's Party defeated in national and provincial elections.

27 New Zealand. Jim Bolger's National party wins general election.
EC. Meeting of heads of state and government agree, with UK expressing reservations, that stage two of economic and monetary union should start on 1 Jan. 1994.

28 Tanzania. Ali Hassan Mwinyi returned in presidential elections.
USA. Agreement reached on compromise budget.

Nov. 3 Norway. Minority Labour government under Gro Brundtland.

6 USA. In mid-term elections Democrats keep their majority in Senate and House of Representatives.

7 India. Prime Minister Singh resigns afer a vote of no confidence.
Ireland. Mary Robinson elected first woman president.

9 Nepal. King Birendra promulgates democratic constitution.

12 Japan. Coronation of Emperor Akihito.

19 CSCE. Second meeting of Conference on Security and Co-operation in Europe leads to treaty between NATO and Warsaw Pact countries for the reduction of conventional arms in Europe.

22 UK. Resignation of Prime Minister Margaret Thatcher after failing to gain a majority in first round of Conservative Party leadership ballot.

28 Liberia. Ceasefire agreed after extraordinary meeting of Economic Community of West African States.
UK. John Major appointed Prime Minister after winning second round of Conservative Party leadership ballot.

29 Iraq. UN Security Council resolution authorizes use of force from 15 Jan. 1991 to restore Kuwaiti sovereignty.

Dec. 1 Chad. President Hissène Habré ousted in military coup.

2 Bulgaria. Resignation of Socialist government.
Germany. Chancellor Kohl's conservative Christian Democratic Union wins victory in first all-German elections for 57 years.

4 Bangladesh. Resignation of President Ershad.

7 GATT. Collapse of Uruguay round talks after failure to reach agreement on farm subsidies.

9 Poland. Lech Wałęsa elected president.

11 Albania. Communist party legalizes opposition parties.

16 South Africa. African National Congress agrees to negotiations with government to end apartheid.

17 Haiti. Father Jean-Bertrand Aristide elected president.

20 USSR. Resignation of Foreign Minister Shevardnadze.

1991

Jan. 6 Guatemala. Centre-right candidate Jorge Serrano elected president.

9 Gulf. Meeting between US Secretary of State James Baker and Iraqi Foreign Minister Tariq Aziz in Geneva ends in stalemate.

CHRONOLOGY—*contd.*

1991		
Jan.	12	Poland. New government under Jan Krzystof Bielecki.
	13	Portugal. Mario Soares re-elected president.
	14	USSR. Valentin Pavlov becomes prime minister.
	15	Gulf. Expiry of UN deadline for Iraqi withdrawal from Kuwait.
	16	Gulf. First airbone attacks by coalition forces.
	17	Norway. Death of Olav V, king since 1957.
	18	Gulf. Iraqi missile attacks on Israel hit Tel Aviv and Haifa.
	27	Somalia. Rebel groups drive out President Siad Barre.
	28	South Africa. Nelson Mandela, of the African National Congress, and Prince Buthelezi, leader of the rival Inkatha Freedom party, issue a joint call for an end to mutual violence.
	30	Gulf. Land battle after Iraqi occupation of Saudi border town of Khafji leads to coalition victory.
Feb.	1	South Africa. President de Klerk announces abolition of Land Act, group Areas Act and Population Registration Act.
	8	UK. Irish Republican army makes unsuccessful mortar bomb attack on UK cabinet in session.
	10	CFE. Conventional Forces in Europe meeting of USA, USSR and European nations in Vienna.
	18	UK. Irish Republican Army bombs at 2 London railway stations.
	22	Gulf. Coalition forces launch land attack to liberate Kuwait. Thailand. Military coup ends three years of democracy.
	24	Gulf. Coalition forces enter Iraq to isolate Iraqi army in Kuwait.
	26	Gulf. Coalition forces drive Iraqis back across Iraqi border.
	27	Gulf. USA calls ceasefire.
	28	Bangladesh. Khaleda Zia's Bangladesh National Party wins just under half the votes in general election.
March	1	Gulf. Meeting of coalition and Iraqi leaders to discuss ceasefire.
	2	Iraq. Rebellion of Shi'ites in the south and Kurds in the north. Sri Lanka. Assassination of Defence Minister Wijeratne.
	3	Gulf. Temporary ceasefire agreed.
	6	India. Resignation of Prime Minister Shekhar.
	21	USSR. Referendum shows 76% of voters in 9 republics favour President Gorbachev's proposed new federal union.
	22	UK. Secretary of State for the Environment Michael Heseltine announces abandonment of community charge.
	26	Mali. Military coup deposes President Traoré.
	28	Iraq. Shi'ite rebellion in south defeated by government forces.
	29	Italy. Resignation of Prime Minister Andreotti.
	31	Warsaw Pact. Unified military command dissolved.

ADDENDA

WARSAW PACT. The unified military command was dissolved on 31 March 1991.

ALBANIA. At the elections of March–April 1991 the Communist party won 168 seats, the Democratic Party 74, Omonia (Greek minority) 5 and the Veterans' Union 1.

BENIN. At the presidential elections of March 1991 Nicephore Soglo defeated President Kerekou, gaining 67·6% of votes cast. He was sworn in 4 April.

FINLAND. At the parliamentary elections of 17 March 1991 the Centre Party won 55 seats, the Social Democrats 48, the Conservatives 40, the Left Alliance 19, the Swedish Liberals 11 and the Greens 10. Esko Aho (Centre Party) was forming a new government in April 1991.

IRAQ. Taha Yassin Ramadan was appointed Vice-President 23 March 1991 and a new cabinet was announced. *Prime Minister:* Saadun Hammadi. *Deputy Prime Ministers:* Tariq Aziz; Mohammed Hamza Zubeidi. *Interior:* Ali Hassan Al Majid. *Foreign:* Ahmed Hussein Al Khudayer. *Agriculture and Irrigation:* Abdel Al Sabbagh. *Waqfs and Religious Affairs:* Abdallah Fadel Abbas. *Planning:* Samal Majid Faraj. *Trade:* Mohamed Mehdi Saleh. *Industry and Oil:* Col. Hussein Kamel Hassan. *Defence:* Gen. Hussein Kamel Hassan. *Culture and Information:* Hamed Yusef Hammadi. *Justice:* Shebib Al Maliki. *Labour and Social Affairs:* Umid Midhat Mubarak. *Health:* Abdessalam Mohammad Said. *Construction:* Mahmud Diab Al Ahmed. *Finance:* Majid Abed Jaafar. *Higher Education:* Abderrazzak Al Hashimi. *Education:* Hikmat Al Baddal. *Transport and Communications:* Abdessattar Al Maini.

On 11 April Iraq accepted a UN Security Council resolution for a permanent ceasefire following its military expulsion from Kuwait. Provisions included: Iraq to respect the Kuwaiti border; the UN to guarantee the border and to deploy a peace-keeping force in a demilitarized zone along it; Iraq to be liable for damages and accept destruction of its chemical and biological weapons. Coalition forces began their withdrawal in early April.

ITALY. Prime Minister Andreotti was forming a new government in April 1991.

KUWAIT. A new government was formed in April 1991.

MALI. On 26 March 1991 President Moussa Traoré was deposed in a military coup. Lieut.-Col. Amadou Touré was named head of a Transitional Committee of Public Safety. *Prime Minister:* Soumana Sacko.

SENEGAL. A new government under Habib Thiam was formed in April 1991.

USSR. At a referendum of 17 March 1991 turn-out was 80% of the electorate in the 9 republics which took part. 76% of voters favoured remaining within a reformed federal union. 6 republics (Armenia, Estonia, Georgia, Latvia, Lithuania and Moldavia) boycotted the referendum.

WESTERN SAMOA. The general election of April 1991 was conducted by universal adult suffrage. The Human Rights Protection Party won 26 seats, the Samoan National Development Party, 18, and independents, 3.

ZAIRE. Lunda Bululu and his government resigned on 14 March 1991. Mulumba Lukoji became caretaker prime minister with the task of introducing multi-party democracy.

PART I

INTERNATIONAL ORGANIZATIONS

THE UNITED NATIONS

The United Nations is an association of states which have pledged themselves, through signing the Charter, to maintain international peace and security and to co-operate in establishing political, economic and social conditions under which this task can be securely achieved. Nothing contained in the Charter authorizes the organization to intervene in matters which are essentially within the domestic jurisdiction of any state.

The United Nations Charter originated from proposals agreed upon at discussions held at Dumbarton Oaks (Washington, D.C.) between the USSR, US and UK from 21 Aug. to 28 Sept., and between US, UK and China from 29 Sept. to 7 Oct. 1944. These proposals were laid before the United Nations Conference on International Organization, held at San Francisco from 25 April to 26 June 1945, and (after amendments had been made to the original proposals) the Charter of the United Nations was signed on 26 June 1945 by the delegates of 50 countries. Ratification of all the signatures had been received by 31 Dec. 1945. (For the complete text of the Charter *see* THE STATESMAN'S YEAR-BOOK, 1946, pp. xxi–xxxii.)

The United Nations formally came into existence on 24 Oct. 1945, with the deposit of the requisite number of ratifications of the Charter with the US Department of State. The official languages of the United Nations are Arabic, Chinese, English, French, Russian and Spanish.

The headquarters of the United Nations is in New York City, USA.

Flag: UN emblem in white centred on a light blue ground.

Membership. Membership is open to all peace-loving states whose admission will be effected by the General Assembly upon recommendation of the Security Council. The table on pp. 7–8 shows the 159 member states of the United Nations.

The Principal Organs of the United Nations are: 1. The General Assembly. 2. The Security Council. 3. The Economic and Social Council. 4. The Trusteeship Council. 5. The International Court of Justice. 6. The Secretariat.

1. **The General Assembly** consists of all the members of the United Nations. Each member has only 1 vote. The General Assembly meets regularly once a year, commencing on the third Tuesday in Sept.; the session normally lasts until mid-December and is resumed for some weeks in the new year if this is required. Special sessions may be convoked by the Secretary-General if requested by the Security Council, by a majority of the members of the United Nations or by 1 member concurred with by the majority of the members. The Assembly also meets in emergency special session. The General Assembly elects its President for each session.

The first regular session was held in London from 10 Jan. to 14 Feb. and in New York from 23 Oct. to 16 Dec. 1946.

Special sessions have been held on Palestine (1947, 1948), Tunisia (1961), Financial Situation of UN (1963), South West Africa, Peace-Keeping, Postponement of Outer Space Conference (1967), Raw Materials and Development (1974), New International Economic Order (1975), Peace-keeping force in the Lebanon, Namibia, Disarmament (1978, 1982), Economic Issues (1980); Emergency Special sessions were held on Suez, Hungary (1956), Lebanon-Jordan-United Arab Republic dispute (1958), Congo (1960), Middle East (1967), Afghanistan, Palestine (1980, resumed 1982), Namibia (1981), Economic Situation in Africa (1986), Namibia (1986) and Third Special Session on Disarmament (1988).

The work of the General Assembly is divided between 7 Main Committees, on which every member state is represented. These are: First committee (disarmament and related international security matters); special political committee; second committee (economic and financial matters); third committee (social, humanitarian and cultural matters); fourth committee (decolonisation matters); fifth committee (administrative and budgetary matters); sixth committee (legal matters).

In addition there is a General Committee charged with the task of co-ordinating the proceedings of the Assembly and its Committees; and a Credentials Committee which verifies the credentials of the delegates. The General Committee consists of 29 members, comprising the President of the General Assembly, its 17 Vice-Presidents and the Chairmen of the 7 Main Committees. The Credentials Committee consists of 9 members, elected at the beginning of each session of the General Assembly. The Assembly has 2 standing committees—an Advisory Committee on Administrative and Budgetary Questions, and a Committee on Contributions. The General Assembly establishes subsidiary and *ad hoc* bodies when necessary to deal with specific matters. These include: Special Committee on Peace-keeping Operations (33 members), Commission on Human Rights (43 members), Committee on the peaceful uses of outer space (53 members), Conciliation Commission for Palestine (3 members), Conference on Disarmament (40 members), International Law Commission (34 members), Scientific Committee on the effects of atomic radiation (20 members), Special Committee on the implementation of the declaration on the granting of independence to colonial countries and peoples (24 members), Special Committee on the policies of Apartheid of the Government of the Republic of South Africa (18 members) and UN Commission on International Trade Law (36 members).

The General Assembly may discuss any matters within the scope of the Charter, and, with the exception of any situation or dispute on the agenda of the Security Council, may make recommendations on any such questions or matters. For decisions on important questions a two-thirds majority is required, on other questions a simple majority of members present and voting. In addition, the Assembly at its fifth session, in 1950, decided that if the Security Council, because of lack of unanimity of the permanent members, fails to exercise its primary responsibility for the maintenance of international peace and security in any case where there appears to be a threat to the peace, breach of the peace or act of aggression, the General Assembly shall consider the matter immediately with a view to making appropriate recommendations to members for collective measures, including in the case of a breach of the peace or act of aggression the use of armed force when necessary, to maintain or restore international peace and security.

The General Assembly receives and considers reports from the other organs of the United Nations, including the Security Council. The Secretary-General makes an annual report to it on the work of the Organization.

2. **The Security Council** consists of 15 members, each of which has 1 vote. There are 5 permanent and 10 non-permanent members elected for a 2-year term by a two-thirds majority of the General Assembly.

Retiring members are not eligible for immediate re-election. Any other member of the United Nations may be invited to participate without vote in the discussion of questions specially affecting its interests.

The Security Council bears the primary responsibility for the maintenance of peace and security. It is also responsible for the functions of the UN in trust territories classed as 'strategic areas'. Decisions on procedural questions are made by an affirmative vote of 9 members. On all other matters the affirmative vote of 9 members must include the concurring votes of all permanent members (in practice, however, an abstention by a permanent member is not considered a veto), subject to the provision that when the Security Council is considering methods for the peaceful settlement of a dispute, parties to the dispute abstain from voting.

For the maintenance of international peace and security the Security Council can, in accordance with special agreements to be concluded, call on armed forces, assistance and facilities of the member states. It is assisted by a Military Staff Committee consisting of the Chiefs of Staff of the permanent members of the Security Council or their representatives.

The Presidency of the Security Council is held for 1 month in rotation by the member states in the English alphabetical order of their names.

The Security Council functions continuously. Its members are permanently represented at the seat of the organization, but it may meet at any place that will best facilitate its work.

The Council has 2 standing committees of Experts and on the Admission of New Members. In addition, from time to time, it establishes *ad hoc* committees and commissions such as the Truce Supervision Organization in Palestine.

Permanent Members: China, France, USSR, UK, USA.

Non-Permanent Members: Cuba, Côte d'Ivoire, Yemen, Romania, Zaïre (until 31 Dec. 1991); Austria, Belgium, Ecuador, India and Zimbabwe (until 31 Dec. 1992).

3. **The Economic and Social Council** is responsible under the General Assembly for carrying out the functions of the United Nations with regard to international economic, social, cultural, educational, health and related matters.

By Nov. 1977, 15 'specialized' inter-governmental agencies working in these fields had been brought into relationship with the United Nations. The Economic and Social Council may also make arrangements for consultation with international non-governmental organizations and, after consultation with the member concerned, with national organizations; by 1983 over 600 non-governmental organizations had been granted consultative status.

The Economic and Social Council consists of 54 Member States elected by a two-thirds majority of the General Assembly. Forty-two are elected each year for an 18-year term. Retiring members are eligible for immediate re-election. Each member has 1 vote. Decisions are made by a majority of the members present and voting.

The Council nominally holds 2 sessions a year, and special sessions may be held if required. The President is elected for 1 year and is eligible for immediate re-election.

The Economic and Social Council has the following commissions:

Regional Economic Commissions: ECE (Economic Commission for Europe. Geneva); ESCAP (Economic and Social Commission for Asia and the Pacific. Bangkok); ECLAC (Economic Commission for Latin America and the Caribbean. Santiago, Chile); ECA (Economic Commission for Africa. Addis Ababa). ESCWA (Economic Commission for Western Asia. Baghdad). These Commissions have been established to enable the nations of the major regions of the world to co-operate on common problems and also to produce economic information.

Six functional commissions, including: (1) a Statistical Commission with sub-commission on Statistical Sampling. (2) Commission on Human Rights; with sub-commission on Prevention of Discrimination and Protection of Minorities; (3) Social Development Commission; (4) Commission on the Status of Women; (5) Commission on Narcotic Drugs; (6) Population Commission.

The Economic and Social Council has the following standing committees: The Economic Committee, Social Committee, Co-ordination Committee, Committee on Non-Governmental Organizations, Interim Committee on Programme of Conferences, Committee for Industrial Development, Advisory Committee on the Application of Science and Technology to Development, Committee on Housing, Building and Planning.

Other special bodies are the International Narcotics Control Board, the Interim Co-ordinating Committee for International Commodity Arrangements and the Administrative Committee on Co-ordination to ensure (1) the most effective implementation of the agreements entered into between the United Nations and the specialized agencies and (2) co-ordination of activities.

Membership: Belize, Bolivia, Bulgaria, Canada, China, Denmark, Iran, Norway, Oman, Poland, Rwanda, Somalia, Sri Lanka, Sudan, USSR, United Kingdom, Uruguay, Zaïre (until 31 Dec. 1989). Colombia, Cuba, France, Federal Republic of Germany, Ghana, Greece, Guinea, India, Ireland, Japan, Lesotho, Liberia, Libya, Portugal, Saudi Arabia, Trinidad and Tobago, Venezuela, Yugoslavia (until 31 Dec. 1990); Bahamas, Brazil, Cameroon, Czechoslovakia, Indonesia, Iraq, Italy, Jordan, Kenya, Netherlands, New Zealand, Nicaragua, Niger, Thailand, Tunisia, Ukraine, USA, Zambia (until 31 Dec. 1991).

4. **The Trusteeship Council.** The Charter provides for an international trusteeship system to safeguard the interests of the inhabitants of territories which are not yet fully self-governing and which may be placed thereunder by individual trusteeship agreements. These are called trust territories.

All of the original 11 trust territories except one, the Pacific Islands (Micronesia), administered by the USA, have become independent or joined independent countries. The Trusteeship Council consists of the 1 member administering trust territories: USA; the permanent members of the Security Council that are not administering trust territories: China, France, USSR and UK. Decisions of the Council are made by a majority of the members present and voting, each member having 1 vote. The Council holds one regular session each year, and special sessions if required.

5. **The International Court of Justice** was created by an international treaty, the Statute of the Court, which forms an integral part of the United Nations Charter. All members of the United Nations are *ipso facto* parties to the Statute of the Court.

The Court is composed of independent judges, elected regardless of their nationality, who possess the qualifications required in their countries for appointment to the highest judicial offices, or are jurisconsults of recognized competence in international law. There are 15 judges, no 2 of whom may be nationals of the same state. They are elected by the Security Council and the General Assembly of the United Nations sitting independently. Candidates are chosen from a list of persons nominated by the national groups in the Permanent Court of Arbitration established by the Hague Conventions of 1899 and 1907. In the case of members of the United Nations not represented in the Permanent Court of Arbitration, candidates are nominated by national groups appointed for the purpose by their governments. The judges are elected for a 9-year term and are eligible for immediate re-election. When engaged on business of the Court, they enjoy diplomatic privileges and immunities.

The Court elects its own *President* and *Vice-President* for 3 years and remains permanently in session, except for judicial vacations. The full court of 15 judges normally sits, but a quorum of 9 judges is sufficient to constitute the Court. It may form chambers of 3 or more judges for dealing with a particular case or particular categories of cases. Sir Robert Jennings (UK) and Shigeru Oda (Japan) are, respectively, President and Vice-President of the Court until 1994.

Competence and Jurisdiction. Only states may be parties in cases before the Court, which is open to the states parties to its Statute. The conditions under which the Court will be open to other states are laid down by the Security Council. The Court exercises its jurisdiction in all cases which the parties refer to it and in all matters provided for in the Charter, or in treaties and conventions in force. Disputes concerning the jurisdiction of the Court are settled by the Court's own decision.

The Court may apply in its decision: *(a)* international conventions; *(b)* international custom; *(c)* the general principles of law recognized by civilized nations; and *(d)* as subsidiary means for the determination of the rules of law, judicial decisions and the teachings of highly qualified publicists. If the parties agree, the Court may decide a case *ex aequo et bono*. The Court may also give advisory opinions on legal questions to the General Assembly, the Security Council, certain other organs of the UN and a number of international organizations.

Procedure. The official languages of the Court are French and English. All questions are decided by a majority of the judges present. If the votes are equal, the President has a casting vote. The judgment is final and without appeal, but a revision may be applied for within 10 years from the date of the judgment on the ground of a new decisive factor. No court fees are paid by parties to the Statute.

Judges. The judges of the Court, elected by the Security Council and the General Assembly, are as follows: (1) To serve until 5 Feb. 1994: Taslim Olawale Elias (Nigeria), Manfred Lachs (Poland), Jens Evensen (Norway), Shigeru Oda (Japan), Ni Zhengyu (China). (2) To serve until 5 Feb. 1997: Roberto Ago (Italy), Mohamed Shahabuddeen (Guyana), Stephen Schwebel (USA), Mohammed Bedjaoui (Algeria), Nikolaï K. Tarasov (USSR). (3) To serve until 5 Feb. 2000: Sir Robert

Jennings (UK), Gilbert Guillaume (France), Andrés Aguilar Mawdsley (Venezuela), Christopher G. Weeramantry (Sri Lanka), Raymond Ranjeva (Madagascar).

If there is no judge on the bench of the nationality of a party to a case, that party has the right to choose a person to sit as judge for that case. Such judges take part in the decision on terms of complete equality with their colleagues.

The Court has its seat at The Hague, but may sit elsewhere whenever it considers this desirable. The expenses of the Court are borne by the UN.

Registrar: Eduardo Valencia-Ospina (Colombia).

6. **The Secretariat** is composed of the Secretary-General, who is the chief administrative officer of the organization, and an international staff appointed by him under regulations established by the General Assembly. However, the Secretary-General, the High Commissioner for Refugees and the Managing Director of the Fund are appointed by the General Assembly. The first Secretary-General was Trygve Lie (Norway), 1946–53; the second, Dag Hammarskjöld (Sweden), 1953–61; the third, U. Thant (Burma), 1961–71; the fourth, Kurt Waldheim (Austria), 1972–81.

The Secretary-General acts as chief administrative officer in all meetings of the General Assembly, the Security Council, the Economic and Social Council and the Trusteeship Council.

The financial year coincides with the calendar year; accountancy is in US$. Budget for 1988–89, $1,400m.

Secretary-General: Javier Pérez de Cuéllar (Peru), re-appointed 1 Jan. 1986 for a 5-year term.

The Secretary-General is assisted by Under-Secretaries-General and Assistant Secretaries-General.

MEMBER STATES OF THE UN

(as in 1990 with percentage scale of contribution)

Afghanistan	0·01	1946
Albania	0·01	1955
Algeria	0·14	1962
Angola	0·01	1976
Antigua and Barbuda	0·01	1981
Argentina [1]	0·62	1945
Australia [1]	1·66	1945
Austria	0·74	1955
Bahamas	0·01	1973
Bahrain	0·02	1971
Bangladesh	0·02	1974
Barbados	0·01	1966
Belgium [1]	1·18	1945
Belize	0·01	1981
Belorussia [1]	0·34	1945
Benin	0·01	1960
Bhutan	0·01	1971
Bolivia [1]	0·01	1945
Botswana	0·01	1966
Brazil [1]	1·40	1945
Brunei Darussalam	0·04	1984
Bulgaria	0·16	1955
Burkina Faso	0·01	1960
Burma	0·01	1948
Burundi	0·01	1962
Cambodia	0·01	1955
Cameroon	0·01	1960
Canada [1]	3·06	1945
Cape Verde	0·01	1975
Central African Rep.	0·01	1960
Chad	0·01	1960
Chile [1]	0·07	1945
China [1]	0·79	1945
Colombia [1]	0·13	1945
Comoros	0·01	1975
Congo	0·01	1960
Costa Rica [1]	0·02	1945
Côte d'Ivoire	0·02	1960
Cuba [1]	0·09	1945
Cyprus	0·02	1960
Czechoslovakia [1]	0·70	1945
Denmark [1]	0·72	1945
Djibouti	0·01	1977
Dominica	0·01	1978
Dominican Republic [1]	0·03	1945
Ecuador [1]	0·03	1945
Egypt [1]	0·07	1945
El Salvador [1]	0·01	1945
Equatorial Guinea	0·01	1968
Ethiopia [1]	0·01	1945
Fiji	0·01	1970
Finland	0·50	1955
France [1]	6·37	1945
Gabon	0·03	1960
Gambia	0·01	1965
Germany	9·59	1973
Ghana	0·01	1957
Greece [1]	0·44	1945
Grenada	0·01	1974
Guatemala [1]	0·02	1945

Guinea	0·01	1958	Peru [1]	0·07	1945
Guinea-Bissau	0·01	1974	Philippines [1]	0·10	1945
Guyana	0·01	1966	Poland [1]	0·64	1945
Haiti [1]	0·01	1945	Portugal	0·18	1955
Honduras [1]	0·01	1945	Qatar	0·04	1971
Hungary	0·22	1955	Romania	0·19	1955
Iceland	0·03	1946	Rwanda	0·01	1962
India [1]	0·35	1945	St Christopher and Nevis	0·01	1983
Indonesia	0·14	1950	St Lucia	0·01	1979
Iran [1]	0·63	1945	St Vincent and the Grenadines	0·01	1980
Iraq [1]	0·12	1945	Samoa, Western	0·01	1976
Ireland	0·18	1955	São Tomé and Principe	0·01	1975
Israel	0·22	1949	Saudi Arabia [1]	0·97	1945
Italy	3·79	1955	Senegal	0·01	1960
Jamaica	0·02	1962	Seychelles	0·01	1976
Japan	10·84	1956	Sierra Leone	0·01	1961
Jordan	0·01	1955	Singapore	0·10	1965
Kenya	0·01	1963	Solomon Islands	0·01	1978
Kuwait	0·29	1963	Somalia	0·01	1960
Laos People's Dem. Rep.	0·01	1955	South Africa [1]	0·44	1945
Lebanon [1]	0·01	1945	Spain	2·03	1955
Lesotho	0·01	1966	Sri Lanka	0·01	1955
Liberia [1]	0·01	1945	Sudan	0·01	1956
Libyan Arab Jamahiriya	0·26	1955	Suriname	0·01	1975
Liechtenstein	0·01	1990	Swaziland	0·01	1968
Luxembourg [1]	0·05	1945	Sweden	1·25	1946
Madagascar	0·01	1960	Syrian Arab Rep.[1]	0·04	1945
Malawi	0·01	1964	Tanzania	0·01	1961
Malaysia	0·10	1957	Thailand	0·09	1946
Maldives	0·01	1965	Togo	0·01	1960
Mali	0·01	1960	Trinidad and Tobago	0·04	1962
Malta	0·01	1964	Tunisia	0·03	1956
Mauritania	0·01	1961	Turkey [1]	0·34	1945
Mauritius	0·01	1968	Uganda	0·01	1962
Mexico [1]	0·89	1945	Ukrainian Soviet Socialist Rep.[1]	1·28	1945
Mongolia	0·01	1961	USSR [1]	10·20	1945
Morocco	0·05	1956	United Arab Emirates	0·18	1971
Mozambique	0·01	1975	UK [1]	4·86	1945
Nepal	0·01	1955	USA [1]	25·00	1945
Netherlands [1]	1·74	1945	Uruguay [1]	0·04	1945
New Zealand [1]	0·24	1945	Vanuatu	0·01	1981
Nicaragua [1]	0·01	1945	Venezuela [1]	0·60	1945
Niger	0·01	1960	Vietnam	0·01	1977
Nigeria	0·19	1960	Yemen	0·02	1947
Norway [1]	0·54	1945	Yugoslavia [1]	0·46	1945
Oman	0·02	1971	Zaïre	0·01	1960
Pakistan	0·06	1947	Zambia	0·01	1964
Panama [1]	0·02	1945	Zimbabwe	0·02	1980
Papua New Guinea	0·01	1975			
Paraguay [1]	0·02	1945			

[1] Original member.

Further Reading

Yearbook of the United Nations. New York, 1947 ff. Annual
United Nations Chronicle. Quarterly
Monthly Bulletin of Statistics
General Assembly: Official-Records: Resolutions
Reports of the Secretary-General of the United Nations on the Work of the Organization. 1946 ff.
Documents of the United Nations Conference on International Organization, San Francisco, 1945. 16 vols.
Charter of the United Nations and Statute of the International Court of Justice. Text in English, French, Chinese, Russian and Spanish.
Repertory of Practice of UN's Organs. 5 vols. New York, 1955
Official Records of the Security Council, the Economic and Social Council, Trusteeship Council and the Disarmament Commission

Demographic Yearbook, 1948 ff. New York, 1969
Everyone's United Nations. New York. 10th ed., 1986
Statistical Yearbook. New York, 1947 ff.
United Nations Handbook 1987. New Zealand Ministry of Foreign Affairs, Wellington, 1987
Yearbook of International Statistics. New York, 1950 ff.
World Economic Survey. New York, 1947 ff.
Economic Survey of Asia and the Far East. New York, 1946 ff.
Economic Survey of Latin America. New York, 1948 ff.
Economic Survey of Europe. New York, 1948 ff.
Economic Survey of Africa. New York, 1960 ff.
Foote, W., *Dag Hammarskjöld—Servant of Peace.* London, 1962
Forsythe, D., *United Nations Peacemaking: The Conciliation Commission for Palestine.* Johns Hopkins Univ. Press, 1973
Humana, C., *World Human Rights Guide.* 2nd ed. London, 1986
Lie, T., *In the Cause of Peace.* London, 1954
Luard, E., *A History of the United Nations.* Vol. 1. London, 1982
Osmanczyk, E., *Encyclopaedia of the United Nations.* London, 1985
Peterson, M. J., *The General Assembly in World Politics.* Winchester, Mass, 1986
Thant, U., *Towards World Peace.* New York, 1964
Walters, F. P., *A History of the League of Nations.* 2 vols. London, 1952
Williams, D., *The Specialised Agencies of the United Nations.* London, 1987
Witthauer, K., *Die Bevölkerung der Erde: Verteilung und Dynamik.* Gotha, 1958.—*Distribution and Dynamics Relating to World Population.* Gotha, 1969

United Nations Information Centre. 20 Buckingham Gate, London SW1E 6LB

UNITED NATIONS SYSTEM

The bulk of the work of the UN, measured in terms of money and personnel, is aimed at achieving the pledge made in Article 55 of the Charter to 'promote higher standards of living, full employment and conditions of economic and social progress and development'.

In addition to the 18 independent specialized agencies, there are some 14 major United Nations programmes and funds devoted to achieving economic and social progress in the developing countries.

Total contributions to the funds and programmes of the UN and specialized agencies for development activities amounted to $1,100m. (not including contributions to the World Bank group) in 1987. The highest total contributions in 1989 went to the UN Development Programme (UNDP – $1,200m.) the UN Children's Fund (UNICEF – $290m.) and the UN Fund for Population Activities (UNFPA – $167m.). The World Food Programme, which provides food aid to support development projects and emergency relief operations, provided aid worth $900m. in 1983, making it the largest single source of development assistance in the UN system, apart from the World Bank.

The *United Nations Development Programme* (UNDP) is the world's largest agency for multilateral technical and pre-investment co-operation. It is the funding source for most of the technical assistance provided by the United Nations system, and UNDP is active in 152 countries and territories and in virtually every economic and social sector. UNDP assistance is provided only at the request of Governments and in response to their priority needs, integrated into over-all national and regional plans.

There were (1988) 5,900 UNDP-supported projects currently in operation at the national, regional, inter-regional and global levels, all aimed at helping developing countries make better use of their assets, improve living standards and expand productivity. The volume of such work was $1,200m. in 1988.

UNICEF, established in 1946 to deliver post-war relief to children, now concentrates its assistance on development activities aimed at improving the quality of life for children and mothers in developing countries. During 1983, UNICEF was working in over 110 countries with a child population of some 1,300m., concentrating on basic services for children and maternal health care, nutrition, water supply and sanitation and education. *The State of the World's Children Report*, published annually by UNICEF, has helped to spread acceptance by local and national leaders of a strategy for child health and nutrition which UNICEF estimates could save the lives of 7m. children. UNICEF has focused on popularising four primary health care techniques which are low in cost and produce results in a relatively short time. These include: Oral rehydration therapy to fight the effects of diarrhoeal infections, which kill some 4m. children each year; expanded immunization against the 6 most common childhood diseases; child growth monitoring, and promotion of breast-feeding. The World Health Organization and UNICEF work closely together, providing training, equipment and the services of health care professionals. UNICEF is the world's largest supplier of vaccines and the 'cold chain' equipment needed to deliver them, as well as oral rehydration salts.

Executive Director: James P. Grant (USA).

The UN Population Fund (UNFPA) carries out programmes in over 130 countries and territories. The Fund's aims are to build up capacity to respond to needs in population and family planning; to promote awareness of population problems in both developed and developing countries and possible strategies to deal with them; to assist developing countries at their request in dealing with population problems. More than 25% of international population assistance to developing countries is channeled through UNFPA.

Executive Director: Dr Nafis Sadik (Philippines).

An International Conference on Population was convened by the United Nations in 1984 in Mexico City to review the World Population Plan of Action adopted by the 1974 population conference, and make recommendations for its future implementation.

Humanitarian relief to refugees and victims of natural and man-made disasters is also an important function of the UN system. Among the organizations involved in such relief activities are the Office of the UN Disaster Relief Co-ordinator (UNDRO), the Office of the UN High Commissioner for Refugees (UNHCR) and the UN Relief and Works Agency for Palestine Refugees in the Near East (UNRWA).

UNRWA was created by the General Assembly in 1949 as a temporary, non-political agency to provide relief to the nearly 750,000 people who became refugees as a result of the disturbances during and after the creation of the State of Israel in the former British Mandate territory of Palestine. 'Palestine refugees', as defined by UNRWA's mandate, are persons or descendants of persons whose normal residence was Palestine for at least 2 years prior to the 1948 conflict and who, as a result of the conflict, lost their homes and means of livelihood. UNRWA has also been called upon to assist persons displaced as a result of renewed hostilities in the Middle East in 1967. The situation of Palestine refugees in south Lebanon was of special concern to the Agency in 1984 which has carried out an emergency relief programme in that area for Palestine refugees affected in the aftermath of the Israeli invasion of Lebanon in 1982.

Over 2m. refugees are registered with the Agency which provides education, health care, supplementary feeding and relief services. Education and basic health care account for over 80% of the Agency's budget, which is financed by voluntary contributions from Governments. In 1986 its operating budget amounted to $230m., while cash contributions were expected to total only $194m.

Commissioner-General: Giorgio Giacomelli.

The *Office of the United Nations High Commissioner for Refugees* (UNHCR) was established by the UN General Assembly with effect from 1 Jan. 1951, originally for three years. Since 1954, its mandate has been renewed for successive five-year periods.

The work of UNHCR is of a purely humanitarian and non-political character. The main functions of the Office are to provide international protection for refugees and to seek permanent solutions to their problems through voluntary repatriation, local integration into the country of first asylum or resettlement in other countries.

UNHCR may also be called upon to provide emergency relief and on-going material assistance where necessary.

UNHCR concerns itself with refugees who have been determined to come within its mandate under the Statute, and with persons in analogous circumstances whom it assists under the terms of the 'good offices' resolutions adopted by the General Assembly.

The High Commissioner is elected by the General Assembly and follows policy directives given by the General Assembly or the Economic and Social Council, mainly through the Geneva-based Executive Committee of the High Commissioner's Programme.

International protection is the primary function of UNHCR. Its main objective is to promote and safeguard the rights and interests of refugees. In so doing UNHCR devotes special attention to promoting a generous policy of asylum on the part of Governments and seeks to improve the status of refugees in their country of residence. It also helps them to cease being refugees through the acquisition of the nationality of their country of residence when voluntary repatriation is not possible. UNHCR pursues its objectives in the field of protection by encouraging the conclusion of intergovernmental legal instruments in favour of refugees, by supervising the implementation of their provisions and by encouraging Governments to adopt legislation and administrative procedures for the benefit of refugees.

UNHCR also provides material assistance to refugees, largely in camps and settlements, and seeks to promote their self-sufficiency leading to the attainment of durable solutions for their plight. Since 1951 UNHCR has assisted and found solutions for an estimated 30 million refugees and displaced persons.

In 1989 a number of major movements occurred in Africa and there were repatriations from the Sudan to Ethiopia and Uganda and of Ethiopians from Somalia and Djibouti. Afghans, estimated at 3m. in Pakistan and 2m. in Iran, remained the largest single refugee population in the world. An international Conference on Indo-Chinese refugees which took place in June 1984 adopted a comprehensive Plan of Action (CPA) which presents a package of inter-related measures covering such aspects of the problem as clandestine departures, regular departure programmes, reception of new arrivals, determination of the status of asylum-seekers and resettlement. The objective is to rechannel, to the extent possible, departures through legal means, while limiting entitlement to resettlement to recognized and *bona fide* refugees and encouraging voluntary return to countries of origin of rejected cases.

In Oct. 1990 the 43-member *Executive Committee* of the High Commissioner's Programme approved a budget of US$345m. for general programmes in 1990. Member countries' contributions are voluntary. Inability to collect the full revenue projected for 1990 led to a closure of 19 of the 100 regional bureaux.

The UNHCR was awarded the Nobel Peace Prize in 1955 and 1981.

Headquarters: Palais des Nations, 1211, Geneva 10, Switzerland.
UK Office: 36 Westminster Palace Gardens, London, SW1P 1RR.

High Commissioner: Sadako Ogata (till Dec. 1993).

UN funds and programmes participating in the 1984 pledging conference for development activities:
UN Development Programme; Special Measures Fund for the Least Developed Countries; UN Development Programme Energy Account; UN Capital Development Fund; UN Special Fund for Land-Locked Developing Countries; UN Revolving Fund for National Resources Exploration; Special Voluntary Fund for the UN Volunteers; UN Financing System for Science and Technology for Development; UN Trust Fund for Sudano-Sahelian Activities; UN Children's Fund; UN Fund for Population Activities; UN Industrial Development Fund; UN Trust Fund for African Development Activities; Voluntary Fund for the UN Decade for Women; UN Trust Fund for the International Research and Training Institute for the Advancement of Women; UN Centre for Human Settlements (Habitat): UN Habitat and Human Settlements Foundation; UN Trust Fund for the Transport and Communications Decade in Africa; Trust Fund for the UN Centre on Transnational

Corporations; UN Institute for Training and Research; UN Fund for Drug Abuse Control; UN Trust Fund for Social Defence; UN Development Programme Study Programme; Fund of the UN Environment Programme.

SPECIALIZED AGENCIES OF THE UN

INTERNATIONAL ATOMIC ENERGY AGENCY (IAEA)

Origin. The International Atomic Energy Agency came into existence on 29 July 1957. Its statute had been approved on 26 Oct. 1956, at an international conference held at UN Headquarters, New York. A relationship agreement links it with the United Nations. The IAEA had 112 member states in 1990.

Functions. (1) To accelerate and enlarge the contribution of atomic energy to peace, health and prosperity throughout the world, and (2) to ensure that assistance provided by it or at its request or under its supervision or control is not used in such a way as to further any military purpose. In addition, under the terms of the Non-Proliferation Treaty, the Treaty of Tlatelolco and the Treaty of Rarotonga, to verify states' obligation to prevent diversion of nuclear energy from peaceful uses to nuclear weapons or other nuclear explosive devices.

The IAEA gives advice and technical assistance to developing countries on nuclear power development, on nuclear safety, on radioactive waste management, on legal aspects of the use of atomic energy, and on prospecting for and exploiting nuclear raw materials; in addition it promotes the use of radiation and isotopes in agriculture, industry, medicine and hydrology through expert services, training courses and fellowships, grants of equipment and supplies, research contracts, scientific meetings and publications. During 1989, a total of 1,135 projects were operational of which 165 were completed and 106 training courses were held. These activities involved 2,144 expert assignments while 1,975 persons received training abroad. The IAEA has research laboratories in Austria and Monaco. At Trieste, the International Centre for Theoretical Physics was established in 1964 which is now operated jointly by UNESCO and IAEA.

In Dec. 1989, a total of 172 safeguards agreements were in force with 101 states. Safeguards are the technical means applied by the IAEA to verify that nuclear equipment or materials are used exclusively for peaceful purposes. IAEA safeguards cover more than 95% of the civilian nuclear installations outside the 5 nuclear-weapon states (China, France, UK, USA and USSR). All nuclear-weapon states have opened all (UK, USA, USSR) or some (China, France) of their civilian nuclear plants to IAEA safeguards inspection. Installations in non-nuclear-weapon states under safeguards or containing safeguarded material at 31 Dec. 1989 were 183 power reactors, 173 research reactors and critical assemblies, 8 conversion plants, 43 fuel fabrication plants, 5 reprocessing plants, 7 enrichment plants, and 405 other installations.

Organization. The Statute provides for an annual General Conference, a Board of Governors of 35 members and a Secretariat headed by a Director-General.

Headquarters: Vienna International Centre, PO Box 100, A-1400 Vienna, Austria.
Director-General: Hans Blix (Sweden).

INTERNATIONAL LABOUR ORGANISATION (ILO)

Origin. The ILO, established in 1919 as an autonomous part of the League of Nations, is an intergovernmental agency with a tripartite structure, in which representatives of governments, employers and workers participate. It seeks through international action to improve labour conditions, raise living standards and promote productive employment. In 1946 the ILO was recognized by the United Nations as a specialized agency. In 1969 it was awarded the Nobel Peace Prize. In 1990 it numbered 148 members.

Functions. One of the ILO's principal functions is the formulation of international standards in the form of International Labour Conventions and Recommendations. Member countries are required to submit Conventions to their competent national authorities with a view to ratification. If a country ratifies a Convention it agrees to bring its laws into line with its terms and to report periodically how these regulations are being applied. More than 5,500 ratifications of 171 Conventions had been deposited by mid-1989. Machinery is available to ascertain whether Conventions thus ratified are effectively applied.

Recommendations do not require ratification, but member states are obliged to consider them with a view to giving effect to their provisions by legislation or other action. By the end of 1990 the International Labour Conference had adopted 178 recommendations.

Organization. The ILO consists of the International Labour Conference, the Governing Body and the International Labour Office.

The Conference is the supreme deliberative organ of the ILO; it meets annually at Geneva. National delegations are composed of 2 government delegates, 1 employers' delegate and 1 workers' delegate.

The Governing Body, elected by the Conference, is the executive council. It is composed of 28 government members, 14 workers' members and 14 employers' members.

Ten governments hold permanent seats on the Governing Body because of their industrial importance, namely, Brazil, China, Germany, France, India, Italy, Japan, USA, USSR and UK. The remaining 18 government seats were, at the end of 1990, held by Australia, Bangladesh, Belgium, Belorussia, Bulgaria, Cameroon, Canada, Costa Rica, Lesotho, Madagascar, Mexico, Morocco, Nigeria, Philippines, Togo, United Arab Emirates, Uruguay and Venezuela.

The Office serves as secretariat, operational headquarters, research centre and publishing house.

The ILO budget for 1990–91 amounted to US$330m.

Activities. In addition to its research and advisory activities, the ILO extends technical co-operation to governments under its regular budget and under the UN Development Programme and Funds-in-Trust in the fields of employment promotion, human resources development (including vocational and management training), development of social institutions, small-scale industries, rural development, social security, industrial safety and hygiene, productivity, etc. Technical co-operation also includes expert missions and a fellowship programme. Over $140m. was spent on technical co-operation in 1989. Projects were in progress in some 115 countries and about 900 experts involved.

Major emphasis is being given to the ILO's World Employment Programme, launched in 1969 with the purpose of stimulating national and international efforts to increase the volume of productive employment, and so to counter the problem of rising unemployment in developing countries. A World Employment Conference in 1976 linked employment generation to the satisfaction of over-all basic human needs. Employment strategy missions have provided policy guidance to numerous developing countries while practical assistance continues through regional teams of specialists in Africa, Asia and Latin America, backed by an intensive programme of world-wide research. The Programme is currently focusing on instructional efforts—in which the major financial institutions are involved—to mitigate the social consequences of economic structural adjustment.

The International Labour Conference (Geneva, June 1990) adopted Conventions concerning night work and the use of chemicals at work, and began the two-year process of setting new standards relating to working conditions in hotels and restaurants.

In 1960 the ILO established in Geneva the International Institute for Labour Studies. The Institute specializes in advanced education and research on social and labour policy. It brings together for group study experienced persons from all parts of the world—government administrators, trade-union officials, industrial experts, management, university and other specialists.

A training institution was opened by the ILO in Turin, Italy, in 1965—the International Centre for Advanced Technical and Vocational Training. The Centre provides opportunities for technical, vocational and management training for individuals who have advanced beyond the facilities available in their own countries. Courses are geared particularly to the needs of developing countries.

Headquarters: International Labour Office, CH-1211 Geneva 22, Switzerland.
Director-General: Gerd Muhr (Germany).
Chairman of the Governing Body: Douglas G. Poulter (Australia).
London Branch Office: Vincent House, Vincent Square, London, SW1P 2NB.

The ILO has regional offices in Abidjan (for Africa), Bangkok (for Asia and the Pacific), Lima (for Latin America and the Caribbean) and Geneva (for Arab States).

Further Reading

Publications: Regular periodicals in English, French and Spanish include the *International Labour Review, Labour Law Documents, Bulletin of Labour Statistics, Year Book of Labour Statistics, Official Bulletin* and *Labour Education.* The *Social and Labour Bulletin* are issued in English and French.

New volumes published in 1990 included: *Year Book of Labour Statistics: Retrospective Edition on Population Censuses, 1945–89; Year Book of Labour Statistics, 1989/90; Conditions of Work Digest: Telework, Civil Service Pay in Africa; Computer Integrated Manufacturing: The Social Dimension; Expert Systems: A Manager's Guide; International Directory of Occupational Safety and Health Institutions; Unemployment and Labour Market Flexibility: Finland; Women and Social Security: Progress Towards Equality of Treatment; Health Insurance in Development Countries: The Social Security Approach.*

FOOD AND AGRICULTURE ORGANIZATION OF THE UNITED NATIONS (FAO)

Origin. The UN Conference on Food and Agriculture in May 1943, at Hot Springs, Virginia, set up an Interim Commission in Washington in July 1943 to plan the Organization, which came into being on 16 Oct. 1945.

Aims and Activities. The aims of FAO are to raise levels of nutrition and standards of living; to improve the production and distribution of all food and agricultural products from farms, forests and fisheries; to improve the living conditions of rural populations; and, by these means, to eliminate hunger.

In carrying out these aims, FAO promotes investment in agriculture, better soil and water management, improved yields of crops and livestock, agricultural research, and the transfer of technology to developing countries. FAO promotes the conservation of natural resources and the rational use of fertilizers and pesticides. The Organization combats animal diseases, promotes the development of marine and inland fisheries, and encourages the sustainable management of forest resources. Technical assistance is provided in all these fields and others such as nutrition, agricultural engineering, agrarian reform, development communications, remote sensing for climate and vegetation, and the prevention of post-harvest food losses.

Special FAO programmes help countries prepare for, and provide relief in the event of, emergency food situations, in particular through the setting up of food reserves. Since the early 1980s, Africa has needed special emphasis and FAO created a special task force for that continent. The Agricultural Rehabitation Plan for Africa, begun in 1985, channelled some US$287m. to projects in 25 countries during its two years of operation. The Global Information and Early Warning System provides current information on the world food situation and identifies countries threatened by shortages to guide potential donors.

The Organization also has a major rôle in the collection, analysis and dissemination of information on agricultural production, including commodities.

FAO sponsors the World Food Programme (WFP) with the UN; WFP uses food commodities, cash and services contributed by member States of the UN to back programmes of social and economic development, as well as for relief in emergency situations.

Finance and Administration. The FAO Conference, composed of all member states, meets every other year to determine the policy and approve the budget and work programme of FAO. The Council, consisting of 49 member nations elected by the Conference, serves as FAO's governing body between Sessions of the Conference. At its 25th Session in Nov. 1989, the Conference approved a total working budget for the 1990-91 biennium, of US$568·8m. However outstanding contributions by member nations totalled US$175m., of which US$142m. were owed by the Organization's largest contributor, the United States. The working budget of FAO's Regular Programme, financed by contributions from member governments, covers the cost of the Organization's secretariat, its Technical Cooperation Programme (TCP) and part of the costs of several special programmes.

The technical assistance programme, however, is funded from extra-budgetary sources. The single largest contributor is the United Nations Development Programme (UNDP), which in 1989 accounted for US$164·3m., or 46% of field project expenditures. Equally important are the trust funds that come mainly from donor countries and international financing institutions, totalling US$163·8m., or 45·7% of technical assistance funds. FAO's contribution under its TCP was some US$29·9m., or 8·4%. FAO's total field programme expenditure for 1989 was an estimated US$358m. An estimated 50% of the expenditure was in Africa, 24% in Asia and the Pacific, 13% in the Near East, 8% in Latin America and the Caribbean, 1% in Europe, and 4% on interregional or global projects.

Headquarters: Via delle Terme di Caracalla, 00100 Rome, Italy.
Director-General: Dr Edouard Saouma (Lebanon).

Further Reading

FAO publications include: Ceres (bi-monthly); *Unasylva* (quarterly); *The State of Food and Agriculture* (annual), 1947 ff.; *Animal Health Yearbook* (annual), 1957 ff.; *Production Yearbook* (annual), 1947 ff.; *Trade Yearbook* (annual), 1947 ff.; *FAO Commodity Review* (annual), 1961 ff.; *Yearbook of Forest Products Statistics* (annual), 1947 ff.; *Yearbook of Fishery Statistics* (in two volumes). *FAO Fertilizer Yearbook, FAO Plant Protection Bulletin* (quarterly).

UNITED NATIONS EDUCATIONAL, SCIENTIFIC AND CULTURAL ORGANIZATION (UNESCO)

Origin. A Conference for the establishment of an Educational, Scientific and Cultural Organization of the United Nations was convened by the Government of the UK in association with the Government of France, and met in London, 1–16 Nov. 1945. UNESCO came into being on 4 Nov. 1946.

Functions. The purpose of UNESCO is to contribute to peace and security by promoting collaboration among the nations through education, science and culture in order to further universal respect for justice, for the rule of law and for the human rights and fundamental freedoms which are affirmed for the peoples of the world, without distinction of race, sex, language or religion, by the Charter of the United Nations.

Activities. The education programme has four main objectives: The extension of education; the improvement of education; and life-long education for living in a world community.

To train teachers specialized in the techniques of fundamental education UNESCO is helping to establish regional and national training centres. A centre for Latin America was opened in Mexico in 1951, one for the Arab States was set up in Egypt in 1953. UNESCO seeks to promote the progressive application of the right to free and compulsory education for all and to improve the quality of education everywhere.

In the natural sciences, UNESCO seeks to promote international scientific co-operation, such as the International Hydrological Programme which began in 1966. It encourages scientific research designed to improve the living conditions of mankind. Science co-operation offices have been set up in Montevideo, Cairo, New Delhi, Nairobi and Jakarta.

In the field of communication, UNESCO endeavours, by disseminating information, carrying out research and providing advice, to increase the scope and quality of press, film and radio services throughout the world.

In the cultural field, UNESCO assists member states in studying and preserving both the physical and the non-physical heritage of each society.

In the social sciences UNESCO helps in the development of research and teaching facilities and focuses on questions concerning Peace, Human Rights, Philosophy, Youth and Development Studies.

Organization. The organs of UNESCO are a General Conference (composed of representatives from each member state), an Executive Board (consisting of 51 government representatives elected by the General Conference) and a Secretariat. UNESCO had 158 members in 1988.

National commissions act as liaison groups between UNESCO and the educational, scientific and cultural life of their own countries.

Budget for 1988–89: $350,386,000.

Headquarters: UNESCO House, 7 Place de Fontenoy, Paris.
Director-General: Federico Mayor (Spain).

Further Reading

Periodicals. Museum (quarterly, English and French); *International Social Science Journal* (quarterly, English and French); *Impact of Science on Society* (quarterly, English and French); *Unesco Courier* (monthly, English, French and Spanish); *Prospects* (quarterly, English, French and Spanish); *Copyright Bulletin* (twice-yearly, English and French); *Unesco News* (English and French); *Nature and Resources* (quarterly, English, French and Spanish).

Hajnal, P. I., *Guide to UNESCO*. London and New York, 1983

WORLD HEALTH ORGANIZATION (WHO)

Origin. An International Conference, convened by the UN Economic and Social Council, to consider a single health organization resulted in the adoption on 22 July 1946 of the constitution of the World Health Organization. This constitution came into force on 7 April 1948.

Structure. The principal organs of WHO are the World Health Assembly, the Executive Board and the Secretariat. Each of the 166 member states has the right to be represented at the Assembly, which meets annually usually in Geneva, Switzerland. The 31-member Executive Board is composed of technically qualified health experts designated by as many member states elected by the Assembly. The Secretariat consists of technical and administrative staff headed by a Director-General. Health activities in member countries are carried out through regional organizations which have been established in Africa (regional office, Brazzaville), South-East Asia (New Delhi), Europe (Copenhagen), Eastern Mediterranean (Alexandria) and Western Pacific (Manila). The Pan American Sanitary Bureau in Washington serves as the Regional Office of WHO for the Americas.

Functions. WHO's objective, as stated in the first article of the Constitution is 'the attainment by all peoples of the highest possible level of health'. As the directing and co-ordinating authority on international health it establishes and maintains collaboration with the UN, specialized agencies, government health administrations, professional and other groups concerned with health. The Constitution also directs WHO to assist governments to strengthen their health services, to stimulate and advance work to eradicate diseases, to promote maternal and child health, mental health, medical research and the prevention of accidents; to improve standards of teaching and training in the health professions, and of nutrition, housing, sanitation, working conditions and other aspects of environment health. The Organization also is empowered to propose conventions, agreements and regulations and make recommendations about international health matters; to revise the international nomenclature of diseases, causes of death and public health practices; to develop, establish and promote international standards concerning foods, biological, pharmaceutical and similar substances.

Methods of work. Co-operation in country projects is undertaken only on the request of the government concerned, through the 6 regional offices of the Organization. Worldwide technical services are made available by headquarters. Expert committees whose members are chosen from the 54 advisory panels of experts meet to advise the Director-General on a given subject. Scientific groups and consultative meetings are called for similar purposes. To further the education of health personnel of all categories, seminars, technical conferences and training courses are organized and advisors, consultants and lecturers are provided. WHO awards fellowships for study to nationals of member countries.

Activities. The main thrust of WHO's activities in recent years has been towards promoting national, regional and global strategies for the attainment of the main social target of the Member States for the coming years: 'Health for All by the Year 2000', or the attainment by all citizens of the world of a level of health that will permit them to lead a socially and economically productive life.

Almost all countries indicated a high level of political commitment to this goal, and guiding principles for formulating corresponding strategies and plans of action were prepared.

The 42nd World Health Assembly which met in May 1989 approved a biennial budget of US$653·74m. for 1990-91. Extrabudgetary funds amounting to approximately US$700m. in voluntary contributions are also expected for the biennium. The Assembly called on the international community to increase substantially co-operation particularly with countries in greatest need.

Namibia. The Assembly welcomed the admission of Namibia to WHO and emphasized the urgent need to mobilize international support for the reconstruction and development of the health sector in Namibia.

Improving technical co-operation among developing countries. The Assembly commended WHO for the action taken to intensity international technical co-operation for accelerated implementation of primary health care in developing countries facing serious economic difficulties and debt problems.

Protecting, promoting and supporting breast-feeding. Reiterating its concern over the decreasing prevalence and duration of breast-feeding in many countries, the Assembly urged WHO's Member States to protect and promote breast-feeding, as an essential component of their overall food and nutrition policies and programmes on behalf of women and children, so as to enable all women exclusively to breast-feed their infants during the first four to six months of life.

Elimination of iodine deficiency disorders by the year 2000. In view of the progress already achieved and the promising potential of current and planned national prevention and control programmes, WHO shall aim at eliminating iodine deficiency disorders (still affecting one thousand million people on all continents) as a major public health problem in all countries by the year 2000.

Women, children and AIDS. The Assembly urged Member States to ensure that programmes for the control of HIV infection/AIDS are co-ordinated or integrated with other programmes for women, children and families, particularly maternal and child health, family planning, and sexually transmitted disease control.

Reduction in demand for illicit drugs. The World Ministerial Summit to Reduce Demand for Drugs and to Combat the Cocaine Threat, held in London in April 1990, gave emphasis to health issues. WHO was asked to intensity its action to prevent the spread of drug abuse in individuals, families, communities and countries, and to develop effective approaches to the treatment of drug dependence and associated diseases.

Hazardous wastes management. WHO was commended by the Assembly for establishing the WHO Commission on Health and Environment, which will examine the subject of hazardous wastes and their potential effects on human health.

Action programme on essential drugs. The Assembly recognized with satisfaction that essential drug lists for the different levels of health services exist in more than

100 countries, and about 50 countries have formulated, or are formulating, national drug policies, taking into account the WHO essential drug concept.

Tobacco or Health. The Assembly felt encouraged by the continuing decline in tobacco consumption wherever comprehensive smoking control policies have been adopted. It was deeply concerned however by increasing evidence of the dangers to health posed by 'passive smoking' or smoke inhaled by non-smokers. A new WHO estimate showed that, unless current smoking rates decrease, there will be three million tobacco-related deaths per year in the 1990s and that this figure will quickly rise to 10 million deaths per year by the 2020s.

Tropical Diseases Research. Tropical diseases – and especially malaria – have continued to escalate in some countries to the extent that malaria is once again one of the leading causes of morbidity. The Assembly appealed to the pharmaceutical industry to increase research and development in tropical diseases and to intensity its collaboration with the WHO Special Programme, dealing with malaria, schistosomiasis, filiariasis (including onchocerciasis), African trypanosomiasis, Chagas disease, leishmaniasis and leprosy.

Palestine Issue. The Assembly adopted a resolution requesting the Director-General to continue his studies on the Palestine request for admission as a member of WHO.

Technical Discussions. Being held in the framework of the Assembly, this year the Technical Discussions have dealt with the Role of Health Research in the Strategy for Health for All by the Year 2000.

World Health Day. World Health Day, 7 April 1990, was devoted to the theme of the environment and health. The theme chosen for 1991 is disaster preparedness.

Headquarters: 1211 Geneva 27, Switzerland.
Director-General: Hiroshi Nakajima (Japan).

Further Reading

Basic Documents. 37th ed., 1988 (Arabic, Chinese, English, French, Russian, Spanish)
Handbook of Resolutions and Decisions. Vol. I, 1973, Vol. II, 1985 and Vol. III, 1 ed., 1987 (Arabic, English, French, Russian, Spanish)
World Health Forum (from 1980, quarterly: Arabic, Chinese, English, French, Russian and Spanish)
Bulletin of WHO (quarterly, 1947–51; 6 issues a year from 1978; bilingual English/French)
International Digest of Health Legislation (quarterly, from 1948; English and French)
World Health, the Magazine of WHO. 1957 ff. (6 issues a year; English, French, German, Portuguese, Russian and Spanish; and 4 issues a year. Arabic and Persian)
WHO Technical Report Series, 1950 ff. (Arabic, Chinese, English, French, Russian, Spanish)
Public Health Papers, 1959 ff. (Arabic, Chinese, English, French, Russian, Spanish)
World Health Statistics Annual (from 1952; English, French and Russian)
World Health Statistics Quarterly (monthly, 1947–76 then quarterly; bilingual English/ French)
Weekly Epidemiological Record (from 1926; bilingual English/French)
WHO Drug Information (from 1987, quarterly; English and French)
Publications of the WHO, 1948–89; Catalogue of New Books, 1986–1990
World Directories:
Medical Schools, 1987; Schools of Public Health and Postgraduate Training Programmes in Public Health (1985); Schools for Medical Assistants, 1973 (1976); *Auxiliary Sanitarians 1973* (1978); *Dental Auxiliaries 1973* (1977); *Medical Lab. Technicians and Assistants, 1973* (1977)
The International Pharmacopoeia. 3rd. ed., 3 vols, 1979, 1981, 1987 (English, French and Spanish)
Manual of the International Statistical Classification of Diseases, Injuries and Causes of Death. 9th rev. (1977; English, French, Russian, Spanish)
IARC Monographs on the Evaluation of Carcinogenic Risk of Chemicals to Humans. 1967 *ff.* (English)
Report on the World Health Situation. 1959 ff. (Arabic, Chinese, English, French, Russian, Spanish); Seventh report (1987)
The Work of WHO, 1988–89: Biennial Report of the Director-General (1990) (Arabic, Chinese, English, French, Russian, Spanish)
International Health Regulations (1969). 3rd annotated ed., 1983 (Arabic, English, French, Russian, Spanish)

INTERNATIONAL MONETARY FUND (IMF)

The International Monetary Fund was established on 27 Dec. 1945 as an independent international organization and began operations on 1 March 1947; its relationship with the UN is defined in an agreement of mutual co-operation which came into force on 15 Nov. 1947. The first amendment to the Fund's articles creating the special drawing right (SDR; ISO code, XDR) took effect on 28 July 1969 and the second amendment took effect on 1 April 1978.

The capital resources of the Fund comprise SDRs and currencies that the members pay under quotas calculated for them when they join the Fund. Members' quotas in the Fund, in 1990, amounted to SDR 91,102·6m. and are closely related to (*i*) subscription to the Fund, (*ii*) their drawing rights on the Fund under both regular and special facilities, (*iii*) their voting power, and (*iv*) their share of any allocations of SDRs. Every Fund member is required to subscribe to the Fund an amount equal to its quota. An amount not exceeding 25% of the quota has to be paid in reserve assets, the balance in the member's own currency. The ranking of the top subscribers was changed in May 1990 and is now: 1st, the USA; joint 2nd, Germany and Japan; joint 4th, France and the UK.

The Fund is authorized under its Articles of Agreement to supplement its resources by borrowing. In Jan. 1962, a 4-year agreement was concluded with 10 industrial members (Belgium, Canada, France, Federal Republic of Germany, Italy, Japan, Netherlands, Sweden, UK, USA) who undertook to lend the Fund up to $6,000m. in their own currencies, if this should be needed to forestall or cope with an impairment of the international monetary system. Switzerland subsequently joined the group. These arrangements, known as the General Arrangements to Borrow (GAB), have been extended several times and the most recent 5-year renewal was to end in Dec. 1993. In early 1983 agreement was reached to increase the credit arrangements under the GAB to SDR 17,000m.; to permit use of GAB resources in transactions with Fund members that are not GAB participants; to authorize Swiss participation; and to permit borrowing arrangements with non-participating members to be associated with the GAB. Saudi Arabia and the Fund have entered into such an arrangement under which the Fund will be able to borrow up to SDR 1,500m. to assist in financing purchases by any member for the same purpose and under the same circumstances as in the GAB. The changes became effective by 26 Dec. 1983. The Fund has also borrowed from member countries and official institutions for two oil facilities and a supplementary financing facility.

Purposes: To promote international monetary co-operation, the expansion of international trade and exchange rate stability; to assist in the removal of exchange restrictions and the establishment of a multilateral system of payments; and to alleviate any serious disequilibrium in members' international balance of payments by making the financial resources of the Fund available to them, usually subject to conditions to ensure the revolving nature of Fund resources.

Activities. Each member of the Fund undertakes a broad obligation to collaborate with the Fund and other members to ensure the existence of orderly exchange arrangements and to promote a system of stable exchange rates. In addition, members are subject to certain obligations relating to domestic and external policies that can affect the balance of payments and the exchange rate. The Fund makes its resources available, under proper safeguards, to its members to meet short-term or medium-term payments difficulties. The first allocation of special drawing rights was made on 1 Jan. 1970 with five SDR allocations since then. SDRs in existence now total SDR 21,400m. To further enhance its balance of payments assistance to its members the Fund established a compensatory financing facility on 27 Feb. 1963, temporary oil facilities in 1974 and 1975, a trust fund in 1976, and an extended facility for medium-term assistance to members with special balance of payments problems on 13 Sept. 1974 with additional financing now provided through a policy of enlarged access. In March 1986, it established the structural adjustment facility to provide assistance to low-income countries. In Dec. 1987, the Fund established the enhanced structural adjustment facility to provide further assistance to low-income countries facing high levels of indebtedness. In Aug.

1988, the compensatory and contingency financing facility was established, succeeding the compensatory financing facility; the new facility provides broader protection to members pursuing Fund-supported adjustment programmes.

The Committee on Reform of the International Monetary System and Related Issues, generally known as the Committee of Twenty, held its first session at the 1972 annual meeting, with the mandate to advise and report to the Board of Governors on all aspects of the international monetary system, including proposals for any amendments of the Articles of Agreement. The Committee of Twenty disbanded after submitting its final report in 1974. An Interim Committee of the Board of Governors on the International Monetary System and a Joint Ministerial Committee of the Boards of Governors of the World Bank and the Fund on the Transfer of Real Resources to Developing Countries (Development Committee) were established and held their initial meetings in Jan. 1975 and since then have met on a semi-annual basis. Details of the reform of the international monetary system were incorporated in the second amendment of the Fund's Articles of Agreement, effective April 1978. In order to oversee the compliance of members with their obligations under the Articles of Agreement, the Fund is required to exercise firm surveillance over their exchange rate policies.

Organization. The highest authority in the Fund is exercised by the Board of Governors on which each member government is represented. Normally the Governors meet once a year, although the Governors may take votes by mail or other means between annual meetings. The Board of Governors has delegated many of its powers to the executive directors in Washington, of whom there are 22, of which 6 are appointed by individual members and the other 16 elected by groups of countries. Each appointed director has voting power proportionate to the quota of the government he represents, while each elected director casts all the votes of the countries which elected him. The 6 appointed executive directors represent the US, UK, France, Federal Republic of Germany, Japan and Saudi Arabia.

The managing director is selected by the executive directors; he presides as chairman at their meetings, but may not vote except in case of a tie. His term is for 5 years, but may be extended or terminated at the discretion of the executive directors. He is responsible for the ordinary business of the Fund, under general control of the executive directors, and supervises a staff of about 1,900.

There were 152 members of the IMF in 1990.

Headquarters: 700 19th St. NW, Washington, D.C., 20431. Offices in Paris and Geneva.

Managing Director: Michel Camdessus (France).

Further Reading

Publications. Summary Proceedings of Annual Meetings of the Board of Governors.—Annual Report of the Executive Board.—Selected Decisions of the International Monetary Fund and Selected Documents.—International Financial Statistics (monthly).—*IMF Survey* (bi-weekly).—*Balance of Payments Statistics.* Washington, monthly.—*IMF Staff Papers* (four times a year). Washington, from Feb. 1950.—*IMF Occasional Papers.—IMF Pamphlets.—Annual Report on Exchange Arrangements and Exchange Restrictions.* Washington, 1950 ff.—*Finance and Development.* Washington, from June 1964 (quarterly).—*Direction of Trade Statistics.* Washington (monthly). *IMF World Economic and Financial Surveys.* Washington. *Government Finance Statistics Yearbook. The International Monetary Fund, 1945–65: Twenty Years of International Monetary Co-operation.* 3 vols. Washington D.C. 1969

de Vries, M. G., *The International Monetary Fund, 1966–1971: The System Under Stress.* 2 vols. Washington D.C. 1976.—*The International Monetary Fund 1972–1978: Co-operation on Trial.* 3 vols. Washington D.C., 1985

INTERNATIONAL BANK FOR RECONSTRUCTION AND DEVELOPMENT (IBRD)

Conceived at the Bretton Woods Conference, July 1944, the 'World Bank' began operations in June 1946. Its purpose is to provide funds and technical assistance to facilitate economic development in its porer member countries.

The Bank obtains its funds from the following sources: Capital paid in by member countries; sales of its own securities; sales of parts of its loans; repayments; and net earnings. The subscribed capital of the Bank amounted to $115,668m. at 30 June 1989. On 27 April 1988, the Board of Governors adopted a resolution that increased the authorized capital stock of the Bank by $171,400m. This represented an increase of approximately $40,000m. The resolution provides that the paid-in portion of the shares authorized to be subscribed under it will be 3%. Outstanding medium- and long-term borrowings had reached $79,750m. by 30 June 1989. The Bank is self-supporting. Its net earnings for year ending 30 June 1989 amounted to $1,004m.

By 30 June 1989 the Bank had made 3,055 loans totalling $171,482m. in 103 of its 151 member countries. Lending was for the following purposes: Agriculture and rural development, $34,117m.; Development Finance Companies, $17,675m.; education, $6,052m.; energy, $37,738m.; industry (including tourism), $12,832m.; non-project, $13,334m.; population, health and nutrition, $1,251m.; small-scale enterprizes, $4,476m.; telecommunications, $2,596m.; transportation, $26,235m.; urban development, $7,148m.; water supply and sewerage, $7,698m., and technical assistance, $330m. In order to eliminate wasteful overlapping of development assistance and to ensure that the funds available are used to the best possible effect, the Bank has organized consortia or consultative groups of aidgiving nations for the following countries: Bangladesh, Bolivia, Burma, Colombia, Côte d'Ivoire, Egypt, Ethiopia, Ghana, Guinea, Guinea-Bissau, India, Kenya, Korea, Madagascar, Malaŵi, Mauritania, Mauritius, Morocco, Mozambique, Nepál, Nigeria, Pakistan, Papua New Guinea, Peru, the Philippines, Senegal, Somalia, Sri Lanka, Sudan, Tanzania, Thailand, Togo, Tunisia, Uganda, Zaïre, Zambia and the Caribbean Group for Co-operation in Economic Development. The Bank furnishes a wide variety of technical assistance. It acts as executing agency for a number of pre-investment surveys financed by the UN Development Programme. Resident missions have been established in 40 developing member countries as well as 3 regional missions in East and West Africa and Thailand primarily to assist in the preparation of projects. The Bank helps member countries to identify and prepare projects for the development of agriculture, education and water supply by drawing on the expertise of the FAO, WHO, UNIDO and UNESCO through its co-operative agreements with these organizations. The Bank maintains a staff college, the Economic Development Institute in Washington, D.C., for senior officials of the member countries.

Headquarters: 1818 H St., NW, Washington, D.C., 20433, USA. *European office:* 66 avenue d'Iéna, 75116 Paris, France. *London office:* New Zealand House, Haymarket, SW1Y 4TE, England. *Tokyo office:* Kokusai Building, 1–1, Marunouchi 3-chome, Chiyoda-ku, Tokyo 100, Japan.

President: Barber B. Conable, Jr., (USA).

Further Reading

Publications. Annual Reports. 1946 ff.—*Summary Proceedings of Annual Meetings.* 1947 ff.—*The World Bank & International Finance Company.* 1986.—*The World Bank Atlas.* 1967 ff.—*Catalog of Publications,* 1986 ff.—*World Development Report.* 1978 ff.

Payer, C., *The World Bank: A Critical Analysis.* London, 1982

INTERNATIONAL DEVELOPMENT ASSOCIATION (IDA)

A lending agency which came into existence on 24 Sept. 1960. Administered by the World Bank, IDA is open to all members of the Bank.

IDA concentrates its assistance on those countries with an annual *per capita* gross national product of less than $481 (1987 rate). Its resources consist mostly of subscriptions, general replenishments from its more industrialized and developed members, special contributions, and transfers from the net earnings of the Bank. IDA credits are made to Governments only. It had committed $52,700m. for 1,904 development projects in 84 countries, by 30 June 1989.

INTERNATIONAL FINANCE CORPORATION (IFC)

The Corporation, an affiliate of the World Bank, was established in July 1956. Paid-in capital at 30 June 1990 was $1,100m., subscribed by 135 member countries. In addition, it has accumulated earnings of $792m. IFC supplements the activities of the World Bank by encouraging the growth of productive private enterprises in developing member countries. Chiefly, IFC makes investments in the form of subscriptions to the share capital of privately owned companies, or long-term loans, or both. The Corporation will help finance new ventures and assist established enterprises to expand, improve or diversify. It also provides a variety of advisory services to public and private sector clients.

At 30 June 1990 IFC had investments of $11,438m. in over 90 countries.

President: Barber B. Conable, Jr., (USA).
Executive Vice-President: Sir William Ryrie (UK).

Publications. Annual Reports. 1956 ff.—*What IFC Does.* 1988,—*How to Work with IFC,* 1988

INTERNATIONAL CIVIL AVIATION ORGANIZATION (ICAO)

Origin. The Convention providing for the establishment of the International Civil Aviation Organization was drawn up by the International Civil Aviation Conference held in Chicago from 1 Nov. to 7 Dec. 1944. A Provisional International Civil Aviation Organization (PICAO) operated for 20 months until the formal establishment of ICAO on 4 April 1947.

The Convention on International Civil Aviation superseded the provisions of the Paris Convention of 1919, which established the International Commission for Air Navigation (ICAN), and the Pan American Convention on Air Navigation drawn up at Havana in 1928.

Functions. It assists international civil aviation by establishing technical standards for safety and efficiency of air navigation and promoting simpler procedures at borders; develops regional plans for ground facilities and services needed for international flying; disseminates air-transport statistics and prepares studies on aviation economics; fosters the development of air law conventions. As part of the UN Development Programme it provides technical assistance to States in developing civil aviation programmes.

Organization. The principal organs of ICAO are an Assembly, consisting of all members of the Organization, and a Council, which is composed of 33 states elected by the Assembly, for 3 years, and meets in virtually continuous session. In electing these states, the Assembly must give adequate representation to: (1) states of major importance in air transport; (2) states which make the largest contribution to the provision of facilities for the international civil air navigation; (3) those states not otherwise included whose election will ensure that all major geographical areas of the world are represented. The main subsidiary bodies are: The Air Navigation Commission, composed of 15 members appointed by the Council; Air Transport Committee, open to council members; and the Legal Committee, on which all members of ICAO may be represented. There are 161 members. Budget for 1990: US$34m.

Headquarters: 1000 Sherbroke St. West, Montreal, Quebec, Canada H3A 2R2.
President: Dr Assad Kotaite (Lebanon).
Secretary-General: Dr Shivinder Singh Sidhu (India).

Annual Report of the Council. (English, French, Russian, Spanish)
ICAO Journal (Monthly)

UNIVERSAL POSTAL UNION (UPU)

Origin. The UPU was established on 1 July 1875, when the Universal Postal Convention adopted by the Postal Congress of Berne on 9 Oct. 1874 came into force. The UPU was known at first as the General Postal Union, its name being changed at the Congress of Paris in 1878. In 1990 there were 169 member countries.

Functions. The aim of the UPU is to assure the organization and perfection of the various postal services and to promote, in this field, the development of international collaboration. To this end, the members of UPU are united in a single postal territory for the reciprocal exchange of correspondence.

Organization. The UPU is composed of a Universal Postal Congress which usually meets every 5 years, a permanent Executive Council consisting of 40 members, a consultative Committee, which consists of 35 members elected on a geographical basis by each Congress, and an International Bureau, which functions as the permanent secretariat.

A specialized agency of the UN since 1948, the Union is governed by the Constitution of the UPU adopted at the 1964 Vienna Congress, and amended by the 1969 (Tokyo), 1974 (Lausanne), 1984 (Hamburg) and 1989 (Washington) Additional Protocols.

Budget for 1990: US$18m.

Headquarters: Weltpoststrasse 4, 3000, Berne 15, Switzerland.
Director-General: Adwaldo Cardoso Botto de Barros (Brazil).

Further Reading

Acts of the Universal Postal Union: revised at Hamburg in 1984 and annotated by the International Bureau. vols 1–4.—*The Postal Union* (quarterly, Arabic, Chinese, English, French, German, Spanish, Russian).—*The UPU: Its Foundation and Development.* Bern, 1959.

INTERNATIONAL TELECOMMUNICATION UNION (ITU)

Origin. In 1932, at Madrid, the Union decided to merge the Telegraph Convention adopted in 1865 and the Radiotelegraph Convention adopted in 1906 into a single International Telecommunication Convention within annex, the Telephone, Telegraph and Radio Regulations. It also decided to change its name to International Telecommunication Union to better reflect all its new responsibilities. The ITU has been governed since 1 Jan. 1984 by the International Telecommunication Convention adopted in Nairobi in 1982.

Functions. (1) to maintain and extend international co-operation for the improvement and rational use of telecommunications of all kinds, as well as to promote and to offer technical assistance to developing countries in the field of telecommunications; (2) to promote the development of technical facilities and their most efficient operation with a view to improving the efficiency of telecommunication services, increasing their usefulness and making them, so far as possible, generally available to the public; (3) to harmonize the actions of nations in the attainment of those ends.

Organization. The ITU consists of the Plenipotentiary Conference, Administrative Conferences, the Administrative Council of 43 members, and of 5 permanent organs (the General Secretariat, the International Frequency Registration Board, and 2 international consultative committees, one for radio and one for telephone and telegraph and the Telecommunications Development Bureau).

Budget for 1989: Sw.Frs.132,087,000.

Headquarters: Place des Nations, CH-1211 Geneva 20, Switzerland.
Secretary-General: Dr Pekka Tarjanne (Finland).

WORLD METEOROLOGICAL ORGANIZATION (WMO)

Origin. A Conference of Directors of the International Meteorological Organization (set up in 1873), meeting in Washington in 1947, adopted a Convention creating the World Meteorological Organization. The WMO Convention became effective on 23 March 1950, and WMO was formally established on 19 March 1951, when the first session of its Congress was convened in Paris. An agreement to bring WMO into relationship with the United Nations was approved by this Congress and came into force on 21 Dec. 1951 with its approval by the General Assembly of the United Nations.

Functions. (1) To facilitate world-wide co-operation in the establishment of networks of stations for the making of meteorological observations as well as hydrological or other geophysical observations related to meteorology, and to promote the establishment and maintenance of meteorological centres charged with the provision of meteorological and related services; (2) to promote the establishment and maintenance of systems for the rapid exchange of meteorological and related information; (3) to promote standardization of meteorological and related observations and to ensure the uniform publication of observations and statistics; (4) to further the application of meteorology to aviation, shipping, water problems, agriculture and other human activities; (5) to promote activities in operational hydrology and to further close co-operation between meteorological and hydrological services; and (6) to encourage research and training in meteorology and, as appropriate, to assist in co-ordinating the international aspects of such research and training.

Organization. WMO is an inter-governmental organization of 154 member states and 5 member territories responsible for the operation of their own meteorological services. Constituent bodies of WMO are the World Meteorological Congress which meets every 4 years, the executive council composed of 36 members elected in their personal capacity and including the President and 3 Vice-Presidents of the Organization, 6 regional associations of members and 8 technical commissions established by the Congress. A permanent secretariat is maintained in Geneva.

Budget for 1988–91: Sw.Frs.170m.

Headquarters: Case postale No. 2300, CH-1211, Geneva 2, Switzerland.
Secretary-General: G. O. P. Obasi (Nigeria).

Publications. *WMO Bulletin.* 1952 ff.—*Meteorological Services of the World.* 1985. —*Publications of the World Meteorological Organization, 1951–1986.*

INTERNATIONAL MARITIME ORGANIZATION (IMO)

Origin. The International Maritime Organization, until 1982 known as Inter-Governmental Maritime Consultative Organization (IMCO), was established as a specialized agency of the UN by a convention drawn up at the UN Maritime Conference held at Geneva in Feb./March 1948. The Convention became effective on 17 March 1958 when it had been ratified by 21 countries, including 7 with at least 1m. gross tons of shipping each. The International Maritime Organization started operations in Jan. 1959.

Functions. To facilitate co-operation among governments on technical matters affecting merchant shipping, especially concerning safety at sea; to prevent and control marine pollution caused by ships; to facilitate international maritime traffic. The International Maritime Organization is responsible for convening international maritime conferences and for drafting international maritime conventions. It also provides technical assistance to countries wishing to develop their maritime activities.

Organization. The International Maritime Organization had 134 members (and 2 associate members) in 1991. The Assembly, composed of all member states, normally meets every 2 years. The Council of 32 member states acts as governing body between Assembly sessions. The Maritime Safety Committee deals with all technical questions relating to maritime safety. It has established several sub-committees to deal with specific problems and like the Marine Environment Protection Committee, Legal Committee, Facilitation Committee and Committee on Technical Co-operation is open to all International Maritime Organization members. The Secretariat is composed of international civil servants.

The International Maritime Organization is depositary authority for the International Convention for the Safety of Life at Sea, 1960, and the Regulations for Preventing Collisions at Sea, 1948 and 1960; the International Convention for the Prevention of Pollution of the Sea by Oil, 1954, as amended in 1962 and 1969; the Convention on Facilitation of International Maritime Traffic, 1965; the International Convention on Load Lines, 1966; the International Convention on Tonnage Measurement of Ships, 1969; the International Convention relating to Intervention on the High Seas in cases of Oil Pollution Casualties, 1969; the International Convention on Civil Liability for Oil Pollution Damage, 1969; Convention on International Compensation Fund for Oil Pollution Damage, 1971; Special Trade Passenger Ships Agreement, 1971; Convention on International Regulations for Preventing Collisions at Sea, 1972; the International Convention for Safe Containers, 1972; the International Convention on Prevention of Pollution from Ships, 1973 as modified by the Protocol of 1978; the International Convention for the Safety of Life at Sea, 1974; Athens Convention relating to the Carriage of Passengers and their Luggage by Sea, 1974; Convention on the International Maritime Satellite Organization, 1976; Convention on Limitation of Maritime Claims, 1976; Torremolinos International Convention for the Safety of Fishing Vessels, 1977; International Convention on Standards of Training, Certification and Watchkeeping for Seafarers, 1978; International Convention on Maritime Search and Rescue, 1979; International Convention on Sabotage, 1979; Convention for the Suppression of Unlawful Acts Against the Safety of Maritime Navigation, 1988; International Convention on Salvage, 1989.

Headquarters: 4 Albert Embankment, London SE1 7SR.
Secretary-General: William O'Neil (Canada).

IMO News

GENERAL AGREEMENT ON TARIFFS AND TRADE (GATT)

Origin. The General Agreement on Tariffs and Trade was negotiated in 1947 and entered into force on 1 Jan. 1948. Its 23 original signatories were members of a Preparatory Committee appointed by the UN Economic and Social Council to draft the charter for a proposed International Trade Organization. Since this charter was never ratified, the General Agreement, intended as an interim arrangement, has instead remained as the only international instrument laying down trade rules accepted by countries responsible for nearly 90% of the world's trade. In Dec. 1990 there were 100 contracting parties, with one country acceding provisionally, and a further 28 countries applying GATT rules on a *de facto* basis.

Functions. GATT functions both as a multilateral treaty that lays down a common code of conduct in international trade and trade relations and as a forum for negotiation and consultation to overcome trade problems and reduce trade barriers. Key provisions of the Agreement guarantee most-favoured-nation treatment (exceptions being granted to customs unions and free trade areas, and for certain preferences in favour of developing countries); require that protection be given to domestic industry only through tariffs (apart from specified exceptions); provide for negotiations to reduce tariffs (which are then 'bound' against subsequent increase) and other trade distortions; and lay down principles (particularly in Part IV of the Agreement, added in 1965) to assist the trade of developing countries. The Agreement also provides for consultation on, and settlement of, disputes, for 'waivers' (the grant of authorization, when warranted, to derogate from specific GATT obligations) and for emergency action in defined circumstances.

Seven 'rounds' of multilateral trade negotiations, including the Kennedy Round of 1964–67, have been completed in GATT. The latest in this series, the Tokyo Round, although held in Geneva, was so called because it was launched at a Ministerial meeting in the Japanese capital in Sept. 1973.

Ninety-nine countries participated in the Tokyo Round. In Nov. 1979, the negotiations were concluded with agreements covering: An improved legal framework for the conduct of world trade (which includes recognition of tariff and nontariff treatment in favour of and among developing countries as a permanent legal feature of the world trading system); non-tariff measures (subsidies and countervailing duties; technical barriers to trade; government procurement; customs valuation; import licensing procedures; and a revision of the 1967 GATT anti-dumping code); bovine meat; dairy products; tropical products; and an agreement on free trade in civil aircraft. The agreements contain provisions for special and more favourable treatment for developing countries.

Participating countries also agreed to reduce tariffs on thousands of industrial and agricultural products, for the most part over a period of 7 years ending on 1 Jan. 1987. As a result of these concessions, industrialized countries reduced the average level of their import duties on manufactures by about 34%, a cut comparable to that achieved in the Kennedy Round.

The agreements providing an improved framework for the conduct of world trade took effect in Nov. 1979. The other agreements took effect on 1 Jan. 1980, except for those covering government procurement and customs valuation, which took effect on 1 Jan. 1981, and the concessions on tropical products which began as early as 1977. Committees were established to supervise implementation of each of the Tokyo Round agreements.

On 20 Sept. 1986, agreement was reached to launch the Uruguay Round of multilateral trade negotiations. In Dec. 1990, there were 106 states participating in the negotiations.

The Declaration is divided into two sections. The first covers negotiations on trade in goods. Its objectives are to bring about further liberalization and expansion of world trade; to strengthen the role of GATT and improve the multilateral trading system; to increase the responsiveness of GATT to the evolving international economic environment; and to encourage co-operation in strengthening the inter-relationship between trade and other economic policies affecting growth and development.

In the area of trade in goods, Ministers committed themselves to a 'standstill' on new trade measures inconsistent with their GATT obligations and to a 'rollback' programme aimed at phasing out existing inconsistent measures. Negotiations are being undertaken in the following areas: Tariffs, non-tariff measures, tropical products, natural resource-based products, textiles and clothing, agriculture, subsidies, safeguards, trade-related aspects of intellectual property rights, including trade in counterfeit goods, and trade-related investment measures. Participants are reviewing certain GATT Articles, attempting to improve and strengthen the dispute settlement procedure, and negotiating to improve, clarify or expand the agreements reached during the Tokyo Round. One part of the negotiation is devoted to the functioning of the GATT system itself. The second part of the Declaration covers a negotiation on trade in services.

The first three years of the Uruguay Round were marked by intensive activity, both in Geneva, where the negotiations take place, and in the capitals of the participating countries. During this time the groups responsible for the negotiations held around 300 formal meetings and around 1,500 negotiating proposals and working papers were tabled.

In Dec. 1988, ministers met in Montreal for the Mid-term Review meeting of the Trade Negotiations Committee. Agreements on the future conduct of the Round were reached in 11 of the 15 negotiating areas. At the same time, ministers were able to agree a package of concessions on tropical products covering trade worth around US$20,000m.; a series of measures to streamline the disputes settlement system and a new trade policy review mechanism under which the trade policies of individual GATT contracting countries are subject to regular assessment. Each of these was implemented provisionally in 1989. In April 1989, a Trade Negotiations Committee meeting in Geneva succeeded in securing Mid-term agreements on the remaining 4 negotiating areas: Agriculture (covering both short-term commitments and long-term objectives), safeguards, textiles and clothing and intellectual property. Meetings of the Round held in Dec. 1990, in Brussels, were unable to reach agreement owing to differences over the EC's Common Agricultural Policy. Talks were resumed in Feb. 1991.

To assist the trade of developing countries, GATT established in 1964 the *International Trade Centre* (since 1968 operated jointly with the UN, the latter acting through the UN Conference on Trade and Development) to provide information and training on export markets and marketing techniques. Other GATT action in favour of developing countries includes training courses on trade policy questions, organization of seminars and briefings, and technical assistance to delegations in the form of data and background documentation.

Budget for 1990: Sw. Frs. 74,571,000.

Headquarters: Centre William Rappard, 154 rue de Lausanne, 1211 Geneva 21, Switzerland.

Director-General: Arthur Dunkel (Switzerland).

Further Reading

Publications. Basic Instruments and Selected Documents. 4 vols. and 34 supplements 1952–87.—*International Trade* [i.e., annual review], 1952 ff. Annually from 1953.—*Review of Development in the Trading System.* Semi-annually from 1987.—*GATT, What It Is, What It Does.*—*GATT Activities,* 1960 ff. Annually from 1972.—*GATT Focus.* From Feb. 1981 (10 issues a year).—*News of the Uruguay Round.* Monthly from March 1987.—*GATT Studies in International Trade.* 1971 ff. (irregular series).—*The Tokyo Round of Multilateral Trade Negotiations.* Report of the Director-General, 2 vols., 1979.—*Textile and Clothing in the World Economy,* 1984.—*The World Markets for Dairy Products.* Annually from 1981.—*The International Markets for Meat.* Annually from 1981.—*Trade in Natural Resource Products: Aluminium* (1987), *Lead* (1987), *Zinc* (1988), *Nickel* (1990).

Casadio, G. P., *Transatlantic Trade: USA–EEC Confrontation in the GATT Negotiations.* Farnborough, 1973

Dam, K. W., *The GATT: Law and International Economic Organization.* Chicago and London, 1970

Golt, S., *The GATT Negotiations, 1973–75: A Guide to the Issues.* London, 1974

Hudec, R. E., *The GATT Legal System and World Trade Diplomacy.* New York, 1975

Long, O., *Law and its Limitations in the GATT Multilateral Trade System.* Dordrecht, 1985

WORLD INTELLECTUAL PROPERTY ORGANIZATION (WIPO)

Origin. The Convention establishing WIPO was signed at Stockholm in 1967 by 51 countries, and entered into force in April 1970. In Dec. 1974 WIPO became a specialized agency of the UN. *Inter alia* it took over the functions of the United International Bureaux for the Protection of Intellectual Property, also known as BIRPI (the French acronym of that name), which were established in 1893 to administer the affairs of the two principal international intellectual property treaties – the Paris Convention for the Protection of Industrial Property of 1883 and the Berne Convention for the Protection of Literary and Artistic Works of 1886.

Functions. WIPO is responsible for the promotion of the protection of intellectual property throughout the world. Intellectual property comprises two main branches: Industrial property (patents and other rights in technological inventions, rights in trademarks, industrial designs, appellations of origin, etc.) and copyright and neighbouring rights (in literary, musical and artistic works, in films and performances of performing artists, phonograms, etc.). WIPO administers various international treaties, of which the most important are the Paris Convention for the Protection of Industrial Property and the Berne Convention for the Protection of Literary and Artistic Works. WIPO carries out a substantial programme of activities to promote creative intellectual activity, protection of intellectual property, international co-operation and the transfer of technology, especially to and among developing countries.

Membership of WIPO is open to any State which is a member of at least one of the Unions created by the Paris Convention and the Berne Convention and to other States which are members of the organizations of the United Nations system, are party to the Statute of the International Court of Justice, or are invited to join by the General Assembly of WIPO. Membership of the Unions is open to any State. The number of member states of WIPO was 125 on 1 Jan. 1991; in addition, 9 States are party to treaties administered by WIPO but have not yet become members of WIPO.

Organization. The bodies of WIPO are: The *General Assembly* consisting of all member states of WIPO which are members of any of the Unions. Among its other functions, the General Assembly appoints and gives instructions to the Director General, reviews and approves his reports and adopts the biennial budget of expenses common to the Unions. The *Conference,* consisting of all States members of WIPO whether or not they are members of any of the Unions. Among its functions, the Conference adopts its biennial budget and establishes the biennial programme of legal-technical assistance. The *Co-ordination Committee,* consisting of the States members of WIPO which are members of the Executive Committees of the Paris or Berne Unions.

In addition, the Paris and Berne Unions have Assemblies and Executive Committees, with functions similar to those of the WIPO bodies in respect of the biennial budgets and programmes of the Unions.

The *WIPO Permanent Committees for Development Co-operation Related to Industrial Property* and *Related to Copyright and Neighbouring Rights* plan and review activities in the said fields; the *WIPO Permanent Committee on Industrial Property Information* is responsible for intergovernmental co-operation in industrial property documentation and information matters such as the standardization and exchange of patent documents.

WIPO has an international staff of 375. The working languages of the Organization are: Arabic, English, French, Russian and Spanish.

Headquarters: 34, chemin des Colombettes, 1211 Geneva 20, Switzerland.
Director-General: Dr Arpad Bogsch (USA).

Further Reading

Periodicals. Industrial Property (monthly, in English and French; quarterly, in Spanish).—*Copyright* (monthly, in English and French; quarterly, in Spanish).—*Les Marques internationales* (monthly, in French).—*International Designs Bulletin* (monthly, in English and French)—*Newsletter* (irregular, in Arabic, English, French, Portuguese, Russian and Spanish)—*PCT Gazette* (fortnightly, in English and French)—*Les appellations d'origine* (irregular)—*Intellectual Property in Asia and the Pacific* (quarterly). *Collection of Industrial Property and Copyright Laws and Treaties.*

INTERNATIONAL FUND FOR AGRICULTURAL DEVELOPMENT (IFAD)

The establishment of IFAD was one of the major actions proposed by the 1974 World Food Conference. The agreement for IFAD entered into force on 30 Nov. 1977, and the agency began its operations the following month. By the end of 1990 the Fund had invested US$3·2m. in financing 294 projects in 94 developing countries. IFAD's purpose is to mobilise additional funds for agricultural and rural development in developing countries through projects and programmes directly benefiting the poorest rural populations while preserving their natural resource base. In line with the Fund's focus on the rural poor, its resources are being made available mainly in highly concessional loans as well as grants.

Organization. The Governing Council, consisting of the entire membership, directs the Fund's operations. The chief executive is the President, who is also the Chairman of the 18-member Executive Board.

President: Idriss Jazairy (Algeria).
Headquarters: 107 Via del Serafico, Rome, 00142, Italy.

THE COMMONWEALTH

The Commonwealth is a free association of sovereign independent states, numbering 50 at the beginning of 1991. There is no charter, treaty or constitution; the association is expressed in co-operation, consultation and mutual assistance for which the Commonwealth Secretariat is the central co-ordinating body.

The Commonwealth was first defined by the Imperial Conference of 1926 as a group of 'autonomous Communities within the British Empire, equal in status, in no way subordinate one to another in any aspect of their domestic or external affairs, though united by a common allegiance to the Crown, and freely associated as members of the British Commonwealth of Nations'. The basis of the association changed from one owing allegiance to a common Crown, and the modern Commonwealth was born in 1949 when the member countries accepted India's intention of becoming a republic at the same time continuing 'her full membership of the Commonwealth of Nations and her acceptance of the King as the symbol of the free association of its independent member nations and as such the Head of the Commonwealth'. There were (1991) 17 Queen's realms, 28 republics, and 5 indigenous monarchies in the Commonwealth. All acknowledge the Queen symbolically as Head of the Commonwealth.

The Queen's legal title rests on the statute of 12 and 13 Will. III, c. 3, by which the succession to the Crown of Great Britain and Ireland was settled on the Princess Sophia of Hanover and the 'heirs of her body being Protestants'. By proclamation of 17 July 1917 the royal family became known as the House and Family of Windsor. On 8 Feb. 1960 the Queen issued a declaration varying her confirmatory declaration of 9 April 1952 to the effect that while the Queen and her children should continue to be known as the House of Windsor, her descendants, other than descendants entitled to the style of Royal Highness and the title of Prince or Princess, and female descendants who marry and their descendants should bear the name of Mountbatten-Windsor. The Royal Style and Titles of Queen Elizabeth are: In *Antigua and Barbuda* 'Elizabeth the Second, by the Grace of God, Queen of Antigua and Barbuda and of Her other Realms and Territories, Head of the Commonwealth'. In *Australia*: 'Elizabeth the Second, by the Grace of God Queen of Australia and Her other Realms and Territories, Head of the Commonwealth'. In the *Bahamas*: 'Elizabeth the Second, by the Grace of God, Queen of the Commonwealth of the Bahamas and of Her other Realms and Territories, Head of the Commonwealth'. In *Barbados*: 'Elizabeth the Second, by the Grace of God, Queen of Barbados and of Her other Realms and Territories, Head of the Commonwealth'. In *Belize*: 'Elizabeth the Second, by the Grace of God, Queen of Belize and of Her Other Realms and Territories, Head of the Commonwealth'. In *Canada*: 'Elizabeth the Second, by the Grace of God of the United Kingdom, Canada and Her other Realms and Territories Queen, Head of the Commonwealth, Defender of the Faith'. In *Grenada*: 'Elizabeth the Second, by the Grace of God, Queen of the United Kingdom of Great Britain and Northern Ireland and of Grenada and Her other Realms and Territories, Head of the Commonwealth'. In *Jamaica*: 'Elizabeth the Second, by the Grace of God of Jamaica and of Her other Realms and Territories Queen, Head of the Commonwealth'. In *Mauritius*: 'Elizabeth the Second, Queen of Mauritius and of Her other Realms and Territories, Head of the Commonwealth'. In *New Zealand*: 'Elizabeth the Second, by the Grace of God Queen of New Zealand and Her Other Realms and Territories, Head of the Commonwealth, Defender of the Faith'. In *Papua New Guinea*: 'Elizabeth the Second, Queen of Papua New Guinea and Her other Realms and Territories, Head of the Commonwealth'. In *Saint Christopher and Nevis*: 'Elizabeth the Second, by the Grace of God, Queen of Saint Christopher and Nevis and Her other Realms and Territories, Head of the Commonwealth'. In *Saint Lucia*: 'Elizabeth the Second, by the Grace of God, Queen of Saint Lucia and of Her other Realms and Territories, Head of Commonwealth'. In *Saint Vincent and the Grenadines*: 'Elizabeth the Second, by the Grace of God, Queen of Saint Vincent and the Grenadines and of Her other Realms and Territories, Head of the Commonwealth'. In *Solomon Islands*: 'Elizabeth the Second by the Grace of God Queen of Solomon Islands and of Her other Realms and Territories, Head of the Commonwealth'. In *Tuvalu*: 'Elizabeth the Second by the Grace of God Queen of Tuvalu and of Her other Realms and Territories, Head of the Commonwealth'. In the *United Kingdom*: 'Elizabeth the Second, by the Grace of God of the United Kingdom of Great Britain and Northern Ireland and of Her other Realms and Territories Queen, Head of the Commonwealth, Defender of the Faith'.

A number of territories, formerly under British jurisdiction or mandate did not join the Commonwealth: Egypt, Iraq, Transjordan, Burma, Palestine, Sudan, British Somaliland, South Cameroons, and Aden. 3 countries, Ireland in 1948, the Republic of South Africa in 1961 and Pakistan in 1972, have left the Commonwealth. Fiji's membership lapsed with the emergence of its Republic in 1987. Pakistan was re-admitted to the Commonwealth on 1 Oct. 1989.

Nauru and Tuvalu are special members, with the right to participate in all functional Commonwealth meetings and activities but not to attend meetings of Commonwealth Heads of Government.

Member States. The following are the member countries, with their dates of independence, and, where appropriate, the date on which they became republics: *United Kingdom*; *Canada* 1 July 1867[1]; *Australia* 1 Jan. 1901[1]; *New Zealand* 26 Sept. 1907[1]; *India* 15 Aug. 1947 (Republic on 26 Jan. 1950); *Sri Lanka* 4 Feb. 1948 (Republic on 22 May 1972); *Ghana* 6 March 1957 (Republic on 1 July 1960); *Malaysia* 31 Aug. 1957 as Federation of Malaya, 16 Sept. 1963 as Federation of Malaysia; *Cyprus* 16 Aug. 1960 (Republic on independence; joined Commonwealth on 13 March 1961); *Nigeria* 1 Oct. 1960 (Republic on 1 Oct. 1963); *Sierra Leone* 27 April 1961 (Republic on 19 April 1971); *Tanzania*–Tanganyika 9 Dec. 1961 (Republic on 9 Dec. 1962), Zanzibar 10 Dec. 1963 (Republic on 12 Jan. 1964), United Republic of Tanganyika and Zanzibar 26 April 1964; renamed United Republic of Tanzania 29 Oct. 1964; *Western Samoa* 1 Jan. 1962 (joined Commonwealth on 28 Aug. 1970); *Jamaica* 6 Aug. 1962; *Trinidad and Tobago* 31 Aug. 1962 (Republic on 1 Aug. 1976); *Uganda* 9 Oct. 1962 (Republic 8 Sept. 1967, second republic 25 Jan. 1971); *Kenya* 12 Dec. 1963 (Republic on 12 Dec. 1964); *Malaŵi* 6 July 1964 (Republic on 6 July 1966); *Malta* 21 Sept. 1964 (Republic on 13 Dec. 1974); *Zambia* 24 Oct. 1964 (Republic on independence); *The Gambia* 18 Feb. 1965 (Republic on 24 April 1970); *Maldives* 26 July 1965 (Republic on independence, joined Commonwealth on 9 July 1982); *Singapore* 16 Sept. 1963 as a state in the Federation of Malaysia, 9 Aug. 1965 as an independent state and republic not part of Malaysia; *Guyana* 26 May 1966 (Republic on 23 Feb. 1970); *Botswana* 30 Sept. 1966 (Republic on independence); *Lesotho* 4 Oct. 1966; *Barbados* 30 Nov. 1966; *Nauru* [2] 31 Jan. 1968 (Republic on independence); *Mauritius* 12 March 1968; *Swaziland* 6 Sept. 1968; *Tonga* [3] 4 June 1970; *Bangladesh* seceded from Pakistan as Republic 16 Dec. 1971, recognized by United Kingdom 4 Feb. 1972 (joined Commonwealth on 18 April 1972); *Bahamas* 10 July 1973; *Grenada* 7 Feb. 1974; *Papua New Guinea* 16 Sept. 1975; *Seychelles* 29 June 1976 (Republic on independence); *Solomon Islands* 7 July 1978; *Tuvalu* 1 Oct. 1978; *Dominica* 3 Nov. 1978 (Republic on independence); *Saint Lucia* 22 Feb. 1979; *Kiribati* 12 July 1979 (Republic on independence); *Saint Vincent and the Grenadines* 27 Oct. 1979; *Zimbabwe* 18 April 1980 (Republic on independence); *Vanuatu* 30 July 1980 (Republic on independence); *Belize* 21 Sept. 1981; *Antigua* and *Barbuda* 1 Nov. 1981; *Saint Christopher and Nevis* 19 Sept. 1983; *Brunei* [2] 1 Jan 1984; *Pakistan* 15 Aug. 1947 (Republic on 23 March 1956); left Commonwealth 30 Jan. 1972, re-admitted 1 Oct. 1989; *Namibia* 21 March 1990 (Republic on independence).

[1] These are the effective dates of independence, given legal effect by the Statute of Westminster 1931.

[2] Nauru had been first a Mandate, then a Trust territory.

[3] Brunei and Tonga had been sovereign states in treaty relationship with the UK, whereby the UK was responsible for the conduct of external affairs and had a consultative responsibility for defence.

Dependent Territories and Associated States. There are 15 British dependent territories, 7 Australian external territories, 2 New Zealand dependent territories and 2 New Zealand associated states. A dependent territory is a territory belonging by settlement, conquest or annexation to the British, Australian or New Zealand Crown.

United Kingdom dependent territories administered through the Foreign and Commonwealth Office comprise, in the Far East: Hong Kong; in the Indian Ocean: British Indian Ocean Territory; in the Mediterranean: Gibraltar; in the Atlantic Ocean: Bermuda, Falkland Islands, South Georgia and the South Sandwich Islands, British Antarctic Territory, St Helena, St Helena Dependencies (Ascension and Tristan da Cunha); in the Caribbean: Montserrat, British Virgin Islands, Cayman Islands, Turks and Caicos Islands, Anguilla; in the Western Pacific: Pitcairn Group of Islands. The Australian external territories are: Coral Sea Islands Territory, Cocos (Keeling) Islands, Christmas Island, Heard Island and McDonald Islands, Norfolk

Island, Australian Antarctic Territory and the Territory of Ashmore and Cartier Islands. The New Zealand dependent territories are: Tokelau and Ross Dependency. The New Zealand associated states are: Cook Islands and Niue.

While constitutional responsibility to Parliament for the government of the British dependent territories rests with the Secretary of State for Foreign and Commonwealth Affairs, the administration of the territories is carried out by the Governments of the territories themselves.

British Government Department. With effect from 17 Oct. 1968, the Secretary of State for Foreign and Commonwealth Affairs is responsible for the conduct of relations with members of the Commonwealth as well as with foreign countries, and for the administration of British dependent territories.

Commonwealth Secretariat. The Commonwealth Secretariat is an international body at the service of all 50 member countries. It provides the central organization for joint consultation and co-operation in many fields. It was established in 1965 by Commonwealth Heads of Government and has observer status at the UN General Assembly.

The Secretariat disseminates information on matters of common concern, organizes and services meetings and conferences, co-ordinates many Commonwealth activities, and provides expert technical assistance for economic and social development through the multilateral Commonwealth Fund for Technical Cooperation. The Secretariat is organized in divisions and sections which correspond to its main areas of operation: International affairs, economic affairs, food production and rural development, youth, education, information, applied studies in government, science and technology, law and health. Within this structure the Secretariat organizes the biennial meetings of Commonwealth Heads of Government, annual meetings of Finance Ministers of member countries, and regular meetings of Ministers of Education, Law, Health, and others as appropriate.

To emphasize the multilateral nature of the association, meetings are held in different cities and regions within the Commonwealth. Heads of Government decided that the Secretariat should work from London as it has the widest range of communications of any Commonwealth city, as well as the largest assembly of diplomatic missions.

The Commonwealth Secretary-General, who has access to Heads of Government, is the head of the Secretariat which is staffed by officers from member countries and financed by contributions from member governments.

Commonwealth Day is observed throughout the Commonwealth on the second Monday in March.

Flag: Royal blue with the emblem of a globe surrounded by 49 rays, all in gold.

Headquarters: Marlborough House, Pall Mall, London, SW1Y 5HX.

Secretary-General: Emeka Anyaoku (Nigeria).

Further Reading

The Commonwealth Year-Book, HMSO, Annual

The Cambridge History of the British Empire. 8 vols. CUP, 1929 ff.

Austin, D., *The Commonwealth and Britain*. London, 1988

Burns, Sir Alan, *In Defence of Colonies*. London, 1957

Chadwick, J., *The Unofficial Commonwealth*. London, 1982

Dale, W., *The Modern Commonwealth*. London, 1983

Garner, J., *The Commonwealth Office, 1925–1968*. London, 1978

Hailey, Lord, *An African Survey*. Rev. ed. Oxford, 1957.—*Native Administration in the British African Territories*. 5 vols. HMSO, 1951 ff.

Hall, H. D., *Commonwealth: A History of the British Commonwealth*. London and New York, 1971

Judd, D. and Slinn, P., *The Evolution of the Modern Commonwealth*. London, 1982

Keeton, G. W. (ed.) *The British Commonwealth: Its Laws and Constitutions*. 9 vols. London, 1951 ff.

Mansergh, N., *The Commonwealth Experience*. 2 vols. London, 1982

Maxwell, W. H. and L. F., *A Legal Bibliography of the British Commonwealth of Nations*. 2nd ed. London, 1956

Moore, R. J., *Making the New Commonwealth*. Oxford, 1987
Papadopoulos, A. N., *Multilateral Diplomacy within the Commonwealth: A Decade of Expansion*. The Hague, 1982
Smith, A. and Sanger, C., *Stitches in Time: The Commonwealth in World Politics*. New York, 1983
Wade, E. C. S. and Phillips, G. G., *Constitutional Law: An Outline of the Law and Practice of the Constitution, Including Central and Local Government and the Constitutional Relations of the British Commonwealth and Empire*. 8th ed. London, 1970

WORLD COUNCIL OF CHURCHES

The World Council of Churches was formally constituted on 23 Aug. 1948, at Amsterdam, by an assembly representing 147 churches from 44 countries. By 1990 the member churches numbered over 300, from more than 100 countries.

The basis of membership (1975) states: 'The World Council of Churches is a fellowship of Churches which confess the Lord Jesus Christ as God and Saviour according to the Scriptures and therefore seek to fulfil together their common calling to the glory of the one God, Father, Son and Holy Spirit.' Membership is open to Churches which express their agreement with this basis and satisfy such criteria as the Assembly or Central Committee may prescribe. Today 312 Churches of Protestant, Anglican, Orthodox, Old Catholic and Pentecostal confessions belong to this fellowship.

The World Council was founded by the coming together of several diverse Christian movements. These included the overseas mission groups gathered from 1921 in the International Missionary Council, the Faith and Order Movement founded by American Episcopal Bishop Charles Brent, and the Life and Work Movement led by Swedish Lutheran Archbishop Nathan Söderblom.

On 13 May 1938 at Utrecht a provisional committee was appointed to prepare for the formation of a World Council of Churches. It was under the chairmanship of William Temple, then Archbishop of York.

Assembly. The governing body of the World Council, consisting of delegates specially appointed by the member Churches. It meets every 7 or 8 years to frame policy and to consider some main theme. The Assembly has no legislative powers and depends for the implementation of its decisions upon the action of the member Churches. Assemblies have been held in Amsterdam (1948), Evanston (1954), New Delhi (1961), Uppsala (1968), Nairobi (1975) and Vancouver (1983). The 1991 Assembly was scheduled to meet in Canberra with the theme 'Come, Holy Spirit – Renew the Whole Creation'. In between assemblies, a 150-member Central Committee meets annually to carry out the assembly mandate, with a smaller 22-member Executive Committee meeting twice a year.

Presidents: Dame R. Nita Barrow (Barbados), Dr Marga Bührig (Switzerland), Metropolitan Paulos Mar Gregorios (India), Bishop Johannes Hempel (German Democratic Republic), Patriarch Ignatios IV (Syria), Most Rev. W. P. K. Makhulu (Botswana), Very Rev. Dr Lois Wilson (Canada).

WCC programmes are organized from headquarters in Geneva, Switzerland, by a staff of 307 and a range of supervisory committees drawn from member churches. The 3 programme units are:

(i) Faith and Witness includes the Commission on Faith and Order, World Mission and Evangelism, Church and Society and the sub-unit on Dialogue with People of Living Faiths.

(ii) Justice and Service which includes Inter-Church Aid, Refugee and World Service (channelling over $35m. from member churches to areas of need); the Commission on the Churches' Participation in Development; the Commission of the Churches on International Affairs, the Programme to Combat Racism and the Christian Medical Commission.

(iii) Education and Renewal includes sections dealing with renewal and congregational life, women, youth, church-related education, biblical studies, family ministry and the Programme on Theological Education.

A General Secretariat with a Communication Department, a Finance Department and a Library co-ordinates the work of the 3 Programme Units and supervises the work of Ecumenical Institute Céligny (Switzerland).

Since 1975 the WCC has held several major world conferences on such diverse themes as 'Faith, Science and the Future', 'Your Kingdom Come', 'Family Power and Social Change', 'Strategies for Churches Combating Racism in the 1980's', 'The Community of Women and Men in the Church', 'Giving an Account of the Hope that is in Us', 'Called to be Neighbours' and 'Your Will be Done—Mission in Christ's Way'.

Officers of the Central and Executive Committees: *Moderator:* Rev. Dr Heinz J. Held (Federal Republic of Germany). *Vice-moderators:* Dr Sylvia Ross Talbot (USA), Metropolitan Chrysostomos of Myra (Turkey). *General Secretary:* The Rev. Dr Emilio Castro.

Office: PO Box 2100, 150 route de Ferney, 1211 Geneva 2, Switzerland.

Further Reading

Official Reports: The First [. . . *etc.*] *Assembly* (London, 1948, 1955, 1962, Geneva, 1968, 1975, 1983)
Directory of Christian Councils. 1985
New Delhi to Uppsala 1961–68. Geneva, 1968
Uppsala to Nairobi 1968–75. Geneva, 1975
Nairobi to Vancouver. Geneva, 1983
Official Reports of the Faith and Order Conferences at Lausanne 1927, Edinburgh 1937, Lund 1952, Montreal 1963, Meeting of Faith and Order Commission, Louvain 1971, Accra 1974, Bangalore 1978, Vancouver 1983
Minutes of the Central Committee. Geneva, 1949 to date
Howell, L., *Acting in Faith: The World Council of Churches since 1975*. London, 1982
Potter, P., *Life in all its Fullness*. Geneva, 1981
van der Bent, A. J., *What in the World is the World Council of Churches?* Geneva, 1978.—*Handbook of Member Churches of the World Council of Churches*. Geneva, 1985
Vermaat, J. A. A., *The World Council of Churches and Politics*. New York, 1989
Visser 't Hooft, W. A., *The Genesis and Formation of the World Council of Churches*. Geneva, 1982

INTERNATIONAL TRADE UNIONISM

There are three main international trade union confederations *(i)* the International Confederation of Free Trade Unions (ICFTU) which has in membership most of the national trade union confederations in the Western industrialized countries, unions in Czechoslovakia and Poland and national organizations in Asia, Africa, and Latin America; *(ii)* the World Federation of Trade Unions (WFTU) which until 1989 drew its support mainly from Eastern Europe, but which now has one affiliated organization in Poland and one in the USSR, an affiliate in France and affiliates in Cuba and other developing countries; and *(iii)* the World Confederation of Labour (WCL) which has affiliates in Western Europe, Latin America and a small number of African and Asian countries. In addition, national trade unions are frequently members of international trade union federations, set up to protect the interests of working people in particular industries or trades, which are associated with the international confederations. The International Trade Secretariats (ITS) are associated with the ICFTU; Trade Union Internationals (TUI) with the WFTU; and the International Trade Federations (ITF) with the WCL.

History. The international trade union structure between 1945 and 1989 was shaped mainly by political factors. In 1945 the WFTU was set up with world-wide membership. Attempts by trade unions in Eastern Europe to turn the WFTU into an organization voicing unquestioning support for the policies of the USSR led most of the affiliates in the Western European countries to break away from the WFTU and to form the ICFTU in 1949.

EUROPEAN TRADE UNION CONFEDERATION. In Feb. 1973 the European Trade Union Confederation was formed by trade unionists in 15 Western European countries to deal with questions of interest to European working people arising inside and outside the EC. All the founding organizations were ICFTU affiliates but subsequently they accepted into membership European WCL affiliates, the Irish Congress of Trade Unions and the Italian Communist and Socialist trade union centre (CGIL) and other national organizations. The ETUC Congress meets every 3 years and the Executive Committee 5 times a year. The membership was (June 1990) about 45m. from 39 centres in 21 countries.

General Secretary: Mathias Hinterscheid.
Headquarters: Rue Montagne aux Herbes Potagères 37, 1000 Brussels.

INTERNATIONAL CONFEDERATION OF FREE TRADE UNIONS. The first congress of ICFTU was held in London in Dec. 1949. The constitution as amended provides for co-operation with the United Nations and the International Labour Organization and for regional organizations to promote free trade unionism, especially in less-developed countries.

Organization. The Congress meets every 4 years. It elects the Executive Board of 37 members nominated on an area basis for a 4-year period; 1 seat is reserved for a woman nominated by the Women's Committee; the Board meets at least twice a year. Various committees cover policy *vis-à-vis* such problems as those connected with nuclear energy and also the administration of the International Solidarity Fund. There are joint ICFTU–ITS committees for co-ordinating activities.

Headquarters: 37–41, rue Montagne aux Herbes Potagères, Brussels 1000, Belgium.

General Secretary: John Vanderveken.

Regional organizations exist in America, office in Mexico City; Asia, office in New Delhi; and Africa, office in Sierre Leone.

Membership. The ICFTU had in Dec. 1990 144 affiliated organizations in 101 countries, which together represent about 99m. workers. The largest organizations were the American Federation of Labor and Congress of Industrial Organizations (13·7m.), the British Trades Union Congress (8·5m.), the Japanese Confederation of Labour, Rengo (8m.), the German Deutscher Gewerkschaftsbund (7·1m.), the Confederazione Italiana Sindacati Lavoratori (3·1m.), the Swedish Landsorganisationen (2·1m.), the Indian National Trade Union Congress (4·7m.), the Argentinian Confederacion General de Trabajo (6m.), the Czechoslovak CSKOS (6m.) and the Indian Hind Mazdoor Sabha (2·6m.).

Publications (in 4 languages). *Free Labour World* (fortnightly).

THE WORLD FEDERATION OF TRADE UNIONS. The WFTU formally came into existence on 3 Oct. 1945, representing trade-union organizations in more than 50 countries of the world, both Communist and non-Communist, excluding Federal Republic of Germany and Japan, as well as a number of lesser and colonial territories. Representation from the USA was limited to the Congress of Industrial Organizations, as the American Federation of Labor declined to participate.

In Jan. 1949 the British, USA and Netherlands trade unions withdrew from WFTU, which had come under complete Communist control; and by June 1951 all non-Communist trade-unions, and the Yugoslav Federation, had left WFTU.

Organization. The Congress meets every 4 years. In between, the General Council, of 134 members (including deputies), is the governing body, meeting (in theory) at least once a year. The Bureau controls the activities of WFTU between meetings of the General Council; it consists of the President, the General Secretary and members from different continents, the total number being decided at each Congress. The Bureau is elected by the General Council. Regional bureaux were instituted in 1990 as a move towards decentralization.

President: I. Zakaria (Sudan).
General Secretary: Aleksandr Zharikov (USSR).

Membership. With the collapse of many Communist-type trade union organizations membership became very fluid in 1990. 106 organizations were members in 1991, including the former official unions of the USSR and Poland, and the French Confederation of Labour (CGT).

The headquarters was in Prague until 1991.

Publications. World Trade Union Movement (monthly, in 9 languages); *Trade Union Press* (fortnightly, in 6 languages).

WORLD CONFEDERATION OF LABOUR. The first congress of the International Federation of Christian Trade Unions (IFCTU), as the WCL was then called, met in 1920; but a large proportion of its 3·4m. members were in Italy and Germany, where affiliated unions were suppressed by the Fascist and Nazi régimes, and in 1940 IFCTU went out of existence. It was reconstituted in 1945, and declined to merge with WFTU and, later, with ICFTU. The policy of IFCTU was based on the papal encyclicals *Rerum novarum* (1891) and *Quadragesimo anno* (1931), but in 1968, when the Federation became the WCL, it was broadened to include other concepts. The WCL now has Protestant, Buddhist and Moslem member confederations as well as its mainly Roman Catholic members.

Organization. The WCL is organized on a federative basis which leaves wide discretion to its autonomous constituent unions. Its governing body is the Congress, which meets every 4 years. The Congress appoints (or re-appoints) the Secretary-General at each 4-yearly meeting. The General Council which meets at least once a year, is composed of the members of the Confederal Board (at least 22 members, elected by the Congress) and representatives of national confederations, international trade federations, and trade union organizations where there is no confederation affiliated to the WCL. The Confederal Board is responsible for the general leadership of the WCL, in accordance with the decisions and directives of the Council and Congress. Headquarters: 71 rue Joseph II, Brussels 1040, Belgium.

Secretary-General: Carlos Luís Custer.

There are regional organizations in Latin America (office in Caracas), Africa (office in Banjul, Gambia) and Asia (office in Manila) There is also a liaison centre in Montreal.

Membership. A total membership of 11m. in about 90 countries is claimed. The biggest group is the Confederation of Christian Trade Unions of Belgium (1·2m.).

Publication. Labour Press and Information (11 each year, in 5 languages).

ORGANISATION FOR ECONOMIC CO-OPERATION AND DEVELOPMENT (OECD)

History and Membership. On 30 Sept. 1961 the Organisation for European Economic Co-operation (OEEC), after a history of 13 years (*see* THE STATESMAN'S YEAR-BOOK , 1961, p. 32), was replaced by the Organisation for Economic Co-operation and Development. The change of title marks the Organisation's altered status and functions: With the accession of Canada and USA as full members it ceased to be a purely European body; while at the same time it added development aid to the list of its other activities. The member countries are now Australia, Austria, Belgium, Canada, Denmark, Finland, France, Germany, Greece, Iceland, Ireland, Italy, Japan, Luxembourg, the Netherlands, New Zealand, Norway, Portugal, Spain, Sweden, Switzerland, Turkey, UK and USA. Yugoslavia participates in the Organisation's activities with a special status. The Commission of the European Communities generally takes part in OECD's work.

Objectives. To promote economic and social welfare throughout the OECD area by assisting its member governments in the formulation of policies designed to this end and by co-ordinating these policies; and to stimulate and harmonize its members' efforts in favour of developing countries.

Organs. The supreme body of the Organisation is the Council composed of one representative for each member country. It meets either at Heads of Delegations level (about twice a month) under the Chairmanship of the Secretary-General, or at Ministerial level (usually once a year) under the Chairmanship of a Minister of a country elected annually to assume these functions. Decisions and Recommendations are adopted by mutual agreement of all members of the Council.

The Council is assisted by an Executive Committee composed of 14 members of the Council designated annually by the latter. The major part of the Organisation's work is, however, prepared and carried out in numerous specialized committees, working parties and sub-groups, of which there exist over 200. Thus, the Organisation comprises Committees for Economic Policy; Economic and Development Review; Development Assistance (DAC); Commodities; Trade; Capital Movements and Invisible Transactions; Financial Markets; Fiscal Affairs; Competition Law and Policy; Consumer Policy; Maritime Transport; International Investment and Multinational Enterprises; Tourism; Energy Policy; Industry; Steel; Scientific and Technological Policy; Information, Computer and Communications Policy; Road Transport Research; Education; Manpower and Social Affairs; Environment; Urban Affairs; Control of Chemicals; Agriculture; Fisheries, etc.

In 1990 the Centre for Co-operation with European Economics in Transition (CCEET) was established to act as OECD's point of contact for Central and East European countries seeking guidance in moving towards a market economy.

Four autonomous or semi-autonomous bodies also belong to the Organisation: The International Energy Agency (IEA); the Nuclear Energy Agency (NEA); the Development Centre and the Centre for Educational Research and Innovation (CERI). Each one of these bodies has its own governing committee.

The Council, the committees and the other bodies are serviced by an international Secretariat headed by the Secretary-General of the Organisation.

All member countries have established permanent Delegations to OECD, each headed by an Ambassador.

Chairman of the Council (ministerial): A minister from the country elected (annually) to assume this function.

Chairman of the Council (official level): The Secretary-General.

Secretary-General: Jean-Claude Paye (France).

Deputy Secretaries-General: Robert A. Cornell (USA), Pierre Vinde (Sweden), Makoto Taniguchi (Japan).

Executive Director of the International Energy Agency: Helga Steeg (Federal Republic of Germany).

Headquarters: 2, rue André Pascal, 75775 Paris Cedex 16, France.

Further Reading

OECD publishes numerous reports and statistical papers. Regular features include:

Activities of OECD. Annual
News from OECD. Monthly
Main Economic Indicators. Monthly
The OECD Observer. Bi-monthly
The OECD Economic Outlook. Semi-annual
OEEC/OECD Economic Surveys of Member Countries.
OECD Employment Outlook. Annual
Geographical Distribution of Financial Flows to Developing Countries. Annual
Development Co-operation Report. Annual
Tourism Policy and International Tourism in OECD Member Countries.
Maritime Transport. Annual
Energy Policies and Programmes of the IEA Member Countries.

NORTH ATLANTIC TREATY ORGANIZATION (NATO)

Western perceptions of the political situation in Europe following World War II gave rise, in 1947, to 2 major US initiatives – the Truman Doctrine and the Marshall Plan. These policies were designed to increase the ability of Western European countries to resist outside pressure and to assist them in bringing about their economic recovery. By 1948, on the initiative of the Foreign Secretary of the UK Ernest Bevin, 5 Western European nations had also entered into a treaty of mutual assistance in which they pledged themselves to come to each other's aid in the event of armed aggression against them (Brussels Treaty, 17 March 1948). The idea of a single mutual defence system involving North America as well as the European signatories of the Brussels Treaty was put forward by the Canadian Secretary of State for External Affairs in April 1948. It led, via the Vandenberg Resolution which enabled the US constitutionally to participate, to the creation of the Atlantic Alliance.

On 4 April 1949 the foreign ministers of Belgium, Canada, Denmark, France, Iceland, Italy, Luxembourg, the Netherlands, Norway, Portugal, the UK and the USA met in Washington and signed a treaty, the main clauses of which read as follows:

Article 1. The parties undertake, as set forth in the Charter of the United Nations, to settle any international disputes in which they may be involved by peaceful means in such a manner that international peace and security and justice are not endangered, and to refrain in their international relations from the threat or use of force in any manner inconsistent with the purposes of the United Nations.

Article 2. The parties will contribute toward the further development of peaceful and friendly international relations by strengthening their free institutions, by bringing about a better understanding of the principles upon which these institutions are founded, and by promoting conditions of stability and well-being. They will seek to eliminate conflict in their international economic policies and will encourage economic collaboration between any or all of them.

Article 3. In order more effectively to achieve the objectives of this treaty, the parties, separately and jointly by means of continuous and effective self-help and mutual aid, will maintain and develop their individual and collective capacity to resist armed attack.

Article 4. The parties will consult together whenever, in the opinion of any of them, the territorial integrity, political independence or security of any of the parties is threatened.

Article 5. The parties agree that an armed attack against one or more of them in Europe or North America shall be considered an attack against them all and consequently they agree that, if such an armed attack occurs, each of them, in exercise of the right of individual or collective self-defence recognized by article 51 of the Charter of the United Nations, will assist the party or parties so attacked by taking forthwith, individually and in concert with the other parties, such action as it deems necessary, including the use of armed force, to restore and maintain the security of the North Atlantic area. Any such armed attack and all measures taken as a result thereof shall immediately be reported to the Security Council. Such measures shall be terminated when the Security Council has taken the measures necessary to restore and maintain international peace and security.

Article 6. For the purpose of Article 5 an armed attack on one or more of the parties is deemed to include an armed attack *(i)* on the territory of any of the parties in Europe or North America, on the Algerian Departments of France, on the territory of Turkey or on the islands under the jurisdiction of any of the parties in the North Atlantic area north of the Tropic of Cancer; *(ii)* on the forces, vessels or aircraft of any of the parties, when in or over these territories or any other area in Europe in which occupation forces of any of the parties were stationed on the date when the treaty entered into force or the Mediterranean Sea or the North Atlantic area north of the Tropic of Cancer.

Article 8. Each party declares that none of the international engagements now in force between it and any other of the parties or any third state is in conflict with the provisions of this treaty, and undertakes not to enter into any international engagement in conflict with this treaty.

Article 10. The parties may, by unanimous agreement, invite any other European state in a position to further the principles of this treaty and to contribute to the security of the North Atlantic area to accede to this treaty. Any state so invited may become a party to the treaty by depositing its instrument of accession with the government of the United States of America. The government of the United States of America will inform each of the parties of the deposit

Article 12. After the treaty has been in force for 10 years, or at any time thereafter, the parties shall, if any of them so requests, consult together for the purpose of reviewing the treaty, having regard for the factors then affecting peace and security in the North Atlantic area, including the development of universal as well as regional arrangements under the Charter of the United Nations for the maintenance of international peace and security.

Article 13. After the treaty has been in force for 20 years, any party may cease to be a party one year after its notice of denunciation has been given to the government of the United States of America, which will inform the governments of the other parties of the deposit of each notice of denunciation.

The treaty came into force on 24 Aug. 1949. Greece and Turkey were admitted as parties to the treaty in 1952, the Federal Republic of Germany in 1955 and Spain in 1982. Since 1990 the USSR had diplomatic representation at NATO. Hungary gained associate membership in Jan. 1991.

In their London Declaration of June 1990 the member states noted that Europe had 'entered a new, promising era' and 'as a consequence, this Alliance can and will adapt'; it was resolved to 'remain a defensive alliance' but to 'enhance the political component', and to propose to Warsaw Pact members a 'joint declaration in which we solemnly state that we are no longer adversaries'. It was further proposed that the Conference on Security and Co-operation in Europe (CSCE) should be instititutionalized.

NATO is an organization of sovereign states equal in status. Decisions taken are expressions of the collective will of member governments arrived at by common consent.

The *North Atlantic Council* is composed of representatives of the 16 member countries. At Ministerial Meetings of the Council, member nations are represented by Ministers of Foreign Affairs. These meetings are held twice a year. The Council also meets on occasion at the level of Heads of State and Government. In permanent session, at the level of Ambassadors, the Council meets at least once a week.

The *Defence Planning Committee* is composed of representatives of all member countries except France. Like the Council, it meets both in permanent session at the level of Ambassadors and twice a year at Ministerial level. At Ministerial Meetings member nations are represented by Defence Ministers.

The Council and Defence Planning Committee are chaired by the Secretary General of NATO at whatever level they meet. Opening sessions of Ministerial Meetings of the Council are presided over by the President, an honorary position held annually by the Foreign Minister of one of the member nations.

Nuclear matters are discussed by the *Nuclear Planning Group* in which 15 countries now participate. It meets regularly at the level of Permanent Representatives (Ambassadors) and twice a year at the level of Ministers of Defence.

The Permanent Representatives of member countries are supported by the National Delegations located at NATO Headquarters. The Delegations are composed of advisors and officials qualified to represent their countries on the various committees created by the Council. The Committees are supported by the International Staff responsible to the Secretary General.

Headquarters: 1110 Brussels, Belgium.
Secretary-General: Manfred Wörner (Federal Republic of Germany).
Flag: Dark blue with a white compass rose of 4 points in the centre.

The *Military Committee* is responsible for making recommendations to the Council and the Defence Planning Committee on military matters and for supplying guidance to the Allied Commanders. Composed of the Chiefs-of-Staff of all member countries except France and Iceland (which has no military forces), the Committee is assisted by an International Military Staff. It meets at Chiefs-of-Staff level at least twice a year but remains in permanent session at the level of national military representatives. Liaison between the Military Committee and the French High Command is effected through the French Mission to the Military Committee. The chairman of the Military Committee is elected by the Chiefs-of-Staff for a period of 2–3 years. The present chairman is Gen. Wolfgang Altenburg (Federal Republic of Germany), appointed Oct. 1986.

The area covered by the North Atlantic Treaty is divided among three commands:

The Atlantic Ocean Command, the European Command and the Channel Command. Defence plans for the North American area are developed by the Canada–US Regional Planning Group.

The NATO commanders are responsible for the development of defence plans for their respective areas, for the determination of force requirements and for the deployment and exercise of the forces under their command.

The *Allied Command Europe* (ACE) covers the area extending from the North Cape to the Mediterranean and from the Atlantic to the eastern border of Turkey. Responsibilities relating to the defence of Portugal and the UK are included but these come within the purview of more than one NATO Command. The European area, which is subdivided into a number of subordinate commands, is under the Supreme Allied Commander Europe (SACEUR) whose Headquarters, near Mons in Belgium, are known as SHAPE (Supreme Headquarters Allied Powers Europe).

SACEUR has also under his orders the ACE Mobile Force, composed of both land and air force units from different member countries, which can be ready for action at very short notice in any threatened area. The present SACEUR is Gen. John R. Galvin (USA).

Under the Supreme Allied Commander Atlantic (SACLANT) the *Atlantic Command* extends from the North Pole to the Tropic of Cancer and from the coastal waters of North America to those of Europe and Africa, but excludes the Channel and the British Isles. SACLANT, who would have the primary task in wartime of ensuring the security of the sea lanes in the whole Atlantic area, is an operational rather than an administrative commander. Under his direct command is the Standing Naval Force Atlantic (STANAVFORLANT) which is a permanent international squadron of ships drawn from NATO navies which normally operate in the Atlantic. The present SACLANT, whose Headquarters are in Norfolk (USA), is Admiral Frank B. Kelso II (US), appointed Nov. 1988.

The *Channel Command* covers the English Channel and the southern North Sea. Under the Allied Commander-in-Chief Channel (CINCHAN) its mission is to control and protect merchant shipping in the area, co-operating with SACEUR in the air defence of the Channel. The forces earmarked to the Command in emergency are predominantly naval but include maritime air forces. CINCHAN also has under his command the NATO Standing Naval Force Channel (STANAVFORCHAN) which is a permanent force comprizing mine counter-measure ships of different NATO countries. The present CINCHAN, with Headquarters at Northwood (UK), is Admiral Sir Benjamin Bathurst, KCB (UK), appointed May 1987.

The *Canada–US Regional Planning Group*, which covers the North American area, develops and recommends to the Military Committee plans for the defence of this area. It meets alternately in Washington and Ottawa.

Further Reading

The NATO Information Service publishes documentation, reference material and information brochures including: *The NATO Handbook; NATO: Facts and Figures; The NATO Review* (periodical); economic and scientific publications.

Cook, D., *The Forging of an Alliance*. London, 1989
De Staercke, A., *Nato's Anxious Birth: The Prophetic Vision of the 1940's*. London, 1985
Godson, J., *Challenges to the Western Alliance*. London,1986
Goldstein, W., *Reagan's Leadership and the Atlantic Alliance*. New York, 1986
Hanning, H., *NATO–Our Guarantee for Peace*. London, 1986
Henderson, N., *The Birth of NATO*. London, 1982
Sloan, S. R., *NATO in the 1990s*. Washington, 1989
Smith, J. (ed.) *The Origins of NATO*. Exeter Univ. Press, 1990
Williams, G. and Lee, A., *The European Defence Initiative*. London, 1986

WESTERN EUROPEAN UNION

On 17 March 1948 a 50-year treaty 'for collaboration in economic, social and cultural matters and for collective self-defence' was signed in Brussels by the Foreign

Ministers of the UK, France, the Netherlands, Belgium and Luxembourg. (*See* THE STATESMAN'S YEAR-BOOK, 1954, pp. 32 f.)

On 20 Dec. 1950 the functions of the Western Union defence organization were transferred to the North Atlantic Treaty command, but it was decided that the reorganization of the military machinery should not affect the right of the Western Union Defence Ministers and the Chiefs of Staff to meet as they please to consider matters of mutual concern to the Brussels Treaty powers.

After the breakdown of the European Defence Community on 30 Aug. 1954 a conference was held in London from 28 Sept. to 3 Oct. 1954, attended by Belgium, Canada, France, the Federal Republic of Germany, Italy, Luxembourg, the Netherlands, the UK and the USA, at which it was decided to invite the Federal Republic of Germany and Italy to accede to the Brussels Treaty, to end the occupation of Western Germany and to invite the latter to accede to the North Atlantic Treaty; the Federal Republic agreed that it would voluntarily limit its arms production, and provision was made for the setting up of an agency to control the armaments of the 7 Brussels Treaty powers; the UK undertook not to withdraw from the Continent her 4 divisions and the Tactical Air Force assigned to the Supreme Allied Commander against the wishes of a majority, *i.e.*, 4 of the Brussels Treaty powers, except in the event of an acute overseas emergency.

At a Conference of Ministers held in Paris from 20 to 23 Oct. 1954 these decisions were embodied in 4 Protocols modifying the Brussels Treaty which were signed in Paris on 23 Oct. 1954 and came into force on 6 May 1955.

At a meeting of the Foreign and Defence Ministers of WEU members held in Rome on 26–27 Oct. 1984, the Council adopted the 'Rome Declaration' and a document on institutional reform. Member Governments support the reactivation of the Organization as a means of strengthening the European contribution to the North Atlantic Alliance and improving defence co-operation among the countries of Western Europe.

Since the 1984 reforms, the WEU *Council of Ministers* (Foreign and Defence) meets twice a year in the capital of the presiding country. The presidency rotates annually. The *Permanent Council*, which consists of the member states' ambassadors to the UK and an official of the UK Foreign and Commonwealth Office, meets regularly at the seat of the Secretariat-General. The WEU *Assembly* in Paris comprises 108 parliamentarians of the member states and meets twice a year.

On 14 Nov. 1988, Spain and Portugal became members.

In Feb. 1991 the member nations were: Belgium, France, Germany, Italy, Luxembourg, the Netherlands, Portugal, Spain and the UK.

Secretariat-General: 9 Grosvenor Place, London, SW1X 7HL.

Secretary-General: Willem van Eekelen.

COUNCIL OF EUROPE

In 1948 the 'Congress of Europe', bringing together at The Hague nearly 1,000 influential Europeans from 26 countries, called for the creation of a united Europe, including a European Assembly. This proposal, examined first by the Ministerial Council of the Brussels Treaty Organization, then by a conference of ambassadors, was at the origin of the Council of Europe, which is, with its 25 member States, the widest organization bringing together all European democracies. The Statute of the Council was signed at London on 5 May 1949 and came into force 2 months later. The founder members were Belgium, Denmark, France, Ireland, Italy, Luxembourg, the Netherlands, Norway, Sweden and the UK. Turkey and Greece joined in 1949, Iceland in 1950, the Federal Republic of Germany in 1951 (having been an associate since 1950), Austria in 1956, Cyprus in 1961, Switzerland in 1963, Malta in 1965, Portugal in 1976, Spain in 1977, Liechtenstein in 1978, San Marino in 1988, Finland in 1989, Hungary in 1990 and Czechoslovakia in 1991.

Membership is limited to European States which 'accept the principles of the rule of law and of the enjoyment by all persons within [their] jurisdiction of human rights and fundamental freedoms'. The Statute provides for both withdrawal (Art. 7) and suspension (Arts. 8 and 9). Greece withdrew from the Council in Dec. 1969 and rejoined in Nov. 1974.

Structure. Under the Statute two organs were set up: An inter-governmental *Committee of* [*Foreign*] *Ministers* with powers of decision and of recommendation to governments, and an inter-parliamentary deliberative body, the *Parliamentary Assembly* (referred to in the Statute as the *Consultative Assembly*)—both of which are served by the Secretariat. In addition, a large number of committees of experts have been established, two of them, the Council for Cultural Co-operation and the Committee on Legal Co-operation, having a measure of autonomy; on municipal matters the Committee of Ministers receives recommendations from the Standing Conference of Local and Regional Authorities of Europe.

The Committee of Ministers meets usually twice a year, their deputies 12 times a year.

The Parliamentary Assembly normally consists of 184 parliamentarians elected or appointed by their national parliaments (Austria 6, Belgium 7, Cyprus 3, Denmark 5, Finland 5, France 18, Federal Republic of Germany 18, Greece 7, Hungary 7, Iceland 3, Ireland 4, Italy 18, Liechtenstein 2, Luxembourg 3, Malta 3, Netherlands 7, Norway 5, Portugal 7, San Marino 2, Spain 12, Sweden 6, Switzerland 6, Turkey 12, UK 18); it meets 3 times a year for approximately a week. The work of the Assembly is prepared by parliamentary committees. Since June 1989 representatives of Poland, the USSR and Yugoslavia have been permitted to attend as non-voting members.

The *Joint Committee* acts as an organ of co-ordination and liaison between representatives of the Committee of Ministers and members of the Parliamentary Assembly and gives members an opportunity to exchange views on matters of important European interest.

The European Convention on Human Rights, signed in 1950, set up special machinery to guarantee internationally fundamental rights and freedoms. The *European Commission of Human Rights* investigates alleged violations of the Convention submitted to it either by States or, in most cases, by individuals. Its findings can then be examined by the *European Court on Human Rights* (set up in 1959), whose obligatory jurisdiction has been recognized by 23 States, or by the Committee of Ministers, empowered to take binding decisions by two-thirds majority vote.

The Social Development Fund, formerly the Resettlement Fund was created in 1956. The main purpose of the Fund is to give financial aid, particularly in the spheres of housing, vocational training, regional planning and development. Since 1956 the Fund has granted loans totalling ECU 7,000m.

In 1970 the Council set up a European Youth Centre at Strasbourg, where young people can discuss their own approach to international co-operation. More recently, a European Youth Foundation was created, and which provides money to subsidize activities by European Youth Organizations in their own countries.

Aims and Achievements. Art. 1 of the Statute states that the Council's aim is 'to achieve a greater unity between its members for the purpose of safeguarding and realising the ideals and principles which are their common heritage and facilitating their economic and social progress'; 'this aim shall be pursued. . . by discussion of questions of common concern and by agreements and common action'. The only limitation is provided by Art. 1 *(d)*, which excludes 'matters relating to national defence'.

Although without legislative powers, the Assembly acts as the power-house of the Council, initiating European action in key areas by making recommendations to the Committee of Ministers. As the widest parliamentary forum in Western Europe, the Assembly also acts as the conscience of the area by voicing its opinions on important current issues. These are embodied in resolutions. The Ministers' rôle is to translate the Assembly's recommendations into action, particularly as regards lowering the barriers between the European countries, harmonizing their legislation or introducing where possible common European laws, abolishing discrimination on grounds of nationality and undertaking certain tasks on a joint European basis.

In May 1976 the first plan of intergovernmental co-operation to be undertaken by the Council of Europe was adopted by the Committee of Ministers. The third one, adopted in Nov. 1986, will run until Dec. 1991. The plan takes account of political developments and progress achieved, and covers 9 key areas: Human rights, the media, social and socio-economic questions, education, culture and sport, youth, public health, heritage and environment, local and regional government, and legal co-operation.

Some 137 Conventions and Agreements have been concluded covering such matters as social security, cultural affairs, conservation of European wild life and natural habitats, protection of archaeological heritage, extradition, medical treatment, equivalence of degrees and diplomas, the protection of television broadcasts, adoption of children and transportation of animals. Treaties in the legal field include the adoption of the European Convention on the Suppression of Terrorism, the European Convention on the Legal Status of Migrant Workers and the Transfer of Sentenced Persons. The Committee of Ministers adopted a European Convention for the protection of individuals with regard to the automatic processing of personal data (1981), a Convention on the compensation of victims of violent crimes (1983), a Convention on spectator violence and misbehaviour at sport events and in particular at football matches (1985), the European Charter of Local Government (1985), and a Convention for the Prevention of Torture and Inhuman or Degrading Treatment or Punishment (1987). The European Social Charter of 1965 sets out the social and economic rights which all member governments agree to guarantee to their citizens.

The official languages are English and French.

Chairman of the Committee of Ministers: (held in rotation).
President of the Parliamentary Assembly: Anders Bjorck (Sweden).
President of the European Court on Human Rights: Rolv Ryssdal (Norway).
President of the European Commission of Human Rights: Carl Aage Nørgaard (Denmark).
Secretary-General: Catherine Lalumière.
Headquarters: Palais de l'Europe, 67006, Strasbourg, Cedex, France.
Flag: Blue with a ring of 12 gold stars in the centre.

Further Reading

The Information Department, Council of Europe, BP 431, R6-67006 Strasbourg-Cedex.
European Yearbook. The Hague, from 1955
Forum. Strasbourg, from 1978, 4 times a year
Yearbook on the Convention on Human Rights. Strasbourg, from 1958
Cook, C. and Paxton, J., *European Political Facts, 1918–84.* London, 1986

EUROPEAN COMMUNITIES

In May 1950 Belgium, France, the Federal Republic of Germany, Italy, Luxembourg and the Netherlands started negotiations with the aim of ensuring continual peace by a merging of their essential interests. The negotiations culminated in the signing in 1951 of the Treaty of Paris creating the European Coal and Steel Community (ECSC). Two more communities with the aims of gradually integrating the economies of the 6 nations and of moving towards closer political unity, the European Economic Community (EEC) and the European Atomic Energy Community (EAEC or Euratom) were created in 1957 by the signing of the Treaties of Rome.

On 30 June 1970 membership negotiations began between the Six and the UK, Denmark, Ireland and Norway. On 22 Jan. 1972 those 4 countries signed a Treaty of Accession, although this was rejected by Norway in a referendum in Nov. 1972. On 1 Jan. 1973 the UK, Denmark and Ireland became full members. Greece joined the Community on 1 Jan. 1981; Spain and Portugal on 1 Jan. 1986, although Community legislation will only apply to them entirely after a transitional period. In Dec. 1985 the Treaties were amended again by the Single Act of Luxembourg. Turkey applied for membership in April 1987, but is unlikely to be accepted in the near future. The territory of the former German Democratic Republic entered into full membership on re-unification with Federal Germany in Oct. 1990. Malta formally applied for membership in July 1990 and an application from Cyprus is in prospect. In Dec. 1990 the Swedish parliament voted to apply for membership; a formal application would follow in 1991. The membership of Austria has been put in question by its commitment under the 1955 State Treaty to permanent neutrality, but it made a formal application early in 1990. Hungary has expressed a desire for associate membership.

Greenland exercised its autonomy under the Danish Crown to secede in 1985.

The institutional arrangements of the Communities provide an independent executive with powers of proposal (the Commission), various consultative bodies, and a decision-making body drawn from the Governments (the Council). Until 1967 the 3 Communities were completely distinct, although they shared some nondecision-making bodies: From that date the executives were merged in the European Commission, and the decision-taking bodies in the Council. The institutions and organs of the Communities are as follows:

The *Commission* consists of 17 members appointed by the member states to serve for 4 years. The Commission acts independently of any country in the interests of the Community as a whole, with as its mandate the implementation and guardianship of the Treaties. In this it has the right of initiative (putting proposals to the Council for action); and execution (once the Council has decided); and can take the other institutions or individual countries before the Court of Justice (see below) should any of these renege upon its responsibilities. The Commission operates through 23 Directorates-General.

Flag: Blue with a ring of 12 gold stars.
President: Jacques Delors.
Address: 200 rue de la Loi, 1049, Brussels, Belgium.

The *Council of Ministers* consists of foreign ministers from the 12 national governments and represents the national as opposed to the Community interests. It is the body which takes decisions under the Treaties. Since the adoption of the Single Act of Luxembourg, an increasing number of its decisions are taken by majority vote, though some areas (e.g. taxation) are still reserved to unanimity. Specialist Councils (e.g. the *Agriculture Council*) meet to discuss matters related to individual policies. The Single Act also formalizes the meetings of Heads of State and Government in the *European Council*, which meets 3 times a year; and of Foreign Ministers in *Political Co-operation*, to discuss co-operation outside the framework of the Treaties. The Presidency of the Council is held for a 6-month term in the following order: Belgium, Denmark, Federal Republic of Germany, Greece, Spain, France, Ireland, Italy, Luxembourg, Netherlands, Portugal, UK.

Address: 170 rue de la Loi, 1048, Brussels.

The *European Parliament* consists of 518 members, directly elected from all Member States. France, Germany, Italy and the UK return 81 members each, Spain 60, the Netherlands 25, Belgium, Greece and Portugal 24, Denmark 16, Ireland 15 and Luxembourg 6. Party representation in Parliament was as follows: Socialists, 180; European People's Party (Christian Democratic Group), 121; Liberal, Democratic and Reform Group 49; European Democrats (formerly European Conservatives), 34; Greens, 29; European United Left, 28; European Democratic Alliance, 22; the European Right, 17; the 'Rainbow' group (a group of mixed tendencies), 14; Left Unity, 14; Independents, 10. The Parliament has a right to be consulted on a wide range of legislative proposals, and forms one arm of the Community's Budgetary Authority. Since the Single Act it has an increased role in legislation, through the 'concertation' procedure, under which it can reject certain Council drafts in a second reading procedure. Elections were held in June 1989 for a 5-year mandate.

President: Baron Crespo.
Address: Centre européen du Kirchberg, Luxembourg.

Lodge, J. (ed.) *The 1989 Election of the European Parliament.* London, 1990

The *Economic and Social Committee* has an advisory role and consists of 189 representatives, employers, trade unions, consumers, etc. The *Consultative Committee*, of 96 members, performs a similar role for the ECSC.

President: François Staedelin.
Address: 2, rue Ravenstein, 1000 Brussels.

The *European Court of Justice* is composed of 13 judges and 6 advocates-general, is responsible for the adjudication of disputes arising out of the application of the treaties, and its findings are enforceable in all member countries. A Court of First Instance was created in 1989.

President: Ole Due.
Address: Palais de la Cour de Justice, Kirchberg, Luxembourg.

The *Court of Auditors* was established by a Treaty signed on 22 July 1975 which took effect on 1 June 1977. It consists of 12 members, and replaced the former *Audit Board*. It audits all income and current and past expenditure of the European Communities.

President: Aldo Angioi.
Address: 29 Rue Aldringen, Luxembourg.

Annual Report of the Court of Auditors, from 1977

The *European Investment Bank* (EIB) was created by the EEC Treaty to which its statute is annexed. Its governing body is the Board of Governors consisting of ministers designated by member states. Its main task is to contribute to the balanced development of the common market in the interest of the Community by financing projects: Developing less-developed regions; for modernizing or converting undertakings; or developing new activities.

Governor: Günter Bröder.
Address: 100, Boulevard Konrad Adenauer, Plateau du Kirchberg, Luxembourg.

Annual Report of the European Investment Bank

Community Law. Provisions of the Treaties and secondary legislation may be either directly applicable in Member States or only applicable after Member States have enacted their own implementing legislation. Secondary legislation consists of: Regulations, which are of general application and binding in their entirety and directly applicable in all member states; directives which are binding upon each Member State as to the result to be achieved within a given time, but leave the national authority the choice of form and method of achieving this result; decisions, which are binding in their entirety on their addressees. In addition the Council and Commission can issue recommendations and opinions, which have no binding force.

The Community's Legislative Process starts with a proposal from the Commission (either at the suggestion of its services or in pursuit of its declared political aims) to the Council. The Council generally seeks the views of the European Parliament on the proposal, and the Parliament adopts a formal Opinion, after consideration of the matter by its specialist Committees. The Council may also (and in some cases is obliged to) consult the Economic and Social Committee, which similarly delivers an opinion. When these opinions have been received, the Council will decide. Most decisions are taken on a majority basis, but will take account of reserves expressed by individual member states. The text eventually approved may differ substantially from the original Commission proposal.

Community Finances. Revenue for financial years in ECU1m.:

	1989	*1990*	*1991*
Own resources	41,881	42,160	53,237
Surpluses	1,162	3,645	1,371
Miscellaneous Community taxes, levies and dues	226,293	248,633	265,515
Administrative operation of the institutions	69,970	32,720	40,269
Total	45,900	46,928	55,556

Expenditure for 1991 was ECU55,556m.

The resources of the Community (the levies and duties mentioned above, and up to a 1·4% VAT charge) have been surrendered to it by Treaty. The Budget is made by the Council and the Parliament acting jointly as the Budgetary Authority. The Parliament has control, within a certain margin, of non-obligatory expenditure (*i.e.*, expenditure where the amount to be spent is not set out in the legislation concerned), and can also reject the Budget. Otherwise, the Council decides. ECSC operations are partly funded by a turnover levy (1988: 0·31%) on the coal and steel industries of the Community, partly from the general budget. The ECSC operating budget for 1988 was ECU432m.

THE EUROPEAN COAL AND STEEL COMMUNITY. The ECSC was the first of the 3 Communities, coming into existence on 10 Aug. 1952 following the signature of the Treaty of Paris on 18 April 1951. Its aim was to contribute towards economic expansion, growth of employment and a rising standard of living in Member States, through common action in the coal and steel sector, in a Community open to other nations. Since 1957 it has had the same membership as the other Communities.

THE EUROPEAN ECONOMIC COMMUNITY (EEC) or COMMON MARKET

Based on the Treaty of Rome of 25 March 1957 the EEC came into being on 1 Jan. 1958 with the same original members as the ECSC. The Treaty guarantees certain rights to the citizens of all Member States (*e.g.*, the outlawing of economic discrimination by nationality, and equal pay for equal work as between men and women) and sets out certain other areas where secondary legislation is to fill in the details. The most important policy areas are as follows:

Freedom of movement for persons, goods and capital. Under the Treaty individuals or companies from one Member State may establish themselves in another country (for the purposes of economic activity) or sell goods or services there on the same basis as nationals of that country. With a few exceptions, restrictions on the movement of capital have also been ended. Under the Single Act the Member States bound themselves to achieve the suppression of all barriers to free movement of persons, goods and services by 31 Dec. 1992.

Customs Union and External Trade Relations. Goods or Services originating in one Member State have free circulation within the EEC, which implies common arrangements for trade with the rest of the world. Member States can no longer make bilateral trade agreements with third countries: This power has been ceded to the Community. The Customs Union was achieved in July 1968, with the abolition of internal customs tariffs (or equivalents) and quantitative restrictions, and the establishment of the Common External Tariff. Denmark, Ireland and the UK adopted these from July 1977; Greece from Jan. 1986.

Following the 1973 accessions the Community made a series of agreements with the member states of EFTA to form an industrial free trade zone and to start the liberalization of agricultural trade. A new impetutus was given by the 1984 Luxembourg agreement, and the EFTA countries are now seeking to co-operate in the achievement of the Internal Market. Association agreements which could lead to accession or customs union have been made with Cyprus, Malta and Turkey; and commercial, industrial, technical and financial aid agreements with Algeria, Egypt, Israel, Jordan, Lebanon, Morocco, Syria, Tunisia and Yugoslavia. In 1976 Canada signed a framework agreement for co-operation in industrial trade, science and natural resources. Co-operation agreements also exist with a number of Latin American countries and groupings (e.g. the Andean Group) and with Arab and Asian countries; and an economic and commercial agreement has been signed with ASEAN.

In the *Development Aid* sector, the Community has an agreement (the Lomé Convention, originally signed in 1975 but renewed and enlarged in 1979 and 1984) with some 60 African, Caribbean and Pacific countries which removes customs duties without reciprocal arrangements for most of their imports to the Community, and under which ECU8,760m. of aid was granted between 1986–90. An economic and commercial agreement has also been signed with ASEAN.

The Common Agricultural Policy (CAP). The objectives set out in the Treaty are to increase agricultural productivity, to ensure a fair standard of living for the agricultural community, to stabilise markets, to assure supplies, and to ensure reasonable consumer prices. In Dec. 1960 the Council laid down the fundamental principles on which the CAP is based: A single market, which calls for common prices, stable currency parities and the harmonising of health and veterinary legislation; Community preference, which protects the single Community market from imports; common financing, through the European Agricultural Guidance and Guarantee Fund (EAGGF), which seeks to improve agriculture through its Guidance section, and to stabilise markets against world price fluctuations through market intervention, with levies and refunds on exports. At present common market organizations cover over 95% of EEC agricultural production. Greece is bringing its agricultural prices into line with the Community over a period of up to 7 years.

Following the disappearance of stable currency parities, artificial currency levels have been applied in the CAP. This factor, together with over-production due to high producer prices, means that the CAP consumes about two-thirds of the Communities' budget. In Jan. 1991 the European Commission began discussion of plans to reform the CAP.

The European Monetary System (EMS). Founded in March 1979 to control inflation, protect European trade from international disturbances and ultimately promote convergence between the European economies. The *Exchange Rate Mechanism (ERM)* is run by the finance ministries and central banks of the EC countries on a day-to-day basis; monthly reviews are carried out by the EC Monetary Committee (finance ministries) and the EC Committee of Central Bankers. All EC countries are members of EMS, but only Belgium, Denmark, France, Germany, Italy, Luxembourg, the Netherlands, Spain and the UK are in the ERM. Members are obliged to restrict the fluctuations in the value of their currencies to a variation 'band', usually of 2·25% (though this may be widened to 6% on a country's initial joining) higher or lower than a central rate established by comparing all the currencies in the ERM and the European Currency Unit, the Ecu (XEU). If a currency reaches its top or bottom limits, central banks are obliged to buy or sell currency on the foreign exchanges. Further stabilization measures would involve adjustment of national interest rates, central bank borrowing from other central banks or withdrawal of reserves from the European Monetary Co-operation Fund. The adjustment of last resort is re- or devaluation.

Dod's European Companion. Hurst Green, East Sussex, 1990

Competition. The Competition (anti-trust) law of the Community is based on 2 principles: That businesses should not seek to nullify the creation of the common market by the erection of artificial national (or other) barriers to the free movement of goods; and against the abuse of dominant positions in any market. These two principles have led among other things to the outlawing of prohibitions on exports to other Member States, of price-fixing agreements and of refusal to supply; and to the refusal by the Commission to allow mergers or take-overs by dominant undertakings in specific cases. Increasingly heavy fines are imposed on offenders.

THE EUROPEAN ATOMIC ENERGY COMMUNITY (EURATOM)

Like the EEC, Euratom came into being on 1 Jan. 1958 following a Treaty signed in Rome on 25 March 1957, and it had the same Member States as the EEC. Its task is to promote common efforts between its members in the development of nuclear energy for peaceful purposes, and for this purpose it has monopoly powers of acquisition of fissile materials for civil purposes. It is in no way concerned with military uses of nuclear power.

The execution of the Treaty now rests with the European Commission, which is advised by the Scientific and Technical Committee (28 members). Major decisions rest with the Council. Euratom has 1 substantial research institute of its own, at Ispra, in Italy; it does other work in co-operation with research institutes in the Member States, or in joint and international undertakings.

A common market for nuclear materials and equipment came into force, and external tariffs were suspended, in Jan. 1959.

European Community Delegation to the US: 2111 M Street NW (Suite 707), Washington DC 20037.
Head of Delegation: Andreas van Agt.
US Delegation to the European Community: 40 Boulevard du Régent, 1000 Brussels.
Head of Delegation: Thomas M. T. Niles.
European Community Delegation to the United Nations: 1 Dag Hammarskjöld Plaza, 245 East 47th Street, New York NY 10017.
Head of Delegation: Jean-Pierre Derisbourg.

Further Reading

Official Journal of the European Communities.—General Report on the Activities of the European Communities (annual, from 1967).—*The Agricultural Situation in the Community.* (annual).—*The Social Situation in the Community.* (annual).—*Report on Competition Policy in the European Community.* (annual).—*Basic Statistics of the Community* (annual).— *Bulletin of the European Community* (monthly).—*Register of Current Community Legal Instruments.* 1983
Europe (monthly), obtainable from the Information Office of the European Commission, 8 Storey's Gate, London, SW1P 3AT
Arbuthnott, H. and Edwards, G. (eds.) *A Common Man's Guide to the Common Market.* London, 1979
Cook, C. and Francis, M., *The First European Elections.* London, 1979
Drew, J., *Doing Business with the European Community.* London, 1979
Fennell, R., *The Common Agricultural Policy of the European Community.* London, 1979
Fitzmaurice, J., *The European Parliament.* London, 1982
Hallstein, W., *Europe in the Making.* London, 1973
Lodge, J., *The European Community: Bibliographical Excursions.* London, 1983
Mayne, R., *Postwar Europe.* London, 1983
Morris, B. *and Boehm, K., The European Community: A Practical Directory and Guide for Business, Industry and Trade.* London, 2nd ed. 1986
Palmer, D. M., *Sources of Information on the European Communities.* London, 1979
Parry, A. and Dinnage, J., *EEC Law.* London, 1982
Paxton, J., *The Developing Common Market.* London, 1976.—*A Dictionary of the European Communities.* 2nd ed. London, 1982
Twitchett, C. C., *Harmonisation in the EEC.* London, 1981
Wallace, W. and Herreman, I. (eds.) *A Community of Twelve?* Bruges, 1978
Walsh, A. E. and Paxton, J., *Competition Policy.* London, 1975

EUROPEAN FREE TRADE ASSOCIATION (EFTA)

The European Free Trade Association has 6 member countries: Austria, Finland (an associate member from 1961–1985), Iceland, Norway, Sweden and Switzerland. The Stockholm Convention establishing the Association entered into force on 3 May 1960 and Finland became associated on 27 March 1961. Iceland joined EFTA on 1 March 1970 and was immediately granted duty-free entry for industrial goods exported to EFTA countries, while being given 10 years to abolish her own existing protective duties. The UK and Denmark, both founder members, left EFTA on 31 Dec. 1972 to join the EEC as did Portugal, also a founder member, on 31 Dec. 1985.

When the Association was created it had three objectives: To achieve free trade in industrial products between member countries, to assist in the creation of a single market embracing the countries of Western Europe, and to contribute to the expansion of world trade in general.

The first objective was achieved on 31 Dec. 1966, when virtually all inter-EFTA tariffs were removed. This was 3 years earlier than originally planned. Finland removed her remaining EFTA tariffs a year later on 31 Dec. 1967 and Iceland removed her tariffs on 31 Dec. 1979.

The fulfilment of the second aim was secured in 1972. On 22 Jan. 1972 the UK and Denmark signed the Treaty of Accession to the EEC whereby they became members of the enlarged Community from 1 Jan. 1973. On 22 July 1972, 5 other EFTA countries, Austria, Iceland, Portugal, Sweden and Switzerland signed Free Trade Agreements with the enlarged EEC. A similar agreement negotiated with Finland was signed on 5 Oct. 1973. Norway, whose intention of joining the EEC was reversed following a referendum, signed a similar agreement on 14 May 1973. The agreements now also apply to trade between the EFTA countries and the 3 countries which joined the EC at later dates: Greece (1 Jan. 1981) and Spain and Portugal (1 Jan. 1986). The Luxembourg Declaration of April 1984 which followed the final abolition of tariffs on EFTA-EC trade in industrial goods set out the guidelines for strengthening and developing EFTA-EC co-operation, with the aim of creating the European Economic Area (EEA) comprising all the countries in the European free trade system. Since 1989 the main preoccupation of EFTA has been to work for a more structured partnership with the EC. The aim is to have an EEA treaty enter into force by 1 Jan. 1993, to coincide with the completion of the EC's internal market.

The third objective was to contribute to the expansion of world trade. In 1959 trade between the countries now in EFTA amounted to US$705·6m. and total exports from these countries were US$6,562m. In 1989 the respective figures were US$25,890m. and US$187,339m. More than half EFTA trade is with the EC.

EFTA tariff treatment applies to those industrial products which are of EFTA origin, and these are traded freely between member countries. Each EFTA country remains free, however, to impose its own rates of duty on products entering from outside either EFTA or the EC.

Generally, agricultural products do not come under the provisions for free trade, but bilateral agreements have been negotiated to increase trade in these products.

The operation of the Convention is the responsibility of a Council assisted by a small secretariat. Each EFTA country holds the chairmanship of the Council for 6 months.

Secretary-General: Georg Reisch (Austria).

Headquarters: 9–11 rue de Varembé, 1211 Geneva 20, Switzerland.

Brussels Office: 118 rue d'Arlon, B-1040, Brussels.

Convention Establishing the European Free Trade Association
EFTA Bulletin (Four issues a year)
EFTA What it is, What it does
The European Free Trade Association

CONFERENCE ON SECURITY AND CO-OPERATION IN EUROPE (CSCE)

Initiatives from both NATO and the Warsaw Pact culminated in the first summit CSCE of heads of state and government in Helsinki on 30 July–1 Aug. 1975, which adopted a 'Final Act' laying down 10 principles concerning human rights, self-determination and the inter-relations of the participant states. Conferences followed in Belgrade (1977–78), Madrid (1980–83), Stockholm (1984–86) and Vienna (1986–89). At the Paris summit of 19–21 Nov. 1990 the members of NATO and the Warsaw Pact signed a Treaty on the Reduction of Conventional Forces in Europe (CFE) and a declaration that they are 'no longer adversaries' and do not intend to 'use force against the territorial integrity or political independence of any state'. All the 34 participants adopted the Confidence and Security-Building Measures (CSBMs), which pertain to the exchange of military information, verification of military installations, objection to unusual military activities etc., and signed the Charter of Paris.

The signatories of the Charter comprised the USA, Canada and all the sovereign states of Europe (except Albania, which had observer status), viz., Austria, Belgium, Bulgaria, Cyprus, Czechoslovakia, Denmark, Finland, France, Germany,

Greece, Hungary, Iceland, Ireland, Italy, Liechtenstein, Luxembourg, Malta, Monaco, the Netherlands, Norway, Poland, Portugal, Romania, San Marino, Spain, Sweden, Switzerland, Turkey, USSR, UK, Vatican and Yugoslavia.

The Charter sets out principles of human rights, democracy and the rule of law to which all the signatories undertake to adhere, lays down the bases for east-west co-operation and other future action, and institutionalizes the CSCE, establishing a *Secretariat* in Prague, a *Conflict Prevention Centre* in Vienna and an *Election Observation Office* in Warsaw. An 'Assembly of Europe' is also envisaged made up of representatives from national parliaments and meeting at the Council of Europe Assembly in Strasbourg. The foreign minsiters of the signatories will meet at least once a year, and the heads of state or government every 2 years, starting in 1992.

THE WARSAW PACT

On 14 May 1955 the USSR, Albania, Bulgaria, Czechoslovakia, the German Democratic Republic, Hungary, Poland and Romania signed, in Warsaw, a 20-year treaty of friendship and collaboration, after the USSR annulled treaties of alliance with the UK and France. The treaty was extended for 10 years in July 1975 and renewed for 20 years in April 1985. After 1985 the Pact's Political Consultative Committee met annually in member countries in turn. It established a Committee of Defence Ministers (1969), a Military Council (1969), a Technical Committee (1969) and a Committee of Foreign Ministers.

The main provisions of the treaty were:

Article 4. In case of armed aggression in Europe against one or several States party to the pact by a State or group of States, each State member of the pact. . . will afford to the State or States which are the object of such aggression immediate assistance. . . with all means which appear necessary, including the use of armed force. . . These measures will cease as soon as the Security Council takes measures necessary for establishing and preserving international peace and security.

Article 5. The contracting Powers agree to set up a joint command of their armed forces to be allotted by agreement between the Powers, at the disposal of this command and used on the basis of jointly established principles. They will also take over agreed measures necessary to strengthen their defences.

Article 9. The present treaty is open to other States, irrespective of their social or Government regime, who declare their readiness to abide by the terms of the treaty in order to safeguard peace and security of the peoples.

Article 11. In the event of a system of collective security being set up in Europe and a pact to this effect being signed—to which each party to this treaty will direct its efforts—the present treaty will lapse from the day such a collective security treaty comes into force.

In a document signed on 25 Feb. 1991 Bulgaria, Czechoslovakia, Hungary, Poland, Romania and the USSR (the remaining original signatories, Albania having left the Pact in 1968, and the German Democratic Republic having been reunified with the Federal Republic of Germany in 1990) agreed to dismantle all 'military organs, institutions and activities' by 31 March 1991. Pending final dissolution, the Pact's political structure has been transformed into a voluntary consultative body. A joint communiqué declared that the 'legacy of confrontation and a divided Europe is now over', and all future security issues would reflect each sovereign nation's 'freedom of choice'.

Further Reading

Fodor, N., *The Warsaw Treaty Organization: a Political and Organizational Analysis*. London, 1990

Sword, K. (ed.) *The Times Guide to Eastern Europe: the Changing Face of the Warsaw Pact – a Comprehensive Handbook*. London, 1990

ORGANIZATION FOR INTERNATIONAL ECONOMIC CO-OPERATION (OIEC)

The Council for Mutual Economic Assistance (COMECON, CMEA) was established in Jan. 1949 on a Soviet initiative with Bulgaria, Czechoslovakia, Hungary, Poland and Romania as the other founder members. The German Democratic Republic, Mongolia, Cuba and Vietman joined later, and Yugoslavia had associate status. Its ostensible purpose was to create a common market amongst its members and promote the co-ordination and integration of their economies. For an account of its charter, structure and subordinate institutions *see* THE STATESMAN'S YEAR-BOOK, 1990–91, pp. 48–50. With the transition of its members from command to market economies, and the commencement of their mutual trade in convertible currency from 1 Jan. 1991, COMECON lost its raison d'être as constituted, and in 1991 its Executive Committee agreed a statute for a successor organization named the 'Organization for International Economic Co-operation'. This has largely an advisory and consultative role though it will deal with questions of residual tariffs and quotas, and the development of relations with other organizations, including the EEC. Membership is open to the countries of Europe, Cuba, Mongolia and Vietnam. Members are committed to market principles and integration into the world economy. A much-reduced secretariat and a meeting of representatives of members' governments constitute the only formal structure. Initial funding was 6·8m. rubles.

The headquarters of COMECON were: Prospekt Kalinina, 56, Moscow G-205.

Associated with it were:

The **International Bank for Economic Co-operation** was founded in 1963 with a capital of 300m. transferable roubles (i.e., used for intra-CMEA clearing accounts only) and started operating on 1 Jan. 1964. It undertakes multilateral settlements and advances credits to finance trading and other operations.

The **International Investments Bank** was founded in 1970 and went into operation on 1 Jan. 1971 with a capital of 1,071m. transferable roubles.

Economic relations. Trading accounts between members of COMECON were settled in 'transferable roubles', but a decision to proceed towards currency convertibility was taken at the 1987 Council, and since 1 Jan. 1991 members have been trading in convertible currency at world prices.

EUROPEAN BANK FOR RECONSTRUCTION AND DEVELOPMENT (EBRD, BERD)

History and Membership. A treaty to establish the EBRD was signed May 1990; it was inaugurated on 15 April 1991. It has 41 original members: the European Commission, the European Investment Bank, all the EEC countries and all the countries of East Europe except Albania.

Its founding capital was of ecu 10m., of which the USA contributed 10%, the UK, France, Germany, Italy, Japan 8·5% each, and the USSR 6%.

Objectives. It was set up to lend funds at market rates to East European companies and countries 'which are committed to, and applying, the principles of multi-party democracy and market economics'. The USSR will be eligible for lending, but for an initial 3-year period only up to the amount of its capital, and for private projects.

The *Board* has 23 seats.

Headquarters: London.

President: Jacques Attali.

General Secretary: Bart le Blanc.

COLOMBO PLAN

History: Founded in 1950 to promote the development of newly independent Asian member countries, the Colombo Plan has grown from its modest beginning as a group of seven Commonwealth nations into an international organization of 26 countries.

Originally the Plan was conceived for a period of six years. Its life has since been extended from time to time, generally at five-year intervals. The Consultative Committee, the Plan's highest deliberative body, at its meeting in Jakarta in 1980, gave the Plan an indefinite span of life; its need and relevance will henceforth be examined only if considered necessary.

The Plan is multilateral in approach but bilateral in operation: Multilateral in that it takes cognizance of the problems of development of member countries in the Asia and Pacific region and endeavours to deal with them in a co-ordinated way; bilateral because negotiations for assistance are made direct between a donor and a recipient country.

Aims: The aims of the Colombo Plan are: *(a)* to promote interest in and support for the economic and social development in Asia and the Pacific; *(b)* to keep under review economic and social progress in the region and help accelerate development through co-operative effort; and *(c)* to facilitate development assistance to and within the region.

Member Countries: Afghanistan, Australia, Bangladesh, Bhután, Burma, Cambodia, Canada, Fiji, India, Indonesia, Iran, Japan, Republic of Korea, Lao People's Democratic Republic, Malaysia, Maldives, Nepál, New Zealand, Pakistan, Papua New Guinea, Philippines, Singapore, Sri Lanka, Thailand, UK and USA.

Development Assistance: Colombo Plan aid covers all fields of socio-economic development and amounted to US$6,729·3m. in 1988. It takes three principal forms:

(i) *Capital Aid* including grants and loans for national projects mainly from the six developed member countries of the Plan.
The total amount of capital aid and technical co-operation assistance provided by the developed donors under the plan in 1986 was as follows:

	US$1m.
Japan	4,404·1
USA	1,035·4
Australia	461·3
Canada	420·0
UK	399·0
New Zealand	9·5
Total	6,729·3

(ii) *Technical Co-operation:* Assistance is provided in the form of services of experts and volunteers, fellowships, and equipment for training and research. During 1988, 35,002 students and trainees received training, 8,226 experts and 1,615 volunteers were sent out. Total disbursements on technical co-operation by the developed member countries in 1988 amounted to $1,020·7m.

(iii) *Technical Co-operation Among Developing Countries (TCDC):* The promotion of TCDC is a major objective of the Plan. Under TCDC programmes in 1988, 2,356 students and trainees received training and 69 experts were sent out. TCDC expenditures during 1986 amounted to $9·8m.

Structure: There are four organs which give focus to the Plan:

Consultative Committee: The Committee is the highest deliberative body of the Plan and consists of Ministers of member Governments who meet once in two years. The Ministerial meeting is preceded by a meeting of senior officials who are directly concerned with the operation of the Plan in various countries.

Colombo Plan Council: The Council is also a deliberative body which meets several times a year in Colombo, where most member countries have resident diplomatic missions, to review the economic and social development of the Asia-Pacific region and promote co-operation among member countries.

Colombo Plan Bureau: Its functions include servicing the meetings of the Colombo Plan Council and the Consultative Committee, carrying out research, and dissemination of statistical and other information relating to activities under the Plan. Since 1973 the Bureau has been operating a Drug Advisory Programme to assist national and regional efforts to eliminate the causes and ameliorate the effects of drug abuse.

Colombo Plan Staff College: The Colombo Plan Staff College for Technician Education, established in 1975, transferred from Singapore to the Philippines in 1987. The College helps member countries in developing their systems of technician education, mainly through training courses, seminars and consultancies. It is separately financed by most Colombo Plan member countries and functions under the guidance of its own Governing Board consisting of the heads of member countries' diplomatic missions resident in Singapore.

Flag: Dark blue with a central white disc containing the Colombo Plan logo in black.

Headquarters: Colombo Plan Bureau, 12 Melbourne Avenue, PO Box 596, Colombo 4, Sri Lanka.

The Colombo Plan (Cmd. 8080). HMSO, 1950; reprinted 1952.—*Annual Report.* HMSO 1952 to 1971 followed by Colombo Plan Bureau, Sri Lanka, 1971–86

Reports of the Council for Technical Co-operation. HMSO annually until 1966–67 followed by the Colombo Plan Bureau, Sri Lanka, 1967–68 to date

ASSOCIATION OF SOUTH EAST ASIAN NATIONS (ASEAN)

History and Membership. The Association of South East Asian Nations is a regional organization formed by the governments of Indonesia, Malaysia, the Philippines, Singapore and Thailand through the Bangkok Declaration which was signed by the Foreign Ministers of ASEAN countries on 8 Aug. 1967. Brunei joined in 1984.

Objectives. The main objectives are to accelerate economic growth, social progress and cultural development, to promote active collaboration and mutual assistance in matters of common interest, to ensure the stability of the South East Asian region and to maintain close co-operation with existing international and regional organizations with similar aims. Principal projects concern economic co-operation and development, with the intensification of intra-ASEAN trade and trade between the region and the rest of the world; joint research and technological programmes; co-operation in transportation and communications; promotion of tourism and South East Asian studies; including cultural, scientific, educational and administrative exchanges.

Organs. The highest authority in ASEAN are the Heads of Government of the Member Countries who meet as and when necessary to give directions to ASEAN. The highest policy-making body is the Meeting of Foreign Ministers, commonly known as the Annual Ministerial Meeting, which convenes in each of the ASEAN member countries on a rotational basis in alphabetical order. The Standing Committee, comprising the Foreign Minister of the country hosting the Ministerial Meeting in that particular year and the accredited ambassadors of the other member countries, carries out the work of the Association in between the Ministerial Meetings and handles the routine matters to ensure continuity and to make decisions based on the guidelines or policies set by the Ministerial Meetings and submit for the consideration of the Foreign Ministers all reports and recommendations of the various ASEAN committees. There are five economic committees under the ASEAN Economic Ministers and three non-economic committees that recommend and draw up programmes for ASEAN co-operation. These committees are responsible for the operation and implementation of ASEAN projects in their respective fields. Each ASEAN capital has an ASEAN National Secretariat. The central secretariat for

ASEAN is located in Jakarta, Indonesia, and is headed by the Secretary General, a post that revolves among the member states in alphabetical order every 3 years. Bureau directors and other officers of the ASEAN Secretariat remain in office for 3 years.

Secretary-General: Roderick Yong (Brunei Darussalam).

Further Reading

Broinowski, A., *Understanding ASEAN*. London, 1982;—(ed.) *ASEAN into the 1990s*. London, 1990.

Wawn, B., *The Economies of the ASEAN Countries*. London, 1982

ORGANIZATION OF AMERICAN STATES

On 14 April 1890 representatives of the American republics, meeting in Washington at the First International Conference of American States, established an 'International Union of American Republics' and, as its central office, a 'Commercial Bureau of American Republics', which later became the Pan American Union. This international organization's object was to foster mutual understanding and co-operation among the nations of the western hemisphere. Since that time, successive inter-American conferences have greatly broadened the scope of work of the organization.

This led to the adoption on 30 April 1948 by the Ninth International Conference of American States, at Bogotá, Colombia, of the Charter of the Organization of American States. This co-ordinated the work of all the former independent official entities in the inter-American system and defined their mutual relationships. The purposes of the OAS are to achieve an order of peace and justice, promote American solidarity, strengthen collaboration among the member states and defend their sovereignty, territorial integrity and independence. The OAS is a regional organization of the United Nations for the maintenance of peace and security.

Membership is on a basis of absolute equality. Each country has one vote in the Council of the Organization and its organs. The member countries were (1991): Antigua and Barbuda, Argentina, Bahamas, Barbados, Belize, Bolivia, Brazil, Canada, Chile, Colombia, Costa Rica, Cuba, Commonwealth of Dominica, Dominican Republic, Ecuador, El Salvador, Grenada, Guatemala, Haiti, Honduras, Jamaica, Mexico, Nicaragua, Panama, Paraguay, Peru, Saint Christopher (Kitts) and Nevis, Saint Lucia, Saint Vincent and the Grenadines, Suriname, Trinidad and Tobago, USA, Uruguay, Venezuela.

The OAS has been concerned increasingly in recent years with programmes to promote Latin American economic and social development. The OAS provides specialized training for thousands of Latin Americans each year in a wide variety of development-related fields. It also carries out many missions projects each year in response to requests from member governments.

Under the amended Charter, the OAS accomplishes its purposes by means of:

(a) The *General Assembly*, which meets annually in various countries of the member states.

(b) The *Meeting of Consultation of Ministers of Foreign Affairs*, held to consider problems of an urgent nature and of common interest.

(c) Three councils of equal rank: the *Permanent Council*, which replaces the old OAS Council; the *Inter-American Economic and Social Council*; and the *Inter-American Council for Education, Science and Culture*. Functions are to direct and co-ordinate work in the areas of their competence and render the governments such specialized services as they may request. Each council is composed of 1 representative from each member state, appointed by his government.

(d) The *Inter-American Juridical Committee* which acts as an advisory body to the OAS on juridical matters and promotes the development and codification of international law. Eleven jurists, elected every 4 years by the General Assembly, represent all the American States.

(e) The *Inter-American Commission on Human Rights* which oversees the obser-

vance and protection of human rights. Seven members represent all the OAS member states.

(f) The *General Secretariat* is the central and permanent organ of the OAS.

(g) The *Specialized Conferences*, meeting to deal with special technical matters or to develop specific aspects of inter-American co-operation.

(h) The *Specialized Organizations*, inter-governmental organizations established by multilateral agreements to discharge specific functions in their respective fields of action, such as women's affairs, agriculture, child welfare, Indian affairs, geography and history, and health.

Secretary General: João Clemente Baena Soares (Brazil).
Assistant Secretary-General: Christopher Thomas (Trinidad and Tobago).

The Secretary-General and the Assistant Secretary-General are elected by the General Assembly for 5-year terms. The General Assembly approves the annual budget for the Organization, which is financed by quotas contributed by the member governments.

General Secretariat: Washington, D.C., 20006, USA.
Flag: Light blue with the OAS seal in colour in the centre.

Further Reading

Publications of the OAS General Secretariat include:

Charter of the Organization of American States. 1948.—*As Amended by the Protocol of Buenos Aires in 1967 and the Protocol of Cartagena de Indias in 1985*
Americas. Illustrated bi-monthly, from 1949 (Spanish and English edition)
Organization of American States, a Handbook. Rev. ed. 1977
Organization of American States. Directory. Quarterly, from 1951
Report on the Tenth Inter-American Conference, Caracas 1954. 1955
Inter-American Review of Bibliography. Quarterly, from 1951
Annual Report of the Secretary-General
Status of Inter-American Treaties and Conventions. Annual
The Alliance for Progress: The Charter of Punta del Este. 1962
The Americas in the 1980s: An Agenda for the Decade Ahead. 1982

Publications on Latin America (*see also* the bibliographical notes appended to each country):

Revenue, Expenditure and Public Debts of the Latin American Republics. Division of Financial Information, US Department of Commerce. Annual
Boundaries of the Latin American Republics: An Annotated List of Documents, 1493–1943. Department of State, Office of the Geographer. Washington, 1944
Burgin, M. (ed.) *Handbook of Latin American Studies*. Gainesville, Fla., 1935 ff.
Hirschman, A. O., *Latin American Issues:* [11] *Essays and Comments*. New York, 1961
Plaza, G., *The Organization of American States: Instrument for Hemispheric Development*. Washington, 1969.—*Latin America Today and Tomorrow*. Washington, 1971
Steward, J. H. (ed.) *Handbook of the South American Indian*. 7 vols. Washington, 1946–59
Thomas, A. V. W. and A. J., *The Organization of American States*. Southern Methodist Univ. Press, 1963

LATIN AMERICAN ECONOMIC GROUPINGS

Latin American Integration Association (LAIA) /*Asociación Latinoamericana de Integración* (ALADI). The Association took over from the Latin American Free Trade Area (LAFTA) on 1 Jan. 1981 which was created in 1960 to further trade between the member states and promote regional integration. Members: Argentina, Bolivia, Brazil, Chile, Colombia, Ecuador, Mexico, Paraguay, Peru, Uruguay and Venezuela.

Headquarters: Cebollati 1461, Casilla 577, Montevideo, Uruguay.

Síntesis ALADI (monthly, Spanish)
Newsletter (six issues a year, Spanish)

Central American Common Market (CACM) /*Mercado Común Centroamericano*. In Dec. 1960 El Salvador, Guatemala, Honduras and Nicaragua concluded the General Treaty of Central American Economic Integration *(Tratado General de Integración Económica Centroamericana)* under the auspices of the Organization of Central American States (ODECA) in Managua. Costa Rica acceded in 1962. Members: Costa Rica, El Salvador, Guatemala, Honduras and Nicaragua.

Headquarters: 4a Avda 10–25, Zona 14, Apdo 1237, Guatemala City, Guatemala.

Carta Informativa (monthly)
Anuario Estadística Centroamericano de Comercio Exterior (annual)

The Andean Group (Grupo Andino). On 26 May 1969 an agreement was signed by Bolivia, Chile, Colombia, Ecuador and Peru creating the Andean Group. Venezuela was initially actively involved but did not sign the agreement until 1973. Chile withdrew from the Group in 1977. Members: Bolivia, Colombia, Ecuador, Peru and Venezuela.

Headquarters: Avda Paseo de la Republica 3895, Casilla 18–1177, Lima 27, Peru.

Latin American Economic System/Sistema Económico Latinoamericano (SELA). SELA was created by 25 Latin American and Caribbean countries (Suriname joined in 1979) meeting in Panama, 17 Oct. 1975. The System provides member countries with permanent institutional machinery for joint consultation, coordination, co-operation and promotion in economic and social matters at both intraregional and extraregional levels.

Headquarters: Apdo 17035, El Conde, Caracas 1010, Venezuela.

Latin American Association of Development Financing Institutions/Asociación Latinoamericana de Instituciones Financieros de Desarrollo (ALIDE). Founded in 1968 to promote co-operation among regional development financing organizations.

Headquarters: Paseo de la Republica 3211, POB 3988, Lima, Peru.

Latin American Banking Federation/Federación Latinoamericana de Bancos (FELABAN). Established to co-ordinate efforts towards a wider and accelerated economic development in Latin American countries.

Headquarters: Apdo Aereo 091959, Bogotá, DE8, Colombia.

Organization of the Cooperatives of America/Organización de las Cooperativas de América. Founded in 1963 to improve social, economic, cultural and moral conditions through the co-operative system.

Headquarters: POB 13568–24163, Calle 97A no. 11–31, Oficina 201, Bogotá, Colombia.

Cooperativa America (six times a year, Spanish)

Further Reading

British Bulletin of Publications on Latin America, the Caribbean, Portugal and Spain. London, from June 1949 (half-yearly)
South America, Central America and the Caribbean, 1988. London, 1987
The Latin America and Caribbean Review, 1989. Saffron Walden, 1988
Angarita, C. and Coffey, P., *Europe and the Andean Countries: A Comparison of Economic Policies and Institutions.* London, 1988
Box, B., (ed.) *1990 South American Handbook.* Bath (annual)
Bulmer-Thomas, V., *The Political Economy of Central America since 1920.* CUP, 1987. —*Britain and Latin America: A Changing Relationship,* 1989
Duran, E., *European Interests in Latin America.* London, 1985
Ferguson, J. and Pearce, J., *The Thatcher Years: Britain and Latin America.* London, 1988
Inter-American Development Bank, *Economic and Social Progress in Latin America: Economic Integration.* Washington, 1984

CARIBBEAN COMMUNITY (CARICOM)

Establishment and Functions. The Treaty establishing the Caribbean Community, including the Caribbean Common Market, and the Agreement establishing the

Common External Tariff for the Caribbean Common Market, was signed by the Prime Ministers of Barbados, Guyana, Jamaica and Trinidad and Tobago at Chaguaramas, Trinidad, on 4 July 1973, and entered into force on 1 Aug. 1973. Six less developed countries of CARIFTA signed the Treaty of Chaguaramas on 17 April 1974. They were Belize, Dominica, Grenada, Saint Lucia, St Vincent and Montserrat, and the Treaty came into effect for those countries on 1 May 1974. Antigua acceded to membership on 4 July 1974 and on 26 July the Associated State of St Kitts–Nevis–Anguilla signed the Treaty of Chaguaramas in Kingston, Jamaica, and became a member of the Caribbean Community, Bahamas became a member of the Community but not of the Common Market on 4 July 1983.

The Caribbean Community has 3 areas of activity: *(i)* economic co-operation through the Caribbean Common Market; *(ii)* co-ordination of foreign policy; *(iii)* functional co-operation in areas such as health, education and culture, youth and sports, science and technology, and tax administration.

The Caribbean Common Market provides for the establishment of a Common External Tariff, a common protective policy and the progressive co-ordination of external trade policies; the adoption of a scheme for the harmonization of fiscal incentives to industry; double taxation arrangements among member countries; the co-ordination of economic policies and development planning; and a special regime for the less developed countries of the community.

In 1990 a target date of 1994 for the creation of a common market was agreed. A common tariff on imports from third countries will be applied by some member countries from the beginning of 1991; other members will implement it later. By mid-1991 all barriers to intra-CARICOM trade were scheduled for removal.

Membership: Antigua and Barbuda, Bahamas, Barbados, Belize, Dominica, Grenada, Guyana, Jamaica, Montserrat, St Kitts–Nevis, Saint Lucia, St Vincent and the Grenadines, and Trinidad and Tobago. Turks and Caicos Islands and the British Virgin Islands.

Structure: The *Conference of Heads of Government* is the principal organ of the Community, and its primary responsibility is to determine the policy of the Community. It is the final authority of the Community and the Common Market, and for the conclusion of treaties and relationships between the Community and international organizations and States. It is responsible for financial arrangements for meeting the expenses of the Community.

The *Common Market Council* is the principal organ of the Common Market and consists of a Minister of Government designated by each member state. Decisions in both the Conference and the Council are in the main taken on the basis of unanimity.

The *Secretariat*, successor to the Commonwealth Caribbean Regional Secretariat, is the principal administrative organ of the Community and of the Common Market. The Secretary-General is appointed by the Conference on the recommendation of the Council for a term not exceeding 5 years and may be reappointed. The Secretary-General shall act in that capacity in all meetings of the Conference, the Council, and of the institutions of the Community.

Institutions of the Community, established by the Heads of Government Conference, are: Conference of Ministers responsible for Health; Standing Committees of Ministers responsible for Education, Tourism, Labour, Foreign Affairs, Finance, Agriculture, Energy, Mines and Natural Resources, Industry, Science and Technology, Transport and Legal Affairs, respectively.

Associate Institutions: Caribbean Development Bank; Caribbean Examinations Council; Council of Legal Education; University of the West Indies; University of Guyana; Caribbean Meteorological Organization; West Indies Shipping Corporation.

Flag: Divided horizontally light blue over dark blue; in the centre a white disc bearing the linked letters CC in light blue and dark blue respectively.

Secretary-General: Roderick Rainford.

Deputy Secretary-General: Frank Abdulah.

Headquarters: Bank of Guyana Building, PO Box 10827, Georgetown, Guyana.

The language of the Community is English.

Further Reading

CARICOM Bibliography. Georgetown, CARICOM Secretariat, annual
CARICOM Perspective. (3 times a year). Georgetown, CARICOM Secretariat
CARICOM Secretary-General's Report. Georgetown, annual *Treaty Establishing the Caribbean Community*. Georgetown, CARICOM Secretariat, 1982
Axline, A. W., *Caribbean Integration: The Politics of Regionalism*. London and New York, 1979
Parry, J. H., *et. al. A Short History of the West Indies*. Rev. ed. London, 1987
Payne, A. J., *The Politics of the Caribbean Community 1961–79*. Manchester Univ. Press, 1980

SOUTH PACIFIC FORUM

The South Pacific Forum held its first meeting of Heads of Government in New Zealand in 1971. Membership (and year of adhesion): Australia (1971), Cook Islands (1971), the Federated States of Micronesia (1987), Fiji (1971), Kiribati (1979), Nauru (1971), New Zealand (1971), Niue (1975), Papua New Guinea (1974), the Republic of the Marshall Islands (1987), Solomon Islands (1978), Tonga (1971), Tuvalu (1978), Vanuatu (1980) and Western Samoa (1971).

In 1985 the Forum adopted a treaty for a nuclear-free zone in the South Pacific, and in 1987 a treaty on fisheries with the USA; and in 1978, 1986 and 1989 conventions on fishery and protection of marine resources.

THE LEAGUE OF ARAB STATES

Origin. The formation of the League of Arab States in 1945 was largely inspired by the Arab awakening of the 19th century. This movement sought to re-create and reintegrate the Arab community which, though for 400 years a part of the Ottoman Empire, had preserved its identity as a separate national group held together by memories of a common past, a common religion and a common language, as well as by the consciousness of being part of a common cultural heritage. The leaders of the Arab movement in the 19th century and of the Arab revolt against Turkey in the First World War sought to achieve these aims through secession from the Ottoman Empire into a united and independent Arab state comprising all the Arab countries in Asia. However the 1919 peace settlement divided the Arab world in Asia (with the exception of Saudi Arabia and the Yemen) into British and French spheres of influence and established in them a number of separate states and administrations (Syria, Lebanon, Iraq, Jordan and Palestine) under temporary mandatory control.

By 1943, however, 7 of these countries had substantially achieved their independence. An Arab conference therefore met in Alexandria in the autumn of 1944; it formulated the 'Alexandria Protocol', which delineated the outlines of the Arab League. It was found that neither a unitary state nor a federation could be achieved, but only a league of sovereign states. A covenant, establishing such a league, was signed in Cairo on 22 March 1945 by the representatives of Egypt, Iraq, Saudi Arabia, Syria, Lebanon, Jordan and Yemen. There were (1991) 20 members of the League: Algeria, Bahrain, Djibouti, Iraq, Jordan, Kuwait, Lebanon, Libya, Mauritania, Morocco, Oman, the Palestine Liberation Organization, Qatar, Saudi Arabia, Somalia, Sudan, Syria, Tunisia, United Arab Emirates and Yemen.

In the Charter's Special Annex on Palestine, the signatories considered the special circumstances of Palestine and decided that until the country can effectively exercise its independence, the Council of the League should take charge in the selection of an Arab representative from Palestine to take part in its work.

Egypt's membership of the League was suspended in March 1979 and the secretariat moved from Cairo to Tunis. This action was taken in response to the signing of a bilateral peace treaty between Egypt and Israel. Egypt was readmitted in May 1989 and the secretariat again moved to Cairo.

Organization. The machinery of the League consists of a Council, a number of Special Committees and a Permanent Secretariat. On the Council each state has one vote. The Council may meet in any of the Arab capitals. Its functions include mediation in any dispute between any of the League states or a League state and a country outside the League. The Council has a Political Committee consisting of the Foreign Ministers of the Arab states. There are also 22 specialized agencies.

The Permanent Secretariat of the League, under a Secretary-General (who enjoys, along with his senior colleagues, full diplomatic status), has its seat in Cairo.

The League considers itself a regional organization within the framework of the United Nations at which its secretary-general is an observer.

Secretary-General: vacant.

Flag: Dark green with the seal of the Arab League in white in the centre.

Arab Common Market. The Arab Common Market came into operation on 1 Jan. 1965. The agreement, reached on 13 Aug. 1964 and open to all the Arab League states, has been signed by Iraq, Jordan, Syria and Egypt. The agreement provides for the abolition of customs duties on agricultural products and natural resources within 5 years, by reducing tariffs at an annual rate of 20%. Customs duties on industrial products are to be reduced by 10% annually. The agreement also provides for the free movement of capital and labour between member countries, the establishment of common external tariffs, the co-ordination of economical development and the framing of a common foreign economic policy.

Further Reading

Arab Maritime Data, 1979–80. London, 1979

Gomaa, A. M., *The Foundation of the League of Arab States.* London, 1977

ORGANIZATION OF THE PETROLEUM EXPORTING COUNTRIES (OPEC)

Aims. The Organization was founded in Baghdad, Iraq, in 1960 with the following founder members, Iran, Iraq, Kuwait, Saudi Arabia and Venezuela. The principal aims are unifying the petroleum policies of member countries and determining the best means for safeguarding their interests, individually and collectively; to devise ways and means of ensuring the stabilization of prices in international oil markets with a view to eliminating harmful and unnecessary fluctuations; and to secure a steady income for the producing countries, an efficient, economic and regular supply of petroleum to consuming nations, and a fair return on their capital to those investing in the petroleum industry.

Membership (1989). Algeria, Ecuador, Gabon, Indonesia, Iran, Iraq, Kuwait, Libya, Nigeria, Qatar, Saudi Arabia, United Arab Emirates and Venezuela. Membership is open to any other country having substantial net exports of crude petroleum, which has fundamentally similar interests to those of member countries.

OPEC Fund for International Development: The Fund was established in 1976 to provide financial aid to developing countries, other than OPEC members, on advantageous terms.

Secretary-General: Dr Subroto.

Deputy Secretary-General: Vacant.

Headquarters: Obere Donaustrasse 93, A–1020 Vienna, Austria.

Flag: Light blue with the Opec logo in white in the centre.

Further Reading

OPEC publications include: *Annual Statistical Bulletin. Annual Report. OPEC Bulletin* (monthly). *OPEC Review* (quarterly).

Ahrari, M. E., *Opec: The Failing Giant.* Univ. Press of Kentucky, 1986

Al-Chalabi, F., *OPEC and the International Oil Industry: A Changing Structure*. OUP, 1980
El Mallakh, R., *OPEC: Twenty Years and Beyond*. London, 1982
Griffin, J. and Teece, D. J., *OPEC Behaviour and World Oil Prices*. London and Boston, 1982
Skeet, *OPEC: Twenty-five years of Prices and Policies*. CUP, 1988

ORGANIZATION OF AFRICAN UNITY

On 25 May 1963 the heads of state or government of 32 African countries, at a conference in Addis Ababa, signed a charter establishing an 'Organization of African Unity'. It had 51 members in 1990.

Its chief objects are the furtherance of African unity and solidarity; the co-ordination of the political, economic, cultural, health, scientific and defence policies and the elimination of colonialism in Africa.

The organs of the Organization are: (1) the assembly of the heads of state and government; (2) the council of ministers; (3) the general secretariat; (4) a commission of mediation, conciliation and arbitration. Arabic, French, Portuguese and English are recognized as working languages.

Chairman: Yoweri Museveni (Uganda).

Secretary-General: Salim Ahmed Salim.

Headquarters: Addis Ababa.

Flag: Horizontally green, white, green, with the white fimbriated yellow, and the seal of the OAU in the centre.

DANUBE COMMISSION

The Danube Commission was constituted in 1949 based on the Convention regarding the regime of navigation on the Danube, which was signed in Belgrade on 18 Aug. 1948. The Belgrade Convention reaffirmed that navigation on the Danube from Ulm to the Black Sea, with access to the sea through the Sulina arm and the Sulina Canal, is equally free and open to the nationals, merchant shipping and merchandise of all states as to harbour and navigation fees as well as conditions of merchant navigation.

The Danube Commission is composed of representatives from the countries on the Danube (1 for each of these countries), namely, Austria, Bulgaria, Hungary, Romania, Czechoslovakia, USSR and Yugoslavia. Since 1957, representatives of the Ministry of Transport from the Federal Republic of Germany have attended the meetings of the Commission as guests of the Secretariat.

The functions of the Danube Commission are to check that the provisions of the Convention are carried out, to establish a uniform buoying system on all the Danube's navigable waterways and to establish the basic regulations for navigation on the river. The Commission co-ordinates the regulations for river, customs and sanitation control as well as the hydrometeorological service and collects statistical data concerning navigation on the Danube.

The Danube Commission enjoys legal status. It has its own seal and flag. The members of the Commission and elected officers enjoy diplomatic immunity. The Commission's official buildings, archives and documents are inviolable. French and Russian are the official languages of the Commission.

Since 1954 the headquarters of the Commission have been in Budapest.

Flag: Blue, with a red strip fimbriated white along the bottom edge, and the initials of the Commission within a wreath in the canton—Latin letters on obverse Cyrillic on reverse.

Further Reading

Danube Commission's publications include: Compilation of Agreements on Danube Navigation; Basic Regulations of Navigation; Recommendations relating to the establishment of the dimensions of the channel and hydrotechnical and other works (1969; 1975; 1979; 1988 Editions); Recommendations on the Prevention of Water Pollution by Navigation; Recommendations on the Use of Radiocommunications on the Danube; Plan of basic works aiming at obtaining the dimensions of the channel and hydrotechnical and other works recommended on the Danube for the period 1980–1990 (1984 ed.); Danubian Bridges; Danubian Ships; Danube Maintenance; Danube Profile; Mileage Charts; Pilots' Charts; Sailing Direction; Hydrological Yearbooks; Hydrological Manuals; Statistical Yearbooks; Statistical Manuals; Recommendations on unified rules for sanitary, veterinary, plant protection and customs control; Rules of Procedure and other organization documents of the Danube Commission; Proceedings of Sessions; General Information on the Danube Commission and on its activity (with the text of the Convention regarding the regime of navigation on the Danube in annex).

ANTARCTIC TREATY

Antarctica is an island continent some 15·5m. sq. km in area which lies almost entirely within the Antarctic Circle. Its surface is composed of an ice sheet over rock, and it is uninhabited except for research and other workers in the course of duty. It is in general ownerless; for countries with territorial claims, *see* Argentina (p. 92), Australian Antarctic Territory (p. 125), British Antarctic Territory (p. 238), Chile (p. 348), French Southern and Antarctic Territories (p. 510), the Ross dependency, New Zealand (p. 931) and Queen Maud Land, Norway (p. 963).

12 countries which had maintained research stations in Antarctica during International Geophysical Year, 1957–58, (Argentina, Australia, Belgium, Chile, France, Japan, New Zealand, Norway, South Africa, the USSR, the UK and the USA) signed the Antarctic Treaty on 1 Dec. 1959. Austria, Brazil, Bulgaria, Canada, China, Colombia, Cuba, Czechoslovakia, Denmark, Ecuador, Finland, Germany, Greece, Hungary, India, Italy, South Korea, North Korea, the Netherlands, Papua New Guinea, Peru, Poland, Romania, Spain, Sweden, Switzerland and Uruguay have subsequently acceded to the Treaty. The Treaty reserves the Antarctic area south of 60° S. lat. for peaceful purposes, provides for international co-operation in scientific investigation and research, and preserves, for the duration of the Treaty, the *status quo* with regard to territorial sovereignty, rights and claims. The Treaty entered into force on 23 June 1961. The 39 nations party to the Treaty meet biennially. Decisions taken by the signatories of the 1959 Washington Treaty must be unanimous.

In June 1988 a Convention on the Regulation of Antarctic Mineral Resource Activities was initialled which would regulate the commercial exploitation of mineral resources. In order to come into force, the convention requires ratification by 16 of the nations party to the Treaty by 1992. However, discussion is still proceeding on an alternative of a total ban on mining.

PART II

COUNTRIES OF THE WORLD

A—Z

AFGHANISTAN

Capital: Kabul
Population: 15·81m. (1989)
GNP per capita: US$250 (1985)

Jamhuria Afghanistan

(Republic of Afghanistan)

HISTORY. A military coup on 17 July 1973 overthrew the monarchy of King Zahir Shah. The coup was led by the King's cousin and brother-in-law Mohammad Daoud who declared a Republic. King Zahir abdicated on 24 Aug. 1973. President Daoud was killed in a military coup in April 1978 which led to the establishment of a pro-Soviet government of the People's Democratic Party of Afghanistan (PDPA).

In Dec. 1979 Soviet troops invaded Afghanistan and Hafizullah Amin was deposed and replaced by Babrak Karmal. The pretext for the airlift of combat troops to Kabul was the Treaty of Friendship signed in Dec. 1978 between the USSR and Afghanistan. In May 1986 Karmal was replaced as General Secretary of the PDPA by Dr Sayid Mohammed Najibullah who was elected President in Sept. 1987 at a special session of the Revolutionary Council. In early 1988 there were some 115,000 Soviet troops in Afghanistan but under the Geneva accords signed in April 1988 all Soviet troops were withdrawn by 15 Feb. 1989.

AREA AND POPULATION. Afghanistan is bounded in the north by the USSR, east and south by Pakistan and west by Iran.

The area is 251,773 sq. miles (652,090 sq. km). Population according to the last (1979) census was 15,551,358, of which some 2·5m. were nomadic tribes. Estimate (1989, excluding nomads) 15·81m. (21% urban). Approximately 3m. Afghans have sought refuge in Pakistan, over 1m. in Iran and several hundred thousand have been killed since 1979. Infant mortality rates, averaged over 1985–90, were 172 per 1,000 live births; annual growth rate, 2·6%; expectation of life, 41·5 years. The population of Kabul is over 2m. There are no current reliable population figures for other cities and major towns.

Census (1979), Kabul 913,164; Kandahar, 178,409; Herat, 140,323; Mazar-i-Sharif, 103,372; Jalalabad, 53,915; Kunduz, 53,251; Baghlan, 39,228; Maimana, 38,251; Pul-i-Khumri, 31,101; Ghazni, 30,425; Charikar, 22,424; Shiberghan, 18,955; Gardez, 9,550; Faizabad, 9,098; Qala-i-nau, 5,340; Uiback, 4,938; Meterlam, 3,987; Cheghcheran, 2,974.

The main ethnic group are the Pathans. Other ethnic groups include the Tajiks, the Hazaras, the Turkomans and the Uzbeks.

CLIMATE. The climate is arid, with a big annual range of temperature and very little rain, apart from the period Jan. to April. Winters are very cold, with considerable snowfall, which may last the year round on mountain summits. Kabul. Jan. 27°F (–2·8°C), July 76°F (24·4°C). Annual rainfall 13" (338 mm).

CONSTITUTION AND GOVERNMENT. A new Constitution was approved in Nov. 1987. The PDPA remains the leading political force in the country. It is governed by a Central Committee (112 full members and 63 alternate members), which elects a Political Bureau, currently of 14 full, and 4 alternate, members to decide policy. At that time, the name of the country was changed from the Democratic Republic of Afghanistan to the Republic of Afghanistan.

A State of Emergency was declared on 19 Feb. 1989 following the withdrawal of Soviet forces and a Military Council headed by President Najibullah (b. 1947) was announced. On 20 Feb. the Prime Minister Dr Mohammed Hasan Sharq resigned when the 20-man Supreme Military Council for the Defence of the Homeland took over full control of economic, political and military policy. The state of emergency was lifted in May 1990.

The *Loya Jirga* (Grand Assembly) was convened on 21 May 1989 following elections on 17 May.

In May 1990 Fazal Haq Khaliqyar (PDPA) was appointed *Prime Minister* and Sultan Ali Keshtmand *Vice-President.*

In June 1990 the PDPA adopted new rules and renamed itself the Fatherland Party. An Executive Committee of 15 and a Central Committee of 14 replaced the Politburo and former Central Committee.

National flag: Three equal horizontal stripes of red, black and green, with the national arms in the canton.

The official languages are Pushtu and Dari (Persian).

Local Government: There are 31 provinces each administered by an appointed governor.

DEFENCE. Conscription is currently for a period of 2 years, followed soon after by another period of 2 years for non-graduates.

Army. The Army is organized in 3 armoured and 16 infantry divisions, 1 special guard division, 1 mechanized infantry brigade, 1 artillery brigade, 5 commando brigades and 3 independent special guard brigades. Equipment includes 50 T-34, 400 T-54/-55 and 170 T-62 battle tanks. Strength was (1991) about 50,000, but most units of the Army are well below strength, largely as a result of desertions.

Air Force. The Air Force, which is Soviet-equipped, had (1989) about 180 combat aircraft and 5,000 officers and men. Nominal strength comprises 3 squadrons of Su-7 and Su-20 attack aircraft, 3 squadrons of MiG-21 interceptors (about 40 aircraft), 3 squadrons of MiG-17s and 3 squadrons of MiG-23s, a helicopter attack force of at least 50 Mi-24s, a transport wing with 6-8 An-12s, 12 twin-turboprop An-26s, about 10 piston-engined An-2s, 50 Mi-8 and 10 Mi-4 helicopters and 2 turboprop Il-18s, and Yak-18, Aero L-39 and MiG-15UTI trainers. The main fighter station is Bagram, with facilities for the largest jet transports and bombers. There is a fighter-bomber station at Shindand, a training station at Mazar-i-Sharif and an air academy at Sherpur. Large numbers of SA-2 and SA-3 surface-to-air missiles are operational. The Soviet Union is withdrawing its aviation units but is leaving aircraft behind for the national Air Force.

Police and Militia. In addition to the Army and Air Force there are a number of paramilitary units, including a 50,000-strong gendarmerie, secret police and 'Defence of the Revolution' forces.

INTERNATIONAL RELATIONS

Membership. Afghanistan is a member of the UN and Colombo Plan.

ECONOMY

Planning. A 5-year plan was adopted in 1986 to cover 1986–1991. Emphasis is on reconstruction of agriculture and irrigation systems as well as exploitation of natural gas resources.

Budget. In 1983–84 the budget envisaged expenditure of Afs. 49,941m. and revenue of Afs. 34,120m.

Currency. The unit of currency is the *afghani* (AFA) of 100 *puls*. Rates of exchange are fixed (1991) Afs. 99·25 = £1; Afs. 52·32 = US$1; unofficial rates are: Afs. 345 = £1; Afs. 225 = US$1. Inflation was 56·8% in 1989.

Banking and Finance. The Afghan State Bank *(Da Afghanistan Bank)* is the largest of the 3 main banks and also undertakes the functions of a central bank, holding the exclusive right of note issue. Total assets of the 3 main banks were: Da Afghanistan Bank (1981), Afs. 22,839m.; Pashtany Tejaraty Bank (1981), Afs. 6,997m.; Bank-i-Milli (1981), Afs. 3,087m. Foreign banks have been permitted to operate since May 1990.

Weights and Measures. Weights and measures used in Kabul are: Weights: 1 *khurd* = 0·244 lb.; 1 *pao* = 0·974 lb.; 1 *charak* = 3·896 lb.; 1 *sere* = 16 lb.; 1 *kharwár* = 1,280 lb. or 16 maunds of 80 lb. each. Long measure: 1 yard or *gaz* = 40 in. The metric system is in increasingly common use. Square measures: 1 *jaríb* = 60 x 60 kábuli yd or $^1/_2$ acre; 1 *kulbá* = 40 jaríbs (area in which $2^1/_2$ kharwárs of seed can be sown); 1 jaríb yd = 29 in. Local weights and measures are in use in the provinces.

ENERGY AND NATURAL RESOURCES

Electricity. Hydro-electric plants have been constructed at Sarobi, Nangarhar, Naghlu, Mahipar, Pul-i-Khumri and Kandahar. Production (1986) 1,390m. kwh. Supply 220 volts; 50 Hz.

Natural gas. Production (1985) 2,400m. cu. metres. Natural gas is found in northern Afghanistan around Shiberghan and Sar-i-Pol; over 2,000m. cu. metres, about 95% of production, is piped to the USSR annually.

Minerals. Mineral resources are scattered and little developed. Coal is mined at Karkar in Pul-i-Khumri, Ishpushta near Doshi, north of Kabul and Dar-i-Suf south of Mazar (total production, 1983–84, 145,300 tonnes). Rich, but as yet unexploited, deposits of iron ore exist in the Hajigak hills about 100 miles west of Kabul; beryllium has been found in the Kunar valley and barite in Bamian province. Other deposits include gold; silver (now unexploited, in the Panjshir valley); lapis lazuli (in the Panjshir valley and Badakhshan); asbestos; mica; sulphur (near Maimana); chrome (in the Logar valley and near Herat); and copper (in the north).

Agriculture. Although the greater part of Afghanistan is more or less mountainous and a good deal of the country is too dry and rocky for successful cultivation, there are many fertile plains and valleys, which, with the assistance of irrigation from small rivers or wells, yield very satisfactory crops of fruit, vegetables and cereals. It is estimated that there are 14m. ha of cultivable land in the country, of which only 6% of the total land was being cultivated in 1982–83 (5·34m. ha of this being irrigated land). Before 1979 Afghanistan was virtually self-supporting in foodstuffs but in 1989 it was estimated that 33% of the land had been destroyed by war. The castor-oil plant, madder and the asafœtida plant abound.

Fruit forms a staple food (with bread) of many people throughout the year, both in the fresh and preserved state, and in the latter condition is exported in great quantities. The fat-tailed sheep furnish the principal meat diet, and the grease of the tail is a substitute for butter. Wool and skins provide material for warm apparel and one of the more important articles of export. Persian lambskins (Karakuls) are one of the chief exports.

Production, 1988, in 1,000 tonnes: Wheat, 2,035; barley, 274; maize, 587; rice, 343.

Livestock (1988): Cattle, 2·7m.; horses, donkeys and mules (1986), 1·69m.; sheep, 19m.; goats (1986), 3m.; chickens, 5·9m.

INDUSTRY.

At Kabul there are factories for the manufacture of cotton and woollen textiles, leather, boots, marble-ware, furniture, glass, bicycles, prefabricated houses and plastics. A large machine shop has been constructed and equipped by the USSR, with a capability of manufacturing motor spares. There is a wool factory and there are several cotton-ginning plants; a small cotton factory at Jabal-us-Seraj and a larger one at Pul-i-Khumri; a cotton-seed oil extraction plant at Lashkargah; a cotton textile factory at Gulbahar, and a cotton plant at Balkh.

An ordnance factory manufactures arms and ammunition, boots and clothing, etc. for the Army. There is a beet sugar plant at Baghlan and a fruit-canning factory in Kandahar.

Industries include cement, coalmining, cotton textiles, small vehicle assembly plants, fruit canning, carpet making, leather tanning, footwear manufacture, sugar manufacture, preparation of hides and skins, and building. Most of these are relatively small and, with the exception of hides and skins, carpets and fruits, do not meet domestic requirements.

FOREIGN ECONOMIC RELATIONS. Foreign debt was US$4,850m. in 1985. Trade has been supervised by the Ministries of Commerce and Finance and the Da Afghanistan Bank, but it was announced in May 1990 that trade was to be deregulated. The Government monopoly controls the import of petrol and oil, sugar, cigarettes and tobacco, motor vehicles and consignment goods from bilateral trading countries. The principal surface routes for imports to Afghanistan are via the Soviet rail system and the border posts at Torghundi and Hairatan; and from Karachi via the border post at Torkham.

Commerce. In 1988 imports totalled US$1,558m. and exports US$558m. Main export commodities in 1985 were karakul skins (US$13·5m.), raw cotton (US$12·5m.), dried fruit and nuts (US$141m.), fresh fruit (US$53·3m.) and natural gas (US$302·4m.). Main items imported in 1985 were petroleum products (US$164m.), textiles (US$122·5m.). The USSR supplied 58·1% of imports in 1988 and received 49·1% of exports.

Total trade between Afghanistan and UK (in £1,000 sterling, British Department of Trade returns):

	1986	*1987*	*1988*	*1989*	*1990*
Imports to UK	11,913	11,289	11,501	4,813	9,194
Exports and re-exports from UK	11,444	10,735	12,109	5,376	7,815

Tourism. Owing to internal political instability there has been negligible tourism since 1979.

COMMUNICATIONS

Roads. There were in 1986 22,000 km of roads. The Americans asphalted the Kandahar–Chaman and Kabul–Torkham roads. The Russians constructed a road and tunnel through the Salang pass (over 11,000 ft) which was opened in Sept. 1964 and cut 120 miles off the old road from Kabul to the north; they continued this road to Kunduz and Sherkhan Bandar (Qizil Qala) on the Oxus. In addition, the Americans in 1966 completed the road between Kabul and Kandahar and the Russians constructed a concrete road between Kandahar and Herat. In 1968 the Americans completed an asphalt road from Herat to the Iranian frontier at Islam Qala. With Soviet assistance a metalled road from Pul-i-Khumri to Mazar-i-Sharif was completed in 1969 and Mazar-i-Sharif to Shiberghan in 1971. A Soviet-built road and rail bridge across the Oxus (Amu Darya) River was opened in May 1982. There are about 90,000 cars and commercial vehicles registered in Kabul. All roads, particularly outside the towns, are in a very poor state of repair as a result of the war.

Railways. There are no railways in the country, but the Oxus bridge opened in 1982, brought Soviet Railways' track into the country. A 200 km line of 1,520 mm gauge has been authorized from Termez to Pul-i-Khumri.

Aviation. On 29 June 1956 Afghanistan signed an agreement with the USA for the development of civil aviation, including the construction of the international airport at Kandahar, comprising a loan of $5m. and a grant of $9·56m. Kabul airport has been expanded with Soviet assistance. New runways at Kabul and Kandahar airports have been completed. Provincial all-weather airports have been constructed at Herat, Qunduz, Jalalabad and Mazar-i-Sharif.

Bakhtar Afghan Airlines (the domestic national airline) began operations on 8 Feb. 1968 and regularly serves the main internal airfields, which, from 1985 was merged with Ariana Afghan Airlines (the national airline) operating regular services to New Delhi, Prague, Tashkent and Moscow.

Shipping. There are practically no navigable rivers, and timber is the only article of commerce conveyed by water, floated down the Kunar and Kabul rivers from Chitral on rafts. A port has been built at Qizil Qala on the Oxus; barge traffic is increasing on the Oxus. Three river ports on the Amu Darya have been built at Sherkhan Bandar, Tashguzar and Hairatan, linked by road to Kabul.

Telecommunications. Telephones, installed in most of the large towns, numbered 31,200 in 1978. There is telegraphic communication between all the larger towns and with other parts of the world. Kabul Radio broadcasts in Pushtu, Persian, Urdu, English, French, Russian and German. In 1986 there were 823,000 radio receivers and 12,800 television receivers.

Newspapers. In 1983 there were 3 daily newspapers with a circulation of 67,000.

JUSTICE, RELIGION, EDUCATION AND WELFARE

Justice. A Supreme Court was established in June 1978. If no provision exists in the Constitution or in the general laws of the State, the courts follow the Hanafi jurisprudence of Islamic law.

Religion. The predominant religion is Islam, mostly of the Sunni sect, though there is a minority of Shia Moslems.

Education. Some 25% of the population were estimated to be literate in 1990. There are elementary schools throughout the country, but secondary schools exist only in Kabul and provincial capitals. Both elementary and secondary education are free. In 1985 there were 580,000 pupils (16,000 teachers) in primary education and 105,000 pupils (5,700 teachers) in secondary education. There are 3 teacher-training institutions in Kabul and 11 elsewhere; UNESCO is supporting an expansion programme. Technical, art, commercial and medical schools exist for higher education. Kabul University was founded in 1932 and has 9 faculties (medicine, science, agriculture, engineering, law and political science, letters, economics, theology, pharmacology). The University of Nangarhar in Jalalabad was founded in 1963. A Polytechnic in Kabul was completed in 1968. In 1982 there were 13,115 students in higher education, 4,427 in teacher-training schools and 1,230 in technical schools.

Health. In 1982 there were 1,215 doctors and 6,875 hospital beds. Two-thirds of the doctors and half the beds were in Kabul.

DIPLOMATIC REPRESENTATIVES

Of Afghanistan in Great Britain (31 Prince's Gate, London, SW7 1QQ)
Chargé d'Affaires: Taza Khan Wial.

Of Great Britain in Afghanistan (Karte Parwan, Kabul)
Staff temporarily withdrawn.

Of Afghanistan in the USA (2341 Wyoming Ave., NW, Washington, D.C., 20008)
Chargé d'Affaires: M. Miagol.

Of the USA in Afghanistan (Wazir Akbar Khan Mina, Kabul)
Ambassador: Vacant.

Of Afghanistan to the United Nations
Ambassador: Noor Ahmad Noor.

Further Reading

Arney, G., *Afghanistan.* London, 1990
Bradsher, H. S., *Afghanistan and the Soviet Union.* Duke Univ. Press, 1983
Ghaus, A. S., *The Fall of Afghanistan: An Insider's Account.* Oxford, 1988
Gilbertson, G. W., *Pakkhto Idiom Dictionary.* 2 vols. London, 1932
Giradet, E. R., *Afghanistan: The Soviet War.* London, 1985
Hammond, T. T., *Red Star over Afghanistan.* Boulder and London, 1984
Hanifi, M. J., *Historical and Cultural Dictionary of Afghanistan.* Metuchen, 1976
Hyman, A., *Afghanistan under Soviet Domination 1964–83.* London, 1984
Roy, O., *Islam and Resistance in Afghanistan.* 2nd ed. CUP, 1990
Saikal, A. and Maley, W., *The Soviet withdrawal from Afghanistan.* CUP, 1989
Sykes, P. M., *A History of Afghanistan.* 2 vols. New York, 1975

ALBANIA

Capital: Tirana
Population: 3·2m. (1989)
GNP per capita: US$930 (1986)

Republika Popullore Socialiste e Shqipërisë

HISTORY. For the history of Albania before the Second World War *see* THE STATESMAN'S YEAR-BOOK 1985–86, p. 66. During the years 1939–44 the country was overrun by Italians and Germans. The official Albanian date of the liberation is 29 Nov. 1944.

On 10 Nov. 1945 the British, US and USSR Governments recognized a Provisional Government under Gen. Enver Hoxha, on the understanding that it would hold free elections. The elections of 2 Dec. 1945 resulted in a Communist-controlled assembly, which on 11 Jan. 1946 proclaimed Albania a republic.

In 1946 Great Britain and the USA broke off relations with Albania and vetoed its admission to the UN. Albania was finally admitted in 1955.

Because of Albania's Stalinist and pro-Chinese attitudes diplomatic relations with USSR were broken off in 1961. In 1977 Albania terminated its special relationship with China.

Beginning in July 1990 there were several demonstrations against the government often led by students. In Dec. the Communist Party dismissed 5 members of its Politburo and the People's Assembly adopted a decree legalizing opposition parties. On 20 Feb. 1991 the President assumed direct control of government. Several thousand refugees found asylum abroad.

AREA AND POPULATION. Albania is bounded in the north and east by Yugoslavia, south by Greece and west by the Adriatic. The area of the country is 28,748 sq. km (11,101 sq. miles). By the peace treaty Italy restored the island of Sazan (Saseno) to Albania. At the census of 1982 the population was, 2,786,100. The population in 1988 was 3,138,100 (1,522,000 female; 1,111,440 urban). Population in 1989, 3·2m. (34% urban in 1987; density 109·2 per sq. km). The capital is Tirana (population in 1990, 210,000); other large towns are Durrës (Durazzo) (72), Shkodër (Scutari) (71), Elbasan (70), Vlorë (Vlonë, Valona) (61), Korçë (Koritza) (57), Fier (37), Berat (37), Lushnjë (24), Kavajë (23) and Gjirokastër (Argyrocastro) (21).

Ethnic minorities (mainly Greeks) numbered some 300,000 in 1990.

Vital statistics, 1988: Marriages, 28,174; births, 80,241; deaths, 17,027; divorces, 2,597. Rates (per 1,000, 1988): Births, 25·5; deaths, 5·4; marriages, 9; divorces, 0·8; natural increase, 20·1 per thousand. Life expectancy in 1988 was 69·4 years, males; 74·9, females. In 1988 33% of the population were under 15. 20,000 persons emigrated legally in 1990.

The country is administratively divided into 26 districts (*rreth*) (*see* map in THE STATESMAN'S YEAR-BOOK, 1962. N.B. The district of Ersekë has been renamed Kolonjë), 66 towns, 306 town boroughs, 537 village unions and 2,844 villages.

Districts	*Area (sq. km)*	*Population (in 1,000) (1988)*	*Districts*	*Area (sq. km)*	*Population (in 1,000) (1988)*
Berat	1,027	173·7	Lushnjë	712	132·2
Dibrë	1,568	148·2	Mat	1,028	75·9
Durrës	848	242·5	Mirditë	867	49·7
Elbasan	1,481	238·6	Permet	929	39·4
Fier	1,175	239·7	Pogradec	725	70·5
Gjirokastër	1,137	65·5	Pukë	1,034	48·2
Gramsh	695	43·8	Sarandë	1,097	86·6
Kolonjë	805	24·6	Shkodër	2,528	233·0
Korçë	2,181	213·2	Skrapar	775	45·8
Krujë	607	105·3	Tepelenë	817	49·1
Kukës	1,330	99·4	Tirana	1,238	363·1
Lezhë	479	61·6	Tropojë	1,043	44·2
Librazhd	1,013	70·8	Vlorë	1,609	174·0

Districts are named after their capitals; exceptions: Tropojë, capital—Bajram Curri; Mat—Burrel; Mirditë—Rrëshen; Skrapar—Çorovodë; Dibrë—Peshkopi; Kolonjë—Ersekë.

The Albanian language is divided into two dialects—Gheg, north of the river Shkumbi, and Tosk in the south. Many places therefore have two forms of name: Vlonë (Gheg), Vlorë (Tosk), etc., and many are known also by an Italian name, *e.g.*, Valona. Since 1945 the official language has been based on Tosk.

CLIMATE. Mediterranean-type, with rainfall mainly in winter, but thunderstorms are frequent and severe in the great heat of the plains in summer. Winters in the highlands can be severe, with much snow. Tirana. Jan. 44°F (6·8°C), July 75°F (23·9°C). Annual rainfall 54" (1,353 mm). Shkodër. Jan. 39°F (3·9°C), July 77°F (25°C). Annual rainfall 57" (1,425 mm).

CONSTITUTION AND GOVERNMENT. The political structure derived from the Constitution of 14 March 1946 as amended in 1950, 1955, 1960 and 1963. In Dec. 1976 a new Constitution was adopted, by which Albania became a 'Socialist People's Republic'. The supreme legislative body is the single-chamber People's Assembly of 250 deputies, which meets twice a year, and delegates its day-to-day functions to a Presidium. Election to the People's Assembly is by universal suffrage (at 18) every 4 years.

A law of Nov. 1990 permitted independent candidates to stand in secret-ballot elections. In Dec. an opposition Democratic Party was allowed to form.

In the elections of 1 Feb. 1987 a 100% turnout of the electorate of 1,830,653 was claimed to vote for the 250 candidates (73 women) on the single list of the Democratic Front. (There was 1 vote against). The next, multi-party, elections were scheduled for 31 March 1991.

The Government consisted of a Council of Ministers, of 22 members, including the Chairman (Prime Minister) and 3 Deputies.

Effective rule was exercised by the Albanian Labour (*i.e.*, Communist) Party, founded 8 Nov. 1941, between 1945 and 1990, during which period it enjoyed a monopoly of political power. Its governing body is its Politburo, which in Feb. 1991 consisted of Ramiz Alia (*First Secretary of the Central Committee of the Party*), Besnik Bekteshi, Adil Çarçani, Vangjel Çerava, Xhelil Gjonj, Hekuran Isai, Pali Miska, Kiço Mustaqi,and 3 candidate members: Xhemal Dymylia, Llambi Gegprifti, Niko Gjyzarč.

In 1981 the Party had 122,600 full members and candidates (in 1979 37·5% workers, 29% farmers, 27% women).

Titular Head of State, Chairman of the Presidium of the People's Assembly: Ramiz Alia, elected Nov. 1982; *Deputy Chairmen:* Xhafer Spahiu, Emine Guri; *Secretary:* Sihat Tozaj.

Following a wave of demonstrations against the government which began in July 1990, Ramiz Alia assumed direct presidential control of government on 20 Feb. 1991, having dismissed all except 4 of the previous ministers. An 8-member Presidential Council was set up, chaired by Fatos Nano.

Local government is carried out by People's Councils at village, village union, town borough, town and district level. Councillors are elected for 3 years. Elections were held in May 1989; turn-out was 99·99%.

National flag: Red, with a black double-headed eagle and a red, gold-edged 5-pointed star above it. *Mercantile flag:* Red, black, red (horizontal) with a red yellow-edged star in the centre.

National anthem: Rreth Flamurit te per bashkuar (The flag that united us in the struggle).

DEFENCE. Albania withdrew from the Warsaw Pact in 1968 in protest against the invasion of Czechoslovakia. The Constitution precludes the stationing of foreign troops in Albania. Conscription is for 2 years.

Army. The Army consists of 1 tank brigade, 4 infantry brigades, 1 engineer, and 3 artillery regiments. Equipment includes 190 T-34 and T-54 main battle tanks. Strength (1990) 35,000 (including 20,000 conscripts) and reserves number 150,000. There are also paramilitary internal security forces (5,000 men) and frontier guards (7,000).

Navy. The combatant navy includes 2 submarines, 2 offshore patrol craft, 29 hydrofoil torpedo boats, 6 inshore patrol craft and 1 fleet minesweeper. Auxiliaries include 1 tanker and about 10 service craft. Navy personnel in 1990 totalled 2,000 officers and ratings, including 400 coastal defence guards. Service for ratings is 3 years. There are naval bases at Durrës and Vlorë.

Air Force. The Air Force, controlled by the Army, had (1990) about 11,000 officers and men (1,400 conscripts), and in 1991 operated 95 combat aircraft, of which about 80 had been received before relations with China were broken. The force included 20 Chinese-built F-7s and 30 F-6s, and 3 ground attack squadrons of F-2s and F-4s. Transport and training types include 3 Il-14s, 10 An-2s, Mi-4 helicopters, Yak-18s and MiG-15UTIs.

INTERNATIONAL RELATIONS

Membership. Albania is a member of the UN. In 1990 Albania applied for observer status in the CSCE and agreed to sign the Non-Proliferation of Nuclear Weapons Treaty.

ECONOMY

Policy. For the first seven 5-year plans *see* THE STATESMAN'S YEAR-BOOK, 1989–90. Cautious moves towards 'economic logic', a recognition of market forces were made in 1989. Targets of the eighth 5-year plan (1986–90): Social production, 30–32%; national income, 34–36%; industry, 29–31%; agriculture, 34–36%.

Budget. Budget figures for 1989: Revenue, 9,550m. leks; expenditure, 9,500m. leks. Revenue in 1988 (in 1m. leks): Centralized state income, 3,880; from enterprises, 2,850; social insurance, 889. Expenditure: Economy, 4,211; social 2,725; defence, 955 (998 in 1986); administration, 155.

Currency. The monetary unit is the *lek* (ALL) of 100 *qintars*. It replaced the gold franc *(franc ar)* in July 1947. In Aug. 1965 a new *lek* was introduced: 10 old *leks* = 1 new *lek*. There are 5, 10, 20 and 50 *qintar* coins and a 1 *lek* coin; notes are for 1, 3, 5, 10, 25, 50 and 100 *leks*. Exchange rates, March 1991: US$1 = 5·31 *leks*; £1 = 10·08.

Banking and Finance. The Albanian State Bank was founded in 1925 with Italian aid. Its *Director General* is Niko Gjyzari. In 1988 savings deposits amounted to 1,478m. leks. In 1970 the Agricultural Bank was set up as a credit institution for agricultural co-operatives.

Weights and Measures. The metric system is in force.

ENERGY AND NATURAL RESOURCES

Electricity. Albania is rich in hydro-electric potential. Electric power production in 1988 was 3,984m. kwh. 2,000m. kwh. were exported in 1984 to Yugoslavia, Bulgaria, Romania and Greece.

Oil. Oil reserves are some 20m. tonnes. Output in 1989: Crude, 3m. tonnes; refined (1973), 1,596,000 tonnes. Refining capacity in 1970 was over 1m. tonnes. Oil is produced chiefly at Qytet Stalin which a pipeline connects to the port of Vlorë. Natural gas is extracted. Reserves: 8,000m. cu. metres; 1985 production, 420m. cu. metres.

Minerals. The mineral wealth of Albania is considerable and includes lignite, oil, chrome and ferro-nickel ores, but it is only recently being developed. Production (in

1,000 tonnes), (1988): Lignite, 2,184; chromium ore, 1,109; copper ore, 1,087; iron-nickel ore, 1,067.

Agriculture. The country for the greater part is rugged, wild and mountainous, the exceptions being along the Adriatic littoral and the Korçë (Koritza) Basin, which are fertile. In 1988 the cultivated area was 714,200 ha, of which 589,800 ha were sown to crops, 59,600 ha were orchards, 44,500 ha olive groves and 20,300 ha vineyards. There were 403,000 ha of pasture. 58·2% of arable land was irrigated.

Land is held by the State (largely forests and non-agricultural), state farms (50 in 1982 averaging 3,000 ha of arable land) and co-operatives (460 in 1989 covering 528,700 ha). In 1989 co-operatives were permitted to fix their own prices and keep any profits surplus to plan. There is a pension scheme for collective farmers. As of July 1990 peasants were permitted personal plots of up to 2,000 square metres, and had the right to raise cattle on them. In 1988 there were 21,033 tractors (in 15HP units).

Production (in 1,000 tonnes) (and sown area in 1,000 ha) of the main crops in 1988: Wheat, 589 (199); sugarbeet, 360 (7·4); maize, 306 (72·1); potatoes, 137 (12·9); fruit, 216; grapes, 88; oats, 30; sorghum, 38; seed cotton, 14 (14·5); barley, 40; sunflower seeds, 27 (25·6); wine, 25; rice, 11 (3·2); tobacco, 29 (32).

Livestock, 1988: Cattle, 696,000 (including 284,000 milch cows); sheep, 1,525,000; goats, 1,076,000; pigs, 197,000; horses and mules, 176,000; poultry, 5m; beehives, 82,000.

Forestry. Forests covered 1,046,150 ha in 1988, mainly oak, elm, pine and birch. Some 40,000 ha per annum are afforested or improved. In 1988 171,000 cubic metres of sawn timber were produced.

Fisheries. The catch in 1988 was 4,000 tonnes.

INDUSTRY. Industry is nationalized, but since July 1990 individuals have been permitted to own craft businesses. Family members may work in these, but not hired labour. Output is small, and the principal industries are agricultural product processing, textiles, oil products and cement. Chemical and engineering industries are being built up.

Production. In 1988 (in 1,000 tonnes): Blister copper, 15; copper cable, 11·6; carbonic ferrochrome, 38·7; coke, 291; rolled steel, 96; phosphate fertilizer, 165; ammonium nitrate, 96; urea, 77; sulphuric acid, 81; caustic soda, 31; soda ash, 22; cement, 746; machinery (in 1m. lek) 496; 16,500 TV sets; 25,000 radio sets; 5·4m. pairs of footwear.

Labour. In 1988 the workforce was 811,000 (46·8% women), of whom 51·7% worked in agriculture, 22·9% in industry, 7% in building, 4·8% in trade, 4·5% in education and culture, 2·9% in transport and communications and 2·9% in the health service.

Minimum wages (450 leks per month in 1990) may not fall below one-third of maximum. Hours of labour: 8-hour day, 6-day week and 12 days yearly paid holiday. Retirement age is 60 for men and 55 for women. Wage increases of up to 20% were introduced in Oct. 1990. Average monthly wage, 1990: 570 leks.

FOREIGN ECONOMIC RELATIONS. Yugoslavia is Albania's main trading partner: in Nov. 1985 a 5-year agreement provided for a 20% increase in trade. Trade links with China were reestablished in 1983, and a 5-year agreement was signed in Dec. 1985. Foreign investment was legalized in Nov. 1990.

Commerce. Exports in 1988 totalled 2,709m. leks; imports, 3,218m. leks. In 1988 exports included 39·8% minerals, 16·1% plant and animal products, 8·7% processed foodstuffs, 7·3% electricity; imports: 28·5% machinery, 25·2% fuels and minerals, 14% plant and animal raw materials, 13·1% chemical products.

Share of export market in 1988: Czechoslovakia, 10%; Romania, 9·7%; Bulgaria, 9·4%; German Democratic Republic, 8·2%, Poland, 7·5%; Yugoslavia, 7·1%; Italy, 6·3%; Hungary, 5·9%; Austria, 5·4%; China, 5·1%.

Total trade between Albania and UK (British Department of Trade returns, in £1,000 sterling):

	1986	*1987*	*1988*	*1989*	*1990*
Imports to UK	129	91	2,764	605	413
Exports and re-exports from UK	2,887	2,565	1,126	1,957	4,542

Tourism. The right of Albanian citizens to apply for a passport was announced in May 1990.

COMMUNICATIONS

Roads. There were, in 1981, 21,000 km of roads suitable for motor traffic. The mountain districts of the north are still often inaccessible for wheeled vehicles. Motor vehicles in 1970: Cars, 3,500; lorries and buses, 11,000. Road traffic carried 77·29m. passengers in 1988; goods carried, 76·98m. tonnes. Private ownership of motor vehicles became legal in Feb. 1991.

Railways. Total length, in 1988 was 417 km. They comprise the lines from Durrës to Tirana, Vlorë, Ballsh, Korcë, Shkodër and across the Yugoslav border to Titograd. In 1990 the Milot-Klos line was completed. 10·97m. passengers and 7·66m. tonnes of freight were carried in 1988.

Aviation. There are regular scheduled flights from Tirana (Rinas Airport) to Belgrade, Bucharest, Budapest, Berlin and Zurich. Olympic Airways operate a weekly flight from Athens to Tirana. In 1990 Albania opened its air space to foreign commercial aircraft.

Shipping. In 1986 there were 20 ships totalling 56,133 GRT. The main ports are the Enver Hoxha Port of Durrës, Vlorë, Sarandë and Shëngjin. There is a ferry service from Trieste to Durrës. 1·1m. tonnes of freight were carried in 1988 (769,000 tonnes overseas).

Telecommunications. Number of post and telegraph offices (1988), 635; telephones (1990), 6,000. In 1987 there were 32 radio and 216 TV transmitting stations. Radio Tirana operates a foreign service in 18 languages. Radio receiving sets (1983), 210,000; television sets, 20,500. Regular television broadcasting began in 1971. There were 7 TV stations in 1984.

Cinemas and Theatres. In 1988 there were 106 cinemas with an attendance of 3·03m. and 28 theatres with an attendance of 1·84m. 14 full-length films were produced in 1980.

Newspapers and Books. In 1988 there were 42 newspapers with an annual circulation of 62·4m. and 74 periodicals. 1,018 book titles were published in 1981. There were 45 public libraries in 1988.

JUSTICE, RELIGION, EDUCATION AND WELFARE

Justice is administered by People's Courts. Minor crimes are tried by tribunals. Judges of the Supreme Court are elected by the People's Assembly for 4-year terms. The Office of the Procurator-General oversees the administration of justice. In 1983 an Investigator's Office was set up, separate from the Ministry of the Interior and answerable to the People's Assembly. A Ministry of Justice was re-established in 1990 and a Bar Council set up. In May 1990 capital offences were reduced from 34 to 11 and the death penalty abolished for women.

Religion. Albania is constitutionally an atheist state but in 1990 the ban on religious propaganda was lifted. In 1967 the Government closed all mosques and churches; they were permitted to re-open in 1990. For details of the situation before 1967 *see* THE STATESMAN'S YEAR-BOOK, 1969–70. The population had been 70% Moslem, 20% Orthodox and 10% Roman Catholic. There were 32 Roman Catholic priests in 1990.

Education. Primary education is free and compulsory in 8-year schools from 7 to 15 years. Secondary education is available in 12-year (general), technical-professional or lower vocational schools. Periods of productive work and military service are intermingled with full-time education. There were, in 1988, 3,251 nursery schools with 121,000 pupils and 5,299 teachers, 1,691 primary schools with 547,000 pupils (5,000 part-time) and 27,862 teachers, 485 secondary schools with 194,000 pupils (63,000 part-time) and 9,004 teachers (including 442 vocational secondary schools with 135,000 pupils and 7,221 teachers), and 8 tertiary institutions, with 25,000 students (5,000 part-time) and 1,659 lecturers. There were 19,953 (10,143 female) full-time students and 5,248 (2,524 female) part-time students in higher education in 1988, including 13,329 at the University of Tirana. An Albanian Academy was founded in 1972.

Welfare. 981m. leks were expended on pensions in 1988.

Health. Medical services are free, though medicines are charged for. In 1988 there were 158 hospitals with 12,350 beds. There were 5,497 doctors and dentists. In 1988 there were 3,210 out-patient clinics and 630 maternity homes.

DIPLOMATIC REPRESENTATIVE

Talks on the re-establishment of relations began in Dec. 1990 between Great Britain and Albania. Diplomatic relations were resumed between the USA and Albania on 15 March 1991.

Of Albania to the United Nations
Ambassador: Bashkim Pitarka.

Further Reading

Vjetari Statistikor i R.P.S. të Shqipërisë/Statistical Yearbook of P.S.R. of Albania, 1989 [In English and Albanian]. Tirana, 1989
35 vjet Shqipëri socialiste (statistical handbook). Tirana, 1979
History of the Labour Party of Albania 1966–1980. Tirana, 1981
Portrait of Albania. Tirana, 1982
Bertolino, J., *Albanie: la Citadelle de Staline*. Paris, 1979
Bland, W. B., *Albania*. [Bibliography] Oxford and Santa Barbara, 1988
Duro, I. and Hysa, R., *Albanian-English Dictionary*. Tirana, 1981
Halliday, J., (ed.) *The Artful Albanian: The Memoirs of Enver Hoxha*. London, 1986
Hetzer, A. and Roman, V. S. *Albania: A Bibliographic Research Survey*. Munich, 1983
Hoxha, E., *Speeches, Conversations and Articles, 1969–1970*. Tirana, 1980.—*The Khrushchevites: Memoirs*. Tirana, 1980.—*The Anglo-American Threat to Albania*. Tirana, 1982.—*Selected works*. Tirana, 1982.
Lendvai, P., *Das einsame Albanien*. Zurich, 1985
Logoreci, A., *The Albanians: Europe's Forgotten Survivors*. London, 1977
Marmullaku, R., *Albania and the Albanians*. London, 1975
Martin, N., *La Forteresse Albanaise: un Communisme National*. Paris, 1979
Pollo, S. and Arben, P., *The History of Albania*. London, 1981
Prifti, P. R., *Socialist Albania since 1944*. Cambridge, Mass., 1978
Schnytzer, A., *Stalinist Economic Strategy in Practice: The Case of Albania*. OUP, 1982

ALGERIA

Capital: Algiers
Population: 25·36m. (1990)
GNP per capita: US$2,450 (1988)

Al-Jumhuriya al-Jazairiya ad-Dimuqratiya ash-Shabiya

(People's Democratic Republic of Algeria)

HISTORY. On 1 Nov. 1954 the National Liberation Front (FLN) went over to open warfare against the French administration and armed forces. For details of history 1958–62 *see* p. 76 THE STATESMAN'S YEAR-BOOK, 1982–83. A cease-fire agreement was reached on 18 March 1962, and Gen. de Gaulle declared Algeria independent on 3 July 1962; the Republic was declared on 25 Sept. 1962.

The Government was overthrown by a junta of army officers which, on 19 June 1965, established a Revolutionary Council under Col. Houari Boumédienne.

AREA AND POPULATION. Algeria is bounded west by Morocco and Western Sahara, south-west by Mauritania and Mali, south-east by Niger, east by Libya and Tunisia, and north by the Mediterranean Sea. It has an area of 2,381,741 sq. km (919,595 sq. miles). Population (census 1987) 22,971,558; estimate (1990) 25·36m. (44·3% urban). Population density (1988), 10 per sq. km. Annual growth rate (averaged over 1985–90), 3·1%; infant mortality, 74 per 1,000; expectation of life, 62·5 years. Some 2m. Algerians live abroad.

In 1987, 49% lived in urban areas and 46% were under 15 years of age. 83% speak Arabic, 17% Berber; French is widely spoken. A law of Dec. 1990 makes Arabic the sole official language.

The populations (1987 Census) of the 48 *wilayat* were as follows:

Adrar	216,931	Mila	511,047
Ain Defla	536,205	Mostaganem	504,124
Ain Témouchent	271,454	M'Sila	605,578
Annaba (Bône)	453,951	Naâma	112,858
Batna	757,059	Ouahran (Oran)	916,578
al-Bayadh	155,494	Ouargla	286,696
Béchar	183,896	al-Oued	379,512
Béjaia (Bougie)	697,669	Oum al-Bouaghi	402,683
Biskra	429,217	Qacentina (Constantine)	662,330
Bordj Bou Arreridj	429,009	Relizane	545,061
Bouira	525,460	Saida	235,240
al-Boulaida (Blida)	704,462	Setif	997,482
Boumerdes	646,870	Sidi bel-Abbès	444,047
Cheliff (Orléansville)	679,717	Skikda	619,094
Djelfa	490,240	Souk Ahras	298,236
Guelma	353,329	Tamanrasset	94,219
Ghardaia	215,955	at-Tarf	276,836
Illizi	19,698	Tébessa	409,317
al-Jaza'ir (Algiers)	1,687,579	Tiaret	574,786
Jijel	471,319	Tindouf	16,339[1]
Khenchela	243,733	Tipaza	615,140
Laghouat	215,183	Tissemsilt	227,542
Mascara	562,806	Tizi-Ouzou	931,501
Médéa	650,623	Tlemcen	707,453

[1] Excluding Saharawi refugees (170,000 in 1988) in camps.

The capital is Algiers (1987 population, 1,507,000). Other major towns (with 1983 populations): Oran, 663,504; Constantine, 448,578; Annaba, 348,322; Blida,

191,314; Sétif, 186,978; Sidi-Bel-Abbès, 186,978; Tlemcen, 146,089; Skikda,141,159; Bejaia, 124,122; Batna, 122,788; al Asnam, 118,996; Tizi-Ouzou, 100,749; Médéa, 84,292.

CLIMATE. Coastal areas have a warm temperate climate, with most rain in winter, which is mild, while summers are hot and dry. Inland, conditions become more arid beyond the Atlas Mountains. Algiers. Jan. 54°F (12·2°C), July 76°F (24·4°C). Annual rainfall 30" (762 mm). Biskra. Jan. 52°F (11·1°C), July 93°F (33·9°C). Annual rainfall 6" (158 mm). Oran. Jan. 54°F (12·2°C), July 76°F (24·4°C). Annual rainfall 15" (376 mm).

CONSTITUTION AND GOVERNMENT. A Constitution was approved by referendum in Feb. 1989. There was a turnout of 83% and 92% of the voters approved of the constitutional reforms which included the beginning of the separation of the National Liberation Front (FLN) from the State in that the Prime Minister is to be responsible to the National Assembly rather than the FLN, the legalization of opposition parties and the omission of references to socialism.

The President of the Republic is Head of State, Head of the Armed Forces, and Head of Government. He is elected by universal suffrage for 5-year terms (renewable).

President of the Republic, General Secretary of the FLN, Minister of Defence: Bendjedid Chadli (sworn in 9 Feb. 1979, re-elected in 1984 and 1989).

The President appoints a Prime Minister and other Ministers, and presides over meetings of the Council of Ministers.

The Council of Ministers in Dec. 1990 consisted of:

Prime Minister: Mouloud Hamrouche.

Foreign Affairs: Sid-Ahmed Ghozali. *Interior:* Mohammed Saleh Mohammedi. *Defence:* Maj.-Gen. Khaled Nezzar. *Religious Affairs:* Said Chibane. *Economy:* Ghazi Hidouci. *Education:* Mohamed el-Mili Brahimi. *Youth:* Abdelkader Boudjemaa. *Justice:* Ali Benflis. *Social Affairs:* Mohamed Ghrib. *Equipment:* Cherif Rahmani. *Mines:* Saddek Boussena. *Transport:* Hassan Kahlouche. *Agriculture:* Abdelkader Bendaoud. *Public Health:* Akli Kheddis. *Posts and Telecommunications:* Hamid Sidi Said. *Ministers Delegate:* Benali Henni (*Local Authorities*), Abdessalem Ali-Rachedi (*Universities*), Abdennour Keramane (*Professional Training*), Smail Goumeziane (*Organization of Commerce*), Amar Kara Mohamed (*Employment*). *Secretary of State for Maghreb Affairs:* Abdelaziz Khellef. *Secretary-General of the Government:* Ahmed Medjhouda.

Legislative power is held by the National People's Assembly, whose 295 members were elected for a 5-year term by universal suffrage from the single list of the FLN who nominate 3 candidates for each single-member seat. Beginning in 1989 the political system was being liberalized. Proportional representation was adopted in March 1990. Elections were due in June 1991.

National flag: Vertically green and white, a red crescent and star over all in centre.

Local government: There are 48 provincial councils and 1,539 local authorities. At elections in June 1990 turn-out was 65%. The Islamic Salvation Front (FIS) gained control of 32 provincial and 853 local councils, the FLN of 14 and 487.

DEFENCE. Conscription is for a period of 6 months at the age of 19.

Army. The Army had a strength of 107,000 (70,000 conscripts) in 1991, organized in 3 armoured, 8 mechanized and 9 motorized brigades; 31 infantry, 4 paratroop, 5 artillery, 5 air defence and 4 engineer battalions; and 12 companies of desert troops. Equipment includes 113 T-34, 390 T-54/-55, 300 T-62 and 100 T-72 main battle tanks.

Navy. The Naval combatant force, largely supplied from the USSR, consists of 4 diesel powered patrol submarines, 3 frigates, 3 missile-armed corvettes, 11 fast missile craft, 11 fast patrol craft, 1 ocean minesweeper, 2 tank landing ships, and 1 tank landing craft. There are some 10 auxiliaries. An associated coastguard operates 16 fast cutters. Naval personnel in 1990 totalled 6,500. There are naval bases at Algiers, Annaba and Mers el Kebir.

Air Force. Five MiG-15 jet-fighters were delivered in 1962 as the nucleus of an Algerian Air Force. Since then many more aircraft of Soviet design have followed, and the Air Force had (1990) about 300 combat aircraft and 12,000 personnel. Training and technical assistance have been given by Egypt and the Soviet Union. There are 8 squadrons of MiG-21s, 3 squadrons of MiG-23 variable-geometry interceptors and fighter-bombers, 3 squadrons of Su-7 and Su-20 variable-geometry attack aircraft, 2 squadrons with MiG-25 fighter and reconnaissance aircraft, more than 40 Mi-24 assault helicopters and gunships, 17 C-130H Hercules, 3 F.27, 4 Il-76 and 6 An-12 transports, an Il-18 and a variety of smaller transports, a wing of 4 Mi-6, 30 Mi-8, about 30 Mi-4, 5 Puma, 6 Alouette III and 6 Hughes 269 helicopters, and training units equipped with CM.170 Magister armed jet counter-insurgency/trainers (20), 8 Beech Queen Air twin-engine/instrument trainers, MiG-15UTIs and MiG-17s, and two-seat versions of operational types. Surface-to-air missile units have Soviet-built 'Guidelines', 'Goas', 'Gainfuls' and 'Gaskins'.

INTERNATIONAL RELATIONS

Membership. Algeria is a member of UN, OAU, the Arab League and OPEC.

ECONOMY

Planning. The fourth development plan (1985–89) envisaged expenditure of DA 550,000m. primarily on housing, agriculture and water resources.

Budget. Administrative expenditure for 1988 was DA 63,000m.

Currency. The unit of currency is the *Algerian dinar* (DZD) of 100 *centimes*. There are in circulation banknotes of DA 5, 10, 50 and 100 and coins of 1, 2, 5, 20 and 50 centimes and DA 1, 5 and 10. Inflation was 9·2% in 1989. In March 1991, £1 = 31·01 DA; US$1 = 16·35 DA.

Banking and Finance. The Central Bank and bank of issue is the Banque Centrale d'Algérie. The *Governor* is Abderrahmane Hadj Nacer. Other banks operating in Algeria are Banque National d'Algérie, Crédit Populaire d'Algérie, Banque Extérieure d'Algérie, Caisse Algérienne de Développement, Banque Algérienne de Développement, Banque de l'Agriculture et du Développement.

Weights and Measures. The metric system is in use.

ENERGY AND NATURAL RESOURCES

Electricity. Production (1986) 12,410m. kwh. Supply 127 and 220 volts; 50 Hz.

Oil. Two large oilfields went into production in 1957 around Edjéle and Hassi Messaoud and in 1959 at El Gassi. In 1960 about 200 wells were productive. Natural gas was discovered at Djebel Berga in 1954 and at Hassi-R'Mel in 1956. Oil pipelines from Edjéle to Skirra (Tunisia) and from Hassi Messaoud to Béjaia, and a gas pipeline from Hassi Messaoud *via* Hassi-R'Mel to Mostaganem–Oran–Algiers, have been completed. Oil production in 1989, 52m. tonnes.

Gas. Production of natural gas in 1985 was 50,000m. cu. metres. Proven reserves are 3,700,000m. cu. metres.

Minerals. Algeria possesses deposits of iron, zinc, lead, mercury, silver, copper and antimony. Kaolin, marble and onyx, salt and coal are also found. Mineral output in 1985 (1,000 tonnes): Iron ore, 3,370; copper, 0·9; lead, 3·6; phosphates (1988), 1,207; barite, 100; clay, 58; sulphur, 10; zinc, 10; coal, 8.

Agriculture. The greater part of Algeria is of limited value for agricultural purposes. In the northern portion the mountains are generally better adapted to grazing and forestry than agriculture. There were an estimated 7·5m. ha of agricultural land in 1978–79, of which 6·8m. ha were arable, 200,000 ha under vine and 31·7m. ha pastures and brushlands. In 1987 the government sold back to the private sector land which had been nationalized on the declaration of independence in 1962; a further 0·5m. ha, expropriated in 1973, were returned to some 30,000 small landowners in 1990. There were 86,000 tractors and 9,000 combine harvesters in 1987.

The chief crops in 1988 were (in 1,000 tonnes): Wheat, 1,150; barley, 556; dates, 182; potatoes, 950; oranges, 190; mandarins and tangerines, 83; watermelons, 320; wine, 100; tomatoes, 490; olives, 170; onions, 175; oats, 58.

Livestock, 1988: 187,000 horses, 635,000 mules and asses, 361,000 cattle, 14,325,000 sheep, 3,570,000 goats and 130,000 camels.

Forestry. Forests cover 4·7m. ha or 2% of the land area. The greater part of the state forests are mere brushwood, but there are very large areas covered with cork-oak trees, Aleppo pine, evergreen oak and cedar. The dwarf-palm is grown on the plains, alfa on the table-land. Timber is cut for firewood, also for industrial purposes, for railway sleepers, telegraph poles, etc., and for bark for tanning. Considerable portions of the forest area are also leased for tillage, or for pasturage for cattle and sheep.

Fisheries. There are extensive fisheries for sardines, anchovies, sprats, tunny fish, etc., and also shellfish. Fish taken in 1986 amounted to 70,000 tonnes.

INDUSTRY. In 1981, 10·5m. tonnes of petroleum products were refined. Production of cement (1981) 4·45m. tonnes, crude steel (1988) 1,710,000 tonnes.

Labour. In 1989 the economically active population was estimated at 5·61m. In 1985 41% of the active population worked in services, 32·1% in industry and 26·9% in agriculture. Unemployment was 22% in 1989.

Trade Unions. The General Union of Algerian Workers (leader, Abdelhak Benhammouda) had in 1982 about 1m. members in 8 affiliated groups, while the National Union of Algerian Peasants had 700,000. The Islamic Federation of Trade Unions was formed in July 1990.

FOREIGN ECONOMIC RELATIONS. In Feb. 1990 Algeria signed a treaty of economic co-operation with the other countries of the Maghreb: Libya, Mauritania, Morocco and Tunisia.

Foreign debt was US$25,300m. in 1990.

Foreign investors are permitted to hold 100% of the equity of companies,and to repatriate all profits.

Commerce. The foreign trade of Algeria was as follows (in DA 1m.):

	1985	*1986*	*1987*	*1990 (estimate)*
Imports	49,491	43,415	34,196	US$10,500m.
Exports	64,564	36,890	39,000	US$13,200m.

Main trade partners in 1990, with percentages of total trade: France (exports, 13·5%; imports, 24·7%); Italy (20·3%; 14·5%); USA (18·8%; 9·3%); Federal Germany (7·4%; 9·5%). In 1988 oil and gas made up 94·7% of exports.

Total trade between Algeria and UK (British Department of Trade returns, in £1,000 sterling):

	1986	*1987*	*1988*	*1989*	*1990*
Imports to UK	140,860	172,927	159,748	177,546	259,959
Exports and re-exports from UK	129,624	73,115	86,615	74,368	73,831

Tourism. In 1986, there were 150,000 visitors.

COMMUNICATIONS

Roads. There were in 1986, 78,410 km of national highway including 45,070 km of concrete or bituminous roads. The mountainous regions are accessible only with difficulty. Motor vehicles in 1980 included 472,483 passenger cars and 283,966 commercial vehicles.

Railways. In 1988 there were 3,836 km of which 2,698 km is of 1,435mm gauge

(299 km electrified) and 1,138 km of 1,055mm gauge railway open for traffic. In 1989 the railways carried 12·06m. tonnes of freight and 52·5m. passengers.

Aviation. There are 5 international airports as well as another 65 airfields controlled by government and 135 owned by petroleum companies. Air Algeria serves the main Algerian cities, and an international network. Algeria is also served by Swissair, Royal Air Maroc and United Arab Airline. In 1980 the airports handled 2·84m. passengers and 22,479 tonnes of freight. In May 1990 the Maghreb countries (Algeria, Libya, Mauritania, Morocco and Tunisia) agreed to merge their national airlines into Air Maghreb.

Shipping. In 1982, 69·4m. tonnes of goods were handled at Algerian ports.

A state shipping line, Compagnie Nationale Algérienne de Navigation, was formed in Jan. 1964.

Telecommunications. There were, in 1980, 1,534 post offices; number of telephones (1985), 769,000. In 1982 *Radiodiffusion Télévision Algérienne* broadcast in Arabic, French and Kabyle (Berber) from 16 radio stations to (1986) 3·3m. radio receivers and from 16 television stations to about (1986) 1·54m. receivers.

Newspapers (1989). There were 6 daily newspapers, with a combined circulation of 1m.

JUSTICE, RELIGION, EDUCATION AND WELFARE

Justice. There are appeal courts at Algiers, Constantine and Oran; and in the *arrondissements* are 17 courts of first instance. There are also commercial courts and justices of the peace with extensive powers. Criminal justice is organized as in France. The Supreme Court is at the same time Council of State and High Court of Appeal.

Religion. Virtually the whole population are Sunni Moslems. There are about 150,000 Christians, mainly Roman Catholic.

Education. Literacy was some 54% in 1987. In 1987 there were 11,692 state primary schools with 133,250 teachers and 3,625,000 pupils; 1,900 secondary schools with 95,000 teachers and 1,877,000 pupils; and 71 technical and teacher-training colleges with 2,528 teachers and (1982) 12,903 students in technical education and 1,124 teachers and 13,315 students in teacher-training.

In 1981 there were 72,200 students in higher education including universities at Algiers (with 17,086 students), Oran (9,000), Constantine (8,340), Annaba (6,126), Sétif (5,800) and Boumerdes. There are also Universities of Science and Technology at Algiers (11,500) and Oran (5,800) and university centres at Tlemcen, Tizi-Ouzou, Batna, Tiaret, Constantine, Mostaganem, Sidi-Bel-Abbés and Boulaida.

Health. There were in 1986, 49,280 hospital beds; there were 15,361 doctors. There were also 1,422 dispensaries and consulting rooms, 747 health centres and 175 specializing centres for tuberculosis, venereal disease and trachoma in 1980.

DIPLOMATIC REPRESENTATIVES

Of Algeria in Great Britain (54 Holland Park, London, W11 3RS)
Ambassador: Abdelkrim Gheraieb.

Of Great Britain in Algeria (Résidence Cassiopée, 7 Chemin des Glycines, Algiers)
Ambassador: C. C. R. Battiscombe.

Of Algeria in the USA (2118 Kalorama Rd., NW, Washington, D.C., 20008)
Ambassador: Abderrahmane Bensid.

Of the USA in Algeria (4 Chemin Cheich Bachir Ibrahimi, Algiers)
Ambassador: Christopher W. S. Ross.

Of Algeria to the United Nations
Ambassador: Hocine Djoudi.

Further Reading

Statistical Information: The Service de Statistique Générale publishes the annual *Statistique Générale de l'Algérie, Documents statistiques sur le commerce de l'Algérie* (from 1902).

Ageron, C.-R., *A History of Modern Algeria*. London, 1988
Bennoune, M., *The Making of Contempory Algeria, 1830–1987*. CUP, 1988
Horne, A., *A Savage War of Peace: Algeria 1954–1962*. London, 1977
Knapp, W., *North West Africa: A Political and Economic Survey*. OUP, 1977
Lawless, R. I., *Algeria*. [Bibliography] Oxford and Santa Barbara, 1981

ANDORRA

Capital: Andorra-la-Vella
Population: 51,400 (1988)

Principat d'Andorra

HISTORY. The political status of Andorra was regulated by the *Paréage* of 1278 which placed Andorra under the joint suzerainty of the Comte de Foix and of the Bishop of Urgel. The rights vested in the house of Foix passed by marriage to that of Bearn and, on the accession of Henri IV, to the French crown.

AREA AND POPULATION. The co-principality of Andorra is situated in the eastern Pyrenees on the French–Spanish border. The country consists of gorges, narrow valleys and defiles, surrounded by high mountain peaks varying between 1,880 and 3,000 metres. Its maximum length is 30 km and its width 20 km; it has an area of 468 sq. km (181 sq. miles) and a population (census, 1986) of 46,976 (65% urban); estimate (1988) 51,400, scattered in 7 parishes (*parròquia*). The chief towns (1986) are Andorra-la-Vella, the capital (15,639) and its suburb Escaldes-Engordany (11,955).

Catalan is the official language and was spoken by 30% of the population in 1986 but 59% spoke Spanish and 6% French.

CLIMATE. Escaldes-Engordany. Jan. 36°F (2·3°C), July 67°F (19·3°C). Annual rainfall 32" (808 mm).

CONSTITUTION AND GOVERNMENT. Sovereignty is exercised jointly by the President of the French Republic and the Bishop of Urgel. The co-princes are represented in Andorra by the *'Viguier français'* and the *'Viguier Episcopal'*. Each co-prince has set up a Permanent Delegation for Andorran affairs; the Prefect of the Eastern Pyrenees is the French Permanent Delegate.

The valleys pay every second year a due of 960 francs to France and 460 pesetas to the bishop.

The *General Council of the Valleys* is an elected assembly which submits motions and proposals to the Permanent Delegations. Its 28 members are elected for 4 years; half of the council is renewed every 2 years. The Council nominates as its Chairman a First Syndic from among its members and a Second Syndic from outside. In 1982 an *Executive Council* was appointed and legislative and executive powers were separated. Elections to the General Council were held in Dec. 1989. Electorate, 7,185 (most residents are classified as 'foreign' and ineligible to vote). Turn-out was 80%.

First Syndic: Albert Gelabert (elected 15 Feb. 1991).
Head of Government: Oscar Ribas Reig.
Finance, Commerce and Industry: Jaume Bartumeu Cassany. *Agriculture and Natural Heritage:* Guillem Benazet Riba. *Public Works:* Joan Santamaria Tarre. *Tourism and Sport:* Candid Naudi Mora. *Labour and Social Welfare:* Antui Armengol Aleix.

National flag: Three vertical strips of blue, yellow, red, with the arms of Andorra in the centre.

INTERNATIONAL RELATIONS. Andorra's foreign affairs are conducted by France.

ECONOMY

Budget. In 1986 the budget balanced at 6,655m. pesetas.

Currency. French and Spanish currency are both in use.

ENERGY AND NATURAL RESOURCES

Electricity. Production (1986) 140m. kwh. Andorra imported another 200m. kwh from Spain.

Agriculture. In 1988 there were some 1,000 ha of arable land, 10,000 ha of forests and 25,000 ha of pasture. In 1981, 472 tonnes of potatoes and 264 tonnes of tobacco were produced.

Livestock (1982): 9,000 sheep, 1,115 cattle, 217 horses.

FOREIGN ECONOMIC RELATIONS. Andorra is a member of the EEC Customs Union for industrial goods, and a third country for agricultural produce.

Commerce. In 1986, imports amounted to 74,313m. pesetas (42% from Spain and 27% from France) and exports to 2,325m. pesetas (54% to France and 33% to Spain).

Total trade between Andorra and UK (British Department of Trade returns, in £1,000 sterling):

	1988	*1989*	*1990*
Imports to UK	46	236	9
Exports and re-exports from UK	10,780	10,493	15,763

Tourism. Tourism is the main industry, and over 6m. people visited Andorra in 1982.

COMMUNICATIONS

Roads. There are 220 km of roads (120 km paved). A good road connects the Spanish and French frontiers by way of Sant Julia, Andorra-la-Vella, Escaldes-Engordany, Encamp, Canillo and Soldeu: it crosses the Col d'Envalira (2,400 metres). Another road connects Andorra-la-Vella with La Massana and Ordino. Motor vehicles (1983) 24,789.

Aviation. The nearest airports are at Seo de Urgel, Barcelona and Perpignan.

Telecommunications. Number of telephones (1982) 17,719. Number of receivers (1986), radio, 8,000; TV, 4,000.

JUSTICE, RELIGION, EDUCATION AND WELFARE

Justice. Judicial power is exercised in civil matters in the first instance, according to the plaintiff's choice, by either the *Bayle Français* or the *Bayle Episcopal*, who are nominated by the respective co-princes. The judge of appeal is nominated alternately for 5 years by each co-prince; the third instance *(Tercera Sala)* is either the supreme court of Andorra at Perpignan or the supreme court of the Bishop at Urgel.

Criminal justice is administered by the *Corts* consisting of the 2 Viguiers, the judge of appeal, 2 *rahonadors* elected by the general council of the valleys, a general attorney and an attorney nominated for 5 years alternatively by each of the co-princes. The accused may be assisted by a barrister.

Religion. The prevailing religious denomination is Roman Catholic.

Education. In 1986–87 there were 1,866 pupils at infant schools, 3,458 at primary schools, 3,271 at secondary schools, 230 at technical schools and 46 at special schools.

Health. In 1988 there were 112 doctors and 113 hospital beds.

Further Reading

Corts Peyret, J., *Geografia e Historia de Andorra*. Barcelona, 1945
Llobet, S., *El medio y la vida en Andorra*. Barcelona, 1947
Riberaygua-Argelich, B., *Les Valls d'Andorra*. Barcelona, 1946

ANGOLA

Capital: Luanda
Population: 10·02m. (1990)
GNP per capita: US$500 (1985)

República Popular de Angola

HISTORY. The first Europeans to arrive in Angola were the Portuguese in 1482, and the first settlers arrived there in 1491. Luanda was founded in 1575. Apart from a brief period of Dutch occupation from 1641 to 1648, Angola remained a Portuguese colony until 11 June 1951, when it became an Overseas Province of Portugal. On 11 Nov. 1975 Angola became fully independent as the People's Republic of Angola. The People's Liberation Movement of Angola (MPLA) and the National Union for the Total Independence of Angola (UNITA) committed themselves to putting their rival claims to power to a popular vote, but the agreement broke down in battles which left MPLA in control of the capital and the other factions banished to the countryside. In 1990 MPLA and UNITA began peace talks.

AREA AND POPULATION. Angola is bounded by Congo on the north, Zaïre on the north and north-east, Zambia on the east, Namibia on the south and the Atlantic ocean on the west. The area is 1,246,700 sq. km (481,351 sq. miles) including the 7,107 sq. km province of Cabinda, an enclave of territory separated by 30 km of Zaïre. The population at census, 1970, was 5,646,166, of whom 14% urban. Estimate (1990) 10,015,000, including (in 1988) 114,000 in Cabinda. Urban population (1986) 30% of whom 38% speak Umbundu, 27% Kimbundu, 13% Lunda and 11% Kikongo. Portuguese remains the official language. There were (1986) about 30,000 Europeans (mostly Portuguese) in Angola. Refugees living in Angola totalled 90,458 (1988) of whom 69,000 were Namibians.

The most important towns (with 1970 populations) are Luanda, the capital (480,613; 1988, 1·2m.), Huambo (61,885), Lobito (59,258), Benguela (40,996), Lubango (31,674; 1984, 105,000), Malange (31,559) and Namibe (formerly Moçâmedes, 23,145; 1981, 100,000).

CLIMATE. The climate is tropical, with low rainfall in the west but increasing inland. Temperatures are constant over the year and most rain falls in March and April. Luanda. Jan. 78°F (25·6°C), July 69°F (20·6°C). Annual rainfall 13" (323 mm). Lobito. Jan. 77°F (25°C), July 68°F (20°C). Annual rainfall 14" (353 mm).

CONSTITUTION AND GOVERNMENT. Under the Constitution adopted at independence, the sole legal party is the MPLA. In Dec. 1990, however, MPLA announced that the Constitution would be revised to permit opposition parties by March 1991. The supreme organ of state is the unicameral National People's Assembly, whose members were first elected in Aug. 1980 for a 3-year term. In 1987 the Assembly had 206 members. There is an executive President elected for renewable terms of 5 years, who appoints a Council of Ministers to assist him.

Substantial parts of the country are, however, under the control of the anti-government forces of UNITA.

The Council of Ministers in Nov. 1990 was as follows:

President: José Eduardo dos Santos (re-elected 9 Dec. 1985).

Ministers of State: Zeferino Kassa Yombo *(Petroleum and Energy)*, Kundi Paihama *(Inspection and Control, State Security)*.

Planning: António Henriques da Silva. *Defence:* Col.-Gen. Pedro Maria Tonha (Pedalé). *External Relations:* Lieut.-Col. Pedro de Castro Van-Dúnem. *Justice:* Fernando José França Van-Dúnem. *Education:* Augusto Lopes Teixeira (Tutu). *Health:* Flavio João Fernandes. *Finance:* Augusto Teixeira de Matos. *Foreign Trade:* Domingo das Chagas Simoes Rangel. *Internal Trade:* Joaquim Guerreiro

Dias. *Industry:* Henrique de Carvalho dos Santos (Onambwe). *Transport and Communications:* Carlos António Fernandes. *Labour and Social Security:* Diogo Jorge de Jesus. *Agriculture:* Fernando Faustino Muteka. *Interior:* Francisco Magalhaes Paiva. *Construction:* João Henriques Garcia. *Fisheries:* José Ramos da Cruz.

Flag: Horizontally red over black, with a star and an arc of cogwheel crossed by a machete, all yellow over all in the centre.

Local government: Angola is divided into 18 provinces divided into 139 districts – (Cabinda, Zaïre, Uíge, Luanda, Cuanza Norte, Cuanza Sul, Malange, Lunda Norte, Lunda Sul, Benguela, Huambo, Bié, Moxico, Cuando-Cubango, Namibe, Huíla, Cunene and Bengo) each under a Provincial Commissioner, appointed by the President and an elected legislative of from 55 to 85 members.

DEFENCE. Conscription is for a period of 2 years.

Army. The Army has 70 brigades, each with infantry, tank, armoured personnel carriers, artillery and anti-aircraft units; and 10 SAM batteries. Total strength (1990) 91,500. Equipment includes Soviet 100 T-34, 300 T-54/55 and more than 100 T-62 and PT-76 tanks.

Navy. 20 Portuguese naval craft were transferred on independence in 1975 of which most have been discarded, and 9 vessels were acquired from the Soviet Navy in 1977-79. There are 6 fast missile boats, 5 fast torpedo boats, 9 inshore patrol boats, 2 mine-hunters, 2 landing ships and 11 landing craft, and 11 auxiliary vessels. Naval personnel in 1990 totalled 1,500.

Air Force. The Angolan People's Air Force (FAPA) was formed in 1976. The combat force has been expanded since 1983 with Soviet assistance. It included (1989) 50 MiG-21, 30 MiG-23 and 40 Su-22 fighters, plus 25 Mi-24 and 6 Gazelle gunships. (The MiG-17 is being withdrawn from service.) There are 10 An-2, 20 An-26, 12 Islander, 4 Turbo-Porter, 8 Aviocar and 2 F.27 transports, 2 Embraer EMB-111 maritime surveillance aircraft, 4 PC-9,12 PC-7 and 3 MiG-15UTI trainers, and 40 Mi-8, 15 Mi-17, 6 Dauphin, 2 Lama and 40 Alouette III helicopters. Personnel (1990) 7,000.

INTERNATIONAL RELATIONS

Membership. Angola is a member of the UN, OAU and is an ACP state of the EEC.

ECONOMY

Policy. Reforms are in train to introduce a market economy and restore private property.

Budget. The 1986 budget included 90,400m. kwanza for capital and current expenditure and revenue at 78,500m. kwanza.

Currency. The unit of currency is the *kwanza* (AOK) of 100 *lwei*. Coins are of 50 *lwei*, 1, 2, 5, 10 and 20 *kwanza*; notes are of 20, 50, 100, 500 and 1,000 *kwanza*. In March 1991, £1 = 59·39 *kwanza*; US$1 = 31·31 *kwanza*.

Banking and Finance. All banking was nationalized in 1975. The *Banco Nacional de Angola* is the central bank and bank of issue, while the *Banco Popular de Angola* handles all commercial activities throughout the country.

Weights and Measures. The metric system is in force.

ENERGY AND NATURAL RESOURCES

Electricity. Production (1986) totalled 851m. kwh, mainly hydro-electricity. In Nov. 1984 an agreement was signed with Brazil and USSR to construct a hydro-electric plant at Kapanda on the river Kwanza, 250 miles south of Luanda.

Oil. Total production (1989) about 24m. tonnes.

Minerals. Production of diamonds during 1985 totalled 625,000 carats. Production (1985) of salt, 10,000 tonnes. There has been no production of iron ore since 1975, but the mines at Kassinga were restarted in 1985. Phosphate mining commenced in the north in 1981. Manganese and copper deposits exist.

Agriculture. The principal cash crops (with 1988 production, in 1,000 tonnes): Sugar-cane (330), coffee (15), bananas (280), palm oil (40), palm kernels (12), seed cotton (33); others include tobacco, citrus fruit and sisal. Food crops comprise cassava (1,980), maize (270), sweet potatoes (180) and dry beans (40).

Livestock (1988): 3·4m. cattle, 265,000 sheep, 975,000 goats, 480,000 pigs.

Forestry. In 1988 there were 53·1m. ha of forests, representing 43% of the land area. Mahogany and other hardwoods are exported, chiefly from the tropical rain forests of the north, especially Cabinda. Production (1986) 10m. cu. metres.

Fisheries. Total catch (1984) 70,700 tonnes.

INDUSTRY. In 1985, 10,000 tonnes of steel were produced and 350,000 tonnes of cement.

FOREIGN ECONOMIC RELATIONS. In 1988 foreign debt was sone US$6,000m.

Commerce. Imports and exports for 4 calendar years in 1m. Kwanza.

	1982	*1983*	*1984* [1]	*1985* [1]
Imports	25,946	20,197	19,448	41,240
Exports	48,736	54,508	60,112	59,280

[1] Provisional.

The chief imports are textiles, transport equipment, foodstuffs, pig-iron and steel; chief exports are crude oil, coffee, diamonds, sisal, fish, maize, palm-oil. In 1983, crude petroleum represented 85% of exports, petroleum products, 5·6%, coffee 3·9% and diamonds 5·6%. In 1985 Portugal provided 13% of imports, France 12%, the USA 11%, and Brazil 11%, while 45% of exports went to the USA, 14% to Spain and 11% (all diamonds) to the Bahamas.

Total trade between Angola and UK (British Department of Trade returns, in £1,000 sterling):

	1987	*1988*	*1989*	*1990*
Imports to UK	2,312	10,036	1,286	5,142
Exports and re-exports from UK	29,573	20,154	24,785	29,284

COMMUNICATIONS

Roads. There were, in 1986, 73,830 km of roads, and in 1984, 56,625 cars and 29,000 commercial vehicles.

Railways. The length of railways open for traffic in 1987 was 2,952 km comprising 2,798 km of 1,067 mm gauge and 154 km of 600 mm gauge. The Benguela Railway runs from Lobito to the Zaïre border at Dilolo where it connects with the National Railways of Zaïre. Other lines link Luanda with Malange; Gunza with Gabela; and Namibe with Menongue. In 1986 Angola's railways carried 4·1m. passengers and 2·5m. tonnes of freight.

Aviation. Luanda had international air links to Lisbon, Rome, Paris, Moscow, Budapest, Brazzaville, Saõ Tomé, Lusaka, Maputo, Sal (Cape Verde Islands), Havana, Kinshasa, Libreville, Berlin, Tripoli, Lagos, Algiers, Niamey, Sofia, Malta, Rio de Janeiro and São Paulo, but most were inoperative during the civil war.

Shipping. In 1975, 2·85m. tonnes were discharged and 16m. tonnes loaded in Angolan ports. In 1986 there were 100 merchant vessels (over 100 GRT) totalling 127,000 GRT.

Telecommunications. Angola is connected by cable with east, west and south African telegraph systems. There were, in 1973, 1,808 km of telegraph lines, 77 telephone stations (with 40,000 instruments in 1982), 162 telegraph stations and 31 wireless stations.

Rádio Nacional de Angola is the largest of the 18 stations operating on medium- and short-waves. *Rádio Nacional* transmits 3 programmes as well as operating 2 regional stations. Number of radio receivers (1988) 1·2m. and television receivers 200,000.

Cinemas. There were, in 1972, 47 cinemas with seating capacity of 35,142.

Newspaper. The national daily newspaper is *Jornal de Angola*, with a circulation of 41,000 in 1988.

JUSTICE, RELIGION, EDUCATION AND WELFARE

Justice. The Supreme Court and Court of Appeal are in Luanda.

Religion. Article 7 of the Constitution of the People's Republic of Angola states that: 'The People's Republic of Angola is a secular state, where there is a complete separation of religious institutions from the state'. All religions will be respected.

In 1988 there were 8·45m. Christians, the remainder following traditional animist religion.

Education. In 1983 there were 2·4m. pupils in primary schools, 153,000 in secondary schools and 4,746 students in higher education. The *Universidade de Angola* (founded 1963) at Luanda with faculties at Huambo and Lubango, had 3,500 students in 1982.

Health. In 1980 there were 436 doctors and 20,700 hospital beds and in 1973, 87 pharmacists, 284 midwives and 3,115 nursing personnel.

DIPLOMATIC REPRESENTATIVES

Of Angola in Great Britain (10 Fife Road, London, SW14)
Ambassador: Luis Neto-Kiambata.

Of Great Britain in Angola (Rua Diogo Cão, 4, Luanda)
Ambassador: J. G. Flynn.

Of Angola to the United Nations
Ambassador: Manuel Pedro Pacavlra.

Further Reading

Anuário Estatistico de Angola. Luanda, from 1897
Araújo, A. Correia de, *Aspectos do desenvolvimento económico e social de Angola*. Lisbon, 1964
Bender, G. J., *Angola under the Portuguese: Myth and Reality*. London, 1979
Bhagavan, M. R., *Angola's Political Economy 1975–1985*. Uppsala, 1986
Davidson, B., *In the Eye of the Storm*. London, 1972
Marcrum, J., *The Angolan Revolution*. (2 vols.) MIT Press, 1969 and 1978
Somerville, K., *Angola: Politics, Economics and Society*. London and Boulder, 1986
Wheeler, D. L. and Pélissier, R., *Angola*. London, 1971

ANGUILLA

Capital: The Valley
Population: 7,019 (1989)

HISTORY. Anguilla was probably given its name by the Spaniards because of its eel-like shape. After British settlements in the 17th century, the territory was administered as part of the Leeward Islands. From 1825 it became more closely associated with St Kitts and ultimately incorporated in the colony of St Kitts-Nevis-Anguilla. Opposition to this association grew and finally in 1967 the island seceded unilaterally. Following direct intervention by the UK in 1969 Anguilla became *de facto* a separate dependency of Britain; and this was formalized on 19 Dec. 1980 under the Anguilla Act 1980. A new Constitution came into effect in April 1982.

AREA AND POPULATION. Anguilla is the most northerly of the Leeward Islands, some 70 miles (112 km) to the north-west of St Kitts and 5 miles (8 km) to the north of St Martin/St Maarten. The territory also comprises the island of Sombrero and several other off-shore islets or cays. The total area of the territory is about 60 sq. miles (155 sq. km). Census population (1984) was 6,987. Estimate, 1989, 7,019. The capital is The Valley.

CONSTITUTION AND GOVERNMENT. The House of Assembly consists of a Speaker, 7 elected members, 2 nominated members and 2 official members.

Executive power is vested in the Governor who is appointed by HM The Queen. Apart from his special responsibilities (External Affairs, Defence, Internal Security, including the Police, and the Public Service) and his reserve powers in respect of legislation, the Governor discharges his executive powers on the advice of an Executive Council comprising a Chief Minister, 3 Ministers and 2 official members: Attorney-General and Permanent Secretary, Finance.

Governor: B. G. J. Canty.
Chief Minister: Emile Gumbs.

ECONOMY

Budget. In 1989, the budget was: Expenditure EC$26·76m.; revenue EC$28·2m. Anguilla finances its recurrent budget and a small part of its capital budget but for the most part aid for capital projects comes from UK and other donors.

Currency. The currency is the Eastern Caribbean *dollar*.

ENERGY AND NATURAL RESOURCES

Electricity. Production (1988) 4m. kwh.

Agriculture. Because of low rainfall agriculture potential is limited. Main crops are pigeon peas, corn and sweet potatoes. Livestock consists of sheep, goats, cattle and poultry.

Fisheries. Fishing is a thriving industry with exports to neighbouring islands.

FOREIGN ECONOMIC RELATIONS

Commerce. Total trade between Anguilla and UK (British Department of Trade returns, in £1,000 sterling):

	1987	*1988*	*1989*	*1990*
Imports to UK	188	68	1,402	122
Exports and re-exports from UK	1,328	1,372	1,952	1,853

Tourism. There are a few hotels of international standing and others are under construction. There are also several locally-owned hotels, guest houses and apartments. In 1988 there were 69,482 tourists, of which 41,275 were day visitors.

COMMUNICATIONS

Roads. There are about 43 miles of tarred roads and 25 miles of secondary roads. In 1985 there were 973 passenger cars and 239 commercial vehicles.

Aviation. There is a 3,600 ft surfaced runway at Wallblake Airport. Apart from regular air taxi and charter flights WINAIR (subsidiary of ALM) provides daily scheduled services between Juliana International Airport, St Martin and Anguilla. WINAIR, LIAT and American Eagle operate direct flights from San Juan, Puerto Rico. Air BVI flies from Tortola and St Thomas to Anguilla.

Shipping. The main seaports are Road Bay and Blowing Point, the latter serving passenger and cargo traffic to and from St Martin.

Telecommunications. There is a modern internal telephone service with (1986–87) 1,825 exchange lines; and international telegraph, telex and telephone services, all operated by Cable & Wireless. In 1986 there were 2,200 radio receivers.

Newspapers. In 1988 there was 1 daily newspaper.

RELIGION, EDUCATION AND WELFARE

Religion. There were in 1988 Anglicans, Roman Catholics, Methodists, Seventh Day Adventists, Church of God and Baptists.

Education. There are 6 government primary schools with (1989) 1,290 pupils and 1 comprehensive school with (1989) 883 pupils. Tertiary education is provided at regional universities and similar institutions.

Health. There is a 24-bed cottage hospital, clinics and a modern dental clinic. There were (1987) 4 doctors and 1 dentist.

Further Reading

Petty, C. L., *Anguilla: Where there's a Will, there's a Way.* Anguilla, 1984

ANTIGUA AND BARBUDA

Capital: St John's
Population: 85,000 (1990)
GNP per capita: US$ 2,800 (1988)

HISTORY. Antigua was discovered by Colombus in 1493 and named by him after a church in Seville (Spain). It was first colonized by English settlers in 1632; nearby Barbuda was colonized in 1661 from Antigua. Formed part of the Leeward Islands Federation from 1871 until 30 June 1956, when Antigua became a separate Crown Colony, which was part of the West Indies Federation from 3 Jan. 1958 until 31 May 1962. It became an Associated State of the UK on 27 Feb. 1967 and obtained independence on 1 Nov. 1981.

AREA AND POPULATION. Antigua and Barbuda comprises 3 islands of the Lesser Antilles situated in the Eastern Caribbean with a total land area of 442 sq. km (171 sq. miles); it consists of Antigua (280 sq. km), Barbuda, 40 km to the north (161 sq. km) and uninhabited Redonda, 40 km to the southwest (1 sq. km).

The population at the Census of 7 April 1970 was 65,525. In 1990 the estimated population was 85,000 of whom 31·8% were urban. 1,500 lived in Barbuda in 1986. The chief towns are St John's, the capital on Antigua (30,000 inhabitants in 1982) and Codrington, the only settlement on Barbuda.

CLIMATE. A tropical climate, but drier than most West Indies islands. The hot season is from May to Nov., when rainfall is greater. Mean annual rainfall is 40" (1,000 mm).

CONSTITUTION AND GOVERNMENT. H.M. Queen Elizabeth, as Head of State, is represented by a Governor-General appointed by her on the advice of the Prime Minister. There is a bicameral legislature, comprising a 17-member Senate appointed by the Governor-General and a 17-member House of Representatives elected by universal suffrage for a 5-year term. The Governor-General appoints a Prime Minister and, on the latter's advice, other members of the Cabinet.

Governor-General: Sir Wilfred Ebenezer Jacobs, GCMG, GCVO, OBE, QC.

Prime Minister and Finance: Right Hon. Vere C. Bird, Sen., PC.

Deputy Prime Minister, Foreign Affairs, Economic Development, Tourism and Energy: Lester Bryant Bird. *Finance:* John E. St Luce. *Attorney-General and Minister of Legal Affairs:* Keith B. Ford. *Public Utilities and Aviation:* Robin Yearwood. *Agriculture, Fisheries, Lands and Housing:* Hillroy Humphries. *Home Affairs:* Christopher Manasseh O'Mard. *Education, Culture and Youth Affairs:* Reuben H. Harris. *Labour and Health:* Adolphus Eleazer Freeland. *Trade, Industry and Commerce:* Hugh Marshall. *Public Works and Communications:* Eustace Cochrane. *Ministers without Portfolio:* Donald Christian, Donald Shepherd, Hugh Marshall, Henderson Simon, Molwyn Joseph.

At the general elections held on 17 April 1984, the ruling Antigua Labour Party won all 16 seats on Antigua and there was one independent (representing Barbuda).

Flag: Red, with a triangle based on the top edge, divided horizontally black, blue, white, with a rising sun in gold on the black portion.

DEFENCE. The defence force has a strength of about 700. A coastguard service has been formed.

INTERNATIONAL RELATIONS

Membership. Antigua and Barbuda is a member of UN, the Commonwealth, CARICOM and is an ACP state of the EEC.

ECONOMY

Budget. The budget for 1988 envisaged revenue at EC$217m. and expenditure of EC$231·7m.

Currency. The unit of currency is the *Eastern Caribbean dollar* (XCD). In March 1991, £1 = EC$5·12; US$1 = EC$2·70.

Banking. Barclays Bank International, Royal Bank of Canada, Canadian Imperial Bank of Commerce, the Virgin Islands National Bank, the Antilles International Trust Co. and the Bank of Nova Scotia have branches at St John's. There is also the Antigua Co-operative Bank and a government savings bank.

ENERGY AND NATURAL RESOURCES

Electricity. Production (1986) 63·8m. kwh.

Agriculture. Cotton and fruits are the main crops. Production (1988) of fruits, 10,000 tonnes. There were 70,000 tonnes of cotton produced in 1985.

Livestock (1988): Cattle, 18,000; pigs, 4,000; sheep, 13,000; goats, 13,000.

Fisheries. Catch (1983) 1,013 tonnes.

INDUSTRY. An oil refinery was opened in 1982. Manufactures include toilet tissue, stoves, refrigerators, blenders, fans, garments and rum (molasses imported from Guyana).

Labour. In 1985 the workforce numbered 32,254, and there was 21% unemployment.

FOREIGN ECONOMIC RELATIONS

Commerce. Imports in 1984 amounted to EC$356·1m. and exports to EC$47·5m. of which the major amount came from bunkering provided to ships. The main trading partners were the USA, the UK and Canada.

Total trade between Antigua and Barbuda and UK (British Department of Trade returns, in £1,000 sterling):

	1987	*1988*	*1989*	*1990*
Imports to UK	4,271	10,845	3,447	2,931
Exports and re-exports from UK	19,334	20,755	23,954	17,980

Tourism. There were 149,000 tourists (excluding cruise passengers) in 1986.

COMMUNICATIONS

Roads. There are 600 miles of roads (150 miles main road). In 1985 there were 10,000 passenger cars and 15,000 commercial vehicles.

Aviation. There is an international airport (V. C. Bird) on Antigua, and a small airstrip at Codrington on Barbuda.

Shipping. The main harbour is the St John's deep water harbour. There are 2 tugs for the berthing of ships and all modern and efficient general cargo handling equipment. The harbour can also accommodate 3 large cruise ships simultaneously.

Telecommunications. In 1983 there were 10,470 telephones. In 1983 there were 20,000 radios and 17,000 television sets.

RELIGION, EDUCATION AND WELFARE

Religion. The vast majority of the population are Christian, preponderantly Anglican.

Education. In 1985 there were 10,551 pupils and 436 teachers in 48 primary schools, and 5,106 pupils and 304 teachers in (1983) 16 secondary schools.

Health. There is a general hospital (Holberton) with 215 beds, a mental hospital with 200 beds, a geriatric unit with 150 beds, 4 health centres and 16 dispensaries.

DIPLOMATIC REPRESENTATIVES

Of Antigua and Barbuda in Great Britain (15 Thayer St., London, W1M 5LD)
High Commissioner: James A. E. Thomas.

Of Great Britain in Antigua and Barbuda (38 St Mary's St., St John's)
High Commissioner: E. T. Davies, CMG (resides in Bridgetown).

Of Antigua and Barbuda in the USA (3400 International Dr., NW, Washington, D.C., 20008)
Ambassador: Edmund Hawkins Lake.

Of the USA in Antigua and Barbuda (FPO Miami 34054, St. Johns)
Ambassador: (Vacant)

Of Antigua and Barbuda to the United Nations
Ambassador: Lionel Alexander Hurst.

Further Reading

Dyde, B., *Antigua and Barbuda: The Heart of the Caribbean.* London, 1986

ARGENTINA

Capital: Buenos Aires
Population: 32·69m. (1990)
GNP per capita: US$2,640 (1988)

República Argentina

HISTORY. In 1515 Juan Díaz de Solis discovered the Río de La Plata. In 1534 Pedro de Mendoza was sent by the King of Spain to take charge of the 'Gobernación y Capitanía de las tierras del Rio de La Plata', and in Feb. 1536 he founded the city of the 'Puerto de Santa María del Buen Aire'. In 1810 the population rose against Spanish rule, and in 1816 Argentina proclaimed its independence. Civil wars and anarchy followed until, in 1853, stable government was established.

Military leaders supported by the Navy and Air Force staged a *coup d'état* on 24 March 1976, and The Junta of Commanders in Chief deposed Isobel Perón and her Government elected in 1972. The Commander in Chief of the Army, Lieut-Gen. Videla, was appointed President. The previous Constitution remained in force in so far as it was consistent with the statutes and objectives of the Junta. Return to civilian rule took place on 10 Dec. 1983. For details of earlier history and Constitutions *see* THE STATESMAN'S YEAR-BOOK, 1982–83 and 1985–86.

AREA AND POPULATION. The Argentine Republic is bounded in the north by Bolivia, in the north-east by Paraguay, in the east by Brazil, Uruguay and the Atlantic Ocean and the west by Chile. The republic consists of 22 provinces, 1 federal district and the National Territories of Tierra del Fuego, the Antarctic and the South Atlantic Islands (census of 1980) as follows:

Provinces	*Area: Sq. km. 1960*	*Population Estimate 1989*	*Capital*	*Population census, 1980 (1,000)*
Litoral				
Federal Capital	200	2,900,794	Buenos Aires	2,908
Buenos Aires	307,571	12,604,018	La Plata	455
Corrientes	88,199	748,834	Corrientes	180
Entre Ríos	78,781	1,005,885	Paraná	160
Chaco	99,633	824,447	Resistencia	218
Santa Fé	133,007	2,765,678	Santa Fé	287
Formosa	72,066	354,512	Formosa	95
Misiones	29,801	723,839	Posadas	140
Norte				
Jujuy	53,219	502,694	San Salvador de Jujuy	124
Salta	154,775	822,378	Salta	260
Santiago del Estero	135,254	641,273	Santiago del Estero	148
Tucumán	22,524	1,134,309	San Miguel de Tucumán	393
Centro				
Córdoba	168,766	2,748,006	Córdoba	969
La Pampa	143,440	237,386	Santa Rosa	52
San Luis	76,748	246,087	San Luis	71
Andina				
Catamarca	100,967	232,523	Catamarca	78
La Rioja	89,680	191,468	La Rioja	67
Mendoza	148,827	1,387,914	Mendoza	118
San Juan	89,651	528,838	San Juan	118
Neuquén	94,078	326,313	Neuquén	90
Patagonia				
Chubut	224,686	327,780	Rawson	13
Rio Negro	203,013	466,713	Viedma	24
Santa Cruz	243,943	147,928	Rio Gallegos	43
Tierra del Fuego	21,263	27,358	Ushuaia	11

The total area is 2,780,092 sq. km excluding the claimed 'Antarctic Sector' and the population at the 1980 Census was 27,947,446; estimate (1990) 32,686,000. In 1980, 95% spoke the national language, Spanish, while 3% spoke Italian, 1% Guaraní and 1% other languages. In 1983, 83% lived in urban areas and 17% rural, while 98% were white and 2% mestizo (mixed).

The official census including the 'Antarctic Sector', and stated to comprise the 'Malvinas' (Falklands), South Orcadas (Orkneys), South Georgias, South Sandwich Islands and the 'sovereign territories of Argentina in the Antarctic': population 3,300.

The principal metropolitan areas (1980 Census) are Buenos Aires (9,927,404), Córdoba (982,018), Rosario (954,606), Mendoza (596,796), La Plata (560,341), San Miguel de Tucumán (496,914), Mar del Plata (407,024), and San Juan (290,479). The suburbs of Buenos Aires, outside the Federal District, include San Justo (946,715), Morón (596,769), Lomas de Zamora (508,620), General Sarmiento (499,648), Lanus (465,891), Quilmes (441,780), General San Martín (384,306), Caseros (340,343), Almirante Brown (332,548), Avellaneda (330,654), Vicente López (289,815), San Isidro (287,048), Merlo (282,828), Tigre (205,926), Berazategui (200,926), and Esteban Echeverría (187,969).

Other large cities (1980 Census) are Rosario (875,664), Mar del Plata (407,024), Bahía Blanca (220,765), Guaymallén (157,334), Godoy Cruz (141,553), Rio Cuarto (110,254), Comodoro Rivadavia (98,985), San Nicolás (96,313) and Concordia (93,618).

In April 1990 the National Congress declared that the Falklands and other British-held islands in the South Atlantic were part of a new province of Tierra del Fuego.

CLIMATE. The climate is warm temperate over the pampas, where rainfall occurs at all seasons, but diminishes towards the west. In the north and west, the climate is more arid, with high summer temperatures, while in the extreme south conditions are also dry, but much cooler. Buenos Aires. Jan. 74°F (23·3°C), July 50°F (10°C). Annual rainfall 37" (950 mm). Bahía Blanca. Jan. 74°F (23·3°C), July 48°F (8·9°C). Annual rainfall 21" (523 mm). Mendoza. Jan. 75°F (23·9°C), July 47°F (8·3°C). Annual rainfall 8" (190 mm). Rosario. Jan. 76°F (24·4°C), July 51°F (10·6°C). Annual rainfall 35" (869 mm). San Juan. Jan. 78°F (25·6°C), July 50°F (10°C). Annual rainfall 4" (89 mm). San Miguel de Tucumán. Jan. 79°F (26·1°C), July 56°F (13·3°C). Annual rainfall 38" (970 mm). Ushuaia. Jan. 50°F (10°C), July 34°F (1·1°C). Annual rainfall 19" (475 mm).

CONSTITUTION AND GOVERNMENT. Presidential, congressional and municipal elections took place on 30 Oct. 1983 and a return to civilian rule took place on 10 Dec. 1983. With the return to constitutional rule the Constitution of 1853 (as amended up to 1898) is again in effect. The President and Vice-President are elected by a 600-member electoral college (directly elected by popular vote) for 6-year terms; both must be Roman Catholics of Argentine birth. The President is Commander-in-Chief of the Armed Services, and appoints to all civil and judicial offices.

The following is a list of Presidents from 1973 onwards:

Gen. Juan Domingo Perón. 12 Oct. 1973–1 July 1974.
Maria Estela (Isabel) Martinez Perón. 1 July 1974 (*a.i.* from 29 June 1974)–23 March 1976. (Deposed.)
Gen. Jorge Rafael Videla. 29 March 1976–29 March 1981.
Gen. Roberto Viola, 29 March–22 Dec. 1981.
Gen. Leopoldo Fortunato Galtieri, 22 Dec. 1981–17 June 1982.
Gen. Reynaldo Benito Antonio Bignone, 1 July 1982–10 Dec. 1983.
Dr Raúl Alfonsín, 10 Dec. 1983–30 June 1989.

The National Congress consists of a Senate and a House of Deputies: The Senate comprises 46 members, 2 nominated by each provincial legislature and 2 from the Federal District for 9 years (one-third retiring every 3 years). The House of Deputies comprises 254 members directly elected by universal suffrage (at age 18).

In the presidential elections held on 14 May 1989 Carlos Saúl Menem of the Justicalist Party won the support of 310 electors in the 600-member electoral college.

President of the Republic: Carlos Saúl Menem (sworn in 8 July 1989).

Vice-President: Eduardo Duhalde.

The Cabinet in Jan. 1990 was composed as follows:

Defence: Antonio Erman González. *Economy:* Domingo Cavallo. *Education:* Antonio Francisco Salonia. *Foreign Relations:* Guido José Maria di Tella. *Interior:* Eduardo Bauãá. *Labour and Social Security:* Rodolfo Diaz. *Public Health and Social Action:* Avelino Porto. *Secretary-General of the Presidency:* Alberto Kohan. *Justice:* Raúl Granillo Ocampo.

National flag: Three horizontal stripes of light blue, white and light blue, with the gold Sun of May in the centre.

National anthem: Oid, mortales, el grito sagrado Libertad ('Hear, mortals, the sacred cry of Liberty'; words by V. López y Planes, 1813; tune by J. Blas Parera).

Local Government. In Oct. 1983 the governors were elected by the people.

DEFENCE

Army. There are 5 military regions. The Army is organized in 4 army corps; it consists of 2 armoured, 2 mechanized infantry, 2 mountain, 1 motorized infantry, 1 jungle and 1 mixed infantry brigades; 2 engineering, 1 aviation and 1 air defence battalions. Equipment in 1990 includd 350 100 M-4 Sherman and 250 TAM main battle tanks and 60 AMX-13 light tanks.

In 1990 the Army was 40,000 strong, of whom 10,000 were conscripts.

The trained reserve numbers about 250,000, of whom 200,000 belong to the National Guard and 50,000 to the Territorial Guard.

Navy. The flagship of the Armada Republica Argentina is the light aircraft carrier *Veinticinco de Mayo* displacing 20,200 tonnes full load, and embarking an air group of 4 Super-Etendard, 3 S-2 Tracker and 4 S-61D Sea King aircraft. Originally the British *Venerable* (completed in 1948) she served in the Royal Netherlands Navy as *Karel Doorman*, from 1956 to 1968. She is currently undergoing major refit including re-engining. Of the two cruisers, the *General Belgrano*, ex-*Phoenix*, purchased from the USA in 1951 was sunk by the British submarine *Conqueror* in May 1982, while her sister ship *Nueve de Julio* (*ex*-USS *Bloise*) was withdrawn from service in 1980.

Other combatant forces include 4 German-built diesel submarines, 4 modern German-built destroyers, 2 British-built guided missile destroyers (Type 42), 4 German-designed and 3 French-built frigates, 2 old training frigates, 2 fast torpedo craft, 11 patrol ships, 4 coastal minesweepers, 2 minehunters and 1 tank landing ship. Auxiliaries include 2 survey ships, 2 training ships, 3 transports, 1 icebreaker and numerous harbour and service craft.

The new construction programme includes 2 diesel submarines (both building – but slowly) and 2 small frigates.

The Naval Aviation Service has some 60 combat aircraft and helicopters with (1990) 2,000 personnel, in 5 wings. Aircraft include 12 Super-Etendard strike aircraft, 11 EMB-326 and 5 EMB-339A light jet armed trainers, 1 Lockheed Electra maritime surveillance aircraft and 6 S-2E carrier-adapted Tracker anti-submarine aircraft, plus varied training, transport and general purpose aircraft. There is a squadron of S-60 anti-submarine helicopters plus some 8 Alouettes. A variable mix of Super Etendards, Skyhawks and Trackers plus Sea King and Alouette helicopters will operate from the aircraft carrier if her refit is completed.

Main bases are at Buenos Aires, Puerto Belgrano (HQ and Dockyard), Mar del Plata and Ushuaia.

The active personnel of the navy in 1989 comprised 25,000, 4,000 of whom were conscripts, and including 5,000 marines.

The Prefectura Naval Argentina (PNA) for Coast Guard and rescue duties operates 5 new 910-tonne corvettes with helicopter and hangar, an ex-whaler of 700 tonnes, and 23 patrol vessels.

Air Force. The Air Force is organized into Air Operations, Air Regions, Materiel and Personnel Commands. Air Operations Command, responsible for all operational flying, is made up of air brigades, each with 1 to 4 squadrons, usually operating from a single base. No. I Air Brigade is a military air transport service, with responsibility also for LADE (state airline) operations into areas of Argentina not served by civilian companies. Its equipment includes 6 C-130E/H Hercules and 10 F.27 Friendship/Troopship turboprop transports, 2 KC-130H Hercules tanker/transports, 4 twin-turbofan F.28 Fellowship freighters, 7 Twin Otters, 15 Guarani IIs, the Presidential Boeing 707-320B and 707-320C, 4 more 707s, 2 VIP Fellowships, and many older or smaller types. No. II Air Brigade has 4 Canberra twin-jet bombers and 2 Canberra trainers; a photographic squadron with Guarani IIs and Learjets. No. III Air Brigade has 2 squadrons of IA 58 Pucara twin-turboprop COIN aircraft. No. IV Air Brigade comprises 2 ground attack squadrons equipped with about 30 Paris light jet combat and liaison aircraft, now being replaced by IA 63 Pampas, and one squadron with Mirage IIIs. No. V Air Brigade comprises 2 squadrons with a total of about 30 A-4P Skyhawk strike aircraft. No. VI Air Brigade has 40 Dagger (Israeli-built Mirage III) fighters, equipping 2 squadrons, and 1 squadron with 15 Mirage IIIE fighter-bombers and 4 Mirage IIID trainers. No. VII Air Brigade has 2 helicopter squadrons with 12 armed Hughes 500M, 8 Bell 212, 6 Bell UH-1 and 2 Chinook helicopters. No. X Air Brigade has 1 squadron of Mirage IIIC/5 fighters. There is a flying school at Córdoba, equipped with turboprop-powered Embraer Tucanos and Paris jets. There were (1990) about 15,000 personnel and about 150 combat aircraft.

INTERNATIONAL RELATIONS

Membership. Argentina is a member of the UN, OAS and LAIA.

ECONOMY

Policy. In 1990, to reduce the public deficit (US$5,000m. in 1989), the government introduced a programme privatizing some 40 public enterprises.

Budget. The financial year commences on 1 Jan. Budget receipts in 1988 were 151,208m. australes and expenditure, 156,029m. australes.

Currency. The monetary unit is the *austral* (ARA) divided into 100 *centavos*. Circulation consists chiefly of notes (issued since 1897) ranging from 50,000 *australes* down to 1 *austral*. The coins actually circulating, 1988, were steel-nickel, 1, 5, 10 and 50 centavos. In March 1991, US$1 = 9,822·64 *austral*; £1 = 18,633·55 *austral*.

Banking. In 1988 there were 36 government banks, 109 private banks and 33 foreign banks. The *Governor* of the Central Bank is Roberto Alemán.

Weights and Measures. Since 1 Jan. 1887 the use of the metric system has been compulsory.

ENERGY AND NATURAL RESOURCES

Electricity. Electric power production (1988) was 48,965m. kwh. Supply 220 volts; 50 Hz.

Oil. Crude oil production (1989) 23m. tonnes. The oil industry was deregulated in Jan. 1991.

Gas. Natural gas production (1983) 13,500,000m. cu. metres. New offshore fields were reported in 1988.

Minerals. Argentina produced 505,000 tonnes of washed coal in 1988. Gold, silver and copper are worked in Catamarca, where there are also 2 tin-mines, and gold and copper in San Juan, La Rioja and the south-western territories. Iron ore (654,800 tonnes in 1988), tungsten, beryllium, clay, marble, lead (39,400 tonnes in 1988), barites, zinc (73,300 tonnes in 1988), borate (245,000 tonnes in 1988), bentonite and granite are produced. Primary aluminium production was 162,000 tonnes in 1989.

Agriculture. Argentina has an area of about 670,251,000 acres, of which about 41% is pasture land, 32% woodland and 11% (73·73m. acres) cultivated.

Livestock (1988): Cattle 50,782,000; sheep, 29,202,000; pigs, 4·1m.; horses, 3·1m. The Province of Buenos Aires has 37% of the cattle. Wool production, 1988, was 138,000 tonnes.

Wheat production (1988) 7,769,000 tonnes from 4,617,000 ha.

Argentina's meat exports are calculated in terms of actual weight; not 'carcase weight', as is the international practice.

Cotton, potatoes, vine, tobacco, citrus fruit, olives, rice, soya, and yerba maté (Paraguayan tea) are also cultivated. There are 36 cane-sugar mills and 1 beet-sugar factory; cane-sugar production, 1988, 14,773,000 tonnes. Potato production, 1988, amounted to 2·19m. tonnes. The area under tobacco, 1988, was 55,000 ha; output 74,000 tonnes.

Sunflower seed (production (1988) 2,915,000 tonnes), first grown by Russian immigrants in 1900, now furnishes the country's most popular edible oil. There are more than 10m. olive trees. 443,000 tonnes of groundnuts were produced in 1988 (mainly in Córdoba). Argentina is the world's largest source of tannin.

Forestry. In 1989 woodland covered 22% of the land area (59·5m. ha).

Fisheries. Fish landings in 1986 amounted to 420,300 tonnes.

INDUSTRY. Production (1988 in tonnes) Paper, 761,393; steel (1986), 2·85m.; sulphuric acid, 258,024; cement (1987), 6,302,065. Motor vehicles produced totalled, 131,253; television receivers, 454,429.

FOREIGN ECONOMIC RELATIONS. In April 1990 Argentina signed a treaty of trade and co-operation with the EEC. In Dec. 1990 Argentina and the UK signed a treaty protecting investments.

Commerce. Import values include charges for carriage, insurance and freight; export values are on a f.o.b. basis. Real values of foreign trade (in US$1m.):

	1986	*1987*	*1988*
Imports	4,724	5,818	5,322
Exports	6,852	6,360	9,135

Total trade between Argentina and UK (British Department of Trade returns, in £1,000 sterling):

	1986	*1987*	*1988*	*1989*	*1990*
Imports to UK	28,635	64,595	66,281	98,490	144,205
Exports and re-exports from UK	10,115	10,267	12,991	13,585	35,953

Tourism. In 1988, 2,119,140 tourists visited Argentina.

COMMUNICATIONS

Roads. In 1983 there were 220,093 km of national and provincial highways. The 4 main roads constituting Argentina's portion of the Pan-American Highway were opened to traffic in 1942. In 1985 there were 5·08m. cars and commercial vehicles.

Railways. The system based on the 1949 amalgamation of 18 government, British and French-owned railways, comprises 7 railways with a total route-km in 1989 of 34,509 km (210 km electrified) on metre, 1,435 mm and 1,676 mm gauges. In 1989 railways carried 8,274m. tonne-km and 10,651m. passenger-km. In 1988 parts of the network were being prepared for privatization.

Aviation. 85% of the former state-owned airline, Aerolineas, was privatized in July 1990. There were (1986) 10 international airports and 54 other airports.

Shipping. The merchant fleet, 1988, consisted of 451 vessels of 2,834,000 DWT.

Telecommunications. The nationalized telephone service Entel was privatized in Nov. 1990. Instruments numbered 3,250,000 in 1984. There were (1984) 122 radio stations and 4 television channels in Buenos Aires. In 1986 there were 6m. radio receivers and 5·9m. television receivers.

Newspapers (1985). Daily newspapers numbered 227 with a circulation of 2·7m.

JUSTICE, RELIGION, EDUCATION AND WELFARE

Justice. Justice is administered by federal and provincial courts. The former deal only with cases of a national character, or in which different provinces or inhabitants of different provinces are parties. The chief federal court is the Supreme Court, with 5 judges at Buenos Aires. Other federal courts are the appeal courts, at Buenos Aires, Bahía Blanca, La Plata, Córdoba, Mendoza, Tucumán and Resistencia. Each province has its own judicial system, with a Supreme Court (generally so designated) and several minor chambers. Trial by jury is established by the Constitution for criminal cases, but never practised, except occasionally in the provinces of Buenos Aires and Córdoba.

The death penalty was re-introduced in 1976 for the killing of government, military police and judicial officials, and for participation in terrorist activities.

The police force is centralized under the Federal Security Council.

Religion. The Roman Catholic religion is supported by the State and membership was 26m. in 1986. There are several Protestant denominations with a total congregation (1983) of 500,000. The Jewish congregation numbered 300,000 in 1983.

Education. In 1984 the primary schools had 218,520 teachers and 4,430,513 pupils; secondary schools had 86,874 teachers and 656,521 pupils, vocational schools had 119,309 teachers and 905,755 pupils.

There are National Universities at Buenos Aires (2), Córdoba (2), La Plata, Tucumán, Santa Fé (Litoral), Rosario, Corrientes (Nordeste), Mendoza (Cuyo), Bahía Blanca (Sur), Catamarca, Tandil, Neuquén (Comahue), San Salvador de Jujuy, Salta, Santa Rosa (La Pampa), Mar del Plata, Comodoro Rivadavia (Patagonia), Río Cuarto, Entre Ríos, Resistencia, San Juan and Santiago del Estero. There are also private universities in Buenos Aires (6), Mendoza (3), Córdoba, Comodoro Rivadavia, La Plata, Morón, Tucumán, Salta, Santa Fé and Santiago del Estero. In 1981 universities had 525,688 students and 54,039 lecturers.

Health. Free medical attention is obtainable from public hospitals. Many trade unions provide medical, dental and maternity services for their members and dependants. In 1980 there were 151,568 hospital beds and 72,762 doctors.

DIPLOMATIC REPRESENTATIVES

Of Argentina in Great Britain (53, Hans Place, London, SW1X 0LA)
Ambassador: Mario Cámpora.

Of Great Britain in Argentina (Dr Luis Agote 2412/52, 1425 Buenos Aires)
Ambassador: The Hon. Humphrey Maud, CMG.

Of Argentina in the USA (1600 New Hampshire Ave., NW, Washington, D.C., 20009)
Ambassador: Vacant.

Of the USA in Argentina (4300 Colombia, 1425, Buenos Aires)
Ambassador: Terence A. Todman.

Of Argentina to the United Nations
Ambassador: Dr Jorge Vazquez.

Further Reading

Boletin del comercio exterio Argentino y estadisticas económicas retrospectivas. Annual
Anuario de comercio exterior de la República Argentina. Annual
Economic Review, Banco de la Nación. Buenos Aires

Sintesis Estadistica Mensual. Dirección General de Estadistica. Buenos Aires, 1947 ff.
Boletin Internacional de Bibliografia Argentina. Ministry of Foreign Relations. Buenos Aires. Monthly
Geografia de la República Argentino. Ed. by the Sociedad Argentina de Estudios Geográficos. 7 vols. Buenos Aires. 1945–53
Biggins, A., *Argentina*. [Bibliography]. Oxford and Santa Barbara, 1990
Crawley, E., *A House Divided: Argentina 1880–1980*. London, 1984
Ferns, H. S., *Britain and Argentina in the 19th Century*. OUP, 1960.—*The Argentine Republic 1516–1971*. Newton Abbot, 1973
Graham-Yooll, A., *The Forgotten Colony: A History of the English-Speaking Communities in Argentina*. London, 1981
Lewis, P., *The Crisis of Argentine Capitalism*. North Carolina Univ. Press, 1990
Rock, D., *Argentina 1516–1982*. London, 1986
Santillán, Diego A. de (ed.) *Gran Enciclopedia Argentina*. 9 vols. 1956–64
Simpson, J. and Bennett, J., *The Disappeared: Voices from a Secret War*. London, 1985
Wynia, G. W., *Argentina*. Hoddesdon, 1986

AUSTRALIA

Commonwealth of Australia

Capital: Canberra
Population: 17·1m. (1990)
GNP per capita: US$12,390 (1988)

HISTORY. On 1 Jan. 1901 the former British colonies of New South Wales, Victoria, Queensland, South Australia, Western Australia and Tasmania were federated under the name of the 'Commonwealth of Australia', the designation of 'colonies' being at the same time changed into that of 'states'—except in the case of Northern Territory, which was transferred from South Australia to the Commonwealth as a 'territory' on 1 Jan. 1911.

In 1911 the Commonwealth acquired from the State of New South Wales the Canberra site for the Australian capital.

Territories under the administration of Australia in Jan. 1987, but not included in it, comprise Norfolk Island, the territory of Ashmore and Cartier Islands, and the Australian Antarctic Territory (acquired 24 Aug. 1936), comprising all the islands and territory, other than Adélie Land, situated south of 60° S. lat. and between 160° and 45° E. long. The Coral Sea Islands became an External Territory in 1969.

The British Government transferred sovereignty in the Heard Island and McDonald Islands to the Australian Government on 26 Dec. 1947. Cocos (Keeling) Islands on 23 Nov. 1955 and Christmas Island on 1 Oct. 1958 were also transferred to Australian jurisdiction.

AREA AND POPULATION. Australia, including Tasmania but excluding external territories, covers a land area of 7,682,300 sq. km, extending from Cape York (10° 41' S) in the north some 3,680 km to Tasmania (43° 39' S), and from Cape Byron (153° 39' E) in the east some 4,000 km west to Western Australia (113° 9' E). Growth in Census population has been:

1901	3,774,310	1947	7,579,358	1971	12,755,638
1911	4,455,005	1954	8,986,530	1976	13,915,500
1921	5,435,734	1961	10,508,186	1981	15,053,600
1933	6,629,839	1966	11,599,498	1986	15,763,000

The next census was due to be held on 6 Aug. 1991.

Area and resident population (estimate), 30 June 1990, 17,086,197 (8,554,994 females), divided as follows:

States and Territories	*Area (sq. km)*	*Total*	*Per sq. km*
New South Wales (NSW)	801,600	5,827,373	7·0
Victoria (Vic.)	227,600	4,379,981	18·5
Queensland (Qld.)	1,727,200	2,906,838	1·5
South Australia (SA)	984,000	1,439,157	1·4
Western Australia (WA)	2,525,500	1,633,896	0·6
Tasmania (Tas.)	67,800	456,663	6·6
Northern Territory (NT)	1,346,200	157,304	0·1
Australian Capital Territory (ACT)	2,400	284,985	110·9
Total	7,682,300	17,086,197	2·2

Rate of population increase (per 1,000) in 1989: 7·9 (natural), 16·2 (with migration).

85·4% of the population was urban in 1986. Resident population (estimate) in State capitals and other major cities (statistical districts), 30 June 1988:

Capitals	*State*	*Population*	*Statistical district*	*State*	*Population*
Canberra [1]	ACT	297,300	Darwin	NT	72,900
Sydney	NSW	3,596,000	Newcastle	NSW	422,100
Melbourne	Vic.	3,002,300	Wollongong	NSW	235,300
Brisbane	Qld.	1,240,300	Gold Coast [2]	Qld.	235,600
Adelaide	SA	1,023,700	Geelong	Vic.	148,300
Perth	WA	1,118,800	Townsville	Qld.	109,700
Hobart	Tas.	179,900			

[1] Includes Queanbeyan (20,450). [2] Includes Tweed Heads.

At 30 June 1990 the age-group distribution was: Under 15, 3,741,699; 15-64, 11,436,918; 65 and over, 1,907,580. Life expectancy in 1986 was 72·9 (males), 79·2 (females).

Australians born overseas (30 June 1990), 3·85m., of whom 1·2m. came from the UK and Ireland; 1·16m. from continental Europe; 814,295 from Asia and 288,900 from New Zealand.

Aboriginals have been included in population statistics only since 1967. At the 1986 census they numbered 227,645.

Vital statistics for 1988:

States and Territories	*Marriages*	*Divorces*	*Births*	*Deaths*	*Infant deaths*
New South Wales	40,812	11,880	84,647	44,676	775
Victoria	30,687	10,250	62,134	30,726	486
Queensland	18,850	7,690	40,561	18,803	339
South Australia	10,128	4,031	19,155	10,690	152
Western Australia	10,578	3,964	25,143	9,532	214
Tasmania	3,053	1,220	6,779	3,547	65
Northern Territory	782	275	3,439	876	66
ACT	1,944	1,697	4,335	1,016	35
Total	116,816	41,007	246,193	119,866	2,132
Rate [1]	7·1	2·1	14·8	7·8	9·2 [2]

[1] Resident (estimate). [2] Per 1,000 live births registered.

There were 251,000 births in 1989.

Overseas arrivals and departures:

	1987	*1988*
Arrivals	3,592,900	4,141,100
of whom long-term	221,620	253,860
(including settlers)	(128,290)	(151,550)
Departures	3,421,300	3,976,500
of whom long-term	97,770	104,760
(including former settlers and other residents)	(20,410)	(20,320)

There were 133,500 immigrants in 1989. The 1990–91 quota for settlers was 126,000. The Migration Act of Dec. 1989 sought to curb illegal entry and ensure that annual immigrant intakes were met but not exceeded. Provisions for temporary visitors to become permanent were restricted.

Australian Bureau of Statistics, *Australian Demographic Statistics*. Quarterly. Canberra, June 1979 to date

National Population Inquiry, Population and Australia: Recent Demographic Trends and their Implications. Canberra, 1978

CLIMATE. Over most of the continent, four seasons may be recognised. Spring is from Sept. to Nov., Summer from Dec. to Feb., Autumn from March to May and Winter from June to Aug., but because of its great size there are climates that range from tropical monsoon to cool temperate, with large areas of desert as well. In Northern Australia there are only two seasons, the wet one lasting from Nov. to March, but rainfall amounts diminish markedly from the coast to the interior. Central and southern Queensland are subtropical, north and central New South Wales are warm temperate, as are parts of Victoria, Western Australia and Tasmania, where most rain falls in winter. Canberra. Jan. 68°F (20°C), July 42°F (5·6°C). Annual rainfall 23" (629 mm). Adelaide. Jan. 73°F (22·8°C), July 52°F (11·1°C).

Annual rainfall 21" (528 mm). Brisbane. Jan. 77°F (25°C), July 58°F (14·4°C). Annual rainfall 45" (1,153 mm). Darwin. Jan. 83°F (28·3°C), July 77°F (25°C). Annual rainfall 59" (1,536 mm). Hobart. Jan. 62°F (16·7°C), July 46°F (7·8°C). Annual rainfall 24" (629 mm). Melbourne. Jan. 67°F (19·4°C), July 49°F (9·4°C). Annual rainfall 26" (659 mm). Perth. Jan. 74°F (23·3°C), July 55°F (12·8°C). Annual rainfall 35" (873 mm). Sydney. Jan. 71°F (21·7°C), July 53°F (11·7°C). Annual rainfall 47" (1,215 mm).

CONSTITUTION AND GOVERNMENT. *Federal Government:* Under the Constitution legislative power is vested in a Federal Parliament, consisting of the Queen, represented by a Governor-General, a Senate and a House of Representatives. Under the terms of the constitution there must be a session of parliament at least once a year.

The *Senate* comprises 76 Senators (12 for each State voting as one electorate and as from Aug. 1974, 2 Senators respectively for the Australian Capital Territory and the Northern Territory). Senators representing the States are chosen for 6 years. The terms of Senators representing the Territories expire at the close of the day next preceding the polling day for the general elections of the House of Representatives. In general, the Senate is renewed to the extent of one-half every 3 years, but in case of disagreement with the House of Representatives, it, together with the House of Representatives, may be dissolved, and an entirely new Senate elected. The *House of Representatives* consists, as nearly as practicable, of twice as many Members as there are Senators, the numbers chosen in the several States being in proportion to population as shown by the latest statistics, but not less than 5 for any original State. The numerical size of the House after the election in 1990 was 000, including the Members for Northern Territory and the Australian Capital Territory. The Northern Territory has been represented by 1 Member in the House of Representatives since 1922, and the Australian Capital Territory by 1 Member since 1949 and 2 Members since May 1974. The Member for the Australian Capital Territory was given full voting rights as from the Parliament elected in Nov. 1966. The Member for the Northern Territory was given full voting rights in 1968. The House of Representatives continues for 3 years from the date of its first meeting, unless sooner dissolved. The annual salary of both Senators and Representatives is $A55,000, with increments for holders of office.

Every Senator or Member of the House of Representatives must be a subject of the Queen, be of full age, possess electoral qualifications and have resided for 3 years within Australia. The franchise for both Houses is the same and is based on universal (males and females aged 18 years) suffrage. Compulsory voting was introduced in 1925. If a Member of a State Parliament wishes to be a candidate in a federal election, he must first resign his State seat.

Executive power is vested in the *Governor-General* advised by an Executive Council. The Governor-General presides over the Council, and its members hold office at his pleasure. All Ministers of State, who are members of the party or parties commanding a majority in the lower House, are members of the Executive Council under summons. A record of proceedings of meetings is kept by the Secretary to the Council. At Executive Council meetings the decisions of the Cabinet are (where necessary) given legal form, appointments made, resignations accepted, proclamations, regulations and the like made.

The policy of a ministry is, in practice, determined by the Ministers of State meeting without the Governor-General under the chairmanship of the Prime Minister. This group is known as the *Cabinet*. There are 11 Standing Committees of the Cabinet comprising varying numbers of Cabinet and non-Cabinet Ministers. In Labour Governments all Ministers have been members of Cabinet. In Liberal and National Country Party Governments, only the senior ministers. Cabinet meetings are private and deliberative and records of meetings are not made public. The Cabinet does not form part of the legal mechanisms of Government; the decisions it takes have, in themselves, no legal effect. The Cabinet substantially controls, in ordinary circumstances, not only the general legislative programme of Parliament but the whole course of Parliamentary proceedings. In effect, though not in form, the Cabinet, by reason of the fact that all Ministers are members of the Executive Council, is also the dominant element in the executive government of the country.

The legislative powers of the Federal Parliament embrace trade and commerce, shipping, etc.; taxation, finance, banking, currency, bills of exchange, bankruptcy, insurance; defence; external affairs, naturalization and aliens, quarantine, immigration and emigration; the people of any race for whom it is deemed necessary to make special laws; postal, telegraph and like services; census and statistics; weights and measures; astronomical and meteorological observations; copyrights; railways; conciliation and arbitration in disputes extending beyond the limits of any one State; social services; marriage, divorce etc.; service and execution of the civil and criminal process; recognition of the laws, Acts and records, and judicial proceedings of the States. The Senate may not originate or amend money bills; and disagreement with the House of Representatives may result in dissolution and, in the last resort, a joint sitting of the two Houses. No religion may be established by the Commonwealth. The Federal Parliament has limited and enumerated powers, the several State parliaments retaining the residuary power of government over their respective territories. If a State law is inconsistent with a Commonwealth law, the latter prevails.

The Constitution also provides for the admission or creation of new States. Proposed laws for the alteration of the Constitution must be submitted to the electors, and they can be enacted only if approved by a majority of the States and by a majority of all the electors voting.

The Australia Acts 1986 removed residual powers of the British government to intervene in the government of Australia or the individual states.

The 36th Parliament was elected on 24 March 1990.

House of Representatives (1991): Australian Labor Party, 77 seats; Liberal Party, 56; National Party, 14; independent, 1.

Senate (1991): Australian Labor Party, 32; Liberal Party, 29; Australian Democratic Party, 8; National Party, 5; independent, 2.

Governor-General: Sir William George Hayden.

The following is a list of former Governors-General of the Commonwealth:

Earl of Hopetoun	1901–02	HRH the Duke of Gloucester	1945–47
Lord Tennyson	1902–04	Sir William McKell	1947–53
Lord Northcote	1904–08	Viscount Slim	1953–60
Earl of Dudley	1908–11	Viscount Dunrossil	1960–61
Lord Denman	1911–14	Viscount De L'Isle	1961–65
Viscount Novar	1914–20	Lord Casey	1965–69
Lord Forster	1920–25	Sir Paul Hasluck	1969–74
Lord Stonehaven	1925–31	Sir John Kerr	1974–77
Sir Isaac Isaacs	1931–36	Sir Zelman Cowen	1977–82
Earl Gowrie	1936–45	Sir Ninian Stephen	1982–89

National flag: The British Blue Ensign with a large star of 7 points beneath the Union Flag, and in the fly 5 stars of the Southern Cross, all in white.

National Anthem: 'Advance Australia Fair' (adopted 19 April 1984). The 'Royal Anthem' (i.e. 'God Save the Queen') is used in the presence of the British Royal Family.

The cabinet of the Labour administration in Feb. 1991 was composed as follows:

Prime Minister: Robert Hawke.
Treasurer: Paul Keating.
Industry, Technology and Commerce: John Button.
Foreign Affairs and Trade: Gareth Evans.
Trade Negotiations: Neil Blewitt.
Finance: Ralph Willis.
Employment, Education and Training: John Dawkins.
Attorney General: Michael Duffy.
Transport and Communications: Kim Beazley.

Primary Industries and Energy: John Kerin.
Community Services and Health: Brian Howe.
Social Security: Graham Richardson.
Defence: Robert Ray.
Immigration, Local Government and Ethnic Affairs: Gerry Hand.
Arts, Sport, the Environment, Tourism and Territories: Rosalind Kelly.
Industrial Relations: Peter Cook.
Administrative Services: Nick Bolkus.

The leader of the Liberal Party is John Hewson; of the National Party, Tim Fischer.

The Acts of the Parliament of the Commonwealth of Australia Passed from 1901 to 1973. 12 vols. Annual volumes, 1974 to date
The Australian Constitution Annotated. Attorney-General's Department, Canberra, 1980
Parliamentary Handbook of the Commonwealth of Australia. Canberra, 1915 to date
Commonwealth of Australia Directory [1921–1958 The Federal Guide; 1961–72 *Commonwealth Directory;* 1973–75 *Australian Government Directory*]. Prime Minister's Department. Canberra, 1924 to date
Crisp, L. F., *Australian National Government.* 3rd ed. Melbourne and London, 1975
Hughes, C. A. and Graham, B. D., *A Handbook of Australian Government and Politics.* Canberra, 1968
Odgers, J. R., *Australian Senate Practice.* 5th ed. Canberra, 1976
Paton, Sir George (ed.) *The Commonwealth of Australia: its Laws and Constitution.* London, 1952
Pettifer, J. A., *House of Representatives Practice.* Canberra, 1981
Sawer, G., *Australian Federal Politics and Law 1901–1929, 1929–1949.* 2 vols. Melbourne, 1974.—*Australian Government To-day.* 11th ed. Melbourne, 1973
Wynes, W. A., *Executive and Judicial Powers in Australia.* 5th ed. Sydney, 1976

State Government: In each of the 6 States (New South Wales, Victoria, Queensland, South Australia, Western Australia, Tasmania) there is a State government whose constitution, powers and laws continue, subject to changes embodied in the Australian Constitution and subsequent alterations and agreements, as they were before federation. The system of government is basically the same as that described above for the Commonwealth—*i.e.*, the Sovereign, her representative (in this case a Governor), an upper and lower house of Parliament (except in Queensland, where the upper house was abolished in 1922), a cabinet led by the Premier and an Executive Council. Among the more important functions of the State governments are those relating to education, health, hospitals and charities, law, order and public safety, business undertakings such as railways and tramways, and public utilities such as water supply and sewerage. In the domains of education, hospitals, justice, the police, penal establishments, and railway and tramway operation, State government activity predominates. Care of the public health and recreative activities are shared with local government authorities and the Federal Government, social services other than those referred to above are now primarily the concern of the Federal Government, and the operation of public utilities is shared with local and semi-government authorities.

Administration of Territories. Since 1911, responsibility for administration and development of the Australian Capital Territory (ACT) has been vested in Federal Ministers and Departments. The ACT became self-governing on 11 May 1989.

The ACT House of Assembly has been accorded the forms of a legislature, but continues to perform an advisory function for the Minister for the Capital Territory.

On 1 July 1978 the Northern Territory of Australia became a self-governing Territory with expenditure responsibilities and revenue-raising powers broadly approximating those of a State.

Local Government. The system of municipal government is broadly the same throughout Australia, although local government legislation is a State matter.

Each State is sub-divided into areas known variously as municipalities, cities, boroughs, towns, shires or district councils, totalling about 900. Within these areas the management of road, street and bridge construction, health, sanitary and garbage services, water supply and sewerage, and electric light and gas undertakings, hospitals, fire brigades, tramways and omnibus services and harbours is generally part of the functions of elected aldermen and councillors. State governments may also be responsible for some services.

In some instances, *e.g.*, in New South Wales, a number of local government authorities combine to conduct a public undertaking such as the supply of water or electricity. Local taxation revenue was $A93,632m. in 1987–88.

DEFENCE. The Minister for Defence has responsibility under legislation for the control and administration of the Defence Force. The Chief of Defence Force Staff is vested with command of the Defence Force. He is the principal military adviser to the Minister. The Secretary, Department of Defence is the Permanent Head of the Department. He is the principal civilian adviser to the Minister and has statutory responsibility for financial administration of the Defence outlay. The Chief of Defence Force Staff and the Secretary are jointly responsible for the administration of the Defence Force except with respect to matters falling within the command of the Defence Force or any other matter specified by the Minister.

The Chief of Naval Staff, the Chief of the General Staff and the Chief of the Air Staff command the Navy, Army and Air Force respectively. They have delegated authority from the Chief of Defence Force Staff and the Secretary to administer matters relating to their particular Service.

The structure of Defence is characterized by 3 organizational types: *(i)* A Central Office comprising 5 groups of functional orientated Divisions: Strategic Policy and Force Development; Supply and Support; Manpower and Financial Services; Management and Infrastructure Services; and, Defence Science and Technology; *(ii)* the 3 Armed Services of the Defence Force, each having a Service Office element in addition to the command structure; and *(iii)* a small number of outrider organizations concerned with such specialist fields as intelligence and natural disasters.

Defence Support. The Department of Defence Support purchases goods and services for defence purposes; provides technical expertise and other assistance to the defence industry; involves Australian industry in defence equipment to the maximum practical extent; administers the Australian Offsets Program so as to stimulate technological advancement and broaden the capabilities of strategic industries; within overall defence policies helps the capacity, efficiency and capability of Australian industry to design and export defence materiel; manages the Government's munitions and aircraft factories, and dockyards; markets defence and allied products and services to help maintain strategic industries.

In 1988 the Department employed 14,189 civilians.

Army. Overall organization and financial control of the Australian Army is vested in the Chief of General Staff. Under the Defence Force Re-organisation Act, which received the Royal Assent on 9 Sept. 1975, the Military Board, which was previously the controlling body of the Army, was abolished. The Act became effective on 1 Feb. 1976. A functional command structure, Headquarters Field Force Command, Headquarters Logistic Command, and Headquarters Training Command, with Headquarters in military districts, was introduced in 1973.

The strength of the Army was 31,300 in 1990. The Command troops consist of 1 regiment each of Air Defence, engineering, aviation and Special Air Service; the 1 infantry division is composed of 1 mechanized and 2 infantry brigades, 3 artillery regiments, and 1 regiment each of reconnaissance, armoured personnel carriers, engineering and aviation. Equipment included 103 Leopard 1A3 main battle tanks. The Army Aviation Corps has 22 GAF N22-B Missionmaster and 14 Turbo-Porter transports, and 73 helicopters.

The effective strength of the Army Reserve in 1990 was 23,400.

Staff and command training is carried out at the Command and Staff College, Queenscliff, Victoria, and the Land Warfare Centre, Canungra, Queensland.

In Jan. 1986 the Australian Defence Force Academy, Canberra, accepted its first officer cadets for the 3 Services. Cadets will study at the academy for degrees in arts, science and engineering. During semester breaks they will carry out military training with their particular Services.

At the end of 3 years at the academy, army officer cadets will undertake a year of military training at the Royal Military College, Duntroon. This will culminate with commissioning as a lieutenant.

From 1986 the Royal Military College have taken officer cadets for commssioning who previously would have attended the Officer Cadet School, Portsea, and the Women's Officer Cadet School, Sydney.

Navy. The Chief of Naval Staff is assisted by the Deputy Chief of Naval Staff and Assistant Chiefs for Personnel, Operational Requirements and Plans, Material and Logistics. The command, operation and administration of the Fleet is now vested in the Maritime Commander, Australia (previously known as the Commander, Australian Fleet) headquartered at Sydney.

Combatants include 6 UK-built Oxley class diesel submarines, 3 US-built guided missile destroyers, 4 US-built guided missile frigates, commissioned 1980-84 and 5 older frigates, 3 minehunters, 1 tank landing ship, 3 tank landing craft and 22 inshore patrol craft. Major auxiliaries include 2 fleet replenishment tankers, 1 training ship, 3 survey ships, and there are some 85 minor auxiliaries and service craft.

New procurement includes 6 replacement submarines of Swedish design, with construction of the first recently begun, 2 guided-missile frigates and 8 German-designed frigates, construction of which should start in 1991.

The Fleet Air Arm operates a shore-based anti-submarine helicopter squadron of 7 Sea Kings, and has acquired 3 S-70B Lamps-III helicopters for the Guided Missile frigates which are having their flight decks extended to operate them. There are additionally 2 transport aircraft and 17 transport and utility helicopters.

The fleet main base is at Sydney, with subsidiary bases at Garden Island, Cairns and Darwin.

The all-volunteer Navy was (1990) 15,650 strong including 1,200 Fleet Air Arm.

Air Force. Command of the Royal Australian Air Force is vested in the Chief of the Air Staff (CAS) assisted by the Deputy Chief of the Air Staff, Chief of Air Force Operations and Plans, Chief of Air Force Materiel, Chief of Air Force Personnel, Chief of Air Force Technical Services, Director-General Supply—Air Force and Assistant Secretary Resources Planning.

The CAS administers and controls RAAF units through two commands: Operational Command and Support Command. Operational Command is responsible to the CAS for the command of operational units and the conduct of their operations within Australia and overseas. Support Command is responsible to the CAS for training of personnel, and the supply and maintenance of service equipment.

Flying establishment comprises 16 squadrons, of which 2 are equipped with 24 F-111 strike/reconnaissance aircraft. Of the others, 3 are equipped with missile-armed F-18 Hornet interceptors and 2 with Orion maritime reconnaissance aircraft. There are eight transport squadrons, 2 with Hercules turboprop transports, 2 with Caribou STOL transports, 1 with a mix of Ecureuil and Iroquois helicopters, 1 with Boeing Vertol CH-47C medium lift helicopters, 1 with Black Hawk helicopters, and a special transport squadron equipped with BAC One-Eleven, Mystère 20 and HS 748 aircraft. There is also one squadron operating B707 aircraft. Training aircraft include piston-engined Airtrainers, built in New Zealand, Aermacchi MB 326H jets for pilot training, and HS 748 aircraft for navigator training. A training unit has F-18 Hornets for crew conversion.

Training for commissioned rank is carried out at the RAAF Academy and Officers' Training School, both located at Point Cook, Victoria. Other major training activities which lead to commissioned rank include basic aircrew training and technical and commercial cadet schemes. Basic ground training to tradesman level is conducted at RAAF technical training schools. Higher command and staff training is, in the main, carried out at the RAAF Staff College, Fairbairn, ACT.

Personnel (1990) 22,600. There is also an Australian Air Force Reserve.

Long, G. (ed.) *Australia in the War of 1939–45*. 22 vols. Canberra, 1952 ff.
O'Neil, R. and Horner, D. M., *Australian Defence Policy for the 1980s*. Univ. of Queensland Press, 1983

INTERNATIONAL RELATIONS

Membership. Australia is a member of the UN, the Commonwealth, GATT, OECD, Colombo Plan, the South Pacific Commission and the South Pacific Bureau for Economic Co-operation.

ECONOMY

Financial relations with the States. Since 1942 the Federal Government alone has levied taxes on incomes. In return for vacating this field of taxation, the State Governments are reimbursed by grants from the Federal Government out of revenue received. Payments to the States represent about one-third of Federal Government outlays, and in turn the payments State Governments receive from the Federal Government account for nearly half of their revenues.

The Financial Agreement of 1927 established the Australian Loan Council which represents the Federal and six State Governments, and co-ordinates domestic and overseas borrowings by these governments, including annual borrowing programmes. The Federal Government acts as a central borrowing agency in raising loans to finance the major part of those programmes. The Loan Council in 1984 agreed upon arrangements for the co-ordination of borrowings by semi-government and local authorities and government-owned companies.

Budget. In 1929, under a financial agreement between the Federal Government and States, approved by a referendum, the Federal Government took over all State debts existing on 30 June 1927 and agreed to pay $A15·17m. a year for 58 years towards the interest charges thereon, and to make substantial contributions towards a sinking fund on State debt. The Sinking Fund arrangements were revised under an amendment to the agreement in 1976.

Outlays and revenues of the Commonwealth Government for years ending 30 June (in $A1m.):

	1987–88	*1988-89*	*1989–90* [1]
Total outlays	78,764	82,128	86,753
including			
Assistance to States and NT	14,248	12,543	12,825
Assistance to the aged	7,240	7,870	8,786
Interest	5,850	5,370	5,328
Assistance to the disabled	2,481	2,736	3,015
Medical services and benefits	3,455	3,723	4,181
Hospitals	1,695	3,740	4,026
Assistance to unemployed and sick	3,886	3,689	3,794
Assistance to veterans	3,128	3,187	3,404
Defence personnel	3,102	3,290	3,384
Tertiary education	2,841	2,913	3,369
Schools	1,950	2,120	2,190
Total revenue	80,829	88,030	95,875
including			
PAYE income tax	37,751	43,976	46,730
Company tax	8,801	10,265	11,360
Sales tax	7,547	9,402	10,500
Other individual tax	8,251	7,712	9,300
Excise duty	9,668	8,603	9,264
Customs duty	3,683	3,802	4,082

[1]Estimates.

Foreign currency reserves were $A20,410m. in 1989.

Gross foreign debt at 30 June 1989 was $A37,046m.

The Consumer Price Index rose by 8% over the year to Sept. 1989.

Australian National Accounts. Australian Bureau of Statistics. 1953–54 to date
Public Authority Finance: Commonwealth Government Finance, Australia. Australian Bureau of Statistics, 1962–63 to date
Public Authority Finance: State and Local Government Finance, Australia. Australian Bureau of Statistics, 1971–72 to date
National Income and Expenditure. Australian Bureau of Statistics. Canberra, 1946 to date
Treasury Information Bulletin (and Supplements). Canberra Treasury Dept., 1956 to date (quarterly)
Hagger, A. J., *A Guide to Australian Economic and Social Statistics*. Sydney, 1983

Currency. On 14 Feb. 1966 Australia adopted a system of decimal currency. The currency unit, the *Australian dollar* (AUD) is divided into 100 *cents*. Decimal notes are issued in denominations of $A1, 2, 5, 10, 20, 50 and 100. Coins are issued in denominations of 1, 2, 5, 10, 20 and 50 cents and $A1.

Money in circulation in June 1989, $A12,193m. In March 1991, US$1 = 1·29 *dollars*; £1 = 2·44 *dollars*.

The underlying inflation rate for the year ending Sept. 1989 was 5·8%.

Banking and Finance. The banking system in Australia comprises:

(a) The Reserve Bank of Australia is the central bank and bank of issue. The *Governor* is Bernie Fraser. Its Rural Credits Department provides short-term credit for the marketing of primary produce. Its assets were $A26,073m. in June 1987 and its liabilities $A26,541m., of which notes on issue, $9,801m.; deposits by trading banks, $3,472m.; deposits by Commonwealth Government, $2,090m.; assets $26,541m. of which gold and foreign exchange (including IMF Special Drawing Rights), $17,120m., treasury notes $1,657m., other Commonwealth Government securities $6,638m. Its functions and responsibilities derive from the Reserve Bank Act 1959, the Banking Act 1959, and the Financial Corporations Act 1974. For the history of the Reserve Bank *see* THE STATESMAN'S YEAR-BOOK 1986–87, p. 104.

(b) Four major trading banks: (i) The Commonwealth Bank of Australia; (ii) 3 private trading banks: The Australia and New Zealand Banking Group Ltd, Westpac Banking Corporation and the National Commercial Banking Corporation of Australia Ltd.

(c) Other trading banks: (i) 3 State Government banks—The State Bank of New South Wales, The State Bank of South Australia, and the Rural and Industries Bank of Western Australia; (ii) one joint stock bank—The Bank of Queensland Ltd, formerly The Brisbane Permanent Building and Banking Co. Ltd, which has specialized business in one district only; (iii) The Australian Bank Ltd; (iv) branches of 17 overseas banks—the restrictions on foreign banks operating in Australia, and on foreign investment in the merchant banks, were lifted in 1984–85.

(d) The Commonwealth Development Bank of Australia commenced operations on 14 Jan. 1960. Its function is to provide finance for primary production and small business.

(e) The Australian Resources Development Bank Ltd opened on 29 March 1968, to assist Australian enterprises in developing Australia's natural resources, through direct loans and equity investment or by re-financing loans made by trading banks. The bank is jointly owned by the 4 major Australian trading banks.

(f) The Primary Industry Bank of Australia Ltd commenced operations on 22 Sept. 1978. The equity capital of the bank consists of eight shares. Seven shares are held by the Australian Government and the major trading banks while the eighth share is held equally by the 4 State banks. The main objective of the bank is to facilitate the provision of loans to primary producers on longer terms than are otherwise generally available. The role of the bank is restricted to re-financing loans made by banks and other financial institutions.

(g) Savings banks, with total deposits of $71,567m. at 30 June 1989 ($61,783m. in 1988). In 1989 16 savings banks were operating in Australia. These comprise subsidiaries of the four major trading banks; four State-owned banks, six private banks, one trustee bank and one overseas bank. At 30 June 1988 these savings banks had 6,005 branches and 8,028 agencies.

Treasury Information Bulletin. Department of the Treasury. Canberra, 1956 to date (quarterly)

At June 30 1988 there were 62 building societies with assets of $S21,680m. Building societies are permitted to have up to 50% of their assets in non-home loans. 3 major societies collapsed in June 1990.

There is an Australian Stock Exchange (ASX).

Weights and Measures. Conversion to the metric system is in progress.

ENERGY AND NATURAL RESOURCES

Electricity. Electricity supply is the responsibility of the State governments. Production 1988–89, 144,854m. kwh (13,949m. hydro-electric in 1988). Supply 240 and 250 volts; 50 Hz.

Oil and gas. The main fields are Gippsland (Vic.) and Carnarvon (WA). Crude oil production was 31,264m. litres in 1987-88, natural gas, 15,249,000m. litres.

Minerals. Australia is a leading producer of bauxite (41·4% of world production in 1988) and diamonds (40·7%). Coal is Australia's major source of energy. Reserves are large (1987 estimate: 50,000m. tonnes) and easily worked. The main fields are in New South Wales and Queensland. Production in 1988-89 was 183·86m. tonnes. Brown coal (lignite) reserves are mainly in Victoria and were estimated 41,900m. tonnes in 1988. Production, 1988-89: 46·11m. tonnes.

Production of other major minerals in 1988-89 (1,000 tonnes): Bauxite, 37,355; copper ore, 77,556; iron ore, 97,618; lead-copper concentrate, 30,988; lead-zinc concentrate, 90,103; manganese ore, 1,907; tungsten, 2,378; nickel ore, 1,921; silver concentrate, 5,117; uranium concentrate, 4,193 (1987–88); 216,872 kg of gold bullion. Gross value of coal and lignite production, 1988-89, $A5,389m.; metallic minerals, $A8,790m.; oil and gas, $A3,448m.

Agriculture. In 1987 there were about 169,700 farms. Farms in 1988 covered 472m. ha. 424m. ha were grazing or fallow, 18·36m. ha sown to crops, of which the most important are wheat (12·29m. tonnes from 9m. ha in 1988); sugar cane (24·83m. from 387,000 ha); barley (3·42m. from 2·35m. ha); oats (1·7m. from 1·28m. ha) and rice (740,000 from 106,000 ha). Vineyards (57,000 ha) produced 372m. litres of wine from 512,000 tonnes of grapes in 1987; grapes in 1988, 799,000 tonnes.

Gross value of agricultural production in 1988-89, $A21,983m., including (in $A1m.): Crops, 9,260; livestock slaughtering, 4,912; wool, 5,794; other livestock products, 2,008. Wool taxes were raised in 1990 in order to combat price falls caused by over-production.

In 1989 74,005 farms had cattle and 63,138 sheep.

Livestock (in 1,000) at 31 March 1989:

	NSW	*Vic.*	*Qld*	*SA*	*WA*	*Tas.*	*NT*	*ACT*	*Australia*
Cattle	5,329	3,509	8,994	943	1,702	560	1,388	11	22,434
Sheep	59,109	28,067	14,880	17,414	37,090	4,933	—	111	161,603
Pigs	855	423	611	450	285	45	3	—	2,671
Poultry	25,972	10,130	10,467	4,840	5,275	833	221	219	57,957

Livestock products (in 1,000 tonnes) for the year ending 30 June 1989: Beef, 1,459; veal, 32; lamb and mutton, 542; pigmeat, 312; poultry meat, 359; milk, 6,289m. litres, 171,790 sheep were shorn, producing 768,718 tonnes of wool.

Forestry. The Federal Government is responsible for forestry at the national level. Each State is responsible for the management of publicly-owned forests. Total forest area was 40·84m. ha in 1987, of which 29·94m. ha were publicly-owned. The major part of wood supplies derives from coniferous plantations, of which there were 832,172 ha in 1986. Timber production was 3·09m. cubic metres in 1986-87.

INDUSTRY. Statistics of manufacturing industries, 1987–88: Number of firms, 31,606; persons employed, 1,063,792; salaries paid, $A23,949·8m.; turnover, $A133,819·6m. (excludes small single-establishment enterprises employing fewer than 4 persons).

Manufacturing by sector as at June 1988:

	No. of firms	*Persons employed*	*Salaries in $A1m.*	*Turnover in $A1m.*
Food, beverages and tobacco	3,938	175,514	3,866·0	27,764·7
Textiles	731	35,417	754·7	3,891·0
Clothing and footwear	2,332	75,194	1,217·2	4,672·1
Wood, wood products and furniture	4,688	81,993	1,503·3	7,006·5
Paper, paper products, printing and publishing	3,356	109,544	2,680·2	12,018·3
Chemical, petroleum and coal products	960	54,316	1,566·2	12,877·3
Non-metallic mineral products	1,863	40,454	1,006·2	6,020·8
Basic metal products	582	74,708	2,150·3	16,358·2
Fabricated metal products	4,848	104,815	2,197·6	10,113·0
Transport equipment	1,494	111,338	2,561·9	12,763·8
Other machinery equipment	4,220	135,031	3,035·9	13,088·4
Miscellaneous manufacturing	2,594	65,468	1,410·4	7,245·5

Manufactured products in 1988-89 included: Beer, 1,951m. litres; bricks, 2,142m.; cement, 6·9m. tonnes; carpets, 44·8m. square metres; confectionery, 156,800 tonnes; electric motors, 2·6m.; washing machines, 397,000; refrigerators, 380,000; TV sets, 162,000; cars, 360,000; caravans, 5,600; pig iron, 5·88m. tonnes; crude steel, 6·65m. tonnes; sulphuric acid, 1·9m. tonnes; superphosphates, 3·68m. tonnes; tobacco, 27,100 tonnes; woollen wove, 9·6m. square metres; woollen yarn, 21,500 tonnes; scoured wool, 100,900 tonnes.

Labour. In Aug. 1989 the total workforce (persons aged 15 and over) numbered (in 1,000s) 8,197, of whom there were employed: 7,728, including women, 3,156 (of whom married, 1,927). In 1988 the labour force included 378,900 employers, 6,143,000 wage and salary earners and 741,700 self-employed. The majority of wage and salary earners have their minimum wages and conditions of work prescribed in awards of industrial arbitration authorities established under federal and State legislation. In some States, some conditions of work (*e.g.*, weekly hours of work, leave) are set down in State legislation. Average weekly wage, May 1989: A$442·20 (women, A$339). Average working week, 1988: 36 hours (males 40·6; females 29·3). 4 weeks annual leave is standard.

Employees in all States are covered by workers' compensation legislation and by certain industrial award provisions relating to work injuries.

During 1988 industrial disputes involving stoppages of work of 10 working days or more accounted for 1,641,400 working days lost. In these disputes 894,400 workers were involved.

The following table shows the distribution of employed persons by industry in 1988, by sex and average weekly hours worked, and total persons in 1989:

Industry	*1988* Numbers (in 1,000) Persons	(Females)	Hours worked Persons	(Females)	*1989* Persons
Agriculture, forestry, fishing and hunting	431·0	(123·8)	42·0	(27·3)	432·4
Mining	96·7	(8·0)	41·2	(37·2)	98·0
Manufacturing	1,199·4	(316·4)	38·5	(33·0)	185·2
Food, beverages and tobacco	163·3	(48·1)	37·5	(32·6)	203·7
Metal products	205·9	(23·1)	40·4	(31·9)	829·6
Other manufacturing	830·2	(245·2)	38·2	(33·1)	1,218·5
Electricity, gas and water	113·8	(11·4)	33·5	(30·0)	119·4
Construction	526·2	(66·9)	38·0	(21·1)	567·5
Wholesale and retail trade	1,496·1	(660·9)	35·1	(27·5)	1,552·7
Transport and storage	376·7	(73·1)	38·3	(30·2)	384·6
Communication	134·2	(35·4)	33·2	(29·8)	137·8
Finance, property and business services	801·1	(400·0)	36·7	(31·3)	830·0
Public administration and defence	321·6	(121·6)	34·4	(31·4)	324·9
Community services	1,304·9	(844·0)	32·9	(29·5)	1,330·4
Recreation, personal and other services	528·3	(304·4)	32·4	(27·6)	539·9
Totals	7,330·1	(2,965·8)	36·0	(29·3)	7,540·3

In June 1988 1,739,800 wage and salary earners worked in the public sector and 4,198,900 in the private sector.

The following table shows the distribution of employed persons in 1988 according to the *Australian Standard Classification of Occupations*:

Occupation	*Employed persons (in 1,000)* Persons	(Females)
Managers and administrators	820·5	(163·0)
Professionals	905·3	(361·2)
Para-professionals	444·9	(188·3)
Tradespersons	1,171·4	(105·9)
Clerks	1,255·1	(698·5)
Salespersons and personnel service	1,025·0	(660·5)
Plant and machine operators, and drivers	584·1	(102·0)
Labourers and related workers	1,123·7	(383·2)
	7,330·1	(2,965·8)

In Aug. 1989 469,400 persons (5·7% of the labour force) were unemployed, (including 208,700 females of whom 99,300 persons were seeking part-time work. In Aug. 1988, 153,400 persons had been unemployed for more than one year. In May 1988 there were 58,500 job vacancies. In the year ended June 1989 689,981 unemployment beneficiaries received a total of $A3,136m., 110,369 sickness beneficiaries received a total of $A553m. and 133,275 special beneficiaries received a total of $A178·3m. 380,000 persons were unemployed in Aug. 1990.

Trade Unions. In June 1988 there were 308 trade unions with 3,213,000 members (1,122,300 females). About 53% of wage and salary earners (43% females) were estimated to be members of unions. In 1988 there were 37 unions with fewer than 100 members and 9 unions with 80,000 or more members. Many of the larger trade unions are affiliated with central labour organizations, the oldest and by far the largest being the Australian Council of Trade Unions formed in 1927. In an agreement of Nov. 1990 the government agreed to increase tax cuts in exchange for wage restraint.

Labour Statistics 1987. Australian Bureau of Statistics. Canberra, 1988
Portus, J. H., *The Development of Australian Trade Union Law*. Melbourne, 1958
Rawson, D. W., *A Handbook of Australian Trade Unions and Employees' Associations*. Canberra, 1977

FOREIGN ECONOMIC RELATIONS. In 1990 Australia and New Zealand completed a Closer Economic Relations agreement (initiated in 1983) which establishes free trade in goods. External debt was $A103,500m. in Dec. 1990.

Commerce. Merchandise imports and exports for years ending 30 June, in $A1m.:

	Imports	*Exports*
1986–87	36,988	35,806
1987–88	40,591	40,946
1988–89	47,073	43,409

The Australian customs tariff provides for preferences to goods produced in and shipped from certain countries as a result of reciprocal trade agreements. These include UK, New Zealand, Canada and Ireland.

Exports and imports, 1988-89 (in $A1m.):

	Exports	*Imports*
Live animals	301·7	156·4
Meat and preparations	2,247·8	30·3
Dairy goods and eggs	568·5	91·1
Fish, shellfish and their preparations	592·5	437·5
Cereals and preparations	2,804·4	72·1
Vegetables and fruit	525·2	382·5
Sugar and honey	917·9	43·6
Coffee, tea, cocoa, spices and their manufacturers	64·7	352·3

	Exports	*Imports*
Animal feed (excl. unmilled cereal)	266·7	73·0
Miscellaneous edible products	95·0	201·3
Beverages	227·2	281·5
Tobacco and manufactures	20·5	92·4
Raw hides and skins	500·7	12·5
Oil seeds and fruit	70·1	49·8
Crude rubber (incl. synthetic and reclaimed)	9·4	113·8
Cork and wood	422·9	561·0
Pulp and waste paper	36·9	224·1
Textile fibres (not wool tops)	6,243·9	179·4
Crude fertilizers, minerals (not coal, petroleum, gems)	238·2	282·5
Metal ores and scrap	6,335·0	77·8
Crude animal and vegetable materials	123·6	107·6
Coal, coke and briquettes	4,742·0	11·1
Petroleum and products	1,464·4	2,002·3
Gas, natural and manufactured	161·3	3·7
Animal oils and fats	105·0	2·9
Fixed vegetable oils and fats	10·7	101·5
Processed oils and fats, waxes thereof	10·6	12·9
Organic chemicals	96·9	1,165·4
Inorganic chemicals	92·9	683·2
Dyeing, colouring and tanning materials	104·4	217·4
Medicinal and pharmaceutical products	232·2	694·1
Essential oils, perfume and cleansing preparations	94·4	262·0
Manufactured fertilizers	7·1	213·5
Plastics in primary forms	147·9	717·0
Plastics in non-primary forms	59·7	444·9
Chemical materials and products	194·9	560·0
Leather and manufactures, dressed furskins	148·7	150·7
Rubber manufactures	65·7	682·3
Cork and wood manufactures (not furniture)	11·4	233·3
Paper, board and pulp	123·1	1,296·5
Textile yarn, fabrics and products	151·7	1,999·5
Non-metallic mineral goods	337·7	966·0
Iron and steel	498·3	1,077·9
Non-ferrous metals	4,162·5	358·7
Metal manufactures	325·6	1,191·8
Power generators	310·4	1,126·0
Special machinery, industrial	337·1	2.361·1
Metalworking machinery	37·4	375·8
General machinery and parts, industrial	331·8	2,522·3
Office machines and data-processing equipment	397·5	3,326·2
Telecommunications and sound equipment	163·9	1,717·8
Electrical machinery and parts	285·9	2,358·9
Road vehicles (inc. air-cushion vehicles)	404·4	4,806·4
Other transport equipment	421·4	2,038·8
Sanitary, plumbing, heating and lighting fittings	27·2	124·6
Furniture and parts	36·8	284·9
Travel goods, handbags etc.	4·8	190·5
Clothing and accessories	63·9	759·1
Footwear	15·4	338·1

	Exports	Imports
Professional, scientific and controlling instruments	195·9	1,066·0
Photographic and optical goods, watches and clocks	262·9	782·2
Miscellaneous manufactured articles	437·6	2,882·9
Other commodities and transactions	3,677·2	1,110·0
Gold and other coin	243·9	20·1
Non-mometary gold	2,487·5	150·6
Confidential items	795·4	186·8
Total trade	43,409·2	47,072·6

Trade in 1988–89:

	Exports		Imports	
	$A1m.	*%*	*$A1m.*	*%*
ASEAN	3,866	8·9	2,813	6·0
Indonesia	745	1·7	419	0·9
Malaysia	742	1·7	687	1·5
Singapore	1,482	3·4	1,090	2·3
Other	896	2·1	617	1·3
Canada	705	1·6	1,067	2·3
China	1,210	2·8	1,027	2·2
EEC	5,997	13·8	10,783	22·9
France	973	2·2	1,276	2·7
Germany, Federal Republic of	1,071	2·5	2,951	6·3
Italy	1,017	2·3	1,382	2·9
Netherlands	659	1·5	601	1·3
UK	1,521	3·5	3,454	7·3
Other	756	1·7	1,119	2·4
Hong Kong	1,888	4·3	891	1·9
Japan	11,840	27·3	9,766	20·7
Korea, South	2,174	5·0	1,262	2·7
New Zealand	2,210	5·1	1,970	4·2
Papua New Guinea	784	1·8	105	0·2
Saudi Arabia	250	0·6	460	1·0
Switzerland	349	0·8	496	1·1
Taiwan	1,565	3·6	1,920	4·1
USA	4,412	10·2	10,129	21·5
USSR	1,010	2·3	5·4	0·1
Other countries	5,195	12·0	4,812	10·2
	43,409	100·0	47,073	100·0

Overseas Trade. Australian Bureau of Statistics. Canberra, 1906 to date

Net customs revenue, 1988–89: $A3,687m.; net excise revenue, $A8,616m.

Total trade between UK and Australia (British Department of Trade returns, in £1,000 sterling):

	1986	*1987*	*1988*	*1989*	*1990*
Imports to UK	643,238	673,837	745,570	864,965	1,039,080
Exports and re-exports from UK	1,227,647	1,223,613	1,377,997	1,711,241	1,645,620

Tourism. During 1987, 1·7m. overseas visitors arrived in Australia intending to stay for less than 12 months; tourists spent $A3,700m.

Australian Bureau of Statistics, Canberra: *Rural Industries*. 1962–63 to date.—*Manufacturing Establishments: Details of Operations*. 1968–69 to date.—*Non-rural Primary Industries*. 1967–68 and 1968–69.—*Value of Production*. 1964–65 to 1968–69.—*Manufacturing Industry*. 1963–64 to 1967–68.—*Manufacturing Commodities*. 1963–64 and 1964–65.— *Building and Construction*. 1964–65 to date

Quarterly Review of Agricultural Economics. Bureau of Agricultural Economics. Canberra, 1948 to date

Developments in Australian Manufacturing Industry. Department of Trade. Melbourne, 1954–55 to date (annual)

The Australian Mineral Industry Review. Department of National Development—Bureau of Mineral Resources, Geology and Geophysics. Canberra, 1948 to date

Australian Economy. Department of the Treasury. Canberra, 1956 to date
Australasian Institute of Mining and Metallurgy. *Proceedings: New Series*. Melbourne, 1912 to date

COMMUNICATIONS

Roads. In 1987 there were 38,124 km of state highways and freeways, 38,090 km of trunk roads, 31,673 km of ordinary main roads and 36,338 km of other roads.

At 30 June 1988, 7,243,600 cars, 1,977,600 vans, trucks and buses and 323,300 motor cycles were registered. New registrations, 1987-88, include 384,283 cars, 86,617 vans, trucks and buses and 18,532 motor cycles.

463·67m. passenger journeys were made by bus in 1986-87.

In 1987 there were 25,500 road accidents in which 2,772 persons were killed.

Railways. There are six government-owned railway systems. Statistics for the year ended 30 June 1987:

System	*Route length in km* [4]	*Passenger journeys, 1,000*	*Goods carried, (1,000 tonnes)*	*Gross earnings, ($A1m.)*
State:				
New South Wales	9,907	224,300	54,600	1,121·2
Victoria	5,257	97,822	10,597	481·3
Queensland	10,210	44,334	75,169	1,028·9
South Australia [3]	149	11,798	...	14·4
Western Australia	5,553	10,051	21,264	258·2
Australian National [1, 2]	7,315	329	12,900	283·3
	38,393	388,634	174,530	3,187·3

[1] The Australian National Railways operates services of the former Commonwealth Railways, the non-metropolitan South Australian Railways and the Tasmanian Railways.
[2] Excludes Adelaide metropolitan rail passenger services and the Tasmanian Region.
[3] The South Australian State Transport Authority operates services in the Adelaide metropolitan area.
[4] Inter system traffic is included in the total for each system over which it passes.

The State railway gauges are: New South Wales, 1,435 mm; Victoria, 1,600 mm (325 km 1,435 mm); Queensland, 1,067 mm (111 km 1,435 mm); South Australia, 1,600 mm for 2,533 km, 1,824 km 1,435 mm and the rest 1,067 mm; West Australia, 137 km, 1,435 mm and the rest 1,067 mm, and Tasmania, 1,067 mm. Of the Australian National Railways, the gauge of the Trans-Australian and Australian Capital Territory is 1,435 mm, and for the Central Australia 1,067 mm for 869 km and 1,435 mm for 350 km. Under various Commonwealth–State standardization agreements, all the State capitals are now linked by 1,435 mm gauge track. The Central Australia railway extends as far north as Alice Springs (now standard gauge on new alignment from Tarcoola to Alice Springs).

There are also private industrial and tourist railways.

Aviation. With effect from 1 July 1988 the Civil Aviation Authority has been responsible for aviation safety under the Civil Aviation Act, 1988.

In 1988 Australia had air service agreements with 26 countries, and 32 international airlines were operating scheduled services. Qantas Airways, Australia's international airline, operated 25 Boeing 747s and 7 Boeing 767s. All shares in Qantas are owned by the Commonwealth Government. In 1986-87 6·14m. passengers and 263,989 tonnes of freight were flown on international flights. The major international airports are Adelaide, Brisbane, Darwin, Melbourne, Perth, Sydney and Townsville.

Internal airlines carried 13·7m. passengers and 147,939 tonnes of freight in 1987-88. Domestic airlines were deregulated in Oct. 1990.

At 30 June 1988 there were 430 licensed aerodromes (67 owned by the Commonwealth Government) and 9 helicopter pads.

Shipping. The chief ports are Sydney, Newcastle, Port Kembla (NSW); Melbourne, Geelong, Westernport (Vic.); Hay Point, Gladstone, Brisbane (Qld.); Port Hedland,

Dampier, Port Walcott, Fremantle (WA). As at 30 June 1988 the Australian merchant marine (vessels of 150 tonnes gross and over) consisted of 63 coastal vessels of 876,276 tonnes gross and 30 overseas vessels of 1,293,187 tonnes gross.

Arrivals and departures of vessels engaged in overseas trade:

	Arrivals			*Departures*		
	No of port visits [1]	*DWT (1,000 tonnes)*	*Cargo discharged (1,000 tonnes gross)*	*No. of port visits* [1]	*DWT (1,000 tonnes)*	*Cargo loaded (1,000 tonnes gross)*
1987–88	11,932	458,614	6,738	11,848	456,694	268,236
1988-89	12,153	465,978	36,603	12,029	458,595	267,230

[1] Before 1987–88 figures were given for direct arrivals or departures only.

46·89m. tonnes of cargo were carried by coastal shipping in 1986-87.

Telecommunications. Postal services are operated by Australia Post, established by the Postal Services Act, 1975. Revenue was $A1,656·4m. in 1987-88, expenditure $A1,601·4m. There were 4,489 post offices and other agencies in 1988. 3,662m. postal items were handled.

Telecommunications are operated by Telecom Australia under the Telecommunications Act, 1975. Revenue was $A7,199·5m. in 1987-88, expenditure $A6,423·3m. There were 7,091,549 telephones. Services to other countries are operated by the Overseas Telecommunications Commission Australia (OTC), established by the Overseas Telecommmunications Act, 1946.

Australia's National Satellite System is owned and operated by AUSSAT Pty Ltd under the Satellite Communications Act, 1984. 75% of its shares are owned by the Commonwealth Government and the rest by Telecom Australia; 3 satellites are in orbit covering the entire continent.

Broadcasting is regulated by the Broadcasting Act, 1942 and the Broadcasting Ownership and Control Acts, 1987. Foreign ownership of commercial radio and TV companies is restricted to 20%. The National Broadcasting Service is provided by the Australian Broadcasting Corporation (ABC), which at 30 June 1988 operated 100 MW, 141 FM and 6 high-frequency radio stations. In addition, 133 MW and 9 FM, commercial stations and 9 MW and 66 public stations were operating. The short-wave international service Radio Australia broadcasts in English, Bahasa Malay, Cantonese, Chinese, French, Japanese, Thai, Tok Pisin and Vietnamese.

The National Television Service is provided by the ABC, which at 30 June 1988 operated 366 transmitter stations. In addition, 50 commercial companies operated 288 transmitters.

In 1989 there were estimated to be 7·17m. radios and 6m. TV sets in use.

Cinemas In 1985 there were 444 cinemas and 172 drive-in cinemas.

Newspapers (1981). There was 1 national newspaper (average daily circulation 126,000) and 14 metropolitan daily newspapers in Australia with a combined daily circulation of 3·6m. Of these, 3 papers published in Melbourne accounted for 1·3m. and 4 published in Sydney for 1·2m.

Australian Transport. Sydney, Institute of Transport, 1937 to date (quarterly)

JUSTICE, RELIGION, EDUCATION AND WELFARE

Justice. The judicial power of the Commonwealth of Australia is vested in the High Court of Australia (the Federal Supreme Court), in the Federal courts created by the Federal Parliament (the Federal Court of Australia and the Family Court of Australia) and in the State courts invested by Parliament with Federal jurisdiction.

High Court. The High Court consists of a Chief Justice and 6 other Justices, appointed by the Governor-General in Council. The Constitution confers on the High Court original jurisdiction, *inter alia*, in all matters arising under treaties or affecting consuls or other foreign representatives, matters between the States of the Commonwealth, matters to which the Commonwealth is a party and matters between residents of different States. Federal Parliament may make laws conferring original jurisdiction on the High Court, *inter alia*, in matters arising under the Constitution or under any laws made by the Parliament. It has in fact conferred jurisdiction on the High Court in matters arising under the Constitution and in matters arising under certain laws made by Parliament.

The High Court may hear and determine appeals from its own Justices exercising original jurisdiction, from any other Federal Court, from a Court exercising Federal jurisdiction and from the Supreme Courts of the States. It also has jurisdiction to hear and determine appeals from the Supreme Courts of the Territories. The right of appeal from the High Court to the Privy Council was abolished in 1986.

Other Federal Courts. Since 1924, 4 other Federal courts have been created to exercise special Federal jurisdiction, *i.e.* the Federal Court of Australia, the Family Court of Australia, the Australian Industrial Court and the Federal Court of Bankruptcy. The Federal Court of Australia was created by the Federal Court of Australia Act 1976 and began to exercise jurisdiction on 1 Feb. 1977. It exercises such original jurisdiction as is invested in it by laws made by the Federal Parliament including jurisdiction formerly exercised by the Australian Industrial Court and the Federal Court of Bankruptcy, and in some matters previously invested in either the High Court or State and Territory Supreme Courts. The Federal Court also acts as a court of appeal from State and Territory courts in relation to Federal matters. Appeal from the Federal Court to the High Court will be by way of special leave only. The State Supreme Courts have also been invested with Federal jurisdiction in bankruptcy.

State Courts. The general Federal jurisdiction of the State courts extends, subject to certain restrictions and exceptions, to all matters in which the High Court has jurisdiction or in which jurisdiction may be conferred upon it.

Industrial Tribunals. The chief federal industrial tribunal is the Australian Conciliation and Arbitration Commission, constituted by presidential members (with the status of judges) and commissioners. The Commission's functions include settling industrial disputes, making awards, determining the standard hours of work and wage fixation. Questions of law, the judicial interpretation of awards and imposition of penalties in relation to industrial matters, are dealt with by the Industrial Division of the Federal Court.

Australian Digest of Reported Decisions of the Australian Courts and of Australian Appeals to the Privy Council. 2nd ed. Sydney, Law Book Co. 1963—Supplements 1964 ff.
Baalman, J., *Outline of Law in Australia*. 4th ed. Sydney, 1979
Bates, N., *Introduction to Legal Studies*. 3rd ed. Melbourne, 1980
Benjafield, D. G. and Whitmore, H., *Principles of Australian Administrative Law*. 3rd ed. Sydney, 1966
Cowen, Z., *Federal Jurisdiction in Australia*. 2nd ed. Melbourne, 1978
Fleming, J. G., *The Law of Torts*. 5th ed. Sydney, 1977
Gunn, J. A. L., *Australian Income Tax Law and Practice*. 9th ed. by F. C. Bock and E. F. Mannix, Sydney, 1969, and *Butterworth's Taxation Service* to date
Howard, C., *Criminal Law*. 3rd ed. Sydney, 1975
Mills, C. P. and Sorrell, G. H., *Federal Industrial Law. (Nolan and Cohen.)* 5th ed. Sydney, 1975
O'Connell, D. P. (ed.) *International Law in Australia*. Sydney, 1966
Paterson, W. E. and Ednie, H. H., *Australian Company Law*. 2nd ed. Sydney, 1976, and *Butterworth's Company Service* to date
Sawer, G., *The Australian and the Law*. Melbourne, 1976
Twyford, J., *The Layman and the Law in Australia*. 2nd ed. Sydney, 1980
Wynes, A., *Legislative, Executive and Judicial Powers in Australia*. 5th ed. Sydney, 1976
Yorston, R. K. and Fortescue, E. E., *Australian Mercantile Law*. 14th ed. Sydney, 1971

Religion. Under the Constitution the Commonwealth cannot make any law to establish any religion, to impose any religious observance or to prohibit the free exercise of any religion, nor can it require a religious test as qualification for office or public trust under the Commonwealth. The following percentages refer to those religions with the largest number of adherents at the census of 1986. The census question on religion was not obligatory, however.

Christian, 73% of population; Catholic, 26%; Anglican, 23·9%; Uniting, 7·6%;

Presbyterian, 3·6%; Orthodox, 2·7%; Baptist, 1·3%; Lutheran, 1·3%; Church of Christ, 0·6%; Religion other than Christian 2·%, No religion 12·7%, No statement 12·3%.

Education. The Governments of the Australian States and the Northern Territory have the major responsibility for education, including the administration and substantial funding of primary, secondary, and technical and further education. In most States, a single Education Department is responsible for these three levels, but in New South Wales and South Australia there is a separate department responsible solely for technical and further education and in Victoria, a Technical and Further Education Board. Furthermore, in New South Wales an Education Commission advises the Minister on primary, secondary and post-secondary education.

The Australian Government is responsible for education in Norfolk Island, Christmas Island and the Cocos (Keeling) Islands. It also provides supplementary finance to the States and is responsible for the total funding of universities and colleges of advanced education. It has special responsibilities for student assistance, education programmes for Aboriginal people and children from non-English-speaking backgrounds, and for international relations in education.

The Australian Constitution empowers the Federal Government to make grants to the States and to place conditions upon such grants. There are two national Education Commissions which advise the Federal Government on the financial needs of educational institutions. The Commonwealth Schools Commission, established in 1973, advises on financial assistance to the States for schools. The Commonwealth Tertiary Education Commission advises on providing the States with total funding for universities and colleges of advanced education, and supplementary assistance for their institutions of technical and further education.

In 1984 legislation was passed to reactivate the national Curriculum Development Centre (CDC) within the framework of the Commonwealth Schools Commission. The CDC's functions are to concentrate on co-ordination and dissemination and on sponsoring the development of materials through contract arrangements with other agencies.

School attendance is compulsory between the ages of 6 and 15 years (16 years in Tasmania), at either a government school or a recognized non-government educational institution. Many children attend pre-schools for a year before entering school (usually in sessions of 2-3 hours, for 2-5 days per week). Government schools are usually co-educational and comprehensive. Non-government schools have been traditionally single-sex, particularly in secondary schools, but there is a trend towards co-education. Tuition is free at government schools, but fees are normally charged at non-government schools.

Primary and secondary schools at July 1989:

	Schools		*Teachers* [1]		*Pupils* [2]	
States and Territories	*Government*	*Non-government*	*Government schools*	*Non-government schools*	*Government schools*	*Non-government schools*
New South Wales	2,200	858	45,812	17,281	749,263	284,330
Victoria	2,059	719	40,737	16,400	527,700	257,407
Queensland	1,300	394	24,257	7,367	387,438	126,418
South Australia	708	183	13,376	3,550	185,769	56,363
Western Australia	753	241	13,243	4,227	212,461	67,503
Tasmania	254	66	4,732	1,180	64,977	18,394
Northern Territory	143	25	1,997	393	25,987	6,025
ACT	96	37	2,804	1,214	40,760	20,592
Australia	7,513	2,523	146,957	51,611	2,194,355	837,032

[1] Full-time teachers plus the full-time equivalent of part-time teaching.
[2] Full-time pupils only.

In post-secondary education, tuition fees were abolished in 1974 and student allowances are provided for full-time students subject to a means test. Universities are autonomous institutions, as are the substantial majority of colleges of advanced education. While both offer degree courses, colleges also offer diploma and associate diploma courses; these tend to be vocational. The major part of technical and further education is provided in government-administered technical and further education institutions (TAFE). These had 1,430,925 students in 1987. Other institutes of advanced education had 225,528 students (126,204 full-time) and 10,711 teachers in 1988.

There were 19 universities in 1988. They were, with numbers of academic staff (and students): Sydney, 1,588 (18,236); New South Wales (including the Australian Defence Force Academy), 1,292 (19,771); New England, 477 (9,427); Newcastle, 384 (6,375); Macquarie, 595 (11,194); Wollongong, 499 (7,964); Melbourne, 2,076 (16,733); Monash, 1,274 (14,768); La Trobe, 962 (13,128); Deakin, 287 (7,209); Queensland, 1,359 (18,233); James Cook, 384 (4,244); Griffith, 279 (5,339); Adelaide, 860 (9,177); Flinders, 417 (6,028); Western Australian, 828 (10,063); Murdoch, 279 (5,196); Tasmania, 418 (5,376); Australian National, 947 (6,651).

The Victoria University of Technology was founded in 1990, and also a Catholic University under the sponsorship of La Trobe. A private university in Queensland, the Bond University, was founded in 1989 with 800 students.

Teacher education usually takes place in colleges of advanced education, though a substantial number of secondary teachers and a few primary teachers receive their pre-service education in a university.

The Australian Government provides assistance for students. The Secondary Allowances Scheme aims to help parents with a limited income to keep their children at school for the final 2 years of secondary education. The Assistance for Isolated Children Scheme provides special support to families whose children are isolated from schooling or are handicapped. The Adult Secondary Education Assistance Scheme provides assistance for mature-age students undertaking a full-time one-year matriculation level programme or a two-year programme if studies beyond the tenth year in the Australian secondary school system have not previously been undertaken. The Tertiary Education Assistance Scheme is a means-tested scheme to assist students enrolled for full-time study in approved courses at post-secondary institutions. Allowances are also available for post-graduate study and overseas study. Aboriginal students are eligible for assistance under the Aboriginal Secondary Grants Scheme and the Aboriginal Study Grants Scheme. The States also offer various schemes of assistance, principally at the primary and secondary levels.

National bodies with a co-ordinating, planning or funding rôle include: the Australian Education Council, comprising the Federal and State Ministers of Education, the Conference of Directors-General of Education and an advisory body, the National Aboriginal Education Committee.

Total expenditure on education in Australia (public and private sectors) in 1983–84 was estimated at $A10,805m.

Australian Education Directory. Canberra, 1983
Directory of Higher Education Courses 1982. Canberra, 1982
Primary and Secondary Schooling in Australia. Canberra, 1977
Schools Commission, *Triennium 1982–84. Report for 1982*. Canberra, 1981
Tertiary Education Commission, *Report for 1982–84, Triennium Vol. 2: Recommendations for 1982*. Canberra, 1981

Health. In 1987 there were an average 5·4 hospital beds per 1,000 population. There were 1,053 hospitals (general). The Royal Flying Doctor Service serves remote areas.

Social Security and Welfare. All Commonwealth Government social security pensions, benefits and allowances are financed from the Commonwealth Government's general revenue. In addition, assistance is provided for welfare services.

Expenditure on main programmes, 1987–88, $A22,599m.

The following summarizes the conditions of the major benefits.

Age and invalid pensions—age pensions are payable to men 65 years of age or more and women 60 years of age or more who have lived in Australia for a specified period and, unless permanently blind, also satisfy an income test. Persons over 16 years of age who are permanently blind or permanently incapacitated for work to the extent of at least 85% may receive an invalid pension. There is no residence qualification for an invalid pension if the permanent incapacity or blindness occurred within Australia or during temporary absence from Australia. An income test must be satisfied for an invalid pension unless permanently blind. Additional amounts are paid to pensioners with dependent children. Supplementary assistance may be paid to a pensioner paying rent or private lodging subject to an income test. Remote area allowance is payable to pensioners living in income tax zone A, except for those aged 70 or more receiving the special rate of age pension. Supplementary assistance, additional pension for children, mother's/guardian's allowance and remote area allowance are not taxable.

In 1987-88 1,328,814 age pensioners received a total of $A6,972m., and 296,913 invalid pensioners received $A2,188m.

Wife's pension—payable to the wife of an age or invalid pensioner if she is not eligible for a pension in her own right. The maximum rate and the income test are identical to those for age and invalid pensioners.

Spouse carer's pension—payable to the husband of an age or invalid pensioner who is providing constant care and attention at home for his wife if he is not eligible for pension in his own right. The maximum rate and the income test are identical to those for age and invalid pensions.

Widow's pension—widows, divorcees, certain deserted wives, women who have been the dependant of a man for 3 years immediately prior to his death and women whose husbands have been convicted of an offence and have been imprisoned for not less than 6 months may, if they satisfy a residence requirement and an income test, receive a widow's pension. If they have any dependent children they also receive a mother's/ guardian's allowance plus an additional allowance for each child. Persons who pay private rent may also receive supplementary assistance subject to an income test. Pensions are subject to income tax, but not mother's allowances, additional pension for children, supplementary assistance, or remote area allowance.

In 1987-88 143,451 widow pensioners received a total of $A1,002m.

Supporting parents benefit—sole parents who have custody, care and control of any dependent children may, if they satisfy a residence requirement and an income test, receive supporting parents benefit. It is payable at the same rate as the widow's pension and is subject to the same income test. Mother's/guardian's allowance, additional pension for each dependent child, supplementary assistance and remote area allowance are also payable.

In 1988-89 239,469 beneficiaries received a total of $A2,226m.

Sheltered employment allowance—is payable to disabled persons under age—pension age engaged in approved sheltered employment who are qualified to receive invalid pension. The rates of payment and allowances and income test are the same as invalid pension.

Rehabilitation allowance—persons undertaking a rehabilitation programme with the Commonwealth Rehabilitation Service who are eligible for a social security pension or benefit are eligible to receive a non taxable rehabilitation allowance during treatment or training and for up to 6 months thereafter. The allowance is equivalent to the invalid pension and is subject to the same income test.

Family Allowance—is paid without income test to assist families with children under 16 years or dependent full-time students aged 16 years to under 25 years. It is not subject to income tax.

In 1988-89 1,927,015 families comprising 3,760,462 children received a total of $A1,315m.

Family income supplement—payable subject to an income test to families with one or more children eligible for family allowances so long as they are not in receipt of any Commonwealth pension, benefit or allowance which provides additional payment for dependent children; this is not taxable.

In 1987-88 141,336 families received a total $A214m.

Child disability allowance—payable to parents or guardians of severely physically or mentally handicapped children in the family home and needing constant care and attention. The allowance is free of an income test but is subject to a residence qualification similar to that for family allowance.

In 1988-89 36,777 allowances totalling $A50·9m. were paid.

Double orphan's pension—the guardian of a child under 16 years of age or of a full-time student under 25, both of whose parents are dead, or one of whose parents is dead and the whereabouts of the other parent unknown, and for refugee children where both parents are outside Australia, may receive double orphan's pension. The payment is not subject to an income test nor is it taxable.

Unemployment and sickness benefits—are paid, subject to an income test, to persons between the ages of 18 and 16 respectively and age pension age who are unemployed, able and willing to work and making efforts to obtain work, or temporarily unable to work because of sickness or injury. The 1990 Budget abolished the existing indefinite benefits of $A105 per week in favour of a 'job search allowance' of $A57 per week for up to one year. To be granted benefit a person must have resided in Australia for at least 12 months preceding his claim or intend to remain in Australia permanently. For unemployment benefit purposes unemployment must not be due to industrial action by that person or by members of a union to which that person is a member. Special benefits may be granted to persons not qualified above. For numbers of beneficiaries and amounts paid *see* **Labour** p. 108.

Service Pensions are paid by the Department of Veterans' Affairs, similar to the age and invalid pensions provided by the Department of Social Security. Male Veterans who have reached the age of 60 years or are permanently unemployable, and who served in a theatre of war, are eligible subject to an income test. Female Veterans who served abroad and who have reached the age of 55 or are permanently unemployable, are also eligible. Wives of service pensioners are also eligible provided that they do not receive a pension from the Department of Social Security. *Disability pension* is a compensatory payment in respect of incapacity attributable to war service. It is paid at a rate commensurate with the degree of incapacity and is free of any income test. A separate allowance may be paid to dependents. In 1988-89 396,439 pensioners received a total of $A2,055m.

In addition to cash benefits, welfare services are provided either directly or through State and Local government authorities and voluntary agencies, for people with special needs.

Medicare. On 1 Feb. 1984 the Commonwealth Government introduced a universal health scheme known as Medicare. This covers: Automatic entitlement under a single public health fund to medical and optometrical benefits of 85% of the Medical Benefits Schedule fee, with a maximum patient payment for any service where the Schedule fee is charged; access without direct charge to public hospital accommodation and to inpatient and outpatient treatment by doctors appointed by the hospital; the restoration of funds for community health to approximately the same real level as 1975; a reduction in charges for private treatment in shared wards of public hospitals, and increases in the daily bed subsidy payable to private hospitals.

The Medicare programme is financed in part by a 1·25% levy on taxable incomes, with low income cut-off points, which were $A8,980 p.a. for a single person in 1989 and $A15,090 p.a. for a family with a $A2,100 reduction for each child. The Commonwealth Government subsidises registered health insurance organizations by contributing to the Health Benefits, and makes an annual contribution to the Reinsurance Trust Fund of $A20m. for payments of benefits to patients with hospital treatment in excess of 35 days.

Medicare benefits are available to all persons ordinarily resident in Australia. Visitors from UK, New Zealand and Malta have immediate access to necessary medical treatment, as do all visitors staying more than 6 months.

Medical Benefits. The Health Insurance Act provides for a Medical Benefits Schedule which lists medical services and the Schedule (standard) fee applicable in each

State in respect of each medical service. Schedule fees are set and updated by an independent fees tribunal appointed by the Government. The fees so determined are to apply for Medicare benefits purposes.

Home and Community Care Program was introduced in 1985 to provide support services to enable aged and disabled persons to live at home. It is jointly funded by the Commonwealth and State or Territory Governments. Commonwealth funding was $A168m. in 11987-88.

DIPLOMATIC REPRESENTATIVES

Of Australia in Great Britain (Australia House, Strand, London, WC2B 4LA)
High Commissioner: R. J. Smith.

Of Great Britain in Australia (Commonwealth Ave., Canberra)
High Commissioner: Brian Barder.

Of Australia in the USA (1601 Massachusetts Ave., NW, Washington, D.C., 20036)
Ambassador: Michael John Cork.

Of the USA in Australia (Moonah Pl., Canberra)
Ambassador: Melvin F. Sembler.

Of Australia to the United Nations
Ambassador: Dr Peter Stephen Wilenski, AO.

Further Reading

Statistical Information: The Australian Bureau of Statistics (Cameron Offices, Belconnen, A.C.T., 2616) was established in 1906. All the activities of the Bureau are covered by the Census and Statistics Act, which confers authority to collect information and contains secrecy provisions to ensure that individual particulars obtained are not divulged. Under the provisions of the Statistics (Arrangements with States) Act which became law on 12 May 1956, the statistical services of all the States have been integrated with the Australian Bureau. An outline of the development of statistics in Australia is published in the *Official Year Book*, No. 51, 1965. *Australian Statistician:* Dr Ian Castles.

The principal publications of the Bureau are:

Year Book Australia. 1907 to date
Pocket Year Book, Australia. 1913 to date
Monthly Summary of Statistics Australia. Oct. 1937 to date
Digest of Current Economic Statistics Australia. Aug. 1959 to date
Catalogue of Publications, 1976 to date

Other Official Publications

Atlas of Australian Resources. Dept. of Resources and Energy, Division of National Mapping
Climatological Atlas of Australia. Bureau of Meteorology. Melbourne, 1940
Norfolk Island—Annual Report. Dept. of Territories and Local Government
Cocos (Keeling) Islands—Annual Report. Dept. of Territories and Local Government
Christmas Island—Annual Report. Dept. of Territories and Local Government
Australian Books: Select List of Works About or Published in Australia. National Library of Australia, Canberra, 1934 to date
Australian National Bibliography. Canberra, 1936 to date
Historical Records of Australia. 34 vols. National Library, Canberra, 1914–25
Australia Handbook. Dept. of Administrative Services. Australian Information Services
Annual Report. Dept. of Foreign Affairs, Canberra, 1932 to date
Australian Foreign Affairs Record. Dept. of Foreign Affairs, Canberra, 1936 to date
Australian Treaty List. Dept. of Foreign Affairs, Canberra, consolidated volume from Federation to 1970 with supplements to date
Coxon, H., *Australian Official Publications*. Oxford, 1981
Documents on Australian Foreign Policy 1937–49. Vols. I–VI. Dept. of Foreign Affairs, Canberra, 1975–83
Diplomatic List. Dept. of Foreign Affairs, Canberra. 1949 to date
Consular and Trade Representatives. Dept. of Foreign Affairs, Canberra. 1936 to date

Non-Official Publications

Australian Encyclopædia. 12 vols. Sydney, 1983
Australian Quarterly: A Quarterly Review of Australian Affairs. Sydney, 1929 to date
Blainey, G., *The Tyranny of Distance: How Distance Shaped Australia's History*. Melbourne, 1982
Caves, P. E. and Krause, L. B., *The Australian Economy: A View from the North*. Sydney, 1984
Clark, M., *A Short History of Australia*. Melbourne, 1981
Deery, S. and Plowman, D., *Australian Industrial Relations*. Sydney, 1985
Gilbert, A. D. and Inglis, K. S. (eds.) *Australians: A Historical Library*. 5 vols. CUP, 1988
Hancock, K. (ed.) *Australian Society*. Cambridge Univ. Press, 1990
Hocking, B. (ed.) *Australia towards 2000* London, 1990
Howard, C., *Australia's Constitution*. Melbourne, 1985
Hurst, J., *Hawke P. M.* Sydney, 1983
Inglis, K., *This is the ABC: The Australian Broadcasting Commission*. Melbourne, 1983
Jupp, J., *Party Politics: Australia, 1966–1981*. Sydney, 1982
Kepars, I., *Australia*. [Bibliography] Oxford and Santa Barbara, 1984
Lucy, R., *The Australian Form of Government*. Melbourne, 1985
Moore, D. and Hall, R., *Australia: Image of a Nation*. London, 1983
Oxford History of Australia. vol 5: 1942–88. OUP, 1990
Serle, P., *Dictionary of Australian Biography*. 2 vols. Sydney, 1949
Solomon, D., *Australia's Government and Parliament*. Melbourne, 1981
Spann, R. N., *Government Administration in Australia*. Sydney, 1979
Who's Who in Australia. Melbourne, 1906 to date
Wilson, R. K., *Australia's Resources and their Development*. Univ. of Sydney, 1980

National Library: The National Library, Canberra, A.C.T. *Director-General:* Harrison Bryan.

AUSTRALIAN TERRITORIES

AUSTRALIAN CAPITAL TERRITORY

HISTORY. The area, now the Australian Capital Territory (ACT), was first visited by Europeans in 1820 and settlement commenced in 1824. Until its selection as the seat of government it was a quiet pastoral and agricultural community.

AREA AND POPULATION. The area of the Australian Capital Territory is 2,432 sq. km (including Jervis Bay area). The population (estimate) at 31 March 1988 was 271,900. Previous census population:

	Males	*Females*	*Total*		*Males*	*Females*	*Total*
1911	992	722	1,714	1966	49,991	46,041	96,032
1921	1,567	1,005	2,572	1971	73,589	70,474	144,063
1933	4,805	4,142	8,947	1976	100,103	95,519	197,622
1947	9,092	7,813	16,905	1981	110,415	111,194	221,609
1954	16,229	14,086	30,315	1986	132,100	132,300	264,400
1961	30,858	27,970	58,828				

(Figures before 1961 exclude particulars of full-blood Aborigines.)

CONSTITUTION AND GOVERNMENT. The Constitution of Australia provided (Sec. 125) that the seat of government should be selected by parliament and that it should be within New South Wales, distance not less than 160 km from Sydney. The present area was surrendered by New South Wales and accepted by the Australian Government from 1 Jan. 1911. In 1915 an additional 73 sq. km at Jervis Bay was transferred from New South Wales to serve as a port. In 1911 an international competition was held for the city plan. The plan chosen was that of W. Burley Griffin, of Chicago. Construction, delayed by the First World War, began in 1923 and on 9 May 1927 Parliament was opened and Canberra became the seat of government. Most Australian Government departments now have their headquarters in Canberra.

The general administration lies with the ACT Administration, responsible to the Federal Minister for the Arts, Sport, Environment, Tourism and Territories. The Administration provides all municipal and Territorial services except police and courts (responsibility of the Federal Attorney-General).

The Australian Capital Territory Representation (House of Representatives) Act, 1973, provided for the representation of residents of the Territory by 2 elected members in the House of Representatives. The Senate (Representation of Territories) Act 1973 provided for the election of 2 Senators from the Territory. Elections took place on 1 Dec. 1984. The ACT became self-governing on 11 May 1989.

FINANCE. In 1987–88 the ACT was given its own budget. It is treated equitably with the States regarding local revenue raising, expenditure and assistance by the Commonwealth government.

PRODUCTION. Outside Canberra the Territory is mainly reserved for forestry and nature conservation (Namadgi National Park is 94,000 hectares). A considerable amount of reafforestation (mostly pine) has been undertaken, the total area of coniferous plantations at 30 June 1988 being 16,194 hectares. Farming is mainly in grazing: Livestock (1988), 12,422 cattle, 116,851 sheep, and 1,948 horses.

EDUCATION. In July 1989 there were 96 government schools comprising 66 primary schools, 24 secondary schools and colleges, 1 combined primary/secondary school and 5 special schools. Non-government schools numbered 37 of which there were 23 primary schools, 6 secondary schools and 8 schools with both primary and secondary enrolments. Students enrolled full-time in government schools in 1989 numbered 22,188 and 18,096 in primary and secondary school levels respectively. Enrolments at non-government schools comprised 10,278 primary school students and 10,314 secondary school students. Pre-school education was provided at 73 centres with a total enrolment of 4,360. There is an Institute of Technical and Further Education and a Canberra Institute of the Arts.

The Canberra College of Advanced Education commenced operation in 1970. Enrolments (1988) 6,582. The Australian National University is situated in Canberra. Enrolments (1988) 6,645.

Further Reading

Australian Capital Territory Statistical Summary. Australian Bureau of Statistics. From 1960
Wigmore, L., *Canberra: A History of Australia's National Capital*. 2nd ed. Canberra, 1971

NORTHERN TERRITORY

HISTORY. The Northern Territory, after forming part of New South Wales, was annexed on 6 July 1863 to South Australia and in 1901 entered the Commonwealth as a corporate part of South Australia. The Commonwealth Constitution Act of 1900 made provision for the surrender to the Commonwealth of any territory by any state, and under this provision an agreement was entered into on 7 Dec. 1907 for the transfer of the Northern Territory to the Commonwealth, and it formally passed under the control of the Commonwealth Government on 1 Jan. 1911. For details of Constitutional development until 1978 *see* THE STATESMAN'S YEAR-BOOK 1980–81 pp. 123–24. The Commonwealth Government retained responsibility until Self-Government was granted on 1 July 1978.

AREA AND POPULATION. The Northern Territory is bounded by the 26th parallel of S. lat. and 129° and 138° E. long. Its total area is 1,346, 200 sq. km. The coastline is about 6,200 km in length, and the Territory includes adjacent islands between 129° and 138° E. long. The greater part of the interior consists of a tableland rising gradually from the coast to a height of about 700 metres. On this tableland there are large areas of excellent pasturage. The southern part of the Territory is generally sandy and has a small rainfall, but water may be obtained by means of sub-artesian bores.

The population of the Territory in June 1990 was 157,304. The capital, seat of Government and principal port is Darwin, on the north coast; population 73,300 in

June 1990. Other main centres include Katherine (7,500), 330 km south of Darwin; Alice Springs (24,000), in Central Australia; Tennant Creek (3,000), a rich mining centre 500 km north of Alice Springs; Nhulunbuy (3,400), a bauxite mining centre on the Gove Peninsula in eastern Arnhem Land; and Jabiru, a model town built to serve the rich Uranium Province in eastern Arnhem Land with a planned population of 6,000 (actual, 1986, 1,410). Palmerston is a Darwin satellite town (1990, 7,900); Yulara (1,158) is a resort village serving Uluru National Park and Ayers Rock. There also are a number of large self-contained Aboriginal communities. Aboriginals were 34,739 at the 1986 Census. On 31 July 1984, 26,692,400 ha were designated Aboriginal Land under the Aboriginal Land Rights (N.T.) Act 1976.

Vital statistics for 1989: Births, 3,379; deaths, 787; marriages (1988), 782.

CONSTITUTION AND GOVERNMENT. The Northern Territory (Self-Government) Act 1978 established the Northern Territory as a body politic as from 1 July 1978, with Ministers having control over and responsibility for Territory finances and the administration of the functions of government as specified by the Federal Government. Regulations have been made conferring executive authority for the bulk of administrative functions. At 31 Dec. 1979 the only important powers retained by the Commonwealth related to rights in respect of Aboriginal land, some significant National Parks and the mining of uranium and other substances prescribed in the Atomic Energy Act. Proposed laws passed by the Legislative Assembly require the assent of the Administrator, who may assent, withhold assent, return them with recommended amendments or reserve them for the Governor-General's pleasure. The Governor-General may disallow any law assented to by the Administrator within 6 months of the Administrator's assent.

The Northern Territory has federal representation, electing 1 member to the House of Representatives and 2 members to the Senate.

The Legislative Assembly has 25 members, directly elected for a period of 4 years. The Chief Minister, Deputy Chief Minister and Speaker are elected by, and from, the members. The *Administrator* (J. H. Muirhead, QC) appoints Ministers on the advice of the Leader of the majority party.

The Legislative Assembly, elected in 1990, in Feb. 1991 comprised: Country Liberal Party, 14; Australian Labor Party, 9; Independents, 2.

The Country Liberal Party Cabinet was as follows in Feb. 1991:

Chief Minister and Treasurer: Marshall Perron.

Deputy Chief Minister, Mines and Energy and Industries and Development: Barry Coulter. *Attorney-General, Lands and Housing and Conservation:* Daryl Manzie. *Education, the Arts and Cultural Affairs:* Tom Harris. *Health and Community Services, Conservation:* Steve Hatton. *Transport and Works, Gaming and Racing:* Fred Finch. *Labour, Administrative Services and Local Government and Minister Assisting on Aboriginal Affairs:* Terry McCarthy. *Tourism, Youth, Sport, Ethnic Affairs and Minister Assisting on Central Australian Affairs:* Eric Poole. *Primary Industry and Fisheries, Correctional Services:* Mike Reed.

Local Government: Local government was established in Darwin in 1957 and later in 5 regional centres. These are each managed by a mayor and a municipal council elected at intervals of not more than 4 years by universal adult franchise. Provision has been made for a limited form of local government for smaller communities.

FINANCE. Budgets in $A1m.:

	1987–88	*1988–89*	*1989–90*	*1990–91*
Revenue	1,506·5	1,666·9	1,756·6	1,861·0
Expenditure	1,506·2	1,666·8	1,749·1	1,861·0

The revenue in 1990–91 comprised $A1,038·3m. in grants and allowances to the Northern Territory from the Commonwealth, as established by agreement at the time of self-government, together with $A948m. raised by the Northern Territory which included $A162·1m. through state-like taxes.

Expenditure during 1990–91 included $A294m. for education; $A189m. for housing and community amenities; $A203m. for health; $A124m. for public order and safety; $A225m. for energy.

ENERGY AND NATURAL RESOURCES

Oil and Gas. Significant oil and gas reserves have been discovered offshore in the Joseph Bonaparte Gulf and Timor Sea areas and onshore in the Amadeus Basin. In July 1990 offshore production was some 80,000 bbls a day. Total value of oil and gas production in 1988–89 was $A350m. Natural gas is piped from the Amadeus Basin to Darwin.

Minerals. The most important natural resources are minerals, and mining is the largest industry. Uranium, gold, manganese, bauxite, lead, silver, zinc and copper production dominated the minerals sector in 1988–89. Gross value of output, $A950m. in 1988-89.

The Northern Territory has large reserves of uranium. It has the world's largest manganese mine at Groote Eyland, and the world's largest known deposit of lead, silver and zinc at McArthur River. Bauxite is mined at Gove, and alumina is produced and exported to Europe, the USA, Canada, the USSR and China. The Territory is Australia's third largest producer of gold and has major deposits of platinum and palladium.

Agriculture. Cattle and buffalo production constitute the largest farming industry in the Northern Territory. Value of live cattle exports, 1989-90, $A15·5m.; total value of beef cattle industry, 1989-90, $A118m. Total value of the buffalo industry in 1989–90 was $A8·2m.

The USA is the largest importer of Territory beef, followed by Taiwan and the EEC.

There are 243 pastoral stations in the Northern Territory which produce cattle for Australian and overseas markets. They vary from smalls tations of 270 sq. km. to huge properties like Wave Hill Station which runs cattle over 12,359 sq. km.

Other animal industries contribute approximately $A12m. per annum. This sector consists of dairying, poultry and pig production, as well as crocodile farming for hides and meat. The horticultural industry is valued at $A20m. per annum and is increasing in importance. The main commodities in value are mangoes, rock melons and grapes. Some 800 ha are under sesame and mung beans, and cattle feeds including sorghum, rice and maize.

Fisheries. The total value of fish products landed in 1989-90 was $A28·2m. Of this, prawns contributed $A25·7m. and barramundi $A0·5m. Mud crabs, threadfin salmon, shark, mackerel, mother of pearl, bay lobster and molluscs made up most of the remainder. An expanding aquaculture industry produces crayfish, prawns, giant clams and beta carotene extraction.

INDUSTRY. In 1988–89 there were 158 manufacturing establishments (with 4 or more persons employed). Turnover was $A542m. 3,280 persons were employed in these factories. The labour force totalled 82,100 in 1990. In 1989, 71 trade unions had 19,300 members.

Tourism. In 1988-89, 835,000 people travelled to the Territory and tourism generated approximately $A415m. to the economy.

National Parks and Reserves. There are 74 areas totalling more than 2,350,326 ha set aside as National Parks or Conservation Reserves, and many other areas are managed by the Conservation Commission.

COMMUNICATIONS

Roads. There were (in 1988) 5,528 km of sealed road and 5,450 km of gravel and crushed stone road within the Northern Territory. They include three major interstate links: The Stuart Highway from Darwin to Adelaide (1,486 km), the Barkly Highway, Tennant Creek to the Queensland border (636 km), and the Victoria

Highway, Katherine to the Western Australian border (468 km). In addition to this there are 4,758 km of formed roads and 4,194 km of unformed roads or tracks, totalling approximately 19,931 km of roads. In 1989–90 74,600 motor vehicles were registered.

Railways. In 1980 Alice Springs was linked to the Trans-continental network by a standard (1,435 mm) gauge railway to Tarcoola (831 km). Direct services from Sydney started in 1984. The standard gauge railway is to be extended to Darwin, providing Australia with its first north-south rail link.

Aviation. There are daily flights from Darwin to Alice Springs with connexions to all Australian capital cities by 2 major domestic carriers, Australian Airlines and Ansett Airlines. Darwin is a first port of call for international aircraft flying in from Asia and a departure point for flights to such places as Singapore, Bali, Brunei and Timor.

Shipping. Regular freight shipping services connect Darwin with Western Australia, the eastern States and overseas. Passenger vessels also call at Darwin at irregular intervals.

The Port of Darwin is 997 km in extent; it is equipped to handle bulk, container and roll-on-roll-off traffic. There is a cyclone shelter for fishing vessels.

The ports of Melville Bay (Gove) and Milner Bay (Groote Eylandt) are connected with Darwin, the eastern States and overseas by regular shipping freight services.

The inland and coastal communities around the coast are provided with regular freight barge services from Darwin. Some of these communities also receive a barge freight-transhipment service out of a Brisbane vessel which calls at Melville and Milner Bays.

Telecommunications. Darwin's radio services include four ABC stations, one commercial station and a public station. In 1991 a second commercial FM station is to be established.

Darwin has one commercial and one ABC television service.

Alice Springs radio services include three ABC stations, one commercial and two public stations. It has one commercial and one ABC television service.

The rest of the Northern Territory is serviced through the AUSSAT satellite which provides one commercial and one ABC television station. The ABC provides two radio services to all other major regional centres.

EDUCATION AND WELFARE

Education. Education is compulsory from the age of 6-15 years. There were (1989) about 32,000 pre-school, primary and secondary students enrolled in about 165 Government and non-Government schools. The proportion of migrant and Aboriginal students in the Territory is high with the latter comprising about 30% of total school enrolments. Schools range from single classrooms and transportable units catering for the needs of small Aboriginal communities and pastoral properties to urban high schools and secondary colleges (years 11–12) catering for over 1,000 pupils. Bilingual programmes operate in some Aboriginal communities where traditional Aboriginal culture prevails. Secondary education extends from school years 8 to 12. The Northern Territory University was founded in 1989 by amalgamating the existing University College of the Northern Territory and the Darwin Institute of Technology, with the technical and further education courses hitherto offered by the latter to be conducted by an Institute of Technical and Further Education within the new University. The Alice Springs College of TAFE, the Katherine Rural College, the Northern Territory Open College and Batchelor College (a tertiary institution providing courses for Aboriginal people) offer a wide range of specialized courses.

Health. In 1990 there were 6 hospitals. Community health services are provided from urban and rural Health Centres including mobile units. Remote communities are served by the Aerial Medical Service and by resident Aboriginal health workers.

Further Reading

The Northern Territory: Annual Report. Dept. of Territories, Canberra, from 1911. Dept. of the Interior, Canberra, from 1966–67. Dept. of Northern Territory, from 1972

Australian Territories, Dept. of Territories, Canberra, 1960 to 1973. Dept. of Special Minister of State, Canberra, 1973–75. Department of Administrative Services, 1976

Northern Territory Statistical Summary. Australian Bureau of Statistics, Canberra, from 1960

Donovan, P. F., *A Land Full of Possibilities: A History of South Australia's Northern Territory 1863–1911*. 1981.—*At the Other End of Australia: The Commonwealth and the Northern Territory 1911–1978*. Univ. of Queensland Press, 1984

Heatley, A., *The Government of the Northern Territory*. Univ. of Queensland Press, 1979.—*Almost Australians: the Politics of Northern Territory Self-Government*. Australian National Univ. Press, 1990

Mills, C. M., *A Bibliography of the Northern Territory*. Canberra, 1977

Powell, A., *Far Country: A Short History of the Northern Territory*. Melbourne Univ. Press, 1982

AUSTRALIAN EXTERNAL TERRITORIES

AUSTRALIAN ANTARCTIC TERRITORY. An Imperial Order in Council of 7 Feb. 1933 placed under Australian authority all the islands and territories other than Adélie Land situated south of 60° S. lat. and lying between 160° E. long. and 45° E. long. The Order came into force with a Proclamation issued by the Governor-General on 24 Aug. 1936 after the passage of the Australian Antarctic Territory Acceptance Act 1933. The boundaries of Adélie Land were definitively fixed by a French Decree of 1 April 1938 as the islands and territories south of 60° S. lat. lying between 136° E. long. and 142° E. long. The Australian Antarctic Territory Act 1954 declared that the laws in force in the Australian Capital Territory are, so far as they are applicable and are not inconsistent with any ordinance made under the Act, in force in the Australian Antarctic Territory.

The area of the territory is estimated at 6,119,818 sq. km (2,362,875 sq. miles).

On 13 Feb. 1954 the Australian National Antarctic Research Expeditions (ANARE) established a station on MacRobertson Land at lat. 67° 37' S. and long. 62° 52' E. The station was named Mawson in honour of the late Sir Douglas Mawson. Meteorological and other scientific research is conducted at Mawson, which is the centre for coastal and inland survey expeditions.

A second Australian scientific research station was established on the coast of Princess Elizabeth Land on 13 Jan. 1957 at lat. 68° 34' S. and long. 77° 58' E. The station was named Davis in honour of Capt. John King Davis, Mawson's second-in-command on 2 expeditions. The station was temporarily closed down in Jan. 1965 and re-opened in Feb. 1969.

In Feb. 1959 the Australian Government accepted from the US Government custody of Wilkes Station, which was established by the US on 16 Jan. 1957 on the Budd Coast of Wilkes Land, at lat. 66° 15' S. and long. 110° 32' E. The station was named in honour of Lieut. Charles Wilkes, who commanded the 1838–40 US expedition to the area, and was closed in Feb. 1969. Operations were then transferred to the new station, Casey. Construction commenced on Casey station in Jan. 1965 and was continued, mainly during summer visits, until Feb. 1969, when it was opened. The station, specially designed to withstand blizzard winds and prevent inundation by snow, is situated 2·4 km south of Wilkes at lat. 66° 17' S. and long. 110° 32' E. The Antarctic Division has also operated a station, since March 1948, at Macquarie Island, about 1,360 km south-east of Hobart. Macquarie Island is part of the State of Tasmania.

COCOS (KEELING) ISLANDS. The Cocos (Keeling) Islands are 2 separate atolls comprising some 27 small coral islands with a total area of about 14·2 sq. km, and are situated in the Indian Ocean at 12° 05' S. lat. and 96° 53' E. long. They lie 2,768 km north-west of Perth and 3,685 km west of Darwin, while Colombo is 2,255 km to the north-west of the group.

The main islands in this Australian Territory are West Island (the largest, about

10 km from north to south) on which is an airport and an animal quarantine station, and most of the European community; Home Island, occupied by the Cocos Malay community; Direction, South and Horsburgh Islands, and North Keeling Island, 24 km to the north of the group.

Although the islands were discovered in 1609 by Capt. William Keeling of the East India Company, they remained uninhabited until 1826, when the first settlement was established on the main atoll by an Englishman, Alexander Hare, with a group of followers, predominantly of Malay origin. Hare left the islands in 1831, by which time a second settlement had been formed on the main atoll by John Clunies-Ross, a Scottish seaman and adventurer, who began commercial development of the islands' coconut palms.

In 1857 the islands were annexed to the Crown; in 1878 responsibility was transferred from the Colonial Office to the Government of Ceylon, and in 1886 to the Government of the Straits Settlement. By indenture in 1886 Queen Victoria granted all land in the islands to George Clunies-Ross and his heirs in perpetuity (with certain rights reserved to the Crown). In 1903 the islands were incorporated in the Settlement of Singapore and in 1942–46 temporarily placed under the Governor of Ceylon. In 1946 a Resident Administrator, responsible to the Governor of Singapore, was appointed.

On 23 Nov. 1955 the Cocos Islands were placed under the authority of the Australian Government as the Territory of Cocos (Keeling) Islands. An Administrator, appointed by the Governor-General, is the Government's representative in the Territory and is responsible to the Minister for Territories and Local Government. The Cocos (Keeling) Islands Council, established as the elected body of the Cocos Malay community in July 1979, advises the Administrator on all issues affecting the Territory.

In 1978 the Australian Government purchased the Clunies-Ross family's entire interests in the islands, except for the family residence. A Cocos Malay co-operative has been established to take over the running of the Clunies-Ross copra plantation (118 tonnes of copra were exported in 1985–86) and to engage in other business with the Commonwealth in the Territory, including construction projects.

The population of the Territory at 30 June 1986 was 616, distributed between Home Island (414) and West Island (202).

The islands are low-lying, flat and thickly covered by coconut palms, and surround a lagoon in which ships drawing up to 7 metres may be anchored, but which is extremely difficult for navigation.

An equable and pleasant climate, affected for much of the year by the south-east trade winds. Temperatures range over the year from 68° F (20° C) to 88° F (31·1° C) and rainfall averages 80" (2,000 mm) a year.

The Cocos (Keeling) Islands Act 1955 is the basis of the Territory's administrative, legislative and judicial systems. Under section 8 of this Act, those laws which were in force in the Territory immediately before the transfer continued in force there.

Roads. There are 24 km of roads.

Telecommunications. In 1986 there were 150 radio receivers and (1985) 180 telephones.

Religion. About 58% are Moslems and 22% Christians.

Education. In 1986 there were 2 primary schools (on Home Island and West Island) with 105 pupils and 8 teachers, a secondary school (on West Island) with 30 pupils and 5 staff, and a technical school with 9 pupils.

Health. In 1985 there was a doctor and 4 nursing personnel, with 5 beds in clinics.

Administrator: C. M. Stuart.

CHRISTMAS ISLAND is an isolated peak in the Indian Ocean, lat. 10° 25' 22" S., long. 105° 39' 59" E. It lies 360 km S., 8° E. of Java Head, and 417 km N. 79° E. from Cocos Islands, 1,310 km from Singapore and 2,623 km from Fremantle.

Area about 135 sq. km. The climate is tropical with temperatures varying little over the year at 27° C. The wet season lasts from Nov. to April with an annual total of about 2,673 mm. The island was formally annexed by the UK on 6 June 1888, placed under the administration of the Governor of the Straits Settlements in 1889, and incorporated with the Settlement of Singapore in 1900. Sovereignty was transferred to the Australian Government on 1 Oct. 1958. The population (Census, 1981) was 2,871; estimate (1986) 2,000 of whom 1,300 were of Chinese, 600 of Malay and 100 of Australian/European origin.

The legislative, judicial and administrative systems are regulated by the Christmas Island Act, 1958–73. They are the responsibility of the Commonwealth Government and operated by an Administrator. The laws of Singapore which were in force before the transfer have been continued but can be amended, repealed or substituted by ordinances made by the Governor-General. The first Island Assembly was elected in Sept. 1985.

Extraction and export of rock phosphate dust was the island's only industry until 1987. In Dec. 1948 Australia and New Zealand bought the lease rights of the Christmas Island Phosphate Co. and set up the Christmas Island Phosphate Commission (CIPC), which conducted the mining operation until mid-1981. The Phosphate Mining Co. of Christmas Island Ltd (PMCI) acted as managing agents for the CIPC until the Commission was wound up and then mined in its own right. The Commonwealth Government appointed liquidators on 11 Nov. 1987, with a view to ending all mining.

Electricity. Production (1985) 33m. kwh.

Roads. There are 32 km of roads, 759 passenger cars and 383 commercial vehicles.

Railways. There is a 20 km railway to serve the phosphate mines.

Aviation. There are weekly flights to Perth (Western Australia) and to Singapore.

Shipping. In 1985, 1·2m. tonnes (mostly phosphates) were loaded and 46,000 tonnes discharged at the port.

Telecommunications. There are 2 post offices and (1986) 2,500 radio receivers.

Religion. About 35% are Buddhists, 25% Muslims and 20% Christians.

Education. In 1985 there were 261 pupils in 2 primary schools, 114 pupils in a secondary school and 60 students in a technical school.

Health. In 1985 there were 2 doctors, a dentist, a pharmacist and a hospital with 35 beds.

Administrator: T. F. Paterson.

NORFOLK ISLAND. 29° 02' S. lat. 167° 57' E. long., area 3,455 hectares, population, (June 1986), 1,977. The island was formerly part of the colony of New South Wales and then of Van Diemen's Land. It was a penal colony 1788–1814 and 1825–55. In 1856 it received all 194 descendants of the *Bounty* mutineers from Pitcairn Island. It has been a distinct settlement since 1856, under the jurisdiction of the state of New South Wales; and finally by the passage of the Norfolk Island Act 1913, it was accepted as a Territory of the Australian Government. The Norfolk Island Act 1957 is the basis of the Territory's legislative, administrative and judicial systems. An Administrator, appointed by the Governor-General and responsible to the Minister for Territories and Local Government, is the senior government representative in the Territory.

The Norfolk Island Act 1979 gives Norfolk Island responsible legislative and executive government to enable it to run its own affairs to the greatest practicable extent. Wide powers are exercised by the Norfolk Island Legislative Assembly of 9 elected members, and by an Executive Council, comprising the executive members of the Legislative Assembly who have ministerial-type responsibilities. The seat of administration is Kingston, the only major settlement. The Act preserves the Commonwealth's responsibility for Norfolk Island as a Territory under its authority, indicating Parliament's intention that consideration would be given to an extension of the powers of the Legislative Assembly and the political and administrative institutions of Norfolk Island within 5 years. Some powers were transferred in 1985 and further transfers are being considered.

The Territory Administration is financed from local revenue which for 1987–88 totalled $A4,872,000; expenditure, $A4,840,128.

Public revenue is derived mainly from tourism, the sale of postage stamps, customs duties, liquor sales and company registration and licence fees. Residents are not liable for income tax on earnings within the Territory, nor are death and personal stamp duties levied.

In 1986, 29,428 visitors travelled to Norfolk. Descendants of the *Bounty* mutineer families constitute the 'original' settlers and are known locally as 'Islanders', while later settlers, mostly from Australia, New Zealand and UK, are identified as 'mainlanders'. Over the years the Islanders have preserved their own lifestyle and customs, and their language remains a mixture of West Country English, Gaelic and Tahitian.

Roads. There are 72 km of roads (53 km paved), 1,802 passenger cars and 90 commercial vehicles.

Telecommunications. There is one post office and (1984) 1,090 telephones, 400 television and (1987) 1,500 radio receivers.

JUSTICE, RELIGION, EDUCATION AND WELFARE

Justice. The island's Supreme Court sits as required and a Court of Petty Sessions exercises both civil and criminal juristiction.

Religion. 40% of the population are Anglicans.

Education. In 1986 there were 2 primary schools with 120 pupils and a secondary school with 111 pupils.

Health. In 1985 there were 2 doctors, a pharmacist and a hospital with 20 beds.

Administrator: Commodore J. A. Matthew, CVO, MBE.
Chief Minister: David E. Buffett.

HEARD AND McDONALD ISLANDS. These islands, about 2,500 miles south-west of Fremantle, were transferred from UK to Australian control as from 26 Dec. 1947. Heard Island is about 43 km long and 21 km wide; Shag Island is about 8 km north of Heard. The total area is 412 sq. km (159 sq. miles). The McDonald Islands are 42 km to the west of Heard.

TERRITORY OF ASHMORE AND CARTIER ISLANDS. By Imperial Order in Council of 23 July 1931, Ashmore Islands (known as Middle, East and West Islands) and Cartier Island, situated in the Indian Ocean, some 320 km off the north-west coast of Australia (area, 5 sq. km), were placed under the authority of the Commonwealth.

Under the Ashmore and Cartier Islands Acceptance Act, 1933, the islands were accepted by the Commonwealth under the name of the Territory of Ashmore and Cartier Islands, and the effective date was proclaimed by the Governor-General to be 10 May 1934. It was the intention that the Territory should be administered by the State of Western Australia, but owing to administrative difficulties the Territory was annexed to and deemed to form part of the Northern Territory of Australia (by amendment to the Act in 1938) with relevant laws of the Northern Territory, applying to the Territory of Ashmore and Cartier Islands. Responsibility for the administration of Ashmore and Cartier Islands rests with the Minister for the Arts, Sport, the Environment, Tourism and Territories.

On 16 Aug. 1983 a national nature reserve was declared over Ashmore Reef and the area so declared is now known as Ashmore Reef National Nature Reserve.

The islands are uninhabited but Indonesian fishing boats, which have traditionally plied the area, fish within the Territory and land to collect water in accordance with an agreement between the governments of Australia and Indonesia.

Periodic visits are made to the islands by ships of the Royal Australian Navy, and aircraft of the Royal Australian Air Force make aerial surveys of the islands and neighbouring waters.

TERRITORY OF CORAL SEA ISLANDS. The Coral Sea Islands became a Territory of the Commonwealth of Australia under the Coral Sea Islands Act 1969. It comprises scattered reefs and islands over a sea area of about 1m. sq. km. The Territory is uninhabited apart from a manned meteorological station on Willis Island.

NEW SOUTH WALES

HISTORY. New South Wales became a British possession in 1770; the first settlement was established at Port Jackson in 1788; a partially elective Council was established in 1843, and an elective Parliament and responsible government in 1856. New South Wales federated with the other Australian states to form the Commonwealth of Australia in 1901.

AREA AND POPULATION. New South Wales is situated between the 29th and 38th parallels of S. lat. and 141st and 154th meridians of E. long., and comprises 309,433 sq. miles (801,428 sq. km), inclusive of Lord Howe Island, 6 sq. miles (17 sq. km), but exclusive of the Australian Capital Territory (911 sq. miles, 2,359 sq. km) and 28 sq. miles (73 sq. km) at Jervis Bay.

Lord Howe Island, 31° 33' 4" S., 159° 4' 26" E., which is part of New South Wales, is situated about 702 km north-east of Sydney; area, 1,654 hectares, of which only about 120 hectares are arable; resident population, estimate (30 June 1987), 290. The Island, which was discovered in 1788, is of volcanic origin. Mount Gower, the highest point, reaches a height of 866 metres.

The Lord Howe Island Board manages the affairs of the Island and supervises the Kentia palm-seed industry.

Census population of New South Wales (including full-blood Aboriginals from 1966):

	Males	*Females*	*Persons*	*Population per sq. km*	*Average annual increase % since previous census*
1901	710,264	645,091	1,355,355	2	1·86
1911	857,698	789,036	1,646,734	2	1·97
1921	1,071,501	1,028,870	2,100,371	3	2·46
1933	1,318,471	1,282,376	2,600,847	3	1·76
1947	1,492,211	1,492,627	2,984,838	4	0·99
1954	1,720,860	1,702,669	3,423,529	4	1·98
1961	1,972,909	1,944,104	3,917,013	5	1·94
1966	2,126,652	2,111,249	4,237,901	5	1·58
1971	2,307,210	2,293,970	4,601,180	6	1·66
1976	2,380,172	2,396,931	4,777,103	6	0·75
1981	2,548,984	2,577,233	5,126,217	6	1·42
1986	2,684,570	2,717,311	5,401,881	7	1·05

At 30 June 1988 the estimated resident population was 5,701,500 (2,861,300 female); Sydney Statistical Division, 3,596,000; Newcastle Statistical Subdivision, 422,100; Wollongong Statistical Subdivision, 253,200. Population of principal municipalities outside Sydney, 1987 (and 1985): Albury, 39,610 (39,180); Armidale, 20,920 (20,680); Bathurst, 25,620 (25,300); Broken Hill, 24,170 (25,170); Casino, 10,820 (10,770); Cessnock, 43,170 (42,700); Dubbo, 31,290 (31,040); Goulburn, 21,700 (21,780); Grafton, 16,230 (16,380); Greater Lithgow, 20,070 (20,170); Greater Taree, 36,960 (36,310); Hastings, 42,220 (41,170); Kiama, 14,080 (13,740); Lake Macquarie, 159,300 (158,300); Lismore, 38,130 (37,480); Maitland, 46,130 (45,410); Newcastle, 132,240 (132,940); Orange, 32,520 (32,340); Queanbeyan, 23,880 (23,180); Shellharbour, 45,550 (45,250);

Shoalhaven, 59,470 (57,670); Tamworth, 33,830 (33,710); Wagga Wagga, 50,930 (50,380); Wollongong, 174,020 (173,520).

Vital statistics for calendar years:

	Live births	*Marriages*	*Divorces*	*Deaths (excluding still-births)*	*Infantile mortality per 1,000 live births*
1986	84,531	41,319	11,661	42,167	9·0
1987	86,093	40,650	12,044	42,189	8·5
1988	84,647	40,812	11,880	44,676	9·2

The annual rates per 1,000 of mean estimated resident population in 1988 were: Births, 14·8; deaths, 7·8; marriages, 7·2.

CONSTITUTION AND GOVERNMENT. Within the State there are three levels of government: The Commonwealth Government, with authority derived from a written constitution; the State Government with residual powers; the local government authorities with powers based upon a State Act of Parliament, operating within incorporated areas extending over almost 90% of the State.

The Constitution of New South Wales is drawn from several diverse sources; certain Imperial statutes such as the Commonwealth of Australia Constitution Act (1900); the Australian States Constitution Act (1907); an element of inherited English law; amendments to the Commonwealth of Australia Constitution Act; the (State) Constitution Act; the Australia Acts of 1986; the Constitution (Amendment) Act 1987 and certain other State Statutes; numerous legal decisions; and a large amount of English and local convention.

The Parliament of New South Wales may legislate for the peace, welfare and good government of the State in all matters not specifically reserved to the Commonwealth Government.

The State Legislature consists of the Sovereign, represented by the Governor, and two Houses of Parliament, the Legislative Council (upper house) and the Legislative Assembly (lower house).

Australian citizens aged 18 and over, and other British subjects who were enrolled prior to 25 Jan. 1984, men and women aged 18 years and over, are entitled to the franchise. Voting is compulsory. The optional preferential method of voting is used for both houses.

The Legislative Council has 45 members elected for a term of office equivalent to three terms of the Legislative Assembly, with 15 members retiring at the same time as the Legislative Assembly elections. The whole State constitutes a single electoral district. In Oct. 1988, the Council consisted of the following parties: Australian Labor Party (ALP), 21; Liberal Party of Australia (Lib), 12; National Party of Australia (NP), 7; Call to Australia Group (CTA), 3; Australian Democrats (AD), 2.

The President of the Legislative Council has an annual salary (1988) of $A77,985; the Leader of the Opposition members, the Chairman of Committees and the Deputy Leader of the Government members (if not a Minister), $A58,771 each; the Deputy Leader of the Opposition members and Government and Opposition Whips, $A54,388 each. The President is paid an annual expense allowance of $A12,977; the Leader of the Opposition members, the Chairman of Committees, the Deputy Leader of the Government members (if not a Minister) and the Deputy Leader of the Opposition members (when a leader of a party), $A7,133 each; the Deputy Leader of the Opposition members (when not a leader of a party) and Government and Opposition Whips, $A2,861 each. Other members who are not Ministers receive an annual salary of $A48,750. All members receive an annual electoral allowance of $A16,180.

The Legislative Assembly has 109 members elected in single seat electoral districts for a maximum period of 4 years. The Legislative Assembly, elected on 19 March 1988, consisted in Feb. 1991 of the following parties: ALP, 43; Lib, 39; NP, 20; Independents, 7.

The Speaker of the Legislative Assembly and the Leader of the Opposition members receive a salary of (1988) $A77,985 each; the Chairman of Committees and Deputy Leader of the Opposition members, $A58,771 each; Government and Opposition Whips, $A55,383 each. The Speaker and the Leader of the Opposition members also receive an expense allowance of $A12,977 each; the Chairman of Committees and Deputy Leader of the Opposition members, $A7,133 each; Government and Opposition Whips, and Deputy Leader of the National Party, $A3,367 each. Members who are not Ministers receive an annual salary of $A48,750. All members receive an annual electoral allowance ranging from $A16,180 to $A31,359 according to the location of their constituencies.

Executive power is vested in the Governor, who is appointed by the Crown, and an Executive Council consisting of members of the Cabinet. Ministers receive the following annual salaries (1988): Premier, $A96,946; Deputy Premier, $A87,585; the Leader of the Government members in the Legislative Council, $A88,537; Deputy Leader of Government members in the Legislative Council, $A84,477; other Ministers, $A82,869. Ministers also receive an expense allowance (Premier, $A27,777; Deputy Premier, $A13,888; other Ministers, $A12,977 each). Ministers also receive an electoral allowance ranging from $A16,180 to $A27,221 to members of the Legislative Assembly, according to the location of their electorate; and $A16,180 to each member of the Legislative Council.

Governor: Rear-Adm. Peter Sinclair, AO.

The New South Wales Ministry, in Oct. 1990, was as follows:

Premier, Treasurer and Minister for Ethnic Affairs: The Hon. N. F. Greiner, MP.

Deputy Prime Minister, Minister for State Development and Minister for Public Works: The Hon. W. T. J. Murray, MP. *Minister for Health and Minister for the Arts:* The Hon. P. E. J. Collins, MP. *Minister for Agriculture and Rural Affairs:* The Hon. I. M. Armstrong, OBE, MP. *Attorney-General:* The Hon. J. R. A. Dowd, MP. *Minister for Housing:* The Hon. J. J. Schipp, MP. *Minister for the Environment and Assistant Minister for Transport:* The Hon. T. J. Moore, MP. *Chief Secretary and Minister for Tourism:* The Hon. G. B. West, MP. *Minister for Police and Emergency Services and Vice-President of the Executive Council:* The Hon. E. P. Pickering, MLC. *Minister for Sport, Recreation and Racing:* The Hon. R. B. R. Smith, MLC. *Minister for Family and Community Services:* The Hon. Virginia Chadwick, MLC. *Minister for Education and Youth Affairs:* The Hon. T. A. Metherell, MP. *Minister for Transport:* The Hon. B. G. Baird, MP. *Minister for Administrative Services and Assistant Minister for Transport:* The Hon. Matthew Singleton, MP. *Minister for Business and Consumer Affairs:* The Hon. G. B. P. Peacocke, MP. *Minister for Mineral Resources and Minister for Energy:* The Hon. N. E. W. Pickard, MP. *Minister for Industrial Relations and Employment and Minister Assisting the Premier:* The Hon. J. J. Fahey, MP. *Minister for Natural Resources:* The Hon. I. R. Causley, MP. *Minister for Local Government and Minister for Planning:* The Hon. D. A. Hay, MP. *Minister for Corrective Services:* The Hon. M. R. Yabsley, MP.

Agent-General in London: Norman Brunsdon (66 Strand, WC2N 5LZ).

Local Government. A system of local government extends over most of the State, including the whole of the Eastern and Central land divisions and almost three-quarters of the sparsely populated Western division. At 26 Sept. 1988 there were 65 municipalities, and 110 corporate bodies called shires. A number of the municipalities and shires have combined to form 41 county councils, which administer electricity or water supply undertakings or render other services of common benefit.

ECONOMY

Budget. State Consolidated Fund: Statement of receipts and expenditure (in $A1m.) for financial years ending 30 June:

	1984–85	*1985–86*	*1986–87*	*1987–88*
Receipts: Recurrent	7,348	8,220	10,657	12,379
Capital	654	659	1,508	1,384
Total Receipts	8,002	8,879	12,165	13,763

	1984–85	1985–86	1986–87	1987–88
Expenditure: Recurrent	7,511	8,305	10,634	11,871
Capital	491	573	1,531	1,592
Revenue Equalization	...	...	...	...
Total Expenditure	8,002	8,879	12,165	13,519
Surplus/deficit	—	—	—	245

State Government receipts (in $A1m.) for 1987–88 included receipts from loan raisings, 114; Commonwealth general revenue grant, 4,269; and state taxation, 5,423. Expenditure included capital works and services, 1,592; education, 2,646; health, 3,137; and public debt charges, 750.

Public Debt. The long term debt of the State has three components. Debt outstanding at 30 June 1988 (in $A1m.) for each of these components was:

Debt of statutory bodies under State Government guarantee	18,142·1
Loan liability to the Commonwealth under the 1927 Financial Agreement	5,962·7
Loan liability to the Commonwealth outside the Financial Agreement	3,178·0
Total debt	27,282·8

Since 1983, access to the capital markets for borrowings has been principally through the New South Wales Treasury Corporation which acts as the central borrowing authority of the State.

Banking. There were 27 trading banks operating in New South Wales at 30 June 1988, including the Commonwealth Bank of Australia and the State Bank of New South Wales (Government banks). The trading bank business is transacted chiefly by the Commonwealth Bank of Australia, the State Bank of New South Wales and 3 private banks. At 30 June 1988 the 27 banks operated 1,960 branches and 293 agencies in New South Wales.

The weekly average amount of deposits held in New South Wales by the 27 banks was $A25,778·7m. in June 1988, consisting of $A19,219·1m. bearing interest and $A6,559·6m. not bearing interest. Bank advances, overdrafts, bills discounted, etc., amounted to $A30,669·7m. A statement of other assets and liabilities of the banks in New South Wales is of little significance, as banking business is conducted on an Australia-wide basis.

Savings bank deposits at the end of June 1988 amounted to $A20,155·9m., representing $A3,548 per head of population.

ENERGY AND NATURAL RESOURCES

Electricity. At 30 June 1989 the total nominal capacity of the Electricity Commission of New South Wales system was 11,950 mw.

Minerals. New South Wales contains extensive mineral deposits. The most important minerals mined are: Coal (which accounted for 66% of the value of the State's mineral production in 1987–88); silver–lead–zinc (13%); construction materials (sand, gravel, stone, etc., 10%); and mineral sands (rutile, zircon, etc., 1%). At 30 June 1988, there were 440 mining establishments. Average employment in mining, 1986–87, was 26,005 persons. During 1987–88, wages and salaries paid were $A938m., and value added was $A2,086m. Mine production of coal and metallic minerals (gross content) is shown below:

	1984–85	1985–86	1986–87	1987–88
Antimony (tonnes)	1,409	1,264	1,202	1,146
Cadmium (tonnes)	1,735	1,216	1,113	952
Coal (1,000 tonnes)	70,034	64,082	73,312	63,945
Cobalt (tonnes)	66	55	55	74
Copper (tonnes)	23,038	26,733	32,400	31,378
Gold (kg)	1,464	1,015	2,227	5,224
Lead (tonnes)	251,595	233,270	206,139	223,953
Manganese (tonnes)	...	3,897	3,858	3,413
Silver (kg)	355,827	367,751	408,829	428,123

	1984–85	1985–86	1986–87	1987–88
Sulphur (tonnes)	248,681	253,800	264,631	293,008
Tin (tonnes)	1,306	1,280	249	3
Titanium dioxide (tonnes)	41,283	47,240	58,066	59,961
Zinc (tonnes)	385,075	355,443	362,180	373,520
Zircon (tonnes)	47,113	53,607	50,234	49,885

The value of output in mining and quarrying in 1987–88 was $A3,222m.

Agriculture. Area under cultivation (in hectares) during 3 years (ended 31 March) and the principal crops (in tonnes) produced were as follows (Data relates to farms whose estimated value of agricultural operations was $A20,000 or more at the census):

	1985	1986	1987	1988
Area under cultivation	5,712,279	5,925,308	5,325,305	4,908,459

		1986		1987		1988	
Principal crops		*Sown area*	*Production*	*Sown area*	*Production*	*Sown area*	*Production*
Wheat	Grain	3,647,638	5,898,015	3,098,826	4,855,244	2,463,707	3,996,913
	Hay	15,112	46,611	19,237	55,456	20,128	57,915
Barley	Grain	538,754	811,780	408,315	613,646	464,746	744,000
	Hay	1,393	3,277	1,801	4,574	...	8,000
Oats	Grain	422,250	530,726	482,257	635,185	525,798	707,000
	Hay	25,200	71,009	39,066	111,344	43,305	120,391
Grain Sorghum		159,407	298,380	188,062	391,582	174,669	...
Potatoes		5,840	108,085	6,225	121,573	6,440	119,875
Lucerne (hay)		63,731	309,325	71,710	341,859	77,208	369,823
Rice		102,805	701,472	92,281	589,074	101,825	721,000
Cotton (raw and seed)		135,820	738,875	125,026	676,428	163,631	757,419
Oilseeds		205,589	206,712	149,760	156,452	109,258	115,392

In 1987–88, 15,992 ha of sugar-cane were cut for crushing, the production being 1,631,921 tonnes. The total area under grapes was 12,068 (including 566 not bearing) ha; the production of table grapes was 8,017 tonnes; of wine, 126,782 tonnes; for drying, 48,216 tonnes (fresh weight).

In 1987–88, there were 4,333 ha of banana plantations; production, 66,201 tonnes; there were 30,372 ha of orchard fruit.

At 31 March 1988 the State had 54,932,000 sheep and lambs, 4,962,000 cattle and 853,000 pigs. The production of shorn and crutched wool in 1987–88 was 251,610 tonnes (greasy). In the year ended 30 June 1988 production of butter was 1,057 tonnes; cheese, 13,142 tonnes, and bacon and ham, 32,343 tonnes.

Forestry. The estimated area of Crown and private lands is 15m. hectares. The total area of State forests amounts to 3·2m. hectares, and 223,000 hectares have been set apart as timber reserves.

In 1986–87, 3,466,000 cu. metres of timber (excluding firewood) were produced, including 1,214,000 cu. metres of forest hardwoood and 1,323,000 cu. metres of pulpwoods.

INDUSTRY AND TRADE

Industry. Some 17% of employed persons are in manufacturing.

A wide range of manufacturing is undertaken in the Sydney area, and there are large iron and steel works near the coalfields at Newcastle and Port Kembla.

Manufacturing establishments' operations, 1987–88:

Industry	*No. of establishments* [1]	*Persons employed (1,000)* [2]	*Wages and salaries* [3] *($A1m.)*	*Turnover ($A1m.)*
Food, beverages and tobacco	1,266	53,787	1,236·0	8,117·8
Textiles	345	9,512	210·7	1,162·3
Clothing and footwear	1,077	23,360	368·1	1,676·1
Wood, wood products and furniture	2,388	26,958	497·5	2,411·1
Paper, paper products, printing and publishing	1,954	40,815	1,019·7	4,654·2
Chemical, petroleum and coal products	496	24,757	742·5	5,780·7

Industry	No. of establishments [1]	Persons employed (1,000) [2]	Wages and salaries [3] ($A1m.)	Turnover ($A1m.)
Non-metallic mineral products	799	13,848	352·8	2,023·9
Basic metal products	228	36,606	1,064·6	6,846·2
Fabricated metal products	2,789	38,069	820·4	3,729·8
Transport equipment	704	28,932	688·5	2,295·2
Other machinery and equipment	2,325	57,980	1,314·8	5,564·8
Miscellaneous manufacturing	1,535	24,378	529·6	2,695·1
Total manufacturing	15,906	379,002	8,845·6	46,957·2

[1] Operating at 30 June 1988. Excludes single-establishment manufacturing enterprises with less than 4 persons employed.
[2] Persons employed at 30 June 1988, including working proprietors.
[3] Excludes drawings of working proprietors.

Some of the principal articles manufactured in 1988–89 were:

Article	Quantity	Article	Quantity
Flour (1,000 tonnes)	552	Ready mixed concrete (1,000 cu. metres)	5,177
Footwear (1,000 pairs)	6,492	Clay bricks (1m.) [1]	786
Raw steel (1,000 tonnes)	5,259	Electricity (1m. kwh.) [1]	51,813

[1] Includes the Australian Capital Territory.

Value of building jobs, 1988–89:

Commenced	Under construction	Completed
$A10,499m.	$A11,580	$A7,984

Value of building work, 1988–89; private sector, $A8,116m.; public sector, $A1,344m.

Labour. In Aug. 1989 2,580,600 persons (57·5% of the civil population over 14) were employed out of a total workforce of 2,744,300: 552,400 in wholesale and retail trade; 436,900 in community services and 418,200 in manufacturing.

Industrial tribunals are authorized to fix minimum rates of wages and other conditions of employment. Their awards may be enforced by law, as may be industrial agreements between employers and organizations of employees, when registered.

The principal State arbitration and conciliation tribunal is the Industrial Commission of New South Wales. The Commission is empowered to exercise all the powers conferred on subsidiary tribunals, and has in addition authority to determine any widely defined 'industrial matter', to adjudicate in case of illegal strikes and lockouts, to investigate union ballots when irregularities are alleged and to hear appeals from subsidiary tribunals. Subsidiary tribunals are Conciliation Committees for various industries, each having an equal number representing employers and employees and a Conciliation Commissioner as chairman.

Trade Unions. Registration of trade unions is effected under the New South Wales Trade Union Act 1881, which follows substantially the Trade Union Acts of 1871 and 1876 of England. Registration confers a quasi-corporate existence with power to hold property, to sue and be sued, etc., and the various classes of employees covered by the union are required to be prescribed by the constitution of the union. For the purpose of bringing an industry under the review of the State industrial tribunals, or participating in proceedings relating to disputes before Commonwealth tribunals, employees and employers must be registered as industrial unions, under State or Commonwealth industrial legislation respectively. At 30 June 1988, there were 170 trade unions with a total membership of 1,179,800. Approximately 55% (estimate) of wage and salary earners were members of trade unions.

Commerce. External commerce, exclusive of inter-state trade, is included in the statement of the commerce of Australia (*see* pp. 109–11). Overseas commerce of New South Wales in $A1m. for years ending 30 June:

	Imports	Exports		Imports	Exports
1984–85	12,478·4	6,674·0	1987–88	18,087·4	10,582·1
1985–86	15,129·9	7,363·2	1988–89	20,873·9	10,903·7
1986–87	16,055·9	8,364·2			

The major commodities exported from New South Wales in 1988–89 (in $A1m.) were coal, coke and briquettes (1,841·8), sheep's and lamb's wool (1,629·8) and aluminium (924·0). Principal imports were computers (1,664·1), road vehicles (1,443·1) and electrical equipment (1,082·8).

Principal destinations of all exports from New South Wales in 1988–89 (in $A1m.) were Japan (3,355·8), Hong Kong (896·1), Republic of Korea (698·0), New Zealand (683·6), USA (676·2), Taiwan (532·7). Major sources of supply were USA (4,935·7), Japan (4,186·5), UK (1,650·1), Federal Republic of Germany (1,196·0), New Zealand (947·5), Taiwan (874·8).

Tourism. In the year ended 30 June 1989, 1·06m. overseas visitors arrived for short term visits. At 30 June 1989 there were 1,592 hotels providing 45,962 rooms, and 815 caravan parks.

COMMUNICATIONS

Roads. In 1987 there were some 205,000 km of public roads of all sorts. The Roads and Traffic Authority of New South Wales is responsible for the administration and upkeep of major roads. In 1989 there were 38,988 km of roads under its control, including 10,397 km of state highways, 25,124 km of main roads and 292 km of secondary roads.

The number of registered motor vehicles (excluding tractors and trailers) at 30 June 1989 was 3,153,300, including 2,365,100 cars and station wagons, 189,800 utilities, 227,700 panel vans, 214,300 trucks, 56,900 buses and 99,400 motor cycles.

Railways. At 30 June 1988, 9,917 km of government railway were open (616 km electrified). The revenue (including supplements) in 1987–88 was $A2,065m.; the expenditure from revenue, $A2,065m. In 1989 249·3 passengers were carried and 50·2m. tonnes of freight. Also open for traffic are 325 km of Victorian Government railways which extend over the border; 68 km of private railways (mainly in mining districts) and 53 km of Commonwealth Government-owned track.

Aviation. Sydney is the major airport in New South Wales and Australia's principal international air terminal. Durlng the year ended 31 Dec. 1987 scheduled aircraft movements at Sydney totalled 114,632. Passengers totalled 7,006,689 on domestic services and 3,462,604 on international services. Freight handled on domestic and international services was 61,232 tonnes and 153,337 tonnes respectively.

Shipping. The main ports are at Sydney, Newcastle, Port Kembla and Port Botany. Arrivals of vessels engaged in overseas trade in the ports of New South Wales in 1989 totalled 3,953 (84·78m. GRT). The number of overseas vessels which entered in 1989 was 1,602.

JUSTICE, RELIGION, EDUCATION AND WELFARE

Justice. Legal processes may be conducted in Local Courts presided over by magistrates or in higher courts (District Court or Supreme Court) presided over by judges. There is also an appellate jurisdiction. Persons charged with the more serious crimes must be tried before a higher court.

Children's Courts have been established with the object of removing children as far as possible from the atmosphere of a public court. There are also a number of tribunals exercising special jurisdiction, *e.g.*, the Industrial Commission and the Compensation Court.

At 30 June 1989 there were 5,304 persons in prison.

Religion. There is no established church in New South Wales, and freedom of worship is accorded to all.

The following table shows the statistics of the religious denominations in New South Wales at the census in 1986, and of ministers of religion registered for the celebration of marriages in 1987:

Denomination	*Ministers*	*Adherents*	*Denomination*	*Ministers*	*Adherents*
Catholic	1,701	1,529,176	Other Christian	1,496	288,865
Anglican	1,008	1,519,806	Muslim	11	57,551
Uniting Church	603	327,360	Jewish	29	28,236
Presbyterian	228	227,663	Other Non-Christian	38	57,079
Orthodox	66	165,659	Others	...	1,101,409 [1]
Baptist	443	67,187			
Lutheran	38	31,890	Total	5,661	5,401,881

[1] Comprises 539,467 'no religion' and 561,942 'religion not stated' or 'inadequately described' (this is not a compulsory question in the census schedule).

Education. The State Government maintains a system of free primary and secondary education, and attendance at school is compulsory from 6 to 15 years of age. Non-government schools are subject to government inspection.

In 1989 there were 2,200 government schools with 749,263 students and 45,812 teachers, including 1,659 primary (434,098 students and 21,593 teachers), 381 secondary and 62 combined primary and secondary (310,765 students and 23,345 teachers), and 98 special schools (4,400 students and 875 teachers); and 858 non-government schools, with 284,330 students and 17,281 teachers, including 542 primary (148,819 students and 7,129 teachers), 152 secondary and 132 combined primary and secondary (134,662 students and 9,983 teachers), and 32 special schools (849 students and 169 teachers). Non-government schools included 601 Catholic (with 215,538 students and 12,197 teachers) and 37 Anglican (with 22,082 students and 1,666 teachers).

The University of Sydney, founded in 1850, had 18,236 students in 1988. There are 7 colleges providing residential facilities at the university. The University of New England at Armidale, previously affiliated with the University of Sydney, was incorporated in 1954, and in 1988 had 9,427 students.

The University of New South Wales was established in 1949. Enrolments in 1988 numbered 18,706. There are 7 colleges providing residential facilities at the university. The University of Newcastle, previously affiliated with the University of New South Wales, was granted autonomy from 1965, and in 1988 had 6,375 students. The University of Wollongong, also previously associated with the University of New South Wales, became autonomous in 1975, and in 1988 had 7,964 students. Macquarie University in Sydney, established in 1964, had 11,194 students in 1988.

Advanced education courses at colleges of advanced education and other institutions provide tertiary training with a vocational emphasis. In 1988 there were 61,077 students enrolled in these courses.

Post-school technical and further education is provided at State technical and further education colleges. Enrolments in 1988 totalled 474,051 (87% being part-time).

State Government expenditure (including capital expenditure and federal grants) on education in 1985–86 was $A3,787m.

Social Welfare. The Commonwealth Government makes provision for social benefits, such as age and invalid pensions, widows' pensions, supporting parents' benefits, family allowances, and unemployment, sickness and special benefits.

The number of age and invalid pensions (including wives' and carers' pensions) current in New South Wales on 30 June 1988 was: Age, 488,751; invalid, 128,806. Expenditure for the year ended 30 June 1988 was $A2,549m. for age pensions and $A735m. for invalid pensions.

In addition there were 50,607 widows' pensions current in New South Wales at 30 June 1988. Expenditure on widows' pensions totalled $A353m. in 1987–88. Supporting parents' benefits at 30 June 1988 numbered 68,387; expenditure in 1987–88 was $A579m.

Under the Family Allowance scheme, which commenced in 1976, payments to families and approved institutions for children under 16 years and full-time students under 18 years (under 25 in special circumstances) during 1987–88 amounted to $A478m. The scheme covered 1,402,413 children and students at 30 June 1987.

Unemployment, sickness and special benefits commenced in 1945. During the year 1987–88 claims totalling $A1,599m. were paid in New South Wales. At 30

June 1988 unemployment benefit was being paid to 181,445 persons, sickness benefits to 33,329 persons and special benefits to 9,379 persons.

Direct State Government social welfare services are limited, for the most part, to the assistance of persons not eligible for Commonwealth Government pensions or benefits and the provision of certain forms of assistance not available from the Commonwealth Government. The State also subsidizes many approved services for needy persons.

Health. At 30 June 1988 there were 19,212 medical practitioners. At 30 June 1989 there were 3,652 dentists and 68,833 nurses. In 1989 there were 245 public hospitals with 29,483 beds and 97 private hospitals with 6,218 beds.

Further Reading

Statistical Information: The NSW Government Statistician's Office was established in 1886, and in 1957 was integrated with the Commonwealth Bureau of Census and Statistics (now called the Australian Bureau of Statistics). *Deputy Commonwealth Statistician:* John Wilson. Its principal publications are:

New South Wales Year Book (1886/87–1900/01 under the title *Wealth and Progress of New South Wales*). Annual
Regional Statistics: latest issue, 1991
New South Wales Pocket Year Book. Published since 1913; latest issue, 1991
Monthly Summary of Statistics. Published since May 1931
New South Wales in Brief. 1991

New South Wales Dept. of Business and Consumer Affairs, *New South Wales Business Handbook.* Sydney, 1987
New South Wales Department of Environment and Planning, *Sydney Into Its Third Century: Metropolitan Strategy for the Sydney Region.* Sydney, 1988
New South Wales Government Information Service, *New South Wales Government Directory.* 5th ed. Sydney, 1987

State Library: The State Library of NSW, Macquarie St., Sydney. *State Librarian:* Alison Crook, BA (Hons), MBA, Dip Lib, Dip Ed, ALAA, AAIM.

QUEENSLAND

AREA AND POPULATION. Queensland comprises the whole northeastern portion of the Australian continent, including the adjacent islands in the Pacific Ocean and in the Gulf of Carpentaria. Estimated area 1,727,000 sq. km.

The increase in the population as shown by the censuses since 1901 has been as follows:

	Census counts			*Intercensal increase*	
Year	*Males*	*Females*	*Total*	*Numerical*	*Rate per annum %*
1901	277,003	221,126	498,129	—	—
1911	329,506	276,307	605,813	107,684	1·98
1921	398,969	357,003	755,972	150,159	2·24
1933	497,217	450,317	947,534	191,562	1·86
1947	567,471	538,944	1,106,415	158,881	1·11
1954	676,252	642,007	1,318,259	211,844	2·53
1961	774,579	744,249	1,518,828	200,569	2·04
1966	849,390 [1]	824,934 [1]	1,674,324 [1]	144,857	1·84
1971	921,665 [1]	905,400 [1]	1,827,065 [1]	152,741 [1]	1·76 [1]
1976	1,024,611 [1]	1,012,586 [1]	2,037,197 [1]	210,132 [1]	2·20 [1]
1981	1,153,404 [1]	1,141,719 [1]	2,295,123 [1]	257,926 [1]	2·41 [1]
1986	1,295,630 [1]	1,291,685 [1]	2,587,315 [1]	292,192 [1]	2·43 [1]

[1] Including Aboriginals.

Since the 1981 census, official population estimates are according to place of usual residence and are referred to as estimated resident population. Estimated resident population at 30 June 1989, 2,830,198.

Statistics on birthplaces from the 1986 census are as follows: Australia, 2,162,995 (83·6%); UK and Ireland, 158,949 (6·1%); other countries, 229,760 (8·9%); at sea and not stated, 35,611 (1·4%).

Vital statistics (including Aboriginals) for calendar years:

	Total births	*Marriages*	*Divorces*	*Deaths*
1986	40,371	18,030	7,042	17,861
1987	39,365	18,265	6,918	18,861
1988	40,561	18,850	7,690	18,803

The annual rates per 1,000 population in 1988 were: Marriages, 6·9; births, 14·8; deaths, 6·9. The infant death rate was 8·4 per 1,000 births.

Brisbane, the capital, had at 30 June 1988 (estimate) a resident population of 1,240,286 (Statistical Division). The resident populations of the other major centres (Statistical Districts) at the same date were: Gold Coast-Tweed, 207,966; Townsville, 109,699; Sunshine Coast, 95,683; Toowoomba, 79,934; Cairns, 76,475; Rockhampton, 61,124; Mackay, 50,301; Bundaberg, 43,837 and Gladstone, 30,623. Other cities included Mount Isa, 24,104; Maryborough, 22,986; Hervey Bay, 21,151.

CONSTITUTION AND GOVERNMENT. Queensland, formerly a portion of New South Wales, was formed into a separate colony in 1859, and responsible government was conferred. The power of making laws and imposing taxes is vested in a Parliament of one House—the Legislative Assembly, which comprises 89 members, returned from 4 electoral zones for 3 years, elected for single-member constituencies at compulsory ballot. Members are entitled to $A54,500 per annum, with individual electorate allowances for travelling, postage, etc., of from $A21,525 to $A43,884.

At the general election of 1 Nov. 1986 there were 1,563,294 persons registered as qualified to vote under the Elections Act 1983. This Act provides franchise for all males and females, 18 years of age and over, qualified by 6 months' residence in Australia and 3 months in the electoral district.

At the elections to the Legislative Assembly of 2 Dec. 1989 the Australian Labor Party won 51 seats, the National Party, 29 and the Liberals, 3. (Previous Assembly: National, 49; Labor, 30; Liberal, 10).

Governor of Queensland: Sir Walter Benjamin Campbell, QC (assumed office 22 July 1985).

The Executive Council of Ministers in Feb. 1991 consisted of:

Premier, Minister for Economic and Trade Development and Minister for the Arts: Wayne Goss

Deputy Premier, Minister for Housing and Local Government: Tom Burns. *Police and Emergency Services:* Terry Mackenroth. *Treasurer and Minister for Regional Development:* Keith De Lacy. *Tourism, Sport and Racing:* Robert Gibbs. *Transport and Minister Assisting the Premier on Economic and Trade Development:* David Hamill. *Employment, Training and Industrial Relations:* Neville Warburton. *Resource Industries:* Kenneth Vaughan. *Primary Industries:* Ed Casey. *Health:* Kenneth McElligott. *Education:* Paul Braddy. *Environment and Heritage:* Pat Comben. *Attorney-General:* Deane Wells. *Family Services and Aboriginal and Islander Affairs:* Anne Warner. *Justice and Corrective Services:* Glen Milliner. *Administrative Services:* Ronald McLean. *Manufacturing and Commerce:* Geoffrey Smith. *Land Management:* Bill Eaton.

Ministers have a salary of $A88,229, the Premier receives $A111,524, the Deputy Premier, $A95,941, and the Leader of the Opposition, $A79,666.

Agent-General in London: Hon. D. T. McVeigh (392–3 Strand, WC2R 0LZ).

Local Government. Provision is made for local government by the subdivision of the State into cities, towns and shires. These are under the management of aldermen or councillors, who are elected by all persons 18 years and over. Local Authorities are charged with the control of all matters of a parochial nature, such as sewerage, cleansing and sanitary services, health services, domestic water supplies, and roads and bridges within their allotted areas. In addition to Government grants and subsidies, Local Authority revenue is derived from general rates, paid by landowners on the unimproved capital value of land, and by charging for some specific services.

For the year ended 30 June 1988, the receipts and expenditure (including loans) for the 134 Local Authorities were $A2,047·6m. and $A2,018·6m. respectively and their rateable values amounted to $A27,601·2m.

ECONOMY

Budget. Revenue and expenditure of the Consolidated Revenue Fund of Queensland during 5 years ending 30 June (in $A1,000):

	1983–84	*1984–85*	*1985–86*	*1986–87*	*1987–88*
Revenue	4,212,842	4,681,674	5,190,941	5,649,027	6,308,439
Expenditure	4,211,919	4,682,431	5,190,727	5,648,701	6,270,305

Total receipts of the Queensland Government Authorities in 1987–88 were $A8,116·2m., of which Taxation and Federal Government grants amounted to $A5,896·8m. Expenditure from these funds included: Education, $A1,959·9m.; fuel and energy, $A441m.; transport and communications, $A942·1m.; health, $A1,080m.

Revenue and expenditure of Commonwealth Government departments on account of Queensland are not included.

Debt. The public debt of the State at 30 June 1989 was $A2,420·3m.

Banking. The major national trading and savings banks dominate banking operations in Queensland. The Bank of Queensland, which is a privately owned bank with its head office in Queensland, and several licensed foreign banks also provide trading and savings bank facilities. In June 1989 the average of weekly deposits held in trading banks in Queensland amounted to $A10,197m. while the average of advances owing to the banks was $A9,321m. The total depositors' balances held in savings banks in Queensland at 30 June 1989 was $A9,687m.

ENERGY AND NATURAL RESOURCES

Electricity. During 1988–89, 96·7% of the State's generation of 23,774m. kwh was derived from coal-fuelled steam power stations. The hydro-electric stations located in north Queensland provided 3·2% of the State's electricity needs with the remainder being produced by gas turbine and internal combustion generation using light fuel oil and natural gas.

Minerals. Principal minerals produced during 1987–88 were: Copper, 158,000 tonnes; coal, 65,189,000 tonnes; lead, 202,000 tonnes; zinc, 242,000 tonnes; silver, 525,000 kg; tin, 386 tonnes; gold, 19,000 kg; bauxite, 8,449,000 tonnes; mineral sands concentrates, 464,000 tonnes; nickel, 29,000 tonnes; liquid petroleum, 1,685,000 kilolitres. Value of output, at the mine, was $A4,107m. The chief mines are at Mount Isa (copper, silver, lead, zinc), Weipa (bauxite), Kidston, Mount Leyshon, Mount Morgan, Red Dame, Pajingo and Cracow (gold), Moreton and Bowen Basin (coal), Greenvale (nickel), Cooper-Eromanga Basin (petroleum) and North Stradbroke Island (mineral sands).

Land Settlement. At 30 June 1989, of the 172·7m. hectares of the State, 121·5m. hectares was Crown leasehold, 20·5m. hectares was in process of freeholding and the remaining 30·7m. hectares was roads, reserves, freehold, mining tenures and vacant land.

In the western portion of the State water is comparatively easily found by sinking artesian bores. At 30 June 1988, 3,700 such bores had been drilled, of which 2,595 were flowing.

Agriculture. Livestock on farms and stations at 31 March 1988 numbered 8·83m. cattle, 14·37m. sheep and 617,000 pigs. The wool production (greasy) was, in 1987–88, 78m. kg, valued at $A477m. The total area under crops during 1987–88 was 2·9m. hectares.

Crop	Area (hectares) 1986–87	1987–88	Production (tonnes) 1986–87	1987–88
Sugar-cane, crushed	286,967	291,169	23,466,026	23,199,753
Wheat	794,582	646,140	833,138	718,395
Maize	38,348	36,930	118,017	124,209
Sorghum	624,902	565,174	1,018,807	1,213,117
Barley	167,917	169,427	275,855	244,173
Oats	20,315	19,486	18,793	13,566
Potatoes	6,335	6,617	132,729	120,048
Pumpkins	3,602	3,538	33,122	33,071
Tomatoes	3,570	3,424	78,778	81,411
Peanuts	32,843	31,137	44,470	35,651
Tobacco	2,942	2,816	7,572	7,105
Apples [1]	2,804	2,669	36,591	33,640
Grapes [2]	1,059	982	4,191	4,190
Citrus [1]	1,689	1,546	46,507	46,651
Bananas [2]	3,408	3,505	64,298	79,183
Pineapples [2]	3,758	3,764	142,288	146,463
Green fodder [3]	580,203	582,100	...	...
Hay (all kinds)	51,643	62,722	228,583	258,026
Cotton (raw)	30,996	80,918	40,248	72,099

[1] Area of trees 6 years and over. [2] Bearing area only.
[3] Excluding lucerne and other pastures.

Forestry. A considerable area consists of natural forest, eucalyptus, pine and cabinet woods being the timbers mostly in evidence; a large quantity of ornamental woods is utilized by cabinet makers. The amount of timber processed, including plantation and imported, in 1988–89 was (in cu. metres): Conifers, 947,768; hardwoods, structural timbers and cabinet woods, 620,760.

INDUSTRY AND TRADE

Industry. In 1987–88, there were 4,624 establishments, with four or more workers, employing 97,335 males and 30,209 females, and producing goods and services worth $A17,255m. The manufacturing establishments contributing most to the overall production during 1987–88 were those predominantly engaged in the processing of food, beverages and tobacco.

The gross value of Queensland agricultural commodity production (in $A1,000) during 1987–88, amounted to 3,935,009, which included crops, 1,824,024; livestock disposals, 1,405,716; livestock products, 705,270.

Labour. In 1989 the labour force comprised 1·4m. persons, 63% of the 2·2m. civilian population aged 15 years and older, and the unemployment rate was 6·6%. Major industries employing people were wholesale and retail trade (22%), community services (16%) and manufacturing (13%).

Trade Unions. Unions both of employees and employers must be registered with the State or Australian Commission. There were 130 trade unions operating at June 1988 with 435,400 members (about 50% of total employees).

Commerce. The overseas commerce of Queensland is included in the statement of the commerce of Australia (*see* pp. 109–11).

Total value of the direct overseas imports and exports of Queensland (in $A1,000) f.o.b. port of shipment for both imports and exports:

	1983–84	*1984–85*	*1985–86*	*1986–87*	*1987–88*	*1988–89*
Imports	2,114,900	2,315,492	2,649,953	2,503,854	2,844,208	3,788,296
Exports	5,559,161 [1]	6,602,936 [1]	7,737,046 [1]	7,928,406 [1]	8,289,659 [1]	9,083,994 [1]

[1] State of origin.

In 1988–89 interstate exports totalled $A3,532·7m. and imports $A8,317·8m. The chief exports overseas are minerals including alumina, coal, meat (preserved or frozen), sugar, wool, cereal grains, copper and lead, and manufactured goods. Principal overseas imports are machinery, motor vehicles, mineral fuels (including lubricants, etc.), chemicals and manufactured goods classified by material. Chief sources of imports in 1988–89 were Japan ($A961·1m.), USA ($A912·9m.), UK ($A157·9m.), EEC, excluding UK ($A362·4m.); exports went chiefly to Japan ($A3,371·6m.), USA ($A730·7m.), UK ($A556·8m.), EEC, excluding UK ($A875·1m.).

COMMUNICATIONS

Roads. At 30 June 1988 there were 169,589 km of roads; of these, 152,952 km were formed roads, of which 56,700 km were surfaced with sealed pavement.

At 30 June 1988 motor vehicles registered in Queensland totalled 1,616,201, comprising 1,159,196 cars and station wagons, 220,652 utilities, 86,918 panel vans, 9,998 buses, 71,756 trucks and 67,681 motor cycles.

Railways. Practically all the railways are owned by the State Government. Total length of line at 30 June 1990 was 10,094 km, of which 1,707 km were electrified. In 1989–90, 44·1m. passengers and 82·5m. tonnes of goods and livestock were carried.

Aviation. Queensland is well served with a network of air services, with overseas and interstate connexions. Subsidiary companies provide planes for taxi and charter work, and the Flying Doctor Service operates throughout western Queensland.

Shipping. In 1987–88, cargo discharged was 2·6m. GWT and cargo loaded was 70·8m. GWT.

Telecommunications. At 30 June 1988, 113 broadcasting and 98 television and translator stations were in operation throughout Queensland.

JUSTICE, RELIGION, EDUCATION AND WELFARE

Justice. Justice is administered by Higher Courts (Supreme and District), Magistrates' Courts and Children's Courts. The Supreme Court comprises a Chief Justice, a senior puisne judge, 18 puisne judges and 2 masters; the District Courts, 24 district court judges of whom 1 is chairman. Stipendiary magistrates preside over the Magistrates' and Children's Courts, except in the smaller centres, where justices of the peace officiate. A parole board may recommend prisoners for release.

The total number of appearances resulting in conviction as the most serious outcome in the Higher Courts in 1987–88 was 2,817; summary convictions in Magistrates' Courts totalled 131,721 and proven offences in Children's Courts numbered 4,728. There were, at 30 June 1988, 5 prisons, 2 prison farms conducted on the honour system and 1 prison for criminally-insane patients, with 2,304 male and 114 female prisoners. The total police force was 5,322 at 30 June 1988.

Religion. There is no State Church. Membership, census 1986: Anglican, 640,867; Catholic, 628,906; Uniting Church, 255,287; Presbyterian, 120,239; Lutheran, 56,910; Baptist, 39,099; other Christian, 211,316; Buddhist, 5,769; Muslim, 3,731; Hebrew, 2,631; all others (including not stated and no religion), 622,560.

Education. Education in Queensland ranges from pre-school level through to tertiary level. In addition, child care, kindergarten and adult education facilities are available. Education is compulsory between the ages of 6 and 15 years and is provided free in government schools. Expenditure on education by State and local government authorities for 1986–87 was $A1,954·6m.

At July 1988, pre-school education and child care was provided at 1,397 centres with 4,803 staff and 80,381 children.

Primary and secondary education comprises 12 years of full-time formal schooling and is provided by both the government and non-government sectors. At July 1989, the State administered 995 primary, 70 primary/secondary, and 170 secondary schools with 242,183 primary students and 141,712 secondary students. In addition, 65 special schools provided educational programmes for 3,543 children. State education programmes were provided by 12,982 primary, 10,465 secondary and 810 special school teachers. Non-government enrolments at July 1989 were 63,933 primary students and 62,416 secondary students at 240 primary, 66 primary/

secondary and 86 secondary schools. Educational programmes at non-government schools were provided by 7,367 teachers.

Post-secondary education in Queensland involves technical and further education, advanced education and university education. In 1987, enrolments in TAFE courses totalled 179,423. At 30 April 1988, 34,976 students were enrolled in advanced education courses and 27,816 students were enrolled in university courses.

Social Welfare. Public hospitals are maintained by State and Federal Government endowment, supplemented by fees from patients not in standard wards. Welfare institutions providing shelter and social care for the aged, the handicapped, and children, are maintained or assisted by the State. A child health service is provided throughout the State. Age, invalid, widows', disability and war service pensions, family allowances, and unemployment and sickness benefits are paid by the Federal Government. Age pensioners in the State at 30 June 1988 numbered 210,818; invalid pensioners, 44,313; disability and service pensioners, 144,784 (including dependants).

There were 22,744 widows' pensions current at 30 June 1988, and at the same date family allowances were being paid to 336,796 families in respect of 663,731 children under 16 years and eligible students aged 16 to 24 years. In addition, family allowances were paid to 2,907 children and students in institutions.

Further Reading

Statistical Information: The Statistical Office (313 Adelaide St., Brisbane) was set up in 1859. *Deputy Commonwealth Statistician:* J. K. Cornish. *A Queensland Official Year Book* was issued in 1901, the annual *ABC of Queensland Statistics* from 1905 to 1936 with exception of 1918 and 1922. Present publications include: *Queensland Year Book*. Annual, from 1937 (omitting 1942, 1943, 1944, 1987, 1991).—*Queensland Pocket Year Book*. Annual from 1950.—*Monthly Summary of Statistics, Queensland*. From Jan. 1961

Australian Sugar Year Book. Brisbane, from 1941

Endean, R., *Australia's Great Barrier Reef*. Brisbane, 1982

Johnston, W. R., *A Bibliography of Queensland History*. Brisbane, 1981.—*The Call of the Land: A History of Queensland to the Present Day*. Brisbane, 1982

Johnston, W. R. and Zerner, M., *Guide to the History of Queensland*. Brisbane, 1985

Queensland State Public Relations Bureau, *Queensland Resources Atlas*, Brisbane, 1980

Queensland Department of Commercial and Industrial Development, *Resources and Industry of Far North Queensland*, Brisbane, 1980

State Library: The State Library of Queensland, Queensland Cultural Centre, South Bank, South Brisbane. *State Librarian:* D. H. Stephens.

SOUTH AUSTRALIA

AREA AND POPULATION. The total area of South Australia is 380,070 sq. miles (984,377 sq. km). The settled part is divided into counties and hundreds. There are 49 counties proclaimed, covering 23m. ha, of which 19m. ha are occupied. Outside this area there are extensive pastoral districts, covering 76m. ha, 43m. of which are under pastoral leases.

Census population (exclusive of full-blood Aboriginals before 1966):

	Males	*Females*	*Total*		*Males*	*Females*	*Total*
1901	180,485	177,861	358,346	1966	550,196	544,788	1,094,984
1911	207,358	201,200	408,558	1971	586,051	587,656	1,173,707
1921	248,267	246,893	495,160	1976	620,162	624,594	1,244,756
1933	290,962	289,987	580,949	1981	635,696	649,337	1,285,033
1947	320,031	326,042	646,073	1986	665,960	679,985	1,345,945
1961	490,225	479,115	969,340				

The number of Aboriginals and Torres Strait Islanders (as reported on Census schedules) in the State at the Census of 30 June 1986 was 14,291.

Vital statistics for calendar years:

	Live Births	*Marriages*	*Divorces*	*Deaths*
1986	19,741	9,878	3,776	10,328
1987	19,235	9,695	4,050	10,565
1988	19,155	10,128	4,031	10,690
1989	19,610	9,769	3,740	11,348

The infant mortality rate in 1989 was 7·45 per 1,000 live births.

The Adelaide Statistical Division had 1,037,702 inhabitants at 30 June 1989 in 22 cities and 8 municipalities and other districts. Cities outside this area (with populations at 30 June 1989) are Whyalla (26,731), Mount Gambier (22,214), Port Augusta (15,766), Port Pirie (15,224) and Port Lincoln (12,953).

CONSTITUTION AND GOVERNMENT. South Australia was formed into a British province by letters patent of Feb. 1836, and a partially elective Legislative Council was established in 1851. The present Constitution bears date 24 Oct. 1856. It vests the legislative power in an elected Parliament, consisting of a Legislative Council and a House of Assembly. The former is composed of 22 members. Every 4 years half the members retire, and the resulting vacancies are filled at a general election on the basis of proportional representation with the State as one multi-member electorate. The qualifications of an elector are, to be an Australian citizen, or a British subject who on 25 Jan. 1984 was enrolled on a Commonwealth electoral roll and/or at some time between 26 Oct. 1983 and 25 Jan. 1984 inclusive was enrolled on an electoral roll for a South Australian Assembly district or a Commonwealth electoral roll in any State. The person must be of at least 18 years of age and have lived continuously in Australia for at least 6 months, in South Australia for at least 3 months and in the sub-division for which he is enrolled at least 1 month. War service may substitute for residential qualifications in some cases. By the Constitution Act Amendment Act, 1894, the franchise was extended to women, who voted for the first time at the general election of 25 April 1896. The qualifications for election as a member of both Houses are the same as for an elector. Certain persons are ineligible for election to either House.

The House of Assembly consists of 47 members elected for 4 years, representing single electorates. Election of members of both Houses takes place by preferential secret ballot. Voting is compulsory for those on the Electoral Roll.

The House of Assembly, elected on 25 Nov. 1989, consists (preliminary figures) of the following members: Liberal Party of Australia, 22; Australian Labor Party, 22; Independent Labor, 2. The Legislative Council consists of 9 Liberal Party of Australia, 11 Labor and 2 Australian Democrat members.

Each member of Parliament receives $A53,289 per annum with allowances of $A14,639–44,606 according to location of electorate, a free pass over government railways and superannuation rights. Electors enrolled (Sept. 1990) numbered 962,642.

The executive power is vested in a Governor appointed by the Crown and an Executive Council, consisting of the Governor and the Ministers of the Crown. The Governor has the power to dissolve the House of Assembly but not the Legislative Council unless that Chamber has twice consecutively with an election intervening defeated the same or substantially the same Bill passed in the House of Assembly by an absolute majority.

Governor: Dame Hon. Roma Mitchell, AC, DBE.

The South Australian Labor Ministry, in Aug. 1990 was as follows:

Premier, Treasurer and Minister of State Development: John Charles Bannon, MP.

Deputy Premier, Minister of Health, Minister of Family and Community Services and Minister for the Aged: Donald Jack Hopgood, MP. *Attorney-General, Minister of Crime Prevention and Minister of Corporate Affairs:* Christopher John Sumner, MLC. *Minister of Industry, Trade and Technology, Minister of Agriculture, Minister of Fisheries and Minister of Ethnic Affairs:* Lynn Maurice Ferguson Arnold, MP. *Minister of Education and Minister of Children's Services:* Gregory John Crafter, MP. *Minister of Transport, Minister of Correctional Services and Minister of*

Finance: Frank Trevor Blevins, MP. *Minister of Tourism, Minister of Consumer Affairs and Minister of Small Business:* Barbara Jean Wiese, MLC. *Minister of Housing and Construction, Minister of Public Works and Minister of Recreation and Sport:* Milton Kym Mayes, MP. *Minister of Environment and Planning, Minister of Water Resources and Minister of Lands:* Susan Mary Lenehan, MP. *Minister of Emergency Services, Minister of Mines and Energy and Minister of Forests:* John Heinz Cornelis Klunder, MP. *Minister of Labour, Minister of Occupational Health and Safety and Minister of Marine:* Robert John Gregory, MP. *Minister of Local Government, Minister for the Arts and Minister of State Services:* Judith Anne Winstanley Levy, MLC. *Minister of Employment and Further Education, Minister of Youth Affairs, Minister of Aboriginal Affairs and Minister Assisting the Minister of Ethnic Affairs:* Michael David Rann, MP.

Ministers are jointly and individually responsible to the legislature for all their official acts, as in the UK.

Agent-General in London: G. Walls (50 Strand, WC2N 5LW).

Local Government. The closely settled part of the State (mainly near the sea-coast and the River Murray) is incorporated into local government areas, and sub-divided into district councils (rural areas only), municipal corporations (mainly metropolitan, but including larger country towns) and cities (more densely populated areas with a qualification of 15,000 residents in the Adelaide metropolitan area, and 10,000 in the country). The main functions of councils are the construction and maintenance of roads and bridges, sport and recreational facilities and garbage collection and disposal.

The number and area of the sub-divisions, together with expenditure (in $A1,000) for the year ended 30 June 1989, were:

	No.	*Area (1,000 ha)*	*Roads and bridges*	*Recreation and culture*	*All other*	*Total expenditure*
Adelaide statistical division	30	189·3	63,897	70,737	250,322	384,956
Other municipal corporations and district councils	91	15,223·4	53,901	20,589	111,106	185,596
Total	121	15,412·7	117,798	91,326	361,428	570,552

ECONOMY

Budget. Recurrent revenue and expenditure (in $A1,000) for years ended 30 June:

	1985	*1986*	*1987*	*1988*	*1989*	*1990*
Revenue	2,639,937	2,966,345	3,217,176	4,225,669	4,123,056	4,554·600
Expenditure	2,626,240	2,955,350	3,214,926	4,215,265	4,206,418	4,483·600

Banking. In June 1990 the average weekly balance of deposits held by all banks was $A12,074m. The average weekly balance of loans, advances and bills discounted was $A13,771m.

NATURAL RESOURCES

Minerals. The value of minerals produced in 1988–89 was $A1,080·8m. The principal minerals produced are opals, natural gas, iron ore, copper, gypsum, salt, talc, clays, limestone, dolomite and sub-bituminous coal.

Agriculture. Of the total area of South Australia (984,377 sq. km), 260,742 sq. km were alienated, 490,150 sq. km were held under lease and 233,485 sq. km were unoccupied. Area used for agricultural purposes, at 31 March 1989, was 580,286 sq. km.

Soil Conservation. Under the direction of special officers in the Department of Agriculture, determined efforts are made to deal with the problems of erosion and soil conservation. Included in the programme are the planting of cereal rye, perennial rye and other grasses to check sand drifts; contour-furrowing and contour banking; contour planting with vines and fruit trees and several water-diversion schemes.

Irrigation. For the year ended 31 March 1987, 91,765 ha were under irrigated culture, being used as follows: Vineyards, 16,418; orchards, 11,865; vegetables, 6,244, and other crops and pasture, 57,238. Most of these areas are along the river Murray.

Gross value of agricultural production (in $A1,000), 1988–89: Crops, 1,102,959; livestock slaughtering, 433,308; livestock products, 731,888. Total gross value, 2,268,155; local value (*i.e.* less marketing costs), 2,064,223.

	1987–88		*1988–89*	
Chief crops	*Ha*	*Tonnes*	*Ha*	*Tonnes*
Wheat	1,555,573	1,803,041	1,520,012	1,361,138
Barley	876,298	1,260,520	836,641	1,032,927
Oats	131,752	134,574	155,513	131,426
Hay	180,186	535,106	195,026	528,913
Vines	...	210,359,000 [1]	...	259,127,000 [1]

[1] Litres of wine.

Fruit culture is extensively carried on, and in 1988–89, 237,967 tonnes of fresh fruit were produced. Other products, in addition to all kinds of root crops and vegetables, are grass seeds and oil seeds. Livestock, March 1989: 942,504 cattle, 17,413,880 sheep and 449,893 pigs. In 1988–89, 120,600 tonnes of wool and 371m. litres of milk were produced.

INDUSTRY AND TRADE

Industry. The turnover for manufacturing industries for 1988–89 was $A13,076m.

Industry sub-division	*Establish-ments (No.)*	*Persons employed (No.)*	*Wages and salaries ($A1m.)*	*Turnover ($A1m.)*
Food, beverages and tobacco	381	16,307	348	2,471
Textiles	48	2,493	55	378
Clothing and footwear	107	4,293	76	282
Wood, wood products and furniture	394	7,977	152	725
Paper, paper products, printing and publishing	239	7,841	197	831
Chemical, petroleum and coal products	50	2,333	62	514
Non-metallic mineral products	126	3,890	96	549
Basic metal products	48	7,675	218	1,440
Fabricated metal products	419	8,883	181	853
Transport equipment	148	18,752	444	2,884
Other machinery and equipment	372	15,344	331	1,409
Miscellaneous manufacturing	211	7,308	154	740
Total	2,543	103,096	2,315	13,076

Practically all forms of secondary industry are to be found, the most important being, motor vehicle manufacture, saw-milling and the manufacture of household appliances, basic iron and steel, meat and meat products, and wine and brandy.

Labour. Two systems of industrial arbitration and conciliation for the adjustment of industrial relations between employers and employees are in operation—the State system, which operates when industrial disputes are confined to the territorial limits of the State, and the Federal system, which applies when disputes involve other parts of Australia as well as South Australia.

The industrial tribunals are authorized to fix minimum rates of wages and other conditions of employment, and their awards may be enforced by law. Industrial agreements between employers and organizations of employees, when registered, may be enforced in the same manner as awards. In March 1989 the minimum wage under State awards was $A204.10.

Commerce. The commerce of South Australia, exclusive of inter-state trade, is comprised in the statement of the commerce of Australia given under the heading of the Commonwealth, *see* pp. 109–11.

Overseas imports and exports in $A1m. (year ending 30 June):

	1985–86	*1986–87*	*1987–88*	*1988–89*	*1989–90*
Imports	1,737·5	1,503·4	1,804·6	1,861·4	2,049·9
Exports	1,987·3	2,044·2	2,263·3	2,441·3	2,841·3

Principal exports in 1989–90 were (in $A1m.): Wheat, 431·9; barley, 243·4; meat and meat preparations, 241·1; copper, 118·4; petroleum and petroleum products, 117·9; wool, 271·3.

Principal imports in 1989–90 were (in $A1m.): Transport equipment, 544·5; machinery, 352·3; petroleum and petroleum products, 203·6.

In 1989–90 the leading suppliers of imports were (in $A1m.): Japan (530·2), USA (432·3), Saudi Arabia (132·4), UK, (118); Federal Republic of Germany (114·1); main exports went to Japan (353·1), New Zealand (293·9), USA (238·8), Iran (197·3), Saudi Arabia (136·2), UK, (118·3).

Tourism. In June 1990 there were 372 hotels and motels with 10,316 rooms; 210 caravan parks had a total of 23,342 sites.

COMMUNICATIONS

Roads. At 30 June 1989, of the roads customarily used by the public, there were 2,460 km of national roads, 9,792 km of arterial roads and 82,560 km of local roads, totalling 94,812 km. Lengths of road classified by surface were as follows: Sealed, 23,712 km; unsealed, 71,100 km. Costs of construction and maintenance are shared by the State and Commonwealth governments and by the councils of the local areas. Motor vehicles registered at 30 June 1990 included 574,617 cars, 122,807 station wagons, 153,714 commercial vehicles and 29,629 cycles.

Railways. At 30 June 1990, Australian National Railways operated 5,952 km of railway in country areas. The State Transport Authority operated 127 km of railway in the metropolitan area of Adelaide. All public freight and non-metropolitan passenger services are operated by Australian National.

Aviation. For the year ended 30 June 1989 there were 2,299,084 passengers and 23,946 tonnes of freight handled by 47,647 aircraft movements at Adelaide, South Australia's principal airport (including Adelaide International). On 30 June 1990 there were 5 government and 30 licensed aerodromes.

Shipping. There are several good harbours, of which Port Adelaide is the principal one. In 1988, 701 vessels conducting overseas trade entered South Australia with 2,216,000 import tonnes of cargo and left with 5,328,000 export tonnes.

Telecommunications. At 30 June 1989, there were 521 post offices. Telephone services connected totalled 709,998 on 30 June 1989. There were 48 radio and 31 television stations at 30 June 1989.

JUSTICE, RELIGION, EDUCATION AND WELFARE

Justice. There is a Supreme Court, which incorporates admiralty, civil, criminal, land and valuation, and testamentary jurisdiction; district criminal courts, which have jurisdiction in many indictable offences; local courts and courts of summary jurisdiction. Circuit courts are held at several places. In the year ended 31 Dec. 1988, 2,639 criminal matters were proven in higher courts. During the year 1988-89 there were 1,327 sequestrations and schemes under the Bankruptcy Act. There were 3,117 prisoners received under sentence in 1988-89 with a daily average prison population of 658.

Religion. At the Census of 1986 the religious distribution of the population (as reported on Census schedules) was as follows: Catholic, 267,137; Anglican, 242,722; Uniting Church, 176,980; Lutheran, 64,851; Orthodox, 37,149; Baptist, 21,415; Presbyterian, 18,566; other Christians, 108,048; non-Christian, 13,843; indefinite, 5,458; no religion, 227,564; not stated, 162,212.

Education. Education is secular and is compulsory for children 6–15 years of age.

Primary and secondary education at government schools is free. In 1989 there were 708 government schools, comprising 517 primary, 67 primary and secondary, 100 secondary schools and 24 special schools. There were 185,769 full-time students. The Department of Technical and Further Education is responsible for technical, adult and vocational education. In 1989 there were 20 colleges of technical and further education, among the facilities are an adult migrant education service, a further education, a centre for performing arts and schools of music, maritime and external studies. Tertiary education, including teacher education, is provided by the 3 universities. There were 183 non-government schools and colleges, most of which are associated with religious denominations (56,363 students). In 1989 there were 419 pre-school centres with an enrolment of 24,415 pre-school children.

Social Welfare. Age, invalidity, war, unemployment, etc., pensions are paid by the Commonwealth Government. The number of pensioners in South Australia at 30 June 1989 was: Disability and service, 72,393; age, 137,992; invalid, 32,037; unemployment, 42,878. There are schemes for family allowances, widows, supporting parents and sickness and hospital and pharmaceutical benefits.

Further Reading

Statistical Information: The State branch of the Australian Bureau of Statistics is at 41 Currie St., Adelaide (GPO Box 2272). *Deputy Commonwealth Statistician:* R. J. Rogers. Although the first printed statistical publication was the *Statistics of South Australia, 1854* with the title altered to *Statistical Register* in 1859, there is a written volume for each year back to 1838. These contain simple records of trade, demography, production, etc. and were prepared only for the use of the Colonial Office; one copy was retained in the State.

The publications of the State branch include the *South Australian Year Book*, the *Pocket Year Book of South Australia* and a *Monthly Summary of Statistics, South Australia*, a quarterly bulletin of building activity, a quarterly bulletin of tourist accommodation and approximately 40 special bulletins issued each year as particulars of various sections of statistics become available.

South Australia: Premier's Department, Adelaide, 1980
Douglas, J., *South Australia from Space.* Adelaide, 1980
Finlayson, H. H., *The Red Centre: Man and Beast in the Heart of Australia.* 2nd ed. Sydney, 1952
Gibbs, R. M., *A History of South Australia: From Colonial Days to the Present.* Adelaide, 1984
Whitelock, D., *Adelaide, 1836–1976: A History of Difference.* Univ. of Queensland Press, 1977

State Library: The State Library of S.A., North Terrace, Adelaide. *State Librarian:* E. M. Miller, MA (Hons), Dip. NZLS, ANZLA, ALAA.

TASMANIA

HISTORY. Abel Janzoon Tasman discovered Van Diemen's Land (Tasmania) on 24 Nov. 1642. The island became a British settlement in 1803 as a dependency of New South Wales; in 1825 its connexion with New South Wales was terminated; in 1851 a partially elective Legislative Council was established, and in 1856 responsible government came into operation. On 1 Jan. 1901 Tasmania was federated with the other Australian states into the Commonwealth of Australia.

AREA AND POPULATION. Tasmania is an island separated from the mainland by the Bass Strait with an area (including islands) of 68,331 sq. km, or 6·83m. hectares, of which 6,441,000 hectares form the area of the main island. The population at 10 consecutive censuses was:

	Population	*Increase % per annum*		*Population*	*Increase % per annum*
1921	213,780	1·12	1966	371,436	1·18
1933	227,599	0·52	1971	398,100 [1]	0·99
1947	257,078	0·87	1976	412,300 [1]	0·70 [2]
1954	308,752	2·65	1981	427,200 [1]	0·72 [2]
1961	350,340	1·82	1986	436,353	...

[1] Resident population. [2] Not comparable with previous censuses.

At the census of 30 June 1986, 5·32% were born in the UK and Ireland, 2·68% in other European countries and 88·61% in Australia. The last full-blooded Tasmanian Aboriginal died in 1876.

Vital statistics for calendar years:

	Marriages	*Divorces*	*Births*	*Deaths*
1987	3,141	1,115	6,753	3,596
1988	3,034	1,220	6,771	3,529
1989	3,070	1,269	6,885	3,735

The largest cities and towns (with populations at the 1986 Census) are Hobart (175,082), Launceston (88,486), Devonport (1981, 21,424) and Burnie (20,585).

CONSTITUTION AND GOVERNMENT. Parliament consists of the Governor, the Legislative Council and the House of Assembly. The Council has 19 members, elected by adults with 6 months' residence. Members sit for 6 years, 3 retiring annually and 4 every sixth year. There is no power to dissolve the Council. Vacancies are filled by by-elections. The House of Assembly has 35 members; the maximum term for the House of Assembly is 4 years. Members of both Houses are paid a basic salary of $A45,687 (Oct. 1990), plus an electorate allowance, according to the division represented. The annual allowance payable is calculated as a percentage of basic salary. The amounts vary from $A5,025 (11%) to $A15,990 (35%). Women received the right to vote in 1903. Proportional representation was adopted in 1907, the method now being the single transferable vote in 7-member constituencies. Casual vacancies in the House of Assembly are determined by a transfer of the preference of the vacating member's ballot papers to consenting candidates who were unsuccessful at the last general election.

A Minister must have a seat in one of the two Houses; all present Ministers are members of the House of Assembly.

In addition to the salary paid to Ministers as members of either House, the following allowances are payable: Premier, in conjunction with a ministerial office, $A47,160; Deputy Premier, in conjunction with a ministerial office, $A32,069; other Ministers, $A26,410. The Leader of the Opposition in the House of Assembly receives an allowance of $A26,410. The holders of some other offices receive allowances ranging from $A2,264 to $A12,576.

An election in May 1989 resulted in a 'hung parliament' with 17 Liberals, 13 Labor and 5 Independents. The most likely result was predicted to be a minority Liberal government, however, the final outcome was a Labor Party Government in an alliance with the 5 Independents.

The Legislative Council is predominantly independent without formal party allegiance; 1 member is Labor-endorsed.

Governor: Gen. Sir Phillip Bennett, AC, KBE, DSO.

The Labor Party Cabinet was composed as follows in Aug. 1990:

Premier, Minister for Finance, Treasurer, Minister for State Development: M. W. Field.

Deputy Premier, Justice and Attorney-General, Education and the Arts: P. J. Patmore. *Environment and Planning, Employment, Industrial Relations and Training, Minister Assisting Premier on Youth Affairs:* M. A. Aird. *Administrative Services, Consumer Affairs and Minister Assisting Premier on Status of Women:* F. M. Bladel. *Tourism, Sport and Recreation:* H. N. Holgate. *Community Services, Parks, Wildlife and Heritage:* J. L. Jackson. *Primary Industry, Forests:* D. E. Llewellyn. *Resources and Energy, Construction:* M. W. Weldon. *Health, Minister Assisting the Premier on Aboriginal Affairs and on Multicultural Affairs:* J. C. White. *Roads and Transport, Police and Emergency Services:* K. S. Wriedt.

Local Government. For the purposes of local government, the State is divided into 46 municipal areas comprising the cities of Hobart, Launceston, Glenorchy and Devonport and 42 municipalities. The number of municipalities was reduced from

45 in May 1985 because of the amalgamation of 2 municipalities with the City of Launceston. The cities and municipalities are managed by elected aldermen and councillors, respectively, with reference to local matters such as sanitation and health services, domestic water supplies and roads and bridges within each particular area. The chief source of revenue is rates (based on assessed annual value) levied on owners of property.

Tasmanian Islands. Three inhabited Tasmanian islands (Bruny, King and Flinders) are organized as municipalities. Nearly 1,360 km south-east lies Macquarie Island (230 sq. km), part of the State, and used only as an Australian research base and meteorological station.

ECONOMY

Budget. The revenue is derived chiefly from taxation (pay-roll, motor, lottery and land tax, business franchises and stamp duties), and from grants and reimbursements from the Commonwealth Government. Customs, excise, sales and income tax are levied by the Commonwealth Government, which makes grants to Tasmania for both revenue and capital purposes. Commonwealth payments to Tasmania in 1989–90 totalled $A1,014·9m. These included General Revenue Funds, $A501·1m.; Specific Purpose Payments, $A486·1m. and Capital Funds, $A27·7m.

Specific Purpose Grants are mainly used to provide essential services such as hospitals, housing, roads and educational services, while General Purpose Revenue Funds have been paid since 1942 to compensate the State for the loss of income tax to the federal government.

Consolidated Revenue Fund receipts and expenditure, in $A1,000, for financial years ending 30 June:

	1984–85	*1985–86*	*1986–87*	*1987–88*	*1988–89*	*1989–90*
Revenue	953,209	1,024,697	1,107,870	1,201,397	1,259,754	1,674,955
Expenditure	952,922	1,036,954	1,106,608	1,201,175	1,258,945	1,684,849

The public debt at current exchange rates amounted to $A1,218m. at 30 June 1990.

In 1989–90 State taxation revenue amounted to $A408m., of which pay-roll tax provided $A128·9m.; motor tax, $A20m.; stamp duties, $A84m.; business franchises, $A77·9m., and lottery tax, $A19m.

Banking. Trading bank activity in Tasmania is divided between 3 private banks and the Commonwealth Trading Bank. For the month of Dec. 1988 liabilities represented by depositors' balances averaged $A749m. and assets represented by advances, $A929m. The 6 savings banks operating in Tasmania are the Commonwealth Savings Bank, 2 trustee savings banks and 3 private savings banks operated by trading banks. At 31 Dec. 1988 total savings bank deposits were $A1,761m.

ENERGY AND NATURAL RESOURCES

Electricity. Tasmania has good supplies of hydro-electric power because of assured rainfall and high level water storages (natural and artificial). The Hydro-Electric Commission, Tasmania's sole commercial supplier of electricity, has been surveying water power resources of the State for many years and it is estimated that about 3m. kw. can be economically developed. With the addition of the Reece Dam, 2,315,000 kw. of generating plant was in commission in 1989–90. In 1989–90 the peak loading was 1,427,000 kw. The Pieman River Power Development, comprising 3 stations, was completed in 1987. The Gordon River Power Development Stage 2 (the Gordon-below-Franklin scheme) was halted by a High Court decision.

Minerals. The assayed content of principal metallic minerals contained in locally produced concentrates for 1988–89 was (in tonnes): Zinc, 107,439; iron pellets, 1,556,000; copper, 22,257; lead, 42,915; tin, 6,820; gold, 1,926 kg; silver, 110,950 kg. Coal production, 356,282 tonnes.

Primary Industries. The estimated gross value of recorded production from agriculture in 1988–89 was (in $A1m.): Livestock products, 248·4; livestock slaughterings and other disposals, 122·3; crops, 233·4; total gross value, 604·1. Estimated gross value of fisheries was $A91m. in 1986-87.

Agriculture. From 1986–87 the scope of the Census includes only those establishments undertaking agricultural activity and having an EVAO (Estimated Value of Agricultural Operations) of $A20,000 or more. The scope of previous Censuses was establishments undertaking agricultural activity having an EVAO of $A2,500 or more.

The area occupied by the 3,600 holdings in 1988–89 totalled 1,883,500 ha, of which 934,600 were devoted to crops and sown pasture. The following table shows the area and production, in tonnes, of the principal crops:

	1986–87		*1987–88*		*1988–89*	
	Ha	*Production*	*Ha*	*Production*	*Ha*	*Production*
Wheat	1,729	4,739	1,179	3,815	771	2,199
Barley	8,487	20,681	8,024	21,549	7,820	22,022
Oats	7,765	11,215	9,560	15,552	10,233	17,925
Green peas	6,714	22,683	6,211	28,552	6,329	29,585
Potatoes	5,744	223,425	6,380	248,303	6,001	256,849
Hay	45,116	200,363	41,162	163,434	56,752	272,893
Hops (bearing) (dry)	854	1,165	821	1,563	809	1,752

Livestock at 31 March 1989: Sheep, 4·9m.; cattle, 560,400; pigs, 44,900.

Wool produced during 1988–89 was 22,315 tonnes, valued at $A154·7m. In 1989–90 butter production was 5,051 tonnes; cheese, 18,172 tonnes.

Forestry. Indigenous forests cover a considerable part of the State, and the saw-milling and woodchipping industries are very important. Production of sawn timber in 1989–90 was 337,100 cu. metres. 948,700 cu. metres of logs were used for milling in 1988–89 and a further 3,619,300 cu. metres were used for chipping, grinding or flaking. Newsprint and paper are produced from native hardwoods, principally eucalypts.

INDUSTRY AND TRADE

Industry. The most important manufactures for export are refined metals, newsprint and other paper manufactures, pigments, woollen goods, fruit pulp, confectionery, butter, cheese, preserved and dried vegetables, sawn timber, and processed fish products. The electrolytic-zinc works at Risdon near Hobart treat large quantities of local and imported ore, and produce zinc, sulphuric acid, superphosphate, sulphate of ammonia, cadmium and other by-products. At George Town, large-scale plants produce refined aluminium and manganese alloys. During 1989–90, 3,798,600 tonnes (green weight) of woodchips were produced. In 1986–87 the average employment in manufacturing establishments employing 4 or more persons was 24,327; wages and salaries (excluding proprietors' drawings), $A526m.; turnover, $A3,050m.; value added, $A1,236m.; and number operating at 30 June 1987, 633.

Labour. The Commonwealth Industrial Court (judicial powers) and Commonwealth Conciliation and Arbitration Commission (arbitral powers) have jurisdiction over federal unions, *i.e.*, with interstate membership. Most Tasmanian employees are covered by federal awards.

State Industrial Boards, established for the various trades by resolution of Parliament or proclamation of the Governor, cover most of the remaining employees. Each Board consists of a Chairman appointed by the Governor with equal representation of employers and employees. The Boards have authority over minimum rates for wages or piecework, number of working hours for which the wage is payable, conditions of apprenticeship, annual leave and adjustment of wage and piecework rates. Industrial Boards follow to a large extent the wage rates fixed by the Conciliation and Arbitration Commission.

Commerce. In 1988–89 exports totalled $A1,351,099,778 to overseas countries. The principal countries of destination (with values in $A1m.) for overseas exports were: Japan, 514·5; USA, 136·5; Malaysia, 96·1; Indonesia, 71·7; and Taiwan, 84·4. In 1988–89 imports totalled $A348,578,460 from overseas countries. The principal countries of origin (with values in $A1m.) for overseas imports were: Canada, 35; Japan, 53·9; USA, 51·2; New Zealand, 24·5; Taiwan 11·6; Federal Republic of Germany, 13·8; Singapore, 29·9; China, 3·2 and Malaysia, 0·68.

The main commodities by value (with values in $A1m.) exported to overseas countries during 1987–88 were: Non-ferrous metals (mainly copper, lead, tin and tungsten), 294; iron and steel, 40; metalliferous ores and metal scrap, 202; fish, crustaceans and molluscs, 72; and meat and meat preparations, 49. Other main exports, for which details are not available for separate publication were woodchips, newsprint, printing and writing papers, refined aluminium, ferro-alloys and chocolate confectionery. The main imports from overseas countries in 1987–88 (with values in $A1m.) were: Coffee, tea, cocoa and spices, 20; pulp and waste paper, 42; petroleum products, 14; road vehicles, 14; and chemicals and related products, 26.

Tourism. In 1988, 681,500 passengers arrived in Tasmania by sea and air from interstate and New Zealand of whom 406,000 or just over 59% were visitors.

COMMUNICATIONS

Roads. The total road length at 30 June 1987 was 22,715 km, consisting of a classified road system of 3,701 km maintained by the State Department of Main Roads, and the remainder maintained by local government authorities, the Forestry Commission and the Hydro-Electric Commission. Motor vehicles registered at 30 June 1988 comprised 209,400 cars and station wagons, 62,700 other vehicles and 6,000 motor cycles.

Railways. There is an 840-km network of 1,067-mm gauge lines linking Hobart and Launceston with coastal and country areas, part of Australian National Railways. A private railway of 130 km, operated by the Emu Bay Railway Co. Ltd, connects Burnie with the mining settlements on the west coast.

Aviation. Regular daily passenger and freight air services connect the south, north and north-west of the State with the mainland of Australia. In 1988 there was a total of 31,809 scheduled aircraft movements at Tasmanian airports; a total of 1·13m. passengers and 39,153 tonnes of freight, including mail, was carried.

Shipping. In 1987–88 there were, 1,736 ship visits to Tasmania with 11,066,913 mass tonnes of cargo carried through Tasmanian ports.

For posts and telegraphs, *see* p. 113.

JUSTICE, RELIGION, EDUCATION AND WELFARE

Justice. The Supreme Court of Tasmania, with civil, criminal, ecclesiastical, admiralty and matrimonial jurisdiction, established by Royal Charter on 13 Oct. 1823, is a superior court of record, with both original and appellate jurisdiction, and consists of a Chief Justice and 6 puisne judges. There are also inferior civil courts with limited jurisdiction, licensing courts, mining courts, courts of petty sessions and coroners' courts.

During the year 1989, 23,463 offences were finalized in the lower courts, 1,124 in the higher courts and 3,242 in the children's courts. The total police force at Oct. 1989 was 1,073. There was 1 gaol, with 854 imprisonments in 1987-88.

Religion. There is no State Church. At the census of 1986 the following numbers of adherents of the principal religions were recorded:

Anglican Church	154,748	Other religions	33,625
Roman Catholic	80,479	No religion	47,852
Methodist / Uniting Church	36,724	Not stated	61,742
Presbyterian	12,084	Total	435,346
Baptist	8,092		

Education. Education is controlled by the State and is free, secular and compulsory between the ages of 6 and 16. At 1 July 1989 government schools had a total enrolment of 64,977 pupils, including 27,432 at secondary level; private schools had a total enrolment of 18,394 pupils, including 8,417 at secondary level.

Technical and further education is conducted at technical and community colleges in the major centres throughout the state. In 1987 there were 20,523 students enrolled in the Division of Technical and Further Education, 21,982 students in the Division of Adult Education.

Tertiary education is offered at the University of Tasmania in Hobart, the Tasmanian State Institute of Technology and the Australian Maritime College, in Launceston. The University (established 1890) had (1989) 3,999 full-time and 1,619 part-time students, and 385 full-time teachers. There were 2,015 full-time and 715 part-time students enrolled in advanced education courses in 1988.

Social Welfare. Old Age, Invalid, War Service and Widows' Pensions are paid by the Commonwealth Government. The number of pensioners in Tasmania on 30 June 1989 was: Age (including wife and carer pensioners), 37,855; invalid, 9,038; war (service), 16,162; widows, 2,195. Benefit payments totalled $A637m. (including payments to wives).

Further Reading

Statistical Information: The State Government Statistical Office (Commonwealth Government Centre, Hobart), established in 1877, became in 1924 the Tasmanian Office of the Australian Bureau of Statistics, but continues to serve State statistical needs as required.

Deputy Commonwealth Statistician and Government Statistician of Tasmania: Stuart Jackson.

Main publications: *Annual Statistical Bulletins (e.g., Demography, Courts, Agricultural Industry, Finance, Manufacturing Establishments* etc.).—*Tasmanian Pocket Year Book.* Annual (from 1913).—*Tasmanian Year Book.* Annual (from 1967).—*Monthly Summary of Statistics* (from July 1945).

Tasmanian Development Authority, *Tasmanian Manufacturers Directory.* Hobart, 1985
Angus, M., *The World of Olegas Truchanas.* Hobart, 1975
Green, F. C. (ed.) *A Century of Responsible Government.* Hobart, 1956
Phillips, D., *Making more Adequate Provisions: State Education in Tasmania 1839–1985.* Hobart, 1985
Robson, L., *A History of Tasmania. Volume 1: Van Diemen's Land from the Earliest Times to 1855.* Melbourne, 1983
Townsley, W. A., *The Government of Tasmania.* Brisbane, 1976

State Library: The State Library of Tasmania, Hobart. *State Librarian:* D. W. Dunstan.

VICTORIA

AREA AND POPULATION. The State has an area of 227,600 sq. km, and a resident population (estimate) of 4,261,945 at 31 Dec. 1988.

The population is estimated within 13 'Statistical Local Areas' or 'Statistical Divisions' as follows (with 1988 population in 1,000): Melbourne (3,001); Barwon (218·7); South Western (102·8); Central Highlands (133·2); Wimmera (53·7); Northern Mallee (76·5); Loddon-Campaspe (171·4); Goulburn (147·7); North Eastern (87·1); East Gippsland (64·7); Central Gippsland (149); East Central (54·3).

The census count (exclusive of full-blood aboriginals prior to 1971) was:

Date of census enumeration	*Population*			*On previous census*	
	Males	*Females*	*Total*	*Numerical increase*	*Increase %*
5 April 1891	598,222	541,866	1,140,088	278,522	32·33
31 March 1901	603,720	597,350	1,201,070	60,982	5·35
3 April 1911	655,591	659,960	1,315,551	114,481	9·53
4 April 1921	754,724	776,556	1,531,280	215,729	16·40
30 June 1933	903,244	917,017	1,820,261	288,981	18·87
30 June 1947	1,013,867	1,040,834	2,054,701	234,440	12·88
30 June 1954	1,231,099	1,221,242	2,452,341	397,640	19·35
30 June 1961	1,474,395	1,455,718	2,930,113	477,772	19·48
30 June 1966	1,614,240	1,605,977	3,220,217	290,104	9·90
30 June 1971	1,750,061	1,752,290	3,502,351	282,134	8·76
30 June 1976	1,814,783	1,832,192	3,646,975	144,624	4·13
30 June 1981	1,901,411	1,931,032	3,832,443	185,468	5·09
30 June 1986	1,991,469	2,028,009	4,019,478	187,035	4·88

The count for the Melbourne Statistical Division (S.D.) on 30 June 1986 was 2,942,600. The count for the Geelong S.D. was 139,792; Ballarat S.D., 75,210; Bendigo S.D., 62,380; Shepparton-Mooroopna S.D., 37,086; and the Victorian component of Albury-Wodonga S.D., 35,183. Other urban centres: Warrnambool, 22,706; Traralgon, 19,233; Morwell, 16,387; Wangaratta, 16,598; Mildura, 18,382; Sale, 13,559; Horsham, 12,174; Colac, 9,532; Hamilton, 9,969; Bairnsdale, 10,328; Portland, 10,934; Swan Hill, 8,831; Ararat, 8,015; Benalla, 8,490; Maryborough, 7,705; Castlemaine, 6,603.

Vital statistics for calendar years:

	Births	*Marriages*	*Divorces*	*Deaths*
1986	60,152	29,390	9,670	30,175
1987	61,507	29,682	9,626	31,549
1988	62,134	30,687	10,250	30,726

The annual rates per 1,000 of the mean resident population (estimate) in 1988 were: Marriages, 7·2; births, 14·6; deaths, 7·2; divorces, 2·4.

CONSTITUTION AND GOVERNMENT. Victoria, formerly a portion of New South Wales, was, in 1851, proclaimed a separate colony, with a partially elective Legislative Council. In 1856 responsible government was conferred, the legislative power being vested in a parliament of two Houses, the Legislative Council and the Legislative Assembly. At present the Council consists of 44 members who are elected for 2 terms of the Assembly, one-half retiring at each election. The Assembly consists of 88 members, elected for 4 years from the date of its first meeting unless sooner dissolved by the Governor. Members and electors of both Houses must be aged 18 years and Australian citizens or those British subjects previously enrolled as electors, according to the Constitution Act 1975. No property qualification is required, but judges, members of the Commonwealth Parliament, undischarged bankrupts and persons convicted of an offence which is punishable by life imprisonment, may not be members of either House. Single voting (one elector one vote) and compulsory preferential voting apply to Council and Assembly elections. Enrolment for Council and Assembly electors is compulsory. The Council may not initiate or amend money bills, but may suggest amendments in such bills other than amendments which would increase any charge. A bill shall not become law unless passed by both Houses.

Private members of both Houses receive salaries of $A54,500 per annum.

Members holding the following offices receive an additional salary and in some cases an expense allowance. The President of the Council, $A36,510 salary and $A5,355 expense allowance; the Speaker of the Assembly, $A36,510 salary and $A5,355 expense allowance; the Chairman of Committees of the Council, $A15,578 salary and $A1,947 expense allowance; the Chairman of Committees of the Assembly, $A15,578 salary and $A1,947 expense allowance; the Leader of the Opposition in the Assembly, $A36,510 salary and $A8,762 expense allowance; the Deputy Leader of the Opposition in the Assembly, $A15,578 salary and $A2,921 expense allowance; the Leader of the Third Party, $A15,578 salary and $A2,921 expense allowance; a member of either House who is the Parliamentary Secretary of the Cabinet, $A15,578 salary and $A2,921 expense allowance; the Government Whip in the Assembly, $A8,762 salary; the Whip of any recognized Party which consists of at least 12 members of Parliament, of which Party no member is a responsible Minister, $A8,762 salary. Members receive electorate allowances, residential allowances and allowances for attending Parliament and Parliamentary Standing Committees.

The Legislative Assembly, elected on 1 Oct. 1988, is composed as follows: Labor Party, 46; Liberal Party, 33; National Party, 9.

Governor: Dr J. Davis McCaughey, AC.

In the exercise of the executive power the Governor is advised by a Cabinet of responsible Ministers. Section 50 of the Constitution Act 1975 provides that the number of Ministers shall not at any one time exceed 18, of whom not more than 6 may sit in the Legislative Council and not more than 13 may sit in the Legislative

Assembly. No Minister may hold office for more than 3 months unless he or she is or becomes a member of the Council or the Assembly.

Responsible Ministers receive the following amounts: The Premier, $A48,680 salary and $A20,446 expense allowance; the Deputy Premier, $A41,378 salary and $A10,223 expense allowance; 16 other Ministers, $A36,510 salary and $A8,762 expense allowance. The President, Speaker, Chairman of Committees in the Assembly and in the Council, Parliamentary Secretary of the Cabinet, Leader and Deputy Leader of the Opposition in the Assembly, Leader of the Opposition in the Council and Leader in the Assembly of the Third Party, also receive a travelling allowance when travelling on official business. The Premier, Deputy Premier, a Minister or office holder or Member, also receive a travelling allowance when travelling on official business.

The Cabinet was as follows in Feb. 1991:

Prime Minister, Minister for Ethnic Affairs, Minister for Women's Affairs: Joan Kirner.

Deputy Prime Minister, Attorney-General: Jim Kennan. *Minister for Conservation and the Environment, Minister for Tourism:* Steve Crabb. *Health:* C. Hogg. *Minister for Local Government, Minister for the Aged:* M. Lyster. *Minister for Planning and Urban Growth, Minister for the Arts:* A. McCutcheon. *Minister for Consumer Affairs, Minister for Prices, Minister for Aboriginal Affairs:* B. Mier. *Minister for Labour, Minister for Youth Affairs:* N. Pope. *Housing and Construction:* B. Pullen. *Treasurer:* Tom Roper. *Agriculture and Rural Affairs:* B. Rome. *Minister for Police and Emergency Services, Minister for Corrections:* M. Sandon. *Community Services:* K. Setches. *Transport:* P. Spyker. *Sport and Recreation:* N. Trezise. *Property and Services:* R. Walsh. *Industry and Economic Planning:* David White.

Agent-General in London: Ian Haig (Victoria House, Melbourne Place, Strand, London, WC28 4LG).

Local Government. With the exception of Yallourn Works area (26·9 sq. km) and the unincorporated areas—French Island (154 sq. km), Lady Julia Percy Island (1·3 sq. km), the Bass Strait Islands and part of Gippsland Lakes (312·8 sq. km) and Tower Hill Lake Reserve (5 sq. km), the State is divided (in Oct. 1988) into 210 municipal districts, namely 68 cities, 5 towns, 6 boroughs and 132 shires. The constitution of cities, towns, boroughs and shires is based on statutory requirements concerning population, rate revenue and net annual value of rateable property.

ECONOMY

Budget. State and local government outlays and receipts (excluding financial enterprises e.g. government savings banks, insurance offices, etc.) for 1987–88 (in $A1m.):

State: Current outlays, 11,637·6; capital outlays, 2,689·9. Revenue, 12,053·4. State expenditure included (with expenditure on new fixed assets): Education, 2,924·3 (226·6); health, 2,021·7 (161·1); general services, 700·4 (10·9); public order and safety, 605·1 (144·2). Revenue included: Property taxes, 1,361·5; payroll taxes, 1,230·8; taxes on financial transactions, 1,118·2; taxes on goods and services, 829·9. The 1990–91 budget increased taxes by $A580m., and cut expenditure by $A508m.

Local: Outlays, 1,947·3, including roads, 431; recreation and culture, 350·9; administration, 348·1; amenities, 247·2; welfare, 179. Revenue, 2,029·6, including rates, 956·2; other charges, 210·2; state government grants, 398·8.

Banking. The State Bank of Victoria, the largest bank in the State, provides a full range of domestic and international banking services for both business and personal customers and is the largest supplier of housing finance in Victoria. In 1990 it ran into debt and was acquired by the Commonwealth from the Victorian government in Sept. 1990.

There are 4 major trading banks in Victoria (Commonwealth Bank of Australia,

Australia and New Zealand Banking Group Ltd, Westpac Banking Corporation and National Australia Bank) with a total of 1,218 branches and 168 agencies between them at 30 June 1987, and 4 other trading banks. Private savings banks had 1,102 branches and 246 agencies at 30 June 1987. On 30 June 1986 there were 8·8m. operative accounts (excluding school bank accounts) in savings banks in Victoria. The total credit due to depositors at 30 June 1987 amounted to $A19,670m., made up of State Savings Bank, $A9,197·4m.; Commonwealth Savings Bank, $A2,862·1m.; private savings banks, $A7,610·6m.

The weekly average of deposits and advances of trading banks operating in Victoria during June 1987 were as follows: Deposits, not bearing interest, $A3,874m.; deposits, bearing interest, $A9,791m.; total deposits, $A13,665m.; loans, advances, and bills discounted, $A15,427m. The weekly average of debits to customers' accounts (excluding debits to Federal and State Government accounts at City branches in State capitals) for the same period totalled $A26,514m.

ENERGY AND NATURAL RESOURCES

Electricity. Electricity is supplied by the State Electricity Commission of Victoria either directly or through 11 metropolitan councils which buy in bulk and distribute electricity through their own systems.

Electricity production in 1988–89 was 36,139,000 kwh.

About 75% of the power generated for the state system is supplied by brown-coal fired generating stations, Yallourn, Morwell, Hazelwood and Loy Yang, located in the La Trobe Valley on one of the largest single brown coal deposits in the world 140 to 180 km east of Melbourne in Central Gippsland.

There are 2 other thermal stations and 3 hydro-electric stations in north east Victoria. Victoria is also entitled to approximately 30% of the output of the Snowy Mountains hydro-electric scheme and half the output of the Hume hydro-electric station, both of which are in New South Wales.

Oil and Natural Gas. Crude oil in commercially recoverable quantities was first discovered by the Esso/BHP partnership in 1967 in 2 large fields offshore in East Gippsland in Bass Strait between 65 and 80 km from land. These fields, Halibut and Kingfish, with 10 other fields since discovered—Marlin, Snapper, Barracouta, Mackerel, Tuna, Cobia, Flounder, Fortescue, Bream and Seahorse have been assessed as containing initial recoverable reserves of more than 2,930m. bbls of treated crude oil. Estimated reserves of crude oil (1987) 161m. cu. metres; of gas (1987), 159m. cu. metres.

In 1987-88 Gippsland Basin produced 84% of Australia's crude oil and 39% of its natural gas. Depletion of production from the 2 major fields, Kingfish and Halibut and the smaller Barracouta field, was expected to occur in the late-1980s. Production of crude oil (1988) 133,194,000 bbls.

Natural gas was discovered offshore in East Gippsland in 1965. The initial recoverable reserves of treated gas are 220,400m. cu. metres. Reserves are sufficient for at least 30 years. Following an extensive development and distribution programme, natural gas was first connected to homes and industry in Victoria in April 1969. All gas consumers in Melbourne, Geelong, Ballarat, Bendigo, Shepparton, Euroa, Benalla, Wangaratta, Wodonga, Albury and a number of towns near Melbourne, in the La Trobe Valley and in East Gippsland, are now using natural gas. At 30 June 1985 a total of 1,013,455 consumers were being supplied with it.

Natural gas and crude oil are conveyed from the producing fields to a large treatment plant at Longford in East Gippsland from where both hydrocarbons are distributed by a network of transmission lines to tank farms and city gate distribution points.

The crude oil is then distributed to refineries in Victoria by pipeline and to other States by seagoing tankers. Natural gas is distributed to residential and industrial consumers through a network of approximately 20,289 km of mains.

Liquefied petroleum gas is now being produced after extraction of the propane and butane fractions from the untreated oil and gas.

Brown Coal. Major deposits of brown coal are located in the Central Gippsland region and comprise approximately 94% of the total resources in Victoria. The resource is estimated to be 202,000 megatonnes, of which about 31,000 megatonnes are regarded as readily accessible reserves. It is young and soft with a water content of 60% to 70%. In the La Trobe Valley section of the region, the thick brown coal seams underlie an area from 10 to 30 km wide extending over approximately 70 kilometres from Yallourn in the west to the south of Sale in the east. It can be won continuously in large quantities and at low cost by specialized mechanical plant.

The primary use of these reserves is to fuel the major base load electricity generating stations located at Morwell and Yallourn. Production of brown coal in 1987-88 was 43,481,000 tonnes, value $A312,031,000.

Minerals. Production of certain metals and minerals, 1987–88: Gold, 1,634 kg, value $A32,868,000; kaolin, 45,000 tonnes, value $A6,625,000; gypsum, 196,000 tonnes, value $A1,306,000; bauxite, 7,345 tonnes, value $A198,000; clays, 1,720,000 tones, value $A5,708,000; limestone, 2,393,000 tonnes, value $A12,757,000.

Land Settlement. Of the total area of Victoria (22·76m. ha), 13,973,915 ha on 30 June 1984 were either alienated or in process of alienation. The remainder (8,786,085) constituted Crown land as follows: Perpetual leases, grazing and other leases and licences, 2,160,352; reservations including forest and timber reserves, water, catchment and drainage purposes, national parks, wildlife reserves, water frontages and other reserves, plus unoccupied and unreserved including areas set aside for roads, 6,625,733.

Agriculture. In 1987-88 the total area of land utilized for agricultural activity was 13,086,000 ha, and the gross value of agricultural commodities produced was $A4,607·7m. The following table shows the area under the principal crops and the produce of each for 3 seasons (in 1,000 units) [1]:

Season	*Total crop area*	*Wheat*		*Oats*		*Barley*		*Potatoes*		*Hay*	
	Ha	*Ha*	*Tonnes*	*Ha*	*Tonnes*	*Ha*	*Tonnes*	*Ha*	*Tonnes*	*Ha*	*Tonnes*
1985–86	2,510	1,488	2,225	204	290	378	464	14	365	390	1,524
1986–87	2,340	1,364	2,795	215	356	265	444	13	364	483	1,932
1987–88	2,001	1,026	1,882	216	325	366	529	14	398	379	1,458

[1] Excluding establishments with an estimated value of agricultural operations less than $A20,000.

In 1987–88 there were 18,763 ha of vineyards with 17,591 ha of bearing vines, yielding 78,407 tonnes of grapes for wine-making and 250,789 tonnes of grapes for drying or for table use. The area planted with fruit, nuts and berries was 20,194 ha; production of nuts was 1,762 tonnes. Production of tobacco was 5,102 tonnes (dry) and hops 695 tonnes (dried weight) from 382 ha. Fruit production, 1988, included pears, 138,814 tonnes; apples, 83,451 tonnes; oranges, 63,154 tonnes, and strawberries, 1,747,881 kg.

At March 1989 there were in the State 3,516,000 head of cattle, 28,071,000 sheep and 423,000 pigs. In 1987–88, mutton production was 73,000 tonnes; lamb, 126,000 tonnes. Wool produced in the season 1987–88 amounted to 160,251 tonnes. Milk production in 1988-89, 3,793m. litres; butter, 83,000 tonnes; cheese, 111,000 tonnes. Egg production, 1987-88, 50,566,000 dozen; honey, 1988, 3,824 tonnes.

INDUSTRY AND TRADE

Industry. At 30 June 1988 there were 9,858 manufacturing establishments employing 4 or more persons. Selected articles manufactured (1987–88, in tonnes): Beef and veal, 291,000; lamb, 111,000; butter, 83,282; cheese, 114,871; white flour, 259,702; cotton yarn, 9,604; wool yarn, 15,967; cotton cloth, 18,389,000 sq. metres; wool cloth, 2,924,000 sq. metres; 186,000 cars and station wagons; plastic and synthetic resins, 472,000; 439m. clay bricks; ready mixed concrete, 4,344,000 cu. metres.

Labour. In Aug. 1989 there were 2,049,800 employed persons (61% of the civilian population aged 15 years and over): Agriculture, forestry, fishing and hunting, 98,700; mining, 6,800; manufacturing, 402,900; electricity, gas and water, 31,900; construction, 158,100; wholesale and retail trade, 406,100; transport and storage, 102,100; communication, 41,600; finance, property and business services, 233,300; public administration and defence, 84,100; community services, 349,200; recreation, personal and other services, 135,100. There were 93,600 unemployed persons in Aug. 1989 (4·4% of the labour force).

Trade Unions. There were 166 trade unions with a total membership of 883,500 operating in Victoria in June 1988.

Commerce. The commerce of Victoria, exclusive of inter-state trade, is included in the statement of the commerce of Australia, *see* pp. 109–11.

The total value of the overseas imports and exports of Victoria, including bullion and specie but excluding inter-state trade, was as follows (in $A1m.):

	1983–84	*1984–85*	*1985–86*	*1986–87*	*1987–88*	*1988–89*
Imports	8,186	10,501	12,409	13,473	14,015	15,968
Exports [1]	4,708	6,452	6,806	7,398	9,051	8,519

[1] Includes re-exports.

The chief exports in 1988–89 (in $A1m.) were: Textile fibres and their wastes, 1,917; non-ferrous metals, 1,140; dairy products and birds' eggs, 481; petroleum, petroleum products and related materials, 474; hides, skins, and fur skins (raw), 209; power generating machinery and equipment, 181; road vehicles, 160. Exports in 1988–89 went mainly to Japan ($A1,791m.), USA ($A824m.) and New Zealand ($A619m.).

The chief imports in 1988–89 (in $A1m.) were: Road vehicles, 1,676; general industrial machinery, equipment and machine parts, 1,058; textile yarns, fabrics, made-up articles and related products, 1,013. Imports in 1988–89 came mainly from the USA ($A3,323m.); Japan ($A3,172m.) and the Federal Republic of Germany ($A1,325m.).

COMMUNICATIONS

Roads. In 1987–88 there were 160,398 km of roads open for general traffic, consisting of 7,537 km of state highways and freeways, 14,793 km of main roads, 1,848 km of tourist and forest roads and 136,220 km of other roads and streets. The number of registered motor vehicles (other than tractors) at 30 June 1989 was 2,585,200.

Railways. All the railways are the property of the State and are under the management of the Public Transport Corporation, responsible to the Victorian Government.

At 30 June 1989, 5,047 km of government railway were open. 9·9m. tonnes of freight and 5·8m. passengers (non-urban) were carried. Melbourne's suburban railways carried 94m. passengers.

Aviation. There were (1988) 70,047 domestic and 13,864 international aircraft movements at Essendon and Melbourne airports. Passengers totalled (1988) 6,033,785 on domestic flights and 1,525,368 on international flights. Freight handled (1988) 96,883 tonnes on domestic flights and 82,297 tonnes on international flights.

Post and Broadcasting. In 1988 there were 2,772,000 telephones. In 1988 there were 52 broadcasting stations and 19 television stations.

JUSTICE, RELIGION, EDUCATION AND WELFARE

Justice. There is a Supreme Court with a Chief Justice and 21 puisne judges. There are a county court, magistrates' courts, a court of licensing, and a bankruptcy court, etc.

Major crime in Victoria during 1987–88: 310,534 offences were reported to the police; 70,494 offences were cleared and 31,610 people were proceeded against.

At 30 June 1988 there were 13 prisons and 2,064 prisoners in custody.

Religion. There is no State Church in Victoria, and no State assistance has been given to religion since 1875. At the date of the 1986 census the following were the enumerated numbers of each of the principal religions: Catholic,[1] 1,104,044; Church of England, 715,414; Uniting, 280,262 (including Methodist); Orthodox, 177,565; Presbyterian, 138,000; Protestant (undefined), 87,557; other Christian, 90,756; Moslem, 37,965; Hebrew, 32,387; no religion, 557,939; no reply, 574,712; other groups, 222,877.

[1] So described on individual census schedules.

Education. Education establishments in Victoria consist of 4 universities, established under special Acts and opened in 1855, 1961, 1967 and 1977; Colleges of Advanced Education; government schools (primary, primary-secondary, high and secondary technical, and further education colleges), and non-government schools.

Total full-time teaching and research staff at the 4 universities in 1988, 3,540. The University of Melbourne, founded in 1853, had, in 1988, 16,733 students: Monash University, founded in 1958 in an eastern suburb of Melbourne, had, in 1988, 14,768 students; La Trobe University, founded in 1964 in a northern suburb of Melbourne, had 13,128 students in 1988; Deakin University (1974) near Melbourne had 7,209 students in 1988.

On 1 July 1988 there were 2,064 government schools with 532,217 pupils and 40,311 full-time teaching staff plus full-time equivalents of part-time teaching staff: 292,686 pupils were in primary schools, 234,615 in secondary schools and 4,196 attended special schools. In 1987 there were 232,467 students (excluding adult education programmes) enrolled in technical and further education schools and colleges, and (1988) 68,395 students enrolled in advanced education courses.

Non-government Schools. There were at 1 July 1988, 730 non-government schools, excluding commercial colleges, with 16,458 teaching staff (FTE) and 256,712 pupils enrolled. Of these schools, more than 66% were Roman Catholic.

Health. At 30 June 1987 there were 285 approved hospitals with 20,978 beds, of which 119 with 6,132 beds were private.

Social Services. Victoria was the first State of Australia to make a statutory provision for the payment of Age Pensions. The Act providing for the payment of such pensions came into operation on 18 Jan. 1901, and continued until 1 July 1909, when the Australian Invalid and Old Age Pension Act came into force. The Social Services Consolidation Act, which came into operation on 1 July 1947, repealed the various legislative enactments relating to age (previously old-age) and invalid pensions, maternity allowances, child endowment, and unemployment, and sickness benefits and while following in general the Acts repealed, considerably liberalized many of their provisions: it has since been amended. On 30 June 1988 there were 344,675 aged and 77,501 invalid pensioners, and the amount paid in pensions, including payments to wives and spouse carers of aged and invalid pensioners, during 1987–88 was $A2,343,434,000.

Under the Australian Unemployment and Sickness Benefit Act 1944, there were 101,193 unemployment, sickness, and special benefits granted during 1987-88 and the amount paid in benefits totalled $A708,333,000 during 1987-88. Unemployment benefits accounted for 80% of both benefits granted and benefits paid.

The number of widows' pensions in force at 30 June 1988 was 36,226, and the total amount paid in allowances during 1987-88 was $A255,417,000.

The number of family allowances in force in 1987-88 was 966,737. In addition, endowment was being paid in respect of 1,249 children who were being maintained in approved institutions. The total amount paid in family allowances and endowment in 1987-88 was $A345,688,000. In 1987-88, $A291,613,000 was paid in supporting parent's benefits to 36,045 beneficiaries, $A12·49m. in handicapped child's allowances for 7,989 children and $A43,715,000 in family income supplement to 29,754 families with 75,635 children.

Further Reading

Statistical Information: Australian Bureau of Statistics (The Rialto Building, 525 Collins Street, Melbourne, 3000). *Deputy Commonwealth Statistician:* Erle Bourke.

Victorian Year Book. (Annually since 1873)
Summary of Statistics, Victoria, 1991
Monthly Summary of Statistics, Victoria (from Jan. 1960)

Historical Records of Victoria. Victorian Government Printing Office, Melbourne (From 1981)
Victoria: The First Century. Official History of Victoria. Melbourne, 1934
Victorian Municipal Directory. Melbourne, (From 1866)
Broome, R., *The Victorians: Arriving.* New South Wales, 1984
Christie, M. F., *Aborigines in Colonial Victoria, 1835–86.* Sydney Univ. Press, 1979
Dingle, T., *The Victorians: Settling.* New South Wales, 1984
Dunstan, D., *Governing the Metropolis: Politics, Technology, and Social Change in a Victorian City: Melbourne 1850–1891.* Melbourne Univ. Press, 1984
Grant, J. and Serle, G., *The Melbourne Scene 1803–1956.* Melbourne Univ. Press, 1956
Pratt, A., *The Centenary History of Victoria.* Melbourne, 1934
Priestley, S., *The Victorians: Making Their Mark.* Melbourne, 1984

State Library: The State Library of Victoria, 328 Swanston St., Melbourne, 3000. *State Librarian:* W. Horton, BA, ALAA.

WESTERN AUSTRALIA

HISTORY. In 1791 Vancouver, in the *Discovery*, took formal possession of the country about King George Sound. In 1826 the Government of New South Wales sent 20 convicts and a detachment of soldiers to King George Sound and formed a settlement then called Frederickstown. In 1827 Captain (afterwards Sir) James Stirling surveyed the coast from King George Sound to the Swan River, and in May 1829 Captain (afterwards Sir) Charles Fremantle took possession of the territory. In June 1829 Captain Stirling, newly appointed Lieut.-Governor, founded the colony now known as the State of Western Australia. On 1 Jan. 1901 Western Australia became one of the 6 federated States within the Commonwealth of Australia.

AREA AND POPULATION. Western Australia lies between 113° 09' and 129° E. long. and 13° 44' and 35° 08' S. lat.; its area is 2,525,500 sq. km.

The population at each census from 1947 was as follows [1]:

	Males	*Females*	*Total*		*Males*	*Females*	*Total*
1947	258,076	244,404	502,480	1971	539,332	514,502	1,053,834
1954	330,358	309,413	639,771	1976	599,959	578,383	1,178,342
1961	375,452	361,177	736,629	1981	659,249	642,807	1,300,056
1966	432,569	415,531	848,100	1986	736,131	722,888	1,459,019

[1] 1961 and earlier exclude persons of predominantly Aboriginal descent; from 1966 figures refer to total population (*i.e.*, including Aborigines). Figures from 1971 are based on estimated resident population.

The population count at the 1986 census was 1,406,929 (707,569 males and 699,360 females). Of these 1,020,362 were born in Australia. Married persons numbered 617,382 (308,974 males and 308,408 females); widowers, 10,787; widows, 49,776; divorced, 23,505 males and 28,268 females; never married, 348,343 males and 294,771 females. The number of males under 21 was 247,826 and of females 235,620.

Perth, the capital, had an estimated resident population of 1,158,387 at June 1989. Of this, the area administered by the City of Perth had a population of 82,413 while the population in the area for which the City of Fremantle is responsible (which includes the chief port of the State) was 23,981.

Principal local government areas outside the metropolitan area, with population at 30 June 1989 (estimate): Bunbury, 26,398; Geraldton, 20,968; Mandurah, 23,107; Roebourne, 16,537; Port Hedland, 13,820; Albany, 14,958; Busselton, 13,422; Kalgoorlie-Boulder, 26,813.

Vital statistics for calendar years [1]:

	Births	Ex-nuptial births	Marriages	Divorces	Deaths
1987	23,332	4,623	10,150	4,044	8,880
1988	25,143	5,314	10,578	3,964	9,532
1989	24,693	5,377	10,739	4,089	9,543

[1] Figures are on State of usual residence basis.

CONSTITUTION AND GOVERNMENT. In 1870 partially representative government was instituted, and in 1890 the administration was vested in the Governor, a Legislative Council and a Legislative Assembly. The Legislative Council was, in the first instance, nominated by the Governor, but it was provided that in the event of the population of the colony reaching 60,000, it should be elective. In 1893 this limit of population being reached, the Colonial Parliament amended the Constitution accordingly.

The Legislative Council consists of 34 members, 2, representing each of the 17 electoral regions. Each member is elected for a term of 4 years.

There are 57 members of the Legislative Assembly, each member representing one of the 57 electoral districts of the State. Members are elected for the duration of the Parliament, normally 4 years. The qualifications applying to candidates and electors are identical for the Legislative Council and the Legislative Assembly. A candidate must have resided in Western Australia for a minimum of 12 months, be at least 18 years of age and free from legal incapacity, be an Australian citizen, and be enrolled, or qualified for enrolment, as an elector. A judge of the Supreme Court, the Sheriff of Western Australia, an undischarged bankrupt or a debtor against whose estate there is a subsisting order in bankruptcy may not be elected to Parliament. No person may hold office as a member of the Legislative Assembly and the Legislative Council at the same time. An elector must be at least 18 years of age, be an Australian citizen free from legal incapacity, must have resided in the Commonwealth of Australia for 6 and in Western Australia for 3 months continuously and in the electoral district for which he or she claims enrolment for a continuous period of 1 month immediately preceding the date of his or her claim. Enrolment is compulsory for all qualified persons except Aboriginal natives of Australia, who are entitled but not required to enrol. Voting at elections is on the preferential system and is compulsory for all enrolled persons.

Ordinary members of the legislature are paid a salary of $A64,150 a year with an additional electorate allowance, ranging from $A16,431 to $A29,819 a year according to location of the electorate. All members of Parliament also receive a basic postage and lettergram allowance of $A4,310 a year.

In addition to the basic Member's salary, electorate and postage allowances, the Premier receives a salary and expense of office allowances of $A80,376. On the same basis the Deputy Premier receives $A50,288; the Leader of the Government in the Legislative Council $A44,000; and other Ministers $A37,010.

The Legislative Assembly representation as at Aug 1990 was: Australian Labor Party, 31; Liberal Party, 19; National Party of Australia, 6; Independent, 1. The Legislative Council was 16 Australian Labor Party, 15 Liberal Party, 3 National Party of Australia.

Governor: His Excellency the Hon Sir Francis Burt, AC, KCMG, QC.

Lieut-Governor: The Honourable David Kingsley Malcolm.

The Australian Labor Party Cabinet was at August 1990:

Premier, Treasurer, Public Sector Management, The Family, Aboriginal Affairs, Multicultural and Ethnic Affairs, Women's Interests: Hon. Carmen Mary Lawrence, MLA.

Deputy Premier, Finance and Economic Development, Trade, Goldfields: Hon. Ian F. Taylor, MLA. *Attorney General, Resources, Corrective Services, Leader of the Government in the Legislative Council:* Hon. Joseph Max Berinson, MLC. *Planning, Lands, Heritage, The Arts, Deputy Leader of the Government in the Legislative Council:* Hon. Elsie Kay Hallahan, MLC. *Transport, Racing and Gaming, Tourism:* Hon. Pamela Anne Beggs, MLA. *Agriculture, Water Resources, North-West:* Hon.

Ernest Francis Bridge, MLA. *Mines, Fuel and Energy, Mid-West:* Hon. Jeffrey Phillip Carr, MLA. *Police, Emergency Services, The Aged:* Hon. Graham John Edwards, MLC. *Consumer Affairs, Housing:* Hon. Yvonne Daphne Henderson, MLA. *Local Government, Fisheries, Sport and Recreation, Youth, Minister assisting the Minister for Multicultural and Ethnic Affairs:* Hon. Gordon Leslie Hill, MLA. *Environment, Leader of the House in the Legislative Assembly:* Hon. Robert John Pearce, MLA. *Community Services, Justice, South-West:* Hon. David Lawrence Smith, MLA. *Productivity and Labour Relations, Minister assisting the Minister for Education with TAFE, Minister assisting the Minister for Public Sector Management:* Hon. Gavan John Troy, MLA. *Health:* Hon. Keith James Wilson, MLA. *Parliamentary Secretary of the Cabinet:* William Ian Thomas, MLA. *Works, Services, Regional Development, Minister assisting the Minister for Aboriginal Affiars:* Hon P.A. Buchanan, MLA.

Agent-General in London: D. Fischer (Western Australia House, 115 Strand, WC2R 0AJ).

Local Government. The only unincorporated area in mainland Western Australia is King's Park, a public reserve of about 403 ha. in Perth. Including the lord-mayoralty of Perth there were 19 cities, 10 towns and 99 shires at 30 June 1990. The executive body in each of these districts is normally an elective council, presided over by a mayor (city and town) or a president (shire), but in certain circumstances it may be a commissioner appointed by the Governor. Their functions include road construction and repair, the provision of parks and recreation grounds, the administration of building controls and local services such as health and library services. Finance is derived largely from rates levied on property owners as well as charges for services and government grants (mainly for road construction).

ECONOMY

Budget. Revenue and expenditure (in $A), as reported in the Consolidated Revenue Fund, in years ended 30 June:

	1988	*1989*	*1990*	*1991*[1]
Revenue	3,810,401,671	4,270,268,532	4,838,556,662	5,072,500,000
Expenditure	3,807,340,069	4,269,990,881	4,838,256,430	5,072,500,000

[1] Estimates.

Main items of revenue in 1989–90: Railways ($A275,101,375), taxation ($A1,300,918,315), lands, timber and mining ($A427,841,917), from Federal funds ($A1,962,993,167). Western Australia had a net public debt of $A1,538,099,306 on 30 June 1989, the charge for that year being $A194,305,932.

Banking. There are 20 trading banks in Western Australia including the Commonwealth Trading Bank and The Rural and Industries Bank of Western Australia. In Dec. 1988, the average of customers' balances was $A6,729m. and average advances $A6,798m.

At 31 Dec. 1988, the 8 savings banks held deposits of $A5,865m., in 2,666,229 accounts.

ENERGY AND NATURAL RESOURCES

Minerals. The mining industry has been for many years of considerable significance in the Western Australian economy. Until the mid-1960s the major mineral produced was gold. It was then replaced by iron ore in terms of value, and has at various times fallen behind nickel concentrates, bauxite, oil, mineral sands and salt. In the latter half of the 1980s it enjoyed a resurgence and in 1987-88 exceeded iron ore in value terms.

The total ex-mine value of minerals from mining and quarrying in the State in 1987–88 was $A5,935·5m. Principal minerals produced in 1987–88 were: Iron ore, 98·0m. tonnes, value $A1,669·8m.; bauxite, 21·0m. tonnes; gold bullion, 106·8m. grammes, value $A1,839·5m.; nickel concentrates, 389,000 tonnes; tin concentrates,

434 tonnes; black coal, 3·7m. tonnes; crude oil, 3,100m.; natural gas, 3,887,000m. kilolitres; salt, 5·5m. tonnes, value $A107·2m.; diamonds, 30·2m. carats, value $A248·2m.; mineral sands concentrates valued at $A196·9m. (1986–87).

Agriculture.

	1987–88		*1988–89*	
	Area	*Production*	*Area*	*Production*
Crop	*1,000 ha*	*1,000 tonnes*	*1,000 ha*	*1,000 tonnes*
Wheat	3,312	3,882	3,297	5,225
Oats	373	502	389	618
Barley	461	617	383	552
Hay	243	778	248	873
Potatoes	2	72	2	78
Cauliflower	1	14	1	18

	1987–88		*1988–89*	
	No. Trees	*Production*	*No. Trees*	*Production*
Crop	*(1,000)*	*Tonnes*	*(1,000)*	*Tonnes*
Apples	702	40,196	667	46,695
Pears	132	6,604	143	6,974
Oranges	179	5,217	198	5,087

Irrigation has been established by the Government along the south-western coastal plain and in the north of the State. Reservoirs with an aggregate capacity of 6,207m. cu. metres provided irrigation water for 20,402 ha in 6 districts during 1985–86.

Livestock at 31 March 1989 included 1,702,000 cattle, 37,090,000 sheep and 285,000 pigs.

The wool clip in 1988–89 was 203,173 tonnes.

Forestry. The area of State forests and timber reserves at 30 June 1989 was 1,892,266 ha; 1988–89 production of sawn timber was 335,191 cu. metres, principally Jarrah and Karri hardwoods.

Fisheries. The catch of fish, crustaceans and molluscs in Western Australia in 1988–89 totalled 35,392 tonnes for a gross value of $A242·4m. Of this, rock lobsters, with a total catch of 11,776 tonnes accounted for $A177·9m.

Value of Agricultural Commodities Produced. The estimated gross values of Western Australian agricultural commodities during 1988–89 were: Crops and pastures, $A1,799·7m.; livestock slaughterings and other disposals, $A424·9m.; livestock products, $A1,495·0m.

INDUSTRY AND TRADE

Industry. Heavy industry in Western Australia is concentrated in the South-West of the state, and is largely tied to export-orientated mineral processing, especially alumina and nickel. Other significant manufacturing industries include meat and seafood processing, production of timber and wood products, metal fabrication and production of industrial and mining machinery. The North West Shelf development has stimulated recent growth in industries involved in providing materials and equipment during the construction phase, as well as in new and existing industries using gas in processing.

The following table shows manufacturing industry statistics for 1988–89 [1]:

Industry sub-division	*Number of establishments operating at 30 June*	*Persons employed [2] 1,000*	*Wages and salaries $Am.*	*Turnover $Am.*
Food, beverages and tobacco	364	12·1	274	2,217
Textiles	41	1·3	23	117
Clothing and footwear	69	1·8	30	80
Wood, wood products and furniture	451	9·0	182	847
Paper, paper products, printing and publishing	255	7·9	161	684
Chemical, petroleum and coal products	75	3·2	94	826

Industry sub-division	Number of establishments operating at 30 June	Persons employed [2] 1,000	Wages and salaries $Am.	Turnover $Am.
Non-metallic mineral products	144	5·1	130	804
Basic metal products	43	5·7	193	2,194
Fabricated metal products	466	9·9	230	1,138
Transport equipment	179	5·0	116	402
Other machinery and equipment	378	8·5	206	835
Miscellaneous manufacturing	186	3·2	70	434
Total	2,651	72·7	1,710	10,579

[1] Excludes single establishment enterprises with less than 4 persons employed.
[2] At 30 June. Includes working proprietors.

Labour. A Court of Arbitration was established in Western Australia in 1901 under the provisions of the 'Industrial Conciliation and Arbitration Act 1900'. The Court of Arbitration was replaced, with effect from 1 Feb. 1964, by the Western Australian Industrial Appeal Court and The Western Australian Industrial Commission, authorities constituted in terms of the *Industrial Arbitration Act 1912*. These authorities continue to operate under the provisions of the *Industrial Relations Act 1979* which was proclaimed on 1 March 1980.

The Western Australian Industrial Appeal Court consists of 3 Judges, one of whom is the Presiding Judge. The members are nominated by the Chief Justice of Western Australia. An appeal lies to the Court from decisions of the President of the Western Australian Industrial Commission, the Full Bench or the Commission in Court Session but only on the ground that the decision is erroneous in law or is in excess of jurisdiction.

The Western Australian Industrial Commission consists of a President, a Chief Industrial Commissioner, a Senior Commissioner, and 'such number of other Commissioners as may, from time to time, be necessary'. There were 8 'other Commissioners' at Oct. 1989. A person shall not be appointed as President unless he is qualified to be a Judge, and on appointment he is entitled to the status of a Puisne Judge. The President or a Commissioner sitting or acting alone constitutes the Commission and may exercise the appropriate powers of the Commission.

The Commission can inquire into any industrial matter and make an award, order or declaration relating to such matter. 'Industrial matter' means any matter affecting or relating to the work, privileges, rights, or duties of employers or employees in any industry and includes any matter relating to the wages, salaries, allowances, or other remuneration of employees or the prices to be paid in respect of their employment; the hours of employment, sex, age, qualification or status of employees and the mode, terms and conditions of employment including conditions which are to take effect after the termination of employment. The Commission may also make inquiries where industrial action has occurred or is likely to occur.

The Commission in Court Session is constituted by not less than 3 Commissioners sitting or acting together, and may make General Orders, hear matters referred by the Commission, and hear appeals from decisions of Boards of Reference.

The Full Bench is constituted by not less than 3 members of the Commission, 1 of whom is the President, and may hear matters referred by the Commission on questions of law, and appeals from decisions of the Commission and Industrial Magistrates.

The following table shows details of the number of industrial awards, unions and members registered with The Western Australian Industrial Commission.

At 30 June	1985	1987	1988	1989	1990
Awards in force	608	592	610	628	610
Employee organizations:					
Number	72	69	70	69	72
Membership	176,769	189,770	186,608	187,206	174,312
Employer organizations:					
Number	15	15	15	16	15
Membership	3,561	2,690	2,825	2,817	2,180

Commerce. The external commerce of Western Australia, exclusive of interstate trade, is comprised in the statement of the commerce of Australia, *see* pp. 109–11.

The total value of imports and exports, including interstate trade, but excluding interstate value of horses, in 5 years (30 June) is, in $A1m., as follows:

	1984–85	*1985–86*	*1986–87*	*1987–88*	*1988–89*
Imports	6,446·5	6,984·9	7,878·2	8,621·5	10,012·5
Exports [1]	7,535·8	8,149·6	8,721·4	9,300·3	10,633·7

[1] Including ships' stores.

Selected overseas exports (in $A million) for 1989–90: Iron ore and concentrates, 2,246; wheat, 1,001; wool, 769; petroleum and petroleum products, 601; gold bullion, 325; live sheep and lambs, 62; beef and veal, 103; salt, 120; mutton and lamb, 57; barley, 64; prawns, 29; hides and skins (including fur skins), 39; whole rock lobsters, 109; fruit and nuts (fresh or dried), 10; oats, 18.

Selected overseas imports (in $A million) for 1989–90: Petroleum and petroleum products, 672; machinery, 942; transport equipment, 704; iron and steel, 94; chemicals, 277; food, 99; crude fertilizer, 35; rubber manufactures, 103.

The chief countries exporting to Western Australia in 1989–90 were (in $A million): Japan, 798; USA, 639; United Arab Emirates, 370; UK, 259; Federal Republic of Germany, 219; Canada, 173; Singapore, 145.

Western Australia's exports in 1989–90 (in $A million) went chiefly to: Japan, 2,695; USA, 1,684; China, 495; Republic of Korea, 494; Singapore, 454 Indonesia, 345; Taiwan, 271.

Tourism. In 1986–87, 216,000 international visitors contributed $A237m. to the economy; 444,200 interstate tourists contributed $274m.; 4,617,000 intrastate tourists contributed $A932m.

COMMUNICATIONS

Roads. At 30 June 1988 there were 122,380 km of prepared and formed roads in Western Australia comprising 41,585 km of bituminous surface, 40,635 km other constructed surfaces and 40,159 km formed but not metalled or otherwise prepared. In addition, there are 19,539 km of roads unprepared except for clearing which are used for general traffic.

New motor vehicles registered in Western Australia during the year ended 30 June 1990 were 59,338.

Railways. At 30 June 1989 the State had 5,553 km of State government railway and 731 km of Federal line, the latter being the western portion of the Trans-Australian line (Kalgoorlie–Port Pirie), which links the State railway system to those of the other States of the Commonwealth. At 30 June 1989, mining companies operated 1,198 km of private railways for the transport of ore to ports on the north-west coast. In 1988–89 state railways carried 24·5m. tonnes and 0·5m. passengers. Perth suburban lines (63 km), controlled by a separate authority, carried 9·4m. passengers.

Aviation. An extensive system of regular air services operates in Western Australia for the transport of passengers, freight and mail. During the year ended 31 Dec. 1988, Perth Airport handled 22,062 aircraft movements and 2,185,227 passengers on domestic and international services.

Shipping. In 1988–89, the number of overseas direct vessels through the major ports was: Port of Fremantle, 1,123 entered, 1,122 cleared; Port Hedland, 367 entered, 357 cleared; other ports, 1,183 entered, 1,210 cleared. The gross weight (in tonnes) of overseas cargo through those ports was: Port of Fremantle, 29,902,254 discharged, 29,303,629 loaded; Port Hedland, 38,260,602 discharged, 36,020,485 loaded; other ports, 86,438 313 discharged, 87,438,808 loaded.

Post and Broadcasting. Postal, telephone and telegraph facilities are afforded at 397 offices. Telephone services connected totalled 676,800 at 30 June 1989.

There were 96 radio broadcasting and 96 television stations, including translator stations, in operation at 30 June 1988.

JUSTICE, RELIGION, EDUCATION AND WELFARE

Justice. In Western Australia justice is administered by a Supreme Court, consisting of a Chief Justice, 11 puisne judges and 3 masters; a District Court comprising a chief judge and 14 other judges; a Magistrates Court, a Chief Stipendiary Magistrate, 36 Stipendiary Magistrates and Justices of the Peace, as at 30 June 1990. All courts exercise both civil and criminal jurisdiction except Justices of the Peace who deal with summary criminal matters only. Juvenile offenders are dealt with by the Children's Court. Overall responsibility for the Children's Court is vested in a President, who has the status of a District Court Judge. A children's court may be constituted by a judge, a magistrate or 2 lay members. Each has different sentencing powers. For certain offences involving first offenders under the age of 16 years who have pleaded guilty, such cases may be dealt with by the Children's (suspended Proceedings) Panel which comprises a representative from the Department for Community Services and one from the Police Department. The Family Court also forms part of the justice system and comprises a Chief Judge, 4 other judges, 7 magistrates/registrars and exercises both State and Federal jurisdictions.

Offences against law	*1984–85*	*1985–86*	*1986–87*	*1987–88*
Charges	115,739 [1]	...	211,966	...
Lower Court convictions [2]	105,025 [1]	...	190,372	...
Higher Court convictions	3,369	4,142	3,912	5,239

[1] Excludes Perth and East Perth Lower Courts.

[2] Includes convictions for traffic offences: 43,851 in 1984–85; 87,140 in 1986–87. In addition, small fines were imposed for minor traffic offences as follows: 1984, 373,662; 1985, 416,774; 1986, 401,415; 1987, 533,012; 1988, 525,581; 1989, 516,362.

Persons in prison at 30 June 1989 numbered 1,494 males and 92 females.

Religion. There is no State Church, and freedom of worship is accorded to all. At the census, 30 June 1986, the principal denominations were: Anglican, 371,302; Catholic, 347,695; Uniting, 82,876; Presbyterian, 31,641; Baptist, 16,869; Orthodox, 16,722; other Christian, 110,922; Buddhist, 7,178; all other, including not stated and no religion, 421,724.

Education. School attendance is compulsory from the age of 6 until the end of the year in which the child attains 15 years. A non-compulsory year of education is available to children from the beginning of the year in which they reach 5 years of age, at pre-primary centres attached to most government primary schools or at community-based and privately owned pre-school centres, and at some non-government schools. Children may be enrolled during their fourth year where vacancies exist. In 1990 there were 761 government primary and secondary schools providing free education to 217,441 students and 249 non-government primary and secondary schools providing education, for which fees are charged, to 69,547 students.

Technical and Further Education (TAFE) is offered by the Department of TAFE, a sub-department of the Ministry of Education, and by three independent regional colleges. The latter also provide higher education facilities. Additionally, higher education is available through a multi-campus college of advanced education and three universities.

Tertiary education:

	Teaching Staff [1]	*Students Enrolled*
University of Western Australia [2]	703	10,423
Murdoch University [3]	276	6,014
Curtin University of Technology [3]	799	15,615
Western Australian College of Advanced Education [2]	683	14,108

[1] Full-time staff and part-time staff on the basis of equivalent full-time staff.
[2] March 1989. [3] April 1989.

State Government expenditure from consolidated revenue on education during the year ended 30 June 1990, amounted to $A1,064,679,000.

Social Welfare. At 30 June 1989 there were 89 acute public hospitals, 20 acute private hospitals, 5 public nursing homes, 100 private nursing homes and 7 permanent/extended care units attached to public hospitals.

The Health Department of Western Australia Psychiatric Services comprised 4 approved psychiatric hospitals, 7 outpatient clinics for adults, 1 rehabilitation unit, 5 psychiatric extended care units, 2 other residential units, 1 halfway-house, 2 specialist units, 2 full-time country clinics, 4 sessional country clinics, 4 occupational day clinics and 1 rehabilitation hostel. Specifically for children are: 3 outpatient clinics and 4 in-patient clinics. The Authority for the Intellectually Handicapped comprised 20 hostels and 27 group homes.

The Department for Community Services is responsible for the provision of welfare and community services throughout the State. There were 10 directorates in the Department on 30 June 1990. Six were regionally based, 3 in the Perth metropolitan area and 3 were in the country. These are concerned with direct service delivery, which is provided through 22 divisional and 33 district offices. The remaining 4 directorates provide central support and administrative functions.

Direct services provided to the community include emergency financial assistance, family and substitute care, and counselling and psychological services. The Department supervises children's Day Care Centres. There is a 24-hour emergency welfare service provided through the Crisis Care Unit. Specialist units work in the areas of child abuse, adoptions, youth activities and Family Court counselling.

The Department provides residential facilities for the temporary accommodation, care and training of children, is responsible for young offenders recommended for detention or remand by a Court and also supervises young offenders subject to non-custodial court orders.

Age, invalid, widows', disability and service pensions, and unemployment benefits are paid by the Federal Government. The number of pensioners in Western Australia at 30 June 1989 was: Age, 104,816; invalid, 29,706; widows, 6,901; disability, 30,761; service, 36,246; and sole parents, 23,357. There were 31,697 recipients of unemployment benefits at 30 June 1989.

During 1989–90 the department provided emergency assistance in 69,250 cases. This assistance, valued at $A4,690,000, was in the form of cash, vouchers to purchase goods and services, and payment on behalf of individuals.

Further Reading

Statistical Information: The State Government Statistician's Office was established in 1897 and now functions as the Western Australian Office of the Australian Bureau of Statistics (Merlin Centre, 30 Terrace Road, Perth). *Deputy Commonwealth Statistician and Government Statistician:* B. N. Pink. Its principal publications are: *Western Australian Year Book* (new series, from 1957). *Western Australia: Facts and Figures* (from 1989). *Monthly Summary of Statistics* (from 1958)

Battye, J. S., *Western Australia: A History from its Discovery to the Inauguration of the Commonwealth.* Oxford, 1924.—*The Cyclopedia of Western Australia.* Adelaide, Vol. 1 (1912), Vol. 2 (1913)
Crowley, F. K., *Australia's Western Third: A History of Western Australia from the First Settlements to Modern Times.* (Rev. ed.). Melbourne, 1970
Kimberly, W. B., *History of Western Australia: A Narrative of Her Past.* Melbourne, 1897
Stannage, C. T. (ed.) *A New History of Western Australia.* Perth, 1980
Stephenson, G. and Hepburn, J. A., *Plan for the Metropolitan Region: Perth and Fremantle.* Perth, 1955

State Library: Alexander Library Building, Perth. *State Librarian:* Lynn Allen, BA (Hon.), MA, PhD, ALAA, AIMM.

AUSTRIA

Republik Österreich

Capital: Vienna
Population: 7·6m. (1989)
GNP per capita: US$16,462 (1989)

HISTORY. Following the break-up of the Austro–Hungarian Empire, the Republic of Austria was proclaimed on 12 Nov. 1918. On 12 March 1938 Austria was forcibly absorbed in the German Reich as *Ostmark* until it was liberated by the Allied armies in 1945. On 27 April 1945 a provisional government was set up and was recognized by the Allies on 20 Oct. 1945. Austria recovered its full independence by the Austrian State Treaty, (signed on 15 May 1955).

AREA AND POPULATION. Austria is a land-locked country bounded north by the Federal Republic of Germany and Czechoslovakia, east by Hungary, south by Yugoslavia and Italy, and west by Switzerland and Liechtenstein. It has an area of 83,857 sq. km (32,377 sq. miles) and its population at recent censuses has been as follows:

1923	6,534,481	1951	6,933,905	1971	7,456,403
1934	6,760,233	1961	7,073,807	1981	7,555,338

Estimate (1989) 7,623,600. In 1981, 65% were urban and 96% were German-speaking, with linguistic minorities of Slovenes (19,000), Croats (26,000), Hungarians (16,000) and Czechs (7,000). The areas, populations and capitals of the 9 federal states are as follows:

Federal States	*Area sq. km*	*Population (1989)*	*State capitals*
Vienna (Wien)	415	1,487,600	Vienna
Lower Austria (Niederösterreich)	19,174	1,430,200	St Pölten
Burgenland	3,965	267,200	Eisenstadt
Upper Austria (Oberösterreich)	11,980	1,366,600	Linz
Salzburg	7,154	468,400	Salzburg
Styria (Steiermark)	16,387	1,180,400	Graz
Carinthia (Kärnten)	9,533	542,300	Klagenfurt
Tirol	12,647	619,600	Innsbruck
Vorarlberg	2,601	321,400	Bregenz

Vital statistics for calendar years:

	Live births	*Still births*	*Deaths* [1]	*Marriages*	*Divorces*
1986	86,964	385	87,071	45,821	14,679
1987	86,503	289	84,907	76,205	14,639
1988	88,052	325	83,263	35,361	14,924
1989	88,759	347	83,407	42,523	15,489

[1] Excluding still births.

The populations of the principal towns (excluding Vienna), according to the census of 12 May 1981 (area, 1 Jan. 1989) were as follows:

Graz	243,166	Steyr	38,942	Feldkirch	23,745	Mödling	19,276
Linz	199,910	Dornbirn	38,641	Baden	23,140	Lustenau	17,401
Salzburg	139,426	Wiener Neustadt	35,006	Krems a.d.D.	23,056	Braunau am Inn	16,318
Innsbruck	117,287	Leoben	31,989	Klosterneuburg	22,975	Ternitz	16,104
Klagenfurt	87,321	Wolfsberg	28,097	Amstetten	21,989	Hallein	15,377
Villach	52,692	Kapfenberg	25,716	Traun	21,464	Bruck an der Mur	15,068
Wels	51,060	Bregenz	24,561	Leonding	19,389		
St Pölten	50,419						

CLIMATE. Climate ranges from cool temperate to mountain type according to situation. Winters are cold, with considerable snowfall, but summers are very warm. The wettest months are May to August.

Vienna, Jan. 28°F (–2°C), July 67°F (19·5°C). Annual rainfall 25·6" (640 mm). Graz, Jan. 28°F (–2°C), July 67°F (19·5°C). Annual rainfall 34" (849 mm). Innsbruck, Jan. 27°F (–2·7°C), July 66°F (18·8°C). Annual rainfall 34·7" (868 mm). Salzburg, Jan. 28°F (–2·0°C), July 65°F (18·3°C). Annual rainfall 50·6" (1,266 mm).

CONSTITUTION AND GOVERNMENT. Austria recovered its sovereignty and independence on 27 July 1955 by the coming into force of the Austrian State Treaty between the UK, the USA, the USSR and France on the one part and the Republic of Austria on the other part (signed on 15 May).

The Constitution of 1 Oct. 1920 was restored on 27 April 1945. Austria is a democratic federal republic comprising 9 states *(Länder)*, with a federal President *(Bundespräsident)* directly elected for not more than 2 successive 6-year terms, and a bicameral National Assembly which comprises a National Council and a Federal Council.

The National Council *(Nationalrat)* comprises 183 members directly elected for a 4-year term by proportional representation on a national basis. At the General Elections of 7 Oct. 1990 the electorate was 6·4m. and turn-out was 86·14%. The Socialist Party (SPÖ) won 80 seats (with 42·8% of the vote), the People's Party (ÖVP), 60 seats (32·06%), the Freedom Party (FPÖ), 33 seats (16·63%) and the Greens (VGÖ), 10 seats (4·78%). The Federal Council *(Bundesrat)* 63 members appointed by the 9 states for the duration of the individual State Assemblies' terms; in 1987 the ÖVP held 33 seats and the SPÖ 30 seats.

The head of government is a Federal Chancellor, who is appointed by the President from the party winning the most seats in National Council elections. The Chancellor nominates a Vice-Chancellor and other Ministers for the President to appoint to a Council of Ministers which the Chancellor leads.

Federal President: Dr Kurt Waldheim (elected 8 June 1986; took office 8 July).

The coalition government was formed on 17 Dec. 1990 by the SPÖ and ÖVP and was composed as follows:

Chancellor: Dr Franz Vranitzky. (SPÖ)

Vice Chancellor and Federalism and Administrative Reform: Dr Josef Riegler (ÖVP). *Foreign Affairs:* Dr Alois Mock (ÖVP). *Economic Affairs:* Dr Wolfgang Schüssel (ÖVP). *Employment and Social Affairs:* Josef Hesoun [1] (SPÖ). *Finance:* Ferdinand Lacina. *Health and Sport:* Harald Ettl (SPÖ). *Interior:* Dr Franz Löschnak (SPÖ). *Justice:* Nikolaus Michalek [1] (Ind). *National Defence:* Werner Fasslabend [1] (ÖVP). *Agriculture and Forestry:* Dr Franz Fischler (ÖVP). *Environment, Youth and Family:* Dr Marilies Flemming. *Education:* Rudolf Scholten [1] (SPÖ). *Public Economy and Transport:* Dr Rudolf Streicher (SPÖ). *Science and Research:* Dr Erhard Busek (ÖVP). *Women's Affairs:* Johanna Dohnal [1] (SPÖ). *Secretaries of State:* Peter Jankowitsch [1] (SPÖ; *Europe and Integration*); Peter Kostelka [1] (SPÖ; *Civil Service*); Günter Stummvoll (ÖVP; *Finance*); Maria Fekter [1] (ÖVP; *Construction and Tourism*).

The *Speaker* is Heinz Fischer.

[1] Holds office for the first time.

The Federal Council *(Bundesrat)* which represents the federal provinces has 63 members and (1987) the Socialist Party had 30 members and the People's Party 33. The *Nationalrat* and *Bundesrat* together form the National Assembly.

National flag: Three horizontal stripes of red, white, red.

National anthem: Land der Berge, Land am Strome (words by Paula Preradovic; tune by W. A. Mozart).

The official language is German.

Local Government. The Republic of Austria comprises 9 Federal States (Vienna, Lower Austria, Upper Austria, Salzburg, Styria, Carinthia, Tirol, Vorarlberg, Burgenland). There is in every province an elected Provincial Assembly.

Every community has a Council, which chooses one of its number to be head of the Community (burgomaster) and a committee for the administration and execution of its resolutions.

DEFENCE. Conscription is for a 6-month period, with liability for 60 days reservist refresher training spread over 15 years.

Army. The Army consists of an alert force *(Bereitschaftstruppe)*, mainly the 1st Armoured Division organized in 3 armoured infantry brigades; 1 air-missile and mountain battalion; field units with 3 artillery, 2 anti-aircraft, 1 anti-tank and 2 engineering battalions; and territorial troops, comprising 26 regiments and security companies. Strength was (1991) 38,000 (20,000 conscripts).

Army Aviation. *(Heeresfliegerkräfte):* The Division comprises 10 squadrons with about 4,500 personnel and about 200 aircraft, organized in three Aviation Regiments each of which including air defence battalions. PC-7 Turbo-trainers are also in service. Some 24 Draken interceptors equip 2 squadrons of a surveillance wing responsible for defence of Austrian airspace and a fighter-bomber wing of two squadrons. Helicopters equip six squadrons for transport/support, communications, observation, search and rescue duties. Types in service include 24 Alouette III, 12 armed Kiowa, JetRanger, 36 Agusta-Bell AB.204, AB.206 and AB.212s. Fixed-wing transports comprise two Skyvans and 12 Turbo-Porters.

INTERNATIONAL RELATIONS. Following the peace treaty signed with France, the USSR, the UK and the USA in May 1955, the National Assembly adopted a statute of permanent neutrality in Oct.

Membership. Austria is a member of UN, OECD and EFTA. With Czechoslovakia, Hungary, Italy and Yugoslavia, Austria was an inaugural member of the Pentagonale meeting on economic and political co-operation in July 1990.

ECONOMY

Budget. The budget for calendar years provided revenue and expenditure (ordinary and extraordinary) as follows (in 1m. schilling):

	1984	*1985*	*1986*	*1987*	*1988*	*1989* [1]	*1990* [2]
Revenue	344,901	372,895	391,675	409,556	451,393	477,597	486,081
Expenditure	435,135	464,673	498,390	514,461	517,824	540,303	549,038

[1] Preliminary. [2] Estimates.

External debt. The budgetary external debt was (1989) 132,300m. schilling.

Currency. The unit of currency is the *schilling* (ATS) of 100 *groschen*. The rate of exchange in March 1991, £1 = 20·48 *schilling*, US$1 = 10·79 *schilling*.

Banking and Finance. The National Bank of Austria, opened on 2 Jan. 1923, was taken over by the German Reichsbank on 17 March 1938. It was re-established on 3 July 1945. Its *President* is Maria Schaumayer. At 31 Dec. 1989 foreign exchange amounted to 94,296m. and note circulation to 112,761m. schilling.

Principal banks with total assets (in 1m. schilling 1989): Creditanstalt-Bankverein, 429,474; Girozentrale und Bank der Österreichischen Sparkassen (the central financial institution for savings banks), 301,773; Österreichische National Bank, 238,371; Österreichische Länderbank, 220,559; Zentralsparkasse und Kommerzialbank, 235,776; Österreichische Kontrollbank, 204,940; Bank für Arbeit und Wirtschaft, 188,550; Raiffeisen Zentralbank Österreich, 176,966; Österreichische Postsparkasse, 180,368; Die Erste Österreichische Spar-Casse-Bank, 146,642; Österreichische Volksbanken, 62,081; Österreichische Investitionskredit AG, 46,274; Bank für Oberösterreich und Salzburg, 50,582; Österreichisches Credit Institut, 39,846; Raiffeisenbank für Wien und Nö, 38,301. The state has a 51% stake in Creditanstalt-Landverein and Österreichische Länderbank.

There is a stock exchange in Vienna.

Weights and Measures. The metric system of weights and measures has been in force since 1872.

ENERGY AND NATURAL RESOURCES

Electricity. In 1990 there were 8 nationalised electricity supply companies. Electric energy produced (1m. kwh.): 1989, 50,167; 1988, 49,014; 1987, 50,518; 1986, 44,653; 1985, 44,534. Supply 220 volts; 50 Hz.

Oil. The commercial production of petroleum began in the early 1930s. Production of crude oil (in tonnes): 1960, 2,448,391; 1971, 2,798,237; 1985, 1,146,958; 1986, 1,115,924; 1987, 1,060,367; 1988, 1,175,186; 1989, 1,323,431.

Gas. Production of natural gas (in 1,000 cu. metres): 1987, 1,167,340; 1988, 1,264,564.

Minerals. The mineral production (in tonnes) was as follows:

	1988	*1989*		*1988*	*1989*
Lignite	2,129,258	2,065,815	Pig-iron	3,664,805	3,822,549
Iron ore	2,300,000	2,410,000	Raw steel	4,560,072	4,717,596
Lead and zinc ore [1]	372,393	274,748	Rolled steel	3,751,956	3,731,810
Raw magnesite [1]	1,121,585	1,204,942	Gypsum	721,745	000,000

[1] Including recovery from slag.

Austria is one of the world's largest sources of high-grade graphite. Production, which averaged 20,000 tonnes yearly from 1929 to 1944, dropped to 246 in 1946, but rose to 102,237 in 1964, and fell again to 23,992 in 1970, 37,199 in 1980, 24,451 in 1982, 40,418 in 1983, 43,789 in 1984, 30,764 in 1985, 36,167 in 1986, 39,391 in 1987, 7,577 in 1988, and 15,307 in 1989.

Agriculture. In 1989 the total area cultivated amounted to 3,548,239 ha.

The chief products (area in hectares, yield in tonnes) were as follows:

	1987		*1988*		*1989*	
	Area	*Yield*	*Area*	*Yield*	*Area*	*Yield*
Wheat	320,366	1,450,731	291,938	1,559,993	278,068	1,362,951
Rye	85,415	309,327	87,889	355,888	91,019	381,188
Barley	291,496	1,178,686	292,384	1,366,424	291,876	1,421,645
Oats	69,373	245,728	69,145	273,067	67,150	249,063
Potatoes	34,128	879,497	33,115	1,001,044	32,395	845,466

Production of raw sugar in 1949, 66,700; 1955, 219,300; 1960, 308,000; refined sugar: 1970, 298,000; 1980, 419,800; 1982, 563,472; 1983, 354,479; 1984, 426,544; 1985, 430,730; 1986, 282,576; 1987, 358,951; 1988, 327,270; 1989, 422,877 tonnes.

Livestock (1989): Cattle, 2,562,393; pigs, 3,372,724; sheep, 288,928; goats, 36,440; horses, 47,923; poultry, 14,145,110.

Forestry. Forested area in 1988, 3·2m. ha (46% of the land area) of which 75% coniferous. Felled timber, in cu. metres: 1960, 10,015,925; 1970, 11,122,896; 1980, 12,732,507; 1987, 11,759,643; 1988, 12,032,399; 1989, 13,822.

INDUSTRY. On 26 July 1946 the Austrian parliament passed a government bill, nationalizing some 70 industrial concerns. As from 17 Sept. 1946 ownership of the 3 largest commercial banks, most oil-producing and refining companies and the principal firms in the following industries devolved upon the Austrian state: River navigation; coal extraction; non-ferrous mining and refining; iron-ore mining; pig-iron and steel production; manufacture of iron and steel products, including structural material, machinery, railroad equipment and repairs, and shipbuilding; electrical machinery and appliances. Six companies supplying electric power were nationalized in accordance with a law of 26 March 1947.

In 1989, 9,393 industrial establishments (including 2,021 sawmills) employed 550,907 persons, producing a value of 720,997m. schillings (excluding value added tax).

Labour. In June 1990 there were 2·93m. employed persons; the unemployment rate was 4·3%. There were 67,722 job vacancies.

The number of foreigners who may be employed in Austria is limited to 10% of the potential workforce.

FOREIGN ECONOMIC RELATIONS

Commerce. Imports and exports are as follows (excluding coined gold):

	Imports			Exports		
	1987	*1988*	*1989*	*1987*	*1988*	*1989*
Quantity (1,000 tonnes)	39,680	40,974	41,829	18,718	20,038	20,980
Value (1m. sch.)	411,859	451,442	514,680	342,433	383,213	429,310

The total trade between Austria and UK (British Department of Trade returns, in £1,000 sterling):

	1986	*1987*	*1988*	*1989*	*1990*
Imports to UK	705,732	781,986	824,616	933,971	957,789
Exports and re-exports from UK	403,000	463,187	509,991	598,099	705,850

Tourism. Tourism is an important industry. In 1989, 19,992 hotels and boarding-houses had a total of 656,936 beds available; 18,201,763 foreigners visited Austria; of these 863,554 came from the UK and 676,035 from the USA. Revenue was 123,200m. schillings.

COMMUNICATIONS

Roads. On 31 Dec. 1989 federal roads had a total length of 10,320 km, 1,405 km autobahn; provincial roads, 22,914 km. On 31 Dec. 1989 there were registered 4,185,692 motor vehicles, including 2,902,949 passenger cars, 246,823 lorries, 386,876 tractors and 326,227 trailers.

Railways. Austrian railways have been nationalized since before the First World War. Length of route in 1990, 5,641 km, of which 3,238 km were electrified. Nineteen private railways have a total length of 566 km. Passengers in 1989 numbered 163m., and 58·6m. tonnes of freight were carried.

Aviation. Austrian Airlines is being privatized. In April 1990 the state's stake was reduced to 51·9%. Austria has 6 airports in Vienna (Schwechat), Linz, Salzburg, Graz, Klagenfurt and Innsbruck. In 1989, 116,923 commercial aircraft and 6,629,262 passengers arrived and departed at Austrian airports; 59,342 tonnes of freight, 14,091 tonnes of transit freight and 6,744 tonnes of mail were handled.

Shipping. Austria has no sea frontiers, but the Danube is an important waterway. Goods traffic (in tonnes): 7,619,115 in 1985; 7,708,311 in 1986; 8,027,360 in 1987; 8,832,907 in 1988; 9,145,423 in 1989. Ore and metal, coal and coke and iron ore comprise in bulk more than two-thirds of these cargoes. The Danube Steamship Co. (DDSG) is the main Austrian shipping company.

Post and Broadcasting. All postal, telegraph and telephone services are run by the State. In 1989 there were 3,102,814 telephones.

The 'Österreichische Rundfunk' transmits 2 national and 9 regional programmes. In the local area of Vienna there is an additional special service in English and French; there is also a 24 hour foreign service (short wave). All broadcasting is financed by licence payments and advertisements. There were 2·7m. registered listeners in Dec. 1989. Television was inaugurated in summer 1955 and 2 programmes are transmitted, both in colour, with 2·5m. licences in Dec. 1989.

Cinemas (1988). There were 413 cinemas.

Newspapers (1989). There were 29 daily newspapers (7 of them in Vienna) and a circulation of 2·8m. of all Austrian daily newspapers.

JUSTICE, RELIGION, EDUCATION AND WELFARE

Justice. The Supreme Court of Justice *(Oberster Gerichtshof)* in Vienna is the highest court in the land. Besides there are 4 higher provincial courts *(Oberlandesgerichte)*, 21 provincial and district courts *(Landes- und Kreisgerichte)* and 206 local courts *(Bezirksgerichte)* (1989).

Religion. In 1981 there were 6,372,645 Roman Catholics (84·3%), 423,162 Protestants (5·6%), 118,866 others (1·6%), 452,039 without religious allegiance (6%) and 79,017 (1%) unknown. The Roman Catholic Church has 2 archbishoprics and 7 bishoprics. There were (1988) 60,000 Moslems in Austria.

Education (1989–90). There were in Austria 5,087 elementary and special schools with 68,442 teachers and 646,961 pupils. Of all kinds of secondary schools there were 1,505 with 485,483 pupils.

There were also 114 commercial academies with 36,570 students and 4,666 teachers. There were 275 schools of technical and industrial training (including schools of hotel management and catering) with 6,604 teachers and 66,850 pupils; 55 higher schools of women's professions (secondary level) with 14,343 pupils; 9 training colleges of social workers with 807 pupils. 120 trade schools had 13,228 pupils.

Austria has 12 universities and 6 colleges of arts maintained by the State: Universities at Vienna (3,231 teachers, 64,628 students), Graz (1,206 teachers, 23,098 students), Innsbruck (1,528 teachers, 20,259 students) and Salzburg (523 teachers, 10,036 students). There are also technical universities at Vienna (1,288 teachers, 18,323 students) and Graz (645 teachers, 9,741 students), a mining university at Leoben (151 teachers, 1,914 students), an agricultural university at Vienna (357 teachers, 5,774 students), a veterinary university at Vienna (172 teachers, 2,517 students), a commercial university at Vienna (297 teachers, 19,115 students), a university for social and economic sciences at Linz (404 teachers, 9,825 students) and a university for educational science at Klagenfurt (156 teachers, 3,078 students). There is an academy of fine arts at Vienna (159 teachers, 514 students), a college of applied arts at Vienna (265 teachers, 1,011 students), 3 colleges of music and dramatic art at Vienna (590 teachers, 2,120 students), 'Mozarteum' Salzburg (352 teachers, 1,358 students) and Graz (325 teachers, 1,205 students); the college for industrial design at Linz (124 teachers, 451 students).

Health and Welfare. In 1989 there were 24,895 doctors, 332 hospitals and 81,619 hospital beds. Maternity leave is for 2 years, and applies to mothers or fathers.

DIPLOMATIC REPRESENTATIVES

Of Austria in Great Britain (18 Belgrave Mews West, London, SW1X 8HU)
Ambassador: Dr Walter F. Magrutsch (accredited 11 Feb. 1988).

Of Great Britain in Austria (Jaurèsgasse 12, 1030 Vienna)
Ambassador: Brian Lee Crowe, CMG (accredited 2 June 1989).

Of Austria in the USA (2343 Massachusetts Ave., NW, Washington, D.C., 20008)
Ambassador: Dr Friedrich Hoess (accredited 21 Dec. 1988).

Of the USA in Austria (Boltzmanngasse, 16, A-1091 Vienna)
Ambassador: Roy M. Huffington.

Of Austria to the United Nations
Ambassador: Dr Peter Hohenfellner (accredited 24 Feb. 1988).

Further Reading

Statistical Information: The Austrian Central Statistical Office was founded in 1829. *Address:* Hintere Zollamtsstrasze 2b, 1033 Vienna. *President:* Mag. Erich Bader.

Main publications:

Statistisches Handbuch für die Republik Österreich. New Series from 1950. Annually
Statistische Nachrichten. Monthly
Beiträge zur österreichischen Statistik (970 vols.)
Statistik in Österreich 1918–1938. [Bibliography] Vienna, 1985
Veröffentlichtungen des Österr. Statist. Zentralamtes 1945-1985. [Bibliography] Vienna, 1986

Bobek, H. (ed.) *Atlas de Republik Österreich.* 3 vols. Vienna, 1961 ff.
Fitzmaurice, J., *Austrian Politics and Society Today: in Defence of Austria.* London, 1990
Salt, D., *Austria.* [Bibliography] Oxford and Santa Barbara, 1986
Sotriffer, K., *Greater Austria: 100 Years of Intellectual and Social Life from 1800 to the Present Time.* Vienna, 1982
Sully, M. A., *A Contemporary History of Austria.* London, 1990

National Library: Österreichische Nationalbibliothek, Vienna. *Director General:* Dr Magda Strebl.

BAHAMAS

Capital: Nassau
Population: 256,000 (1990)
GNP per capita: US$10,570 (1988)

Commonwealth of the Bahamas

HISTORY. The Bahamas were discovered by Columbus in 1492 but the Spanish did not make a permanent settlement. British settlers arrived in the 17th century and it was occupied by Britain, except for a short period in the 18th century, until it gained independence. Internal self-government with cabinet responsibility was introduced on 7 Jan. 1964 and full independence achieved on 10 July 1973.

AREA AND POPULATION. The Commonwealth of The Bahamas consists of 700 islands and more than 1,000 cays off the south-east coast of Florida. They are the surface protuberances of two oceanic banks, the Little Bahama Bank and the Great Bahama Bank. Land area, 5,353 sq. miles (13,864 sq. km).

The areas and populations of the major islands are as follows:

	Sq. km	*1980*		*Sq. km*	*1980*
Grand Bahama	1,373	33,102	San Salvador	163	825
Abaco	1,681	7,271	Rum Cay	78	
Bimini Islands	23	1,411	Long Island	448	3,404
Berry Islands	31	509	Ragged Island	23	164
New Providence	207	135,437	Crooked Island	238	518
Andros	5,957	8,307	Long Cay	23	33
Eleuthera	518	8,331	Acklins Island	389	618
Cat Island	388	2,215	Mayaguana	110	464
Exuma Islands	290	3,670	Inagua Islands	1,671	924

The capital is Nassau on New Providence Island (135,437 inhabitants in 1980) and the only other large town is Freeport (24,423) on Grand Bahama. About 13% of the population were (1980) of British extraction, the rest being of African and mixed descent.

Vital statistics, 1987: Births, 4,018; deaths, 1,212 (excluding still-births); marriages, 1,830.

CLIMATE. Winters are mild and summers pleasantly warm. Most rain falls in May, June, Sept. and Oct., and thunderstorms are frequent in summer. Rainfall amounts vary over the islands from 30" (750 mm) to 60" (1,500 mm). Nassau. Jan. 71°F (21·7°C), July 81°F (27·2°C). Annual rainfall 47" (1,179 mm).

CONSTITUTION AND GOVERNMENT. The Commonwealth of The Bahamas is a free and democratic sovereign state. Executive power rests with Her Majesty the Queen, who appoints a Governor-General to represent her, advised by a Cabinet whom he appoints. There is a bicameral legislature. The Senate comprises 16 members all appointed by the Governor-General, 9 on the advice of the Prime Minister, 4 on the advice of the Leader of the Opposition, and 3 after consultation with both of them. The House of Assembly consists of 49 members elected from single-member constituencies for a maximum term of 5 years. At the general election of 19 June 1987, the Progressive Liberal Party obtained 31 seats, the Free National Movement 16 seats and 2 independents.

Independence from Britain took place on 10 July 1973.

Governor-General: Sir Henry Taylor.

The Cabinet in Feb. 1991 was composed as follows:

Prime Minister, Tourism: Rt. Hon. Sir Lynden O. Pindling, KCMG.

Deputy Prime Minister, Foreign Affairs and Public Personnel: Sir Clement T. Maynard. *Finance:* Paul L. Adderley. *National Security:* Darrell E. Rolle. *Employ-*

ment and Immigration: Alfred T. Maycock. *Works and Lands:* Phillip M. Bethel. *Ministry of Youth, Sports and Community Affairs:* Norman N. Cay. *Minister of Housing and National Insurance:* George W. Mackey. *Health:* Charles Carter. *Education:* Bernard J. Nottage. *Transport:* Peter J. Bethell. *Attorney-General:* Sean McWeeny. *Agriculture, Trade and Industry:* Perry Christie. *Local Government:* Marvin Pinder. *Consumer Affairs:* Vincent Peet.

National flag: Three horizontal stripes of aquamarine, gold, aquamarine, with a black triangle on the hoist.

DEFENCE. The Royal Bahamian Defence Force is a maritime force tasked with naval patrols and protection duties in the extensive waters of the archipelago. Equipment comprises a sea-going fleet of 3 108-foot patrol craft, 13 smaller patrol craft and high speed craft for shallow water duty. There are 3 Jetstream Commander light reconnaissance aircraft. Personnel in 1990 numbered 750, and the base is at Coral Harbour on New Providence Island.

INTERNATIONAL RELATIONS

Membership. The Commonwealth of The Bahamas is a member of UN, OAS, the Commonwealth, CARICOM and an ACP state of the EEC.

ECONOMY

Budget (in B$):

	1987	*1988*	*1989*
Revenue	468,849,335	515,807,454	555,279,397
Expenditure	478,199,453	511,921,218	564,214,210

The main sources of revenue were customs duties and receipts from fees, post office and public utilities.

Currency. The unit of currency is the *Bahamian dollar* (BSD) of 100 *cents.* Notes: B$0.50, 1, 3, 5, 10, 20, 50, 100; coins: 1, 5, 10, 15, 25, 50 cents, $1, 2, 5. American currency is generally accepted. In March 1991, £1 = B$1.90; US$1 = B$1.00.

Banking. The Central Bank of The Bahamas was established in June 1974. Its Governor is James Smith. At June 1989, it had assets of B$244·36m. and capital and reserves of B$55·76m. On 30 June 1989 there were 382 institutions licensed to carry on banking and/or trust business under the Bank and Trust Companies Regulations Act. There were 19 designated institutions by the Exchange Control Department as authorized dealers and agents. Among these were the Royal Bank of Canada, the Bank of Nova Scotia, the Bank of Bahamas, Chase Manhattan Bank, Barclays Bank, the Canadian Imperial Bank of Commerce and Citibank. While the majority of banks are located in Nassau, there are branches on several of the other islands. The Bahamas Development Bank was established in 1974 and began operations in Jan. 1978. At June 1989 it had total assets of B$20·3m. and paid-up capital of B$7·25m.

The Post Office Savings Bank, 31 Dec. 1984, had deposits of B$2·7m.

Weights and Measures. The UK (Imperial) system is in force.

ENERGY AND NATURAL RESOURCES

Electricity. Electricity is provided primarily by The Bahamas Electricity Corporation in conjunction with a few private franchises in the Family Islands. As at 31 Dec. 1987, total generated capacity was 306·1 mw; total units generated, 8,570 mwh and total number of consumers, 67,525. Supply 115 volts; 60 Hz.

Agriculture. In 1988 agricultural production was B$28·83m. (1973, B$17·5m.). Chicken and poultry production was estimated at 15·2m. lb in 1988, (16·9m. lb in 1987). Egg production (1988) declined to 3·6m. dozen. Production of sheep, goats and pigs in 1988: 129 sheep, 165 goats and 2,236 pigs were slaughtered. Beef production increased, with 27 beef cattle slaughtered.

Total agricultural production including fisheries was valued at B$62·1m. in 1988, with fisheries accounting for B$33·3m. Production, 1988 (in 1,000 tonnes): Sugar-cane, 240; vegetables, 27; fruit, 14.

The quantity of meat derived from livestock in 1988 was: Mutton, 4,441 lb; goat meat, 6,559 lb; beef, 13,000 lb; pork, 158,770 lb.

Livestock (1988): Cattle, 5,000; sheep, 40,000; goats, 19,000; pigs, 20,000; poultry, 1m.

Fisheries. Studies were undertaken in 1986 to assess the viability of a stone crab industry. Aquaculture of red fish and marine shrimp have proved to be important.

INDUSTRY. Two industrial sites, one in New Providence and the other in Grand Bahama, have been developed as part of the industrialization programme. Industries include garment manufacturing, ice, furniture, purified water, plastic containers, perfumes, industrial gases, jewellery and others. Larger industrial activities in The Bahamas include manufacture of alcoholic beverages, pharmaceuticals, aragonite mining and solar salt production.

Trade Unions. In 1986 there were 36 unions, the largest is The Bahamas Hotel Catering and Allied Workers' Union (5,000 members) and The Bahamas Public Services Union (over 4,000 members).

FOREIGN ECONOMIC RELATIONS

Commerce. The principal exports in 1985 were hormones, rum, salt, crawfish, cement and aragonite.

The principal imports in 1985 were: Food, drink and tobacco, raw materials and articles mainly unmanufactured and articles wholly or mainly manufactured. Exports of spiny lobster and snappers in 1988 were B$26,954,490. (B$24·6m. in 1987). Imports of fish in 1987 were B$4,971,284. (B$4·5m. in 1986).

Imports and exports (excluding bullion and specie) for 7 calendar years in B$:

	Imports	*Exports*		*Imports*	*Exports*
1980	5,506,577	4,836,366	1984	4,224,175	3,539,428
1981	4,203,000	3,515,000	1985	3,081,116	3,033,142
1982	3,051,000	2,444,000	1986	3,323,437	2,702,162
1983	4,616,251	3,970,319			

Total trade in £1,000 sterling, between Bahamas and UK (British Department of Trade returns):

	1986	*1987*	*1988*	*1989*	*1990*
Imports to UK	10,266	15,943	24,781	17,681	15,053
Exports and re-exports from UK	95,816	27,063	20,708	22,543	22,917

Tourism. Tourism is the most important industry. In 1988 there were just under 3m. foreign arrivals.

COMMUNICATIONS

Roads. There are 245 miles of paved roads in New Providence, and approximately 885 miles in Grand Bahama and the Family Islands. In 1987, 74,062 motor vehicles were registered. There are no railroads.

Aviation. There are international airports at Nassau and Freeport (Grand Bahama Island). Scheduled flights are operated by Air Canada (Montreal and Toronto to Nassau); Bahamasair (Nassau to Miami, Newark, Orlando and Tampa); Delta Airlines (Nassau to Dallas, Fort Lauderdale, Atlanta, Boston and New York); Eastern Airlines (Nassau to Miami, Freeport to Miami); British Airways (London to Nassau); Midway Airlines (Nassau to Fort Lauderdale and Chicago); Pan-Am (Nassau to New York and Freeport to Miami); Aero Coach (Freeport to Fort Lauderdale and West Palm Beach); Carnival Airlines (Nassau to Miami and Fort Lauderdale). There are 58 airstrips on the various Family Islands. During 1986, 1,343,324 passengers landed at Nassau from 61,431 aircraft arrivals. At Freeport in 1986, 618,555 passengers landed from 33,157 aircraft arrivals.

Shipping. In 1987, 2,279 cruise liners cleared Nassau carrying 1,540,000 passengers. In 1984, 542 cargo vessels discharged 757,737 tons of cargo at Nassau. There are indirect cargo services with UK and Canada *via* the USA and passenger services with the USA only.

Telecommunications. In 1985 there were 127 post offices. New Providence and most of the other major islands have modern automatic telephone systems in operation, interconnected by an extensive multi-channel radio network, while local distribution within the islands is by overhead and underground cables. The total number of telephones in use at 31 Dec. 1987 was approximately 119,061. International telecommunications service is provided by a submarine cable system to Florida, USA, and an INTELSAT Standard 'A' Earth Station. International operator assisted and direct dialling telephone services are available to all major countries. There is an automatic Telex system and a packet switching system for data transmission, and land mobile and marine telephone services. The Bahamas Broadcasting Corporation operates radio broadcasting stations on AM and FM in New Providence and Grand Bahama and a TV station in New Providence. In 1986 there were 40,000 television and 120,000 radio receivers.

Cinemas (1990). There is 1 cinema.

Newspapers (1988). There are 2 daily and 1 weekly newspapers in Nassau.

JUSTICE, RELIGION, EDUCATION AND WELFARE

Justice (1986). 32,878 cases (traffic, 11,334; criminal, 17,970; civil, 2,178; domestic, 1,396) were dealt with in the magistrates' court, and civil, 1,561; divorce, 516; criminal, 200 in the Supreme Court. The strength of the police force (1988) was 1,665 officers and other ranks.

Religion. Over 94% of the population is Christian, with 26% being Roman Catholic, 21% Anglican and 48% other Protestants.

Education. Education is under the jurisdiction of the Ministry of Education and Culture. In 1986–87 there were 230 schools, and of these, 190 are fully maintained by Government and 39 are independent schools. Total school enrolment, 60,189. There are 38 government-owned schools in New Providence and 151 on the Family Islands. 26 independent schools are located on New Providence and 14 on the Family Islands. 280 students attended 5 special schools, 3 on New Providence and 2 on Grand Bahama; total staff, 49. Free education is available in ministry schools in New Providence and the Family Islands. Courses lead to the Bahamas Junior Certificate and the General Certificate of Education (GCE). Independent schools provide education at primary, secondary and higher levels.

The College of The Bahamas, officially opened in 1975, is the only publicly-funded tertiary level institution. It offers a wide range of programmes leading to the associate degree, advanced level GCE (London), college diplomas and certificates. Degree programmes in education are offered in conjunction with the University of the West Indies and the University of Miami. Total enrolment (1987) 5,866 with a staff of 128.

The Hotel Training College offers a wide range of subjects up to middle management level in aspects of hotel work. Enrolment in this institution includes Bahamian as well as regional and international students. Several schools of continuing education offer secretarial and academic courses. The Government-operated Princess Margaret Hospital offers a nursing course at two levels.

Health. In 1988 there was a government general hospital (454 beds) and a psychiatric/geriatric care centre (457 beds) in Nassau, and a hospital in Freeport (74 beds). The Family Islands, comprising 20 health districts, had 13 health centres, 38 main clinics and 52 satellite clinics. There was 1 private hospital (24 beds) in Nassau.

DIPLOMATIC REPRESENTATIVES

Of The Bahamas in Great Britain (10 Chesterfield St., London, W1X 8AH)
High Commissioner: Dr Patricia Rodgers.

Of Great Britain in The Bahamas (Bitco Bldg., East St., Nassau)
High Commissioner: Colin Mays, CMG.

Of The Bahamas in the USA (600 New Hampshire Ave., NW, Washington, D.C., 20037)
Ambassador: Margaret MacDonald, CVO, CBE.

Of the USA in The Bahamas (Mosmar Bldg., Queen St., Nassau)
Ambassador: Chic Hecht.

Of The Bahamas to the United Nations
Ambassador: James B. Moultrie.

Further Reading

Bahamas Handbook and Businessman's Annual (Annual)
Albury, P., *The Story of the Bahamas*. London, 1975.—*Paradise Island Story*. London, 1984
Barrett, P. J. H., *Grand Bahama*. London, 1982
Boultbee, P. G., *Bahamas*. [Bibliography] Oxford and Santa Barbara, 1989
Craton, M. A., *A History of the Bahamas*. London, 1962
Hughes, C. A., *Race and Politics in the Bahamas*. Univ. of Queensland Press, 1981
Hunte, G., *The Bahamas*. London, 1975
Stevenson, C. St. J., *The Bahamas Reference Annual*. Annual

Library: Nassau Public Library.

BAHRAIN

Capital: Manama
Population: 486,000 (1990)
GNP per capita: US$6,610 (1987)

Dawlat al Bahrayn

(State of Bahrain)

HISTORY. Treaties with Britain of 1882 and 1892 were replaced by a treaty of friendship which was signed on 15 Aug. 1971. Under the earlier treaties Britain had been responsible for Bahrain's defence and foreign relations. On the same day the State of Bahrain declared its independence.

AREA AND POPULATION. The State of Bahrain forms an archipelago of about 33 small islands in the Arabian Gulf, between the Qatar peninsula and the mainland of Saudi Arabia. The total area is about 265·5 sq. miles (687·75 sq. km). Bahrain ('Two Seas'), is 30 miles long and 10 miles wide (578 sq. km). It is connected by a causeway nearly 1·5 miles long, carrying a motor road, with the second largest island, Muharraq, 4 miles long and 1 mile wide, to the north-east, and by a causeway with Sitra, an island 3 miles long and 1 mile wide, to the east. In Nov. 1986 a causeway linking Bahrain with Saudi Arabia was officially opened. Other islands are Umm Al-Nassan, 3 miles by 2 miles, and Jidda, 1 mile by 0·5 mile, both to the west; Nabih Saleh, to the east; the Hawar group of 16 small islands off Qatar, to the south-east, and several islets, some uninhabited. From Sitra oil pipelines and a causeway carrying a road extend out to sea for 3 miles to a deep-water anchorage. The islands are low-lying, the highest ground being a hill in the centre of Bahrain, 450 ft. (122·4 metres) high.

The population in 1981 (census) was 350,798. Estimate (1990) 486,000, including some 155,000 resident foreigners. The majority of the people are Moslem arabs.

Arabic is the official language. English is widely used in business.

Manama, the capital of the state and the commercial centre, is situated at the northern end of the largest island and extends for 1·5 miles along the shore. It has a population 1988, of 151,500 (1981 census, 108,684). Other towns are Muharraq, 1988, 78,000 (46,061); Jidhafs, 48,000 (7,232); Rifa'a, 28,150 (22,408); Isa Town (21,275) and Hidd (7,111).

CLIMATE. The climate is pleasantly warm between Dec. and March but from June to Sept. the conditions are very hot and humid. The period June to Nov. is virtually rainless. Bahrain. Jan. 66°F (19°C), July 97°F (36°C). Annual rainfall 5·2" (130 mm).

CONSTITUTION AND GOVERNMENT. A Constitution was ratified in June 1973 providing for a National Assembly of 30 members, popularly elected for a 4-year term, together with all members of the Cabinet (appointed by the Amir). Elections took place in Dec. 1973, but in Aug. 1975 the Amir dissolved the Assembly and has since ruled through the Cabinet alone.

Reigning Amir: The ruling family is the Al Khalifa, an Arab dynasty, who have been in power since 1782. The present Amir, HH Shaikh Isa bin Sulman Al-Khalifa (born 1933) succeeded on 2 Nov. 1961. *Crown Prince:* Shaikh Hamad bin Isa Al-Khalifa.

In 1990 the cabinet was composed as follows:

Prime Minister: Shaikh Khalifa bin Sulman Al-Khalifa.

Defence: Shaikh Khalifa bin Ahmed Al-Khalifa. *Transport:* Ibrahim Mohammed Hassan Homaidan. *Housing:* Shaikh Khalid bin Abdulla Al-Khalifa. *Information:*

Tariq Abdulrahman Almoayed. *Education:* Dr Ali Fakhro. *Health:* Jawad Salim Al-Arrayed. *Justice and Islamic Affairs:* Shaikh Abdullah bin Khalid Al-Khalifa. *Labour and Social Affairs:* Shaikh Khalifa bin Sulman bin Mohammed Al-Khalifa. *Works, Power and Water:* Majid Jawad Al Jishi. *Interior:* Shaikh Mohammed bin Khalifa Al-Khalifa. *Foreign Affairs:* Shaikh Mohammed bin Mubarak Al-Khalifa. *Finance and National Economy:* Ibrahim Abdul-Karim. *Development and Industry:* Yousuf Ahmed Al-Shirawi. *Commerce and Agriculture:* Habib Ahmed Kassim. *Acting Minister of State for Cabinet Affairs:* Yousuf Ahmed Al-Shirawi. *Minister of State for Legal Affairs:* Dr Hussain Al Baharna.

Flag: Red, with white serrated vertical strip on hoist.

DEFENCE

Army. The Army consists of 2 infantry and 1 tank battalion, 1 armoured car squadron, 2 artillery and 2 mortar batteries with a personnel strength of 5,000 (1991). Equipment included 54 M-60 A3 main battle tanks, 8 Saladin armoured cars, 22 AML-90 and 8 Ferret scout cars.

Navy. The Naval force consists of 2 West German-built missile corvettes with helicopter facilities, 4 fast missile craft and 7 fast patrol craft. Personnel in 1990 numbered 600. There is also a Coast Guard of 250 with 6 coastal patrol craft and 4 other vessels.

Air Force. An independent Air Force was created in 1985 as the successor to the Air Wing of the Army (Bahrain Defence Force). A fighter squadron operates 12 F-5E/F Tiger IIs, while 16 F-16s are on order for delivery in 1990–91. Three MBB BO 105 helicopters are also in use. Police and security forces both also operate helicopters. Personnel (1989) 200.

INTERNATIONAL RELATIONS

Membership. Bahrain is a member of UN, the Arab League, the Gulf Co-operation Council and OAPEC.

ECONOMY

Budget. The revenue of the State is derived from oil royalties and from customs duties, which are 10% *ad valorem* for luxury goods and 5% for essential goods. The exceptions are motor vehicles (20%); tobacco (30%); alcoholic beverages (100%); fresh fruit and vegetables (7%). Total revenues in 1988, BD 490m. (of which oil BD 252m.) and expenditure BD 365m.

On 2 Jan. 1958 Manama was declared a free transit port and the former 2% transit duty was abolished, but storage charges are levied.

Currency. The unit of currency is the *Bahraini dinar* (BHD), divided into 1,000 *fils*. The Bahrain currency board issues notes of 20, 10, 5 and 1 *dinars*, and 500 *fils*, and coins of 100, 50, 25, 10, 5 and 1 *fils*. £1 = BD 0·70 in March 1991; US$1 = BD 0·37.

Banking. The Bahrain Monetary Agency has central banking powers. Since Nov. 1984 it has been responsible for licensing and monitoring the activities of money changers. There were (1988) 20 full commercial banks (including Bahrain Islamic Bank), 6 of which are locally incorporated and the rest branches of foreign banks. Total assets at 31 Dec. 1988, BD 2,184·9m. Two types of offshore banking units were operating in 1988: 15 locally incorporated banks (including 4 Islamic) with headquarters in Bahrain, and 50 branches of foreign banks. Total assets at 31 Dec. 1988 US$68,100m. There are 15 investment banks (3 Islamic), with assets of US$1,750m. in Dec. 1985. The state-owned Housing Bank provides financing for construction, development of real estate and reclamation of land.

Weights and Measures. The metric system of weights and measures is officially in use.

ENERGY AND NATURAL RESOURCES

Electricity. Production (1988) 2,996·1m. kwh. Supply 230 volts; 50 Hz.

Oil. In 1931 oil was discovered. Operations were conducted by the Bahrain Petroleum Co., registered in Canada but owned by US interests, under a concession granted by the Shaikh. Production of crude oil in 1989 was 2·15m. tonnes. A large oil refinery on Bahrain Island, besides treating crude oil produced locally, also processes oil from Saudi Arabia transported by pipeline.

In 1975 the Bahrain Government assumed a direct 60% interest in the Bahrain oilfield and related crude oil facilities of BAPCO.

Bahrain's proven oil reserves in 1988 were 150m. bbls.

Gas. There is an abundant supply of natural gas with known reserves of 7·1m. cu. ft. in 1987. Production, 1987, 252,431m. cu. ft. Bahrain's gas reserves are 100% government-owned.

Water. Water is obtained from artesian wells and desalination plants and there is a piped supply to Manama, Muharraq, Isa Town, Rifa'a and most villages. In 1987 total water production was about 60m. gallons per day; daily consumption 59·7m. gallons by Aug. 1987. A further desalination plant with a capacity of 10m. gallons per day was due on stream in 1988.

Agriculture. The 6-year agricultural plan, commissioned in 1982, aimed to increase food production from 6–16% of total domestic requirements and to improve conservation of natural water and irrigation techniques.

There are about 900 farms and small holdings (average 2·5 hectares) operated by about 2,500 farmers who produce a wide variety of fruits (49,000 tonnes in 1988) and vegetables (12,000 tonnes in 1988). The major crop is alfalfa for animal fodder. Ninety tonnes of dates a year are processed and a new processing plant produced a further 300 tonnes in 1986.

Thirty-two poultry farms produced about 3,000 tonnes of domestic poultry in 1987. 95% of egg requirements are met by domestic production of 90m. eggs a year, and 30% of broiler needs.

Livestock (1988): Cattle, 6,000; camels, 1,000; sheep, 8,000; goats, 16,000; poultry 1m.

Fisheries. The government operates a fleet of 2 large and 5 smaller trawlers. In 1987 total landings weighed 7,841·5 tonnes.

INDUSTRY. Bahrain is being developed as a major manufacturing state, the first important enterprise being the Aluminium Bahrain (ALBA), a company whose original shareholders included the Bahrain Government and British, Swedish, Federal German and US interests. In 1975, the government acquired a majority shareholding in the enterprise. The aluminium smelter operation is the largest non-oil industry in the Gulf; output, 1987, 180,000 tonnes. Ancillary industries developed around aluminium smelting include the production of aluminium powder. A plant producing aluminium alloys went on stream in 1987. The Gulf Aluminium Rolling Mill Company (GARMCO), a joint venture between Bahrain, Saudi Arabia, Kuwait, Iraq, Oman and Qatar, was inaugurated in Feb. 1986. The Arab Shipbuilding and Repair Yard (ASRY), commissioned in 1977, is now in service. The dry dock can handle up to 50 tankers (500,000 DWT each) annually. A US$207m. iron ore pelletizing plant was inaugurated in Dec. 1984 (output, 1985, 680,000 tonnes) and a US$400m. petrochemical complex started operations in 1985.

In addition to the traditional minor industries such as boat-building, weaving, pottery, etc., other modern industries have developed, which include electronics assembly and the production of building materials, furniture, syringes and other medical items, matches, asbestos pipes and plastics, foodstuffs and textiles.

The pearling industry for which Bahrain used to be famous has considerably declined.

Labour. Total work force in the private sector (estimate 1987) 85,979, of which 25·2% Bahraini. The non-national workforce (1987) was 79,550.

FOREIGN ECONOMIC RELATIONS

Commerce. In 1988 total imports were BD974·6m. and total exports were BD874·5m. Refined petroleum accounted for almost 78% of exports; crude oil accounted for 41·9% of merchandise imports.

The major non-oil imports in 1988 were machinery and transport, BD198·1m.; classified manufactured goods, including Alumina, BD111·5m.; chemicals, BD64·5m.; food and live animals, BD81·2m., and miscellaneous manufactured articles, BD78·2m. The chief sources of supply (in BD1,000) were UK (116,115); USA (62,566); Japan (58,850); Federal Republic of Germany (35,573), and Australia (33,615).

The chief non-oil exports in 1988 were classified manufactured goods, including aluminium, BD135·5m., and machinery and transport, BD31m. The main markets (in BD1m.) were Saudi Arabia (42·9); Japan (27·7); United Arab Emirates (26·3); USA (14·4), and Kuwait (11·3).

Import of arms and ammunition and telecommunication equipment is subject to special permission; the sale of alcoholic liquor is restricted and the import of cultured pearls is forbidden.

Total trade between Bahrain and UK (British Department of Trade returns, in £1,000 sterling):

	1986	*1987*	*1988*	*1989*	*1990*
Imports to UK	19,732	60,687	75,786	61,018	48,459
Exports and re-exports from UK	130,991	125,189	138,150	138,529	127,309

Tourism. More than 165,000 tourists from the Gulf area arrived in 1985.

COMMUNICATIONS

Roads. The 25 km causeway links Bahrain with Saudi Arabia. In 1987 there were 112,520 registered vehicles.

Aviation. The airport, situated at Muharraq, can take the largest aircraft and is considered one of the most modern and efficient in the Middle East, used by 2,486,582 arriving and 2,512,882 departing passengers in 1987. British Airways, Gulf Air, Middle East Airlines, Pakistan International Airways, Qantas, Kuwait Airways, Air India International, Singapore Airlines, UTA, Saudi Arabian Airlines, KLM, Air Lanka, Cathay Pacific Airways, Iraqi Airways, Korean Airways, Philippine Airlines, Thai Airways International, Trans-Mediterranean Airways, Egyptair, Alia, Cyprus Airways, Ethiopia Airlines and Sudan Airways also operate to and from Bahrain. Bahrain International Airport is the Arabian Gulf's main air communication centre.

Shipping. Bahrain's traditional position as the entrepôt of the Southern Gulf has been supplemented by the development of Mina Sulman—the new modern harbour—as a free transit and industrial area. Local and international companies have developed industries in this area, which is also used as a storage centre for firms selling elsewhere in the Gulf. The facilities offered by Mina Sulman include engineering and ship repairing yards; the Basrec slipway is probably the largest between Rotterdam and Hong Kong.

Telecommunications. There were, at Dec. 1987, 120,000 telephones. There is a state-operated radio and television station and in 1983 there were 150,500 radio and 120,000 television receivers. There were 3 public service satellite stations in 1988.

Cinemas. There were 6 cinemas in 1987.

Newspapers. In 1988 there were several Arabic newspapers, and 1 English language daily newspaper, published in Manama.

JUSTICE, RELIGION, EDUCATION AND WELFARE

Justice. Criminal law is codified, based on English jurisprudence.

Religion. Islam is the State religion. In 1981 85% of the population were Moslem (60% Shi'ite in 1990) and 7·3% Christian. There are also Jewish, Bahai, Hindu and Parsee minorities.

Education. Government schools provide free education from primary to technical college level. There were, in 1987, 143 schools for boys and girls with 4,967 teachers and 88,132 pupils. In 1984, 5 boys' general and commercial schools had 2,177 pupils; 3 boys' industrial schools at secondary level, had 1,306 pupils. In addition there were 7 private schools. The Men's Teacher Training College (established 1966) and the Women's Teacher Training College (established 1967) give 2-year courses. In 1987, 1,665 Bahrainis were in higher education abroad. The Gulf Technical College opened in Bahrain in Sept. 1968 and Bahrain University in 1978. In 1987, 6,922 adult education centres were open throughout Bahrain.

Health. There is a free medical service for all residents of Bahrain. In 1987, there were 4 government hospitals and 19 health centres, an American mission hospital, an oil company hospital, a military hospital and an international hospital.

Social Security. In Oct. 1976, pensions, sickness and industrial injury benefits, unemployment, maternity and family allowances were established.

DIPLOMATIC REPRESENTATIVES

Of Bahrain in Great Britain (98 Gloucester Rd., London, SW7 4AU)
Ambassador: Karim Ebrahim Al-Shakar.

Of Great Britain in Bahrain (21 Government Ave., P.O. Box 114, Manama, 306)
Ambassador: J. A. Shepherd, CMG.

Of Bahrain in the USA (3502 International Dr., NW, Washington D.C., 20008)
Ambassador: Ghazi Mohammed Al-Gosaibi.

Of the USA in Bahrain (Road No. 3119, P.O. Box 26431, Manama)
Ambassador: Charles W. Hostler.

Of Bahrain to the United Nations
Ambassador: Muhammad Abdul Ghaffar.

Further Reading

Bahrain Business Directory. Manama (annual)
Statistical and General Information: Ministry of Information, PO Box 253, Manama
Statistical Abstract. Central Statistics Organisation (annual)

Lawson, F. H., *Bahrain: The Modernization of Autocracy*. Boulder, 1989
Rumaihi, M. G., *Bahrain: Social and Political Change since the First World War*. New York and London, 1976
Unwin, P. T. H., *Bahrain*. [Bibliography]. London and Santa Barbara, 1984

BANGLADESH

Capital: Dhaka
Population: 113·34m. (1990)
GNP per capita: US$170 (1988)

Gana Prajatantri Bangladesh

(People's Republic of Bangladesh)

HISTORY. The state was formerly the Eastern Province of Pakistan. In Dec. 1970 Sheikh Mujibur Rahman's Awami League Party gained 167 seats out of 300 at the Pakistan general election and immediately made known their wish for greater independence for the then Eastern Province. Martial law was imposed following disturbances in Dhaka, and civil war developed in March 1971. The war ended in Dec. 1971 and Bangladesh was proclaimed an independent state.

For developments between Jan. 1975 and March 1982, *see* THE STATESMAN'S YEAR-BOOK, 1986–87, pp. 186–187.

On 23 March 1982 there was a bloodless military coup, by which Lieut.-Gen. Hossain Mohammad Ershad became chief martial law administrator. President Sattar was deposed. The Constitution was suspended and parliament ceased to function. Assanuddin Chowdhury was sworn in as civilian president on 27 March. Lieut-Gen. Ershad assumed the presidency on 11 Dec. 1983. He was re-elected on 15 Oct. 1986.

Martial law ended on 10 Nov. 1986. The Constitution (Seventh Amendment) Act restored the constitution but protected the legality of President Ershad's decrees under martial law.

Following popular unrest President Ershad declared a state of emergency on 27 Nov. 1990, but was forced to resign on 4 Dec. and arrested on 12 Dec.

AREA AND POPULATION. Bangladesh is bounded west and north by India, east by India and Burma and south by the Bay of Bengal. The area is 55,598 sq. miles (143,998 sq. km). At the 1981 census the population was enumerated as 87,120,000. An adjustment for under enumeration produced a revised figure of 89,912,000 (46·3m. male, 14·09m. urban). Population estimate, 1988, 106·6m. (51·7m. female); density, 740 per sq. km; 1990, 113,335,000. In 1987 the birth-rate was 33·3 per 1,000 population; death-rate, 11·85; marriage rate, 11·6; infant mortality, 111 per 1,000 live births. Growth rate was 2·8% in 1986-87. Life expectancy, 1987; Males, 55·6; females, 54·9. The capital is Dhaka (population, 1987, 4·77m. The other major cities are Chittagong (1·84m.), Khulna (860,000) and Rajshahi (430,000). The country is administratively divided into 4 divisions, subdivided into 21 regions of 64 districts:

		Area (sq. km)	Population 1981
Dinajpur	(3 districts)	6,566	3,198,000
Rangpur	(5)	9,593	6,510,000
Bogra	(2)	3,888	2,728,000
Rajshahi	(4)	9,456	5,270,000
Pabna	(2)	4,732	3,424,000
Rajshahi division		*34,238*	*21,132,000*
Tangail	(1)	3,403	2,444,000
Mymensingh	(3)	9,668	6,568,000
Jamalpur	(2)	3,349	2,452,000
Dhaka	(6)	7,470	10,014,000
Faridpur	(5)	6,882	4,764,000
Dhaka division		*30,772*	*26,242,000*

		Area (sq. km)	Population 1981
Kushtia	(3)	3,440	2,292,000
Jessore	(4)	6,573	4,020,000
Khulna	(3)	12,168	4,329,000
Barisal	(4)	7,299	4,667,000
Patuakhali	(2)	4,095	1,843,000
Khulna division		*33,575*	*17,151,000*
Sylhet	(4)	12,718	5,656,000
Comilla	(3)	6,599	6,881,000
Noakhali	(3)	5,460	3,816,000
Chittagong	(2)	7,457	5,491,000
Chittagong Hill Tracts	(2)	8,679	580,000
Bandarban	(1)	4,501	171,000
Chittagong division		*45,414*	*22,595,000*

The official language is Bangla. (Bengali). English is also in use for official, legal and commercial purposes.

CLIMATE. A tropical monsoon climate with heat, extreme humidity and heavy rainfall in the monsoon season, from June to Oct. The short winter season (Nov.-Feb.) is mild and dry. Rainfall varies between 50" (1,250 mm) in the west to 100" (2,500 mm) in the south-east and up to 200" (5,000 mm) in the north-east. Dhaka. Jan. 66°F (19°C), July 84°F (28·9°C). Annual rainfall 81" (2,025 mm). Chittagong. Jan. 66°F (19°C), July 81°F (27·2°C). Annual rainfall 108" (2,831 mm).

CONSTITUTION AND GOVERNMENT. Bangladesh is a unitary republic. The Constitution came into force on 16 Dec. 1972 and provides for a parliamentary democracy.

The head of state is the *President*, directly elected every five years. He appoints a *Vice-President.*

There is a *Council of Ministers* to assist and advise the President. The President appoints the Prime Minister from among the members of Parliament who appears to him to command the support of a majority of members; he also appoints the other ministers.

Parliament has one chamber of 300 members directly elected every 5 years by citizens over 18. There are 30 seats reserved for women members elected by Parliament.

Following the enforced resignation of Lieut.-Gen. Hossain Mohammad Ershad as president, a caretaker government was appointed with Shahabuddin Ahmed as interim president.

At the elections of Feb. 1991 the Bangladesh National Party (BNP) won 140 seats, the Awami League 95, the Jatiya Party (led by Hossain Ershad) 35 and Jamit-e-Islami 18.

Prime Minister: Khaleda Zia.

Local government: Elections were held in March 1990.

National flag: Bottle green with a red disc in the centre.

National anthem: Amar Sonar Bangla, ami tomay bhalobashi (My golden Bengal, I love you). Words by Rabindranath Tagore.

DEFENCE. The supreme command of defence services is vested in the President.

Army. There are 6 infantry divisional headquarters, with 14 infantry brigades, and 2 armoured and 6 artillery regiments, and 6 engineer battalions. Strength (1990) 90,000, with an additional 55,000 paramilitary volunteers, including an armed police reserve and the Bangladesh Rifles. Equipment includes 30 Soviet T-54 and 20 Chinese Type-59 tanks.

Navy. Naval bases are at Chittagong, Kaptai, Khulna and Dhaka.

The fleet comprises 1 new Chinese-built missile-armed frigate, 3 ex-British frigates, 8 new Chinese-built 390-tonne fast attack craft, 8 Chinese-built fast missile craft, 8 Chinese-built fast torpedo boats, 2 ex-Yugoslav 200-tonne patrol craft, 8 ex-Chinese 155-tonne fast gunboats, 2 ex-Indian 150-tonne patrol craft, 1 British-built 140-tonne patrol craft, 5 indigenously built 70-tonne river gunboats, 1 oiler, 1 repair vessel, 12 auxiliaries and 1 training ship of 710 tons.

The manpower of the Navy in 1990 was 7,500.

Air Force. Deliveries, from the Soviet Union and China successively, comprise 6 MiG-21 interceptors and about 20 J-6 (MiG-19) fighter-bombers; 1 An-24 and 3 An-26 turboprop transports; over 30 Mi-8, Bell 212, Bell 206L and Alouette III helicopters; 10 Chinese CJ-6 piston-engined primary trainers, FT-2 (MiG-15UTI) jet advanced trainers, 6 Magister armed jet trainers and some light aircraft. Personnel strength, (1990) 6,000.

INTERNATIONAL RELATIONS

Membership. Bangladesh is a member of the Commonwealth, the Asian Development Bank, the Organisation for South Asian Regional Co-operation, the UN and all its related agencies, the Colombo Plan and the Islamic Conference.

External Debt. Estimated debt, June 1985, US$6,000m. Most of this was in loans from the Western aid group through the World Bank.

Treaties. Bangladesh signed an economic and technical co-operation agreement with China on 4 Jan. 1977. The amended constitution of 1977 states that Bangladesh seeks fraternal relations with Moslem countries based on Islamic solidarity.

ECONOMY

Planning. The third 5-year development plan, 1985–90, envisages an annual growth rate of 5·4%, and an industrial growth rate of 10·1% annually; of industrial development funds, 55% is for the private sector. Agriculture receives 30% of total plan expenditure, and the plan aims at self-sufficiency in food by 1990.

Budget. In 1986-87 total Government receipts were Tk.92,764m., of which Tk.45,594m. were revenue receipts, and total expenditure was Tk.82,301m., divided into Tk.40,218m. revenue expenditure and Tk.42,083m. development expenditure. In 1987-88 revenue receipts were Tk.49,150m., revenue expenditure Tk.45,693m. and development expenditure Tk.42,083m. Revenue receipts included (in Tk.1m.) 40,731 from taxation (33,310 indirect). Expenditures: Education, 9,254; administration, 9,107; defence, 7,695; debt servicing, 5,179; justice, 3,992.

Currency. The unit of currency is the *taka* (BDT) of 100 *paisas,* which was floated in 1976. There are 1, 5, 10, 25, 50 and 100 paisa coins and 1, 2, 5, 10, 20, 50, 100 and 500 taka notes. Money supply, 1988: Tk.50,477m. (of which Tk.24,150m. were in circulation). Foreign exchange reserves: Tk.26,963m. (Tk.67·00 = £1 and Tk.35·32 = US$1 in March 1991).

Banking and Finance. Bangladesh Bank is the central bank. There are 4 nationalized commercial banks, 9 private commercial banks, 3 specialized banks and 7 foreign commercial banks. In May 1988 the Bangladesh Bank had Tk.19,971m. deposits; Tk.25,886m. foreign liabilities, Tk.52,709m. assets. The scheduled banks had Tk.131,764m. deposits, Tk.32,210m. assets and Tk.24,313m. borrowings from the Bangladesh Bank. Post office savings deposits were Tk.1,070m. in 1987.

Weights and Measures. The metric system was introduced from July 1982, but imperial measures are still in use. Weight is in the *seer* (1 *seer* = 2 lb.); the *maund* (1 *maund* = 40 *seers*) and the ton.

ENERGY AND NATURAL RESOURCES

Electricity. Electric power is generated and distributed by the Bangladesh Power Development Board and the Rural Electrification Board. Installed capacity, June 1987, 1,757 mw.; electricity generated, 1986–87, 5,288·01m. kwh.; consumption, 3,479·38m. kwh. Supply 220 volts; 50 Hz.

Oil. Supplies have been located in the Bay of Bengal. Drilling is in progress.

Gas. There are 14 natural gas fields with recoverable reserves of 12,610,000m. cu. ft. Production, 1987–88, 147,454m. cu. ft. Consumption, 140,600 cu. ft.

Water. India and Bangladesh are working towards agreement on sharing the water of the river Ganges. The flow will be monitored daily at the Farakka barrage and two other points.

Minerals. The principal minerals are lignite, limestone, china clay and glass sand. Production, 1986–87: Limestone, 44,660m. tons (value Tk.13·34m.); china clay, 12,272m. tons (Tk.17·2m.).

Agriculture. At the 1983-84 census of agriculture there were 10·05m. farm holdings (7·07m. under 2·5 acres; 2·48m. of 2·5 to 7·5 acres; 496,000 over 7·5 acres. 28·3% of households had no cultivable land. Agriculture contributed 41% of GDP in 1987–88. The cultivable area was 22·84m. acres in 1987, of which 21·88m. acres were cropped (26·2m. under rice, 1·4m. wheat and 1·9m. jute). About 5·43m. acres (1987) is irrigated; 2·4m. by tubewells and another 1·63m. by power pump.

Bangladesh produces about 70% of the world's jute which is the principal foreign exchange earner. Production, 1987-88, 839,000 tonnes.

Rice is the most important food crop; production in 1987–88, 15·74m. tonnes. Other crops (1,000 tonnes): Sugar-cane, 7,093; wheat, 1,031; tobacco, 117; pulses, 530; oilseeds, 442; spices, 343; tea, 89·54m. lbs.; potatoes, 1,255.

Fertilizers used (1986–87), 1·32m. tonnes, of which 915m. tonnes was urea.

Livestock in 1988 (1,000): Poultry, 113,000; cattle, 22,789; goats, 10,700; sheep, 1,140; buffalo, 1,950. Livestock products in 1988 (tonnes): Beef and veal, 137,000; cow and buffalo milk, 750,000; goats' milk, 224,000; eggs, 110,000.

Forestry. The area under forests in 1988 was 2·1m. ha (16% of the land area). Output of timber, 1986-87, was 12·76m. cu. ft.

Fisheries. Being bounded on the south by the Bay of Bengal and having numerous inland waterways, Bangladesh is a major producer of fish and products. In 1987-88 there were 497,000 sea- and 752,000 inland-fishermen, with 1,249 mechanized boats, including 52 trawlers, and 3,317 motor boats. Inland catch was 610,000 tonnes, sea, 227,000 tonnes.

INDUSTRY. Industry contributed 8·9% of GDP in 1987-88. The principal industries are jute and cotton textiles, tea, paper, newsprint, cement, chemical fertilizers and light engineering. In 1986-87 there were 4,386 factories (including 881 textile, 801 food and 564 chemical). New government policy in 1982 aimed to restore public-sector jute and textile mills to private ownership and encourage the private sector. Arms and ammunition, atomic energy, forestry, air transport, communications and electrical industries would remain in the public sector.

Production, 1987–88: Jute goods, 529,000 tonnes; cotton yarn, 103m. lb.; cotton cloth, 68m. yards; cement, 310,000 tonnes; sugar, 175,000 tonnes; vegetable products, 6,337 tonnes; fertilizer, 729,000 tonnes, newsprint, 49,000 tonnes; bicycles 19,749; 8,039 motor cycles; 121,000 radios.

Labour. In 1985–86, the labour force was 27·7m. (3·2m. female), of whom 27·4m. (3·1m.) were employed (2·8m. children between 10 and 14 years were also employed). 57·6% worked in agriculture and fishery, 11·5% in trade and 7·1% in production and transport. Average daily industrial wage, 1987-88: Skilled, Tk.49; unskilled, Tk.31.

FOREIGN ECONOMIC RELATIONS

Commerce. The main exports are jute and jute goods, tea, hides and skins, newsprint, fish and garments, and the main imports are machinery, transport equipment, manufactured goods, minerals, fuels and lubricants. In 1987–88 exports were valued at Tk.41,161m., and imports at Tk.91,588m.

Main sources of imports in 1987-88: Japan (mainly machinery and vehicles), Tk.10,098m.; USA (foodstuffs), Tk.8,161m.; Singapore (petroleum), Tk.6,327m.; Hong Kong, Tk.4,271m.; UK, 4,197m. Main export markets: USA, Tk.12,045m.; Italy, Tk.3,677m.; UK, Tk.2,433m. Federal Germany, Tk.2,306m.

Total trade between Bangladesh and UK (British Department of Trade returns, in £1,000 sterling):

	1987	*1988*	*1989*	*1990*
Imports to UK	35,454	50,249	52,527	72,515
Exports and re-exports from UK	54,382	64,018	78,270	70,534

Foreign investment is encouraged and legally protected. The Board of Investment must approve joint ventures if the foreign participation exceeds 49%. There is a duty-free Export Processing Zone at Chittagong.

Tourism. In 1987 there were 106,765 visitors to Bangladesh of whom 47,390 were from India. Foreign exchange earnings, Tk.192·4m.

COMMUNICATIONS

Roads. In 1986 there were 4,039 miles of roads with cement, concrete or bitumen surfaces. In 1987 there were 8,827 buses, 16,375 lorries and 27,120 private cars.

Railways. In 1988 there were 2,745 km of railways, comprising 923 km of 1,676 mm gauge and 1,822 km of metre gauge. They carried 2·5m. tonnes of freight and 53m. passengers.

Aviation. There are international airports at Dhaka (Zia), Chittagong and Sylhet, and 7 domestic airports. Bangladesh Biman (Bangladesh Airways) had 11 aircraft in 1988 and has domestic flights from Zia International Airport and services to Calcutta, Kathmandu, Bombay, Dubai, Abu Dhabi, Jeddah, Bangkok, Singapore, London, Doha, Kuwait, Amsterdam, Rome, Karachi, Kuala Lumpur, Bahrain, Tripoli, Athens and Muscat. In 1987 Zia handled 1·18m. passengers out of a total of 1·6m. Freight and mail handled, Zia, 32,413 tons; total, 34,376: Aircraft movements, Zia, 29,393; total, 55,051.

Shipping. There are sea ports at Chittagong and Mongla, and inland ports at Dhaka, Chandpur, Barisal, Khulna and five other towns. There are 5,000 miles of navigable channels. The three principle navigable rivers, the Padma, Brahmaputra and Meghna serve areas where railways cannot be economically constructed. The Bangladesh Shipping Corporation owned 21 ships in 1987. There are also 881 private cargo and 1,506 passenger vessels. In 1986–87 the port of Chittagong handled 5·8m. tons of imports and 402,000 tons of exports; total, all ports 7·4m. tons of imports and 1·1m. tons of exports. Vessels entered (all ports) 1,792 and cleared, 1,770. The Bangladesh Inland Water Transport Corporation had 430 vessels in 1988.

Telecommunications. There were 7,810 post offices and 187,650 telephones in 1988. International communications are by the Indian Ocean Intelsat IV satellite.

There are radio and TV stations at Dhaka, Chittagong, Khulna, Rangpur, Sylhet, and Rangamati; radio stations at Comilla and Thakurgaon; and TV stations at Natore, Mymensingh, Noakhali, Satkhira and Cox's Bazar. Radio broadcasting is in Bangla, English, Urdu, Hindi, Arabic and Nepali. In 1987 there were 435,000 radios and 426,000 TV sets.

Cinema. In 1987 there were 681 cinemas with 363,000 seats. 75 full-length films were made.

Newspapers and Books. In 1987 there were 49 daily newspapers in Bangla with a circulation of 736,000 and 10 in English with a circualtion of 112,000. There were 171 other periodicals (15 in English) with a circulation of 737,000. Most papers are published in Dhaka. The Government has set up a paper *(Dainik Barta-at Rajshahi)* to stimulate a regional press. There is a Press Institute. In 1987 1,022 book titles were published (90 in English).

JUSTICE, RELIGION, EDUCATION AND WELFARE

Justice. The Supreme Court comprises an Appellate and a High court Division, the latter having control over all subordinate courts. There are benches at Comilla, Rangpur, Jessore, Barisal, Chittagong and Sylhet, and courts at District level. The Chief Justice and other judges of the High Court are appointed by the President and must retire at 62 years.

Religion. Islam is the State Religion. Some 80% of the population are Moslem and the rest Hindus, Buddhists and Christians.

Education. About 29·2% of the population over 15 was literate in 1989 (male 39·7%, female 18%). The Government has taken over school administration. The compulsory primary education scheme has been replaced by model primary education.

In 1987–88 there were 44,502 primary schools (6,864 private), with 11·08m. pupils (4·83m. female) and 186,597 teachers (33,575 female); 10,157 secondary schools (9,895 private), with 2·81m. pupils (927,000 female) and 116,835 teachers (11,432 female); 812 colleges of further education (630 private), with 792,000 students (183,000 female) and 17,215 teachers (2,268 female); and 77 technical colleges with 17,360 students (996 female) and 1,307 teachers (46 female). There is an Islamic University (891 students and 19 teachers in 1987-88) and universities at Dhaka (16,622 and 973), Rajshahi (11,755 and 469), Chittagong (6,025 and 420) and Jahingirnagar (2,660 and 181). There are also universities of agriculture (4,573 and 379) and engineering (3,758 and 349). There were 10 teacher-training colleges in 1987-88, with 3,624 students (1,040 female) and 160 teachers (47 female), and 53 primary training institutes with 6,893 students (4,122 female) and 532 teachers (106 female).

Health. In 1987 there were 608 state and 267 private hospitals with a total of 33,038 beds. There were 16,929 doctors. State expenditure on health, Tk.3,540m. There are 10 medical schools.

DIPLOMATIC REPRESENTATIVES

Of Bangladesh in Great Britain (28 Queen's Gate, London, SW7)
High Commissioner: Maj.-Gen. K. M. Safiullah.
(There are also Assistant High Commissioners in Birmingham and Manchester)

Of Great Britain in Bangladesh (Abu Bakr Hse., Gulshan, Dhaka 12)
High Commissioner: C. H. Imray, CMG.

Of Bangladesh in the USA (2201 Wisconsin Ave., NW, Washington, D.C., 20007)
Ambassador: A. H. S. Ataul Karim.

Of the USA in Bangladesh (Madani Ave., Baridhara, Dhaka 1212)
Ambassador: William B. Millam.

Of Bangladesh to the United Nations
Ambassador: A. H. G. Mohiuddin.

Further Reading

Official statistics are issued by the Bangladesh Bureau of Statistics (Director-General A. M. A. Rahim). Publications include: *Statistical Yearbook of Bangladesh*. 1976; 1979 to date. *Statistical Pocket Book of Bangladesh*. 1980 to date.

Bangladesh Planning Commission, *The First Five Year Plan—The Second Five Year Plan.*
Abdullah, T. and Zeidenstein, S., *Village Women of Bangladesh: Prospects for Change.* Oxford, 1981
Baxter, C., *Bangladesh: A New Nation in an Old Setting.* Boulder, 1986
Chowdhury, R., *The Genesis of Bangladesh.* London, 1972
Dutt, K., *Bangladesh Economy: An Analytical Study.* New Delhi, 1973
Franda, M., *Bangladesh: The First Decade.* New Delhi, 1982
Hartmann, B. and Boyce, J., *A Quiet Violence: View from a Bangladesh Village.* London, 1983
Kamal, K. A., *Sheikh Mujibur Rahman.* 2nd ed. Dhaka, 1970
Khan, A. R., *The Economy of Bangladesh.* London, 1972
de Lucia, R. J. and Jacoby, H. D., *Energy Planning for Developing Countries: A Study of Bangladesh.* John Hopkins Univ. Press, 1982
de Vylder, S., *Agriculture in Chains. Bangladesh: A Case Study in Contradictions and Constraints.* London, 1982
O'Donnell, C. P., *Bangladesh: Biography of a Muslim Nation.* Boulder, 1986
Rahman, M., *Bangladesh Today: An Indictment and a Lament.* London, 1978

BARBADOS

Capital: Bridgetown
Population: 260,000 (1990)
GNP per capita: US$5,990 (1988)

HISTORY. Barbados was occupied by the British in 1627 and during its colonial history never changed hands. Full internal self-government was attained in 1961. Barbados became an independent sovereign state within the Commonwealth on 30 Nov. 1966.

AREA AND POPULATION. Barbados lies to the east of the Windward Islands. Area 166 sq. miles (430 sq. km). In 1980 the census population was 248,983. Estimate (1990) 260,000 (44·2% urban). Bridgetown is the principal city: Population, 7,466 in 1987.

Growth rate (1985–90), 6 per 1,000; infant mortality, 11 per 1,000; expectation of life, 73·9 years.

CLIMATE. An equable climate in winter, but the wet season, from June to Nov., is more humid. Rainfall varies from 50" (1,250 mm) on the coast to 75" (1,875 mm) in the higher interior. Bridgetown. Jan. 76°F (24·4°C), July 80°F (26·7°C). Annual rainfall 51" (1,275 mm).

CONSTITUTION AND GOVERNMENT. The Legislature consists of the Governor-General, a Senate and a House of Assembly. The Senate comprises 21 members appointed by the Governor-General, 12 being appointed on the advice of the Prime Minister, 2 on the advice of the leader of the opposition and 7 in the Governor-General's discretion. The House of Assembly comprises 28 members elected every 5 years. In 1963 the voting age was reduced to 18.

The Privy Council is appointed by the Governor-General after consultation with the Prime Minister. It consists of 12 members and the Governor-General as chairman. It advises the Governor-General in the exercise of the royal prerogative of mercy and in the exercise of his disciplinary powers over members of the public and police services.

In the general election of Jan. 1991 the Democratic Labour Party gained 18 seats and the Barbados Labour Party 10 seats. Turn out was 62%.

Governor-General: Dame Nita Barrow.

The Cabinet, in March 1991, was composed as follows:

Prime Minister, Minister of Finance and Economic Affairs and Minister of the Civil Service: Erskine Sandiford.

Deputy Prime Minister, International Transport, Transport and Works, Immigration and Telecommunications, Leader of the House of Assembly: Philip Greaves. *Attorney-General, Foreign Affairs:* Maurice A. King, QC. *Labour, Consumer Affairs and the Environment:* Warwick O. Franklyn. *Agriculture, Food and Fisheries, Leader of the Senate:* L. V. Harcourt Lewis. *Health:* Brandford Taitt. *Housing and Lands:* E. Evelyn Greaves. *Tourism and Sport:* Wesley Hall. *Trade, Industry and Commerce:* Dr Carl Clarke. *Education:* Cyril Walker. *Justice and Public Safety:* Keith Simmons. *Community Development and Culture:* David J. H. Thompson. There was one Minister of State.

National flag: Three vertical strips of blue, gold, blue, with a black trident in the centre.

INTERNATIONAL RELATIONS

Membership. Barbados is a member of UN, OAS, CARICOM, the Commonwealth and an ACP state of the EEC.

ECONOMY

Budget. The budget for 1987–88 envisaged capital expenditure of BD$176·5 and current expenditure of BD$814·1.

Currency. The unit of currency is the *Barbados dollar* (BBD) of 100 *cents*. Inflation was an annualized 4·8% in 1989. In March 1991, £1 = BD$3.82; US$1 = 2.01.

Banking and Finance. Barclays Bank International, the Royal Bank of Canada, Canadian Imperial Bank of Commerce, the Bank of Nova Scotia, Chase Manhattan Bank, Caribbean Commercial Bank, The Barbados National Bank, Bank of Credit and Commerce International have offices.

Barbados is headquarters for the Caribbean Development Bank. The Barbados Development Bank opened on 15 April 1969 and Barbados became a member of the Inter-American Development Bank on 19 March 1969.

There is a stock exchange.

NATURAL RESOURCES

Electricity. Production (1987) 425m. kwh. Supply 150 volts; 50 Hz.

Oil. Crude oil production (1989) 60,000 tonnes and reserves (1987), 3·24m. bbls.

Gas. Output of gas (1987) 936m. cu. ft and reserves 18,618m. cu. metres.

Agriculture. Of the total area of 106,240 acres, about 55,000 acres are arable land. The land is intensely cultivated. In 1988, 12,000 ha of sugar-cane were harvested. Cotton was successfully replanted in 1983 and 91 bales were harvested from 300 acres in 1985. The agricultural sector accounted for 7·1% (provisional) of GDP in 1985 (1946, 45%; 1967, 24%). In 1985, 6·9% of the total labour force were employed in agriculture. In 1988, 83,000 tonnes of sugar were produced. There are 6 sugar factories and 2 rum refineries in production. In 1988, 2,000 tonnes of yams and 4,000 tonnes of sweet potatoes were produced. Hot peppers, eggplants, watermelons, breadfruit and red ginger lilies are also grown for export.

Livestock (1988): Cattle, 18,000; sheep, 56,000; goats, 33,000; pigs, 49,000; poultry, 1m.

Fisheries. There are about 745 (1987) powered boats and many men and women are employed during the flying-fish season. Large numbers of these boats are laid up from July to Oct. The fish catch in 1987 was 9,800 tonnes.

INDUSTRY. Industrial establishments operating in Barbados in 1987 numbered approximately 330 and ranged from the manufacture of processed food to small specialized products such as garment manufacturing, furniture and household appliances, electrical components, plastic products and electronic parts.

FOREIGN ECONOMIC RELATIONS

Commerce. Total trade for calendar years in BD$1,000:

	1984	*1985*	*1986*	*1987*	*1988*
Domestic Imports [1]	1,324,623	1,221,595	1,181,075	1,035,891	1,170,316
Domestic Exports [1]	583,667	496,471	420,614	214,511	242,738

[1] Exclusive of bullion and specie.

In 1988 the principal imports (BD$1m.) were: Machinery and transport equipment, 275·7; manufactured goods, 360·5; food and live animals, 181·9; lubricants, mineral fuels, etc., 110·5; chemicals, 125·9; crude minerals, 36·2; beverages and tobacco, 29; animal and vegetable oils and fats, 12·9. In 1988 the principal domestic exports (BD$1m.) were: Sugar, 57·7; electronic components, 42·8; clothing, 30·4.

Total trade between Barbados and UK (British Department of Trade returns, in £1,000 sterling):

	1986	*1987*	*1988*	*1989*	*1990*
Imports from UK	11,661	23,320	19,487	22,304	24,294
Exports and re-exports to UK	38,338	33,067	32,061	38,136	35,811

Tourism. In 1988, 449,761 tourists visited Barbados spending BD$914·7m. The industry employs over 10,000 people.

COMMUNICATIONS

Roads. There are 1,035 miles of road open to traffic, of which 855 miles are all-weather roads. In Dec. 1987 there were 34,740 private cars, 2,266 hired cars and taxis, 470 buses including minibuses and 7,855 other vehicles including motor-cycles.

Aviation. There is an international airport at Seawell, Christ Church, Barbados, served by British Airways, BWIA, Leeward Islands Air Transport, PANAM, American Airlines, Wardair, Air Martinique Cruziero (SC), Air Canada, Caribbean Airways and Eastern Airlines, Cubana Airlines, Venezuelan Airlines.

Shipping. A deep-water harbour opened in 1961 at Bridgetown provides 8 berths for ships 500–600 ft in length, including one specially designed for bulk sugar loading. The number of merchant vessels entering in 1986 was 1,961 of 6,452,000 net tons.

Telecommunications. There is a general post office in Bridgetown and 16 branches on the island. In 1987 there were 94,338 telephones in service. In 1986 there were 200,000 radios and 62,000 television sets.

Cinemas. There were (1985) 3 cinemas and 2 drive-in cinemas for 600 cars.

Newspapers. In 1987 there were 2 daily newspapers with a total circulation of 41,000.

JUSTICE, RELIGION, EDUCATION AND WELFARE

Justice. Justice is administered by the Supreme Court and by magistrates' courts. All have both civil and criminal jurisdiction. There is a Chief Justice and 3 puisne judges of the Supreme Court and 8 magistrates.

Religion. The majority (about 70%) of the population are Anglicans, the remainder mainly Methodists, Moravians and Roman Catholics.

Education. In 1984–85 children in 105 government primary schools numbered 29,392; in 21 secondary schools, 21,501; in 5 vocational centres, 967; in 15 assisted private approved secondary schools, 4,227. There are 23 independent primary schools with 3,547 pupils and a number of independent schools for which no accurate figures are available. Education is free in all government-owned and maintained institutions from primary to university level.

The University of the West Indies in Barbados was opened in Sept. 1963 and Cave Hill campus in 1967 and in 1985 had 1,932 students. In 1984–85, 186 students attended Erdiston College and 1,617 students attended the Cave Hill campus. The Barbados Community College for higher education had in 1984–85, 1,806 students (full and part-time).

Health. In 1986 there were 2,054 hospital beds and 243 doctors.

DIPLOMATIC REPRESENTATIVES

Of Barbados in Great Britain (1 Great Russell St., London, WC1B 3NH)
High Commissioner: Sir Roy Marshall, CBE.

Of Great Britain in Barbados (Lower Collymore Rock, Bridgetown)
High Commissioner: E. T. Davies, CMG.

Of Barbados in the USA (2144 Wyoming Ave., NW, Washington, D.C. 20008)
Ambassador: Sir William Douglas, KCMG.

Of the USA in Barbados (PO Box 302, Bridgetown)
Ambassador: (Vacant)

Of Barbados to the United Nations
Ambassador: E. Besley Maycock.

Further Reading

Statistical Information: The Barbados Statistical Service (NIS Bldg, Fairchild St, St Michael) produces selected monthly statistics and annual abstracts. *Director:* Eric Straughn.

Beckles, H., *A History of Barbados: from Amerindian Settlement to Nation-State*. Cambridge Univ. Press, 1990

Dann, G., *The Quality of Life in Barbados*. London, 1984

Hoyos, F. A., *Barbados: A History from the Amerindians to Independence*. London, 1978.—*Barbados: A Visitor's Guide*. London, 1983.—*Tom Adams: A Biography*. London, 1988

Potter, R. B. and Dann, G. M. S., *Barbados* [Bibliography]. Oxford and Santa Barbara, 1987

Warren, A. and Frazer, H., *The Barbados Carollna Connection*. London, 1989

Worrell, D., *The Economy of Barbados 1946–1980*. Bridgetown, 1982

Library: The Barbados Public Library, Bridgetown. *Acting Chief Librarian:* Edwin Ifill.

BELGIUM

Capital: Brussels
Population: 9·93m. (1989)
GNP per capita: US$14,550 (1988)

Royaume de Belgique—Koninkrijk België

(Kingdom of Belgium)

HISTORY. The kingdom of Belgium formed itself into an independent state in 1830, having from 1815 been part of the Netherlands. The secession was decreed on 4 Oct. 1830 by a provisional government, established in consequence of a revolution which broke out at Brussels, on 25 Aug. 1830. A National Congress elected Prince Leopold of Saxe-Coburg King of the Belgians on 4 June 1831; he ascended the throne 21 July 1831.

By the Treaty of London, 15 Nov. 1831, the neutrality of Belgium was guaranteed by Austria, Russia, Great Britain and Prussia. It was not until after the signing of the Treaty of London, 19 April 1839, which established peace between King Leopold I and the King of the Netherlands, that all the states of Europe recognized the kingdom of Belgium. In the Treaty of Versailles (28 June 1919) it is stated that as the treaties of 1839 'no longer conform to the requirements of the situation', these are abrogated and will be replaced by other treaties.

AREA AND POPULATION. Belgium is bounded in the north by the Netherlands, north-west by the North Sea, west and south by France, east by Germany and Luxembourg. Belgium has an area of 30,518 sq. km (11,778 sq. miles). The Belgian exclave of Baarle-Hertog in the Netherlands has an area of 7 sq. km, and a population (1 Jan. 1989) of 1,083 males and 1,007 females.

Dutch (Flemish) is spoken by the Flemish section of the population in the north, French by the Wallon south. The linguistic frontier bisects Brussels, which is bilingual. Some German is spoken in the east.

Percentage of the population in the language communities was on 1 Jan. 1989: Flemish, 57·6; French, 31·9; bilingual, 9·8; German, 0·7. Each language has official status in its own community. (*See* map in THE STATESMAN'S YEAR-BOOK, 1967–68). Bracketed names below contain French or Dutch alternatives.

Census	*Population*	*Increase % per annum*	*Census*	*Population*	*Increase % per annum*
1900	6,693,548	1·03	1947	8,512,195	0·36
1910	7,423,784	1·09	1961	9,189,741	0·52
1920	7,405,569	0·06	1970	9,650,944	0·55
1930	8,092,004	0·84	1981	9,848,647	0·18

Provinces	*Provincial capitals*	*Area (ha)*	*Estimated population (1 Jan.) 1970* [1]	*1988*	*1989*
Antwerp	Antwerp	286,726	1,533,249	1,587,450	1,592,437
Brabant	Brussels	335,811	2,176,373	2,221,818	2,240,926
Flanders West	Bruges (Brugge)	313,439	1,054,429	1,095,193	1,099,384
Flanders East	Ghent	298,167	1,310,117	1,328,779	1,329,830
Hainaut	Mons (Bergen)	378,669	1,317,453	1,271,649	1,278,255
Liège (Luik)	Liège	386,213	1,008,905	992,068	987,364
Limbourg	Hasselt	242,231	652,547	736,981	740,974
Luxembourg	Arlon	444,114	217,310	226,452	229,587
Namur (Namen)	Namur	366,501	380,561	415,326	418,855
Total		3,051,871	9,650,944	9,875,716	9,917,612

[1] Census.

In 1988 there were 5,078,668 females. On 1 Jan. 1989 there were 868,757 resident foreigners.

Vital statistics:

	Births	*Deaths*	*Marriages*	*Divorces*	*Immigration*	*Emigration*
1985	114,283	112,691	57,630	18,530	47,042	54,021
1986	117,271	111,671	56,657	18,434	48,959	53,793
1987	117,448	105,840	56,588	19,830	49,750	57,033
1988	118,764	104,551	59,075	20,809	54,048	54,621

The most populous towns, with estimated population on 1 Jan. 1989:

Brussels and suburbs [1]	970,501	St Niklaas (St Nicolas)	67,941
Antwerp and suburbs [2]	473,082	Tournai (Doornik)	67,669
Ghent	230,822	Hasselt	65,851
Charleroi	208,021	Genk	61,217
Liège (Luik)	199,020	Seraing	61,091
Brugge (Bruges)	117,653	Verviers	53,665
Namur (Namen)	103,131	Mouscron (Moeskroen)	53,504
Mons (Bergen)	91,650	Roeselare (Roulers)	52,450
Leuven (Louvain)	85,947	Turnhout	37,587
Aalst (Alost)	76,441	Herstal	36,343
Kortrijk (Courtrai)	76,279	Lokeren	34,784
La Louvière	76,200	Vilvoorde (Vilvorde)	32,852
Mechelen (Malines)	75,514	Lier (Lierre)	30,856
Ostend	68,370		

[1] The suburbs comprise 18 communes: Anderlecht, Etterbeek, Forest, Ixelles, Jette, Koekelberg, Molenbeek St Jean, St Gilles, St Josse-ten-Noode, Schaerbeek, Uccle, Woluwe-St Lambert, Auderghem, Watermael-Boitsfort, Woluwe-St Pierre, Berchem Ste Agathe, Evere and Ganshoren.

[2] Including Berchem, Borgerhout, Deurne, Hoboken, Merksem and Wilrijk.

CLIMATE. Cool temperate climate, influenced by the sea, giving mild winters and cool summers. Brussels. Jan. 36°F (2·2°C), July 64°F (17·8°C). Annual rainfall 33" (825 mm). Ostend. Jan. 38°F (3·3°C), July 62°F (16·7°C). Annual rainfall 31" (775 mm).

KING. Baudouin, born 7 Sept. 1930, succeeded his father, Leopold III, on 17 July 1951, when he took the oath on the constitution before the two Chambers: Married on 15 Dec. 1960 to Fabiola de Mora y Aragón, daughter of the Conde de Mora and Marqués de Casa Riera.

Brother and Sister of the King. (1) Josephine Charlotte, Princess of Belgium, born 11 Oct. 1927; married to Prince Jean of Luxembourg, 9 April 1953; (2) Albert, Prince of Liège, born 6 June 1934; married to Paola Ruffo di Calabria, 2 July 1959; *offspring:* Prince Philippe, born 15 April 1960; Princess Astrid, born 5 June 1962; married to Archduke Lorenz of Austria, 22 Sept. 1984; Prince Laurent, born 19 Oct. 1963. *Half-brother and half-sisters of the King.* Prince Alexandre, born 18 July 1942; Princess Marie Christine, born 6 Feb. 1951; Princess Maria-Esmeralda, born 30 Sept. 1956.

Aunt of the King. Princess Marie-José, born 4 Aug. 1906, married to Prince Umberto (King Umberto II of Italy in 1946) on 8 Jan. 1930.

BELGIAN SOVEREIGNS

Leopold I	1831–65	Leopold III	1934–44, 1950–51
Leopold II	1865–1909	Regency	1944–50
Albert	1909–34	Baudouin	1951–

CONSTITUTION AND GOVERNMENT. According to the constitution of 1831, Belgium is a constitutional, representative and hereditary monarchy. The legislative power is vested in the King, the Senate and the Chamber of Representatives. The royal succession is in direct male line in the order of primogeniture. By marriage without the King's consent, however, the right of succession is forfeited, but may be restored by the King with the consent of the two Chambers. No act of the King can have effect unless countersigned by one of his Ministers, who thus becomes responsible for it. The King convokes, prorogues and dissolves the Chambers. In default of male heirs, the King may nominate his successor with the consent of the Chambers. If the successor be under 18 years of age the two Chambers meet together for the purpose of nominating a regent during the minority.

National flag: Three vertical strips of black, yellow, red.

National anthem: Après des siècles d'esclavage ('After centuries of slavery'; La Brabançonne; words by Jenneval, 1830; tune by F. van Campenhout, 1930).

Those sections of the Belgian Constitution which regulate the organization of the legislative power were revised in Oct. 1921. For both Senate and Chamber all elections are held on the principle of universal suffrage.

The Senate consists of members elected for 4 years, partly directly and partly indirectly. The number elected directly is equal to half the number of members of the Chamber of Representatives. The constituent body is similar to that which elects deputies to the Chamber; the minimum age of electors is 18 years. Women were given the suffrage at parliamentary elections on 24 March 1948. In the direct elections of members of both the Senate and Chamber of Representatives the principle of proportional representation was introduced by law of 29 Dec. 1899.

Senators are elected indirectly by the provincial councils, on the basis of 1 for 200,000 inhabitants. Every addition of 125,000 inhabitants gives the right to 1 senator more. Each provincial council elects at least 3 senators. There are at present 51 provincial senators. No one, during 2 years preceding the election, must have been a member of the council appointing him. Senators are elected by the Senate itself in the proportion of half the preceding category. The senators belonging to these two latter categories are also elected by the method of proportional representation. All senators must be at least 40 years of age. They receive about 2m. francs per annum. Sons of the King, or failing these, Belgian princes of the reigning branch of the royal family, are by right senators at the age of 18, but have no voice in the deliberations till the age of 25 years; this prerogative is hardly ever used.

The members of the Chamber of Representatives are elected by the electoral body. Their number, at present 212 (law of 3 April 1965), is proportional to the population, and cannot exceed one for every 40,000 inhabitants. They sit for 4 years. Deputies must be not less than 25 years of age, and resident in Belgium.

Each deputy has an annual allowance of about 2m. francs. Senators and deputies have also free railway passes.

The Senate and Chamber meet annually in October and must sit for at least 40 days; but the King has the power of convoking extraordinary sessions and of dissolving them either simultaneously or separately. In the latter case a new election must take place within 40 days and a meeting of the chambers within 2 months.

An adjournment cannot be made for a period exceeding 1 month without the consent of the Chambers.

Constitutional legislation of Dec. 1970, July 1971, July 1974 and Aug. 1980 has led to the establishment of 3 regions with considerable autonomy: Brussels; Flanders (Dutch-speaking, seat of government at Ghent); and Wallonia (French-speaking, seat of government at Namur), all with Regional Councils and the two latter with Community Councils).

Elections were held on 13 Dec. 1987, the Flemish Christian Social Party (CVP) won 43 seats, Francophone Socialist Party (FS) 40, Flemish Socialist Party (SP) 32, Liberal Flemish Freedom and Progress Party (PVV) 25, Francophone Liberal Reform Party (PRL) 23, Francophone Christian Social Party (PSC) 19, Flemish Peoples' Union (VU) 16, Others, 14.

A 5-party coalition government was as follows in Feb. 1991:

Prime Minister: Wilfried Martens (CVP).

Deputy Prime Ministers: Philippe Moureaux, (PS) (*Restructuring of Francophone National Education and Institutional Reform*); Willy Claes, (SP) *(Economic Affairs and Planning, Restructuring of Flemish National Education)*; Jean-Luc Dehaene, (CVP) *(Communications and Institutional Reform)*; Melchior Wathelet, (PSC) *(Justice and Middle Classes)*; Hugo Schiltz, (VU) *(Budget and Scientific Policy).*

Foreign Affairs: Mark Eyskens (CVP). *Finance:* Philippe Maystadt (PSC). *Foreign Trade:* Robert Urbain (PS). *Public Affairs:* Raymond Langendries (PSC). *Post and Telecommunications:* Marcel Colla (SP). *Social Affairs:* Philippe Busquin (PS). *National Defence:* Guy Coëme (PS). *Public Works:* Paula D'Hondt Van Opdenbosch (CVP). *Interior, Modernization of Public Services, and National Scientific and Cultural Institutions:* Louis Tobback (SP). *Co-operation and Development:* André Geens (SP). *Pensions:* Gilbert Mottard (PS). *Employment and Work:* Luc Van den Brande (CVP).

There are thirteen Secretaries of State.

Local Government. Belgium has 9 provinces and since the so-called 'Amalgamation Law' of 30 Dec. 1975, 589 communes (instead of 2,359). They have a large measure of autonomous government. According to the law of 9 June 1982, all Belgians over 18 years of age, who are recorded in the registers of population of the commune have the right to vote in the communal elections. Proportional representation is applied to the communal elections, and communal councils are to be renewed every 6 years. In each commune there is a college composed of the burgomaster as the president and a certain number of aldermen.

DEFENCE. According to the Law of 30 April 1962, the Belgian Armed Forces are recruited by annual calls to the colours and by voluntary enlistments.

Military service is 10 months for conscripts serving in the Federal Republic of Germany and 12 months for those serving in Belgium, 13 months for voluntary reserve officers and 15 for the paracommando regiment. Duration of military obligation varies between 8 and 15 years for soldiers called for compulsory service.

The Medical Service has a strength of 5,785 personnel. Beside the medical units and detachments in the Armed Forces, the medical service manages 6 military hospitals and a central pharmacy.

Army. The Army comprises as major units 1 armoured and 3 mechanized brigades (2 of which are deployed as the Belgian divisions in the Belgian corps area in the Federal Republic of Germany) and 1 paracommando regiment. There are also 2 reconnaissance, 4 air defence, 1 missile, 4 engineering, 2 artillery and 2 tank battalions. Total strength (1990) 62,300. *Gendarmerie,* 15,900.

Equipment includes nearly 334 LEOPARD Main Battle Tanks, 133 SCORPION Light Tanks, 153 SCIMITAR Armoured Fighting Vehicles, 1,267 Armoured Personnel Carriers and 80 JPK 90mm Self-Propelled Anti-Tank Guns; Artillery Battalions are equipped with 155mm and 203mm Self-Propelled Howitzers, LANCE Surface-to-Surface Missiles, HAWK Surface-to-Air Missiles and GEPARD Armoured Vehicles with 35mm Anti-Aircraft Guns.

Other equipment in use: MILAN Anti-Tank Guided Weapon, STRIKER Armoured Fighting Vehicle with SWINGFIRE Anti-Tank Guided Weapon, Islander aircraft, Alouette II helicopters, Epervier Remotely Piloted Vehicle.

Navy. The naval forces, based mainly at Ostend, include 4 frigates (Navy designed and Belgian built), 6 ocean minehunters, 2 command and logistic support ships, 9 coastal tripartite minehunters (1 more building), 4 coastal minesweepers, 8 inshore minesweepers, 2 research ships, 1 ammunition transport, 6 tugs and 2 service craft. Naval personnel in 1990 totalled 4,500 officers and ratings.

The naval air arm comprises 2 Alouette SA-318 general utility helicopters.

Air Force. The Air Force has a strength of (1990) 19,900 personnel and more than 230 aircraft in 12 operational squadrons and support units. There are 5 flying wings. The all-weather fighter wing consists of 2 squadrons of F-16s. One fighter-bomber wing has 2 squadrons of F-16s. Another fighter-bomber wing operates 2 squadrons of F-16s. The fourth wing operates Mirage 5, 1 squadron fighter bomber attack and 1 squadron tactical reconnaissance fighter. The transport wing consists of 1 squadron equipped with 12 C-130H Hercules turboprop transports, and 1 squadron flying 2 Boeing 727s, 3 HS 748 twin-turboprop transports, 5 Swearingen Merlin III light turboprop transports and 2 light twin-jet Falcons. Other types in service include Sea King Mk 48 search and rescue helicopters, SIAI-Marchetti SF.260M and Alpha Jet training aircraft. Two surface-to-air missile squadrons, stationed in Germany, are equipped with Nike Hercules missiles.

INTERNATIONAL RELATIONS

Membership. Belgium is a member of the UN, EC, Benelux Economic Union, Council of Europe, NATO, OECD and WEU. The Schengen Accord of June 1990 abolished border controls between Belgium, France, Germany, Luxembourg and the Netherlands. Italy also acceded in Nov. 1990.

ECONOMY

Budget. Revenue and expenditure for both national and community and regional sectors (in 1,000m. francs):

	1984	*1985*	*1986*	*1987*	*1988*	*1989*
Receipts						
Current	1,400·1	1,487·6	1,509·6	1,567·0	1,608·8	1,638·4
Capital [1]	418·3	436·2	250·4	393·4	504·6	427·0
Total	1,818·4	1,923·8	1,760·0	1,954·4	2,113·4	2,065·4
Expenditure						
Current [2]	1,821·6	1,902·2	1,945·6	1,916·2	1,951·0	2,015·7
Capital	213·9	212·0	213·0	194·2	194·0	171·8
Total	2,035·5	2,114·0	2,158·6	2,110·4	2,145·0	2,187·5

[1] Including bond issues [2] Including debt discharges

On 31 Dec. 1989 the public debt consisted of (in 1,000m. francs): Internal debt consolidated, 3,794·7; short and middle terms, 1,760·4; at sight, 105·1.

Currency. The unit of currency is the *Belgian franc* (BEF) of 100 *centimes*.

In May 1990 the Belgian franc was pegged to operate within a very narrow band against the German Deutschmark within the European Monetary System. Note circulation 31 Dec. 1989, 442,541m. francs.

In March 1991 £1 = BFr59·95; US$1 = BFr31·60.

Banking and Finance. The bank of issue is the National Bank (*Governor*, Alfons Verplaetse), instituted in 1850. It is the cashier of the State, and is authorized to carry on the usual banking operations. Its articles of association were modified in 1948 to strengthen public control.

Savings banks: The General Savings and Superannuation Bank (*Caisse Générale d'Epargne et de Retraite*), a state institution under the authority of the Minister of Finance, consists of a unit (the Caisse d'Epargne) which performs the whole range of banking activities and a further unit which embodies the funds engaged in social security and insurance activities. It co-operates with the postal service, obviating the need of a postal-savings system. The savings deposits and savings bonds of the Caisse d'Epargne amounted to BFr1,122,937m. on 31 Dec. 1989. The Banking and Finance Commission supervises the financial situation and the activities of the Caisse d'Epargne, and also of the private savings banks, whose liabilities expressed in savings accounts and bonds amounted to BFr1,226,011m. on 31 Dec. 1989.

There is a stock exchange in Brussels. Stock exchange reforms of Jan. 1991 provided for the formation of stockbroking firms into limited companies (which may be owned by banks or insurance companies), and set new strict rules on capital adequacy. The Banking and Finance Commission (formerly the Banking Commission) was renamed and given wider powers.

Weights and Measures. The metric system is in force.

ENERGY AND NATURAL RESOURCES

Electricity. The production of electricity amounted to 61,913m. kwh. in 1988. In 1990 66% of electricity was nuclear-produced. Supply 127 and 220 volts; 50 Hz.

Gas. Production of gas (in 1m. cu. metres): 675 in 1980; 690 in 1981; 594 in 1982; 623 in 1983; 717 in 1984; 716 in 1985; 636 in 1986; 674 in 1987; 689 in 1988.

Minerals. Output (in tonnes) for 4 calendar years:

	1986	*1987*	*1988*	*1989*
Coal	5,589,208	4,356,455	2,487,217	1,892,600
Coke	5,130,229	5,226,272	5,548,724	5,458,820
Cast iron	8,047,635	8,242,366	9,146,905	8,862,655
Wrought steel	9,764,551	9,786,422	11,220,497	10,952,815
Finished steel	7,359,316	7,415,200	8,771,198	8,599,877

Agriculture. There were, in 1989, 1,361,820 ha under cultivation, of which 349,599 were under cereals, 30,979 vegetables, 122,930 industrial plants, 150,069 root crops, 637,542 pastures and meadows.

Chief	*Area in ha*			*Produce in tonnes*		
crops	*1987*	*1988*	*1989*	*1987*	*1988*	*1989*
Wheat	185,349	186,258	202,784	1,046,523	1,251,782	1,402,100
Barley	122,878	120,292	107,725	678,104	737,760	646,986
Oats	14,667	15,728	12,737	60,430	54,892	44,708
Rye	4,145	3,365	3,133	16,663	14,299	12,531
Potatoes	44,574	41,104	41,529	1,620,310	1,613,659	1,442,703
Beet (sugar)	106,189	109,316	105,800	5,425,174	6,108,603	6,061,292
Beet (fodder)	13,614	12,332	11,939	1,145,379	1,163,938	1,114,052
Tobacco	398	415	439	1,097	1,461	1,623

In 1989 there were 21,189 horses, 3,126,844 cattle, 187,789 sheep, 8,614 goats and 6,474,110 pigs.

Forestry. In 1989 forest covered 610,156 ha (20% of the land surface).

Fisheries. Fish landed, 1989: 29,255 tonnes valued at 3,020m. francs. The fishing fleet had a total tonnage of 25,445 gross tons.

INDUSTRY. Output in 1989 of sugar factories and refineries, 1,311,832 tonnes; 8 distilleries, 40,473 hectolitres of alcohol; 128 breweries, 13·16m. hectolitres of beer; margarine factories, 185,741 tonnes.

Six trusts control the greater part of Belgian industry: The Société Générale (founded in 1822) owns about 40% of coal, 50% of steel, 65% of non-ferrous metals and 35% of electricity; Brufina-Confinindus operates in steel, coal, electricity and heavy engineering; the Groupe Solvay rules the chemical industry; the Groupe Copée has interests in steel and coal; Empain controls tramways and electrical equipment; the Banque Lambert owns petroleum firms and their accessories.

FOREIGN ECONOMIC RELATIONS. By the convention concluded at Brussels on 25 July 1921 between Belgium and Luxembourg and ratified on 5 March 1922 an economic union was formed by the two countries, and the customs frontier between them was abolished on 1 May 1922. Dissolved in Aug. 1940, the union was re-established on 1 May 1945. On 14 March 1947, in execution of an agreement signed in London on 5 Sept. 1944, there was concluded a customs union between Belgium and Luxembourg, on the one hand, and the Netherlands, on the other. The union came into force on 1 Jan. 1948, and is now known as the *Benelux Economic Union.* A joint tariff has been adopted and import duties are no longer levied at the Netherlands frontier, but import licences may still be required. A full economic union of the three countries came into operation on 1 Nov. 1960.

Benelux information is supplied by the Secretariat General of the Benelux Economic Union, Rue de la Régence, 39, 1000 Brussels. It publishes *Benelux. Bulletin Trimestriel de Statistique; Statistisch Kwartaalbericht* (1955 ff.).

External debt was 1,131,100m. francs in 1990.

Commerce. Trade by selected countries (in 1,000 Belgian francs):

	Imports from 1987	1988	1989	Exports to 1987	1988	1989
France	487,806,590	522,017,828	578,609,236	633,879,572	675,428,913	804,065,350
USA	147,642,847	144,308,070	178,777,786	161,264,087	168,334,379	189,721,061
UK	244,250,202	258,982,640	305,983,040	261,011,649	315,503,055	370,114,274
Netherlands	533,407,032	602,058,448	682,275,534	465,960,727	496,597,430	540,272,029
German Dem. Rep.	7,190,164	7,275,266	8,113,111	4,760,106	5,637,680	5,425,247
Germany, Fed. Rep.	755,713,195	829,074,083	912,440,898	614,626,364	657,665,780	744,524,669
Argentina	7,321,373	9,621,813	11,696,051	2,557,859	2,725,186	1,814,051
Italy	132,439,516	144,480,019	164,462,883	197,522,718	210,426,308	251,028,430
Switzerland	60,519,623	61,273,525	63,210,391	70,898,295	77,240,373	89,594,751
Zaïre	23,934,164	31,286,766	34,297,520	10,425,291	11,312,419	12,648,337
Denmark	18,613,319	20,849,828	22,728,744	32,846,697	32,096,727	35,022,549
USSR	48,008,183	45,927,319	46,542,983	18,351,712	19,324,636	21,229,429
India	12,474,942	19,415,820	27,878,475	38,463,192	50,780,290	63,955,655
Rep. of S. Africa	14,362,466	20,687,750	28,827,991	10,205,743	13,541,472	15,192,328
Canada	21,623,568	23,241,765	25,824,494	15,070,357	17,205,073	19,045,127
Brazil	17,524,444	19,045,975	22,857,779	5,259,733	4,148,598	6,091,029
Australia	9,697,209	14,487,917	17,751,942	8,400,324	9,610,003	13,322,368

Imports and exports for 6 calendar years (in 1,000 Belgian francs):

	Imports	Exports		Imports	Exports
1984	3,195,768,712	2,992,116,161	1987	3,110,090,284	3,100,148,807
1985	3,317,811,996	3,167,691,043	1988	3,386,496,188	3,381,088,190
1986	3,065,238,630	3,070,326,871	1989	3,879,400,943	3,940,072,459

The total trade between Belgium-Luxembourg and the UK was as follows (British Department of Trade returns, in £1,000 sterling):

	1986	1987	1988	1989	1990
Imports to UK	4,083,883	4,362,463	4,956,037	5,700,534	5,732,427
Exports and re-exports from UK	3,832,605	3,857,717	4,251,961	4,872,641	5,648,625

Principal Belgian-Luxembourg exports to UK in 1989[1] (tonnes; francs): Textiles (182,102; 32,481m.); metals (897,597; 37,542m.); chemical and pharmaceutical products (647,070; 32,245m.); precious stones and manufactures thereof (374; 47,889m.).

Principal Belgian-Luxembourg imports from the UK in 1989[1] (tonnes; francs): Machinery and electrical apparatus (107,758; 57,512m.); vehicles, chiefly motor cars, and aircraft (140,563; 28,528m.); textiles (51,008; 12,588m.); precious stones (107; 95,447m.); base metals and manufactures thereof (375,049; 16,715m.).

[1] Provisional.

Tourism. In 1989 receipts totalled 120·7m. francs.

COMMUNICATIONS

Roads. Length of roads, 1990: Motorways,1,631 km; other state roads, 12,885 km; provincial roads, 1,360 km. The number of motor vehicles registered on 1 Aug. 1990 was 4,594,058, including 3,864,159 passenger cars, 15,644 buses, 343,241 lorries, 37,138 non-agricultural tractors, 152,696 agricultural tractors, 139,174 motor cycles and 42,006 special vehicles.

Railways. The main Belgian lines were a State enterprise from their inception in 1834. In 1926 the *Société Nationale des Chemins de Fer Belges (SNCB)* was formed to take over the railways. The State is sole holder of the ordinary shares of SNCB, which carry the majority vote at General Meetings. The length of railway operated in 1990 was 3,513 km, (electrified, 2,266 km). Revenue (1989), 68,604m. francs; expenditure, 67,816m. francs. In 1989, 65·9m. tonnes of freight and 142m. passengers were carried.

The *Société Nationale des Chemins de Vicinaux (SNCV)* operates electrified light railways around Charleroi (97 km) and from De Panne to Knokke (68 km). There is also a metro and tramway in Brussels, and tramways in Antwerp and Ghent.

Aviation. The national Belgian airline SABENA (*Société anonyme belge d'exploitation de la navigation aérienne*) was set up in 1923. Its capital is 750m. francs. It was announced in Nov. 1990 that it was to be partially privatized, the state retaining a 25% stake. In addition to its European network, SABENA operates different routes to North and South America, to North, Central and South Africa and to the Near, the Middle and the Far East. In 1989 its airfleet comprised 30 aircraft. In 1989 SABENA flew 72m. km, carrying 2,811,792 passengers and 662 tonne/km of freight.

Shipping. [1] On 1 Jan. 1990 the merchant fleet was composed of 69 vessels of 1,914,560 tons. There were 36 shipping companies.

[1] Belgian shipping returns are given in the official 'Moorsom tons', which may be converted into net tons by deducting 19·85% from the Moorsom total.

The navigation at the port of Antwerp in 1989 was as follows: Number of vessels entered, 15,581; tonnage, 131,623,000. Number of vessels cleared, 15,689; tonnage, 132,641,000.

The total length of navigable waterways was 1,569·3 km in 1989.

Telecommunications. On 31 Dec. 1989 there were 1,832 post offices. The gross revenue of the post office in the year 1989 amounted to 35,159m. francs.

In 1989 there were 5,138,282 telephones, 3,711,641 telephone subscribers, 32,639 mobile telephone subscribers, 60,331 subscribers to the paging service and 20,934 telex subscribers. There were 33,581 data transmission lines.

Radio-Television belge de la Communauté française (RTBF) and *Belgische Radio en Televisie* (BRT) are public institutions broadcasting in French and Dutch respectively. BRT has 5 radio programmes: BRT 1 is for service and information, documentary programmes, radio drama and light music; BRT 2 is for regional entertainment from each of the Flemish provinces. Both stations broadcast on medium-wave and on FM (stereo). BRT 3, on FM (stereo) is the cultural station; Studio Brussels (medium-wave and FM) gives information and light music for young listeners; the International Service (short- and medium-wave) aims at reaching Flemings living abroad and at presenting a picture of Flemish cultural life.

RTBF has 5 radio programmes: Radio I (medium-wave) for information; Radio II (FM stereo) for entertainment and local information; Radio III (FM stereo) for classical music; Radio 21 (FM stereo) a young people's popular music and news programme; *Radio quatre internationale* (short-wave) which broadcasts to Africa.

Each body has 2 television channels, one general and one mainly for sport, special events, cultural events, feature films; broadcasting is by PAL standards. Commercial advertising is not allowed on BRT radio or television, which are financed by the Flemish Council. In 1988 the Flemish community had 3·2m. radio receivers and 1·9m. television sets of which 85·5% were colour sets; the French-speaking community had 1·7m. radio receivers and 1·2m. television sets of which 72% were colour sets; 83·2% of the Flemish and 89% of the French-speaking households were connected to a television cable-network. Number of receivers (1989), radio, 2,161,742; TV, 3,274,236 (including 2,852,087 colour).

Cinemas (1989). There were 442 cinemas, with a seating capacity of 113,870.

Newspapers (1989). There are 35 daily newspapers (some of them only regional or local editions of larger dailies), of which 19 are in French, 15 in Dutch and 1 in German.

JUSTICE, RELIGION, EDUCATION AND WELFARE

Justice. Judges are appointed for life. There is a court of cassation, 5 courts of appeal, and assize courts for political and criminal cases. There are 27 judicial districts, each with a court of first instance. In each of the 222 cantons is a justice and judge of the peace. There are, besides, various special tribunals. There is trial by jury in assize courts.

Religion. Of the inhabitants professing a religion the majority are Roman Catholic, but no inquiry as to the profession of faith is now made at the censuses. There are, however, statistics concerning the clergy, and according to these there were in 1988: Roman Catholic higher clergy, 139; inferior clergy, 6,945; Protestant pastors, 95; Anglican Church, 12 chaplains; Jews (rabbis and ministers), 30. The State does not interfere in any way with the internal affairs of any church. There is full religious liberty, and part of the income of the ministers of all denominations is paid by the State. There are 8 Roman Catholic dioceses subdivided into 260 deaneries.

Estimated number of Protestants, 24,000; of Jews, 35,000; of Moslems, 285,000.

The Protestant (Evangelical) Church is under a synod. There is also a Central Jewish Consistory, a Central Committee of the Anglican Church and a Free Protestant Church.

Education. Following the constitutional reform of 1988, education is the responsibility of the Flemish and Wallon communities, who in 1990 received respectively BFr165,000m. and BFr135,000m.

Higher Education (1988–89). Higher education is given in state universities: Ghent (12,840 students), Liège (9,824 students), Mons (1,994 students), the Polytechnic Faculty in Mons (1,002 students), the Antwerp State University Centre (1,990 students), the Gembloux Faculty of Agronomical Sciences (886 students), the Royal Military School in Brussels (800 students) and in the private universities: Catholic University of Louvain (40,433 students), the Free University of Brussels (22,088), University Institution Antwerp (1,818 students), St Ignatius Antwerp (3,690 students), Our Lady of Peace in Namur (3,968 students), Catholic University Faculty in Mons (1,256 students), St Louis in Brussels (1,139 students), St Aloysius in Brussels (884 students), the Limbourg University Centre (728 students) and the Protestant Faculty of Theology in Brussels (123 students). The total number of students in university colleges, faculties and institutes was 105,463.

There are 5 royal academies of fine arts and 5 royal conservatoires at Brussels, Liège, Ghent, Antwerp and Mons.

Secondary Education. 2,107 (1988–89) middle schools had a total of 89,673 pupils in the general classes and 127,521 in the technical classes in the traditional system and 605,918 pupils in the new system.

Elementary Education. There were 4,439 (1988–89) primary schools, with 755,609 pupils and 4,125 (1988–89) infant schools, with 369,398 pupils.

Normal Schools. Under the French and German linguistic systems there were 23 (1988–89) schools for training secondary teachers (2,148 students); 31 for training elementary teachers (2,365 students); 20 technical normal schools with 757 students and 16 normal infant schools with 1,598 pupils.

Health. In 1989 there were 32,571 physicians (including 456 dentists), 6,448 other dentists and 11,629 pharmacists. Hospital beds numbered 51,081 on 1 Jan. 1988.

Social Security. Social security is based on the law of Dec. 1944. It applies to all workers subject to an employment contract, and is administered by the Central National Office of Social Security (ONSS), which collects from employers and employees all contributions referring to family allowances, health insurance, old age insurance, holidays and unemployment. These sums are distributed by the Central Office to the various institutions concerned with these benefits. Insurance against unemployment is organized through a common fund, which also undertakes to retrain the unemployed for another employment while providing for their families. Since 1944 further laws have increased allowances, made fresh provisions for housing (1945), injuries while working, professional illnesses, etc. (1948).

Apart from private charity, the poor are assisted by the communes through the agency of the *Centre Public d'Aide Sociale* in French-speaking parts of the country and *Openbaar Centrum voor Maatschappelijk Welzijn* in Dutch-speaking areas. Provisions of a national character have been made for looking after war orphans and men disabled in the war. Certain other establishments, either state or provincial, provide for the needs of the deaf-mutes and the blind, and of children who are placed under the control of the courts. Provision is also made for repressing begging and providing shelter for the homeless.

DIPLOMATIC REPRESENTATIVES

Of Belgium in Great Britain (103 Eaton Sq., London, SW1W 9AB)
Ambassador: Herman Dehennin.

Of Great Britain in Belgium (Britannia Hse., rue Joseph II 28, 1040 Brussels)
Ambassador: Robert James O'Neill, CMG.

Of Belgium in the USA (3330 Garfield St., NW, Washington, D.C., 20008)
Ambassador: J. Cassiers.

Of the USA in Belgium (Blvd. du Régent 27, 1000 Brussels)
Ambassador: Bruce Gelb.

Of Belgium to the United Nations
Ambassador: P. Noterdaeme.

Further Reading

Statistical Information: The Institut National de Statistique (44 rue de Louvain, Brussels) was established on 24 Jan. 1831, under the designation of Bureau de Statistique Générale; after several changes, it received its present name on 2 May 1946. *Director-General (in charge):* L. Diels. *Main publications:*

Statistiques du commerce extérieur (monthly)
Bulletin de Statistique. Bi-monthly
Annuaire Statistique de la Belgique (from 1870).—*Annuaire statistique de poche* (from 1965)
Statistiques Agricoles. Irregular

Annuaire administratif et judiciaire de Belgique. Annual. Brussels
L'économie belge. Ministère des Affaires Economiques. Annual (from 1947)
Guide des Ministères: Revue de l'Administration Belge. Brussels, Annual
Riley, R. C., *Belgium*. [Bibliography] Oxford and Santa Barbara, 1989

BELIZE

Capital: Belmopan
Population: 193,000 (1990)
GNP per capita: US$1,460 (1988)

HISTORY. The early settlement of the territory was probably effected by British woodcutters about 1638; from that date to 1798, in spite of armed opposition from the Spaniards, settlers held their own and prospered. In 1780 the Home Government appointed a superintendent, and in 1862 the settlement was declared a colony, subordinate to Jamaica. It became an independent colony in 1884. Self-government was attained in 1964. Independence was achieved on 21 Sept. 1981.

AREA AND POPULATION. Belize is bounded in the north by Mexico, west and south by Guatemala and east by the Caribbean. Fringing the coast there are 3 atolls and some 400 islets (cays) in the world's second longest barrier reef (140 miles). Area, 22,963 sq. km. There are 6 districts:

	Sq. km	*Population census, 1980*		*Sq. km*	*Population census, 1980*
Corozal	1,860	22,902	Cayo	5,338	22,337
Belize	4,204	50,801	Stann Creek	2,176	14,181
Orange Walk	4,737	22,870	Toledo	4,649	11,762

Total population (census, 1980) 145,353. Estimate (1990) 193,000. In 1989 the birth rate per 1,000 was 37·2 and the death rate 4·2; infantile mortality 19·4 per 1,000 births and there were 1,138 marriages.

English is the official language. Spanish is spoken by 31·6% of the population. The main ethnic groups are Creole (African descent), Mestizo (Spanish-Maya) and Garifuna (Caribs).

Main city, Belize City; population, census 1980, 39,771. Estimate (1989) 43,621. Following the severe hurricane which struck the territory on 31 Oct. 1961 the then capital Belmopan was moved to a new site 50 miles inland; construction began in Jan. 1967 and it became the seat of government on 3 Aug. 1970 (population, 1989, 5,276). *See* map in the 1978–79 edition of THE STATESMAN'S YEAR-BOOK.

CLIMATE. A tropical climate with high rainfall and small annual range of temperature. The driest months are Feb. and March. Belize, Jan. 74°F (23·3°C), July 81°F (27·2°C). Annual rainfall 76" (1,890 mm).

CONSTITUTION AND GOVERNMENT. Having achieved self-government in Jan. 1964 delays occurred in achieving independence because of the outstanding territorial claim by Guatemala. Attempts to reach agreement on the claim finally failed prior to independence being granted, but guarantees were given by Britain that a military force would remain.

The Constitution, which came into force on 21 Sept. 1981, provided for a National Assembly, with a 5-year term, comprising a 28-member House of Representatives elected by universal adult suffrage, and a Senate consisting of 8 members appointed by the Governor-General on the advice of the Prime Minister, 2 on the advice of the Leader of the Opposition and 1 on the advice of the Belize Advisory Council.

At the general election in Sept. 1989 the People's United Party won 15 seats in the House of Representatives and the United Democratic Party 13.

Governor-General: Dame Elmira Minita Gordon, GCMG, GCVO.

The cabinet in Oct. 1990 was composed as follows:

Prime Minister and Minister of Finance, Trade, Commerce, Home Affairs and Defence: The Rt Hon. George Cadle Price.

Deputy Prime Minister and Minister of Natural Resources: Florencio Marin. *Foreign Affairs, Economic Development and Education:* Said Musa. *Industry, Hous-*

ing and Co-operatives: Leopoldo Briceño. *Works:* Samuel Waight. *Health and Urban Development:* Dr Theodore Aranda. *Attorney-General and Minister of Tourism and the Environment:* Glenn Godfrey. *Social Services and Community Development:* Remijio Montejo. *Agriculture and Fisheries:* Michael Espat. *Labour, Public Service and Local Government:* Valdemar Castillo. *Energy and Communications:* Carlos Diaz.

There are 5 Ministers of State.

Flag: Blue with red band along the top and bottom edges. In the centre a white disc containing the coat of arms surrounded by a green garland.

DEFENCE. In June 1990 Belize assumed full responsibility for the Belize Defence Force, which consists of 1 infantry battalion, with 4 active and 3 reserve companies. The Air Wing operates two twin-engined BN-2B Defenders for maritime patrol and transport duties. There is also a Maritime wing of the Belize Defence Force. It operates 2 armed Wasp patrol vessels and a number of smaller vessels utilized for anti-smuggling and coast guard duties. Naval personnel (1991) 50. British Army Forces in Belize number about 1,500, including a detachment of the Royal Air Force which deploys Harrier V/STOL ground attack/reconnaissance aircraft. Personnel (1991) 300.

INTERNATIONAL RELATIONS

Membership. Belize is a member of the UN, the Commonwealth, OAS, CARICOM and is an ACP state of the EEC.

ECONOMY

Budget. In 1990–91 envisaged expenditure of $B260·9m., of which $B37·4m. were earmarked for administration, $B27·5m. for law and order and defence, $B66·5m. for social services, $B40m. for education, $B30·7m. for agriculture and $B45·9m. for transport and communications.

Public external debt, 31 Dec. 1988, US$116·1m.

Currency. The unit of currency is the *Belize dolar* (BZD) of 100 *cents*. There are notes of $B100, 20, 10, 5 and 1, and coins of 1-, 5-, 10-, 25- and 50-cent and $B1. In March 1991, £1 = $B3·80 and US$1 = $B2.

Banking. A Central Bank was established in 1981. There were (1987) 4 commercial banks with a total of 14 branches: Belize Bank, Barclays Bank PLC, Bank of Nova Scotia and the locally incorporated Atlantic Bank. The Development Finance Corporation provides long-term credit for development of agriculture and industry. There were (1985) 7 government savings banks and 17 insurance companies, and (1989) 40 registered credit unions. Amendments to the Banking Ordinance permit offshore banking.

ENERGY AND NATURAL RESOURCES

Electricity. Production (1988) 90·5m. kwh. Supply 110 and 220 volts; 60 Hz.

Oil. Several oil companies were (1990) exploring for oil both off-shore and on-shore. Oil was discovered in the north in 1981 but not in commercial quantities.

Agriculture. In 1986 agriculture provided 65% of total foreign exchange earnings and employed 30% of the total labour force. The main agricultural export is sugar, followed by citrus fruit, chiefly grapefruit and oranges processed into oil, squash and concentrates. Citrus production, 1989, 1,447,834 boxes of oranges, 889,092 boxes of grapefruit. Sugar-cane production in 1989 was 867,267 tonnes. Bananas are the third export crop; production, 1989, 1,440,099 boxes. [Ed. note: Box of grapefruit, 80 lb., oranges, 90 lb., bananas, 42 lb.]. Cacao is becoming increasingly important as an export crop. Mangoes are also grown commercially; production, 1989, 200 tonnes. Main cultivated food crops (with production, 1989) are maize (51,104,859 lb), rice (11,115,000 lb) and red kidney beans (9,279,925 lb). Belize is self-sufficient in fresh beef and pork, poultry and eggs. A dairy plant (daily milk processing capacity 400 gallons) began operations in 1986. Beekeeping co-operatives produced 206,216 lb of honey in 1989.

Livestock (1988): Cattle, 54,025; sheep, 2,585; pigs, 16,417; poultry, 2·5m.

Forestry. 1m. ha, 44% of the total land area, were under forests in 1988, which include mahogany, cedar, Santa Maria, pine and rosewood, and many secondary hardwoods of known or probable market value, as well as woods suitable for pulp production. Exports of forest produce in 1989 amounted to $B4·7m.

Fisheries. There were (1988) 8 registered fishing co-operatives. Food and game fish are plentiful, and domestic consumption is heavy. Main export markets for scale fish are in the USA, Mexico and Jamaica. Fish products exported in 1989 to the USA were valued at $B12.8m. Turtles—Hawksbill, Loggerhead and Green—are plentiful but as yet are not exported. There were 747 fishing vessels in 1988.

INDUSTRY. In 1989 production of the major commodities was: Sugar, 90,934 tonnes; molasses, 28,440 tonnes; cigarettes, 97·1m.; beer, 740,000 gallons; batteries, 8,835; wheat flour, 21·5m. lb.; rum 15,000 proof gallons; fertilizer, 8,954 tonnes; garments, 3,492,000; citrus concentrates, 3,029,000 gallons; soft drinks, 881,000 cases.

Labour. The labour market alternates between full employment, often accompanied by local shortages in the citrus and sugar-cane harvesting (Jan.–July), and under-employment during the wet season (Aug.–Dec.), aggravated by the seasonal nature of the major industries.

Trade Unions. There are 14 accredited unions with an estimated membership of 8,200.

FOREIGN ECONOMIC RELATIONS

Commerce. In 1989 total imports amounted to $B431·4m. Total exports, $B248·1m. The principal domestic exports were timber ($B4·7m.), 78,750 long tons of sugar ($B68·1m.), fish products ($B38·9m.), garments, 1988 ($B37·3m.), 56·6m. lbs of bananas, 1·85m. gallons of citrus products ($B57·6m.), molasses ($B1·3m.) and honey ($B200,000).

Total trade between Belize and UK (British Department of Trade returns, in £1,000 sterling):

	1986	*1987*	*1988*	*1989*	*1990*
Imports to UK	17,954	22,757	22,461	24,272	22,734
Exports and re-exports from UK	8,232	7,543	12,064	11,842	12,439

Tourism. Tourists totalled 216,187 in 1989 spending US$35m.

COMMUNICATIONS

Roads. There are four major highways and all principal towns and villages are linked by road to Belmopan and Belize City. In 1988, there were 14,014 licensed vehicles.

Aviation. The Philip Goldson International Airport is 14 km from Belize City. In 1989, 5 airlines maintained international services to and from the USA, Central America and Mexico. In 1988, 765,430 passengers arrived and departed on international flights. Domestic air services provide connections to all main towns and 3 of the main offshore islands.

Shipping. The main port is Belize City, with a modern deep water port able to handle containerized shipping. During 1989, 276 port calls were made by cargo vessels carrying 304,960 short tons of cargo. The second largest port, Commerce Bight just south of Dangriga, can accommodate vessels up to 23 ft draft.

Telecommunications. Number of telephones (1990), 15,917 (8,628 in Belize City). Belize Telecommunications Ltd has instituted a country-wide fully automatic telephone dialling facility. There are 7 main post offices and 61 sub-post offices.

In Aug. 1990, the Belize Broadcasting Network became the Broadcasting Corporation of Belize (BCB). The BCB broadcasts daily. Proportion of programmes; 70% in English: 25% in Spanish and 5% in the Maya, Mopan, Maya Ketchi and Garifuna dialects. In 1989 there were 12 television stations. There are satellite links with Bermuda, the USA and the UK, and radio links with Central America.

Cinemas (1988). There were 5 cinemas with seating capacity of 5,000.

Newspapers. There were 4 weekly newspapers and 2 monthly magazines in 1990.

JUSTICE, RELIGION, EDUCATION AND WELFARE

Justice. Each of the 6 judicial districts has summary jurisdiction courts (criminal) and district courts (civil), both of which are presided over by magistrates. There is a Supreme Court, a Court of Appeal and a Family Court was established in May 1989 to deal with domestic and juvenile cases. There is a Director of Public Prosecutions, a Chief Justice and 2 Puisne Judges.

Religion. In 1986 about 62% of the population was Roman Catholic and 28% Protestant, including Anglican, Methodist, Seventh Day Adventist, Mennonite, Nazarene, Jehovah's Witness, Pentecostal and Baptist. There was a small group of Bahai.

Education. State education is managed by the main religious groups, Roman Catholic and Anglican. It is compulsory for children between 6-14 years and primary education is free. In 1989, 228 primary schools had a total enrolment of 44,000 pupils with 1,861 teachers; 31 secondary schools, 8,814 pupils with, in 1988, 576 teachers; (1987) 8 other technical schools, 932 students with 69 teachers. The Belize Teachers' College offers courses for primary and secondary school teachers. The 2-year course leads to a teachers' diploma. The University College of Belize opened in 1986. There is 1 government-maintained special school for handicapped children. The University of the West Indies maintains an extra-mural department in Belize City.

93% literacy was claimed in 1991.

Health. In 1990 there were 7 government hospitals (1 in Belmopan, 1 in Belize City and 1 in each of the other 5 districts) and an infirmary for geriatric and chronically ill patients, with 94 doctors and 525 hospital beds. Medical services in rural areas are provided by health care centres and mobile clinics.

DIPLOMATIC REPRESENTATIVES

Of Belize in Great Britain (200 Sutherland Ave., London, W9 1RX)
High Commissioner: David MacKilligan.

Of Great Britain in Belize (P.O. Box 91, Belmopan)
High Commissioner: P. A. B. Thomson, CVO.

Of Belize in the USA (3400 International Dr., NW, Washington, D.C., 20008)
Ambassador: James Hyde.

Of the USA in Belize (Gabourel Lane and Hutson St., Belize City)
Ambassador: Richard G. Rich, Jr.

Of Belize to the United Nations
Ambassador: Carl Lindberg B. Rogers.

Further Reading

Abstract of Statistics 1981. Government Printer, Belize City, 1982
Belize Today. Government Printer, monthly
Bianchi, W. J., *Belize: The Controversy Between Guatemala and Great Britain.* New York, 1959
Dobson, D., *A History of Belize.* Belize, 1973
Fernandez, J., *Belize: Case Study for Democracy in Central America.* Aldershot, 1989
Grant, C. H., *The Making of Modern Belize.* CUP, 1976
Setzekorn, W. D., *Formerly British Honduras: A Profile of the New Nation of Belize.* Ohio Univ. Press, 1981
Woodward, R. L., Jr, *Belize.* [Bibliography] Oxford and Santa Barbara, 1980

BENIN

Capital: Porto-Novo
Population: 4·76m. (1990)
GNP per capita: US$340 (1988)

République du Bénin

HISTORY. The territory of the present State was occupied by France in 1892 and was constituted a division of French West Africa in 1904 under the name of Dahomey. It became an independent republic within the French Community on 4 Dec. 1958, and acquired full independence on 1 Aug. 1960.

In the sixth coup since independence, Maj. Mathieu (now Ahmed) Kerekou came to power on 26 Oct. 1972 and proclaimed a Marxist–Leninist state, whose name was altered from Dahomey to Benin on 1 Dec. 1975.

In Dec. 1989 the leadership abandoned Marxism-Leninism and called a national conference in Feb. 1990 to steer the country towards pluralist democracy.

AREA AND POPULATION. Benin is bounded east by Nigeria, north by Niger and Burkina Faso, west by Togo and south by the Gulf of Guinea. The area is 112,622 sq. km, and the population, census 1979, 3,338,240. Estimate (1990) 4,758,000.

Vital statistics, 1985–90: Growth rate, 3·2%; infant mortality, 110 per 1,000; expectation of life, 40·6 years.

The seat of government is Porto-Novo (208,258 inhabitants in 1982); the chief port and business centre is Cotonou (487,020 in 1982); other important towns (1982) are Parakou (65,945), Natitingou (50,800, 1979), Abomey (54,418), Kandi (53,000) and Ouidah. On 1 Jan. 1988 there were 3,033 refugees in Benin, primarily from Chad.

The areas, populations and capitals of the 6 provinces are as follows:

Province	*Sq. km*	*Census 1979*	*Estimate 1987*	*Capital*
Atakora	31,200	479,604	622,000	Natitingou
Borgou	51,000	490,669	630,000	Parakou
Zou	18,700	570,433	731,000	Abomey
Mono	3,800	477,378	610,000	Lokossa
Atlantique	3,200	686,258	909,000	Cotonou
Ouéme	4,700	626,868	806,000	Porto-Novo

French is the official language, while 47% of the people speak Fon, 12% Adja, 10% Bariba, 9% Yoruba, 6% Fulani, 5% Somba and 5% Aizo.

CLIMATE. In coastal parts there is an equatorial climate, with a long rainy season from March to July and a short rainy season in Oct. and Nov. The dry season increases in length from the coast, with inland areas having rain only between May and Sept. Porto Novo. Jan. 82°F (27·8°C), July 78°F (25·6°C). Annual rainfall 52" (1,300 mm). Cotonou. Jan. 81°F (27·2°C), July 77°F (25°C). Annual rainfall 53" (1,325 mm).

CONSTITUTION AND GOVERNMENT. The Benin Party of Popular Revolution (PRPB) held a monopoly of power from 1977 to 1989 in the unicameral 64-member National Revolutionary Assembly.

In Feb. 1990 a 'National Conference of the Vital Elements (*'Vives forces'*) of the Nation proclaimed its sovereignty and appointed Nicéphore Soglo *Prime Minister* of a provisional government. At the elections of Feb. 1991 24 of the 34 legal parties fielded candidates and 17 gained seats.

The office of the *President*, Brig.-Gen. Ahmed Kerekou, became largely ceremonial in 1990. Presidential elections were due in March 1991.

National flag: Horizontally yellow over red with a green vertical strip in the hoist.

Local Government. The 6 provinces, each governed by an appointed Prefect and a Provincial Revolutionary Council, are divided into 84 districts.

DEFENCE. National service is for a period of 18 months.

Army. The Army consists of 3 infantry, 1 para-commando and 1 engineer battalions, 1 armoured reconnaissance squadron and 1 artillery battery. Strength (1991) 3,800, with an additional 2,000-strong paramilitary gendarmerie.

Navy. A naval force was formed in 1979 with 2 Soviet torpedo craft and 4 inshore patrol craft. A new French inshore patrol craft was delivered in 1987, but all are now believed unserviceable. Personnel in 1990 numbered 200, and the force is based at Cotonou.

Air Force. The Air Force had a strength of (1990) about 350 officers and men, 2 twin-turboprop An-26 and 2 C-47 transports, 1 Cessna Skymaster, 1 Aero Commander 500, 2 Broussard communications aircraft and 2 Ecureuil helicopters.

INTERNATIONAL RELATIONS

Membership. Benin is a member of the UN, OAU and is an ACP state of EEC.

ECONOMY

Policy. A 10-year development plan (1981–90) envisaged an expenditure of 958,800m. francs CFA.

Budget. In 1987 revenue, 51,929m. francs CFA and expenditure, 53,737m. francs CFA.

Currency. The monetary unit is the *franc CFA* (XOF), with a parity value of 50 *francs CFA* to 1 French *franc*. There are coins of 1, 2, 5, 10, 25, 50 and 100 *francs CFA*, and banknotes of 50, 100, 500, 1,000, 5,000 and 10,000 *francs CFA*. In March 1991, £1 = 496·13 *francs CFA*; US$1 = 261·53 *francs CFA*.

Banking and Finance. The *Banque Centrale des Etats de l'Afrique de l'Ouest* is the bank of issue and the central bank. The *Banque Commerciale du Bénin*, in Cotonou, conducts all government business.

ENERGY AND NATURAL RESOURCES

Electricity. *Société Béninoise d'Electricité et d'Eau*, produced 172m. kwh in 1985 from generating plants at Cotonou, Porto-Novo and Parakou. Major development of hydro-electric resources along the Mono river are being conducted jointly with Togo. Supply 220 volts; 50 Hz.

Oil. The Semé oilfield, located 10 miles offshore, was discovered in 1968. Production commenced in 1982 and reached 200,000 tonnes in 1989.

Agriculture. 90% of the population subsist by agriculture. The chief products, 1988 (in 1,000 tonnes) were: Cassava, 725; yams, 850; maize, 432; sorghum, 105; groundnuts, 67; dry beans, 45; rice, 9; and sweet potatoes, 34, while cash crops were palm kernels, 20, and palm oil, 40. Cotton cultivation has been successfully introduced in the north; coffee cultivation has given good results in the south.

Livestock (1988 in 1,000): Cattle (914), sheep (860), goats (960), pigs (648), poultry (23,000), horses (6), asses (1).

Forestry. There were (1988) 3·6m ha of forest (43% of the land area), mainly in the north. Roundwood production in 1986 was 4·5m. cu. metres.

Fisheries. Total catch in 1986 was 23,500 tonnes (68% from inland and lagoon waters).

INDUSTRY. Industrial plants are few, limited mainly to palm-oil processing and brewing. There is a sugar complex at Savé, a cement plant at Onigbolo and textile mills at Cotonou and Parakou. Production (1985) included 51,000 tonnes of sugar, 37,000 tonnes of palm oil and 318,000 tonnes of cement.

Labour. In 1973 the small trade unions were amalgamated to form a single body, now named the *Union Nationale des Syndicats des Travailleurs du Bénin.*

FOREIGN ECONOMIC RELATIONS.

Foreign debt was some US$1,005m. in 1988.

Commerce. Imports in 1983, US$113m.; exports, US$78m. The main exports are palm oil and kernels, cocoa, cotton and sugar. In 1984, 32% of exports were to Spain, 21% to Federal Republic of Germany and 16% to France, which provided the largest share (23%) of imports.

Total trade between Benin and UK (British Department of Trade returns, in £1,000 sterling):

	1986	*1987*	*1988*	*1989*	*1990*
Imports to UK	4,910	2,930	2,450	356	1,197
Exports and re-exports from UK	6,728	7,207	8,169	7,294	6,130

Tourism. There were 72,000 foreign tourists in 1985.

COMMUNICATIONS

Roads. There were 7,445 km of roads in 1985, 2,740 passenger cars and 567 goods vehicles.

Railways. There are 579 km of metre-gauge railway. One line connects Cotonou with Parakou (438 km) and is being extended to Dosso (in Niger); the second runs from Cotonou *via* Porto-Novo to Pobé (107 km); and the third from Cotonou *via* Ouidah to Segboroué on the Togo frontier (34 km), continuing to Lomé. In 1988 1·5m. passengers and 184m. tonne-km of freight were carried.

Aviation. In 1981, 80,400 passengers and 9,763 tonnes of freight passed through Cotonou airport.There are other airports at Abomey, Natitingou, Kandi and Parakou.

Shipping. In 1983, 736,000 tonnes were unloaded and 64,400 tonnes loaded at the port of Cotonou. There were (1986) 15 vessels of 4,887 GRT registered in Benin.

Telecommunications. There were, in 1985, 8,650 telephones. Telegraph lines connect Cotonou with Togo, Niger and Senegal. In 1984 there were 68,000 radios and 17,250 television receivers.

Cinemas. In 1976 there were 4 cinemas with a seating capacity of 4,400.

Newspapers. In 1990 there were 31 daily newspapers.

JUSTICE, RELIGION, EDUCATION AND WELFARE

Justice. The Supreme Court is at Cotonou. There are Magistrates Courts in Cotonou, Porto-Novo, Natitingou, Abomey, Kandi, Ouidah and Parakou, and a *tribunal de conciliation* in each district.

Religion. 61% of the population follow animist beliefs, chiefly Voodoo, about 22% are Christian, mainly Roman Catholic, and 15% Moslem.

Education. There were, in 1988, 471,016 pupils in 2,850 primary schools and 97,000 in 184 secondary schools. The University of Benin (Cotonou) had 6,302 students in 1983. Adult literacy (1980) 28%.

Health. In 1982 there were 6 hospitals, 31 health centres, 186 dispensaries and 65 maternity clinics with (1978, combined) 4,968 beds, and in 1979 there were 204 doctors, 13 dentists, 55 pharmacists and 1,294 midwives.

DIPLOMATIC REPRESENTATIVES

Of Benin in Great Britain
Ambassador: Souler Issoufou Idrissou (resides in Paris).

Of Great Britain in Benin
Ambassador: B. L. Barder (resides in Lagos).

Of Benin in the USA (2737 Cathedral Ave., NW, Washington, D.C., 20008)
Ambassador: Theophile Nata.

Of the USA in Benin (Rue Caporal Anani Bernard, Cotonou)
Ambassador: Harriet W. Isom.

Of Benin to the United Nations
Ambassador: René Valéry Mongbe.

BERMUDA

Capital: Hamilton
Population: 59,066 (1989)
GNP per capita: US$21,300 (1989)

HISTORY. The Spaniards visited the islands in 1515, but, according to a 17th-century French cartographer, they were discovered in 1503 by Juan Bermudez, after whom they were named. No settlement was made, and they were uninhabited until a party of colonists under Sir George Somers was wrecked there in 1609. A company was formed for the 'Plantation of the Somers' Islands', as they were called at first, and in 1684 the Crown took over the government.

AREA AND POPULATION. Bermuda consists of a group of some 150 small islands (about 20 inhabited), situated in the western Atlantic (32° 18' N. lat., 64° 46' W. long.); the nearest point of the mainland, about 570 miles distant, is Cape Hatteras, N.C., and 690 miles from New York.

The area is 20·59 sq. miles (53·3 sq. km), of which 2·3 sq. miles were leased in 1941 for 99 years to the US Government for naval and air bases. The civil population (i.e., excluding British and American military, naval and air force personnel) in 1980 (Census) was 54,893. Estimate (1989) 59,066.

Chief town, Hamilton; population, about 3,000.

In 1988 there were 935 live births, 868 marriages and 399 deaths; infantile mortality rate was 3·2 per 1,000 live births.

CLIMATE. A pleasantly warm and humid climate, with up to 60" (1,500 mm) of rain, spread evenly throughout the year. Hamilton. Jan. 63°F (17·2°C), July 79°F (26·1°C). Annual rainfall 58" (1,463 mm).

CONSTITUTION AND GOVERNMENT. Bermuda is a colony with representative government. Under the constitution of 8 June 1968 the Governor, appointed by the Crown, is normally bound to accept the advice of the Cabinet in matters other than external affairs, defence, internal security and the police, for which he retains special responsibility. The Cabinet is appointed from among members of the bicameral legislature, on the recommendation of the Premier. The Senate, of whom one or two members may serve on Cabinet, consists of 11 members. As a result of a Constitutional Conference held in Feb. 1979, it was decided that 5 Senators would be appointed by the Governor on the recommendation of the Premier, 3 by the Governor on the recommendation of the Opposition Leader and 3 by the Governor in his own discretion. The 40 members of the House of Assembly are elected 2 from each of 20 constituencies under full universal, adult suffrage. A general election was held in Feb. 1989. The United Bermuda Party won 23 seats, the Progressive Labour Party 15, and others, 2.

Governor: Sir Desmond Langley, KCVO, MBE.
Premier: Sir John W. D. Swan, KBE.
Flag: The British Red Ensign with the badge of the Colony in the fly.

DEFENCE. The Bermuda Regiment had 734 men and women in 1989.

ECONOMY

Budget. Revenue and expenditure in BD$1,000 for years ending 31 March:

	1986–87	*1987–88*	*1988–89*	*1989–90*	*1990–91*
Revenue	231,509	251,550	297,639	307,439	347,294
Expenditure	200,706	220,172	245,542	274,738	314,010

Expenditure in BD$1,000 (excluding capital items) was earmarked as follows:

	1985–86	*1986–87*	*1987–88*	*1988–89*	*1989–90*
Education	25,585	27,853	30,063	32,775	35,409
Health and Social Services	434,100	491,600	565,783	801,500	854,000
Public Works	20,195	21,427	25,713	27,226	30,958
Police	15,970	17,204	18,589	20,572	22,715
Tourism	17,793	19,383	22,316	25,508	26,230
Marine and Ports Services	5,127	5,852	6,809	7,246	7,527
Public Transportation	93,200	77,800	3,932	5,318	4,887
Agriculture and Fisheries	5,719	6,126	6,747	7,647	8,292
Post Office	5,022	5,991	6,724	6,828	7,804

The estimated chief sources of revenue in 1988–89 were: Customs duties, $115m.; employment tax, $23·9m.; land tax, $12m.; hospital levy, $30m.; vehicle licenses, $9,513,000; stamp duties, $13m.; passenger taxes, $10·4m. Public debt, as at 31 March 1989, was nil.

Currency. Decimal currency based on a *Bermuda dollar* (BMD) of 100 *cents* was introduced 6 Feb. 1970. The Bermuda Monetary Authority issues notes in denominations of BD$100, 50, 20, 10, 5 and 1, and coins in values of BD$5, 1, 50c, 25c, 10c, 5c and 1c. In March 1991 £1 = BD$1.90 and US$1 = BD$1.

Banking. There are 3 banks, the Bank of Bermuda, Ltd, the Bank of N. T. Butterfield and Son, Ltd, and the Bermuda Commercial Bank, Ltd, with correspondent banks and representatives in either New York, London, Canada or Hong Kong.

Weights and Measures. Metric, except that US and Imperial (British) measures are used in certain fields.

ENERGY AND NATURAL RESOURCES

Electricity. Production (1989) 418m. kwh. Supply 115 volts; 60 Hz.

Agriculture. The chief products are fresh vegetables, bananas and citrus fruit. In 1989, 845 acres were being used for pasture, forage or fallow. 6,555 persons were employed in agriculture, fishing and quarrying.

In 1989, total value of agricultural products was BD$10,612,290.

Livestock (1988): Cattle, 1,000; pigs, 2,000; goats, 1,000.

INDUSTRY

Trade Unions. Legislation providing for trade unions was enacted in Oct. 1946, and there are 9 trade unions with a total membership (1989) of 8,278.

FOREIGN ECONOMIC RELATIONS. The visible adverse balance of trade is more than compensated for by invisible exports, including tourism and offshore insurance business.

Commerce. Imports and exports in BD$:

	1987	*1988*	*1989*
Imports	419,939,867	488,285,238	534,409,715
Exports	29,218,856	30,815,235	50,398,458

Imports in 1988 from USA, $303m.; UK, $48m.; Canada, $31m; Japan, $29m.

In 1988 the principal imports were food, drink and tobacco ($98m.); electric equipment ($50m.); clothing ($37m.), transport equipment ($37m.). The bulk of exports comprise sales of fuel to aircraft and ships, and re-exports of pharmaceuticals.

Total trade between Bermuda and UK, in £1,000 sterling (British Department of Trade returns):

	1986	*1987*	*1988*	*1989*	*1990*
Imports to UK	1,262	1,208	6,767	4,517	12,849
Exports and re-exports from UK	26,180	25,383	24,995	27,122	28,114

Tourism. In 1989, 547,371 tourists visited Bermuda.

COMMUNICATIONS

Roads. In 1948 the railway service was discontinued and a government-operated bus service introduced.

Between 1908 and Aug. 1946 the use of motor vehicles, with the exception of ambulances, fire engines and other essential services, was prohibited. In 1988, out of 44,518 registered vehicles, 18,339 were private cars.

Aviation. Bermuda is served on a regularly scheduled basis by Air Canada, British Airways, American Airlines, Delta Airlines, Eastern Airlines, Pan American World Airways, Continental and Piedmont. Bermuda is connected by direct flights to Toronto, Canada; New York, Newark, Baltimore, Boston, Raleigh Durham, Tampa, Philadelphia and Atlanta in the USA; and London. The Caribbean is reached through scheduled connexions in the USA and Europe is reached through Gatwick.

Shipping. In 1989, there were 172 visits by cruise ships, 239 visits by cargo ships and 24 visits by oil and gas tankers.

Telecommunications (1989). There are 15 post offices. The Bermuda Telephone Company is privately owned. There is International Direct Dialling to over 140 countries. Cable and Wireless Ltd provide external communications including telephone, telex, packet-switching, facsimile and electronic mail in conjunction with the Bermuda Telephone Company, and an International Database Access Service. Radio and television broadcasting is commercial.

Newspapers (1989). There is 1 daily newspaper with a circulation of 17,961 and 3 weeklies with a total circulation of 27,500.

JUSTICE, EDUCATION AND WELFARE

Justice. There are 3 magistrates' courts, 3 Supreme Courts and a court of appeal. The police had a strength of 476 men and women in 1989.

Education. Education is compulsory between the ages of 5 and 16, and government assistance is given by the payment of grants, and, where necessary, of school fees. In 1988, there were 18 primary schools, 14 secondary schools (of which 5 are private, including 2 denominational schools and one run by the US Armed Forces in Bermuda), 4 special schools at the primary and secondary levels for handicapped persons aged 14–21, and 11 pre–schools. There were 428 full-time students attending the Bermuda College in 1988. Extra-mural courses are available from Queen's University in Canada and the University of Maryland in the USA.

Health. In 1988 there were 2 hospitals, 57 doctors, 23 dentists, 643 nurses and 35 pharmacists.

Further Reading

Report of the Manpower Survey 1989. Hamilton, 1989
Bermuda Report, Second Edition 1985–88. Hamilton, 1988
Bermuda Historical Quarterly. 1944 ff.
Hayward, S. J., Holt-Gomez, V. and Sterrer, W.,, *Bermuda's Delicate Balance: People and the Environment*. Hamilton, 1981
Warwick, J. B., (ed.) *Who's Who in Bermuda 1980–81*. Hamilton, 1982
Wilkinson, H. C., *Bermuda from Sail to Steam*. OUP, 1973
Zuill, W. S., *The Story of Bermuda and Her People*. London, 1973

National Library: The Bermuda Library, Hamilton. *Head Librarian:* Cyril O. Packwood.

BHUTAN

Capital: Thimphu
Population: 1·4m. (1990)
GNP per capita: US$217 (1989)

Druk-yul

(Kingdom of Bhutan)

HISTORY. In 1774 the East India Company concluded a treaty with the ruler of Bhutan. Under a treaty signed in Nov. 1865 the Bhutan Government was granted an annual subsidy. By an amending treaty concluded in Jan. 1910 the British Government undertook to exercise no interference in the internal affairs of Bhutan, and the Bhutan Government agreed to be guided by the advice of the British Government in regard to its external relations.

The Government of India concluded a fresh treaty with Bhutan on 8 Aug. 1949. Under this treaty the Government of Bhutan continues to be guided by the Government of India in regard to its external relations, and the Government of India have undertaken not to interfere in the internal administration of Bhutan. The subsidy paid to Bhutan has been increased to Rs 500,000, and the Government of India agreed to retrocede to Bhutan an area of about 32 sq. miles in the territory known as Dewangiri, which was annexed in 1865.

AREA AND POPULATION. Bhutan is situated in the eastern Himalayas, bounded in the north by China and on all other sides by India. Extreme length from east to west 190 miles: extreme breadth 90 miles. Area about 18,000 sq. miles (46,500 sq. km); population estimated at approximately 1,400,000 (1988). A Nepali minority makes up 25%-30% of the population, mainly in the south. Life expectancy (1985) was 48 years. The capital is at Thimphu (1987, 15,000 population).

CLIMATE. The climate is largely controlled by altitude. The mountainous north is cold, with perpetual snow on the summits, but the centre has a more moderate climate, though winters are cold, with rainfall under 40" (1,000 mm). In the south, the climate is humid sub-tropical and rainfall approaches 200" (5,000 mm).

KING. Jigme Singye Wangchuck, succeeded his father Jigme Dorji Wangchuck who died 21 July 1972.

In 1907 the Tongsa Penlop (the governor of the province of Tongsa in central Bhutan), Sir Ugyen Wangchuk, GCIE, KCSI, was elected as the first hereditary Maharaja of Bhutan. The Bhutanese title is Druk Gyalpo, and his successor is now addressed as King of Bhutan.

CONSTITUTION AND GOVERNMENT. From Oct. 1969 the absolute monarchy was changed to a form of 'democratic monarchy'. The National Assembly (*Tshogdu*) was reinstituted in 1953. It has 151 members and meets twice a year. Two-thirds are representatives of the people and are elected for a 3-year term. All Bhutanese over 25 years may be candidates. Ten monastic representatives are elected by the central and regional ecclesiastical bodies, while the remaining members are nominated by the King, and include members of the Council of Ministers (the Cabinet) and the Royal Advisory Council.

The official languages are Dzongkha, English and Nepali.

National flag: Diagonally yellow over orange, over all in the centre a white dragon.

Local government: There are 18 districts, each under a district officer *(dzongda)* responsible to the Royal Civil Service Commission through the Home Ministry.

DEFENCE

Army. There was (1991) an Army of 5,000 men. 3 to 5 weeks militia training was introduced in May 1989 for senior students and government officials, and for the general population in Oct. 1990.

INTERNATIONAL RELATIONS

Membership. Bhutan is a member of the UN.

ECONOMY

Policy. The revised 6th development plan (1987–92) allows for expenditure of Nu9,559m. Forest and mineral wealth is to be exploited and educational and medical facilities extended.

Budget. The preliminary budget for 1990–91 envisaged expenditure of Nu2,229m. and internal revenue of Nu1,211m.

Currency. Paper currency known as the *Ngultrum* was introduced in the early 1970s. Cupronickel and bronze currency coinage is known as *Chetrum* (100 *Chetrum* = 1 *Ngultrum*). Indian currency is also legal tender. In March 1991, £1 = Nu36·50; US$1 = Nu19·24.

Banking and Finance. The Bank of Bhutan was established in 1968. The headquarters are at Phuntsholing with 25 branches throughout the country. The Royal Monetary Authority, Thimphu, was founded in 1982 to act as Bhutan's central bank. Deposits (Dec. 1987) Nu828m.

ENERGY AND NATURAL RESOURCES

Electricity. Installed capacity at June 1990 was 348·4 mw (of which 342 mw were hydro-electric) with maximum generation of 1,557m. units. Production (1986) 1,950m. kwh, and 23 towns and 93 villages had electricity.

Minerals. Large deposits of limestone, marble, dolomite, slate, graphite, lead, copper, slate, coal, talc, gypsum, beryl, mica, pyrites and tufa have been found. Most mining activity (principally limestone, coal, slate and dolomite is small-scale).

Agriculture. The area under cultivation in 1988 was some 0·13m. ha. The chief products (1988 production in 1,000 tonnes) are rice (80), millet (7), wheat (16), barley (4), maize (81), cardamom, potatoes (50), oranges (51), apples (4), handloom cloth, timber and yaks.

Livestock (1988): Cattle, 362,000; yaks, 36,000; pigs, 66,000; sheep and goats, 84,000; poultry, 237,000; horses, 26,000.

Forestry. In 1988, 3·3m. ha were forested (70% of the land area).

INDUSTRY. In 1986 there were 349 manufacturing and mining firms (14 government-owned). 249 were in the food industry, mostly with fewer than 10 employees. There are a cement plant, a tea-chest ply veneer factory, a resin and turpentine factory, a salt iodization plant and 3 distilleries.

FOREIGN ECONOMIC RELATIONS. The cumulative outstanding convertible currency debt at 30 June 1990 was some US$73·62m. (about 28·3% of GNP), together with a rupee debt of some Rs1,000m. To the same date, debt service payments totalled US$6·76m.

Financial support is received from India, the UN and other international aid organizations.

Commerce. Trade with India dominates but timber, cardamom and liquor are also exported to the Middle East, Singapore and Western Europe.

Total trade between Bhutan and UK (British Department of Trade returns, in £1,000 sterling):

	1987	*1988*	*1989*	*1990*
Imports to UK	14	175	328	111
Exports and re-exports from UK	411	12,464	363	778

Tourism. Tourism is the largest source of foreign exchange (1989, US$1·95m. gross). In 1989, 1,480 tourists visited Bhutan (2,197 in 1988).

COMMUNICATIONS

Roads. In 1989 there were about 2,280 km of roads and 7,002 registered vehicles, including 4,567 private cars, jeeps or scooters, and 1,370 were heavy vehicles.

Aviation. In 1991 Druk-Air made 1 flight weekly between Paro and Calcutta, 2 weekly flights to Delhi, 2 weekly services to Bangkok via Dhaka and 1 weekly flight to Kathmandu using a 78-seater BAe-146.

Telecommunications. A modern postal system was introduced in 1962. In 1988 there were 2 general post offices, 55 post offices and 28 branch post offices. In 1987 there were 943 km of telephone lines, 13 automatic exchanges and 1,945 telephones.

An international microwave link connects Thimphu to the Calcutta and Delhi satellite connexions. A telecommunications link between Thimphu and London by Intelsat-satellite was inaugurated in 1990. Thimphu and Phuntsholing are connected by telex to Delhi.

In 1988 there were 39 radio stations for internal administrative communications, and 13 hydro-met stations, with an estimated 15,000 radio receivers. Bhutan Broadcasting Service, Thimphu, broadcasts a daily programme in English, Sharchopkha, Dzongkha and Nepali.

Cinemas. There are two, in Thimpu.

Newspapers. The only weekly newspaper, *Kuensel*, began publication in Aug. 1986 to replace the government weekly bulletin. It is published in English, Dzongkha and Nepali. Total circulation (1990) about 7,770.

JUSTICE, RELIGION, EDUCATION AND WELFARE

Justice. The High Court consists of 8 judges (2 elected by the National Assembly for 5-year terms) appointed by the King. There is a Magistrate's Court in each district, under a *Thrimpon*, from which appeal is to the High Court at Thimphu.

Religion. In 1990 there were some 1,500 monks in the Central Monastic Body (Thimphu and Punakha) and 2,120 in the District Monk Bodies. The monks are headed by an elected Je Khenpo (Head Abbot). The majority of the people are Mahayana Buddhists of the Drukpa subsect of the Kagyud School which was first introduced from Tibet during the 12th century. Hindus of Nepalese origin represent approximately 25-30% of the population.

Education. In April 1990 there were 3,978 pupils an 85 teachers in extension classrooms, 48,051 pupils and 1,672 teachers in primary schools, 15,984 pupils and 662 teachers in junior high and high schools and 2,341 pupils and 206 teachers in technical, vocational and tertiary-level schools. Many students receive higher technical training in India, as well as under the UN Development Programme, the Colombo Plan, etc., in Australia, Germany, New Zealand, Japan, Singapore, the USA and the UK. In Oct. 1990 140 students were receiving university education in India.

Health. There were (1988) 28 hospitals (2 indigenous), 46 dispensaries, 69 basic health units, 6 indigenous dispensaries, 5 leprosy hospitals, 1 mobile hospital, 1 health school and 15 malaria eradication centres. In 1988 beds totalled 932; there were 142 doctors and 674 paramedics.

DIPLOMATIC REPRESENTATIVE

Of Bhutan to the United Nations
Ambassador: Ugyen Tshering.

Further Reading

Bhutan, Himalayan Kingdom. Bhutan Government, Thimphu, 1979
Aris, M., *Bhutan: The Early History of an Himalayan Kingdom.* Warminster, 1979
Chakravarti, B., *A Cultural History of Bhutan.* 2nd rev. ed., 2 vols. Chitteranjan, 1981
Collister, P., *Bhutan and the British.* London, 1987
Das, N., *The Dragon Country.* New Delhi, 1973
Dogra, R. C., *Bhutan:* [Bibliography]. Oxford and Santa Barbara, 1991
Edmunds, T. O., *Bhutan: Land of the Thunder Dragon.* London, 1988
Hickman, K., *Dreams of the Peaceful Dragon: a Journey through Bhutan.* London, 1987
Mehra, G. N., *Bhutan: Land of the Peaceful Dragon.* Rev. ed. New Delhi, 1985

Misra, H. N., *Bhutan: Problems and Policies*. New Delhi, 1988
Rahul, R., *Royal Bhutan*. New Delhi, 1983
Ronaldshay, the Earl of, *Lands of the Thunderbolt*. 2nd ed. London, 1931
Rose, L. E., *The Politics of Bhutan*. Cornell Univ. Press, 1977
Rustomji, N., *Bhutan: The Dragon Kingdom in Crisis*. OUP, 1978
Strydonck, G. van, *et al*, *Bhutan: a Kingdom of the Eastern Himalayas*. Geneva and London, 1984
Verma, R., *India's Role in the Emergence of Contemporary Bhutan*. Delhi, 1988

BOLIVIA

República de Bolivia

Capital: Sucre
Seat of Government: La Paz
Population: 6·41m. (1989)
GNP per capita: US$570 (1988)

HISTORY. Until 1884, when Bolivia was defeated by Chile, she had a strip bordering on the Pacific which contains extensive nitrate beds and at that time the port of Cobija (which no longer exists). She lost this area to Chile; but in Sept. 1953 Chile declared Arica a free port and, although it is no longer a free port for Bolivian imports, Bolivia still has certain privileges.

AREA AND POPULATION. Bolivia is a landlocked state bounded north and east by Brazil, south by Paraguay and Argentina and west by Chile and Peru, with an area of some 424,165 sq. miles (1,098,581 sq. km).

Population estimate, 1989: 6·41m. Area and population of the departments (capitals in brackets) at the 1982 census and in 1988:

Departments	*Area (sq. km)*	*Census 1982*	*Estimated population, 1988 (in 1,000)*	*Per sq. km 1988*
La Paz (La Paz)	133,985	1,913,184	1,926·2	14·3
Cochabamba (Cochabamba)	55,631	908,674	982·0	17·6
Potosí (Potosí)	118,218	823,485	667·8	5·6
Santa Cruz (Santa Cruz)	370,621	942,986	1,110·1	2·9
Chuquisaca (Sucre)	51,524	435,406	442·6	8·5
Tarija (Tarija)	37,623	246,691	246·6	6·5
Oruro (Oruro)	53,588	385,121	388·3	7·2
Beni (Trinidad)	213,564	217,700	215·4	1·0
Pando (Cobija)	63,827	42,594	41·0	0·6
Total	1,098,581	5,915,841	6,405·1	5·8

Population (1988 estimate, in 1,000) of the principal towns: La Paz, 669·4; Santa Cruz, 529·2; Cochabamba, 403·6; El Alto, 307·4; Oruro, 176·7; Sucre, 105·8; Tarija, 66·9.

Spanish is the official and commercial language. The Amerindian languages Aymara and Quechua are spoken exclusively by 22% and 5·2% of the population respectively.

CLIMATE. The very varied geography of Bolivia produces several different climates. The two most significant are the low-lying areas in the Amazon Basin, which are very warm and damp throughout the year, with heavy rainfall from Nov. to March, and the alti-plano, which is generally dry between May and Nov. with abundant sunshine, but the nights are cold in June and July, while the months from Dec. to March are the wettest. La Paz. Jan. 53°F (11·7°C), July 47°F (8·3°C). Annual rainfall 23" (574 mm). Sucre. Jan. 55°F (13°C), July 49°F (9·4°C). Annual rainfall 27" (675 mm).

CONSTITUTION AND GOVERNMENT. The Republic of Bolivia was proclaimed on 6 Aug. 1825; its first constitution was adopted on 19 Nov. 1826.

La Paz is the actual capital and seat of the Government, but Sucre is the legal capital and the seat of the judiciary.

Presidents since 1966 and the date on which they took office:

Gen. René Barrientos Ortuño (Constitutional President killed in air accident), 6 Aug. 1966–27 April 1969.
Dr Luis Adolfo Siles Salinas (deposed), 27 April 1969–26 Sept. 1969.
Gen. Alfredo Ovando Candia, 26 Sept. 1969–6 Oct. 1970.
Gen. Juan José Torres, 7 Oct. 1970–21 Aug. 1971.
Gen. Hugo Banzer Suarez, 21 Aug. 1971–21 July 1978.
Gen. Juan Pereda Asbun, 21 July 1978–24 Nov. 1978.
Gen. David Padilla Arancibia, 24 Nov. 1978–8 Aug. 1979.
Dr Walter Guevara Arze (deposed), 8 Aug. 1979–1 Nov. 1979.
Dr Lydia Gueiler Tejada (deposed), 16 Nov. 1979–17 July 1980.
Maj.-Gen. Luis García Meza Tejada (resigned), 18 July 1980–4 Aug. 1981.
Military Junta, 4 Aug. 1981–4 Sept. 1981.
Gen. Celso Torrelio Villa, (resigned), 4 Sept. 1981–19 July 1982.
Brig.-Gen. Guido Vildoso Calderón, 21 July 1982–10 Oct. 1982.
Dr Hernan Siles Zuazo, 10 Oct. 1982–6 Aug. 1985.
Dr Victor Paz Esstensoro, 6 Aug. 1985–6 Aug. 1989

The President and Vice-President are elected by universal suffrage for a 4-year term. The President appoints the members of his Cabinet. There is a bicameral legislature; the Senate comprises 27 members, 3 from each department, and the Chamber of Deputies 130 members, all elected for 4 years.

The Cabinet was composed as follows in March 1991:

President: Jaime Paz Zamora (sworn in 6 Aug. 1989).

Foreign Affairs and Worship: Carlos Iturralde Ballivían. *Interior, Migration and Justice:* Carlos Saavedra Bruno. *Defence:* Héctor Ormachea Peñaranda. *Finance:* Miguel Angel Sabalo. *Planning and Coordination:* Enrique Garcia Rodriquez. *Industry, Commerce and Tourism:* Guido Céspedes Argandoña. *Mining and Metallurgy:* Walter Soriano Lea Plaza. *Energy and Hydrocarbons:* Angel Zanil Claros. *Agriculture and Peasant Affairs:* Mauro Bertero Gutiérrez. *Labour and Labour Development:* Oscar Zamora Medinacelli. *Education and Culture:* Mariano Bapista Gumucio. *Housing and Urban Affairs:* Elena Velasco de Urresti. *Transport and Communications:* Willy Vargas Vacaflor. *Without Portfolio:* Guillermo Fortún Suárez.

National flag: Three horizontal stripes of red, yellow, and green.

National anthem: Bolivianos, el hado propicio ('Bolivians, the propitious fate'; words by I. de Sanjinés; tune by B. Vincenti).

Local Government: The republic is divided into 9 departments, established in Jan. 1826, with 108 provinces administered by sub-prefects, and 1,713 cantons administered by corregidores. The supreme authority in each department is vested in a prefect appointed by the President.

DEFENCE. Bolivia is divided into 6 military regions; regional HQ are located at La Paz, Sucre, Tarija, Potosí, Trinidad and Cobija. There is selective conscription for 12 months at the age of 18 years.

Army. The Army consists of 8 cavalry groups, 1 motorized infantry regiment, 22 infantry, 1 artillery, 1 airborne and 6 engineer battalions. Equipment, 36 Kuerassier SK105 light tanks and 24 EE-9 Cascavel armoured cars. Strength (1991) 22,000 (15,000 conscripts).

Navy. A small force exists for river and lake patrol duties, comprising 10 patrol craft operating on Lake Titicaca, and in the 6,000-mile Beni and Bolivia-Paraguay river systems. 1 ocean-going transport for use to and from Bolivian free zones in Argentina and Uruguay and 2 17-tonne hospital craft on Lake Titicaca complete the inventory.

Personnel in 1990 totalled 3,800, including 2,000 marines. Most training of officers and petty officers is carried out in Argentina while junior ratings are almost entirely re-trained soldiers.

Air Force. The Air Force, established in 1923, has 3 combat-capable Groups, 2 equipped with T-33 armed jet trainers, and one with armed T-6s, SF.260s and

Hughes 500 helicopters, for counter-insurgency operations. A search and rescue helicopter Group has 15 Brazilian-assembled Lamas and 20 UH-1 Iroquois. Other types in service include Brazilian T-23 Uirapuru and American T-41 primary trainers and Swiss turboprop-powered Pilatus PC-7 basic trainers, 1 Electra four-turboprop transport, 6 Fokker F.27 and 2 Israeli-built Arava twin-turboprop light transports, 2 Convair transports, 8 C-130H/L-100 Hercules, 6 C-47s, 15 Turbo-Porters and about 35 Cessna single- and twin-engined light aircraft. Personnel strength (1991) about 4,000 (2,200 conscripts).

INTERNATIONAL RELATIONS

Membership. Bolivia is a member of the UN, OAS, GATT, LAIA, the Andean Group and the Amazon Pact.

ECONOMY

Budget. Expenditure in 1984 was envisaged at 6,891,200m. *pesos bolivianos.*

Currency. On 1 Jan. 1987 the *boliviano* ($b. equal to 1m. *pesos*) was introduced. Exchange rates were $b.3·49 = US$1 and $b.6·61 = £1 in March 1991.

Banking and Finance. In 1990 the principal banks were Banco Central de Bolivia, Banco del Estado, Banco de Santa Cruz de la Sierra, Banco Agricola de Bolivia, Banco Boliviano Americano, Banco Hipotecario Nacional, Banco Mercantil, Banco Minero de Bolivia, Banco Nacional de Bolivia, Banco de Cochabamba, Banco de la Paz, Banco de Inversión Boliviano, Banco Ganadero de Beni, Banco Industrial, Banco Real, Banco de la Nacion Argentina, Banco Popular del Peru, Banco Industrial S.A., First National City Bank, Banco del Progreso Nacional and Bank of America.

A stock exchange opened in La Paz in 1989.

Weights and Measures. The metric system of weights and measures is used by the administration and prescribed by law, but the old Spanish system is also employed.

ENERGY AND NATURAL RESOURCES

Electricity. Electric power production is expanding. Installed capacity was estimated at 490,000 kw. in 1985. Estimated production from all sources (1986), 2,080m. kwh. Supply 110 volts in La Paz but 220 volts in most other cities; 60 Hz.

Oil and Gas. There are petroleum and natural gas deposits in the Santa Cruz-Camiri areas. A pipeline for crude oil connects Caranda (Santa Cruz) with the Pacific coast at Arica (Chile) and a natural gas pipeline to Argentina was inaugurated in May 1972. All production, refining and internal distribution is now in the hands of *Yacimientos Petroliferos Fiscales Bolivianos* (the State Petroleum Organization). Total production of crude oil in 1989 was estimated at 900,000 tonnes. Production of natural gas in 1981 was estimated at 175,478m. cu. ft.

Minerals. Mining is the most important industry, accounting for about 69% of the foreign-exchange earnings. About half the mineral mined is tin. Tin mines are at altitudes of from 12,000 to 18,000 ft, where few except native Indians can stand the conditions; transport is costly. Bolivian tin is extracted by shaft-mining, frequently very deep; the ore yields only 0·7% or less of tin and is very refractory; tin is exported in concentrates called *barrilla,* through Pacific ports for refining. Smelting capacity was increased in 1980 and it is planned to smelt all the ores from the State Mining Co. but complex ores still have to be exported for smelting. Tin production in 1984 was 17,875 tonnes.

Alluvial gold deposits in the Alto Beni region are being exploited. Production (1987) 2·7 tonne.

Agriculture. The extensive and still largely undeveloped region east of the Andes comprises about three-quarters of the entire area of the country, and since the agrarian reform of 1953 sugar-cane, rice and cotton have been grown in this *Oriente* in increasing abundance, reaching self-sufficiency in all these products. Output in 1,000 tonnes in 1988 was: Sugar-cane, 2,000; rice, 171; coffee, 26; maize, 446; potatoes, 700; wheat, 63; cotton (lint), 4; cocoa, 3. Coca is the largest crop. In 1990 Bolivia received US$18m. of US aid for destroying coca (the source of cocaine). Some 60,000 coca farmers received US$2,000 for every ha destroyed.

Livestock: In 1988 there were 5·45m. head of cattle, mostly in the Santa Cruz and Beni departments; some are exported to Peru; horses, 315,000; asses, 620,000; pigs, 1·75m.; sheep, 9·6m.; goats, 2·35m.; poultry, 12m.

Forestry. Forests cover 55·8m. hectares (51% of the land area). Tropical forests with woods ranging from the 'iron tree' to the light *palo de balsa* are beginning to be exploited.

INDUSTRY. There are few industrial establishments.

FOREIGN ECONOMIC RELATIONS. Bolivia relies on imports for the supply of many consumer goods. However an investment law passed in 1971 provides incentives and protection for new foreign investment, and for reinvestment in various fields including manufacturing industry, mining, agriculture, construction and tourism.

Commerce. The value of imports and exports in US$1,000 has been as follows:

	1982	*1983*	*1984*	*1985*	*1986*	*1987*
Imports	496,300	451,100	713,800	551,900	711,500	776,000
Exports	898,500	786,700	609,500	672,500	637,500	569,600

Chief exports: Natural gas, tin, silver, zinc, wolfram, coffee, sugar.

Chief imports: Raw materials for industry, capital goods for industry, consumer goods, transport equipment and construction materials.

Imports (in US$1m.), by country, 1989: USA, 86; Brazil, 63·4; Argentina, 40·9; Federal Germany, 21·7; Chile, 21·5; Peru, 9·1; UK, 5·6; Belgium, 2·9; Switzerland, 2·9; France, 2·4.

Total exports, 1984, of all minerals, in concentrates, ingots or solder, were valued at US$363·9m.

Bolivia having no seaport, imports and exports pass chiefly through the ports of Arica and Antofagasta in Chile, Mollendo-Matarani in Peru, through La Quiaca on the Bolivian-Argentine border and through river-ports on the rivers flowing into the Amazon.

Total trade between Bolivia and UK (British Department of Trade returns in £1,000 sterling):

	1986	*1987*	*1988*	*1989*	*1990*
Imports to UK	10,225	14,799	13,224	17,666	12,387
Exports and re-exports from UK	3,663	3,658	6,029	6,148	6,234

Tourism. There were 133,000 visitors in 1986.

COMMUNICATIONS

Roads. A highway, in poor condition, 497 km long, runs from Cochabamba to the lowland farming region of Santa Cruz. La Paz and Oruro are also connected by a metalled road. Of other main highways (unmetalled) there is one from La Paz through Guaqui into Peru, another from La Paz, *via* Oruro, Potosí, Tarija and Bermejo, into Argentina, with branches to Cochabamba, Sucre and Camiri, passable throughout the year except at the height of the rainy season, and others from Villazón to Villa Montes *via* Tarija, passable during the dry season. The total length of the road system is 41,000 km (1984). Motor vehicles in use in 1984, 168,600, including 43,677 cars.

Railways. In 1964 Bolivian National Railways (ENFE) was formed by the amalgamation of the Bolivian Government Railways, Bolivian Railway Co. and the Bolivian section of the Antofagasta (Chili) & Bolivia Railway. The Guaqui-La Paz Railway, formerly operated by Peru, became part of ENFE in 1973 and the privately-owned Marchacamarca Uncia mineral line was taken over in 1987. Access to the Pacific is by 3 routes: To Antofagasta and Arica in Chile, and to Mollendo in Peru *via* Guaqui, the Lake Titicaca train ferry to Puno (Peru), then rail to the coast. Construction began in 1978 of a 150-km line linking Puno with Desaguadero on the Bolivian border which would by-pass the train ferry, though gauge difference would still prevent through running to Peru. Current network totals 3,642 km of metre gauge, comprising unconnected Eastern (1,386 km) and Western (2,257 km) systems. In 1989 the railways carried 1·1m. passengers and 1m. tonnes of freight.

Aviation. The 2 international airports are El Alto (8½ miles from La Paz) and Viru Viru (10 miles from Santa Cruz). The national airline is Lloyd Aéreo Boliviano. The airline runs regular services between La Paz and Lima, São Paulo, Buenos Aires, Miami, Caracas, Salta and Arica as well as many internal services. Eastern Airways runs regular flights between La Paz, Buenos Aires, Santiago and Asunción linking Bolivia to the USA. Lufthansa links Bolivia with Europe. Other airlines serving Bolivia are Aerolineas Argentinas, Cruzeiro, Aero Peru and Lan Chile.

Shipping. Traffic on Lake Titicaca between Guaqui and Puno is carried on by the steamers of the Peruvian Corporation. About 12,000 miles of rivers, in 4 main systems (Beni, Pilcomayo, Titicaca-Desaguadero, Mamoré), are open to navigation by light-draught vessels.

Telecommunications. In Bolivia there were, in 1978, 458 post offices, of these, 205 provided telegraph and telephone services together with a further 245 offices for telegraph and telephone service only. There is telephone service in the cities of La Paz, Cochabamba, Oruro, Sucre, Potosí, Santa Cruz, Tarija, Camiri, Tupiza, Villazon, Riberalta and Trinidad with (1983), 204,747 telephones. There were (1987) about 85 radio stations, the majority of which are local and commercial. There is a commercial government television service. There are 4 private television stations and 1 University station (educational channel) in La Paz.

Cinemas. In 1989 there were 30 cinemas in La Paz and 50 in other cities.

Newspapers. There were (1984) 7 daily newspapers in La Paz, 2 in Oruro, and 1 in Cochabamba. Several other towns have regular newspapers devoted to local news, but most of them appear only a few times a week. An economic monthly journal *Revista Economica* and 4 daily newspapers are produced in Santa Cruz.

JUSTICE, RELIGION, EDUCATION AND WELFARE

Justice. Justice is administered by the Supreme Court, superior district courts (of 5 or 7 judges) and courts of local justice. The Supreme Court, with headquarters at Sucre, is divided into two sections, civil and criminal, of 5 justices each, with the Chief Justice presiding over both. Members of the Supreme Court are chosen on a two-thirds vote of Congress.

Religion. The Roman Catholic is the recognized religion of the state; the free exercise of other forms of worship is permitted. The Catholic Church is under a cardinal (in Sucre), an archbishop (in La Paz), 6 bishops (Cochabamba, Santa Cruz, Oruro, Potosí, Riberalta and Tarija) and vicars apostolic (titular bishops resident in Cueva, Trinidad, San Ignacio de Velasco, Riberalta and Rurrenabaque).

By a law of 11 Oct. 1911 all marriages must be celebrated by the civil authorities. Divorce is permitted by a law enacted on 15 April 1932.

Education. Primary instruction is free and obligatory between the ages of 6 and 14 years. In 1986 there were 1·4m. pupils and 51,000 teachers in 9,093 primary and elementary schools, and 225,000 pupils, 10,400 teachers in 2,300 secondary schools.

At Sucre, Oruro, Potosí, Cochabamba, Santa Cruz, Tarija, Trinidad and La Paz are universities; La Paz is the most important of them while the San Francisco Xavier University at Sucre is one of the oldest in America, founded in 1624.

Health. In 1972 there were 2,143 doctors.

DIPLOMATIC REPRESENTATIVES

Of Bolivia in Great Britain (106 Eaton Sq., London, SW1W 9AD)
Ambassador: Gary Prado.

Of Great Britain in Bolivia (Avenida Arce 2732–2754, La Paz)
Ambassador: M. F. Daly, CMG.

Of Bolivia in the USA (3014 Massachusetts Ave, NW, Washington, D.C., 20008)
Ambassador: Jorge Crespo Velasco.

Of the USA in Bolivia (Banco Popular Del Peru Bldg, La Paz)
Ambassador: Robert S. Gelbard.

Of Bolivia to the United Nations
Ambassador: Hugo Navajas-Mogro.

Further Reading

Anuario Geográfico y Estadístico de la República de Bolivia
Anuario del Comercia Exterior de Bolivia
Boletín Mensual de Información Estadistica
Dunkerley, J., *Rebellion in the Veins: Political Struggle in Bolivia 1952–1982*. London, 1984
Fifer, J. V., *Bolivia: Land, Location and Politics Since 1825*. CUP, 1972
Guillermo, L., *A History of the Bolivian Labour Movement 1848–1971*. CUP, 1977
Klein, H., *Bolivia: The Evolution of a Multi-Ethnic Society*. OUP, 1982
Yeager, G. M., *Bolivia*. [Bibliography] Oxford and Santa Barbara, 1988

BOTSWANA

Capital: Gaborone
Population: 1·26m. (1989)
GNP per capita: US$1,050 (1988)

Republic of Botswana

HISTORY. In 1885 the territory was declared to be within the British sphere; in 1889 it was included in the sphere of the British South Africa Company, but was never administered by the company; in 1890 a Resident Commissioner was appointed, and in 1895, on the annexation of the Crown Colony of British Bechuanaland to the Cape of Good Hope, the British Government was in favour of transferring the Protectorate to the BSA Company, but the three major chiefs of the Bakwena, the Bangwaketse and the Bamangwato went to England to protest against this proposal, and agreement was reached that their country should remain a British Protectorate if they ceded a strip of land on the eastern side of the country for railway construction. This railway was built in 1896–97.

On 30 Sept. 1966 the Bechuanaland Protectorate became an independent and sovereign member of the Commonwealth under the name of the Republic of Botswana.

AREA AND POPULATION. Botswana is bounded west and north by Namibia, north-east by Zambia and Zimbabwe and east and south by the Republic of South Africa. Area about 222,000 sq. miles (582,000 sq. km); population, estimate 1989, was 1,255,749 (census, 1981, 941,027).

The main business centres (with estimated population, 1989) are Gaborone (120,239), Mahalapye (104,450), Serowe (95,041), Tutume (86,405), Bobonong (55,060), Francistown (52,725), Selebi-Phikwe (49,542), Boteti (32,711), Lobatse (26,841), Palapye (16,959), Jwaneng (13,895), Tlokweng (11,760), Orapa (8,894).

The seat of government is at Gaborone.

The official language is English; the national language is Setswana.

CLIMATE. Most of the country is sub-tropical, but there are arid areas in the south and west. In winter, days are warm and nights cold, with occasional frosts. Summer heat is tempered by prevailing north-east winds. Rainfall comes mainly in summer, from Oct. to April, while the rest of the year is almost completely dry with very high sunshine amounts. Gaborone. Jan. 79°F (26·1°C), July 55°F (12·8°C). Annual rainfall 21" (538 mm).

CONSTITUTION AND GOVERNMENT. The Constitution adopted on 30 Sept. 1966 provides for a republican form of government headed by the President with 3 main organs: The Legislature, the Executive and the Judiciary.

The executive rests with the President of the Republic who is responsible to the National Assembly.

The National Assembly consists of 38 members, 34 elected by universal suffrage. The general election, held in Oct. 1989, returned 31 members of the Botswana Democratic Party and 3 Botswana National Front.

The President is an *ex-officio* member of the Assembly. If the President is already a member of the National Assembly, a by-election will be held in that constituency.

There is also a House of Chiefs to advise the Government. It consists of the Chiefs of the 8 tribes who were autonomous during the days of the British protectorate, and 4 members elected by and from among the sub-chiefs in 4 districts.

The first President of Botswana, who was re-elected 3 times, was Sir Seretse Khama, KBE, who died 13 July 1980.

President of the Republic: Dr Quett Ketumile Joni Masire (re-elected 1989).

In Dec. 1990 the Cabinet was as follows:
Vice President and Minister of Local Government and Lands: P. S. Mmusi. *Presi-*

dential Affairs and Public Administration: Lieut.-Gen. Mompati Merafhe. *External Affairs:* Gaositwe K. T. Chiepe. *Health:* Kebatlamang P. Morake. *Works, Transport and Communications:* C. J. Butale. *Commerce and Industry:* Ponatshego Kedikilwe. *Mineral Resources and Water Affairs:* Archie M. Mogwe. *Education:* Ray Molombo. *Finance and Development Planning:* Festus Mogae. *Labour and Home Affairs:* Patrick Balopi.

National flag: Light blue with a horizontal black stripe, edged white, across the centre.

Local Government. Local government is carried out by 10 district councils and 5 town councils. Revenue is obtained mainly from sales taxes; from rates in the towns and from central government subventions in the districts.

DEFENCE

Army. A defence force has been created for border control and comprises 5 infantry, 1 armoured car, 1 reconnaissance and 1 engineer companies. Personnel (includes Air Force) in 1991, 4,500.

Air Force. Equipment includes 8 BAC Strikemaster light strike aircraft, 5 Britten-Norman Defender armed light transports for border patrol, counter-insurgency and casualty evacuation duties, 5 Bulldog piston-engined basic trainers, 2 CN-235 turboprop-powered medium transports, 2 Skyvan turboprop passenger/cargo transports, 2 Trislander 3-engined transports, 2 Ecureuil and 3 Bell 412 helicopters and 2 Cessna 152 light aircraft.

INTERNATIONAL RELATIONS

Membership. Botswana is a member of UN, OAU, SADCC, the Non-Aligned Movement, the Commonwealth and is an ACP state of the EEC.

ECONOMY

Policy. The Development Plan for 1985–91 envisaged capital expenditure of P1,200m.

Budget. The 1989–90 budget envisaged expenditure of P2,164m., revenue was envisaged at P1,032m.

Currency. The unit of currency is the *pula* (BWP) of 100 *thebe*, which superseded the South African rand in Aug. 1976 (P3·59 = £1 sterling and P1·89 = US$1 in March 1991).

Banking. There were (1986) 3 commercial banks (Barclays Bank of Botswana Ltd, Standard Chartered Bank Botswana Ltd and Bank of Credit and Commerce (Botswana) Ltd) with 34 branches and sub-branches, and 44 agencies. The Bank of Botswana, established in 1976, is the central bank. The National Development Bank, founded in 1964, has 6 regional offices and agricultural, industrial and commercial development divisions. The government-owned Botswana Savings Bank operates through 64 post offices.

Total assets and liabilities of the 3 commercial banks at 31 March 1989, P897m. and of the Bank of Botswana, P4,785·1m.

ENERGY AND NATURAL RESOURCES

Electricity. The coal-fired power station at Morupule supplies all major cities. Production (1986) 533m. kwh. Supply 220 volts; 50 Hz.

Water. Surface water resources are about 18,000m. cu. metres a year. Nearly all flows into northern districts from Angola through the Okavango and Kwando river systems. The Zambezi, also in the north, provides irrigation in Chobe District. In the south-east, there are dams to exploit the ephemeral flow of the tributaries of the Limpopo. 80% of the land has no surface water, and must be served by boreholes.

Minerals. An important part of government revenue comes from the diamond mines at Orapa and Jwaneng and the nickel–copper complex at Selebi-Phikwe. An open-pit coalmine has been developed at Morupule. Mineral production 1988: Diamonds, 15,229,000 carats; copper–nickel, 43,238 tonnes (value P81,374,000); coal, 612,713 tonnes (P11,300,000).

Mineral resources in north-east Botswana are being investigated, including salt and soda ash on the Sua Pan of the Makgadikgadi Salt Pans, nickel–copper at Selkirk and Phoenix, copper south of Maun and close to Ghanzi, and coal at Mmamabula.

Agriculture. Cattle-rearing is the chief industry, and the country is more a pastoral than an agricultural one, crops depending entirely upon the rainfall. In 1987, 295,000 ha were planted with crops. In 1988 the number of cattle was 2·35m.; goats, 1m.; sheep, 220,000; poultry, 1m. Meat and meat products (1986) exported P144,157,165, sold locally P7,469,859.

Production (1988, in 1,000 tonnes): Maize, 12; sorghum, 40; groundnuts, 1; millet, 3; wheat, 1; roots and tubers, 7; sunflower seeds, 1; pulses, 14; seed cotton, 3; vegetables, 16; fruit, 11.

Forestry. There are forest nurseries and plantations. Concessions have been granted to harvest 7,500 cu. metres in Kasane and Chobe Forest Reserves and up to 2,500 cu. metres in the Masame area.

Conservation. About 17% of land is set aside for wildlife preservation. In 1986 there were 4 national parks, 6 game reserves, 3 game sanctuaries and 40 controlled hunting areas for photographic and game viewing safaris and recreational (safari) and subsistence hunting.

INDUSTRY. In 1987 there were 80,449 Batswana employed in the mines of the Republic of South Africa. The estimated total number of paid employees in all sectors in Botswana in Sept. 1987 was 150,200.

FOREIGN ECONOMIC RELATIONS. Botswana is a member of the South African customs union with Lesotho, the Republic of South Africa and Swaziland.

Commerce. In 1987 imports totalled P1,572,456 and exports P2,663,802. Of imports, 79·6% came from the South African customs area, 7·7% from other African countries. Exports are mainly diamonds (to Switzerland), copper–nickel matte (to USA), beef and beef products (to EEC).

Imports (1987 in P1,000) included vehicles and transport equipment, 242,785; food, beverages and tobacco, 253,422; machinery and electrical equipment, 260,370: Exports were mainly diamonds, 2,252,453. Imports in 1987 were mainly from the South African customs area (P1,250,954,000) and exports mainly to Europe (P2,412,152,000).

Total trade between Botswana and UK (British Department of Trade returns, in £1,000 sterling):

	1986	*1987*	*1988*	*1989*	*1990*
Imports to UK	16,652	11,836	6,942	13,135	18,854
Exports and re-exports from UK	8,629	10,275	26,763	34,582	24,777

Tourism. There were 432,323 foreign visitors in 1987.

COMMUNICATIONS

Roads. On 31 Dec. 1985, 1,914 km of road were bitumen-surfaced, 1,255 km gravel and about 4,860 km earth. In 1988 there were 46,560 registered motor vehicles including 14,199 cars, 16,350 light delivery vans and 6,895 lorries.

Railways. The main line from Mafikeng in Bophuthatswana to Bulawayo in Zimbabwe traverses Botswana. With two short branches the total was (1989) 705 km. These lines, formerly operated by National Railways of Zimbabwe, were taken over by the new Botswana Railways organization in 1987. In 1988–89 railways carried 0·4m. passengers and 2·1m. tonnes of freight.

Aviation. The Seretse Khama International Airport at Gaborone opened in 1984.

Regular international flights are flown by Air Botswana, Air Zimbabwe, Royal Swazi Air, Air Zambia, Air Tanzania, Air Malawi, Kenya Airways, Lesotho Airways, South African Airways and British Airways into Gaborone. In 1988, 77,250 passengers arrived by air, 65,519 departed and 4,056 were in transit.

Telecommunications. In 1986 there were 66 post offices and 72 agencies. There were 12,511 telephones installed in 1987. Radio Botswana broadcasts 119 hours a week in English and Setswana.

Newspapers. In 1987 there was 1 daily newspaper, the bilingual (Setswana-English) *Daily News*, which is published by the Department of Information and Broadcasting; circulation, 36,000. There are 3 other privately-owned newspapers.

JUSTICE, RELIGION, EDUCATION AND WELFARE

Justice. The Botswana Court of Appeal was established in 1954. It has jurisdiction in respect of criminal and civil appeals emanating from the High Court of Botswana and has jurisdiction in all criminal and civil causes and proceedings. Subordinate courts and traditional courts are in each of the 12 administrative districts. The police force was 2,359 in 1985.

Religion. Freedom of worship is guaranteed under the Constitution. Christian denominations include the United Congregational Church of Southern Africa, the Catholic Church, Anglican, Lutheran, Dutch Reformed, Seventh Day Adventist, Assemblies of God, Methodist and Quaker groups. Non-Christian religions include Bahais, Moslems and Hindus.

Education. Primary education has been free since 1980 and secondary education from 1988. In 1988 enrolment in primary schools was 259,152 with (1987) 7,704 teachers, and in secondary schools 40,000 with (1987) 1,682 teachers. In 1987 there were 1,316 students with 78 teachers in teacher training colleges and 2,261 students with 328 instructors in vocational and technical training. There is a Polytechnic and an Auto Trades Training School. Throughout the country, Brigades provide lower level vocational training. The Department of Non-Formal Education offers secondary level correspondence courses and is the executing agency for the National Literacy Programme. The University of Botswana had 1,884 full-time students and 250 academic staff in 1987.

In 1987, 63% of those over 15 years could read and write.

Health (1986). There were 13 general hospitals, a mental hospital, 7 health centres, 81 clinics and 246 health posts. There were also 438 stops for mobile health teams. In 1986 there were 156 registered medical practitioners, 14 dentists, and 1,530 nurses. The health facilities are the concern of central and local government, medical missions, mining companies and voluntary organizations.

DIPLOMATIC REPRESENTATIVES

Of Botswana in Great Britain (6 Stratford Pl., London, W1N 9AE)
High Commissioner: Margaret Nasha.

Of Great Britain in Botswana (Private Bag 0023, Gaborone)
High Commissioner: Brian Smith, OBE.

Of Botswana in the USA (4301 Connecticut Ave., NW, Washington, D.C., 20008)
Ambassador: Kingsele Sebele.

Of the USA in Botswana (PO Box 90, Gaborone)
Ambassador: David Passage.

Of Botswana to the United Nations
Ambassador: Legwaila Joseph Legwaila.

Further Reading

General Information: The Director of Information and Broadcasting, PO Box 0060, Gaborone, Botswana publishes *Botswana Handbook*, the monthly *Kutlwano, The Botswana Daily News, Botswana in Brief* and *Botswana Up To Date*.

Botswana '86: An Official Handbook. Department of Information and Broadcasting, Gaborone, 1986
Statistical Bulletins. Quarterly. Central Statistical Office, Gaborone
Report on the Population Census, 1981. Government Printer, Gaborone, 1982
Campbell, A. C., *The Guide to Botswana*. Gaborone, 1980
Colclough, C. and McCarthy, S., *The Political Economy of Botswana*. OUP, 1980
Harvey, C., (ed.) *Papers on the Economy of Botswana*. London and Nairobi, 1981
Parson, J., *Botswana: Liberal Democracy and Labour Reserve in Southern Africa*. Aldershot, 1984

BRAZIL

Capital: Brasília, (Federal District)
Population: 155·6m. (1990)
GNP per capita: US$2,280 (1988)

República Federativa do Brasil

HISTORY. Brazil was discovered on 22 April 1500 by the Portuguese Admiral Pedro Alvares Cabral, and thus became a Portuguese settlement; in 1815 the colony was declared 'a kingdom', and it was proclaimed an independent Empire in 1822. The monarchy was overthrown in 1889 and a republic declared. Following a coup in 1964 the armed forces retained overall control until civilian government was restored on 15 March 1985.

AREA AND POPULATION. Brazil is bounded east by the Atlantic and on its northern, western and southern borders by all the South American countries except Chile and Ecuador. The area is 8,511,996 sq. km (3,286,485 sq. miles) including 55,457 sq. km of inland water. Population as at 1 Sept. 1980 (census) and 1 July 1990 (estimate):

Federal Unit and Capital	*Area (sq. km)*	*Census 1980*	*Estimate 1990*
North	3,851,560	5,880,268	10,581,561
Rondônia (Pôrto Velho)	238,379	491,069	1,125,118
Acre (Rio Branco)	153,698	301,303	434,708
Amazonas (Manaus)	1,567,954	1,430,089	2,213,966
Roraima (Boa Vista)	225,017	79,159	135,956
Pará (Belém)	1,246,833	3,403,391	5,391,864
Amapá (Macapá)	142,359	175,257	267,576
Tocantins (Palmas)	277,322	–	1,012,373
North-east	1,556,001 [1]	34,812,356	44,429,181
Maranhão (São Luís)	329,556	3,996,404	5,274,797
Piaui (Teresina)	251,273	2,139,021	2,799,919
Ceará (Fortaleza)	145,694	5,288,253	6,666,651
Rio Grande do Norte (Natal)	53,167	1,898,172	2,451,076
Paraíba (João Pessoa)	53,958	2,770,176	3,420,340
Pernambuco (Recife) [2]	101,023	6,141,993	7,603,176
Alagoas (Maceió)	29,107	1,982,591	2,522,197
Sergipe (Aracajú)	21,863	1,140,121	1,516,064
Bahia (Salvador)	566,979	9,454,346	12,174,961
South-east:	924,266	51,734,125	67,067,873
Minas Gerais (Belo Horizonte)	586,624	13,378,553	16,854,745
Espírito Santo [3] (Vitória)	45,733	2,023,340	2,635,307
Rio de Janeiro (Rio de Janeiro) [4]	43,653	11,291,520	14,061,694
São Paulo (São Paulo)	248,256	25,040,712	33,516,127
South	575,316	19,031,162	23,393,001
Parana (Curitiba)	199,324	7,629,392	9,341,569
Santa Catarina (Florianópolis)	95,318	3,627,933	4,601,500
Rio Grande do Sul (Pôrto Alegre)	280,674	7,773,837	9,449,932
Central West	1,604,852	7,544,795	10,091,301
Mato Grosso (Cuiabá) [5]	901,421	1,138,691	2,118,197
Mato Grosso do Sul (Campo Grande) [5]	357,472	1,369,567	1,881,211
Goiás (Goiânia)	340,166	3,859,602	4,288,415
Distrito Federal (Brasília)	5,794	1,176,935	1,803,478
Total	8,511,996	119,002,706	155,562,917

For notes *see* p. 230.

Population (1990) 155,562,917; density, 18 per sq. km. The 1980 census showed 59,123,361 males and 59,879,345 females. The urban population comprised 74·4% in 1989.

The language is Portuguese.

Population of principal cities (1980 census):

São Paulo	7,032,547	Brasília	410,999	São José dos Campos	268,034
Rio de Janeiro	5,090,700	Santos	410,933	Olinda	266,751
Salvador	1,491,642	Guarulhos	426,693	Londrina	257,899
Belo Horizonte	1,441,567	Niterói	382,736	Sorocaba	254,672
Recife	1,183,391	São Bernardo do Campo	381,097	Uberlândia	230,185
Pôrto Alegre	1,114,867	Natal	376,446	Diadema	228,660
Curitiba	842,818	Maceió	375,771	Feira de Santana	227,004
Belém	755,984	Teresina	339,042	Campina Grande	222,102
Goiânia	702,858	Duque de Caxias	306,243	Jundiaí	221,888
Fortaleza	647,917	Ribeirao Prêto	300,828	São Gonçalo	221,591
Manaus	611,763	Juiz de Fora	299,432	Joinville	216,986
Campinas	566,627	João Pessoa	290,247	Canoas	213,999
Santo André	549,556	Aracajú	287,934	São João de Meriti	210,574
Nova Iguaçu	491,766	Campo Grande	282,857	Mauá	205,740
Osasco	474,543				

The principal metropolitan areas (estimate, 1990) were São Paulo (17,112,712), Rio de Janeiro (11,205,567), Belo Horizonte (3,615,234), Porto Alegre (2,906,472), Recife (2,814,795), Salvador (2,424,878), Fortaleza (2,119,774), Curitiba (1,966,426) and Belém (1,418,061).

CLIMATE. Because of its latitude, the climate is predominantly tropical, but factors such as altitude, prevailing winds and distance from the sea cause certain variations, though temperatures are not notably extreme. In tropical parts, winters are dry and summers wet, while in Amazonia conditions are constantly warm and humid. The N.E. sertao is hot and arid, with frequent droughts. In the south and east, spring and autumn are sunny and warm, summers are hot, but winters can be cold when polar air-masses impinge. Brasilia. Jan. 72°F (22·2°C), July 64°F (17·8°C). Annual rainfall 64" (1,600 mm). Bahia. Jan. 80°F (26·7°C), July 74°F (23·3°C). Annual rainfall 76" (1,900 mm). Belém. Jan. 79°F (26°C), July 79°F (26°C). Annual rainfall 97" (2,438 mm). Manaus. Jan. 81°F (27·2°C), July 82°F (27·8°C). Annual rainfall 72" (1,811 mm). Recife. Jan. 81°F (27·2°C), July 75°F (24°C). Annual rainfall 64" (1,610 mm). Rio de Janeiro. Jan. 78°F (25·6°C), July 69°F (20·6°C). Annual rainfall 43" (1,082 mm).

CONSTITUTION AND GOVERNMENT. The present Constitution came into force on 5 Oct. 1988, the eighth since independence from the Portuguese in 1822. President and Vice-President are elected for a 5-year term and are not immediately re-eligible. To be elected candidates must secure 51% of the votes, otherwise a second round of voting is held to elect the President between the two most voted candidates. Voting is compulsory for men and women between the ages of 18 and 70 and optional for: illiterates, persons from 16 to 18 years old and persons over 70.

Congress consists of a 91-member Senate (3 Senators per state) and a 503-member Chamber of Deputies. The Senate is two-thirds directly elected (50% of these elected for 8 years in rotation) and one-third indirectly elected. The Chamber of

---

[1] Including litigious area between states of Piauí and Ceará (3,382 sq. km).

[2] The State of Fernando de Noronha (census 1980 population 1,279) was integrated into the State of Pernambuco by the Constitution of 1988.

[3] Including the islands of Trindade and Martin Vaz.

[4] The former States of Rio de Janeiro and Guanabara were consolidated, from 15 March 1975, into a single State of Rio de Janeiro.

[5] The former state of Mato Grosso was divided into 2 new states from 1 Jan 1979.

Deputies is elected by universal franchise for 4 years. The two Chambers of Congress are to become a constituent body in 1993. Elections were held in Oct. 1990 for the governors of the 27 states, territories and federal district, 27 senators (one-third of the Senate), 503 federal deputies and 1,049 state deputies. Some 70,000 candidates from 22 parties stood. The electorate was 84m.

Voting is voluntary from 16 and compulsory for men and women between the ages of 18 and 65 and optional for persons over 65. Enlisted men (who numbered 339,849 at the 1980 census) may not vote. The Constitutional Amendment number 25 of 15 May 1985 granted illiterate persons (until then disenfranchised) the right to vote and also provided for the direct election of the President.

Former Presidents since 1961 have been as follows:

João Belchior Marques Goulart, 7 Sept. 1961–31 March 1964 (deposed).

Marshal Humberto de Alencar Castello Branco, 15 April 1964–15 March 1967.

Gen. Arthur da Costa e Silva, 15 March 1967–31 Aug. 1969 (resigned).

Gen. Emilio Garrastazu Medici, 30 Oct. 1969–15 March 1974.

Gen. Ernesto Geisel, 15 March 1974–15 March 1979.

Gen. João Baptista de Oliveira Figueiredo, 15 March 1979–21 March 1985.

José Sarney, 21 March 1985–15 March 1990.

President of the Republic: Fernando Collor de Mello (b. 1949), assumed office 15 March 1990; *Vice-President:* Itamar Franco.

In Feb. 1991 the government consisted of the following ministers: *Foreign Relations*, José Francisco Resek; *Economy*, Zélia Cardoso de Mello; *Infrastructure*, Eduardo Texeira; *Labour*, Antônio Magri; *Social Security*, Margarida Procópio; *Education*, Carlos Chiarelli; *Agriculture*, Antônio Cabrera; *Navy*, Adm. Mario Flores; *Armed Forces*, Gen. Carlos Ribeiro Gomes; *Air Force*, Brig. Sócrates da Costa Monteiro; *Justice*, Jarbas Passarinho; *Health*, Alceni Guerra.

National flag: Green, with yellow lozenge on which is placed a blue sphere, containing 23 white stars and crossed with a band bearing the motto *Ordem e Progresso*.

National anthem: Ouviram do Ipiranga. . . ('They hear the river Ipiranga' words by J. O. Duque Estrada; tune by F. M. da Silva).

Local Government. Brazil consists of 26 states and 1 federal district. Each state has its distinct administrative, legislative and judicial authorities, its own constitution and laws, which must, however, agree with the constitutional principles of the Union. Taxes on interstate commerce, levied by individual states, are prohibited. The governors and members of the legislatures are elected for 4-year terms, but magistrates are appointed and are not removable from office save by judicial sentence. The country is sub-divided into 4,491 *municípios*, each under an elected mayor *(prefeito)* and municipal council, and then further sub-divided into *distritos*. The Federal District is the national capital, inaugurated in 1960; it is divided into 13 administrative Regions, the first Region being Brasília. Gubernatorial elections were held for all 27 states etc. in Oct.–Nov. 1990.

DEFENCE

Army. The Army is organized in 8 divisions, each with 4 armoured, 4 mechanized cavalry brigades and 12 motorized infantry brigades; in addition there are 7 light 'jungle' infantry battalions, 28 artillery groups and 2 engineer groups; total strength (1991) over 223,000 (143,000 conscripts). An Aviation Corps is being formed.

Navy. The principal ship of the Brazilian Navy is the 20,200 tonne Light Aircraft Carrier *Minas Gerais*, formerly the British *Vengeance*, completed in 1945, purchased in 1956, and capable of operating an air group of 8 S-2E Tracker anti-submarine aircraft, and 8 ASH-3H anti-submarine Sea King helicopters. She is currently non-operational.

There are also 7 diesel submarines (1 built in Germany, 3 British Oberon-class and 3 old ex-US), 11 frigates including 4 ex-US Garcia class leased in 1989 for 5 years, 6 built to two variants of a British design in the 1970s, and the first of a class of 4 locally designed and built. The fleet still includes 9 old ex-US Gearing class destroyers, but some of these have begun to decommission following acquisition of the Garcias. There are also 6 coastal minesweepers and a patrol force of 9 tug/trawler types, 6 ex-US inshore craft and a number for work on the rivers. Major auxiliaries include 1 oiler, 1 repair ship, 4 transports, 5 survey and rescue, 1 training frigate and 5 tugs. There are some 70 minor auxiliaries. Amphibious forces consist of 2 recently-acquired ex-US landing ships and 1 tank landing ship. A further 2 diesel submarines and 3 small frigates are being built, and there is a long term project to build a nuclear-powered submarine.

Fleet Air Arm personnel only fly helicopters, the 11 S-2E Tracker anti-submarine aircraft held for carrier operations and the 21 shore-based maritime patrol EMB-110A and EMB-111 being operated by the Air Force. Naval aircraft include 10 ASH-3 Sea King for carrier service, 8 Lynx, 7 Wasp and 8 Esquilo for embarkation in the smaller ships. Utility and sea-air reconaissance duties are performed by 16 Bell 206B Sea Ranger, and 4 Super Puma helicopters. Naval bases are at Rio de Janeiro, Aratu (Bahia), Belém, Natal, Rio Grande do Sul, and Salvador, with river bases at Ladario and Manaus.

Active personnel in 1990 totalled 50,500, including 15,000 Marines and 700 Naval Aviation.

Air Force. The Air Force is organized in 6 zones, centred on Belém, Recife, Rio de Janeiro, São Paulo, Porto Alegre and Brasília. The 1a ALADA (air defence wing) has 16 Mirage IIIE fighters and 5 Mirage IIID trainers, integrated with Roland mobile short-range surface-to-air missile systems deployed by the Army, and a radar/communications/computer network. Two fighter groups have 3 squadrons of F-5E Tiger II supersonic fighter-bombers and two-seat F-5Bs; 4 others operate AT-26 (Aermacchi MB 326G) Xavante light jet attack/trainers, licence-built by Embraer in Brazil. Counter-insurgency squadrons are also equipped with Neiva Regente lightplanes, Universal armed piston-engined trainers, Super Puma transports and UH-1D/H Iroquois and armed Ecureuil helicopters for liaison and observation. There is an ASW group of S-2A/E Trackers for shore-based and carrier-based operations; a maritime patrol group (2 squadrons) with 12 EMB-111 (P-95) twin-turboprop aircraft developed from the Embraer Bandeirante transport and 3 Lear jets; and 2 air-sea rescue units with Bandeirantes. Equipment of transport units includes 1 squadron of C-130E/H Hercules transports; 1 squadron of Boeing 707 and KC-130H Hercules tanker/transports; 1 group made up of a squadron of HS 748 and a second squadron of Bandeirante turboprop transports; 2 troop-carrier groups with DHC-5 Buffaloes; 1 group with Bandeirantes; and 7 independent squadrons with Bandeirantes and Buffaloes. Light aircraft for liaison duties include 30 Embraer U-7s (licence-built Piper Senecas) and 7 Cessna Caravans. The VIP transport group has 2 Boeing 737s, 11 HS 125 twin-jet light transports, several Embraer Brasilias, 6 Embraer Xingu (VU-9) twin-turboprop pressurized transports and Ecureuil and JetRanger helicopters. Training is performed primarily on locally-built T-25 Universal and turboprop T-27 Tucano (EMB-312) basic trainers, and AT-26 Xavante armed jet basic trainers. New equipment will include 79 AM-X jet attack aircraft, produced jointly by Embraer and Aeritalia/Aermacchi of Italy, of which deliveries began late in 1989.

Personnel strength (1991) about 50,700, with more than 600 aircraft of all types.

INTERNATIONAL RELATIONS

Membership. Brazil is a member of the UN, OAS, SELA and LAIA.

ECONOMY

Policy. In order to contain inflation, private savings were frozen until late 1991.

Budget. In 1988 the budget balanced at 4,667,963,808,000m. cruzeiros.

Internal federal debt, Dec. 1988 was NCz$56,295·5m. Internal states and municipalities (main securities outstanding), Dec. 1988, NCz$3,834·2m.

Currency. The *cruzeiro* (BRC) is the monetary unit which was introduced in

March 1990 at parity with the former *cruzado*. The exchange rate in March 1991 was US$1 = Cr$226·04; £1 = Cr$428·80.

Banking and Finance. The Bank of Brazil (founded in 1853 and reorganized in 1906) is a state-owned commercial bank; it had 2,535 branches in 1988 throughout the republic. On 31 Dec. 1987 deposits were Cr$837,912,257,000.

On 31 Dec. 1964 the Banco Central do Brasil (*President*, Ibrahim Eris) was founded as the national bank of issue; assets (1985) Cr$639,424m.

There are stock exchanges in Rio de Janeiro and São Paulo.

Weights and Measures. The metric system has been compulsory since 1872.

ENERGY AND NATURAL RESOURCES

Electricity. Brazil's hydro-electric potential capacity for electric power production was estimated at 106,500 mw per year in Dec. 1987, one of the largest in the world, of which 34% belongs to the Amazon hydro-electric basin. Installed capacity (1988) 53,166 mw of which 45,871 mw hydro-electric. Production (1988) 231,951m. kwh (217,162m. kwh hydro-electric). Supply 110, 127 and 220 volts; 60 Hz.

Oil. There are 13 oil refineries, of which 11 are state owned. Crude oil production (1989) 30m. tonnes; (1988) 28·92m. tonnes of which 68% was from the continental shelf. Promising results have been obtained with the exploration of that area.

The country imported substantial amounts of oil in 1989: 29,180,116 tonnes (value f.o.b. US$3,390m.). Imports came mainly from Saudi Arabia and Iraq.

In Dec. 1984 a major oil field was reported on the fringes of the existing Campos Basin oil field; reserves are estimated at 4,000m. bbls. Total proven reserves (1986) 2,194m. bbls.

Gas. Production (1988) 5,844,106 cu. metres; proven reserves (1986) 93,000m. cu. metres.

Minerals. Brazil is the only source of high-grade quartz crystal in commercial quantities; output, 1987, 209,034 tonnes raw, 7,062 tonnes processed. It is a major producer of chrome ore (reserves of 9·6m. tonnes; output, 1987, 829,739 tonnes); other minerals are mica (15 tonnes in 1987); zirconium, 26,040; beryllium 10; graphite 525,164; titanium ore 3,344,318 tonnes, and magnesite 860,163 tonnes. Along the coasts of the states of Rio de Janeiro, Espírito Santo and Bahia are found monazite sands containing thorium; output, 1987, 4,956 tonnes; reserves are estimated at 37,000 tonnes. Manganese ores of high content are important (reserves in 1987 were estimated at 75·3m. tonnes); output, 1987, 3,045,564 tonnes. Output of bauxite, 1987, 10,318,682 tonnes; mineral salt (1987), 951,645; tungsten ore, 346,557, unrough, 1,364; lead, 180,269; asbestos, 3,176,231; coal (1983), 21,367,472. Primary aluminium production in 1989 was 888,000 tonnes. Deposits of coal exist in Rio Grande do Sul, Santa Catarina and Paraná. Total reserves were estimated at 4,159·5m. tonnes in 1984.

Iron is found chiefly in Minas Gerais, notably the Cauê Peak at Itabira. The Government is now opening up what is believed to be one of the richest iron-ore deposits in the world, situated in Carajás, in the northern state of Para, with estimated reserves of 35,000m. tonnes, representing the largest concentration of high-grade (66%) iron ore in the world. Total output of iron ore, 1987, mainly from the Cia. Vale do Rio Doce mine at Itabira, was 182,744,974 tonnes.

Production of tin ore (cassiterite, processed) was 40,324 tonnes in 1987. Output of barytes, 99,424 tonnes. Output of phosphate rock, 28·1m. tonnes.

Gold is chiefly from Pará (12,590 kg in 1987), Mato Grosso (5,219 kg) and Minas Gerais (7,787 kg); total production (1987), 34,996 kg processed. Silver output (processed in 1987) 2,064 kg. Diamond output in 1987 was 522,437 carats (203,900 carats from Minas Gerais, 307,800 carats from Mato Grosso).

Agriculture. In 1985, 23,273,517 people were employed in agriculture, and there were 5·83m. farms. Production (in tonnes):

	1988	1989 [1]		1988	1989 [1]
Bananas (1,000 bunches)	515,585	550,163	Tomatoes	1,838,334	2,173,278
Beans	2,900,754	2,308,355	Grapes	764,524	691,972
Cassava	21,611,540	23,616,442	Coconut	374,868	...
Castor beans	145,478	128,079	Coffee	2,704,216	3,064,670
Oranges (1,000 fruits)	75,549,274	88,867,897	Cotton	2,535,127	1,844,254
			Jute	16,054	8,328
			Maize	24,749,550	26,589,867
Potatoes	2,299,499	2,129,334	Soya	18,020,677	24,051,673
Rice	11,806,451	11,029,804	Sugar-cane	258,448,735	252,290,181
Sisal	189,654	221,231	Wheat	5,751,219	5,555,544

[1] Preliminary.

Harvested coffee area, 1989, 3,041,387 ha, principally in the 4 states of São Paulo, Paraná, Espírito Santo and Minas Gerais. Harvested cocoa area, 1989, 659,522 ha. Bahia furnished 84% of the output in 1989. Two crops a year are grown. Harvested castor-bean area, 1989, 268,618 ha. Tobacco output was 443,869 tonnes in 1989 and 365,000 tonnes in 1990, grown chiefly in Rio Grande do Sul and Santa Catarina.

In March 1990 the Government abolished the Brazilian Coffee Institute and the privileges (support prices, regulated foreign exchange rates) previously accorded the coffee trade. Minimum support prices for beans, maize and rice were raised in 1990. In Nov. 1990 the Government ended its monopoly of wheat distribution, though retaining control of imports.

Rubber is produced chiefly in the states of Acre, Amazonas, Rondônia and Pará. Output, 1987, 26,555 tonnes (natural). Brazilian consumption of rubber in 1987, was 415,332 tonnes. Tobacco output, 1988, 430,437 tonnes; 1989 (preliminary), 443,869 tonnes. Plantations of tung trees were established in 1930; output, 1988, 4,137 tonnes. Soyabean production was estimated at 19·4m. tonnes (from 10·2m. ha) in 1990.

Livestock (in 1,000): 1989, 139,599 cattle, 32,121 swine, 20,085 sheep, 11,313 goats, 5,971 horses, 1,304 asses and 1,984 mules. In 1989, 13,462,000 cattle, 9,695,000 swine, 871,000 sheep and lambs, 773,000 goats and 844,723,000 poultry were slaughtered for meat.

Forestry. Roundwood production (1987) 93,679,451 cu. metres.

Fisheries. The fishing industry had a 1988 catch of 830,102 tonnes.

INDUSTRY. The value of production was Cr$1,132m. in 1985.

The National Iron and Steel Co. at Volta Redonda, State of Rio de Janeiro, furnishes a substantial part of Brazil's steel. Total output, 1989: Pig-iron, 24,381,100 tonnes; crude steel, 25,017,300 tonnes.

Cement output, 1989, was 25,917,000 tonnes. Output of paper, 1988, was 4,683,952 tonnes. Production (1989) of rubber tyres for motor vehicles, 29·22m. units; motor vehicles, 998,681.

Labour. The work force in 1988 numbered 61,047,954, of whom 14,233,308 were in agriculture. 5,608,704 worked in industry in 1985.

Trade Unions. The main union is the United Workers' Centre (CUT).

FOREIGN ECONOMIC RELATIONS. In 1990 Brazil repealed most of its protectionist legislation.

Foreign debt (including states and municipalities) on 30 Sept. 1988 amounted to US$99,558·4m.

Commerce. Imports and exports for calendar years in Cr$1m.:

	1985	1986	1987	1988
Imports	84,815,017	207,785,180	597,938,989	4,019,592,744
Exports	148,571,718	319,271,108	947,658,530	7,357,336,278

Principal imports in 1988 were (in US$1m.): Mineral products, 5,334; chemical products, 2,562; machinery and mechanical appliances, electrical equipment, 3,878; vegetable products (1986), 1,195.

Principal exports in 1989 were (in US$1m.): Coffee (green), 1,610; soybean bran, 2,136; iron ore (1985), 1,101; soya, 1,154; orange juice, 1,019; footwear, 1,312; cocoa beans, 134; pig iron, 361.

Of exports (in US$1m.) in 1988, USA took 8,715; Japan, 2,274; Netherlands, 2,585; Germany (Fed. Rep.), 1,424; Italy, 1,378; France, 850; Argentina, 975; UK, 1,065; China, 718. Of 1989 imports, USA furnished 3,349; Germany (Fed. Rep.), 1,530; Iraq, 1,358; Japan, 1,058; Saudi Arabia, 1,090; Argentina, 739.

Total trade between Brazil and UK (according to British Department of Trade returns, in £1,000 sterling):

	1987	*1988*	*1989*	*1990*
Imports to UK	636,675	742,145	817,545	719,849
Exports and re-exports from UK	347,916	304,735	338,634	328,234

Tourism. In 1987, 1,929,053 tourists visited Brazil. 499,011 were Argentinian, 251,958 US citizens, 221,265 Uruguayan, 113,643 Paraguayan, 92,410 German, 79,497 Italian, 63,230 French, 55,721 Bolivian, 55,589 Spanish, 47,282 Chilean, 40,796 UK citizens, 37,802 Swiss, 33,666 Portuguese, 30,543 Japanese.

COMMUNICATIONS

Roads. There were (1988) 1,673,735 km of highways. In 1985 there were 13,026,154 motor vehicles, including 9,527,296 passenger cars, 1,884,296 commercial vehicles and 130,719 buses and minibuses.

Railways. Public railways are operated by two administrations, the Federal Railways (RFFSA) formed in 1957 and São Paulo Railways (FEPASA) formed in 1971, which is confined to the state of São Paulo. RFFSA had a route-length of 22,067 km (82 km electrified) in 1988 and FEPASA 5,072 km (1,527 km electrified). An RFFSA subsidiary CBTU (the Brazilian Urban Train Company) runs passenger services in the principal cities. Principal gauges are metre (24,373 km) and 1,600 mm (3,449 km). Traffic moved by RFFSA in 1989 amounted to 81·3m. tonnes of freight and 525m. passengers. FEPASA carried 23·8m. tonnes and 109m. passengers.

There are several important independent freight railways, including the Vitoria à Minas (798 km in 1987), the Carajas (opened 1985, 1,153 km in 1987) and the Amapa (194 km). There are rapid-transit railways (metros) operating in São Paulo (from 1975), Rio de Janeiro city (1979), Belo Horizonte, Pôrto Alegre (both in 1985), and small systems in Fortaleza and Salvador.

Aviation. There were 34 companies (30 foreign) operating in 1985. The 4 Brazilian companies cover the whole territory and in 1987 they carried 16,144,000 passengers (14,067,000 in domestic traffic). Their commercial fleet consisted of 248 aircraft on 31 Dec. 1984. There were 243 taxiplane companies on 31 Dec. 1985. The 4 airlines are Viação Aérea Rio Grande do Sul (VARIG), Cruzeiro do Sul, Trans Brasil and VASP. In 1986 there were 126 airports with scheduled flights.

Shipping. Inland waterways, mostly rivers, are open to navigation over some 43,000 km; number of vessels in 1984, 1,348. Santos and Rio de Janeiro are the 2 leading ports; there are 19 other large ports. During 1988, 41,112 vessels entered and cleared the Brazilian ports. 320m. tonnes of cargo were loaded and unloaded in 1990. Port services were deregulated and privatized in 1991. Brazilian shipping, 1984 amounted to 1,636 vessels of 10,001,356 DWT. Petrobrás, the government oil monopoly, took over the government tanker fleet of 26 vessels in 1958; total tanker fleet in 1984 was 70 vessels of 5,090,494 DWT (private and government-owned).

Telecommunications. Of the telegraph system of the country, about half, including all interstate lines, is under control of the Government. There were 12,687 post and telegraph offices in 1988. There were 13,905,290 telephones in 1988 (São Paulo, 5,102,604; Rio de Janeiro, 2,042,652; Brasília, 358,793). In 1986 there were 2,073 radio and 177 television stations, with 75m. radio and 34m. television receivers.

Cinemas (1985). Cinemas numbered 1,623.

Newspapers (1985). There were 322 daily newspapers with a total yearly circulation of 1,699m. Foreigners and corporations (except political parties) are not allowed to own or control newspapers or wireless stations.

JUSTICE, RELIGION, EDUCATION AND WELFARE

Justice. There is a Supreme Federal Court of Justice at Brasília composed of 11 judges, and a Supreme Court of Justice; all judges are appointed by the President with the approval of the Senate. There are also Regional Federal Courts, Labour Courts, Electoral Courts and Military Courts. Each state organizes its own courts and judicial system in accordance with the federal Constitution.

Religion. At the 1980 census Roman Catholics numbered 105,861,113 (89% of the total), Protestants, 7,885,846 (6·6%) and Spiritualists, 1,538,230.

Education. Elementary education is compulsory. In 1989 there were 76,058,259 persons aged 15 years or over who could read and write; this was 78% of that age group (78·09% among men; 78·04% among women).

In 1984 there were 37,348 pre-primary schools with 2,493,381 pupils and 107,338 teachers. In 1988 there were 201,541 primary schools, with 26,821,134 pupils and 1,119,907 teachers; 10,174 secondary schools, with 3,339,930 pupils and 229,183 teachers; and 871 higher education institutions, with 1,921,878 pupils and 138,016 teachers. This tertiary level comprises 83 universities and 788 other institutions.

Of the 83 universities, 19 are in the state of São Paulo, 11 in Rio Grande do Sul and 9 in Rio de Janeiro. There are also foundations in Niterói, Belo Horizonte, João Pessoa, Salvador, Pôrto Alegre, Recife, Manaus, Curitiba, Fortaleza and Natal. There are federal, state and private universities; the largest state university is that of São Paulo (founded 1934), and there are 2 Municipal universities.

The private universities include 11 Catholic universities in Rio de Janeiro, São Paulo, Pôrto Alegre, Campinas, Recife, Belo Horizonte, Goiânia, Curitiba, Pelotas, Salvador and Petrópolis.

Health. In 1987 there were 32,450 hospitals and clinics (12,276 private) of which 7,062 were for inpatients (5,359 private). In 1987 there were 206,382 doctors, 28,772 dentists, 6,094 pharmacists and 29,082 nurses.

DIPLOMATIC REPRESENTATIVES

Of Brazil in Great Britain (32 Green St., London, W1Y 4AT)
Ambassador: Paulo Tarso Flecha de Lima.

Of Great Britain in Brazil (Setor de Embaixadas Sul, Quadra 801, Conjunto K, 70.408, Brasília, D.F.)
Ambassador: M. J. Newington, CMG.

Of Brazil in the USA (3006 Massachusetts Ave., NW, Washington, D.C., 20008)
Ambassador: Marcílio Marques Moreira.

Of the USA in Brazil (Av. das Nações, Lote 03, Brasília, D.F.)
Ambassador: Richard Melton.

Of Brazil to the United Nations
Ambassador: Luís Augusto Saint Brisson de Araujo Castro.

Further Reading

Anuário do Transporte Aéreo. Ministério da Aeronáutica, DAC. Rio de Janeiro, 1986
Anuário Estatístico do Brasil. Vol. 49. Fundação Instituto Brasileiro de Geografia e Estatística, Rio de Janeiro, 1989
Anuário Estatístico do Transporte Aquaviário. 1987
Anuário Mineral Brasileiro. Departamento Nacional da Produção Mineral. Brasília, 1988
Boletim do Banco Central do Brasil. Banco Central do Brasil. Brasília. Monthly
Indicadores – IBGE. Monthly
Estatísticas da Saúde – 1987 IBGE
Bruneau, T. C., *The Church in Brazil: The Politics of Religion.* Univ. of Texas Press, 1982
Bryant, S. V., *Brazil* [Bibliography] Oxford and Santa Barbara, 1985

Burns, E. B., *A History of Brazil*. 2nd ed. Columbia Univ. Press, 1980
Falk, P. S. and Fleischer, D. V., *Brazil's Economic and Political Future*. Boulder, 1988
Font, M. A., *Coffee, Contention and Change in the Making of Modern Brazil*. Oxford, 1990
Hanbury-Tenison, R., *A Question of Survival for the Indians of Brazil*. London, 1973
Lees, F. A. *et al*. (eds.), *Banking and Financial Deepening in Brazil*. London, 1990
McDonough, P., *Power and Ideology in Brazil*. Princeton Univ. Press, 1981
Mainwaring, S., *The Catholic Church and Politics in Brazil, 1916–86*. Stanford Univ. Press, 1986
Micallef, J., (ed.) *Brazil: Country with a Future*. London, 1982
Moraes, R. Borba de., *Bibliographia Brasiliana (1504–1900)*. 2 vols. 1958
Trebat, T. J., *Brazil's State-Owned Enterprises*. CUP, 1983
Tyler, W. G., *The Brazilian Industrial Economy*. Aldershot, 1981
Young, J. M., *Brazil: Emerging World Power*. Malabar, 1982

National Library: Biblioteca Nacional Avenida Rio Branco 219–39, Rio de Janeiro, RJ.

BRITISH ANTARCTIC TERRITORY

HISTORY. The British Antarctic Territory was established on 3 March 1962, as a consequence of the entry into force of the Antarctic Treaty (*see* p. 60), to separate those areas of the then Falkland Islands Dependencies which lay within the Treaty area from those which did not (i.e. South Georgia and the South Sandwich Islands see p. 1113).

AREA AND POPULATION. The territory encompasses the lands and islands within the area south of 60°S latitude lying between 20°W and 80°W longitude (approximately due south of the Falkland Islands and the Dependencies). It covers an area of some 660,000 sq. miles, and its principal components are the South Orkney and South Shetland Islands, the Antarctic Peninsula (Palmer Land and Graham Land) the Filchner and Ronne Ice Shelves and Coats Land.

The British Antarctic Territory has no indigenous or permanently resident population. There is however an itinerant population of scientists and logistics staff of about 300, manning a number of research stations.

The territory was administered by a High Commissioner resident in Port Stanley, Falkland Islands until 1989 and thereafter by the Foreign and Commonwealth Office in London. Designated personnel of the scientific stations of the British Antarctic Survey are appointed to exercise certain legal and administrative functions.

Commissioner: M. S. Baker-Bates.
Administrator: Dr. J. A. Heap.

Fox, R., *Antarctica and the South Atlantic*. London, 1985
Parsons, A., *Antarctica: The Next Decade*. CUP, 1987

BRITISH INDIAN OCEAN TERRITORY

HISTORY. This territory was established by an Order in Council on 8 Nov. 1965, consisting then of the Chagos Archipelago (formerly administered from Mauritius) and the islands of Aldabra, Desroches and Farquhar (all formerly administered from Seychelles). The latter islands became part of Seychelles when that country achieved independence on 29 June 1976.

AREA AND POPULATION. The group, with a total land area of 23 sq. miles (60 sq. km) comprises 5 coral atolls (Diego Garcia, Peros Banhos, Salomon, Eagle and Egmont) of which the largest and southern-most, Diego Garcia, covers 17 sq. miles (44 sq. km) and lies 450 miles (724 km) south of the Maldives. The British Indian Ocean Territory was established to meet UK and US defence requirements in the Indian Ocean. In accordance with the terms of Exchanges of Notes between the UK and US governments in 1966 and 1976, a US Navy support facility has been established on Diego Garcia. There is no permanent population in the British Indian Ocean Territory.

Commissioner: R. J. S. Edis (non-resident).
Administrator: R. G. Wells (non-resident).
Commissioner's Representative: Cdr R. A. Hornshaw, JP, RN.
Flag: Blue and white wavy stripes with the Union Flag in the canton and a crowned palm-tree in the fly.

BRUNEI

Capital: Bandar Seri Begawan
Population: 267,000 (1990)
GNP per capita: US$14,120 (1987)

Negara Brunei Darussalam

HISTORY. The Sultanate of Brunei was a powerful state in the early 16th century, with authority over the whole of the island of Borneo and some parts of the Sulu Islands and the Philippines. At the end of the 16th century its power had begun to decline and various cessions were made to Great Britain, the Rajah of Sarawak and the British North Borneo Company in the 19th century to combat piracy and anarchy. By the middle of the 19th century the State had been reduced to its present limits. In 1847 the Sultan of Brunei entered into a treaty with Great Britain for the furtherance of commercial relations and the suppression of piracy, and in 1888, by a further treaty, the State was placed under the protection of Great Britain. As a result of negotiations in June 1978, the Sultan and the British Government signed a new treaty on 7 Jan. 1979 under which Brunei became a fully sovereign and independent State on 31 Dec. 1983.

AREA AND POPULATION. Brunei, on the northwest coast of Borneo, is bounded on all sides by Sarawak territory, which splits the State into two separate parts, with the smaller portion forming Temburong district. Area, about 2,226 sq. miles (5,765 sq. km), with a coastline of about 100 miles. Population (1981 census) was 192,832; estimate (1990) 267,000 (124,600 males and 116,800 females in 1988). Malays (105,700), Chinese (43,400). The 4 districts are Brunei/Muara (147,300), Belait (56,000), Tutong (28,500), Temburong (about 9,000). The capital is Bandar Seri Begawan (census, 1981) 49,902, 9 miles from the mouth of Brunei River; other large towns are Seria (23,415) and Kuala Belait (19,335). 50% of the population speak Malay and 26% Chinese.

CLIMATE. The climate is tropical marine, hot and moist, but nights are cool. Humidity is high and rainfall heavy, varying from 100" (2,500 mm) on the coast to 200" (5,000 mm) inland. There is no dry season. Bandar Seri Begawan. Jan. 80°F (26·7°C), July 82°F (27·8°C). Annual rainfall 131" (3,275 mm).

RULER. The Sultan and Yang Di Pertuan of Brunei Darussalam is HM Paduka Seri Baginda Sultan Haji Hassanal Bolkiah Mu'izzadin Waddaulah. He succeeded on 5 Oct. 1967 at his father's abdication and was crowned on 1 Aug. 1968.

CONSTITUTION AND GOVERNMENT. On 29 Sept. 1959 the Sultan promulgated a Constitution, but parts of it have been in abeyance since Dec. 1962. At independence, the Privy Council, Council of Ministers, and the posts of Chief Minister and State Secretary were abolished. There is no legislature (the 33-member Legislative Council was dissolved in Feb. 1984) and supreme political powers are vested in the Sultan.

The Council of Ministers was composed as follows in Dec. 1990:

Prime Minister, Minister of Defence: HM The Sultan and Yang Di Pertuan of Brunei Darussalam.

Foreign Affairs: Prince Haji Mohammad Bolkiah. *Finance:* Prince Haji Jefri Bolkiah. *Special Adviser to HM The Sultan and Yang Di Pertuan of Brunei Darussalam in the Prime Minister's Department, Home Affairs:* Pehin Dato Haji Isa. *Education:* Pehin Dato Haji Abdul Aziz. *Law:* Pengiran Haji Bahrin. *Industry and Primary Resources:* Pehin Dato Haji Abdul Rahman. *Religious Affairs:* Pehin Dato Dr Haji Mohammad Zain. *Development:* Pengiran Dato Dr Haji Ismail. *Culture, Youth and Sports:* Pehin Dato Haji Hussain. *Health:* Dato Dr Haji Johar. *Communications:* Dato Haji Zakaria.

The official language is Malay, but English may be used for other purposes. The Chinese community mainly use the Hokkien dialect.

Flag: Yellow, with 2 diagonal strips of white over black with the national arms in red placed over all in the centre.

DEFENCE

Army. The armed forces are known as the Task Force and contain the naval and air elements. Strength (1991) 3,400. Military units include 2 infantry battalions, 1 armoured reconnaissance squadron, 1 engineer squadron and 1 surface-to-air missile battalion. Equipment includes 16 Scorpion light tanks, 24 Sankey AT-104 armoured personnel carriers and 12 Rapier missiles.

Navy. The Royal Brunei Armed Forces Flotilla comprises 3 fast missile-armed attack craft of 200 tonnes and 3 coastal patrol boats. There are also 2 landing craft, 2 utility craft and 3 small patrol boats. The River Division operates 24 fast assault boats. The order for 3 much larger offshore patrol craft in 1989 was deferred. Personnel in 1990 numbered 500.

Two coastal patrol craft operate with 7 smaller boats for the Marine Police.

Air Wing. The Air Wing of the Royal Brunei Armed Forces was formed in 1965. Current equipment includes 6 MBB BO 105, 2 Bell 206B JetRanger, 1 Bell 214, 2 Sikorsky S-70 and 11 Bell 212 helicopters, and 2 SF.260M piston-engined trainers. Personnel (1991), 300.

Police. The Royal Brunei Police numbers 1,750 officers and men (1991). In addition, there are 500 additional police officers mostly employed on static guard duties.

INTERNATIONAL RELATIONS

Membership. Brunei is a member of the UN, the Commonwealth and ASEAN.

ECONOMY

Policy. A fifth Five-Year National Development Plan (1986–90) aimed to further improve the economic, social and cultural life of the people.

Budget. The budget for 1988 envisaged expenditure of B$2,487m. and revenue of B$2,721m.

Currency. The unit of currency is the *Brunei dollar* (BRD) of 100 *cents*, with a par value of 0·290 299 gramme of gold. In March 1991, £1 = B$3·29; US$1 = B$1·73.

Banking. In 1988 there were 7 banks (1 incorporated in Brunei) with a total of 28 branches.

ENERGY AND NATURAL RESOURCES

Electricity. Electric power production (1988) was 1,114m. kwh. installed capacity, 387,000 kw, consumption, 1,081m. kwh. Supply 240 volts; 50 Hz.

Oil. The Seria oilfield, discovered in 1929, has passed its peak production. The high level of crude oil production is maintained through the increase of offshore oilfields production, which exceeds onshore oilfields production. There were 564 producing wells at 31 Dec. 1988. Production was 7·5m. tonnes in 1989. The crude oil is exported directly, and only a small amount is refined at Seria for domestic uses.

Gas. Natural gas is produced (8,544m. cu. metres in 1988) at one of the largest liquefied natural gas plants in the world and is exported to Japan.

Agriculture. The main crops produced in 1988 were, rice (1,422 tonnes), vegetables (848 tonnes), arable crops (523 tonnes) and fruits (3,300 tonnes).

Production, 1988 (in tonnes): Buffalo meat, 212; beef, 57; goat meat, 4·8; pork, 3,193; broilers, 3,750; and 59m. eggs.

Livestock in 1988: Cattle, 3,000; buffaloes, 10,000; pigs, 14,000; goats, 1,000; chickens, 2m.

Forestry. Most of the interior is under forest, containing large potential supplies of serviceable timber. In 1988 production of round timber was 140,800 cu. metres; sawn timber, 72,500 cu. metres.

INDUSTRY. Brunei depends primarily on its oil industry, which employs more than 7% of the entire working population. Other minor products are rubber, pepper, sawn timber, gravel and animal hides. Local industries include boat-building, cloth weaving and the manufacture of brass- and silverware.

FOREIGN ECONOMIC RELATIONS

Commerce. Liquefied natural gas accounts for 50% of the total value of the exports. The second main export is crude oil, which contributes 42% and petroleum products 6%. In 1988 (estimate) imports totalled B$1,451m.; exports (including re-exports), B$3,460m. In 1986 Singapore supplied 24% of imports, the USA 15·2% and Japan 20%. Japan took 68% of all exports.

Total trade between Brunei and UK (British Department of Trade returns, in £1,000 sterling):

	1986	*1987*	*1988*	*1989*	*1990*
Imports to UK	71,624	34,144	142,461	186,110	158,516
Exports and re-exports from UK	154,146	204,129	171,556	264,371	224,562

Tourism. There were 85,358 visitors in 1987.

COMMUNICATIONS

Roads. There were (1988) 1,956 km of road, of which 1,015 miles are bituminous surfaced. The main road connects Bandar Seri Begawan with Kuala Belait and Seria. In 1989 there were 93,000 passenger cars and 17,512 commercial vehicles.

Aviation. Brunei International Airport serves 400,000 passengers annually. Royal Brunei Airlines (RBA) and Singapore Airlines provide daily services linking Brunei and Singapore. RBA also operates services to Bangkok, Manila, Kuala Lumpur, Kuching, Kota Kinabalu, Hong Kong, Darwin, Jakarta, Taipei and Dubai (*via* Singapore). Cathay Pacific Airways also operates to Brunei and on to Western Australia from Hong Kong. British Airways provides a weekly service between Brunei and UK. Malaysian Airlines System has air connections from neighbouring regions. In 1985 Brunei International Airport handled 380,000 passengers and 8,500 tons of freight.

Shipping. Regular shipping services operate from Singapore, Hong Kong, and from ports in Sarawak and Sabah to Bandar Seri Begawan. Private companies operate a passenger ferry service between Bandar Seri Begawan and Labuan daily.

Telecommunications. There are 12 post offices (1988) and a telephone network (44,619 telephones in 1988) linking the main centres. Radio Brunei, operates on medium- and shortwaves in Malay, English, Chinese and Nepali. Number of receivers (1988): Radio 87,000 and television 58,500.

JUSTICE, RELIGION, EDUCATION AND WELFARE

Justice. The Supreme Court comprises a High Court and a Court of Appeal and the Magistrates' Courts. The High Court receives appeals from subordinate courts in the districts and is itself a court of first instance for criminal and civil cases. Appeal from the High Court is to a Court of Appeal. The Judicial Committee of the Privy Council in London is the final court of appeal. Shariah Courts deal with Islamic law.

Religion. The official religion is Islam. In 1986, 66% of the population were Moslem (mostly Malays), 12% Buddhists and 9% Christian.

Education (1989). The government provides free education to all Brunei citizens from pre-school up to the highest level at local and overseas universities and institutions. In 1989 there were about 144 government schools and educational institutions (including one university) with about 53,000 students, and 40 non-government schools with about 16,000 students.

The University of Brunei Darussalam opened in 1985 with an enrolment of 176 students, and enables locals to pursue degree courses in the state. For courses not available at the university, scholarships are awarded to qualify Brunei citizns to study in Britain, the USA, New Zealand, Australia, Canada, Malaysia, Singapore and Egypt.

Health. Medical and health services are free to Brunei citizens and those in government service and their dependants. Citizens are sent overseas at government expense for medical care not available in Brunei. Flying medical services are provided to remote areas. In 1989 there were 8 hospitals with 893 beds; there were also 171 doctors, 31 dentists, 8 pharmacists, 185 midwives and 779 nursing personnel.

DIPLOMATIC REPRESENTATIVES

Of Brunei in Great Britain (49 Cromwell Rd, London, SW7 2ED)
High Commissioner: Pengiran Haji Mustapha.

Of Great Britain in Brunei (Hong Kong Bank Chambers, Bandar Seri Begawan 2085)
High Commissioner: Roger Westbrook, CMG.

Of Brunei in the USA (2600 Virginia Ave., NW, Washington, D.C., 20037)
Ambassador: Haji Mohammad Suni bin Haji Idriss.

Of the USA in Brunei (Teck Guan Plaza, Bandar Seri Begawan 2085)
Ambassador: Christopher H. Phillips.

Of Brunei to the United Nations
Ambassador: Dato Paduka Haji Jaya Bin Abdul Latif.

Further Reading

Krausse, S. C. E. and G. H., *Brunei.* [Bibliography] Oxford and Santa Barbara, 1988

BULGARIA

Republika Bulgaria

Capital: Sofia
Population: 8·97m. (1988)
GNP per capita: US$6,460 (1985)

HISTORY. The Bulgarian state was founded in 681, but fell under Turkish rule in 1396. By the Treaty of Berlin (1878), the Principality of Bulgaria and the Autonomous Province of Eastern Rumelia, both under Turkish suzerainty, were constituted. In 1885 Rumelia was reunited with Bulgaria. On 5 Oct. 1908 Bulgaria declared her independence of Turkey.

In 1941 Bulgaria signed the Three Power Pact and the Anti-Comintern Pact. After a referendum which abolished the monarchy (for details *see* THE STATESMAN'S YEAR-BOOK, 1986–87) the Fatherland Front government asked for an armistice, which was signed on 28 Oct. 1944 by the USSR, the UK and the USA. A People's Republic was proclaimed on 15 Sept. 1946. The peace treaty was signed in Paris on 10 Feb. 1947. It restored the frontiers as on 1 Jan. 1941.

Following demonstrations in Sofia in Nov. 1989 which were occasioned by the Helsinki Agreement ecological conference, but broadened into demands for political reform, Todor Zhivkov was replaced as Communist Party leader and head of state by the foreign minister Petūr Mladenov. In Dec. the National Assembly approved 21 measures of constitutional reform, including the abolition of the Communist Party's sole right to govern. The government resigned in Feb. 1990 but was succeeded by the Communist government of Andrei Lukanov as opposition parties declined to join a coalition. President Mladenov resigned in July 1990 following allegations that he brutally suppressed a demonstration in Dec. 1989. Following demonstrations and a general strike Lukanov's government resigned in Nov. 1990 and was replaced by a caretaker government.

AREA AND POPULATION. The area of Bulgaria is 110,994 sq. km (42,855 sq. miles) and is bounded in the north by Romania, east by the Black Sea, south by Turkey and Greece and west by Yugoslavia.

The country is divided into 9 regions (*oblast*) formed from amalgamations of 28 former provinces in 1987 (for these *see* THE STATESMAN'S YEAR-BOOK 1989-90, p. 243). Area and population in 1987:

Region	*Area (sq km)*	*Pop. 1,000*	*Region*	*Area (sq. km)*	*Pop. 1,000*
Burgas	14,657	872·7	Razgrad	10,842	850·0
Khaskovo	13,892	1,044·4	Sofia (city)	1,331	1,208·2
Lovech	15,150	1,072·1	Sofia (region)	18,979	1,017·0
Mikhailovgrad	10,607	668·2	Varna	11,929	980·1
Plovdiv	13,628	1,258·0			

The capital, Sofia, has regional status. The population at the census of Dec. 1985 was 8,942,976 (females, 4,515,936). Population on 1 Jan. 1988 was 8,973,600 (4·4m. males; 66% urban). Population density 80·9 per sq. km.

Ethnic minorities are not identified officially, but there are some 1·2m. Moslem Turks. Attempts forcibly to Bulgarianize these led to an exodus of some 300,000 of them into Turkey in 1989. There are also some 300,000 Moslem 'Pomaks' of Bulgarian origin. Both groups were granted linguistic and religious freedom in Dec. 1989. The use of Turkish in schools was authorized in Feb. 1991. There are also Gipsies, Jews, Romanians and Armenians.

Population of principal towns (1987): Sofia, 1,128,859; Plovdiv, 356,596; Varna, 305,891; Ruse, 190,450; Burgas, 197,555; Stara Zagora, 156,441; Pleven, 133,747; Shumen, 106,496; Tolbukhin, 111,037; Sliven, 106,610; Pernik, 97,225; Yambol, 94,951; Khaskovo, 91,409; Gabrovo, 81,554; Pazardzhik, 81,513.

Vital statistics, 1987: Live births, 116,672; deaths, 107,213; marriages, 64,429; divorces, 11,687; birth rate, 13 per 1,000 population; death rate, 12; infant mortality, 14·7 per 1,000; growth rate, 1. Abortions, 1987: 134,097.

Expectation of life in 1986 was 71·19 years.

CLIMATE. The southern parts have a Mediterranean climate, with winters mild and moist and summers hot and dry, but further north the conditions become more continental, with a larger range of temperature and greater amounts of rainfall in summer and early autumn. Sofia. Jan. 28°F (–2·2°C), July 69°F (20·6°C). Annual rainfall 25·4" (635 mm).

CONSTITUTION AND GOVERNMENT. The 'Tŭrnovo' Constitution of 1879 was replaced by the 'Dimitrov' Constitution in 1947. This was in turn replaced by a new constitution on 18 May 1971. For an account of the political structure of the Communist régime *see* THE STATESMAN'S YEAR-BOOK, 1990-91, p. 244.

The National Assembly has 400 seats. The June 1990 elections were held in two rounds, the first for 200 seats on a first-past-the-post system, the second for the remaining 200 seats by proportional representation. The electorate was 6·5m.; turnout was 91% in the first round, 74% in the second. 3,098 candidates stood. Entry was over a 4% threshold. Seats gained: Bulgarian Socialist Party (BSP; formerly Communists), 211; Union of Democratic Forces (UDF; a grouping of 16 opposition movements), 144; Movement for Rights and Freedoms (in fact representing ethnic Turkish interests), 23; Agrarian Party, 16; Fatherland Union, 2; Social Democrats, 1; Fatherland Labour Party, 1; independents, 2.

The government is a constituent assembly elected for a period of 18 months which it can extend.

In Aug. 1990 Zhelyu Zhelev was elected unopposed by the National Assembly as *President* of the Republic by 284 votes, The *Vice-President* is Atanas Semerdzhiev. The *Speaker* of the National Assembly is Nikolai Todorov.

The BSP government elected in June 1990 was replaced in Nov. by a caretaker government headed by Dimitŭr Popov (ind).

The country was renamed 'Republic of Bulgaria' (from 'People's Republic...') on 15 Nov. 1990.

Elections were scheduled for May 1991.

National flag: Three horizontal stripes of white, green, red, with the national emblem in the canton.

National anthem: An arrangement of Mila Rodino (Dear Fatherland), a popular patriotic song, was declared the national anthem in 1964.

Local Government. People's Councils for the 9 regions, 29 urban areas and 299 other districts are elected for 30 months. In addition to their civic functions they supervise the management of publicly owned enterprises. The Councils' executive organs are Permanent Committees. Elections were held on 28 Feb. 1988, for the first time with multiple candidacies; 25·87% of the 65,455 councillors elected were non-party, 23·75% women. Local elections were scheduled for Feb. 1991.

DEFENCE. There is a compulsory service of 18 months in the Army and Air Force (3 years in the Navy). Defence spending was cut by 12% in 1989.

Army. In 1990 the Army had a strength of 97,000, including 65,000 conscripts, and is organized in 8 motor rifle divisions and 5 tank brigades. Bulgaria is divided into 3 Military Districts, based on Sofia, Plovdiv and Sliven. Equipment includes 862 T-34, 1,612 T-54/-55, 334 T-72 and 80 T-62 tanks (in store). Paramilitary forces, including border guards, security police and People's Territorial Militia, number some 178,000.

Navy. The reducing number of Navy combatants, all ex-Soviet, comprise 2 operational and 2 reserve 'Romeo' class diesel submarines, 2 'Riga' class small frigates, 5 'Poti' class corvettes, 6 'Osa' class missile craft, 10 patrol vessels, 6 torpedo craft, 5 coastal minesweepers and 28 inshore minesweepers. There are two medium landing ships and 23 craft. Major auxiliaries include 2 oilers, 2 research ships, an electronic intelligence gatherer and a training ship. There are some 20 minor auxiliaries and service craft. There are 2 regiments of coastal artillery including some missile-armed, and some 6 shore-based helicopters. The naval headquarters is at Varna, and there are bases at Burgas and Sozopol. Personnel in 1990 totalled 8,000 of whom half were conscripts.

Air Force. The large tactical Air Force had (1987) about 250 Soviet-built combat aircraft and (1991) 22,000 personnel (16,000 conscripts). There are 3 regiments of MiG-21 and MiG-23 interceptors; 2 regiments of fighter/ground attack MiG-23s and MiG-17s; 2 reconnaissance squadrons of MiG-17s and MiG-21s; some Mi-24 helicopter gunships; a total of about 35 Tu-134, Il-14, An-2 and An-24/26 transport aircraft; a total of about 60 Mi-4, Mi-2, Ka-26, and Mi-8 helicopters; and L-29 Delfin, L-39 Albatros, MiG-15UTI, Zlin 42 and MiG-21UTI trainers. Soviet-built 'Guideline', 'Goa' and 'Ganef' surface-to-air missiles have also been supplied to Bulgaria.

INTERNATIONAL RELATIONS

Membership. Bulgaria is a member of the UN, OIEC, IMF and the Warsaw Pact.

ECONOMY

Policy. For planning until 1990 *see* THE STATESMAN'S YEAR-BOOK, 1990-91, p. 245.

Budget. The revenue and expenditure of Bulgaria for calendar years were as follows (in 1m. leva):

	1977	*1980*	*1981*	*1982*	*1983*	*1984*	*1985*	*1986*	*1987*
Revenue	9,498	13,187	15,385	15,824	16,812	17,754	18,097	19,506	20,672
Expenditure	9,477	13,167	15,370	15,809	16,663	17,392	18,087	19,491	20,662

Of the 1984 revenue 92% came from the national economy. 1983 expenditure was: National economy, 8,630m. leva; education, 2,945m.; social security, 2,846m.

Currency. The unit of currency is the *lev* (BGL) of 100 *stotinki*. Notes are issued for 1, 2, 5, 10 and 20 *leva* and coins for 1, 2, 5, 10, 20, 50 *stotinki* and 1, 2 and 5 *leva*. In March 1991, £1 = 5·48 leva; US$1 = 2·89 leva.

Banking and Finance. Under a 1987 reform the National Bank (*Governor*, Todor Vŭlchev) remains the central bank and is responsible for issuing currency. The Foreign Trade Bank (founded 1964) and the State Savings Bank also remain, the latter now serving local enterprises as well as the public. In 1986, 10·48m. depositors had savings totalling 13,954m. leva. Five commercial banks serving various specific industrial sectors, and three more broadly-based (the Economic Bank, the Agricultural Bank and the Bank for Economic Initiative) have been set up. The first private bank opened in Aug. 1990.

Weights and Measures. The metric system is in general use. On 1 April 1916 the Gregorian calendar came into force.

ENERGY AND NATURAL RESOURCES

Energy. Bulgaria has little oil, gas or high-grade coal and energy policy is based on the exploitation of its low-grade coal and hydro-electric resources, which produce 20% of the electricity supply. Supply 220 volts; 50 Hz.

Electricity. In 1987 there were 135 power stations with a potential of 10·7m. kw. (thermal, (46) 6·5m. kw.; hydroelectric, (88) 2m. kw.; nuclear, (1) 2·26m. kw.). Output, 1987, 43,464m. kwh. Domestic consumption was rationed in 1987–88, and remained in short supply thereafter.

Oil. Oil is extracted in the Balchik district on the Black Sea, in an area 100 km north of Varna and at Dolni Dubnik near Pleven. There are refineries at Burgas (annual capacity 5m. tonnes) and Dolni Dubnik (7m. tonnes). Total crude oil production (1989) 280,000 tonnes.

Minerals. Ore production 1987: Manganese, 10,900 tonnes; iron, 559,000 tonnes.

38·5m. tonnes of coal including 372,000 tonnes of hard coal and 31·4m. tonnes of lignite were mined in 1987. 92 tonnes of salt were extracted in 1987.

Agriculture. In 1987 agricultural land covered 6,165,300 ha, of which 4,650,300 ha were arable.

Collective and state farms had been incorporated into 'agricultural-industrial complexes'. There were 285 of these in 1987.

A law of Feb. 1991 provides for the redistribution of collectivized land to its former owners up to 30 ha. Landless peasants receive state land or compensation in lieu. Foreigners and Bulgarians resident abroad may not acquire such land. It may be rented out, but not sold for 3 years.

Production in 1988 (in 1,000 tonnes): Wheat, 4,713; maize, 1,625; barley, 1,306; sugar beet, 677; sunflower seed, 367; seed cotton, 14; tobacco, 117; tomatoes, 809; potatoes, 359; grapes, 929. Bulgaria produces 80% of the world supply of attar of roses; annual production, 1,200 kg. Other products (in 1,000 tonnes) in 1988: Meat, 788; wool, 30·3; honey, 10·2; eggs, 162·2; milk, 2,585.

Livestock (1988, in 1,000s): 123 horses, 1,649 cattle, including 646 milch cows, 8,886 sheep, 4,034 pigs, 41,424 poultry and 608 beehives.

In Oct. 1990 there was a Federation of Independent Agricultural Trade Unions.

Forestry. Forest area, 1987, was 3,868,000 ha (34% coniferous, 25% oak). 46,041 ha were afforested in 1987 and 6·7m. cu. metres of timber were cut.

Fisheries. Catch, 1982: 115,600 tonnes (15,600 tonnes freshwater).

INDUSTRY. All industry was nationalized in 1947 and is divided into 11 associations of up to 150 linked enterprises. A Labour Code of 1986 provides for the self-management of enterprises and the election of management by the workforce.

Industrial production	*1982*	*1983*	*1984*	*1985*	*1986*	*1987*
Crude steel (1,000 tonnes)	2,584	2,831	2,878	2,944	2,965	3,045
Pig-iron (1,000 tonnes)	1,558	1,623	1,578	1,702	1,615	1,652
Cement (1,000 tonnes)	5,614	5,644	5,717	5,296	5,700	5,494
Sulphuric acid (1,000 tonnes)	916	861	908	810	807	689

In 1987 there were also produced (in 1,000 tonnes): Coke, 1,314; rolled steel, 3,325; artificial fertilizers, 2,003; calcinated soda, 689; sugar, 416; cotton fabrics, 352m. metres; woollens, 43m. metres.

Labour. There is 42½-hour 5-day working week. The average wage (excluding peasantry) was 3,300 leva per annum in 1990. Population of working age (males 16–60; females 16–55), 1985, 5·02m. (2·7m. males). The labour force (excluding peasantry) in 1987 was 4,112,674 (49·8% female), of whom 2,811,334 (44·9%) were manual labourers. 1,422,215 worked in industry, 350,711 in building and 875,202 in agriculture and forestry.

Trade Unions. An independent white-collar trade union movement, Podkrepa, was formed in Nov. 1989. It claimed 100,000 members in July 190. The former official Central Council of Trade Unions reconstituted itself in 1990 as the Executive Committee of Independent Trade Unions.

FOREIGN ECONOMIC RELATIONS. Joint Western-Bulgarian industrial ventures have been permitted since 1980. Western share participation may exceed 50%. There were 6 in operation in 1985. In Oct. 1987 the Bulgarian government offered to repurchase Bulgarian bonds. Indebtedness to the West was US$9,000m. in 1989.

A trade pact was signed with the EEC in May 1990.

Commerce. Foreign trade is controlled by the Ministry of Foreign Trade. Bulgarian trade has developed as follows (in 1m. foreign exchange leva):

	1983	*1984*	*1985*	*1986*	*1987*
Imports	11,966	12,842	14,067	14,353	14,067
Exports	11,818	12,987	13,739	13,351	13,802

Proportion of major exports in 1987: Production machinery, 59%; foods, 11%; industrial consumer goods, 10%. Imports: Production machinery, 44%; fuels, 32%; chemicals, 6%.

Main exports are food products, tobacco, non-ferrous metals, cast iron, leather articles, textiles and (to Communist countries) machinery; main imports are machinery, oil, natural gas, steel, cellulose and timber.

Total trade between Bulgaria and UK (British Department of Trade returns, in £1,000 sterling):

	1986	*1987*	*1988*	*1989*	*1990*
Imports to UK	32,459	24,249	28,068	34,272	32,787
Exports and re-exports from UK	80,504	88,761	82,156	86,209	45,022

Tourism. Since 1988 5-year passports have been issued instead of ad hoc exeats. Exit visas were abolished in Jan. 1991. Bulgaria received 7·59m. foreign visitors in 1987 and 540,000 Bulgarians made visits abroad.

COMMUNICATIONS

Roads. In 1987 there were 36,908 km of roads, including 242 km of motorways and 2,938 km of main roads. 940m. passengers and 917m. tonnes of freight were carried.

Railways. In 1987 there were 4,294 km of standard gauge railway, including 2,510 km electrified. 110m. passengers and 83m. tonnes of freight were carried.

Aviation. BALKAN (Bulgarian Airlines) operates internal flights from Sofia (airport: Vrazhdebna) and international flights to Algiers, Amsterdam, Athens, Baghdad, Bratislava, Belgrade, Benghazi, Berlin, Brussels, Bucharest, Budapest, Cairo, Casablanca, Copenhagen, Damascus, Dresden, Frankfurt, Istanbul, London, Madrid, Moscow, Nicosia, Paris, Prague, Rome, Stockholm, Syktyvkar, Tunis, Vienna, Warsaw and Zurich. There are also flights from Burgas to Leningrad and Kiev, and from Varna to Leningrad, Kuwait, Athens and Stockholm. In 1990 BALKAN had 48 aircraft, all Soviet. In 1987 BALKAN carried 2·8m. passengers and 24,213 tonnes of freight.

Shipping. Ports, shipping and shipbuilding are controlled by the Bulgarian United Shipping and Shipbuilding Corporation. In 1982 it had 194 ocean-going vessels with a loading capacity of 1·6m. DWT. Burgas is a fishing and oil-port open to tankers of 20,000 tons. Varna is the other important port. There is a rail ferry between Varna and Ilitchovsk (USSR). In 1987 Bulgaria set up an exclusive economic zone extending 200 miles into the Black Sea. In 1987, 460,000 passengers and 26m. tonnes of cargo were carried by sea-borne shipping, and 299,000 passengers and 4·08m. tonnes of freight by inland waterways.

Pipeline. Conveyed 21m. tonnes in 1987.

Telecommunications. In 1987 there were 4,053 post and telecommunications offices, 2,228,681 telephones, 80 radio transmitters and 43 television transmitters. Radio Sofia transmits 2 TV programmes and 2 radio programmes on medium- and short-waves. A service for tourists is broadcast *via* the Varna II transmitter on 1,124 kHz. Bulgaria participates in the East European TV link 'Intervision', and receives transmissions from the French satellite channel TV5. Colour programmes by SECAM system. Radio receiving sets licensed in 1987, 1,982,929; television, 1,692,711.

Cinemas and Theatres (1987). There were 37 theatres, 20 puppet theatres, 8 opera houses, 1 operetta house and 3,305 cinemas. 705 films were made (35 full-length).

Newspapers and Books. In 1987 there were 17 dailies with a circulation of 2·2m. and 377 other periodicals. 3,786 book titles were published in 1987.

JUSTICE, RELIGION, EDUCATION AND WELFARE

Justice. A law of Nov. 1982 provides for the election (and recall) of all judges by the National Assembly. There are a Supreme Court, 28 provincial courts (including

Sofia), 105 regional courts and 'Comrades' Courts' for minor offences. Jurors are elected at the local government elections.

The maximum term of imprisonment is 20 years. 'Exceptionally dangerous crimes' carry the death penalty. In 1985 harsh penalties were imposed for terrorist acts and drug smuggling following incidences of both.

The Prosecutor General who is elected by the National Assembly for 5 years and subordinate to it alone, exercises supreme control over the observance of the law by all government bodies, officials and citizens. He appoints and discharges all Prosecutors of every grade. The powers of this office were extended and redefined by a law of 1980 to put a greater emphasis on crime prevention and the rights of citizens.

Religion. 'The traditional church of the Bulgarian people' (as it is officially described), is that of the Eastern Orthodox Church. It was disestablished under the 1947 Constitution. In 1953 the Bulgarian Patriarchate was revived. The present Patriarch is Metropolitan Maksim of Lovech (enthroned 1971). The seat of the Patriarch is at Sofia. There are 11 dioceses, each under a Metropolitan, 10 bishops, 2,600 parishes, 1,700 priests, 400 monks and nuns, 3,700 churches and chapels, one seminary and one theological college.

The Constitution provides for freedom of conscience and belief but forbids propaganda against the Government. The State provides 17% of Church funds.

Churches may not maintain schools or colleges, except theological seminaries, or organize youth movements.

In 1990 there were some 70,000 Roman Catholics with 53 priests, in 2 bishoprics. In 1987 there were 10,000 Uniates with 20 priests. In 1984 there were 5 Protestant groups: Pentecostals (10,000 members, 120 churches, 30 pastors); Baptists (1,000 members, 20 churches); Methodists; Congregationalists; Adventists. There were estimated to be about 700,000 practising Moslems in 1984 under a Chief Mufti elected by 7 regional muftis. There were about 1,000 mosques in 1987.

Education. Education is free, and compulsory for children between the ages of 7 and 16. The gradual introduction of unified secondary polytechnical schools offering compulsory education for all children from the ages of 7 to 17 was begun in 1973–74. Complete literacy is claimed. Schools are classified according to which years of schooling they offer: Elementary (1–3), primary (1–8), preparatory (4–8), secondary (9–11), complete secondary (1–11).

Educational statistics for 1987–88: 4,840 kindergartens (344,396 children, 28,652 teachers); 732 elementary schools; 2,159 primary schools; 44 preparatory schools; 72 secondary schools; 482 complete secondary schools. Numbers of teachers and pupils: School years 1 to 3, 24,442 and 412,520; 4 to 8, 37,612 and 679,677; 9 to 11, 9,837 and 167,845. There were also 4 vocational-technical schools (51 teachers, 1,343 students), 261 secondary vocational-technical schools (7,405 teachers, 106,564 students), 248 technical colleges (10,619 teachers, 115,036 students), 16 post-secondary institutions (780 teachers, 11,019 students) and 30 institutes of higher education (15,941 teachers, 116,407 students). University entrance is by competitive examination. Failure rate was 65% in 1985. There are 3 universities: the Kliment Ohrid University in Sofia (founded 1888) had 1,502 teachers and 15,501 students (in 1987–88); the Kirill i Metodii University in Veliko Tŭrnovo (founded 1971) had 417 teachers and 5,042 students and the Paisi Hilendarski University in Plovdiv (founded 1961) had 487 teachers and 5,117 students.

The Academy of Sciences was founded in 1869.

Social Welfare. Retirement and disablement pensions and temporary sick pay are calculated as a percentage of previous wages (respectively 55–80%, 35–100%, 69–90%) and according to the nature of the employment.

Monthly family allowances for children under 16: 15 leva for 1 child, 60 leva for 2 children and 115 leva for 3 children.

In 1986, 2·25m. persons received pensions totalling 2,650m. leva.

All medical services are free. In 1987 there were 185 hospitals (including 15 mental hospitals and addiction treatment centres) and 85,804 beds. There were 27,107 doctors and 5,229 dentists.

DIPLOMATIC REPRESENTATIVES

Of Bulgaria in Great Britain (186 Queen's Gate, London, SW7 5HL)
Ambassador: Ivan Stancioff.

Of Great Britain in Bulgaria (Blvd. Marshal Tolbukhin 65–67, Sofia)
Ambassador: Richard Thomas, CMG.

Of Bulgaria in the USA (1621 22nd St., NW, Washington, D.C., 20008)
Ambassador: Velichko Velichkov.

Of the USA in Bulgaria (1 Stamboliski Blvd., Sofia)
Ambassador: Kenneth Hill.

Of Bulgaria to the United Nations
Ambassador: Dimitŭr T. Kostov.

Further Reading

Kratka Bŭlgarska Entsiklopediia (Short Bulgarian Encyclopaedia), 5 vols. Sofia, 1963–69
Statistical Reference Book: PR of Bulgaria. Sofia, annual from 1988
Statisticheski Godishnik (Statistical Yearbook). Sofia from 1956
Constitution of the People's Republic of Bulgaria. Sofia, 1971
Modern Bulgaria: History, Politics, Economy, Culture. Sofia, 1981
Normative Acts of the Foreign Economic Relations of the People's Republic of Bulgaria. Sofia, 1982
Atanasova, T., *et al., Bulgarian-English Dictionary.* Sofia, 1975
Bell, J. D., *The Bulgarian Communist Party from Blagoev to Zhivkov.* Stanford, 1985
Crampton, R. J., *A Short History of Modern Bulgaria.* CUP, 1987.—*Bulgaria.* [Bibliography] Oxford and Santa Barbara, 1989
Feiwel, G. R., *Growth and Reforms in Centrally Planned Economies: the Lessons of the Bulgarian Experience.* New York, 1977
Lampe, J. R., *The Bulgarian Economy in the Twentieth Century.* London, 1986

BURKINA FASO

Capital: Ouagadougou
Population: 8·76m. (1990)
GNP per capita: US$230 (1988)

République Démocratique Populaire de Burkina Faso

HISTORY. A separate colony of Upper Volta was in 1919 carved out of the colony of Upper Senegal and Niger, which had been established in 1904. In 1932 it was abolished and most of its territory transferred to Ivory Coast, with small parts added to French Sudan and Niger, but it was re-constituted with its former borders on 4 Sept. 1947. Upper Volta became an autonomous republic within the French Community on 11 Dec. 1958 and reached full independence on 5 Aug. 1960.

On 3 Jan. 1966 the government of Maurice Yameogo was overthrown by a military coupled by Lieut-Col. Sangoulé Lamizana, who assumed the Presidency. In a further coup on 25 Nov. 1980, President Lamizana was overthrown and a military regime assumed power. Further coups took place on 7 Nov. 1982, 4 Aug. 1983 and 15 Oct. 1987 and 18 Sept. 1989. The name of the country was changed to Burkina Faso in 1984.

AREA AND POPULATION. Burkina Faso is bounded north and west by Mali, east by Niger, south by Benin, Togo, Ghana and the Côte d'Ivoire. The republic covers an area of 274,122 sq. km; population (census, 1985) 7,967,019 (3,846,518 males). Estimate (1990) 8·76m. (8·8% urban). Vital statistics (1985–90): rate, 2·7%; infant mortality, 138 per 1,000 live births; expectation of life, 47·2 years. The largest cities (1985 census) are Ouagadougou, the capital (442,223), Bobo-Dioulasso (231,162), Koudougou (51,670), Ouahigouya (38,604), Banfora (35,204), Kaya (25,799), Fada N'Gourma and Tenkodogo.

The areas and populations of the 30 provinces were:

Province	*Sq. km*	*Census 1985*	*Province*	*Sq. km*	*Census 1985*
Bam	4,017	164,263	Nahouri	3,843	105,273
Bazéga	5,313	306,976	Namentenga	7,755	198,798
Bougouriba	7,087	221,522	Oubritenga	4,693	303,229
Boulgou	9,033	403,358	Oudalan	10,046	105,715
Boulkiemde	4,138	363,594	Passoré	4,078	225,115
Comoé	18,393	250,510	Poni	10,361	234,501
Ganzourgou	4,087	196,006	Sanguie	5,165	218,289
Gnagna	8,600	229,249	Sanmatenga	9,213	368,365
Gourma	26,613	294,123	Sèno	13,473	230,043
Houet	16,472	585,031	Sissili	13,736	246,844
Kadiogo	1,169	459,138	Soum	13,350	190,464
Kénédougou	8,307	139,722	Sourou	9,487	267,770
Kossi	13,177	330,413	Tapoa	14,780	159,121
Kouritenga	1,627	197,027	Yatenga	12,292	537,205
Mouhoun	10,442	289,213	Zoundwéogo	3,453	155,142

The principal ethnic groups are the Mossi (48%), Fulani (10%), Lobi-Dagari (7%), Mandé (7%), Bobo (7%), Sénoufo (6%), Gourounsi (5%), Bissa (5%), Gourmantché (5%). French is the official language.

CLIMATE. A tropical climate with a wet season from May to Nov. and a dry season from Dec. to April. Rainfall decreases from south to north. Ouagadougou. Jan. 76°F (24·4°C), July 83°F (28·3°C). Annual rainfall 36" (894 mm).

CONSTITUTION AND GOVERNMENT. Following the coup of 15 Oct. 1987, when President Sankara was killed, the ruling National Recovery Council was dissolved and the government re-shuffled. A new Military Council was formed on 31 Oct. 1987.

Head of State and Government: Capt. Blaise Compaoré.

The ruling Popular Front appointed a Council of Ministers, composed in Sept. 1988 as follows:

Popular Defence and Security: Maj. Jean-Baptiste Boukary Lingani. *External Relations:* Jean Marc Palm. *Justice:* Salif Sampegbo. *Economic Development:* Capt. Henri Zongo. *Health and Social Welfare:* Alain Zougba. *Secondary and Higher Education and Scientific Research:* Clément Oumarou Ouedraogo. *Planning and Co-operation:* Youssouf Ouedraogo. *Territorial Administration:* Jean-Léonard Compaoré. *Information and Culture:* Serge Théophile Balima. *Environment and Tourism:* Beatrice Damiba. *Commerce and People's Supply:* Frederic Korsaga. *Transport and Communications:* Issa Konate. *Peasant Co-operatives:* Capt. Laurent Sedgho. *Equipment:* Capt. Kambou Daprou. *Sports:* Capt. Hein Théodore Kilimite. *Labour, Social Security and Civil Service:* Nabou Kanidoua. *Finance:* Bintou Sanogo. *Agriculture and Livestock:* Albert Guigma. *Water Resources:* Alfred Nombre. *Primary Education and Mass Literacy:* Alice Tiendrebeogo. *Secretary-Gen. of the Revolutionary Committees:* Capt. Arsène Ye Bognessan. *Secretary-Gen. of the Council of Ministers:* Prosper Vocouma.

There are also 7 Secretaries of State.

National flag: Horizontally red over green with a yellow star over all in the centre.

Local government: The country is divided into 30 provinces and 250 districts.

DEFENCE

Army. The Army consists of 5 infantry regiments, 1 airborne regiment and tank, artillery and engineer support units. Equipment includes about 83 armoured cars. Strength (1991), 7,000 with a further 1,000 men in paramilitary forces.

Air Force. Creation of a small air arm to support the land forces began, with French assistance, in 1964. Combat equipment includes 5 MiG-21 fighters and MiG-21U trainers and 10 SF.260W Warrior light strike aircraft. Other equipment comprises 2 HS.748 twin-turboprop freighters, 1 C-47, 2 twin-turboprop Nord 262s, an Aero Commander 500, 2 Broussard and 1 Reims/Cessna Super Skymaster for transport and liaison duties, 1 Cessna 172 trainer, and 2 Dauphin and 1 Alouette III helicopters. Personnel total (1991) 200.

INTERNATIONAL RELATIONS

Membership. Burkina Faso is a member of the UN, OAU and is an ACP state of the EEC.

ECONOMY

Policy. A 5-year Development Plan (1986–90) aimed at economic sufficiency and envisaged expenditure of 630,000m. francs CFA.

Budget. Government revenue in 1988 was 90,295m. francs CFA and expenditure 96,285m. francs CFA.

Currency. The unit of currency is the *franc CFA* (XOF) with a parity rate of 50 *francs* CFA to 1 French *franc*. In March 1991, £1 = 496·13 *francs*; US$1 = 261·53 *francs*.

Banking. The *Banque Centrale des Etats de l'Afrique de l'Ouest* is the bank of issue. The main commercial bank is the *Banque Internationale du Burkina*. In Dec. 1982 it had deposits of 32,046m. francs CFA.

ENERGY AND NATURAL RESOURCES

Electricity. Production of electricity (1986) was 159m. kwh.

Minerals. There are deposits of manganese near Tambao in the north, but exploitation is limited by existing transport facilities. Magnetite, bauxite, zinc, lead, nickel and phosphates have been found in the same area. Gold was discovered in 1987 at Assakan, near the Malian border.

Agriculture. Production (1989, in 1,000 tonnes): Sorghum, 991; millet, 649; sugar-cane, 340; maize, 257; groundnuts, 131; rice, 42; seed cotton, 179; sesame, 11. Rice and groundnuts are of increasing importance.

Livestock (1988): 2,809,000 cattle, 2,972,000 sheep, 5,198,000 goats, 70,000 horses, 200,000 donkeys.

Forestry. In 1988, 25% of the land was forested, chiefly in the deep river valleys of the Mouhoun (Black Volta), Nakambe, (White Volta) and Nazinon (Red Volta). Production (1986), 6·93m. cu. metres.

Fisheries. River fishing produced 7,000 tonnes in 1986.

INDUSTRY. In 1982 gross manufacturing (including energy) was 68,146,600 francs CFA, of which textiles (3,666,600 francs CFA) and metal products (2,795,100 francs CFA).

Labour. In 1985 the labour force was 3,421,000.

Trade Unions. The trade union federation is the *Confédération syndicale burkinabe*.

FOREIGN ECONOMIC RELATIONS

Commerce. In 1986 imports totalled 139,640m. francs CFA and exports 28,665m. francs CFA. The major exports were cotton (37%) and karite nuts (7%). In 1983 France provided 28%, the Côte d'Ivoire 24% and USA 9% of imports, while the Côte d'Ivoire took 9%, France 12%, Taiwan 27%, China 11% and UK 8% of exports.

Total trade between Burkina Faso and UK (British Department of Trade returns, in £1,000 sterling):

	1987	*1988*	*1989*	*1990*
Imports to UK	462	546	954	967
Exports and re-exports from UK	4,168	3,732	4,647	6,557

Tourism. There were 68,304 tourists in 1987 spending 2,300m. francs CFA.

COMMUNICATIONS

Roads. The road system comprises 13,134 km, of which 4,396 km are national, 1,744 km departmental, 2,364 km regional and 1,940 km unclassified roads. In 1982 there were 33,769 vehicles, comprising 16,463 private cars, 419 buses, 14,852 commercial vehicles, 411 special vehicles and 1,123 tractors.

Railway. An independent Burkina Faso railway organization was established in 1988 to run the portion in Burkina (495 km of metre-gauge) of the former Abidjan-Niger Railway. An extension was under construction (1990) from the terminus at Ouagadougou to Kaya (107 km).

Aviation. Ouagadougou and Bobo-Dioulasso are regularly served by UTA and Air Afrique and in 1982 dealt with 120,684 passengers and 6,778 tonnes of freight. Air Burkina operates all internal flights to 47 domestic airports.

Telecommunications. There were, in 1982, some 42 post offices and (1984) 14,000 telephones. There are radio stations at Ouagadougou and Bobo-Dioulasso and (1984) 116,000 receivers. The state television service, Télévision Nationale du Burkina, broadcasts 6 days a week in Ouagadougou; there were (1984) 20,000 receivers.

Cinemas. In 1982 there were 12 cinemas with 14,000 seats.

Newspapers. Four daily newspapers were published in Ouagadougou in 1986.

JUSTICE, RELIGION, EDUCATION AND WELFARE

Justice. There is a Supreme Court in Ouagadougou and Courts of Appeal at Ouagadougou and Bobo-Dioulasso. Revolutionary People's Tribunals have replaced the former lower courts.

Religion. In 1980 45% of the population followed animist religions; 43% were Moslem and 12% Christian (mainly Roman Catholic).

Education. There were (in 1986) 351,807 pupils and 6,091 teachers in 1,758 primary schools, 48,875 pupils and 1,514 teachers in 107 secondary schools, 4,808 students with 421 teachers in 18 technical schools and 347 students in a teacher-training establishment. The Université d'Ouagadougou had 3,869 students and 325 teaching staff in 1986.

Health (1980). There were 5 hospitals, 254 dispensaries, 11 medical centres, 65 regional clinics and 167 mobile clinics with a total of 4,587 beds. There were 119 doctors, 14 surgeons, 52 pharmacists, 163 health assistants, 229 midwives and 1,345 nursing personnel.

A 10-year health programme started in 1979, providing for 7,000 village health centres, 515 district health centres, regional and sub-regional medical centres, 10 departmental hospitals, 2 national hospitals and a university centre of health sciences in Ouagadougou.

DIPLOMATIC REPRESENTATIVES

Of Burkina Faso in Great Britain
Ambassador: Vacant; resides in Brussels.

Of Great Britain in Burkina Faso
Ambassador: Vacant; resides in Abidjan.

Of Burkina Faso in the USA (2340 Massachusetts Ave., NW, Washington, D.C., 20008)
Ambassador: Paul-Désiré Kabore.

Of the USA in Burkina Faso (PO Box 35, Ouagadougou)
Ambassador: Edward P. Brynn.

Of Burkina Faso to the United Nations
Ambassador: Gaëtan Rimwanguiya Ouedraogo.

Further Reading

MacFarlane, D. M., *Historical Dictionary of Upper Volta.* Metuchen, 1978

BURMA

Capital: Rangoon (Yangon)
Population: 39·3m. (1990)
GNP per capita: US$200 (1986)

Pyidaungsu Myanma Naingngandaw

(Union of Myanmar)

HISTORY. The Union of Burma came formally into existence on 4 Jan. 1948 and became the Socialist Republic of the Union of Burma in 1974. In 1948 Sir Hubert Rance, the last British Governor, handed over authority to Sao Shwe Thaike, the first President of the Burmese Republic, and Parliament ratified the treaty with Great Britain providing for the independence of Burma as a country not within His Britannic Majesty's dominions and not entitled to His Britannic Majesty's protection. This treaty was signed in London on 17 Oct. 1947 and enacted by the British Parliament on 10 Dec. 1947. On 19 June 1989 the military government changed the official name of the country in English to the Union of Myanmar.

For the history of Burma's connexion with Great Britain *see* THE STATESMAN'S YEAR-BOOK, 1950, p. 836.

AREA AND POPULATION. Burma is bounded east by China, Laos and Thailand, west by the Indian ocean, Bangladesh and India. The total area of the Union is 261,228 sq. miles (676,577 sq. km). The population in 1983 (census) was 35,313,905. Estimate (1990) 39,297,000. Birth rate (1989 estimate), 28·5 per 1,000; death rate, 8·8 per 1,000; infant deaths, 47·1 per 1,000 live births. The leading towns are: Rangoon (Yangon), the capital (1983), 2,458,712; other towns, Mandalay, 532,985; Moulmein, 219,991; Pegu, 150,447; Bassein, 144,092; Sittwe (Akyab), 107,907; Taunggye, 107,607; Monywa, 106,873.

The population of the 7 States and 7 Divisions at the 1983 census (provisional): Kachin State, 903,982; Kayah State, 168,355; Karen State, 1,057,505; Chin State, 368,985; Sagaing Division, 3,855,991; Tenasserim Division, 917,628; Pegu Division, 3,800,240; Magwe Division, 3,241,103; Mandalay Division, 4,580,923; Mon State, 1,682,041; Rakhine State, 2,045,891; Rangoon Division, 3,973,782; Shan State, 3,718,706; Irrawaddy Division, 4,991,057.

The Burmese belong to the Tibeto-Chinese (or Tibeto-Burman) family.

CLIMATE. The climate is equatorial in coastal areas, changing to tropical monsoon over most of the interior, but humid temperate in the extreme north, where there is a more significant range of temperature and a dry season lasting from Nov. to April. In coastal parts, the dry season is shorter. Very heavy rains occur in the monsoon months May to Sept. Rangoon. Jan. 77°F (25°C), July 80°F (26·7°C). Annual rainfall 104" (2,616 mm). Akyab. Jan. 70°F (21·1°C), July 81°F (27·2°C). Annual rainfall 206" (5,154 mm). Mandalay. Jan. 68°F (20°C), July 85°F (29·4°C). Annual rainfall 33" (828 mm).

CONSTITUTION AND GOVERNMENT. On 18 Sept. 1988, the Armed Forces, under Chief of Defence Staff Gen. Saw Maung, seized power and set up a State Law and Order Restoration Council, with Gen. Saw Maung as Chairman.

In Oct. 1990 the government comprised:

Prime Minister, Defence, Foreign Affairs: Gen. Saw Maung.

Planning and Finance, Trade: Brig.-Gen. D. O. Abel. *Energy and Mines:* Vice-Adm. Maung Maung Khin. *Transport and Communications, Social Welfare and Labour:* Lieut.-Gen. Tin Tun. *Construction, Co-operatives:* Lieut.-Gen. Aung Ye Kyaw. *Home and Religious Affairs, Information and Culture:* Maj.-Gen. Phone Myint. *Health, Education:* Col. Pe Thein. *Industry:* Maj.-Gen. Sein Aung. *Livestock and Fisheries, Agriculture and Forests:* Lieut.-Gen. Chit Swe.

In elections in May 1990 the opposition National League for Democracy (NLD), led by Aung San Suu Kyi, won 392 of the 485 People's Assembly seats contested with some 60% of the valid vote. Turn-out was 72%, but 12·4% of ballots cast were declared invalid. The ruling State Law and Order Restoration Council at first said it would hand over power after the People's Assembly had agreed on a new constitution, but in July 1990 it stipulated that any such constitution must conform to guidelines which it would itself prescribe. By Oct. 1990 most of the NLD leaders had been arrested.

National flag: Red with a blue canton bearing 2 ears of rice within a cog-wheel and a ring of 14 stars, all in white.

Language: The official language is Burmese; the use of English is permitted.

Local government: Burma is divided into 7 states and 7 administrative divisions; these are sub-divided into 314 townships and thence into villages and wards.

DEFENCE

Army. The strength of the Army (1991) was 212,000. The Army is organized into 9 regional commands comprising 9 light infantry divisions. Combat units comprise 2 armoured, 175 independent infantry and 4 artillery battalions, and 1 anti-aircraft battery. Equipment includes over 26 Comet tanks, 40 Humber armoured cars and 45 Ferret scout cars. In addition, there are 2 paramilitary units: People's Police Force (50,000) and People's Militia (35,000).

Navy. The fleet includes 2 old escort patrol vessels (ex-USA PCE and MSF types), 2 small indigenously built coastal patrol craft, 21 patrol craft, and 5 river gunboats. Auxiliaries include 1 patrol craft support ship, 1 survey ship and 13 small landing craft. Personnel in 1990 totalled 9,000 including 800 naval infantry.

The Fishery Protection Service (under the Pearl and Fishery Department) operates 3 coastal and 9 inshore patrol craft.

Air Force. The Air Force is intended primarily for internal security duties. Its combat force comprises about 5 T-33A jet fighter/trainers supplied under MAP, supplemented by 15 SIAI-Marchetti SF.260W light piston-engined attack/trainers. Other training aircraft include 20 turboprop Pilatus PC-7s and PC-9s, and 10 jet-powered T-37Cs. Transport and second-line units are equipped with 4 FH-227, 7 Turbo-Porter, 1 Citation and 6 Cessna 180 aircraft, 10 Japanese-built Bell 47 (H-13), 12 Bell UH-1, and 10 Alouette III helicopters. Personnel (1991) 9,000.

INTERNATIONAL RELATIONS

Membership. Burma is a member of the UN and Colombo Plan.

ECONOMY

Policy. The Development Plan, 1986–90, envisaged a total investment of K.14,000m.

Budget. Estimates for 1990–91: Revenue, K.35,570m.; expenditure, K.51,990m.

The largest items, in 1986–87, of revenue were commodities and service tax (K.5,778m.) and customs (K.4,208m.); of expenditure, processing and manufacturing (K.2,490m.); trade (K.1,000m.); mining (2,841m.).

Currency. The unit of currency is the *kyat* (BUK) of 100 *pyas*. There are notes of *kyat* 200, 90, 45, 15, 10, 5 and 1, and coins of *kyat* 1 and *pyas* 50, 25, 10, 5 and 1.

In March 1991, £1 = K.11·46 and US$1 = K.6·04.

Banking and Finance. A Central Bank was established in July 1990. Other banks include the Myanmar Economic Bank, the Myanmar Foreign Trade Bank, the Myanmar Investment and Commercial Bank and the Myanmar Agricultural and Rural Development Bank. The state insurance company is the Myanmar Insurance Corporation.

ENERGY AND NATURAL RESOURCES

Electricity. In 1988–89 the total installed capacity of the Electric Power Enterprise was 983,000 kw, of which 229,000 was hydro-electricity, 92,000 thermal, 302,000 natural gas and 84,000 diesel. Production (1988–89) was 2,226m. kwh. Supply 220 volts; 50 Hz.

Oil. Production (1989) of crude oil was 700,000 tonnes; natural gas, 39,085m. cu. feet.

Minerals. Production in 1988–89 (in tonnes): Zinc concentrates, 4,975; nickel speiss, 101; antimonial lead, 160; refined tin metal, 110; refined lead, 3,198; tin concentrates, 180; tungsten concentrates, 26; tin, tungsten and scheelite mixed, 938. Refined silver, 220,000 fine oz.; gold, 994 troy oz; in 1987–88: Refined copper, 234; steel billets, 16,000; steel grinding balls, 3,000.

Agriculture. Production (1988–89) in 1,000 tonnes: Paddy, 13,164; sugar-cane, 2,197; maize, 193; jute, 47; cotton, 60; wheat, 230; butter beans, 34; soya beans, 27; rubber, 14.

Livestock (1987–88): Cattle, 9·9m.; buffaloes, 2·2m.; pigs, 3·1m.; sheep and goats, 1·5m.; poultry, 39·5m.

In 1988–89 the area irrigated by government-controlled irrigation works was 2,516,289 acres.

Forestry. The area of reserved forests in 1989 was 38,841 sq. miles. Teak extracted in 1988–89, 291,000 cu. tons; hardwood, 4,543,000 cu. tons. All the teak is from the state sector. Other forest products included 17,383,000 cu. tons of firewood and 761,000 cu. tons of charcoal.

Fisheries. In 1988–89 sea fishing produced 343·84m. *viss* and freshwater fisheries 73·56m. *viss*. [Ed. note 1 *viss* = 3·6 lb.].

INDUSTRY.

Production (1988–89) in 1,000 tonnes: Cement, 310; fertilizers, 214; sugar, 29; paper, 8·8; cotton yarn, 7·25. 900 motor cars, 220 tractors and 7,427 bicycles.

Labour. Economically active persons in 1989–90: 15·22m., of whom 66% were employed in agriculture, 9% in trade, 7% in manufacturing and 4% in administration.

FOREIGN ECONOMIC RELATIONS.

Foreign debt was some US$4,200m. in 1990, of which US$2,000m. was owed to Japan. A law of 1989 permitted joint ventures, with foreign companies or individuals able to hold 100% of the shares.

Commerce. All imports and exports are controlled by the government trading organizations.

Imports and exports (K.1m.) for 1987–88: Imports 4,100 and exports 2,098·7.

Total trade between Burma and UK (British Department of Trade returns, in £1,000 sterling):

	1986	*1987*	*1988*	*1989*	*1990*
Imports to UK	5,092	3,826	4,427	3,484	4,582
Exports and re-exports from UK	10,835	24,715	11,685	12,217	15,951

Tourism. There were 2,854 tourists in 1989, and 22,252 in 1988.

COMMUNICATIONS

Roads. There were 14,533 miles of road in 1987–88, of which 2,452 miles were union highway.

Railways. In 1989 there were 2,791 miles of route on metre gauge. In 1988–89 the railway carried 1·27m. tons of freight and 39·2m. passengers.

Aviation. Myanma Airways maintains international services only to Bangkok and Singapore. There were, in 1990, 37 civil airfields. In 1988–89 290,000 passengers were carried on domestic, and 18,000 on international, flights.

Shipping. There are 60 miles of navigable canals. The Irrawaddy is navigable up to Myitkyina, 900 miles from the sea, and its tributary, the Chindwin, is navigable for 390 miles. The Irrawaddy delta has nearly 2,000 miles of navigable water. The Salween, the Attaran and the G'yne provide about 250 miles of navigable waters around Moulmein. In 1988–89 14·54m. passengers and 1·84m. tons of freight were carried on inland waterways and 52,000 passengers and 566,000 tons of freight coastally and overseas.

Telecommunications. There were 1,115 post offices in 1988–89. Number of telephones was 66,172 in 1988–89. The government runs a TV and a radio station. In 1985 there were 725,000 radio and 35,000 television receivers.

Newspapers. 1 newspaper is published, by the government, in Burmese and English versions.

JUSTICE, RELIGION, EDUCATION AND WELFARE

Justice. The highest judicial authority is the Chief Judge, appointed by the State Law and Order Restoration Council.

Religion. Religious freedom is allowed. At the 1983 census, 68% of the population was Buddhist.

Education. The medium of instruction in all schools is Burmese; English is taught as a compulsory second language from kindergarten level.

Education is free in the primary, junior secondary and vocational schools; fees are charged in senior secondary schools and universities.

In 1988–89 there were 726 state high schools with 284,892 pupils, 1,702 state middle schools with 1,134,303 pupils and 31,499 state primary schools with 5,159,330 pupils; the total teaching staff was 218,444, of whom 166,950 were in primary schools.

Beside the Arts and Science University, there are independent degree-giving institutes of engineering, education, medicine, agriculture, economics and commerce, and veterinary sciences. A foreign-languages institute in Rangoon had (1987) 1,127 students learning English, French, German, Russian, Japanese, Chinese and Italian.

There are intermediate colleges at Taunggyi, Magwe, Akyab and Myitkyina, and degree colleges at Moulmein and Bassein, and several technical and agricultural institutes at higher and middle level. 7,040 school teachers were being trained in 16 training colleges in 1986–87. Technical high schools had 5,414 students; agricultural schools, 1,675; other vocational colleges, 4,639, and university colleges 91,748. Universities were closed in 1988, but medical schools re-opened in Jan. 1991.

Health. In 1988–89 there were 10,559 doctors and 631 hospitals with 25,309 beds.

DIPLOMATIC REPRESENTATIVES

Of Burma in Great Britain (19A Charles St., London, W1X 8ER)
Ambassador: U Tin Hlaing (accredited 15 June 1989).

Of Great Britain in Burma (80 Strand Rd., Rangoon)
Ambassador: Julian D. N. Hartland-Swann.

Of Burma in the USA (2300 S. St., NW, Washington, D.C., 20008)
Ambassador: U Myo Aung.

Of the USA in Burma (581 Merchant St., Rangoon)
Chargé d'affaires: Franklin P. Huddle, Jr.

Of Burma to the United Nations
Ambassador: Kyaw Min.

Further Reading

Burma: Treaty between the Government of the United Kingdom and the Provisional Government of Burma. (Treaty Series No. 16, 1948.) HMSO, 1948

Cornyn, W. S. and Musgrave, J. K., *Burmese Glossary.* New York, 1958

Herbert, P., *Burma* [bibliography]. Santa Barbara and Oxford, 1991
Lehman, F. K., *The Structure of Chin Society*. Univ. of Illinois Press, 1963
Lintner, B., *Outrage: Burma's Struggle for Democracy*. 2nd ed. London, 1990
Silverstein, J., *Burma: Military Rule and the Politics of Stagnation*. Cornell Univ. Press, 1978.
—*Burmese Politics: The Dilemma of National Unity*. Rutgers Univ. Press, 1980
Steinberg, D. I., *Burma*. Boulder, 1982
Stewart, J. A. and Dunn, C. W., *Burmese–English Dictionary*. London, 1940 ff.
Taylor, R. H., *The State in Burma*. London, 1988

BURUNDI

Capital: Bujumbura
Population: 5·54m. (1989)
GNP per capita: US$230 (1988)

Republika y'Uburundi

HISTORY. Tradition recounts the establishment of a Tutsi kingdom under successive Mwamis as early as the 16th century. German military occupation in 1890 incorporated the territory into German East Africa. From 1919 Burundi formed part of Ruanda-Urundi administered by the Belgians, first as a League of Nations mandate and then as a UN trust territory. Internal self-government was granted on 1 Jan. 1962, followed by independence on 1 July 1962.

On 8 July 1966 Prince Charles Ndizeye deposed his father Mwami Mwambutsa IV, suspended the constitution and made Capt. Michel Micombero Prime Minister. On 1 Sept. Prince Charles was enthroned as Mwami Ntare V. On 28 Nov., while the Mwami was attending a Head of States Conference in Kinshasa (Congo), Micombero declared Burundi a republic with himself as president.

On 31 March 1972 Prince Charles returned to Burundi from Uganda and was placed under house arrest. On 29 April 1972 President Micombero dissolved the Council of Ministers and took full power; that night heavy fighting broke out between rebels from both Burundi and neighbouring countries, and the ruling Tutsi, apparently with the intention of destroying the Tutsi hegemony. Prince Charles was killed during the fighting and it was estimated that up to 120,000 were killed. On 14 July 1972 President Micombero reinstated a Government with a Prime Minister. On 1 Nov. 1976 President Micombero was deposed by the Army. as was President Bagaza on 3 Sept. 1987. Pierre Buyoya assumed the presidency on 1 Oct. 1987.

AREA AND POPULATION. Burundi is bounded north by Rwanda, east and south by Tanzania and west by Zaïre, and has an area of 27,834 sq. km (10,759 sq. miles).

The population at the census in 1986 was 4,782,406; estimate (1989) 5·54m. There are three ethnic groups—Hutu (Bantu, forming over 83% of the total): Tutsi (Nilotic, less than 15%); Twa (pygmoids, less than 1%). There are some 3,500 Europeans and 1,500 Asians. In 1988 some 270,000 Tutsi refugees were living in Burundi, the majority from Rwanda.

Bujumbura, the capital, had (1986 census) 272,600 inhabitants. Gitega (95,300) was formerly the royal residence.

The local language is Kirundi, a Bantu language. French is also an official language. Kiswahili is spoken in the commercial centres.

CLIMATE. An equatorial climate, modified by altitude. The eastern plateau is generally cool, the easternmost savanna several degrees hotter. The wet seasons are from March to May and Sept. to Dec. Bujumbura. Jan. 73°F (22·8°C), July 73°F (22·8°C). Annual rainfall 33" (825 mm).

CONSTITUTION AND GOVERNMENT. A new Constitution promulgated on 21 Nov. 1981 provided for a one-party state. It was suspended following the coup of Sept. 1987. A new 20-member government was set up under Pierre Buyoya as President, only candidate as leader of the sole party, the Party of Unity and National Progress (UPRONA).

In May 1990 President Buyoya promised a 'democratic constitution under one-party government' to end his military rule, and a referendum on a charter to unify Tutsi and Hutu tribes. In Jan. 1991 UPRONA unanimously adopted a charter of national unity to be submitted to a referendum in Feb. 1991 proposing a new constitution which would legalize opposition parties.

President of the Republic, Minister of Defence: Major Pierre Buyoya (assumed office 1 Oct. 1987).

Foreign Affairs and Co-operation: Cyprien Mbonimpa. *Finance:* Gerard Niyibigira.

Flag: White diagonal cross dividing triangles of red and green, in the centre a white disc bearing 3 red green-bordered 6-pointed stars.

Local Government: There are 15 provinces, each under a military governor, and sub-divided into 114 districts and then into communes.

DEFENCE. The national armed forces total (1991), 7,200 (there are also about 1,500 in paramilitary units) and include a small naval flotilla and air force flight of 3 SF 260, 3 Cessna 150 and 1 DO27 liaison aircraft, 4 Alouette III and 2 armed Gazelle helicopters. The Army comprises 2 infantry battalions, 1 parachute battalion, 1 commando battalion and 1 armoured-car company.

INTERNATIONAL RELATIONS

Membership. Burundi is a member of the UN and OAU and is an ACP state of EEC.

ECONOMY

Policy. The 5th, 5-year economic and social development plan, 1988-92 envisages investment of 159,000 Burundi francs.

Budget. The 1989 budget envisaged receipts of 28,679m. Burundi francs and expenditure at 34,790m. Burundi francs.

Currency. The unit of currency is the *Burundi franc* (BIF) of 100 *centimes*. There are coins of 1, 5 and 10 *francs* and bank notes of 10, 20, 50, 100, 500, 1,000 and 5,000 *francs*. The exchange rate was 317·51 *Burundi francs* = £1 and 167·37 *Burundi francs* = US$1 in March 1991.

Banking and Finance. The Bank of the Republic of Burundi is the central bank and 4 commercial banks have headquarters in Bujumbura.

Weights and Measures. The metric system operates.

ENERGY AND NATURAL RESOURCES

Electricity. Electricity production was (1986) 44m. kwh. The majority of the electricity is supplied by Zaïre. Supply 220 volts; 50 Hz.

Minerals. Mineral ores such as bastnasite and cassenite were formerly mined but output is now insignificant. Gold is mined on a small scale. Deposits of nickel (280m. tonnes) and vanadium remain to be exploited.

Agriculture. The main economic activity and 85% of employment is subsistence agriculture. Beans, cassava, maize, sweet potatoes, groundnuts, peas, sorghum and bananas are grown according to the climate and the region.

The main cash crop is coffee, of which about 95% is arabica. It accounts for 90% of exports and taxes and levies on coffee constitute a major source of revenue. A coffee board (OCIBU) manages the grading and export of the crop. Production (1988) 33,000 tonnes. The main food crops (production 1988, in 1,000 tonnes) are cassava (620), yams (10), bananas (1,480), dry beans (316), maize (170), sorghum (251), groundnuts (85) and peas (40). Other cash crops are cotton (8) and tea (5).

Cattle play an important traditional role, and there were about 340,000 head in 1988. There were (1988) some 750,000 goats, 350,000 sheep and 80,000 pigs.

Forestry. Production (1985) 3·6m. cu. metres. For most of the population wood is the main form of energy.

Fisheries. There is a small commercial fishing industry on Lake Tanganyika. The catch in 1985 totalled 14,900 tonnes.

INDUSTRY. Industrial development is rudimentary. In Bujumbura there are plants for the processing of coffee and by-products of cotton, a brewery, cement works, a textile factory, a soap factory, a shoe factory and small metal workshops.

FOREIGN ECONOMIC RELATIONS

Commerce. The total value of exports in 1986 was US$184·6m., and of imports, US$245·4m. Main exports in 1986 were coffee and tea. Main imports, petrol products, food, vehicles and textiles. In 1984, 34% of exports were to the Federal Republic of Germany, while Belgium supplied 15% and France 14% of imports.

Total trade between Burundi and the UK (British Department of Trade returns, in £1,000 sterling):

	1986	*1987*	*1988*	*1989*	*1990*
Imports to UK	3,074	1,330	1,807	1,974	541
Exports and re-exports from UK	2,324	2,867	2,922	2,738	2,804

Tourism. Tourism is developing and there were 66,000 visitors in 1986.

COMMUNICATIONS

Roads. There is a road network of 5,144 km connecting with Rwanda, Zaïre and Tanzania. In 1984 there were 7,533 cars and 4,364 commercial vehicles.

Aviation. In 1984, 38,141 passengers arrived or departed through Bujumbura International airport, and there are local airports at Gitega, Nyanza-Lac, Kiofi and Nyakagunda.

Shipping. There are lake services from Bujumbura to Kigoma (Tanzania) and Kalémie (Zaïre). The main route for exports and imports is *via* Kigoma, and thence by rail to Dar es Salaam.

Telecommunications. In 1983 there were 38 post offices and 6,033 telephones. In 1986 there were 4,000 television and 230,000 radio sets.

Cinemas. In 1980 there were 7 cinemas with 2,000 seats.

Newspapers. There was (1984) one daily newspaper *(Le Renouveau)* with a circulation of 20,000.

JUSTICE, RELIGION, EDUCATION AND WELFARE

Justice. There is a Supreme Court, an appeal court and a *tribunal de première instance* at Bujumbura and provincial tribunals in each provincial capital.

Religion. About 60% of the population is Roman Catholic; there is a Roman Catholic archbishop and 3 bishops. About 3% are Pentecostal, 1% Anglican and 1% Moslem, while the balance follow traditional tribal beliefs.

Education. In 1984 there were 387,710 pupils in 1,023 primary schools, 13,037 in 62 secondary schools, 12,902 in 47 technical schools and 2,783 students in higher education.

Health. In 1983 there were 216 doctors, 6 dentists, 24 pharmacists, 1,126 nursing personnel and 33 hospitals with 5,709 beds.

DIPLOMATIC REPRESENTATIVES

Of Burundi in Great Britain
Ambassador: Julien Nahayo, resides in Brussels (accredited 26 July 1989).

Of Great Britain in Burundi
Ambassador: R. L. B. Cormack, CMG (resides in Kinshasa).

Of Burundi in the USA (2233 Wisconsin Ave., NW, Washington, D.C., 20007)
Ambassador: Julien Kavakure.

Of the USA in Burundi (PO Box 1720, Ave. du Zaïre, Bujumbura)
Ambassador: Cynthia S. Perry.

Of Burundi to the United Nations
Ambassador: Benoît Seburyamo.

Further Reading

Lemarchand, R., *Rwanda and Burundi*. London, 1970
Weinstein, W., *Historical Dictionary of Burundi*. Metuchen, 1976

CAMBODIA

Capital: Phnom Penh
Population: 8·3m. (1990)

State of Cambodia

HISTORY. The recorded history of Cambodia starts at the beginning of the Christian era with the Kingdom of Fou-Nan, whose territories at one time included parts of Thailand, Malaya, Cochin-China and Laos. The religious, cultural and administrative inspirations of this state came from India. The Kingdom was absorbed at the end of the 6th century by the Khmers, under whose monarchs was built, between the 9th and 13th centuries, the splendid complex of shrines and temples at Angkor. Attacked on either side by the Vietnamese and the Thai from the 15th century on, Cambodia was saved from annihilation by the establishment of a French protectorate in 1863. Thailand eventually recognized the protectorate and renounced all claims to suzerainty in exchange for Cambodia's north-western provinces of Battambang and Siem Reap, which were, however, returned under a Franco-Thai convention of 1907, confirmed in the Franco-Thai treaty of 1937. In 1904 the province of Stung Treng, formerly administered as part of Laos, was attached to Cambodia. For history to 1969 *see* THE STATESMAN'S YEAR-BOOK, 1973–74, p. 1112.

Prince Sihanouk was deposed in March 1970 and on 9 Oct. 1970 the Kingdom of Cambodia became the Khmer Republic. From 1970 hostilities extended throughout most of the country involving North and South Vietnamese and US forces as well as Republican and anti-Republican Khmer troops. During 1973 direct American and North Vietnamese participation in the fighting came to an end, leaving a civil war situation between the forces of the Khmer Republic supported by American arms and economic aid and the forces of the United National Cambodian Front including 'Khmer Rouge' communists supported by North Vietnam and China. The Khmer Rouge captured Phnom Penh in April 1975, and instituted a harsh and highly regimented régime, cutting the country off from normal contact with the world and expelling all foreigners. All towns were forcibly evacuated and the population set to work in the fields.

The régime had difficulties with the Vietnamese from 1975 and this escalated into full-scale fighting in 1977–78. On 7 Jan. 1979, Phnom Penh was captured by the Vietnamese, and the Khmer Rouge government under Pol Pot was ousted. The Vietnam-backed Kampuchean National United Front for National Salvation (KNUFNS) proclaimed a People's Republic on 8 Jan. 1979.

In June 1982 the Khmer Rouge (who claim to have abandoned their Communist ideology and to have disbanded their Communist Party) entered into a coalition with Son Sann's Khmer People's National Liberation Front and Prince Sihanouk's group. This 'Coalition Government of Democratic Kampuchea' occupied Cambodia's seat at the UN.

In 1988 there were unofficial talks in Jakarta between the 4 Cambodian factions with the aim of obtaining a settlement of the political situation. From 30 July-30 Aug. 1989 an international conference, held in Paris, aiming to solve the political problems of Cambodia, was unsuccessful. The last Vietnamese forces withdrew in Sept. 1989. In Mid-1990 the Khmer Rouge still had about 25,000 resistance fighters.

In Aug. 1990 the UN Security Council agreed to set up a Supreme National Council (SNC) in Cambodia, and to place the foreign, defence, interior, finance and information ministries under UN control until elections could be held. The SNC was at first to consist of six members from the Government, and two from each group in the guerilla coalition: the Khmer Rouge, the Khmer People's National Liberation Front and Prince Norodom Sihanouk's group. The first meeting of the SNC in Sept. was unable to agree a chairman, and Prince Sihanouk proposed himself as chairman and the allocation of an extra seat, raising the total to fourteen.

On 15 Oct. 1990 the UN General Assembly adopted the Security Council resolution by consensus. On 26 Nov. Indonesia and the 5 permanent members of the Security Council agreed a plan for a ceasefire and elections under UN supervision. Talks continued throughout 1990 without agreement being reached.

AREA AND POPULATION. Cambodia is bounded in the north by Laos and Thailand, west by Thailand, east by Vietnam and south by the Gulf of Thailand. It has an area of about 181,035 sq. km (69,898 sq. miles).

The total population was 5,756,141 (census, 1981) of whom 93% were Khmer, 4% Vietnamese and 3% Chinese. Estimate (1990), 8·3m.

The capital, Phnom Penh is located at the junction of the Mekong and Tonle Sap rivers. Populations of major towns have fluctuated greatly since 1970 by flows of refugees from rural areas and from one town to another. Phnom Penh formerly had a population of at least 2·5m. but a 1990 estimate puts it at 800,000. Other cities are Kompong Cham and Battambang. Khmer is the official language.

CLIMATE. A tropical climate, with high temperatures all the year. Phnom Penh. Jan. 78°F (25·6°C), July 84°F (28·9°C). Annual rainfall 52" (1,308 mm).

CONSTITUTION AND GOVERNMENT. The Kampuchean National United Front for National Salvation (KNUFNS) on 8 Jan. 1979 proclaimed a People's Republic of Kampuchea, and established a People's Revolutionary Council to administer the country. A 117-member National Assembly was elected on 1 May 1981 for a 5-year term, which was extended by its own decision in Feb. 1986; in June 1981 it ratified a new Constitution under which it appointed a 7-member Council of State and a 16-member Council of Ministers, replacing the Revolutionary Council. A new Constitution of 1989 renamed the country the State of Cambodia. Real power lies with the Kampuchean People's Revolutionary Party (Communists), whose Secretary General is Heng Samrin.

President of the Council of State: Heng Samrin.

Prime Minister: Hun Sen (b. 1950). *Deputy Prime Ministers:* Say Chum; Hor Nam Hong; *Minister of Agriculture:* Nguon Nhel. *Speaker of the National Assembly:* Cheam Sim.

National flag: Divided red over blue with a depiction of the temple of Angkor Vat in yellow over all in the centre.

DEFENCE

Army. Strength (1990) 55,500 including 6 infantry divisions and some 50 supporting units. Equipment reported includes 100 T-54/-55 and 10 PT-76 tanks. There are also provincial (22,500) and district (32,000) forces, and paramilitary local forces of some 50,000.

Navy. The navy is believed to include 2 ex-Soviet hydrofoil torpedo craft, 9 inshore patrol craft and a miscellany of riverine and support craft. Naval personnel in 1989 did not exceed 1,000.

Air Force. Aviation operations were resumed in 1988 under the aegis of the Army, equipment includes a newly-formed fighter squadron with MiG-21s and a small number of Mil Mi-8 transport helicopters and Mi-24 gunships.

ECONOMY

Policy. Reforms of 1989 permit a much greater role for the private sector.

Currency. Under the Khmer Rouge money was abolished, but in 1980 the use of money was restored by the People's Republic of Kampuchea. The unit of currency is the *riel* (KHR) of 100 *sen*. There are banknotes of 5, 50 and 100 *riel*. The riel was devalued three times in 1990. In March 1991, £1 = 872·62 *riel*; US$1 = 460 *riel*.

Banking. In 1964 all bank functions were taken over by the Government bank.

ENERGY AND NATURAL RESOURCES

Electricity. Production (1986) 142m. kwh. Supply 120 and 220 volts; 50 Hz.

Minerals. A phosphate factory, jointly controlled by the State and private interests, was set up in 1966 near a deposit of an estimated 350,000 tons. Another deposit of about the same size is earmarked for exploitation. High-grade iron-ore deposits (possibly as much as 2·5m. tons) exist in Northern Cambodia, but are not exploited commercially because of transportation difficulties. Some small-scale gold panning (6,687 troy oz. in 1963) and gem (mainly zircon) mining is carried out at Pailin where there is potential for considerable expansion.

Agriculture. The overwhelming majority of the population is normally engaged in agriculture, fishing or forestry. Some 8m. ha of the total land area are cultivable. In 1980, 1·5m. ha were cultivated. Before the spread of war the high productivity provided for a low, but well-fed standard of living for the peasant farmers, the majority of whom owned the land they worked before agriculture was collectivised. A relatively small proportion of the food production entered the cash economy. The war and unwise pricing policies have led to a disastrous reduction in production to a stage in which the country had become a net importer of rice. Private ownership of land was restored by the 1989 Constitution.

A crop of about 2m. tonnes of paddy was produced in 1988. Rubber production in 1988 amounted to 25,000 tonnes. Production of other crops (1988 in tonnes): Maize, 100,000; dry beans, 36,000; soybeans, 2,000.

Livestock (1988): Cattle, 1·95m.; buffaloes, 700,000; sheep, 1,000; pigs, 1·5m.; horses, 15,000; poultry, 10m.

Forestry. Some 8m. ha of the land area are covered by potentially valuable forests, 3·8m. ha of which are reserved by the Government to be awarded to concessionaires, and are not at present worked to an appreciable extent. The remainder is available for exploitation by the local residents, and as a result some areas are over-exploited and conservation is not practised. There are substantial reserves of pitch pine. Roundwood production (1982), 5·1m. cu. metres.

Fisheries. There are very large freshwater fish resources. Production in 1982 was 84,700 tonnes.

INDUSTRY. Some development of industry had taken place before the spread of open warfare in 1970, but little was in operation in 1990 except rubber processing, sea-food processing, jute sack making and cigarette manufacture. In the private sector there are about 3,200 manufacturing enterprises, producing a wide range of goods; most of them are small family concerns.

FOREIGN ECONOMIC RELATIONS. Foreign investment has been encouraged since 1989.

Commerce. Principal imports by order of value (1972) were petroleum products, metals and machinery (including vehicles), general foodstuffs and chemicals.

The only recorded export in 1972 was 7,328 tonnes of rubber. Much of the country's trade is with Hong Kong and Singapore.

Total trade between Cambodia and UK (British Department of Trade returns, in £1,000 sterling):

	1986	*1987*	*1988*	*1989*	*1990*
Imports to UK	58	268	55	219	56
Exports and re-exports from UK	217	435	322	530	478

COMMUNICATIONS

Roads. There were, in 1981, 2,670 km of asphalt roads (including the 'Khmer-American Friendship Highway' from outside Phnom Penh to close to Kompong Som, built under the US aid programme and opened in July 1959), and 10,680 km of unsurfaced roads.

Railways. A line of 385 km (metre gauge) links Phnom Penh to Poipet (Thai frontier). In 1988 0·9m. passengers and 0·2m. tonnes of freight were carried. Work was completed during 1969 on a line Phnom Penh-Kompong Som *via* Takeo and Kampot. Total length, 649 km but by 1973 only a short stretch between Battambang and the Thai border remained in operation, the remainder having been closed by military action. Irregular passenger and freight trains were running over all the network in 1988.

Aviation. Pochentong airport is 10 km from Phnom Penh. Air Kampuchea has three aircraft. There are regular services to Hanoi and Vientiane (weekly), Ho Chi Minh City (twice weekly) and Moscow (three a month) by Air Kampuchea, Air Vietnam, Air Lao and Aeroflot.

Shipping. The port of Phnom Penh can be reached by the Mekong (through Vietnam) by ships of between 3,000 and 4,000 tons. In 1970, 97 ocean-going vessels imported 51,300 tons of cargo at Phnom Penh and exported 86,400 tons.

A new ocean port has been built under the French aid programme at Kompong Som (formerly Sihanoukville) on the Gulf of Siam and is being increasingly used by long-distance shipping.

Telecommunications. There were 58 post offices functioning in 1968. There are telephone exchanges in all the main towns; number of telephones in 1981, 7,315. There is an International Telex network in Phnom Penh and direct telephone and telegraphic links with Singapore. In 1986 there were 6 radio stations and 200,000 receivers, and 2 television stations with 52,000 receivers.

Newspapers. In 1984 there were 16 daily newspapers.

RELIGION, EDUCATION AND WELFARE

Religion. The majority of the population practises Theravada Buddhism. The Constitution of 1989 reinstated Buddhism as the state religion. There are small Roman Catholic and Moslem minorities.

Education. In 1984 there were 1,504,840 pupils in primary schools, 147,730 in secondary schools and 7,334 in vocational establishments. Phnom Penh University reopened in 1988.

Health. In 1984 there were 200 doctors, 130 pharmacists and 146 hospitals and clinics with 16,200 beds.

DIPLOMATIC REPRESENTATIVES

UK and USA Embassies have been closed as have Cambodian Embassies in London and Washington.

Of the Coalition Government of Democratic Kampuchea to the United Nations
Ambassador: Thiounn Prasith.

Further Reading

Ablin, D. A. and Hood, M., (eds.) *The Cambodian Agony*. London and New York, 1987
Barron, J. and Paul, A., *Murder of a Gentle Land.* New York, 1977.—*Peace with Horror.* London, 1977
Debré, F., *La Révolution de la Forêt*. Paris, 1976
Etcheson, C., *The Rise and Demise of Democratic Kampuchea*. London, 1984
Kiljunen, K., (ed.) *Kampuchea: Decade of the Genocide*. London, 1984
McDonald, M., *Angkor*. London, 1958
Ponchaud, F., *Cambodia, Year Zero*. London, 1978
Vickery, M., *Cambodia: 1975–1982*. London, 1984

CAMEROON

Capital: Yaoundé
Population: 11·54m. (1990)
GNP per capita: US$1,010 (1988)

République du Cameroun—Republic of Cameroon

HISTORY. The former German colony of Kamerun was occupied by French and British troops in 1916. The greater portion of the territory (422,673 sq. km) was in 1919 placed under French administration, excluding the territory ceded to Germany in 1911, which reverted to French Equatorial Africa. The portion under French trusteeship was granted full internal autonomy on 1 Jan. 1959 and complete independence was proclaimed on 1 Jan. 1960.

The portion assigned to British trusteeship consisted of 2 parts where separate plebiscites were held in Feb. 1961. The northern part decided in favour of joining Nigeria, while the southern part decided to join the Cameroon Republic. This was implemented on 1 Oct. 1961 with the formation of a Federal Republic of Cameroon. As a result of a national referendum, Cameroon became a unitary republic on 2 June 1972. In Jan. 1984 the country was renamed the Republic of Cameroon.

AREA AND POPULATION. Cameroon is bounded west by the Gulf of Guinea, north-west by Nigeria and east by Chad, with Lake Chad at its northern tip, and the Central African Republic, and south by Congo, Gabon and Equatorial Guinea. The total area is 475,440 sq. km. Population (1976 census) 7,663,246 (28·5% urban). Estimate (1988) 11,540,000; density, 24·3 per sq. km. Population growth rate (1985–90): 2·6%; infant mortality, 94 per 1,000 live births; expectation of life, 51 years.

The areas, populations and chief towns of the 10 provinces were:

Province	*Sq. km*	*Census 1976*	*Chief town*	*Estimate 1981*
Adamaoua	63,691	359,227	Ngaoundéré	47,508
Centre	68,926	1,176,206	Yaoundé	653,670 [1]
Est	109,011	366,235	Bertoua	18,254
Extrême-Nord	34,246	1,394,958	Maroua	81,861
Littoral	20,239	935,166	Douala	1,029,731 [1]
Nord (Bénoué)	65,576	479,072	Garoua	77,856
Nord-Ouest	17,810	980,531	Bamenda	58,697
Ouest	13,872	1,035,597	Bafoussam	75,832
Sud	47,110	315,739	Ebolowa	22,222
Sud-Ouest	24,471	620,515	Buéa	29,953

[1] 1986.

Other large towns (1981): Nkongsamba (86,870), Kumba (53,823), Foumban (41,358), Limbe (32,917), Edéa (31,016), Mbalmayo (26,934) and Dschang (21,705).

The population is composed of Sudanic-speaking people in the north (Fulani, Sao and others) and Bantu-speaking groups, mainly Bamileke, Beti, Bulu, Tikar, Bassa, Duala, in the rest of the country. The official languages are French and English.

CLIMATE. An equatorial climate, with high temperatures and plentiful rain, especially from March to June and Sept. to Nov. Further inland, rain occurs at all seasons. Yaoundé. Jan. 76°F (24·4°C), July 73°F (22·8°C). Annual rainfall 62" (1,555 mm). Douala. Jan. 79°F (26·1°C), July 75°F (23·9°C). Annual rainfall 160" (4,026 mm).

CONSTITUTION AND GOVERNMENT. The 1972 Constitution, subsequently amended, provides for a President as head of state and government and commander of the armed forces. He is directly elected for a 5-year term, and there is a Council of Ministers whose members must not be members of parliament.

The National Assembly, elected by universal adult suffrage for 5 years, consists of 180 representatives. Elections took place in April 1988. Since 1966 the sole legal party has been the Cameroon People's Democratic Movement (RDPC), which is administered by a 65-member Central Committee and a 12-member Political Bureau. However, in Dec. 1990 the National Assembly legalized opposition parties.

The Council of Ministers in Oct. 1990 comprised:

President: Paul Biya (assumed office 6 Nov. 1982, re-elected April 1988).

Minister-Delegate at the Presidency, Defence: Michel Meva'a M'Eboutou. *Territorial Administration:* Ibrahim Mbomo Njoya. *Social and Women's Affairs:* Aissatou Yaou. *Agriculture:* John Niba Ngu. *Special Duties at the Presidency:* Ogork Ebot Ntui. *Industrial and Commercial Development:* Joseph Tsanga Abanda. *National Education:* Joseph Mbui. *Livestock, Fisheries and Animal Industries:* Dr Hamadjoda Adjoudji. *Higher Education, Computer Services and Scientific Research:* Abdoulaye Babale. *Finance:* Sadou Hayatou. *Public Service and State Control:* Joseph Owona. *Information and Culture:* Henri Bandolo. *Youth and Sports:* Dr Joseph Fofe. *Justice, Keeper of the Seals:* Adolphe Moudiki. *Water Resources and Energy:* Francis Nkwain. *Plan and Regional Development:* Elisabeth Tankeu. *Posts and Telecommunications:* Oumarou Sanda. *External Relations:* Jacques-Roger Booh Booh. *Public Health:* Joseph Mbede. *Public Works and Transport:* Claude Tchepanou. *Labour and Social Welfare:* Jean Baptiste Bokam. *Town Planning and Housing:* Ferdinand Leopold Oyono. *Tourism:* Benjamin Itoue.

There were 7 Secretaries of State.

The *Speaker* of the National Assembly is Lawrence Fonka Shang.

National flag: Three vertical strips of green, red, yellow, with a gold star in the centre.

National anthem: O Cameroon, Thou Cradle of our Fathers.

Local Government: The 10 provinces are each administered by a governor appointed by the President. They are sub-divided into 49 *départements* (each under a *préfet*) and then into *arrondissements* (each under a *sous-préfet*).

DEFENCE

Army. The Army consists of 1 armoured car, 1 para-commando, 1 engineer and 5 infantry battalions and 5 artillery and 1 anti-aircraft batteries. Equipment includes 8 Ferret scout cars. Total strength (1991) 6,600; there are an additional 4,000 paramilitary troops.

Navy. The Navy, all French-built, operates 1 missile craft and 3 inshore patrol vessels. There are some 7 landing craft and 32 auxiliaries and service craft. Personnel in 1990 numbered 700.

The marine wing of the Gendarmerie operates 1 coastal and 12 inshore patrol craft.

Air Force. The Air Force has 3 C-130H Hercules turboprop transports, 4 Buffalo and 1 Caribou STOL transports, 3 C-47s for transport and communications duties, 3 Broussard liaison aircraft, 10 Magister armed jet basic trainers, 5 Alpha Jet close support/trainers, and 5 Alouette helicopters. Some of 4 Gazelle light helicopters are armed with anti-tank missiles. A small VIP transport fleet, maintained in civil markings, comprises 1 Boeing 727 jet aircraft, 1 Gulfstream III and 3 Aerospatiale helicopters. Radar-equipped Dornier 128-6 twin-turboprop aircraft serve for off-shore patrol. Personnel (1991), 300.

INTERNATIONAL RELATIONS

Membership. Cameroon is a member of the UN, OAU, the Non-Aligned Movement and is an ACP state of the EEC.

ECONOMY

Policy. The Sixth 5-year Development Plan (from 1 July 1986 to 30 June 1991) gives priority to rural development and food self-sufficiency.

Budget. The budget for 1990 balanced at 600,000m. francs CFA.

Currency. The unit of currency is the *franc CFA* (XAF), with a parity rate of 50 *francs CFA* to 1 French *franc*. In March 1991, £1 = 496·13 *francs CFA*; US$1 = 261·53 *francs CFA*.

Banking and Finance. The Banque des Etats de l'Afrique Centrale is the sole bank of issue. The commercial banks are Banque Internationale pour l'Afrique Occidentale, Société Camerounaise de Banque, Société Générale de Banque au Cameroun, Banque International pour le Commerce et l'Industrie du Cameroun, Cameroon Bank, Banque Camerounaise de Développement, Bank of Credit and Commerce Cameroon, Paribas Cameroun, Boston Bank Cameroon Ltd, Chase Bank Cameroon Ltd and Bank of America Cameroon. Most of the banks operate in all the large cities and towns throughout the Republic.

ENERGY AND NATURAL RESOURCES

Electricity. There are 3 hydro-electric power stations at Edéa on the Sanaga river with a capacity of 180,000 kw. Total production (1986) 4,200m. kwh. Supply 127 and 220 volts; 50 Hz.

Oil. Production (estimate, 1989) mainly from Kole oilfield was 9m. tonnes.

Minerals. There are considerable deposits of bauxite and kyanite around Ngaoundéré. Further deposits of bauxite and cassiterite remain to be exploited in the Adamaoua plateau.

Agriculture. The main food crops (with 1988 production in 1,000 tonnes): Cassava, 680; millet, 410; maize, 380; plantains, 1,100; yams, 420; groundnuts, 142; bananas, 68. Cash crops include palm oil, 110; palm kernels, 27; cocoa, 130; coffee, 138; rubber, 26; cotton lint, 47; raw sugar, 80.

Livestock (1988): 4·5m. cattle, 2·9m. sheep, 2·9m. goats, 1·2m. pigs.

Forestry. Forests cover 24·9m. hectares, 53% of the land area, ranging from tropical rain forests in the south (producing hardwoods such as mahogany, ebony and sapele) to semi-deciduous forests in the centre and wooded savannah in the north. Production in 1986 amounted to 12·2m. cu. metres.

Fisheries. In 1986 the total catch was 84,000 tonnes.

INDUSTRY. There is a major aluminium smelting complex at Edéa; aluminium production in 1983 amounted to 77,600 tonnes. Production of cement totalled 227,000 tonnes in 1980. There are also factories producing shoes, beer, soap, oil and food products, cigarettes. Agro-industrial production (1984–85, in tonnes): Rubber, 17,679; palm-oil, 76,954; sugar, 73,717; oil palm, 14,849; tea, 2,279.

Labour. In 1982 the work-force numbered 3,543,000 of whom 73% were occupied in agriculture.

Trade Unions. The principal trade union federation is the *Organisation des syndicats des travailleurs camerounais* (OSTC) established on 7 Dec. 1985 to replace the former body, the UNTC.

FOREIGN ECONOMIC RELATIONS

Commerce. Imports and exports in 1m. francs CFA were as follows:

	1984–85	*1985–86*	*1986–87*
Imports	482,297	513,898	558,265
Exports	822,041	816,912	508,200

In 1984–85, exports (in 1m. francs CFA) went mainly to the Netherlands (136,057), France (127,966), Italy (58,333), Federal Republic of Germany (35,089),

USA (30,098) and Spain (25,517), while imports were mainly from France (193,176), USA (51,687), Japan (36,354), Federal Republic of Germany (31,220) and Italy (26,610); the main exports were crude oils (123,398), coffee and by-products (111,201) and cocoa and by-products (105,858).

Total trade between Cameroon and UK (British Department of Trade returns, in £1,000 sterling):

	1986	*1987*	*1988*	*1989*	*1990*
Imports to UK	7,634	14,201	16,180	11,362	8,241
Exports and re-exports from UK	34,368	28,057	20,472	24,838	20,652

Tourism. There were an estimated 115,203 foreign visitors in 1987.

COMMUNICATIONS

Roads. In 1986 there were 66,910 km of roads, of which 2,922 km were tarmac. In 1984–85 there were 73,963 passenger cars and 43,165 commercial vehicles.

Railways. Cameroon Railways, *Regifercam* (1,115 km in 1985) link Douala with Nkongsamba and Ngaoundéré, with branches M'Banga–Kumba and Makak–M'Balmayo. In 1987–88 railways carried 2·4m. passengers and 1·4m. tonnes of freight.

Aviation. Douala is the main international airport; other airports are at Yaoundé and Garoua. Camair, the national airline, serve 7 domestic airports. In 1981–82, 644,000 passengers and 14,600 tonnes of freight passed through the airports.

Shipping. The merchant-marine consisted (1986) of 48 vessels (over 100 GRT) of 76,433 GRT. The major port of Douala handled (1984) 3m. tonnes of imports and 1m. tonnes of exports and in 1984–85, 671 cargo ships and 2,582 other ships entered the port. Timber is exported mainly through the south-west ports of Kribi and Campo. Other ports are Bota, Tiko, Limbe and Garoua.

Telecommunications. There were (1975) 150 post offices supplemented by a mobile postal service; telephones (1984), 47,200; radio stations, 10 with 785,000 receivers. Television was introduced in 1985.

Cinemas. There were (1979) 52 cinemas with a capacity of 29,000 seats.

Newspapers. There was (1984) 1 daily newspaper with a circulation of 20,000. It was announced in Dec. 1990 that press censorship would be lifted.

JUSTICE, RELIGION, EDUCATION AND WELFARE

Justice. The Supreme Court sits at Yaoundé, as does the High Court of Justice (consisting of 9 titular judges and 6 surrogates all appointed by the National Assembly). There are magistrates' courts situated in the provinces.

Religion. In 1980, 21% of the population was Roman Catholic, 22% Moslem, 18% Protestant, while 39% followed traditional (animist) religions.

Education (1986–87). There were 1,795,254 pupils and 35,728 teachers in primary schools, 291,842 pupils and 9,017 teachers in general secondary schools and 90,666 pupils and 3,714 teachers in technical secondary schools. In 1984–85 there were 13,753 students and 572 teaching staff at higher education institutions of the University of Yaoundé. 59% literacy was claimed in 1987.

Health. In 1981 there were 1,003 hospitals and health centres with 24,541 beds; there were also (1982) 604 doctors and 17 dentists, 96 pharmacists, 399 midwives and 1,086 nursing personnel.

DIPLOMATIC REPRESENTATIVES

Of Cameroon in Great Britain (84 Holland Pk., London, W11 3SB)
Ambassador: Dr Gibering Bol-Alima.

Of Great Britain in Cameroon (Ave. Winston Churchill, BP 547, Yaoundé)
Ambassador: William Quantrill.

Of Cameroon in the USA (2349 Massachusetts Ave., NW, Washington, D.C., 20008)
Ambassador: Vincent Paul-Thomas Pondi.

Of the USA in Cameroon (Rue Nachtigal, BP 817, Yaoundé)
Ambassador: Frances D. Cook.

Of Cameroon to the United Nations
Ambassador: M. Pascal Biloa Tang.

Further Reading

Statistical Information: The Service de la Statistique Générale, at Douala, set up in 1945, publishes a monthly bulletin (from Nov. 1950)

DeLancey, M. W., *Cameroon: Dependence and Independence.* London, 1989
DeLancey, M. W. and Schraeder, P. J., *Cameroon.* [Bibliography] Oxford and Santa Barbara, 1986
Ndongko, W. A., *Planning for Economic Development in a Federal State: The Case of Cameroon, 1960–71.* New York, 1975
Rubin, N., *Cameroon.* New York, 1972

CANADA

Capital: Ottawa
Population: 26·6m. (1990)
GNP per capita: US$16,760 (1988)

HISTORY. The territories which now constitute Canada came under British power at various times by settlement, conquest or cession. Nova Scotia was occupied in 1628 by settlement at Port Royal, was ceded back to France in 1632 and was finally ceded by France in 1713 to England, by the Treaty of Utrecht; the Hudson's Bay Company's charter, conferring rights over all the territory draining into Hudson Bay, was granted in 1670; Canada, with all its dependencies, including New Brunswick and Prince Edward Island, was formally ceded to Great Britain by France in 1763; Vancouver Island was acknowledged to be British by the Oregon Boundary Treaty of 1846, and British Columbia was established as a separate colony in 1858. As originally constituted, Canada was composed of Upper and Lower Canada (now Ontario and Quebec), Nova Scotia and New Brunswick. They were united under an Act of the Imperial Parliament, 'The British North America Act, 1867', which came into operation on 1 July 1867 by royal proclamation. The Act provided that the constitution of Canada should be 'similar in principle to that of the United Kingdom'; that the executive authority shall be vested in the Sovereign, and carried on in his name by a Governor-General and Privy Council; and that the legislative power shall be exercised by a Parliament of two Houses, called the 'Senate' and the 'House of Commons'.

On 30 June 1931 the British House of Commons approved the enactment of the Statute of Westminster freeing the Provinces as well as the Dominion from the operation of the Colonial Laws Validity Act, and thus removing what legal limitations existed as regards Canada's legislative autonomy. A joint address of the Senate and the House of Commons was sent to the Governor-General for transmission to London on 10 July 1931. The statute received the royal assent on 12 Dec. 1931.

Provision was made in the British North America Act for the admission of British Columbia, Prince Edward Island, Newfoundland, Rupert's Land and Northwest Territory into the Union. In 1869 Rupert's Land, or the Northwest Territories, was purchased from the Hudson's Bay Company. On 15 July 1870, Rupert's Land and the Northwest Territory were annexed to Canada and named the Northwest Territories, Canada having agreed to pay the Hudson's Bay Company in cash and land for its relinquishing of claims to the territory. By the same action the Province of Manitoba was created from a small portion of this territory and they were admitted into the Confederation on 15 July 1870. On 20 July 1871 the province of British Columbia was admitted, and Prince Edward Island on 1 July 1873. The provinces of Alberta and Saskatchewan were formed from the provisional districts of Alberta, Athabaska, Assiniboia and Saskatchewan and originally parts of the Northwest Territories and admitted on 1 Sept. 1905. Newfoundland formally joined Canada as its tenth province on 31 March 1949.

In Feb. 1931 Norway formally recognized the Canadian title to the Sverdrup group of Arctic islands. Canada thus holds sovereignty in the whole Arctic sector north of the Canadian mainland.

In Nov. 1981 the Canadian government agreed on the provisions of an amended constitution, to the end that it should replace the British North America Act and that its future amendment should be the prerogative of Canada. These proposals were adopted by the Parliament of Canada and were enacted by the UK Parliament as the Canada Act of 1982.

The enactment of the Canada Act was the final act of the UK Parliament in Canadian constitutional development. The Act gave to Canada the power to amend the Constitution according to procedures determined by the Constitutional Act 1982, which was proclaimed in force by the Queen on 17 April 1982. The Constitution Act 1982 added to the Canadian Constitution a charter of Rights and Freedoms, and provisions which recognize the nation's multi-cultural heritage, affirm the existing rights of native peoples, confirm the principle of equalization of benefits among the provinces, and strengthen provincial ownership of natural resources.

AREA AND POPULATION. Canada is bounded north-west by the Beaufort Sea, north by the Arctic Ocean, north-east by Baffin Bay, east by the Davis Strait, Labrador Sea and Atlantic Ocean, south by the USA and west by the Pacific Ocean and USA (Alaska). Population of the area now included in Canada:

1851	2,436,297	1901	5,371,315	1951 [1]	4,009,429
1861	3,229,633	1911	7,206,643	1961	18,238,247
1871	3,689,257	1921	8,787,949	1971	21,568,311
1881	4,324,810	1931	10,376,786	1981	24,343,181
1891	4,833,239	1941	11,506,655		

[1] From 1951 figures include Newfoundland.

Population (census), 3 June 1986, was 25,354,064. Estimate (1990) 26·6m.

Areas of the provinces, etc. (in sq. km) and population at recent censuses:

Province	*Land area*	*Fresh water area*	*Total land and fresh water area*	*Population, 1976*	*Population, 1981*	*Population, 1986* [1]
Newfoundland	371,690	34,030	405,720	557,725	567,681	568,349
Prince Edward Island	5,660	—	5,660	118,229	122,506	126,646
Nova Scotia	52,840	2,650	55,490	828,571	847,442	873,199
New Brunswick	72,090	1,350	73,440	677,250	696,403	710,442
Quebec	1,356,790	183,890	1,540,680	6,234,445	6,438,403	6,540,276
Ontario	891,190	177,390	1,068,580	8,264,465	8,625,107	9,113,515
Manitoba	548,360	101,590	649,950	1,021,506	1,026,241	1,071,232
Saskatchewan	570,700	81,630	652,330	921,323	968,313	1,010,198
Alberta	644,390	16,800	661,190	1,838,037	2,237,724	2,375,278
British Columbia	929,730	18,070	947,800	2,466,608	2,744,467	2,889,207
Yukon	478,970	4,480	483,450	21,836	23,153	23,504
Northwest Territories	3,293,020	133,300	3,426,320	42,609	45,471	52,238
Total	9,215,430	755,180	9,970,610	22,992,604	24,343,181	25,354,064

[1] Including estimates of incompletely enumerated Indian reserves and Indian settlements.

Of the total population in 1986, 21,113,855 were Canadian born, 3,908,150 foreign born, 282,025 of the latter being USA born and 2,435,100 European born.

The population (1986) born outside Canada in the provinces was in the following ratio (%): Newfoundland, 1·6; Prince Edward Island, 3·5; Nova Scotia, 4·7; New Brunswick, 3·8; Quebec, 8·3; Ontario, 23·1; Manitoba, 13·6; Saskatchewan, 7·2; Alberta, 15·6; British Columbia, 22·1; Yukon, 11·5; Northwest Territories, 5·4.

In 1986, figures for the population, according to origin, were [1]:

Single origins	18,035,665	Portuguese	199,595
Austrian	24,900	Romanian	18,745
Belgian	28,395	Russian	32,080
British	6,332,725	Scandinavian	171,715
Czech and Slovak	55,535	Spanish	57,125
Chinese	360,320	Swiss	19,130
Dutch (Netherlands)	351,765	Ukrainian	420,210
Finnish	40,565	Other single origins:	99,025
French [2]	6,093,160		
German	896,720	*Multiple origins:*	6,986,345
Greek	143,780	Other multiple origins	616,000
Hungarian	97,850	British and French	1,139,345
Italian	709,590	British and Other	2,262,525
Japanese	40,245	French and Other	325,655
Polish	222,260		

[1] Data on ethnic origins for the 1986 Census excludes the population on incompletely enumerated Indian reserves and settlements. For Canada there were 136 such reserves and settlements and the total population was estimated to be about 45,000 in 1986.

[2] Includes the single origins of French, Acadian, French Canadian and Québécois.

In April 1990 62·1% of the population gave their mother tongue as English, 25·1% as French, 16·2% stated themselves bilingual.

The total aboriginal population single origins numbered 373,265 in 1986 and the Inuit population was 27,290 in 1986.

Populations of Census Metropolitan Areas (CMA) and Cities (proper), 1986 census:

	CMA	City proper		CMA	City proper
Toronto	3,427,168	612,289	Halifax	295,990	113,577
Montreal	2,921,357	1,015,420	Victoria	255,547	66,303
Vancouver	1,380,729	431,147	Windsor	253,988	193,111
Ottawa-Hull	819,263	—	Oshawa	203,543	123,651
Ottawa	—	300,763	Saskatoon	200,665	177,641
Hull	—	58,722	Regina	186,521	175,064
Edmonton	785,465	573,982	St John's	161,901	96,216
Calgary	671,326	636,104	Chicoutimi-Jonquière	158,468	—
Winnipeg	623,304	594,551	Chicoutimi	—	61,083
Quebec	603,267	164,580	Jonquière	—	58,467
Hamilton	557,029	306,728	Sudbury	148,877	88,717
St Catharines-Niagara	343,258	—	Sherbrooke	129,960	74,438
St Catharines	—	123,455	Trois Rivières	128,888	50,122
Niagara Falls	—	72,107	Thunder Bay	122,217	112,272
London	342,302	269,140	Saint John	121,265	76,381
Kitchener	311,195	150,604			

The total 'urban' population of Canada in 1986 was 19,352,085, against 18,435,927 in 1989.

While the registration of births, marriages and deaths is under provincial control, the statistics are compiled on a uniform system by Statistics Canada.

The following table gives the results for the year 1989:

Province	Live births Number	Marriages Number	Deaths Number
Newfoundland	7,310	3,420	3,660
Prince Edward Island	1,970	1,020	1,190
Nova Scotia	12,290	6,660	7,510
New Brunswick	9,730	4,820	5,570
Quebec	91,200	31,820	48,740
Ontario	135,960	76,520	70,360
Manitoba	17,140	7,820	9,120
Saskatchewan	17,120	6,360	8,000
Alberta	43,780	18,940	13,910
British Columbia	42,590	24,100	22,760
Yukon Territory	510	210	120
N.W. Territories	1,440	240	210
	381,040	181,930	191,150

Immigrant arrivals by country of last permanent residence:

Country	1987	1988	1989
UK	8,547	9,172	8,419
France	2,290	2,589	2,883
Germany	1,906	1,696	2,025
Netherlands	575	821	824
Greece	771	579	771
Italy	1,031	860	1,036
Portugal	5,977	6,467	5,415
Other Europe	16,466	17,728	30,715
Asia	67,337	81,136	93,202
Australia	530	745	626
USA	7,967	6,537	6,927
Caribbean	11,227	9,439	10,902
All other	27,474	24,160	28,227
Total	152,098	161,929	191,971

CLIMATE. The climate ranges from polar conditions in the north to cool temperate in the south, but with considerable differences between east coast, west coast and the interior, affecting temperatures, rainfall amounts and seasonal distribution. Winters are very severe over much of the country, but summers can be very hot inland. *See* individual provinces for climatic details.

CONSTITUTION AND GOVERNMENT. Parliament consists of the Senate and the House of Commons. The members of the *Senate* are appointed until age 75 by summons of the Governor-General under the Great Seal of Canada. Members appointed before 2 June 1965 may remain in office for life. The Senate consists of 104 senators, namely, 24 from Ontario, 24 from Quebec, 10 from Nova Scotia, 10 from New Brunswick, 4 from Prince Edward Island, 6 from Manitoba, 6 from British Columbia, 6 from Alberta, 6 from Saskatchewan, 6 from Newfoundland, 1 from the Yukon Territory and 1 from the Northwest Territories. Each senator must be at least 30 years of age, be a subject of the Queen, reside in the province for which he or she is appointed and have a total net worth of at least $4,000. The *House of Commons* is elected by universal secret suffrage, for 5 years, unless sooner dissolved. From 1867 to the election of 1945 representation was based on Quebec having 65 seats and the other provinces the same proportion of 65 which their population had to the population of Quebec. In the General Election of 1949 readjustments were based on the population of all the provinces taken as a whole. Generally speaking, this format for representation has prevailed in all subsequent elections with readjustments made after each decennial census. Under the Constitution Act, 1986 (Representation), effective March 1986, the formula contained in section 51 of the Constitution Act, 1867 dealing with the number of seats in the House of Commons and their distribution throughout the country, was changed.

In Jan. 1991 a 12-member commission, the Citizen's Forum on Canada's Future, started sounding public opinion on the constitutional future of Canada.

The thirty-fourth Parliament, elected in Nov. 1988, comprises 295 members and the provincial and territorial representation are: Ontario, 99; Quebec, 75; Nova Scotia, 11; New Brunswick, 10; Manitoba, 14; British Columbia, 32; Prince Edward Island, 4; Saskatchewan 14; Alberta, 26; Newfoundland, 7; Yukon, 1; Northwest Territories, 2.

State of the parties in the Senate (Sept. 1990): Liberals, 52; Progressive Conservatives, 41; Independent, 4; Independent Liberal, 1; Reform Party, 1; Vacant, 5; total 104.

State of the parties in the House of Commons (Aug. 1990): Progressive Conservatives, 161; Liberals, 78; New Democratic Party, 44; Reform Party, 1; Independent, 9; Vacant, 2; total, 295.

The following is a list of Governors-General of Canada:

Viscount Monck	1867–1868	Viscount Willington	1926–1931
Lord Lisgar	1868–1872	Earl of Bessborough	1931–1935
Earl of Dufferin	1872–1878	Lord Tweedsmuir	1935–1940
Marquess of Lorne	1878–1883	Earl of Athlone	1940–1946
Marquess of Lansdowne	1883–1888	Field-Marshal Viscount	
Lord Stanley of Preston	1888–1893	Alexander of Tunis	1946–1952
Earl of Aberdeen	1893–1898	Vincent Massey	1952–1959
Earl of Minto	1898–1904	Georges Philias Vanier	1959–1967
Earl Grey	1904–1911	Roland Michener	1967–1974
HRH the Duke of Connaught	1911–1916	Jules Léger	1974–1979
Duke of Devonshire	1916–1921	Edward Schreyer	1979–1984
Viscount Byng of Vimy	1921–1926	Jeanne Sauvé	1984–1989

Governor-General: Hon. Ramon Hnatyshyn.

National flag: Vertically red, white, red with the white of double width and bearing a stylized red maple leaf.

The office and appointment of the Governor-General are regulated by letters patent, signed by the King on 8 Sept. 1947, which came into force on 1 Oct. 1947. In 1977 the Queen approved the transfer to the Governor-General of functions discharged by the Sovereign. He is assisted in his functions, under the provisions of the Act of 1867, by a Privy Council composed of Cabinet Ministers.

The following is the list of the Conservative Cabinet in July 1990, in order of precedence, which attaches generally rather to the person than to the office:

Prime Minister: The Rt. Hon. Martin Brian Mulroney.
Secretary of State for External Affairs: The Rt. Hon. Charles Joseph Clark.
Minister for International Trade: The Hon. John Carnell Crosbie.

Deputy Prime Minister, President of the Privy Council and Minister for Agriculture: The Hon. Donald Frank Mazankowski.
Minister of Public Works and Minister for the Atlantic Canada Opportunities Agency: The Hon. Elmer MacIntosh Mackay.
Minister of Energy, Mines and Resources: The Hon. Arthur Jacob Epp.
President of the Treasury Board and Acting Minister of the Environment: The Hon. Robert R. de Cotret.
Minister of National Health and Welfare: The Hon. Henry Perrin Beatty.
Minister of Finance: The Hon. Michael Holcombe Wilson.
Minister of State and Leader of the Government in the House of Commons: The Hon. Harvie Andre.
Minister of National Revenue: The Hon. Otto John Jelinek.
Minister of Indian Affairs and Northern Development: The Hon. Thomas Edward Siddon.
Minister of Western Economic Diversification and Minister of State (Grains and Oilseeds): The Hon. Charles James Mayer.
Minister of National Defence: The Hon. William Hunter McKnight.
Minister of Industry, Science and Technology: The Hon. Benoit Bouchard.
Minister of Communications: The Hon. Marcel Masse.
Minister of Employment and Immigration: The Hon. Barbara Jean McDougall.
Minister of Veterans Affairs: The Hon. Gerald S. Merrithew.
Minister of State (Employment and Immigration) and Minister of State (Seniors): The Hon. Monique Vézina.
Minister of Forestry: The Hon. Frank Oberle.
Leader of the Government in the Senate and Minister of State (Federal-Provincial Relations): The Hon. Lowell Murray.
Minister of Supply and Services: The Hon. Paul Wyatt Dick.
Solicitor-General of Canada: The Hon. Pierre H. Cadieux.
Minister of State (Small Businesses and Tourism): The Hon. Thomas Hockin.
Minister of External Relations: The Hon. Monique Landry.
Minister of Fisheries and Oceans: The Hon. Bernard Valcourt.
Secretary of State of Canada and Minister of State (Multiculturalism and Citizenship): The Hon. Gerry Weiner.
Minister of Transport: The Hon. Douglas Grinsdale Lewis.
Minister of Consumer and Corporate Affairs and Minister of State (Agriculture): The Hon. Pierre Blais.
Minister of State (Privatization and Regulatory Affairs): The Hon. John McDermid.
Minister of State (Indian Affairs and Northern Development): The Hon. Shirley Martin.
Associate Minister of National Defence and Minister Responsible for the Status of Women: The Hon. Mary Collins.
Minister of State (Housing): Vacant.
Minister for Science: The Hon. William Winegard.
Minister of Justice and Attorney-General of Canada: The Hon. Kim Campbell.
Minister of Labour and Minister of State: The Hon. Jean Corbeil.
Minister of State (Finance): The Hon. Gilles Loiselle.
Minister of State (Youth) and Minister of State (Fitness and Amateur Sport) and Deputy Leader of the Government in the House of Commons: The Hon. Marcel Danis.

The salary of a member of the House of Commons (Jan. 1990) is $62,100 with a tax-free allowance ranging from $20,600 to $27,200. The salary of a senator is $62,100 with a tax-free allowance of $9,800. The salary and allowances of the Prime Minister total $153,700, that of the Speaker of the House of Commons is $134,100; of the Speaker of the Senate is $105,000; of the Opposition Leader is $132,100 and of the National Democratic Party Leader is $115,900.

An Act to provide retiring allowances, on a contributory basis, to members of the House of Commons was given the Royal Assent on 4 July 1952. Subsequent amendments provide allowances for surviving spouses and for former Prime Ministers or their surviving spouses.

Guide to Federal Programs and Services 1990. 10th ed. Supply and Services Canada, Ottawa
A consolidation of the *The Constitution Acts 1867 to 1982*. Department of Justice Canada. Ottawa, 1989
Bureaucracy in Canadian Government: selected readings. 2nd edition, edited by W. D. K. Kernashan, Toronto, 1973
Laskin's Canadian Constitutional Law. 5th ed., Vol. 2, Neil Finkelstein. Toronto: Carswell, 1986
Leading Constitutional decisions: Cases on the British North America Act. Edited and with an introduction by Peter H. Russell, 4th edition. Ottawa, 1987
The Canadian Parliamentary Guide. Annual. Ottawa
Report of the Royal Commission on Dominion–Provincial Relations, Canada 1867–1939. 3 vols. Ottawa, 1940
Bayehsky, A. F., *Canada's Constitution Act 1982 and Amendments: a Documentary History*. 2 vols. Toronto, 1989
Bejermi, J., *Canadian Parliamentary Handbook*. Ottawa, 1986
Byers, R. B. (ed.) *Canada Challenged: The Viability of the Confederation*. Toronto, 1979
Cheffins, R. I. and Johnson, P. A., *The Revised Canadian Constitution, Politics as law*. Toronto, 1986
Fox, P. W., and White, G., *Politics Canada*. 6th ed. Toronto, 1987
Franks, C. E. S., *The Parliament of Canada*. Univ. of Toronto Press, 1987
Hogg, P. W., *Constitutional Law of Canada*. 2nd ed. Toronto, 1985
Kennedy, W. F. M., *Statutes, Treaties and Documents of the Canadian Constitution, 1713–1929*. Toronto, 1939
Morton, W. L., *The Kingdom of Canada; A General History From Earliest Times*. Toronto, 1969

DEFENCE. The Department of National Defence was created by the National Defence Act, 1922, which established one civil Department of Government in place of the previous Departments of Militia and Defence, Naval Service and the Air Board. The Department now operates under authority of RSC 1970, c.N1-4. The Minister of National Defence has the control and management of the Canadian Forces and all matters relating to national defence establishments and works for the defence of Canada. He is the Minister responsible for presenting before the Cabinet matters of major defence policy for which Cabinet direction is required. He is also responsible for the emergency measures organization known since 1 July 1986 as 'Emergency Preparedness Canada'.

In Dec. 1976, the Minister of National Defence was named as minister responsible for all aspects of air Search and Rescue (SAR) in the areas of Canadian SAR responsibility, and for the overall co-ordination of marine Search and Rescue including provision of air resources for marine SAR within Canadian territorial waters and in designated oceanic areas off the Pacific and Atlantic Coasts in accordance with agreements made with the United States Coast Guard. A group from Transport Canada, the Department of National Defence and the Department of Fisheries and Oceans was set up at the same time, as a co-ordinating body.

Since September 1985 the Minister has shared his responsibilities with an Associate Minister of National Defence.

The Canadian Forces (CF) are the military element of the Canadian government and are part of the Department of National Defence (DND). Government policy concerning the CF takes into account national and foreign policy. The roles of the CF are developed within this framework. They are:

- the protection of Canada and Canadian national interests at home and abroad; this includes the provision of aid of the civil power and national development;
- the defence of North America in co-operation with the United States' military forces;
- the fulfillment of such North Atlantic Treaty Organization (NATO) commitments to security as may be agreed upon; the performance of such international peacekeeping roles as Canada may from time to time assume.

Personnel and Budget

The 1989-90 Department of National Defence budget main estimate was \$11,300m. or 8·7% of the government's budget.

The strength of the Regular Force for 1990 was approximately 88,000.

Command Structure. The missions and roles of the CF are undertaken by functional and regional commands. Commands and major organizations report directly to National Defence Headquarters (NDHQ) in Ottawa, Ontario from headquarters situated as follows:

- Mobile Command, St Hubert, Quebec;
- Maritime Command, Halifax, Nova Scotia;
- Air Command, Winnipeg, Manitoba;
- Canadian Forces Training System, Trenton, Ontario;
- Canadian Forces Communication Command, Ottawa, Ontario;
- Canadian Forces Europe, Lahr, Federal Republic of Germany (FRG); and
- Northern Region, Yellowknife, NWT.

1. *Mobile Command.* Mobile Command (FMC) maintains combat ready land forces to meet Canada's defence commitments.

Defence of North America

Mobile Command is prepared to undertake defence of North America operations in conjunction with the forces of the United States. Under the Canada-United States Basic Defence Agreement, a number of mutual defence treaties exist. One that directly concerns Mobile Command is Canada-United States Land Operations (CANUS LANDOP). It is designed to provide the co-ordination of the land defence of Canada, Alaska, and the continental United States. Under this plan, Mobile Command is responsible for co-ordinating the land defence of Canada by both Canadian and US forces, if required, and must be prepared to assist US forces in the defence of Alaska and the United States. Both this and the National Security task force involves Mobile Command in maintaining a presence in the Canadian North through surveillance and patrols and numerous exercises.

NATO Commitment

Mobile Command (FMC) provides forces in support of several NATO commitments. FMC NATO commitments include:

(a) A division to Central Army Group (CENTAG) in Europe. In 1989 5e Groupe-brigade du Canada (5 GBC), located in Quebec, 4 Canadian Mechanized Brigade Group (4 CMBG) in Lahr (in Germany), and various support groups were consolidated into 1 Canadian Division, committed to Central Europe. The commitment of the Canadian Air/Sea Transportable (CAST) Brigade to northern Norway ceased in 1989 with the operational tasking of 1 Canadian Division.

(b) The first battalion, Princess Patricia's Canadian Light Infantry, based on Calgary, would deploy to Norway in time of crisis to reinforce NATO's northern flank as part of either the Allied Command Europe (ACE) Mobile Force or the NATO Composite Force.

Although the land force units located in Europe are part of Canadian Forces Europe, FMC provides trained replacements through individual, sub-unit and unit rotations to sustain peacetime manning requirements.

International Peacekeeping or Stability Operations

Mobile Command is committed to providing forces for international peacekeeping or stability operations. In 1990, its UN involvement included commitments in Cyprus, on the Golan Heights and in Namibia, Iran-Iraq, and Afghanistan. Non-UN commitments included the Multi-National Peacekeeping Force (MFO) in the Sinai and a group of engineers in Pakistan teaching Afghan refugees mine recognition.

Budget and Personnel

In 1989–90, the FMC budget was approximately $370m. for operations and maintenance costs. This excluded salaries. Expenditures in support of British, German and US Army units training on FMC bases were recovered from the nations concerned.

Personnel included approximately 18,800 Regular Force, 22,000 Militia and 5,500 civilians.

2. *Maritime Command.* The Maritime Command (MARCOM) role is to maintain combat-ready general purpose maritime forces to meet Canada's defence commit-

ments. This role is fulfilled using MARCOM resources and designated Air Command aircraft under MARCOM control.

Maritime Command comprises operational maritime forces, headquarters and supporting units located primarily on the east and west coasts of Canada, but also extending as far north as Iqaluit, Northwest Territories and as far south as Bermuda.

Operational forces include 19 destroyers, 6 coastal patrol boats, 3 submarines, 2 mine counter-measures vessels, 3 operational support ships, 1 diving support ship, 3 research vessels and 12 tugboats. In addition there are more than 30 minor vessels located at Reserve Training Units on both coasts. The first of the new Canadian Patrol Frigates was scheduled for delivery in 1990.

Protection of Canada and National Interests

Maritime Command conducts military surveillance of Canadian territorial waters on both coasts. Surveillance patrols in support of Canadian national interests are conducted in the 370 km economic zone by surface and air units. Fisheries patrols are conducted on both coasts.

Operations and Training

The air, surface and sub-surface resources of MARCOM maintain a high level of combat readiness through operations, tactical research, joint exercises and planned maintenance. Training is conducted on both coasts through exercises run by the destroyer squadrons. Advanced training, designed to maintain combat readiness and evaluate new tactics, is accomplished through Maritime co-ordinated exercises.

NATO Exercises

Canada is continuously represented in NATO's Standing Naval Force Atlantic (STANAVFORLANT) by a destroyer. This multi-national squadron provides a highly visible demonstration of NATO solidarity. The squadron visits ports throughout Europe, the Mediterranean and the east coast of North America, strengthening ties with NATO'S member countries. On the east coast destroyers participate in the NATO Squadron and are involved in a number of exercises on both sides of the Atlantic. West coast ships conduct national exercises on a regular basis.

Personnel and Budget

MARCOM's budget for fiscal year 1989–90 was $237m. for operations and maintenance, naval reserve, cadets and miscellaneous. Personnel included approximately 10,000 Regular Force, 4,000 Naval Reserve and 7,000 civilians.

3. *Air Command.* Air Command's six functional groups provide combat-ready air forces to meet Canada's defence commitments.

Functional Organization

Air Command is divided into six functional air groups. The Commander, Air Command, delegates operational control to the commanders of the air groups over their assigned resources. The Commander retains responsibility for flight safety, as well as air doctrine and standards relating to flying operations throughout the Canadian Forces, including units located outside Canada. The air groups are:

(a) Fighter Group (North Bay, Ontario) maintains the sovereignty of Canada's airspace, supports Mobile and Maritime Command training and operations, and fulfills Canada's commitments to NATO and NORAD.

(b) Air Transport Group (Trenton, Ontario) provides airlift resources and Search and Rescue (SAR) forces for the CF.

(c) Maritime Air Group (MAG) (Halifax, Nova Scotia) provides operationally ready air forces to MARCOM in areas including anti-submarine warfare, surveillance, sovereignty, fisheries and pollution monitoring.

(d) 10 Tactical Air Group (St. Hubert, Quebec) provides combat-ready tactical aviation forces for operational employment in support of Mobile Command operations, training and other defence commitments.

(e) 14 Training Group (Winnipeg, Manitoba) trains aircrew and other air personnel to initial classification and trade specifications, and provides other training as directed.

(*f*) Air Reserve Group (Winnipeg, Manitoba) provides support to Air Command by provision of reserve operational units and individual augmentees.

Personnel and Budget

Air Command consists of 21,629 Regular Force members, 1,350 Air Reserves and 6,868 civilians for a total of 29,847 members. The operations and maintenance budget for 1989–90 was $510m. including aviation fuel and operations and maintenance costs.

4. *Canadian Forces Training System.* The role of the Canadian Forces Training System is to plan, organize, conduct and control the training of service personnel whose trade is required by more than one command. As such, CFTS is a joint formation manned by personnel from FMC, MARCOM and air command. The commander of CFTS exercises command over 20 schools located on five CFTS bases and two schools located on bases assigned to other commands.

Training

Canadian Forces Training System plans, controls and conducts all basic recruit and officer training as well as occupational training for 18 of 36 officer classifications and 53 of 100 non-commissioned member trades that are common to more than one operational command. Additionally, CFTS conducts specialty and advanced training for most members of the Canadian Forces. This role was expanded in 1989, when CFTS assumed command of the Canadian Forces Management Development School.

Personnel and Budget

In 1989 CFTS included 4,578 military personnel, of whom almost 1,800 were instructors. CFTS employed 3,679 civilian personnel. The CFTS budget is $123·7m., which included operations and maintenance, dependent education, cadets, travel and base utilities.

5. *Canadian Forces Communication Command (CFCC).* Canadian Forces Communication Command (CFCC) provides strategic communication services, including communications research message handling and data transfer, telephone systems and high frequency radio direction-finding services for the CF. To effect these services CFCC operates and maintains several data networks and voice communications systems.

It is implicit in the provision of strategic communications for the CF and emergency government that the organization be capable of extending services to the various military and civil headquarters during a national emergency. As well, it must supply reliable strategic communications from Canada to CF combat elements anywhere in the world. To these ends, Communication Command personnel exercise their equipment and procedures regularly.

Personnel and Budget

The Canadian Forces Communication Command's (CFCC) 5,700 personnel includes a regular force contingent of 3,300 members, a Communication Reserve of 1,800 and a civilian force of approximately 600.

The 1989 command budget was $117·4m. Of that budget, 77% was expended on strategic communications services with the remainder to operation of the Communication Reserve, command operations and maintenance and miscellaneous.

6. *Canadian Forces Europe (CFE).* Throughout 1989 Canadian Forces Europe (CFE) continued to provide, maintain and support European-based, combat-ready land and air forces to Supreme Allied Commander Europe in accordance with Canada's NATO commitment. The two formations stationed permanently in Central Europe, 4 Canadian Mechanized Brigade Group (4 CMBG) and 1 Canadian Air Group (1 CAG), completed challenging and realistic training programmes to maintain their operational readiness at the highest possible state. Support for the two formations was provided by Canadian Forces Bases Lahr and Baden-Soellingen in Germany.

Personnel and Budget

During 1989 service personnel at CFE numbered 8,000. There were approximately 4,400 civilian employees and a total of about 21,500 Canadian military and civilian personnel and their dependents.

During the fiscal year 1988–89, CFE was allocated an operations and maintenance budget of $186m., which includes civilian salaries but not military pay or new construction.

7. *Northern Region Headquarters.* Situated in Yellowknife, NWT, the Northern Region Headquarters (NRHQ) was formed on 15 May 1970 to assist in maintaining Canadian sovereignty and support ongoing Canadian Forces activities in the North.

Training

During 1989, NRHQ continued to provide planning advice and liaison support to territorial governments and military units for exercises 'north of 60'.

Regional organization. A regional structure is superimposed over the functional organization to most effectively respond to support requirements within Canada. This was accomplished by dividing Canada into six geographic regions and appointing the senior commander in each region as the region commander. Thus the following interrelationship of functional command/region/geographical area exists: *Maritime Command* – Atlantic Region (Newfoundland, New Brunswick, Nova Scotia and Prince Edward Island); *Mobile Command* – Eastern Region (Quebec); *Training System* – Central Region (Ontario); *Air Command* – Prairie Region (Manitoba, Saskatchewan, and Alberta); *Maritime Forces Pacific* – Pacific Region (British Columbia); and *Northern Region Headquarters* – Northern Region (Yukon and Northwest Territories). In 1989, a move was made to transfer the operational responsibilities from the regions to Mobile Command. Central Region operations was the first affected; others will be transferred in the future. Operational responsibilities include vital points defence, aid of the civil power, explosive ordinance disposal and many others. Responsibilities remaining with the regions include medical, dental, support to cadets, civilian personnel administration, etc.

The *Reserve Force* consists of officers and non-commissioned members who are enrolled for other than continuing full-time military service. The sub-components of the Reserve Force are the Primary Reserve, the Supplementary Ready Reserve, the Supplementary Holding Reserve, the Cadet Instructors List and the Canadian Rangers.

The elements of the Primary Reserve are the Naval Reserve, Militia, Air Reserve and Communication Reserve. Funded personnel levels for these four elements are 4,011, 18,768, 1,350 and 1,706, respectively. Officers and non-commissioned members of the Primary Reserve undergo part-time training at local armouries or collective training at central locations, often during the summer months.

The Supplementary Ready Reserve consists of former Regular and Reserve Force officers and non-commissioned members who are militarily fit and current, and prepared to report for duty when required in an emergency. The Supplementary Holding Reserve includes former members required to report for such duty only when the entire Supplementary Reserve was put on active service.

The Cadet Instructors List consists of commissioned officers whose primary duty is the supervision, administration and training of cadets.

The Canadian Rangers consists of officers and non-commissioned members who volunteer to hold themselves in readiness for service but are not required to undergo annual training. Their role is to provide a military force in sparsely settled, northern coastal and isolated areas of Canada.

Royal Canadian Mounted Police. The Royal Canadian Mounted Police is a civil force maintained by the federal government. It was established in 1873, as the North-West Mounted Police for service in what was then the North-West Territories and, in recognition of its services, was granted the use of the prefix 'Royal' by King Edward VII in 1904. Its sphere of operations was expanded in 1918 to include all of Canada west of Thunder Bay. In 1920 the force absorbed the Dominion

Police, its headquarters was transferred from Regina to Ottawa, and its title was changed to Royal Canadian Mounted Police. The force is responsible to the Solicitor-General of Canada and is controlled and managed by a Commissioner who holds the rank and status of a Deputy Minister. The Commissioner is empowered under the Royal Canadian Mounted Police Act to appoint members to be peace officers in all provinces and territories of Canada.

The responsibilities of the Royal Canadian Mounted Police are national in scope. The administration of justice within the provinces, including the enforcement of the Criminal Code of Canada, is part of the power and duty delegated to the provincial governments.

All provinces except Ontario and Quebec have entered into contracts with the Royal Canadian Mounted Police to enforce criminal and provincial laws under the direction of the respective Attorneys-General. In addition, in these 8 provinces the Force is under agreement to provide police services to 191 municipalities, thereby assuming the enforcement responsibility of municipal as well as criminal and provincial laws within these communities. The Royal Canadian Mounted Police is also responsible for all police work in the Yukon and Northwest Territories enforcing federal law and territorial ordinances. The 13 Divisions, alphabetically designated, make up the strength of the Force across Canada; they comprise 52 sub-divisions which include 723 detachments. Headquarters Division, as well as the Office of the Commissioner, is located in Ottawa. The Force maintains liaison officers in 18 countries and represents Canada in the International Criminal Police Organization (Interpol) which has its headquarters in Paris.

Thorough training is emphasized for members of the Force. Recruits receive 6 months of basic training at the Royal Canadian Mounted Police Academy in Regina. This is followed by a further 6 months of supervised on-the-job training. The RCMP also operates the Canadian Police College at which its members and selected representatives of other Canadian and foreign police forces may study the latest advances in the fields of crime prevention and detection.

Many of these advances have been incorporated into the operation of the Force. A modern communications system links the widespread divisional headquarters with the administrative centre at Ottawa and a network of fixed and mobile radio units operates within the provinces. Assisting the criminal investigation work of the Force is the Directorate of Identification Services; its services, together with those of divisional and sub-divisional units, and of 8 Crime Detection Laboratories, are available to police forces throughout Canada. The Canadian Police Information Centre at RCMP Headquarters, a national computer network, is staffed and operated by the Force. Law Enforcement agencies throughout Canada have access via remote terminals to information on stolen vehicles, licences and wanted persons.

In Oct. 1990, the Force had a total strength of 21,050 including regular members, special constables, civilian members and public service employees. It maintained 6,984 motor vehicles, 87 police service dogs and 156 horses.

The Force has 13 divisions actively engaged in law enforcement, 1 Headquarters Division and 1 training division. Maritime services are divisional responsibilities and the Force currently has 394 boats at various points across Canada. The Air Directorate has stations throughout the country and maintains a fleet of 26 fixed-wing aircraft and 8 helicopters.

INTERNATIONAL RELATIONS

Membership. Canada is a member of the UN, Commonwealth, OAS, OECD, NATO and Colombo Plan.

ECONOMY

Budget. Budgetary revenue and expenditure of the Government of Canada for years ended 31 March (in $1m.):

	1986–87	*1987–88*	*1988–89*	*1989–90*	*1990–91* [1]
Revenue	85,784	97,452	103,981	113,715	119,300
Expenditure	116,389	125,535	132,715	142,657	147,775

[1] Estimate.

Main items of revenue in 1989–90 (estimates in $1m.):

Unemployment contributions	10,738	Customs import duties	4,592
Income tax, personal	51,895	Non-resident tax	1,361
Income tax, corporate	13,021	Return on investments	5,839
Sales tax	17,671		

Main items of expenditure in 1989–90 (in $1m.): Old age security benefits, guaranteed income supplements and spouses' benefits, 16,154; unemployment benefit, 11,694; family allowances, 2,654; medical care, 6,663; Canada Assistance Plan, 5,006; education support, 2,166; defence, 11,454; external affairs and aid, 3,786; public debt charges, 38,836.

On 31 March 1990 the net public debt was $357,961m.

On 1 Jan. 1991 a 7% Goods and Services Tax (GST) was introduced, superseding a 13·5% manufacturers' sales tax.

Canadian Tax Foundation. *The National Finances: An Analysis of the Revenues and Expenditures of the Government of Canada*. Toronto. Annual

Currency. The unit of currency is the *Canadian dollar* (CAD) of 100 *cents*. There are coins of 1, 5, 10, 25, 50 cents and $1, and notes of $2, $5, $10, $20, $50, $100 and $1,000. The $1 note was withdrawn in 1989. The monetary standard is gold of 900 millesimal fineness (23·22 grains of pure gold equal to 1 gold dollar). The Currency Act provides for gold coins in the denominations of $5, $10 and $20, which are legal tender. The British and US gold coins are also legal tender, at the par rate of exchange. The legal equivalent of the British sovereign is $4.86²/₃.

Since 1935 the Bank of Canada has the sole right to issue paper money for circulation in Canada. Restrictions introduced by the 1944 revisions of the Bank Act cancelled the right of chartered banks to issue or re-issue notes after 1 Jan. 1945; and in Jan. 1950 the chartered banks' liability for such of their notes as then remained outstanding was transferred to the Bank of Canada in return for payment of a like sum to the Bank of Canada. On 31 May 1970 the Canadian dollar which was stabilized at 92·50 US cents was allowed to fluctuate. The value of the US$ in Canadian funds was $1·16 and £1 sterling = Canadian $2·19 in March 1991.

The Ottawa Mint was established in 1908 as a branch of the Royal Mint, in pursuance of the Ottawa Mint Act, 1901. In Dec. 1931 control of the Mint was passed over to the Canadian Government, and since that time it has operated as the Royal Canadian Mint. The Mint issues nickel, bronze and cupronickel coins for circulation in Canada. In 1967, in celebration of Canada's Centennial of Confederation, a $20 gold piece was minted, the first gold coin struck since 1919. In 1935, on the occasion of His Majesty's Silver Jubilee, the Royal Canadian Mint issued the first Canadian silver dollar. Commemorative dollars were also issued in 1939 on the occasion of the visit of King George VI and Queen Elizabeth to Canada; in 1949, when Newfoundland became the tenth Province of Canada; in 1958, the one-hundredth anniversary of the establishment of the Colony of British Columbia; in 1964, the centennial of the Charlottetown and Quebec Conferences which paved the way to confederation. The silver dollar bearing the design of the canoe manned by an Indian and a Voyageur has been issued in the years 1935–38, 1945–48, 1950–57, 1959–63, 1965 and 1966. In 1968, the coin bore the same design but its composition changed from silver to nickel. This composition remained for all the following years. The design was used again in 1969, 1972, 1975–87. For centennial year the Canada goose replaced the usual canoe design on the silver dollar. Because of a world-wide shortage of silver, the Government, in Aug. 1967, authorized the Mint to change the metal content of the 25-cent and 10-cent coins. Commencing in Sept. 1968, 10-cent, 25-cent, 50-cent and $1 coins were minted in pure nickel. Gold refining is one of the principal activities of the Mint. On average the Mint refines about 70% of Canada's total gold production. In 1989 the Mint refined over 4·58m. troy ounces of gold. Coins issued (1987): Gold bullion 2,468,495 pieces.

Banking and Finance. Commercial banks in Canada are known as chartered banks and are incorporated under the terms of the Bank Act, which imposes strict conditions as to capital, returns to the Federal government, types of lending operations and other matters. In Aug. 1990 there were 64 chartered banks (8 domestic banks and 56 foreign bank subsidiaries) incorporated under the provisions of the Bank Act; the 8 had 6,884 branches serving 1,700 communities in all provinces in Canada and 262 branches in other countries. The foreign bank subsidiaries operate 295 offices in Canada including 57 head offices. The Bank Act is subject to revision by Parliament every 10 years. Bank charters expire every 10 years and are renewed at each decennial revision of the Bank Act. The chartered banks make detailed monthly and yearly returns to the Minister of Finance and are subject to periodic inspection by the Superintendent of Financial Institutions, an official appointed by the Government.

The Bank of Canada Act, effective from 3 July 1934, provided for the establishment of a central bank for the Dominion. This bank commenced operations on 11 March 1935 with a paid-up capital of $5m. By reason of certain changes introduced into the composition of stockholders of the bank (for which *see* THE STATESMAN'S YEAR-BOOK, 1944 pp. 322–23), the Minister of Finance on behalf of Canada is the sole registered owner of the capital stock of the bank. The revised Bank Act, which came into force on 1 Dec. 1980, requires chartered banks to maintain a statutory primary reserve of 10% on demand deposits, 3% on foreign-currency deposits and 2% on notice deposits, with an additional 1% on the portion of notice deposits exceeding $500m. This reserve is required to be maintained in the form of notes and deposits with the Bank of Canada. A secondary reserve of 4% in the form of treasury bills, government bonds, etc., is also required. All gold held in Canada by the chartered banks was transferred to the Bank of Canada along with the gold held by the Government as reserve against Dominion notes outstanding at the time of the commencement of operations of the Bank of Canada. The liability of the Dominion notes outstanding at the commencement of business of the Bank of Canada was assumed by the bank. The *Governor* of the Bank of Canada is John Crow.

Weights and Measures. The legal weights and measures are in transition from the Imperial to the International system of units. The Metric Commission, established in June 1971, co-ordinates Canada's conversion to the metric system.

ENERGY AND NATURAL RESOURCES

Electricity. Electricity generation in 1989 was 483,741,000 mwh., of which 433,067,000 was used to meet domestic demand. Of the total, 59·6% was from hydro generation, 24·8% from thermal generation and 15·6% nuclear. Supply 115 volts; 60 Hz.

Oil and Natural Gas. Production of marketable crude and equivalent oil, 1989, 97·38m. cu. metres; natural gas, 1989, 96,116m. cu. metres, and natural gas by-products 16·35m. cu. metres.

Minerals. Alberta and Ontario accounted for 60·3% of the value of mineral products in 1989. Total value of minerals produced in 1989 (preliminary) was $36,474m. Principal minerals produced in 1989 (preliminary):

	Quantity (1,000)	*Value ($1m.)*
Metallics		
Copper (kg)	706,117	2,415
Nickel (kg)	196,133	3,080
Zinc (kg)	1,315,274	2,844
Iron ore (tonnes)	40,773	1,493
Gold (grammes)	158,440	2,298
Lead (kg)	275,800	287
Silver (kg)	1,262	263
Uranium 'U' (kg)	11,564	990
Others	...	659
Total metallics	...	14,329

	Quantity (1,000)	Value ($1m.)
Non-metallics		
Asbestos (tonnes)	691	259
Potash (K_2O) (tonnes)	7,036	947
Salt (tonnes)	11,350	270
Sulphur, elemental (tonnes)	5,183	441
Others	…	623
Total non-metallics	…	2,540
Fuels		
Crude petroleum (cu. metres)	97,379	11,745
Natural gas (1,000 cu. metres)	96,116	5,395
Natural gas by-products (cu. metres)	16,345	728
Coal (tonnes)	70,473	1,836
Total fuels	…	19,713
Structural materials		
Cement (tonnes)	12,550	998
Sand and gravel (tonnes)	277,122	383
Stone (tonnes)	116,657	633
Others	…	877
Total structural materials	…	2,891

Value (in $1m.) of mineral production by provinces:

Provinces	*1988*	*1989* [1]	*Provinces*	*1988*	*1989* [1]
Newfoundland	864	959	Saskatchewan	3,043	3,068
Pr. Ed. Island	2	2	Alberta	15,062	16,498
Nova Scotia	453	443	British Columbia	3,943	4,090
New Brunswick	911	910	Yukon Territory	492	540
Quebec	2,711	2,812	N.W. Territories	957	1,155
Ontario	6,896	7,309			
Manitoba	1,627	1,688	Total	36,961	39,474

[1] Preliminary.

Agriculture. According to the census of 1986 the total land area is 2,278·6m. acres of which 167·6m. acres are agricultural land.

Grain growing, dairy farming, fruit farming, ranching and fur farming are all carried on successfully. Total farm cash receipts (1989) $22,415·6m.

The following table shows the value of farm cash receipts for 1989, for selected agricultural commodities, in $1,000:

Wheat	2,186,397	Tobacco	297,367
Oats and barley	820,275	Cattle and calves	3,904,968
Canola	896,173	Hogs	1,787,732
Potatoes	423,483	Sheep and lambs	28,408
Vegetables	660,840	Dairy products	3,075,015
Fruit	316,052	Poultry and eggs	1,721,878

Number of occupied farms (census of 1986) was 293,089; average farm size, 571·8 acres.

Field Crops. The estimated acreage and yield of the principal field crops, by provinces, in 1989 were:

Provinces	*Wheat* 1,000 acres	1,000 bushels	*Tame hay* 1,000 acres	1,000 bushels	*Oats* 1,000 acres	1,000 bushels
Newfoundland	—	—	12	25	—	—
Prince Edward Island	14	740	139	420	23	1,700
Nova Scotia	7	430	173	510	17	1,000
New Brunswick	10	500	174	470	31	1,880
Quebec	126	5,840	2,449	6,870	309	19,130
Ontario	740	40,200	2,570	8,100	360	22,000
Manitoba	5,175	147,300	1,600	2,800	500	22,000
Saskatchewan	19,870	457,700	2,050	2,700	1,200	52,000
Alberta	7,600	236,800	4,600	9,800	1,700	105,000
British Columbia	130	4,600	870	2,300	80	5,300
Total, Canada	33,672	894,110	14,637	33,995	4,220	230,010

Provinces	*Barley* 1,000 acres	1,000 bushels	*Rye* 1,000 acres	1,000 bushels	*Corn for Grain* 1,000 acres	1,000 bushels
Prince Edward Island	70	4,800	—	—	—	—
Nova Scotia	14	830	—	—	4	330
New Brunswick	32	2,080	—	—	—	—
Quebec	381	22,280	—	—	642	62,900
Ontario	480	28,100	50	1,700	1,740	183,000
Manitoba	1,600	71,000	230	7,800	85	4,300
Saskatchewan	3,788	138,000	700	17,300	—	—
Alberta	5,100	262,000	250	7,300	19	550
British Columbia	135	6,700	9	300	—	—
Total, Canada	11,512	535,790	1,239	34,400	2,480	251,170

Provinces	*Canola* 1,000 acres	1,000 bushels	*Mixed grains* 1,000 acres	1,000 bushels	*Soybeans* 1,000 acres	1,000 bushels
Prince Edward Island	—	—	54	4,000	—	—
Nova Scotia	—	—	—	—	—	—
New Brunswick	—	—	—	—	—	—
Quebec	—	—	69	3,674	43	1,580
Ontario	50	1,400	490	30,300	1,290	43,200
Manitoba	1,150	17,600	70	3,000	—	—
Saskatchewan	3,200	57,000	70	2,200	—	—
Alberta	2,700	59,000	180	9,000	—	—
British Columbia	75	1,500	10	550	—	—
Total, Canada	7,175	136,500	943	52,724	1,333	44,780

Livestock. In parts of Saskatchewan and Alberta stockraising is still carried on as a primary industry, but the livestock industry of the country at large is mainly a subsidiary of mixed farming. The following table shows the numbers of livestock (in 1,000) by provinces in July 1990:

Provinces	*Milch cows*	*Other cattle and calves*	*Sheep and lambs*	*Swine*
Newfoundland	4·6	4·2	7·2	16·0
Prince Edward Island	20·1	76·9	5·0	117·0
Nova Scotia	33·2	94·8	33·5	135·0
New Brunswick	26·4	78·6	9·5	84·0
Quebec	540·0	873·0	118·0	2,975·0
Ontario	440·0	1,810·0	215·0	3,181·0
Manitoba	64·0	1,011·0	24·0	1,240·0
Saskatchewan	52·0	2,108·0	56·0	790·0
Alberta	123·0	4,187·0	233·0	1,760·0
British Columbia	76·0	664·0	58·0	234·0
Total	1,379·3	10,907·5	759·2	10,532·0

Net production of farm eggs in 1989, 477m. doz. ($524·5m.). Wool production in 1989, 1,317 tonnes.

Dairying. In 1986 [1], the dairy products industry (which includes fluid milk industries and other dairy products industries) reported 393 for the number of establishments. The number of employees for the same period was 14,839. Production, 1989: Butter, 98,531 tonnes; cheddar cheese, 114,820 tonnes [2]; concentrated whole milk products, 58,998 tonnes; concentrated milk by-products, 93,476 tonnes.

[1] The number of establishments/employees are based on the 1980 Standard Industrial Classification.
[2] Includes cheddar used to make processed cheese.

Fruit Farming. The value of fruit production (excluding apples) in 1989 was (in $1,000): Ontario, 86,705; British Columbia, 69,228; Quebec, 29,349; New Brunswick, 6,124; Newfoundland, 2,365; Prince Edward Island, 1,626. Total apple production in Canada in 1988 was 500,749 tonnes, value $121,189,000; in 1989, 536,700 tonnes.

Tobacco. Commercial production of tobacco is confined to Ontario, Quebec and the eastern provinces. Farm cash receipts for 1989 totalled $297·4m.

Forestry. As of 1986, the total area of land covered by forests is estimated at about 453·3m. ha, of which 260·1m. ha are classed as productive forest land.

The values of shipments from forestry-related industries in 1987 were: Logging, $6,668m.; sawmill and planing mill products, $8,862m.; shingle and shale, $227m.; veneer and plywood, $1,147m.; pulp and paper, $18,385m.; paper and allied products, $23,993m.

Fur Trade. In 1988–89, 3,019,658 pelts valued at $75,821,116, were taken (4,640,276 pelts in 1987–88). In wild-life pelt production marten led in total value; in fur farm production, mink. The value of mink pelts from fur farms in 1988-89 was $35,043,614 ($49,748,431 in 1987–88). There were, in 1989, 980 fur farms reporting fox and 477 mink.

Fisheries. During 1988, landings in commercial fisheries reached 1,652,528 tonnes. The landed value was $1,628m. and the estimated market value was $3,189m. The landed value of principal fish in 1988 was (in $1,000): Salmon, 316,731; cod, 245,035; lobster, 264,881; herring, 127,244; scallops, 85,236; freshwater fish, 82,000; halibut, 34,066.

Canadian Mines Handbook. Annual. Toronto, from 1931
Canadian Fisheries, Highlights 1987. Dept. of Fisheries and Oceans, 1988

INDUSTRY. Industry groups ranked by value of shipments, survey of 1986 (based on 1980 Standard Industrial Classification):

Industry	*Production workers*	*Wages ($1,000)*	*Cost of materials ($1,000)*	*Value of shipments ($1,000)*
Food industries	137,261	2,939,976	22,968,140	34,143,605
Beverage industries	17,200	516,127	2,144,602	5,045,073
Tobacco products	4,069	138,082	854,707	1,623,215
Rubber products	18,589	497,174	1,257,440	2,643,613
Plastic products	33,527	639,069	2,353,279	4,384,722
Leather and allied industries	20,192	302,557	660,889	1,324,840
Primary textile industries	20,011	421,166	1,514,506	2,957,500
Textile products	27,011	459,052	1,616,227	2,892,955
Clothing industries	102,032	1,419,854	3,020,998	6,015,636
Wood industries	94,888	2,295,282	6,658,611	12,432,604
Furniture and fixtures	48,393	888,608	1,933,909	4,011,972
Paper and allied industries	88,880	2,892,539	9,357,461	20,066,737
Printing, publishing and allied industries	77,725	1,969,558	3,849,150	10,370,848
Primary metal industries	78,149	2,633,458	8,722,055	17,108,965
Metal fabricating industries	121,520	2,809,825	7,655,455	15,024,300

Industry	*Production workers*	*Wages ($1,000)*	*Cost of materials ($1,000)*	*Value of shipments ($1,000)*
Machinery industries	57,510	1,399,526	4,080,054	8,098,978
Transport equipment industries	165,383	4,936,210	30,139,909	44,399,837
Electrical and electronic products	88,899	2,129,961	7,215,734	14,304,033
Non-metallic mineral products	42,011	1,121,461	2,630,675	6,632,011
Refined petroleum and coal prods.	6,359	265,156	12,798,291	15,756,364
Chemical and chemical prods.	47,288	1,356,794	9,109,639	18,639,240
Other manufacturing	54,666	1,050,258	2,794,417	5,533,506
All industries	1,351,563	33,081,693	143,336,148	253,410,556

Labour. In 1988 (annual average) the industrial distribution of the employed was estimated as follows (in 1,000): Community, business and personal services, 4,062; manufacturing, 2,104; trade, 2,168; transport, communication and other utilities, 904; construction, 726; public administration, 815; finance, insurance and real estate, 728; agriculture, 444; non-agriculture, 11,801; other primary industries, 294; total employed, 12,245; unemployed, 1,030. Unemployment was 8·3% in Aug. 1990 (1·14m.).

Certain specific minimum standards in regard to working conditions are set by law, for the most part by provincial labour legislation. Minimum wages, maximum hours of work or an overtime rate of pay after a specified number of hours, minimum weekly rest periods, annual vacations with pay, statutory holidays, maternity protection and parental leave and notice of termination of employment are established for the majority of workers.

Trade Unions. Union returns filed for 1987 in compliance with the Corporations and Returns Act (1962), show 459 labour organizations reporting on 15,173 local union branches. Union membership in 1987 was 3·67m. 51·8% of the membership belonged to national unions, with 58·6% of the membership affiliated to the Canadian Labour Congress.

It is generally established by legislation, both federal and provincial, that a trade union to which the majority of employees in a unit suitable for collective bargaining belong, is given certain rights and duties. An employer is required to meet and negotiate with such a trade union to determine wage-rates and other working conditions of his employees. The employer, the trade union and the employees affected are bound by the resulting agreement. If an impasse is reached in negotiation conciliation services provided by the appropriate government board are available. Generally, work stoppages do not take place until an established conciliation or mediation procedure has been carried out and are prohibited while an agreement is in effect.

Freedom of association is a civil right, and under common law workers are at liberty to join unions and participate in their activities. This right has also been guaranteed by statutes which make it an offence to interfere with freedom of association.

FOREIGN ECONOMIC RELATIONS. Canada is one of the signatories of the General Agreement on Tariffs and Trade (GATT) and an active participant in the subsequent GATT negotiations. On 1 Jan. 1989, the Canada-US Free Trade Agreement came into effect. The Agreement, which provides for the phased removal of tariffs and other barriers, is consistent with Canada's obligation to its trading partners.

Commerce. Imports and domestic exports (in $1,000) for calendar years:

	Imports	*Exports*		*Imports*	*Exports*
1960	5,842,695	5,255,575	1986	112,511,445	116,733,385
1970	13,951,903	16,820,098	1987	116,238,614	121,462,342
1980	69,273,844	74,445,976	1988	131,554,000	137,695,000
1985	104,355,196	116,145,111	1989	135,033,000	138,339,000

Exports (domestic) by countries in 1989 (in $1m.):

Commonwealth countries

Australia	1,101
Bahamas	29
Bangladesh	65
Barbados	47
Belize	5
Bermuda	39
Cyprus	5
Ghana	33
Guyana	4
Hong Kong	1,076
India	311
Jamaica	132
Kenya	6
Malawi	5
Malaysia	223
Malta	3
New Zealand	170
Nigeria	33
Pakistan	69
Singapore	265
Sri Lanka	11
Tanzania	21
Trinidad and Tobago	58
Uganda	5
UK	3,551
Zambia	19
Zimbabwe	17

Non-Commonwealth countries

Algeria	298
Angola	11
Argentina	39
Austria	112
Bahrain	6
Belgium	1,425
Bolivia	7
Brazil	529
Cameroon	38
Chile	113
China	1,145
Colombia	202
Costa Rica	23
Côte d'Ivoire	11
Cuba	160
Czechoslovakia	13
Denmark	151
Dominican Republic	62
Ecuador	34
Egypt	61
El Salvador	11
Ethiopia	25
Fiji	2
Finland	140
France	1,318
Gabon	6
German Democratic Rep.	100
Germany, Fed. Rep. of	1,871
Greece	60
Greenland	10
Guatemala	21
Guinea	4
Haiti	19
Honduras	14
Hungary	6
Iceland	11
Indonesia	311
Iran	299
Iraq	377
Ireland	165
Israel	131
Italy	1,128
Japan	8,850
Jordan	6
Korea, South	1,695
Kuwait	26
Lebanon	6
Liberia	4
Libya	62
Luxembourg	4
Mexico	622
Morocco	120
Mozambique	10
Netherlands	1,590
Netherlands Antilles	12
Nicaragua	23
Norway	642
Panama	19
Peru	58
Philippines	221
Poland	37
Portugal	154
Puerto Rico	203
Qatar	5
Romania	41
St Pierre and Miquelon	29
Saudi Arabia	340
Senegal	18
Somalia	3
South Africa	105
Spain	404
Sudan	9
Sweden	337
Switzerland	737
Syria	5
Taiwan	973
Thailand	345
Togo	4
Tunisia	40
Turkey	161
USSR	688
United Arab Emirates	33
USA	101,411
US Virgin Islands	4
Uruguay	26
Venezuela	163
Vietnam	2
Yemen (South)	2
Yugoslavia	50
Zaïre	19

Imports by countries in 1988 (in $1m.):

Commonwealth countries			
Australia	618	German Democratic Rep.	40
Bahamas	32	Germany, Fed. Rep. of	3,709
Bangladesh	23	Greece	69
Barbados	13	Guatemala	41
Belize	8	Guinea	18
Bermuda	3	Haiti	12
Ghana	5	Honduras	25
Guyana	19	Hungary	44
Hong Kong	1,160	Iceland	9
India	233	Indonesia	191
Jamaica	188	Iran	163
Kenya	14	Iraq	61
Malaysia	320	Ireland	167
Malta	16	Israel	148
Mauritius	7	Italy	2,015
New Zealand	216	Japan	9,571
Nigeria	505	Korea, South	2,441
Pakistan	79	Lebanon	3
Sierra Leone	15	Liberia	6
Singapore	502	Libya	5
Sri Lanka	33	Luxembourg	24
Trinidad and Tobago	22	Mexico	1,704
Uganda	6	Morocco	39
UK	4.562	Netherlands	822
Zimbabwe	6	Netherlands Antilles	16
		Nicaragua	74
		Norway	784
Non-Commonwealth countries		Panama	18
Algeria	29	Peru	89
Angola	88	Philippines	204
Argentina	132	Poland	88
Austria	376	Portugal	161
Bahrain	7	Puerto Rico	340
Belgium	540	Romania	102
Bolivia	6	Saudi Arabia	253
Brazil	1,129	South Africa	206
Chile	174	Spain	565
China	1,112	Sweden	939
Colombia	157	Switzerland	599
Costa Rica	57	Taiwan	2,381
Côte d'Ivoire	29	Thailand	419
Cuba	62	Togo	41
Czechoslovakia	69	Turkey	81
Denmark	254	USSR	117
Dominican Republic	40	United Arab Emirates	36
Ecuador	107	USA	88,017
Egypt	5	US Virgin Islands	11
El Salvador	28	Uruguay	79
Ethiopia	8	Venezuela	596
Fiji	15	Vietnam	14
Finland	372	Yugoslavia	93
France	2,019	Zaïre	18

Categories of imports in 1989, estimate (in $1,000):

Live animals	139,970	Fabricated materials, inedible	26,243,275
Food, feed, beverages and tobacco	7,412,036	End products, inedible	90,529,067
Crude materials, inedible	7,974,851	Special transactions	2,835,693

Categories of exports (Canadian produce) in 1989, estimate (in $1,000):

Live animals	563,253	Fabricated materials, inedible	47,111,357
Food, feed, beverages and tobacco	9,300,883	End products, inedible	58,061,636
Crude materials, inedible	18,027,014	Special transactions	706,344

Crude oil exports were 37,548,000 cu. metres in 1989; imports, 28,247,000 cu. metres. Natural gas exports were 37,547m. cu. metres in 1989.

Export of fishery products in 1988 were valued at $2,701m.

Total trade of Canada with UK (British Department of Trade returns, in £1,000 sterling):

	1986	*1987*	*1988*	*1989*	*1990*
Imports to UK	1,470,434	1,470,434	2,038,245	2,174,334	2,259,099
Exports and re-exports from UK	1,698,156	1,938,237	2,038,433	2,165,731	1,901,939

Tourism. The number of visitors to Canada in 1988 was 39,252,915 (1989, 37,981,925). In 1988, 36,147,055 came from the USA (1989, 34,705,087).

COMMUNICATIONS

Roads. The total length of federal and provincial territorial roads and highways at the end of March 1986 was 280,251 km. Expenditures by these two levels of government on roads and highways during the fiscal year 1985–86 amounted to approximately $5,347·7m.

In general highways are controlled and maintained by the provinces who also have the responsiblity of providing assistance to their municipalities and townships. Federal expenditures are directed largely to the maintenance of national park highways, Indian Reserve roads and designated provincial/territorial highway construction in projects. The Alaska Highway is part of the Canadian highway system. For the Trans-Canada Highway *see* map in THE STATESMAN'S YEAR-BOOK, 1962.

In 1988 intercity and rural bus services carried 18m. passengers 156m. km, earning $332·8m.

Registered motor vehicles totalled 16,366,261 in 1988; they included 12,086,001 passenger cars and taxis, 3,765,866 trucks and buses and 369,758 motor cycles.

Railways. The total length of track in 1988 was 91,365 km, including: Mainline track, 38,922 km; branch line, 27,287 km and industrial and siding track, 25,155 km.

Canada has 2 great trans-continental systems: The Canadian National Railway system (CN), a government-owned body which operates 48,753 km (1988) of track, and the Canadian Pacific Railway (CP), a joint-stock corporation operating 32,638 km (1988). From 1 April 1978, a government-funded organization known as Via Rail took over passenger services formerly operated by CP and CN; 5·9m. passengers were carried in 1987.

There are metros in Montreal, Toronto and Vancouver, and tram/light rail systems in Calgary, Edmonton and Toronto. In 1987 urban transit systems carried 1,515m. passengers for an operating revenue of $2,581·8m.

Selected statistics for 1988: Passenger revenue $276·8m.; freight revenue, $6,571m.; total railway operating revenues, $8,003·1m.; total operating expenses, $6,979m.

Aviation. Civil aviation is under the jurisdiction of the federal government. The technical and administrative aspects are supervised by Transport Canada, while the economic functions are assigned to the National Transportation agency.

In 1989 Canadian airports handled 45,339,760 revenue passengers on major scheduled services and 714,071 tonnes of cargo. Operating revenue for commercial air carriers (1989) was $5,604·5m.; operating expenditure, $5,622·9m.

The 2 major airlines are Air Canada (privatized in July 1989) and Canadian Airlines International. Air Canada had 105 aircraft in 1991.

Shipping. Total vessel arrivals and departures at Canadian ports in domestic shipping was 56,801 in 1989, totalling a cumulative GRT of 224,433,364. A total of 58,297 vessel movements in international shipping at Canadian ports in 1989 loaded and unloaded 236m. tonnes of cargo, totalling a GRT of 592,231,671.

The major canals in Canada are those of the St Lawrence–Great Lakes waterway with their 7 locks, providing navigation for vessels of 26-ft draught from Montreal to Lake Ontario; the Welland Canal by-passing the Niagara River between Lake

Ontario and Lake Erie with its 8 locks; and the Sault Ste Marie Canal and lock between Lake Huron and Lake Superior. These 16 locks overcome a drop of 582 ft from the head of the lakes to Montreal. The St Lawrence Seaway was opened to navigation on 1 April 1959 (*see* map in THE STATESMAN'S YEAR-BOOK, 1957). In 1989, traffic on the Montreal–Lake Ontario Section of the Seaway numbered 2,768 transits carrying 37·1m. cargo tonnes; on the Welland Canal Section, 3,598 transits with 39·9m. cargo tonnes. Value of fixed assets was $533,447,000 and investments, $44,872,000 at 31 March 1990.

Coast Guard. The Canadian Coast Guard (formed in 1962) is responsible to the Minister of Transport. In 1989 it comprised 8 heavy icebreakers; 11 medium icebreakers; 1 light icebreaker/navigational aid tender; 7 ice-strengthened/navigational aid tenders; 16 navigational aid tenders; 1 hydraulic survey and sounding vessel; 80 search and rescue vessels; 4 hovercraft; 35 helicopters and 1 fixed-wing aircraft (DC-3).

Telecommunications. In 1989–90 there were 16,749 retail postal outlets in operation. Total revenue (1989–90) was $3,756m.; total expenditure, $3,607m. (excluding amortization of extraordinary restructuring costs).

There were 14·5m. telephone access lines reported by major telephone companies in 1989.

There were 831 originating stations operating at 31 March 1990, of which 385 were AM radio stations, 317 FM radio stations and 129 television stations.

Cinemas. (1988). There were 675 cinemas and 146 drive-in theatres.

Newspapers. In 1988 there were 96 dailies in English (total circulation, 4·95m.) and 11 in French (1m.).

JUSTICE, RELIGION, EDUCATION AND WELFARE

Justice. There is a Supreme Court in Ottawa, having general appellate jurisdiction in civil and criminal cases throughout Canada. The Exchequer Court (established in 1875) was replaced by the Federal Court in 1971. This has a Trial Division, consisting of the Associate Chief Justice and 9 other judges, and an Appeal Division, consisting of the Chief Justice and 3 other judges. Its seat is in Ottawa, but each Division may sit in any place in Canada. Decisions of the Trial Division may be appealed to the Appeal Division, those of the latter to the Supreme Court. There is a Superior Court in each province and county courts, with limited jurisdiction, in most of the provinces, all the judges in these courts being appointed by the Governor-General. Police, magistrates and justices of the peace are appointed by the provincial governments.

For the year ended 31 Dec. 1989, 2,431,428 Criminal Code Offences were reported and 418,863 adults were charged.

Canadian Legal and Directory. Toronto. Annual

Religion. The *Yearbook of American and Canadian Churches*, published by the National Council of the Churches of Christ in the USA, New York, presents the latest figures available (1988) from official statisticians of church bodies:

Religious body	*Inclusive membership*	*Number of churches*	*Number of clergy*
Anglican Church of Canada	805,521	3,105	3,300
Canadian Baptist Federation	122,247	1,136	1,298
Evangelical Lutheran Church	208,149	652	817
Pentecostal Assemblies of Canada	191,607	1,068	...
Presbyterian Church	213,690	1,033	1,168
Roman Catholic Church	11,375,914	5,878	11,838
Ukrainian Greek Orthodox	120,000	258	91
United Church of Canada	2,052,342	4,138	3,795

Membership of other denominations: Mormons (1987), 118,000; Jewish (1981), 296,425; Jehovah's Witnesses (1989), 94,605; Lutheran Church – Canada (1988), 90,944; Salvation Army (1988), 88,899.

Education. Under the Constitution the various provincial legislatures have powers over education. These are subject to certain qualifications respecting the rights of denominational and minority language schools. Newfoundland and Quebec legislations provide for Roman Catholic and Protestant school boards. School Acts in Ontario, Saskatchewan and Alberta provide tax support for both public and separate schools. School board revenues derive from local taxation on real property and government grants from general provincial revenue.

Statistics for 1988–89 (estimates) of all elementary and secondary schools, public, federal and private:

Province	*Schools*	*Teachers*	*Pupils*
Newfoundland	546	7,982	130,503
Prince Edward Island	72	1,336	24,804
Nova Scotia	566	10,284	169,561
New Brunswick	463	7,755	136,402
Quebec	2,880	64,448	1,139,491
Ontario	5,332	112,514	1,974,487
Manitoba	838	12,692	219,172
Saskatchewan	1,004	11,487	212,547
Alberta	1,709	25,199	491,433
British Columbia	1,951	28,623	556,100
Yukon	25	310	5,150
Northwest Territories	77	810	13,732
National Defence (overseas)	8	260	3,722
Total	15,461	283,710	5,077,104

Enrolment for Indian and Inuit children, 1989-90: Federal schools, 11,764; band operated schools, 34,674; provincial schools, 41,720.

In 1989–90, 514,422 full-time regular students (graduates and undergraduates) were enrolled in universities. In 1989 105,239 received first degrees of which 16,954 were in education; 12,837 in humanities; 7,916 in engineering and applied sciences; 3,375 in fine and applied arts; 40,404 in social sciences; 7,282 in agriculture/biological sciences; 7,309 in health professions; 6,784 in mathematics/physical sciences; and 2,378 were unclassified.

Health. Constitutional responsibility for health care services rests with the ten provinces and two territories of Canada. Accordingly, Canada's national health insurance system consists of an interlocking set of provincial and territorial hospital and medical insurance plans conforming to certain national standards rather than a single national programme. These national standards, which are set out in the Canada Health Act, include: Provision of a comprehensive range of hospital and medical benefits; universal population coverage; access to necessary services on uniform terms and conditions; portability of benefits; and public administration of provincial and territorial insurance plans.

Provinces and territories satisfying these national standards are eligible for federal financial transfer payments according to the provisions of the Federal-Provincial Fiscal Arrangements and Federal Post-Secondary Education and Health Contributions Act. Under this Act, the provinces and territories are entitled to receive equal-per-capita federal health contributions escalated annually by the three year average increase in nominal Gross National Product. These federal contributions, estimated at $13,000m. in 1990, are paid in the form of a combination of tax point and cash transfers. Over and above these health transfers, the federal government also provides financial support for such provincial and territorial extended health care service programmes as nursing home care, certain home care services, ambulatory health care services and adult residential care services. These supplementary equal-per-capita cash payments, estimated at $1,360m. in 1990, are also escalated annually by increases to nominal GNP.

The national health insurance programmes were introduced in stages. The Hospital Insurance and Diagnostic Services Act was passed in 1958, providing prepaid coverage to all Canadians for in-patient and, at the option of each province and territory, out-patient hospital services. The Medical Care Act was introduced in 1968 to extend universal coverage to all medically equipped services provided by medical practitioners. The Canada Health Act, which took effect 1 April 1984, consolidated the original federal health insurance legislation and clarified the national standards provinces and territories are required to meet in order to qualify for full federal health contributions.

The approach taken by Canada is one of state-sponsored health insurance. Accordingly, the advent of insurance programmes produced little change in the ownership of hospitals, almost all of which are owned by non-government non-profit corporations, or in the rights and privileges of private medical practice. Patients are free to choose their own general practitioner. Except for 0·5% of the population whose care is provided for under other legislation (such as serving members of the Canadian Armed Forces and inmates of federal penitentiaries), all residents are eligible, regardless of whether they are in the work force. Benefits are available without upper limit so long as they are medically necessary, provided any registration obligations are met. Benefits are also portable during any temporary absence from Canada anywhere in the world—subject to any limitation a province or territory may impose upon treatment electively sought outside the particular province or territory without prior approval.

In addition to the benefits qualifying for federal contributions, provinces and territories provide additional benefits at their own discretion. All provinces and territories provide benefits covering a variety of services (*e.g.*, optometric care, children's dental care, drug benefits). Most fund their portion of health costs out of general provincial and territorial revenues. Two provinces levy health premiums which meet part of the provincial and territorial costs, 2 provinces impose a levy on employers, and 2 provinces utilize a tax or surcharge, based on personal income tax, for this purpose, and 1 province utilizes a payroll tax paid by employers. There are no co-charges for medically necessary short-term hospital care or medical care. Most provinces and territories have charges for long-term chronic hospital care geared, approximately, to the room and board portion of this OAS–GIS payment mentioned under Social Welfare. In 1989, total health expenditures were about $51·7m., representing 8·9% of GNP. Public sector spending accounts for about 75% of total national health expenditure.

Social Welfare. The social security system provides financial benefits and social services to individuals and their families through a variety of programmes administered by federal, provincial and municipal governments, and voluntary organizations. Federally, the Department of Health and Welfare Canada is responsible for research into the areas of health and social issues, provision of grants and contributions for various social services, improvement and construction of health facilities, the administration of several of Canada's income security programmes and the development and promotion of measures designed to improve the health and well-being of Canadians. These programmes are: The Family Allowances programme, introduced in 1945 and amended in 1973; the Old Age Security programme, introduced in 1952 and to which were added the Guaranteed Income Supplement in 1967 and the Spouse's Allowance in 1975; and the Canada Pension Plan and Canada Assistance Plan which came into being in 1966.

The 1973 Family Allowances Act provides for the payment of a monthly Family Allowance ($33.33 in 1990) in respect of a dependent child under the age of 18 who is a resident of Canada and is wholly or substantially maintained by a parent or guardian. At least one parent must be a Canadian citizen, or admitted to Canada as a permanent resident under the Immigration Act, or admitted to Canada for a period of not less than 1 year, if during that time his or her income is subject to Canadian income tax. Benefits are also paid under prescribed circumstances to Canadian citizens living abroad. Eligibility for Family Allowances (FA) is a precondition for receipt of the refundable Child Tax Credit discussed below. A Special Allowance ($49.72 monthly in 1990) is paid on behalf of a child under the age of 18 who is maintained by a welfare agency, a government department or an institution. In some cases, payment is made directly to a foster parent.

The Family Allowances Act specifies that a provincial government may request the federal government to vary the allowance rates payable within the province by age and/or family size subject to the fulfillment of stipulated conditions. Only the provinces of Alberta and Quebec have exercised this option. During the month of Oct. 1990, over 3·7m. Canadian families (including 6·6m. eligible children) received Family Allowances; the Special Allowance was paid on behalf of 31,000 of these children. The total bill for FA and Special Allowances for 1990–91 was $2,621m.

The Old Age Security (OAS) pension is payable to persons 65 years of age and over who satisfy the residence requirements stipulated in the Old Age Security Act. The amount payable, whether full or partial, is also governed by stipulated conditions, as is the payment of an OAS pension to a recipient who absents himself from Canada. OAS pensioners with little or no income apart from OAS may, upon application, receive a full or partial supplement known as the Guaranteed Income Supplement (GIS). Entitlement is normally based on the pensioner's income in the preceding year, calculated in accordance with the Income Tax Act. The spouse of an OAS pensioner, aged 60 to 64, meeting the same residence requirements as those stipulated for OAS, may be eligible for a full or partial Spouse's Allowance (SPA). SPA is payable, on application, depending on the annual combined income of the couple (not including the pensioner spouse's basic OAS pension or GIS). In 1979, the SPA programme was expanded to include a spouse, who is eligible for SPA in the month the pensioner spouse dies, until the age of 65 or until remarriage (Extended Spouse's Allowance). Since Sept. 1985, SPA has also been available to low income widow(er)s aged 60–64 regardless of the age of their spouse at death. For the fourth quarter of 1990, the basic OAS pension was $351·41 monthly; the maximum Guaranteed Income Supplement was $417·61 monthly for a single pensioner or a married pensioner whose spouse was not receiving a pension or a Spouse's Allowance, and $272·9 monthly for each spouse of a married couple where both were pensioners. The maximum Spouse's Allowance for the same quarter was $623·42 monthly (equal to the basic pension plus the maximum GIS married rate), and $688·26 for widow(er)s. Total OAS/GIS/SPA benefit expenditures for 1989–90 were $7,641m.; in July 1990, over 3m. Canadians received benefits through these programmes.

The Canada Pension Plan (CPP) is designed to provide workers with a basic level of income protection in the event of retirement, disability or death. Benefits may be payable to a contributor, a surviving spouse or an eligible child. As of 1 Jan. 1987, payment of actuarially adjusted retirement benefits may begin as early as age 60 or as late as age 70. Benefits are determined by the contributor's earnings and contributions made to the Plan. Contribution is compulsory for most employed and self-employed Canadians 18 to 65 years of age. The Canada Pension Plan does not operate in Quebec, which has exercised its constitutional prerogative to establish a similar plan, the Quebec Pension Plan (QPP), to operate in lieu of CPP; there is reciprocity between the two to ensure coverage for all adult Canadians in the labour force. In 1990, the maximum retirement pension payable under CPP and QPP was $577.08, the maximum disability pension was $709.52, and the maximum surviving spouse's pension was $346.25 (for survivors 65 years of age and over). For survivors under 65 years of age CPP pays a reduced flat rate while QPP pays varied rates depending on the age of the survivor. In 1990 both CPP and QPP were funded by equal contributions of 2·2% of pensionable earnings from the employer and 2·2% from the employee (self-employed persons contribute the full 4·4%), in addition to the interest on the investment of excess funds. In 1990, the range of yearly pensionable earnings was from $2,800 to $28,900; a person who earned and contributed at less than the maximum level receives monthly benefits at rates lower than the maximum allowable under CPP/QPP. In Oct. 1990, over 3·3m. Canadians received Canada or Quebec Pension Plan benefits. Total expenditures in 1990–91 for CPP were about $10,618m.

Social security programme agreements co-ordinate the operation of the Old Age Security programme and the Canada Pension Plan with the comparable programmes of another country in order to accomplish four basic objectives: To remove restrictions, based on nationality, which may otherwise prevent Canadians from receiving benefits under the legislation of the other country; to ease or eliminate restrictions on the payment of social security benefits abroad; to eliminate situations in which a worker may have to contribute to the social security programmes of both countries for the same work; to assist migrants in qualifying for benefits based on the periods they have lived or worked in each country. Such agreements are in force with Italy, France, Portugal, the USA, Greece, Jamaica, Barbados, Belgium, Denmark, Norway, Sweden, Austria, St Lucia, Spain, Australia, Dominica, Luxembourg, the Netherlands, Germany, Finland and Iceland. In addition, agreements have been signed with Cyprus and Ireland.

Ismael, J. S., (ed.) *Canadian Welfare State: Evolution and Transition.* Univ. of Alberta Press, 1987

DIPLOMATIC REPRESENTATIVES

Of Canada in Great Britain (Macdonald House., Grosvenor Sq., London, W1X 0AB)
High Commissioner: The Hon. Donald S. Macdonald, PC (accredited 11 Nov. 1988).

Of Great Britain in Canada (80 Elgin St., Ottawa, K1P 5K7)
High Commissioner: Brian J. P. Fall, CMG.

Of Canada in the USA (501 Pennsylvania Ave., NW, Washington, D.C., 20001)
Ambassador: Derek H. Burney.

Of the USA in Canada (100 Wellington St., Ottawa, K1P 5TI)
Ambassador: Edward N. Ney.

Of Canada to the United Nations
Ambassador: Yves Fortier, QC.

Further Reading

Statistical Information: Statistics Canada, Ottawa, has been the official central statistical organization for Canada since 1918. The Agency, which reports to Parliament through the Minister responsible for the Department of Regional Industrial Expansion, serves as the statistical agency for federal government departments; co-ordinates the statistics of the provincial governments along national lines; and channels all Canadian statistical data to internal organizations. *Chief Statistician of Canada:* Dr I. P. Fellegi.

Publications of Statistics Canada are classified as periodical (issued more frequently than once a year), annual, biennial and occasional publications. The occasional publications frequently supplement the annual reports and usually contain historical information. A complete list is contained in the Statistics Canada catalogue 1988–89, available at a nominal cost. Reference publications include:

The Canada Year Book. Biennial, from 1905
Canada: A Portrait. Biennial, from 1980
Canadian Economic Observer. Monthly, with annual historical supplements, from 1988
Twelfth Decennial Census of Canada, 1981. Ottawa, 1982
Atlas and Gazetteer of Canada. Dept. of Energy, Mines and Resources. Ottawa, 1969
Cambridge History of the British Empire. Vol. VI. Canada and Newfoundland. Cambridge, 1930
Canadian Almanac and Directory. Toronto. Annual
Canadian Annual Review. Annual, from 1960
Canadian Dictionary: French–English. Toronto, 1970
Canadian Encyclopedia. 3 vols. Edmonton, 1985
Canadiana; A List of Publications of Canadian Interest. National Library, Ottawa. Monthly, with annual cumulation. 1951 ff.
Cook, R., *French-Canadian Nationalism; An Anthology.* Toronto, 1970.—*The Maple Leaf Forever; Essays on Nationalism and Politics in Canada.* Toronto, 1971
Creighton, D. G., *Canada's First Century.* Toronto, 1970.—*Towards the Discovery of Canada.* Toronto, 1974

Dewitt, D. B. and Kirton, J. J., *Canada as a Principal Power: A Study in Foreign Policy.* Toronto, 1983
Dictionnaire Bélisle de la langue française au Canada; dictionnaire Oxford. 1970
Dictionnaire canadien; français–anglais–français. Toronto, 1962
Encyclopedia Canadiana. 10 vols. Rev. ed. Ottawa, 1967
Granatstein, J. L., *Twentieth Century Canada.* Toronto, 1983
Hardy, W. G., *From Sea to Sea; Canada, 1850–1920: The Road to Nationhood.* Toronto, 1960
Harris, R. C., (ed.) *Historical Atlas of Canada.* Vol 1. Univ. of Toronto, 1987
Hockin, T. A., *Government in Canada.* London, 1976
Ingles, E., *Canada.* [Bibliography] Oxford and Santa Barbara, 1990
Jackson, R. J., *Politics in Canada: Culture, Institutions, Behaviour and Public Policy.* 2nd ed. Scarborough, Ont., 1990
Kerr, D. G. G., *Historical Atlas of Canada.* Toronto, 1960
Leacy, F. H., (ed.) *Historical Statistics of Canada.* Government Printer, Ottawa, 1983
Lower, A. R. M., *Colony to Nation: A History of Canada.* 4th ed. Toronto, 1964
McCann, L. D., (ed.) *Heartland and Hinterland: A Geography of Canada.* Scarborough, Ontario, 1982
Mallory, J. R., *The Structure of Canadian Government.* Toronto, 1971
Moir, J. and Saunders, R., *Northern Destiny: A History of Canada.* Toronto, 1970
Nurgitz, N. and Segal, H., *No Small Measure: The Progressive Conservatives and the Constitution.* Ottawa, 1983
Smith, D. L., (ed.) *History of Canada: An Annotated Bibliography.* Oxford and Santa Barbara, 1983
White, W. L. *Introduction to Canadian Politics and Government.* 5th ed. Toronto, 1990

National Library: The National Library of Canada, Ottawa, Ontario. *Librarian:* Marianne Scott.

CANADIAN PROVINCES

The 10 provinces have each a separate parliament and administration, with a Lieut.-Governor, appointed by the Governor-General in Council at the head of the executive. They have full powers to regulate their own local affairs and dispose of their revenues, provided only they do not interfere with the action and policy of the central administration. Among the subjects assigned exclusively to the provincial legislatures are: The amendment of the provincial constitution, except as regards the office of the Lieut.-Governor; property and civil rights; direct taxation for revenue purposes; borrowing; management and sale of Crown lands; provincial hospitals, reformatories, etc.; shop, saloon, tavern, auctioneer and other licences for local or provincial purposes; local works and undertakings, except lines of ships, railways, canals, telegraphs, etc., extending beyond the province or connecting with other provinces, and excepting also such works as the Canadian Parliament declares are for the general good; marriages, administration of justice within the province; education.

Local Government. Under the terms of the British North America Act the provinces are given full powers over local government. All local government institutions are, therefore, supervised by the provinces, and are incorporated and function under provincial acts.

The acts under which municipalities operate vary from province to province. A municipal corporation is usually administered by an elected council headed by a mayor or reeve, whose powers to administer affairs and to raise funds by taxation and other methods are set forth in provincial laws, as is the scope of its obligations to, and on behalf of, the citizens. Similarly, the types of municipal corporations, their official designations and the requirements for their incorporation vary between provinces. The following table sets out the classifications as at 1 Jan. 1988.

Type and size of group	*Nfld.*	*PEI*	*NS*	*NB*	*Que.*	*Ont.*	*Man.*
Type:							
Regional municipalities	—	—	—	—	98	39	—
Metropolitan and regional municipalities [1]	—	—	—	—	3	12	—
Counties and regional districts	—	—	—	—	95	27	—
Unitary municipalities	170	86	66	114	1,500	792	184
Cities [2]	3	1	3	6	65	50	5
Towns	167	8	39	25	193	145	35
Villages	—	—	—	83	233	119	39
Rural municipalities [3]	—	77	24	—	1,009	478	105
Quasi-municipalities [4]	143	—	—	—	—	8	17
Total	313	86	66	114	1,598	839	201
Population size group (1986 census):							
Unitary municipalities—							
Over 100,000	—	—	2	—	4	18	1
50,000 to 99,999	1	—	1	2	16	14	—
10,000 to 49,999	4	1	18	4	80	81	4
Under 10,000	165	85	45	108	1,400	679	179
Total	170	86	66	114	1,500	792	184

Type and size of group	*Sask.*	*Alta.*	*BC*	*YT*	*NWT*	*Canada*
Type:						
Regional municipalities	—	—	28	—	—	165
Metropolitan and regional municipalities [1]	—	—	—	—	—	15
Counties and regional districts	—	—	28	—	—	150
Unitary municipalities	821	345	144	8	8	4,238
Cities [2]	12	15	37	2	1	200
Towns	146	108	12	2	5	885
Villages	364	172	48	4	2	1,064
Rural municipalities [3]:	299	50	47	—	—	2,089
Quasi-municipalities [4]	14	19	—	—	30	231
Total	835	364	172	8	38	4,634
Population size group (1986 census):						
Unitary municipalities—						
Over 100,000	2	2	4	—	—	33
50,000 to 99,999	—	—	10	—	—	44
10,000 to 49,999	7	18	29	1	1	248
Under 10,000	812	325	101	7	7	3,913
Total	821	345	144	8	8	4,238

[1] Includes urban communities in Quebec; and Metropolitan Toronto, regional municipalities and the district municipality of Muskoka in Ontario. [2] Includes the borough of East York. [3] Includes municipalities in Nova Scotia; parishes, townships, united townships and municipalities without designation in Quebec; townships in Ontario; rural municipalities in Manitoba and Saskatchewan; municipal districts and counties in Alberta; and districts in British Columbia. [4] Includes local government communities and the metropolitan area in Newfoundland; improvement districts in Ontario and Alberta; local government districts in Manitoba; and hamlets in the Northwest Territories.

ALBERTA

HISTORY. The southern half of the province of Alberta was part of Rupert's land which was granted by royal charter in 1670 to the Hudson's Bay Company. The intervention by the North West Company in the fur trade after 1783 led to the establishment of trading posts. In 1869 Rupert's land was transferred from the Hudson's Bay Company (which had absorbed its rival in 1821) to the new Dominion, and in the following year this land was combined with the former Crown land of the North Western Territories to form the Northwest Territories.

In 1882 'Alberta' first appeared as a provisional 'district', consisting of the southern half of the present province. In 1905 the Athabasca district to the north was added when provincial status was granted to Alberta.

Four parties have held office: The Liberals 1905–21; the United Farmers 1921–35; Social Credit 1935–71, and Progressive Conservative since Sept. 1971.

AREA AND POPULATION. The area of the province is 661,185 sq. km; 644,389 sq. km being land area and 16,796 sq. km water area. The population (estimate 1 July 1990) was 2,472,500; the urban population (1986), centres of 1,000 or over, was 1,877,758 and the rural 488,067. Population (30 June 1990) of the 16 cities (*see below under* Local Government for definition): Calgary, 692,885; Edmonton, 605,538; Lethbridge, 60,614; Red Deer, 56,922; Medicine Hat, 42,929; St Albert, 40,707; Fort McMurray, 33,698; Grande Prairie, 27,558; Leduc, 13,566; Camrose, 12,968; Spruce Grove, 12,403; Fort Saskatchewan, 11,753; Airdrie, 11,904; Lloydminster (Alberta portion), 10,201; Wetaskiwin, 10,203; Drumheller, 6,366.

Vital statistics, *see* p. 273.

CLIMATE. A continental climate: Long, cold winters and mild summers. Rainfall amounts are greatest between May and Sept. Edmonton. Jan. 5°F (–15°C), July 63°F (17°C). Annual rainfall 13·6" (345·6 mm).

CONSTITUTION AND GOVERNMENT. The constitution of Alberta is contained in the British North America Act of 1867, and amending Acts; also in the Alberta Act of 1905, passed by the Parliament of the Dominion of Canada, which created the province out of the then Northwest Territories. All the provisions of the British North America Act, except those with respect to school lands and the public domain, were made to apply to Alberta as they apply to the older provinces of Canada. On 1 Oct. 1930 the natural resources were transferred from the Dominion to provincial government control. The province is represented by 6 members in the Senate and 26 in the House of Commons of Canada.

The executive is vested nominally in the Lieut.-Governor, who is appointed by the federal government, but actually in the Executive Council or the Cabinet of the legislature. Legislative power is vested in the Assembly in the name of the Queen.

Members of the Legislative Assembly are elected by the universal vote of adults over the age of 18 years.

There are 83 members in the legislature (elected 20 March 1989): 59 Progressive Conservative, 16 New Democratic Party, 8 Liberal.

Lieut.-Governor: Hon. Helen Hunley (sworn in 22 Jan. 1985).

Flag: Blue with the shield of the province in the centre.

The members of the Ministry were as follows in Oct. 1989:

Premier, President of Executive Council: Hon. D. R. Getty.

Deputy Premier and Minister of Federal and Intergovernmental Affairs: Hon. J. Horsman. *Transportation and Utilities:* Hon. J. A. Adair. *Consumer and Corporate Affairs:* Hon. D. Anderson. *Health:* Hon. N. Betkowski. *Education:* Hon. J. Dinning. *Economic Development and Trade:* Hon. J. Elzinga. *Forestry, Lands and Wildlife:* Hon. E. L. Fjordbotten. *Solicitor General:* Hon. D. Fowler. *Advanced Education:* Hon. J. Gogo. *Agriculture:* Hon. E. Isley. *Provincial Treasurer:* Hon. A. D. Johnston. *Environment:* Hon. R. Klein. *Public Works, Supply and Services:* Hon. K. Kowalski. *Culture and Multiculturalism:* Hon. D. Main. *Labour:* Hon. E. McCoy. *Family and Social Services:* Hon. J. Oldring. *Energy:* Hon. R. Orman. *Attorney-General:* Hon. K. Rostad. *Tourism:* Hon. D. Sparrow. *Municipal Affairs:* Hon. R. Speaker. *Technology, Research and Telecommunications:* Hon. F. Stewart. *Occupational Health and Safety:* Hon. P. Trynchy. *Career Development and Employment:* Hon. N. Weiss. *Recreation and Parks:* Hon. S. West.

Local Government. The local government units are City, Town, New Town, Village, Summer Village, County, Municipal District and Improvement District.

There are 16 cities (*see* Area and Population, above). These cities operate under the Municipal Government Act. The governing body consists of a mayor and a council of from 6 to 20 members. A city can be incorporated by order of the Lieut.-Governor-in-Council. A population of 10,000 is required on incorporation.

There are no limits of area specified in the statutes for any of the different local government units. The population requirement for a Town as specified in the Municipal Government Act is 1,000 people, and the area at incorporation is that of the original village.

A Village must contain 75 separate and occupied dwellings. The Municipal Government Act requires each dwelling to have been occupied continuously for a period of at least 6 months. A Summer Village must contain 50 separate dwellings.

A rural county area is an area incorporated through an order of the Lieut.-Governor-in-Council under the provisions of the County Act. One board of councillors deal with both municipal and school affairs.

A rural Municipal District is an area which has been incorporated under the Municipal Government Act. In Municipal Districts separate boards control municipal and school affairs.

Areas not incorporated as counties or Municipal Districts are termed Improvement Districts or Special Areas. Sparsely populated, such districts are administered and taxed by the Department of Municipal Affairs of the provincial government. There are no requirements as to the minimum number of residents of a County or Municipal District.

FINANCE. The budgetary revenue and expenditure (in $1m.) for years ending 31 March were as follows:

	1987–88	*1988–89*	*1989–90* [1]
Revenue	9,466	9,106	11,420
Expenditure	10,399	10,889	12,200

[1] Estimates.

Personal income *per capita* (1988), $19,947.

ENERGY AND NATURAL RESOURCES

Oil. In 1988, 76,958,000 cu. metres of crude oil were produced with gross sales value of $7,710,659,000. Alberta produced 82% of Canada's crude petroleum output in 1988. Production of natural gas by-products was 21,699,000 cu. metres, valued at $1,542,377,000.

Oil sands underlie some 60,000 sq. km of Alberta, the 4 major deposits being: The Athabasca, Cold Lake, Peace River and Buffalo Head Hills deposits. Some 7% (3,250 sq. km) of the Athabasca deposit can be exploited through open-pit mining. The rest of the Athabasca, and all the deposits in the other areas, are deeper reserves which must be developed through in situ techniques. These reserves reach depths of 760 metres.

Two oil sands mining plants in the Fort McMurray area produced 11·7m. cu. metres of synthetic crude oil in 1988.

Gas. Natural gas is found in abundance in numerous localities. In 1988, 77,995m. cu. metres valued at $4,584,528,000 were produced.

Minerals. Coal reserves are estimated at 2,600,000m. tonnes, of which 800,000m. tonnes are recoverable. Production (1988) 29·47m. tonnes valued at $459m.

Value of total mineral production decreased from $17,079,970,000 in 1987 to $15,061,958,000 in 1988.

Agriculture. Total area of farms (1986) 51,040,463 acres; improved land, 31,891,516; (under crops, 22,641,092; improved pasture, 3,402,183; summer fallow, 5,255,965; other improved land, 592,276); unimproved land, 19,148,947; (unimproved pasture, 16,057,185; woodland, 713,699; other unimproved land, 2,378,063). Number of farms (1986) 57,777.

For particulars of agricultural production and livestock *see* pp. 000–00. Farm cash receipts in 1989 totalled $4,368,271,000, of which crops contributed $1,179,558,000; livestock and products, $2,033,222,000, and direct payments, $555,491,000.

Forestry. Forest land in 1990 covered some 202,000 sq. km. In 1988–89 9,645,039 cu. metres were cut from land managed by the Crown.

Fisheries. The largest catch in commercial fishing is whitefish. Perch, tullibee, walley, pike and lake trout are also caught in smaller quantities. In 1984 a provincial fish marketing policy was implemented and a new commercial fishery licensing system was implemented in 1987. Commercial fish production in 1988–89 was 2,548 tonnes, value $2·8m.

INDUSTRY. The leading manufacturing industries are food and beverages, petroleum refining, metal fabricating, wood industries, primary metal, chemical and chemical products and non-metallic mineral products industries. There were in 1987 2,590 manufacturing establishments, in which were employed 78,220 persons, who earned in salaries and wages $2,278,685,000.

Manufacturing shipments had a total value of $18,612m. in 1989. Chief among these shipments were: Food and beverages, $4·411m.; chemicals and chemical products, $3·298m.; refined petroleum and coal products, $3,029m.; primary metals, $1,120m.; fabricated metal products, $1,075m.; wood, $930m.; printing, publishing and allied products, $755m.; machinery, $746m.; paper and allied products, $587m.; non-metal mineral products, $546m.; transport equipment, $506m.

Total retail sales (1989) $19,219m.

Tourism is of increasing importance and in 1989 contributed $2,580m. to the economy.

COMMUNICATIONS

Roads. In 1990 there were 153,873 km of roads and highways, including 109,763 km gravelled and 20,550 km paved.

At 31 March 1990 there were 1,899,973 motor vehicles registered, including 1,439,004 passenger cars.

Railways. In 1990 the length of main railway lines was 10,200 km. There are rail local transit networks in Edmonton (11·2 km) and Calgary (29·2 km).

Telecommunications. The telephone system is owned and operated by the Telus Corporation (in which the Alberta Government holds 44% of the shares), except in the city of Edmonton (owned and operated by the City Council). There were 1,379,588 telephone subscriber lines in service in April 1990.

JUSTICE AND EDUCATION

Justice. The Supreme Judicial authority of the province is the Court of Appeal. Judges of the Court of Appeal and Court of Queen's Bench are appointed by the Federal Government and hold office until retirement at the age of 75. There are courts of lesser jurisdiction in both civil and criminal matters. The Court of Queen's Bench has full jurisdiction over civil proceedings. A Provincial Court which has jurisdiction in civil matters up to $2,000 is presided over by provincially appointed judges. Youth Courts have power to try boys and girls 12–17 years old inclusive for offences against the Young Offenders Act.

The jurisdiction of all criminal courts in Alberta is enacted in the provisions of the Criminal Code. The system of procedure in civil and criminal cases conforms as nearly as possible to the English system.

Education. Schools of all grades are included under the term of public school (including those in the separate school system which are publicly supported). The same board of trustees controls the schools from kindergarten to university entrance. In 1988–89 there were 432,718 pupils enrolled in grades 1-12, including private schools and special education programmes. The University of Alberta (in

Edmonton), organized in 1907, had, in 1988–89, 25,024 full-time students. The University of Calgary, formerly part of the University of Alberta and autonomous from April 1966, had in 1988–89, 17,302 full-time students. The University of Lethbridge, organized in 1966, had in 1988–89, 3,165 full-time students. The Athabasca University had in 1988–89, 10,936 part-time students. Banff Centre for Continuing Education had in 1988–89, 1,130 part-time students. The full-time enrolment at Alberta's 11 public colleges totalled 19,861 students in 1988–89.

Further Reading

Statistical Information: The Alberta Bureau of Statistics (Dept. of Treasury, Edmonton), which was established in 1939, collects, compiles and distributes information relative to Alberta. Among its publications are: *Alberta Statistical Review* (Quarterly).—*Alberta Economic Accounts* (Annual).—*Alberta Facts* (Annual).—*Population Projections, Alberta* (Occasional).—*Alberta Population Growth* (Quarterly).

Dept. of Economic Development and Trade, *Alberta Industry and Resources Database.* Edmonton, (Biannual)

MacGregor, J. G., *A History of Alberta.* 2nd ed. Edmonton, 1981
Masson, J., *Alberta's Local Governments and their Politics.* Univ. of Alberta Press, 1985
Richards, J., *Prairie Capitalism: Power and Influence in the New West.* Toronto, 1979
Wiebe, Rudy., *Alberta, a Celebration.* Edmonton, 1979

BRITISH COLUMBIA

HISTORY. Vancouver Island was organized as a colony in 1849; the mainland as far as the watershed of the Rocky Mountains was organized as a colony following a gold rush on the Fraser River in 1859. The two were united as the colony of British Columbia in 1866; this became a Canadian Province in 1871.

AREA AND POPULATION. British Columbia has an area of 952,263 sq. km. The capital is Victoria. The province is bordered westerly by the Pacific ocean and Alaska Panhandle, northerly by the Yukon and Northwest Territories, easterly by the Province of Alberta and southerly by the USA along the 49th parallel. A chain of islands, the largest of which are Vancouver Island and the Queen Charlotte Islands, affords protection to the mainland coast.

The 1986 census population was 2,889,207; estimate (1990) 3,130,400.

The principal cities and their 1989 estimated populations are as follows: Metropolitan Vancouver, 1,498,980; Metropolitan Victoria, 273,242; Kelowna, 67,027; Prince George, 65,451; Kamloops, 62,261; Matsqui, 59,717; Nanaimo, 53,788; Chilliwack, 45,643; Penticton, 25,312; Vernon, 20,678; Campbell River, 19,501; Prince Rupert, 15,059; Cranbrook, 15,024; Fort St. John, 12,660.

Vital statistics, *see* p. 273.

CLIMATE. The climate is cool temperate, but mountain influences affect temperatures and rainfall very considerably. Driest months occur in summer. Vancouver. Jan. 36°F (2·2°C), July 64°F (17·8°C). Annual rainfall 58" (1,458 mm).

CONSTITUTION AND GOVERNMENT. British Columbia (then known as New Caledonia) originally formed part of the Hudson's Bay Company's concession. In 1849 Vancouver Island and in 1858 British Columbia were constituted Crown Colonies; in 1866 the two colonies amalgamated. The British North America Act of 1867 provided for eventual admission into Canadian Confederation, and on 20 July 1871 British Columbia became the sixth province of the Dominion.

British Columbia has a unicameral legislature of 69 elected members. Government policy is determined by the Executive Council responsible to the Legislature. The Lieut.-Governor is appointed by the Governor-General of Canada, usually for a term of 5 years, and is the head of the executive government of the province.

Lieut.-Governor: The Hon. David See-Chai Lam.

Flag: A banner of the arms, *i.e.*, blue and white wavy stripes charged with a setting sun in gold, across the top of a Union Flag with a gold coronet in the centre.

The Legislative Assembly is elected for a maximum term of 5 years. Every male or female Canadian citizen 19 years and over, having resided a minimum of 6 months in the province, duly registered, is entitled to vote. Representation of the parties in Dec. 1989: Social Credit Party, 38; New Democratic Party, 26; Independent, 5.

The province is represented in the Federal Parliament by 32 members in the House of Commons, and 6 Senators.

The Executive Council was composed as follows, June 1990:

Premier and President of the Executive Council: Hon. William N. Vander Zalm.

Advanced Education, Training and Technology: Hon. Bruce Strachan. *Agriculture and Fisheries:* Hon. John Savage. *Attorney-General and Solicitor General:* Hon. Russell Fraser. *Crown Lands:* Hon. David Parker. *Education:* Hon. Anthony Brummet. *Energy, Mines and Petroleum Resources:* Hon. Jack Davis. *Environment:* Hon. John Reynolds. *Finance and Corporate Relations:* Hon. Mel Couvelier. *Forests:* Hon. Claude Richmond. *Government Management Services and Minister responsible for Women's Programs:* Hon. Carol Gran. *Health, responsible for Seniors:* Hon. John Jansen. *International Business and Immigration:* Hon. Elwood Veitch. *Labour and Consumer Services and Minister of Social Services and Housing:* Hon. Norman Jacobsen. *Municipal Affairs, Recreation and Culture:* Hon. Lyall Hanson. *Native Affairs:* Hon. Jack Weisgerber. *Parks:* Hon. Ivan Messmer. *Provincial Secretary:* Hon. Howard Dirks. *Regional and Economic Development:* Hon. Stan Hagen. *Tourism:* Hon. Cliff Michael. *Transportation and Highways:* Hon. Rita Johnston.

Agent-General in London: Garde Gardom (British Columbia House, 1 Regent St., London, SW1Y 4NS).

Local Government. Vancouver City was incorporated by statute and operates under the provisions of the Vancouver Charter of 1953 and amendments. This is the only incorporated area in British Columbia not operating under the provisions of the Municipal Act. Under this Act municipalities are divided into the following classes: *(a)* a village with a population between 500 and 2,500, governed by a council consisting of a mayor and 4 aldermen; *(b)* a town with a population between 2,500 and 5,000, governed by a council consisting of a mayor and 4 aldermen; *(c)* a city where the population exceeds 5,000 governed by a council consisting of a mayor and 6 or 8 aldermen depending on population; *(d)* a district where the area exceeds 810 hectares and the average density is less than 5 persons per hectare, governed by a council consisting of a mayor and 6 or 8 aldermen depending on population; *(e)* an Indian government district.

There are 3 other forms of local government: There are 8 Development Regions each represented in Cabinet by a Minister of State; the regional district covering a number of areas both incorporated and unincorporated, governed by a board of directors; and the improvement district governed by a board of 3 trustees.

Revenue for municipal services is derived mainly from real-property taxation, although additional revenue is derived from licence fees, business taxes, fines, public utility projects and grants-in-aid from the provincial government.

ECONOMY

Budget. Current provincial revenue and expenditure, including all capital expenditures, in Canadian $1m. for fiscal years ending 31 March:

	1987–88	*1988–89*	*1989–90* [1]	*1990–91* [2]
Revenue	10,247·1	11,605·9	13,502·0	15,260·0
Expenditure	11,038·0	11,935·4	13,362·0	15,260·0

[1] Forecast [2] Estimate

The main sources of current revenue are the income taxes, contributions from the federal government, and privileges, licences and natural resources taxes and royalties.

The main items of expenditure in 1990–91 (estimate) are as follows: Health, $4,891·4m.; education, $4,137·1m.; social services, $1,608·9m.; transportation, $1,216·9m.; natural resources and economic development, $1,138·5m.; debt servicing, $482·2m.

Banking. On 31 Oct. 1990, Canadian chartered banks maintained 819 branches and had total assets of $42·400m. in British Columbia; credit unions at 114 locations had total assets of $9·378m. Several foreign banks have Canadian head offices in Vancouver and several others have branches.

ENERGY AND NATURAL RESOURCES

Electricity. Generation in 1989 totalled 57,655m. kwh. of which a net 2,082m. kwh. were exported. Consumption within the province was 55,572m. kwh.

Minerals. Copper, coal, natural gas, crude oil, gold and silver are the most important minerals produced. The 1989 total of mineral production was estimated at $4,163m. Total value of mineral fuels produced in 1989 was estimated at: Coal, $1,040m.; oil and gas, $944m.

Agriculture. Only 2·4m. ha or 4% of the total land area is arable or potentially arable. Farm cash receipts, in 1989, were $1,153m. of which livestock and products $703m., crops, $374m.

Forestry. About 46% of British Columbia's land is productive forest land, with 43·3m. hectares bearing commercial forest. Over 94% of the forest area is owned or administered by the provincial government. The total cut from forests in 1989 was 87·4m. cu. metres. Output of forest-based products, 1989: Lumber, 35,952,000 cu. metres; plywood, 1,829,000 cu. metres; pulp, 6·99m. tonnes; paper and paperboard, 1,173,000 tonnes; newsprint, 1,679,000 tonnes.

Fisheries. In 1989, the total value of the catch was $409m.

INDUSTRY AND TRADE

Industry. The selling value of factory shipments from all manufacturing industries reached an estimated $25,877m. in 1989.

Labour. The labour force averaged 1,578,000 persons in 1989 with 1,435,000 employed, of which 511,000 were in service industries, 271,000 in trade, 175,000 in manufacturing, 120,000 in transportation, communication and other utilities, 90,000 in finance, insurance and real estate, 86,000 in public administration, 99,000 in construction, 30,000 in agriculture, 28,000 in forestry, 18,000 in mining and 8,000 in fishing and trapping.

Commerce. Exports of British Columbia origin during 1989 totalled $17,762m. in value, while imports amounted to $13,888m. USA is the largest market for products exported through British Columbia customs ports ($7,442·8m. in 1988) followed by Japan ($5,094m.).

The leading exports were: Lumber, $4,048m.; pulp, $3,719m.; coal, $1,513m.; paper and newsprint, $969m.

Tourism. In 1989, 14·7m. tourists spent $3,974m.

COMMUNICATIONS

Roads. At 31 March 1989 there were 42,105·1 km of provincial roads and rights of way in the province, of which 21,905 km were paved. In 1989, 1,393,530 passenger cars and 490,941 commercial vehicles were licensed.

Railways. The province is served by two transcontinental railways, the Canadian

Pacific Railway and the Canadian National Railway. Passenger service is provided by VIA Rail, a Crown Corporation. British Columbia is also served by the publicly owned British Columbia Railway, the Railway Freight Service of the B.C. Hydro and Power Authority, the Northern Alberta Railways Company and the Burlington Northern Inc. The combined route-mileage of mainline track operated by the CPR, CNR and BCR totals 7,500 km. The system also includes CPR and CNR wagon ferry connections to Vancouver Island, between Prince Rupert and Alaska, and interchanges with American railways at southern border points. A metro line was opened in Vancouver in 1986.

Aviation. International airports are located at Vancouver and Victoria. Daily interprovincial and intraprovincial flights serve all main population centres. Small public and private airstrips are located throughout the province. Total passenger arrivals and departures on scheduled services (1989) 9,651,000.

Shipping. The major ports are Vancouver, New Westminster, Victoria, Nanaimo and Prince Rupert. The volume of domestic cargo handled through the port of Vancouver during 1988 was 46·7m. tonnes; international cargo, 64·6m. tonnes.

The British Columbia Ferries connect Vancouver Island with the mainland and also provide service to other coastal points; in 1989, 19·2m. passengers and 7·5m. vehicles were carried. Service by other ferry systems is also provided between Vancouver Island and the USA. The Alaska State Ferries connect Prince Rupert with centres in Alaska.

Telecommunications. The British Columbia Telephone Company had (1989) approximately 1·8m. telephones in service. In March 1989 there were 91 radio and 10 television stations originating in British Columbia. In addition there were 259 rebroadcasting stations in the province.

JUSTICE, EDUCATION AND WELFARE

Justice. The judicial system is composed of the Court of Appeal, the Supreme Court, County Courts, and various Provincial Courts, including Magistrates' Courts and Small Claims Courts. The federal courts include the Supreme Court of Canada and the Federal Court of Canada.

Education. Education, free up to Grade XII levels, is financed jointly from municipal and provincial government revenues. Attendance is compulsory from the age of 7 to 15. There were 512,926 pupils enrolled in 1,589 public schools from kindergarten to Grade XII in Sept. 1989.

The universities had a full-time enrolment of approximately 38,941 for 1989–90. They include University of British Columbia, Vancouver; University of Victoria, Victoria and Simon Fraser University, Burnaby. The regional colleges are Camosun College, Victoria; Capilano College, North Vancouver; Cariboo College, Kamloops; College of New Caledonia, Prince George; Douglas College, New Westminster; East Kootenay Community College, Cranbrook; Fraser Valley College, Chilliwack/Abbotsford; Kwantlen College, Surrey; Malaspina College, Nanaimo; North Island College, Comox; Northern Lights College, Dawson Creek/Fort St John; Northwest Community College, Terrace/Prince Rupert; Okanagan College, Kelowna with branches at Salmon Arm and Vernon; Selkirk College, Castlegar; Vancouver Community College, Vancouver.

There are also the British Columbia Institute of Technology, Burnaby; Emily Carr College of Art and Design, Vancouver; Justice Institute of British Columbia, Vancouver; Open Learning Institute, Richmond; Pacific Marine Training Institute, North Vancouver; Pacific Vocational Institute, Burnaby/Maple Ridge/ Richmond. A televised distance education and special programmes through KNOW, the Knowledge Network of the West is provided.

Health. The Government operates a hospital insurance scheme giving universal coverage after a qualifying period of 3 months' residence in the province. The province has come under a national medicare scheme which is partially subsidized by the provincial government and partially by the federal government.

Further Reading

Statistical Information: Planning and Statistics Division (Ministry of Finance and Corporate Relations, Hon. Mel Couvelier—Minister, Parliament Buildings, Victoria, B.C., V8V 1X4), collects, compiles and distributes information relative to the Province.

Publications include *Manufacturers' Directory; External Trade Report* (annual); *British Columbia Economic Accounts* (annual); *British Columbia Population Forecast* (annual).

Ministry of Finance, *British Columbia Economic and Statistical Review.* Victoria, B.C. (annual)
Morley, J. T., *The Reins of Power: Governing British Columbia.* Vancouver, 1983
Ormsby, M., *British Columbia: A History.* Vancouver, 1958

MANITOBA

HISTORY. The Hudson's Bay Company formed a colony on the Red River in 1812, which was part of territory annexed to Canada in 1870. The Metis colonists (part-Indian, mostly French-speaking, Catholic) objected to the arrangements for the purchase of the Company territory by Canada and the province of Manitoba was created to accommodate them. It was extended northwards and westwards in 1881 and to Hudson Bay in 1912.

AREA AND POPULATION. The area of the province is 250,946 sq. miles (649,047 sq. km), of which 211,721 sq. miles are land and 39,225 sq. miles water. From north to south it is 1,225 km and at the widest point it is 793 km.

The population (census, 1986) was 1,071,232. Estimate (1988), 1,084,800. Population of Winnipeg, the capital (June 1986), 625,304; other principal cities (census, 1986): Brandon, 38,708; Thompson, 14,701; Portage la Prairie, 13,198; Selkirk, 10,013; Flin Flon (Manitoba portion), 7,243.

Vital statistics, *see* p. 273.

CLIMATE. The climate is cold continental, with very severe winters but pleasantly warm summers. Rainfall amounts are greatest in the months May to Sept. Winnipeg. Jan. –3°F (–19·3°C), July 67°F (19·6°C). Annual rainfall 21" (539 mm).

CONSTITUTION AND GOVERNMENT. Manitoba was known as the Red River Settlement before its entry into the Dominion in 1870. The provincial government is administered by a *Lieut.-Governor* assisted by an *Executive Council* (Cabinet) which is appointed from and responsible to a *Legislative Assembly* of 57 members elected for 5 years. Women were enfranchised in 1916. The Electoral Division Act, 1955, created 57 single-member constituencies and abolished the transferable vote. There are 28 rural electoral divisions, and 29 urban electoral divisions. The province is represented by 6 members in the Senate and 14 in the House of Commons of Canada.

Lieut.-Governor: Dr George Johnson (sworn in 12 Dec. 1986).
Flag: The British Red Ensign with the shield of the province in the fly.

Elections to the Legislative Assembly were held on 11 Sept. 1990: the Progressive Conservative Party gained 30 seats (with 42% of votes cast), the New Democratic Party, 20 (29%) and the Liberal Party, 7 (28%).

The members of the Progressive Conservative Ministry (sworn in 9 Sept. 1990) were:

President of the Executive Council, Minister of Federal-Provincial Relations, Chairman of the Treasury Board: Gary Albert Filmon.

Deputy-President, Minister of Northern Affairs, Minister responsible for Native Affairs, the Communities Economic Development Fund Act, Channel Area Loggers Ltd, Moose Lake Loggers Ltd, A. E. MacKenzie Company Ltd, Seniors: James Erwin

Downey. *Health:* Donald Warder Orchard. *Highways and Transportation, Government Services:* Albert Driedger. *Finance, Minister responsible for the Crown Corporations Accountability Act, and the Manitoba Data Services Act:* Clayton Sidney Manness. *Family Services:* Harold Gilleshammer. *Natural Resources:* Harry John Enns. *Deputy Premier, Minister responsible for the Manitoba Public Insurance Corporation Act, and Jobs Fund, Environment:* James Glen Cummings. *Justice and Attorney-General, Minister responsible for Corrections, Constitutional Affairs, Liquor Control Act, Keeper of the Great Seal:* James Collus McCrae. *Minister responsible for the Workers Compensation Act, Co-operative, Consumer and Corporate Affairs:* Edward James Connery. *Industry, Trade and Tourism, Minister responsible for the Development Corporation Act, Sport, Minister responsible for Fitness and Amateur Sport, Boxing and Wrestling Commission Act, Manitoba Forestry Resources Ltd:* James Arthur Ernst. *Agriculture, Minister responsible for the Manitoba Telephone Act:* Glen Marshall Findlay. *Education and Training:* Leonard Derkach. *Urban Affairs, Housing:* Gerald Ducharme. *Culture, Heritage and Recreation, Multicultural Affairs and the Status of Women, Minister responsible for the Manitoba Lotteries Foundation Act:* Bonnie Elizabeth Mitchelson. *Rural Development:* John (Jack) Penner. *Energy and Mines, Minister responsible for the Manitoba Hydro Act:* Harold Johan Neufeld. *Labour, Minister responsible for the Status of Women, the Civil Service Superannuation Act, the Civil Service Special Supplementary Severance Benefit Act, the Public Servants Insurance Act:* Darren Praznik.

Local Government. Rural Manitoba is organized into rural municipalities which vary widely in size. Some have only 4 townships (a township is 6 sq. miles), while the largest has 22 townships. The province has 105 rural municipalities, as well as 35 incorporated towns, 39 incorporated villages and 5 incorporated cities.

On 1 Jan. 1972, the cities and towns comprising the metropolitan area of Winnipeg were amalgamated to form the City of Winnipeg. A mayor and council are elected to a central government, but councillors also sit on 'community committees' which represent the areas or wards they serve. These committees are advised by non-elected residents of the area on provision of municipal services within the community committee jurisdiction. Taxing powers and overall budgeting rest with the central council. The mayor is elected at the same time as the councillors in a city-wide vote. Revisions to the City of Winnipeg Act came into effect with the municipal elections held in Oct. 1977.

Since Jan. 1945, 17 Local Government Districts have been formed in the less densely populated areas of the province. They are administered by a provincially appointed person, who acts on the advice of locally elected councils.

In the extreme north, many communities have locally elected councils, while others are administered directly by the Department of Northern Affairs. This department provides most of the funding in all these northern settlements.

FINANCE. Provincial revenue and expenditure (current account) for fiscal years ending 31 March (in Canadian $):

	1986–87	*1987–88*	*1988–89*	*1989–90* [1]	*1990–91* [2]
Revenue	3,385,800,000	3,772,600,000	4,678,670,300	4,658,000,000	4,800,000,000
Expenditure	3,945,600,000	4,187,900,000	4,766,060,500	4,802,000,000	5,100,000,000

[1] Preliminary unaudited. [2] Budgeted.

ENERGY AND NATURAL RESOURCES

Electricity. The total generating capacity of Manitoba's power stations is 4·1m. kw. The Manitoba Hydro system, owned by the province, provides most of this power, while the city-owned Winnipeg Hydro provides about 190,000 kw. The systems have about 452,000 customers and consumption was 14·3m. kwh. in 1988.

Oil. Crude oil production in 1986 was valued at $195m. for the 825,000 cu. metres produced.

Minerals. Total value of minerals in 1988 was about $1,679m. Principal minerals mined are nickel, zinc, copper, and small quantities of gold and silver. Manitoba has the world's largest deposits of caesium ore.

Agriculture. Rich farmland is the main primary resource, although the area of Manitoba in farms is only about 14% of the total land area. In 1988 the total value of agricultural production in Manitoba was $1,800m., with $954m. from crops, $810m. from livestock and from the sale of other products including furs, hides and honey.

Forestry. About 51% of the land area is wooded, of which 334,440 sq. km is productive forest land. Total sales of wood-using industries (1988, estimate) $500m.

Fur Trade. Value of fur production to the trapper was $5m. in 1986.

Fisheries. From 57,000 sq. km of rivers and lakes fisheries production was about $28·3m. in 1987–88. Whitefish, sauger, pickerel and pike are the principal varieties of fish caught.

INDUSTRY AND TRADE

Industry. Manufacturing, the largest industry in the province, encompasses almost every major industrial activity in Canada. Estimated shipments in 1988 totalled $6,239m. Manufacturing employed about 63,000 persons. Due to the agricultural base of the province, the food and beverage group of industries is by far the largest, valued at $1,736m. in 1988. The next largest segments are transportation equipment, $608m., printing and publishing, $454m. and fabricated metals, $390m.

Trade. Products grown and manufactured in Manitoba find ready markets in other parts of Canada, in the USA, particularly the upper midwest region, and in other countries. Export shipments to foreign countries from Manitoba in 1988 were valued at $2,867m. Of total exports, $912·2m. were raw materials and $1,465·7m. processed and manufactured products.

Tourism. In 1986, non-Manitoban tourists numbered 2·4m. All tourists including Manitobans contributed $657m. to the economy.

COMMUNICATIONS

Roads. Highways and provincial roads totalled 19,721 km in 1989.

Railways. At 30 June 1988 the province had 6,600 km of track, not including industrial track, yards and sidings.

Aviation. A total of 108 licensed commercial air carriers operate from bases in Manitoba, as well as 5 regularly scheduled major national and international airlines.

Telecommunications. All of the Manitoba Telephone System's 535,000 (1988) telephones are dialoperated. There are some privately-owned fixtures and extension phones; all service is operated by MTS.

EDUCATION. Education is controlled through locally elected school divisions. There are about 199,000 children enrolled in the province's elementary and secondary schools. Manitoba has 3 universities with an enrolment of about 43,500 during the 1987–88 year; the University of Manitoba, founded in 1877, in Winnipeg, the University of Winnipeg, and Brandon University. Expenditure (estimate) on education in the 1987–88 fiscal year was $747m.

Three community colleges, in Brandon, The Pas and Winnipeg, offer 2-year diploma courses in a number of fields, as well as specialized training in many trades. They also give a large number and variety of shorter courses, both at their campuses and in many communities throughout the province.

Further Reading

General Information: Inquiries may be addressed to the Information Services Branch, Room 29, Legislative Building, Winnipeg, R3C OV8.

The Department of Agriculture publishes: *Year Book of Manitoba Agriculture*
Information Services Branch publishes: *Manitoba Facts*
Manitoba Statistical Review. Manitoba Bureau of Statistics, Quarterly
Twelfth Census of Canada: Manitoba. Statistics Canada, 1981
Jackson, J. A., *The Centennial History of Manitoba*. Toronto, 1970
Morton, W. L., *Manitoba: A History*. Univ. of Toronto Press, 1967

NEW BRUNSWICK

HISTORY. Touched by Jacques Cartier in 1534, New Brunswick was first explored by Samuel de Champlain in 1604. It was ceded by the French in the Treaty of Utrecht in 1713 and became a permanent British possession in 1763. It was separated from Nova Scotia and became a province in June 1784, as a result of the great influx of United Empire Loyalists. Responsible government came into being in 1848, and consisted of an executive council, a legislative council (later abolished) and a House of Assembly.

AREA AND POPULATION. The area of the province is 28,354 sq. miles (73,440 sq. km), of which 27,633 sq. miles (71,569 sq. km) are land area. The population (census 1986) was 710,422. Estimate (1990) 723,900. Of the individuals identifying a single ethnic origin (at the 1986 census), 46·9% were British and 33·3% French. Other significant ethnic groups were German, Dutch and Scandinavian. Among those who provided a multiple response 9·9% were of British and French descent and 4·3% British and other. In 1986 there were 9,375 Native People or Native People and other. Census 1986 population of urban centres: Saint John, 76,381; Moncton, 55,468; Fredericton (capital), 44,352; Bathurst, 14,683; Edmundston, 11,497; Campbellton, 9,073.

Vital statistics, *see* p. 273.

CLIMATE. A cool temperate climate, with rain at all seasons but temperatures modified by the influence of the Gulf Stream. Saint John. Jan. 14°F (–10°C), July 63°F (17·2°C). Annual rainfall 51" (1,278 mm).

CONSTITUTION AND GOVERNMENT. The government is vested in a Lieut.-Governor and a Legislative Assembly of 58 members each of whom is individually elected to represent the voters in one constituency or riding. A simultaneous translation system is used in the Assembly. Any Canadian subject of full age and 6 months' residence is entitled to vote. As a result of the provincial election held on 13 Oct. 1987 and subsequent by-elections, the Assembly is composed of 58 Liberal Party members. The province has 10 members in the Canadian Senate and 10 members in the federal House of Commons.

Lieut.-Governor: Hon. Gilbert Finn (appointed Aug. 1987).

Flag: A banner of the Arms, *i.e.*, yellow charged with a black heraldic ship on wavy lines of blue and white; across the top a red band with a gold lion.

The members of the Liberal government are as follows (Sept. 1990):

Premier and Minister responsible for the Advisory Council on the Status of Women, and for Regional Development: Hon. Francis J. McKenna.

President of the Executive Council and Intergovernmental Affairs: Hon. Aldéa Landry.

Attorney General and Justice: Hon. James Lockyer. *Finance and responsibility for the New Brunswick Liquor Corporation:* Hon. Allan Maher. *Chairman of Board of Management:* Hon. Gérald Clavette. *Supply and Services:* Hon. Bruce Smith. *Transportation:* Hon. Sheldon Lee. *Natural Resources and Energy:* Hon. Morris Green. *Agriculture:* Hon. Alan Graham. *Health and Community Services:* Hon. Ray Frenette. *Income Assistance:* Hon. Laureen Jarrett. *Labour and responsibility for Multiculturalism:* Hon. Michael McKee. *Education:* Hon. Shirley Dysart. *Advanced Education and Training:* Hon. Russell King, MD. *Municipal Affairs:* Hon. Hubert Seamans. *Environment:* Hon. Vaughn Blaney. *Commerce and Technology:* Hon. A. W. Lacey. *Fisheries and Aquaculture:* Hon. Denis Losier. *Tourism, Recreation and Heritage:* Hon. Roland Beaulieu. *Housing:* Hon. Peter Trites. *Chairman of the New Brunswick Electric Power Commission:* Hon. Rayburn Doucett. *Solicitor General:* Hon. Conrad Landry. *Mines:* Hon. Edmond Blanchard. *Childhood Services:* Hon. Jane Barry.

Local Government. Under the reforms introduced in 1967 the province has assumed complete administrative and financial responsibility for education, health, welfare and administration of justice. Local government is now restricted to provision of services of a strictly local nature. Under the new municipal structure, units include existing and new cities, towns and villages. Counties have disappeared as municipal units. Areas with limited populations have become local service districts. The former local improvement districts have become towns, villages or local service districts depending on their size.

FINANCE. The ordinary budget (in Canadian $) is shown as follows (financial years ended 31 March):

	1987	*1988*	*1989*	*1990*
Gross revenue	2,770,035,356	3,024,858,732	3,322,730,180	3590·7
Gross expenditure	2,890,963,016	3,131,700,768	3,253,858,361	3471·1

Funded debt and capital loans outstanding (exclusive of Treasury Bills) as of 31 March 1990 was $4,331m. Sinking funds held by the province at 31 March 1990, $1,393m. The ordinary budget excludes capital spending.

ENERGY AND NATURAL RESOURCES

Electricity. Hydro-electric, thermal and nuclear generating stations of the New Brunswick Electric Power Commission had an installed capacity of 3,221,976 kw. at 31 March 1990, consisting of 14 generating stations. The Mactaquac hydro-electric development near Fredericton, has a name plate capacity of 653,400 kw. The largest thermal generating station, Coleson Cove, near Saint John, has over 1m. kw. of installed capacity. Atlantic Canada's first nuclear generating station, a 630,000 kw. plant on a promontory in the Bay of Fundy, near Saint John, went into operation in 1983. New Brunswick is electrically inter-connected with utilities in neighbouring provinces of Quebec, Nova Scotia and Prince Edward Island, as well as the New England States of the USA. Electricity exports accounted for over 30% of revenue in 1989–90; imports, mainly from the large Hydro Quebec system, supplied only 3% of in-province energy requirements. This was due mainly to low water reservoirs and higher loads in Quebec.

Minerals. In 1989, a total of 20 different metals, minerals and commodities were produced. These included lead, zinc, copper, cadmium, bismuth, gold, silver, antimony, potash, salt, limestone, oil, gas, coal, oil shales, sand, gravel, clay, peat and marl. The total value of minerals produced in 1989 reached a record high of $91·0m. The largest contributors to mineral production are zinc, silver and lead accounting for over 65% of total value in 1989. These 3 minerals recorded significant increases in price in late 1986 which continued into 1988. In Canada in 1989, New Brunswick ranked first in the production of antimony and bismuth, second in lead, third in zinc, fourth in silver and fifth in the production of copper. Antimony is mined at Lake George and production resumed at the Durham Resources mine near Fredericton in 1985. Peat, rapidly becoming a major industry, is produced from 18 operations in the north. Two potash mines are in operation in the Sussex area, including the Denison-Potacan mine where production commenced in 1985. Oil and natural gas continue to be produced in the Stoney Creek and Hillsborough areas. Gordex Minerals produced its first gold in 1986 using the heap leach process. Coal is strip-mined at Grand Lake, producing some 530,000 tonnes annually. Not all of the province's minerals have been explored sufficiently and research continues. Provincial government programmes are being supplemented by a 5-year, $22m. Mineral Development Agreement between the Canada Department of Energy, Mines and Resources and the province. Federal and Provincial agencies are co-operating on field, laboratory and other projects.

Agriculture. The total area under crops is estimated at 129,475 ha. Farms numbered 3,554 and averaged 115 ha each (census 1986). Potatoes account for 28% of total farm cash income. Mixed farming is common throughout the province. Dairy farming is centred around the larger urban areas, and is located mainly along the Saint John River Valley and in the south-eastern sections of the province. Income from dairy operations provides about 22% of farm cash income. New Brunswick is self-sufficient in fluid milk and supplies a processing industry. For particulars of agricultural production and livestock, *see under* CANADA, pp. 000–00. Farm cash receipts in 1989 were $272m.

Forestry. New Brunswick contains some 62,000 sq. km of productive forest lands. The gross value of forest production was over $2,396·1m. in 1989, and it accounts for almost 40% of all goods produced in the province. The pulp and paper and allied industry group is the largest component of the industry contributing about 85% of the value of output. Timber-using plants employ about 16,000 people for all aspects of the forest industry, including harvesting, processing and transportation. Practically all forest products are exported from the province's numerous ports and harbours near which many of the mills are located or sent by road or rail to the USA.

Fisheries. Commercial fishing is one of the most important primary industries of the province, employing 7,903. Nearly 50 commercial species of fish and shellfish are landed, including scallop, shrimp, crab, herring and cod. Landings in 1989 (150,846 tonnes) amounted to $87·7m. In 1990 there were 167 fish processing plants employing nearly 8,000 people in peak periods. In 1989 molluscs and crustaceans ranked first with a value of $59·9m., 68% of the total landed value; pelagic fish second, 20%, and groundfish third, 11%. Exports (1989) $231m., mainly to the USA and Japan.

INDUSTRY. In 1989 there were 1,625 manufacturing and processing establishments, employing about 46,800 persons. New Brunswick's location, with deepwater harbours open throughout the year and container facilities at Saint John, makes it ideal for exporting. Industries include food and beverages, paper and allied industries, timber products. About 20% of the industrial labour force work in Saint John.

TOURISM. Tourism is one of the leading contributors to the economy. In 1989, 2·5m. non-resident and over 2·55m. resident travellers spent approximately $520m.

COMMUNICATIONS

Roads. There are about 1,541·9 km of arterial highways and 2,381·7 km of collector roads, all of which are hard-surfaced. 12,279·9 km of local roads provide access to most areas in the province. The main highway system, including 596·4 km of the Trans-Canada Highway, links the province with the principal roads in Quebec, Nova Scotia, and Prince Edward Island, as well as the Interstate Highway System in the eastern seaboard states of the USA. Passenger vehicles, 31 March 1989, numbered 300,836; commercial vehicles, 129,809; motor cycles, 11,290.

Railways. New Brunswick is served by main lines of both Canadian Pacific and Canadian National railways.

Telecommunications. In 1989 the New Brunswick Telephone Co. Ltd had 523,406 telephones in service. The province is served by 21 radio stations. Sixteen are privately owned and 3 owned by the Canadian Broadcasting Corporation and 2 are university stations. Three stations broadcast in the French language, 3 are bilingual and the CBC International Service broadcasts in several languages from its station at Sackville. The province is served by 4 television stations, 1 of which broadcasts in French.

Newspapers. New Brunswick had (1989) 4 daily newspapers, 1 in French, and 24 weekly newspapers, 7 in French or bilingual.

EDUCATION. Public education is free and non-sectarian. There are 4 universities. The University of New Brunswick at Fredericton (founded 13 Dec. 1785 by the Loyalists, elevated to university status in 1823, reorganized as the University of New Brunswick in 1859) had 6,977 full-time students at the Fredericton campus and 1,232 full-time students at the Saint John campus (1989–90); Mount Allison University at Sackville had 1,869 full-time students; the Université de Moncton at Moncton, 3,608 full-time students, with 308 and 557 full-time students respectively at its satellite campuses at Shippegan and Edmundston; St Thomas University at Fredericton, 1,358 full-time students. During the period 1 July 1988 to 30 June 1989, there were 18,142 students enrolled full-time at 10 Community College campuses and at various campus training centres.

There were, in Sept. 1989, 134,592 students and 7,920 full-time (equivalent) teachers in the province's 423 schools. There are 42 school boards.

Further Reading

Industrial Information: Dept. of Commerce and Technology, Fredericton. *Economic Information:* Dept. of Finance, New Brunswick Statistics Agency, Fredericton. *General Information:* Communications New Brunswick, Fredericton.

Directory of Products and Manufacturers. Department of Commerce and Development; Annual

Thompson, C., *New Brunswick Inside Out.* Ottawa, 1977

Trueman, S., *The Fascinating World of New Brunswick.* Fredericton, 1973

NEWFOUNDLAND AND LABRADOR

HISTORY. Archaeological finds at L'Anse-au-Meadow in northern Newfoundland show that the Vikings had established a colony there at about A.D. 1000. This site is the only known Viking colony in North America. Newfoundland was discovered by John Cabot 24 June 1497, and was soon frequented in the summer months by the Portuguese, Spanish and French for its fisheries. It was formally occupied in Aug. 1583 by Sir Humphrey Gilbert on behalf of the English Crown, but various attempts to colonize the island remained unsuccessful. Although British sovereignty was recognized in 1713 by the Treaty of Utrecht, disputes over fishing rights with the French were not finally settled till 1904. By the Anglo-French Convention of 1904, France renounced her exclusive fishing rights along part of the coast, granted under the Treaty of Utrecht, but retained sovereignty of the offshore islands of St Pierre and Miquelon.

AREA AND POPULATION. Area, 143,501 sq. miles (371,690 sq. km) of which freshwater, 13,139 sq. miles (34,030 sq. km). In March 1927 the Privy Council decided the boundary between Canada and Newfoundland in Labrador. This area, now part of the Province of Newfoundland and Labrador, is 102,699 sq. miles. The coastline is extremely irregular. Bays, fiords and inlets are numerous and there are many good harbours with deep water close to shore. The coast is rugged with bold rocky cliffs from 200 to 400 ft high; in the Bay of Islands some of the islands rise 500 ft, with the adjacent shore 1,000 ft above tide level. The interior is a plateau of moderate elevation and the chief relief features trend north-east and south-west. Long Range, the most notable of these, begins at Cape Ray and extends north-east for 200 miles, the highest peak reaching 2,673 ft. Approximately one-third of the area is covered by water. Grand Lake, the largest body of water, has an area of about 200 sq. miles. The principal rivers flow towards the north-east. On the borders of the lakes and water-courses good land is generally found, particularly in the valleys of the Terra Nova River, the Gander River, the Exploits River and the Humber River, which are also heavily timbered.

Census population, 1986, was 568,349.

The capital of Newfoundland is the City of St John's (161,901, metropolitan area). The other cities are Corner Brook (22,719), Mt Pearl (20,293); important towns are Labrador City (8,664), Gander (10,207), Conception Bay South (15,531), Stephenville (7,994), Grand Falls (9,121), Happy Valley–Goose Bay (7,248), Marystown (6,660), Channel-Port aux Basques (5,901), Windsor (5,545), Carbonear (5,337), Bonavista (4,605), Wabana (4,057), Wabush (2,637).

Vital statistics, *see* p. 273.

CLIMATE. The cool temperate climate is marked by heavy precipitation, distributed evenly over the year, a cool summer and frequent fogs in spring. St. John's. Jan. 23°F (–5°C), July 59°F (15°C). Annual rainfall 54" (1,367 mm).

CONSTITUTION AND GOVERNMENT. Until 1832 Newfoundland was ruled by the Governor under instructions of the Colonial Office. In that year a Legislature was brought into existence, but the Governor and his Executive Council were not responsible to it. Under the constitution of 1855, which lasted until its suspension in 1934, the government was administered by the Governor appointed by the Crown with an Executive Council responsible to the House of Assembly of 27 elected members and a Legislative Council of 24 members nominated for life by the Governor in Council. Women were enfranchised in 1925. At the Imperial Conference of 1917 Newfoundland was constituted as a Dominion.

In 1933 the financial situation had become so critical that the Government of Newfoundland asked the Government of the UK to appoint a Royal Commission to investigate conditions. On the strength of their recommendations, the parliamentary form of government was suspended and Government by Commission was inaugurated on 16 Feb. 1934.

A National Convention, elected in 1946, made, in 1948, recommendations to H.M. Government in Great Britain as to the possible forms of future government to be submitted to the people at a national referendum. Two referenda were held. In the first referendum (June 1948) the three forms of government submitted to the people were: Commission of government for 5 years, confederation with Canada and responsible government as it existed in 1933. No one form of government received a clear majority of the votes polled, and commission of government, receiving the fewest votes, was eliminated. In the second referendum (July 1948) confederation with Canada received 78,408 and responsible government 71,464 votes.

In the Canadian Senate on 18 Feb. 1949 Royal assent was given to the terms of union of Newfoundland and Labrador with Canada, and on 23 March 1949, in the House of Lords, London, Royal assent was given to an amendment to the British North America Act made necessary by the inclusion of Newfoundland and Labrador as the tenth Province of Canada.

Under the terms of union of Newfoundland and Labrador with Canada, which was signed at Ottawa on 11 Dec. 1948, the constitution of the Legislature of Newfoundland and Labrador as it existed immediately prior to 16 Feb. 1934 shall, subject to the terms of the British North America Acts, 1867 to 1946, continue as the constitution of the Legislature of the Province of Newfoundland and Labrador until altered under the authority of the said Acts.

The franchise was in 1965 extended to all male and female residents who have attained the age of 19 years and are otherwise qualified as electors.

The House of Assembly (Amendment) Act, 1979, established 52 electoral districts and 52 members of the Legislature.

In April 1989 there were 32 Liberals and 20 Progressive-Conservatives.

The province is represented by 6 members in the Senate and by 7 members in the House of Commons of Canada.

Lieut.-Governor: Hon. James W. McGrath (assumed office 5 Sept. 1986).

Flag: White, in the hoist 4 solid blue triangles; in the fly 2 red triangles voided white, and between them a yellow tongue bordered in red.

The Liberal Executive Council was, in May 1989, composed as follows:

Premier: Clyde Kirby Wells.

President of Executive Council and President of Treasury Board: Richard Winston Baker. *Fisheries:* Walter Carmichael Carter. *Employment and Labour Relations:* Patricia Anne Cowan. *Health:* Christopher Robert Decker. *Justice:* Paul David Dicks. *Social Services:* Reuben John Efford. *Forestry and Agriculture:* Graham Ralph Flight. *Development:* Charles Joseph Furey. *Mines and Energy:* Dr Rex Vincent Gibbons. *Works, Services and Transportation:* David Samuel Gilbert. *Municipal and Provincial Affairs:* Eric Augustus Gullage. *Environment and Lands:* Otto Paul James Kelland. *Finance:* Dr Hubert William Kitchen. *Education:* Dr Philip John Warren. *Speaker of the House of Assembly:* Thomas Lush.

Agent-General in London: H. Watson Jamer (60 Trafalgar Sq., WC2).

FINANCE. Budget[1] in Canadian $1,000 for fiscal years ended 31 March:

	1985–86	*1986–87*	*1987–88*	*1988–89*	*1989–90* [2]	*1990–91* [3]
Gross revenue	2,072,581	2,233,339	2,424,887	2,600,429	2,827,500	2,962,081
Gross expenditure	2,117,012	2,260,845	2,456,146	2,601,221	2,789,656	2,951,838

Capital account:

	1987–88	*1988–89*	*1989–90* [2]	*1990–91* [3]
Gross revenue	120,670,000	63,968,000	93,057,000	108,767,000
Gross expenditure	287,235,000	289,101,000	352,634,000	367,519,000

[1] Current amount only. [2] Revised estimates. [3] Estimates.

Public debenture debt as at 31 March 1990 (preliminary) was $4,424·5m.; sinking fund, $1,453·5m.

ENERGY AND NATURAL RESOURCES

Electricity. The electrical energy requirements of the province are met mainly by hydro-electric power, with petroleum fuels being utilized to provide the balance. The total amount of energy generated in the province in 1988 was 41,274,782 mwh., of which 96% was derived from hydro-electric facilities. The greater part of the energy produced in 1988 came from Churchill Falls, of which 30,727,113 mwh. was sold to Hydro-Quebec under the terms of a long-term contract. Energy consumed in the province during 1988 totalled 10,520,669 mwh., with 8,997,007 mwh., or 86%, coming from hydro-electric facilities.

At Dec. 1988 total electrical generating capacity in the province was 7,426 mw., with hydro-electric plants accounting for 6,652 mw., or 90%. It is estimated that potential additional hydro-electric generating capacity of up to 4·5m. kw. can be developed at various sites in Labrador.

Oil. Since 1965, 138 wells have been drilled on the Continental Margin of the Province. In 1989 offshore exploration expenditures were $91·5m. (preliminary).

By 31 Dec. 1985 there had been 20 significant hydrocarbon discoveries off Newfoundland and delineation drilling had been initiated or was ongoing at 6: Terra Nova, Ben Nevis, Whiterose, North Ben Nevis and Mara. In 1986 only the Hibernia discovery had commercial capability and the Canada-Newfoundland Offshore Petroleum Board approved Mobil Oil Canada's development plan for the Hibernia Project, with production starting in the early 1990's. In Sept. 1990 the governments of Canada and Newfoundland and a development consortium signed an agreement to start developing the Hibernia discovery from Oct. 1990.

In 1979, a discovery of oil was made on the Hibernia geological structure located 164 nautical miles east of Cape Spear. The discovery well, Hibernia P–15, tested medium gravity, sweet crude from several intervals with a reported total producing capability in excess of 20,000 bbls of oil per day.

Minerals. The mineral resources are vast but only partially documented. Large deposits of iron ore, with an ore reserve of over 5,000m. tons at Labrador City, Wabush City and in the Knob Lake area are supplying approximately half of Canada's production. Other large deposits of iron ore are known to exist in the Julienne Lake area.

There are a variety of other minerals being produced in the province in more limited amounts.

Uranium deposits in the Kaipokak Bay area near Makkovik in Labrador are presently being studied by Brinex. The Central Mineral Belt, which extends from the Smallwood Reservoir to the Atlantic coast near Makkovik, holds uranium, copper, beryllium and molybdenite potential.

In 1986 a gold mine was being developed at Hope Brook on the south coast east of Port aux Basques. Full production from an underground operation using conventional carbon-in-pulp gold processing is planned to start in late 1988.

Production in 1989 (preliminary): Iron ore, 20,119,000 tonnes ($788,239,000); zinc, 29,767,000 kg ($64,357,000); asbestos, 64,000 tonnes ($24,175,000); sand and gravel, 5,096,000m. tonnes ($17,479,000); stone, 590,000 tonnes ($4,707,000); peat, 1,000 tonnes ($44,000).

Agriculture. The estimated value of agricultural products sold, including livestock, 1989, was $55·2m.

Forestry. The forestry economy in the province is mainly dependent on the operation of 3 newsprint mills. In 1989 the gross value of newsprint exported from these 3 mills totalled $490·3m. Lumber mills and saw-log operations produced 49m. flat board metres in 1989–90.

Fisheries. The principal fish landings are cod, flounder, redfish, Queen crabs, lobster, salmon and herring. In 1988 (preliminary) a yearly average of some 10,400 persons were employed by the fish-processing industry and there were 29,023 licensed full-, part-time and casual fishermen engaged in harvesting operations. 241 processing operations were licensed in 1989. The production of fresh and frozen fish products was $620m. (estimate) in 1989.

The total catch in 1989 (preliminary) was 501,923 tonnes valued at $258,173,000, which comprised: Cod, 259,187 tonnes ($118,327,000); flounders and soles, 48,080 ($20,186,000); herring, 20,532 tonnes ($2,656,000); redfish, 14,932 ($4,449,000); lobster, 3,021 ($17,339,000); salmon, 831 ($3,488,000); capelin, 87,935 ($19,604,000); crab, 8,117 ($10,005,000); other, 59,328 ($62,119,000).

INDUSTRY. The total value of manufacturing shipments in 1989 was $1,365m. This consists largely of first-stage processing of primary resource products with two of the largest components being paper and fish products.

TRADE UNIONS. There were 540 unions in 1989 representing 80,429 members of international and national unions and government employee associations.

COMMUNICATIONS

Roads. In 1987 there were 8,238 km, of which 5,671 were paved.

Railways. In 1989 the Quebec North Shore and Labrador Railway operated 576 km of standard-gauge main railway track. The route runs from Sept-Iles, Quebec, to Shefferville, Quebec, with a branch at Ross Bay Junction to Wabush, Labrador.

Aviation. The province is linked to the rest of Canada by regular air services provided by Air Canada, Canadian International Airways, Quebecair and a number of smaller air carriers.

Shipping. At 31 Dec. 1989 there were 1,612 ships registered in Newfoundland. In 1989 Marine Atlantic provided a freight and passenger service all year round to the south of the island and during the ice-free season as far north as Nain. There is a year-round ferry from Port-aux-Basques to North Sydney, Nova Scotia, and seasonal ferries connect Argentia with North Sydney, and Lewisporte with Goosebay, Labrador.

Post. There were 466 post offices in 1989. Telephone access lines numbered 221,198 in 1988 (170,335 private). There were 2,935 public pay phones.

EDUCATION. The number of schools in 1989–90 was 549. The enrolment was 130,724; full-time teachers numbered 7,920. The Memorial University, offering courses in arts, science, engineering, education, nursing and medicine, had 16,621 full- and part-time students in 1989–90. Total expenditure for education by the Government in 1990–91 (estimate) was $758·4m.

Further Reading

Blackburn, R. H. (ed.) *Encyclopaedia of Canada: Newfoundland Supplement.* Toronto, 1949
Horwood, H., *Newfoundland.* Toronto, 1969
Loture, R. de, *Histoire de la grande pêche de Terre-Neuve.* Paris, 1949
Mercer, G. A., *The Province of Newfoundland and Labrador: Geographical Aspects.* Ottawa, 1970
Perlin, A. B., *The Story of Newfoundland, 1497–1959.* St John's, 1959
Tanner, V., *Outlines of Geography. Life and Customs of Newfoundland–Labrador.* 2 vols. Helsinki, 1944, and Toronto, 1947
Taylor, T. G., *Newfoundland: A Study of Settlement.* Toronto, 1946

NOVA SCOTIA

HISTORY. The first permanent settlement was made by the French early in the 17th century, and the province was called Acadia until finally ceded to the British by the Treaty of Utrecht in 1713.

AREA AND POPULATION. The area of the province is 21,425 sq. miles (55,000 sq. km), of which 20,401 sq. miles are land area, 1,024 sq. miles water area. The population (census 1986) was 873,199; (estimate 1990) 891,600.

Population of the principal cities and towns (census 1986): Halifax, 113,577; Dartmouth 65,243; Sydney, 27,754; Glace Bay, 20,467; Truro, 12,124; New Glasgow, 10,022; Amherst, 9,671; New Waterford, 8,326; Sydney Mines, 8,063; Bedford, 8,010; North Sydney, 7,472; Yarmouth, 7,617.

Vital statistics, *see* p. 273.

CLIMATE. A cool temperate climate, with rainfall occurring evenly over the year. The Gulf Stream moderates the temperatures in winter so that ports remain ice-free. Halifax. Jan. 23°F (–5°C), July 64°F (17·8°C). Annual rainfall 56" (1,412 mm).

CONSTITUTION AND GOVERNMENT. Under the British North America Act of 1867 the legislature of Nova Scotia may exclusively make laws in relation to local matters, including direct taxation within the province, education and the administration of justice. The legislature of Nova Scotia consists of a Lieut.-Governor, appointed and paid by the federal government, and holding office for 5 years, and a House of Assembly of 52 members, chosen by popular vote at least every 5 years. The province is represented in the Canadian Senate by 10 members, and in the House of Commons by 11.

The franchise and eligibility to the legislature are granted to every person, male or female, if of age (19 years), a British subject or Canadian citizen, and a resident in the province for 1 year and 2 months before the date of the writ of election in the county or electoral district of which the polling district forms part, and if not by law otherwise disqualified. State of parties in Feb. 1991: 26 Progressive Conservatives, 22 Liberals, 2 New Democrats, 1 independent, 1 vacant.

Lieut.-Governor: Lloyd Crouse.

Flag: A banner of the Arms, *i.e.*, white with a blue diagonal cross, bearing in the centre the royal shield of Scotland.

The members of the Progressive Conservative Ministry were as follows in Feb. 1991:

Premier, President of the Executive Council, Minister of Intergovernmental Affairs, Minister responsible for Sydney Steel Corporation: Hon. Donald Cameron.

Deputy Premier, Deputy President of the Executive Council, Minister of Industry, Trade and Technology, Chairman of the Policy Board, Minister responsible for the Administration of the Nova Scotia Research Foundation Corporation Act, for the Nova Scotia business Capital Corporation Act, for Small Business Development Corporation, for Voluntary Planning Act, for Youth: Hon. Tom McInnis. *Tourism and Culture, Minister responsible for the Heritage Property Act:* Hon. Terry Donahoe. *Transport and Communications:* Hon. Kenneth Streatch. *Education:* Hon. Ronald Giffin, QC. *Finance, Chairman of the Management Board, Minister in charge of the Lottery Act, Minister responsible for the Civil Service Act:* Hon. Greg Kerr. *Attorney-General, Solicitor-General, Provincial Secretary, Minister for the Administration of the Human Rights Act, Minister in charge of the Regulations Act:* Hon. Joel Matheson, QC. *Education, Advanced Education and Job Training:* Hon. Ron Giffin. *Labour:* Hon. Leroy Legere. *Environment, responsible for the Emergency Measures Organization Act:* Hon. John Leefe. *Health and Fitness, Registrar General, Minister in charge of the Administration of the Drug Dependency Act:* Hon. George C. Moody. *Community Services, Minister responsible for reporting on Disabled Persons, responsible for the Administration of the Advisory Council on the Status of Women Act:* Hon. Marie Dechman. *Municipal Affairs:* Hon. Brian Young. *Minister of Fisheries, Minister responsible for Acadian Affairs, responsible for Aboriginal Affairs:* Hon. Guy LeBlanc. *Consumer Affairs, Minister in charge of the Residential Tenancies Act, responsible for the Housing Development Act:* Hon. Don McInnes. *Agriculture and Marketing:* Hon. George Archibald. *Lands and Forests, responsible for Tidal Power Corporation:* Hon. Charles MacNeil. *Minister of Government Services, responsible for the Sport and Recreation Commission, for the Administration of the Liquor Control Act, for the Communications and Information Act:* Hon. Neil LeBlanc.

Agent-General in the UK: Donald M. Smith, (14 Pall Mall, London, SW1Y 5LU).

Representative in the USA: Wendell Sandford, (4 Copley Place, Boston, Mass. 02116).

Local Government. The main divisions of the province for governmental purposes are the 3 cities, the 39 towns and the 24 rural municipalities, each governed by a council and a mayor or warden. The cities have independent charters, and the various towns take their powers from and are limited by The Towns Act, and the various municipalities take their powers from and are limited by The Municipal Act as revised in 1967. The majority of municipalities comprise 1 county, but 6 counties are divided into 2 municipalities each. In no case do the boundaries of any municipality overlap county lines. The 18 counties as such have no administrative functions.

Any city (of which there are 3) or incorporated town (of which there are 39) that lies within the boundaries of a municipality is excluded from any jurisdiction by the municipal council and has its own government.

FINANCE. Revenue is derived from provincial sources, payments from the federal government under the Federal-Provincial Fiscal Arrangements and Established Programs Financing Act. Recoveries consist generally of amounts received under various federal cost-shared programmes. Main sources of provincial revenues include income and sales taxes.

Revenue, expenditure and debt (in Canadian $1m.) for fiscal years ending 31 March:

	1987	*1988*	*1989*	*1990* [1]	*1991* [2]
Budgetary Transactions					
Current Expenditure	3,093·1	3,283·6	3,526·6	3,753·5	4,010·3
Current Revenues and Recoveries	2,903·9	3,164·5	3,465·5	3,706·0	3,982·9
Operating Deficit (Surplus)	189·2	119·1	61·1	47·5	27·4
Sinking Fund Instalments and Serial Retirements	87·3	86·5	90·9	98·5	100·0
Net Capital Expenditures	198·5	219·3	297·9	331·8	285·4
Net Budgetary Transactions	475·0	421·1	449·9	477·9	412·8
Non-Budgetary Transactions					
Capital Expenditures	0·9	2·5	2·7	3·0	1·0
Net Increase (Decrease) in Advances and Investments	28·1	(18·9)	7·8	51·4	29·0
Net Other Transactions	7·2	7·2	4·5	7·7	1·6
Non-Budgetary Transactions	36·2	(9·0)	15·0	62·1	31·6
	511·2	418·3	464·9	540·0	444·4

[1] Forecast. [2] Estimate.

Banking. All major Canadian banks are represented with numerous branch locations throughout the Province. In March 1990 total deposits with chartered banks in Nova Scotia totalled $4,654m.

NATURAL RESOURCES

Minerals. Principal minerals in 1989 were: Coal, 3·6m. tonnes, valued at $207·3m.; gypsum, 6·3m. tonnes, valued at $59·3m.; sand and gravel, 8m. tonnes, valued at $23·7m. Total value of mineral production in 1989 was about $406·6m.

Agriculture. Dairying, poultry and egg production, livestock and fruit growing are the most important branches. Farm cash receipts for 1989 were estimated at $315·1m., with an additional $3·8m. going to persons on farms as income in kind.

Cash receipts from sale of dairy products were $85·4m., with total milk and cream sales of 175,517,000 litres.

The production of poultry meat in 1989 was 22,553 tonnes, of which 19,421 tonnes were chickens and fowls and 3,132 tonnes were turkeys. Egg production was 19·2m. dozen.

The main 1989 fruit crops were apples, 43,817 tonnes; blueberries, 7,717 tonnes; and strawberries, 2,268 tonnes.

Forestry. The estimated forest area of Nova Scotia is 15,555 sq. miles (40,298 sq. km), of which about 25% is owned by the province. The principal trees are spruce, balsam fir, hemlock, pine, larch, birch, oak, maple, poplar and ash. 4,322,147 cu. metres of round forest products were produced in 1988.

Fisheries. The fisheries of the province in 1989 had a landed value of $410·8m. of sea fish including scallop fishery, $79·2m., and lobster fishery, $137·3m. In 1987 there were 7,225 employees in the fish processing industry; the value of shipment of goods was $1,139·4m.

INDUSTRY. The number of manufacturing establishments was 721 in 1987; the number of employees was 37,715; wages and salaries, $905m. The value of shipments in 1989, was $4,784m., and the leading industries were food, paper and allied industries and transportation equipment.

TRADE UNIONS. Total union membership in 1989 was 107,533 belonging to 94 unions comprised of 631 individual locals. The largest union membership was in the service sector followed by public administration and defence.

COMMUNICATIONS

Roads. In 1989 there were 26,053 km of highways; paved included 128 km freeway, 2,667 km arterial, 4,916 km collector and 5,454 km local. 12,888 km of highway are unpaved.

Railways. The province is covered with a network of 1,100 km of mainline track.

Aviation. There is direct air service to all major Canadian points and international scheduled service to Boston, New York, Bermuda, London, Glasgow and Amsterdam. There are winter charter services to Florida and the Caribbean.

Shipping. Ferry services connect Nova Scotia with Newfoundland, Prince Edward Island, New Brunswick and Maine. Direct service by container vessels is provided from the Port of Halifax to ports in the USA (east and west coast), Europe, Asia, Australia/New Zealand and the Caribbean.

JUSTICE AND EDUCATION

Justice. The Supreme Court (Trial Division and Appeal Division) is the superior court of Nova Scotia and has original and appellate jurisdiction in all civil and criminal matters unless they have been specifically assigned to another court by Statute. An appeal from the Supreme Court, Appeal Division, is to the Supreme Court of Canada. The other courts in the Province are the Provincial Court, which hears criminal matters only, the Small Claims Court, which has limited monetary jurisdiction, Probate Court, County Court, which has jurisdiction in criminal matters as well as original jurisdiction over actions not exceeding $50,000, and Family Court. Young offenders are tried in the Family Court or the Provincial Court.

For the year ending 31 March 1990 there were 3,509 adult admissions to provincial custody; of these, 1,993 were sentenced.

Education. Public education in Nova Scotia is free, compulsory and undenominational through elementary and high school. Attendance is compulsory to the age of 16. In addition to 530 public schools there are the Atlantic Provinces Resource Centres for the Hearing Handicapped and for the Visually Impaired; the Shelburne Youth Centre for young offenders and the Nova Scotia Residential Centre for delinquent children; and the Nova Scotia Youth Training Centre for mentally handicapped children. The province has 19 universities, colleges and technical institutions, of which the largest is Dalhousie University in Halifax. The Nova Scotia Agricultural College and the Nova Scotia Teachers' College are located at Truro. The Technical University of Nova Scotia at Halifax grants degrees in engineering and architecture.

The Department of Vocational and Technical Training administers 2 institutes of technology, a nautical institute and 14 other facilities under the system of Community colleges. It also provides in-school training for the Department of Labour Apprenticeship programme.

The Nova Scotia government offers financial support and organizational assistance to local school boards for provision of weekend and evening courses in academic and avocational subjects, and citizenship for new Canadians. It also provides local authorities with specialist support services to assist them in providing community workshops and it operates a correspondence study service for children and adults.

Total estimated expenditure on all levels of education for the year 1990-91 was $1,428·6m., of which 69% was borne by the provincial government. In 1990–91, classrooms operated in 530 elementary-secondary schools, with 9,890 teachers and 165,150 pupils.

Further Reading

Nova Scotia Fact Book. N.S. Department of Industry, Trade and Technology, Halifax, 1988
Nova Scotia Resource Atlas. N.S. Department of Industry, Trade and Technology, Halifax, 1986

Atlantic Provinces Economic Council. *The Atlantic Vision, 1990.* Halifax, 1979
Public Archives of Nova Scotia. *Place Names and Places of Nova Scotia.* Halifax, 1967
Beck, M., *The Evolution of Municipal Government in Nova Scotia, 1749–1973.* 1973
Fergusson, C. B., *Nova Scotia in Encyclopedia Canadiana,* Vol. VII. Toronto, 1968
Hamilton, W. B., *The Nova Scotia Traveller.* Toronto, 1981
McCormick, P., *A Guide to Halifax.* Tantallon, 1984
McCreath, P. and Leefe, J., *History of Early Nova Scotia.* Halifax, 1982
Vaison, R., *Nova Scotia Past and Present: A Bibliography and Guide.* Halifax, 1976

ONTARIO

HISTORY. The French explorer Samuel de Champlain explored the Ottawa River from 1613. The area was governed by the French, first under a joint stock company and then as a royal province, from 1627 and was ceded to Great Britain in 1763. A constitutional act of 1791 created there the province of Upper Canada, largely to accommodate loyalists of English descent who had immigrated after the United States war of independence. Upper Canada entered the Confederation as Ontario in 1867.

AREA AND POPULATION. The total area is about 412,582 sq. miles (1,068,630 sq. km), of which some 344,100 sq. miles (891,200 sq. km) are land area and some 64,490 sq. miles (189,196 sq. km) are lakes and fresh water rivers.

The province extends 1,050 miles (1,690 km) from east to west and 1,075 miles (1,730 km) from north to south.

Ontario is bounded on the north by the waters of Hudson and James Bay, on the east by Quebec, on the west by Manitoba, and on the south by the states of New York, Pennsylvania, Ohio, Michigan, Wisconsin and Minnesota.

The population of the province (census, 1 June 1981) was 8,625,107. Estimate (1988) 9·1m. Population of the principal cities (1985): Hamilton, 307,690 (city), 421,264 (metropolitan area); Kitchener, 147,439 (city), 287,801 (census metropolitan area); London, 276,000 (city); Ottawa (federal capital), 304,448 (city), 562,782 (census metropolitan area); Sudbury, 90,453 (city), 154,387 (regional municipality); Toronto (provincial capital), 606,247 (city), 2,998,947 (census metropolitan area); Windsor, 195,028 (city).

There are some 0·5m. French speakers.

Vital statistics, *see* p. 273.

CLIMATE. A temperate continental climate, but conditions are quite severe in winter, though proximity to the Great Lakes has a moderating influence on temperatures. Ottawa. Jan. 12°F (–11·1°C), July 69°F (20·6°C). Annual rainfall 35" (871 mm). Toronto. Jan. 23°F (–5°C), July 69°F (20·6°C). Annual rainfall 33" (815 mm).

CONSTITUTION AND GOVERNMENT. The provincial government is administered by a *Lieut.-Governor*, a cabinet and a single-chamber 130-member legislature elected by a general franchise for a period of 5 years. The minimum voting age is 18 years.

At the elections of Sept. 1990 to the provincial legislature, the New Democratic Party won 74 seats, the Liberal Party, 36, and the Progressive Conservative Party, 20.

Lieut.-Governor: Right Hon. Lincoln M. Alexander, PC, QC (appointed Sept. 1985).

Flag: The British Red Ensign with the shield of Ontario in the fly.

The members of the Executive Council in Feb. 1991 were as follows:

Premier and Minister of Intergovernmental Affairs: Hon. Bob Rae.

Deputy Premier: Hon. Floyd Laughren. *Agriculture and Food:* Hon. Elmer Buchanan. *Attorney-General:* Hon. Howard Hampton. *Citizenship:* Hon. Elaine Ziemba. *Colleges and Universities:* Hon. Richard Allen. *Community and Social Services:* Hon. Zanana Akande. *Consumer and Commercial Relations:* Hon. Peter Kormos. *Correctional Services:* Hon. Mike Farnan. *Culture and Communications:* Hon. Rosario Marchese. *Education:* Hon. Marion Boyd. *Energy:* Hon. Jenny Carter. *Environment:* Hon. Ruth Grier. *Financial Institutions:* Hon. Peter Kormos. *Francophone Affairs:* Hon. Gilles Pouliot. *Government Services:* Hon. Frances Lankin. *Health:* Hon. Evelyn Gigantes. *Housing:* Hon. Dave Cook. *Industry, Trade and Technology:* Hon. Allan Pilkey. *Labour:* Hon. Bob MacKenzie. *Mines:* Hon. Gilles Pouliot. *Municipal Affairs:* Hon. Dave Cook. *Native Affairs, Natural Resources:* Hon. Bud Wildman. *Northern Development:* Hon. Shelly Martel. *Revenue:* Hon. Shelly Wark-Martyn. *Solicitor General:* Hon. Mike Farnan. *Tourism and Recreation:* Hon. Peter North. *Transportation:* Hon. Ed Philip. *Ministers Without Portfolio:* Hon. Shirley Coppen, Hon. Anne Swarbrick (Responsible for Women's Issues).

Local Government. Local government in Ontario is divided into two branches, one covering municipal institutions and the other education.

The present municipal system dates from The Municipal Corporations Act enacted by The Province of Canada in 1849. It has been considerably modified in recent years with the creation of the Municipality of Metropolitan Toronto in 1954 and the launching of the Government of Ontario's local government restructuring programme in 1968. Generally, there are two levels of municipal government in Ontario. The upper level consists of 27 counties plus 12 restructured regional municipalities. The local level comprises more than 800 cities, towns and townships. Cities in the traditional county system function independently of the county in which they lie, as do 4 towns which have been separated for municipal purposes. There are no separated municipal units in regional governments.

Ontario's local municipalities are governed by councils elected by popular vote.

A city council usually consists of a mayor, aldermen and, sometimes, an executive committee known as a board of control.

Councils of towns, villages and townships usually consist of a mayor, reeve, deputy reeve, councillors and, in the case of the newer regional municipalities, one or more regional councillors who represent the area municipalities on the regional council.

County and regional government councils are federated assemblies.

A county council consists of the reeves and deputy reeves of the towns, villages and townships. The head of the county council is the warden, who is elected by the council from among its own members.

A regional council consists of the heads of council of the local municipalities, as well as a varying number of regional councillors, who are elected on the basis of representation, either directly or indirectly. The head of the regional council is the chairman who is elected by council but who, unlike a county warden, need not have been a council member.

No municipality in Ontario may incur long-term debts without the sanction of the tribunal created by the Provincial Legislature and known as the Ontario Municipal Board. Debenture obligations incurred by municipalities for utility undertakings (water-works and electric light and power systems) are discharged ordinarily out of revenues derived from the sale of utility services and do not fall upon the ratepayers.

Municipal councils have no jurisdiction for education beyond the collection of taxes for school purposes. Responsibility for providing, operating and maintaining school facilities, and for the supply of teachers, rests with local education authorities known as Boards of Education or School Boards. These Boards are now generally organized on a county or regional basis. Apart from some of the larger cities, local municipal school boards no longer exist.

Municipal institutions come under the jurisdiction of the Provincial Ministry of Intergovernmental Affairs. One of the principal functions of the Ministry is to advise and assist municipalities on such matters as accounting, reporting, auditing, budgeting and planning. Educational support and guidance at the provincial level is the responsibility of the Ministry of Education, which deals with the training of teachers and the formulation of curriculum. (At the university and community college level, education support services are provided by the Ministry of Colleges and Universities.)

There are considerable areas in the northernmost parts of Ontario where as yet there is little or no settlement of population. In such areas no municipal organization exists, and control for all purposes over such areas remains in the hands of the Provincial Government.

FINANCE. The gross revenue and expenditure and the net cash requirements (in Canadian $1,000) for years ending 31 March were as follows:

	1984–85	*1985–86*	*1986–87*	*1987–88*	*1989–90*
Gross revenue	23,765	26,228	28,454	33,866	40,713
Gross expenditure	26,430	32,562	31,031	34,846	41,290
Net cash requirement	1,701	2,134	1,544	980	577

Gross revenue and expenditure figures include all non-budgetary transactions, *i.e.*, the lending and investment activity of the Government to Crown corporations, agencies and municipalities as well as the repayment of these loans or recovery of investments. Transactions on behalf of Ontario Hydro are excluded.

ENERGY AND NATURAL RESOURCES

Electricity (1989). Ontario Hydro recorded for the calendar year an installed generating capacity of 33,854m. kw. and a net energy output generated and purchased of 143,062m. kwh.

Minerals (1989). The total value of shipments from mines was $7,200m. Important commodities (in $1m.) were: Nickel, 20,030; copper, 893; uranium, 461; gold, 1,170; zinc, 578. The mining industry employed about 25,000 people in 1989.

Agriculture. In 1989, 3·5m. ha were under field crops with total farm receipts of $5,663m.

Forestry. According to the most recent inventory (1988) the total area of productive forest is 39·9m. ha, comprising: Softwoods, 26·3m.; hardwoods, 13·6m. The growing stock equals 5,102m. cu. metres. The estimated value of shipments by the forest products industry (including logging) was (1988) $10,220m.

INDUSTRY AND TRADE

Industry (1989). Ontario is Canada's most highly industrialized province. About 73% of value added in commodity-producing industries is accounted for by manufacturing. Construction is next with 7%.

In 1989, the labour force was 5,214,000. Total labour income was $138,433m. The 1989 Gross Provincial Product (GPP) was $269,997m.

The leading manufacturing industries are motor vehicles and parts, iron and steel, meat and meat preparations, dairy products, paper and paperboard, chemical products, petroleum and coal products, machinery and equipment, metal stamping and pressing and communications equipment.

Trade. In 1989 Ontario exported 49% ($67,425m.) of Canada's total foreign trade.

COMMUNICATIONS

Roads. There were, in 1989, 156,390·3 km of roads. Motor licences (on the road) numbered (1989) 7,415,894, of which 4,701,949. were passenger cars, 1,081,659 commercial vehicles, 28,909 buses, 1,089,548 trailers, 131,230 motor cycles and 308,373 snow vehicles.

Railways. The provincially-owned Ontario Northland Railway has about 550 miles of track and the Algoma Central Railway 325 miles. The Canadian National and Canadian Pacific Railways operate a total of about 9,500 miles in Ontario. There is a metro and tramway network in Toronto.

Post (1987). Telephone service is provided by 30 independent systems (178,527 telephones) and Bell Canada (10m. telephones).

EDUCATION. There is a complete provincial system of elementary and secondary schools as well as private schools. In 1989 publicly financed elementary and secondary schools had a total enrolment of 1,867,431 pupils.

In 1965 Ontario established Colleges of Applied Arts and Technology (CAATS). There are now 23 of these publicly owned colleges with full-time enrolment (1988) of 110,718 in full-time academic courses.

The University of Toronto, founded in 1827 (full-time enrolment, 1989, 31,765), and 14 other universities (total full-time enrolment, 1989, 187,763), all receive provincial grants. The general expenditure of the provincial ministries of education and colleges and universities for 1988-89 was $7,780m.

Further Reading

Statistical Information: Annual publications of the Ontario Ministry of Treasury and Economics include: *Ontario Statistics; Ontario Budget; Public Accounts; Financial Report.*
Guillet, E. C., *Pioneer Days in Upper Canada.* Toronto, 1933
McDonald, D. C. (ed.) *The Government and Politics of Ontario.* 2nd ed. Toronto, 1980
Middleton, J. E., *The Province of Ontario: A History 1615–1927.* Toronto, 1927, 4 vols.
Schull, J., *Ontario since 1867.* Toronto, 1978

PRINCE EDWARD ISLAND

HISTORY. After 10 millennia of Amerindian settlement, the first recorded European visit was by Jacques Cartier in 1534, who named it Isle St-Jean. In 1719 it was settled by the French, but was taken from them in 1758, annexed to Nova Scotia in 1763, and constituted a separate colony in 1769. Named Prince Edward Island in honour of Prince Edward, Duke of Kent, in 1799, it entered the Canadian Confederation on 1 July 1873.

AREA AND POPULATION. The province lies in the Gulf of St Lawrence, and is separated from the mainland of New Brunswick and Nova Scotia by Northumberland Strait. The area of the island is 2,185 sq. miles (5,660 sq. km). Total population (census, 1986), 126,646; (estimate, 1990), 130,400. Population of the principal cities: Charlottetown (capital), 15,776; Summerside, 8,020.

Vital statistics, *see* p. 273.

CLIMATE. The cool temperate climate is affected in winter by the freezing of the St. Lawrence, which reduces winter temperatures. Charlottetown. Jan. 19°F (–7·2°C), July 67°F (19·4°C). Annual rainfall 43" (1,077 mm).

CONSTITUTION AND GOVERNMENT. The provincial government is administered by a Lieut.-Governor-in-Council (Cabinet) and a Legislative Assembly of 32 members who are elected for up to 5 years. In June 1989, parties in the Legislative Assembly were: Liberals, 30; Progressive Conservatives, 2.

Lieut.-Governor: Marion L. Reid (sworn in 16 Aug. 1990).

The Executive Council was composed as follows in Feb. 1991:

Premier, President of the Executive Council, Minister of Justice and Attorney-General: Hon. Joseph A. Ghiz, QC.

Finance and Environment: Hon. Gilbert R. Clements. *Community and Cultural Affairs and Fisheries and Aquaculture:* Hon. J. G. Leonce Bernard. *Industry:* Hon. Robert J. Morrissey. *Health and Social Services:* Hon. Wayne D. Cheverie, QC. *Transportation and Public Works:* Hon. Gordon MacInnis. *Agriculture:* Hon. Keith Milligan. *Education:* Hon. Paul Connolly. *Energy and Forestry:* Hon. Barry Hicken. *Tourism and Parks:* Hon. Nancy Guptill. *Labour:* Hon. Roberta Hubley.

Flag: A banner of the arms, *i.e.*, a white field bearing 3 small trees and a larger tree on a compartment, all green, and at the top a red band with a golden lion; on 3 sides a border of red and white rectangles.

Local Government. The Municipalities Act, 1983, provides for the incorporation of Towns and Communities. The City of Charlottetown and the town of Summerside are incorporated under private Acts of the Legislature.

FINANCE. Revenue and expenditure (in Canadian $) for 5 financial years ending 31 March:

	1986–87	*1987–88*	*1988–89*	*1989–90*	*1990–91*
Revenue	490,913,588	533,231,248	600,319,801	656,622,400	684,881,400
Expenditure	509,867,825	546,010,988	605,092,077	654,338,000	678,679,000

ENERGY AND NATURAL RESOURCES

Electricity. Electric power is supplied to 100% of the population. In 1989, total supply of electric energy was 726,766 mwh; net generation, 104,408 mwh. An undersea cable links the island with New Brunswick and the Maritime Power Grid. Electricity received from other provinces in 1989 totalled 619,511 mwh. In 1989, 85·6% of power requirements were supplied through this system.

Agriculture. Total area of farms occupied approximately 673,000 acres in 1989 out of the total land area of 1,399,040 acres. Farm cash receipts in 1989 were $256·1m. with cash receipts from potatoes accounting for 46·5% of the total. Cash receipts from dairy products, cattle and hogs followed in importance. For particulars of agricultural production and livestock, *see* pp. 000–00.

Forestry. Forested lands cover 278,000 ha. During 1989, 100,000 cords of roundwood were burnt for heating, and 22m. board feet of timber, worth some $7m., were sawn.

Fisheries. The catch in 1989 had a landed value of $72·4m. Lobsters and shellfish accounted for 83% of the total. Value of groundfish landings accounted for 8·3%; ocean and estuarial, 4·1%; Irish moss, 4·6%.

INDUSTRY AND TRADE

Industry. Value of manufacturing shipments for all industries in 1989 was $391·0m.

Labour. Per capita personal income rose from $13,126 in 1987 to $14,411 in 1988. The average weekly wage (industrial aggregate) rose from $379·26 in 1988 to $400·07 in 1989. The labour force averaged 63,000 in 1989, while employment averaged 54,000.

In 1989, provincial GDP in constant prices for manufacturing was $71·7m.; construction, $138·4m. In 1989 the total value of retail trade was $731·9m.

Tourism. The value of the tourist industry was estimated at $98·3m. in 1989 with 249,725 tourist parties.

COMMUNICATIONS

Roads. At the end of 1989 there were 5,295 km of road, including 3,780 km of paved highway. A bus service operates 3 times daily to the mainland.

Railways. Rail service closed on 31 Dec. 1989.

Aviation. In 1989 15 daily return flights for passengers, mail and freight were operated by 4 airlines between Charlottetown and Halifax. Daily non-stop service between Charlottetown and Toronto was also provided.

Shipping. Access to the mainland for passengers and road traffic is provided by a year-round ferry service between the island and New Brunswick, employing 4 ferries which make approximately 20 return crossings a day. A second ferry service for passengers and road vehicles operates between the island and Nova Scotia from May until mid-December providing up to 19 crossings a day with 4 vessels. Ferry service is also provided between Prince Edward Island and the Magdalen Islands, Quebec, on daily or twice-daily schedules from April till the end of January. There are 4 commercial ports handling mainly potato exports and petroleum products. These ports are iced up in winter; 2 of the ferries are ice-breakers.

Telecommunications. In 1989 there were 91,495 telephones.

EDUCATION (1989–90). Under the regional school boards there were 66 public schools, 1,447 teaching positions and 24,744 students. There is one undergraduate university (2,322 full-time students), and a veterinary college (184 students), both in Charlottetown. A college of applied arts and technology in centres across the province served 8,520 students (full-time and continuing education programmes), which equated to 2,800 full-time equivalent students. Total expenditure on education in the year ending 31 March 1990 was $145,589,300.

Further Reading

Baldwin, D. O., *Abegweit: Land of the Red Soil.* Charlottetown, 1985
Bolger, F. W. P., *Canada's Smallest Province.* Charlottetown, 1973
Clark, A. H., *Three Centuries and the Island.* Toronto, 1959
Hocking, A., *Prince Edward Island.* Toronto, 1978
MacKinnon, F., *The Government of Prince Edward Island.* Toronto, 1951

QUEBEC—QUÉBEC

HISTORY. Quebec was formerly known as New France or Canada from 1534 to 1763; as the province of Quebec from 1763 to 1790; as Lower Canada from 1791 to 1846; as Canada East from 1846 to 1867, and when, by the union of the four original provinces, the Confederation of the Dominion of Canada was formed, it again became known as the province of Quebec (Québec).

The Quebec Act, passed by the British Parliament in 1774, guaranteed to the people of the newly conquered French territory in North America security in their religion and language, their customs and tenures, under their own civil laws.

In the referendum held 20 May 1980, 59·5% voted against and 40·5% for 'separatism'.

AREA AND POPULATION. The area of Quebec (as amended by the Labrador Boundary Award) is 1,667,926 sq. km (594,860 sq. miles), of which 1,315,134 sq. km is land area and 352,792 sq. km water. Of this extent, 911,106 sq. km represent the Territory of Ungava, annexed in 1912 under the Quebec Boundaries Extension Act. The population (census 1986) was 6,532,461. Estimate (1989) 6,688,700.

Principal cities (1986): Quebec (capital), 164,580; Montreal, 1,015,420; Laval, 284,164; Sherbrooke, 74,438; Verdun, 60,246; Hull, 58,722; Trois-Rivières, 50,122.

Vital statistics, *see* p. 273.

CLIMATE. Cool temperate in the south, but conditions are more extreme towards the north. Winters are severe and snowfall considerable, but summer temperatures are quite warm. Rain occurs at all seasons. Quebec. Jan. 10°F (−12·2°C), July 66°F

(18·9°C). Annual rainfall 40" (1,008 mm). Montreal. Jan. 11°F (–11·7°C), July 67°F (19·4°C). Annual rainfall 30" (776 mm).

CONSTITUTION AND GOVERNMENT. There is a Legislative Assembly consisting of 125 members, elected in 125 electoral districts for 4 years. At the provincial general elections held Sept. 1989, Liberals won 92 seats, *Parti Québecois*, 29 and *Parti Egalité*, 4.

Lieut.-Governor: The Hon. Martial Asselin.

Flag: The Fleurdelysé flag, blue with a white cross, and in each quarter a white fleur-de-lis.

Members of the Executive Council as in Feb. 1991, included:

Prime Minister: Robert Bourassa.

Deputy Prime Minister and Energy and Resources: Lise Bacon. *Finance:* Gérard D. Lévesque. *Education:* Claude Ryan. *Justice:* Gil Rémillard. *Communications:* Lawrence Cannon. *Cultural Affairs:* Liza Frulla-Hébert. *International Affairs:* John Claccia. *Autochthonous Affairs:* Christos Sirros. *Transport:* Sam Elkas. *Public Security:* Claude Ryan.

General-delegate in London: Reed Scowen (59 Pall Mall, London SW1Y 5JH).

General-delegate in New York: Léo Paré (17 West 50th St., Rockefeller Center, New York 10020).

General-delegate in Paris: Marcel Bergeron (66 Pergolèse, Paris 75116).

ECONOMY

Budget. Ordinary revenue and expenditure (in Canadian $1,000) for fiscal years ending 31 March:

	1984–85	*1985–86*	*1986–87*	*1987–88*	*1988–89*
Revenue	23,310,027	24,080,778	25,646,247	28,363,891	29,967,892
Expenditure	25,542,499	27,222,178	28,465,454	30,738,141	31,578,118

The total net debt at 31 March 1989 was $25,386,320,000.

ENERGY AND NATURAL RESOURCES

Electricity. Water power is one of the most important natural resources of the province of Quebec. Its turbine installation represents about 40% of the aggregate of Canada. At the end of 1988 the installed generating capacity was 32,713 mw. Production, 1989, was 144,898 gwh.

Minerals (1989). The estimated value of the mineral production (metal mines only) was $2,814,450,000. Chief minerals: Iron ore, (confidential); copper, $205,915,000; gold, $521,351,000; zinc, $202,261,000.

The second major iron-ore development in northern Quebec is, like the one at Knob Lake which gave birth to Schefferville, based on the Quebec–Labrador Trough which extends from Lac Jeannine to the northern tip of Ungava peninsula. The port of Sept-Iles and the railway connecting it with Schefferville allow easy shipment to the furnaces and steel mills of Canada, the USA and Europe.

Non-metallic minerals produced include: Asbestos ($176,716,000; about 68·3% of Canadian production), titane-dioxide (confidential), industrial lime, dolomite and brucite, quartz and pyrite. Among the building materials produced were: Stone, $220,639,000; cement, $186,900,000; sand and gravel, $80,078,000; lime, (confidential).

Agriculture. In 1989 the total area (estimate) of the principal field crops was 2,032,400 ha. The yield of the principal crops was (1989 in 1,000 tonnes):

Crops	*Yield*	*Crops*	*Yield*
Tame hay	6,320	Fodder corn	1,720
Oats for grain	295	Maize for grain	1,570
Potatoes	370	Barley	485
Mixed grains	75	Buckwheat	10

The farm cash receipts from farming operations estimated in 1989 amounted to $3,672,709,000. The principal items being: Livestock and products, $2,484,134,000; crops, $679,360,000; dairy supplements payments, $129,670,000, forest and maple products, $93,375,000.

Forestry. Forests cover an area of 912,123 sq. km. About 734,316 sq. km are classified as productive forests, of which 664,289 sq. km are provincial forest land and 66,866 sq. km are privately owned. Quebec leads the Canadian provinces in pulp and paper production, having nearly half of the Canadian estimated total.

In 1988 production of lumber was softwood and hardwood, 11,560,695 cu. metres; pulp and paper, 7,873,000 tonnes.

Fisheries. The principal fish are cod, herring, red fish, lobster and salmon. Total catch of sea fish, 1989, 79,101 tonnes, valued at $79,467,000.

INDUSTRY AND TRADE

Industry. In 1987 there were 11,183 industrial establishments in the province; employees, 520,459; salaries and wages, $13,443,485,000; cost of materials, $40,411,645,000; value of shipments, $72,608,303,000. Among the leading industries are petroleum refining, pulp and paper mills, smelting and refining, dairy products, slaughtering and meat processing, motor vehicle manufacturing, women's clothing, saw-mills and planing mills, iron and steel mills, commercial printing.

Commerce. In 1989 the value of Canadian exports through Quebec custom ports was $22,875,103,000; value of imports, $24,735,807,000.

COMMUNICATIONS

Roads. In 1989 there were 59,844 km of roads and 3,884,825 registered motor vehicles.

Railways. There were (1989) 8,475 km of railway. There is a metro system in Montreal.

Aviation. In 1989 Quebec had 2 international airports, Dorval (Montreal) with landing runway of 8·4 km and Mirabel (Montreal) with 7·3 km.

Post and Broadcasting. Telephones numbered 3,526,581 in 1988 and there were 34 television and 117 radio stations.

Newspapers (1989). There were 10 French- and 2 English-language daily newspapers.

EDUCATION. The province has 7 universities: 3 English-language universities, McGill (Montreal) founded in 1821, Bishop (Lennoxville) founded in 1845 and the Concordia University (Montreal) granted a charter in 1975; 4 French-language universities: Laval (Quebec) founded in 1852, Montreal University, opened in 1876 as a branch of Laval and became independent in 1920, Sherbrooke University founded in 1954 and University of Quebec founded in 1968.

In 1988–89 there were 118,864 full-time university students and 122,169 part-time students.

In 1988–89, in pre-kindergartens, there were 6,554 pupils; in kindergartens, 87,446; primary schools, 587,075; in secondary schools, 454,489; in colleges (post-secondary, non-university), 154,058; and in classes for children with special needs, 142,165. The school boards had a total of 60,101 teachers.

Expenditure of the Departments of Education for 1988–89, $8,102,888,000 net. This included $1,330,493,000 for universities, $5,054,902,000 for public primary and secondary schools, $259,170,000 for private primary and secondary schools and $1,142,205,000 for colleges.

Further Reading

Statistical Information: The Quebec Bureau of Statistics was established in 1912. The Bureau, which reports to the Finance Dept. since March 1983, collects, compiles and distributes statistical information relative to Quebec. *Director:* Luc Bessette.

A statistical information list is available on request. Among the most important publications are: *Le Québec Statistique, Statistiques* (quarterly), *Comptes économiques du Québec* (annual), *Situation démographique* (annual), *Commerce international du Québec* (annual), *Investissements privés et publics* (annual).

Baudoin, L., *Le Droit civil de la province de Québec.* Montreal, 1953
Blanchard, R., *Canada-français.* Paris, 1959
Hamelin, J., *Histoire du Québec.* St-Hyacinthe, 1978
Jacobs, J., *The Question of Separatism: Quebec and the Struggle for Sovereignty.* London, 1981
McWhinney, E., *Quebec and the Constitution.* Univ. of Toronto Press, 1979
Ouellet, F., *Histoire de la Chambre de Commerce de Québec, 1809–1959.* Québec, 1959
Raynauld, A., *Croissance et structure économiques de la province de Québec.* Québec, 1961
Trofimenkoff, S. M., *Action Française.* Univ. of Toronto Press, 1975
Wade, F. M., *The French Canadians, 1760–1967.* Toronto, 1968.—*Canadian Dualism: Studies of French–English Relations.* Quebec–Toronto, 1960

SASKATCHEWAN

HISTORY. Saskatchewan derives its name from its major river system, which the Cree Indians called ‘Kis-is-ska-tche-wan’, meaning ‘swift flowing’. It officially became a province when it joined the Confederation on 1 Sept. 1905.

In 1670 King Charles II granted to Prince Rupert and his friends a charter covering exclusive trading rights in ‘all the land drained by streams finding their outlet in the Hudson Bay’. This included what is now Saskatchewan. The trading company was first known as The Governor and Company of Adventurers of England; later as the Hudson’s Bay Company. In 1869 the Northwest Territories was formed, and this included Saskatchewan. In 1882 the District of Saskatchewan was formed. By 1885 the North-West Mounted Police had been inaugurated, with headquarters in Regina (now the capital), and the Canadian Pacific Railway’s transcontinental line had been completed, bringing a stream of immigrants to southern Saskatchewan. The Hudson’s Bay Company surrendered its claim to territory in return for cash and land around the existing trading posts. Legislative government was introduced.

AREA AND POPULATION. Saskatchewan is bounded on the west by Alberta, on the east by Manitoba, to the north by the Northwest Territories; to the south it is bordered by the US states of Montana and North Dakota. The area of the province is 251,700 sq. miles (570,113 sq. km), of which 220,182 sq. miles is land area and 31,518 sq. miles is water. The population, 1986 census, was 1,010,198. Population of cities, 1986 census: Regina (capital), 175,064; Saskatoon, 177,641; Moose Jaw, 35,073; Prince Albert, 33,686; Yorkton, 15,574; Swift Current, 15,666; North Battleford, 14,876; Estevan, 10,161; Weyburn, 10,153; Lloydminster, 7,155; Melfort, 6,078; Melville, 5,123.

Vital statistics, *see* p. 273.

CLIMATE. A cold continental climate, with severe winters and warm summers. Rainfall amounts are greatest from May to Aug. Regina. Jan. 0°F (–17·8°C), July 65°F (18·3°C). Annual rainfall 15" (373 mm).

CONSTITUTION AND GOVERNMENT. The provincial government is vested in a Lieut.-Governor, an Executive Council and a Legislative Assembly, elected for 5 years. Women were given the franchise in 1916 and are also eligible for election to the legislature. State of parties in Oct. 1990: Progressive Conservative, 36; New Democratic Party, 26; Vacancies, 2.

Lieut.-Governor: Hon. Sylvia O. Fedoruk.
Flag: Green over gold, with the shield of the province in the canton, and a green and red prairie lily in the fly.

The Progressive Conservative Ministry in Oct. 1990 was composed as follows:

Premier, Agriculture and Food: Grant Divine.
Deputy Premier, Urban Affairs, Minister responsible for the Status of Women: Pat Smith. *Health:* George McLeod. *Finance, Crown Management Board:* Lorne Hepworth. *Justice and Attorney-General, Provincial Secretary, Telephones:* Gary Lane. *Rural Development:* Neil Hardy. *Environment and Public Safety, Indian and Native Affairs:* Grant Hodgins. *Human Resources, Labour and Employment, Minister of Economic Diversification and Trade:* Grant Schmidt. *Consumer and Commercial Affairs:* Jack Klein. *Associate Minister of Economic Diversification and Trade:* John Gerich. *Associate Minister of Agriculture and Food:* Harold Martens. *Education, Science and Technology:* Ray Meiklejohn. *Highways and Transportation:* Sherwin Peterson. *Energy and Mines:* Richard Swenson. *Parks and Renewable Resources, Northern Affairs:* Lorne Kopelchuk. *Family, Minister responsible for Seniors, Minister of Culture, Multiculturism and Recreation:* Beattie Martin. *Social Services:* William Neudorf. *Associate Minister of Health:* John Wolfe.

Agent-General in London: Paul Rousseau, 21 Pall Mall, SW1Y 5LP.

Local Government. The organization of a city requires a minimum population of 5,000 persons; that of a town, 500; that of a village, 100 people. No requirements as to population exist for the rural municipality.

Cities, towns, villages and rural municipalities are governed by elected councils, which consist of a mayor and 6–20 aldermen in a city; a mayor and 6 councillors in a town; a mayor and 2 other members in a village; a reeve and a councillor for each division in a rural municipality (usually 6).

FINANCE. Budget and net assets (years ending 31 March) in Canadian $1,000:

	1987–88	*1988–89*	*1989–90*	*1990–91*
Budgetary revenue	3,202,508	3,607,683	4,083,400	4,278,200
Budgetary expenditure	3,779,743	3,935,896	4,309,460	4,641,345

ENERGY AND NATURAL RESOURCES. Agriculture used to dominate the history and economics of Saskatchewan, but the 'prairie province' is now a rapidly developing mining and manufacturing area. It is a major supplier of oil; has the world's largest deposits of potash; and net value of non-agricultural production accounts for (1989 estimate) 89·5% of the provincial economy.

Electricity. The Saskatchewan Power Corporation generated 13,224m. kwh. in 1989.

Minerals. The 1989 mineral sales were valued at $2,940,369,034, including (in $1m.): Petroleum, 1,169·6; natural gas, 206·9; coal and others, 141·0; gold, 44·9; copper, 2·1; zinc, 1·9; potash, 880·9; salt, 19·9; uranium, 380·1; sodium sulphate, 23·1.

Agriculture. Saskatchewan normally produces about two-thirds of Canada's wheat. Wheat production in 1989 (in 1,000 tonnes), was 12,457 from 19·9m. acres; oats, 802 from 1·2m. acres; barley, 3,005 from 3·7m. acres; rye, 406 from 660,000 acres; rapeseed, 1,273 from 3·2m. acres; flax, 254 from 750,000 acres. Livestock (1 July 1989): Cattle and calves, 2·13m.; swine, 830,000; sheep and lambs, 52,000. Poultry in 1989: Chickens, 12,116,000; turkeys 744,000. Cash income from the sale of farm products in 1989 was $4,475m. At the June 1986 census there were 63,431 farms in the province, each being a holding of 1 acre or more with sales of agricultural products during the previous 12 months of $250 or more.

The South Saskatchewan River irrigation project, whose main feature is the Gardiner Dam, was completed in 1967. It will ultimately provide for an area of 200,000 to 500,000 acres of irrigated cultivation in Central Saskatchewan. As of

1989, 218,203 acres are irrigated. Total irrigated land in the province, 309,848 acres.

Forestry. Half of Saskatchewan's area is forested, but only 115,000 sq. km are of commercial value at present. Forest products valued at $366m. were produced in 1989. The province's first pulp-mill, at Prince Albert, went into production in 1968; its daily capacity is 1,000 tons of high-grade kraft pulp.

Fur Production. In 1988–89 wild fur production was estimated at $1,810,746. Ranch-raised fur production amounted to $98,220.

Fisheries. The lakeside value of the 1988–89 commercial fish catch of 3·3m. kg was $3·4m.

INDUSTRY. In 1987 Saskatchewan had 810 manufacturing establishments, employing 19,772 persons. Manufacturing contributed $1,222m., construction $846m. to the total gross domestic product at factor cost of $19,414m. in 1989.

TOURISM. An estimated 1·7m. out of province tourists spent $278m. in 1989.

COMMUNICATIONS

Roads. In 1989 there were 25,463 km of provincial highways, 160,000 km of municipal roads (including prairie trails). Motor vehicles registered totalled (1989) 715,000. Bus services are provided by 2 major lines.

Railways. There were (1989) approximately 11,746 km of main railway track.

Aviation. Saskatchewan had 2 major airports, 176 airports and landing strips in 1987.

Telecommunications. There were (1989) 598 post offices (excluding sub-post offices), 82 TV and re-broadcasting stations and 51 AM and FM radio stations. There were 553,137 telephone network access services to the Saskatchewan Telecommunications system in 1989.

EDUCATION. The University of Saskatchewan was established at Saskatoon on 3 April 1907. In 1989–90 it had 14,200 full-time students, 3,700 part-time students and 1,200 full-time staff. The University of Regina was established 1 July 1974; in 1989–90 it had 6,708 full-time and 4,410 part-time students and 499 full-time staff.

The Saskatchewan education system in 1989–90 consisted of 111 school divisions and 5 comprehensive school boards, of which 22 are Roman Catholic separate school divisions, serving 141,137 elementary pupils, 56,637 high-school students and 2,737 students enrolled in special classes. In addition, provincial technical and vocational schools had 50,212 students enrolled in 1989. In addition there are 10 regional colleges with an enrolment of approximately 29,470 students in the 1989–90 school year.

Further Reading

Tourist and industrial publications, descriptive of the Government's programme, are obtainable from the Department of Industry and Commerce; other government publications from Government Information Services (Legislative Building, Regina).

Saskatchewan Economic Review. Executive Council, Regina. Annual

Archer, J. H., *Saskatchewan: A History*. Saskatoon, 1980

Arora, V., *The Saskatchewan Bibliography*. Regina, 1980

Richards, J. S. and Fung, K. I. (eds.) *Atlas of Saskatchewan*. Univ. of Saskatchewan, 1969

THE NORTHWEST TERRITORIES

HISTORY. The Territory was developed by the Hudson's Bay Company and the North West Company (of Montreal) from the 17th century. The Canadian Government bought out the Hudson's Bay Company in 1869 and the Territory was annexed to Canada in 1870. The Arctic Islands lying north of the Canadian mainland were annexed to Canada in 1880 by Queen Victoria.

AREA AND POPULATION. The total area of the Territories is 1,304,903 sq. miles (3,376,698 sq. km), divided into 5 administrative regions: Fort Smith, Inuvik, Kitikmeot, Keewatin and Baffin. The population in June 1989 was 52,730, 37% of whom were Inuit (Eskimo) and 17% Dene (Indian) and Metis. The capital is Yellowknife, population (1989); 13,511. Other main centres (with population in 1989): Iqaluit (3,126), Hay River (2,885), Inuvik (2,773), Fort Smith (2,512), Rankin Inlet (1,440), Rae-Edzo (1,431) and Arviat (1,321).

CLIMATE. Conditions range from cold continental to polar, with long hard winters and short cool summers. Precipitation is low. Yellowknife. Jan. mean high –24·7°C, low –33°C; July mean high 20·7°C, low 11·8°C. Annual rainfall 26·7 cm.

CONSTITUTION AND GOVERNMENT. The Northwest Territories comprises all that portion of Canada lying north of the 60th parallel of N. lat. except those portions within the Yukon Territory and the Provinces of Quebec and Newfoundland: It also includes the islands in Hudson Bay, James Bay and Ungava Bay except those within the Provinces of Manitoba, Ontario and Quebec.

The Northwest Territories is governed by a Government Leader, with a 7-member cabinet and a Legislative Assembly. The Assembly is composed of 24 members elected for a 4-year term of office. A Commissioner of the Northwest Territories acts as a lieutenant-governor and is the federal government's senior representative in the Territorial government. The seat of government was transferred from Ottawa to Yellowknife when it was named Territorial capital on 18 Jan. 1967.

Government Leader: Dennis Patterson.

Commissioner: Daniel L. Norris.

Flag: Vertically, blue, white, blue, with the white of double width and bearing the shield of the Territory.

Legislative powers are exercised by the Executive Council on such matters as taxation within the Territories in order to raise revenue, maintenance of justice, licences, solemnization of marriages, education, public health, property, civil rights and generally all matters of a local nature.

The Territorial Government has assumed most of the responsibility for the administration of the Northwest Territories but political control of Crown lands and non-renewable resources still rests with the Federal Government. On 6 Sept. 1988, the Federal and Territorial Governments signed an agreement for the transfer of management responsibilities for oil and gas resources, located on- and off-shore, in the Northwest Territories to the Territorial Government. In a Territory-wide plebiscite in April 1982, a majority of residents voted in favour of dividing the Northwest Territories into two jurisdictions, east and west. Two forums for each jurisdiction have been created to develop constitutions for the proposed new territories and to negotiate a dividing boundary.

ENERGY AND NATURAL RESOURCES

Oil and Gas. As of Dec. 1988, 27 licences for oil and gas exploration were held for 3·9m. hectares, 17 production licences were held for 62,245 hectares and 78 significant discovery licences were retained on 600,000 hectares.

Crude oil is produced at Norman Wells and piped to Alberta. In 1986, oil production was 117,520 cu. metres.

Minerals. Mineral production in 1987 was valued at $810,005,000, 7% of Canada's total. The Northwest Territories yielded 34% of lead, 25% of zinc, 10% of gold, 7% of cadmium and 8% of silver produced in Canada in 1987.

Trapping and Game. The 71,000 pelts, furs and hides sold by Northwest Territories hunters and trappers in the 1988–89 season were valued at $4·4m. The pelts of highest value are those of the marten, mink, polar bear and lynx. There are some

1·5m. barren-ground caribou, 60,000 muskox and 12,500 polar bears. There are protected herds of wood bison.

Forestry. The principal trees are white and black spruce, jack-pine, tamarack, balsam poplar, aspen and birch. In 1988–89, 39,963 cu. metres of timber, valued at $2·2m., was produced.

Fisheries. Commercial fishing, principally on Great Slave Lake, in 1987–88 produced 3·6m. lbs of fish valued at $2·7m., principally trout, arctic char and whitefish.

CO-OPERATIVES. There are 39 active co-operatives, including 2 housing co-operatives and one central organization to service local co-operatives, in the Northwest Territories. They are active in handicrafts, furs, fisheries, retail stores, hotels and print shops. Total revenue in 1988 was about $41m.

COMMUNICATIONS

Roads. The Mackenzie Route connects Grimshaw, Alberta, with Hay River, Pine Point, Fort Smith, Fort Providence, Rae-Edzo and Yellowknife. The Mackenzie Highway extension to Fort Simpson and a road between Pine Point and Fort Resolution have both been opened.

Highway service to Inuvik in the Mackenzie Delta was opened in spring 1980, extending north from Dawson, Yukon as the Dempster Highway. The Liard Highway connecting the communities of the Liard River valley to British Columbia opened in 1984.

Railways. There is one small railway system in the north which runs from Hay River, on the south shore of Great Slave Lake, 435 miles south to Grimshaw, Alberta, where it connects with the Canadian National Railways, but it is not in use.

Aviation (1988). Fourteen certified airports are operated by the federal Department of Transport and there are 25 certified and 13 uncertified airports operated by the Government of the Northwest Territories. Numerous certified and uncertified airports are operated privately in support of military operations, mining and resource exploration, and tourism. There are 20 privately-owned float plane bases. Major communities receive daily jet service to southern points. Most smaller communities are served by scheduled jet-prop air service several times weekly.

Shipping. A direct inland-water transportation route for about 1,700 miles is provided by the Mackenzie River and its tributaries, the Athabasca and Slave rivers. Subsidiary routes on Lake Athabasca, Great Slave Lake and Great Bear Lake total more than 800 miles.

Telecommunications (1989). There were 60 post offices. The CBC northern service operated radio stations at Yellowknife, Inuvik, Frobisher Bay and Rankin Inlet. Virtually all communities of 150 or over were receiving television *via* satellite. Telephone service is provided by common carriers to nearly all communities in the Northwest Territories. Those few communities without service have high frequency or very high frequency radios for emergency use.

EDUCATION AND WELFARE

Education. In 1989-90 there were six divisional boards of education. Two other regions were working towards divisional board status, which provides for more local and regional control of education. There were also three independent boards of education operating in Yellowknife: A separate school board, a public school board and a board of secondary education.

In 1989-90 there were 76 schools operating, with 837 teachers for 13,618 enrolled students. Residences in regional larger communities provide accommodation for students from smaller communities that cannot provide all education services up to grade 12. There is a full range of courses available in the school system: Academic, French immersion, native language and culture, commercial, technical and occupational training. Post secondary programmes include the 6-campus Arctic

College, which offers a variety of certificate and diploma programmes, along with a first-year general arts university programme. Financial assistance (from the territorial government) is available to qualifying students for post-secondary studies.

Health. In April 1988 responsibility for health services was transferred to the territorial government by the Government of Canada. In 1989 the Department of Health, Government of the Northwest Territories, was responsible for six hospitals (Yellowknife, Hay River, Inuvik, Churchill, Winnepeg, Montreal), six public health centres (Yellowknife, Hay River, Inuvik, Rae, Fort Simpson, Fort Smith) and six satellite health centres.

Welfare. Welfare services are provided by professional social workers. Facilities included (1989) for children: 8 group homes, 1 receiving home, 3 residential treatment centres, 3 secure custody facilities for young offenders, 3 open custody young offender centres and 4 homes for the aged.

Further Reading

Annual Report of the Government of the Northwest Territories
Government Activities in the North, 1983–84. Indian and Northern Affairs, Canada
NWT Data Book 86/87. Yellowknife, 1986
Dawson, C. A., *The New North-West*. Toronto, 1947
MacKay, D., *The Honorable Company*. Toronto, 1949
Zaslow, M., *The Opening of the Canadian North 1870–1914*. Toronto, 1971

YUKON TERRITORY

HISTORY. Formerly part of the Northwest Territories, the Yukon was joined to the Dominion as a separate territory on 13 June 1898.

AREA AND POPULATION. The Yukon is situated in the extreme north-western section of Canada and comprises 482,515 sq. km. of which 4,481 fresh water. The census population in 1981 was 23,153; 1990 (estimate), 29,199. Principal centres are Whitehorse (capital), 20,721; Watson Lake, 1,651; Dawson City, 1,718; Faro, 1,475; Mayo-Elsa, 520.

Vital statistics, *see* p. 273.

CLIMATE. A cold climate in winter with moderate temperatures in summer provide a considerable annual range of temperature and moderate rainfall. Whitehorse. Jan. 5°F (–15°C), July 56°F (13·3°C). Annual rainfall 10" (250 mm). Dawson City. Jan. –22°F (–30°C), July 57°F (13·9°C). Annual rainfall 13" (mm).

CONSTITUTION AND GOVERNMENT. The Yukon Territory was constituted a separate territory in June 1898. It is governed by a 5-member Executive Council (Cabinet) appointed from the majority party in the 16-member elected Legislative Assembly. The members are elected for a 4-year term. The seat of government is at Whitehorse. A federally appointed Commissioner has the final signing authority for all legislation passed by the Assembly.

Commissioner: Ken McKinnon (appointed 27 March 1986)
Flag: Vertically green, white, blue, in the proportions 2 : 3 : 2, charged in the centre with the arms of the Territory.

The legislative authority of the Assembly includes direct taxation, education, property and civil rights, territorial civil service, municipalities and generally all matters of local or private nature. All other major administration including federal Crown lands, and natural resources is federally controlled. Discussions are continuing between the federal and territorial governments on the transfer of certain federal programmes to the Yukon government. A formula financing agreement allows the Yukon government to determine how it will spend funds transferred from the federal government.

ECONOMY

Activities. GDP grew at a rate of 8·8% in 1989, reaching an estimated $840m. Territorial government expenditures were just over $302m. The main sectors of the economy are mining and tourism. Renewable resource industries' production was estimated at $10m. in 1989, a reduction of $5m. over 1988 owing to a weak fur market, closure of a lumber mill and a smaller salmon harvest. Processing of renewable resources is an important source of economic diversification. In the manufacturing sector, manufacturers' shipments were valued at $15–20m. in 1989.

Finance. The Territorial Government's revenue and expenditure (in $1,000) for years ended 31 March was:

	1987–88	*1988–89*	*1989–90*	*1990–91*[1]
Revenue	276,000	305,000	334,699	353,498
Expenditure	278,800	322,800	334,004	346,602

[1] Estimates

ENERGY AND NATURAL RESOURCES

Electricity. Hydro generated power is supplied through plants at Whitehorse Rapids, Aishihik and Mayo. Diesel-generated power is supplied to several other communities (Dawson City, Watson Lake, Old Crow, Teslin). Current capacity is 78 mw hydro and 44 mw diesel-generated power.

Oil. Dome Petroleum, Gulf, Esso Resources, Petro Canada and Shell had been exploring (1986) extensively for oil in the Beaufort Sea but falling world oil prices resulted in much of this exploration being curtailed after 1987.

Minerals. Mining remains the main industry. Lead, zinc, silver and gold are the chief minerals. Production figures for year ending 31 Dec. 1989 (provisional) in tonnes were: Lead, 117,058; zinc, 143,939; silver, 340; gold, 5. The value of mining production sales in 1988 was $486·83m.; in 1989 (provisional) $534·46m.

Agriculture. There are areas where the climate is suitable for the production of forage crops (occupying the largest acreage and used as feed for the estimated 2,500 horses), early maturing varieties of cereals and grains and vegetables. In 1984 cereal crop and forage fertility trials were initiated and the Yukon New Crop Development Project began in 1985. In 1989 there were 30 full-time and 75 part-time farmers. The total improved area was 8,000 acres and the estimated value of agricultural products (farm gate not retail) $2·5m.

Forestry. The forests are part of the great Boreal forest region of Canada which stretches from the east coast of Canada into Alaska and north well above the Arctic Circle. Vast areas are covered by coniferous stands in the southern portion of Yukon with white spruce and lodgepole pine forming pure stands on wet sites and in northern aspects. Deciduous species form pure stands or occur mixed with conifers throughout forest areas.

The value of forest production in 1989 was approximately $3m.

Fisheries. Commercial fishing concentrates on chinook salmon, chum salmon, lake trout and whitefish. The value of fish processed in 1988 was between $3m. and $4m.

Game and Furs. The country abounds with big game, such as moose, goat, caribou, mountain sheep and bear (grizzly and black). The fur trapping industry is considered vital to rural and remote residents and especially native people wishing to maintain a traditional lifestyle. In 1989, 19,813 pelts were taken for a market value of $1,067,916. Marten was the most valuable fur and made up 63% of the total harvest bringing in $670,807 in revenues.

TOURISM. In 1989 tourists spent an estimated $50m. Some 180,000 tourists visited in 1988.

COMMUNICATIONS

Roads. The Alaska Highway and its side roads connect Yukon's main communities with Alaska and the provinces and with adjacent mining centres. Interior roads connect the mining communities of Elsa (silver–lead), Faro (lead–zinc–silver) and Dawson City (gold) and mineral exploration properties (lead–zinc and tungsten) north of Ross River. The 727 km Dempster Highway north of Dawson City connects with Inuvik, on the Arctic coast; this highway, the first public road to be built to the Arctic ocean, was opened in Aug. 1979. The Carcross–Skagway road was opened in May 1979, providing a new access to the Pacific Ocean. There are 4,688 km of roads in the Territory, of which about 250 km are paved. The other major roads, including the Alaska Highway, have received a new surface treatment which resembles pavement and the rest are all-weather gravel of which 1,364 km are accessible during the summer months only.

Railways. The 176-km White Pass and Yukon Railway connected Whitehorse with year-round ocean shipping at Skagway, Alaska, but was closed in 1982. A modified passenger service was restarted in 1988 to take cruise ship tourists from Skagway to the White Pass summit and back. There are no plans to run the service all the way to Whitehorse.

Aviation. In 1990 one commercial airline provided regular daily service between Whitehorse, Watson Lake, Edmonton and Vancouver. A second airline provided a summer service from Whitehorse to Vancouver in 1990. Regularly scheduled air services extend from Whitehorse to interior communities of Faro, Mayo, Dawson City, Old Crow, Ross River and Watson Lake as well as to Yellowknife in the Northwest Territories and to Juneau and Fairbanks in Alaska, with connecting service to Anchorage and other points in Alaska, and Seattle (USA). There are several commercial operations offering charter services.

Shipping. The majority of goods are shipped into the Territory by truck over the Alaska and Stewart–Cassiar Highways. Some goods are shipped by barge to Skagway and Haines, Alaska, and then trucked to Whitehorse, for distribution throughout the Territory. The majority of goods are transported by road within the Territory, while a modest amount is shipped by air. Although navigable, the rivers are no longer used for shipping.

Telecommunications. There are 3 radio stations in Whitehorse and 12 low-power relay radio transmitters operated by CBC, as well as 3 operated by the Yukon Govenrment. CHON-FM, operated by Northern Native Broadcasting Society offers 12 hours of programming, 5 days a week, and is transmitted to virtually all Yukon communities by satellite. Dawson City has its own community run radio station, CFYT, which provides 15 hours of local programming 7 days a week. There are also 10 basic and 6 extended pay-cable TV channels in Whitehorse, and private cable operations in Faro and Watson Lake. Live CBC national television is provided by the Anik satellite to all communities in the Territory. All telephone and telecommunications in the Territory are provided by Northwestel, a subsidiary of Bell Canada Enterprises. Microwave stations and satellite ground stations now provide most of the telephone transmissions services to the communities.

Newspapers. In 1990 there were 2 newspapers, 1 published 5 days a week and 1 twice a week, in Whitehorse, and monthly papers in Faro and Dawson City. *Dann Zha*, a publication for native people, is a monthly. Other publications include a monthly newspaper aimed at the Francophone population, a quarterly produced by a women's organization in Whitehorse, and a private monthly magazine which is distributed free.

EDUCATION AND WELFARE

Education. The Yukon Department of Education owns and operates the Territory's 26 schools, both public and separate, from nursery school to grade 12. There are no private schools. In Sept. 1990 there were 366 teachers and 4,915 pupils. A separate francophone school opened in Sept. 1988. French immersion schooling is also offered at 2 schools. Yukon College provides post-secondary training at the main campus at Whitehorse and 13 community campuses throughout the territory. In Oct. 1990 some 600 full-time students were enrolled, and about 2,500 part-time. The Yukon government provides financial assistance to students whether they study at the College or outside the territory. Financial assistance is available to students of aboriginal descent from the federal Department of Indian Affairs and Northern Development.

Health. The health care system provides all residents with the care demanded by illness or accident. The federal government operates 1 general hospital at Whitehorse, 3 cottage hospitals, 2 nursing stations, with a total of 160 beds, 11 health centres and 4 health stations. The territorial government also operates a medical evacuation programme to send patients to Edmonton or Vancouver for specialized treatment not available in the Territory.

Further Reading

Annual Report of the Government of the Yukon.
Yukon Executive Council, *Statistical Review.*
Berton, P., *Klondike.* (Rev. ed.) Toronto, 1987
Coates, K. and Morrison, W., *Land of the Midnight Sun: A History of the Yukon.* Edmonton, 1988
Coults, R., *Yukon Places and Names.* Sidney, 1980
McClelland, C., *Part of the Land, Part of the Water.* Vancouver, 1987
Minter, R., *White Pass: Gateway to the Klondike.* Toronto, 1987

There is a Yukon Archive at Yukon College, Whitehorse.

CAPE VERDE

República de Cabo Verde

Capital: Praia
Population: 369,000 (1990)
GNP per capita: US$460 (1986)

HISTORY. The Cape Verde Islands were discovered in 1460 by Diogo Gomes, the first settlers arriving in 1462. In 1587 its administration was unified under a Portuguese governor. The colony became an Overseas Province on 11 June 1951.

On 30 Dec. 1974 Portugal transferred power to a transitional government headed by the Portuguese High Commissioner. Full independence was granted on 5 July 1975.

AREA AND POPULATION. Cape Verde is situated in the Atlantic Ocean 620 km WNW of Senegal and consists of 10 islands and 5 islets. Praia is the capital. The islands are divided into 2 groups, named Barlavento (windward) and Sotavento (leeward). The total area is 4,033 sq. km (1,557 sq. miles). The population (census, 1980) was 295,703. Estimate (1990) 369,000. About 600,000 Cape Verdeans live abroad.

The areas and populations (1980, census) of the islands are:

	Sq. km	*Population*		*Sq. km*	*Population*
Santo Antão	779	43,321	Maio	269	4,098
São Vicente [1]	227	41,594	São Tiago	991	145,957
São Nicolau	388	13,572	Fogo	476	30,978
Sal	216	5,826	Brava	67	6,985
Boa Vista	620	3,372			
			Sotavento	1,803	188,018
Barlovento	2,230	107,685			
			Total	4,033	295,703

[1] Includes Santa Luzia which is uninhabited.

The main towns (1980 census) are Praia, the capital (37,676) on São Tiago; and Mindelo (36,746) on São Vicente. 70% of the inhabitants are of mixed origins, and another 28% are black. Crioulo serves as the common language of the islands, although the official language is Portuguese.

Vital statistics (1985): Births, 10,949; deaths, 2,804.

CLIMATE. The climate is arid, with a cool dry season from Dec. to June and warm dry conditions for the rest of the year. Rainfall is sparse, rarely exceeding 5" (127 mm) in the northern islands or 12" (304 mm) in the southern ones. There are periodic severe droughts. Praia. Jan. 72°F (22·2°C), July 77°F (25°C). Annual rainfall 10" (250 mm).

CONSTITUTION AND GOVERNMENT. The Constitution adopted on 12 Feb. 1981 removed all reference to possible future union with Guinea-Bissau, and the *Partido Africano da Independencia de Cabo Verde* (PAICV), founded 20 Jan. 1981, became the sole legal party. The legislature consisted of a unicameral People's National Assembly of 83 members elected for 5 years by universal suffrage; it elects the President, who appoints and leads a Council of Ministers. Elections were held on 7 Dec. 1985.

In Sept. 1990 the People's National Assembly abolished the PAICV's sole right to rule.

Past President: Arístides Maria Pereira (assumed office 5 July 1975; re-elected 1981 and 1986).

Multi-party elections for a new National Assembly of 79 members were held in Jan. 1991. The electorate was 165,000. The Movement for Democracy (MPD) gained some 68% of votes cast and obtained 56 seats; the PAICV won 23 seats.

Presidential elections took place on 17 Feb. 1991. Antonio Mascarenhas Monteiro (b. 1943) was elected by 72% of votes cast, defeating the incumbent President Pereira.

Prime Minister: Carlos Veiga (MPD; b. 1949).

National flag: Horizontally yellow over green, with a vertical red strip in the hoist charged slightly above the centre with a black star surrounded by a wreath of maize, and beneath this a yellow clam shell.

Local government: There are 2 districts (Barlavento and Sotavento) sub-divided into 14 *conçelhos*. Barlavento comprises: Ribeira Grande, Paúl, Porto Novo (these 3 covering Santo Antão island), São Vicente (including Santa Luzia), São Nicolau, Sal, Boa Vista. Sotavento comprises: Maio, Praia, Santa Catarina, Tarrafal, Santa Cruz (these 4 covering São Tiago island), Fogo and Brava.

DEFENCE

Army. The Popular Revolutionary Armed Forces had a strength of 1,000 in 1991.

Navy. There are 5 fast patrol craft and 3 attack boats, all ex-Soviet, and 1 small hydrographic survey vessel. Personnel (1990), 200.

Air Force. An embryo air force operates two survivors of three An-26 twin-turboprop transports and has (1991) under 100 personnel.

INTERNATIONAL RELATIONS

Membership. Cape Verde is a member of the UN, OAU and an ACP state of the EEC.

ECONOMY

Budget. In 1984, the budget included revenue of 1,630m. escudos and expenditure, 2,134·5m.

Currency. The unit of currency is the *Cape Verde escudo* (CVE) of 100 *centavos*. There are coins of 20 and 50 *centavos* and of 1, 2½, 10, 20 and 50 *escudos*, and banknotes of 100, 500 and 1,000 *escudos*. In March 1991, 122·52 *Escudo* = £1 and 64·58 *Escudo* = US$1.

Banking and Finance. The Banco de Cabo Verde is the bank of issue and commercial bank, with branches at Praia, Mindelo and Espargos airport (Sal).

ENERGY AND NATURAL RESOURCES

Electricity. Production in 1986 amounted to 18m. kwh; capacity (1986), 14,000 kw.

Minerals. Salt is obtained on the islands of Sal, Boa Vista and Maio. Volcanic rock (pozzolana) is mined for export.

Agriculture. Mostly confined to irrigated inland valleys, the chief crops (production, 1988, in 1,000 tonnes) are: Coconuts, 10; sugar-cane, 16; bananas, 5; potatoes, 3; cassava, 4; sweet potatoes, 6; maize, 8; beans, groundnuts and coffee. Bananas and coffee are mainly for export.

Livestock (1988): 80,000 goats, 13,000 cattle, 70,000 pigs and 6,000 asses.

Fisheries. The catch in 1985 was 10,200 tonnes, of which tuna comprised 46%. About 200 tonnes of lobsters are caught annually.

FOREIGN ECONOMIC RELATIONS

Commerce. Imports in 1985 totalled 7,445m. escudos of which 27% came from Portugal, 22% from the Netherlands; exports in 1985 totalled 462m. escudos Caboverdianos, of which 31% went to Algeria, 30% to Portugal, 14% to Italy. In 1983, expatriated earnings from Cape Verdeans abroad totalled 2,800m. escudos. Exports: Fish, salt and bananas.

Total trade of Cape Verde with UK (British Department of Trade returns, in £1,000 sterling):

	1986	*1987*	*1988*	*1989*	*1990*
Imports to UK	426	301	132	178	336
Exports and re-exports from UK	1,618	1,208	1,812	2,301	1,537

COMMUNICATIONS

Roads. There were 2,250 km of roads (660 km paved) in 1984 and there were 3,000 private cars and 750 commercial vehicles.

Aviation. Amilcar Cabral International Airport, at Espargos on Sal, is a major refuelling point on flights to Africa and Latin America. Transportes Aéros de Cabo Verde provides regular services to smaller airports on most of the other islands.

Shipping. The main ports are Mindelo and Praia. In 1982 the ports handled 371,812 tonnes of imports and 146,822 tonnes of exports. In 1986, the merchant marine comprised 25 vessels of 14,095 GRT.

Telecommunications. There are 2 radio stations, at Praia and Mindelo; both are government-owned. There were (1985) 50,000 radio and 500 television receivers and (1984) 2,384 telephones.

JUSTICE, RELIGION, EDUCATION AND WELFARE

Justice. There is a network of People's Tribunals, with a Supreme Court in Praia.

Religion. In 1982, over 98% of the population were Roman Catholic.

Education. In 1987 there were 49,703 pupils and 1,464 teachers at 347 primary schools, 10,304 pupils and 321 teachers at 16 preparatory schools, 5,026 pupils and 170 teachers at 4 secondary schools, and 531 students and 52 teachers at a technical school. There were 211 students and 53 teachers in 3 teacher-training colleges and about 500 students were at foreign universities.

In 1981, 49% of the adult population were literate.

Health. In 1980 there were 21 hospitals and dispensaries with 632 beds; there were also 51 doctors, 3 dentists, 7 pharmacists, 9 midwives and 184 nursing personnel.

DIPLOMATIC REPRESENTATIVES

Of Cape Verde in Great Britain
Ambassador: Luis Fonseca (resides in The Hague).

Of Great Britain in Cape Verde
Ambassador: R. C. Beetham, LVO (resides in Dakar).

Of Cape Verde in the USA (3415 Massachusetts Ave., NW, Washington, D.C., 20007)
Ambassador: José Luis Fernandes Lopes.

Of the USA in Cape Verde (Rua Hojl Ya Yenna 81, Praia)
Ambassador: Francis T. McNamara.

Of Cape Verde to the United Nations
Ambassador: Humberto Bettencourt Santos.

Further Reading

Annuario Estatistico de Cabo Verde. Praia. Annual
Carreira, A., *The People of the Cape Verde Islands*. London, 1982
Foy, C., *Cape Verde: Politics, Economics and Society*. London, 1988
Shaw, C., *Cape Verde Islands:* [Bibliography]. Oxford and Santa Barbara, 1990

CAYMAN ISLANDS

Capital: George Town
Population: 25,355 (1990)
GNP per capita: US$18,000 (1990)

HISTORY. The islands were discovered by Columbus on 10 May 1503 and (with Jamaica) were recognized as British possessions by the Treaty of Madrid in 1670. Grand Cayman was settled in 1734 and the other islands in 1833. They became a separate Crown Colony on 4 July 1959, administered by the same governor as Jamaica until the latter's independence on 6 Aug. 1962 when they received their own Administrator (From 1972 a governor).

AREA AND POPULATION. Cayman Islands consist of Grand Cayman, Little Cayman and Cayman Brac. Situated in the Caribbean Sea, about 200 miles NW of Jamaica. Area, 100 sq. miles (260 sq. km). Census population of 1989, 25,355 (13,202 Caymanians by birth). The spoken language is English. The chief town is George Town, census (1989) 12,921. Vital statistics (1989): Births, 438; marriages, 267; deaths, 113.

The areas and populations of the islands are:

	Sq. km	*Census 1979*	*Census 1989*
Grand Cayman	197	15,000	23,881
Cayman Brac	36	1,607	1,441
Little Cayman	26	70	33

CLIMATE. The climate is tropical maritime, with a cool season from Nov. to March and temperatures some 10°F warmer for the remaining months. Rainfall averages 56" (1,400 mm) a year at George Town. Hurricanes may be experienced between July and Nov.

CONSTITUTION AND GOVERNMENT. A new Constitution came into force in Aug. 1972. The Legislative Assembly consists of the Governor (as President), 3 official members, and 12 elected members.

The Executive Council consists of the Governor (as Chairman), the 3 official members and 4 elected members elected by the elected members of the Legislative Assembly.

Governor: A. J. Scott, CVO, CBE.

Flag: British Blue Ensign with the arms of the Colony on a white disc in the fly.

ECONOMY

Budget. Revenue 1990, CI$112m.; expenditure, CI$110·8m. Public debt (31 Dec. 1989), CI$19·4m.; total reserves, CI$18·2m.

Currency. The unit of currency is the *Cayman Island dollar* (KYD), divided into 100 *cents*. In March 1991, £1 = 1·58 CI$; US$1 = 0·83.

Banking and Finance. 540 commercial banks and trust companies held licences in Oct. 1990, which permit the holders to offer services to the public, over 30 domestically. Barclays Bank PLC has offices at George Town and Cayman Brac. Financial services are the Islands' chief industry.

INDUSTRY

Electricity. Production (1989) 182·1m. kwh.

Industry. In 1990 over 21,000 companies were registered in the islands.

FOREIGN ECONOMIC RELATIONS

Commerce. Exports, 1989 (f.o.b.), totalled CI$2·1m. Imports, (c.i.f.), CI$215·6m.; principally foodstuffs, manufactured items, textiles, building materials, automobiles and petroleum products.

Total trade between Cayman Islands and UK (British Department of Trade returns, in £1,000 sterling):

	1987	*1988*	*1989*	*1990*
Imports to UK	1,318	9,858	8,693	2,262
Exports and re-exports from UK	6,442	5,051	5,174	13,394

Tourism. Tourism is the chief industry, after financial services, and there were (1989) 2,476 beds in hotels and 2,702 in apartments, guesthouses and cottages. There were 617,769 visitors in 1989, including 203,818 by air, an increase of 15% over 1988.

COMMUNICATIONS

Roads. There were (1990) about 150 miles of road and 12,154 (1989) motor vehicles.

Aviation. Cayman Airways provides regular services between Grand Cayman and Miami, Houston, Tampa, Atlanta, New York and Jamaica. Pan American, American and Northwest Airlines provide a daily service between Miami and Grand Cayman. CAL provides a regular inter-island service. Air Jamaica also provides services between Grand Cayman and Jamaica.

Shipping. Motor vessels ply regularly between the Cayman Islands, Jamaica, Costa Rica and Florida. Shipping registered at George Town, 450 vessels (June 1990).

Telecommunications. There were 18,153 telephones in 1989 and there are 2 radio broadcasting stations in the islands, with (1989) an estimated 20,000 receivers.

Newspapers. The *Caymanian Compass* is published 5 days a week and *The New Caymanian*, weekly.

JUSTICE, RELIGION, EDUCATION AND WELFARE

Justice. There is a Grand Court, sitting 6 times a year for criminal sessions at George Town under a Chief Justice and 2 puisne judges. There are 2 Magistrates presiding over the Summary Court, which sits at other times.

Religion. There are Anglican, Roman Catholic, Presbyterian and other Christian communities represented in the islands.

Education. In 1989 there were 10 government primary schools with 1,407 pupils, 6 private elementary schools with 956 pupils and 3 private secondary schools with 323 pupils. Post-primary education at the government high schools and the government middle school was attended by 1,811 pupils. There is also a private institution for tertiary education; a government school for special educational needs; a government-operated community college offering technical, vocational and business studies, as well as adult, educational and recreational courses; and a centre for training of handicapped persons.

Health. In 1989 there was a fully-equipped general hospital in George Town with 21 doctors, a dental clinic, 4 district clinics and a hospital in Cayman Brac.

Further Reading

Annual Report, 1990. Cayman Islands Government, 1990
Statistical Abstract of the Cayman Islands, 1989. Cayman Islands Government Statistics Unit, 1989

CENTRAL AFRICAN REPUBLIC

Capital: Bangui
Population: 2·9m. (1988)
GNP per capita: US$390 (1988)

République Centrafricaine

HISTORY. Central African Republic became independent on 13 Aug. 1960, after having been one of the 4 territories of French Equatorial Africa (under the name of Ubangi Shari) and from 1 Dec. 1958 a member state of the French Community. A new Constitution was adopted in 1976 and it provided for the country to be a parliamentary democracy and to be known as the Central African Empire. President Bokassa became Emperor Bokassa I. The Emperor was overthrown in a coup on 20–21 Sept. 1979 and the empire was abolished. On 15 March 1981 David Dacko was re-elected President but Army Chief General André Kolingba took power in a bloodless coup on 1 Sept. 1981 at the head of a Military Committee for National Recovery (CMRN), which held supreme power until 21 Sept. 1985 when President Kolingba dissolved it and initiated a return towards constitutional rule.

AREA AND POPULATION. The Central African Republic is bounded north by Chad, east by Sudan, south by Zaïre and Congo, and west by Cameroon. The area covers 622,436 sq. km (240,324 sq. miles); its population in 1975 (census), 2,054,610 and estimate in 1988 was 2,899,376 of which 37% urban. The capital is Bangui (596,776 inhabitants in 1988).

The areas, populations and capitals of the prefectures are as follows:

Prefecture	*Sq. km*	*Estimate 1988*	*Capital*	*Estimate 1988*
Bangui [1]	67	596,776	Bangui	596,776
Ombella-M'poko	31,835	137,469	Boali	...
Lobaye	19,235	174,134	M'baiki	29,495
Sangha [2]	19,412	62,977	Nola	...
Haute-Sangha	30,203	253,717	Berbérati	45,432
Nana-Mambere	26,600	213,630	Bouar	49,166
Ouham-Pende	32,100	258,166	Bozoum	22,600
Ouham	50,250	292,132	Bossangoa	41,877
Gribingui [2]	19,996	92,558	Kaga-Bandoro	19,774
Bamingui-Bangoran	58,200	31,082	Ndele	...
Vakaga	46,500	25,629	Birao	...
Kemo-Gribingui	17,204	84,884	Sibut	22,214
Ouaka	49,900	235,277	Bambari	52,092
Basse-Kotto	17,604	199,830	Mobaye	...
Haute-Kotto	86,650	57,583	Bria	24,620
M'bomou	61,150	143,971	Bangassou	36,254
Haut-M'bomou	55,530	39,560	Obo	...

[1] Autonomous commune. [2] Economic prefecture.

French is the official language.

CLIMATE. A tropical climate with little variation in temperature. The wet months are May, June, Oct. and Nov. Bangui. Jan. 80°F (26·5°C), July 77°F (25°C). Annual rainfall 61" (1,525 mm). Ndeie. Jan. 83°F (28·3°C), July 77°F (25°C). Annual rainfall 57" (1,417 mm).

CONSTITUTION AND GOVERNMENT. Under the Constitution adopted by a national referendum on 21 Nov. 1986, the sole legal political party is the *Rassemblement Démocratique Centrafricaine (RDC)*. Legislative elections for the 52-member National Assembly were held on 31 July 1987. The President is elected by popular vote for a term of 6 years, and appoints and leads a Council of Ministers.

The Council of Ministers in Jan. 1991 was composed as follows:

President of the Republic and of the RDC, Minister of Defence. Gen. André Kolingba (assumed office 1 Sept. 1981, re-elected 21 Nov. 1986).

Prime Minister: Edouard Frank.

Foreign Affairs: Michel Gbezera-Bria. *Interior, Territorial Administration:* Christophe Grelombe. *Economy, Finance, Planning and International Co-operation:* Dieudonné Wazoua. *National and Higher Education:* Jean Louis Psimhis. *Transport and Civil Aviation:* Pierre Gonifei-Ngaibounanou. *Civil Service, Labour, Social Security and Professional Training:* Daniel Sehoulia. *Justice, Keeper of the Seals:* Thomas Mapouka. *Public Health and Social Affairs:* Jean Willybiro-Sako. *Rural Development:* Théodore Bagayambo. *Energy and Mines, Geology and Hydrology:* Michel Salle. *Tourism, Water Resources, Forestry, Hunting and Fishing:* Raymond Mbitikon. *Trade and Industry, Small and Medium-sized Enterprises:* Thimothée Marboua. *Posts and Telecommunications:* Hugues Dobozendji. *Public Works and Territorial Planning:* Jacques Kithe. *Information, Arts and Culture:* Jean Bengue. *Parliamentary Relations, Secretary to Council of Ministers:* Edouard Franck.

There are also 5 Secretaries of State.

National flag: Four horizontal stripes of blue, white, green, yellow; over all in the centre a vertical red strip, and in the canton a yellow star.

Local Government: Central African Republic is divided into 14 prefectures (sub-divided into 50 sub-prefectures); 2 'economic prefectures' and the autonomous commune of Bangui (the capital).

DEFENCE. Selective national service for a 2-year period is in force. There are some 2,700 personnel in the para-military gendarmerie. Some 1,200 French military personnel were stationed in 1991.

Army. The Army consisted (1991) of about 3,500 men, comprising a Republican Guard, a territorial defence and combined arms regiments. Equipment includes 4 T-55 tanks, 39 armoured personnel carriers and 10 Ferret scout cars.

Navy. The naval wing of the army has 9 river patrol craft and (1990) 85 personnel.

Air Force. The Air Force has 2 Rallye Guerrier armed light aircraft, 1 twin-jet Caravelle, 1 DC-4 and 2 C-47 transports, 2 Reims-Cessna 337, 6 Aermacchi AL.60 and 5 Broussard liaison aircraft, 1 Alouette and 1 Ecureuil helicopters. It also maintains and operates the government's Caravelle and Falcon 20 twin-jet VIP aircraft. Personnel strength (1991) about 300.

INTERNATIONAL RELATIONS

Membership. Central African Republic is a member of the UN, OAU and an ACP state of the EEC.

ECONOMY

Policy. The new recovery plan (1983–86) provided for expenditure of 31,300m. francs CFA for development of agriculture, transport and infrastructure.

Budget. The budget for 1987 provided for expenditure of 56,610m. francs CFA, and for revenue of 46,230m. francs CFA.

Currency. The unit of currency is the *franc CFA* with a parity of 50 *francs CFA* to 1 French *franc*. There are coins of 1, 2, 5, 10, 25, 50, 100 and 500 *francs CFA*, and banknotes of 100, 500, 1,000, 5,000 and 10,000 *francs CFA*. In March 1991, £1 = 496·13 *francs CFA*; US$1 = 261·53 *francs CFA*.

Banking. The *Banque des Etats de l'Afrique Centrale* is the bank of issue.

ENERGY AND NATURAL RESOURCES

Electricity. Production in 1987 totalled 92m. kwh. Supply 220 volts; 50 Hz.

Minerals. In 1986 258,701 carats of gem diamonds, 98,678 carats of industrial diamonds and (1987) 224 kg of gold were mined. There are significant regions of uranium in the Bakouma area.

Agriculture. Over 86% of the working population is occupied in subsistence agriculture. The main crops (production 1988, in 1,000 tonnes) are cassava, 400; groundnuts, 85; bananas, 86; plantains, 66; millet, 50; maize, 64; seed cotton, 43; coffee, 22; rice, 12.

Livestock (1988): Cattle, 2,313,000; goats, 1,159,000; sheep, 120,000; pigs, 382,000.

Forestry. There are 35·8m. ha of forest, representing 58% of the land area. The extensive hardwood forests, particularly in the south-west, provide mahogany, obeche and limba for export. Production (1985) 3·42m. cu. metres.

Fisheries. Catch (1983) 13,000 tonnes.

INDUSTRY. The small industrial sector includes factories producing cotton fabrics, footwear, beer and radios.

FOREIGN ECONOMIC RELATIONS

Commerce. Imports and exports in 1m. francs CFA:

	1984	*1985*	*1986*	*1987*
Imports	77,700	90,370	96,677	...
Exports	50,057	58,720	44,960	39,180

In 1983, France took 30% of exports and provided 46% of imports. Of all exports, coffee comprised 29% (by value), diamonds 24%, timber 19% and cotton 13%.

Total trade of Central African Republic with UK (British Department of Trade returns, in £1,000 sterling):

	1987	*1988*	*1989*	*1990*
Imports to UK	233	195	418	58
Exports and re-exports from UK	1,127	733	1,630	1,669

Tourism. There were about 4,000 visitors in 1986.

COMMUNICATIONS

Roads. In 1986 there were 20,286 km of roads, of which 442 km bitumenized and (1984) 46,982 vehicles in use.

Railways. There are no railways, but a proposal existed (1985) for an 800 km line (1,435 mm gauge) from Bangui through Cameroon and Congo to connect with the Trans-Gabon railway at Belinga.

Aviation. There are international airports at Mpoko, near Bangui, and Berbérati. Air Centrafrique operates extensive internal services to several airstrips.

Shipping. Timber and barges are taken to Brazzaville (Congo).

Telecommunications. There were (1982) 1,200 television and (1986) 125,000 radio receivers and 3,323 telephones.

Cinemas. In 1987 there were 5 cinemas.

Newspapers. In 1984 there was one daily newspaper.

JUSTICE, RELIGION, EDUCATION AND WELFARE

Justice. The Criminal Court and Supreme Court are situated in Bangui. There are 16 high courts throughout the country.

Religion. About 57% of the population follow animist beliefs, 20% are Roman Catholic, 15% Protestant and 8% Moslem.

Education. The University of Bangui was founded in 1970 and had 1,489 students in 1980. In 1986-87 there were 274,179 pupils at primary schools and 44,804 at secondary schools; technical schools (1984-85) had 2,514 students, while (1982) 327 were at the 2 teacher-training establishments.

Health. In 1984 there were 104 hospitals and health centres with 3,774 beds; there were also 112 doctors, 6 dentists, 16 pharmacists, 168 midwives and 710 nursing personnel.

DIPLOMATIC REPRESENTATIVES

Of Central African Republic in Great Britain
Ambassador: (Vacant).

Of Great Britain in Central African Republic
Ambassador: M. Reith (resides in Yaoundé).

Of Central African Republic in the USA (1618 22nd St., NW, Washington, D.C. 20008)
Ambassador: Jean-Pierre Sohahong-Kombet.

Of the USA in Central African Republic (Ave. President Dacko, Bangui)
Ambassador: Daniel H. Simpson.

Of Central African Republic to the United Nations
Ambassador: Jean-Pierre Sohahong-Kombet.

Further Reading

Kalck, H. P., *Historical Dictionary of the Central African Republic*. Metuchen, 1980

CHAD

Capital: N'djaména
Population: 5·54m. (1990)
GNP per capita: US$160 (1988)

République du Tchad

HISTORY. France proclaimed a protectorate over Chad on 5 Sept. 1900, and in July 1908 the territory was incorporated into French Equatorial Africa. It became a separate colony March 1920, and in 1946 one of the four constituent territories of French Equatorial Africa. On 28 Nov. 1958 Chad became an autonomous republic within the French Community and achieved full independence on 11 Aug. 1960, although the northern prefecture of Borkou-Ennedi-Tibesti remained under French military administration until 1965.

Conflicts between the central government and secessionist groups, particularly in the Moslem north and centre of Chad, began in 1965 and flared into a prolonged and confused civil war that continued under different protagonists, with occasional pauses during attempts at reconciliation. On 7 June 1982 the *Forces Armées du Nord* (FAN) led by Hissène Habré gained control of the country. In June 1983 the Libyan-backed forces of former President Goukouni Oueddei re-occupied Bourkou-Ennedi-Tibesti, but by April 1987 most of the rebels rallied to the government side, which then forced the Libyans back into the Aozou Strip, a 114,000 sq. km region in the extreme north of Chad occupied by Libyan forces since 1973. A ceasefire took effect on 11 Sept. 1987. There was an attempted coup on 1 April 1989.

Rebel forces of the Popular Salvation Movement led by Idriss Deby entered Chad from Sudan in Nov. 1990 and, meeting little resistance, overcame the government forces of President Hissène Habré, who took refuge in Cameroon. On 4 Dec. 1990 Deby declared himself President.

AREA AND POPULATION. Chad is bounded west by Cameroon, Nigeria and Niger, north by Libya, east by Sudan and south by the Central African Republic. Area, 1,284,000 sq. km; its population in 1990 was estimated at 5,540,000 (32% urban; census 1975, 4,029,917). The capital is N'djaména with 594,700 inhabitants in 1988, other large towns being Sarh (113,400), Moundou (102,800), Abéché (83,000), Bongor (35,600) and Doba (34,000).

The areas, populations and chief towns of the 14 prefectures were:

Préfecture	*sq. km*	*Population Estimate 1988*	*Capital*
Borkou-Ennedi-Tibesti	600,350	109,000	Faya (Largeau)
Biltine	46,850	216,000	Biltine
Ouaddaï	76,240	422,000	Abéché
Batha	88,800	431,000	Ati
Kanem	114,520	245,000	Mao
Lac	22,320	165,000	Bol
Chari-Baguirmi	82,910	844,000	N'djaména
Guéra	58,950	254,000	Mongo
Salamat	63,000	131,000	Am Timan
Moyen-Chari	45,180	646,000	Sarh
Logone Oriental	28,035	377,000	Doba
Logone Occidental	8,695	365,000	Moundou
Tandjilé	18,045	371,000	Laï
Mayo-Kabbi	30,105	852,000	Bongor

The official languages are French and Arabic, but more than 100 different languages and dialects are spoken. The largest ethnic group is the Sara of southern Chad.

CLIMATE. A tropical climate, with adequate rainfall in the south, though Nov. to April are virtually rainless months. Further north, desert conditions prevail. N'djaména. Jan. 75°F (23·9°C), July 82°F (27·8°C). Annual rainfall 30" (744 mm).

CONSTITUTION AND GOVERNMENT. Hissène Habré was sworn in as President on 21 Oct. 1982 and appointed a Council of Ministers. A provisional constitution had been promulgated on 29 Sept. 1982, under which an official political party was established in 1984, the *Union nationale pour l'independence et la révolution* (UNIR). A National Consultative Assembly was set up on 21 Oct. 1982. On 10 Dec. 1989, in a referendum, the electorate adopted a new Constitution and voted for the President to continue in office for a further 7 years. In July 1990 a Legislative Assembly of 123 deputies replaced the National Consultative Assembly.

After overthrowing the regime of Hissène Habré, Idriss Deby proclaimed himself *President* and was sworn in on 4 March 1991.

A National Salvation Council and a State Council have been set up. In March 1991 the National Salvation Council introduced a national charter to be in force for 30 months. This provides for a 31-member consultative Provisional Republican Council.

Prime Minister: Jean Alingué Bawoyeu.

National flag: Three vertical strips of blue, yellow, red.

Local Government: The 14 *préfectures* are divided into 53 *sous-préfectures.*

DEFENCE

Army. The Army includes 3 infantry and 1 armoured battalions with 2 artillery batteries. Equipment includes 63 armoured fighting vehicles. In 1991 the strength was over 17,000 and there was a paramilitary force of 5,700.

Air Force. The Air Force has 3 C-130 Hercules, 1 VIP Caravelle, 1 C-54, 2 Aviocar and 6 C-47 transports, 4 Reims-Cessna F337 light aircraft, 2 Turbo-Porters, 2 Broussard communications aircraft, 2 Gazelle helicopters, 2 armed PC-7 aircraft and 2 SF.260W Warrior trainers. Personnel (1991) about 200.

INTERNATIONAL RELATIONS

Membership. Chad is a member of the UN, OAU and is an ACP state of the EEC.

ECONOMY

Budget. The budget for 1990 envisaged expenditure of 39,705m. francs CFA and revenue, 33,400m. francs CFA.

Currency. The unit of currency is the *franc CFA* with a parity value of 50 *francs CFA* to 1 French *franc*. In March 1991, £1 = 496·13 *francs*; US$1 = 261·53 *francs*.

Banking. The *Banque des Etats de l'Afrique Centrale* is the bank of issue, and the principal commercial banks are the *Banque de Développement du Tchad* and the *Banque Tchadienne de Crédit et de Dépôts*.

ENERGY AND NATURAL RESOURCES

Electricity. Production (1989) amounted to 80m. kwh. Supply 220 volts; 50 Hz.

Oil. The oilfield in Kanem préfecture has been linked by pipeline to a new refinery at Laï (in Tandjilé) but production has remained minimal due to war disruption.

Minerals. Salt (about 4,000 tonnes per annum) is mined around Lake Chad, and deposits of uranium, gold and bauxite are to be exploited.

Agriculture. Cotton growing (in the south) and animal husbandry (in the central zone) are the most important industries. Production (1988, in 1,000 tonnes) was: Millet, 695; sugar-cane, 290; yams, 240; seed cotton, 112; groundnuts, 78; cassava, 330; rice, 52; dry beans, 42; sweet potatoes, 46; mangoes, 32; dates, 32; maize, 47; cotton lint, 37; cotton seed, 68.

Livestock: Cattle (1990), 4,299,205; sheep (1988), 2·25m.; goats, 2·25m.; chickens, 4m.

Fisheries. Fish production from Lake Chad and the Chari and Logone rivers, was estimated at 110,000 tonnes in 1986.

INDUSTRY. Cotton ginning is the principal activity, undertaken in 51 mills.

Sugar refineries produced 37,309 tonnes in 1989. A textile factory produced 10·3m. metres of woven fabric in 1989, a brewery 114,700 hectolitres of beer and a cigarette factory 186m. cigarettes. There are also rice and flour mills and other factories involved in food processing or light industry.

FOREIGN ECONOMIC RELATIONS

Commerce. Trade (in 1m. francs CFA):

	1988	*1989*	*1990*
Imports	68,029	75,103	77,743
Exports	42,901	46,571	51,502

The main trading partners are France and Nigeria. Cotton formed 91% of exports in 1983.

Total trade with UK (British Department of Trade returns, in £1,000 sterling):

	1986	*1987*	*1988*	*1989*	*1990*
Imports to UK	2,806	1,101	1,764	822	369
Exports and re-exports from UK	1,250	1,006	639	3,462	1,567

COMMUNICATIONS

Roads. In 1983 there were 40,000 km of roads, of which only 400 km are surfaced. In 1985 there were 3,000 private cars and 4,000 lorries and buses.

Aviation. There is an international airport at N'djaména, from which UTA and Air Afrique run 4 flights per week to Paris; there are also flights to Bangui and Kinshasa. Air Tchad operates internal services to 12 secondary airports.

Telecommunications. In 1978 there were 3,850 telephones and (1985), 1·1m. radios in use.

JUSTICE, RELIGION, EDUCATION AND WELFARE

Justice. There are criminal courts and magistrates courts in N'djaména, Moundou, Sarh and Abéché, with a Court of Appeal situated in N'djaména.

Religion. The northern and central parts of the country are predominantly Moslem (44% of the total population) and the southern part is mainly animist (38%) or Christian (17%).

Education. In 1987 there were 300,000 pupils in primary schools, 42,000 in secondary schools, and 4,000 in technical schools and teacher-training establishments. The University of Chad (founded 1971) at N'djaména had (1984) 1,643 students and 141 teaching staff.

Health. There were 33 hospitals with 3,353 beds in 1977 and in 1978 90 doctors, 4 dentists, 9 pharmacists, 98 midwives and 993 nursing personnel.

DIPLOMATIC REPRESENTATIVES

Of Chad in Great Britain
Ambassador: Abdoulaye Lamana (resides in Brussels).

Of Great Britain in Chad
Chargé d'affaires: J. Cummins, MBE (resides in London).

Of Chad in the USA (2002 R. St., NW, Washington, D.C., 20009)
Ambassador: Mahamat Ali Adoum.

Of the USA in Chad (Ave., Felix Eboue, N'djaména)
Ambassador: Richard W. Bogosian.

Of Chad to the United Nations
Ambassador: Mahamat Ali Adoum.

Further Reading

Kelley, M. P., *Conditions of the State's Survival.* Oxford, 1986
Thompson, V. and Adloff, R., *Conflict in Chad.* London and Berkeley, 1981
Westebbe, R., *Chad: Development Potential and Constraints.* Washington, D.C., 1974

CHILE

República de Chile

Capital: Santiago
Population: 12·96m. (1990)
GNP per capita: US$1,510 (1988)

HISTORY. The Republic of Chile threw off allegiance to the crown of Spain, constituting a national government on 18 Sept. 1810, finally freeing itself from Spanish rule in 1818.

The Marxist coalition government of President Salvador Allende Gossens was ousted on 11 Sept. 1973 by the armed services, which formed a government headed by a junta of the four Commanders-in-Chief. Gen. Augusto Pinochet Ugarte, Commander-in-Chief of the Army, took over the presidency. President Allende committed suicide on the day of the coup.

The new government assumed wide-ranging powers. A constitution of 1981 provided for an eventual return to democracy. Gen. Pinochet was rejected as president in a plebiscite in 1988. Patricio Aylwyn Azócar was elected president in Dec. 1989.

AREA AND POPULATION. Chile is bounded in the north by Peru, east by Bolivia and Argentina, and south and west by the Pacific ocean.

Chile has an area of 736,905 sq. km (284,520 sq. miles) excluding the claimed Antarctic territory. Many islands to the west and south belong to Chile: The Islas Juan Fernández (179 sq. km with 516 inhabitants in 1982) lie about 600 km west of Valparaíso, and the volcanic Isla de Pascua (Easter Island or Rapa Nui, 118 sq. km with 1,867 inhabitants in 1982), discovered in 1722, lies about 3,000 km WNW of Valparaíso. Small uninhabited dependencies include Sala y Goméz (400 km east of Easter Is.), San Ambrosio and San Félix (1,000 km northwest of Valparaíso, and 20 km apart) and Islas Diego Ramírez (100 km SW of Cape Horn).

In 1940 Chile declared, and in each subsequent year has reaffirmed, its ownership of the sector of the Antarctic lying between 53° and 90° W. long.; and asserted that the British claim to the sector between the meridians 20° and 80° W. long. overlapped the Chilean by 27°. Seven Chilean bases exist in Antarctica. A law promulgated 21 July 1955 put the Intendente (*now* Gobernador) of the Province (*now* Region) of Magallanes in charge of the 'Chilean Antarctic Territory' which has an area of 1,269,723 sq. km. and a population (1982) of 1,368.

The total population at the census in 1982 was 11,275,440. Estimate (1990) 12,958,000.

The areas of the 13 regions and their populations (census, 1982) were as follows:

Region	*Sq. km*	*Census 1982*	*Capital*	*Estimate 1987*
Tarapacá	58,786	273,427	Iquique	132,948
Antofagasta	125,253	341,203	Antofagasta	204,577
Atacama	74,705	183,071	Copiapó	70,241 [1]
Coquimbo	40,656	419,178	La Serena	106,617
Aconcagua	16,396	1,204,693	Valparaíso	278,762
Metropolitan	15,549	4,294,938	Santiago	4,858,342
Liberador	16,456	584,989	Rancagua	172,489
Maule	30,518	723,224	Talca	164,482
Bíobío	36,939	1,516,552	Concepción	294,375
Araucanía	31,946	692,924	Temuco	217,789
Los Lagos	67,247	843,430	Puerto Montt	113,488
Aisén	108,997	65,478	Coihaique	31,167 [1]
Magallanes	132,034	132,333	Punta Arenas	111,724

[1] Census, 1982

Vital statistics (1984): Birth rate 21·2 per 1,000 population; death rate, 6·3; marriage rate, 7 (1982); infantile mortality rate, 20·1 per 1,000 live births. Life expectancy (1981): Men, 65·4 years, women, 70·1.

Over 92% of the population is mixed or *mestizo*; only about 2% are European immigrants and their descendants, while the remainder are indigenous Amerindians of the Araucanian, Fuegian and Chango groups. Language and culture remain of European origin, with the 675,000 Araucanian-speaking (mainly Mapuche) Indians the only sizeable minority.

Other large towns (estimate, 1987) are: Viña del Mar (297,294), Talcahuano (231,356), Arica (169,774), San Bernardo (168,534), Puente Alto (165,534), Chillán (148,805), Los Angeles (126,122), Osorno (122,462), Valdívia (117,205), Calama (109,645), Coquimbo (105,252) and Quilpué (103,004).

CLIMATE. With its enormous range of latitude and the influence of the Andean Cordillera, the climate of Chile is very complex, ranging from extreme aridity in the north, through a Mediterranean climate in Central Chile, where winters are wet and summers dry, to a cool temperate zone in the south, with rain at all seasons. In the extreme south, conditions are very wet and stormy. Santiago. Jan. 67°F (19·5°C), July 46°F (8°C). Annual rainfall 15" (375 mm). Antofagasta. Jan. 69°F (20·6°C), July 57°F (14°C). Annual rainfall 0·5" (12·7 mm). Valparaíso. Jan. 64°F (17·8°C), July 53°F (11·7°C). Annual rainfall 20" (505 mm).

CONSTITUTION AND GOVERNMENT. The Government of President Pinochet had assumed wide-ranging powers but the 'state of siege' ended in March 1978. A new Constitution was approved by 67·5% of the voters on 11 Sept. 1980 and came into force on 11 March 1981. It provided for a return to democracy after a minimum period of 8 years. Gen. Pinochet would remain in office during this period after which the Government would nominate a single candidate for President.

A plebiscite was held on 5 Oct. 1988 with President Pinochet as the candidate to be approved or rejected by the people, to continue for 8 more years. Votes against 54·6%, votes in favour 43·31%.

The following is a list of the presidents since 1946:

Gabriel González Videla, 3 Nov. 1946–3 Nov. 1952.
Carlos Ibáñez del Campo, 3 Nov. 1952–3 Nov. 1958.
Jorge Alessandri Rodriguez, 3 Nov. 1958–3 Nov. 1964.
Eduardo Frei Montalva, 3 Nov. 1964–3 Nov. 1970.
Salvador Allende Gossens, 3 Nov. 1970–11 Sept. 1973 (deposed).
Gen. Augusto Pinochet, 17 Dec. 1974-11 March 1990.

President of the Republic: At the presidential elections of 14 Dec. 1989 Patricio Aylwyn Azócar obtained 55·2% of the vote. He assumed office on 11 March 1990.

In Feb. 1991 the Cabinet comprised *Foreign Affairs:* Enrique Silva Cimma. *Agriculture:* Juan Agustin Figueroa. *Interior:* Enrique Krauss. *Justice:* Francisco Cumplido. *Defence:* Patricio Rojas. *Finance:* Alejandro Foxley. *Labour:* Rene Cortázar. *Health:* Jorge Jiménez. *Mining:* Juan Hamilton. *National Planning:* Serglo Molina. *Presidential Secretary:* Edgardo Boeninger. *General Secretary of the Government:* Enrique Correa. *Economy:* Carlos Ominami. *Education:* Ricardo Lagos. *Transportation:* Germán Correa. *National Property:* Luis Alvarado. *Energy:* Jaime Toha. *Public Works:* Carlos Hurtado. *Corporation for Promotion of Production:* Rene Abeliuk. *Housing:* Alberto Etchegaray.

National flag: Two horizontal bands, white, red, with a white star on blue square in top sixth next to staff.

National anthem: Dulce patria, recibe los votos ('Sweet Fatherland, receive the vows'; words by E. Lillo, 1847; tune by Ramón Carnicer, 1828).

Local Government. For the purposes of local government the Military Junta in pursuance of its policy of administrative decentralization divided the republic into 13 regions (12 and Greater Santiago). Each region is presided over by an intendent, while the provinces (51) included in it are in charge of a governor who represents the central government. The provinces are divided into municipalities under a mayor. All these officials are appointed by the President.

DEFENCE. Military service is for a period of 2 years at the age of 19.

Army. The Army is organized in 6 divisions, each with infantry, armoured cavalry, artillery, mountain and engineer regiments; and 1 helicopter-borne ranger unit. Equipment includes 60 M-4A3, 150 M-51 and 21 AMX-30 tanks, 157 light tanks and 500 armoured personnel carriers. The service operates over 80 aircraft. Strength (1991) 54,000 (30,800 conscripts) with 80,000 reserves.

Navy. The principal ships of the Chilean Navy are the 1937-vintage ex-US cruiser *O'Higgins*, of 13,700 tonnes, armed with 9 152mm guns and 8 127mm. She carries one light helicopter. There are also 4 ex-British 'County'-class guided missile armed destroyers renamed *Capitan Prat, Almirante Cochrane, Almirante Latorre,* and *Blanco Encalada*, purchased on their disposal from the Royal Navy between 1982 and 1987. The last named has had the Sea Slug launcher removed and replaced with an extended helicopter hangar and flight deck.

There are also 2 small modern West German-built diesel submarines, 2 British Oberon class submarines, 4 other destroyers (2 British-built in 1960, and 2 ex-US dating from 1944), 2 British Leander class frigates, 2 fast missile craft, 4 torpedo boats, 5 offshore patrol vessels and 26 coastal craft. There are 3 French-built medium landing ships. Major auxiliaries include 2 tankers, 1 submarine support vessel, 2 landing craft, 1 survey ship, 4 transports, 2 training ships and 1 Antarctic patrol ship.

The Naval Air Service has 4 squadrons of maritime patrol aircraft, transports, anti-submarine helicopters and trainers.

Naval personnel in 1990 totalled 29,000 all ranks (3,000 conscripts) including 5,200 marines and 500 in the naval air service.

A separate Coast Guard numbering 1,600 operates 13 patrol craft and a helicopter.

Air Force. Strength (1991) is 12,800 personnel (800 conscripts), with (1987) 105 first-line and 150 second-line aircraft, divided among 12 groups, each comprising 1 squadron, within 4 combat and support wings. Groups 1 and 12 have twin-jet A-37Bs, from a total of 34 acquired for light strike/reconnaissance duties. Group 2 is equipped for photo-reconnaissance with 2 Canberras. Group 4 has 13 Mirage 50 fighters. Group 5 has 14 Twin Otters for light transport and survey duties. Group 7 has 12 F-5E Tiger II fighter-bombers and 2 F-5F trainers. Groups 8 and 9 are also fighter-bomber units, with a total of 30 Hunter F.71s, ex-RAF FGA.9s, and T.72s. Group 10 is a transport wing, with 2 C-130H Hercules, 2 Boeing 707s, 3 Douglas piston-engined transports and various helicopters. An aerial survey unit has 2 Learjets and 3 Beech twin-engined aircraft. Training aircraft include piston-engined Piper Dakota and T-35 Pillan basic trainers and licence-built CASA C-101BB Aviojets. CASA C-101CC Aviojet light strike aircraft were being delivered in 1989.

INTERNATIONAL RELATIONS

Membership. Chile is a member of the UN, OAS and LAIA (formerly LAFTA).

ECONOMY

Budget. In 1987 revenue was US$8,469·8m. and expenditure, US$8,421·6m.

Currency. The unit of currency is the *Chilean peso* (CLP) of 100 *centavos*.

On 31 Dec. 1987 notes and coins in circulation were 161,337m. pesos.

In March 1991 there were 640·20 *pesos* = £1 and 337·48 *pesos* = US$1.

Banking. There is a Central Bank and State Bank and in 1988 18 domestic and 24 foreign banks were operating. The Central Bank was made independent of government control in March 1990.

In 1988 deposits in foreign currency totalled US$866·9m. and deposits in local currency, 1,745,545m. pesos.

Weights and Measures. The metric system has been legally established in Chile since 1865, but the old Spanish weights and measures are still in use to some extent.

ENERGY AND NATURAL RESOURCES

Electricity. In 1987 production of electricity was 14,821m. kwh, of which 80% hydro-electric. Supply 220 volts; 50 Hz.

Oil. Petroleum was discovered in 1945 in the southern area of Magallanes. Production (1989) 1·25m. tonnes.

Gas. Production (1987) 4,352·6m. cu. metres.

Minerals. The wealth of the country consists chiefly in its minerals, especially in the northern provinces of Atacama and Tarapacá.

Copper is the most important source of foreign exchange (about 41% of exports in 1987) and government revenues (almost 40%). The copper industry's output in 1987 was 1,417,780 tonnes. Exports during 1987 were valued at US$2,100·5m. Copper production will increase by up to 30% in 1991 when the Escondida mine begins production.

Nitrate of soda is found in the Atacama deserts. Exports were US$98·8m. in 1987. Production was 870,000 tonnes in 1985. Iodine is a by-product: 1985 production totalled 2,760 tonnes. The use of solar evaporation as a means of reducing costs has developed the production of potassium salts as an additional by-product.

Iron ore, of which high-grade deposits estimated at over 1,000m. tonnes exist in the provinces of Atacama and Coquimbo, has overtaken nitrate as Chile's second mineral. Production in 1987 was 6,690,168 tonnes, plus 3,684,590 tonnes processed into pellet form.

Coal reserves exceed 2,000m. tons, partially low in thermal unit. Net 1987 production was 1,736,152 tonnes.

In 1987 other minerals included molybdenum (16,941 tonnes, pure), zinc (19,618 tonnes), manganese (31,803 tonnes), lead (829 tonnes).

Agriculture. Total area of land available for agricultural use in 1986 was 29m. ha, of which 12% was sown crops, 38% grassland and 15% forested.

Some principal crops were as follows:

Crop	*Area harvested, 1,000 ha 1988*	*Production, 1,000 tonnes 1988*	Crop	*Area harvested, 1,000 ha 1988*	*Production, 1,000 tonnes 1988*
Wheat	577	1,874	Potatoes	62	727
Oats	61	127	Dry beans	77	81
Barley	24	48	Lentils	39	25
Maize	90	617	Green peas	7	24
Rice	39	147	Sugar-beet	47	2,650

In 1987 fruit plantations had expanded to 119,600 ha with 9 types of fruit, mainly apples and table grapes. Production, 1988 (in 1,000 tonnes): Apples, 592; grapes, 440; pears, 80; peaches and nectarines, 78; plums, 72; oranges, 70; lemons and limes, 50. Exports in the season ended May 1988 totalled 90m. cases valued at US$527m.

Production of animal products in 1987 was (in 1,000 tonnes): Cattle, 174·6; sheep, 14·5; pork, 88·3; poultry, 89·5. Eggs, 1,790m.; milk, 1,100m. litres.

Livestock (1988): Cattle, 3,371,000; horses, 490,000; asses, 28,000; sheep, 6·54m.; goats, 600,000; pigs, 1·36m.; poultry, 21m.

Forestry. In 1987, there were 1,150,000 ha of cultivated forests from Maule to Magallanes, the most important species being the pine (*pinus radiata*) which covers almost 930,000 ha. Eucalyptus and poplar cover some 92,000 ha. Native species of importance amounted to 9·4m. ha in 1983.

Production during 1988 amounted to about 2·7m. cu. metres of sawn timber. Exports of forestry products in 1987 were valued at US$587m.

Fisheries. Chile has 4,200 km of coastline and exclusive fishing rights to 1·6 m. sq. km. There are 220 species of edible fish. Catch of fish and shellfish in 1987 was 4·9m. tonnes; shellfish, 167,000 tonnes. Exports of seafood in 1987 were US$654·3m., of which fishmeal accounted for US$375m. The industry employs 70,000 (1·5% of the working population).

INDUSTRY. A nationally-owned steel plant operates from Huachipato, near Concepción. Output, 1987, 689,800 tonnes of steel ingots. Cellulose and wood-pulp are two industries which are rapidly developing; in 1987, 673,100 tonnes of cellulose were produced. Cement (1·5m. tonnes) and fishmeal (469,400 tonnes) are also important.

Labour. In Dec. 1987 the total workforce numbered 4·01m., of which 837,000 were employed in agriculture, 208,000 in construction, 607,000 in manufacturing industries, 690,000 in trade, 81,000 in mining and 253,000 in transport and communications. A methanol plant with production capacity of 750,000 tonnes a year began operations in 1988 in Punta Arenas.

Trade unions began in the middle 1880s.

FOREIGN ECONOMIC RELATIONS

Commerce. Imports and exports in US$1m.:

	1982	*1983*	*1984*	*1985*	*1986*	*1987*
Imports	3,580	2,969	3,357	2,955	3,099	3,967
Exports	3,798	3,835	3,650	3,743	4,199	5,046

In 1987 imports (in US$1m.) from USA, were valued at 773; Venezuela, 144; Brazil, 380; Japan, 387; Federal Republic of Germany, 335; Argentina, 159; Spain, 117; France, 129; UK, 128; Italy, 96.

In 1987 the principal imports were (in US$1m.): Fuels, 460; chemicals, 740; industrial equipment, 718; transport equipment, 260; tools, 38, live animals, 4; foodstuffs, 40. The principal exports in 1987 were (in US$1m.): Copper, 2,100; paper and pulp, 365; gold, 165; fresh fruit, 527; fish meal, 375; nitrate, 99.

Total trade between Chile and UK (British Department of Trade returns, in £1,000 sterling):

	1986	*1987*	*1988*	*1989*	*1990*
Imports to UK	128,007	112,843	179,628	193,280	222,469
Exports and re-exports from UK	67,459	105,838	80,901	96,003	128,056

Tourism. Some 560,000 tourists visited Chile in 1987.

COMMUNICATIONS

Roads. In 1986 there were in Chile 78,025 km of highways. There were in 1986 (estimate), 850,000 automobiles, 185,000 goods vehicles and 22,500 buses.

Railways. The total length of state railway lines was (1989) 3,494 km, including 1,169 km electrified, of broad- and metre-gauge. In 1989 the State Railways carried 6·4m. tonnes and 8·1m. passengers, including freight traffic on the Northern Railway (1,429 km of metre-gauge) which was taken over by a mixed corporation in 1989. Further electrification is in progress between Concepción and Puerto Montt (600 km). An underground railway in Santiago was opened in Sept. 1975. The Antofagasta (Chili) and Bolivia Railway (702 km, metre-gauge) links the port of Antofagasta with Bolivia and Argentina and carried 1·4m. tonnes in 1987.

Aviation. There are 7 international airports, 16 domestic airports and about 300 landing grounds. Chile is served by 19 commercial air companies (2 Chilean). In 1986, 999,000 passengers were carried.

Shipping. The mercantile marine has consisted since 1982 of 60 ships of over 100 tons (825,076 DWT) but most of the fleet operates under flags of convenience. Valparaíso is the chief port. The free ports of Magallanes, Chiloé and Aysén serve the southern provinces.

Telecommunications. There are 1,486 post offices and agencies. In 1983 there were 608,200 (Santiago, 360,053) telephones in use.

In 1988 there were 30m. radio receivers and 3·5m. television receivers.

Cinemas (1986). Cinemas numbered 170; 60 of them are in Santiago.

Newspapers (1986). There were 65 daily newspapers and 100 magazines.

JUSTICE, RELIGION, EDUCATION AND WELFARE

Justice. There are a High Court of Justice in the capital, 12 courts of appeal distributed over the republic, tribunals of first instance in the departmental capitals and second-class judges in the sub-delegations.

Religion. 89·5% of the population are Catholics. There are 1 cardinal-archbishop, 5 archbishops, 22 bishops and 2 vicars apostolic. Latest estimates show 6·7m. Roman Catholics, 880,500 Protestants and 25,000 Jews.

Education. Education is in 3 stages: Basic (6–14 years), Middle (15–18) and University (19–23). Enrolment (1987): 2,065,400 pupils in the basic schools, 752,000 pupils in the middle schools and 224,000 students in higher education, including universities.

University education is provided in the state university, University of Chile (founded in 1842), the Catholic University at Santiago (1888), the University of Concepción (1919), the Catholic University at Valparaíso (1928), the Universidad Técnica Federico Santa María at Valparaíso (1930), the Universidad Técnica del Estado (1952), Universidad Austral, Valdivia (1954) and Universidad del Norte, Antofagasta (1957).

Health. In 1982 there were 5,416 doctors, 1,644 dentists, 201 pharmacists, 1,930 midwives and 25,889 nursing personnel. 205 hospitals, 296 health centres and 888 emergency posts.

DIPLOMATIC REPRESENTATIVES

Of Chile in Great Britain (12 Devonshire St., London, W1N 2FS)
Ambassador: German Riesco.

Of Great Britain in Chile (La Concepción 177, Casilla 72-D, Santiago)
Ambassador: Richard Neilson, CMG, LVO.

Of Chile in the USA (1732 Massachusetts Ave., NW, Washington, D.C., 20036)
Ambassador: Patricio Silva.

Of the USA in Chile (Agustinas 1343, Santiago)
Ambassador: Charles A. Gillespie Jr.

Of Chile to the United Nations
Ambassador: Juan Somavia.

Further Reading

Statistical Information: The Instituto Nacional de Estadística (Santiago), was founded 17 Sept. 1847. *Director General:* Alvaro Vial Donoso. Principal publications: *Anuario Estadística* and the bi-monthly *Estadística Chilena.*

Other sources are: *Geografía Económica,* by the Corporación de Fomento de la Production, and *Boletín Mensual,* by the Banco Central de Chile.

Blakemore, H., *Chile.* [Bibliography] Oxford and Santa Barbara, 1988
Davis, N., *The Last Two Years of Salvador Allende.* London, 1985
Falcoff, M., *et al Chile: Prospects for Democracy.* New York, 1988
Garretón, M. A., *The Chilean Political Process.* London and Boston, 1989
Heyerdahl, T., *Easter Island: The Mystery Solved.* New York and London, 1989
Horne, A., *Small Earthquake in Chile. A Visit to Allende's South America.* London, 1972
Smith, B. H., *Church and Politics in Chile: Challenges to Modern Catholicism.* Princeton Univ. Press, 1983

CHINA

Capital: Beijing (Peking)
Population: 1,114m. (1990)
GNP per capita: US$330 (1988)

Zhonghua Renmin Gonghe Guo

(People's Republic of China)

HISTORY. In the course of 1949 the Communists obtained full control of the mainland of China, and in 1950 also over most islands off the coast (but not Taiwan, *see* p. 366-67).

On 1 Oct. 1949 Mao Zedong (Tse-tung) proclaimed the establishment of the People's Republic of China. In mid-1966 Mao launched the 'Great Proletarian Cultural Revolution', which lasted until April 1969. For details of the factional disputes which followed *see* THE STATESMAN'S YEAR-BOOK for 1989-90, p. 358. In April 1976 Hua Guofeng became Prime Minister and also, on the death of Mao on 9 Sept., Party Chairman (later General Secretary). Hua was replaced as Prime Minister by Zhao Ziyang in Sept. 1980 and as Party General Secretary by Hu Yaobang in June 1981. Hu was himself forced to resign following student demonstrations in Jan. 1987. Most prominent leader during this period was sometime Party Leader Deng Xiaoping, who resigned from the Politburo in Nov. 1987 and from the chairmanship of the Military Commissions in Nov.1989.

The funeral of Hu Yaobang on 15 April 1989 sparked off mass student demonstrations which escalated into a popular 'pro-democracy' movement in Beijing, Shanghai and other provincial centres demanding reforms. Despite Government appeals to disperse the demonstrations gathered strength during the summit visit of the Soviet President Gorbachev (15-17 May) and culminated in a sit-in in Tiananmen Square, Beijing. This was confronted by army units, at first peacefully. However, on 4 June troops opened fire on the demonstrators and tanks were sent in to disperse them. The official casualty figures are: 'over 200' demonstrators and 'dozens' of soldiers killed, and some 9,000 injured.

A hard-line faction assumed control in the Party Politburo which replaced Zhao Ziyang by Jiang Zemin as General Secretary. Martial law was imposed from May 1989 to Jan. 1990, and several prominent demonstrators were executed.

The visit of President Gorbachev marked the culmination of a process of gradual normalization of Sino-Soviet relations. It was announced that 'both sides favoured a reasonable settlement of the boundary question'.

AREA AND POPULATION. China is bounded north by the USSR and Mongolia, east by Korea, the Yellow Sea and the East China Sea, with Hong Kong and Macao as enclaves on the south-east coast; south by Vietnam, Laos, Burma, India, Bhutan and Nepal; west by India, Pakistan, Afghanistan and the USSR.

The capital is Beijing (Peking).

The total area (including Taiwan) is estimated at 9,572,900 sq. km (3,696,100 sq. miles).

At the 1990 census the population was 1,133,682,501 (51·6% male). Ethnic minorities numbered some 91m. There are 55 ethnic minorities; those numbering more than 3m. were: Zhuang, Hui, Uighur, Yi, Miao, Manchu, Tibetan and Mongolian.

1979 regulations restricting married couples to a single child, a policy enforced by compulsory abortions and economic sanctions, have been widely ignored, and it was admitted in 1988 that the population target of 1,200m. by 2000 would have to be revised to 1,270m. Since 1988 peasant couples have been permitted a second child after 4 years if the first born is a girl, a measure to combat infanticide.

Vital statistics, 1988: Birth rate (per 1,000), 20·78; death rate, 6·58; growth rate, 14·2. Population density, 113 per sq. km. in 1987. There were 8,290,588 marriages and 457,938 divorces in 1985. Expectation of life was 67 in 1985.

Estimates of persons of Chinese race outside China, Taiwan and Hong Kong in 1980 varied from 15m. to 20m. Since 1982 China has permitted the emigration of a limited number of persons to Hong Kong.

A number of widely divergent varieties of Chinese are spoken. The official 'Modern Standard Chinese' is based on the dialect of North China. The ideographic writing system of 'characters' is uniform throughout the country, and has undergone systematic simplification. In 1958 a phonetic alphabet (*Pinyin*) was devised to transcribe the characters, and in 1979 this was officially adopted for use in all texts in the Roman alphabet. The previous transcription scheme (Wade) is still used in Taiwan.

China is administratively divided into 22 provinces, 5 autonomous regions (originally entirely or largely inhabited by ethnic minorities, though in some regions now outnumbered by Han immigrants) and 3 government-controlled municipalities. These are in turn divided into 151 prefectures, 431 cities (of which 183 are at prefecture level and the remainder at county level), 1,936 counties and 647 urban districts. (For earlier administrative divisions *see* THE STATESMAN'S YEAR-BOOK 1986–87).

Government-controlled municipalities	*Area (in 1,000 sq. km)*	*Population in 1987 (in 1,000s)*	*Density per sq. km*	*Capital*
Beijing	17·8	9,750	580	—
Tianjin	4·0	8,190	725	—
Shanghai	5·8	12,320	1,987	—
Provinces				
Hebei	202·7	56,170	299	Shijiazhuang
Shanxi	157·1	26,550	170	Taiyuan
Liaoning	151·0	37,260	256	Shenyang
Jilin	187·0	23,150	124	Changchun
Heilongjiang	463·6	33,320	71	Harbin
Jiangsu	102·2	62,130	611	Nanjing
Zhejiang	101·8	40,700	400	Hangzhou
Anhui	139·9	52,170	374	Hefei
Fujian	123·1	27,490	227	Fuzhou
Jiangxi	164·8	35,090	211	Nanchang
Shandong	153·3	77,760	507	Jinan
Henan	167·0	78,080	468	Zhengzhou
Hubei	187·5	49,890	266	Wuhan
Hunan	210·5	56,960	271	Changsha
Guangdong	231·4	63,640	299	Guangzhou
Hainan	...	2,098	...	...
Sichuan	569·0	103,200	182	Chengdu
Guizhou	174·0	30,080	171	Guiyang
Yunnan	436·2	34,560	88	Kunming
Shaanxi	195·8	30,430	148	Xian
Gansu	530·0	20,710	46	Lanzhou
Qinghai	721·0	4,120	6	Xining
Autonomous regions				
Inner Mongolia	450·0	20,290	17	Hohhot
Guangxi	220·4	39,460	167	Nanning
Tibet [1]	1,221·6	2,030	2	Lhasa
Ningxia	170.0	4,240	64	Yinchuan
Xinjiang	1,646·8	13,840	9	Urumqi

[1] See also paragraph on Tibet below.

Population of largest cities in 1989: Shanghai, 7·33m.; Beijing (Peking), 6·8m.; Tianjin, 5·62m.; Shenyang, 4·44m.; Wuhan, 3·64m.; Guangzhou (Canton), 3·49m.; Harbin, 2·93m.; Chongqing, 2·75m.; Chengdu, 2·74m.; Zibo, 2·4m.; Xian, 2·65m.; Nanjing, 2·43m.; Taiyuan, 2·01m.; Changchun, 2·02m.; Dalian, 2·33m.; Zhengzhou, 1·63m.; Kunming, 1·48m.; Jinan, 2·18m.; Tangshan, 1·46m.; Guiyang, 1·46m.; Lanzhou, 1·45m.; Fushun, 1·32m.; Qiqihar, 1·35m.; Anshan, 1·35m.; Hangzhou,

1·31m.; Qingdao, 2·01m.; Fuzhou, 1·25m.; Changsha, 1·26m.; Shijazhuang, 1·26m.; Nanchang, 1·29m.; Jilin, 1·23m.; Baotou, 1·16m.; Huainan, 1·14.; Luoyang, 1·13m.; Urumqi, 1·07m.; Ningbo, 1·06m.; Datong, 1·06m.; Handan, 1·06m.; Nanning, 1·03m.

Tibet. For events before and after the revolt of 1959 *see* THE STATESMAN'S YEAR-BOOK, 1964–65 (under TIBET), and 1988–89. On 9 Sept. 1965 Tibet became an Autonomous Region. 301 delegates were elected to the first People's Congress, of whom 226 were Tibetans. The Chief of Government is Gyaincain Norbu. The senior spiritual leader, the Dalai Lama, is in exile. He was awarded the Nobel Peace Prize in 1989. The Banqen Lama died in Jan. 1989. In 1988 the Tibetan population of Tibet was 2,123,000, Han 79,800. Population of the capital, Lhasa, in 1987 was 130,000. Expectation of life was 45 years in 1985. 2m. Tibetans live outside Tibet, in China, and in India and Nepal. Chinese efforts to modernize Tibet include irrigation, road-building and the establishment of light industry: in 1985 296 small and medium-sized factories and mines were producing electric power, coal, building materials, lumber, textiles, chemicals and animal products.

In 1979, 1·6m. were engaged in agriculture, including 0·5m. nomadic herdsmen. By 1984, a large measure of autonomy for the peasantry had been re-introduced: Compulsory deliveries and some taxes were abolished and private ownership of livestock and 30-year disposition of land were granted. There were 23m. cattle in 1984. In 1975 Tibet became self-sufficient in grain. There are now 21,600 km of highways, and air routes link Lhasa with Chengdu, Xian and Kathmandu. Six more were opened in 1987. 30,000 tourists visited Tibet in 1986.

The borders were opened for trade with neighbouring countries in 1980. In July 1988 Tibetan was reinstated as a 'major official language', competence in which is required of all administrative officials.

Since 1980 178 monasteries and 743 shrines have been renovated and reopened. There were some 15,000 monks and nuns in 1987. In 1984 a Buddhist seminary in Lhasa opened with 200 students. Circulation of the Tibetan-language *Xizang Daily* now totals 38,000. In 1988 there were 2,437 primary schools, 67 secondary schools, 14 technical schools and 3 higher education institutes. The total number of students was 166,000. A university was established in 1985. In 1987 there were 7,048 medical personnel (of whom 59% were Tibetan) and 957 medical institutions, with a total of 4,738 beds.

Since 1987 there have been several anti-Chinese demonstrations in which a number of people have been killed. Martial law, declared on 8 March 1989, was lifted in April 1990

Batchelor, S., *The Tibet Guide*. London, 1987
The Dalai Lama, *My Land and My People* (ed. D. Howarth). London, 1962:-*Freedom in Exile*. London, 1990.
Grunfeld, A. T., *The Making of Modern Tibet*. London, 1987
Jäschke, H. A., *A Tibetan–English Dictionary*. London, 1934
Levenson, C. B., *The Dalai Lama: A Biography*. London, 1988
Shakabpa, T. W. D., *Tibet: A Political History*. New York, 1984
Sharabati, D., *Tibet and its History*. London, 1986

CLIMATE. Most of China has a temperate climate but, with such a large country, extending far inland and embracing a wide range of latitude as well as containing large areas at high altitude, many parts experience extremes of climate, especially in winter. Most rain falls during the summer, from May to Sept., though amounts decrease inland. Peking (Beijing). Jan. 24°F (–4·4°C), July 79°F (26°C). Annual rainfall 24·9" (623 mm). Chongqing. Jan. 45°F (7·2°C), July 84°F (28·9°C). Annual rainfall 43·7" (1,092 mm). Shanghai. Jan. 39°F (3·9°C), July 82°F (27·8°C). Annual rainfall 45·4" (1,135 mm). Tianjin. Jan. 24°F (–4·4°C), July 81°F (27·2°C). Annual rainfall 21·5" (533·4 mm).

CONSTITUTION AND GOVERNMENT. On 21 Sept. 1949 the 'Chinese People's Political Consultative Conference' met in Peking, convened by the Chinese Communist Party. The Conference adopted a 'Common Programme' of 60 articles and the 'Organic Law of the Central People's Government' (31 articles).

Both became the basis of the Constitution adopted on 20 Sept. 1954 by the 1st National People's Congress, the supreme legislative body. The Consultative Conference continued to exist after 1954 as an advisory body. In 1988 it had 2,083 members.

New Constitutions were adopted in 1975 and 1978 (for details *see* THE STATESMAN'S YEAR-BOOK 1986-87).

A further Constitution was adopted in 1982. It defines 'socialist modernisation' as China's basic task and restores the post of State President (*i.e.* Head of State). Constitutional amendments of 1988 legalized private companies and sanction the renting out of 'land-use' rights.

The *National People's Congress* can amend the Constitution, elects and has power to remove from office the highest State dignitaries, decides on the national economic plan, etc. The Congress elects a *Standing Committee* (which supervises the State Council) and the *State President* for a 5-year term: Yang Shangkun was elected in April 1988. *Vice-President:* Wang Zhen.

Congress is elected for a 5-year term and meets once a year for 2 or 3 weeks. When not in session, its business is carried on by its *Standing Committee*. It is composed of deputies elected on a constituency basis by direct secret ballot. Any voter, and certain organizations, may nominate candidates. Nominations may exceed seats by 50-100%. 2,978 deputies were elected to the 7th Congress in March-April 1988.

In March 1991 the government included: *Prime Minister:* Li Peng. *Chairman of the Commission for Economic Restructure:* Chen Jinhua. *Deputy Prime Ministers:* Tian Jiyun, Yao Yilin, Wu Xueqian. Other ministers included: Qian Qichen *(Foreign Affairs)*, Zheng Tuobin *(Foreign Trade)*, Liu Zhongyi (*Agriculture*), Qin Jiwei *(Defence)*, Wang Bingqian *(Finance)*, Zou Jiahua *(Chairman, State Planning Commission)* and Tao Siju *(Public Security)*.

State emblem: 5 stars above Peking's Gate of Heavenly Peace, surrounded by a border of ears of grain entwined with drapings, which form a knot in the centre of a cogwheel at the base; the colours are red and gold.

National flag: Red with a large star and 4 smaller stars all in yellow in the canton.

National anthem: 'March of the Volunteers' composed 1935 by Tien Han. (Replacing the 1978 version).

De facto power is in the hands of the Communist Party of China, which had 48m. members in 1989. A purge of members was instituted following the events of June 1989. There are 8 other parties, all members of the Chinese People's Political Consultative Conference. The members of the Politburo in March 1991 (the first 6 constituting its Standing Committee) were Jiang Zemin (*General Secretary*; b. 1926), Li Peng, Qiao Shi, Song Ping, Li Ruihuan, Yao Yilin, Wan Li, Tian Jiyun, Li Tieying, Li Ximing, Yang Rudai, Yang Shangkun, Wu Xueqian, Qin Jiwei, Hu Qili; candidate member, Ding Guangen. Deng Xiaoping has no formal post but is officially still a member of the 'second-generation leadership.'

Local Government. There are 4 administrative levels: (1) Provinces, Autonomous Regions and the municipalities directly administered by the Government; (2) prefectures and autonomous prefectures (*zhou*); (3) counties, autonomous counties and municipalities; (4) towns. Local government organs ('congresses') exist at provincial, county and township levels and in national minority autonomous prefectures, but not in ordinary prefectures which are just agencies of the provincial government. Up to county level congresses are elected directly. Elections take place every 3 years. Any person proposed by 10 electors may stand after political vetting. There are quotas for party members and women. Multiple candidacies are permitted at local elections.

DEFENCE. In Nov. 1989 Jiang Zemin took over from Deng Xiaoping as chairman of the State and Party's Military Commissions. China is divided into 7 military regions. The military commander also commands the air, naval and civilian militia forces assigned to each region.

Conscription is compulsory but for organizational reasons selective: Only some

10% of potential recruits are called up. Service is 3 years with the Army and 4 years with the Air Force and Navy.

A Defence University to train senior officers in modern warfare was established in 1985.

Army. The Army (PLA: 'People's Liberation Army') is divided into main and local forces. Main forces, administered by the 7 military regions in which they are stationed but commanded by the Ministry of Defence, are available for operation anywhere and are better equipped. Local forces concentrate on the defence of their own regions. There are 24 Integrated Group Armies comprising 80 infantry, 10 armoured and 6 artillery divisions; and 50 engineer regiments. Land-based missile forces consisted of (1990 estimate): 8 intercontinental and 60 intermediate range. Total strength in 1990 was 2·3m. including 1m. conscripts.

There is a para-military force of 12m., including 1,850,000 People's armed police.

Navy. The warship construction programme remains slow, with emphasis on foreign sales. Despite technical backwardness, the naval arm of the People's Liberation Army remains an important factor in the balance of power in the eastern hemisphere.

Strength comprises 1 nuclear-powered ballistic missile armed submarine, 4 nuclear-propelled fleet submarines, 1 diesel cruise missile submarine and some 85 old patrol submarines (of which probably no more than 40 are operational). Surface combatant forces include 18 destroyers, 37 frigates, some 215 missile craft and 160 torpedo craft. There is a mixed coastal and inshore patrol force of some 500 vessels and 50 riverine craft. The mine warfare force consists of 35 ex-Soviet offshore minesweepers, some 12 inshore, and about 60 unmanned drones. There are 58 landing ships of various types and some 400 craft. Major auxiliaries number over 100, including 3 oilers and 1 fleet stores ship, and there are several hundred minor auxiliaries, yard craft and service vessels.

The land-based naval air force of almost 900 combat aircraft, primarily for defensive and anti-submarine service, is organized into 3 bomber and 6 fighter divisions. The force includes some 50 H-6 bombers and 130 H-5 torpedo bombers, about 100 Q-5 fighter/ground attack aircraft and 600 fighters including J-5 (MiG-17), J-6 (MiG-19), and J-7 (MiG-21) types. Maritime patrol tasks are performed by 10 Be-6 flying boats, and anti-submarine operations by 50 Z-5, and 12 Super Frelon helicopters from shore and about 6 Z-9 afloat. There are also about 60 communications, research, training and transport aircraft.

Main naval bases are at Qingdao (North Sea Fleet), Shanghai (East Sea Fleet), and Zhanjiang (South Sea Fleet).

Active personnel continue to reduce slowly as tasks are handed over to the militia; in 1990 there were some 250,000, including 25,000 in the naval air force, 27,000 coastal defence troops and 6,000 marines.

Air Force. In 1984 the Air Force was estimated at 4,500 front-line aircraft, organized in over 100 regiments of jet-fighters and about 12 regiments of tactical bombers, plus reconnaissance, transport and helicopter units. Each regiment is made up of 3 or 4 squadrons (each 12 aircraft), and 3 regiments form a division.

Equipment includes about 500 J-7 (MiG-21), 2,000 J-6 (MiG-19) and 750 J-4 and J-5 (MiG-17) interceptors and fighter-bombers, with about 500 H-5 (Il-28) jet-bombers, about 120 H-6 Chinese-built copies of the Soviet Tu-16 twin-jet strategic bomber, plus 500 Q-5 twin-jet fighter-bombers, evolved from the MiG-19. In service in small numbers is a locally-developed fighter designated J-8 (known in the west as 'Finback'). Transport aircraft include about 500 Y-5 (An-2), Y-8 (An-12), Y-12, An-24/26, Li-2, Il-14 and three-turbofan Trident fixed-wing types, plus 300 Z-5 (Mi-4) and Z-6 (Mi-8) helicopters. The MiG fighters and Antonov transports have been manufactured in China, initially under licence, and other types have been assembled there, including several hundred JJ-5 (2-seat MiG-17) trainers. Small quantities of Western aircraft have been procured in the past few years, including 24 Black Hawk and 6 Super Puma transport helicopters, 8 Gazelle armed helicopters and 5 Challenger VIP transports. The US Government is providing technical assistance in developing the J-8 fighter. Total strength (1990) 470,000, including 220,000 in air defence organization.

Joffe, E., *The Chinese Army after Mao*. London, 1987

INTERNATIONAL RELATIONS

Membership. The People's Republic of China is a member of UN (and its Security Council), the IMF, the Asian Development Bank, and is an observer at GATT.

ECONOMY

Policy. For planning history 1953–73 *see* THE STATESMAN'S YEAR-BOOK, 1973–74, p. 817.

A programme for fundamental reform of the urban economy was introduced in 1985. State planning was reduced in scope and enterprises gained a degree of freedom in deciding their production and marketing a portion of it. Wages were varied according to work performed, and prices adjusted to reflect market conditions. However, the end of 1988 saw a return to more central economic planning as a response to declining production, inflation, a foreign trade imbalance and unequal regional development. Further measures of state control were introduced in Dec. 1989. 'Key enterprises' (metals, coal, timber) were to be completely government managed, and other firms not meeting production quotas have their supplies reduced. A national economic plan published in Jan. 1990 aimed to reduce inflation, balance state revenue and expenditure and reduce internal debt. Public sector industry received preferential treatment in terms of subsidies and credit terms.

An eighth 5-year plan covers 1991–95; there is also a 10-year plan to 2000.

Budget. 1988 revenue was 258,780m. yuan; expenditure, 266,831m. yuan. Estimates for 1989: Revenue, 285,680m. yuan; expenditure, 293,080m. yuan.

Sources of revenue, 1989 (in million yuan): Tax receipts, 255,710; subsidies for enterprise losses, 52,140; construction funds, 20,500; foreign loans, 16,500. Expenditure: Capital construction, 62,790; education, science and health, 51,380; subsidies, 40,960; defence, 24,550; administration, 22,660; agriculture, 17,390; technical renovation of enterprises, 15,580; urban maintenance, 10,300; debt service, 9,560.

China's foreign exchange reserves in March 1988 were US$17,100m. Gold reserves in 1988 were 12·67m. troy oz. of gold. Inflation was 18·8% in 1989 (27·9% in 1988).

Currency. The currency is called Renminbi (*i.e.*, People's Currency). The unit of currency is the *yuan* (CNY) which is divided into 10 *jiao*, the *jiao*, into 10 *fen*. In Nov. 1990 the *yuan* was devalued by 9·57%. Inflation was 5·3% in Nov. 1990. The official rate of exchange in March 1991 was £1 = 9·99 *yuan*; US$1 = 5·27 *yuan*.

Notes are issued for 1, 2 and 5 *jiao* and 1, 2, 5 and 10 *yuan* and coins for 1, 2 and 5 *fen*.

Banking and Finance. A re-organization of the banking system in 1983 resulted in the People's Bank of China assuming the role of a Central Bank (*Director:* Li Guixian). Its former commercial role has been taken over by the Industrial and Commercial Bank. Other specialized banks include the Agricultural Bank of China, the China Investment Bank and the Chinese People's Construction Bank. The Bank of China will continue to be responsible for foreign banking operations. It has branches in London, New York, Singapore, Luxembourg, Macao and Hong Kong, and agencies in Tokyo and Paris.

Savings bank deposits were 3,807,000m. yuan in 1988.

Stock exchanges opened in the Shenzhen special economic zone in 1987 and in Shanghai in 1990. A securities trading system linking 6 cities (Securities Automated Quotations System) was inaugurated in 1990 for trading in government bonds.

Weights and Measures. The metric system is in general use alongside traditional units of measurement, for which *see* THE STATESMAN'S YEAR-BOOK, 1975–76, p. 826 and 1954, pp. 877–88.

ENERGY AND NATURAL RESOURCES

Electricity. Sources of energy in 1988: Coal 73·1%; oil, 20·4%; hydroelectric power, 4·5%; gas, 2%. Hydroelectric potential is 676m. kw. Generating is not centralized; local units range between 30 and 60 mw of output. Output in 1990: 615,000m. kwh. Supply 220 volts; 50 Hz. There is a nuclear energy plant at Shanghai. Plans to build further nuclear power plants have been abandoned.

Oil. There are on-shore fields at Daqing, Shengli, Dagang and Karamai, and 10 provinces south of the Yangtze River have been opened for exploration in co-operation with foreign companies. Crude oil production was 138m. tonnes in 1989.

Gas. Natural gas is available from fields near Canton and Shanghai and in Sichuan province. Production was 13,890m. cu. metres in 1987, but is only used locally.

Minerals. *Coal.* Most provinces contain coal, and there are 70 major production centres, of which the largest are in Hebei, Shanxi, Shandong, Jilin and Anhui. Coal reserves are estimated at 873,719m. tonnes. Coal production was 1,090m. tonnes in 1990.

Iron. Iron ore deposits are estimated at 49,731m. tonnes and are abundant in the anthracite field of Shanxi, in Hebei and in Shandong and are found in conjunction with coal and worked in the north-east. Estimated output of iron ore in 1984, 122m. tonnes. The biggest steel bases are at Anshan with a capacity of 6m. tons, Wuhan (capacity 3·5m. tonnes), Baotou and Maanshan (both 2·5m. tonnes) and Baoshan near Shanghai.

Tin. Tin ore is plentiful in Yunnan, where the tin-mining industry has long existed. Tin production was 40,000 tonnes in 1989.

Tungsten. China is the world's principal producer of wolfram (tungsten ore), producing 14,000 tonnes in 1981. Mining of wolfram is carried on in Hunan, Guangdong and Yunnan.

Production of other minerals in 1989 (in 1,000 tonnes): Aluminium, 770; copper, 540; nickel, 30; lead, 270; zinc, 430. Other minerals produced: Barite, bismuth, gold, graphite, gypsum, mercury, molybdenum, silver. Reserves (in tonnes) of phosphate ore 15,032m.; sylvite, 272·47m.; salt, 275,579m.

Agriculture. China remains essentially an agricultural country. 95·72m. ha were cultivated in 1989. Intensive agriculture and horticulture have been practised for millennia. Present-day policy aims to avert the traditional threats from floods and droughts by soil conservancy, afforestation, irrigation and drainage projects, and to increase the 'high stable yields' areas by introducing fertilizers, pesticides and improved crops. 44·4m. ha were irrigated in 1988, and 17·99m. tonnes of chemical fertilizer were applied.

Since 1979 agricultural communes have shed the administrative functions which they had in the Maoist period to become 'rural economic associations', whose members manage them jointly and share the costs and benefits. There were 470,600 associations in 1989, with 4,339,500 members. There were also 232,800 agricultural township and village enterprises, engaging 95,454,600 persons. There were 2,126 state farms in 1988 with 4·68m. workers, and 180m. peasant households in 1989.

The 1988 harvest fell short of targets. Reasons for the shortfall included the greater profitability in devoting land to cash crops and stock-breeding and the migration of 60m. peasants to industry. Net *per capita* annual peasant income, 1987: 460 yuan.

In 1988 there were 870,187 large and medium-sized tractors and in 1986 34,573 combine harvesters.

Agricultural production (in 1m. tonnes), 1988: Rice, 172·37; wheat, 87·5; maize, 73·82; soybeans, 10·92; roots and tubers, 144·93; tea, 0·57; cotton, 4·2; oilseed crops, 13·2; sugar-cane, 49·08; fruit, 16·62. The gross value of agricultural output in 1988 was 586,500m. yuan.

Livestock, 1988: Horses, 10,691,000; cattle, 73,963,000; goats, 77,894,000; pigs, 334,862,000; sheep, 102,655,000. Meat production in 1987 was 19·21m. tonnes.

Forestry. Forest area in 1989 was 124·65. ha, including 2·6m. ha of timber forest. Timber reserves were 102,600m. cu. metres in 1985. The chief forested areas are in Heilongjiang, Sichuan and Yunnan. Timber output in 1988 was 63m. cu. metres.

Fisheries. Total catch, 1988: 10·46m. tonnes. There were 172,582 motor fishing vessels in 1985.

INDUSTRY. 'Cottage' industries persist into the late 20th century. Modern industrial development began with the manufacture of cotton textiles, and the establishment of silk filatures, steel plants, flour-mills and match factories. In 1988 there were 8,105,600 industrial enterprises, of which 10,800 were classified as 'large or medium', 99,000 were state-owned, 1,853,000 were collectives and 6,148,100 were individually owned. In 1988 2,597,100 enterprises were engaged in heavy industry. A law of Aug. 1988 ends direct state control of firms and provides for the possibility of bankruptcy. Expanding sectors of manufacture are: Steel, chemicals, cement, agricultural implements, plastics and lorries.

Output of major products, 1988 (in tonnes): Cotton yarn, 4·54m.; paper, 12·1m.; sugar, 4·55m.; salt, 22m.; synthetic detergents, 1·29m.; aluminium ware, 87,500; steel, 59·18m.; rolled steel, 46·98m.; cement, 203m.; sulphuric acid, 10·98m.; chemical fertilizers, 17·67m.; civil shipping, 1·4m.; cotton cloth, 17,600m. metres; woollen fabrics, 265m. metres; bicycles, 41·22m.; TV sets, 24·85m.; tape recorders, 23·44m.; cameras, 2·92m.; washing machines, 10·46m.; refrigerators, 7·4m.; motor vehicles, 646,700; tractors, 52,100; locomotives, 843.

The gross value of industrial output in 1988 was 1,822,400m. yuan.

Labour. Workforce (excluding peasantry), 1989: 543·34m. (36·9% female), including 323m. rural workers, 97m. industrial workers, 28m. workers in service trades and commerce, 25m. in building and 14m. in transport and telecommunications. 19m. worked in private businesses in 1989. At the 1990 census there was a floating population of 21m. internal migrants who tour the country seeking seasonal employment. There were 2·96m. unemployed in 1988. Average annual non-agricultural wage in 1988: 1,747 yuan. There is a 6-day 48-hour working week.

Trade Unions. The All-China Federation of Trade Unions is headed by Zhu Houze.

FOREIGN ECONOMIC RELATIONS. In 1991 there were six Special Economic Zones at Shanghai and in the provinces of Guangdong and Fujian, in which concessions are made to foreign businessmen. In 1984 14 coastal cities and Hainan Island were opened for technological imports, and in 1988 Hainan was also designated a Special Economic Zone. Since 1979 joint ventures with foreign firms have been permitted. By 1987 4,040 equity joint ventures, 4,864 contractual joint ventures and 176 wholly-owned foreign subsidiaries had been launched. About 80% of the investment was from Hong Kong. There is no maximum limit on the foreign share of the holdings; the minimum limit is 25%. Contracts between Chinese and foreign firms are only legally valid if in writing and approved by the appropriate higher authority. IMF loans of US$780m. were suspended after the events of June 1989.

In May 1989 the UK and China signed a 6-year trade agreement worth US$3,000m.

In 1988 Japan and China signed an investment protection treaty, putting Japanese firms in China on the same footing as local firms.

In 1978 a most-favoured-nation agreement was signed with the EEC, and in 1980 the EEC extended preferential tariffs to China. In Oct. 1990 the EEC lifted sanctions imposed after the events of June 1989.

In Feb. 1991 China and India resumed cross-border trade, which had ceased in 1962.

Commerce. Trade in 1988: Imports, US$55,250m.; exports, US$47,540m.

Major exports in 1987 (in 1,000 tonnes): Crude oil, 32,170; grain, 7,080; tea, 174; raw silk, 9·2; tungsten ore, 23·1; cotton cloth, 2,342m. metres; imports: Wheat, 13,200; rolled steel, 12,400; motor vehicles, 90,239 units; chemical fertilizers, 10,900.

In 1984 only 7·2% of China's trade was with Communist countries (2·5% with the USSR), but trade with the USSR reached some US$2,800m. in 1988. Japan is China's biggest trading partner. Other major partners are Hong Kong, USA, Germany and Canada. Customs duties with Taiwan were abolished in 1980.

Total trade between China and UK (British Department of Trade returns, in £1,000 sterling):

	1986	*1987*	*1988*	*1989*	*1990*
Imports to UK	327,032	391,766	443,698	530,720	583,425
Exports and re-exports from UK	535,943	416,012	411,563	417,911	465,585

China agreed to settle by 1990 British claims for assets totalling £23·4m. confiscated by the present Chinese Government when it took power in 1949.

Tourism. 31·69m. foreigners visited China in 1988. Tourist numbers dropped by 50% after the events of June 1989. Restrictions on Chinese wishing to travel abroad were eased in Feb. 1986.

COMMUNICATIONS

Roads. The total road length was 995,600 km in 1988. Highways are well graded but mostly unmetalled. In 1988 there were 3·19m. lorries and 1m. passenger vehicles, 152,899 of the latter were privately owned. The use of bicycles is very widespread.

In 1988, 7,323·15m. tonnes of freight and 6,504·73m. persons were transported by road.

Railways. In 1988 there were 52,800 km of railway including 5,700 km electrified. Gauge is standard except for some 600 mm track in Yunnan.

The principal railways are:

(1) The great north–south trunk lines: (*a*) Beijing–Canton Railway (over 2,300 km), *via* Zhengzhou–Wuhan–Zhuzhou–Hengyang. (*b*) Tianjin–Shanghai Railway (1,500 km), *via* Pukow and Nanjing. (*c*) Baoji–Chongqing Railway, *via* Chengdu (1,174 km). Chongqing with the east–west route from Hengyang to the Vietnam border, and to Kunming, connecting there with the Yunnan Railway to the Vietnam border. Two further lines connect Baoji.

(2) Great east–west trunk lines: (*a*) Longhai Railway; Lianyungkang–Xuzhou–Zhengzhou (on the Beijing–Canton line) –Xian–Baoji–Tianshui–Lanzhou (1,500 km). (*b*) Lanzhou–Xinjiang Railway: Lanzhou–Yumen–Hami–Turfan–Urumqi (1,800 km); (c) Shanghai–Youyiguan (Vietnam border) *via* Hangzhou, Nanchang, Hengyang (on the Beijing–Canton line), Guilin, Liuzhou and Nanning. (*d*) Beijing–Lanzhou *via* Xining (from which a branch connects with the lines through Mongolia to the Trans–Siberian Railway), Dadong (from which a branch serves the province of Shanxi), Baotou and Yinchuan (Ningxia). (*e*) Zhuzhou–Guiyang (632 km). (*f*) Xiangfan–Chongqing.

Branches link coastal areas (*e.g.,* Fujian province) and the smaller inland centres with the main parts of the system. Surveys have been made for a new 500-km railway, linking the trunk line with the oilfield of Karamai in Xinjiang.

(3) The Manchurian system: (*a*) Chinese Eastern (Changchun) Railway (2,370 km), from Manzhouli on the Soviet border through northern Inner Mongolia and Manchuria *via* Qiqihar, Harbin and Mudanjiang to the Soviet border near Vladivostok. (*b*) South Manchuria Railway (705 km, 1,120 km with branches), Changchun–Shenyang–Luda. (*c*) Beijing–Shenyang Railway, with branches in Manchuria (854 km, 1,350 km with branches).

The Beijing–Lanzhou line connects through a branch with the Trans–Siberian Railway in the USSR. A line from Xinjiang across the border to Soviet Kazakhstan is due for completion in 1991.

In 1988 the railways carried 1,449·48 tonnes of freight and 1,226·45m. passengers.

Aviation. Since 1985 the Civil Aviation Administration of China has become the administrative body for 5 new airlines: Air China (based on Beijing); Eastern Airways (Shanghai); Southern Airways (Canton); South-Western Airways (Chengdu) and the Capital Helicopter Company. There were 410 civil aircraft in 1988, including 7 Boeing 747s, 21 737s, 10 707s and 5 Airbus A310s, and 81 Soviet aircraft. There are services to Sharjah, Vancouver, Toronto, Rome, Stockholm, Nagasaki, Pyongyang, Hanoi, Rangoon, Singapore, Bangkok, Karachi, Tokyo, Moscow, Ulan Bator, Teheran, Addis Ababa, Bucharest, Belgrade, Zürich, Paris, Frankfurt, Manila, New York, San Francisco, London, Sydney and Hong Kong. Route lengths in 1988, 373,800 km, of which 128,300 km were international. British Airways have a direct flight London-Beijing. Japan Airlines have a route from Tokyo to Beijing (*via* Osaka and Shanghai), Air France Paris to Beijing (*via* Athens and Karachi), Pakistan Airlines Karachi to Beijing, Aeroflot Moscow to Beijing, Ethiopian Airlines Addis Ababa to Shanghai, Tarom Bucharest to Beijing, Swissair Geneva to Beijing and Shanghai, Iran Air Paris to Beijing and PANAM Beijing *via* Tokyo. Singapore Airlines Singapore to Beijing and Thai Airways Bangkok to Beijing.

In 1988 CAAC carried 21·4 person/km and 0·74 tonne/km of freight.

Shipping. In 1980 the ocean-going merchant fleet consisted of 431 vessels with a total DWT of 7·92m.

Cargo handled by the major ports in 1985 (in tonnes): Shanghai, 113m.; Dalian, 44m.; Qinhuangdao, 44m.; Qingdao, 26m.; Huangpu, 18m.; Tianjin, 18m.; Zhanjiang, 12m. In 1987 79·8m. tonnes of freight were carried.

Inland waterways totalled 109,400 km in 1988. 858m. tonnes of freight and 458m. passengers were carried.

Pipeline. A pipeline links the Daqing oilfield to the port of Luda and to refineries in Peking. There is a pipeline from Lanzhou to Lhasa. There were 14,300 km of pipeline in 1988 which carried a load of 156·2m. tonnes.

Telecommunications. There were 52,900 post offices in 1988. There were 10m. telephones and some 10,000 fax machines in 1990. The use of *Pinyin* transcription of place names has been requested for mail to addresses in China (*e.g.*, 'Beijing' *not* 'Peking').

In 1988 there were 461 radio and 422 television stations. In 1981 there were 9·02m. TV receivers.

Cinemas and Theatres. There were 8,331 cinemas, 135,719 film projection units and 2,094 theatres in 1987. 158 feature films were made in 1988.

Newspapers and books. In 1987 there were 850 newspapers with a circulation of 20,490m. and 5,687 periodicals. The Party newspaper is *Renmin Ribao* (People's Daily). In 1979 it had a daily circulation of 7m. 60,193 book titles were produced in 62,500m. copies in 1987. There were 2,479 public libraries in 1988.

JUSTICE, RELIGION, EDUCATION AND WELFARE

Justice. Six new codes of law (including criminal and electoral) came into force in 1980, to regularize the legal unorthodoxy of previous years. There is no provision for *habeas corpus*. An anti-crime campaign was launched in Aug. 1983 which, it was claimed in 1985, had cut the crime rate sharply; by 1986 624,000 sentences of death or long-term imprisonment had been imposed. The death penalty has been extended from treason and murder to include rape, embezzlement, smuggling, drug-dealing, bribery and robbery with violence. Courts will no longer be subject to the intervention of other state bodies, and their decisions will be reversible only by higher courts. 'People's courts' are divided into some 30 higher, 200 intermediate and 2,000 basic-level courts, and headed by the Supreme People's Court. The latter tries cases, hears appeals and supervises the people's courts.

People's courts are composed of a president, vice-presidents, judges and 'people's assessors' who are the equivalent of jurors. 'People's conciliation committees' are charged with settling minor disputes.

There are also special military courts.

Procuratorial powers and functions are exercised by the Supreme People's Procuracy and local procuracies.

Religion. Confucianism, Buddhism and Taoism have long been practised. Confucianism has no ecclesiastical organization and appears rather as a philosophy of ethics and government. Taoism—of Chinese origin—copied Buddhist ceremonial soon after the arrival of Buddhism two millennia ago. Buddhism in return adopted many Taoist beliefs and practices. It is no longer possible to estimate the number of adherents to these faiths. A more tolerant attitude towards religion had emerged by 1979, and the Government's Bureau of Religious Affairs was reactivated.

Ceremonies of reverence to ancestors have been observed by the whole population regardless of philosophical or religious beliefs.

Moslems are found in every province of China, being most numerous in the Ningxia–Hui Autonomous Region, Yunnan, Shaanxi, Gansu, Hebei, Honan, Shandong, Sichuan, Xinjiang and Shanxi. They totalled 14m. in 1986.

Roman Catholicism has had a footing in China for more than 3 centuries. In 1985 there were about 3m. Catholics who are members of the Patriotic Catholic Association, which declared its independence of Rome in 1958. In 1979 there were about 1,000 priests. In 1977 there were 78 bishops and 4 apostolic administrators, not all of whom were permitted to undertake religious activity. This figure included 46 'democratically elected' bishops not recognized by the Vatican. A bishop of Beijing was consecrated in 1979 without the consent of the Vatican and 2 auxiliary bishops of Shanghai in 1984. Archbishop Gong Pinmei, arrested in 1955, was freed in 1988. Protestants are members of the All-China Conference of Protestant Churches. 2 Protestant bishops were installed in 1988, the first for 30 years.

Education. In 1988 220m. people (70% women) were illiterate. In 1986 90% of school-age children attended school. In 1987 there were 176,775 kindergartens with 18·1m. children and 941,000 teachers. An educational reform of 1985 is phasing in compulsory 9-year education consisting of six years of primary schooling and three years of secondary schooling, to replace a previous 5-year system. In 1987 there were 807,406 primary schools with 6·09m. teachers and 128·4m. pupils, and 105,151 secondary schools, with 4·55m. teachers and 54·03m. pupils. There were 1,063 institutes of higher education, with 969,000 teachers and 1·95m. students.

University entry is dependent upon entrance examinations and students are funded by competitive scholarships. Following student demonstrations in Jan. 1987 political education courses and periods of labour service were restored to university curricula, and political criteria of selection re-applied. In 1989 the number of university places was cut by 30,000 to 610,000, and a compulsory year of military service inserted before student enrolment. First degree courses usually last 4 years. A further year of labour is obligatory before proceeding to postgraduate studies. In 1988 there were 149,000 full-time postgraduate and 670,000 undergraduate students.

There is an Academy of Sciences with provincial branches. An Academy of Social Sciences was established in 1977.

Among the universities are the following: People's University of China, Peking (founded 1912 by Dr Sun Yat-sen; reorganized 1950; about 3,000 students); Peking University, Peking (1898, enlarged 1945; about 10,000 students); Xiamen University, Fujian (1921 and 1937); Fudan University, Shanghai (1905); Inner Mongolia University, Hohhot; Lanzhou University, Lanzhou (Gansu Prov.); Nankai University, Tianjin (1919); Nanjing University, Nanjing (1888 and 1928); Jilin University, Changchun (Jilin Prov.); North-West University, Xian (Shanxi Prov.); Shandong University, Qingdao (1926); Sun Yat-sen University, Canton (founded 1924 by Dr Sun Yat-sen); Sichuan University, Chengdu (1931); Qinghua University, Peking, Wuhan University, Wuhan (Hubei Prov.; 1905 and 1928); Yunnan University, Kunming. In 1987 some 36,000 students were studying abroad, but in 1988 the number has reduced to 3,000 a year (600 only to USA).

Chen, T. H., *Chinese Education since 1949*. Oxford, 1981
Heyhoe, R., (ed.) *Contemporary Chinese Education*. London, 1984

Health. Medical treatment is free only for certain groups of employees, but where costs are incurred they are partly borne by the patient's employing organization. In 1988 there were 1,618,000 doctors, of whom 1,096,000 practised Chinese medicine. About 10% of doctors are in private practice.

In 1987 there were 60,429 hospitals (including 348 mental hospitals) and in 1988 2·5m. hospital beds.

DIPLOMATIC REPRESENTATIVES

Of China in Great Britain (49 Portland Pl., London, W1N 3AH)
Ambassador: (vacant).

Of Great Britain in China (Guang Hua Lu 11, Jian Guo Men Wai, Beijing)
Ambassador: Robin McLaren.

Of China in the USA (2300 Connecticut Ave., NW, Washington, D.C., 20008)
Ambassador: Zhu Qizhen.

Of the USA in China (Xiu Shui Bei Jie 3, Beijing)
Ambassador: James R. Lilley.

Of China to the United Nations
Ambassador: Li Daoyu.

Further Reading

Beijing Review. Beijing, weekly
China Daily [European ed.]. London, from 1986
China Directory [in Pinyin and Chinese]. Tokyo, annual
The China Quarterly. London, from 1960
China Reconstructs. Beijing, monthly
China's Foreign Trade. Bimonthly. Beijing, from 1966
People's Republic of China Yearbook. Beijing, from 1983
China Statistical Yearbook, 1989. Beijing and the Univ. of Illinois, 1990
The Population Atlas of China. OUP, 1988
Barnett, A. D., *The Making of Foreign Policy in China*. London, 1985
Barnett, A. D. and Clough, R., (eds.) *Modernizing China: Post-Mao Reform and Development*. Boulder, 1986
Bartke, W. (ed.) *Who's Who in the People's Republic of China*. 2nd ed. New York, 1986
Bartke, W. and Schier, P., *China's New Party Leadership: Biographies and Analysis*. London, 1985
Blecher, M., *China: Politics, Economics and Sociology*. London, 1986
Bonavia, D., *The Chinese*. New York, 1980.—*The Chinese: A Portrait*. London, 1981
Boorman, H. L. and Howard, R. C., (eds.) *Biographical Dictionary of Republican China*. 5 vols. Columbia Univ. Press, 1967–79
Brady, J. P., *Justice and Politics in People's China: Legal Order or Continuing Revolution?* London, 1982
Brown, D. G., *Partnership with China: Sino-foreign Joint Ventures in Historical Perspective*. Boulder, 1985
Bullard, M., *China's Political-Military Evolution*. Boulder, 1985
The Cambridge History of China. 14 vols. CUP, 1978 ff.
Chang, D. W., *China under Deng Xiao-ping: Political and Economic Reforms*. London, 1989
Cheng, P., *China*. [Bibliography] Oxford and Santa Barbara, 1983
Chow, G. C., *The Chinese Economy*. New York, 1985
Chu, G. C. and Hsu, F. L., (eds.) *China's New Social Fabric*. London, 1983
Cotterell, A., *China: A Concise Cultural History*. London, 1989
Deng Xiaoping, *Speeches and Writings*. 2nd ed. Oxford, 1987
Dietrich, C., *People's China: A Brief History*. OUP, 1986
Domes, J., *The Government and Politics of the PRC*. Boulder, 1985
Fairbank, J. K., *The Great Chinese Revolution 1800–1985*. London, 1987
Fathers, M. and Higgins, A., *Tiananmen: The Rape of Peking*. London and New York, 1989
Grummit, K., *China Economic Handbook*. London, 1986
Guide to China's Foreign Economic Relations and Trade. Hong Kong, 1984

Harding, H. (ed.) *China's Foreign Relations in the 1980's*. Yale Univ. Press, 1984.—*China's Second Revolution*. Washington, 1987
Hinton, H. C. (ed.) *The People's Republic of China 1949–1979*. 5 vols. Wilmington, 1980
Hook, B. (ed.) *The Cambridge Encyclopaedia of China*. CUP, 1982
Hsieh, C. M., *Atlas of China*. New York, 1973
Jingrong, W. (ed.) *The Pinyin-Chinese Dictionary*. Beijing and San Francisco, 1979
Kaplan, F. M. (ed.) *Encyclopedia of China Today*. 3rd ed. London, 1982
Kapur, H., *China and the European Economic Community*. Dordrecht, 1986
Kim, S. S. (ed.) *China and the World: Chinese Foreign Policy in the Post-Mao Era*. Boulder, 1984
Klein, D. W. and Clark, A. B., *Biographic Dictionary of Chinese Communism, 1921–1965*. Harvard Univ. Press, 1971
Lamb, M., *Directory of Officials and Organizations in China, 1968–1983*. Armonk, 1984
Lardy, N. R., *Agriculture in China's Modern Economic Development*. CUP, 1983
Leeming, F., *Rural China Today*. London, 1985
Lippit, V. D., *The Economic Development of China*. Armonk, 1987
Mabbett, I., *Modern China: The Mirage of Modernity*. New York, 1985
McCormick, B. L. *Political Reform in Post-Mao China: Democracy and Bureaucracy in a Leninist State*. California Univ. Press, 1990
Mancall, M., *China at the Center: 300 Years of Foreign Policy*. New York, 1984
Marshall, M., *Organizations and Growth in Rural China*. London, 1985
Maxwell, N. and McFarlane, B. (eds.) *China's Changed Road to Development*. Oxford, 1984
Moise, E. E., *Modern China: A History*. London, 1986
Moser, L. J., *The Chinese Mosaic: the Peoples and Provinces of China*. Boulder, 1985
Nathan, A. J., *Chinese Democracy*. London, 1986;-*China's Crisis: Dilemmas of Reform and Prospects for Democracy*. Columbia Univ. Press, 1990
Pan, L., *The New Chinese Revolution*. London, 1987
Pannell, C. W. and Laurence, J. C., *China: the Geography of Development and Modernization*. London, 1983
Riskin, C., *China's Political Economy: The Quest for Development since 1949*. OUP, 1987
Rodzinski, W., *A History of China*. Oxford, 1981–84
Schram, S. R. (ed.) *The Scope of State Power in China*. London, 1985
Segal, G., *Defending China*. OUP, 1985
Segal, G. and Tow, W. T. (eds.) *Chinese Defence Policy*. London, 1984
Song, J., *et al*, *Population Control in China*. New York, 1985
Spence, J. D., *The Search for Modern China*. London, 1990
The Times Atlas of China. London, 1974
Wong, K. and Chu, D. (eds.) *Modernization in China: The Case of the Shenzhen Special Economic Zone*. OUP, 1986
Yahuda, M. B., *Towards the End of Isolationism: China's Foreign Policy after Mao*. London, 1983
Yin, J., *Government of Socialist China*. Lanham, 1984
Young, G. (ed.) *China: Dilemmas of Modernisation*. London, 1985

TAIWAN [1]

'Republic of China'

Capital: Taipei
Population: 20·3m. (1990)
GNP per capita: US$7,992 (1990)

HISTORY. The island of Taiwan (Formosa) was ceded to Japan by China by the Treaty of Shimonoseki on 8 May 1895. After the Second World War the island was surrendered to Gen. Chiang Kai-shek in Sept. 1945 and was placed under Chinese administration on 25 Oct. 1945. USA broke off diplomatic relations with Taiwan on 1 Jan. 1979 on establishing diplomatic relations with the Peking Government. Relations between the USA and Taiwan are maintained through the American Institute on Taiwan and the Co-ordination Council for North American Affairs in the USA, set up in 1979 and accorded diplomatic status in Oct. 1980.

[1] See note on transcription of names p. 355.

AREA AND POPULATION. Taiwan lies between the East and South China Seas about 100 miles from the coast of Fujian. The total area of Taiwan Island, the Penghu Archipelago and the Kinma area is 13,969 sq. miles (36,179 sq. km). Population (1990), 20·3m., of whom some 2m. are mainland Chinese who came with the Nationalist Government. There are also 337,342 aboriginals. Population density: 562 per sq. km.

In 1989, birth rate was 1·46%; death rate, 0·43%; rate of growth, 1·03% per annum (2000 target: 0·72% per annum). Life expectancy, 1989: Males, 71 years; females, 76·2 years.

Taiwan is divided into two special municipalities (Taipei, the capital, population 2·71m. in 1989 and Kaohsiung, population 1·38m. in 1989), 5 municipalities (Taichung, Keelung, Tainan, Chiayi and Hsinchu) and 16 counties (*hsien*): Changhwa, Chiayi, Hsinchu, Hualien, Ilan, Kaohsiung, Miaoli, Nantou, Penghu, Pingtung, Taichung, Tainan, Taipei, Taitung, Taoyuan, Yunlin. The seat of the provincial government is at Chunghsing New Village.

CLIMATE. A tropical climate with hot, humid conditions and heavy rainfall in the summer months but cooler from Nov. to March when rainfall amounts are not so great. Typhoons may be experienced. Taipei. Jan. 59°F (15·3°C), July 83°F (29·2°C). Annual rainfall 100" (2,500 mm).

CONSTITUTION AND GOVERNMENT. Taiwan is controlled by the remnants of the Nationalist Government. On 1 March 1950, Chiang Kai-shek resumed the presidency of the 'Republic of China'. He died 5 April 1975. His son Chiang Ching-kuo was president from March 1978 to his death in Jan. 1988. He was succeeded by Lee Teng-hui, who on 21 March 1990 was re-elected unopposed as *President* for a 6-year term by the National Assembly by 641 votes to 47. The *Vice-President* is Li Yuan-zu.

The *National Assembly* was elected in 1947. In 1990 it had 648 delegates. Government is conducted through 5 councils (Executive, Legislative, Judicial, Examination, and Control *Yuan*). The highest administrative organ is the Executive Yuan, headed by the Prime Minister, which includes a number of ministers. The highest legislative body is the *Legislative Yuan*, elected in 1948, which in 1990 numbered 251 members. *Speaker:* Liang Su-yung. The National Assembly, Legislative Yuan and Control Yuan are elected bodies. Their terms of office have been extended indefinitely. As the number of original delegates dwindled, regulations introduced in 1966 and 1972 provided for the election of additional members to the National Assembly and Legislative Yuan, and elections were held in 1969, 1972, 1975, 1980, 1983 and 1986. In Feb. 1990 payments were introduced as an incentive for Mainland deputies to step down. Martial law, in force since 1949, was lifted in July 1987, and a ban on opposition parties was dropped in Jan. 1989. A new Democratic Progress Party (DPP) was formed in Oct. 1986 and a Democratic Liberal Party in Sept. 1987. In Dec. 1989 elections were held for 101 of the 261 seats in the Legislative Yuan, the remainder being Mainland deputies (122) or Presidential appointees. The Kuomintang (KMT) (membership, 2·44m. in 1990) won 60% of the vote, the DPP 30%, the latter winning 21 seats. In simultaneous *local elections* for 21 county executives and city mayors, the DPP won 6 posts with 40% of the vote. At the local authority elections of 1990 the KMT won 60% of the vote, the DPP, 30%.

State emblem: A 12-pointed white sun in a blue sky.

National flag: Red with a blue first quarter bearing the state emblem in white.

National anthem: 'San Min Chu I', words by Dr Sun Yat-sen; tune by Cheng Mao-yun.

The cabinet included the following in March 1991:

Prime Minister: Hau Pei-tsun (b. 1920).

Vice-Premier: Shih Chi-yang. *Foreign Minister:* Frederick F. Chien. *Minister of National Defence:* Chen Li-an. *Minister of the Interior:* Hsu Shui-teh. *Minister of Finance:* Wang Chien-hsien. *Minister of Education:* Mao Kao-wen. *Minister of Economic Affairs:* Vincent C. Sien. *Minister of Communications:* Clement C. P. Chang. *Chairman, Mongolian and Tibetan Affairs Commission:* Wu Hua-peng.

Chairman, Overseas Chinese Affairs Commission: Tseng Kwang-shun. The *Governor of Taiwan Province* was Lien Chan.

DEFENCE

Army. The Army, which was formed on the forces which escaped to Taiwan under Chiang Kai-shek at the end of the civil war in 1949, numbered about 270,000 in 1990. It was reorganized, re-equipped and trained by the USA and in 1990 consisted of 12 heavy and 6 light infantry divisions, 2 armoured infantry and 1 airborne brigades, 4 tank groups, 22 field artillery and 5 SAM battalions. The aviation element has about 118 helicopters. There is a conscription system for 2 years and reserve liability. Equipment includes 309 M-48A5 and 100 M-48H tanks and 275 M-24 and 675 M-41 light tanks.

Navy. The Taiwan navy consists principally of former US Navy ships over 40 years old and well overdue for replacement. A major programme of renewal has been initiated with new submarines, frigates and support ships on order. Current fleet strength is 2 new Netherlands-built diesel submarines, 24 ex-US 1940s destroyers, 10 frigates, 3 corvettes (ex-fleet minesweepers), 52 fast missile craft, 21 other patrol craft and 8 coastal minesweepers. The amphibious force includes 1 amphibious flagship, 1 dock landing ship, 25 landing ships and about 280 amphibious craft. Auxiliary craft include 4 support tankers, 2 repair and salvage ships, 6 tugs and 1 survey ship.

Main bases are at Tsoying, Makung and Keelung.

Active personnel in 1990 totalled 35,500 in the Navy and 30,000 in the Marine Corps. There are over 60,000 naval and marine reservists.

The Naval Air Command operates 12 small anti-submarine helicopters from the destroyers, 6 search and rescue helicopters and 32 S-2 Tracker anti-submarine aircraft are based ashore.

The Customs service operates 5 offshore cutters and 8 fast boats.

Air Force. The Nationalist Air Force is equipped mainly with aircraft of US design, including F-5E fighters built in Taiwan. It has 11 front-line squadrons of F-5E/F Tiger IIs, 3 of F-104G Starfighters and 1 tactical reconnaissance squadron of RF-104G Starfighters. The 6 transport squadrons are equipped with a VIP Boeing 720, 4 Boeing 727s, 12 Beech 1900s, 20 C-47s, about 40 C-119Gs, 12 C-130H Hercules and 10 C-123 Providers. There is a naval co-operation squadron with S-2A/E Trackers. Search and rescue units operate S-70 and Iroquois helicopters, and there are other helicopter and large training elements, some equipped with AT-3 twin-jet trainers designed and built in Taiwan and others with US-supplied T-34Cs. Total strength in 1990: 70,000 personnel.

INTERNATIONAL RELATIONS. By a treaty of 1 Dec. 1954 the USA was pledged to protect Taiwan, but this treaty lapsed 1 year after the USA established diplomatic relations with the People's Republic of China on 1 Jan. 1979. In April 1979 the Taiwan Relations Act was passed by the US Congress to maintain commercial, cultural and other relations between USA and Taiwan.

The People's Republic took over the China seat in the UN from the Nationalists on 25 Oct. 1971.

In May 1991 Taiwan ended its formal state of war with the People's Republic.

ECONOMY

Policy. There have been a series of development plans. The tenth (1990–93), aims at a growth rate of 7% (industry 6%, agriculture 1·5%).

Budget. There are 2 budgets, the national together with a special defence budget (partly secret) and the provincial (*i.e.,* for Taiwan proper). For the fiscal year July 1990–June 1991 the national budget is scheduled for NT$1,056,858m. Expenditure planned: 31·6% on defence; 20·1% on economic development; 17·5% on welfare; 21·7% on education, science and culture. Foreign exchange reserves were US$63,631m. in June 1990.

Currency. The unit of currency is the *New Taiwan dollar* (TWD), of 100 *cents*. There are coins of NT$ 0·5, 1, 5 and 10 and notes of NT$ 10, 50, 100, 500 and 1,000. Gold reserves were 13·6m. oz. July 1990. Exchange rates (March 1991): £1 = NT$51·35; US$1 = NT$27·07.

Banking and Finance. The Central Bank of China (reactivated in 1961) regulates the money supply, manages foreign exchange and issues currency. *Governor:* Samuel Shieh.

The Bank of Taiwan is the largest commercial bank and the fiscal agent of the Government. In addition, there are 15 domestic commercial banks and 38 local branches of foreign banks.

There is a stock exchange in Taipei.

ENERGY AND NATURAL RESOURCES

Electricity. Output of electricity in 1989 was 76,913m. kwh.; total generating capacity was 16·6m. kw. There are 3 nuclear power-stations (capacities 1m., 1m. and 0·6m. kw.) and a fourth is envisaged. Supply 110 volts; 60 Hz.

Minerals. There are reserves of coal (171m. tonnes), gold (1·1m. tonnes), copper (4·7m. tonnes), oil (0·5m. kl.) and natural gas (14·85m. cu. metres). In 1989, coal production was 0·8m. tonnes; refined oil, 2·5m. kl.; natural gas, 1,158m. cu. metres. Crude oil production (1989) 140,000 tonnes.

Agriculture. The cultivated area was 894,601 ha in 1989, of which 483,514 ha were paddy fields. Production in 1,000 tonnes, in 1989: Rice, 1,865; tea, 22; bananas, 198; pineapples, 231; sugar-cane, 6,628; sweet potatoes, 206; soybeans, 11; peanuts, 65.

Livestock (1989): Cattle, 165,136; pigs, 7,783,276; goats, 179,003.

Forestry. Forest area, 1989: 1,865,141 ha; forest reserves, 326,421,397 cu. metres; timber production, 191,215 cu. metres.

Fisheries. The fleet comprised 6,073 vessels over 20 GRT in 1989; the catch was 1,360,868 tonnes in 1988.

INDUSTRY. Output (in tonnes) in 1988 (and 1989): Steel bars, 3·6m. (4·3m.); pig-iron, 25,092 (29,904); shipbuilding, 662,508 (1,201,549); sugar, 575,403 (500,511); cement, 17·3m. (18m.); fertilizers, 1·24m. (1·36m.); paper, 787,617 (879,844); cotton fabrics, 745m. metres (786m.).

Labour. In 1989 the labour force was 8·39m., of whom 1·07m. worked in agriculture, forestry and fisheries, 3·49m. in industry (including 2·8m. in manufacturing and 630,000 in building), 1·61m. in commerce, 450,000 in transport and communications, and 1·64m. in other services. 139,000 were registered unemployed in 1988.

FOREIGN ECONOMIC RELATIONS

Commerce. Foreign trade affairs are handled by the China External Trade Development Council (founded 1970), which operates branches in 20 countries mostly under the name of Far East Trade Service. Principal exports: Textiles, electronic products, agricultural products, metal goods, plastic products. Principal imports: Oil, chemicals, machinery, electronic products. Total trade, in US$1m.:

	1984	*1985*	*1986*	*1987*	*1988*	*1989*
Imports	21,959	20,102	24,165	34,957	49,656	52,249
Exports	30,456	30,723	39,789	53,538	60,585	66,201

The USA, Japan and Hong Kong are Taiwan's major trade partners followed by Germany, UK and Canada. A mounting trade surplus has caused friction with the USA and a sharp appreciation of the Taiwan dollar. Economic liberalisation measures are being undertaken to improve the position.

Principal exports in 1989, in US$1,000m. (and percentage of total exports): Machinery and electrical equipment, 21·83 (33%); textiles, 10·33 (15·6%); metal and metalware, 5·19 (7·8%); footwear, headwear and umbrellas, 4·47 (6·8%); plastic and rubber goods, 4·33 (6·5%); toys, games, sports equipment, 3·03 (4·6%); vehicles and aircraft, 3·01 (4·6%); animals and products, 1·79 (2·7%); precision instruments, 1·68 (2·5%); leather and fur goods, 1·49 (2·3%).

Total trade between Taiwan and UK (British Department of Trade returns, in £1,000 sterling):

	1986	*1987*	*1988*	*1989*	*1990*
Imports to UK	705,775	1,006,880	1,150,392	1,351,695	1,211,968
Exports and re-exports from UK	192,492	292,275	355,786	407,432	430,643

Tourism. In 1989 2,004,126 tourists visited Taiwan, and 2,107,813 Taiwanese made visits abroad. The ban on Taiwanese travel to Communist China was lifted in 1987.

COMMUNICATIONS

Roads. In 1989 there were 19,998 km of roads (16,984 km surfaced). 10,205,185 motor vehicles were registered including 1,969,291 passenger cars, 21,852 buses, 573,576 trucks and 7,619,038 motor cycles. 1,754m. passengers and 244m. tonnes of freight were transported (excluding urban buses).

Railways. Total route length in 1989 was 2,502 km (1,067 mm to 762 mm gauge), of which a large proportion is owned by the Taiwan Sugar Corporation and other concerns. The state network consisted of 1,072 km. Freight traffic amounted to 18·1m. tonnes and passenger traffic to 127·3m.

Aviation. There are 2 international airports: Chiang Kai-shek at Taoyuan near Taipei, and Kaohsiung which operates daily flights to Hong Kong. There are 9 domestic airlines, including China Airlines (CAL), which also operates international services to Bangkok, Hong Kong, Jakarta, Kuala Lumpur, Manila, Seoul, Singapore, Amsterdam, Saudi Arabia, Japan and USA. In 1989 17·21m. passengers and 608,580 tonnes of freight were flown.

Shipping. The merchant marine in 1989 comprised 6 passenger ships, 79 container ships, 37 bulk carriers, 15 tankers and 127 mixed service ships, with a total DWT of 8·23m.

There are 4 international ports: Kaohsiung, Keelung, Hwalien and Taichung. The first two are container centres. Suao port is an auxiliary port to Keelung.

Telecommunications. In 1989 there were 12,441 post offices. In 1989 there were 5,822,663 telephone subscribers and 7,834,910 stations for telephone service. There are 3 TV networks.

Cinemas (1990). Cinemas numbered 623.

Newspapers and Books. There were 130 daily papers and 4,046 periodicals in 1989. 38,003 book titles were published in 1989.

RELIGION, EDUCATION AND WELFARE

Religion. There were 2·68m. Taoists in 1989 with 7,959 temples and 27,499 priests, 4·48m. Buddhists with 4,011 temples and 8,925 priests, 428,162 Protestants and 289,303 Catholics.

Education. Since 1968 there has been compulsory education for 9 years (6–15) with free tuition. In that year the curriculum was modernized to give more emphasis to science while retaining the traditional basis of Confucian ethics. Since 1983 school-leavers aged 15-18 receive part-time vocational education. There were, in 1989–90, 2,484 primary schools with 80,849 teachers and 2,384,801 pupils; 1,073 secondary schools with 81,986 teachers and 1,767,835 students; 116 schools of higher education, including 41 universities and colleges, with 25,581 full-time teachers and 535,064 students.

Health. In 1989 there were 86,646 medical personnel, including 18,529 doctors,

4,865 dentists and 3,353 doctors of Chinese medicine. There were 94 public hospitals with 34,489 beds and 771 private hospitals with 47,262 beds.

Further Reading

Statistical Yearbook of the Republic of China. Taipei, annual
Republic of China: A Reference Book. Taipei, annual
Taiwan Statistical Data Book. Taipei, annual
Annual Review of Government Administration, Republic of China. Taipei, annual
Gälli, A., *Taiwan ROC: A Chinese Challenge to the World*. London, 1987
Gold, T. B., *State and Society in the Taiwan Miracle*. Armonk, 1986
Hsieh, C. C., *Strategy for Survival: The Foreign Policy and External Relations of the Republic of China on Taiwan 1949–1979*. London, 1985
Kuo, S. W., *The Taiwan Economy in Transition*. Boulder, 1983
Lee, S.-Y., *Money and Finance in the Economic Development of Taiwan*. London, 1990
Lee, W.-C., *Taiwan:* [Bibliography]. Oxford and Santa Barbara, 1990
Liu, A. P. L., *Phoenix and the Lame Lion: Modernization in Taiwan and Mainland China, 1950–1980*. Stanford, 1987
Simon, D. F. S., *Taiwan, Technology Transfer, and Transnationalism*. Boulder, 1983

National Library: National Central Library, Taipei (established 1986). *Director:* Wang Chen-ku.

COLOMBIA

Capital: Bogotá
Population: 33m. (1990)
GNP per capita: US$1,280 (1989)

República de Colombia

HISTORY. The Vice-royalty of New Granada gained its independence of Spain in 1819, and was officially constituted 17 Dec. 1819, together with the present territories of Panama, Venezuela and Ecuador, as the state of 'Greater Colombia', which continued for about 12 years. It then split up into Venezuela, Ecuador and the republic of New Granada in 1830. The constitution of 22 May 1858 changed New Granada into a confederation of 8 states, under the name of Confederación Granadina. Under the constitution of 8 May 1863 the country was renamed 'Estados Unidos de Colombia', which were 9 in number. The revolution of 1885 led the National Council of Bogotá, composed of 2 delegates from each state, to promulgate the constitution of 5 Aug. 1886, forming the Republic of Colombia, which abolished the sovereignty of the states, converting them into departments, with governors appointed by the President of the Republic, though they retained some of their old rights, such as the management of their own finances.

AREA AND POPULATION. Colombia is bounded north by the Caribbean sea, north-west by Panama, west by the Pacific ocean, south-west by Ecuador and Peru, north-east by Venezuela and south-east by Brazil. The estimated area is 1,141,748 sq. km (440,829 sq. miles). It has a coastline of about 2,900 km, of which 1,600 km are on the Caribbean sea and 1,300 km on the Pacific ocean. Population census, (1985) 29,481,852; estimate (1990) 32,978,172. Bogotá, the capital, (census, 1985) 4,185,174; estimate (1990) 4,819,696.

The following table gives the officially adjusted figures for the 1985 census of population.

Departments	*Area (sq. km)*	*Population census 1985*	*Capital*	*Population census 1985*
Antioquia	63,612	4,067,664	Medellín	1,480,382
Atlántico	3,388	1,478,213	Barranquilla	927,233
Bolívar	25,978	1,288,985	Cartagena	563,949
Boyacá	23,189	1,209,739	Tunja	94,451
Caldas	7,888	883,024	Manizales	308,784
Caquetá	88,965	264,507	Florencia	87,342
Cauca	29,308	857,731	Popayán	164,809
César	22,905	699,428	Valledupar	223,637
Chocó	46,530	313,567	Quibdó	93,806
Córdoba	25,020	1,013,247	Montería	242,515
Cundinamarca [1]	22,478	1,512,928	Bogotá	4,227,706
La Guajira	20,848	299,995	Riohacha	85,621
Huila	19,890	693,713	Neiva	199,567
La Magdalena	23,188	890,934	Santa Marta	233,632
Meta	85,635	474,046	Villavicencio	191,001
Nariño	33,268	1,085,173	Pasto	136,646
Norte de Santander	21,658	913,491	Cúcuta	388,397
Quindío	1,845	392,208	Armenia	195,453
Risaralda	4,140	652,872	Pereira	300,224
Santander	30,537	1,511,392	Bucaramanga	377,585
Sucre	10,917	561,649	Sincelejo	141,012
Tolima	23,562	1,142,220	Ibagué	314,934
Valle	22,140	3,027,247	Cali	1,429,026

[1] Excluding Bogotá.

Intendencias	*Area (sq. km)*	*Population census 1985*	*Capital*	*Population census 1985*
Arauca	23,818	89,972	Arauca	26,736
Casanare	44,460	147,472	Yopal	29,707
Putumayo	24,885	174,219	Mocoa	27,153
San Andrés y Providencia	287	35,818	San Andrés	32,142

Comisarías	*Area (sq. km)*	*Population census 1985*	*Capital*	*Population census 1985*
Amazonas	109,665	39,937	Leticia	24,092
Guainía	72,238	12,345	Obando (Puerto Inírida)	12,345
Guaviare	42,327	47,073	San José del Guaviare	41,476
Vaupés	54,135	26,178	Mitú	18,007
Vichada	100,242	18,702	Puerto Carreño	10,758

Estimated population, 1990: 32,978,172 (females, 16,607,452). Deaths, 1987: 145,218 (infantile, 15,218).

The bulk of the population lives at altitudes of from 4,000 to 9,000 ft above sea-level. It is divided broadly into: 68% mestizo, 20% white, 7% Indio and 5% Negro.

The official language is Spanish.

CLIMATE. The climate includes equatorial and tropical conditions, according to situation and altitude. In tropical areas, the wettest months are March to May and Oct. to Nov. Bogotá. Jan. 58°F (14·4°C), July 57°F (13·9°C). Annual rainfall 42" (1,052 mm). Baranquilla. Jan. 80°F (26·7°C), July 82°F (27·8°C). Annual rainfall 32" (799 mm). Cali. Jan. 75°F (23·9°C), July 75°F (23·9°C). Annual rainfall 37" (915 mm). Medellin. Jan. 71°F (21·7°C), July 72°F (22·2°C). Annual rainfall 64" (1,606 mm).

CONSTITUTION AND GOVERNMENT. The legislative power rests with a *Congress* of 2 houses, the *Senate*, of 112 members, and the *House of Representatives*, of 199 members, both elected for 4 years. Congress meets annually at Bogotá on 20 July. Women were given the vote on 25 Aug. 1954.

The President is elected by direct vote of the people for a term of 4 years, and is not eligible for re-election until 4 years afterwards. Congress elects, for a term of 2 years, one substitute to occupy the presidency in the event of a vacancy during a presidential term.

A National Economic Council, functioning since May 1935, went through several transformations, becoming in 1954 a Directorate of Planning.

National Flag: Three horizontal stripes of yellow, blue, red with the yellow of double width.

National anthem: Oh! Gloria inmarcesible ('Oh Glory unfading!'; words by R. Núñez; tune by O. Síndici).

The following is a list of presidents since 1953:

Gen. Gustavo Rojas Pinilla, 13 June 1953–10 May 1957.
Military Junta, Maj.-Gen. Gabriel París and 4 others, 10 May 1957–7 Aug. 1958.
Dr Alberto Lleras Camargo (Lib.), 7 Aug. 1958–7 Aug. 1962.
Dr Guillermo León Valencia (Cons.), 7 Aug. 1962–7 Aug. 1966.
Dr Carlos Lleras Restrepo (Lib.), 7 Aug. 1966–7 Aug. 1970.
Dr Misael Pastrana Borrero (Cons.), 7 Aug 1970–7 Aug. 1974.
Dr Alfonso López Michelsen (Cons./Lib.), 7 Aug. 1974–7 Aug. 1978.
Dr Julio Cesar Turbay Ayala (Lib.), 7 Aug. 1978–7 Aug. 1982.
Dr Belisario Betancur Cuartas (Cons.), 7 Aug. 1982–7 Aug. 1986.
Dr Virgilio Barco Vargas (Lib.), 7 Aug. 1986–7 Aug. 1990.

President: At the presidential elections of May 1990 César Gaviria Trujillo was elected by 47% of the vote (turn-out was 45%). He took office on 7 Aug. 1990.

Simultaneously with the presidential elections, a referendum was held in which 7m. votes were cast for the establishment of a special assembly to draft a new constitution. Elections were held on 9 Dec. 1990 for this 70-member 'Constitutional Assembly' which was scheduled to operate from Feb. to July 1991. The electorate was 14·2m.; turn-out was 3·7m. The Liberals gained 24 seats, M-19 (a former guerilla organization), 19.

The Cabinet was composed as follows in Feb. 1991:

Defence: Gen. Oscar Botero. *Interior:* Humberto de la Calle. *Finance:* Rudolph Hommes. *Agriculture:* Gabriel Rosas Vega. *Economic Development:* Ernesto Samper. *Labour and Social Security:* Maria Teresa Forero de Saade. *Health:* Antonio Navarro Wolff. *Mines and Energy:* Margarita Mena de Quevado. *Educa-*

tion: Manuel F. Becera. *Public Works and Transport:* Priscila Ceballos Ordoñez. *Government:* Raul Orujuela Bueno. *Justice:* Carlos Lemos Simmonds. *Foreign Affairs:* Luis Fernando Jaramillo.

Local government: The country is divided into 23 *departamentos*, 4 *intendencias*, 5 *comisarías* and a Special District of Bogotá. The governor of each is appointed by the President, but each has also a directly-elected legislature. The *departamentos* are subdivided into municipalities. The mayors of these, and the Special District of Bogotá, are elected by direct vote for a 2-year term.

DEFENCE. Men become liable for 1 year's military service at age 18, although the system is applied selectively. *Ex*-conscripts remain in the reserve, divided into 3 classes, until age 45.

Army. The Army consists of 14 infantry brigades, artillery, cavalry, engineer and motorized troops and the usual services. Personnel (1990) 111,400 men (conscripts, 38,000); reserves 100,000. Number of national police (1990) 80,000.

Navy. Colombia has 2 Federal German-built 1,200-ton diesel-electric powered patrol submarines completed in 1975, 2 Italian-built midget submarines; 4 small German-built missile-armed frigates with helicopter decks and 2 fast patrol craft. There are 3 river gunboats and 10 riverine patrol craft. Auxiliaries include 2 surveying vessels, 2 small transports, 1 training ship, 5 service craft and 10 tugs. Personnel in 1989 totalled 6,000, plus a brigade of marines numbering 6,000. An air arm was formed in 1984 and operates 4 BO-105 helicopters for ship-based ASW and SAR duties.

Air Force. Formed in 1922, the Air Force has been independent of the Army and Navy since 1943, when its reorganization began with US assistance. In 1986 it had about 300 aircraft, including a squadron of Mirage 5-COA fighter-bombers, 5-COR reconnaissance aircraft and 5-COD two-seat operational trainers; 2 squadrons of A-37B jets for counter-insurgency duties, a transport group equipped with 3 C-130, 12 C-47s, 3 C-54s, 4 DC-6s and a small number of Arava, Beaver and Turbo-Porter light transports; a presidential F-28 Fellowship jet transport; 1 Boeing 707, UH-1B/H utility helicopters; and a reconnaissance unit with Iroquois, Lama, Hughes OH-6A, 300C and TH-55 helicopters. Eight more C-47s, 2 C-54s, 1 F-28 and 4 HS.748 transports are flown by the Air Force operated airline SATENA. Thirty Cessna T-41D primary trainer/light transports were delivered in 1968 and were followed by 10 T-37C jet advanced trainers to supplement piston-engined T-34s and T-33A armed jet trainers. Total strength (1990) 7,000 personnel.

INTERNATIONAL RELATIONS

Membership. Colombia is a member of the UN, OAS, the Andean Group and LAIA.

ECONOMY

Policy. The 1986–90 Development Plan gave priority to the eradication of poverty.

Budget. Revenue and expenditure of central government in 1989: Revenue, 2,234,095m. pesos; expenditure, 2,131,124m. pesos. External public debt, 30 June 1989, US$13,296m.

Currency. Coins include 1, 2, 5, 10, 20 and 50 *pesos*. There are also notes representing 100, 200, 500, 1,000, 2,000 and 5,000 *gold pesos*. Money in circulation, Feb. 1989: 410,705m. pesos. Exchange rate, March 1991: 1111·15 *pesos* = £1 sterling; 585·74 *pesos* = US$1.

Banking and Finance. On 23 July 1923 the Bank of the Republic was inaugurated as a semi-official central bank, with the exclusive privilege of issuing bank-notes in Colombia; its charter, in 1951, was extended to 1973. Its note issues must be covered by a reserve in gold of foreign exchange of 25% of their value. Its international reserves in Feb. 1989 were US$3,635·6m. Total assets (Dec. 1988) 2,858,364m.

There are 25 commercial banks, of which 12 are privately owned, 8 jointly owned by Colombian and foreign interest and 5 official in nature, with total assets of 3,483,559 pesos as of June 1988.

There are stock exchanges in Bogotá, Medellín and Cali.

Weights and Measures. The metric system was introduced in 1857, but in ordinary commerce Spanish weights and measures are generally used; according to new definitions by the Ministry of Development, *e.g.*, *botella* (750 grammes), *galón* (5 *botellas*), *vara* (70 cm), *arroba* (25 lb., of 500 grammes; 4 *arrobas* = 1 quintal).

ENERGY AND NATURAL RESOURCES

Electricity. Capacity of electric power (1989) was 8·85m. kw. Electric power produced in 1987, 29,650m. kwh. Supply 110, 120 and 150 volts; 60 Hz.

Oil. Production in 1989 was 20·3m. tonnes.

Minerals. Colombia is rich in minerals; gold is found chiefly in Antioquia and moderately in Cauca, Caldas, Tolima, Nariño and Chocó; output in 1989, 948,626 troy oz.

Other minerals are silver (220,139 troy oz. in 1989), copper, lead, mercury, manganese, emeralds (of which Colombia accounts for about half of world production) and platinum; production of platinum, 1989, 31,281 troy oz. The chief emerald mines are those of Muzo and Chivor.

The Government holds the monopoly, which is leased to the Banco de la República, for extracting salts from the outstanding Zipaquirá mines (several hundred feet in depth and several hundred square miles in area) and for evaporating many sea salt pans; salt production in 1989 was 190,380 tonnes of land salt from the Zipaquirá mines and 471,140 tonnes of sea salt from Manaure and Galerazamba on the Caribe coast. Coal reserves were estimated at 20,963m. tonnes in 1986; production (1990, provisional) 20·5m. tonnes.

Agriculture. Very little of the country is under cultivation, but much of the soil is fertile and is coming into use as roads improve. The range of climate and crops is extraordinary; the agricultural colleges have different courses for 'cold-climate farming' and 'warm-climate farming'. In 1990 there were 2,461,960 ha under temporary cultivation and 1,340,010 under permanent.

Coffee area harvested (1988) 1m. ha; production (1990) 11,066,000 60 kg. sacks. Crops are grown by smallholders, and are picked all the year round. Production (1990, in 1,000 tonnes): Potatoes, 2,797·6; rice, 2,100·5; maize, 1,187·8; sorghum, 757·8.

The rubber tree grows wild but is also cultivated. Fibres are being exploited, notably the 'fique' fibre, which furnishes all the country's requirements for sacks and cordage; output (1990 estimate) 23,460 tonnes.

Livestock (1988): 24,307,000 cattle, 2,586,000 pigs, 2,652,000 sheep, 152·4m. poultry.

Fisheries. Total catch (1987) 83,569 tonnes.

INDUSTRY

Production (1989): Iron, 567,353 tons; cement, 6,643,473 tons; motor cars, 40,203; industrial vehicles, 13,573. In 1987 there were 6,927 manufacturing establishments.

Labour. In 1987 477,170 persons were employed in manufacturing (145,644 women).

FOREIGN ECONOMIC RELATIONS

Commerce. Imports (c.i.f. values) and exports (f.o.b. values) (excluding export tax) for calendar years (in US$1m.):

	1985	*1986*	*1987*	*1988*	*1989*
Imports	4,131	3,852	4,228	5,005	5,010
Exports	3,552	5,108	5,024	5,026	5,739

Important articles of export in 1989 (in US$1m.) were coffee (1,524), bananas

(260), flowers (105), clothing and textiles (148), crude oil (1,045), bituminous (447), fuel oil (304), precious stones and gems (102). The chief imports are machinery, vehicles, tractors, metals and manufactures, rubber, chemical products, wheat, fertilizers and wool.

Imports in 1989 (in US$1,000) from USA were valued at 1,566,210; Japan, 496,462; Federal Republic of Germany, 352,477; Brazil, 201,145; Venezuela, 196,634. Exports in 1989 (in US$1,000) to USA, 2,343,184; Federal Germany, 496,318; Japan, 259,211; Netherlands, 328,814; Panama, 229,513; Venezuela (1988), 220,729.

Total trade between Colombia and UK (British Department of Trade returns, in £1,000 sterling):

	1986	*1987*	*1988*	*1989*	*1990*
Imports to UK	94,112	65,331	61,835	71,658	82,507
Exports and re-exports from UK	58,084	61,385	53,132	63,525	60,469

Tourism. Foreign visitors totalled 828,903 in 1988.

COMMUNICATIONS

Roads. Owing to the mountainous character of the country, the construction of arterial roads and railways is costly and difficult. Total length of highways, about 75,000 km in 1983. Of the 2,300-mile Simón Bolívar highway, which runs from Caracas in Venezuela to Guayaquil in Ecuador, the Colombian portion is complete. Buenaventura and Cali are linked by a highway (Carreterra al Mar). Motor vehicles in 1989 numbered 1,433,956, of which 231,306 were passenger cars and 272,882 lorries. In 1988 4,917m. passengers were carried by road transport.

Railways. There are 5 divisions of the State Railway with a total length of 2,622 km in 1985 and a gauge of 914 mm. The Pacific Railway connects Bogotá with the port of Buenaventura. The Atlantic line from Bogotá to Sta. Marta was opened in July 1961. Three connecting links are planned to improve the operating efficiency of the network. Total railway traffic, 1989, was 866,743 passengers and 654,104 tonnes of freight. By 1990 the State Railway was in liquidation, and 3 new public companies were preparing to take over services and obligations in 1992. A metro is scheduled to open in Medellín in 1992.

Aviation. There are 670 landing grounds of all kinds. In 1989 the national airports moved 5,625,000 passengers and 88,784 tonnes of cargo. There were 1,026,000 international passengers and 113,131 tonnes of international cargo.

Shipping. Vessels entering Colombian ports in 1989 unloaded 5,581,000 tonnes of imports and loaded 17,893,000 tonnes of exports.

The Magdelena River is subject to drought, and navigation is always impeded during the dry season, but it is an important artery of passenger and goods traffic. The river is navigable for 900 miles; steamers ascend to La Dorada, 592 miles from Barranquilla. 1,124,537 passengers, 149,852 head of cattle and 3,040 tonnes of freight were carried by inland waterways in 1988.

Telecommunications. The length of telephone lines in service in 1989 was 943,076 km (Bogotá), nationally, 1,976,618 km.; instruments in use, 1 Jan. 1984, 2,547,222. The cable company is government owned. Television was established in 1954 and in 1978 there were 1·75m. sets in use. In 1983 there were 485 radio stations, of which 50 were in Bogotá.

Cinemas (1987). There were 657 cinemas, of which 64 were in Bogotá.

Newspapers (1984). There were 31 daily newspapers, with daily circulation totalling 1·5m.

JUSTICE, RELIGION, EDUCATION AND WELFARE

Justice. The Supreme Court, at Bogotá, of 20 members, is divided into 3 chambers—civil cassation (6), criminal cassation (8), labour cassation (6). Each of the 61 judicial districts has a superior court with various sub-dependent tribunals of lower juridical grade. 257,511 crimes were reported in 1988.

Religion. The religion is Roman Catholic, with the Cardinal Archbishop of Bogotá as Primate of Colombia, the Cardinal Archbishop of Cartagena and 8 other archbishops in Manizales, Medellín, Nueva Pamplona, Popayán, Cali, Bucaramanga, Ibagué, Barranquilla, Santa Fé de Antioquia and Tunja. There are also 44 bishops, 8 apostolic vicars, 5 apostolic prefects and 2 prelates. In 1990 there were 1,546 parishes and 4,020 priests. Other forms of religion are permitted so long as their exercise is 'not contrary to Christian morals or the law.'

Education. Primary education is free but not compulsory, and facilities are limited. Schools are both state and privately controlled. In 1988 there were 7,759 pre-primary schools with 14,918 teachers and 340,244 pupils, 37,948 primary schools with 136,549 teachers and 4,044,220 pupils and 6,134 secondary schools with 99,392 teachers and 2,076,455 pupils. There were 235 higher education establishments with 457,680 students.

In 1987 there were 60 institutes of higher education with 79,743 students, 42 technological institutes with 29,729 students and 60 institutes for professional training with 28,891 students.

There are 73 universities including the National University in Bogotá (founded 1886). In 1988 there were 319,319 students.

Health. In 1988 there were 926 hospitals and clinics. There were also 861 health centres.

DIPLOMATIC REPRESENTATIVES

Of Colombia in Great Britain (3 Hans Cres., London, SW1X 0LR)
Ambassador: Virgilio Barco Vargas.

Of Great Britain in Colombia (Calle 98, No. 9–03 Piso 4, Bogotá)
Ambassador: K. Elliott Hedley Morris.

Of Colombia in the USA (2118 Leroy Pl., NW, Washington, D.C., 20008)
Ambassador: Dr Jaime Garcia Parrz.

Of the USA in Colombia (Calle 38, 8-61, Bogotá)
Ambassador: Thomas E. McNamara.

Of Colombia to the United Nations
Ambassador: Dr Enrique Peñalosa Carnargo.

Further Reading

Anuario de Comercio Exterior de Colombia. Departamento Administrativo Nacional de Estadística (DANE)
Anuario de Industria Manufactura. DANE
Anuario Estadístico Bogotá D. E. Bogotá
Boletín Mensual de Estadística. DANE, monthly
Colombia Estadística. DANE, annual
Economía y Estadística. DANE, occasional
Estadística del Sector Agropecuario. Ministerio de Agricultura, annual
Informe Financiero del Contralor General. Annual
Informe del Gerente de la Caja de Crédito Agrario, Industrial y Minero. Annual
Memorias (13) de los Ministros al Congreso Nacional. Annual
Braun, H., *The Assassination of Gaitán: Public Life and Urban Violence in Colombia.* Univ. of Wisconsin Press, 1985
Hartlyn, J., *The Politics of Coalition Rule in Colombia.* CUP, 1988
Morairetz, D., *Why the Emperor's New Clothes are not made in Colombia.* OUP, 1982

COMOROS

Capital: Moroni
Population: 503,000 (1990)
GNP per capita: US$440 (1988)

République Fédérale Islamique des Comores

HISTORY. The 3 islands forming the present state became French protectorates at the end of the 19th century, and were proclaimed colonies on 25 July 1912. With neighbouring Mayotte they were administratively attached to Madagascar from 1914 until 1947, when the 4 islands became a French Overseas Territory, achieving internal self-government in Dec. 1961.

In referenda held on each island on 22 Dec. 1974, the 3 western islands voted overwhelmingly for independence, while Mayotte voted to remain French. The Comoran Chamber of Deputies unilaterally declared the islands' independence on 6 July 1975, but Mayotte remained a French dependency.

The first government of Ahmed Abdallah was overthrown on 3 Aug. 1975 by a coup led by Ali Soilih (who assumed the Presidency on 2 Jan. 1976), but Ahmed Abdallah regained the Presidency after a second coup ousted Ali Soilih in May 1978. In Nov. 1989 President Abdallah was assassinated. The revolt was helped by mercenaries led by Bob Dinard who finally left the Comoros on 15 Dec. 1989.

AREA AND POPULATION. The Comoros consists of 3 islands in the Indian ocean between the African mainland and Madagascar with a total area of 1,862 sq. km (719 sq. miles). Population (estimate, 1990) 503,000.

	Area sq. km	*Population census 1980*	*Chief town*	*Population census 1980*
Njazídja (Grande Comore)	1,148	192,177	Moroni	20,112
Mwali (Mohéli)	290	17,194	Fomboni	5,663
Nzwani (Anjouan)	424	137,621	Mutsamudu	12,518
	1,862	346,992		

The indigenous population are a mixture of Malagasy, African, Malay and Arab peoples; the vast majority speak Comoran, an Arabised dialect of Swahili, but a small proportion speak Makua (a bantu language), French or Arabic. In 1990, 27·1% of the population were urban.

CLIMATE. There is a tropical climate, affected by Indian monsoon winds from the north, which gives a wet season from Nov. to April. Moroni. Jan. 81°F (27·2°C), July 75°F (23·9°C). Annual rainfall, 113" (2,825 mm).

CONSTITUTION AND GOVERNMENT. Under the new Constitution approved by referendum on 1 Oct. 1978 (amended 1983), the Comoros are a Federal Islamic Republic. Mayotte has the right to join when it so chooses.

The *President* is Head of State, directly elected for a 6-year term (renewable once). He appoints up to 9 other Ministers to form the Council of Government, on which each island's Governor has a non-voting seat. There is a 42-member unicameral Federal Assembly, directly elected for 5 years. Each of the 3 islands is administered by a Governor (nominated by the President), up to 4 Commissioners whom he appoints to assist him, and a *Legislative Council* directly elected for 5 years.

At the presidential elections of March 1990 Said Mohamed Djohar gained 55% of votes cast, against one opponent.

President: Said Mohamed Djohar, assumed office in March 1990.

National flag: Green with a crescent and 4 stars all in white in the centre, tilted towards the lower fly.

DEFENCE

Army. The army had a strength of about 700 in 1988.

Navy. An ex-British landing craft built in 1945 was transferred from France in 1976 and another vessel, with ramps, was purchased in 1981. Two small patrol boats were supplied by Japan in 1982. Personnel in 1990 numbered about 200.

Air Arm. In 1988 only 1 Cessna 402B communications aircraft and an Ecureuil helicopter were in operation.

INTERNATIONAL RELATIONS

Membership. Comoros is a member of UN and an ACP state of EEC.

ECONOMY

Budget. In 1986, current revenue amounted to 5,816m. Comorian francs and current expenditure to 10,380m. Comorian francs; the separate capital budget totalled 17,400m. Comorian francs revenue against 17,400m. Comorian francs expenditure.

Currency. The unit of currency is the *Comorian franc* (KMF). There are banknotes of 500, 1,000, and 5,000 *Comorian francs*. In March 1991, £1 = CF496·13; US$1 = CF261·53.

Banking. The Institut d'émission des Comores was established as the new bank of issue in 1975. The chief commercial banks are the Banque des Comores, established in 1974 by the separation of the former Comoran section of the Banque de Madagascar et des Comores and the Banque de Développement des Comores.

Weights and Measures. The metric system is in force.

ENERGY AND NATURAL RESOURCES

Electricity. Production (1986) 5m. kwh.

Agriculture. The chief product was formerly sugar-cane, but now vanilla, copra, maize and other food crops, cloves and essential oils (citronella, ylang, lemongrass) are the most important products. Production (1988 in tonnes): Cassava, 95,000; coconuts, 53,000; bananas, 39,000; sweet potatoes, 19,000; rice, 18,000; maize, 6,000 and copra, 3,000.

Livestock (1988): Cattle, 85,000; sheep, 10,000; goats, 96,000; asses, 4,000.

Forestry. Njazídja has a fine forest and produces timber for building.

Fisheries. In 1983 the catch was (estimate) 4,000 tonnes.

FOREIGN ECONOMIC RELATIONS

Commerce. Imports in 1985 amounted to 16,481m. Comorian francs, exports to 7,048m. Comorian francs. France provided 41% of imports and took 66% of exports. The main exports (1985) were vanilla (67% of value), cloves (20%), ylang-ylang (9%), essences, copra and coffee.

Trade between Comoros and UK (British Department of Trade returns, in £1,000 sterling):

	1986	*1987*	*1988*	*1989*	*1990*
Imports to UK	...	91	33	60	54
Exports and re-exports from UK	307	527	333	419	236

Tourism. In 1986 there were about 5,000 visitors.

COMMUNICATIONS

Roads. In 1983 there were 750 km of classified roads, of which 262 km were tarmac. There were 3,600 passenger cars and about 2,000 commercial vehicles.

Aviation. There is an international airport at Hahaya (on Njazídja). Air Comores have twice-weekly flights to Antananarivo, Dar es Salaam and Mombasa. Air

France and Air Madagascar also have twice-weekly flights to Antananarivo. Air Comores has daily internal flights between Moroni and Nzwani, and 5 per week between Moroni and Mwali.

Shipping. In 1982, vessels entering Comoran ports (excluding internal traffic) discharged 39,000 tonnes and loaded 15,000 tonnes.

Telecommunications. There were 496 telephones in 1983. *Comores-Inter* broadcasts in French and Comorian on short-wave and FM for approximately 8 hours a day. Number of radios (1988) 40,000.

JUSTICE, RELIGION, EDUCATION AND WELFARE

Justice. French and Moslem law is in a new consolidated code.The Supreme Court comprises 7 members, 2 each appointed by the President and the Federal Assembly, and 1 by each island's Legislative Council.

Religion. Islam is the official religion, and over 99% of the population are Sunni Moslems; there are about 1,300 Christians.

Education. In 1981 there were 59,709 pupils and 1,292 teachers in 236 primary schools; 32 secondary schools had 13,528 pupils and 432 teachers, 2 technical schools held 151 students with 9 teachers, and a teacher-training college had 119 students and 8 teachers.

Health. In 1978 there were 20 doctors, 1 dentist, 2 pharmacists, 35 midwives and 124 nursing personnel. In 1980 there were 17 hospitals and clinics with 763 beds.

DIPLOMATIC REPRESENTATIVES

Of Great Britain in Comoros
Ambassador: M. E. Howell, CMG, OBE (resides in Port Louis).

Of the Comoros in the USA
Ambassador: Amini Al Moumin.

Of the USA in the Comoros
Ambassador: Harry K. Walker. (resides in Antananarivo).

Of the Comoros to the United Nations
Ambassador: Amini Ali Moumin.

Further Reading

Newitt, N., *The Comoro Islands*. London, 1985

CONGO

Capital: Brazzaville
Population: 2·26m. (1990)
GNP per capita: US$930 (1988)

République Populaire du Congo

HISTORY. First occupied by France in 1882, the Congo became (as 'Middle Congo') a territory of French Equatorial Africa from 1910–58, when it became a member state of the French Community. It became an independent Republic on 15 Aug. 1960.

The first President, Fulbert Youlou, was deposed on 15 Aug. 1963 by a *coup* led by Alphonse Massemba-Débat, who became President on 19 Dec. Following a second *coup* in Aug. 1968, the Army took power under the leadership of Major Marien Ngouabi, whose colleague, Major Alfred Raoul, was appointed President from 3 Sept. until 1 Jan. 1969, when Ngouabi himself became President.

The country's present name was established on 3 Jan. 1970, when a Marxist-Leninist state was introduced. Ngouabi was assassinated on 18 March 1977, and succeeded by Col. Joachim Yhombi-Opango, who in turn was replaced on 5 Feb. 1979 by Col. Denis Sassou-Nguesso.

AREA AND POPULATION. The Congo is bounded by Cameroon and the Central African Republic in the north, Zaïre to the east and south, Angola and the Atlantic Ocean to the south-west and Gabon to the west, and covers 341,821 sq. km. At the census of 1984 the population was 1,909,248, including the towns of Brazzaville, the capital (585,812), Pointe-Noire, the main port and oil centre (294,203), Nkayi (formerly Jacob) (35,540) and Loubomo (formerly Dolisie) (49,134). Over 51% were urban.

Estimated population in 1990, 2,264,300 (Brazzaville, 760,300; Pointe-Noire, 387,774; Loubomo, 62,073; Nkayi, 40,019; Mossendjo, 15,570; Ouesso, 14,587).

Area, estimated population and capitals of the regions in 1990 were:

Region	*Sq. km*	*1990*	*Capital*	*Region*	*Sq. km*	*1990*	*Capital*
Kouilou	13,650	83,156	Pointe-Noire	Capital District	65	760,300	Brazzaville
Niari	25,918	120,057	Loubomo	Plateaux	38,400	114,629	Djambala
Lékoumou	20,950	71,248	Sibiti	Cuvette	71,248	144,427	Owando
Bouenza	12,258	165,967	N'kayi	Sangha	55,796	34,851	Ouesso
Pool	33,955	188,285	Kinkala	Likouala	66,044	61,358	Impfondo

In 1984, 45% spoke Kongo dialects, chiefly in the south and south-west; 20% were Teke (in the south-east); 15% Sanka and 16% Ubangi chiefly inhabit the north. There are also about 12,000 pygmies and 12,000 Europeans (mainly French). French is the official language, but 2 local *patois*, Monokutuba (west of Brazzaville) and Lingala (north of Brazzaville), serve as lingua francas.

CLIMATE. An equatorial climate, with moderate rainfall and a small range of temperature. There is a long dry season from May to Oct. in the S.W. plateaux, but the Congo Basin in the N.E. is more humid, with rainfall approaching 100" (2,500 mm). Brazzaville. Jan. 78°F (25·6°C), July 73°F (22·8°C). Annual rainfall 59" (1,473 mm).

CONSTITUTION AND GOVERNMENT. In July 1979 a new Constitution was approved by referendum. Executive power was vested in the President, elected for a 5-year term by the National Congress of the *Parti congolais du travail* (the sole legal party since 1969). The President is assisted by a Council of Ministers, appointed and led by him. The PCT Congress elects a Central Committee of 75 members and a Political Bureau of 10 to administer it; it nominates all candidates for the 153-member People's National Assembly and for the regional, district and local councils, all of which were last elected on 11 Aug. 1984. In 1984 a constitutional amendment made the President Head of Government and reduced the role of the Prime Minister to that of a co-ordinator. In Dec. 1990 the President announced that on 25 Feb. 1991 a national conference would convene to consider the Congo's constitutional future, set up a provisional government and fix dates for presidential and parliamentary elections.

The Council of Ministers in Jan. 1991 was composed as follows:

President, Head of Government, Minister of Defence and Security: Col. Denis Sassou-Nguesso.

Prime Minister: Gen. Louis Sylvain Goma.

Planning and Economy: Pierre Moussa. *Youth and Rural Development:* Gabriel Oba-Apounou. *Ngollo Forestry:* Col. Raymond Damas. *Foreign Affairs and Co-operation:* Antoine Ndinga Oba. *Information:* Paul Ngatse. *Territorial Adminstration and People's Power:* Celestin Ngoma-Foutou. *Equipment, with responsibility for the Environment:* Florent Tsiba. *Health and Social Affairs:* Ossebi Douniam. *Mines and Energy, Posts and Telecommunications:* Aimé Emmanuel Yoka. *Secondary and Higher Education, with responsibility for Scientific Research:* Rodolphe Adada. *Basic Education and Literacy:* Pierre-Damien Bassoukou-Boumba. *Physical Education and Sport:* Jean-Claude Ganga. *Culture and Arts:* Jean-Baptiste Tati-Loutard. *Trade and Small and Medium-Sized Enterprises:* Alphonse Boudenesa. *Fishing, Industry and Handicrafts, with responsibility for Tourism:* Hilaire Babassana. *Labour and Social Security:* Jeanne Dambenzet. *Minister in the Presidency, with responbsibility for State Control:* Auxence Ickonga. *Finance and Budget:* Edouard Ngakosso. *Justice, Keeper of the Seals, with responsibility for Administrative Reforms:* Alphonse Nzoungou. *Transport and Civil Aviation:* François Bita.

National flag: Red, in the canton the national emblem of a crossed hoe and mattock, a green wreath and a gold star.

Local Government: The capital district of Brazzaville and the 9 regions are under an appointed Commissioner and an elected Council, and are sub-divided into 46 districts and 6 communes: Brazzaville, Pointe-Noire, Loubomo, Nkayi, Mossendjo and Ouesso.

DEFENCE

Army. The Army consists of 8 battalions, 2 armoured, 1 artillery and 3 infantry, 1 engineering, and 1 paracommando. Equipment includes 35 T-54/-55 and 15 T-59 tanks. Total personnel (1991) 8,000.

Navy. The combatant flotilla includes 3 modern Spanish-built, 6 ex-Soviet and 3 ex-Chinese inshore patrol craft. There are also 2 French-built tugs and numerous boats. Personnel in 1990 totalled 300.

Air Force. The Air Force had (1991) about 500 personnel, 15 MiG-17 jet fighters, 6 Antonov An-24/26 turboprop transports, 2 C-47, 2 Nord 262, and 2 Noratlas piston-engined transports, 3 Broussard communications aircraft, 4 L-39 jet trainers and 2 Alouette II and 2 Alouette III light helicopters.

INTERNATIONAL RELATIONS

Membership. Congo is a member of the UN, OAU and is an ACP state of the EEC.

ECONOMY

Budget. The 1988 Budget provided for revenue of 251,800m. francs CFA (over 50% from overseas funding) and expenditure of 283,976m. francs CFA, of which 252,800m. were for administration and 31,976m. for investment.

Currency. The unit of currency is the *franc CFA* (BEAC) with a parity value of 50 *francs CFA* to 1 French franc. There are coins of 1, 2, 5, 10, 25, 50, 100 and 500 *francs* CFA, and banknotes of 100, 500, 1,000, 5,000 and 10,000 *francs* CFA. In March 1991, £1 = 496·13 *francs*; US$1 = 261·53 *francs*.

Banking and Finance. The *Banque des États de l'Afrique Centrale* is the bank of issue. There are 4 commercial banks situated in Brazzaville, including the *Banque Commerciale Congolaise* and the *Union Congolaise de Banques*.

ENERGY AND NATURAL RESOURCES

Electricity. Total production in 1989 was 397m. kwh from a hydro-electric plant at Djoué near Brazzaville. Supply 220 volts; 50 Hz.

Oil. Oil reserves are estimated at 500–1,000m. tonnes. Output in 1989 was 7,969,300 tonnes from the 26 offshore oil platforms operated by Elf Congo and Agip Congo. There is a refinery at Pointe-Noire.

Minerals. Lead, copper, zinc and gold (5 kg in 1985) are the main minerals. 800 kg of gold were mined in 1989. There are reserves of phosphates, bauxite and iron.

Agriculture. Production (1988, in 1,000 tonnes): Cassava, 700; sugar-cane, 400; pineapples, 114; bananas, 32; plantains, 65; yams, 15; maize, 9; groundnuts, 17; palm-oil, 16; coffee, 2; cocoa, 2; rice, 2; sweet potatoes, 14.

Livestock (1988): Cattle, 70,000; pigs, 48,000; sheep, 64,000; goats, 186,000; poultry, 1m.

Forestry. In 1988 equatorial forests cover 21m. hectares (62% of the total land area) from which (in 1983) 2,238,000 cu. metres of timber were produced, mainly okoumé from the south and sapele from the north. Hardwoods (mainly mahogany) are also exported.

Fisheries. In 1986 the catch amounted to 30,000 tonnes.

INDUSTRY. There is a growing manufacturing sector, located mainly in the 4 major towns, producing processed foods, textiles, cement, metal industries and chemicals; in 1981 it employed 26% of the labour force. Production in 1989: Printed cloth, 11·55m. metres; cement, 121,000 tonnes; shoes, 14,670 pairs.

Trade Unions. In 1964 the existing unions merged into one national body, the *Confédération Syndicale Congolaise*.

FOREIGN ECONOMIC RELATIONS

Commerce. Imports in 1989 (in 1m. francs CFA) totalled 160,967m. francs CFA (mainly machinery, 63,985) and exports 290,275m. (mainly oil products, 238,879). Exports to the USA in 1989, 113,356; to France, 49,.952; to Spain, 11,999.

Total trade between the Congo and UK (British Department of Trade returns, in £1,000 sterling):

	1986	*1987*	*1988*	*1989*	*1990*
Imports to UK	2,444	1,930	2,016	3,442	2,563
Exports and re-exports from UK	9,165	19,219	8,521	5,258	9,211

Tourism. There were 39,000 tourists in 1986.

COMMUNICATIONS

Roads. In 1986 there were 8,410 km of all-weather roads, of which 1,218 km were bitumenized. In 1982 there were 30,500 cars and 18,600 commercial vehicles. 4,237 cars were registered in 1988.

Railways. A railway (610 km, 1,067 mm gauge) and a telegraph line connect Brazzaville with Pointe-Noire via Loubomo and Bilinga and a 285 km branch links Mont-Belo with Mbinda on the Gabon border. In 1989 railways carried 434m. passenger-km and 1,037m. tonne-km of freight.

Aviation. The principal airports are at Brazzaville (Maya Maya) and Pointe-Noire (A. A. Neto). In addition there are 24 airfields served by the national airline, Lina-Congo and other companies.

Shipping. The main port is Pointe-Noire, which handled 10·2m. tonnes of freight in 1988. There were (1985) 21 vessels of 8,458 GWT registered. There are hydrofoil connexions from Brazzaville to Kinshasa (30 km across the River Congo).

Telecommunications. Telephones (1983) numbered 18,093. In 1985 there were 99,000 radios and 5,000 TV sets in use.

Newspapers. In 1986 there were 3 daily newspapers with a combined circulation of 24,000.

JUSTICE, RELIGION, EDUCATION AND WELFARE

Justice. The Supreme Court, Court of Appeal and a criminal court are situated in Brazzaville, with a network of *tribunaux de grande instance* and *tribunaux d'instance* in the regions.

Religion. In 1980, 54% of the population were Roman Catholic, 24% Protestant, 19% followed animist beliefs and 3% were Moslem.

Education. In 1985 there were 475,805 pupils and 7,745 teachers in 1,558 primary schools, 197,491 pupils and 4,773 teachers in secondary schools, 25,142 students with 1,549 teachers in technical schools and teacher-training establishments. The Université Marien-Ngouabi (founded 1972) in Brazzaville had 9,385 students and 565 teaching staff in 1985. Adult literacy (1980) 56%.

Health. There were (1978) 274 doctors, 2 dentists, 28 pharmacists, 413 midwives, 1,915 nursing personnel and 473 hospitals and dispensaries with 6,876 beds.

DIPLOMATIC REPRESENTATIVES

Of the Congo in Great Britain
Ambassador: Jean-Marie Ewengue (resides in Paris).

Of Great Britain in the Congo (Ave. du General de Gaulle, Plateau, Brazzaville)
Ambassador: Peter W. Chandley, MVO.

Of the Congo in the USA (4891 Colorado Ave., NW, Washington D.C., 20011)
Ambassador: M. Ikourou-Yoka.

Of the USA in the Congo (PO Box 1015, Brazzaville)
Ambassador: James D. Phillips.

Of the Congo to the United Nations
Ambassador: Dr Martin Adouki.

Further Reading

Thompson, V. and Adloff, R., *Historical Dictionary of the People's Republic of the Congo.* 2nd ed. Metuchen, 1984

COSTA RICA

Capital: San José
Population: 2·91m. (1990)
GNP per capita: US$1,760 (1988)

República de Costa Rica

HISTORY. Part of the Spanish Viceroyalty of New Spain from 1540, Costa Rica (the 'Rich Coast') formed part of Central America when the latter acquired independence on 15 Sept. 1821. Central America seceded to Mexico on 5 Jan. 1822 until 1 July 1823, when it became an independent confederation as the United Provinces of Central America. The province of Guanacaste was acquired from Nicaragua in 1825. Costa Rica left the confederation and achieved full independence in 1838. The first Constitution was promulgated on 7 Dec. 1871.

AREA AND POPULATION. Costa Rica is bounded north by Nicaragua, east by the Caribbean, southeast by Panama, and south and west by the Pacific. The area is estimated at 51,100 sq. km (19,730 sq. miles). The population at the census of 1 June 1984 was 2,416,809. Estimate (1990) 2,914,000.

The area and census of population for 1 June 1984 was as follows:

Province	*Area (sq. km)*	*Population*	*Capital*	*Population*
San José	4,959·63	1,055,611	San José	284,550
Alajuela	9,753·23	512,886	Alajuela	42,047
Cartago	3,124·67	324,299	Cartago	28,588
Heredia	2,656·27	233,185	Heredia	25,812
Guanacaste	10,140·71	232.414	Liberia	27,637[1]
Puntarenas	11,276·97	321,920	Puntarenas	35,603[1]
Limón	9,188·52	206,675	Limón	64,406[1]

[1] District

In 1988, 44% lived in urban areas, and 36% were aged under 15; population density 56·5 per sq. km.

Vital statistics for calendar years:

	Marriages	*Births*	*Deaths*
1987	21,743	80,326	10,687
1988	22,918	81,376	10,944

The population is mainly of Spanish and mixed descent. There are some 15,000 West Indians, mostly in Limón province. The indigenous Amerindian population is dwindling and is now estimated at 1,200. There were (1988) some 23,100 refugees (19,000 from Nicaragua).

Spanish is the official language.

CLIMATE. The climate is tropical, with a small range of temperature and abundant rains. The dry season is from Dec. to April. San José. Jan. 66°F (18·9°C), July 69°F (20·6°C). Annual rainfall 72" (1,793 mm).

CONSTITUTION AND GOVERNMENT. The Constitution was promulgated in Nov. 1949. It forbids the establishment or maintenance of an army. The legislative power is normally vested in a single chamber called the Legislative Assembly, which since 1962 consists of 57 deputies, 1 for every 49,000 inhabitants, elected for 4 years. The President and 2 Vice-Presidents are elected for 4 years; the candidate receiving the largest vote, provided it is over 40% of the total, is declared elected, but a second ballot is required if no candidate gets 40% of the total. Suffrage is universal, there being no exemption for reasons of economic status, race or sex. The vote is direct by secret ballot for all nationals of 18 years or over. Elections are normally held on the first Sunday in February. Voting for President, Deputies and Municipal Councillors is secret and compulsory for all men under 70 years of age. Independent non-party candidates are barred from the ballot.

Presidential elections took place on 4 Feb. 1990 and Rafael Angel Calderón of the Social Christian Unity Party defeated Dr Carlos Manuel Castillo of the ruling National Liberation Party by a 3% margin.

President: Rafael Angel Calderón (b. 1949; assumed office 8 May 1990).

The powers of the President are limited by the constitution, which leaves him the power to appoint and remove at will members of his cabinet. All other public appointments are made jointly in the names of the President and of the minister in charge of the department concerned.

National flag: Five unequal stripes of blue, white, red, white, blue, with the national arms on a white disc near the hoist.

National anthem: Noble patria, tu hermosa bandera (words by J. M. Zeledón, 1903; tune by M. M. Gutiérrez, 1851).

DEFENCE

Army. The Army was abolished in 1948, and replaced by a Civil Guard 4,600 strong in 1991.

Navy. The para-military Civil Guard flotilla includes 1 fast patrol craft and 5 small coastguard cutters. Personnel (1990), 100 officers and men.

Air Wing. The Civil Guard operates a small air wing equipped with 16 light planes and helicopters.

INTERNATIONAL RELATIONS

Membership. Costa Rica is a member of the UN, CACM and OAS.

ECONOMY

Policy. An austerity programme was introduced in June 1990, including an increase in income tax, rises in public utility prices and a devaluation of the currency.

Budget. The 1985 Budget provided for revenue of 41,101·6m. colones and expenditure of 43,135·5m. colones.

Currency. The unit of currency is the *Costa Rican colón* (CRC) of 100 *céntimos*. The official rate is used for all imports on an essential list and by the Government and autonomous institutions and a free rate is used for all other transactions. The currency was devalued in June 1990. The official rate in March 1991 was ₡111·54 = US$1; 211·59 = £1.

The currency is chiefly notes. The Central Bank issue notes for 5, 10, 20, 50, 100, 500 and 1,000 colones. Silver coins of 1 colon, 50 centimos and 25 centimos were in 1935 replaced by coins (2 and 1 colones and 50 and 25 centimos) made up of 3 parts copper and 1 part nickel, and given the same value as the subsidiary silver currency. There are copper coins (and chromium stainless steel coins) of 10 and 5 centimos.

Banking and Finance. The Central Bank was established in 1950 for the organization and direction of the national monetary system and of dealings in foreign exchange, the promotion of facilities for credit and the supervision of all banking operations in the country. The bank has a board of 7 directors appointed by the Government, including *ex officio* the Minister of Finance and the Planning Office Director. The *Governor* is Jorge Guaradia.

The National Insurance Institute *(Instituto Nacional de Seguros)* is a Government organization, created in 1924, which has a monopoly of new insurance business.

Weights and Measures. The metric system is legally established; but in the country districts the following old Spanish weights and measures are found: *libra* =

1·014 lb. avoirdupois; *arroba* = 25·35 lb. avoirdupois; *quintal* = 101·40 lb. avoirdupois, and *fanega* = 11 Imperial bushels.

ENERGY AND NATURAL RESOURCES

Electricity. Electricity, derived from water power in the highlands, is increasingly used as motive power. Output, 1986, was 2,770m. kwh. Supply 120 volts; 60 Hz.

Minerals. Gold output is about 3,000 troy oz. per year. Salt production from sea water is about 10,000 tonnes annually. Haematite ore was discovered on the Nicoya Peninsula late in 1960 and sulphur near San Carlos in 1966.

Agriculture. Agriculture is the principal industry. The cultivated area is about 1m. acres; grass lands cover 1·8m. acres. The principal agricultural products are coffee, bananas, sugar and cattle. Coffee production was some 138,000 tonnes in 1990.

Coffee production in 1988 was 145,000 tonnes; sugar-cane, 2·73m.; bananas, 1·05m.; cocoa, 4,000; maize, 105,000; tobacco, 2,000; rice, 194,000; potatoes, 40,000.

In 1988 cattle numbered 2·19m. and pigs 223,000.

Forestry. In 1988 there were 1·6m. hectares of woodlands, representing 32% of the land surface. There are thousands of square miles of public lands that have never been cleared on which can be found quantities of rosewood, cedar, mahogany and other cabinet woods.

Fisheries. Total catch (1986) 21,000 tonnes.

INDUSTRY. The main manufactured goods are foodstuffs, textiles, fertilizers, pharmaceuticals, furniture, cement, tyres, canning, clothing, plastic goods, plywood and electrical equipment.

Trade Unions. As Costa Rica is still essentially an agricultural country, the organization of labour has made progress only in the larger centres of population, and even there it is not a strong movement. There are two main trade unions, *Rerum Novarum* (anti-Communist) and *Confederación General de Trabajadores Costarricenses* (Communist).

FOREIGN ECONOMIC RELATIONS

Commerce. The value of imports into and exports from Costa Rica in 5 years was as follows in US$:

	1982	*1983*	*1984*	*1985*	*1986*
Imports	867,000,000	987,826,445	1,093,739,311	1,098,178,489	1,147,500,000
Exports	870,800,000	559,951,375	1,006,389,617	1,084,100,000	1,106,000,000

The values (in US$1m.) of the principal imports in 1984 were: Machinery, including transport equipment, 219·6; manufactures, 317·5; chemicals, 250·1; fuel and mineral oils, 166·7; foodstuffs, 9.

Chief exports (in US$1m.) in 1984 were: Manufactured goods and other products, 450·6; coffee, 267·8 (mostly to Federal Republic of Germany, USA, UK and Italy); bananas, 251 (to USA); sugar, 35·5; cocoa, 1·5.

Total trade between Costa Rica and UK (British Department of Trade returns in £1,000 sterling):

	1986	*1987*	*1988*	*1989*	*1990*
Imports to UK	30,318	16,752	16,902	24,113	17,468
Exports and re-exports from UK	12,007	14,407	11,390	12,780	14,556

Tourism. There was a total of 261,000 tourists in 1986.

COMMUNICATIONS

Roads. In 1987 there were about 35,000 km of all-weather motor roads open. On the Costa Rica section of the Inter-American Highway it is possible to motor to Panama during the dry season. The Pan-American Highway into Nicaragua is metalled for most of the way and there is now a good highway open almost to Puntarenas. Motor vehicles, 1985, numbered 186,046.

Railways. The nationalized railway system *(Incofer)*, totalling 828·5 km (128 km electrified) of 1,067 mm gauge, connects San José with Limón, the Atlantic port, and San José with Puntarenas, the Pacific port. Total railway traffic in 1988 was 1m. tonnes of freight and 1·3m. passengers.

Aviation. There were 92 airports (59 private) in service in 1984. Passenger movement in and out of Costa Rica is almost entirely by air *via* the local company, LACSA, PANAM and TACA. Passengers carried, 1984, 1,014,559. LACSA links San José by daily services with all the more important towns.

Shipping. In 1981, 1,221 ships entered and cleared the ports of the republic (Puerto Limón, Puntarenas and Golfito).

Telecommunications. There were 281,042 telephones in 1983.

The commercial wireless telegraph stations are operated by *Cia Radiográfica Internacional de Costa Rica*. The stations are located at Cartago, Limón, Puntarenas, Quepos and Golfito. The Government has 19 wireless telegraph stations in its local network. The principal or central station at San José also maintains international radio-telegraph circuits to Nicaragua, Honduras, San Salvador and Mexico. The Government has 202 telegraph offices and 88 official telephone stations. In 1986 there were 200,000 radio and 470,000 television receivers.

Cinemas (1979). Cinemas numbered 106, with seating capacity of 105,000.

Newspapers (1984). There were 4 daily newspapers all published in San José.

JUSTICE, RELIGION, EDUCATION AND WELFARE

Justice. Justice is administered by the Supreme Court, 5 appeal courts divided into 5 chambers; the Court of Cassation, the Higher and Lower Criminal Courts, and the Higher and Lower Civil Courts. There are also subordinate courts in the separate provinces and local justices throughout the republic. Capital punishment may not be inflicted.

Religion. Roman Catholicism is the religion of the State, which contributes to its maintenance but controls the Church Patronage and insists on lay instruction in history, economics and similar subjects; there is entire religious liberty under the constitution, but religious appeals are forbidden in current political discussions. The Archbishop of Costa Rica has 4 bishops at Alajuela, Limón, San Isidro el General and Tilarán.

Protestants number about 40,000.

Education. Costa Rica has a very low illiteracy rate. Elementary instruction is compulsory and free; secondary education (since 1949) is also free. Elementary schools are provided and maintained by local school councils, while the national government pays the teachers, besides making subventions in aid of local funds. In 1986 there were 3,107 public primary schools with 13,500 teachers and administrative staff and 380,000 enrolled pupils; there were 241 public and private secondary schools with 8,926 teachers and 141,691 pupils. The University of Costa Rica, founded in San José in 1843, had (1980) 2,337 professors in 13 faculties and 38,629 students.

Health. In 1982 there were 1,929 doctors and 39 hospitals with 7,706 beds. In 1979 there were 239 dentists.

DIPLOMATIC REPRESENTATIVES

Of Costa Rica in Great Britain (14 Lancaster Gate, London, W2 3LW)
Ambassador: Luís Rafael Tinoco.

Of Great Britain in Costa Rica (Edificio Centro Colón, Apartado 815, San José)
Ambassador and Consul-General: William Marsden.

Of Costa Rica in the USA (1825 Connecticut Ave., NW Washington D.C., 20009)
Ambassador: Danilo Jiménez.

Of the USA in Costa Rica (Pavas, San José)
Ambassador: (vacant).

Of Costa Rica to the United Nations
Ambassador: Cristián Tattenbach.

Further Reading

Statistical Information: Official statistics are issued by the Director General de Estadística (Ministerio de Industria y Comercio, San José) as they become available. The compilation of statistics was started in 1861.

Ameringer, C. D., *Democracy in Costa Rica*. New York, 1982
Biesanz, R., *(et al), The Costa Ricans*. Hemel Hempstead, 1982
Bird, L., *Costa Rica: Unarmed Democracy*. London, 1984
Fernandez Guardia, L., *Historia de Costa Rica*. 2nd ed., 2 vols. San José, 1941
Seligson, M. A., *Peasants of Costa Rica and the Development of Agrarian Capitalism*. Univ. of Wisconsin Press, 1980
Stansifer, C., *Costa Rica*. [Bibliography] Oxford and Santa Barbara, 1988

CÔTE D'IVOIRE

Capital: Abidjan
Population: 12·10m. (1990)
GNP per capita: US$740 (1988)

République de la Côte d'Ivoire

(Republic of the Ivory Coast)

HISTORY. France obtained rights on the coast in 1842, but did not actively and continuously occupy the territory till 1882. On 10 Jan. 1889 Ivory Coast was declared a French protectorate, and it became a colony on 10 March 1893; in 1904 it became a territory of French West Africa. On 1 Jan. 1933 most of the territory of Upper Volta was added to the Ivory Coast, but on 1 Jan. 1948 this area was returned to the re-constituted Upper Volta, now Burkina Faso. The Ivory Coast became an autonomous republic within the French Community on 4 Dec. 1958 and achieved full independence on 7 Aug. 1960. From 1 Jan. 1986 the French version of the name of the country became the only correct title.

AREA AND POPULATION. Côte d'Ivoire is bounded west by Liberia and Guinea, north by Mali and Burkina Faso, east by Ghana, and south by the Gulf of Guinea. It has an area of 322,463 sq. km and a population at the 1975 census of 6,702,866 (of whom 31·8% were urban). Estimate (1990) 12,100,000 (45·6% urban).

The areas and populations of the 34 departments were:

Department	*Sq. km*	*Census 1975*	*Department*	*Sq. km*	*Census 1975*
Abengourou	6,900	177,692	Ferkéssédougou	17,728	90,423
Abidjan	14,200	1,389,141	Gagnoa	4,500	174,018
Aboisso	6,250	148,823	Guiglo	14,150	137,672
Adzopé	5,230	162,837	Issia	3,590	104,081
Agboville	3,850	141,970	Katiola	9,420	77,875
Biankouma	4,950	75,711	Korhogo	12,500	276,816
Bondoukou	16,530	296,551	Lakota	2,730	76,105
Bongouanou	5,570	216,907	Man	7,050	278,659
Bouaflé	5,670	164,817	Mankono	10,660	82,358
Bouaké	23,800	808,048	Odienné	20,600	124,010
Bouna	21,470	84,290	Oumé	2,400	85,486
Boundiali	7,895	96,449	Sassandra	17,530	116,644
Dabakala	9,670	56,230	Séguéla	11,240	75,181
Daloa	11,610	265,529	Soubré	8,270	75,350
Danané	4,600	170,249	Tingréla	2,200	35,829
Dimbokro	8,530	258,116	Touba	8,720	77,786
Divo	7,920	202,511	Zuénoula	2,830	98,792

The principal cities (populations, census 1975) are the capital, Abidjan (951,216; estimate 1982, 1·85m.), Bouaké (175,264), Daloa (60,837), Man (50,288), Korhogo (45,250) and Gagnoa (42,362). The new capital will be at Yamoussoukro (120,000 in 1984).

The principal ethnic groups are the Akan-speaking peoples of the south-east (Baule, 12% and Anyi, 11%) and the Bete (20%) and Kru of the south-west; in the north-east are Voltaic groups including Senufo (14%), while Malinké (7%) and other Mandé peoples inhabit the north-west.

French is the official language and there were (1985) about 50,000 French residents.

CLIMATE. A tropical climate, affected by distance from the sea. In coastal areas, there are wet seasons from May to July and in Oct. and Nov., but in central areas the periods are March to May and July to Nov. In the north, there is one wet season from June to Oct. Abidjan. Jan. 81°F (27·2°C), July 75°F (23·9°C). Annual rainfall 84" (2,100 mm). Bouaké. Jan. 81°F (27·2°C), July 77°F (25°C). Annual rainfall 48" (1,200 mm).

CONSTITUTION AND GOVERNMENT. The 1960 Constitution was amended in 1971, 1975, 1980, 1985 and 1986. The sole legal Party has been the Democratic Party of Côte d'Ivoire, but opposition parties were legalized in May 1990. There is a 175-member *National Assembly* elected by universal suffrage for a 5-year term. The President is also directly elected for a 5-year term (renewable). He appoints and leads a Council of Ministers who assist him. At the elections of Oct. 1990 Félix Houphouët-Boigny (b. 1905) was elected president for a seventh 5-year term by 81·68% of the votes cast, against one opponent.

In Nov. 1990 the National Assembly voted that its Speaker should become president in the event of the latter's incapacity, and created the post of prime minister to be appointed by the president.

At the National Assembly elections of Nov. 1990 490 candidates stood. The electorate was 4·7m.; turn-out was 60%. The Democratic Party won 163 seats; the Ivorian Popular Front, 9; the Workers' Party, 1; independents, 2.

A new government was formed in Nov. 1990 of 20 ministers including:

Prime Minister: Alassane Ouattara (b. 1952).

Minister of the Economy and Finance: Daniel Duncan. *Minister for Raw Materials:* Guy Gauze.

The *Speaker* is Henri Konan Bedie.

National flag: Three vertical strips of orange, white, green.

Local government: There are 34 departments, each under an appointed Prefect and an elected Conseil-Général, sub-divided into 163 sub-prefectures. At the elections of Dec. 1990 turn-out was low. The Democratic Party won 123 out of 132 authorities; the Ivorian Popular Front, 6; independents, 3.

DEFENCE

Army. The Army consisted in 1990 of 1 armoured battalion, 3 infantry battalions and support units. Equipment includes 5 AMX-13 light tanks and 7 ERC-90 armoured cars. Total strength (1991), 5,500. Paramilitary forces, 7,800.

Navy. Offshore, riverine and coastal patrol squadrons include 2 fast missile craft, 2 patrol vessels, 1 riverine defence craft, 1 light transport and 2 minor landing craft. Personnel in 1990 totalled 700 and the force is based at Locodjo (Abidjan).

Air Force. The Air Force, formed in 1962, has 6 Alpha Jet advanced trainers, with combat potential, 1 turbofan Fokker 100, 1 Super-King Air, 1 Cessna 421, 1 Gulfstream transport, 2 Reims-Cessna 150s, 6 Beech F-33Cs and 4 SA330 Puma, 4 Dauphin 2, 1 Alouette III and 3 Gazelle helicopters. Personnel (1991) 900.

INTERNATIONAL RELATIONS

Membership. Côte d'Ivoire is a member of the UN, OAU and is an ACP state of the EEC.

ECONOMY

Policy. Austerity measures were introduced in May 1990.

Budget. The budget for 1988 totalled 493,500m. francs CFA and for recurrent expenditure and 143,600m. francs CFA for investment. Capital expenditure 145,879 francs CFA.

Currency. The currency is the *franc CFA* with a parity rate of 50 *francs CFA* to 1 French *franc*. In March 1991, £1 sterling = 496·13 francs CFA; US$1 = 261·53 francs CFA.

Banking. The *Banque Centrale des Etats de l'Afrique de l'Ouest* is the bank of issue. Numerous foreign and domestic banks have offices in Abidjan, and *Société Générale de Banque, Société Ivoirienne de Banque, Banque Internationale pour le Commerce et l'Industrie de la Côte d'Ivoire* and *Banque Internationale pour l'Afrique Occidentale* maintain wide branch networks throughout the country.

ENERGY AND NATURAL RESOURCES

Electricity. The electricity industry was privatized in 1990. Production in 1985 amounted to 2,162m. kwh mostly from new hydroelectric projects at Kassou and Taabo on the Bandama river, Buyo on the Sassandra river, and from 2 older dams on the Bia river. Supply 220 volts; 50 Hz.

Oil. Petroleum has been produced (offshore) since Oct. 1977. Production (1989) 350,000 tonnes.

Minerals. Diamond extraction was 700,000 carats in 1985. There are iron ore deposits at Bangolo and gold-mining began in Jan. 1990, reserves are estimated at 4,500 kg.

Agriculture. The main crops (production, 1988 in 1,000 tonnes) are coffee (187), bananas (130), pineapples (265), palm oil (235), palm kernels (42), seed cotton (256), rubber (54), yams (2,452), cassava (1,333), plantains (1,076), rice (597), maize (448), millet (42), sugar-cane (1,500) and groundnuts (119).

Cocoa production was 720,000 tonnes in 1990 (820,000 tonnes in 1989).

Livestock, 1988: 960,000 cattle, 1·5m. sheep, 1·5m. goats, 450,000 pigs, 1,000 horses and 1,000 donkeys.

Forestry. Equatorial rain forests, especially in the south, cover 3m. hectares and produce over 30 commercially valuable species including teak, mahogany and ebony. Production in 1986 was 11·9m. cu. metres.

Fisheries. The catch in 1986 amounted to 97,200.

INDUSTRY. Industrialization has developed rapidly since independence, particularly food processing, textiles and sawmills. Several factories produce palm-oil, fruit preserves and fruit juice.

Trade Unions. The main trade union is the *Union Générale des Travailleurs de Côte d'Ivoire*, with over 100,000 members.

FOREIGN ECONOMIC RELATIONS. External debt was US$15,000m. in 1990.

Commerce. Trade for calendar years in 1m. francs CFA:

	1981	*1982*	*1983*	*1984*	*1985*
Imports	681,464	718,593	714,828	658,569	772,987
Exports	689,298	747,452	796,774	1,184,347	1,318,059

In 1985 exports of coffee furnished 21% of exports, cocoa 30%, timber 7% and petroleum products, 9%. Of the total 17% went to France, 17% to the Netherlands, 12% to the USA and 9% to Italy. Of the imports, France supplied 32% and Nigeria, 11%.

Total trade between the Côte d'Ivoire and UK (British Department of Trade returns, in £1,000 sterling):

	1986	*1987*	*1988*	*1989*	*1990*
Imports to UK	117,058	90,246	64,041	65,943	69,849
Exports and re-exports from UK	34,266	26,834	31,172	29,434	26,941

Tourism. In 1986 there were 187,000 foreign tourists.

COMMUNICATIONS

Roads. In 1984 roads totalled 53,736 km (including 128 km of motorway) and there were 182,956 private cars and 43,001 commercial vehicles.

Railways. From Abidjan a metre-gauge railway runs to Léraba on the border with Burkina Faso (655 km), and thence through Burkina Faso to Ouagadougou. Operation of the railway as a single entity ended in 1986, and in 1988 separate organizations were established in each country. In 1986–87 the railways carried 1·6m. passengers and 684,000 tonnes of freight.

Aviation. The international airport is at Abidjan-Port-Buet. In 1981 it handled 870,000 passengers and 33,000 tonnes of freight and mail. Air Ivoire provides regular domestic services to 10 regional airports and 15 landing strips.

Shipping. The main ports are Abidjan and San Pedro. In 1981 Abidjan port handled 5·8m. tonnes and San Pedro 1·5m. tonnes. In 1986 the merchant marine comprised 61 vessels of 141,674 tons gross.

Telecommunications. There were 87,700 telephones in 1984 and 1,800 telex machines. In 1986 there were 550,000 television and 1·2m. radio receivers.

Newspapers. In 1984 there was 1 daily newspaper, *Fraternité-Matin.*

JUSTICE, RELIGION, EDUCATION AND WELFARE

Justice. There are 28 courts of first instance and 3 assize courts in Abidjan, Bouaké and Daloa, 2 courts of appeal in Abidjan and Bouaké, and a supreme court in Abidjan.

Religion. In 1980, 24% were Moslems (mainly in the north), 32% Christians (chiefly Roman Catholics in the south), and 44% animists.

Education. There were, in 1984, 1,179,456 pupils in primary schools, 245,342 pupils in secondary schools and (1979) 22,437 in technical schools. The *Université Nationale de Côte d'Ivoire,* at Abidjan (founded 1964), had 12,755 students in 1984.

Health. In 1978 there were 9,962 hospital beds, 429 doctors, 36 dentists, 615 midwives, 3,052 nurses and 76 pharmacists.

DIPLOMATIC REPRESENTATIVES

Of the Côte d'Ivoire in Great Britain (2 Upper Belgrave St., London, SW1X 8BJ)
Ambassador: Gervais Attoungbré.

Of Great Britain in the Côte d'Ivoire (Immeuble 'Les Harmonies', Blvd. Carde, Abidjan)
Ambassador: (vacant).

Of the Côte d'Ivoire in the USA (2424 Massachusetts Ave., NW, Washington, D.C., 20008)
Ambassador: Charles Gomis.

Of the USA in the Côte d'Ivoire (5 Rue Jesse Owens, Abidjan)
Ambassador: Kenneth L. Brown.

Of the Côte d'Ivoire to the United Nations
Ambassador: Amara Essy.

Further Reading

Statistical Information: Service de la Statistique, Abidjan. It publishes *Bulletin Statistique Mensuel and Inventoire Économique de la Côte d'Ivoire.*

Sugar, H., *Ivory Coast.* [Bibliography] Oxford and Santa Barbara, 1990
Zartman, I. W. and Delgado, C., *The Political Economy of Ivory Coast.* New York, 1984
Zolberg, A. R., *One-Party Government in the Ivory Coast.* Rev. ed. Princeton Univ. Press, 1974

CUBA

República de Cuba

Capital: Havana
Population: 10·58m. (1989)
GNP per capita: US$2,696 (1981)

HISTORY. Cuba, except for the brief British occupancy in 1762–63, remained a Spanish possession from its discovery by Columbus in 1492 until 10 Dec. 1898, when the sovereignty was relinquished under the terms of the Treaty of Paris, which ended the struggle of the Cubans against Spanish rule. Cuba thus became an independent republic, but the United States stipulated under the 'Platt Amendment' (abrogated by Roosevelt in 1934) that Cuba must enter into no treaty relations with a foreign power, which might endanger its independence.

The revolutionary movement against the Batista dictatorship, led by Dr Fidel Castro Ruíz, started on 26 July 1953 (now a national holiday). It achieved power on 1 Jan. 1959 when Batista fled the country.

An invasion force of émigrés and adventurers landed in Cuba on 17 April 1961; the main body was defeated at the Bay of Pigs (Mantanzas province) and mopped up by 20 April.

The US Navy blockaded Cuba from 22 Oct. to 22 Nov. 1962.

AREA AND POPULATION. The island of Cuba forms the largest and most westerly of the Greater Antilles group and lies 135 miles south of the tip of Florida, USA. The Republic of Cuba has an area of 110,860 sq. km, and comprises the island of Cuba, (104,945 sq. km.); the Isle of Youth (Isla de la Juventud, formerly the Isle of Pines; 2,200 sq. km.), and some 1,600 small isles ('cays'; 3,715 sq. km.). Census (1981) 9,723,605; estimate, 1989, 10,577,000 (in 1988 there were 5,270,800 males and 5,197,800 females).

The area, population and density of population of the 14 provinces and the special Municipality of the Isle of Youth were as follows (1989 estimate):

	Area sq. km	*Population*		*Area sq. km.*	*Population*
Pinar del Río	10,860	681,500	Camagüey	14,134	727,700
La Habana	5,671	633,400	Las Tunas	6,373	481,500
Ciudad de La Habana	727	2,068,600	Holguín	9,105	927,700
Matanzas	11,669	599,500	Granma	8,452	777,300
Cienfuegos	4,149	356,700	Santiago de Cuba	6,343	974,100
Villa Clara	8,069	788,800	Guantánamo	6,366	487,900
Sancti Spíritus	6,737	422,300			
Ciego de Avila	6,485	355,500	Isla de la Juventud	2,199	70,900

The chief cities (1986, estimate) were Havana, the capital (2,014,800), Santiago de Cuba (358,800), Camagüey (260,800), Holguín (194,700), Santa Clara (178,300), Guantánamo (174,400), Cienfuegos (109,300), Matanzas (105,400), Bayamo (105,300), Pinar del Río (100,900), Las Tunas (91,400), Ciego de Avila (80,500) and Sancti Spíritus (75,600).

Infant mortality (1989) 11·1 per 1,000 live births.

CLIMATE. Situated in the sub-tropical zone, Cuba has a generally rainy climate, affected by the Gulf Stream and the N.E. Trades, though winters are comparatively dry after the heaviest rains in Sept. and Oct. Hurricanes are liable to occur between June and Nov. Havana. Jan. 72°F (22·2°C), July 82°F (27·8°C). Annual rainfall 48" (1,224 mm).

CONSTITUTION AND GOVERNMENT. The previous Constitution was suspended in Jan. 1959. The first socialist Constitution came into force on 24 Feb. 1976.

Since 1940 the following have been Presidents of the Republic:

	Took office		*Took office*
Gen. Fulgencio Batista y Zaldívar	10 Oct. 1940	Gen. Fulgencio Batista y Zaldívar	10 March 1952
Dr Ramón Grau San Martín	10 Oct. 1944	Dr Manuel Urratia Lleo	2 Jan. 1959
Dr Carlos Prío Socarrás	10 Oct. 1948	Osvaldo Dórticos Torrado	17 July 1959

Legislative power is vested in the National Assembly of People's Power, consisting of 499 deputies elected for a 5-year term by the Municipal Assemblies; elections were held in 1976, 1981 and 1986. The National Assembly elects a 31-member Council of State as its permanent organ. The Council of State's President, who is head of state and of government, nominates and leads a Council of Ministers approved by the National Assembly.

President: Dr Fidel Castro Ruíz became President of the Council of State on 3 Dec. 1976. He is also President of the Council of Ministers, First Secretary of the Cuban Communist Party and C.-in-C. of the Revolutionary Armed Forces.

First Vice-President of the Council of State and of the Council of Ministers, Minister of the Revolutionary Armed Forces: Raúl Castro Ruíz. *Foreign Affairs:* Isidoro Octavio Malmierca Peoli. *Interior:* Gen. Abelardo Colome. *Justice:* Juan Escalona Reguera. *Foreign Trade:* Ricardo Cabrisas Ruíz.

The Council of Ministers also includes 10 other Vice-Presidents, the Presidents of 10 State Planning Committees and 17 other Ministers.

Dr Castro on 2 Dec. 1961 proclaimed 'a Marxist–Leninist programme adapted to the precise objective conditions existing in our country'. The provisional *Organizaciones Revolucionarias Integradas* (ORI) were established as an intermediate stage towards a single (communist) party, and gave way to the *Partido Unido de la Revolución Socialista* (PURS). This brought together the *Partido Socialista Popular, Movimiento de 26 Julio* and (Students') *Directorio Revolucionario*. The PURS in turn became (3 Oct. 1965) the *Partido Comunista de Cuba.*

The Congress of the PCC elects a Central Committee of 146 full and 79 alternate (non-voting) members, which in turn appoints a Political Bureau comprising 14 full and 10 alternate members.

National flag: 3 blue, 2 white stripes (horizontal); a white 5-pointed star in a red triangle at the hoist.

National anthem: Al combate corred bayameses (words and tune by P. Figueredo, 1868).

Local Government. The country is divided into 14 provinces, the special Municipality (the Isle of Youth) and 169 municipalities. Local Government is the responsibility of the organizations of Peoples' Power. Elections were held in 1976, 1979, 1981, 1984 and 1987 for delegates to the Municipal Assemblies by universal suffrage for 2½ year terms; the Municipal Assemblies then elected the Provincial Assemblies for similar terms.

DEFENCE. On 13 Nov. 1963 conscription was introduced for all men between the ages of 16 and 45, later raised to 50 (3 years); women of the 17–35 age groups may volunteer (for 2 years).

Army. The strength was 145,000 officers and men (60,000 conscripts) in 1991. Reserves are estimated at 130,000. The Army is organized in 4 corps, 3 armoured divisions, 9 mechanized infantry divisions, 13 infantry divisions and air defence regiments. Equipment includes 800 T-54/-55, 300 T-62 tanks and 60 PT-76 light tanks. Para-military forces total 69,000 and the new Territorial Militia, 1·3m. including reservists, all armed.

Navy. Naval combatants, all ex-Soviet, include 3 'Foxtrot' class diesel submarines, 3 'Koni' class frigates, 18 fast missile craft, 9 patrol hydrofoils, 29 inshore patrol craft, 4 coastal minehunters and 10 inshore minesweepers. There are 2 medium landing ships and 6 craft. The major auxiliaries include 1 tanker, 1 electronic intelligence gatherer, 1 tug and 1 training ship. Some 20 minor auxiliaries and service craft complete the total.

Personnel in 1990 totalled 13,500 (8,500 conscripts) including marines and coastguard. Main bases are at Cienfuegos, Havana and Mariel. The USA still occupies the Guantánamo naval base, but the Cuban Government refuses to accept the nominal rent of US$5,000 per annum.

A separate coast guard division of the Frontier Guards operates 4 inshore patrol craft.

Air Force. The Air Force has been extensively re-equipped with aircraft supplied by USSR and in 1991 had a strength of some 22,000 officers and men (11,000 conscripts) and 300 combat aircraft. About 12 interceptor and 4 ground-attack squadrons fly MiG-23, MiG-21 and MiG-17 jet fighters. There is a squadron of An-26 twin-turboprop transports, some An-24 twin-turboprop transports, piston-engined Il-14s, and about 100 Mi-24 gunship, Mi-8 (some armed), Mi-17 and Mi-4 helicopters, Zlin 326 piston-engined trainers and L-39, MiG-15UTI, MiG-21U and MiG-23U jet trainers. An-2M biplanes are operated by the Air Force, mainly on agricultural and liaison duties. Soviet-built surface-to-air ('Guideline', 'Goa' and 'Gainful') and coastal defence ('Samlet') missiles are in service.

INTERNATIONAL RELATIONS

Membership. Cuba is a member of the UN, SELA, the Non-Aligned Movement and OIEC.

ECONOMY

Policy. The economy is still centrally planned. Food was rationed in Nov. 1990.

Budget. Revenue in 1989 11,900m. pesos and expenditure, 13,500m. pesos.

Currency. The unit of currency is the *Cuban peso* (CUP) of 100 *centavos*, which is not convertible although an official exchange rate is announced daily reflecting any changes in the strength of the US$. In March 1991 £1 = 1·31 *pesos*; US$1 = 0·80 *pesos*.

Copper-nickel coins of 1 *peso* and 20, 5, 2 and 1 *centavo* are issued. Notes are for 100, 50, 20, 10, 5, 3 and 1 *peso*.

Banking and Finance. The central bank was created in 1948 (with capital of US$10m.) and began operating on 27 April 1950.

On 14 Oct. 1960 all banks were nationalized, except the Royal Bank of Canada and the Bank of Nova Scotia, which were bought out later. All banking is now carried out by the National Bank of Cuba through its 250 agencies, or via the Banco Financiero.

All insurance business was nationalized in Jan. 1964. A National Savings Bank was established in 1983.

Weights and Measures. The metric system of weights and measures is legally compulsory, but the American and old Spanish systems are much used. The sugar industry uses the Spanish long ton (1·03 tonnes) and short ton (0·92 tonne). Cuba sugar sack = 329·59 lb. or 149·49 kg. Land is measured in *caballerías* (of 13·4 ha or 33 acres).

ENERGY AND NATURAL RESOURCES

Electricity. Production in 1989 was 15,237m. kwh. Supply 115 and 120 volts; 60 Hz.

Oil. Crude oil production (1989) 800,000 tonnes.

Minerals. Iron ore abounds, with deposits estimated at 3,500m. tons, of which 90% were held as reserves by American steel interests but are now controlled by the Cuban Ministry of Basic Industry; output (tonnes), 1,180. Output of copper concentrate (1989) was 2,800 tonnes; refractory chrome (1987), 52,400 tonnes. Other minerals are nickel and cobalt (1989, 46,500 tonnes), silica and barytes. Gold and silver are also worked. Salt output from the solar evaporation of sea water was 114,900 tonnes in 1989.

Agriculture. In May 1959 all land over 30 *caballerías* was nationalized and has since been turned into state farms. In Oct. 1963 private holdings were reduced to a maximum of 5 *caballerías* (approximately 67 ha).

In Sept. 1984 there were 1,472 co-operatives comprising 70,000 *caballerías* of land. The total cultivated land (1982) included state-owned, 3,398,200 ha, and in the private sector, 475,400 ha.

The most important product is sugar and its by-products. The 1989-90 crop was estimated at 8·04m. tonnes. Tobacco, coffee, cotton, maize, rice, potatoes and citrus fruit are grown.

Production of other important crops in 1989 was (in tonnes): Tobacco, 42,900; rice, 532,400; coffee, 22,500; maize (1988), 95,000.

Tobacco is grown mainly in the Vuelta–Abajo district, near Pinar del Río. Coffee is grown chiefly in the province of Oriente.

A fast-growing fibre, *kenaf*, originally from India, soft in texture, is replacing jute for sacking (production, 1986, 13,468 tonnes); the tobacco industry uses *majagua*, another local fibre, while a third fibre, *yarey*, from palms is also used. Rice cultivation is highly mechanized and the sown area produces two crops a year.

In 1987 citrus fruit production was 885,510 tonnes. In 1989 production of pineapples was 20,600 tonnes, tomatoes 244,400 tonnes and potatoes, 281,400 tonnes.

In 1989 the livestock included 1,292,000 pigs; 665,300 horses; 853,100 sheep and goats; 4·98m. head of cattle (in 1988).

Forestry. Cuba has 2·7m ha of forests representing 25% of the land area. These forests contain valuable cabinet woods, such as mahogany and cedar, besides dyewoods, fibres, gums, resins and oils. Cedar is used locally for cigar-boxes, and mahogany is exported. Cedars, mahogany, *majagua*, teca, etc., are also raised. In 1989 182·4m. saplings were planted, which included eucalyptus, pine, majagua, mahogany, cedar and casuarina.

Fisheries. Fishing is the third most important export industry, after sugar and nickel. Catch (1989) 191,889 tonnes.

INDUSTRY. Production in 1989 was: Textiles, 218·6m. sq. metres (cotton fabrics 182·6m. sq. metres); cement (1989), 3,800m. tonnes; wheat flour, 398,000 tonnes; fuel oil (1989), 4,152,800 tonnes; diesel oil (1989), 1,178,500 tonnes; processed crude oil, 7,916,000 tonnes; steel, 314,200 tonnes; steel bars, 367,100 tonnes; nickel and cobalt, 46,500 tonnes; copper, 2,759,100 tonnes; 314,700 tyres; 231,200 inner tubes; leather shoes, 11·00m. pairs; paint (1989), 121,000 hectolitres; soft drinks (1989), 2,396,500 hectolitres; 308,500m. cigars; 16,519,700m. cigarettes; fertilizers, 898,600 tonnes; 2,345 buses; 172,700 radios; 70,500 TVs; 9,100 refrigerators; sulphuric acid, 381,500 tonnes; fine salt, 114,900 tonnes.

Labour. In 1989 the monthly average salary was 188 pesos.

Trade Unions. The Workers' Central Union of Cuba, to which 23 unions are affiliated, had 2m. members in 1978.

FOREIGN ECONOMIC RELATIONS. In 1989 Cuba's hard currency reserves were US$100m. Foreign debt was US$6,200m.

Commerce. Imports and exports (including bullion and specie) for calendar years (in 1m. pesos):

	1985	*1986*	*1987*	*1988*	*1989*
Imports	7,983	7,569	7,612	4,549	7,580
Exports	7,209	6,702	5,401	5,518	5,519

The principal exports are sugar, minerals, tobacco, citrus fruit and fish. In 1988 exports included (in tonnes): Sugar, 6·9m.; fish, 23,700; citrus fruits, 536,000; alcoholic beverages (excluding wine), 92,500 hectolitres and 69·4m. cigars.

In 1988 imports included (in tonnes): Wheat flour, 18,600; steel sections, 696,400; coke, 66,000; urea, 257,000; medicines, 48·2m. pesos; sawn wood, 477,100 cu. metres; tractors, 8,889; buses, 460; dump trucks, 1,390.

In 1985 the USSR provided 67% of imports (by value) and took 75% of exports; in 1984 sugar formed 75% of all exports.

Total trade between Cuba and UK (British Department of Trade returns, in £1,000 sterling):

	1986	*1987*	*1988*	*1989*	*1990*
Imports to UK	8,555	12,776	28,489	34,388	30,294
Exports and re-exports from UK	58,760	41,510	31,162	53,255	37,568

Tourism. In 1989 there were 514,500 visitors. Revenue amounted to 4,230·8m. pesos.

COMMUNICATIONS

Roads. In 1986 there were 16,740 km of paved highways open to traffic, traversing the island for 760 miles from Pinar del Río to Santiago. In 1983 there were 49,841 hire cars (including coaches and buses).

Railways. There were (1986) 4,881 km of public railway (mainly 1,435 mm gauge) of which 152 km is electrified. In 1987 it carried 2,189m. passenger-km and 13·2m. tonnes of freight. In addition, the large sugar estates have 7,773 km of lines on 1,435, 914 and 760 mm gauges.

Aviation. The state airline CUBANA operates all internal services, and from Havana to Mexico City, Madrid, Moscow and East Berlin, Montreal, Prague, Paris and Brussels, and also to Lima, Panama, Kingston, Bridgetown, Port of Spain, Georgetown and Managua. The other regular foreign services are Mexican, Spanish, Soviet, Czech, East German and Canadian.

Shipping. The coastline is over 3,500 miles long and has many fine harbours. The merchant marine, in 1989, consisted of 117 sea-going vessels of 1,400,000 DWT.

Telecommunications. There are 3,545 miles of public and 8,902 miles of private telegraph wires. Cuba has 103 radio broadcasting stations and 2 television stations. Radio receiving sets, 1985, numbered 2·14m.; television sets, 1·53m. The national telephone system (1989) had 311,100 lines in use.

Cinemas and Theatres. In 1987 there were 535 (35mm) and 905 (16mm) cinemas. In 1989, 99 films were made, there were 44·8m. cinema attendances; there were 49 theatres and 1,387,700 attendances.

Newspapers. Since Oct. 1990 *Granma* has been the only national daily newspaper due, it was stated, to shortage of paper.

JUSTICE, RELIGION, EDUCATION AND WELFARE

Justice. There is a Supreme Court in Havana and 7 regional courts of appeal. The provinces are divided into judicial districts, with courts for civil and criminal actions, with municipal courts for minor offences. The civil code guarantees aliens the same property and personal rights as are enjoyed by nationals.

The 1959 Agrarian Reform Law and the Urban Reform Law passed on 14 Oct. 1960 have placed certain restrictions on both. Revolutionary Summary Tribunals have wide powers.

Religion. There is no state Church, though Roman Catholics predominate. There is a bishop of the American Episcopal Church in Havana; there are congregations of Methodists in Havana and in the provinces as well as Baptists and other denominations.

Education. Education is compulsory (between the ages of 6 and 14) and free, and now available everywhere. In 1964 illiteracy was officially declared to have been completely eliminated.

In 1987–88 the universities had 262,225 students and 22,492 teaching staff. In 1989 there were 899,900 pupils and 73,200 teachers at 9,522 primary schools, 800,300 pupils and 77,800 teachers at 1,540 intermediate schools and in 1988 there were 164,891 students at adult primary schools.

In 1989 there were 18,000 foreign pupils from over 30 developing countries attending international secondary/pre-university schools free of charge, including 7 Angolan schools (3,581 pupils) and 4 Mozambiquan schools (2,231 pupils), and about 30,000 foreign students attending polytechnics, teacher training colleges and universities at an annual cost of US$40m. Cuba sends teachers abroad to more than 40 countries.

Health. There were (1989) 34,752 doctors, 6,482 dentists, 58,589 nursing personnel and 264 hospitals with 74,407 beds. The 1989 health and education budget was 2,906·2m. pesos.

Free medical services are provided by the state polyclinics, though a few doctors still have private practices. All serious tropical diseases are effectively kept under control, and virtually all children under the age of 15 have been vaccinated against poliomyelitis.

DIPLOMATIC REPRESENTATIVES

Of Cuba in Great Britain (167 High Holborn, London, WC1)
Ambassador: María de los Angeles Florez.

Of Great Britain in Cuba (Edificio Bolivar, Carcel 101–103, Havana)
Ambassador: Leycester Coltman.

Of Cuba to the United Nations
Ambassador: Ricardo Alarcón de Quesada.

The USA broke off diplomatic relations with Cuba on 3 Jan. 1961 but in 1977 Interest Sections were opened, officially attached to the Swiss Embassy in Havana and to the Czech Embassy in Washington respectively.

Further Reading

Anuario azucarero de Cuba. Havana, from 1937
Anuario Estadístico de a República de Cuba. Havana
Boletín Oficial, Ministerio de Comercio. Monthly
Estadística General: Commercio Exterior. Quarterly and Annual.—*Movimiento de Población*. Monthly and Annual. Havana
Brundenius, C., *Revolutionary Cuba: The Challenge of Economic Growth with Equity*. Oxford, 1984
Domínguez, J. I., *Cuba: Order and Revolution*. Harvard Univ. Press, 1978
Gravette, A. G., *Cuba: Official Guide*. London, 1988
Guerra y Sánchez, R. and others, *Historia de la Nación Cubana*. 10 vols. Havana, 1952
MacEwan, A., *Revolution and Economic Development in Cuba*. London, 1981
Mesa-Lago, C., *The Economy of Socialist Cuba: A Two-Decade Appraisal*. Univ. of New Mexico Press, 1981
O'Connor, J., *The Origins of Socialism in Cuba*. London, Cornell Univ. Press, 1970
Ritter, A. R. M., *The Economic Development of Revolutionary Cuba: Strategy and Performance*. New York, 1974
Ruttin, P., *Capitalism and Socialism in Cuba: a Study of Dependency, Development and Underdevelopment*. London, 1990
Thomas, H., *The Cuban Revolution: 25 Years Later*. Epping, 1984
Zimbalist, A. and Brundenius, C., *The Cuban Economy: Measurement and Analysis of Socialist Performance*. Johns Hopkins Univ. Press, 1990

CYPRUS

Capital: Nicosia
Population: 698,800 (1989)
GNP per capita government controlled area: US$6,260 (1988)

Kypriaki Dimokratia—Kibris Çumhuriyeti

(Republic of Cyprus)

HISTORY. For the history of Cyprus to 1974 *see* THE STATESMAN'S YEAR-BOOK, 1990–91, p. 400.

On 15 July 1974 a coup was staged by supporters of the Greek ruling junta for the overthrow of President Makarios. The President left the island and the coup was short-lived. The Speaker of the House of Representatives acted as President until the return of President Makarios on Dec. 7 1974.

Turkey invaded the island on 20 July 1974, eventually occupying the northern part of Cyprus. As a result 200,000 Greek Cypriots fled to live as refugees in the south. The UN General Assembly unanimously adopted resolutions calling for the withdrawal of all foreign troops from Cyprus and the return of refugees to their homes, but without result.

On 13 Feb. 1975 at a special meeting of the executive council and legislative assembly of the Autonomous Turkish Cypriot Administration a Turkish Cypriot Federated State was proclaimed. Rauf Denktash was appointed President and he declared that the state would not seek international recognition. The proclamation was denounced by President Makarios and the Greek Prime Minister but welcomed by the Turkish Prime Minister. On 15 Nov. 1983 the Turkish state unilaterally proclaimed itself the 'Turkish Republic of Northern Cyprus'. In Nov. 1983 and May 1984 the UN Security Council declared all secessionist actions illegal. UN-inspired talks on a possible federal state failed in Jan. 1985. On 15 Sept. 1988 the first meeting between President Vassiliou and Rauf Denktash took place following a UN initiative in Aug. to restart substantive talks. A further initiative by the UN Secretary-General was made in July 1989, without success.

AREA AND POPULATION. The island lies in the eastern Mediterranean, about 50 miles off the south coast of Turkey and (at the nearest points) 65 miles off the coast of Syria. Area 3,572 sq. miles (9,251 sq. km); greatest length from east to west about 150 miles, and greatest breadth from north to south about 60 miles. The Turkish occupied area is 3,400 sq. km (about 37% of the total area). Population by ethnic group:

Ethnic group	*1946*	*1960*	*1973*	*1988*	*1989*
Greek Orthodox	361,199	441,656	498,511	550,400	556,400
Turkish Moslem	80,548	104,942	116,000	128,200	129,600
Others	8,367	26,968	17,267	8,900	9,000
Total	450,114	573,566	631,778	687,500	695,000

Population estimate (June 1989) 695,000, of which 80% are Greek Cypriot (Armenian, Maronite and Latin minorities included), 19% Turkish Cypriot and 1% other, mainly British. Principal towns with populations (Dec. 1989 estimate): Nicosia (the capital), 168,800 (Government controlled area); Limassol, 132,100; Larnaca, 60,900; Paphos, 27,800.

As a result of the Turkish invasion and the occupation of part of Cyprus, 200,000 Greek Cypriots were displaced and forced to find refuge in the south of the island. The urban centres of Famagusta, Kyrenia and Morphou were completely evacuated. See p. 405 for details of the 'Turkish Republic of Northern Cyprus'.

Vital statistics. The birth rate per 1,000 population in 1989 was 18·3; death rate, 8·6; infantile mortality per 1,000 live births, 11.

CLIMATE. The climate is Mediterranean, with very hot, dry summers and variable winters. Maximum temperatures may reach 112°F (44·5°C) in July and Aug., but minimum figures may fall to 22°F (–5·5°C) in the mountains in winter when snow is experienced. Rainfall is generally between 10" and 27" (250 and 675 mm) and occurs mainly in the winter months, but it may reach 48" (1,200 mm) in the Troodos mountains. Nicosia. Jan. 50°F (10·0°C), July 83°F (28·3°C). Annual rainfall 15" (371 mm).

CONSTITUTION AND GOVERNMENT. Under the 1960 Constitution executive power is vested in a President elected for a 5-year term by universal suffrage and exercised through a Council of Ministers appointed by him. Ministers may be appointed from outside the House of Representatives. The House of Representatives exercises legislative power. It is elected by universal suffrage for 5-year terms, and consists of 80 members, of whom 56 were elected by the Greek community and 24 by the Turkish community. As from Dec. 1963 the Turkish members have ceased to attend.

Former Presidents: Archbishop Makarios, 1959–77; Spyros Kyprianou, 1977–88. In 1988 George Vassiliou was installed as President following elections held on 14 Feb.

The Speaker of the House of Representatives is Vassos Lyssarides.

Flag: White with a copper-coloured outline of the island with 2 green olive-branches beneath.

The elections held on 8 Dec. 1985 returned 16 Democratic Party, 15 Akel Party (Communists), 6 EDEK (Socialist Party), 19 Democratic Rally.

The Council of Ministers in Jan. 1991 was as follows:

Foreign Affairs: George Iacovou. *Interior:* Christodoulos Veniamin. *Defence:* Andreas Aloneftis. *Agriculture and Natural Resources:* Andreas Gavrielides. *Commerce and Industry:* Takis Nemitsas. *Health:* Panikos Papageorghiou. *Communications and Works:* Pavlos Savvides. *Finance:* George Syrimis. *Education:* Christoforos Christofides. *Labour and Social Insurance:* Iacovos Aristedou. *Justice:* Nicos Papaioannou.

DEFENCE

Army. Total strength (1989) 13,000 organized in 2 mechanized, 1 armoured, 1 artillery and 1 commando battalions. The National Guard has a twin-engined Maritime Islander light transport, 4 PC-9 trainers and 6 armed Gazelle helicopters. There is also a para-military force of 3,700 armed police.

The Turkish-Cypriot Security Force: 35,000 Turkish mainland troops, 5,000 Turkish Cypriots, and some T-34 tanks are stationed in occupied Cyprus (see p. 406).

INTERNATIONAL RELATIONS

Membership. Cyprus is a member of UN, the Commonwealth, the Council of Europe and the Non-Aligned Movement.

ECONOMY

Policy. There is a Central Planning Commission, headed by the President of the Republic and including five ministers. Its administrative arm is the Planning Bureau.

Budget. Revenue and expenditure for calendar years (in £C1m.):

	1984	*1985*	*1986*	*1987*	*1988*	*1989*
Expenditure	418	448	491	535	600	664
Revenue	344	390	427	462	536	633

Main sources of ordinary revenue in 1989 (in £C1m.) were: Import duties, 117 (including 25 temporary refugee levy on imports); excise duties, 78; income tax, 124; rents, royalties and interest, 26; sales of goods and services, 30; other duties and taxes, 61; social security contributions, 96.

Main divisions of ordinary expenditure in 1989 (in £C1m.): Wages and salaries,

204; pensions and gratuities, 19; commodity subsidies, 36; expenditures on goods and services, 30; public debt charges, 183; social insurance benefits, 100.

Development expenditure for 1989 (in £C1m.) included 12 for water development, 6 for agriculture, forests and fisheries, 4 for rural development, 27 for roads and 2 for airports. (An independent Ports Authority with its own funds was set up in 1977.)

The outstanding long-term public debt as at 31 Dec. 1989 was £C675m. Outstanding loans as at 31 Dec. 1989 totalled £C62·5m. Foreign debt (1989) public and private, £C734m.

Currency. The *Cyprus pound* (CYP) is divided into 100 *cents*. Notes of the following denominations are in circulation: £C10, £C5, 50 cents. Coins in circulation: 20, 5, 2, 1 cent and ½ cent. Rate of exchange, March 1991: £1 = £C0·83; US$1 = £C0·44.

Banking. There is a Central and Issuing Bank exercising monetary functions, and the Cyprus Development Bank Ltd established by the Government as a major source of loan funds for industrial development. Commercial banks operating in Cyprus are: Bank of Cyprus Ltd, Turkish Bank Ltd, Cyprus Popular Bank Ltd, Barclays Bank International, National Bank of Greece, Hellenic Bank Ltd, Arab Bank Ltd and Turkiye Is Bankasi. There are 2 central co-operative banks (Co-operative Central Bank Ltd and the Cyprus Turkish Co-operative Central Bank) and 3 specialized financial institutions (Mortgage Bank of Cyprus Ltd, Lombard Natwest Banking Ltd and Housing Finance Corporation). Seventeen offshore banking units were in operation in 1989.

The Central Bank of Cyprus, established in 1963, is responsible for the issue of currency, the regulation of money supply and credit, administration of the exchange control law and the foreign-exchange reserves of the republic. The Bank also acts as a banker of the banks operating in Cyprus and of the Government and acts as supervisor of the banking system.

At the end of Dec. 1988 total deposits in banks were £C1,679m. The country's foreign exchange reserves at the end of Dec. 1988 were £C572m.

Weights and Measures. The metric (SI) system was introduced in 1986 and is now widely applied.

ENERGY AND NATURAL RESOURCES

Electricity. Production (1989) 1,845m. kwh. Supply 240 volts; 50 Hz.

Water Resources. In 1988 £C20·9m. was spent on water dams, water supplies, hydrological research and geophysical surveys. Existing dams had (1989) a capacity of 297m. cu. metres as against 6m. cu. metres before independence.

Minerals. The principal minerals extracted in 1989 were (in tonnes): Flotation pyrites, 57,455; copper concentrates, 1,752; copper precipitates, 1,080. Mining is a declining industry.

Agriculture. Chief agricultural products in 1989 (1,000 tonnes): Grapes, 212; potatoes, 190; milk, 132; cereals (wheat and barley), 148; citrus fruit, 169; meat, 63; carobs, 9; fresh fruit, 27; olives, 9; other vegetables, 124; eggs, 12m. dozen.

Of the island's 2·3m. acres, approximately 1m. are cultivated. About 13·2% (1989) of the economically active population are engaged in agriculture.

Livestock in 1989 (in 1,000): Cattle, 49; sheep, 325; goats, 208; pigs, 281; poultry, 2,475.

Forestry. By Dec. 1982, the reforesting of burnt areas in the Paphos Forest was completed and an area of 7,492 ha (56,000 donums) was reforested. Reforestation work in other bare areas of state forests was carried out in an area of 6,464 ha (42,318 donums). Total forest area, 1,345 sq. km.

In 1989 the chief forest products were timber, 48,895 cu. metres valued at £C922,000; firewood, £C160,000; figures relate to the area of Cyprus not occupied by Turkey.

Fisheries. Catch (1989) 2,647 tonnes.

INDUSTRY AND TRADE

Industry. The most important industries (in £C1m.) in 1988 were: Food, beverages and tobacco, 245·1; textiles, wearing apparel and leather, 202·7; chemicals and chemical petroleum, rubber and plastic products, 130·1; metal products, machinery and equipment, 110·0; wood and wood products including furniture, 76·7. Manufacturing industry in 1989 contributed about £C334·0m. to the GDP and gave employment to 48,000 of the economically active population.

The highest increases in output in 1989 were production of wearing apparel, metal products and machinery and equipment. Industrial exports rose to £C189·1m. in 1989 and accounted for 77% of total domestic exports.

Trade Unions and Associations. About 80% of the workforce is organized and the majority of workers belong either to the Pancyprian Federation of Labour or the Cyprus Workers Confederation.

Commerce. The commerce and the shipping, exclusive of coasting trade, for calendar years were (in £C1,000):

	1985	*1986*	*1987*	*1988*	*1989*
Imports	762,311	659,073	711,419	866,765	1,130,298
Exports [1]	290,611	260,158	297,992	330,861	393,049

[1] Including re-exports and ships' stores.

Chief civil imports, 1989 (in £C1m.):

Live animals and animal products	26·0
Vegetable products	46·3
Prepared foodstuffs, beverages and tobacco	66·6
Mineral products	112·6
Products of chemical or allied industries	68·8
Plastics and rubber and articles thereof	43·7
Pulp, waste paper and paperboard and articles thereof	37·7
Textiles and textile articles	108·2
Footwear, headgear, umbrellas, prepared feathers, etc.	6·3
Articles of stone, plaster, cement, etc., ceramic and glass products	22·6
Machinery, electrical equipment, sound and television recorders	189·7
Vehicles, aircraft, vessels and equipment	210·5
Optical, photographic, medical, musical and other instruments, clocks and watches	24·7
Raw hides and skins, leather and articles, travel goods	11·6
Wood and articles, charcoal, cork and articles, basketware, etc.	18·6
Pearls, precious stones and metals, semi-precious stones and articles	16·4

Chief domestic exports, 1989 (in £C1,000):

Grapes	5,209
Citrus fruit	17,009
Potatoes	20,692
Wine	4,616
Fruit, preserved and juices	10,807
Cigarettes	6,971
Paper products	3,726
Cement	6,569
Clothing	69,515
Footwear	15,502
Medicinal and pharmaceutical products	6,701

In 1989 the EEC countries supplied 55·8% of the imports; Arab countries, 5·4%; others, 38·8%. Of the exports (1989), 28·0% went to Arab countries; 46·1% to EEC countries; 5·7% to Eastern Europe and 20·2% to other countries.

Total trade between Cyprus and UK (British Department of Trade returns, in £1,000 sterling):

	1986	*1987*	*1988*	*1989*	*1990*
Imports to UK	124,198	118,250	121,828	145,047	154,065
Exports and re-exports from UK	140,387	141,129	159,788	173,092	204,857

Tourism. Foreign visitors (1988), 1,311,591 (1,111,818 tourists and 199,773 excursionists).

COMMUNICATIONS

Roads. In 1989 the total length of roads in the Government controlled area was 9,824 km, of which 5,240 km were bituminous and 4,584 km were earth or gravel roads. The asphalted roads maintained by the Ministry of Communications and Works (Public Works Department) by the end of 1989 totalled 2,071 km, of which

260 km were within the municipal areas. Roads improved or constructed and asphalted in 1989 totalled 175 km. On 31 Dec. 1988, there were 326,327 motor vehicles including 2,604 buses, 71,848 goods vehicles, 47,188 motorcycles, and 11,696 tractors etc.

The area controlled by the Government of the Republic and that occupied by Turkey are now served by separate transport systems, and there are no services linking the two areas.

Aviation. Nicosia airport has been closed since Aug. 1974. In 1989, 32 international airlines operated scheduled services between Cyprus and Europe, Africa and the Middle East, and another 28 airlines operated non-scheduled services. During 1989, 2,881,000 persons travelled and 28,431 tonnes of commercial air-freight was handled through Larnaca and Paphos international airports.

Shipping. The 3 main ports are Limassol, Larnaca and Paphos. In 1989, 5,678 ships of 14,793,384 net tons entered Cyprus ports. Ships under Cyprus registry at the end of 1989, numbered 1,952 of 17,890,061 GRT. Famagusta has been closed to international traffic since Aug. 1974. In 1989, 5,674 vessels with a total net registered tonnage of 14,732,000 visited Cyprus carrying 7,348 tonnes of cargo from, to, and via Cyprus.

Telecommunications. In 1989 there were 55 post offices and 713 postal agencies. In 1989, (including Turkish occupied areas) there were some 333,600 telephone instruments and 232,057 lines (39·3% per 100 population). Wireless licences issued (1981) were 247,000, including television licences.

Cyprus Broadcasting Corporation broadcasts mainly in Greek, but also in Turkish, English, and Armenian on medium-waves. The corporation also broadcasts on one TV channel. A law of June 1990 permits the operation of commercial radio and TV stations. There are also 2 foreign broadcasting stations.

Cinemas (1990). In the government-controlled area there were 6 cinemas.

Newspapers (1990). There were 10 Greek, 8 Turkish and 1 English daily newspapers and 3 Greek, 3 Turkish weeklies and 1 English weekly.

JUSTICE, RELIGION, EDUCATION AND WELFARE

Justice. The administration of justice is exercised by a separate and independent judiciary. There is a Supreme Court, Assize Courts and District Courts.

The Supreme Court is composed of 13 judges one of whom is the President of the Court (in 1990, Andreas Nicolas Loizou). There is an Assize Court and a District Court for each district. The Assize Courts have unlimited criminal jurisdiction and may order the payment of compensation up to £C3,000. The District Courts exercise original civil and criminal jurisdiction, the extent of which varies with the composition of the Bench.

There is a Supreme Council of Judicature, consisting of the President and Judges of the Supreme Court, entrusted with the appointment, promotion, transfers, termination of appointment and disciplinary control over all judicial officers, other than the Judges of the Supreme Court.

The Attorney-General (in 1991, Michalakis Triantafyllides) is head of the independent Law Office and legal advisor to the President and his Ministers.

Religion. *See* Area and Population, p. 400.

Education. Until 31 March 1965 each community managed its own schooling through its respective Communal Chamber. Intercommunal education had been placed under the Minister of the Interior, assisted by a Board of Education for Intercommunal Schools, of which the Minister was the Chairman. In 1965 the Greek Communal Chamber was dissolved and a Ministry of Education was established to take its place. Intercommunal education has been placed under this Ministry.

Greek-Cypriot Education. Elementary education is compulsory and is provided free in 6 grades to children between 5½ and 11½ years of age. In some towns and large villages there are separate junior schools consisting of the first three grades. Apart from schools for the deaf and blind, there are also 9 schools for handicapped children. In 1989–90 the Ministry ran 198 kindergartens for children in the age group $2^1/_2$-5; there were 342 privately run pre-primary schools. There were 378 primary schools with 60,841 pupils and 2,824 teachers in 1989–90.

Secondary education is also free and attendance for the first cycle is compulsory. The secondary school is 6 years, 3 years at the gymnasium followed by 3 years at the *lykeion* (lyceum). In 1978–79 the lyceums of optional subjects were introduced, in which students can choose one of the 5 main fields of specialization: Classical, science, economics, commercial/secretarial and foreign languages. There are 3-year technical schools. In 1989–90 there were 108 secondary schools with 3,526 teachers and 43,219 pupils.

Post-secondary education is provided at the Pedagogical Academy, which organizes 3-year courses for the training of pre-primary and primary school teachers, and at the Higher Technical Institute, which provides 3–4-year courses for technicians in civil, electrical, mechanical and marine engineering. There is also a 2-year Forestry College (administered by the Ministry of Agriculture), a Hotel and Catering Institute, the Mediterranean Institute of Management (Ministry of Labour and Social Insurance) and a 1–3-year Nurses' School (Ministry of Health). Adult education is conducted through youth centres in rural areas, foreign language institutes in the towns and private institutions offering courses in business administration and secretarial work.

In 1988–89, 9,410 students were studying in universities abroad, mainly in Greece, the USA, UK, Federal Republic of Germany and Italy.

Greek is the language of 82% of the population and Turkish of 18%. English is widely spoken. English and French are compulsory subjects in secondary schools. Illiteracy is largely confined to older people.

Social Security. The administration of the social-security services in Cyprus is in the hands of the Ministry of Labour and Social Insurance, with the Ministry of Health providing medical services through public clinics and hospitals on a means test, except medical treatment for employment accidents, which is given free to all insured employees and financed by the Social Insurance Scheme.

DIPLOMATIC REPRESENTATIVES

Of Cyprus in Great Britain (93 Park St., London, W1Y 4ET)
High Commissioner: Angelos M. Angelides.

Of Great Britain in Cyprus (Alexander Pallis St., Nicosia)
High Commissioner: D. J. M. Dain.

Of Cyprus in the USA (2211 R. St., NW, Washington, D.C., 20008)
Ambassador: Michael Sherifis.

Of the USA in Cyprus (Therissos St., Nicosia)
Ambassador: (Vacant).

Of Cyprus to the United Nations
Ambassador: Andreas Mavrommatis.

'TURKISH REPUBLIC OF NORTHERN CYPRUS'

HISTORY. *See* p. 400.

AREA AND POPULATION. The Turkish Republic of Northern Cyprus occupies 3,355 sq. km (about 37% of the island of Cyprus) and its population in 1990, was approximately 165,000. Population of principal towns (1985): Nicosia, 37,400; Famagusta, 19,428; Kyrenia, 6,902; Morphou, 10,179; Lefka, 3,785. Ethnic groups: Turks, 158,225; Greeks, 733; Maronites, 368; Others, 961. Passport formalities with Turkey were abolished in July 1990.

CONSTITUTION AND GOVERNMENT. The Turkish Republic of Northern Cyprus was proclaimed on 15 Nov. 1983. Rauf Denktash was re-elected President in April 1990 by 68·6% of the vote. A 50-seat Legislative Assembly was elected in May 1990. The National Unity Party won 34 seats, the Communal Liberation Party, 7, the Republican Turkish Party, 7, and the New Dawn Party, 2. The Council of Ministers comprised in Feb. 1991 of:

Prime Minister: Derviş Eroğlu.

Foreign Affairs and Defence: Kenan Atakol. *Economy and Finance:* Nazif Borman. *Interior, Rural Affairs and Environment:* Serder Denktas. *Education and Culture:* Esber Serakinci. *Agriculture and Forests:* Ilkay Kamil. *Communications, Works and Tourism:* Mehmet Bayram. *Trade and Industry:* Atay A. Rasit. *Health and Social Welfare:* Ertugrul Hasipoglu. *Housing:* Erkan Enekci.

The Speaker of the Leglislative Assembly is Hakki Atun.

Flag: White with horizontal bars of red set near the top and bottom; between these a crescent and star in red.

Budget. The 1991 Budget balanced at 300,000m. Turkish lira.

Currency. The Turkish lira is used throughout Northern Cyprus.

Banking Turkish Bank Ltd, Turkiye Is Bankasi and the Cyprus Turkish Co-operative Central Bank Ltd are operating in the Turkish occupied area and no control is exercised by the Central Bank of Cyprus.

Agriculture. Agriculture accounted for 11·8% of GNP in 1990.

Foreign Economic Relations. Exports earned US$55m. in 1989. Imports in 1986 amounted to TL102,461m. and exports to TL35,018m. Customs barriers with Turkey were abolished in July 1990.

Tourism. There were over 350,000 tourists in 1989, including 60,000 from Europe. Tourist earnings totalled US$130m.

Aviation. A new international airport was constructed in 1975 at Evcan. Flights operate to Europe, the Middle East and the Gulf via Istanbul and Ankara. There is another international airport (1985) at Geçitkale.

Telecommunications. The local radio, Radio Bayrak (BRTK) broadcasts in several languages incuding Arabic, English and French. BRT Television broadcasts for an average of 3½ hours a day.

Newspapers. In 1990 there were 8 daily, and 6 weekly newspapers.

Education. In 1987 there were 20,781 pupils and 751 teachers in primary schools, 11,103 pupils and 706 teachers in secondary schools, 1,748 students and 192 teachers in technical schools, and 1,649 students with 84 teaching staff in higher education. There are 4 universities.

Health. In 1989 there were over 300 doctors and 3 state hospitals.

Further Reading

Statistical Information: Statistics and Research Department, Nicosia.
North Cyprus Almanack, London, 1987
Denktash, R., *The Cyprus Triangle*. London, 1982
Ertekün, N. M., *The Cyprus Dispute*. Nicosia North, 1984
Georghallides, G. S., *A Political and Administrative History of Cyprus 1918–1926*. Nicosia, 1979
Halil, K., *The Rape of Cyprus*. London, 1982
Hill, Sir George F., *A History of Cyprus*. 4 vols. Cambridge, 1940–52
Hitchins, C., *Cyprus*. London, 1984
Hunt, D., *Footprints in Cyprus*. London, 1982
Kitromilides, P. M. and Evriviades, M. L., *Cyprus*, [Bibliography]. Oxford and Santa Barbara, 1982
Kyle, K., *Cyprus*. London, 1984
Loizos, P., *The Heart Grows Bitter: A Chronicle of Cypriot War Refugees*. CUP, 1982
Mayes, S., *Makarios*. London, 1981
Necatigil, Z. M., *Our Republic in Perspective*. Nicosia, 1985
Reddaway, J., *Burdened With Cyprus*. London, 1986
St John-Jones, L. W., *The Population of Cyprus*. London, 1983

CZECHOSLOVAKIA

Capital: Prague
Population: 15·62m. (1989)
GNP per capita: US$8,700 (1985)

Česká a Slovenská Federátivní Republika

(Czech and Slovak Federative Republic)

HISTORY. The Czechoslovak State came into existence on 28 Oct. 1918, when the Czech *Národni Výbor* (National Committee) took over the government of the Czech lands upon the dissolution of Austria–Hungary. Two days later the Slovak National Council manifested its desire to unite politically with the Czechs. On 14 Nov. 1918 the first Czechoslovak National Assembly declared the Czechoslovak State to be a republic with T. G. Masaryk as President (1918–35).

The Treaty of St Germain-en-Laye (1919) recognized the Czechoslovak Republic, consisting of the Czech lands (Bohemia, Moravia, part of Silesia) and Slovakia. To these lands were added as a trust the autonomous province of Subcarpathian Ruthenia.

This territory was broken up for the benefit of Germany, Poland and Hungary by the Munich agreement (29 Sept. 1938) between UK, France, Germany and Italy.

In March 1939 the German-sponsored Slovak government proclaimed Slovakia independent, and Germany incorporated the Czech lands into the Reich as the 'Protectorate of Bohemia and Moravia'. A government-in-exile, headed by Dr Beneš, was set up in London in July 1940.

Liberation by the Soviet Army and US Forces was completed by May 1945.

Territories taken by Germans, Poles and Hungarians were restored to Czechoslovak sovereignty. Subcarpathian Ruthenia was transferred to the USSR.

Elections were held in May 1946, at which the Communist Party obtained about 38% of the votes.

A coalition government under a Communist Prime Minister, Klement Gottwald, remained in power until 20 Feb. 1948, when 12 of the non-Communist ministers resigned in protest against infiltration of Communists into the police.

In Feb. a predominantly Communist government was formed by Gottwald. In May elections resulted in an 89% majority for the government and President Beneš resigned.

In 1968 pressure for liberalization culminated in the overthrow of the Stalinist leader, Antonín Novotný, and his associates. The Communist Party introduced an 'Action Programme' of far-reaching reforms.

Soviet pressure to abandon this programme was exerted between May and Aug. 1968, and finally, Warsaw Pact forces occupied Czechoslovakia on 21 Aug. The Czechoslovak government was compelled to accept a policy of 'normalization' (*i.e.*, abandonment of most reforms) and the stationing of Soviet forces.

A Czechoslovak–Soviet 20-year Treaty of Friendship was signed in 1970.

In 1974 the German Federal Republic and Czechoslovakia annulled the Munich agreement of 1938.

Mass demonstrations demanding political reform began in Nov. 1989. After the authorities' use of violence to break up a demonstration on 17 Nov., the Communist Party leader, Miloš Jakeš, and the entire Politburo resigned. On 30 Nov. the Federal Assembly abolished the Communist Party's sole right to govern, and a new Government was formed on 3 Dec. The protest movement, focussed on the recently-established Civic Forum, in which prominent Charter 77 dissidents were active, continued to grow, and on 10 Dec. another Government was formed. Gustáv Husák resigned as President of the Republic, and was replaced by Václav Havel on the unanimous vote of 323 members of the Federal Assembly on 29 Dec.

In Dec. 1989 the Communist Party denounced the Warsaw Pact invasion of 1968 as 'unjustified and incorrect'.

AREA AND POPULATION. Czechoslovakia is bounded north-west by the German Democratic Republic, north by Poland, east by the USSR, south by Hungary and Austria and south-west by the Federal Republic of Germany. At the census of 11 Nov. 1980 the population was 15,283,095 (4,991,168 in Slovakia; 7·9m. females). Population in 1989, 15,624,021 (Slovakia, 5,263,541; females 8m. in 1987). There are 12 administrative regions *(Kraj)*, one of which is the capital, Prague (Praha) and one the capital of Slovakia, Bratislava.

Region	*Chief city*	*Area in sq. km*	*Population 1989*
Czech			
Prague	—	496	1,211,106
Středočeský	Prague (Praha)	10,994	1,122,023
Jihočeský	Ceské Budějovice	11,345	697,785
Západočeský	Plzeň (Pilsen)	10,875	869,592
Severočeský	Ustí nad Labem	7,819	1,190,606
Východočeský	Hradec Králove	11,240	1,240,847
Jihomoravský	Brno	15,028	2,058,530
Severomoravský	Ostrava	11,067	1,969,991
Slovak			
Bratislava	—	368	435,499
Západoslovenský	Bratislava	14,492	1,725,766
Stredoslovenský	Banská Bystrica	17,982	1,608,192
Východoslovenský	Košice	16,193	1,494,084

The area of Czechoslovakia is 127,899 sq. km (Slovakia, 49,035 sq. km). Population density in 1989: 122 per sq. km. Growth rate in 1988, 2·4 per 1,000. Expectation of life in 1985 was 67 (males); 74 (females).

Ethnic minorities have equal political and cultural rights. In 1987 there were (in 1,000): Czechs, 9,804; Slovaks, 4,953; Hungarians, 597; Poles, 73; Germans, 54; Ukrainians, 48; Russians, 7. There were 303,000 gipsies in 1983.

The official languages are Czech in the Czech lands and Slovak in Slovakia; minority languages may be used for official business if its speakers make up at least 20% of the population.

The population of the principal towns in 1989 was as follows (in 1,000):

Prague (Praha)	1,211	Liberec	104	Gottwaldov	87
Bratislava	435	Hradec Králové	100	Banská Bystrica	87
Brno	390	Ceské Budějovice	97	Kladno	73
Ostrava	331	Zilina	96	Trnava	72
Košice	232	Pardubice	96	Karviná	72
Plzeň	175	Havírov	92	Most	70
Olomouc	107	Nitra	89	Frýdek-Místek	65
Ustí nad Labem	106	Prešov	87	Martin	65

Vital statistics for calendar years:

	Live births	*Marriages*	*Divorces*	*Deaths*
1986	220,494	119,979	37,885	185,718
1987	214,927	122,168	39,522	179,224
1988 [1]	216,158	118,956	38,922	178,229

[1] Provisional

Infant mortality in 1988 (per 1,000 live births), 4·6. Abortion rate per 1,000 live births, in 1985: Czech Lands, 728; Slovakia, 504. Abortion law was liberalized in 1986.

CLIMATE. A humid continental climate, with warm summers and cold winters. Precipitation is generally greater in summer, with thunderstorms. Autumn, with dry, clear weather and spring, which is damp, are each of short duration. Prague. Jan. 29·5°F (–1·5°C), July 67°F (19·4°C). Annual rainfall 19·3" (483mm). Brno. Jan. 31°F (–0·6°C), July 67°F (19·4°C). Annual rainfall 21" (525mm).

CONSTITUTION AND GOVERNMENT. For details of previous constitutions, *see* THE STATESMAN'S YEAR-BOOK, 1990–91, pp. 408–9.

Czechoslovakia is a federal republic consisting of two nations of equal rights: The Czech Republic (the Czech lands, previously Bohemia, Moravia and part of Silesia), and the Slovak Republic (Slovakia). A law of 12 Dec. 1990 defines the respective competences of the Czech and Slovak Republics and devolves most of former federal administratove and economic authority to them. Religious and ethnic affairs remain a federal responsibility. Each Republic is governed by a National Council (the Czech with 200 deputies, the Slovak with 150), which delegates to an overall Federal Assembly responsibility for constitutional and foreign affairs, defence and important economic decisions. The Federal Assembly has two chambers which have equal status, and usually meet in joint session: the Chamber of the People which has 101 Czech and 49 Slovak delegates, and the Chamber of the Nations, which has 75 Czech and 75 Slovak delegates. Both Chambers are elected by direct universal suffrage. Minimum age of voters is 18; of deputies, 21 years.

Elections were held in June 1990. Turn-out was 95% of the 11,247,000 electorate. Voting was by proportional representation. 22 parties took part, but to gain entry to any chamber needed 5% of the vote. Percentages of vote gained for the Chamber of the People (and Nations): Civic Forum, together with its Slovak ally, Public Against Violence, 46·6% (46·9%); Communist Party, 13·6% (13·7%); Christian Democratic Union, 12% (11·3%); Moravian-Silesian Society, 5·4% (6·2%); Slovak Nationalist Party, 3·5% (3·6%); Coexistence, 2·8% (2·7%).

Seats gained in the Chamber of the People (and Nations): Civic Forum, together with Public Against Violence, 87 (83); Communist Party, 23 (24); Christian Democratic Union, 20 (20); Moravian-Silesian Society, 9 (7); Slovak Nationalist Party, 6 (7); Coexistence, 5 (7). The next elections are due in 1992.

President of the Republic: Václav Havel, elected on 5 July 1990 for a two-year period by the Federal Assembly by 234 votes to 50. *Speaker of the Federal Assembly:* Alexander Dubček (b. 1921).

In March 1991 the Government consisted of: *Chancellor:* Karel Schwarzenberg; *Commandant of the Military Office:* Lt.-Gen. Ladislav Tomeček; *Chairman of the Council of Consultants:* Milan Šimečka; *Prime Minister:* Marián Čalfa (b. 1946); *Deputy Prime Ministers (in charge of),* Václav Valeš *(Economic Reform),* Jiří Dienstbier *(Foreign Affairs),* Jozef Mikloško *(Human Rights, Religion and Culture),* Pavel Rychetský *(Legislation)*; *Cabinet Ministers: Economic Control,* Květoslava Kořínková; *Defence,* Luboš Dobrovský; *Economic Affairs,* Vladimír Dlouhý; *Environment,* Josef Vavroušek; *Finance,* Václav Klaus; *Interior,* Ján Langoš; *Labour and Social Affairs,* Petr Miller; *Strategic Planning,* Pavel Hoffman; *Transport,* Jiří Nezval; *Telecommunications,* Theodor Petřík; *Federal Bureau for Economic Competition:* Imrich Flasík.

The Chairman of the Czech National Council is Dagmar Burešová; of the Slovak, František Mikloško. The Czech Prime Minister is Peter Pithart; the Slovak, Vladimír Mečiar.

Local government. At elections in Nov. 1990 turn-out was 75% in the Czech Republic and 63·75% in Slovakia. In the Czech Republic Civic Forum gained 35·6% of the vote, and the Communist Party, 17·2%. In Slovakia the Christian Democratic Movement gained 28·4% of the vote, Public Against Violence, 20·4%. The former National Committees have been replaced by district bureaux with the power to raise local taxes and with responsibility for roads, schools, utilities and public health.

National flag: White and red (horizontal), with a blue triangle of full depth at the hoist, point to the fly.

National anthem: Kde domov můj ('Where is my homeland'; Czech anthem, words by J. K. Tyl); combined with, Nad Tatru sa blýska ('Over Tatra it lightens'; Slovak anthem, words by J. Matuška).

DEFENCE. Conscription is for 12 months.

Soviet troops in the country, legalized by an agreement which followed the Warsaw Pact invasion of Aug. 1968, began to withdraw in 1990.

Army. The Army had a strength (1990) of 148,600 (100,000 conscripts). It consists of 3 tank, 5 motor rifle and 1 artillery divisions; 2 anti-tank regiments, 3 *Scud*, 6 engineer and 1 airborne brigades and 5 regiments of Civil Defence troops. Equipment includes 4,585 T-54/-55/-72 tanks. There are also 2 paramilitary forces: Border Troops (11,000) and People's Militia (120,000).

Air Force. The Air Force is organized as a tactical force, under overall army command, and had a strength of some 44,800 personnel (18,000 conscripts) and 450 combat aircraft in 1990. Three interceptor regiments (each 3 squadrons of 14 aircraft) are equipped with MiG-29, MiG-23 and MiG-21 jets, and MiG-29 are coming into service. There are 4 regiments of Su-22, Su-25, MiG-23 and MiG-21 ground attack aircraft, as well as Mi-24 gunship helicopters. MiG-21s and modified L-39 Albatros jet trainers are used for tactical reconnaissance. Transport units have a total of 60 Let L-410, An-24/26, Il-14 and Tu-134 aircraft and about 100 Mil Mi-2 (some armed), Mi-4, Mi-8 and Mi-17 helicopters. Training units are equipped with 2-seat MiG-23s and MiG-21s and Czech-built aircraft, including L-29 and L-39 Albatros jet advanced trainers and Zlin primary trainers. Surface-to-air ('Guideline', 'Goa', 'Ganef', 'Gainful' and 'Gaskin') missile units are operational.

INTERNATIONAL RELATIONS

Membership. Czechoslovakia is a member of the UN, OIEC, Council of Europe, Warsaw Pact and IMF, and with Austria, Hungary, Italy and Yugoslavia was an inaugural member of the 'Pentagonale' meeting on economic and political co-operation in July 1990.

ECONOMY

Policy. For planning under the Communist régime *see* THE STATESMAN'S YEAR-BOOK, 1990–91, p. 410. The Government is pursuing a programme of reallocation of ownership of enterprises. Federal Government will retain control of defence, telecommunications, transport and mining; light and service industries will devolve to the Czech and Slovak Republics, and local public services to municipal control. Small businesses will be privatized first. Subsequently large firms will be denationalized and ownership transferred to companies through the National Assets Foundation. Citizens' shares in companies will be mediated through a voucher system. Sales of some 100,000 small businesses began in Dec. 1990. A law of Feb. 1991 restores property confiscated by the Communist regime.

Budget. Budgets for calendar years (in Kčs. 1m.):

	1982	*1983*	*1984*	*1985*	*1986*	*1987*	*1988*
Revenue	314,203	324,127	343,805	359,692	368,696	383,732	404,045
Expenditure	314,046	323,890	342,192	358,028	365,949	382,151	401,199

Main items of the 1988 budget were (in Kčs. 1,000m.): Revenue: From the economy, 258; direct taxes, 47. Expenditure: National economy, 90; health and social services, 96; defence, 27; administration, 4.

Currency. The monetary unit is the *koruna* (CSK) or crown of 100 *haler*. Notes in circulation: Kčs. 10, 20, 50, 100, 500, 1,000. Coin: 5, 10, 20, 50 *halers*, and Kčs. 1, 2, 5. Gold reserves were US$1,832m. in 1987. The crown became fully internally convertible in 1990. It was devalued by 75% in Dec. 1989 and again by 35·3% in Oct. 1990. A single exchange rate for the crown was set in Dec. 1990 and it became convertible on 1 Jan. 1991. Official rates of exchange (March 1991): £1 = Kčs. 51·39; US$1 = Kčs. 27·09.

Banking and Finance. For previous banking history *see* THE STATESMAN'S YEAR-BOOK, 1990–91, p. 410. The central bank and bank of issue is the State Bank (Statní Banka). The Governorship alternates annually between a Czech and a Slovak. There were 20·2m. savings accounts totalling 265,569m. Kčs in 1988.

Weights and Measures. The metric system is in force.

ENERGY AND NATURAL RESOURCES

Electricity. Production of electricity in 1988: 87,374m. kwh. In 1990 there were two nuclear power stations, producing 28% of all electricity. Two more were under construction. Supply 120 and 220 volts; 50 Hz.

Oil. Production (1989 estimate) 130,000 tonnes. There is an oil pipeline from the USSR with branches to Bratislava and Zaluzi.

Gas. A natural gas pipeline from the USSR supplies the German Federal and Democratic Republics, Austria and Italy as well as Czechoslovakia. A second is under construction.

Minerals. Czechoslovakia is not rich in minerals. There are hard and soft coal reserves (chief coalfields: Most, Chomutov, Kladno, Ostrava and Sokolov). There is also uranium, glass sand and salt, and small quantities of iron ore, graphite, copper and lead. Gold deposits were found near Prague in 1985. Production in 1988 (in 1,000 tonnes): Coal, 25,504; lignite and brown coal, 96,361.

Agriculture. In 1988 there were 6·8m. ha of agricultural land (4·8m. ha arable, 0·8m. meadow, 0·8m. pasture), of which 4·3m. were held by collective farms, 2·1m. by state farms and 67,000 as private plots (maximum size 1 ha).

In 1988 there were 1,657 collective farms with 1,004,517 members and 238 state farms with 173,725 employees. Crop production in 1988 (in 1,000 tonnes): Sugar-beet, 5,418; wheat, 6,547; potatoes, 3,659; barley, 3,411; maize, 996; rye, 534.

Livestock. In 1988: Cattle, 5,075,000 (including 1,815,000 milch cows); horses, 44,000; pigs, 7,384,000; sheep, 1,047,000; poultry, 49m. In 1988 production of meat was 1,846,980 tonnes (live weight); milk, 6,754m. litres; 5,596m. eggs. In 1988 there were 141,191 tractors. 36,470 ha were irrigated in 1988.

Forestry. Forest area in 1989 was 4,606,673 ha (50% spruce, 16% beech and pine, 7% oak) representing 37% of the land area. The area reafforested in 1988 was 17,630 ha. The timber yield was 18·1m. cu. metres in 1988.

Fisheries. Total catch was 21·25m. tonnes in 1988.

INDUSTRY. Industrialization was well developed before the Communist régime, under which all industry was nationalized.

Output in 1988 (in 1,000 tonnes): Pig-iron, 9,706; crude steel, 15,319; coke, 10,586; rolled-steel products, 11,420; cement, 10,974; paper, 974; sulphuric acid, 1,249; nitrogenous fertilizers, 594; phosphate fertilizers, 313; plastics, 1,192; synthetic fibres, 204; sugar, 707; beer, 22·7m. hectolitres; cars, 163,834 (no.).

Textile production (in 1m. metres) in 1988: Cotton, 591; llnen, 105; woollen, 59; shoes, 119·1m. pairs (55·3m. leather).

Labour. There were 8,882,691 persons of employable age in 1988 (*i.e.*, males, 15–59; females 15–54), of whom 7·5m. (46% women) were employed: 5·8m. in production (industry, 2·9m.; agriculture, 838,902; building, 694,425); and 2m. in services.

A 5-day 42-hour week with 4 weeks annual holiday is standard. Average monthly wage in 1989: Kčs. 3,300.

Trade Unions. The former offical trade union organization ROH dissolved itself in March 1990. The Czechoslovak Confederation of Trade Unions (Chairman, Igor Pleskot), evolved from strike committees set up in 1989. It claimed 6m. members in 1990.

FOREIGN ECONOMIC RELATIONS. A trade pact was signed with the EEC in May 1990. External debt was some US$8,000m. in 1990. Foreign currency reserves were US$4,832m. in 1987. Joint venture law permits foreign investors 100% ownership and exemption from state planning regulations.

Commerce. Total trade (in Kčs. 1m.) for calendar years:

	1983	1984	1985	1986	1987	1988
Imports	103,012	113,737	120,323	125,449	127,259	129,134
Exports	103,838	114,230	119,818	121,777	125,875	132,781

In 1988, trade with Communist countries amounted to 205,560m. Kčs. (109,200m. Kčs. with the USSR, 25,354m. Kčs. with the German Democratic Republic, 27,486m. Kčs. with Poland). The UK was Czechoslovakia's third biggest non-Communist trade partner after the Federal German Republic and Austria.

Market share (1989) of exports: USSR, 30·5%; Poland, 8·5%; Federal Germany, 8·3%; GDR, 6·6%; Austria, 4·6%. Imports: USSR, 29·7%; Federal Germany, 9·3%; Poland, 8·6%; GDR, 7·8%; Austria, 5·5%.

Total trade between Czechoslovakia and UK for calendar years (British Department of Trade returns, in £1,000 sterling):

	1986	1987	1988	1989	1990
Imports to UK	125,399	141,472	148,248	156,649	135,988
Exports and re-exports from UK	108,841	114,101	130,420	131,418	133,158

Tourism. In 1988, 14·03m. tourists visited Czechoslovakia (1·1m. from the West) and 6·3m. Czechoslovak tourists made visits abroad (346,000 to the West). Visa-free travel to the West has been permited since Dec. 1989.

COMMUNICATIONS

Roads. In 1988 there were 73,540 km of motorways and first-class roads (660 km of motorways in 1988). In 1984 there were 2,639,564 private cars (figures have not been given since). In 1988 state road transport carried 2,343m. passengers and 339m. tonnes of freight. In 1988 there were 109,521 accidents with 1,246 fatalities.

Railways. In 1988 the length of railway routes was 13,103 km. Of this, 3,798 km were electrified. In 1988, 415·4m. passengers and 294·8m. tonnes of freight were carried.

Aviation. Air transport is run by ČSA (Czechoslovak Airlines), which had 32 aircraft in 1990. The main airports are: Prague (Ruzyně), Brno (Cernovice), Bratislava (Vajnory), Olomouc (Holice), Košice (Barca). In 1988, 1·5m. passengers and 28,066 tonnes of freight were flown. There are 6 internal and 53 international flights from Prague. British Airways operates air traffic London–Prague, Air France Paris–Prague–Bucharest.

Shipping. In 1988 Czechoslovak Maritime Shipping had 14 freighters totalling 227,638 DWT, based on Szczecin. In 1988, 1·63m. tonnes of cargo were carried.

There are 475 km of inland waterways. Freight transport totalled 15·21m. tonnes in 1988. 537,000 passengers were carried in 1988.

Czechoslovak Danube Shipping operate 5 ships totalling 244,000 DWT in the Mediterranean from Bratislava, and Czechoslovak Elbe-Oder Shipping had a fleet of 284,500 DWT in 1985.

Telecommunications. There were 5,137 post offices in 1988. Number of telephones in 1990 was 4m. *Československy Rozhlas*, the governmental broadcasting station, broadcasts on 2 networks; 1 from Prague with 3 programmes in Czech and Slovak and 1 from Bratislava with 2 programmes in Slovak and additional broadcasts in Hungarian and Ukrainian. *Československa Televise* broadcast 2 television programmes nation-wide, including colour broadcasts. In 1988, 4·23m. people held radio and 4·66m. TV licences.

Cinemas and Theatres (1988). There were 2,778 cinemas and 86 theatres. 42 full-length films were made.

Newspapers and Books (1988). There were 30 daily newspapers, including 12 in Slovak, and 1,057 other periodicals. 6,977 book titles were published in 102·7m. copies. There were 9,014 public libraries.

JUSTICE, RELIGION, EDUCATION AND WELFARE

Justice. The criminal and criminal procedure codes date from 1 Jan. 1962, as amended in April 1973.

There is a Federal Supreme Court and federal military courts, with judges electeu by the Federal Assembly. Both republics have Supreme Courts and a network of regional and district courts whose professional judges are elected by the republican National Councils. Lay judges are elected by regional or district local authorities. Local authorities and social organizations may participate in the decision-making of the courts. An amnesty for some 30,000 of the 40,000 persons in prison was announced in Jan. 1990.

Religion. Official surveys suggest that 20% of the population are religious believers. In 1987 there were 18 different faiths with 5,500 clergy and 7,500 churches. The largest single church is the Roman Catholic (3·7m. members, 4,336 parishes 5,085 churches and 3,175 priests, 1985): Its main support is in Slovakia. Cardinal František Tomašek was installed as archbishop of Prague in 1978. The archbishopric of Trnava is held by a bishop and that of Olomouc by an administrator. Most of the remaining 10 dioceses are directed by Government-appointed capitulary vicars but 3 bishops were consecrated in 1988, the first since 1973. There were 2 seminaries and 6 theological faculties in 1989.

In 1986 there were 1·3m. non-Catholic church members, including 475,000 Hussites, 81,000 Czech Brethren with 670 congregations, 370,000 Slovak Lutherans in 2 districts with 15 associations of parishes, 36,000 Silesian Lutherans and 120,000 Reformed Christians with 7 associations of parishes. In 1981 there were 15,000 Jews (mainly in Prague, where there is a synagogue and, since 1984, a rabbi). In 1986 there were 150,000 Orthodox with 100 congregations in 4 dioceses. The Uniate Church was suppressed in 1950 but maintained a clandestine existence.

Education. In 1988–89 there were 11,393 kindergartens for children from 3 to 6 years, with 50,483 teachers and 651,365 pupils. Education is free and compulsory for 10 years. Children of 6 to 14 years attend primary school (grades 1 to 9). Selection then takes place for secondary schools (4 years), vocational secondary schools (4 years) or apprentice centres (2-4 years). University entrance is mainly from secondary schools. In 1988–89 there were 6,216 primary schools with 2,013,910 pupils and 97,853 teachers, 349 secondary schools with 145,532 pupils and 10,378 teachers and 561 secondary vocational schools with 271,014 students and 16,857 teachers. In higher education in 1988–89, there were 136,656 (60,606 women) full-time students, and 20,434 teachers. There are 36 institutions of higher education, with 112 faculties. These include 5 universities—the Charles University in Prague (founded 1348); the Masaryk (formerly Purkyně) University in Brno (1919); the Comenius University in Bratislava (1919); the Palacký University in Olomouc (1573); the Šafárik University in Košice (1959); and 12 technical universities or institutes.

Welfare. Medical care is free. In 1988 Kčs. 32,190m. were spent on health insurance benefits. There were, in 1988, 231 hospitals with a total of 123,844 beds, and 57,112 doctors and dentists. Family allowances (Kčs. per month): 1 child, 200; 2 children, 650; 3, 1,210. Old age pensions averaging 67% of salary are paid at the age of 60 (men), 53–57 (women).

DIPLOMATIC REPRESENTATIVES

Of Czechoslovakia in Great Britain (25 Kensington Palace Gdns., London, W8 4QY)
Ambassador: Karel Duda.

Of Great Britain in Czechoslovakia (Thunovská 14, 11800 Prague 1)
Ambassador: P. L. O'Keeffe, CMG, CVO.

Of Czechoslovakia in the USA (3900 Linnean Ave., NW, Washington, D.C., 20008)
Ambassador: Rita Klimová.

Of the USA in Czechoslovakia (Tržiste 15–12548 Praha, Prague)
Ambassador: Eduard Kukan.

Of Czechoslovakia to the United Nations
Ambassador: Evžen Zápotocký.

Further Reading

The Constitution of the Czechoslovak Socialist Republic. Prague, 1960
Statistická ročenka CSSR [Statistical Yearbook]. Prague, annual since 1958
Historická statistická ročenka CSSR. Prague, 1985
Czechoslovak Foreign Trade. Prague, monthly
Batt, J., *Economic Reform and Political Change in Eastern Europe: A Comparison of the Czechoslovak and Hungarian Experiences.* Basingstoke, 1988
Bradley, J. F. N. *Politics in Czechoslovakia, 1945–1971.* Lanham, 1981
Czechoslovak Chamber of Commerce and Industry. *Facts on Czechoslovak Foreign Trade.* Prague, annual since 1965.—*Your Trade Partners in Czechoslovakia.* Prague, 1986
Demek, J. and others, *Geography of Czechoslovakia.* Prague, 1971
Havel, V., *Disturbing the Peace.* London, 1990.—*Living in Truth: Twenty-Two Essays.* London, 1990
Hermann, A. H., *A History of the Czechs.* London, 1975
Hejzlar, Z. and Kusin, V. V., *Czechoslovakia, 1968–1969.* New York, 1975
Kalvoda, J., *The Genesis of Czechoslovakia.* New York, 1986
Kaplan, K., *The Communist Party in Power: A Profile of Party Politics in Czechoslovakia.* Boulder, 1987
Kolafova, V. and Slaba, D. *Czech-English and English-Czech dictionary.* Prague, 1979
Korbel, J., *Twentieth-Century Czechoslovakia: The Meanings of its History.* Columbia Univ. Press, 1977
Krystufek, Z., *The Soviet Régime in Czechoslovakia.* Columbia Univ. Press, 1981
Kusin, V. V., *From Dubček to Charter 77.* Edinburgh, 1978
Leff, C. S., *National Conflict in Czechoslovakia: The Making and Remaking of a State, 1918–1987.* Princeton, 1988
Mamatey, V. S. and Luža, R. (eds.) *A History of the Czechoslovak Republic 1918–1948.* Princeton Univ. Press, 1973
Mlynař, Z., *Night Frost in Prague: the End of Humane Socialism.* New York, 1980
Procházka, J., *English–Czech and Czech–English Dictionary.* 16th ed. London, 1959
Sejna, J. *We Will Bury You.* London, 1982
Short, D., *Czechoslovakia.* [Bibliography] Oxford and Santa Barbara, 1986
Stone, N. and Strouhal, E., (eds.) *Czechoslovakia: Crossroads and Crises, 1918-88.* London, 1989
Teichova, A., *The Czechoslovak Economy, 1918–1980.* London, 1988
Wallace, W. V., *Czechoslovakia.* London, 1977

DENMARK

Kongeriget Danmark

(Kingdom of Denmark)

Capital: Copenhagen
Population: 5·14m. (1990)
GNP per capita: US$18,470 (1988)

HISTORY. First organized as a unified state in the 10th century, Denmark acquired approximately its present boundaries in 1815, having ceded Norway to Sweden and its north German territory to Prussia. Denmark became a constitutional monarchy in 1849.

AREA AND POPULATION. According to the census held on 9 Nov. 1970 the area of Denmark proper was 43,075 sq. km (16,631 sq. miles) and the population 4,937,579. Population, Jan. 1990: 5,135,409.

Administrative divisions		*Area (sq. km) 1990*	*Population 1970*	*Population 1990*	*Population 1990 per sq. km.*
København (Copenhagen)	(city)	88	622,773	466,723	5,288·6
Frederiksberg	(borough)	9	101,874	85,611	9,761·8
Københavns	(county)	526	615,343	600,889	1,142·5
Frederiksborg	,,	1,347	259,442	341,067	253·1
Roskilde	,,	891	153,199	216,964	243·4
Vestsjælland	,,	2,984	259,057	283,641	95·0
Storstrøm	,,	3,398	252,363	256,912	75·6
Bornholm	,,	588	47,239	45,900	78·0
Fyn	,,	3,486	432,699	459,354	131·8
Sønderjylland	,,	3,938	238,062	250,612	63·6
Ribe	,,	3,131	197,843	218,582	69·8
Vejle	,,	2,997	306,263	330,398	110·3
Ringkøbing	,,	4,853	241,327	267,295	55·1
Aarhus	,,	4,561	533,190	597,143	130·9
Viborg	,,	4,123	220,734	229,775	55·7
Nordjylland	,,	6,173	456,171	484,543	78·5
Total		43,093	4,937,579	5,135,409	119·2

The population is almost entirely Scandinavian; in Jan. 1990, of the inhabitants of Denmark proper, 95·7% were born in Denmark, including Faroe Islands and Greenland.

On 1 Jan. 1990 the population of the capital, Copenhagen (comprising Copenhagen, Frederiksberg and Gentofte municipalities), was 617,637 (including suburbs, 1,337,114); Aarhus, 261,437; Odense, 176,133; Aalborg, 155,019; Esbjerg, 81,504; Randers, 61,020; Kolding, 57,285; Helsingør, 56,701; Herning, 56,687; Horsens, 55,210.

Vital statistics for calendar years:

	Living births	*Still births*	*Marriages*	*Divorces*	*Deaths*	*Emigration*	*Immigration*
1984	51,800	230	28,624	14,490	57,109	25,053	29,035
1985	53,749	240	29,322	14,385	58,378	26,715	36,214
1986	55,312	242	30,773	14,490	58,100	27,928	38,932
1987	56,221	288	31,132	14,381	58,136	30,123	36,296
1988	58,904	292	32,080	14,717	59,034	34,544	35,051

Illegitimate births: 1983, 40·6%; 1984, 41·9%; 1985, 43%; 1986, 43·9%; 1987, 44·7%.

CLIMATE. The climate is much modified by marine influences, and the effect of the Gulf Stream, to give winters that are cold and cloudy but warm and sunny summers. In general, the east is drier than the west, though few places have more than 27" (675 mm) of rain a year. Long periods of calm weather are exceptional and windy conditions are common. Copenhagen. Jan. 33°F (0·5°C), July 63°F (17°C). Annual rainfall 22·8" (571 mm). Esbjerg. Jan. 33°F (0·5°C), July 59°F (15°C). Annual rainfall 32" (800 mm).

REIGNING QUEEN. Margrethe II, born 16 April 1940; married 10 June 1967 to Prince Henrik, born Count de Monpezat; *offspring:* Crown Prince Frederik, born 26 May 1968; Prince Joachim, born 7 June 1969. She succeeded to the throne on the death of her father, King Frederik IX, on 14 Jan. 1972.

Mother of the Queen: Queen Ingrid, born Princess of Sweden, 28 March 1910.
Sisters of the Queen: Princess Benedikte, born 29 April 1944 (married 3 Feb. 1968 to Prince Richard of Sayn-Wittgenstein-Berleburg); Princess Anne-Marie, born 30 Aug. 1946 (married 18 Sept. 1964 to King Constantine of Greece).

The crown of Denmark was elective from the earliest times. In 1448 after the death of the last male descendant of Swein Estridsen the Danish Diet elected to the throne Christian I, Count of Oldenburg, in whose family the royal dignity remained for more than 4 centuries, although the crown was not rendered hereditary by right till 1660. The direct male line of the house of Oldenburg became extinct with King Frederik VII on 15 Nov. 1863. In view of the death of the king, without direct heirs, the Great Powers signed a treaty at London on 8 May 1852, by the terms of which the succession to the crown of Denmark was made over to Prince Christian of Schleswig-Holstein-Sonderburg-Glücksburg, and to the direct male descendants of his union with the Princess Louise of Hesse-Cassel, niece of King Christian VIII of Denmark. In accordance with this treaty, a law concerning the succession to the Danish crown was adopted by the Diet, and obtained the royal sanction 31 July 1853. Linked to the constitution of 5 June 1953, a new law of succession, dated 27 March 1953, has come into force, which restricts the right of succession to the descendants of King Christian X and Queen Alexandrine, and admits the sovereign's daughters to the line of succession, ranking after the sovereign's sons.

Subjoined is a list of the kings of Denmark, with the dates of their accession, from the time of election of Christian I of Oldenburg:

House of Oldenburg

Christian I	1448	Christian IV	1588	Frederik V	1746
Hans	1481	Frederik III	1648	Christian VII	1766
Christian II	1513	Christian V	1670	Frederik VI	1808
Frederik I	1523	Frederik IV	1699	Christian VIII	1839
Christian III	1534	Christian VI	1730	Frederik VII	1848
Frederik II	1559				

House of Schleswig-Holstein-Sonderburg-Glücksburg

Christian IX	1863	Christian X	1912	Margrethe II	1972
Frederik VIII	1906	Frederik IX	1947		

CONSTITUTION AND GOVERNMENT. The present constitution of Denmark is founded upon the 'Grundlov' (charter) of 5 June 1953.

The legislative power lies with the Queen and the *Folketing* (Diet) jointly. The executive power is vested in the Queen, who exercises her authority through the ministers. The judicial power is with the courts. The Queen must be a member of the Evangelical-Lutheran Church, the official Church of the State. The Queen cannot assume major international obligations without the consent of the *Folketing*. The *Folketing* consists of one chamber. All men and women of Danish nationality of more than 18 years of age and permanently resident in Denmark possess the franchise and are eligible for election to the *Folketing*, which is at present composed of 179 members; 135 members are elected by the method of proportional representation in 17 constituencies. In order to attain an equal representation of the different parties, 40 *tillægsmandater* (additional seats) are divided among such parties which have not obtained sufficient returns at the constituency elections. Two members are elected for the Faroe Islands and 2 for Greenland. The term of the legislature is 4 years, but a general election may be called at any time.

The *Folketing* must meet every year on the first Tuesday in October. Besides its legislative functions, it appoints every 6 years judges who, together with the ordinary members of the Supreme Court *(Højesteret)*, form the *Rigsret*, a tribunal which can alone try parliamentary impeachments. The ministers have free access to the House, but can vote only if they are members.

Folketing: At the elections of 12 Dec. 1990 Social Democrats won 69 seats (with 37·4% of votes cast), Conservatives (C) 30 (16%), Liberals (L) 29 (15·8%), Socialist People's Party 15 (8·3%), Progress Party 12 (6·4%), Centre Democrats 9 (5·1%), Radical Liberals 7 (3·5%), Christian People's Party 4 (2·3%). 2 members were elected for the Faroe Islands and 2 for Greenland.

A coalition government of Conservatives and Liberals was formed on 17 Dec. 1990:

Prime Minister: Poul Schlüter (C).

Foreign Affairs: Uffe Ellemann-Jensen (L). *Finance:* Henning Dyremose (C). *Economic and Fiscal Affairs:* Anders Fogh Rasmussen (L). *Justice:* Hans Engell (L). *Environment:* Per Stig Møller (C). *Education and Research:* Bertel Haarder (L). *Social Affairs:* Else Winther Andersen (L). *Ecclesiastical Affairs and Communications:* Torben Rechendorff (C). *Energy:* Jens Bilgrav Nielsen. *Labour:* Knud Erik Kirkegaard (C). *Fisheries:* Kent Kirk (C). *Industry and Energy:* Anne Birgitte Lundhoff (C). *Culture:* Grethe Rostbøll (C). *Health:* Ester Larsen (L). *Agriculture:* Laurits Tørnœs (L). *Defence:* Knud Enggaard (L). *Housing:* Svend Erik Hovmand (L). *Interior and Nordic Affairs:* Thor Pedersen (L). *Transport:* Kaj Ikast (C).

The ministers are individually and collectively responsible for their acts, and if impeached and found guilty, cannot be pardoned without the consent of the *Folketing*.

In 1948 a separate legislature *(Lagting)* and executive *(Landsstyre)* were established for the Faroe Islands, to deal with specified local matters and in 1979 a separate legislature *(Landsting)* and executive *(Landsstyre)* were established for Greenland, also to deal with specified local matters.

National flag: Red with white Scandinavian cross (Dannebrog).

National anthems: Kong Kristian stod ved højen Mast (words by J. Ewald, 1778; tune by J. E. Hartmann, 1780) and Der er et yndigt land.

Local Government. For administrative purposes Denmark is divided into 275 municipalities *(kommuner)*; each of them has a district council of between 7 and 31 members, headed by an elected mayor. The city of Copenhagen forms a district by itself and is governed by a city council of 55 members, elected every 4 years, and an executive *(magistraten)*, consisting of the chief burgomaster *(overborgmesteren)* and 6 burgomasters, appointed by the city council for 4 years. There are 14 counties *(amtskommuner)*, each of which is administered by a county council *(amstråd)* of between 13 and 31 members, headed by an elected mayor. All councils are elected directly by universal suffrage and proportional representation for 4-year terms.

The counties and Copenhagen are superintended by the Ministry of Interior Affairs. The municipalities are superintended by 14 local supervision committees, headed by a state county prefect *(statsamtmand)* who is a civil servant appointed by the Queen.

DEFENCE. Military defence is organized in accordance with the Defence Act of May 1982 as amended in April 1990, and the overall organization of the Danish Armed Forces comprises the Defence Command, the Army, the Navy, the Air Force and interservice authorities and institutions. To this should be added the Home Guard, which is an indispensable part of Danish military defence. The Home Guard is based on the Home Guard Act of May 1982.

In accordance with the Defence Act the Chief of Defence has full command of the three services: The Army, the Navy and the Air Force. The Chief of Defence, and the Defence Staff constitute the Defence Command.

The Constitution of 1849 declared it the duty of every fit man to contribute to the national defence, and this provision is still in force. According to the Personnel Act of May 1982, the military personnel comprises officers, n.c.o.s and privates. Private personnel are provided by enlistment and by recruiting of volunteers. Selection of conscripts takes place at the age of 18–19 years, and the conscripts are normally called up for service ½–1½ years later. Afterwards conscripts may be recalled for refresher training or musters. The initial training period for conscripts is between 4 and 12 months.

Army. The Army comprises field army formations and the local defence forces. The field army formations are organized in a covering force and in reserve units. The covering force numbers about 17,000 men and comprises a standing force (regulars and conscripts with more than six months' service), and a supplementary force consisting of men newly released from service. The standing force are organized in standing brigade units, headquarters units and support units. The brigade units are organized in 5 mechanized infantry brigades. The field army is equipped with 210 medium battle tanks, 52 light tanks and about 530 armoured personnel carriers as well as artillery including 76 self-propelled howitzers. The Army has 14 Hughes 500 helicopters and 8 Supporter aircraft for observation and liaison. The local defence units consist of about 18,000 men organized in 9 infantry battalions and some artillery battalions. The men of the latest annual service groups form the troops of the line, while those of the previous years form the local defence, the reserve and the reserve for the Home Guard. There are 55,000 Army reservists.

Navy. The Navy, in 1991, 7,100 strong (810 conscripts) is supported by 5,700 reservists and 4,100 Naval Home Guard. The fleet includes 5 small submarines, 3 frigates, 5 offshore patrol vessels, 5 coastal patrol craft, 10 fast missile craft, 4 ocean minelayers, 2 coastal minelayers and 3 coastal minesweepers. Major auxiliaries include 2 tankers, and the Royal Yacht; and there are some 21 minor auxiliaries. The Naval Air Arm comprises 8 Lynx helicopters (one is carried in each of the offshore patrol craft), and the Home Guard operates 37 inshore patrol craft.

Coastal Defence forces man 2 permanent fortresses armed with 150mm guns.

Additional forces of a para-military nature include 4 icebreakers maintained by the navy at the main base at Frederikshavn.

Air Force. The operational units of the Air Force comprise 8 surface-to-air missile squadrons and 6 flying squadrons.

The air defence force consists of the 8 Hawk surface-to-air missile squadrons and 4 all-weather air-defence squadrons with a total of 57 F-16s. All squadrons have an air-defence and a fighter-bomber rôle.

The fighter bomber force comprises 2 squadrons with a total of 32 F 35 Drakens, one unit having a secondary reconnaissance role.

In addition the Air Force has a number of supplementary units, including 1 transport squadron (C-130 Hercules and Gulfstream III), 1 helicopter rescue squadron (S-61As), and a control and warning system.

Total strength of the Air Force is about 9,100, and the mobilization force about 10,000 men.

Home Guard. The overall Home Guard organization comprises the Home Guard Command, the Army Home Guard, the Naval Home Guard, the Air Force Home Guard and the Service Corps.

The personnel of the Home Guard is recruited on a voluntary basis. The personnel establishment of the Home Guard is at present about 70,700 persons (55,400 in the Army Home Guard, 4,100 in the Navy Home Guard, 9,100 in the Air Force Home Guard and 2,100 in the Service Corps.).

INTERNATIONAL RELATIONS

Membership. Denmark is a member of the UN, NATO, OECD and the European Communities.

ECONOMY

Budget. The budget *(Finanslovforslag)* must be laid before the Parliament *(Folketing)* not later than 4 months before the beginning of a new fiscal year.

The following shows the actual revenue and expenditure as shown in central government accounts for the calendar years 1986, 1987 and 1988, the approved budget figures for 1989 and the budget for 1990 (in 1,000 kroner):

	1988	*1989*	*1990*	*1991*
Revenue	199,758,658	208,441,215	221,460,257	291,392,600
Expenditure	213,249,915	227,138,309	228,485,205	307,527,100

Receipts and expenditures of special government funds and expenditures on public works are included.

The 1991 budget envisaged revenue of 133,776m. kroner from income and property taxes and 121,791m. from consumer taxes.

The central government debt on 31 Dec. 1988 amounted to 435,786m. kroner.

Currency. The monetary unit is the *Danish krone* (DKK) of 100 *øre*.

There are notes of 1,000, 500, 100 and 50 kroner, and coins of 20, 10, 5 and 1 krone and 50 and 25 øre. In March 1991, £1 = 11·19 *kroner*; US$1 = 5·90 *kroner*.

Banking and Finance. On 31 Dec. 1988 the accounts of the National Bank balanced at 148,871m. kroner. The assets included official net foreign reserves of 76,239m. kroner. The liabilities included notes and coin of 23,870m. kroner. On 31 Dec. 1989 there were 75 commercial banks, with deposits of 352,491m. kroner, and 152 savings banks, with deposits of 142,423m. kroner. On 31 Dec. 1988 the money supply was 376,158m. kroner.

There is a stock exchange in Copenhagen.

Weights and Measures. The metric system has been obligatory since 1912.

ENERGY AND NATURAL RESOURCES

Electricity. Production (1989), 20,993m. kwh. Supply 220 volts; Hz 50.

Oil. Production (1989) 5·4m. tonnes.

Agriculture. Land ownership is widely distributed. In June 1989 there were 81,267 holdings with at least 5 ha of agricultural area (or at least a production equivalent to that from 5 ha of barley). About 8,000 holdings were below the sample threshold. There were 14,749 small holdings (with less than 10 ha), 50,953 medium-sized holdings (10–50 ha) and 15,565 holdings with more than 50 ha.

There were 23,709 agricultural workers in 1989.

In 1989 the cultivated area was (in 1,000 ha): Grain, 1,562; peas and beans, 123; root crops, 208; other crops, 329; green fodder and grass, 550; fallow, 5; total cultivated area, 2,774.

	Area (1,000 ha)			*Production (in 1,000 tonnes)*		
Chief crops	*1987*	*1988*	*1989*	*1987*	*1988*	*1989*
Wheat	399	308	444	2,285	2,080	2,320
Rye	137	80	100	512	366	487
Barley	954	1,154	988	4,292	5,419	4,959
Oats [1]	21	44	30	94	202	125
Potatoes	30	33	34	957	1,246	1,238
Other root crops	180	178	124	8,314	10,391	10,217

[1] Including mixed grain.

Livestock, 1989: Horses, 35,000; cattle, 2,221,000; pigs, 9,190,000; poultry, 16,266,000.

Production (in 1,000 tonnes) in 1989: Milk, 4,747; butter, 92; cheese, 277; beef, 236; pork and bacon, 1,218; eggs, 82.

In 1989 tractors numbered 165,908 and combine harvesters, 33,863.

Fisheries. The total value of the fish caught was (in 1m. kroner): 1950, 156; 1955, 252; 1960, 376; 1965, 650; 1970, 854; 1975, 1,442; 1980, 2,888; 1984, 3,645; 1985, 3,542; 1986, 3,576; 1987, 3,510; 1988, 3,476; 1989, 3,623.

INDUSTRY. The following table sets forth the gross factor income (in 1m. kroner) by industrial origin in 3 calendar years:

	1987		*1988*		*1989*	
	Current Prices	*1980 Prices*	*Current Prices*	*1980 Prices*	*Current Prices*	*1980 Prices*
Agriculture, fur-farming, forestry, etc.	25,173	19,923	24,440	20,433	28,344	21,620
Fishing	2,152	1,414	2,097	1,307	2,458	1,470
Total	27,324	21,337	26,537	21,740	30,803	23,090
Mining and quarrying	5,360	9,641	4,681	10,227	6,515	11,740
Manufacturing	115,176	70,729	121,788	70,612	125,953	72,263
Electricity, gas and water	8,212	5,825	9,537	6,025	11,138	6,476
Construction	40,133	25,528	40,984	24,726	42,729	23,873
Total	171,881	111,723	176,960	111,593	186,335	114,352
Wholesale and retail trade	79,338	51,194	81,457	50,312	87,055	51,665
Restaurants and hotels	8,581	4,507	8,884	4,489	9,148	4,490
Transport and storage	37,181	23,489	39,717	25,321	42,373	26,404
Communication	8,777	4,986	9,515	5,298	10,592	5,407
Financing and insurance	21,609	13,466	20,312	12,101	21,170	11,764
Dwellings	51,674	29,532	52,782	30,069	59,026	30,762
Business services	32,310	19,731	34,952	20,201	39,136	20,611
Market services of education, health	7,044	4,285	7,474	4,281	7,740	4,225
Recreational and cultural services	5,413	3,523	5,760	3,664	6,958	4,216
Household services, incl. auto repair	16,866	9,217	18,303	9,349	20,050	9,587
Total	268,794	163,979	279,167	165,065	303,248	169,195
Other producers, excl. government	4,145	2,464	4,446	2,561	4,790	2,497
Producers of government services	131,770	83,261	142,112	83,907	187,380	83,564
Total	135,915	85,725	146,558	86,468	152,170	86,061
Imputed bank service charges	–22,048	–13,592	–20,300	–12,056	–21,669	–11,821
Gross domestic product at factor cost	581,366	369,173	608,421	372,810	650,886	380,877
Plus indirect taxes	135,982	69,711	140,081	65,354	139,289	63,080
Less subsidies	22,011		24,455		24,806	
Gross domestic product at market prices	695,837	438,884	724,047	438,163	765,369	443,957

Some 37,000 manufacturing enterprises registered for value-added tax in 1985. In the following table 'number of wage-earners' refers to 7,200 establishments with 6 employees or more (1989), while 'gross-output' and 'value-added' cover 3,298 enterprises with 20 employees or more (1989).

Branch of industry	*Number of wage-earners (1,000)*	*Gross output in factor values (1m. kroner)*	*Value added in factor values (1m. kroner)*
Mining and quarrying	0·9	815	630
Food products	49·1	95,310	25,130
Beverages	4·6	7,541	4,517
Tobacco	1·4	2,577	1,633
Textiles	10·2	8,695	3,929

Branch of industry	*Number of wage-earners (1,000)*	*Gross output in factor values (1m. kroner)*	*Value added in factor values (1m. kroner)*
Wearing apparel	006·6	003,192	001,596
Leather and products	0·5	409	162
Footwear	0·8	1,056	347
Wood products	8·4	6,413	2,888
Furniture and fixtures	12·0	7,199	3,714
Paper and products	7·1	8,364	3,878
Printing, publishing	14·9	14,529	9,538
Industrial chemicals	12·4	29,221	15,466
Other chemical products, petroleum refineries, petroleum coal products and rubber	2·9	11,440	3,156
Plastic products	7·5	6,613	3,554
Pottery, china, glass and products	3·3	1,778	1,075
Non-metal products	9·1	9,869	5,897
Iron, steel and non-ferrous metals	4·5	4,891	2,138
Metal products	27·7	21,676	10,281
Machinery	40·4	33,779	17,685
Electrical machinery	15·1	15,126	7,798
Transport equipment	16·4	13,950	6,113
Controlling equipment	6·8	6,528	4,015
Other industries	4·5	4,829	2,841
Total manufacturing	267·1	315,799	138,522

Labour. In 1989, 6% of the working population lived on agriculture, forestry and fishery, 20% on industries and handicrafts, 7% on construction, 14% on commerce, etc., 7% on transport and communication, and 46% on administration, professional services, etc.

FOREIGN ECONOMIC RELATIONS

Commerce. The following table shows the value, in 1,000 kroner, of special trade imports and exports (including trade with the Faroe Islands and Greenland) for calendar years:

	1985	*1986*	*1987*	*1988*	*1989* [1]
Imports	191,562,564	184,732,811	174,066,090	174,428,775	194,567,327
Exports	179,577,142	171,790,740	175,302,411	182,414,968	204,833,792

[1] Preliminary.

Imports and exports (in 1m. kroner) for calendar years:

Leading commodities	*1988 Imports*	*1988 Exports*	*1989* [1] *Imports*	*1989* [1] *Exports*
Live animals, meat, etc.	1,140	18,778	1,476	21,324
Dairy products, eggs	915	6,609	982	7,762
Fish and fish preparations	5,594	10,765	6,205	11,625
Cereals and cereal preparations	1,205	4,465	1,270	4,683
Sugar and sugar preparations	745	1,332	637	1,546
Coffee, tea, cocoa, etc.	1,752	397	1,838	529
Feeding stuff for animals	3,998	1,681	4,395	2,064
Wood, lumber and cork	2,567	600	2,876	692
Textiles, fibres, yarns, fabrics, etc.	5,993	4,268	6,179	4,529
Fuels, lubricants, etc.	10,764	3,838	12,998	5,812
Pharmaceutical products	2,902	6,223	2,953	7,123
Fertilizers, etc.	1,912	1,148	2,044	1,141
Metals, manufactures of metals	16,477	8,861	19,096	9,968
Machinery, electrical, equipment, etc.	37,006	37,538	40,567	43,100
Transport equipment	13,272	9,201	18,064	9,608

[1] Provisional.

Distribution of Danish foreign trade (in 1,000 kroner) according to countries of origin and destination, for calendar years:

Countries	Imports 1987	1988	1989[1]	Exports 1987	1988	1989[1]
Belgium	5,996,888	5,933,826	6,321,300	3,573,618	3,671,209	4,106,524
Finland	5,433,310	5,435,364	5,656,129	4,006,170	4,545,625	5,608,593
France	9,273,109	8,642,431	9,677,817	9,713,865	10,426,090	12,368,277
Germany (Fed. Rep.)	41,006,430	39,907,494	43,252,421	29,718,704	31,934,335	35,789,484
Norway	7,377,149	7,798,472	8,524,849	12,971,518	12,412,741	11,683,754
Sweden	21,267,090	21,377,630	23,482,809	20,114,801	20,958,329	25,015,731
Switzerland	3,730,737	3,802,755	3,919,350	4,094,550	4,170,381	4,447,241
UK	13,272,660	12,320,004	13,514,520	20,194,965	21,746,325	24,838,786
USA	9,305,670	10,471,953	13,384,615	12,385,059	10,670,988	11,432,593

[1] Provisional.

Total trade between Denmark (without the Faroe Islands) and UK (British Department of Trade returns, in £1,000 sterling):

	1986	1987	1988	1989	1990
Imports to UK	1,752,174	1,873,495	2,028,089	2,229,340	2,278,569
Exports and re-exports from UK	1,211,637	1,231,097	1,170,853	1,209,220	1,413,713

Tourism. In 1989, foreigners visiting Denmark spent some 16,898m. kroner. In 1989 foreigners spent 4·84m. nights in hotels and 3·24m. nights at camping sites.

Industrial Statistics. Danmarks Statistik. Copenhagen (annually)
Quarterly Statistics for the Industry: Commodity Statistics. Danmarks Statistik, Copenhagen
Statistics on Agriculture, Horticulture and Forestry. Danmarks Statistik. Copenhagen (annually)
Agricultural Statistics 1900–1965. Vol. I: *Agricultural Area and Harvest and Utilization of Fertilizers*.—Vol. II: *Livestock and Livestock Products, and Consumption of Feeding Stuffs*. Danmarks Statistik. Copenhagen, 1968–69
External Trade of Denmark. Danmarks Statistik, Copenhagen
Danish Industry in Facts and Figures. Federation of Danish Industries. Copenhagen (annually)
Energy Supply of Denmark, 1900–58 and *1948–65*. Danmarks Statistik. Copenhagen, 1959, 1967. Annual Supplements 1966–75 have been published in Statistical News
Report on Fisheries. Ministry of Fisheries, Copenhagen (annually)

COMMUNICATIONS

Roads. Denmark proper had (1 Jan. 1990), 601 km of motorways, 3,968 km of other state roads, 7,037 km of provincial roads and 59,168 km of commercial roads. Motor vehicles registered at 31 Dec. 1988 comprised 1,581,344 passenger cars, 293,543 lorries, 11,784 taxicabs (including 5,256 for private hire), 8,093 buses and 42,450 cycles.

Railways. In 1988 there were 2,344 km of State railways (199 km electrified), which carried 4,797m. passenger-km and 1,657m. tonne-km. There were also 494 km of private railways.

Aviation. On 1 Oct. 1950 the 3 Scandinavian airlines, Det Danske Luftfartsselskab, ABA and DNL, combined in Scandinavian Airlines System. In 1989 SAS flew 169m. km and carried 13,341,000 passengers.

SAS inaugurated its transpolar routes Copenhagen–Los Angeles on 15 Nov. 1954 and Copenhagen–Tokyo on 25 Feb. 1957, and its trans-Asian express route Copenhagen–Bangkok–Singapore *via* Tashkent on 4 Nov. 1967.

Shipping. On 31 Dec. 1989 the merchant fleet consisted of 2,882 vessels (above 20 GRT) of 4,625,307 GRT.

In 1989, 34,978 vessels of 58m. GRT entered Danish ports, unloading 42m. tonnes and loading 25m. tonnes of cargo; traffic by passenger ships and ferries is not included.

Telecommunications. There were, in 1988, 1,280 post offices. On 31 Dec. 1988 the length of telephone circuits of private companies was 17,093,855 km. On 31 Dec. 1988 there were 4,508,572 telephones. Postal revenues, 1988, 12,554m. kroner; expenditure, 10,623m. kroner.

Danmarks Radio is the government broadcasting station and is financed by licence fees. Television is broadcast by *Danmarks Radio* and *TV2* with colour programmes by PAL system. Number of receivers (1989): TV, 1·95m., including 1·76m. colour sets; radio, 2·02m.

Cinemas. In 1989 there were 357 auditoria with a seating capacity of 58,704.

Newspapers. In 1989 there were 46 daily newspapers with a combined circulation of 1·85m. on weekdays.

JUSTICE, RELIGION, EDUCATION AND WELFARE

Justice. The lowest courts of justice are organized in 82 tribunals *(underretter)*, where minor cases are dealt with by a single judge. The tribunals at Copenhagen have 33 judges and Aarhus 12; the other tribunals have 1 to 9. Cases of greater consequence are dealt with by the superior courts *(Landsretterne)*; these courts are also courts of appeal for the above-named minor cases. Of superior courts there are two: *Østre Landsret* in Copenhagen with 45 judges, *Vestre Landret* in Viborg with 22 judges. From these an appeal lies to the Supreme Court *(Højesteret)* in Copenhagen, composed of 15 judges. Judges under 65 years of age can be removed only by judicial sentence.

In 1989, 15,263 men and 1,955 women were convicted of violations of the criminal code, fines not included. In 1988, the daily average population in penal institutions was 3,360 men and 164 women, of whom 813 men and 55 women were on remand.

Religion. At the Reformation in 1536 the Danish Church ceased to exist as a legally independent unit, a part of the Roman Catholic Church, and became instead a Lutheran Church under the direction of the State. Since that time the State has, in one form or another, continued to exercise supreme authority in the affairs of the Church, and has regulated these by the passing of laws, by royal decree, or other appropriate means. The great majority of Danish citizens (about 90%) belongs to the National Church. Administratively, Denmark is divided into 10 dioceses each with a Bishop who, within the framework of the law, is the supreme diocesan authority in ecclesiastical affairs. The Bishop together with the Chief Administrative Officer of the county make up the diocesan governing body, responsible for all matters of ecclesiastical local finance and general administration. Bishops are appointed by the Crown after an election at which the clergy and parish council members of the diocese have had the opportunity of voting for the candidates nominated. Each diocese is divided into a number of deaneries (107 in the whole country) each with its Dean and Deanery Committee, who have certain financial powers. Local government at parish level (there are about 2,100 parishes in all) is in the hands of Parish Councils, who are elected for a 4-year period of office.

Since the Constitution of 1849 complete religious toleration is extended to every sect, and no civil disabilities attach to Dissenters.

Education. Education has been compulsory since 1814. The *folkeskole* (public primary and lower secondary school) comprises a pre-school class *(børnehaveklasse)*, a 9-year basic school corresponding to the period of compulsory education and a 1-year voluntary tenth form. Compulsory education may be fulfilled either through attending the *folkeskole* or private schools or through home-instruction, on the condition that the instruction given is comparable to that given in the *folkeskole. The folkeskole* is mainly a municipal school and no fees are paid. In the year 1988–89, 2,269 primary and lower secondary schools had 651,233 pupils and employed 62,700 teachers. 17% of the total number of schools were private schools and they were attended by 10% of the total number of pupils. The 9-year basic school is in practice not streamed. However, a certain differentiation may take place in the eighth and ninth forms.

On completion of the eighth and ninth forms the pupils may sit for the leaving examination of the *folkeskole (folkeskolens afgangsprøve)*. On completion of the tenth form the pupils may sit for either the leaving examination of the *folkeskole (folkeskolens afgangsprøve)* or the advanced leaving examination of the *folkeskole (folkeskolens udvidede afgangsprøve)*.

For 14–18 year olds there is an alternative of completing compulsory education at continuation schools, with the same leaving examinations as in the *folkeskole*. In the year 1988–89 there were 200 continuation schools with 15,584 pupils.

Under certain conditions the pupils may continue school either in the 3-year gymnasium (upper secondary school) or 2-year *studenterkursus* (adult upper secondary school) ending with *studentereksamen* (upper secondary school leaving examination) or in the 2-year higher preparatory examination course ending with the *højere forberedelseseksamen*. There were (1988–89) 155 of these upper secondary schools with 71,685 pupils.

Vocational education and training consists of apprenticeship training, *lærlingeuddannelse*; vocational education, *EFG-uddannelse*, consisting of a 1-year basic course, *EFG-basisår*, followed by a second part, *EFG-2.del*, and courses preparing for a vocation, leading to a diploma.

Vocational education and training cover courses in commerce and trade, iron and metal industry, chemical industry, construction industry, graphic industry, service trades, food industry, agriculture, horticulture, forestry and fishery, transport and communication, and health related auxiliary programmes.

In 1988–89 70,805 students were enrolled within trade and commerce, of whom 7,321 were in apprenticeship training and 44,389 in vocational education. 84,966 students were enrolled within technical education, of whom 35,276 were in apprenticeship training and 37,103 in vocational education. 19,095 students were admitted to the diploma courses within the field of trade and commerce, and 12,587 students were admitted to the technical diploma courses.

Tertiary education comprises all education after the 12th year of education, no matter whether the 3 years after the 9th form of the *folkeskole* have been spent on a course preparing for continued studies *(studentereksamen* or *højere forberedelseseksamen)*, or a course preparing for a vocation (*lærlingeuddannelse, EFG-uddannelse*, etc.). Tertiary education can be divided into 2 main groups, short courses of further education and long courses of higher education. There was a total of 27,641 students at short courses of further education.

There were 27 teacher-training colleges with 5,849 students and 26 colleges for training of teachers for kindergartens and leisure-time activities with 4,823 students.

Degree-courses in engineering: The Technical University of Denmark had 5,438 students. The Engineering Academy had 2,326 students and 9 engineering colleges had 7,639 students.

Universities: The University of Copenhagen (founded 1479) 23,933 students. The University of Aarhus (founded in 1928) 12,638 students. The University of Odense (founded in 1964) 5,984 students. Roskilde University Centre (founded in 1972) 2,927 students. Aalborg University Centre (founded in 1974) 5,873 students.

Other types of post-secondary education: The Royal Veterinary and Agricultural University had 2,637 students. The two dental colleges had 657 students. The Danish School of Pharmacy had 901 students. The 11 colleges of economics, business administration and modern languages had 25,245 students. The 2 schools of architecture had 1,645 students. Five academies of music had 816 students. Two schools of librarianship had 604 students. The Royal Danish School of Educational Studies had 2,378 students. The 5 schools of social work had 781 students. The Danish School of Journalism had 778 students. Ten colleges of physical therapy had 1,361 students. Two schools of Midwifery Education had 91 students. Two colleges of home economics had 365 students. The School of Visual Arts had 149 students. Two schools of nursing had 416 students. Three military academies had 348 students.

Among adult education the most well-known are *Folkeskolehøjskoler*, folk high schools. Adult education in general programmes, single subjects (since 1978) and courses for semi-skilled workers and for skilled workers is organized by counties.

Andreseén, A., *The Danish Folk High School To-day*. Copenhagen, 1981

Struve, K., *Schools and Education in Denmark.* Copenhagen, 1981
Thorsen, L., *Public Libraries in Denmark.* English and French eds., Copenhagen, 1972

Social Security. The main body of Danish social welfare legislation is consolidated in 7 acts concerning (1) public health security, (2) sick-day benefits, (3) social pensions (for early retirement and old age), (4) employment injuries insurance, (5) employment services and unemployment insurance, (6) social assistance including assistance to handicapped, rehabilitation, child and juvenile guidance, day-care institutions, care of the aged and sick, and (7) family allowances.

Public health security, covering the entire population, provides free medical care, substantial subsidies for certain essential medicines together with some dental care and a funeral allowance. Hospitals are primarily municipal and the hospital treatment is normally free. All employed workers are granted daily sickness allowances, others can have limited daily sickness allowances. Daily cash benefits are granted in the case of temporary incapacity for work because of illness, injury or child-birth to all persons who earn an income derived from personal work. The benefit is paid at the rate of 90% of the average weekly earnings. There was a maximum rate of 2,457 kroner a week in 1990.

Social pensions cover the entire population. Entitlement to old-age pensions at the full rates is subject to the condition that the beneficiary has been ordinarily resident in Denmark for a number of years (40). For a shorter period of residence, the benefits are reduced proportionally. The basic amount of the old-age pension in July 1990 was 84,816 kroner a year to married couples and 44,508 to single persons. Various supplementary allowances, depending on age and income, may be payable with the basic amount. Persons aged 55–66 may, depending on health and income, apply for an early-retirement pension. Persons over 67 years of age are entitled to the basic amount. The pensions to a married couple are calculated and paid to the husband and the wife separately. Early retirement pension to a disabled person is payable, having regard to the degree of disability, at a rate of up to 104,544 kroner to a single person. Early-retirement pensions may be subject to income regulation. The same applies to the basic amount of the old age pension to persons aged 67–69.

Employment injuries insurance provides for disablement or survivors' pensions and compensations. The scheme covers practically all employees.

Employment services are provided by regional public employment agencies. The insurance against unemployment provides daily allowances. The unemployment insurance funds had in Dec. 1989 a membership of 2,018,846.

The *Social Assistance Act* applies to the field of social legislation which rules the individually granted benefits in contrast to the other fields of social legislation which apply to fixed benefits.

Total social expenditure, including hospital and health services, statutory pensions, etc, amounted in the financial year 1986 to 185,440m. kroner.

Bibliography of Foreign Language Literature on Industrial Relations and Social Services in Denmark. Ministries of Labour and Social Affairs, Copenhagen, 1975
Social Conditions in Denmark. Vols. 1–8. Ministries of Labour and Social Affairs, Copenhagen
Marcussen, E., *Social Welfare in Denmark.* 4th ed. Copenhagen, 1980

THE FAROE ISLANDS
Føroyar/Færøerne

HISTORY. A Norwegian province to the peace treaty of 14 January 1814, the islands have been represented by 2 members in the Danish parliament since 1851, and in 1852 they obtained an elected assembly of their own, called *løgting,* which in 1948 secured a certain degree of home-rule within the Danish realm. The islands are not included in the EEC, but left EFTA together with Denmark on 31 Dec. 1972.

AREA AND POPULATION. The archipelago is situated due north of Scotland, 300 km from the Shetland Islands, 675 km from Norway and 450 km from Iceland, with a total land area of 1,399 sq. km (540 sq. miles). There are 17 inhabited islands (the main ones being Stremoy, Eysturoy, Vágoy, Suðuroy, Sandoy and Borðoy) and numerous islets, all mountainous and of volcanic origin. The census population in 1977 was 41,969; estimate (31 Dec. 1988) 47,663. The capital is Tórshavn (14,547 inhabitants on 31 Dec. 1988) on Stremoy. The inhabitants speak Faroese (føroyskt), a Scandinavian language which since 1948 has been the official language of the islands along with Danish.

CONSTITUTION AND GOVERNMENT. The parliament *(løgting)*, comprises 32 members elected by proportional representation by universal suffrage at age 18. The *løgting* elected in Nov. 1990 includes 10 Social Democratic Party, 7 People's Party, 6 Unionist Party, 4 Republican Party. Parliament elects a government *(Landsstýri)* of at least 3 members which administers the home rule. Denmark is represented in the *løgting* by the chief administrator (*ríkisumboðsmaður*).

Chief Minister (Løgmaður): Jøgvan Sundstein.

Local government is vested in the 50 *kommunur*, which have 29 or more inhabitants and income taxes of their own.

Flag: White with a red blue-edged Scandinavian cross.

ECONOMY

Budget. The 1988 Budget balanced at 3,151m. kr.

Currency. Since 1940 the currency has been the Faroese *krøna* (kr.) which remains freely interchangeable with the Danish krone.

ENERGY AND NATURAL RESOURCES

Electricity. There are 5 hydro-electric stations at Vestmanna on Stremoy and one at Eiði on Eysturoy. Total production (1988) 215·6m. kwh, of which hydro-electric 60·2m. kwh.

Agriculture. Only 2% of the surface is cultivated. The chief use is for grazing, the traditional mainstay of the economy. A small amount of potatoes is grown for home consumption. Livestock (1988): Sheep, 55,503; cattle, 2,176.

Fisheries. Deep sea fishing now forms the most important sector of the economy, primarily in the 200-mile exclusive zone but also off Greenland, Iceland, Svalbard and Newfoundland and in the Barents Sea. Total catch (1988) 357,000 tonnes, primarily cod, blue whiting, coalfish, prawns, mackerel and herring.

COMMERCE. The main industry is fishery. Exports, mainly fresh, frozen, filleted and salted fish, amounted to 2,345m. kr. in 1988; imports to 3,221m. kr. In 1988 Denmark supplied 39·6% of imports, Norway 21·1%, UK 8·2%, Sweden 6·3% and Federal Republic of Germany 5·8%; exports were mainly to Denmark (18·6%), UK (11·5%), Federal Republic of Germany (5·7%), USA (9·1%) and Norway (8%).

Total trade with UK (British Department of Trade returns, in £1,000 sterling):

	1985	*1986*	*1987*	*1988*	*1989*	*1990*
Imports to UK		21,380	19,239	23,141	31,042	34,396
Exports and re-exports from UK		5,709	7,165	4,445	6,353	7,882

COMMUNICATIONS

Roads. In 1988 there were 433 km of roads, 14,232 passenger cars and 3,445 commercial vehicles.

Aviation. The airport is on Vágoy, from which there are regular services to Copenhagen and Reykjavík.

Shipping. The chief port is Tórshavn, with smaller ports at Klaksvik, Vestmanna, Skálafjørður, Tvøroyri, Vágur and Fuglafjørður.

Post and Broadcasting. In 1988 there were 20,816 telephones. *Utvarp Føroya* broadcasts from Tórshavn about 40 hours a week on 4 transmitters. In 1988 there were 17,000 radio and 11,000 television receivers.

RELIGION, EDUCATION AND WELFARE

Religion. About 80% are Evangelical Lutherans and 20% are Plymouth Brethren or belong to small communities of Roman Catholics, Pentecostal, Adventists, Jehovah Witnesses and Bahai.

Education. In 1988–89 there were 5,440 primary and 2,979 secondary school pupils with 601 teachers.

Health. In 1988 there were 87 doctors, 39 dentists, 10 pharmacists, 17 midwives and 344 nursing personnel. In 1989 there were 3 hospitals with 369 beds.

Further Reading

Årbog for Færøerne. 1986
Føroya landsstýri: Arsfrágreiðing 1988. Tórshavn 1989
Faroes in Figures. Thorshavn, annual, from 1956
Rutherford, G. K., (ed.) *The Physical Environment of the Færoe Islands*. The Hague, 1982
Wang, Z., *Stjórnmálafrøði*. Tórshavn, 1989
West, J. F., *Faroe*. London, 1973
Wylie, J., *The Faroe Islands: Interpretations of History*. Lexington, 1987
Young, G. V. C. and Clewer, C. R., *Faroese-English Dictionary*. Peel, 1985

GREENLAND
Grønland/Kalaallit Nunaat

HISTORY. A Danish possession since 1380, Greenland became on 5 June 1953 an integral part of the Danish kingdom. Following a referendum in Jan. 1979, home rule was introduced from 1 May 1979, and full internal self-government was attained in Jan. 1981 after a transitional period.

AREA AND POPULATION. Area 2,186,000 sq. km (844,000 sq. miles), made up of 1,802,400 sq. km of ice cap and 383,600 sq. km of ice-free land. The population, 1 Jan. 1990, numbered 55,558; West Greenland, 50,217; East Greenland, 3,443; North Greenland (Thule), 843, and 1,052 not belonging to any specific municipality. Of the total, 9,416 were born outside Greenland. The capital is Nuuk (Godthåb), with a population in 1990 of 12,217.

CONSTITUTION. At the introduction of home rule, the council *(Landsråd)* was replaced by a 27-member parliament *(Landsting)*. At the elections of March 1991 the *Siumut* gained 11 seats with 37% of votes cast, the *Atassut*, 8 seats, the *Inuit Ataqatigiit*, 5 seats. The *Prime Minister* is Lars-Emil Johansen. There is a 5-member administration, the *Landsstyre*. Denmark is represented by an appointed commissioner. There are 18 local government divisions.

ECONOMY

Budget. The Budget for 1989 balanced at 5,037m. kroner.

Currency. The Danish kroner remains the legal currency.

ENERGY AND NATURAL RESOURCES

Electricity. Production (1989) 161·3m. kwh.

Fisheries. In 1989 the catch totalled 214,200 tonnes.

INDUSTRY. Until the beginning of this century, the hunting of land and sea mammals, especially seals, was the main occupation of the population; now fishing is most important. Fish-processing industries, construction and trade are also important occupations.

Production of lead and zinc concentrates was in 1989 about 35,500 tonnes and 130,500 tonnes respectively. The mine is now worked out.

A hydro-electric power station is under construction 40 miles south of Nuuk.

COMMERCE. Imports (c.i.f. Greenland) (in 1m. kroner): 1987, 3,471; 1988, 3,495; 1989, 2,879 (provisional). Exports (f.o.b. Greenland) (in 1m. kroner): 1987, 2,370; 1988, 2,630; 1989, 2,930 (provisional). Trade is mainly with Denmark.

Total trade with UK (British Department of Trade returns, in £1,000 sterling):

	1986	*1987*	*1988*	*1989*	*1990*
Imports to UK	4,789	838	1,430	3,793	10,322
Exports and re-exports from UK	452	735	1,151	1,487	2,256

COMMUNICATIONS

Roads. There were (1970) 150 km of roads, of which 60 km were paved.

Aviation. There is an international airport at Søndre Srømfjord, and 12 local airports with scheduled services.

Telecommunications. Greenland Radio (Kalaallit Nunaata Radioa) broadcasts in Greenlandic and Danish. Several towns have local television stations. In 1989 there were 16,561 telephones, (1984) 10,000 television sets and (1984) 13,500 radio sets.

JUSTICE, RELIGION, EDUCATION AND WELFARE

Justice. The High Court in Nuuk comprises one professional judge and 2 lay magistrates, while there are 18 district courts under lay assessors.

Religion. About 98% of the population are Evangelical Lutherans.

Education. There were (1988–89) 8,967 pupils in primary comprehensive schools, of whom 7,459 were in the course of compulsory education (9 years). On 1 Sept. 1988, 2,297 students were enrolled in vocational training.

Health. The medical service is free to all inhabitants. There is a central hospital in Nuuk and 16 smaller district hospitals. In 1989 there were 78 doctors and 444 hospital beds.

Further Reading

The Danish Prime Minister's Office, Greenland Section, has published a yearbook since 1989, *Grønland/Kalaallit Nunaat.*

Statistiske Efterretninger (Statistical News), from 1983 special series: *Færøerne og Grønland* (Faroe Islands and Greenland)

Gad, F., *A History of Greenland.* 2 vols. London, 1970–1973

Hertling, K. (ed.) *Greenland Past and Present.* Copenhagen, 1970

Greenland National Library, P.O. Box 1011, DK-3900, Nuuk

DIPLOMATIC REPRESENTATIVES

Of Denmark in Great Britain (55 Sloane St., London, SW1X 9SR)
Ambassador: Rudolph Thorning-Petersen.

Of Great Britain in Denmark (36–40 Kastelsvej, DK-2100, Copenhagen)
Ambassador: N. C. R. Williams, CMG.

Of Denmark in the USA (3200 Whitehaven St., NW, Washington, D.C., 20008)
Ambassador: Peter Pedersen Dyvig.

Of the USA in Denmark (Dag Hammarskjolds Alle 24, Copenhagen)
Ambassador: Keith L. Brown.

Of Denmark to the United Nations
Ambassador: Kjeld Vilhelm Mortensen.

Further Reading

Statistical Information: Danmarks Statistik (Sejrøgade 11, 2100 Copenhagen Ø.) was founded in 1849 and reorganized in 1966 as an independent institution; it is administratively placed under the Minister of Economic Affairs. *Chief:* N. V. Skak-Nielsen. Its main publications are: *Statistisk Årbog* (Statistical Yearbook). From 1896; *Statistiske Efterretninger* (Statistical News). *Statistiske Månedsoversigt* Monthly Review of Statistics), *Statistisk hårsoversigt* (Statistical Ten-Year Review).

Ministry of Foreign Affairs, *Danish Foreign Office Journal. Commercial and General Review.—Denmark.* 1961.—*Economic Survey of Denmark* (annual).—*Facts About Denmark.* 1959.—Hæstrup, J., *From Occupied to Ally: the Danish Resistance Movement.* 1963
Bibliografi over Danmarks Offentlige Publikationer. Institut for International Udveksling, Copenhagen. Annual
Dania polyglotta. Annual Bibliography of Books ... in Foreign Languages Printed in Denmark. State Library, Copenhagen. Annual
Kongelig Dansk Hof og Statskalender. Copenhagen. Annual
Brynildsen, F., *A Dictionary of the English and Dano-Norwegian Languages.* 2 vols. Copenhagen, 1902–07
Danstrup, J., *History of Denmark.* 2nd ed. Copenhagen, 1949
Johansen, H. C., *The Danish Economy in the Twentieth Century.* London, 1987
Krabbe, L., *Histoire de Danemark.* Copenhagen and Paris, 1950
Miller, K. E., *Denmark.* [Bibliography] Oxford and Santa Barbara, 1987
Nielsen, B. K., *Engelsk–Dansk Ordbog.* Copenhagen, 1964
Trap, J. P., *Kongeriget Danmark.* 5th ed. 11 vols. Copenhagen, 1953 ff.
Vinterberg, H. and Bodelsen, C. A., *Dansk-Engelsk Ordbog.* Copenhagen, 1966

National Library: Det kongelige Bibliotek, P.O.B. 2149, DK-1016 Copenhagen K. *Director:* Erland Kolding Nielsen.

DJIBOUTI

Capital: Djibouti
Population: 484,000 (1988)
GNP per capita: US$760 (1984)

Jumhouriyya Djibouti

(Republic of Djibouti)

HISTORY. At a referendum held on 19 March 1967, 60% of the electorate voted for continued association with France rather than independence and the new statute for the territory came into being on 5 July 1967. In Jan. 1976, following discussions between Ali Aref and President Giscard d'Estaing, it was announced that the French Government affirmed that the Territory of the Afars and the Issas was destined for independence but no date was fixed. Legislative elections were held on 8 May and independence as the Republic of Djibouti was achieved on 27 June 1977.

AREA AND POPULATION. Djibouti is bounded north-east by the Gulf of Aden, south-east by Somalia and all other sides by Ethiopia.

Djibouti has an area of 23,200 sq. km (8,958 sq. miles). The population was estimated in 1988 at 484,000, of whom 47% were Somali (Issa), 37% Afar, 8% European (mainly French) and 6% Arab. There were (1987) about 13,000 refugees from Ethiopia. Djibouti, the seat of government, had (1988) 290,000 inhabitants; other towns are Tadjoura, Obock, Dikhil and Ali-Sabieh. There are 5 administrative districts.

CLIMATE. Conditions are hot throughout the year, with very little rain. Djibouti. Jan. 78°F (25·6°C), July 96°F (35·6°C). Annual rainfall 5" (130 mm).

CONSTITUTION AND GOVERNMENT. Under an organic law approved by the Constituent Assembly on 10 Feb. 1981, the President is directly elected for a 6-year term (renewable once) and the Constituent Assembly became a 65-member Chamber of Deputies, with a 5-year term. In Oct. 1981, the Assembly declared Djibouti a one-Party state, the ruling Party being the *Rassemblement Populaire pour le Progrès*. Elections for the Chamber of Deputies were held 21 May 1982, when 26 Somali, 23 Afar and 16 Arab members were elected.

President: Hassan Gouled Aptidon (elected 1977 and re-elected 1981 and 1987).

The Council of Ministers in Oct. 1989 was composed as follows:

Prime Minister, Planning and Land Development: Barkat Gourad Hamadou.

Interior, Posts and Telecommunications: Khaireh Alleleh Hared. *Justice and Islamic Affairs:* Elaf Orbiss Ali. *Foreign Affairs and Co-operation:* Moumin Bahdon Farah. *Defence:* Hussein Barkad Siraj. *Commerce:* Moussa Bourale Roble. *Finance:* Muhammad Djama Elabe. *Civil Service:* Ismail Ali Youssouf. *Industry:* Salem Abdou. *Labour:* Ahmed Ibrahim Ardi. *Education:* Suleiman Farah Lodon. *Agriculture:* Muhammad Moussa Chehem. *Public Works:* Ahmed Aden Youssouf. *Health:* Ougoure Hassan Ibrahim. *Ports:* Bourhan Ali Warki. *Youth:* Omar Chirdon Abass.

National flag: Horisontally blue over green, with a white triangle based on the hoist charged with a red star.

DEFENCE

Army. The Army comprises 1 infantry battalion, 1 armoured squadron, 1 support battalion, 1 border commando battalion and 1 parachute company. Equipment includes 45 armoured cars. The strength of the Army (of which the Navy and Air

Force form part) was (1991) 2,700 men. There is also a paramilitary gendarmerie of some 1,200 men.

Navy. A coastal patrol is maintained consisting of 6 inshore patrol craft. Personnel (1990) 90.

Air Force. There is a small air force, all equipment *via* French aid. There are 2 CASA Aviocar and 2 Noratlas transports, 1 Falcon 20 VIP aircraft, 1 Cessna 206 for liaison, 1 Rallye trainer, and 5 helicopters (Alouette II and Ecureuil). Personnel (1991) 100.

INTERNATIONAL RELATIONS

Membership. Djibouti is a member of the UN, OAU, the Arab League and is an ACP state of the EEC.

ECONOMY

Budget. Revenue for 1986 was 24,494m. Djibouti francs and expenditure 23,133m.

Currency. The currency is the *Djibouti franc* (DJB). In March 1991, £1 = 330 *Djibouti francs*; US$1 = 173·96 *Djibouti francs.*

Banking. The Banque Nationale de Djibouti is the bank of issue. There are 6 commercial banks.

ENERGY AND NATURAL RESOURCES

Electricity. Production (1986) 140m. kwh. Installed capacity 80,100 kw.

Minerals. Minerals supposed to exist are gypsum, mica, amethyst and sulphur.

Agriculture. Mainly market gardening at the oasis of Ambouli and near urban areas. Tomato production (1988) 1,000 tonnes. Livestock (1988): 70,000 cattle, 414,000 sheep, 500,000 goats, 8,000 donkeys, 58,000 camels.

Fisheries. The catch in 1984 was 426 tonnes.

INDUSTRY

Labour. In 1986 there were 2,134 persons employed in construction and 1,235 in manufacturing.

FOREIGN ECONOMIC RELATIONS

Commerce. The main economic activity is the operation of the port. The chief imports are cotton goods, sugar, cement, flour, fuel oil and vehicles; the chief exports are hides, cattle and coffee (transit from Ethiopia). Trade in 1m. Djibouti francs:

	1983	*1984*	*1985*	*1986*
Imports	39,307	39,425	35,670	33,106
Exports	1,919	2,362	2,488	3,628

Total trade between Djibouti and UK (British Department of Trade returns, in £1,000 sterling):

	1986	*1987*	*1988*	*1989*	*1990*
Imports to UK	53	175	169	489	174
Exports and re-exports from UK	12,537	12,501	8,479	10,555	14,962

Tourism. There were 21,790 visitors in 1987.

COMMUNICATIONS

Roads. There were (1987) 3,037 km of roads, of which 412 km were hard-surfaced. In 1987 there were 11,799 passenger cars and 1,501 commercial vehicles.

Railway. For the line Djibouti–Addis Ababa, of which 106 km lies within Djibouti *see* p. 464. Traffic carried is mainly in transit to and from Ethiopia.

Aviation. Air Djibouti provides services to Addis Ababa, Nairobi, Jidda and the Gulf. Other airlines serving Djibouti international airport (Ambouli) are Ethiopian Airlines, Air France, Air Tanzania and Yemen Airways Corporation. In 1987, 67,856 passengers and 6,036 tonnes of freight arrived at Ambouli, and 61,518 passengers and 1,612 tonnes of freight departed.

Shipping. In 1986 there entered at Djibouti 1,723 vessels, unloading 466,000 tonnes and loading 155,000 tonnes of merchandise. In 1981 the merchant marine comprised 8 vessels of 3,185 GRT. Djibouti became a free port in 1981.

Telecommunications. Number of telephones (1987), 4,452. *Radiodiffusion-Télévision de Djibouti* broadcasts on medium- and short-waves in French, Somali, Afar and Arabic. There is a television transmitter in Djibouti, broadcasting for 36 hours a week. Number of receivers (1985): Radio, 30,000; TV, 10,000.

JUSTICE, RELIGION, EDUCATION AND WELFARE

Justice. There is a Court of First Instance and a Court of Appeal in the capital. The judicial system is based on Islamic law.

Religion. The vast majority of the population is Moslem, with about 24,000 Roman Catholics.

Education. In 1987–88 there were 26,173 pupils and 592 teachers at primary schools, 6,327 pupils and 307 teachers at secondary and technical schools. There were 117 students in teacher training with 13 lecturers.

Health. In 1987 there were 29 hospitals and dispensaries with 1,285 beds, 89 physicians, 10 dentists and 15 pharmacists.

DIPLOMATIC REPRESENTATIVES

Of Djibouti in Great Britain
Chargé d'Affaires: Foudha Abdoulatif (resides in Paris).

Of Great Britain in Djibouti
Ambassador: M. A. Marshall (resides in San'a).

Of the USA in Djibouti (Plateau du Serpent Blvd., Djibouti)
Ambassador: Robert S. Barrett IV.

Of Djibouti to the United Nations and in the USA
Ambassador: Roble Olhaye.

Further Reading

Poinsot, J.-P., *Djibouti et la Côte française des Somalis*. Paris, 1965
Schraeder, P. J., *Djibouti*. [Bibliography] Oxford and Santa Barbara, 1990
Thompson, V. and Adloff, R., *Djibouti and the Horn of Africa*. Stanford Univ. Press, 1967

DOMINICA

Capital: Roseau
Population: 81,200 (1988)
GNP per capita: US$1,650 (1988)

Commonwealth of Dominica

HISTORY. Dominica was discovered by Columbus. It was a British possession from 1805, a member of the Federation of the West Indies 1958–62, an Associated State of the UK, 1967–78 and became an independent republic as the Commonwealth of Dominica on 3 Nov. 1978.

AREA AND POPULATION. Dominica is an island in the Windward group of the West Indies situated between Martinique and Guadeloupe. It has an area of 751 sq. km (290 sq. miles) and a population at the 1981 Census of 74,851; estimate (1988) 81,200. The chief town, Roseau, had 8,279 inhabitants in 1981.

The population is mainly of African and mixed origins, with small white and Asian minorities. There is a Carib settlement of about 500, almost entirely of mixed blood.

CLIMATE. A tropical climate, with pleasant conditions between Dec. and March, but there is a rainy season from June to Oct., when hurricanes may occur. Rainfall is heavy, with coastal areas having 70" (1,750 mm) but the mountains may have up to 2250" (6,250 mm). Roseau. Jan. 76°F (24·2°C), July 81°F (27·2°C). Annual rainfall 78" (1,956 mm).

CONSTITUTION AND GOVERNMENT. The House of Assembly has 21 elected and 9 nominated members. The Speaker is elected from among the members of the House or from outside. The Cabinet is presided over by the Prime Minister and consists of 6 other Ministers including the Attorney-General (official member). Elections were held in May 1990. The Dominica Freedom Party won 11 seats, the United Dominica Labour Party 6 seats and the Dominica Labour Party, 4.

President: Sir Clarence Seignoret GCB, OBE.
The Cabinet in Jan. 1991 was composed as follows:

Prime Minister and Minister of Finance, and Economic Affairs: Mary Eugenia Charles (b. 1919).

Minister for Legal Affairs, Information and Public Relations: Jenner Armour. *External Affairs and Organization of Eastern Caribbean States' Unity:* Brian Alleyne. *Trade, Industry and Tourism:* Charles Maynard. *Education and Sports:* Rupert Sorhaindo Sen. *Community Development and Social Affairs:* Henry George. *Health and Social Security:* Allan Guye. *Labour and Immigration:* Heskeith Alexander. *Communications, Works and Housing:* Alleyne Carbon. *Agriculture:* Maynard Joseph. *Without Portfolio:* Dermott Southwell.

National flag: Green with a cross over all of yellow, black, and white pieces, and in the centre a red disc charged with a Sisserou parrot in natural colours facing the hoist within a ring of 10 green yellow-bordered stars.

INTERNATIONAL RELATIONS

Membership. Dominica is a member of the UN, OAS, CARICOM, the Commonwealth and is an ACP state of the EEC.

ECONOMY

Budget. In 1988-89 revenue, EC$105·9m. and expenditure, EC$101·4m.

Currency. The French *franc,* the £ sterling and the *East Caribbean dollar* are legal tender. In March 1991, EC$2·70 = US$1 and EC$5·12 = £1.

Banking. Savings bank (Dec. 1982), 2,862 depositors, with $593,659 deposits. There are branches of Barclays Bank International and Royal Bank of Canada in Roseau, and branches of Barclays and National Commercial and Development Bank at Portsmouth. The National Commercial and Development Bank was opened in 1977 and Banque Française Commerciale opened in 1979.

ENERGY AND NATURAL RESOURCES

Electricity. Production (1987) 16m. kwh.

Agriculture. Production (1988): Bananas, 66,000 tonnes; coconuts, 14,000; beef (1987) 439; pork (1987) 420. Livestock (1988): Cattle, 9,000; pigs, 5,000; sheep, 9,000; goats, 10,000; poultry (1986), 115,000.

FOREIGN ECONOMIC RELATIONS

Commerce (1987). Imports, EC$179,215,824; exports and re-exports, EC$129,590,586. Chief products: Bananas, soap, fruit juices, essential oils, coconuts, vegetables, fruit and fruit preparations, and alcoholic drinks.

Total trade between Dominica and UK (British Department of Trade returns, in £1,000 sterling):

	1987	*1988*	*1989*	*1990*
Imports to UK	37,083	32,423	23,709	23,483
Exports and re-exports from UK	10,431	8,416	8,727	9,707

Tourism. Tourists (1987) totalled 41,200.

COMMUNICATIONS

Roads. In 1988 there were 470 miles of road and 280 miles of track. Vehicles totalled (Oct. 1988) 6,933.

Telecommunications. Telephone lines, 210 route miles; number of telephones, 7,700 (Oct. 1988). Radio receivers (1982) 13,405.

Cinemas. In 1987 there was 1 cinema with a seating capacity of 1,000.

JUSTICE, RELIGION, EDUCATION AND WELFARE

Justice. There are 12 magistrates' courts. There is also a supreme court which dealt with 60 criminal and 307 civil cases in 1987–88. The police force consists of 10 officers and 431 other ranks.

Religion. 80% of the population is Roman Catholic.

Education. In 1987–88 there were 65 primary schools with 15,262 pupils and 10 secondary schools with 3,251 pupils, and 2 colleges of higher education.

Health. In Sept. 1988 there were 3 hospitals with 245 beds, 31 doctors, 4 dentists, 10 pharmacists, 273 nursing personnel, 7 health centres and 44 health clinics.

DIPLOMATIC REPRESENTATIVES

Of Dominica in Great Britain and to the United Nations
High Comm. Ambassador: Franklin Andrew Baron (resides in Roseau; London office: 1, Collingham Gardens, London, SW5 0HW).

Of Great Britain in Dominica
High Commissioner: E. T. Davies, CMG (resides in Bridgetown).

Of Dominica in the USA
Ambassador: McDonald P. Benjamin.

Further Reading

Myers, R. A., *Dominica*. [Bibliography] Oxford and Santa Barbara, 1987
Library: Public Library, Roseau. *Librarian:* Mrs. C. Williams.

DOMINICAN REPUBLIC

Capital: Santo Domingo
Population: 7·2m. (1990)
GNP per capita: US$680 (1988)

República Dominicana

HISTORY. On 5 Dec. 1492 Columbus discovered the island of Santo Domingo, which he called La Española; for a time it was called Hispaniola. The city of Santo Domingo, founded by his brother, Bartholomew, in 1496, is the oldest city in the Americas. The western third of the island—now the Republic of Haiti—was later occupied and colonized by the French, to whom the Spanish colony of Santo Domingo was also ceded in 1795. In 1808 the Dominican population, under the command of Gen. Juan Sánchez Ramirez, routed an important French military force commanded by Gen. Ferrand, at the famous battle of Palo Hincado. This battle was the beginning of the end for French rule in Santo Domingo and culminated in the successful siege of the capital. Eventually, with the aid of a British naval squadron, the French were forced to capitulate and the colony returned again to Spanish rule, from which it declared its independence in 1821. It was invaded and held by the Haitians from 1822 to 1844, when they were expelled, and the Dominican Republic was founded and a constitution adopted. Independence day 27 Feb. 1844. Great Britain, in 1850, was the first country to recognize the Dominican Republic. The country was occupied by American Marines from 1916 until 1924. In 1936 the name of the capital city was changed from Santo Domingo to Ciudad Trujillo; and back again in 1961.

AREA AND POPULATION. The Dominican Republic occupies the eastern portion (about two-thirds) of the island of Hispaniola, Quisqueya or Santo Domingo, the western division forming the Republic of Haiti.

Area is 48,442 sq. km (18,700 sq. miles) with 870 miles of coastline, 193 miles of frontier line with Haiti (marked out in 1936).

The populations of the 26 provinces and National District at the 1981 census, and the 3 new provinces with estimates for 1987, were:

Province	Population	Province	Population
La Altagracia	100,112	Pedernales	17,006
Azua	142,770	Peravia	168,123
Bahoruco	78,636	Puerto Plata	206,757
Barahona	137,160	La Romana	109,769
Dajabón	57,709	Salcedo	99,191
Districto Nacional	1,550,739	Samaná	65,699
Duarte	235,544	Sánchez Ramírez	126,567
Espaillat	164,017	San Cristóbal	446,132
La Estrelleta	65,384	San Juan	239,957
Hato Mayor	76,023 [1]	San Pedro de Macorís	152,890
Independencia	38,768	Santiago	550,372
María Trinidad Sánchez	112,629	Santiago Rodríguez	55,411
Monseñor Nouel	121,906 [1]	El Seibo	157,866
Monte Cristi	83,407	Valverde	100,319
Monte Plata	170,758 [1]	La Vega	385,043

[1] Estimate, 1987.

Census (1981) 5,647,977. Estimate (1990) 7,176,000.

Population of the principal municipalities (Census 1981): Santo Domingo, the capital, 1,313,172; Santiago de los Caballeros, 278,638; La Romana, 91,571; San Pedro de Macoris, 78,562; San Francisco de Macoris, 64,906; La Vega, 52,432; San Juan de la Managuana, 49,764; Barahona, 49,334; Puerto Plata, 45,348.

The population is partly of Spanish descent, but is mainly composed of a mixed race of European and African blood.

CLIMATE. A tropical maritime climate with most rain falling in the summer months. The rainy season extends from May to Nov. and amounts are greatest in the north and east. Hurricanes may occur from June to Nov. Santo Domingo. Jan. 75°F (23·9°C), July 81°F (27·2°C). Annual rainfall 56" (1,400 mm).

CONSTITUTION AND GOVERNMENT. A new Constitution was promulgated on 28 Nov. 1966.

The President is elected for 4 years, by direct vote. In case of death, resignation or disability, he is succeeded by the Vice-president. There are 12 secretaries of state, a judicial adviser with secretary-of-state rank and 2 ministers without portfolio in charge of departments. Citizens are entitled to vote at the age of 18, or less when married.

At the general elections held in May 1986, 56 seats were won by the *Partido Reformista Social Cristiano*, 48 by the *Partido Revolucionario Dominicano*, and 16 seats by the *Partido de la Liberación Dominicana*.

At the presidential elections of May 1990 Joaquín Balaguer (b. 1907; Social Christian Reform Party) was elected for a second term by 678,568 votes to 653,423.

There is a bicameral legislature, comprising a 27-member Senate and a 120-member Chamber of Deputies, both elected for 4-year terms at the same date as the President.

President: Dr Joaquín Balaguer (elected May 1990).
Foreign Affairs: Joaquín Ricardo García.

National flag: Blue, red; quartered by a white cross.
National anthem: Quisqueyanos valientes, alzemos (words by E. Prud'homme; tune by J. Reyes, 1883).

Local Government: The republic consists of a National District (containing the capital, Santo Domingo, and surrounding areas) and 29 provinces, divided into 97 municipalities.

DEFENCE

Army. The Army has a strength (1991) of about 15,000. It is organized in 4 infantry brigades and 1 artillery, 1 engineer and 1 armoured battalions. There were (1991) 14 light tanks and 20 armoured cars.

Navy. The Navy largely comprises former US vessels. The combatant force consists of 1 frigate (built 1944) acting as the flagship, 3 offshore and 11 inshore patrol craft. There is 1 utility landing craft and support is provided by 2 small oilers, 1 ocean tug, and some 12 harbour and service craft. Personnel in 1990 totalled 4,000 officers and men.

Air Force. The Air Force, with HQ at San Isidoro, has 1 combat squadron with 8 Cessna A-37s; 1 squadron with a total of about 12 Bell 205A-1, OH-6A and Alouette II/III helicopters; 1 transport squadron with 3 C-47s and some smaller communications aircraft; a Presidential Dauphin 2 helicopter; and an assortment of trainers, including 10 T-34B Mentors, 5 Cessna T-41s and 2 T-6 Texans. Personnel strength was (1991) 3,800.

INTERNATIONAL RELATIONS

Membership. The Dominican Republic is a member of the UN and OAS.

ECONOMY

Budget. Expenditure (1986) RD$2,251m. and revenue RD$2,113m. In 1985 external debt was RD$3,551m.

Currency. The unit of currency is the *Dominica peso* (DOP), of 100 *centavos*.

There are silver coins for 50, 25 and 10 centavos, a copper-nickel 5-centavo piece and a copper 1-centavo piece.

The currency was devalued by 30% in Sept. 1990.
In March 1991, £1 = RD$28·52; US$1 = RD$15·04.

Banking. There are 4 foreign banks—the Royal Bank of Canada with 12 branches, the Bank of Nova Scotia with 11 branches, the Citibank with 6 branches, the Chase Manhattan Bank with 7 branches and the Bank of America with 4 branches. An agricultural and mortgage bank, with paid-up capital of RD$500,000, was established in 1945; in 1950 its capital was increased to RD$5m. In 1947 the Central Bank of the Dominican Republic was established. A Banco Popular Dominicano, with an authorized capital of RD$5m., opened in Jan. 1964.

Weights and Measures. The metric system was nominally adopted on 1 Aug. 1913, but English and Spanish units have remained in common use in ordinary commercial transactions; on 17 Sept. 1954 a more drastic law requiring the decimal metric system was passed.

ENERGY AND NATURAL RESOURCES

Electricity. In 1986, 3,800m. kwh. of electricity was generated. There was a severe shortagae in 1990. Supply 110 and 220 volts; 60 Hz.

Minerals. Bauxite output in 1982 was 152,250 tonnes. Silver and platinum have been found, and near Neiba there are several hills of rock salt. Ferronickel production (1986) 58,000 tonnes. Production of gold (1986) 285,458 troy oz.; silver, 1,356,000.

Agriculture. Agriculture and its processing industries are the chief source of wealth, sugar cultivation being the principal industry. Of the total area (1984) meadows and pastures, 43%; permanant cultivation, 30%; forestry 13%.

Livestock in 1988: 2,129,000 cattle, 409,000 pigs, 100,000 sheep.

Sugar-cane production, 1988, was 8·3m. tonnes. Coffee is exported mainly to USA. Output, 1988, 54,000 tonnes. Production of rice for home consumption and export is fostered; output, 1988, 463,000 tonnes. Cocoa is the second principal crop and covers 2m. *tareas* (340,000 acres); output in 1988, 39,000 tonnes. There are useful crops of yucca and beans for local consumption. Scientific growing of bananas (1988: 391,000 tonnes) and of leaf tobacco (1988: 30,000 tonnes) is progressing.

Fisheries. The total catch (1986) was 17,200 tonnes.

INDUSTRY. Important products are sugar (89,100 of refined sugar in 1985), cement (960,000 tonnes in 1981). Value of textile manufactures (1983), RD$30·4m.; tobacco products, RD$63·5m.

FOREIGN ECONOMIC RELATIONS. Foreign debt was some US$4,500m. in 1990.

Commerce. Total imports and exports in RD$1m. (equal to US$1m.):

	1981	*1982*	*1983*	*1984*	*1985*
Imports	1,450·2	1,255·8	1,297·0	1,257·1	1,285·9
Exports	1,188·0	767·7	785·9	868·1	739·3

The principal exports in 1983 were (in RD$1m.): Sugar, 263·5; coffee, 76·3; ferronickel, 83·5; Doré, 164·5.

Total trade between the Dominican Republic and UK (British Department of Trade returns, in £1,000 sterling):

	1986	*1987*	*1988*	*1989*	*1990*
Imports to UK	7,599	8,637	8,523	11,223	17,440
Exports and re-exports from UK	15,178	23,887	17,235	25,519	19,668

Tourism. About 1m. tourists visited the Dominican Republic in 1987.

COMMUNICATIONS

Roads. Total length of roads (1985) 17,120 km. There were 102,000 cars and 61,000 commercial vehicles in 1984.

Railways. Some 142 km of the Dominican Government Railway remains in use between La Vega and the port of Sánchez. Twelve lines, including the Central Romana Railway, exist to serve the sugar industry, totalling 1,600 km.

Aviation. The country is reached from the American continent and the Caribbean islands by 8 international airlines and in 1987 there were 4 airports. Two local aviation companies provide interior services and connect Santo Domingo with San Juan in Puerto Rico, Curaçao, Aruba and Miami.

Shipping. Santo Domingo is the leading port; Puerto Plata ranks next. In 1971, vessels of 9,833,000 tons entered the ports to discharge 3,009,000 tonnes of cargo, and vessels of 5,276,000 tons cleared the ports having loaded 1,986,000 tonnes.

Telecommunications. Number of telephone instruments (1983), 175,054, of which 138,169 in Santo Domingo. The telegraph has a total length of about 500 km, privately owned; they have been leased to All-America Cables, Inc., which also controls submarine cables connecting, in the north, Puerto Plata with Puerto Rico and New York, and in the south, Santo Domingo with Puerto Rico, Cuba and Curaçao.

There were (1989) more than 90 broadcasting stations in Santo Domingo and other towns; this includes the 2 government stations. There are 4 television stations. In 1986 there were 800,000 radio and 500,000 television receivers.

Newspapers (1985). There were 9 daily newspapers with a circulation of 208,000.

JUSTICE, RELIGION, EDUCATION AND WELFARE

Justice. The judicial power resides in the Supreme Court of Justice, the courts of appeal, the courts of first instance, the communal courts and other tribunals created by special laws, such as the land courts. The Supreme Court consists of a president and 8 judges chosen by the Senate, and the procurator-general, appointed by the executive; it supervises the lower courts. Each province forms a judicial district, as does the *Distrito Nacional*, and each has its own procurator fiscal and court of first instance; these districts are subdivided, in all, into 72 municipalities and 18 municipal districts, each with one or more local justices. The death penalty was abolished in 1924.

Religion. The religion of the state is Roman Catholic; other forms of religion are permitted.

Education. Primary instruction (5,956 schools) is free and obligatory for children between 7 and 14 years of age; there are also secondary, normal, vocational and special schools, all of which are either wholly maintained by the State or state-aided; in 1985, primary schools had 28,000 teachers and 1,220,000 pupils and there were 11,754 teachers and 438,922 pupils in secondary schools.

The University of Santo Domingo (founded 1538) and 5 other universities had 88,000 students in 1985–86.

Health. There were, in 1980, 2,142 doctors and 8,953 hospital beds.

DIPLOMATIC REPRESENTATIVES

Of Dominican Republic in Great Britain
Ambassador: (Vacant).

Of Great Britain in the Dominican Republic
Ambassador: Giles Fitzherbert, CMG (resides in Caracas).

Of the Dominican Republic in the USA (1715 22nd St., NW, Washington, D.C., 20008)
Ambassador: Carlos A. Morales.

Of the USA in the Dominican Republic (Calle Cesar Nicolas Penson, Santo Domingo)
Ambassador: Paul D. Taylor.

Of the Dominican Republic to the United Nations
Ambassador: (Vacant).

Further Reading

Anuario estadístico de la República Dominicana, 1944–45. Ciudad Trujillo. 1949. This has been succeeded by separate annual reports covering foreign trade, vital statistics, banking, insurance, housing and communications.

Official Guide to the Dominican Republic, 79–80. Tourist Information Center, Santo Domingo, 1980

Atkins, G. P., *Arms and Politics in the Dominican Republic.* London, 1981

Bell, I., *The Dominican Republic.* London, 1980

Black, J. K., *The Dominican Republic: Politics and Development in an Unsovereign State.* London, 1986

Diederich, B., *Trujillo: The Death of the Goat.* London, 1978

Schoenhals, K., *Dominican Republic:* [Bibliography]. London and Santa Barbara, 1990

Wiarda, H. J. and Kryzanek, M. J., *The Dominican Republic: A Caribbean Crucible.* Boulder, 1982

ECUADOR

Capital: Quito
Population: 10·49m. (1989)
GNP per capita: US$681 (1988)

República del Ecuador

HISTORY. The Spaniards under Francisco Pizarro founded a colony after their victory at Cajamarca (16 Nov. 1532). Their rule was first challenged by the rising of 10 Aug. 1809. Marshal Sucre defeated the Spaniards at Pichincha in 1822, and in 1822 Bolívar persuaded the new republic to join the federation of Gran Colombia. The Presidency of Quito became the Republic of Ecuador by amicable secession 13 May 1830.

AREA AND POPULATION. Ecuador is bounded on the north by Colombia, on the east and south by Peru, on the west by the Pacific ocean. The frontier with Peru has long been a source of dispute between the two countries. The latest delimitation of it was in the treaty of Rio, 29 Jan. 1942, when, after being invaded by Peru, Ecuador lost over half her Amazonian territories. Ecuador unilaterally denounced this treaty in Sept. 1961. *See* map in THE STATESMAN'S YEAR-BOOK, 1942. Fighting between Peru and Ecuador began again in Jan. 1981 over this border issue but a ceasefire was agreed in early Feb.

No definite figure of the area of the country can yet be given, as a portion of the frontier has not been delimited. One estimate of the area of Ecuador is 270,670 sq. km, excluding the litigation zone between Peru and Ecuador, which is 190,807 sq. km, but including the Galápagos Islands (7,844 sq. km).

Mainland Ecuador has 3 distinct zones: the *Sierra* or uplands of the Andes, consisting of high mountain ridges with valleys, with 3·76m. of the population and high-priced farming land; the *Costa*, the coastal plain between the Andes and the Pacific, with 4·03m., whose permanent plantations furnish bananas, cacao, coffee, sugar-cane and many other crops; the *Oriente*, the upper Amazon basin on the east and the site of the main oilfields, consisting of tropical jungles threaded by large rivers (0·26m.).

The population is predominantly of Mestizos and Amerindians, with some proportion of people of European or African descent.

The official language is Spanish. The Amerindians of the highlands also speak the Quechua language; in the Oriental Region various tribes have languages of their own.

Census population in 1982, 8,072,702. Estimate (1989) 10·49m.

The population 28 Nov. 1982 was distributed by provinces as follows:

Province	*Sq. km*	*Census 1982*	*Capital*	*Census 1982*
Azuay	8,092	443,044	Cuenca	272,397
Bolívar	4,142	141,566	Guaranda	14,155 [1]
Cañar	3,481	174,674	Azogues	13,840 [1]
Carchi	3,744	125,452	Tulcán	33,635 [1]
Chimborazo	6,056	320,268	Riobamba	149,757
Cotopaxi	5,198	279,765	Latacunga	55,979
El Oro	5,908	337,818	Machala	117,243
Esmeraldas	15,162	247,311	Esmeraldas	141,030
Guayas	21,382	2,047,001	Guayaquil	1,300,868
Imbabura	4,976	245,745	Ibarra	60,719 [1]
Loja	11,472 [2]	358,952	Loja	86,196
Los Ríos	6,370	457,065	Babahoyo	42,583 [1]
Manabi	18,105	858,780	Portoviejo	167,070
Pichincha	16,587	1,376,831	Quito	1,110,248
Tungurahua	3,110	324,286	Ambato	221,392
Napo [3]	52,318 [2]	115,110	Tena	4,735 [1]
Pastaza [3]	30,269 [2]	31,779	Puyo	...
Morona-Santiago [3]	26,418 [2]	70,217	Macas	...
Zamora-Chinchipa [3]	18,394 [2]	46,691	Zamora	6,365
Colon (Galápagos)	7,994	6,119	Baquerizo Moreno	...

[1] 1983 estimate. [2] Excluding Peru-Ecuador litigation zone.
[3] Comprising 'Región Oriental'.

Vital statistics for calendar years: Births, (1985) 209,974; deaths, (1985) 51,134.

CLIMATE. The climate varies from equatorial, through warm temperate to mountain conditions, according to altitude which affects temperatures and rainfall. In coastal areas, the dry season is from May to Dec., but only from June to Sept. in mountainous parts, where temperatures may be 20°F colder than on the coast. Quito Jan. 59°F (15°C), July 58°F (14·4°C). Annual rainfall 44" (1,115 mm). Guayaquil. Jan. 79°F (26·1°C), July 75°F (23·9°C). Annual rainfall 39" (986 mm).

CONSTITUTION AND GOVERNMENT. A new Constitution came into force on 10 Aug. 1979. It provides for an executive President and a Vice-President to be directly elected for a non-renewable 4-year term by universal suffrage, with a further 'run-off' ballot being held between the two leading candidates where no-one has secured an absolute majority of the votes cast. The President appoints and leads a Council of Ministers.

Legislative power is vested in a unicameral 71-member National Congress, also directly elected for a 4-year term, 12 members on a national basis and 59 on a provincial basis. Voting is obligatory for all literate citizens of 18 years and over. Congressional elections were held in June 1990 for 60 seats.

The following is a list of the presidents and provisional executives since 1948:

Galo Plaza Lasso, 1 Sept. 1948–31 Aug. 1952.
Dr José María Velasco Ibarra, 1 Sept. 1952–31 Aug. 1956.
Dr Camilo Ponce Enríquez, 1 Sept. 1956–31 Aug. 1960.
Dr José María Velasco Ibarra, 1 Sept. 1960–8 Nov. 1961 (withdrew).
Dr Carlos Julio Arosemena Monroy, 8 Nov. 1961–11 July 1963 (deposed).
Military Junta, 11 July 1963–31 March 1966.
Clemente Yerovi Indaburu, 31 March–16 Nov. 1966 (interim).
Dr Otto Arosemena Gómez, 17 Nov. 1966–1 Sept. 1968.
Dr José María Velasco Ibarra, 1 Sept. 1968–15 Feb. 1972 (deposed).
Gen. Guillermo Rodriguez Lara, 16 Feb. 1972–11 Jan. 1976 (resigned).
Adm. Alfredo Poveda Burbano, 11 Jan. 1976–10 Aug. 1979.
Jaime Roldós Aguilera, 10 Aug. 1979–24 May 1981.
Osvaldo Hurtado Larrea, 24 May 1981–10 Aug. 1984.
León Febres Codero Rivadeneira, 10 Aug. 1984–10 Aug. 1988.

President: Rodrigo Borja Cevallos (elected 9 May 1988; installed 10 Aug. 1988).

The Cabinet in Feb. 1991 was composed as follows:

Government and Justice: César Verduga. *Defence:* Gen. Jorge Félix. *Education and Culture:* Andrés Vera. *Agriculture and Livestock:* Alfredo Saltos Guale. *Public Works and Communications:* Raúl Carrasco. *Finance and Public Credit:* Jorge Gallardo. *Foreign Affairs:* Diego Cordóvez. *Industry, Commerce and Integration:* Jacinto Jouvin Marquez de la Plata. *Public Health:* Plutarco Naranjo. *Social Welfare:* Raúl Baco Carbo. *Secretary General for Administration:* Washington Herrera. *Energy:* Diego Tamariz. *Labour and Human Resources:* Roberto Gómez. *Secretary General for Public Information:* Leopoldo Barriga.

National flag: Three horizontal stripes of yellow, blue, red, with the yellow of double width, and in the centre over all the national arms.

National anthem: Indignados tus hijos del yugo ('Indignant thy sons of the yoke'; words by J. L. Mera; music by A. Neumann, 1866).

Local Government. The country is divided politically into 21 provinces; 5 of them comprise the 'Región Oriental' and one the Archipelago of Galápagos, situated in the Pacific ocean about 600 miles to the west of Ecuador and comprising 15 islands. The provinces are administered by governors, appointed by the Government; their sub-divisions, or cantons, by political chiefs and elected cantonal councillors; and the parishes by political lieutenants. The Galápagos Archipelago is administered by the Ministry of National Defence. The 21 provinces are made up of 115 cantons, 212 urban parishes and 715 rural parishes. Elections for 50 provincial and 528 municipal councillors were held in June 1990.

DEFENCE. Military service is selective, with a 1-year period of conscription. The country is divided into 4 military zones, with headquarters at Quito, Guayaquil, Cuenca and Pastaza.

Army. The Army consists of 5 infantry, 1 armoured and 3 'jungle' brigades. Strength (1991) 50,000, with about 80,000 reservists. Equipment includes 45 American M-3 and 108 French AMX-13 light tanks. The aviation element has 3 survey aircraft, and 36 transport aircraft (19 helicopters).

Navy. Navy combatant forces include 2 German-built diesel submarines; 1 ex-US Gearing class destroyer, 6 Italian-built missile corvettes (with helicopter deck), 6 fast missile craft and 6 inshore patrol craft. Amphibious capability is 1 landing ship and 6 small craft. Auxiliaries consist of 1 small tanker, 1 survey ship, 2 tugs and a training ship plus some 8 harbour and service vessels. The Maritime Air Force has 10 aircraft, including 4 Cessna light aircraft, 3 T-34C trainers and 1 Alouette III helicopter. Naval personnel in 1990 totalled 4,800 officers and men including some 1,000 marines.

There are 6 inshore Coast Guard cutters and some 12 boats.

Air Force. The Air Force, formed with Italian assistance in 1920, was reorganized and re-equipped with US aircraft after Ecuador signed the Rio Pact of Mutual Defence in 1947 but latest equipment acquired from Europe and Brazil. 1991 strength of about 3,000 personnel and 70 combat aircraft includes a strike squadron equipped with 9 single-seat and 2 two-seat Jaguars; an interceptor squadron of 14 single-seat and 1 two-seat Mirage F.1; an interceptor squadron with 11 Kfirs; 3 counter-insurgency units equipped with 11 Cessna A-37B, 25T-33 and 12 Strikemaster light jet attack and training aircraft, 1 squadron with 2 C-130, 2 Buffalo and 4 HS 748 turboprop transports; Alouette III, AS 332 Super Puma, SA 330 Puma, Bell 47, Bell 212, UH-1 Iroquois and SA 315B Lama helicopters; and Cessna 150, T-34C-1 and T-41A/D trainers. Other transports are operated by the military airline TAME.

INTERNATIONAL RELATIONS

Membership. Ecuador is a member of the UN, OAS, the Andean Group and LAIA.

ECONOMY

Budget. Estimated revenue in 1988 was 812,000m. sucres and expenditure, 804,000m. sucres.

Net international reserves, 31 Dec. 1988, were US$176m.

Currency. The monetary unit is the *sucre* (ECS), divided into 100 *centavos*. In circulation are coins of 1, 5, 10, 20 and 50 *sucres*. The currency consists mainly of the notes of the Central Bank in denominations of 100, 500, 1,000 and 5,000 sucres. In March 1991, US$1 = 979·12; £1 = 1,857·40.

Banking and Finance. The Central Bank of Ecuador, at Quito, with a capital and reserves of 2,815m. sucres at 31 Aug. 1989, is modelled after the Federal Reserve Banks of US: through branches opened in 16 towns it now deals in mortgage bonds. All commercial banks must be affiliated to the Central Bank. American and European banks include the Bank of London and Canada with branches in Quito and Guayaquil.

Weights and Measures. By a law of 6 Dec. 1856 the metric system was made the legal standard but the Spanish measures are in general use. The quintal is equivalent to 101·4 lb.

The meridian of Quito has been adopted as the official time.

ENERGY AND NATURAL RESOURCES

Electricity. In 1989, total capacity of hydraulic and thermal plants was 1,814,700 kw. Estimated output was 5,352m. kwh in 1988. Supply 110,120 and 220 volts; 60 Hz.

Oil. Production of crude oil in 1989 was 14·7m. tonnes. In 1988 management of oil companies was taken over by the government.

Gas. In 1987, natural gas production was 460,778·9m. cu. metres.

Minerals. Production (1983): Silver, 3,137·6 troy oz; gold, 607·6 troy oz; copper, 7,900 kg; zinc, 14,820 kg. The country also has some iron, uranium, lead and coal.

Agriculture. Ecuador is divided into two agricultural zones: The coast and lower river valleys, where tropical farming is carried on in an average temperature of from 18° to 25°C.; and the Andean highlands with a temperate climate, adapted to grazing, dairying and the production of cereals, potatoes, pyrethrum and other flowers, and vegetables suitable to temperate climes. Some wheat has to be imported.

In 1989, some 3,284,000 persons depended for their living upon agriculture, of whom 993,000 were economically active.

124,000 acres of rich virgin land in the Santo Domingo de los Colorados area has been set aside for settlement of smallholders.

The staple export products are bananas, cacao and coffee. Main crops, in 1,000 tonnes, in 1988: Rice, 420; potatoes, 301; maize, 387; coffee, 136; barley, 41; cocoa, 77; bananas, 2,238.

Livestock (1988): Cattle, 4,007,000; sheep, 1,707,000; pigs, 4·16m.; horses, 438,000; poultry, 48m.

Forestry. Excepting the two agricultural zones and a few arid spots on the Pacific coast, Ecuador is a vast forest. In 1988, 11·8m. ha, 43% of the land area, was forested. In 1981, 4·5m. cu. metres of timber were cut, but much of the forest is not commercially accessible.

Fisheries. Fisheries and fish product exports were valued at US$387·6m. in 1986 (268,000 tonnes).

INDUSTRY. Production in 1987: Sugar, 3,000 tonnes; cement 2·87m. tonnes.

FOREIGN ECONOMIC RELATIONS

Commerce. Imports and exports for calendar years, in US$1m.:

	1984	*1985*	*1986*	*1987*	*1988*
Imports (f.o.b.)	1,567	1,611	1,631	1,888	1,517
Exports (f.o.b.)	2,622	2,905	2,186	1,928	2,193

Of the total exports (1988); petroleum, US$875m.; bananas, US$298m.; cocoa, US$298m.; coffee, US$152m.

Total trade between Ecuador and UK (British Department of Trade returns, in £1,000 sterling):

	1986	*1987*	*1988*	*1989*	*1990*
Imports to UK	11,339	14,002	13,120	19,319	19,572
Exports and re-exports from UK	46,673	37,934	50,417	29,410	30,155

Tourism. There were 252,443 visitors in 1986, spending US$170m.

COMMUNICATIONS

Roads. In 1985, there were 36,187 km of roads of all types in this mountainous country. A trunk highway through the coastal plain is under construction which will link Machala in the extreme south-west with Esmeraldas in the north-west and with Quito and the northern section of the Pan-American Highway. In 1984, there were 314,360 cars and 32,379 commercial vehicles.

Railways. A 1,067 mm gauge line runs from San Lorenzo through Quito to Guayaquil and Cuenca, total 971 km.

Aviation. There are 2 international airports. The following international lines operate: Air France, Avianca, Eastern, Ecuatoriana de Aviación, KLM, Lufthansa, Pan-Am, Iberia, LAN Chile, Aerovías Peruanas, Aereolinas Argentinas, Air Panama and Varig. They connect Quito with North and Central America, other countries in

South America and Europe. All the leading towns are connected by an almost daily service.

Shipping. Ecuador has 3 major seaports, of which Guayaquil is the chief and 6 minor ones. The merchant navy comprises 39,964 tons of seagoing and 21,232 tons of river craft. In 1980 ships totalling 26·58m. GRT entered Ecuadorean ports, unloading 2·28m. tons, and loading 8·59m. tons.

There is river communication, improved by dredging, throughout the principal agricultural districts on the low ground to the west of the Cordillera by the rivers Guayas, Daule and Vinces (navigable for 200 miles by river steamers in the rainy season).

Post and Telecommunications. In 1985 there were 339,040 telephones in use, 104,000 in Quito and 104,000 in Guayaquil; most were operated by the Government; 99% were automatic. Television was inaugurated in 1960 in Guayaquil, in 1961 in Quito and in 1967 in Cuenca. In 1985 there were 1·9m. radio receivers and 600,000 television receivers.

Newspapers (1984). There were 22 daily newspapers with an aggregate daily circulation of 526,000; 7 papers in Quito and Guayaquil have the bulk of the circulation.

JUSTICE, RELIGION, EDUCATION AND WELFARE

Justice. The Supreme Court in Quito, consisting of a President and 15 Justices, comprises 5 chambers each of 3 Justices. There is a Superior Court in each province, comprising chambers (as appointed by the Supreme Court) of 3 magistrates each. There are numerous lower and special courts. Capital punishment and all forms of torture are prohibited by the constitution, as are imprisonment for debt and contracts involving personal servitude or slavery.

Religion. The state recognizes no religion and grants freedom of worship to all. In 1984, 92% of the population were Roman Catholics. Divorce is permitted. Illegitimate children have the same rights as legitimate ones with respect to education and inheritance.

Education. Primary education is free and obligatory. Private schools, both primary and secondary, are under some state supervision. In 1986, 14,190 primary schools had 1·8m. pupils; 2,207 secondary schools with 744,000 pupils. There were (1989) 21 universities and polytechnics.

Health. In 1984 there were 11,000 doctors and 337 hospitals with 15,455 beds. In 1979 there were 795 dentists and 505 pharmacists.

DIPLOMATIC REPRESENTATIVES

Of Ecuador in Great Britain (3 Hans Cres., London, SW1X 0LS)
Ambassador: Dr José Antonio Correa (accredited 7 Feb. 1989).

Of Great Britain in Ecuador (Calle Gonzalez Suarez 111, Quito)
Ambassador: F. B. Wheeler, CMG.

Of Ecuador in the USA (2535 15th St., NW, Washington, D.C., 20009)
Ambassador: Jaime Moncayo García.

Of the USA in Ecuador (Avenida 12 de Octubre y Avenida Patria, Quito)
Ambassador: Paul C. Lambert.

Of Ecuador to the United Nations
Ambassador: Dr José Ayala Lasso.

Further Reading

Anuario de Legislación Ecuadoriana. Quito. Annual
Boletín del Banco Central. Quito

Boletín General de Estadistica. Tri-monthly
Boletín Mensual del Ministerio de Obras Públicas. Monthly
Informes Ministeriales. Quito. Annual
Bibliografia Nacional, 1756–1941. Quito, 1942
Invest in Ecuador. Banco Central del Ecuador, Quito, 1980
Buitrón, A. and Collier, Jr, J., *The Awakening Valley: Study of the Otavalo Indians*. New York, 1950
Corkill, D., *Ecuador*. [Bibliography] Oxford and Santa Barbara, 1989
Cueva, A., *The Process of Political Domination in Ecuador*. London, 1982
Hickman, J., *The Enchanted Islands: The Galapagos Discovered*. Oswestry, 1985
Martz, J. D., *Ecuador: Conflicting Political Culture and the Quest for Progress*. Boston, 1972.—*Politics and Petroleum in Ecuador*. New Brunswick, 1987
Middleton, A., *Class, Power and the Distribution of Credit in Ecuador*. Glasgow, 1981

EGYPT

Capital: Cairo
Population: 50·74m. (1989)
GNP per capita: US$650 (1988)

Jumhuriyat Misr al-Arabiya

(Arab Republic of Egypt)

HISTORY. Part of the Ottoman Empire from 1517 until Dec. 1914 when it became a British protectorate, Egypt became an independent monarchy on 28 Feb. 1922. Following a revolution on 23 July 1952, a Republic was proclaimed on 18 June 1953. Egypt merged with Syria on 22 Feb. 1958 to form the United Arab Republic, retaining that name when Syria broke away from the union on 28 Sept. 1961, finally re-adopting the name of Egypt on 2 Sept. 1971.

AREA AND POPULATION. Egypt is bounded east by Israel, the Gulf of Aqaba and the Red Sea, south by Sudan, west by Libya and north by the Mediterranean. The total area is 1,002,000 sq. km (386,900 sq. miles), but the cultivated and settled area, that is, the Nile valley, delta and oases, covers only about 35,580 sq. km.

The area, population (1976 Census and 1985 estimate) and capitals of the governorates are:

Governorate	*Sq. km*	*1976 census*	*1985 estimate*	*Capital*
Sinai al-Janûbîya	33,140	10,104	24,000	At-Tur
Sinai ash-Shamâlîya	25,574		152,000	Al-Arish
Suez	17,840	194,001	254,000	Suez
Ismailia	1,442	351,889	465,000	Ismâilya
Port Said	72	262,620	374,000	Port Said
Sharqîya	4,180	2,621,208	3,318,000	Zaqâziq
Daqahlîya	3,471	2,732,756	3,469,000	Mansûra
Damietta	589	557,115	728,000	Damietta
Kafr el Sheikh	3,437	1,403,468	1,795,000	Kafr el-Sheikh
Alexandria	2,679	2,318,655	2,821,000	Alexandria
Behera	10,130	2,517,292	3,199,000	Damanhur
Gharbîya	1,942	2,294,303	2,847,000	Tanta
Menûfîya	1,532	1,710,982	2,157,000	Shibin el-Kom
Qalyûbîya	1,001	1,674,006	2,186,000	Benha
Cairo	214	5,084,463	6,205,000	Cairo
Gîza	85,105	2,419,247	3,159,000	Gîza
Faiyûm	1,827	1,140,245	1,495,000	Faiyûm
Beni Suef	1,322	1,108,615	1,424,000	Beni-Suef
Minya	2,262	2,055,739	2,692,000	Minyâ
Asyût	1,530	1,695,378	2,179,000	Asyût
Sohag	1,547	1,924,960	2,455,000	Sohag
Qena	1,851	1,705,594	2,159,000	Qinâ
Aswân	679	619,932	781,000	Aswân
al-Bahr al-Ahmar	203,685	56,191	70,000	Al-Ghurdaqah
al-Wadi al-Jadid	376,505	84,645	113,000	Al-Kharijah
Mersa Matruh	212,112	112,772	173,000	Matruh
Total		36,656,180	46,694,000	

The principal towns, with their (estimate) 1986 populations, were:

Cairo	6,325,000	Asyût	291,300	Sani Suwayf	162,500
Alexandria	2,893,000	Zagâziq	274,400	Uqsur (Luxor)	147,900
Gaza	1,670,800	Suez	265,000	Qinâ	141,700
Shubrâ al-Khayma	533,300	Kafr ad-Dawwar	240,000	Sawhâj	141,500
Mahalla al-Kubrâ	385,300	Ismâiliya	236,300	Shibin al-Kawm	135,900
Port Said	382,000	Fayyûm	227,300	Dumyât	121,200
Tantâ	373,500	Damanhûr	225,900	Banhâ	120,200
Mansûra	357,800	Minyâ	203,300	Kafr ash-Shaykh	104,200
Hulwan	352,300	Aswân	195,700		

Population (1989) 50·74m. and of Greater Cairo 13·3m.

The official language is Arabic, although French and English are widely spoken.

CLIMATE. The climate is mainly dry, but there are winter rains along the Mediterranean coast. Elsewhere, rainfall is very low and erratic in its distribution. Winter temperatures are everywhere comfortable, but summer temperatures are very high, especially in the south. Cairo. Jan. 56°F (13·3°C), July 83°F (28·3°C). Annual rainfall 1·2" (28 mm). Alexandria. Jan. 58°F (14·4°C), July 79°F (26·1°C). Annual rainfall 7" (178 mm). Aswân. Jan. 62°F (16·7°C), July 92°F (33·3°C). Annual rainfall trace. Giza. Jan. 55°F (12·8°C), July 78°F (25·6°C). Annual rainfall 16" (389 mm). Ismailia. Jan. 56°F (13·3°C), July 84°F (28·9°C). Annual rainfall 1·5" (37 mm). Luxor. Jan. 59°F (15°C), July 86°F (30°C). Annual rainfall trace. Port Said. Jan. 58°F (14·4°C), July 78°F (27·2°C). Annual rainfall 3" (76 mm).

CONSTITUTION AND GOVERNMENT. The Constitution was approved by referendum on 11 Sept. 1971. It defines Egypt as 'an Arab Republic with a democratic, socialist system' and the Egyptian people as 'part of the Arab nation' with Islam as the state religion and Arabic as the official language.

The *President* of the Republic is nominated by the People's Assembly and confirmed by plebiscite for a 6-year term. He is the supreme commander of the armed forces and presides over the defence council.

Presidents since the establishment of the Republic have been:

Gen. Mohamed Neguib, 18 June 1953–14 Nov. 1954 (deposed).
Col. Gamal Abdel Nasser, 14 Nov. 1954–28 Sept. 1970 (died).
Col. Muhammad Anwar Sadat, 28 Sept. 1970–6 Oct. 1981 (assassinated).
Lieut.-Gen. Muhammad Hosni Mubarak, 7 Oct. 1981–.

The *People's Assembly* is a unicameral legislature consisting of 454 members directly elected for a 5-year term; the President of the Republic may appoint up to 10 additional members. Following a ruling in June 1990 by the Constitutional High Court that proportional representation was unconstitutional general elections were held in 2 rounds in Nov. and Dec. 1990. 2,681 candidates stood, but the New Wafd Party and Socialist Labour Party abstained. The National Democratic Party (NDP) won 270 seats, the Progressive Unionist Rally 6; the remainder went to independents, more than 80 of whom were NPD members.

The President may appoint one or more Vice-Presidents, and appoints a Prime Minister and a Council of Ministers, whom he may remove as he wishes.

A 210-member consultative body, the Shura Council, was established in 1980. Two-thirds of its members are elected and one-third appointed by the President.

President of the Republic: Hosni Mubarak, sworn in for second 6-year term Oct. 1987.

The Council of Ministers in Jan. 1991 was composed as follows:

Prime Minister: Dr Atef Mohamed Naguib Sidki.

Defence and Military Production: Gen. Youssef Sabri Abu Taleb. *Economy and Foreign Trade:* Youssri Mustafa. *Finance:* Mohammed Ahmed al Razaz. *Foreign Affairs and Deputy Prime Minister:* Ahmed Esmat Abdel Meguid. *Interior:* Mohammed Abdul-Halim Moussa.

National flag: Three horizontal stripes of red, white, black, with the national emblem in the centre in gold.

Local Government. There are 26 governorates: 16 provinces, 5 cities and 5 frontier districts.

DEFENCE. Conscription is for 3 years, between the ages of 20 and 35. Graduates serve for 1 year.

Army. The Army comprises 4 armoured and 8 mechanized infantry divisions; 1 Republican Guard, 1 independent armoured, 3 independent infantry, 4 independent mechanized, 2 airmobile, 1 parachute, 14 artillery and 2 heavy mortar brigades; 7

commando groups; and 2 surface-to-surface missile regiments. Strength (1991) 320,000 (180,000 conscripts) and about 500,000 reservists. Equipment includes 1,040 T-54/-55, 600 T-62 and 1,550 M-60 tanks.

Navy. 4 of the current submarine force of 10 old ex-Soviet and ex-Chinese 'Romeo' class submarines are to be modernized and 2 larger modernized ex-British Oberon class are to be added. Major surface combatants include 1 old destroyer, 2 Spanish-built and 2 Chinese-built missile armed frigates. There are also 21 missile craft of mixed British, Soviet and Chinese origin and 18 coastal and inshore patrol craft. A small shore-based naval aviation branch operates 5 Sea King and 12 Gazelle helicopters. Mine warfare forces include 4 coastal and 2 inshore minesweepers. 3 ex-Soviet medium landing ships provide amphibious lift supported by 11 minor landing craft. There are 6 major auxiliaries and some 14 minor service vessels. There are naval bases at Alexandria, Port Said, Mersa Matruh, Port Tewfik, Hurghada and Safaqa. Naval personnel in 1990 totalled 20,000 plus reserves of 14,000. An associated para-military coastguard about 2,000 strong operates 32 inshore cutters and numerous boats.

Air Force. Until 1979, the Air Force was equipped largely with aircraft of USSR design, but subsequent re-equipment involves aircraft bought in the West, as well as some supplied by China. Strength (1991) is about 30,000 personnel (10,000 conscripts) and 500 combat aircraft, of which the interceptors are operated by an independent Air Defence Command, in conjunction with many 'Guideline', 'Goa', 'Gainful', Hawk and Crotale missile batteries. There are about 12 Tu-16 twin-jet strategic bombers, some equipped to carry 'Kelt' air-to-surface missiles. Other interceptor/ground attack fighter divisions are equipped with 75 F-16 Fighting Falcons, 50 Mirage 5s, 33 F-4E Phantoms, 20 Mirage 2000s, 80 F-6s (Chinese-built MiG-19s), 15 Alpha Jets, 50 Su-7s, more than 120 MiG-21s, and 60 F-7s (Chinese-built MiG-21s). Airborne early warning capability is provided by 5 E-2C Hawkeyes. Transport units have 19 C-130H Hercules turboprop heavy freighters, 12 An-12s, 9 twin-turboprop Buffaloes, 6 Beech 1900s, and up to 175 Gazelle, Mi-4, Mi-6, Mi-8, Sea King/Commando and Agusta-built CH-47C helicopters; some Commando helicopters and 2 EC-130H Hercules are equipped for electronic warfare duties. Training units are equipped with Gomhouria piston-engined trainers, Embraer Tucanos, Czech-built L-29 Delfin and French-designed Alpha Jet jet trainers, two-seat versions of the MiG-15, MiG-17s, two-seat FT-6s, Mirage 5s, MiG-21Us and Su-7Us, and UH-12E helicopters. Main aircrew training centre is the EAF Academy at Bilbeis.

INTERNATIONAL RELATIONS

Membership. Egypt is a member of the UN, OAU, Arab League and OAPEC.

ECONOMY

Policy. A 5-year development plan runs 1987/88–1991–92 and envisages investments totalling £E46,500m.

Budget. Ordinary revenue and expenditure for fiscal years ending 30 June, in £E1m.:

	1985–86	*1986–87*	*1987–88*
Revenue	15,010	14,451	17,910
Expenditure	19,910	20,246	23,060

Currency. The monetary unit is the *Egyptian pound* (EGP) of 100 *piastres* of 10 *millièmes.* Coins in circulation are 20, 10, 5, 2 piastres (silver); 2, 1 piastre, 5 millièmes, 1 millième (bronze). The Treasury issues 5- and 10-piastre currency notes. Bank-notes are issued by the National Bank in denominations of 5, 10, 25 and 50 piastres, £E1, 5, 10, 20, and 100. In Feb. 1991 the oficial exchange rate was abolished, leaving a free rate, and a rate set by a panel of bankers.

In March 1991, £1 sterling = £E6·13; US$1 = £E3·23.

Banking. On 18 Aug. 1960 a Central Bank of Egypt was established by decree. It manages the note issue, the Government's banking operations and the control of commercial banks. At the same date the National Bank founded in 1898 ceased to be the central bank and became a purely commercial bank. In 1986 there were 27 commercial banks, 33 business and investment banks (joint ventures and 22 foreign currency branches) and 4 specialized banks. There were also 29 representative offices of foreign banks.

Weights and Measures. In 1951 the metric system was made official with the exception of the feddân and its subdivisions.

Capacity. Kadah = 1/96th ardeb = 3·36 pints. *Rob* = 4 kadahs = 1·815 gallons. *Keila* = 8 kadahs = 3·63 gallons. *Ardeb* = 96 kadahs = 43·555 gallons, or 5·44439 bu., or 198 cu. decimetres.

Weights. Rotl = 144 dirhems = 0·9905 lb. *Oke* = 400 dirhems = 2·75137 lb. *Qantâr* or 100 rotls or 36 okes = 99·0493 lb. 1 *Qantâr* of unginned cotton = 315 lb. 1 *Qantâr* of ginned cotton = 99·05 lb. The approximate weight of the ardeb is as follows: Wheat, 150 kg; beans, 155 kg; barley, 120 kg; maize, 140 kg; cotton seed, 121 kg.

Surface. Feddân, the unit of measure for land = 4,200·8 sq. metres = 7,468·148 sq. pics = 1·03805 acres. 1 sq. pic = 6·0547 sq. ft = 0·5625 sq. metre.

ENERGY AND NATURAL RESOURCES

Electricity. Electricity generated in 1986 was 40,600m. kwh. Supply 110 and 220 volts; 50 Hz.

Oil. The first commercial discovery of oil in the Middle East outside Iran was made in Egypt in 1909, but production long remained low and often insufficient to meet Egypt's domestic requirements. Policy is controlled by the Egyptian General Petroleum Corporation (EGPC) a wholly state-owned corporation answerable to the Minister of Petroleum. EGPC is whole or part-owner of the various production and refining companies and controls supplies to the domestic marketing companies. With the agreement of EGPC several foreign oil companies were exploring for oil in 1986.

Production 1989, was 45m. tonnes of crude oil. Net oil earnings (1983–84) US$2,340m.

Gas. The first gas field, at Abu Madi in the Nile delta, became operational in 1974 and produced 4,306,000 tonnes in 1986. The 2 other fields are at Abu Gharadeq in the Western Desert and Abu Qir near Alexandria.

Water. The Aswân High Dam, completed in 1970, allows for a perennial irrigation system.

Minerals. Production (1986 in tonnes): Phosphate rock, 1·2m.; iron ore, 2,135,000; marine salt, 1,040,000. Other minerals discovered include manganese, chrome, tantalum, molybdenum and uranium.

Agriculture. The cultivated area of Egypt proper was estimated in 1982 at 11·17m. feddâns (1 feddân = 1·038 acres) and of this, 4,945,000 feddâns were under winter crops, 5,017,000 under summer crops, 818,000 under Nile crops and 390,000 under orchards.

Irrigation occupies a predominant place in the economic development of the country. An intricate irrigation system now reaches most cultivated areas but only about 6·5% of the total land area is arable. The 'vertical' development policy calls for improved methods, better drainage and the introduction of stiff penalties for encroachment of farmland. Under the first phase of the 'horizontal' expansion programme, which aims to add 2·8m. feddâns to the arable area over 20 years, 24,000 feddâns are being added near Alexandria. Export earnings from agriculture have fallen and Egypt is no longer self sufficient in food production partly due to the increase in population. No priority has been given in government planning and because of inadequate investment earnings have fallen for its three most important export crops, cotton, oranges and rice.

In 1985–86 the area sown with cotton rose 7% to 440,705 ha; output increased 8% to 1,985,000 bales.

The major summer crops are cotton, rice, maize and sorghum. Berseem (Egyptian clover), wheat and beans are the main winter crops.

Production (1988, in 1,000 tonnes): Sugar cane, 9,750; maize, 4,088; tomatoes, 5,000; rice, 1,900; wheat, 2,839; potatoes, 1,700; oranges, 1,400; lint cotton, 348.

Livestock (1988): 1·92m. cattle, 2·6m. buffaloes, 1,165,000 sheep, 1·62m. goats, 70,000 camels and 15,000 pigs.

Forestry. In 1986 total removal of roundwood was 2·06m. cu. metres of which 2m. was fuel wood.

Fisheries. The catch of the Egyptian sea, Nile and lake fisheries in 1986 amounted to 138,800 tonnes.

INDUSTRY. (1987) Almost all large-scale enterprises are in the public sector and these account for about two-thirds of total output. The private sector, dominated by food processing and textiles, consists of about 150,000 small and medium businesses, most employing less than 50 workers. A car industry is being established.

Production in 1985–86 (in 1,000 tonnes) included: Phosphates, 766; fertilizer phosphates, 100·1; fertilizer nitrates, 4,482; cement, 7,735; cotton yarn, 225; cotton fabrics, 608,000 metres.

FOREIGN ECONOMIC RELATIONS

Commerce. Imports and exports for 5 years (in £E1,000):

	1982	*1983*	*1984*	*1985*	*1986*
Imports	6,354,517	7,192,657	7,536,100	6,276,300	8,051,400
Exports	2,184,122	2,250,295	2,197,900	2,600,000	1,243,700

In 1985 major exports (in £E1m.) included: Crude petroleum, 1,402·1; refined petroleum, 362·5; cotton, 299. Major imports (1984–85) included: Machinery and transport equipment, 1,915·2; foodstuffs, 1,848·5.

Exports, 1985 (in US$1m.), were mainly to Italy (656·6), Israel (462), Romania (434·2), France (430), USSR (177·8), Netherlands (152·1), Greece (119·2), Japan (113·8), Spain (100·2) and Republic of Korea (99·7); imports were mainly from USA (1,295·7), Federal Republic of Germany (953·8), Italy (757·3), France (700·9), Japan (514·7), UK (425·3), Spain (390·1), Romania (369·7), Netherlands (356·5) and Australia (335·7).

Total trade between Egypt and UK (British Department of Trade returns, in £1,000 sterling):

	1986	*1987*	*1988*	*1989*	*1990*
Imports to UK	328,053	127,261	163,038	212,727	145,323
Exports and re-exports from UK	371,007	342,195	289,309	296,272	298,262

Tourism. In 1986 there were 1·36m. tourists (43% from Arab countries) spending £E251·3m.

COMMUNICATIONS

Roads. In 1980, the total length of roads was 21,637 km, of which 16,182 km were paved. Motor vehicles, in 1981, 580,000 private cars, 165,000 commercial vehicles (including buses).

Railways. In 1988 there were 4,548 km of state railways (1,435 mm gauge), of which 42 km were electrified. 44·9m. passengers and 9·4m. tonnes of freight were carried. An underground rail system was opened in Cairo in 1987.

Aviation. There is an international airport at Cairo. There are 95 airfields (77 unusable). The national airline Egyptair operates scheduled flights connecting Cairo with Athens, Rome, Frankfurt, Zürich, London, Khartoum, Tokyo, Bombay, Aden, Jeddah, Doha, Dharan, Kuwait, Beirut, Baghdad, Tripoli, Benghazi, Algiers, Entebbe, Nairobi, Dar-es-Salaam, Kano, Lagos, Accra, Abidjan, Damascus, Amman, Manilla, Paris, Munich, Copenhagen, Nicosia, Karachi, Aleppo, Bahrain,

Abu Dhabi, Dubai, Sharjah, Sanaa and Vienna. In addition, Egyptair operates scheduled flights on a widespread domestic network connecting Cairo with Port Said, Mersa Matruh, Asyût, Luxor, Aswân. In 1982, 62,000 tonnes of cargo were carried.

Shipping. The Egyptian merchant navy in 1980 consisted of 75 steamers of 387,460 tons.

In 1977, 3,050 ships of 11,432,000 tons entered the port of Alexandria and 876 ships of 4,583,000 tons entered Port Said.

Suez Canal. The Suez Canal was opened for navigation on 17 Nov. 1869. By the convention of Constantinople of 29 Oct. 1888 the canal is open to vessels of all nations and is free from blockade, except in time of war, but the UAR Government did not allow Israeli ships to use the canal until May 1979. It is 173 km long (excluding 11 km of approach channels to the harbours), connecting the Mediterranean with the Red Sea. It is being deepened from 17 to 22 metres and widened from 365 to 415 metres to permit the passage of oil-tankers of 250,000 tonnes.

In 1976 a 2-stage development project was started. The first stage which was completed in 1980 allowing vessels, of up to 150,000 tons, fully loaded, and up to 370,000 tons in ballast to pass through the canal and give a draught of 53 ft.

During the war with Israel in June 1967 the Canal was blocked. The canal was cleared and re-opened to shipping on 5 June 1975. This is part of a programme to develop and rebuild the whole area of Suez to make it one of the largest tax-free industrial zones. In 1987 17,541 vessels (347m. tons) went through the canal. The first tunnel below the canal, located 10 miles north of Suez City, was completed on 30 April 1980 and the first phase of a £E4,000m. development plan, to widen and deepen the canal, was completed in 1980.

Telecommunications. There were, in 1980–81, 1,821 postal agencies, 1,812 mobile offices (1978), 1,747 government and 2,956 private post offices. Number of telephones in 1984, 600,000. Number of wireless licences in 1984, 12m. and 4m. TV licences.

The internal telecommunications system is owned and operated by the Telecommunications Organization. Government landlines connect with those of the Gaza sector and the Sudan.

Newspapers. In 1984 there were 11 dailies published in Cairo and 6 in Alexandria.

JUSTICE, RELIGION, EDUCATION AND WELFARE

Justice. The National Courts in 1981 were as follows: Court of Cassation with a bench of 5 judges which constitutes the highest court of appeal in both criminal and civil cases; Courts of Appeal with 3 judges situated in Cairo and 4 other cities; Assize Courts with 3 judges which deal with all cases of serious crime; Central Tribunals with 3 judges which deal with ordinary civil and commercial cases; Summary Tribunals presided over by a single judge which hear civil disputes in matters up to the value of £E3,250, and criminal offences punishable by a fine or imprisonment of up to 3 years.

Religion. In 1986 about 90% of the population were Moslems, mostly of the Sunni sect, and about 7% Coptic Christians, the remainder being Roman Catholics, Protestants or Greek Orthodox, with a small number of Jews.

There are in Egypt large numbers of native Christians connected with the various Oriental Churches; of these, the largest and most influential are the Copts, who adopted Christianity in the 1st century. Their head is the Coptic Patriarch. There are 25 metropolitans and bishops in Egypt; 4 metropolitans for Ethiopia, Jerusalem, Khartoum and Omdurman, and 12 bishops in Ethiopia. Priests must be married before ordination, but celibacy is imposed on monks and high dignitaries. The Copts use the Diocletian (or Martyrs') calendar, which begins in A.D. 284.

Education. Primary education (6 years) was made free in 1944, secondary and technical education in 1950. Compulsory education is provided in primary schools (6 years).

In 1982–83 there were 503 nurseries and kindergartens with 84,539 pupils. In 1982–83 there were in basic education (6–15 years) 5,036,608 primary stage pupils in 12,013 schools and 1,769,768 preparatory stage pupils in 3,151 schools. In secondary education there were 517,998 general secondary pupils in 823 schools; 441,636 commercial secondary pupils in 639 schools; 208,468 industrial secondary pupils in 170 schools and 84,527 agricultural secondary pupils in 65 schools. Ninety-two teacher training schools had 63,429 pupils and 144 rehabilitation schools had 8,215 pupils.

El Azhar institutes educate students who join the faculties of El Azhar University after graduation. In 1982–83, 1,287 institutes had 308,370 students.

Government experimental language schools, which teach in foreign languages, had 5,000 nursery and kindergarten pupils in 1982–83, and 2,700 primary stage pupils in 1983–84.

Higher education: In 1982, there were 64,870 students in 17 higher commercial institutes and 22,341 students in 16 industrial institutions.

There were 11 universities in Egypt (apart from El Azhar University), with 558,527 students and 74,945 graduates in 1980–81. El Azhar University had 65,451 students and 5,346 graduates in 1980–81.

Health. In 1983–84 there were about 73,300 doctors and 85,350 hospital beds.

DIPLOMATIC REPRESENTATIVES

Of Egypt in Great Britain (26 South St., London, W1Y 8EL)
Ambassador: Mohamed I. Shaker.

Of Great Britain in Egypt (Ahmed Ragheb St., Garden City, Cairo)
Ambassador: Sir William Adams, KCMG.

Of Egypt in the USA (2310 Decatur Pl., NW, Washington, D.C., 20008)
Ambassador: Abdel Raouf El-Ridy.

Of the USA in Egypt (Lazougi St., Garden City, Cairo)
Ambassador: Frank G. Wisner.

Of Egypt to the United Nations
Ambassador: Amre M. Moussa.

Further Reading

The Egyptian Almanac. Annual
Le Mondain Egyptien (Who's Who). Cairo. Annual
Aliboni, R., *(et al) Egypt's Economic Potential*. London, 1984
Ansari, H., *Egypt: The Stalled Society*. New York, 1986
Hart, V., *Modern Egypt*. Cairo, 1984
Heikal, M., *Autumn of Fury: Assassination of Sadat*. London, 1983
Hopwood, D., *Egypt: Politics and Society 1945–1981*. London, 1982
Kepel, G., *Muslim Extremism in Egypt*. Univ. of California Press, 1986
McDermott, A., *Egypt: From Nasser to Mubarak*. London, 1988
Makar, R. N., *Egypt*. [Bibliography] Oxford and Santa Barbara, 1988
Vatikiotis, P. J., *History of Modern Egypt: from Muhammad Ali to Mubarak*. London, 1991
Waterbury, J., *The Egypt of Nasser and Sadat*. Princeton Univ. Press, 1983

EL SALVADOR

Capital: San Salvador
Population: 5·21m. (1990)
GNP per capita: US$950 (1988)

República de El Salvador

HISTORY. In 1839 the Central American Federation, which had comprised the states of Guatemala, El Salvador, Honduras, Nicaragua and Costa Rica, was dissolved, and El Salvador declared itself formally an independent republic in 1841.

Throughout the 1980s the Marti National Liberation Front (FMLN) waged guerilla war against the government.

AREA AND POPULATION. El Salvador is the smallest and most densely populated (256 inhabitants per sq. km) of the Central American states. Its area (including 247 sq. km of inland lakes) is estimated at 21,393 sq. km (8,236 sq. miles) with population estimate (1990) 5,210,000 (44·1% urban).

The republic is divided into 14 departments, each under an appointed governor. Their areas and populations in 1981 were:

Department	*Sq. km*	*1981*	*Chief town*	*1985*
Ahuachapán	1,281	241,323	Ahuachapán	71,846
Sonsonate	1,133	321,989	Sonsonate	47,489 [1]
Santa Ana	1,829	445,462	Santa Ana	208,322
La Libertad	1,650	388,538	Nueva San Salvador	52,226 [1]
San Salvador	892	979,683	San Salvador	972,810
Chalatenango	2,507	235,757	Chalatenango	28,675 [2]
Cuscatlán	766	203,978	Cojutepeque	31,108 [1]
La Paz	1,155	249,635	Zacatecoluca	81,035
San Vicente	1,175	206,959 [2]	San Vicente	65,462
Cabañas	1,075	179,909	Sensuntepeque	50,448 [2]
Usulután	1,780	399,912	Usulután	69,355
San Miguel	2,532	434,047	San Miguel	161,156
Morazan	1,364	215,163	San Francisco	13,015 [2]
La Unión	1,738	309,879	La Unión	27,186 [1]

[1] 1984. [2] 1980.

CLIMATE. Despite its proximity to the equator, the climate is warm rather than hot and nights are cool inland. Light rains occur in the dry season from Nov. to April while the rest of the year has heavy rains, especially on the coastal plain. San Salvador. Jan. 71°F (21·7°C), July 75°F (23·9°C). Annual rainfall 71" (1,775 mm). San Miguel. Jan. 77°F (25°C), July 83°F (28·3°C). Annual rainfall 68" (1,700 mm).

CONSTITUTION AND GOVERNMENT. A new Constitution was enacted in Dec. 1983. The Executive Power is vested in a President elected for a non-renewable term of 5 years, with Ministers and Under-Secretaries appointed by him. The Legislative power is an Assembly of 84 members elected by universal suffrage and proportional representation for a term of 3 years. The judicial power is vested in a Supreme Court, of a President and 9 magistrates elected by the Legislative Assembly for renewable terms of 3 years; and subordinate courts. For governments, 1961–79 *see* THE STATESMAN'S YEAR-BOOK 1982–83, p. 436.

At the March 1991 elections turn-out was 50%. The Alianza Republicana Nacionalista (ARENA) won 39 seats, the Christian Democratic Party 26, the Party of National Conciliation 9 and Democratic Convergence 8.

President: Alfredo Felix Cristiani Burkard (sworn in 1 June 1989).

In June 1990 the Cabinet was composed as follows:

Foreign Affairs: José Manuel Pacas Castro. *Planning and Co-ordination of Economic and Social Development:* Mirna Liévano de Márquez. *Interior:* Col. Juan Antonio Martinez Varela. *Justice:* Dr Oscar Santamaría. *Finance:* Rafael Alvarado Cano. *Economics:* Arturo Zablah. *Education:* Dr Réné Hernández Valiente.

Defence and Public Safety: Col. René Emilio Ponce. *Labour and Social Security:* Mauricio González Dubón. *Public Health and Social Welfare:* Dr Lisandro Vásquez Sosa. *Agriculture and Livestock:* Antonio Cabrales. *Works:* Mauricio Stubig.

National flag: Blue, white, blue (horizontal): the white stripe charged with the arms of the republic.

National anthem: Saludemos la patria orgullosos ('We proudly salute the Fatherland'; words by J. J. Cañas, tune by J. Aberle).

DEFENCE. There is selective national service for 2 years.

Army. The Army comprises 6 infantry brigades, 1 mechanized cavalry regiment, 1 artillery brigade, 1 engineer, 1 anti-aircraft, 1 parachute and 6 counter-insurgency battalions. Equipment includes 5 M-3A1 light tanks and 12 AML-90 armoured cars. Strength was (1991) 40,000. There are also National Guard, National Police and Treasury Police, paramilitary units, numbering (1991) about 13,000 and a territorial civil defence force of up to 12,500.

Navy. A small coastguard force based at Acajutla, with 700 (1990) personnel, operates 6 inshore patrol craft, 3 landing craft and numerous boats. There were also (1990) 1,300 marines, and 200 'Commandos'.

Air Force. The Air Force underwent a major re-equipment programme in 1974–75, with most aircraft coming from Israel and US aid for transport units, but lost 18 aircraft in a guerrilla attack in Jan. 1982. Counter-insurgency equipment includes 8 A-37B and 6 Magister attack aircraft, 6 armed C-47 transports and 4 Hughes 500MD helicopters. Other aircraft are 6 C-47, 3 Arava, 1 DC-6 and 2 C-123 transports, 6 Cessna O-2 patrol aircraft, plus 3 Lamas, 3 Alouette III and 50 UH-1H helicopters. Training types include about 15 piston-engined T-41Cs, T-6s and T-34s. Strength totalled about 2,400 personnel in 1991.

INTERNATIONAL RELATIONS

Membership. El Salvador is a member of the UN, CACM and OAS.

ECONOMY

Policy. An economic liberalization programme aims at raising exports, foreign investment and domestic savings.

Budget. Revenue and expenditure for fiscal years ending 31 Dec., in ₡1,000:

	1984	*1985*	*1986*	*1987*	*1988*
Revenue	2,817,730	2,391,010	3,508,159	3,232,628	3,175,573
Expenditure	2,685,009	2,276,052	3,481,152	3,397,276	3,428,129

Currency. The monetary unit is the *colón* (SVC) of 100 *centavos*. The *colón* (₡) is issued in denominations of 1, 2, 5, 10, 25 and 100 *colones*; 25 and 50 *centavos* and 1 *colón* (silver); 1, 2, 5 and 10 *centavos* (copper–nickel and copper–zinc); 1 centavo (nickel). In March 1991, £1 = ₡15·23; US$1 = ₡8·03.

Banking and Finance. It is planned to privatize banks and financial institutions. Individual private holdings may not exceed 5% of the total equity. There are 10 native commercial banks, including the Banco Salvadoreño (paid-up capital, ₡6m.). The Citibank Bank of America and the Bank of Santander and Panama S. A. are the only foreign institutions. The Central Reserve Bank of El Salvador, formed in 1934 from the Banco Agricola Comercial, was nationalized on 20 April 1961.

Weights and Measures. On 1 Jan. 1886 the metric system was made obligatory. But other units are still commonly in use, of which the principal are as follows: *Libra* = 1·014 lb. av.; *quintal* = 101·4 lb. av.; *arroba* = 25·35 lb. av.; *fanega* = 1·5745 bushels.

ENERGY AND NATURAL RESOURCES

Electricity. A 200 ft high dam completed in 1954 was constructed across the (unnavigable) Lempa River, 35 miles north-east of San Salvador, with an annual capacity of 344m. kwh. The San Lorenzo dam, completed in 1983, has an annual capacity of 722m. kwh. Production in 1987, 1,971m. kwh.; consumption (1987), 1,672m. kwh. Supply 120 and 240 volts; 60 Hz.

Oil. Production of petroleum derivatives during 1988 totalled ₡1,076,639,000.

Minerals. The mineral output of the republic is now negligible, but the Ministry of Public Works has recently started to investigate 2 new silver mines in the department of Morazán.

Agriculture. El Salvador is predominantly agricultural; 32·5% of its total area is used for crops and 30·2% for pasture. Area devoted to coffee (1982–83) was about 516,615 acres, entirely owned by nationals. In 1981, 35·5% of the working population was engaged in farming.

Production (1988, in 1,000 tonnes): Coffee, 152; seed cotton, 27; maize, 589; dry beans, 56; rice, 57; sorghum, 152; sugar-cane, 3,407. A little rubber is exported.

Livestock (1988): 1,144,000 cattle, 442,000 pigs, 5,000 sheep, 15,000 goats.

Forestry. In the national forests are found dye woods and such woods as mahogany, cedar and walnut. Balsam trees also abound: El Salvador is the world's principal source of this medicinal gum. Sawn wood production, 1986, 38,000 cu. metres.

Fisheries. Total catch 1986, 12,500 tonnes.

INDUSTRY. Total production was valued at ₡4,579,322m. in 1984, which included (in ₡1,000): Food, ₡1,827,983; textiles, ₡273,573; chemicals, ₡310,922; footwear and clothing, ₡218,287; beverages, ₡352,224.

FOREIGN ECONOMIC RELATIONS. External debt amounted to US$1,826m. in 1989.

Commerce. Imports (including parcels post) and exports in calendar years in ₡1,000:

	1984	*1985*	*1986*	*1987*	*1988*
Imports	2,443,575	2,403,444	4,284,000	4,970,335	5,034,860
Exports	1,793,432	1,697,420	2,524,700	2,954,705	2,982,095

Of total exports (1988), coffee furnished about 34·9% by weight and 58·4% by value. The coffee is of the 'mild' variety; it is sold in bags of 60 kg, but trade statistics use a bag of 69 kg. An estimated 162,000 tonnes were exported in 1990 (96,000 tonnes in 1989).

In 1988 the USA took ₡904,433,000 of exports and furnished ₡1,417,720,000 of imports. The chief imports in 1988 were manufactured goods (28%), chemical and pharmaceutical products (18·1%), non-edible crude materials, mainly crude oil (8%), electric machinery, tools and appliances and transport equipment (25·6%). The other Central American Republics, Germany, Japan, Canada, Mexico, Spain, France and the Netherlands are also important trading partners.

Total trade between El Salvador and UK (British Department of Trade returns, in £1,000 sterling):

	1986	*1987*	*1988*	*1989*	*1990*
Imports to UK	1,323	1,890	2,961	2,133	1,261
Exports and re-exports from UK	6,917	9,595	8,186	9,594	10,415

Tourism. There were 125,000 visitors in 1987.

COMMUNICATIONS

Roads. In 1985 there were 12,164 km of national roads in the republic, including 1,706 km of main paved roads; 3,421 km main asphalted roads; other roads, 7,038 km. Vehicles registered, 1987: Cars, 138,000; buses, 7,000 and goods vehicles, 17,000.

Railways. All railways (602 km) came under the control of National Railways of El Salvador *(Fenadesal)* in 1975. Lines run from Acajutla to San Salvador; Cutuco to

San Salvador; between San Salvador and Santa Ana, San Miguel and Sonsonate; there is also a link to the Guatemalan system. Total railway traffic in 1989 was 216,000 tonnes of freight and 345,000 passengers.

Aviation. The airport at Ilopango, 8 km from San Salvador, now a military airport, and the new international airport at Cuscatlán, 40 km from San Salvador, opened in 1979. In 1985, 170,510 passengers arrived and 179,827 departed.

Shipping. The principal ports are La Unión, La Libertad and Acajutla, all on the Pacific. Passengers (and some freight) use the Guatemalan port of Puerto Barrios on the Atlantic, reaching El Salvador by rail or road.

Telecommunications. The telephone and telegraph systems are government-owned; the radio-telephone systems are partly private, partly government-owned. In 1989 there were 94,691 telephones. There were (1986) over 50 radio stations. Radio El Salvador is state-owned. There were (1988) 4 commercial television channels and 2 educational channels sponsored by the Ministry of Education. In 1985 there were 1·9m. radio receivers and (1986) 242,000 television sets.

Cinemas (1976). Cinemas numbered 65.

Newspapers (1990). There are 5 daily newspapers in San Salvador and 1 in Santa Ana.

JUSTICE, RELIGION, EDUCATION AND WELFARE

Justice. Justice is administered by the Supreme Court of Justice, courts of first and second instance, and minor tribunals. Magistrates of the Supreme Court and courts of second instance are elected by the Legislative Assembly for a renewable 3-year term.

An anti-Communist law, effective 29 Sept. 1962, has made the propagation of totalitarian or Communist doctrines an offence punishable by imprisonment; supplementary offences, contrary to democratic principles, are punished by prison terms of from 3 to 7 years.

Religion. About 90% of the population is Roman Catholic. Under the 1962 Constitution churches are exempted from the property tax; the Catholic Church is recognized as a legal person, and other churches are entitled to secure similar recognition. There is an archbishop in San Salvador and bishops at Santa Ana, San Miguel, San Vicente, Santiago de María, Usulután, Sonsonate and Zacatecoluca. There are about 200,000 Protestants.

Education. Education is free and obligatory. In 1929 the State took over control of all schools, public and private, but the provision that the teaching in government schools must be wholly secular was removed in 1945.

In 1986 there were 72,500 pupils in nursery schools, 1,140,000 in primary and secondary schools and 73,500 students receiving higher education.

Social Welfare. The Social Security Institute now administers the sickness, old age and death insurance, covering industrial workers and employees earning up to ₡700 a month. Employees in other private institutions with salaries over this amount are included but are excluded from the medical and hospital benefits.

DIPLOMATIC REPRESENTATIVES

Of El Salvador in Great Britain (62 Welbeck St., London, W1)
Ambassador: Dr Mauricio Rosales-Rivera.

Of Great Britain in El Salvador
Ambassador and Consul General: P. J. Streams, CMG. (resides in Tegucigalpa).

Of El Salvador in the USA (2308 California St., NW, Washington, DC., 20008)
Ambassador: Dr Miguel Angel Salaverria.

Of the USA in El Salvador (25 Ave. Norte, Colonia Dueñas, San Salvador)
Ambassador: William G. Walker.

Of El Salvador to the United Nations
Ambassador: Dr Ricardo G. Castaneda-Cornejo.

Further Reading

Statistical Information: The Dirección General de Estadistica y Censos (Villa Fermina, Calle Arce, San Salvador) dates from 1937. *Director General:* Lieut.-Col. José Castro Meléndez. Its publications include *Anuario Estadistico.* Annual from 1911.—*Boletin Estadístico.* Quarterly.—*El Salvador en Gráficas.* Annual.—*Atlas Censal de El Salvador.* 1955 only.—Revista Mensual, Banco Central de Reserva de El Salvador.

Angel Gallardo, M., *Cuatro Constituciones Federales de Centro América y Las Constituciones Politicas de El Salvador.* San Salvador, 1945
Armstrong, R. and Shenk, J., *El Salvador: The Face of Revolution.* London, 1982
Baloyra, E. A., *El Salvador in Transition.* Univ. of North Carolina Press, 1982
Bevan, J., *El Salvador. Education and Repression.* London, 1981
Browning, D., *El Salvador: Landscape and Society.* OUP, 1971
Devire, F. J., *El Salvador: Embassy under Attack.* New York, 1981
Didion, J., *Salvador.* London, 1983
Erdozain, P., *Archbishop Romero: Martyr of El Salvador.* Guildford, 1981
Montgomery, T.S., *Revolution in El Salvador: Origins and Evolution.* Boulder, 1982
North, L., *Bitter Grounds: Roots of Revolt in El Salvador.* London, 1981
Schmidt, S. W., *El Salvador: America's Next Vietnam.* Salisbury (N.C.), 1983
Woodward, R. L., *El Salvador.* [Bibliography] Oxford and Santa Barbara, 1988

EQUATORIAL GUINEA

Capital: Malabo
Population: 417,000 (1990)
GNP per capita: US$350 (1988)

República de Guinea Ecuatorial

HISTORY. Equatorial Guinea was a Spanish colony (Territorios Españoles del Golfo de Guinea) until 1 April 1960, the territory was then divided into two Spanish provinces with a status comparable to the metropolitan provinces until 20 Dec. 1963, when they were re-joined as an autonomous Equatorial Region. It became an independent Republic on 12 Oct. 1968 as a federation of the two provinces, and a unitary state was established on 4 Aug. 1973. The first President, Francisco Macías Nguema, was declared President-for-Life on 14 July 1972, but was overthrown by a military coup on 3 Aug. 1979. A Supreme Military Council then created was the sole political body until constitutional rule was resumed on 12 Oct. 1982.

AREA AND POPULATION. The mainland part of Equatorial Guinea is bounded north by Cameroon, east and south by Gabon, and west by the Gulf of Guinea in which lie the islands of Bioko (formerly Macías Nguema, formerly Fernando Póo) and Annobón (called Pagalu from 1973 to 1979). The total area is 28,051 sq. km (10,831 sq. miles) and the population at the 1983 census was 300,000. Estimate (1990) 417,000. Another 110,000 are estimated to remain in exile abroad.

The 7 provinces are grouped into 2 regions, Continental (C), chief town Bata and Insular (I), chief town Malabo, with areas and populations as follows:

	Sq. km	*Census 1983*	*Chief town*
Annobón (I)	17	2,006	San Antonio de Palea
Bioko Norte (I)	776	46,221	Malabo
Bioko Sur (I)	1,241	10,969	Luba
Centro Sur (C)	9,931	52,393	Evinayong
Kié-Ntem (C)	3,943	70,202	Ebebiyin
Litoral (C)	6,665 [1]	66,370	Bata
Wele-Nzas (C)	5,478	51,839	Mongomo

[1] Including the adjacent islets of Corisco, Elobey Grande and Elobey Chico (17 sq. km).

In 1986 the largest towns were Bata (17,000) and the capital Malabo (10,000).

The main ethnic group on the mainland is the Fang; there are several minority groups along the coast and adjacent islets. On Bioko the indigenous inhabitants (Bubis) constitute 60% of the population there, the balance being mainly Fang and coast people; the formerly numerous immigrant workers from Nigeria and Cameroon have mostly been repatriated. On Annobón the indigenous inhabitants are the descendents of Portuguese slaves and still speak a Portuguese patois. The official language is Spanish.

CLIMATE. The climate is equatorial, with alternate wet and dry seasons. In Río Muni, the wet season lasts from Dec. to Feb.

CONSTITUTION AND GOVERNMENT. A new Constitution was approved in Aug. 1982 by 95% of the votes cast in a plebiscite, which also confirmed the President in office for a further 7-year term. It provides for an 11-member Council of State, and for a 41-member House of Representatives of the People, the latter being directly elected on 28 Aug. 1983 for a 5-year term and re-elected on 10 July 1988. The President appoints and leads a Council of Ministers.

On 12 Oct. 1987 a single new political party was formed as the *Partido Democrático de Guinea Ecuatorial*.

President of the Supreme Military Council, Defence: Brig.-Gen. Teodoro Obiang Nguema Mbasogo.

Prime Minister: Cristino Seriche Bioko.

Foreign Affairs: Marcelino Nguema Ongueme. *Economy and Finance:* Antonio Fernando Nve. *Justice and Religion:* Angel Ndong Micha.

National flag: Three horizontal stripes of green, white, red; a blue triangle based on the hoist; in the centre the national arms.

DEFENCE

Army. The Army consists of 3 infantry battalions with (1991) 1,100 personnel. There is also a paramilitary force of some 2,000.

Navy. A small force, numbering 100 in 1990, and based at Malabo, operate 4 in-shore patrol craft.

INTERNATIONAL RELATIONS

Membership. Equatorial Guinea is a member of the UN, OAU and is an ACP state of the EEC.

ECONOMY

Budget. The 1988 budget envisaged income at 7,147m. francs CFA and expenditure at 7,894m. francs CFA.

Currency. On 2 Jan. 1985 the country joined the franc zone and the *ekuele* was replaced by the *franc CFA* with a parity value of 50 *francs* CFA to 1 French franc. There are coins of 1, 2, 5, 10, 25, 50, 100 and 500 *francs* CFA, and banknotes of 100, 500, 1,000, 5,000 and 10,000 *francs* CFA. In March 1991, £1 = 496.13 *francs* CFA; US$1 = 261.53 *francs* CFA.

Banking. The *Banque des Etats de l'Afrique Centrale* became the bank of issue in Jan. 1985. There are 2 commercial banks.

ENERGY AND NATURAL RESOURCES

Electricity. Production (1986) 17m. kwh.

Agriculture. The chief products are cocoa (74,000 ha in 1988) and coffee (19,000 ha). Production (in 1,000 tonnes in 1988): Cocoa, 17; coffee 7; palm oil, 5; palm kernels, 3; bananas, 20; cassava, 56; sweet potatoes, 37. Plantations in the hinterland have been abandoned by their Spanish owners and except for cocoa, commercial agriculture is under serious difficulties.

Livestock (1988): Cattle, 5,000; sheep, 35,000; goats, 8,000; pigs, 5,000.

Forestry. In 1988, 1·3m. ha, 46% of the land area was forested. Production: 1981, 465,000 cu. metres.

Fisheries. Catch (1986) 4,400 tonnes.

INDUSTRY. Bioko has very few industries. The mainland has no industry except lumbering. Post-independence political conditions have not been conducive to private investment.

FOREIGN ECONOMIC RELATIONS

Commerce. In 1981 imports amounted to 7,982m. Bikuele (of which 80% came from Spain) and exports to 2,502m. Bikuele (of which Spain took 87%). Cocoa amounted to 71% of all exports and timber to 24%.

Total trade between Equatorial Guinea and UK (British Department of Trade returns, in £1,000 sterling):

	1986	*1987*	*1988*	*1989*	*1990*
Imports to UK	1	...	...	2	10
Exports and re-exports from UK	633	1,572	1,029	640	1,159

COMMUNICATIONS

Roads. Length (1982) 2,760 km of which 330 km surfaced.

Aviation. There are international airports at Malabo and Bata. The line Madrid–Malabo–Bata is subsidized by Spain. Links with Douala (from Malabo) and Libreville (Gabon) exist.

Shipping. Malabo is the main port. The other ports are Luba, formerly San Carlos (bananas, cocoa) in Bioko and Bata, Evinayong and Mbini (wood) on the mainland. A new harbour in Bata has been completed. In 1981 47,731 tonnes were unloaded and 50,843 loaded.

Telecommunications. In Feb. 1989 the radio stations began broadcasting in French in addition to Spanish. Estimated number of telephones (1969), 1,451. In 1985 there were 100,000 radio and 2,200 TV receivers.

JUSTICE, RELIGION, EDUCATION AND WELFARE

Justice. The Constitution guarantees an independent judiciary. The Supreme Tribunal is the highest court of appeal and is located at Malabo. There are Courts of First Instance and Courts of Appeal at Malabo and Bata.

Religion. The population of Equatorial Guinea is nominally Roman Catholic with influential Protestant groups in Malabo and the mainland.

Education. There were in 1981 about 40,110 pupils and 647 teachers in 511 primary schools and 3,013 pupils and 288 teachers in 14 secondary schools.

DIPLOMATIC REPRESENTATIVES

Of Equatorial Guinea in Great Britain
Ambassador: (Vacant).

Of Great Britain in Equatorial Guinea
Ambassador and Consul-General: M. Reith (resides in Yaoundé).

Of the USA in Equatorial Guinea (Calle de Los Ministros, Malabo)
Ambassador: Chester E. Norris Jr.

Of Equatorial Guinea to the USA and the United Nations
Ambassador: Dámaso-Obiang Ndong.

Further Reading

Atlas Historico y Geográfico de Africa Española. Madrid, 1955

Plan de Desarrollo Económico de la Guinea Ecuatorial. Presidencia del Gobierno. Madrid, 1963

Berman, S., *Spanish Guinea: An Annotated Bibliography.* Microfilm Service, Catholic University. Washington, D.C. 1961

Liniger-Goumaz, M., *La Guinée équatoriale un pays méconnu.* Paris, 1980.—*Connaître la Guinée Equatoriale.* Paris, 1986.—*Guinea Ecuatorial: Bibliografía General.* vols 1-7. Geneva, 1974-91

Pélissier, R., *Les Territoires espagnols d'Afrique.* Paris, 1963.—*Los territorios españoles de Africa.* Madrid, 1964.—*Etudes Hispano-Guinéennes.* Orgeval, 1969

ETHIOPIA

Capital: Addis Ababa
Population: 50m. (1989)
GNP per capita: US$120 (1988)

People's Democratic Republic of Ethiopia

HISTORY. The empire of Ethiopia had its origin in the centuries before and after the birth of Christ, at Aksum in the north, as a result of Semitic immigration from South Arabia. The immigrants imposed their language and culture on a basic Hamitic stock. Ethiopia's subsequent history is one of sporadic expansion southwards and eastwards. Modern Ethiopia dates from the reign of the Emperor Theodore (1855–68).

Menelik II (1889–1913) defeated the Italians in 1896 and thereby safeguarded the empire's independence in the scramble for Africa. By successful campaigns in neighbouring kingdoms within Ethiopia (Jimma, Kaffa, Harar, etc.) he united the country under his rule.

In 1936 Ethiopia was conquered by the Italians, who were in turn defeated by the Allied forces in 1941 when the Emperor returned.

The former Italian colony of Eritrea was in accordance with a resolution of the General Assembly of the UN, dated 2 Dec. 1950, handed over to Ethiopia on 15 Sept. 1952. Eritrea thereby became an autonomous unit within the federation of Ethiopia and Eritrea.

This federation became a unitary state on 14 Nov. 1962 when Eritrea was fully integrated with Ethiopia. The Federation gave rise to an Eritrean secessionist movement which has since pursued a campaign of military resistance. The government engaged in preliminary peace talks with the rebels in Sept. 1989 and former president Carter of the USA also acted as mediator. Fierce fighting commenced in Tigre in late 1989.

A provisional military government assumed power on 12 Sept. 1974, deposed the Emperor and executed 60 former military and civilian leaders.

In Feb. 1977 Lieut.-Col. Mengistu Haile Mariam became Chairman of the Provisional Military Administrative Council, and in Sept. 1987 he was elected President of the newly-inaugurated People's Democratic Republic.

For the war with Somalia *see* THE STATESMAN'S YEAR-BOOK, 1989-90, p.462.

AREA AND POPULATION. Ethiopia is bounded north-east by the Red Sea, east by Djibouti and Somalia, south by Kenya and west by Sudan. It has a total area of 1,221,900 sq. km (471,800 sq. miles). The first census was carried out in 1984: Population (preliminary) 42,019,418. Estimate (1989), 50m. Growth rate was 2·9% in 1989; expectation of life, 40·9 years. There were 265,000 refugees in Ethiopia in Jan. 1988.

The dominant race of Ethiopia, the Amhara, inhabit the central Ethiopian highlands. To the north of them are the Tigréans, akin to the Amhara and belonging to the same Christian church, but speaking a different, though related, language. Both these races are of mixed Hamitic and Semitic origin, and further mixed by intermarriage with Oromo (Galla) and other races. The Oromos, some of whom are Christian, some Moslem and some pagan, comprise about 40% of the entire population, and are a pastoral and agricultural people of Hamitic origin. Somalis, another Hamitic race, inhabit the south-east of Ethiopia, in particular the Ogaden desert region. These like the closely related Afar people, are Moslem. The Afar stretch northwards from Wollo region into Eritrea.

Region	Area (sq. km)	Population May 1984	Chief town	Population May 1984
Addis Ababa	218	1,412,575	—	—
Arussi	23,500	1,662,233	Assela	36,720
Bale	124,600	1,006,491	Goba	22,963
Eritrea	117,600	2,614,700	Asmara	275,385
Gemu Gofa	39,500	1,248,034	Arba Minch	23,030
Gojjam	61,600	3,244,882	Debre Markos	39,808
Gondar (Begemdir)	74,200	2,905,362	Gondar	68,958
Hararge	259,700	4,151,706	Harar	62,160
Illubabor	47,400	963,327	Mattu	12,491
Kefa	54,600	2,450,369	Jimma	60,992
Shoa	85,200	8,090,565	—	—
Sidamo	117,300	3,790,579	Awassa	36,169
Tigre	65,900	2,409,700	Mekele	61,583
Wollega	71,200	2,369,677	Lekemti	28,824
Wollo	79,400	3,609,918	Dessie	68,848

Other large towns (population, May 1984): Dire Dawa, in Hararge, 98,104; Nazret, in Shoa, 76,284; Bahr Dar, 54,800; Debre Zeit, 51,143.

The official language is Amharic.

CLIMATE. The wide range of latitude produces many climatic variations between the high, temperate plateaus and the hot, humid lowlands. The main rainy season lasts from June to Aug., with light rains from Feb. to April, but the country is very vulnerable to drought. Addis Ababa. Jan. 59°F (15°C), July 59°F (15°C). Annual rainfall 50" (1,237 mm). Harar. Jan. 65°F (18·3°C), July 64°F (17·8°C). Annual rainfall 35" (897 mm). Massawa. Jan. 78°F (25·6°C), July 94°F (34·4°C). Annual rainfall 8" (193 mm).

CONSTITUTION AND GOVERNMENT. The People's Democratic Republic of Ethiopia was inaugurated on 10 Sept. 1987 at the first meeting of the newly elected National Assembly. A new Constitution, on a Marxist model, was approved on 1 Feb. 1987 in a referendum. On 14 June 1987 Ethiopia held its first parliamentary election when 813 members belonging to the single political party the Workers' Party of Ethiopia were elected to the new civilian legislature.

President: Mengistu Haile Mariam (elected Sept. 1987).
Vice President: Fisseha Desta.
Acting Prime Minister: Hailu Yimenu; *Foreign:* Tesfaye Dinka.

National flag: Three horizontal stripes of green, yellow and red.
National anthem: Ityopya, Ityopia Kidemi (tune by Daniel Yohannes, 1975).

Local Government. Since 1987 the country has been divided into 24 administrative and 5 autonomous regions. Each region is governed by a regional assembly.

DEFENCE. President Mengistu is Commander in chief of the armed forces which are large, experienced and capable in comparison with most other Sub-Saharan nations. The army is the largest in Africa and the Navy and Air Force rank only second to South Africa in numbers of personnel.

Army. The Army expanded from 35,000 to 240,000 men between 1975 and 1981, then fell to some 180,000 between 1981 and 1983. National military service was revived in 1984 and the major military setbacks of early 1988 and 1989 accelerated conscription to the extent that the Army's strength now lies at around 300,000. Army HQ is in Addis Ababa. Four revolutionary Armies are made up of over 23 infantry, 4 mechanized and one airborne divisions. Each regular infantry division normally has four brigades plus support units varying from 4–10,000 men. The divisions include three types of soldier: members of the People's Militia; conscripts and the regular army volunteer. Equipment includes 100 T-62, 600 T-54/-55, 20 T-34 and 30 M-47 tanks.

Navy. The Navy, almost all of Soviet origin, consists nominally of 2 small frigates,

8 fast missile craft, 6 fast torpedo craft and 6 patrol craft. There are also 2 medium landing ships and 6 craft. Major auxiliaries comprise 1 transport and a training ship.

The main base and training establishments were at Massawa, and there are other bases at Assab, and in the Dahlak Islands. Since Massawa was in the hands of the Eritrean People's Liberation Front in 1991, and the condition of the ships is poor because of inadequate operating funds and limited maintenance facilities, the effectiveness of the force is in doubt.

Personnel in 1990 are believed to have numbered 1,800.

Air Force. President Mengistu's authority as Commander in Chief of the Armed Forces is passed through the Defence Minister to the Air Force Commander at Debre Zeyit Air Base. The Air Force has expanded from 53 assorted aircraft and 2,100 men in 1973 to over 350 aircraft and 4,500 men in 1988. There are fighter, transport, trainer, reconnaissance and air rescue units at Debre Zeyit and fighter units only at Asmara, Gode, Dire Dawa and Deke airfields. Prior to the large-scale Soviet supply of equipment, Ethiopia received arms from the United States, but the US-supplied fighters, reconnaissance aircraft and trainers are very short of spares and are rarely flown. The large quantities of late-model MIG-21 and MIG–23 fighters and AN-12/AN-26 transports are thought to be in fair operating condition.

INTERNATIONAL RELATIONS

Membership. Ethiopia is a member of the UN, OAU and is an ACP state of the EEC.

ECONOMY

Policy. The economy is centrally planned and organized. GDP growth 1974–85 averaged 1·2%.

Budget. Revenue for 1985–86 was EB4,356m. and expenditure EB4,392m.

Of the estimated revenue in 1985–86, EB1,620m. came from taxes.

Currency. The *Ethiopian birr* (ETB), of 100 *cents*, is the unit of currency; it is based on 5·52 grains of fine gold. It consists of notes of EB1, 2, 10, 50 and 100 denominations, and bronze 1-, 5-, 10-, 25- and 50-cent coins. In March 1991 *birr* 3·90 = £1 sterling; *birr* 2·05 = US$1.

Banking and Finance. The State Bank is the National Bank of Ethiopia. The Investment Bank of Ethiopia, was established in 1963 with a capital of EB10m., of which the Government held the majority of shares. In Sept. 1965 it became the Ethiopian Investment Corporation, which is a substantial shareholder in a number of industrial and other ventures. There is also the Agricultural and Industrial Development Bank, SC.

On 1 Jan. 1975 the Government nationalized all banks, mortgage and insurance companies.

Weights and Measures. The metric system of weights and measures is officially in use. Traditional weights and measures vary considerably in the various provinces: the principal ones are: *Frasilla* = approximately 37½ lb.; *gasha*, the principal unit of land measure, which is normally about 100 acres but can vary between 80 and 300 acres, depending on the quality of the land.

ENERGY AND NATURAL RESOURCES

Electricity. Production in 1986 totalled 722m. kwh. Supply 220 volts; 50 Hz. Over 92% of energy supply is from firewood, charcoal, dung and crop residues. The main power source is hydro-electricity although imported fuel supplies 22% of public power systems.

Oil. A Soviet built state-owned oil refinery at Assab came on stream in 1967 with a capacity of 750,000 tonnes of crude per annum.

Minerals. Ethiopia has little proved mineral wealth. Salt is produced mainly in Eritrea, while a placer goldmine is worked by the Government of Adola in the south. Gold production, in 1985–86, was 923 kg. A new mine was under development at Lega Dembi in 1989. Small quantities of other minerals are produced including platinum.

Agriculture. In 1990 farmers were permitted to vote on the dissolution of co-operatives. Land remains the property of the state, but individuals are granted rights of usage which can be passed to their children, and produce may be sold on the open market instead of compulsorily to the state Agriculture Marketing Corporation at low fixed prices.

Coffee is by far the most important source of rural income. Teff (*Eragrastis abyssinica*) is the principal food grain, followed by barley, wheat, maize and durra. Cane sugar is an important crop.

Production (1988 in 1,000 tonnes): Maize, 1,650; sorghum, 1,100; barley, 1,050; pulses, 987.

Livestock (1989): 27m. cattle, 26m. sheep, 17m. goats; smaller numbers of donkeys, horses, mules and camels. Hides and skins and butter (ghee) are important for home consumption and export. Sheep, cattle and chickens are the main providers of meat. In 1989 85% of the population were engaged in agriculture, producing 43% of GDP. The droughts of 1989–90 have brought famine.

Forestry. In 1988 forests covered 27·4m. ha, representing 25% of the land area. Sawnwood production (1983) 45,000 cu. metres.

Fisheries. Catch (1986) 4,100 tonnes.

INDUSTRY. Industrial output is controlled by the State and most public industrial enterprizes are controlled by the Ministry of Industry. Most individual activity is centred around Addis Ababa and Asmara, although Asmara has been severely hit by the civil war in Eritrea.

FOREIGN ECONOMIC RELATIONS

Commerce. Imports and exports (in EB1m.) for 4 years.

	1983	*1984*	*1985*	*1986*
Imports	1,810	1,601	1,734	1,822
Exports	863	866	689	702

Coffee exports accounted for 90% of foreign earnings in 1989.

Total trade between Ethiopia and UK (British Department of Trade returns, in £1,000 sterling):

	1986	*1987*	*1988*	*1989*	*1990*
Imports to UK	22,343	12,875	8,451	12,772	19,465
Exports and re-exports from UK	50,049	46,146	47,661	44,148	41,403

Tourism. There were 59,000 tourists in 1986. This figure has substantially decreased due to the civil war and general unrest.

COMMUNICATIONS

Roads. There were (1989) 3,508 km of ashphalt roads and 9,687 km of rural and gravel roads.

Motor vehicles (1984): Cars, 41,300; lorries and trucks, 8,800; buses, 3,041.

Railways. The former Franco-Ethiopian Railway Co. (782 km, metre-gauge) became the Ethiopian-Djibouti Railway Corp. in 1981, when the remaining France-owned shares were bought out. In 1989 the railway carried 128m. tonne-km of freight and 297m. passenger-km.

Aviation. Ethiopian Air Lines, formed in 1946, carried 470,000 passengers in 1988, using Boeing 767s on its long-haul flights. There are international airports at Addis Ababa, Dire Dawa and Asmara (the latter closed to international traffic because of the civil war in Eritrea).

Shipping. A state shipping line was established in 1964. The ports unloaded 1·75m. tonnes in 1982 and loaded 547,000.

Telecommunications. The postal system serves 301 offices, mainly by air-mail. All the main centres are connected with Addis Ababa by telephone or radio telegraph. International telephone services are available at certain hours to most countries in Europe, North America and India. Number of telephones (1986), 162,000.

The Ethiopian Broadcasting Service makes sound broadcasts on the medium and short waves in English, Amharic and in the vernacular languages spoken within the country. There were about 45,000 television sets and 2m. radio receivers in 1986.

Cinemas (1974). There were 31 cinemas, with seating capacity of about 25,600.

Newspapers. There were (1991) 4 government-controlled daily newspapers with a combined circulation of about 60,000.

JUSTICE, RELIGION, EDUCATION AND WELFARE

Justice. The legal system is said to be based on the Justinian Code. A new penal code came into force in 1958 and Special Penal Law in 1974. Codes of criminal procedure, civil, commercial and maritime codes have since been promulgated.

The extra-territorial rights formerly enjoyed by foreigners have been abolished, but any person accused in an Ethiopian court has the right to have his case transferred to the High Court, provided he asks for this before any evidence has been taken in the court of first instance.

Provincial and district courts have been established, and High Court judges visit the provincial courts on circuit. The Supreme Court at Addis Ababa is presided over by the Chief Justice.

Religion. About 45% of the population are Moslem and 40% Christian, mainly belonging to the Ethiopian Orthodox Church.

Education. Primary education commences at 7 years and continues with optional secondary education at 13 years. In the academic year 1988–89 there were more than 2·5m. pupils in primary schools and in secondary schools there were 500,000 students. Higher education is co-ordinated under the National University, chartered in 1961; in 1979–80, there were 14,562 students. The University College, the Engineering, Building and Theological Colleges are in Addis Ababa, the Agricultural College in Harar and the Public Health College in Gondar.

Adult literacy was 62·5% in 1990.

Health. In 1987 there were about 90 hospitals with 11,000 beds.

DIPLOMATIC REPRESENTATIVES

Of Ethiopia in Great Britain (17 Prince's Gate, London, SW7 1PZ)
Ambassador: Ato Teferra Haile-Selassie (accredited 24 June 1985).

Of Great Britain in Ethiopia (Fikre Mariam Abatechan St., Addis Ababa)
Ambassador: M. J. C. Glaze, CMG.

Of Ethiopia in the USA (2134 Kalorama Rd., NW, Washington D.C., 20008)
Chargé d'Affaires: Girma Amare.

Of the USA in Ethiopia (Entoto St., Addis Ababa)
Chargé d'Affaires: James R. Cheek.

Of Ethiopia to the United Nations
Ambassador: Tesfaye Tadesse.

Further Reading

Clapham, C., *Transformation and Continuity in Revolutionary Ethiopia*. CUP, 1988
Halliday, F. and Molyneaux, M., *The Ethiopian Revolution*. London, 1981
Hancock, G., *Ethiopia: The Challenge of Hunger*. London, 1985
Keller, E. J. *Revolutionary Ethiopia: From Empire to People's Republic*. Indiana Univ. Press, 1989
Monro-Hay, S. and Pankhurst, R., *Ethiopia:* [Bibliography]. Oxford and Santa Barbara, 1991
Pool, D., *Eritrea: Africa's Longest War*. London, 1982
Schwab, P., *Ethiopia: Politics, Economics and Society*. Boulder, 1985.

FALKLAND ISLANDS

Capital: Stanley
Population: 1,916 (1986)

HISTORY. France established a settlement in 1764 and Britain a second settlement in 1765. In 1770 Spain bought out the French and drove off the British. This action on the part of Spain brought that country and Britain to the verge of war. The Spanish restored the settlement to the British in 1771, but the settlement was withdrawn on economic grounds in 1774. In 1806 Spanish rule was overthrown in Argentina, and the Argentine claimed to succeed Spain in the French and British settlements in 1820. The British objected and reclaimed their settlement in 1832 as a Crown Colony.

On 2 April 1982 Argentine forces invaded the Falkland Islands and the Governor was expelled. At a meeting of the UN Security Council, held on 3 April, the voting was 10 to 1 in favour of the resolution calling for Argentina to withdraw. Britain regained possession on 14–15 June after Argentina surrendered.

In April 1990 Argentina's Congress declared the Falkland and other British-held South Atlantic islands part of the new Argentine province of Tierra del Fuego.

AREA AND POPULATION. The Crown Colony is situated in the South Atlantic Ocean about 480 miles north-east of Cape Horn. The numerous islands cover 4,700 sq. miles. The main East Falkland Island, 2,610 sq. miles; the West Falkland, 2,090 sq. miles, including the adjacent small islands. The open country is called 'The Camp'.

The population of the Falkland Islands at census 1986 was 1,916. The only town is Stanley, in East Falkland, with a population of just over 1,200. The population of the Falkland Islands is nearly all of British descent, with about 67% born in the islands. A large garrison of British servicemen was stationed near Stanley in 1987.

CLIMATE. A cool temperate climate, much affected by strong winds, particularly in spring. Stanley. Jan. 49°F (9·4°C), July 35°F (1·7°C). Annual rainfall 27" (681 mm).

CONSTITUTION AND GOVERNMENT. A new Constitution came into force on 3 Oct. 1985. This incorporated a chapter protecting fundamental human rights and in the preamble recalled the provisions on the right of self-determination contained in international covenants.

Executive power is vested in the Governor who must consult the Executive Council except on urgent or trivial matters. He must consult the Commander British Forces on matters relating to defence and internal security (except police).

There is a Legislative Council consisting of 8 elected members and 2 *ex officio* members, the Chief Executive and Financial Secretary. Only elected members have a vote. The Commander British Forces has a right to attend and take part in its proceedings but has no vote. The Attorney General also has a similar right to take part in proceedings with the consent of the person presiding. The Governor presides over sittings. He also presides over sittings of the Executive Council which consists of 3 elected members (elected by and from the elected members of Legislative Council) and the Chief Executive and Financial Secretary (*ex officio*). The Commander British Forces and Attorney General have a right to attend but may not vote.

Offices in the Public Service are constituted by the Governor and he makes appointments and is responsible for discipline. The Constitution allows for the establishment of a public service commission.

Governor: W. H. Fullerton, CMG.
Chief Executive: R. Sampson.
Financial Secretary: J. H. Buckland-James.
Attorney General: D. G. Lang.
Government Secretary: C. F. Redston.

Flag: British Blue Ensign with arms of Colony on a white disc in the fly.

DEFENCE. Since 1982 the Islands have been defended by a large garrison of British servicemen. The Commander British Forces is responsible for all military matters in the Islands. He liaises with the Governor on civilian and political matters, and advises him on matters of defence and internal security, except police. In addition there is a local volunteer defence force.

ECONOMY

Policy. The Falkland Islands Development Corporation was established by statute in June 1984 with the aim of encouraging economic development. The first projects assisted by the Corporation include inshore and offshore fisheries surveys to establish potential catch size and value, agricultural improvement schemes to encourage investment in the land, a wool spinning and knitting factory to process a portion of the islands' main product, a new dairy and a hydroponic market garden.

Budget. Revenue and expenditure (in £ sterling) for fiscal years ending 30 June:

	1983–84	*1984–85*	*1985–86*	*1986–87*	*1987–88* [1]	*1988–89* [1]
Revenue	5,314,000	5,163,000	6,003,315	19,646,310	22,774,680	35,761,900
Expenditure	3,867,000	4,358,000	5,344,048	12,212,805	21,968,150	28,646,190

[1] Estimate

Revenue from licences to fish illex squid is a major component, amounting to some £30m. in 1990.

Currency. The unit of currency is the *Falkland Islands pound* (FKP) of 100 *pence*, at parity with £1 sterling.

Banking. The Standard Chartered Bank provides a full range of banking facilities.

Agriculture. The economy was formerly based solely on agriculture, principally sheep farming; much of the land area is divided into large sheep runs. Subdivision into smaller family units is actively being pursued. There were 78 farms in 1991. In Feb. 1991 it was announced that the Falklands Islands Co. was to sell its agricultural holdings, about 27% of the total area. Wool is the principal product, but hides are exported. In 1988 there were 704,602 sheep, 5,969 cattle and 1,837 horses in the islands.

Fisheries. Since the establishment of a 150-mile interim conservation and management zone around the Islands in 1986 and the consequent introduction, on 1 Feb. 1987, of a licensing regime for vessels fishing within the zone, income from the associated fishing activities is now the largest source of revenue.

On 26 Dec. 1990 the UK and Argentina agreed to enforce a ban on fishing in further 50-mile semi-circular area to the east of this zone. A UK-Argentine South Atlantic Fisheries Commission was set up in 1990; it meets at least twice a year. Some 0·5m. tonnes of illex squid are caught annually.

TRADE. Total trade between the Falkland Islands and UK (British Department of Trade returns, in £1,000 sterling):

	1987	*1988*	*1989*	*1990*
Imports to UK	8,148	4,209	5,375	4,817
Exports and re-exports from UK	7,353	9,037	10,200	11,309

COMMUNICATIONS

Roads. There are 27 km of made-up roads in and around Stanley and another 54 km of all-weather road between Stanley and Mount Pleasant Airport. Other settlements outside Stanley are linked by tracks, which are passable, with high axle clearing four-wheel drive vehicles in all but the worst weather. Work has recently recommenced on the construction of an all-weather track linking the Estancia Farm with the Stanley to Mount Pleasant Road which help towards opening up the north of East Falkland. The Government is also providing assistance to farms which wish to improve tracks and bridges to their immediate area.

Aviation. Air communication is currently via Ascension Island. A new airport, completed in 1986, is sited at Mount Pleasant on East Falkland. RAF Tristar aircraft operate a twice-weekly service between the Falklands and the UK. Internal air links are provided by the government-operated air service, which carries passengers, mail, freight and medical patients between the settlements and Stanley on non-scheduled flights in Islander aircraft. A Chilean airline runs a fortnightly service to Punta Arenas.

Shipping. A charter vessel calls 4 or 5 times a year to/from the UK. There is occasional direct communication with South Georgia, the South Sandwich Islands and British Antarctic Territory by research ships and the ice-patrol vessel HMS *Endurance*. Vessels of the Royal Fleet Auxiliary run regularly to South Georgia. Sea links with Chile and Uruguay began in 1989.

Telecommunications. Number of telephones (1987) 560. International direct dialling is available, as are international telex and facsimile links. Cable and Wireless plc signed a contract with the Falkland Islands Government in Sept. 1988 for the complete replacement of the telecommunications network with a modern system. There is a government-operated broadcasting station at Stanley and television broadcasts began in 1988.

JUSTICE, EDUCATION AND WELFARE

Justice. There is a Supreme Court, and a Court of Appeal sits in the United Kingdom; appeals may go from that court to the judicial committee of the Privy Council. Judges have security of tenure and may only be removed for inability or misbehaviour on the advice of the judicial committee of the Privy Council. The senior resident judicial officer is the Senior Magistrate. There is an Attorney General and a Crown Counsel and a firm of solicitors established an office in Stanley in 1988.

Education. Education is compulsory between the ages of 5 and 15 years. In Sept. 1989 there were 375 children receiving education in the Colony. Almost 75% attended schools in Stanley, the others were taught in settlement schools or by itinerant teachers. Expenditure on education and training from own funds 1988-89 was £1,031,050.

Health. The Government Medical Department is responsible for all medical services to civilians. Expenditure (1988-89) £1,224,440. The Chief Medical Officer advises the Government on policy, and is chairman of the Board of Health responsible for public health. Medical services for the Islands are run from a temporary hospital; a new hospital and some sheltered accommodation was completed in March 1987. Services include all primary care for Stanley and the flying doctor service for outlying farm settlements.

WILD LIFE. The Falkland Islands are noted for their outstanding wild life, including penguin and seal. Four Nature Reserves have been declared and 18 Wild Animal and Bird Sanctuaries gazetted. The brown trout introduced between 1947 and 1952 can now be found in nearly all the rivers and there are good runs of sea-trout during spring and autumn.

Further Reading

Falkland Islands: The Facts. HMSO, London, 1982
Falkland Islands Journal. Stanley, from 1967
Falkland Islands Review [Franks Report] Cmnd. 8787. HMSO, London, 1983
Falklands/Malvinas, Whose Crisis? Latin American Bureau, London, 1982
Calvert, P., *The Falklands Crisis: The Rights and the Wrongs*. London, 1982
Hanrahan, B. and Fox, R., *'I counted them all out and I counted them all back'*. London, 1982
Hastings, M. and Jenkins, S., *The Battle for the Falklands*. London, 1983
Hoffmann, F. L. and Hoffmann, O. M., *Sovereignty in Dispute*. London, 1984
Phipps, C., *What Future for the Falklands?* London, 1977
Shackleton, E., *Falkland Islands Economic Study 1982*. HMSO, London, 1982
Strange, I. J., *The Falkland Islands*. 3rd ed. Newton Abbot, 1983.—*The Falkland Islands and their Natural History*. Newton Abbot, 1987

FIJI

Capital: Suva
Population: 727,104 (1989)
GNP per capita: US$1,540 (1988)

Republic of Fiji

HISTORY. The first European discovery of the Fiji Islands was by the Dutch navigator Abel Tasman in 1643, and they were recorded in detail by Capt. Bligh after the mutiny of the *Bounty* (1789). In the 19th century the search for sandalwood, in which enormous profits were made, brought many ships. The influence of the deserters, shipwrecked sailors and missionaries who settled on the islands disrupted the pattern of life of the indigenous Fijians and gave rise to inter-tribal wars until Fiji was ceded to Britain on 10 Oct. 1874. Fiji became an independent state within the Commonwealth on 10 Oct. 1970. Following the electoral defeat of the Fijian-dominated National Alliance Party by an Indian-supported coalition in April 1987, Brig. Sitiveni Rabuka seized power after two coups, and declared Fiji a republic in Oct.; membership of the Commonwealth lapsed.

AREA AND POPULATION. Fiji comprises about 332 islands and islets (about 110 inhabited) lying between 15° and 22° S. lat. and 174° E. and 177° W. long. The largest is Viti Levu, area 10,429 sq. km (4,027 sq. miles), next is Vanua Levu, area 5,556 sq. km (2,145 sq. miles). The island of Rotuma (47 sq. km, 18 sq. miles), about 12° 30' S. lat., 178° E. long., was added to the colony in 1881. Total area, 7,078 sq. miles (18,333 sq. km).

A population census is taken every 10 years. Total population (census, Aug. 1986), 715,375; average annual increase about 2%. The 1989 estimated total population of 727,104 consisted of the following: 351,966 (48·4%) Fijians; 337,557 (46·4%) Indians (whose ancestors had been introduced as field workers by the British); 37,581 (5·2%) were of other races.

Suva, the capital, is on the south coast of Viti Levu; population (census, 1986), 71,608. Suva was proclaimed a city on 2 Oct. 1953. Lautoka had 28,728 in 1986.

Vital statistics, 1987: Crude birth rate per 1,000 population, Fijian, 30·7, Indian, 25·6; crude death rate per 1,000 population, Fijian, 5·4, Indian, 5·2. Average life expectancy (1989) 68 years.

CLIMATE. A tropical climate, but oceanic influences prevent undue extremes of heat or humidity. The S.E. Trades blow from May to Nov., during which time nights are cool and rainfall amounts least. Suva. Jan. 80°F (26·7°C), July 73°F (22·8°C). Annual rainfall 117" (2,974 mm).

CONSTITUTION AND GOVERNMENT. On 25 July 1990 a new constitution was promulgated giving 'indigenous Fijians' the right to hold the prime ministership and a guaranteed 37 seats in the 70-seat House of Representatives. Fijian citizens of Indian descent have 27 seats, other races 5, and the Polynesian island of Rotuma, 1. The Upper House has 24 seats for Fijians, 9 for other races and 1 for Rotuma.

President: Ratu Sir Penaia Ganilau, GCMG, KCVO, KBE, DSO.

Prime Minister and Minister for Home and Foreign Affairs: Ratu Sir Kamisese Mara, GCMG, KBE.

Attorney-General and Justice: Sailosi Kepa. *Finance and Economic Planning:* Josevata Kamikamica. *Education, Youth and Sport:* Filipe Bole. *Primary Industries and Co-operatives:* Viliame Gonelevu. *Health:* Dr Apenisa Kurisaqila. *Indian Affairs:* Irene Jai Narayan. *Fijian Affairs and Rural Development:* Col. Vatiliai Navunisaravi. *Tourism, Civil Aviation and Energy:* David Pickering. *Women and Social Welfare:* Adi Finau Tabakaucoro. *Forests:* Ratu Sir Josaia Tavaiqia. *Lands and Mineral Resources:* Ratu William Toganivalu. *Infrastructure and Public Utilities:* Apisai Tora. *Housing and Urban Development:* Tomasi Vakatora. *Employment and Industrial Relations:* Taniela Veitata. *Trade and Commerce:*

Berenado Vunibobo. *Information, Broadcasting, Television and Telecommunications:* Ratu Inoke Kubuabola.

Flag: Light blue with the Union Flag in the canton and the shield of Fiji in the fly.

Local Government. Fiji is divided into 14 provinces, each with its own council under which 188 Tikina Councils have been established. The number of Tikina Councils within a province varies from 4 to 22. Tikina Councils have wide powers to make by-laws and levy rates to raise revenue. 50% of the rates collected is credited to the Provincial Council treasury for the running of the Council and 50% is used for the financing of the Tikina and village projects.

DEFENCE. The Fiji Military Forces are for the defence of Fiji, maintenance of law and order and provision of forces to international peace-keeping agencies overseas. The forces have two overseas battalions (in Egypt and Lebanon) and regular and territorial units at home. Total active strength (1991), 4,700 (reserves, 5,000).

Navy. A naval division of the armed forces was formed in 1974 to perform miscellaneous offshore duties. Present strength is 3 ex-US coastal patrol craft (1 with a helicopter deck) and 2 inshore craft. There is also 1 survey ship. Naval personnel in 1990 numbered 300. The naval base is in Suva.

INTERNATIONAL RELATIONS

Membership. Fiji is a member of the UN, the Colombo Plan, the South Pacific Forum and is an ACP state of the EEC.

ECONOMY

Budget. The financial year corresponds with the calendar year. All figures are in $1m. Fijian.

	1985	*1986*	*1987*	*1988*	*1989*
Revenue	349·9	348·1	341·2	389·7	390·0
Expenditure	349·3	370·9	393·9	434·6	539·0

Currency. The unit of currency is the *Fiji dollar* (FJD) of 100 *cents.* In March 1991, £1 = $F2·74; US$ = $F1·44.

Banking and Finance. The National Bank of Fiji had, in 1985, deposits amounting to $F62·3m. due to 241,375 accounts. The headquarters are at Suva, and there are 11 branches, 35 postal agencies and 9 private agencies throughout Fiji. The Westpac Banking Corporation has 9 branches, 2 sub-branches and 18 agencies; the Bank of New Zealand has 8 branches, and 18 agencies; the Australia and New Zealand Bank has 9 branches and 7 agencies and the Bank of Baroda has 8 branches and 3 agencies in Fiji.

ENERGY AND NATURAL RESOURCES

Electricity. Production (1986) 220m. kwh. Supply 240 volts; 50 Hz.

Agriculture. Some 600,000 acres of land are in agricultural use. Sugar-cane is the principal cash crop (production, 1988, 3·1m. tonnes); one quarter of the population depend on it directly for their livelihood. Copra, Fiji's second major cash crop (output, 1988, 13,000 tonnes), provides coconut oil and other products for export. Ginger is the third major export crop replacing bananas which has declined through disease and hurricane. Production, 1988 (in 1,000 tonnes): Rice, 31; maize, 2; fruit, 23; vegetables, 10. Tobacco and cocoa are also cultivated. There is a small, but fast developing, livestock industry.

Livestock (1988): Cattle, 159,000; horses, 42,000; goats, 60,000; pigs, 29,000; poultry, 2m.

Forestry. In 1987 there were 1·2m. ha of forests and woodland; 65% of the land area. Fiji supplies the bulk of its own timber requirements. A comprehensive pine scheme has been implemented.

Fisheries. Catch (1985) 15,900 tonnes. Exports (1986) F$20m.

INDUSTRY. Major industries include 4 large sugar-mills, the goldmines (2,647 kg in 1987) and 2 mills which process copra into coconut oil and coconut meal. There is a great variety of light industries.

Trade Unions. In 1987 there were 46 trade unions operating with about 45,000 members.

FOREIGN ECONOMIC RELATIONS

Commerce. Exports in 1987, $F408,815,000 (including re-exports). Imports, $F465,583,000. Exports in 1989 were worth US$388m. Chief exports, 1989: Sugar, 36%, gold, 13%, clothing, 9% and canned fish, 7%.

Total trade between Fiji and UK (British Department of Trade returns, in £1,000 sterling):

	1986	*1987*	*1988*	*1989*	*1990*
Imports to UK	66,500	53,062	65,273	69,558	61,863
Exports and re-exports from UK	8,775	7,381	6,358	10,221	8,168

Tourism. In 1988, there were 208,155 visitors. Earnings (1988) $F180·6m. There were some 0·25m. visitors in 1989.

COMMUNICATIONS

Roads. Total road mileage is 2,996, of which 376 are sealed (paved), 2,534 are gravelled and 86 are unimproved. In 1987, there were 70,206 vehicles including 29,262 private cars, 23,029 goods vehicles, 1,289 buses, 4,499 tractors, 2,236 taxis and 2,882 rental and hire cars and others.

Railway. Fiji Sugar Cane Corporation runs 600 mm gauge railways at four of its mills on Viti Levu and Vanua Levu, totalling 595 km.

Aviation. Fiji provides an essential staging point for long-haul trunk-route aircraft operating between North America, Australia and New Zealand. Under the South Pacific Air Transport Council, which comprises the UK, Australia, New Zealand and Fiji, the international airport at Nadi has been developed and administered. Eighteen other airports are in use for domestic services. In 1985, 257,646 passengers arrived at airports.

Shipping. The 3 ports of entry are Suva, Lautoka and Leuuka. In 1985, 1,313 vessels called at Suva, 780 at Lautoka and 1,004 at Leuuka. Local shipping provides services to scattered outer islands of the group.

Telecommunications. There were (1988) 50 post offices and 185 postal agencies. Overseas telephone and telegram services are available through the Commonwealth cable to most countries except those in the South Pacific, which are served by direct radio circuits. The automatic telex network operates through New Zealand into the international telex system. There are ship-to-shore radio facilities. There were 60,017 telephones in 1987. In 1983 there were 400,000 radio receivers.

Newspapers. In 1988 there were 2 daily newspapers (circulation 40,000).

JUSTICE, RELIGION, EDUCATION AND WELFARE

Justice. An independent Judiciary is guaranteed under the Constitution of Fiji. The Constitution allows for a High Court of Fiji which has unlimited original jurisdiction to hear and determine any civil or criminal proceedings under any law.

The High Court also has jurisdiction to hear and determine constitutional and electoral questions including the membership of members of the House of Representatives.

The Chief Justice of Fiji is appointed by the President acting after consultation with the Prime Minister.

The Fiji Court of Appeal of which the Chief Justice is *ex officio* President is formed by three specially appointed Justices of Appeal. The Justices of Appeal are appointed by the President acting after consultation with the Judicial and Legal Services Commission. Generally any person convicted of any offence has a right of appeal from the High Court to the Fiji Court of Appeal. The final appellant court is the Supreme Court. Most matters coming before the Superior Courts originate in Magistrates' Courts.

Police. The Royal Fiji Police Force had (1987) a total strength of 1,561.

Religion. The 1986 census showed: Christians, 378,452; Hindus, 273,088; Sikhs, 4,674; Moslems, 56,001; Confucians, 82.

Education (1987). School attendance is not compulsory in Fiji. There were 815 schools scattered over 56 islands, staffed by 7,082 teachers, of whom about 99·3% were trained. There were also 236 pre-schools. The 674 primary and 141 secondary schools had 180,514 pupils. The technical and vocational schools had 4,039 students and the teachers' college 205. There were 3 teacher-training colleges, 1 medical and 2 agricultural schools.

The University of the South Pacific (USP) opened in Feb. 1968 at Laucala Bay in Suva. In 1987 there were about 2,344 students enrolled in courses on campus and about 4,085 enrolments in extension services. The University has an operating budget of $F12·13m. a year provided by the 11 countries it serves.

Total government expenditure on education in 1987 (including USP) was $F76,184,852.

Health. In 1987 there were 25 hospitals with 1,721 beds, 271 doctors, 48 dentists and 1,543 nurses.

DIPLOMATIC REPRESENTATIVES

Of Fiji in Great Britain (34 Hyde Park Gate, London, SW7 5DN)
Ambassador: Brig.-Gen. Ratu Epeli Nailatikau, LVO, OBE.

Of Great Britain in Fiji (47 Gladstone Rd., Suva)
Ambassador: A. B. Peter Smart, CMG.

Of Fiji in the USA (2233 Wisconsin Ave., NW, Washington, D.C., 20007)
Chargé d'Affaires: Abdul Yusuf.

Of the USA in Fiji (31 Loftus St., Suva)
Ambassador: Evelyn I. H. Teegen.

Of Fiji to the United Nations
Ambassador: Winston Thompson.

Further Reading

Statistical Information: A Bureau of Statistics was set up in 1950 (Government Buildings, Suva).
Trade Report. Annual (from 1887 [covering 1883–86]). Bureau of Statistics, Suva.
Journal of the Fiji Legislative Council. Annual (from 1914 [under different title from 1885]). Suva
Fiji Today. Suva, Annual
Fiji Facts and Figures. Suva, 1986
Report of Commission of Inquiry Into Natural Resources and Population Trends in Fiji. Suva, Government Press, 1960
Ali, A., *Plantations to Politics, studies on Fiji Indians.* Suva, 1980
Bain, K., *Fiji at the Crossroads.* London, 1989
Capell, A., *New Fijian Dictionary.* 2nd ed. Glasgow, 1957
Ravuvu, A., *Vaka i Taukei: The Fijian Way of Life.* Suva, 1983
Scarr, D., *Fiji, A Short History.* Sydney, 1984
Wright, R., *On Fiji Islands.* London, 1987

FINLAND

Capital: Helsinki
Population: 4·97m. (1989)
GNP per capita: US$23,196 (1989)

Suomen Tasavalta—Republiken Finland

HISTORY. Since the Middle Ages Finland was a part of the realm of Sweden. In the 18th century parts of south-eastern Finland were conquered by Russia, and the rest of the country was ceded to Russia by the peace treaty of Hamina in 1809. Finland became an autonomous grand-duchy which retained its previous laws and institutions under its Grand Duke, the Emperor of Russia. After the Russian revolution Finland declared itself independent on 6 Dec. 1917. The Civil War began in Jan. 1918 between the 'whites' and 'reds', the latter being supported by Russian bolshevik troops. The defeat of the red guards in May 1918 consequently meant freeing the country from Russian troops. A peace treaty with Soviet Russia was signed in 1920.

On 30 Nov. 1939 Soviet troops invaded Finland, after Finland had rejected territorial concessions demanded by the USSR. These, however, had to be made in the peace treaty of 12 March 1940, amounting to 32,806 sq. km and including the Carelian Isthmus, Viipuri and the shores of Lake Ladoga.

When the German attack on the USSR was launched in June 1941 Finland again became involved in the war against the USSR. On 19 Sept. 1944 an armistice was signed in Moscow. Finland agreed to cede to Russia the Petsamo area in addition to cessions made in 1940 (total 42,934 sq. km) and to lease to Russia for 50 years the Porkkala headland to be used as a military base. Further, Finland undertook to pay 300m. gold dollars in reparations within 6 years (later extended to 8 years). The peace treaty was signed in Paris on 10 Feb. 1947. The payment of reparations was completed on 19 Sept. 1952. The military base of Porkkala was returned to Finland on 26 Jan. 1956.

AREA AND POPULATION. Finland is bounded north-west and north by Norway, east by the USSR, south by the Baltic Sea and west by the Gulf of Bothnia and Sweden. The area and the population of Finland on 31 Dec. 1989 (Swedish names in brackets):

Province	*Area (sq. km)* [1]	*Population* [2]	*Population per sq. km* [2]
Uusimaa (Nyland)	9,898	1,235,460	124·8
Turku-Pori (Åbo-Björneborg)	22,170	716,639	32·3
Ahvenanmaa (Åland)	1,527	24,231	15·9
Häme (Tavastehus)	17,010	688,267	40·5
Kymi (Kymmene)	10,783	335,466	31·1
Mikkeli (St Michel)	16,342	208,156	12·7
Pohjois-Karjala (Norra Karelen)	17,782	176,566	9·9
Kuopio	16,509	256,381	15·5
Keski-Suomi (Mellersta Finland)	16,230	251,206	15·5
Vaasa (Vasa)	26,447	444,624	16·8
Oulu (Uleåborg)	56,868	437,414	7·7
Lappi (Lappland)	93,057	199,973	2·1
Total	304,623	4,974,383	16·3

[1] Excluding inland water area which totals 33,522 sq. km. [2] Resident population.

The growth of the population, which was 421,500 in 1750, has been:

End of year	*Urban*	*Rural*	*Total*	*Percentage urban*
1800	46,600	786,100	832,700	5·6
1900	333,300	2,322,600	2,655,900	12·5
1950	1,302,400	2,727,400	4,029,800	32·3
1960	1,707,000	2,739,200	4,446,200	38·4
1970	2,340,300	2,258,000	4,598,300	50·9
1980	2,865,100	1,922,700	4,787,800	59·8
1989	3,067,000	1,907,400	4,974,400	61·7

The population on 31 Dec. 1988 by language primarily spoken: Finnish, 4,638,941; Swedish, 297,155; other languages, 16,535; Lappish, 1,728.

The principal towns with resident census population, 31 Dec. 1989, are (Swedish names in brackets):

Helsinki (Helsingfors)—capital	490,629	Kajaani	36,099
(metropolitan area)	993,704	Kokkola (Gamlakarleby)	34,566
Tampere (Tammerfors)	171,561	Imatra	33,832
(metropolitan area)	261,914	Rovaniemi	33,041
Turku (Åbo)	159,469	Mikkeli (St Michel)	31,785
(metropolitan area)	264,854	Kouvola	31,632
Espoo (Esbo)	169,851	Järvenpää	30,819
Vantaa (Vanda)	152,262	Rauma (Raumo)	29,937
Oulu (Uleåborg)	100,281	Savonlinna (Nyslott)	28,524
Lahti	93,132	Seinäjoki	27,505
Kuopio	80,002	Kerava	27,155
Pori (Björneborg)	76,456	Nokia	25,807
Jyväskylä	66,387	Kemi	25,565
Kotka	65,933	Riihimäki	24,880
Lappeenranta (Villmanstrand)	54,804	Varkaus	24,596
Vaasa (Vasa)	53,364	Iisalmi	23,830
Joensuu	47,204	Tornio	22,698
Hämeenlinna (Tavastehus)	43,098	Valkeakoski	22,042
Hyvinkää (Hyvinge)	39,992	Kuusankoski	21,788

Vital statistics in calendar years:

	Living births	*Of which illegitimate*	*Still-born*	*Marriages*	*Deaths (exclusive of still-born)*	*Emigration*
1982	66,106	9,007	263	30,459	43,408	7,403
1983	66,076	9,386	268	29,474	45,388	6,822
1984	65,076	9,825	260	28,550	45,098	7,467
1985	62,796	10,931	241	25,751	48,198	7,739
1986	60,632	10,292	193	25,820	47,135	8,269
1987	59,827	11,467	314	26,267	47,949	8,475
1988	63,313	...	334	26,453	49,026	8,447
1989	63,388	...	...	25,043	49,072	11,086

In 1988 the rate per 1,000 was: Births, 12·8; marriages, 5; deaths, 9·8, and infantile deaths (per 1,000 live births), 6·1.

Population Census 1985. 5 vols. Helsinki, 1988
Population. Annual. Helsinki

CLIMATE. The climate is severe in winter, which lasts about 6 months, but mean temperatures in south and south-west are less harsh, 21°F (–6°C). In the north, mean temperatures may fall to 8·5°F (–13°C). Snow covers the ground for three months in the south and for over six months in the far north. Summers are short but quite warm, with occasional very hot days. Precipitation is light throughout the country, with one third falling as snow, the remainder mainly as convectional rain in summer and autumn. Helsinki (Helsingfors). Jan. 21°F (–6°C), July 62°F (16·5°C). Annual rainfall 24·7" (618 mm).

CONSTITUTION AND GOVERNMENT. Finland is a republic according to the Constitution of 17 July 1919.

Parliament consists of one chamber of 200 members chosen by direct and proportional election in which all Finnish citizens (men or women) who are 18 years have the vote (since 1972). The country is divided into 15 electoral districts with a representation proportional to their population. Every citizen over the age of 18 is eligible for Parliament, which is elected for 4 years, but can be dissolved sooner by the President.

The President is elected for 6 years by direct popular vote or, if no presidential candidate wins an absolute majority, by a college of 301 electors, elected by the votes of the citizens in the same way as the members of Parliament.

President of Finland: Dr Mauno Koivisto (elected 1982, re-elected 1988).

State of Parties for Parliament elected on 15–16 March 1987: Conservative 53; Swedish Party, 13 (including 1 for Coalition of Åland); Centre, 40; Rural, 9; Social Democratic Party, 56; People's Democratic League, 16; Christian League, 5; the Greens, 4; Democratic Alternative, 4.

The Council of State (Cabinet), composed as follows in Aug. 1990:

Prime Minister: Harri Holkeri.

Foreign Affairs: Pertti Paasio. *Finance:* Matti Louekoski. *Finance (Deputy):* Ulla Puolanne. *Education:* Ole Norrback. *Education (Deputy):* Anna-Liisa Kasurinen. *Social Affairs and Health:* Mauri Miettinen. *Social Affairs and Health (Deputy):* Tuulikki Hämäläinen. *Justice:* Tarja Halonen. *Agriculture and Forestry:* Toivo T. Pohjala. *Transport and Communication:* Ilkka Kanerva. *Labour:* Matti Puhakka. *Trade and Industry:* Ilkka Suominen. *Defence:* Elisabeth Rehn. *Environment:* Kaj Bärlund. *Interior:* Jarmo Rantanen. *Foreign Trade:* Pertti Salolainen.

National flag: White with a blue Scandinavian cross.

National anthem: Maamme; Swedish: Vårt land (words by J. L. Runeberg, 1843; tune by F. Pacius, 1848).

Finnish and Swedish are the official languages of Finland.

Local Government. For administrative purposes Finland is divided into 12 provinces (*lääni*, Sw.: *län*). The administration of each province is entrusted to a governor (*maaherra*, Sw.: *landshövding*) appointed by the President. He directs the activities of the provincial office (*lääninhallitus*, Sw.: *länsstyrelse*) and of local sheriffs (*nimismies*, Sw.: *länsman*). In 1989 the number of sheriff districts was 224.

The unit of local government is the commune. Main fields of communal activities are local planning, roads and harbours, sanitary services, education, health services and social aid. The communes raise taxes independent from state taxation. Two different kinds of communes are distinguished: Urban communes (*kaupunki*, Sw.: *stad*) and rural communes. In 1990 there were altogether 460 communes of which 94 were urban and 366 rural. In all communes communal councils are elected for terms of 4 years; all inhabitants (men and women) of the commune who have reached their 18th year are entitled to vote and eligible. The executive power is in each commune vested in a board which consists of members elected by the council and one or a few chief officials of the commune. Several communes often form an association for the administration of some common institution, *e.g.*, a hospital or a vocational school.

The autonomous county *(landskap)* of Åland has a county council *(landsting)* of one chamber, elected according to rule corresponding to those for parliamentary elections. In addition to its provincial governor it has a county board with executive power in matters within the field of the autonomy of the county.

Constitution Act and Parliament Act of Finland. Helsinki, 1978

DEFENCE. The period of military training is 240, 285 or 330 days and refresher training obligation 40 to 100 days between conscript service and age 50 (officers and NCOs age 60). Total strength of trained and equipped reserves is about 700,000.

Army. The country is divided into 7 military areas. The Army consisted in 1991 of 1 armoured brigade, 8 infantry brigades, 4 independent infantry battalions, 1 artillery regiment, 2 coastal artillery regiments, 3 independent coastal artillery battalions, 4 anti-aircraft regiments, and 2 engineering battalions, making a total strength, in 1991, of 27,800 (22,300 conscripts).

Navy. The Navy, which operates a mixture of indigenous and Soviet ships and weapons, is divided into 4 functional squadrons. About 50% of the combatant units are kept manned, with the others in short-notice reserve and re-activated on a regular basis. The inventory comprises 2 anti-submarine corvettes, 9 missile craft (of which 4 are indigenous Helsinki class), 11 inshore patrol craft, 2 minelayers, and 6 inshore minesweepers. There are 14 landing craft of various types and some 30 minor auxiliaries and tenders. There are also 9 civil-manned icebreakers.

Naval bases exist at Upinniemi (near Helsinki) and Turku. Total personnel strength (1990) was 1,400 of whom 1,400 are conscripts, and there are about 12,000 reserves.

Air Force. The Air Force has 3 fighter squadrons, 1 transport squadron, an air academy, a technical school, a signal school and a depot. The fighter squadrons have 60 MiG-21bis and Saab J35 Draken S and F aircraft. Other equipment includes 28 Valmet Vinka piston-engined primary trainers of Finnish design, 63 Hawk MK.51, MiG-21U and Saab J35B and C advanced jet trainers, 3 Fokker F.27 Friendship transport aircraft, 3 Gates Learjet 35A/S aircraft, Piper Arrow liaison aircraft, Piper Chieftain utility transports, and 7 Mi-8 and 2 Hughes 500 Ds helicopters. Personnel (1991), 1,800 (800 conscripts) officers and men.

Frontier Guard. Comprises 5 large patrol craft, 9 coastal craft and 34 coastal patrol boats. Personnel (1990) 4,200.

INTERNATIONAL RELATIONS. Finland's role in international relations has been one of neutrality.

Membership. Finland is a member of UN, the Nordic Council, OECD, EFTA and the Council of Europe.

Treaties. A Treaty of friendship, co-operation and mutual assistance between Finland and the USSR was concluded in Moscow on 6 April 1948 for 10 years, extended on 19 Sept. 1955 to cover a period of 20 years, extended on 19 July 1970 for a further period of 20 years and extended again on 6 June 1983 for a further period of 20 years.

ECONOMY

Budget. Actual revenue and expenditure for the calendar years 1984–89, the ordinary budget for 1990 and the proposed budget for 1991 in 1m. marks:

	1984	*1985*	*1986*	*1987*	*1988*	*1989*	*1990*	*1991*
Revenue	86,611	96,408	96,769	108,650	119,551	134,828	141,661	157,655
Expenditure	85,748	95,803	95,172	106,988	117,275	129,459	141,609	157,653

Of the total revenue, 1989, 32% derived from sales tax, 29% from income and property tax, 11% from excise duties, 14% from other taxes and similar revenue, 3% from loans (net) and 12% from miscellaneous sources. Of the total expenditure, 1989, 18% went to education and culture, 18% to social security, 8% to transport, 8% to agriculture and forestry, 10% to general administration, public order and safety, 9% to health, 5% to communities and housing policy, 5% to defence, 3% to promotion of industry and 16% to other expenditures.

At the end of Dec. 1989 the foreign loans totalled 22,786m. marks. The internal loans amounted to 30,126m. marks. The cash surplus was 3,842m. marks. The total public debt was 52,912m. marks.

Currency. The unit of currency is the *markka* (FIM) or mark of 100 *pennis*. There are coins of 1, 5, 10, 20 and 50 pennis and 1 and 5 marks, and notes of 10, 50, 100, 500 and 1,000 marks. Exchange rate in March 1991: 7·03 marks = £1; 3·71 marks = US$1.

Banking and Finance. The Bank of Finland (founded in 1811) is owned by the State and under the guarantee and supervision of Parliament. It is the only bank of issue, and the limit of its right to issue notes is fixed equal to the value of its assets of gold and foreign holdings plus 500m. marks. Notes in circulation at the end of 1987 amounted to 9,117m. marks.

At the end of 1989 the deposits in banking institutions totalled 306,699m. marks and the loans granted by them 243,800m. marks. The most important groups of banking institutions in 1990 were:

	Number of institutions	*Number of offices*	*Deposits (1m. marks)*	*Loans (1m. marks)*
Commercial banks	10	1,020	110,063	134,339
Savings banks	178	1,307	71,225	79,993
Co-operative banks	361	1,198	61,166	69,871

The 5 largest banks are Kansallis-Osake-Pannki, Union Bank of Finland, Skopbank, Okobank and the state-owned Postipannki.

There is a stock exchange in Helsinki.

Weights and Measures. The metric system is legal.

ENERGY AND NATURAL RESOURCES

Electricity. Electricity production was (in 1m. kwh.) 52,564 in 1987; 53,066 in 1988, of which 25% was hydro-electric; 50,765 in 1989 (preliminary). Supply 220 volts; 50 Hz.

Minerals. The most important mines, Outokumpu (copper) and Otanmäki (iron) were exhausted and closed in 1990 and 1985 respectively. Notable of the remaining mines are Pyhäsalmi and Vihanti (zinc), Enonkoski (nickel) and Kemi (chromium). In 1989 (preliminary) the metal content (in tonnes) of the output of copper concentrates was 22,101, of zinc concentrates 58,218, of nickel concentrates 9,233 and of lead concentrates 2,522.

Agriculture. The cultivated area covers only 9% of the land and of the economically active population 9% were employed in agriculture and forestry in 1989. The arable area was divided in 1988 into 189,049 farms, and the distribution of this area by the size of the farms was: Less than 5 ha cultivated, 53,925 farms; 5–20 ha, 99,657 farms; 20–50 ha, 31,609 farms; 50–100 ha, 3,456 farms; over 100 ha, 402 farms.

The principal crops (area in 1,000 ha, yield in tonnes) were in 1989:

Crop	*Area*	*Yield*	*Crop*	*Area*	*Yield*
Rye	69	195,900	Oats	440	1,443,800
Barley	517	1,629,900	Potatoes	45	981,300
Wheat	51	507,200	Hay	294	1,238,100

The total area under cultivation in 1990 was 2,049,800 ha, including (in 1,000 ha): Rye, 81; barley, 486; wheat, 180; oats, 453; potatoes, 41; hay, 286. Production of dairy butter in 1989 was 63,900 tonnes, and of cheese, 90,500 tonnes.

Livestock (1990): Horses, 15,600; cattle, 1,357,400; pigs, 1,298,000; poultry, 6,138,000; reindeer (1989), 407,000.

Forestry. The total forest land amounts to 30–31m. ha. The productive forest land covers 19·73m. ha.

In 1989 there were exported: Round timber, 584m. cu. metres; sawn wood, 4,472m. cu. metres; plywood and veneers, 537m. cu. metres.

INDUSTRY. The following data cover establishments with a total personnel of 5 or more in 1989 [1]:

Industry	*Establishments* [2]	*Personnel* [3]	*Value of production* Gross (1m. marks)	*Value of production* Value added (1m. marks)
Mining and quarrying	134	4,226	3,268	1,950
Metal ore mining	7	1,356	1,409	950
Other mining	126	2,864	1,886	1,022
Manufacturing	6,315	441,154	279,132	102,252
Manufacture of food, beverages and tobacco	931	53,953	49,049	12,197
Textile, wearing apparel and leather industries	707	34,711	8,868	4,048
Manufacture of textiles	239	11,995	3,757	1,718
Manufacture of wearing apparel, except footwear	339	17,239	3,597	1,694
Manufacture of wood and wood products, incl. furniture	905	42,763	20,571	7,541
Manufacture of paper and paper prod., printing, publishing	845	86,026	65,048	24,558
Manufacture of paper and paper products	151	45,523	47,817	16,763
Printing, publishing, etc.	694	40,471	17,242	7,853

[1] Preliminary. [2] 1988. [3] Working proprietors, salaried employees and wage earners.

Industry	Establishments[2]	Personnel[3]	Value of production: Gross (1m. marks)	Value of production: Value added (1m. marks)
Manufacture of chemicals and chemical, petroleum, coal, rubber and plastic products	440	37,579	32,566	12,473
Manufacture of industrial chemicals	152	13,701	13,758	5,341
Manufacture of other chemical products	89	10,042	5,768	2,660
Petroleum refineries	4	3,236	7,897	2,182
Manufacture of non-metallic mineral products	405	19,596	9,846	4,909
Basic metal industries	75	17,183	22,687	6,015
Iron and steel basic industries	50	12,493	13,795	4,048
Non-ferrous metal basic industries	25	4,687	8,893	1,966
Manufacture of fabricated metal products, machinery, etc.	1,909	145,089	68,884	29,827
Manufacture of fabricated metal products, excl. machinery	732	32,035	14,379	6,623
Manufacture of machinery, except electrical	614	50,294	25,318	11,097
Manufacture of electrical machinery, apparatus, etc.	228	25,870	12,601	5,901
Manufacture of transport equipment	246	31,111	14,285	5,003
Other manufacturing industries	98	3,977	1,275	656
Electricity, gas and water	522	27,322	30,073	12,572
All industry	6,971	472,702	312,473	116,773

[2] 1988. [3] Working proprietors, salaried employees and wage earners.

GDP (at market prices) *per capita* (1989) 99,807 marks.

FOREIGN ECONOMIC RELATIONS

Commerce. Imports and exports for calendar years, in 1m. marks:

	1985	*1986*	*1987*	*1988*	*1989*
Imports	81,520	77,602	86,696	88,229	105,519
Exports	84,028	82,579	87,564	90,854	99,782

The trade with some principal import and export countries was (in 1,000 marks):

Country	*Imports 1988*	*Imports 1989*	*Exports 1988*	*Exports 1989*
Australia	364,801	378,112	1,020,388	1,206,870
Austria	1,089,422	1,294,584	914,700	1,174,735
Belgium–Luxembourg	2,231,679	2,931,881	1,789,335	1,946,555
Brazil	566,311	632,235	220,441	368,140
Canada	637,535	919,228	1,099,169	1,359,087
China	567,532	688,372	463,440	337,582
Colombia	336,178	329,334	65,601	78,156
Czechoslovakia	449,647	515,067	278,851	353,608
Denmark	2,588,561	3,289,709	3,204,122	3,257,060
France	3,589,745	4,417,460	4,835,190	5,453,347
German Dem. Rep.	484,562	530,372	385,205	534,176
Germany (Fed. Rep.)	14,859,667	18,233,665	9,842,401	10,784,550
Greece	246,740	299,580	511,883	639,661
Hungary	370,389	422,531	276,384	314,086
Iran	8,808	10,619	169,065	238,564
Iraq	365	93	42,184	90,921
Ireland	381,773	503,401	536,005	542,006
Israel	157,760	162,691	321,732	323,581
Italy	3,924,293	4,900,237	2,462,806	2,989,072
Japan	6,522,497	7,695,320	1,649,197	2,033,231
Netherlands	2,867,562	3,416,063	3,312,774	3,961,202
Norway	2,096,425	2,456,563	3,137,309	2,919,976
Poland	852,327	1,065,181	290,235	306,014
Portugal	759,403	884,052	392,304	506,483
Saudi Arabia	394,715	377,995	423,404	285,832

Country	Imports 1988	Imports 1989	Exports 1988	Exports 1989
Spain	979,573	1,129,257	1,418,562	1,830,757
Sweden	11,765,250	14,314,190	12,835,219	14,313,992
Switzerland	1,639,199	1,829,138	1,553,718	1,680,398
USSR	10,592,193	12,152,159	11,863,809	14,495,880
UK	5,941,908	6,897,931	13,562,872	11,957,969
USA	5,615,962	6,669,113	5,245,131	6,387,682

Principal imports 1989 (in 1m. marks): Machinery, apparatus and appliances, 42,490; mineral fuels, lubricants, etc., 10,365; chemicals, 11,039; food and live animals, 4,700; road vehicles, 11,554; crude materials, inedible, except fuels, 5,900; textile yarn, fabrics, etc., 3,102; iron and steel, 4,023.

Principal exports in 1989 (in 1m. marks): Paper and paper-board, 26,604; machinery and transport equipment, 28,820; wood shaped or simply worked, 4,614; wood pulp, 5,268; ships, 3,951; clothing, 2,088; veneers, plywood, etc., and other wood manufactures, 2,338; food and live animals, 1,779; road vehicles, 3,358.

Timber exports in 1989 (in 1m. cu. metres): Round timber, 584; sawn wood, 4,472; plywood and veneers, 537.

Total trade between Finland and UK (British Department of Trade returns, in £1,000 sterling):

	1986	1987	1988	1989	1990
Imports to UK	1,346,058	1,539,011	1,813,549	1,893,163	1,775,766
Exports and re-exports from UK	664,451	797,236	824,951	925,784	1,041,739

Tourism. In 1989 the total revenue from tourism was 4,484m. marks and the total expenditure 8,958m. marks.

COMMUNICATIONS

Roads. In Jan. 1990 there were 77,258 km of public roads, of which 45,693 km were paved. At the end of 1988 there were 1,795,908 registered cars, 52,736 lorries, 160,301 vans and pick-ups, 9,229 buses and coaches and 15,392 special automobiles.

Railways. On 31 Dec. 1989 the total length of the line operated was 5,863 km (1,636 km electrified), of which all was owned by the State. The gauge is 1,524 mm. In 1989 45·5m. passengers and 33·6m. tonnes of freight were carried. The total revenue in 1989 was 3,361m. marks and the total expenditure 4,386m. marks.

Aviation. The scheduled traffic of Finnish airlines covered 55m. km in 1989. The number of passengers was 4·3m. and the number of passenger-km 4,625,000. The air transport of freight and mail amounted to 137m. tonne-km.

Shipping. The total registered mercantile marine on 31 Dec. 1989 was 441 vessels of 1,053,405 gross tons. In 1989 the total number of vessels arriving in Finland from abroad was 18,938 and the goods discharged amounted to 33·6m. tonnes. The goods loaded for export from Finland ports amounted to 22·4m. tonnes.

The lakes, rivers and canals are navigable for about 6,160 km. Timber floating is important, and there are about 9,460 km of floatable inland waterways. In 1989 bundle floating was about 4·2m. tonnes and free floating 1m. tonnes.

On 27 Aug. 1963 the USSR leased to Finland the Russian part of the canal connecting Lake Saimaa with the Gulf of Finland. After extensive rebuilding the canal was opened for traffic in 1968. The Saimaa Canal and deepwater channels on Lake Saimaa (770 km) can be used by vessels with dimensions not larger than as follows: Length 82 metres, width 11·8 metres, draught 4·2 metres and height of mast 24·5 metres.

Telecommunications. In 1989 there were 3,377 post offices and 255 telecommunications offices. The total length of telegraph wires was 582,000 km and that of domestic trunk and net group telephone wires 9·6m. km. The number of telephone subscriber lines (1989), 2·58m. All post and telegraph systems are administered by the State jointly with a large part of the telephone services. The total revenues from postal services were 4,050m. marks and from (wire and radio) telegraph services 4,182m. marks.

On 31 Dec. 1989 the number of television licences was 1,879,249, of which licences for colour television, 1,731,922. *Oy Yleisradio AB* broadcasts 4 programmes (1 in Swedish), covering the whole country on long-, medium- and short-waves, and on FM. Four TV programmes (1 commercial) are broadcast.

Cinemas. In Dec. 1989 there were 344 cinema halls with a seating capacity of 67,000.

Newspapers. In 1989 the number of newspapers published more often than 3 times a week was 67, of which 9 were in Swedish.

JUSTICE, RELIGION, EDUCATION AND WELFARE

Justice. The lowest courts of justice are the municipal courts in towns and district courts in the country. Municipal courts are held by the burgomaster and at least 2 members of court, district court by judge and 5 jurors, the judge alone deciding, unless the jurors unanimously differ from him, when their decision prevails. From these courts an appeal lies to the courts of appeal *(Hovioikeus)* in Turku, Vaasa, Kuopio, Helsinki, Kouvola and Rovaniemi. The Supreme Court *(Korkein oikeus)* sits in Helsinki. Appeals from the decisions of administrative authorities are in the final instance decided by the Supreme Administrative Court *(Korkein hallintooikeus)*, also in Helsinki. Judges can be removed only by judicial sentence.

Two functionaries, the *Oikeuskansleri* or Chancellor of Justice, and the *Oikeusasiamies* (ombudsman), or Solicitor-General, exercise control over the administration of justice. The former acts also as counsel and public prosecutor for the Government; while the latter, who is appointed by the Parliament, exerts a general control over all courts of law and public administration.

At the end of 1989 the prison population numbered 3,410 men and 112 women; the preliminary number of convictions in 1987 was 365,312, of which 340,962 were for minor offences with maximum penalty of fines and 24,220 with penalty of imprisonment. 10,255 of the prison sentences were unconditional.

Religion. Liberty of conscience is guaranteed to members of all religions. National churches are the Lutheran National Church and the Greek Orthodox Church of Finland. The Lutheran Church is divided into 8 bishoprics (Turku being the archiepiscopal see), 79 provostships and 598 parishes. The Greek Orthodox Church is divided into 3 bishoprics (Kuopio being the archiepiscopal see) and 27 parishes, in addition to which there are a monastery and a convent.

Percentage of the total population at the end of 1988: Lutherans, 88·4; Greek Orthodox, 1·1; others, 0·6; not members of any religion, 9·9.

Education (1988–89). *Primary and Secondary Education:*

	Number of institutions	*Teachers*	*Students*
First-level Education (Lower sections of the comprehensive schools, grades I–VI)			387,951
Second-level Education General education (Upper sections of the comprehensive schools, grades VII–IX, and senior secondary schools)	5,336	42,506	285,135
Vocational education	542	17,662	110,598

Higher Education. Education at the third level (including universities and third level education at vocational colleges) was provided for 151,083 students. Education at universities was provided at 20 institutions with 7,650 teachers and 103,895 students.

University Education. Universities and university-type institutions with the number of teachers and students in 1988–89:

	Founded	Teachers	Students Total	Students Women
Universities				
Helsinki	1640	1,800	27,494	15,984
Turku (Swedish)	1919	312	4,585	2,625
Turku (Finnish)	1922	781	10,220	6,123
Jyväskylä	1958	545	7,000	4,461
Oulu	1958	850	8,600	4,092
Tampere	1966	582	10,337	6,323
Joensuu	1969	337	4,524	2,806
Kuopio	1972	294	2,732	1,708
Lapland	1979	123	1,374	727
Vaasa	1968	113	1,959	997
Universities of Technology				
Lappeenranta	1969	156	1,895	297
Helsinki	1849	586	9,659	1,693
Tampere	1972	272	4,111	591
College of Veterinary Medicine, Helsinki	1946	51	306	240
Schools of Economics and Business Administration				
Helsinki (Finnish)	1911	154	3,321	1,501
Helsinki (Swedish)	1927	98	1,792	783
Turku (Finnish)	1950	74	1,628	798
Universities of Art				
Sibelius Academy	1939	293	1,130	661
University of Industrial Arts	1949	167	988	636
Theatre Academy	1979	62	235	108

General adult education (at civic institutes, folk high schools and study centres) had 844,000 students in 1987–88.

Health. In 1988 there were 9,614 physicians, 3,746 dentists and (1987) 67,246 hospital beds.

Social Security. The Social Insurance Institution administers general systems of old age pensions (to all persons over 65 years of age and disabled younger persons) and of health insurance. An additional system of compulsory old age pensions paid for by the employers is in force and works through the Central Pension Security Institute. Systems for child welfare, care of vagrants, alcoholics and drug addicts and other public aid are administered by the communes and supervised by the National Social Board and the Ministry of Social Affairs and Health.

The total cost of social security amounted to 113,899m. marks in 1988. Out of this 33,170m. (29·1%) was spent for health, 2,150m. (1·9%) for industrial accidents, 6,616m. (5·8%) for unemployment, 44,286m. (38·9%) old age and disability, 18,065m. (15·9%) for family allowances and child welfare, 1,270m. (1·1%) for general welfare purposes, 2,782m. (2·4%) for war-disabled, etc., 1,543m. (1·4%) as tax reductions for children. Out of the total expenditure 29% was financed by the State, 16% by local authorities, 43% by employers, 8% by the beneficiaries and 4% by users.

DIPLOMATIC REPRESENTATIVES

Of Finland in Great Britain (38 Chesham Pl., London, SW1X 8HW)
Ambassador: (Vacant).

Of Great Britain in Finland (16–20 Uudenmaankatu, Helsinki 00120)
Ambassador: G. Neil Smith, CMG.

Of Finland in the USA (3216 New Mexico Ave., NW, Washington, D.C., 20016)
Ambassador: Jukka Valtasaari.

Of the USA in Finland (Itäinen Puistotie 14A, Helsinki 00140)
Ambassador: John Giffen Weinmann.

Of Finland to the United Nations
Ambassador: Dr Klaus Törnudd.

Further Reading

Statistical Information: The Central Statistical Office (Tilastokeskus, Swedish: Statistikcentralen; address: PO Box 504, SF-00101 Helsinki 10) was founded in 1865 to replace earlier official statistical services dating from 1749 (in united Sweden–Finland). Statistics on foreign trade, agriculture, forestry, navigation, health and social welfare are produced by other state authorities. Its publications include: *Statistical Yearbook of Finland* (from 1879) and *Bulletin of Statistics* (monthly, from 1924). A bibliography of all official statistics of Finland was published in Finnish, Swedish and English in *Statistical publications 1856–1979*. Helsinki, 1980.

Constitution Act and Parliament Act of Finland. Helsinki, 1984
Suomen valtiokalenteri–Finlands statskalender (State Calendar of Finland). Helsinki. Annual
Facts About Finland. Helsinki. Annual (Union Bank of Finland)
Facts about Finland. Helsinki, 1988
Finland in Figures. Helsinki, Annual
Finland in Maps. Helsinki, 1979
Finnish Press Laws. Helsinki, 1984
Making and Applying Law in Finland. Ministry of Justice, 1983
Statistical Yearbook of Finland. Helsinki, Annual
Yearbook of Finnish Foreign Policy. Helsinki, Annual
The Finnish Banking System. Helsinki, 1987
Finnish Industry. Helsinki, 1988
Finnish Local Government. Helsinki, 1983
Health Care in Finland. Helsinki, 1987
Arter, D., *Politics and Policy-Making in Finland*. Brighton, 1987
Hurme-Malin-Syväoja, *Finnish-English General Dictionary*. Helsinki, 1984
Hurme-Pesonen, *English–Finnish General Dictionary*. Helsinki, 1982
Jakobson, M. *Myth and Reality*. Helsinki, 1987
Jutikkala, E. and Pirinen, K., *A History of Finland*. 3rd ed. New York, 1979
Kekkonen, U., *President's View*. London, 1982
Kirby, D. G., *Finland in the Twentieth Century*. 2nd ed. London, 1984
Klinge, M., *A Brief History of Finland*. Helsinki, 1987
Paasivirta, J., *Finland and Europe. The Period of Autonomy and the International Crises 1808–1914*. London, 1981
Polvinen, T., *Between East and West – Finland in International Politics 1944–1947*. Minnesota Univ. Press, 1986
Puntila, L. A., *The Political History of Finland, 1809–1966*. Helsinki, 1974
Screen, J. E. O., *Finland*. [Bibliography] Oxford and Santa Barbara, 1981
Singleton, F., *The Economy of Finland in the Twentieth Century*. Univ. of Bradford Press, 1987
University of Turku, *Political Parties in Finland*. Turku, 1987

FRANCE

Capital: Paris
Population: 56·18m. (1989)
GNP per capita: US$16,080 (1988)

République Française

HISTORY. The republic proclaimed on the fall of the Bourbon monarchy in 1792 lasted until the First Empire, under Napoleon I, was established in 1804. The Bourbon monarchy was restored in 1814 and (with an interval during 1815) lasted until the abdication of Louis Philippe in 1848. The Second Republic was established on 12 March 1848, the Second Empire (under Louis Napoleon) on 2 Dec. 1852. The Third Republic was established on 4 Sept. 1870 following the capture and imprisonment of Louis Napoleon in the Franco-Prussian war, and lasted until the German occupation of 1940. Power during the occupation was nominally exercised by the Vichy regime of Marshal Pétain. Following the liberation of 1944, the Fourth Republic was established on 24 Dec. 1946 but was dogged throughout by weak governments with unstable parliamentary support. It collapsed on 4 Oct. 1958 under the impetus of military revolt in Algeria, following which General de Gaulle assumed power. He subsequently inspired the constitution of the Fifth Republic, now in force.

AREA AND POPULATION. France is bounded in the north by the English Channel *(La Manche)*, north-east by Belgium and Luxembourg, east by Germany, Switzerland and Italy, south by the Mediterranean (with Monaco as a coastal enclave), south-west by Spain and Andorra, and west by the Atlantic Ocean The total area is 543,965 sq. km (210,033 sq. miles).

The population (present in actual boundaries) at successive censuses has been:

1801	27,349,003	1881	37,672,048	Mar. 1946	40,506,639
1821	30,461,875	1891	38,342,948	May 1954	42,777,174
1841	34,230,178	1901	38,961,945	Mar. 1962	46,519,997
1861	37,386,313	1911	39,604,992	Mar. 1968	49,778,540
1866	38,067,064	1921	39,209,518	Feb. 1975	52,655,802
1872	36,102,921	1931	41,834,923	Mar. 1982	54,334,871

The 1982 total included 3,680,100 foreigners, of whom 795,920 were Algerian, 764,860 Portuguese, 431,120 Moroccan, 333,740 Italian and 321,440 Spanish.

Population estimate (Oct. 1989) is 56,184,000.

Vital statistics for calendar years:

	Marriages	*Live births*	*Deaths*
1985	269,300	768,431	552,500
1986	265,340	778,940	546,880
1987	265,177	767,828	527,466
1988	271,124	770,690	524,600

Live birth rate in 1988 was 13·8 per 1,000 inhabitants; death rate, 9·4; marriage rate, 4·9; divorce rate (1986), 2; infant mortality (1987), 7·6 per 1,000 live births. Life expectation at birth (1987); men, 72; women, 80·3. Population growth rate (1986), 4·2 per 1,000. Average density (1988) 102·7 persons per sq. km.

The areas, populations and chief towns of the 22 Metropolitan regions were as follows:

Regions	*Area (sq. km)*	*Census March 1982*	*Estimate Jan. 1987*	*Chief town*
Alsace	8,280	1,566,048	1,605,300	Strasbourg
Aquitaine	41,308	2,656,544	2,723,600	Bordeaux
Auvergne	26,013	1,332,678	1,329,200	Clermont-Ferrand
Basse-Normandie	17,589	1,350,979	1,379,400	Caen
Bourgogne (Burgundy)	31,582	1,596,054	1,610,600	Dijon
Bretagne (Brittany)	27,208	2,707,886	2,763,100	Rennes
Centre	39,151	2,264,164	2,333,800	Orléans

Regions	Area (sq. km)	Census March 1982	Estimate Jan. 1987	Chief town
Champagne-Ardenne	25,606	1,345,935	1,357,900	Reims
Corse (Corsica)	8,680	240,178	246,000	Ajaccio
Franche-Comté	16,202	1,084,049	1,088,000	Besançon
Haute-Normandie	12,317	1,655,362	1,699,600	Rouen
Île-de-France	12,012	10,073,059	10,259,400	Paris
Languedoc-Roussillon	27,376	1,926,514	2,053,600	Montpellier
Limousin	16,942	737,153	734,700	Limoges
Lorraine	23,547	2,319,905	2,326,900	Nancy
Midi-Pyrénées	45,348	2,325,319	2,369,500	Toulouse
Nord-Pas-de-Calais	12,414	3,932,939	3,931,500	Lille
Pays de la Loire	32,082	2,930,398	3,042,500	Nantes
Picardie	19,399	1,740,321	1,776,400	Amiens
Poitou-Charentes	25,810	1,568,230	1,591,500	Poitiers
Provence-Alpes-Côte d'Azur	31,400	3,965,209	4,112,500	Marseille
Rhône-Alpes	43,698	5,015,947	5,174,800	Lyon

Populations of the principal conurbations and towns at Census 1982:

	Conurbation	Town		Conurbation	Town
Paris	8,706,963 [1]	2,188,918	Limoges	171,689	144,082
Lyon	1,220,844 [2]	418,476	Mantes-la-Jolie	170,265	43,585
Marseille	1,110,511	878,689	Amiens	154,498	136,358
Lille	936,295 [3]	174,039	Thionville	138,034	41,448
Bordeaux	640,012	211,197	Perpignan	137,915	113,646
Toulouse	541,271	354,289	Nîmes	132,343	129,924
Nantes	464,857	247,227	Pau	131,265	85,766
Nice	449,496	338,486	Saint-Nazaire	130,271	68,947
Toulon	410,393	181,985	Montbéliard	128,194	33,362
Grenoble	392,021	159,503	Bayonne	127,477	42,970
Rouen	379,879	105,083	Aix-en-Provence	126,552	124,550
Strasbourg	373,470	252,264	Troyes	125,240	64,769
Valenciennes	349,505	40,881	Besançon	120,772	119,687
Lens	327,383	38,307	Hagondange-Briey	119,669	9,091
Saint-Étienne	317,228	206,688	Annecy	112,632	51,593
Nancy	306,982	99,307	Valence	106,041	68,157
Cannes	295,525	72,787	Maubeuge	105,714	36,156
Tours	262,786	136,483	Lorient	104,025	64,675
Béthune	258,383	26,105	Angoulême	103,552	50,151
Clermont-Ferrand	256,189	151,092	Poitiers	103,204	82,884
Le Havre	254,595	200,411	La Rochelle	102,143	78,231
Rennes	234,418	200,390	Calais	100,823	76,935
Montpellier	221,307	201,067	Forbach	99,606	27,321
Mulhouse	220,613	113,794	Boulogne-sur-Mer	98,566	48,349
Orléans	220,478	105,589	Chambéry	96,163	54,896
Dijon	215,865	145,569	Bourges	92,202	79,408
Douai	202,366	44,515	Cherbourg	85,485	30,112
Brest	201,145	160,355	Saint-Brieuc	83,900	51,399
Reims	199,388	181,985	Creil	82,505	36,128
Angers	195,859	141,143	Melun	82,479	36,218
Dunkerque	195,705	73,618	Colmar	82,468	63,764
Le Mans	191,080	150,331	Saint-Chamond	82,059	40,571
Metz	186,437	118,502	Roanne	81,786	49,638
Caen	183,526	117,119	Béziers	81,347	78,477
Avignon	174,264	91,474	Arras	80,477	45,364

[1] Including towns of Boulogne-Billancourt (102,595), Argenteuil (96,045), Versailles (95,240), Montreuil (93,394), Saint-Denis (91,275), Nanterre (90,371) and Vitry-sur-Seine (85,820).
[2] Including towns of Villeurbanne (118,330) and Vénissieux (64,982).
[3] Including towns of Roubaix (101,836) and Tourcoing (97,121).

The official language is French. Regional languages are also spoken. In 1990 the Conseil Supérieur de la Langue Française (established 1989) recommended minor orthographic changes, to be introduced in schools in 1991.

CLIMATE. The north-west has a moderate maritime climate, with small temperature range and abundant rainfall, but inland, rainfall becomes more seasonal, with a summer maximum, and the annual range of temperature increases. Southern

France has a Mediterranean climate, with mild moist winters and hot dry summers. Eastern France has a continental climate and a rainfall maximum in summer, with thunderstorms prevalent.

Paris. Jan. 37°F (3°C), July 64°F (18°C). Annual rainfall 22·9" (573 mm). Bordeaux. Jan. 41°F (5°C), July 68°F (20°C). Annual rainfall 31·4" (786 mm). Lyon. Jan. 37°F (3°C), July 68°F (20°C). Annual rainfall 31·8" (794 mm).

CONSTITUTION AND GOVERNMENT. The Constitution of the Fifth Republic, superseding that of 1946, came into force on 4 Oct. 1958. It consists of a preamble, dealing with the Rights of Man, and 92 articles.

France is a Republic, indivisible, secular, democratic and social; all citizens are equal before the law (Art. 2). National sovereignty resides with the people, who exercise it through their representatives and by referenda (Art. 3). Political parties carry out their activities freely, but must respect the principles of national sovereignty and democracy (Art. 4).

The *President* of the Republic sees that the Constitution is respected; he ensures the regular functioning of the public authorities, as well as the continuity of the state. He is the protector of national independence and territorial integrity (Art. 5). He is elected for 7 years by direct universal suffrage (Art. 6). He appoints a Prime Minister and, on the latter's advice, appoints and dismisses the other members of the Government (Art. 8). He presides over the Council of Ministers (Art. 9). He can dissolve the National Assembly, after consultation with the Prime Minister and the Presidents of the two Houses (Art. 12). He appoints to the civil and military offices of the state (Art. 13). In times of crisis, he may take such emergency powers as the circumstances demand; the National Assembly cannot be dissolved during such a period (Art. 16). The President's salary is 35,663 francs a month.

Previous Presidents of the Fifth Republic:

General Charles André Joseph de Gaulle, 8 Jan. 1959–28 April 1969 (resigned); Alain Poher (interim), 28 April 1969–20 June 1969; Georges Jean Raymond Pompidou, 20 June 1969–2 April 1974 (died); Alain Poher (interim), 2 April 1974–27 May 1974; Valéry Giscard d'Estaing, 27 May 1974–21 May 1981.

President of the Republic: François Mitterrand (elected 10 May 1981; took office 21 May 1981; re-elected 8 May 1988).

The government determines and conducts the policy of the nation (Art. 20). The Prime Minister directs the operation of the Government, is responsible for national defence and ensures the execution of laws (Art. 21). Members of the Government must not be members of Parliament (Art. 23).

The Council of Ministers was composed as follows in March 1991:

Prime Minister: Michel Rocard (PS).
National Education, Youth and Sport: Lionel Jospin (PS).
Economy, Finance and Budget: Pierre Bérégovoy (PS).
Equipment and Housing: Maurice Faure (MRG).
Foreign Affairs: Roland Dumas (PS).
Ministers:
Justice, Keeper of the Seals: Henri Nallet (PS).
Defence: Jean-Pierre Chevènement (PS).
Interior: Pierre Joxe (PS).
Industry and Regional Planning: Roger Fauroux (non-party).
European Affairs: Elizabeth Guigou.
Transport and Sea: Michel Delebarre (PS).
Civil Service and Administrative Reform: Michel Durafour (UDF-Rad.).
Labour, Employment and Vocational Training: Jean-Pierre Soisson (UDF-PR).
Co-operation and Overseas Development: Jacques Pelletier (UDF-Rad.).
Culture, Communication, Major Works and the Bicentenary: Jack Lang (PS).
Overseas Departments and Territories and Government Spokesman: Louis Le Pensec (PS).
Agriculture and Forestry: Louis Mermaz.
Postal Services, Telecommunications and Space: Paul Quilès (PS).

Relations with Parliament: Jean Poperen (PS).
Solidarity, Health and Social Protection: Claude Evin (PS).
Research and Technology: Hubert Curien (PS).
Foreign Trade: Jean-Marie Rausch (UDF-CDS).
Ministers-Delegate: Michel Charasse (PS) *(Budget)*, Olivier Stirn (PS) *(Tourism)*, Alain Decaux (non-party) *(Relations with Francophone countries)*, Jacques Mellick (PS) *(Sea)*, Jacques Chérèque (PS) *(Regional Planning and Redeployment)*, Théo Braun (PS) *(Elderly)*, Edwige Avice (PS) *(Foreign Affairs)*, François Doubin (MRG) *(Trade and Artisan Industries)*, Catherine Tasca (non-party) *(Communication)*.
There were also 17 Secretaries of State.

Parliament consists of the *National Assembly* and the *Senate*; the National Assembly is elected by direct suffrage and the Senate by indirect suffrage (Art. 24). It convenes as of right in two ordinary sessions per year, the first on 2 Oct. for 80 days and the second on 2 April for not more than 90 days (Art. 28).

The National Assembly comprises 577 Deputies, elected for a 5-year term from single-member constituencies – 555 in Metropolitan France and 22 in the various overseas departments and dependencies. The General Election, held in June 1988, resulted in a composition (by group, including 'affiliates') of 275 Socialist Party (PS) (including 9 Leftwing Radicals Movement (MRG) and 6 other 'affiliates'), 40 Centre Union (Social Democrats Centre), 132 *Rassemblement Pour la République* (RPR; Gaullists), 90 Union of French Democracy (UDF) (of which 58 Republican Party), 25 Communist Party (PCF) and 15 others. The *Speaker* is Laurent Fabius.

The Senate comprises 319 Senators elected for 9-year terms (one-third every 3 years) by an electoral college in each Department or overseas dependency, made up of all members of the Departmental Council or its equivalent in overseas dependencies, together with all members of Municipal Councils within that area; there are 296 Senators for Metropolitan France, 13 for the Overseas Departments and dependencies, and 10 for French citizens residing outside France and its dependencies. Following the partial elections held in Sept. 1986, the Senate was composed of (by group, including 'affiliates') 154 UDF, 77 RPR, 73 Socialist Group (including 9 MRG) and 15 Communist Group.

The Constitutional Council is composed of 9 members whose term of office is 9 years (non-renewable), one-third every 3 years; 3 are appointed by the President of the Republic, 3 by the President of the National Assembly, and 3 by the President of the Senate; in addition, former Presidents of the Republic are, by right, life members of the Constitutional Council (Art. 56). It oversees the fairness of the elections of the President (Art. 58) and Parliament (Art. 59) and of referenda (Art. 60), and acts as a guardian of the Constitution (Art. 61).

The Economic and Social Council advises on Government and Private Members' Bills (Art. 69). It comprises representatives of employers', workers' and farmers' organizations in each Department and Overseas Territory.

National flag: The Tricolour of three vertical stripes of blue, white, red.

National anthem: La Marseillaise (words and music by C. Rouget de Lisle, 1792).

Local Government: France is divided into 22 regions for national development, planning and budgetary policy. Many of these regions are broadly comparable with the provinces of pre-revolutionary France, and give a measure of recognition to the distinctive personalities of peripheral areas such as Alsace and Brittany. In March 1982 state-appointed Regional Prefects were abolished and their executive powers transferred to the Presidents of the Regional Councils, which are directly elected. Measures of limited autonomy for Corsica were proposed in 1991.

There are 96 *départements* within the 22 regions each governed by a directly-elected *Conseil Général*. From 1982 their Presidents' powers were extended to take over local administration and expenditure from the former Departmental prefects, now called 'Commissioners of the Republic' with responsibility for public order. The *arrondissement* (325 in 1982) and the *canton* (3,714 in 1982), have little administrative significance.

The unit of local government is the *commune*, the size and population of which vary very much. There were, in 1982, in the 96 metropolitan departments, 36,433 communes. Most of them (31,122) had less than 1,500 inhabitants, and 16,144 had less than 300, while 227 communes had more than 30,000 inhabitants. The local affairs of the commune are under a Municipal Council, composed of from 9 to 36 members, elected by universal suffrage for 6 years by French citizens of 21 years or over after 6 months' residence. Each Municipal Council elects a mayor, who is both the representative of the commune and the agent of the central government.

At the local elections of March 1990 the Socialist Party made most gains, winning 22 towns with populations over 20,000. The Communist Party lost control of 15 such towns.

Under a local taxation reform of 1990, some 11,000m. francs out of a total revenue of 42,000m. francs were based on income rather than rental values.

In Paris the *Conseil de Paris* is composed of 109 members elected from the 20 *arrondissements*. It combines the functions of departmental *Conseil Général* and Municipal Council.

DEFENCE. The President of the Republic exercises command over the Armed Forces. He is assisted by the High Council of Defence *(Conseil Supérieur de Défense)*, which studies defence problems, and by two Committees *(Comité de Défense* and *Comité de Défense restreint)* which formulate directives. The Prime Minister is responsible for national defence; he exercises his military responsibilities and co-ordinates inter-ministry defence activities through the General Secretariat of National Defence (SGDN). Under the Prime Minister's authority, the Minister of Defence is responsible for the execution of military policy, in particular the organization and administration of the Armed Forces.

On 5 July 1969 the Ministry of Defence assumed responsibility from the former individual service Ministries for the Army, Air Force and Navy. The Ministry prepares general directives for negotiations relating to defence. The preparation and control of the Armed Forces is exercised by the Chief of Staff of the Armed Forces, the Chiefs of Staff of the 3 services—Army, Navy and Air—and the head of the *Gendarmerie*.

French forces are not formally under the NATO command structure. About 48,000 French service personnel are stationed in the Federal Republic of Germany, with a further 15,000 stationed in other overseas locations.

The General Directorate for Armament (DGA) is responsible for all aspects of the procurement of defence equipment. It employs about 73,000 personnel, and co-ordinates another 217,000 others employed in the defence industry.

Army. The Army consisted in 1991 of 288,550 personnel, of whom 6,000 were women and 180,500 are conscripts. Conscripts may not serve abroad unless war is declared.

The Territorial Defence Forces consist of 7 zone brigades, 23 joint-services divisional regiments (RIAD), an infantry division and a Rhine division. They provide the main operational defence of French territory.

The peace-time tactical units comprise the Mechanized Armoured Corps (CBM) and the Rapid Intervention Force (FAR). The CBM forms the 1st Army of 170,000 men, with headquarters in Strasbourg, and is organized, equipped and trained for action in the Central Europe theatre; it consists of 6 armoured divisions, 2 light armoured divisions and 2 motorized rifle divisions, plus artillery, engineering, signals, parachute, transport, supply and naval infantry and artillery units. It also includes 5 nuclear artillery regiments equipped with 30 launchers for 'Pluton' missiles.

The headquarters of the FAR are at Maisons-Laffite. It comprises 47,000 men organized, equipped and trained for rapid engagement either in Europe or over large distances elsewhere; it includes a parachute division, an air-portable marine division, a light armoured division, an alpine division and an air-mobile division, together with various specialized units.

Equipment includes 1,400 AMX-30 and 230 AMX-13 main battle tanks, 284 AMX-10 armoured vehicles, 823 other armoured vehicles, 556 155-mm guns, 183

Roland anti-aircraft missile systems and 1,440 *Milan* anti-tank weapons.

The *Aviation Légère de l'Armée de Terre* (ALAT) with about 7,000 personnel is an integral part of the Army, equipped with 700 helicopters of various types for observation, reconnaissance, combat area transport, liaison and supply duties.

The *Foreign Legion* was formed in 1831 for duty in North Africa. It is officered by French nationals and based at Aubagne, near Marseilles. About half the other ranks are French. It numbered 8,500 in 1991.

Gendarmerie. The para-military police force exists to ensure public security and maintain law and order, as well as participate in the operational defence of French territory as part of the armed forces. It consists of (1991) 91,800 personnel including 10,700 conscripts, 1,400 women and 967 civilians. It comprises a mobile force of over 18,000 personnel and 120 departmental forces with over 51,000 personnel, together with specialised units. It is equipped with 28 VBC-90 armoured guncarriers, 121 light armoured cars, 155 armoured vehicles and 33 troop transport vehicles, as well as 42 helicopters and 6 light aircraft.

Navy. The missions of the French Navy are to provide the prime element of the French independent nuclear deterrent through its force of strategic submarines, to assure the security of the French offshore zones so as to contribute to NATO's logistic transatlantic re-supply, and to provide on-station and deployment forces overseas in support of French interests.

French territorial seas and economic zones are organized into 3 maritime regions, each under the authority of a Maritime Prefect (with headquarters in Cherbourg, Brest and Toulon). Offshore, the seas and oceans are divided into 5 zones: Atlantic, Mediterranean, Indian Ocean, Pacific and Antilles-Guyana. Home-based forces are commanded by Commanders-in-Chief based in Brest and Toulon, those in the Indian Ocean and Pacific by Flag Officers based afloat in the Indian Ocean, and at Nouméa (in New Caledonia). Naval forces in the Caribbean come under a joint force commander based at Cayenne.

The following is a summary of the strength of the fleet at the end of the years shown:

	1984	*1985*	*1986*	*1987*	*1988*	*1989*	*1990*
Aircraft carriers	2	2	2	2	2	2	2
Strategic-missile submarines	6	6	6	6	6	6	6
Other submarines	20	16	17	18	16	14	13
Cruisers	2	2	2	2	2	2	2
Destroyers	4	4	4	4	4	4	5
Frigates	40	37	38	38	36	36	35

The Navy operates 6 nuclear-powered strategic-missile submarines. The first 5 were of the Le Redoutable class, (*Redoutable, Terrible, Foudroyant, Indomptable* and *Tonnant*), 9,100 tonnes, completed between 1971 and 1980, and deploying 16 M-20 ballistic missiles. 3 have been, and a further 1 is being converted to carry 16 M-4 missiles, which are also fitted in an intermediate ship, *L'Inflexible*, 9,100 tonnes, completed in 1985. A new, much larger class, (14,200 tonnes) is being built, of which the first, *Le Triomphant*, was laid down in 1988 for completion in 1995, and will deploy 16 M-4/5 missiles.

There are also 4 small (2,700 tonne) nuclear-powered submarines of the Rubis class commissioned 1983-87, and 13 diesel submarines.

The principal surface ships are the aircraft carriers *Clemenceau* and *Foch* of 33,300 tonnes each, completed in 1961 and 1963, and 2 cruisers. The 2 carriers embark an air group typically comprising 16 Super-Etendard strike aircraft, 2 Etandard reconnaissance, 7 F-8E Crusader, 6 Alize anti-submarine and warning, plus a flight of 4 utility helicopters. They are due to be withdrawn from service in 1998 and 2002, when nuclear-powered replacements are planned. The first of these, *Charles de Gaulle*, was laid down at Brest in 1988. The guided-missile cruiser *Colbert*, of 11,500 tonnes, completed in 1959, is armed with a twin Masurca surface-to-air missile launcher, 4 Exocet anti-ship missiles, and 4,100mm guns. The helicopter cruiser *Jeanne d'Arc*, of 12,600 tonnes completed in 1963 is used in peacetime as a training vessel, but could perform amphibious or anti-submarine tasks in war. In these roles she could accommodate up to 8 Lynx helicopters, and 700 men. Her armament comprises 6 Exocet and 4 100mm guns.

Other surface combatants include 5 destroyers and 35 frigates. A modern mine countermeasure force consists of 10 tripartite coastal minehunters and 5 others, 4 old coastal minesweepers and 4 diver support vessels. The amphibious force includes 4 dock landing ships of which one is assigned to the Pacific nuclear test centre, 5 medium landing ships, and some 28 craft. Patrol forces include 1 ship (usually deployed in the South Indian Ocean), 21 coastal and 2 inshore patrol vessels. The Navy deploys a substantial support force which includes 8 large and 2 small tankers, 16 other maintenance and logistic ships, 5 weapon system trials ships and 7 survey and research ships. There are several hundred minor auxiliaries.

All warships, and a proportion of naval weapons, are produced by the government armaments service, of which the naval element, *Direction des Constructions Navales*, operates the shipbuilding yards as well as dockyards. Building takes place at Cherbourg, Brest and Lorient. In addition to units already mentioned, 2 more nuclear-powered fleet submarines, 5 frigates are being built. Fiscal restraints have caused many of these programmes to be slowed down.

The naval air arm, known as *Aeronavale*, numbers some 11,000. Operational aircraft include 40 Super-Etendard nuclear-capable strike aircraft, 20 Etendard reconnaissance aircraft, 30 US-built Crusader F-8E all-weather fighters, 28 Alize turboprop anti-submarine aircraft, 30 Atlantic and 5 Gardian maritime reconnaissance aircraft. The *Aeronavale* faces a problem with its fighter aircraft as the Crusaders' fatigue safe life expires in mid-1993, while the replacement, the maritime version of the Rafale, is unlikely to enter service before 1998. A programme has been launched to extend the Crusaders' life, but there are unlikely to be enough serviceable aircraft available for both carriers. Rotary wing strength includes 16 commando Super Frelon, and 38 anti-submarine and search-and-rescue Lynx helicopters. Numerous training, utility and transport aircraft bring the total strength to about 375 comprising 275 fixed-wing aircraft and 100 helicopters.

A small Marine force of 2,600 'Fusiliers Marins' provides 4 assault groups, plus numerous naval base protection units.

Personnel in 1990 numbered 65,000 including 19,000 conscripts (term of service 12 months) and a growing number of women, currently 1,800.

Air Force. Formed as the *Service Aéronautique* in April 1910, the *Armeé de l'Air* is organized in 7 major commands. The *Commandement des Forces Aériennes Stratégiques* (CFAS) commands the airborne nuclear deterrent force. The *Commandement de la Force Aérienne Tactique* (FATAC) directs the tactical air forces and is responsible for support of the ground forces. Under FATAC the 1st *Commandement Aérien Tactique* (1° CATAC) controls tactical air units based in eastern France; the 2nd *Commandement Aérien Tactique* (2° CATAC) controls the reserve forces and the air component of the *Force d'Intervention*. The *Commandement du Transport Aérien Militaire* (COTAM) is responsible for air transport operations and participates also in the training and transport of airborne forces. The *Commandement de la Défense Aérienne* (DA) controls French airspace. The *Commandement des Écoles de l'Armée de l'Air* (CEAA) is responsible for training the personnel for all branches of the Air Force. The *Commandement des Transmissions* has responsibility for communications and electronic warfare. Finally, the *Commandement du Génie de l'Air,* made up mainly of Army personnel, undertakes airbase construction and maintenance under Air Force control.

The home-based French Air Force is divided territorially among 4 metropolitan air regions (Metz, Villacoublay, Bordeaux, Aix-en-Provence); overseas, small air units are integrated into the local joint-service commands. There are about 40 combat squadrons plus about 30 transport, helicopter and support squadrons, and the Air Force uses a total of 60 bases.

The strategic, tactical and air defence forces are equipped entirely with jet aircraft. The CFAS has 20 Mirage IV supersonic nuclear bombers, deployed in 2 squadrons supported by 11 C-135F in-flight refuelling tanker transports. The FATAC deploys 6 wings (18 squadrons), with about 105 Mirage III-E and 5F ground-attack fighters, 30 Mirage 2000N, and 120 Jaguar strike aircraft, 3 reconnaissance squadrons with Mirage F1-CRs, and operational conversion units equipped with Mirage III-Bs and Jaguars. The air defence forces have 4 wings, comprising 8 squadrons with 120 Mirage F1-C and 4 squadrons with 60 Mirage 2000C interceptors. The COTAM is organized into 3 wings, equipped with 74 Transall C.160 turboprop transports, 5 DC-8s, 10 C-130s and 105 helicopters. Training aircraft include CAP-10/20/230 piston-engined primary trainers, Epsilon piston-engined and Fouga-Magister jet basic trainers, Mirage F1Bs, Mirage III-Bs, Mirage 2000Bs and two-seat Jaguars in wings for operational transformation; 25 Embraer 121-Xingus bought from Brazil are dual-purpose training/liaison aircraft. Total officers and other ranks (1991) 93,100 (5,600 women; 35,650 conscripts); 450 combat aircraft.

INTERNATIONAL RELATIONS

Membership. France is a member of the UN, the Council of Europe, NATO, WEU and the EC.

The Schengen Accord of June 1990 abolished border controls between France, Belgium, Germany, Luxembourg and the Netherlands. Italy acceded in Nov. 1990.

France is the focus of the *French Community* which formally links France with many of its former colonies in Africa. A wide range of agreements both with formal members of the Community and with other French-speaking countries extend to economic and technical matters and in particular to the disbursement of overseas aid.

ECONOMY

Policy. For the history of planning in France from 1947 to 1980, *see* THE STATESMAN'S YEAR-BOOK, 1982–83, p. 474. The Eighth Plan, covering the 1981–85 period, was set aside after the change of government in May 1981 and replaced by an interim plan for 1982–83, followed by a new Ninth Plan for 1984–88.

Budget. Receipts and expenditure in 1m. francs:

Receipts	*1989*	*1990*
Taxation	1,279,747	1,381,161
Income tax	243,830	261,850
Corporation tax	134,863	161,092
Payroll tax	29,983	32,078
Taxes on consumption		
V.A.T.	564,067	612,223
Non fiscal receipts	96,359	105,237
Receipts from special allocations account	71,541	77,205
Internal taxes on petroleum products	113,483	118,377
Total gross budget receipts	1,376,106	1,486,398

Proportion of 1990 gross receipts of largest categories: V.A.T., 41·2%; income tax, 17·6%; corporation tax, 10·8%; internal taxes on petroleum products, 8%; non-fiscal receipts, 7·1%.

Net receipts, 1990, (after payment of EEC levies, 187,232m. francs, and fiscal reimbursements, 169,705m. francs) were 1,129,461m. francs.

Expenditure	*1989*	*1990*
Public debt	117,337	137,995
Administration	382,965	412,270
Subsidies	350,599	357,424
Civil investment	79,614	81,984
Defence	221,807	230,766
Special allocations	11,704	13,439
Total expenditure	1,624,026	1,233,878

The accounts of revenue and expenditure are examined by a special administrative tribunal (*Cour des Comptes*), instituted in 1807.

Currency. The unit of currency is the *franc* (FRF) of 100 *centimes*. Coins are issued for 5, 10, 20 and 50 centimes, 1, 2, 5 and 10 francs; and bank-notes for 10, 20, 50, 100, 200 and 500 francs. In March 1991, £1 sterling = 9·92 *francs*; US$1 = 5·23 *francs*.

Banking and Finance. The Banque de France, founded in 1800, and nationalized on 2 Dec. 1945, has the monopoly (since 1848) of issuing bank-notes throughout France. Note circulation at 31 Dec. 1981 was 151,900m. francs. As a central bank, it puts monetary policy into effect and supervises its application. Its *Governor* is Jacques de Larosière.

The National Credit Council, formed in 1945 to regulate banking activity and consulted in all political decisions on monetary policy, comprises 45 members nominated by the Government; its president is the Minister for the Economy, its vice-president is the Governor of the Banque de France. Four principal deposit banks were nationalized in 1945 and the remainder in 1982 but the latter were privatized in 1987. The 10 chief banks in 1990 in order of their capital assets were: Crédit Agricole; Paribas (investment); Banque Nationale de Paris (state-owned); Crédit Lyonnais (state-owned); Société Générale; Caisses d'Epargne Ecureuil; Banques Populaires; CIC; Indosuez (investment); Crédit Commercial de France. Total deposits and short- and medium-term held bills by the banks at 31 Dec. 1981 was 1,302,800m. francs.

The state savings organization Caisse Nationale d'Epargne is administered by the post office on a giro system. On 31 Dec. 1981 the private savings banks (*Caisses d'epargne et de prévoyance*), numbering about 500 had 434,000m. francs in deposits; the state savings banks had 206,300m. francs in deposits. Deposited funds are centralized by a non-banking body, the *Caisse de Dépôts et Consignations*, which finances a large number of local authorities and state aided housing projects, and carries an important portfolio of transferable securities.

There is a stock exchange (Bourse) in Paris.

Weights and Measures. The metric system is in general use.

ENERGY AND NATURAL RESOURCES

Electricity. In 1990 there were 54 nuclear reactors in operation and 2 under construction, and some 75% of the electricity output was nuclear-produced, providing 33% of France's total energy consumption; a further 30% came from oil, 12% from gas and 8% from hydro-electric sources. Production (in 1m. kwh.): 1987, 360,744, of which 72,061 was hydroelectric and 288,683 nuclear. Supply 127 and 220 volts; 50 Hz.

Oil. In 1989 3·2m. tonnes of crude oil were produced. The greater part came from the Parentis oilfield in the Landes. Reserves (1985) total 221m. bbls. France has an important oil-refining industry, chiefly utilizing imported crude oil. The principal plants are situated in Seine-Maritime and in Bouches-du-Rhône. In 1985, 72·49m. tonnes of petroleum products were refined. There are 7,802 km of pipelines.

There has been considerable development of the production of natural gas and sulphur in the region of Lacq in the foothills of the Pyrenees. Production of natural gas was 10,574m. cu. metres in 1984; reserves (1985) 41,000m. cu. metres.

Minerals. Principal minerals and metals produced in 1983, in 1,000 tonnes: Coal, 33,396; crude steel, 17,616; iron ore, 15,972; pig iron, 13,752; bauxite, 1,660; potash salts, 1,651.

Agriculture. Of the total area of France (54·9m. ha), the utilized agricultural area comprised 31·4m. ha in 1987, 18m. ha (57·1%) were arable, 11·9m. ha (37·9%) were pasture, and 1·3m. ha (4·2%) were under permanent crops including vines (0·98m. ha). In 1986 there were 1,484,900 tractors in use. In 1987 there were 981,722 holdings and in 1988 1·48m. persons (6·8% of the employed civilian workforce) were employed in agriculture, hunting, fishing and forestry.

The following table shows the area under the leading crops and the production for 3 years:

	Area (1,000 ha)			Produce (1,000 tonnes)		
	1986	1987	1988	1986	1987	1988
Wheat	4,859	4,932	4,825	26,475	27,415	29,677
Rye	81	82	79	229	299	276
Barley	2,090	1,992	1,916	10,063	10,489	10,086
Oats	312	281	273	1,066	1,122	1,074
Potatoes	201	197	183	6,267	6,720	6,344
Sugar-beet	448	446	432	25,830	26,471	28,606
Maize	1,884	1,743	1,936	11,641	12,470	13,996

Production (1988, in 1,000 tonnes): Centrifugal raw sugar, 4,424; beef and veal, 1,832; pork, 1,740; lamb and mutton, 152; poultry, 1,429; milk, 29,012; eggs, 0·94m.; wine, 69·34m. hectolitres.

The production of fruits (other than for cider making) for 3 years was (in 1,000 tonnes) as follows:

	1986	1987	1988		1986	1987	1988
Apples	2,739	2,424	2,357	Melons	274	286	275
Pears	370	439	355	Nuts	50	50	51
Plums	209	203	222	Grapes	9,340	9,164	7,419
Peaches	473	488	472	Strawberries	92	99	95
Apricots	121	98	97	Oranges	3	3	3

Livestock (in 1,000) in 1988 (and 1989): Horses, 292; cattle, 21,052 (20,122); sheep, 10,221; goats, 1,003; pigs, 11,915 (11,706); poultry, 220,000.

Forestry. In 1990 forest (36% coniferous, 31% oak) covered some 13·9m. ha, about 27% of the land area. 1·7m. ha are state property. Timber sold (1988), 32·9m. cu. metres valued at 10,500m. francs. 0·55m. persons were employed in forestry in 1990.

Fisheries. (1987). There were 23,426 fishermen, and 9,620 sailing-boats, steamers and motor-boats. Catch (in tonnes): Fish, total, 513,367; crustaceans, 24,111; shell fish, 226,890.

INDUSTRY. Industrial production (in 1,000 tonnes) for 3 years was as follows:

	1986	1987	1988
Sulphuric acid	3,956	3,960	4,081
Caustic acid	1,517	1,430	1,494
Sulphur	1,170	1,092	1,022
Polystyrene	501	527	536
Polyvinyl	880	933	1,017
Polyethylene	1,133	1,156	1,135
Wool	48	43	43
Cotton	139	136	136
Linen	1.2	1·2	1·0
Silk	66	67	73
Jute	4.8	4·9	4·6
Cheese	1,289	1,321	…
Chocolate	325	373	…
Biscuits	404	416	…
Sugar	3,410	3,655	…
Fish preparations	107	104	…
Jams and jellies	144	151	…
Cement and lime	22,596	23,557	30,863

Engineering production (in 1,000 units) for 3 years:

	1986	1987	1988
Motor vehicles	3,195	3,493	3,699
Television sets	1,869	2,015	2,081
Radio sets	…	2,132	1,983
Tyres	51,138	56,450	60,366

Labour (1987). Out of an economically active population of 24,084,300 persons, 1,465,300 were engaged in agriculture, forestry and fishing, 1,521,900 in building, 1,183,100 in manufacturing industries, 897,900 in transport, 602,300 in banking and insurance, 4,228,700 in services, 2,592,500 in commerce. At 31 Dec. 1987, there were 21,230,200 employed.

Trade Unions. The main confederations recognized as nationally representative are: the CGT (Confédération Générale du Travail), founded in 1895; the CGT-FO (Confédération Générale du Travail–Force Ouvrière) which broke away from the CGT in 1948 as a protest against Communist influence therein; the CFTC (Confédération Française des Travailleurs Chrétiens), which was founded in 1919 and divided in 1964, with a breakaway group retaining the old name and the main body continuing under the new name of CFDT (Confédération Française Démocratique du Travail); and the CGC (Confédération Générale des Cadres) formed in 1944 which only represents managerial and supervisory staff.

Membership is estimated because unions are not required to publish figures; but at elections held on 8 Dec. 1982 for labour tribunals, the CGT was supported by 2·8m. members, the CGT–FO by 1·4m., the CFDT by 1·8m., the CFTC by 650,000 and the CGC by 740,000. Except for the CGC unions operate within the framework of industries and not of trades.

FOREIGN ECONOMIC RELATIONS

Commerce. Imports (c.i.f.) and exports (f.o.b.) in 1m. francs for 5 calendar years were (including gold):

	1983	*1984*	*1985*	*1986*	*1987*
Imports	799,754	903,664	962,747	887,502	944,999
Exports	694,659	813,031	870,811	825,417	857,936

The chief imports for home use and exports of home goods are to and from the following countries, in 1m. francs (including gold):

	Imports (c.i.f)		*Exports (f.o.b.)*	
Countries	*1986*	*1987*	*1986*	*1987*
Belgium-Luxembourg	83,917	88,681	74,895	79,873
Germany, Fed. Rep. of	172,324	186,666	133,107	142,713
Italy	103,289	110,811	97,059	103,637
Netherlands	32,204	36,063	11,157	13,225
Japan	50,997	53,270	40,665	43,602
Spain	36,941	41,241	33,781	45,500
Switzerland	22,167	23,624	37,727	36,787
UK	57,684	67,178	72,622	75,524
USA	66,995	67,592	61,091	62,527

Foreign trade by sector, 1987, in 1m. francs:

	Imports (c.i.f)	*Exports (f.o.b.)*
Agriculture and agri-food industry	119,036	148,570
Energy	100,274	18,540
Raw materials and semi-products	246,431	230,023
Capital goods	229,838	212,039
Surface transport equipment	92,852	115,769
Consumer goods	153,325	127,306

Total trade between France and UK (British Department of Trade returns, in £1,000 sterling):

	1986	*1987*	*1988*	*1989*	*1990*
Imports to UK	7,348,574	8,381,984	9,390,207	10,785,429	11,758,481
Exports and re-exports from UK	6,210,216	7,781,546	8,270,408	9,461,648	10,885,803

Tourism. In 1987 there were 31·9m. tourists.

COMMUNICATIONS

Roads. In 1986 there were 345,000 km of departmental road network and, in 1988, 36,800 km of national road network of which 8,590 km were motorway. In 1987 there were 5,364,251 registered vehicles, including 4,373,675 private and commercial vehicles, 6,988 coaches and buses, 600,000 lorries and vans and 231,035 motorcycles.

Railways. As from 1 Jan. 1938 all the independent railway companies were merged with the existing state railway system in a Société Nationale des Chemins de Fer Français (SNCF), which became a public industrial and commercial establishment in 1983.

In 1988, SNCF totalled 34,322 km (12,433 km electrified) and carried 146m. tonnes of freight and 825m. passengers. A new railway for high-speed trains (TGV) was completed in 1983 between Paris and Lyon. 2 further routes opened in 1989 to Le Mans to serve Britanny and in 1990 to Tours to serve the south-west.

The Paris transport network consisted in 1989 of 551 km of underground railway (métro) and regional express railways. In 1989 it carried 1,551m. passengers.

Boring of the Channel tunnel began in March 1988. A network (TGV Nord) is under construction linking Paris to the tunnel as well as to Lille, and this network will also connect Paris and the tunnel to Brussels and be extended to the Netherlands and the Germany.

Aviation. Air France, UTA and Air Inter, the national airlines, merged in 1990 to control 97% of French air traffic. In 1990 they operated some 200 aircraft, servicing Europe, North America, Central and South America, West and East Africa, Madagascar, the Near, Middle and Far East. 9 European routes were closed down in 1990. There are local networks in the West Indies and Central America. In 1988 Air France, UTA and Air Inter flew 3,693m. tonne-km (excluding mail) and 447,389m. passenger-km. There were (1984) 60 airports with scheduled services.

Shipping. Merchant ships, in 1988, numbered 261 vessels of 4,389,000 GRT (241 in 1989). During 1987, 186·87m. tonnes of cargo were unloaded, of which 92·2m. tonnes were crude and refined petroleum products, and 61·93m. tonnes were loaded; total passenger traffic, 21·5m.

In 1988 there were 8,500 km of navigable rivers, waterways and canals (of which 1,647 km accessible to vessels over 3,000 tons), with a total traffic in 1987 of 60·72m. tonnes.

Telecommunications. In 1988 the telephone system (government-owned) had 24,635,000 subscribers, and there were 17,028 post offices. In Jan. 1991 France Télécom was removed from the control of the Ministry of Posts and Telecommunications and is now run as a state-owned service company.

Some 5m. Minitel videotext terminals have been distributed free to the public.

Radio and television broadcasting was reorganized under the Act of 7 Aug. 1974 which replaced the Office de Radiodiffusion Télévision Française with 4 broadcasting companies, a production company and an audio-visual institute. The broadcasting authority is the *Conseil Supérieur de l'Audiovisuel*. In 1988 radio programmes are broadcast from 874 VHF transmitters of which 418 belong to 4 stations: *France Info, France Inter, France Musique* and *France Culture*. Television programmes are broadcast from 541 transmitters and 9,378 relay stations. TV broadcasts must contain at least 60% EC-generated programmes and 50% of these must be French. There were about 20m. radio and 17·95m. TV sets in use in 1986.

Cinemas (1987). There were 5,063 cinemas; attendances totalled 132·5m.

Newspapers (1987). There were 72 daily papers published in the provinces with a circulation of 6·7m. copies, and 14 published in Paris with a national circulation of 2·5m. Among Paris dailies *France-Soir* sells 539,000; *Le Monde* 445,000; *Le Parisien Libéré* 421,000 and *Le Figaro* 465,000. Among provincial dailies *Ouest-France* (Rennes) sells 783,000; *Le Progrés* (Lyon) 447,000; *La Voix du Nord* (Lille) 372,000; *Sud-Ouest* (Bordeaux) 430,000; *La Dauphine Libérée* (Grenoble) 401,000 and *Le Provençal* (Marseilles) 345,000.

JUSTICE, RELIGION, EDUCATION AND WELFARE

Justice. The system of justice is divided into 2 jurisdictions: the judicial, and the administrative.

Within the judicial jurisdiction are common law courts including 473 lower courts (*tribunaux d'instance*, including 11 in overseas departments), 186 higher courts (*tribunaux de grande instance*, including 5 *tribunaux de première instance* in the overseas territories), and 454 police courts (*tribunaux de police*, including 11 in overseas departments).

The *tribunaux d'instance* are presided over by a single judge. The *tribunaux de grande instance* usually have a collegiate composition, although may be presided over by a single judge in some civil cases. The police courts, presided over by a judge on duty in the *tribunal d'instance*, deal with petty offences (*contraventions*); correctional chambers (*chambres correctionelles*, of which there is at least one in each *tribunal de grande instance*) deal with graver offences (*délits*), including cases involving imprisonment up to 5 years. Correctional chambers consist of 3 judges of a *tribunal de grande instance* (a single judge in some cases). Sometimes in cases of *délit*, and in all cases of more serious *crimes*, a preliminary inquiry is made in secrecy by one of 569 examining magistrates (*juges d'instruction*), who either dismisses the case or sends it for trial before a public prosecutor.

Still within the judicial jurisdiction are various specialised courts, including 229 commercial courts (*tribunaux de commerce*), composed of tradesmen and manufacturers elected for 2 years initially and then for 4 years; 282 conciliation boards (*conseils de prud'hommes*), composed of an equal number of employers and employees elected for 5 years to deal with labour disputes; 437 courts for settling rural landholding disputes (*tribunaux paritaires des baux ruraux*, including 11 in overseas departments); and 110 social security courts (*tribunaux des affaires de sécurité sociale*).

When the decisions of any of these courts are susceptible of appeal, the case goes to one of the 35 courts of appeal (*cours d'appel*) composed each of a president and a variable number of members. There are 102 courts of assize (*cours d'assises*), each composed of a president who is a member of the court of appeal, and 2 other magistrates, and assisted by a lay jury of 9 members. These try crimes involving imprisonment of over 5 years. The decisions of the courts of appeal and the courts of assize are final, However, the Court of Cassation (*Cour de cassation*) has discretion to verify if the law has been correctly interpreted and if the rules of procedure have been followed exactly. The Court of Cassation may annul any judgment, following which the cases must be retried by a court of appeal or a court of assizes.

The administrative jurisdiction exists to resolve conflicts arising between citizens and central and local government authorities. It consists of 33 administrative courts (*tribunaux administratifs*, including 7 in overseas departments and territories) and 5 administrative courts of appeal (*cours administratives d'appel*). The Council of State is the final court of appeal in administrative cases, though it may also act as a court of first instance.

Cases of doubt as to whether the judicial or administrative jurisdiction is competent in any case are resolved by a *Tribunal de conflits* composed in equal measure of members of the Court of Cassation and the Council of State.

Capital punishment was abolished in Aug. 1981.

On 24 Jan. 1973 the first Ombudsman (*médiateur*) was appointed for a 6-year period.

The French penal institutions consist of: (1) *maisons d'arrêt* and *de correction*, where persons awaiting trial as well as those condemned to short periods of imprisonment are kept; (2) central prisons (*maisons centrales*) for those sentenced to long imprisonment; (3) special establishments, namely (*a*) schools for young adults, (*b*) hostels for old and disabled offenders, (*c*) hospitals for the sick and psychopaths. Special attention is being paid to classified treatment and the rehabilitation and vocational re-education of prisoners including work in open-air and semi-free establishments. There is 1 penal institution for women.

Juvenile delinquents go before special judges in 133 (11 in overseas departments) juvenile courts (*tribunaux pour enfants*); they are sent to public or private institutions of supervision and re-education.

The population at 1 Oct. 1990 of all penal establishments was 46,223 men and 2,054 women.

Religion. No religion is officially recognized by the State. Under the law promulgated on 9 Dec. 1905, which separated Church and State, the adherents of all creeds are authorized to form associations for public worship (*associations culturelles*).

The law of 2 Jan. 1907 provided that, failing *associations culturelles*, the buildings for public worship, together with their furniture, would continue at the disposition of the ministers of religion and the worshippers for the exercise of their religion; but in each case there was required an administrative act drawn up by the *préfet* as regards buildings belonging to the State or the departments and by the *maire* as regards buildings belonging to the communes.

There were (1985) 125 archbishops and bishops of the Roman Catholic Church, with (1974) 43,557 clergy of various grades and (1986) 42·35m. members. The Protestants of the Augsburg confession are, in their religious affairs, governed by a General Consistory, while the Reformed Church is under a Council of Administration, the seat of which is in Paris. In 1988 there were about 800,000 Protestants and 1·9m. Moslems.

Education. The primary, secondary and higher state schools constitute the 'Université de France'. The Supreme Council of 84 members has deliberative, administrative and judiciary functions, and as a consultative committee advises respecting the working of the school system, the inspectors-general are in direct communication with the Minister. For local education administration France is divided into 25 academic areas, each of which has an Academic Council whose members include a certain number elected by the professors or teachers. The Academic Council deals with all grades of education. Each is under a Rector, and each is provided with academy inspectors, 1 for each department.

Compulsory education is now provided for children of 6–16. The educational stages are as follows:

1. Non-compulsory pre-school instruction for children aged 2–5, to be given in infant schools or infant classes attached to primary schools.

2. Compulsory elementary instruction for children aged 6–11, to be given in primary schools and certain classes of the *lycées*. It consists of 3 courses: Preparatory (1 year), elementary (2 years), intermediary (2 years). Physically or mentally handicapped children are cared for in special institutions or special classes of primary schools.

3. Lower secondary education (*Enseignement du premier cycle du Second Degré*) for pupils aged 11–15, consists of 4 years of study in the *lycées* (grammar schools), *Collèges d'Enseignement Technique* or *Collèges d'Enseignement Général*.

4. Upper secondary education (*Enseignement du second cycle du Second Degré*) for pupils aged 15–18:

Long, général or *professionel* provided by the *lycées* and leading to the *baccalauréat* or to the *baccalauréat de technicien* after 3 years.

Court, professional courses of 3, 2 and 1 year are taught in the *lycées d'enseignement professionel*, or the specialized sections of the *lycées*, CES or CEG.

The following table shows the number of schools in 1987–88 and the numbers of pupils in full-time education:

	State		*Private*	
	Schools	*Pupils*	*Schools*	*Pupils*
Nursery	17,900	5,732,931	385	930,853
Primary	40,235		6,038	
Secondary	7,342	4,481,797	3,905	1,192,813

Higher Instruction is supplied by the State in the universities and in special schools, and by private individuals in the free faculties and schools. The law of 12 July 1875 provided for higher education free of charge. This law was modified by that of 18 March 1880, which granted the state faculties the exclusive right to confer degrees. A decree of 28 Dec. 1885 created a general council of the faculties, and the creation of universities, each consisting of several faculties, was accomplished in 1897, in virtue of the law of 10 July 1896.

The law of 12 Nov. 1968 laying down future guidelines for higher education redefined the activities and working of universities. Bringing several disciplines together, 780 units for teaching and research (UER–Unités d'Enseignement et de

Recherche) were formed which decided their own teaching activities, research programmes and procedures for checking the level of knowledge gained. They and the other parts of each university must respect the rules designed to maintain the national standard of qualifications.

The UERs form the basic units of 69 Universities and 3 National Polytechnic Institutes (with university status), grouped into 25 *académies* with 980,404 students in 1987.

There are also Catholic university facilities in Paris, Angers, Lille, Lyon and Toulouse with (1981–82) 34,118 students and private universities with (1984–85) 17,646 students.

Outside the university system, higher education (academic, professional and technical) is provided by over 400 schools and institutes, including the 177 Grandes Écoles, highly-selective public or private institutions offering mainly technological or commercial curricula, with an annual output of about 17,000 graduates. In 1984–85 there were 139,827 students in state establishments and 61,996 in private establishments. In 1986–87 there were also 48,811 students in preparatory classes leading to the Grandes Écoles, 129,942 in the Sections de Techniciens Supérieurs and 47,300 in the Écoles d'ingénieurs; there were also (1984-85) 18,951 students in Écoles normales d'instituteurs (teacher-training).

Health. On 1 Jan. 1988 there were 138,825 doctors, (1987) 49,610 chemists, (1986) 34,946 dentists, (1986) 294,260 nurses and (1986) 9,725 midwives. On 1 Jan. 1987 there were 3,730 hospitals with 574,000 beds.

Social Welfare. An order of 4 Oct. 1945 laid down the framework of a comprehensive plan of Social Security and created a single organization which superseded the various laws relating to social insurance, workmen's compensation, health insurance, family allowances, etc. All previous matters relating to Social Security are dealt with in the Social Security Code, 1956; this has been revised several times.

Contributions. All wage-earning workers or those of equivalent status are insured regardless of the amount or the nature of the salary or earnings. The funds for the general scheme are raised mainly from professional contributions, these being fixed within the limits of a ceiling and calculated as a percentage of the salaries. The calculation of contributions payable for family allowances, old age and industrial injuries relates only to this amount; on the other hand, the amount payable for sickness, maternity expenses, disability and death is calculated partly within the limit of the 'ceiling' and partly on the whole salary. These contributions are the responsibility of both employer and employee, except in the case of family allowances or industrial injuries, where they are the sole responsibility of the employer.

Self-employed Workers. From 17 Jan. 1948 allowances and old-age pensions were paid to self-employed workers by independent insurance funds set up within their own profession, trade or business. Schemes of compulsory insurance for sickness were instituted in 1961 for farmers and in 1966, with modifications in 1970, for other non-wage-earning workers.

Social Insurance. The orders laid down in Aug. 1967 ensure that the whole population can benefit from the Social Security Scheme; at present all elderly persons who have been engaged in the professions, as well as the surviving spouse, are entitled to claim an old-age benefit.

Sickness Insurance refunds the costs of treatment required by the insured and the needs of dependants.

Maternity Insurance covers the costs of medical treatment relating to the pregnancy, confinement and lying-in period; the beneficiaries being the insured person or the spouse.

Insurance for Invalids is divided into 3 categories: (1) those who are capable of working; (2) those who cannot work; (3) those who, in addition, are in need of the help of another person. According to the category, the pension rate varies from 30 to 50% of the average salary for the last 10 years, with additional allowance for home help for the third category.

Old-age Pensions for workers were introduced in 1910 and are now fixed by the Social Security Code of 28 Jan. 1972. Since 1983 people who have paid insurance for at least 37½ years (150 quarters) receive at 60 a pension equal to 60% of basic salary. People who have paid insurance for less than 37½ years but no less than 15 years can expect a pension equal to as many 1/150ths of the full pension as their quarterly payments justify. In the event of death of the insured person, the husband or wife of the deceased person receives half the pension received by the latter. Compulsory supplementary schemes ensure benefits equal to 70% of previous earnings.

Family Allowances. The system comprises: (*a*) Family allowances proper, equivalent to 25·5% of the basic monthly salary (1,246 francs) for 2 dependent children, 46% for the third child, 41% for the fourth child, and 39% for the fifth and each subsequent child; a supplement equivalent to 9% of the basic monthly salary for the second and each subsequent dependent child more than 10 years old and 16% for each dependent child over 15 years. (*b*) Family supplement (519 francs) for persons with at least 3 children or one child aged less than 3 years. (*c*) Antenatal grants. (*d*) Maternity grant equal to 260% of basic salary; increase for multiple births or adoptions, 198%; increase for birth or adoption of third or subsequent child, 457%. (*e*) Allowance for specialized education of handicapped children. (*f*) Allowance for orphans. (*g*) Single parent allowance. (*h*) Allowance for opening of school term. (*i*) Allowance for accommodation, under certain circumstances. (*j*) Minimum family income for those with at least 3 children. Allowances (*b*), (*g*), (*h*) and (*j*) only apply to those whose annual income falls below a specified level.

Workmen's Compensation. The law passed by the National Assembly on 30 Oct. 1946 forms part of the Social Security Code and is administered by the Social Security Organization. Employers are invited to take preventive measures. The application of these measures is supervised by consulting engineers (assessors) of the local funds dealing with sickness insurance, who may compel employers who do not respect these measures to make additional contributions; they may, in like manner, grant rebates to employers who have in operation suitable preventive measures. The injured person receives free treatment, the insurance fund reimburses the practitioners, hospitals and suppliers chosen freely by the injured. In cases of temporary disablement the daily payments are equal to half the total daily wage received by the injured. In case of permanent disablement the injured person receives a pension, the amount of which varies according to the degree of disablement and the salary received during the past 12 months.

Unemployment Benefits vary according to circumstances (full or partial unemployment) which are means-tested. Since 1926 unemployment benefits have been paid from public funds.

DIPLOMATIC REPRESENTATIVES

Of France in Great Britain (58 Knightsbridge, London, SW1X 7JT)
Ambassador: Bernard Dorin.

Of Great Britain in France (35 rue du Faubourg St Honoré, 75383 Paris)
Ambassador: Sir Ewen Fergusson, KCMG.

Of France in the USA (4101 Reservoir Rd., NW, Washington, D.C., 20007)
Ambassador: Jacques Andreani.

Of the USA in France (2 Ave. Gabriel, Paris)
Ambassador: Walter J. Curley.

Of France to the United Nations
Ambassador: Jean-Bernard Mérimée.

Further Reading

Statistical Information: The Institut National de la Statistique et des Études économiques (18, Boulevard Adolphe Pinard, 75014 Paris) is the central office of statistics. It was established by a law of 27 April 1946, which amalgamated the Service National des Statistiques (created in 1941 by merging the Direction de la Statistique générale de la France and the Service de la Démographie) with the Institut de Conjoncture (set up in 1938) and some statistical services of the Ministry of National Economy. The Institut comprises the following departments: Metropolitan statistics, Overseas statistics, Market research and economic studies, Documentation, Research statistics and economics, Informatics, Foreign Economic Studies.

The main publications of the Institut include:

Annuaire statistique de la France (from 1878)
Annuaire statistique des Territoires d'Outre-Mer (from 1959)
Bulletin mensuel de statistique (monthly)
Documentation économique (bi-monthly)
Données statistiques africaines et Malgaches (quarterly)
Economie et Statistique (monthly)
Tableaux de l'Economie Française (biennially, from 1956)
Tendances de la Conjoncture (monthly)

Braudel, F., *The Identity of France*. 2 vols. London, 1988-90
Caron, F., *An Economic History of Modern France*. London, 1979
Chambers, F. J., *France*. [Bibliography] Oxford and Santa Barbara, (rev. ed.) 1990
Crozier, M., *A Strategy for Change: The Future of French Society*. MIT Press, 1982
Monnier, A., *La Population de la France*. Paris, 1990
Peyrefitte, A., *The Trouble with France*. New York, 1981
Pinchemel, P., *France: A Geographical, Social and Economic Survey*. CUP, 1987
Weston, M., *English Reader's Guide to the French Legal System*. Oxford, 1991
Who's Who in France [in French]. Paris, annual

OVERSEAS DEPARTMENTS

On 19 March 1946 the French colonies of Guadeloupe, French Guiana, Martinique and Réunion each became an Overseas Department of France, with the same status as the departments comprising Metropolitan France. The former territory of Saint Pierre and Miquelon held a similar status from July 1976 until June 1985, when it became a *collectivité territorial*.

GUADELOUPE

HISTORY. Discovered by Columbus in Nov. 1493, the two main islands were then known as *Karukera* (Isle of Beautiful Waters) to the Carib inhabitants, who resisted Spanish attempts to colonize. A French colony was established on 28 June 1635, and apart from short periods of occupancy by British forces, Guadeloupe has since remained a French possession. On 19 March 1946 Guadeloupe became an Overseas Department; in 1974 it additionally became an administrative region.

AREA AND POPULATION. Guadeloupe consists of a group of islands in the Lesser Antilles. The two main islands, Basse-Terre to the west and Grande-Terre to the east, are separated by a narrow channel, called Rivière Salée. Adjacent to these are the islands of Marie Galante *(Ceyre* to the Caribs) to the south-east, La Désirade to the east, and the Îles des Saintes to the south. The islands of St Martin and St Barthélemy lie 250 km to the north-west.

	Area in sq. km	*Census 1974*	*Census 1982*	*Chief town*
St Martin [1]	54 [2]	6,191	8,072	Marigot
St Barthélemy	21	2,491	3,059	Gustavia
Basse-Terre	848	135,746	135,341	Basse-Terre
Grande-Terre	590	159,424	163,668	Pointe-à-Pitre
Îles des Saintes	13	3,084	2,901	Terre-de-Bas
La Désirade	20	1,682	1,602	Grande Anse
Marie-Galante	158	15,912	13,757	Grand-Bourg
	1,705	324,530	328,400	

[1]Northern part only; the southern third is Dutch. [2]Includes uninhabited Tintamarre.

Population (estimate, 1988) 336,300. 77% are mulatto, 10% black and 10% mestizo, but the populations of St Barthélemy and Les Saintes are still mainly descended from 17th-century Breton and Norman settlers. French is the official language, but a Creole dialect is spoken by the vast majority except on St Martin.

The seat of government is Basse-Terre (13,656 inhabitants in 1982) at the south-west end of that island but the largest towns are Pointe-à-Pitre (25,310 inhabitants), the economic centre and main port, and its suburb, Les Abymes (51,837 inhabitants).

Vital statistics (1987): Live births, 6,855; deaths, 2,244; marriages, 1,880.

CLIMATE. Warm and humid. Pointe-à-Pitre. Jan. 74°F (23·4°C), July 80°F (26·7°C). Annual rainfall 71" (1,814 mm).

CONSTITUTION AND GOVERNMENT. Guadeloupe is administered by a *Conseil Général* of 42 members (assisted by an Economic and Social Committee of 40 members) and a Regional Council of 39 members, both directly elected for terms of 6 years. It is represented in the National Assembly by 4 deputies, in the Senate by 2 senators and on the Economic and Social Council by 2 councillors. There are 3 *arrondissements,* sub-divided into 34 communes, each administered by an elected municipal council. The French government is represented by an appointed Commissioner.

Commissioner: Yves Bonnet.

President of the Conseil Général: Dominique Larifla.

President of the Regional Council: Félix Proto.

ECONOMY

Budget. The budget for 1983 balanced at 1,633m. francs.

Banking. The main commercial banks are the Banque des Antilles Françaises (with 6 branches), the Banque Populaire de la Guadeloupe (with 6 branches), the Banque Nationale de Paris (14 branches), the Crédit Agricole (26), the Banque Française Commerciale (8), the Société Generale de Banque aux Antilles (5) and the Chase Manhattan Bank (1). The Caisse Centrale de Coopération économique is the official bank of the department and issues its bank-notes.

ENERGY AND NATURAL RESOURCES

Electricity. Production in 1986 totalled 315m. kwh.

Agriculture. Chief products (1988) are bananas (120,000 tonnes), sugar-cane (891,000 tonnes), rum (64,883 hectolitres of pure alcohol in 1984). Other fruits and vegetables are grown for domestic consumption. 11·8m. flowers were grown in 1984.

Livestock (1988): Cattle, 74,000; goats, 33,000; sheep, 4,000; pigs, 43,000.

Forestry. In 1985, there were 395 sq. km of forests. In 1984, 51,848 cu. metres of wood were produced.

Fisheries. The catch in 1984 was 8,500 tonnes; crustacea (120 tonnes), shell fish (300 tonnes).

COMMERCE. Trade for 1985 (in 1m. francs) was imports 5,745 and exports 669, 60% of imports were from France, while 63% of exports went to France and 18% to Martinique. In 1985 bananas formed 43% of the exports, sugar 10% and rum 7%. St Martin and St Barthélemy are free ports.

Total trade between Guadeloupe and UK (British Department of Trade returns, £1,000 sterling):

	1989	*1990*
Imports to UK	119	53
Exports and re-exports from UK	4,381	5,084

Tourism. Tourism is the chief economic activity, producing some 2,000m. francs in

1989. 320,000 tourists visited in 1989, of which 70% were French, 15% North American and 10% German.

COMMUNICATIONS

Roads. In 1984 there were 3,500 km of roads. There were 87,785 passenger cars and 33,350 commercial vehicles in 1981.

Aviation. Air France and 7 other airlines call at Guadeloupe. In 1984 there were 31,451 arrivals and departures of aircraft and 1,325,500 passengers at Raizet (Pointe-à-Pitre) airport and, 6,682 aircraft movements and 116,000 passengers at Marie-Galante airport.

Shipping. Guadeloupe is in direct communication with France by means of 12 steam navigation companies. In 1983, 1,239 vessels arrived to disembark 74,921 passengers and 1,035,800 tonnes of freight and to embark 74,999 passengers and 470,600 tonnes of freight.

Telecommunications. In 1984 there were 47 post offices and 64,916 telephones. RFO broadcasts for 17 hours a day in French and television broadcasts for 6 hours a day. There were (1983) 25,000 radio and (1981) 32,886 TV receivers.

Newspapers. There was (1984) 1 daily newspaper *(France-Antilles)* with a circulation of 25,000.

JUSTICE, RELIGION, EDUCATION AND WELFARE

Justice. There are 4 *tribunaux d'instance* and 2 *tribunaux de grande instance* at Basse-Terre and Pointe-à-Pitre; there is also a court of appeal and a court of assizes at Basse-Terre.

Religion. The majority of the population are Roman Catholic.

Education. In 1984 there were 62,303 pupils at 284 primary schools and 45,843 at secondary schools. The University Antilles-Guyane had 4,809 students in 1984–85, of which Guadeloupe itself had 1,870.

Health. The medical services in 1985 included 11 public hospitals (2,891 beds) and 18 private clinics (1,256 beds). There were 416 physicians, 127 dentists, 127 pharmacists, 70 midwives and 1,131 nursing personnel.

Further Reading

Information: Office du Tourisme du départemente, Point-à-Pitre. *Director:* Eric W. Rotin.

Lasserre, G., *La Guadeloupe, étude géographique.* 2 vols. Bordeaux, 1961

GUIANA

Guyane Française

HISTORY. A French settlement on the island of Cayenne was established in 1604 and the territory between the Maroni and Oyapock rivers finally became a French possession in 1817. Convicts settlements were established from 1852, that on off-shore Devil's Island being most notorious; all were closed by 1945. On 19 March 1946 the status of Guiana was changed to that of an Overseas Department and in 1974 also became an administrative region.

AREA AND POPULATION. French Guiana is situated on the north-east coast of South America, and has an area of about 83,533 sq. km (32,252 sq. miles) and a population at the 1982 Census of 73,800, of whom 3,000 were tribal Indians; estimate (1989) 93,540. The chief towns (1982 populations) are Cayenne, the capital (38,093), Kourou (7,061) and Saint-Laurent-du-Maroni (6,971). These figures exclude the floating population of miners, officials and troops and about 7,000 Surinamese refugees since 1986.

In 1982, 43% of the inhabitants were of Creole origin, 14% Chinese, 11% from Metropolitan France and 8% Haitian. 90% of the population speak Creole.

Vital statistics (1988): Live births, 2,700; deaths, 562; marriages (1987), 365.

CONSTITUTION AND GOVERNMENT. French Guiana is administered by a General Council of 19 members and a Regional Council of 31 members, both directly elected for terms of 6 years. It is represented in the National Assembly by 2 deputies and in the Senate by 1 senator. The French government is represented by a Prefect. There are 2 *arrondissements* (Cayenne and SaintLaurent-du-Maroni) subdivided into 21 communes.

Prefect: Jean-Pierre Lacroix.
President of the General Council: Elie Castor.
President of the Regional Council: Georges Othily.

ECONOMY

Budget. The budget for 1987 balanced at 847m. francs, excluding duplicated items and national expenditure.

Banking. The Banque de la Guyane has a capital of 10m. francs and reserve fund of 2·39m. francs. Loans totalled 2,762m. francs in 1987. Other banks include Banque National de Paris-Guyane, Crédit Populaire Guyanais and Banque Française Commerciale.

ENERGY AND NATURAL RESOURCES

Electricity. Production in 1988 totalled 243m. kwh. Supply 220 volts; 50 Hz.

Agriculture. Only 12,581 hectares are under cultivation. The crops (1988, in tonnes) consist of rice (14,000), manioc (6,263) and sugar-cane (1,740).

Livestock (1988): 15,000 cattle, 9,000 swine and (1987) 117,000 poultry.

Forestry. The country has immense forests (about 66,700 sq. km in 1988) rich in many kinds of timber. Roundwood production (1988) 101,273 cu. metres.

Fisheries. The fishing fleet for shrimps comprises 31 US and 41 French boats. The catch in 1988 totalled 4,256 tonnes of shrimps and 1,024 tonnes of fish. Production of *Macrobrachium Rosenbergii* (an edible river shrimp) totalled 62·8 tonnes.

COMMERCE. Trade in 1m. francs:

	1985	*1986*	*1987*	*1988*
Imports	2,287	2,065	2,371	2,742
Exports	300	255	323	325

In 1986, 8% of imports came from Trinidad and Tobago, 65% from France and 11% from the EEC, while 36% of exports went to the USA, 16% to Japan, 22% to the French West Indies and 23% to France. In 1985, shrimps formed 53% of exports and timber, 9%.

Total trade between Guiana and UK (British Department of Trade returns, in £1,000 sterling):

	1986	*1987*	*1988*	*1989*	*1990*
Imports to UK	55	380	1,148	9,009	4,048
Exports and re-exports from UK	1,052	1,134	4,232	4,559	11,939

TOURISM. There were 14,500 tourists in 1987.

COMMUNICATIONS

Roads. Three chief and some secondary roads connect the capital with most of the coastal area by motor-car services. There are (1986) 372 km of national and 341 km of departmental roads. In 1989 there were 23,520 passenger cars, 1,568 trucks and 121 buses. Connexions with the interior are made by waterways which, despite rapids, are navigable by local craft.

Aviation. In 1988, 123,792 passengers and 3,632 tonnes of freight arrived and

121,575 passengers and 1,572 tonnes of freight departed by air at Rochambeau International Airport (Cayenne). There are regular internal flights to 7 other airports.

The base of the European Space Agency (ESA) is located near Kourou and has been operational since 1979.

Shipping. The chief ports are: Cayenne, St-Laurent-du-Maroni and Kourou. Dégrad des Cannes (the port of Cayenne) is visited regularly by ships of the Compagnie Général Maritime, the Compagnie Maritime des Chargeurs Réunis and Marseille Fret. In 1988, 706 vessels arrived and departed. 189,000 tonnes of petroleum products arrived and 333,000 tonnes of other freight arrived and departed.

Telecommunications. Number of telephones (1989), 26,146. There are wireless stations at Cayenne, Oyapoc, Régina, St-Laurent-du-Maroni and numerous other locations.

RFO-Guyane (Guiana Radio) broadcasts for 133 hours each week on medium- and short-waves and FM in French. Television is broadcast for 135 hours each week on 2 channels. In 1986 there were 44,000 radio and 6,500 TV receivers.

Newspapers. There was (1988) 1 daily newspaper *(Presse de la Guyane)* with a circulation of 1,000 and a paper published 4 times a week *(France-Guyane)* with a circulation of 5,500.

JUSTICE, RELIGION, EDUCATION AND WELFARE

Justice. At Cayenne there is a *tribunal d'instance* and a *tribunal de grande instance*, from which appeal is to the regional *cour d'appel* in Martinique.

Religion. In 1984, 77·6% of the population was Roman Catholic and 4% Protestant.

Education. Primary education has been free since 1889 in lay schools for the two sexes in the communes and many villages. In 1988 public primary schools had 18,024 pupils and (1986) 890 teachers, 10,897 pupils and (1986) 793, the *lycées* and *collèges d'enseignement secondaire*, 793 teachers and 9,085 pupils. Private schools had 152 teachers and 2,224 pupils. The *Institut Henri Visioz* forms part of the *Université des Antilles-Guyane,* with 253 students.

Health. There were (1986) 160 physicians, 44 dentists, 33 pharmacists, 29 midwives and 496 nursing personnel. In 1987 there were 3 hospitals with 748 beds and 3 private clinics with 162 beds.

MARTINIQUE

HISTORY. Discovered by Columbus in 1493, the island was known to its inhabitants as *Madinina*, from which its present name was corrupted. A French colony was established in 1635 and, apart from brief periods of British occupation the island has since remained under French control. On 19 March 1946 its status was altered to that of an Overseas Department, and in 1974 it also became an administrative region.

AREA AND POPULATION. The island, situated in the Lesser Antilles between Dominica and St Lucia, occupies an area of 1,079 sq. km (417 sq. miles). The population, 1982 Census, was 328,566 (estimate, 1990, 359,000), of whom in 1988 99,844 lived in Fort-de-France, the capital and chief commercial town, which has a landlocked harbour nearly 40 sq. km in extent. Other towns (1982) are Lamentin (26,367), Schoelcher (19,375) and La Trinité (10,076).

French is the official language, but the majority of the population use a Creole dialect.

Vital statistics (1988): Live births 6,397; deaths 2,099; marriages 1,537.

CLIMATE. Fort-de-France. Jan. 74°F (23·5°C), July 78°F (25·6°C). Annual rainfall 72" (1,840 mm).

CONSTITUTION AND GOVERNMENT. The island is administered by a General Council of 45 members and a Regional Council of 41 members, both directly elected for terms of 6 years. The French government is represented by an appointed Commissioner. There are 3 *arrondissements*, sub-divided into 34 communes, each administered by an elected municipal council. Martinique is represented in the National Assembly by 4 deputies, in the Senate by 2 senators and on the Economic and Social Council by 2 councillors.

At the Regional Council elections of Oct. 1990, the electorate was 223,658. 91,433 votes were cast. The Progressive Martinique Party (PPM) won 14 seats with 29,961 votes; the UDF-RPR 9, with 20,364 votes; the Martinique Independence Movement (MIM) 7, with 15,090 votes. 5 seats went to a left-wing, and 4 to a right-wing, coalition, and 2 to independents.

Commissioner: Jean-Claude Roure.
President of the General Council: Émile Maurice.
President of the Regional Council: Camille Darsieres.

ECONOMY

Budget. The budget, 1988, balanced at 2,451m. francs.

Banking. The Institut d'Émission des Départements d'Outre-Mer is the official bank of the department. The Caisse Centrale de Coopération Économique is used by the Government in assisting the economic development of the department.

The Banque des Antilles Françaises (with a capital of 32·5m. francs), the Crédit Martiniquais (30·4m. francs), the Société Générale de Banque aux Antilles (15m. francs), the Banque Française Commerciale (49m. francs), the Banque Nationale de Paris and the Crédit Agricole are operating in Fort-de-France.

ENERGY AND NATURAL RESOURCES

Electricity. Production in 1987 totalled 513m. kwh.

Agriculture. Bananas, sugar and rum are the chief products, followed by pineapples, food and vegetables. In 1988 there were 3,458 hectares under sugar-cane, 8,290 hectares under bananas and 400 hectares under pineapples. Production (1988): Sugar, 7,500 tonnes; rum, 85,987 hectolitres; cane for sugar, 93,535 tonnes; cane for rum, 121,835 tonnes; bananas 200,000 tonnes; pineapples, 24,000 tonnes.

Livestock (1988): 43,000 cattle, 90,000 sheep, 48,000 pigs, 46,000 goats and 2,000 horses.

Forestry. Production (1985) 11,000 cu. metres. Forests comprise 26% of the land area.

Fisheries. The catch in 1988 was 3,000 tonnes.

COMMERCE. Trade in 1m. francs:

	1985	*1986*	*1987*	*1988*
Imports	6,050	6,065	6,708	7,722
Exports	1,300	1,496	1,163	1,172

In 1987 the main items of import were crude petroleum and foodstuffs; main items of export were petroleum products (14%), bananas (46%) and rum (13%); 65% of imports came from France and 64% of exports went to France and 24% to Guadeloupe.

Total trade between Martinique and UK (British Department of Trade returns, in £1,000 sterling):

	1986	*1987*	*1988*	*1989*	*1990*
Imports to UK	14	712	83	158	1,071
Exports and re-exports from UK	21,230	10,705	3,886	8,815	26,315

Tourism. In 1988 there were 665,500 tourists, including 385,500 cruise visitors.

COMMUNICATIONS

Roads. In 1989 there were 7 km of motorway, 260 km of national roads, 620 km of district roads and 803 km of local roads. In 1987 there were 10,065 passenger cars and 2,361 commercial vehicles registered.

Aviation. In 1988, 1,273,376 passengers arrived and departed by air at Fort-de-France–Lamentin airport.

Shipping. The island is visited regularly by French, American and other lines. In 1987, 1,330 commercial vessels called at Martinique and discharged 8,970 passengers and (1988) 1,573,400 tonnes of freight and embarked 7,744 passengers and (1988) 711,000 tonnes of freight, excluding about 150,000 passengers calling in transit.

Telecommunications. There were, in 1985, 46 post offices and, 81,985 telephones. Radio-telephone service to Europe is available. In 1984 there were 46,000 radio and 42,500 TV receivers.

Newspapers. In 1989 there was 1 daily newspaper with a circulation of 19,000.

JUSTICE, RELIGION, EDUCATION AND WELFARE

Justice. Justice is administered by 2 lower courts (*tribunaux d'instance*), a higher court (*tribunal de grande instance*), a regional court of appeal, a commercial court, a court of assizes and an administrative court. For definitions *see* pp.494-95.

Religion. In 1982, 94% of the population was Roman Catholic.

Education. Education is compulsory between the ages of 6 and 16 years. In 1988, there were 18,923 pupils in nursery schools, 32,986 pupils in primary schools, 31,234 pupils in comprehensive schools, 8,035 students at technical college and 7,000 pupils in sixth-form colleges. The *Institut Henri Visioz* forms part of the *Université des Antilles-Guyane*, which had (1986-87) 5,551 students.

Health. There were (1986) 3,427 hospital beds, 519 doctors, 160 pharmacists, 110 dentists and 134 midwives.

Further Reading

Annuaire statistique I.N.S.E.E. 1977–80. Martinique, 1982
La Martinique en quelques chiffres. Martinique, 1982
Guide Economique des D.O.M.-T.O.M., Paris, 1982

RÉUNION

HISTORY. Réunion (formerly Île Bourbon) became a French possession in 1638 and remained so until 19 March 1946, when its status was altered to that of an Overseas Department; in 1974 it also became an administrative region.

AREA AND POPULATION. The island of Réunion lies in the Indian Ocean, about 640 km east of Madagascar and 180 km south west of Mauritius. It has an area of 2,512 sq. km (968·5 sq. miles) and had a population of 515,798 (at the 1982 census) and of an estimated 596,000 in 1990. The capital is Saint-Denis (population, 1990: 109,072); the other town is Saint-Pierre, (population, 1990: 50,082). The official language is French. There is a creole vernacular.

Vital statistics (1989): Live births, 10,574; deaths, 3,306; marriages, (1988) 3,354.

The islands of Juan de Nova, Europa, Bassas da India, Iles Glorieuses and Tromelin, with a combined area of 32 sq. km, are uninhabited and lie at various points in the Indian Ocean adjacent to Madagascar. They remained French after Madagascar's independence in 1960, and are now administered by Réunion. Both Mauritius and the Seychelles claim Tromelin (transferred by the UK from the Seychelles to France in 1954), and Madagascar claims all 5 islands.

CLIMATE. A sub-tropical maritime climate, free from extremes of weather, though the island lies in the cyclone belt of the Indian Ocean. Conditions are generally humid and there is no well-defined dry season. Saint-Denis. Jan. 80°F (26·7°C), July 70°F (21·1°C). Annual rainfall 56" (1,400 mm).

CONSTITUTION AND GOVERNMENT. Réunion is administered by a General Council (*Conseil Général*) of 44 members and a Regional Council of 45 members, both directly elected for terms of 6 years. Réunion is represented in the National Assembly in Paris by 5 deputies, in the Senate by 3 senators, and in the Economic and Social Council by 1 councillor. There are 4 *arrondissements*, sub-divided into 24 communes each administered by an elected municipal council. The French government is represented by an appointed Commissioner.

Commissioner: Daniel Constantin.
President of the General Council: Eric Boyer.
President of the Regional Council: Pierre Lagourgue.

ECONOMY

Production. GDP was estimated at 22·7m francs in 1988.

Budget. The budget for 1987 balanced at 2,938m. French francs.

Banking. The Institut d'émission des Départements d'Outre-mer has the right to issue bank-notes. Banks operating in Réunion are the Banque de la Réunion (Crédit Lyonnais), the Banque Nationale de Paris Internationale, the Caisse Régionale de Crédit Agricole Mutuel de la Réunion, the Banque Française Commerciale (BFC) CCP, Trésorerie Générale, and the Banque de la Réunion pour l'Economie et la Développement.

ENERGY AND NATURAL RESOURCES

Electricity. Production (1988) 762·8m. kwh.

Agriculture Production in tonnes: Sugar, 1989: 252,400; molasses, (1988): 79,500, bananas, 1988: 4,520; rum, 1989: 73,622 hectolitres; maize, 1988: 13,019; potatoes, 1989: 10,182; onions, 1989: 3,315; pineapples, 1989: 4,770; tomatoes, 1988: 3,155; vanilla, 1989: 250; tobacco, 1989: 102; geranium oil, 1989: 14·6.

Livestock (1988): 20,000 cattle, 75,000 pigs, 3,000 sheep, 44,000 goats and 4m. poultry.

Forestry. There were (1989) 100,392 ha. of forest. Roundwood production (1985) 75,000 cu. metres.

Fisheries. In 1989 the catch was 1,180 tonnes.

INDUSTRY

Labour. The workforce was 220,000 in 1989. The sugar industry employed 3,844.

COMMERCE. Trade in 1m. French francs:

	1983	*1984*	*1985*	*1986*	*1987*	*1988*
Imports	6,410	6,895	7,457	7,861	8,751	9,839
Exports	662	695	802	930	887	1,058

The chief export is sugar, forming (1989) 94% by value. In 1989 (by value) 25·5% of imports were from, and 80% of exports to, France.

Total trade between Réunion and UK (British Department of Trade returns, in £1,000 sterling):

	1987	*1988*	*1989*	*1990*
Imports to UK	1,056	1,372	4,389	1,204
Exports and re-exports from UK	8,624	8,536	7,529	11,732

Tourism. There were 182,000 visitors in 1989, including 132,000 from France and 143,600 tourists.

COMMUNICATIONS

Roads. There were, in 1989, 2,719 km of roads. There were some 126,000 registered vehicles in 1989.

Aviation. Réunion is served by Air France (up to 15 flights a week) and 7 other airlines including South African Airways, Air Mauritius and Air Madagascar. In 1989, 368,170 passengers and 12,959 tonnes of freight arrived at, and 370,215 passengers and 3,429 tonnes of freight departed from Saint-Denis-Gillot airport.

Shipping. 6 shipping lines serve the island. In 1989, 455 vessels visited the island, unloading 1,712,653 tonnes of freight and loading 68,355 tonnes at Pointe-des-Galets.

Telecommunications. There are telephone and telegraph connexions with Mauritius, Madagascar and metropolitan France. There are 648 post offices and a central telephone office; number of telephones (1990), 170,000.

RFO broadcast in French on medium- and short-waves for more than 18 hours a day. There are 2 television channels broadcasting for 70 hours a week and one independent channel.

Cinemas. In 1990 there were 17 cinemas.

Newspapers. There were (1990) 3 daily newspapers, 3 weeklies and 3 monthlies.

JUSTICE, RELIGION, EDUCATION AND WELFARE

Justice. There are 3 lower courts (*tribunaux d'instance*), 2 higher courts (*tribunaux de grande instance*), 1 appeal, 1 administrative court and 1 conciliation board. For definitions *see* pp.494-95.

Religion. In 1990, 95% of the population was Roman Catholic.

Education. In 1989-90 there were 115,000 pupils in primary, and 75,000 pupils in secondary, education. Secondary education was provided in (1989–90) 7 *lycées,* 52 *collèges,* and 12 technical *lycées.* There were 18 primary and secondary private schools, with 306 teachers, and 8,827 pupils. The *Université Française de l'Océan Indien* (founded 1971) had 4,750 students in 1989–90.

Health. In 1989 there were 19 hospitals with 3,270 beds, 928 physicians, 250 dentists, 185 pharmacists, 140 midwives and 2,070 nursing personnel.

Further Reading

Institut National de la Statistique et des Etudes Economiques. *Tableau Economique de la Réunion.* Paris, 1989

Bulletin de la Chambre de Commerce et de l'Industrie de la Réunion

Bertile, W., *Atlas Thématique et Régional.* Réunion, 1990

TERRITORIAL COLLECTIVITIES

MAYOTTE

HISTORY. Mayotte was a French colony from 1843 until 1914, when it was attached, with the other Comoro islands, to the government-general of Madagascar. The Comoro group was granted administrative autonomy within the French Republic and became an Overseas Territory.

When the other 3 islands voted to become independent (as the Comoro state) in 1974, Mayotte voted against this and remained a French dependency. In Dec. 1976, it became (following a further referendum) a Territorial Collectivity.

AREA AND POPULATION. Mayotte, east of the Comoro Islands, consists of a main island (362 sq. km) with 57,363 inhabitants at the 1985 Census, containing the chief town, Mamoundzou (12,119); and the smaller island of Pamanzi (11 sq. km) lying 2 km to the east, with 9,775 inhabitants in 1985, containing the old capital of Dzaoudzi (5,675). The whole territory covers 373 sq. km (144 sq. miles) and had a 1985 Census population of 67,138; estimate (1988) 77,300. The spoken language is Mahorian (akin to Comoran, an Arabized dialect of Swahili), but French remains the official and commercial language.

CONSTITUTION AND GOVERNMENT. The island is administered by a *Conseil Général* of 17 members, directly elected for a 6-year term. The French government is represented by an appointed Commissioner. Mayotte is represented by 1 deputy in the National Assembly and by 1 member in the Senate. There are 17 communes, including 2 on Pamanzi.

Commissioner: Akli Khider.
President of the Conseil Général: Younoussa Bamana.

ECONOMY

Budget. In 1984, revenue was 137·1m. francs (44% being subsidies from France) and expenditure 148·4m. francs. The 1985 Budget balanced at 313m. francs.

Currency. Since Feb. 1976 the currency has been the (metropolitan) *French franc*.

Banking. The *Institut d'Emission d'Outre-mer* and the *Banque Française Commerciale* both have branches in Dzaoudzi.

ENERGY AND NATURAL RESOURCES

Electricity. Production (1982) 5m. kwh.

Agriculture. The main food crops (1983 production in tonnes) are mangoes (1,500), bananas (1,300), breadfruit (700), cassava (500) and pineapples (200). The chief cash crops are ylang-ylang, vanilla, coffee, copra, cinnamon and cloves.

Livestock (1982): Cattle, 3,000; goats, 10,000; pigs, 2,000.

Fisheries. A lobster and shrimp industry has recently been created. Annual catch is about 2,000 tonnes.

COMMERCE. In 1984, exports totalled 34m. francs (57% to France in 1983) and imports 182·8m. francs (53% from France). Ylang-ylang formed 48% of exports, vanilla 33% and coffee 12%. Total trade between Mayotte and UK (1984): Imports to UK, £67,000 and exports and re-exports from UK, £343,000.

Total trade between Mayotte and UK (British Department of Trade returns, in £1,000 sterling):

	1987	*1988*	*1989*	*1990*
Imports to UK	185	654	117	103
Exports and re-exports from UK	2,352	3,123	5,059	2,474

COMMUNICATIONS

Roads. In 1984 there were 93 km of main roads and 137 km of local roads, with 1,528 motor vehicles.

Aviation. In 1985, 17,426 passengers and 172 tonnes of freight arrived and departed by air.

Post and Broadcasting. In 1984 there were 6,000 radio receivers. Telephones (1981) 400.

Newspapers. There is 1 daily newspaper, *le Journal de Mayotte*.

JUSTICE, RELIGION, EDUCATION AND WELFARE

Justice. There is a *tribunal de première instance* and a *tribunal supérieur d'appel*.

Religion. The population is 97% Sunni Moslem, with a small Christian (mainly Roman Catholic) minority.

Education. In 1984 there were 14,992 pupils and 407 teachers in 72 primary schools; 1,374 pupils in 1 secondary school; and 475 students in 2 technical and teacher-training establishments.

Health. In 1980 there were 9 doctors, 1 dentist, 1 pharmacist, 2 midwives and 51 nursing personnel. In 1981 there were 2 hospitals with 86 beds.

ST PIERRE AND MIQUELON

Îles Saint-Pierre et Miquelon

HISTORY. The only remaining fragment of the once-extensive French possessions in North America, the archipelago was settled from France in the 17th century. It was a French territory from 1816 until 1976, an overseas department until 1985, and is now a territorial collectivity.

AREA AND POPULATION. The archipelago consists of 8 small islands off the south coast of Newfoundland, with a total area of 242 sq. km, comprising the Saint-Pierre group (26 sq. km) and the Miquelon-Langlade group (216 sq. km). The population (census, 1990) was 6,392 of whom 5,683 were on Saint-Pierre and 709 on Miquelon. The chief town is St Pierre.

Vital statistics (1989): Births, 77; marriages, 23; deaths, 43.

CONSTITUTION AND GOVERNMENT. The dependency is administered by a General Council of 19 members, directly elected for a 6-year term. It is represented in the National Assembly in Paris by 1 deputy, in the Senate by 1 senator and in the Economic and Social Council by 1 councillor. The French government is represented by an appointed Commissioner.

Commissioner: Jean-Pierre Marquie.
President of the General Council: Marc Plantegenest.

ECONOMY

Budget. The ordinary budget for 1989 balanced at 87·4m. francs.

Currency. The French franc is in use.

Banking. Banks include the Banque des Îles Saint-Pierre et Miquelon and the Crédit Saint-Pierrais.

ENERGY AND NATURAL RESOURCES

Electricity. Production (1989) 45·5m. kwh.

Agriculture. The islands, being mostly barren rock, are unsuited for agriculture, but some vegetables are grown and livestock kept for local consumption.

Fisheries. The catch (the islands' main industry) amounted in 1989 to 9,202 tonnes, chiefly cod.

COMMERCE. Trade in 1m. francs:

	1985	*1986*	*1987*	*1988*	*1989*
Imports	358·4	348·3	343·5	366·7	533·1
Exports	106·7	163·1	186·7	143·5	200·8

In 1989, 47% of imports came from Canada, while 25% of exports were to France, 16% to EEC and 12% to Canada.

The main exports are fish (73%), shellfish (20%) and fishmeal (7%).

Total trade between St Pierre and Miquelon and UK (British Department of Trade returns in £1,000 sterling):

	1986	*1987*	*1988*	*1989*	*1990*
Imports to UK	474	77	159	164	719
Exports and re-exports from UK	367	604	470	533	450

Tourism. There were (1989) 14,100 visitors.

COMMUNICATIONS

Roads. In 1988 there were 120 km of roads, of which 50 km were paved. In 1989 there were 1,917 passenger cars and 717 commercial vehicles.

Aviation. Air Saint-Pierre connects St Pierre with Montreal, with Halifax and Sydney (Nova Scotia), and there are occasional flights to and from St John's (Newfoundland).

Shipping. St Pierre has regular services to Fortune and Halifax in Canada. In 1989, 119,440 tonnes of freight were unloaded and 66,817 tonnes loaded, while 1,232 ships (of 1·85m. gross tonnage) entered the harbour.

Telecommunications. There were 2,997 telephones in 1989. RFO broadcasts in French on medium-waves. St Pierre is connected by radio-telecommunication with most countries of the world.

Cinemas. There were (1988) 2 cinemas with a seating capacity of 760.

JUSTICE, RELIGION, EDUCATION AND WELFARE

Justice. There is a court of first instance and a higher court of appeal at St Pierre. For definitions *see* pp.494-95.

Religion. The population is chiefly Roman Catholic.

Education. Primary instruction is free. There were, in 1990, 5 nursery and 5 primary schools with 791 pupils and 4 secondary schools (including 2 technical schools) with 690 pupils.

Health. There was (1988) 1 hospital on St Pierre with 100 beds; 12 doctors and 4 dentists.

Further Reading

De Curton, E., *Saint-Pierre et Miquelon.* Paris, 1944
De La Rüe, E. A., *Saint-Pierre et Miquelon.* Paris, 1963
Ribault, J. Y., *Histoire de Saint-Pierre et Miquelon: Des Origines à 1814.* St Pierre, 1962

OVERSEAS TERRITORIES

Among the 7 French Overseas Territories remaining since Algerian independence in 1962, the Comoro Islands declared their independence on 6 July 1975 (recognized by France on 31 Dec.), but the island of Mayotte remained French and in Dec. 1976 was classed as a 'territorial collectivity'. The territory of Saint Pierre and Miquelon became a fifth Overseas Department in July 1976, but in June 1985 it acquired the same status as Mayotte. The former French Somaliland (subsequently Territory of the Afars and Issas) became independent on 27 June 1977 as the Republic of Djibouti. The remaining French Overseas Territories are New Caledonia (with its dependancies), French Polynesia, Wallis and Futuna, and the French Southern and Antarctic Territories.

SOUTHERN AND ANTARCTIC TERRITORIES

Terres Australes et Antarctiques Françaises (TAAF)

The Territory of the TAAF was created on 6 Aug. 1955. It comprises the Kerguelen and Crozet archipelagoes, the islands of Saint Paul and Amsterdam (formerly Nouvelle Amsterdam), all in the southern Indian ocean, and Terre Adélie.

The Administrator is assisted by a 7-member consultative council which meets twice yearly in Paris; its members are nominated by the Government for 5 years. The 12 members of the Scientific Council are appointed by the Senior Administrator after approval by the Minister in charge of scientific research. A 15-member Consultative Committee on the Environment, created in Nov. 1982, meets at least once a year to discuss all problems relating to the preservation of the environment. The administration has its seat in Paris.

Administrateur supérieur: Bernard de Gouttes.

The staff of the permanent scientific stations of the TAAF (180 in 1990) is renewed annually and forms the only population.

Kerguelen islands, situated 48–50° S. lat., 68–70° E. long., consists of 1 large and 85 smaller islands and over 200 islets and rocks with a total area of 7,215 sq. km (2,786 sq. miles), of which Grande Terre occupies 6,675 sq. km (2,577 sq. miles). It was discovered in 1772 by Yves de Kerguelen, but was effectively occupied by France only in 1949. Port-aux-Français has several scientific research stations (75 members). Reindeer, trout and sheep have been acclimatized.

Crozet islands, situated 46° S. lat., 50–52° E. long., consists of 5 larger and 15 tiny islands, with a total area of 505 sq. km (195 sq. miles); the western group includes Apostles, Pigs and Penguins islands; the eastern group, Possession and Eastern islands. The archipelago was discovered in 1772 by Marion Dufresne, whose mate, Crozet, annexed it for Louis XV. A meteorological and scientific station (35 members) at Base Alfred-Faure on Possession Island was built in 1964.

Amsterdam Island and **Saint-Paul Island,** situated 38–39° S. lat., 77° E. long. Amsterdam, with an area of 54 sq. km (21 sq. miles) was discovered in 1522 by Magellan's companions; Saint-Paul, lying about 100 km to the south, with an area of 7 sq. km (2·7 sq. miles), was probably discovered in 1559 by Portuguese sailors. Both were first visited in 1633 by the Dutch explorer, Van Diemen, and were annexed by France in 1843. They are both extinct volcanoes. The only inhabitants are at Base Martin de Vivies, established in 1949 on Amsterdam Island, with several scientific research stations, hospital, communication and other facilities (35 members). Crayfish are caught commercially on Amsterdam.

Terre Adélie comprises that section of the Antarctic continent between 136° and 142° E. long., south of 60° S. lat. The ice-covered plateau has an area of about 432,000 sq. km (166,800 sq. miles), and was discovered in 1840 by Dumont d'Urville. A research station (30 members) is situated at Base Dumont d'Urville, which is maintained by the French Polar Expeditions.

NEW CALEDONIA

Nouvelle Calédonie et Dépendances

HISTORY. New Caledonia was annexed by France in 1853 and, together with most of its former dependencies, became an overseas territory in 1958.

AREA AND POPULATION. The territory comprises the island of New Caledonia and various outlying islands, all situated in the south-west Pacific with a total land area of 18,576 sq. km (7,172 sq. miles). In 1989 the population (census) was 164,173, including 55,085 Europeans (majority French), 73,598 Melanesians (Kanaks), 7,652 Vietnamese and Indonesians, 4,750 Polynesians, 14,186 Wallisians, 8,902 others. The capital, Nouméa had (1989) 65,110 inhabitants. Vital statistics (1989): Live births, 3,945; deaths, 990.

The main islands are:

1. The island of New Caledonia with an area of 16,372 sq. km, has a total length of about 400 km, and an average breadth of 50 km, and a population (census, 1989) of 144,051. The east coast is predominantly Melanesian, the Nouméa region predominantly European, and the rest of the west coast of mixed population.

2. The Loyalty Islands, 100 km (60 miles) east of New Caledonia, consisting of 3 large islands, Maré, Lifou and Uvéa, and many small islands with a total area of 1,981 sq. km and a population (census, 1989) of 17,912, nearly all Melanesians except on Uvéa, which is partly Polynesian. The chief culture in the islands is that of coconuts and the chief export, copra.
3. The Isle of Pines, 50 km (30 miles) to the south-east of Nouméa, with an area of 152 sq. km and a population of 1,465 (census 1989), is a tourist and fishing centre.
4. The Bélep Archipelago, about 50 km north-west of New Caledonia, with an area of 70 sq. km and a population of 745 (census 1989).

The remaining islands are all very small and none have permanent inhabitants. The largest are the Chesterfield Islands, a group of 11 well-wooded coral islets with a combined area of 10 sq. km, about 550 km west of the Bélep Archipelago. The Huon Islands, a group of 4 barren coral islets with a combined area of just 65 ha, are 225 km north of the Bélep Archipelago. Walpole, a limestone coral island of 1 sq. km, lies 150 km east of the Isle of Pines; Matthew Island (20 ha.) and Hunter Island (2 sq. km), respectively 250 km and 330 km east of Walpole, are spasmodically active volcanic islands also claimed by Vanuatu.

CLIMATE. Nouméa. Jan. 78°F (25·6°C), July 67°F (19·4°C). Annual rainfall 43" (1,083 mm).

CONSTITUTION AND GOVERNMENT. Following constitutional changes introduced by the French government in 1985 and 1988, the Territory is administered by a High Commissioner assisted by a 4-member Consultative Committee, consisting of the President of the Territorial Congress (as President) and the Presidents of the 3 Provincial Assemblies. The French government is represented by the appointed High Commissioner. In Sept. 1987 the electorate voted in favour of remaining a French possession.

There is a 54-member Territorial Congress consisting of the complete membership of the 3 Provincial Assemblies.

New Caledonia is represented in the National Assembly by 2 deputies, in the Senate by 1 senator and in the Economic and Social Council by 1 councillor.

The Territory is divided into 3 provinces, Nord, Sud and Iles Loyauté, each under a directly-elected Regional Council. They are sub-divided into 32 communes administered by locally-elected councils and mayors.

Agreement was reached in June 1988 between the French government and representatives of both the European and Melanesian communities on New Caledonia, and confirmed in Nov. 1988 by plebiscites in both France and New Caledonia, under which the territory has been divided into 3 autonomous provinces, and a further referendum on full independence will be held in 1998.

High Commissioner: Bernard Grasset.

ECONOMY

Budget. The budget for 1989 balanced at 51,786m. francs CFP.

Currency. The unit of currency is the *CFP franc* (XPF), with a parity of 18·18 to the French franc.

Banking. There are branches of the Westpac Banking Corporation, the Banque Nationale de Paris, the Banque de Paris et des Pays-Bas, the Société Générale, and the Banque de la Nouvelle-Calédonie (Crédit Lyonnais).

ENERGY AND NATURAL RESOURCES

Electricity. In 1989, production totalled 1,192m. kwh.

Minerals. The mineral resources are very great; nickel, chrome and iron abound; silver, gold, cobalt, lead, manganese, iron and copper have been mined at different times. The nickel deposits are of special value, being without arsenic. Production of nickel ore in 1989, 4·92m. tonnes and chrome ore 113,705 tonnes. In 1989 the furnaces produced 10,650 tonnes of matte nickel and 36,285 tonnes of ferro-nickel.

Agriculture. In 1989 7,646 persons worked in agriculture. 271,864 ha are pasture land; about 10,035 ha are commercially cultivated. The chief products are beef, pork, poultry, coffee, copra, maize, fruit and vegetables.

Livestock (1988): Cattle, 124,000; pigs, 47,000; goats, 21,000.

Forestry. There are about 250,000 ha of forest. Roundwood production (1988) 5,118 cu. metres.

Fisheries. The catch in 1987 totalled 5,775 tonnes.

INDUSTRY. Local industries include chlorine and oxygen plants, cement, soft drinks, barbed wire, nails, pleasure and fishing boats, clothing, pasta, household cleaners and confectionery.

Labour. The working population (1989 census) was 54,230.

COMMERCE. Imports and exports in 1m. CFP francs:

	1985	*1986*	*1987*	*1988*	*1989*
Imports	55,931	62,939	63,349	65,386	88,608
Exports	43,938	26,249	20,653	50,805	77,900

In 1988, 47·9% of the imports came from France and 10·3% from Australia, while 38·4% of the exports went to France. Refined minerals (mainly ferro-nickel and nickel) formed 81·2% of exports by value, nickel ore 10·2% and chrome ore 1·7%. Imports to the UK (British Department of Trade returns, £1,000 sterling) 2,528; exports from the UK, 8,051.

Tourism. Tourists, 1989, 75,621 (14·7% French, 35·2% Japanese).

COMMUNICATIONS

Roads. There were, in 1987, 6,340 km of roads, of which 1,823·5 km were paved. There were (1989) 62,000 vehicles.

Aviation. New Caledonia is connected by air routes with France and Tahiti (by UTA and Minerve), Australia (UTA and Qantas), New Zealand (UTA and Air New Zealand), Fiji and Wallis and Futuna (by Air Cal International), Vanuatu (by UTA), and Nauru (by Air Nauru). In 1989, 124,097 passengers arrived and 123,313 departed *via* La Tontouta airport, near Nouméa. Internal services connect Nouméa with 21 domestic air fields.

Shipping. In 1989, 543 vessels entered Nouméa unloading 977,000 tonnes of goods and loading 2·22m. tonnes of which 1m. tonnes comprised mineral exports.

Telecommunications. There were (1989) 46 post offices and telex, telephone, radio and television services. There were (1989) 24,000 telephones. RFO broadcasts in French on medium- and short-wave radio (there are also 9 private stations) and on 2 television channels for 95 hours a week. There were 85,000 radios in 1986 and 28,077 TV sets in 1989.

Cinemas. In 1990 there were 11 cinemas.

Newspapers. In 1990 there was 1 daily newspaper with a circulation of 20,000.

JUSTICE, RELIGION, EDUCATION AND WELFARE

Justice. There is a *Tribunal de Première Instance* and a *Cour d'Appel* in Nouméa.

Religion. In 1980 over 72% of the population was Roman Catholic, 16% Protestant and 4% Moslem.

Education. In 1989, there were 33,872 pupils and 1,660 teachers in 278 primary schools, 13,675 pupils in 44 secondary schools, 6,477 students in 29 technical and vocational schools, and 1,392 students and 141 teaching staff in 6 higher education establishments. The University of the Pacific had 465 students and 84 academic staff in 1989.

Health. In 1988 there were 173 physicians, 37 dentists, 29 pharmacists, 20 midwives and 761 paramedical personnel; 6 hospitals and 24 dispensaries had a total of 1,081 beds.

Further Reading

Journal Officiel de la Nouvelle Calédonie
Tableaux de l'Economie Caledonienne, 1988
Information statistiques rapides. (monthly)

FRENCH POLYNESIA

Territoire de la Polynésie Française

HISTORY. French protectorates since 1843, these islands were annexed to France 1880–82 to form 'French Settlements in Oceania', which opted in Nov. 1958 for the status of an overseas territory within the French Community.

AREA AND POPULATION. The total land area of these 5 archipelagoes, scattered over a wide area in the Eastern Pacific is 3,265 sq. km (1,260 sq. miles). The population, Census, 1983, was 166,753; census (1988) 188,814.

The official languages are French and Tahitian.

Vital statistics (1987): Births, 5,384; marriages, 1,251; deaths, 980.

The islands are administratively divided into 5 *circonscriptions:*

1. The **Windward Islands** (Îles du Vent) (140,341 inhabitants in 1988) comprise Tahiti with an area of 1,042 sq. km and 115,820 inhabitants; Moorea with an area of 132 sq. km and 7,059 inhabitants; Maio (Tubuai Manu) with an area of 9 sq. km and 190 inhabitants, and the smaller Mehetia and Tetiaroa. The capital is Papeete (78,814 inhabitants including suburbs).

2. The **Leeward Islands** (Îles sous le Vent), comprise the volcanic islands of Raiatéa, Tahaa, Huahine, Bora-Bora and Maupiti, together with 4 small atolls, the group having a total land area of 404 sq. km and 22,232 inhabitants in 1988. The chief town is Uturoa on Raiatéa.

The Windward and Leeward Islands together are called the Society Archipelago (Archipel de la Société). Tahitian, a Polynesian language, is spoken throughout the archipelago and used as a *lingua franca* in the rest of the territory.

3. The **Tuamotu Archipelago**, consisting of two parallel ranges of 78 atolls lying north and east of the Society Archipelago, have a total area of 690 sq. km; the most populous atolls are Rangiroa, Hao and Turéia. Mururoa and Fangataufa atolls in the south-east of the group have been used by France for nuclear tests since 1966, having been ceded to France in 1964 by the Territorial Assembly.

The *circonscription* (12,374 inhabitants in 1988) also includes the **Gambier Islands** further east (of which Mangareva is the principal), with an area of 36 sq. km and a population of 582; the chief centre is Rikitea on Mangareva.

4. The **Austral or Tubuai Islands**, lying south of the Society Archipelago, comprise a 1,300 km chain of volcanic islands and reefs. They include Rimatara, Rurutu, Tubuai, Raivaevae and, 500 km to the south, Rapa-Iti, with a combined area of 148 sq. km and 6,509 (1988) inhabitants; the chief centre is Mataura on Tubuai.

5. The **Marquesas Islands**, lying north of the Tuamotu Archipelago, with a total area of 1,049 sq. km and 7,538 (1988) inhabitants, comprise Nukuhiva, Uapu, Uahuka, Hivaoa, Tahuata, Fatuhiva and 4 smaller (uninhabited) islands; the chief centre is Taiohae on Nukuhiva.

CLIMATE. Papeete. Jan. 81°F (27·1°C), July 75°F (24°C). Annual rainfall 83" (2,106 mm).

CONSTITUTION AND GOVERNMENT. Under the 1984 Constitution, the Territory is administered by a Council of Ministers, whose President is elected by the Territorial Assembly from among its own members; he appoints a Vice-President and 9 other ministers. There is an advisory Economic and Social Committee. French Polynesia is represented in the French Assembly by 2 deputies, in the Senate by 1 senator, and in the Economic and Social Council by 1 councillor. The French government is represented by a High Commissioner. The Territorial Assembly comprises 41 members elected every 5 years by universal suffrage.

At the elections held in March 1986, the *Tahoeraa Huiraatiraa* (Gaullists) won 22 seats, the *Amuitahiraa No Porinesia* 5 seats, Nationalists 5 seats and others 9 seats.

High Commissioner: Jean Montpezat.
President of the Council of Ministers: Alexandre Leontieff.

Flag: Three horizontal stripes of red, white, red, with the white of double width containing the emblem of French Polynesia in yellow.

ECONOMY

Budget. The ordinary budget for 1987 balanced at 52,135m. francs CFP.

Currency. The unit of currency is the *franc CFP* (XPF), with a parity of *CFP francs* 18·18 to the French *franc*.

Banking. There are 5 commercial banks, the Bank Indosuez, the Bank of Tahiti, the Banque de Polynésie, Paribas Pacifique and Société de Crédit et de Développement de l'Océanie.

ENERGY AND NATURAL RESOURCES

Electricity. Production in 1987 amounted to 265m. kwh (18% hydro-electric).

Agriculture. An important product is copra (coconut trees covering the coastal plains of the mountainous islands and the greater part of the low-lying islands), production (1988) 15,000 tonnes. Tropical fruits, such as bananas, pineapples, oranges, etc., are grown only for local consumption.

Livestock (1988): Cattle, 10,000; horses, 2,000; pigs, 54,000; sheep, 2,000; goats, 3,000; poultry, 1m.

Fisheries. The catch in 1986 amounted to 1,703 tonnes of fish.

COMMERCE. Trade in 1m. francs CFP:

	1983	*1984*	*1985*	*1986*	*1987*
Imports	74,241	85,622	88,864	92,666	90,544
Exports	4,823	5,084	6,564	5,106	8,986

Total trade between French Polynesia and UK (British Department of Trade returns, in £1,000 sterling):

	1986	*1987*	*1988*	*1989*	*1990*
Imports to UK	95	18	56	416	16
Exports and re-exports from UK	4,890	5,275	3,421	3,996	4,763

Chief exports are coconut oil and cultured pearls. In 1987, France provided 52% of imports and USA 13%, while (1985) 44% of exports went to France and 21% to USA.

Tourism. Tourism is very important, earning almost half as much as the visible exports. There were 143,000 tourists in 1987.

COMMUNICATIONS

Roads. In 1985 there were 797 km of roads and 44,000 vehicles.

Aviation. Seven international airlines connect Tahiti with Paris, Los Angeles and many Pacific locations. There is also a regular air service between Faaa airport (on Tahiti), Moorea and the Leeward Isles with occasional connexions to the other groups. In 1987, 194,218 international passengers arrived and 197,301 departed *via* the airports at Faaa and on Mooréa and Bora-Bora. Thirty other airfields have regular domestic services.

Shipping. Several shipping companies connect France, San Francisco, New Zealand, Japan, Australia, South East Asia and most Pacific locations with Papeete.

Telecommunications. Number of telephones (1985), 28,192. *Radio Tele Tahiti* belongs to *Société de Radiodiffusion et de Télévision pour l'Outre-mer* (RFO) and broadcasts in French, Tahitian and English on medium- and short-waves and also broadcasts 1 television programme *via* 5 transmitters. There are also 9 private radio stations. Number of receivers (1986): Radio, 84,000; TV, 26,400.

Cinemas. In 1986 there were 8 cinemas in Papeete.

Newspapers. In 1988 there were 2 daily newspapers.

JUSTICE, RELIGION, EDUCATION AND WELFARE

Justice. There is a *tribunal de première instance* and a *cour d'appel* at Papeete.

Religion. In 1980 it was estimated that 46·5% of the inhabitants were Protestants, 39·4% Roman Catholic and 5·1% Mormon.

Education. There were, in 1987-88, 42,735 pupils in 264 primary schools, 15,002 pupils in 41 secondary schools, and 4,156 pupils in technical schools and teacher-training colleges.

Health. There were (1987) 273 physicians, 88 dentists, 35 pharmacists, 24 midwives and 464 nursing personnel. There was (1987) a main hospital at Mamao (on Tahiti), 7 secondary hospitals, 2 private clinics, 9 medical centres and 18 infirmaries, with together 1,048 beds.

DEPENDENCY. The uninhabited Clipperton Island, 1,000 km off the west coast of Mexico, is administered by the High Commissioner for French Polynesia but does not form part of the Territory; it is an atoll with an area of 5 sq. km.

Further Reading

Journal Officiel des Etablissements Françaises de l'Océanie, and *Supplement Containing Statistics of Commerce and Navigation*. Papeete
Andrews, E., *Comparative Dictionary of the Tahitian Language*. Chicago, 1944
Bounds, J. H., *Tahiti*. Bend, Oregon, 1978
Luke, Sir Harry, *The Islands of the South Pacific*. London, 1961
O'Reilly, P. and Reitman, E., *Bibliographie de Tahiti et de la Polynésie française*. Paris, 1967
O'Reilly, P. and Teissier, R., *Tahitiens. Répertoire bio-bibliographique de la Polynésie française*. Paris, 1963

WALLIS AND FUTUNA

HISTORY. French dependencies since 1842, the inhabitants of these islands voted on 22 Dec. 1959 by 4,307 votes out of 4,576 in favour of exchanging their status to that of an overseas territory, which took effect from 29 July 1961.

AREA AND POPULATION. The territory comprises two groups of islands (total area 274 sq. km) in the central Pacific, The Îles de Hoorn lie 240 km north-east of Fiji and consist of 2 main islands–Futuna (64 sq. km) and uninhabited Alofi (51 sq. km). The Wallis Archipelago lies another 160 km further north-east, and comprises one main island – Uvea (159 sq. km), with a surrounding coral reef. The capital is Mata-Utu (815 inhabitants, 1983) on Uvea.

The resident population, census March 1985, was 12,408 (Uvea, 8,084; Futuna, 4,324) (estimate, 1988, 15,400), comprising 7,843 on Uvea and 4,100 on Futuna. In 1990 11,943 Wallisians lived in New Caledonia. Wallisian and Futunian are distinct Polynesian languages.

CONSTITUTION AND GOVERNMENT. The Senior Administrator represents the French government and carries out the duties of head of the territory, assisted by a 20-member Territorial Assembly, directly elected for a 5-year term, and a 6-member Territorial Council, comprising the 3 traditional chiefs and 3 nominees of the Senior Administrator agreed by the Territorial Assembly. The territory is represented in Paris by 1 deputy in the National Assembly, by 1 senator in the Senate, and by 1 member on the Economic and Social Council. There are 3 districts: Singave and Alo (both on Futuna) and Wallis. In each tribal kings exercise customary powers assisted by ministers and district and village chiefs.

Senior Administrator: Jacques Le Illénaff.

President of the Territorial Assembly: Falakiko Gata.

ECONOMY

Policy. A development plan was adopted in 1986.

Budget. The 1982 budget provided for expenditure of 303·8m. francs CFP.

Currency. The unit of currency is the *CFP franc* (XPF), with a parity of 18·18 to the French franc.

Banking. There is a branch of Indosuez at Mata-Utu.

ENERGY AND NATURAL RESOURCES

Electricity. There is a thermal power station at Mata-Utu. Supply is 220 volts; 50 Hz.

Agriculture. The chief products are copra, cassava, yams, taro roots and bananas.

Livestock: Pigs, 30,000 (1988); goats, 8,000 (1988).

COMMERCE. Imports (1984) amounted to 1,302m. CFP francs. There are few exports.

COMMUNICATIONS

Roads. In 1977 there were 100 km of roads on Uvea.

Aviation. 3 flights a week link Wallis and Futuna. Air Calédonie International operates 2 flights a week to Nouméa.

Shipping. A regular cargo service links Mata-Utu (Wallis) and Singave (Futuna) with Nouméa (New Caledonia).

Telecommunications. In 1986 there were 2 radio stations and 6 post offices. In 1985 there were 340 telephones.

JUSTICE, RELIGION, EDUCATION AND WELFARE

Justice. There is a court of first instance, from which appeals can be made to the court of appeal in New Caledonia. For definitions *see* pp.494-95.

Religion. The majority of the population is Roman Catholic.

Education. In 1989, there were 4,080 pupils in primary classes and 542 in (some 90% of school-age children) lower secondary classes. Further education is available in New Caledonia.

Health. In 1990 there was 1 hospital with 45 beds and 4 dispensaries.

GABON

Capital: Libreville
Population: 1·22m. (1988)
GNP per capita: US$3,300 (1990)

République Gabonaise

HISTORY. First colonized by France in the mid-19th century, Gabon was annexed to French Congo in 1888 and became a separate colony in 1910 as one of the 4 territories of French Equatorial Africa. It became an autonomous republic within the French Community on 28 Nov. 1958 and achieved independence on 17 Aug. 1960.

AREA AND POPULATION. Gabon is bounded west by the Atlantic ocean, north by Equatorial Guinea and Cameroon and east and south by Congo. The area covers 267,667 sq. km; its population at the 1970 census was 950,007; estimate (1988) is 1,226,000. The capital is Libreville (350,000 inhabitants, 1983), other large towns being Port-Gentil (123,300), Masuku (formerly Franceville, 38,030), Lambaréné (26,257 in 1978) and Mouanda (22,909 in 1978).

Vital statistics (1975): Birth rate, 3·22%; death rate, 2·22%.

Provincial areas, populations (estimate 1978, in 1,000) and capitals are as follows:

Province	*Sq. km*	*1978*	*Capital*	*Province*	*Sq. km*	*1978*	*Capital*
Estuaire	20,740	359	Libreville	Nyanga	21,285	98	Tchibanga
Woleu-Ntem	38,465	166	Oyem	Ngounié	37,750	118	Mouila
Ogooué-Ivindo	46,075	53	Makokou	Ogooué-Lolo	25,380	49	Koulamoutou
Moyen-Ogooué	18,535	49	Lambaréné	Haut-Ogooué	36,547	213	Masuku
Ogooué-Maritime	22,890	194	Port-Gentil				

The largest ethnic groups are the Fang (30%) in the north, Eshira (25%) in the south-west, and the Adouma (17%) in the south-east. French is the official language.

CLIMATE. The climate is equatorial, with high temperatures and considerable rainfall. Mid-May to mid-Sept. is the long dry season, followed by a short rainy season, then a dry season again from mid-Dec. to mid-Feb., and finally a long rainy season once more. Libreville. Jan. 80°F (26·7°C), July 75°F (23·9°C). Annual rainfall 99" (2,510 mm).

CONSTITUTION AND GOVERNMENT. The 1967 Constitution (as subsequently revised) provides for an Executive President directly elected for a 7-year term, who appoints a Council of Ministers to assist him. The unicameral National Assembly consists of 120 members, directly elected for a 5-year term. Opposition parties were legalized in May 1990. Elections were held in Sept. 1990, but because of irregularities the results were partially anulled and a second round of voting took-place in Oct. In the final result the Gabonese Democratic Party (the former sole party permitted) won 63 seats. There are 7 opposition parties, including Morena-Bûcheron, with 20 seats, and the Gabonese Progress party, with 18.

Former President: Leon M'ba (17 Aug. 1960–died 30 Nov. 1967).

President: Omar Bongo (succeeded 2 Dec. 1967, re-elected in 1973, 1979 and 1986).

The Council of Ministers in Dec. 1990 consisted of 26 ministers and 10 secretaries of state.

Prime Minister: Casimir Oyé Mba.

Flag: Three horizontal stripes of green, yellow, blue.

Local government: The 9 provinces, each administered by a governor appointed by the President, are divided into 37 *départements*, each under a prefect.

DEFENCE

Army. The Army consists of 1 all-arms Presidential Guard battalion group with support units, totalling (1991), 3,250 men. There is also a paramilitary force of 2,000 personnel. France maintains a 550-strong marine infantry battalion.

Navy. The small naval flotilla in 1990 consisted of 1 French-built fast missile craft, 1 coastal and 4 inshore patrol craft. The flagship is a French-built medium landing ship, and there are about 3 minor service tenders. A separate Coast Guard operates some 10 small launches. Personnel in 1990 totalled 350 officers and men.

Air Force. The Air Force has 6 single-seat, 3 two-seat Mirage 5 and 3 Magister ground-attack aircraft, and 1 EMB-111 maritime patrol aircraft. Transport duties are performed primarily by 3 Hercules and 1 EMB-110 Bandeirante turboprop aircraft, 3 Nord 262s. Single Falcon 900, Gulfstream III DC-8 aircraft are used for VIP duties. Three T-34C-1 armed turboprop aircraft and an EMB-110 Bandeirante are operated for *La Garde Présidentiale*. Also in service are 2 Puma, 1 Bell 212, 1 Bel 412 and 2 Alouette III helicopters. Personnel (1991) 1,000.

INTERNATIONAL RELATIONS

Membership. Gabon is a member of the UN, OAU and OPEC and is an ACP state of the EEC.

ECONOMY.

Planning. The Fifth 5-year Plan (1984–88, later extended to 1990) envisaged public expenditure of 1,228,478m. francs CFA, of which 595,662m. were to develop the infrastructure.

Budget. The 1989 budget provided for expenditure of 358,000m. francs CFA and revenue of 260,000m.

Currency. The unit of currency is the franc CFA, with a parity value of 50 francs CFA to 1 French franc. There are coins of 1, 2, 5, 10, 25, 50, 100 and 500 *francs* CFA, and banknotes of 100, 500, 1,000, 5,000 and 10,000 *francs* CFA. In March 1991 £1 = 496·12 *francs* CFA; US$1 = 261·53 *francs* CFA.

Banking and Finance. The *Banque des États de l'Afrique Centrale* is the bank of issue. There are 9 commercial banks situated in Gabon. The *Banque Gabonaise de Développement* and the *Union Gabonaise de Banque* are Gabonese controlled.

ENERGY AND NATURAL RESOURCES

Electricity. The semi-public *Société d'energie et d'eau du Gabon* produced 886m. kwh. in 1986, mainly from thermal plants but increasingly from hydro-electric schemes at Kinguélé (near Libreville), Tchimbélé and Poubara (near Masuku). Supply 220 volts; 50 Hz.

Oil. Extraction from offshore fields totalled 11m. tonnes in 1989. Gabon operates 2 refineries, at Port-Gentil and at nearby Pointe Clairette. Proven reserves (1984) 490m. bbls.

Gas. Natural gas production (1985) was 201m. cu. metres.

Minerals. Production (1988) of manganese ore (from deposits around Moanda in the south-east) amounted to 2·25m. tonnes. Uranium is mined nearby at Mounana (850 tonnes in 1988). An estimated 850m. tonnes of iron ore deposits, discovered 1971 at Mékambo (near Bélinga in the north-east) await completion of the branch railway line to be exploited. Gold (18 kg in 1982), zinc and phosphates also occur.

Agriculture. The major crops (production, 1988, in 1,000 tonnes) are: Sugar-cane, 155; cassava, 265; plantains, 180; maize, 10; groundnuts, 9; bananas, 8; palm oil, 3·8; cocoa, 2; coffee, 2 and rice, 1.

Livestock (1988): 9,000 cattle, 84,000 sheep, 63,000 goats, 154,000 pigs.

Forestry. Equatorial forests cover 85% of the land area. Softwood production was

1·38m. cu. metres in 1985. Hardwoods (mahogany, ebony and walnut) are also produced.

Fisheries. The total catch (1986) amounted to 20,400 tonnes.

INDUSTRY.

A sugar refinery at Masuku produced (1984) 15,000 tonnes raw sugar. Most manufacturing is based on the processing of food, timber and mineral resources.

Labour. The workforce in 1986 numbered 522,000 of whom 71% were agricultural.

FOREIGN ECONOMIC RELATIONS.

Foreign debt was US$2,500m. in 1990.

Commerce. In 1985 imports totalled 384,000m. francs CFA and exports 876,000m. francs CFA. France and USA are Gabon's principal trading partners. In 1983 petroleum made up 83·5% of exports; metals, 7·5% and timber, 7%.

Total trade between Gabon and the UK (British Department of Trade returns, in £1,000 sterling):

	1986	*1987*	*1988*	*1989*	*1990*
Imports to UK	36,642	5,357	5,091	2,389	1,809
Exports and re-exports from UK	16,627	11,962	18,808	14,945	17,563

COMMUNICATIONS

Roads. There were (1987) 6,898 km of roads and in 1985 there were 16,093 passenger cars and 10,506 commercial vehicles.

Railways. A 1,435-mm gauge (Transgabonais) railway runs from Owendo *via* N'Djole to Booué and Lastourville, Mouanda and Masuku, opened throughout in 1986. Total 649 km of 1,437 mm gauge. In 1986, 134,000 passengers and 662,000 tonnes of freight were transported.

Aviation. There are 3 international airports at Port-Gentil, Masuku, and Libreville; internal services link these to 65 domestic airfields.

Shipping. Owendo (near Libreville), Mayumba and Port-Gentil are the main ports. In 1987 there were 23 merchant vessels of 97,967 GNT. In 1986, 5·9m. tonnes were loaded and 968,000 tonnes unloaded at the ports.

Telecommunications. In 1985 there were 11,700 telephones, and (1986) 23,000 television and 117,000 radio licences.

Newspapers. There were (1984) 2 newspapers published in Libreville; *Gabon-Matin* (daily) has a circulation of 18,000 and *L'Union* (weekly) 15,000.

JUSTICE, RELIGION, EDUCATION AND WELFARE

Justice. There are *tribunaux de grande instance* at Libreville, Port-Gentil, Lambaréné, Mouila, Oyem, Masuku and Koulamoutou, from which cases move progressively to a central Criminal Court, Court of Appeal and Supreme Court, all 3 located in Libreville. Civil police number about 900.

Religion. 84% of the population is Christian (65% Roman Catholic), the majority of the balance following animist beliefs. There are about 10,000 Moslems.

Education. Education is compulsory between 6–16 years. In 1984–85 there were 178,111 pupils with 3,837 teachers in 940 primary schools; 25,815 pupils with 1,894 teachers in 51 secondary schools; 13,529 students with 720 teachers in 29 technical and teacher-training establishments.

The Université Omar Bongo, founded in 1970 in Libreville, had (1983–84) 3,228 students and 616 teaching staff.

Health. In 1985 there were 565 doctors, and in 1977, 20 dentists, 28 pharmacists, 99 midwives and 823 nursing personnel. In 1981 there were 16 hospitals and 87 medical centres, with a total of 4,815 beds, as well as 258 local dispensaries.

DIPLOMATIC REPRESENTATIVES

Of Gabon in Great Britain (27 Elvaston Place, London, SW7 5NL)
Ambassador: Vincent Boulé.

Of Great Britain in Gabon (Immeuble CK2, Blvd de l'Indépendence, Libreville)
Ambassador: P. J. Priestley.

Of Gabon in the USA (2034 20th St., NW, Washington, D.C., 20009)
Ambassador: Jean Robert Odzaga.

Of the USA in Gabon (Blvd de la Mer, Libreville)
Ambassador: Keith L. Wauchope.

Of Gabon to the United Nations
Ambassador: Denis Dangue Rewaka.

Further Reading

Bory, P., *The New Gabon*. Monaco, 1978
Remy, M., *Gabon Today*. Paris, 1977
Saint Paul, M. A., *Gabon: The Development of a Nation*. London, 1989

THE GAMBIA

Capital: Banjul
Population: 875,000 (1990)
GNP per capita: US$290 (1989)

Republic of the Gambia

HISTORY. The Gambia was discovered by the early Portuguese navigators, but they made no settlement. During the 17th century various companies of merchants obtained trading charters and established a settlement on the river, which, from 1807, was controlled from Sierra Leone; in 1843 it was made an independent Crown Colony; in 1866 it formed part of the West African Settlements, but in Dec. 1888 it again became a separate Crown Colony. The boundaries were delimited only after 1890. The Gambia achieved full internal self-government on 4 Oct. 1963 and became an independent member of the Commonwealth on 18 Feb. 1965. The Gambia became a republic within the Commonwealth on 24 April 1970. The Gambia, with Senegal formed the Confederation of Senegambia on 1 Feb. 1982.

AREA AND POPULATION. The Gambia takes its name from the River Gambia, and consists of a strip of territory never wider than 10 km on both banks. It is bounded in the west by the Atlantic Ocean and on all other sides by Senegal. Area of Banjul (formerly Bathurst) and environs, 87·8 sq. km. In the provinces (area, 10,601·5 sq. km) the settled population (1971) was 275,469, not including temporary immigrants. Total population (census, April 1983), 687,817; (estimate, 1990) 875,000. The largest tribe is the Mandingo (251,997), followed by the Fulas (117,092), Woloffs (91,004), Jolas (64,494) and Sarahulis (51,137). The country is administratively divided into the capital, Banjul, 1983 census (44,188), and the surrounding urban area, Kombo St Mary (101,504), and 5 divisions (with chief town): Lower River (Mansa Konko); MacCarthy Island (Georgetown); North Bank (Kerewan); Upper River (Basse Santa Su); Western (Brikama; population, 19,584 in 1983). Other principal towns are Serekunda (68,433), Bakau (19,309), Sukuta (7,227), Gunjur (7,115) and Farafenni (10,168).

Birth rate (1983) 49 per 1,000; death rate, 21.

CLIMATE. The climate is characterized by two very different seasons. The dry season lasts from Nov. to May, when precipitation is very light and humidity moderate. Days are warm but nights quite cool. The SW monsoon is likely to set in with spectacular storms and produces considerable rainfall from July to Oct., with increased humidity. Banjul. Jan. 73°F (22·8°C), July 80°F (26·7°C). Annual rainfall 52" (1,295 mm).

CONSTITUTION AND GOVERNMENT. Parliament consists of the House of Representatives which consists of a Speaker, Deputy Speaker and 36 elected members; in addition, 5 Chiefs are elected by the Chiefs in Assembly; 7 nominated members are without votes and the Attorney-General is appointed and has no vote. *See* Senegal for details about Senegambia.

A general election was held March 1987. State of parties (Jan. 1988): The People's Progressive Party 31 and the National Convention Party 5.

The Government was in Feb. 1991 composed as follows:

President and Minister of Defence: Sir Dawda Kairaba Jawara.

Vice-President, Education, Youth, Sports and Culture: Bakary B. Darbo. *External Affairs:* Alhaji Omar Sey. *Finance and Economic Affairs:* Saikou Sabally. *Agriculture:* Omar A. Jallow. *Health, Labour, Social Welfare and Environment:* Louise Njie. *Works and Communications:* Matthew Yaya Baldeh Cadi Cham. *Industry and Employment:* Mbemba Jatta. *Justice and Attorney-General:* Hassan Jallow. *Water Resources:* Sarjo Touray. *Information and Tourism:* Alkali James Gaye. *Interior:* Alhaji Lamin kiti Jabang. *Local Government and Lands:* Landing Jallow Sonko.

National flag: Three wide horizontal stripes of red, blue, green, with narrower stripes of white between them.

Local Administration. The Gambia is divided into 35 districts, each traditionally under a Chief, assisted by Village Heads and advisers. These districts are grouped into 6 Area Councils containing a majority of elected members, with the Chiefs of the district as *ex-officio* members. The city of Banjul is administered by a City Council.

DEFENCE. The Gambia National Army, 900 strong, has four infantry companies and an engineer squadron.

The marine unit of the Army consisted in 1990 of 600 personnel operating 2 ex-Chinese and 1 British-built inshore patrol craft based at Banjul.

INTERNATIONAL RELATIONS

Membership. The Gambia is a member of UN, OAU, the Commonwealth, ECOWAS, the Non-Aligned Conference and is an ACP state of EEC.

ECONOMY

Budget. Revenue and expenditure for years ending 30 June are (in dalasi):

	1983–84	*1984–85*	*1985–86*	*1986–87*
Revenue	150,500,000	172,300,050	218,080,000	266,730,000
Expenditure	164,908,621	189,279,550	207,524,639	262,531,520

Currency. The currency is the *dalasi* (GMD) and is divided into 100 *butut*. 13·91 *dalasi* = £1 sterling; 7·33 *dalasi* = US$1 (March 1991).

Banking. There are 4 banks in the Gambia, the Standard Chartered Bank of Gambia Ltd, Central Bank of the Gambia, Commercial and Development Bank and la Banque Internationale pour le Commerce et l'Industrie (BICI). On 30 Nov. 1978 the government savings bank had about 36,000 depositors holding approximately 992,496 dalasi.

ENERGY AND NATURAL RESOURCES

Electricity. Production (1986) 63m. kwh. Supply 230 volts; 50 Hz.

Minerals. Heavy minerals, including ilmenite, zircon and rutile, have been discovered (1m. tons up to 31 Dec. 1980) in Sanyang, Batokunku and Kartong areas.

Agriculture. Almost all commercial activity centres upon the marketing of groundnuts, which is the only export crop of financial significance; in 1988, 110,000 tonnes were produced. Cotton is also exported on a limited scale. Rice is of increasing importance for local consumption; production (1988) 30,000 tonnes.

Livestock (1988): 300,000 cattle, 200,000 goats, 200,000 sheep, 13,000 pigs and (1982) 300,000 poultry.

Forestry. Forests cover 200,000 ha, 17% of the land area.

Fisheries. Total catch (1986) 10,700 tonnes, of which 2,700 tonnes were from inland waters.

FOREIGN ECONOMIC RELATIONS

Commerce. Chief items of imports are textiles and clothing, vehicles and machinery, metal goods and petroleum products.

Imports and exports, in 1,000 dalasi:

	1984–85	*1985–86*	*1986–87*	*1987–88* [1]
Imports	358,569	567,631	797,568	844,973
Exports	163,890	204,195	221,319	245,621

[1] Provisional.

Chief items of export (1985–86, in 1,000 dalasi): Groundnuts shelled, 33,570; groundnut oil, 15,132; groundnut cake, 4,142; cotton lint, 3,862; fish and fish preparations, 2,507; hides and skins, 1,652. Main imports: Food and live animals,

175,280; basic manufactured goods, 113,916; machinery and transport equipment, 97,850; mineral fuels and lubricants, 56,630.

Total trade between the Gambia and UK (British Department of Trade returns, in £1,000 sterling):

	1986	*1987*	*1988*	*1989*	*1990*
Imports to UK	2,273	3,038	2,927	2,340	3,158
Exports and re-exports from UK	16,707	19,765	19,236	16,583	17,815

TOURISM. In 1988–89, 120,000 tourists visited the Gambia.

COMMUNICATIONS

Roads. There are 2,990 km of motorable roads, of which 1,718 km rank as all-weather roads including 306 km of bituminous surface and 531 km of laterite gravel. Number of licensed motor vehicles (1985): 5,200 private cars, 700 buses, lorries and coaches, 2,000 motorcycles, scooters and mopeds.

Aviation. The Gambia is served by Gambia Air Shuttle, Minerve, British Airways, Ghana Airways and Nigeria Airways. The number of aircraft landing at Yundum Airport in 1984–85 was 1,576.

Shipping. The chief port is Banjul. In 1985–86, 125,959 tonnes of goods were loaded and 300,212 tonnes unloaded. Internal communication is maintained by steamers and launches. The Gambia River Development Organization was founded in 1978 as a joint project with Senegal to develop the river and its basin. Guinea and Guinea-Bissau were also members in 1984.

Telecommunications. There are several post offices and agencies; postal facilities are also afforded to all river towns. Telephones numbered 3,476 in Jan. 1980.

Radio Gambia, a government station, broadcasts for about 15 hours a day; Radio Syd, a commercial station, broadcasts for 20 hours. Number of radio receivers (1986, estimate), 110,000.

Cinemas. In 1984 there were 14 cinemas.

Newspapers. There is an official newspaper and several news-sheets.

JUSTICE, RELIGION, EDUCATION AND WELFARE

Justice. Justice is administered by a Supreme Court consisting of a chief justice and puisne judges. It has unlimited jurisdiction but there is a Court of Appeal. Two magistrates' courts and divisional courts are supplemented by a system of resident divisional magistrates. There are also Moslem courts, group tribunals dealing with cases concerned with customs and traditions, and one juvenile court.

Religion. About 90% of the population is Moslem. Banjul is the seat of an Anglican and a Roman Catholic bishop. There are some Methodist missions. Some sections of the population retain their original animist beliefs.

Education (1984–85). There were 189 primary schools (2,640 teachers, 66,257 pupils), 16 secondary technical schools (502 teachers, 10,102 pupils), 8 secondary high schools (235 teachers, 4,348 pupils). In 1982–83 there were 8 post-secondary schools (179 teachers, 1,489 pupils). Gambia College, which replaced Yundum College as a teacher-training and vocational centre, opened for agricultural and health students in 1979.

Health. In 1980 there were 43 government doctors, 23 private doctors and about 635 hospital beds.

DIPLOMATIC REPRESENTATIVES

Of the Gambia in Great Britain (57 Kensington Ct., London, W8 5DG)
High Commissioner: Horace R. Monday, Jr.

Of Great Britain in the Gambia (48 Atlantic Rd., Fajara, Banjul)
High Commissioner: A. J. Pover, CMG.

Of the Gambia in USA (1030, 15th St, NW, Washington, D.C. 2005)
Ambassador: Ousman Ahmodu Sallah, also *Ambassador* to the United Nations.

Of the USA in the Gambia (Fajara (East), Kairaba Ave., Banjul)
Ambassador: Arlene Render.

Further Reading

The Gambia since Independence 1965–1980. Banjul, 1980
Gamble, D. P., *The Gambia*. [Bibliography] Oxford and Santa Barbara, 1988
Tomkinson, M., *The Gambia: A Holiday Guide*. London, 1983

GERMANY

Capital: Berlin
Seat of Government: Bonn
Population: 79·07m. (1990)
GNP per capita: US$20,311 (1988)

Bundesrepublik Deutschland

(Federal Republic of Germany)

For the former **GERMAN DEMOCRATIC REPUBLIC (GDR)** *as an independent state see* THE STATESMAN'S YEAR-BOOK, 1990–91, pp. 526–32.

HISTORY. Following the unconditional surrender of the German armed forces on 8 May 1945 there was no central authority whose writ ran in the whole of Germany, and consequently no peace treaty was signed. France, the USSR, the UK and the USA assumed supreme authority over Germany by the Berlin Declaration of 5 June 1945. Each of the 4 signatories was allotted an occupation zone, in which the supreme power was to be exercised by the commander-in-chief in that zone (*see* map in THE STATESMAN'S YEAR-BOOK, 1947). Jointly these 4 commanders-in-chief constituted the Allied Control Council in Berlin, which was to be competent in all 'matters affecting Germany as a whole'. The territory of Greater Berlin, divided into 4 sectors, was to be governed as an entity by the 4 occupying powers.

At the Potsdam Conference (July–Aug. 1945) the northern part of the province of East Prussia, including its capital Königsberg (renamed Kaliningrad), was transferred to the USSR, and it was agreed that Poland should administer those parts of Germany east of a line running from the Baltic Sea west of Swinemünde along the river Oder to its confluence with the Western Neisse and thence along the Western Neisse to the Czechoslovak frontier (the 'Oder-Neisse line').

In June 1948 USA, UK and France agreed on a central government for the 3 western zones. An Occupation Statute, which came into force on 30 Sept. 1949, reduced the responsibilities of the occupation authorities. Formally, the Federal Republic of Germany came into existence on 21 Sept. 1949. The Petersberg Agreement of 22 Nov. 1949 freed the Federal Republic of numerous restrictions of the Occupation Statute. In 1951 the USA, the UK and France as well as other states terminated the state of war with Germany; the USSR followed on 25 Jan. 1955. On 5 May 1955 the High Commissioners of the USA, the UK and France signed a proclamation revoking the Occupation Statute. On the same day, the Paris and London treaties, signed in Oct. 1954, came into force and the Federal Republic of Germany became a sovereign independent country.

The eastern zone was administered by the USSR through a military government. A 'People's Chamber' (Volkskammer) was set up which promulgated a Soviet-type constitution in Oct. 1949 and proclaimed the German Democratic Republic. The GDR attained sovereignty in 1954 and obtained *de facto* diplomatic recognition from most countries. In 1961 the GDR built the mined and guarded 'Berlin Wall' to separate East from West Berlin. A treaty of 21 Dec. 1972 between the GDR and the Federal Republic agreed the basis of relations between the two countries.

Following public demonstrations in the GDR in favour of the democratization of political life in the autumn of 1989, and a mounting exodus of refugees to Federal Germany, Erich Honecker was replaced as Communist Party leader on 18 Oct. by Egon Krenz.

Exit restrictions were progressively eased until the border with Federal Germany, including the Berlin Wall, was opened on 9 Nov. On 13 Nov. the Volkskammer elected Hans Modrow as Prime Minister in place of Willi Stoph, and other Communist leaders were replaced. On 30 Nov. Egon Krenz and the entire Communist Party leadership resigned, amidst revelations of corruption under the former régime. Gregor Gysi was elected Party leader on 11 Dec.

On 1 Feb. 1990 Hans Modrow said 'Germany should again become the unified fatherland of all citizens of the German nation'.

Following the reforms in the GDR in Nov. 1989 the Federal Chancellor Helmut Kohl issued a 10-point plan for German confederation. The ambassadors of the 4 war-time allies met in Berlin in Dec. After talks with Chancellor Kohl on 11 Feb. 1990, President Gorbachev said the USSR had no objection to German re-unification in principle. On 13 Feb. 1990 Federal Germany, the GDR and the war-time allies agreed a formula ('two-plus-four') for re-unification talks to begin after the GDR elections on 18 March. 'Two-plus-four' talks began on 5 May 1990. On 18 May Federal Germany and the GDR signed a treaty transferring Federal Germany's currency, and its economic, monetary and social legislation, to the GDR as of 1 July. On 23 Aug. the Volkskammer by 294 votes to 62 'declared its accession to the jurisdiction of the Federal Republic as from 3 Oct. according to article 23 of the Basic Law', which provided for the Länder of pre-war Germany to accede to the Federal Republic.

On 12 Sept. the Treaty on the Final Settlement with Respect to Germany was signed by Federal Germany, the GDR and the 4 war-time allies: France, the USSR, the UK and the USA. This was ratified by the Volkskammer (by 200 votes to 80), the Bundestag (442 to 47) and the Bundesrat (unanimously). The treaty states *inter alia* 'that the unification of Germany as a state with definitive borders is a significant contribution to peace and stability in Europe' and that 'with the unification of Germany as a democratic and peaceful state, the rights and responsibilities of the Four Powers relating to Berlin and to Germany as a whole lose their function (Preamble); that the 'united Germany shall comprise the territory of the Federal Republic, the GDR and the whole of Berlin. Its external borders shall be the borders of the Federal Republic and the GDR' (Article 1.1); that 'the united Germany and Poland shall confirm the existing border between them in a treaty that is binding under international law' (Article 1.2); that 'the united Germany has no territorial claims whatsoever against other states and shall not assert any in the future' (Article 1.3); that the Federal Republic and the GDR declare 'that only peace will emanate from German soil' and 'acts to disturb peaceful relations between nations are unconstitutional and a punishable offence' (Article 2); that France, the USSR, the UK and the USA 'terminate their rights and responsibilities relating to Berlin and to Germany as a whole. As a result, the corresponding related quadripartite agreements, decisions and practices are dissolved' (Article 7.1); and that 'the united Germany shall have accordingly full sovereignty over its internal and external affairs' (Article 7.2).

AREA AND POPULATION. Germany is bounded in the north by Denmark and the North and Baltic Seas, east by Poland, east and south-east by Czechoslovakia, south-east and south by Austria, south by Switzerland and west by France, Luxembourg, Belgium and the Netherlands. Area: 356,945 sq. km. Population estimate, 1990: 79,070,000; density, 222 per sq. km. *In West Germany* there were 26·22m. households in 1987; 8·77m. were single-person, and 8·28m. had a female principal breadwinner. There were 778,000 unmarried couple households. 9·34m. persons were over 65 in 1987. *In the GDR* population at the census of 31 Dec. 1981 was 16,705,635. Population in 1988 was 16,674,632 (7·97m. male; 12·8m. urban). There were some 110,000 Sorbs, a Slav minority, in 1985.

On 14 Nov. 1990 Germany and Poland signed a treaty confirming Poland's existing western frontier and renouncing German claims to territory lost as a result of the Second World War.

The capital is Berlin; after re-unification the seat of government remained at Bonn.

The Federation comprises 16 Länder (states). Area and population:

Länder	*Area in sq. km*	*Population (in 1,000's) 1987 census*	*1990 estimate*	*Per sq. km*
Baden-Württemberg	35,751	9,286	9,619	269
Bavaria	70,554	10,903	11,221	159
Berlin [1]	883	...	3,410	3,862
Brandenburg [2]	29,059	...	2,641	91
Bremen	404	660	674	1,668
Hamburg	755	1,593	1,626	2,154

[1] 1987 census population of West Berlin: 2,013,000 [2] Reconstituted in 1990 in the GDR

Länder	Area in sq. km	Population (in 1,000's) 1987 census	1990 estimate	Per sq. km
Hessen	21,114	5,508	5,661	268
Lower Saxony	47,344	7,162	7,238	153
Mecklenburg-West Pomerania [2]	23,838	...	1,964	82
North Rhine-Westphalia	34,070	16,712	17,104	502
Rhineland-Palatinate	19,849	3,631	3,702	186
Saarland	2,570	1,056	1,065	414
Saxony [2]	18,337	...	4,901	267
Saxony-Anhalt [2]	20,445	...	2,965	145
Schleswig-Holstein	15,729	2,554	2,595	165
Thuringia [2]	16,251	...	2,684	165

[1] 1987 census population of West Berlin: 2,013,000 [2] Reconstituted in 1990 in the GDR

Birth rate in 1989, 11·1 per 1,000; death rate, 11·4.

Vital statistics *for West Germany:*

	Marriages	Live births	Of these to single parents	Deaths	Divorces
1986	372,008	625,963	59,808	701,890	122,581
1987	382,564	642,010	62,358	687,419	129,850
1988	397,595	677,259	67,957	687,516	...

Vital statistics *for the GDR:*

	Live births	Marriages	Divorces	Deaths
1985	227,648	131,514	51,240	225,353
1986	222,269	137,208	52,439	223,536
1987	225,959	141,283	50,640	213,872
1988	215,734	137,165	49,380	213,111

Rates per 1,000, 1988: Birth, 12·9; marriage, 8·2; divorce, 3; death, 12·8; infant mortality: 5 stillborn, 8·1 under 1 year. Expectation of life, 1987: Men, 69·8; women, 75·9. 74,515 births were to unmarried mothers in 1987.

Marriage rate in 1988 was 6·5 per 1,000 population; infantile mortality 7·6; growth rate, –0·2.

In 1988 there were 4,489,100 resident foreigners (1,956,200 female) *in West Germany*. 37,810 persons were naturalized in 1987.

In 1987 there were 400,932 emigrants and 614,603 immigrants. 842,227 refugees entered in 1989 (345,581 in 1988). These comprised 720,909 ethnic Germans (including 343,854 from GDR, 250,340 from Poland, 98,134 from USSR and 23,387 from Romania) and 121,318 non-Germans (mainly from Poland, Turkey, Yugoslavia, Sri Lanka, Lebanon and Iran). In 1990 ethnic German emigrants from East Europe numbered some 397,000, including 148,000 from the USSR, 133,000 from Poland and 111,000 from Romania.

Populations of towns of over 100,000 inhabitants in 1988 (in '000):

Town	Land	Population	Town	Land	Population
Berlin	Berlin	3,410·0 [1]	Chemnitz	Saxony	301·9 [1]
Hamburg	Hamburg	1,597·5	Mannheim	Baden-Württ.	298·8
Munich	Bavaria	1,206·4	Magdeburg	Saxony	288·4 [1]
Cologne	N. Rhine-Westph.	934·4	Gelsenkirchen	N. Rhine-Westph.	286·7
Frankfurt am Main	Hessen	623·7	Bonn	N. Rhine-Westph.	279·7
			Karlsruhe	Baden-Württ.	263·1
Essen	N. Rhine-Westph.	620·0	Wiesbaden	Hessen	253·4
Dortmund	N. Rhine-Westph.	584·6	Rostock	Meckl.-W. Pom.	253·0 [1]
Düsseldorf	N. Rhine-Westph.	564·4	Braunschweig	Lower Saxony	252·9
Stuttgart	Baden-Württ.	560·1	Mönchengladbach	N. Rhine-Westph.	251·6
Bremen	Bremen	533·8			
Leipzig	Thuringia	530·0 [1]	Münster	N. Rhine-Westph.	246·7
Duisburg	N. Rhine-Westph.	525·1	Augsburg	Bavaria	245·6
Dresden	Saxony	501·4 [1]	Kiel	Schleswig-Holstein	239·2
Hanover	Lower Saxony	497·2	Krefeld	N. Rhine-Westph.	233·9
Nuremberg	Bavaria	477·0	Aachen	N. Rhine-Westph.	232·0
Bochum	N. Rhine-Westph.	386·9	Halle	Saxony-Anhalt	230·7 [1]
Wuppertal	N. Rhine-Westph.	368·2	Oberhausen	N. Rhine-Westph.	220·4
Bielefeld	N. Rhine-Westph.	309·0	Erfurt	Thuringia	217·0 [1]

Town	Land	Population	Town	Land	Population
Lübeck	Schleswig-Holstein	210·4	Wolfsburg	Lower Saxony	125·4
Hagen	N. Rhine-Westph.	209·1	Würzburg	Bavaria	125·0
Kassel	Hessen	188·2	Remscheid	N. Rhine-Westph.	120·3
Saarbrücken	Saarland.	188·2	Recklinghausen	N. Rhine-Westph.	119·3
Freiburg im Breisgau	Baden-Württ.	182·0	Zwickau	Saxony	118·9 [1]
			Regensburg	Bavaria	118·7
Mülheim a.d. Ruhr	N. Rhine-Westph.	175·2	Göttingen	Lower Saxony	117·1
			Bottrop	N. Rhine-Westph.	115·3
Herne	N. Rhine-Westph.	174·3	Paderborn	N. Rhine-Westph.	112·9
Mainz	Rhinel.-Pal.	173·7	Offenbach am Main	Hessen	111·9
Hamm	N. Rhine-Westph.	172·0			
Solingen	N. Rhine-Westph.	159·9	Heilbronn	Baden-Württ.	111·9
Ludwigshafen am Rhein	Rhinel.-Pal.	158·0	Salzgitter	Lower Saxony	111·4
			Pforzheim	Baden-Württ.	108·4
Leverkusen	N. Rhine-Westph.	155·8	Koblenz	Rhine-Pal.	107·4
Osnabrück	Lower Saxony	151·2	Siegen	N. Rhine-Westph.	106·1
Neuss	N. Rhine-Westph.	143·3	Jena	Thuringia	105·8 [1]
Potsdam	Brandenburg	141·4	Ulm	Baden-Württ.	105·4
Oldenburg	Lower Saxony	140·4	Hildesheim	Lower Saxony	103·2
Darmstadt	Hessen.	135·3	Witten	N. Rhine-Westph.	103·2
Gera	Thuringia	132·3 [1]	Bergisch Gladbach	N. Rhine-Westph.	101·5
Heidelberg	Baden-Württ.	129·6			
Schwerin	Meckl.-W. Pom.	129·5 [1]	Moers	N. Rhine-Westph.	101·3
Cottbus	Brandenburg	128·9 [1]	Dessau	Saxony-Anhalt	101·3 [1]
Bremerhaven	Bremen	126·6	Erlangen	Bavaria	100·0 [1]

[1] Population in 1989

CLIMATE. Oceanic influences are only found in the north-west where winters are quite mild but stormy. Elsewhere a continental climate is general. To the east and south, winter temperatures are lower, with bright frosty weather and considerable snowfall. Summer temperatures are fairly uniform throughout. Berlin. Jan. 31°F (–0·5°C), July 66°F (19°C). Annual rainfall 22·5" (563 mm). Dresden. Jan. 30°F (–0·1°C), July 65°F (18·5°C). Annual rainfall 27·2" (680 mm). Frankfurt. Jan. 33°F (0·6°C), July 66°F (18·9°C). Annual rainfall 24" (601 mm). Hamburg. Jan. 31°F (–0·6°C), July 63°F (17·2°C). Annual rainfall 29" (726 mm). Hanover. Jan. 33°F (0·6°C), July 64°F (17·8°C). Annual rainfall 24" (604 mm). Köln. Jan. 36°F (2·2°C), July 66°F (18·9°C). Annual rainfall 27" (676 mm). Munich. Jan. 28°F (–2·2°C), July 63°F (17·2°C). Annual rainfall 34" (855 mm). Stuttgart. Jan. 33°F (0·6°C), July 66°F (18·9°C). Annual rainfall 27" (677 mm).

CONSTITUTION. The Constituent Assembly (known as the 'Parliamentary Council') met in Bonn on 1 Sept. 1948, and worked out a Basic Law (*Grundgesetz*) which was approved by a two-thirds majority of the parliaments of the participating Länder and came into force on 23 May 1949. It is to remain in force until 'a constitution adopted by a free decision of the German people comes into being'.

The Basic Law consists of a preamble and 146 articles. There have been 35 amendments. The first section deals with the basic rights which are legally binding for legislation, administration and jurisdiction.

The Federal Republic is a democratic and social constitutional state on a parliamentary basis. The federation is constituted by the 16 Länder (states) (*see* p. 527). The Basic Law decrees that the general rules of international law form part of the federal law. The constitutions of the Länder must conform to the principles of a republican, democratic and social state based on the rule of law. Executive power is vested in the Länder, unless the Basic Law prescribes or permits otherwise. Federal law takes precedence over state law.

Legislative power is vested in the *Bundestag* (Federal Assembly) and the *Bundesrat* (Federal Council).

The Bundestag is composed of 662 members and is elected in universal, free, equal and secret elections for a term of 4 years. A party must gain 5% of total votes cast in order to gain representation in the Bundestag. The electoral system combines relative-majority and proportional voting; each voter has 2 votes, the first for the direct constituency representative, the second for the competing party lists in the Länder. This second proportional vote determines each party's share of the Bundestag seats.

The Bundesrat consists of 68 members appointed by the governments of the Länder in proportions determined by the number of inhabitants. Each Land has at least 3 votes.

The Head of State is the Federal President *(Bundespräsident)* who is elected for a 5-year term by a Federal Convention specially convened for this purpose. This Convention consists of all the members of the Bundestag and an equal number of members elected by the Länder parliaments in accordance with party strengths, but who need not themselves be members of the parliaments. No president may serve more than two terms. Presidents since 1949: Theodor Heuss (1949-59); Heinrich Lübke (1959-69); Gustav Heinemann (1969-74); Walter Scheel (1974-1979); Karl Castens (1979–84).

Executive power is vested in the Federal Government, which consists of the Federal Chancellor, elected by the Bundestag on the proposal of the Federal President, and the Federal Ministers, who are appointed and dismissed by the Federal President upon the proposal of the Federal Chancellor.

The Federal Republic has exclusive legislation on: (1) foreign affairs (2) federal citizenship; (3) freedom of movement, passports, immigration and emigration, and extradition; (4) currency, money and coinage, weights and measures, and regulation of time and calendar; (5) customs, commercial and navigation agreements, traffic in goods and payments with foreign countries, including customs and frontier protection; (6) federal railways and air traffic; (7) post and telecommunications; (8) the legal status of persons in the employment of the Federation and of public law corporations under direct supervision of the Federal Government; (9) trade marks, copyright and publishing rights; (10) co-operation of the Federal Republic and the Länder in the criminal police and in matters concerning the protection of the constitution, the establishment of a Federal Office of Criminal Police, as well as the combating of international crime; (11) federal statistics.

For concurrent legislation in which the Länder have legislative rights if and as far as the Federal Republic does not exercise its legislative powers, *see* THE STATESMAN'S YEAR-BOOK, 1956, p. 1038.

Federal laws are passed by the Bundestag and after their adoption submitted to the Bundesrat, which has a limited veto. The Basic Law may be amended only upon the approval of two-thirds of the members of the Bundestag and two-thirds of the votes of the Bundesrat.

The foreign service, federal finance, railways, postal services, waterways and shipping are under direct federal administration.

In the field of finance the Federal Republic has exclusive legislation on customs and financial monopolies and concurrent legislation on: (1) excise taxes and taxes on transactions, in particular, taxes on real-estate acquisition, incremented value and on fire protection; (2) taxes on income, property, inheritance and donations; (3) real estate, industrial and trade taxes, with the exception of the determining of the tax rates.

The Federal Republic can, by federal law, claim part of the income and corporation taxes to cover its expenditures not covered by other revenues. Financial jurisdiction is uniformly regulated by federal legislation.

National flag: Three horizontal stripes of black, red, gold.

National anthem: Einigkeit und Recht und Freiheit ('Unity and right and freedom' words by H. Hoffmann, 1841; tune by J. Haydn, 1797).

Local Government. Below *Land* level local government is carried on by elected councils to counties *(Landkreise)* and county boroughs *(Kreisfreie Städte)*, which form the electoral districts for the *Land* governments, and are subdivided into communities *(Gemeinden)*.

GOVERNMENT. The 12th Bundestag was elected on 2 Dec. 1990. A special 5% threshold was applied to constituencies in the former GDR. Electoral turnout was 78·5%. The government is formed by a coalition of the Christian Democrat/Christian Socialist (CDU/CSU) alliance with the Free Democrats (FDP). (The CSU is a Bavarian party where the CDU does not stand). Percentage votes, and seats gained (1987 electoral results in brackets): CDU/CSU 43·8%, 319 (44·3%, 223); Social Democratic Party (SPD), 33·5%, 239 (37%, 186); FDP, 11%, 79 (9·1%, 46); Democratic Socialists (former Communists), 2·4%, 17; Alliance '90/Greens, 1·2%, 8.

After the *Länder* elections of Oct. 1990 the Bundesrat had 35 CDU and 33 SPD members.

Federal President: Dr Richard von Weizsäcker (sworn in 1 July 1984); elected for a second term 23 May 1989).
Speaker of the Bundestag: Rita Süssmuth (elected Nov. 1988).

A new Cabinet was formed in Jan. 1991 as follows:

Chancellor: Dr Helmut Kohl (CDU).
Deputy Chancellor, Minister of Foreign Affairs: Hans-Dietrich Genscher (FDP).
Interior: Wolfgang Schäuble (CDU).
Justice: Klaus Kinkel (ind).
Finance: Theo Waigel (CSU).
Economy: Jürgen Mölleman (FDP).
Defence: Dr Gerhard Stoltenberg (CDU).
Transport: Günther Krause (CDU).
Family and Elderly: Hannelore Rönsch (CDU).
Minister at the Chancellery: Rudolf Seiters (CDU).
Women and Youth: Angela Merkel (CDU).
Food, Agriculture and Forestry: Ignaz Kiechle (CSU).
Labour and Social Affairs: Dr Norbert Blüm (CDU).
Health: Gerda Hasselfeldt (CDU).
Environment, Nature Conservation and Reactor Safety: Klaus Töpfer (CDU).
Posts and Telecommunications: Dr Christian Schwarz-Schilling (CDU).
Construction: Irmgard Adam-Schwätzer (CSU).
Research and Technology: Dr Heinz Riesenhuber (CDU).
Education and Science: Rainer Ortleb (FDP).
Economic Co-operation: Carl-Dieter Spranger (CSU).

At the ultimate elections to the *GDR* Volkskammer in March 1990 turn-out was 93%. Percentage votes, and seats gained: Alliance for Germany (CDU, German Social Union and Democratic Awakening), 48·1%, 193; SPD, 21·8%, 87; Party of Democratic Socialism (former Communists), 16%, 65; Alliance of Free Democrats (German Forum Party, Liberal Democratic Party and Free Democratic Party), 5·3%, 21; Alliance '90, 2·9%, 12; Democratic Farmers, 2·2%, 9; Greens, 2%, 8; National Democrats, 0·4%, 2. 3 other parties won 1 seat each.

Lothar de Maizière (CDU) formed a government.

At the *GDR local elections* in May 1990 turn-out was 80%. The CDU gained 34·3% of the vote, the SPD 21·2%, the Party of Democratic Socialism, 14·5%, the Liberal Democratic Party, 6·6%, and the German Social Union, 3·4%.

DEFENCE. The Paris Treaties, which entered into force in May 1955, stipulated a contribution of the Federal Republic to western defence within the framework of NATO and the Western European Union. On 30 Oct. 1990 the Bundestag ratified 2 treaties providing for the withdrawal of all Soviet forces from the territory of the former GDR by 1994. The German government is defraying part of the expenses of this operation. There were some 380,000 Soviet troops in the GDR.

The Federal Armed Forces *(Bundeswehr)* had a total strength (1988) of 488,400 all ranks (223,450 conscripts) and a further 750,000 reserves. Conscription was reduced from 15 to 12 months in Oct. 1990. Defence expenditure was DM 53,700m. in 1990 and a scheduled DM 52,600m. in 1991.

On re-unification the GDR's forces (see THE STATESMAN'S YEAR-BOOK, 1990–91, p. 528) were reduced from 170,000 to 50,000, and these latter were integrated into the Federal forces.

Army. The *West German* Army is divided into the Field Army, containing the units assigned to NATO in event of war, and the Territorial Army. The Field Army is organized in 3 corps, comprising 6 armoured, 4 armoured infantry, 1 mountain and 1 airborne divisions. Equipment includes 650 M-48, 2,130 Leopard I and 2,000 Leopard II tanks. An air component operates 210 BO 105P anti-armour helicopters, 108 CH-53G and 87 UH-1D Iroquois transport helicopters, plus 138 Alouette II and 97 BO 105M liaison/observation helicopters. The Territorial Army is organized into 5 Military Districts, under 3 Territorial Commands. Its main task is to defend rear areas and remains under national control even in wartime. Total strength was (1990) 340,700 (conscripts 175,900); Territorial Army 41,700.

Navy. The Federal Navy is tasked to maritime operations in support of the central European theatre in the Baltic and North Sea environments. The emphasis is thus on coastal and shallow-seas warfare. The Fleet Commander operates from a modern Maritime Headquarters at Glücksburg, close to the Danish border.

The fleet includes 24 diesel coastal submarines, 3 US-built guided-missile and 3 other destroyers, 8 frigates, 5 anti-submarine corvettes and 40 fast missile craft. There is a large mine-warfare force of 53 vessels, comprising 2 minelayer/transports, 34 coastal minesweepers and hunters of which 2 are new combined minelayer/hunters and 6 control ships for TROIKA minesweeping drones, and 18 inshore minesweepers. Major auxiliaries include 4 tankers, 2 repair ships, 5 oilers, 7 minesweeper/patrol craft support and HQ ships, 8 logistic transports, 8 large tugs, 3 intelligence collectors, 2 trial ships and a sail training vessel. There are several dozen minor auxiliaries and service craft, as well as, in early 1991, the units inherited from the GDR's navy.

The main naval bases are at Wilhemshaven, Bremerhaven, Kiel and Olpenitz; there are several lesser bases.

The Naval Air Arm, 6,700 strong, is organized into 4 wings and comprises 104 missile-armed Tornado strike aircraft. 19 Atlantic long range, plus 19 Dornier-28 coastal patrol aircraft, 22 shore-based Sea King helicopters and 19 Lynx (12 frigate-based) complete the inventory.

Procurement of 4 new frigates and 16 further replacement mine warfare craft is in hand. Modernization of the existing force proceeds. Personnel in mid-1990 numbered 38,000 including the Naval Air Arm.

The 15,000 strength of the GDR navy in 1989 had shrunk to some 9,000 when Germany was re-unified in October 1990. Of these, about half were conscripts, but some 4-5,000 long service officers and men were eligible for incorporation into the Federal Germany Navy. The means by which this is to be achieved had not (in Dec. 1990) been fully determined, as the total naval ceiling strength of the reformed *Bundeswehr* remained to be announced. The Federal Navy has no operational requirement for the ships of the former GDR navy, and apart from 12 of the newer units which are to be retained temporarily for training, the remainder, numbering some 3 frigates and two dozen patrol and coastal combatants, are to be sold or scrapped. The former East German Maritime Border Guards are being disbanded.

Air Force. Since 1970, the *West German Luftwaffe* has comprised the following commands: German Air Force Tactical Command, German Air Force Support Command (including two German Air Force Regional Support Commands—North and South) and General Air Force Office. Its strength in 1990 was approximately 106,000 officers and other ranks and over 550 first-line combat aircraft. Combat units, including 12 heavy fighter-bomber squadrons, 7 light ground attack/reconnaissance squadrons, 4 reconnaissance squadrons, 8 surface-to-surface missile squadrons, and an air defence force of 4 interceptor squadrons, 24 batteries of *Nike-Hercules* and 36 batteries of *Improved Hawk* surface-to-air missiles, are assigned to NATO. There are 4 F-4F Phantom interceptor squadrons, 8 Tornado attack squadrons, 4 attack squadrons of F-4Fs, 4 RF-4E Phantom reconnaissance squadrons, and 7 light attack/reconnaissance squadrons of Alpha Jets. Four transport squadrons (each 15 aircraft) with turboprop Transall C-160 aircraft and 1 wing of 5 helicopter squadrons with UH-1D Iroquois add to the air mobility of the *Bundeswehr*. There are also VIP, support and light transport aircraft. Guided weapons in service include

8 squadrons of *Pershing* surface-to-surface missiles and 6 battalions of *Nike-Hercules* and 9 battalions of *Improved Hawk* surface-to-air missiles.

INTERNATIONAL RELATIONS

Membership. Germany is a member of the UN, OECD, EC, WEU, NATO and the Council of Europe. The Schengen Accord of June 1990 abolished border controls between Germany, Belgium, France, Luxembourg and the Netherlands. Italy acceded in Nov. 1990.

ECONOMY

Budget. Since 1 Jan. 1979 tax revenues have been distributed as follows: Federal Government. Income tax, 42·5%; capital yield and corporation tax, 50%; turnover tax, 67·5%; trade tax, 15%; capital gains, insurance and accounts taxes, 100%; excise duties (other than on beer), 100%. Länder. Income tax, 42·5%; capital yield and corporation tax, 50%; turnover tax, 32·5%; trade tax, 15%; other taxes, 100%. Local authorities. Income tax, 15%; trade tax, 70%; local taxes, 100%. Income tax was reduced in 1990.

Budgets for 1988, 1989 and 1990 (in DM1m.):

	All public authorities		*Federal portion*	
Revenue	*1988*	*1989*	*1989*	*1990*
		Current		
Taxes	456,967	513,698	249,789	257,051
Economic activities	28,235	34,280	11,408	13,654
Interest	1,892	2,938	1,201	1,202
Current allocations and subsidies	110,338	118,865	1,812	1,506
Other receipts	32,297	33,677	4,485	5,408
minus equalising payments	99,346	106,841	...	...
	539,383	596,607	268,695	278,821
		Capital		
Sale of assets	9,083	7,944	572	793
Allocations for investment	23,068	24,523	20	11
Repayment of loans	5,585	8,661	3,079	2,456
Public sector borrowing	2,859	2,978	...	...
minus equalising payments	22,190	23,869	...	...
	18,405	20,237	3,671	3,260
Totals	557,788	616,844	272,366	282,081
Expenditure		*Current*		
Staff	190,807	195,430	41,339	43,592
Materials	92,880	97,470	40,856	42,805
Interest	60,034	61,135	32,099	33,307
Allocations and subsidies	270,863	290,681	140,810	153,693
minus equalising payments	99,346	106,842	...	...
	515,238	537,874	255,103	273,397
		Capital		
Construction	39,708	42,064	6,177	6,941
Acquisition of property	12,197	13,585	1,851	2,069
Allocations and subsidies	44,122	49,956	19,496	21,923
Loans	16,095	19,130	8,478	7,629
Acquisition of shares	3,331	3,264	1,331	1,384
Repayments in the public sector	1,437	1,476	...	...
minus equalising payments	22,190	23,869	...	...
	94,700	105,606	37,333	39,946
Totals	609,938	643,480	292,436	314,538

Major areas of expenditure in 1987 (and 1988) in DM1,000m.: Social, 87·2 (89·2); defence, 53·6 (53·9); transport and communications, 13·1 (12·9); economy, 10·2 (11·6). Supplementary budgets were drawn up in 1990 to cover the costs of reunification, and a further tax rise, including 7·5% on income tax, was imposed in July 1991 for 1 year.

Government expenditure was budgetted at DM324,000m. for 1991.

The budget of *the GDR* was as follows (in M 1m.) for calendar years:

	1983	*1984*	*1985*	*1986*	*1987*	*1988*
Revenue	192,410	213,535	235,535	247,013	260,449	269,699
Expenditure	191,689	211,778	234,392	246,368	260,167	269,466

Of 1988 expenditure, M 49,811m. went on price subsidies, M 36,275m. on social benefits and pensions, M 19,376m. on education and culture, M 17,801m. on health and social services, M 15,654m. on defence. Revenue included M 20,816m. from taxes and M 18,822m. from social insurance.

Currency. The unit of currency is the *deutsche Mark* (DEM) of 100 *pfennig* (pf.). There are 1, 2, 5, 10, 50 pf., 1, 2, 5 and 10 DM coins and 5, 10, 20, 50, 100, 200, 500 and 1,000 DM notes. Money in circulation in 1989, DM 154,538m. The deutsche Mark became the sole German currency on 2 July 1990, replacing the GDR's Mark at parity. In March 1991, £1 = 2·91 DM; US$1 = 1·54.

Banking and Finance. In 1948 the Bank deutscher Länder was established in Frankfurt as the central bank. This and the Berlin central bank were merged on 1 Aug. 1957 to form the Deutsche Bundesbank (German Federal Bank). The central bank's duty is to protect the stability of the currency. It is independent of the government but obliged to support the government's general policy. The *Governor* is Karl Otto Pöhl. Its assets were DM 308,571m. in 1989. The largest private banks are the Deutsche Bank, Dresdner Bank and Commerzbank. The public sector banks consist of 583 retail savings banks and 11 Landesbanken which represent them in the wholesale markets. The former GDR central bank Staatsbank has become a public commercial bank. Its former credit arm Deutsche Kreditbank has been taken over by Deutsche Bank and Dresdner Bank.

Savings deposits were DM 715,236m. in 1989.

There are stock exchanges in Frankfurt and Berlin.

Weights and Measures. The metric system is in force.

ENERGY AND NATURAL RESOURCES

Electricity. In 1990 some 50% of electricity was produced from coal in *West Germany*, and 34% from nuclear power. There is a moratorium on further nuclear plant construction. In 1988, 431,200m. kwh. were produced. In *the GDR* in 1989 sources of energy included 73% lignite (85% in 1988) and 9·9% nuclear power from a single plant which was closed in 1990. Production, 1988: 118,328 kwh. Supply 220 volts; 50 Hz.

Oil and Gas. The chief oilfields are in Emsland (Lower Saxony). In 1988, 13·94m. tonnes of crude, 9·72m. tonnes of petroleum, and 11·71m. tonnes of diesel oil were produced. Gas production was 14,783m. cu metres.

Minerals. The main production areas of *West Germany* are: North Rhine-Westphalia (for coal, iron and metal smelting-works), Central Germany (for brown coal), and Lower Saxony (Salzgitter for iron ore; the Harz for metal ore).

Production (in 1,000 tonnes):

Minerals	*1984*	*1985*	*1986*	*1987*	*1988*	*1989*
Coal	79,426	82,398	80,801	76,300	73,304	71,428
Lignite	126,739	120,667	114,310	108,799	108,563	110,081
Potash	29,543	29,248	24,775	25,795	27,030	26,002

Production of iron and steel (in 1,000 tonnes):

	1984	*1985*	*1986*	*1987*	*1988*	*1989*
Pig-iron	30,203	31,919	29,443	28,918	33,016	32,777
Steel	39,389	40,497	37,134	36,248	41,023	41,073
Rolled products finished	27,962	28,919	27,409	27,437	30,385	31,702

The former *GDR* was a major producer of lignite (production in 1989: 311m. tonnes).

Agriculture. Area cultivated in *West Germany*, 1989: 11·89m. ha (arable, 7·27m.; pasture, 4·52m.).

In 1989 the number of agricultural holdings classified by area farmed was:

	Total	1–5 ha	5–20 ha	20–100 ha	Over 100 ha
Schleswig-Holstein	28,423	6,231	5,108	15,571	1,513
Hamburg	1,173	700	263	198	12
Lower Saxony	100,220	25,608	26,688	45,494	2,430
Bremen	384	116	93	167	8
North Rhine-Westphalia	83,436	25,511	27,776	29,493	656
Hessen	48,347	16,876	18,331	12,802	338
Rhineland-Palatinate	49,055	20,153	17,037	11,573	292
Baden-Württemberg	109,438	42,798	42,300	23,896	444
Bavaria	224,794	57,082	108,567	58,429	716
Saarland	3,393	1,317	1,001	998	77
Berlin (West)	109	60	29	20	...
Federal Republic	*648,772*	*196,453*	*247,193*	*198,640*	*6,486*

Area (in 1,000 ha) and yield (in 1,000 tonnes) of the main crops:

	Area				Yield			
	1986	*1987*	*1988*	*1989*	*1986*	*1987*	*1988*	*1989*
Wheat	1,648	1,671	1,743	1,777	10,406	9,932	11,922	11,031
Rye	414	412	378	382	1,768	1,599	1,579	1,797
Barley	1,947	1,849	1,836	1,746	9,377	8,571	9,588	9,716
Oats	506	459	474	419	2,276	2,008	2,039	1,533
Potatoes	210	206	199	201	7,390	6,836	7,433	7,451
Sugar-beet	391	376	379	383	20,260	19,049	18,590	20,767

4·52m. tonnes of fertilizers were used in Oct. 1987-Sept. 1988.

Wine production (in 1,000 hectolitres): 15,352 in 1988; 15,094 in 1989.

Livestock (in 1,000s), 1989: Cattle, 14,828 (including 4,922 milch cows); sheep, 2,015; pigs, 22,548; horses (1988), 375; poultry (1988), 72,035. Milk production was 3·74m. tonnes in 1989.

In 1987 there were 1·73m. tractors.

In *the GDR* in 1989 the agricultural area was 6·2m. ha including 4·7m. ha arable and 1·26m. ha grassland. There were 3,855 collective farms with 5·3m. ha of arable land, and 465 state farms with 448,895 ha of land in 1988. In 1987 private plots accounted for 9% of production. In 1988 there were 167,529 tractors and 18,404 combine harvesters.

The yield of the main crops in 1988 was as follows (in 1,000 tonnes): Potatoes, 11,546; sugar-beet, 4,625; barley, 3,798; wheat, 3,699; rye, 1,785; oats, 507.

Livestock (in 1,000) in 1988: Cattle, 5,710 (including 2,009 milch cows); pigs, 12,464; sheep, 2,634; poultry, 49,430. 2·8m. tonnes of meat, 8m. tonnes of milk and 5,720m. eggs were produced.

Forestry. Forestry is of great importance, conducted under the guidance of the State on scientific lines. In recent years enormous depredation has occurred through pollution with acid rain. Forest area in *West Germany* in 1989 was 5·3m. ha, of which 2·25m. were owned by the State. In 1988 29·51m. cu. metres of timber were cut. In *the GDR* in 1988 there were 2,981,303 ha of forest. Timber production was 10·9m. cu. metres.

Fisheries. In *West Germany* in 1989 the yield of sea fishing was 166,495 tonnes live weight. The fishing fleet consisted of 15 trawlers (26,624 GRT) and 613 cutters. In *the GDR* in 1988 the sea catch was 244,900 tonnes; inland, 26,524 tonnes.

INDUSTRY. Public limited companies are managed on the 'co-determination' principle, and have 3 statutory bodies: a board of directors, a works council elected by employees, and a supervisory council which includes employee representatives but has an in-built management majority.

In *West Germany* in 1988 there were 50,849 firms (with 20 and more employees) employing 8·24m. persons, made up of 282,000 in energy and water services, 197,000 in mining, 1·37m. in raw materials processing, 3·77m. in the manufacture of producers' goods, 1·26m. in the manufacture of consumer goods, 461,000 in food and tobacco and 898,000 in building.

Production of major industrial products:

Products (1,000 tonnes)	*1985*	*1986*	*1987*	*1988*	*1989*
Aluminium	745	765	793	753	734
Artificial fertilizers	1,651	1,425	1,449	1,274	1,179
Sulphuric acid, SO_3	3,428	3,351	3,323	3,308	3,288
Soda, Na_2CO_3	1,412	1,442	1,448	1,404	1,443
Cement	25,758	26,580	25,268	26,215	28,499
Plastics	7,666	7,941	8,546	9,218	9,176
Cotton yarn	131	128	142	126	124
Woollen yarn	42	41	40	38	36
Passenger cars (1,000)	3,867	3,952	4,008	3,980	4,106
TV sets (1,000)	3,738	3,895	3,537	3,737	3,236

In *the GDR* industry produced about 70% of the national income in 1989. The major industries were energy, chemicals, metallurgy, mechanical and electrical engineering, electronics and instruments.

1988 production (in 1,000 tonnes): Rolled steel, 9,472; sulphuric acid, 799; chemical fertilizers, 5,192; petrol, 4,765; diesel fuel, 6,301; caustic soda, 627; plastics and synthetic resins, 1,149; cement, 12,510; antibiotics, 84·9 tonnes; passenger cars (no.), 218,045; television receivers (no.), 774,100; shoes, 91m. pairs.

Labour. In *West Germany* 27·74m. persons were employed in 1988, including 10·79m. women and 1·69m. foreign workers. Major categories: Manufacturing industries, 11·33m.; services, 10·39m.; commerce and transport, 4·97m.; self-employed, 2·46m.; agriculture, forestry and fishing, 1·04m. Unemployed 2·03m.; unfilled vacancies, 251,415; part-time workers, 107,873.

In *the GDR* in 1988 the workforce was 8·59m. (4·2m. females), of whom 7·59m. were employees, 629,100 worked on collective farms, 164,000 in co-operative workshops and 181,700 were self-employed. Workforce distribution by activity, 1988: Industry, 37·4%; services, 21·4%; agriculture, 10·8%; commerce, 10·3%; building, 6·6%; transport, 5·9%; handicrafts, 3·1%; posts and telecommunications, 1·5%; other products, 3%.

Trade Unions. The majority of trade unions belong to the *Deutscher Gewerkschaftsbund* (DGB, German Trade Union Federation), which had (women in brackets) 7·8m. (1·83m.) members in 1989, including 5·22m. (895,876) manual workers, 1·83m. (818,410) white-collar workers and 807,409 (168,270) civil servants. DGB unions are organized in industrial branches such that only one union operates within each enterprise. Outside the DGB lie several smaller unions: The *Deutscher Beamtenbund* (DBB) or civil servants union with 793,607 (216,252) members, the *Deutsche Angestellten-Gewerkschaft* (DAG) or union of salaried staff with 503,528 (227,317 members and the *Christlicher Gewerkschaftsbund Deutschlands* (CGD, Christian Trade Union Federation of Germany) with 304,741 (75,821) members.

Strikes are not legal unless called by a union with the backing of 75% of members. Certain public service employees are contractually not permitted to strike. 100,409 working days were lost through strikes in 1989.

The official GDR trade union organization (FDGB) was dissolved in Sept. 1990 and the 21 branch unions were merged in the Deutscher Gewerkschaftsbund.

FOREIGN ECONOMIC RELATIONS

Commerce. *West German* imports and exports in DM 1m.:

Imports				*Exports*			
1986	*1987*	*1988*	*1989*	*1986*	*1987*	*1988*	*1989*
413,744	409,641	439,768	506,648	526,363	527,377	567,750	641,342

Distribution of imports and exports by categories of countries in 1989 (in DM 1m.): EEC, 252,781, 352,961; developing countries, 62,291, 61,742; Communist countries, 24,972, 29,314 (USSR, 8,392, 11,528; China, 5,796, 4,619). Most important trading partners in 1989 (trade figures in DM 1m.) Imports: France, 60,422; Netherlands, 51,972; Italy, 45,197; USA, 38,266; Belgium with Luxembourg, 34,975; UK, 34,698; Japan, 32,186; Switzerland, 21,249; Austria, 20,995. Exports:

France, 84,358; Italy, 59,830; UK, 59,364; Netherlands, 54,422; USA, 46,659; Belgium with Luxembourg, 45,979; Switzerland, 38,149; Austria, 32,275.

Distribution by commodities in 1988 (in DM 1m.) Imports and exports: Live animals, 725,000, 1,036; foodstuffs, 47,211, 26,060; luxury foods and tobacco, 8,204, 4,948; raw materials, 32,177, 7,476; semi-finished products, 63,117, 36,255; manufactures, 346,865, 563,506.

Trade with the former German Democratic Republic was not categorized as 'foreign'. In 1988 goods supplied were worth DM 7·23m. and goods received DM 6·79m.

Total trade between the Federal Republic of Germany and UK (British Department of Trade returns, in £1,000 sterling):

	1986	*1987*	*1988*	*1989*	*1990*
Imports to UK	14,139,097	15,783,904	17,667,097	20,005,276	19,907,062
Exports and re-exports from UK	8,542,196	9,404,257	9,521,851	11,110,623	13,169,405

Total trade between the former *GDR* and UK (British Department of Trade returns, in £1,000 sterling):

	1986	*1987*	*1988*	*1989*	*1990*
Imports to UK	195,513	180,299	152,977	168,742	128,498
Exports and re-exports from UK	81,276	81,489	113,239	106,445	57,013

Tourism. In 1989 there were 48,000 places of accommodation with 1·8m. beds (including 10,168 hotels with 570,541 beds). In the summer of 1989 155·25m. overnight stays (21·18m. by foreigners) were registered.

COMMUNICATIONS

Roads. In *West Germany* in 1989 the total length of classified roads was 173,652 km, including 8,721 km of motorway *(Autobahn)*, 35,344 km of federal highways, 63,441 km first-class and 70,382 km second-class country roads. Motor vehicles licensed on 1 July 1989: 34,704,300 (including 29,755,400 passenger cars, 1,378,500 trucks and 70,200 buses. In 1989 414m. tonnes of freight (113·4m. tonne-kilometres) and 5,294m. passengers were transported by long-distance road traffic.

Road casualties in 1988 totalled 448,223 injured and 8,213 killed.

In *the GDR* there were, in 1988, 47,203 km of classified roads including 1,855 km of motorways. 3,531m. passengers and 143m. tonnes of goods were carried by public road transport. There were 3,743,554 cars, 228,872 lorries, 1,318,571 motorcycles and 60,744 buses. There were 46,804 road accidents in 1988, with 1,441 fatalities.

Railways. Length of railway in 1989 was 41,034 km (1,435 mm gauge) of which 15,136 km was electrified. West German railways in 1989 carried 1,127m. passengers and 315m. tonnes of freight. There were also 2,845 km of privately-owned and other minor railways.

In the *GDR* in 1989 592m. passengers and 339m. tonnes of freight were carried.

Aviation. Lufthansa was set up in 1953 with a capital of DM 900m. In 1990 51% was state-owned.

Lufthansa flies to 181 destinations in 86 countries, including 8 in Germany, London, Moscow and 11 other European cities, Tokyo and New York.

In *West Germany* in 1989 civil aviation had 242 aircraft over 20 tonnes. In 1989 there were 33·3m. passenger arrivals and 33·49m. departures. 56m. passengers were carried (16,638 person-kilometres), including 21·60m. to destinations abroad. Major international airports include Frankfurt am Main, Düsseldorf, Munich, Hamburg and 2 at Berlin (Tegel and Schönefeld).

In the *GDR* in 1988 1·58m. passengers and 31,300 tonnes of freight were carried. The GDR carrier, Interflug, had 32 aircraft.

Shipping. In 1988 the mercantile marine comprised 1,642 ocean-going vessels of 5,347,556 GRT.

Navigable inland waterways have a total length of 6,717 km.

The inland-waterways fleet on 31 Dec. 1988 included 2,030 motor freight vessels totalling 1·92m. tonnes and 438 tankers of 580,042 tonnes.

Sea-going ships in 1989 carried 155·7m. tonnes of cargo. Inland waterways carried 255·3m. tonnes in 1988.

Pipeline. In 1989 there were 3,038 km of pipeline. 58·8m. tonnes of oil were transported in *West Germany*. In the *GDR* 37m. tonnes of material were transported in 1988.

Telecommunications. Telecommunications were deregulated in 1989.

In *West Germany* in 1989 there were 17,482 post offices, 43·1m. telephones and 411,095 fax transmitters.

The post office savings banks had, in 1989, 22,427,000 depositors with DM 40,885m. to their credit.

In 1989 postal revenues amounted to DM 59,848m. and expenditure to DM 56,672m.

There were 9 regional broadcasting stations. The *Arbeitsgemeinschaft der öffentlich-rechtlichen Rundfunkanstalten der Bundesrepublik Deutschland* (ARD) organizes co-operation between them and also broadcasts a federal-wide TV programme of its own. Number of wireless licences, (1989) 27·43m.; of television licences, 24·14m.

In the *GDR* in 1988 there were 11,971 post offices, 3,976,844 telephones and 17,363 telex subscribers. There were 6·78m. radio and 6·2m. TV licences.

Cinemas and Theatres. In 1988 there were 4,054 cinemas and 532 theatres with seating capacities of 851,453 and 210,392 respectively. 57 feature films were made in 1988 in *West Germany*.

Newspapers and Books. In *West Germany* in 1988, 356 newspapers and 7,711 periodicals were published with respective circulations of 24·53m. and 300·28m. 68,611 book titles were published. In 1988 there were 1,011 learned libraries, and 11,378 public libraries, the latter with 6·68m. users.

In the *GDR* there were 542 newspapers and periodicals in 1988. 6,590 book titles were published in 149·6m. copies.

JUSTICE, RELIGION, EDUCATION AND WELFARE

Justice. Justice is administered by the federal courts and by the courts of the Länder. In criminal procedures, civil cases and procedures of non-contentious jurisdiction the courts on the Land level are the local courts *(Amtsgerichte)*, the regional courts *(Landgerichte)* and the courts of appeal *(Oberlandesgerichte)*. Constitutional federal disputes are dealt with by the Federal Constitutional Court *(Bundesverfassungsgericht)* elected by the Bundestag and Bundesrat. The Länder also have constitutional courts. In labour law disputes the courts of the first and second instance are the labour courts and the Land labour courts and in the third instance, the Federal Labour Court *(Bundesarbeitsgericht)*. Disputes about public law in matters of social security, unemployment insurance, maintenance of war victims and similar cases are dealt with in the first and second instances by the social courts and the Land social courts and in the third instance by the Federal Social Court *(Bundessozialgericht)*. In most tax matters the finance courts of the Länder are competent and in the second instance, the Federal Finance Court *(Bundesfinanzhof)*. Other controversies of public law in non-constitutional matters are decided in the first and second instance by the administrative and the higher administrative courts *(Oberverwaltungsgerichte)* of the Länder, and in the third instance by the Federal Administrative Court *(Bundesverwaltungsgericht)*.

For the inquiry into maritime accidents the admiralty courts *(Seeämter)* are competent on the Land level and in the second instance the Federal Admiralty Court *(Bundesoberseeamt)* in Hamburg.

The death sentence has been abolished.

Religion. In *West Germany* at the 1987 census there were 26,232,000 (13,822,000 female) Roman Catholics, 25,412,600 Protestants (13,784,000 female) and 1,651,000 Moslems (722,700 females).

The Evangelical (Protestant) Church (EKD) consists of 24 member-churches including 7 Lutheran Churches, 8 United-Lutheran-Reformed, 2 Reformed Churches and 1 Confederation of United member Churches: 'Church of the Union'. Its organs are the Synod, the Church Conference and the Council under the chairmanship of Bishop Dr Eduard Lohse (Hanover). There are also some 12 Evangelical Free Churches. In 1988 there were 10,729 parishes, 18,729 priests and 25·2m. members in *West Germany*.

In *West Germany* in 1988 there were 26·48m. Catholics. There are 5 Catholic archbishoprics (Bamberg, Cologne, Freiburg, Munich and Freising, Paderborn) and 17 bishoprics. Chairman of the German Bishops' Conference is Cardinal Joseph Höffner, Archbishop of Cologne. A concordat between Germany and the Holy See dates from 10 Sept. 1933.

There were 27,711 Jews in 1989 with 53 synagogues and 13 rabbis.

In the *GDR* according to the census of 1950, 80·5% of the population were Protestants and 11% were Roman Catholics. The Synod of Lutheran Churches was founded in 1969 and embraces 8 regional churches. There were some 1·5m. Lutherans in 1989 in 7,200 parishes with 4,300 priests. The Catholic Church is organized in 2 dioceses, 3 episcopal districts and one apostolic administration. In 1989 there were 1·05m. Catholics in 916 parishes with 1,155 priests. There were 300 monasteries. There were also 40 Free and other churches, including Methodists, Quakers and Seventh-Day Adventists. In 1989 there were 8 synagogues.

Education. Education is compulsory for children aged 6 to 15. After the first 4 (or 6) years at primary school *(Grundschulen)* children attend post-primary *(Hauptschulen)*, secondary modern *(Realschulen)*, grammar *(Gymnasien)*, or comprehensive schools *(Integrierte Gesamtschulen)*. Secondary modern school comprises 6, grammar school 9, years. Entry to higher education is by the final Grammar School Certificate (Abitur-Higher School Certificate). There are special schools *(Sonderschulen)* for handicapped or maladjusted children.

In *West Germany* in 1988–89 there were 3,199 kindergartens with 66,559 pupils and 4,252 teachers, 13,595 primary schools with 2,363,178 pupils and 7,118 post-primary schools with 1,289,387 pupils. There were 229,974 teachers at primary and post-primary schools. There were also 2,770 special schools with 247,965 pupils and 41,991 teachers, 2,580 secondary modern schools with 875,049 pupils and 57,698 teachers; 2,460 grammar schools with 1,562,966 pupils and 122,354 teachers; 407 comprehensive schools with 257,593 pupils and 30,172 teachers.

Vocational education is provided in part-time, full-time and advanced vocational schools (*Berufs-*, *Berufsaufbau-*, *Berufsfach-* and *Fachschulen*, including *Fachschulen für Technik* and *Schulen des Gesundheitswesens*). Occupation-related, part-time vocational training of 6 to 12 hours per week is compulsory for all (including unemployed) up to the age of 18 years or until the completion of the practical vocational training. Full-time vocational schools comprise courses of at least one year. They prepare for commercial and domestic occupations as well as specialized occupations in the field of handicrafts. Advanced full-time vocational schools are attended by pupils over 18. Courses vary from 6 months to 3 or more years.

In 1988–89 there were 7,543 full- and part-time vocational schools with 2,401,090 pupils (1,088,426 female) and 90,716 teachers.

Higher Education. In *West Germany* in 1989–90 there were 62 institutes of university status: Universities proper at Augsburg, Bamberg, Bayreuth, Berlin (West), Bielefeld, Bochum, Bonn, Bremen, Cologne, Dortmund, Düsseldorf, Erlangen-Nuremberg, Frankfurt am Main, Freiburg im Breisgau, Giessen, Göttingen, Hamburg, Hanover, Heidelberg, Hohenheim, Kaiserslautern, Karlsruhe, Kiel, Konstanz, Mainz, Mannheim, Marburg, Munich, Münster, Oldenburg, Osnabrück, Passau, Regensburg, Saarbrücken, Stuttgart, Trier, Tübingen, Ulm and Würzburg; technical universities at Berlin (West), Braunschweig, Clausthal, Hamburg-Harburg and Munich; military universities at Hamburg and Munich; a medical university at Lübeck; a Catholic university at Eichstatt; a private Nordic university at Flensburg; and advanced schools *(Hochschulen)* at Aachen, Cologne (sport), Darmstadt (technical), Hamburg (economics and politics), Hanover (medical, veterinary), Hildesheim, Koblenz (private business), Lüneberg, Rhineland-Palatinate (education),

Speyer (administration) and Witten-Herdecke (private). There were 182 other institutes of higher education.

Academic staff in 1988–89: Universities including teacher training and theological colleges, 113,235; other institutes, 37,744.

Students in 1989–90: Universities, 1,004,755 (416,821 women); other institutes, 503,486.

In the *GDR* 10-year comprehensive schooling had been compulsory and free. In 1988 764,423 children were in 13,402 pre-school educational institutions. General education schools numbered 5,907 with 167,207 teachers and 2,054,817 pupils. Of these schools 5,207 with 1,953,012 pupils offered 10 years schooling and the remainder 12.

In addition there were 955 vocational schools *(Berufsschulen)* with 16,256 teachers and 359,308 trainees, and 237 technical schools with 157,513 students. There were also 9 universities and 44 other higher education institutes with 132,423 full-time students, including 65,152 women.

Health. In 1989 there were 218,640 doctors (including 87,515 in *West German* hospitals) and 41,576 dentists. There were 3,612 hospitals (including 975 private) with 838,784 beds.

Social Welfare (figures are for *West Germany*). *Social Health Insurance* (introduced in 1883). Wage-earners and apprentices, salaried employees with an income below a certain limit and socialinsurance pensioners are compulsorily insured. Voluntary insurance is also possible.

Benefits: Medical treatment, medicines, hospital and nursing care, maternity benefits, death benefits for the insured and their families, sickness payments and out-patients' allowances.

37·00m. persons were insured in 1988 (21·84m. compulsorily) and 10·8m. persons (including 6·7m. women) were drawing pensions. Number of cases of incapacity for work totalled 26·50m., and 413·29m. working days were lost. Total disbursements DM 134,376m.

Accident Insurance (introduced in 1884). Those insured are all persons in employment or service, apprentices and the majority of the self-employed and the unpaid family workers.

Benefits in the case of industrial injuries and occupational diseases: Medical treatment and nursing care, sickness payments, pensions and other payments in cash and in kind, surviving dependants' pensions.

Number of insured in 1988, 39·72m.; number of current pensions, 938,671; total disbursements, DM 14,038m.

Workers' and Employees' Old-Age Insurance Scheme (introduced in 1889). All wage-earners and salaried employees, the members of certain liberal professions and—subject to certain conditions—self-employed craftsmen are compulsorily insured. The insured may voluntarily continue to insure when no longer liable to do so or increase the insurance.

Benefits: Measures designed to maintain, improve and restore the earning capacity; pensions paid to persons incapable of work, old age and surviving dependants' pensions.

Number of insured in 1989, 32·73m. (15·79m. women); number of current pensions, 1988: 14·12m.; pensions to widows and widowers, 3·97m. Total disbursements in 1988, DM 207,238m.

There are also special retirement and unemployment pension schemes for miners and farmers, assistance for war victims and compensation payments to members of German minorities in East European countries expelled after the Second World War and persons who suffered damage because of the war or in connexion with the currency reform. Special benefits for refugees from the GDR were abolished in July 1990.

Family Allowances. The monthly allowance for the first child is DM 50, for the second, DM 70-100 (varying according to income), for the third DM 140-220 and the fourth DM 140-240. DM 10,117m. were dispersed to 6·17m. recipients in 1989.

Unemployment Allowances. In 1989 888,000 persons (433,000 women) were receiving unemployment benefit and 496,000 (147,000 women) earnings-related benefit. Total expenditure on these and similar benefits (e.g. short-working supplement, job creation schemes) was DM 39,833m. in 1989.

Accommodation Allowances averaging DM 148 a month were paid in 1988 to 1·9m. persons.

Public Welfare (introduced in 1962). In 1988 DM 27·01m. were distributed to 3·35m. recipients (1·86m. women).

Public Youth Welfare. For supervision of foster children, official guardianship, assistance with adoptions and affiliations, social assistance in juvenile courts, educational assistance and correctional education under a court order. Total expenditure in 1988, DM 9,258m.

DIPLOMATIC REPRESENTATIVES

Of Germany in Great Britain (23 Belgrave Sq., London, SW1X 8PZ)
Ambassador: Baron Hermann von Richthofen.

Of Great Britain in Germany (Friedrich-Ebert-Allee 77, 5300 Bonn 1)
Ambassador: Sir Christopher Mallaby, KCMG.

Of Germany in the USA (4645 Reservoir Rd, NW, Washington, D.C., 20007)
Ambassador: Juergen Ruhfus.

Of the USA in Germany (Deichmanns Ave., 5300, Bonn)
Ambassador: Gen. Vernon A. Walters.

Of Germany to the United Nations
Ambassador: Dr Hans Otto Bräutigam.

Further Reading

Statistical Information: The central statistical agency is the Statistisches Bundesamt, 62 Wiesbaden 1, Gustav Stresemann Ring 11. *President:* Egon Hölder. Its publications include:

Statistisches Jahrbuch für die Bundesrepublik Deutschland; Wirtschaft und Statistik (monthly, from 1949); *Das Arbeitsgebiet der Bundesstatistik* (latest issue 1988; Abridged English version: *Survey of German Federal Statistics*).

Ardagh, J., *Germany and the Germans.* London, 1987
Bark, D. L. and Gress, D. R., *A History of West Germany, 1945-1988.* 2 vols. Oxford, 1989
Berghahn, V. R., *Modern Germany: Society, Economy and Politics in the Twentieth Century.* CUP, 1982
Beyme, K. von, *The Political System of the Federal Republic of Germany.* New York, 1983
Die Bundesrepublik Deutschland: Staatshandbuch. Cologne, annual
Burdick, C., *et al.* (eds.) *Contemporary Germany: Politics and Culture*, Boulder, 1984
Childs, D., *Germany since 1918.* 2nd ed. New York, 1980
Conradt, D. P., *The German Polity.* 2nd ed. New York, 1982
Craig, G. A., *Germany, 1866–1945.* Oxford Univ. Press, 1981—*The Germans.* Harmondsworth, 1984
Dennis, M., *German Democratic Republic.* London, 1987
Detwiler, D. S. and Detwiler, I. E., *West Germany.* [Bibliography] Oxford and Santa Barbara, 1988
Dittmers, M., *The Green Party in West Germany.* 2nd ed. Buckingham, 1988
Edinger, L. J., *West German Politics.* New York, 1986
Eley, G., *From Unification to Nazism: Reinterpreting the German Past.* London, 1986
Friese, F-J., *Investment and Business Establishments in the Federal Republic of Germany: A Guide for the Foreign Investor.* Frankfurt-am-Main, 1988
Hardach, K., *The Political Economy of Germany in the Twentieth Century.* California Univ. Press, 1980
Hucko, E. M. (ed.) *The Democratic Tradition* [Texts of German Constitutions]. Leamington Spa, 1987
James, H. A., *A German Identity.* rev. ed. London, 1990
Johnson, N., *State and Government in the Federal Republic of Germany: the Executive at Work.* 2nd ed. Oxford, 1983
Jonas, M., *The United States and Germany: A Diplomatic History.* Cornell Univ. Press, 1984

Koch, H. W., *A Constitutional History of Germany in the Nineteenth and Twentieth Centuries*. London, 1984
Kohl, W. L. and Basevi, G., *West Germany: A European and Global Power*. London, 1982
Kolinsky, E., *Parties, Opposition and Society in West Germany*. London, 1984
König, K., *et al.* (eds.) *Public Administration in the Federal Republic of Germany*. Boston, 1983
Leaman, J., *The Political Economy of West Germany, 1945–1985*. Basingstoke, 1987
Marsh, D., *The New Germany: at the Crossroads*. London, 1990
Marshall, B., *The Origins of Post-War German Politics*. London, 1988
Pasley, M. (ed.) *Germany: a Companion to German Studies*. 2nd ed. London, 1982
Schweitzer, D.-C., (ed.) *Politics and Government in the Federal Republic of Germany: Basic Documents*. Leamington Spa, 1984
Smith, G., *Democracy in Western Germany*. 3rd ed. Aldershot, 1986
Thomaneck, J. and Mellis, J., (eds.) *Politics, Society and Government in the German Democratic Republic: Basic Documents*. Oxford, 1989
Wallace, I., *East Germany: the German Democratic Republic*. [Bibliography]. Oxford and Santa Barbara, 1987
Wallach, P. and Romoser, G. K. (eds.) *West German Politics in the Mid-Eighties: Crisis and Continuity*. New York, 1985
Weizsäcker, R. von, *A Voice from Germany: Speeches*. London, 1986
Wild, T. (ed) *Urban and Rural Change in West Germany*. London, 1983

National Libraries: Deutsche Bibliothek, Zeppelinallee 4–8; Frankfurt-am-Main. *Director:* K.-D. Lehmann; (Berliner) Staatsbibliothek Preussischer Kulturbesitz, Potsdamer Str., Postfach 1407 D-1000 Berlin 30. *Director:* Dr. Richard Landwehrmeyer.

THE LÄNDER

BADEN–WÜRTTEMBERG

AREA AND POPULATION. Baden-Württemberg comprises 35,751 sq. km, with a population (at 1 Jan. 1990) of 9,648,696 (4,670,168 males, 4,948,528 females).

The Land is administratively divided into 4 areas, 9 urban and 35 rural districts, and numbers 1,111 communes. The capital is Stuttgart.

Vital statistics for calendar years:

	Live births	*Marriages*	*Divorces*	*Deaths*
1987	103,590	56,780	16,781	91,587
1988	110,627	58,939	17,204	92,418
1989	111,600	58,835	16,953	94,262

CONSTITUTION. The Land Baden-Württemberg is a merger of the 3 Länder, Baden, Württemberg-Baden and Württemberg-Hohenzollern, which were formed in 1945. The merger was approved by a plebiscite held on 9 Dec. 1951, when 70% of the population voted in its favour. It has 7 seats in the Bundesrat.

At the elections to the Diet of Jan. 1991, turn-out was 71%. The Social Democrats won 40·8% of the vote; the Christian Democrats, 40·2%; the Greens, 8·8% and the Free Democrats, 7·4%. The Social Democrats (SPD) won a 2-seat majority.

The Government is formed by Social Democrats and Greens, with Hans Eichel (SPD) as *Prime Minister*.

AGRICULTURE. Area and yield of the most important crops:

	Area (in 1,000 ha)			*Yield (in 1,000 tonnes)*		
	1987	*1988*	*1989*	*1987*	*1988*	*1989*
Rye	16·2	16·3	16·1	64·0	73·9	73·8
Wheat	220·1	214·0	216·9	1,071·0	1,326·8	1,315·3
Barley	190·2	202·7	201·6	809·8	1,025·4	1,022·1
Oats	74·2	77·6	72·0	332·9	406·5	325·8
Potatoes	14·0	12·4	10·8	304·6	399·6	338·9
Sugar-beet	22·4	22·6	22·1	1,219·7	1,215·1	1,192·9

Livestock (3 Dec. 1989): Cattle, 1,625,000 (including 599,800 milch cows); horses (1988), 52,904; pigs, 2,227,200; sheep, 250,900; poultry (1988), 5,925,231.

INDUSTRY. In 1989 9,185 establishments (with 20 and more employees) employed 1,457,114 persons; of these, 268,439 were employed in machine construction (excluding office machines, data processing equipment and facilities); 65,025 in textile industry; 257,175 in electrical engineering; 229,447 in car building.

LABOUR. The economically active persons totalled 4,447,000 at the 1%-EC-sample survey of April 1989. Of the total 486,900 were self-employed (including family workers), 3,960,100 employees; 142,500 were engaged in agriculture and forestry; 2,099,700 in power supply, mining, manufacturing and building, 664,700 in commerce and transport, 1,540,100 in other industries and services.

ROADS. On 1 Jan. 1990 there were 27,979 km of 'classified' roads, including 978 km of autobahn, 5,006 km of federal roads, 10,118 km of first-class and 11,877 km of second-class highways. Motor vehicles, at 1 Jan. 1990, numbered 5,665,098, including, 4,841,033 passenger cars, 9,444 buses, 208,300 lorries, 317,660 tractors and 220,194 motor cycles.

JUSTICE. There are a constitutional court *(Staatsgerichtshof)*, 2 courts of appeal, 17 regional courts, 108 local courts, a Land labour court, 9 labour courts, a Land social court, 8 social courts, a finance court, a higher administrative court *(Verwaltungsgerichtshof)*, 4 administrative courts.

RELIGION. On 1 Jan. 1989, 41·1% of the population were Protestants and in 1987 45·3% were Roman Catholics.

EDUCATION. In 1989–90 there were 2,608 primary schools *(Grund* and *Hauptschule)* with 31,845 teachers and 563,859 pupils; 537 special schools with 8,240 teachers and 42,769 pupils; 444 intermediate schools with 11,159 teachers and 170,273 pupils; 417 high schools with 18,628 teachers and 230,087 pupils; 31 *Freie Waldorf* schools with 1,172 teachers and 15,827 pupils. Other schools together had 729 teachers and 10,070 pupils; there were also 40 *Fachhochschulen* (colleges of engineering and others) with 48,897 students.

In the winter term 1989–90 there were 9 universities (Freiburg, 22,931 students; Heidelberg, 26,709; Konstanz, 8,325; Tübingen, 23,865; Karlsruhe, 20,214; Stuttgart, 20,111; Hohenheim, 5,730; Mannheim, 12,241; Ulm, 5,424); 6 teacher-training colleges with 9,145 students; 5 colleges of music with 2,965 students and 2 colleges of fine arts with 1,027 students.

Statistical Information: Statistisches Landesamt Baden-Württemberg (P.O.B. 10 60 33, D7000 Stuttgart 10) (*President:* Prof. Dr. Max Wingen), publishes: *'Baden-Württemberg in Wort und Zahl'* (monthly); *Jahrbücher für Statistik und Landeskunde von Baden-Württemberg; Statistik von Baden-Württemberg* (series); *Statistisch-prognostischer Bericht* (latest issue 1988–89); *Statistisches Taschenbuch* (latest issue 1988–89).

State Library: Württembergische Landesbibliothek, Konrad-Adenauer-Str. 8, 7000 Stuttgart 1. *Director:* Dr Hans-Peter Geh. Badische Landesbibliothek Karlsruhe, Lamm-Str. 16, 7500 Karlsruhe 1. *Director:* Dr Römer.

BAVARIA

Bayern

AREA AND POPULATION. Bavaria has an area of 70,554 sq. km. The capital is Munich. There are 7 areas, 96 urban and rural districts and 2,051 communes. The population (31 Dec. 1988) numbered 11,049,263 (5,322,555 males, 5,726,708 females).

Vital statistics for calendar years:

	Live births	*Marriages*	*Divorces*	*Deaths*
1986	118,439	67,061	18,352	120,489
1987	119,623	70,035	19,846	119,662
1988	126,409	71,742	19,496	118,450

CONSTITUTION. The Constituent Assembly, elected on 30 June 1946, passed a constitution on the lines of the democratic constitution of 1919, but with greater emphasis on state rights; this was agreed upon by the Christian Social Union (CSU) and the Social Democrats (SPD). Bavaria has 7 seats in the Bundesrat. The CSU replaces the Christian Democratic Party in Bavaria.

At the Diet elections of Oct. 1990 the CSU won 127 seats with 54·9% of the vote, the SPD, 58 with 26%, the Greens, 12 with 6·4% and the Free Democrats 7 with 5·2%. The *Prime Minister* is Max Streibl.

AGRICULTURE. Area and yield of the most important products:

	Area (in 1,000 hectares)			*Yield (in 1,000 tonnes)*		
	1987	*1988*	*1989* [1]	*1987*	*1988*	*1989* [1]
Wheat	501·0	511·6	501·3	2,686·1	3,865·0	3,298·6
Rye	53·5	51·5	57·7	189·1	225·4	267·0
Barley	500·3	516·9	510·6	2,028·2	2,707·9	2,901·3
Oats	114·0	114·0	105·6	468·4	505·4	440·4
Potatoes	68·1	65·2	62·1	1,849·1	2,587·3	2,228·1
Sugar-beet	77·0	77·6	79·4	4,216·2	4,256·6	...

[1] Preliminary figures.

Livestock (2 Dec. 1988): 4,939,800 cattle (including 1,890,200 milch cows); 64,900 horses; 340,800 sheep; 3,781,900 pigs; 12,089,600 poultry.

INDUSTRY. In 1988, 9,290 establishments (with 20 or more employees) employed 1,355,802 persons; of these, 254,386 were employed in electrical engineering; 184,495 in mechanical engineering; 113,473 in clothing and textile industries.

LABOUR. The economically active persons totalled 5,344,800 at the 1% sample survey of the microcensus of April 1988. Of the total, 528,600 were self-employed, 255,500 unpaid family workers, 4,560,700 employees; 2,239,400 in power supply, mining, manufacturing and building; 880,900 in commerce and transport; 1,831,100 in other industries and services.

ROADS. There were, on 1 Jan. 1989, 41,154 km of 'classified' roads, including 2,015 km of autobahn, 7,126 km of federal roads, 13,800 km of first-class and 18,213 km of second-class highways. Number of motor vehicles, at 1 July 1989, was 6,725,647, including 5,489,445 passenger cars, 246,188 lorries, 13,441 buses, 586,006 tractors, 312,826 motor cycles.

JUSTICE. There are a constitutional court *(Verfassungsgerichtshof)*, a supreme Land court *(Oberstes Landesgericht)*, 3 courts of appeal, 22 regional courts, 72 local courts, 2 Land labour courts, 11 labour courts, a Land social court, 7 social courts, 2 finance courts, a higher administrative court *(Verwaltungsgerichtshof)*, 6 administrative courts.

RELIGION. At the census of 25 May 1987 there were 67·2% Roman Catholics and 23·9% Protestants.

EDUCATION. In 1988–89 there were 2,806 primary schools with 44,015 teachers and 716,178 pupils; 382 special schools with 6,294 teachers and 39,800 pupils; 336 intermediate schools with 8,787 teachers and 121,720 pupils; 395 high schools with 20,227 teachers and 269,102 pupils; 259 part-time vocational schools with 8,042 teachers and 327,852 pupils, including 51 special part-time vocational schools with 573 teachers and 8,162 pupils; 557 full-time vocational schools with 3,851 teachers and 49,874 pupils including 228 schools for public health occupations with 1,052 teachers and 15,498 pupils; 300 advanced full-time vocational schools with 2,294 teachers and 26,768 pupils; 84 vocational high schools *(Berufsoberschulen, Fachoberschulen)* with 1,913 teachers and 29,647 pupils.

In the winter term 1988–89 there were 11 universities with 175,971 students (Augsburg, 10,012; Bamberg, 6,036; Bayreuth, 6,437; Eichstätt, 2,113; Erlangen–Nürnberg, 27,066; München, 63,471; Passau, 6,160; Regensburg, 12,879; Würzburg, 17,803; the Technical University of München, 22,787; München University of the Federal Armed Forces (Universität der Bundeswehr), 2,162); the college of philosophy, München, 347 and 2 philosophical-theological colleges with together 442 students (Benediktbeuern, 132; Neuendettelsau, 310). There were also 2 colleges of music, 2 colleges of fine arts and 1 college of television and film, with together 2,408 students; 13 vocational colleges *(Fachhochschulen)* with 56,032 students including one for the civil service *(Bayerische Beamtenfachhochschule)* with 4,970 students.

Statistical Information: Bayerisches Landesamt für Statistik und Datenverarbeitung, 51 Neuhauser Str. 8000 Munich, was founded in 1833. *President:* Dr Hans Helmut Schiedermaier. It publishes: *Statistisches Jahrbuch für Bayern.* 1894 ff.—*Bayern in Zahlen.* Monthly (from Jan. 1947).—*Zeitschrift des Bayerischen Statistischen Landesamts.* July 1869–1943; 1948 ff.—*Beiträge zur Statistik Bayerns.* 1850 ff.—*Statistische Berichte.* 1951 ff.—*Schaubilderhefte.* 1951 ff.—*Kreisdaten.* 1972 ff.—*Gemeindedaten.* 1973 ff.

Nawiasky, H. and Luesser, C., *Die Verfassung des Freistaates Bayern vom 2. Dez. 1946.* Munich, 1948; supplement, by H. Nawiasky and H. Lechner, Munich, 1953

State Library: Bayerische Staatsbibliothek, Munich 22. *Director:* Dr Franz G. Kaltwasser.

BERLIN

Except for the population total, figures refer only to the former West Berlin.

HISTORY. Greater Berlin was under 4-power (France, USSR, UK and USA) Allied government (the *Kommandatura*) from 5 June 1945 until 1 July 1948, when the Soviet element withdrew. On 30 Nov. 1948 a separate municipal government was set up in the Soviet sector. The French, UK and US sectors coalesced to form the administrative unit of 'West Berlin', covering 480 sq. km. With the establishment of the German Democratic Republic, the Soviet sector ('East Berlin', 403 sq. km) was designated its capital.

East and West Berlin were amalgamated on the re-unification of Germany in Oct. 1990.

AREA AND POPULATION. The area is 883 sq. km. Population, 1990, 3·41m.

Vital statistics for calendar years:

	Live births	*Marriages*	*Divorces*	*Deaths*
1987	19,554	11,961	6,230	30,719
1988	20,980	12,385	5,995	30,021
1989	21,159	12,743	6,157	30,045

CONSTITUTION AND GOVERNMENT. According to the constitution of 1 Sept. 1950, Berlin is simultaneously a Land of the Federal Republic and a city. It is governed by a House of Representatives (of at least 200 members); executive power is vested in a Senate, consisting of the Governing Mayor, the Mayor and not more than 16 senators.

Berlin has 5 seats in the Bundesrat.

At the elections of Dec. 1990 the Christian Democrats won 100 seats in the House of Representatives with 40·3% of the vote; the Social Democrats, 76, with 30·5%; the Party of Democratic Socialism (former Communists), 23, with 9·2%; the Free Democrats, 18, with 7·1%; the Greens, 12, with 5%; Alliance '90/Greens, 11, with 4·4%.

In the Senate, the Christian Democrats gained 8 seats and the Social Democrats, 7. A coalition government was formed.

Governing Mayor: Eberhard Diepgen (Christian Democrat).

ECONOMY

Banking. On 20 March 1949 when the DM (West) became the only legal tender of the Western Sectors, the Zentralbank of Berlin was established. Its functions were similar to those of the Zentralbanks of the Länder of the Federal Republic. The Berlin Central Bank was merged with the Bank deutscher Länder as from 1 Aug. 1957, when the latter became the Deutsche Bundesbank.

AGRICULTURE. Agricultural area (April 1989), 1,245 ha, including 930 ha of arable land and 84 ha of gardens, orchards and nurseries.

Livestock (Dec. 1988): Cattle, 657; pigs, 3,027; horses, 3,461; sheep, 1,241.

INDUSTRY. In 1989 (monthly averages), 1,125 establishments (with 20 or more employees) employed 165,960 persons; of these, 55,603 were employed in electrical engineering, 4,413 in steel construction, 3,776 in textiles. In 1988, 15,312 persons were employed in machine construction and 12,849, in the manufacture of chemicals.

LABOUR. The economically active persons totalled 994,800 at the 1%-sample survey of the microcensus of April 1989. Of the total, 89,300 were self-employed including unpaid family workers, 905,500 employees; 7,500 were engaged in agriculture and forestry; 300,900 in power supply, manufacturing and building; 189,800 in commerce and transport; 496,600 in other industries and services.

ROADS. There were, on 1 Jan. 1990, 146·96 km of 'classified' roads, including 46·9 km of autobahn and 100·5 km of federal roads. On 1 July 1989, 820,323 motor vehicles were registered, including 646,399 passenger cars, 45,747 lorries, 37,712 motor cycles, and 2,138 buses (1988).

JUSTICE. There are a court of appeal *(Kammergericht)*, a regional court, 7 local courts, a Land Labour court, a labour court, a Land social court, a social court, a higher administrative court, an administrative court and a finance court.

EDUCATION. In 1989–90 (preliminary figures) there were 453 schools providing general education (excluding special schools) with 186,381 pupils; 55 special schools with 6,264 pupils. There were a further 179 vocational schools with 55,496 pupils.

In the winter term 1989–90 there was 1 university (58,181 students); 1 technical university (34,540); 1 theological (evangelical) college (508); 1 college of fine arts with 4,649 students; 1 vocational college (for economics) (1,695); 2 colleges for social work (1,406); 1 technical college (6,605), 1 college of the Federal postal administration (535) and 2 colleges for public administration (2,739).

Statistical Information: The Statistisches Landesamt Berlin was founded in 1862 (Fehrbelliner Platz 1, 1000 Berlin 31). *Director:* Prof. Günther Appel. It publishes: *Statistisches Jahrbuch* (from 1867): *Berliner Statistik* (monthly, from 1947).—*100 Jahre Berliner Statistik* (1962).

Childs, D. and Johnson, J., *West Berlin: Politics and Society.* London, 1981
Hillenbrand, M. J., *The Future of Berlin.* Monclair, 1981

State Library: Amerika-Gedenkbibliothek-Berliner Zentralbibliothek-, Blücherplatz 1, D1000 Berlin 61. *Director:* Dr Klaus Bock.

BRANDENBURG

AREA AND POPULATION. The area is 29,059 sq. km. Population in 1990 was 2·64m. The capital is Potsdam.

CONSTITUTION AND GOVERNMENT. The Land was reconstituted on former GDR territory in 1990. Brandenburg has 4 seats in the Bundesrat.

At the Diet elections of Oct. 1990 the Social Democrats won 36 seats with 38·3% of the vote; the Christian Democrats, 27, with 29·4%; the Party of Democratic Socialism (former Communists), 13, with 13·4%; the Free Democrats, 6, with 6·4%; Alliance '90, 6 with 6%.

The *Prime Minister* is Manfred Stolpe (Social Democrat).

BREMEN

Freie Hansestadt Bremen

AREA AND POPULATION. The area of the Land, consisting of the towns and ports of Bremen and Bremerhaven, is 404 sq. km. Population, 31 Dec. 1989, 673,684 (320,682 males, 353,002 females).

Vital statistics for calendar years:

	Live births	*Marriages*	*Divorces*	*Deaths*
1987	5,773	3,951	2,210	8,489
1988	6,420	4,230	2,037	8,712
1989	6,513	4,156	1,919	8,463

CONSTITUTION. Political power is vested in the House of Burgesses *(Bürgerschaft)* which appoints the executive, called the Senate. Bremen has 3 seats in the Bundesrat.

The elections of 13 Sept. 1987 had the following result: 54 Social Democratic Party, 25 Christian Democrats, 10 Free Democratic Party, 10 Die Grünen, 1 Deutsche Volksunion. The Senate is formed only by Social Democrats; its president is Klaus Wedemeier (Social Democrat).

AGRICULTURE. Agricultural area comprised (1989), 10,048 ha: yield of grain crops (1987), 6,059 tonnes; potatoes, 155 tonnes.

Livestock (2 Dec. 1988): 15,588 cattle (including 4,464 milch cows); 3,859 pigs; 540 sheep; 1,045 horses; 22,970 poultry.

INDUSTRY. In 1989, 332 establishments (20 and more employees) employed 77,089 persons; of these, 6,854 were employed in shipbuilding (except naval engineering); 7,318 in machine construction; 9,083 in electrical engineering; 2,229 in coffee and tea processing.

LABOUR. The economically active persons totalled 276,000 at the microcensus of April 1989. Of the total, 22,000 were self-employed, 252,000 employees; 74,000 in commerce and transport, 111,000 in other industries and services. In 1987; 89,000 in power supply, mining, manufacturing and building, and 2,000 in agriculture and fishing.

ROADS. On 1 Jan. 1988 there were 108 km of 'classified' roads, including 46 km of autobahn, 62 km of federal roads. Registered motor vehicles on 1 July 1989 numbered 304,718, including 274,618 passenger cars, 13,569 trucks, 2,503 tractors, 627 buses and 9,351 motor cycles.

SHIPPING. Vessels entered in 1989, 9,915 of 43,808,000 net tons; cleared, 9,806 of 43,789,000 net tons. Sea traffic, 1989, incoming 19,774,000 tonnes; outgoing, 12,683,000 tonnes.

JUSTICE. There are a constitutional court *(Staatsgerichtshof)*, a court of appeal, a regional court, 3 local courts, a Land labour court, 2 labour courts, a Land social court, a social court, a finance court, a higher administrative court, an administrative court.

RELIGION. On 25 May 1987 (census) there were 61% Protestants and 10% Roman Catholics.

EDUCATION. In 1989 there were 309 new system schools with 5,185 teachers and 62,550 pupils; 26 special schools with 545 teachers and 2,641 pupils; 24 part-time vocational schools with 25,550 pupils; 33 full-time vocational schools with 5,427 pupils; 8 advanced vocational schools (including institutions for the training of technicians) with 744 pupils; 10 schools for public health occupations with 935 pupils.

In the winter term 1989–90 12,284 students were enrolled at the university. In addition to the university there were 4 other colleges in 1989–90 with 7,334 students.

Statistical Information: Statistisches Landesamt Bremen (An der Weide 14–16 (P.B. 101309), D2800 Bremen 1), founded in 1850. *Director:* Ltd Reg. Dir. Volker Hannemann. Its current publications include: *Statistische Mitteilungen Freie Hansestadt Bremen* (from 1948).—*Monatliche Zwischenberichte* (1949–53); *Statistische Monatsberichte* (from 1954).—*Statistische Berichte* (from 1956).—*Statistisches Handbuch für das Land Freie Hansestadt Bremen (1950–60,* 1961; *1960–64,* 1967; *1965–69,* 1971; *1970–74,* 1975; *1975–80,* 1982; *1981–85,* 1987).—*Bremen im statistischen Zeitvergleich 1950–1976.* 1977.—*Bremen in Zahlen.* 1989.

State and University Library: Bibliotheks Str., D2800 Bremen 33. *Director:* Prof. Dr Hans-Albrecht Koch.

HAMBURG

Freie und Hansestadt Hamburg

AREA AND POPULATION. In 1938 the territory of the town was reorganized by the amalgamation of the city and its 18 rural districts with 3 urban and 27 rural districts ceded by Prussia. Total area, 755·3 sq. km (1989), including the islands Neuwerk and Scharhörn (7·6 sq. km). Population (31 Dec. 1989), 1,626,220 (767,167 males, 859,053 females).

Vital statistics for calendar years:

	Live births	*Marriages*	*Divorces*	*Deaths*
1987	14,259	9,565	4,825	21,516
1988	15,359	9,787	4,549	21,186
1989	15,335	9,484	4,245	21,241

CONSTITUTION. The constitution of 6 June 1952 vests the supreme power in the House of Burgesses *(Bürgerschaft)* of 120 members. The executive is in the hands of the Senate, whose members are elected by the Bürgerschaft. Hamburg has 3 seats in the Bundesrat.

The elections of 17 May. 1987 had the following results: Social Democrats, 55; Christian Democrats, 49; Green Alternatives, 8; Free Democrats, 8. The First Burgomaster is Dr Henning Voscherau (Social Democrat).

The territory has been divided into 7 administrative districts.

AGRICULTURE. The agricultural area comprised 14,986 ha in 1989. Yield, in tonnes, of cereals, 20,132; potatoes, 885.

Livestock (3 Dec. 1988): Cattle, 10,912 (including 2,500 milch cows); pigs, 5,101; horses, 2,748; sheep, 2,624; poultry, 57,497.

FISHERIES. In 1989 the yield of sea and coastal fishing was 228 tonnes valued at DM 0·6m.

INDUSTRY. In June 1989, 758 establishments (with 20 and more employees) employed 133,174 persons; of these, 20,978 were employed in electrical engineering; 17,044 in machine construction; 7,076 in shipbuilding (except naval engineering); 13,033 in chemical industry.

LABOUR. The economically active persons totalled 740,600 at the 1%-sample survey of the microcensus of April 1989. Of the total, 70,200 were self-employed, 5,500 unpaid family workers, 670,400 employees or were engaged in agriculture and forestry, 194,000 in power supply, mining, manufacturing and building, 208,500 in commerce and transport, 332,600 in other industries and services.

ROADS. On 31 Dec. 1989 there were 3,889 km of roads, including 79 km of autobahn, 153 km of federal roads. Number of motor vehicles (1 July 1990), 752,996, including 678,760 passenger cars, 36,333 lorries, 1,523 buses, 5,245 tractors, 20,397 motor cycles and 10,738 other motor vehicles.

SHIPPING. Hamburg is the largest port in the Federal Republic.

Vessels		*1987*	*1988*	*1989*
Entered:	Number	14,154	13,374	12,710
	Tonnage	55,192,622	55,249,906	55,063,073
Cleared:	Number	14,099	13,406	12,736
	Tonnage	54,975,740	55,138,397	54,371,078

JUSTICE. There is a constitutional court *(Verfassungsgericht)*, a court of appeal *(Oberlandesgericht)*, a regional court *(Landgericht)*, 6 local courts *(Amtsgerichte)*, a Land labour court, a labour court, a Land social court, a social court, a finance court, a higher administrative court, an administrative court.

RELIGION. On 25 May 1987 (census) Evangelical Church and Free Churches 50·2%, Roman Catholic Church 8·6%.

EDUCATION. In 1988 there were about 360 schools of general education (not including *Internationale Schule*) with nearly 11,400 teachers and 153,280 pupils; 60 special schools with 769 teachers and 6,534 pupils; 43 part-time vocational schools with 45,871 pupils; 14 schools with 1,334 pupils in their vocational preparatory year; 21 schools with 2,120 pupils in manual instruction classes; 51 full-time vocational schools with 9,627 pupils; 10 economic secondary schools with 2,418 pupils; 2 technical *Gymnasien* with 417 pupils; 22 advanced vocational schools with 3,372 pupils; 35 schools for public health occupations with 2,723 pupils; 7 vocational introducing schools with 241 pupils and 20 technical superior schools with 2,588 pupils; all these vocational and technical schools have a total number of 2,714 teachers.

In the summer term 1989 there was 1 university with 41,240 students; 1 technical university with 900 students; 1 college of music and 1 college of fine arts with together 1,610 students; 1 university of the *Bundeswehr* with 1,190 students; 1 professional high school *(Fachhochschule)* with 13,380 students; 1 high school for economics and politics with 2,030 students; 1 high school of public administration with 950 students, as well as 1 private professional high school with 150 students.

Statistical Information: The Statistisches Landesamt der Freien und Hansestadt Hamburg (Steckelhörn 12, D2000 Hamburg 11) publishes: *Hamburg in Zahlen, Statistische Berichte, Statistisches Taschenbuch, Statistik des Hamburgischen Staates.*

Klessmann, E., *Geschichte der Stadt Hamburg*. Hamburg, 1981
Meyer-Marwitz, B., *Das Hamburg Buch*. Hamburg, 1981
Möller, J., *Hamburg-Länderprofile*. Hamburg, 1985
Plagemann, V., *Industriekultur in Hamburg*. Hamburg, 1984
Studt, B. and Olsen, H., *Hamburg—eine kurzgefaßte Geschichte der Stadt*. Hamburg, 1964

State Library: Staats- und Universitätsbibliothek, Carl von Ossietzky, Von-Melle-Park 3, D2000 Hamburg 13. *Director:* Prof. Dr Horst Gronemeyer.

HESSEN

AREA AND POPULATION. The state of Hessen comprehends the areas of the former Prussian provinces Kurhessen and Nassau (excluding the exclaves belonging to Hessen and the rural counties of Westerwaldkreis and Rhine-Lahn) and of the former Volksstaat Hessen, the provinces Starkenburg (including the parts of Rheinhessen east of the river Rhine) and Oberhessen. Hessen has an area of 21,114 sq. km. Its capital is Wiesbaden. Since 1 Jan. 1981 there have been 3 areas with 5 urban and 21 rural districts and 421 communes. Population, 31 Dec 1989, was 5,660,619 (2,711,376 males, 2,919,243 females).

Vital statistics for calendar years:

	Live births	*Marriages*	*Divorces*	*Deaths*
1987	54,814	33,705	12,448	61,698
1988	57,643	35,280	12,035	62,128
1989	58,803	35,124	12,089	62,873

CONSTITUTION. The constitution was put into force by popular referendum on 1 Dec. 1946. Hessen has 6 seats in the Bundesrat. The Diet, elected in Jan. 1991, consists of 46 Christian Democrats, 46 Social Democrats, 10 Greens and 8 Free Democrats.

The Christian Democrat cabinet is headed by *Prime Minister* Walter Wallmann (CDU).

AGRICULTURE. Area and yield of the most important crops:

	Area (in 1,000 ha)			*Yield (in 1,000 tonnes)*		
	1987	*1988*	*1989*	*1987*	*1988*	*1989*
Wheat	143·1	148·0	149·7	825·5	932·7	885·1
Rye	29·5	26·2	26·7	125·2	118·8	131·6
Barley	138·2	139·6	128·2	648·4	748·5	764·9
Oats	49·5	46·4	41·0	212·1	178·7	145·3
Potatoes	8·3	7·3	6·8	227·5	245·6	206·0
Sugar-beet	21·5	20·9	21·6	1,063·6	1,023·3	1,090·9
Rape	36·9	40·1	46·3	108·7	124·7	145·7

Livestock, Dec. 1989: Cattle, 721,890 (including 242,006 milch cows); pigs 1·03m.; sheep, 149,867. Dec. 1988: Horses, 32,108; poultry, 3·24m.

INDUSTRY. In June 1990, 3,823 establishments (with 20 and more employees) employed 651,861 persons; of these, 101,562 were employed in chemical industry; 93,275 in electrical engineering; 95,551 in car building; 81,168 in machine construction; 32,736 in food industry.

LABOUR. The economically active persons totalled 2·56m. at the 1% sample survey of the microcensus of April 1989. Of the total, 215,300 were self-employed, 38,300 unpaid family workers, 2,307,600 employees; 66,900 were engaged in agriculture and forestry, 978,300 in power supply, mining, manufacturing and building, 501,400 in commerce and transport, 1,014,600 in other services.

ROADS. On 1 Jan. 1990 there were 16,648 km of 'classified' roads, including 930 km of autobahn, 3,492 km of federal highways, 7,186 km of first-class highways and 5,041 km of second-class highways. Motor vehicles licensed on 1 July 1990 totalled 3,396,324, including 2,969,165 passenger cars, 6,289 buses, 124,887 trucks, 142,012 tractors and 116,290 motor cycles.

JUSTICE. There are a constitutional court *(Staatsgerichtshof)*, a court of appeal, 9 regional courts, 58 local courts, a Land labour court, 12 labour courts, a Land social court, 7 social courts, a finance court, a higher administrative court *(Verwaltungsgerichtshof)*, 5 administrative courts.

RELIGION. In 1987 (census) there were 52·7% Protestants and 30·4% Roman Catholics.

EDUCATION. In 1989 there were 1,255 primary schools with 14,897 teachers and 260,618 pupils (including *Förderstufen*); 232 special schools with 2,640 teachers and 17,078 pupils; 161 intermediate schools with 2,385 teachers and 42,152 pupils; 158 high schools with 8,895 teachers and 121,289 pupils; 193 *Gesamtschulen* (comprehensive schools) with 10,428 teachers and 143,663 pupils; 120 part-time vocational schools with 4,589 teachers and 146,838 pupils; 254 full-time vocational schools with 2,411 teachers and 32,992 pupils; 106 advanced vocational schools with 626 teachers and 10,482 pupils; in 1988 there were 168 schools for public health occupations with 9,295 pupils.

In the winter term 1989–90 there were 3 universities (Frankfurt/Main, 31,209 students; Giessen, 17,873; Marburg–Lahn, 14,852); 1 technical university in Darmstadt (15,340); 1 private *Wissenschaftliche Hochschule,* 707; 1 *Gesamthochschule* (12,675); 14 *Fachhochschulen* (42,320); 2 Roman Catholic theological colleges and 1 Protestant theological college with together 422 students; 1 college of music and 2 colleges of fine arts with together 1,314 students.

Statistical Information: The Hessisches Statistisches Landesamt (Rheinstr. 35–37, D6200 Wiesbaden). *President:* Götz Steppuhn. Main publications: *Statistisches Taschenbuch für das Land Hessen* (zweijährlich; 1980–81 ff.).—*Staat und Wirtschaft in Hessen* (monthly).—*Beiträge zur Statistik Hessens.—Statistische Berichte.* —*Hessische Gemeindestatistik 1960–61* (5 vols., 1963 ff.).—*Hessische Gemeindestatistik 1970* (5 vols., 1972 ff.).—*Hessische Gemeindestatistik* (annual, 1980 ff.).

State Library: Hessische Landesbibliothek, Rheinstr. 55–57, D6200 Wiesbaden.

LOWER SAXONY

Niedersachsen

AREA AND POPULATION. Lower Saxony (excluding the town of Bremerhaven, and the districts on the right bank of the Elbe in the Soviet Zone) comprises 47,439 sq. km, and is divided into 4 administrative districts, 38 rural districts, 9 towns and 1,019 communes; capital, Hanover.

Estimated population, on 31 Dec. 1989, was 7,283,795 (3,526,598 males, 3,757,197 females).

Vital statistics for calendar years:

	Live births	*Marriages*	*Divorces*	*Deaths*
1987	73,037	43,730	13,780	82,964
1988	76,036	46,500	13,500	82,920
1989	76,696	47,021	13,172	83,945

GOVERNMENT. The Land Niedersachsen was formed on 1 Nov. 1946 by merging the former Prussian province of Hanover and the *Länder* Brunswick, Oldenburg and Schaumburg-Lippe. Lower Saxony has 7 seats in the Bundesrat. The Diet, elected on 13 May 1990, consists of 67 Christian Democrats, 77 Social Democrats; Free Democrats, 9 and Greens, 8.

The cabinet of the Christian Democratic Union is headed by *Prime Minister* Gerhard Schröder (SPD).

AGRICULTURE. Area and yield of the most important crops:

	Area (in 1,000 ha)			*Yield (in 1,000 tonnes)*		
	1987	*1988*	*1989*	*1987*	*1988*	*1989*
Wheat	301	347	1,989	2,066	2,293	1,892
Rye	178	155	158	690	587	726
Barley	425	411	380	2,071	1,983	1,945
Oats	95	99	83	448	379	255
Potatoes	82	83	89	3,282	3,019	3,506
Sugar-beet	139	140	143	6,264	5,929	6,728

Livestock, 1 Dec. 1989: Cattle, 3,243,661 (including 990,044 milch cows); pigs, 7,172,004; sheep, 215,543; (in Dec. 1988): horses, 77,073; poultry, 36,059,020.

FISHERIES. In 1988 the yield of sea and coastal fishing was 65,332 tonnes valued at DM 113m.

INDUSTRY. In Sept. 1989, 4,222 establishments (with 20 and more employees) employed 663,512 persons; of these 62,495 were employed in machine construction; 69,602 in electrical engineering: (in 1988) 145,979 in car building.

LABOUR. The economically active persons totalled 3,111,500 in 1989. Of the total 271,100 were self-employed, 76,000 unpaid family workers, 2,764,400 employees; 181,500 were engaged in agriculture and forestry, 1,176,300 in power supply, mining, manufacturing and building, 562,000 in commerce and transport, 1,194,700 in other industries and services.

ROADS. At 1 Jan. 1989 there were 27,993 km of 'classified' roads, including 1,176 km of autobahn, 4,857 km of federal roads, 8,780 km of first-class and 13,180 km of second-class highways.

Number of motor vehicles, 1 Jan. 1990, was 4,083,574 including 3,489,460 passenger cars, 153,170 lorries, 8,705 buses, 247,565 tractors, 138,043 motor cycles.

JUSTICE. There are a constitutional court *(Staatsgerichtshof)*, 3 courts of appeal, 11 regional courts, 79 local courts, a Land labour court, 15 labour courts, a Land social court, 8 social courts, a finance court, a higher administrative court (together with Schleswig-Holstein), 4 administrative courts.

RELIGION. On 25 May 1987 (census) there were 66·12% Protestants and 19·6% Roman Catholics.

EDUCATION. In 1989 there were 1,845 primary schools with 16,841 teachers and 286,800 pupils; 291 special schools with 4,511 teachers and 25,824 pupils; 320 stages of orientation with 9,049 teachers and 121,995 pupils; 398 intermediate schools with 6,876 teachers and 76,367 pupils; 392 secondary schools with 7,142 teachers and 95,715 pupils; 241 grammar schools with 12,680 teachers and 140,380 pupils; 5 evening high schools with 104 teachers and 935 pupils; 14 integrated comprehensive schools with 1,662 teachers and 15,594 pupils; 17 co-operative comprehensive schools with 1,562 teachers and 17,815 pupils. In 1988 there were 139 part-time vocational schools with 212,418 pupils; 120 year of basic vocational training with 18,864 pupils; 640 full-time vocational schools with 37,672 pupils; 94 *Fachgymnasien* with 11,935 pupils; 147 *Fachoberschulen* with 9,145 pupils (full-time vocational schools leading up to vocational colleges); 219 advanced full-time vocational schools (including schools for technicians) with 11,142 pupils; 239 public health schools with 14,391 pupils.

In the winter term 1989–90 there were 6 universities (Göttingen, 29,608 students; Hanover, 27,546; Oldenburg, 9,359; Osnabrück, 10,094; Hildesheim, 2,550; Lüneburg, 3,880); 2 technical universities (Braunschweig, 16,384; Clausthal, 3,751); the medical college of Hanover (3,671), the veterinary college in Hanover (1,944).

Statistical Information: The Niedersächsisches Landesverwaltungsamt—Statistik' (Geibelstr. 65, D3000 Hanover 1) fulfils the function of the 'Statistisches Landesamt für Niedersachsen'. *Head of Division:* Abteilungsdirektor Dr Günter Koop. Main publications are: *Statistisches Jahrbuch Niedersachsen* (from 1950).—*Statistische Monatshefte Niedersachsen* (from 1947).—*Statistik Niedersachsen.*

State Library: Niedersächsische Staats- und Universitätsbibliothek, Prinzenstr. 1, 3400, Göttingen. *Director:* Helmut Vogt; Niedersächsische Landesbibliothek, Waterloostr. 8, D3000 Hannover 1. *Director:* Dr W. Dittrich.

MECKLENBURG-WEST POMERANIA

Mecklenburg-Vorpommern

AREA AND POPULATION. The area is 23,838 sq. km. Population in 1990 was 1·96m. The capital is Schwerin.

CONSTITUTION AND GOVERNMENT. The Land was reconstituted on former GDR territory in 1990. It has 4 seats in the Bundesrat.

At the Diet elections of Oct. 1990, the Christian Democrats won 29 seats with 38·3% of the vote; the Social Democrats, 21, with 27%; the Party of Democratic Socialism (former Communists), 12, with 15·7%; and the Free Democrats, 4, with 5·5%. The *Prime Minister* is J. Gomolka (Christian Democrats).

NORTH RHINE-WESTPHALIA

Nordrhein-Westfalen

AREA AND POPULATION. The Land comprises 34,068 sq. km. It is divided into 5 areas, 23 urban and 31 rural districts. Capital Düsseldorf. Population, 31 Dec. 1989, 17,103,588 (8,227,115 males, 8,876,473 females).

Vital statistics for calendar years:

	Live births	*Marriages*	*Divorces*	*Deaths*
1987	177,109	105,446	37,810	185,565
1988	185,877	109,236	37,919	186,987
1989	186,714	111,420	37,116	190,078

GOVERNMENT. The Land Nordrhein-Westfalen has 8 seats in the Bundesrat. It is governed by Social Democrats; *Prime Minister*, Johannes Rau (SPD). The Diet, elected on 13 May 1990, consists of 122 Social Democrats (50% of votes cast), 89 Christian Democrats (36·7%), 14 Free Democrats (5·8%) and 12 Greens (5%).

AGRICULTURE. Area and yield of the most important crops:

	Area (in 1,000 ha)			*Yield (in 1,000 tonnes)*		
	1987	*1988*	*1989*	*1987*	*1988*	*1989*
Wheat	240·9	257·8	268·6	1,551·3	1,772·7	1,673·8
Rye	52·9	53·0	51·7	228·5	224·6	244·9
Barley	328·3	305·1	281·2	1,677·1	1,694·9	1,723·9
Oats	66·1	66·0	56·6	296·8	263·5	164·3
Potatoes	17·4	16·5	17·1	702·0	720·7	658·0
Sugar-beet	78·1	78·7	79·4	3,997·6	4,195·8	4,262·1

Livestock, 3 Dec. 1989: Cattle, 1,944,202 (including 550,567 milch cows); pigs, 5,995,593; sheep, 175,590; horses (2 Dec. 1988), 82,301; poultry (2 Dec. 1988), 11,844,939.

INDUSTRY. In Sept. 1989, 10,964 establishments (with 20 and more employees) employed 1,984,632 persons; of these, 139,747 were employed in mining; 283,349 in machine construction; 131,245 in iron and steel production; 197,042 in chemical industry; 196,725 in electrical engineering; 58,449 in textile industry.

Output and/or production in 1,000 tonnes, 1989: Hard coal, 61,526; lignite, 104,210; pig-iron, 17,723; raw steel ingots, 23,654; rolled steel, 16,795; castings (iron and steel castings), 1,293; cement, 10,522; fireproof products, 1,102; sulphuric acid (including production of cokeries), 1,691; staple fibres and rayon, 318; metal-working machines, 111; equipment for smelting works and rolling mills, 71; machines for mining industry, 151; cranes and hoisting machinery, 71; installation implements, 1,730,992,736 (pieces); cables and electric lines, 301; springs of all kinds, 223; chains of all kinds, 93; locks and fittings, 416; spun yarns, 162; electric power, 168,463m. kwh. Of the total population, 11·6% were engaged in industry.

LABOUR. The economically active persons totalled 6,972,500 at the 1%-sample survey of the microcensus of April 1989. Of the total, 557,900 were self-employed, 64,600 unpaid family workers, 6·35m. employees; 128,900 were engaged in agriculture and forestry, 3,029,500 in power supply, mining, manufacturing and building, 1,276,900 in commerce and transport, 2,537,200 in other industries and services.

ROADS. There were (1 Jan. 1990) 29,851 km of 'classified' roads, including 2,062 km of autobahn, 5,460 km of federal roads, 12,393 km of first-class and 9,937 km of second-class highways. Number of motor vehicles, 1 July 1990, 9,106,247, including 7,239,830 passenger cars, 878,488 lorries, 349,150 motor lorries/trucks, 17,360 buses, 213,329 tractors and 313,873 motor cycles.

JUSTICE. There are a constitutional court *(Verfassungsgerichtshof)*, 3 courts of appeal, 19 regional courts, 130 local courts, 3 Land labour courts, 30 labour courts, a Land social court, 8 social courts, 3 finance courts, a higher administrative court, 7 administrative courts.

RELIGION. On 25 May 1987 (census) there were 35·2% Protestants and 49·4% Roman Catholics.

EDUCATION. In 1989 there were 4,444 primary schools with 60,606 teachers and 1,002,906 pupils; 716 special schools with 12,245 teachers and 76,791 pupils; 530 intermediate schools with 14,904 teachers and 235,802 pupils; 167 *Gesamtschulen* (comprehensive schools) with 9,865 teachers and 110,222 pupils; 631 high schools with 36,315 teachers and 472,931 pupils; in 1989 there were 285 part-time vocational schools with 416,226 pupils; vocational preparatory year 190 schools with 9,730 pupils; 305 full-time vocational schools with 76,581 pupils; 5 schools offering upgrading courses to raise the general level of education and quality for vocational colleges with 94 pupils; 211 full-time vocational schools leading up to vocational colleges with 21,527 pupils; 169 advanced full-time vocational schools with 25,412 pupils; 578 schools for public health occupations with 11,755 teachers and 31,497 pupils; 26 schools within the scope of a pilot system of courses with 60,391 pupils and 2,444 teachers.

In the winter term 1989–90 there were 8 universities (Bielefeld, 13,902 students; Bochum, 33,990; Bonn, 37,437; Dortmund, 19,807; Düsseldorf, 15,961; Cologne, 48,845; Münster, 43,260; Witten, 416); the Technical University of Aachen (36,091); 4 Roman Catholic and 2 Protestant theological colleges with together 1,147 students. There were also 4 colleges of music, 2 colleges of fine arts and the college for physical education in Cologne with together 10,651 students; 20 *Fachhochschulen* (vocational colleges) with 104,905 students, and 6 *Universitäten-Gesamthochschulen* with together 95,674 students.

Statistical Information: The Landesamt für Datenverarbeitung und Statistik Nordrhein-Westfalen (Mauerstr. 51, D4000 Düsseldorf 30) was founded in 1946, by amalgamating the provincial statistical offices of Rhineland and Westphalia. *President:* A. Benker. The Landesamt publishes: *Statistisches Jahrbuch Nordrhein-Westfalen.* From 1946. More than 550 other publications yearly.

Först, W., *Kleine Geschichte Nordrhein-Westfalens.* Münster, 1986.

Land Library: Universitätsbibliothek, Universitätsstr. 1, D4000 Düsseldorf. *Director:* Dr G. Gattermann.

RHINELAND-PALATINATE

Rheinland-Pfalz

AREA AND POPULATION. Rhineland-Pfalz comprises 19,848 sq. km. Capital Mainz. Population (at 31 Dec. 1989), 3,701,661 (1,788,739 males, 1,912,922 females).

Vital statistics for calendar years:

	Live births	*Marriages*	*Divorces*	*Deaths*
1987	37,778	23,905	7,516	42,016
1988	39,850	24,899	7,463	41,882
1989	39,650	24,261	7,467	42,536

CONSTITUTION. The constitution of the Land Rheinland-Pfalz was approved by the Consultative Assembly on 25 April 1947 and by referendum on 18 May 1947, when 579,002 voted for and 514,338 against its acceptance. It has 5 seats in the Bundesrat.

The elections of 17 May 1987 returned 48 Christian Democrats, 40 Social Democrats, 7 Free Democrats and 5 Green Party.

The cabinet is headed by Carl Ludwig Wagner (Christian Democrat).

AGRICULTURE. Area and yield of the most important products:

	Area (1,000 ha)			*Yield (1,000 tonnes)*		
	1987	*1988*	*1989*	*1987*	*1988*	*1989*
Wheat	103·8	100·3	1,020·0	552·5	601·8	583·9
Rye	27·7	25·0	23·5	108·5	109·7	111·0
Barley	128·4	141·0	1,365·0	541·0	657·1	592·1
Oats	35·7	36·1	32·7	140·4	142·6	96·2
Potatoes	11·4	10·9	10·3	336·8	334·2	331·5
Sugar-beet	21·8	22·0	22·2	1,234·6	1,177·2	1,200·7
Wine (1,000 hectolitres)	61·2	61·0	61·1	6,323·0	6,090·9	8,664·6

Livestock (3 Dec. 1989): Cattle, 551,700 (including 191,800 milch cows); horses, 20,900 (1988); sheep, 132,400; pigs, 533,000; poultry, 3,142,700 (1988).

INDUSTRY. In Sept. 1989, 2,672 establishments (with 20 and more employees) employed 380,779 persons; of these 78,173 were employed in chemical industry; electrical equipment, 20,588; 13,254 in production of leather goods and footwear; 50,675 in machine construction; 14,020 in processing stones and earthenware.

LABOUR. The economically active persons totalled 1,571,363 at the census of May 1987. Of the total, 140,854 were self-employed, 38,551 unpaid family workers, 1,391,958 employees; 71,949 were engaged in agriculture and forestry, 649,894 in power supply, mining, manufacturing and building, 264,485 in commerce and transport, 585,035 in other industries and services.

ROADS. There were (1 Jan. 1990) 18,406 km of 'classified' roads, including 790 km of autobahn, 3,229 km of federal roads, 6,976 km of first-class and 7,412 km of second-class highways. Number of motor vehicles, 1 July 1990, was 2,248,047, including 1,900,556 passenger cars, 82,870 lorries, 5,479 buses, 141,021 tractors and 90,718 motor cycles.

JUSTICE. There are a constitutional court *(Verfassungsgerichtshof)*, 2 courts of appeal, 8 regional courts, 47 local courts, a Land labour court, 5 labour courts, a Land social court, 4 social courts, a finance court, a higher administrative court, 4 administrative courts.

RELIGION. On 25 May 1987 (census) there were 37·7% Protestants and 54·5% Roman Catholics.

EDUCATION. In 1989 there were 1,184 primary schools with 14,221 teachers and 227,007 pupils; 154 special schools with 1,745 teachers and 11,709 pupils; 108 intermediate schools with 3,106 teachers and 46,617 pupils; 136 high schools with 6,970 teachers and 93,426 pupils; 88 vocational schools with 94,826 pupils; 152 advanced vocational schools and institutions for the training of technicians (full- and part-time) with 7,815 pupils; 108 schools for public health occupations with 366 teachers and 6,186 pupils.

In the winter term 1989–90 there were the University of Mainz (25,339 students), the University of Kaiserslautern (8,742 students), the University of Trier (8,452 students), the *Hochschule für Verwaltungswissenschaften* in Speyer (470 students), the Koblenz School of Corporate Management *(Wissenschaftliche Hochschule für Unternahmensführung Koblenz in Vallendar)* with 198 students, the Roman Catholic Theological College in Trier (189 students) and the Roman Catholic College in Vallendar (77 students). There were also the Teacher-Training College of the Land

Rheinland-Pfalz *(Erziehungswissenschaftliche Hochschule)* with 3,663 students, the *Fachhochschule des Landes Rheinland-Pfalz* (college of engineering) with 17,814 students and 4 *Verwaltungsfachhochschulen* with 2,523 students; also 2 private colleges for social-pedagogy (873 students).

Statistical Information: The Statistisches Landesamt Rheinland-Pfalz (Mainzer Str., 14–16, D5427 Bad Ems) was established in 1948. *President:* Dr Weis. Its publications include: *Statistisches Jahrbuch für Rheinland-Pfalz* (from 1948); *Statistische Monatshefte Rheinland-Pfalz* (from 1958); *Statistik von Rheinland-Pfalz* (from 1949) 325 vols. to date; *Rheinland-Pfalz im Spiegel der Statistik* (from 1968); *Die kreisfreien Städte und Landkreise in Rheinland-Pfalz* (from 1977); *Rheinland-Pfalz heute* (from 1973); *Benutzerhandbuch des Landesinformationssystems* (1981); *Rheinland-Pfalz heute und morgen* (Mainz, 1985); *Raumordnungsbericht 1985 der Landesregierung Rheinland-Pfalz* (Mainz, 1985). *Landesentwicklungsprogramm 1980* (Mainz, 1980).

Klöpper, R. and Korber, J., *Rheinland-Pfalz in seiner Gliederung nach zentralörtlichen Bereichen.* Remagen, 1957

SAARLAND

HISTORY. In 1919 the Saar territory was placed under the control of the League of Nations. Following a plebiscite, the territory reverted to Germany in 1935. In 1945 the territory became part of the French Zone of occupation, and was in 1947 accorded an international status inside an economic union with France. In pursuance of the German–French agreement signed in Luxembourg on 27 Oct. 1956 the territory returned to Germany on 1 Jan. 1957. Its re-integration with Germany was completed by 5 July 1959.

AREA AND POPULATION. Saarland has an area of 2,570 sq. km. Population, 31 Dec. 1989, 1,064,906 (512,889 males, 552,017 females). The capital is Saarbrücken.

Vital statistics for calendar years:

	Live births	*Marriages*	*Divorces*	*Deaths*
1987	10,517	7,021	2,481	12,318
1988	10,748	7,446	2,781	12,388
1989	10,661	7,249	2,585	12,398

CONSTITUTION. Saarland has 3 seats in the Bundesrat.

The Saar Diet, elected on 28 Jan. 1990, is composed as follows: 30 Social Democrats, 18 Christian Democrats, 3 Free Democrats.

Saarland is governed by Social Democrats in Parliament. *Prime Minister*: Oskar Lafontaine (Social Democrat).

AGRICULTURE AND FORESTRY. The cultivated area (1989) occupied 118,793 ha or 46·2% of the total area; the forest area comprises nearly 33% of the total (256,991 ha).

Area and yield of the most important crops:

	Area (in 1,000 ha)			*Yield (in 1,000 tonnes)*		
	1987	*1988*	*1989*	*1987*	*1988*	*1989*
Wheat	7·0	7·1	7·0	31·1	36·0	36·8
Rye	6·1	5·7	5·6	24·0	23·4	25·5
Barley	10·0	9·9	9·9	42·2	44·2	42·7
Oats	5·4	5·6	5·3	22·4	22·7	19·2
Potatoes	0·4	0·4	0·4	11·4	13·0	13·0

Livestock, Dec. 1989: Cattle, 67,528 (including 22,399 milch cows); pigs, 35,419; sheep, 14,707. Dec. 1988: Horses, 3,958; poultry, 263,420.

INDUSTRY. In June 1990, 607 establishments (with 20 and more employees) employed 140,606 persons; of these 20,094 were engaged in coalmining, 21,566 in manufacturing motor vehicles, parts, accessories, 16,655 in iron and steel production, 15,024 in machine construction, 9,423 in electrical engineering, 7,583 in steel construction. In 1989 the coalmines produced 9·5m. tonnes of coal. 5 blast furnaces and 6 steel furnaces produced 4·1m. tonnes of pig-iron and 4·9m. tonnes of crude steel.

LABOUR. The economically active persons totalled 428,000 at the 1%-sample survey of the microcensus of April 1989. Of the total, 31,500 were self-employed, 392,200 employees; 4,300 were engaged in agriculture and forestry, 179,000 in power supply, mining, manufacturing and building, 81,000 in commerce and transport, 163,700 in other industries and services.

ROADS. At 1 Jan. 1990 there were 2,199 km of 'classified' roads, including 216 km of autobahn, 374 km of federal roads, 813 km of first-class and 786 km of second-class highways. Number of motor vehicles, 31 Dec. 1989, 605,888, including 538,549 passenger cars, 22,819 lorries, 1,607 buses, 13,540 tractors and 23,885 motor cycles.

JUSTICE. There are a constitutional court *(Verfassungsgerichtshof)*, a court of appeal, a regional court, 11 local courts, a Land labour court, 3 labour courts, a Land social court, a social court, a finance court, a higher administrative court, an administrative court.

RELIGION. On 25 May 1987 (census) 72·7% of the population were Roman Catholics and 21·9% were Protestants.

EDUCATION. In 1989–90 there were 322 primary schools with 3,567 teachers and 56,478 pupils; 47 special schools with 466 teachers and 2,678 pupils; 35 intermediate schools with 1,006 teachers and 13,166 pupils; 36 high schools with 1,879 teachers and 23,949 pupils; 11 comprehensive high schools with 481 teachers and 5,196 pupils; 2 *Freie Waldorfschulen* with 66 teachers and 783 pupils; 4 evening intermediate schools with 235 pupils; 2 evening high schools and 1 Saarland College with 427 pupils; 43 part-time vocational schools with 25,354 pupils; year of commercial basic training: 70 institutions with 2,091 pupils; 21 advanced full-time vocational schools and schools for technicians with 3,293 pupils; 52 full-time vocational schools with 4,918 pupils; 10 *Berufsaufbauschulen* (vocational extension schools) with 496 pupils; 29 *Fachoberschulen* (full-time vocational schools leading up to vocational colleges) with 2,863 pupils; 42 schools for public health occupations with 2,043 pupils. The number of pupils visiting the vocational schools amounts to 41,200. They are instructed by 3,118 teachers.

In the winter term 1989–90 there was the University of the Saarland with 19,099 students; 1 academy of music with 305 students; 1 vocational college (economics and engineering) with 3,157 students; 1 vocational college for social affairs with 209 students; 1 vocational college for public administration with 122 students; and 1 academy of fine art with 178 students.

Statistical Information: The Statistisches Amt des Saarlandes (Hardenbergstrasse 3, D6600 Saarbrücken 1) was established on 1 April 1938. As from 1 June 1935, it was an independent agency; its predecessor, 1920–35, was the Statistical Office of the Government Commission of the Saar. *Chief:* Direktor Josef Mailänder. The most important publications are: *Statistisches Handbuch für das Saarland,* from 1950.—*Statistisches Taschenbuch für das Saarland,* from 1959.—*Saarländische Bevölkerungs-und Wirtschaftszahlen.* Quarterly, from 1949.—*Saarland in Zahlen* (special issues).—*Einzelschriften zur Statistik des Saarlandes,* from 1950—*Statistische Nachrichten,* from 1981.

Fischer, P., *Die Saar zwischen Deutschland und Frankreich.* Frankfurt, 1959
Osang, R.M., *Saarland ABC.* Saarbrücken, 1975
Schmidt, R. H., *Saarpolitik 1945–57.* 3 vols. Berlin, 1959–62

SAXONY

Sachsen

AREA AND POPULATION. The area is 18,337 sq. km. Population in 1990 was 4·9m. The capital is Dresden.

CONSTITUTION AND GOVERNMENT. The Land was reconstituted on former GDR territory in 1990. It has 5 seats in the Bundesrat.

At the Diet elections of Oct. 1990 the Christian Democrats won 92 seats, with 53·8% of the vote; the Social Democrats, 32, with 19·1%; the Party of Democratic Socialism (former Communists), 17, with 10·2%; New Forum/Alliance '90/Greens, 10, with 8%; and the Free Democrats, 9, with 5·3%.

The *Prime Minister* is Kurt Biedenkopf (Christian Democrat).

SAXONY-ANHALT

Sachsen-Anhalt

AREA AND POPULATION. The area is 20,445 sq. km. Population in 1990 was 2·97m. The capital is Halle.

CONSTITUTION AND GOVERNMENT. The Land was reconstituted on former GDR territory in 1990. It has 4 seats in the Bundesrat.

At the Diet elections of Oct. 1990 the Christian Democrats won 48 seats, with 39% of the vote; the Social Democrats, 27, with 26%; the Free Democrats, 14, with 13·5%; the Party of Democratic Socialism (former Communists), 12 with 12%; Alliance '90/Greens, 5, with 9·5%.

The *Prime Minister* is Gerd Gies.

SCHLESWIG-HOLSTEIN

AREA AND POPULATION. The area of Schleswig-Holstein is 15,728 sq. km; it is divided into 4 urban and 11 rural districts and 1,131 communes. The capital is Kiel. The population (estimate, 31 Dec. 1989) numbered 2,594,606 (1,255,014 males, 1,339,592 females).

Vital statistics for calendar years:

	Live births	*Marriages*	*Divorces*	*Deaths*
1987	25,956	16,464	5,937	30,885
1988	27,310	17,273	5,495	30,424
1989	27,377	17,238	5,428	30,546

GOVERNMENT. The Land has 4 seats in the Bundesrat. The elections of 8 May 1988 gave the Christian Democrats 27, the Social Democratic Party 46 and the South Schleswig Association 1 seat.

Prime Minister: Björn Engholm.

AGRICULTURE. Area and yield of the most important crops:

	Area (in 1,000 ha)			*Yield (in 1,000 tonnes)*		
	1987	*1988*	*1989*	*1987*	*1988*	*1989*
Wheat	152·8	176·6	0,000·0	1,135·4	1,394·6	1,332·7
Rye	47·3	44·5	00·0	164·6	210·7	210·4
Barley	127·6	113·0	000·0	743·7	740·5	709·6
Oats	18·2	29·3	00·0	85·1	137·8	85·1
Potatoes	3·9	3·6	0·0	120·9	113·3	141·4
Sugar-beet	15·9	16·7	00·0	493·6	756·5	752·9

Livestock, 3 Dec. 1989: 1,487,748 cattle (including 480,272 milch cows), 1,446,288 pigs, 224,456 sheep; (and in 1988) 33,392 horses, 3,293,080 poultry.

FISHERIES. In 1989 the yield of small-scale deep-sea and inshore fisheries was 38,788 tonnes valued at DM86·6m.

INDUSTRY. In 1989 (average), 1,580 establishments (with 20 and more employees) employed 169,350 persons; of these, 8,440 were employed in shipbuilding (except naval engineering); 33,136 in machine construction; 22,530 in food and kindred industry; 18,170 in electrical engineering.

LABOUR. The economically active persons totalled 1,166,000 in 1989. Of the total, 107,500 were self-employed, 17,700 unpaid family workers, 1,040,800 employees; 52,200 were engaged in agriculture and forestry, 348,700 in power supply, mining, manufacturing and building, 242,300 in commerce and transport, 522,800 in other industries and services.

ROADS. There were (1 Jan. 1990) 9,846·7 km of 'classified' roads, including 421·1 km of autobahn, 1,934·3 km of federal roads, 3,503·8 km of first-class and 3,987·6 km of second-class highways. Number of motor vehicles, 1 Jan. 1990, was 1,438,364, including 1,237,412 passenger cars, 55,951 lorries, 2,896 buses, 73,758 tractors, 49,407 motor cycles.

SHIPPING. The Kiel Canal, 98·7 km (51 miles) long, is on Schleswig-Holstein territory. In 1938, 53,530 vessels of 22·6m. net tons passed through it; in 1981, 52,641 vessels of 53·3m. net tons; in 1989, 46,603 vessels of 44·9m. net tons.

JUSTICE. There are a court of appeal, 4 regional courts, 30 local courts, a Land labour court, 6 labour courts, a Land social court, 4 social courts, a finance court, an administrative court.

RELIGION. On 25 May 1987 (census) there were 73·3% Protestants and 6·2% Roman Catholics.

EDUCATION. In 1989–90 there were 685 primary schools with 4,760 teachers and 136,028 pupils; 163 special schools with 1,238 teachers and 12,291 pupils; 173 intermediate schools with 2,409 teachers and 49,392 pupils; 99 high schools with 3,576 teachers and 63,503 pupils; 10 integrated comprehensive schools with 313 teachers and 5,528 pupils; 42 part-time vocational schools with 1,604 teachers and 75,766 pupils; 141 full-time vocational schools with 446 teachers and 10,049 pupils; 56 advanced vocational schools for foreigners with 285 teachers and 5,627 pupils; 60 schools for public health occupations with 4,006 pupils; 62 vocational grammar schools with 404 teachers and 7,161 pupils; 6 vocational colleges with 15,465 pupils in the summer term of 1990.

In the summer term of 1990 the University of Kiel had 17,216 students, 2 teacher-training colleges had 2,293 students; 1 music college had 373 students, 1 Medical University in Lübeck had 1,128 students.

Statistical Information: Statistisches Landesamt Schleswig-Holstein (Fröbel Str. 15–17, D2300 Kiel 1). *Director:* Dr Mohr. Publications: *Statistisches Taschenbuch Schleswig-Holstein,* since 1954.—*Statistisches Jahrbuch Schleswig-Holstein,* since 1951.—*Statistische Monatshefte Schleswig-Holstein,* since 1949.—*Statistische Berichte,* since 1947.—*Beitrage zur historischen Statistik Schleswig-Holstein,* from 1967.—*Lange Reihen,* from 1977.

Baxter, R. R., *The Law of International Waterways.* Harvard Univ. Press, 1964
Brandt, O., *Grundriss der Geschichte Schleswig-Holsteins.* 5th ed. Kiel, 1957
Handbuch für Schleswig-Holstein. 24th ed. Kiel, 1988

State Library: Schleswig-Holsteinische Landesbibliothek, Kiel, Schloss. *Director:* Prof. Dr Dieter Lohmeier.

THURINGIA

Thüringen

AREA AND POPULATION. The area is 16,251 sq. km. Population in 1990 was 2·68m. The capital is Erfurt.

CONSTITUTION AND GOVERNMENT. The Land was reconstituted on former GDR territory in 1990. It has 4 seats in the Bundesrat.

At the Diet elections of Oct. 1990 the Christian Democrats won 44 seats, with 45·4% of the vote; the SPD, 21 with 22·8%; the Party of Democratic Socialism, 9, with 9·7%; the Free Democrats, 9, with 9·3%; New Forum/Greens/Democracy Now, 6 with 7·2%.

The *Prime Minister* is M. Duchac.

GHANA

Capital: Accra
Population: 14·9m. (1990)
GNP per capita: US$400 (1988)

Republic of Ghana

HISTORY. The State of Ghana came into existence on 6 March 1957 when the former Colony of the Gold Coast and the Trusteeship Territory of Togoland attained Dominion status. The name of the country recalls a powerful monarchy which from the 4th to the 13th century A.D. ruled the region of the middle Niger.

The Ghana Independence Act received the royal assent on 7 Feb. 1957. The General Assembly of the United Nations in Dec. 1956 approved the termination of British administration in Togoland and the union of Togoland with the Gold Coast on the latter's attainment of independence.

The country was declared a Republic within the Commonwealth on 1 July 1960 with Dr Kwame Nkrumah as the first President. On 24 Feb. 1966 the Nkrumah regime was overthrown in a military *coup* and ruled by the National Liberation Council until 1 Oct. 1969 when the military regime handed over power to a civilian regime under a new constitution. Dr K. A. Busia was the Prime Minister of the Second Republic. On 13 Jan. 1972 the armed forces and police took over power again from the civilian regime in a *coup*.

In Oct. 1975 the National Redemption Council was subordinated to a Supreme Military Council (SMC). In 1979 the SMC was toppled in a *coup* led by Flight-Lieut. J. J. Rawlings. The new government permitted elections already scheduled and these resulted in a victory for Dr Hilla Limann and his People's National Party. However on 31 Dec. 1981 another *coup* led by Flight-Lieut. Rawlings dismissed the government and Parliament, suspended the Constitution and established a Provisional National Defence Council to exercise all government powers.

AREA AND POPULATION. Ghana is bounded west by the Côte d'Ivoire, north by Burkina Faso, east by Togo and south by the Gulf of Guinea. The area of Ghana is 92,456 sq. miles (239,460 sq. km); census population 1984, 12,296,081. Estimate (1990) 14,925,000.

Ghana is divided into 10 regions:

Regions	*Area (sq. km)*	*Population census 1984*	*Capital*	*Population census 1984*
Eastern	19,977	1,680,890	Koforidua	58,731
Western	23,921	1,157,807	Sekondi-Takoradi	93,400
Central	9,826	1,142,335	Cape Coast	57,224
Ashanti	24,390	2,090,100	Kumasi	376,246
Brong-Ahafo	39,557	1,206,608	Sunyani	38,834
Northern	70,383	1,164,583	Tamale	135,952
Volta	20,572	1,211,907	Ho	37,777
Upper East	8,842	772,744	Bolgatanga	32,495
Upper West	18,477	438,008	Wa	
Greater Accra	2,593	1,431,099	Accra	867,459

The capital is Accra, other chief towns (population, census, 1970); Asamankese, 101,144; Tema, 99,608 (1984); Nsawam, 57,350; Tarkwa, 50,570; Oda, 40,740; Obuasi, 40,001; Winneba, 36,104; Keta, 27,461; Agona Swedru, 23,843.

Vital statistics (1985): Birth rate, 47 per 1,000; death rate 15 per 1,000.

In the south and centre of Ghana, the people are of the Kwa ethno-linguistic group, mainly Akan (Ashanti, Fante, etc.), Ewe (in the Volta region) and Ga, while the 20% living in the north belong to Gur peoples (Dagbane, Gurma and Grusi).

CLIMATE. The climate ranges from the equatorial type on the coast to savannah in the north and is typified by the existence of well-marked dry and wet seasons. Temperatures are relatively high throughout the year. The amount, duration and seasonal distribution of rain is very marked, from the south, with over 80" (2,000 mm) to the north, with under 50" (1,250 mm). In the extreme north, the wet season is from March to Aug., but further south it lasts until Oct. Near Kumasi, two wet seasons occur, in May and June and again in Oct. and this is repeated, with greater amounts, along the coast of Ghana. Accra. Jan. 80°F (26·7°C), July 77°F (25°C). Annual rainfall 29" (724 mm). Kumasi. Jan. 77°F (25°C), July 76°F (24·4°C). Annual rainfall 58" (1,402 mm). Sekondi-Takoradi. Jan. 79°F (25°C), July 76°F (24·4°C). Annual rainfall 47" (1,181 mm). Tamale. Jan. 82°F (27·8°C), July 78°F (25·6°C). Annual rainfall 41" (1,026 mm).

CONSTITUTION AND GOVERNMENT. Since the coup of 31 Dec. 1981, supreme power is vested in the Provisional National Defence Council (PNDC), which in Sept. 1990 consisted of: *Chairman:* Flight-Lieut. Jerry John Rawlings. *Vice Chairman:* Justice Daniel Annan. Mary Grant. Ebo Tawiah. Mahama Iddrisu. P. V. Obeng. Capt. Kojo Tsikata. Lieut.-Gen. Arnold Quainoo. Maj.-Gen. W. M. Mensa-Wood.

In Feb. 1991 PNDC Secretaries (Ministers) included: *Foreign Affairs:* Obed Y. Asamoah. *Internal Affairs:* Nii Okaija Adamafio. *Finance and Economic Planning:* Dr Kwesi Botchwey. *Justice and Attorney-General:* E. G. Tanoh. *Defence:* Mahama Iddrisu. *Trade and Tourism:* Huudu Yahaya. *Cocoa:* Adjei Marfo. *Information:* Kofi Totobi Quakyi.

National flag: Red, gold, green (horizontal); a black star in the centre.

National anthem: Hail the name of Ghana.

Local government: The 10 Regions, each under a Regional Secretary appointed by the PNDC, are divided into 110 districts.

DEFENCE.

Army. The Ghana Army consists of 7 infantry battalions, 1 reconnaissance battalion, 1 field engineer battalion, 1 parachute battalion, 1 mortar battalion, with armoured cars and ancillary units. Total strength, (1991) 10,000.

Navy. The Ghana Navy, based at Sekondi and Tema comprises 2 German-built coastal patrol, 4 inshore patrol craft and 2 small service craft. Naval strength in 1990 numbered 1,400 including support personnel.

Air Force. The Ghana Air Force was formed in 1959, when an Air Force Training School was established at Accra. Its first combat unit has 4 Italian-built Aermacchi M.B.326K light ground attack jets ordered in 1976. It has, for training, transport, search and rescue, and air survey operations, 4 Fokker Friendship twin-turboprop transports, a C-212 Aviocar and a twin-turbofan Fokker Fellowship for Presidential use, all built in the Netherlands, 8 Islander piston-engined light transports, 6 Shorts Skyvan twinturboprop STOL transports, and 10 Bulldog primary trainers, all built in the UK; 2 Bell 212 helicopters built in the US; 4 French-built Alouette III helicopters, and 5 Aermacchi M.B.326F and 2 M.B.339 jet trainers. There are air bases at Takoradi and Tamale. Personnel strength (1991) about 800.

INTERNATIONAL RELATIONS

Membership. Ghana is a member of the UN, the Commonwealth, OAU, ECOWAS and is an ACP state of EEC.

ECONOMY

Budget. In 1989 budget provided for revenue estimated at ₵ 204,617m. and expenditure estimated at ₵ 196,191m.

Currency. The monetary unit is the *cedi* (GHC) of 100 *pesewas* (P). Notes are issued of 1, 2, 5, 10, 50, 200 and 500 ₵; cupro-nickel coins of 2½, 5, 10 and 20 P and 1₵. In March 1991, £1 = ₵ 662·55; US$1 = ₵ 349·26.

Banking and Finance. The Bank of Ghana was established in Feb. 1957 as the central bank of the country. The Ghana Commercial Bank, also established in Feb. 1957, is a purely commercial institution with agricultural financing as one of its priorities. It had 150 full branches in Sept. 1987, 1 in London and 1 subsidiary in

Lomé (Togo). Barclays Bank of Ghana Ltd has 39 branches and agencies and the Standard Bank (Ghana) Ltd has 38 branches.

The National Investment Bank, established in 1963, is an autonomous joint state-private development finance institution. The former post office savings bank has been transformed into the National Savings and Credit Bank. The Bank for Housing and Construction opened in 1973; The Merchant Bank (Ghana) Ltd in 1972; The Ghana Co-operative Bank was established and re-organized in 1974; The Agricultural Development Bank in 1967; The Consolidated Discount House Ltd in Nov. 1987.

ENERGY AND NATURAL RESOURCES

Electricity. Production (1986) 4,372m. kwh, mainly from 2 hydro-electric stations operated by the Volta River Authority, Akosombo (6 units) and Kpong (4 units), with a total capacity of 1,072 mw. Supply 240 volts; 50 Hz.

Oil. The Government announced in Jan. 1978 that oil had been found in commercial quantities with known reserves (1980) 7m. bbls and in Oct. 1983 formed the Ghanaian National Petroleum Corporation with exploration rights in all areas not covered by existing agreements.

Minerals. In 1987 gold production was 323,496 fine oz.; diamonds, 396,720 carats; manganese, 235,123 tonnes; bauxite, 226,415 tonnes.

Agriculture. In southern and central Ghana main food crops are maize, rice, cassava, plantain, groundnuts, yam and cocoyam, and in northern Ghana groundnuts, rice, maize, sorghum, millet and yams.

Production of main food crops (1988 in 1,000 tonnes) was: Maize, 630; rice, 116; millet, 140; sorghum, 175; cassava, 3,300; cocoyam, 650; yam, 1,000; plantain, 700.

Cocoa is by far Ghana's main cash crop. Production (1988) 290,000 tonnes. Output has fallen considerably since the 1970s, and Ghana has lost its long-held position as the world's leading producer to the Côte d'Ivoire. While there is smuggling to that country, Ghana's low cocoa production was due to ageing trees and declining interest in cocoa growing because of poor prices. Since 1982 the PNDC has carried out a rehabilitation programme for cocoa as well as increased producer prices for farmers, which has halted the decline and raised production considerably.

Among other cash crops, tobacco and coffee are important, and improved types of palm oil and coconuts are being planted on an increased scale; progress has been made with clonal rubber in the south-west; pepper, ginger, pineapple, avocado, citrus and other crops are being grown for export, and efforts are being made to increase local supplies of cotton, kenaf, tobacco, palm oil, mango, pineapple and sugar-cane for local industries.

Livestock, 1988: Cattle, 1·3m.; sheep, 2·5m.; goats, 3m.; horses, 4,000; pigs, 750,000; poultry, 12m.

Forestry. In 1988 the closed forest zone covered 8,225,900 hectares (36% of the land area), of which 2,559,400 hectares were reserves and 46,600 hectares unreserved forest lands. In 1986, 221,000 cu. metres of logs and 104,000 cu. metres of sawn timber were exported. Production (1987) 493,543 cu. metres.

Fisheries. Catch (1987) 324,630 tonnes (54,630 from inland waters).

INDUSTRY. The aluminium smelter at Tema is the centre of industrial development, mainly concentrated on Accra/Tema, Kumasi and Takoradi/Sekondi. In 1984 the Volta Aluminium Company (VALCO), which operates the smelter, reached an agreement with the government on the use of Volta dam electricity. Production (1986) 120,000 tonnes.

FOREIGN ECONOMIC RELATIONS

Commerce. In 1989 exports were US$880m.; imports, US$1,200m. Exports went mainly to USA, UK, Japan and Federal Republic of Germany. Imports came from

Nigeria, UK, USA and Federal Republic of Germany. Principal exports: Cocoa, timber and gold; imports were raw materials, capital equipment, petroleum and food.

Total trade between Ghana and UK (British Department of Trade returns, in £1,000 sterling):

	1986	*1987*	*1988*	*1989*	*1990*
Imports to UK	103,480	113,859	106,314	92,208	105,118
Exports and re-exports from UK	113,218	138,081	126,148	121,076	162,057

Tourism. In 1987 there were 103,440 tourists.

COMMUNICATIONS

Roads. In 1988 agencies of the Ministry of Roads and Highways maintained about 14,514 km of trunk roads, 14,000 km of feeder and 10,000 km of other rural roads, and 1,700 km of city and municipal roads. The number of vehicles in use (1986) was 54,196, of which private cars, 26,590.

Railways. Total length of railways in 1989 was 947 km of 1,067 mm gauge. In 1989 railways carried 0·76m. tonnes of freight and 3·3m. passengers.

Aviation. There is an international airport at Accra, domestic airports at Takoradi, Kumasi, Tamale and Sunyani and airstrips at Wa, Navrongo and Ho. Services are operated by Ghana Airways, Nigeria Airways, Swissair, KLM, British Airways, Egypt Air, Air India, Aeroflot, Air Afrique and Bulgarian Airlines. Total aircraft freight in 1986 was 8,661,971 tonnes.

Shipping. The chief ports are Takoradi and Tema. In 1983, 1,299,146 tonnes of cargo were imported and 1,682,519 tonnes were exported by 663 ships.

Telecommunications. There were 444 telephone exchanges and 666 call offices with (1987) 74,935 telephones in use. There are internal wireless stations at Accra, Kumasi, Bawku, Lawra, Kete-Krachi, Tamale, Yendi, Kpandu, Tumu and Sekondi-Takoradi. In 1988 there were over 2·9m. radio and 175,000 television receivers.

Cinemas. In 1987 there were 83 cinemas with an average seating capacity of 1,200.

Newspapers. There were (1989) 3 daily newspapers (circulation 180,000).

JUSTICE, RELIGION, EDUCATION AND WELFARE

Justice. The Courts were constituted as follows:

Supreme Court. The Supreme Court consists of the Chief Justice who is also the President and not less than 4 other Justices of the Supreme Court. The Supreme Court is the final court of appeal in Ghana. The final interpretation of the provisions of the constitution has been entrusted to the Supreme Court.

Court of Appeal. The Court of Appeal consists of the Chief Justice together with not less than 5 other Justices of the Appeal court and such other Justices of Superior Courts as the Chief Justice may nominate. The Court of Appeal is duly constituted by 3 Justices. The Court of Appeal is bound by its own previous decisions and all courts inferior to the Court of Appeal are bound to follow the decisions of the Court of Appeal on questions of law. Divisions of the Appeal Court may be created, subject to the discretion of the Chief Justice.

High Court of Justice. The Court has jurisdiction in civil and criminal matters as well as those relating to industrial and labour disputes including administrative complaints. The High Court of Justice has supervisory jurisdiction over all inferior Courts and any adjudicating authority and in exercise of its supervisory jurisdiction has power to issue such directions, orders or writs including writs or orders in the nature of habeas corpus, certiorari, mandamus, prohibition and quo qarrantto. The High Court of Justice has no jurisdiction in cases of treason. The High Court consists of the Chief Justice and not less than 12 other judges and such other Justices of the Superior Court as the Chief Justice may appoint.

The PNDC has established Public Tribunals in addition to the traditional courts of justice.

There is a Public Tribunal Board consisting of not less than 5 members and not more than 15 members of the public appointed by the PNDC, at least one of whom shall be a lawyer of not less than 5 years' standing as a lawyer. The Board is responsible for the administration of all tribunals.

A tribunal consists of at least three persons and not more than five persons, selected by the Board from among persons appointed by the Council as members of public tribunals.

Religion. In 1988 Christians represented 52% of the population (Protestant, 37%; Roman Catholic, 15%), Moslem, 13%, others, 30%.

Education. In 1985–86 there were 2,399 kindergartens for the age-groups 4–6 years with 171,182 pupils. Primary schools are free and attendance is compulsory. In 1985–86 there were 9,004 primary schools with 1,491,162 pupils. In 1986 there were 5,310 middle schools with 617,613 pupils; 110 junior secondary schools with 18,372 pupils and 233 secondary schools with 133,435 students. In 1986 there were 45 training colleges with 15,210 students and 26 vocational-technical schools with 19,547 students at the beginning of the academic year. In 1987–88 there were 8,847 students at the 3 universities (University of Ghana, the University of Science and Technology at Kumasi, and the University of Cape Coast). University education is free.

Health. In 1988 medical facilities included 46 government hospitals, 252 health centres and posts, 3 university hospitals, 3 mental hospitals, 35 mission hospitals, 34 mission clinics and 40 private hospitals. In addition, there are 26 nurses and midwives training schools. There were 600 doctors, 5,190 nurses and 2,830 midwives in 1986.

DIPLOMATIC REPRESENTATIVES

Of Ghana in Great Britain (13 Belgrave Sq., London, SW1X 8PR)
High Commissioner: (Vacant).

Of Great Britain in Ghana (Osu Link, off Gamel Abdul Nasser Ave., Accra)
High Commissioner: A. M. Goodenough, CMG.

Of Ghana in the USA (3512 International Dr., NW, Washington, D.C., 20008)
Ambassador: Eric K. Otoo.

Of the USA in Ghana (Ring Rd. East, Accra)
Ambassador: Raymond C. Ewing.

Of Ghana to the United Nations
Ambassador: Dr. Kofi Nyidevu Awoonor.

Further Reading

Digest of Statistics. Accra. Quarterly (from May 1953)
Ghana. Official Handbook. Annual
Davidson, B., *Black Star*. London, 1973
Jones, T., *Ghana's First Republic 1960–1966*. London, 1975
Killick, T., *Development Economics in Action: A Study of Economic Policies in Ghana*. London, 1978
Myers, R. A., *Ghana:* [Bibliography]. Oxford and Santa Barbara, 1991
Ray, D. I., *Ghana: Politics, Economics and Society*. London, 1986

GIBRALTAR

Population: 30,689 (1989)
GNP per capita: US$4,370 (1985)

HISTORY. The Rock of Gibraltar was settled by Moors in 711; they named it after their chief Jebel Tariq, 'the Mountain of Tarik'. In 1462 it was taken by the Spaniards, from Granada. It was captured by Admiral Sir George Rooke on 24 July 1704, and ceded to Great Britain by the Treaty of Utrecht, 1713. The cession was confirmed by the treaties of Paris (1763) and Versailles (1783).

On 10 Sept. 1967, in pursuance of a United Nations resolution on the decolonization of Gibraltar, a referendum was held in Gibraltar in order to ascertain whether the people of Gibraltar believed that their interests lay in retaining their link with Britain or in passing under Spanish sovereignty. Out of a total electorate of 12,762, 12,138 voted to retain the British connexion, while 44 voted for Spain.

On 15 Dec. 1982 the border between Gibraltar and Spain was re-opened for Spaniards and Gibraltarian pedestrians who are residents of Gibraltar. The border had been closed by Spain in June 1969. Following an agreement signed in Brussels in Nov. 1984 the border was fully opened on 5 Feb. 1985.

AREA AND POPULATION. Area, 2½ sq. miles (6·5 sq. km). Total population, including port and harbour (census, 1981), 28,719. Estimate (31 Dec. 1989) 30,689 (of which 20,425 were British Gibraltarian, 5,782 Other British and 4,482 Non-British). The population is mostly of Genoese, Portuguese and Maltese as well as Spanish descent.

Vital statistics (1989): Births, 530; marriages, 754; deaths, 219.

CLIMATE. The climate is warm temperate, with westerly winds in winter bringing rain. Summers are pleasantly warm and rainfall is low. Frost or snow is very rare. Jan. 57°F (13·7°C), July 75°F (23·9°C). Annual rainfall 23" (584 mm).

CONSTITUTION AND GOVERNMENT. Following a Constitutional Conference held in July 1968, a new Constitution was introduced in 1969. The Legislative and City Councils were merged to produce an enlarged legislature known as the Gibraltar House of Assembly. Executive authority is exercised by the Governor, who is also Commander-in-Chief. The Governor, while retaining certain reserved powers, is normally required to act in accordance with the advice of the Gibraltar Council, which consists of 4 *ex-officio* members (the Deputy Governor, the Deputy Fortress Commander, the Attorney-General and the Financial and Development Secretary) together with 5 elected members of the House of Assembly appointed by the Governor after consultation with the Chief Minister. Matters of primarily domestic concern are devolved to elected Ministers, with Britain responsible for other matters, including external affairs, defence and internal security. There is a Council of Ministers presided over by the Chief Minister.

The House of Assembly consists of a Speaker appointed by the Governor, 15 elected and 2 *ex-officio* members (the Attorney-General and the Financial and Development Secretary).

A Mayor of Gibraltar is elected by the elected members of the Assembly.

Governor and C.-in-C.: Adm. Sir Derek Reffell, KCB.
Chief Minister: Joseph John Bossano.
Flag: White with a red strip along the bottom, a red triple-towered castle with a gold key depending from the gateway.

DEFENCE. The Gibraltar Regiment is a part-time unit consisting of 1 infantry company, 1 battery of 105 mm light guns and an air defence troop equipped with blowpipe missiles with a small regular cadre. There is also a resident battalion from the British Army, an RAF Base and a Naval Base.

ECONOMY

Budget. Revenue and expenditure (in £ sterling):

	1987–88	*1988–89*	*1989–90*	*1990–91*
Revenue	78,343,477	82,124,000	87,421,000	85,597,000
Expenditure	82,063,600	81,904,000	91,388,000	90,246,000

Currency. The unit of currency is the Gibraltar pound (GIP). There are Gibraltar Government notes in denominations of Gib£50, £20, £10, £5 and £1 and Gibraltar Government coinage. The amount in notes in circulation at 31 March 1990 was £12·01m. In March 1991 £1 = Gib£1; US$ = Gib£0·53.

Banking. Domestic and offshore banking services are provided by 14 banks: Barclays Bank PLC (with 3 branches), Lloyds Bank PLC, Hambros Bank (Gibraltar) Ltd, Bank of Credit and Commerce Gibraltar Ltd, United Bank of Gibraltar Ltd, Algemene Bank Gibraltar Ltd, Banque Indosuez, Banco Espanol de Credito SA, Jyske Bank (Gibraltar) Ltd, Banco de Bilbao (Gibraltar) Ltd, Banco Central SA, National Westminster Bank PLC, National Westminster Bank Finance (Gibraltar) Ltd and Royal Bank of Scotland (Gibraltar) Ltd. In addition there are 10 offshore banks: Gibraltar and Iberian Bank Ltd, Hong Kong Bank and Trust Co. Ltd, Hambros Bank (Gibraltar) Ltd, Gibraltar Private Bank Ltd, Republic National Bank of New York (Gibraltar) Ltd, Gibraltar Trust Bank Ltd, Banco Hispano Americano SA and Abbey National (Gibraltar) Ltd, Republic National Bank of New York (International) Ltd, Varde Bank International (Gibraltar) Ltd. Total assets of commercial banks were £2,216·4m. in Dec. 1989.

INDUSTRY. There are a number of relatively small industrial concerns engaged in the bottling of beer and mineral waters, etc., mainly for local consumption. There is a small but important commercial ship-repair yard with 3 dry docks for vessels of up to 75,000 DWT, and a yacht repair yard.

Labour. The total insured labour force at 31 Dec. 1989, was 14,311. There were (1989) 8 registered trade unions and 9 employers associations. Approximately 45% of the local labour force is employed by the UK departments of the Gibraltar Government. In the private sector the main sources of employment are the construction industry, ship repairing, hotel and catering services, shipping services, trading agencies and retail distribution.

FOREIGN ECONOMIC RELATIONS

Commerce. Imports and exports (in £ sterling):

	1986	*1987*	*1988*	*1989*
Imports	111,700,000	140,962,000	144,787,000	200,493,000
Exports	44,300,000	51,731,000	46,093,000	76,138,000

Britain and the Commonwealth provide the bulk of imports, but fresh vegetables and fruit come mainly from Morocco and Spain. Foodstuffs accounted for 12% of total imports (about £24m.) in 1988. About 44% of non-fuel imports originate from the UK. Other sources include Japan, Spain and USA. Value of non-fuel imports, 1989, £165m. Exports are mainly re-exports of petroleum and petroleum products supplied to shipping. Gibraltar depends largely on tourism, offshore banking and other financial sector activity, the entrepôt trade and the provision of supplies to visiting ships. Exports of local produce are negligible.

Total trade between Gibraltar and UK (British Department of Trade returns, in £1,000 sterling):

	1987	*1988*	*1989*	*1990*
Imports to UK	3,367	4,537	4,560	5,048
Exports and re-exports from UK	49,986	67,944	69,350	69,073

Tourism. The number of tourists in 1989 was 3,984,177 of which 162,438 arrived by air, 78,104 by sea and 3,743,725 by land.

COMMUNICATIONS

Roads. There are 31 miles of roads including 4·25 miles of pedestrian way.

Aviation. Schedule flights are operated by Air Europe and GB Airways to London and Manchester and GB Airways, from Oct. 1990 also operates flights to Tangier.

Shipping. Gibraltar has a government-owned ship repair yard of strategic importance. There is a deep Admiralty harbour of 440 acres. A total of 3,445 merchant ships, 36,179,242 GRT, entered the port during 1989, including 1,932 deep-sea ships of 35,790,002 GRT. In 1989, 4,972 calls were made by yachts, 146,170 GRT and 68 cruise liners called during 1989.

Post and Broadcasting. The local Telephone Service is operated by Gibraltar Nynez Communications, a joint venture of the Government of Gibraltar and Nynez International. The number of telephones (1989) was 14,000. A new Digital System X Exchange became operational in April 1990 with capacity for 14,000 lines. International direct dialling is available to over 130 countries *via* the Gibraltar Telecommunications Ltd (Gibtel) Earth Station and other international circuits. A direct airmail service between Gibraltar and Tangier is run by GB Airways Ltd. Radio Gibraltar broadcasts for 24 hours daily, in English and Spanish, and GBC Television operates for 5 hours daily in English. Number of receivers (31 Dec. 1989), TV, 7,302.

Newspapers. There were (1989) 1 daily and 4 weeklies.

JUSTICE, RELIGION, EDUCATION AND WELFARE

Justice. The judicial system is based on the English system. There is a Court of Appeal, a Supreme Court, presided over by the Chief Justice, a court of first instance and a magistrates' court.

Religion. Religion of civil population mostly Roman Catholic; 1 Anglican and 1 Roman Catholic cathedral and 2 Anglican and 6 Roman Catholic churches; 1 Presbyterian and 1 Methodist church and 4 synagogues; annual subsidy to each communion, £500.

Education. Free compulsory education is provided for children between ages 4 and 15 years. Scholarships are made available for universities, teacher-training and other higher education in Britain. The comprehensive system was introduced in Sept. 1972. There were (1989) 12 primary and 2 comprehensive schools. Primary schools are mixed and divided into first schools for children aged 4-8 years and middle schools for children aged 8-12 years. The comprehensives are single-sex. In addition, there are 2 Services primary schools and 1 private primary school. A new purpose-built Special School for severely handicapped children aged 2-16 years was opened in 1977, and there are 3 Special Units for children with special educational needs (1 attached to a first school, 1 to a middle school and 1 at secondary level), 2 nurseries for children aged 3-4 years and an occupational therapy centre for handicapped adults. Technical education is available at the Gibraltar College of Further Education managed by the Gibraltar Government. In Sept. 1989, there were 1,335 pupils at government first schools, 1,404 at government middle schools, 172 at private and 706 at services schools; 18 at the special school; 975 at the boy's comprehensive school and 907 at the girls' comprehensive. In addition there were 114 full-time and 363 part-time students in the Gibraltar College of Further Education. In 1988–89, government expenditure on education was £6,322,000.

Health. In 1989 there were 2 hospitals with 252 beds and 29 doctors. Total expenditure on medical and health services during year ended 31 March 1989 was £10,000,286.

Further Reading

Gibraltar Year Book. Gibraltar, (Annual)
Ellicott, D., *Our Gibraltar*. Gibraltar, 1975
Green, M. M., *A Gibraltar Bibliography*. London, 1980.—*Supplement*. London, 1982
Hills, G., *Rock of Contention: A History of Gibraltar*. London, 1974
Jackson, W. G. F., *The Rock of the Gibraltarians*. Farleigh Dickinson Univ. Press, 1987
Magauran, H. C., *Rock Siege: The Difficulties with Spain 1964–85*. Gibraltar, 1986
Shields, G. J., *Gibraltar*. [Bibliography] Oxford and Santa Barbara, 1988

GREECE

Capital: Athens
Population: 10·14m. (1990)
GNP per capita: US$5,430 (1990)

Elliniki Dimokratia

(Hellenic Republic)

HISTORY. Greece gained her independence from Turkey in 1821–29, and by the Protocol of London, of 3 Feb. 1830, was declared a kingdom, under the guarantee of Great Britain, France and Russia. For details of the subsequent history to 1947 *see* THE STATESMAN'S YEAR-BOOK, 1957, pp. 1069–70. A coup took place on 21 April 1967, and a military government was formed which suspended the 1952 constitution. King Constantine went abroad in 1967, and a republic was established after referenda in 1973 and 1974. (For details of the monarchy *see* THE STATESMAN'S YEAR-BOOK, 1973–74, p. 1000).

The military government collapsed on 23 July 1974 and a new constitution was introduced in June 1975.

AREA AND POPULATION. Greece is bounded in the north by Albania, Yugoslavia and Bulgaria, east by Turkey and the Aegean Sea, south by the Mediterranean and west by the Ionian Sea. The total area is 131,957 sq. km (50,949 sq. miles), of which the inhabited islands account for 25,042 sq. km (9,669 sq. miles).

The population was 9,740,417 according to the census of 5 April 1981. Estimate (1990) 10,139,000.

Athens is the capital; population of Greater Athens, in 1981, 3,027,331.

The following table shows the prefectures *(Nomoi)* and their population at the time of the 1981 census:

Nomoi	*Area in sq. km*	*Population 1981*	*Capital*	*Population 1981*
Greater Athens [1]	*427*	*3,027,331*	Athens	885,737
			(Piraeus)	196,389
Central Greece and Euboea [2]	*24,391*	*1,099,841*		
Aetolia and Acarnania	5,461	219,764	Missolonghi	10,164
Attica [2]	3,381	342,093	Athens	885,737
Boeotia	2,952	117,175	Levadeia	16,864
Euboea	4,167	188,410	Chalcis	44,867
Evrytania	1,869	26,182	Karpenissi	5,100
Phthiotis	4,441	161,995	Lamia	41,667
Phokis	2,120	44,222	Amphissa	7,156
Peloponnese	*21,379*	*1,012,528*		
Argolis	2,154	93,020	Nauplion	10,609
Arcadia	4,419	107,932	Tripolis	21,311
Achaia	3,271	275,193	Patras	141,529
Elia	2,618	160,305	Pyrgos	21,958
Corinth	2,290	123,042	Corinth	22,658
Laconia	3,636	93,218	Sparta	11,911
Messenia	2,991	159,818	Calamata	41,911
Ionian Islands	*2,307*	*182,651*		
Zante	406	30,014	Zante	9,764
Corfu	641	99,477	Corfu	33,561
Cephalonia	904	31,297	Argostoli	6,788
Leucas	356	21,863	Leucas	6,415

[1] Comprising parts of Attica (2,551,027) and Piraeus (476,304) prefectures.
[2] Excluding figures for the parts of Attica and Piraeus prefectures within Greater Athens.

Nomoi	Area in sq. km	Population 1981	Capital	Population 1981
Epirus	*9,203*	*324,541*		
Arta	1,662	80,044	Arta	18,283
Thesprotia	1,515	41,278	Hegoumenitsa	5,879
Ioannina	4,990	147,304	Ioannina	44,829
Preveza	1,036	55,915	Preveza	12,662
Thessaly	*14,037*	*695,654*		
Karditsa	2,636	124,930	Karditsa	27,291
Larissa	5,381	254,295	Larissa	102,048
Magnesia	2,636	182,222	Volo	71,378
Trikala	3,384	134,207	Trikala	40,857
Macedonia	*34,177*	*2,121,953*		
Grevena	2,291	36,421	Grevena	7,433
Drama	3,468	94,772	Drama	36,109
Imathia	1,701	133,750	Veroia	37,087
Thessaloniki	3,683	871,580	Thessaloniki	406,413
Cavalla	2,111	135,218	Cavalla	56,375
Kastoria	1,720	53,169	Kastoria	17,133
Kilkis	2,519	81,562	Kilkis	11,148
Kozani	3,516	147,051	Kozani	30,994
Pella	2,506	132,386	Edessa	16,054
Pieria	1,516	106,859	Katerini	38,016
Serres	3,968	196,247	Serres	45,213
Florina	1,924	52,430	Florina	12,562
Chalkidiki	2,918	79,036	Polygyros	4,075
Aghion Oros (Mount Athos)	336	1,472	Karyai (locality)	235
Thrace	*8,578*	*345,220*		
Evros	4,242	148,486	Alexandroupolis	34,535
Xanthi	1,793	88,777	Xanthi	31,541
Rhodope	2,543	107,957	Comotini	34,051
Aegean Islands	*9,122*	*428,533*		
Cyclades	2,572	88,458	Hermoupolis	13,876
Lesbos	2,154	104,620	Mytilene	24,115
Samos	778	40,519	Samos	5,575
Chios	904	49,865	Chios	24,070
Dodecanese	2,714	145,071	Rhodes	40,392
Crete	*8,336*	*502,165*		
Heraklion	2,641	243,622	Heraklion	101,634
Lassithi	1,823	70,053	Aghios Nikolaos	8,130
Rethymnon	1,496	62,634	Rethymnon	17,736
Canea	2,376	125,856	Canea	47,338

In 1990 the territory of Greece was administratively reorganized into 13 *regions* comprising in all 51 departments as follows (with their chief towns):

Aegean North (Mytilene): Chios (Chios), Lesbos (Mytilene), Samos (Samos);

Aegean South (Hermoupolis): Cyclades (Hermoupolis), Dodecanese (Rhodes);

Attica (Athens): (Attica is both region and department);

Crete (Heraklion): Canea (Canea), Heraklion (Heraklion), Lassithi (Aghios Nikolaos), Rethymnon (Rethymnon);

Epirus (Ioannina): Arta (Arta), Ioannina (Ioannina), Preveza (Preveza), Thesprotia (Hegoumenitsa);

Greece Central (Lamia): Boeotia (Levadeia), Euboea (Chalcis), Evrytania (Karpenissi), Phokis (Amphissa), Phthiotis (Lamia);

Greece West (Patras): Achaia (Patras), Elia (Pyrgos), Aetolia-Acarnania (Missolonghi);

Ionian Islands (Corfu): Cephalonia (Argostoli); Corfu (Corfu); Leucas (Leucas), Zante (Zante);

Macedonia Central (Thessaloniki): Chalkidiki (Polygyros), Imathia (Veroia), Kilkis (Kilkis), Pella (Edessa), Pieria (Katerini), Serres (Serres), Thessaloniki (Thessaloniki);

Macedonia East and Thrace (Comotini): Cavalla (Cavalla), Drama (Drama), Evros (Alexandroupolis), Rhodope (Comotini), Xanthi (Xanthi);

Macedonia West (Kozani): Florina (Florina), Grevena (Grevena), Kastoria (Kastoria), Kozani (Kozani);

Peloponnese (Tripolis): Arcadia (Tripolis), Argolis (Nauplion), Corinth (Corinth), Laconia (Sparta), Messenia (Calamata);

Thessaly (Larissa): Karditsa (Karditsa), Larissa (Larissa), Magnesia (Volo), Trikala (Trikala).

In 1981 cities (*i.e.*, communes of more than 10,000 inhabitants, including Greater Athens) had 5,475,997 inhabitants (56·2%), towns (*i.e.*, communes with between 2,000 and 9,999 inhabitants), 1,154,567 (11·9%), villages and rural communities (under 2,000 inhabitants), 3,109,853 (31·9%).

The *Monastic Republic of Mount Athos*, the easternmost of the three prongs of the peninsula of Chalcidice, is a self-governing community composed of 20 monasteries. (*See* THE STATESMAN'S YEAR-BOOK, 1945, p. 983.) For centuries the peninsula has been administered by a Council of 4 members and an Assembly of 20 members, 1 deputy from each monastery. The Greek Government on 10 Sept. 1926 recognized this autonomous form of government; Articles 109–112 of the Constitution of 1927 gave legal sanction to the Charter of Mount Athos, drawn up by representatives of the 20 monasteries on 20 May 1924. Article 103 of the 1952 Constitution and Article 105 of the 1975 Constitution confirmed the special status of Mount Athos.

Vital statistics (1988): 107,505 live births; 736 still births; 2,219 illegitimate live births; 47,873 marriages; 92,407 deaths.

The Greek language consists of 2 branches, *katharevousa*, a conscious revival of classical Greek and *demotiki*. Demotiki is the official language both spoken and written.

CLIMATE. Coastal regions and the islands have typical Mediterranean conditions, with mild, rainy winters and hot, dry, sunny summers. Rainfall comes almost entirely in the winter months, though amounts vary widely according to position and relief. Continental conditions affect the northern mountainous areas, with severe winters, deep snow cover and heavy precipitation, but summers are hot. Athens. Jan. 48°F (8·6°C), July 82·5°F (28·2°C). Annual rainfall 16·6" (414·3 mm).

CONSTITUTION AND GOVERNMENT. Voting took place on 29 July 1973 in the referendum to change Greece from a monarchy to a republic and to elect a president. 77·2% of the valid votes were cast for a republican régime.

On 25 Nov. 1973, in a bloodless coup, President Papadopoulos was overthrown and Lieut.-Gen. Phaedon Ghizikis was sworn in. The military dictatorship collapsed on 23 July 1974 and the 1952 Constitution was reintroduced in a modified form. A new Constitution was introduced in June 1975. Parliamentary elections took place on 12 Nov. 1974. A further referendum on the Monarchy took place on 8 Dec. 1974 and 69·2% of the valid votes were cast for an 'uncrowned democracy'.

President: Constantine Karamanlis (b. 1907), elected for 5 years in May 1990.

Parliamentary elections were held in April 1990; 6·45m. votes were cast. Seats gained (and % of vote): New Democracy, 150 (46·9); Pasok (i.e. Panhellenic Socialist Movement), 123 (38·6); Left Coalition, 19 (10·3); independents, 4 (1) and 4 others (2·2), with the support of one of whom New Democracy formed a government. In Feb. 1991 the Cabinet comprised: *Prime Minister, Minister of the Economy*, Constantine Mitsotakis; *Deputy Prime Minister, Minister of Culture,* Tzannis Tzannetakis; *Deputy Prime Minister, Minister of Justice,* Athanassios Kanellopoulos; *Minister to the Prime Minister*, Miltiades Evert; *Foreign Affairs,* Antonis Samaras. *Defence,* Ioannis Varvitsiotis; *Interior,* Sotiris Kouvelas; *Finance,* Ioannis Palaiokrassas; *Agriculture,* Mihalis Papakonstantinou; *Labour,* Aristides Kalatzakos; *Health, Welfare and Social Security,* Marietta Ioannakou; *Education and Religious Affairs,* George Souflias; *Public Order,* Ioannis Vassiliadis; *Industry, Energy and Technology,* Stavros Dimas; *Commerce,* Athanassios Xarhas; *Transport and Communications,* Nikolaos Gelesthasis; *Environment,* Stefanos Manos; *Macedonia and Thrace,* Georgios Tzitzikostas; *Aegean,* Georgios Misailides; Mikis Theodorakis, without portfolio.

National flag: Nine horizontal stripes of blue and white, with a canton of blue with a white cross.

National anthem: Hymn to Freedom, Imnos eis tin Eleftherian (words by Dionysios Solomos, 1824; tune by N. Mantzaros, 1828).

Local government: There are 359 large towns and 5,600 wards with fewer than 10,000 inhabitants. Elections for mayors were held in Nov. 1990. New Democracy won an overall majority.

DEFENCE. In Aug. 1950 the Ministries of War, Marine and Military Aviation were fused into a single Ministry of National Defence. The General Staff of National Defence is directly responsible to the Minister on general defence questions, besides the special staffs for Army, Navy and Air Force. Military service in the Armed Forces is compulsory and universal. Liability begins in the 21st year and lasts up to the 50th. The normal terms of service are Army 21 months, Navy 25 months, Air Force 23 months, followed by 19 years in the First Reserve and 10 years in the Second Reserve.

Army. The Army is organized into 3 Military Regions, comprising 1 armoured, 1 mechanized, 1 para-commando, 6 parachute and 10 infantry divisions; 5 armoured brigades; 2 mechanized brigades, 18 field artillery, 10 anti-aircraft, 2 surface-to-air missile, and 3 army aviation battalions; and 1 independent aviation company. Equipment includes 390 M-47, 1,300 M-48, 149 AMX-30 and 106 Leopard 1A3 main battle tanks. Hellenic Army Aviation has over 150 helicopters, including 43 AB-205 and 64 UH-1H Iroquois, 8 Chinooks, 20 Nardi-Hughes 300s, and 15 Cessna U-17A observation aircraft, 2 Aero Commander and 2 Super King Air transports. Strength (1991) 117,000 (101,000 conscripts), with a further 350,000 reserves. There is also a paramiltary gendarmerie of 26,500 men.

Navy. The Hellenic Navy consists mostly of ex-US ships dating from the 1940s. Current strength includes 10 diesel submarines, 14 destroyers, 7 frigates (2 built in the Netherlands, and commissioned 1981 and 1982) and 16 missile craft dating from the 1970s. Smaller units include 10 fast torpedo craft, 2 coastal and 10 inshore patrol craft, 2 minelayers and 14 mine countermeasure vessels. Substantial amphibious lift is provided by 1 dock landing ship, 7 tank landing ships and 5 medium landing ships plus about 70 landing craft. Major auxiliaries include 2 small replenishment tankers, 1 ammunition transport, 1 water tanker and a purpose-built training ship. There are about 40 minor auxiliaries and service craft. Main bases are at Salamis, Patras, and Soudha Bay (Crete).

The Air Force operates 12 HU-16 Albatross maritime patrol amphibians on naval tasks; and the Navy 14 AB-212 anti-submarine helicopters and 4 Alouettes for search-and-rescue operations and liaison.

Replacement equipment on order includes new frigates to the West German 'MEKO' design, new amphibious ships, and a modernization programme for the submarines.

Personnel in 1990 totalled 19,500 of whom 11,400 were conscripts, on 2 years compulsory service.

The Coastguard and Customs service, 4,000 strong, operate about 100 small patrol craft.

Air Force. The Hellenic Air Force had a strength (1991) of about 26,000 officers and men and 300 combat aircraft, consisting of 3 squadrons of F-4E Phantom air-superiority fighters, 2 squadrons of F-104G Starfighters, 2 squadrons of Mirage F.1 fighters, 3 squadrons of A-7H Corsair II attack aircraft, 3 squadrons of F-5 fighters, 1 squadron of RF-4E reconnaissance fighters and 1 squadron of HU-16B Albatross ASW amphibians (under Navy control). There are also transport squadrons equipped with C-130H Hercules (12), Noratlas, NAMC YS-11, DO28 and C-47 aircraft, 12 Canadair CL-215 twin-engined amphibians, 36 T-2E Buckeye training/attack aircraft, other training and helicopter equipment, and anti-aircraft units equipped with Nike-Hercules and Hawk surface-to-air missiles. Forty F-16 Fighting Falcon and 40 Mirage 2000 fighters are being delivered (1989-90).

The HAF is organized into Tactical, Training and Air Materiel Commands.

INTERNATIONAL RELATIONS

Membership. Greece is a member of UN, EEC, the Council of Europe and the military and political wings of NATO.

ECONOMY

Policy. In 1990 the Government embarked on a large-scale privatization of state industries.

Budget. The 1990 budget was delivered after a 6-month delay in May 1990: Estimated revenue Dr 3,460,000m.; expenditure, Dr 5,530,000m.

Currency. On 11 Nov. 1944 the Greek currency was stabilized at 1 new *drachma* equalling 50,000m. old *drachmai*. Further readjustments took place in 1946, 1949 and 1953. A 'new issue' of notes and coins was put into circulation on 1 May 1954, 1 new drachma equalling 1,000 old drachmai (72 drachmai = £1; 30 drachmai = US$1). The 'new issue' comprises notes of 50, 100, 500 and 1,000 drachmai and metal coins of 1, 2, 5, 10 and 20 drachmai and 10, 20 and 50 *lepta*. Rate of exchange, March 1991, £1 = 314·05 drachmai; US$1 = 165·55.

Banking and Finance. The Bank of Greece *(Trapeza Tis Ellados)* is the bank of issue.

The National Investment Bank for industrial development was set up in Dec. 1963; of its capital of 180m. drachmai, the National Bank provided 60%.

Other important banks are the Ionian and Popular Bank of Greece, the Commercial Bank of Greece, the National Mortgage Bank, the Hellenic Industrial Development Bank, the Investment Bank, the Commercial Credit Bank, the Agricultural Bank, the Bank of Central Greece and the General Bank of Greece.

There is a stock exchange in Athens.

Weights and Measures. The metric system was made obligatory in 1959; the use of other systems is prohibited. The Gregorian calendar was adopted in Feb. 1923.

ENERGY AND NATURAL RESOURCES

Electricity. Total installed capacity of the Public Power Corporation was 7,759,121 kw as at 31 Dec. 1986. Total net production in 1988 was 29,967m. kwh. Supply 220 volts; 50 Hz.

Minerals. Greece produces a variety of ores and minerals, including (with production, 1986, in tonnes) iron-pyrites (150,340), bauxite (2,231,360), nickel (2,196,843), magnesite (943,759), asbestos (3,928,030), chromite (217,979), barytes, marble (white and coloured) and various other earths, chiefly from the Laurium district, Thessaly, Euboea and the Aegean islands. There is little coal, and lignite of indifferent quality (38·41m. tonnes, 1986). Salt production (1986) 160,917 tonnes.

Agriculture. Of the total area (131,957 sq. km) 39,452 sq. km is arable and fallow. Another 52,550 sq. km is grazing land, 29,511 sq. km is forest.
Production (1988, in 1,000 tonnes):

Wheat	2,550	Grapes	1,565
Tobacco	142	Wine	450
Seed cotton	700	Citrus fruit	1,012
Sugar-beet	1,900	Other fruit	2,947
Raisins	160	Milk	1,704
Olive oil	290	Meat	524

Olive production (1988) about 1·5m. tonnes.

Rice is cultivated in Macedonia, the Peloponnese, Epirus and Central Greece. Successful experiments have been made in growing rice on alkaline land previously regarded as unfit for cultivation. The main kinds of cheese produced are white cheese in brine (commercially known as Fetta) and hard cheese, such as Kefalotyri.

Livestock (1988): 800,000 cattle, 1,000 buffaloes, 1,190,000 pigs, 10,816,000 sheep, 3,488,000 goats, 60,000 horses, 83,000 mules, 175,000 asses, 31m. poultry.

Fisheries. In 1987, 15,299 fishermen were active and landed 121,751 tonnes of fish. 10,000 kg of sponges were produced in 1987.

INDUSTRY. Manufacturing contributed 1,145,527m. drachmai to GDP in 1988. The main products are canned vegetables and fruit, fruit juice, beer, wine, alcoholic beverages, cigarettes, textiles, yarn, leather, shoes, synthetic timber, paper, plastics, rubber products, chemical acids, pigments, pharmaceutical products, cosmetics, soap, disinfectants, fertilizers, glassware, porcelain sanitary items, wire and power coils and household instruments.

Production, 1986 (1,000 tonnes): Textile yarns, 230; cement, 12,494; fertilizers, 1,448; ammonia, 294; iron (concrete-reinforcing bars), 857; alumina, 470; aluminium, 176; beer, 310; bottled wine, 112; chemical acids, 1,789; iron wire, 106; glass products, 141; packing materials, 200; cigarettes (1,000 pieces) 27,118; petroleum, 12,369; detergents, 127.

Labour. Of the economically active population in 1987, 970,700 were engaged in agriculture. 715,600 in manufacturing and 1,911,200 in other employment.

Trade Unions. The status of trade unions in Greece is regulated by the Associations Act 1914. Trade-union liberties are guaranteed under the Constitution, and a law of June 1982 altered the unions' right to strike.

The national body of trade unions in Greece is the Greek General Confederation of Labour.

FOREIGN ECONOMIC RELATIONS

Commerce. In 1988 exports totalled (in 1m. drachmai) 776,433·6 including: Clothing, 176,183·1; textile yarn, 40,017·2; petroleum products, 33,161; tobacco, 32,780·5; prepared fruits, 22,758·3; olive oil, 27,763·5; cements, 18,350·6. Imports totalling 1,751,997·8 including: Petroleum oils, crude, 67,660; meat, 24,632; agricultural machinery, 17,394·5; medicines, 12,337.

Exports in 1987 (in 1m. drachmai) were mainly to the Federal Republic of Germany (214,452·6), Italy (142,298·9), France (75,909·4), UK (72,521·7) and USA (59,861·9). Imports were mainly from the Federal Republic of Germany (389,888·6), Italy (215,568·8), France (137,573·7) and the Netherlands (123,752·3).

Total trade between Greece and UK (British Department of Trade returns, in £1,000 sterling):

	1986	*1987*	*1988*	*1989*	*1990*
Imports to UK	308,644	355,320	356,974	395,086	400,476
Exports and re-exports from UK	356,020	444,500	468,032	571,409	682,887

Tourism. Tourists visiting Greece in 1986 numbered 7,025,000. In 1988 they spent the equivalent of US$2,396m.

COMMUNICATIONS

Roads. There were, in 1987, 38,106 km of roads, of which 8,945 were national and 29,161 provincial roads.

Number of motor vehicles in Dec. 1988: 2,215,923, of which 1,507,952 were passenger cars, 688,894 goods vehicles, 19,077 buses.

Railways. In 1987 the State network, Hellenic Railways (OSE), totalled 2,479 km comprising 1,565 km of 1,435 mm gauge, 892 km of 1,000 mm gauge, and 22 km of 750 mm gauge, and carried 3·8m. tonnes of freight and 11·8m. passengers.

Aviation. In 1991 the state-owned Olympic Airways had 38 aircraft, including 6 Boeing 737-400s and 3 Boeing 727s. 6·7m. passengers were carried in 1989. It operates routes from Athens to all important cities of the country, Europe, the Middle East and USA. 34 foreign companies fly to Athens.

Shipping. In Dec. 1988 the merchant navy comprised 2,015 vessels of 21,368,976 GRT. Greek-owned ships under foreign flags totalled 4,164,000 GRT in July 1988.

There is a canal (opened 9 Nov. 1893) across the Isthmus of Corinth (about 4 miles).

Telecommunications. In 1988 there were 3,779 telephone exchanges and 4,300,634 telephones.

Elliniki Radiophonia Tileorasis (ERT), the Hellenic National Radio and Television Institute, is the government broadcasting station. ERT broadcasts 2 TV programmes. Number of receivers: Radio, 5m.; television, 1·4m.

Cinemas (1981). There were 1,150 cinemas.

Newspapers (1987). There were 33 daily newspapers published in Athens, 6 in Piraeus and 100 elsewhere.

JUSTICE, RELIGION, EDUCATION AND WELFARE

Justice. Under the 1975 Constitution judges are appointed for life by the President of the Republic, after consultation with the judicial council. Judges enjoy personal and functional independence. There are three divisions of the courts: Administrative, civil and criminal and they must not give decisions which are contrary to the Constitution. Final jurisdiction lies with a Special Supreme Tribunal.

Some laws, passed before the 1975 Constitution came into force, and which are not contrary to it, remain in force.

Religion. The Christian Eastern Orthodox faith is the established religion to which 98% of the population belong.

The Greek Orthodox Church is under an archbishop and 67 metropolitans, 1 archbishop and 7 metropolitans in Crete, and 4 metropolitans in the Dodecanese. The Roman Catholics have 3 archbishops (in Naxos and Corfu and, not recognized by the State, in Athens) and 1 bishop (for Syra and Santorin). The Exarchs of the Greek Catholics and the Armenians are not recognized by the State.

Complete religious freedom is recognized by the Constitution of 1968, but proselytizing from, and interference with, the Greek Orthodox Church is forbidden.

Education. Public education is provided in nursery, primary and secondary schools, starting at 6 years of age and since 1963 free at all levels.

In 1986–87 there were 5,281 nursery schools with 7,774 teachers and 155,527 pupils; 8,361 primary schools with 37,947 teachers and 865,660 pupils; 1,708 high schools with 25,821 teachers and 450,270 pupils; 1,057 lycea with 17,976 teachers and 267,138 pupils and 506 technical and vocational schools with 7,909 teachers and 118,437 pupils. There were also 7 teacher training schools with 60 teachers and 4,929 students; 12 technical education schools with 4,474 teachers and 73,150 students; 47 vocational and ecclesiastical schools with 675 teachers and 3,760 students and 16 higher education schools with 7,141 teachers and 115,969 students.

In 1982–83 there were 13 universities with 94,574 students and 7,638 lecturers.

Health (1987). There were 454 hospitals and sanatoria with a total of 51,745 beds. There were 33,290 doctors and 9,104 dentists.

DIPLOMATIC REPRESENTATIVES

Of Greece in Great Britain (1A Holland Park, London, W11 3TP)
Ambassador: George D. Papoulias.

Of Great Britain in Greece (1 Ploutarchou St., 106 75 Athens)
Ambassador: Sir David Miers, KBE, CMG.

Of Greece in the USA (2221 Massachusetts Ave., NW, Washington, D.C., 20008)
Ambassador: Christos Zacharakis.

Of the USA in Greece (91 Vasilissis Sophias Blvd., 10160 Athens)
Ambassador: Michael G. Sotirhos.

Of Greece to the United Nations
Ambassador: Constantine Zepos.

Further Reading

Clogg, R., *Greece in the 1980s.* London, 1983
Clogg, M. J. and R., *Greece.* [Bibliography] Oxford and Santa Barbara, 1980

Freris, A. F., *The Greek Economy in the Twentieth Century*. London, 1986
Holden, D., *Greece Without Columns: The Making of the Modern Greeks*. London, 1972
Kousoulas, D. G., *Revolution and Defeat: The Story of the Greek Communist Party*. OUP, 1965
Kykkotis, I., *English–Modern Greek and Modern Greek–English Dictionary*. 3rd ed. London, 1957
Mouzelis, N. P., *Modern Greece*. London, 1978
Pring, J. T., *The Oxford Dictionary of Modern Greek, Greek-English, English-Greek*. OUP, 1965–82
Sarafis, M. and Eve, M. (eds.) *Background to Contemporary Greece*. London, 1990
Tsoukalis, L., *Greece and the European Community*. Farnborough, 1979
Woodhouse, C. M., *The Struggle for Greece, 1941–1949*. London, 1976.—*Karamanlis: The Restorer of Greek Democracy*. OUP, 1982
Xydis, S. G., *Greece and the Great Powers, 1944–47*. Thessaloniki, 1963

GRENADA

Capital: St George's
Population: 110,000 (1989)
GNP per capita: US$1,265 (1988)

HISTORY. Grenada became an independent nation within the Commonwealth on 7 Feb. 1974. Grenada was formerly an Associated State under the West Indies Act, 1967. The 1973 Constitution was suspended in 1979 following a revolution.

On 19 Oct. 1983 the army took control after a power struggle led to the killing of Maurice Bishop the Prime Minister. At the request of a group of Caribbean countries, Grenada was invaded by US-led forces on 24–28 Oct. On 1 Nov. a State of Emergency was imposed which ended on 15 Nov. when an interim government headed by Nicholas Brathwaite was installed.

AREA AND POPULATION. Grenada is the most southerly island of the Windward Islands with an area of 133 sq. miles (344 sq. km); the state also includes the Southern Grenadine Islands to the north, chiefly Carriacou and Petite Martinique, with an area of 13 sq. miles (34 sq. km). The total population (Census, 1988) was 99,205. Estimate (1989), 110,000. The Borough of St. George's, the capital, had 35,742 inhabitants in 1989. In 1989, 84% of the people were black and a further 12% of mixed origins.

Vital statistics (1987): Births, 3,102; deaths, 781.

CLIMATE. The tropical climate is very agreeable in the dry season, from Jan. to May, when days are warm and nights quite cool, but in the wet season there is very little difference between day and night temperatures. On the coast, annual rainfall is about 60" (1,500 mm) but it is as high as 150–200" (3,750–5,000 mm) in the mountains.

CONSTITUTION AND GOVERNMENT. The British sovereign is represented by an appointed Governor-General. There is a bicameral legislature, consisting of a 13-member Senate, appointed by the Governor-General, and a 15-member House of Representatives, elected by universal suffrage. Elections were held for the 15-seat House of Representatives on 13 March 1990. The National Democratic Congress led by Nicholas Brathwaite won 7 seats; Grenada United Labour Party won 4; the National Party, 2 and the New National Party, 2.

Governor-General: Sir Paul Scoon, GCMG, GCVO, OBE.

Prime Minister: Hon. Nicholas Alexander Brathwaite.

National flag: Divided into 4 triangles of yellow, top and bottom, and green, hoist and fly; in the centre a red disc bearing a gold star; along the top and bottom edged red stripes each bearing 3 gold stars; on the green triangle near the hoist a pod of nutmeg.

Local government: There are 7 district councils (including 1 for Carriacou/Petite Martinique) and the Borough Council of St. George's. Local Government Bills had their first reading in Parliament on 24 Oct. 1986. The second reading and final stages of the Bills were postponed. The Department of Local Government has subsequently submitted new proposals for the re-establishment of elected local councils in Grenada, Carriacou and Petite Martinique.

DEFENCE

Army. A People's Revolutionary Army was created in 1979. Personnel about 6,500, organized into 3 infantry battalions and an artillery battery.

There is a Special Services Unit created in 1985.

INTERNATIONAL RELATIONS

Membership. Grenada is a member of the UN, OAS, Caricom, the Commonwealth and is an ACP state of EEC.

ECONOMY

Budget. The 1987 estimates balanced at EC$231·6m. Value added tax has replaced income tax.

Currency. The unit of currency is the *Eastern Caribbean dollar* (XCD). In March 1991, £1 = EC$5·12; US$ = EC$2·70.

Banking. In 1990 there were 5 commercial banks in Grenada: The National Commercial Bank, Barclays Bank International, Grenada Bank of Commerce, Bank of Nova Scotia and the Grenada Co-operative Bank. The Grenada Agricultural Bank was established in 1965 to encourage agricultural development; in 1975 it became the Grenada Agricultural and Industrial Development Corporation. In 1987, bank deposits were EC$269·2m.

ENERGY AND NATURAL RESOURCES

Electricity. Production (1984) 40·5m. kwh.

Agriculture. The principal crops (1988 production in 1,000 lb.) are: Cocoa (3,665), nutmegs (5,510), bananas (21,116), mace (567) and coconuts (540); corn and pigeon peas, citrus, sugar-cane, root-crops and vegetables are also grown, in addition to small scattered cultivations of cotton, cloves, cinnamon, pimento, coffee and fruit trees.

Livestock (1988): Cattle, 5,000; sheep, 17,000; goats, 11,000; pigs, 11,000; poultry (1982), 260,000.

Fisheries. The catch (1989) was 3,769 081 lbs.

FOREIGN ECONOMIC RELATIONS

Commerce. (1987). Total value of imports, EC$239·4m. The exports are cocoa (EC$10·8m.), nutmegs (EC$39·4m.), bananas (EC$11·1m.), mace (EC$7·2m.) and fruit (EC$7m.).

Of exports in 1987, UK took 22·8%; Netherlands, 24·8%; Trinidad, 9·3%; Federal Republic of Germany, 17·9%, Canada, 3·5%; USA, 5%. Of 1987 imports, Trinidad furnished 11·9%; USA, 26·2%; UK, 16·9%; Canada, 6·5%; Netherlands, 2·5%; Federal Republic of Germany, 1·7%.

Total trade between Grenada and UK (British Department of Trade returns, in £1,000 sterling):

	1986	*1987*	*1988*	*1989*	*1990*
Imports to UK	7,011	6,302	6,115	5,924	4,778
Exports and re-exports to UK	8,628	8,772	7,162	9,058	7,822

Tourism. In 1990, there were 307,422 visitors; including 198,320 cruise ship passengers.

COMMUNICATIONS

Roads. The scheduled road mileage is 577, of which 377 have an oiled surface and 210 are graded as third- and fourth-class roads. Vehicles registered (1988) 12,198.

Aviation. A new international airport was inaugurated in Oct. 1984 at Point Salines and has daily connexions to London, New York, Miami and South America *via* nearby islands. Pearls Airport is closed to international air traffic and is only occasionally used for crop spraying purposes. There is a small airstrip on Carriacou.

Shipping. Total shipping for 1987 was 1,004 motor and steamships and 140 sailing and auxiliary vessels, with a total net tonnage of 869,235 and 7,253 respectively.

Telecommunications. A joint company was being formed in 1988 between the Government of Grenada and Cable and Wireless (W.I.) Ltd to replace both the Grenada Telephone Co. Ltd and the Cable and Wireless branch in Grenada. The system is fully digitalized. At 31 Oct. 1990 there were 11,632 lines and 10,930 stations connected. There were (1978) 63,500 radios.

JUSTICE, RELIGION, EDUCATION AND WELFARE

Justice. The Grenada Supreme Court, situated in St George's, comprises a High Court of Justice, a Court of Magisterial Appeal (which hears appeals from the lower Magistrates' Courts exercising summary jurisdiction) and an Itinerant Court of Appeal (to hear appeals from the High Court). The Royal Grenada Police Force numbered 632 in 1990.

Religion. The majority of the population are Roman Catholic; the Anglican and Methodist churches are also well represented.

Education. In 1989 there were 71 pre-primary schools with 3,660 pupils, 58 primary schools with 19,963 pupils, 18 secondary schools with 6,437 pupils, 2 schools for special education and 5 day care centres. The Grenada National College, established in July 1988, incorporates the Institute for Further Education, the Grenada Teachers' College, the Grenada Technical and Vocational Institute, the School of Nursing, the Mirabeau Farm Institute, the Science and Technological Council, the Continuing Education Programme, the Public Service Training Division and the School of Pharmacy. There is also a branch of the University of the West Indies.

Health. In 1990 there was 1 main hospital with 2 subsidiaries. In 1990 there were 36 clinics, 52 doctors, 7 dentists, 28 pharmacists, 36 midwives, 296 nursing personnel and 28 medical technologists (laboratory, radiography and biomedical).

DIPLOMATIC REPRESENTATIVES

Of Grenada in Great Britain (1 Collingham Gdns., London, SW5)
High Commissioner: L. C. Noel.

Of Great Britain in Grenada
High Commissioner: E. T. Davies, CMG (resides in Bridgetown).

Of Grenada in the USA (1701 New Hampshire Ave., NW, Washington, D.C., 20009)
Ambassador: Denneth Modeste.

Of the USA in Grenada (P.O. Box 54, St George's)
Chargé d'Affaires: James Ford Cooper.

Of Grenada to the United Nations
Ambassador: Eugene M. Pursoo.

Further Reading

Davidson, J. S., *Grenada: A Study in Politics and the Limits of International Law.* London, 1987
Ferguson, J., *Grenada: Revolution in Reverse.* London, 1991
Gilmore, W. G., *The Grenada Intervention: Analysis and Documentation.* London, 1984
Heine, J. (ed) *A Revolution Aborted: the Lessons of Grenada.* Pittsburgh Univ. Press, 1990
O'Shaughnessy, H., *Grenada: Revolution, Invasion and Aftermath.* London, 1984
Page, A., Sutton, P. and Thorndike, T., *Grenada and Invasion.* London, 1984
Sandford, G. and Vigilante, R., *Grenada: The Untold Story.* London, 1988
Schoenhals, K., *Grenada*: [Bibliography]. Oxford and Santa Barbara, 1990
Searle, C., *Grenada: The Struggle against Destabilization.* London, 1983
Searle, C. and Rojas, D. (eds) *To Construct from Morning.* Grenada, 1982
Sinclair, N., *Grenada: Isle of Spice.* London, 1987
Thorndike, T., *Grenada: Politics, Economics and Society.* London, 1985

GUATEMALA

Capital: Guatemala City
Population: 9m. (1989)
GNP per capita: US$880 (1988)

República de Guatemala

HISTORY. From 1524 to 1821 Guatemala was a Spanish captaincy-general, comprising the whole of Central America. It became independent from Spain in 1821 and formed part of the Confederation of Central America from 1823 to 1839, when Rafael Carrera dissolved the Confederation and Guatemala became independent.

AREA AND POPULATION. Guatemala is bounded on the north and west by Mexico, south by the Pacific ocean and east by El Salvador, Honduras and Belize, and the area is 108,889 sq. km (42,042 sq. miles). In March 1936 Guatemala, El Salvador and Honduras agreed to accept the peak of Mount Montecristo as the common boundary point.

The census population was 6,054,227 in 1981. Estimate (1989) 9m. (41·6% urban). In 1983, 53% were Amerindian, of 21 different groups descended from the Maya; most of the remainder are mixed Amerindian and Spanish. 45% of the population in 1990 spoke Mayan languages. Density of population, 1989, 82 per sq. km.

Vital statistics, 1984: Births, 302,921; deaths, 75,462; marriages, 31,351.

Guatemala is administratively divided into 22 departments, each with a governor appointed by the President. Population, 1985:

Departments	*Area (sq. km)*	*Population*	*Departments*	*Area (sq. km)*	*Population*
Alta Verapaz	8,686	393,446	Petén	35,854	118,116
Baja Verapaz	3,124	160,567	Quezaltenango	1,951	478,030
Chimaltenango	1,979	283,887	Quiché	8,378	460,956
Chiquimula	2,376	220,067	Retalhuleu	1,858	228,563
El Progreso	1,922	106,115	Sacatepéquez	465	148,574
Escuintla	4,384	565,215	San Marcos	3,791	590,152
Guatemala	2,126	2,050,673	Santa Rosa	2,955	263,060
Huehuetenango	7,403	571,292	Sololá	1,061	181,816
Izabal	9,038	330,546	Suchitepéquez	2,510	327,763
Jalapa	2,063	171,542	Totonicapán	1,061	249,067
Jutiapa	3,219	348,032	Zacapa	2,690	155,496

The capital is Guatemala City with about 2m. inhabitants (1989). Other towns are Quezaltenango (246,000), Puerto Barrios (338,000), Mazatenango (38,319), Antigua (26,631), Zacapa (35,769) and Cobán (120,000).

CLIMATE. A tropical climate, with little variation in temperature and a well marked wet season from May to Oct. Guatemala City. Jan. 63°F (17·2°C), July 69°F (20·6°C). Annual rainfall 53" (1,316 mm).

CONSTITUTION AND GOVERNMENT. A new Constitution, drawn up by the Constituent Assembly elected on 1 July 1984, was promulgated in June 1985 and came into force on 14 Jan. 1986. The President and Vice-President are elected for a term of 5 years by direct election (with a second round of voting if no candidate secures 50% of the first-round votes). The unicameral Legislative Assembly comprises 100 members. At the first round of the presidential elections in Nov. 1990 4 candidates stood: Jorge Carpio (National Centre Union, UCN) gained 25·7% of the votes cast, Jorge Serrano (Movement of Solidarity Action, MAS), gained 24·2%. At the second round in Jan. 1991 some 50% of the 3·2m. electorate voted. Serrano gained the presidency with 68% of the votes.

At the general elections in Nov. 1990 the UCN won 41 of the 116 seats; the Christian Democrats, 29; and MAS, 19. Jorge Serrano formed a government of national unity in Jan. 1991.

President: Jorge Serrano (sworn in 15 Jan. 1991).
Foreign Relations: Alvaro Arzu (Party of National Progress, PAN). *Labour:* Mario Solorzano (Social Democrat). *Defence:* Gen. Luís Mendoza.

National flag: Three vertical strips of blue, white, blue, with the national arms in the centre.
National anthem: ¡Guatemala! Feliz ('Happy Guatemala' words by J. J. Palma; tune by R. Alvarez).

DEFENCE. There is selective conscription into the armed forces for 30 months.

Army. The Army numbered (1991) 41,000, organized in 36 infantry, 2 airborne, 2 air defence, 6 strategic reserve and 1 engineer battalions. Equipment includes light tanks and armoured cars. Reserves, 1991, 35,000. Territorial militia, 600,000.

Navy. A naval element of the combined armed forces operates 9 inshore patrol craft, plus 30 river patrol boats. The force was (1990) 1,200 strong of whom 700 are marines for maintenance of riverine security. Main bases are Puerto Barrios (on the Atlantic Coast), Puerto Quetzal and Puerto San José (Pacific).

Air Force. There is a small Air Force with 10 A-37B and 2 T-33 light attack aircraft, 1DC-6, 10 C-47, 3 F.27 and 7 Israeli-built Arava transports, 10 Pilatus PC-7 turboprop trainers, and a number of Cessna light aircraft and Bell helicopters, including a few armed UH-1 Iroquois. Strength was (1991) about 1,300 personnel and 80 aircraft.

INTERNATIONAL RELATIONS

Membership. Guatemala is a member of the UN, OAS and CACM.

ECONOMY

Planning. The 1988 National Economic Development Plan, called 'Guatemala 2000', calls for sustained GDP growth of at least 6% per annum until 2000.

Budget. 1991 budget estimates balance at Q5,500m.

Currency. The unit of currency is the *quetzal* (CTQ) of 100 *centavos*, established 7 May 1925. There are coins of 25, 10, 5 and 1 *centavos* and notes of 100, 50, 20, 10, 5, 1 and ½ *quetzales* (50 *centavos*). In March 1991, £1 = Q.9·62; US$1 = Q.5·07.

Banking. On 4 Feb. 1946 the Central Bank of Guatemala (founded in 1926 as a mixed central and commercial bank) was superseded by a new institution, the Banco de Guatemala, to operate solely as a central bank. Savings and term deposits at commercial banks were Q.3,885·2m. at 31 July 1988. Total currency in circulation on 31 July 1989 was Q.1,785m.; total net international reserves amounted to Q.50m. on 31 July 1989.

There are 24 banks, including the Banco de Guatemala, Banco Nacional de Desarollo, set up in 1971 to promote agricultural development, its counterpart for small industries (Banco de los Trabajadores) set up in Jan. 1966 with initial capital of US$1·3m. and a subsidiary of Lloyds Bank plc.

Weights and Measures. The metric system has been officially adopted, but is little used in local commerce.

Libra of 16 oz.	=1·014 lb.	*League*	=3 miles
Arroba of 25 libras	=25·35 lb.	*Vara*	=32 in.
Quintal of 4 arrobas	=101·40 lb.	*Manzana*	=100 varas sq.
Tonelada of 20 quintals	=20·28 cwt	*Caballeria* of 64 manzanas	=110 acres
Fanega	=1½ Imp. bushels		

ENERGY AND NATURAL RESOURCES

Electricity. 2,800m. kwh. of electricity were generated in 1989. A large hydro-electric plant was inaugurated in Dec. 1985. Supply 110 and 220 volts; 60 Hz.

Oil. Guatemala began exporting crude oil in 1980; exports, 1984, were valued at US$34m. Production is from wells in Alta Verapaz department from where the oil is piped to Santo Tomas de Castilla. Further exploration is proceeding in the Petén.

Minerals. Mineral production includes zinc and lead concentrates, some antimony and tungsten, a small amount of cadmium and silver; some copper is also being mined. Exports (1988) Q.2m.

Agriculture. The Cordilleras divide Guatemala into two unequal drainage areas, of which the Atlantic is much the greater. The Pacific slope, though comparatively narrow, is exceptionally well watered and fertile between the altitudes of 1,000 and 5,000 ft, and is the most densely settled part of the republic. The Atlantic slope is sparsely populated, and has little of commercial importance beyond the chicle and timber-cutting of the Petén, coffee cultivation of Cobán region and banana-raising of the Motagua Valley and Lake Izabal district. Soil erosion is serious and a single week of heavy rains suffices to cause flooding of fields and much crop destruction.

The principal crop is coffee; there are about 12,000 coffee plantations with 138m. coffee trees on about 338,000 acres, but 80% of the crop comes from 1,500 large coffee farms employing 426,000 workers. Production (1988) 156,000 tonnes. Estimated production, 1990–91: 204,000 tonnes. Banana production was 780,000 tonnes in 1989. Cotton lint production was 44,000 tonnes in 1988. Guatemala is a major producer of chicle gum (used for chewing-gum manufacture in USA). Rubber development schemes are under way, assisted by US funds. Guatemala is one of the largest sources of essential oils (citronella and lemon grass).

Livestock (1988): Cattle, 2·14m.; pigs, 615,000; sheep, 660,000; horses, 112,000; poultry, 15m.

Forestry. The forest area had (1989) an extent of 4m. ha, 37% of the land area. The department of Petén is rich in mahogany and other woods. Production (1980) 11·23m. cu. metres.

Fisheries. Exports were about Q.11·8m. in 1984.

INDUSTRY. The principal industries are food and beverages, tobacco, chemicals, hides and skins, textiles, garments and non-metallic minerals. New industries include electrical goods, plastic sheet and metal furniture.

Trade Unions. There are 3 federations for private sector workers.

FOREIGN ECONOMIC RELATIONS. External debt was US$2,500m. in 1989.

Commerce. Values in US$1,000 were:

	1986	*1987*	*1988*	*1989*
Imports (c.i.f.)	804	1,230	1,250	1,695
Exports (f.o.b.)	825	824	875	1,155

Coffee exports in 1987 were valued at US$400m. mainly to USA and Federal Republic of Germany.

Bananas are still an important export crop, but exports have at times been seriously reduced, partly by labour troubles and by hurricanes. Exports in 1987 were worth US$67m.

Cotton exports in 1984 were valued at US$70·4m. Other important exports (1984) were sugar, US$74·5m.; beef, US$11·6m.

Exports of essential oils were worth US$1·7m. in 1984. Cardamom exports (mainly to Arab countries) were worth US$40m. in 1987).

Total trade between Guatemala and UK (British Department of Trade returns, in £1,000 sterling):

	1986	*1987*	*1988*	*1989*	*1990*
Imports to UK	8,098	7,536	10,678	6,950	42,034
Exports and re-exports from UK	9,288	13,926	15,387	52,324	17,551

Tourism. There were 287,000 foreign visitors in 1986.

COMMUNICATIONS

Roads. In 1989 there were 18,000 km of roads, of which 2,850 are paved. There is a highway from coast to coast via Guatemala City. There are 2 highways from the Mexican to the Salvadorean frontier: the Pacific Highway serving the fertile coastal plain and the Pan-American Highway running through the highlands and Guatemala City. Motor vehicles numbered about 300,000 in 1989.

Railways. The railway system is the government-owned *Ferrocarriles de Guatemala*. All railways are of 914 mm gauge. Total length of all lines was (1989) 953 km. Passengers carried, 1989, numbered 293,000, and freight carried, 426,000 tonnes.

Aviation. The part-government-owned airline, Aviateca, and 2 private airlines furnish both domestic and international services; 6 other airlines handle international traffic from La Aurora airport in Guatemala City.

Shipping. The chief ports on the Atlantic coast are Puerto Barrios and Santo Tomás de Castilla: on the Pacific coast, Puerto Quetzal and Champerico. Total tonnage handled was, 1987, 7m. tons.

Post and Broadcasting. The Government own and operate the telegraph and telephone services; there were 180,000 telephones in Sept. 1988. There are some 70 broadcasting stations. Radio receiving sets in use, 1988, numbered about 1m. There are 4 commercial TV stations, 1 government station and about 250,000 TV receivers. There is also reception by US television satellite.

Cinemas (1989). Cinemas numbered approximately 100.

Newspapers (1989). There are 4 daily newspapers.

JUSTICE, RELIGION, EDUCATION AND WELFARE

Justice. Justice is administered in a Constitution Court, a Supreme Court, 6 appeal courts and 28 courts of first instance. Supreme Court and appeal court judges are elected by Congress. Judges of first instance are appointed by the Supreme Court.

All holders of public office have to show on entering office, and again on leaving, a full account of their private property and income.

Religion. Roman Catholicism is the prevailing faith; but all other creeds have complete liberty of worship. Guatemala has a Roman Catholic archbishopric.

Education. In 1988 there were 11,587 schools with 45,611 teachers and an attendance of 1,331,294 pupils; these figures include private schools. There are 1,237 secondary and other schools having 13,891 teachers and an attendance of 194,484 pupils; the state-supported but autonomous University of San Carlos de Borromeo, founded in 1678, was reopened in 1910 with 7 faculties and schools and there are 4 private universities. Students at the state university (1989) numbered approximately 65,000. All education is in theory free, but owing to a grave shortage of state schools private schools flourish. The 1988 census estimates that 63% of those 10 years of age and older were illiterate.

Social Welfare. A comprehensive system of social security was outlined in a law of 30 Oct. 1946. Medical personnel include about 1,250 doctors and 275 dentists for the whole republic. There are about 60 public hospitals and about 100 dispensaries.

DIPLOMATIC REPRESENTATIVES

Of Guatemala in Great Britain (13 Fawcett St., London, SW10 9HN)
Ambassador: Dr Erwin Blandon.

Of Great Britain in Guatemala (7a Avenida 5-10, Zona 4, Guatemala City)
Ambassador: Justin Nason.

Of Guatemala in the USA (2220 R. St., NW, Washington, D.C., 20008)
Ambassador: John Schwank.

Of the USA in Guatemala (7–01 Avenida de la Reforma, Zone 10, Guatemala City)
Ambassador: Thomas Frank Stroock.

Of Guatemala to the United Nations
Ambassador: Francisco Villagrán DeLeon.

Further Reading

The official gazette is called *Diario de Centro America.*

Banco de Guatemala, *Memoria annual, Estudio económico* and *Boletín Estadístico*
Bloomfield, L. M., *The British Honduras–Guatemala Dispute.* Toronto, 1953
Franklin, W. B., *Guatemala.* [Bibliography] Oxford and Santa Barbara, 1981
Glassman, P., *Guatemala Guide.* Dallas, 1977
Immerman, R. H., *The CIA in Guatemala: The Foreign Policy of Intervention.* Univ. of Texas Press, 1982
Mendoza, J. L., *Britain and Her Treaties on Belize.* Guatemala, 1946
Morton, F., *Xeláhuh.* London, 1959
Plant, R., *Guatemala: Unnatural Disaster.* London, 1978
Schlesinger, S. and Kinzer, S., *Bitter Front: The Untold Story of the American Coup in Guatemala.* London and New York, 1982

National Library: Biblioteca Nacional, 5a Avenida y 8a Calle, Zona 1, Guatemala City.

GUINEA

Capital: Conakry
Population: 6·71m. (1989)
GNP per capita: US$350 (1988)

République de Guinée

HISTORY. Guinea was proclaimed a French protectorate in 1888 and a colony in 1893. It became a constituent territory of French West Africa in 1904. The independent republic of Guinea was proclaimed on 2 Oct. 1958, after the territory of French Guinea had decided at the referendum of 28 Sept. to leave the French Community. Following the death of the first President, Ahmed Sekou Touré on 27 March 1984, the armed forces staged a coup and dissolved the National Assembly.

AREA AND POPULATION. Guinea, a coastal state of West Africa, is bounded north-west by Guinea-Bissau and Senegal, north-east by Mali, south-east by the Côte d'Ivoire, south by Liberia and Sierra Leone, and west by the Atlantic Ocean.

The area is 245,857 sq. km (94,926 sq. miles), and the population, census, 1983, was 5,781,014; estimate, 1989, 6,710,000. The capital is Conakry. In 1989, 22% were urban.

The areas, populations and chief towns of the major divisions are:

	Sq. km	*Census 1983*	*Chief town*	*Census 1983*
Conakry (city)	308	705,280	Conakry	705,280
Guinée-Maritime	43,980	1,147,301	Kindia	55,904
Moyenne-Guinée	51,710	1,595,007	Labé	65,439
Haute-Guinée	92,535	1,086,679	Kankan	88,760
Guinée-Forestière	57,324	1,246,747	Nzérékoré	23,000 [1]

[1] 1972.

The ethnic composition is Fulani (40·3%, predominant in Moyenne-Guinée), Malinké (or Mandingo, 25·8%, prominent in Haute-Guinée), Susu (11%, prominent in Guinée-Maritime), Kissi (6·5%) and Kpelle (4·8%) in Guinée-Forestière, and Dialonka, Loma and others (11·6%).

CLIMATE. A tropical climate, with high rainfall near the coast and constant heat, but conditions are a little cooler on the plateau. The wet season on the coast lasts from May to Nov., but only to Oct. inland. Conakry. Jan. 80°F (26·7°C), July 77°F (25°C). Annual rainfall 172" (4,293 mm).

CONSTITUTION AND GOVERNMENT. Following the coup of 3 April 1984, supreme power rests with a *Comité Militaire de Redressement National*, ruling through a Council of Ministers appointed by the President composed as follows in 1989:

President and Head of CMRN: Brig-Gen. Lansana Conté.

Ministers-Delegate to Presidency: Major Henri Tofani *(National Defence)*, Hervé Vincent Bangoura *(Information, Culture and Tourism)*, Major Henri Foula *(Economy and Finance)*.

Resident (Regional) Ministers: Major Abou Camara *(Guinée-Maritime)*, Lieut.-Col. Sory Doumbouya *(Moyenne-Guinée)*, Major Alpha Oumar Barou Diallo *(Haute-Guinée)*, Major Alhousseini Fofana *(Guinée-Forestière)*.

Local Government: The administrative division comprises the capital Conakry and 33 provinces divided into 175 districts, grouped into 4 regions which correspond to the 4 major geographical and ethnic areas: Guinée-Maritime; Moyenne-Guinée; Haute-Guinée and Guinée-Forestière.

National flag: Three vertical strips of red, gold, green.

Besides French, there are 8 official languages taught in schools: Fulani, Malinké, Susu, Kissi, Kpelle, Loma, Basari and Koniagi.

DEFENCE

Army. The Army of 8,500 men (1991), comprises 1 armoured, 5 infantry, 1 commando and 1 engineer, 1 artillery, 1 air defence and 1 special force battalions. Equipment includes 30 T-34, 8 T-54 and 20 PT-76 tanks. There are also 3 paramilitary forces: People's Militia (7,000), Gendarmerie (1,000) and Republican Guard (1,600).

Navy. A small force of 600 (1990) operate 2 French-built and 7 Soviet-built inshore patrol craft, as well as a number of riverine boats and 2 small landing craft; bases are at Conakry and Kakanda.

Air Force. The Air Force, formed with Soviet assistance, is reported to be equipped with 6 MiG-17 jet-fighters and 2 MiG-15UTI trainers, 4 An-14 and 4 Il-14 piston-engined transports and a Yak-40 jet aircraft for VIP duties, all Russian built, plus a few French-supplied helicopters, piston-engined Yak-18 and L-29 jet trainers. Personnel (1991) 800.

INTERNATIONAL RELATIONS

Membership. Guinea is a member of the UN, OAU and is an ACP state of the EEC.

ECONOMY

Budget. The budget for 1987: balanced at 377,000m. *Guinea francs.*

Currency. The monetary unit is the *Guinea franc*. There are banknotes of 25, 50, 100, 500, 1,000 and 5,000 *Guinea francs*. In March 1991, £1 = 569·31 *francs*; US$1 = 620·22 *francs*.

Banking. In 1986 the Central Bank was restructured and commercial banking returned to the private sector.

ENERGY AND NATURAL RESOURCES

Electricity. Production of electrical energy was 236m. kwh. in 1986.

Minerals. Bauxite is mined at Fria, Boké and Kindia; output (1986) 14·7m. tonnes, alumina 580,000 tonnes. Production of iron ore from the Nimba and Simandou mountains commenced in 1981, following exhaustion of the Kaloum peninsula deposits. Diamond mining output (1985) 105,000 carats of gem diamonds and 7,000 carats of industrial diamonds.

Agriculture. The chief crops (production, 1988, in 1,000 tonnes) are: Cassava, 530; rice, 486; plantains, 350; sugar-cane, 175; bananas, 110; groundnuts, 75; sweet potatoes, 75; yams, 62; maize, 45; palm-oil, 45; palm kernels, 40; pineapples, 20; pulses, 50; coffee, 15; coconuts, 15.

Livestock (1988): Cattle, 1·8m.; sheep, 460,000; goats, 460,000; pigs, 50,000.

Forestry: In 1988, 41% of the country was forested (10m. ha). Round-wood production (1986) 4·4m. cu. metres.

Fisheries: Catch (1986) 30,000 tonnes.

FOREIGN ECONOMIC RELATIONS

Commerce. In 1984 imports totalled 7,542m. *Guinea francs* (32% from France) and exports 11,009m. *Guinea francs* (28% to the USA). Alumina forms about 30% and bauxite 58% of the exports.

Total trade between Guinea and the UK (British Department of Trade returns, in £1,000 sterling):

	1986	*1987*	*1988*	*1989*	*1990*
Imports to UK	23,892	19,538	7,582	10,657	11,508
Exports and re-exports from UK	10,679	10,675	10,106	13,937	11,368

COMMUNICATIONS

Roads. There are 29,000 km of roads and tracks, of which 520 km are bitumenized. In 1985 there were 106,000 cars and 113,000 commercial vehicles.

Railways. A railway connects Conakry with Kankan (662 km) and is to be extended to Bougouni in Mali. A line 134 km long linking bauxite deposits at Sangaredi with Port Kamsar was opened in 1973 (carried 12·3m. tonnes in 1988) and a third line links Conakry and Fria (144 km).

Aviation. There are airports at Conakry and Kankan; in 1982, 131,000 passengers disembarked and embarked.

Shipping. There are ports at Conakry and for bauxite exports at Kamsar (opened 1973). There were (1983) 18 vessels of 6,944 GRT registered in Guinea.

Telecommunications. Telephones, 1981, numbered about 10,000. There were 200,000 radio receivers and 10,000 television receivers in 1986.

Newspapers. In 1979 there was 1 daily newspaper (circulation 20,000).

JUSTICE, RELIGION, EDUCATION AND WELFARE

Justice. There are *tribunaux du premier degré* at Conakry and Kankan, and a *juge de paix* at Nzérékoré. The High Court, Court of Appeal and Superior Tribunal of Cassation are at Conakry.

Religion. In 1980, about 69% of the population was Moslem, 1% Christian (mainly Roman Catholic) and 30% followed tribal religions.

Education. In 1987–88, 290,000 pupils and 7,239 teachers in primary schools, 76,000 pupils and 3,600 teachers in secondary schools, 4,700 students in technical schools and 1,200 in teacher-training colleges and 5,915 in higher education.

Health. In 1976 there were 314 hospitals and dispensaries with 7,650 beds; there were also 277 doctors, 21 dentists, 159 pharmacists, 394 midwives and 1,533 nursing personnel.

DIPLOMATIC REPRESENTATIVES

Of Guinea in Great Britain (resides in Paris)
Ambassador: (Vacant).

Of Great Britain in Guinea
Ambassador: J. E. C. Macrae, CMG (resides in Dakar).

Of Guinea in the USA (2112 Leroy Pl., NW, Washington, D.C., 20008)
Ambassador: Dr Kekoura Camara.

Of the USA in Guinea (2nd Blvd. and 9th Ave., Conakry)
Ambassador: Samuel E. Lupo.

Of Guinea to the United Nations
Ambassador: Zainoul Abidine Sanoussi.

Further Reading

Bulletin Statistique et Economique de la Guinée. Monthly. Conakry
Adamolekun, L., *Sékou Touré's Guinea*. London, 1976
Camara, S. S., *La Guinée sans la France*. Paris, 1976
Taylor, F. W., *A Fulani-English Dictionary*. Oxford, 1932

GUINEA-BISSAU

Capital: Bissau
Population: 966,000 (1990)
GNP per capita: US$190 (1988)

Republica da Guiné-Bissau

HISTORY. Guinea-Bissau, formerly Portuguese Guinea, on the coast of Guinea, was discovered in 1446 by Nuno Tristão. It became a separate colony in 1879. It is bounded by the limits fixed by the convention of 12 May 1886 with France. In 1951 Guinea-Bissau became an overseas province of Portugal. The struggle against colonial rule began in 1963. Independence was declared on 24 Sept. 1973. In 1974 Portugal formally recognized the independence of Guinea-Bissau.

AREA AND POPULATION. Guinea-Bissau is bounded by Senegal in the north, the Atlantic ocean in the west and by Guinea in the east and south. It includes the adjacent archipelago of Bijagós. Area, 36,125 sq. km (13,948 sq. miles); population (census, 1979), 767,739, of whom 125,000 (estimate, 1988) resided in the capital, Bissau; (estimate, 1990) 966,000. Density, 26·7 per sq. km; 30% urban. Annual growth rate (1985–90), 2·1%; infant mortality, 132 per 1,000 live births; expectation of life, 45 years.

The areas and populations (census 1979) of the regions were as follows:

Region	*Sq. km*	*Census 1979*	*Region*	*Sq. km*	*Census 1979*
Bissau City	78	109,214	Gabú	9,150	104,315
Bafatá	5,981	116,032	Oio	5,403	135,114
Biombo	838	56,463	Quinara	3,138	35,532
Bolama-Bijagós	2,624	25,473	Tombali	3,736	55,099
Cacheu	5,175	130,227			

The main ethnic groups were (1979) the Balante (27%), Fulani (23%), Malinké 12%), Mandjako (11%) and Pepel (10%). Portuguese remains the official language, but Crioulo is spoken throughout the country.

CLIMATE. The tropical climate has a wet season from June to Nov., when rains are abundant, but the hot, dry Harmattan wind blows from Dec. to May. Bissau. Jan. 76°F (24·4°C), July 80°F (26·7°C). Annual rainfall 78" (1,950 mm).

CONSTITUTION AND GOVERNMENT. A new Constitution was promulgated on 16 May 1984. The Revolutionary Council, established following the 1980 coup, was replaced by a 15-member Council of State, while in April 1984 a new National People's Assembly was elected comprising 150 Representatives elected by and from the directly-elected regional councils. The sole political movement is the *Partido Africano da Independencia da Guiné e Cabo Verde* (PAIGC), but in Dec. 1990 a policy of 'integral multi-partyism' was announced. The President is Head of State and Government, leading a Council of Ministers which in Oct. 1989 was composed as follows:

President: Brig-Gen. João Bernardo Vieira.
Ministers of State: Col. Iafai Camara *(Armed Forces)*, Dr Vasco Cabral *(Justice)*, Carlos Correia *(Rural Development and Fisheries)*, Tiago Alelua Lopes *(Presidency)*.
Foreign Affairs: Júlio Semedo. *Education, Culture and Sports:* Dr Fidelis Cabral d'Almada. *Commerce and Tourism:* Maj. Manuel dos Santos. *Public Works:* Avito da Silva. *National Security and Public Order:* Maj. José Pereira. *Natural Resources and Industry:* Filinto de Barros. *Finance:* Dr Vítor Freire Monteiro. *Public Health:* Adelino Nunes Correia. *Planning:* (Vacant). *Civil Service and Labour:* Henriqueta Godinho Gomes. *Information and Telecommunications:* Mussa Djassi. *Minister-Governor of Central Bank:* Dr Pedro A. Godinho Gomes.
There are 11 Secretaries of State.

National flag: Horizontally yellow over green with red vertical strip in the hoist bearing a black star.

Local government: The administrative division is in 8 regions (each under an elected regional council), in turn subdivided into 37 sectors; and the city of Bissau, an autonomous sector treated as a separate region.

DEFENCE

Army. The Army consisted in 1991 of 1 artillery and 5 infantry battalions, 1 engineer unit and 1 tank squadron. Equipment includes 10 T-34 tanks. Personnel, 6,800.

Navy. The naval flotilla, based at Bissau, is equipped with 13 inshore patrol craft of diverse origins; Soviet, Chinese and European. Personnel in 1990 totalled 300 officers and men.

Air Force. Formation of a small Air Force began in 1978 with the delivery of a French-built Cessna FTB-337 twin-engined counter-insurgency and general-purpose light transport. It has been followed by 2 Alouette III helicopters and 2 Dornier Do 27 utility aircraft. Personnel (1991) 100.

INTERNATIONAL RELATIONS

Membership. Guinea-Bissau is a member of the UN, OAU and is an ACP state of the EEC.

ECONOMY

Planning. The Development Plan ending 1990 aims at self-sufficiency in food.

Budget. The budget for 1985 balanced at 1,000m. pesos.

Currency. The monetary unit is the *peso* (GWP) of 100 *centavos*. There are coins of 50 *centavos* and 1, 2, 5 and 20 *pesos*, and banknotes of 50, 100, 500 and 1,000 *pesos*. In March 1991, £1 = 1,233·50 *pesos*; US$1 = 650·24 *pesos*.

Banking and Finance. The Banco Nacional da Guiné-Bissau, founded 1976, is the bank of issue and also the commercial bank. There are also state-owned savings institutions.

ENERGY AND NATURAL RESOURCES

Electricity. Production (1986) 28m. kwh.

Minerals. Mining is very little developed although bauxite (200m. tonnes) has been located in the Boé area.

Agriculture. Chief crops (production, 1988, in 1,000 tonnes) are: Groundnuts, 30; sugar-cane, 6; plantains, 25; coconuts, 25; rice, 145; rubber, 23 (1981); palm kernels, 14; millet, 25; palm-oil, 3; sorghum, 35; maize, 15; cashew nuts, 10; timber, hides, seeds and wax.

Livestock (1988): Cattle, 340,000; sheep, 205,000; goats, 210,000; pigs, 290,000; poultry, 1m.

Forestry. Production (1985) 559,000 cu. metres. 33% of the country is forested.

Fisheries. Total catch (1986) 3,620 tonnes. Fishing is an important export industry.

FOREIGN ECONOMIC RELATIONS.

Foreign debt totalled approximately US$423m. in 1989.

Commerce. Imports in 1983, 1,586m. pesos of which 33% from Portugal; exports, 358m. of which 66% went to Portugal, 11% to Senegal and 10% to Guinea. In 1980, fish formed 33% of exports, groundnuts, 24% and coconuts, 17%.

Total trade between Guinea-Bissau and UK (British Department of Trade returns, in £1,000 sterling):

	1986	*1987*	*1988*	*1989*	*1990*
Imports to UK	214	17	22	29	833
Exports and re-exports from UK	1,319	1,152	925	1,185	924

COMMUNICATIONS

Roads. There were (1982) 5,058 km of roads and 4,100 vehicles.

Aviation. There is an international airport serving Bissau at Bissalanca.

Shipping. The main port is Bissau; minor ports are Boloma, Cacheu and Catió. In 1985 vessels entering the ports unloaded 129,000 tonnes.

Telecommunications. In 1986 there were 3,000 telephones and 26,000 radio receivers.

Cinemas. There were 4 cinemas (1988) with a seating capacity of 950.

Newspapers (1984). There was one weekly newspaper, with a circulation of 3,000.

RELIGION, EDUCATION AND WELFARE

Religion. In 1985 about 30% of the population were Moslem and about 5% Christian (mainly Roman Catholic).

Education. There were, in 1984, 81,444 pupils in 658 primary schools with 3,153 teachers; 11,710 pupils in 12 secondary schools with 718 teachers and 1,027 students in 4 technical schools and teacher-training establishments with 107 teachers.

Health. In 1981 there were 17 hospitals and clinics with 1,570 beds and in 1980 there were 108 doctors, 2 dentists, 3 pharmacists, 2 midwives and 56 nursing personnel.

DIPLOMATIC REPRESENTATIVES

Of Guinea-Bissau in Great Britain (resides in Brussels)
Ambassador: (Vacant).

Of Great Britain in Guinea-Bissau
Ambassador: R. C. Beetham, LVO.

Of Guinea-Bissau in the USA
Ambassador: Alfredo Lopes Cabral.

Of the USA in Guinea-Bissau (Ave. Domingos Ramos, Bissau)
Ambassador: William L. Jacobsen, Jr.

Of Guinea-Bissau to the United Nations
Ambassador: Boubacar Toure.

Further Reading

Relatório e Mapas do Movimento Comercial e Maritimo da Guiné. Bolama, Annual
Cabral, A., *Revolution in Guinea*. London, 1969.—*Return to the Source*. New York, 1973
Davidson, B., *Growing from the Grass Roots*. London, 1974
Galli, R., *Guinea-Bissau:* [Bibliography]. Oxford and Santa Barbara, 1991
Gjerstad, O. and Sarrazin, C., *Sowing the First Harvest: National Reconstruction in Guinea-Bissau*. Oakland, 1978
Rudebeck, L., *Guinea-Bissau: A Study of Political Mobilization*. Uppsala, 1974

GUYANA

Capital: Georgetown
Population: 990,000 (1989)
GNP per capita: US$410 (1988)

Co-operative Republic of Guyana

HISTORY. The territory, including the counties of Demerara, Essequibo and Berbice, named from the 3 rivers, was first partially settled by the Dutch West Indian Company about 1620. The Dutch retained their hold until 1796, when it was captured by the English. It was finally ceded to Great Britain in 1814 and named British Guiana. On 26 May 1966 British Guiana became an independent member of the Commonwealth under the name of Guyana and the world's first Co-operative Republic on 23 Feb. 1970.

AREA AND POPULATION. Guyana is situated on the north-east coast of South America on the Atlantic ocean, with Suriname on the east, Venezuela on the west and Brazil on the south and west. Area, 83,000 sq. miles (214,969 sq. km). Estimated population (1989), 990,000. The official language is English, and in 1980 the population comprised 51% (East) Indians, 30% Africans, 10% mixed race, 5% Amerindian and 4% others. The capital is Georgetown, whose metropolitan area had 188,000 inhabitants in 1983; other towns are New Amsterdam, Linden, Rose Hall and Corriverton.

Vital statistics (1988): Birth rate 26·1%; death rate 8%.

Venezuela demanded the return of the Essequibo region in 1963. It was finally agreed in March 1983 that the UN Secretary-General should mediate. There was also an unresolved claim (1984) by Suriname for the return of an area between the New river and the Corentyne river.

CLIMATE. A tropical climate, with rainy seasons from April to July and Nov. to Jan. Humidity is high all the year but temperatures are moderated by sea-breezes. Rainfall increases from 90" (2,280 mm) on the coast to 140" (3,560 mm) in the forest zone. Georgetown. Jan. 79°F (26·1°C), July 81°F (27·2°C). Annual rainfall 87" (2,175 mm).

CONSTITUTION AND GOVERNMENT. A new Constitution was promulgated in Oct. 1980. The National Assembly consists of 65 elected members. Elections are held under the single-list system of proportional representation, with the whole of the country forming one electoral area and each voter casting his vote for a party list of candidates. The legislature is elected for 5 years unless earlier dissolved.

The elections held on 9 Dec. 1985 gave the People's National Congress 42 seats, the People's Progressive Party 8 seats, the United Force 2 seats and the Working People's Alliance 1 seat.

The Cabinet was in Jan. 1991 composed as follows:

President: H. Desmond Hoyte.

First Vice-President and Prime Minister: Hamilton Green.

Vice-President, Deputy Prime Minister, Culture and Social Affairs: Viola Burnham. *Attorney-General:* Keith Massiah. *Deputy Prime Ministers:* Robert H. O. Corbin (*Public Utilities*); William H. Parris (*Planning and Development*). *Foreign Affairs:* Rashleigh Jackson. *Finance:* Carl Greenidge. *Travel and Tourism:* Winston Murray.

National flag: Green with a yellow triangle based on the hoist, edged in white, charged with a red triangle edged in black.

Local government: There are 10 administrative regions: Barima/Waini, Pomeroon/Supernaam, Essequibo Islands/West Demerara, Demerara/Mahaica, Mahaica/Berbice, East Berbice/Corentyne, Cuyuni/Mazaruni, Potaro/Siparuni, Upper Takutu/Upper Essequibo, Upper Demerara/Berbice.

DEFENCE

Army. The Guyana Army had (1991) a strength of 5,100. It comprises 2 infantry, 1 guards, 1 special forces, 1 support weapons and 1 engineer battalions.

Navy. The Maritime Corps is an integral part of the Guyana Defence Force. In 1989 it had 150 personnel and comprised 1 fast inshore patrol craft, a number of armed boats and a utility landing craft.

Air Force. The Air Command has no combat aircraft. It is equipped with light aircraft and helicopters, including 1 Super King Air 200 twin-turboprop transport, 6 Islander twin-engined STOL transports, a Cessna U206F utility lightplane, and 4 Bell 206/212/412 and 2 Mi-8 helicopters. Personnel (1991) 300.

INTERNATIONAL RELATIONS

Membership. Guyana is a member of the UN, Commonwealth, CARICOM, the Non-Aligned Movement and is an ACP state of the EEC.

ECONOMY

Budget. Revenue and expenditure for calendar years (in G$1,000):

	1984	*1985*	*1986*	*1987*	*1988*	*1989*
Revenue	1,537,928	1,200,208	1,667,708	2,004,391	2,296,587	7,012,345
Expenditure	1,585,840	1,562,858	2,551,380	2,976,517	3,528,120	8,796,129

Currency. The unit of currency is the *Guyana dollar* (GYD) of 100 *cents*. There are notes of $1, 5, 10, 20 and 100 and coins of 1-, 5-, 10-, 25- and 50-cent pieces. In March 1991: £1 = 84·38 G$; US$1 = 44·48 G$.

Banking and Finance. The bank of issue is the Bank of Guyana. Of the 5 commercial banks operating in Guyana 2 are foreign-owned (Bank of Baroda and Bank of Nova Scotia) and 3 locally controlled (Guyana National Co-operative Bank, the National Bank of Industry and Commerce and the Republic Bank). The Guyana Agricultural and Industrial Development Bank (Gaibank) for farmers and agri-based industries and the Guyana Co-operative Mortgage Finance Bank for housing. Barclays Bank plc became Guyana Bank of Trade and Commerce in 1988.

ENERGY AND NATURAL RESOURCES

Electricity. Production (1986) 500m. kwh. Supply 110 volts; 60 Hz and 240 volts; 50 Hz.

Minerals. Placer gold mining commenced in 1884, and was followed by diamond mining in 1887. Output of gold was 18,803 oz. in 1988. Production of diamonds was 36,717 stones in 1988. Total production of the 4 grades of bauxite (calcined, chemical, metallurgical and abrasive) was 1·39m. tonnes in 1988. Full-scale production of manganese began in 1960 and other minerals include uranium, oil, copper and molybdenum.

Agriculture. Production, 1989: Sugar, 164,800 tonnes (154,000 tonnes in 1990); rice, 133,900 tonnes. Important products are coconuts, 30,800 tonnes, 1989 and citrus, 7·4m. tonnes. Other tropical fruits and vegetables are grown mostly in scattered plantings; they include mangoes, papaws, avocado pears, melons, bananas and gooseberries. Other important crops are tomatoes, cabbages, black-eye peas, peanuts, carrots, onions, turmeric, ginger, pineapples, red kidney beans, soybeans, eschallot and tobacco. Large areas of unimproved land in the coastal region, which vary in width up to about 30 miles from the sea, are still available for agricultural and cattle-grazing projects.

Livestock estimate (1988): Cattle, 210,000; pigs, 185,000; sheep, 120,000; goats, 77,000; poultry, 15m.

Forestry. In 1988, 16·4m. hectares of the land area (83%) was forested. Production (1986) 4·7m. cu. ft.

Fisheries. Production (1989) of fish, 40,300 tons and shrimp, 1,872 tons.

FOREIGN ECONOMIC RELATIONS

Commerce. Imports and exports (in G$) for calendar years:

	1982	*1983*	*1984*	*1985*	*1986*
Imports	840,442,362	745,000,000	821,300,000	959,500,000	1,618,000,000
Exports	775,544,161	580,000,000	831,300,000	914,400,000	1,092,000,000

Chief imports (1983): Fuel and lubricants, 19,367,367 kg, $272,513,835; milk, 1,386,887 kg, $8,674,714.

Chief domestic exports (1983): Sugar, 210,734 tonnes, $195,814,993; rice, 41,721 tonnes, $64,939,971; bauxite, dried, 779,768 tonnes, $66,629,072; bauxite, calcined, 340,709 tonnes, $136,201,592; alumina, 29,301 tonnes, $7,019,133; rum, 20,442,180 litres, $6,987,107; timber, 49,720 cu. metres, $10,837,689; molasses, 53,938,864 litres, $2,019,371; shrimps, 7,318,145 kg, $14,067,860.

Imports (exclusive of transhipments), 1981, from CARICOM Territories, 35%; from USA, 25%; from UK, 16%; from Canada, 4%; exports (exclusive of transhipments) to UK, 26%; to CARICOM Territories, 17%; to Canada, 5%.

Total trade between Guyana and UK (British Department of Trade returns, in £1,000 sterling):

	1986	*1987*	*1988*	*1989*	*1990*
Imports to UK	55,535	58,502	43,518	54,523	53,892
Exports and re-exports from UK	13,737	15,371	10,590	13,216	15,294

COMMUNICATIONS

Roads. Roads and vehicular trails in the national, provincial and urban systems amount to 8,870 km. Motor vehicles, as of 31 Dec. 1987, totalled 53,446, including 8,401 passenger cars, 3,682 lorries and vans, 8,958 tractors and trailers, and 15,893 motor cycles. The main road on the Atlantic Coast, some 290 km (180 miles) long extends from Charity on the Pomeroon River to Crabwood Creek on the Corentyne, there are two unbridged gaps made by the Berbice and Essequibo Rivers, and the banks of the Demerara River are linked by a 1,853 metre (6,074 ft) floating bridge.

Railways. There is a government-owned railway in the North West District, while the Guyana Mining Enterprise operates a standard gauge railway of 133 km from Linden on the Demerara River to Ituni and Coomacka.

Aviation. Guyana Airways Corporation operates 11 flights weekly on its international service and 21 flights locally. In 1985 Guyana Airways Corporation carried 108,936 passengers on its international service and 59,113 passengers locally. Other services in operation: British Airways 4 times weekly to the Caribbean, Europe and North America: PANAM 3 times weekly to North, Central and South America: Air France, to and from Guadeloupe, Paramaribo and Cayenne 4 times a week; British West Indian Airways, Ltd, to and from Trinidad twice a week, providing direct connexion with New York and London; Cubana Airlines once a fortnight; Suriname Airways and Tropical Airways once weekly. The International Airport at Timehri serves Arrow Air Airlines, BWIA, Cubana Airways, and Suriname Airways.

Shipping. There are 217 nautical miles of river navigation. There are ferry services across the mouths of the Demerara, Berbice and Essequibo rivers, the last providing a link between the islands of Leguan and Wakenaam and the mainland at Adventure, and a number of coastal and river-boat services carrying both passengers and cargo. A number of launch services are operated in the more remote areas by private concerns.

Georgetown harbour, about ½ mile wide and 2½ miles long, has a minimum depth of 24 ft. New Amsterdam harbour is situated at the mouth of the Berbice River;

there are wharves for coastal vessels only. Bauxite is loaded on ocean-going freighters at Mackenzie, 67 miles up the Demerara River, and at Everton on the Berbice River, about 10 miles from the mouth of the waterway. The Essequibo River has several timber-loading berths ranging from 20 to 40 ft. Springlands on the Corentyne River is the point of entry and departure of passengers travelling by launch services to and from Suriname. In 1984 the merchant marine comprised 84 vessels of 20,248 GRT.

Telecommunications. The inland public telegraph and radio communication services are operated and maintained by the Telecommunication Corporation. On 31 Aug. 1988 there were 57 post offices and 28 agencies.

The telephone exchanges had at 31 Aug. 1988 a total of 28,450 direct exchange lines with (1988), 20,000 telephone instruments. The number of route miles in the coastal and inland areas was 2,982 km. 39 land-line stations were maintained at post offices in the coastal area, and 8 telegraph stations in the interior provide communication with the coastal area through a central telegraph office in Georgetown.

The Guyana Broadcasting Corporation, which came into operation on 1 July 1980, has 2 channels. In 1985 there were 350,000 radio receivers.

Cinemas (1989). There are 51 cinemas.

Newspapers (1989). There is 1 daily newspaper with a circulation of 60,000, 1 twice-weekly paper with an estimated circulation of 40,000 and 4 weekly papers with a combined circulation of 40,000.

JUSTICE, RELIGION, EDUCATION AND WELFARE

Justice. The law, both civil and criminal, is based on the common and statute law of England, save that the principles of the Roman–Dutch law have been retained in respect of the registration, conveyance and mortgaging of land.

The Supreme Court of Judicature consists of a Court of Appeal and a High Court.

Religion. In 1980, 34% of the population were Hindu, 34% Protestant, 18% Roman Catholic and 9% Moslem.

Education. In Sept. 1976 the Government assumed total responsibility for education from nursery school to university. Private education was abolished. In Sept. 1988, the total number of schools was 866: Nursery, 351; primary, 432; community high, 37; general secondary, 55.

There are now 3 technical and vocational schools and 2 schools for the teaching of home economics and domestic crafts. Training in co-operatives is provided by the Kuru-Kuru Co-operative College and agriculture by the Guyana School of Agriculture and there is one teacher training complex, the Cyril Potter College of Education. In 1986-87 there were 6,440 students at these post-secondary institutions. Higher education is also provided by the University of Guyana which was established in 1963 with faculties of medicine, natural science, social science, art, technology and education as well as first year students in law. There were 2,250 students in 1987–88. The total number of pupils in all schools was 211,315 in 1986-87.

Health. In 1989 there were 213 health facilities including hospitals. There were (1989) 111 doctors, 15 dentists, 29 pharmacists, 172 midwives and 854 nursing personnel.

DIPLOMATIC REPRESENTATIVES

Of Guyana in Great Britain (3 Palace Ct., London, W2 4LP)
High Commissioner: Cecil S. Pilgrim (accredited 5 Dec. 1986).

Of Great Britain in Guyana (44 Main St., Georgetown)
High Commissioner: R. D. Gordon.

Of Guyana in the USA (2490 Tracy Pl., NW, Washington, D.C., 20008)
Ambassador: Dr Cedric Hilburn Grant.

Of the USA in Guyana (31 Main St., Georgetown)
Ambassador: Theresa A. Tull.

Of Guyana to the United Nations
Ambassador: Samuel R. Insanally.

Further Reading

Baber, C. and Jeffrey, H. B., *Guyana: Politics, Economics and Society.* London, 1986

Braveboy-Wagner, J. A., *The Venezuela-Guyana Border Dispute: Britain's Colonial Legacy in Latin America.* London, 1984

Chambers, F., *Guyana.* [Bibliography] Oxford and Santa Barbara, 1989

Daly, P. H., *From Revolution to Republic.* Georgetown, 1970

Daly, V. T., *A Short History of the Guyanese People.* Rev. ed. London, 1975

Hope, K. R., *Development Policy in Guyana: Planning, Finance and Administration.* London, 1979

Latin American Bureau, *Guyana: Fraudulent Revolution.* London, 1984

Sanders, A., *The Powerless People.* London, 1987

Spinner, T. J., *A Political and Social History of Guyana, 1945–83.* Epping, 1985

HAITI

Capital: Port-au-Prince
Population: 5·7m. (1988)
GNP per capita: US$352 (1988)

République d'Haïti

HISTORY. Haiti occupies the western third of the large island of Hispaniola which was discovered by Christopher Columbus in 1492. The Spanish colony was ceded to France in 1697 and became her most prosperous colony. After the extirpation of the Indians by the Spaniards (by 1533) large numbers of African slaves were imported whose descendants now populate the country. The slaves obtained their liberation following the French Revolution, but subsequently Napoleon sent his brother-in-law, Gen. Leclerc, to restore French authority and re-impose slavery. Toussaint Louverture, the leader of the slaves who had been appointed a French general and governor, was kidnapped and sent to France, where he died in gaol. However, the resistance of the Haitian troops and the ravages of yellow fever forced the French to evacuate the island and surrender to a blockading British squadron.

The country declared its independence on 1 Jan. 1804, and its successful leader, Gen. Jean-Jacques Dessalines, proclaimed himself Emperor of the newly-named Haiti. After the assassination of Dessalines (1806) a separate régime was set up in the north under Henri Christophe, a Black general who in 1811 had himself proclaimed King Henry. In the south and west a republic was constituted, with Alexander Pétion as its first President. Pétion died in 1818 and was succeeded by Jean-Pierre Boyer, under whom the country became re-united after Henry had committed suicide in 1820. From 1822 to 1844 Haiti and the eastern part of the island (later the Dominican Republic) were united. After one more monarchical interlude, under the Emperor Faustin (1847–59), Haiti has been a republic. From 1915 to 1934 Haiti was under United States occupation.

Following a military coup in 1950, and subsequent uprisings, Dr François Duvalier was elected President on 22 Oct. 1957 and subsequently became President for Life in 1964. He died on 21 April 1971 and was succeeded as president for life by his son, Jean-Claude Duvalier who fled the country on 7 Feb. 1986. Gen. Henry Namphy formed a Council of Government. In Jan. 1988 Leslie Manigat was elected president, but Namphy again seized power in June 1988. In Sept. 1988 he was deposed and replaced by the military government of Lieut.-Gen. Prosper Avril. In March 1990 Ertha Pascal-Trouillot became head of an interim government. Father Jean-Bertrand Aristide was elected president in Dec. 1990

A former Tonton Macoute chief, Roger Lafontant, attempted a coup on 7 Jan. 1991.

AREA AND POPULATION. The area is 27,750 sq. km (10,700 sq. miles), of which about three-quarters is mountainous. The population at the census in 1982 was 5,053,792 of which 21% urban and 48·5% male. Estimate (1988) 5,658,124, of which 28% urban.

The areas and populations of the 9 *départements* are as follows:

Département	*Sq. km*	*1988*	*Chief town*	*1988*
Nord-Ouest	2,094	326,361	Port-de-Paix	135,374
Nord	2,175	610,282	Cap Haïtien	133,233
Nord-Est	1,698	199,336	Fort-Liberté	34,043
L'Artibonite	4,895	801,115	Gonaïves	144,081
Centre	3,597	406,608	Hinche	122,003
Ouest	4,595	1,869,805	Port-au-Prince	1,143,626
Sud-Est	2,077	393,554	Jacmel	216,600
Sud	2,602	531,255	Les Cayes	214,606
Grande Anse	3,100	519,808	Jérémie	152,081

The Île de la Gonave, some 40 miles long, lies in the gulf of the same name. Among other islands is La Tortue, off the north peninsula. 95% of the population is black, with an important minority of mulattoes and only about 5,000 white residents, almost all foreign.

The official language is French, but 90% of the people speak Créole.

CLIMATE. A tropical climate, but the central mountains can cause semi-arid conditions in their lee. There are rainy seasons from April to June and Aug. to Nov. Hurricanes and severe thunderstorms can occur. The annual temperature range is small. Port-au-Prince. Jan. 77°F (25°C), July 84°F (28·9°C). Annual rainfall 53" (1,321 mm).

CONSTITUTION AND GOVERNMENT. The 1987 Constitution, ratified by a referendum, provides for a bicameral legislature (*Chamber of Deputies, Senate*), and an executive *President*.

At the presidential, parliamentary and local elections of Dec. 1990 the electorate was some 3m.; turn-out was estimated at 55% by international observers. Father Jean-Bertrand Aristide (b. 1957) was elected president by about 66% of votes cast. He was sworn in on 7 Feb. 1991.

Prime Minister, Interior, Defence: René Préval. *Foreign:* Marie-Louise Fabien-Jean-Louis. *Finance and Economy:* Marie-Michèle Rey. *Information and Coordination:* Marie-Laurence Lassègue. *Justice:* Bayard Vincent. *Public Works, Transport and Communications:* Frantz Verella. *Agriculture:* François Séverin. *Commerce and Industry:* Smarck Michel. *Planning, External Co-operation and Civil Service:* Renaud Bernardin. *Public Health and Population:* Daniel Henrys.

National flag: Horizontally blue over red with the national arms on a white panel in the centre.

National anthem: 'La Dessalinienne': Pour le pays, pour les ancêtres ('For the country, for the ancestors'; words by J. Lhérisson; tune by N. Geffrard, 1903).

DEFENCE. The Haitian Defence Force (*Forces Armées d'Haiti*) totalling about 7,600 men, was divided into Army, Navy, and Air Force. The President is Commander-in-Chief and appoints the officers.

Army. Total strength, about 7,000 (1991), organized into 9 military departments. Three of the Departments are in Port-au-Prince and consist of the Presidential Guard, 1 infantry battalion, 1 airport security company, 2 artillery battalions and 6 artillery elements.

Navy. The Coast Guard of (1990) 150 personnel operates 2 coastal patrol craft and some boats; all are based at Port-au-Prince.

Air Force. Personnel strength was (1991) about 150, with (1987) about 30 aircraft of some 12 varieties. They include 7 Summit/Cessna O2-337 Sentry twin piston-engined counter-insurgency aircraft, 1 DC-3, 6 light transports, 14 training and liaison aircraft, including 4 S.211 jet trainers and 4 turboprop-powered SF.260 TPs.

INTERNATIONAL RELATIONS

Membership. Haiti is a member of UN and OAS and is an ACP state of the EEC.

ECONOMY

Budget. The budget for the fiscal year ending 30 Sept. 1991 is 1,350m. gourdes.

Currency. The unit of currency is the *gourde* (HTG) of 100 *centimes*. Its value is fixed at 5 *gourdes* = US$1. In March 1991, £1 = 9·49 *gourdes*. There are copper–nickel coins for 50, 20, 10 and 5 *centimes* and copper–zinc–nickel coins of 10 and 5 centimes.

Banking and Finance. Banque Nationale de Credit, owned by the State, was established in 1982. US dollars may be included in the minimum required reserves. The Citibank, the Bank of Nova Scotia, the Bank of Boston, the Banque de l'Union Haïtienne (mainly local capital with participation from American, Canadian and Dominican Republic Banks), Banque Nationale de Paris and SOGEBANK (formerly the Royal Bank of Canada, now Haitian-owned) have branches. The Banque Nationale de la République d'Haïti is the central bank and bank of issue.

Weights and Measures. The metric system and British imperial and US measures are in use.

ENERGY AND NATURAL RESOURCES

Electricity. Production (1988) 337m. kwh. Supply 110 and 220 volts; 60 Hz.

Minerals. Copper exists but is at present uneconomic to exploit. Haiti may possess undeveloped mineral resources of oil, gold, silver, antimony, sulphur, coal and lignite, nickel, gypsum and porphyry.

Agriculture. Only one-third of the country is arable and most people own the tiny plots they farm; the resulting pressure of population is the main cause of rural poverty.

The occupations of Haiti are 90% agricultural, carried on in 7 large plains, from 200,000 to 25,000 acres, and in 15 smaller plains down to 2,000 acres. Irrigation is used in some areas. Haiti's most important product is coffee of good quality, classified as 'mild', and grown by peasants. Production in 1989 totalled about 38,400 tonnes. The second most important crop is sugar-cane, used to make sugar and rum and other spirits. Sisal is grown, much of it for export as or for cordage. New types of cotton are being tried with success. New varieties of rice should significantly boost future production, especially in the Artibonite Valley. Output in 1989 (in 1,000 tonnes): Plantains, 499; sorghum, 142; rice, 119; beans, 57; cocoa, 2; and in 1988: Sugar-cane, 3,000; mangoes, 355; maize, 145; bananas, 230; sisal, 5; cotton, 6; sweet potatoes, 300.

Essential oils from vetiver, neroli and amyris are important. Cattle and horse breeding are encouraged.

Livestock (1988); Cattle, 1,545,000; sheep, 94,000; goats, 1·2m.; horses, 430,000; poultry, 12m.

Fisheries. Production (1986) 8,000 tonnes.

INDUSTRY. Light manufacturing industries assembling or finishing goods (mainly clothing, leather goods and electrical/electronic components) for re-export constitute the fastest growing sector. Soap factories produce laundry soap, toilet soap and detergent. A cement factory located near the capital produced 265,000 tonnes in 1987. A steel plant making rods, beams and angles was opened in 1974. There are also a pharmaceutical plant, a tannery, a plastics plant, 2 paint works, 5 shoe factories, a large factory producing enamel cookingware, 2 pastamaking factories, a tomato cannery and a flour-mill, all located in or near Port-au-Prince.

FOREIGN ECONOMIC RELATIONS

Commerce. In 1989 exports were US$184m. and imports, US$314m. The leading imports are petroleum products, foodstuffs, textiles, machinery, animal and vegetable oils, chemicals, pharmaceuticals, raw materials for transformation industries and vehicles.

Total trade between Haiti and UK (British Department of Trade returns, in £1,000 sterling):

	1986	*1987*	*1988*	*1989*	*1990*
Imports to UK	899	621	844	803	1,271
Exports and re-exports from UK	5,147	5,327	6,760	6,566	6,807

Tourism. In 1989, 68,000 tourists visited Haiti.

COMMUNICATIONS

Roads. Total length of roads is some 4,000 km, little of which is practicable in ordinary motors in the rainy season. There were (1984) about 50,000 vehicles.

Railways. The only railway is owned by the Haitian American Sugar Company.

Aviation. An airport capable of handling jets was opened at Port-au-Prince in 1965. US and French carriers provide daily direct services to New York, Miami, Jamaica, Puerto Rico and the French Antilles. There are also services to the Dominican Republic and the Netherlands Antilles. A Haitian company provides a cargo service to the US and Puerto Rico. Air services connecting Port-au-Prince with other Haitian towns are operated by Haiti Air Inter.

Shipping. US, French, German, Dutch, British, Canadian and Japanese lines connect Haiti with the USA, Latin America (except Cuba), Canada, Jamaica, Europe and the Far East.

Telecommunications. Most principal towns are connected by the government telegraph system, telephones and wireless.

The telephone company, of which the Haitian Government is now the majority stockholder, is in process of being modernized. Telephone subscribers totalled 34,000 in 1984.

In 1982 there were 105,000 radio and 65,000 television receivers.

Cinemas (1984). There were 10 cinemas in Port-au-Prince.

Newspapers (1989). There were 6 daily newspapers in Port-au-Prince, also a monthly in English and 1 weekly newspaper in Cap Haïtien.

JUSTICE, RELIGION, EDUCATION AND WELFARE

Justice. Judges, both of the lower courts and the court of appeal, are appointed by the President. The legal system is basically French. The divorce law has recently been amended to permit parties to obtain 'quick and painless' divorces at a moderate cost, in the hope of attracting the US trade, now that the Mexican 'divorce mills' have closed down. This has developed a useful flow of dollar revenue.

Police. The Police number about 1,200 in Port-au-Prince and are part of the armed forces.

Religion. Since the Concordat of 1860, the official religion is Roman Catholicism, under an archbishop with 5 suffragan bishops. There are still quite a number of foreigners, French and French Canadians mainly, among the clergy but the first Haitian archbishop took office in 1966. The Episcopal Church now has its first Haitian bishop who was consecrated in 1971. Other Christian churches number perhaps 10% of the population. The folk religion is Voodoo.

Education. Education is divided into primary (6 years, compulsory), secondary (7 years) and university/higher education. The school system is based on the French system and instruction is in French. In 1990 Educational Reform calling for basic schooling (9 years, compulsory) using Creole and French, with a 3-year secondary cycle, was being implemented.

In 1988 primary schools had 24,800 teachers and 983,000 pupils and 455 secondary schools had 8,400 teachers and 177,000 pupils.

Higher education is offered at the University of Haiti with 5,000 students in 1988.

Health. There were, in 1989, 944 doctors and 98 dentists in practice, and 87 hospitals and health centres with 4,566 beds.

DIPLOMATIC REPRESENTATIVES

Of Haiti in Great Britain. The Embassy closed on 30 March 1987.

Of Great Britain in Haiti
Ambassador: D. F. Milton, CMG (resides in Kingston).

Of Haiti in the USA (2311 Massachusetts Ave., NW, Washington, D.C., 20008)
Ambassador: Louis Harold Joseph.

Of the USA in Haiti (Harry Truman Blvd., Port-au-Prince)
Ambassador: Alvin P. Adams, Jr.

Of Haiti to the United Nations
Ambassador: (Vacant).

Further Reading

The official gazette is *Le Moniteur*.

Revue Agricole d'Haïti. From 1946. Quarterly
Bellegarde, D., *Histoire du Peuple Haïtien*. Port-au-Prince, 1953
Chambers, F. J., *Haiti*. [Bibliography] Oxford and Santa Barbara, 1983
Ferguson, J., *Papa Doc, Baby Doc: Haiti and the Duvaliers*. Oxford, 1987
Laguerre, M. S., *The Complete Haitiana*. [Bibliography] London and New York, 1982.—*Voodoo and Politics in Haiti*. London, 1989
Lawless, R., *Haiti: a Research Guide*. New York, 1990
Lundahl, M., *The Haitian Economy: Man, Land and Markets*. London, 1983
Nicholls, D., *From Dessalines to Duvalier: Race, Colour and National Independence in Haiti*. CUP, rev., 1988.—*Haiti in Caribbean Context: Ethnicity, Economy and Revolt*. London, 1985
Wilentz, A., *The Rainy Season: Haiti since Duvalier*. New York, 1989

National Library: Bibliothèque Nationale, Rue du Centre, Port-au-Prince.

HONDURAS

Capital: Tegucigalpa
Population: 4·44m. (1988)
GNP per capita: US$530 (1990)

República de Honduras

HISTORY. Honduras celebrates 15 Sept. as the anniversary of its national independence from Spain in 1821. On 5 Nov. 1838 Honduras declared itself an independent sovereign state, free from the Federation of Central America, of which it had formed a part.

AREA AND POPULATION. Honduras is bounded in the north by the Caribbean, east and south-east by Nicaragua, west by Guatemala, south-west by El Salvador and south by the Pacific ocean. The area is 112,088 sq. km (43,277 sq. miles). At the Census of 1988 the population was 4,443,721 (2,237,498 female). 1·68m. of the population was urban in 1988. Population density, 37·2 per sq. km. in 1988.

The chief cities (populations in 1,000, 1988) were Tegucigalpa, the capital (678·7), San Pedro Sula (460·6), El Progreso (64·7), Choluteca (68·5), Danlí (20·2) and the Atlantic coast ports of La Ceiba (68·2), Puerto Cortés (43·3) and Tela (28·4); other towns include Olanchito (14·1), Juticalpa (14·3), Comayagua (32·9), Siguatepeque (27·7) and Santa Rosa de Copán (21·2).

Areas and 1988 census populations of the 18 departments and the Central District (Tegucigalpa):

Department	*Sq. km*	*1988*	*Department*	*Sq. km*	*1988*
Atlántida	4,251	238,742	Islas de la Bahía	261	22,062
Choluteca	4,211	295,484	La Paz	2,331	105,927
Colón	8,875	149,677	Lempira	4,290	177,055
Comayagua	5,196	239,859	Ocotepeque	1,680	74,276
Copán	3,203	219,455	Olancho	24,350	283,852
Cortés	3,954	662,772	Santa Bárbara	5,115	278,868
El Paraíso	7,218	254,295	Valle	1,565	119,645
Francisco Morazán	6,298	828,274	Yoro	7,939	333,508
Gracias a Dios	16,630	34,970	Central District	1,648	576,661
Intibucá	3,072	124,681			

The official language is Spanish. The Spanish-speaking population is of mixed Spanish and Amerindian descent. There are some 35,000 aborigines, mainly Miskito, Paya and Xicaque Indians with some African admixture.

Over the period 1974-88, population growth has averaged 3%: Infant mortality rate in 1985 was 70 per 1,000 live births; life expectancy, 62.

CLIMATE. The climate is tropical, with a small annual range of temperature but with high rainfall. Upland areas have two wet seasons, from May to July and in Sept. and Oct. The Caribbean Coast has most rain in Dec. and Jan. and temperatures are generally higher than inland. Tegucigalpa. Jan. 66°F (19°C), July 74°F (23·3°C). Annual rainfall 64" (1,621 mm).

CONSTITUTION AND GOVERNMENT. The Executive, Legislature and Judiciary have formally separate powers but the system is strongly Presidential in character. The present Constitution came into force in 1982.

The President is elected for a 4-year term. Members of the National Congress and municipal councillors are elected on a proportional basis, according to votes cast for the Presidential candidate of their party.

The Nov. 1989 election was won by Rafael Leonardo Callejas (sworn in on 27 Jan. 1990) for the National Party. The National Party gained 71 seats in the National Congress, the Liberals 55 and PINU-SD 2.

National flag: Three horizontal stripes of blue, white, blue, with 5 blue stars in the centre.

National anthem: Tu bandera ('Thy Banner'; words by A. C. Coello; tune by C. Hartling).

Local government: Honduras comprises a Central District (containing the cities of Tegucigalpa and Comayaguela) and 18 departments *'departamentos'*; (each administered by an appointed Governor), sub-divided into 289 municipalities.

DEFENCE. Conscription is for 24 months.

Army. The Army consists of 4 infantry and 1 artillery brigade and 1 engineer, 1 special forces and 1 air defence battalion. Equipment includes 12 Scorpion light tanks. Strength (1991) 15,600 (11,500 conscripts). There is also a paramilitary Public Security Force of 5,000 men.

Navy. A small flotilla operates 5 US-built fast inshore patrol craft, some 6 other inshore craft, a utility landing craft and a number of boats. Personnel (1990), 1,200, of whom 900 are conscripts, and the total includes 600 marines. Bases are at Puerto Cortés and Amapala.

Air Force. Equipment includes 12 F-5E/F Tiger IIs and a few F-86 fighters, 12 A-37B jet light attack aircraft, 4 Spanish-built CASA C-101BB armed jet trainers, 3 four-engined Douglas and Lockheed transports, 6 C-47, 4 Israeli-built Arava and 2 Westwind transports, about 30 helicopters and Tucano and T-41A trainers. Total strength was (1991) about 2,100 personnel (800 conscripts), of whom many are civilian maintenance staff.

INTERNATIONAL RELATIONS

Membership. Honduras is a member of the UN and OAS.

ECONOMY

Budget. Expenditure approved for 1990 was 3,504m. lempiras.

Total external debt (31 Dec. 1989) was US$3,300m.

Currency. The unit of the monetary system is the *lempira* (HNL) also known as a *peso*, comprising 100 *centavos*. Notes are issued by the Banco Central de Honduras which has the sole right to issue, in denominations of 100, 50, 20, 10, 5, 2 and 1 *lempiras*. Coins in circulation are 50 and 20 *centavos* in silver, 10 and 5 *centavos* in cupro-nickel and 2 and 1 *centavos* in copper. There was a devaluation of 50% in 1990.

Rate of exchange, March 1991: £1 = 10·06 *lempiras;* US$1 = 5·30 *lempiras.*

Banking. The central bank of issue is the Banco Central de Honduras. Sixteen other banks belong to the central clearing system. Banco Atlántida is the largest. Banco de Londres y Montreal has branches in Tegucigalpa, San Pedro Sula, Comayaguela and La Ceiba. Banco de Honduras is controlled by Citibank. The Central American Bank for Economic Integration (BCIE) has its head office in Tegucigalpa.

Weights and Measures. The metric system has been legal since 1 April 1897, although there are still some minor traces of the Imperial and old Spanish systems.

ENERGY AND NATURAL RESOURCES

Electricity. Production (1989) 1,886m. kwh. Supply 110 volts; 60 Hz. The El Cajón hydro-electric station at Rio Lindo serves the central and north coast areas. Capacity: 290 mw.

Minerals. Lead, zinc and silver are the main minerals exported.

Agriculture. Honduras is primarily an agricultural country, but only a quarter of the total land area is cultivated and by far the larger portion of this is on the Caribbean and Pacific coastal plains. The main agricultural crops are grains, bananas, coffee and sugar. Coffee production was 108,000 tonnes in 1989–90.

Livestock (1988): Cattle, 2,824,000; sheep, 7,000; pigs, 600,000; goats, 25,000; horses, 170,000; poultry, 8m.

Forestry. Forests in 1988 covered 31% of the total land area, but are not effectively exploited and deforestation is becoming a severe problem. Large stands of mahogany and other hard-woods—granadino, guayacán, walnut and rosewood—grow in the north-eastern part of the country, in the interior valleys, and near the southern coast. Stands of pine occur almost everywhere in the interior, but are severely damaged by bark beetle and fires.

Fisheries. Commercial fishing in territorial waters is restricted to Honduran nationals and Honduran-controlled companies. Shrimps and lobsters are important catches.

INDUSTRY. Small-scale local industries include beer and mineral waters, cement, flour, vegetable lard, coconut oil, sweets, cigarettes, cigars, textiles and clothing, panama hats, plastics, nails, matches, plywood, furniture, paper bags, soap, candles, fruit juices and household chemicals.

Labour. The workforce was (in 1,000) 1,218·2 in 1988, of whom 640·5 worked in agriculture, hunting and fishery; 160·6 in manufacturing; 117·5 in trade; 54·8 in building; 48·1 in transport and communications and 14·1 in finance. A 'Charter of Labour' was granted in Feb. 1955 and an advanced Labour Code and Social Security Bill passed into law in May 1959.

Trade Unions. The organization of trade unions was begun in 1954 with the assistance of ORIT (Inter-American Regional Organization) sponsored by the US trade unions. In 1988 there were 236 active trade unions with about 160,000 members.

FOREIGN ECONOMIC RELATIONS.

Commerce. Imports in 1986 were valued at 1,940m. lempiras and exports at 1,800m. lempiras.

Imports (1985) in 1m. lempiras: Fuel and lubricants, (1986) 565; consumer goods, 426; raw materials, 576; capital goods, 432.

Exports (1986) in 1m. lempiras: Bananas, 530; coffee, 612; timber, 74; refrigerated meats, 40; shrimp and lobster, 88.

Trade with main countries in 1m. lempiras (1986) was: USA, 1,518·8; Japan, 302·2; Federal Republic of Germany, 297·2; Italy, 157·1; Netherlands, 89; Belgium, 85·6; Spain, 55·2; UK, 49.

Total trade between Honduras and UK (British Department of Trade returns, in £1,000 sterling):

	1986	*1987*	*1988*	*1989*	*1990*
Imports to UK	5,280	4,703	8,295	12,121	11,661
Exports and re-exports from UK	9,213	10,449	7,891	5,518	7,345

Tourism. There were 218,253 foreign visitors in 1988; 154,880 Hondurans went abroad.

COMMUNICATIONS

Roads. Honduras is connected with Guatemala, El Salvador and Nicaragua by the Pan-American Highway. Out of a total of 18,494 km of road (1988), 2,262 were asphalted and 9,099 were unpaved but of all-weather construction. There are asphalted highways between Puerto Cortés in the north and Choluteca in the south passing through San Pedro Sula and Tegucigalpa with branches to Guatemala and El Salvador. In 1988 there were 129,115 motor vehicles.

Railways. The small railway system was built to serve the banana industry and is confined to the northern coastal region. it is run by a government agency. The total railways operating in 1986 were 955 km of 1,067 mm and 914 mm gauge, which carried 1m. passengers and 1·2m. tonnes of freight.

Aviation. There are international airports at Tegucigalpa and San Pedro Sula and a domestic one at La Ceiba, with over 30 smaller airstrips in various parts of the country.

Shipping. Sailings to the Atlantic coast port of Puerto Cortés from Europe are frequent, mainly operated by the Harrison Line, Cia Generale Transatlantique, the Royal Netherlands Steamships Co., Hapag Lloyd and vessels owned or chartered by the Tela Railroad Co., a subsidiary of Chiquita International, and the Standard Fruit Co.

Telecommunications. Hondutel, a govenrment agency, had exchanges with a capacity of 121,000 lines in 1988. Some 66,000 telephones were in operation. The telegraph remains important and there were 364 offices in the country in 1988.

In 1988, there were 9 TV channels and 287 radio stations (mostly local) operating.

Cinemas (1982). Cinemas numbered about 60 with seating capacity of some 60,000.

Newspapers (1990). The 4 national daily papers are *El Heraldo* and *La Tribuna* in Tegucigalpa, *La Prensa* and *El Tiempo* in San Pedro Sula. Several local papers exist but their circulation is low and their influence is very limited.

JUSTICE, RELIGION, EDUCATION AND WELFARE

Justice. Judicial power is vested in the Supreme Court, with 9 judges elected by the National Congress for 4 years; it appoints the judges of the courts of appeal, and justices of the peace.

Religion. Roman Catholicism is the prevailing religion, but the constitution guarantees freedom to all creeds, and the State does not contribute to the support of any. Evangelical movements from North America are spreading their influence.

Education. Instruction is free, formally compulsory (from 7 to 13 years of age) and secular. There is a high drop out rate after the first years in Primary education. In 1986 the 6,710 primary schools had 805,504 children (20,732 teachers); the 354 secondary, normal and technical schools had 130,247 pupils (6,945 teachers); the teachers' training college had 3,389 students in 1986. In 1986, the three universities had a total of 31,455 students.

The illiteracy rate was 40% of those 10 years of age and older in 1983.

Health. In 1990 there were about 2,900 doctors. In 1988 there were 21 public hospitals and 25 private, with 5,601 beds, and 617 health centres.

DIPLOMATIC REPRESENTATIVES

Of Honduras in Great Britain (115 Gloucester Pl., London, W1H 3PJ)
Ambassador: Max Velásquez-Diaz (accredited 7 June 1984).

Of Great Britain in Honduras (Edificio Palmira, 3er Piso, Colonia Palmira, Tegucigalpa)
Ambassador: Peter John Streams, CMG (accredited 22 Aug. 1989).

Of Honduras in the USA (3007 Tilden St., NW, Washington, D.C., 20008)
Ambassador: Dr Jorge Ramón Hernandez-Alcerro.

Of the USA in Honduras (Av. La Paz, Tegucigalpa)
Ambassador: Cresencio S. Arcos.

Of Honduras to the United Nations
Ambassador: Flores Bermudez.

Further Reading

The *Anuario Estadístico* (latest issue, *Comercio Exterior de Honduras*, 1983) is published by the Dirección de Estadísticas y Censos, Tegucigalpa. *Director:* Elizabeth Zavala de Turcios.

Monthly Bulletin.—Honduras en Cifras. Banco Central de Honduras, 1986-88
Anderson, T. P., *Politics in Central America.* Boston, Mass., 1988
Howard, P., *Honduras [bibliography].* Oxford and Santa Barbara, 1991
Morris, J. A., *Honduras: Caudillo Politics and Military Rulers.* Boulder, 1984
Rubio Melhado, A., *Geografia General de la República de Honduras.* Tegucigalpa, 1953
Sheehan, E. R. F., *Agony in the garden. A Stranger in Central America.* New York, 1989

HONG KONG

Population: 5·76m. (1989)
GDP per capita: US$9,642 (1988)

HISTORY. Hong Kong Island and the southern tip of the Kowloon peninsula were ceded by China to Britain after the first and second Anglo-Chinese Wars by the Treaty of Nanking 1842 and the Convention of Peking 1860. Northern Kowloon was leased to Britain for 99 years by China in 1898. Since then, Hong Kong has been under British administration, except from Dec. 1941 to Aug. 1945 during the Japanese occupation. Talks began in Sept. 1982 between Britain and China over the future of Hong Kong after the lease expiry in 1997. On 19 Dec. 1984, the two countries signed a joint declaration whereby China would recover sovereignty over Hong Kong (comprising Hong Kong Island, Kowloon and the New Territories) from 1 July 1997 and establish it as a Special Administrative Region where the existing social and economic systems, and the present life-style, would remain unchanged for another 50 years. This 'one country, two systems' principle was embodied in the Basic Law of 1990, and allows Hong Kong after 1997 to keep control of its external economic relations, to remain a separate customs area and retain the status of an international financial centre, with foreign exchange markets and a convertible currency. Hong Kong will also retain a legislature and judiciary.

AREA AND POPULATION. Hong Kong island is 32 km east of the mouth of the Pearl River and 130 km south-east of Guangzhou. The area of the island is 79·45 sq. km. It is separated from the mainland by a fine natural harbour. On the opposite side is the peninsula of Kowloon (11·44 sq. km), which was added to the Territory by the Convention of Peking, 1860. By a further convention, signed at Peking on 9 June 1898, about 979·23 sq. km, consisting of all the immediately adjacent mainland and numerous islands in the vicinity, were leased to Great Britain by China for 99 years. This area is known as the New Territories. Total area of the Territory is 1,071 sq. km (including recent reclamations), a large part of it being steep and unproductive hillside. Some 40% of the Territory is conserved as country parks. Shortage of land suitable for development for housing and industry is a serious problem. Since 1945, the Government has reclaimed about 2,396·8 hectares from the sea, principally from the seafronts of Hong Kong and Kowloon, facing the harbour. In the New Territories, the new town of Tsuen Wan, incorporating Tsuen Wan, Kwai Chung and Tsing Yi, already houses 690,000 of its planned ultimate population of 860,000. The construction of 7 further new towns at Sha Tin, Tuen Mun, Tai Po, Fanling, Yuen Long, Tseung Kwan O and Tin Shui Wai is now well underway, with planned ultimate population of about 750,000, 562,000, 306,000, 280,000, 190,000, 440,000 and 140,000 respectively.

The population was 5,613,000 at 1987 census. Estimate (30 June 1989) 5,761,400. During the war years the population of Hong Kong fluctuated sharply. In Sept. 1945, at the end of the Japanese occupation, it was about 600,000. In mid-1950 it was estimated at 2·24m. From mid-1976 to mid-1989 the average annual growth rate has been 1·9%. Of the present population about 21·8% are under 15 years of age. About 59% of the population was born in Hong Kong. There were 56,810 Vietnamese refugees/boat people on 26 Oct. 1989.

CLIMATE. The climate is warm sub-tropical being much affected by monsoons, the winter being cool and dry and the summer hot and humid, May to Sept. being the wettest months. Jan. 60°F (15·6°C), July 83°F (28·6°C). Annual rainfall 85" (2,224·7 mm).

CONSTITUTION AND GOVERNMENT. The administration is in the hands of a Governor, aided by an Executive Council, composed of the Chief Secretary, the Commander British Forces, the Financial Secretary, the Attorney General (who are members *ex officio*) and such other members as may be appointed by the Queen upon the Governor's nomination. In Nov. 1990 there were, in addition to the 4 *ex-officio* members, 1 nominated official and 9 appointed members. There is also a Legislative Council, presided over by the Governor. In 1990 it consisted of 3 *ex-officio* members, namely the Chief Secretary, the Financial Secretary, the Attorney-General, 7 official members, 20 appointed members and 26 elected members. Chinese and English are the official languages. Two municipal councils with elected members are responsible on a regional basis for environmental hygiene, public health, recreational and cultural matters. Consultative district boards with 274 elected members were set up in 1982 in the 19 administrative districts. At the March 1991 elections turn-out was 32·5%. Pro-democracy candidates won 80 seats. A first political party, the United Democratic Party, led by Martin Lee, was formed in April 1990.

Governor and C.-in-C.: Sir David Wilson, GCMG.

Commander British Forces: Maj.-Gen. Peter Royson Duffell, CBE, MC.

Chief Secretary: Sir David Ford, KBE, LVO, JP.

Flag: British Blue Ensign with the arms of the Territory on a white disc in the fly.

DEFENCE. The Hong Kong garrison, under the Commander British Forces, comprises units of all three services. Its principal rôle is to assist the Hong Kong Government in maintaining security and stability.

Army. The Army constitutes the bulk of the garrison. It comprises a UK battalion, based at Stanley Fort, and 3 Gurkha infantry battalions, all based in the New Territories; supporting units include the Queen's Gurkha Engineers, the Queen's Gurkha Signals, the Gurkha Transport Regiment, and 660 Squadron Army Air Corps.

Navy. The Royal Naval Hong Kong Squadron, partly funded by the Hong Kong government, comprises 3 Peacock class patrol craft and is based at HMS *Tamar* at Victoria.

Air Force. The Royal Air Force is based at Shek Kong. No. 28 (Army Cooperation) Squadron operates Wessex helicopters. In addition to its operational rôle in support of the army and navy, the RAF carries out search and rescue and medical evacuation tasks. It is also responsible for air traffic control services at Shek Kong, and provides a territory-wide air traffic advisory service.

Auxiliary Forces. The local auxiliary defence units, consisting of the Royal Hong Kong Regiment and the Royal Hong Kong Auxiliary Air Force, are administered by the Hong Kong Government, but, if called out, would come under the command of the Commander British Forces. The Royal Hong Kong Regiment (The Volunteers) has a strength of about 950. It is fully mobile and its rôle is to operate in support of regular army battalions stationed in Hong Kong. The Royal Hong Kong Auxiliary Air Force is intended mainly for internal security and air-sea rescue duties. It has a strength of about 171, operating a fleet of 9 aircraft – 2 twin-engined Beech King Air 200s, 4 Slingsby T-67 trainers, and 3 Aérospatiale Dauphin 365C1 helicopters.

ECONOMY

Budget. The public revenue and expenditure for financial years ending 31 March were as follows (in HK$):

	1986–87	*1987–88*	*1988–89*	*1989–90* [1]
Revenue	43,870,000,000	55,641,000,000	72,658,000,000	80,539,000,000
Expenditure	39,928,000,000	44,022,000,000	56,591,000,000	69,065,000,000

[1] Estimate.

The revenue is derived chiefly from rates, licences, tax on earnings and profits, land sales, duties on tobacco, hydrocarbon oils, methyl alcohol, intoxicating liquor, non-intoxicating liquor, non-alcoholic beverages and cosmetics and various duties.

Currency. The unit of currency is the *Hong Kong dollar* (HKD) of 100 *cents*. Banknotes (of denominations of $10 upwards) are issued by the Hongkong and Shanghai Banking Corporation, and the Standard Chartered Bank. Their combined note issue was, at 31 Dec. 1988, HK$31,826m. Subsidiary currency consisting of HK$5, HK$2, HK$1, 50-cent, 20-cent, 10-cent, 5-cent alloy coins and 1-cent notes is issued by the Hong Kong Government and at 31 Dec. 1988 totalled HK$1,889m.

Since Oct. 1983 the HK$ has been linked to the US$1 at a fixed exchange rate of US$1 = HK$7·78. In March 1991, £1 = HK$14·76.

The Hong Kong Government has issued a set of 14 Hong Kong commemorative HK$1,000 gold coins over the years. The set comprises 2 coins commemorating the Queen's visit to Hong Kong in 1975 and in 1986 and 12 coins depicting the animals of the Chinese lunar calendar. The last coin in the lunar series was issued in 1987 to commemorate the Year of the Rabbit.

Banking. At 31 Dec. 1988: There were 160 banks licensed under the Banking Ordinance with a total of 1,397 banking offices, and 152 representative offices of foreign banks; bank deposits were HK$778,989m. and loans and advances HK$866,486m.; there were 216 deposit taking companies registered, and 35 licensed, under the Banking Ordinance with total deposits of HK$66,531.

Weights and Measures. Metric, British Imperial, Chinese and US units are all in current use in Hong Kong. However Government departments have now effectively adopted metric units; all new legislation uses metric terminology and existing legislation is being progressively metricated. Metrication is also proceeding in the private sector.

The statutory equivalent for the *chek* is 14 5/8 inches. The variation of the size of the *chek* with usage still persists in Hong Kong but the *chek* and derived units are now used much less than in the past.

ENERGY AND NATURAL RESOURCES

Electricity. Production (1988) 23,956m. kwh. Supply 220 volts; 50 Hz.

Water. The provision of sufficient reservoir capacity to store the summer rainfall in order to meet supply requirements has always been a serious problem. Over the years no less than 17 impounding reservoirs have been constructed with a total capacity of 586m. cu. metres. The major among these are the Plover Cove Reservoir (230m. cu. metres) finally completed in 1973 and the High Island Reservoir (281m. cu. metres) completed in 1978, both involving the conversion of sea water inlets into fresh water lakes.

There are no sites remaining in Hong Kong suitable for development as storage reservoirs. Consequently the purchase of water from China has been of increasing importance and the future needs of Hong Kong will be met to a large extent from this source. In 1988-89 water purchased from China was in the order of 644m. cu. metres. The agreement with China allows for annual increases up to a total figure of 660m. cu. metres per annum by 1994–95 which will represent 60% of Hong Kong's demand.

These resources can be further supplemented when necessary by up to 181,000 cu. metres of fresh water a day from a desalting plant completed in 1976 and now considered as a reserve resource.

Agriculture. Only 9% of the total land area is suitable for crop farming and most vegetables are produced through intensive market gardening cultivation, with 34% self-sufficiency. In 1988, 132,000 tonnes of vegetables and 2,020 tonnes of fruit were produced. Poultry production was 42,890 tonnes, with 37% self-sufficiency. Livestock (1988): Cattle, 750; pigs, 629,110.

Fisheries. The fishing fleet of 4,900 vessels supplies 74% of fresh marine fish consumed locally. In 1988 the total catch was 228,100 tonnes, valued at HK$2,039m. Inland freshwater farming and coastal marine farming provided 6,640 tonnes of freshwater fish valued at HK$85m. and 3,280 tonnes of marine products valued at HK$222m.

INDUSTRY.

An economic policy based on free enterprise and free trade; an industrious work force; an efficient and aggressive commercial infrastructure; modern and efficient sea-port (including container shipping terminals) and airport facilities; its geographical position relative to markets in North America and its traditional trading links with Britain have all contributed to Hong Kong's success as a modern industrial territory.

In Dec. 1988, there were 49,843 factories employing 837,072 people out of a total population of over 5·7m. The type of factory involved ranges from the small subcontractor type to large highly complex modern establishments. Given the scarcity of land it is most common for light industry to operate in multi-storey buildings specially designed for this purpose. The main industry is textiles and clothing, which employed 43% of the total industrial workforce and accounted for 38% of total domestic exports in 1988. Other major light manufacturing industries include electronic products, clocks and watches, toys, plastic products, electrical products, metalware, footwear, cameras and travel goods. Heavy industry includes shipbuilding, ship-repairing, aircraft engineering and the manufacture of machinery.

Labour. In 1988 the labour force totalled 2·78m., including 837,000 in manufacturing, 521,000 in wholesale, retail and export/import trade, 236,000 in finance, real estate and business services, and 191,000 in hotels and restaurants.

FOREIGN ECONOMIC RELATIONS

Commerce. Hong Kong's industries are mainly export oriented. The total value of domestic exports in 1988 was HK$217,664m. The major markets were USA (33·5%), China (17·5%), Federal Republic of Germany (7·4%), UK (7·1%), Japan (5·3%), Canada (2·7%), Netherlands (2·4%) and Singapore (2·3%). There is also a sizeable and flourishing entrepôt trade which accounted for another HK$275,405m. in 1988.

The total value of imports in 1988 was HK$498,798m., mainly from China (31·2%), Japan (18·6%), Taiwan (8·9%), USA (8·3%), Republic of Korea (5·3%) and Singapore (3·7%).

The chief import items were machinery and transport equipment (28·8%), manufactured goods (26·4%), chemicals (9%), foodstuffs (6·3%), mineral fuel, lubricants and related materials (1·9%).

Duties are levied only on tobacco, hydrocarbon oils, methyl alcohol, alcoholic liquors, non-alcoholic beverages and cosmetics, whether imported into or manufactured in Hong Kong for local consumption.

All imports (apart from foodstuffs, which are subject to a flat declaration charge irrespective of the value of the consignment) and exports are subject to an *ad valorem* declaration charge at the rate of HK50 cents for every $1,000 value (or part thereof) of the goods shipped.

Visible trade normally carries an adverse balance which is offset by a favourable balance of invisible trade, in particular transactions in connexion with air transportation, shipping, tourism and banking services.

Hong Kong has a free exchange market. Foreign merchants may remit profits or repatriate capital. Import and export controls are kept to the minimum, consistent with strategic requirements.

Total trade between Hong Kong and UK (British Department of Trade returns, in £1,000 sterling) is given as follows:

	1986	*1987*	*1988*	*1989*	*1990*
Imports to UK	1,530,786	1,531,681	1,788,631	2,036,976	1,972,154
Exports and re-exports from UK	960,956	1,013,038	1,030,725	1,111,517	1,238,023

Tourism. 5·36m. tourists (1·13m. from Taiwan) spent HK$36,900m. in Hong Kong during 1989.

COMMUNICATIONS

Roads. In March 1989 there were 1,446 km of roads, distributed as follows: Hong Kong Island, 397; Kowloon, 372, and New Territories, 677. A cross-harbour tunnel, 1·8 km in length, opened to traffic in Aug. 1972, now links Hong Kong Island with the Kowloon peninsula. In Sept. 1989, another cross-harbour tunnel, the Eastern Harbour Tunnel, was opened, linking the eastern part of both Hong Kong Island and the Kowloon peninsula. The 1·4 km twin-tube Lion Rock Tunnel, which links Kowloon with Sha Tin New Town and other areas of the north-eastern New Territories, became fully operational in Oct. 1978. The 1·8 km twin-tube Aberdeen Tunnel, which connects Aberdeen and Wan Chai, became operational in March 1983.

Railways. There is an electric tramway with a total track length of 30·4 km, and a cable tramway connecting the Peak district with the lower levels in Victoria. The electrified Kowloon-Canton Railway runs for 34 km from the terminus at Hung Hom in Kowloon to the border point at Lo Wu. It carried 171m. passengers and 4·5m. tonnes of freight in 1989. A light rail system operated by the Kowloon-Canton Railway opened in the Tuen Mun area in Sept. 1988.

An underground Mass Transit Railway system, comprising 43·2 km with 38 stations, is now in operation. The system consists of 4 lines, one linking the Central District of Hong Kong Island with Tsuen Wan in the west of Kowloon, the second linking Quarry Bay on Hong Kong Island with Kwun Tong in East Kowloon with Yau Ma Tei in Nathan Road, the third linking Sheung Wan and Chai Wan on Hong Kong Island. It carried 688m. passengers in 1989.

Aviation. Hong Kong International Airport is situated on the north shore of Kowloon Bay. It is regularly used by some 40 airlines and many charter airlines which provide frequent services throughout the Far East to Europe, North America, Africa, the Middle East, Australia and New Zealand. British Airways operates 17 flights per week via India or the Gulf to the UK. Cathay Pacific Airways, one of the two Hong Kong-based airlines, operates more than 400 passenger and cargo services weekly to Europe (including 14 passenger and 5 cargo services per week to the UK), the Far and Middle East, Australia and North America. Hong Kong Dragon Airlines Ltd, which was set up in July 1985, operates B-737 scheduled and non-scheduled services between Hong Kong and a number of cities in Asia, the People's Republic of China and Micronesia. Air Hong Kong, an all-cargo operator, provides a scheduled twice-weekly service to Manchester, UK, and operates non-scheduled services around the region. About 1,000 scheduled flights are operated weekly to and from Hong Kong by various airlines. In 1988, 8,700 aircraft arrived and departed on international flights, carrying 15·3m. passengers and 700,000 tonnes of freight.

Shipping. The port of Hong Kong, which ranks among the top three container ports in the world, handled 4·03m. 20-ft equivalent units in 1988. The Kwai Chung Container Port has 8 berths with more than 3,000 metres of quay backed by about 120 hectares of cargo handling area. In 1988, some 17,089 ocean-going vessels called at Hong Kong and loaded and discharged some 81m. tonnes of cargo.

Telecommunications. There were 106 post offices in 1988; postal revenue totalled HK$1,450·9m.; expenditure, HK$940·7m in the 1988–89 financial year; 747·9m. letters and parcels were handled. Telephone service is provided by the Hong Kong Telephone Co. Ltd. It provides local, and in association with Cable and Wireless (HK) Ltd., international voice, data and facsimile transmission services for Hong Kong. At 31 Dec. 1988 there were over 2·9m. telephones served by 2·2m. lines. Cable and Wireless (HK) Ltd. provides the international telecommunication services as well as local telegram and telex services. These include public telegram, telex, telephone, television programmes transmission and reception, leased circuits, facsimile, switched data, ship-shore and air-ground communications. International facilities are provided through submarine cables, microwave and satellite radio systems. Hong Kong Telephone Co. Ltd. and Cable and Wireless (HK) Ltd. are wholly-owned subsidiaries of Hong Kong Telecommunications Ltd. which is jointly owned by the Cable and Wireless World Wide Communications Group, Hong Kong Government and public shareholders.

There is a government broadcasting station, Radio Television Hong Kong, which broadcasts through 3 FM and 4 AM channels (3 Chinese, 1 English and 2 bi-lingual services and 1 dedicated to BBC world service), 4 of which provide 24-hour service. A commercial station, the Commercial Broadcasting Co. Ltd, transmits daily in English and Cantonese. It operates 3 channels which provide 24-hour service.

Television Broadcasts Ltd and Asia Television Ltd transmit commercial television in English and Chinese on 4 channels, in colour.

Cinemas. In Oct. 1989 there were 148 cinemas with a seating capacity in excess of 125,000.

Newspapers. In June 1989 there were 63 daily or weekly newspapers, registered and in circulation, including 15 English-language papers, one bilingual paper, 46 Chinese-language dailies, one Japanese-language paper and a number of news agency bulletins.

JUSTICE, EDUCATION AND WELFARE

Justice. There is a Supreme Court which comprises the Court of Appeal and the High Court. While the Court of Appeal hears appeals on all matters, civil and criminal from the lower courts, the High Court has unlimited jurisdiction in both civil and criminal matters including bankruptcy, company winding-up, adoptions, probate and lunacy matters. The District Court has civil jurisdiction to hear monetary claims up to HK$120,000 or, where the claims are for recovery of land, the annual rent or rateable value does not exceed HK$100,000. In its criminal jurisdiction, it may try more serious offences except murder, manslaughter and rape; the maximum term of imprisonment it can impose is seven years. The Magistrates' Court exercises criminal jurisdiction over a wide range of indictable and summary offences. Its powers of punishment are generally restricted to a maximum of two years' imprisonment, or a fine of HK$10,000, though cumulative sentences of imprisonment up to three years may be imposed. The Coroner's Court inquires into the identity of a deceased person and the cause of death. The Juvenile Court has jurisdiction to hear charges against young people aged under 16 for any offence other than homicide. Children under the age of seven are not deemed to have reached the age of criminal responsibility. The Lands Tribunal determines on statutory claims for compensation over land and certain landlord and tenant matters. The Labour Tribunal provides inexpensive and speedy settlements to individual monetary claims arising from disputes between employers and employees. The Small Claims Tribunal deals with monetary claims involving amounts not exceeding HK$15,000. The Obscene Articles Tribunal, established in 1987, has two judicial functions. It has exclusive jurisdiction to determine whether an article referred to it by a court or a magistrate is an obscene or indecent article and where the matter publicly displayed is indecent and it also has power to classify an article as Class I (neither obscene nor indecent), Class II (an indecent article) or Class III (an obscene article).

Police. At the end of 1989, the establishment of the Royal Hong Kong Police Force was 28,000. In addition, there were over 5,800 auxiliary officers. Overall crime has averaged about 80,000 reported for the past 10 years and the detection rate stands at 46·5%

The Marine Police Region is responsible for patrolling some 1,850 sq. km of territorial waters and involved in the control of some 33,000 local craft with a maritime population of about 100,000. At the end of 1989, it consisted of a disciplined staff of more than 3,200 and a fleet of over 150 vessels.

Education. The majority of schools have to be registered with the Education Department under the Education Ordinance. They are required to comply with regulations as to staff, building, fire and health requirements. From Sept. 1971, free and compulsory primary education was introduced in government and the majority of government-aided schools. Free junior secondary education of 3 years' duration was introduced in 1978 and it was made compulsory in Sept. 1979.

In Sept. 1988 there were 214,703 pupils in kindergartens (all private), another 535,037 in primary schools and 443,901 in secondary schools.

There are 8 technical institutes and 16 training centres with a total enrolment of 80,000, 1 technical teachers' college and 3 colleges of education with a total enrolment of 4,839.

The University of Hong Kong had a total enrolment of 8,654 students in academic year 1988-89 and the Chinese University of Hong Kong, inaugurated in Oct. 1963, had a total of 7,900 students. The Hong Kong University of Science and Technology, established in 1989, will admit its first intakes in 1991-92 with 700 students. The Hong Kong Polytechnic, 1988-89, had about 26,000 students. In Oct. 1984, the City Polytechnic of Hong Kong was opened and had a total of 6,900 students in 1988-89. The Hong Kong Baptist College had 2,700 full-time students in 1988-89.

Health. In March 1989 there were 5,636 doctors and about 25,057 hospital beds.

Social Security. The Government co-ordinates and implements expanding programmes in social welfare, which include social security, family services, child care, services for the elderly, youth and community work, probation and corrections and rehabilitation. 159 voluntary welfare agencies are subsidized by public funds.

The Government gives non-contributory cash assistance to needy families, unemployed able-bodied adults, the severely disabled and the elderly. Caseload in Sept. 1989 totalled 394,360. Victims of natural disasters, crimes of violence and traffic accidents are financially assisted.

Further Reading

Statistical Information: The Census and Statistics Department is responsible for the preparation and collation of Government statistics. These statistics are published mainly in the *Hong Kong Monthly Digest of Statistics* which is also available in a collected annual edition. The Department also publishes monthly trade statistics, economic indicators, annual review of overseas trade, etc. Statistical information is also published in the annual reports of Government departments. *Hong Kong 1989*, and other government publications, are available from the Hong Kong Government Publications Centre, GPO Building, Connaught Place, Hong Kong, and the Hong Kong Government Office in London, 6 Grafton Street, London, W1X 3LB.

The Hong Kong Trade Development Council, Convention Plaza, Tower Rd, Wan Chai, Hong Kong, issues a monthly *Hong Kong Enterprise* and other publications.

Hong Kong 1989. Hong Kong Government Press, 1989
Beazer, W. F., *The Commercial Future of Hong Kong*. New York, 1978
Benton, G., *The Hong Kong Crisis*. London, 1983
Bonavia, D., *Hong Kong 1997*. London, 1984
Cheng, J. Y. S. (ed.) *Hong Kong: In Search of a Future*. OUP, 1984
Chill, H., *et al* (eds.) *The Future of Hong Kong: Toward 1997 and Beyond*. Westport, 1987
Endacott, G. B., *A History of Hong Kong*. 2nd ed. OUP, 1973.–*Government and People in Hong Kong, 1841–1962. A Constitutional History*. OUP, 1965
Hopkins, K., *Hong Kong: The Industrial Colony*. OUP, 1971
Morris, J., *Hong Kong: Xianggang*. London, 1988
Patrikeeff, F., *Mouldering Pearl: Hong Kong at the Crossroads*. London, 1989
Scott, I., *Hong Kong:* [Bibliography]. Oxford and Santa Barbara, 1990
Tregear, E. R., *Land Use in Hong Kong*. Hong Kong Univ. Press, 1958.—*Hong Kong Gazetteer*. Hong Kong Univ. Press, 1958.—*The Development of Hong Kong as Told in Maps*. Hong Kong Univ. Press, 1959
Wacks, R., *Civil Liberties in Hong Kong*. OUP, 1988
Wilson, D., *Hong Kong, Hong Kong*. London, 1991
Youngson, A. J., *Hong Kong: Economic Growth and Policy*. OUP, 1982

HUNGARY

Capital: Budapest
Population: 10·59m. (1989)
GNP per capita: US$2,460 (1988)

Magyar Köztársaság (Hungarian Republic)

HISTORY. Hungary first became an independent kingdom in 1001. For events to 1956 *see* THE STATESMAN'S YEAR-BOOK, 1957.

On 23 Oct. 1956 an anti-Stalinist revolution broke out, and the newly-formed coalition government of Imre Nagy on 1 Nov. withdrew from the Warsaw Pact and asked the UN for protection. János Kádár, formed a counter-government on 3 Nov. and asked the USSR for support. Soviet troops suppressed the revolution and abducted Nagy and his ministers; Nagy was secretly executed in 1958.

On 7 Sept. 1967 a second Soviet-Hungarian treaty of friendship was concluded for 20 years with subsequent automatic 5-year renewals.

A gathering reformist tendency within the Hungarian Socialist Workers' (i.e. Communist) Party led by Imre Pozsgay culminated in its self-dissolution in Oct. 1989 and reconstitution as the Hungarian Socialist Party.

Hungary was proclaimed the 'Hungarian Republic' on 23 Oct. 1989.

Nagy was reburied with state honours on 16 Aug. 1989.

AREA AND POPULATION. Hungary is bounded north by Czechoslovakia, north-east by the USSR, east by Romania, south by Yugoslavia and west by Austria. The peace treaty of 10 Feb. 1947 restored the frontiers as of 1 Jan. 1938. The area of Hungary is 93,032 sq. km (35,911 sq. miles).

The official language is Hungarian (Magyar).

At the census of 1 Jan. 1980 the population was 10,709,550 (5,195,300 males). Population in 1989: 10,590,000 (males, 5,107,000). Ethnic miorities, 1984: Germans, 1·6%; Slovaks, 1·1%; Romanians, 0·2%; others, 0·5%. There were 400,000 Gypsies in 1990 with a Gypsy Council.

60% of the population is urban (20% in Budapest). Population density, 114 per sq. km. Birth rate, 1988, 11·7 per 1,000; death rate, 13·1 per 1,000. Since 1981 the population has been decreasing, by 1·4 per 1,000 in 1988; expectation of life (1987): males, 66; females, 74. There is a world-wide Hungarian diaspora, of 1·5m. in 1988 (730,000 in US; 220,000 in Israel; 140,000 in Canada), and Hungarian minorities (3·5m. in 1988) in Romania, Yugoslavia and Czechoslovakia.

Vital statistics, 1988: Births, 124,348; marriages, 65,932 (of which 19,277 remarriages); divorces, 25,000 (estimate); deaths, 139,142; abortions, 87,000 (approx.); infant mortality, 15·8 per 1,000 live births. There were 4,494 suicides in 1988.

Hungary is divided into 19 counties (*megyék*) and the capital, Budapest, which has county status.

Area (in sq. km) and population (in 1,000) of counties and county towns:

Counties (1989)	*Area*	*Population*	*Chief town (1989)*	*Population*
Baranya	4,487	434	Pécs	183
Bács-Kiskun	8,362	552	Kecskemét	106
Békés	5,632	413	Békéscsaba	71
Borsod-Abaúj-Zemplén	7,247	772	Miskolc	208
Csongrád	4,263	456	Szeged	189
Fejér	4,373	426	Székesfehérvár	114
Győr-Sopron	4,012	426	Győr	132
Hajdú-Bihar	6,211	550	Debrecen	220
Heves	3,637	336	Eger	67
Komárom-Esztergom	2,251	320	Tatabánya	77
Nógrád	2,544	227	Salgótarján	49
Pest	6,394	989	Budapest	2,115
Somogy	6,036	348	Kaposvár	74
Szabolcs-Szatmár-Bereg	5,938	564	Nyíregyháza	119
Szolnok [1]	5,607	427	Szolnok	82
Tolna	3,704	262	Szekszárd	39

Counties (1989)	*Area*	*Population*	*Chief town (1989)*	*Population*
Vas	3,337	276	Szombathely	88
Veszprém	4,689	387	Veszprém	66
Zala	3,784	310	Zalaegerszeg	64
Budapest	525	2,115	(has county status)	

[1] Renamed Jasz-Nagykun-Szolnok in 1990

CLIMATE. A humid continental climate, with warm summers and cold winters. Precipitation is generally greater in summer, with thunderstorms. Dry, clear weather is likely in autumn, but spring is damp and both seasons are of short duration. Budapest. Jan. 32°F (0°C), July 71°F (21·5°C). Annual rainfall 25" (625 mm). Pécs. Jan. 30°F (–0·7°C), July 71°F (21·5°C). Annual rainfall 26·4" (661 mm).

CONSTITUTION AND GOVERNMENT. On 1 Feb. 1946 the National Assembly proclaimed a republic.

The People's Republic was established by the constitution of 18 Aug. 1949 (for details see THE STATESMAN'S YEAR-BOOK, 1989-90, p. 615).

On 18 Oct. 1989 Parliament approved by an 88% majority a new constitution which abolished the People's Republic. The preamble states 'The Hungarian Republic is an independent, democratic, law-based state in which the values of bourgeois democracy and democratic socialism hold good in equal measure. All power belongs to the people, which they exercise directly and through the elected representatives of popular sovereignty... No party may direct any organs of state'.

Ethnic minorities have equal rights and education in their own tongue.

The single-chamber National Assembly has 386 members, made up of 176 individual constituency winners, 120 allotted by proportional representation and 90 from a national list. It is elected for 4-year terms.

Elections were held in two rounds in March and April 1990. The Hungarian Democratic Forum (MDF) won 165 seats; the Alliance of Free Democrats, 92; the Independent Smallholders (ISP), 43; the Hungarian Socialist Party (former Communists), 33; the Federation of Young Democrats, 21; the Christian Democratic People's Party (KDNP), 21; others, 5; independents, 6.

An MDF-ISP-KDNP coalition government was formed, which in Feb. 1991 consisted of:

Prime Minister: József Antall (MDF).

Minister of Agriculture: Elemér Gergátz (ISP). *Culture and Education:* Bertalan Andrásfalvy (MDF). *Defence:* Lajos Für (MDF). *Environment:* Sándor Keresztes (MDF). *Finance:* Mihály Kupa (ind). *Foreign Affairs:* Géza Jeszenszky (MDF). *Industry and Commerce:* Péter Bod (MDF). *Interior:* Péter Boross (ind). *International Economic Relations:* Béla Kádár (ind). *Justice:* István Balsai (MDF). *Labour:* Gyula Kiss (ISP). *Public Welfare:* László Surján (KDNP). *Transport and Communications:* Csaba Siklós (MDF). *Without portfolio:* Katalin Botos (MDF); András Gálszéosy (ind); Balázs Horváth (MDF); Ferenc Mádl (ind); Ferenc Nagy (ISP); Ernö Pungor (ind). *Government Spokesman:* László Balász (MDF).

The *Speaker* is György Szabad.

The head of state is the *President* of the Republic. Referenda of Nov. 1989 and July 1990 established that the president is elected for a 4-year term by the National Assembly.

On 3 Aug. 1990 Árpád Göncz (b. 1922; Alliance of Free Democrats) was elected President by 295 votes to 13 with no opponent.

National flag: Three horizontal stripes of red, white, green.

National anthem: Isten áldd meg a magyart–God bless the Hungarians (words by Ferenc Kölcsey, tune by Ferenc Erkel).

Local Government. Elections were held in Sept. 1990 to replace the former Soviet-style councils with multi-party self-governing bodies. Turn-out at 36% failed to reach a mandatory 40%, entailing a second round at which turn-out was 28%. The Alliance of Free Democrats gained 20·2% of the vote, the MDF, 18·3% and the Federation of Young Democrats, 15·2%.

DEFENCE. The President of the Republic is Commander-in-Chief of the armed forces.

Men between the ages of 18 and 23 are liable for 18 months' conscription in the Army, 24 months in the Air Force. Compulsory military service age-limits are 18 to 55 (18 to 45 women).

The Workers' Militia was disbanded in 1989.

The USSR has agreed to withdraw its forces by 1991.

Army. Hungary is divided into 4 army districts: Budapest, Debrecen, Kiskunfélegyháza, Pécs. The strength of the Army was (1991) 72,000 (including 42,500 conscripts). It is organized in 4 tank brigades, 12 motor rifle brigades, 1 artillery and 1 surface-to-surface missile brigade, 1 anti-aircraft regiment, 3 surface-to-air missile regiments and 1 airborne battalion. Equipment includes 1,287 T-54/-55 and 138 T-72 tanks.

Navy. The Danube Flotilla, the maritime wing of the Army, in 1990 consisted of some 500 personnel operating 6 river minesweepers and numerous boats and special-purpose vessels.

Air Force. The Air Force is an integral part of the Army, with a strength (1991) of about 22,000 officers and men (8,000 conscripts) and 200 combat aircraft. The combat aircraft strength comprises 1 regiment of MiG-23 fighters, 1 of MiG-21 interceptors, 1 of Su-22 fighter-bombers, 1 of Su-25 ground attack aircraft, and a regiment of Mi-8 and Mi-24 armed helicopters. Transport units are equipped with An-2, An-24 and An-26 aircraft. Other types in service include Ka-26, Mi-2 and Mi-8 helicopters and L-29 Delfin trainers. 'Guideline' and 'Goa' surface-to-air missiles are also operational.

INTERNATIONAL RELATIONS

Membership. Hungary is a member of the UN, the Council of Europe, the Warsaw Pact, OIEC, IMF, IBRD and is an associate of NATO's North Atlantic Council. With Austria, Czechoslovakia, Italy and Yugoslavia, Hungary was an inaugural member of the 'Pentagonale' meeting on economic and political co-operation in July 1990.

ECONOMY

Policy. For planning under the Communist government *see* THE STATESMAN'S YEAR-BOOK, 1989-90, p. 616-17. An emergency budget in Dec. 1989 opened the economy to market mechanisms, and called for drastic cuts in Government spending, the abolition of price subsidies and the closure of loss-making state industries. It is envisaged that one-third of industry will be privatized by 1992. Enterprise councils, which were established in 1984, are being transformed into limited companies; the State retains 20% of shares while the rest are for sale. Income tax and VAT were introduced in Jan. 1988. Inflation was 18% in 1988. A State Property Agency is overseeing privatization. Retail price index, 1989 (1987 = 100): House purchase, 123·4; rent, 114; clothing, 119·8; household energy, 112·4; food, 110·4; transport, 100.

Budget. The budget for calendar years was as follows (in 1,000 forints):

	1982	*1983*	*1984*	*1985*	*1986*	*1987*	*1991* [1]
Revenue	485,792	543,735	572,920	632,800	682,000	760,600	931,000
Expenditure	498,007	549,822	576,580	646,600	727,300	795,000	931,000

[1] Estimate

1987 revenue included (1,000m. forints): Payments by enterprises, 469·4; consumer taxes, 122·3; payments by the population, 79·3. Expenditure included: Support of enterprises, 150·7; social security, 154·7; consumer price supports, 66·7; capital expenditure, 99·9; education and culture, 65·0; defence, 45·4. The defence budget was cut by 17% in 1989.

Currency. A decree of 26 July 1946 instituted a new monetary unit, the *forint*

(HUF) of 100 *fillér*. There are coins of 10, 20 and 50 fillér and 1, 2, 5, 10, 20 forints, and notes of 10, 20, 50, 100, 500, 1,000 and 5,000 forints. The forint was made fully convertible in Jan. 1991. It was devalued by 15%. Inflation was 30% at the end of 1990. The rate of exchange (March 1991) 135·24 forints to the £1 sterling, 71·29 forints = US$1.

Banking and Finance. In 1987 a two-tier system was established. The National Bank (*Director,* György Surányi) remained the central state financial institution, responsible for the circulation of money and foreign currency exchange, but also became a central clearing bank, with general (but not operational) control over 5 new second-tier commercial banks and 10 specialized development banks. 9 other commercial banks were set up in 1985 to finance development. In 1987 the State Development Institute was established to issue Government bonds to cover the budgetary deficit. A stock exchange was opened in Jan. 1989.

The Hungarian International Trade Bank opened in London in 1973. In 1980 the Central European International Bank was set up in Budapest with 7 Western banks holding 66% of the shares. The National Savings Bank handles local government as well as personal accounts. Deposits in 1988: 296,827m. forints.

Weights and Measures. The metric system is in use.

ENERGY AND NATURAL RESOURCES

Electricity. Supply 220 volts; 50 Hz. Sources of energy in 1988: Oil, 31·6%, gas, 26·8%; coal and lignite, 23·2%; others, 18·4%. Imported, 50·8%. Capacity of power stations was 7,092 mw. There is an 880-mw nuclear power station at Paks. A 750-kv power line links up with the Soviet grid. 29,217m. kwh were produced in 1988 (13,445 kwh by nuclear power), and 13,615m. kwh imported. In May 1989 Hungary withdrew from the Czech-Austrian-Hungarian hydroelectric project on the Danube at Nagymáros.

Oil. Oil and natural gas are found in the Szeged basin and Zala county. Production in 1989: Oil, 1·9m. tonnes; gas (1988), 6,327m. cu. m.

Minerals. Production in 1988 (in 1,000 tonnes): Coal, 2,255; lignite, 5,634; brown coal, 12,986; bauxite, 2,906.

Agriculture. Agricultural land was collectivized in 1950. It was announced in 1990 that land would be restored to its pre-collectivization owners if they wished to cultivate it.

In 1988 the agricultural area was (in 1,000 ha) 6,497, of which 4,712 were arable, 1,210 meadows and pastures, 338 market gardens, and 237 orchards and vineyards.

In 1988 there were 133 state farms (self-governing under the Ministry of Agriculture) with 905,200 ha of land, 1,253 collective farms with 5m. ha of land (including 281,500 ha of household plots) and 1,375 private farms with 529,300 ha. Structure of production, 1987: Co-operative, 48·4%; private, 36·4%; state, 15·2%. The irrigated area was 177,000 ha; 53,000 tractors were in use.

Sown area, 1988: 4·64m. ha (cereals, 2·8m.; industrial crops, 643,000; pulses, 165,000; potatoes, 48,000)

Crop production (in 1,000 tonnes) in 1988 (and 1987): Wheat, 6,962 (5,685); rye, 245 (182); barley, 1,168 (783); oats, 134 (95); maize, 6,027 (7,007); sugar-beet, 4,504 (4,255); sunflower seed, 705, (790); potatoes, 887 (694).

Livestock in 1988 was (in 1,000 head) as follows: Cattle, 1,690; pigs, 8,327; poultry, 35,607; sheep, 2,216; horses, 76,000.

Livestock products (1988): Eggs, 4,695m.; milk, 2,788m. litres; wool, 9,600 tonnes; animals for slaughter, 2,312,000 tonnes.

The north shore of Lake Balaton and the Tokaj area are important wine-producing districts. Wine production in 1988 (and 1987) was 430m. (320m.) litres.

Forestry. 18% of Hungary is under forest: 1·68m. ha in 1988. 35,000 ha were afforested and 7·96m. cu. metres of timber were cut.

Fisheries. There are fisheries in the rivers Danube and Tisza and Lake Balaton. In

1988 there were 26,500 ha of commercial fishponds. Fish production was 25,000 tonnes.

INDUSTRY. In 1988 there were 1,156 state industrial enterprises (employing an average of 1,206 persons), 1,662 industrial co-operatives (195) and 46,995 private business (70). Creditors may proceed against insolvent companies which may be liquidated.

Production (in 1,000 tonnes) in 1988 (and 1987): Pig iron, 2,093 (2,107); steel, 6,373 (6,452); alumina, 873 (858); aluminium, 75 (74); aluminium semi-finished products, 192 (184); cement, 3,873 (4,153); sulphuric acid, 512 (573); petrol, 2,864 (2,977); plastics, 581 (545); chemical fertilizers, 922 (1,067); synthetic fibres, 38 (34); buses (units), 12,340 (12,956); lorries, 703 (577); TV receivers, 393,000 (446,000); refrigerators, 398,000 (399,000).

Labour. In 1988 there were 4,844,800 wage-earners (2,220,800 female) in the following categories: Working-class, 60·8%; white-collar, 26·3%; co-operative peasantry, 7·7%; self-employed tradesmen, 5·2%. 4,550,400 worked in the socialist sector. Percentage distributions of the workforce: Industry, 30·9; agriculture, 18·8; social and cultural services, 12·6; trade, 10·7; transport and communications, 8·3; building, 7·1. A 40-hour 5-day week was introduced in 1984. Average monthly wages in 1988: 7,015 forints. Minimum subsistence level, 1988, was 3,470 forints per month. There were some 30,000 unemployed in 1988. Unemployment benefit for one year became payable from Jan. 1989. Wilful unemployment is a criminal offence. Retirement age: Men, 60; women, 55. Leave entitlement, 15-24 days in 1985.

Trade Unions. The former official communist organizations (National Council of Trade Unions), renamed the Confederation of Hungarian Trade Unions, claimed 2·5m. members in 1990. 16 other unions form the Democratic League for Independent Trade Unions, which claimed 100,000, mainly white-collar, members in 1991. Other unions operate outside these federations.

FOREIGN ECONOMIC RELATIONS. Foreign debt was US$21,000m. in 1990. An EEC loan of £700m. was granted in Oct. 1989.

Commerce. The economy is heavily dependent on foreign trade. Trade for calendar years (in 1m. forints):

	1982	*1983*	*1984*	*1985*	*1986*	*1987*	*1988*
Imports	324,800	365,000	390,500	410,100	439,700	463,100	472,500
Exports	324,500	374,100	414,000	424,600	420,300	450,100	504,100

In 1988 Hungary's trade with communist countries (in 1,000m. forints): Imports, 231·6; exports, 254·9. In 1988 USSR was Hungary's major trading partner (25·0% of imports, 27·6% of exports), ahead of the Federal Republic of Germany (13·9%, 11·0%) and Austria (7·2%, 5·7%).

Commodity structure of foreign trade (%), 1988:

	Imports		*Exports*	
	Communist countries	*Other countries*	*Communist countries*	*Other countries*
Fuels and electricity	27·4	2·3	0·4	3·9
Raw materials	12·9	13·8	2·3	12·0
Semi-finished products	14·3	33·9	9·5	26·4
Spare parts	8·3	14·8	10·3	3·9
Machinery and capital goods	20·9	13·7	47·5	12·5
Industrial consumer goods	13·6	10·2	16·6	15·5
Agricultural produce	0·5	3·7	3·9	10·0
Food industry products	2·1	7·6	9·6	15·8

In 1989 the US granted Hungary most-favoured-nation status. In 1988 a trade agreement was signed with the EEC which will lower quotas by 1995.

Total trade between Hungary and UK (British Department of Trade returns, in £1,000 sterling):

	1986	1987	1988	1989	1990
Imports to UK	77,229	83,267	96,288	105,221	102,741
Exports and re-exports from UK	101,557	101,300	131,212	117,947	121,837

Tourism. In 1988, 17·97m. foreigners visited Hungary (6·38m. from the West), of whom 10·56m. were tourists (3·09m. from the West); and 10·78m. Hungarians travelled abroad (3·33m. to the West) of whom 6·75m. (1·27m.) were tourists.

COMMUNICATIONS

Roads. In 1988 there were 29,701 km of roads, including motorways, 218 km; highways, 93 km and other first class main roads, 1,886 km. Passenger cars numbered 1,789,600 (1,747,300 private), lorries 179,203 and buses 26,569. 211m. tonnes of freight and 629m. passengers were transported by road (excluding intra-urban passengers). In 1988 there were 21,315 road accidents with 1,706 fatalities.

Railways. Route length of public lines in 1989, 7,619 km, of which 2,079 km were electrified. 104m. tonnes of freight and 225m. passengers were carried.

Aviation. Budapest airport (Ferihegy) handled 2·48m. passengers in 1988. In 1989 Hungarian Air Lines (Malév) flew 40 routes to Europe, the Middle East and North America. 1·3m. passengers were carried. Malév had 12 TU154s, 6 TU134s and leased 6 Boeing 737s in 1991. British Airways, PANAM, Air France, SABENA, Swissair, OS, Lufthansa and KLM as well as Aeroflot and East European lines have services to Budapest. TNT operates an express freight service.

Shipping. Navigable waterways have a length of 1,688 km. In 1988 5·34m. tonnes of cargo and 4·22m. passengers were carried. The Hungarian Shipping Company (MAHART) has agencies at Amsterdam, Alexandria, Algiers, Beirut, Rijeka and Trieste. It has 17 sea-going ships.

Pipeline. Length of network, 1988: Oil, 1,204 km; gas, 4,317. Quantity transported, 21·59m. tonnes (5,334m. tonne-kilometres).

Telecommunications. In 1988 there were 3,196 post offices, 858,200 telephones, (593,100 private), and 12,614 telex subscribers. TV licences, (1987) 2,958,000. *Magyar Rádio* broadcasts 3 programmes on medium-waves and FM and also regional programmes, including transmissions in German, Romanian and Serbo-Croat. *Magyar Televizsió* operates 2 TV channels. Colour transmissions use the SECAM system.

Cinemas and Theatres (1988). There were 2,943 cinemas; attendance 51m. 40 full-length feature films were made. There were 41 theatres; attendance 5·55m.

Newspapers and Publishing. In 1988 there were 29 dailies, circulating in 952m. copies and 1,692 other periodicals. 7,562 book titles were published in 1988 in 99·3m. copies.

JUSTICE, RELIGION, EDUCATION AND WELFARE

Justice. The administration of justice is the responsibility of the Procurator-General, elected by Parliament for 6 years. There are 108 regional courts and courts of labour, 20 county courts, 5 district courts and a Supreme Court. Criminal proceedings are dealt with by the regional courts through 3-member councils and by the county courts and the Supreme Court in 5-member councils. A new Civil Code was adopted in 1978 and a new Criminal Code in 1979.

Regional courts act as courts of first instance; county courts as either courts of first instance or of appeal. The Supreme Court acts normally as an appeal court, but may act as a court of first instance in cases submitted to it by the Public Prosecutor. All courts, when acting as courts of first instance, consist of 1 professional judge and 2 lay assessors, and, as courts of appeal, of 3 professional judges. Local government Executive Committees may try petty offences.

Regional and county judges and assessors are elected by the appropriate local councils; members of the Supreme Court by Parliament.

There are also military courts of the first instance. Military cases of the second instance go before the Supreme Court.

The death penalty was abolished in Oct. 1990.

61,977 sentences were imposed on adults in 1988, including 22,820 of imprisonment. Juvenile convictions: 6,220.

Religion. The Office for Church Affairs was replaced by the Secretariat for Church Policies in May 1989. 8·5m. of the population professed a religious faith in 1976; the number of active church members was put between 1m. and 1·5m.

In 1976 there were 5·25m. Roman Catholics with 4,400 churches, and 500,000 Uniates. In 1979 there were 3 seminaries and 1 Uniate seminary, a theological academy, and 8 secondary schools. There were 2,400 Roman Catholic priests in 1986. There are also lay co-operators of both sexes who perform some priestly duties. The Primate of Hungary is Archbishop László Pacskai, appointed Aug. 1986. There are 11 dioceses, all with bishops or archbishops. There is one Uniate bishopric.

In 1976 there were 2m. Calvinists with 4 dioceses, 1,300 ministers and 1,567 churches. There were 2 theological colleges (20% of students female) with 16 teachers, and 1 secondary school. There were 500,000 Lutherans with 16 dioceses, 374 ministers and 673 churches. There is a theological college with 6 teachers. The 10 denominations in the Association of Free Churches had 37,000 members, 230 ministers and 675 churches. There are 4 Orthodox denominations with 40,000 members in 1979. The Unitarian Church has 10,000 members, 11 ministers and 6 churches. In 1991 there were 100,000 Jews (825,000 in 1939) with 136 synagogues, 26 rabbis and a rabbinical college which enrols 10 students a year.

Optional religious education was introduced in schools in 1990.

Education. Education is free and compulsory from 6 to 14. Primary schooling ends at 14; thereafter education may be continued at secondary, secondary technical or secondary vocational schools, which offer diplomas entitling students to apply for higher education, or at vocational training schools which offer tradesmen's diplomas. Students at the latter may also take the secondary school diploma examinations after 2 years of evening or correspondence study.

In 1988–89 there were 4,772 kindergartens with 33,876 teachers and 393,735 pupils; 3,526 primary schools with 90,620 teachers and 1,242,700 pupils; 645 secondary schools with 20,084 teachers and 248,300 pupils; and 294 vocational training schools with 11,745 teachers and 186,700 trainees. There are 4 universities proper (Budapest, Pécs, Szeged, Debrecen), and 14 specialized universities (6 technical, 4 medical, 3 arts, 1 economics). At these and at 40 other institutions of higher education there were 16,242 teachers and 71,700 full-time students (10% of the 18-22 year-old population). Corvin University, a private institution, was preparing to open in Budapest in 1990.

Libraries and Museums. In 1988 there were 4,503 public and 4,456 trade union libraries. The Széchenyi Library is the national library. In 1988 there were 734 museums with 18·34m. visitors.

Health. In 1988 there were 36,059 doctors and dentists and 104,832 hospital beds. Main causes of death, 1988: Heart disease, 37,457; neoplasms, 28,997; cerebrovascular diseases, 21,219. 8 cases of AIDS were reported.

Average daily consumption per head of population, 1988: 13,750 kilojoules.

Social Security. Medical treatment is free. Patients bear 15% of the cost of medicines. Sickness benefit is 75% of wages, old age pensions (at 60 for men, 55 for women) 60–70%. In 1987, 162,000m. forints were paid out in social insurance benefits including 23,182m. in family allowances, 13,400m. in sick pay and 129,966m. in pensions. Benefits were raised in Dec. 1989. There were 2·42m. pensioners in 1988. In 1988 family allowances were paid to 1,327,000 families. Monthly allowances (in forints) are: One child, 1,620; two, 3,240; three, 5,250; four, 7,000 (more for single parents).

DIPLOMATIC REPRESENTATIVES

Of Hungary in Great Britain (35 Eaton Pl., London, SW1X 8BY)
Ambassador: Tibor Antalpéter.

Of Great Britain in Hungary (Harmincad Utca 6, Budapest V)
Ambassador: J. A. Birch, CMG.

Of Hungary in the USA (3910 Shoemaker St., NW, Washington, D.C., 20008)
Ambassador: (Vacant).

Of the USA in Hungary (Szabadság Tér 12, Budapest V)
Ambassador: Charles Thomas.

Of Hungary to the United Nations
Ambassador: Endre Erdos.

Further Reading

Statisztikai Évkönyv. Budapest, annual; since 1871, abridged English version, *Statistical Year-Book*
Statistical Pocket Book of Hungary (in English). Budapest, annual from 1959
State Budget. Budapest, annual from 1983
The Hungarian Economy: a Quarterly Economic and Business Review. Budapest, since 1972
Hungary 66 (67 etc.). Budapest, annual from 1966
Managers in Hungary: A Biographical Directory. Budapest, 1986
Marketing in Hungary. Budapest, quarterly
Quarterly Review of the National Bank of Hungary. From 1983
Information Hungary. Budapest, 1980

Bako, E., *Guide to Hungarian Studies*. 2 vols. Stanford Univ. Press, 1973
Batt, J., *Economic Reform and Political Change in Eastern Europe: A Comparison of the Czechoslovak and Hungarian Experiences*. Basingstoke, 1988
Berend, I. T. and Ranki, G., *Hungary: A Century of Economic Development*. New York and Newton Abbot, 1974.—*Underdevelopment and Economic Growth: Studies in Hungarian Social and Economic History*. Budapest, 1979.—*The Hungarian Economy in the Twentieth Century*. London, 1985
Bernat, T., (ed.) *An Economic Geography of Hungary*. Budapest, 1985
Bölöny, J., *Magyarország Kormányai, 1848–1975*. Budapest, 1978. [Lists governments and politicians]
Brown, D. M., *Towards a Radical Democracy: The Political Economy of the Budapest School*. Cambridge, 1988
Fekete, J., *Back to the Realities: Reflections of a Hungarian Banker*. Budapest, 1982
Hann, C. M. (ed.), *Market Economy and Civil Society in Hungary*. London, 1990
Hegedüs, A., *The Structure of Socialist Society*. London, 1977
Heinrich, H.-G., *Hungary: Politics, Economics and Society*. London, 1986
Kabdebó, T., *Hungary*. [Bibliography] Oxford and Santa Barbara, 1980
Kornai, J., *The Road to a Free Economy: Shifting from a Socialist System—the Example of Hungary*. New York and London, 1990
Lendvai, P., *Hungary: The Art of Survival*. London, 1989
Macartney, C. A., *Hungary: A Short History*. London, 1962
Pamlényi, E. (ed.) *A History of Hungary*. Budapest, 1975
Pécsi, M. and Sárfalvi, B., *Physical and Economic Geography of Hungary*. 2nd ed. Budapest, 1979
Sugar, P. F. (ed.) *A History of Hungary*. London, 1991
Vasary, I., *Beyond the Plan: Social Change in a Hungarian Village*. Boulder, 1987

ICELAND

Capital: Reykjavík
Population: 253,500 (1989)
GNP per capita: US$19,383 (1989)

Lyðveldið Ísland

(Republic of Iceland)

HISTORY. The first settlers came to Iceland in 874. Between 930 and 1264 Iceland was an independent republic, but by the 'Old Treaty' of 1263 the country recognized the rule of the King of Norway. In 1381 Iceland, together with Norway, came under the rule of the Danish kings, but when Norway was separated from Denmark in 1814, Iceland remained under the rule of Denmark. Since 1 Dec. 1918 it has been acknowledged as a sovereign state. It was united with Denmark only through the common sovereign until it was proclaimed an independent republic on 17 June 1944.

AREA AND POPULATION. Iceland is a large island in the North Atlantic, close to the Arctic Circle, and comprises an area of about 103,000 sq. km (39,758 sq. miles), with its extreme northern point (the Rifstangi) lying in 66° 32' N. lat., and its most southerly point (Kötlutangi) in 63° 23' N. lat., not including the islands north and south of the land; if these are included, the country extends from 67° 10' N. (the Kolbeinsey) to 63° 17' N. (Surtsey, one of the Westman Islands). It stretches from 13° 30' (the Gerpir) to 24° 32' W. long. (Látrabjarg). The skerry *Hvalbakur* (The Whaleback) lies 13° 16' W. long.

There are 8 regions:

Region	*Inhabited land (sq. km)*	*Mountain pasture (sq. km)*	*Waste-land (sq. km)*	*Total area (sq. km)*	*Population (1 Dec. 1989)*
Capital area	1,266	716	—	1,982	143,864
Southwest Peninsula					15,082
West	5,011	3,415	275	8,711	14,685
Western Peninsula	4,130	3,698	1,652	9,470	9,840
Northland West	4,867	5,278	2,948	13,093	10,450
Northland East	9,890	6,727	5,751	22,368	26,107
East	16,921	17,929	12,555	21,991	13,243
South				25,214	20,229
Iceland	42,085	37,553	23,181	102,819	253,500

The census population (1980) was 229,187. In 1989, 24,116 were domiciled in rural districts and 229,384 in towns and villages (of over 200 inhabitants). The population is almost entirely Icelandic.

In 1989 foreigners numbered 4,774; of these 1,079 were Danish, 803 US, 501 British, 342 Norwegian and 328 German nationals.

The capital, Reykjavík, had on 1 Dec. 1989, a population of 96,708; other towns were Akranes, 5,362; Akureyri, 14,091; Bolungarvík, 1,215; Dalvík, 1,458; Eskifjörður, 1,095; Garðabær, 6,885; Grindavík, 2,161; Hafnarfjörður, 14,541; Húsavík, 2,487; Ísafjörður, 3,478; Keflavík, 7,423; Kópavogur, 15,900; Neskaupstaður, 1,754; Njarðvík, 2,392; Ólafsfjörður, 1,193; Sauðárkrókur, 2,508; Selfoss, 3,847; Seltjarnarnes, 4,088; Seyðisfjörður, 997; Siglufjörður, 1,806; Vestmannaeyjar, 4,860.

Vital statistics for calendar years:

	Living births	*Still-born*	*Marriages*	*Divorces*	*Deaths*	*Infant deaths*
1987	4,193	15	1,160	477	1,725	30
1988	4,673	18	1,294	459	1,818	29
1989	4,560	6	1,176	520	1,715	24

The official language is Icelandic *(íslenska)*.

CLIMATE. The climate is cool temperate oceanic and rather changeable, but mild for its latitude because of the Gulf Stream and prevailing S.W. winds. Precipitation is high in upland areas, mainly in the form of snow. Reykjavik. Jan. 34°F (1°C), July 52°F (11°C). Annual rainfall 34" (860 mm).

CONSTITUTION AND GOVERNMENT. On 24 May 1944 the people of Iceland decided in a referendum to sever all ties with the Danish Crown. The voters were asked whether they were in favour of the abrogation of the Union Act, and whether they approved of the bill for a republican constitution: 70,725 voters were for severance of all political ties with Denmark and only 370 against it; 69,048 were in favour of the republican constitution, 1,042 against it and 2,505 votes were invalid. On 17 June 1944 the republic was formally proclaimed, and as the republic's first president the Alþingi elected Sveinn Björnsson for a 1-year term (re-elected 1945 and 1949; died 25 Jan. 1952). The President is now elected by direct, popular vote for a period of 4 years.

President of the Republic of Iceland: Vigdís Finnbogadóttir (elected 29 June 1980, with 43,611 out of 129,049 valid votes, inaugurated 1 Aug. 1980); re-elected unopposed in 1984; re-elected in 1988 with 94% of the valid votes.

National flag: Blue with a red white-bordered Scandinavian cross.

National anthem: Ó Guð vors lands (words by M. Jochumsson, 1874; tune by S. Sveinbjörnsson).

The *Alþingi* (Parliament) is divided into two Houses, the Upper House and the Lower House. The former is composed of one-third of the members elected by the whole Alþingi in common sitting. The remaining two-thirds of the members form the Lower House. The members of the Alþingi receive payment for their services.

The budget bills must be laid before the two Houses in joint session, but all other bills can be introduced in either of the Houses. If the Houses do not agree, they assemble in a common sitting and the final decision is given by a majority of two-thirds of the voters, with the exception of budget bills, where a simple majority is sufficient. The ministers have free access to both Houses, but can vote only in the House of which they are members.

The electoral law enacted in 1984 provides for an Alþingi of 63 members. Of these, 54 seats are distributed among the 8 constituencies as follows: 14 seats are allotted to Reykjavík, 8 to Reykjanes (i.e. the South-west excluding Reykjavík) and 5 or 6 to each of the remaining 6. From the 9 seats then left, 8 are divided beforehand among the constituencies according to the number of registered voters in the preceding elections. Finally, one seat is given to a constituency after the elections, to compensate the party with the fewest seats as compared to its number of votes.

At the elections held on 25 April 1987 the following parties were returned: Independence Party, 18; Progressives, 13; Social Democrats, 10; People's Alliance, 8; Citizen's Party, 7; Women's Alliance, 6; Association for Equality and Social Justice, 1. Elections were due on 20 April 1991.

The executive power is exercised under the President by the Cabinet. The coalition Cabinet, as constituted in Jan. 1991, was as follows:

Prime Minister: Steingrímur Hermannsson (Progress).

Foreign Affairs: Jón Baldvin Hannibalsson (Soc. Dem.). *Finance:* Ólafur Ragnar Grímsson (People's Alliance). *Social Affairs:* Jóhanna Sigurðardóttir (Soc. Dem.). *Fisheries:* Halldór Ásgrímsson (Progress). *Justice and Church:* Óli P. Guðbjartsson (Citizens' Party). *Agriculture and Communications:* Steingrímur J. Sigfússon (People's Alliance). *Health and Social Security:* Guðmundur Bjarnason (Progress). *Commerce, Energy and Industry:* Jón Sigurðsson (Soc. Dem.). *Education:* Svavar Gestsson (People's Alliance). *Environment:* Júlíus Sólnes.

Local Administration. Iceland was on 1 Dec. 1988 divided into 217 communes, of which 30 had the status of a town. The commune councils are elected by universal suffrage (men and women 18 years of age and over), in towns and other urban communes by proportional representation, in rural communes by simple majority. For general co-operation the communes are free to form district councils, of which there were 174 in 1990. All the communes except 10 towns are members in 20 district councils. The communes appoint one or more representatives to the district councils according to their population size. The commune councils are supervised by the Ministry of Social Affairs. For national government there are 27 divisions (*lögsagnarumdæmi*), consisting of towns and counties, single or combined, with the exception of Keflavík Airport (also a NATO base), which is a separate national government division consisting of parts of 5 communes. In the capital the different branches of national government are independent (jurisdictional power and executive power, i.e. courts, police, customs etc.), while in other national government divisions they are the charge of the sheriffs, also residing as the local magistrates.

Elections were held in May 1990 for all 30 town councils (there are 250 councillors including 81 women) and for 119 of the 174 district councils.

DEFENCE. Iceland possesses neither an army nor a navy. Under the North Atlantic Treaty, US forces are stationed in Iceland as the Iceland Defence Force. 4 armed offshore patrol craft for fishery protection vessels are maintained by the Icelandic National Coastguard, with 1 patrol aircraft and 1 helicopter. Coastguard Service personnel in 1990 totalled about 150.

INTERNATIONAL RELATIONS

Membership. Iceland is a member of the UN, EFTA, OECD, the Council of Europe, NATO and the Nordic Council.

ECONOMY

Budget. Total revenue and expenditure for calendar years (in 1m. kr.):

	1983	*1984*	*1985*	*1986*	*1987*	*1988*
Revenue	16,282	22,088	28,746	40,176	52,324	71,287
Expenditure	17,717	20,474	30,617	46,374	53,582	73,415

Main items of the Treasury accounts for 1988 (in 1m. kr.):

Revenue		*Expenditure*	
Direct taxes	13,342	Administration, justice and police	6,606
Indirect taxes	53,272	Foreign service	573
Other	4,673	Education, culture and State Church	12,047
		Health and social security	30,791
		Subsidies	3,924
		Agriculture	2,990
		Fisheries	1,650
		Manufacturing and energy	1,338
		Communications	4,727
		Other	8,769

Central government debt was on 31 Dec. 1989, 97,113m. kr, of which the foreign debt amounted to 58,512m. kr.

Currency. The unit of currency is the *Icelandic króna* (ISK) of 100 *aurar*, (singular: *eyrir*). In March 1991, US$1 = kr. 56·01; £1 = kr. 106·25. Note and coin circulation, 31 Dec. 1989, was 2,975m. kr.

Banking. The *Seðlabanki Íslands* (The Central Bank of Iceland; *Governor:* Johannes Nordal), established in 1961, is responsible for note issue and carries out the central banking functions which before 1961 were carried out by the *Landsbanki Íslands* (The National Bank of Iceland, owned entirely by the State), currently (1991) the largest commercial bank. There are 2 other private, commercial banks: Íslandsbanki (The Iceland Bank Ltd), created in Jan. 1990 by a merger of 4 banks, and *Búnaðarbanki Íslands* (The Agricultural Bank of Iceland), founded in 1930. Banking is being deregulated in stages to come into line with the EEC's internal market in Jan. 1993.

On 31 Dec. 1989 the accounts of the Central Bank balanced at 43,529m. kr.; commercial bank deposits were 90,893m. kr.; deposits in the 34 savings banks, 17,650m. kr.

There is a stock exchange.

Weights and Measures. The metric system of weights and measures is obligatory.

ENERGY AND NATURAL RESOURCES

Electricity. The installed capacity of public electrical power plants at the end of 1989 totalled 928,543 kw., of which 752,000 kw. comprised hydro-electric plants. Total electricity production in public-owned plants in 1989 amounted to 4,475m. kwh.; in privately-owned plants, 5m. kwh. Supply 220 volts; 50 Hz.

Agriculture. Of the total area of Iceland, about six-sevenths is unproductive, but only about 1·3% is under cultivation, which is largely confined to hay, potatoes and turnips. In 1989 the total hay crop was 3,222,058 cu. metres; the crop of potatoes, 8,382 tonnes, and of turnips (1988) 10,288 tonnes. At the end of 1989 the livestock was as follows: Horses, 69,238; cattle, 72,789 (including 31,490 milch cows); sheep, 560,920; pigs, 3,247; poultry, 231,997.

Fisheries. Fishing vessels at the end of 1989 numbered 966 with a gross tonnage of 125,797. Total catch in 1988, 1,758,000 tonnes; 1989, 1,506,000 tonnes.

The Icelandic Government announced that the fishery limits off Iceland were extended from 12 to 50 nautical miles from Sept. 1972. An interim agreement for 2 years signed by the UK and Iceland in Nov. 1973 expired in Nov. 1975.

On 15 July 1975 the Icelandic Government issued a decree that from 15 Oct. 1975 the fishery limits of Iceland were extended from 50 to 200 nautical miles. The Icelandic Government maintain that this extension is necessary to protect the fish stocks in Icelandic waters because the fishing industry is of vital importance to the national economy.

INDUSTRY. Production, 1989, in 1,000 tonnes: Aluminium, 88·5; diatomite, 24·9; fertilizer, 47·9; ferro-silicon, 72·0. Sales of cement, 1989, 103·7 tonnes.

Labour. In Nov. 1990, 1·3% of the total labour force was registered as unemployed.

FOREIGN ECONOMIC RELATIONS.

The economy is heavily trade-dependent.

Commerce. Total value of imports (c.i.f.) and exports (f.o.b.) in 1,000 kr.:

	1985	*1986*	*1987*	*1988*	*1989*
Imports	37,600,289	45,905,230	61,231,629	68,723,300	80,249,900
Exports	33,749,626	44,967,770	53,053,078	61,666,700	80,071,700

Leading exports (in 1,000 kg and 1,000 kr.):

	1988		*1989*	
	Quantity	*Value*	*Quantity*	*Value*
Marine products	689,735	43,826,200	637,971	56,811,800
Aluminium	81,071	6,626,400	89,657	10,289,600
Ferro-silicon	73,236	2,418,100	64,192	3,026,800

Leading imports (in 1,000 tonnes and 1,000 kr.):

	1988		*1989*	
	Quantity	*Value*	*Quantity*	*Value*
Ships (number)	34	5,427,600	18	2,770,400
Fuel oil	90,221	351,900	96,074	546,500
Gas oils	270,739	1,741,500	301,113	2,681,900
Jet fuel	69,085	469,100	109,143	1,151,400
Cereals	13,120	223,300	9,694	225,300
Animal feed	51,443	523,900	57,947	869,500
Gasoline	122,850	909,200	110,284	1,257,800
Motor vehicles (number)	14,702	5,115,700	7,430	3,485,100
Fishing nets and other gear	828	379,700	632	365,200

Value of trade with principal countries for 3 years (in 1,000 kr.):

	1987		1988		1989	
	Imports (c.i.f.)	*Exports (f.o.b.)*	*Imports (c.i.f.)*	*Exports (f.o.b.)*	*Imports (c.i.f.)*	*Exports (f.o.b.)*
Austria	460,175	43,839	474,100	63,500	633,000	77,200
Belgium	1,600,741	632,743	1,326,900	480,100	1,509,800	630,200
Brazil	303,435	57,002	250,500	70,900	256,800	262,600
Canada	253,273	155,191	290,900	174,000	429,600	429,600
Czechoslovakia	222,441	52,707	268,300	85,700	306,000	206,700
Denmark	5,623,103	2,049,506	6,357,700	2,032,600	7,262,800	2,927,400
Faroe Islands	51,019	332,770	9,500	544,500	19,600	1,042,500
Finland	1,437,854	901,293	1,693,300	763,700	1,617,800	1,200,200
France	2,067,547	2,853,565	2,150,100	2,978,700	2,496,300	4,594,900
German Dem. Rep.	180,419	29,249	117,500	81,200	164,200	8,900
Germany, Fed. Rep. of	9,309,949	5,301,154	9,783,700	6,367,000	10,497,700	9,506,300
Greece	47,455	544,769	58,500	483,800	74,800	819,900
Hungary	17,822	13,875	23,100	118,100	37,800	57,700
India	33,958	—	56,900	—	53,900	300
Ireland	182,098	96,422	233,300	29,100	307,300	6,900
Israel	29,488	4,277	31,900	1,200	142,500	66,500
Italy	1,922,360	1,612,898	3,010,200	1,560,300	2,486,600	2,552,500
Japan	5,012,566	4,139,386	4,756,500	4,706,500	3,916,900	5,674,800
Netherlands	4,956,247	493,084	5,607,300	704,300	8,358,300	1,373,300
Nigeria	416	796,702	400	241,800	—	347,900
Norway	5,052,542	957,056	6,166,200	1,489,400	5,295,800	1,742,400
Poland	532,591	483,555	979,900	851,700	1,313,900	1,192,500
Portugal	485,120	4,967,089	611,200	5,240,100	658,400	3,447,000
Spain	643,754	1,575,506	651,100	2,113,000	798,600	2,698,100
Sweden	5,032,051	1,014,228	6,025,000	1,094,200	6,592,400	1,384,600
Switzerland	659,240	1,429,739	785,900	2,783,600	1,155,300	4,409,700
USSR	2,573,564	1,932,899	2,396,400	2,194,100	3,382,600	2,489,700
UK	5,032,757	10,321,470	5,608,000	14,340,900	6,508,800	16,630,800
USA	4,367,065	9,677,945	5,185,800	8,372,600	8,823,300	11,435,500

Total trade between Iceland and UK (British Department of Trade returns, in £1,000 sterling):

	1986	*1987*	*1988*	*1989*	*1990*
Imports to UK	173,140	178,314	198,365	196,678	259,438
Exports and re-exports from UK	73,640	84,866	87,100	69,497	88,537

Tourism. There were 130,498 visitors to Iceland in 1989.

COMMUNICATIONS

Roads. On 31 Dec. 1989 the length of the public roads (including roads in towns) was 12,473 km. Of these 8,256 km were national main roads and 3,117 km were provincial roads. Total length of surfaced roads was 2,300 km. A ring road of 1,400 km runs just inland from much of the coast; about 60% of it is smooth-surfaced. Motor vehicles registered at the end of 1989 numbered 138,784, of which 125,559 were passenger cars and 12,152 trucks; there were also 1,073 motor cycles.

Aviation. Icelandair and Eagle Air maintain regular domestic services from Reykjavík. (Icelandair 1989: 252,237 passengers). Icelandair is the only international carrier. It serves 14 destinations in west Europe and 3 in the USA. In 1991 it had 4 Boeing 737-400s, 3 757-200s and 3 757-400s. In 1989 Icelandair carried in scheduled foreign flights 432,304 passengers. There are international airports at Reykjavík and Keflavík (Leifsstöd).

Shipping. Total registered vessels, 1,112 (190,000 GRT) on 31 Dec. 1989, of these 966 were sea-going fishing vessels.

Telecommunications. At the end of 1989 the number of post offices was 130 and telephone and telegraph offices 84; number of telephone subscribers, 125,000. The State Broadcasting Service, *Rikisútvarpid*, broadcasts 2 radio channels and 1 TV channel. On 1 Jan. 1986 the state monopoly on broadcasting was abolished by law and the field opened to others, if they fulfilled certain conditions. Besides *Rikisútvarpid* 3 privately owned radio stations and 1 TV station were in operation in 1989. Number of licensed receivers (1989): Radio, about 85,000; television, about 79,000.

Cinemas (1988). In the capital area there were 6 cinemas (19 cinema halls) with a seating capacity of about 4,655.

Newspapers (1988). There are 6 daily newspapers, 5 in Reykjavík and one in Akureyri, with a combined circulation of about 100,000.

JUSTICE, RELIGION, EDUCATION AND WELFARE

Justice. The lower courts of justice are those of the provincial magistrates (*sýslumenn*) and town judges (*bœjarfógetar*). From these there is an appeal to the Supreme Court (*hœstiréttur*) in Reykjavík, which has 8 judges.

Religion. The national church, and the only one endowed by the State, is Evangelical Lutheran. But there is complete religious liberty, and no civil disabilities are attached to those not of the national religion. The affairs of the national church are under the superintendence of a bishop. In 1989, 6,303 persons (2·5%) were Dissenters and 3,364 persons (1·3%) did not belong to any religious community.

Education. Compulsory education for children began in 1907, and a university was founded in Reykjavík in 1911. There is in Reykjavík a teachers' training college and a technical high school; various specialized institutions of learning and a number of second-level schools are scattered throughout the country. There are many part-time schools of cultural activities, including music.

Compulsory education comprises 9 classes, 7-15 years of age. After completion of a facultative 9th class, attended by 93%-95% of the relevant age group, there is access to further schooling free of charge. Some 53%-74% of the age groups 16-19 years old attend schools. Around 15%-20% of each age group go into handicraft apprenticeship. About 30% pass matriculation examination, generally at the age of 20. Approximately one third-level student out of every four goes abroad for studies, two-thirds of them to Scandinavia, the rest mainly to English- and German-speaking countries.

Immatriculation in Iceland in autumn 1989: Preceding the first level, 4,400. First-level (1st-6th class) 25,500. Second-level first stage (7th-9th class) 12,400. Second-level second stage (4-year courses) 16,700. Third-level studies, 5,400.

Social Welfare. The main body of the Icelandic social welfare legislation is consolidated in six main acts:

(i) The social security legislation (a) health insurance, including sickness benefits; *(b)* social security pensions, mainly consisting of old age pension, disablement pension and widows' pension, and also children's pension; *(c)* employment injuries insurance.

(ii) The unemployment insurance legislation, where daily allowances are paid to those who have met certain conditions.

(iii) The subsistence legislation. This is controlled by municipal government, and social assistance is granted under special circumstances, when payments from other sources are not sufficient.

(iv) The tax legislation. Prior to 1988 children's support was included in the tax legislation, according to which a certain amount for each child in a family was subtracted from income taxes or paid out to the family. Since 1988 family allowances are paid directly to all children age 0-15 years. The amount is increased with the second child in the family, and children under the age of 7 get additional benefits. Single parents receive additional allowances.

(v) The rehabilitation legislation.

(vi) Child and juvenile guidance.

Health insurance covers the entire population. Citizenship is not demanded and there is no waiting period. Most hospitals are both municipally and state run, a few solely state run and all offer free medical help. Medical treatment out of hospitals is partly paid by the patient, the same applies to medicines, except medicines of life-long necessary use, which are paid in full by the health insurance. Dental care is free for the age groups 6-15, but is paid 75% for those five years or younger and the age group 16 but 50% for old age and disabled pensioners. Sickness benefits are paid to those who lose income because of periodical illness. The daily amount is fixed and paid from the 11th day of illness.

The pension system is composed of the public social security system and some 90 private pension funds. The social security system pays basic old age and disablement pensions of a fixed amount regardless of past or present income, as well as supplementary pensions to individuals with low present income. The pensions are index-linked, i.e. are changed in line with changes in wage and salary rates in the labour market. The private pension funds pay pensions that depend on past payments of premiums that are a fixed proportion of earnings. The payment of pension fund premiums is compulsory for all wage and salary earners. The pensions paid by the funds differ considerably between the individual funds, but are generally index-linked. In the public social security system, entitlement to old age and disablement pensions at the full rates is subject to the condition that the beneficiary has been resident in Iceland for 40 years at the age period of 16–67. For shorter period of residence, the benefits are reduced proportionally. Entitled to old age pension are all those who are 67 years old, and have been residents in Iceland for 3 years of the age period of 16–67. Entitled to disablement pension are those who have lost 75% of their working capacity and have been residents in Iceland for 3 years before application or have had full working capacity at the time when they became residents. Old age and disablement pension are of equally high amount, in the year 1989 the total sum was 122,296 kr. for an individual. Married pensioners are paid 90% of two individuals' pensions. In addition to the basic amount, supplementary allowances are paid according to social circumstances and income possibilities. Widows' pensions are the same amount as old age and disablement pension, provided the applicant is over 60 when she becomes widowed. Women at the age 50–60 get reduced pension. Women under 50 are not entitled to widows' pensions.

The employment injuries insurance covers medical care, daily allowances, disablement pension and survivors' pension and is applicable to practically all employees.

Social assistance is primarily municipal and granted in cases outside the social security legislation. Domestic assistance to old people and disabled is granted within this legislation, besides other services.

Child and juvenile guidance is performed by chosen committees according to special laws, such as home guidance and family assistance. In cases of parents' disablement the committees take over the guidance of the children involved.

DIPLOMATIC REPRESENTATIVES

Of Iceland in Great Britain (1 Eaton Terrace, London, SW1W 8EY)
Ambassador: Helgi Ágústsson (accredited 13 Dec. 1989).

Of Great Britain in Iceland (Laufásvegur 49, 101 Reykjavík)
Ambassador and Consul-General: Sir Richard Best, CBE.

Of Iceland in the USA (2022 Connecticut Ave., NW, Washington, D.C., 20008)
Ambassador: Tómas Á. Tómasson.

Of the USA in Iceland (Laufásvegur 21, 101 Reykjavík)
Ambassador: Charles E. Cobb Jr.

Of Iceland to the United Nations
Ambassador: Benedikt Gröndal.

Further Reading

Statistical Information: The Statistical Bureau of Iceland, Hagstofa Íslands (Reykjavík) was founded in 1914. *Director:* Hallgrímur Snorrason. Its main publications are:

Tölfræðihandbók. Statistical Abstract of Iceland (latest issue 1984)
Hagskýrslur Íslands. Statistics of Iceland (from 1912)

Hagtíðindi (Statistical Bulletin) (from 1916)
Hagtólur mánaðarins. Monthly Bulletin (from 1973). Central Bank of Iceland
Economic Statistics Quarterly. Central Bank of Iceland (quarterly from 1980)
Heilbrigðisskýrslur. Public Health in Iceland (latest issue for 1984-85; published 1989)
Yearbook of Nordic Statistics. Nordic Council of Ministers and the Nordic Statistical Secretariat, Copenhagen.
Cleasby, R., *An Icelandic-English Dictionary*. 2nd ed. Oxford, 1957
Einarsson, P. and Lacy, T. G., *Ensk-íslensk viðskiptaorðabók*. English-Icelandic Dictionary of Business Terms. Reykjavík, 1989
Foss, H. (ed.) *Directory of Iceland*. Annual. Reykjavík, 1907–40, 1948 ff.
Hermannsson, Halldór, *Islandica*. An annual relating to Iceland and the Fiske Icelandic Collection in Cornell University Library. Ithaca (from 1908)
Horton, J. J., *Iceland*. [Bibliography] Oxford and Santa Barbara, 1983
Magnússon, S. A., *Northern Sphinx: Iceland and the Icelanders from the Settlement to the Present*. London, 1977
Nordal, J. and Kristinsson, V. (eds) *Iceland 1986*. Central Bank of Iceland, Reykjavík, 1987
Þórðarson, Matthias, *The Althing, Iceland's Thousand-Year-Old Parliament, 930–1930*. Reykjavík, 1930
Zoëga, G. T., *Íslensk-ensk (and Ensk-íslensk) orðabók*. 3rd ed. 2 vols. Reykjavík, 1932–51

National Library: Landsbókasafnið, Reykjavík, *Librarian:* Dr Finnbogi Guðmundsson.

INDIA

Bharat

(Republic of India)

Capital: New Delhi
Population: 843·93m. (1991)
GDP per capita: US$330 (1988)

HISTORY. The Indus civilization was fully developed by *c.* 2500 B.C., and collapsed *c.* 1750 B.C. An Aryan civilization spread from the west as far as the Ganges valley by 500 B.C.; separate kingdoms were established and many of these were united under the Mauryan dynasty established by Chandragupta in *c.* 320 B.C. The Mauryan Empire was succeeded by numerous small kingdoms. The Gupta dynasty (A.D. 320–600) was followed by the first Arabic invasions of the north-west. Moslem, Hindu and Buddhist states developed together with frequent conflict until the establishment of the Mogul dynasty in 1526. The first settlements by the East India Company were made after 1600 and the company established a formal system of government for Bengal in 1700. During the decline of the Moguls frequent wars between the Company, the French and the native princes led to the Company's being brought under British Government control in 1784; the first Governor-General of India was appointed in 1786. The powers of the Company were abolished by the India Act, 1858, and its functions and forces transferred to the British Crown. Representative government was introduced in 1909, and the first parliament in 1919. The separate dominions of India and Pakistan became independent within the Commonwealth in 1947 and India became a republic in 1950.

AREA AND POPULATION. India is bounded north-west by Pakistan, north by China, Tibet, Nepal and Bhutan, east by Burma, south-east, south and south west by the Indian ocean. The far eastern states and territories are almost separated from the rest by Bangladesh as it extends northwards from the Bay of Bengal. The area of the Indian Union (excluding the Pakistan and China-occupied parts of Jammu and Kashmir) is 3,166,829 sq. km. Its population according to the 1991 census was 843,930,861 (excluding the occupied area of Jammu and Kashmir). Population at the 1981 census was 685,184,692. Sex ratio was 933 females per 1,000 males (929 in 1971); density of population, 216 per sq. km. About 23·3% of the population was urban in 1981 (in Maharashtra, 35%; in Himachal Pradesh, 7·6%). Estimated mid-year population, 1988–89, 797m.

Many births and deaths go unregistered. Data from the office of the Registrar General of India suggest that the birth rate for 1988-89 was about 31·3 per 1,000 population, the death rate 10.9 per 1,000. In 1981 (census) the age-group 0–14 years represented 39·5% of the population and only 6·5% were over 60. In 1981 expectation of life 54·4 years.

Marriages and divorces are not registered. The minimum age for a civil marriage is 18 for women and 21 for men; for a sacramental marriage, 14 for girls and 18 for youths.

The main details of the census of 1 March 1971 and of 1 March 1981 are:

Name of State	*Land area in sq. km (1981)*	*Population 1971*	*Population 1981*
States			
Andhra Pradesh	275,608	43,502,708	53,549,673
Assam	78,438	14,625,152	19,896,843
Bihar	173,877	56,353,369	69,914,734
Gujarat	195,024	26,697,475	34,085,799
Haryana	44,212	10,036,808	12,922,618
Himachal Pradesh	55,673	3,460,434	4,280,818
Jammu and Kashmir[1]	101,387	4,616,632	5,987,389
Karnataka	191,791	29,299,014	37,135,714
Kerala	38,863	21,347,375	25,453,680
Madhya Pradesh	443,446	41,654,119	52,178,844

[1] Excludes the Pakistan-occupied area.

Name of State	Land area in sq. km (1981)	Population 1971	Population 1981
Maharashtra	307,690	50,412,235	62,684,171
Manipur	22,429	1,072,753	1,420,953
Meghalaya	22,429	1,011,699	1,325,819
Nagaland	16,579	516,449	774,930
Orissa	155,707	21,944,615	26,370,271
Punjab	50,362	13,551,060	16,788,915
Rajasthan	342,239	25,765,806	34,261,862
Sikkim	7,096	209.845	316,385
Tamil Nadu	130,058	41,199,168	48,408,077
Tripura	10,486	1,556,342	2,053,058
Uttar Pradesh	294,411	88,341,144	110,862,013
West Bengal	87,852	44,312,011	54,580,647
Union Territories			
Andaman and Nicobar Islands	8,249	115,133	188,741
Arunachal Pradesh [1]	83,743	467,511	631,839
Chandigarh	114	257,251	450,610
Dadra and Nagar Haveli	491	74,170	103,676
Daman and Diu	112	62,648	78,981
Delhi	1,483	4,065,698	6,220,406
Goa [2]	3,702	795,123	1,007,749
Lakshadweep	32	31,810	40,249
Mizoram [1]	21,081	332,390	493,797
Pondicherry	492	471,707	604,471
Grand total	3,166,829	548,159,052	685,184,692

[1] Achieved statehood 1986. [2] Achieved statehood 1987.

Greatest density occurs in Delhi (4,194 per sq. km), Chandigarh (3,961), Lakshadweep (1,258) and Pondicherry (1,229). The lowest occurs in Arunachal Pradesh (8).

There were (1981) 343,930,423 males and 321,357,426 females.

In 1981, 525m. were rural (76·7%) and 160m. were urban.

Cities and Urban Agglomerations (with states in brackets) having more than 250,000 population at the 1981 census were (1,000):

Agra (U.P.)	694
Ahmedabad (Guj.)	2,159
Ajmer (Raj.)	376
Aligarh (U.P.)	321
Allahabad (U.P.)	620
Amravati (Mah.)	261
Amritsar (Pun.)	595
Aurangabad (Mah.)	299
Bangalore (Kar.)	2,629
Bareilly (U.P.)	395
Bhatpara (W.B.)	265
Belgaum (Kar.)	274
Bhavnagar (Guj.)	309
Bhilainagar (M.P)	319
Bhopal (M.P.)	671
Bikaner (Raj.)	256
Bombay (Mah.)[2]	8,243
Calcutta (W.B.)[3]	9,196
Calicut (Ker.)	394
Chandigarh (Ch.)	423
Cochin (Ker.)	552
Coimbatore (T.N.)	705
Cuttack (Ori.)	295
Dehra Dun (U.P.)	221
Delhi	4,884
Dhanbad (Bih.)	578
Durgapur (W.B.)	312
Durg-Bhilainagar (M.P.)	490
Erode (T.N.)	275
Faridabad agglomeration (Har.)	331
Ghaziabad (U.P)	276
Gorakhpur (U.P.)	308
Guntur (A.P.)	368
Gwalior (M.P.)	539
Haora (W.B)	744
Hubli-Dharwar (Kar.)	527
Hyderabad (A.P.)	2,187
Indore (M.P.)	829
Jabalpur (M.P.)	649
Jadavpur (W.B)	252
Jaipur (Raj.)	977
Jalandhar (Pun.)	408
Jamnagar (Guj.)	294
Jamshedpur (Bih.)	457
Jodhpur (Raj.)	506
Kanpur (U.P.)	1,486
Kolhapur (Mah.)	341
Kotah (Raj.)	358
Lucknow (U.P.)	917
Ludhiana (Pun.)	607
Madras (T.N.)	3,277
Madurai (T.N.)	821
Meerut (U.P.)	417
Moradabad (U.P.)	330
Mysore (Kar.)	479
Nagpur (Mah.)	1,219
Nasik (Mah.)	262
New Delhi (Del.)	273
Patna (Bih.)	814
Pune (Mah.)	1,203
Raipur (M.P.)	338
Rajahmundry (A.P.)	268
Rajkot (Guj.)	445
Ranchi (Bih.)	490
Saharanpur (U.P.)	295
Salem (T.N.)	361
Sholapur (Mah.)	515
South Suburban (W.B)	395
Srinagar (J. & K.)	595[1]
Surat (Guj.)	777
Thane (Mah.)	310
Tiruchirapalli (T.N.)	362
Tirunelveli (T.N.)	323
Trivandrum (Ker.)	500
Ujjain (M.P.)	282
Ulhasnagar (Mah.)	274
Vadodara (Guj.)	734
Varanasi (U.P.)	721
Vijayawada (A.P.)	462
Visakhapatnam (A.P.)	584
Warangal (A.P.)	335

[1] Estimate. [2] Greater Bombay. [3] Urban agglomeration.

Report of the Officials of the Government of India and the People's Republic of China on the Boundary Question. New Delhi, Ministry of External Affairs, 1961
Census of India: Reports and Papers, Decennial Series. (Government of India.)
Annual Report on the Working of Indian Migration. Government of India, from 1956
Report of the Commissioner for Scheduled Castes and Scheduled Tribes. Government of India. Annual
Public Health. Report of the Public Health Commission with the Government of India. Annual
Agarwala, S. N., *India's Population Problems*. New York, 1973

CLIMATE. India has a variety of climatic sub-divisions. In general, there are four seasons. The cool one lasts from Dec. to March, the hot season is in April and May, the rainy season is June to Sept., followed by a further dry season till Nov. Rainfall, however, varies considerably, from 4" (100 mm) in the N.W. desert to over 400" (10,000 mm) in parts of Assam.

Range of temperature and rainfall: New Delhi. Jan. 57°F (13·9°C), July 88°F (31·1°C). Annual rainfall 26" (640 mm). Bombay. Jan. 75°F (23·9°C), July 81°F (27·2°C). Annual rainfall 72" (1,809 mm). Calcutta. Jan. 67°F (19·4°C), July 84°F (28·9°C). Annual rainfall 64" (1,600 mm). Cherrapunji. Jan. 53°F (11·7°C), July 68°F (20°C). Annual rainfall 432" (10,798 mm). Cochin. Jan. 80°F (26·7°C), July 79°F (26·1°C). Annual rainfall 117" (2,929 mm). Darjeeling. Jan. 41°F (5°C), July 62°F (16·7°C). Annual rainfall 121" (3,035 mm). Hyderabad. Jan. 72°F (22·2°C), July 80°F (26·7°C). Annual rainfall 30" (752 mm). Madras. Jan. 76°F (24·4°C), July 87°F (30·6°C). Annual rainfall 51" (1,270 mm). Patna. Jan. 63°F (17·2°C), July 90°F (32·2°C). Annual rainfall 46" (1,150 mm).

CONSTITUTION AND GOVERNMENT. On 26 Jan. 1950 India became a sovereign democratic republic. India's relations with the British Commonwealth of Nations were defined at the London conference of Prime Ministers on 27 April 1949.

Unanimous agreement was reached to the effect that the Republic of India remains a full member of the Commonwealth and accepts the Queen as 'the symbol of the free association of its independent member nations and, as such, the head of the Commonwealth'. This agreement was ratified by the Constituent Assembly of India on 17 May 1949.

The constitution was passed by the Constituent Assembly on 26 Nov. 1949 and came into force on 26 Jan. 1950. It has since been amended 67 times.

India is a Union of States and comprises 25 States and 7 Union territories. Each State is administered by a Governor appointed by the President for a term of 5 years while each Union territory is administered by the President through an administrator appointed by him.

The capital is New Delhi.

Presidency. The head of the Union is the President in whom all executive power is vested, to be exercised on the advice of ministers responsible to Parliament. He is elected by an electoral college consisting of all the elected members of Parliament and of the various state legislative assemblies. He holds office for 5 years and is eligible for re-election. He must be an Indian citizen at least 35 years old and eligible for election to the Lower House. He can be removed from office by impeachment for violation of the constitution.

There is also a Vice-President who is *ex-officio* chairman of the Upper House of Parliament.

Central Legislature. The Parliament for the Union consists of the President, the Council of States *(Rajya Sabha)* and the House of the People *(Lok Sabha)*. The Council of States, or the Upper House, consists of not more than 250 members; in Nov. 1990 there were 233 elected members and 12 members nominated by the President. The election to this house is indirect; the representatives of each State are elected by the elected members of the Legislative Assembly of that State. The Council of States is a permanent body not liable to dissolution, but one-third of the members retire every second year. The House of the People, or the Lower House, consists of 545 members, 530 directly elected on the basis of adult suffrage from territorial constituencies in the States, and 13 members to represent the Union territories, chosen in such manner as the Parliament may by law provide; in Jan. 1991 there were 513 elected members, 2 members nominated by the President and 30 vacancies. The House of the People unless sooner dissolved continues for a period of 5 years from the date appointed for its first meeting; in emergency, Parliament can extend the term by 1 year.

State Legislatures. For every State there is a legislature which consists of the Governor, and *(a)* 2 Houses, a Legislative Assembly and a Legislative Council, in the States of Bihar, Jammu and Kashmir, Karnataka, Madhya Pradesh (where it is provided for but not in operation), Maharashtra and Uttar Pradesh, and *(b)* 1 House, a Legislative Assembly, in the other States. Every Legislative Assembly, unless sooner dissolved, continues for 5 years from the date appointed for its first meeting. In emergency the term can be extended by 1 year. Every State Legislative Council is a permanent body and is not subject to dissolution, but one-third of the members retire every second year. Parliament can, however, abolish an existing Legislative Council or create a new one, if the proposal is supported by a resolution of the Legislative Assembly concerned.

Legislation. The various subjects of legislation are enumerated in three lists in the seventh schedule to the constitution. List I, the Union List, consists of 97 subjects (including defence, foreign affairs, communications, currency and coinage, banking and customs) with respect to which the Union Parliament has exclusive power to make laws. The State legislature has exclusive power to make laws with respect to the 66 subjects in list II, the State List; these include police and public order, agriculture and irrigation, education, public health and local government. The powers to make laws with respect to the 47 subjects (including economic and social planning, legal questions and labour and price control) in list III, the Concurrent List, are held by both Union and State governments, though the former prevails. But Parliament may legislate with respect to any subject in the State List in circumstances when the subject assumes national importance or during emergencies.

Other provisions deal with the administrative relations between the Union and the States, interstate trade and commerce, distribution of revenues between the States and the Union, official language, etc.

Fundamental Rights. Two chapters of the constitution deal with fundamental rights and 'Directive Principles of State Policy'. 'Untouchability' is abolished, and its practice in any form is punishable. The fundamental rights can be enforced through the ordinary courts of law and through the Supreme Court of the Union. The directive principles cannot be enforced through the courts of law; they are nevertheless fundamental in the governance of the country.

Citizenship. Under the Constitution, every person who was on the 26 Jan. 1950, domiciled in India and *(a)* was born in India or *(b)* either of whose parents was born in India or *(c)* who has been ordinarily resident in the territory of India for not less than 5 years immediately preceding that date became a citizen of India. Special provision is made for migrants from Pakistan and for Indians resident abroad. Under the Citizenship Act, 1955, which supplemented the provisions of the Constitution, Indian citizenship is acquired by birth, by descent, by registration and by naturalization. The Act also provides for loss of citizenship by renunciation, termination and deprivation. The right to vote is granted to every person who is a citizen of India and who is not less than 21 years of age on a fixed date and is not otherwise disqualified.

Parliament. Parliament and the state legislatures are organized according to the following schedule (figures show distribution of seats in Nov. 1990):

	Parliament		State Legislatures	
	House of the People (Lok Sabha)	*Council of States (Rajya Sabha)*	*Legislative Assemblies (Vidhan Sabhas)*	*Legislative Councils (Vidhan Parishads)*
States:				
Andhra Pradesh	42	18	294	–
Arunachal Pradesh	2	1	60	–
Assam	14	7	126	–
Bihar	54	22	324	96
Goa	2	–	40	–
Gujarat	26	11	182	–
Haryana	10	5	90	–
Himachal Pradesh	4	3	68	–
Jammu and Kashmir	6	4	76[2]	36[4]
Karnataka	28	12	224	75
Kerala	20	9	140	–
Madhya Pradesh	40	16	320	–
Maharashtra	48	19	288	63
Manipur	2	1	60	–
Meghalaya	2	1	60	–
Mizoram	1	1	40	–
Nagaland	1	1	60	–
Orissa	21	10	147	–
Punjab	13	7	117	–
Rajasthan	25	10	200	–
Sikkim	1	1	32	–
Tamil Nadu	39	18	234	–
Tripura	2	1	60	–
Uttar Pradesh	85	34	425	108
West Bengal	42	16	294	–
Union Territories:				
Andaman and Nicobar Islands	1	–	–	–
Chandigarh	1	–	–	–
Dadra and Nagar Haveli	1	–	–	–
Delhi	7	3	56	–
Daman and Diu	1	–	–	–
Lakshadweep	1	–	–	–
Pondicherry	1	1	30	–
Nominated by the President under Article 80 (1) (a) of the Constitution	–	12	–	–
Total	545[1]	244	4,047	378

[1] Includes 2 nominated members to represent Anglo-Indians.
[2] Excludes 24 seats for Pakistan-occupied areas of the State which are in abeyance.
[3] Nominated by the President. [4] Excludes seats for the Pakistan-occupied areas.

The number of seats allotted to scheduled castes and scheduled tribes in the House of the People is 79 and 41 respectively. Out of the 4,047 seats allotted to the Legislative Assemblies, 557 are reserved for scheduled castes and 527 for scheduled tribes.

Composition of the House of the People after the election held in Nov. 1989: Congress (I) 193; Janata Dal, 141; Bharatiya Janata Party, 88; CPI (Marxist, 32; CPI, 12; AIADMK (All India Anna Dravida Munnetra Kazagam), 11; Akali Dal (Mann), 6; Revolutionary Socialist Party, 4; Bahujan Samaj Party, 3; Forward Bloc, 3; Jharkhand Mukti Morcha, 3; J. & K. National Conference, 3; Muslim League, 2; Telugu Desam, 2; Independent and others, 22; nominated, 2; vacant, 18.

Composition of the Council of States in Feb. 1991: Congress (I) 108; Communist Party of India (Marxist), 17; All-India Anna DMK, 4; Janata Dal, 23; Bharatiya Janata, 17; Janata, 1; Telugu Desam, 10; Dravida Munnetra Kazagam, 10; Asom Gana Parishad, 5; Revolutionary Socialist Party, 2; J. & K. National Conference, 2; Communist Party, 3; Ind, 12; Janata Dal (S), 15, nominated, 5; vacant, 2.

National flag: Three horizontal stripes of saffron (orange), white and green, with the wheel of Asoka in the centre in blue.

National anthem: Jana-gana-mana ('Thou art the ruler of the minds of all people'; words by Rabindranath Tagore).

Indian Independence Act, 1947. (Ch. 30.) London, 1947
The Constitution of India (Modified up to 15 April 1967). Delhi, 1967
Appadorai, A., *Indian Political Thinking in the Twentieth Century: From Naoroji to Nehru.* OUP, 1971.—*Documents on Political Thought in Modern India.* OUP, 1974
Austin, G., *The Indian Constitution.* OUP, 1972
Mansergh, N., (ed.) *The Transfer of Power 1942–47.* 5 vols. HMSO, 1970–75
Pylee, M. V., *Constitutional Government in India.* 2nd ed. Bombay, 1965
Rao, K. V., *Parliamentary Democracy of India.* 2nd ed. Calcutta, 1965
Seervali, H. M., *Constitutional Law of India.* Bombay, 1967

Language. The Constitution provides that the official language of the Union shall be Hindi in the Devanagari script. It was originally provided that English should continue to be used for all official purposes until 1965. But the Official Languages Act 1963 provides that, after the expiry of this period of 15 years from the coming into force of the Constitution, English might continue to be used, in addition to Hindi, for all official purposes of the Union for which it was being used immediately before that day, and for the transaction of business in Parliament. According to the Official Languages (Use for official purposes of the Union) Rules 1976, an employee may record in Hindi or in English without being required to furnish a translation thereof in the other language and no employee possessing a working knowledge of Hindi may ask for an English translation of any document in Hindi except in the case of legal or technical documents.

The 58th amendment to the Constitution (26 Nov. 1987) authorised the preparation of a Constitution text in Hindi.

The following 15 languages are included in the Eighth Schedule to the Constitution: Assamese, Bengali, Gujarati, Hindi, Kannada, Kashmiri, Malayalam, Marathi, Oriya, Punjabi, Sanskrit, Sindhi, Tamil, Telugu, Urdu.

There are numerous mother tongues grouped under each language. Hindi, Bengali, Telugu, Tamil and Marathi languages (including mother tongues grouped under each) are spoken by 264·2m., 51·5m., 54·2m., 44·7m. and 49·6m. of the population respectively.

Ferozsons English–Urdu, Urdu–English Dictionary. 2 vols. 4th ed. Lahore, 1961
Fallon, S. W., *A New English–Hindustani Dictionary.* Lahore, 1941
Grierson, Sir G. A., *Linguistic Survey of India.* 11 vols. (in 19 parts). Delhi, 1903-28
Mitra, S. C., *Student's Bengali–English Dictionary.* 2nd ed. Calcutta, 1923
Scholberg, H. C., *Concise Grammar of the Hindi Language.* 3rd ed. London, 1955
University of Madras, *Tamil Lexicon.* 7 vols. Madras, 1924-39
Vyas, V. G. and Patel, S. G., *Standard English–Gujarati Dictionary.* 2 vols. Bombay, 1923

Government. *President of the Republic:* R. Venkataraman (sworn in 25 July 1987). *Vice-President:* Shankar Dayal Sharma (elected 21 Aug. 1987).

There is a *Council of Ministers* to aid and advise the President of the Republic in the exercise of his functions; this comprises Ministers who are members of the Cabinet and Ministers of State who are not. A Minister who for any period of 6 consecutive months is not a member of either House of Parliament ceases to be a Minister at the expiration of that period. The Prime Minister is appointed by the President; other Ministers are appointed by the President on the Prime Minister's advice.

The salary of each Minister is Rs 27,000 per annum, and that of each Deputy Minister is Rs 21,000 per annum. Each Minister is entitled to the free use of a furnished residence and a chauffeur-driven car throughout his term of office. A Cabinet Minister has a sumptuary allowance of Rs 1,000 per month, Ministers of State, Rs 500 and Deputy Ministers, Rs 300. At the administrative head of each Ministry is a Secretary of the Government.

After losing a vote of confidence V.P. Singh was replaced in Nov. 1990 by Chandra Shekhar (Janata Dal Secular Party) as *Prime Minister*.

The Cabinet consisted of the following portfolios in Nov. 1990:

Portfolios held by the Prime Minister assisted by Ministers of State: *Defence, Science and Technology, Atomic Energy, Personnel, Space, Home Affairs, Ocean Development, Public Grievances and Pensions, Electronics, Information and Broadcasting, Industry, Labour, Welfare, Planning and Programme Implementation, and other portfolios not allocated to any other Minister.*

Deputy Prime Minister and Agriculture and Tourism; Finance; External Affairs; Commerce, Law and Justice; Urban Development; Steel and Mines; Energy; Communications; Health, Family Welfare; Petroleum and Chemicals, Parliamentary Affairs; Food and Civil Supplies; Railways; Textiles, Food Processing Industries; Human Resources Development; Water Resources, Surface Transport.

There were also 3 Ministers of State with independent responsibilities and 12 Ministers of State.

On 6 March 1991 Chandra Shekhar and his government resigned, remaining in office only long enough to see through the budget.

Elections were expected to be held late in May 1991.

Local Government. There were in 1989-90, 72 municipal corporations, 1,770 municipal committees/boards/councils, 663 town area committees and 337 notified area committees. The municipal bodies have the care of the roads, water supply, drainage, sanitation, medical relief, vaccination, education, street lighting, etc. Their main sources of revenue are taxes on the annual rental value of land and buildings, octroi and terminal, vehicle and other taxes. The municipal councils enact their own bye-laws and frame their budgets, which in the case of municipal bodies other than corporations generally require the sanction of the State government. All municipal councils are elected on the principle of adult franchise.

For rural areas there is a 3-tier system of *panchayati raj* at village, block and district level, although the 3-tier structure may undergo some changes in State legislation to suit local conditions. All *panchayati raj* bodies are organically linked, and representation is given to special interests. Elected directly by and from among villagers, the *panchayats* are responsible for agricultural production, rural industries, medical relief, maternity and child welfare, common grazing grounds, village roads, tanks and wells, and maintenance of sanitation. In some places they also look after primary education, maintenance of village records and collection of land revenue. They have their own powers of taxation. There are some judicial *panchayats* or village courts.

Panchayati raj now cover almost all the States and Union Territories with variations in structural pattern. *Panchayati raj* involvels a 3-tier arrangement: Village level, block level and district level. Tenure of *Panchayati raj* institutions range from 3–5 years.

The powers and responsibilities of *Panchayati raj* institutions are derived from State Legislatures, and from the executive orders of State governments.

NAGARLOK (Municipal Affairs Quarterly). Quarterly. Institute of Public Administration. Delhi

Proceedings of the 13th Meeting of the Central Council of Local Self Government. Delhi, 1970

Report of the Committee on Budgetary Reforms in Municipal Administration. Delhi, 1974

State Machinery for Municipal Supervision. Institute of Public Administration. Delhi, 1970

Statistical Abstract of India. Annual. Delhi.

DEFENCE. The Supreme Command of the Armed Forces vests in the President of the Indian Republic. Policy is decided at different levels by a number of committees, including the Political Affairs Committee presided over by the Prime Minister and the Defence Minister's Committee. Administrative and operational control rests in the respective Service Headquarters, under the control of the Ministry of Defence.

The Ministry of Defence is the central agency for formulating defence policy and for co-ordinating the work of the three services. Among the organizations directly administered by the Ministry are the Research and Development Organization, the Production Organization, the National Defence College, the National Cadet Corps and the Directorate-General of Armed Forces Medical Services.

The Research and Development Organization (headed by the Scientific Adviser to the Minister) has under it about 30 research establishments. The Production Organization controls 8 public-sector undertakings and 38 ordnance factories.

The National Defence College, New Delhi, was established in 1960 on the pattern of the Imperial Defence College (UK): the 1-year course is for officers of the rank of brigadier or equivalent and for senior civil servants. The Defence Services Staff College, Wellington, trains officers of the three Services for higher command for staff appointments. There is an Armed Forces Medical College at Pune.

The National Defence Academy, Khadakvasla, gives a 3-year basic training course to officer cadets of the three Services prior to advanced training at the respective Service establishments.

Army. The Army Headquarters functioning directly under the Chief of the Army Staff is divided into the following main branches: General Staff Branch; Adjutant General's Branch; Quartermaster-General's Branch; Master-General of Ordnance Branch; Engineer-in-Chief's Branch; Military Secretary's Branch.

The Army is organized into 5 commands each divided into areas, which in turn are subdivided into sub-areas. Recruitment of permanent commissioned officers is through the Indian Military Academy, Dehra Dun. It conducts courses for ex-National Defence Academy, National Cadet Corps and direct-entry cadets, and for serving personnel and technical graduates.

The Territorial Army came into being in Sept. 1949, its role being to: (1) relieve the regular Army of static duties and, if required, support civil power; (2) provide anti-aircraft units, and (3) if and when called upon, provide units for the regular Army. The Territorial Army is composed of practically all arms of the Services.

The authorized strength of the Army was (1991) 1·1m., that of the Territorial Army, 160,000. There are 2 armoured, 1 mechanized, 19 infantry and 11 mountain divisions, 5 independent armoured brigades, 7 independent infantry, 3 independent artillery brigades, 1 parachute brigade, 1 mountain brigade, 6 air defence brigades and 4 engineer brigades. An Aviation Corps was formed in 1986 and operates locally-built Alouette and Lama helicopters.

Equipment includes some 800 T-55, 700 T-72/-M1 and 1,700 Vijayanta main battle tanks and 100 PT-76 light tanks.

Navy. The Navy has 3 commands; Eastern, Western and Southern, the latter a training and support command. The fleet is divided into two elements, Eastern and Western; and well-trained, all volunteer personnel operate a mix of Soviet and Western vessels.

The principal ships of the Indian Navy are the two light aircraft carriers, *Viraat* and *Vikrant*. The *Viraat*, formerly HMS *Hermes*, is of 29,000 tonnes and was completed in 1959. Having earlier been converted to vertical/short take-off and landing aircraft operations, she was transferred to the Indian Navy in 1987. Her normal air group is 8 to 10 Sea Harrier fighters, and 8 Sea King anti-submarine helicopters. *Vikrant*, 19,800 tonnes, is the former HMS *Hercules*, and was transferred to India in 1961, and completed conversion to the vertical/short take-off and landing role in 1990. She will embark an air group similar to Viraat.

In addition to the 2 carriers, there is a leased Soviet nuclear-powered missile submarine, *Chakra*, of the Soviet 'Charlie-1' class. The fleet also includes 8 'Kilo' and 8 'Foxtrot' Soviet-built diesel submarines and 2 smaller German-built. 5 new Soviet-built missile armed destroyers, 3 heavily modified and 6 rather less modified 'Leander' class frigates, all built in India, and 14 other frigates form the main surface force. Coastal forces include 10 Soviet-designed missile corvettes, 12 fast missile craft and 11 inshore patrol craft. There are 12 Soviet-built offshore minesweepers, and 8 much smaller inshore vessels. Amphibious lift for the 1,000 strong marine force is provided by 1 tank landing ship and 9 medium landing ships, as well as about 10 craft. Support forces include 3 tankers, 1 submarine depot ship, 1 transport, 10 survey and research, 2 tugs and one training ship.

The Naval Air force, 5,000 strong, operates 18 Sea Harriers, 3 Il-38 'May', 5 Tu-142M 'Bear' and 9 Britten-Norman Islander maritime patrol aircraft. The small squadron of 4 Alize anti-submarine aircraft is now based ashore. Armed helicopters include 10 Chetak, 5 Ka-25, 18 Ka-27 and 40 Sea King, and the inventory is completed with some 22 training and communications aircraft.

Main bases are at Bombay (HQ Western Fleet, and main dockyard), Goa, Vishakhapatnam (HQ Eastern Fleet) and Calcutta on the sub-continent, and Port Blair in the Andaman Islands. HQ Southern Command is at Cochin.

Naval personnel in 1990 numbered 52,000 including 5,000 Naval Air Arm and 1,000 marines.

The Coast Guard is an independent para-military service 2,500 strong in 1990, which functions under Defence Ministry control, but is funded by the Revenue Department. The force comprises 8 offshore patrol vessels and 29 inshore patrol craft. Its 22 aircraft are of Dornier-228, Fokker F-27 and Britten-Norman Islander types.

Air Force. The Indian Air Force Act was passed in 1932, and the first flight was formed in 1933.

The Air Headquarters, under the Chief of Air Staff, consists of 4 main branches, viz., Air Staff, Administration, Policy and Plans, and Maintenance. Units of the IAF are organized into 5 operational commands–Western at Delhi, Central at Allahabad, Eastern at Shillong, Southern at Trivandrum and South-Western at Jodhpur. Training Command HQ is at Bangalore, Maintenance Command at Nagpur. Nominal strength in 1991 was 110,000 personnel and 735 aircraft of all types, in over 50 squadrons of aircraft and helicopters and about 30 squadrons of 'Guideline' and 'Goa' surface-to-air missiles, and close-range missiles such as 'Gainful' and Tigercat.

Air defence units include 2 squadrons of MiG-23 variable-geometry interceptors, 2 squadrons of MiG-29s, 18 squadrons of MiG-21s and 3 of Mirage 2000s. Initial delivery of MiG-21s from the Soviet Union was followed by large-scale licence production in India. Other combat units include 8 squadrons of MiG-27s, 2 of Canberras, 4 of Jaguars, 4 of MiG-23 supersonic fighter-bombers and one of MiG-25 reconnaissance aircraft plus a MiG-25U two seat trainer. Currently the main re-equipment programmes involve the licence-production of MiG-27 and Jaguar strike aircraft.

The large transport force includes An-12s, An-32s, Il-76s, Do 228s, HS 748s, 2 Boeing 737s, and smaller aircraft and helicopters for VIP and other duties. Helicopter units have Mi-8s and Mi-17s (10 squadrons), Mi-26s, and Mi-25 gunships, but the bulk of the Air Force's Chetaks (Alouette IIIs) and Cheetahs (Lamas) have been transferred to Army control, main training types are the Hindustan HPT-32 and Kiran, Polish-built TS-11 Iskra, Hunter T.66, MiG-21UT1 and MiG-23U.

Primary flying training is provided at the Elementary Flying School, Bidar, and advanced flying training at the Air Force Academy, Dundigal, Hyderabad. There is a Navigation and Signals School at Begumpet. The IAF Technical College, Jalahalli, imparts technical training, while the IAF Administrative College, Coimbatore, trains officers of the ground duty branch. There are also land-air warfare, flying instructors' and medical schools.

INTERNATIONAL RELATIONS

Membership. India is a member of the UN, the Commonwealth and the Colombo Plan.

External Debt. At the end of March 1990 India's external public debt was estimated at Rs 799,820m.

Treaties. India pursues a general policy of non-alignment; the exception is a Treaty of Peace, Friendship and Cooperation with the USSR, 1971; the parties agreed to mutual support short of force in the event of either being attacked by a third party.

ECONOMY

Policy. The highest economic decision-making body is the *National Development Council*. There is also a *Planning Commission*.

The eighth 5-year plan (1990–95) emphasizes job creation and increases rural investment, and aims at an annual growth of 5·5% of GDP, 3% in employment and a savings rate of 22% of GDP.

As a first step towards partial privatization of the 248 state-owned corporations, selected public sector enterprises are being allowed to raise funds through equity issues.

Requirements for government approval of investment decisions were reduced in 1990. The eighth plan (1990–95) envisages an outlay of Rs 6,100,000m., with the public sector contributing Rs 3,350,000m. Central plan outlay (1991–92), Rs 421,480m.

Ministry of Agriculture. *Serving the Small Farmer: Policy Choices in Indian Agricultural Development.* 1975

Dutt, A. K. (ed.) *India: Resources, Potentialities and Planning.* Rev. ed. Dubuque, India, 1973

Singh, T., *India's Development Experience.* London, 1975

Budget. Revenue and expenditure (on revenue account) of the central government for years ending 31 March, in crores of rupees:

	1989–90	*1990–91*	*1991–92* [2]
Revenue	52,296	45,294	63,584
Expenditure	52,137	56,671	64,304

[1] Revised. [2] Budget estimates.

Important items of revenue and expenditure on the revenue account of the central government for 1990–91 (estimates), in Rs 1m.:

Revenue		*Expenditure*	
Net tax revenue	377,980	General Services	398,400
Non-tax revenue	118,370	Defence	109,480
		Major subsidies	85,160

Total capital account receipts (1991–92 budget), Rs 366,060m.; capital account disbursements, Rs 288,170m. Total (revenue and capital) receipts, Rs 1,001,900m.; disbursements, Rs 1,101,670m.

Under the Constitution (Part XII and 7th Schedule), the power to raise funds has been divided between the central government and the states. Generally, the sources of revenue are mutually exclusive. Certain taxes are levied by the Union for the sake of uniformity and distributed to the states. The Finance Commission (Art. 280 of the Constitution) advises the President on the distribution of the taxes which are distributable between the centre and the states, and on the principles on which grants should be made out of Union revenues to the states. The main sources of central revenue are: customs duties; those excise duties levied by the central government; corporation, income and wealth taxes; estate and succession duties on non-agricultural assets and property, and revenues from the railways and posts and telegraphs. The main heads of revenue in the states are: taxes and duties levied by the state governments (including land revenues and agricultural income tax); civil administration and civil works; state undertakings; taxes shared with the centre; and grants received from the centre.

Currency. A decimal system of coinage was introduced in 1957. The Indian *rupee* (INR) is divided into 100 *paise*. There are coins of 1, 2, 3, 5, 10, 20, 25 and 50 *paise*. The paper currency consists of: (1) Reserve Bank notes in denominations of Rs 2, 5, 10, 20, 50, 100 and 500; and (2) Government of India currency notes of denominations of Re 1 deemed to be included in the expression 'rupee coin' for the purposes of the Reserve Bank of India Act, 1934.

According to the Reserve Bank of India, the total money supply with the public on the last Friday of March 1990 was Rs 46,564 crores. Foreign exchange reserves, Aug. 1990, Rs 32,031m.

The rupee is valued in relation to a package of main currencies. The £ is the currency of intervention. In March 1991 Rs 36.50 = £1; Rs 19.24 = US$1.

1 *crore* = Rs 10m.; 1 *lakh* = Rs 100,000.

Banking and Finance. The Reserve Bank, the central bank for India, was established in 1934 and started functioning on 1 April 1935 as a shareholder's bank; it became a nationalized institution on 1 Jan. 1949. It has the sole right of issuing currency notes. The Bank acts as adviser to the Government on financial problems and is the banker for central and state governments, commercial banks and some other financial institutions. The Bank manages the rupee public debt of central and state governments. It is the custodian of the country's exchange reserve and supervises repatriation of export proceeds and payments for imports. The Bank gives short-term loans to state governments and scheduled banks and short and medium-term loans to state co-operative banks and industrial finance institutions. The Bank has extensive powers of regulation of the banking system, directly under the Banking Regulation Act, 1949, and indirectly by the use of variations in Bank rate, variation in reserve ratios, selective credit controls and open market operations. Bank rate was raised to 10% in July 1981.

Except refinance for food credit and export credit, the Reserve Bank's refinance facility to commercial banks has been placed on a discretionary basis. The net profit of the Reserve Bank of India for the year ended June 1986, after making the usual or necessary provisions, amounted to Rs 210 crores.

The commercial banking system consisted of 274 scheduled banks (*i.e.*, banks which are included in the 2nd schedule to the Reserve Bank Act) and 4 non-scheduled banks on 30 June 1988; scheduled banks included 196 Regional Rural Banks. Total deposits in commercial banks, March 1990, stood at Rs 172,759 crores. The business of non-scheduled banks forms less than 0·1% of commercial bank business. Of the 274 scheduled banks, 22 are foreign banks which specialize in financing foreign trade but also compete for domestic business. The largest scheduled bank is the State Bank of India, constituted by nationalizing the Imperial Bank of India in 1955. The State Bank acts as the agent of the Reserve Bank and the subsidiaries of the State Bank act as the agents of the State Bank for transacting government business as well as undertaking commercial functions. Fourteen banks with aggregate deposits of not less than Rs 50 crores were nationalized on 19 July 1969. Six banks were nationalized in April 1980. The 28 public sector banks (which comprise the State Bank of India and its seven associate banks and 20 nationalised banks) account for over 88·5% of deposits and bank credit of all scheduled commercial banks.

There are stock exchanges in Ahmedabad, Bombay, Calcutta, Delhi and Madras.

Reserve Bank of India: Report on Currency and Finance.—Report on the Trend and Progress of Banking in India.—Report of the Central Board of Directors. Annual. Bombay

Weights and Measures. Uniform standards of weights and measures, based on the metric system, were established for the first time by the Standards of Weights and Measures Act, 1956, which provided for a transition period of 10 years. So far the system has been fully adopted in trade transactions but there are a few fields such as engineering, survey and land records and the building and construction industry where it has not; efforts are being made to complete the change as early as possible.

In order to align this legislation with the latest international trends an expert committee (Weights and Measures (Law Revision) Committee) was set up by the central government to suggest a revised Bill which was passed by Parliament in April 1976. The new Standards of Weights and Measures Act, 1976, has recognized the International System of Units and other units recommended by the General Conference on Weights and Measures and is in line with the recommendations of the International Organisation of Legal Metrology (OIML). The new Act also covers the system of numeration, the approval of models of weights and measures, regulation and control of inter-state trade in relation to weights and measures. The Act also protects consumers through proper indication of weight, quantity, identity, source, date and price on packaged goods. A draft Standards of Weights and Measures (Enforcement) Bill has also been prepared by the committee for adoption either by Parliament or State legislatures, as enforcement is now in the 'concurrent' list of legislation.

The provisions of the 1976 Act came into force in Sept. 1977, as did the accompanying Standards of Weights and Measures (Packaged Commodities) Rules, 1977.

While the Standards of Weights and Measures are laid down in the Central Act, enforcement of weights and measures laws is entrusted to the state governments; the central Directorate of Weights and Measures is responsible for co-ordinating activities so as to ensure national uniformity.

An Indian Institute of Legal Metrology trains officials of the Weights and Measures departments of India and different developing countries. The Institute is being modernized with technical assistance from the Federal Republic of Germany.

There are 2 Regional Reference Standards laboratories at Ahmedabad and Bhubaneswar which (besides calibrating secondary standards of physical measurements) also provide testing facilities in metrological and industrial measurements. These laboratories are equipped with Standards next in line to the National Standards of physical measurements which are maintained at the National Physical Laboratory in New Delhi.

For weights previously in legal use under the Standards of Weight Act, 1956, *see* THE STATESMAN'S YEAR-BOOK, 1961, p. 171.

Calendar. The dates of the Saka era (named after the north Indian dynasty of the first century A.D.) are being used alongside Gregorian dates in issues of the *Gazette of India*, news broadcasts by All-India Radio and government-issued calendars, from 22 March 1957, a date which corresponds with the first day of the year 1879 in the Saka era.

ENERGY AND NATURAL RESOURCES

Electricity. In Nov. 1990 460,536 villages out of 575,938 had electricity. Production of electricity in 1988–89 was 221,120m. kwh., of which 163,330m. kwh. came from thermal and nuclear stations and 57,790m. kwh from hydro-electric stations. Supply 230 and 250 volts; 50 Hz.

Oil and Gas. The Oil and Natural Gas Commission, Oil India Ltd and the Assam Oil Co. are the only producers of crude oil. Production 1988-89, 32·04m. tonnes, about 60% of consumption. The main fields are in Assam and offshore in the Gulf of Cambay (the Bombay High field). Natural gas production, 1988–89, 13,217m. cu. metres.

Water. The net area of 63·3m. ha (1987-88) under irrigation exceeds that of any other country except China, and equals about 38% of the total area under cultivation. Irrigation projects have formed an important part of all three Five-Year Plans. The possibilities of diverting rivers into canals being nearly exhausted, the emphasis is now on damming the monsoon surplus flow and diverting that. Ultimate potential of irrigation is assessed at 107m. ha, total cultivated land being 142m. ha. In 1985 India and Bangladesh reached an agreement to monitor the water of the Ganges at the Farakka barrage.

1987 was a year of severe drought, affecting both agriculture and water-supplies to cities.

Minerals. Bihar, West Bengal and Madhya Pradesh produce 42%, 25% and 19% of all coal, respectively. The coal industry was nationalized in 1973. Production, 1989–90, 200m. tonnes; reserves (including lignite) are estimated at 176,330m. tonnes. Production of other minerals, 1988-90 (in 1,000 tonnes): Iron ore, 51,657; bauxite, 4,480; chromite 1,038; copper ore, 5,211; manganese ore, 1,305; gold, 1,754 kg. Other important minerals are lead, zinc, limestone, apatite and phosphorite, dolomite, magnesite and silver. Value of mineral production, 1989, Rs 141,760m. of which mineral fuels produced Rs 121,670m., metallic minerals Rs 8,840m. and non-metallic Rs 11,250m.

Agriculture. The chief industry of India has always been agriculture. About 70% of the people are dependent on the land for their living. In 1988-89 it provided about 35% of net national product.

In 1989–90 agricultural commodities accounted for about 9·5% by value of Indian exports. In 1984–85 agricultural commodities, machinery and fertilizers accounted for about 20% of imports. Tea accounted for about 30% of agricultural exports.

An increase in food production of at least 2% per annum is necessary to keep pace with the rising population. Foodgrain production, 1989-90 (estimate) 171m. tonnes.

The Indian Council of Agricultural Research works through 46 institutes, 20 national research centres, 9 project directorates, and 75 national research projects. There are 4 national research bureaux and 23 agricultural universities.

The farming year runs from July to June through three crop seasons: Kharif (monsoon); rabi (winter) and summer.

Agricultural production, 1989-90 (in 1,000 tonnes): Rice, 74,053; wheat, 49,652; total foodgrains, 170,626·5; maize, 9,410; pulses, 12,615; sugar-cane 222,628; oil-seeds, 18,033; cotton, 11·4m. bales (of 180 kg); jute is grown in West Bengal (70% of total yield), Bihar and Assam, total yield, 7·1m. bales (of 180 kg). The coffee industry is growing: The main cash varieties are Arabica and Robusta (main growing areas Karnataka, Kerala and Tamil Nadu).

The tea industry is important, with production concentrated in Assam, West Bengal, Tamil Nadu and Kerala. Total crop in 1989–90, 702,810 tonnes from 414,232 ha.

Livestock (1988): Cattle, 193m.; sheep, 51,684,000; pigs, 10·3m.; horses, 953,000; asses, 1,328,000m.; goats, 105m.; buffaloes, 72m.

Fertilizer consumption in 1989–90 was 11·6m. tonnes.

Land Tenure. There are three main traditional systems of land tenure: *Ryotwari* tenure, where the individual holders, usually peasant proprietors, are responsible for the payment of land revenues; *zamindari* tenure, where one or more persons own large estates and are responsible for payment (in this system there may be a number of intermediary holders); and *mahalwari* tenure, where village communities jointly hold an estate and are jointly and severally responsible for payment.

Agrarian reform, initiated in the first Five-Year Plan, being undertaken by the state governments includes: (1) The abolition of intermediaries under *zamindari* tenure. (2) Tenancy legislation designed to scale down rents to $^1/_4$-$^1/_5$ of the value of the produce, to give permanent rights to tenants (subject to the landlord's right to resume a minimum holding for his personal cultivation), and to enable tenants to acquire ownership of their holdings (subject to the landlord's right of resumption for personal cultivation) on payment of compensation over a number of years. (3) Fixing of ceilings on existing holdings and on future acquisition; the holding of a family is between 4·05 and 7·28 ha if it has assured irrigation to produce two crops a year; 10·93 ha for land with irrigation facilities for only one crop a year; and 21·85 ha for all other categories of land. Tea, coffee, cocoa and cardamom plantations have been exempted. (4) The consolidation of holdings in community project areas and the prevention of fragmentation of holdings by reform of inheritance laws. (5) Promotion of farming by co-operative village management (*see* p. 644).

The average size of holding for the whole of India is 2·63 ha. Andhra Pradesh, 2·87; Assam, 1·46; Bihar, 1·53; Gujarat, 4·49; Jammu and Kashmir, 1·43; Karnataka, 4·11; Kerala, 0·75; Madhya Pradesh, 3·99; Maharashtra, 4·65; Orissa, 1·98; Punjab, 3·85; Rajasthan, 5·5; Tamil Nadu, 1·49; Uttar Pradesh, 1·78; West Bengal, 1·56.

Of the total 71m. rural households possessing operational holdings, 34% hold on the average less than 0·20 ha of land each.

Opium. By international agreement the poppy is cultivated under licence, and all raw opium is sold to the central government. Opium, other than for wholly medical use, is available only to registered addicts.

Fisheries. Total catch (1988–89) was 3·15m. tons, of which Kerala, Tamil Nadu, and Maharashtra produced about half. Of the total catch, 1·82m. tonnes were marine fish. There were 225 deep-sea (20 metres and above) fishing boats in Oct. 1989. There were 23,500 mechanised boats (1987–88). There were 8,530 fishermen's co-operatives with 912,000 members in 1987–88; total sales, Rs 743m.

Forestry. The lands under the control of the state forest departments are classified as 'reserved forests' (forests intended to be permanently maintained for the supply of timber, etc., or for the protection of water supply, etc.), 'protected forests' and 'unclassed' forest land.

In 1988 the total forest area was 67·1m. ha. Main types are teak and sal. About 16% of the area is inaccessible, of which about 45% is potentially productive. In 1985–86 3m. saplings were planted. Some states have encouraged planting small areas around villages.

INDUSTRY. Railways, air transport, armaments and atomic energy are government monopolies. In a number of industries (including the manufacture of iron and steel and mineral oils, shipbuilding and the mining of coal, iron and manganese ores, gypsum, gold and diamonds) new units are set up only by the state. In a further group of industries (road transport, manufacture of chemicals such as drugs, dyestuffs, plastics and fertilizers) the state established new undertakings, but private enterprise may develop either on its own or with state backing, which may take the form of loans or purchase of equity capital. Nationalized industries employed 4m. in 1981. Under the Industries (Development and Regulation) Act, 1951, as amended, industrial undertakings are required to be licensed; 162 industries are within the scope of the Act. The Government are authorized to examine the working of any undertaking, to issue directions to it and to take over its control if this be deemed necessary. A Central Advisory Council has been set up consisting of representatives of industry, labour, consumers and primary producers. There are Development Councils for individual industries and (1981) 4 national development banks.

Oil refinery installed capacity, April 1989, was 49·85m. tonnes; production of petroleum refinery products (1988–89), 45·7m. tonnes. The Indian Oil Corporation was established in 1964 and had (1990) most of the market.

Industry, particularly steel, has suffered from a shortage of power and coal. There is expansion in petrochemicals, based on the oil and associated gas of the Bombay High field, and gas from Bassein field. Small industries numbering 1·7m., (initial outlay on capital equipment of less than Rs 6m.) are important; they employ about 11·3m. and produced (1988–89) goods worth Rs 824,000m.

Industrial production, 1988-89 (in 1,000 tonnes): Pig-iron and ferro-alloys, 12,253; steel ingots, 14,194; finished steel, 11,118; aluminium, 332; 166,920 motor cycles, mopeds and scooters; 115,788 commercial vehicles; petroleum products, 45,696; cement, 44,292; board and paper, 2,072; nitrogen fertilizer, 6,600; phosphate fertilizer, 2,316; jute goods, 1,388; man-made fibre and yarn, 261; diesel engines, 1,854,000 engines; electric motors, 5·3m. h.p.; 201,936 passenger cars and jeeps; 21,384 railway wagons.

Lal, V. B., (et al) *The Aluminium Industry in India: Promise, Prospects, Constraints and Impact*. New Delhi, 1985

Labour. At the 1981 census there were 222·5m. workers, of whom 92·5m. were cultivators, 55·5m. agricultural labourers; in 1987-88 there were 6·3m. in manufacturing, 10·03m. in social, community and personal services, 1·3m. in construction and 3·07m. in transport, communications and storage. The bond labour system was abolished in 1975. Man-days lost by industrial disputes, 1989, 15·18m., of which 2·94m. were in the public sector. An ordnance of July 1981 gave the government power to ban strikes in essential services; the ordnance was to remain in force for six months and would then be renewable.

Companies. The total number of companies limited by shares at work in India, 31 Dec. 1989, was 192,999; aggregate paid-up capital was Rs 54,499 crores. There were 20,425 public limited companies with an aggregate paid-up capital of Rs 23,206 crores, and 172,574 private limited companies (Rs 31,293 crores). There were also 324 companies with unlimited liability and (at 31 March) 1,954 companies limited by guarantee and association not for profit.

During 1988–89, 21,891 new limited companies were registered in the Indian Union under the Companies Act 1956 with a total authorized capital of Rs 4,795 crores; 1,099 were public limited companies (Rs 2,045 crores) and 20,792 were private limited companies (Rs 2,750 crores). There were 10 private companies with unlimited liability and 76 companies with liability limited by guarantee and association not for profit also registered in 1988–89. Of the new non-government limited companies, 390 had an authorized capital of Rs 1 crore and above, and 375 of between Rs 50 lakhs and Rs 1 crore. During 1988–89, 131 companies with an aggregate paid-up capital of Rs 14·64 crores went into liquidation and 68 companies (Rs 0·89 crores) were struck off the register.

On 31 March 1989 there were 1,134 government companies at work with a total paid-up capital of Rs 40,607 crores; 533 were public limited companies and 601 were private limited companies.

On 31 March 1989, 420 companies incorporated elsewhere were reported to have a place of business in India; 127 were of UK and 88 of USA origin.

Department of Company Affairs, Govt. of India. *Annual Report on the Working and Administration of the Companies Act, 1956*. New Delhi, 1989

Co-operative Movement. On 30 June 1989 there were about 350,000 co-operative societies with a total membership of 150m. These included Primary Cooperative Marketing Societies, State Co-operative Marketing Federations and the National Agricultural Co-operative Marketing Federation of India. There were also State Co-operative Commodity Marketing Federations, and 29 general purpose and 16 Special Commodites Marketing Federations.

There were, in 1986-87, 29 State Co-operative Banks, 353 Central Co-operative Banks, 115,781 Primary Agricultural Credit Societies, 19 State Land Development Banks, and 899 primary Land Development Banks/branches which provide long-term investment credit.

Total agricultural credit disbursed by Co-operatives in 1988–89 was Rs 5,442 crores including Rs 3,833 crores in short-term credit, Rs 381 crores in medium-term credit and Rs 731 crores in long-term credit.

Value of agricultural produce marketed by Co-operatives in 1988–89 was about Rs 5,416 crores.

In 1988–89 there were 2,422 agro-processing units; 214 sugar factories produced 5·07m. tons; 108 spinning mills (capacity 2·86m. spindles) produced 179m. kg. of yarn; there were 112 oilseed processing units; total storage capacity was 10·94m. tons.

In 1988–89 there were 67,000 retail depots distributing 3·5m. tons of fertilizers.

Co-operative Movement in India, Statistical Statements Relating to. Annual. Reserve Bank of India, Bombay

FOREIGN ECONOMIC RELATIONS. Foreign investment is encouraged by a tax holiday on income up to 6% of capital employed for 5 years. There are special depreciation allowances, and customs and excise concessions, for export industries. Proposals for investment ventures involving more than 40% foreign equity require government approval. In Feb. 1991 India resumed trans-frontier trade with China, which had ceased in 1962.

Commerce. The external trade of India (excluding land-borne trade with Tibet and Bhutan) was as follows (in 100,000 rupees):

	Imports	*Exports and Re-exports*
1987–88	2,224,374	1,567,366
1988-89	2,819,365	2,029,515
1989–90 [1]	3,541,188	2,768,147

[1]Provisional.

The distribution of commerce by countries and areas was as follows in the year ended 31 March 1989 (in 100,000 rupees):

Countries	*Exports to*	*Imports from*
Afghánistán	3,950	1,683
Argentina	378	9,905
Australia	26,603	70,184
Austria	5,381	10,975
Bahrain	3,850	23,411
Bangladesh	26,193	1,453
Belgium	88,591	203,768
Brazil	5,401	33,311
Bulgaria	3,667	3,477
Burma	225	7,738
Canada	19,722	42,693
Czechoslovakia	18,495	12,603
Denmark	6,990	5,100
Egypt	8,550	7,337
Finland	2,537	14,486
France	43,191	82,160
German Dem. Republic	18,305	13,339

Countries	*Exports to*	*Imports from*
Federal Rep. of Germany	123,660	247,191
Ghana	824	1,353
Hong Kong	82,059	17,525
Hungary	7,000	10,572
Indonesia	4,561	9,140
Iran	8,936	12,915
Iraq	5,286	19,384
Italy	54,058	50,322
Japan	216,226	263,354
Jordan	2,348	19,589
Kenya	5,086	1,371
Korea, Republic of	18,282	43,323
Kuwait	15,536	52,158
Malaysia	13,033	79,214
Morocco	1,460	30,557
Nepál	9,861	3,474
Netherlands	40,411	53,607
New Zealand	3,051	4,845
Nigeria	6,989	789
Norway	2,515	7,241
Pakistan	3,642	7,258
Poland	14,590	6,645
Qatar	2,166	5,140
Romania	3,767	7,175
Saudi Arabia	32,618	189,452
Singapore	32,551	62,750
Spain	12,677	13,984
Sri Lanka	14,703	2,754
Sudan	2,683	3,273
Sweden	7,474	23,547
Switzerland	27,113	28,514
Tanzania	3,194	5,111
Thailand	19,168	22,153
Turkey	2,424	23,928
United Arab Emirates	42,600	88,128
USSR	260,921	125,806
UK	116,489	240,060
USA	373,628	319,653
Yugoslavia	8,885	15,132
Zaïre	288	8,401
Zambia	2,614	17,764

The value (in 100,000 rupees) of the leading articles of merchandise was as follows in the year ended 31 March 1989 (provisional):

Exports	*Value*
Meat and meat preparations	9,447
Marine products	63,250
Processed foods (miscellaneous)	12,112
Rice	33,147
Vegetables and fruits	44,160
Coffee and coffee substitutes	27,971
Tea and mate	59,896
Spices	25,080
Oilcake	37,043
Tobacco unmanufactured and tobacco refuse	10,293
Raw cotton	2,802
Iron ore	67,250
Ores and minerals (excluding iron, mica and coal)	31,330
Cotton yarn, fabrics and madeup articles	113,130
Readymade garments	209,753
Jute manufactures including twist and yarn	24,991
Leather and leather manufactures	148,950
Natural silk textiles	18,588
Man-made textiles	17,095
Carpets, mill made	9,171
Plastic and manufactures thereof	9,710
Sports goods	7,881
Gems and jewellery	439,899
Works of art	32,562
Handmade carpets	46,956
Engineering goods	232,166
Petroleum products	50,496
Chemicals and allied products	143,691

Imports	*Value*
Wheat	37,816
Rice	19,346
Raw wool	15,753
Pulp and waste paper	25,280
Crude rubber including synthetic and reclaimed	17,264
Synthetic and regenerated fibre	3,743
Fertilizers, crude	18,509
Sulphur and unroasted iron pyrites	24,959
Metalliferous ores and metal scrap	67,742
Petroleum, petroleum products and related materials	437,404

Imports	*Value*
Edible oil	72,701
Organic chemicals	112,701
Inorganic chemicals	81,283
Medical and pharmaceutical products	20,209
Fertilizers, manufactured	49,295
Artificial resins, plastic materials etc	81,014
Chemical materials and products	20,409
Paper, paper board and manufactures thereof	30,570
Textile yarn, fabrics and madeup articles	28,734
Pearls, precious and semi-precious stones	317,521
Non-metallic mineral manufactures exclg. pearls	16,583
Iron and steel	193,726
Non-ferrous metal	78,582
Manufactures of metal	19,385
Machinery other than electric	437,090
Electrical machinery	160,802
Transport equipment	76,666
Professional, scientific, controlling instruments, photographic, optical goods, watches and clocks	69,574

Total trade between India and UK (British Department of Trade returns, in £1,000 sterling):

	1986	*1987*	*1988*	*1989*	*1990*
Imports to UK	440,681	536,704	559,684	701,985	799,438
Exports and re-exports from UK	941,169	1,090,146	1,111,740	1,382,436	1,264,189

Annual Statement of the Foreign Trade of India. 2 vols. Calcutta
Monthly Statistics of the Foreign Trade of India. Calcutta
Review of the Trade of India. Annual. Delhi
India–Handbook of Commercial Information. 3 vols. Calcutta
Guide to Official Statistics of Trade, Shipping, Customs and Excise Revenue of India. Rev. ed. Calcutta

Tourism. There were 1·34m. visitors (excluding nationals of Pakistan and Bangladesh) in 1989 bringing about Rs 24,560m. in foreign exchange; 229,496 from UK, 134,314 from USA, 67,680 from Sri Lanka.

COMMUNICATIONS

Roads. In 1988–89 there were about 2m. km of roads, of which about 840,000 km were surfaced. Roads are divided into 5 main administrative classes, namely, national highways, state highways, major district roads, other district roads and village roads. The national highways (33,612 km in 1989) connect capitals of states, major ports and foreign highways. The national highway system is linked with the ESCAP (Economic and Social Commission for Asia and the Pacific) international highway system. The state highways are the main trunk roads of the states, while the major district roads connect subsidiary areas of production and markets with distribution centres, and form the main link between headquarters and neighbouring districts.

There were (31 March 1989) 16,488,000 motor vehicles in India, comprising 2,284,000 private cars, taxis and jeeps, 10·7m. motor cycles and scooters, 293,000 buses and 1,140,000 goods vehicles.

Railways. The Indian railway system is government-owned and (under the control of the Railway Board) is divided into 9 zones; route-km at 31 March 1989:

Zone	*Headquarters*	*Route-km*
Central	Bombay	6,846 km (1,202 km elec.)
Eastern	Calcutta	4,291 km (1,246 km)
Northern	Delhi	10,980 km (884 km)
North Eastern	Gorakhpur	5,145 km
North East Frontier	Maligaon (Guwahati)	3,760 km
Southern	Madras	6,758 km (598 km)
South Central	Secunderabad	7,204 km (733 km)
South Eastern	Calcutta	7,115 km (2,065 km)
Western	Bombay	9,886 km (1,427 km)

Principal gauges are 1,676 mm. and metre, with networks also of 762 and 610 mm. gauge.

Passengers carried in 1989–90 were approximately 3,655m.; revenue earning freight, 309·6m. tonnes. Revenue (1989–90) from passengers, Rs 2,623 crores; from goods, Rs 7,632 crores.

Indian Railways pay to the central government a fixed dividend of 4·5% on capital-at-charge. Railway finance in Rs 1m.:

Financial years	*Gross traffic receipts*	*Working expenses*	*Net revenues (traffic and miscellaneous)*	*Net surplus or deficit (after dividend)*
1986–87	75,057	69,006	6,051	+102
1987–88	84,353	78,030	6,323	+843
1988–89	92,593	86,330	7,373	+217

Aviation. Air transport was nationalized in 1953 with the formation of 2 Air Corporations: Air India for long-distance international air services, and Indian Airlines for air services within India and to adjacent countries. A third airline, Vayudoot, was formed in 1981 as an internal feeder. There are 92 airports.

Air India runs Boeing 747s and 747 Combis, Airbus A-300 and A-310s; it operates from Bombay, Delhi, Madras, Trivandrum, Hyderabad, Goa and Calcutta to Africa (Nairobi, Lagos, Seychelles, Mauritius, Dar es Salaam, Lusaka and Harare); to Europe (London, Paris, Frankfurt, Geneva, Moscow and Rome); to western Asia (Doha, Abu Dhabi, Dharan, Dubai, Bahrain, Kuwait, Muscat, Jeddah, Ras al Khaymah, Sharjah, Tashkent, Tehran, Riyadh and Baghdad); to east Asia (Bangkok, Hong Kong, Tokyo, Osaka, Kuala Lumpur and Singapore); to North America (New York). In addition, freight services are operated to Zurich and Luxembourg. Air India carried 2·12m. passengers in 1988-89 and made a profit of Rs 433·1m.

Indian Airlines has a fleet of 60 aircraft consisting of Airbus A-300, Airbus-320, Boeing 737, F-27, and HS-748. During 1988–89 they carried 10·11m. passengers; net profit Rs 10·68 crores. Flights cover over 85,000 unduplicated route km. 9·85m passengers were carried in 1989-90. Vayudoot serves remote areas of India; it has a network of 55 stations.

The National Airports Authority maintains and operates 88 civil aerodromes and 28 civil enclaves. The management of the 4 international airports at Bombay, Calcutta, Delhi and Madras is vested in the International Airports Authority of India.

Shipping. In Dec. 1990, 405 ships totalling 5·92m. GRT were on the Indian Register; of these, 151 ships of 0·48m. GRT were engaged in coastal trade, and 254 ships of 5·44m. GRT in overseas trade. Traffic of major ports, 1989–90, was as follows:

Port	*Ships cleared*	*Imports (1m. tonnes)*	*Exports (1m. tonnes)*
Kandla	976	10·52	1·90
Bombay	2,035	11·19	6·92
Mormugao	387	0·92	12·54
New Mangalore	398	0·83	6·37
Cochin	676	2·49	0·56
Tuticorin	514	1·50	0·42
Madras	1,471	7·76	8·05
Vizag	781	7·82	7·81
Paradip	244	2·46	2·41
Haldia	583	6·25	0·38
Calcutta	750	2·78	0·75
Jawaharlal Nehru	99	0·52	0·18

The Hindustan shipyard at Vishakhapatnam is capable of building vessels of a maximum of 42,750 DWT. Present capacity is about 118,250 DWT per year. The Mazagon dock in Bombay and Goa shipyard build vessels primarily for defence purposes. The Cochin Shipyard can build ships of 85,000 DWT each and repair ships up to 100,000 DWT. The installed capacity of the shipyard is 84,000 DWT new construction and 1m. GRT ship repair, per annum. Garden Reach Shipbuilders and Engineers are building bulk carriers of 26,000 DWT, ferry ships (6,000 DWT), hydrographic research ships, tugs and fast patrol craft.

There are about 5,200 km of major rivers navigable by motorized craft, of which 1,700 km are used. Canals, 4,300 km, of which 485 km are navigable by motorized craft (335 km are used).

Telecommunications. On 31 March 1989 there were 145,238 post offices and 37,578 telegraph offices.

The telephone system is in the hands of the Telecommunications Department, except in Delhi, served by public corporation. In April 1989 the Department had 4·17m. telephones, 285 telex exchanges and 42,464 subscribers.

There were 102 radio stations in Sept. 1990, and programmes were sent out from 180 transmitters. In 1990 television covered 76% of the population, through a network of 508 transmitters. Entertainment films occupy 27% of broadcasting time, news and current affairs, 45%. A communications satellite ('APPLE') went into operation in July 1981.

Cinemas. In 1988-89 there were 13,355 cinemas and about 750 feature films were produced.

Newspapers. In 1988 the total number of newspapers and periodicals was 25,536; about 30% were published in Delhi, Bombay, Calcutta and Madras. There were 2,281 daily and 7,813 weekly papers. Circulation of newspapers and periodicals (1988), 54·87m. Hindi papers have the highest number and circulation, followed by English, then Bengali, Urdu and Marathi.

Annual Report of the Register of Newspapers for India. New Delhi

JUSTICE, RELIGION, EDUCATION AND WELFARE

Justice. All courts form a single hierarchy, with the Supreme Court at the head, which constitutes the highest court of appeal. Immediately below it are the High Courts and subordinate courts in each state. Every court in this chain, subject to the usual pecuniary and local limits, administers the whole law of the country, whether made by Parliament or by the state legislatures.

The states of Andhra Pradesh, Assam (in common with Nagaland, Meghalaya, Manipur, Mizoram, Tripura and Arunachal Pradesh), Bihar, Gujarat, Himachal Pradesh, Jammu and Kashmir, Karnataka, Kerala, Madhya Pradesh, Maharashtra (in common with Goa and the Union Territories of Daman and Diu and Dadra and Nagar Haveli), Orissa, Punjab (in common with the state of Haryana and the Union Territory of Chandigarh), Rajasthan, Tamil Nadu, Uttar Pradesh, West Bengal and Sikkim have each a High Court. There is a separate High Court for Delhi. For the Andaman and Nicobar Islands the Calcutta High Court, for Pondicherry the High Court of Madras and for Lakshadweep the High Court of Kerala are the highest judicial authorities. The Allahabad High Court has a Bench at Lucknow, the Bombay High Court has Benches at Nagpur, Aurangabad and Panaji, the Gauhati High Court has Benches at Kohima and Aizwal, the Madhya Pradesh High Court has Benches at Gwalior and Indore, the Patna High Court has a Bench at Ranchi and the Rajasthan High Court has a Bench at Jaipur. Judges and Division Courts of the Gauhati High Court also sit in Meghalaya, Manipur and Tripura. Below the High Court each state is divided into a number of districts under the jurisdiction of district judges who preside over civil courts and courts of sessions. There are a number of judicial authorities subordinate to the district civil courts. On the criminal side magistrates of various classes act under the overall supervision of the High Court.

The Code of Criminal Procedure, 1898, has been replaced by the Code of Criminal Procedure, 1973 (2 of 1974), which came into force with effect from 1 April 1974. The new Code provides for complete separation of the Judiciary from the Executive throughout India.

Police. The states control their own police force through the state Home Ministers. The Home Minister of the central government co-ordinates the work of the states and controls the Central Detective Training School, the Central Forensic Laboratory, the Central Fingerprint Laboratory as well as the National Police Academy at Mount Abu (Rajasthan) where the Indian Police Service is trained. This service is recruited by competitive examination of university graduates and provides all senior officers for the state police forces. The Central Bureau of Investigation functions under the control of the Cabinet Secretariat.

The cities of Pune, Ahmedabad, Nagpur, Bangalore, Calcutta, Madras, Bombay, Delhi and Hyderabad have separate police commissionerates.

Sarkar, P. C., *Civil Laws of India and Pakistan*. 2 vols. Calcutta, 1953.—*Criminal Laws of India and Pakistan*. 2nd ed. 2 vols. Calcutta, 1956

Setalvad, M. C., *The Common Law of India*. London, 1960

Sharma, S. R., *Supreme Court in the Indian Constitution*. Delhi, 1959

Religion. The principal religions in 1981 (census) were: Hindus, 549·7m. (82·63%); Moslems, 75·6m. (11·36%); Christians, 16·2m. (2·43%); Sikhs, 13·1m. (1·96%); Buddhists, 4·7m. (0·7%); Jains, 3·2m. (0·48%).

Education. Literacy. According to the 1981 census the literacy percentage in the country (excluding age-group, 0-4) was 36·23 (34·45 in 1971): 46·74% among males, 24·88% among females. Of the states and territories, Chandigarh and Kerala have the highest rates.

Educational Organization. Education is the concurrent responsibility of state and Union governments. In the union territories it is the responsibility of the central government. The Union Government is also directly responsible for the central universities and all institutions declared by parliament to be of national importance; the promotion of Hindi as the federal language; coordinating and maintaining standards in higher education, research, science and technology. Professional education rests with the Ministry or Department concerned, e.g., medical education, the Ministry or Department of Health. The Department of Education is a part of the Union Ministry of Human Resource Development, headed by a cabinet minister. There are several autonomous organizations attached to the Department of Education. These include the University Grants Commission, the National Institute of Educational Planning and Administration and the National Council of Educational Research and Training. There is a Central Advisory Board of Education to advise the Union and the State Governments on any educational question which may be referred to it.

School Education. The school system in India can be divided into four stages: Primary, middle, secondary and senior secondary.

Primary education is imparted either at independent primary (or junior basic) schools or primary classes attached to middle or secondary schools. The period of instruction in this stage varies from 4 to 5 years and the medium of instruction is in most cases the mother tongue of the child or the regional language. Free primary education is available for all children. Legislation for compulsory education has been passed by some state governments and Union Territories but it is not practicable to enforce compulsion when the reasons for non-attendance are socioeconomic. Residential schools are planned for country children.

The period for the middle stage varies from 2 to 3 years.

Higher Education. Higher education is given in arts, science or professional colleges, universities and all-India educational or research institutions. In 1988–89 there were 144 universities, 10 institutions of national importance and 25 institutions deemed as universities. Of the universities, 9 are central: Aligarh Muslim University; Banaras Hindu University; University of Delhi; University of Hyderabad; Jawaharlal Nehru University; North Eastern Hill University; Visva Bharati; Pondicherry; Indira Gandhi National Open. The rest are state universities. Total enrolment at universities, 1988–89, 3,947,922, of which 3,474,171 were undergraduates. Women students, 1,251,491.

Grants are paid through the University Grants Commission to the central universities and institutions deemed to be universities for their maintenance and development and to state universities for their development projects only; their maintenance is the concern of state governments. During 1988–89 the University Grants Commission sanctioned grants of Rs 194·33 crores.

Technical Education. The number of institutions awarding degrees in engineering and technology in 1988-89 was 267 (in 1947: 38), and those awarding diplomas in engineering and technology numbered 818 (in 1947: 53); the former admitted

205,282, the latter 286,397 students. Girls' Polytechnics had 32,137 students. For training high-level engineers and technologists 5 Institutes of Technology and the Indian Institute of Science, Bangalore. There are (1986) 4 national Management Institutions and 42 other management units, admitting about 3,000 annually.

Adult Education. In spite of the improvement in the literacy rate, the number of adult illiterates over 14 was over 424·26m. in 1981. Adult education is, therefore, being accorded a high priority; it formed part of the Minimum Needs Programme under the seventh Five-Year Plan (1985–90). The National Literacy Mission aims to cover all illiterate persons in the age-group 15–35 by 1990. The Directorate of Adult Education, established in 1971, is the national resource centre; with state resource centres it is responsible for producing teaching/learning materials, training and orientation, monitoring and evaluating the programme.

Educational statistics for the year 1988–89:

Type of recognized institution	*No. of institutions*	*No. of students on rolls*	*No. of teachers*
Primary/junior basic schools	548,059	95,739,976	1,603,058
Middle/senior basic schools	144,145	30,940,062	1,032,534
High/higher secondary schools[1]	68,665	16,229,942	1,235,530
Training schools and colleges	1,477	191,562[2]	–
Arts, Science and Commerce colleges	4,670	3,474,171[3]	194,095

[1] Including Junior Colleges.
[2] Enrolment by stages of teachers' training courses at school and college level.
[3] Enrolment by stages of all post-graduate and graduate courses.

Expenditure. Total public expenditure on education 1988–89 is estimated at Rs 9,889 crores. Total public expenditure on education, sport, arts and youth welfare during the Seventh Plan, Rs 6,382·65 crores; Seventh Plan spending on adult education, Rs 130 crores in the central and Rs 230 crores in the state sectors.

Health. Health programmes are primarily the responsibility of the state governments. The Union Government has sponsored and supported major schemes for disease prevention and control which are implemented nationally. These include the prevention and control of malaria, filaria, tuberculosis, leprosy, venereal diseases, smallpox, trachoma and cancer. There are also Union Government schemes in connexion with water supply and sanitation, and with nutrition. The Nutrition Advisory Committee of the Indian Council of Medical Research sponsors schemes for research and advises the Government. The National Nutrition Advisory Committee is to formulate a national nutrition policy and recommend measures for improving national standards.

Medical relief and service is primarily the responsibility of the states. Medical education is also a state responsibility, but there is a co-ordinating Central Health Educational Bureau. Family planning is centrally sponsored and locally implemented. The goal is to reduce the birth-rate by means of education in family planning methods.

Total expenditure on health and family welfare in 1988-89 was Rs 5,048 crores.

DIPLOMATIC REPRESENTATIVES

Of India in Great Britain (India House, Aldwych, London, WC2B 4NA)
High Commissioner: Dr L. M. Singhvi.

Of Great Britain in India (Chanakyapuri, New Delhi 110021)
High Commissioner: Sir David Goodall, KCMG.

Of India in the USA (2107 Massachusetts Ave., NW, Washington, D.C., 20008)
Ambassador: Abid Hussain.

Of the USA in India (Shanti Path, Chanakyapuri, New Delhi 110021)
Ambassador: William Clark, Jr.

Of India to the United Nations
Ambassador: Chinmaya Rajaninath Gharekhan.

Further Reading

Special works relating to States are shown under their separate headings.

India: A Reference Annual. Delhi Govt. Printer. Annual
New Cambridge History of India. 4 vols. CUP, 1988–90
The Times of India Directory and Yearbook. Bombay and London. Annual
Akbar, M. J., *India: The Siege Within.* Harmondsworth, 1985
Balasubramanyam, V. N., *The Economy of India.* London, 1985
Bardham, P., *The Political Economy of Development in India.* Oxford, 1984
Brown, J., *Modern India: The Origins of an Asian Democracy.* OUP, 1985
Fishlock, T., *India File: Inside the Subcontinent.* London, 1983
Fürer-Haimendorf, C. von, *Tribes of India: the Struggle for Survival.* Univ. of California Press, 1983
Gupta, B. K. and Kharbas, D. S., *India.* [Bibliography] Oxford and Santa Barbara, 1984
Hall, A., *The Emergence of Modern India.* Columbia Univ. Press, 1981
Hart, D., *Nuclear Power in India: a Comparative Analysis.* London, 1983
Kesavan, B. S. and Kulkarni, V. Y. (eds) *The National Bibliography of Indian Literature, 1901–53,* New Delhi, 1963 ff.
Kulke, H. and Rothermund, D., *A History of India.* rev. ed. London, 1990
Majumdar, R. C., Raychandhuri, H. C. and Datta, K., *An Advanced History of India.* 2nd ed. London, 1950
Mehra, P., *A Dictionary of Modern Indian History, 1707–1947.* Delhi, 1987
Mitra, H. N., *The Indian Annual Register.* Calcutta, from 1953
Moon, P., *The British Conquest and Dominion of India.* London and Indiana Univ. Press, 1989
Moore, R. J., *Making the New Commonwealth.* Oxford, 1987
Nanda, B. R. (ed.) *Socialism in India.* Delhi, Bombay, Bangalore, Kanpur, London, 1972
Pachauri, R. K., *Energy and Economic Development in India.* New York, 1977
Philips, C. H. (ed.) *The Evolution of India and Pakistan: Select Documents.* OUP, 1962 ff.—*Politics and Society in India.* London, 1963
Poplai, S. L. (ed.) *India, 1947–50* (select documents). 2 vols. Bombay and London, 1959
Ray, R. K., *Industrialisation of India.* OUP, 1983
Roach, J. R., (ed.) *India 2000: The Next Fifteen Years.* Riverdale, My, 1986
Smith, V. E., *Oxford History of India.* 3rd ed. OUP, 1958
Spear, P., *India: A Modern History.* 2nd ed. Univ. of Michigan Press, 1972
Sutton, S. C., *Guide to the India Office Library (founded in 1801).* HMSO, 1952
Thomas, R., *India's Emergence as an Industrial Power.* Royal Institute of International Affairs, London, 1982

STATES AND TERRITORIES

The Republic of India is composed of the following 25 States and 7 centrally administered Union Territories:

States	*Capital*	*States*	*Capital*
Andhra Pradesh	Hyderabad	Manipur	Imphal
Arunachal Pradesh	Itanagar	Meghalaya	Shillong
Assam	Dispur	Mizoram	Aizawl
Bihar	Patna	Nagaland	Kohima
Goa	Panaji	Orissa	Bhubaneswar
Gujarat	Ahmedabad	Punjab	Chandigarh
Haryana	Chandigarh	Rajasthan	Jaipur
Himachal Pradesh	Shimla	Sikkim	Gangtok
Jammu and Kashmir	Srinagar	Tamil Nadu	Madras
Karnataka	Bangalore	Tripura	Agartala
Kerala	Trivandrum	Uttar Pradesh	Lucknow
Madhya Pradesh	Bhopal	West Bengal	Calcutta
Maharashtra	Bombay		

Union Territories

Andaman and Nicobar Islands; Chandigarh; Dadra and Nagar Haveli; Delhi; Daman and Diu; Lakshadweep; Pondicherry.

States Reorganization. The Constitution, which came into force on 26 Jan. 1950, provided for 9 Part A States (Assam, Bihar, Bombay, Madhya Pradesh, Madras, Orissa, Punjab, Uttar Pradesh and West Bengal) which corresponded to the previous governors' provinces; 8 Part B States (Hyderabad, Jammu and Kashmir,

Madhya Bharat, Mysore, Patalia-East Punjab (PEPSU), Rajasthan, Saurashtra and Travancore-Cochin) which corresponded to Indian states or unions of states; 10 Part C States (Ajmer, Bhopal, Bilaspur, Coorg, Delhi, Himachal Pradesh, Kutch, Manipur, Tripura and Vindhya Pradesh) which corresponded to the chief commissioners' provinces; and Part D Territories and other areas (*e.g.,* Andaman and Nicobar Island). Part A States (under governors) and Part B States (under rajpramukhs) had provincial autonomy with a ministry and elected assembly. Part C States (under chief commissioners) were the direct responsibility of the Union Government, although Kutch, Manipur and Tripura had legislatures with limited powers. Andhra was formed as a Part A State on its separation from Madras in 1953. Bilaspur was merged with Himachal Pradesh in 1954.

The States Reorganization Act, 1956, abolished the distinction between Parts A, B and C States and established two categories for the units of the Indian Union to be called States and Territories. The following were the main territorial changes: the Telugu districts of Hyderabad were merged with Andhra; Mysore absorbed the whole Kannada-speaking area (including Coorg, the greater part of 4 districts of Bombay, 3 districts of Hyderabad and 1 district of Madras); Bhopal, Vindhya Pradesh and Madhya Bharat were merged with Madhya Pradesh, which ceded 8 Marathi-speaking districts to Bombay; the new state of Kerala, comprising the majority of Malayalam-speaking peoples, was formed from Travancore-Cochin with a small area from Madras; Patalia-East Punjab was included in Punjab; Kutch and Saurashtra in Bombay; and Ajmer in Rajasthan; Hyderabad ceased to exist.

On 1 May 1960 Bombay State was divided into two parts: 17 districts (including Saurashtra and Kutch) in the north and west became the new state of Gujarat; the remainder was renamed the state of Maharashtra.

In Aug. 1961 the former Portuguese territories of Dadra and Nagar Haveli became a Union territory. The Portuguese territory of Goa and the smaller territories of Daman and Diu, occupied by India in Dec. 1961, were constituted a Union territory in March 1962. In Aug. 1962 the former French territories of Pondicherry, Karikal, Mahé and Yanaon were formally transferred to India and became a Union territory. In Sept. 1962 the Naga Hills Tuensang Area was constituted a separate state under the name of Nagaland. On 1 Nov. 1966, under the Punjab Reorganization Act 1966, a new state of Haryana and a new Union Territory of Chandigarh were created from parts of Punjab (India); for details, *see* pp. 662 and 695. On 26 Jan. 1971 Himachal Pradesh became a state. In 1972 the North East Frontier Agency and Mizo hill district were made Union territories (as Arunachal Pradesh and Mizoram) and Manipur, Meghalaya and Tripura full states. Sikkim became a state in 1975. Statehood for Mizoram was passed by parliament in July 1986; for Arunachal Pradesh in Dec. 1986; for Goa in May 1987.

Report of the States Reorganization Commission. Government of India. Delhi, 1956

ANDHRA PRADESH

HISTORY. Andhra was constituted a separate state on 1 Oct. 1953, on its partition from Madras, and consisted of the undisputed Telugu-speaking area of that state. To this region was added, on 1 Nov. 1956, the Telangana area of the former Hyderabad State, comprising the districts of Hyderabad, Medak, Nizamabad, Karimnaga, Warangal, Khammam, Nalgonda and Mahbubnaga, parts of the Adilabad district and some taluks of the Raichur, Gulbarga and Bidar districts, and some revenue circles of the Nanded district. On 1 April 1960, 221·4 sq. miles in the Chingleput and Salem districts of Madras were transferred to Andhra Pradesh in exchange for 410 sq. miles from Chittoor district. The district of Prakasam was formed on 2 Feb. 1970. Hyderabad was split into 2 districts on 15 Aug. 1978, (Ranga Reddy and Hyderabad). A new district, Vizianagaram, was formed in 1979.

AREA AND POPULATION. Andhra Pradesh is in south India and is bounded south by Tamil Nadu, west by Karnataka, north and northwest by Maharashtra, northeast by Madhya Pradesh and Orissa, east by the Bay of Bengal.

The state has an area of 275,068 sq. km and a population (1981 census) of 53·5m. Density, 195 per sq. km. Growth rate 1971–81, 23·19%. The principal language is Telugu. Cities with over 250,000 population (1981 census), see p. 629. Other large cities (1981): Nellore (237,065); Kakinada (226,409); Kurnool (206,362); Nizamabad (183,061); Eluru (168,154); Machilipatnam (138,503); Anantapur (119,531); Tenali (119,257); Tirupati (115,292); Vizianagaram (114,806); Adoni (108,939); Proddatur (107,070); Cuddapah (103,125); Bheemavaram (101,894).

CONSTITUTION AND GOVERNMENT. Andhra Pradesh has a unicameral legislature; the Legislative Council was abolished in June 1985. There are 295 seats in the Legislative Assembly. At the election of Nov. 1989, the Congress I party took office.

For administrative purposes there are 23 districts in the state. The capital is Hyderabad.

Governor: Krishna Kant.

Chief Minister: N. Janardhan Reddy.

BUDGET. Budget estimate, 1990–91: receipts on revenue account, Rs 4,915·29 crores; expenditure, Rs 5,239·3 crores. Plan outlay, 1991-92: Rs 1,410 crores.

ENERGY AND NATURAL RESOURCES

Electricity. There are 6 hydro-electric plants including Machkund, Upper Sileru and Nizam Sagar and 5 thermal stations including Nellore and Kothagudam. Installed capacity, 1989–90, 4,542 mw., power generated 15,031m. kwh. In 1989–90 there were 27,379 electrified villages and 1·1m. electric pump sets.

Gas. Natural gas has been found in the Krishna–Godavari basin, where 3 gas-powered generating stations are proposed.

Water. In 1989–90, 15 large and 36 medium irrigation projects were in hand. The Telugu Ganga joint project with Tamil Nadu, now in execution, will irrigate about 233,000 hectares, besides supplying drinking water to Madras city (Tamil Nadu).

Minerals The state is an important producer of asbestos and barytes. Other important minerals are copper ore, coal, iron and limestone, steatlte, mica and manganese.

Agriculture. There were (1987–88) about 12·1m. ha of cropped land, of which 3·87m. ha were under food-grains. Production in 1989–90 (in tonnes): Foodgrains, 12·68m.; rice, 9·7m..; wheat, 7,500; pulses, 0·7m., sugar-cane, 11·7m.; oil seeds, 2·2m.

Livestock (1983 provisional): Cattle, 13·12m.; buffaloes, 8·7m.; goats, 5·5m.; sheep, 7·5m.

Forests. In 1989 it was estimated that forests occupy 23·2% of the total area of the state or 63,771 sq. km; main forest products are teak, eucalyuptus, cashew, casuarina, softwoods and bamboo.

Fisheries. Production 1989–90, 111,000 tonnes of marine fish and 134,000 tonnes of inland water fish. The state has a coastline of 974 km.

INDUSTRY. The main industries are textile manufacture, sugar-milling machine tools, pharmaceuticals, cement, chemicals, glass, fertilizers, electronic equipment, heavy electrical machinery, aircraft parts and paper-making. There is an oil refinery at Vishakhapatnam, where India's major shipbuilding yards are situated. In 1990 a steel plant was inaugurated at Vishakhapatnam and a railway repair shop at Tirupathi is functioning.

Cottage industry includes the manufacture of carpets, wooden and lacquer toys, brocades, bidriware, filigree and lace-work. The wooden toys of Nirmal and Kondapalli are particularly well known. Sericulture is developing rapidly. District Industries Centres have been set up to promote small-scale industry.

Tourism is growing; the main centres are Hyderabad, Nagarjunasagar, Warangal, Araku Valley, Horsley Hills and Tirupathi.

COMMUNICATIONS

Roads. In 1989–90 there were 2,587 km of national highways, 8,985 km of state highways and 25,267 km of major district roads. Number of vehicles during 1988–89 were 1,089,286 out of which were 849,332 motor cycles and scooters, 79,479 cars and jeeps, 59,504 goods vehicles and 14,587 buses.

Railways. In 1988–89 there were 5,021 route-km of railway, of which 3,032 km were broad gauge.

Aviation. There are airports at Hyderabad, Tirupathi, Vijayawada and Vishakapatnam, with regular scheduled services to Bombay, Delhi, Calcutta, Bangalore and Madras. A feeder airline serves Rajahmundry and Cuddapah.

Shipping. The chief port is Vishakhapatnam. There are minor ports at Kakinada, Machilipatnam, Bheemunipatnam, Narsapur, Krishnapatnam, Vadarevu and Kalingapatnam.

JUSTICE, RELIGION, EDUCATION AND WELFARE

Justice. The high court of Judicature at Hyderabad has a Chief Justice and 25 puisne judges.

Religion. At the 1981 census Hindus numbered 47,525,681; Moslems, 4,533,700; Christians, 1,433,327; Jains 18,642; Sikhs, 16,222; Buddhists, 12,930.

Education. In 1981, 29·94% of the population were literate (39·13% of men and 20·52% of women). There were, in 1988–89 46,891 primary schools (5,684,237 students); 5,878 upper primary (1,879,838); 5,329 high schools (2,347,522). Education is free for children up to 14.

In 1988–89 there were 931 junior colleges (221,400 students); 368 degree colleges (303,000 students); 54 oriental colleges (6,021 students) and 13 universities: Osmania University, Hyderabad; Andhra University, Waltair; Sri Venkateswara University, Tirupathi; Kakatiya University, Warangal; Nagarjuna University, Guntur; Sri Jawaharlal Nehru Technological University, Hyderabad; Central Institute of English and Foreign Languages, Hyderabad; A.P. Agricultural University, Hyderabad; Sri Krishnadevaraya University, Anantapur; Smt. Padmarathi Mahila Vishwavidyalayam (University for Women), Tirupathi; A. P. Open University, Hyderabad; Telugu University, Hyderabad and A. P. Medical University, Vijayawada.

Health. There were (1989-90) 1,486 allopathic hospitals and dispensaries, 348 Ayurvedic hospitals and dispensaries, 196 Unani and 284 homeopathy dispensaries. There were also 181 nature cure hospitals (1988), and 1,243 primary health centres. Number of beds in hospitals was 29,263 (1988).

ARUNACHAL PRADESH

HISTORY. In Jan. 1972 the former North East Frontier Agency of Assam was created a Union Territory. In Dec. 1986, by the Constitution (55th Amendment) and State of Arunachal Pradesh Acts, the Territory became the 24th state of India.

AREA AND POPULATION. The state is in north-east India and is bounded by Assam, Bhutan, China and Burma; it has 11 districts and comprises the former frontier divisions of Kameng, Tirap, Subansiri, Siang and Lohit; it has an area of 83,743 sq. km and a population (1981 census) of 631,839; growth, 1971–81, 34·34%; density, 7 per sq. km.

The state is mainly tribal; there are over 80 tribes using about 50 tribal dialects.

CONSTITUTION AND GOVERNMENT. There is a Legislative Assembly of 60 members. The capital is Itanagar.

Governor: Surendranath Dwivedi.
Chief Minister: Gegong Apang.

ENERGY AND NATURAL RESOURCES

Electricity. Power generated (1988): 42·01m. units. 1,108 out of 3,257 villages have electricity.

Oil and Coal. Crude oil reserves are estimated at 1·5m. tonnes and coal 850,000 tonnes.

Agriculture. Production of foodgrains, 1988–89, 194,000 tonnes.

Forestry. Area under forest, 51,540 sq. km; revenue from forestry (1988) Rs 141m.

Industries. The state has a light roofing-sheet factory, a fruit processing plant and a cement plant. There are 15 medium and 1,887 small industries. Most of the medium industries are forest-based.

Roads. Total length of roads maintained by the Public Works Department 7,923 km. The state has 330 km of national highway.

EDUCATION AND WELFARE

Education. There were (1988–89) 1,079 primary schools with 103,313 students, 228 middle schools with 22,522 students, 99 high and higher secondary schools with 12,319 students and 4 colleges. Arunachal University was established in 1985.

Health. There are (1990) 13 hospials, 5 community health centres, 20 primary health centres and 125 sub-centres. There are also 2 TB hospitals and 4 leprosy hospitals. Total number of beds, 2,158.

ASSAM

HISTORY. Assam first became a British Protectorate at the close of the first Burmese War in 1826. In 1832 Cachar was annexed; in 1835 the Jaintia Hills were included in the East India Company's dominions, and in 1839 Assam was annexed to Bengal. In 1874 Assam was detached from Bengal and made a separate chief commissionership. On the partition of Bengal in 1905, it was united to the Eastern Districts of Bengal under a Lieut.-Governor. From 1912 the chief commissionership of Assam was revived, and in 1921 a governorship was created. On the partition of India almost the whole of the predominantly Moslem district of Sylhet was merged with East Bengal (Pakistan). Dewangiri in North Kamrup was ceded to Bhután in 1951. The Naga Hill district, administered by the Union Government since 1957, became part of Nagaland in 1962. The autonomous state of Meghalaya within Assam, comprising the districts of Garo Hills and Khasi and Jaintia Hills, came into existence on 2 April 1970, and achieved full independent statehood in Jan. 1972, when it was also decided to form a Union Territory, Mizoram (now a state), from the Mizo Hills district.

AREA AND POPULATION. Assam is in eastern India, almost separated from central India by Bangladesh. It is bounded west by West Bengal, north by Bhutan and Arunachal Pradesh, east by Nagaland, Manipur and Burma, south by Meghalaya, Bangladesh, Mizoram and Tripura. The area of the state is now 78,438 sq. km. Population estimate, 19·9m. Density, 254 per sq. km. Growth rate since 1971, 36·09%. Principal towns with population (1971) are; Guwahati, 122,981; Dibrugarh, 80,344; Tinsukia, 55,392; Nowgong, 52,892; Silchar, 52,612. The principal language is Assamese.

The central government is surveying the line of a proposed boundary fence to prevent illegal entry from Bangladesh.

CONSTITUTION AND GOVERNMENT. Assam has a unicameral legislature of 126 members. In Dec. 1985 elections were held and an Asom Gana Parishad government was returned. Presidential rule was imposed in Nov. 1990. The temporary capital is Dispur. The state has 23 districts.

Governor: Lok Nath Mishra.
Chief Minister: (Vacant).

BUDGET. The budget estimates for 1990–91 showed receipts of Rs 4,111 crores. and expenditure of Rs 4,400 crores. Plan allocation, 1991-92, Rs 2,251 crores.

ENERGY AND NATURAL RESOURCES

Electricity. In 1987–88 there was an installed capacity of 503 mw and 17,897 villages (out of 21,995) with electricity. New power stations are under construction at Lakwa, and Karbi-Langpi hydro-electricity project.

Oil and Gas. Assam contains important oilfields and produces about 50% of India's crude oil. Production (1986-87): Crude oil, 4·97m. tonnes; gas, 1,003m. cu. metres.

Water. In 1987–88, 222,451 hectares were irrigated; 2 major and 11 medium projects were in hand.

Minerals. Coal production (1988), 1,017,103 tonnes. The state also has limestone, refractory clay, dolomite, and corundum.

Agriculture. There are 844 tea plantations, and growing tea is the principal industry. Production in 1988-89, 369m. kg, over 50% of Indian tea. Over 72% of the cultivated area is under food crops, of which the most important is rice. Total foodgrains, 1988–89, 2·6m. tonnes. Main cash crops: Jute, tea, cotton, oilseeds, sugarcane, fruit and potatoes. Wheat production 122,300 tonnes in 1988–89; rice, 2·44m. tonnes; pulses, 51,100 tonnes. Cattle are important.

Forestry. There are 17,409 sq. km of reserved forests under the administration of the Forest Department and 10,063·81 sq. km of unclassed forests, altogether about 30% of the total area of the state. Revenue from forests, 1987–88, Rs 1,721·66 lakhs.

INDUSTRY. Sericulture and hand-loom weaving, both silk and cotton, are important home industries together with the manufacture of brass, cane and bamboo articles. Hand-loom weaving of silk is stimulated by state and central development schemes. There are two silk-spinning mills and 26 cotton-mills. The main heavy industry is petro-chemicals; there are 3 oil refineries with 1 under construction in 1990. Other industries include manufacturing paper, nylon, fertilizers, sugar, jute and plywood products, rice and oil milling.

COMMUNICATIONS

Roads. In 1984–85 there were 26,352 km of road maintained by the Public Works Department. There were 2,035 km of national highway in 1990. There were 216,475 motor vehicles in the state in 1988.

Railways. The route km of railways in 1988 was 2,338 km, of which 262·09 km are broad gauge.

Aviation. Daily scheduled flights connect the principal towns with the rest of India. There are airports at Guwahati, Tezpur, Jorhat, North Lakhimpur, Silchar and Dibrugarh.

Shipping. Water transport is important in Lower Assam; the main waterway is the Brahmaputra River. Cargo carried in 1986 was 65,000 tonnes.

JUSTICE, RELIGION, EDUCATION AND WELFARE

Justice. The seat of the High Court is Guwahati. It has a Chief Justice and 6 puisne judges.

Religion. At the 1971 census Hindus numbered 10,604,618; Moslems, 3,592,124; Christians, 381,010; Buddhists, 22,565; Jains, 12,914; Sikhs, 11,920.

Education. In 1988–89 there were 28,807 primary/junior basic schools with 3,433,077 students; 5,635 middle/senior basic schools with 1,231,297 students;

3,110 high/higher secondary schools with 601,523 students. There were 175 colleges for general education, 3 medical colleges, 3 engineering and 1 agricultural, 9 teacher-training colleges and 3 universities. The universities are Assam Agricultural University, Jorhat, Dibrugarh University, Dibrugarh and Gauhati University, Gauhati. There is a fisheries college at Raha.

Health. In 1988 there were 100 hospitals (9,520 beds) and 835 primary health centres.

BIHAR

The state contains the ethnic areas of North Bihar, Santhalpargana and Chota Nagpur. In 1956 certain areas of Purnea and Manbhum districts were transferred to West Bengal.

AREA AND POPULATION. Bihar is in north India and is bounded north by Nepal, east by West Bengal, south by Orissa, south-west by Madhya Pradesh and west by Uttar Pradesh. The area of Bihar is 173,877 sq. km and its population (1981 census), 69,914,734, a density of 402 per sq. km. Growth rate since 1971, 24·06%. Population of principal towns, *see* p. 629. Other large towns (1981): Muzaffarpur, 190,416; Darbhanga, 176,301; Biharsharif, 151,343; Munger, 129,260; Arrah, 125,111; Katihar, 122,005; Dhanbad, 120,221; Chapra, 111,564; Purnea, 109,649; Bermo, 101,502.

The official language is Hindi (55·8m. speakers at the 1981 census), the second, Urdu (6·9m.), the third, Bengali (2m.).

CONSTITUTION AND GOVERNMENT. Bihar has a bicameral legislature. The Legislative Assembly consists of 324 elected members and the Council, 96. After the elections in Feb. 1990 a Januata Dal government, supported by Bharatiya Janata Party, Communist Party of India, Jharkhand Mukti Morcha and Communist-Marxist, came to power. Total seats, 324: Janata Dal, 122; Congress-I, 71; Bharatiya Janata Party, 37; Communist Party of India, 23; Jharkhand Mukti Morcha, 19; Communist-Marxist, 6; Indian People's Front, 7; Independent and others, 36; vacant, 3. For the purposes of administration the state is divided into 10 divisions covering 42 districts. The capital is Patna.

Governor: Mohammed Shafi Qureshi.
Chief Minister: Lallu Prasad Yadav.

BUDGET. The budget estimates for 1990–91 show total receipts of Rs 56,256·9m and expenditure of Rs 59,875·9m. Plan allocation, 1991–92, Rs 22,510m.

ENERGY AND NATURAL RESOURCES

Electricity. Installed capacity (1988–89) 1,530 mw. Power generated (1988–89), 4,539m. kw.; there were 43,214 villages with electricity. Hydro-electric projects in hand will add about 149·2mw. capacity.

Minerals. Bihar is very rich in minerals, with about 40% of national production. There are huge deposits of copper, capatite and kyanite and sizeable deposits of coal, mica and china clay. Bihar is a principal producer of iron ore. Other important minerals: Manganese, limestone, graphite, chromite, asbestos, barytes, dolomite, feldspar, columbite, pyrites, saltpetre, glass sands, slate, lead, silver, building stones and radio-active minerals. Value of production (1987) Rs 16,280m.

Agriculture. About 26% of the cultivable area is irrigated. Cultivable land, 11·6m. ha, of a total area of 17·4m. ha. Total cropped area, 1987–88, 8·5m. ha. Production (1988–89): Rice, 6·1m. tonnes; wheat, 3·5m.; total foodgrains, 11·7m. Other food crops are maize, rabi and pulses. Main cash crops are jute, sugar-cane, oilseeds, tobacco and potato.

Forests in 1990 covered 2·9m. ha. There are 12 protected forests.

INDUSTRY. Main plants are the Tata Iron and Steel Co., the Tata Engineering and Locomotive Co., the steel plant at Bokaro, oil refinery at Barauni, Heavy Engineering Corporation and Foundry Forge project at Ranchi, and aluminium plant at Muri. Other important industries are machine tools, fertilizers, electrical engineering, sugar-milling, paper-milling, silk-spinning, manufacturing explosives and cement. There is a copper smelter at Ghatsila and a zinc plant at Tundo. There were 54,396 small industries in 1985.

TOURISM. The main tourist centres are Bodh Gaya, Patna, Nalanda, Jamshedpur, Sasaram, Betla, Hazaribagh and Vaishali.

COMMUNICATIONS

Roads. In March 1989 the state had 35,411 km of metalled roads, including 2,118 km of national highway, and 50,259 km of unmetalled roads. Passenger transport has been nationalized in 7 districts. There were 289,717 motor vehicles in March 1988.

Railways. The North Eastern, South Eastern and Eastern railways traverse the state; route-km, 1987–88, 5,305.

Aviation. There are airports at Patna and Ranchi with regular scheduled services to Calcutta and Delhi.

Shipping. The length of waterways open for navigation is 900 miles.

JUSTICE, RELIGION, EDUCATION AND WELFARE

Justice. There is a High Court (constituted in 1916) at Patna, and a bench at Ranchi, with a Chief Justice, 32 puisne judges and 4 additional judges.

Police. The police force is under a Director General of Police; in 1986 there were 1,036 police stations.

Religion. At the 1981 census Hindus numbered 58,011,070; Moslems, 9,874,993; Christians, 740,186; Sikhs, 77,704; Jains, 27,613; Buddhists, 3,003.

Education. At the census of 1981 the number of literates was 18·32m. (26·2%: males 38·11%; females, 13·62%). There were, 1988–89, 3,875 high and higher secondary schools with 820,687m. pupils, 12,530 middle schools with 1·94m. pupils, 52,181 primary schools with 8,301,386 pupils. Education is free for children aged 6-11.

There were 10 universities in 1990: Patna University (founded 1917) with 18,895 students (1984–85); Bihar University, Muzaffarpur (1952) with 60 constituent colleges, 7 affiliated colleges and 75,370 students (1984–85); Bhagalpur University (1960) with 50,473 students (1985–86); Ranchi University (1960) with 88,771 students (1985–86); Kameswar Singh Darbhanga Sanskrit University (1961); Magadha University, Gaya (1962) and Lalit Narayan Mithila University (1972), Darbhanga, Bisra Agricultural University, Ranchi (1980), Rajendra Agricultural University, Samastipur (1970), Nalanda Open University, Nalanda.

Health. In 1985 there were 1,289 hospitals and dispensaries.

Das, A. N., *Agrarian Movements in India: Studies in 20th Century Bihar*. London, 1982

GOA

HISTORY. The coastal area was captured by the Portuguese in 1510 and the inland area was added in the 18th century. In Dec. 1961 Portuguese rule was ended and Goa incorporated into the Indian Union as a Territory together with Daman and Diu. Goa was granted statehood as a separate unit on 30 May 1987. Daman and Diu remained Union Territories (see p. 696).

AREA AND POPULATION. Goa, bounded on the north by Maharashtra and on the east and south by Karnataka, has a coastline of 105 km. The area is 3,702 sq.

km. (Population, 1981 census, 1,007,749). Density, 272 per sq. km. Panaji is the largest town; population (urban agglomeration, 1981) 76,839. The languages spoken are Konkani (official language), Marathi, Hindi, English.

GOVERNMENT. The Indian Parliament passed legislation in March 1962 by which Goa became a Union Territory with retrospective effect from 20 Dec. 1961. On 30 May 1987 Goa attained statehood. It is represented by 2 elected and 2 nominated representatives in Parliament. There is a Legislative Assembly of 40 members. The Capital is Panaji. The state has 2 districts. There are 183 village Panchayats.

Governor: Kurshid Alam Khan.
Chief Minister: Ravi Naik.

BUDGET. The total budget for 1990–91 was Rs 488·87 crores. Annual plan 1991–92, Rs 172·50 crores.

ENERGY AND NATURAL RESOURCES

Electricity. Fifteen towns and 377 villages were supplied with electric power by March 1990. Goa receives its power supply from the states of Maharashtra, Karnataka and Madhya Pradesh.

Minerals. Resources include manganese ore and iron ore, both of which are exported. Iron ore production (1989-90) 9,873,333 tonnes. There are also reserves of ferro-manganese, bauxite, lime stone and clay.

Agriculture. Agriculture is the main occupation, important crops are rice, pulses, ragi, mango, cashew and coconuts. Area under high yielding variety paddy (1989–90) 43,825 ha; production, 207,069 tonnes. Area under pulses 10,705 ha, sugar-cane 1,700 ha, groundnut 997 ha. Total production of foodgrains, 1988–89, 0·13m. tonnes.

Government poultry and dairy farming schemes produced 92m. eggs and 27,000m. litres of milk in 1989–90.

Fisheries. Fish is the state's staple food. In 1989–90 the catch of seafish was 54,550 tonnes (value Rs 2,019·81 lakhs). There is a coastline of about 104 km and about 4,442 active fishing vessels.

INDUSTRY. In 1989–90 there were 42 large and medium industrial projects and 4,552 small units registered. Production included: Nylon fishing nets, ready made clothing, electronic goods, pesticides, pharmaceuticals, tyres and footwear.

In 1989-90 4552 small-scale industry units employed 28,822 persons.

ROADS. In 1989-90 there were 4,163 km of motorable roads (National Highway, 224 km).

JUSTICE, EDUCATION AND WELFARE

Justice. There is a bench of the Bombay High Court at Panaji.

Education. In 1989-90 there were 1,250 primary schools (144,227 students in 1988–89), 436 middle schools (81,493 students in 1988–89) and 368 high and higher secondary schools (53,595 students in 1988–89). There were also 2 engineering colleges, 1 medical college, 1 teacher-training college and 22 other colleges. Goa University, Bambolin (1985) has 28 colleges affiliated to it.

Health. There were (1989-90) 119 hospitals (3,834 beds), 251 rural medical dispensaries, health and sub-health centres and 261 family planning units.

Hutt, A., *Goa: A Traveller's Historical and Architectural Guide*. Buckhurst Hill, 1988

GUJARAT

HISTORY. On 1 May 1960, as a result of the Bombay Reorganization Act, 1960, the state of Gujarat was formed from the north and west (predominantly Gujarati-speaking) portion of Bombay State, the remainder being renamed the state of Maharashtra. Gujarat consists of the following districts of the former state of Bombay: Banas Kantha, Mehsana, Sabar Kantha, Ahmedabad, Kaira, Panch Mahals, Vadodara, Bharuch, Surat, Dangs, Amreli, Surendranagar, Rajkot, Jamnagar, Junagadh, Bhavnagar, Kutch, Gandhinagar and Bulsar.

AREA AND POPULATION. Gujarat is in western India and is bounded north by Pakistan and Rajasthan, east by Madhya Pradesh, south-east by Maharashtra, south and west by the Indian ocean and Arabian sea. The area of the state is 196,024 sq. km and the population at the 1981 census (revised) was 34,086,000; a density of 174 per sq. km. Growth rate 1971–81, 27·2%. The chief cities, *see* p. 629. Gujarati and Hindi in the Devanagari script are the official languages.

CONSTITUTION AND GOVERNMENT. Gujarat has a unicameral legislature, the Legislative Assembly, which has 182 elected members. After the elections in Feb. 1990 a coalition government of Janata Dal and Bharatiya Janata Party came to power. Total seats, 182: Janata Dal, 4; Janata Dal (S), 66; Bharatiya Janata Party, 67; Congress (I), 33; Independents, 12.

The capital is Gandhinagar. There are 19 districts.

Governor: Mahipal Shastri.
Chief Minister: Chimanbhai Patel.

BUDGET. The budget estimates for 1990–91 showed revenue receipts of Rs 3,784·03 crores and revenue expenditure of Rs 3,792·15 crores. Plan outlay for 1990–91, Rs 1,451 crores.

ENERGY AND NATURAL RESOURCES

Electricity. In 1988 the total generating capacity was 3,526 mw of electricity, serving 338,046 towns and villages.

Water. The Karjan Dam, under construction, will provide a reservoir of 630m. cu. metres capacity; it is designed to irrigate 56,000 hectares through 2 main canals.

Oil and Gas. There were crude oil and gas reserves in 23 fields in 1982–83. Production: Crude oil, 4·53m. tonnes; gas, 685m. cu. metres in 1986.

Minerals. Chief minerals produced in 1986 (in tonnes) included lime stone (5·2m.), agate stone (849), calcite (1,089), quartz and silica (212,316), bauxite (467,447), crude china clay (15,427), refined china clays (7,233), dolomite (249,893), crude fluorite (121,262), calcareous and sea sand (537,000) and lignite (1·07m.). Value of production (1987) Rs 9,150m. Enormous reserves of coal were found under the Kalol and Mehsana oil and gas fields in May 1980. The deposit, mixed with crude petroleum, is estimated at 100,000m. tonnes, extending over 500 km.

Agriculture. In 1985–86 drought was exceptionally severe. Cropped area, 1983–84, was 11·9m. ha. Production of principal crops, 1988–89: Rice, 566,000 tonnes from 536,000 ha; foodgrains, 5·3m. tonnes (wheat, 1,512,000 tonnes), pulses, 490,000 tonnes.

Livestock (1982): Buffaloes, 4·43m.; other cattle, 6·93m.; sheep, 2·33m.; goats, 3·26m.; horses and ponies, 24,000.

Fisheries. There were (1987) 80,204 people engaged in fisheries. There were 13,811 fishing vessels (5,313 motor vessels). The catch for 1988–89 was 381,000 tonnes.

INDUSTRY. Gujarat is one of the 4 most industrialized states. In 1985 there were more than 70,000 small-scale units and 13,000 factories including 1,328 textile factories. There were 167 industrial estates. Principal industries are textiles, general and electrical engineering, petrochemicals, machine tools, heavy chemicals, pharmaceuticals, dyes, sugar, soda ash, cement, man-made fibres, salt, sulphuric acid, paper and paperboard. Large fertilizer plants have been set up and there is an oil refinery at Koyali near Vadodara, with a developing petro-chemical complex.

State production of soda-ash is 90·4% of national output, and of salt, about 60%. Salt production (1986) 6·6m. tonnes; cement production, 2·4m. tonnes.

COMMUNICATIONS

Roads. In 1988-89 there were 62,142 km of roads. Gujarat State Transport Corporation operated 14,609 routes. Number of vehicles, 1,239,141.

Railways. In 1988 the state had 5,553 route km of railway line.

Aviation. Ahmedabad is the main airport. There are regular services between Ahmedabad and Bombay, Jaipur and Delhi. There are 8 other airports: Baroda, Bhavnagar, Bhuj, Jamnagar, Kandla, Keshod, Porbandar and Rajkot.

Shipping. The largest port is Kandla. There are 39 other ports, 11 intermediate, 28 minor.

Post. There were (March 1984–85) 9,000 post offices, 2,000 telegraph offices. Ahmedabad has direct dialling telephone connexion (or night S.T.D.) with 273 cities and 16 foreign countries. There were 227,000 telephone connexions in the state.

JUSTICE, RELIGION, EDUCATION AND WELFARE

Justice. The High Court of Judicature at Ahmedabad has a Chief Justice and 18 puisne judges.

Religion. At the 1981 census Hindus numbered 30,518,500; Moslems, 2,907,744; Jains, 467,768; Christians, 132,703; Sikhs, 22,438; Buddhists, 7,550.

Education. In 1981 the number of literates was 14·85m. (43·7%). Primary and secondary education up to Standard XI are free. Education above Standard XII is free for girls. In 1988–89 there were 13,100 primary schools with 5,337,000 students and 16,700 middle/senior basic schools with 1,524,300 students. There were 4,870 secondary schools with 1,004,000 students including 1,320 higher secondary schools.

There are 9 universities in the state. Gujarat University, Ahmedabad, founded in 1949, is teaching and affiliating; it has 147 affiliated colleges. The Maharaja Sayajirao University of Vadodara (1949) is residential and teaching. The Sardar Patel University, Vallabh-Vidyanagar, (1955) has 16 constituent and affiliated colleges, Saurashtra University at Rajkot with 64 affiliated colleges, and South Gujarat at Surat with 39. Bhavnagar University (1978) is residential and teaching with 8 affiliated colleges. North Gujarat University was established at Patan in 1986. Gujarat Vidyapith at Ahmedabad is deemed a university under the University Grants Commission Act. There are also Gujarat Agricultural University, Banaskantha and Gujarat Ayurved University, Jamnagar.

There are 11 engineering colleges, 24 polytechnics, 6 medical colleges, 6 agricultural, 3 pharmaceutical and 2 veterinary. There are also 223 arts, science and commerce colleges and 40 teacher-training colleges.

Health. In 1987 there were 1,854 hospitals (22,595 beds), 457 primary health centres and 5,551 sub-centres.

Rushbrook Williams, L. F., *The Black Hills: Kutch in History and Legend.* London, 1958
Desai, I. F., *Untouchability in Rural Gujarat.* Bombay, 1977

HARYANA

HISTORY. The state of Haryana, created on 1 Nov. 1966 under the Punjab Reorganization Act, 1966, was formed from the Hindi-speaking parts of the state of Punjab (India). It comprises the districts of Hissar, Mohindergarh, Gurgaon, Rohtak and Karnal; Bhiwani, Faridabad, Jind, Kurukshetra, Sirsa, Sonipat, Ambala.

AREA AND POPULATION. Haryana is in north India and is bounded north by Himachal Pradesh, east by Uttar Pradesh, south and west by Rajasthan and north-west by Punjab. Delhi forms an enclave on its eastern boundary. The state has an area of 44,212 sq. km and a population (1981) of 12,922,618; density, 291 per sq. km. Growth rate, 1971–81, 28·75%. The principal language is Hindi.

CONSTITUTION AND GOVERNMENT. The state has a unicameral legislature with 90 members. In Feb. 1991 Janata Dal (S) held 41 seats; Bharatiya Janata, 17; Congress (I), 4; others, 5; vacant, 1. The state shares with Punjab (India) a High Court, a university and certain public services. The capital (shared with Punjab) is Chandigarh (*see* p. 693). Its transfer to Punjab, intended for 1986, has been postponed. There are 12 districts.

Governor: Dhanik Lal Mandal.
Chief Minister: Om Prakash Chautala.

BUDGET. Budget estimates for 1989–90 show income of Rs 1,666 crores and expenditure of Rs 1,623 crores. Annual plan 1990–91, Rs 700 crores.

ENERGY AND NATURAL RESOURCES

Electricity. Approximately 1,000 mw are supplied to Haryana, mainly from the Bhakra Nangar system. In 1988–89 installed capacity was 2,177 mw and all the villages had electric power.

Minerals. Minerals include placer gold, barytes and rare earths. Value of production, 1987–88, Rs 40m.

Agriculture. Haryana has sandy soil and erratic rainfall, but the state shares the benefit of the Sutlej-Beas scheme. Agriculture employs over 82% of the working population; in 1981 there were about 900,000 holdings (average 3·7 ha), and the gross irrigated area was 2·04m. ha. Area under high-yielding varieties of foodgrains, 1988–89, 2·76m. ha; foodgrain production was 9·48m. tonnes (rice 1·4m. tonnes, wheat 6·2m. tonnes); pulses 672,000 tonnes; sugar (gur) and oilseeds are important.

Forests cover 3·3% of the state.

INDUSTRY. Haryana has a large market for consumer goods in neighbouring Delhi. In 1988–89 there were 394 large and medium scale industries employing 120,000 and producing goods worth over Rs 10,000m. There were 86,200 small units. The main industries are cotton textiles, agricultural machinery, woollen textiles, scientific instruments, glass, cement, paper and sugar milling, cars, tyres and tubes, motor cycles, bicycles, steel tubes, engineering goods, electrical and electronic goods. An oil refinery is being set up at Karnal, capital outlay, Rs 1,300 crores.

COMMUNICATIONS

Roads. There were (1988–89) 21,250 km of metalled roads, linking all villages. Road transport is nationalized. There were 282,294 motor vehicles in 1986–87.

Railways. The state is crossed by lines from Delhi to Agra, Ajmer, Ferozepur and Chandigarh. Route km, 1987–88, 1,500. The main stations are at Ambala and Kurukshetra.

Aviation. There is no airport within the state but Delhi is on its eastern boundary.

JUSTICE, EDUCATION AND WELFARE

Justice. Haryana shares the High Court of Punjab and Haryana at Chandigarh.

Education. In 1981 the number of literates was 4·67m. In 1988-89 there were 5,032 primary schools with 1,628,716 students, 2,118 high and higher secondary schools with 366,741 students, 1,232 middle schools with 686,718 students and 114 colleges of arts, science and commerce, 3 engineering colleges and 2 medical colleges. There are 3 universities. The universities are Haryana Agricultural University, Hisar, Kurukshetra University, Kurukshetra and Maharshi Dayanand University, Rohtak.

Health. There were (1988-89) 77 hospitals (10,621 beds), 33 health centres, 124 dispensaries and 333 primary health centres.

HIMACHAL PRADESH

HISTORY. The territory came into being on 15 April 1948 and comprised 30 former Hill States. The state of Bilaspur was merged with Himachal Pradesh in 1954. The 6 districts were: Mahasu, Sirmur, Mandi, Chamba, Bilaspur and Kinnuar. On 1 Nov. 1966, under the Punjab Reorganization Act, 1966, certain parts of the State of Punjab (India) were transferred to Himachal Pradesh. These comprise the districts of Shimla, Kullu, Kangra, and Lahaul and Spiti; and parts of Hoshiarpur, Ambala and Gurdaspur districts.

AREA AND POPULATION. Himachal Pradesh is in north India and is bounded north by Kashmir, east by Tibet, south-east by Uttar Pradesh, south by Haryana, south-west and west by Punjab. The area of the state is 55,673 sq. km and it had a population at the 1981 census of 4,280,818. Density, 77 per sq. km. Growth rate, 1971–81, 23·71%. Principal languages are Hindi and Pahari.

CONSTITUTION AND GOVERNMENT. Full statehood was attained, as the 18th state of the Union, on 25 Jan. 1971.

On 1 Sept. 1972 districts were reorganized and 2 new districts created, Hamirpur and Una, making a total of 12. The capital is Shimla.

There is a unicameral legislature. After the elections in Feb. 1990 a Bharatiya Janata Party government came to power. Total seats, 68: Bharatiya Janata Party, 44; Janata Dal, 11; Congress (I), 8; Independents and others, 2; vacant, 3.

Governor: Virendra Verma.
Chief Minister: Shanta Kumar.

BUDGET. Budget estimates for 1991–92 showed revenue receipts of Rs 936·4 crores and expenditure on revenue account of Rs 1,009 crores. Annual plan, 1991–92, Rs 410 crores.

ENERGY AND NATURAL RESOURCES

Electricity. In 1990, all the 16,807 villages had electricity. Power generation is the first priority of the 7th five-year plan.

Water. An artificial confluence of the Sutlej and Beas rivers has been made, directing their united flow into Govind Sagar Lake. Other major rivers are Ravi, Chenab and Yamuna.

Minerals. The state has rock salt, slate, gypsum, limestone, barytes, dolomite and pyrites.

Agriculture. Farming employs 71% of the people. Irrigated area is 17% of the area sown. Main crops are seed potatoes, wheat, maize, rice and fruits such as apples, peaches, apricots, nuts, pomegranates.

Production of foodgrains (1988-89) 1·14m. tonnes (rice, 89,800 tonnes, wheat, 512,500 tonnes), pulses, 7,300 tonnes.

Livestock (1982 census): Buffaloes, 617,000; other cattle, 2,174,000; goats and sheep, 2·15m.

Forestry. (1989) Himachal Pradesh forests cover 38·3% of the state and supply the largest quantities of coniferous timber in northern India. The forests also ensure the safety of the catchment areas of the Yamuna, Sutlej, Beas, Ravi and Chenab rivers. Commercial felling of green trees has been totally halted and forest working nationalized. Efforts are being made to bring 50% of the area of the state under forests by the turn of the century.

INDUSTRY. The main sources of employment are the forests and their related industries; there are factories making turpentine and rosin. The state also makes fertilizers, cement and TV sets. There is a foundry and a brewery. Other industries include salt production and handicrafts, including weaving. The state has 118 large and medium units, 18,900 small scale units and 5 industrial estates.

COMMUNICATIONS

Roads. The national highway from Chandigarh runs through Shimla; other main highways from Shimla serve Kullu, Manali, Kangra, Chemba and Pathankot. The rest are minor roads. Pathankot is also on national highways from Punjab to Kashmir. Length of roads (1987) 20,279 km, number of vehicles 5,194.

Railways. There is a line from Chandigarh to Shimla, and the Jammu-Delhi line runs through Pathankot. A Nangal-Talwara rail link has been approved by the central government and was in an advanced stage of completion in 1989.

Aviation. The state has airports at Bhuntar near Kullu and at Jubbarharthi near Shimla. Another airport, at Gaggal in Kangra district, was nearing completion in 1989.

JUSTICE, EDUCATION AND WELFARE

Justice. The state has its own High Court at Shimla.

Education. There were (1988-89) 7,182 primary schools with 663,000 students, 1,066 middle schools with 337,200 students, 941 high and higher secondary schools with 153,300 students, 39 arts, science and commerce colleges, 1 engineering college, 1 medical college, 2 teacher training colleges and 3 universities. The universities are Himachal Pradesh University, Shimla (1970) with 27 affiliated colleges, Himachal Pradesh Agricultural University, Palanpur (1978) and Dr Y. S. Parmar University of Horticulture and Forestry, Solan (1985). In 1981, 42·48% of the population was literate.

Health. There were (1987) 68 hospitals (7,036 beds), 180 primary health centres and 646 allopathic and Ayurvedic dispensaries.

JAMMU AND KASHMIR

HISTORY. The state of Jammu and Kashmir, which had earlier been under Hindu rulers and Moslem sultans, became part of the Mogul Empire under Akbar from 1586. After a period of Afghan rule from 1756, it was annexed to the Sikh kingdom of the Punjab in 1819. In 1820 Ranjit Singh made over the territory of Jammu to Gulab Singh. After the decisive battle of Sobraon in 1846 Kashmir also was made over to Gulab Singh under the Treaty of Amritsar. British supremacy was recognized until the Indian Independence Act, 1947, when all states decided on accession to India or Pakistan. Kashmir asked for standstill agreements with both. Pakistan agreed, but India desired further discussion with the Government of Jammu and Kashmir State. In the meantime the state became subject to armed attack from the territory of Pakistan and the Maharajah acceded to India on 26 Oct. 1947, by signing the Instrument of Accession. India approached the UN in Jan. 1948; India-Pakistan conflict ended by ceasefire in Jan. 1949. Further conflict in 1965 was followed by the Tashkent Declaration of Jan. 1966. Following further hostilities between India and Pakistan a ceasefire came into effect on 17 Dec. 1971, followed by the Simla Agreement in July 1972, whereby a new line of control was delineated bilaterally through negotiations between India and Pakistan and came into force on 17 Dec. 1972.

AREA AND POPULATION. The state is in the extreme north and is bounded north by China, east by Tibet, south by Himachal Pradesh and Punjab and west by Pakistan. The area is 222,236 sq. km, of which about 78,932 sq. km is occupied by Pakistan and 42,735 sq. km by China; the population of the territory on the Indian side of the line, 1981 census, was 5,987,389. Growth rate, 1971–81, 29·57%. The official language is Urdu; other commonly spoken languages are

Kashmiri (3·1m. speakers at 1981 census), Hindi (1m.), Dogri, Balti, Ladakhi and Punjabi.

CONSTITUTION AND GOVERNMENT. The Maharajah's son, Yuvraj Karan Singh, took over as Regent in 1950 and, on the ending of hereditary rule (17 Oct. 1952), was sworn in as Sadar-i-Riyasat. On his father's death (26 April 1961) Yuvraj Karan Singh was recognized as Maharajah by the Indian Government; he decided not to use the title while he was elected head of state.

The permanent Constitution of the state came into force in part on 17 Nov. 1956 and fully on 26 Jan. 1957. There is a bicameral legislature; the Legislative Council has 36 members and the Legislative Assembly has 76. Since the 1967 elections the 6 representatives of Jammu and Kashmir in the central House of the People are directly elected; there are 4 representatives in the Council of States. After a period of President's rule, a National Conference–Indira Congress coalition government was formed in March 1987. The government was dismissed and the state was brought under President's rule on 18 July 1990.

Kashmir Province has 8 districts and Jammu Province has 6 districts. Srinagar (population, 1981, 586,038) is the summer and Jammu (206,135) the winter capital.

Governor: Girish Saksena.
Chief Minister: (Vacant).

BUDGET. Total expenditure (1990-91) Rs 2,427 crores; total revenue, Rs 1,881·6 crores.

ENERGY AND NATURAL RESOURCES

Electricity. Installed capacity (1987–88) 212 mw.; 5,976 villages had electricity.

Minerals. Minerals include coal, bauxite and gypsum.

Agriculture. About 80% of the population are supported by agriculture. Rice, wheat and maize are the major cereals. The total area under food crops (1984-85) was estimated at 872,000 ha. Total foodgrains produced, 1988–89, 1·3m. tonnes (rice, 579,600 tonnes; wheat, 245,600 tonnes), pulses, 24,600 tonnes. Fruit is important; production, 1985–86, 800,000 tonnes; exports, Rs 2,000m.

The Agrarian Reforms Act came into force in July 1978; the Debtors Relief Act and the Restriction of Mortgage Properties Act also alleviate rural distress. The redistribution of land to cultivators is continuing.

Livestock (1982): Cattle, 2,325,200; buffaloes, 5,631,000; goats, 1,003,900; sheep, 1,908,700; horses, 973,000, and poultry, 2,406,760.

Forestry. Forests cover about 20,891·89 sq. km., forming an important source of revenue, besides providing employment to a large section of the population. About 20,174 sq. km of forests yield valuable timber; state income in 1985–86 was Rs 477m.

INDUSTRY. There are 2 central public sector industries and 30 medium-scale (latter employing 6,468 in 1984). The largest industrial complex is the Bari Brahmara estate in Jammu which covers 320 acres and accommodates diverse manufacturing, as does the Khanmuh estate. The Sopore industrial area in Kashmir Division is intended for industries based on horticulture. There are 26,332 small units (1988–89) employing 115,243. The main traditional handicraft industries are silk spinning, wood-carving, papier-maché and carpet-weaving.

COMMUNICATIONS

Roads. Kashmir is linked with the rest of India by the motorable Jammu-Pathankot road. The Jawahar Tunnel, through the Banihal mountain, connects Srinagar and Jammu, and maintains road communication with the Kashmir Valley during the winter months. In 1988-89 there were 10,260 km of roads.

There were 104,864 motor vehicles in 1989.

Railways. Kashmir is linked with the Indian railway system by the line between Jammu and Pathankot; route km of railways in the state, 1987–88, 77 km.

Aviation. Major airports, with daily service from Delhi, are at Srinagar and Jammu. There is a third airport at Leh. Srinagar airport is being developed as an international airport.

Post. There were 1,457 post offices in 1985, 82 telephone exchanges and approximately 18,000 private telephones.

JUSTICE, RELIGION, EDUCATION AND WELFARE

Justice. The High Court, at Srinagar and Jammu, has a Chief Justice and 4 puisne judges.

Religion. The majority of the population, except in Jammu, are Moslems. At the 1981 census Moslems numbered 3,843,451; Hindus, 1,930,448; Sikhs, 133,675; Buddhists, 69,706; Christians, 8,481; Jains, 1,576.

Education. The proportion of literates was 27% in 1981. Education is free. There were (1988–89) 1,097 secondary schools with 181,313 students, 2,320 middle schools with 291,738 students and 8,712 primary schools with 738,760 students. Jammu University (1969) has 3 constituent and 11 affiliated colleges, with 8,903 students (1985–86); Kashmir University (1948) has 6 constituent, 15 affiliated and 6 oriental institutions (11,900 students); the third university is Sher-E-Kashmir University of Agricultural Sciences and Technology. There are 2 medical colleges, 4 engineering and technology colleges, 2 polytechnics, 8 oriental colleges and an Ayurvedic college, and 3 teacher training colleges.

Health. In 1984–85 there were 50 hospitals, 93 primary health centres and 425 units, 679 clinics and dispensaries, and 483 other units. There were (1986) 3,442 doctors. There is a National Institute of Medical Sciences.

Bamzai, P. N. K., *A History of Kashmir*. Delhi, 1962
Gupta, S., *Kashmir: A Study in IndiaPakistan Relations*. London, 1967

KARNATAKA

HISTORY. The state of Karnataka, constituted as Mysore under the States Reorganization Act, 1956, brought together the Kannada-speaking people distributed in 5 states, and consisted of the territories of the old states of Mysore and Coorg, the Bijapur, Kanara and Dharwar districts and the Belgaum district (except one taluk) in former Bombay, the major portions of the Gulbarga, Raichur and Bidar districts in former Hyderabad, and South Kanara district (apart from the Kasaragod taluk) and the Kollegal taluk of the Coimbatore district in Madras. The state was renamed Karnataka in 1973.

AREA AND POPULATION. The state is in south India and is bounded north by Maharashtra, east by Andhra Pradesh, south by Tamil Nadu and Kerala, west by the Indian ocean and north-east by Goa. The area of the state is 191,791 sq. km, and its population (1981 census), 37,135,714, an increase of 26·43% since 1971. Density, 194 per sq. km. Kannada is the language of administration and is spoken by about 66% of the people. Other languages include Telugu (8·17%), Urdu (9%), Marathi (4·5%), Tamil (3·6%), Tulu and Konkani. Principal cities, *see* p. 629.

CONSTITUTION AND GOVERNMENT. Karnataka has a bicameral legislature. The Legislative Council has 75 members. The Legislative Assembly consists of 224 elected members. After elections in Nov. 1989 the Congress-I party formed a government.

The state has 20 districts (of which Bangalore Rural is one) in 4 divisions: Bangalore, Mysore, Belgaum and Gulbarga. The capital is Bangalore.

Governor: Kurshid Alam Khan.
Chief Minister: S. Bangarappa.

BUDGET. Budget estimates, 1989–90: receipts, Rs 3,429·24 crores; expenditure, Rs, 3,551·41 crores. Plan allocation 1991-92, Rs 1,510 crores.

ENERGY AND NATURAL RESOURCES

Electricity. In 1987 the state's installed capacity was 2,530 mw. Electricity generated, 1987–88, 7,434m. kwh.

Water. About 2·25m. ha were irrigated in 1986-87.

Minerals. Karnataka is an important source of gold and silver. The estimated reserves of high grade iron ore are 5,000m. tonnes. These reserves are found mainly in the Chitradurga belt. The National Mineral Development Corporation of India has indicated total reserves of nearly 1,000m. tonnes of magnesite and iron ore (with an iron content ranging from 25 to 40) which have been found in Kudremukh Ganga-Mula region in Chickmagalur District. Value of production (1987-88) Rs 138 crores. The estimated reserves of manganese are over 275m. tonnes.

Limestone is found in many regions; deposits (1986) are about 4,248m. tonnes.

Karnataka is the largest producer of chromite. It is one of the only two states of India producing magnesite. The other minerals of industrial importance are corundum and garnet.

Agriculture. Agriculture forms the main occupation of more than three-quarters of the population. Physically, Karnataka divides itself into four regions–the coastal region, the southern and northern 'maidan' or plain country, comprising roughly the districts of Bangalore, Tumkur, Chitaldrug, Kolar, Bellary, Mandya and Mysore, and the 'malnad' or hill country, comprising the districts of Chickmagalur, Hassan and Shimoga. Rainfall is heavy in the 'malnad' tracts, and in this area there is dense forest. The greater part of the 'maidan' country is cultivated. Coorg district is essentially agricultural.

The main food crops are rice and jowar, and ragi which is also about 30% of the national crop. Total foodgrains production (1988–89), 6·72m. tonnes of which rice 2·4m. tonnes, wheat 161,700 tonnes, pulses 516,400 tonnes. Sugar, groundnut, castor-seed, safflower, mulberry silk and cotton are important cash crops. The state grows about 70% of the national coffee crop.

Production, 1987–88 (1,000 tonnes): Sugar-cane, 14,464; cotton, 576 bales (170 kg).

Livestock (1986): Buffaloes, 3,647,967; other cattle, 11,300,223; sheep, 4,791,650; goats, 4,546,928.

Forestry. Total forest in the state (1986–87) is 3,060,840 acres, producing sandal wood, bamboo and other timbers, and ivory.

Fisheries. Production, 1987–88, 176,000 tonnes, of which marine fish 130,000 tonnes.

INDUSTRY. There were 12,436 factories employing 803,285 in March 1988. The Vishweswaraya Iron and Steel Works is situated at Bhadravati, while at Bangalore are national undertakings for the manufacture of aircraft, machine tools, light engineering and electronics goods. Other industries include textiles, vehicle manufacture, cement, chemicals, sugar, paper, porcelain and soap. In addition, much of the world's sandalwood is processed, the oil being one of the most valuable productions of the state. Sericulture is a more important cottage industry giving employment, directly or indirectly, to about 2·7m. persons; production of raw silk, 1986–87, 4,671 tonnes, over two-thirds of national production.

COMMUNICATIONS

Roads. In 1987–88 the state had 110,947 km of roads, including 1,968 km of national highway. There were (31 March 1988) 1,031,131 motor vehicles.

Railways. In 1987 there were 3,029 km of railway (including 154 km of narrow gauge) in the state.

Aviation. There are airports at Bangalore, Mangalore, Bellary and Belgaum, with regular scheduled services to Bombay, Calcutta, Delhi and Madras.

Shipping. Mangalore is a deep-water port for the export of mineral ores. Karwar is being developed as an intermediate port.

JUSTICE, RELIGION, EDUCATION AND WELFARE

Justice. The seat of the High Court is at Bangalore. It has a Chief Justice and 24 puisne judges.

Religion. At the 1981 census there were 31,906,793 Hindus; 4,104,616 Moslems; 764,449 Christians; 297,974 Jains; 42,147 Buddhists; 6,401 Sikhs.

Education. The number of literates, according to the 1981 census, was 38·5m. In 1988–89 the state had 23,337 primary schools with 5,428,714 students, 15,725 middle schools with 1,687,515 students, 4,799 high and higher secondary schools with 829,205 students, 173 polytechnic and 18 medical colleges, 50 engineering and technology colleges, 403 arts, science and commerce colleges and 8 universities. Education is free up to pre-university level.

Universities: Mysore (1916); Karnatak (1950) at Dharwar; University of Agricultural Sciences (1964) at Hebbal, Bangalore; Gulbarga, and Mangalore; University of Agricultural Sciences, Dharwad; Kuvempu University, Shimoga. Mysore has 6 university and 117 affiliated colleges (1983–84); Karnatak, 5 and 115; Bangalore, 126 affiliated; Hebbal, 8 constituent colleges.

The Indian Institute of Science, Bangalore, has the status of a university.

Health. There were in 1987, 2,872 hospitals, dispensaries and family welfare centres.

KERALA

HISTORY. The state of Kerala, created under the States Reorganization Act, 1956, consists of the previous state of Travancore-Cochin, except for 4 taluks of the Thiruvananthapuram (Trivandrum) district and a part of the Shencottah taluk of Kollam (Quilon) district. It took over the Malabar district (apart from the Laccadive and Minicoy Islands) and the Kasaragod taluk of South Kanara (apart from the Amindivi Islands) from Madras State.

AREA AND POPULATION. Kerala is in south India and is bounded north by Karnataka, east and south-east by Tamil Nadu, south-west and west by the Indian ocean. The state has an area of 38,863 sq. km. The 1981 census showed a population of 25,453,680; density of population was 655 per sq. km (highest of any state). Growth rate, 1971–81, 19%. Population of principal cities, *see* p. 629.

Languages spoken in the state are Malayalam, Tamil and Kannada.

The physical features of the land fall into three well-marked divisions: (1) the hilly tracts undulating from the Western Ghats in the east and marked by long spurs, extensive ravines and dense forests; (2) the cultivated plains intersected by numerous rivers and streams; and (3) the coastal belt with dense coconut plantations and rice fields.

CONSTITUTION AND GOVERNMENT. The state has a unicameral legislature of 140 elected (and one nominated) members including the Speaker. After the elections of March 1987 the Indian National (I) Congress Party and allies held 59 seats, the Left Front (CPI, CPI (M) and allies), 79 and independents, 2.

The state has 14 districts. The capital is Thiruvananthapuram (Trivandrum).

Governor: B. Rachiah.
Chief Minister: E. K. Nayanar.

BUDGET. Budget estimates for 1990–91 showed total receipts of Rs 2,236 crores, expenditure Rs 2,596 crores. Annual Plan expenditure, 1991–92, Rs 807 crores.

ENERGY AND NATURAL RESOURCES

Electricity. Installed capacity (March 1988), 1,476·5 mw.; energy generated in 1987–88 was 4,094m. kw. The Idukki hydro-electric plant produced 2,314·4m. kwh, the Sabarigiri scheme 962·99m.

Minerals. The beach sands of Kerala contain monazite, ilmenite, rutile, zircon, sillimanite, etc. There are extensive whiteclay deposits; other minerals of commercial importance include mica, graphite, limestone, quartz sand and lignite. Iron ore has been found at Kozhikode (Calicut).

Agriculture. Area under irrigation in 1986-87 was 299,264 ha, 19 irrigation projects were under execution in 1987-88. The chief agricultural products are rice, tapioca, coconut, arecanut, cashewnut, oilseeds, pepper, sugar-cane, rubber, tea, coffee and cardamom. About 98% of Indian black pepper and about 95% of Indian rubber is produced in Kerala. Area and production of principal crops, 1986–87 (in 1,000 ha and 1,000 tonnes): Rice, 664, 1,134; black pepper, 129, 30·4; arecanut, 58, 10,563 (million nuts); coconuts, 706, 3,173 (million nuts); tea, 34·6, 50·33; coffee, 65·6, 23·5; rubber, 348, 202; tapioca, 194, 3,292.

Livestock (1982, provisional); Buffaloes, 408,584; other cattle, 3·1m.; goats, 2m. In 1985–86 milk production was 1·34m. tonnes. Egg production, 1,397m.

Forestry. Forest occupied 1,081,509 ha in 1987. About 24% of the area is comprised of forests, including teak, sandal wood, ebony and blackwood and varieties of softwood. Net forest revenue, 1986–87, Rs 48·18 crores, from timber, bamboos, reeds and ivory.

Fisheries. Fishing is a flourishing industry; the catch in 1988-89 was about 365,400 tonnes. Fish exports, Rs 183·94 crores in 1987-88.

INDUSTRIES. Most of the major industrial concerns are either owned or sponsored by the Government. Among the privately owned factories are the numerous cashew and coir factories. Other important factory industries are rubber, tea, tiles, oil, textiles, ceramics, fertilizers and chemicals, zinc-smelting, sugar, cement, rayon, glass, matches, pencils, monazite, ilmenite, titanium oxide, rare earths, aluminium, electrical goods, paper, shark-liver oil, etc.

The number of factories registered under the Factories Act 1948 on 1 July 1990 was 12,557, with daily average employment of 292,000.

Among the cottage industries, coir-spinning and handloom-weaving are the most important, forming the means of livelihood of a large section of the people. Other industries are the village oil industry, ivory carving, furniture-making, bell metal, brass and copper ware, leather goods, screw-pines, mat-making, rattan work, bee-keeping, pottery, etc. These have been organized on a co-operative basis.

COMMUNICATIONS

Roads. In 1986–87 there were 110,649 km of roads in the state; national highways, 839 km. There were 581,054 motor vehicles at 31 March 1990.

Railways. There is a coastal line from Mangalore in Karnataka which serves Kannur (Cannanore), Mahé, Kozhikode (Calicut), Ernakulam (for Kochi (Cochin)), Aleppuzha (Aleppy), Kollam (Quilon) and Thiruvananthapuram (Trivandrum), and connects them with main towns in Tamil Nadu. In 1988–89 there were 1,097 route-km of track.

Aviation. There are airports at Kozhikode, Kochi and Thiruvananthapuram with regular scheduled services to Delhi, Bombay and Madras; international flights leave from Thiruvananthapuram.

Shipping. Port Kochi, administered by the central government, is one of India's major ports; in 1983 it became the out-port for the Inland Container Depot at Coimbatore in Tamil Nadu. There are 13 other ports and harbours.

JUSTICE, RELIGION, EDUCATION AND WELFARE

Justice. The High Court at Ernakulam has a Chief Justice and 14 puisne judges and 3 additional judges.

Religion. At the 1981 census there were 14,801,347 Hindus; 5,409,687 Moslems; 5,233,865 Christians; 3,605 Jains; 1,295 Sikhs.

Education. Kerala is the most literate Indian State with 17m. literates at the 1981 census (70·7%). Education is free up to the age of 14.

In 1988–89 there were 6,817 primary schools with 3.22m. students, 2,885 middle schools with 1.76m students and 2,456 high schools with 0.89m students.

Kerala University (established 1937) at Trivandrum, is affiliating and teaching; in 1986–87 it had 43 affiliated arts and science colleges. The University of Cochin is federal, and for post-graduate studies only. The University of Calicut (established 1968) is teaching and affiliating and has 92 affiliated colleges. Kerala Agricultural University (established 1971) has 8 constituent colleges. Mahatma Gandhi University at Kottayam was established in 1983 and has 56 affiliated colleges.

Health. There were 140 allopathic, 101 Ayurvedic and 279 homeo hospitals, and 881 health centres in 1990.

MADHYA PRADESH

HISTORY. Under the provisions of the States Reorganization Act, 1956, the State of Madhya Pradesh was formed on 1 Nov. 1956. It consists of the 17 Hindi districts of the previous state of that name, the former state of Madhya Bharat (except the Sunel enclave of Mandsaur district), the former state of Bhopal and Vindhya Pradesh and the Sironj subdivision of Kotah district, which was an enclave of Rajasthan in Madhya Pradesh.

For information on the former states, *see* THE STATESMAN'S YEAR-BOOK , 1958, pp. 180–84.

AREA AND POPULATION. The state is in central India and is bounded north by Rajasthan and Uttar Pradesh, east by Bihar and Orissa, south by Andhra Pradesh and Maharashtra, west by Gujarat. Madhya Pradesh is the largest Indian state in size, with an area of 443,446 sq. km. In respect of population it ranks sixth. Population (1981 census), 52,178,844, an increase of 25·15% since 1971. Density, 118 per sq. km.

Cities with over 250,000 population, *see* p. 629. Other large cities (1981): Sagar, 174,770; Ratlam, 155,578; Burhanpur, 140,886; Durg, 118,507; Khandwa, 114,725; Rewa, 100,641.

The number of persons speaking each of the more prevalent languages (1981 census) were: Hindi, 43,870,242; Urdu, 1,131,288; Marathi, 1,184,128; Gujarati, 581,084. In April 1990 Hindi became the sole official language.

CONSTITUTION AND GOVERNMENT. Madhya Pradesh is one of the 9 states for which the Constitution provides a bicameral legislature, but the Vidhan Parishad or Upper House (to consist of 90 members) has yet to be formed. The Vidhan Sabha or Lower House has 320 elected members. Following the election of Feb. 1990, a Bharatiya Janata Party government was returned, with 220 out of 320 seats; Congress (I), 56; Janata Dal, 28; Independents and others, 15; vacant 1.

For administrative purposes the state has been split into 12 divisions with a Commissioner at the head of each; the headquarters of these are located at Bhopal, Bilaspur, Chambal, Gwalior, Hoshangabad, Indore, Jabalpur, Jagdalpur, Raipur, Rewa, Sagar and Ujjain. There are 45 districts.

The seat of government is at Bhopal.

Governor: Kunwar Mahmood Ali Khan.
Chief Minister: Sundarlal Patwa.

BUDGET. Budget estimates for 1990–91 showed total revenue of Rs 5,005·75 crores and expenditure of Rs 6,196·12 crores. Annual plan, 1991–92, Rs 2,426 crores.

ENERGY AND NATURAL RESOURCES

Electricity. Madhya Pradesh is rich in low-grade coal suitable for power generation, and also has immense potential hydro-electric energy. Power generated, 29,470m. kwh. in 1990–91. The thermal power stations are at Korba in Bilaspur district, Amarkantak in Shahdol district and Satpura in Betul district; new stations are being built. The only hydro-electric power station is at Gandhi Sagar lake in Mandsaur district; this, with a maximum water surface of 165 sq. miles, is the biggest man-made lake in Asia.

Water. Major irrigation projects include the Chambal Valley scheme (started in 1952 with Rajasthan), the Tawa project in Hoshangabad district, the Barna and Hasdeo schemes, the Mahanadi canal system and schemes in the Narmada valley at Bargi and Narmadasagar.

Minerals. The state has extensive mineral deposits including coal (35% of national deposits), iron ore (30%) and manganese (50%), bauxite (44%), ochre, sillimanite, limestone, dolomite, rock phosphate, copper, lead, tin, fluorite, barytes, china clay and fireclay, corundum, gold, diamonds, pyrophyllite and diaspore, lepidolite, asbestos, vermiculite, mica, glass sand, quartz, felspars, bentonite and building stone. New and very large reserves of copper were found in the Malanjkhand area in 1986.

In 1987 the output of major minerals was (in tonnes): Coal, 34·2m.; limestone, 11·2m.; diamonds, 15,000 carats; iron ore, 7·7m.; manganese ore, 200,000. Value of production, 1987, Rs 11,120m.

Agriculture. Agriculture is the mainstay of the state's economy and 80% of the people are rural. 43·9% of the land area is cultivable, of which 14% is irrigated. The Malwa region abounds in rich black cotton soil, the low-lying areas of Gwalior, Bundelkhand and Baghelkhand and the Chhatisgarh plains have a lighter sandy soil, while the Narmada valley is formed of deep rich alluvial deposits. Production of principal crops, 1988–89 (in tonnes): Foodgrains, 16m. of which rice, 4·9m.; wheat 4.6m., pulses 2.7m.

Livestock (1988–89): Buffaloes, 7,263,715; other cattle, 27,270,700; sheep, 885,308; goats, 7,484,586; horses and ponies, 92,433.

Forestry. In 1982 155,411 sq. km, or about 35% of the state's area was covered by forests. The forests are chiefly of sal, saja, bija, bamboo and teak. They are the chief source in India of best-quality teak; they also provide firewood for about 60% of domestic fuel needs, and form valuable watershed protection. Forest revenue, 1986–87, Rs 3,070m.

INDUSTRY. The major industries are the steel plant at Bhilai, Bharat Heavy Electricals at Bhopal, the aluminium plant at Korba, the security paper mills at Hoshangabad, the Bank Note Press at Dewas, the newsprint mill at Nepanagar and alkaloid factory at Neemuch, cement factories, vehicle factory, ordnance factory, and gun carriage factory. There are also 23 textile mills, 7 of them nationalized.

The Bhilai steel plant near Durg is one of the 6 major steel mills. A power station at Korba (Bilaspur) with a capacity of 420 mw serves Bhilai, the aluminium plant and the Korba coalfield.

The heavy electrical factory was set up by the Government of India at Bhopal during the second-plan period. This is India's first heavy electrical equipment factory.

Other industries include cement, sugar, fertilizers, straw board, paper, vegetable oil, refractories, potteries, textile machinery, steel casting and rerolling, industrial gases, synthetic fibres, drugs, biscuit manufacturing, engineering, tools, rayon and art silk. The number of heavy and medium industries in the state is 518, with 181 ancillary industries; the number of small-scale establishments in production is 275,000. 39 out of 45 districts in the state are categorized as industrially backward.

There are 22 'growth centres' in operation.

The main industrial development agencies are Madhya Pradesh Financial Corporation, Madhya Pradesh Audyogik Vikas Nigam Ltd, Madhya Pradesh State Industries Corporation, Madhya Pradesh Laghu Udyog Nigam, Madhya Pradesh State Textile Corporation, Madhya Pradesh Handicrafts Board, Khadi and Village Industries Board and Madhya Pradesh State Mining Corporation.

The state is known for its traditional village and home crafts such as handloom weaving, best developed at Chanderi and Maheshwar, toys, pottery, lacework, woodwork, zari work, leather work and metal utensils. The ancillary industries of dyeing, calico printing and bleaching are centred in areas of textile production.

COMMUNICATIONS

Roads. Total length of roads in 1989–90 was 857,000 km, of which 680,000 km were surfaced. In 1989–90 there were 1,251,411 motor vehicles.

Railways. Bhopal, Bilaspur, Katni, Khandwar and Ratlam are junctions for the central, south-eastern and western networks. Route km of railways (1988–89), 5,764 km.

Aviation. There are airports at Bhopal, Indore, Khajuraho and Raipur with regular scheduled services to Bombay and Delhi.

JUSTICE, RELIGION AND EDUCATION

Justice. The High Court of Judicature at Jabalpur has a Chief Justice and 24 puisne judges.

Religion. At the 1981 census Hindus numbered 48,504,575; Moslems, 2,501,919; Christians, 351,972; Buddhists, 75,312; Sikhs, 143,020, Jains, 444,960.

Education. The 1981 census showed 14·5m. people to be literate. Education is free for children aged up to 14.

In 1988–89 there were 65,897 primary schools with 7,744,492 students, 13,453 middle schools with 2,523,520 students and 3,449 secondary schools with 1,005,837 students.

There are 12 universities in Madhya Pradesh: Dr. Hari Singh Gour University (established 1946), at Sagar, had 92 affiliated colleges and 30,487 students in 1990–91; Rani Durgavati University at Jabalpur (1957) had 36 affiliated colleges and 20,101 students; Vikram University (1957), at Ujjain, had 80 affiliated colleges and 24,226 students; Indira Kala Sangeet Vishwavidyalaya (1956), at Khairagarh, had 33 affiliated colleges and 6,720 students on roll (this university teaches music and fine arts); Devi Ahilya University at Indore (1964) had 26 affiliated colleges and 20,332 students; Jiwaji University (1963), at Gwalior, had 58 affiliated colleges and 25,766 students; Jawaharlal Nehru Krishi University (1964), at Jabalpur, had 10 constituent colleges and 2,994 students in 1985–86; Ravishankar University (1964), at Raipur, had 84 affiliated colleges; Indira Gandhi Krishi Vishwa Vidyalaya, Raipur; A. P. Singh University, Rewa; Barkatullah Vishwavidyalaya, Bhopal; Guru Ghasidas University, Bilaspur. In 1990-91 there were 554 colleges of arts, science and commerce, 19 teacher-training colleges, and 13 engineering and technology colleges, 6 medical colleges, 32 polytechnics and 63 technical-industrial arts and craft schools.

MAHARASHTRA

HISTORY. Under the States Reorganization Act, 1956, Bombay State was formed by merging the states of Kutch and Saurashtra and the Marathi-speaking areas of Hyderabad (commonly known as Marathwada) and Madhya Pradesh (also called Vidarbha) in the old state of Bombay, after the transfer from that state of the Kannada-speaking areas of the Belgaum, Bijapur, Kanara and Dharwar districts which were added to the state of Mysore, and the Abu Road taluka of Banaskantha district, which went to the state of Rajasthan.

By the Bombay Reorganization Act, 1960, which came into force 1 May 1960, 17 districts (predominantly Gujarati-speaking) in the north and west of Bombay State became the new state of Gujarat, and the remainder was renamed Maharashtra.

The state of Maharashtra consists of the following districts of the former Bombay State: Ahmednagar, Akola, Amravati, Aurangabad, Bhandara, Bhir, Buldana, Chanda, Dhulia (West Khandesh), Greater Bombay, Jalgaon (East Khandesh), Kolaba, Kolhapur, Nagpur, Nanded, Nasik, Osmanabad, Parbhani, Pune, Ratnagiri, Sangli, Satara, Sholapur, Thana, Wardha, Yeotmal; certain portions of Thana and Dhulia districts have become part of Gujarat.

AREA AND POPULATION. Maharashtra is in central India and is bounded north and east by Madhya Pradesh, south by Andhra Pradesh, Karnataka and Goa, west by the Indian ocean and north-west by Daman and Gujarat. The state has an area of 307,690 sq. km. The population at the 1981 census (revised) was 62,784,171 (an increase of 24·36% since 1971), of whom about 30m. were Marathi-speaking. Density, 204 per sq. km. The area of Greater Bombay was 603 sq. km. and its population 8,227,000. For other principal cities, *see* p. 629.

CONSTITUTION AND GOVERNMENT. Maharashtra has a bicameral legislature. The Legislative Council has 78 members. The Legislative Assembly has 288 elected members and 1 member nominated by the Governor to represent the Anglo-Indian community. Following the election of Feb. 1990 Congress (I) retained power with the support of some independent members. Total seats, 288: Congress (I), 141; Shiv Shena, 52; Bharatiya Janata Party, 42; Janata Dal, 24; People's and Workers' Party, 8; Independents and others, 21.

The Council of Ministers consists of the Chief Minister, 16 other Ministers, and 19 Ministers of State.

The capital is Bombay. The state has 30 districts.

Governor: C. Subramaniam

Chief Minister: Sharad Pawar.

BUDGET. Budget estimates, 1990–91: receipts, Rs 10,843·42 crores; expenditure; Rs 10,853·6 crores. Plan outlay, 1991-92, Rs 3,000 crores.

ENERGY AND NATURAL RESOURCES

Electricity. Installed capacity, 31 March 1989, 7,658 mw. (5,634 mw. thermal, 1,436 mw. hydro-electricity and 160 mw. nuclear).

Minerals. Value of main mineral production, 1987, Rs 313 crores. The state has coal, silica, sand, dolomite, kyanite, sillimanite, limestone, iron ore, manganese, bauxite.

Agriculture. About 23·43% of the cropped area is irrigated. In 1988–89 there was heavy rain in 16 of the state's 30 districts. The monsoon-season harvest was feeble, and the winter-season harvest was good.

In normal seasons the main food crops are rice, wheat, jowar, bajri and pulses. Main cash crops: Cotton, sugar-cane, groundnuts. Production, 1988-89 (in tonnes): Foodgrains, 11.1m. of which rice, 2.65m. and wheat, 1.04m.; pulses, 1.73m.

Livestock (1982 census): Buffaloes, 3,972,000; other cattle, 16,162,000; sheep, 2,671,000; goats, 7,705,000; horses and ponies, 49,000; poultry, 19,844,000.

Forestry. Forests occupy 20·8% of the state.

INDUSTRY. Industry is concentrated mainly in Bombay, Pune and Thane. The main groups are chemicals and products, textiles, electrical and non-electrical machinery, petroleum and products, aircraft, rubber and plastic products, transport equipment and food products. The state industrial development corporation had invested Rs 5,600 crores in 8,800 industrial units by 1989.

COMMUNICATIONS

Roads. On 31 March 1989 there were 169,921 km of roads, of which 121,207 km were surfaced. There were 2,056,357 motor vehicles on 31 March 1989, of which

557,142 were in Greater Bombay. Passenger and freight transport has been nationalized.

Railways. The total length of railway on 31 March 1988 was 5,440 km; 61% was broad gauge, 18% metre gauge and 20% narrow gauge. The main junctions and termini are Bombay, Manmad, Akola, Nagpur, Pune and Sholapur.

Aviation. The main airport is Bombay, which has national and international flights. Nagpur airport is on the route from Bombay to Calcutta and there are also airports at Pune and Aurangabad.

Shipping. Maharashtra has a coastline of 720 km. Bombay is the major port, and there are 48 minor ports.

JUSTICE, RELIGION, EDUCATION AND WELFARE

Justice. The High Court has a Chief Justice and 45 judges. The seat of the High Court is Bombay, but it has benches at Nagpur, Aurangabad and Panaji (Goa).

Religion. At the 1981 census Hindus numbered 51,109,457; Moslems, 5,805,785; Buddhists, 3,946,149; Christians, 795,464; Jains, 939,392; Sikhs, 107,255. Other religions, 155,692; religion not stated, 1,394.

Education. The number of literates, according to the 1981 census, was 29.6m. In 1988–89, there were 9,248 high and higher secondary schools with 2,135,000 pupils; 17,550 middle schools with 3,364,000 pupils, and 38,623 primary schools, with 9,986,000 pupils. There are 75 engineering and technology colleges, 16 medical colleges, 88 teacher training colleges, 140 polytechnics and 540 arts, science and commerce colleges.

Bombay University, founded in 1857, is mainly an affiliating university. It has 159 colleges with a total (1988–89) of 162,000 students. Colleges in Goa can affiliate to Bombay University. Nagpur University (1923) is both teaching and affiliating. It has 117 colleges with 55,000 students. Pune University, founded in 1948, is teaching and affiliating; it has 191 colleges and 97,000 students. The SNDT Women's University had 25 colleges with a total of 26,000 students. Marathwada University, Aurangabad, was founded in 1958 as a teaching and affiliating body to control colleges in the Marathwada or Marathi-speaking area, previously under Osmania University; it has 133 colleges and 55,000 students. Shiwaji University, Kolhapur, was established in 1963 to control affiliated colleges previously under Pune University. It has 138 colleges and 56,000 students. Amravati University has 88 colleges and 35,000 students.Other universities are: Marathwada Krishi Vidyapeeth, Parbhani; Y. Chavan Maharashtra Open University, Nashik; North Maharashtra University, Jalgaon; Tilak Vidyapeeth, Pune.

Health. In 1987 there were 768 hospitals (100,363 beds), 1,799 dispensaries and 1,539 primary health centres.

Statistical Information: The Director of Publicity, Sachivalaya, Bombay.
Tindall, G., *City of Gold*, London, 1982

MANIPUR

HISTORY. Formerly a state under the political control of the Government of India, Manipur, on 15 Aug. 1947, entered into interim arrangements with the Indian Union and the political agency was abolished. The administration was taken over by the Government of India on 15 Oct. 1949 under a merger agreement, and it is centrally administered by the Government of India through a Chief Commissioner. In 1950–51 an Advisory form of Government was introduced. In 1957 this was replaced by a Territorial Council of 30 elected and 2 nominated members. Later in 1963 a Legislative Assembly of 30 elected and 3 nominated members was established under the Government of Union Territories Act 1963. Because of the unstable party position in the Assembly, it had to be dissolved on 16 Oct. 1969 and President's Rule introduced. The status of the administrator was raised from Chief

Commissioner to Lieut.-Governor with effect from 19 Dec. 1969. On the 21 Jan. 1972 Manipur became a state and the status of the administrator was changed from Lieut.-Governor to Governor.

AREA AND POPULATION. The state is in north-east India and is bounded north by Nagaland, east by Burma, south by Burma and Mizoram, and west by Assam. Manipur has an area of 22,327 sq. km and a population (1981) of 1,420,953. Density, 64 per sq. km. Growth rate, 1971–81, 32·46%. The valley, which is about 1,813 sq. km, is 2,600 ft above sea-level. The hills rise in places to nearly 10,000 ft, but are mostly about 5,000–6,000 ft. The average annual rainfall is 65 in. The hill areas are inhabited by various hill tribes who constitute about one-third of the total population of the state. There are about 40 tribes and sub-tribes falling into two main groups of Nagas and Kukis. Manipuri and English are the official languages. A large number of dialects are spoken, while Hindi is gradually becoming prevalent.

CONSTITUTION AND GOVERNMENT. With the attainment of statehood, Manipur has a Legislative Assembly of 60 members, of which 19 are from reserved tribal constituencies. There are 8 districts. Capital, Imphal (population, 1981, 155,639). Presidential rule was imposed in Feb. 1981. Following the election in Feb. 1990, a United Legislature Front government led by Manipur People's Party came to power. Total seats, 60: Congress (I), 26; Manipur People's Party, 10; Janata Dal, 10; Congress (S), 6; Independents and others, 6; vacant, 2.

Governor: Chintamani Panigrahi.
Chief Minister: R. K. Ranvir Singh.

BUDGET. Budget estimates for 1988–89 show revenue of Rs 3,540m. and expenditure of Rs 3,460m. Plan allocation 1991–92, Rs 1,950m.

ENERGY AND NATURAL RESOURCES

Electricity. Installed capacity (1988-89) is 10,715 Kw. from diesel and hydro-electric generators. This has been augmented since 1981 by the North Eastern Regional Grid. In 1989-90 there were 1,292 villages with electricity.

Water. The main power, irrigation and flood-control schemes are the Loktak Lift Irrigation scheme (irrigation potential, 40,000 ha; the Singda scheme (potential 4,000 ha, and improved water supply for Imphal); the Thoubal scheme (potential 34,000 ha, 7·5 mw. of electricity and 10 MGD of water supply), and four other large projects. By 1986–87 more than 43,500 ha had been irrigated.

Agriculture. Rice is the principal crop; with wheat, maize and pulses. Total food-grains, 1988–89, 331,900 tonnes (rice 319,700 tonnes).

Agricultural work force, about 348,000. Only 210,000 ha are cultivable, of which 186,000 are under paddy. Fruit and vegetables are important in the valley, including pineapple, oranges, bananas, mangoes, pears, peaches and plums. Soil erosion, produced by shifting cultivation, is being halted by terracing.

Forests. Forests occupy about 15,154 sq km. The main products are teak, jurjan, pine; there are also large areas of bamboo and cane, especially in the Jiri and Barak river drainage areas, yielding about 300,000 tonnes annually. Total revenue from forests, 1987–88, Rs 17·1m.

Fisheries. Landings in 1981–82, 3,450 tonnes.

INDUSTRY. Handloom weaving is a cottage industry. Larger-scale industries include the manufacture of bicycles and TV sets, sugar, cement, starch, vegetable oil and glucose. Sericulture produces about 45 tonnes of raw silk annually. Estimated non-agricultural work force, 240,000.

COMMUNICATIONS. A national highway from Kazirangar (Assam) runs through Imphal to the Burmese frontier. A railway link was opened in 1990. There is an airport at Imphal with regular scheduled services to Delhi and Calcutta. Length of road (1987) 3,971 km; number of vehicles (1988) 29,760.

EDUCATION AND HEALTH

Education. The 1981 census gave the number of literates as 587,618. In 1988–89 there were 2,771 primary schools with 268,800 students, 443 middle schools with 73,000 students, 388 high and higher secondary schools and 33 colleges with 50,400 students, 1 medical college, 3 teacher training colleges, 1 polytechnic as well as Manipur University.

Health. In 1987–88 there were 11 hospitals, 52 dispensaries, 8 community health centres, 49 primary health centres and 389 sub-centres.

MEGHALAYA

HISTORY. The state was created under the Assam Reorganization (Meghalaya) Act 1969 and inaugurated on 2 April 1970. Its status was that of a state within the State of Assam until 21 Jan. 1972 when it became a fully-fledged state of the Union. It consists of the former Garo Hills district and United Khasi and Jaintia Hills district of Assam.

AREA AND POPULATION. Meghalaya is bounded north and east by Assam, south and west by Bangladesh. In 1981 (census figure) the area was 22,429 sq. km and the population 1,335,819. Density 60 per sq. km. Growth rate, 1971–81, 31·04%. The people are mainly of the Khasi, Jaintia and Garo tribes.

CONSTITUTION AND GOVERNMENT. Meghalaya has a unicameral legislature. The Legislative Assembly has 60 seats. Party position in Nov. 1990: Meghalaya United Parliamentary Party, 32; United Meghalaya Parliamentary Forum, 27.

There are 5 districts. The capital is Shillong (population, 1981, 109,244).

Governor: Madhukar Dighe.
Chief Minister: B. B. Lyngdoh.

BUDGET. Budget estimates for 1986–87 showed revenue receipts of Rs 2,177m. and expenditure of Rs 1,639m. Annual Plan expenditure, 1991–92, Rs 1,750m.

ENERGY AND NATURAL RESOURCES

Electricity. Total installed capacity (1988–89) was 128.72 mw. 1,397 villages had electricity.

Minerals. The East and West Khasi and Jaintia Hills districts produce coal, sillimanite (95% of India's total output), limestone, fire clay, dolomite, felspar, quartz and glass sand. The state also has deposits of coal (estimated reserves 500m. tonnes), limestone (4,000m.), fire clay (100,000) and sandstone which are virtually untapped because of transport difficulties.

Agriculture. About 80% of the people depend on agriculture. Principal crops are rice, maize, potatoes, cotton, oranges, ginger, tezpata, areca nuts, jute, mesta, bananas and pineapples. Production 1988–89 (in tonnes) of principal crops: Rice, 105,600; potatoes, 71,100; maize, 20,600; jute, 37,300; wheat, 6,700; cotton, 4,200; rape and mustard, 3,400; pulses, 2,300.

Forest products are the state's chief resources.

INDUSTRY. Apart from agriculture the main source of employment is the extraction and processing of minerals; there are also important timber processing mills. The state has a plywood factory, a cement factory (production capacity, 930 tonnes per day), a beverage plant and watch and match splint factories. Meghalaya Industrial Development Corporation has set up industrial units. There is a new industrial area in Byrnihat, and two industrial estates in Shillong and Mendipathar. Tantalum capacitors are manufactured in the Khwan Industrial Area near Shillong. In 1988–89 there were 58 registered factories and 1,231 small-scale industries.

COMMUNICATIONS. Three national highways run through the state. The state has no railways. Umroi airport (20 km from Shillong) connects the state with main air services. In 1989 there were 461 km of national highway and (1988-89) 5,399 km of surfaced and unsurfaced roads.

JUSTICE, EDUCATION AND WELFARE

Justice. The Guwahati High Court is common to Assam, Meghalaya, Nagaland, Manipur, Mizoram, Tripura and Arunachal Pradesh. There is a bench of the Guwahati High Court at Shillong.

Education. In 1988–89 the state had 4,175 primary schools with 239,291 students, 749 middle schools with 68,370 students, 342 high schools with 42,260 students, 1 teacher training college, 1 polytechnic and 23 colleges. The North-eastern Hill University started functioning at Shillong in 1973.

Health. In 1989–90 there were 8 government hospitals, 56 primary health centres, 24 government dispensaries and 247 sub-centres. Total beds (hospitals and health centres), 1,714.

MIZORAM

HISTORY. On 21 Jan. 1972 the former Mizo Hills District of Assam was created a Union Territory. A long dispute between the Mizo National Front (originally Seperatist) and the central government was resolved in 1985. Mizoram became a state by the Constitution (53rd Amendment) and the State of Mizoram Acts, July 1986.

AREA AND POPULATION. Mizoram is one of the eastern-most Indian states, lying between Bangladesh and Burma, and having on its northern boundaries Tripura, Assam and Manipur. The area is 21,081 sq. km and the population (1981 census) 493,757. Denslty, 23 per sq. km; growth rate 1971–81, 48·55%.

CONSTITUTION AND GOVERNMENT. Mizoram has a unicameral Legislative Assembly with 40 seats: Congress I, 22; Mizo National Front, 14; others, 4. The capital is Aizawl.

Governor: Swaraj Kaushal.
Chief Minister: Lalthnahawla.

BUDGET. Annual plan outlay (1991-92) Rs 150 crores.

ELECTRICITY. Installed capacity (1986–87), 16,109 kw. Work was in progress (1988) on one diesel and two hydro-electric generators.

AGRICULTURE. About 90% of the people are engaged in agriculture, either on terraced holdings or in shifting cultivation. Area under rice, 1988–89, 49,400 ha; production, 53,000 tonnes.

Total forest area, 15,935 sq. km.

INDUSTRY. Hand loom weaving and other cottage industries are important.

COMMUNICATIONS. Aizawl is connected by road and air with Silchar in Assam.

RELIGION. The mainly tribal population is 83·81% Christian.

EDUCATION. In 1988–89 there were 1,053 primary schools with 106,176 students, 498 middle schools with 33,750 students and 185 high schools with 12,436 students; there were 13 colleges and one university.

HEALTH. In 1986–87 there were 9 hospitals, 22 primary and 25 subsidiary health centres. Total beds, 893.

NAGALAND

HISTORY. The territory was constituted by the Union Government in Sept. 1962. It comprises the former Naga Hills district of Assam and the former Tuensang Frontier division of the North-East Frontier Agency; these had been made a Centrally Administered Area in 1957, administered by the President through the Governor of Assam. In Jan. 1961 the area was renamed and given the status of a state of the Indian Union, which was officially inaugurated on 1 Dec. 1963.

For some years a section of the Naga leaders sought independence. Military operations from 1960 and the prospect of self-government within the Indian Union led to a general reconciliation, but rebel activity continued. A 2-month amnesty in mid 1963 had little effect. A 'ceasefire' in Sept. 1964 was followed by talks between a Government of India delegation and rebel leaders. The peace period was extended and the 'Revolutionary Government of Nagaland' (a breakaway group from the Naga Federal Government) was dissolved in 1973. Further talks with the Naga underground movement resulted in the Shillong Peace Agreement of Nov. 1975.

AREA AND POPULATION. The state is in the extreme north-east and is bounded west and north by Assam, east by Burma and south by Manipur. Nagaland has an area of 16,579 sq. km and a population (1981) census of 774,930. Density 47 per sq. km. Growth rate, 1971–81, 50·05%. Towns include Kohima, Mokokchung, Tuensang and Dimapur. The chief tribes in numerical order are: Angami, Ao, Sema, Konyak, Chakhesang, Lotha, Phom, Khiamngan, Chang, Yimchunger, Zeliang-Kuki, Rengma and Sangtam.

CONSTITUTION AND GOVERNMENT. An Interim Body (Legislative Assembly) of 42 members elected by the Naga people and an Executive Council (Council of Ministers) of 5 members were formed in 1961, and continued until the State Assembly was elected in Jan. 1964. The Assembly has 60 members, and includes: Congress I, 24; Nagaland People's Council, 17. The Governor has extraordinary powers, which include special responsibility for law and order.

The state has 7 districts (Kohima, Mon, Zunheboto, Wokha, Phek, Mokokchung and Tuensang). The capital is Kohima.

Governor: M. M. Thomas.
Chief Minister: S. Vamuzo.

BUDGET. Budget estimates 1988–89, revenue receipts, Rs 4,090m., expenditure, Rs 4,100m. Annual Plan, 1991–92, Rs 170 crores.

ENERGY AND NATURAL RESOURCES

Electricity. Installed capacity (1984) 5·12 mw; all towns and villages are electrified.

Agriculture. 90% of the people derive their livelihood from agriculture. The Angamis, in Kohima district, practise a fixed agriculture in the shape of terraced slopes, and wet paddy cultivation in the lowlands. In the other two districts a traditional form of shifting cultivation (*jhumming*) still predominates, but some farmers have begun tea and coffee plantations and horticulture. About 27,133 ha were under terrace cultivation and 76,512 ha under *jhumming* in 1988–89. Production of rice (1988–89) was 130,000 tonnes, total foodgrains 153,300 tonnes, pulses 4,000 tonnes.

Forests covered 2,875 sq. km in 1988.

INDUSTRY. There is a forest products factory at Tijit; a paper-mill (100 tonnes daily capacity) at Tuli, a distillery unit and a sugar-mill (1,000 tonnes daily capacity) at Dimapur. Bricks and TV sets are also made, and there are over 1,000 small units. Oil has been located in 3 districts. Other minerals include: Coal, limestone, clay, glass sand and slate.

COMMUNICATIONS. There is a national highway from Kaziranga (Assam) to Kohima and on to Manipur. There are state highways connecting Kohima with the district headquarters. Total length of roads in 1989, 9,345 km.; 1,538 km were surfaced in 1988. Dimapur has a rail-head and a daily air service to Calcutta.

RELIGION, EDUCATION AND WELFARE

Religion. At the 1981 census there were 621,590 Christians; 111,266 Hindus; 11,806 Moslems; 1,153 Jains; 743 Sikhs.

Education. The 1981 census records 329,000 literates, or 42·57%: 50·06% of men and 33·89% of women. In 1988-89 there were 1,286 primary schools with 153,800 students, 343 middle schools with 48,000 students, 120 high schools with 17,500 students, 20 colleges, 1 teacher training college and 1 polytechnic. The North Eastern Hill University opened at Kohima in 1978.

Health. In 1988 there were 33 hospitals (1,409 beds), 23 primary and 3 community health centres, 73 dispensaries, 218 sub-centres.

Aram, M., *Peace in Nagaland,* New Delhi, 1974

ORISSA

HISTORY. Orissa, ceded to the Mahrattas by Alivardi Khan in 1751, was conquered by the British in 1803. In 1803 a board of 2 commissioners was appointed to administer the province, but in 1805 it was designated the district of Cuttack and was placed in charge of a collector, judge and magistrate. In 1829 it was split up into 3 regulation districts of Cuttack, Balasore and Puri, and the non-regulation tributary states which were administered by their own chiefs under the aegis of the British Government. Angul, one of these tributary states, was annexed in 1847, and with the Khondmals, ceded in 1835 by the tributary chief of the Boudh state, constituted a separate non-regulation district. Sambalpur was transferred from the Central Provinces to Orissa in 1905. These districts formed an outlying tract of the Bengal Presidency till 1912, when they were transferred to Bihar, constituting one of its divisions under a commissioner. Orissa was constituted a separate province on 1 April 1936, some portions of the Central Provinces and Madras being transferred to the old Orissa division.

The rulers of 25 Orissa states surrendered all jurisdiction and authority to the Government of India on 1 Jan. 1948, on which date the Provincial Government took over the administration. The administration of 2 states, viz., Seraikella and Kharswan, was transferred to the Government of Bihar in May 1948. By an agreement with the Dominion Government, Mayurbhanj State was finally merged with the province on 1 Jan. 1949. By the States Merger (Governors' Provinces) Order, 1949, the states were completely merged with the state of Orissa on 19 Aug. 1949.

AREA AND POPULATION. Orissa is in eastern India and is bounded north by Bihar, north-east by West Bengal, east by the Bay of Bengal, south by Andhra Pradesh and west by Madhya Pradesh. The area of the state is 155,707 sq. km, and its population (1981 census), 26,370,271, density 169 per sq. km. Growth rate, 1971–81, 20·17%. The largest cities are Cuttack (295,268 in 1988), Rourkela (214,521) and Berhampur (162,550). The principal and official language is Oriya.

CONSTITUTION AND GOVERNMENT. The Legislative Assembly has 147 members. After the election in Feb 1990 a Janata Dal government came to power. Total seats, 147: Janata Dal, 123; Congress (I), 10; Communist Party of India, 5; Independents and others, 9.

The state consists of 16 districts.

Union government was enabled to impose a state of emergency on the Punjab for a period of up to 3 years. The state is under President's rule.

There are 12 districts. The capital is Chandigarh (*see* p. 695). There are 106 municipalities, 118 community development blocks and 9,331 elected village *panchayats*.

Governor: Gen. O. P. Malhotra.

BUDGET. Budget estimates, 1990–91, showed revenue receipts of Rs 20,727.9m. and revenue expenditure of Rs 25,408.4m. Plan outlay, 1991-92, Rs 10,000m.

ENERGY AND NATURAL RESOURCES

Electricity. Installed capacity, 1987–88, was 2,661 mw; all villages had electricity.

Agriculture. About 75% of the population depends on agriculture which is technically advanced. The irrigated area rose from 2·21m. ha in 1950–51 to 6·7m. ha in 1986–87. In 1988–89,wheat production was 11.6m. tonnes, rice, 4.9m.; maize, 292,000; oilseeds (1987-88), 178,000.

Livestock (1977 census): Buffaloes, 4,110,000; other cattle, 3·31m.; sheep and goats, 1,219,600; horses and ponies, 75,900; poultry, 5·5m.

Forestry. In 1988–89 there were 284,237 ha of forest land, of which 134,804 ha belonged to the Forest Department.

INDUSTRY. In March 1987 the number of registered industrial units in the Punjab (India) was 122,766, employing about 800,000 people. On 31 March 1988 there were (provisional) 135,305 small industrial units, investment Rs 937 crores. The chief manufactures are textiles (especially hosiery), sewing machines, sports goods, sugar, bicycles, electronic goods, machine tools, hand tools, vehicle parts, surgical goods and vegetable oils. Recent (1989) large projects include food processing, electronics, railway coaches, paper and newsprint.

COMMUNICATIONS

Roads. The total length of metalled roads on 31 March 1988 was 35,964 km. State transport services cover 815,380 route km daily with a fleet of 3,422 buses carrying a daily average of over 1m. passengers. Coverage by private operators is estimated as 40%.

Railways. The Punjab possesses an extensive system of railway communications, served by the Northern Railway. Route-km (1988) 2,145 km.

Aviation. There is an airport at Amritsar, and Chandigarh airport is on the north-eastern boundary; both have regular scheduled services to Delhi, Jammu, Srinagar and Leh. There are also Vayudoot services to Ludhiana and Kulu.

JUSTICE, RELIGION, EDUCATION AND WELFARE

Justice. The Punjab and Haryana High Court exercises jurisdiction over the states of Punjab and Haryana and the territory of Chandigarh. It is located in Chandigarh. It consists (1988) of a Chief Justice and 21 puisne judges.

Religion. At the 1981 census Hindus numbered 6,200,195; Sikhs, 10,199,141; Moslems, 168,094; Christians, 184,934; Jains, 27,049.

Education. Compulsory education was introduced in April 1961; at the same time free education was introduced up to 8th class for boys and 9th class for girls as well as fee concessions. The aim is education for all children of 6-11.

In 1988-89 there were 12,357 primary schools with 2,092,295 students, 1,413 middle schools with 809,795 students, 2,353 high schools with 373,124 students and 387 senior secondary schools with 165,112 students.

Punjab University was established in 1947 at Chandigarh as an examining, teaching and affiliating body. In 1962 Punjabi University was established at Patiala and Punjab Agricultural University at Ludhiana. Guru Nanak Dev University has been established at Amritsar to mark the 500th anniversary celebrations for Guru Nanak Dev, first Guru of the Sikhs. Altogether there are 197 affiliated colleges, 171 for arts and science, 18 for teacher training, 5 medical, 3 engineering and 11 for other studies.

Health. Punjab claims the longest life expectancy (60·6 years for women, 60·7 for men) and lowest death rate (9 per 1,000). There were (1988) 268 hospitals, 528 Ayurvedic and Unani hospitals and dispensaries, 170 primary health centres, 2,702 sub-centres and 1,839 dispensaries.

Singh, Khushwant, *A History of the Sikhs*. 2 vols. Princeton and OUP, 1964–67

RAJASTHAN

HISTORY. As a result of the implementation of the States Reorganization Act, 1956, the erstwhile state of Ajmer, Abu Taluka of Bombay State and the Sunel Tappa enclave of the former state of Madhya Bharat were transferred to the state of Rajasthan on 1 Nov. 1956, whereas the Sironj subdivision of Rajasthan was transferred to the state of Madhya Pradesh.

EVENTS. An instance of *suttee* on 4 Sept. 1987 brought about state legislation (Rajasthan Sati (Prevention) Ordinance) promulgated on 1 Oct., and the central government's Sati Prevention Act (strengthening existing penalties) in Dec. 1987.

AREA AND POPULATION. Rajasthan is in north-west India and is bounded north by Punjab, north-east by Haryana and Uttar Pradesh, east by Madhya Pradesh, south by Gujarat and west by Pakistan. The area of the state is 342,239 sq. km and its population (census 1981, revised), 34,261,862, density 100 per sq. km. Growth rate, 1971–81, 32·36%. The chief cities, *see* p. 629.

CONSTITUTION AND GOVERNMENT. There is a unicameral legislature, the Legislative Assembly, having 200 members. After the election in Feb 1990 a coalition government of Bharatiya Janata Party and Janata Dal come to power. Bharatiya Janata party, 85; Janata Dal, 54; Congress (I), 50; Independents and others, 10; vacant, 1..

The capital is Jaipur. There are 27 districts.

Governor: Dr Debi Prasad Chattopadhyay.
Chief Minister: Bhairon Singh Shekhawat.

BUDGET. Estimates for 1991–92 show total revenue receipts of Rs 38,254.4m., and expenditure of Rs 40,200.4m. Annual plan 1991–92, Rs 11,660m.

ENERGY AND NATURAL RESOURCES

Electricity. Installed capacity in Feb. 1988, 1,978 mw.; 24,882 villages and 318,000 wells had electric power.

Water. In 1984 the Bhakra Canal irrigated 300,000 hectares, the Chambal Canal, 200,000 and the Rajasthan Canal, 450,000. The Rajasthan (now the Indira Gandhi canal) is the main canal system, of which (1984) 189 km. of main canal and 2,950 km of distributors had been built. Cost, at 1 March 1984, Rs 419 crores. There were 28,739 villages with drinking water in March 1987, out of 34,968.

Minerals. The state is rich in minerals. In 1987, 1·7m. tonnes of gypsum and 300,000 tonnes of rock phosphate were produced. Other minerals include silver (21,550 kg., 1987 estimate), asbestos, felspar, copper, limestone and salt. Total sale value of mineral production in 1987 (estimate) was about Rs 350 crores. Lead-zinc reserves have been found near Rampura-Agucha, estimated at 61m. tonnes.

Agriculture. The state has suffered drought and encroaching desert for several years. The cultivable area is (1988–89) about 26·6m. ha, of which 4.3m. is irrigated.

Production of principal crops (in tonnes), 1988–89: Pulses, 1.6m.; rice, 185,800; wheat, 3.97m. Total foodgrains (1988–89) 10.7m. tonnes.

Livestock (1983): Buffaloes, 6,034,743; other cattle, 13,466,474; sheep, 15,389,100; goats, 15,397,993; horses and ponies, 45,381; camels, 7,528,287.

INDUSTRY. In Dec. 1987 there were 9,665 registered factories and 122,304 small industrial units. There were 171 industrial estates. Total capital investment Rs 4,750·7m. Chief manufactures are textiles, cement, glass, sugar, sodium, oxygen and acetylene units, pesticides, insecticides, dyes, caustic soda, calcium, carbide, nylon tyre cords and refined copper.

COMMUNICATIONS

Roads. In 1988-89 there were 55,123 km of roads including 42,478 km of good and surfaced roads in Rajasthan; there were 2,521 km of national highway. Motor vehicles numbered 719,364 in Dec. 1987.

Railways. Jodhpur, Marwar, Udaipur, Ajmer, Jaipur, Kota, Bikaner and Sawai Madhopur are important junctions of the north-western network. Route km (1989) 5,611.

Aviation. There are airports at Jaipur, Jodhpur, Kota and Udaipur with regular scheduled services by Indian Airlines.

JUSTICE, RELIGION, EDUCATION AND WELFARE

Justice. The seat of the High Court is at Jodhpur. There is a Chief Justice and 11 puisne judges. There is also a bench of High Court judges at Jaipur.

Religion. At the 1981 census Hindus numbered 30,603,970; Moslems, 2,492,145; Jains, 624,317; Sikhs, 492,818; Christians, 39,568; Buddhists, 4,427.

Education. The proportion of literates to the total population was 24·39% at the 1981 census.

In 1988–89 there were 28,507 primary schools with 4,399,839 students, 8,355 middle schools with 1,252,350 students, 2,171 high schools with 492,653 students and 897 higher secondary schools with 133,143 students. Elementary education is free but not compulsory.

In 1988–89 there were 179 colleges. Rajasthan University, established at Jaipur in 1947, is teaching and affiliating (6 affiliated colleges); Jodhpur University and Udaipur University were founded in 1962. There are 6 other universities: Rajasthan Vidyapeeth, Udaipur; Rajasthan Agricultural University, Bikaner; Mohanlal Sukhadia University, Udaipur; Ajmer University, Ajmer; Banasthali Vidyapith, Banasthali; Kota Open University, Kota. There are also 5 medical and nursing colleges, 3 engineering colleges, 21,436 adult and other education centres, 32 sanskrit institutions, 33 teacher-training colleges and 14 polytechnics.

Health. In 1987 there were 899 hospitals and dispensaries, 498 primary health centres. In addition there were 3,228 Ayurvedic, Unani, homoepathic and naturopathy hospitals. There were 116 maternity centres.

SIKKIM

HISTORY. Sikkim became the twenty-second state of the Indian Union in May 1975. It is inhabited chiefly by the Lepchas, who are a tribe indigenous to Sikkim with their own dress and language, the Bhutias, who originally came from Tibet, and the Nepalis, who entered from Nepal in large numbers in the late 19th and early 20th century. The main languages spoken are Bhutia, Lepcha and Nepali. Being a small country Sikkim had frequently been involved in struggles over her territory, and as a result her boundaries have been very much reduced over the centuries. In particular the Darjeeling district was acquired from Sikkim by the British East India

Company in 1839. The Namgyal dynasty had been ruling Sikkim since the 14th century; the first consecrated ruler was Phuntsog Namgya I who was consecrated in 1642 and given the title of 'Chogyal', meaning 'King ruling in accordance with religious laws', derived from Cho–religion and Gyalpo–king. The last Chogyal was deposed in 1975 and died in America in 1982.

Sikkim is a land of wide variation in altitude, climate and vegetation, and is known for the great number and variety of birds, butterflies, wild flowers and orchids to be found in the different regions. It is a fertile land and to the Sikkimese is known as Denjong, The Valley of Rice.

AREA AND POPULATION. Sikkim is in the Eastern Himalayas and is bounded north by Tibet, east by Tibet and Bhutan, south by West Bengal and west Nepal. Area, 7,096 sq. km. Census population (1981), 316,385, of whom 36,768 lived in the capital, Gangtok. Density 43 per sq km. Growth rate, 1971–81, 50·01%.

CONSTITUTION AND GOVERNMENT. Sikkim was joined to the British Empire by a treaty in 1886 until 1947, but that relationship ceased when Britain withdrew from India in 1947. Thereafter there was a standstill agreement between India and Sikkim until a treaty was signed on 5 Dec. 1950 between India and Sikkim by which Sikkim became a protectorate of India and India undertook to be responsible for Sikkim's defence, external relations and strategic communications. The Chogyal had governed Sikkim with the help of the Sikkim Council, consisting of 18 elected members and 6 members nominated by the Chogyal. Sikkim parties represented were: National Party, Sikkim National Congress and, later, Sikkim Janta Congress.

Political reforms were demanded by the National Congress and the Janta Congress in March-April 1973 and Indian police took over control of law and order at the request of the Chogyal. On 13 April it was announced that the Chogyal had agreed to meet most of the political demands. Elections were held in April 1974 to a popularly-elected assembly. By the Government of Sikkim Act, June 1974, the Chogyal became a constitutional monarch with power of assent to the Assembly's legislation. By the Constitution (Thirty-Sixth Amendment) Act 1974 Sikkim became a state associated with the Indian Union. The office of Chogyal was abolished in April 1975. By the Constitution (Thirty-Eighth Amendment) Act 1975 Sikkim became the twenty-second state of the Indian Union. The Assembly has 32 members. After the election of Nov. 1989 the Sangram Parishad government continued in power.

Governor: Adm. R. H. Tahiliani.
Chief Minister: Nar Bahadur Bhandari.

The official language of the Government is English. Lepcha, Bhutia, Nepali and Limboo have also been declared official languages.

Sikkim is divided into 4 districts for administration purposes, Gangtok, Mangan, Namchi and Gyalshing being the headquarters for the Eastern, Northern, Southern and Western districts respectively. Each district is administered by a District Collector. Within this framework are the Panchayats or Village Councils.

ECONOMY

Budget. Budget estimates for 1991-92 show revenue receipt of Rs 216·85 crores and total disbursements of Rs 229·93 crores. Annual plan outlay for 1991-92 is Rs 950m.

ENERGY AND NATURAL RESOURCES

Electricity. There are 4 operational hydro-electric power stations; the Lagyap project is also being implemented by the Government of India as aid to meet the growing demand for electrical power for new industries. The first of its two 6 mv generators was commissioned 1 Sept. 1979.

Agriculture. The economy is mainly agricultural; main food crops are rice, maize, millet, wheat and barley; cash crops are cardamom (a spice), mandarin oranges, apples, potatoes, and buckwheat. Foodgrain production, 1988-89, 112,300 tonnes (rice 18,600 tonnes, wheat 17,600 tonnes); pulses, 12,300 tonnes. A tea plantation has recently been started. Forests occupy about 1,000 sq. km. of the land area (excluding hill pastures) and the potential for a timber and wood-pulp industry is being explored. Some medicinal herbs are exported.

INDUSTRY AND TRADE

Industry. There is a state Industrial Development Investment Corporation and an Industrial Training Institute offering 7 trades. There are two cigarette factories (at Gangtok and Rangpo), two distilleries and a tannery at Rangpo and a fruit preserving factory at Singtam. Copper, zinc and lead are mined by the Sikkim Mining Corporation. A recent survey by the Geological Survey of India and the Indian Bureau of Mines has confirmed further deposits of copper, zinc, silver and gold in Dikchu, North Sikkim. There is a jewel-bearing factory for the production of industrial jewels. A watch factory has been set up in collaboration with Hindustan Machine Tools (India). A number of small manufacturing units for leather, wire nails, storage cells batteries, candles, safety matches and carpets, are already producing in the private sector. Local crafts include carpet weaving, making handmade paper, wood carving and silverwork. To encourage trading in indigenous products, particularly agricultural produce, the State Trading Corporation of Sikkim has been established.

Tourism. There is great potential for the tourist industry; a 78-bed lodge at Gangtok and a 50-bed tourist lodge in West Sikkim have been opened. Tourism has been stimulated by the opening of new roads from Pemayangtse to Yuksam in West Sikkim and from Yuksam to the Dzongri Glacier.

COMMUNICATIONS

Roads. There are 1,456 km. of roads, all on mountainous terrain, and 18 major bridges under the Public Works Department. Public transport and road haulage is nationalized.

Railways. The nearest railhead is at Siliguri (115 km from Gangtok).

Aviation. The nearest airport is at Bagdogra (128 km from Gangtok), linked to Gangtok by helicopter service.

Post and Broadcasting. There are 1,445 telephones (1987) and 37 wireless stations. A radio broadcasting station, Akashvani Gangtok, was built in 1982, and a permanent station in 1983. Gangtok also has a low-power TV transmitter.

RELIGION, EDUCATION AND WELFARE

Religion. At the 1981 census there were 212,780 Hindus; 3,241 Moslems; 7,015 Christians; 90,848 Buddhists; 322 Sikhs; 108 Jains.

Education. At the 1981 census there were 100,000 literates. Sikkim had (1988-89) 528 pre-primary schools with 17,981 students, 489 primary schools with 62,917 students, 123 middle schools with 15,226 students, 54 high schools with 5,139 students and 14 higher secondary schools with 1,490 students. Education is free up to class XII; text books are free up to class V. There are 500 adult education centres. There is also a training institute for primary teachers and a degree college.

Health. There are (1983) 4 district hospitals at Singtam, Gyalshing, Namchi and Mangan, and one central referral hospital at Gangtok, besides 20 primary health centres, 109 sub-centres and 8 dispensaries, a maternity ward, chest clinic and 2 blocks for tuberculosis patients. There is a blood bank at Gangtok. There are 110 doctors. Medical and hospital treatment is free; there is a health centre for every 20,000 of the population. Small-pox and Kala-azar have been completely eliminated and many schemes for the provision of safe drinking water to villages and bazaars have been implemented. A leprosy hospital (20 beds) has been built near Gangtok.

TAMIL NADU

HISTORY. The first trading establishment made by the British in the Madras State was at Peddapali (now Nizampatnam) in 1611 and then at Masulipatnam. In 1639 the English were permitted to make a settlement at the place which is now Madras, and Fort St George was founded. By 1801 the whole of the country from the Northern Circars to Cape Comorin (with the exception of certain French and Danish settlements) had been brought under British rule.

Under the provisions of the States Reorganization Act, 1956, the Malabar district (excluding the islands of Laccadive and Minicoy) and the Kasaragod district taluk of South Kanara were transferred to the new state of Kerala; the South Kanara district (excluding Kasaragod taluk and the Amindivi Islands) and the Kollegal taluk of the Coimbatore district were transferred to the new state of Mysore; and the Laccadive, Amindivi and Minicoy Islands were constituted a separate Territory. Four taluks of the Trivandrum district and the Shencottah taluk of Quilon district were transferred from Travancore-Cochin to the new Madras State. On 1 April 1960, 405 sq. miles from the Chittoor district of Andhra Pradesh were transferred to Madras in exchange for 326 sq. miles from the Chingleput and Salem districts. In Aug. 1968 the state was renamed Tamil Nadu.

AREA AND POPULATION. Tamil Nadu is in south India and is bounded north by Karnataka and Andhra Pradesh, east and south by the Indian ocean and west by Kerala. Area, 130,058 sq. km. Population (1981 census), 48,408,077, density of 372 per sq. km. Growth rate, 1971–81, 17·5%. Tamil is the principal language and has been adopted as the state language with effect from 14 Jan. 1958. The principal towns, *see* p. 629. There are 21 districts. The capital is Madras.

CONSTITUTION AND GOVERNMENT. The Governor is aided by a Council of 16 ministers. There is a unicameral legislature; the Legislative Assembly has 235 members: DMK, 144; AIADMK, 29; Congress I, 26; others, 36.

Presidential rule was imposed in Jan. 1991 and the Assembly was dissolved.

Governor: Bishma Narain Singh.

BUDGET. Budget estimates for 1991-92, total receipts, Rs 5,585 crores, total expenditure, Rs 5,955 crores. Annual plan 1991–92, Rs 1,600 crores.

ENERGY AND NATURAL RESOURCES

Electricity. Installed capacity 1987–88 amounted to 4,558 mw of which 1,799 mw was hydro-electricity and 2,408 mw thermal. 99·9% of villages were supplied with electricity. The Kalpakkam nuclear power plant became operational in 1983; capacity, 350 mw.

Water. A joint project with Andhra Pradesh was agreed in 1983, to supply Madras with water from the Krishna river, also providing irrigation, *en route*, for Andhra Pradesh. In 1986–87 2·84m. ha were irrigated.

Minerals. Value of mineral production, 1987, Rs 176 crores. The state has magnesite, salt, coal, chromite, bauxite, limestone, manganese, mica, quartz, gypsum and feldspar.

Agriculture. In 1981 there were 5·5m. cultivators and 5·9m. agricultural labourers. The land is a fertile plain watered by rivers flowing east from the Western Ghats, particularly the Cauvery and the Tambaraparani. Temperature ranges between 6°C. and 39°C., rainfall between 442 mm. and 1,307 mm. Of the total land area (13m. ha), 6,508,349 ha were cropped and 298,659 ha of waste were cultivable. The staple food crops grown are paddy, maize, jawar, bajra, pulses and millets. Important commercial crops are sugar-cane, oilseeds, cashew-nuts, cotton, tobacco, coffee, tea, rubber and pepper. Production 1989–90, in 1,000 tonnes, (and area, 1,000 ha): Rice 5,850 (1,950); small millet 158 (154); sugar-cane 2,420 (200); pulses 455 (1,059); cotton 520 (244).

Livestock (1982 census): Buffaloes, 3,212,242; other cattle, 10,365,500; sheep, 5,536,514; goats, 5,246,192; swine, 693,735; horses, ponies, mules, camels and donkeys, 90,632; poultry, 18,283,720.

Forestry. Forest area, 1986–87, 2,250,670 ha, of which 1,854,944 ha were reserved forest. Forests cover about 27% of land area. Main products are teak, soft wood, wattle, sandalwood, pulp wood, cashew and cinchona bark.

Fisheries. There were 105,466 active marine fishermen working the 1,000 km coastline in 1987–88.

INDUSTRY AND TRADE

Industry. The number of working factories was 12,599 in 1989, employing 813,290 workers. The consumption of power in the industrial sector was 43% of total state consumption in 1982–83. The biggest central sector project is Salem steel plant.

Cotton textiles is one of the major industries. There are nearly 180 cotton textile mills and many spinning mills supplying yarn to the decentralized handloom industry. Other important industries are cement, sugar, manufacture of textile machinery, power-driven pumps, bicycles, electrical machinery, tractors, motor-cars, rubber tyres and tubes, bricks and tiles and silk.

Public sector undertakings include the Neyveli lignite complex, petrochemicals, integral coach factory, high-pressure boiler plant, photographic film factory, surgical instruments factory, teleprinter factory, oil refinery, continuous casting plant and defence vehicles manufacture. Main exports: Cotton goods, tea, coffee, spices, engineering goods, motor-car ancillaries, leather and granite.

In 1988 there were 4,468 registered trade unions. Man-days lost by strikes, 2,618,993; by lockouts, 631,230.

Tourism. In 1989, 369,883 foreign tourists visited the state.

COMMUNICATIONS

Roads. On 31 March 1987 the state had approximately 170,652 km of national and state highways, major and other district roads. In 1988 there were 1,005,240 registered motor vehicles.

Railways. On 31 March 1989 there were 6,555·45 km of railway track (3,937 route km). Madras and Madurai are the main centres.

Aviation. There are airports at Madras, Tiruchirapalli and Madurai, with regular scheduled services to Bombay, Calcutta and Delhi. Madras is the main centre of airline routes in South India.

Shipping. Madras and Tuticorin are the chief ports. Important minor ports are Cuddalore and Nagapattinam. Madras handled 23·9m. tonnes of cargo in 1988-89, Tuticorin, 5·2m. The Inland Container Depot at Coimbatore has a capacity of 50,000 tonnes of export traffic; it is linked to Cochin (Kerala).

JUSTICE, RELIGION, EDUCATION AND WELFARE

Justice. There is a High Court at Madras with a Chief Justice and 16 judges. *Police:* Strength of police force, 1 Jan. 1990, 67,094.

Religion. At the 1981 census Hindus numbered 43,016,546 (88·86%), Christians, 2,798,048 (5·78%); Moslems, 2,519,947 (5·21%).

Education. At the 1981 census 22·6m. people were literate (14·3m. males).

Education is free up to pre-university level. In 1989-90 there were 40,091 schools for general education, 12·3m. students and 297,918 teachers. There were 212 general colleges (203,215 students and (1986–87) 15,155 teachers); 119 professional colleges (62,498 and 14,759); (1986–87) 19 special education colleges (2,366 and 316).

There are 14 universities. Madras University (founded in 1857) is affiliating and teaching. Annamalai University, Annamalainagar (founded 1928) is residential; Madurai Kamaraj University (founded 1966) is an affiliating and teaching university; 11 others include one agricultural and one rural university, Mother Theresa Women's University, and Tamil University, Tanjavur.

Health. There were (1988-89) 410 hospitals, 1,160 dispensaries, 1,094 primary health centres and 8,243 health sub-centres.

Statistical Information: The Department of Statistics (Fort St George, Madras) was established in 1948 and reorganized in 1953. *Director:* C. Sethu. Main publications: *Annual Statistical Abstract; Decennial Statistical Atlas; Season and Crop Report; Quinquennial Wages Census; Quarterly Abstract of Statistics.*

TRIPURA

HISTORY. A Hindu state of great antiquity having been ruled by the Maharajahs for 1,300 years before its accession to the Indian Union on 15 Oct. 1949. With the reorganization of states on 1 Sept. 1956 Tripura became a Union Territory, and was so declared on 1 Nov. 1957. The Territory was made a State on 21 Jan. 1972.

EVENTS. Tripura National Volunteers (tribal guerillas) signed an agreement with Union and State governments in Aug. 1988, to end an 8-month campaign of insurgency.

AREA AND POPULATION. Tripura is bounded by Bangladesh, except in the north-east where it joins Assam and Mizoram. The major portion of the state is hilly and mainly jungle. It has an area of 10,486 sq. km and a population of 2,053,058 (1981 census); Density, 196 per sq. km. Growth rate, 1971-81, 32·37%.

The official languages are Bengali and Kokbarak. Manipuri is also spoken.

CONSTITUTION AND GOVERNMENT. There is a Legislative Assembly of 60 members. The election of Jan. 1983 was won by the Communist Party of India (Marxist). The territory has 3 districts, divided into 10 administrative subdivisions, namely, Sadar, Khowai, Kailasahar, Dharmanagar, Sonamura, Udaipur, Belonia, Kamalpur, Sabroom and Amarpur.

The capital is Agartala (population, 1981, 132,186).

Governor: Raghunath Reddy.

Chief Minister: Sudhir Ranjan Majumdar.

BUDGET. Budget estimates 1988-89, receipts Rs 428 crores and expenditure Rs 452 crores. Annual plan outlay for 1991-92 is Rs 225 crores.

ENERGY AND NATURAL RESOURCES

Electricity. Installed capacity (1988), 25 mw; there were (1988) 2,292 electrified villages.

Agriculture. About 24% of the land area is cultivable. The tribes practise shifting cultivation, but this is being replaced by modern methods. The main crops are rice, wheat, jute, mesta, potatoes, oilseeds and sugar-cane. Foodgrain production (1987-88), about 442,100 tonnes. There are 54 registered tea gardens producing 3,339,000 kg. per year, and employing 8,945.

Forestry. Forests cover about 55% of the land area. They have been much depleted by clearance for shifting cultivation and, recently, for refugee settlements of Bangladeshis. About 8% of the forest area still consists of dense natural forest; losses elsewhere are being replaced by plantation. Commercial rubber plantation has also been encouraged. In 1988, 7,597 ha were under new rubber plantations.

INDUSTRY. Tea is the main industry. There is also a jute mill producing about 15 tonnes per day and employing about 2,000. The main small industries: Aluminium utensils, rubber, saw-milling, soap, piping, fruit canning, handloom weaving and sericulture. Handloom weaving products (1983–84) were valued at Rs 9·75 crores.

COMMUNICATIONS

Roads. Total length of motorable roads (1989) 6,348 km, of which 2,731 km were surfaced. Vehicles registered, 31 March 1988, 13,963, of which 3,542 were lorries.

Railways. There is a railway between Dharmanagar and Kalkalighat (Assam).

Aviation. There is 1 airport and 2 airstrips. The airport (Agartala) has regular scheduled services to Calcutta.

EDUCATION AND WELFARE

Education. In 1988-89 there were 1,989 primary schools (371,372 pupils); 419 middle schools (116,998); 381 high and higher secondary schools (66,142). There were 13 colleges of general education, 1 engineering college, 1 teacher training college and 1 polytechnic.

Health. There were (1988) 21 hospitals, with 1,810 beds, 317 dispensaries, 539 doctors and 618 nurses. There were 47 primary health centres and 66 family planning centres.

UTTAR PRADESH

HISTORY. In 1833 the then Bengal Presidency was divided into two parts, one of which became the Presidency of Agra. In 1836 the Agra area was styled the North-West Province and placed under a Lieut.-Governor. The two provinces of Agra and Oudh were placed, in 1877, under one administrator, styled Lieut.-Governor of the North-West Province and Chief Commissioner of Oudh. In 1902 the name was changed to 'United Provinces of Agra and Oudh', under a Lieut.-Governor, and the Lieut.-Governorship was altered to a Governorship in 1921. In 1935 the name was shortened to 'United Provinces'. On Independence, the states of Rampur, Banaras and Tehri-Garwhal were merged with United Provinces. In 1950 the name of the United Provinces was changed to Uttar Pradesh.

AREA AND POPULATION. Uttar Pradesh is in north India and is bounded north by Himachal Pradesh, Tibet and Nepál, east by Bihar, south by Madhya Pradesh and west by Rajasthan, Haryana and Delhi. The area of the state is 294,411 sq. km. Population (1981 census), 110,862,013, a density of 377 per sq. km. Growth rate, 1971–81, 25·52%. Cities with more than 250,000 population, *see* p. 629. The sole official language has been Hindi since April 1990.

CONSTITUTION AND GOVERNMENT. Uttar Pradesh has had an autonomous system of government since 1937. There is a bicameral legislature. The Legislative Council has 108 members; the Legislative Assembly has 426, of which 425 are elected. After the elections in Nov. 1989 a Janata Dal government was returned.

There are 13 administrative divisions, each under a Commissioner, and 63 districts.

The capital is Lucknow.

Governor: B. Satya Narain Reddy.
Chief Minister: Mulayan Singh Yadav.

BUDGET. Budget estimates 1991–92 show revenue and capital receipts of Rs 131,876m.; revenue and capital account expenditure, Rs 143,845m. Annual plan outlay (1991-92) Rs 37,100m.

ENERGY AND NATURAL RESOURCES

Electricity. The State Electricity Board had, 1988–89, an installed capacity of 5,376·35 mw. There were 78,749 villages with electricity in March 1989, out of a total 112,566.

Minerals. The state has magnesite, fire-clay, coal, copper, dolomite, limestone, soapstone, gypsum, bauxite, diaspore, ochre, phosphorite, pyrophyllite, silica sand and steatite among others.

Agriculture. Agriculture occupies 78% of the work force. 10·13m. ha are irrigated. The state is India's largest producer of foodgrains; production (1988–89), 35·7m. tonnes (rice 9·6m. tonnes, wheat 19·7m. tonnes); pulses, 2·66m. tonnes. The state is one of India's main producers of sugar; production of sugar-cane (1987-88), 8·82m. tonnes. There were (1987-88) 1,605 veterinary centres for cattle.

Forests cover (1987) about 5·13m. sq. km.

The state government in 1985 began a management programme for the ravines of the Chambal river catchment area. The programme includes stabilizing ravines, soil conservation, afforestation, pasture development and ravine reclamation. Estimated cost of a six-year programme, Rs 453·96m.

INDUSTRY. Sugar production is important; other industries include edible oils, textiles, distilleries, brewing, leather working, agricultural engineering, paper and chemicals. There is an aluminium smelter at Renukoot. An oil refinery at Mathura has capacity of 6m. tonnes per annum. Large public-sector enterprises have been set up in electrical engineering, pharmaceuticals, locomotive building, general engineering, electronics and aeronautics. Village and small-scale industries are important; there were 130,061 small units in 1987-88. A petrochemical complex and a fertilizer complex are being implemented at Auriya and Shahjahanpur respectively. About one-third of cloth output is from hand-looms. Total working population (1981) 30·8m., of whom 6·8m. were non-agricultural.

COMMUNICATIONS

Roads. There were, 31 March 1989, 97,559 km of motorable roads. In 1987-88 there were 1,240,939 motor vehicles of which 829,230 were motorcycles.

Railways. Lucknow is the main junction of the northern network; other important junctions are Agra, Kanpur, Allahabad, Mughal Sarai, Dehra Dun and Varanasi.

Aviation. There are airports at Lucknow, Kanpur, Varanasi, Allahabad, Agra and Gorakhpur.

JUSTICE, RELIGION, EDUCATION AND WELFARE

Justice. The High Court of Judicature at Allahabad (with a bench at Lucknow) has a Chief Justice and 49 puisne judges including additional judges. There are 56 sessions divisions in the state.

Religion. At the 1981 census Hindus numbered 92,365,968; Moslems, 17,657,735; Sikhs, 458,647; Christians, 162,199; Jains, 141,549; Buddhists, 54,542.

Education. At the 1981 census 30·1m. people were literate. In 1988–89 there were 74,705 primary schools with 12,618,000 students, 16,652 middle schools with 3,931,000 students, 2,366 high schools with 1,935,514 students and 3,380 intermediate/junior colleges with 2,436,531 students.

Uttar Pradesh has 19 universities: Allahabad University (founded 1887); Agra University (1927); the Banaras Hindu University, Varanasi (1916); Lucknow University (1921); Aligarh Muslim University (1920); Roorkee University (1948), formerly Thomason College of Civil Engineering (established in 1847); Gorakhpur University (1957); Sampurnanand Sanskrit Vishwavidyalaya, Varanasi (1958). Kanpur University and Meerut University were founded in 1966. Govind Ballabh Pant University of Agriculture and Technology, Pantnagar (1960); H. N. Bahuguna Garhwal University, Srinagar, (1973). C. S. Azad University of Agriculture and

Technology, Kaupur, and Narendra Deva University of Agriculture and Technology, Faizabad, were founded in 1974–75 and Avadh, Kumaon, Rohilkhand and Bundelkhand Universities in 1975. Jaunpur University (Purvanchal Vishwavidyalaya) was founded in 1987.

There are also 3 institutions with university status: Gurukul Kangri Vishwavidyalaya, Hardwar, Kashi Vidyapith, Varanasi and Dayal Bagh Educational Institute. There are 8 medical colleges, 3 engineering colleges, 13 teacher-training colleges and 407 arts, science and commerce colleges.

Health. In 1987–88 there were 4,034 allopathic, 2,448 ayurvedic and unani and 980 homoepathic hospitals. There were also TB hospitals and clinics.

WEST BENGAL

HISTORY. For the history of Bengal under British rule, from 1633 to 1947, *see* THE STATESMAN'S YEAR-BOOK , 1952, p. 183.

Under the terms of the Indian Independence Act, 1947, the Province of Bengal ceased to exist. The Moslem majority districts of East Bengal, consisting of the Chittagong and Dacca Divisions and portions of the Presidency and Rajshahi Divisions, became what was then East Pakistan (now Bangladesh).

EVENTS. Gorkha seperatists have campaigned for a Gorkha state in the hill areas; there has been strike and terrorist action. In Aug. 1988 an agreement was signed establishing a Darjeeling Gorkha Hill Council with limited autonomy.

AREA AND POPULATION. West Bengal is in north-east India and is bounded north by Sikkim and Bhután, east by Assam and Bangladesh, south by the Bay of Bengal and Orissa, west by Bihar and north-west by Nepál. The total area of West Bengal is 88,752 sq. km. At the 1981 census its population was 54,580,647, an increase of 23·17% since 1971, the density of population 621 per sq. km. Population of chief cities, *see* p. 629. The principal language is Bengali.

CONSTITUTION AND GOVERNMENT. The state of West Bengal came into existence as a result of the Indian Independence Act, 1947. The territory of Cooch-Behar State was merged with West Bengal on 1 Jan. 1950, and the former French possession of Chandernagore became part of the state on 2 Oct. 1954. Under the States Reorganization Act, 1956, certain portions of Bihar State (an area of 3,157 sq. miles with a population of 1,446,385) were transferred to West Bengal.

The Legislative Assembly has 295 seats. Distribution, Nov. 1990: Communist Party of India (Marxist), 184; Forward Bloc, 27; Revolutionary Socialist Party, 19; Communist Party of India, 10; Revolutionary Communist Party of India, 1; Forward Bloc (Marxist), 2; Democratic Socialist Party, 2; Socialist Party, 4; Indian National Congress, 38; Socialist Unity Centre, 2; Moslem League, 1; nominated, 1; vacant, 5.

The capital is Calcutta.

For administrative purposes there are 3 divisions (Jalpaiguri, Burdwan and Presidency), under which there are 17 districts, including Calcutta. The Calcutta Metropolitan Development Authority has been set up to co-ordinate development in the metropolitan area (1,350 sq. km). For the purposes of local self-government there are 15 *zila parishads* (district boards) excluding Darjeeling, 331 *panchayat samities* (regional boards), and 3,346 *gram* (village) *panchayats*. There are 111 municipalities, 3 Corporations and 9 Notified Areas. The Calcutta Corporation has a mayor and deputy mayor, a commissioner, aldermen and standing committees.

Governor: Nurul Hasan.
Chief Minister: Jyoti Basu.

BUDGET. Budget estimates for 1990–91, revenue receipts Rs 41,770·5m. and expenditure Rs 56,157m. Plan outlay for 1990-91 was Rs 14,860m.

ENERGY AND NATURAL RESOURCES

Electricity. Installed capacity, 1989–90, 3,653 mw; 24,858 villages had electricity at 31 March 1990.

Water. The largest irrigation and power scheme under construction is the Teesta barrage (9,000 ha). Other major irrigation schemes are the Mayurakshi Reservoir, Kansabati Reservoir, Mahananda Barrage and Aqueduct and Damodar Valley. At March 1988 there were 10,896 tubewells and 3,198 riverlift irrigation schemes.

Minerals. Value of production, 1988, Rs 6,278m. The state has coal (the Raniganj field is one of the 3 biggest in India) including coking coal. Coal production (1988) 21·56m. tonnes.

Agriculture. About 11m. ha were under rice-paddy in 1988-89. Total foodgrain production, 1988–89, 11·5m. tonnes (rice 10·6m. tonnes, wheat 625,000 tonnes); pulses 208,000 tonnes; oilseeds, 403,600 tonnes; jute, 4·53m. tonnes; wheat, 0·62m. tonnes; tea, 150·93m. kg. The state produces 59·5% of the national output of jute and *mesta*.

Livestock (1976 census): 11,968,000 cattle, 758,000 buffaloes; 1981 census, 758,000 sheep and goats, and 15,052,000 poultry.

Forests cover 13·4% of the state.

Fisheries. Landings, 1989–90, about 523,000 tonnes. During 1986–87 Rs 78m. was invested in fishery schemes.

INDUSTRY. The total number of registered factories, 1988, was 8,573; average daily employment in public sector industries, 1988, 2·1m. The coalmining industry, 1987, had 115 units with average daily employment of 121,000.

There is a large automobile factory at Uttarpara, and there are aluminium rolling-mills at Belur and Asansol. Durgapur has a large steel plant and other industries under the state sector—a thermal power plant, coke oven plant, fertilizer factory, alloy steel plant and ophthalmic glass plant. There are a locomotive factory and cable factory at Chittaranjan and Rupnarayanpur. A refinery and fertilizer factory are operating at Haldia. Other industries include chemicals, engineering goods, electronics, textiles, automobile tyres, paper, cigarettes, distillery and aluminium foil.

Small industries, including the silk industry, are important; 308,305 units were registered at 31 Dec. 1989, (estimated employment, 1·6m.).

COMMUNICATIONS

Roads. In 1987–88 the length of national highway was 1,631 km. On 31 March 1989 the state had 776,301 motor vehicles.

Railways. The route-km of railways within the state (1988–89) is 3,867 km. The main centres are Howrah, Sealdah, Kharagpur, Asansol and New Jalpaiguri. The Calcutta Metro is under construction.

Aviation. The main airport is Calcutta which has national and international flights. The second airport is at Bagdogra in the extreme north, which has regular scheduled services to Calcutta. Vayudoot domestic airline also operates in the state.

Shipping. Calcutta is the chief port: A barrage has been built at Farakka to control the flow of the Ganges and to provide a rail and road link between North and South Bengal. A second port is being developed at Haldia, halfway between the present port and the sea, which is intended mainly for bulk cargoes. West Bengal possesses 779 km of navigable canals.

JUSTICE, RELIGION, EDUCATION AND WELFARE

Justice. The High Court of Judicature at Calcutta has a Chief Justice and 44 puisne judges. The Andaman and Nicobar Islands *(see below)* come under its jurisdiction.

Police. In 1989 the police force numbered 57,599, under a director-general and an inspector-general. Calcutta has a separate force under a commissioner directly responsible to the Government; its strength was 21,535 at 1 Oct. 1989.

Religion. At the 1981 census Hindus numbered 42,007,159; Moslems, 11,743,259; Christians, 319,670; Buddhists, 156,296; Sikhs, 49,054; Jains, 38,663.

Education. At the 1981 census 22·2m. people were literate. In 1988–89 there were 50,827 primary schools with 9,274,121 students, 4,179 junior high schools with 2,742,767 students and 6,804 high and higher secondary schools with 1,598,616 students. Education is free up to higher secondary stage. There are 8 universities.

The University of Calcutta (founded 1857) is affiliating and teaching; in 1983–84 it had 150,000 students. Visva Bharati, Santiniketan, was established in 1951 and is residential and teaching; it had 3,943 students in 1985–86. The University of Jadavpur, Calcutta (1955), had 6,000 students in 1990–91. Burdwan University was established in 1960; in 1985–86 there were 84,095 students. Kalyani University was established in 1960 (2,306 students in 1985–86). The University of North Bengal (1962) had 22,504 students in 1984–85. Rabindra Bharati University had 4,273 students in 1985–86. Bidhan Chandra Krishi Viswavidyalaya (1974) had 540 students in 1985–86. There is also Vidyasagar University, Medinipur. There are 9 engineering and technology colleges, 10 medical colleges, 43 teacher training colleges, 46 polytechnics and 302 arts, science and commerce colleges.

Health. There were (1988) 410 hospitals, 1,177 clinics, 1,177 health centres and 551 dispensaries.

UNION TERRITORIES

ANDAMAN AND NICOBAR ISLANDS. The Andaman and Nicobar Islands are administered by the President of the Republic of India acting through a Lieut.-Governor. There is a 30-member Pradesh Council, 5 members of which are selected by the Administrator as advisory counsellors. The seat of administration is at Port Blair, which is connected with Calcutta (1,255 km away) and Madras (1,190 km) by steamer service which calls about every 10 days; there are air services from Calcutta and Madras. Roads in the islands, 733 km black-topped and 48 km others. There are 2 districts.

The population (1981 census) was 188,741; Area, 8,249 sq. km; density 23 per sq. km. Port Blair (1981), 49,634.

The climate is tropical, with little variation in temperature. Heavy rain (125" annually) is mainly brought by the south-west monsoon. Humidity is high.

Budget figures for 1989–90 show total revenue receipts of Rs 23·67 lakhs, and total expenditure on revenue account of Rs 142·33 lakhs. Plan outlay, 1990-91, Rs 970m.

In 1988-89 there were 185 primary schools with 37,176 students, 42 middle schools with 17,451 students, 29 high schools with 7,877 students and 31 higher secondary schools with 3,450 students. There is a teachers' training college, a polytechnic and a college. Literacy (1981 census), 51·56%.

Lieut.-Governor: Lieut.-Gen. R. S. Dayal.

The **Andaman Islands** lie in the Bay of Bengal, 193 km from Cape Negrais in Burma, 1,255 from Calcutta and 1,190 from Madras. Five large islands grouped together are called the Great Andamans, and to the south is the island of Little Andaman. There are some 204 islets, the two principal groups being the Ritchie Archipelago and the Labyrinth Islands. The Great Andaman group is about 467 km long and, at the widest, 51 km broad.

The original inhabitants live in the forests by hunting and fishing; they are of a small Negrito type and their civilization is about that of the Stone Age. Their exact numbers are not known, as they avoid all contact with civilization. The total population of the Andaman Islands (including about 430 aboriginals) was 158,287 in 1981. Main aboriginal tribes, Andamanese, Onges, Jarawas and Sentinelese. Under a central government scheme started in 1953, some 4,000 displaced families, mostly from East Pakistan, had been settled in the islands by May 1967.

Japanese forces occupied the Andaman Islands on 23 March 1942. Civil administration of the islands was resumed on 8 Oct. 1945.

From 1857 to March 1942 the islands were used by the Government of India as a penal settlement for life and long-term convicts, but the penal settlement was abolished on re-occupation in Oct. 1945.

The Great Andaman group, densely wooded, contains many valuable trees, both hardwood and softwood. The best known of the hardwoods is the *padauk* or Andaman redwood; *gurjan* is in great demand for the manufacture of plywood. Large quantities of softwood are supplied to match factories. Annually the Forest Department export about 25,000 tons of timber to the mainland. Coconut, coffee and rubber are cultivated. The islands are slowly being made self-sufficient in paddy and rice, and now grow approximately half their annual requirements. Livestock (1982): 27,400 cattle, 9,720 buffaloes, 17,600 goats and 21,220 pigs. Fishing is important. There is a sawmill at Port Blair and a coconut-oil mill. Little Andaman has a palm-oil mill.

The islands possess a number of harbours and safe anchorages, notably Port Blair in the south, Port Cornwallis in the north and Elphinstone and Mayabandar in the middle.

The **Nicobar Islands** are situated to the south of the Andamans, 121 km from Little Andaman. The British were in possession 1869–1947. There are 19 islands, 7 uninhabited; total area, 1,841 sq. km. The islands are usually divided into 3 sub-groups (southern, central and northern), the chief islands in each being respectively, Great Nicobar, Camotra with Nancowrie and Car Nicobar. There is a fine land-locked harbour between the islands of Camotra and Nancowrie, known as Nancowrie Harbour.

The population numbered, in 1981, 30,454, including about 22,200 of Nicobarese and Shompen tribes. The coconut and arecanut are the main items of trade, and coconuts are a major item in the people's diet.

The Nicobar Islands were occupied by the Japanese in July 1942; and Car Nicobar was developed as a big supply base. The Allies reoccupied the islands on 8 Oct. 1945.

CHANDIGARH. On 1 Nov. 1966 the city of Chandigarh and the area surrounding it was constituted a Union Territory. Population (1981), 451,610; density, 3,948 per sq. km.; growth rate, 1971–81, 74·9%. Area, 114 sq. km. It serves as the joint capital of both Punjab (India) and the state of Haryana, and is the seat of a High Court and of a university serving both states. The city will ultimately be the capital of just the Punjab; joint status is to last while a new capital is built for Haryana.

There is some cultivated land and some forest (27·5% of the territory).

Administrator: Gen. O. P. Malhotra.

DADRA AND NAGAR HAVELI. Formerly Portuguese, the territories of Dadra and Nagar Haveli were occupied in July 1954 by nationalists, and a pro-India administration was formed; this body made a request for incorporation into the Union, 1 June 1961. By the 10th amendment to the constitution the territories became a centrally administered Union Territory with effect from 11 Aug. 1961, forming an enclave at the southernmost point of the border between Gujarat and Maharashtra. Area 491 sq. km.; population (1981), 103,676 (males 52,515, females 51,161); density 211 per sq. km; growth rate, 1971–81, 39·78%. There is an Administrator appointed by the Government of India. The day-to-day business is done by various departments, co-ordinated by the Administrator's secretary and headed by a Collector. Headquarters are at Silvassa. The territory and 78·82% of the population is tribal and organized in 72 villages. Languages used are Bhilli, Gujarati, Bhilodi (91·1%), Marathi and Hindi.

Administrator: Bhanu Prakash Singh.
Chief Secretary: R. P. Rai.

Electricity. Electricity is supplied by Gujarat, and all villages have been electrified.

Water. As the result of a joint project with the governments of Gujarat, Goa, Daman and Diu there is a reservoir at Damanganga with irrigation potential of 8,280 ha.

Agriculture. Farming is the chief occupation, and about 25,000 hectares were under crops in 1988–89. Much of the land is terraced and there is a 100% subsidy for soil conservation. The major food crops are rice and ragi; wheat, small millets and pulses are also grown. There is little irrigation (1,280 hectares). There are 9 veterinary centres, a veterinary hospital, an agricultural research centre and breeding centres to improve strains of cattle and poultry. During 1988–89 the Administration distributed 250 tonnes of high yielding paddy seed, and high yielding wheat seed, and 611 tonnes of fertilizer.

Forests. About 20,311 hectares or 41·2% of the total area is forest, mainly of teak, sadad and khair. Timber production provides the largest simple contribution to the territory's revenue. There was (1985) a moratorium on commercial felling, to preserve the environmental function of the forests and ensure local supplies of firewood, timber and fodder.

Industry. There is no heavy industry, and the Territory is a ''No Industry District''. Industrial estates for small and medium units have been set up at Piparia, Masat and Khadoli. There were (1989) 322 small units, and 89 medium scale, employing about 7,000. Concessions (25% subsidy, 15 years' sales tax holiday) are available for small industries.

Communications. There are (1989) 326 km of motorable road. The railway line from Bombay to Ahmedabad runs through Vapi near Silvassa. The nearest airport is Bombay.

Tourism. The territory is a rural area between the industrial centres of Bombay and Surat-.Vapi. The Tourism Department is developing areas of natural beauty to promote acceptable tourism.

Justice. The territory is under the jurisdiction of the Bombay (Maharashtra) High Court. There is a District and Sessions Court and one Junior Division Civil Court at Silvassa.

Education. Literacy was 26·67% of the population at the 1981 census. In 1988–89 there were 150 adult education centres (4,500 students); there were 122 primary schools, 39 middle schools (4,058 students); 3 higher secondary schools and 5 high schools. Total primary enrolment was 15,002; high-school and higher secondary, 1,905.

Health. The territory had (1989) 1 cottage hospital, 5 primary health centres and 4 dispensaries; there is also a mobile dispensary.

DAMAN AND DIU. Daman (Damão) on the Gujarat coast, 100 miles (160 km) north of Bombay, was seized by the Portuguese in 1531 and ceded to them (1539) by the Shar of Gujarat. The island of Diu, captured in 1534, lies off the south-east coast of Kathiawar (Gujarat); there is a small coastal area. Former Portuguese forts on either side of the entrance to the Gulf of Cambay, in Dec. 1961 the territories were occupied by India and incorporated into the Indian Union; they were administered as one unit together with Goa, to which they were attached until 30 May 1987, when Goa was seperated from them and became a state.

Area and Population. Daman, 72 sq. km, population (1981) 48,560; Diu, 40 sq. km, population 30,421. The main language spoken is Gujarati.

The chief towns are Daman (population, 1981, 21,003) and Diu (8,020).

Daman and Diu have been governed as parts of a Union Territory since Dec. 1961, becoming the whole of that Territory on 30 May 1987.

The main activities are tourism, fishing and tapping the toddy palm. In Daman there is rice-growing, some wheat and dairying. Diu has fine tourist beaches, grows coconuts and pearl millet, and processes salt.

Administrator: Bhanu Prakash Singh.

Education. In 1988-89 there were 39 primary schools with 10,345 students, 39 middle schools with 7,695 students, 17 high schools with 4,650 students and 2 higher secondary schools with 819 students. There is a degree college.

DELHI. Delhi became a Union Territory on 1 Nov. 1956.

Area and Population. The territory forms an enclave inside the eastern frontier of Haryana in north India. Delhi has an area of 1,483 sq. km. At the 1981 census its population was 6,220,406 (density per sq. km, 4,194). Estimate, 1 July 1987, 8·04m. Growth rate, 1971–81, 53%. In the rural area of Delhi there are 214 inhabited and 17 deserted villages and 27 census towns. They are distributed in 5 community development blocks.

Government. The Lieut-Governor is the Administrator. Delhi Metropolitan Council stands dissolved with effect from 13 Jan. 1990 and the Chief Executive Councillor and other Executive Councillors ceased to hold their offices. The Territory is covered by 3 local bodies: Delhi Municipal Corporation, New Delhi Municipal Committee and Delhi Cantonment Board.

Lieut.-Governor: Markendaya Singh.

Budget. Revised estimates 1989–90 show total revenue of Rs 11,729m. and expenditure including plan expenditure: Rs 15,123m. of which plan, Rs 6,373m.; power, Rs 1,676m.; transport, Rs 852m.; water and sewerage, Rs 930m.; urban development, Rs 814m.; medical services and public health, Rs 584m. Plan outlay (1991-92) Rs 9,200m.

Agriculture. The contribution to the economy is not significant. In 1988-89 about 77,087 ha were cropped (of which 57,509 are irrigated). Animal husbandry is increasing and mixed farms are common. Chief crops are wheat, jowar, bajra, grain, sugar-cane and vegetables.

Industry. The modern city is the largest commercial centre in northern India and an important industrial centre. Since 1947 a large number of industrial concerns have been established; these include factories for the manufacture of razor blades, sports goods, radios and television and parts, bicycles and parts, plastic and PVC goods including footwear, textiles, chemicals, fertilizers, medicines, hosiery, leather goods, soft drinks, hand tools. There are also metal forging, casting, galvanising, electroplating and printing enterprises. The number of industrial units functioning was about 77,000 in 1988–89; average number of workers employed was 693,000. Production was worth Rs 40,500m. and investment was about Rs 15,000m.

Some traditional handicrafts, for which Delhi was formerly famous, still flourish; among them are ivory carving, miniature painting, gold and silver jewellery and papier mâché work. The handwoven textiles of Delhi are particularly fine; this craft is being successfully revived.

Delhi publishes major daily newspapers, including the *Times of India, Hindustan Times, The Hindu*, *Indian Express*, *National Herald*, *Patriot*, *Economic Times*, *Financial Express* and *Statesman* (all in English); *Nav Bharat Times, Jansatta* and *Hindustan* (in Hindi), and 3 Urdu dailies.

Roads. Five national highways pass through the city. There were (1989) 1,589,795 registered motor vehicles in Delhi. The Transport Corporation had 4,399 buses in daily service in 1989-90.

Railways. Delhi is an important rail junction with three main stations: Delhi, New Delhi, Hazarat Nizamuddin. There is an electric ring railway for commuters.

Aviation. Indira Gandhi International Airport operates international flights; Palam airport operates internal flights.

Religion. At the 1981 census Hindus numbered 5,200,432; Sikhs, 393,921; Moslems, 481,802; Jains, 73,917; Christians, 61,609; Buddhists, 7,117; others, 1,608.

Education. The proportion of literates to the total population was 61·54% at the

1981 census (68·4% of males and 53·07% of females). In 1988-89 there were 1,849 primary schools with 888,417 students, 384 middle schools with 479,095 students, 282 high schools with 226,394 students and 735 higher secondary schools with 129,786 students. There are 2 engineering and technology colleges, 4 medical colleges and 5 polytechnics.

The University of Delhi was founded in 1922; it had 69 constituent colleges and institutions in 1988–89, and a total of 121,445 students in 1987-88. There are also Jawaharlal Nehru University, Indira Gandhi National Open University and the Jamia Millia Islamia University; the Indian Institute of Technology at Haus Khas; the Indian Agricultural Research Institute at Pusa; the All India Institute of Medical Science at Ansari Nagar and the Indian Institute of Public Administration are the other important institutions.

Health. In 1989 there were 79 hospitals including 43 general, 27 special, 5 Ayurvedic, 2 Unani, 2 Homeopathic. There were 609 dispensaries.

LAKSHADWEEP. The territory consists of an archipelago of 36 islands (10 inhabited), about 300 km off the west coast of Kerala. It was constituted a Union Territory in 1956 as the Laccadive, Minicoy and Amindivi Islands, and renamed in Nov. 1973. The total area of the islands is 32 sq. km. The northern portion is called the Amindivis. The remaining islands are called the Laccadives (except Minicoy Island). The inhabited islands are: Androth (the largest), Amini, Agatti, Bitra, Chetlat, Kadmat, Kalpeni, Kavaratti, Kiltan and Minicoy. Androth is 4·8 sq. km, and is nearest to Kerala. An Advisory Committee associated with the Union Home Minister and an Advisory Council to the Administrator assist in the administration of the islands; these are constituted annually. Population (1981 census), 40,249, nearly all Moslems. Density, 1,258 per sq. km.; growth rate, 1971–81, 26·53%. The language is Malayalam, but the language in Minicoy is Mahl. Plan outlay, 1990-91, Rs 211·3m. There were, in 1988-89, 9 high schools (1,181 students) and 9 nursery schools (932 students), 19 junior basic schools (8,418 students), 4 senior basic schools (3,087 students) and 2 junior colleges. There are 2 hospitals and 7 primary health centres. The staple products are copra and fish. There is a tourist resort at Bangarem, an uninhabited island with an extensive lagoon. Headquarters of administration, Kavaratti Island. An airport, with Vayudoot services, opened on Agatti island in April 1988. The islands are also served by ship from the mainland and have helicopter inter-island services.

Administrator: Pradeep Singh.

PONDICHERRY. Formerly the chief French settlement in India, Pondicherry was founded by the French in 1674, taken by the Dutch in 1693 and restored to the French in 1699. The English took it in 1761, restored it in 1765, re-took it in 1778, restored it a second time in 1785, retook it a third time in 1793 and finally restored it to the French in 1814. Administration was transferred to India on 1 Nov. 1954. A Treaty of Cession (together with Karikal, Mahé and Yanam) was signed on 28 May 1956; instruments of ratification were signed on 16 Aug. 1962 from which date (by the 14th amendment to the Indian Constitution) Pondicherry, comprising the 4 territories, became a Union Territory.

Area and Population. The territory is composed of enclaves on the Coromandel Coast of Tamil Nadu and Andhra Pradesh, with Mahé forming an enclave on the coast of Kerala. The total area of Pondicherry is 492 sq. km, divided into 4 Districts. On Tamil Nadu coast: Pondicherry (293 sq. km; population, 1981 census, 444,417), Karikal (160; 120,010). On Kerala coast: Mahé (9; 28,413). On Andhra Pradesh coast: Yanam (30; 11,631). Total population (1981 census), 604,471; density, 1,228 per sq. km.; growth rate, 1971–81, 28·14%. Pondicherry Municipality had (1981) 162,639 inhabitants. The principal languages spoken are Tamil, Telugu, Malayalam, French and English.

Government. By the Government of Union Territories Act 1963 Pondicherry is governed by a Lieut.-Governor, appointed by the President, and a Council of Ministers responsible to a Legislative Assembly. Led by Dravida Munnetra Kazagam (DMK), a DMK-Janata Dal ministry was formed after the election in Feb 1990. Total seats, 30: Congress (I), 11; DMK, 9; Janata Dal, 4; All India Anna DMK, 3; Independents and others, 3.

Presidential rule was imposed in Jan. 1991.

Lieut.-Governor: Swarup Singh.

Planning. Approved outlay for 1989–90 was Rs 630m. Of this, Rs 24m. was for agriculture, Rs 16m. for rural development, Rs 10m. for co-operatives, Rs 128m. for education, Rs 12m. for public works, Rs 85m. for electricity, Rs 12m. for fisheries.

Budget. Budget estimates for 1991–92 show revenue receipts of Rs 2,272.2m. and expenditure of Rs 2,272·2m. Plan outlay, 1991-92, Rs 850m.

Electricity. Power is bought from neighbouring states. All 292 villages have electricity. Consumption, 1988–89, 361 units per head. Peak demand, 88 mw.; total consumption, 360·74m. units.

Agriculture. Nearly 45% of the population is engaged in agriculture and allied pursuits; 90% of the cultivated area is irrigated. The main food crop is rice. Foodgrain production, 65,800 tonnes from 31,315 ha in 1988–89, of which 62,000 tonnes was paddy; cash crops include oilseeds, cotton (7,700 bales of 180 kg) and sugar-cane (325,325 tonnes).

Industry. There are (1989) 13 large and 42 medium-scale industries manufacturing consumer goods such as textiles, sugar, cotton yarn, paper, spirits and beer, potassium chlorate, rice bran oil, vehicle parts and soap. There were also 3,322 small industrial units engaged in varied manufacturing.

Roads. There were (1988-89) 2,371 km of roads of which 1,218 km were surfaced. Motor vehicles (1986) 47,817.

Railways. Pondicherry is connected to Villupuram Junction.

Aviation. The nearest airport is Madras.

Education. There were, in 1988-89, 110 pre-primary schools (7,289 pupils), 351 primary schools (96,883), 101 middle schools (47,186), 72 high schools (19,326) and 24 higher secondary schools (6,024). There were 6 general education colleges; a medical college, a law college, an engineering college and 3 polytechnics.

Health. On 31 March 1988 there were 8 hospitals, 59 health centres and dispensaries and 70 sub-centres. In 1987 family schemes had reduced the birth rate to 22·4 per 1,000 and the infant mortality rate to 35·5 per 1,000 live births.

INDONESIA

Capital: Jakarta
Population: 179·1m. (1989)
GNP per capita: US$430 (1988)

Republik Indonesia

HISTORY. In the 16th century Portuguese traders in quest of spices settled in some of the islands, but were ejected by the British, who in turn were ousted by the Dutch (1595). From 1602 the Netherlands East India Company conquered the Netherlands East Indies, and ruled them until the dissolution of the company in 1798. Thereafter the Netherlands Government ruled the colony from 1816 to 1941, when it was occupied by the Japanese until 1945. An independent republic was proclaimed by Dr Sukarno and Dr Hatta on 17 Aug. 1945.

Complete and unconditional sovereignty was transferred to the Republic of the United States of Indonesia on 27 Dec. 1949, except for the western part of New Guinea, the status of which was to be determined through negotiations between Indonesia and the Netherlands within one year after the transfer of sovereignty. A union was created to regulate the relationship between the two countries. A settlement of the New Guinea (Irian Jaya) question was, however, delayed until 15 Aug. 1962, when, through the good offices of the United Nations, an agreement was concluded for the transfer of the territory to Indonesia on 1 May 1963. In Feb. 1956 Indonesia abrogated the union and in Aug. 1956 repudiated Indonesia's debt to the Netherlands.

During 1950 the federal system which had sprung up in 1946–48 (*see* THE STATESMAN'S YEAR-BOOK, 1950, p. 1233) was abolished, and Indonesia was again made a unitary state. The provisional constitution was passed by the Provisional House of Representatives on 14 and came into force on 17 Aug. 1950. On 5 July 1959 by Presidential decree, the Constitution of 1945 was reinstated and the Constituent Assembly dissolved. For history 1960–66 *see* THE STATESMAN'S YEAR-BOOK, 1982–83, p. 678.

On 11–12 March 1966 the military commanders under the leadership of Lieut.-Gen. Suharto took over the executive power while leaving President Sukarno as the head of State. The Communist Party was at once outlawed and the National Front was dissolved in Oct. 1966. On 22 Feb. 1967 Sukarno handed over all his powers to Gen. Suharto.

AREA AND POPULATION. Indonesia, covering a total land area of 741,098 sq. miles (1,919,443 sq. km), consists of 13,677 islands (6,000 of which are inhabited) extending about 3,200 miles east to west through three time-zones (East, Central and West Indonesian Standard time) and 1,250 miles north to south. The largest islands are Sumatra, Java, Kalimantan (Indonesian Borneo), Sulawesi (Celebes) and Irian Jaya (the western part of New Guinea). Most of the smaller islands except Madura and Bali are grouped together. The two largest groups of islands are Maluku (the Moluccas) and Nusa Tenggara (the Lesser Sundas).

Population at the 1980 census was 147,490,298. For breakdown by province, *see* THE STATESMAN'S YEAR-BOOK, 1990-91, p. 700.

The estimated population in 1989 was 179,136,110, distributed as follows:

Province	*Sq. km*	*Estimate 1989*	*Chief town*	*Census 1980*
Aceh (D.I.)	55,392	3,323,664	Banda Aceh	72,090
Sumatera Utara	70,787	10,330,091	Medan	1,378,955
Sumatera Barat	49,778	3,904,725	Padang	480,922
Riau	94,562	2,882,826	Pakanbaru	186,262
Jambi	44,924	2,022,560	Telanaipura	230,373
Sumatera Selatan	103,688	6,072,526	Palembang	787,187
Bengkulu	21,168	1,114,219	Bengkulu	64,783
Lampung	33,307	7,231,379	Tanjungkarang	284,275
Sumatera	473,606	36,881,990		

Province	*Sq. km*	*Estimate 1989*	*Chief town*	*Census 1980*
Jakarta Raya (D.C.I.)	590	9,104,786	Jakarta	6,503,449
Jawa Barat	46,300	33,769,422	Bandung	1,462,637
Jawa Tengah	34,206	28,644,330	Semarang	1,026,671
Yogyakarta (D.I.)	3,169	3,126,969	Yogyakarta	398,727
Jawa Timur	47,922	32,868,291	Surabaya	2,027,913
Jawa and Madura	132,187	107,513,798		
Kalimantan Barat	146,760	3,148,169	Pontianak	304,778
Kalimantan Tengah	152,600	1,273,948	Palangkaraya	60,447
Kalimantan Selatan	37,660	2,463,782	Banjarmasin	381,286
Kalimantan Timur	202,440	1,791,560	Samarinda	264,718
Kalimantan	539,460	8,677,459		
Sulawesi Utara	19,023	2,472,942	Menado	217,159
Sulawesi Tengah	69,726	1,734,229	Palu	298,584
Sulawesi Selatan	72,781	7,001,751	Ujung Padang	709,038
Sulawesi Tenggara	27,686	1,298,728	Kendari	41,021
Sulawesi	189,216	12,507,650		
Bali	5,561	2,782,038	Denpasar	261,263
Nusa Tenggara Barat	20,177	3,305,006	Mataram	68,964
Nusa Tenggara Timur	47,876	3,383,490	Kupang	403,110
Timor Timur [1]	14,874	714,847	Dili	60,150
Maluku	74,505	1,814,150	Amboina	208,898
Irian Jaya	421,981	1,555,682	Jayapura	149,618
Pulau–Pulau Lain	584,974	13,555,213		

[1] Formerly Portuguese East Timor.

Other major cities (census 1980): Malang, 511,780; Surakarta, 469,888; Bogor, 247,409; Cirebon, 223,776; Kediri, 221,830; Madiun, 150,562; Pematangsiantar, 150,376; Pekalongan, 132,558; Tegal, 131,728; Magelang, 123,484; Jember, 122,712; Sukabumi, 109,994 and Probolinggo, 100,296 (all on Java); Balikpapan (on Kalimantan), 280,875.

Vital statistics, 1988: Birth rate, 28·7 per 1,000; death rate, 7·9.

The principal ethnic groups are the Acehnese, Bataks and Minangkabaus in Sumatra, the Javanese and Sundanese in Java, the Madurese in Madura, the Balinese in Bali, the Sasaks in Lombok, the Menadonese, Minahasans, Torajas and Buginese in Sulawesi, the Dayaks in Kalimantan, Irianese in Irian Jaya, the Ambonese in the Moluccas and Timorese in Timor Timur. There were some 6m. Chinese resident in 1991.

Bahasa Indonesia, a Malay dialect, is the official language of the Republic although Dutch is spoken as an unofficial language.

CLIMATE. Conditions vary greatly over this spread of islands, but generally the climate is tropical monsoon, with a dry season from June to Sept. and a wet one from Oct. to April. Temperatures are high all the year and rainfall varies according to situation on lee or windward shores. Jakarta. Jan. 78°F (25·6°C), July 78°F (25·6°C). Annual rainfall 71" (1,775 mm). Padang. Jan. 79°F (26·7°C), July 79°F (26·7°C). Annual rainfall 177" (4,427 mm). Surabaya. Jan. 79°F (27·2°C), July 78°F (25·6°C). Annual rainfall 51" (1,285 mm).

CONSTITUTION AND GOVERNMENT. Indonesia is a sovereign, independent republic.

The People's Consultative Assembly is the supreme power. It has 1,000 members and it sits at least once every 5 years. The House of People's Representatives has 500 members, 400 of them elected, 100 as representatives from various groupings, and sits for a 5-year term.

General elections to the 400 elected seats in the House of Representatives were held on 23 April 1987 and 299 seats were won by the Golkar Party.

The Cabinet was as follows in Nov. 1990:

President, Prime Minister and Minister of Defence: Gen. Suharto, elected by the People's Consultative Assembly in 1968 and re-elected in 1973, 1978, 1983 and 1988.

Vice-President: Sudharmono. *Internal Affairs:* Rudini. *Foreign Affairs:* Ali Alatas. *Defence and Security:* L. B. Murdani. *Justice:* Ismail Saleh. *Information:* Harmoko. *Finance:* Dr J. B. Sumarlin. *Trade:* Dr Arifin Siregar. *Industry:* Hartarto. *Agriculture:* Wardoyo. *Mines and Energy:* Dr Ginandjar Kartasasmita. *Public Works:* Radinal Mochtar. *Communications:* Azwar Anas. *Co-operatives:* Bustanil Arifin. *Manpower:* Cosmas Batubara. *Transmigration:* Sugiarto. *Tourism, Post and Telecommunications:* Susilo Sudarman. *Education and Culture:* Dr Fuad Hassan. *Health:* Dr Adhyatma. *Religious Affairs:* H. Munawir Sjadzali. *Social Affairs:* Dr Haryati Soebadio. *Forestry:* Hasrul Harahap. *Co-ordinator Minister of Political and Security Affairs:* Sudomo. *Co-ordinator Minister of Economic, Financial and Industrial Affairs and Development Supervision:* Radius Prawiro. *Co-ordinator Minister of People's Welfare:* Supardjo Rustam. *State Minister and Secretary of State:* Moerdiono. *State Minister of National Development Planning and Chairman of the National Development Planning Board:* Dr Saleh Afiff. *State Minister of Population Affairs and Environment:* Dr Emil Salim. *State Minister of Housing Affairs:* Siswono Yudohusodo. *State Minister of Youth Affairs and Sports:* Akbar Tandjung. *State Minister of Research and Technology and Chairman of the Agency for the Assessment and Application of Technology:* Dr B. J. Habibe. *State Minister of Administrative Reform:* Sarwono Kusumaatmadja. *State Minister of Women's Affairs:* Sulasikin Murpratomo. *Commander-in-Chief of the Armed Forces:* Gen. Try Sutrisno. *Attorney-General:* Sukarton Marmosudjono. *Governor of Central Bank:* Dr Adrianus Moy.

There are 6 junior ministers.

National flag: Horizontally red over white.

National anthem: Indonesia Raya ('Indonesia the Great'; tune by Wage Rudolf Supratman, 1928).

Local government: There are 27 provinces, 3 of which are special territories (the capital city of Jakarta, Yogyakarta and Aceh), each administered by a Governor appointed by the President; they are divided into 246 districts (*kabupatens*), each under a district head (*bupati*), and 55 municipalities (*kotamadya*), each under a mayor (*wali kota*). The districts are divided into 3,592 sub-districts (*kecamtans*), each headed by a *camat*. There are 66,594 villages (1988).

DEFENCE. The Indonesian Armed Forces were formally set up on 5 Oct. 1945. On 11 Oct. 1967 the Army, Navy, Air Force and Police were integrated under the Department of Defence and Security. Their commanders no longer hold cabinet rank. There is selective military service.

Army. There are 2 infantry divisions and another forming: 1 armoured cavalry brigade, 3 infantry brigades, 3 airborne infantry brigades, 3 artillery regiments, 1 air defence regiment, 2 engineer battalions and 4 special warfare groups. There are 63 independent infantry battalions, 17 independent artillery battalions and 8 independent cavalry battalions. Equipment includes 100 AMX-13 and 41 PT-76 light tanks. The Army has over 80 aircraft, including 1 Islander, 2 C-47s and 25 other fixed-wing types, 16 Bell 205, 13 BO 105, 20 Hughes 300, 28 helicopters and locally-built Bell 412 helicopters. Total strength in 1991 was 215,000.

Navy. The Indonesian navy in 1990 numbered 43,000, including 12,000 in the Commando Corps, and 1,000 in the Naval Air Arm. Combatant strength includes 2 German-built diesel submarines and 15 frigates of which 6 are former Dutch Van Speijk class, and 3 former British Ashanti class. There are also 4 fast missile craft, 2 torpedo-armed craft and 21 miscellaneous patrol craft as well as 2 Dutch-built tripartite coastal minehunters. Amphibious lift is provided by 15 tank landing ships

(4 with helicopter facilities) and 64 craft. The auxiliary force includes 1 tanker, 8 surveying vessels, 2 command and submarine support ships, 1 repair ship, 3 training ships and some dozens of minor auxiliaries and service craft.

The Naval Air Arm operates 60 aircraft, including 18 Searchmaster maritime reconnaissance, and 12 anti-submarine helicopters plus miscellaneous communications and utility aircraft.

A separate Military Sealift Command operates about 15 inter-island transport ships (which number includes 3 of the tank landing ships in the navy listing) totalling approximately 30,000 tonnes. The Maritime Security Agency operates 10 cutters, the Customs about 70 and the armed Marine Police 60 craft.

Air Force. Operational combat units comprise two squadrons of A-4E Skyhawk attack aircraft, and single squadrons of F-5E Tiger II and of F-16 fighters and OV-10F Bronco twin-turboprop counter-insurgency aircraft. There are 3 transport squadrons, equipped with turboprop C-130 Hercules, Nurtanio/CASA NC-212 Aviocar and F27 Friendship aircraft, and piston-engined C-47s, plus 3 specially-equipped Boeing 737 dual-purpose maritime surveillance/transports; and an assortment of other aircraft in transport, helicopter and training units including 16 Hawk attack/trainers, 25 T-34C-1 armed turboprop trainers, and 40 Swiss-built AS 202 Bravo piston-engined primary trainers. On order are 32 CN-235 twin-turboprop transports and Bell 412 helicopters, from IPTN of Indonesia. Personnel (1991) approximately 25,000.

INTERNATIONAL RELATIONS

Membership. Indonesia is a member of the UN, OPEC and ASEAN.

ECONOMY

Policy. The fifth Five-Year Development Plan (1990-94) constitutes the final 5 years of the Government's first 25-Year Long Term Development Plan. It places emphasis on the structural diversification of the economy to reduce dependence on crude oil and, in particular, it places importance on the development of export-oriented and labour-intensive industries in the agricultural and manufacturing sectors.

Budget. The budget (in Rp.) in 1989–90, envisaged expenditure of 36,574,900m. (development 11,325,100m.) and expenditure revenue of 25,249,800m.

Currency. The monetary unit is the *rupiah* (IDR) of 100 *sen*. There are banknotes of 1, 2·5, 5, 10, 25, 50, 100, 500, 1,000, 5,000 and 10,000 rupiahs and aluminium coins of 1, 5, 10, 25 and cupro-nickel coins of 50 sen.

In March 1991 there were 3,657 rupiahs = £1 sterling; 1,928 rupiahs = US$1.

Banking and Finance. The Bank Indonesia, successor to De Javasche Bank established by the Dutch in 1828, was made the central bank of Indonesia on 1 July 1953. It had an original capital of Rp. 25m.; a reserve fund of Rp. 18m. and a special reserve of Rp. 84m. Total assets and liabilities at 31 March 1988, Rp. 36,252,000m.

There are 117 commercial banks, 28 development banks and other financial institutions, 8 development finance companies and 9 joint venture merchant banks. Commercial banking is dominated by 5 state-owned banks: Bank Rakyat Indonesia provides services to smallholder agriculture and rural development; Bank Bumi Daya, estate agriculture and forestry; Bank Negara Indonesia 1946, industry; Bank Dagang Negara, mining; and Bank Expor-Impor Indonesia, export commodity sector. All state banks are authorized to deal in foreign exchange.

There are 70 private commercial banks owned and operated by Indonesians. The 11 foreign banks, which specialize in foreign exchange transactions and direct lending operations to foreign joint ventures, include the Chartered Bank, the Hongkong and Shanghai Banking Corporation, the Bank of America, the City Bank, the Bank of Tokyo, Chase Manhattan and the American Express International Banking Corporation. The government owns one Savings Bank, Bank Tabungan Negara, and

1,000 Post Office Savings Banks. There are also over 3,500 rural and village savings bank and credit co-operatives.

The state-run stock exchange in Jakarta was scheduled for privatization in 1991.

Weights and Measures. The metric system is is use.

The following are the old weights and measures: *Pikol* = 136·16 lb. avoirdupois; *Katti* = 1·36 lb. avoirdupois; *Bau* = 1·7536 acres; *Square Pal* = 227 hectares = 561·16 acres; *Jengkal* = 4 yd; *Pal* (Java) = 1,506 metres; *Pal* (Sumatra) = 1,852 metres.

ENERGY AND NATURAL RESOURCES

Electricity. There were 7 hydro-electric plants in 1989; 19,044 out of 66,594 villages are supplied with electricity in Java and Sumatra. Electricity produced (1986) 30,000m. kwh. Supply 127 and 220 volts; 50 Hz.

Oil. Indonesia is the principal producer of petroleum in the Far East, production coming from Sumatra, Kalimantan (Indonesian Borneo) and Java. Proven reserves (1986) 8,500m. bbls. The 1989 output of crude oil was 66m. tonnes.

Gas. Pertamina, the state oil company, started to pump natural gas to Jakarta in 1979. Production (1988–89) 1,787,000m. cu. ft.

Water. In 1988–89, 23,677 ha of new irrigation networks were constructed and 377,461 ha rehabilitated and maintained.

Minerals. The high cost of extraction means that little of the large mineral resources outside Java is exploited; however, there is copper mining in Irian Jaya, nickel mining and processing on Sulawesi, aluminium smelting in northern Sumatra. Coal production (1988–89) 7,792,700 tonnes; bauxite (1988–89), 514,100 tonnes. Output (in 1,000 tonnes, 1988–89) of iron ore was 210·5; copper, 302·7; silver (1987–88), 5,178·6 kg; gold, 5,050 kg; nickel ore, 1,881·6. In 1988–89 tin production was 28,900 tonnes.

Agriculture. Production (1988, in 1,000 tonnes): Rice, 41,769; cassava, 15,166; maize, 6,229; sweet potatoes, 2,166; sugar-cane, 20,800; coconuts and copra, 12,750; palm oil, 1,370; soybeans, 1,260; rubber, 1,094; coffee, 358; groundnuts, 585; vegetables, 3,180; fruits, 5,598; tea, 144; tobacco, 147.

Livestock (1988): Cattle, 6·5m.; buffaloes, 3m.; horses, 722,000; sheep, 5·4m.; goats, 12·7m.; pigs, 6·5m.; poultry, 439m.

Forestry. The forest area was (1988) 122m. ha, 67% of the land area. Production (1988–89), provisional: Sawn timber, 4·3m. cu. metres; plywood, 7·5m. cu. metres. Exports (1988–89, provisional) of sawn timber, 2,874,000 cu. metres; plywood, 6·86m. cu. metres.

Fisheries. In 1988 the catch of sea fish was 2,166,000 tonnes; inland fish was 715,000 tonnes. In 1988 there were 117,526 motorized and 222,233 other fishing vessels. Exports (1988, provisional) included 56,552 tonnes of shrimps, 59,049 tonnes of fresh fish and 955 tonnes of ornamental fish.

INDUSTRY. There are shipyards at Jakarta Raya, Surabaya, Semarang and Amboina. There were (1985) more than 2,000 textile factories (total production in 1987–88, 2,925·6m. metres), large paper factories (817,200 tonnes, 1986–87), match factories, automobile and bicycle assembly works, large construction works, tyre factories, glass factories, a caustic soda and other chemical factories. Production (1987–88): Cement, 22,419,000 tonnes; fertilizers, 5,811,000 tonnes; 160,372 motor vehicles and 249,573 motorcycles; 2·36m. boxes of matches; glasses and bottles, 126,060 tonnes; steel ingots, 1,337,000 tonnes; 640 TV sets and 159,020 refrigerators.

Labour. In 1985 there were 62,457,138 people employed: 34,141,809 in agriculture; 9,345,210 in commerce; 8,317,285 in public services; 5,795,919 in industry; 2,095,577 in construction; 1,958,333 in transport and communications; 415,512 in mining and quarrying; 250,481 in finance and insurance; 69,715 in electricity, gas and water.

Trade Unions. Workers have a constitutional right to organize. Unions are expected to affiliate to the All Indonesia Labour Federation (FBSI) which enjoys government approval, but in Nov. 1990 an independent union, Setia Kawan (Solidarity) was set up. About 40% of the labour force belong to unions. Strikes are forbidden by law.

FOREIGN ECONOMIC RELATIONS

Commerce. Imports and exports (including oil and gas) in US$1m. for year ending March:

	1985–86	*1986–87*	*1987–88*	*1988–89*
Imports f.o.b.	12,522	11,451	12,952	14,311
Exports f.o.b.	18,612	13,697	18,343	19,824

The main export items (in US$1m.) in 1987 were: Gas and oil, 8,556; forestry products, 2,504; manufactured goods, 1,262; rubber, 961; coffee, 535; fishery products, 430; copper, 159; tin, 155; pepper, 148; palm products, 144; tea, 119. Exports went mainly to Japan (43·1%), USA (19·5%), Singapore (8·4%), Netherlands (2·9%), Federal Republic of Germany (2·1%) and Australia (2·1%).

The main import items are non-crude oil, rice, consumer goods, fertilizer, chemicals, weaving yarn, iron and steel, industrial and business machinery. In 1987 imports came mainly from Japan (28·7%), USA (11·3%), Singapore (8·7%), Federal Republic of Germany (6·7%), Australia (4·4%), Taiwan (3·7%), China (3·3%) and France (3·1%).

Total trade between Indonesia and UK (British Department of Trade returns, in £1,000 sterling):

	1986	*1987*	*1988*	*1989*	*1990*
Imports to UK	141,242	144,819	233,807	273,102	327,877
Exports and re-exports from UK	196,629	236,027	203,275	184,032	194,274

Tourism. In 1988 1,301,249 tourists visited Indonesia.

COMMUNICATIONS

Roads. The total length of the artery and connecting road network in 1988-89 was 44,552 km, of which 27,480 km were in good condition. Motor vehicles, at 31 Dec. 1989, totalled 9,674,246.

Railways. In 1987 the State Railways totalled 6,458 km of 1,067 mm gauge, comprising 4,967 km on Java (of which 125 km electrified) and 1,491 km on Sumatra. In 1989–90 they carried 55·3m. passengers and 12·2m. tonnes of freight. In addition some narrow gauge lines are still operated.

Aviation. In 1988-89 there were 797 aircraft in operation with 175 scheduled and 622 non-scheduled flights. The total number of passengers carried was 6,679,438, total freight 76,486 tonnes. Domestic airlines are operated by Garuda Indonesia, Merpati Nusantara, Mandala and Bouraq Indonesia Airlines.

Shipping. There are 16 ports for oceangoing ships, the largest of which is Tanjung Priok, which serves the Jakarta area and has a container terminal. The national shipping company Pelajaran Nasional Indonesia (PELNI) maintains interinsular communications. The Jakarta Lloyd maintains regular services between Jakarta, Amsterdam, Hamburg and London. In 1988–89, 35 ocean-going ships with a capacity of 446,980 DWT carried 17,887,500 tonnes of freight.

Telecommunications. In 1979 the postal and telegraph services of Indonesia included 2,796 post offices. There were 660 telegraph offices which handled 3·9m. domestic and 488,000 international cables. Post offices handled 396·63m. letters, Rp. 388,700m. in money orders and 4,550,000m. in postal cheques in 1987–88. Deposits with post office savings accounts, Rp. 31,210m. Number of telephones (1988), 999,321.

Radio Republik Indonesia, under the Department of Information, operates 49 stations. In 1988–89 there were 8,948,195 TV receivers, and 54,318 public TV sets had been placed in villages within reach of the state-owned Televisi Republik Indonesia telecast.

Newspapers (1986–87). There were about 252 newspaper publishers with estimated circulation (1988-89) of 10,783,009, of which 3,716,056 daily newspapers. There were 270 publishers of weekly papers and magazines with a circulation (1988–89) of 3,444,802 and 1,721,130 respectively.

JUSTICE, RELIGION, EDUCATION AND WELFARE

Justice. There are courts of first instance, high courts of appeal in every provincial capital and a Supreme Court of Justice for the whole of Indonesia in Jakarta. Administrative matters on judicial organization are under the direction of the Department of Justice.

In civil law the population is divided into three main groups: Indonesians, Europeans and foreign Orientals, to whom different law systems are applicable. When, however, people from different groups are involved, a system of so-called 'intergentile' law is applied.

The present criminal law, which has been in force since 1918, is codified and is based on European penal law. This law is equally applicable to all groups of the population. For private and commercial law, however, there are various systems applicable for the various groups of the population. For the Indonesians, a system of private and agrarian law is applicable; this is called Adat Law, and is mainly uncodified. For the other groups the prevailing private and commercial law system is codified in the Private Law Act (1847) and the Commercial Law Act (1847). These Acts have their origins in the French *Code Civile* and *Code du Commerce* through the similar Dutch codifications. These Acts are entirely applicable to Indonesian citizens and to Europeans, whereas to foreign Orientals they are applicable with some exceptions, mainly in the fields of family law and inheritance. Penal law was in the process of being codified in 1981.

Religion. Religious liberty is granted to all denominations. About 87% of the Indonesians were Moslems in 1988 and 9% Christians. There are also about 1·6m. Buddhists, probably for the greater part Chinese. Hinduism has 3·5m. members, of whom 2·5m. are on Bali.

Education. In 1987–88 there were 30,960,000 pupils in primary schools and, in 1988–89, 6,679,700 students in junior high schools and 4,146,900 students in senior high schools, vocational schools, higher training and sports teachers' training colleges.

English is the first foreign language taught in schools. Literacy rate was 72% in 1984.

Total number of students in higher education (1988–89) 1,663,900. In 1987–88 there were 49 state and 637 private universities and technical institutes.

Health. In 1988 there were 23,084 doctors, 64,087 nurses, 5,472 public health centres, 12,562 sub-public health centres and 3,521 mobile units.

DIPLOMATIC REPRESENTATIVES

Of Indonesia in Great Britain (38 Grosvenor Sq., London W1X 9AD)
Ambassador: T.M Hadi Thayeb.

Of Great Britain in Indonesia (Jalan M.H. Thamrin 75, Jakarta 10310)
Ambassador: R. J. Carrick, CMG, LVO.

Of Indonesia in the USA (2020 Massachusetts Ave., NW, Washington, D.C., 20036)
Ambassador: A. R. Ramly.

Of the USA in Indonesia (Medan Merdeka Selatan 5, Jakarta)
Ambassador: John C. Monjo.

Of Indonesia to the United Nations
Ambassador: Nana Sutresna.

Further Reading

Indonesia 1989. Department of Information, Jakarta, 1989
Bee, O. J., *The Petroleum Resources of Indonesia*. OUP, 1982
Bemmelen, R. W. van, *Geology of Indonesia*. 2 vols. The Hague, 1949
Echols, J. M. and Shadily, H., *An Indonesian–English Dictionary*. 3rd ed. Cornell Univ. Press, 1989
International Commission of Jurists, *Indonesia and the Rule of Law*. London, 1987
Leifer, M., *Indonesia's Foreign Policy*. London, 1983
McDonald, H., *Suharto's Indonesia*. Univ. Press of Hawaii, 1981
Palmier, L., *Understanding Indonesia*. London, 1986
Papenek, G., *The Indonesian Economy*. Eastbourne, 1980
Polomka, P., *Indonesia Since Sukarno*. London, 1971
Robison, R., *Indonesia: The Rise of Capital*. Sydney, 1986
Thoolen, H., *Indonesia and the Rule of Law*. London, 1987

IRAN

Capital: Tehran
Population: 53·92m. (1988)
GNP per capita: US$1,690 (1986)

Jomhori-e-Islami-e-Irân

(Islamic Republic of Iran)

HISTORY. Persia was ruled by the Shahs as an absolute monarchy until 30 Dec. 1906 when the first Constitution was granted. Reza Khan took control after a coup on 31 Oct. 1925 deposed the last Shah of the Qajar Dynasty, and became Reza Shah Pahlavi on 12 Dec. 1925. The country's name was changed to Iran on 21 March 1935. Reza Shah abdicated on 16 Sept. 1941 in favour of his son, Mohammad Reza Pahlavi.

Following widespread civil unrest, the Shah left Iran on 17 Jan. 1979. The Ayatollah Ruhollah Khomeini, spiritual leader of the Shi'a Moslem community, returned from 15 years' exile on 1 Feb. 1979 and appointed a provisional government on 5 Feb. An Islamic Republic was proclaimed on 1 Apr. 1979.

In Sept. 1980 war began with Iraq with destruction of some Iranian towns and damage to the oil installations at Abadan. A UN-arranged ceasefire took place on 20 Aug. 1988 and UN-sponsored peace talks continued in 1989. On 15 Aug. 1990 the Iraqi President Saddam Hussein offered peace terms and began the withdrawal of Iraqi forces. Iran and Iraq exchanged prisoners of war in the last quarter of 1990.

AREA AND POPULATION. Iran is bounded north by the USSR and the Caspian Sea, east by Afghanistan and Pakistan, south by the Gulf of Oman and the Persian Gulf, and west by Iraq and Turkey. It has an area of 1,648,000 sq. km (634,724 sq. miles), but a vast portion is desert, and the average density is only (1987) 31 inhabitants to the sq. km. Refugees in Iran (Jan. 1988) 2·6m. (of which 2·2m. Afghans).

The population at recent censuses was as follows: (1956) 18,944,821; (1966) 25,781,090; (1976) 33,708,744; (1986) 49,445,010. Population estimate in 1988 (tentative because of unquantified losses in the war with Iraq): 53·92m.

The areas, populations and capitals of the 24 provinces *(ostan)* were:

Province	*Area (sq. km)*	*Census 1976*	*Census 1986*	*Capital*
Azarbaijan, East	67,102	3,197,685	4,114,084	Tabriz
Azarbaijan, West	38,850	1,407,604	1,971,677	Orumiyeh [2]
Bakhtaran [1]	23,667	1,030,714	1,462,965	Bakhtaran [3]
Boyer ahmadi and Kohkiluyeh	14,261	244,370	411,828	Yasuj
Bushehr	27,653	347,863	612,183	Bushehr
Chahar Mahal and Bakhtiari	14,870	394,357	631,179	Shahr-e-Kord
Esfahan	104,650	2,176,694	3,294,916	Esfahan
Fars	133,298	2,035,582	3,193,769	Shiraz
Gilan	14,709	1,581,872	2,081,037	Rasht
Hamadan	19,784	1,088,024	1,505,826	Hamadan
Hormozgan	66,870	462,440	762,206	Bandar-e-Abbas
Ilam	19,044	246,024	382,091	Ilam
Kerman	179,916	1,091,148	1,622,958	Kerman
Khorasan	313,337	3,264,398	5,280,605	Mashhad
Khuzestan	67,282	2,187,118	2,681,978	Ahvaz
Kordestan	24,998	782,440	1,078,415	Sanandaj
Lorestan	28,803	933,939	1,367,029	Khorramabad
Markazi	29,080	796,754	1,082,109	Arak
Mazandaran	46,456	2,387,171	3,419,346	Sari
Semnan	90,905	289,463	417,035	Semnan
Sistan and Baluchestan	181,578	664,292	1,197,059	Zahedan
Tehran (formed from Markazi)	29,993	5,624,784	8,712,087	Tehran
Yazd	70,011	356,849	574,028	Yazd
Zanjan	36,398	1,117,157	1,588,600	Zanjan

[1] Formerly Kermanshahan. [2] Formerly Rezayeh. [3] Formerly Kermanshah.

The principal cities were:

	Census 1976	Census 1986		Census 1976	Census 1986
Tehran	4,530,223	6,042,584	Ardabil	147,865	281,973
Esfahan	661,510	986,753	Khorramshahr	140,490	...
Mashhad	667,770	1,463,508	Kerman	140,761	257,284
Tabriz	597,976	971,482	Karaj	137,926	275,100
Shiraz	425,813	848,289	Qazvin	139,258	248,591
Ahvaz	334,399	579,826	Yazd	135,925	230,483
Abadan	294,068	...	Arak	116,832	265,349
Bakhtaran	290,600	560,514	Desful	121,251	151,420
Qom	247,219	543,139	Khorramabad	104,912	208,592
Rasht	188,957	290,897	Borujerd	101,345	183,879
Orumiyeh	164,419	300,746	Zanjan	100,351	215,261
Hamadan	165,785	272,499			

The national language is Farsi or Persian, spoken by 45% of the population. 23% spoke related languages, including Kurdish and Luri in the west and Baluchi in the south-east, while 26% spoke Turkic languages, primarily the Azerbaijani-speaking peoples of the north-west and the Turkomen of Khorasan in the north-east.

CLIMATE. Mainly a desert climate, but with more temperate conditions on the shores of the Caspian Sea. Seasonal range of temperature is considerable. Abadan. Jan. 54°F (12·2°C), July 97°F (36·1°C). Annual rainfall 8" (204 mm). Tehran. Jan. 36°F (2·2°C), July 85°F (29·4°C). Annual rainfall 10" (246 mm).

CONSTITUTION AND GOVERNMENT. The Constitution of the Islamic Republic was approved by a national referendum in Dec. 1979. It gives supreme authority to the *Spiritual Leader* (*wali faqih*), which position was held by Ayatollah Khomeini until his death on 3 June 1989. Seyed Ali Khamenei was elected to succeed him on 4 June 1989.

The 83-member *Assembly of Experts* was established in 1982. it is popularly elected every 8 years. Its mandate is to interpret the constitution and select the Spiritual Leader. Candidates for election are examined by the Council of Guardians. At the elections of Oct. 1990 turn-out was 46%.

The *President* of the Republic is popularly-elected for a 4-year term and is head of the executive; he appoints a Prime Minister and other Ministers, subject to approval by the *Majlis*.

Presidents since the establishment of the Islamic Republic:

Abolhassan Bani-Sadr. 4 Feb. 1980–22 June 1981 (deposed).

Mohammad Ali Raja'i, 24 July 1981–30 Aug. 1981 (assassinated).

Sayed Ali Khamenei, 12 Oct. 1981-4 June 1989.

The Cabinet was composed as follows in 1990:

President: Hojatolislam Ali Akbar Hashemi Rafsanjani (sworn in on 3 Aug. 1989).

Vice President: Hassan Habibi.

Foreign Affairs: Ali Akbar Vellayati. *Oil:* Gholamreza Aghazadeh. *Interior:* Abdollah Nouri. *Economic Affairs and Finance:* Mohsen Nourbakhsh. *Agriculture and Rural Affairs:* Isa Kalantari. *Commerce:* Abdol-Hossein Vahaji. *Energy:* Namdar Zanganeh. *Roads and Transport:* Mohammed Saeedi Kya. *Construction Jihad:* Gholamreza Foruzesh. *Heavy Industries:* Mohammad Hadi Nezhad-Hosseinian. *Industry:* Mohammad Reza Nematzadeh. *Housing and Urban Development:* Sarajuddin Kazeruni. *Labour and Social Affairs:* Hossein Kamali. *Posts, Telephones and Telegraphs:* Mohammed Gharazi. *Health, Treatment and Medical Education:* Iraj Fazel. *Education and Training:* Mohammad Ali Najafi. *Higher Education and Culture:* Mostafa Moin. *Justice:* Hojatolislam Ismail Shostari. *Defence and Armed Forces Logistics:* Akbar Torkan. *Intelligence and Security:* Hojatolislam Ali Fallahiyan. *Culture and Islamic Guidance:* Seyyed Mohammad Khatami. *Mines and Metals:* Mohammad Hossein Mahloji.

Legislative power is held by the 270-member *(Majlis)* Islamic Consultative Assembly, directly elected on a non-party basis for a 4-year term in May-April 1988. The *Speaker* is Hojatoleslam Karrubi. All legislation is subject to approval by a 12-member *Council of Guardians* who ensure it is in accordance with the Islamic code and with the Constitution. Six members are appointed by the *Spiritual Leader* and six by the judiciary.

National flag: Three horizontal stripes of green, white and red; on the borders of the green and red stripes the legend *Allah Akbar* in white Kufi script repeated 22 times in all; in the centre of the white stripe the national emblem in red.

Local Government. The country is divided into 24 provinces *(ostan)*, these are sub-divided into 195 *shahrestan* (counties), each under a *farmandar* (governor) and thence into 500 *bakhsh* (districts), each under a *bakhshdar*. The districts are sub-divided into *dehistan* (groups of villages) each under a *dehdar*, each village having its elected *kadkhoda* (headman).

DEFENCE. Two years' military service is compulsory.

Army. The Army consisted (1991) of 305,000 men (about 250,000 conscripts), with some 350,000 reservists. It is organized in 4 mechanized, 1 special force, 6 infantry and 1 airborne divisions, and auxiliary units. Equipment includes T-54/-55/-62, T-72, Chieftain, M-47/-48 and M-60A1 main battle tanks. There is also a 300,000-strong Revolutionary Guard Corps. The Army operates 40 Cessna and some 500 helicopters but the full strength is not known.

Navy. The Navy is slowly recovering from the effects of the war with Iraq, but remains weakened by shortages of spares and technical support. The combatant fleet is currently believed to comprise 1 ex-British 'Battle' class and 2 ex-US Sumner class destroyers, 3 UK-built frigates, 2 old ex-US patrol frigates and about 10 missile craft (for which there may be no missiles). Other units include 19 inshore patrol craft (some of them hovercraft), 3 small minesweepers and a substantial amphibious force of 7 tank landing ships and 4 tank landing craft. Auxiliaries include 3 tankers, 1 repair ship, 2 water tankers and 2 accommodation ships.

Naval Aviation comprises 1 anti-submarine helicopter squadron with perhaps 9 Sea King and AB-212 helicopters, a mine counter-measures squadron with 2 RH-53D helicopters and a transport squadron with about a dozen various aircraft. Main naval bases are at Bandar-e-Abbas, Bushehr and Chah Bahar.

The naval forces of the Revolutionary Guard were organizationally separate, but some integration may have followed the appointment in Nov. 1989 of a former Revolutionary Guard leader as Commander of the Navy. Integrated operations are now exercised. The Revolutionary Guard operate some 40-60 fast boats armed with portable weapons, exercise control of the offshore oil rigs used as bases, and control coastal artillery and missile batteries.

Air Force. In Aug. 1955 the Air Force became a separate and independent arm, and had a strength of about 23 first-line squadrons (each 15 aircraft, plus reserves), with 100,000 personnel before the 1979 revolution. Strength (1991) was estimated at 35,000 personnel and 185 serviceable combat aircraft. The latter include some MiG-19/Chinese-built F-6 fighter-bombers, supplied via North Korea, and surviving US fighters that include F-14 Tomcat, F-5E Tiger II and F-4D/E Phantom II fighter-bombers, plus a few RF-4E reconnaissance-fighters. Transport aircraft include F27s, C-130 Hercules, PC-6 Turbo-Porters, Boeing 707s and 747s, some equipped as flight refuelling tankers. The status of the large fleet of CH-47C Chinook, Bell Model 214 and other helicopters is not known; but two P-3F Orion maritime patrol aircraft remain operational. Training aircraft include Bonanza basic trainers and 35 turboprop PC-7 Turbo-Trainers.

INTERNATIONAL RELATIONS

Membership. Iran is a member of the UN, OPEC and the Colombo Plan.

ECONOMY

Budget. The budget for 1988–89 balanced at 9·8m. *rials*.

Currency. The unit of currency is the *rial* (IRR) of 100 *dinars*.

Notes in circulation are of denominations of 100, 200, 500, 1,000, 2,000, 5,000 and 10,000 *rials*. Coins in circulation are bronze–aluminium and copper, 50 *dinar*; silver alloy, 1, 2, 5, 10, 20 and 50 *rials*. In March 1991, US$1 = 65·47 *rials*; £1 = 124·20 *rials*.

Banking and Finance. The *Bank Markazi Iran* was established in 1960 as the note-issuing authority and government bank. All other banks and insurance companies were nationalized in June 1979, and re-organized into 8 new state banking corporations. The 'Law for Usury-Free Banking' was given final approval in Aug.-Sept. 1983. From 21 March 1985 interest on accounts was abolished.

Weights and Measures. The metric system is in force.

The Iranian year is a solar year running from 21 March to 20 March; the Hejira year 1362 corresponds to the Christian year 21 March 1984–20 March 1985.

ENERGY AND NATURAL RESOURCES

Electricity. Capacity of generators installed at institutions affiliated to Ministry of Energy, 1985, was 12,369,000 kw., and 36,720m. kwh. was generated. Supply 220 volts; 50 Hz.

Oil. For a history of Iran's oil industry 1951–79, *see* THE STATESMAN'S YEAR-BOOK, 1982–83.

The petroleum industry was seriously disrupted by the 1979 revolution, and many facilities, including the vast refinery at Abadan, the new refinery at Bandar Khomeini and the tanker terminal at Kharg Island, have been destroyed or put out of action during the Gulf war with Iraq. All operating companies were nationalized in 1979 and operations are now run by the National Petrochemical Company.

Crude oil production, 145m. tonnes, 1989.

Gas. Natural gas production (1985) was 30,900m. cu. metres.

Minerals. Iran has substantial mineral deposits relatively underdeveloped. Production figures for 1985 (in 1,000 tonnes): Iron ore, 2,099; coal, 674; zinc and lead, 56; manganese, 46; chromite, 56; salt, 618.

Agriculture. In 1982, cultivatable land totalled 14,867,000 ha, of which 5,664,000 were irrigated and 4,929,000 ha fallow land. Forests totalled 12·7m. ha and pastures 90m.

Crop production for 1988 (in 1,000 tonnes): Wheat, 8,200; barley, 2,500; rice, 1,757; sugar-beet, 3,500; sugar-cane, 2,035; tobacco, 22.

Wool comes principally from Khorasan, Bakhtaran, Mazandaran and Azarbaijan. Production, 1988, 16,000 tonnes greasy, 8,800 tonnes scoured.

Rice is grown largely on the Caspian shores.

Cigarette tobacco is grown mainly in Hormozgan, Bushehr and West Azarbaijan *ostans*. It is purchased by the Tobacco Monopoly and manufactured in the government factory at Tehran.

Opium, until 1955, was an important export commodity in Iran. On 7 Oct. 1955 an Act was approved by Parliament to prohibit the cultivation and usage of opium.

Livestock (1988): 34·5m. sheep, 13·62m. goats, 8·35m. cattle, 316,000 horses, 27,000 camels, (1984) 20,000 pigs, 230,000 buffaloes, and 1·8m. donkeys.

Fisheries. The Caspian Fisheries Co. (Shilat) is a government monopoly. Total catch (1986) 152,000 tonnes.

INDUSTRY. Production of industrial goods, 1984: Vegetable oil, 444,192 tonnes; sugar, 639,514 tonnes; finished cloth, 661,961,229 metres; footwear, 66,290,969 pairs; bricks, 10,824,612; cement, 12,064,027 tonnes; tractors, 14,513; combines, 612; tillers and threshers, 18,637; agricultural discs, 25,136; small vans,

68,644; trucks and small trucks, 14,932; private cars, 57,790; buses, 2,532; mini-buses, 8,170; ambulances, 559; motor cycles, 199,782. In 1984 there were 7,513 large-scale manufacturing establishments and the labour force was 619,332.

FOREIGN ECONOMIC RELATIONS.

FOREIGN ECONOMIC RELATIONS. In May 1990 Iran and the USA signed a US$50m. agreement to settle 2,750 US small claims arising from the Iranian revolution in 1979.

EEC sanctions were lifted in Oct. 1990.

Commerce. Imports totalled 799,555m. rials in 1987. Exports totalled 81,107m. rials in 1987, excluding oil and hydrocarbon solvents obtained from oil.

Total trade between Iran and UK (British Department of Trade returns, in £1,000 sterling):

	1986	*1987*	*1988*	*1989*	*1990*
Imports to UK	100,303	187,572	140,207	250,548	279,135
Exports and re-exports from UK	399,373	307,853	247,768	257,149	384,713

Tourism. Total number of visitors (1987) 171,837.

COMMUNICATIONS

Roads. In 1985 the total length of roads was 139,368 km, of which 504 km were freeways, 16,346 km main roads, 35,930 km by-roads, 33,618 km rural roads and 52,366 km other roads.

In 1984 private motor vehicles numbered 2,246,143; rented vehicles, 377,745; government vehicles, 144,248.

Railways. The State Railways totalled 4,567 km of main lines in 1985, of which 146 km electrified. In 1988 the railways carried 6·8m. passengers and 13m. tonnes of freight. Construction began in 1983 of a link from Kerman to Zahedan to connect the network to Pakistan.

Aviation. In 1985, 1,470,000 passengers arrived at Mehrabad Airport (1,157,000 on domestic flights and 313,000 on international flights) and 1,516,000 passengers departed (1,155,000 domestic and 361,000 international). The state airline carried 3,166,000 passengers and 52,303 tons of cargo and mail in 1983.

Shipping. In 1985, 1,345 ships, capacity 11,998,000 tonnes, entered commercial ports, unloading 12,660,000 tonnes and loading 447,000 tonnes of goods (excluding oil products).

Telecommunications. Postal, telegraph and telephone services are administered by the Ministry of Posts, Telegraphs and Telephones.

In 1985 the number of telephones was 1,305,122, of which some 488,516 were in Tehran province. Radio sets numbered 10m. in 1986, and television sets 2·1m.

Cinemas (1983). There were 277 cinemas with 174,366 seats.

Newspapers. There were in 1982, 17 daily papers in Tehran and other cities. Their circulation is relatively small, *Ettela'at* and *Kayhan* leading with about 220,000 and 350,000 respectively.

JUSTICE, RELIGION, EDUCATION AND WELFARE

Justice. A new legal system based on Islamic law was introduced by the new constitution in 1979. The President of the Supreme Court and the public Prosecutor-General are appointed by the Spiritual Leader. The Supreme Court has 16 branches and 109 offences carry the death penalty. To these were added economic crimes in July 1990.

Religion. The official religion is the Shi'a branch of Islam, known as the *Ithna-Ashariyya,* which recognizes 12 Imams or spiritual successors of the Prophet Mohammad. Of the total population, 96% are Shi'a, 3% are Sunni and 1% non-Moslem.

Education. The great majority of primary and secondary schools are state schools.

Elementary education in state schools and university education are free; small fees are charged for state-run secondary schools. Text-books are issued free of charge to pupils in the first 4 grades of elementary schools.

In 1984 there were 634,200 pupils in elementary schools, 2,021,520 in orientation schools and 901,056 in general secondary schools; there were 184,520 students in technical and vocational schools, 37,247 in teacher-training schools, 18,590 gifted children, and 182,239 in adult education courses. Universities and other institutes of higher education had 145,809 students in 1984. The Free Islamic University was established after the revolution and in 1983 the International University of Islamic Studies was being organized.

A literacy movement was established in 1981 and by 1985, 3m. citizens had participated.

Health. In 1984 70,152 hospital beds were available in 589 hospitals. Medical personnel included 15,945 physicians and 2,340 dentists in 1982.

DIPLOMATIC REPRESENTATIVES

Diplomatic links between Great Britain and Iran, broken in March 1989, were resumed in Oct. 1990.

Of Iran in Great Britain (27 Prince's Gate, London, SW7 1PX)
Chargé d'Affaires: Seyed Shamseddin Khareghani.

Of Great Britain in Iran (Ave. Ferdowski Tehran)
Chargé d'Affaires: David Reddaway, MBE.

Of Iran in the USA (3005 Massachusetts Ave., NW, Washington, D.C., 20008)
Ambassador: (Vacant).

Of the USA in Iran (260 Takhte Jamshid Ave., Tehran)
Ambassador: (Vacant).

Of Iran to the United Nations
Ambassador: Dr Kamal Kharrazi.

Further Reading

Statistical Information. Statistical Centre of Iran, Dr Fakemi Avenue, Tehran, Iran, 14144.

Afshar, H., *Iran: A Revolution in Turmoil.* London, 1985
Arberry, A. J. (ed.) *The Cambridge History of Iran.* 8 vols. CUP, 1968ff.
Bakhash, S., *The Reign of the Ayatollahs.* London, 1984
Benard, C. and Zalmay, K., *'The Government of God': Iran's Islamic Republic.* Columbia Univ. Press, 1984
Haim, S., *Shorter Persian–English Dictionary.* Tehran, 1958
Heikal, M., *Iran: The Untold Story.* New York, 1982
Hiro, D., *Iran under the Ayatollahs.* London, 1985
Hussain, A., *Islamic Iran: Revolution and Counter-Revolution.* London, 1985
Karshenas, M., *Oil, State and Industry in Iran.* CUP, 1990
Katouzian, H., *The Political Economy of Iran.* London, 1981
Keddie, N., *Roots of Revolution.* Yale Univ. Press, 1981
Nashat, G., *Women and Revolution in Iran.* Boulder, 1983
Navabpour, A. R., *Iran.* [Bibliography] Oxford and Santa Barbara, 1988
Rahnema, A. and Nomani, F., *The Secular Miracle: Religion, Politics and Economic Activity.* London, 1990
Sick, G., *All Fall Down.* London, 1985
Steinglass, F. J., *A Comprehensive Persian–English Dictionary.* 2nd ed. London, 1930
Stempel, J. D., *Inside the Iranian Revolution.* Indiana Univ. Press, 1981
Zabih, S., *Iran's Revolutionary Upheaval: An Interpretive Essay.* San Francisco, 1979.—*The Mosadegh Era: Roots of the Iranian Revolution.* Chicago, 1982.—*Iran since the Revolution.* London, 1982.—*The Left in Contemporary Iran.* London and Stamford, 1986

IRAQ

Capital: Baghdad
Population: 17·06m. (1988)
GNP per capita: US$2,140 (1986)

Jumhouriya al 'Iraqia

(Republic of Iraq)

HISTORY. Part of the Ottoman Empire from the 16th century, Iraq was captured by British forces in 1916 and became in 1921 a Kingdom under a League of Nations mandate, administered by Britain. It became independent on 3 Oct. 1932 under the Hashemite Dynasty, which was overthrown on 14 July 1958 by a military coup which established a Republic under Gen. Qassim. In 1963 Qassim was overthrown and Gen. Abdul Salam Aref became President, to be succeeded in 1966 by his brother Abdul Rahman Aref. In 1968 a successful coup was mounted by the Ba'th Party, which brought Gen. Ahmed Al Bakr to the Presidency. His Vice-President, from 1969, Saddam Hussein, became President in a peaceful transfer of power in 1979.

The Revolutionary Command Council formed after the 17 July 1968 coup announced in 1970 a complete and constitutional settlement of the Kurdish secessionist uprising in the north-east, but fighting has continued.

In Sept. 1980 Iraq invaded Iran in a dispute over territorial rights in the Shatt-al-Arab waterway which developed into a full-scale war. A UN-arranged ceasefire took place on 20 Aug. 1988 and UN sponsored peace talks continued in 1989. On 15 Aug. 1990 President Saddam offered peace terms to Iran and began the withdrawal of troops from Iranian soil. Iraq and Iran exchanged prisoners of war during the last quarter of 1990.

Early on 2 Aug. 1990 Iraqi forces without warning invaded and rapidly overran Kuwait, meeting little resistance. The Amir escaped to Saudi Arabia. President Saddam declared the annexation of Kuwait on 8 Aug. Numbers of foreign nationals resident in Kuwait were transferred to Baghdad as hostages, but all were released by Dec. 1990.

On 6 Aug. the UN Security Council voted by 13 to nil with 2 abstentions (Cuba and Yemen) to impose total economic sanctions on Iraq until it withdrew from Kuwait. On 7 Aug. the USA announced it was sending a large military force to Saudi Arabia at the latter's request to prevent a further Iraqi invasion of the area, and the UK made a similar commitment the following day. Various other countries announced the despatch of forces and equipment to this coalition force, including 12 Arab League countries on 10 Aug.

Measures to secure Iraq's withdrawal from Kuwait were given international legal sanction by a UN Security Council resolution of 25 Aug. (by 13 votes to nil), authorizing a naval blockade of Iraq under UN auspices. Further Security Council resolutions included (25 Sept., by 14 votes to 1) an air embargo of Iraq and (29 Oct., 13-nil) a call for compensation to be paid by Iraq to states for losses resulting from the invasion of Kuwait. A 12th resolution of 29 Nov. (12 in favour, Cuba and Yemen against, China abstaining) authorized the use of military force if Iraq did not withdraw by 15 Jan. 1991.

Iraq accepted an offer of talks between its Foreign Minister and the US Secretary of State at Geneva on 9 Jan. 1991. Following the failure of these talks to secure Iraq's withdrawal from Kuwait, the UN Secretary-General went to Baghdad, but was unable to secure a peaceful solution.

On the night of 16-17 Jan. coalition forces began an air attack on strategic targets in Iraq. Iraqi counter-attacks included missile strikes against Israel, which caused fatal casualties.

After a last-minute Soviet peace initiative had failed to secure an unconditional Iraqi withdrawal from Kuwait, coalition forces launched a land offensive on 24 Feb. The Iraqi army was routed and sustained massive destruction. Kuwait City was liberated on 27 Feb. and on 28 Feb. Iraq agreed to the conditions of a provisional ceasefire, including withdrawal from Kuwait. Coalition forces advanced into Iraq and held positions up to the lower River Euphrates.

A UN resolution of 2 March setting out the conditions of a permanent ceasefire was carried by 11 votes to 1 (Cuba) with 3 abstentions (China, India, Yemen). Iraq accepted it.

AREA AND POPULATION. Iraq is bounded north by Turkey, east by Iran, south-east by the Gulf, south by Kuwait and Saudi Arabia, and west by Jordan and Syria. The country has an area of 434,924 sq. km (167,925 sq. miles) and its population census (1977) was 12,000,497 and (estimate) 1988, 17,064,000.

The areas, populations (1977) and capitals of the governorates were:

Governorate	*sq. km*	*Estimate 1985*	*Capital*	*Estimate 1985*
Al-Anbar	137,723	582,058	Ar-Ramadi	137,388
Babil (Babylon)	5,258	739,031	Al-Hillah	215,249
Baghdad	5,159	4,648,609	Baghdad	4,648,609
al-Basrah	19,070	1,304,153	Al-Basrah	616,700
Dahuk [1]	6,120	330,356	Dahuk	19,736 [3]
Dhi Qar	13,626	725,913	an-Nasiriyah	138,842
Diyala	19,292	691,350	Ba'qubah	114,516
Irbil [1]	14,471	742,682	Irbil	333,903
Karbala	5,034	329,234	Karbala	184,574
Maysan	14,103	411,843	Al-Amarah	131,758
Al-Muthanna	51,029	253,816	As-Samawah	33,473 [2]
an-Najaf	27,844	472,103	An-Najaf	242,603
Ninawa (Nineveh)	37,698	1,358,082	Mosul	570,926
al-Qadisiyah	8,507	511,799	Ad-Diwaniyah	60,553 [2]
Salah ad-Din	29,004	442,782	Samarra	62,008 [3]
As-Sulaymaniyah [1]	15,756	906,495	As-Sulaymaniyah	279,424
Ta'mim	10,391	650,965	Kirkuk	207,852 [3]
Wasit	17,308	483,716	Al-Kut	58,647 [3]

[1] Forming Kurdish Autonomous Region. [2] Census 1965. [3] Estimate 1970.

The national language is Arabic, spoken by 81% of the population. There is a major minority group of Kurdish-speakers in the north-east (15·5%) and smaller groups speaking Turkic, Aramaic and Iranian languages.

CLIMATE. The climate is mainly arid, with small and unreliable rainfall and a large annual range of temperature. Summers are very hot and winters cold, al-Basrah. Jan. 55°F (12·8°C), July 92°F (33·3°C). Annual rainfall 7" (175 mm). Baghdad. Jan. 50°F (10°C), July 95°F (35°C). Annual rainfall 6" (140 mm). Mosul. Jan. 44°F (6·7°C), July 90°F (32·2°C). Annual rainfall 15" (384 mm).

CONSTITUTION AND GOVERNMENT. The Provisional Constitution was published on 22 Sept. 1968 and promulgated on 16 July 1970. The highest state authority remains the 6-member Revolutionary Command Council (RCC) but some legislative power has now been given to the 250-member National Assembly, elected in April 1989 for a 4-year term.

The only legal political grouping is the National Progressive Front (founded July 1973) comprising the Arab Socialist Renaissance (Ba'th) Party and various Kurdish parties; the Iraqi Communist Party left the Front in March 1979.

The President and Vice-President are elected by the RCC; the President appoints and leads a Council of Ministers responsible for administration.

President: Saddam Hussein at-Takriti (assumed office 17 July 1979).

In March 1991 the *Deputy President* was Sadoun Hammadi; *Foreign Minister:* Tariq Aziz; *Defence*, Lieut.-Gen. Saadi Tu'ma Abbas al-Jabouri.

National flag: Three horizontal stripes of red, white, black, with 3 green stars on the white stripe.

Local Government. Iraq is divided into 18 governorates *(liwa)*, each administered by an appointed Governor; three of the governorates form a (Kurdish) Autonomous Region, with an elected 57-member Kurdish Legislative Council. Each governorate is divided into *qadhas* (under Qaimaqams) and *nahiyahs* (under Mudirs).

DEFENCE. Reliable data was not available after the losses sustained by the Iraqi forces during their expulsion from Kuwait in Feb. 1991. The figures below reflect strengths at the end of 1990. Peace-time conscription is 21-24 months at age 18.

Army. The Army is organized into 7 armoured/mechanized and 40 infantry divisions including People's Army and Reserve brigades; 6 Republican Guard divisions, 20 special forces and 2 missile brigades. Equipment includes 1,500 T-54/-55/-77, 1,500 Chinese T-59/-69, 1,500 T-62, 1,000 T-72 and 30 Chieftian main battle tanks, and 100 PT-76 light tanks. Strength (1990 estimate) 955,000, including 480,000 active reserves.

Navy. The navy is an insignificant force, and it played little part in the war with Iran. A major order for 11 new ships was placed in Italy in 1981; the completed ships remain impounded in Italy, originally due to difficulties over payment. These ships are 4 frigates, 4 missile corvettes, and a tanker. Apart from these the force comprises 1 modern frigate/training ship, 8 ex-Soviet missile craft, 6 ex-Soviet torpedo boats, and 20 inshore patrol craft. There are also 3 Danish-built Ro-Ro ships used as tank landing ships, 3 medium landing ships, and 2 presidential yachts.

In 1990 naval personnel totalled 5,000 officers and ratings. The main base at Basra remains unusable, due to mines and obstructions in the Shatt al 'Arab, but that at Um Qasr could be used before 1991.

Air Force. Except for some 40 Bell 214ST helicopters from the USA and 100 Mirage F.1E/B fighters, about 40 Alouette III, 10 Super Frelon, 40 Puma and 59 Gazelle helicopters acquired from France, the combat and transport squadrons are equipped primarily with aircraft of Soviet design, including 6 Tu-22 supersonic medium bombers, 30 Su-7 and 70 Su-20 fighter-bombers, some MiG-29 and 90 MiG-23 interceptors and fighter-bombers, and 100 Chinese-built F-7 and MiG-21 interceptors, 60 Chinese-built F-6 (MiG-19) fighters, 40 Mi-24 gunship helicopters, 100 Mi-8 helicopters, and four-turbofan Il-76, turboprop An-12 and An-24/26 transports. USSR was also reported (1987) to have supplied Su-25 ground attack aircraft. Total strength (1990) 40,000 personnel (including 10,000 air defence) and 689 combat aircraft. Soviet 'Guideline', 'Goa', 'Gainful', 'Gaskin' and Roland surface-to-air missiles are operational.

INTERNATIONAL RELATIONS

Membership. Iraq is a member of UN, Arab League and the Non-Aligned Movement.

ECONOMY

Budget. Revenue and expenditure for 1989 balanced at I.D. 19,434m.

Oil revenues account for nearly 50%, customs and excise for about 26% of the total revenue.

Currency. The monetary unit is the *Iraqi dinar* (IQD) of 1,000 *fils*. Silver alloy coins for 100 and 50 fils (*dirham*) and 25 fils are in circulation, and other coins for 10, 5 and 1 fils. Notes are for ¼, ½ and 1 dinar, and for 5 and 10 dinars. In March 1991, £1 = 0·59 *dinar*; US$1 = 0·31 *dinar*.

Banking. All banks were nationalized on 14 July 1964. The Central Bank of Iraq is the sole bank of issue. In 1941 the Rafidain Bank, financed by the Iraqi Government, was instituted to carry out normal banking transactions. Its head office is in Baghdad and it has 239 branches, 11 abroad, including London. Its assets were US$47,000m. in Sept. 1990. In addition, there are 4 government banks which are authorized to issue loans to companies and individuals: the Industrial Bank, the Agricultural Bank, the Estate Bank, and the Mortgage Bank.

Weights and Measures. The metric system is in general use.

ENERGY AND NATURAL RESOURCES

Electricity. Production in 1986 amounted to 22,560m. kwh. Supply 220 volts; 50 Hz.

Oil. Following the nationalization of the Iraqi oil industry in June 1972, the Iraqi National Oil Company (INOC) is responsible for the exploration, production, transport and marketing of Iraqi crude oil and oil products.

The total crude petroleum production was (1989) 138m. tonnes and of natural gas (1980) 1,760m. cu. ft. Oil exports are essential for the economy but oil terminals in the Gulf were destroyed in 1980 and the trans-Syria pipeline closed in 1982. Iraq is now wholly reliant on the 625 mile pipeline from Kirkuk to the Mediterranean *via* Turkey.

Agriculture. In 1990 there were 17m. ha of arable land, but only 13% was cultivated. In Sept. 1990 farmers were ordered by the government to plant 80% of their land with wheat. The chief winter crops (1988) are wheat, 1·2m. tonnes and barley, 1·25m. tonnes. The chief summer crop is rice, 250,000 tonnes. The date crop is important (350,000 tonnes), the country furnishing about 80% of the world's trade in dates; the chief producing area is the totally irrigated riverain belt of the Shatt-el-Arab. Wool and cotton are also important exports.

Livestock (1988): Cattle, 1·6m.; buffaloes, 145,000; sheep, 9·2m.; goats, 1·55m.; horses, 55,000; camels, 55,000; chickens, 76m.

Fisheries. Catch (1986) 20,600 tonnes.

INDUSTRY. Iraq is still relatively under-developed industrially but work has begun on new industrial plants.

FOREIGN ECONOMIC RELATIONS

Commerce. Imports and exports for 4 calendar years were (in US$1m.):

	1981	*1982*	*1983*	*1984*
Imports	10,530	10,250	9,785	11,260
Exports	20,922	21,728	12,275	11,720

In 1983, crude oil formed 98·6% of all exports, of which 23% to Brazil and 12·5% to Italy. 13·8% of imports came from Federal Republic of Germany and 11% from Kuwait.

Total trade between Iraq and UK (British Department of Trade returns, in £1,000 sterling):

	1986	*1987*	*1988*	*1989*	*1990*
Imports to UK	66,129	33,871	43,406	55,175	101,557
Exports and re-exports from UK	443,890	271,655	412,091	450,495	293,393

Tourism. About 1,004,000 tourists visited Iraq in 1986.

COMMUNICATIONS

Roads. There were 25,500 km of main roads in 1985. Vehicles registered in 1986 totalled 492,000 passenger cars and 246,000 commercial vehicles.

Railways. Following closure of metre-gauge operations in 1988, Iraqi Republic Railways comprised in 1989 2,032 km of 1,435 mm gauge route. In 1989 it carried 1,643m. passenger-km and 2,678m. tonne-km.

Aviation. Baghdad airport is served by British Airways, Lufthansa, Alitalia, SAS, Swissair, KLM, Middle East Air Lines, PIA, Iraqi Airways, Air Liban, United Arab Airlines and Aeroflot. In 1982 passenger-km were 1,476m. and cargo, 37·5m. tonne-km.

Shipping. The merchant fleet in 1980 comprised 142 vessels (over 100 gross tons) with a total tonnage of 1,465,949. The ports of Basra and Um Qasr have been closed since Sept. 1980.

Telecommunications. Wireless telegraph services exist with UK, USA, UAR, Lebanon and Saudi Arabia, and wireless telephone services with UK, USA, Italy, UAR and USSR. Telephones, 1983, 624,685 (Baghdad, 302,219). In 1986 there were 2·5m. radio and 750,000 television receivers.

Newspapers (1989). In Baghdad there are 4 main daily newspapers (one of which is in English with a circulation of 550,000).

JUSTICE, RELIGION, EDUCATION AND WELFARE

Justice. The courts are established throughout the country as follows: For civil matters: The court of cassation in Baghdad; 6 courts of appeal at Baghdad (2), Basra, Babylon, Mosul and Kirkuk; 18 courts of first instance with unlimited powers and 150 courts of first instance with limited powers, all being courts of single judges. In addition, 6 peace courts have peace court jurisdiction only. 'Revolutionary courts' deal with cases affecting state security.

For *Shara'* (religious) matters: The Shara' courts at all places where there are civil courts, constituted in some places of specially appointed Qadhis (religious judges) and in other places of the judges of the civil courts. For criminal matters: The court of cassation; 6 sessions courts (2 being presided over by the judge of the local court of first instance and 4 being identical with the courts of appeal). Magistrates' courts at all places where there are civil courts, constituted of civil judges exercising magisterial powers of the first and second class. There are also a number of third-class magistrates' courts, powers for this purpose being granted to municipal councils and a number of administrative officials. Some administrative officials are granted the powers of a peace judge to deal with cases of debts due from cultivators.

Religion. The population is about 60% Shi'ite Moslem. The constitution proclaims Islam the state religion, but also stipulates freedom of religious belief and expression. In 1990 there were some 1·2m. Christians in 14 sects, including: 0·75m. Chaldean Church, with some 100 priests; 0·25m. Apostolic Assyrian (Nestorian) Church, with 29 priests and 70,000 Syriac Orthodox. There were some 10,000 in various Protestant sects.

Education. Primary and secondary education is free and primary education became compulsory in Sept. 1976. Primary school age is 6–12. Secondary education is for 6 years, of which the first 3 are termed intermediate. The medium of instruction is Arabic; Kurdish is used in primary schools in northern districts.

There were, in 1987, 8,210 primary schools with 2,917,474 pupils, and 2,315 secondary schools with 1,012,426 pupils. 245 vocational schools had 133,568 students and 43 teacher-training colleges had 28,164 students.

There were (1987) 6 universities with 110,173 students and 19 other higher educational establishments with 32,322 students.

Health. In 1981 there were 7,634 doctors, and 25,443 hospital beds.

DIPLOMATIC REPRESENTATIVES

Of Iraq in Great Britain (21 Queen's Gate, London, SW7 5JG)
On 6 Feb. 1991 Iraq broke off diplomatic relations with Great Britain.

Of Great Britain in Iraq (Zukaq 12, Mahala 218, Hai Al Khelood, Baghdad)

Of Iraq in the USA (1801 P. St., NW, Washington, D.C., 20036)
On 6 Feb. 1991 Iraq broke off diplomatic relations with the USA.

Of the USA in Iraq (PO Box 2447, Alwiyah, Baghdad)

Of Iraq to the United Nations
Ambassador: Dr Abdul Amir A. Al-Anbari.

Further Reading

Statistical Information: The Central Statistical Organization, Ministry of Planning, Baghdad (*President:* Dr Salah Al-Shaikhly) publishes an annual *Statistical Abstract* (latest issue 1973). Foreign Trade statistics are published annually by the Ministry of Planning.

Abdulrahman, A. J., *Iraq* [Bibliography]. Oxford and Santa Barbara, 1984
Al-Khalil, S., *Republic of Fear: the Politics of Modern Iraq*. Univ. of California Press, 1989
Axelgrad, F. W., *Iraq in Transition: A Political, Economic and Strategic Perspective*. London, 1986
Chubin, S. and Tripp, C., *Iran and Iraq at War*. London, 1988
Farouk-Sluglett, M., and Sluglett, P., *Iraq since 1958: from Revolution to Dictatorship*. London, 1991
Ghareeb, E., *The Kurdish Question in Iraq*. Syracuse Univ. Press, 1981
Postgate, E., *Iraq: International Relations and National Development*. London, 1983

IRELAND

Capital: Dublin
Population: 3·54m. (1988)
GNP per capita: US$8,500 (1990)

Éire

HISTORY. In April 1916 an insurrection against British rule took place and a republic was proclaimed. The armed struggle was renewed in 1919 and continued until 1921. The independence of Ireland was reaffirmed in Jan. 1919 by the National Parliament (*Dáil Éireann*), elected in Dec. 1918.

In 1920 an Act was passed by the British Parliament, under which separate Parliaments were set up for 'Southern Ireland' (26 counties) and 'Northern Ireland' (6 counties). The Unionists of the 6 counties accepted this scheme, and a Northern Parliament was duly elected on 24 May 1921. The rest of Ireland, however, ignored the Act.

On 6 Dec. 1921 a treaty was signed between Great Britain and Ireland by which Ireland accepted dominion status subject to the right of Northern Ireland to opt out. This right was exercised, and the border between *Saorstát Éireann* (26 counties) and Northern Ireland (6 counties) was fixed in Dec. 1925 as the outcome of an agreement between Great Britain, the Irish Free State and Northern Ireland. The agreement was ratified by the three parliaments.

Subsequently the constitutional links between *Saorstát Éireann* and the UK were gradually removed by the *Dáil*. The remaining formal association with the British Commonwealth by virtue of the External Relations Act, 1936, was severed when the Republic of Ireland Act, 1948, came into operation on 18 April 1949.

AREA AND POPULATION. The Republic of Ireland lies in the Atlantic ocean, separated from Great Britain by the Irish Sea to the east, and bounded north-east by Northern Ireland.

Counties and county boroughs	*Area in ha* [1]	*Population, 1988*		
		Males	*Females*	*Total*
Province of Leinster				
Carlow	89,635	20,816	20,172	40,988
Dublin County Borough	11,499	237,988	264,761	502,749
Dublin-Belgard	} 80,657	99,163	100,383	199,546
Dublin-Fingal		68,661	69,818	138,479
Dun Laoghaire-Rathdown		86,467	94,208	180,675
Kildare	169,425	59,542	56,705	116,247
Kilkenny	206,167	37,325	35,861	73,186
Laois	171,954	27,531	25,753	53,284
Longford	104,387	16,153	15,343	31,496
Louth	82,334	45,530	46,280	91,810
Meath	233,587	52,931	50,950	103,881
Offaly	199,774	30,819	29,016	59,835
Westmeath	176,290	32,048	31,331	63,379
Wexford	235,143	51,782	50,770	102,552
Wicklow	202,483	46,980	47,562	94,542
Total of Leinster	1,963,335	913,736	938,913	1,852,649
Province of Munster				
Clare	318,784	46,913	44,431	91,344
Cork County Borough	3,731	64,493	68,778	133,271
Cork	742,257	141,977	137,487	279,464
Kerry	470,142	63,293	60,866	124,159
Limerick County Borough	1,904	27,537	28,742	56,279
Limerick	266,676	55,149	53,141	108,290
Tipperary, N. R.	199,622	30,347	29,175	59,522
Tipperary, S. R.	225,836	39,381	37,716	77,097

[1] Exclusive of certain rivers, lakes and tideways.

Counties and county boroughs	Area in ha [1]	Population, 1988 Males	Females	Total
Province of Munster—contd.				
Waterford County Borough	3,809	19,336	20,193	39,529
Waterford	179,977	26,282	25,340	51,622
Total of Munster	2,412,738	514,708	505,869	1,020,577
Province of Connacht				
Galway County Borough	...	22,578	24,526	47,104
Galway	593,966	68,047	63,401	131,448
Leitrim	152,476	14,205	12,830	27,035
Mayo	539,846	58,729	56,455	115,184
Roscommon	246,276	28,351	26,241	54,592
Sligo	179,608	28,184	27,862	56,046
Total of Connacht	1,712,172	220,094	211,315	431,409
Province of Ulster (part of)				
Cavan	189,060	28,202	25,763	53,965
Donegal	483,058	65,906	63,758	129,664
Monaghan	129,093	27,044	25,335	52,379
Total of Ulster (part of)	801,211	121,152	114,856	236,008
Total	6,889,456	1,769,690	1,770,953	3,540,643

[1] Exclusive of certain rivers, lakes and tideways.

The capital is Dublin (Baile Átha Cliath). Town populations, 1986: Greater Dublin including Dún Laoghaire, 920,956; Cork, 173,694; Limerick, 76,557; Galway, 47,104; Waterford, 41,054.

Vital statistics for 6 calendar years:

	Births	Marriages	Deaths		Births	Marriages	Deaths
1984	64,062	18,513	32,076	1987	58,433	18,309	31,413
1985	62,388	18,791	33,213	1988 [1]	54,300	17,936	31,575
1986	61,620	18,573	33,630	1989 [1]	51,659	17,769	31,103

[1] Provisional

In 1989-90, 31,000 people emigrated. Total 1982-90 (estimate) 210,000.

CLIMATE. Influenced by the Gulf Stream, there is an equable climate with mild south-west winds, making temperatures almost uniform over the whole country. The coldest months are Jan. and Feb. (39–45°F, 4–7°C) and the warmest July and Aug. (57–61°F, 14–16°C). May and June are the sunniest months, averaging 5·5 to 6·5 hours each day, but over 7 hours in the extreme S.E. Rainfall is lowest along the eastern coastal strip. The central parts vary between 30–44" (750–1,125 mm), and up to 60" (1,500 mm) may be experienced in low-lying areas in the west. Dublin. Jan. 40°F (4·7°C), July 59°F (15°C). Annual rainfall 30" (750 mm). Cork. Jan. 42°F (5·6°C), July 61°F (16°C). Annual rainfall 41" (1,025 mm).

CONSTITUTION AND GOVERNMENT. Ireland is a sovereign independent, democratic republic. Its parliament exercises jurisdiction in 26 of the 32 counties of Ireland.

The first Constitution of the Irish Free State came into operation on 6 Dec. 1922. Certain provisions which were regarded as contrary to the national sentiments were gradually removed by successive amendments, with the result that at the end of 1936 the text differed considerably from the original document. On 14 June 1937 a new Constitution was approved by Parliament (*Dáil Éireann*) and enacted by a plebiscite on 1 July 1937. This Constitution came into operation on 29 Dec. 1937. Under it the name Ireland (Éire) was restored.

The Constitution provides that, pending the reintegration of the national territory, the laws enacted by the Parliament established by the Constitution shall have the same area and extent of application as those of the Irish Free State.

The head of state is the *President*, whose role is largely ceremonial, but who has the power to refer legislation which might infringe the constitution to the Supreme Court.

The *Oireachtas* or National Parliament consists of a House of Representatives, (*Dáil Éireann*) and a Senate (*Seanad Éireann*). The *Dáil*, consisting of 166 members, is elected by adult suffrage on the Single Transferable Vote system, which involves constituencies of 4 or 5 members. Each elector has the same number of votes as there are seats, and numbers preferences in order. A quota is calculated from the minimum number of votes required to win. When a candidate obtains this quota, further votes are transferred to other candidates according to second and further preferences. Candidates with the least votes are eliminated and their votes redistributed. Of the 60 members of the Senate, 11 are nominated by the *Taoiseach* (Prime Minister), 6 are elected by the universities and the remaining 43 are elected from 5 panels of candidates established on a vocational basis, representing the following public services and interests: (1) national language and culture, literature, art, education and such professional interests as may be defined by law for the purpose of this panel; (2) agricultural and allied interests, and fisheries; (3) labour, whether organized or unorganized; (4) industry and commerce, including banking, finance, accountancy, engineering and architecture; (5) public administration and social services, including voluntary social activities. The electing body is a college of 1,109 members, comprising members of the *Dáil*, Senate, county boroughs and county councils. There are no formal party divisions in the Senate.

A maximum period of 90 days is afforded to the Senate for the consideration or amendment of Bills sent to that House by the *Dáil*, but the Senate has no power to veto legislative proposals.

No amendment of the Constitution can be effected except with the approval of the people given at a referendum.

Irish is the first official language; English is recognized as a second official language. For further details of the Constitution *see* THE STATESMAN'S YEAR-BOOK , 1952, pp. 1123–34.

President: Mary Robinson (b. 1944), elected out of 3 candidates by 817,000 votes to 731,000 on 7 Nov. 1990, inaugurated 3 Dec. 1990.

Former Presidents: Dr Douglas Hyde (1938–45); Seán T. O. Ceallaigh (1945–59; 2 terms); Éamon de Valéra (1959–73; 2 terms); Erskine Childers (1973–74; died in office); Cearbhall Ó Dálaigh (1974–76; resigned). Pádraig Ó hIrighile (Patrick Hillery) (1976–90; 2 terms).

A general election was held in June 1989: Fianna Fáil, 77 (Feb. 1987 election, 81); Fine Gael, 55 (51); Labour Party, 15 (12); Progressive Democrats, 6 (14); Workers' Party, 7 (4); Others 6 (4).

The Government consisted of the following members in March 1991:

Taoiseach (Prime Minister) and Minister for the Gaeltacht: Charles J. Haughey.

Tánaiste (Deputy Prime Minister) and Minister for the Marine: John P. Wilson. *Foreign Affairs:* Gerard Collins. *Finance:* Albert Reynolds. *Agriculture and Food:* Michael O'Kennedy. *Industry and Commerce:* Desmond O'Malley. *Labour:* Bertie Ahern. *Energy:* Bobby Molloy. *Social Welfare:* Dr Michael Woods. *Justice:* Ray Burke. *Environment:* Pádraig Flynn. *Health:* Dr Rory O'Hanlon. *Education:* Mary O'Rourke. *Defence:* Brendan Daly. *Tourism, Transport and Communications:* Séamus Brennan.

There were 15 Ministers of State.

Attorney-General: John L. Murray.

National flag: Three vertical strips of green, white, orange.

National anthem: The Soldier's Song (words by P. Kearney; music by P. Heaney).

Local Government. The elected local authorities comprise 27 county councils, 5 county borough corporations, 6 borough corporations, 49 urban district councils and 26 Boards of Town Commissioners. All the members of these authorities are elected under a system of proportional representation, normally every 5 years. All residents of an area who have reached the age of 18 are entitled to vote in the local election for their area. Elected members are not paid, but provision is made for the payment of travelling expenses and subsistence allowances.

The range of services for which local authorities are responsible is broken down into 4 main programme groups as follows: Housing, Roads, Environment and General Local Services, and Sanitary Services. Because of the small size of their administrative areas the functions carried out by town commissioners and some of the smaller urban district councils have tended to become increasingly limited, and the more important tasks of local government have tended to become the responsibility of the county councils.

The local authorities have a system of government which combines an elected council and a whole-time manager. The elected members have specific functions reserved to them which include the striking of rates (local tax), the borrowing of money, the adoption of development plans, the making, amending or revoking of bye-laws and the nomination of persons to other bodies. The managers, who are paid officers of their authorities, are responsible for the performance of all functions which are not reserved to the elected members, including the employment of staff, making of contracts, management of local authority property, collection of rates and rents and the day-to-day administration of local authority affairs. The manager for a county council is manager also for every borough corporation, urban district council and board of town commissioners whose functional area is wholly within the county.

DEFENCE. Under the direction of the President, and subject to the provisions of the Defence Act, 1954, the military command of the Defence Forces is exercisable by the Government through the Minister for Defence. To aid and counsel the Minister for Defence on all matters in relation to the business of the Department of Defence on which he may consult it, there is a Council of Defence consisting of the Minister of State at the Department of Defence, the Secretary of the Department of Defence, the Chief of Staff, the Adjutant-General and the Quartermaster-General. At present the Permanent Defence Force strength is approximately 13,000 all ranks including the Air Corps and the Naval Service. The Reserve Defence Force strength is approximately 16,100 all ranks. Recruitment is on a voluntary basis. The minimum terms of enlistment are 3 years in the Permanent Defence Force and 6 years in the Reserve. There is no conscription.

Since May 1978 an Irish contingent has formed part of the United Nations force in Lebanon. The contingent now comprises 750 all ranks. 21 Irish officers are at present serving with the UN Truce Supervision Organization in the Middle East. Of these, 1 is seconded to the Office of the Secretary General Afghanistan and Pakistan (OSGAP) which was established early in 1988. 43 Irish officers are serving with the UN Iran/Iraq Military Observer Group (UNIIMOG), established in Aug. 1988. 15 of the officers act as observers and 3 serve with the Military Police Company, which also includes 25 other ranks. 31 Irish officers are serving with the UN Observer Group in Central America (ONUCA) since Dec. 1989, and 8 with the UN force in Cyprus (UNIFICYP).

Army. The Army has 4 infantry brigades and an infantry force of 2 battalions. 3 of the brigades have 2 infantry battalions and 1 brigade has 3 infantry battalions. Each brigade has a field artillery regiment and a squadron/company size unit for each of the support corps. Equipment includes 14 Scorpion light tanks. The current (1990) strength of the Army is 11,456 all ranks.

Navy. The Naval Service comprises 6 offshore patrol vessels and 1 helicopter offshore patrol vessel. The Air Corps operates 2 Dauphin helicopters for use from the helicopter patrol vessel. The Naval Base is at Haulbowline Island, in Cork. The 1990 strength of the Naval Service was 979 all ranks.

Air Corps. The Air Corps has a current (1990) strength of 834 all ranks. It has a total of 43 aircraft, comprised of 6 Fouga Magister armed jet trainers, 9 SF 260W armed piston-engined trainers, 8 Rheims-Cessna Rockets, 8 Alouette III, 5 Dauphin and 2 Gazelle helicopters, 3 twin-turbo prop Beech Super Kingair for coastal fishery patrol, and 1 Gulfstream GIII and 1 British Aerospace HS-125/700 twin turbofan transports.

INTERNATIONAL RELATIONS

Membership. Ireland is a member of the UN, OECD, the Council of Europe and the EC.

ECONOMY

Budget. Current revenue and expenditure (in IR£1m.):

Current revenue	*1989*	*1990*
Customs duties	139	147
Excise duties	1,638	1,684
Capital taxes	60	64
Stamp duties	279	286
Income tax	2,810	2,920
Income levy	—	—
Corporation tax	303	338
Value-added tax	1,943	2,015
Agricultural levies (EC)	13	13
Motor vehicle duties	148	149
Youth employment levy	117	124
Non-Tax Revenue	313	390
Total	7,756	8,130
Current expenditure		
Debt service	2,141	2,310
Industry and Labour	210	224
Agriculture	380	356
Fisheries, Forestry, Tourism	56	54
Health	1,240	1,312
Education	1,239	1,303
Social Welfare	2,690	2,793
Less: Receipts, e.g. social security	(–)1,662	(–)1,837
Total (including other items)	6,294	6,479

Capital expenditure amounted to IR£1,410m. in 1989, and IR£1,695m. in 1990.

On 31 Dec. 1989 the National Debt amounted to IR£24,827·9m. of which IR£15,705·2m. was denominated in Irish pounds and IR£9,122·7m. in foreign currencies and the official external reserves of the Central Bank of Ireland amounted to IR£2,521m.

Currency. The unit of currency is the *Irish pound* (IEP) or *punt Éireannach* of 100 *pence*. From 10 Sept. 1928 when the first Irish legal-tender notes were issued, the Irish currency was linked to Sterling on a one-for-one basis. This relationship was discontinued on 30 March 1979 when, following Ireland's adherence to the European Monetary System, it became inconsistent with Ireland's obligations under that system.

The Central Bank has the sole right of issuing legal tender notes; token coinage is issued by the Minister for Finance through the Bank. In March 1991, £1 = IR£1·09; US$ = IR£0·58.

The volume of legal-tender notes outstanding in June 1990 was £1,229m.

Banking and Finance. The Central Bank, which was established as from 1 Feb. 1943, in accordance with the Central Bank Act, 1942, replaced the Currency Commission, which was set up under the Currency Act, 1927, and had been responsible *inter alia* for the regulation of the note issue. In addition to the powers and functions of the Currency Commission the Central Bank has the power of receiving deposits from banks and public authorities, of rediscounting Exchequer bills and bills of exchange, of making advances to banks against such bills or against Government securities, of fixing and publishing rates of interest for rediscounting bills, or buying and selling certain Government securities and securities of any international bank or financial institution formed wholly or mainly by governments. The Bank also collects and publishes information relating to monetary and credit matters. The Central Bank Acts, 1971 and 1989, give further powers to the Central Bank in the regulation of banking including licensing of banks, the supervision of their operations and control of liquidity and reserve ratios. The capital of the Bank is IR£40,000, of which IR£24,000 has been paid up and is held by the Minister for Finance.

The Board of Directors of the Central Bank consists of a Governor, appointed by the President on the advice of the Government, and 9 directors, all appointed by the Minister for Finance.

The principal independent commercial banks are Allied Irish Banks PLC., Bank of Ireland and two smaller banks, Ulster Bank and National Irish Bank. They operate the branch banking system; on 29 June 1990 their total deposit and current accounts within Ireland amounted to IR£8,082·3m. and their total gross assets in Ireland, IR£17,251m.

There are also 30 Non-Associated Banks of which 21 are merchant and commercial banks and 9 are industrial banks whose main activity is instalment credit. Four of the merchant or commercial banks are subsidiaries of the Associated Banks; 10 are from other EC countries and 5 from outside the EC (mainly US) and the remainder are Irish. On 29 June 1990 their current and deposit accounts and interbank borrowings amounted to IR£11,588m. (47% of total bank resources) and their lending to IR£5,480·9m. (34·6% of lending to residents); total gross assets in Ireland, IR£13,171·8m.

There are two state-owned credit corporations, one industrial and one agricultural, and 9 building societies. There are 2 Trustee Savings Banks and the Post Office Savings Bank which together had deposits of IR£1,072m. in March 1989.

There is a stock exchange in Dublin.

Weights and Measures. Conversion to the metric system is in progress; with some exceptions which are confined to the domestic market, all imperial units of measurement will cease to be legal, for general use, after 31 Dec. 1994.

ENERGY AND NATURAL RESOURCES

Electricity. The total generating capacity was (1989) 3,932 mw. In 1989 the total sales of electricity amounted to 11,169m. units supplied to 1,256,765 customers. Electricity generated by fuel source 1989: Coal, 44%; oil, 5%; gas, 31%; peat, 15%; hydro, 5%. Supply 220 volts; 50 Hz.

Oil. About 618,000 sq. km of the Irish continental shelf has been designated an exploration area for oil and gas; at the furthest point the limit of jurisdiction is 520 nautical miles from the coast. Since 1970, 110 exploratory offshore wells have been drilled. A number of encouraging oil and gas flows have been recorded. In 1990, 53 blocks were held under exclusive offshore exploration licences and offshore petroleum leases.

Gas. (1990) All of Ireland's natural gas requirements are met by the Kinsale Head gas field 50 km off the south coast. In March 1989 additional natural gas was discovered about 10 miles north-west of this field at Ballycotton, a field of modest proportions from which gas was scheduled to flow in late 1991. Existing gas reserves should be depleted in approximately 15 years. Gas Transmission is controlled by the Irish Gas Board (BGE), which sells the gas into electricity generation, fertilizer production, and distribution systems for domestic, commercial and industrial use.

Peat. The country has very little indigenous coal, but possesses large reserves of peat, the development of which is handled largely by Bord na Mona (Peat Board). To date, the Board has acquired over 200,000 acres of bog and has 15 locations around the country. In the year ending 31 March, 1989, the Board sold 157,123 tonnes of sod peat to the domestic market and 68,437 tonnes for use in 4 sod peat electricity generating stations. The Board also sold 3,265,605 tonnes of milled peat for use in 7 milled peat generating stations. A further 967,517 tonnes was used by the Board in its factories to produce 363,000 tonnes of briquettes for sale to the domestic heating market. The Board also sold 1,311,597 cu. metres of horticultural peat.

Minerals. Lead and zinc concentrates are important. Reserves of 0·7m. tonnes of zinc were discovered in 1990. Metal content of production, 1990: Zinc, 168,800 tonnes; lead, 32,100 tonnes. Barytes, gypsum, limestone and aggregates are also important, and there is some coal, silver, quartz, dolomite, silica sand and marble. Exploration activity is centred on base metals, precious metals, industrial minerals and coal and about 45 companies are prospecting.

Agriculture. Although in 1990 17% of the employed workforce made a living from agriculture, population is tending to migrate from rural areas, and in 1990 50% of farmers were over 50 years old. General distribution of surface (in ha) in 1989: Crops and pasture, 4,673,000; other land, including grazed mountain, 2,216,200; total, 6,889,200.

Estimated area (ha) under certain crops calculated from sample returns:

			Area		
Crops	*1985*	*1986*	*1987*	*1988*	*1989*
Wheat	78,100	76,100	56,900	60,400	62,300
Oats	23,300	20,900	20,400	19,600	19,100
Barley	298,400	282,800	276,000	266,100	263,400
Potatoes	33,000	30,500	30,300	28,100	25,900
Sugar-beet	33,900	37,000	37,100	33,300	32,100

Gross agricultural output (including value of changes in stocks) for the year 1989 was valued at £3,357·6m.

Livestock (1989): Cattle, 6,800,500; sheep, 7,697,800; pigs, 995,700; horses and ponies, 51,700; poultry, 8,496,100.

Forestry. The total area under forest at 31 Dec. 1989 was some 0·42m. ha, of which 83% was owned by the Coillte Teoranta (state forestry company) and 17% privately-owned. Timber production, 1990, 1·6m. cu. metres.

Fisheries. In 1989 approximately 13,500 people were engaged full- or part-time in the sea fishing industry; 5,850 full-time and 6,250 part-time in the fish catching, farming and processing industries. The number of vessels engaged in fishing in 1990 was 3,900, of which 1,100 accounted for the greater part of the fishing effort. The quantities and values of fish landed during 1988 were: Demersal fish, 44,450 tonnes, value IR£44,445,000; pelagic fish, 159,023 tonnes; shellfish, 22,783 tonnes. Total quantity: 226,256 tonnes; total value, IR£83,932,000.

INDUSTRY. The census of industrial production for 1987 gives the following details of the values (in IR£1m.) of gross and net output for the principal manufacturing industries. The figures for net output are those of gross output minus cost of materials, including fuel, light and power, repairs to plant and machinery and amounts paid to others in connexion with products made.

	Gross output	*Net output*
Slaughtering, preparing and preserving meat	1,658·9	231·7
Manufacture of dairy products	1,677·6	292·7
Bread, biscuit and flour confectionery	214·8	100·4
Cocoa, chocolate and sugar confectionery	240·4	72·9
Animal and poultry foods	410·7	76·7
Brewing and malting	277·4	187·0
Spirit distilling and compounding	147·3	77·4
Paper and paper products	213·9	82·7
Printing and publishing	387·2	246·9
Manufacture of metal articles	482·4	214·0
Manufacture of non-metallic mineral products	487·4	207·3
Chemicals, including manmade fibres	1,647·9	902·0
Mechanical engineering	403·9	198·7
Office machinery and data-processing machinery	1,772·6	826·3
Electrical engineering	1,206·1	666·1
Manufacture and assembly of motor vehicles, parts and accessories	102·6	47·6

	Gross output	*Net output*
Manufacture of other means of transport	159·5	80·8
Instrument engineering	423·2	251·7
Textiles	443·1	180·7
Manufacture of footwear and clothing	302·9	141·7
Timber and wooden furniture	278·2	116·2
Processing rubber and plastics	417·7	195·7
Mineral oil refining	193·1	28·1
Gas, water and electricity	949·5	639·2
All other industries	2,130·3	1,285·7
Total (all industries)	16,628·6	7,350·2

Labour. The total labour force at mid-April 1989 was about 1,292,000, of which about 202,000 persons were out of work. Of the estimated 1·09m. persons at work, 163,000 were in the agricultural sector, 306,000 in industry and 621,000 in services.

Trade Unions. The number of trade unions in Dec. 1989 was 69; total membership, 487,000. About 229,000 were organized in 3 general unions catering both for white collar and manual workers. There were 16 employers' associations holding negotiation licences, with membership of 11,200.

FOREIGN ECONOMIC RELATIONS

Commerce. Value of imports and exports of merchandise for calendar years (in IR£):

	1986	*1987*	*1988*	*1989*
Imports	8,621,291,016	9,155,206,863	10,214,757,580	12,287,833,068
Exports	9,374,310,355	10,723,497,879	12,304,847,558	14,596,912,275

The values of the chief imports and total exports are shown in the following table (in IR£1,000):

	Imports		*Exports*	
	1988	*1989*	*1988*	*1989*
Live animals and food	1,066,239	1,153,931	2,900,560	3,208,932
Raw materials	338,233	392,411	563,451	642,155
Mineral fuels and lubricants	568,001	674,301	64,548	68,656
Chemicals	1,292,151	1,524,802	1,612,583	2,084,847
Manufactured goods	1,637,605	1,847,176	1,036,052	1,148,765
Machinery and transport equipment	3,516,580	4,649,829	3,840,390	4,652,376
Manufactured articles	1,345,892	1,552,922	1,965,651	1,965,651

Exports, in IR£1m., for 1989 (and 1988): UK, 4,896·1 (4,349·7); Federal Republic of Germany, 1,610·4 (1,368·8); France, 1,455 (1,121); USA, 1,153·4 (949·5); Netherlands, 1,031·1 (861); Belgium and Luxembourg, 661·2 (545); Italy, 646·6 (464·5); Japan, 317·1 (238·7); Spain, 286·9 (209·6); Sweden, 269·1 (231·6); Switzerland, 218·4 (160·3); Norway, 162·7 (148·3); Denmark, 131·7 (95·7). Imports: UK, 5,027·5 (4,303·6); USA, 1,973·2 (1,623·3); Federal Republic of Germany, 1,074·8 (880·8); Japan, 718·9 (496·9); Netherlands, 508·5 (407·5); France, 503·2 (417); Italy, 324·2 (259·5); Belgium and Luxembourg, 267·4 (214); Sweden, 198·7 (160·1); Spain, 151·5 (118·4); Denmark, 114 (93·5).

Total trade between Ireland and UK (British Department of Trade returns, in £1,000 sterling):

	1986	*1987*	*1988*	*1989*	*1990*
Imports to UK	3,053,807	3,488,406	3,876,630	4,279,202	4,498,571
Exports and re-exports from UK	3,558,372	3,831,737	4,057,046	4,714,780	5,311,539

Tourism. Total number of overseas tourists in 1989 was 2,732,000. These, together with cross-border visitors, spent IR£989m.

COMMUNICATIONS

Roads. At 31 Dec. 1989 there were 92,303 km of public roads, consisting of 8 km of motorway, 2,630 km of national primary roads, 2,625 km of national secondary roads, 10,566 km of regional roads, 73,975 km of county roads and 2,499 km of urban roads.

Number of licensed motor vehicles at 30 Sept. 1989: Private cars, 773,396; public-service vehicles, 8,895; goods vehicles, 130,020 agricultural vehicles, 70,125; motor cycles, 24,492; other vehicles, 12,632.

The total number of km run by road motor passenger vehicles of the omnibus type during 1987 was 93·33m. Passengers carried numbered 226,109,000 and the gross receipts from passengers were IR£120,904,000.

Railways. The total length of railway open for traffic at 31 Dec. 1989 was 1,944 km (38 km electrified), all 1,600 mm gauge.

Railway statistics for years ending 31 Dec.	*1988*	*1989*
Passengers (journeys)	24,043,000	25,595,000
Km run by coaching trains	9,288,000	9,534,000
Freight (tonne-km)	544,591,000	555,940,000
Km run by freight trains	3,942,000	4,136,000
Receipts (IR£)	134,220,000	133,464,000
Expenditure (IR£)	129,091,000	124,888,000

Aviation. The state-owned Aer Lingus Group comprises Aer Lingus plc, incorporated in 1936, which operates services within Ireland and between Ireland and Britain and Europe, and Aerlinte Eireann plc, incorporated in 1947, which operates services to the USA. Although separate legal entities, the two companies share a common management and board of directors and their services are integrated under the marketing name of Aer Lingus as the national airline. During the year ended 31 March 1990 Aer Lingus carried 3,595,102 passengers and 28,739 tonnes of cargo/mail on its European services and 474,295 passengers and 21,444 tonnes of cargo/mail on its trans-Atlantic services.

In addition to Aer Lingus, there were in 1990 10 independent air transport operators, the largest of which, Ryanair, operates air services on a number of international routes (Ireland/UK, Ireland/Germany).

The principal airports are at Dublin, Shannon and Cork.

Shipping. The Irish merchant fleet, of vessels of 100 gross tonnes or over, consisted of 67 vessels totalling 125,359 GRT at 30 June 1990. Total cargo traffic passing through the country's ports amounted to 24·9m. tonnes in 1990.

Inland Waterways. The principal inland waterways open to navigation are the Shannon Navigation (130 miles) and the Grand Canal and Barrow Navigation (156 miles). The Office of Public Works is responsible for the waterways system as a public amenity. Merchandise traffic has now ceased and navigation is confined to pleasure craft operated either privately or commercially.

Telecommunications. Telecommunication services are provided by Telecom Eireann, a statutory body set up under the Postal and Telecommunications Services Act, 1983. Number of working lines (March 1990), 916,000; telex lines, 4,480; data lines, over 8,800; Eirpac (public packet-switched network), 2,003 customers; Eircell (mobile telephone network), 13,800 customers; Eirpage (radio paging network), 4,700 customers.

Postal services are provided by An Post, a statutory body established under the Postal and Telecommunications Services Act, 1983. Number of Post Offices as of Dec. 1989, 2,098. Delivery points, 1·17m. Number of items delivered during year ended 31 Dec. 1989, 471·7m. An Post also offers a range of services throughout its Post Office network including National Savings Services and payment of Social Welfare Benefits/Pensions on an agency basis for the State.

Public service broadcasting is provided by Radio Telefis Eireann, a statutory body established under the Broadcasting Authority Acts 1960–79 to provide the national TV and radio services. RTE is financed by advertising and by TV licences. On 31 Dec. 1987 there were 787,501 holders of current TV licences. In 1988 new legislation was enacted to provide for the establishment of independent commercial radio services and an independent TV service. During 1989–90, 20 independent local radio stations and an independent national radio station began broadcasting, and it was expected that the TV service would begin broadcasting in autumn 1991.

Cinemas. There were (1986) 124 cinemas and 169 (estimate) screens.

Newspapers (1986). There are 7 daily newspapers (all in English) with a combined circulation of 647,912; 5 of them are published in Dublin (circulation, 555,282).

JUSTICE, RELIGION, EDUCATION AND WELFARE

Justice. The Constitution provides that justice shall be administered in public in Courts established by law by Judges appointed by the President on the advice of the Government. The jurisdiction and organization of the Courts are dealt with in the Courts (Establishment and Constitution) Act, 1961 and the Courts (Supplemental Provisions) Acts, 1961–88. These Courts consist of Courts of First Instance and a Court of Final Appeal, called the Supreme Court. The Courts of First Instance are the High Court with full original jurisdiction and the Circuit and the District Courts with local and limited jurisdiction. A judge may not be removed from office except for stated misbehaviour or incapacity and then only on resolutions passed by both Houses of the *Oireachtas*. Judges of the Supreme, High and Circuit Courts are appointed from among practising barristers. Judges of the District Court (called District Justices) may be appointed from among practising barristers or practising solicitors.

The Supreme Court, which consists of the Chief Justice (who is *ex officio* an additional judge of the High Court) and 4 ordinary judges, has appellate jurisdiction from all decisions of the High Court. The President may, after consultation with the Council of State, refer a Bill, which has been passed by both Houses of the *Oireachtas* (other than a money bill and certain other bills), to the Supreme Court for a decision on the question as to whether such Bill or any provision thereof is repugnant to the Constitution.

The High Court, which consists of a President (who is *ex officio* an additional Judge of the Supreme Court) and 15 ordinary judges, has full original jurisdiction in and power to determine all matters and questions, whether of law or fact, civil or criminal. In all cases in which questions arise concerning the validity of any law having regard to the provisions of the Constitution, the High Court alone exercises original jurisdiction. The High Court on Circuit acts as an appeal court from the Circuit Court.

The Court of Criminal Appeal consists of the Chief Justice or an ordinary Judge of the Supreme Court, together with either 2 ordinary judges of the High Court or the President and one ordinary judge of the High Court. It deals with appeals by persons convicted on indictment where the appellant obtains a certificate from the trial judge that the case is a fit one for appeal, or, in case such certificate is refused, where the court itself, on appeal from such refusal, grants leave to appeal. The decision of the Court of Criminal Appeal is final, unless that court or the Attorney-General certifies that the decision involves a point of law of exceptional public importance, in which case an appeal is taken to the Supreme Court.

The Offences against the State Act, 1939 provides in Part V for the establishment of Special Criminal Courts. A Special Criminal Court sits without a jury. The rules of evidence that apply in proceedings before a Special Criminal Court are the same as those applicable in trials in the Central Criminal Court. A Special Criminal Court is authorised by the 1939 Act to make rules governing its own practice and procedure. An appeal against conviction or sentence by a Special Criminal Court may be taken to the Court of Criminal Appeal. On 30 May 1972 Orders were made establishing a Special Criminal Court and declaring that offences of a particular class or kind (as set out) were to be scheduled offences for the purposes of Part V of the Act, the effect of which was to give the Special Criminal Court jurisdiction to try persons charged with those offences.

The High Court exercising criminal jurisdiction is known as the Central Criminal Court. It consists of a judge or judges of the High Court, nominated by the President of the High Court. The Court sits in Dublin and tries criminal cases which are outside the jurisdiction of the Circuit Court.

The country is divided into a number of circuits for the purposes of the Circuit Court. The President of the Circuit Court is *ex officio* an additional judge of the High Court. The jurisdiction of the court in civil proceedings is limited to IR£15,000 in contract and tort, IR£15,000 in actions founded on hire-purchase and credit-sale agreements, IR£5,000 in equity and IR£5,000 in probate and administration, save by consent of the parties, in which event the jurisdiction is unlimited. In criminal matters it has jurisdiction in all cases except murder, treason, piracy and allied offences. The Circuit Court acts as an appeal court from the District Court.

The District Court has summary jurisdiction in a large number of criminal cases where the offence is not of a serious nature. In civil matters the Court has jurisdiction in contract and tort (except slander, libel, seduction, slander of title and false imprisonment) where the claim does not exceed IR£2,500; in proceedings founded on hire-purchase and credit-sale agreements, the jurisdiction is IR£2,500.

All criminal cases, except those of a minor nature, and those tried in the Special Criminal Court, are tried by a judge and a jury of 12. A majority vote of the jury (10 must agree) is necessary to determine a verdict.

Religion. According to the census of population taken in 1981 the principal religious professions were as follows:

	Leinster	*Munster*	*Connacht*	*Ulster (part of)*	*Total*
Roman Catholics	1,645,489	949,938	406,811	202,238	3,204,476
Church of Ireland (Anglican)	58,356	18,076	5,973	12,961	95,366
Presbyterians	4,337	542	345	9,031	14,255
Methodists	3,339	1,285	324	842	5,790
Other religious denominations	9,148	2,586	753	483	12,970
Not stated or no religion	69,852	25,888	10,204	4,604	110,548

Cahal Daly (b. 1917) is the Roman Catholic Archbishop of Armagh and Primate of All Ireland.

In May 1990 the General Synod of the Church of Ireland voted to ordain women.

Education. *Elementary.* Elementary education is free and was given in about 3,364 national schools (including 117 special schools) in 1990. The total number of pupils on rolls in 1988–89 was 560,116, including pupils in special schools and classes; the number of teachers of all classes was about 20,362 in 1990, including remedial teachers and teachers of special classes. The estimated state expenditure on elementary education for 1990 was IR£463,487,000, excluding the cost of administration.

Special. Special provision is made for handicapped and deprived children in special schools which are recognized on the same basis as primary schools, in special classes attached to ordinary schools and in certain voluntary centres where educational services appropriate to the needs of the children are provided. Categories of children include visually handicapped, hearing impaired, physically handicapped, mentally handicapped, emotionally disturbed, travelling children and other socially disadvantaged children. Provision is also made, on an increasing scale, for children with dual or multiple handicaps. In each case a programme suited to the needs of a particular handicap is provided. Each class is very much smaller than ordinary classes in a primary school and, because of the size of the catchment areas involved, an extensive system of school transport has been developed. Many handicapped children who have spent some years in a special school or class are integrated into normal schools for part of their school career, if necessary with special additional facilities such as nursing services, special equipment, etc. For others who cannot progress within the ordinary school system the special schools or classes provide both the primary and post-primary level of education. There are also part-time teaching facilities in hospitals, child guidance clinics, rehabilitation workshops, special 'Saturday-morning' centres and home teaching schemes.

Special schools (1990) numbered 117 with approximately 8,500 pupils. There were also some 3,000 pupils enrolled in about 300 special classes, and 857 remedial teachers were employed for backward pupils in ordinary national schools. 36 peripatetic teachers were employed for children with hearing or visual impairments, and for travelling children.

Secondary. Voluntary secondary schools are under private control and are conducted in most cases by religious orders. These schools receive grants from the State and are open to inspection by the Department of Education. The number of recognized secondary schools during the school year 1989–90 was 492, and the number of pupils in attendance was 214,114.

Vocational Education Committee schools provide courses of general and technical education. The number of vocational schools during the school year 1989–90 was 251, and the number of full-time students in attendance was 85,068. These schools are controlled by the local Vocational Education Committees; they are financed mainly by state grants and also by contributions from local rating authorities and VEC receipts.

Comprehensive. Comprehensive schools which are financed by the State combine academic and technical subjects in one broad curriculum so that each pupil may be offered educational options suited to his needs, abilities and interests available to him. Pupils are prepared for State examinations and for entrance to universities and institutes of further education. The number of comprehensive schools during the school year 1989–90 was 16 and the number of students in attendance was 8,842.

Community. Community schools continue to be established through the amalgamation of existing voluntary secondary and Vocational Education Committee schools, where this is found feasible and desirable, and in new areas where a single larger school is considered preferable to 2 smaller schools under separate managements. These schools provide second-level education and also provide adult education facilities for their own areas. They also make facilities available to voluntary organizations and to the adult community generally. The number of community schools during the school year 1989–90 was 47 and the number of students in attendance was 31,298.

The estimated State expenditure for post-primary education for 1990 was IR£450,167,000.

Education Third-Level. University education is provided by the National University of Ireland, founded in Dublin in 1908, by the University of Dublin (Trinity College), founded in 1592, and by the Dublin City University and the University of Limerick established in 1989. The National University comprises 3 constituent colleges–University College, Dublin, University College, Cork, and University College, Galway.

St Patrick's College, Maynooth, Co. Kildare, is a national seminary for Catholic priests and a pontifical university with the power to confer degrees up to doctoral level in philosophy, theology and canon law. It also admits lay students (men and women) to the courses in arts, science and education which it provides as a recognized college of the National University.

Besides the University medical schools, the Royal College of Surgeons in Ireland (a long-established independent medical school) provides medical qualifications which are internationally recognized. Courses to degree level are available at the National College of Art and Design, Dublin.

Regional Technical Colleges in 9 centres (Athlone, Carlow, Cork, Dundalk, Galway, Letterkenny, Sligo, Tralee and Waterford) provide vocational education and training for trade and industry from craft to professional level, operating under the aegis of the Vocational Education Committees (VECs) for their areas. Six colleges in Dublin provide degree and diploma level courses in engineering, architecture, business studies, catering, music, etc., operating under the aegis of the Dublin VEC. A College of Art, Commerce and Technology in Limerick and a School of Art and a School of Music in Cork operate under the aegis respectively of the cities of Limerick and Cork VECs. Total full-time enrolments in 1989–90 were approximately 24,000.

There are 5 Colleges of Education for training primary school teachers. For degree awarding purposes, 3 of these colleges are associated with Trinity College, 2 with University College, Dublin, and one with University College, Cork. Thomond College of Education, Limerick, trains post-primary teachers in the areas of physical education, metal and engineering technology, wood building and technology and commercial and secretarial subjects. There are also 2 Home Economics Colleges for teacher training, one associated with Trinity College and the other with University College, Galway.

The total full-time enrolment at third-level for 1989–90 was approximately 66,350 and estimated State expenditure on third-level education for 1990 was IR£207,808,000. The National Council for Educational Awards, established on a statutory basis in 1979, is the validating and awarding authority for courses in the third-level sector outside the universities.

Agricultural. Teagasc – the Agriculture and Food Development Authority is the agency responsible for providing agricultural advisory, training, research and development services. Full-time instruction in agriculture is provided for all sections of the farming community. There are 4 agricultural colleges for young people, administered by Teagasc, and 7 private Teagasc-aided agricultural colleges, at each of which a 1-year course in agriculture is given. A second-year course in farm machinery is provided at one college. Scholarships tenable at these colleges, all of which are residential, are awarded by Teagasc which also provides a comprehensive agricultural advisory service and operates an intensive programme of short courses for adult farmers in agriculture and horticulture at local centres.

Horticultural. Two of the agricultural colleges mentioned above also provide a commercial horticultural course. A third college aided by Teagasc also provides this course. A 3-year course in amenity horticulture is provided at the National Botanic Gardens in Dublin.

A comprehensive 3-year training programme for young entrants to farming leading to a 'Certificate in Farming', the main training programme for young people entering farming, involving both formal instruction and a period of supervised on-farm work experience, was introduced by ACOT in 1982. Students taking the Certificate in Farming can follow a course in general agriculture, pigs, poultry or horticulture. In the case of horticulture, the major part of this course is taken at one of the three horticultural colleges.

Health Services. There are 3 categories of entitlement, based on a person's income:
(i) Persons on a low income and their dependants, who qualify for the full range of health services, free of charge, i.e. family doctor, drugs and medicines, hospital and specialist services as well as dental, aural and optical services. Maternity care and infant welfare services are also provided. There is no fixed limit, but guidelines laid down by health boards, determine eligibility – each application is considered on its merit. There is provision for hardship cases.
(ii) Persons whose income for the year ended 5 April 1990 was under IR£16,700. They and their dependants are entitled to hospital services, subject to certain charges, both as an in-patient and an out-patient, a full maternity and infant welfare service and assistance towards the cost of prescriptions. The latter limits the nett outlay on medicines used in a calendar month to IR£28.
(iii) Persons whose income for the year ended 5 April 1990 was IR£16,700 or more. They are entitled to in-patient and out-patient hospital services, subject to certain charges, but they are liable for the fees of consultants. They are also entitled to assistance towards the cost of prescriptions. Drugs and medicines are made available free of charge to all persons suffering from specified long-term ailments such as diabetes, multiple sclerosis, epilepsy, etc. Hospital in-patient and out-patient services are free of charge to all children under 16 years of age, suffering from specified long-term conditions such as cystic fibrosis, spina bifida, cerebral palsy, etc. Immunization and diagnostic services as well as hospital services are free of charge to everyone suffering from an infectious disease. A maintenance allowance is also payable in necessitous cases.

From 18 May 1987 persons in categories *(ii)* and *(iii)* are liable for in-patient and out-patient charge. A charge of IR£10 is made for each day or part of a day during which in-patient services are availed of subject to a maximum payment of IR£100 in any period of 12 consecutive months. A charge of IR£10 for out-patient services is made for the first and subsequent instances relating to the same matter. Persons in category *(i)*, women receiving service in respect of motherhood, children suffering from certain diseases etc. are not liable for these charges.

Services for Children: Health Boards are involved, with the co-operation of a wide network of voluntary organizations, in the provision of a range of child care services including adoption, fostering, residential care, day care and social work services for families in need of support.

Welfare Services: There are various services provided for the elderly, the chronic sick, the disabled and families in stress, such as social support service, day care services for children, home helps, home nursing, meals-on-wheels, day centres, cheap fuel, etc. Health Boards also provide disabled persons, without charge, with training for employment and place them in jobs.

Grants and Allowances: Disabled Persons' Maintenance Allowance is payable to the chronically disabled over the age of 16 who are not in long term care. Recipients are entitled to free travel and subject to certain conditions to electricity allowance, free TV licence, telephone rental and fuel vouchers. Mobility allowance is payable to severely disabled persons between 16 and 66 years who are unable to walk. Allowance for the Domiciliary Care of Severely Handicapped Children is payable to the mother of a severely handicapped child, maintained at home, but needing constant care and supervision. Blind welfare allowance: This allowance is in addition to the benefits for the blind operated by the Department of Social Welfare. Grants up to IR£1,500 are paid, subject to a means test, to disabled persons towards the purchase of a car, in order that they might obtain or retain employment.

Health contributions: A health contribution of 1·25% of income up to a ceiling of IR£16,700 is payable by all.

Social Welfare Services. The Department of Social Welfare provides a range of payments and benefits in kind. The payments can be divided into two categories, social insurance and social assistance. The Department also administers a scheme of grants for voluntary organizations working in the social services area.

Social Insurance Payments. Payments under social insurance are funded by employers, their employees and the self-employed. Any deficit in the fund is met by Exchequer subvention. Employees and self-employed people between the ages of 16 and 66 are liable for pay-related social insurance contributions. The majority of employees must pay a contribution which gives cover for the full range of social insurance benefits while self-employed people must pay a contribution which gives cover for widows and orphans pensions and old age contributory pension. Entitlement to social insurance benefits depends on the claimant having a number of contributions paid or credited in a specific time period. The contribution conditions vary according to the different schemes. The social insurance schemes are: Old Age Contributory Pension; Widow's Contributory Pension; Orphan's Contributory Allowance; Disability Benefit; Pay-related Benefit, Dental and Optical Benefit; Retirement Pension; Deserted Wife's Benefit; Invalidity Pension, Unemployment Benefit; Maternity Benefits; Death Grant. There is also a scheme of occupational injuries benefits which is not strictly a social insurance scheme as there are no contribution conditions for entitlement. Expenditure on this scheme is paid from a fund which is financed by employers' contributions and income from investments.

Social Assistance Payments. Social assistance schemes are financed entirely by the Exchequer. One of the basic qualifying conditions for payment is that the applicant satisfies a means test. The social assistance payments are: Old Age Non-Contributory Pension; Blind Person's Pension; Lone Parent's Allowance; Widow's Non-Contributory Pension [1]; Deserted Wife's Allowance [1]; Prisoner's Wife's Allowance [1]; Unemployment Assistance; Supplementary Welfare Allowance; Orphan's Non-Contributory Pension; Single Woman's Allowance [2]; Rent Allowance; Family Income Supplement; Carer's Allowance. Child benefit is payable without a means test in respect of each child under age 16 and children between 16 and 18 who are at school or incapacitated for a prolonged period. it is funded from the Exchequer.

Other Schemes. The Department also provides a range of benefits in kind, principally for the elderly and disabled. These are: Free travel; free electricity allowance; free gas allowance; free telephone rental; free TV licence; fuel allowance.

[1] For certain women who do not qualify for the lone parent's allowance.
[2] For women between ages 58 and 66.

DIPLOMATIC REPRESENTATIVES

Of Ireland in Great Britain (17 Grosvenor Pl., London, SW1X 7HR)
Ambassador: Andrew O'Rourke.

Of Great Britain in Ireland (33 Merrion Rd., Dublin, 4)
Ambassador: Sir Nicholas Fenn, KCMG.

Of Ireland in the USA (2234 Massachusetts Ave., NW, Washington, D.C., 20008)
Ambassador: Padraic N. MacKernan.

Of the USA in Ireland (42 Elgin Rd., Ballsbridge, Dublin)
Ambassador: Richard A. Moore.

Of Ireland to the United Nations
Ambassador: Francis Mahon Hayes.

Further Reading

Statistical Information: The Central Statistics Office (Earlsfort Terrace, Dublin, 2) was established in June 1949, and is attached to the Department of the Taoiseach. *Director:* T. P. Linehan, B.E., B.Sc.

Principal publications of the Central Statistics Office are *National Income and Expenditure* (annually), *Statistical Abstract* (annually), *Census of Population Reports, Census of Industrial Production Reports, Trade and Shipping Statistics* (annually and monthly), *Trend of Employment and Unemployment* (annually), *Reports on Vital Statistics* (annually and quarterly), *Irish Statistical Bulletin* (quarterly), *Labour Force Surveys* (annually), *Trade Statistics* (monthly), *Economic Series* (monthly).

Aspects of Ireland. (Series). Dublin Department of Foreign Affairs.
Atlas of Ireland. Royal Irish Academy, Dublin, 1979
Facts About Ireland. Dublin Department of Foreign Affairs, 6th ed. 1985
The Gill History of Ireland. 11 vols. Dublin
Bartholomew, P. C., *The Irish Judiciary.* Dublin, Institute of Public Administration, 1974
Chubb, B., *The Constitution and Constitutional Change in Ireland.* Dublin, reprinted 1988
Coolahan, J., *Irish Education: Its History and Structure.* Dublin, 1981
Eager, A. R., *A Guide to Irish Bibliographical Material.* 2nd ed. London, 1980
Encyclopaedia of Ireland. Dublin, 1968
Foster, R. F., *Modern Ireland 1600–1972.* London, 1988
Hensey, B., *The Health Services of Ireland.* 4th ed. Dublin, 1988
Hickey, D. J. and Doherty, J. E., *A Dictionary of Irish History since 1800.* Dublin, 1980
Johnston, T. J. and others, *A History of the Church of Ireland.* Dublin, 1953
Lee, J. J., *Ireland 1912-1985: Politics and Society.* CUP, 1989
McDunphy, Michael, *The President of Ireland: His Powers, Functions and Duties.* Dublin, 1945
Maher, D., *The Tortuous Path: The Course of Ireland's Entry into the EEC 1948–73.* Dublin, 1986
Miller, K. A., *Emigrants and Exiles: Ireland and the Irish Exodus to North America.* OUP, 1988
Page, R., *Sources of Economic Information: Ireland.* Dublin, 1985
Shannon, M. O., *Irish Republic.* [Bibliography] Oxford and Santa Barbara, 1986
Thom's Directory of Ireland. 2 vols. (Dublin, Street Directory, Commercial). Dublin, 1979–80
Tobin, F., *Ireland in the 1960s.* Dublin, 1984

ISRAEL

Capital: Jerusalem
Population: 4·82m. (1990)
GNP per capita: US$8,650 (1988)

Medinat Israel

(State of Israel)

HISTORY. During the First World War the then Turkish province of Palestine, populated mainly by Arabs, was occupied by the British, who in 1917 issued the Balfour Declaration, viewing 'with favour the establishment in Palestine of a national home for the Jewish people'. This position was endorsed by the League of Nations; in Nov. 1947 the UN called for the establishment of both a Jewish and an Arab state. Jewish settlement had been taking place throughout the British mandate.

The State of Israel was proclaimed on 14 May 1948. No Arab state was established. Neighbouring Arab states invaded Israel on 15 May without success. At the ceasefire in Jan. 1949 Israel had increased its territory by one-third.

There have been conflicts with Egypt (sometimes with the involvement of other Arab states) in the 1956 Suez crisis; the 1967 'Six-Day War', which left Israel in possession of the Gaza Strip, the West Bank (of the River Jordan) and the Sinai Peninsula; and in 1973. (For details *see* THE STATESMAN'S YEAR-BOOK, 1990–91, p. 734).

Negotiations began between Israel and Egypt at Camp David in the USA in Oct. 1978 and a peace treaty was signed on 26 March 1979. Israel had withdrawn from Sinai by April 1982.

On 18 Jan. 1991, following the air attack on Iraq by the UN-supported coalition enforcing Iraq's withdrawal from Kuwait, Iraq began a series of missile attacks on Israel, causing fatal casualties.

AREA AND POPULATION. The area of Israel, within the boundaries defined by the 1949 armistice agreements with Egypt, Jordan, the Lebanon and Syria, is 20,770 sq. km (8,017 sq. miles), with a population (June 1983 census) of 4,037,600 (estimated, 1990, 4,822,000). Population of areas under Israeli administration as a result of the Six-Day War was, in 1988: Judaea and Samaria (West Bank), 895,000, Gaza Strip, 589,000.

Crude birth rate per 1,000 population of Jewish population (1988), 20·2; non-Jewish: Moslems, 35·5; Christians, 22·9; Druzes and others, 30·5. Crude death rate, Jewish, 7·3; non-Jewish: Moslems, 3·5; Christians, 5·4; Druzes and others, 3·1. Infant mortality rate per 1,000 live births, Jewish, 7·7; non-Jewish: Moslems, 17; Christians, 10·5; Druzes and others, 18·7. Life expectancy (1987): Males, 73·6 years; females, 77. Average population growth rate, 1980–89, 1·8%. Growth rate in 1990 was 5·8%, largely due to increased immigration from the USSR.

Israel is administratively divided into 6 districts:

District	*Area (sq. km)*	*Population* [1]	*Chief town*
Northern	4,501	739,500	Nazareth
Haifa	854	602,800	Haifa
Central	1,242	938,600	Ramla
Tel Aviv	170	1,029,700	Tel Aviv
Jerusalem [2]	627	538,300	Jerusalem
Southern	14,107	529,300	Beersheba

[1] 1988. [2] Includes East Jerusalem.

On 23 Jan. 1950 the Knesset proclaimed Jerusalem the capital of the State and on 14 Dec. 1981 extended Israeli law into the Golan Heights. Population of the main towns (1988): Tel-Aviv/Jaffa, 317,800; Jerusalem, 493,500; Haifa, 222,600; Ramat Gan, 115,700; Bat-Yam, 133,100; Holon, 146,100; Petach-Tikva, 133,600; Beersheba, 113,200.

The official languages are Hebrew and Arabic.

Areas under Israeli occupation as a result of the 6-day war:

The **West Bank** has an area of 5,879 sq. km (2,270 sq. miles) and a population (1988) of 895,000, of whom 97% were Palestinian Arabs. Nearly 85% are Muslims, 7·4% Jewish and 8% Christian. In 1984, the birth rate was 3·9% and the death rate 8%. In 1987, there were 39,091 private cars and 13,710 commercial vehicles registered. There were (1988) 183,041 pupils in primary schools and 105,007 in secondary schools, while (1983) there were 7,066 students in higher education. In 1988 there were 16 hospitals and clinics with 1,336 beds.

The **Gaza Strip** has an area of 363 sq. km (140 sq. miles) and a population (1988) of 589,000. The chief town is Gaza itself, with (1979) 120,000 inhabitants. In 1984, over 98% of the population were Arabic-speaking Muslims; the birth rate was 4·8% and the death rate 0·8%. Citrus fruits, wheat and olives are grown, with farm land covering 193 sq. km (1980) and occupying most of the active workforce. Some 1,600 tonnes of fish (1984) was also caught. In 1987 there were 18,761 private cars and 4,374 commercial vehicles registered. There were (1988) 112,959 pupils in primary schools and 64,699 in secondary schools, with (1983) 2,387 students in higher education. In 1988 there were 7 hospitals and clinics with 895 beds.

Immigration. The following table shows the numbers of Jewish immigrants entering Palestine (Israel), including persons entering as travellers who subsequently registered as immigrants. For a year-by-year breakdown, *see* THE STATESMAN'S YEAR-BOOK, 1951, p. 1167.

1919–48	482,857	1958–68	384,870	1980–88	129,789
1948–57	905,740	1969–79	384,066		

During 1948–68, 45·5% of the immigrants came from Europe and America and 54·5% from Asia and Africa; in 1988, 74% came from Europe and America and 25·7% from Asia and Africa. With the liberalization of Soviet emigration policy, there has been a marked increase in immigrants from the USSR (185,000 in 1990). In all some 360,000 immigrants were expected in 1990–91.

The Jewish Agency, which, in accordance with Article IV of the Palestine Mandate, played a leading role in establishing the State of Israel continues to organize immigration.

CLIMATE. From April to Oct., the summers are long and hot, and almost rainless. From Nov. to March, the weather is generally mild, though colder in hilly areas, and this is the wet season. Jerusalem. Jan. 48°F (9°C), July 73°F (23°C). Annual rainfall 21" (528 mm). Tel Aviv. Jan. 57°F (14°C), July 81°F (27°C). Annual rainfall 22" (550 mm).

CONSTITUTION AND GOVERNMENT. Israel is an independent sovereign republic, established by proclamation on 14 May 1948.

In 1950 the Knesset (*Parliament*), which in 1949 had passed the Transition Law dealing in general terms with the powers of the Knesset, President and Cabinet, resolved to enact from time to time fundamental laws, which eventually, taken together, would form the Constitution. Fundamental laws that have been passed are: The Knesset (1958), Israel Lands (1960), the President (1964), the Government (1968), the State Economy (1975), the Army (1976), Jerusalem, capital of Israel (1980), and the Judicature (1984).

National flag: White with 2 horizontal blue stripes, the blue Shield of David in the centre.

National anthem: Hatikvah (The Hope). Words by N. N. Imber (1878); adopted as the Jewish National Anthem by the first Zionist Congress (1897).

The Knesset, a one-chamber Parliament, consists of 120 members. It is elected for a 4-year term by secret ballot and universal direct suffrage. The system of election is by proportional representation. After the Nov. 1988 elections the Knesset was composed as follows: Likud (Lik), 40; Labour Alignment (Lab), 39; Shas (Oriental Jew Religions), 6; National Religious Party, 5; Agudat Yisrael, 5; Citizens Rights

Movement, 5; Communists, 4; Mapam, 3; Tehiya, 3; Shinui, 2; Moledet, 2; Degel Hatora, 2; Tsomet, 2; Arab Democratic List, 1; Progressive List for Peace, 1. The *President* (head of state) is elected by the Knesset by secret ballot by a simple majority; his term of office is 5 years. He may be re-elected once.

Former Presidents of the State: Chaim Weizmann (1949–52); Izhak Ben-Zvi (1952–63); Zalman Shazar (1963–68); Ephraim Katzir (1968–78); Yitzhak Navon (1978–83).

President: Chaim Herzog, elected 1983; re-elected 1988.

In June 1990 Yitzhak Shamir formed a new Likud government. In Nov. 1990 the government entered into a coalition with Agudat Israel, an orthodox religious party. In Feb. 1991 the Cabinet consisted of:

Prime Minister: Yitzhak Shamir (b. 1916, Lik).

Deputy Prime Minister and Foreign Minister: David Levy (Lik). *Deputy Prime Minister and Minister of Industry and Commerce:* Moshe Nissim (Lik). *Defence:* Moshe Arens (Lik). *Finance:* Yitzhak Moda'i (Zionist Renewal). *Environment:* Ariel Sharon (Lik). *Justice:* Dan Meridor (Lik). *Transport:* Moshe Katzav (Lik). *Economy:* David Magen (Lik). *Police:* Ronni Milo (Lik). *Tourism:* Gideon Patt (Lik). *Health:* Ehud Olmert (Lik). *Education:* Zevulun Hammer (National Religious Party). *Religious Affairs:* Avner Shaki (National Religious Party). *Science and Energy:* Yuval Neeman (Tehiya). *Agriculture:* Raphael Eytan (Tsomet). *Interior:* Arie Der'i (Shas). *Communications:* Raphael Pinhasi (Shas). *Immigration:* Yitzhak Peretz (Shas). *Without portfolio:* Rehavam Ze'evi (Homeland).

Local Government. Local authorities are of three kinds, namely, municipal corporations, local councils and regional councils. Their status, powers and duties are prescribed by statute. Regional councils are local authorities set up in agricultural areas and include all the agricultural settlements in the area under their jurisdiction. All local authorities exercise their authority mainly by means of bye-laws approved by the Minister of the Interior. Their revenue is derived from rates and a surcharge on income tax. Local authorities are elected for a 4-year term of office concurrently with general elections.

There were (1989) 42 municipalities (3 Arab), 136 local councils (63 Arab and Druze) and 54 regional councils.

DEFENCE. The Defence Service Law, provides a compulsory 36-month conscription for men (Jews and Druze only). Unmarried women (Jews only) serve 24 months.

The Israel Defence Force is a unified force, in which army, navy and air force are subordinate to a single chief-of-staff. The Minister of Defence is *de facto* commander-in-chief but from Oct. 1973 the cabinet formed a defence committee with authority to make decisions on military operations.

Army. The Army is organized in 3 armoured divisions, 3 infantry divisions, 5 mechanized infantry brigades, 3 artillery battalions and 1 surface-to-surface missile battalion. The Reserves are organized in 9 armoured divisions, 1 mechanized (air mobile) division, 10 infantry and 4 artillery brigades. Equipment includes 1,080 Centurion, 550 M-48A5, 1,400 M-60/A1/A3, 488 T-54/-55, 110 T-62 and 660 Merkava main battle tanks and 6,000 other armoured fighting vehicles. Strength (1991) 104,000 (conscripts 88,000), rising to 598,000 on mobilization.

Navy. The Navy, tasked primarily for coastal protection and based at Haifa, Ashdod and Eilat, includes 3 small diesel submarines, 26 missile craft, 22 of which are of the evolving SA'AR types, from 250 to 500 tonnes, and 3 missile-armed hydrofoils. There are an additional 37 fast inshore patrol craft, 9 amphibious craft and a few minor auxiliaries.

Planned construction includes 2 corvettes and 2 submarines, to be built through the US foreign military sales programme.

Naval personnel in 1990 totalled 9,000 officers and men, of whom 3,000 are conscripts, including a Naval Cammando of 300. There are also 1,000 naval reservists available on mobilization.

Air Force. The Air Force has a personnel strength (1990) of 28,000 (19,000 conscripts), rising to 37,000 on mobilization, with about 629 first-line aircraft, all jets, of Israeli and US manufacture. There are 3 squadrons with about 50 F-15s, and 6 squadrons with the first 140 of a planned 250 F-16s in an interceptor role; 4 squadrons with 110 F-4E Phantoms, 4 squadrons with about 160 Kfirs, and 3 squadrons with A-4E/H/N Skyhawks in the fighter-bomber/attack role; and 15 RF-4E reconnaissance fighters; supported by 4 E-2C Hawkeye airborne early warning and control aircraft, RC-12 and RU-21 Elint aircraft. There are transport squadrons of turboprop C-130/KC-130 Hercules, C-47, Arava, Islander, and Boeing 707 (some equipped for tanker or ECM duties) aircraft, helicopter squadrons of CH-53, Super Frelon, AH-1 Huey-Cobra, Hughes 500MD/TOW Defender, JetRanger, Dauphin, Agusta-Bell 205, 206 and 212 aircraft, and training units with locally-built Magister jet trainers, which can be used also in a light ground attack role. Missiles in service include surface-to-air Hawks and surface-to-surface Lances.

INTERNATIONAL RELATIONS

Membership. Israel is a member of UN.

ECONOMY

Budget. The budget year runs from 1 April to 31 March. Government revenue in 1987-88 amounted to 44,539m. new shekels; expenditure, 44,021m. new shekels.

Currency. The unit of currency is the *shekel* (ILS) of 100 *agorot*. Currency in circulation on 31 Dec. 1984 was I£161,651m. (bank-notes and coins). In March 1991, £1 = 3·86 *shekel*; US$ = 1·32 *shekel*.

Banking and Finance. The Bank of Israel was established by law in 1954 as Israel's central bank. Its *Governor* is appointed by the President on the recommendation of the Cabinet for a 5-year term. He acts as economic adviser to the Government and has ministerial status. The *Governor* is Michael Bruno. There are 26 commercial banks headed by Bank Leumi Le Israel, Bank Hapoalim and Israel Discount Bank, 2 merchant banks, 1 foreign bank, 15 mortgage banks and 9 lending institutions specifically set up to aid industry and agriculture. The government holds a majority stake in the 4 largest banks, but there are plans to privatize them by 1992.

Weights and Measures. The metric system is in general use. The (metrical) *dunam* = 1,000 sq. metres (about 0·25 acre).

Jewish Year. The Jewish year 5749 corresponds to 12 Sept. 1988–29 Sept. 1989; 5750 30 Sept. 1989–19 Sept. 1990; 5751 20 Sept. 1990–8 Sept. 1991.

ENERGY AND NATURAL RESOURCES

Electricity. Electric-power production amounted during 1988 to 18,761m. kwh. Supply 230 volts; 50 Hz.

Oil and Gas. The only significant indigenous hydrocarbon known to be found is oil shale. In 1988 recoverable potential was estimated to be 250m. tons of oil.

Minerals. The most valuable natural resources of the country are the potash, bromine and other salt deposits of the Dead Sea, which are exploited by the Dead Sea Works, Ltd. Geological research and exploration of the natural resources in the Negev are undertaken by the Israel Mining Corporation. Potash production in 1986 was 2,035,000 tons.

Agriculture. In the coastal plain (Sharon, Emek Hefer and the Shephelah) mixed farming, poultry raising, citriculture and vineyards are the main agricultural activities. The Emek (the Valley of Jezreel) is the main agricultural centre of Israel. Mixed farming is to be found throughout the valleys; the sub-tropical Beisan and Jordan plainlands are also centres of banana plantations and fish breeding. In Galilee mixed farming, olive and tobacco plantations prevail. The Hills of Ephraim are a vineyard centre; many parts of the hill country are under afforestation. In the northern Negev farming has been aided by the Yarkon–Negev water pipeline. This has become part of the overall project of the 'National Water Carrier', which is to take water from the Sea of Galilee (Lake Kinnereth) to the south. The plan includes a number of regional projects such as the Lake Kinnereth–Negev pipeline which came into operation in 1964; it has an annual capacity of 320m. cu. metres.

The area under cultivation (in 1,000 dunams) in 1988 was 4,317, of which 2,156 were under irrigation. Of the total cultivated area 2,361 dunams were under field crops, 422 under vegetables, potatoes, pumpkins and melons, 359 under citrus and plantations, 26 under fish ponds and the rest under miscellaneous crops, including auxiliary farms, nurseries, flowers, etc.

Industrial crops, such as cotton, have successfully been introduced. In 1988 the area under cotton totalled 503,000 dunams.

Production, 1988 (in 1,000 tonnes): Wheat, 211; barley, 20; maize, 25; potatoes, 207; pumpkins, 25; melons, 142; tomatoes, 236; citrus fruit, 1,282; seed cotton, 196.

Livestock (1988) included 307,000 cattle, 394,000 sheep, 125,000 goats, 130,000 pigs, 4,000 horses, 25m. poultry.

Characteristic types of rural settlement are, among others, the following: (1) The *Kibbutz* and *Kvutza* (communal collective settlement), where all property and earnings are collectively owned and work is collectively organized. (126,100 people lived in 270 settlements in 1988). (2) The *Moshav* (workers' co-operative smallholders' settlement) which is founded on the principles of mutual aid and equality of opportunity between the members, all farms being equal in size. (146, 500 in 409). (3) The *Moshav Shitufi* (co-operative settlement), which is based on collective ownership and economy as in the *Kibbutz*, but with each family having its own house and being responsible for its own domestic services. (11,300 in 47). (4) Other rural settlements in which land and property are privately owned and every resident is responsible for his own well-being. In 1988 there were 226 villages with a population of 112,000.

INDUSTRY. A wide range of products is manufactured, processed or finished in the country, including chemicals, metal products, textiles, tyres, diamonds, paper, plastics, leather goods, glass and ceramics, building materials, precision instruments, tobacco, foodstuffs, electrical and electronic equipment.

Labour. The workforce was 1,553,000 in 1989

Trade Unions. The General Federation of Labour (Histadrut) founded in 1920, had, in 1987, 1·6m. members (including 170,000 Arab and Druze members); including workers' families, this membership represents 71·5% of the population covering 87% of all wage-earners. Several trades unions also exist representing other political and religious groups.

FOREIGN ECONOMIC RELATIONS

Commerce. External trade, in US$1m., for calendar years:

	1984	*1985*	*1986*	*1987*	*1988*
Imports	8,257	8,202	9,550	11,916	12,960
Exports	6,242	6,682	7,712	8,475	9,739

The main exportable commodities are citrus fruit and by-products, fruit-juices, flowers, wines and liquor, sweets, polished diamonds, chemicals, tyres, textiles, metal products, machinery, electronic and transportation equipment. The main exports were, in 1988 (US$1m.): Diamonds, 2,837; chemical and oil products, 1,122·6; agricultural products including citrus fruit, 573; manufactured goods, machinery and transport equipment, 4,328. In 1987 64·1% of imports came from Europe, 17·2% from Canada and USA, 8·3% from Africa and Asia. Of exports, 36·4% went to Europe, 33·5% to Canada and USA, 14·2% to Africa and Asia.

Total trade between Israel and UK (British Department of Trade returns, in £1,000 sterling):

	1986	*1987*	*1988*	*1989*	*1990*
Imports to UK	385,164	437,014	460,289	479,840	506,106
Exports and re-exports from UK	452,407	523,591	487,255	502,411	567,712

Tourism. In 1988 there were about 1,165,000 tourists.

COMMUNICATIONS

Roads. There were 12,980 km of paved roads in 1988. Registered motor vehicles in 1988 totalled 952,786, including 8,693 buses, 143,805 trucks and 753,450 private cars.

Railways. Internal communications (1988) are provided by 575 km of standard gauge line. Construction is in progress of 215 km of new line linking Eilat on the Gulf of Aqaba with Sedom and the existing rail network. In 1989, 2·3m. passengers and 6·6m. tonnes of freight were carried.

Aviation. Air communications are centred in the airport of Ben Gurion, near Tel-Aviv. In 1988, 10,757 planes landed at Israeli airports on international flights; 1,705,000 passengers arrived, 1,726,000 departed. In 1988, 91,271 tons of freight were loaded and 82,458 tons unloaded. The Israeli airline El Al maintains regular flights to London, Paris, Rome, Amsterdam, Brussels, Cairo, Madrid, Lisbon, Bucharest, Athens, Vienna, New York, Montreal, Zurich, Munich, Istanbul, Johannesburg, Nairobi, Frankfurt and Copenhagen. In 1986–87 El Al carried 1·5m. passengers.

Shipping. Israel has 3 commercial ports, Haifa, Ashdod and Eilat. In 1987, 3,243 ships departed from Israeli ports; 19m. tons. of freight were handled. The merchant fleet consisted in 1988 of 72 vessels, totalling 1,573,000 GRT.

Telecommunications. The Ministry of Communications controls the postal service, and a public company responsible to the Ministry administers the telecommunications service. In 1986 there were 594 post offices and postal agencies, 50 mobile post offices and (1988) 1·94m. telephones.

Israeli television and the state radio station, *Kol Israel* are controlled by the Israel Broadcasting Authority, established in 1965. Radio licences in 1985 numbered approximately 1·12m. and television licences (1986) 936,000.

Cinemas. In 1987 there were 162 cinemas.

Newspapers (1987). There were 23 daily newspapers.

JUSTICE, RELIGION, EDUCATION AND WELFARE

Justice. *Law.* Under the Law and Administration Ordinance, 5708/1948, the first law passed by the Provisional Council of State, the law of Israel is the law which was obtaining in Palestine on 14 May 1948 in so far as it is not in conflict with that Ordinance or any other law passed by the Israel legislature and with such modifications as result from the establishment of the State and its authorities.

Capital punishment was abolished in 1954, except for support given to the Nazis and for high treason.

The law of Palestine was derived from three main sources, namely, Ottoman law, English law (Common Law and Equity) and the law enacted by the Palestine legislature, which to a great extent was modelled on English law. The Ottoman law in its turn was derived from three main sources, namely, Moslem law which had survived in the Ottoman Empire, French law adapted by the Ottomans and the personal law of the non-Moslem communities.

Civil Courts. Municipal courts, established in certain municipal areas, have criminal jurisdiction over offences against municipal regulations and bye-laws and certain specified offences committed within a municipal area.

Magistrates courts, established in each district and sub-district, have limited jurisdiction in both civil and criminal matters.

District courts, sitting at Jerusalem, Tel-Aviv and Haifa, have jurisdiction, as courts of first instance, in all civil matters not within the jurisdiction of magistrates courts, and in all criminal matters, and as appellate courts from magistrates courts and municipal courts.

The Supreme Court has jurisdiction as a court of first instance (sitting as a High Court of Justice dealing mainly with administrative matters) and as an appellate court from the district courts (sitting as a Court of Civil or of Criminal Appeal).

In addition, there are various tribunals for special classes of cases, such as the Rents Tribunals and the Tribunals for the Prevention of Profiteering and Speculation. Settlement Officers deal with disputes with regard to the ownership or possession of land in settlement areas constituted under the Land (Settlement of Title) Ordinance.

Religious Courts. The rabbinical courts of the Jewish community have exclusive jurisdiction in matters of marriage and divorce, alimony and confirmation of wills of members of their community other than foreigners, concurrent jurisdiction with the civil courts in such matters of members of their community who are foreigners if they consent to the jurisdiction, and concurrent jurisdiction with the civil courts in all other matters of personal status of all members of their community, whether foreigners or not, with the consent of all parties to the action, save that such courts may not grant a decree of dissolution of marriage to a foreign subject.

The courts of the several recognized Christian communities have a similar jurisdiction over members of their respective communities.

The Moslem religious courts have exclusive jurisdiction in all matters of personal status over Moslems who are not foreigners, and over Moslems who are foreigners, if under the law of their nationality they are subject in such matters to the jurisdiction of Moslem religious courts.

Where any action of personal status involves persons of different religious communities, the President of the Supreme Court will decide which court shall have jurisdiction, and whenever a question arises as to whether or not a case is one of personal status within the exclusive jurisdiction of a religious court, the matter must be referred to a special tribunal composed of 2 judges of the Supreme Court and the president of the highest court of the religious community concerned in Israel.

Religion. Religious affairs are under the supervision of a special Ministry, with departments for the Christian and Moslem communities. The religious affairs of each community remain under the full control of the ecclesiastical authorities concerned: in the case of the Jews, the Sephardi and Ashkenazi Chief Rabbis, in the case of the Christians, the heads of the various communities, and in the case of the Moslems, the Qadis. The Druze were officially recognized in 1957 as an autonomous religious community.

In 1988 there were: Jews, 3,659,000; Moslems, 634,600; Christians, 105,000; Druze and others, 78,100.

The Jewish Sabbath and Holy Days are observed as days of rest in the public services. Full provision is, however, made for the free exercise of other faiths, and for the observance by their adherents of their respective days of rest and Holy Days.

Education. Laws passed by the Knesset in 1949 and 1978 provide for free and compulsory education from 5 to 16 years of age. There is free education until 18 years of age.

The State Education Law of 12 Aug. 1953 established a unified state-controlled elementary school system wlth a provlsion for special religious schools. The standard curriculum for all elementary schools is issued by the Ministry with a possibility of adding supplementary subjects comprising not more than 25% of the total syllabus. Most schools in towns are maintained by municipalities, a number are private and some are administered by teachers' co-operatives or trustees.

Statistics relating to schools under government supervision, 1988–89:

Type of School [1]	*Schools*	*Teachers*	*Pupils*
Hebrew Education			
Primary schools	1,323	32,197	482,215
Schools for handicapped children	191	3,162	11,434
Schools of intermediate division	304	13,274	120,339
Secondary schools	536		202,261
Vocational schools	315	24,649	94,454
Agricultural schools	25		5,022
Arab Education			
Primary schools	312	6,424	138,074
Schools for handicapped children	15	220	1,146
Schools of intermediate division	63	1,868	27,230

Type of School [1]	Schools	Teachers	Pupils
Hebrew Education (cont'd)			
Secondary schools	84	2,542	38,237
Vocational schools	42		6,516
Agricultural schools	2		718

[1] Schools providing more than one type of education are included more than once.

There are also a number of private schools maintained by religious foundations—Jewish, Christian and Moslem—and also by private societies.

The Hebrew University of Jerusalem, founded in 1925, comprises faculties of the humanities, social sciences, law, science, medicine and agriculture. In 1988–89 it had 16,000 students. The Technion in Haifa had 8,730 students. The Weizmann Institute of Science in Rehovoth, founded in 1949, had 650 students.

Tel Aviv University had 18,730 students. The religious Bar-Ilan University at Ramat Gan, opened in 1965 had 8,830 students. The Haifa University had 6,540 students. The Ben Gurion University had 5,410 students.

Health. In 1988 Israel had 161 hospitals with 27,842 beds and 9,500 doctors.

The National Insurance Law, which took effect in April 1954, provides for old-age pensions, survivors' insurance, work-injury insurance, maternity insurance, family allowances and unemployment benefits.

DIPLOMATIC REPRESENTATIVES

Of Israel in Great Britain (2 Palace Green, London, W8 4QB)
Ambassador: Yoav Biran (accredited 24 Nov. 1988).

Of Great Britain in Israel (192 Hayarkon St., Tel Aviv 63405)
Ambassador: Mark Elliott, CMG.

Of Israel in the USA (3514 International Dr., NW, Washington, D.C., 20008)
Ambassador: Moshe Arad.

Of the USA in Israel (71 Hayarkon St., Tel Aviv)
Ambassador: William A. Brown.

Of Israel to the United Nations
Ambassador: Yohanan Bein.

Further Reading

Statistical Information: There is a Central Bureau of Statistics at the Prime Minister's Office, Jerusalem. It publishes monthly bulletins of statistics (economic and social), foreign trade statistics and price statistics.
Atlas of Israel. 3rd ed. 1985
Government Yearbook. Government Printer, Jerusalem. 1951 ff. (latest issue, 1971/72)
Facts about Israel. Ministry of Foreign Affairs, Jerusalem, 1985
Statistical Abstract of Israel. Government Printer, Jerusalem (from 1949/50)
Israel Yearbook. Tel-Aviv, 1948–49 ff.
Statistical Bulletin of Israel. 1949 ff.
Reshumoth (Official Gazette)
Middle East Record, ed. Y. Oron. London, 1960 ff.
Laws of the State of Israel. Authorized translation. Government Printer, Jerusalem, 1958 ff.
Alkalay, R., *The Complete English–Hebrew Dictionary.* 4 vols. Tel-Aviv, 1959–61
Ben-Gurion, D., *Ben-Gurion Looks Back.* London, 1965.—*The Jews in Their Land.* London, 1966.—*Israel: A Personal History.* New York, 1971
Gilbert, M., *The Arab-Israeli Conflict: Its History in Maps.* 3rd ed. London, 1981
Harkabi, Y., *Israel's Fateful Decisions.* London, 1989
Harris, W., *Taking Root: Israeli Settlement in the West Bank, The Golan and Gaza Sinai 1967–1980.* Chichester, 1981
Kieval, G. R., *Party Politics in Israel and the Occupied Territories.* Westport, 1983
Louis, W. R. and Stookey, R. W., *The End of the Palestine Mandate.* London, 1986
O'Brien, C. C., *The Siege.* London, 1986
Peri, Y., *Between Battles and Ballots: Israeli Military in Politics.* CUP, 1983
Reich, B., *Israel: Land of Tradition and Conflict.* London, 1986
Sachar, H. M., *A History of Israel.* 2 vols. OUP, 1976 and 1987

Sager, S., *The Parliamentary System of Israel*. Syracuse Univ. Press, 1986
Segev, T., *1949: The First Israelis*. New York, 1986
Sharkansky, I., *The Political Economy of Israel*. Oxford and Santa Barbara, 1986
Shimshoni, D., *Israeli Democracy: The Middle of the Journey*. New York, 1982
Snyder, E. M. and Kreiner, E., *Israel*. [Bibliography] Oxford and Santa Barbara, 1985
Wolffsohn, M., *Politik in Israel*. Opladen, 1983

National Library: The Jewish National and University Library, Jerusalem.

ITALY

Capital: Rome
Population: 57·6m. (1989)
GNP per capita: US$13,320 (1988)

Repubblica Italiana

HISTORY. On 10 June 1946 Italy became a republic on the announcement by the Court of Cassation that a majority of the voters at the referendum held on 2 June had voted for a republic. The final figures, announced on 18 June, showed: For a republic, 12,718,641 (54·3% of the valid votes cast, which numbered 23,437,143); for the retention of the monarchy, 10,718,502 (45·7%); invalid and contested, 1,509,735. Total 24,946,878, or 89·1% of the registered electors, who numbered 28,005,449. For the results of the polling in the 13 leading cities, *see* THE STATESMAN'S YEAR-BOOK , 1951, p. 1175. Voting was compulsory, open to both men and women 21 years of age or older, including members of the Civil Service and the Armed Forces; former active Fascists and a few other categories were excluded.

On 18 June the then Provisional Government without specifically proclaiming the republic, issued an 'Order of the Day' decreeing that all court verdicts should in future be handed down 'in the name of the Italian people', that the *Gazzetta Ufficiale del Regno d'Italia* should be re-named *Gazzetta Ufficiale della Repubblica Italiana,* that all references to the monarchy should be deleted from legal and government statements and that the shield of the House of Savoy should be removed from the Italian flag.

Thus ended the reign of the House of Savoy, whose kings had ruled over Piedmont for 9 centuries and as Kings of Italy since 18 Feb. 1861. (For fuller account of the House of Savoy, *see* THE STATESMAN'S YEAR-BOOK, 1946, p. 1021.) The Crown Prince Umberto, son of King Victor Emmanuel III, became Lieut.-Gen. (*i.e.*, Regent) of the kingdom on 5 June 1944. Following the abdication and retirement to Egypt of his father on 9 May 1946, Umberto was declared King Umberto II; his reign lasted to 13 June, when he left the country. King Victor Emmanuel III died in Alexandria on 28 Dec. 1947.

AREA AND POPULATION. Italy is bounded north by Switzerland and Austria, east by Yugoslavia and the Adriatic Sea, south-east by the Ionian Sea, south by the Mediterranean Sea, south-west by the Tyrrhenian Sea and Ligurian Sea and west by France. The population (present in actual boundaries) at successive censuses were as follows:

31 Dec. 1881	29,277,927	21 April 1936	42,302,680
10 Feb. 1901	33,370,138	4 Nov. 1951	47,158,738
10 June 1911	35,694,582	15 Oct. 1961	49,903,878
1 Dec. 1921	37,403,956	24 Oct. 1971	53,744,737
21 April 1931	40,582,043	25 Oct. 1981	56,243,935

The following table gives area and population of the Regions (census 1981 and estimate, 1988):

Regions	*Area in sq. km (1981)*	*Resident pop. census, 1981*	*Resident pop. estimate, 1989*	*Density per sq. km (1981)*
Piemonte	25,399	4,479,031	4,357,559	175
Valle d'Aosta	3,262	112,353	115,270	35
Lombardia	23,856	8,891,652	8,911,995	373
Trentino-Alto Adige	13,613	873,413	886,679	64
Bolzano-Bozen	*7,400*	*430,568*	*439,765*	*58*
Trento	*6,213*	*442,845*	*446,914*	*71*
Veneto	18,364	4,345,047	4,385,023	235
Friuli-Venezia Giulia	7,846	1,233,984	1,202,877	157
Liguria	5,416	1,807,893	1,727,212	332
Emilia Romagna	22,123	3,957,513	3,921,597	178
Toscana	22,992	3,581,051	3,560,582	155
Umbria	8,456	807,552	820,316	95
Marche	9,694	1,412,404	1,430,726	145
Lazio	17,203	5,001,684	5,170,672	289
Abruzzi	10,794	1,217,791	1,266,448	113
Molise	4,438	328,371	335,348	73

Regions	Area in sq. km (1981)	Resident pop. census, 1981	Resident pop. estimate, 1989	Density per sq. km (1981)
Campania	13,595	5,463,134	5,808,705	398
Puglia	19,347	3,871,617	4,069,359	199
Basilicata	9,992	610,186	623,175	60
Calabria	15,080	2,061,182	2,152,539	135
Sicilia	25,708	4,906,878	5,172,785	189
Sardegna	24,090	1,594,175	1,657,562	66
Total	301,268	56,556,911	57,576,429	187

Vital statistics for calendar years:

	Marriages	Living births: Legitimate	Living births: Illegitimate	Living births: Total	Still-born	Deaths excl. of still-born
1982	312,486	590,042	29,055	619,097	4,757	534,935
1983	303,663	572,641	29,287	601,928	4,396	564,330
1984	300,889	557,773	30,098	587,871	4,175	534,676
1985	298,523	546,224	31,121	577,345	3,871	547,436
1986	297,540	523,876	31,569	555,445	3,584	544,489
1987	306,264	519,406	32,133	551,539	3,483	532,771
1988	318,296	535,266 [1]	33,025 [1]	568,291 [1]	3,504 [1]	539,426
1989 [1]	311,613	521,886	33,800	555,686	3,306	525,960

[1] Provisional.

Emigrants to non-European countries, by sea and air: 1978, 23,589; 1979, 21,302; 1980, 20,360; 1981, 20,628; 1982, 22,324; 1983, 20,443; 1984, 16,776; 1985, 16,151; 1986, 13,215; 1987, 12,796; 1988, 11,457. Since 1960 nearly nine-tenths of these emigrants have gone to Canada, USA and Australia.

Communes of more than 100,000 inhabitants, with population resident at the census of 25 Oct. 1981 and on 31 Dec. 1989:

	1981	1989		1981	1989
Roma (Rome)	2,840,259	2,803,931	Perugia	142,348	149,261
Milano (Milan)	1,604,773	1,449,403	Ravenna	138,034	136,166
Napoli (Naples)	1,212,387	1,204,149	Pescara	131,330	128,695
Torino (Turin)	1,117,154	1,002,863	Reggio nell'E.	130,376	130,825
Genova (Genoa)	762,895	706,754	Rimini	127,813	130,638
Palermo	701,782	731,418	Monza	123,145	123,073
Bologna	459,080	417,410	Bergamo	122,142	117,584
Firenze (Florence)	448,331	413,069	Sassari	119,596	119,717
Catania	380,328	366,226	Siracusa (Syracuse)	117,615	124,606
Bari	371,022	355,352	La Spezia	115,392	104,511
Venezia (Venice)	346,146	320,990	Vicenza	114,598	109,109
Verona	265,932	258,476	Terni	111,564	110,020
Messina	260,233	273,570	Forli	110,806	109,986
Trieste	252,369	233,047	Piacenza	109,039	104,023
Taranto	244,101	244,512	Cosenza	106,801	105,349
Padova (Padua)	234,678	220,358	Ancona	106,498	103,454
Cagliari	233,848	219,095	Bolzano	105,180	100,707
Brescia	206,661	196,935	Pisa	104,509	102,150
Modena	180,312	176,857	Torre del Greco	103,605	103,577
Parma	179,019	174,341	Novara	102,086	103,088
Livorno (Leghorn)	175,741	171,346	Udine	102,021	–
Reggio di C.	173,486	178,620	Catanzaro	100,832	103,521
Prato	160,220	165,888	Alessandria	100,523	–
Salerno	157,385	152,159	Trento	99,179	101,416
Foggia	156,467	159,199	Lecce	91,289	101,957
Ferrara	149,453	141,404			

CLIMATE. The climate varies considerably with latitude. In the south, it is warm temperate, with little rain in the summer months, but the north is cool temperate with rainfall more evenly distributed over the year.

Florence, Jan. 42°F (5·6°C), July 76°F (25°C). Annual rainfall 36" (901 mm). Milan, Jan. 35°F (2°C), July 75°F (24°C). Annual rainfall 32" (802 mm). Naples, Jan. 48°F (8·9°C), July 77°F (25·6°C). Annual rainfall 34" (850 mm). Palermo, Jan. 52°F (11·1°C), July 79°F (26·1°C). Annual rainfall 28" (702 mm). Rome, Jan. 44·5°F (7°C), July 77°F (25°C). Annual rainfall 26" (657 mm). Venice, Jan. 38°F (3·3°C), July 75°F (23·9°C). Annual rainfall 29" (725 mm).

CONSTITUTION AND GOVERNMENT. The new Constitution was passed by the constituent assembly by 453 votes to 62 on 22 Dec. 1947; it came into force on 1 Jan. 1948. The Constitution consists of 139 articles and 18 transitional clauses. Its main dispositions are as follows:

Italy is described as 'a democratic republic founded on work'. Parliament consists of the *Chamber of Deputies* and the *Senate*. The Chamber is elected for 5 years by universal and direct suffrage and it consists of 630 deputies. The Senate is elected for 5 years on a regional basis; each Region having at least 7 senators, consisting of 315 elected senators; the Valle d'Aosta is represented by 1 senator only. The President of the Republic can nominate 5 senators for life from eminent men in the social, scientific, artistic and literary spheres. On the expiry of his term of office, the President of the Republic becomes a senator by right and for life, unless he declines. The *President* of the Republic is elected in a joint session of Chamber and Senate, to which are added 3 delegates from each Regional Council (1 from the Valle d'Aosta). A two-thirds majority is required for the election, but after a third indecisive scrutiny the absolute majority of votes is sufficient. The President must be 50 years or over; his term lasts for 7 years. The President of the Senate acts as his deputy. The President can dissolve the chambers of parliament, except during the last 6 months of his term of office.

The Cabinet can be forced to resign only on a motivated motion of censure; the defeat of a government bill does not involve the resignation of the Government.

The salary of the President in 1990 was 248·41m. lira a year; of the Prime Minister, 240m. lira; and of members of the Chamber of Deputies, 180m. lira.

A Constitutional Court, consisting of 15 judges who are appointed, 5 each, by the President of the Republic, Parliament (in joint session) and the highest law and administrative courts, has rights similar to those of the Supreme Court of the USA. It can decide on the constitutionality of laws and decrees, define the powers of the State and Regions, judge conflicts between the State and Regions and between the Regions, and try the President of the Republic and the Ministers. The court was set up in Dec. 1955.

The reorganization of the Fascist Party is forbidden. Direct male descendants of King Victor Emmanuel are excluded from all public offices, have no right to vote or to be elected, and are banned from Italian territory; their estates are forfeit to the State. Titles of nobility are no longer recognized, but those existing before 28 Oct. 1922 are retained as part of the name.

National flag: Three vertical strips of green, white, red.

National anthem: Fratelli d'Italia ('Brothers of Italy'; words by G. Mameli; tune by M. Novaro, 1847).

Head of State: On 3 July 1985 Chamber and Senate in joint session elected by an absolute majority (752 votes out of 977 votes cast) Francesco Cossiga (Christian Democrat; b. 1928), President of the Republic.

Former Presidents of the Republic: Luigi Einaudi (1948–55); Giovanni Gronchi (1955–62); Antonio Segni (1962–64); Giuseppe Saragat (1964–71); Giovanni Leone (1971–78); Alessandro Pertini (1978–85).

General elections for the Senate and Chamber of Deputies took place on 22 July 1989.

Senate. Christian Democrats, 125; Communists, 101; Socialists, 36; Italian Social Movement, 16; Social Democrats, 5; Republicans, 8; Liberals, 3; other groups, 21. Total: 315.

Chamber. Christian Democrats, 234; Communists, 177; Socialists, 94; Italian Social Movement, 35; Republicans, 21; Social Democrats, 17; Liberals, 11; Radical Party, 13; Green Party, 13; other groups, 15. Total: 630.

The coalition government was composed as follows in Oct. 1990.

Prime Minister: Giulio Andreotti (DC).

Vice Prime Minister: Claudio Martelli (PSI).

Foreign Affairs: Gianni De Michelis (PSI).

Interior: Vincenzo Scotti (DC).

Justice: (Vacant).

Southern Affairs: Giovanni Maroggio (DC).
Treasury: Guido Carli (DC).
Budget: Paolo Cirino Pomicino (DC).
Finance: Rino Formica (PSI).
Defence: Virginio Rognoni (DC).
Education: Gerardo Bianco (DC).
Public Works: Giovanni Prandini (DC).
Agriculture: Vito Saccamandi (DC).
Transport: Carlo Bernini (DC).
Post: Oscar Mammi (PRI).
Industry: Adolfo Battaglia (PRI).
Labour: Carlo Donat Cattin (DC).
Foreign Trade: Renato Ruggiero (PSI).
Merchant Navy: Carlo Vizzini (PSDI).
State Shareholdings: vacant.
Health: Francesco De Lorenzo (PLI).
Tourism: Carlo Tognoli (PSI).
Culture: Ferdinando Facchiano (PSDI)
EEC Affairs: Pierluigi Romita (PSI).
Public Administration: Remo Gaspari (DC).
Scientific Research and Universities: Antonio Ruberti (PSI).
Regional and Institutional Affairs: Antonio Maccanico (PRI).
Relations with Parliament: Egidio Sterpa (PLI).
Civil Protection: Vito Lattanzio (DC).
Ecology: Giorgio Ruffolo (PSI).
Urban Problems: Carmelo Conte (PSI).
Special Affairs: Rosa Russo Jervolino (DC).

Regional Administration. Italy is administratively divided into 15 autonomous regions, 5 autonomous regions with special statute, regions, provinces and municipalities. The regions have their own parliaments (*consiglio regionale*) and governments (*giunta regionale e presidente*) with certain legislative and administrative functions adapted to the circumstances of each region. A government commissioner co-ordinates regional and national activities.

Regional provincial and municipal elections were held in May 1990. Turn-out was 86·3%. Share of votes cast: Christian Democrats, 33·4%; Communists, 24%; Socialists, 15·3%; various regional autonomy movements, 5·6%; Greens, 5%; Italian Social Movement (MSI), 4%. Results were as follows:

Regions	*Election date*	*Christian Democrats*	*Communists*	*Socialists*	*Social Movement*	*Social Democrats*	*Republicans*	*Liberals*	*Others*	*Total*
Piemonte	6 May 1990	18	14	9	2	2	2	2	11	60
Valle d'Aosta [1]	26 June 1988	7	5	3	1	–	1	–	18	35
Lombardia	6 May 1990	25	15	12	2	1	2	1	22	80
Trentino-Alto Adige [1]	20 Nov. 1988	20	4	5	5	1	1	1	32	70
Veneto	6 May 1990	27	10	8	1	1	1	1	11	60
Friuli-Venezia Giulia [1]	26 June 1988	24	11	12	3	2	1	1	8	62
Liguria	6 May 1990	12	12	6	1	1	1	1	6	40
Emilia-Romagna	6 May 1990	13	23	6	1	1	2	1	3	50
Toscana	6 May 1990	14	22	6	1	1	1	1	4	50
Umbria	6 May 1990	9	12	5	1	–	1	–	2	30
Marche	6 May 1990	15	13	5	1	1	1	1	3	40
Lazio	6 May 1990	22	15	9	4	2	3	1	4	60
Abruzzi	6 May 1990	20	8	6	1	1	1	1	2	40
Molise	6 May 1990	19	4	4	1	1	1	–	–	30
Campania	6 May 1990	25	10	12	3	3	3	1	3	60
Puglia	6 May 1990	22	10	10	3	2	1	1	1	50
Basilicata	6 May 1990	15	6	6	1	2	–	–	–	30
Calabria	6 May 1990	16	8	9	2	2	1	1	1	40
Sicilia [1]	22 June 1986	36	19	13	8	4	5	3	2	90
Sardegna [1]	11 June 1989	29	19	12	3	4	3	–	10	80

[1] Autonomous regions with special statute.

DEFENCE. Most of the restrictions imposed upon Italy in Part IV of the peace treaty signed on 10 Feb. 1947 were repudiated by the signatories on 21 Dec. 1951, only the USSR objecting.

Head of the armed forces is the Defence Chief of Staff. In 1947 the ministries of war, navy and air were merged into the ministry of defence. The technical and scientific council for defence directs all research activities.

National service lasts 12 months in the Army and Air Force, and 18 months in the Navy.

Army. The Army consists of 3 corps, one of which is mountain, consisting of 8 mechanized, 4 armoured, 5 mountain and 1 motorized brigades. In addition there is a rapid intervention force, 2 amphibious battalions and a support brigade with missiles. Equipment includes 313 M-47, 300 M-60A1 and 920 Leopard main battle tanks. The Army air corps operates 91 light aircraft and 356 helicopters. Strength (1991) 260,000 (207,000 conscripts), with 584,000 reserves. The paramilitary Carabinieri number 111,400.

Navy. The principal ships of the Navy are the light aircraft carrier *Giuseppe Garibaldi*, the helicopter-carrying cruiser *Vittorio Veneto*, and the guided missile cruiser *Andrea Doria*. The *Giuseppe Garibaldi*, 13,450 tonnes, was completed in 1985 and currently operates an air group of 16 SH-3D Sea King anti-submarine helicopters. She is also armed with 4 Teseo anti-ship missiles. The *Vittorio Veneto*, completed in 1969, is of 9,650 tonnes, and operates a squadron of 6 AB-212 anti-submarine helicopters as well as a twin launcher for ASROC and US Standard SM-1 surface-to-air missiles, and 4 Teseo. The *Andrea Doria* displaces 7,400 tonnes, was completed in 1964, is armed with Standard SM-1 missiles, and operates 3 AB-212 anti-submarine helicopters.

The combatant forces also include 10 diesel submarines, 4 guided-missile destroyers armed with Standard SM-I, 23 frigates, of which 14 carry one or more AB-212 helicopters, 3 corvettes and 7 missile-armed patrol hydrofoils. Mine countermeasure forces comprise 4 ocean minesweepers, 6 coastal minehunters and 5 coastal sweepers. There are 3 new offshore patrol vessels for the protection of economic resources. Amphibious lift for the San Marco commando group (800 men) is provided by 2 dock landing ships and 33 craft. Auxiliaries include 2 replenishment oilers, 5 water carriers, 3 survey ships, 3 trial vessels, 2 training ships and 9 large tugs.

The Naval Air Arm operates 98 anti-submarine and training helicopters. There is a Special Forces commando of some 600 assault swimmers.

Main naval bases are at Spezia, Naples, Taranto and Ancona, with minor bases at Brindisi and Venice. The personnel of the Navy in 1990 numbered 50,000, including the naval air arm (1,500) and the marine battalion.

Paramilitary maritime tasks are carried out by the Financial Guards fleet of some 70 patrol craft and a harbour control force with 25 inshore patrol craft and numerous boats.

Air Force. Control is exercised through 2 regional HQ near Taranto and Milan. Units assigned to NATO comprise the 1st air brigade of Nike-Hercules surface-to-air missiles, 5 fighter-bomber, 2 light attack, 8 interceptor and 2 tactical reconnaissance squadrons, with supporting transport, search and rescue, and training units. Two of the fighter-bomber squadrons have Tornados, others have Aeritalia G91Ys. The light attack squadrons operate AM-X Centauros and MB.339s. F-104S Starfighters have been standardized throughout the interceptor squadrons. The reconnaissance force operates RF-104G Starfighters. A total of 187 AM-X jet aircraft, built jointly by Aeritalia, Aermacchi and Embraer of Brazil, are replacing G91R, G91Y and F-104G/S aircraft in eight squadrons from 1989.

One transport squadron has turboprop C-130H Hercules aircraft; 2 others have turboprop Aeritalia G222s. There is a VIP and personnel transport squadron, equipped with AS-61, DC-9, Gulfstream III and Falcon 50 aircraft. Electronic warfare duties are performed by specially equipped G222s, PD-808s and MB 339s. Two land-based anti-submarine squadrons operate Breguet Atlantics. Search and rescue are performed by 30 Agusta-Sikorsky HH-3F helicopters, Canadair CL-215 amphibians and smaller types. There are also strong support and training elements; some MB 339 jet trainers have armament provisions for secondary close air support and anti-helicopter roles.

Air Force strength in 1991 was about 79,600 (30,000 conscripts), about 425 combat aircraft, 200 fixed-wing second-line aircraft and over 100 helicopters.

INTERNATIONAL RELATIONS

Membership. Italy is a member of the UN, NATO, EC and WEU. With Austria, Czechoslovakia, Hungary and Yugoslavia, Italy was an inaugural member of the 'Pentagonale' meeting on economic and political co-operation in July 1990. In Nov. 1990 Italy acceded to the Schengen Accord of June 1990 which abolished border controls between Belgium, France, Germany, Luxembourg and the Netherlands.

ECONOMY

Budget. Total revenue and expenditure for fiscal years, in 1m. lire:

	Revenue	*Expenditure*		*Revenue*	*Expenditure*
1983	177,142,000	250,203,000	1986	266,301,009	384,344,429
1984	199,986,000	292,348,000	1987	283,875,850	442,965,463
1985	218,973,000	319,099,000	1988	312,790,760	474,587,541

In the revenue for 1988 turnover and other business taxes accounted for 76,829,509m. lire, customs duties and indirect taxes for 27,563,586m. lire.

The public debt at 31 Dec. 1988 totalled 925,607,657m. lire, including consolidated debt of 40,442m. lire and the floating debt 385,793,054m. lire.

Currency. The unit of currency is the *lira* (ITL). From 30 March 1960 the gold standard was formally established as equal to 0·00142187 gramme of gold per lira.

State metal coins are of 5, 10, 20, 50, 100, 200, and 500 lire. There are in circulation bank-notes of 1,000, 2,000, 5,000, 10,000, 20,000, 50,000 and 100,000 lire; they are neither convertible into gold as foreign moneys nor exportable abroad, nor importable from abroad into Italy (except for certain specified small amounts).

Circulation of money at 31 Dec. 1988: State coins and notes, 1,248,900m. lire; bank-notes, 58,935,100m. lire.

Foreign reserves (excluding gold) totalled US$46,700m. in 1989.

In March 1991 the rate of exchange was 1,148 lire = US$1 and 2,178 lire = £1 sterling.

Banking and Finance. The Bank of Italy was founded in 1893 and became the sole bank of issue in 1926. In 1991 it received increased responsibility for the supervision of banking and stock exchange affairs. Its *governor* is Carlo Ciampi. Its gold reserve amounted to 33,664,000m. lire in Dec. 1989; the foreign credit reserves of the Exchange Bureau (*Ufficio Italiano Cambi*) amounted to 50,343,000m. lire at the same date.

Since 1936, all credit institutions have been under the control of a State organ, named 'Inspectorate of Credit'; the Bank of Italy has been converted into a 'public institution', whose capital is held exclusively by corporate bodies of a public nature. Other credit institutions, totalling 1,085, are classified as: (1) 6 chartered banks (Banco di Napoli, Banco di Sicilia, Banca Nazionale del Lavoro, Monte dei Paschi di Siena, Istituto di S. Paolo di Torino, Banca di Sardegna); (2) 3 banks of national interest (Banca Commerciale Italiana in Milan, Credito Italiano in Genoa and Banco di Roma); (3) banks and credit concerns in general, including 146 joint-stock banks and 113 co-operative banks; (4) 82 savings banks and Monti di pegno (institutions granting loans against personal chattels as security); (5) 730 *Casse rurali e agrarie* (agricultural banks, established as co-operative institutions with unlimited liability of associates); (6) 5 Istituti di Categoria.

The 'Amato' law of July 1990 gave public sector banks the right to become joint stock companies and permitted the placing of up to 49% of their equity with private shareholders.

At 31 Dec. 1989 there were 302 credit institutes handling 94% of all deposits and current accounts, with capital and reserves of 87,501,000m. lire.

On 31 Dec. 1989 the post office savings banks had deposits and current accounts of 145,275,000m. lire; credit institutions, 629,392,000m. lire.

Legislation reforming stock markets came into effect in Dec. 1990. There are stock exchanges in Milan, Rome, Turin and Genoa.

Insurance. By a decree of 29 April 1923 life-assurance business is carried on only by the National Insurance Institute and by other institutions, national and foreign, authorized by the Government. At 31 Dec. 1988 the insurances vested in the *Istituto Nazionale delle Assicurazioni* amounted to 26,148,572m. lire, including the decuple of life annuities.

Weights and Measures. The metric system is in general use.

ENERGY AND NATURAL RESOURCES

Electricity. Italy has greatly developed its hydro-electric resources. In 1989 the total power generated was 210,750m. kwh., of which 37,484m. kwh. were generated by hydro-electric plants. Supply 220 volts; 50 Hz and 120, 125, 160 and 260 volts; 60 Hz.

Oil. Production in 1989 amounted to 4,563,424 tonnes, of which 814,859 came from Sicily. Natural gas production (1989) 596,579m. cu. ft.

Minerals. Mining is most developed in Sicily (Caltanissetta), Tuscany (Arezzo, Florence and Grosseto), Sardinia (Cagliari, Sassari and Iglesias), Lombardy (particularly near Bergamo and Brescia) and Piedmont.

Italy's fuel and mineral resources are wholly inadequate. Only sulphur and mercury outputs yield a substantial surplus for exports. In 1989 outputs, in tonnes, of raw steel were 25,180,676; rolled iron, 22,772,238; cast-iron ingots, 11,761,000.

Production of metals and minerals (in tonnes) was as follows:

	1984	*1985*	*1986*	*1987*	*1988*	*1989*
Iron pyrites	442,674	690,395	760,860	784,924	720,132	835,713
Iron ore	273,700	–	–	–	–	–
Manganese	9,528	8,621	6,396	3,802	9,701	5,899
Zinc	81,291	87,380	50,515	67,798	71,979	80,960
Crude sulphur	20,639	4,911	–	–	-	–
Bauxite	–	–	2,250	15,057	17,864	15,864
Lead	37,429	37,051	27,219	58,515	68,946	67,418
Aluminium	230,207	226,300	262,562	258,051	257,995	233,046

Agriculture. The area of Italy in 1988 comprised 301,278 sq. km, of which 262,780 sq. km was agricultural and forest land and 38,498 sq. km was unproductive; the former was mainly distributed as follows (in 1,000 ha): Forage and pasture, 7,881; woods, 6,750; cereals, 4,590; vines, 1,165; olive trees, 994; garden produce, 680; leguminous plants, 289.

At the third general census of agriculture (24 Oct. 1982) agricultural holdings numbered 3,270,560 and covered 23,559,924 ha. 3,063,010 owners (93·6%) farmed directly 16,597,798 ha (70·4%); 152,250 owners (4·7%) worked with hired labour on 6,209,702 ha (26·4%); 130,648 share-croppers (3·6%) tilled 1,271,485 ha (5·1%); the remaining 55,300 holdings (1·7%) of 752,424 ha (3·2%) were operated in other ways.

According to the labour force survey in July 1990 persons engaged in agriculture numbered 1·9m. (1·22m. males and 0·68m. females).

In 1988, 1,362,932 farm tractors were being used.

The production of the principal crops (in 1,000 metric quintals) in 1989: Sugar beet, 168,146; wheat, 74,120; maize, 63,879; tomatoes, 56,609; potatoes, 24,401; oranges, 20,710; rice, 12,459; barley, 16,910; lemons, 6,653; oats, 2,955; olive oil, 5,222; tangerines, mandarines and clementines, 4,490; other citrus fruit, 448; rye, 206.

Production of wine, 1989, 60,327,000 hectolitres; of tobacco, 188,000 tonnes.

In 1988 consumption of chemical fertilizers in Italy was as follows (in 1,000 tons): Perphosphate, 705·7; nitrate of ammonia, 823·3; sulphate of ammonium, 335·5; potash salts, 339·2; nitrate of calcium 15/16, 64·6; deposed slags, 23·9.

Livestock estimated in 1989: Cattle, 8,745,900; pigs, 9,254,300; sheep, 11,568,600; goats, 1,246,000; horses, 269,350; donkeys, 75,660; mules, 43,080.

Fisheries. The Italian fishing fleet comprised in 1988, 19,756 motor boats (1987: 19,831 of 273,679 gross tons) and 6,667 sailing vessels of 8,796 gross tons. The catch in 1988 was 3,881,590 metric quintals.

INDUSTRY. The main branches of industry are: (% of industrial value added at factor cost in 1982) Textiles, clothing, leather and footwear (17·7%), food, beverages and tobacco (10·4%), energy products (7·9%), agricultural and industrial machines (7·7%), metal products except machines and means of transport (7%), mineral and non-metallic mineral products (7%), timber and wooden furniture (6·6%), electric plants and equipment (6·3%), chemicals and pharmaceuticals (6·2%), means of transport (6·1%).

Production, 1989: Steel, 25,180,676 tonnes; motor vehicles, 2,224,602; cement, 39,692,045 tonnes; artificial and synthetic fibres (including staple fibre and waste), 694,594 tonnes; polyethylene resins, 878,394 tonnes.

Labour. In 1988, 20·8m. persons were employed and 2m. unemployed. Unemployment was 12% in 1990.

Trade Unions. There are 4 main groups: Confederazione Generale Italiana del Lavoro (Communist-dominated); Confederazione Italiana Sindacati Lavoratori (Catholic); Unione Italiana del Lavoro and Confederazione Italiana Sindacati Nazionali Lavoratori.

FOREIGN ECONOMIC RELATIONS. Foreign debt was US$74,000m. in Nov. 1990.

Commerce. The territory covered by foreign trade statistics includes Italy, the Republic of San Marino, but excludes the municipalities of Livigno and Campione.

The following table shows the value of Italy's foreign trade (in 1m. lire):

	1983	*1984*	*1985*	*1986*	*1987*	*1988*
Imports	121,978,334	148,162,029	172,809,202	148,993,862	161,596,640	180,064,049
Exports	110,530,106	129,026,980	149,723,608	145,331,231	150,454,324	167,189,222

The following table shows trade by countries in 1m. lire:

	Imports into Italy from			*Exports from Italy to*		
Countries	*1986*	*1987*	*1988*	*1986*	*1987*	*1988*
Argentina	530,980	447,774	591,995	453,949	498,648	453,033
Australia	905,845	862,113	1,272,254	1,049,527	1,135,914	1,298,182
Austria	3,188,037	3,730,502	4,320,180	3,445,688	3,793,928	4,129,405
Belgium-Luxembourg	6,920,226	8,032,085	8,801,012	4,842,513	5,078,461	5,712,674
France	21,654,420	23,592,402	26,733,833	22,704,291	24,570,821	27,677,255
Germany, Fed. Rep. of	30,506,735	34,076,283	39,217,256	26,355,260	27,958,933	30,211,166
Japan	3,119,645	3,457,826	4,549,940	1,966,167	2,403,860	3,165,492
Netherlands	8,771,001	9,035,325	10,299,944	4,755,267	4,640,120	5,136,207
Switzerland	6,485,310	7,718,373	8,062,673	6,607,199	7,082,240	7,868,418
USSR	3,464,909	3,676,009	4,091,736	2,410,783	2,847,165	2,733,745
UK	7,596,570	8,513,763	9,168,468	10,298,981	11,192,851	13,416,658
USA	8,495,617	8,618,939	10,053,542	15,604,645	14,456,025	14,834,391
Yugoslavia	2,004,412	2,367,747	2,959,017	2,020,347	1,867,069	2,041,451

In 1988 the main imports were maize, wood, greasy wool, metal scrap, pit-coal, petroleum, raw oils, meat, paper, rolled iron and steel, copper and alloys, mechanical and electric equipment, motor vehicles. The main exports were fruit and vegetables, fabrics, footwear and other clothing articles, rolled iron and steel, machinery, motor vehicles, plastic materials and petroleum by-products.

Italy's balance of trade (in 1,000m. lire) has been estimated as follows:

	Goods and services			Income from investments and	Net
	Export	*Import*	*Balance*	*work, balance*	*balance*
1980	83,705	94,276	–10,571	790	–9,781
1988	208,816	206,734	+1,482	–7,888	–5,806
1989	241,898	243,664	–1,766	–10,323	–12,089

Remittances from Italians abroad (in US$1m. until 1969 and then 1,000m. lire): 1950, 72; 1960, 214; 1970, 289; 1980, 1,059; 1989, 1,858.

Total trade between Italy and UK (British Department of Trade returns, in £1,000 sterling):

	1986	*1987*	*1988*	*1989*	*1990*
Imports to UK	4,658,036	5,216,751	5,817,445	6,701,683	6,735,496
Exports and re-exports from UK	3,472,364	4,145,659	4,106,417	4,630,896	5,612,751

Tourism. In 1989, 55·1m. foreigners visited Italy; they included 10·1m. German, 10·2m. Swiss, 9·4m. French, 6·1m. Austrian, 5·9m. Yugoslav, 1·9m. British, 1·8m. Dutch and 1·4m. US citizens. They spent about 16,443,000m. lire.

COMMUNICATIONS

Roads. Italy's roads totalled (31 Dec. 1988) 302,403 km, of which 50,843 km were state roads and highways, 109,894 km provincial roads, 141,666 km communal roads. Motor vehicles, Dec. 1987: Cars, 24,320,167m.; buses, 74,114; lorries, 1,994,661; motor cycles, light vans, etc., 6,890,339.

Railways. Railway history in Italy begins in 1839, with a line between Naples and Portici (8 km). Length of railways (31 Dec. 1989), 19,595 km, including 16,030 km of state railways, of which 6,587 had not yet been electrified. The first section of a new high-speed direct railway linking Rome and Florence opened in Feb. 1977. In 1989 the state railways carried 419m. passengers and 67m. tonnes of goods. The Rome Underground opened in Feb. 1980.

Aviation. The Italian airline Alitalia (with a capital of 585,000m. lire, of which 99·1% is owned by the State) operates flights to every part of the world. Airports include 25 international, 36 national and 75 club airports. Domestic and international traffic in 1989 registered 20,784,413 passengers arrived and 20,846,342 departed, while freight and mail (excluding luggage) amounted to 205,842 tonnes unloaded and 229,787 tonnes loaded.

Shipping. The mercantile marine at 31 Dec. 1986 consisted of 2,031 vessels of 8,060,067 gross tons, not including pleasure boats (yachts, etc.), sailing and motor vessels. There were 1,371 motor vessels of 100 gross tons and over.

In 1988, 271,266,000 tonnes of cargo were unloaded, and 104,211,000 tonnes of cargo were loaded in Italian ports.

Telecommunications. On 31 Dec. 1985 there were 14,276 post offices and 13,759 telegraph offices. The maritime radio-telegraph service had 20 coast stations. On 1 Jan. 1987 the telephone service had 26,873,730 apparatus. *Radiotelevisione Italiana* broadcasts 3 programmes and additional regional programmes, including transmissions in English, French, German and Slovenian on medium- and short-waves and on FM. It also broadcasts 2 TV programmes. Radio licences numbered 157,958; television and radio licences, 14,851,310 in 1989.

Cinemas. There were 3,587 cinemas in 1989.

Newspapers. There were (1988) 73 daily newspapers with a combined circulation of 6,005,000 copies; of the papers 12 are published in Rome and 7 in Milan. One daily each is published in German and Slovene.

JUSTICE, RELIGION, EDUCATION AND WELFARE

Justice. Italy has 1 court of cassation, in Rome, and is divided for the administration of justice into 25 appeal court districts (and 1 detached section), subdivided into 160 tribunal *circondari* (districts), and these again into *mandamenti* each with its own magistracy (*Pretura*), 626 in all. There are also 90 first degree assize courts and 26 assize courts of appeal. For civil business, besides the magistracy above mentioned, *Conciliatori* have jurisdiction in petty plaints (those to a maximum amount of 1m. lire).

On 31 Dec. 1989 there were 20,889 male and 1,289 female prisoners in establishments for preventive custody, 6,391 males and 448 females in penal establishments and 1,450 males and 73 females in establishments for the execution of safety measures.

Religion. The treaty between the Holy See and Italy, of 11 Feb. 1929, confirmed by article 7 of the Constitution of the republic, lays down that the Catholic Apostolic Roman Religion is the only religion of the State. Other creeds are permitted, provided they do not profess principles, or follow rites, contrary to public order or moral behaviour.

The appointment of archbishops and of bishops is made by the Holy See; but the Holy See submits to the Italian Government the name of the person to be appointed in order to obtain an assurance that the latter will not raise objections of a political nature.

Catholic religious teaching is given in elementary and intermediate schools. Marriages celebrated before a Catholic priest are automatically transferred to the civil register. Marriages celebrated by clergy of other denominations must be made valid before a registrar. In 1972 there were 279 dioceses with 28,154 parishes and 43,714 priests. There were 187,153 members (154,796 women) of about 20,000 religious houses.

In 1962 there were about 100,000 Protestants and about 50,000 Jews.

Education. Education is compulsory from 6 to 14 years of age. An optional preschool education is given to the children between 3 and 5 years in the preparatory schools (kindergarten schools). Illiteracy of males over 6 years was 2·2% in 1981, of females 3·9%.

Compulsory education can be classified as primary education (5-year course) and junior secondary education (3-year course).

Senior secondary education is subdivided in classical (*ginnasio* and classical *liceo*), scientific (scientific *liceo*), language lyceum, professional institutes and technical education: agricultural, industrial, commercial, technical, nautical institutes, institutes for surveyors, institutes for girls (5-year course) and teacher-training institutes (4-year course).

University education is given in Universities and in University Higher Institutes (4, 5, 6 years, according to degree course).

Statistics for the academic year 1989–90:

Elementary schools	*No.*	*Pupils*
Kindergarten	28,049	1,565,039
Public elementary schools	22,940	2,885,978
Private elementary schools Private elementary recognized schools (*parificate*)	2,276	252,570

Government secondary schools		*Total students*
Junior secondary schools	10,021	2,395,403
Classical lyceum	746	227,628
Lyceum for science	1,019	447,603
Language lyceum	381	46,481
Teachers' schools	188	23,800
Teachers' institutes	657	166,742
Professional institutes	1,706	537,889
Technical institutes, of which:		
Industrial institutes	621	332,247
Commercial institutes	1,305	675,241
Surveyors' institutes	534	161,389
Agricultural institutes Nautical institutes Technical institutes for tourism Managerial institutes Girls technical schools	419	138,680
Artistic studies	286	94,914

Universities and higher institutes	*Date of foundation*	*Students 1988–89*	*Teachers 1988–89*	*Universities and higher institutes*	*Date of foundation*	*Students 1988–89*	*Teachers 1988–89*
Ancona	1965	7,188	377	Modena	1678	8,105	643
Arezzo	1971	1,054	79	Napoli	1224	117,087	4,507
Bari	1924	63,750	1,892	Padova	1222	48,545	2,444
Bergamo	1970	4,295	131	Palermo	1805	42,454	2,236
Bologna	1200	69,749	2,765	Parma	1502	15,982	993
Brescia	1970	7,640	355	Pavia	1390	20,889	1,459
Cagliari	1626	24,935	1,277	Perugia	1276	19,462	1,156
Camerino (Macerata)	1727	4,222	168	Pescara	1965	11,621	241
				Piacenza	1924	607	100
Campobasso	1986	1,311	170	Pisa	1338	29,349	2,029
Cassino (Frosinone)	1968	5,669	270	Potenza	1983	2,214	297
				Reggio di C.	1968	4,323	190
Catania	1434	33,194	1,622	Roma	1303	174,490	6,606
Catanzaro	1983	4,704	163	Salerno	1944	24,853	576
Chieti	1965	4,378	237	Sassari	1677	8,834	534
Cosenza	1972	6,816	493	Siena	1300	11,434	740
Feltre (Belluno)	1969	558	33	Teramo	1965	6,313	147
Ferrara	1391	4,985	598	Torino	1404	66,647	2,729
Firenze	1924	48,074	2,343	Trento	1965	6,458	371
Foggia	1986	732	112	Trieste	1924	15,703	954
Genova	1243	34,328	1,900	Udine	1969	5,798	472
L'Aquila	1956	6,095	591	Urbino	1564	15,666	545
Lecce	1959	10,613	422	Venezia	1868	25,676	710
Macerata	1290	5,721	187	Verona	1969	10,360	638
Messina	1549	28,467	1,446	Viterbo	1980	1,851	82
Milano	1924	149,446	4,183				

Health. The provision of health services is a regional responsibility, but they are funded by central government. Medical consultations are free, but a portion of prescription costs have been payable since April 1989. In 1986 there were 245,116 doctors and (1987) 440,187 hospital beds.

Social Security. Social expenditure is made up of transfers which the central public departments, local departments and social security departments, make to families. Payment is principally for pensions, family allowances and health services. Expenditure on subsidies, public assistance to various classes of people and people injured by political events or national disasters are also included.

State pensions are indexed to prices, 19m. pensions were paid in 1990.

DIPLOMATIC REPRESENTATIVES

Of Italy in Great Britain (14 Three Kings Yard, London, W1Y 2EH)
Ambassador: Boris Biancheri (accredited 11 Nov. 1987).

Of Great Britain in Italy (Via XX Settembre 80A, 00187, Rome)
Ambassador: Sir Stephen Egerton, KCMG.

Of Italy in the USA (1601 Fuller St., NW, Washington, D.C., 20009)
Ambassador: Rinaldo Petrignani.

Of the USA in Italy (Via Veneto 119/A, Rome)
Ambassador: Peter Secchia.

Of Italy to the United Nations
Ambassador: Vieri Traxler.

Further Reading

Statistical Information: The Istituto Nazionale di Statistica (16 Via Cesare Balbo 00100 Rome) was set up by law of 9 July 1926 as the national institute in charge of census and all statistical information. *President:* Prof. Guido Mario Rey. *Director-General:* Vincenzo Siesto. Its publications include:

Annuario statistico italiano. 1989, *Compendio statistico italiano.* 1990, *Bollettino mensile di statistica.* Monthly, from 1950, *Statistiche industriali.* 1987, *Statistiche demografiche.* 1988,

Statistiche agrarie. 1988, *Statistiche della navigazione marittima*. 1990, *Statistiche del commercio interno*. 1990, *Statistiche annuale del commercio con l'estero*. 1988, *Statistiche del commercio con l'estero*. Quarterly, *Statistiche del lavoro*. 1986, *Censimento generale dell'agricoltura*. 1982, *Censimento generale della popolazione, 1981*. Vol. I, II and III, *Censimento generale dell'industria e del commercio*. 1981 *Sommario di statistiche storiche, 1926–1988*.

Italy. Documents and Notes. Servizi delle Informazioni, Rome. 1952 ff.
Italian Books and Periodicals. Bimonthly from 1958
Banco di Roma, *Review of the Economic Condition in Italy* (in English). Bimonthly, 1947 ff.
Credito Italiano, *The Italian Economic Situation*. Bimonthly. Milan, from June 1961 (in Italian), from June 1962 (in English)
Compendio Economico Italiano. Rome, Unione Italiana delle Camere di Commercio. Annually from 1954
Clark, M., *Modern Italy 1871–1982*. London, 1984
Finer, S. E. and Mastropaolo, A. (eds.), *The Italian Party System, 1945–80*. London, 1985
Ginsborg, P., *A History of Contemporary Italy: Society and Politics, 1943–1988*. London, 1990
Smith, D. M., *The Making of Italy 1796–1866*. London, 1988
Spotts, F. and Wieser, T., *Italy: A Difficult Democracy*. CUP, 1986
Woolfe, S. J. (ed.) *The Rebirth of Italy, 1943–50*. New York, 1972

National Library: Biblioteca Nazionale Centrale Vittorio Emanuele II Viale Castro Pretorio, Rome. *Director:* Dr L. M. Crisari.

JAMAICA

Capital: Kingston
Population: 2·4m. (1988)
GNP per capita: US$1,348 (1988)

HISTORY. Jamaica was discovered by Columbus in 1494, and was occupied by the Spaniards between 1509 and 1655, when the island was captured by the English; their possession was confirmed by the Treaty of Madrid, 1670. Self-government was introduced in 1944 and gradually extended until Jamaica achieved complete independence within the Commonwealth on 6 Aug. 1962.

AREA AND POPULATION. The island of Jamaica lies in the Caribbean Sea about 150 km south of Cuba. The area is 4,411 sq. miles (11,425 sq. km). The population at the census of 8 June 1982 was 2,095,878, distributed on the basis of the 14 parishes of the island as follows: Kingston and St Andrew, 565,487; St Thomas, 76,347; Portland, 70,787; St Mary, 101,442; St Ann, 132,475; Trelawny, 65,038; St James, 127,994; Hanover, 60,420; Westmoreland, 116,163; St Elizabeth, 132,353; Manchester, 136,517; St Catherine, 315,970; Clarendon, 194,885.

Chief towns (census, 1982): Kingston and St Andrew, 524,638, metropolitan area; Spanish Town, 89,097; Montego Bay, 70,265; May Pen, 40,962; Mandeville, 34,502.

Estimated population, in 1989, was 2·4m. The population is 76% of African ethnic origin, 3% European and 21% mixed and other groups.

Vital statistics (1989): Births, 59,100 (24·9 per 1,000 population); deaths, 14,300 (6·0); migration loss, 23,305.

CLIMATE. A tropical climate but with considerable variation. High temperatures on the coast are usually mitigated by sea breezes, while upland areas enjoy cooler and less humid conditions. Rainfall is plentiful over most of Jamaica, being heaviest in May and from Aug. to Nov. The island lies in the hurricane zone. Kingston. Jan. 76°F (24·4°C), July 81°F (27·2°C). Annual rainfall 32" (800 mm).

CONSTITUTION AND GOVERNMENT. Under the Constitution of Aug. 1962 the Crown is represented by a Governor-General appointed by the Crown on the advice of the Prime Minister. The Governor-General is assisted by a Privy Council. The Legislature comprises two chambers, an elected House and a nominated Senate. The executive is chosen from both chambers.

The Executive comprises the Prime Minister, who is the leader of the majority party, and Ministers appointed by the Prime Minister. Together they form the Cabinet, which is the highest executive power. An Attorney-General is a member of the House and is legal adviser to the Cabinet.

The Senate consists of 21 senators appointed by the Governor-General, 13 on the advice of the Prime Minister, 8 on the advice of the Leader of the Opposition. The House of Representatives (60 members, Feb. 1991) is elected by universal adult suffrage for a period not exceeding 5 years. Electors and elected must be Jamaican or Commonwealth citizens resident in Jamaica for at least 12 months before registration. The powers and procedure of Parliament correspond to those of the British Parliament.

The Privy Council consists of 6 members appointed by the Governor-General in consultation with the Prime Minister.

Governor-General: Sir Florizel Glasspole, GCMG, GCVO.

National flag: A yellow diagonal cross dividing triangles of green, top and bottom, and black, hoist and fly.

The elections to the House of Representatives, held on 9 Feb. 1989, returned 45 members of the People's National Party and the Jamaica Labour Party, 15 seats.

The Cabinet in Feb. 1991 was comprised as follows:
Prime Minister: Rt. Hon. Michael Manley, P.C.

Deputy Prime Minister and Minister of Finance and Planning: P. J. Patterson, QC. *Foreign Affairs and Foreign Trade:* David Coore, QC. *National Security:* K. D. Knight. *Justice and Attorney-General:* Carl Rattray, QC. *Education:* Carlyle Dunkley. *Health:* Easton Douglas. *Labour, Welfare and Sports:* Portia Simpson. *Construction:* O. D. Ramtallie. *Public Utilities and Transport:* Robert Pickersgill. *Agriculture and Commerce:* Horace Clarke. *Local Government:* Ralph Brown. *Tourism:* Frank Pringle. *Mining and Energy:* Hugh Small, QC. *Youth, Culture and Community Development:* Dr Douglas Manley. *Public Serice, Industry and Leader of the House (with special responsibility for Parliamentary Affairs):* Dr Kenneth McNeil. *Information:* Dr Paul Robertson.

There are 10 Ministers of State.

DEFENCE

Army. The Jamaica Defence Force consists of a Regular and a Reserve Force. The Regular Force is comprised of the 1st battalion, Jamaica Regiment and Support Services which include the Air Wing and Coast Guard. The Coast Guard, numbering 200 in 1990, operates 5 inshore patrol craft based at Port Royal. The Reserve Force consists of the 3rd battalion, Jamaica Regiment. Total strength (all services, 1991), 3,350. Reserves, 870.

Air Force. The Air Wing of the Jamaica Defence Force was formed in July 1963 and has since been expanded and trained successively by the British Army Air Corps and Canadian air force personnel. Equipment for army liaison, search and rescue, police co-operation, survey and transport duties includes 2 Defender armed STOL transports; 1 Beech King Air and 1 Cessna 337 light transports; 4 JetRanger and 2 Bell 212 helicopters. Personnel (1990) 150.

INTERNATIONAL RELATIONS

Membership. Jamaica is a member of UN, the Commonwealth, OAS, CARICOM and is an ACP state of EEC.

ECONOMY

Budget. Revenue and expenditure for fiscal years ending 31 March (in J$1m.):

	1986–87	*1987–88*	*1988–89*	*1989–90*
Revenue	4,467	5,429	6,020	7,895
Expenditure	5,631	6,509	8,199	7,738

The chief heads of recurrent revenue are income tax; consumption, customs and stamp duties. The other major share of current resources is generated by the Bauxite levy.The chief items of recurrent expenditure are public debt, education and health. Total external debt at 31 Dec. 1989, US$4,035m.

Currency. The unit of currency is the *Jamaican dollar* (JMD), divided into 100 *cents*. The Jamaican dollar was floated in Sept. 1990. Currency circulation at 30 June 1989 was J$1,129·8m. In March 1991, £1 = J$14·93; US$1 = J$7·87.

Banking and Finance. The central bank is the Bank of Jamaica. It has the sole right to issue notes and coins, acts as Banker to the Government and to the commercial banks, and administers the island's external reserves and exchange control.

There are 10 commercial banks with about 171 branches and agencies in operation. 6 of these banks are subsidiaries of major British and North American banks, of which 4 are incorporated locally. The Workers' Savings and Loan Bank is owned by the Government, Trade Unions and the private sector. The National Commercial Bank (Jamaica) Ltd, is 49% government-owned. The other 8 banks which operate are: The Bank of Nova Scotia (Jamaica) Ltd, City Bank of North America, Mutual Security Bank, Canadian Imperial Bank of Commerce, Jamaica Citizens Bank Ltd, Eagle Commercial Bank, Bank of Credit and Commerce International and Century National Bank. There is a stock exchange in Kingston.

Total deposits in commercial banks, 30 June 1990, J$11,083·2m., of which J$3,202·1m. were time deposits and J$5,695·8m. (51·4%) were savings.

ENERGY AND NATURAL RESOURCES

Electricity. The Jamaica Public Service Co. is the public supplier of electricity. The bauxite companies, sugar estates and the Caribbean Cement Co. and Goodyear generate their own electricity. Total installed capacity, 1989, 485·7 mw. Production (1989) 1,878m. kwh. Supply 110 and 220 volts; 50 Hz.

Minerals. Bauxite, ceramic clays, marble, silica sand and gypsum are commercially viable. Jamaica has become the world's third largest producer of bauxite and alumina. The bauxite deposits are worked by a Canadian, an American and a Jamaican company. In 1989, 9·6m. tonnes of bauxite ore was mined; gypsum, 178,000 tonnes; marble, 5,000 tonnes; sand and gravel, 900,000 cu. metres; industrial lime, 2·5m. cu. metres.

Agriculture (1989). Production: Sugar-cane, 2,257,000 tons; sugar, 197,000 tons; rum, 5,556,000 proof gallons; molasses, 85,000 tons; bananas, 43,000 tons; citrus fruit, 591,000 boxes; cocoa, 1,442 tons; spices, 1,932 tons; copra, 256 short tons; domestic food crops, 387,652 short tons.

Livestock (1988): Cattle, 290,000; goats, 440,000; pigs, 250,000; poultry, 6m. Slaughtered livestock (1989): Cattle, 62,090 heads: goats, 44,083 heads: pigs, 125,601; poultry, 86,000 lbs.

INDUSTRY. Three bauxite-mining companies also process bauxite into alumina; production, 1989, 2·2m. tonnes. From processing only a few agricultural products—sugar, rum, condensed milk, oils and fats, cigars and cigarettes—the island is now producing clothing, footwear, textiles, paints, building materials (including cement), agricultural machinery and toilet articles. There is an oil refinery in Kingston. In 1989 manufacturing contributed J$4,497·5m. to the total GDP at current prices.

Labour. Average total labour force (1989), 1,062,900, of whom 871,800 were employed. Government and other services employed 247,000; agriculture, forestry and fishing, 247,700; manufacturing, 133,800; construction and installation, 54,900.

FOREIGN ECONOMIC RELATIONS

Commerce. Value of imports and domestic exports for calendar years (in US$1m.):

	1986	*1987*	*1988*	*1989*	*1990*
Imports	969	1,234	1,435	1,826	1,782
Domestic exports	567	692	812	970	1,112

Principal imports in 1990 (in US$1m.): Manufactured goods classified by materials, 289·9 (16·3%); machinery and transport equipment, 469·5 (26·3%); food, 206·7 (11·8%); minerals, fuels, lubricants and related materials, 342·0 (19·2%); chemicals, 206·8 (11·6%).

Principal domestic exports in 1990 (in US$1m.): Crude materials, inedible oils except fuels, 718·5 (64·6%), of which alumina, 632·6 (56·9%) and bauxite, 103·1 (9·3%); food, 174·2 (15·6%), of which sugar, 73·0 (6·5%); miscellaneous materials, 98·7 (8·9%).

Total trade between Jamaica and UK (British Department of Trade returns, in £1,000 sterling):

	1986	*1987*	*1988*	*1989*	*1990*
Imports to UK	87,416	85,655	89,693	95,516	136,535
Exports and re-exports from UK	43,378	54,644	48,855	61,355	58,702

Tourism. In 1990, 1,236,089 tourists arrived in Jamaica, spending about US$700m.

COMMUNICATIONS

Roads (1989). The island has 3,000 miles of main roads, and over 7,000 miles of secondary and tertiary roads. Main roads are constructed and maintained by the Ministry of Construction (Works), while other roads are constructed and maintained by parish councils. In 1989 there were 98,857 licensed vehicles.

Railways. There are 294 km of railway open of 1,435 mm gauge, operated by the Jamaica Railway Corporation. In 1988 the railway carried 38,540 tonnes and in 1989, carried 1·08m. passengers.

Aviation. Scheduled commercial international airlines operate through the Norman Manley and Sangster international airports at Palisadoes and Montego Bay. In 1989 Norman Manley airport had 25,258 aircraft movements, handled 1·18m. passengers and 25,443 tonnes of freight. Sangster had 20,404 movements, with 1·7m. passengers and 4,164 tonnes of freight. Trans-Jamaica Airlines Ltd operates internal flights; in 1987 it carried 37,600 passengers. Air Jamaica, originally set up in conjunction with BOAC and BWIA in 1966, became a new company, Air Jamaica (1968) Ltd, and is affiliated to Air Canada. In 1969 it began operations as Jamaica's national airline. In 1989 Air Jamaica carried 1·13m. passengers.

Shipping. In 1989 there were 2,456 visits to all ports; 11·6m. tons of cargo were handled. Kingston had 1,411 visits and handled 1·9m. tons. The outports had 1,045 visits and handled 9·6m. tons, of which 7·3m. was loaded and 2·3m. landed.

Telecommunications. In 1989 there were 824 postal points. In Dec. 1989 there were 177,808 telephones.

There was (1989) 2 commercial and 1 publicly owned broadcasting stations; the latter also operates a television service.

Cinemas. In 1989 there were 35 cinemas and 2 drive-in cinemas.

JUSTICE, RELIGION, EDUCATION AND WELFARE

Justice. The Judicature comprises a Supreme Court, a court of appeal, resident magistrates' courts, petty sessional courts, coroners' courts, a traffic court and a family court which was instituted in 1975. The Chief Justice is head of the judiciary. All prosecutions are initiated by the Director of Public Prosecutions.

Police. The Constabulary Force in 1989 stood at approximately 5,460 officers, sub-officers and constables (men and women).

Religion. Freedom of worship is guaranteed under the Constitution. The main Christian denominations are Anglican, Baptist, Roman Catholic, Methodist, Church of God, United Church of Jamaica, and Grand Cayman (Presbyterian–Congregational) Moravian, Seventh-Day Adventists, Pentecostal, Salvation Army, Quaker, and Disciples of Christ. Pocomania is a mixture of Christianity and African survivals. Non-Christians include Hindus, Jews, Moslems, Bahai followers and Rastafarians.

Education. In Sept. 1973 education became free for all government grant-aided schools (the majority of all schools) and for all Jamaicans entering the University of the West Indies, the College of Arts, Science and Technology and the Jamaica School of Agriculture. In 1988–89 there were 1,307 pre-primary schools and departments (130,355 pupils); 298 primary schools (172,416 pupils); 493 all-age schools (154,908 pupils).

There were 141 secondary and vocational schools (104,774 students). Teacher-training colleges had 3,190 students; community colleges had 5,508; the College of Arts, Science and Technology had 4,964; the College of Agriculture, 236 and the University of the West Indies, 4,512.

Health. In 1989 the public health service had 3,742 staff in medicine, nursing and pharmacology; 305 in dentistry; 262 public health inspectors; 61 in nutrition. In 1989 there were 359 primary health centres, 5,021 public hospital beds and 282 private beds.

DIPLOMATIC REPRESENTATIVES

Of Jamaica in Great Britain (1-2 Prince Consort Rd., London, SW7 2BZ)
High Commissioner: Ellen Bogle CD (accredited 27 Oct. 1989).

Of Great Britain in Jamaica (Trafalgar Rd., Kingston 10)
High Commissioner: Derek Milton, CMG.

Of Jamaica in the USA (1850 K. St., NW, Washington, D.C., 20006)
Ambassador: Keith Johnson.

Of the USA in Jamaica (2 Oxford Rd., Kingston 5)
Ambassador: Glen A. Holden.

Of Jamaica to the United Nations
Ambassador: Herbert S. Walker.

Further Reading

Statistical Information: The Department of Statistics, now Statistical Institute of Jamaica (25 Dominica Dr., Kingston), was set up in 1945—the nucleus being the Census Office, which undertook the operations of the 1943 Census of Jamaica and its Dependencies. *Director:* Vernon James. Publications of the Institute include the *Bulletin of Statistics on External Trade* and the *Annual Abstract of Statistics.*

Economic and Social Survey, Jamaica. Planning Institute of Jamaica, Kingston (Annual)
Social and Economic Studies. Institute of Social and Economic Research, Univ. of the West Indies. Quarterly
A Review of the Performance of the Jamaican Economy 1981–1983. Jamaica Information Service, 1985
Quarterly Economic Report. Planning Institute of Jamaica, Kingston
Bakan, A. B. *Ideology and Class Conflict in Jamaica: the Politics of Rebellion.* Montreal, 1990
Beckford, G. and Witter, M., *Small Garden... Bitter Weed. The Political Struggle and Change in Jamaica.* 2nd ed. London, 1982
Cassidy, F. G. and Le Page, R. B., *Dictionary of Jamaican English.* CUP, 1966
Floyd, B., *Jamaica: An Island Microcosm.* London, 1979
Goulbourne, H., *Teachers, Education and Politics in Jamaica, 1892–1972.* London, 1988
Ingram, K. E., *Jamaica.* [Bibliography] Oxford and Santa Barbara, 1984
Manley, M., *A Voice at the Work Place.* London, 1975.—*Jamaica: Struggle in the Periphery.* London, 1983
Payne, A. J., *Politics in Jamaica.* London and New York, 1988
Post, K., *Strike the Iron, A Colony at War: Jamaica 1939–1945.* 2 vols. Atlantic Highlands, N.J., 1981
Sherlock, P., *Keeping Company with Jamaica.* London, 1984
Stephens, E. H. and Stephens, J. D., *Democratic Socialism in Jamaica.* London, 1986
Stone, C., *Class, Race and Political Behaviour in Urban Jamaica.* Kingston, 1973—*Democracy and Clientelism in Jamaica.* London and New Brunswick, N.J., 1981
Bibliography of Jamaica, 1900–1963. Jamaica Library Service, 1963

Libraries: National Library of Jamaica, Kingston. Jamaica Library Service, Kingston.

JAPAN

Nippon (*or* Nihon)

Capital: Tokyo
Population: 123·26m. (1989)
GNP per capita: US$23,382 (1988)

HISTORY. The house of Yamato, from about 500 B.C. the rulers of one of several kingdoms, in about A.D. 200 united the nation; the present imperial family are their direct descendants. From 1186 until 1867 successive families of Shoguns exercised the temporal power. In 1867 the Emperor Meiji recovered the imperial power after the abdication on 14 Oct. 1867 of the fifteenth and last Tokugawa Shogun Keiki (in different pronunciation: Yoshinobu). In 1871 the feudal system (Hoken Seido) was abolished; this was the beginning of the rapid westernization.

At San Francisco on 8 Sept. 1951 a Treaty of Peace was signed by Japan and representatives of 48 countries. For details *see* THE STATESMAN'S YEAR-BOOK, 1953, p. 1169. On 26 Oct. 1951 the Japanese Diet ratified the Treaty by 307 votes to 47 votes with 112 abstentions. On the same day the Diet ratified a Security Treaty with the US by 289 votes to 71 votes with 106 abstentions. The treaty provided for the stationing of American troops in Japan until she was able to undertake her own defence. The peace treaty came into force on 28 April 1952, when Japan regained her sovereignty. In 1960 Japan signed the Japan–US Mutual Security Treaty, valid for 10 years, which was renewed in 1970. Of the islands under US administration since 1945, the Bonin (Ogasawara), Volcano, and Daito groups and Marcus Island were returned to Japan in 1968, and the southern Ryukyu Islands (Okinawa) in 1972.

AREA AND POPULATION. Japan consists of 4 major islands, Honshu, Hokkaido, Kyushu and Shikoku, and many small islands, with an area of 377,835 sq. km. Census population (1 Oct. 1985) 121,047,196 (males 59,495,663, females 61,551,553). Estimate (1989) 123,255,000 (males 60,581,000, females 62,673,000). Foreigners registered 31 Dec. 1989 were 984,455, of whom 681,838 were Koreans, 137,499 Chinese, 34,900 Americans, 38,925 Filipinos, 9,272 British, 5,542 Thais, 6,316 Vietnamese, 14,528 Brazilians, 4,172 Canadians, 1,538 stateless persons. In 1988 there were 3,542 Malaysians and 3,222 West Germans.

Japanese overseas, Oct. 1988, 548,404; of these 189,856 lived in USA, 112,979 in Brazil, 13,162 in the UK, 19,620 in Canada, 19,827 in the Federal Republic of Germany, 15,416 in Argentina, 14,761 in France, 11,339 in Australia, 11,156 in Thailand, 11,140 in the Philippines.

The areas, populations and chief cities of the principal islands (and regions) are:

Island/Region	*Sq. km*	*Census 1988*	*Chief cities*
Hokkaido	83,409	5,671,000	Sapporo
Honshu/Tohoku	65,573	9,745,000	Sendai
/Kanto	32,105	37,867,000	Tokyo
/Chubu	65,252	20,858,000	Nagoya
/Kinki	32,814	22,105,000	Osaka
/Chugoku	31,830	7,777,000	Hiroshima
Shikoku	18,780	4,224,000	Matsuyama
Kyushu	42,142	13,319,000	Fukuoka
Okinawa	2,263	1,213,000	Naha

The leading cities, with population, 31 March 1989 (in 1,000), are:

Akashi	264	Fukuyama	364	Ibaraki	250
Akita	296	Funabashi	522	Ichihara	251
Amagasaki	495	Gifu	407	Ichinomiya	260
Aomori	292	Hachioji	439	Ichikawa	419
Asahikawa	362	Hakodate	309	Iwaki	358
Chiba	809	Hamamatsu	526	Kagoshima	529
Fujisawa	341	Higashiosaka	502	Kanazawa	425
Fukui	249	Himeji	450	Kashiwa	296
Fukuoka	1,169	Hirakata	387	Kasugai	261
Fukushima	273	Hiroshima	1,049	Kawagoe	294

Kawaguchi	427	Naha	310	Suita	340
Kawasaki	1,128	Nara	344	Takamatsu	328
Kitakyushu	1,030	Neyagawa	256	Takatsuki	355
Kobe	1,426	Niigata	472	Tokorozawa	292
Kochi	313	Nishinomiya	411	Tokushima	258
Koriyama	306	Oita	397	Tokyo	8,099
Koshigaya	276	Okayama	580	Toyama	317
Kumamoto	559	Okazaki	296	Toyohashi	329
Kurashiki	416	Omiya	390	Toyonaka	403
Kyoto	1,415	Osaka	2,535	Toyota	319
Machida	339	Sagamihara	509	Urawa	401
Maebashi	282	Sakai	806	Utsunomiya	419
Matsudo	446	Sapporo	1,609	Wakayama	400
Matsuyama	437	Sasebo	248	Yao	270
Miyazaki	284	Sendai	879	Yokkaichi	270
Nagano	343	Shimonoseki	259	Yokohama	3,153
Nagasaki	444	Shizuoka	470	Yokosuka	433
Nagoya	2,101				

Vital statistics (in 1,000) for calendar years:

	1982	*1983*	*1984*	*1985*	*1986*	*1987*	*1988*
Births	1,515	1,509	1,490	1,432	1,383	1,347	1,314
Deaths	712	740	740	752	751	751	793

Crude birth rate of Japanese nationals in present area, 1988, was 10·8 per 1,000 population (1947: 34·3); crude death rate, 6·5; crude marriage rate, 5·8; infant mortality rate per 1,000 live births, 4·8. Population growth rate was 3·3 per 1,000 in 1989. Expectation of life was 75·8 years for men, 81·9 years for women.

CLIMATE. The islands of Japan lie in the temperate zone, north-east of the main monsoon region of S.E. Asia. The climate is temperate with warm, humid summers and relatively mild winters except in the island of Hokkaido and northern parts of Honshu facing the Japan Sea. There is a month's rainy season in June-July, but the best seasons are spring and autumn, though Sept. may bring typhoons. There is a summer rainfall maximum. Tokyo. Jan. 40·5°F (4·7°C), July 77·4°F (25·2°C). Annual rainfall 63" (1,460 mm). Hiroshima. Jan. 39·7°F (4·3°C), July 78°F (25·6°C). Annual rainfall 61" (1,603 mm). Nagasaki. Jan. 43·5°F (6·4°C), July 79·7°F (26·5°C). Annual rainfall 77" (2,002 mm). Osaka. Jan. 42·1°F (5·6°C), July 80·6°F (27°C). Annual rainfall 53" (1,400 mm). Sapporo. Jan. 23·2°F (–4·9°C), July 68·4°F (20·2°C). Annual rainfall 47" (1,158 mm).

EMPEROR. The Emperor bears the title of Nihon-koku Tenno ('Emperor of Japan'). **Akihito,** born in Tokyo, 23 Dec. 1933; succeeded his father, Hirohito, 7 Jan. 1989 (enthroned, 12 Nov. 1990); married 10 April 1959, to Michiko Shoda, born 20 Oct. 1934. *Offspring:* Crown Prince Naruhito (Hironomiya), born 23 Feb. 1960; Prince Fumihito (Akishinomiya), born 30 Nov. 1965; Princess Sayako (Norinomiya), born 18 April 1969.

By the Imperial House Law of 11 Feb. 1889, revised on 16 Jan. 1947, the succession to the throne was fixed upon the male descendants.

CONSTITUTION AND GOVERNMENT. Japan's Government is based upon the Constitution of 1947 which superseded the Meiji Constitution of 1889. In it the Japanese people pledge themselves to uphold the ideas of democracy and peace. The Emperor is the symbol of the States and of the unity of the people. Sovereign power rests with the people. The Emperor has no powers related to government. Fundamental human rights are guaranteed.

National flag: White, with a red disc.

National anthem: Kimi ga yo wa (words 9th century, tune by Hiromori Hayashi, 1881).

Legislative power rests with the *Diet*, which consists of the *House of Representatives* (of 512 members), elected by men and women over 20 years of age for a 4-year term, and the *House of Councillors* of 252 members (100 elected by party list system with proportional representation according to the d'Hondt method and 152 from prefectural districts), one-half of its members being elected every 3 years. The House of Representatives controls the budget and approves treaties with foreign powers.

The former House of Peers is replaced by the House of Councillors, whose members, like those of the House of Representatives, are elected as representatives of all the people. The House of Representatives has pre-eminence over the House of Councillors.

In 1990 the Prime Minister's salary was 2,062,280 yen per month.

On 8 Jan. 1991 the House of Representatives consisted of 281 Liberal-Democrats, 140 Socialists, 46 Komeito, 16 Communists, 14 Democratic-Socialists, 12 others.

The Cabinet, as constituted in 1990, was as follows:

Prime Minister: Toshiki Kaifu.
Justice: Megumo Sato.
Foreign Affairs: Taro Nakayama.
Finance: Ryutaro Hashimoto.
Education: Yutaka Inoue.
Health and Welfare: Shinichiro Shimojo.
Agriculture, Forestry and Fishery: Motoji Kondo.
Trade and Industry: Eiichi Nakao.
Transport: Kanezo Muraoka.
Postal Service: Katsutsugu Sekiya.
Labour: Sadatoshi Ozato.
Construction: Yuji Otsuka.
Home Affairs: Akina Fukida.
Science and Technology: Akiko Santo.

Local Government. The country is divided into 47 prefectures (*Todofuken*), including Tokyo-to (the capital), Osaka-fu and Kyoto-fu, Hokkai-do, and 43 *Ken*. Each *Todofuken* has its governor (*Chiji*) elected by the voters in the area. The prefectural government of Tokyo-to is also responsible for the urban part (formerly Tokyo-shi) of the prefecture. Each prefecture, city, town and village has a representative assembly elected by the same franchise as in parliamentary elections. There were 3,268 local authorities in 1990.

DEFENCE. Japan has renounced war as a sovereign right and the threat or the use of force as a means of settling disputes with other nations. Its troops may not serve abroad, a stipulation upheld by the Diet in 1990.

In Jan. 1991 Japan and the USA signed a renewal agreement under which Japan pays 40% of the costs of stationing US forces and 100% of the associated labour costs.

Army. The 'Ground Self-Defence Force' had in 1991 an authorized strength of 156,200 uniformed personnel, plus a reserve of 46,000 men. The Army is organized in 12 infantry divisions, 1 armoured division, 1 airborne brigade, 2 air defence brigades, 1 artillery, 2 combined and 1 helicopter brigades in addition to 4 anti-aircraft artillery groups. Equipment includes 1,222 main battle tanks, approximately 450 anti-tank guided weapons, observation and training helicopters, as well as 22 fixed-wing aircraft.

The Northern Army, stationed in Hokkaido, consists of 4 divisions (1 of which is armoured), an artillery brigade, an anti-aircraft artillery brigade, a tank group and an engineering brigade. The Western Army, stationed in Kyushu, consists of 2 divisions and 1 combined brigade. The North-Eastern Army (2 divisions), the Eastern Army (2 divisions and 1 airborne brigade), the Middle Army (3 divisions and 1 combined brigade). The infantry division establishment is approximately 9,000 with 4 infantry regiments or 7,000 (lower establishment) with 3 infantry regiments. Each infantry division has an artillery regiment, an anti-tank unit, a tank battalion and an engineering battalion in addition to administrative units.

Navy. The 'Maritime Self-Defence Force' is tasked with coastal protection and defence of the sea lanes to 1,000 nautical miles range from Japan. The modern and well-equipped combatant forces are mainly equipped with American weapon systems, which in many cases have been re-engineered and improved in Japan.

The combatant fleet, all home-built, comprises 14 diesel submarines and one trials boat, 6 guided-missile destroyers armed with US Standard SM1 surface to air missiles, 23 helicopter-carrying frigates, with one or more Sea King anti-submarine helicopters, and 35 other frigates of which 6 are employed on non-military tasks. Light forces comprise 5 torpedo craft and 9 small inshore patrol craft. There are 49 mine warfare vessels, 1 minelayer, 1 layer/command ship, 34 coastal minesweepers and 12 smaller vessels. A substantial amphibious capability is provided by 6 tank landing ships supported by some 40 smaller craft. 12 major auxiliaries include 3 combined oiler/ammunition ships, 5 survey vessels and 3 training support vessels, and there are several hundred minor auxiliaries and service craft.

The Air Arm, numbering 7 operational Air Wings, includes 76 Orion and Neptune anti-submarine patrol aircraft, 10 US-1 rescue flying boats, 60 Sea King anti-submarine helicopters, 7 mine countermeasures helicopters plus numerous transport, training and utility aircraft.

The main elements of the fleet are organized into 4 escort flotillas based at Yokosuka (2), Sasebo and Maizuru. The submarines are based at Sasebo and Kure.

Personnel in 1990 numbered 46,400 including about 12,000 in the Naval Air Arm.

The Maritime Safety Agency (coastguard) regulates and safeguards all coastal navigation, providing a comprehensive search-and-rescue and navigation service. It operates 81 offshore patrol vessels, 11 coastal patrol vessels, and some 240 inshore patrol craft, as well as numerous boats and service vessels. There are numerous shore command and support facilities, and 24 fixed-wing aircraft and 38 helicopers complete the equipment inventory. Personnel in 1990 numbered 12,000.

Air Force. An 'Air Self-Defence Force' was inaugurated on 1 July 1954. In 1989 its equipment included 5 interceptor squadrons of F-15J/DJ Eagles (total of 168 aircraft to be acquired by 1992) and 5 of F-4EJ Phantoms; 3 squadrons of Mitsubishi F-1 close-support fighters; 1 squadron of RF-4E reconnaissance fighters; 8 E-2C Hawkeye AWACS aircraft; ECM flight with 2 YS-11Es; 3 squadrons of turbofan Kawasaki C-1 and turboprop C-130H Hercules and NAMC YS-11 transports. About 55 helicopters, mostly KV-107s (to be replaced with CH-47 Chinooks), and MU-2 twin-turboprop aircraft perform search, rescue and general duties. Training units use piston-engined Fuji T-3 basic trainers, Fuji T-1 jet intermediate trainers, T-33 jet trainers and supersonic Mitsubishi T-2 jet advanced trainers. The T-33s are being replaced with Kawasaki T-4s from 1989. Six surface-to-air missile groups (19 squadrons) are in service. Total strength (1991) 387 combat aircraft and 46,400 officers and men.

INTERNATIONAL RELATIONS

Membership. Japan is a member of the UN, Colombo Plan and OECD.

ECONOMY

Policy. The 1988–92 Plan envisages an onward real growth rate of 3·75% and a nominal 4·75%. The real growth rate for 1991 was envisaged at 3·8% and the nominal 5·5%.

Budget. Ordinary revenue and expenditure for fiscal year ending 31 March 1991 balanced at 66,236,800m. yen.

Of the proposed revenue in 1990, 58,004,000m. was to come from taxes and stamps, 5,593,200m. from public bonds. Main items of expenditure: Social security, 11,614,800m.; public works, 6,214,700m.; local government, 15,275,100m.; education, 5,112,900m.; defence, 4,159,300m.

The outstanding national debt incurred by public bonds was estimated in March 1989 to be 159,095,500m. yen, including 500m. yen of Japan's foreign currency bonds.

The estimated 1990 budgets of the prefectures and other local authorities forecast a total revenue of 67,140,000m. yen, to be made up partly by local taxes and partly by government grants and local loans.

Currency. The unit of currency is the *yen* (JPY). Coins of 1, 5, 10, 50, 100 and 500 *yen* are in circulation as well as notes of the Bank of Japan, of 1,000, 5,000 and 10,000 *yen*. Bank-notes for 500 *yen* are still in circulation but are gradually being replaced by coins. In March 1990, £1 = 257 *yen*; US$1 = 135·48 *yen*.

In Dec. 1989 the currency in circulation consisted of 37,420,000m. yen Bank of Japan notes and 3,029,000m. yen subsidiary coins.

Banking and Finance. The modern banking system dates from 1872. The Nippon Ginko (Bank of Japan) was founded in 1882. The Bank of Japan has undertaken to finance the Government and the banks; its function is similar to that of a Central Bank in other countries. The Bank undertakes the actual management of Treasury funds and foreign exchange control. Its *Governor* is Yasushi Mieno.

Gold bullion and cash holdings of the Bank of Japan at 31 Dec. 1989 stood at 430,000m. yen.

There were on 31 Dec. 1989, 13 city banks, 64 regional banks, 7 trust banks, 3 long-term credit banks, 68 Sogo banks (mutual savings and loan banks), 455 Shinkin banks (credit associations), 414 credit co-operatives, and 83 foreign banks. There are also various governmental financial institutions, including postal savings which amounted to 133,488,200m. yen in Sept. 1990. Total savings by individuals, including insurance and securities, stood at 736,458,200m. yen on 30 Sept. 1990, and about 62% of these savings were deposited in banks and the post-office.

Many foreign banks operate branches in Japan including: Bank of Indo-China, Hongkong & Shanghai Banking Corporation, Chartered Bank of India, Australia and China, Bank of India, Mercantile Bank of India, Bank of Korea, Bank of China, Algemene Bank Nederland NV, National Handelsbank NV, Bank of America, National City Bank of New York, Chase Manhattan Bank, Bangkok Bank and American Express Co.

Weights and Measures. The metric system was made obligatory by a law passed in March 1921, and the period of grace for its compulsory use ended on 1 April 1966.

ENERGY AND NATURAL RESOURCES

Electricity. In 1988 generating facilities were capable of an output of 181,708,000 kw.; electricity produced was 753,728m. kwh. There were 38 nuclear power stations in 1990, producing about 30% of electricity. Supply 100 and 200 volts; 50 or 60 Hz.

Oil and Gas. Output of crude petroleum, 1988, was 689,000 tonnes, almost entirely from oilfields on the island of Honshu, but 193,851,000 tonnes crude oil had to be imported. Output of natural gas, 1988, 2,097m. cu. metres.

Minerals. Ore production in tonnes, 1988, of chromite, 9,508; coal, 11,223,000; iron, 97,461; zinc, 47,217; manganese 80; copper, 16,666; lead, 22,899; tungsten, 438; silver, 251,971 kg.; gold, 7,308 kg.

Agriculture. Agricultural workers in 1989 were 5,968,000, including 561,000 subsidiary and seasonal workers; 8·4% (1985) of the labour force as opposed to 24·7% in 1962. The arable land area in 1989 was 5,279,000 ha. Rice is the staple food, but its consumption is declining. Rice cultivation accounted for 2,110,000 ha in 1989. The area planted with industrial crops such as rapeseed, tobacco, tea, rush, etc., was 245,000 ha in 1988.

Average farm size was just over 1 ha in 1990. Farmers are represented by the co-operative organization in Nokyo.

In 1989 there were 4,703,000 power cultivators and tractors and 2,205,000 rice power planters, (1988): 1,408,000 power sprayers and 1,674,000 power dusters.

Output of rice was 11,878,000 in 1984, 11,662,000 in 1985, 11,647,000 in 1986, 10,627,000 in 1987, 9,935,000 in 1988 and 10,347,000 in 1989.

Production in 1989 (in 1,000 tonnes) of barley was 371; wheat, 985; soybeans

(1988), 277. Sweet potatoes, which in the past mitigated the effects of rice famines, have, in view of rice over-production, decreased from 4,955,000 tonnes in 1965 to 1,326,000 tons in 1988. Domestic sugar-beet and sugar-cane production accounted for only 33·2% of requirement in 1988. In 1988, 1,885,000 tonnes were imported, 35·9% of this being imported from Australia, 18·8% from South Africa, 25·6% from Thailand, 17·6% from Cuba.

Fruit production, 1988 (in 1,000 tonnes): Mandarins, 1,998; apples, 1,402; pears, 455; grapes, 296; peaches, 203; and persimmons, 288.

Livestock (1989): 4,682,000 cattle (including about 2m. milch cows), 22,000 horses, 11,866,000 pigs, 30,000 sheep, 37,000 goats, 344m. chickens. Milk (1988), 7·61m. tonnes.

Forestry. Forests and grasslands cover about 25m. ha (nearly 70% of the whole land area), with an estimated timber stand of 2,862m. cu. metres in 1986. In 1987, 38,440,000 cu. metres were felled.

Fisheries. Before the War, Japanese catch represented one-half to two-thirds of the world's total fishing, in 1987 it was 12·8%. The catch in 1988 was 12·79m. tonnes, excluding whaling.

INDUSTRY. Japan's industrial equipment, 1987, numbered 719,908 plants of all sizes, employing 11,371,000 production workers.

Since 1920 there has been a shift from light to heavy industries. The production of electrical appliances and electronic machinery has made great strides: Television sets (1988: 14,560,000), radio sets (1988: 10,969,000), cameras (1988: 15,747,000), computing machines and automation equipment are produced in increasing quantities. The chemical industry ranks third in production value after machinery and metals (1987). Production, 1988, included (in tonnes): Sulphuric acid, 6,767,000; caustic soda, 3,403,000; ammonium sulphate, 1,835,000; calcium superphosphate, 476,000.

Output (1988), in 1,000 tonnes, of pig iron was 79,295; crude steel, 105,681; ordinary rolled steel, 84,100.

In 1988 paper production was 14,343,000 tonnes; paperboard, 10,228,000 tonnes.

Japan's textile industry before the War had 13m. cotton-yarn spindles. After the War she resumed with 2·78m. spindles; in 1964, 8·42m. spindles were operating. Output of cotton yarn, 1988, 464,000 tonnes, and of cotton cloth, 1,885m. sq. metres.

In wool, Japan aims at wool exports sufficient to pay for the imports of raw wool. Output, 1988, 120,000 tonnes of woollen yarns and 353m. sq. metres of woollen fabrics.

Output, 1988, of rayon woven fabrics, 602m. sq. metres; synthetic woven fabrics, 2,672m. sq. metres; silk fabrics, 103m. sq. metres.

Shipbuilding has been decreasing and in 1988, 3,867,000 gross tons were launched, of which 1,417,000 GRT were tankers.

Labour. Total labour force, 1989, was 61·28m., of which 4·2m. were in agriculture and forestry, 440,000 in fishing, 70,000 in mining, 5·8m. in construction, 14·84m. in manufacturing, 16m. in commerce and finance, 3·98m. in transport and other public utilities, 13·36m. in services (including the professions) and 1·89m. in government work. Normal retirement age is 60, but some 40% of the workforce retire earlier.

Trade Unions. In 1989 there were 12,227,000 workers organized in 72,600 unions. The largest federation is the 'Japanese Private Sector Trade Union Confederation' (Rengo) with 5,445,000 members. The 'General Council of Japanese Trade Unions' (Sohyo) had 3,907,000 members. Rengo was organized in Nov. 1987 by dissolving the 'Japanese Confederation of Labour' (Domei Kaigi) and the 'Federation of Independent Unions' (Churitsu Roren).

In 1989, 1·42m. (2·3%) were unemployed. In 1989, 220,000 working days were lost in industrial stoppages.

FOREIGN ECONOMIC RELATIONS

Commerce. Trade (in US$1m.):

	1983	1984	1985	1986	1987	1988	1989
Imports	126,393	136,503	129,539	126,408	149,515	187,354	210,847
Exports	146,927	170,114	175,638	209,151	229,221	264,917	275,175

Distribution of trade by countries (customs clearance basis) (US$1m.):

	Exports		*Imports*	
	1988	*1989*	*1988*	*1989*
Africa	4,806	4,609	3,944	4,078
Australia	6,680	7,805	10,285	11,605
Canada	6,424	6,807	8,308	8,045
China	9,476	8,516	9,859	11,146
Fed. Rep. of Germany	15,793	15,920	8,101	8,995
Hong Kong	11,706	11,526	2,109	2,219
Latin America	9,297	9,381	8,313	8,871
South-east Asia	67,109	73,516	47,802	52,906
Korea, Republic of	15,441	16,561	11,811	12,994
Taiwan	14,354	15,421	8,743	8,979
USSR	3,130	3,082	2,766	3,005
UK	10,632	10,741	4,193	4,466
USA	89,634	93,188	42,037	48,246

Principal items in 1989, with value in 1m. yen were:

Imports, c.i.f.		*Exports, f.o.b.*	
Mineral fuels	5,916,000	Machinery and transport equipment	28,238,000
Foodstuffs	4,264,000	Metals and metal products	2,964,000
Metal ores and scrap	1,280,000	Textile products	994,000
Machinery and transport equipment	4,461,000	Chemicals	2,029,000

Total trade between Japan and UK (British Department of Trade returns, in £1,000 sterling):

	1986	1987	1988	1989	1990
Imports to UK	4,932,497	5,463,116	6,509,137	7,108,441	6,761,592
Exports and re-exports from UK	1,193,933	1,495,111	1,742,747	2,259,823	2,631,326

Tourism. In 1989, 2,985,764 foreigners visited Japan, 538,117 of whom came from USA, 172,833 from UK. Japanese travelling abroad totalled 9,662,752 in 1989.

COMMUNICATIONS

Roads. The total length of roads (including urban and other local roads) was 1,104,282 km at 1 April 1988. There were 46,661 km of national roads, of which 45,589 km were paved. Motor vehicles, at 31 Dec. 1989, numbered 53,948,000, including 32,621,000 passenger cars and 21,085,000 commercial vehicles.

Railways. The first railway was completed in 1872, between Tokyo and Yokohama (29 km). In April 1987 the Japanese National Railways was reorganized into 7 private companies, the Japanese Railways (JR) Group – 6 passenger companies and 1 freight company. Total length of railways, in March 1987, was 25,782 km, of which the national railways had 19,639 km (9,367 km electrified) and private railways, 6,143 km (5,006 km electrified). In 1988 the JR carried 7,761m. passengers (other private, 12,980m.) and 56m. tons of freight (other private, 27m.). An undersea tunnel linking Honshu with Hokkaido was opened to rail services in 1988.

Aviation. The principal airlines are Japan Airlines (JAL) and All Nippon Airways. Japan Airlines, founded in 1953 and privatized in 1987, had 63 Boeing-747s in 1990. It operates international services from Tokyo to the USA, Europe, the Middle East and Southeast Asia, including flights to London over the North Pole and to Moscow by way of Siberia. In 1987 Japanese companies carried 50,045,000 passengers in domestic services and 8,474,000 passengers in international services.

Shipping. On 1 July 1989 the merchant fleet consisted of 7,777 vessels of 100 gross tons and over; total tonnage 26m. gross tons; there were 688 ships for passenger transport (1,283,000 gross tons), 2,541 cargo ships (1,336,000 gross tons) and 1,244 oil tankers (7,951,000 gross tons).

Coastguard. The 'Maritime Safety Agency' (Coastguard) consists of 11 regional MS headquarters, 66 MS offices, 51 MS stations, 14 air stations, 1 special rescue station, 9 district communications centres, 3 traffic advisory service centres, 4 hydrographic observatories and 119 navigation aids offices (with 5,136 navigation aids facilities) and controls 44 large patrol vessels, 47 medium patrol vessels, 11 small patrol vessels, 225 patrol craft, 21 hydrographic service vessels, 5 firefighting vessels, 10 firefighting boats, 69 guard and rescue boats and 79 navigation aids service supply vessels. Personnel in 1990 numbered 12,123 officers and men.

The Coastguard aviation service includes 26 fixed-wing aircraft and 41 helicopters.

Telecommunications. Telephone services have been operated by a private company (NTT) since 1985. In 1988 there were 49·9m. instruments.

On 31 March 1989, 99% of all households owned colour television sets.

Cinemas (1988). Cinemas numbered 1,912 with an annual attendance of 144m. (1960: 1,014m.).

Newspapers (1988). Daily newspapers numbered 124 with aggregate circulation of 71,172,000, including 4 major English-language newspapers.

JUSTICE, RELIGION, EDUCATION AND WELFARE

Justice. The Supreme Court is composed of the Chief Justice and 14 other judges. The Chief Justice is appointed by the Emperor, the other judges by the Cabinet. Every 10 years a justice must submit himself to the electorate. All justices and judges of the lower courts serve until they are 70 years of age.

Below the Supreme Court are 8 regional higher courts, district courts (*Chihosaibansho*) in each prefecture (4 in Hokkaido) and the local courts.

The Supreme Court is authorized to declare unconstitutional any act of the Legislature or the Executive which violates the Constitution.

The police are under central government control.

Religion. There has normally been religious freedom, but Shinto (literally, The Way of the Gods) was given the status of *quasi*-state-religion in the 1930s; in 1945 the Allied Supreme Command ordered the Government to discontinue state support of Shinto. State subsidies have ceased for all religions, and all religious teachings are forbidden in public schools.

In Dec. 1988 Shintoism claimed 111,792,000 adherents, Buddhism 93,109,000; these figures obviously overlap. Christians numbered 1,423,000.

Education. Education is compulsory and free between the ages of 6 and 15. Almost all national and municipal institutions are co-educational. On 1 May 1989 there were 14,995 kindergartens with 100,407 teachers and 2,037,614 pupils; 24,018 elementary schools with 445,450 teachers and 9,606,627 pupils; 11,175 junior high schools with 286,301 teachers and 5,619,297 pupils; 5,342 senior high schools with 284,461 teachers and 5,644,376 pupils; 584 junior colleges with 19,830 teachers and 461,849 pupils.

There were also 845 special schools for handicapped children (43,300 teachers, 95,008 pupils).

Japan has 7 main state universities, formerly known as the Imperial Universities: Tokyo University (1877); Kyoto University (1897); Tohoku University, Sendai (1907); Kyushu University, Fukuoka (1910); Hokkaido University, Sapporo (1918); Osaka University (1931), and Nagoya University (1939). In addition, there are various other state and municipal as well as private universities of high standing, such as Keio (founded in 1859), Waseda, Rikkyo, Meiji universities, and several women's universities, among which Tokyo and Ochanomizu are most notable. There are 499 colleges and universities with (1 May 1989) 2,066,962 students and 121,140 teachers.

Social Welfare. Hospitals on 1 Oct. 1988 numbered 10,034 with 1,634,309 beds. Physicians at the end of 1988 numbered 201,658; dentists, 70,572.

There are in force various types of social security schemes, such as health insurance, unemployment insurance and old-age pensions. The total population come under one or more of these schemes.

In 1988 14,155,099 persons and 8,172,213 households received some form of regular public assistance, the total of which came to 1,433,683m. yen.

14 weeks maternity leave is statutory.

DIPLOMATIC REPRESENTATIVES

Of Japan in Great Britain (101 Piccadilly, London, W1V 9FN)
Ambassador: Hiroshi Kitamura.

Of Great Britain in Japan (1 Ichiban-cho, Chiyoda-ku, Tokyo 102)
Ambassador: Sir John Whitehead, KCMG, CVO.

Of Japan in the USA (2520 Massachusetts Ave., NW, Washington, D.C., 20008)
Ambassador: Ryohei Murata.

Of the USA in Japan (10–1, Akasaka 1-chome, Minato-Ku, Tokyo)
Ambassador: Michael Armacost.

Of Japan to the United Nations
Ambassadors: Yoshio Hatano and Katsumi Sezaki.

Further Reading

Statistics Bureau of the Prime Minister's Office: *Statistical Year-Book* (from 1949).—*Statistical Abstract* (from 1950).—*Statistical Handbook of Japan 1977*.—*Monthly Bulletin* (from April 1950)
Economic Planning Agency: *Economic Survey* (annual), *Economic Statistics* (monthly), *Economic Indicators* (monthly)
Ministry of International Trade: *Foreign Trade of Japan* (annual)
Kodansha Encyclopedia of Japan. 9 vols. Tokyo, 1983
Japan Times Year Book. (I. Year Book of Japan. II. Who's Who in Japan. III. Business Directory of Japan.) Tokyo, first issue 1933
Labor in Tokyo. Tokyo Metropolitan Government, 1986
Treaty of Peace with Japan. (Cmd. 8392). HMSO, 1951; (Cmd. 8601). HMSO, 1952
Allen, G. C., *The Japanese Economy*. London, 1981
Baerwald, H. H., *Japan's Parliament*. CUP, 1974.—*Party Politics in Japan*. Boston, 1986
Beasley, W. T., *The Rise of Modern Japan*. London, 1990
Cambridge History of Japan. vols. 3-5. CUP, 1990
Cortazzi, H., *The Japanese Achievement*. London, 1990
Goodhart, C. A. E. and Sutija, G. (eds.) *Japanese Financial Growth*. London, 1990
Morishima, U. *Why has Japan 'Succeeded'?* CUP, 1984
Murata, K., *An Industrial Geography of Japan*. London, 1980
Nester, W. R., *The Foundation of Japanese Power: Continuities, Changes, Challenges*. London, 1990
Newland, K., (ed.) *The International Relations of Japan*. London, 1990
Nippon: A Chartered Survey of Japan. Tsuneta Yano Memorial Society. Tokyo, annual
Okita, S., *The Developing Economics of Japan: Lessons in Growth*. Univ. of Tokyo Press, 1983
Prindl, A., *Japanese Finance: Guide to Banking in Japan*. Chichester, 1981
Sansom, G. B., *A History of Japan*. 3 vols. London, 1958–64
Shulman, F. J., *Japan*. [Bibliography] Oxford and Santa Barbara, 1990
Steven, R., *Japan's New Imperialism*. London, 1990
Tsoukalis, L., (ed.) *Japan and Western Europe*. London, 1982
Vogel, E. F., *Japan as Number One*. Harvard Univ. Press, 1979
Ward, P., *Japanese Capitals*. Cambridge, 1985

JORDAN

Capital: Amman
Population: 3·17m. (1989)
GNP per capita: US$1,500 (1988)

Al Mamlaka al Urduniya al Hashemiyah

(Hashemite Kingdom of Jordan)

HISTORY. By a Treaty, signed in London on 22 March 1946, Britain recognized Transjordan as a sovereign independent state. On 25 May 1946 the Amir Abdullah assumed the title of King, and when the treaty was ratified on 17 June 1946 the name of the territory was changed to that of 'The Hashemite Kingdom of Jordan' in 1949. A new Anglo-Transjordan treaty was signed in Amman on 15 March 1948. The treaty was to remain in force for 20 years, but by mutual consent was terminated on 13 March 1957.

The Arab Federation between the Kingdoms of Iraq and Jordan, which was concluded on 14 Feb. 1958, lapsed after the revolution in Iraq of 14 July 1958, and was officially terminated by royal decree on 1 Aug. 1958.

Since the occupation of the West Bank in June 1967 by Israeli forces, that part of Palestine has not been administratively controlled by the Jordanian government.

On 31 July 1988, King Hussein announced that Jordan was to abandon its efforts to administer the Israeli-occupied West Bank and surrendered its claims to the territory to the Palestine Liberation Organization.

AREA AND POPULATION. The part of Palestine remaining to the Arabs under the armistice with Israel on 3 April 1949, with the exception of the Gaza strip, was in Dec. 1949 placed under Jordanian rule and formally incorporated in Jordan on 24 April 1950. For the frontier lines *see* map in THE STATESMAN'S YEAR-BOOK, 1951. In June 1967 this territory, known as the West Bank, was occupied by Israeli forces. For details *see* p. 734.

The area formerly administered by the Jordanian government, known as the East Bank, comprised 89,206 sq. km (34,443 sq. miles) following an exchange of territory with Saudi Arabia on 10 Aug. 1965. Its population at the 1979 Census was 2,132,997; latest estimate (1989) 3,165,000. The area and population of the 8 governorates were:

Muhafaza	*1986*	*Muhafaza*	*1986*
Asimah	1,160,000	Ma'an	97,500
Balqa	193,800	Mafraq	98,600
Irbid	680,200	Tafilah	41,400
Karak	120,100	Zarqa	404,500

The largest towns with suburbs, with estimated population, 1986: Amman, the capital, 1,160,000; Irbid, 680,200; Zarqa, 404,500;.

In 1986 registered births numbered 112,451; deaths, 8,853; marriages, 19,397; divorces (1984), 2,652.

CLIMATE. Predominantly a Mediterranean climate, with hot dry summers and cool wet winters, but in hilly parts summers are cooler and winters colder. Those areas below sea-level are very hot in summer and warm in winter. Eastern parts have a desert climate. Amman. Jan. 46°F (7·5°C), July 77°F (24·9°C). Annual rainfall 12" (290 mm). Aqaba. Jan. 61°F (16°C), July 89°F (31·5°C). Annual rainfall 1·5" (35 mm).

KING. The Kingdom is a constitutional monarchy headed by HM King **Hussein**, GCVO, eldest son of King Talal, who, being incapacitated by mental illness, was deposed by Parliament on 11 Aug. 1952 and died 8 July 1972. The King was born 14 Nov. 1935, and married Princess Dina Abdul Hamid on 19 April 1955 (divorced 1957), Toni Avril Gardiner (Muna al Hussein) on 25 May 1961 (divorced 1972), Alia Toukan on 26 Dec. 1972 (died in air crash 1977) and Elizabeth Halaby on 15 June 1978. *Offspring:* Princess Alia, born 13 Feb. 1956; Prince Abdulla, born 30 Jan. 1962; Prince Faisal, born 11 Oct. 1963; Princesses Zein and Aisha, born 23 April 1968; Princess Haya, born 3 May 1974; Prince Ali, born 23 Dec. 1975; Prince Hamzah, born 1 April 1980; Prince Hashem, born 10 June 1981; Princess Iman, born 4 April 1983; Princess Raya, born 9 Feb. 1986. *Crown Prince* (appointed 1 April 1965): Prince Hassan, younger brother of the King.

CONSTITUTION AND GOVERNMENT. The Constitution passed on 7 Nov. 1951 provides that the Cabinet is responsible to Parliament.

The legislature consists of a lower house of 80 members elected by universal suffrage and a senate of 30 members nominated by the King.

On 5 Feb. 1976 both Houses of Parliament approved amendments to the Constitution by which the King was empowered to postpone calling elections until further notice. The lower house was dissolved. This step was taken because no elections could be held in the West Bank which has been under Israeli occupation since June 1967.

Parliament was reconvened on 9 Jan. 1984. By-elections were held in March 1984 and 6 members were nominated for the West Bank bringing Parliament to 60 members. Women voted for the first time in 1984. Elections were held on 8 Nov. 1989; the Moslem Brotherhood won 22 of the 80 seats. A government reshuffle of Jan. 1991 gave them 5 ministries: *Justice, Social Development, Religious Affairs, Health, Education.*

In Jan. 1991 King Hussein approved a national charter legalizing political parties.

Prime Minister and Defence: Modar Badran.
Foreign Minister: Taher Al-Masri.
The *Speaker* of the lower house is Abdul-Latif Arabiyat.

National flag: Three horizontal stripes of black, white, green, with a red triangle based on the hoist, bearing a white 7-pointed star.

The official language of the country is Arabic.

DEFENCE

Army. The Army is organized in 2 armoured and 2 mechanized infantry divisions, 1 Royal Guard and 1 special forces brigade, and 1 field artillery brigade. Equipment includes 1,131 main battle tanks. Total strength (1991) 74,000 men.

Navy. The Jordan Coastal Guard numbered 250 in 1990 and operates 6 small patrol boats.

Air Force. The Air Force has 2 interceptor and 3 ground attack squadrons equipped respectively with Mirage F1 and F-5E Tiger II fighters, and 2-seat F-5Fs, plus an OCU equipped with F-5A fighters and 2-seat F-5Bs. Two anti-armour squadrons have Bell AH-1S Huey Cobra helicopters. There are 6 C-130B/H Hercules and 2 CASA Aviocar turboprop transports, S-70 Blackhawk, S-76, Gazelle, Alouette III and Hughes 500D helicopters, piston-engined Bulldog basic trainers and CASA Aviojet jet trainers. Hawk surface-to-air missiles equip 14 batteries. Strength (1990) about 10,000 officers and men and 104 combat aircraft and 24 armed helicopters.

INTERNATIONAL RELATIONS

Membership. Jordan is a member of the UN and the Arab League.

ECONOMY

Policy. A 5-year plan (1986–90) aimed at improving agriculture and the development of water resources.

Budget. The budget estimates for the year 1989 provide for revenue of JD.907m. and expenditure of JD.1,106m. which included 209m. for defence. External public debt JD.1,868m.

Currency. The unit of currency is the *Jordan dinar,* (JOD) of 1,000 *fils.* The following bank-notes and coins are in circulation: 10, 5 dinars, 1 dinar, 500 fils (notes), 250, 100, 50, 25, 20 fils (cupronickel), 10, 5, 1 fils (bronze). In March 1991, £1 = JD.123·72; US$ = JD.0·65.

Banking and Finance. The Central Bank of Jordan was established in 1964. In 1986 there were 9 local commercial banks including Arab Bank (the largest, with a capital of JD.22m.), 8 foreign commercial banks including Grindlays Bank and 6 foreign banks with representative offices. In 1985 there were 2 investment banks, 5 finance companies, 3 Islamic institutions and 3 real estated-linked savings and loan associations.

Assets and liabilities of the Jordanian banking system (including the Central Bank, commercial banks and the Housing Bank) totalled JD.2,404·34m. in 1984.

Weights and Measures. The metric system is in force.

ENERGY AND NATURAL RESOURCES

Electricity. Production (1986) 2,955m. kwh. Supply 220 volts; 50 Hz.

Oil. Oil was discovered in 1982 at Azraq, 70 km east of Amman and 7 new wells were under development in 1985. Deposits of oil shale, estimated at 10,000m. tonnes, have been discovered at Lajjun.

Minerals. Phosphates production in 1987 was 6·85m. tonnes. Potash is found in the Dead Sea. Reserves, over 800m. tonnes. A potash plant built on the southeast shore to extract compounds by solar evaporation produced 1·2m. tonnes in 1987. Cement production (1987), 2·3m. tonnes.

Agriculture. The country east of the Hejaz Railway line is largely desert; north-western Jordan is potentially of agricultural value and an integrated Jordan Valley project began in 1973. Arable land was 308,000 ha. in 1989; permanent crops, 66,000 ha.; permanent pasture, 791,000 ha. The agricultural cropping pattern for irrigated vegetable cultivation was introduced in 1984 to regulate production and diversify the crops being cultivated. In 1987 Jordan was self-sufficient in the production of potatoes and onions. In 1986 the government began to lease state-owned land in the semi-arid southern regions for agricultural development by private investors, mostly for wheat and barley. Jordan is self-sufficient in poultry meat. The main crops are tomatoes and other vegetables, citrus fruit, wheat and olives.

Production in 1988 included (in tonnes): Tomatoes, 200,000; olives, 30,000; citrus fruit, 113,000; wheat, 80,000.

Livestock (1988): 1·22m. sheep; 460,000 goats; 29,000 cattle; 14,000 camels.

There were 5,673 tractors in 1989.

Forestry. There were 71,000 ha. of forest and woodland in 1989.

INDUSTRY. Production (1987, in tonnes): Phosphates, 6,841,000; petroleum products, 2,229,000; cement, 2,472,000; iron, 219,000; fertilizer, 1,656,000.

Other industries include cigarettes, cosmetics, textiles, shoes, batteries, plastic products, leather tanning, pharmaceutical products, iron pipes, detergents, aluminium and ceramics. Some 50% of industry is based in Amman.

Labour. The economically active population in 1989 was 732,000, of whom 45,000 worked in agriculture.

FOREIGN ECONOMIC RELATIONS

Commerce. Imports in 1987 were valued at JD.915·54m. and exports and re-exports at JD.315·7m. Total remittances from Jordanians working abroad reached US$1,187·5m. in 1984.

Major exports in 1987 (in JD.1m.) included phosphates, 61; chemicals, 69·93; food and live animals, 248·77; manufactured goods, 37·34. Major imports included machinery and transport equipment, 186·29; crude oil, 118·59.

Exports in 1987 (in JD.1m.) were mainly to Iraq, 59·87; Saudi Arabia, 26·2 and India, 22. Imports were mainly from Saudi Arabia, 76·76 and the USA, 93·39.

Total trade between Jordan and UK (British Department of Trade returns, in £1,000 sterling):

	1986	*1987*	*1988*	*1989*	*1990*
Imports to UK	49,766	29,285	21,310	16,462	14,788
Exports and re-exports from UK	130,385	188,998	183,555	110,684	109,483

Tourism. In 1987 there were 1·9m. foreign visitors spending US$600m.

COMMUNICATIONS

Roads. Total length of public highways, 4,095 km. Motor vehicles in 1980 included 73,078 private passenger cars, 11,207 taxis, 1,415 buses, 29,517 goods vehicles, 4,888 motor cycles.

Railways. The 1,050 mm gauge Hejaz Jordan and Aqaba Railway runs from the Syrian border at Nassib to Ma'an and Naqb Ishtar and Aqaba Port (total, 618 km). In 1988 the railways carried some 20,000 passengers and 614m. tonne-km of freight.

Aviation. The Queen Alia International airport, at Zizya, 30 km south of Amman was inaugurated in 1983. There are other international airports at Amman and Aqaba. Jordan is served by over 20 international airlines.

Shipping (1980). The port of Aqaba handled 6,598,591 tons of cargo. JD.65m. was spent between 1980–85 on developing facilities and US$1,000m. is to be provided under the 1986–90 plan on further developments including a special oil terminal and 4 new wharves.

Telecommunications. In 1982 there were 791 post offices and (1987) 189,502 telephones. There were 250,000 TV receivers and 1·1m. radios in 1988.

Newspapers (1988). There were 4 daily (including 1 in English) and 3 weekly papers, with a total circulation (1987) of 188,000. Newspapers were denationalized in 1990, though government institutions still hold majority ownership.

RELIGION, EDUCATION AND WELFARE

Religion. About 80% of the population are Sunni Moslems.

Education (1987). There were 411 pre-primary schools with 1,461 teachers and 31,827 pupils; 1,294 elementary schools with 18,448 teachers and 542,519 pupils; 1,124 preparatory schools with 10,495 teachers and 214,743 pupils; 510 secondary schools with 7,023 teachers and 98,786 pupils and 27 vocational educational schools with 2,180 teachers and 31,770 pupils. The University of Jordan, inaugurated on 15 Dec. 1962 had in 1987, 12,672 students. The Yarmouk University (Irbid) was inaugurated in 1976 with (1987) 11,603 students. The Mu'tah University was inaugurated in 1981 with (1987) 1,349 students. The Jordan University of Science and Technology was inaugurated in 1987 with 2,815 students.

Health (1987). There were 4,500 physicians, 1,041 dentists and 56 hospitals with 5,672 beds.

DIPLOMATIC REPRESENTATIVES

Of Jordan in Great Britain (6 Upper Phillimore Gdns., London, W8 7HB)
Ambassador: Dr Albert Butros.

Of Great Britain in Jordan (Abdoun, Amman)
Ambassador: Anthony Reeve, CMG.

Of Jordan in the USA (3504 International Dr., NW, Washington, D.C., 20008)
Ambassador: Hussein Hamami.

Of the USA in Jordan (Jebel Amman, Amman)
Ambassador: Roger G. Harrison.

Of Jordan to the United Nations
Ambassador: Abdullah Salah.

Further Reading

The Department of Statistics, Ministry of National Economy, publishes a *Statistical Yearbook* (in Arabic and English), latest issue 1968, and a *Statistical Guide*, latest issue 1965.—*External Trade Statistics*, 1968.—*National Accounts and Input-Output Analysis, 1959–65*, 1967

The Constitution of the Hashemite Kingdom of Jordan. Amman, 1952

Gubser, P., *Jordan*. Boulder, 1982

Seccombe, I., *Jordan*. [Bibliography] Oxford and Santa Barbara, 1984

Seton, C. R. W., *Legislation of Transjordan, 1918-30*. London, 1931. [Continued by the Government of Jordan as an annual publication: *Jordan Legislation*. Amman, 1932 ff.]

Toni, Y. T. and Mousa, S., *Jordan: Land and People*. Amman, 1973

Wilson, M. C., *King Abdullah, Britain and the making of Jordan*. CUP, 1987

KENYA

Capital: Nairobi
Population: 24·08m. (1989)
GNP per capita: US$360 (1988)

Jamhuri ya Kenya

(Republic of Kenya)

HISTORY. Until Kenya became independent on 12 Dec. 1963, it consisted of the colony and the protectorate. The protectorate comprised the mainland dominions of the Sultan of Zanzibar, viz., a coastal strip of territory 10 miles wide, to the northern branch of the Tana River; also Mau, Kipini and the Island of Lamu, and all adjacent islands between the rivers Umba and Tana. The Sultan on 8 Oct. 1963 ceded the coastal strip to Kenya with effect from 12 Dec. 1963.

The colony and protectorate, formerly known as the East African Protectorate were, on 1 April 1905, transferred from the Foreign Office to the Colonial Office and in Nov. 1906 the protectorate was placed under the control of a governor and C.-in-C. and (except the Sultan of Zanzibar's dominions) was annexed to the Crown as from 23 July 1920 under the name of the Colony of Kenya, thus becoming a Crown Colony.

The territories on the coast became the Kenya Protectorate.

A Treaty was signed (15 July 1924) with Italy under which Great Britain ceded to Italy the Juba River and a strip from 50 to 100 miles wide on the British side of the river. Cession took place on 29 June 1925. The northern boundary is defined by an agreement with Ethiopia in 1947. A Constitution conferring internal self-government was brought into force on 1 June 1963, and full independence was achieved on 12 Dec. 1963. On 12 Dec. 1964 Kenya became a republic.

AREA AND POPULATION. Kenya is bounded by Sudan and Ethiopia in the north, Uganda in the west, Tanzania in the south and the Somali Republic and the Indian ocean in the east. The total area is 224,960 sq. miles (582,600 sq. km), of which 219,790 sq. miles is land area. In the 1979 census, the population was 15,327,061, of which 15,101,540 were Africans, 78,600 Asians, 39,900 Europeans, 39,140 Arabs. Estimate (1988), 24,078,000 (22·8% urban).

The land areas, populations and capitals of the provinces are:

Province	*Sq. km*	*Census 1979*	*Estimate 1987*	*Capital*	*Census 1979*
Rift Valley	171,108	3,240,402	4,702,400	Nakuru	92,851
Eastern	155,760	2,719,851	3,864,700	Embu	15,986
Nyanza	12,526	2,643,956	3,892,600	Kisumu	152,643
Central	13,173	2,345,833	3,284,800	Nyeri	35,753
Coast	83,040	1,342,794	1,904,100	Mombasa	425,634 [1]
Western	8,223	1,832,663	2,535,900	Kakamega	32,025
Nairobi District	684	827,775	1,288,700	Nairobi	1,103,554 [1]
North-Eastern	126,902	373,787	554,000	Garissa	14,076

[1] Estimate, 1984.

Other towns (1979): Machakos (84,320), Meru (70,439), Eldoret (59,503), Thika (41,324).

Kiswahili is the official language, but 21% speak Kikuyu as their mother tongue, 14% Luhya, 13% Luo, 11% Kamba, 11% Kalenjin, 6% Gusii, 5% Meru and 5% Mijikenda. English is spoken in commercial centres.

CLIMATE. The climate is tropical, with wet and dry seasons, but considerable differences in altitude make for varied conditions between the hot, coastal lowlands and the plateau, where temperatures are very much cooler. Heaviest rains occur in April and May, but in some parts there is a second wet season in Nov. and Dec. Nairobi. Jan. 65°F (18·3°C), July 60°F (15·6°C). Annual rainfall 39" (958 mm). Mombasa. Jan. 81°F (27·2°C), July 76°F (24·4°C). Annual rainfall 47" (1,201 mm).

CONSTITUTION AND GOVERNMENT. There is a unicameral National Assembly of 203 members, comprising 188 elected by universal suffrage for a 5-year term, 12 members appointed by the President, and the Speaker and Attorney-General ex-officio. The President is also directly elected for 5 years; he appoints a Vice-President and other Ministers to a Cabinet over which he presides. The sole legal political party is the Kenya African National Union (KANU). In Dec. 1990 KANU restored the secret ballot and security of tenure for judges, but remained committed to the principle of 'democracy with a sole party'.

Elections to the National Assembly took place by secret ballot on 21 March 1988. Only 123 seats were contested, the rest were unopposed.

President: Daniel T. arap Moi (elected 1978, re-elected 1983 and 1988).

Vice-President and Minister of Finance: George Saitoti. *Environment and Natural Resources:* Nioroge Mungai. *Lands, Housing and Physical Planning:* M Mbela. *Water Development:* John Okwanyo. *Home Affairs and National Heritage:* Davidson Kuguru. *Planning and National Development:* Z. T. Onyonka. *Transport and Communications:* Joseph Kamotho. *Energy:* N. K. Biwott. *Local Government and Physical Planning:* William Ntimama. *Foreign Affairs and International Cooperation:* Wilson Ayah. *Commerce:* Arthur Magugu. *Tourism and Wildlife:* Katana Ngala. *Culture and Social Services:* James Niiru. *Agriculture:* Elijah Mwangale. *Health:* Mwai Kibaki. *Public Works:* Timothy Mibei. *Cooperative Development:* John Cheruiyot. *Labour:* Philip Masinde. *Education:* Peter O Aringo. *Information and Broadcasting:* Nahashon Kanyi. *Livestock Development:* Jeremiah Nvagah. *Industry:* D Otieno. *Research, Science and Technology:* George Muhoko. *Supplies and Marketing:* Wycliffe Mudavadi. *Technical Training and Applied Technology:* S K Ongeri. *Manpower Development and Employment:* vacant. *Reclamation and Development of Arid, Semi-Arid and Wasteland:* G M Ndoto. *Regional Development:* Onyango Midika. *Attorney-General:* Justice Mathew Muli.

National flag: Three horizontal stripes of black, red, green, with the red edged in white; bearing in the centre an African shield in black and white with 2 crossed spears behind.

Administration. The country is divided into the Nairobi Area and 7 provinces and there are 40 districts.

DEFENCE

Army. The Army consists of 1 armoured, 1 engineer and 2 infantry brigades; 2 engineer, 1 air cavalry, airborne, 1 anti-aircraft and 5 infantry batallions. Equipment includes 76 Vickers Mk3 main battle tanks. Total strength (1991) 19,000.

Navy. The Navy, based in Mombasa, in 1990 consisted of 2 56-metre fast missile craft, 4 smaller missile craft, and 1 inshore patrol craft, all built in Britain, and 1 tug. Personnel in 1990 totalled 1,100.

The Marine police and Customs operate an additional 15 patrol boats.

Air Force. An air force, formed 1 June 1964, was built up with RAF assistance and is under Army command. Equipment includes 11 F-5E/F-5F supersonic combat aircraft/trainers, 12 Hawk and 5 BAC 167 Strikemaster light jet attack/trainers, 8 twin-turboprop Buffaloes for transport, air ambulance, anti-locust spraying and security duties, 7 Skyservant light twins, 12 Bulldog piston-engined primary trainers and Puma and Gazelle helicopters. Personnel (1991) 3,500, with 28 combatant aircraft and 38 armed helicopters.

INTERNATIONAL RELATIONS

Membership. Kenya is a member of UN, the Commonwealth, OAU and is an ACP state of EEC.

ECONOMY

Planning. The sixth national development plan (1989-93) aims to expand the economy and create 2m. jobs.

Budget. Ordinary revenue and expenditure for 1988–89: Revenue, KSh.36,298m.; expenditure, KSh.55,504m.

Currency. The monetary unit is the *Kenya shilling* (KES) of 100 *cents*; 20 shillings = K£1. Notes of the Central Bank of Kenya are circulated in denominations of KSh.5, 10, 20, 50, 100, 200 and 500 and coins in denominations of 5, 10 and 50 cents and KSh.1 and 5. Currency in circulation at Dec. 1987: Notes, K£425,080,000; coins, K£13·7m. Inflation was 30% in Sept. 1990. In March 1991, £1 = 47·97 *shilling*; US$1 = 25·29 *shilling*.

Banking and Finance. Banks operating in Kenya: The National & Grindlays Bank International, Ltd; the Standard Bank, Ltd; Barclays Bank of Kenya Ltd; Algemene Bank Nederland NV; Bank of India, Ltd; Bank of Baroda, Ltd; Habib Bank (Overseas), Ltd; Commercial Bank of Africa, Ltd; Citibank; The Co-operative Bank of Kenya, Ltd; National Bank of Kenya, Ltd; Agricultural Finance Corporation; The Kenya Commercial Bank (70% state-owned); The Central Bank of Kenya. In Jan. 1985 there were 43 non-bank finance institutions.

The Kenya Post Office Savings Bank, a state savings bank established in 1978, had 1,250,000 ordinary savings accounts with total deposits of KSh.750m. at 31 Dec. 1984.

There is a stock exchange in Nairobi.

ENERGY AND NATURAL RESOURCES

Electricity. Installed generating capacity was 575 mw in 1987; two-thirds was provided by hydropower from power stations on the Tana river, 30% by oil-fired power stations and the rest by geothermal power. Production (1987) 2,454m. kwh. Supply 220 volts; 50 Hz.

Minerals. Production, 1987 (in 1,000 tonnes): Soda ash, 228; fluorspar ore, 47; salt, 72. Other minerals included gold, raw soda, lime and limestone, diatomite, garnets and vermiculite.

Agriculture. As agriculture is possible from sea-level to altitudes of over 9,000 ft, tropical, sub-tropical and temperate crops can be grown and mixed farming can be advocated. Four-fifths of the country is range-land which produces mainly livestock products and wild game which constitutes the major attraction of the country's tourist industry.

The main areas of crop production are the Central, Rift Valley, Western and Nyanza Provinces and parts of Eastern and Coastal Provinces. Coffee, tea, sisal, pyrethrum, maize and wheat are crops of major importance in the Highlands, while coconuts, cashew nuts, cotton, sugar, sisal and maize are the principal crops grown at the lower altitudes. Production, 1989 (in 1,000 tonnes), of principal food crops: Maize, 2,925; wheat, 258; rice, 50; barley, 20; millet, 60; sorghum, 143; potatoes, 300; sweet potatoes, 550; cassava, 620; sugar-cane, 4,500. Main cash crops (1989): Tobacco, 9; coffee, 119; tea, 181; vegetables, 491; fruit, 764; seed cotton, 24; sisal, 43.

Livestock (1989): Cattle, 13·46m.; sheep, 6·33m.; goats, 7·5m.; pigs, 100,000; poultry, 24m.

Forestry. The total area of gazetted forest reserves in Kenya amounts to 16,800 sq. km, of which the greater part is situated between 6,000 and 11,000 ft above sea-level, mostly on Mount Kenya, the Aberdares, Mount Elgon, Tinderet, Londiani, Mau watershed, Elgeyo and Charangani ranges. These forests may be divided into coniferous, broad-leaved or hardwood and bamboo forests. The upper parts of these forests are mainly bamboo, which occurs mostly between altitudes of 8,000 and 10,000 ft and occupies some 10% of the high-altitude forests.

Fisheries. Landings in 1987 were 118,216 tonnes of fresh water fish, 6,096 tonnes of marine fish, 299 tonnes of crustaceans and 39 tonnes of other marine products; total value K£18,849,000.

INDUSTRY. In 1986 industry accounted for some 13% of GDP and employed about one-fifth of the wage-earning labour force. The main activities were textiles, chemicals, vehicle assembly and transport equipment, leather and footwear, printing and publishing, food and tobacco processing. An important sub-sector was the refining of crude petroleum at Mombasa.

FOREIGN ECONOMIC RELATIONS

Commerce. Total domestic exports (1987, provisional) K£753m.; imports K£1,431m.

Chief imports in 1987 were petroleum and petroleum products (19·7% of total), industrial supplies (32·8%), machinery and other capital equipment (22·4%), food and drink (6·9%) and transport equipment (13·3%). Chief exports were coffee (26%), tea (22%) and petroleum products (12·6%). By 1986 fresh vegetables, fruits and flowers became the fourth largest foreign exchange earner.

Imports in 1987 were mainly from the UK (17%), Japan (10·9%), Federal Republic of Germany (8%) and USA (7·1%). Exports were mainly to the UK (16·8%), Federal Republic of Germany (9·6%), Uganda (8·9%), USA (5·4%) and Pakistan (15·7%).

Total trade between Kenya and UK (British Department of Trade returns, in £1,000 sterling):

	1986	*1987*	*1988*	*1989*	*1990*
Imports to UK	163,745	129,236	142,455	154,313	149,474
Exports and re-exports from UK	170,671	199,059	202,094	208,464	223,080

Tourism. In 1987, about 662,100 tourists visited Kenya and spent KSh.5,840m.

COMMUNICATIONS

Roads. In 1987 there were 6,600 km of bitumen surfaced roads and 45,000 km of gravel-surfaced roads.

Railways. On 11 Feb. 1977 the independent Kenya Railways Corporation was formed following break-up of the East African Railways administration. The network totals 2,654 km of metre-gauge. In 1987, the railways carried 3·8m. passengers and 3m. tonnes of freight.

Aviation. Total number of passengers handled at the 3 main airports (1984) was 2,058,000. Jomo Kenyatta Airport, Nairobi, handles nearly 30 international airlines as well as Kenya Airways. South African Airways began a weekly flight from Johannesburg to Nairobi in Dec. 1990.

Shipping. A national shipping service is planned (1984) to be based in Mombasa, the Kenyan main port at Kilindini on the Indian Ocean. The port handles cargo freight both for Kenya as well as for the neighbouring East African states.

Post and Broadcasting. The Voice of Kenya operates 2 national services (Swahili–English) from Nairobi and regional services in Kisumu, Nairobi and Mombasa. The television service provides programmes mainly in English and Swahili. Telephones (1983) 216,674; television sets (1985) 250,000; radios (1985) 3·4m.

JUSTICE, RELIGION, EDUCATION AND WELFARE

Justice. The courts of Justice comprises the court of Appeal, the High Court and a large number of subsidiary courts.

The court of Appeal is the final Apellant court in the country and is based in Nairobi. It comprises of 7 Judges of Appeal. In the course of its Appellate duties the court of Appeal visits Mombasa, Kisumu, Nakuru and Nyeri.

The High court with full jurisdiction in both civil and criminal matters comprises of a total of 28 puisne Judges. Puisne Judges sit in Nairobi (16), Mombasa (2), Nakuru, Kisumu, Nyeri, Eldoret Meru and Kisii (1 each).

The Magistracy consists of approximately 300 magistrates of various cadres based in all provincial, district and some divisional centres. In addition to the above there are the Kadhi courts established in areas of concentrated Muslim populations:

Mombasa, Nairobi, Malindi, Lamu, Garissa, Kisumu and Marsabit. They exercise limited jurisdiction in matters governed by Islamic Law.

Religion. In 1987, the Roman Catholic Church had nearly 6m. adherents (27% of the population), Protestants 4m. (19%) and other Christian churches over 6m. (27%), while Islam had 1·3m. (6%), traditional tribal religions 4m. (19%) and others 400,000 (2%).

Education. *Primary* (1987). 13,849 primary schools with 5·03m. pupils and 149,151 teachers.

Secondary (1987). There were 2,592 secondary schools with a total enrolment of 522,261 and 24,251 teachers.

Technical (1987). There were 17 Institutes of Science and Technology with 4,200 students and 433 teachers. Kenya, Mombasa and Eldoret Polytechnics and Jomo Kenyatta College of Agriculture and Technology had 7,100 students in 1987.

Teacher training (1987). 17,733 students were training as teachers in 22 colleges with 1,348 lecturers.

Higher Education. In 1987–88 there were 4 public universities and enrolments were: University of Nairobi (inaugurated 1970), 10,841; Moi University (opened 1985), 970; Kenyatta University, 5,135; Egerton University, 1,935 (592 undergraduates and 1,343 diploma students).

Health. In 1987 beds and cots in hospitals (including mission hospitals) totalled 31,356. 2,071 hospitals and health centres, including sub-centres and dispensaries, were in operation. Free medical service for all children and adult out-patients was launched in 1965.

DIPLOMATIC REPRESENTATIVES

Of Kenya in Great Britain (45 Portland Pl., London, W1)
High Commissioner: Dr Sally J. Kosgei.

Of Great Britain in Kenya (Bruce Hse., Standard St., Nairobi)
High Commissioner: Sir William Tomkys, KCMG.

Of Kenya in the USA (2249 R. St., NW, Washington, D.C., 20008)
Ambassador: Denis D. Afande.

Of the USA in Kenya (Moi/Haile Selassie Ave., Nairobi)
Ambassador: Smith Hempstone, Jr.

Of Kenya to the United Nations
Ambassador: Michael George Okeyo.

Further Reading

Kenya Economic Survey, 1988. Nairobi, 1988
Statistical Abstract. Government Printer, Nairobi, 1982
Who's Who in Kenya 1982–1983. London, 1983
Arnold, G., *Kenyatta and the Politics of Kenya.* London, 1974.—*Modern Kenya.* London, 1982
Bigsten, A., *Education and Income Distribution in Kenya.* Brookfield, Vermont, 1984
Collison, R. L., *Kenya.* [Bibliography] London and Santa Barbara, 1982
Harbeson, J. W., *Nation-Building in Kenya: The Role of Land Reform.* Northwestern Univ. Press, 1973
Hazlewood, A., *The Economy of Kenya: The Kenyatta Era.* OUP, 1980
Langdon, S. W., *Multinational Corporations in the Political Economy of Kenya.* London, 1981
Miller, N. N., *Kenya, the Quest for Prosperity.* Boulder and London, 1984
Tomkinson, M., *Kenya: A Holiday Guide.* 5th ed. London and Hammamet, 1981

KIRIBATI

Capital: Tarawa
Population: 66,250 (1987)
GNP per capita: US$650 (1988)

Republic of Kiribati

HISTORY. The Gilbert and Ellice Islands were proclaimed a protectorate in 1892 and annexed (at the request of the native governments) as the Gilbert and Ellice Islands Colony on 10 Nov. 1915 (effective on 12 Jan. 1916). On 1 Oct. 1975 the former Ellice Islands severed its constitutional links with the Gilbert Islands and took a new name Tuvalu.

Internal self-government was obtained on 1 Nov. 1976 and independence achieved on 12 July 1979 as the Republic of Kiribati.

AREA AND POPULATION. Kiribati (pronounced Kiribass) consists of 3 groups of coral atolls and one isolated volcanic island, spread over a large expanse of the Central Pacific with a total land area of 717·1 sq. km (276·9 sq. miles). It comprises Banaba or Ocean Island (5 sq. km), the 16 Gilbert Islands (295 sq. km), the 8 Phœnix Islands (55 sq. km), and 8 of the 11 Line Islands (329 sq. km), the other 3 Line Islands (Jarvis, Palmyra and Kingman Reef) being uninhabited dependencies of the US. Population, 1985 census, 63,848; estimate (1987) 66,250. It was announced in 1988 that 4,700 people are to be resettled on Teraina and Tabuaeran atolls because the main island group is overcrowded. Banaba, all 16 Gilbert Islands, and 3 atolls in the Line Islands (Teraina, Tabuaeran and Kiritimati—formerly Washington, Fanning and Christmas Islands respectively) are inhabited; their populations in 1985 (census) were as follows:

Banaba (Ocean Is.)	189	Abemama	2,966	Onotoa	1,927
Makin	1,777	Kuria	1,052	Tamana	1,348
Butaritari	3,622	Aranuki	984	Arorae	1,470
Marakei	2,693	Nonouti	2,930	Phœnix Island	24
Abaiang	4,386	Tabiteuea	4,493	Teraina	416
Tarawa	24,598	Beru	2,702	Tabuaeran	445
Maiana	2,141	Nikunau	2,061	Kiritimati	1,737

The remaining 13 atolls have no permanent population; the 8 Phœnix Islands comprise Birnie, Rawaki (formerly Phœnix), Enderbury, Kanton (or Abariringa), Manra (formerly Sydney), Orona (formerly Hull), McKean and Nikumaroro (formerly Gardner), while the others are Malden and Starbuck in the Central Line Islands and Caroline, Flint and Vostok in the Southern Line Islands. The population is almost entirely Micronesian.

CLIMATE. The Line Islands, Phœnix Islands and Banaba have a maritime equatorial climate, but the islands further north and south are tropical. Annual and daily ranges of temperature are small and mean annual rainfall ranges from 50" (1,250 mm) near the equator to 120" (3,000 mm) in the north. Tarawa. Jan. 83°F (28·3°C), July 82°F (27·8°C). Annual rainfall 79" (1,977 mm).

CONSTITUTION AND GOVERNMENT. Under the independence Constitution the republic has a unicameral legislature, comprising 36 members elected from 20 constituencies for a 4-year term. The *Beretitenti* (President) is both Head of State and of Government.

In Feb. 1991 the government was composed as follows:

President and Foreign Affairs: Ieremia Tabai, GCMG.

Vice-President, Finance and Economic Planning: Teatao Teannaki. *Home Affairs and Decentralization:* Babera Kirata, OBE. *Trade, Industry and Labour:* Raion Bataroma. *Health and Family Planning:* Rotaria Ataia. *Natural Resource Development:* Taomati Iuta, OBE. *Education:* Ataraoti Bwebwenibure. *Communications:* Uera Rabaua. *Minister for the Line and Phœnix Group of Islands:* Tekinaiti Kaiteie. *Works and Energy:* Baitika Toom. *Attorney-General:* Michael Takabwebwe.

National flag: Red, with blue and white wavy lines in base, and in the centre a gold rising sun and a flying frigate bird.

National anthem: Teirake Kain Kiribati.

INTERNATIONAL RELATIONS

Membership. Kiribati is a member of the Commonwealth, South Pacific Forum and is an ACP state of the EEC.

ECONOMY

Budget. Budget estimates for 1989 show revenue, $A20,648,000; principal items: Fishing licences, $A3·87m.; customs duties, $A5m.; direct taxation, $A2·5m. Expenditure amounted to $A20,648,000.

Currency. The currency in use is the Australian *dollar*.

ENERGY AND NATURAL RESOURCES

Electricity. Electric power production (1986) was 8m. kwh.

Minerals. Phosphate production was discontinued in 1979.

Agriculture. Land under agriculture and permanant cultivation, 50·7%; forest, 2·8%; other, 46·5%. The land is basically coral reefs upon which coral sand has built up, and then been enriched by humus from rotting vegetation and flotsam which has drifted ashore. The principal tree is the coconut, which grows prolifically on all the islands except some of the Phœnix Islands. Other food-bearing trees are the pandanus palm and the breadfruit. As the amount of soil is negligible, the only vegetable which grows in any quantity is a coarse calladium (alocasia) with the local name 'babai', which is cultivated most laboriously in deep pits. Pigs and fowls are kept throughout Kiribati.

Copra production is mainly in the hands of the individual landowner, who collects the coconut products from the trees on his own land. Production (1988) 12,000 tonnes; coconuts, 90,000 tonnes.

Livestock (1988): Pigs, 10,000; poultry (1982), 163,000.

Fisheries. Tuna fishing is an important industry and licenses have been granted to USSR fleets.

FOREIGN ECONOMIC RELATIONS

Commerce. The principal imports (1988, in A$1m.) are: Machinery and transport equipment, 9·3; food, 2·5; manufactured goods, 3·4; fuels, 1·23. The value of exports for 1988 amounted to $A6·7m. Exports are almost exclusively copra.

Total trade between Kiribati and UK (British Department of Trade returns, in £1,000 sterling):

	1987	*1988*	*1989*	*1990*
Imports to UK	8	128	26	21
Exports and re-exports from UK	301	522	378	604

Tourism. Tourism is in the early stages of development and in 1984 total income from the industry was US$1·4m.

COMMUNICATIONS

Roads. There were (1988) 640 km of roads, of which 483 km suitable for vehicles.

Shipping. The main port is at Betio (Tarawa). Other ports of entry are Christmas Island and Banaba. In 1988, 60 vessels were handled at Betio.

Aviation. Air Tungaru is the national carrier. It operates services from Tarawa to the other 15 outer Islands in the Gilbertese Group, services varying between one and four flights each week. There is a charter service weekly to Christmas Island, in the Line Islands, which continues to Honolulu. A fortnightly service operates to Funafuti and weekly to Majuro and Nandi. Air Nauru has a weekly flight between Nauru and Tarawa.

Telecommunications. There were 911 telephones in 1987. Radio Tarawa transmits daily in English and I-Kiribati. A telephone line to Australia was installed in 1981. There were (1989 estimate) 25,000 radio receivers.

Cinemas. In 1989 there were 4 cinemas.

Newspapers. There was (1989) 1 bi-lingual weekly newspaper.

JUSTICE, RELIGION, EDUCATION AND WELFARE

Justice. In 1989 Kiribati had a police force of 232 under the command of a Commissioner of Police. The Commissioner of Police is also responsible for prisons, immigration, fire service (both domestic and airport) and firearms licensing.

Religion. The majority of the population belong to the Roman Catholic or Protestant (Congregational) church; there are small numbers of Seventh-day Adventist, Mormons, Baha'i and Church of God.

Education. In 1987 the government maintained boarding school had an enrolment of 470 pupils and there were 112 primary schools, with a total of 13,192 pupils, 6 secondary schools with 1,649 pupils, and 1 community high school with 232 pupils. The Government also maintains a teachers' training college with 56 students in 1987 and a marine training school which offers training for about 70 merchant seamen each year. The Tarawa Technical Institute at Betio offers a variety of part-time and evening technical and commercial courses and had 389 students in 1986.

In 1986, 85 islanders were in overseas countries for secondary and further education or training.

Welfare. Government maintains free medical and other services. There are few towns, and the people are almost without exception landed proprietors, thus eliminating child vagrancy and housing problems to a large extent, except in the Tarawa urban area. Destitution is almost unknown. There were 16 doctors in 1986. There is a general hospital on Tarawa and dispensaries on other islands, with 283 beds.

DIPLOMATIC REPRESENTATIVES

Of Kiribati in Great Britain
High Commissioner: Peter T. Timeon (resides in Tarawa).

Of Great Britain in Kiribati (Tarawa)
High Commissioner: D. L. White.

Of Kiribati in the USA
Ambassador: Atanraoi Baiteke, OBE (resides in Tarawa).

Further Reading

Kiribati, Aspects of History. Univ. of South Pacific, 1979
Bailey, E., *The Christmas Island Story.* London, 1977
Cowell, R., *Structure of Gilbertese.* Suva, 1950
Grimble, Sir Arthur, *A Pattern of Islands.* London, 1953.—*Return to the Islands.* London, 1957
Maude, H. E., *Of Islands and Men.* London, 1968.—*Evolution of the Gilbertese Boti.* Suva, 1977
Sabatier, E., *Astride the Equator.* Melbourne, 1978
Whincup, T., *Nareau's Nation.* London, 1979

KOREA

Han Kook

(Republic of Korea)

Capital: Seoul
Population: 42·8m. (1990)
GNP per capita: US$3,450 (1988)

HISTORY. Korea was united in a single kingdom under the Silla dynasty from 668. China, which claimed a vague suzerainty over Korea, recognized Korea's independence in 1895. Korea concluded trade agreements with the USA (1882), Great Britain, Germany (1883). After the Russo-Japanese war of 1904–5 Korea was virtually a Japanese protectorate until it was formally annexed by Japan on 29 Aug. 1910 thus ending the rule of the Choson kingdom, which had begun in 1392.

Following the collapse of Japan in 1945, American and Russian forces entered Korea to enforce the surrender of the Japanese troops there, dividing the country for mutual military convenience into two portions separated by the 38th parallel of latitude. Negotiations between the Americans and Russians regarding the future of Korea broke down in May 1946.

On 25 June 1950 the North Korean forces crossed the 38th parallel and invaded South Korea. The same day, the Security Council of the United Nations asked all member states to render assistance to the Republic of Korea. When the UN forces had reached the Manchurian border Chinese troops entered the war on the side of the North Koreans on 26 Nov. 1950 and penetrated deep into the south. By the beginning of April 1951, however, the UN forces had regained the 38th parallel. On 23 June 1951 Y. A. Malik, President of the Security Council, suggested a cease-fire, and on 10 July representatives of Gen. Ridgway met representatives of the North Koreans and of the Chinese Volunteer Army. A cease-fire agreement was signed on 27 July 1953.

For the contributions of member-nations of the United Nations to the war, *see* THE STATESMAN'S YEAR-BOOK, 1954, p. 1195, and 1956, p. 1180.

On 16 Aug. 1953 the USA and Korea signed a mutual defence pact and on 28 Nov. 1956 a treaty of friendship, commerce and navigation.

On 4 July 1972 it was announced in Seoul and Pyongyang (North Korea) that talks had taken place aimed at 'the peaceful unification of the fatherland as early as possible'. In Nov. 1984 agreement was reached to form a joint economic committee.

A North Korean–UN agreement of 6 Sept. 1976 established a joint security area 850 metres in diameter, divided into 2 equal parts to ensure the separation of the two sides.

Several rounds of talks with North Korea have taken place since 1985, including 3 meetings of prime ministers between Sept. and Dec. 1990.

AREA AND POPULATION. South Korea is bounded north by the demilitarized zone (separating it from North Korea), east by the Sea of Japan (East Sea), south by the Korea Strait (separating it from Japan) and west by the Yellow Sea. The area is 99,222 sq. km. The population (census, 1 Nov. 1985) was 40,466,577 (male, 20,280,857). Estimate (1990) 42,800,000. Population growth rate, 1990: 9·7 per 1,000. Life expectancy was 70·8 years in 1990.

The areas (in sq. km) and 1985 census populations of the Regions were as follows:

Region	*sq. km*	*1985*	*Region*	*sq. km*	*1985*
Seoul (city)	627	9,645,824	South Chungchong	8,807	3,001,538
Pusan (city)	433	3,516,768	North Cholla	8,052	2,202,218
Taegu (city)	455	2,030,649	South Cholla	12,189	3,748,442
Inchon (city)	201	1,387,475	North Kyongsang	19,427	3,013,276
Kyonggi	10,875	4,794,240	South Kyongsang	11,850	3,519,121
Kangwon	16,894	1,726,029	Cheju	1,825	489,458
North Chungchong	7,430	1,391,084			

The chief cities (populations, census 1985) are:

Seoul	9,645,824	Kwangchu	905,896	Masan	449,236
Pusan	3,516,768	Taejon	866,303	Seongnam	447,832
Taegu	2,030,649	Ulsan	551,219	Suweon	430,827
Inchon	1,387,475	Puch'on	456,311	Chonchu	426,490

CLIMATE. The extreme south has a humid warm temperate climate while the rest of the country experiences continental temperate conditions. Rainfall is concentrated in the period April to Sept. and ranges from 40" (1,020 mm) to 60" (1,520 mm). Pusan. Jan. 36°F (2·2°C), July 76°F (24·4°C). Annual rainfall 56" (1,407 mm). Seoul. Jan. 23°F (–5°C), July 77°F (25°C). Annual rainfall 50" (1,250 mm).

CONSTITUTION AND GOVERNMENT. A new constitution was approved by national referendum in Oct. 1987 and came into force on 25 Feb. 1988. It provides for a President, to be directly elected for a single 5-year term, a State Council of ministers whom he appoints and leads, and a National Assembly (299 members) directly elected for 4 years (224 from local constituencies and 75 by proportional representation).

The National Assembly was elected on 26 April 1988. In Jan. 1990 the Democratic Justice Party merged with 2 of the 3 opposition parties to form the Democratic Liberal Party with 200 seats in the National Assembly, leaving the Party for Peace and Democracy as the sole opposition party.

President of the Republic: Roh Tae-woo (took office 25 Feb. 1988).

The Cabinet in March 1991 was composed as follows:

Prime Minister: Roh Jae-Bong (b.1936).

Deputy Prime Minister and Minister of National Unification: Choi Ho-Joong. *Foreign Affairs:* Lee Sang-Ok. *Home Affairs:* Kim Tae-Ho. *Finance:* Lee Kyu-Sung. *Economic Planning:* Choi Kak-Kyu. *Justice:* Lee Jong Koo. *National Defence:* Lee Sang-Hoon. *Education:* Yoon Hyong-Sup. *Youth and Sport:* Park Chul-Un. *Agriculture, Forestry and Fisheries:* Cho Kyun Shik. *Commerce and Industry:* Lee Bong-Suh. *Construction:* Lee Jin Sul. *Health and Social Affairs:* Kim Chong-In. *Labour Affairs:* Choe Byung Yul. *Transportation:* Kim Chang-Keun. *Communications:* Lee Woo-Jae. *Culture and Information:* Choi Chang-Yun. *Government Administration:* Kim Yong-Nae. *Science and Technology:* Rhee Sang-Hi. *Minister for State Affairs:* Kim Yung-Chung. *Office of Legislation:* Hyun Hong-Joo. *Patriots and Veterans Affairs Agency:* Lee Sahng-Yeon. *Environment:* Huh Nam Hoon.

National flag: White charged in the centre with the *yang-um* in red and blue and with 4 black *p'algwae* trigrams.

Local government: South Korea is divided into 9 provinces *(Do)* and 6 cities with provincial status (Seoul, Pusan, Taegu, Inchon, Kwangju and Taegeon); the provinces are sub-divided into 137 districts *(Gun)* and 67 cities *(Shi)*.

Local elections were scheduled for 26 March 1991, the first to be held since 1961.

DEFENCE. Military service is compulsory for 30-36 months in all services.

Army. The Army is organized in 19 infantry divisions, 2 mechanized infantry divisions, 7 independent special forces brigades, 2 anti-aircraft artillery brigades, 2 surface-to-air missile brigades, 1 army aviation brigade and 2 surface-to-surface missile battalions. Equipment includes 250 Type 88, 350 M-47 and 950 M-48A5 main battle tanks. Army aviation equipment includes 50 Hughes 500 and 48 AH-1F/-J helicopters for anti-armour operations, observation and liaison, 8CH-47D transport helicopters and 259 utility helicopters. Strength (1991) 650,000, with a Regular Army Reserve of 1·5m. and a Homeland Reserve Defence Force of 3·3m. Para-military Civilian Defence Corps, 3·5m.

Navy. A substantial force of 60,000 (19,000 conscripts) including 25,000 marines (1990), which has hitherto operated very old ex-US ships but is now modernizing rapidly. Current strength includes 3 midget submarines (175 tonnes), 9 aged (1943–46) ex-US destroyers, and 25 locally-built frigates with new US and European weapons, 4 corvettes, 11 fast missile craft, together with a patrol force of 68 inshore craft. There are 9 coastal minesweepers and an amphibious force of 8 tank landing ships, 7 medium landing ships, together with 37 amphibious craft. Major auxiliaries include 3 tankers, 2 large tugs, 4 survey vessels and 35 service craft. The Navy has a small aviation element with 24 shore-based S-2A/F Tracker anti-submarine aircraft and 25 Hughes 500MD and 10 Alouette helicopters, some of which embark in frigates and destroyers.

Three German-designed diesel submarines are under construction; and the squadron may in due course reach a total of 6.

Main bases are at Chinhae, Inchon and Pusan.

The Coastguard numbering some 12,000 (mostly shore-based) operates 14 off-shore and 32 inshore patrol craft as well as 9 light helicopters.

Air Force. With a 1991 strength of about 40,000 men and 469 combatant aircraft, the Air Force is undergoing rapid expansion with US assistance. Its combat aircraft include 36 F-16C/D Fighting Falcons, about 120 F-4D/E Phantoms, 60 F-5A/B tactical fighters, more than 200 F-5E/F tactical fighters, 6 RF-5A reconnaissance fighters, 10 O-2A forward air control aircraft and 10 Hughes 500-D Defender helicopters. There are also 10 C-54 and 10 C-123 piston-engined transports, 4 C-130 Hercules turboprop-engined transports, 2 HS.748s, 1 Boeing 737 and 1 DC-6 for VIP transport; UH-1, Bell 212 and Bell 412 transport helicopters, and T-41, T-28, T-33 and T-37C trainers.

ECONOMY

Policy. Under the sixth 5-year social and economic plan (1987–91) the 1988 growth rate was 12·2% and the forecasted annual rate for 1989–91 is 7·3%.

Budget. The 1991 budget estimates: 27,183,000m. won. Expenditure on welfare in 1990 was 32·7% of total: Housing, US$300m.; health, US$200m.; health insurance, US$870m.

Currency. The unit of currency is the *won* (KRW) of 100 *chon*. Notes are issued by the Bank of Korea in denominations of 10,000, 5,000, 1,000 and 500 *won* and coins in denominations of 500, 100, 50, 10, 5 and 1 *won*. The exchange rate is determined daily by the Bank of Korea. In March 1991, 723·81 *won* = US$1; 1,373·07 *won* = £1 sterling.

Banking and Finance. The central bank is the Bank of Korea (*Governor*, Kim Kun). State-run banks include the Korean Development Bank, the Medium & Small Industry Bank, the Citizen's National Bank, the Korea Exchange Bank, the National Livestock Co-operatives Federation and the Federation of Fisheries Co-operatives serving as banking and credit institutions for farmers and fishermen, the Korea Housing Bank, the Export and Import Bank of Korea.

There are 8 commercial banks: The Bank of Seoul & Trust Co. Ltd, the Cho Heung Bank Ltd, the Commercial Bank of Korea, the Korea First Bank, the Hanil Bank, the Shinhan Bank, the Koram Bank, the Donghwa Bank; and 10 local banks. The Bank of Korea is the central bank and the only note-issuing bank, the authorized purchaser of domestically produced gold.

In addition, there are non-bank financial institutions consisting of 20 insurance companies, the Land Bank of Korea, the Credit Guarantee Fund, 32 short-term financial companies, 237 mutual credit companies, and the Merchant Banking Corporation.

There is a stock exchange in Seoul.

ENERGY AND NATURAL RESOURCES

Electricity. Electricity generated (1988) was 85,462m. kwh. Supply 100 and 220 volts; 60 Hz.

Oil. The KODECO Energy Co. and the Indonesian state-run oil company Pertamin are developing an oil field off the coast of Indonesia's Madura Island. KODECO began drilling operations in 1982 and began producing oil in Sept. 1985 from the Madura field, which contains 22·1m. bbls of proven oil deposits. The state-run Korean Petroleum Development Corp. (PEDCO) and the US company Hadson

Petroleum International are exploring for oil in the southern part of the Fifth Continental Shelf oil mining block off the coast of the Korean Peninsula. Oil worth US$3,788m. was imported in 1988.

Minerals. In 1986, 1,948 mining companies employed 94,811 people. Mineral deposits are mostly small, with the exception of tungsten; the Sangdong mine is one of the world's largest deposits of tungsten. Output, 1988, included (in tonnes): Anthracite coal, 22·7m.; iron ore, 666,000; tungsten ore, 3,433; limestone, 48·5m.; graphite, 104,384; lead ore, 25,806; silver, 12,809; zinc ore, 45,554.

Agriculture. The arable land in South Korea comprised 2,143,430 ha. in 1987, of which 1,351,657 ha. were rice paddies and 791,773 ha. dry fields.

Production (1987, in tonnes) of polished rice was 5,493,343; barley, 263,960; radishes, 1,972,683; Chinese cabbages, 2,433,981; apples, 556,160; grapes, 158,158; tobacco (leaf), 78,039.

In 1987 draught cattle numbered 1,923,121; milk cows, 463,330; pigs, 4,281,315; chickens, 59,323,977; ducks, 585,912.

Fisheries. Fishery exports (1987) US$1,731m. In 1987, 710 Korean deep-sea fishing vessels were operating overseas. In 1987, there was a total of 94,155 boats (911,958 gross tons). The fish catch (inland and marine) was 3,331,825 tonnes in 1987.

INDUSTRY. Manufacturing industry was concentrated primarily in 1988 on oil, petrochemicals, chemical fibres, construction, iron and steel, cement, machinery, shipbuilding, automobiles and electronics.

Output of tobacco manufactures, a government monopoly, was 82,982 tonnes in 1986.

Labour. Manufacturing employed 4,667,000 persons in 1988. There were 1,616 strikes in 1989, and 7m. workdays were lost. Unemployment was 2·2% in 1990.

FOREIGN ECONOMIC RELATIONS. Since March 1991 foreign partners in joint ventures holding less than 50% of the capital have needed only to report, instead of seek approval for, their projects. Tax concessions for foreign investments have been reduced.

Commerce. In 1988 the total exports were US$59,648m., while imports were US$48,203m. In 1988 USA provided 26·5% and Japan 33% of imports; USA received 35·9% of exports, Japan 20·1%.

Major exports are textiles, electronics, iron and steel and machinery, and in 1988 included (in US$1m.): Heavy and chemical products, 32,913; light industrial products, 24,408. Major imports included: Crude oil and raw materials, 27,875; capital goods, 19,033; grain and other goods, 4,900.

Total trade between Korea and UK (British Department of Trade returns, in £1,000 sterling):

	1986	*1987*	*1988*	*1989*	*1990*
Imports to UK	661,975	936,038	1,135,107	1,164,723	963,829
Exports and re-exports from UK	288,421	427,229	1,742,747	493,945	620,690

Tourism. In 1989 there were 2,728,100 foreign tourists. Age limits for foreign travel were lifted in Jan. 1989, and in 1989 1·2m. Koreans travelled abroad.

COMMUNICATIONS

Roads. In 1987 there were 54,689 km of roads. In 1988 motor vehicles totalled 2,035,448 including 635,445 trucks, 259,600 buses, 1,117,999 passenger cars.

Railways. In 1989 the National Railroad totalled 3,120 km of 1,435 mm gauge (525 km electrified) and 46 km of 762 mm gauge. In 1989 railways carried 584m. passengers and 58·7m. tonnes of freight.

Aviation. In 1989, 40 countries maintained aviation agreement with Korea and had 47 air routes with 28 cities in 18 countries. The Ministry of Transportation opened the Seoul-Singapore-Jakarta passenger route in 1989.

In Sept. 1989 Korea had 159 commercial aircraft (62 Korean Air passenger-cargo planes, 9 Asiana Airlines passenger-cargo planes, 38 light planes and 43 helicopters). In 1987, 4·73m. passengers and 337,139 tons of cargo and mail were carried on domestic routes and in 1989 4,095,000 passengers on international routes.

Shipping. In Dec. 1987, there were 25 first-grade ports and 22 second-grade ports, and 8,852,000 gross tons in various vessels. Of the total tonnage, registered vessels accounted for 7,239,000 tons, chartered vessels for 1,613,000 tons. Passenger ships accounted for 54,000 tons, cargo vessels 6,932,000 tons and oil tankers 1,729,000 tons and others 146,000 tons.

Post and Telecommunications. Post offices total 3,199 (1988); telephones were 10,306,000 in 1988. The fifth satellite earth station was opened in June 1988, bringing the number of communications circuits *via* satellite to 2,866. There were 6·1m. television receivers in 1989.

Cinemas. In 1988 there were 696 with a seating capacity of 240,000.

Newspapers (1989). There were 68 daily papers, including 2 in English appearing in Seoul and 2 news agencies.

RELIGION, EDUCATION AND WELFARE

Religion. Basically the religions of Korea have been Shamanism, Buddhism (introduced A.D. 372) and Confucianism, which was the official faith from 1392 to 1910. Catholic converts from China introduced Christianity in the 18th century, but the ban on Roman Catholicism was not lifted until 1882. Protestantism was introduced in the late 19th century. The Christian population in 1985 was 8,343,455.

Education. In 1988 Korea had 4,819,857 pupils enrolled in 6,463 elementary schools, 2,523,515 pupils in 2,371 middle schools and 2,300,582 pupils in 1,653 high schools.

For higher education, 1,312,053 students attended 260 universities, colleges and junior colleges in 1988. There are 251 graduate schools granting master's degrees in 2 years and doctor's degrees in 3 years, where 75,177 students attended in 1988. There are 6 Open Universities.

Health. In 1987 there were 38,611 physicians, 4,426 oriental medical doctors, 6,761 dentists, 6,849 midwives, 186,177 nurses, and 32,855 pharmacists. There were 20,899 hospitals, clinics and health care centres in 1987 with 114,511 beds.

DIPLOMATIC REPRESENTATIVES

Of Korea in Great Britain (4 Palace Gate, London, W8 5NF)
Ambassador: (Vacant).

Of Great Britain in Korea (4 Chung-Dong, Chung-Ku, Seoul)
Ambassador: David J. Wright, LVO.

Of Korea in the USA (2370 Massachusetts Ave., NW, Washington, D.C., 20008)
Ambassador: Park Tong-Jin.

Of the USA in Korea (Sejong-Ro, Seoul)
Ambassador: Donald Gregg.

Of Korea at the United Nations:
Hyun Hong-Choo.

Further Reading

A Handbook of Korea. 4th ed. Seoul, 1982
Guide to Investment in Korea. Economic Planning Board. Seoul, 1980
Korea Annual 1983. 20th ed. Seoul, 1983
Korea Statistical Year Book. Seoul, 1981
Major Economic Indicators, 1979–80. Seoul, 1980
Monthly Statistics of Korea. Seoul
Hastings, M., *The Korean War*. London, 1987
Srivastava, M.P., *The Korean Conflict: Search for Unification*. New Delhi, 1982

NORTH KOREA

Capital: Pyongyang
Population: 22·42m. (1989)
GNP per capita: US$1,180 (1985)

Chosun Minchu-chui Inmin Konghwa-guk

(People's Democratic Republic of Korea)

HISTORY. In northern Korea the Russians, arriving on 8 Aug. 1945, one month ahead of the Americans, established a Communist-led 'Provisional Government'. The newly created Korean Communist Party merged in 1946 with the New National Party into the Korean Workers' Party. In July 1946 the KWP, with the remaining pro-Communist groups and non-party people, formed the United Democratic Patriotic Front. On 25 Aug. 1948 the Communists organized elections for a Supreme People's Assembly, both in Soviet-occupied North Korea (212 deputies) and in US-occupied South Korea (360 deputies, of whom a certain number went to the North and took their seats). A People's Democratic Republic was proclaimed on 9 Sept. 1948. Several proposals for talks between North and South Korea on re-unification have been made since 1980, but have repeatedly broken down. North-South economic talks were held in 1985, and there was an exchange of family visits in 1989. There were 3 meetings of the prime ministers of North and South Korea between Sept. and Dec. 1990.

AREA AND POPULATION. North Korea is bounded north by China, east by the sea of Japan, west by the Yellow Sea and south by South Korea, from which it is separated by a demilitarized zone of 1,262 sq. km. Its area is 120,538 sq. km. Population estimate in 1989, 22·42m. (64% urban). Population density, 186 per sq. km. Rate of population increase, 2·4% per annum; birth rate, 1985, 3%; death rate, 0·6%. Marriage is discouraged before the age of 32 for men and 29 for women. Expectation of life in 1987 was: Males, 65; females, 71 years. Large towns (estimate, 1984): Pyongyang, the capital (2,639,448); Chongjin (754,128); Nampo (691,284); Sinuiju (500,000); Wonsan (350,000); Kaesong (345,642); Kimchaek (281,000); Haeju (131,000); Sariwon (130,000); Hamhung (775,000 in 1981).

CLIMATE. There is a warm temperate climate, though winters can be very cold in the north. Rainfall is concentrated in the summer months. Pyongyang. Jan. 18°F (–7·8°C), July 75°F (23·9°C). Annual rainfall 37" (916 mm).

CONSTITUTION AND GOVERNMENT. The political structure is based upon the Constitution of 27 Dec. 1972. The Constitution provides for a *Supreme People's Assembly* elected every 4 years by universal suffrage. Citizens of 17 years and over can vote and be elected. Elections were held in April 1990. It was claimed that 99·78% of the electorate voted for the list of single candidates presented. There are 687 deputies. The government consists of the *Administration Council* directed by the Central People's Committee (*Secretary,* Chi Chang Ik).

The head of state is the *President*, elected for 4-year terms. On 24 May 1990 the National Assembly unanimously elected Kim Il Sung (b. 1912) for a fifth term.

In practice the country is ruled by the Korean Workers' (*i.e.*, Communist) Party which elects a Central Committee which in turn appoints a Politburo. In March 1991 this was composed of: Marshal Kim Il Sung, *(General Secretary of the Party, President of the Republic, Chairman of the Central People's Committee, Supreme Commander of the Armed Forces)*; Kim Jong Il (b. 1941; Kim Il Sung's son and designated successor) *(Vice-President of the Republic)*; O Jin U *(Armed Forces'*

Minister) (The latter 3 constituting the Politburo's Presidium); Kang Song San; Li Jong Ok *(Vice-President of the Republic)*; Pak Sung Chul *(Vice-President of the Republic)*; So Chol; Kim Yong Nam *(Deputy Prime Minister and Foreign Minister)*; Kim Hwan *(Deputy Prime Minister, Minister of the Chemical Industry)*; Yon Hyong Muk *(Prime Minister)*; O Guk Ryol; So Yun Sok; Ho Dam *(Deputy Prime Minister)*; Hong Song Nam *(First Deputy Prime Minister, Chairman, State Planning Commission)*; Kye Ung Tae. There were also 9 candidate members.

Ministers not full members of the Politburo include Kim Yun Hyok *(Deputy Prime Minister)*; Cho Se Ung *(Deputy Prime Minister)*; Yun Gi Jong *(Finance)*; Chong Song Nam *(Foreign Economic Affairs)*; Kim Bok Sin; Chong Jun Gi, Kim Yun Hyok, Kim Chang Ju *(Deputy Prime Ministers)*; Choe Jong Gun *(Foreign Trade)*; Paek Hak Rim *(Public Security)*.

In 1981 the Party had some 2m. members.

There are also the puppet religious Chongu and Korean Social Democratic Parties and various organizations combined in a Fatherland Front.

National flag: Blue, red and blue horizontal stripes separated by narrow white bands. The red stripe bears a white circle within which is a red 5-pointed star.

National anthem: 'A chi mun bin na ra i gang san' ('Shine bright, o dawn, on this land so fair'). Words by Pak Se Yong; music by Kim Won Gyun.

Local government: The country is divided into 13 administrative units: 4 cities (Pyongyang, Chongjin, Hamhung and Kaesong) and 9 provinces (capitals in brackets): South Pyongan (Nampo), North Pyongan (Sinuiju), Jagang (Kanggye), South Hwanghai (Haeju), North Hwanghai (Sariwon), Kangwon (Wonsan), South Hamgyong (Hamheung), North Hamgyong (Chongjin), Yanggang (Hyesan). These are sub-divided into 152 counties. There are 26,539 deputies in People's Assemblies at city/province, county and commune level. Elections were on 15 Nov. 1987.

DEFENCE. There is a *National Defence Commission* headed by Kim Il Sung. Chief of the General Staff is Choe Gwang (appointed 1988). Military service is compulsory at the age of 16 for periods of 5-8 years in the Army, 5-10 years in the Navy and 3–4 years in the Air Force. In 1987 defence spending was 22% of GNP. North Korea adhered to the 1968 Non-Proliferation Treaty on nuclear weapons in 1985.

Army. The Army is organized in 25 infantry divisions; 15 armoured, 30 motorized infantry and 3 independent infantry brigades; 1 special purpose corps numbering 80,000; and an artillery corps with multiple rocket launchers and 6 surface-to-surface missile battalions. Equipment includes 200 T-34, 1,600 T-54/55, and 175 Type-59 main battle tanks. Strength (1991) 1m., with 0·5m. reserves. There is also a paramilitary militia of some 4m. men and a Ministry of Public Security force of 200,000 including border guards.

Navy. The Navy, principally tasked to coastal patrol and defence, comprises 24 diesel submarines (20 of Chinese design and 4 ex-Soviet). Surface forces include 3 small frigates, (1 missile-armed), 3 corvettes, 34 missile craft, 173 fast torpedo craft, 6 anti-submarine patrol craft and some 150 inshore patrol craft. Amphibious forces consist of some 130 small craft. Support is provided by 2 ex-Soviet ocean tugs and 100 service craft. There is a coastal defence element equipped with some 6 missile batteries and old 122 mm, 130 mm and 152 mm guns. Personnel in 1990 totalled 41,000 officers and men with 40,000 reserves.

Air Force. The Air Force had a total of about 716 combat aircraft and 60 armed helicopters and 70,000 personnel in 1991. Since 1985 the USSR has supplied 50 MiG-23 supersonic and 30 MiG-29 interceptors, 40 Su-25 fighter-bombers and 30 SA3 surface-to-air missiles. Other equipment is believed to include about 160 supersonic MiG-21 interceptors, more than 100 F-6s (Chinese-built MiG-19s), 150 MiG-17s for ground attack and reconnaissance, 30 Su-7 fighter-bombers, 40 Chinese-built A5 fighter-bombers, 60 Il-28 twin-jet light bombers, 200 An-2 light transport aircraft, 40 Mi-4 and Mi-8 transport helicopters and 80 US Hughes 300 and 500 helicopters.

INTERNATIONAL RELATIONS

North Korea is a member of WHO and OIEC and an observer at UN.

ECONOMY

Planning. For previous plans *see* THE STATESMAN'S YEAR-BOOK, 1987–88. After a hiatus it was announced in Oct. 1986 that a third 7-year plan would run from 1987 to 1993. Steel production targets have been reduced (to 10m. tonnes) and more emphasis placed on export items, non-ferrous metals and fishery products.

Budget (in 1m. won) for calendar years:

	1984	*1985*	*1986*	*1987*	*1988*
Revenue	26,305	27,439	28,539	30,337	31,852
Expenditure	26,158	27,329	28,396	30,085	31,852

Defence spending was 13·8% of the budget in 1987 (14% in 1986). Local government revenue in 1987: 4,185m. *won*; expenditure, 3,427m. *won*.

Currency. The monetary unit is the *won* (KPW) of 100 *jun*. There are coins of 1, 5, 10 and 50 *jun* and 1, 5, 10, 50 and 100 *won*. In March 1991, US$1 = 0·97 *won*; £1 = 1·84 *won*.

Weights and Measures. While the metric system is in force traditional measures are in frequent use. The *jungbo* = 1 hectare; the *ri* = 3,927 metres.

ENERGY AND NATURAL RESOURCES

Electricity. There are 3 thermal power stations and 4 hydro-electric plants. A nuclear power plant is being built. Output in 1986, was 50,000m. kwh (29,000m. kwh. hydro-electric). Installed capacity was 6·11m. kw in 1987. Hydro-electric potential exceeds 8m. kw. A hydro-electric plant and dam under construction on the Pukhan near Mount Kumgang has been denounced as a flood threat by the South Koreans, who constructed a defensive 'Peace Dam' in retaliation.

Oil. Oilwells went into production in 1957. An oil pipeline from China came on stream in 1976. Crude oil refining capacity was 70,000 barrels a year in 1986.

Minerals. North Korea is rich in minerals. Estimated reserves in tonnes: Iron ore, 3,300m.; copper, 2·15m.; lead, 6m.; zinc, 12m.; coal, 11,990m.; uranium, 26m.; manganese, 6,500m. 37·5m. tonnes of coal were mined in 1986, 8m. tonnes of iron ore and 15,000 tonnes of copper ore. 1986 production of gold was 160,000 fine troy oz; silver, 1·6m. fine troy oz; salt, 570,000 tonnes.

Agriculture. In 1987 there were 2·36m. ha. of arable land, including 635,000 ha. of paddy fields. In 1982, 38% of the population made a living from agriculture.

Collectivization took place between 1954 and 1958. 90% of the cultivated land is farmed by co-operatives. Land belongs either to the State or to co-operatives, and it is intended gradually to transform the latter into the former, but small individually-tended plots producing for 'farmers' markets' are tolerated as a 'transition measure'. Livestock farming is mainly carried on by large state farms.

There is a large-scale tideland reclamation project. There were 37,600 km of irrigation canals in 1976, making possible 2 rice harvests a year. In 1982 there were 133,000 tractors (15 h.p. units). The technical revolution in agriculture (nearly 95% of ploughing, etc., is mechanized) has considerably increased the yield of grain (sown on 2·3m. *jungbo* of land); rice production, 1988, was 6·35m. tonnes, maize, 2·95m. tonnes; potatoes, 1,975,000m. tonnes; soya beans, 448,000 tonnes.

Livestock, 1988: 1·25m. cattle, 3·1m. pigs, 20m. poultry.

Forestry. Between 1961 and 1970, 800,000 ha. were afforested. 4·6m. cu metres of timber were cut in 1986.

Fisheries. Catch in 1986: 1·7m. tonnes. There is a fishing fleet of 28,000 vessels including 19,000 motor vessels.

INDUSTRY. Industries were intensively developed by the Japanese, notably cotton spinning, hydro-electric power, cotton, silk and rayon weaving, and chemical fertilizers. Production (in tonnes) in 1982: Pig-iron, 4m.; crude steel, 4m.; rolled steel, 3·2m.; lead, 30,000; zinc, 140,000; copper, 48,000; ship-building, 400,000; chemical fertilizers, 620,000; chemicals, 20,000; synthetic resins, 90,000; cement (1986), 9,040; textiles (1986), 600m. metres; woven goods, 600m. metres; shoes, 40m. pairs; motor-cars (1986), 20,000; TV sets (1986), 240,000; refrigerators, 10,000. Annual steel production capacity was 4·3m. tonnes in 1987.

Labour. The economically-active population was 9m. (4·18m. females) in 1985. Industrial workers make up some 60% of the work force. Average monthly wage, 1984: 90 *won*.

FOREIGN ECONOMIC RELATIONS. Joint ventures with foreign firms have been permitted since 1984. In 1990 foreign debt was estimated at US$4,500m. (of which US$3,800m. were to the USSR). The USA imposed sanctions in Jan. 1988 for alleged terrorist activities.

Commerce. Exports in 1989 were US1,800m.; imports, US$2,500m. 58% of trade was with the USSR, 13% with China, 10% with Japan. Total trade in 1989 was 13% below 1988. The chief exports are metal ores and products, the chief imports machinery and petroleum products.

Trade with the USSR is based on 5-year agreements, the last of which was signed in 1986.

Total trade between North Korea and UK (British Department of Trade returns, in £1,000 sterling):

	1986	*1987*	*1988*	*1989*	*1990*
Imports to UK	1,374	641	824	1,095	373
Exports and re-exports from UK	3,331	2,198	3,125	3,087	4,774

Tourism. A 40-year ban on non-Communist tourists was lifted in 1986.

COMMUNICATIONS

Roads. There were 22,000 km of road in 1985, including 240 km of motorways. There were 180,000 motor cars in 1982. A 200 km 4-lane highway began construction in 1988 from Pyongyang to Kaesong.

Railways. The two trunk-lines Pyongyang–Sinuiju and Pyongyang–Myongchon are both electrified, and the Pyongyang–Sariwon trunk is in course of electrification. The 'Wonra' line runs from Wonsan to Rajin and is electrified from Myongchon to Rajin and beyond to Tumangang. The Namdokchon–Toknam line was opened in 1983. Lines are under construction from Pukchong to Toksong, from Palwon to Kujang and Kanggye *via* Hyesan to Musan. In 1987 the Unbong–Cha Song and Huju–Hyesan sections of this latter were opened. In 1988 there were 4,549 km of track, (2,706 km were electrified in 1984). In 1986, 89% of trains were hauled by electricity. In 1987 86% of all freight was transported by rail. A weekly service from Pyongyang to Beijing opened in 1983, and a twice-weekly service to Moscow in 1987.

Aviation. There are services to Moscow, Khabarovsk, Beijing and Hong Kong. An agreement envisaging a service from Pyongyang to Tokyo was signed in 1990. There are domestic flights from Pyongyang to Hamhung and Chongjin.

Shipping. The leading ports are Chongjin, Wonsan and Hungnam. Nampo, the port of Pyongyang, has been dredged and expanded. Pyongyang is connected to Nampo by railway and river. In 1987 the ocean-going merchant fleet numbered 71 vessels totalling 407,253 GRT.

The biggest navigable river is the Yalu, 698 km up to the Hyesan district.

Telecommunications. There is a central TV station at Pyongyang and stations at Kaesong and Mansudae. In 1986 there were some 250,000 television receivers. The central broadcasting station is Radio Pyongyang. There are several local stations and a station for overseas broadcasts. There were some 30,000 telephones in 1985.

An agreement to share in Japan's telecommunications satellites was reached in Sept. 1990.

Newspapers. There were 11 newspapers in 1984. The party newspaper is *Nodong* (or *Rodong*) *Sinmun* (Workers' Daily News). Circulation about 600,000.

JUSTICE, RELIGION, EDUCATION AND WELFARE

Justice. The judiciary consists of the Supreme Court, whose judges are elected by the Assembly for 3 years; provincial courts; and city or county people's courts. The procurator-general, appointed by the Assembly, has supervisory powers over the judiciary and the administration; the Supreme Court controls the judicial administration.

Religion. The Constitution provides for 'freedom of religion as well as the freedom of anti-religious propaganda'. In 1986 there were 3m. Chondoists, 400,000 Buddhists and 200,000 Christians. Another 3m. followed traditional beliefs.

Education. Free compulsory universal technical education lasts 11 years: 1 pre-school year, 4 years primary education starting at the age of 6, followed by 6 years secondary.

In 1988 there were 47,600 kindergartens. In 1980 there were some 10,000 11-year schools. In 1982–83 there were 5·2m. pupils and 110,000 teachers, and nearly 1m. students in higher education. In 1985 there were 216 institutes of higher education, including 3 universities—Kim Il Sung University (founded 1946), Kim Chaek Technical University, Pyongyang Medical School—and an Academy of Sciences (founded 1952).

In 1977–78 Kim Il Sung University had some 17,000 students.

Health. Medical treatment is free. In 1982 there were 1,531 general hospitals, 979 specialized hospitals and 5,414 clinics. There were 24 doctors and 130 hospital beds per 10,000 population in 1983.

DIPLOMATIC REPRESENTATIVE

Of North Korea at the United Nations:
Pak Gil Yon.

Further Reading

North Korea Directory. Tokyo, annual since 1988
An, T. S., *North Korea in Transition*. Westport, 1983;–*North Korea: a Political Handbook*. Washington, 1983
Baik Bong, *Kim Il Sung: Biography*. 3 vols. New York, 1969–70
Chung, C.-S., (ed.) *North Korean Communism: A Comparative Analysis*. Seoul, 1980
Kihl, Y. W., *Politics and Policies in Divided Korea*. Boulder, 1984
Kim Han Gil, *Modern History of Korea*. Pyongyang, 1979
Kim Il Sung, *Works*. Pyongyang, 1980–83
Kim, Y. S., (ed.) *The Economy of the Korean Democratic People's Republic, 1945–1977*. Kiel, 1979
Koh, B. C., *The Foreign Policy Systems of North and South Korea*. Berkeley, 1984
Park, J. K. and Kim, J.-G., *The Politics of North Korea*. Boulder, 1979
Scalapino, R. A. and Lee, C.-S., *Communism in Korea. Part I: The Movement. Part II: The Society*. Univ. of Calif. Press, 1972—and Kim, J-Y. (eds.), *North Korea Today: Strategic and Domestic Issues*. Univ. of California Press, 1983
Suh, D.-S., *Korean Communism, 1945–1980: A Reference Guide to the Political System*. Honolulu, 1981

KUWAIT

Capital: Kuwait
Population: 2·04m. (1990)
GNP per capita: US$13,680 (1988)

Dowlat al Kuwait

(State of Kuwait)

HISTORY. The ruling dynasty was founded by Shaikh Sabah al-Owel (ruled 1756-72). In 1899 Shaikh Mubarak concluded a treaty with the UK: in return for British protection, he undertook not to alienate any of his territory without British agreement. In 1914 the UK recognized Kuwait as an independent government under British protection. On 19 June 1961 an agreement reaffirmed the independence and sovereignty of Kuwait and recognized the Government of Kuwait's responsibility for the conduct of internal and external affairs; the agreement of 1899 was terminated and the UK agreed to assist Kuwait should it request it.

Early on 2 Aug. 1990 Iraqi forces without warning invaded and rapidly overran the country, meeting little resistance. The Amir escaped to Saudi Arabia, but his brother Sheikh Fahd, was killed. President Saddam of Iraq declared the annexation of Kuwait on 8 Aug. The Kuwaiti government established itself in exile at Taif (Saudi Arabia) during the Iraqi occupation.

Following the expiry of the date required by the UN for the withdrawal of Iraqi forces on 15 Jan. 1991, an air offensive was launched by coalition forces against targets in Kuwait, followed by a land attack on 24 Feb. Iraqi forces were routed, and Kuwait City was liberated on 27 Feb. In compliance with the provisional ceasefire of 28 Feb., Iraq withdrew all its forces from Kuwait.

AREA AND POPULATION. Kuwait is bounded east by the Gulf, north and west by Iraq and south and south-west by Saudi Arabia, with an area of about 6,880 sq. miles (17,819 sq. km); the total population at the census of 1985 was 1,697,301, of which about 60% were non-Kuwaitis. Estimate (1990) 2·04m., including 1·1m. non-Kuwaitis. Population density, 110 per sq. km. Over 78% speak Arabic, the official language, 10% speak Kurdish and 4% Iranian (Farsi). English is also used as a second language.

The country is divided into 4 governorates: The capital (comprising Kuwait City, Kuwait's 9 islands and territorial and shared territorial waters), with an area of 983 sq. km (population 167,750 at 1985 census); Hawalli, 620 sq. km (943,250); Ahmadi, 4,665 sq. km (304,662) and Jahra, 11,550 sq. km (279,466).

The chief cities were (census, 1985) Kuwait, the capital (44,335), and its suburbs Hawalli (145,126), as-Salimiya (153,369) and Jahra (111,222).

The Neutral Zone (3,560 sq. miles, 5,700 sq. km), jointly owned and administered by Kuwait and Saudi Arabia from 1922 to 1966, was partitioned between the two countries in May 1966, but the exploitation of the oil and other natural resources will continue to be shared.

CLIMATE. Kuwait has a dry, desert climate which is cool in winter but very hot and humid in summer. Rainfall is extremely light. Kuwait. Jan. 56°F (13·5°C), July 99°F (36·6°C). Annual rainfall 5" (125 mm).

RULER. HH Shaikh Jabir al-Ahmad al-Jabir al-Sabah the 13th Amir of Kuwait, succeeded on 31 Dec. 1977.

CONSTITUTION AND GOVERNMENT. In 1976 the Amir dissolved the Assembly and at the same time parts of the Constitution were suspended. In April 1990 the National Assembly was re-established, consisting of 50 elected members and 25 appointed by the Amir. The franchise, limited to men whose families have been of Kuwaiti nationality for at least one generation, produces an electorate of

62,000. Elections were held in June 1990. Executive authority is vested in the Council of Ministers. Martial law was imposed for 3 months after the Iraqi withdrawal in March 1991.

The Cabinet in Feb. 1991 was composed as follows:

Prime Minister: HRH Crown Prince Shaikh Saad al-Abdullah as Salim as Sabah.

Deputy Prime Minister, Foreign Affairs: Shaikh Sabah al Ahmad al Jabir as Sabah. *Finance and Economy:* Shaikh Ali al Khalifa al Adhibi as Sabah. *Education:* Anwar Abdullah al Nuri. *Waqfs and Islamic Affairs:* Khaled Ahmed Saad al Jasir. *Defence:* Shaikh Nawaf al Ahmad al Jabir as Sabah. *Justice, Legal and Administrative Affairs:* Dari Abdullah al Uthman. *Public Works:* Abdel Rahman Ibrahim al Houti. *Public Health:* Dr Abdurrahman Abdullah al Awadi. *Planning:* Suleiman Mutawa. *Oil:* Rashid Salim al Amiri. *Communications:* Khalid Jumayan Salim al Jumayan. *Electricity and Water:* Mohammed as Saad Abdel Moshin al Rifai. *Information, National Assembly Affairs:* Abdel Rahman al Awad. *Social Affairs and Labour:* Jabir Mubarak al Hamad. *Interior:* Shaikh Salim as Sabah as Salim as Sabah. *Trade and Industry:* Faisal Abdel Razzaq al Khaled.

Flag: Three horizontal stripes of green, white, red, with a black trapezium based on the hoist.

DEFENCE. Military service is compulsory for 24 months (university students, 12 months).

Army. Kuwait maintains a small, well-equipped and mobile army of 2 armoured, 1 artillery and 1 mechanized infantry brigades and 1 surface-to-surface missile battalion. Equipment includes 70 Vickers Mk I, 40 Centurion and 165 Chieftain main battle tanks. Strength (1991) about 16,000 men.

Navy. At the time of the Iraqi invasion in Aug. 1990 the combatant flotilla comprised 8 missile craft (all German-built), 15 inshore patrol craft and some 25 boats. 4 UK and 3 Singapore-built landing craft were used on logistic support tasks. In 1990 personnel totalled 2,100 Bases: El Adami (HQ) and As Shuwaikh. Most of the flotilla escaped to Saudi Arabia after the invasion by Iraq.

Air Force. From a small initial combat force the Air Force has grown rapidly. It has 2 squadrons with 25 Mirage F1-C fighters and 4 Mirage F1-B 2-seat trainers; and 2 squadrons with 30 A-4KU/TA-4KU Skyhawk attack aircraft. Other equipment includes 2 DC-9 jet transports, 4 L-100-30 Hercules turboprop transports and 12 Hawk jet trainers, 10 Puma, 6 Exocet missile-armed Super Puma and 25 missile-armed Gazelle helicopters. Hawk surface-to-air missiles are in service. Personnel strength (1991) about 2,200, with 35 combat aircraft and 18 armed helicopters.

INTERNATIONAL RELATIONS

Membership. Kuwait is a member of the UN, Arab League, Gulf Co-operation Council, OPEC and OAPEC.

ECONOMY

Policy. The 5-year development plan ran from 1986–90.

Budget. In 1985–86 revenue, KD1,979m.; expenditure, KD3,158m.

Currency. The unit of currency is the *Kuwaiti dinar* (KWD) of 1,000 *fils*, which replaced the Indian external rupee on 1 April 1961. Coins in circulation are, 1, 5, 10, 20, 50 and 100 fils and notes of KD, 20, 10, 5, 1, ½ and ¼. Official reserves were some US$80,000m. in 1990. After the Iraqi occupation, the Kuwaiti dinar was phased out in obligatory exchanges with the Iraqi dinar at parity (former exchange rate, KD12 = ID1). In March 1990, £1 sterling = KD 0·491; US$1 = KD 0·294.

Banking and Finance. In addition to the Central Bank, 7 commercial banks (Bank of Kuwait and the Middle East, National Bank of Kuwait, Commercial Bank of Kuwait, Gulf Bank, Al-Ahli Bank, Burgan Bank and Bank of Bahrain and Kuwait) and 3 specialized banks (Credit and Savings Bank, Kuwait Real Estate Bank and Industrial Bank of Kuwait) operate in Kuwait. Late in 1990 the Central Bank began operating from exile in London, mandating the National Bank of Kuwait (also in London) to set up an international settlement system for Kuwaiti banks incapacitated by the Iraqi invasion. The *Governor* of the Central Bank is Shaikh Salem Abdul-Aziz al Sabah. There is also the Kuwait Finance House, which is not subject to the control of the Central Bank.

Weights and Measures. The metric system was adopted in 1962.

ENERGY AND NATURAL RESOURCES

Electricity. 16,360m. kwh. were produced in 1986. Supply 240 volts; 50 Hz.

Oil. The Kuwait Petroleum Corporation (KPC) was set up in 1980 to reorganize, integrate and develop the oil sector. The functions of the operating oil companies have been reallocated: Kuwait Oil Company (KOC) specializes in exploration, drilling and production in all areas; Kuwait National Petroleum Company (KNPC) is responsible for refining, local marketing and gas liquefaction operations; Kuwait Oil Tankers Company (KOTC) is in charge of transporting crude oil, liquefied gas and oil products to various world markets; Petrochemical Industries Company is in charge of use of hydrocarbon resources to set up diverse petrochemical industries, and the International Marketing Department of KPC markets and sells oil and gas worldwide.

Oil revenues in 1983–84 were KD2,787·6m. Crude oil production in 1989, 91m. tonnes. Kuwait is also refining, marketing refined products, and prospecting and producing abroad. About 600 of the approximately 950 oil wells were fired by the Iraqi occupation forces. Production seemed unlikely to resume before 1992.

Gas. Production (1983) 170,200m. cu. ft.

Water. The country depends upon desalination plants. In 1986 there were 5 plants with a daily total capacity of 215m. gallons. Fresh mineral water is pumped and bottled at Rawdhatain. Underground brackish water is used for irrigation, street cleaning and livestock; production, 1985, 18,000m. gallons.

Agriculture. In 1985 the area of cultivated land was 20m. sq. metres and there were 27 dairy farms with a total production capacity of about 30,000 tonnes of fresh milk. Major crops (production, 1988, in tonnes) were melons (6,000), tomatoes (39,000), onions (25,000), dates (1,000), radishes, clover.

Livestock (1988): Cattle, 26,000; sheep, 300,000; goats, 20,000; poultry, 28m.

Fisheries. Shrimp fishing is becoming one of the important non-oil industries.

INDUSTRY. In 1985 there were 600 industrial establishments and 50,000 workers in the industrial sector. Industries, apart from oil, include boat building, fishing, food production, petrochemicals, gases and construction. The manufacture or import of alcoholic drinks is prohibited.

Labour. In 1985 the labour force totalled 670,385, with 530,996 employed.

Trade Unions. In 1986 there were 16 trade unions and 17 labour federations.

FOREIGN ECONOMIC RELATIONS

Commerce. The port of Kuwait formerly served mainly as an entrepôt for goods for the interior, for the export of skins and wool, and for pearl fishing. Entrepôt trade continues but, with the development of the oil industry, is declining in importance. Pearl fishing is now on a small scale. Dhows and launches of traditional construction are still built.

In 1986 total imports were valued at KD1,661m.; exports, (1984) KD3,632m. and oil accounted for 83·5% of exports at KD2,938m.

Major domestic exports include chemical fertilizers and other chemicals, shrimps, metal pipes and building materials, which represent about 33% of total non-oil products. The other 66% come from re-exports, particularly of machinery, transport equipment, foodstuffs and some industrial goods, which go mainly to neighbouring Arab countries.

Main imports include machinery, electrical generators, appliances, cars and medicines.

Total trade between Kuwait and UK (British Department of Trade returns, in £1,000 sterling):

	1986	*1987*	*1988*	*1989*	*1990*
Imports to UK [1]	58,517	81,530	72,318	150,354	109,970
Exports and re-exports from UK	300,586	225,168	237,515	228,711	181,480

[1] Including oil.

Tourism. There were 116,000 visitors in 1985.

COMMUNICATIONS

Roads. In 1986 there were 3,800 km of roads. Number of vehicles (1988) was 585,000 (private cars 469,000; buses, 11,000; lorries, 100,000; motorcycles, 5,000).

Aviation. There were 29,000 scheduled and unscheduled flights to and from Kuwait International Airport in 1985, carrying 2,257,000 passengers and 74,000 tonnes of freight. In Sept. 1990 Iraq announced the dissolution of Kuwait Airways, and Iraqi Airways took possession of 15 aircraft. In Oct. Kuwaiti Airways resumed operations from Cairo with 8 aircraft which were out of the country during the invasion, with services to Jiddah, Bahrain, Dubai, New York, London, Frankfurt and Rome.

Shipping. The largest oil terminal is at Mina Ahmade, which received 348 oil tankers in 1984. Three small oil ports lie to the south of Mina Ahmade: Mina Shuaiba (250 oil tankers in 1984); Mina Abdullah (25) and Mina Al-Zor (40). The main ports for other traffic are at Shuwaikh, where 1,585 ships docked in 1985, discharging 5m. tonnes of goods; Shuiaba, about 3·75m. tonnes were handled in 1985 (3·1m. imported, 650,000 exported), and Doha.

Telecommunications. There were (1984), 419,200 telephones and there is a broadcasting and a television station. In 1986 there were 580,000 TV receivers and 750,000 radios.

Cinemas. In 1984 there were 14 cinemas, including 2 drive-ins.

Newspapers. In 1987 there were 5 daily newspapers in Arabic and 2 in English, with a combined circulation of about 418,000.

JUSTICE, RELIGION, EDUCATION AND WELFARE

Justice. In 1960 Kuwait adopted a unified judicial system covering all levels of courts. These are: Courts of Summary Justice, Courts of the First Instance, Supreme Court of Appeal, Court of Cassation, Constitutional Court and State Security Court. Islamic Sharia is a major source of legislation.

Religion. In 1980 about 78% of the population were Sunni Moslems, 14% Shia Moslems, 6% Christians and 2% others. In 1988 there were 1·43m. Moslems in all.

Education. In 1987–88 there were 33,375 pupils in kindergartens, 119,932 in primary schools, 120,961 in intermediate schools and 93,317 in secondary schools. In 1988 there were 836 students in the Religious Institute and 1,898 in special training institutes. The University of Kuwait had 15,990 students and 877 teachers in 1985–86.

Health. Medical services are free to all residents. There were (1985) 25 hospitals and sanatoria with 5,886 beds, 64 clinics and 25 health centres. In 1985 there were 2,692 doctors, 291 dentists and 8,557 nursing staff.

DIPLOMATIC REPRESENTATIVES

Of Kuwait in Great Britain (45 Queen's Gate, London, SW7)
Ambassador: Ghazi Mohammed Amin Al-Rayes (accredited 12 Feb. 1981).

Of Great Britain in Kuwait (Arabian Gulf St., Kuwait)
Ambassador: Michael Weston.

Of Kuwait in the USA (2940 Tilden St., NW, Washington, D.C., 20008)
Ambassador: Shaikh Saud Nasir Al-Sabah.

Of the USA in Kuwait (PO Box 77, Safat, Kuwait)
Ambassador: Edward Gneim.

Of Kuwait to the United Nations
Ambassador: Mohammad A. Abulhasan.

Further Reading

Arabian Year Book. Kuwait, 1978
Annual Statistical Abstract of Kuwait. Kuwait
Kuwait Facts and Figures 1986. Ministry of Information, 1987
Clements, F. A., *Kuwait.* [Bibliography] Oxford and Santa Barbara, 1985
Girgis, M., (ed.) *Industrial Progress in Small Oil-Exporting Countries: The Prospect for Kuwait.* Harlow, 1984
Sabah, Y. S. F., *The Oil Economy of Kuwait.* London, 1980

LAOS

Capital: Vientiane
Population: 4·05m. (1989)
GNP per capita: US$180 (1988)

(Lao People's Democratic Republic)

HISTORY. The Lao People's Democratic Republic was founded on 2 Dec. 1975. Until that date Laos was a Kingdom, once called Lanxang (the land of a million elephants).

In 1893 Laos became a French protectorate and in 1907 acquired its present frontiers. In 1941 French authority was suppressed by the Japanese. When the Japanese withdrew in 1945 an independence movement known as Lao Issara (Free Laos) set up a government under Prince Phetsarath, the Viceroy of Luang Prabang. This government collapsed with the return of the French in 1946 and the leaders of the movement fled to Thailand.

Under a new Constitution of 1947 Laos became a constitutional monarchy under the Luang Prabang dynasty, and in 1949 became an independent sovereign state within the French Union. Most of the Lao Issara leaders returned to Laos but a few remained in dissidence under Prince Souphanouvong, who allied himself with the Vietminh and subsequently formed the 'Pathet Lao' (Lao State) rebel movement.

The war in Laos from 1953 to 1973 between the Royal Lao Government (supported by American bombing and Thai mercenaries) and the Patriotic Front *Pathet Lao* (supported by large numbers of North Vietnamese troops) ended in 1973 when an agreement and a protocol were signed. A provisional coalition government was formed by the two sides in 1974. However, after the communist victories in neighbouring Vietnam and Cambodia in April 1975, the *Pathet Lao* took over the running of the whole country, although maintaining the façade of a coalition. On 29 Nov. 1975 HM King Savang Vatthana abdicated and a 264-member People's Congress proclaimed a People's Democratic Republic of Laos on 2 Dec. For the history of *Pathet Lao* and the military intervention of the Vietminh, *see* THE STATESMAN'S YEAR-BOOK, 1971–72, pp. 1126–28 and 1975–76 ed., pp. 1115–16.

AREA AND POPULATION. Laos is a landlocked country of about 91,400 sq. miles (236,800 sq. km) bordered on the north by China, the east by Vietnam, the south by Cambodia and the west by Thailand and Burma. Apart from the Mekong River plains along the border of Thailand, the country is mountainous, particularly in the north, and in places densely forested.

The population (census, 1986) was 3,722,000 (1,824,000 male); estimate (1989) 4·05m. Growth rate (1989), 2·9%. The most heavily populated areas are the Mekong River plains by the Thailand border. Otherwise, the population is sparse and scattered, particularly in the northern provinces, and the eastern part of the country has been depopulated by war. The majority of the population is officially divided into 4 groups: about 56% Lao-Lum (Valley-Lao), 34% Lao-Theung (Lao of the mountain sides); and 9% Lao-Soung (Lao of the mountain tops), who comprise the Meo and Yaoe. Other minorities include Vietnamese, Chinese, Europeans, Indians and Pakistanis.

The Lao-Lum and Lao-Tai belong to the Lao branch of the Tai peoples, who migrated into South-East Asia at the time of the Mongol invasion of South China. The Lao-Theungma diverse group consists of many tribes but most belong to the Mon-Khmer group.

The Meo and Yaoe live in northern Laos. Far greater numbers live in both North Vietnam and China, having migrated over the last century. Their religions have strong Confucian and animistic features but some are Christians.

There are 17 provinces. Compared with other parts of Asia, Laos has few towns. The administrative capital and largest town is Vientiane, with a population of census (1985) 377,409. Other important towns (1973) are Luang Prabang, 44,244; Pakse, 44,860, in the extreme south, and Savannakhet, 50,690.

Lao is the official language.

CLIMATE. A tropical monsoon climate, with high temperatures throughout the year and very heavy rains from May to Oct. Vientiane. Jan. 70°F (21·1°C), July 81°F (27·2°C). Annual rainfall 69" (1,715 mm).

CONSTITUTION AND GOVERNMENT. There is a Supreme People's Assembly. In Feb. 1991 the Government included:

Prime Minister, Secretary General of the Lao People's Revolutionary Party (LPRP): Kaysone Phomvihane.

First Deputy Prime Minister, Deputy Secretary General of the Central Committee of the Lao People's Revolutionary Party: Nouhak Phounsavanh. *Deputy Prime Ministers:* Phoumi Vongvichit [1]; Khamtai Siphandon [1] (also *Minister for Defence, Deputy Secretary General of the LPRP*); Phoun Sipaseut [1] (also *Foreign Minister*); Sali Vongkhamsao (also *Minister for Economics, Planning and Finance*).

Other ministers: Asang Laoli, *Defence*; Phao Bounnaphon, *Commerce and Foreign Economic Relations*; Inkong Mahavong, *Agriculture, Forestry, Irrigation and Co-operatives*; Soulivong Daravong, *Industry and Crafts*; Oudom Khatthi-gna, *Transport and Communications*; Saman Vi-guaket, *Education*; Khamkou Sounikay, *Health and Welfare*; Thongsing Thammavong, *Culture*; Kou Souvannamethi, *Justice.*

The Politbureau of the LPRP comprises the above 3 plus: Phoumi Vongvichit [1], Gen. Phoune Sipraseuth [1] *(Minister of Foreign Affairs),* Gen. Khamtai Siphandon [1] *(Minister of National Defence, Supreme Commander of the Lao People's Army)* and Sisomphon Lovansay *(Vice-President of the Supreme People's Assembly).* Ministers not in the Politbureau include Saly Vongkhamsao [1] *(Chairman of State Planning Committee).*

[1] Member of the LPRP Politburo.

National flag: Three horizontal stripes of red, blue, red, with blue of double width with in the centre a large white disc.

National anthem: Peng Sat Lao (Hymn of the Lao People).

Provincial Administration: All provincial administration is in the hands of the Lao People's Revolutionary Party. Orders come from the Central Committee through a series of 'People's Revolutionary Committees' at the province, town and village level.

DEFENCE. Military service is compulsory for 18 months.

Army. The Army is organized in 5 infantry divisions; 3 engineering regiments, 7 independent infantry regiments and 65 independent infantry companies; and 5 artillery and 9 anti-aircraft battalions. Equipment includes 30 T-54/-55 main battle tanks. Strength (1991) about 52,500.

Navy. There is believed to be a riverine force of about 650 personnel organized into 4 squadrons running some 40 river patrol craft for operations on the Mekong.

Air Force. Since 1975, the Air Force has received aircraft from the USSR, including 40 MiG-21 fighters, 6 An-24 and 3 An-26 turboprop transports and 10 Mi-8 helicopters. They may be supplemented by a few of the C-47 and C-123 transports, and UH-1 Iroquois, supplied by the USA to the former régime. Personnel strength, about 2,000 in 1991, with 34 combat aircraft.

INTERNATIONAL RELATIONS

Membership. Laos is a member of the UN.

Aid. Foreign aid in 1986, was US$44m.

ECONOMY

Policy. The priorities of the second Five Year Plan, 1986–90, continued to be infrastructure projects (telecommunications and transport), agriculture (crop diversification and improving paddy production), and agro-industrial processing. In 1989, in an attempt to stimulate the economy, the Government introduced a 'New Economic Management Mechanism' introducing managerial autonomy into state enterprises and a limited increase of private sector activities. Further moves towards a free market were announced in Dec. 1990.

Budget. Total revenue 1986, K.14,127m.; total expenditure, K.24,900m. including capital expenditure of K.12,800m.

Currency. The unit of currency is the *kip* (LAK) of 100 *att*. Coinage, 1, 2 and 5 *att*; banknotes, 1, 5, 10, 20, 50, 100 and 500 *kip*. The official rate of exchange was (March 1991) K.700 = US$1; £1 = K1,328.

Banking and Finance. The head of the State Bank is Pani Vangkhamatou.

ENERGY AND NATURAL RESOURCES

Electricity. Hydro-electric resources are important. Total installed capacity (1985) was 168,000 kw. Transmission lines to Vientiane and to Thailand have been constructed, but few towns have electricity. Production (1986) 900m. kwh. Supply 127 and 220 volts; 50 Hz.

Minerals. Various minerals are found, but only tin is mined to any significant extent at present, and only at 2 mines. Production of tin concentrates (1986) 559 tonnes. There are deposits of high-quality iron in Xieng Khouang province, potash near Vientiane, gypsum and coal.

Agriculture. Agriculture accounts for 60% of GDP. The chief products (1988 output in 1,000 tonnes) are rice (1,003), maize (40), tobacco (4), seed-cotton (21), coffee (8), potatoes and sugar-cane. Opium is produced but its manufacture is controlled by the state.

Livestock (1988): Cattle, 590,000; buffaloes, 1m.; horses, 42,000; pigs, 1·52m.; goats, 76,000; poultry, 9m.

Forestry. The forests, which cover 13m. hectares, representing 56% of the land area, produce valuable woods such as teak.

INDUSTRY. Industry accounts for 14% of GDP. Industry is limited to wood-processing, textiles and light industry. Most factories have been working at limited capacity in recent years.

Labour. The workforce was 1·95m. in 1990. Unemployment was 21%.

FOREIGN ECONOMIC RELATIONS. Since 1988 foreign companies have been permitted to participate in Lao enterprises, but few have done so.

Commerce. In 1989 (and 1988) imports amounted to US$162 (125)m. and exports to US$54 (49)m. The main imports in 1988 (in US$1m.) were: Machinery and raw materials, 8·8; rice and other food, 5·7; petroleum products, 5·3. The chief supplying countries were Thailand and Japan. The main exports in 1988 (in US$1m.) were: Timber, 350; electricity, 11·1; gypsum, 1; tin, 0·9.

Total trade between Laos and UK (British Department of Trade returns, in £1,000 sterling):

	1986	*1987*	*1988*	*1989*	*1990*
Imports to UK	150	621	2	1,369	54
Exports and re-exports from UK	1,460	1,742	1,332	908	1,261

COMMUNICATIONS

Roads. In 1986 the national road network, consisted of 2,350 km paved, 3,250 km gravel and 6,780 km earth roads.

Railways. There is no railway in Laos, but the Thai railway system extends to

Nongkhai, on the Thai bank of the Mekong, which is connected by ferry with Thadeua about 12 miles east of Vientiane.

Aviation. Lao Aviation provides scheduled domestic air services linking major towns in Laos and international services to Bangkok, Phnom Penh and Hanoi. Thai International, Aeroflot and Air Vietnam provide flights from Bangkok, Hanoi, Rangoon, Ho Chi Min City and Moscow.

Shipping. The river Mekong and its tributaries are an important means of transport, but rapids, waterfalls and narrow channels often impede navigation and make transshipments necessary.

Telecommunications. There is a radio network as well as a limited TV service with the main station at Vientiane. There were (1988) about 400,000 radio and 32,000 television receivers. A ground station constructed near Vientiane under the Soviet aid programme enables USSR television programmes to be received in the capital. It also provides a telephone service to Hanoi and Eastern Europe.

In 1985 there were 8,136 telephones.

RELIGION, EDUCATION AND WELFARE

Justice. Criminal legislation of 1990 established a system of courts and a prosecutor's office.

Religion. The majority of the population is Buddhist (Hinayana) but 34% follow tribal religions.

Education. In 1985–86 school year there were 8,000 elementary schools (523,000 pupils); 420 secondary schools (97,000 pupils); 60 senior high schools (4,900 pupils); and 55 vocational schools (6,800 students). There is 1 teachers' training college, 1 college of education, 1 school of medicine, 1 agricultural college and an advanced school of Pali.

Sisavangvong University in Vientiane (founded 1958) had 1,600 students in 1984, and there are regional technical colleges in Luang Prabang, Savannakhét and Champasak.

65% literacy was claimed in 1990.

Health. In 1985 there were 430 doctors and 11,650 hospital beds.

DIPLOMATIC REPRESENTATIVES

Of Laos in Great Britain (resides in Paris)
Ambassador: vacant.

Of Great Britain in Laos
Ambassador: Ramsay Melhuish, CMG (resides in Bangkok).

Of Laos in USA (2222 S. St., NW, Washington, D.C., 20008)
Chargé d'Affaires: Sipaseuth Phounsavanh.

Of USA in Laos (Rue Bartholonie, Vientiane)
Chargé d'Affaires: Charles B. Salmon, Jr.

Of Laos to the United Nations
Ambassador: Saly Khamsy.

Further Reading

Cordell, H., *Laos.* [Bibliography] Oxford and Santa Barbara, 1990

Stuart-Cox, M., *Contemporary Laos.* Univ. of Queensland Press, 1983.—*Laos: Politics, Economics and Society.* London, 1986

Zasloff, J. J., *The Pathet Lao: Leadership and Organization.* Lexington, Toronto and London, 1973 – and Unger, L. (eds.) *Laos: Beyond the Revolution.* London, 1991

LEBANON

Capital: Beirut
Population: 2·8m. (1988)

Al-Jumhouriya al-Lubnaniya

(Republic of Lebanon)

HISTORY. After 20 years as a mandate of France, Lebanon was proclaimed independent on 26 Nov. 1941. The evacuation of foreign troops was completed in Dec. 1946.

For events between the insurrection of 1958 and the intervention of the Arab Deterrent Force *see* THE STATESMAN'S YEAR-BOOK, 1990-91, p.799.

By Nov. 1976 the Syrian-dominated Arab Deterrent Force had ensured sufficient security to permit Lebanon to establish quasi-normal conditions under President Sarkis. Large areas of the country, however, remained outside government control, including West Beirut which was the scene of frequent conflict between opposing militia groups. The South, where the Arab Deterrent Force could not deploy, remained unsettled and subject to frequent Israeli attacks. In March 1978 there was an Israeli invasion following a Palestinian attack inside Israel. Israeli troops eventually withdrew in June, but instead of handing over all their positions to UN Peacekeeping Forces they installed Israeli-controlled Lebanese militia forces in border areas. Severe disruption continued in the South. In June 1982, following on the attempted assassination of the Israeli ambassador in London, Israeli forces once again swept through the country, eventually laying siege to and bombing Beirut. In Sept. Palestinian forces evacuated Beirut.

On 23 Aug. 1982 Bachir Gemayel was elected President of Lebanon. On 14 Sept. he was assassinated. His brother, Amin Gemayel, was elected in his place on 21 Sept. There followed a state of 'no peace, no war' with intermittent clashes between the various forces. Israeli forces began a phased withdrawal in 1985 and have now relinquished control of all but their so-called security zone in the South of the country. The heads of the 3 leading militia forces signed an agreement on political reform and relations with Syria in 1985 but this was never implemented; Syrian forces remain deployed in most areas of Lebanon.

The term of office of President Amin Gemayel expired in September 1988 and efforts to elect a successor failed. Gemayel appointed the Commander of the Army, Gen. Michel Aoun, Prime Minister until such time as a President could be elected. His appointment was disputed by the Moslems and the Syrians, and the existing Prime Minister, Selim Hoss, remained in office heading a rival administration in West Beirut. In 1989 Gen. Aoun launched his 'war of liberation' against the Syrians. The resulting damage and death toll prompted the Arab League to take action and in Oct. 1989 Lebanese parliamentarians gathered in Taif in Saudi Arabia to sign an agreement on political reform and relations with Syria formulated by a tripartite committee of the Arab League. In Nov. 1989 Rene Moawwad was elected President, but he was assassinated later that month and Elias Hrawi elected in his place. Gen. Aoun refused to accept the Taif accords or recognise the legitimacy of the Hrawi presidency. Aoun was dismissed as head of the Lebanese Armed Forces and replaced by Gen. Emile Lahoud. In Feb. 1990 full-scale hostilities broke out between elements of the Lebanese army loyal to Aoun and the principal Christian militia, the Lebanese Forces. As a result Lebanon's remaining commercial and industrial infrastructure was severely damaged. In Sept. 1990 constitutional changes establishing the Second Republic were made, enabling the implementation of the political reform provisions of the Taif accords. In Oct. 1990 Syrian forces in support of the Lebanese government ousted Gen. Aoun, who took refuge in the French embassy. In Nov. and Dec. the various militias which had held sway in Beirut withdrew. A new Government of National Reconciliation was announced on 24 Dec. 1990. In Feb. 1991 the army began to move south.

AREA AND POPULATION. Lebanon is a mountainous country about 135 miles long and varying between 20 and 35 miles wide, bounded on the north and east by Syria, on the west by the Mediterranean and on the south by Israel. Between the two parallel mountain ranges of Lebanon and Anti-Lebanon lies the fertile Bekaa Valley. About one-half of the country lies at an altitude of over 3,000 ft.

The area of Lebanon is estimated at 10,452 sq. km (4,036 sq. miles) and the population at 2·8m. (1988, estimate). The principal towns, with estimated population (1988), are: Beirut (the capital), 1·5m.; Tripoli, 160,000; Zahlé, 45,000; Saida (Sidon), 38,000; Tyre, 14,000.

The official language is Arabic. French and, increasingly, English are widely spoken in official and commercial circles.

CLIMATE. A Mediterranean climate with short, warm winters and long, hot and rainless summers, with high humidity in coastal areas. Rainfall is largely confined to the winter months and can be torrential, with snow on high ground. Beirut. Jan. 55°F (13°C), July 81°F (27°C). Annual rainfall 35·7" (893 mm).

CONSTITUTION AND GOVERNMENT. Lebanon is an independent republic. The first Constitution was established under the French Mandate on 23 May 1926. It has since been amended in 1927, 1929, 1943 (twice), 1947 and 1990. It is a written constitution based on the classical separation of powers, with a President, a single-chamber *National Assembly* elected by universal adult suffrage, and an independent judiciary. The executive consists of the President and a Prime Minister and Cabinet appointed after consulation between the President and the Chamber of Deputies. The system is, however, adapted to the peculiar communal balance on which Lebanese political life depends. This is done by the electoral law which allocates deputies according to the confessional distribution of the population, and by a series of constitutional conventions whereby, *e.g.*, the President is always a Maronite Christian, the Prime Minister a Sunni Moslem and the Speaker of the Assembly a Shia Moslem. There is no highly developed party system other than on religious confessional lines. In Aug. 1990 the National Assembly voted to enlarge itself from 99 to 108 members with equal numbers of Christians and Moslems.

On 21 Sept. President Hrawi formally established the Second Republic by signing constitutional amendments which had been negotiated at Taif (Saudi Arabia) in Oct. 1989. These institute an executive collegium between the President, Prime Minister and Speaker, and remove from the President the right to recall the Prime Minister, dissolve the Assembly and vote in the Council of Ministers.

President of the Republic: Elias Hrawi (Maronite; elected 24 Nov. 1989).
Prime Mnister: Omar Karame.

National flag: Three horizontal stripes of red, white, red, with the white of double width and bearing in the centre a green cedar of Lebanon.

National anthem: Kulluna lil watan lil 'ula lil' alam (words by Rashid Nachleh, tune by Flaïfel brothers).

Local government: The 6 governorates (including the city of Beirut) are subdivided into 26 districts.

Since Sept. 1988 there have been 2 rival cabinets. General Michel Aoun has been acting Prime Minister of the Christian government and Dr Selim Hoss acting Prime Minister of the Moslem government.

DEFENCE

Army. The strength of the Army was about 21,000 in 1991 but it is in a state of flux and most of its units are well below strength. Its equipment includes 105 M-48, 32

AMX-13 tanks and Saladin armoured cars. In addition, there are numerous private militias under arms in Lebanon, divided between the Maronite-Christian factions, notably the Lebanese Forces of some 10,000 men, and others, notably AMAL (Shi'ite), the Progressive Socialist Party (Druze) and Hizballah (Shi'ite fundamentalists).

Navy. The Christian-controlled flotilla of 4 inshore patrol craft and 2 tank-landing craft numbering (1990) 500 was captured by non-government forces in Feb. 1990.

Air Force. The Air Force had (1991) about 800 men and 50 aircraft. In addition to 5 Hunter jet fighter-bombers, it has (in storage) 9 Mirage III supersonic fighters and 1 Mirage 2-seat trainer. Other aircraft include 12 Alouette II and III, 4 Gazelle, 9 Puma and 8 Agusta-Bell 212 helicopters, and 5 Fouga Magister jet and 5 piston-engined Bulldog trainers. Serviceability of most aircraft is low because of the troubled national political situation.

INTERNATIONAL RELATIONS

Membership. Lebanon is a member of the UN and Arab League.

ECONOMY

Budget. The budget for 1986 provided for a total expenditure of £Leb.17,937m.

Currency. The unit of currency is the *Lebanese pound* (LBP) of 100 *piastres*. There is a fluctuating official rate of exchange, fixed monthly (March 1991: £Leb.1,959·10 = £1 sterling; £Leb.1,032·74 US$1), this in practice is used only for the calculation of *ad-valorem* customs duties on Lebanese imports and for import statistics. For other purposes the free market is used.

Banking and Finance. The Bank of Lebanon (*Governor*, Edmond Naim) is the bank of issue. It commenced operating in 1964. As a result of the civil war, Beirut has lost much of its former status as an international and regional banking centre; in general only local offices for banks remain.

Weights and Measures. The use of the metric system is legal. In outlying districts the former weights and measures may still be in use. They are: 1 *okiya* = 0·47 lb.; 6 *okiyas* = 1 *oke* = 2·82 lb.; 2 *okes* = 1 *rottol* = 5·64 lb.; 200 *okes* = 1 *kantar*.

ENERGY AND NATURAL RESOURCES

Electricity. Electric power production (1986) was 2,270m. kwh. Supply 110 and 120 volts; 50 Hz.

Oil. There are 2 oil refineries: at Tripoli, which refines oil brought by ship from Iraq, and at Sidon, which refines oil brought from Saudi Arabia by a pipeline owned by the Trans-Arabian Pipeline Co. These refineries have not been fully active since the late 1970s, and the country depends on imports.

Minerals. Iron ore exists but is difficult to work. Other minerals known to exist are iron pyrites, copper, bituminous shales, asphalt, phosphates, ceramic clays and glass sand; but the available information is of doubtful value.

Agriculture. Lebanon is essentially an agricultural country, although owing to its physical character only about 38% of the total area of the country is at present cultivated.

The estimated production (in 1,000 tonnes) of the main crops in 1988 was as follows: Citrus fruits, 354; apples, 80; grapes, 159; potatoes, 210; sugar-beet, 4; wheat, 19; bananas, 23; olives, 75.

Livestock (estimated, 1988): Goats, 470,000; sheep, 141,000; cattle, 52,000; pigs, 22,000; horses, 2,000; donkeys, 11,000; mules, 4,000.

Forestry. The forests of the past have been denuded by exploitation and in 1988 covered 100,000 hectares, about 8% of the land area.

Fisheries. Total catch (1986) 1,600 tonnes.

INDUSTRY. Industry has suffered badly during the civil war. The manufacturing industry was small but had doubled in size in the 10 years before the war. Some concerns have closed, others are working at reduced capacity.

FOREIGN ECONOMIC RELATIONS. Foreign and domestic trade is the principal source of income. Because of the protectionist policies of some neighbouring countries, this sector has been declining, the sectors to gain being those of banking, real estate, government and services.

Commerce. Total trade between Lebanon and UK (British Department of Trade returns, in £1,000 sterling):

	1986	*1987*	*1988*	*1989*	*1990*
Imports to UK	9,845	9,528	14,172	11,054	6,249
Exports and re-exports from UK	55,867	40,707	55,575	48,474	53,266

COMMUNICATIONS

Roads. There were (1987) 7,000 km of roads of which main roads (2,000 km) are not good by international standards. The surface is normally of asphalt and they are well maintained in normal times.

In 1985 there were about 300,000 cars and taxis.

Railways. There are 3 railway lines, all operated by the *Office des Chemins de Fer de l'Etat Libanais* (CFL): (1) Nakoura–Beirut–Tripoli (standard gauge); (2) a narrow-gauge line running from Beirut to Riyak in the Bekaa Valley and thence to Damascus, Syria; (3) a standard-gauge line from Tripoli to Homs and Aleppo in Syria, providing access to Ankara and Istanbul. From Homs a branch of the CFL line extends south and re-enters Lebanon, terminating at Riyak. The total length is 417 km. Apart from a short section near Beirut these lines have been closed since the civil war began.

Aviation. Beirut International Airport is used by a few international airlines. There are 2 national airlines, Middle East Airlines/Air Liban and Trans-Mediterranean Airways. Over the past few years Beirut airport has been closed several times.

Shipping. Beirut is the largest port, followed by Tripoli, principaly Jounieh and Sidon. Illegal ports sprung up, reducing the legal ports' activity.

Telecommunications. There is an automatic telephone system in Beirut which is being extended to other parts of the country. There are no communications with Israel. Number of telephones (1986), 150,000.

The state radio transmits in Arabic, French, English and Armenian. Teté-Liban, which is 50% government-owned, was the only television station in operation in 1984. There were 450,000 TV sets in 1986 and 1·5m. radios.

Newspapers (1989). There were about 30 daily newspapers in Arabic, 2 in French, 1 in English and 4 in Armenian, and 30 weekly periodicals.

RELIGION, EDUCATION AND WELFARE

Religion. The Christian faith has been indigenous since the earliest times. The Christians include the Maronites, Greek Orthodox, Armenians, Greek and Roman Catholics, Armenian Catholics and the Protestants. Moslems include the Sunnis, the Shi'ites and the Druzes. In 1990 it was estimated that the population was 62% Moslem (including 31% Shi'ite and 27% Sunni) and 38% Christian (including 22% Maronite).

Education. Government schools comprise primary and secondary schools. There were also private primary and secondary schools. There are also 5 universities, namely the Lebanese (State) University, the American University of Beirut, the French University of St Joseph (founded in 1875), the Arab University, a branch of Alexandria University and Beirut University College. The French Government runs the École Supérieure de Lettres and the Centre d'Études Mathématiques. The Maronite monks run the University of the Holy Spirit at Kaslik.

The Lebanese Academy of Fine Arts includes schools of architecture, art, music, political and social science.

Health. There are several government-run hospitals, and many private ones.

DIPLOMATIC REPRESENTATIVES

Of Lebanon in Great Britain (21 Kensington Palace Gdns., London, W8 4QM)
Ambassador: Mahmoud Hammoud.

Of Great Britain in Lebanon (Shamma Bldg., Raouché, Ras Beirut)
Ambassador: D. E. Tatham.

Of Lebanon in the USA (2560 28th St., NW, Washington, D.C., 20008)
Ambassador: Nassib Lahoud.

Of the USA in Lebanon
Ambassador: Ryan Crocker.

Of Lebanon to the United Nations
Acting Ambassador: Khalil Makkawi.

Further Reading

Statistical Information: Import and export figures are produced by the Conseil Supérieur des Douanes. The Service de Statistique Générale (M. A. G. Ayad, *Chef du Service*) publishes a quarterly bulletin (in French and Arabic) covering a wide range of subjects, including foreign trade, production statistics and estimates of the national income.

Cobban, H., *The Making of Modern Lebanon.* London, 1985
Fisk, R., *Pity the Nation: Lebanon at War.* London, 1990
Gilmour, D., *Lebanon: The Fractured Country.* Oxford and New York, 1983
Gordon, D. C., *The Republic of Lebanon: Nation in Jeopardy.* London, 1983
Khairallah, S., *Lebanon.* [Bibliography] Oxford and Santa Barbara, 1979
Norton, A. R., *Amal and the Shi'a: Struggle for the Soul of Lebanon.* Univ. of Texas Press, 1987
Rabanovich, I., *The War for Lebanon, 1970–1983.* Cornell Univ. Press, 1984
Shehadi, N. and Mills, D.H., *Lebanon: A History of Conflict and Consensus.* London, 1988
Weinberger, N. J., *Syrian Intervention in Lebanon.* New York, 1986

National Library: Dar el Kutub, Parliament Sq., Beirut.

LESOTHO

Kingdom of Lesotho

Capital: Maseru
Population: 1·72m. (1989)
GNP per capita: US$410 (1988)

HISTORY. Basutoland first received the protection of Britain in 1868 at the request of Moshoeshoe I, the first paramount chief. In 1871 the territory was annexed to the Cape Colony, but in 1884 it was restored to the direct control of the British Government through the High Commissioner for South Africa.

On 4 Oct. 1966 Basutoland became an independent and sovereign member of the Commonwealth under the name of the Kingdom of Lesotho.

King Moeshoeshoe II was deposed by the Military Council in Nov. 1990 and replaced by King Letsie III.

AREA AND POPULATION. Lesotho, an enclave within the Republic of South Africa is bounded on the west by the Orange Free State, on the north by the Orange Free State and Natal, on the east by Natal, and on the south by Transkei. The altitude varies from 1,500 to 3,482 metres. The area is 11,720 sq. miles (30,355 sq. km). Lesotho is a purely African territory, and the few European residents are government officials, traders, missionaries and artisans.

The census in 1986 showed a total population of 1,577,536 persons. Estimate (1989) 1,724,000. The capital is Maseru (population, 1986, 109,382).

The official languages are Sesotho and English.

CLIMATE. A healthy and pleasant climate, with variable rainfall, but averaging 29" (725 mm) a year over most of the country. The rain falls mainly in the summer months of Oct. to April, while the winters are dry and may produce heavy frosts in lowland areas and frequent snow in the highlands. Temperatures in the lowlands range from a maximum of 90°F (32·2°C) in summer to a minimum of 20°F (–6·7°C) in winter.

CONSTITUTION AND GOVERNMENT. Lesotho is a constitutional monarchy with HM the King as Head of State, but the constitution adopted at independence was suspended and the elections of 27 Jan. 1970 were declared invalid on 31 Jan. 1970. Parliamentary rule, with a National Assembly of nominated members, was reintroduced in April 1973, but the National Assembly was dissolved on 1 Jan. 1985 by the first Prime Minister, Chief Joseph Leabua Jonathan.

Chief Jonathan was deposed in a bloodless military coup on 20 Jan. 1986. HM the King, acts through a *Council of Ministers* on the advice of a *Military Council.*

Ruler: Mohato Seeisa, King Letsie III, (b.1963), eldest son of Moeshoeshoe II, was proclaimed King by an assembly of traditional chiefs on 9 Nov. 1990.

Chairman of the Military Council and Council of Ministers: Maj.-Gen. Justin Lekhanya. *Members:* Col. M. Tsotsetsi; Col. E. Ramaema; Brig. B. Lerotholi; Col. J. Jane; Lieut. Col. M. Mokete.

In Dec. 1990 the Council of Ministers comprised: *Minister of Finance, Planning, Economic and Manpower Development:* The Hon E. R. Sekhonyana. *Foreign Affairs, Information and Broadcasting:* T. Thabane. *Education:* I.B.B.J. Machobane. *Justice, Prisons, Law and Constitutional Affairs:* A. K. Maope. *Water, Energy and Mining:* Col. A. I. Jane. *Employment, Social Security and Pensions:* Col. P. Molapo. *Highlands Water and Energy:* Maj. R. Habi. *Works Transport and Telecommunications:* Col. V. M. Mokone. *Interior, Chieftainship Affairs and Rural Development:* P. Molapo. *Health:* A. I. Thoahlane. *Tourism, Sports and Culture:* I. Matheahra. *Trade and Industry:* M. Mokoroane.

The *College of Chiefs* settles the recognition and succession of Chiefs and adjudicates cases of inefficiency, criminality and absenteeism among them.

National flag: Diagonally white over blue over green with the white of double width charged with a brown Basotho shield in the upper hoist.

Local Government. The country is divided into 10 districts, subdivided into 22 wards, as follows: Maseru, Qacha's Nek, Mokhotlong, Leribe, Butha–Buthe, Teyateyaneng, Mafeteng, Mohale's Hoek, Quthing, Thaba–Tseka. Most of the wards are presided over by hereditary chiefs allied to the Moshoeshoe family.

DEFENCE

The Royal Lesotho Defence Force has 2,000 personnel. Formed in 1978, to facilitate deployment of men and equipment to less accessible regions, the service has 3 Bell 412 and 2 BO-105 helicopters.

INTERNATIONAL RELATIONS

Membership. Lesotho is a member of the UN, OAU, the Commonwealth and is an ACP state of the EEC.

ECONOMY

Budget. Expenditure (1986–87) M463m.; revenue, M385m.

Currency. The unit of currency is the *loti* (plural *maloti*) (LSM) of 100 *lisente* which is at par with the South African *rand*. In March 1991, £1 = 4·92 *maloti*; US$1 = 2·59 *maloti*.

Banking. The Standard Bank of South Africa and Barclays Bank International have branches at Maseru, Mohale's Hoek and Leribe. The Lesotho Bank has branches throughout the country.

ENERGY AND NATURAL RESOURCES

Electricity. Production (1985) 1m. kwh. Supply 230 volts; 50 Hz.

Agriculture. The chief crops were (1988 production in 1,000 tonnes): Wheat, 21; maize, 126; sorghum, 55; barley, oats, beans, peas and other vegetables are also grown. Soil conservation and the improvement of crops and pasture are matters of vital importance.

Livestock (1988): Cattle, 525,000; horses, 119,000; donkeys, 126,000; pigs, 72,000; sheep, 1·43m.; goats, 1·03m.; mules, 1,000; poultry, 1m.

INDUSTRY. Industrial development is progressing under the National Development Corporation.

FOREIGN ECONOMIC RELATIONS. Lesotho, Botswana and Swaziland are members of the South African customs union, by agreement dated 29 June 1910.

Commerce. Total values of imports and exports into and from Lesotho (in Mm.):

	1983	*1984*	*1985*	*1986*
Imports	627	725	797	893
Exports	35	42	50	58

In 1981, 97% of imports came from within the Southern African customs union, while 47% of exports went to the same countries and 42% to Switzerland.

Principal imports were food, livestock, drink and tobacco, machinery and transport equipment, mineral fuels and lubricants; principal exports were wool and mohair and diamonds.

The majority of international trade is with the Republic of South Africa.

Total trade between Lesotho and UK (British Department of Trade returns, in £1,000 sterling):

	1986	*1987*	*1988*	*1989*	*1990*
Imports to UK	277	486	977	734	1,288
Exports and re-exports from UK	2,128	1,112	1,260	795	642

Tourism. In 1986 there were 213,000 visitors.

COMMUNICATIONS

Roads. There were (1988) 572 km of tarred roads and 2,300 km of gravel-surfaced roads. In addition to the main roads there were (1983) 931 km of food aid tracks leading to trading stations and missions. Communications into the mountainous interior are by means of bridlepaths suitable only for riding and pack animals, but a mountain road of 80 miles has been constructed, and some parts are accessible by air transport, which is being used increasingly. In 1983 there were 10,200 commercial vehicles and 4,359 passenger cars.

Railways. A railway built by the South African Railways, 1 mile long, connects Maseru with the Bloemfontein–Natal line at Marseilles.

Aviation. There is a scheduled passenger service between Maseru and Jan Smuts Airport, Johannesburg, operated jointly by Lesotho National Airways and South African Airways. There are also 30 airstrips for light aircraft.

Telecommunications. There were 5,409 telephones in 1983. Radio Lesotho transmits daily in English and Sesotho. Radio receivers (1987), 400,000.

Newspapers. In 1985, 3 daily newspapers had a combined circulation of 44,000.

JUSTICE, RELIGION, EDUCATION AND WELFARE

Justice. The Lesotho High Court and the Court of Appeal are situated in Maseru, and there are Magistrates' Courts in the districts.

Religion. About 93% of the population are Christians, 44% being Roman Catholics.

Education. Education is largely in the hands of the 3 main missions (Paris Evangelical, Roman Catholic and English Church), under the direction of the Ministry of Education. In 1984–85 the total enrolment in 1,141 primary schools was 314,003; in 143 secondary schools, 35,423; in the National Teacher-Training College and 8 technical schools enrolment 2,221. University education is provided at the National University of Lesotho established in 1975 at Roma; enrolment in 1985, 1,119 and 146 teaching staff.

Health. The government medical staff of the territory consists of 1 Permanent Secretary for Health, 1 Director of Health Services, 1 medical superintendent, 8 district medical officers and a total of 102 doctors including 20 specialists.

There are 11 government hospitals staffed by 308 matrons, sisters and nurses. There is accommodation for 2,175 patients in government hospitals.

DIPLOMATIC REPRESENTATIVES

Of Lesotho in Great Britain (10 Collingham Rd., London, SW5 0NR)
High Commissioner: M. K. Tsekoa (accredited 15 Nov. 1989).

Of Great Britain in Lesotho (PO Box Ms 521, Maseru 100)
High Commissioner: J. C. Edwards, CMG.

Of Lesotho in the USA (2511 Massachusetts Ave., NW, Washington, D.C., 20008)
Ambassador: W. T. Van Tonder.

Of the USA in Lesotho (PO Box 333, Maseru, 100)
Ambassador: (Vacant).

Of Lesotho to the United Nations
Ambassador: Monyane P. Phoofolo.

Further Reading

Statistical Information: Bureau of Statistics, PO Box 455, Maseru, Lesotho.
Ashton, H., *The Basuto.* 2nd ed. OUP, 1967
Bardill, J. E. and Cobbe, J. H., *Lesotho: Dilemmas of Dependence in South Africa.* London, 1986
Murray, C., *Families Divided: The Impact of Migrant Labour in Lesotho.* OUP, 1981
Willet, S. M. and Ambrose, D. P., *Lesotho.* [Bibliography] Oxford and Santa Barbara, 1981

LIBERIA

Capital: Monrovia
Population: 2·44m. (1988)
GNP per capita: US$440 (1987)

Republic of Liberia

HISTORY. The Republic of Liberia had its origin in the efforts of several American philanthropic societies to establish freed American slaves in a colony on the West African coast. In 1822 a settlement was formed near the spot where Monrovia now stands. On 26 July 1847 the State was constituted as the Free and Independent Republic of Liberia.

On 12 April 1980, President Tolbert was assassinated and his government overthrown in a coup led by Master-Sergeant Samuel Doe, who was later installed as Head of State and Commander-in-Chief of the army.

At the beginning of 1990 rebel forces entered Liberia from the north and fought their way successfully southwards to confront President Doe's forces in Monrovia. The rebels comprised the National Patriotic Front of Liberia led by Charles Taylor, and the hostile breakaway Independent National Patriotic Front led by Prince Johnson. A peacekeeping force dispatched by the Economic Community of West African States (ECOWAS) disembarked at Monrovia on 25 Aug. 1990, and attempts to form a new provisional government were made.

On 9 Sept. President Doe was assassinated by Prince Johnson's rebels. At an ECOWAS summit at Bamako (Mali) on 28 Nov. government forces and the two rebel factions signed a ceasefire. ECOWAS installed a provisional government led by Amos Sawyer. Charles Taylor also declared himself president, as did the former vice-president, Harry Moniba.

On 13 Feb. 1991 Taylor, Johnson and the commander of the Liberian armed forces signed a second ceasefire and agreed to hold a national conference in March to form a new interim government.

AREA AND POPULATION. Liberia has about 350 miles of coastline, extending from Sierra Leone, on the west, to the Côte d'Ivoire, on the east. It stretches inland to a distance, in some places, of about 250 miles and is bounded in the north by Guinea.

The total area is about 42,989 sq. miles (111,370 sq. km). At the census (1984) population 2,101,628. Estimate (1988) 2,436,000. English is the official language spoken by 15% of the population. The rest belong in the main to 3 linguistic groups: Mande, West Atlantic, and the Kwa. These are in turn subdivided into 16 ethnic groups: Bassa, Bella, Gbandi, Mende, Gio, Dey, Mano, Gola, Kpelle, Kissi, Krahn, Kru, Lorma, Mandingo, Vai and Grebo.

Monrovia, the capital, had (1984) a population of 425,000; other towns include Buchanan (24,000).

There are 13 counties, whose areas, populations (1984 census) and capitals are as follows:

County	*Sq. km*	*1984*	*Chief town*
Bomi	1,955	66,420	Tubmanburg
Bong	8,099	255,813	Gbarnga
Grand Bassa	8,759	159,648	Buchanan
Grand Cape Mount	5,827	79,322	Robertsport
Grand Gedeh	17,029	102,810	Zwedru
Lofa	19,360	247,641	Voinjama
Margibi	3,263	97,992	Kakata
Maryland	5,351	132,058	Harper
Montserrado	2,740	544,878	Bensonville
Nimba	12,043	313,050	Saniquillie
Rivercess	4,385	37,849	Rivercess
Sinoe	10,254	64,147	Greenville

The county of Grand Kru (chief town, Barclayville) was created in 1985 from the former territories of Kru Coast and Sasstown.

CLIMATE. An equatorial climate, with constant high temperatures and plentiful rainfall, though Jan. to May is drier than the rest of the year. Monrovia. Jan. 79°F (26·1°C), July 76°F (24·4°C). Annual rainfall 206" (5,138 mm).

CONSTITUTION AND GOVERNMENT. A new Constitution was approved by referendum in July 1984 and came into force on 6 Jan. 1986. The National Assembly consists of a 26-member Senate and a 64-member House of Representatives. General elections were held on 15 Oct. 1985. The National Democratic Party of Liberia gained 21 seats in the Senate; the Liberal Action Party, 3 seats and the Liberian Unification Party and the Unity Party one each. In the House of Representatives, the NDPL won 45 seats and others 19 seats.

Following the insurrection of 1990 and the assassination of President Doe, in Jan. 1991 3 factions were claiming to be the government.

National flag: Six red and 5 white horizontal stripes alternating. In the upper corner, nearest the staff, is a square of blue covering a depth of 5 stripes. In the centre of this blue field is a 5-pointed white star.

National anthem: All hail, Liberia, hail! (words by President Warner; tune by O. Lucas, 1860).

DEFENCE

Army. The establishment organized on a militia basis numbered 7,300 (1990), divided into 6 infantry battalions with support units.

Navy. A coast-guard force of (1990) about 500 operated 5 inshore patrol craft, none exceeding 50 tonnes.

Air Force. The Air Reconnaissance Unit, supports the Liberian Army. Equipment includes 2 C-47 transports, 4 Israeli-built Arava twin-turboprop light transports, 1 Cessna 208 Caravan transport and a small number of Cessna 172, 185 and 337G light aircraft. Personnel (1990) about 250.

INTERNATIONAL RELATIONS

Membership. Liberia is a member of the UN, OAU, ECOWAS and is an ACP state of the EEC.

ECONOMY

Budget. Revenue and expenditure was as follows (in US$1,000):

	1984–85	*1985–86*	*1986–87*
Revenue	315,000	237,600	366,400
Expenditure	371,000	366,700	366,400

Currency. The legal currency is the *Liberian dollar* (LRD) which is equivalent to US$1 which itself has been in circulation since 3 Nov. 1942, but there is a Liberian coinage in silver and copper. Official accounts are kept in dollars and cents. The Liberian coins are as follows: Silver,$5, $1, 50-, 25-, 10- and 5-cent pieces; alloy, 2-cent and copper 1-cent pieces. The Government has not yet issued paper money. In March 1991, £1 = 1·90 Liberian $; US$1 = 1 Liberian $.

Banking and Finance. The First National City Bank (Liberia) was founded in 1935. An Italian bank, Tradevco, started business in 1955. The International Trust Co. of Liberia opened a commercial banking department at the end of 1960. The Liberian Bank of Development and Investment (LBDI) was founded in 1964 and began operations in 1965. The National Bank of Liberia opened on 22 July 1974, to act as a central bank. The National Housing and Savings Bank opened on 20 Jan. 1972. The Liberian Finance & Trust Corporation was incorporated Oct. 1976 and began operations in May 1977. The Liberian Agricultural and Co-operative Development Bank started operations in 1978. The Bank of Credit & Commerce International opened in Sept. 1978 and Meridien Bank of Liberia in July 1985.

Weights and Measures. Weights and measures are the same as in UK and USA.

ENERGY AND NATURAL RESOURCES

Electricity. Production (1986) was 655m. kwh. Supply 120 volts; 60 Hz.

Minerals. Iron ore production was 8·9m. tonnes in 1985. Gold production (1986) 21,125 oz valued at US$7·3m. and diamond production (1985) 66,000 carats.

Agriculture. Over 65% of the labour force is engaged in agriculture. The soil is productive, but due to excessive rainfall (from 160 to 180 in. per year), there are large swamp areas. Rice, cassava, coffee, citrus and sugar-cane are cultivated. The Government is negotiating the financing of large-scale investment in rice production aimed at making the country self-sufficient in rice production. Coffee, cocoa and palm-kernels are produced mainly by the traditional agricultural sector.

The Liberia Produce Marketing Corporation (LPMC) operates an oil-mill in Monrovia, processing most of the palm-kernels. There were 2 large commercial oil-palm plantations in the country. The Liberia Industrial Co-operative (LBINC) has 6,000 acres of oil-palm (of which 5,000 acres are in production) in Grand Bassa County, and West Africa Agricultural Co. (WAAC) has 4,020 acres in production in Grand Cape Mount County.

Production (1988, in 1,000 tonnes): Rice, 279; cassava, 310; coffee, 5; oranges, 7; sugar-cane, 225; cocoa, 5; palm-kernels, 8.

Livestock (1988): Cattle, 42,000; pigs, 140,000; sheep, 240,000; poultry, 4m.

Forestry. The Firestone Plantation Co. have large rubber plantations, employing over 40,000 men. Their concession comprises about 1m. acres and expires in the year 2025. About 100,000 acres have been planted. Independent producers have a further 65,000 acres planted.

Production in 1986 was 4·75m. cu. metres.

Fisheries. Catch (1986) 16,100 tonnes.

INDUSTRY. There are a number of small factories (brick and tile, soap, nails, mattresses, shoes, plastics, paint, oxygen, acetylene, tyre retreading, a brewery, soft drinks, cement, matches, candy and biscuits).

FOREIGN ECONOMIC RELATIONS

Commerce. Imports in 1986 totalled US$259,037,900 (1985, US$284,377,000) and exports US$408,374,099 (1985, US$435,570,000). Liberia's main trading partners are the USA and the Federal Republic of Germany.

In 1987, iron ore accounted for about 70% of total export earnings, rubber 15% and sawn timber over 5%. Other exports were coffee, cocoa, palm-kernel oil, diamonds and gold.

Total trade between Liberia and UK (British Department of Trade returns, in £1,000 sterling):

	1986	*1987*	*1988*	*1989*	*1990*
Imports to UK	7,574	7,284	9,574	12,776	13,240
Exports and re-exports from UK	22,056	13,538	11,684	15,148	8,639

The figures for exports from the UK include the value of shipping transferred to the Liberian flag; the genuine exports are considerably lower.

COMMUNICATIONS

Roads. In 1981, there were 4,794 miles of public roads (1,165 primary, 366 paved, 799 all-weather, 3,629 secondary and feeder) and 1,474 miles of private roads (93 paved, 1,381 laterite and earth). The principal highway connects Monrovia with the road system of Guinea, with branches leading into the Eastern and Western areas of Liberia. The latter branch reaches the Sierra Leone border and joins the Sierra Leone road system. A bridge over the St Paul River carries road traffic to the iron-ore mines at Bomi Hills.

Railway. A railway (for freight only) was built in 1951, connecting Monrovia with the Bomi Hills iron-ore mines about 69 km distant; this has been extended to the

National Iron Ore Co. area by 79 km. There is a line from Bong to Monrovia (78 km).

Aviation. The airport for Liberia is Roberts International Airport (30 miles from Monrovia). The James Spriggs Payne Airfield, 5 miles from Monrovia, can be used by light aircraft and mini jumbo jets. Air services are maintained by Ghana Airways, Swissair, British Caledonian, Air Guinea, SABENA, Iberia Airlines, Romanian Airlines and Air Liberia.

Shipping. Over 2,000 vessels enter Monrovia each year. The Liberian Government requires only a modest registration fee and an almost nominal annual charge and maintains no control over the operation of ships flying the Liberian flag. In 1990, 1,370 ships were registered totalling 88·3m. DWT, of which some 56m. DWT represented oil tankers.

Telecommunications. There is cable communication with Europe and America via Dakar, and a wireless station is maintained by the Government at Monrovia. There is a telephone service (8,510 telephones, 1983), in Monrovia, which is gradually being extended over the whole country. There were (1988) 570,000 radio and 43,000 television receivers.

JUSTICE, RELIGION, EDUCATION AND WELFARE

Justice. Justice is administered by a Supreme Court of 5 judges, 14 circuit courts and lower courts.

Religion. The main denominations represented in Liberia are Methodist, Baptist, Episcopalian, African Methodist, Pentecostal, Seventh-day Adventist, Lutheran and Roman Catholic, working through missionaries and mission schools. There were (1985) about 670,000 Moslems.

Education. Schools are classified as: (1) Public schools, maintained and run by the Government; (2) Mission schools, supported by foreign Missions and subsidized by the Government, and operated by qualified Missionaries and Liberian teachers; (3) Private schools, maintained by endowments and sometimes subsidized by the Government.

In 1986 there were estimated to be 1,830 schools with 8,744 teachers and 443,786 pupils.

Health. There were 236 doctors in 1981 and about 3,000 hospital beds.

DIPLOMATIC REPRESENTATIVES

Of Liberia in Great Britain (2 Pembridge Pl., London, W2)
Chargé d'affaires ad interim: Stephen Seaman.

Of Great Britain in Liberia (PO Box 10-0120, 1000, Monrovia)
Ambassador and Consul-General: M. E. J. Gore.

Of Liberia in the USA (5201 16th St., NW, Washington, D.C., 20011)
Ambassador: Eugenia Wordsworth-Stevenson.

Of the USA in Liberia (United Nations Drive, Monrovia)
Ambassador: Peter J. de Vos.

Of Liberia to the United Nations
Ambassador: William Bull.

Further Reading

Economic Survey of Liberia, 1981. Ministry of Planning and Economic Affairs
Dunn, D. E., *The Foreign Policy of Liberia during the Tubman Era, 1944–71.* London, 1979
Fraenkel, M., *Tribe and Class in Monrovia.* OUP, 1964
Wilson, C. M., *Liberia: Black Africa in Microcosm.* New York, 1971

LIBYA

Capital: Tripoli
Population: 4m. (1990)
GNP per capita: US$5,410 (1988)

Al-Jamahiriya Al-Arabiya Al-Libiya Al-Shabiya Al-Ishtirakiya Al-Uzma

(Great Socialist People's Libyan Arab Republic)

HISTORY. Tripoli fell under Turkish domination in the 16th century, and though in 1711 the Arab population secured some measure of independence, the country was in 1835 proclaimed a Turkish vilayet. In Sept. 1911 Italy occupied Tripoli and on 17 Oct. 1912, by the Treaty of Ouchy, Turkey recognized the sovereignty of Italy in Tripoli.

After the expulsion of the Germans and Italians in 1942 and 1943, Tripolitania and Cyrenaica were placed under British, and the Fezzan under French, military administration. Britain recognized the Amir Mohammed Idris Al-Senussi as Amir of Cyrenaica in June 1949.

Libya became an independent, sovereign, federal kingdom under the Amir of Cyrenaica, Mohammed Idris Al-Senussi, as King of the United Kingdom of Libya, on 24 Dec. 1951, when the British Residents in Tripolitania and Cyrenaica and the French Resident in the Fezzan transferred their remaining powers to the federal government of Libya, in pursuance of decisions passed by the United Nations in 1949 and 1950.

On 1 Sept. 1969 King Idris was deposed by a group of army officers. Twelve of the group of officers formed the Revolutionary Command Council chaired by Col. Muammar Qadhafi and proclaimed a republic.

AREA AND POPULATION. Libya is bounded north by the Mediterranean Sea, east by Egypt and Sudan, south by Chad and Niger and west by Algeria and Tunisia. The area is estimated at 1,759,540 sq. km (679,358 sq. miles). The population, at the census on 31 July 1984, was 3,637,488; estimate (1990), 4m.

In 1985, 65% of the population was urban. The chief cities (1981) were: Tripoli, the capital (858,000), Benghazi (368,000) and Misurata (117,000).

The populations (1984) of the municipalities were as follows:

Ajdabiya	100,547	Jabal al-Akhdar	120,662	Shati	46,749
Awbari	48,701	Khums	149,642	Surt	110,996
Aziziyah	85,068	Kufrah	25,139	Tarhunah	84,640
Benghazi	485,386	Marzuq	42,294	Tobruk	94,006
Derna	105,031	Misurata	178,295	Tripoli	990,697
Fatah	102,763	Niqat al-Khums	181,584	Yafran	73,420
Ghadames	52,247	Sabha	76,171	Zawia	220,075
Gharyan	117,073	Sawfajjin	45,195	Zlitan	101,107

CLIMATE. The coastal region has a warm temperate climate, with mild wet winters and hot dry summers, though most of the country suffers from aridity. Tripoli. Jan. 52°F (11·1°C), July 81°F (27·2°C). Annual rainfall 16" (400 mm). Benghazi. Jan. 56°F (13·3°C), July 77°F (25°C). Annual rainfall 11" (267 mm).

CONSTITUTION AND GOVERNMENT. In March 1977 a new form of direct democracy, the 'Jamahiriya' (state of the masses) was promulgated and the official name of the country was changed to Socialist Peoples Libyan Arab Jamahiriya. Under this system, every adult is supposed tobe able to share in policy making through the Basic People's Congresses of which there are some 2,000 throughout Libya. These Congresses appoint Popular Committees to execute policy. Provincial and urban affairs are handled by Popular Committees responsible to Municipality People's Congresses, of which there are 13. Officials of these Congresses and Committees form at national level the General People's Congress which now normally meets for about a week early each year (usually in March). This is the highest policy-making body in the country. The General People's Congress appoints its own General Secretariat and the General People's Committee, whose members (the equivalents of ministers under other forms of government) head the 10 government departments which execute policy at national level.

Until 1977 Libya was ruled by a Revolutionary Command Council headed by Col. Muammar Qadhafi. Upon its abolition in that year the 5 surviving members of the RCC became the General Secretariat of the General People's Congress, still under Qadhafi's direction. In 1979 they stood down to be replaced by elected officials. Since then, Col. Qadhafi has retained his position as Leader of the Revolution. But neither he nor his former RCC colleagues have any formal posts in the present administration, although they continue to wield considerable authority.

A new government of 12 members was appointed in Oct. 1990 which included:

Secretary of the General People's Congress (Prime Minister): Abu Zaid Omar Burda.

Foreign Affairs: Ibrahim Mohammed Bishari. *Planing and Economy:* Omar Mustapha Al-Muntasir. *Vocational Training:* Maatooq Mohammed. *Information and Culture:* Ali Milad Abu Jaziyah.

The *Speaker* of the Congress is Abd Al-Raziq Sawsa.

National flag: Plain green.

Arabic is the official language

DEFENCE. There is selective conscription for 2-4 years. Enrolment in the reserves, numbering about 40,000, continues until age 49. On 31 Aug. 1989 it was announced that the traditional armed forces were abolished and in future would be known as the 'Armed People'.

Army. The Army is organized into 1 tank and 2 mechanized infantry divisions in addition to 38 tank battalions, 54 mechanized infantry, 1 National Guard, 41 artillery, 2 anti-aircraft and 12 parachute commando battalions, 7 surface-to-surface and 3 surface-to-air brigades. Equipment includes 2,000 T-54/-55/-62 and 300 T-72 main battle tanks. The Army has an aviation component; with 13 transport and 16 liaison helicopters. Strength (1991) 55,000. The paramilitary Pan-African Islamic Legion numbers approximately 2,500, the Revolutionary Guard, 3,000.

Navy. The fleet, a mixture of Soviet and West European-built ships, comprises 6 Soviet-built diesel submarines, 3 missile-armed frigates, 7 missile-armed corvettes, 23 fast missile craft and 23 inshore patrol craft. There are 2 tank landing ships and 3 medium landing ships as well as 2 landing craft. Auxiliaries include 1 logistic support ship, 1 salvage ship, 1 transport and a diving support ship.

1 Soviet-built missile corvette was sunk and 1 severely damaged by the US Navy in March 1986.

There is a small Naval Aviation wing operating 25 Haze and 12 Super-Frelon helicopters from shore bases.

Personnel in 1990 totalled 8,000, including coastguard. The forces are based at Tarabulus, Benghazi, Darnah, Tobruk, Sidi Bilal and Al Khums.

Air Force. The creation of an Air Force began in 1959. In 1974, delivery was completed of a total of 110 Mirage 5 combat aircraft and trainers, of which about 50 remain. They have been followed by 10 Tu-22 supersonic reconnaissance bombers, 70 MiG-25 interceptors and reconnaissance aircraft, 100 Su-22 ground attack fighters, 94 MiG-21s, and about 140 MiG-23 variable-geometry fighters and fighter-bombers from the USSR. In 1989 the first of 15 Su-2YD supersonic bombers were delivered. Other equipment includes 40 Mirage F1 fighters from France, 6 Mirage F1-B two-seat trainers, 20 Mi-24 gunship helicopters, Mi-14 anti-submarine helicopters, 10 C-130/L-100 Hercules and 20 Aeritalia G222T transports, 8 Super Frelon and 6 Agusta-built CH-47C Chinook heavy-lift helicopters, and a total of 16 Bell 212, Bell 47, Alouette III and Mi-8 helicopters. Training is performed on piston-engined SF.260Ms (some of which are armed for light attack duties) from Italy; L-39 Albatros, Galeb and Magister jet aircraft; and twin-engined L-410s built in Czechoslovakia. Personnel total (1991) about 22,000, with many of the combat aircraft operated by foreign aircrew, with 513 combatant aircraft and 35 armed helicopters.

INTERNATIONAL RELATIONS

Membership. Libya is a member of UN, OAU, OIC, OPEC, Arab Maghreb Union and the Arab League.

ECONOMY

Policy. Declining oil revenues (60% down on 1980 levels) has meant postponing most projects envisaged in the 5-year development plan (1981–85) though the Great-Man-Made River Project has not been affected.

Budget. A budget of LD3,240m. was announced for 1991.

Currency. The unit of currency is the *Libyan dinar* (LYD) of 1,000 *millemes*. Rate of exchange, March 1991: LD 0·5169 = £1; LD 0·2724 = US$1.

Banking and Finance. A National Bank of Libya was established in 1955; it was renamed the Central Bank of Libya in 1972. The *Governor* is Said Al-Zilitny. All foreign banks were nationalized by Dec. 1970. In 1972 the government set up the Libyan Arab Foreign Bank whose function is overseas investment and to participate in multinational banking corporations. The National Agricultural Bank, which has been set up to give loans and subsidies to farmers to develop their land and to assist them in marketing their crops, has offices in Tripoli, Benghazi, Sebha and other agricultural centres.

Weights and Measures. Although the metric system has been officially adopted and is obligatory for all contracts, the following weights and measures are still used: *oke* = 1·282 kg; *kantar* = 51·28 kg; *draa* = 46 cm; *handaza* = 68 cm.

ENERGY AND NATURAL RESOURCES

Electricity. Electricity capacity (1985) 5,615 mw. Production (1986) 2,126m. kwh. Supply 110, 115 and 220 volts; 50 Hz.

Oil. Production (1989) 53m. tonnes. Reserves (1988) 23,000m. bbls. The Libyan National Oil Corporation (NOC) was established in March 1970 to be the state's organization for the exploitation of Libya's oil resources. NOC does not participate in the production of oil but has a majority share in all the operating companies with the exception of two small producers Aquitaine-Libya and Wintershall Libya.

The largest producers are Waha (formerly Oasis, until the withdrawal of US oil companies at the end of June 1986) and AGECO who together produce more than 50% of total production. The other significant producers are Zuweitina (formerly Occidental Libya), AGIP, Sirte Oil Company, and Veba (also known as Mobil Oil Libya, although Mobil Inc. withdrew in July 1982 after EXXON's withdrawal from the Sirte Oil Company in Oct. 1981).

Gas. Reserves (1988) 620,000m. cu. metres. Production (1982) 29,000m. cu. metres. In 1983 a gas pipeline was under construction which will take gas from Brega, along the coast to Misurata. In 1987 agreement was reached with Algeria and Tunisia to construct a gas pipeline to supply western Libya with Algerian gas.

Water. Since 1984 a major project has been under way to bring water from wells in southern Libya to the coast. This scheme, called the 'Great Man-made River', is planned, on completion, to irrigate some 185,000 acres of land with water brought along some 4,000 km of pipes. It is planned that Phase I project will be operational in 1990 at a cost of US$3,300m; Phase II of the project (covering the west of Libya) was announced in Sept. 1989. This contract is valued at US$5,300m. and is expected to last 74 months.

Minerals. Cement production (1987) 2·7m. tonnes. Gypsum output (1982) 172,400 tonnes. Iron ore deposits have been found in the south and uranium has reportedly been found in the region of Ghat in the south-west.

Agriculture. Tripolitania has 3 zones from the coast inland—the Mediterranean, the sub-desert and the desert. The first, which covers an area of about 17,231 sq. miles, is the only one properly suited for agriculture, and may be further subdivided into: (1) the oases along the coast, the richest in North Africa, in which thrive the date palm, the olive, the orange, the peanut and the potato; (2) the steppe district, suitable for cereals (barley and wheat) and pasture; it has olive, almond, vine, orange and mulberry trees and ricinus plants; (3) the dunes, which are being gradually afforested with acacia, robinia, poplar and pine; (4) the Jebel (the mountain district, Tarhuna, Garian, Nalut-Yefren), in which thrive the olive, the fig, the vine and other fruit trees, and which on the east slopes down to the sea with the fertile hills of Msellata. Of some 25m. acres of productive land in Tripolitania, nearly 20m. are used for grazing and about 1m. for static farming. The sub-desert zone produces the alfa plant. The desert zone and the Fezzan contain some fertile oases, such as those of Ghadames, Ghat, Socna, Sebha, Brak.

Cyrenaica has about 10m. acres of potentially productive land, most of which, however, is suitable only for grazing. Certain areas, chief of which is the plateau known as the Barce Plain (about 1,000 ft above sea-level), are suitable for dry farming; in addition, grapes, olives and dates are grown. With improved irrigation, production, particularly of vegetables, could be increased, but stock raising and dry farming will remain of primary importance. About 143,000 acres are used for settled farming; about 272,000 acres are covered by natural forests. The Agricultural Development Authority plans to reclaim 6,000 ha each year for agriculture. In the Fezzan there are about 6,700 acres of irrigated gardens and about 297,000 acres are planted with date palms.

Production (1988, in tonnes): Wheat, 193,000; barley, 99,000; milk, 143,000; meat, 154,000. Olive trees number about 3·4m. and productive date-palm trees about 3m.

Livestock (1988): 5·7m. sheep, 965,000 goats, 215,000 cattle, 37m. poultry.

Fisheries. The catch in 1986 was 7,800 tonnes.

INDUSTRY. Since the revolution there has been an ambitious programme of industrial development aimed at the local manufacture of building materials (steel and aluminium pipes and fittings, electric cables, cement, bricks, glass, etc.), foodstuffs (dairy products, flour, tinned fruits and vegetables, dates, fish processing and canning, etc.), textiles and footwear (ready-made clothing, woollen and cotton cloth, blankets, leather footwear, etc.) and development of mineral deposits (iron ore, phosphates, mineral salts). Many projects have been delayed or reduced in recent years, owing to fall in oil revenues since 1980. Small scale private sector industrialization in the form of partnerships is permitted. From 21 Sept. 1969 all businesses, except oil and banks, were Libyan-owned; subsequently all banks and most oil companies were nationalized.

FOREIGN ECONOMIC RELATIONS. In Feb. 1989 Libya signed a treaty of economic co-operation with the 4 other Maghreb countries, Algeria, Mauritania, Morocco and Tunisia.

Commerce. Total imports in 1987 were valued at US$4,969 (f.o.b.) and exports at US$6,612 (f.o.b.), virtually all crude oil. In 1987, 25% of imports came from Italy, while 33% of exports were to Italy, 16% to the Federal Republic of Germany and 11% to Spain.

Total trade between Libya and UK (British Department of Trade returns, in £1,000 sterling):

	1986	*1987*	*1988*	*1989*	*1990*
Imports to UK	136,390	133,649	111,812	104,546	151,605
Exports and re-exports from UK	260,529	220,626	235,957	239,191	244,850

COMMUNICATIONS

Roads. In 1986 there were 25,675 km of roads. In 1982 there were 415,509 passenger cars and 334,405 commercial vehicles.

Railways. In 1990 there were no operating railways.

Aviation. A national airline, the Libyan Arab Airlines (LAA), was inaugurated on 30 Sept. 1965. Benghazi and Tripoli are linked by LAA and other international airlines to Athens, Rome, Madrid, Malta, Moscow, Frankfurt, Paris, Amsterdam, Vienna and Zurich. In 1990 the 5 Maghreb countries announced they would merge their airlines in an Air Maghreb.

Telecommunications. Tripoli is connected by telegraph cable with Malta and by microwave link with Bengardane (Tunis). There are overseas wireless-telegraph stations at Benghazi and Tripoli, and radio-telephone services connect Libya with most countries of western Europe. In 1982 some 102,000 telephones were in use and in 1983 there were 165,000 radio sets and 170,000 television receivers.

Newspapers. There was (1990) 1 daily in Tripoli with a circulation of about 40,000 and a number of weeklies.

JUSTICE, RELIGION, EDUCATION AND WELFARE

Justice. The Civil, Commercial and Criminal codes are based mainly on the Egyptian model. Matters of personal status of family or succession matters affecting Moslems are dealt with in special courts according to the Moslem law. All other matters, civil, commercial and criminal, are tried in the ordinary courts, which have jurisdiction over everyone.

There are civil and penal courts in Tripoli and Benghazi, with subsidiary courts at Misurata and Derna; courts of assize in Tripoli and Benghazi, and courts of appeal in Tripoli and Benghazi.

Religion. Islam is declared the State religion, but the right of others to practise their religions is provided for. In 1990, 97% were Sunni Moslems.

Education. There were (1981–82) 718,124 pupils in primary schools, 286,414 in preparatory and secondary schools, 44,789 pupils in technical schools and 25,700 students in higher education. There are 3 universities of Al Fatah (in Tripoli), Garyounes (in Benghazi) and Sabha.

Health. In 1981 there were 74 hospitals with 15,375 beds, 4,690 physicians, 314 dentists, 420 pharmacists, 1,080 midwives and 5,346 nursing personnel.

DIPLOMATIC REPRESENTATIVES

UK broke off diplomatic relations with Libya on 22 April 1984. Saudi Arabia looks after Libyan interests in UK and Italy looks after UK's interests in Libya.

USA suspended all embassy activities in Tripoli on 2 May 1980.

Of Libya to the United Nations
Ambassador: Dr Ali Treiki.

Further Reading

Allen, J. A., *Libya: The Experience of Oil*. London and Boulder, 1981.—*Libya since Independence*. London, 1982
Bearman, J., *Qadhafi's Libya*. London, 1986
Blundy, D. and Lycett, A., *Qadhafi and the Libyan Revolution*. London, 1987
Cooley, J. K., *Libyan Sandstorm: The Complete Account of Qaddafi's Revolution*. London and New York, 1983
Davis, J., *Libyan Politics: Tribe and Revolution*. London, 1988
Fergiani, M. B., *The Libyan Jamahiriya*. London, 1984
Hahn, L., *Historical Dictionary of Libya*. London, 1961
Harris, L. C., *Libya: Qadhafi's Revolution and the Modern State*. Boulder and London, 1986
Lawless, R. I., *Libya*. [Bibliography] Oxford and Santa Barbara, 1987
St John, R. B., *Qaddafi's World Design: Libyan Foreign Policy, 1969-1987*. London, 1987
Waddhams, F. C., *The Libyan Oil Industry*. London, 1980
Wright, J., *Libya: A Modern History*. London, 1982.— *Libya, Chad and the Central Sahara*. London, 1969

LIECHTENSTEIN

Capital: Vaduz
Population: 28,181 (1988)

Fürstentum Liechtenstein

(Principality of Liechtenstein)

HISTORY. The Principality of Liechtenstein, situated between the Austrian province of Vorarlberg and the Swiss cantons of St Gallen and Graubünden, is a sovereign state whose history dates back to 3 May 1342, when Count Hartmann III became ruler of the county of Vaduz. Additions were later made to the count's domains, and by 1434 the territory reached its present boundaries. It consists of the two former counties of Schellenberg and Vaduz (until 1806 immediate fiefs of the Roman Empire). The former in 1699 and the latter in 1712 came into the possession of the house of Liechtenstein and, by diploma of 23 Jan. 1719, granted by the Emperor Charles VI, the two counties were constituted as the Principality of Liechtenstein.

AREA AND POPULATION. Liechtenstein is bounded on the east by Austria and the west by Switzerland. Area, 160 sq. km (61·8 sq. miles); population, of Alemannic race (census 1980), 25,215; estimate, 1988, 28,181. In 1988 there were 416 births and 195 deaths. Population of Vaduz (census 1980), 4,606; estimate, 1988, 4,919. The language is German.

REIGNING PRINCE. Hans-Adam II, born 14 Feb. 1945; succeeded his father Prince Francis-Joseph, 13 Nov. 1989 (he exercised the prerogatives to which the Sovereign is entitled from 26 Aug. 1984); married on 30 July 1967 to Countess Marie Kinsky; there are 3 sons, Hereditary Prince Alois (born 11 June 1968), Prince Maximilian (born 16 May 1969) and Prince Constantin (born 15 March 1972), and one daughter, Princess Tatjana (born 10 April 1973). The monarchy is hereditary in the male line.

CONSTITUTION AND GOVERNMENT. Liechtenstein is a constitutional monarchy ruled by the princes of the House of Liechtenstein. The present constitution of 5 Oct. 1921 provided for a unicameral parliament (Diet) of 15 members elected for 4 years, but this was amended to 25 members in 1988. Election is on the basis of proportional representation. The prince can call and dismiss the parliament. On parliamentary recommendation, he appoints the prime minister and the 4 councillors for a 4-year term. Any group of 1,000 persons or any 3 communes may propose legislation (initiative). Bills passed by the parliament may be submitted to popular referendum. A law is valid when it receives a majority approval by the parliament and the prince's signed concurrence. The capital and seat of government is Vaduz and there are 10 more communes all connected by modern roads. The 11 communes are fully independent administrative bodies within the laws of the principality. They levy additional taxes to the state taxes. Since Feb. 1921 Liechtenstein has had the Swiss currency, and since 29 March 1923 has been united with Switzerland in a customs union.

At the elections for the Diet, on 5 March 1989, the Fatherland Union obtained 13 seats, the opposition Progressive Citizens' Party, 12 seats.

Head of Government: Hans Brunhart.

National flag: Horizontally blue over red, with a gold coronet in the first quarter.

National anthem: Oben am jungen Rhein (words by H. H. Jauch, 1850; tune, 'God save the Queen').

INTERNATIONAL RELATIONS

Membership. Liechtenstein is a member of the UN, EFTA, the Council of Europe and the International Court of Justice.

ECONOMY

Budget. Budget estimates for 1989: Revenue, 377,530,000 Swiss francs; expenditure, 371,193,000 Swiss francs. There is no public debt.

Currency. The Swiss *franc*.

Banking. There were (1989) 3 banks: Liechtensteinische Landesbank, Bank in Liechtenstein Ltd, Verwaltungs-und Privatbank Ltd.

Weights and Measures. The metric system is in force.

ENERGY AND NATURAL RESOURCES

Electricity. Electricity produced in 1988 was 60,082,000 kwh.

Agriculture. The rearing of cattle, for which the fine alpine pastures are well suited, is highly developed. In March 1989 there were 6,175 cattle (including 2,847 milk cows), 211 horses, 2,470 sheep, 176 goats, 2,698 pigs. Total production of dairy produce, 1988, 12,968,400 kg.

INDUSTRY. The country has a great variety of light industries (textiles, ceramics, steel screws, precision instruments, canned food, pharmaceutical products, heating appliances, etc.).

Since 1945 Liechtenstein has changed from a predominantly agricultural country to a highly industrialized country. The farming population has gone down from 70% in 1930 to only 2% in 1988. The rapid change-over has led to the immigration of foreign workers (Austrians, Germans, Italians, Spaniards). Industrial undertakings affiliated to the Liechtenstein Chamber of Industry and Commerce in 1988 employed 6,929 workers earning 356m. Swiss francs.

FOREIGN ECONOMIC RELATIONS.

Commerce. Exports of home produce, for firms in membership of the Chamber of Commerce, in 1988 amounted to 1,876m. Swiss francs. 22·3% went to EFTA countries, of which Switzerland took 304m. (16·2%) and 39·6% went to EEC countries.

Total trade with UK is included with Switzerland from 1968.

Tourism. In 1988, 71,633 overnight visitors arrived in Liechtenstein.

COMMUNICATIONS

Roads. There are 250 km of roads. Postal buses are the chief means of public transportation within the country and to Austria and Switzerland.

Railways. The 18·5 km of main railway passing through the country is operated by Austrian Federal Railways.

Telecommunications. In 1988 there were 14,612 telephones, 424 telex, 9,780 radios and 9,155 TV sets. Post and telegraphs are administered by Switzerland.

Cinemas. There were 2 cinemas in 1988.

Newspapers. In 1989 there were 2 daily newspapers with a total circulation of 16,350.

JUSTICE, RELIGION, EDUCATION AND WELFARE

Justice. The principality has its own civil and penal codes. The lowest court is the county court, *Landgericht*, presided over by one judge, which decides minor civil cases and summary criminal offences. The criminal court, *Kriminalgericht*, with a bench of 5 judges is for major crimes. Another court of mixed jurisdiction is the court of assizes (with 3 judges) for misdemeanours. Juvenile cases are treated in the Juvenile Court (with a bench of 3 judges). The superior court, *Obergericht*, and Supreme Court, *Oberster Gerichtshof*, are courts of appeal for civil and criminal cases (both with benches of 5 judges). An administrative court of appeal from government actions and the State Court determines the constitutionality of laws.

The death penalty was abolished in 1989.

Police. The principality has no army. Police force, 45; auxiliary police, 23 (1989).

Religion. In 1988, 87·3% of the population was Roman Catholic and 8·2% was Protestant.

Education (1989–90). In 14 primary, 3 upper, 5 secondary, 1 grammar and 2 (for backward children) schools there were 3,587 pupils and 264 teachers. There is also an evening technical school, a music school and a children's pedagogic-welfare day school.

Health. In 1989 there was 1 hospital, but Liechtenstein has an agreement with the Swiss cantons of St Gallen and Graubünden and the Austrian Federal State of Vorarlberg that her citizens may use certain hospitals.

DIPLOMATIC REPRESENTATIVES

In 1919, Switzerland agreed to represent the interests of Liechtenstein in countries where it has diplomatic missions and where Liechtenstein is not represented in its own right. In so doing Switzerland always acts only on the basis of mandates of a general or specific nature, which it may either accept or refuse, while Liechtenstein is free to enter into direct relations with foreign states or to set up its own additional diplomatic missions.

British Consul-General: T. Bryant, CMG. (resident in Zürich).
USA Consul-General: Ruth N. van Heuven (resident in Zürich).

Of Liechtenstein to the United Nations
Ambassador: Claudia Fritsche

Further Reading

Statistical Information: Amt für Volkswirtschaft, Vaduz.

Rechenschaftsbericht der Fürstlichen Regierung. Vaduz. Annual, from 1922
Jahrbuch des Historischen Vereins. Vaduz. Annual since 1901
Batliner, E. H., *Das Geld- und Kreditwesen des Fürstentums Liechtenstein in Vergangenheit und Gegenwart*. 1959
Green, B., *Valley of Peace*. Vaduz, 1967
Larke, T. A. T., *Index and Thesaurus of Liechtenstein*. 2nd ed. Berkeley, 1984
Malin, G., *Kunstführer Fürstentum Liechtenstein*. Berne, 1977
Raton, P., *Liechtenstein: History and Institutions of the Principality*. Vaduz, 1970
Seger, O., *A Survey of Liechtenstein History*. 4th English ed. Vaduz, 1984
Steger, G., *Fürst und Landtag nach Liechtensteinischem Recht*. Vaduz, 1950

LUXEMBOURG

Capital: Luxembourg
Population: 378,400 (1990)
GNP per capita: US$22,856 (1989)

Grand-Duché de Luxembourg

HISTORY. The country formed part of the Holy Roman Empire until it was conquered by the French in 1795. In 1815 the Grand Duchy of Luxembourg was formed under the house of Orange-Nassau, also sovereigns of the Netherlands. In 1839 the Walloon-speaking area was joined to Belgium. In 1890 the personal union with the Netherlands ended with the accession of a member of another branch of the house of Nassau, Grand Duke Adolphe of Nassau-Weilburg.

AREA AND POPULATION. Luxembourg has an area of 2,586 sq. km (999 sq. miles) and is bounded on the west by Belgium, south by France, east by the Federal Republic of Germany. The population (1990) was 378,400. The capital, Luxembourg, had (1990) 74,400 inhabitants; Esch-Alzette, the centre of the mining district, 23,890; Differdange, 16,050; Dudelange, 14,230, and Petange, 11,900. In 1990 the foreign population was about 104,000.

Vital statistics (1989): 4,665 births, 3,984 deaths, 2,184 marriages.

The official languages are French and German. The national language is Letzebuergesch, spoken by the entire population.

CLIMATE. Cold, raw winters with snow covering the ground for up to a month are features of the upland areas. The remainder resembles Belgium in its climate, with rain evenly distributed throughout the year. Jan. 33·3°F (0·7°C), July 63·5°F (17·5°C). Annual rainfall 30·1" (764 mm).

REIGNING GRAND DUKE. Jean, born 5 Jan. 1921, son of the late Grand Duchess Charlotte and the late Prince Felix of Bourbon-Parma; succeeded 12 Nov. 1964 on the abdication of his mother; married to Princess Joséphine-Charlotte of Belgium, 9 April 1953. *Offspring:* Princess Marie-Astrid, born 17 Feb. 1954, married Christian of Habsbourg-Lorraine 6 Feb. 1982 (*Offspring:* Marie Christine, born 31 July 1983; Imre, born 8 Dec. 1985); Prince Henri, *heir apparent*, born 16 April 1955, married Maria Teresa Mestre 14 Feb. 1981; (*Offspring:* Prince Guillaume, born 11 Nov. 1981, Prince Felix, born 3 June 1984, Prince Louis, born 3 Aug. 1986). Prince Jean, born 15 May 1957, married Hélène Vestur; Princess Margaretha, born 15 May 1957, married Prince Nikolaus of Liechtenstein 20 March 1982; Prince Guillaume, born 1 May 1963.

The civil list is fixed at 300,000 gold francs per annum, to be reconsidered at the beginning of each reign.

On 28 Sept. 1919 a referendum was taken in Luxembourg to decide on the political and economic future of the country. The voting resulted as follows: For the reigning Grand Duchess, 66,811; for the continuance of the Nassau-Braganza dynasty under another Grand Duchess, 1,286; for another dynasty, 889; for a republic, 16,885; for an economic union with France, 60,133; for an economic union with Belgium, 22,242. But France refused in favour of Belgium, and on 22 Dec. 1921 the Chamber of the Grand Duchy passed a Bill for the economic union between Belgium and Luxembourg. The agreement, which is for 60 years, provides for the disappearance of the customs barrier between the two countries and the use of Belgian, in addition to Luxembourg, currency as legal tender in the Grand Duchy. It came into force on 1 May 1922.

The Grand Duchy was under German occupation from 10 May 1940 to 10 Sept. 1944. The Grand Duchess Charlotte and the Government carried on an independent administration in London. Civil government was restored in Oct. 1944.

National flag: Three horizontal stripes of red, white and light blue.

National anthem: Ons Hemecht ('Our Homeland'; words by M. Lentz, 1859; tune by J. A. Zinnen).

CONSTITUTION AND GOVERNMENT. The Grand Duchy of Luxembourg is a constitutional monarchy, the hereditary sovereignty being in the Nassau family. The constitution of 17 Oct. 1868 was revised in 1919, 1948, 1956, 1972, 1979, 1983, 1988 and 1989. The revision of 1948 has abolished the 'perpetually neutral' status of the country and introduced the concepts of right to work, social security, health services, freedom of trade and industry, and recognition of trade unions. The revision of 1956 provides for the devolution of executive, legislative and judicial powers to international institutions.

The country forms 4 electoral districts. An elector must be a citizen (male or female) of Luxembourg and have completed 18 years of age; to be eligible for election the citizen must have completed 21 years of age.

The Chamber of Deputies consists of 22 Christian Social, 18 Socialists, 11 Democrats, 1 Communist, 2 Green Alternatives, 2 Green Ecologists and 4 5/6 Action Committee (elections of 18 June 1989). A maximum of 60 members are elected for 5 years; they receive a salary and a travelling allowance.

The head of the state takes part in the legislative power, exercises the executive power and has a certain part in the judicial power. The constitution leaves to the sovereign the right to organize the Government, which consists of a Minister of State, who is President of the Government, and of at least 3 Ministers.

The Cabinet was, in Dec. 1989, composed as follows:

Prime Minister, Minister of State, Minister for Exchequer, Cultural Affairs: Jacques Santer.

Vice-Prime Minister, Foreign Affairs, Foreign Trade and Cooperation, Armed Forces: Jacques F. Poos. *Family Affairs and Social Solidarity, Middle Classes and Tourism:* Fernand Boden. *Interior, Housing and Town Planning:* Jean Spautz. *Finance, Labour:* Jean-Claude Juncker. *National Education, Justice, Civil Service:* Marc Fischbach. *Health, Social Security, Physical Education and Sports, Youth:* Johny Lahure. *Agriculture, Viticulture and Country Planning:* René Steichen. *Economy, Public Works, Transport:* Robert Goebbels. *Land Planning and Environment, Energy, Communications:* Alex Bodry. *Secretary of State for Foreign Affairs, Foreign Trade and Co-operation, Armed Forces:* Georges Wohlfart. *Secretary of State for Health, Social Security, Physical Education and Sports, Youth:* Mady Delvaux-Stehres.

Besides the Cabinet there is a Council of State. It deliberates on proposed laws and Bills, and on amendments; it also gives administrative decisions and expresses its opinion regarding any other question referred to it by the Grand Duke or the Government. The Council of State is composed of 21 members chosen for life by the sovereign, who also chooses a president from among them each year.

DEFENCE. A law passed by Parliament on 29 June 1967 abolished compulsory service and instituted a battalion-size army of volunteers enlisted for 3 years. Strength (1991) 800. The defence estimates for 1989 amounted to 2,346m. francs. Luxembourg is an original member of NATO and the battalion is committed to NATO ACE mobile force.

INTERNATIONAL RELATIONS

Membership. Luxembourg is a member of the UN, Benelux, the European Communities, OECD, the Council of Europe, NATO and WEU.

The Schengen Accord of June 1990 abolished border controls between Luxembourg, Belgium, France, Germany and the Netherlands. Italy acceded in Nov. 1990.

ECONOMY

Budget. Revenue and expenditure (including extraordinary) for years ending 30 April (in 1m. francs):

	1985	*1986*	*1987*	*1988*	*1989*	*1990* [1]
Revenue	81,363·8	82,385·3	86,313·0	85,047·5	89,593·5	97,162·7
Expenditure	79,536·8	81,863·3	86,239·7	88,913·8	88,922·3	94,414·5

[1] Provisional.

Consolidated debt at 31 Dec. 1989 amounted to 11,088m. francs (long-term) and 3,437m. francs (short-term).

Currency. The unit of currency is the *Luxembourg franc* (LUF), fixed at par value with the Belgian franc on 14 Oct. 1944. Notes of the Belgian National Bank are legal tender in Luxembourg.

Banking and Finance. Luxembourg's equivalent of a central bank is its Monetary Institute (*Director-General*, Pierre Jaans). On 31 Dec. 1989 depositors in the State Savings Bank had a total of 54,949m. francs to their credit. In 1990 there were 180 banks and 24 non-bank credit institutions established in Luxembourg, which has become an international financial centre. There is a stock exchange.

Weights and Measures. The metric system is in force.

ENERGY AND NATURAL RESOURCES

Electricity. Power production was 1,380m. kwh. in 1989.

Minerals. In 1989 production (in tonnes) of pig-iron, 2,683,800; of steel, 3,720,920.

Agriculture. Agriculture is carried on by about 6,200 of the population on (1989) 3,945 farms with an average area of 37·18 ha; 126,514 ha were under cultivation in 1989. Production, 1989 (in tonnes) of main crops: Maize, 385,830; roots and tubers, 36,150; bread crops, 34,900; other crops, 87,340; forage crops, 69,350; pulses, 1,400; grassland, 137,630. Production, 1989 (in 1,000 tonnes) of meat, 21·9; milk, 279·8; butter, 5·9; cheese, 4·1. In 1989, 232,100 hectolitres of wine were produced from 1,288 ha. In 1989 there were 9,781 tractors, 1,428 harvester-threshers, 2,559 manure spreaders and 2,685 gatherer-presses.

Livestock (1989): 1,669 horses, 214,987 cattle, 76,553 pigs, 7,511 sheep.

Forestry. In 1987 there were 88,600 ha of forests, which produced 154,000 cu. metres of broadleaved and 159,050 cu. metres of coniferous wood.

INDUSTRY. Production, 1989 (in 1,000 tonnes); Steel, 3,721; rolled steel products, 4,113. At 1 Nov. 1989 there were 2,074 industrial enterprises.

FOREIGN ECONOMIC RELATIONS. By treaties of 5 Sept. 1944 and 14 March 1947 Luxembourg with Belgium and the Netherlands, became a party to the Benelux Customs Union, which came into force on 1 Jan. 1948. For further particulars *see* p. 000.

Commerce. Trade between Luxembourg and the UK has been included with Belgium since 1974.

Tourism. In 1989 there were 792,322 tourists.

COMMUNICATIONS

Roads. In 1989 there were 5,091 km of roads of which 78 km were motorways. Motor vehicles registered on 1 Jan. 1990 included 183,404 passenger cars, 11,275 trucks, 734 buses, 3,334 motorcycles, 20,546 tractors and special vehicles.

Railways. In 1989 there were 272 km of railway (standard gauge) of which 162 km were electrified. It carried 704m. tonne-km and 280m. passenger-km.

Aviation. Findel is the airport for Luxembourg. 945,454 passengers and 126,933 tonnes of freight were handled in 1989.

Shipping. A shipping register was set up in 1990.

Telecommunications. In 1989 there were 167,363 telephones and 107 post and telegraph offices. *Compagnie Luxembourgeoise de Télédiffusion* broadcasts 1 programme in Letzebuergesch on FM. Powerful transmitters on long-, medium- and short-waves are used for commercial and religious programmes in French, Dutch, German, English and Italian. Ten TV programmes are broadcast. Colour transmission is by the SECAM system. 2 Astra satellites are based on Luxembourg City.

Cinemas (1990). There were 17 cinemas.

Newspapers (1990). There were 5 daily newspapers with a circulation of 130,000.

RELIGION, EDUCATION AND WELFARE

Religion. The population is 95% Roman Catholic. The remaining 5% is mainly Protestant or Jewish, or does not belong to any religion. The Protestant Church is organized on an interdenominational basis.

Education. Education is compulsory for all children between the ages of 6 and 15. In 1988-89 nursery schools had 7,867 pupils; primary schools, 25,725 pupils. In 1988-89 technical secondary schools had 14,367 pupils; secondary schools, 7,885 pupils. In higher eduction the Higher Institute of Technology, 251 students. 174 students were in teacher training, and 572 pursued university studies.

Health. In 1987 there were 666 doctors and 4,661 hospital beds.

DIPLOMATIC REPRESENTATIVES

Of Luxembourg in Great Britain (27 Wilton Crescent, London, SWIX 8SD)
Ambassador: Edouard Molitor, KCMG (accredited 13 June 1989).

Of Great Britain in Luxembourg (14 Blvd Roosevelt, Luxembourg)
Ambassador and Consul-General: Juliet J. d'A. Campbell, CMG.

Of Luxembourg in the USA (2200 Massachusetts Ave., NW, Washington, D.C., 20008)
Ambassador: André Philippe.

Of the USA in Luxembourg (22 Blvd. Emmanuel Servais, Luxembourg)
Ambassador: Edward Morgan Rowell.

Of Luxembourg to the United Nations
Ambassador: Jean Feyder.

Further Reading

Statistical Information: The Service Central de la Statistique et des Études Économiques (STATEC) was founded in 1900 and reorganized in 1962 (19–21 boulevard Royal, C.P. 304 Luxembourg-City). *Director:* Robert Weides. Main publications: *Bulletin du STATEC.—Annuaire statistique.— Cahiers économiques.*

Bulletin de Documentation. Government Information Service. From 1945 (monthly)
The Institutions of the Grand Duchy of Luxembourg. Information and Press Service, Luxembourg, 1989
La Vie Politique au Grand-Duché de Luxembourg. Information and Press Service, Luxembourg, 1990
Als, G., *Le Luxembourg: Statistiques Historiques 1839-1989.* Luxembourg, 1989
Calmes, C., *The Making of a Nation from 1815 up to our Days.* Luxembourg, 1989
Heiderscheid, A., *Aspects de Sociologie Religieuse du Diocèse de Luxembourg.* 2 vols. Luxembourg, 1961
Hury, C. and Christophory, J., *Luxembourg.* [Bibliography] Oxford and Santa Barbara, 1981
Majerus, P., *Le Luxembourg independant.* Luxembourg, 1948.—*L'État Luxembourgeois.* Luxembourg, 1983
Newcomer, J., *The Grand Duchy of Luxembourg: The Evolution of Nationhood, 963 A.D. to 1983.* Washington, 1983
Trausch, G., *The Significance of the Historical Date of 1839.* Luxembourg, 1989

Archives of the State: Luxembourg-City. *Director:* Cornel Meder.
National Library: Luxembourg-City, 37 Boulevard Roosevelt. *Director:* Jules Christophory.

MADAGASCAR

Capital: Antananarivo
Population: 11·44m. (1990)
GNP per capita: US$280 (1988)

Repoblika Demokratika Malagasy

HISTORY. Madagascar was discovered by the Portuguese, Diego Diaz, in 1500. The island was unified under the Imérina monarchy between 1797 and 1861, but French claims to a protectorate led to hostilities culminating in the establishment of a protectorate on 30 Sept. 1895. Madagascar became a French Colony on 6 Aug. 1896 and the monachy was abolished on 26 Feb. 1897.

Madagascar became an Overseas Territory in 1946, and on 14 Oct. 1958, following a referendum, was proclaimed the autonomous Malagasy Republic within the French Community, achieving full independence on 26 June 1960.

The government of Philibert Tsiranana, President from independence, resigned on 18 May 1972 and executive powers were given to Maj.-Gen. Gabriel Ramanantsoa, who replaced Tsiranana as President on 11 Oct. 1972. On 5 Feb. 1975, Col. Richard Ratsimandrava became Head of State, but was assassinated 6 days later. A National Military Directorate under Brig.-Gen. Gilles Andriamahazo was established on 12 Feb. On 15 June it handed over power to a Supreme Revolutionary Council (SRC) under Didier Ratsiraka.

AREA AND POPULATION. Madagascar is situated off the south-east coast of Africa, from which it is separated by the Mozambique channel, the least distance between island and continent being 250 miles (400 km); its length is 980 miles (1,600 km); greatest breadth, 360 miles (570 km).

The area is 587,041 sq. km (226,658 sq. miles). In 1975 (census) the population was 7,603,790. Estimate (1990) 11,443,000.

Province	*Area in Sq. km*	*Population 1990*	*Chief town*	*Population 1990*
Antsiranana	43,046	715,000	Antsiranana	54,418
Mahajanga	150,023	1,253,000	Mahajanga	121,967
Toamasina	71,911	1,585,000	Toamasina	145,431
Antananarivo	58,283	3,811,000	Antananarivo	802,390
Fianarantsoa	102,373	2,420,000	Fianarantsoa	124,489
Toliary	161,405	1,659,000	Toliary	61,460

Vital statistics, 1984: Births, 456,000; deaths, 146,000. Growth rate, 1989: 3 per 1,000.

The indigenous population are of Malayo-Polynesian stock, divided into 18 ethnic groups of which the principal are Merina (26%) of the central plateau, the Betsimisaraka (15%) of the east coast, and the Betsileo (12%) of the southern plateau. Foreign communities include Europeans, mainly French (30,000), Indians (15,000), Chinese (9,000), Comorians and Arabs.

CLIMATE. A tropical climate, but the mountains cause big variations in rainfall, which is very heavy in the east and very light in the west. Antananarivo. Jan. 70°F (21·1°C), July 59°F (15°C). Annual rainfall 54" (1,350 mm). Toamasina. Jan. 80°F (26·7°C), July 70°F (21·1°C). Annual rainfall 128" (3,256 mm).

CONSTITUTION AND GOVERNMENT. The new Constitution of the Democratic Republic of Madagascar was approved by referendum on 21 Dec. 1975 and came into force on 30 Dec. It provides for a National People's Assembly of 137 members elected by universal suffrage for a 5-year term from the single list of the *Front National pour la Défense de la Révolution Socialiste Malgache;* following the general elections held on 28 Aug. 1983, this comprised 117 members of the *Avant-garde de la Révolution Malgache,* 9 of the *Parti du Congrès de l'Indépendence* and

11 others. Executive power is vested in the President, directly elected for 7 years, who appoints a Council of Ministers to assist him, with the guidance of the 27-member Supreme Revolutionary Council.

President: Adm. Didier Ratsiraka (re-elected 12 March 1989).

The Council of Ministers in Nov. 1989 was composed as follows:

Prime Minister, Head of Government: Col. Victor Ramahatra.

Revolutionary Art and Culture: Gisèle Rabesahala. *Defence:* Brig.-Gen. Mahasampo Christophère Bien-Aimé Raveloson. *Keeper of the Seals, Justice:* Joseph Bedo. *Civil Service and Labour:* Georges Ruphin. *Information, Ideological Guidance and Co-operatives:* Jean-Claude Rahaga. *Health:* Dr Jean-Jacques Séraphin. *Planning and Economy:* Jean Robiarivony. *Animal Production, Water Resources and Forestry:* Maxime Zafera. *Finance and Budget:* Léon Rajaobelina. *Posts and Telecommunications:* Simon Pierre. *Interior:* Augustin Ampy Portos. *Higher Education:* Ignace Rakoto. *Commerce:* Georges Solofoson. *Foreign Affairs:* Jean Bemananjara. *Transport, Meteorology and Tourism:* Lucien Zasy. *Secondary and Basic Education:* Aristide Velompanahy. *Industry, Energy and Mines:* Vincent Radanielson. *Public Works:* Jean-Emile Tsaranazy. *Population, Social Welfare, Youth and Sport:* Badhroudine. *Agricultural Production, Agrarian Reform and Land Inheritance:* José Andrianoelison. *Scientific Research and Development:* Zafera Antoine Rabesa.

National flag: Horizontally red over green, in the hoist a vertical white strip.

National anthem: Ry tanindrazanay malala ô!

Malagasy, which is a language of Malayo-Polynesian origin, is the official language. French and English are understood and taught in Malagasy schools.

Local Government: The six provinces (*faritany*) are sub-divided into 111 *fivondronana*, which in turn are divided into 13,476 *fokontany* (the traditional communal divisions). Each level is governed by an elected council.

DEFENCE

Army. The Army is organized in 2 battalion groups, and 1 engineer, 1 signals, 1 service and 7 construction regiments. Equipment includes PT-76 light tanks and M-8 armoured cars. Strength (1991) 20,000 and gendarmerie 7,500.

Navy. In 1989 the small maritime force had a strength of 500 (including 100 marines), and was equipped with 1 250-tonne patrol craft, 1 medium landing ship, a few small landing craft, together with a 600 tonne former trawler used for transport and training.

Air Force. Created in 1961, the Malagasy Air Force received its first combat equipment in 1978, with the arrival of 8 MiG-21 and 4 MiG-17 fighters, plus flying and ground staff instructors, from North Korea. Other equipment includes 5 An-26 turboprop transports, 1 Britten-Norman Defender armed transport, 2 C-47s, 1 HS. 748 and 1 Yak-40 for VIP use, 1 Aztec, 2 Cessna Skymasters, 4 Cessna 172Ms and 6 Mi-8 helicopters. Personnel (1991), 500, with 12 combat aircraft.

INTERNATIONAL RELATIONS

Membership. Madagascar is a member of the UN, OAU and is an ACP state of the EEC.

ECONOMY

Policy. A programme of privatization was launched in 1989.

Budget. The 1990 budget envisaged expenditure of MGFr1,124,400m.

Currency. The unit of currency is the *Malagasy franc* (MGF). There are coins of MGFr1, 2, 5, 10, 50 and 100 and banknotes of MGFr50, 100, 500, 1,000, 5,000 and 10,000. In March 1991, £1 = MGFr2,917; US$1 = MGFr1,538.

Banking and Finance. A Central Bank was formed in 1973, replacing the former

Institut d'Emission Malgache as the central bank of issue. All commercial banking and insurance was nationalized in 1975 and privatized in 1988. Industrial development is financed through the *Bankin'ny Indostria*. Other commercial banking is undertaken by the *Bankin'ny Tantsaha Mpamokatra*, the *Banky Fampandrosoana ny Varotra*. The Malagasy Bank of the Indian Ocean was set up in Sept. 1990 as part of a bank privatization programme.

Weights and Measures. The metric system is in use.

ENERGY AND NATURAL RESOURCES

Electricity. Production (1986) 479m. kwh. Supply 127 and 220 volts; 50 Hz.

Oil. The oil refinery at Toamasina has a capacity of 12,000 bbls a day.

Minerals. Mining production in 1989 included: Graphite, 15,865 tonnes; chromite, 165,397 tonnes; zircon, 220 kg; beryl (industrial), 30,434 kg; mica, 1,182 kg; gold, 61 grammes; industrial garnet, 407 kg.

Agriculture. 80–85% of the workforce is employed in agriculture. The principal agricultural products in 1988 were (in 1,000 tonnes): Rice, 2,380; cassava, 2,277; mangoes, 180; bananas, 217; potatoes, 271; sugar-cane, 1,990; maize, 160; sweet potatoes, 483; coffee, 85; citrus fruits, 81; pineapples, 50; seed cotton, 42; groundnuts, 30; sisal, 20; tobacco, 9.

Cattle breeding and agriculture are the chief occupations. There were, in 1989, 10,243,000 cattle, 1·4m. pigs, 1,950,000 sheep and goats and 30m. poultry.

Forestry. The forests covered (1989) 14·7m. hectares (about 25% of the land surface) and contain many valuable woods, while gum, resins and plants for tanning, dyeing and medicinal purposes abound. Production (1984) 6·26m. cu. metres.

Fisheries. The fish catch in 1984 was 56,000 tonnes.

INDUSTRY. Industry, hitherto confined mainly to the processing of agricultural products, is now extending to cover other fields.

FOREIGN ECONOMIC RELATIONS

Commerce. Trade in MGFr1m.:

	1984	*1985*	*1986*	*1987*	*1988*	*1989*
Imports (c.i.f)	213,531	265,916	238,458	376,792	512,063	545,399
Exports (f.o.b)	192,267	181,630	205,875	348,025	385,080	506,193

Chief exports, in tonnes (and value): Coffee, 1989, 43,105 (MGFr104,080m.); cloves, 1989, 16,449 (MGFr51,408m.); vanilla, 1988, 625 (MGFr58,531m.). In 1985 France took 37% of exports, the USA, 14% and Japan, 11%, while France supplied 33% of imports, the USSR, 9%, Federal Republic of Germany, 6%, Qatar, 6% and the USA, 6%.

Total trade between Madagascar and UK (British Department of Trade returns, in £1,000 sterling):

	1987	*1988*	*1989*	*1990*
Imports to UK	6,925	7,154	5,865	5,952
Exports and re-exports from UK	6,382	4,747	3,352	16,093

Tourism. There were 38,954 tourists in 1989.

COMMUNICATIONS

Roads. In 1986 there were about 50,000 km of roads (10% bitumenized). In 1986 there 42,131 motor vehicles.

Railways. In 1989 there were 883 km of railways, all metre gauge. In 1989, 2·4m. passengers and 528,000m. tonnes of cargo were transported.

Aviation. Air France and Air Madagascar connect Antananarivo (International airport, Ivato) with Paris, Alitalia connects with Rome. Several weekly services operated by Air Madagascar connect the capital with the ports and the chief inland towns. In 1987, 129,736 passengers and 4,734 tonnes of cargo arrived and departed.

Shipping. In 1987, 692,270 tonnes were loaded and 1,261,205 tonnes unloaded at Toamasina, Mahajanga and other ports. In 1980, registered merchant marine was 56 vessels (of more than 100 GRT) with a total of 91,211 GRT.

Telecommunications. There were in 1986, 724 post offices and agencies. There were (1983) 37,100 telephone subscribers, and (1989) 0·8m. radio receivers and 0·15m. television receivers.

Newspapers. In 1985 there were 7 daily newspapers with a total circulation of 68,000.

Cinemas. There were, in 1974, 31 cinemas with a seating capacity of 12,500.

JUSTICE, RELIGION, EDUCATION AND WELFARE

Justice. The Supreme Court and the Court of Appeal are in Antananarivo. In most towns there are Courts of First Instance for civil and commercial cases. For criminal cases there are ordinary criminal courts in most towns.

Religion. In 1989 47% of the population practised the traditional religion; 26% were Roman Catholic, 22% Protestant (mainly belonging to the Fiangonan'i Jesosy Kristy eto Madagaskar) and 1·7% Moslem.

Education. Education is compulsory from 6 to 14 years of age in the primary schools. In 1988-89 there were 1,534,142 pupils and 37,894 teachers in 13,672 primary schools, 257,377 pupils and 11,200 teachers in 1,142 secondary schools and 87,925 students and 4,976 teachers in 366 *lycées*. The University of Madagascar has a main campus at Antananarivo and 5 university centres in the other provincial capitals, with 35,106 students and 884 academic staff in 1987. There are also 4 agricultural schools at Nanisana, Ambatondrazaka, Marovoay and Ivoloina.

Health. In 1980 there were 749 hospitals and dispensaries with 18,485 beds; there were (1985) 1,189 doctors, 100 dentists, 37 pharmacists, 1,638 midwives and 3,323 nursing personnel.

DIPLOMATIC REPRESENTATIVES

Of Madagascar in Great Britain
Ambassador: François de Paul Rabotoson (resides in Paris)

Of Great Britain in Madagascar (Immeuble Ny Havana, Cite de 67 Ha, Antananarivo)
Ambassador: D. O. Amy, OBE.

Of Madagascar in the USA (2374 Massachusetts Ave., NW, Washington, D.C., 20008)
Ambassador: Pierrot J. Rajaonarivelo.

Of the USA in Madagascar (14 rue Rainitovo, Antsahavola, Antananarivo)
Ambassador: Howard K. Walker.

Of Madagascar to the United Nations
Ambassador: Blaise Rabetafika.

Further Reading

Official sources: Publications of the Banque des Donnés de l'Etat include the *Bulletin mensuel de Madagascar* (from 1971); *Situation Économique de Madagascar au 1 Janvier 1988*; *Inventaire Socio-Economique 1976–86* 2 vols; *Recensement Industriel Annuel* (latest 1986). The Government has published an *Annuaire Officiel, 1987–88*.
Brandt, H., *Guide to Madagascar*. Chalfont St Peter, 1988
Brown, M., *Madagascar Rediscovered*. London, 1978
Deschamps, H., *Histoire de Madagascar*. Paris, 4th ed. 1972
Rabetafika, R., *Réforme Fiscal et Révolution Socialiste à Madagascar*. Paris, 1990
Rajoelina, P. and Ramelet, A., *Madagascar, la Grande Ile*. Paris, 1989
Ramahatra, O., *Madagascar: une Economie en Phase d'Ajustement*. Paris, 1989

MALAŴI

Capital: Lilongwe
Population: 7·98m. (1987)
GNP per capita: US$160 (1988)

Republic of Malaŵi

HISTORY. Malaŵi was formerly the Nyasaland (until 1907 British Central Africa) Protectorate, constituted on 15 May 1891.

Nyasaland became a self-governing country on 1 Feb. 1963, and on 6 July 1964 an independent member of the Commonwealth under the name of Malaŵi. It became a republic on 6 July 1966.

AREA AND POPULATION. Malaŵi lies along the southern and western shores of Lake Malaŵi (the third largest lake in Africa), and is otherwise bounded north by Tanzania, south by Mozambique and west by Zambia. Land area (excluding inland water of Lakes Malombe, Chilwa and Chiuta) 36,325 sq. miles, divided into 3 regions and 24 districts, each administered by a District Commissioner.

Lake Malaŵi waters belonging to Malaŵi are 9,250 sq. miles and the whole Lake Malaŵi (including the waters under Mozambique by an agreement made between the two countries in 1950) is 11,650 sq. miles.

Population at census 1987, 7,982,607. Over 90% of the population live in rural areas.

Population of main towns (census 1987) was as follows: Blantyre, 331,588; Lilongwe, 233,973; Mzuzu, 44,238; Zomba, 42,878.

Population of the regions, census 1987 (and census 1977): Northern, 907,121 (648,853); Central, 3,116,038 (2,143,716); Southern, 3,959,448 (2,754,891).

The official languages are Chichewa, spoken by over 50% of the population, and English.

CLIMATE. The tropical climate is marked by a dry season from May to Oct. and a wet season for the remaining months. Rainfall amounts are variable, within the range of 29–100" (725–2,500 mm), and maximum temperatures average 75–89°F (24–32°C), and minimum temperatures 58–67°F (14·4–19·4°C). Lilongwe. Jan. 73°F (22·8°C), July 60°F (15·6°C). Annual rainfall 36" (900 mm). Blantyre. Jan. 75°F (23·9°C), July 63°F (17·2°C). Annual rainfall 45" (1,125 mm). Zomba. Jan. 73°F (22·8°C), July 63°F (17·2°C). Annual rainfall 54" (1,344 mm).

CONSTITUTION AND GOVERNMENT. The President of the republic is also head of Government and of the Malaŵi Congress Party. Malaŵi is a one-party state. Parliament is composed of 120 members: 104 elected for up to 5 years, and 16 nominated by the President.

Life President, External Affairs, Agriculture, Justice, Works: Ngwazi Dr H. Kamuzu Banda. (Took office 6 July 1966 and became Life President on 6 July 1971).

The Cabinet in Nov. 1990 was composed as follows:

Without Portfolio, Administrative Secretary of Malaŵi Congress Party: Maxwell Pashane. *Labour:* Wadson B. Deleza. *Health:* E. C. Katola Phiri. *Trade, Industry and Tourism:* Robson W. Chirwa. *Finance:* Louis J. Chimango. *Forestry and Natural Resources:* Stanford Demba. *Transport and Communications:* Dalton S. Katopola. *Education and Culture:* Michael Mlambala. *Local Government:* Stanford Demba. *Community Services:* Mfunjo Mwanjasi Mwakikunga.

National flag: Three equal horizontal stripes of black, red, green, with a red rising sun on the centre of the black stripe.

DEFENCE. All services form part of the Army and have a strength (1991) 7,250.

Army. The army is organized into 3 infantry battalions and 1 support battalion. Equipment includes scout cars.

Navy. A single patrol craft and some 3 boats operated by about (1990) 100 personnel based at Chilumba on Lake Nyasa.

Air Wing. To support the infantry battalion, the Air Wing has 1 Do 28D Skyservant and 3 Do 228 light transports, and 2 Puma, 1 Ecureuil, 1 Dauphin, and 1 Alouette III helicopters. An HS 125 jet is used for VIP transport. Personnel (1991), 150.

INTERNATIONAL RELATIONS

Membership. Malaŵi is a member of the UN, the Commonwealth, the Non-Aligned States, OAU, SADCC and is an ACP state of the EEC.

ECONOMY

Policy. The government operates a 3-year 'rolling' public-sector investment programme, revised annually to take into account changing needs and the expected level of resources available. The greatest part of the development programme is annually financed from external aid, and priority in the use of resources has always been given to providing the counterpart contributions to funds received from external sources. The balance of these local resources is used for financing projects commanding high national priority for which no external funds can be secured.

Budget. Revenue Account receipts and expenditure (in K.1,000) for years ending 31 March:

	1987–88	*1988–89*	*1989–90*	*1990–91*
Revenue	583,382	681,800	941,733	1,066,360
Expenditure	728,834	784,300	1,056,606	1,168,738

Currency. The unit of currency is the *kwacha* (MWK) of 100 *tambala*. From 9 June 1975 the kwacha has been pegged to Special Drawing Rights. In March 1991: £1 sterling = K.4·94, US$1 = K.2·60.

Banking and Finance. In July 1964 the Reserve Bank of Malaŵi was set up with a capital of K.1m. to be responsible for the issue of currency and the holding of external reserves and to issue treasury bills and local registered stock on behalf of the Government. Since then, the Reserve Bank has fully assumed the responsibilities of a Central Bank.

The National Bank of Malaŵi has a total of 14 branches in major urban areas and 25 static and 41 mobile agencies in rural areas. The Commercial Bank of Malaŵi Ltd opened in 1970 and has branches at Limbe, Lilongwe, Mzuzu and Zomba and an agency in Dedza and headquarters at Blantyre. It has 4 permanent and 65 mobile agencies.

In 1972 The Investment Development Bank of Malaŵi was established in Blantyre. Its resources are derived from domestic and foreign official sources and its objective is to provide medium and long-term credits to private entities considered of importance to the economy.

The Post Office Savings Bank had (1985) 257 offices conducting savings business throughout the country, and the New Building Society has agencies in Limbe, Mzuzu, Zomba, Muloza and Blantyre with its head office in Lilongwe.

Weights and Measures. The metric system became fully operational in 1982.

ENERGY AND NATURAL RESOURCES

Electricity. The Electricity Supply Commission of Malaŵi is the sole supplier of electrical power and energy and the demand and supply of electricity and power on the inter-connected system was met from the hydro-electric generator sets installed at Tedzani Falls and Nkula Falls stations which together have a total capacity of 124 mw as at 1984. The inter-connected system extends from the Shire River hydro stations and covers most areas of the Southern and Central Regions, and part of the Northern Region. Production (1986) 466m. kwh. Supply 230 volts; 50 Hz.

Thermal plant of 23·8 mw capacity is available on the inter-connected system and there are stations at Blantyre, Lilongwe, Mtunthama, Kasungu, and Mzuzu. The capacity of the isolated station at Karonga was increased to 480 kw with the installation of 120 kw diesel generator set.

Minerals. The main product in 1976 was marble (149,254 tonnes) for the manufacture of cement. Coal mining began in 1985.

Agriculture. Malawî is predominantly an agricultural country. In 1983 agriculture contributed about 43% to the GDP, and agricultural produce accounted for 90% of total exports. Maize is the main subsistence crop and is grown by over 95% of all smallholders; production (1988) 1,455,000 tonnes. Tea cultivation is of growing importance; in 1988, 35,000 tonnes were produced. Almost all the surplus crops produced by smallholders are sold to the Agricultural Development and Marketing Corporation. Production (1988): Tobacco, 56,000 tonnes; sugar-cane, 1·7m. tonnes.

Livestock in 1988: Cattle, 1m.; sheep, 210,000; goats, 950,000; pigs, 210,000.

Forestry. There were (1989) 4·3m. ha of forests; 46% of the land area. In 1983–84, 11,108 cu. metres of sawn timber were removed.

Fisheries. Landings in 1987 were 88,400 tonnes.

INDUSTRY. Index of manufacturing output in 1987 (1984 = 100): manufacturing for domestic consumption, excluding mining and quarrying, 290·8; of this consumer goods were at 109 and intermediate goods for building and construction were at 99·9. Manufacturing for export, 97·4.

FOREIGN ECONOMIC RELATIONS

Commerce. Exports 1987 (in K.1m.): Tobacco, 373·7; tea, 61; sugar, 63·5; pulses, 25·6; groundnuts, 13·2; rice (1985), 3; other crops including manufactures, 41·5.

Trade statistics for calendar years are (in K.1m.):

	1984	*1985*	*1986*	*1987*
Imports	381·5	492·5	480·0	653·9
Exports	446·2	419·6	445·9	602·5

Total trade between Malawî and UK (British Department of Trade returns, in £1,000 sterling):

	1987	*1988*	*1989*	*1990*
Imports to UK	44,223	30,183	27,890	24,666
Exports and re-exports from UK	18,069	27,618	30,604	33,575

Tourism. There were 76,134 visitors to Malawî in 1987.

COMMUNICATIONS

Roads. In 1988 there were 2,701 km of main road, of which 1,857 km were bitumen surfaced and 410 km gravel; 2,782 km of secondary roads, of which 285 km were surfaced and 239 km gravel; 5,354 km of district roads, of which 24 km were surfaced and 16 km gravel, and 8,008 km of earth roads. In 1987 there were 14,911 cars and 15,643 commercial vehicles.

Railways. Malawî Railways (789 km–1,067 mm gauge) operates a main line from Salima to the Mozambique border near Nsanje, from which running powers over the Trans-Zambezia Railway allow access to the port of Beira; a branch opened in 1970 runs eastwards from a point 16 km south of Balaka to the Mozambique border to give a direct route to the deep-water port of Nacala. The 26-km section from Nsanje to the border is operated by the Central Africa Railway Co. Ltd. An extension of 111 km from Salima to the new state capital of Lilongwe was opened in Feb. 1979, and a further extension to Mchinji on the Zambian border (120 km) was completed in 1981. In 1988–89, 71 tonne-km of freight and 112m. passenger-km were carried.

Aviation. In 1983 the Kamuzu International Airport at Lilongwe was inaugurated. It handled (1989-90) 320,505 passengers and 5,646·6 tonnes. In 1989-90 Chileka Airport handled 80,116 passengers and 1,228 tonnes of freight.

Shipping. In 1987–88 lake ships carried 210,103 passengers and 28,983 tonnes of freight.

Telecommunications. Number of telephones (1987) 25,000. The Malawî Broadcasting Corporation broadcasts in English and Chichewa. There were 1m. radio sets in 1983.

Newspapers (1989). *The Daily Times* (English, Monday to Friday); 17,000 copies daily. *Malaŵi News* (English and Chichewa, Saturdays); 23,000 copies weekly. *Odini* (English and Chichewa); 8,500 copies fortnightly. *Boma Lathu* (Chichewa); 80,000 copies monthly. *Za Alimi* (English and Chichewa); 10,000 copies monthly.

JUSTICE, RELIGION, EDUCATION AND WELFARE

Justice. Justice is administered in the High Court, the magistrates' courts and traditional courts. There are 23 magistrates' courts, 176 traditional courts and 23 local appeal courts.

Appeals from traditional courts are dealt with in the traditional appeal courts and in the national traditional appeal court. Appeals from magistrates' courts lie to the High Court, and appeals from the High Court to Malaŵi's Supreme Court of Appeal.

Religion. In 1988 the Roman Catholic Church claimed 1·5m. members; Church of Central Africa Presbyterian, 500,000; Diocese of Southern Malaŵi and Lake Malaŵi (part of the Province of Central Africa (the Anglican Communion) (1983), 70,606; Seventh Day Adventist Church (1984), 59,319. Zambezi Evangelical Church (formerly Zambezi Industrial Mission) (1987), 30,000; Assembly of God, 13,740; Seventh Day Baptist (Central Africa Conference) (1987), 4,861; Church of Christ, 60,000; African Evangelical Church (1983), 6,000. Moslems were estimated to number about 500,000 in 1983.

Education In 1986–87 the number of pupils in primary schools was 1,022,765; in secondary schools, 25,681. There were 25,013 teachers in primary schools and 1,229 in secondary schools. The primary school course is of 8 years' duration, followed by a 4-year secondary course. English is taught from the 1st year and becomes the general medium of instruction from the 4th year. There were 1,802 students in teacher training schools and 777 in government technical schools.

The University of Malaŵi was inaugurated in 1965. In 1988–89 there were 2,323 students taking degree and diploma courses.

Health. In 1989 there were two central hospitals, one general hospital, one mental hospital, two leprosaria and 45 hospitals of which 21 were government district hospitals. In 1986 there were 7,081 hospital beds of which 1,612 were for maternity.

DIPLOMATIC REPRESENTATIVES

Of Malaŵi in Great Britain (33 Grosvenor St., London, W1X 0DE)
High Commissioner: Tony Kandiero.

Of Great Britain in Malaŵi (Lingadzi Hse., Lilongwe, 3)
High Commissioner: W. N. Wenban-Smith.

Of Malaŵi in the USA (2408 Massachusetts Ave., NW, Washington, D.C., 20008)
Ambassador: Robert Mbaya.

Of the USA in Malaŵi (PO Box 30016, Lilongwe, 3)
Ambassador: George A. Trail III.

Of Malaŵi to the United Nations
Ambassador: Robert Mbaya.

Further Reading

General Information: The Chief Information Officer, PO Box 494, Blantyre.

Boeder, R. B., *Malawi.* [Bibliography] Oxford and Santa Barbara, 1980

MALAYSIA

Capital: Kuala Lumpur
Population: 17·81m. (1990)
GNP per capita: US$1,870 (1988)

Federation of Malaysia

HISTORY. On 16 Sept. 1963 Malaysia came into being, consisting of the Federation of Malaya, the State of Singapore and the colonies of North Borneo (renamed Sabah) and Sarawak. The agreement between the UK and the 4 territories was signed on 9 July (Cmnd. 2094); by it, the UK relinquished sovereignty over Singapore, North Borneo and Sarawak from independence day and extended the 1957 defence agreement with Malaya to apply to Malaysia. Malaysia became automatically a member of the Commonwealth of Nations. *See* map in THE STATESMAN'S YEAR-BOOK, 1964–65.

On 9 Aug. 1965, by a mutual agreement dated 7 Aug. 1965 between Malaysia and Singapore, Singapore seceded from Malaysia to become an independent Sovereign nation.

AREA AND POPULATION. The federal state of Malaysia comprises the 11 states and 1 federal territory of Peninsular Malaysia on the Malay Peninsula, bounded in the north by Thailand, and with the island of Singapore as an enclave on its southern tip; and, on the island of Borneo to the east, the state of Sabah (which includes the federal territory of the island of Labuan), and the state of Sarawak, with Brunei as an enclave, both bounded in the south by Indonesia and in the north-west and north-east by the South China and Sulu Seas.

The area of Malaysia is 329,758 sq. km (127,317 sq. miles) and the population (1990 estimate) is 17,812,000. The growth of Census population has been:

Year	*Peninsular Malaysia*	*Sarawak*	*Sabah/Labuan*	*Total Malaysia*
1970	8,809,557	975,918	655,295	10,440,770
1980	11,426,613	1,307,582	1,011,046	13,745,241

The areas, populations and chief towns of the states and federal territories are:

State	*Sq. km*	*Census 1980* [1]	*Capital*	*Census 1980*
Johor	18,985	1,638,229	Johor Baharu	249,880
Kedah	9,425	1,116,140	Alor Setar	71,682
Kelantan	14,931	893,753	Kota Baharu	170,559
Kuala Lumpur [2]	243	977,102	Kuala Lumpur	937,875
Melaka	1,658	464,754	Melaka	88,073
Negeri Sembilan	6,646	573,578	Seremban	136,252
Pahang	35,960	798,782	Kuantan	136,625
Perak	21,005	1,805,198	Ipoh	300,727
Perlis	795	148,276	Kangar	12,956
Pinang	1,033	954,638	Pinang (Georgetown)	250,578
Selangor	7,956	1,515,536	Shah Alam	24,138
Terengganu	12,955	540,627	Kuala Terengganu	186,608
Peninsular Malaysia	131,592	11,426,613		
Labuan [2]	98	26,413	Victoria	...
Sabah	73,613	984,633	Kota Kinabalu	55,997
Sarawak	124,449	1,307,582	Kuching	74,229
East Malaysia	198,160	2,318,628		

[1] Revised figures [2] Federal Territories.

Other large cities (1980 Census): Petaling Jaya (207,805), Kelang (192,080), Taiping (146,002), Sibu (85,231), Sandakan (70,420) and Miri (52,125).

Vital statistics (1988): Crude birth rate 30 per 1,000 population; crude death rate 4·7; infant mortality rate 13·19 per 1,000 live births.

Of the total population in 1980, 47% were Malay, 32% Chinese, 8% Indian and 13% others.

Over 58% speak Bahasa Malaysia, the official language, 9% Chinese, 4% Tamil and 3% Iban.

CLIMATE. Malaysia is affected by the monsoon climate. The N.E. monsoon prevails from Oct. to Feb., bringing rain to the east coast of the peninsula. The S.W. monsoon lasts from mid-May to Sept. and affects the opposite coastline the most. Temperatures are uniform throughout the year. Kuala Lumpur. Jan. 81°F (27·2°C), July 81°F (27·2°C). Annual rainfall 97·6" (2,441 mm). Penang. Jan. 82°F (27·8°C), July 82°F (27·8°C). Annual rainfall 109·4" (2,736 mm).

CONSTITUTION AND GOVERNMENT. The Constitution of Malaysia is based on the Constitution of the former Federation of Malaya, but includes safeguards for the special interests of Sabah and Sarawak. It was amended in 1983.

The federal capital is Kuala Lumpur, established on 1 Feb. 1974 with an area of approximately 94 sq. miles. The official language is Bahasa Malaysia.

The Constitution provides for one of the 9 Rulers of the Malay States to be elected from among themselves to be the *Yang di-Pertuan Agong* (Supreme Head of the Federation). He holds office for a period of 5 years. The Rulers also elect from among themselves a Deputy Supreme Head of State, also for a period of 5 years.

Supreme Head of State (Yang di-Pertuan Agong): HM Sultan Azlan Shah Muhibbuddin Shah ibni Almarhum Sultan Yussuf Izzuddin Ghafarullahu-lahu Shah, DK, DMN, PMN, SPCM, SPMP, elected as 9th *Yang di-Pertuan Agong* from 2 March 1989, succeeded 26 April 1989 and installed 18 Sept. 1989.

Raja of Perlis: HRH Tuanku Syed Putra ibni Al-Marhum Syed Hassan Jamalullail, DK, DKM, DMN, SMN, SPMP, SPDK, acceded 12 March 1949.

Sultan of Kedah: HRH Tuanku Haji Abdul Halim Mu'adzam Shah ibni Al-Marhum Sultan Badlishah, DK, DKH, DKM, DMN, DUK, SPMK, SSDK, acceded 20 Feb. 1959.

Sultan of Johor: HRH Sultan Mahmood Iskandar ibni Al-Marhum Sultan Ismail, DK, SPMJ, SPDK, DK (Brunei), SSIJ, PIS, BSI, acceded 11 May 1981 (Supreme Head of State from 26 April 1984 to 25 April 1989), returned as Sultan of Johor 26 April 1989.

Sultan of Selangor: HRH Sultan Salahuddin Abdul Aziz Shah ibni Al-Marhum Sultan Hisamuddin 'Alam Shah Al-Haj, DK, DMN, SPMS, SPDK, acceded 3 Sept. 1960.

Regent of Perak: HRH Raja Nazrin, appointed April 1989.

Yang di-Pertuan Besar of Negeri Sembilan: HRH Tuanku Ja'afar ibni Al-Marhum Tuanku Abdul Rahman, DMN, DK, acceded 8 April 1968.

Sultan of Kelantan: HRH Sultan Ismail Petra ibni Al-Marhum Sultan Yahya Petra, DK, SPMK, SJMK, SPSM, appointed 29 March 1979.

Sultan of Trengganu: HRH Sultan Mahmud Al-Marhum ibni Al-Marhum Tuanku Al-Sultan Ismail Nasiruddin Shah, DK, SPMT, SPCM, appointed 2 Sept. 1979.

Sultan of Pahang: Sultan Haji Ahmad Shah Al-Musta'in Billah ibni Al-Marhum Sultan Abu Bakar Ri'Ayatuddin Al-Mu'Adzam Shah, DKM, DKP, DK, SSAP, SPCM, SPMJ.

Yang di-Pertua Negeri Paau Pinang: HE Tun Haji Hamdan Sheikh Tahir, appointed 2 May 1989.

Yang di Pertua Negeri Melaka: HE Tun Datuk Seri Utama Syed Ahmad Al-Haj bin Syed Mahmud Shahabudin, SSM, PSM, DUNM, SPMK, SSDK, PGDK, PNBS, JMN, JP, appointed 4 Dec. 1984.

Yang di-Pertua Negeri Sarawak: HE Datuk Patinggi Haji Ahmad Zaidi Adruce bin Muhammed Noor, SSM, DP, DUNM, PNBS, BM Adipradana (Indonesia) appointed 2 April 1985.

Yang di-Pertua Negeri Sabah: HE Tan Sri Datuk Haji Mohd Said bin Keruak, PMN, SPDK, appointed 31 Dec. 1986.

Parliament consists of the *Yang di-Pertuan Agong* and two *Majlis* (Houses of Parliament) known as the *Dewan Negara* (Senate) of 69 members and *Dewan Rakyat* (House of Representatives) of 180 members, allocated by state as follows: Perlis, 2; Kedah, 14; Kalantan, 13; Terengganu, 9; Penang, 11; Perak, 23; Pahang, 10; Selangor, 14; Kuala Lumpur Federal Territory, 7; Negri Sembilan, 7; Melaka, 5; Johor, 18; Labuan Federal Territory, 1; Sabah, 20; Sarawak, 27. Appointment to the Senate is for 3 years. The maximum life of the House of Representatives is 5 years, subject to its dissolution at any time by the *Yang di-Pertuan Agong* on the advice of his Ministers.

National flag: Fourteen horizontal stripes of red and white, with a blue quarter bearing a crescent and a star of 14 points, all in gold.

National Anthem: Negara-Ku.

The elections to the House of Representatives held on 21 Oct, 1990, returned the following members: National Front, 127; opposition, 53 (made up of: Democratic Action Party, 20; Bersatu Sabah Party, 14; S46, 8; Pas, 7; ind, 4.

The Cabinet formed on 26 Oct. 1990 consisted of:

Prime Minister and Minister for Home Affairs: Datuk Seri Dr Mahathir Mohamad.

Deputy Prime Minister and Minister for National and Rural Development: Encik Abdul Ghafar Baba. *Transport:* Datuk Seri Dr Ling Lionel Sik. *Energy, Telecommunications and Posts:* Datuk Seri S. Samy Vellu. *Primary Industries:* Datuk Seri Dr Lim Keng Yaik. *Works:* Datuk Leo Moggie Anak Irok. *International Trade and Industry:* Datuk Seri Rafidah Aziz. *Domestic Trade and Consumer Affairs:* Datuk Abu Hassan Omar. *Agriculture:* Datuk Seri Sanusi Junid. *Education:* Datuk Dr Sulaiman Daud. *Foreign Affairs:* Abdullah Ahmad Badawi. *Finance:* Datuk Seri Anwar Ibrahim. *Health:* Datuk Lee Kim Sai. *Defence:* Datuk Seri Mohd Najib Tun Abdul Razak. *Information:* Datuk Mohamed Bin Rahmat. *Culture, Arts and Tourism:* Datuk Sabbaruddin Chik. *National Unity and Community Development:* Datuk Napsiah Omar. *Public Enterprises:* Datuk Dr Mohamad Yusof Mohamad Nor. *Human Resources:* Datuk Lim Ah Lek. *Science, Technology and Environment:* Law Hieng Ding. *Housing and Local Government:* Dr Ching Tew Peh. *Land and Co-operative Development:* Tan Sri Sakaran Dandai. *Justice:* Syed Hamid Syed Jaafar Albar. *Youth and Sports:* Annuar Musa.

DEFENCE. The Malaysian Constitution provides for the *Yang di-Pertuan Agong* (Supreme Head of State) to be the Supreme Commander of the Armed Forces who exercises his powers and authority in accordance with the advice of the Cabinet. Under the general authority of the Yang di-Pertuan Agong and the Cabinet, there is the Armed Forces Council which is responsible for the command, discipline and administration of all other matters relating to the Armed Forces, other than those relating to their operational use.

The Armed Forces Council is chaired by the Minister of Defence and its membership consists of the chief of the Defence Forces, the 3 Service Chiefs and 2 other senior military officers, the Secretary-General of the Ministry of Defence, a representative of State Rulers and an appointed member.

The chief of the Armed Forces Staff is the professional head of the Armed Forces and the senior military member in the Armed Forces Council. He is the principal adviser to the Minister of Defence on the military aspects of all defence matters. The chief of the Armed Forces Staff's committee, established under the authority of the Armed Forces Council, is the highest level at which joint planning and coordination with the Armed Forces are carried out. The Committee is chaired by the chief of the Armed Forces Staff and its membership consists of the chief of the Army, Navy and Air Force, the chief of Personnel Staff, the chief of logistic Staff and the chief of Staff of the Ministry of Defence.

Army. The Army is organized into 4 divisions, comprising 9 infantry brigades made up of 36 infantry battalions; 4 armoured, 5 field artillery, 5 engineer and 5 signals regiments and 2 anti-aircraft battalions. There is also a special service regiment. Equipment includes 26 Scorpion light tanks. Strength (1991) about 97,000, with as reserves the Malaysian Territorial Army and the regular reservists who have completed their full-time service (45,000).

Navy. The Royal Malaysian Navy is commanded by the Chief of the Navy from the integrated Ministry of Defence in Kuala Lumpur. Main bases are at Lumut, and on Labuan Island which are also the headquarters for the Malay Peninsula and Borneo operational areas respectively. The peace-time tasks include fishery protection and anti-piracy patrols.

The combatants include 2 German-built and 2 British-built frigates all with helicopter platforms, 8 fast missile craft, 2 offshore and 27 inshore patrol craft. There are also 4 Italian-type offshore mine countermeasure vessels and 2 tank landing ships normally employed in support of patrol and missile craft. Auxiliaries include 2 multi-purpose support ships, 1 survey ship, 1 diving support ship and 33 amphibious craft.

A Naval aviation squadron was formed in 1988 and operates 6 ex-British Wasp helicopters. Navy personnel in 1990 totalled 12,500 and 2,200 reserves.

Paramilitary maritime forces include 50 armed patrol launches, 48 operated by the Royal Malaysian Police and 2 by the Government of Sabah which also operates 4 other patrol boats, 1 landing craft and a yacht.

Air Force. Formed on 1 June 1958, the Royal Malaysian Air Force is equipped primarily to provide air defence and air support for the Army, Navy and Police. Its secondary rôle is to render assistance to Government departments and civilian organizations. There were in late 1989 11 squadrons, of which 9 operated transport aircraft and helicopters. Some 35 A-4 Skyhawks, which previously equipped 2 squadrons, have been withdrawn from use and placed in storage. Other equipment includes 14 F-5E Tiger II jet fighterbombers, 2 RF-5E reconnaissance-fighters, and 3 F-5F trainers, 1 F.28 Fellowship and 1 Falcon 900 VIP transports, 9 C-130 Hercules four-engined transport and patrol aircraft, 15 Caribou twin-engined STOL transports, 2 HU-16 amphibians, 33 Sikorsky S-61A-4 Nuri heavy troop and cargo transport helicopters, 20 Alouette III, and 9 Bell 47 helicopters, 10 Cessna 402Bs for twin-engine training and liaison, 44 PC-7 Turbo-Trainers, 11 MB.339 jet trainers, 2 H.S. 125 Merpati twin-jet executive transports and 1 Super Puma VIP transport helicopter. Personnel (1991) totalled about 12,000, with 67 combat aircraft.

Volunteer Forces. The Army Volunteer Force (Territorial Army) consists of first-line infantry, signals, engineer and logistics units able to take the field with the active army, and a second-line organization to provide local defence. There is also a small Naval Volunteer Reserve with Headquarters in Penang and Kuala Lumpur. The Royal Malaysian Air Force Volunteer Reserve has both air and ground elements.

INTERNATIONAL RELATIONS

Membership. Malaysia is a member of the UN, the Commonwealth, Non-Aligned countries, the Colombo Plan, Organization of Islamic Conference and ASEAN.

ECONOMY

Policy. The fifth 5-year plan, 1986–90 envisaged an expenditure of M$74,000m. and aimed the development of manufacturing industries, revitalization of agriculture and improvement of productivity. There are privatization programmes involving telecommunications, railways, airports, electricity and shipping.

Budget. Revenue and expenditure for calendar years, in M$1m.:

	1986	*1987*	*1988*	*1989*	*1990*
Revenue	19,518	18,143	21,967	23,863	24,589
Operating expenditure	20,075	20,185	21,812	23,634	24,148
Development expenditure (net)	6,949	4,111	4,045	5,473	7,857

Sources of revenue in 1990: Income tax, 25·1%, other direct taxes, 22·2%; indirect taxes, 12·5%; import duties, 9·5%; export duties, 4·3%; borrowing, 26·4%. Expenditure: Emoluments, 26·5%; debt service, 20·1%; supply and services, 8·9%; grants to states, 3·9%; pensions, 3·2%; economic services, 15·6%; social services, 7·9%; security, 2·2%.

The 1991 budget abolished export and import taxes on rubber, tin and pepper, reduced corporate taxes from 40% to 35%, and reduced income tax by 1–5%.

Currency. Bank Negara Malaysia (Central Bank of Malaysia) assumed sole currency issuing authority in Malaysia on 12 June 1967. The unit of currency issued by Bank Negara Malaysia is the Malaysian *ringgit* (MYR) of 100 *sen*. Currency notes are of denominations of M$1, 5, 10, 20, 50, 100, 500 and 1,000. Coins are of denominations of 1 *sen*, 5, 10, 20, 50 *sen* and M$1, 5 and 100. Total amount of currency in circulation at 30 June 1988, M$7,497m.

Inflation was 6·7% in 1990 (5·5% in 1989).

In March 1991 £1 = M$5·17; US$1 = M$2·72.

Banking and Finance. Thirty-eight commercial banks were operating at 31 Dec. 1988; of these 22 were incorporated locally, with 911 banking offices. Total deposits with commercial banks at 30 June 1989 were M$69,001m. There were 12 merchant banks at 31 Dec. 1988. Their total income was M$157m. in 1988. The Islamic Bank of Malaysia began operations in July 1983. The National Savings Bank (formerly known as the post office savings bank) held M$973·8m. due to 3,600,948 depositors at 31 Dec. 1978.

There were 47 finance companies with 486 offices in 1988.

There is a stock exchange at Kuala Lumpur.

Weights and Measures. The standard measures are the imperial yard, pound and gallon. The Weights and Measures Act of 1972 provides for a 10-year transition to the metric system, and was completed by 31 Dec. 1981.

ENERGY AND NATURAL RESOURCES

Oil. Production (1989) 28m. tonnes.

Gas. Natural gas reserves, 1987, 1,400,000m. cu. metres. Production of LNG in 1988 was approximately 6·2m. tonnes, most of which was exported to Japan.

Minerals. Production (1986, in 1,000 tonnes): Bauxite, 566; iron ore, 208; copper, 115; tin, 29. Tin production was estimated at 31,000 tonnes in 1990.

Agriculture. Production (1988): Pineapples, 199,000 tonnes; tobacco leaves, 9,000 tonnes from 10,000 ha; cocoa, 220,000 tonnes from 233,000 ha; rubber, 1,612,000 tonnes; sugar-cane, 1·2m. tonnes from 19,000 ha; tea, 18,000 tonnes from 8,000 ha; coconuts, 1,186,000 tonnes; vegetables, 479,000 tonnes. Estimated production (1,000 tonnes) in 1990: Rubber, 1,500; palm oil, 6,500; cocoa, 260.

Livestock (1988): Cattle, 625,000, buffaloes, 220,000; sheep, 99,000; pigs, 2,258,000; goats, 347,000.

Forestry. In 1988 there were 19·6m. ha of forests, 60% of the land area; the total output of saw logs was 34·3m. cu. metres; sawn timber, 6·6m. cu. metres.

Fisheries. Total landings of marine fish, 1987, 515,000 tonnes.

INDUSTRY.

Production, 1989, provisional (1,000 tonnes): Rubber, 1,580; tin, 30; crude palm oil, 5,515; sawlogs, 35,400,000 cu. metres.

Labour. 1989: 6,287,700 were employed: 1,934,600 in agriculture, forestry and fishing; 1,065,900 in manufacturing; 852,700 in government services; 1,548,300 in other services; 38,300 in mining and quarrying; 361,800 in construction; 216,100 in finance, insurance, business services and real estate; 270,000 in transport, storage and communication. Unemployment was 8%.

Trade Unions. Membership was 617,000 in 1988, of which the Malaysian Trades Union Congress, an umbrella organization of 138 unions, accounted for 0·5m.

FOREIGN ECONOMIC RELATIONS.

Privatization policy permits foreign investment of 25–30%.

Commerce. In 1989 (provisional) exports totalled M$66,441m. and imports M$57,710m.

Chief imports (1989, provisional): Machinery and transport equipment,

M$26,352m.; manufactured goods, M$9,278m.; food, beverages and tobacco M$4,763m.; crude petroleum and related products, M$2,405m.

Chief exports (1989, provisional): Manufactured goods (M$36,350m.); crude petroleum (M$7,312m.); palm oil (M$4,473m.); rubber (M$4,320m.); saw logs (M$4,200m.); tin, M$1,173.

In 1988 imports (in M$1m.) came chiefly from Japan (10,170); USA (7,669) and Singapore (5,730). Exports went chiefly to Singapore (10,697), USA (9,611) and Japan (9,395).

Total trade of Malaysia with UK (British Department of Trade returns, in £1,000 sterling):

	1987	*1988*	*1989*	*1990*
Imports to UK	397,122	525,017	676,258	775,667
Exports and re-exports from UK	257,970	310,462	441,762	601,909

COMMUNICATIONS

Aviation. In 1989 there were 4 international airports and 15 other aerodromes at which regular public air transport was operated. About 20 international airlines operate through Kuala Lumpur linking Malaysia with the rest of the world. Malaysia Airlines, the national airline, operates domestic flights within Peninsular Malaysia as well as between Kuala Lumpur and Sabah and Sarawak, and flies to international destinations in Asia, Australia, Europe and the USA. In 1987 there were 204,155 landings and take-offs, carrying 5,445,610 passengers.

Shipping. The major ports are Port Kelang, Labuan, Pulau Pinang, Pasir Gudang, Kuantan, Kota Kinabalu, Sandakan, Kuching, Sibu and Bintulu. The Malaysian International Shipping Corporation operates a fleet of vessels (1,211,954 DWT).

Post and Telecommunications. Postal services are under the Ministry of Energy, Telecommunications and Post and are headed by a Director-General. There were 1·2m. telephone subscribers in 1988. As at 31 Dec. 1986, 525 post offices, 1,586 postal agencies, 236 mobile post offices and 1 riverine postal office were operating.

In 1987, 378,314 radio licences and 1,658,566 television licences were issued.

Newspapers. Papers are published in Malay (1,226,000 daily sales in 1984), English (830,000), Chinese (387,000) and Tamil (19,000). The national news agency Bernama has the sole right to receive and distribute news.

JUSTICE, RELIGION, EDUCATION AND WELFARE

Justice. By virtue of Art. 121(1) of the Federal Constitution judicial power in the Federation is vested on 2 High Courts of co-ordinate jurisdiction and status namely the High Court of Malaya and the High Court of Borneo, and the inferior courts. The Federal Court with its principal registry in Kuala Lumpur is the Supreme Court in the country.

The Lord President as the supreme head of the Judiciary, the 2 Chief Justices of the High Courts and 6 other Judges form the constitution of the Federal Court. Apart from having exclusive jurisdiction to determine appeals from the High Court the Federal Court is also conferred with such original and consultative jurisdiction as is laid out in Articles 128 and 130 of the Constitution.

A panel of 3 Judges or such greater uneven number as may be determined by the Lord President preside in every proceeding in the Federal Court.

The right of appeal to the Yang di-Pertuan Agong (who in turn refers the appeal to the Judicial Committee of the British Privy Council) from a decision of the Federal Court in respect of criminal and constitutional matters was abolished on 1 July 1978.

Religion. Islam is the official religion but there is freedom of worship.

Education. In 1988 there were 2,269,940 pupils enrolled in primary schools, 940,883 in lower secondary and 373,974 in upper secondary schools, 47,543 at pre-university level, 66,837 college students and 47,702 at university.

Health. In 1988 there were 6,274 private and government doctors, (1986) 1,130 dentists, 12,032 government nurses, 101 hospitals and 2,654 government clinics.

Social Security. The Employment Injury Insurance Scheme provides medical and cash benefits and the Invalidity Pension Scheme provides protection to employees against invalidity due to disease or injury from any cause. Other supplementary measures are the Employees' Provident Fund, the pension scheme for government employees, free medical benefits for all who are unable to pay and the provision of medical benefits particularly for workers under the Labour Code.

DIPLOMATIC REPRESENTATIVES

Of Malaysia in Great Britain (45 Belgrave Sq., London, SW1X 8QT)
High Commissioner: Tan Sri Dato Wan Sidek bin Haji Abdul Rahman.

Of Great Britain in Malaysia (185, Jalan Semantan, Ampang, Kuala Lumpur)
High Commissioner: Sir Nicholas Spreckley, KCVO, CMG.

Of Malaysia in the USA (2401 Massachusetts Ave., NW, Washington, D.C., 20008)
Ambassador: Albert S. Talalla.

Of the USA in Malaysia (376 Jalan Tun Razak, Kuala Lumpur)
Ambassador: Paul M. Cleveland.

Of Malaysia to the United Nations
Ambassador: Razali Ismail.

Further Reading

Statistical Information: The Department of Statistics, Malaysia, Kuala Lumpur, was set up in 1963, taking over from the Department of Statistics, States of Malaya. *Chief Statistician:* Khoo Teik Huat. Main publications: *Peninsular Malaysia Monthly* and *Annual Statistics of External Trade; Malaysia External Trade* (quarterly); *Peninsular Malaysia Statistical Bulletin* (monthly); *Rubber Statistics* (monthly); *Rubber Statistics Handbook* (annual); *Oil Palm Statistics* (monthly); *Oil Palm, Coconut and Tea Statistics* (annual). *Malaysia 1985,* The Department of Information, Kuala Lumpur, 1986

Anand, S., *Inequality and Poverty in Malaysia.* OUP, 1983
Brown, I. and Ampalavanar, R., *Malaysia.* [Bibliography] Oxford and Santa Barbara, 1986
Gullick, J., *Malaysia: Economic Expansion and National Unity.* Boulder and London, 1982
Jomo, K. S., *Growth and Structural Change in the Malaysian Economy.* London, 1990
Meerman, J., *Public Expenditure in Malaysia.* OUP, 1980
Snodgrass, D. R., *Inequality and Economic Development in Malaysia.* OUP, 1982
Zakaria, A., *Government and Politics in Malaysia.* OUP, 1987

PENINSULAR MALAYSIA

AREA AND POPULATION. The total area of Peninsular Malaysia is about 50,810 sq. miles (131,598 sq. km). Population (1990 estimate) 14,667,000. The federal capital is Kuala Lumpur (244 sq. km).

CONSTITUTION AND GOVERNMENT. The States of the Federation of Malaya, now known as Peninsular Malaysia, comprises the 11 States of Johor, Pahang, Negeri Sembilan, Selangor, Perak, Kedah, Perlis, Kelantan, Trengganu, Penang and Melaka.

For earlier history of the States and Settlements *see* THE STATESMAN'S YEAR-BOOK, 1957, p. 241.

The Constitution is based on the agreements reached at the London conference of Jan.-Feb. 1956, between HM Government in the UK, the Rulers of the Malay states and the Alliance Party (which at the first federal elections on 27 July 1955 obtained 51 of the 52 elected members), and subsequently worked out by the Constitutional Commission appointed after that conference.

ECONOMY

Budget. See p. 835.

ENERGY AND NATURAL RESOURCES

Electricity. In 1987, 16,287m. kwh. were generated. Supply 240 volts; 50 Hz.

Oil. Production (1987) 23·6m. tonnes of crude oil.

Minerals. Production (in tonnes): Tin-in-concentrates: 1986, 29,134; 1987, 30,388. Iron ore: 1986, 207,963; 1987, 161,287. Bauxite: 1986, 566,170; 1987, 482,125. Copper: 1986, 115,304; 1987, 122,206. Gold: 1986, 2,221 troy oz.; 1987, 2,716.

Agriculture. Production in 1986 (in tonnes): Rice (1985), 1,122,400 from (1986) 627,000 ha; rubber, 1·54m.; palm oil, 4·54m.; palm kernels, 1·34m.; cocoa, 102,000; coconuts, 33,900; (the following all 1985) copra, 216,000; vegetables, 481,000; fruit, 898,000; sugar-cane, 1·2m.; tea, 4,000; cassava, 370,000; sweet potatoes, 50,000; roots and tubers, 505,000; maize, 24,000.

Forestry (1984). Reserved forests, 4·7m. ha. Production of logs (1986), 30m. cu. metres; sawn timber, 5·15m. cu. metres; plywood (1984), 630,000 cu. metres.

Fisheries. Landings in 1983 493,117 tonnes. Fishermen (1985) 87,000; 70% offshore.

INDUSTRY AND TRADE

Trade Unions. There were, in 1987, 311 trade unions with 560,800 members in Peninsular Malaysia.

Tourism. In 1987 there were 3,285,166 tourists.

COMMUNICATIONS

Roads. In 1986 the Public Works Department maintained 39,915 km of roads. In 1985 the 8-mile road bridge between the mainland and Penang island opened.

In 1987, 4,591,472 motor vehicles were registered, including 1,475,760 private cars, 22,134 buses, 316,846 lorries and vans, 2,611,584 motor cycles.

Railways. The Malayan Railway main line runs from Singapore to Butterworth opposite Penang Island. From Bukit Mertajam 8 miles south of Butterworth a branch line connects Peninsular Malaysia with the State Railways of Thailand at the frontier station of Padang Besar. Other branch lines connect the main line with Port of Klang, Teluk Anson, Port Dickson and Ampang. The east-coast line, branching off the main line at Gemas, runs for over 300 miles to Tumpat, Kelantan's northernmost coastal town; a 13-mile branch line linking Pasir Mas with Sungei Golok makes a second connexion with Thailand.

In 1988 there were 1,672 km (metre gauge) which carried 7,300m. passenger-km and 4m. tonnes of freight.

Aviation (1985). International air services are operated into Kuala Lumpur, Johor and Penang airports. The national carrier, Malaysian Airlines System (MAS), began operation on 1 Oct. 1972 to provide both domestic and international services.

Civil aviation statistics for airports in Peninsular Malaysia (1984): Aircraft movements, 97,890; terminal passengers, 6,078,273; freight, 80,232 tonnes; mail, 7,163 tonnes.

Shipping. The major ports of Peninsular Malaysia are Port Kelang, Penang, Johor and Kuantan. In 1984 Port Kelang handled 12,357,262 tonnes of cargo valued at M$16,318·4m., of which imports totalled 7,744,789 tonnes (M$9,532·9m.) and exports 4,612,473 tonnes (M$6,785·5m.). A total of 4,630 ships, GRT 35m. tonnes, called in 1984. In 1984 the Port of Penang handled 7,960,506 tonnes of cargo, of which 5,220,550 tonnes were imports and 2,739,956 tonnes exports. The total cargo handled in all ports during 1984 was 31,986,000 tonnes.

JUSTICE, RELIGION, EDUCATION AND WELFARE

Justice. Unlike the Federal Court and the High Court which were established under the Constitution, the subordinate courts in Peninsular Malaysia comprising the sessions court, the Magistrates' court and the Penghulu's court were established under a Federal Law (the subordinate Courts Act, 1948 (Revised 1972)).

All offences other than those punishable with death are tried before a Sessions

Court President who is empowered to pass any sentence allowed by law other than the sentence of death. In civil matters, the sessions court has jurisdiction to hear all actions and suits where the amount in dispute does not exceed M$25,000.

A First Class Magistrate's criminal jurisdiction is limited to offences for which the maximum term provided by law does not exceed 10 years' imprisonment and to certain specified offences where the term of imprisonment provided for may be extended to 14 years' imprisonment or which are punishable with fine only.

Juvenile courts established under the Juvenile Courts Act, 1947 for juvenile offenders below the age of 18 are presided over by a First Class Magistrate assisted by 2 advisers. There are 30 penal institutions, including Borstal establishments and an open prison camp.

Religion. More than half the population are Moslems, and Islam is the official religion. In 1970 there were 4,673,670 Moslems, 765,250 Hindus, 220,897 Christians and 2,495,739 Buddhists.

Education. In 1987 there were 6,703 state assisted primary schools with 2,325,462 pupils and 103,983 teachers and in 1980, 208 private primary schools with 5,130 pupils and 224 teachers.

In 1986 there were 1,226 secondary schools with 1,329,399 pupils and 60,863 teachers.

There were (1980): 10 special schools with 1,312 pupils and 104 teachers; 401 classes for further education with 10,281 students and 997 teachers; 25 teacher training colleges with over 12,000 students.

In 1989–90 there were 11 institutions of higher education: Utara Malaysia University; University of Malaya, Kuala Lumpur; University of Kebangsaan, Bangi; International Islamic University; University of Science, Penang; University of Agriculture, Serdang; University of Technology, Kuala Lumpur; Ungku Omar Polytechnic, Ipoh; Kuantan Polytechnic; MARA Institute of Technology, Shah Alam; Tunku Ab. Rahman College, Kuala Lumpur.

Health. In 1987 there were 68 hospitals and 1,252 clinics. In 1983 there were 4,082 doctors, 774 dentists, 13,874 midwives and 17,916 nurses.

Further Reading

Morris, M. W., *Local Government in Peninsular Malaysia*. London, 1980
Wilkinson, R. J., *Malay-English Dictionary*. 2 vols. New ed. London, 1956
Winstedt, Sir R., *Malaya and Its History*. 3rd ed. London, 1953.—*An English–Malay Dictionary*. 3rd ed. Singapore, 1949.—*The Malays: A Cultural History*. London, 1959

SABAH

HISTORY. The territory now named Sabah, but until Sept. 1963 known as North Borneo, was in 1877-78 ceded by the Sultans of Brunei and Sulu and various other rulers to a British syndicate, which in 1881 was chartered as the British North Borneo (Chartered) Company. The Company's sovereign rights and assets were transferred to the Crown with effect from 15 July 1946. On that date, the island of Labuan (ceded to Britain in 1846 by the Sultan of Brunei) became part of the new Colony of North Borneo. On 16 Sept. 1963 North Borneo joined the new Federation of Malaysia and became the State of Sabah.

AREA AND POPULATION. Area, about 28,460 sq. miles (73,710 sq. km), with a coastline of 973 miles (1,577 km). The interior is mountainous, Mount Kinabalu being 13,455 ft (4,175 metres) high. Population, 1980 census 1,011,046, of whom 838,141 were Pribumis, 163,996 Chinese, 5,613 Indians, 3,296 others. The native population comprises Kadazans (largest and mainly agricultural, Christians since the 16th century), Bajaus and Bruneis (agriculture and fishing), Muruts (hill tribes), Suluks (mainly seafaring) and several smaller tribes (1989 estimate, 1,443,439). In 1990 there were some 350,000 Filipino and 150,000 Indonesian immigrants, mostly illegal.

The island of Labuan became Federal territory on 16 April 1984, 35 sq. miles (75 sq. km) in area, lying 6 miles (9·66 km) off the north-west coast of Borneo is a free port.

The principal towns are situated on or near the coast. They include Kota Kinabalu, the capital (formerly Jesselton), 1980 census population, 108,725, Tawau (113,708), Sandakan (113,496), Keningau in the hinterland (41,204), and Kudat (38,397).

CLIMATE. The climate is tropical monsoon, but on the whole is equable, with temperatures around 80°F (26·5°C) throughout the year. Annual rainfall varies, according to locality, from 10" (250 mm) to 148" (3,700 mm). The north-east monsoon lasts from Dec. to April and chiefly affects the east coast, while the south-west monsoon from May to Aug. gives the west coast its wet season.

CONSTITUTION AND GOVERNMENT. The Constitution of the State of Sabah provides for a Head of State, called the *Yang Dipertua Negeri Sabah*. Executive authority is vested in the State Cabinet headed by the Chief Minister.

At the elections of July 1990 the electorate was 0·49m. 253 candidates from 9 parties stood. The Bersatu Sabah Party (Christian) won 36 of the 48 electable seats; the United Sabah National Organization (mainly Moslem) won 12.

Head of State: Tan Seri Mohamad Said Keruak.
Chief Minister: Datuk Joseph Pairin Kitingan.
Deputy Chief Minister: Bernard Dompok.

Flag: Three horizontal stripes of blue, white and red with a large light blue canton bearing an outline of Mount Kinabalu in dark blue.

The Legislative Assembly consists of the Speaker, 48 elected members and not more than 6 nominated members.

The official language was English for a period of 10 years from Sept. 1963 but in Aug. 1973 Bahasa Malaysia was introduced and in 1974 was declared the official language. English is widely used especially for business.

ECONOMY

Budget. Budgets (not including the Federal Territory of Labuan) for calendar years, in M$1,000:

Ordinary Budget	*1985*	*1986*	*1987*	*1988*	*1989*
Revenue	1,156,431	1,099,475	1,411,509	2,037,913	1,743,998
Expenditure	1,037,226	1,017,981	1,061,724	1,715,387	1,740,731
Development Budget					
Revenue	202,861	219,067	183,680	333,574	426,665
Expenditure	239,231	206,510	212,710	306,325	409,202

Banking. There are branches of The Chartered Bank at Kota Kinabalu, Sandakan, Tawau, Labuan, Kudat, Tenom and Lahad Datu. The Hongkong and Shanghai Bank has branches at Kota Kinabalu, Sandakan, Labuan, Beaufort, Papar and Tawau. The Hock Hua Bank (S) has branches at Kota Kinabalu, Sandakan and Tawau. The Chung Khiaw Bank has branches at Kota Kinabalu, Tuaran and Sandakan. Malayan Banking Ltd has branches at Kota Kinabalu, Tawau, Semporna and Sandakan. United Overseas Bank and the Overseas Chinese Banking Corporation have each a branch at Kota Kinabalu. Bank Bumiputra Malaysia has branches at Kota Kinabalu. Lahad Datu, Sandakan and Keningau. Overseas Union Bank and the Development and Commercial Bank have each a branch at Sandakan. The Sabah Bank Berhad and Sabah Development Bank were established in Kota Kinabalu in 1979.

The National Savings Bank had (1989) M$45·7m. due to depositors. It also provides additional services to depositors including the granting of loans for housing.

COMMERCE. The main imports are machinery and transport equipment, manufactured goods and food. The main exports are crude oil, saw logs and sawn timber. Statistics for calendar years, in M$1,000:

	1985	*1986*	*1987*	*1988*	*1989*
Imports	4,037,766	3,432,768	3,604,801	4,127,769	5,344,688
Exports	5,546,967	4,967,423	6,477,242	6,809,728	7,640,191

Tourism. In 1989 54,731 tourists visited Sabah, excluding foreign visitors arriving via Peninsular Malaysia, Sarawak and Labuan.

COMMUNICATIONS

Roads (1989). There were 8,978 km of roads, of which 2,567 km were bitumen surfaced, 5,591 km gravel surfaced and 820 km of earth road. Work is in progress on a network of roads, notably the Kota Kinabalu-Sandakan and Sandakan-Lahad Datu road links.

Railways. A metre-gauge railway, 134 km, runs from Kota Kinabalu to Tenom in the interior. It carried 423,600 passengers and 133,300 tonnes of freight in 1989.

Aviation. External communications are provided from the international airport at Kota Kinabalu by Cathay Pacific Airways Ltd to Hong Kong; Malaysian Airways to Hong Kong, Manila, Brunei, Kuching, Singapore, Tokyo, Seoul and Kuala Lumpur; Brunei Airways to Brunei and Kuching and Philippine Airlines to Manila.

The total air traffic handled at Sabah airports during 1989 was 2,673,594 passengers, 23,385 tonnes of freight and 4,482 tonnes of mail.

Shipping (1989). Merchant shipping totalling 19,901,419 NRT used the ports, handling 20,522,971 tonnes of cargo.

Telecommunications. As at 31 Dec. 1989 there were 41 post offices, handling 375,140 parcels. There were 111,049 telephones on 31 Dec. 1989, and 85,548 television licences issued.

JUSTICE, EDUCATION AND WELFARE

Justice. Pursuant to the Subordinate Courts Ordinance (Cap. 20) (1951) Courts of a Magistrate of the First Class, Second Class and Third Class were established to adjudicate upon the administration of civil and criminal law. The civil jurisdiction of a First Class Magistrate is limited to cases where the amount in dispute does not exceed M$1,000. but provision is made for the Chief Justice to enlarge that jurisdiction to M$3,000. This has been established so as to confer this jurisdiction on all stipendiary magistrates. A Second Class Magistrate can only try suits where the amount involved does not exceed M$500 and a Third Class Magistrate where it does not exceed M$100.

The criminal jurisdiction of these Magistrates' Courts is limited to offences of a less serious nature although stipendiary magistrates have enhanced jurisdiction. There are no Juvenile Courts.

There are also Native Courts with jurisdiction to try cases arising from breach of native law and custom (including Moslem Law and custom) where all parties are natives or one of the party is a native (if the matter is a religious, matrimonial or sexual one). Appeals from Native Courts lie to a District Judge or a Native Court of Appeal presided over by a Judge.

In 1989, 3,144 convictions were obtained in 733 cases taken to court.

Education. In 1989, there were 228,789 primary and 110,244 secondary pupils. There are 971 primary schools (798 government, 161 grant-aided and 12 private), and 132 general secondary schools (82 government, 37 grant-aided and 13 private) throughout the State. There were 4 teacher-training colleges, with (1989) 2,345 students.

The Government also runs 6 vocational schools offering carpentry, motor mechanics, electrical installation, fitting/turning, radio and television and heavy plant fitting.

The Department of Education also runs further education classes in most towns and districts. The main medium of instruction in primary schools is Bahasa Malaysia although there are some Chinese medium primary schools. Secondary education is principally English but this is being replaced by Bahasa Malaysia.

Health. The principal diseases are septicaemia, pneumonia and cerebrovascular disease.

As at 31 Dec. 1989 there were 16 hospitals (2,799 beds) and 265 clinics. Sixty-five fixed dispensaries in outlying districts providing in-patient and out-patient care

are staffed by hospital assistants under the supervision of district medical officers. There is one mental hospital at Kota Kinabalu. There are 18 maternity and child health centres throughout the State.

Further Reading

Statistical Information: Director, Federal Department of Information, Kota Kinabalu.

Tregonning, K. G., *North Borneo.* HMSO, 1960

SARAWAK

HISTORY. The Government of part of the present territory was obtained on 24 Sept. 1841 by Sir James Brooke from the Sultan of Brunei. Various accessions were made between 1861 and 1905. In 1888 Sarawak was placed under British protection. On 16 Dec. 1941 Sarawak was occupied by the Japanese. After the liberation the Rajah took over his administration from the British military authorities on 15 April 1946. The Council Negeri, on 17 May 1946, authorized the Act of Cession to the British Crown by 19 to 16 votes, and the Rajah ceded Sarawak to the British Crown on 1 July 1946.

On 16 Sept. 1963 Sarawak joined the Federation of Malaysia.

AREA AND POPULATION. The area is about 48,050 sq. miles (124,449 sq. km), with a coastline of 450 miles and many navigable rivers.

The population at 1980 census was 1,307,582 (1989 estimate, 1,633,069, including 481,960 Ibans; 474,176 Chinese; 339,368 Malays; 136,741 Bidayuhs; 93,946 Melanaus; 88,260 other indigenous; 18,618 others).

The capital, Kuching City, is about 34 km inland, on the Sarawak River (1989 population: 157,000). The other major towns (with 1989 population) are Sibu, 128 km up the Rejang River, which is navigable by large steamers (114,000) and Miri, the headquarters of the Sarawak Shell Ltd (91,000).

CONSTITUTION AND GOVERNMENT. On 24 Sept. 1941 the Rajah began to rule through a constitution. Since 1855 two bodies, known as Majlis Mesyuarat Kerajaan Negeri (Supreme Council) and the Dewan Undangan Negeri (State Legislature), had been in existence. By the constitution of 1941 they were given, by the Rajah, powers roughly corresponding to those of a colonial executive council and legislative council respectively. Sarawak has retained a considerable measure of local autonomy in state affairs. The State or Legislature consists of 56 elected members and sits for 5 years unless sooner dissolved.

A ministerial system of government was introduced in 1963. The Chief Minister presides over the Supreme Council, which contains no more than 8 other Council Negeri members, all of whom are Ministers.

Elections to the State Legislature on 15 and 16 April 1987 returned 28 members of the Sarawak Barisan Nasional comprising the Party Pesaka Bumiputera Bersatu (PBB), the Sarawak United Peoples' Party and the Sarawak National Party.

Sarawak has 27 seats in the Malaysia House of Representatives and 6 seats in the Senate.

Sarawak has 9 divisions each under a Resident.

Head of State: Tun Datuk Patinggi Haji Ahmad Zaidi Adruce bin Muhammed Noor, SMN, SSM, DP, PNBS, Bintang Mahaputera Adipradana (Indonesia), PSLJ (Brunei).

Chief Minister: Datuk Patinggi Tan Sri Haji Abdul Taib Mahmud, DP, PSM, SPMJ, DGSM, PGDK, Kt. WE (Thailand) KOU (Korea), KEPN (Indonesia).

Deputy Chief Ministers: Datuk Amar Tan Sri Sim Kheng Hong, DA, PSM, PGDK, JMN. Datuk Amar Alfred Jabu Anak Numpang, DA, PNBS, KMN. *Environment and Tourism:* Datuk Amar James Wong Kim Min, DA, PNBS. *Infrastructure Development:* Datuk Amar Dr Wong Soon Kai, DA, PNBS, PBS. *Housing:* Datuk Celestine Ujang Anak Jilan, PNBS. *Industrial Development:* Abang Abdul Rahman Zohari bin Tun Datuk Abang Haji Openg, JBS. *Land Devel-*

opment: Datuk Adenan bin Haji Satem, JBS. *Special Functions:* Datuk Dr George Chan Hong Nam, KMN, PBS. *State Secretary:* Tan Sri Datuk Amar Haji Bujang Mohd. Nor, DA, PNBS, JSM, AMN. *Acting State Attorney-General:* Encik Abdul Hamid Mohammed Yusof, PPB. *State Financial Secretary:* Datuk Liang Kim Bang, PNBS, JBS, PPC, KMN.

The official language is Bahasa Malaysia. The use of English as official language in Sarawak was abolished in 1985.

Flag: Yellow with a diagonal stripe divided black over red charged with a yellow star of nine points.

ECONOMY

Planning. The revised fifth Malaysia 5-year development plan (1986-90) provided for Sarawak an expenditure of M$5,458·03m.; of this amount, 25·6% was allocated to energy and public utilities, 20·74% to transport and communication, 18·59% to agriculture and rural development and 10·43% to commerce, industry and urban development.

Budget. In 1990 State revenue was M$1,077,524,630.; expenditure, M$1,432,388,712. The revenue is mainly derived from royalties on oil, timber and gas.

Currency. The monetary unit is the Malaysian *ringgit*.

Banking. The National savings bank had 166,714 depositors in July 1988; the amount to their credit was M$75m. There are branches of Bank Negara Malaysia in Kuching, and branches of the Chartered Bank, the Hongkong & Shanghai Bank, Bank Bumiputera Malaysia, the Overseas Chinese Banking Corporation, the Malayan Bank.

Nine local banks have branches in major towns. Sibu is the centre for local commercial banking with Hock Hua Bank (established in 1951, 13 branches and assets of M$872·4m. in 1983) and Kwong Ming Bank (established in 1964, 8 branches and assets of M$170m. in 1983). Both are locally owned and have branches in Kuala Lumpur and other towns.

INDUSTRY AND TRADE

Industry. Industry includes petroleum and petroleum products, natural gas, timber and timber products and rubber. Emphasis is being given to the development of petro-chemical, timber-based and agro-based industries.

Commerce. The main exports in 1989 were: Saw logs, which accounted for 29·7% of the total, with 14,960,000 cu. metres, value M$2·67m.; liquefied natural gas, 22·9% of the total, with 6,629,000 cu. metres, value, M$2·1m.; crude petroleum, 22·5% of the total, with 5,792,000 tonnes, value M$2·03m.; petroleum products, 6·1% of the total, with 1,302,000 tonnes, value M$549,018; sawn timber, 2·2% of the total, with 27,900 cu. metres, value M$197,060. The major agricultural exports, which together accounted for M$355·9m. or 3·9% of the total in 1989, were pepper, cocoa beans, palm oil and rubber.

Total import value, 1989, M$4,756·9m.

Sarawak's major trading partners in 1989 were Japan (export, 45·5%; import, 15·7%), Peninsular Malaysia (export, 11·4%, import, 41·7%); Republic of Korea (export, 12·1%, import, 0·3%); Singapore (export, 10·9%, import, 0·6%); USA (export, 1·4%, import, 14·1%); Sabah (export, 5·8%, import, 1·2%).

Tourism. In 1989 there were 238,723 visitors.

COMMUNICATIONS

Roads. In 1988 there were 6,902 km of roads, consisting of 2,878 km of bitumen surfaced, 3,062 km of gravel or stone surfaced and 962 km of earth roads. There are no railways.

Aviation. There are daily Malaysian Airline System (MAS) B737 and Airbus flights between Kuching and Kuala Lumpur via Singapore, and also scheduled flights between Kuching, Brunei and Hong Kong. Major towns in Sarawak are linked up by internal air routes.

Shipping. In 1989 Sarawak ports handled a total of 27m. tonnes of cargo. Kuching wharf, operational since 1974, can accommodate vessels up to 15,000 tonnes. The Bintulu Port, the largest in the State, handled more than 11m. tonnes in 1989.

Telecommunications. There are 54 post offices, 18 mobile offices and 209 postal agencies. The Telecommunications department was privatized in 1986 and renamed Syarikat Telekoms Malaysia (STM). A telephone system with 65 automatic exchanges (86,000 telephones) covers the country. There are International Subscribers Dialling (ISD) links with 75 countries and Atur system was introduced in 1985. The government radio and television service had, in 1986, 245 electric radio, 28,693 battery radio and 92,739 TV registered receivers.

Newspapers (1989). There are 2 Malay bi-weekly, 3 English and 8 Chinese dailies. 1 Malay and 1 Iban monthly newspaper are published by the Government.

JUSTICE, RELIGION, EDUCATION AND WELFARE

Justice (1987). In Sarawak there are the High Court and the Subordinate Court. High Court cases go on appeal to the Supreme Court which sits in Sarawak and Sabah twice a year. The Subordinate Courts (Amendment) Act 1987 was extended to Sarawak on 2 Sept. 1987 in which the jurisdiction of the Sessions Court judges and magistrates of the First Class and Second Class was enhanced.

In 1986 a Syariah Court was established, and the Juvenile Court was extended to Sarawak.

Police. There is a Royal Malaysia Police, Sarawak Component, with a total establishment of about 9,000 regular officers and men.

Religion. There is a large Moslem population and many Buddhists. Islam is the national religion. There are Church of England, Roman Catholic, American Methodist, Seventh-day Adventist and Borneo Evangelical missions.

Education (1989). There were 1,266 government and government-aided primary schools with 226,542 pupils and 11,804 teachers, and 129 secondary schools with 125,071 pupils and 5,978 teachers. There were 3 teacher-training centres with 2,945 students and an agricultural university campus conducting pre-university courses. The MARA Institute of Technology campus, established in 1973, had 960 students in 1987 and offers 3-year courses leading to diploma in accountancy, stenography and business studies and a 6-month pre-commerce course.

The Kuching Polytechnic campus, established in 1985, has 211 students and offers 2 and 3-year courses leading to a diploma in accountancy and certificates in book-keeping, general mechanical, civil works, electronic and computer engineering and power engineering.

Health. In 1988 there were 17 government hospitals, 156 static and 119 travelling health centres, clinics and dispensaries, 155 public dental and school dental clinics and 165 maternal and child health centres. There were 358 doctors and 51 registered dentists.

Further Reading

Population and Housing Census of Malaysia, 1980. Dept. of Statistics, Kuala Lumpur
Sarawak Annual of Statistics. Dept. of Statistics, Kuching, 1981
Sarawak Annual External Trade Statistics. Dept. of Statistics, Kuching, 1982
1983 Sarawak Budget. Information Dept., Sarawak
Milne, R. S. and Ratnam, K. J., *Malaysia, New States in a New Nation: Political Development of Sarawak and Sabah in Malaysia.* London, 1974
Runciman, S., *The White Rajahs.* CUP, 1960
Scott, N. C., *Sea Dyak Dictionary.* Govt. Printing Office, Kuching, 1956

National Library: The Sarawak Central Library, Kuching.

MALDIVES

Capital: Malé
Population: 214,139 (1990)
GNP per capita: US$410 (1988)

Divehi Jumhuriya
(Republic of the Maldives)

HISTORY. The islands were under British protection from 1887 until complete independence was achieved on 26 July 1965. Maldives became a republic on 11 Nov. 1968. An attempted coup took place in Nov. 1988.

AREA AND POPULATION. The Republic of Maldives, some 400 miles to the south-west of Sri Lanka, consists of 1,200 low-lying (the highest point is 6 feet above sea-level) coral islands, grouped into 12 clearly defined clusters of atolls 202 are inhabited. Area 115 sq. miles (298 sq. km). According to the preliminary results of 1990 census, the population was 214,139. Males: 110,271. Females: 103,868. Capital, Malé (56,060).

CLIMATE. The islands are hot and humid, and affected by monsoons. Malé: Average temperature 81°F (27°C), annual rainfall 59" (1,500 mm).

CONSTITUTION AND GOVERNMENT. The President is elected every 5 years by universal adult suffrage. He is assisted by the Ministers' *Majlis*, a cabinet of ministers of his own choice whom he may dismiss at will. There is also a Citizens' *Majlis* (Parliament) which consists of 48 members, 8 of whom are nominated by the President and 40 directly elected (2 each from Malé and the 19 administrative districts) for a term of 5 years. There are no political parties.

President, Minister of Defence and National Security: Maumoon Abdul Gayoom (re-elected unopposed for a third term on 23 Sept. 1988).

In Feb. 1991, the Government consisted of: *Home Affairs and Sports:* Umar Zahir. *Education:* Abdulla Hameed. *Health and Welfare:* Abdul Sattar Moosa Didi. *Fisheries and Agriculture:* Abbas Ibrahim. *Tourism:* Ismail Shafeen. *Foreign Affairs:* Fathulla Jameel. *Atolls Administration and the Speaker:* Abdulla Jameel. *Trade and Industries:* Ahmed Mujuthaba. *Justice:* Mohamed Rasheed Ibrahim. *Public Works and Labour:* Abdulla Kamaludeen. *Minister at the President's Office:* Mohamed Zahir Hussain. *Attorney-General:* Ahmed Zahir.

There are 2 Ministers of State.

The official and spoken language is Divehi, which is akin to Elu or old Sinhalese.

National flag: Red with a green panel bearing a white crescent.

Local government: Maldives is divided into the capital and 19 other administrative districts, each under an appointed governor *(verin)* assisted by local chiefs *(katheebun)*, who are also appointed.

INTERNATIONAL RELATIONS

Membership. The Maldives is a member of the UN, the Commonwealth and the Colombo Plan.

ECONOMY

Budget. In 1989 revenue totalled 429·6m. rufiyaas and expenditure 598·4m. rufiyaas.

Currency. The unit of currency is the *rufiyaa* of 100 *laari*. There are notes of 2, 5, 10, 20, 50, 100, 500 *rufiyaa*. In March 1991, £1 = 18·22 *rufiyaa*; US$1 = 9·60 *rufiyaa*.

ENERGY AND NATURAL RESOURCES

Electricity. Production, 1990, 21·4m. kwh.

Minerals. Inshore coral mining has been banned as a measure against the encroachment of the sea.

Agriculture. The islands are covered with coconut palms and yield millet, cassava, yams, melons and other tropical fruit as well as coconut produce.

Production in 1989 included (in 1,000 tonnes): Coconuts, 12; copra, 2.

Fisheries. Catch, 1989, 71,200 tonnes.

INDUSTRY. The main industries are fishing, tourism, shipping, reedware, lacquerwork, coconut processing and garment manufacturing.

FOREIGN ECONOMIC RELATIONS

Commerce. In 1989 imports amounted to 1,963·54m. rufiyaas and exports to 381·36m. rufiyaas. Bonito ('Maldive fish') is the main export commodity. It is exported principally to Thailand, Singapore, Sri Lanka, Japan, and some European markets.

Total trade between the Republic of Maldives and UK (British Department of Trade returns, in £1,000 sterling):

	1986	*1987*	*1988*	*1989*	*1990*
Imports to UK	276	440	1,859	5,224	6,573
Exports and re-exports from UK	1,321	2,772	1,689	3,412	3,458

Tourism. Tourism is the major foreign currency earner. There were 158,488 visitors in 1989.

COMMUNICATIONS

Roads. In 1989 there were 509 cars, 2,388 motorbikes, 934 handcarts, 23,953 bicycles.

Aviation. There are direct flights from Colombo, Trivendram, Dubai, Karachi, Singapore, Paris and Zurich. In 1987, 2,975 aircraft, 292,903 passengers and 3,067,206 kg of freight were handled at Malé International Airport. There are 4 domestic airports. Air Maldives operates domestic flights only.

Shipping. The Maldives Shipping Line operated (1984) 32 vessels.

Telecommunications. There were (1989) 5,467 telephones. There is one AM and one FM radio station broadcasting. There were (1990) 26,201 radio receivers and 5,890 television sets.

Newspapers. There were (1989) 2 daily newspapers, 3 weekly and 8 monthly periodicals.

JUSTICE, RELIGION, EDUCATION AND WELFARE

Justice. Justice is based on the Islamic Shari'ah.

Religion. The State religion is Islam.

Education. Education is not compulsory. In 1987 there were 300 primary schools with 53,412 pupils and 1,134 teachers and 6 secondary schools with 1,313 students and 116 teachers. In 1989, there were 50 government schools (23,375 pupils) and 211 community and private schools (36,504 pupils).

Health. In 1989 there was a 94-bed hospital in Malé, 4 regional hospitals and 225 health centres. In 1987 there were 7 doctors, 1 dentist and 19 nurses.

DIPLOMATIC REPRESENTATIVES

Of Great Britain in the Republic of the Maldives
High Commissioner: D. A. S. Gladstone, CMG (resides in Colombo).

Of the Republic of the Maldives to the United Nations
Ambassador: Hussain Manikufaan.

Further Reading

Bell, H. C. P., *History, Archaeology and Epigraphy of the Maldive Islands.* Ceylon Govt. Press, Colombo, 1940

Bernini, F. and Corbin, G., *Maldives.* Turin, 1973

Forbes, A. D. W., *The Maldives.* [Bibliography] Oxford and Santa Barbara, 1989

MALI

Capital: Bamako
Population: 9·09m. (1989)
GNP per capita: US$230 (1988)

République du Mali

HISTORY. Annexed by France between 1881 and 1895, the region became the territory of French Sudan as a part of French West Africa. It became an autonomous state within the French Community on 24 Nov. 1958, and on 4 April 1959 joined with Senegal to form the Federation of Mali. The Federation achieved independence on 20 June 1960, but Senegal seceded on 22 Aug. and Mali proclaimed itself an independent republic on 22 Sept. The National Assembly was dissolved on 17 Jan. 1968 by President Modibo Keita, whose government was then overthrown by an Army coup on 19 Nov. 1968; power was assumed by a Military Committee for National Liberation led by Lieut. (now General) Moussa Traoré, who became President on 19 Sept. 1969.

AREA AND POPULATION. Mali is a landlocked state, consisting of the Middle and Upper Niger basin in the south, the Upper Senegal basin in the south-west, and the Sahara in the north. It is bounded west by Senegal, north-west by Mauritania, north-east by Algeria, east by Niger and south by Burkina Faso, Côte d'Ivoire and Guinea. The republic covers an area of 1,240,192 sq. km (478,841 sq. miles) and had a population of 7,620,225 at the 1987 Census; estimate (1989) 9,092,000. In 1985, 21% lived in urban areas.

The areas, populations and chief towns of the regions are:

Region	*Sq. km*	*Census 1987*	*Chief town*	*Census 1976*
Kayes	197,760	1,058,575	Kayes	44,736
Koulikoro	89,833	1,180,260	Koulikoro	16,876
Capital District	267	646,153	Bamako	404,022
Sikasso	76,480	1,308,828	Sikasso	47,030
Ségou	56,127	1,328,250	Ségou	64,890
Mopti	88,752	1,261,383	Mopti	53,885
Tombouctou	408,977	453,032	Tombouctou	20,483
Gao	321,996	383,734	Gao	30,714

The various indigenous languages belong chiefly to the Mande group; of these the principal are Bambara (spoken by 60% of the population), Soninké, Malinké and Dogon; non-Mande languages include Fulani, Songhai, Senufo and Tuareg. The official language is French.

CLIMATE. A tropical climate, with adequate rain in the south and west, but conditions become increasingly arid towards the north and east. Bamako. Jan. 76°F (24·4°C), July 80°F (26·7°C). Annual rainfall 45" (1,120 mm). Kayes. Jan. 76°F (24·4°C), July 93°F (33·9°C). Annual rainfall 29" (725 mm). Tombouctou. Jan. 71°F (21·7°C), July 90°F (32·2°C). Annual rainfall 9" (231 mm).

CONSTITUTION AND GOVERNMENT. A new constitution was announced on 26 April 1974 and approved by a national referendum on 2 June; it was amended by the National Assembly on 2 Sept. 1981. The sole legal party is the *Union démocratique du peuple malien* (UDPM), formally constituted on 30 March 1979 and governed by a 17-member Central Executive Bureau responsible to a 137-member National Council who nominate all candidates for election.

The President is directly elected for a term of 6 years. The 82-member National Assembly is also directly elected, for a term of 3 years. Elections were held on 26 June 1988.

The Council of Ministers in Sept. 1990 comprised:

President, Head of Government, Minister of National Defence: Gen. Moussa Traoré (assumed office Sept. 1969, re-elected June 1985).

Secretary-General to the Presidency: Diango Cissoko. *Public Health and Social Affairs:* Abdoulaye Diallo. *Foreign Affairs and International Co-operation:* Ngolo Traoré. *National Education:* Gen. Sékou Ly. *Transport and Tourism:* Zeini Moulaye. *Planning:* Souleymane Dembele. *Agriculture:* Moulaye Mohammed Haidara. *Environment and Animal Husbandry:* Morifing Kone. *Industry, Water Affairs and Energy:* Amadou Deme. *Public Works, Housing and Construction:* Cheikh Oumar Doumbia. *Territorial Administration and Basic Development:* Col. Issa Ongoiba. *Employment and Civil Service:* Diallo Lalla Sy. *Justice:* Mamadou Sissoko. *Information and Telecommunications:* Niamanto Diarra. *Finance and Trade:* Tiena Coulibaly. *Sports, Art and Culture:* Bakary Traoré. *Minister-Delegate for National Defence:* Gen. Abdoulaye Ouologuem.

National flag: Three vertical stripes of green, yellow, red.

Local Government: Mali is divided into the Capital District of Bamako and 7 regions, sub-divided into 46 *cercles* and then into 279 *arrondissements*.

DEFENCE. There is a selective system of 2 years' military service.

Army. The Army consists of 4 infantry battalions, 2 tank, 1 engineer, 1 parachute, 1 special force, 2 artillery battalions and support units. Equipment includes 21 T-34 tanks. Strength (1991) 6,900. There are also paramilitary forces of 7,800 men.

Air Force. The Air Force has 3 MiG-17 jet fighters, 1 MiG-15UTI jet trainer, some Yak-18 piston-engined trainers, 2 An-24, 2 An-26 and 2 An-2 transports, and 3 Mi-8 and Mi-4 helicopters from USSR. A twin-turbofan Corvette is used for VIP transport. Personnel (1991) total about 400, with 26 combat aircraft.

INTERNATIONAL RELATIONS

Membership. Mali is a member of the UN, OAU and is an ACP state of the EEC.

ECONOMY

Budget. The budget for 1988 provided for revenue of 112,100m. francs CFA and expenditure of 146,500m. francs CFA.

Currency. Mali introduced its own currency, the *Mali franc,* in July 1962 but reverted to the *franc CFA* on 1 June 1984 at a rate of 2 *Mali francs* to 1 *franc CFA*. There are coins of 1, 2, 5, 10, 25, 50 and 100 *francs CFA*, and notes of 50, 100, 500, 1,000, 5,000 and 10,000 *francs CFA*.

Banking. The *Banque Centrale du Mali* (founded in 1968) is the bank of issue. There are 4 domestic and 2 French-owned banks.

ENERGY AND NATURAL RESOURCES

Electricity. Production (1986) totalled 161m. kwh. Supply 220 volts; 50 Hz.

Minerals. Mineral resources are limited, but marble (at Bafoulabé) and limestone (at Diamou) are being extracted in the Upper Senegal valley; iron ore deposits in this area await development. Salt is mined at Taoudenni in the far north (4,500 tonnes in 1986) and phosphates at Bouren (10,000 tonnes).

Agriculture. Production in 1988 included (in 1,000 tonnes): Millet, 1,900; sugar-cane, 220; groundnuts, 60; rice, 289; maize, 211; seed cotton, 187; cotton lint, 71; cassava, 73; sweet potatoes, 57.

Livestock, 1988: Cattle, 4,738,000; horses, 62,000; asses, 550,000; sheep, 5·5m.; goats, 5·5m.; camels, 241,000; chickens, 19m.

Forestry. Production (1986) 5·05m. cu. metres. 7% of the land is forested.

Fisheries. In 1986 60,000 tonnes of fish were caught in the rivers.

FOREIGN ECONOMIC RELATIONS

Commerce. Exports in 1985 totalled 77,200m. francs CFA. Chief imports are foodstuffs, automobiles, petrol, building material, sugar, salt and beer. France and Côte d'Ivoire are the main sources of imports. Cotton formed 41% of exports and livestock in 1983; 25% went to Belgium and 16% to France.

Total trade between Mali and UK (British Department of Trade returns, in £1,000 sterling):

	1986	*1987*	*1988*	*1989*	*1990*
Imports to UK	8,282	6,937	2,240	2,305	1,835
Exports and re-exports from UK	4,121	5,573	12,732	7,102	8,819

Tourism. There were 54,000 foreign tourists in 1986.

COMMUNICATIONS

Roads. There were (1985) 15,700 km of roads, 23,209 passenger cars and 6,802 commercial vehicles.

Railways. Mali has a railway from Kayes to Koulikoro by way of Bamako, a continuation of the Dakar–Kayes line in Senegal. Total length 642 km (metre-gauge) and in 1986 carried 756,000 passengers and 503,000 tonnes of freight.

Aviation. Air services connect the republic with Paris, Dakar and Abidjan. There are international airports at Bamako and Mopti, and Air Mali operates domestic services to 10 other airports.

Shipping. For about 7 months in the year small steamboats perform the service from Koulikoro to Tombouctou and Gao, and from Bamako to Kouroussa.

Telecommunications. There were, in 1984, 9,537 telephones and (1986) 300,000 radio and 1,000 television receivers.

JUSTICE, RELIGION, EDUCATION AND WELFARE

Justice. The Supreme Court was established at Bamako in 1969 with both judicial and administrative powers. The Court of Appeal is also at Bamako, at the apex of a system of regional tribunals and local *juges de paix*.

Religion. In 1983, 90% of the population were Sunni Moslems, 9% animists and 1% Christians.

Education. In 1982–83 there were 364,382 pupils and 10,912 teachers in 1,558 primary and intermediate schools, 13,227 pupils and 890 teachers in 20 senior schools, 12,612 students in 11 technical schools. There were 5,792 students and 491 teaching staff in 7 higher educational establishments in 1979.

Health. In 1980 there were 12 hospitals, 327 health centres and 445 dispensaries, with a total of 3,200 beds; there were 319 doctors, 18 surgeons, 14 dentists (1978), 24 pharmacists (1978), 250 midwives and 1,312 nursing personnel.

DIPLOMATIC REPRESENTATIVES

Of Mali in Great Britain (resides in Brussels)
Ambassador: Lamine Keita (accredited 18 Feb. 1988).

Of Great Britain in Mali
Ambassador: R. C. Beetham, LVO (resides in Dakar).

Of Mali in the USA (2130 R. St., NW, Washington, D.C., 20008)
Ambassador: Mohamed Alhousseyni Toure.

Of the USA in Mali (Rue Testard and Rue Mohamed V, Bamako)
Ambassador: Robert M. Pringle.

Of Mali to the United Nations
Ambassador: Noumou Diakite.

MALTA

Capital: Valletta
Population: 354,900 (1990)
GNP per capita: US$5,153 (1989)

Repubblika ta' Malta

HISTORY. Malta was held in turn by Phoenicians, Carthaginians and Romans, and was conquered by Arabs in 870. From 1090 it was subject to the same rulers as Sicily until 1530, when it was handed over to the Knights of St John, who ruled until dispersed by Napoleon in 1798. The Maltese rose in rebellion against the French and the island was subsequently blockaded by the British aided by the Maltese from 1798 to 1800. The Maltese people freely requested the protection of the British Crown in 1802 on condition that their rights and privileges be preserved. The islands were finally annexed to the British Crown by the Treaty of Paris in 1814.

On 15 April 1942, in recognition of the steadfastness and fortitude of the people of Malta during the Second World War, King George VI awarded the George Cross to the island.

Malta became independent on 21 Sept. 1964 and became a republic within the Commonwealth on 13 Dec. 1974. For earlier constitutional and government history *see* THE STATESMAN'S YEAR-BOOK, 1980–81, p. 837.

In 1971 Malta began to follow a policy of non-alignment and closed the NATO base. In March 1972 agreement was reached on the phasing out of the British Military base which was closed down completely on 31 March 1979.

AREA AND POPULATION. The area of Malta is 246 sq. km (94·9 sq. miles); Gozo, 67 sq. km (25·9 sq. miles); Comino, 3 sq. km (1·1 sq. miles); total area, 316 sq. km (121·9 sq. miles). Population, census 16 Nov. 1985, 345,418; estimate (1990) 354,900. Malta island (1988), 323,530; Gozo and Comino, 25,484. Chief town and port, Valletta, population 9,210 but the urban harbour area, 101,210.

Vital statistics, 1989, estimate: Births, 5,584; deaths, 2,610; marriages, 2,531; emigrants, 399; returned emigrants, 722.

CLIMATE. The climate is Mediterranean, with hot, dry and sunny conditions in summer and very little rain from May to Aug. Rainfall is not excessive and falls mainly between Oct. and March. Average daily sunshine in winter is 6 hours and in summer over 10 hours. Valletta. Jan. 55°F (12·8°C), July 78°F (25·6°C). Annual rainfall 23" (578 mm).

CONSTITUTION AND GOVERNMENT. Malta is a democracy. The Constitution provides for a *President* of the Republic, a *House of Representatives* of elected members and a Cabinet consisting of the Prime Minister and such number of Ministers as may be appointed. The Constitution, which is founded on work, makes provision for the protection of fundamental rights and freedom of the individual, and for freedom of conscience and religious worship. In Jan. 1987 the 2 political parties agreed to amend the Constitution to provide that any political party winning more than 50% of all valid votes (but less than 50% of elected members) shall have the number of its members increased in order to have a majority in the House of Representatives. Elections were held in May 1987 in which the Nationalist Party obtained 50·91% of the votes but fewer seats than the Malta Labour Party. As a result of the above Amendment the Nationalist Party now commands a majority with 35 seats to the MLP 34 seats.

Maltese and English are the official languages.

Elections were held on 9 May 1987. State of parties on 31 Dec. 1988: Nationalist Party, 35; Malta Labour Party, 34.

President: Dr Censu Tabone (sworn in April 1989).

The Cabinet (Nationalist Party) was as at Feb. 1991:

Prime Minister: Dr Edward Fenech-Adami.

Deputy Prime Minister, Minister of Foreign Affairs and Justice: Dr Guido de Marco. *Education and the Interior:* Dr Ugo Mifsud-Bonnici. *Social Policy:* Dr Louis Galea. *Finance:* Dr George Bonello Dupuis. *Development of Infrastructure:* Michael Falzon. *Agriculture and Fisheries:* Lawrence Gatt. *Development of Tertiary Sector:* Dr Emmanuel Bonnici. *Gozo:* Anton Tabone. *Economic Affairs:* John Dalli.

National flag: Vertically white and red, with a representation of the George Cross medal in the canton.

DEFENCE. The Armed Forces of Malta in 1991 totalled 1,500 and are organized into 2 regiments, comprising 1 infantry company, 1 airport company, 1 engineer company, 1 general duties company and 1 air defence battery. There is a Helicopter Flight equipped with 4 Augusta Bell 47G light helicopters and 1 AB206A Jet Ranger. The Marine Squadron in 1990 operated 5 inshore patrol craft and a number of boats.

INTERNATIONAL RELATIONS

Membership. Malta is a member of the UN, the Commonwealth and the Council of Europe.

ECONOMY

Policy. After a lengthy commitment to state ownership, overall policy now is to dispose of government shareholdings in non-strategic sectors as rapidly as possible. National economic strategy aims especially at the attraction of new investment and the creation of new employment in the directly productive and market services (tertiary) sectors as a means of stimulating export-oriented growth. The objective is to promote the location in Malta of new manufacturing industry with higher skill production, develop the island as an offshore financial centre, and enter the EEC as a full member under suitable conditions. With this in mind an industrial incentive package has been announced, and a scheme introduced for the retraining of workers for productive employment in the private sector. Besides manufacturing (food, clothing, chemicals and electrical machinery parts), ship repair and shipbuilding and tourism are the mainstays of the economy.

Budget. Revenue and expenditure (in Lm):

	1986	*1987*	*1988*	*1989*
Revenue	225,853,367	221,160,214	308,747,572	291,779,385
Expenditure	240,463,682	263,619,931	274,003,588	320,743,721

The most important sources of revenue are customs and excise duties, income tax, social security and receipts from the Central Bank of Malta.

Currency. The unit of currency is the *Maltese pound* (MTP) of 100 *cents* of 10 *mils*. Central Bank of Malta notes of Lm2, Lm5, Lm10 and Lm20 denominations are in circulation. Malta coins are issued in the following denominations: Lm1, 50, 25, 10, 5, 2 and 1 cents; 5, 3 and 2 *mils*. Total notes and coins in circulation on 31 Oct. 1990, Lm328·8m. In March 1991, £1 sterling = Lm 0·58; US$1 = Lm 0·30.

Banking and Finance. The Central Bank of Malta was founded in 1968. Commercial banking facilities are provided by Bank of Valletta Ltd, Lombard Bank (Malta) Ltd and MidMed Bank Ltd. The other domestic banking institutions are the Investment Finance Bank (long-term industrial loans), the Apostleship of Prayer Savings Bank Ltd, Lohombus Corporation Ltd (house mortgage) and Melita Bank International Ltd (offshore bank).

Malta is developing as a financial and offshore trading centre. The Malta International Business Authority (founded June 1989) had 300 foreign companies registered with it in 1991.

ENERGY AND NATURAL RESOURCES

Electricity. Electricity is generated at 2 interconnected power stations located at Marsa, having a total available generating capacity of 286 mw. The larger station with an installed capacity of 235 mw is also equipped to produce potable water as a co-generation process. Supply 240 volts; 50 Hz.

The gross electricity generated in 1988–89 was 1,095m. kwh.

Oil. The government announced a new offshore exploration campaign in March 1988 and a number of companies were (1991) awarded contracts by the government for the exploration of certain offshore blocks.

Agriculture. In 1989 agriculture and fisheries contributed Lm22·2m. to the Gross Domestic Product as against Lm21·1m. in 1988. (The 1989 figure represents a share of 3·7% in the GDP.) Some 37% of the total land area was arable in 1991 (44% in 1979). In 1989 agriculture employed 2,812 full-timers. A further 13,000 workers were estimated to be engaged in part-time farm work.

In 1989 the value of Malta's main agricultural exports reached Lm1·6m. The 1989 exports consisted mainly of: Potatoes, Lm879,687; seeds, cut-flowers and plants, Lm320,376; vegetables, 103,786; wine, Lm32,798; hides, Lm96,698.

Livestock (1990): Cattle, 21,330; pigs, 61,970; sheep, 5,945; goats 5,094; poultry, 1,612,512.

Fisheries. In 1989 the fishing industry employed 1,164 power propelled and 42 other fishing boats, engaging 227 full-time and 1,021 part-time fishermen. The catch in 1989 was 819 tonnes valued at Lm853,799.

INDUSTRY.

Over 300 state-aided manufacturing enterprises are in operation in various industrial sectors, of which the majority are foreign-owned or have foreign interests. The Malta Development Corporation is the Government agency responsible for promoting and implementing new industrial projects.

Labour. The total labour force in Sept. 1990 was 132,879 (females, 33,439), distributed as follows: Agriculture and fisheries, 3,240; manufacturing, 32,089; building, construction and quarrying, 6,558; services, 43,814; electricity, gas and drydocks, 5,936; government, 31,577; training scheme and auxiliary workers, 3,945. Unemployment was 5,720 in Sept. 1990.

Trade Unions. There were 29 trade unions registered as at 5 Dec. 1990, with a total membership of 66,666 and 21 employers' associations with a total membership of 5,799.

FOREIGN ECONOMIC RELATIONS.

Imports are being gradually liberallzed, and plans are under way to turn Marsaxlokk all weather port into a free port zone for transhipment activities.

Commerce. Imports and exports including bullion and specie (in Lm1,000):

	1984	*1985*	*1986*	*1987*	*1988*	*1989*
Imports	330,489	354,139	347,909	392,874	447,431	515,805
Exports	181,364	187,099	194,668	208,590	235,920	294,405

In 1989 the principal items of imports were: Semi-manufactures, Lm114·8m.; machinery and transport, Lm208·4m.; food, Lm53·4m.; fuels, Lm32·6m.; manufactures, Lm47·1m.; chemicals, Lm36·1m.; others, Lm23·9m. Of domestic exports: Manufactures, Lm95·6m.; machinery and transport, Lm137m.; semi-manufactures, Lm28m.; beverages and tobacco, Lm2·1m.; food, Lm5·1m.; chemicals, Lm3m.

In 1988, Lm99·7m. of the imports came from Italy, Lm79·9m. from UK, Lm66·2m. from Federal Republic of Germany, Lm42·7m. from USA, Lm36·5m. from Asia, Lm13·8m. from the EFTA, Lm14·6m. from Africa, Lm1·8m. from Australia/Oceania, Lm29·1m. from other European countries; of domestic exports, Lm61·2m. to Federal Republic of Germany, Lm61·2m. to UK, Lm40m. to Italy, Lm15m. to Africa, Lm12·2m. to Asia, Lm25·8m. to USA, Lm3·8m. to EFTA and Lm4·9m. to other European countries.

Total trade between Malta and UK (British Department of Trade returns, in £1,000 sterling):

	1986	*1987*	*1988*	*1989*	*1990*
Imports to UK	49,197	52,105	40,189	42,194	50,541
Exports and re-exports from UK	101,877	107,941	121,696	132,287	141,298

Tourism. Tourism is the major foreign currency earner. In 1989 828,311 tourists (59·5% from the UK) produced earnings of Lm135m. Estimated number of tourists in 1990 was 864,000.

COMMUNICATIONS

Roads. Every town and village is served by motor omnibuses. There are ferry services running between Malta and Gozo; cars can be transported on the ferries. In 1990 there were 1,405 km of roads. Motor vehicles registered at 31 Dec. 1990 totalled 139,316, of which 104,863 were private cars, 4,268 hire cars, 21,870 commercial vehicles, 630 buses and minibuses and 7,685 motor cycles.

Aviation. In 1988 the main scheduled airlines, Air Malta, Alitalia, British Airways, Corse Air, Interflug, JAT, KLM, Lufthansa, Libyan Arab Airlines, Balkan Bulgarian Airlines, Czechoslovakian Airlines, Austrian Airlines, Swissair, Aeroflot and Tunisavia, operated scheduled services between Malta and UK, German Democratic Republic, Federal Republic of Germany, France, Italy, Libya, Netherlands, Switzerland, Yugoslavia, Bulgaria, Czechoslovakia, Austria, USSR, Tunisia, Greece and Hungary. In 1990 there were 18,805 civil aircraft movements at Luqa Airport (Valletta). 1,751,897 passengers, 6,792 tonnes of freight and 604 tonnes of mail were handled.

Shipping. The number of yachts and ships registered in Malta on 31 Dec. 1989 was 1,026; 4,347,593 GRT. Ships entering harbour, excluding yachts and fishing vessels, during 1989, 2,469. In 1991 3m. tonnes of international shipping was registered in Malta.

Telecommunications. Telephone services are administered by Telemalta Corporation with exchanges at Malta and Gozo. On 30 Sept. 1990 there were 177,093 telephones, 143,107 television sets and (31 Dec. 1988) 27,226 radio sets.

Cinemas (1989). There were 11 cinemas with a seating capacity of 7,000.

Newspapers. There were (1989) 1 English, 2 Maltese daily newspapers and 7 weekly papers.

JUSTICE, RELIGION, EDUCATION AND WELFARE

Justice. The number of persons convicted of crimes in 1989 was 1,086; those convicted for contraventions against various laws and regulations numbered 4,832. 95 were committed to prison and 5,825 were awarded fines.

Police. On 31 Dec. 1990 police numbered 88 officers and 1,533 other ranks, including 132 women police.

Religion. The majority of the population (98%) belong to the Roman Catholic Church.

Education. Education in Malta is compulsory between the ages of 5 and 16 and free in government schools. Kindergarten education is provided for 3- and 4-year old children. The primary level enrols children between 5 and 11 years in a 6-year course. In 1989, there were 25,142 children (13,095 boys and 12,047 girls) in 80 primary schools. Another 1,306 pupils were enrolled in preparatory (secondary) classes and classes for weaker pupils. Eight Junior Lyceums (6 in Malta and 2 in Gozo) had a total of 8,044 students (3,171 boys, 4,873 girls). There were 28 other secondary schools with a total of 12,427 (6,717 boys, 5,710 girls). Secondary schools run 5-year courses leading to GCE 'O' level. Two-year GCE 'A' level courses leading to university entrance, during which students are paid an allowance and expected to gain work experience, are offered by the New Lyceums, *i.e.* upper secondary schools (2 in Malta and 1 in Gozo, with a total of 1,831 students). A higher Secondary School catering for students at GCE 'O' and 'A' level enrolled 736 students. Enrolment in vocational and technician courses in 3 technical institutes and 5 specialized training centres was 900. Trade schools provide a technical and vocational education at craft level and are open to students who finish their second year of secondary education. Extended skills training schemes are also available for trade school graduates. The number of students of all ages in special education was 441.

There were 80 private schools with a population of 4,385 at the nursery level, 10,200 at the primary level and 6,500 at the secondary level.

About 5,000 students attended evening courses in academic, commercial, technical and practical subjects established in various centres. Other schools run on a mainly part-time basis by the Education Department for adult students are the School of Art, the School of Music and the School of Art and Design.

The University of Malta consists of 10 faculties: Law; Medicine and Surgery; Architecture and Civil Engineering; Dental Surgery; Education; Economics, Management and Accountancy; Mechanical and Electrical Engineering; Theology; Arts; Science. There were 2,209 full-time students in 1989–90.

Social Security. The Social Security Act, 1987, provides cash benefits for marriage, maternity, sickness, unemployment, widowhood, orphanhood, invalidity, old age, children's allowances and industrial injuries.

The total number of persons in receipt of benefits on 31 Dec. 1990 was 158,638, viz., 503 in receipt of sickness benefit, 479 unemployment benefit, 298 special unemployment benefit, 96 injury benefit, 334 disablement benefit, 92 death benefit, 24,562 retirement pensions, 10,110 widows' pensions, 8 widows' special allowance, 9 orphan's allowance, 4,485 invalidity pensions, 51,184 children's allowances and 493 maternity benefit, 14,123 parental allowance and 51,859 family bonus.

The Act further provides for the payment of social assistance, medical assistance and non-contributory pensions to persons over 60 years of age, to blind persons over the age of 14 years and to handicapped persons over the age of 16 years.

The number of households in receipt of social assistance and of medical assistance on 31 Dec. 1990 was 7,685 and 8,976 respectively, and the number of pensioners in receipt of a non-contributory pension was 4,921.

Health. In 1990 there were 785 doctors, 98 dentists, 390 pharmacists, 264 midwives, 3,879 nursing personnel and 6 hospitals with 3,266 beds.

DIPLOMATIC REPRESENTATIVES

Of Malta in Great Britain (16 Kensington Sq., London, W8 5HH)
High Commissioner: Victor Camilleri.

Of Great Britain in Malta (7 St Anne St., Floriana)
High Commissioner: Brian Hitch, CMG, CVO.

Of Malta in the USA (2017 Connecticut Ave., NW, Washington, D.C., 20008)
Ambassador: Salvino J. Stellini.

Of the USA in Malta (Development Hse., St Anne St., Floriana)
Ambassador: Sally J. Novetzke.

Of Malta to the United Nations
Ambassador: Dr Alexander Borg Olivier.

Further Reading

Statistical Information: The Central Office of Statistics (Auberge d'Italie, Valletta) was set up in 1947. It publishes *Statistical Abstracts of the Maltese Islands*, a quarterly digest of statistics, quarterly and annual trade returns, annual vital statistics and annual publications on shipping and aviation, education, agriculture, industry, National Accounts and Balance of Payments.

Government publications: Department of Information (Auberge de Castille, Malta), set up in 1955, publishes *The Malta Government Gazette*, *Malta Information*, *Economic Survey 1990*, *Reports on the Working of Government Departments for the year 1989*, *Malta: Weekly Review of the Press, Report on the Organisation of the Public Service, Acts of Parliament and Subsidiary Legislation for the year 1989, Laws of Malta.*

Annual Reports. Central Bank of Malta
Trade Directory. Chamber of Commerce (annual)
The Year Book. Sliema (annual)
Malta Independence Constitution (Cmnd 2406). HMSO, 1964
Constitution of the Republic of Malta. Department of Information, 1975
Made in Malta. METCO, 1991
Blouet, B., *The Story of Malta.* London, Rev. ed. 1981
Cremona, J. J., *The Malta Constitution of 1835 and its Historical Background.* Malta, 1959.—*The Constitutional Developments of Malta under British Rule.* Malta Univ. Press, 1963.—*Human Rights Documentation in Malta.* Malta Univ. Press, 1966
Gerada, E. and Zuber, C., *Malta: An Island Republic.* Paris, 1979
Price, G. A., *Malta and the Maltese: A Study in 19th-century Migration.* Melbourne, 1954
Thackrah, J. R., *Malta.* [Bibliography] Oxford and Santa Barbara, 1985

MAURITANIA

Capital: Nouakchott
Population: 1·97m. (1989)
GNP per capita: US$480 (1988)

République Islamique de Mauritanie

HISTORY. Mauritania became a French protectorate in 1903 and a colony in 1920. It became an autonomous republic within the French Community on 28 Nov. 1958 and achieved full independence on 28 Nov. 1960. Under its first President, Moktar Ould Daddah, Mauritania became a one-party state in 1964, but following his deposition by a military coup flon 10 July 1978, the ruling *Parti du peuple mauritanien* was dissolved.

Following the Spanish withdrawal from Western Sahara on 28 Feb. 1976, Mauritania occupied the southern part (88,667 sq. km) of this territory and incorporated it under the name of Tiris el Gharbia. In Aug. 1979 Mauritania renounced sovereignty and withdrew from Tiris el Gharbia.

Following the *coup* of 10 July 1978, power was placed in the hands of a Military Committee for National Recovery (CMRN); the constitution was suspended and the 70-member National Assembly dissolved. On 6 April 1979 the CMRN was renamed the Military Committee for National Salvation (CMSN).

AREA AND POPULATION. Mauritania is bounded west by the Atlantic ocean, north by Western Sahara, north-east by Algeria, east and south-east by Mali, and south by Senegal. The total area is 1,030,700 sq. km (398,000 sq. miles) of which 47% is desert, and the population at the Census of 1976 was 1,419,939 including 12,897 in Tiris el Gharbia; latest estimate (1989) 1,969,000. The capital Nouakchott had a population of over 500,000 in 1985; other towns (1976) were Nouâdhibou (21,961), Kaédi (20,848), Zouérate (17,474), Rosso (16,466) and Atâr (16,326).

The areas and populations of the Capital District and 12 Regions are:

Region	*Sq. km*	*Estimate 1982*	*Region*	*Sq. km*	*Estimate 1982*
Nouakchott District	120	150,000	Adrar	215,300	60,000
Hodh ech-Chargui	182,700	235,000	Dakhlet Nouâdhibou	22,300	30,000
Hodh el-Gharbi	53,400	154,000	Tagant	95,200	84,000
Açâba	36,600	152,000	Guidimaka	10,300	102,000
Gorgol	13,600	169,000	Tiris Zemmour	252,900	28,000
Brakna	33,000	171,000	Inchiri	46,800	23,000
Trarza	67,800	242,000			

In 1983, 34% of the population were urban and 25% were nomadic. In 1980 81% of the inhabitants were Moorish, speaking the Hassaniyah dialect of Arabic, while the other 19% consist of Negro peoples, mainly Fulfulde-speaking Tukulor (8%) and Fulani (5%) who together with the Soninike (Sarakole) and Wolof groups all inhabit the Senegal valley in the extreme south.

The official languages are Arabic and French.

CLIMATE. A tropical climate, but conditions are generally arid, even near the coast, where the only appreciable rains come in July to Sept. Nouakchott. Jan. 71°F (21·7°C), July 82°F (27·8°C). Annual rainfall 6" (158 mm).

CONSTITUTION AND GOVERNMENT. The 24-member CMSN wields all executive and legislative powers, working through an appointed Council of Ministers composed as follows in Feb. 1991:

President, Prime Minister, Minister of Defence and Chairman of CMSN: Col. Moaouia Ould Sidi Mohamed Taya (assumed office 12 Dec. 1984).

Foreign Affairs: Hosni Ould Didih. *Finance:* Mohamed Ould Nany.

National flag: Green, with a crescent beneath a star in yellow in the centre.

Local Government: Mauritania is divided into a capital district and 12 regions and sub-divided into 49 *départements*.

DEFENCE

Army. The Army consists of 2 infantry, 1 parachute and 1 artillery battalion, 1 Camel Corps, 3 armoured car squadrons and support units; total strength, 10,500 in 1991.

Navy. The Navy, some 450 strong in 1990, is based at Nouadhibou and consists of 4 fast patrol craft and a few boats.

Air Force. The Air Force has 6 Britten-Norman Defender armed light transports, 2 Maritime Surveillance Cheyennes for coastal patrol, 2 Buffalo and 2 Skyvan transports, 4 Reims-Cessna 337 Milirole twin-engined counter-insurgency, forward air control and training aircraft and 4 Hughes 500 helicopters for communications. Personnel (1991) 150.

INTERNATIONAL RELATIONS

Membership. Mauritania is a member of the UN, OAU, the Arab League and is an ACP state of the EEC.

ECONOMY

Budget. The ordinary budget for 1989 balanced at 22,000m. ouguiyas.

Currency. The monetary unit is the *ouguiya* (MRO) which is divided into 5 *khoums*. Banknotes of 1,000, 500, 200 and 100 *ouguiya* and coins of 20, 10, 5 and 1 *ouguiya* and 1 *khoum* are in circulation. In March 1991, £1 = 144·83 *ouguiya*; US$1 = 76·35 *ouguiya*.

Banking and Finance. *The Banque Centrale de Mauritanie* (created 1973) is the bank of issue, and there are 5 commercial banks situated in Nouakchott.

ENERGY AND NATURAL RESOURCES

Electricity. Production (1986) 74m. kwh.

Minerals. Iron ore production (1984) 9·5m. tonnes. Copper mining at Akjoujt (by the state-owned SOMIMA), suspended in 1978, resumed in 1983.

Agriculture. Agriculture is mainly confined to the south, in the Senegal river valley. Production in tonnes (1988) of millet, 89,000; dates, 13,000; potatoes, 1,000; maize, 8,000; sweet potatoes, 3,000; rice, 15,000; groundnuts, 2,000.

In 1988 there were 810,000 camels, 1·25m. cattle, 149,000 asses, 17,000 horses, 4·1m. sheep, 3·2m. goats.

Forestry. There were 15m. ha of forests, chiefly in the southern regions, where wild acacias yield the main product, gum arabic.

Fisheries. Total catch (1986) 104,100 tonnes.

FOREIGN ECONOMIC RELATIONS. In Feb. 1989 Mauritania signed a treaty of economic co-operation with the 4 other Maghreb countries, Algeria, Libya, Morocco and Tunisia.

Commerce. In 1986 imports totalled 17,392m. ouguiya, and exports, 25,950 ouguiya of which iron ore comprised 40% of exports and salted and dried fish 60%; 24% of all exports went to Italy, 22% to Japan, 18% to Belgium and 15% to France, while France provided 22% of imports and Spain 20%.

Total trade between Mauritania and UK (British Department of Trade returns, in £1,000 sterling):

	1986	*1987*	*1988*	*1989*	*1990*
Imports to UK	2,184	8,724	7,259	15,387	14,525
Exports and re-exports from UK	2,495	3,862	3,048	4,005	2,997

Tourism. In 1986 there were 13,000 tourists.

COMMUNICATIONS

Roads. There were 8,900 km of roads in 1983. In 1985 there were 15,017 passenger cars and 2,188 commercial vehicles.

Railways. A 652-km railway links Zoué rate with the port of Point-Central, 10 km south of Nouâdhibou, and is used primarily for iron ore exports. In 1989 it carried 12·1m. tonnes of freight and (in 1986) 19,353 passengers.

Aviation. There are international airports at Nouakchott, Nouâdhibou and Néma. In 1990 the 5 Maghreb countries agreed to merge their airlines into Air Maghreb.

Shipping. The major ports are at Point-Central (for mineral exports), Nouakchott and Nouâdhibou.

Telecommunications. There were, in 1985, 3,161 telephones and 200,000 radio receivers and about 1,000 television receivers.

JUSTICE, RELIGION, EDUCATION AND WELFARE

Justice. There are *tribunaux de première instance* at Nouakchott, Atâr, Kaédi, Aïoun el Atrouss and Kiffa. The Appeal Court and Supreme Court are situated in Nouakchott. Islamic jurisprudence was adopted in Feb. 1980.

Religion. Over 99% of Mauritanians are Sunni Moslem, mainly of the Qadiriyah sect.

Education. In 1986 there were 150,605 pupils in primary schools, 35,129 in secondary schools, 2,808 in technical schools and teacher-training establishments and 4,830 students in higher education. The University of Nouakchott (founded 1983) had 974 students in 1984.

Health. In 1984 there were 13 hospitals and clinics with 1,325 beds. In 1984 there were 170 doctors, 8 dentists, 16 pharmacists, 129 midwives and 582 nursing personnel.

DIPLOMATIC REPRESENTATIVES

Of Mauritania in Great Britain
Ambassador: Mohamed El Hanchi Ould Mohamed Saleh (resides in Paris).

Of Great Britain in Mauritania
Ambassador: John Macrae, CMG (resides in Rabat).

Of Mauritania in the USA
Ambassador: Abdellah Ould Daddah.

Of the USA in Mauritania (PO Box 222, Nouakchott)
Ambassador: William H. Twaddell.

Of Mauritania to the United Nations
Ambassador: Mohamedou Ould Mohamed Mahmoud.

Further Reading

Stewart, C. C. and Stewart, E. K., *Islam and Social Order in Mauritania.* New York, 1970
Westebbe, R. M., *The Economy of Mauritania.* New York, 1971

MAURITIUS

Capital: Port Louis
Population: 1,081,669 (1989)
GNP per capita: US$1,810 (1988)

HISTORY. Mauritius was known to Arab navigators probably not later than the 10th century. It was probably visited by Malays in the 15th century, and was discovered by the Portuguese between 1507 and 1512, but the Dutch were the first settlers (1598). In 1710 they abandoned the island, which was occupied by the French under the name of Ile de France (1715). The British occupied the island in 1810, and it was formally ceded to Great Britain by the Treaty of Paris, 1814. In 1965 the Chagos Archipelago was transferred to the British Indian Ocean Territory. Mauritius became an independent state and a monarchical member of the Commonwealth on 12 March 1968 after 7 months of internal self-government.

AREA AND POPULATION. Mauritius, the main island, lies 500 miles (800 km) east of Madagascar. Rodrigues (formerly a dependency and now a part of Mauritius) is about 350 miles (560 km) east of Mauritius. The outer islands consist of Agalega and the St Brandon Group. Population estimate (1989) 1,081,669.

Island	*Area in sq. km*	*Census 1983*	*Estimate 1989*
Mauritius	1,865	966,863	1,043,631
Rodrigues	104	33,082	37,538
Dependencies			
Agalega	70	487	500
St Brandon	1	–	–
Total	2,040	1,000,432	1,081,669

Port Louis is the capital (139,038, 1987). Other towns, Beau Bassin-Rose Hill, 93,016; Curepipe, 64,687; Quatre Bornes, 64,668; Vacoas-Phoenix, 55,464.

Vital statistics, 1989: Births, 20,955 (20·4 per 1,000); marriages, 11,040; deaths, 6,946 (6·8 per 1,000).

The official language is English.

CLIMATE. The sub-tropical climate produces quite a difference between summer and winter, though conditions are generally humid. Most rain falls in the summer so that the pleasantest months are Sept. to Nov. Rainfall amounts vary between 40" (1,000 mm) on the coast to 200" (5,000 mm) on the central plateau, though the west coast only has 35" (875 mm). Mauritius lies in the cyclone belt, whose season runs from Nov. to April, but is seldom affected by intense storms. Port Louis. Jan. 73°F (22·8°C), July 81°F (27·2°C). Annual rainfall 40" (1,000 mm).

CONSTITUTION AND GOVERNMENT. The *Governor-General* is the local representative of HM the Queen, who remains the Head of the State.

The *Cabinet* is presided over by the Prime Minister. Each of the other 18 members of the Cabinet is responsible for the administration of specified departments or subjects and is bound by the rule of collective responsibility. 10 Parliamentary Secretaries may also be appointed by the Governor-General on the advice of the Prime Minister.

The *Legislative Assembly* consists of a Speaker, elected from its own members, and 62 elected members (3 each for the 20 constituencies of Mauritius and 2 for Rodrigues) and 8 additional seats in order to ensure a fair and adequate representation of each community within the Assembly. General Elections are held every 5 years on the basis of universal adult suffrage.

The Constitution also provides for the Public Service Commission and the Judicial and Legal Service Commission which have both assumed executive powers for appointments to the Public Service. An Ombudsman assumed office on 2 March 1970.

At the General Election held on 30 Aug. 1987, 41 of the 62 seats were won by the ruling *Alliance* (Mouvement Socialiste Mauricien, 26; Mauritius Labour Party, 9; Parti Mauricien Social-Démocrate, 4; Organisation du Peuple Rodriguais, 2) and 21 by the opposition *Union for the Future* (the Mouvement Militant Mauricien and its allies); of the 8 additional seats awarded to the highest losers in each community, 5 went to the *Alliance* and 3 to the *Union*.

Governor-General: Sir Veerasamy Ringadoo, GCMG, QC.

The Cabinet was composed as follows in Jan. 1991:

Prime Minister, Defence and Internal Security, Information, External Communications, the Outer Islands and Finance: Sir Anerood Jugnauth, QC.

Deputy Prime Minister and Health: Prem Nababsing. *Deputy Prime Minister and Economic Planning and Development:* Dr Beergoonath Ghurburrun. *Education, Arts and Culture:* Armoogum Parsuraman. *Trade and Shipping:* Dwarkanath Gungah. *Energy, Water Resources and Postal Services:* Mahyendrah Utchanah. *Labour and Industrial Relations, Women's Rights and Family Welfare:* Sheilabai Bappoo. *Youth and Sports and Tourism:* Michael James Kevin Glover. *Co-operatives:* Jagdishwar Goburdhun. *Agriculture, Fisheries and Natural Resources:* Murlidas Dulloo. *Social Security and Reform Institutions:* Vishwanath Sajadah. *Works:* Ramduth Jaddoo. *Rodrigues:* Serge Clair. *Industry and New Technology:* Cassam Uteem. *Local Government:* Regis Finette. *Civil Service Affairs and Employment:* Kailash Ruhee. *External Affairs:* Jean-Claude de L'Estrac. *Justice and Housing:* Jayen Cuttaree. *Environment:* Swaley Kasenally.

National flag: Horizontally 4 stripes of red, blue, yellow and green.

Local government: The Island of Mauritius (only) is divided into 9 administrative districts.

DEFENCE. The Mauritius Police, which is responsible for defence, is equipped with arms; its strength was (1990) 6,584 officers and men.

INTERNATIONAL RELATIONS

Membership. Mauritius is a member of the UN, Commonwealth, OAU, Non-Aligned Movement and is an ACP state of the EEC.

ECONOMY

Budget. Revenue and expenditure (in Rs1m.) for years ending 30 June:

	1986–87	*1987–88*	*1988–89*	*1989–90*
Revenue	5,009	6,215	8,065	8,283
Expenditure	4,635	5,813	7,700	8,290

Principal sources of revenue, 1989–90 (estimate): Direct taxes, Rs 1,417·3m.; indirect taxes, Rs 5,742·1m.; receipts from public utilities, Rs 160m.; receipts from public services Rs 180m.; interest and reimbursement, Rs 448m. Capital expenditure was Rs 2,415m. Capital revenue, Rs 1,931m. On 30 June 1990 the public debt of Mauritius was Rs 2,173m.

Currency. The unit of currency is the *Mauritius rupee* (MUR) of 100 *cents*.

The currency consists of: (i) Bank of Mauritius notes of Rs 500, 200, 100, 50, 25, 10 and 5; (ii) Cupro-nickel coins of 5 rupees and 1 rupee; (iii) nickel-plated steel coins of 50 cents and 20 cents; (iv) copper-plated steel coins of 5 cents and 1 cent. In March 1991, £1 = 27·05 *rupees*; US$1 = 14·26.

Banking and Finance. The Bank of Mauritius was established in 1966, with an authorized capital of Rs 10m., to exercise the function of a central bank. The *Governor* is Sir Indurduth Ramphul. There are 13 commercial banks, the Mauritius Commercial Bank Ltd (established 1838), Barclays Bank PLC, the Bank of Baroda Ltd, The HongKong and Shanghai Banking Corporation, the Mauritius Co-operative Central Bank Ltd, Banque Nationale de Paris (Intercontinentale), the Habib Bank Ltd, the State Commercial Bank Ltd, the Bank of Credit and Commerce International SA, Indian Ocean International Bank Ltd, Mauritius Commercial Bank Finance Corporation Ltd, Union International Bank Ltd and Habib Bank (Zurich). Other financial institutions include the Mauritius Housing Corporation, the Development Bank of Mauritius and the Post Office Savings Bank.

On 31 Dec. 1988 the Post Office Savings Bank held deposits amounting to Rs 228·4m., belonging to 246,660 depositors.

ENERGY AND NATURAL RESOURCES

Electricity. Electric power production (1988) was 545m. kwh. Supply 230 volts; 50 Hz.

Agriculture. In 1989 90,000 ha were planted with sugar-cane. There were 19 factories and sugar production (1989 in tonnes) was 568,000, molasses, 165,000.

The main secondary crops in 1989 were tea (3,775 ha from which 5,500 tonnes were produced), tobacco (1,058 tonnes), potatoes (18,210 tonnes) and maize (2,325 tonnes).

In 1989 beef production totalled 784 tonnes, pork 595 tonnes and goat meat 131 tonnes.

Livestock (1989): Cattle, 10,836; goats, 15,892; poultry, 2m.

Forestry. The total forest area was estimated (1989) at 65,400 ha including some 6,775 ha of plantations. In 1988 production totalled 27,954 cu. metres of timber, poles and fuel wood.

Fisheries. Production (1988) 15,872 tonnes.

INDUSTRY. Manufactures include: Knitwear, clothing, footwear, diamond cutting, jewellery, furniture, watchstraps, sunglasses, plastic ware and chemical products.

Labour. In 1989 the labour force was 273,152, of whom 106,765 were employed in manufacturing.

Trade Unions. In 1989 there were 291 registered trade unions and 11 federations with a total membership of about 100,000.

FOREIGN ECONOMIC RELATIONS

Commerce. Total trade (in Rs1m.) for calendar years:

	1986	*1987*	*1988*	*1989*
Imports c.i.f.	9,199	13,042	17,247	20,217
Exports f.o.b.	9,063	11,497	13,454	15,049

In 1989, Rs 2,848m. of the imports came from France, Rs 1,817m. from the Republic of South Africa, Rs 1,284m. from UK, Rs 512m. from Australia. In 1988 Rs 4,799m. of the exports went to UK, Rs 3,025m. to France, Rs 1,793m. to USA and Rs 1,273m. to Federal Republic of Germany.

Sugar exports in 1989 were 646,000 tonnes, Rs 3,561m. Other major exports (1989) included clothing, Rs 7,148m.; tea, Rs 87m. and toys, games and sporting goods, Rs 92m. Major imports included (1987) textiles and fabrics, Rs 3,972m. and (1989) machinery and transport equipment, Rs 4,639m.

Total trade between Mauritius and UK (British Department of Trade returns, in £1,000 sterling):

	1986	*1987*	*1988*	*1989*	*1990*
Imports to UK	153,271	163,271	186,240	216,190	233,936
Exports and re-exports from UK	32,087	44,395	38,553	43,528	50,746

Tourism. In 1989, 379,080 tourists visited Mauritius.

COMMUNICATIONS

Roads. In 1989 there were 29 km of motorway, 856 km of main roads, 816 km of secondary and other roads. At 31 Dec. 1989 there were 27,697 cars, 1,858 buses, 10,271 motor cycles, 35,650 auto cycles and 10,421 lorries and vans.

Aviation. Mauritius is linked by air with Europe, Africa, Asia and Australia by the following airlines: Air France, Air India, Air Madagascar, Air Mauritius, Air Zimbabwe, British Airways, Cathay Pacific Airways, Lufthansa, Malaysian Airline System, Singapore Airlines, South African Airways and Zambia Airways. In addition to passenger services a weekly cargo flight is operated by Air France to Paris. In 1989, 407,933 passengers arrived at Sir Seewoosagur Ramgoolam international airport and 7,500 tonnes of freight were unloaded. Air Mauritius operates a joint regional service with Air Madagascar on the Mauritius–Antananarivo–Moroni–Nairobi route, a twice weekly service jointly with Air India to Bombay, and a joint weekly service to Hong Kong with Cathay Pacific Airlines.

Shipping. In 1989, 1,079 vessels entered Port Louis with a total gross tonnage of 4·2m. tonnes.

Telecommunications. In 1989 there were 33 telephone exchanges and 74,118 individual telephone installations in Mauritius and Rodrigues. Communication with other parts of the world is established *via* satellite.

At 31 Dec. 1989 there were 143,737 television sets.

Cinemas (1988). There were 36 cinemas, with a seating capacity of about 40,000.

Newspapers. There were (1988) 5 French daily papers (with occasional articles in English) and 2 Chinese daily papers with a combined circulation of about 80,000.

RELIGION, EDUCATION AND WELFARE

Religion. At the 1983 Census (excluding Rodrigues) there were 247,723 Roman Catholics, 6,049 Protestants (Church of England and Church of Scotland), 506,270 Hindus and 160,190 Moslems.

Education. Primary education is free and not usually compulsory. About 96% of children aged 5 to 11 years attend schools. In 1989 there were 134,136 pupils at 273 primary schools and 72,389 pupils at 125 secondary schools. There were 8 special schools and 870 students in 3 technical institutions and 5 handicraft training centres and 501 teachers in training in 1989.

In 1989, 1,241 students were enrolled at the University of Mauritius.

Health. In 1989 there were 860 doctors, including 152 specialists, and 2,857 hospital beds.

DIPLOMATIC REPRESENTATIVES

Of Mauritius in Great Britain (32–33 Elvaston Pl., London, SW7)
High Commissioner: Dr Boodhun Teelock (accredited 23 Feb. 1989).

Of Great Britain in Mauritius (King George V Ave., Floreal, Port Louis)
High Commissioner: M. E. Howell, CMG, OBE.

Of Mauritius in the USA (4301 Connecticut Ave., NW, Washington, D.C., 20008)
Ambassador: Chitmansing Jesseramsing.

Of the USA in Mauritius (Rogers Bldg., John Kennedy St., Port Louis)
Ambassador: Penne Percy Korth.

Of Mauritius to the United Nations
Ambassador: Dr S. Peerthum.

Further Reading

Statistical Information: The Central Statistical Information Office (Rose Hill, Mauritius) was founded in July 1945. Its main publication is the *Bi-annual Digest of Statistics.*

Ministry of Information, *Fruits of Political and Social Democracy.—Mauritius Facts and Figures 1980.—The Mauritius Handbook 1989*

Simmons, A. S., *Modern Mauritius: The Politics of Decolonization.* Indiana Univ. Press, 1982

Library: The Mauritius Institute Public Library, Port Louis.

MEXICO

Capital: Mexico City
Population: 81·14m. (1990)
GNP per capita: US$1,820 (1988)

Estados Unidos Mexicanos

(United States of Mexico)

HISTORY. Mexico's history falls into four epochs: the era of the Indian empires (before 1521), the Spanish colonial phase (1521–1810), the period of national formation (1810–1910), which includes the war of independence (1810–21) and the long presidency of Porfirio Díaz (1876–80, 1884–1911), and the present period which began with the social revolution of 1910–21 and is regarded by Mexicans as the period of social and national consolidation.

AREA AND POPULATION. Mexico is bounded in the north by the USA, west and south by the Pacific Ocean, southeast by Guatemala, Belize and the Caribbean Sea, and north-east by the Gulf of Mexico. It comprises 1,958,201 sq. km (756,198 sq. miles), including uninhabited islands (5,073 sq. km) offshore. Population density, 41·25 per sq. km.

Population at recent censuses: 1900, 13,607,272; 1950, 25,791,017; 1960, 34,923,129; 1970, 48,225,288; 1980, 66,846,833; 1990, 81,140,922.

Area population and capitals of the Federal District and 31 states:

	Area (Sq. km)	*Population (1990 census)*	*Population (1989 estimate)*	*Capital*
Federal District	1,479	8,236,960	10,355,347	Mexico City
Aguascalientes	5,471	719,650	702,615	Aguascalientes
Baja California Norte	69,921	1,657,927	1,408,774	Mexicali
Baja California Sur	73,475	317,326	327,389	La Paz
Campeche	50,812	528,824	617,133	Campeche
Chiapas	74,211	3,203,915	2,559,461	Tuxtla Gutiérrez
Chihuahua	244,938	2,439,954	2,253,975	Chihuahua
Coahuila	149,982	1,971,344	1,937,209	Saltillo
Colima	5,191	424,656	426,225	Colima
Durango	123,181	1,352,156	1,402,782	Victoria de Durango
Guanajuato	30,491	3,980,204	3,593,210	Guanajuato
Guerrero	64,281	2,622,067	2,604,947	Chilpancingo
Hidalgo	20,813	1,880,636	1,847,259	Pachuca de Soto
Jalisco	80,836	5,278,987	5,269,816	Guadalajara
México	21,355	9,815,901	12,013,056	Toluca de Lerdo
Michoacán de Ocampo	59,928	3,534,042	3,424,235	Morelia
Morelos	4,950	1,195,381	1,288,875	Cuernavaca
Nayarit	26,979	816,112	857,359	Tepic
Nuevo Léon	64,924	3,086,466	3,202,434	Monterrey
Oaxaca	93,952	3,021,513	2,669,120	Oaxaca de Juárez
Puebla	33,902	4,118,059	4,139,609	Puebla de Zaragoza
Querétaro	11,449	1,044,227	976,548	Querétaro
Quintana Roo	50,212	493,605	414,301	Chetumal
San Luis Potosí	63,068	2,001,966	2,055,364	San Luis Potosí
Sinaloa	58,328	2,210,766	2,425,006	Culiacán Rosales
Sonora	182,052	1,822,247	1,828,390	Hermosillo
Tabasco	25,267	1,501,183	1,322,613	Villahermosa
Tamaulipas	79,384	2,244,208	2,294,680	Ciudad Victoria
Tlaxcala	4,016	763,683	676,446	Tlaxcala
Veracruz	71,699	6,215,142	6,798,109	Jalapa Enríquez
Yucatán	38,402	1,363,540	1,327,298	Mérida
Zacatecas	73,252	1,278,279	1,259,407	Zacatecas

At the 1980 census 33,039,307 were males, 33,807,526 females. Urban population was 66·3% in 1988. The official language is Spanish, the mother tongue of over 92% of the population, but there are 5 indigenous language groups (Náhuatl,Maya, Zapotec, Otomi and Mixtec) from which are derived a total of 59 dialects spoken by 5,181,038 inhabitants (1980 census). In 1980, about 16% of the population were of European ethnic origin, 55% mestizo and 29% Amerindian.

The populations (1990 Census) of the largest cities were:

México [1]	13,636,127	Hermosillo	449,472	Guasave	257,821
Guadalajara [1]	2,846,720	Saltillo	440,845	Tepic	238,101
Monterrey [1]	2,521,697	Victoria de Durango	414,015	Gómez Palacio	232,550
Puebla de Zaragoza	1,054,921	Villa Hermosa	390,161	Coatzacoalcos	232,314
Léon de los Aldama	872,453	Irapuato	362,471	Tapachula	222,282
Ciudad Juárez	797,679	Veracruz Llave	327,522	Nuevo Laredo	217,914
Tijuana	742,686	Celaya	315,577	Uruapán	217,142
Mexicali	602,391	Atizapán de Zaragoza	315,413	Oaxaca de Juárez	212,943
Culiacán Rosales	602,114	Mazatlán	314,249	Ciudad Victoria	207,830
Acapulco de Juárez	592,187	Ciudad Obregón	311,078	Salamanca	206,275
Mérida	557,340	Los Mochis	305,507	Minatitlán	199,840
Chihuahua	530,487	Matamoros	303,392	Pachuca de Soto	179,440
San Luis Potosí	525,819	Tuxtla Gutiérrez	295,615	Monclova	178,023
Aguascalientes	506,384	Jalapa Enríquez	288,331	Campeche	172,208
Morelia	489,758	Cuernavaca	281,752	Ciudad Madero	159,644
Toluca de Lerdo	487,630	Reynosa	281,392	Poza Rica de Hidalgo	151,201
Torreón	459,809	Tampico	271,636	Córdoba	150,428
Querétaro	454,049	Ensenada	260,905		

[1] Metropolitan Area.

Vital statistics for calendar years:

	Births	*Deaths*	*Marriages*	*Divorces*
1988	2,629,292	432,186	623,219	47,924
1989	2,586,708	436,127	618,162	40,414

CLIMATE. Latitude and relief produce a variety of climates. Arid and semi-arid conditions are found in the north, with extreme temperatures, whereas in the south there is a humid tropical climate, with temperatures varying with altitude. Conditions on the shores of the Gulf of Mexico are very warm and humid. In general, the rainy season lasts from May to Nov, Mexico City. Jan. 55°F (12·6°C), July 61°F (16·1°C). Annual rainfall 30" (747 mm). Guadalajara. Jan. 59°F (15·2°C), July 69°F (20·5°C). Annual rainfall 36" (902 mm). La Paz. Jan. 64°F (17·8°C), July 85°F (29·4°C). Annual rainfall 6" (145 mm). Mazatlan Jan. 66°F (18·9°C), July 82°F (27·8°C). Annual rainfall 33" (828 mm). Merida. Jan. 72°F (22·2°C), July 83°F (28·3°C). Annual rainfall 38" (957 mm). Monterrey. Jan. 58°F (14·4°C), July 81°F (27·2°C). Annual rainfall 23" (588 mm). Puebla de Zaragoza. Jan. 54°F (12·2°C), July 63°F (17·2°C). Annual rainfall 34" (850 mm).

CONSTITUTION AND GOVERNMENT. A new Constitution was promulgated on 5 Feb. 1917 and has been amended from time to time. Mexico is a representative, democratic and federal republic, comprising 31 states and a federal district, each state being free and sovereign in all internal affairs, but united in a federation established according to the principals of the Fundamental Law. Citizenship, including the right of suffrage, is vested in all nationals of 18 years of age and older who have 'an honourable means of livelihood'.

There is complete separation of legislative, executive and judicial powers (Art. 49). Legislative power is vested in a General Congress of 2 chambers, a Chamber of Deputies and a Senate (Art.50). The Chamber of Deputies consists of 500 members directly elected for 3 years, 300 of them from single-member constituencies and 200 chosen under a system of proportional representation (Arts.51–55). In July 1990 Congress voted a new Electoral Code by 369 votes to 65. This establishes a body to organize elections (IFE), an electoral court (TFE) to resolve disputes, new electoral rolls and introduces a voter's registration card. Congressional and gubernatorial elections were due in 1991.

At the general elections held on 7 July 1988, 234 of the single-member seats were won by the Institutional Revolutionary Party (PRI), 38 by the Party of National Action (PAN). The PRI held 263 seats in Nov. 1990.

The Senate comprises 64 members, 2 from each state and 2 from the federal district, directly elected for 6 years (Arts.56–58). At the elections of 7 July 1988, the PRI won 60 seats and the FDN 4 seats. Members of both chambers are not immediately re-eligible for election (Art.59). Congress sits from 1 Sept. to 31 Dec. each year; during the recess there is a permanent committee of 15 deputies and 14 senators appointed by the respective chambers.

The President is the supreme executive authority. He appoints the members of the Council of Ministers and the senior military and civilian officers of the state. He is directly elected for a single 6-year term.

The names of the presidents from 1958 are as follows:

Adolfo López Mateos, 1 Dec. 1958–30 Nov. 1964.
Gustavo Díaz Ordaz, 1 Dec. 1964–30 Nov. 1970.
Luis Echeverría Alvarez, 1 Dec. 1970–30 Nov. 1976.
José López Portillo y Pacheco, 1 Dec. 1976–30 Nov. 1982.
Miguel de la Madrid Hurtado, 1 Dec. 1982–30 Nov. 1988.

President: Carlos Salinas de Gortari (b. 1948; assumed office 1 Dec. 1988).

In Nov. 1990 the Council of Ministers was composed as follows:

Interior: Fernando Gutiérrez Barrios. *Foreign Relations:* Fernando Solana Morales. *Defence:* Gen. Antonio Riviello Bazan. *Navy:* Adm. Luis Carlos Ruano Angulo. *Finance and Public Credit:* Dr Pedro Aspe Armella. *Planning and Federal Budget:* Dr Ernesto Cedillo Ponce de León. *Comptroller-General:* María Elena Vásquez Nava. *Energy, Mines and Public Industries:* Fernando Hiriart Balderrama. *Commerce and Industrial Development:* Dr Jaime Serra Puche. *Agriculture and Water Resources:* Carlos Hank González. *Communications and Transport:* Andres Caso Lombardo. *Urban Development and Ecology:* Patricio Chirinos Calero. *Education:* Manuel Bartlett Diaz. *Health:* Dr Jesús Kumate Rodriguez. *Labour and Social Welfare:* Arsenio Farell Cubillas. *Agrarian Reform:* Victor Cervera Pacheco. *Tourism:* Pedro Joaquín Coldwell. *Fisheries:* Maria de los Angeles Moreno Uruegas. *Governor of Federal District:* Manuel Camacho Solis. *Attorney-General:* Enrique Alvárez del Castillo. *Attorney-General of the Federal District:* Ignacio Morales Lechuga. *Chief of the Presidential Staff:* Brig.-Gen. Arturo Cardona Marino. *Director-General of the Technical Cabinet Secretariat:* Dr José Córdoba Montoya. *Presidential Secretary:* Andrés Massieu Berlanga. *Director-General of Legal Affairs of the Presidency:* Ruben Valdés Abascal. *Director-General of Presidential Public Relations:* Otto Granados Roldán.

National flag: Three vertical strips of green, white, red, with the national arms in the centre.

National anthem: Mexicanos, al grito de guerra (words by F. González Bocanegra; tune by Jaime Nunó, 1854).

Local Government. Mexico is divided into 31 states and a Federal District. The latter is co-extensive with Mexico City and is administered by a Governor appointed by the President. Each state has its own constitution, with the right to legislate and to levy taxes (but not inter-state customs duties); its Governor is directly elected for 6 years and its unicameral legislature for 3 years; judicial officers are appointed by the state governments. Mexico City is sub-divided into 16 municipalities and the 31 states into 2,378 municipalities.

DEFENCE

Army. Enlistment into the regular army is voluntary, but there is also one year of conscription by lottery. The army consists of 3 infantry brigades (one of which is mechanized), 3 armoured regiments, a garrison for each of the country's 36 military zones (with motorized cavalry, artillery and infantry), and support units. Equipment includes 45 M-3/-8 tanks and some 140 armoured cars. Strength of the regular army (1991) 105,500; conscripts, 60,000.

Navy. The Navy is primarily equipped and organized for offshore and coastal patrol duties. It comprises 3 ex-US destroyers, 6 modern offshore patrol vessels with small helicopter decks and hangars, and 35 older offshore ships, mostly ex-US. There are also 32 inshore patrol vessels and 20 riverine patrol craft. Auxiliaries include 4 survey ships, 1 repair ship, 2 training ships, 6 tugs and some 24 service craft.

The naval air force, 500 strong, operates 10 Aviocars and 11 HU-16 Albatross amphibians for maritime patrol and rescue, 12 Bo-105 helicopters for service afloat, and some 21 fixed wing and 7 helicopters for transport and liaison duties.

Naval personnel in 1990 totalled 35,000, including the naval air force and 9,000 marines.

Air Force. The Air Force had (1991) a strength of about 8,000 with 113 combatant aircraft and 23 armed helicopters, and has nine operational groups, each with one or two squadrons. No. 1 Group comprises No. 208 Squadron with 9 IAI Aravas for transport, search and rescue and counter-insurgency duties; and No. 209 Squadron with Bell 205A, 206B JetRanger, Alouette III and Puma helicopters. No. 2 Group has two Squadrons (Nos. 206 and 207) of Swiss-built Pilatus PC-7 Turbo-Trainers for light attack duty. No. 3 Group (203 and 204 Squadrons) also operates PC-7s; No. 4 Group (201 and 205 Squadrons) is equipped with PC-7s. No. 5 Group consists of No. 101 communications Squadron and a photo-reconnaissance unit, both equipped with Aero Commander 500S piston-engined light twins. Nos. 301 and 302 Squadrons, in No. 6 Group, operate a total of 8 turboprop-powered Lockheed C-130 Hercules and 5 C-54, 2 C-118A and 1 DC-7 piston-engined transports. The main combat Group, No. 7, comprises No. 401 Squadron with 11 F-5E Tiger II and F-5F 2-seat fighters; and No. 202 Squadron with AT-33A jet trainer/fighter-bombers. No. 8 Group has 7 C-47s in a VIP transport squadron. No. 9 Group operates the Air Force's remaining 12 or more C-47s in Nos. 311 and 312 transport Squadrons. There is a Presidential Squadron with 7 Boeing 727s, 1 757, 2 737s, 1 HS.125, 1 Electra, 1 JetStar, 1 Islander, 2 Super Pumas and 1 Bell 212. Other training aircraft include 20 Mudry CAP-10Bs, 20 Beech Musketeers, 40 Bonanzas, over 30 T-28 Trojans and PC-7 Turbo-Trainers.

INTERNATIONAL RELATIONS

Membership. Mexico is a member of UN, OAS, SELA and LAIA.

ECONOMY

Policy. An economic development plan (1989-94) was announced in June 1989 aimed at restoring growth and improving living standards. A privatization programme includes banks, steel and telecommunications.

Budget. The 1988 budget provided for expenditure of 103,348,500m. pesos and revenue of 65,505,900m. pesos. Budget estimate for 1991: 234,000,000m. pesos.

Currency. The unit of currency is the *Mexican peso* (MXP). There are coins of 1, 5, 10, 20, 50, 100, 200, 500, 1,000 and 5,000 *pesos*; and banknotes of 1,000, 2,000, 5,000, 10,000, 20,000 and 50,000 *pesos*. In Oct. 1990 the annualized rate of inflation was 31·8%. Throughout 1990 the peso was progressively devalued against the US dollar at an annual rate first of 10·5%, then of 5%. International exchange reserves were US$8,410m. in 1990. Total currency in circulation (1988) was 13,164,400m. *pesos*. Rate of exchange (controlled rate), March 1991: 2,965 pesos = US$1; 5,625 pesos = £1. There is a higher rate, for 'essential imports'.

Banking and Finance. The Bank of Mexico, established 1 Sept. 1925, is the central bank of issue; it is modelled on the Federal Reserve system, with large powers to 'manage' the currency. Banks were nationalized in 1982, but in May 1990 the government approved their reprivatization. The state continues to have a majority holding in foreign trade and rural development banks. Foreign holdings are limited to 30%.

There is a stock exchange in Mexico City.

Weights and Measures. The metric system is legal.

ENERGY AND NATURAL RESOURCES

Electricity. Output in 1989 was 109,948 kwh, of which 24,158 kwh was hydro-electric. Supply 120 volts; 50 Hz and some 120 volts; 60 Hz.

Oil. Mexico has the largest oil deposits in Latin America. Crude petroleum output was 144·8m. tonnes in 1989.

Gas. Natural gas production 3,478m. cu. feet in 1988.

Minerals. Mexico is a leading producer of strontium and fluorite. Uranium reserves, 1982: 15,000 tonnes proven, 150,000 tonnes potential. Coal reserves, 5,448m. tonnes, including 1,675m. tonnes (65% cokeable) high-grade coking coal in Coahuila.

A 1990–94 development plan for minerals envisages an expansion of foreign investment and a full inventorization of mineral reserves.

Output, 1989 (in 1,000 tonnes): Lead, 62·8; copper, 42·7; zinc, 81·3; fluorite, 80·6; pig iron, 5,373·1; sulphur, 2,083·3; manganese, 50; barite, 324·2; coal, 6,460; graphite, 40; silver (tonnes), 2,308; gold, 8.

Agriculture. In 1981 Mexico had 21·9m. ha of arable land, 74·4m. ha of meadows and pastures, 48·1m. ha of forests, 1·6m. ha of permanent crops and 40·6m. ha of other land. Agriculture provided 9·2% of GDP in 1987. Some 60% of agricultural land belongs to *ejidos*, communal lands with each member farming his plot independently. *Ejidos* can be inherited but not sold or rented. Other private farmers may not own more than 100 ha of irrigated land or an equivalent in unirrigated land. There is a theoretical legal minimum of 10 ha for holdings, but some 60% of private farms were less than 5 ha in 1990. Grains occupy most of the cultivated land, with about 43% given to maize, 10% to sorghum and 5% to wheat. In 1982 there were 146,083 tractors.

Livestock (1989): Cattle, 35·4m.; sheep, 5·9m.; pigs, 16·2m.; goats, 10·2m.; (1988) horses, 6·16m.; mules, 3·13m.; donkeys, 3,183,000; poultry, 243m.

Production of crops in 1989 (in 1,000 tonnes): Wheat, 4,374; rice, 637; barley, 433; maize, 10,945; sorghum, 4,807; cotton-seed, 255; sugar-cane, 25,112; tomatoes, 1,869; grapes, 569; apples, 499; oranges, 1,166; lemons and limes, 727; mangoes, 860; pineapples, 227; bananas, 1,185; coffee, 421; (1988) potatoes, 960; cotton-yarn, 253.

Forestry. Forests extended over 44m. ha in 1984, representing 23% of the land area, containing pine, spruce, cedar, mahogany, logwood and rosewood. There are 14 forest reserves (nearly 0·8m. ha) and 47 national park forests of 0·75m. ha. In 1989 total roundwood production amounted to 8·58m. cu. metres.

Fisheries. Catch (1989, in 1,000 tonnes), 1,333·7, including: Sardines, 418·1; anchovies, 85·5; shrimp and prawns, 52·1; oysters, 55·7; tuna, 148; dog-fish and shark, 27·3; sea perch (*mojarras*), 84·1; sea bass, 11; freshwater fish, 11·9.

INDUSTRY. In 1989 manufacturing industry provided 22·5% of GDP.

Labour. In 1987 unemployment was estimated to be over 50%.

Trade Unions. The Mexican Labour Congress (CTM), leader Fidel Velazquez (b. 1900), is incorporated into the Institutional Revolutionary Party, and is an umbrella organization numbering some 5m. In 1990 there were attempts to form independent unions. A 'Pact for Economic Stability and Growth' between government, business and labour restrained prices and wages in the private sector throughout 1991.

FOREIGN ECONOMIC RELATIONS. Nominal foreign debt was US$79,000m. in 1990.

Commerce. Trade for calendar years in US$1m.:

	1985	*1986*	*1987*	*1988*	*1989*
Imports	14,014	11,918	12,761	19,720	24,475
Exports	21,866	16,031	20,656	20,565	22,765

Of total imports in 1989, 64·8% came from USA, 5·6% from Federal Republic of Germany and 4·4% from Japan.

Of total exports in 1989, 69·3% went to USA, 5·8% to Japan and 5% to Spain.

The in-bond (*maquiladora*) assembly plants along the US border generate the largest flow of foreign exchange with oil (40% of exports in 1990) and tourism.

Total trade between Mexico and UK (British Department of Trade returns, in £1,000 sterling):

	1986	*1987*	*1988*	*1989*	*1990*
Imports to UK	116,078	244,719	144,947	165,295	172,144
Exports and re-exports from UK	162,328	198,992	190,011	205,130	262,952

Tourism. In 1990, there were 6·6m. tourists; gross revenue, including border visitors, amounted to US$3,000m.

COMMUNICATIONS

Roads. Total length, (1989) 238,006 km, of which 48,164 km were main roads, 60,239 km were secondary roads and 129,603 km by-roads. 6,067,831 motor vehicles were registered in 1989 (5,817,169 private) including 2,606,190 lorries and 218,698 motorcycles.

Railways. The sole common carrier is National Railways, *Ferrocarriles Nacionales de Mexico* (NdeM). It comprises 20,216 km of 1,435 mm gauge and 90 km of 914 mm gauge. In 1989 it carried 53.9m. tonnes of freight and 15.9m. passengers. In Mexico City an urban railway system opened in 1969 had 141 km of route and 8 lines in 1989 and carried 1,543m. passengers.

Aviation. There are 32 international and 41 national airports. Each of the larger states has a local airline which links them with main airports. Thirty-four companies maintained international services, of which *Aeromexíco* and *Mexicana de Aviacíon* are Mexican. In 1989 there were 17·78m. passengers on domestic flights and 8·67m. on international flights.

Shipping. Mexico has 49 ocean ports, of which, on the Gulf coast, the most important include Coatzacoalcos, Carmen (Campeche), Tampico, Veracruz and Tuxpan. On the Pacific Coast are Salina Cruz, Isla de Cedros, Guaymas, Santa Rosalia, Manzanillo, Lázaro Cárdenas and Mazatlán.

Merchant shipping loaded 121·73m. tonnes and unloaded 44·73m. tonnes of cargo in 1989. In 1982, the merchant marine comprised 545 vessels (of over 100 GRT) with a total tonnage of 1,251,630 GRT.

Telecommunications. In 1980 the telegraph and telephone system had 7,140 offices. *Teléfonos de México*, a state-controlled company, controls about 98% of all the telephone service. Telephones in use, Jan. 1985, 7,329,416.

In 1989 there were 1,524 radio stations while (1986) 21m. homes had receiving sets. In 1989 commercial television stations numbered 537; there were 9·5m. homes with receiving sets in 1988.

Cinemas (1987). Cinemas numbered 2,226.

Newspapers (1986). There were 308 dailies with a combined circulation of 10·36m., 25 newspapers of lesser frequency (0·72m.) and 98 journals (16·94m.).

JUSTICE, RELIGION, EDUCATION AND WELFARE

Justice. Magistrates of the Supreme Court are appointed for 6 years by the President and confirmed by the Senate; they can be removed only on impeachment. The courts include the Supreme Court with 21 magistrates, 12 collegiate circuit courts with 3 judges each and 9 unitary circuit courts with 1 judge each, and 68 district courts with 1 judge each.

The penal code of 1 Jan. 1930 abolished the death penalty, except for the armed forces.

Religion. The prevailing religion is the Roman Catholic (92·6% of the population in 1980); with (1983) 3 cardinals, 12 archbishops and 87 bishops, but by the constitution of 1857, the Church was separated from the State, and the constitution of 1917 provided strict regulation of this and all other religions. At the 1980 census there were also 3·3% Protestants, and 4·1% members of other religions.

Education. Primary and secondary education is free and compulsory, and secular. In 1988–89 there were:

	Establishments	*Teachers*	*Students*
Nursery	43,210	96,550	2,668,561
Primary	81,346	468,044	14,656,357
Secondary	18,712	246,035	4,619,424
Preparatory/Vocational	4,953	127,652	1,897,236
Teacher-training	488	8,491	64,700
Higher education	1,717	108,002	1,199,120

The most important university is the Universidad Nacional Autónoma de México (UNAM) in México City which, with its associated institutions, had, in 1982, 136,534 students (excluding post-graduates). UNAM was founded in 1551, re-organized in 1910, and granted full autonomy in 1920. Other universities of particular importance in México City are the Instituto Politécnico Nacional, specializing in technology and applied science, with 52,694 students, and the Universidad Autónoma Metropolitana with 27,452 students, opened in 1973.

Outside México City the principal universities are the Universidad de Guadalajara (in Guadalajara) with 65,799 students; the Universidad Veracruzana (in Jalapa) with 57,755 students; the Universidad Autónoma de Nueva León (in Monterrey) with 48,124 students; the Universidad Autónoma de Puebla (in Puebla) with 39,505 students; the Universidad Auto noma de Sinaloa (in Culiacán) with 33,366 students; and the Universidad Michoacana (in Morelia) with 23,935 students.

Health. In 1986 Mexico had 71,058 physicians; there were 11,072 state and private hospitals and clinics with 57,391 beds.

DIPLOMATIC REPRESENTATIVES

Of Mexico in Great Britain (8 Halkin St., London, SW1X 7DW)
Ambassador: Bernardo Sepúlveda, GCMG.

Of Great Britain in Mexico (Lerma 71, Col. Cuauhtémoc, México City 06500, D.F.)
Ambassador: M. K. O. Simpson-Orlebar, CMG (accredited 13 July 1989).

Of Mexico in the USA (2829 16th St., NW, Washington, D.C., 20009)
Ambassador: Gustavo Petricioli.

Of the USA in Mexico (Paseo de la Reforma 305, México City 5, D.F.)
Ambassador: John D. Negroponte.

Of Mexico to the United Nations
Ambassador: Dr Jorge Montaño

Further Reading

Anuario Estadístico de los Estados Unidos Mexicanos. Annual
Revista de Estadística (Monthly); *Revista de Economia* (Monthly)
Banco de México S.A., Annual report
Banco Nacional de Comercio Exterior. *Comercio Exterior,* monthly.—*Mexico.* Annual (in Spanish or English)
Bailey, J. J., *Governing Mexico: The Statecraft of Crisis Management.* London and New York, 1988
Bazant, J., *A Concise History of Mexico.* CUP, 1977
Grayson, G. W., *Oil and Mexican Foreign Policy.* Univ. of Pittsburgh Press, 1988
Hamilton, N. and Harding, T. F., (eds.) *Mexico: State, Economy and Social Conflict.* London, 1986
Philip, G., (ed.) *Politics in Mexico.* London, 1985
Riding, A., *Distant Neighbours.* London, 1985.—*Mexico: Inside the Volcano.* London, 1987
Robbins, N. C., *Mexico.* [Bibliography] Oxford and Santa Barbara, 1984
Wyman, D. L., (ed) *Mexico's Economic Crisis: Challenges and Opportunities.* San Diego, 1983

MONACO

Capital: Monaco
Population: 29,876 (1990)

Principauté de Monaco

HISTORY. Monaco is a small Principality on the Mediterranean, surrounded by the French Department of Alpes Maritimes except on the side towards the sea. From 1297 it belonged to the house of Grimaldi. In 1731 it passed into the female line, Louise Hippolyte, daughter of Antoine I, heiress of Monaco, marrying Jacques de Goyon Matignon, Count of Torigni, who took the name and arms of Grimaldi. The Principality was placed under the protection of the Kingdom of Sardinia by the Treaty of Vienna, 1815, and under that of France in 1861. Prince Albert I (reigned 1889–1922) acquired fame as an oceanographer; and his son Louis II (1922–49) was instrumental in establishing the International Hydrographic Bureau.

AREA AND POPULATION. The area is 195 ha (481 acres). The Principality is divided into 4 districts: Monaco-Ville, la Condamine, Monte-Carlo and Fontvieille. Population (1990), 29,876, of whom 6,200 were Monegasques. The official language is French.

CLIMATE. A Mediterranean climate, with mild moist winters and hot dry summers. Monaco. Jan. 50°F (10°C), July 74°F (23·3°C). Annual rainfall 30" (758 mm).

REIGNING PRINCE. Rainier III, born 31 May 1923, son of Princess Charlotte, Duchess of Valentinois, daughter of Prince Louis II, 1898–1977 (married 19 March 1920 to Prince Pierre, Comte de Polignac, who had taken the name Grimaldi, from whom she was divorced 18 Feb. 1933). Prince Rainier succeeded his grandfather Louis II, who died on 9 May 1949. He married on 19 April 1956 Miss Grace Kelly, a citizen of the USA (died 14 Sept. 1982). *Issue:* Princess Caroline Louise Marguerite, born 23 Jan. 1957; married Philippe Junot on 28 June 1978, divorced, 9 Oct. 1980, married Stefano Casiraghi on 29 Dec. 1983 (died, 3 Oct. 1990), offspring: Andrea, born 8 June 1984, Charlotte, born 3 Aug. 1986, Pierre, born 7 Sept. 1987. Prince Albert Alexandre Louis Pierre, born 14 March 1958 *(heir apparent).* Princess Stephanie Marie Elisabeth, born 1 Feb. 1965.

CONSTITUTION AND GOVERNMENT. Prince Rainier III on 28 Jan. 1959 suspended the Constitution of 5 Jan. 1911, thereby dissolving the National Council and the Communal Council. On 28 March 1962 the National Council (18 members elected every 5 years, last elections 1988) and the Communal Council (15 members elected every 4 years, last elections 1987) were re-established as elected bodies. On 17 Dec. 1962 a new constitution was promulgated. It maintains the hereditary monarchy, though Prince Rainier renounces the principle of divine right. The supreme tribunal becomes the custodian of fundamental liberties, and guarantees are given for the right of association, trade union freedom and the right to strike. It provides for votes for women and the abolition of the death penalty.

The constitution can be modified only with the approval of the elected National Council. Women were given the vote in 1945.

Monegasque relations with France are based on conventions of 1963. French citizens are treated as if in France.

National flag: Horizontally red over white.

ECONOMY

Planning. A 22-ha site reclaimed from the sea at Fontvieille has been earmarked for office and residential development. The present industrial zone is to be reorganized and developed with a view to attracting new light industry.

Budget. The budget (in 1,000 francs) was as follows:

	1986	*1987*	*1988*	*1989*	*1990*
Revenue	2,139,305	2,232,032	2,542,175	2,436,246	2,666,568
Expenditure	1,999,764	2,229,806	2,494,307	2,427,436	2,657,565

Currency. Monaco is a member of the French Franc Zone.

Banking and Finance. There were 38 banks in 1990. Financial services represent about 35% of economic activity.

Weights and Measures. The metric system is in use.

INDUSTRY. Light industry makes up about 25% of economic activity. There are some 700 small businesses, including chemicals, plastics, electronics, engineering and paper.

Labour. There were 27,940 persons employed on 1 June 1990.

Trade Unions. Membership of trade unions was estimated at 2,000 out of a work force of 25,600 (1989).

EXTERNAL ECONOMIC RELATIONS

Commerce. There is a customs union with France, and international trade is included with France.

Tourism. Tourism is the main industry. There were 245,146 overnight tourists in 1989, who spent a total of 740,566 nights.

COMMUNICATIONS

Roads. There were 50 km of roads in 1989.

Railways. The 1·6 km of main line passing through the country is operated by the French National Railways (SNCF).

Aviation. The nearest airport is at Nice, France. At the Heliport of Monaco (Fontvieille) there were 98,550 passengers in the year ending Sept. 1990 (109,180 in 1989).

Shipping. The harbour has an area of 15 ha; depth at the entrance is 26 metres, and alongside the quays, 7 metres. Length of the quays: 2,290 metres.

Telecommunications. Telephone subscribers numbered 26,240 in 1990 and telex subscribers, 676. Monaco issues its own postage stamps.

Radio Monte Carlo broadcasts FM commercial programmes in French (long- and medium-waves). Radio Monte Carlo owns 55% of Radio Monte Carlo Relay Station on Cyprus. The foreign service is dedicated exclusively to religious broadcasts and is maintained by free-will contributions. It operates in 36 languages under the name 'Trans World Radio' and has relay facilities on Bonaire, West Indies, and is planning to build relay facilities in the southern parts of Africa. *Télé Monté-Carlo* broadcasts TV programmes in French, Italian and English. There is a 30-channel cable service.

Cinemas. In 1989 there were 4 cinemas (one open air) with seating capacity of 1,000.

JUSTICE, RELIGION, EDUCATION AND WELFARE

Justice. There are the following courts, *Juge de Paix*, Tribunal of the First Instance, a Court of Appeal, Criminal Tribunal, *Cour de Révision Judiciaire* and a Supreme Tribunal.

Police: There is an independent police force *(Sûreté Publique)* which comprised (1989) 236 policemen and inspectors.

Religion. There has been since 1887 a Roman Catholic bishop elevated since 1982 to an archbishop, directly dependent on the Holy See.

Education. In 1990 there were 5,523 pupils with over 735 teachers.

Health. In 1990 there were 537 hospital beds and 80 physicians.

DIPLOMATIC REPRESENTATIVES

British Consul-General (resident in Marseilles): John Illman.
British Honorary Consul (resident in Nice): Lieut.-Col. R. W. Challoner, OBE.
Consul-General for Monaco in London: I. S. Ivanovic.

Further Reading

Journal de Monaco. Bulletin Officiel. 1858 ff.
Handley-Taylor, G., *Bibliography of Monaco.* London, 1968
Hudson, G. L. *Monaco*: [Bibliography]. Oxford and Santa Barbara, 1990

MONGOLIA

Capital: Ulan Bator
Population: 2·095m. (1989)
GNP per capita: US$473 (1989)

Bügd Nayramdakh Mongol Ard Uls

(Mongolian People's Republic)

HISTORY. Outer Mongolia was a Chinese province from 1691 to 1911, an autonomous state under Russian protection from 1912 to 1919 and again a Chinese province from 1919 to 1921. On 13 March 1921 a Provisional People's Government was established which declared the independence of Mongolia and on 5 Nov. 1921 signed a treaty with Soviet Russia annulling all previous unequal treaties and establishing friendly relations. On 26 Nov. 1924 the Government proclaimed the country the Mongolian People's Republic.

On 5 Jan. 1946 China recognized the independence of Outer Mongolia after a plebiscite in Mongolia (20 Oct. 1945) had resulted in an overwhelming vote for independence. A Sino-Soviet treaty of 14 Feb. 1950 guaranteed this independence. In Aug. 1986 a consular agreement, in June 1987 a boundary agreement, and in Nov. 1988 a border treaty, were signed with China.

Until 1990 sole power was in the hands of the Mongolian People's Revolutionary (*i.e.*, Communist) Party (MPRP), but an opposition Mongolian Democratic Party, founded in Dec. 1989, achieved tacit recognition and held its first congress in Feb. 1990. Following demonstrations and hunger-strikes, on 12 March the entire MPRP Politburo resigned and political opposition was legalized.

AREA AND POPULATION. Mongolia is bounded north by the USSR, east and south and west by China. Area, 1,567,000 sq. km (604,250 sq. miles). Population (1989 census); 2,095,600 (57% urban; 49·9% male). Density, 1·34 per sq. km. Birth rate, 36·4 per 1,000; death rate, 8·4 per 1,000; marriage rate, 6·6 per 1,000; divorce rate, 0·2 per 1,000. Rate of increase, 28·0 per 1,000. The population is predominantly made up of Mongolian peoples (78·8% Halh). There is a Turkic Kazakh minority (5·9% of the population) and 20 Mongol minorities. The official language is Halh Mongol. Expectation of life in 1987 was 63 years. 44·2% of the population is under 16.

The republic is administratively divided into 3 cities: Ulan Bator, the capital, (1989 population, 560,600), Darhan, (87,400) and Erdenet (57,100), and 18 provinces *(aimag)*. The provinces are sub-divided into 306 districts *(suums)*.

CLIMATE. A very extreme climate, with six months of mean temperatures below freezing, but much higher temperatures occur for a month or two in summer. Rainfall is very low and limited to the months mid-May to mid-Sept. Ulan Bator. Jan. –14°F (–25·6°C), July 61°F (16·1°C). Annual rainfall 8" (208 mm).

CONSTITUTION AND GOVERNMENT. For the Communist régime before 1990 *see* THE STATESMAN'S YEAR-BOOK 1990–91, p. 872.

In accordance with a constitutional amendment of 12 May 1990, the legislature consists of the 430-member *Great People's Hural* elected from 306 rural constituencies (*suums*) and 10,000-strong urban constituencies; and the 50-member *Small State Hural*. Suffrage is universal at 18. The Great Hural meets 4 times in its 5-year term. The Small Hural meets twice a year for 75-day periods during its 5-year term; it is elected partly by the Great Hural and partly directly, and its Chairman is Vice-

President of the Republic. The *President* of the Republic is elected by the Great Hural.

At the election of July 1990 the electorate was 1m.; turn-out was 91·9%. The Mongolian People's Revolutionary Party (Communists) won 357 seats in the Great Hural and 31 in the Small Hural. In the Great Hural the Democratic Party won 20 seats, the National Progress Party, 6, and the Social Democratic Party, 4.

In Sept. 1990 the Great Khural elected Punsalmaagiin Ochirbat (b. 1942) *President* of the Republic, Radnaasumberelin Gonchigdorj (b. 1954) *Vice-President*, and Dashiin Byambasuren (b. 1942) *Prime Minister*.

National flag: Red–sky-blue–red (vertical), with a golden 5-pointed star and under it the golden *soyombo* emblem on the red stripe nearest to the flagpole.

National anthem: Was being revised in 1991 to expunge references to the USSR.

Local government is carried out by 380 People's Deputies' Hurals. Some 13,000 deputies were elected in July 1990.

DEFENCE. Military service is 2 years.

Army. The Army comprises 4 motorized infantry divisions. Equipment includes 650 T-54/-55/-62 main battle tanks. Strength (1991) 21,000, with reserves of 200,000. There is a paramilitary Ministry of Public Security force of about 10,000 men. A civil defence force was set up in 1970.

There were some 12,500 Soviet service personnel in Mongolia in 1991, but these are scheduled for withdrawal by 1992.

Air Force. The Air Force has about 100 pilots and more than 70 aircraft, including 12 MiG-21 and 10 MiG-17 fighters; a total of about 30 An-2, An-24 and An-26 transports used mainly on civil air services; 3 Wilga utility aircraft; 6 Mi-4 and 10 Mi-8 helicopters; and Yakovlev trainers. Personnel (1991), 500 with 28 combatant aircraft and 10 armed helicopters.

INTERNATIONAL RELATIONS

Membership. Mongolia is a member of the UN and OIEC.

ECONOMY

Policy. Mongolia has had for centuries a traditional nomadic pastoral economy, which the Government aims to transform into a market economy.

Budget (in 1m. tugriks):

	1980	*1982*	*1983*	*1985*	*1987*	*1989*
Revenue	4,070	4,830	5,156	5,741·0	6,441·7	6,901·6
Expenditure	4,058	3,131	5,126	5,700·9	6,408·6	7,062·3

Sources of revenue, 1989: Turnover tax, 60%; profits tax, 32%; social insurance, 3·7%. Expenditure: Economy, 47%; social and cultural, 39%.

Currency. The unit of currency is the *tugrik* (MNT) of 100 *möngö*. Notes are issued for 1, 2, 5, 10, 20, 50 and 100 *tugriks*; and coins for 1, 2, 5, 10, 15, 20, 50 *möngö* and 1 *tugrik*. In March 1991, £1 = 6·37 *tugriks*; US$1 = 3·36 *tugriks*.

Banking and Finance. The Mongolian State Bank (established 1924) is the bank of issue, being also a commercial, savings and development bank. It has 21 main branches. There are also a Trade and Industry Bank, an Insurance Bank and a Co-operative Bank. The banking system is being restructured.

Weights and Measures. The metric system is in use.

ENERGY AND NATURAL RESOURCES

Electricity. There are 6 thermal electric power stations. Production of electricity, 1989, 3,568·3m. kwh.

Minerals. There are large deposits of copper, nickel, zinc, molybdenum, phosphorites, tin, wolfram and fluorspar; production of the latter in 1989, 578,200 tonnes, entirely exported to the USSR. The copper/molybdenum ore-dressing plant at Erdenet was completed in 1981. There are major coalmines near Ulan Bator and Darhan. Coal (mainly lignite) production in 1989 was 8m. tonnes.

Agriculture. 70% of agricultural production derives from cattle-raising. In 1989 there were 2,199,600 horses, 2,692,700 cattle, 14,265,200 sheep, 558,300 camels and 4,959,100 goats.

Ownership of livestock (in 1m.) in 1989:

	Collective farms	*State farms*	*Private*
Cattle	1·10	0·28	1·30
Camels	0·47	0·01	0·08
Horses	1·05	0·15	1·00
Sheep	9·75	1·52	2·92
Goats	3·26	0·14	1·55

In 1989 there were 192,100 pigs and 369,900 poultry. 239,600 tonnes of meat and 3·3m. litres of fermented mare's milk. Milk production was 62m. litres. In 1989 there were 255 collective farms, 39 inter-farm associations, 21 fodder supply farms and 52 state farms.

All cultivated land belongs to collective or state farms. The total agricultural area in 1989 was 125·5m. ha, of which 1·3m. were arable (0·8m. sown) and 124·2m. meadows and pastures. 60·5% of the sown area belongs to state farms, 23·5% to collectives. In 1989 80% was sown to cereals, 18% to fodder and 2% to vegetables. The 1989 crop was 686,900 tonnes of wheat; 3,200 tonnes of rye; 38,200 tonnes of oats; 108,500 tonnes of barley. In 1989, 155,500 tonnes of potatoes were harvested. In 1989 there were 7,700 tractors (15 h.p. units) and 2,500 combine harvesters.

Forestry. Forests, chiefly larch, cedar, fir and birch, occupy 13·9m. ha, 9% of the land area. Production, 1989: 2,673,300 cu. metres of sawn wood.

INDUSTRY. Industry though still small in scale and local in character, is being vigorously developed and now accounts for a greater share of GNP than agriculture. The food industry accounts for 25% of industrial production. The main industrial centre is Ulan Bator; others are at Erdenet and Baga-Nur, and a northern territorial industrial complex is being developed based on Darhan and Erdenet to produce copper and molybdenium concentrates, lime, cement, machinery and wood- and metal-worked products. Production figures (1989): Scoured wool, 10,100 tonnes; cement, 512,600 tonnes; leather footwear, 4·1m. pairs; meat, 61,700 tonnes; soap, 4,500 tonnes.

Labour. The labour force was 633,200 in 1989, including 119,600 in industry, 186,000 in agriculture, 41,700 in building, 53,900 in transport and communications and 47,500 in trade. In 1989 53% of the labour force was female. Average wage was 539 tugriks per month in 1989.

Trade Unions. Membership was 0·53m. in 1988.

FOREIGN ECONOMIC RELATIONS. Relations with the USSR have been based on a 1985 treaty of economic co-operation. The USSR is Mongolia's only creditor.

Joint ventures with foreign firms are permitted.

Commerce. Since 1989 some enterprises have been able to trade directly abroad. Trade figures for 1989 (in 1m. tugriks): Exports, 2,148; imports, 2,682. Exports in 1989 included 43% minerals and fuels, 26% food and consumer goods and 19% non-food raw materials. 93% of foreign trade is with communist countries. Main imports are machinery and fuel. Imports from the USSR totalled 534·1m. roubles in 1989, exports to the USSR, 354m. roubles. The main non-Communist trading partner is Japan.

Total trade between Mongolia and UK (British Department of Trade returns, in £1,000 sterling):

	1987	*1988*	*1989*	*1990*
Imports to UK	3,847	1,857	405	1,674
Exports and re-exports from UK	941	1,637	979	1,636

Tourism. 236,500 tourists visited Mongolia in 1989.

COMMUNICATIONS

Roads. There are 1,185 km of surfaced roads running around Ulan Bator, from Ulan Bator to Darhan, at points on the frontier with USSR and towards the south. Truck services run where there are no surfaced roads. 62·0m. tonnes of freight were carried in 1989, and 242·2m. passengers.

Railways. The Trans-Mongolian Railway (1,100 km in 1989) connects Ulan Bator with the Soviet Union and China. The Moscow–Ulan Bator–Beijing express runs each way once a week, and there are services to Irkutsk, Moscow and Beijing. There are spur lines to Erdenet and to the coalmines at Nalayh and Sharin Gol. A separate line connects Choybalsan in the east with Borzya on the Trans-Siberian railway. 2·7m. passengers and 16·8m. tonnes of freight were carried in 1989.

Aviation. Mongolian Airlines (MIAT) operates internal services, a flight to Irkutsk which links with the Soviet airlines (Aeroflot) stopping service to Moscow, and (with Aeroflot) a daily non-stop service to Moscow from Ulan Bator. There are weekly flights to Beijing. 10,000 tons of freight were carried in 1989 and 800,000 passengers. Ulan Bator airport (Buyant Uhaa) was modernized and expanded in 1985.

Shipping. There is a steamer service on the Selenge River and a tug and barge service on Hövsgöl Lake. 60,000 tonnes of freight were carried in 1989.

Telecommunications. There were, in 1989, 429 post offices and 329 telephone exchanges. Number of telephones (1989), 62,600.

There are wireless stations at Ulan Bator, Gobi Altai and Olgii. In 1989 there were 211,700 radio and 132,900 television receivers. Television services began in 1967. A Mongolian television station opened in 1970. Mongolia is a member of the international TV organization Intervision.

Cinemas. In 1989 there were 27 cinemas, 516 mobile cinemas and 28 theatres.

Newspapers and books. In 1989, 35 newspapers and 41 journals were published. 977 book titles were published in 1987 in 7·5m. copies.

JUSTICE, RELIGION, EDUCATION AND WELFARE

Justice. The Procurator-General is appointed, and the Supreme Court elected, by the *Hural* for 5 years. There are also courts at province, town and district level. Lay assessors sit with professional judges.

Religion. Tibetan Buddhist Lamaism was the prevalent form of religion. It was suppressed in the 1930s, 40 monasteries with some 500 lamas (monks) function today.

Education. In 1989 there were 822 nurseries with 88,300 children. Schooling begins at the age of 7. In 1988-89 there were 615 general education schools with 446,700 pupils and 19,800 teachers, 30 specialized secondary schools with 20,500 students and 1,200 teachers and 46 vocational technical schools with 34,100 pupils. There is a state university (founded 1942) at Ulan Bator (6 professors, 277 lecturers and 1,900 students in 1989), and 7 other institutes of higher learning (teacher training, medicine, agriculture, economics, etc.) with 17,600 students in 1989 and 1,192 teachers. The Academy of Sciences (founded 1961) has 15 institutes and 662 research workers. In 1989, 5,400 students were sent to study abroad, principally in the USSR.

In 1946 the Mongolian alphabet was replaced by Cyrillic, but its teaching has now been resumed.

Health and Welfare. In 1989 160·7m. tugriks were spent on maternity benefits.

Annual average per capita consumption (in kilogrammes) of foodstuffs in 1989: Meat, 93; milk and products, 121; sugar, 24; flour, 105; potatoes, 27; fresh vegetables, 22. In 1989 there were 28 doctors and 118 hospital beds per 10,000 population.

DIPLOMATIC REPRESENTATIVES

Of Mongolia in Great Britain (7 Kensington Ct., London, W8 5DL)
Ambassador: Ishetsogyin Ochirbal.

Of Great Britain in Mongolia (30 Enkh Taivny Gudamzh, Ulan Bator)
Ambassador: D. K. Sprague, MVO.

Of Mongolia in the USA
Ambassador: Gendengiin Nyamdoo.

Of the USA in Mongolia
Ambassador: Joseph Edward Lake.

Of Mongolia to the United Nations
Ambassador: Mangalyn Dugersuren.

Further Reading

The Central Statistical Office: *National Economy of the MPR, 1924–1984: Anniversary Statistical Collection*. Ulan Bator, 1984

Bawden, C. R., *The Modern History of Mongolia*. London, 1968
Boberg, F., *Mongolian–English, English–Mongolian Dictionary*. 3 vols. Stockholm, 1954–55
Butler, W. E., (ed.) *The Mongolian Legal System: Contemporary Legislation and Documentation*. The Hague, 1982
Haltod, M. (ed.) *Mongolian–English Dictionary*. Berkeley, Cal., 1961
Jagchid, S. and Hyer, P., *Mongolia's Culture and Society*. Folkestone, 1979
Lattimore, O., *Nationalism and Revolution in Mongolia*. Leiden, 1955.—*Nomads and Commissars*. OUP, 1963
Lörinc, L., *Histoire de la Mongolie des Origines à nos Jours*. Budapest, 1984
News from Mongolia. Ulan Bator, fortnightly, Jan. 1980
Rupen, R. A., *How Mongolia is Really Ruled: A Political History of the Mongolian People's Republic, 1900–1978*. Stanford, 1979
Sanders, A. J. K., *The People's Republic of Mongolia: A General Reference Guide*. OUP, 1968.—*Mongolia: Politics, Economics and Society*. London, 1987
Shirendev, B. and Sanjdorj, M. (eds.) *History of the Mongolian People's Republic*. Vol. 3 (vols. 1 and 2 not translated). Harvard Univ. Press, 1976

MONTSERRAT

Capital: Plymouth
Population: 11,852 (1985)
GNP per capita: US$3,127 (1985)

HISTORY. Montserrat was discovered by Columbus in 1493 and colonized by Britain in 1632 who brought Irish settlers to the island. Montserrat formed part of the federal colony of the Leeward Islands from 1871 until 1956, when it became a separate colony following the dissolution of the Federation. The island's Constitution came into force in 1960 and the title Administrator was changed to that of Governor in 1971. On 17 Sept. 1989 hurricane 'Hugo' caused damage estimated at US$330m.

AREA AND POPULATION. Montserrat is situated in the Caribbean Sea 25 miles south-west of Antigua. The area is 39·5 sq. miles (106 sq. km). Population, 1985, 11,852. Chief town, Plymouth, 3,500 inhabitants.

CLIMATE. A tropical climate but with no well-defined rainy season, though July to Dec. shows slightly more rainfall, with the average for the year being about 60" (1,500 mm). Dec. to March is the cooler season while June to Nov. is the hotter season, when hurricanes may occur. Plymouth. Jan. 76°F (24·4°C), July 81°F (27·2°C). Annual rainfall 65" (1,628 mm).

CONSTITUTION AND GOVERNMENT. Montserrat is a crown colony. The Executive Council is composed of 4 elected Ministers (the Chief Minister and 3 other Ministers) and 2 civil service officials (Attorney-General and Financial Secretary). The Legislative Council consists of 7 elected and 2 civil service officials (the Attorney-General and Financial Secretary) and 2 nominated members. The Executive Council is presided over by the Governor and the Legislative Council by the Speaker.

In elections to the Legislative Council in 1987, 4 seats were won by the People's Liberation Movement, 2 by the National Development Party and 1 by the Progressive Democratic Party.

Governor: David Taylor.
Chief Minister: Hon. John A. Osborne.
Flag: The British Blue Ensign with the shield of Montserrat in the fly.

ECONOMY

Budget. In 1989 the budget expenditure was at EC$35m. (EC$31m. in 1988 of which EC$8·64m. was capital expenditure). In 1981 the territorial budget ceased to be grant-aided by the British Government.

Currency. 100 cents = 1 Eastern Caribbean dollar (XCD). Coins: 1, 2, 5, 25, 50 cents. Notes: 1, 5, 10, 20 and 100 dollars.

Banking and Finance. There is a Bank of Montserrat, a Government Savings Bank; Barclays Bank, the Guardian International Bank and the Royal Bank of Canada maintain branches and the Montserrat Building Society. Responsibility for overseeing offshore banking rests with the Governor.

ENERGY AND NATURAL RESOURCES

Electricity. Production (1987) 16·3m. kwh.

Agriculture. Self-sufficiency in fruit, ground provisions and vegetables though canned and preserved foodstuffs were imported was achieved in 1988. The processing and packaging of tropical fruits and herbal teas for export are being encouraged together with the growing of ornamental plants for export.

Livestock (1988); Cattle, 3,000; pigs, 1,000; sheep and goats, 11,005; poultry, 50,500.

Fisheries. Catch (1988) 100 tonnes.

INDUSTRY. Manufacturing contributes about 6% to GDP and accounts for 10% of employment, but is responsible for up to 85% of exports. It is limited to small scale industries producing light consumer goods such as electronic components, plastic bags, leather goods and various items made from locally grown cotton.

FOREIGN ECONOMIC RELATIONS

Commerce. Imports in 1988 totalled EC$72m.; domestic exports, EC$6m. Chief imports were manufactured goods, food and beverages, machinery and transport equipment and fuel. Chief exports were cotton clothing, electronic parts and lighting fittings.

Total trade between Montserrat and UK (British Department of Trade returns, in £1,000 sterling):

	1986	*1987*	*1988*	*1989*	*1990*
Imports to UK	358	139	125	494	425
Exports and re-exports from UK	3,926	2,432	2,524	3,092	3,515

Tourism. In 1988, 29,736 tourists arrived in Montserrat.

COMMUNICATIONS

Roads. In 1987 there were 290 km of roads, 212 km paved, 1,368 passenger cars and 270 commercial vehicles.

Aviation. At Blackburne airport 4,447 aircraft landed in 1988, disembarking 30,272 passengers and 214 tonnes of cargo.

Shipping. In 1988, 270 cargo vessels arrived, landing 47,026 and loading (1987) 663 tonnes of cargo.

Post and Broadcasting. Number of telephones (1988), 3,938; telex, 46 and 44 facsimile subscribers. In 1984 there were 4,000 radio and 1,100 TV receivers.

JUSTICE, RELIGION, EDUCATION AND WELFARE

Justice. There are 2 magistrates' courts, at Plymouth and Cudjoe Head. Strength of the police force (1987), 2 gazetted officers, 3 inspectorate and 89 other ranks.

Religion. In 1980 (census) there were 1,368 Roman Catholics, 3,676 Anglicans, 2,742 Methodists, 1,041 Seventh Day Adventists, 1,503 Pentecostals and 285 members of the Church of God. There is also a Christian Council of Churches.

Education. There were (1989) 2 day-care centres, 12 nursery schools, 12 primary schools, a comprehensive secondary school with 3 campuses, and a technical training college. Schools are run by the Government, the churches and the private sector. In 1988 there were 460 pupils at nursery schools; 1,403 at primary school, 1,043 at secondary school and 72 at the technical training college. There is an Extra Mural Department of the University of the West Indies in Plymouth with about 200 students and 15 part-time and 1 full-time lecturers.

Health. In 1985 there were 8 doctors and 67 hospital beds.

Further Reading

Population Census 1980. Montserrat
Overseas Trade 1983. Montserrat Government
Vital Statistics Report. Montserrat Government, 1983
Statistical Digest 1984. Montserrat Government
Fergus, H.A., *Montserrat: Emerald Isle of the Caribbean*. London, 1983

Library: Public Library, Plymouth. *Librarian:* Miss Ruth Allen.

MOROCCO

Capital: Rabat
Population: 24.5m. (1989)
GNP per capita: US$750 (1988)

Al-Mamlaka al-Maghrebia
(Kingdom of Morocco)

HISTORY. From 1912 to 1956 Morocco was divided into a French protectorate (established by the treaty of Fez concluded between France and the Sultan on 30 March 1912), a Spanish protectorate (established by the Franco-Spanish convention of 27 Nov. 1912) and the international zone of Tangier (set up by France, Spain and Great Britain on 18 Dec. 1923).

On 2 March 1956 France and the Sultan terminated the treaty of Fez; on 7 April 1956 Spain relinquished her protectorate, and on 29 Oct. 1956 France, Spain, Great Britain, Italy, USA, Belgium, the Netherlands, Sweden and Portugal abolished the international status of the Tangier Zone. The northern strip of Spanish Sahara was ceded by Spain on 10 April 1958, and on 30 June 1969 the former Spanish province of Ifni was returned to Morocco.

A tripartite agreement was announced on 14 Nov. 1975 providing for the transfer of power from Spanish Sahara (Western Sahara) to the Moroccan and Mauritanean governments on 28 Feb. 1976. Spanish troops left El Aaiún on 20 Dec. 1975. On 14 April 1976 a Convention was signed by Mauritania and Morocco in which the 2 countries agreed to partition the former Spanish territory, but on 14 Aug. 1979 Mauritania renounced its claim to its share of the territory (Tiris El-Gharbiya) which was added by Morocco to its area.

AREA AND POPULATION. Morocco is bounded by Algeria to the east and south-east, Western Sahara to the south-west, the Atlantic ocean to the north-west and the Mediterranean to the north. Excluding the Western Saharan territory claimed and occupied since 1976 by Morocco, the total area is 458,730 sq. km and its total population at the Sept. 1982 census was 20,255,687; the latest estimate (1989) is 24.5m. (47.8% urban).

The areas (in sq. km) and populations (census 1982) of the provinces are:

Province	*Sq. km*	*1982*	*Province*	*Sq. km*	*1982*
Agadir	5,910	579,741	Nador	6,130	593,255
Taroudant	16,460	558,501	Ouarzazate	41,550	533,892
Al-Hoceima	3,550	311,298	Oujda	20,700	780,762
Azilal	10,050	387,115	Rabat-Salé [1]	1,275	1,020,001
Beni Mellal	7,075	668,703	Safi	7,285	706,618
Ben Slimane	2,760	174,464	Settat	9,750	692,359
Boulemane	14,395	131,470	Tangier	1,195	436,227
Casablanca-Anfa [1]		923,630	Tan-Tan	17,295	47,040
Aïn Chok-Hay Hassani [1]		298,376	Taounate	5,585	535,972
Ben Msik-Sidi Othmane [1]	1,615	639,558	Tata	25,925	99,950
Hay Mohamed-Aïn Sebâa [1]		421,272	Taza	15,020	613,485
Mohamedia-Znata [1]		153,828	Tétouan	6,025	704,205
Chechaouèn	4,350	309,024	Tiznit	6,960	313,140
El Jadida	6,000	763,351			
El Kelâa-Srarhna	10,070	577,595	Morocco	458,730	20,255,687
Er Rachidia	59,585	421,207			
Es Saouira	6,335	393,683			
Fez	5,400	805,464	Boujdour		
Figuig	55,990	101,359	(Bojador)	100,120	8,481
Guelmim	28,750	128,676	Es Semara		
Kénitra	4,745	715,967	(Smara)	61,760	20,480
Sidi Kacem	4,060	514,127	Laâyoune		
Khémisset	8,305	405,836	(Al Aaiún)	39,360	113,411
Khénifra	12,320	363,716	Oued Ed		
Khouribga	4,250	437,002	Dahab	50,880	21,496
Marrakesh	14,755	1,266,695			
Meknès	3,995	626,868	Sahara	252,120	163,868
Ifrane	3,310	100,255			

[1] Urban prefectures

The chief cities (with Census populations, 1982) are as follows:

Casablanca	2,139,204	Tangier	266,346	Agadir	110,479
Rabat	518,616	Oujda	260,082	Mohammedia	105,120
Fez	448,823	Tétouan	199,615	Beni Mellal	95,003
Marrakesh	439,728	Safi	197,616	Al Jadida	81,455
Meknès	319,783	Kénitra	188,194	Taza	77,216
Salé	289,391	Khouribga	127,181	Ksar al Kabir	73,541

The official language is Arabic, spoken by 75% of the population; the remainder speak Berber. French and Spanish are considered subsidiary languages.

CLIMATE. The climate ranges from semi-arid in the south to warm temperate Mediterranean conditions in the north, but cooler temperatures occur in the mountains. Rabat. Jan. 55°F (12·9°C), July 72°F (22·2°C). Annual rainfall 23" (564 mm). Agadir. Jan. 57°F (13·9°C), July 72°F (22·2°C). Annual rainfall 9" (224 mm). Casablanca. Jan. 54°F (12·2°C), July 72°F (22·2°C). Annual rainfall 16" (404 mm). Marrakesh. Jan. 52°F (11·1°C), July 84°F (28·9°C). Annual rainfall 10" (239 mm). Tangier. Jan. 53°F (11·7°C), July 72°F (22·2°C). Annual rainfall 36" (897 mm).

REIGNING KING. Hassan II, born on 9 July 1929, succeeded on 3 March 1961, on the death of his father Mohammed V, who reigned 1927–61. The royal style was changed from 'His Sherifian Majesty the Sultan' to 'His Majesty the King' on 18 Aug. 1957. *Heir apparent:* Crown Prince Sidi Mohammed, born 21 Aug. 1963.

The King holds supreme civil and religious authority; the latter in his capacity of Emir-el-Muminin or Commander of the Faithful. He resides usually at Rabat, but occasionally in one of the other traditional capitals, Fez (founded in 808), Marrakesh (founded in 1062), or at Skhirat.

CONSTITUTION AND GOVERNMENT. A new Constitution was approved by referendum in March 1972 and amendments were approved by referendum in May 1980. The Kingdom of Morocco is a constitutional monarchy with a legislature of a single chamber composed of 306 deputies. Deputies for 102 seats are elected by indirect vote through an electoral college representing the town councils, the regional assemblies, the chambers of commerce, industry and agriculture, and the trade unions. Deputies for the remaining 204 seats are by general election. The King, as sovereign head of State, appoints the Prime Minister and other Ministers, has the right to dissolve Parliament and approves legislation.

In the General Elections held on 14 Sept. 1984, the new *Union constitutionelle* (founded Jan. 1983) won 83 seats, the *Rassemblement nationale des indépendants* 61 seats, the *Union socialiste des forces populaires* 36 seats, the *Mouvement populaire* 47 seats, *Istiqlal* (Independence) 41 seats; others 38 seats.

Elections due in 1990 have been postponed to 1992.

National flag: Red, with a green pentacle star in the centre.

The cabinet in 1990 was composed as follows:

Prime Minister: N. Azzeddine Laraki.

Justice: Moulay Mustapha Belarbi Alaoui. *Interior:* Driss Basri. *Foreign Affairs, Co-operation and Information:* Abdellatif Filali. *Planning:* Rachid Ghazouani. *National Education:* Mohamed Hilali. *Economic Affairs:* Moulay Zine Zahidi. *Finance:* Abdellatif Jouahri. *Trade, Industry and Tourism:* Abdallah al-Azmani. *Handicrafts and Social Affairs:* Mohamed Labied. *Transport:* Mohamed Bouamoud. *Energy and Mining:* Mohamed Fettah. *Health:* Tayeb Bencheikh. *Maritime Fishing and Merchant Navy:* Bensalem Smili. *Secretary-General of the Government:* Abbas Kaissi. *Cultural Affairs:* Mohamed Benaissa. *Housing and Land Management:* Abderrahmane Boufettas. *Equipment, Executive and Professional Training:* Mohamed Kabbaj. *Posts and Telecommunications:* Mohand Laensar. *Agriculture and Land Reform:* Otman Demnati. *Relations with Parliament:* Tahar Afifi. *Youth and Sports:* Abdellatif Semlali. *Labour:* Hassan Abbadi. *Islamic Affairs:* Abdelkbar Alaoui Medaghri. *Administrative Affairs:* Abderrahim Ben

Abdeljalil. *Saharan Province:* Khali H. Ould Rachid. *Relations with the European Community:* Azzedine Guessous. There was 1 Minister of State.

Local Government: The country is administratively divided into 39 provinces and 8 urban prefectures.

DEFENCE. Military service is compulsory for 18 months.

Army. The Army comprises 1 mechanized infantry and 2 motorized infantry brigades; 2 parachute brigades; 11 mechanized infantry regiments; 10 artillery groups; 7 armoured, 1 Royal Guard, 3 camel corps, 3 desert cavalry, 1 mountain, and 4 engineer battalions. Equipment includes 224 M-48A5 main battle tanks, 50 AMX-13 light tanks and many armoured cars. Strength (1991) 175,000 men. There are also 40,000 paramilitary troops.

Navy. The Navy includes 1 missile-armed Spanish-built frigate, 4 fast missile craft, 9 coastal patrol craft and 10 inshore patrol craft. There are additionally 3 medium landing ships of French origin, 2 transports and 1 Ro-Ro ferry in naval use. Personnel in 1990 numbered 7,000, including a 1,500 strong brigade of Naval Infantry. Bases are located at Casablanca, Agadir, Al-Hoceina and Dakhla.

The Coast Guard wing of the Royal Gendarmerie operates 18 patrol craft.

Air Force. The Air Force was formed in Nov. 1956. Equipment in current use is mainly of US and West European origin. It includes 40 Mirage F1s, a total of 30 F-5A/B/E/F fighter-bombers and RF-5A reconnaissance-fighters, 3 OV-10 Bronco counter-insurgency aircraft, 2 Falcon 20s for electronic warfare, and 24 Gazelle armed helicopters, 24 Alpha Jet advanced trainers, 22 Magister armed jet basic trainers, 12 T-34C-1 turboprop basic trainers, 10 Swiss-built Bravo primary trainers, 2 Mudry CAP 10B aerobatic trainers, 4 Broussard liaison aircraft, 90 Agusta-Bell 205 and 212, Puma and JetRanger helicopters, 2 Do 28D Skyservants for coastal patrol, 11 CH-47C heavy-lift helicopters, 18 C-130H turboprop transport aircraft, 2 KC-130H tanker/transports, a Falcon 50 and a Gulfstream II VIP transport, 2 Boeing 707s and 8 turboprop King Air light transports. Personnel strength (1991) about 13,500, with 93 combatant aircraft and 24 armed helicopters.

INTERNATIONAL RELATIONS

Membership. Morocco is a member of the UN, the Non-Aligned Movement, the Islamic Conference and the Arab League.

ECONOMY

Budget. The budget for 1988 envisaged revenue of 50,547m. DH and expenditure of 59,736m. DH.

Currency. The unit of currency is the *dirham* (MAD) of 100 *centimes*, introduced in 1959. Notes: 10, 50, 100 DH; coins: 0·10, 0·20, 0·50, 1 DH. The exchange rate in March 1991 was £1 sterling = 14·92 DH; US$1 = 7·86 DH.

Banking and Finance. The central bank is the Banque al Maghrib. Authorized banks are: La Banque Marocaine du Commerce Extérieur, La Banque Marocaine pour le Commerce et l'Industrie, La Banque Commerciale du Maroc, Compagnie Marocaine du Crédit et de Banque, Société Générale Marocaine de Banque, Crédit du Maroc, Union Marocaine de Banque, Société de dépôt et de crédits, Arab Bank Ltd, Bank of America, Banco Espagnol en Maruecos, Banque de Paris et des Pays-Bas, First National City Bank, Société Hollandaise de Banque et de Gestion, The British Bank of the Middle East, Société de Dépôt et de Crédits, Wafabank, Citibank, Algemene Bank Nederland and Banque Américano-Suisse pour le Maroc. The Banque Centrale Populaire and regional Banques populaires also provide banking services for small and medium businesses. There are 3 development banks: Banque Nationale du Development Economique, whose major area of investment has been industry; Credit Industrial et Hotelier, which finances housing on easy terms; Caisse Nationale du Credit Agricole, which specializes in agriculture. La

Banque National pour le Développement économique grants loans to the industrial sector. Le Crédit Immobilier et Hôtelier grants loans for construction. La Caisse de Dépôt et de Gestion is responsible for the centralization of savings and their management.

Weights and Measures. The metric system is legal.

ENERGY AND NATURAL RESOURCES

Electricity. Electric power-plants produced 6,920m. kwh. in 1986. Supply 110, 127 and 220 volts; 50 Hz.

Oil. Crude oil production, 17,500 tonnes 1981. Refined oil production (including imported crude), 4·5m. tonnes in 1983.

Minerals. The principal mineral exploited is phosphate, the output of which was 21·4m. tonnes in 1986. Other important minerals (in tonnes, 1985) are: Anthracite (774,500), iron ore (190,258), lead (153,636), copper (59,245), zinc (27,153), manganese (43,690), baryt (463,380), fluorine (74,350), salt (118,173).

Agriculture. Land suitable for cultivation, 1984, 7·7m. ha, of which (in 1,000 hectares): Cereals, 4,500; leguminous vegetables, 400; market gardening, 150; oil-producing and industrial cultivation, 130; fodder, 110; dense fruit plantations, 400; fallows, 2,000.

Production in 1988 (in 1,000 tonnes): Wheat, 4,035; barley, 3,501; maize, 355; fruit, 1,787 (of which citrus fruits, 1,275); pulses, 450; sunflower seeds, 88; groundnuts, 32; sugar beets, 2,770; sugar-cane, 800; olives, 360; potatoes, 550; tomatoes, 400; onions, 272.

Dairy production in 1988 included: Milk, 923,000 tonnes; butter, 13,629 tonnes; cheese, 7,221 tonnes. Meat production (1988) 369,000 tonnes.

Livestock (in 1,000 heads), 1988: Cattle, 3,300; sheep, 15,700; goats, 5,800.

Forestry. Forests covered (1988) 5m. ha (12% of land area) and employed (1984) 50,000. They produce mainly firewood, building and industrial timber, some cork and charcoal.

Fisheries. The industry employed 83,000 workers in 1987. Total catch in 1986 was 591,000 tonnes, value 2,442,404,000 DH. The value of fish exports in 1986 was 2,860,552,000 DH.

INDUSTRY In 1984 industry represented 14% of the GNP. Manufacturing industries are concentrated in Casablanca (metallurgy, car assembly, sugar-producing and pharmaceutical products), Fez, Rabat, Muhammadia (textile), Safi (chemicals, manure, fish treatment) and Agadir (fish treatment, canning factories). There are 8 cement factories, with an output of 3,848,200 tonnes in 1983, when self-sufficiency was achieved.

The agricultural and food industries produce 40% of the whole industrial output. The sugar industry meets 76% of the country's needs and produced 426,800 tonnes of crude sugar in 1983.

Labour. An increase of 15% in the minimum wage was decreed in 1991.

Trade Unions. In 1984 there were 8 trade unions.

FOREIGN ECONOMIC RELATIONS In Feb. 1989 Morocco signed a treaty of economic co-operation with the 4 other Maghrels countries: Algeria Libya, Mauritania and Tunisia.

Foreign debt was US$21,000m. in Sept. 1990.

Commerce. Imports and exports were (in DH1m.):

	1985	*1986*	*1987*
Imports	38,675	34,608	35,271
Exports	21,740	22,103	23,390

Exports (1986) of phosphates 13·7m. tonnes, value DH3,840m.

Exports in 1985 went mainly to France (24%), Spain (7%), Federal Republic of Germany (7%), Italy (6%) and UK (3%). Imports were mainly from France (25%), Spain (14%), Federal Republic of Germany (8%), Italy (6%) and UK (3%).

Total trade between Morocco and UK (British Department of Trade returns, in £1,000 sterling):

	1986	*1987*	*1988*	*1989*	*1990*
Imports to UK	65,419	61,108	78,896	96,138	106,425
Exports and re-exports from UK	84,510	94,487	79,017	84,475	118,599

Tourism. In 1986, 1·47m. visitors came to Morocco, spending (1985) DH6,200m.

COMMUNICATIONS

Roads. In 1983 there were 57,592 km of classified roads, of which 19,099 km were surfaced. A motorway links Rabat to Casablanca. In 1987 there were in use 207,000 commercial vehicles, 554,000 private cars and 19,000 motor cycles.

Railways. In 1989 there were 1,893 km of railways, of which 974 km were electrified. The principal standard-gauge lines are from Casablanca eastward to the Algerian border, forming part of the continuous rail line to Tunis; Casablanca to Marrakesh with 2 important branches, one eastward to Oued Zem tapping the Khouribga phosphate mines, the other westward to the port of Safi. Another branch serves the manganese mines at Bou Arfa. Two new double-track electrified lines are to serve a new deep-water port at Jorf Lasfar.

In 1989 the railways carried 2,168m. passenger-km and 4,519m. tonne-km of freight.

Aviation. There are 15 international airports as well as national airports. The most important, Mohamed V airport in Casablanca, handled 18,154 flights with 1,367,548 passengers and 24,968·8 tonnes of freight including mail in 1983. Total flights, 1983, 44,606 with 3,176,648 passengers and 29,882·7 tonnes of freight including mail. In 1990 the 5 Maghreb countries agreed to merge their national airlines into Air Maghreb

Shipping. In 1983, 17,555 vessels entered and cleared the ports of Morocco and 19,393,000 tonnes of merchandise, including 13,891,500 tonnes of phosphate, were loaded and 11,260,000 tonnes unloaded.

Telecommunications. In 1983 there were 359 post offices. Telephone subscribers totalled 265,672 in 1983.

There are broadcasts in Arabic, Berber, French, Spanish and English from Rabat and Tangier; television in Arabic and French began in 1962. In 1988 there were 4·4m. radio receivers and 1·2m. television receivers.

Newspapers. In 1984 there were 12 daily newspapers (7 Arabic, 5 French) and 18 main weeklies and monthlies (10 Arabic, 8 French).

JUSTICE, RELIGION, EDUCATION AND WELFARE

Justice. A uniform legal system is being organized, based mainly on French and Islamic law codes and French legal procedure. The judiciary consists of a Supreme Court, courts of appeal, regional tribunals and magistrates' courts.

Religion. Islam is the established state religion. 98% are Sunni Moslems of the Malekite school and 2% are Christians, mainly Roman Catholic.

Education. In 1959 a standardization of the various school systems (French, Spanish, Israeli, Moslem, etc.) was begun. Education is compulsory from the age of 7 to 13.

In 1984 there were 2,550,000 pupils and 75,094 teachers in 3,144 state primary schools; 1,050,000 pupils and 51,711 teachers in secondary schools; 10,020 (1981) students in technical schools and 16,148 (1981) students in teacher-training establishments.

The language of instruction in primary and secondary schools is Arabic. Some scientific courses were (1985) still taught in French.

Professional and vocational colleges had 6,942 students in 1983. There were 30,000 students abroad.

There are six universities, Mohamed V at Rabat, Hassan II at Casablanca, Mohamed Ben Abdallah at Fez, Quaraouyine at Fez, Mohamed I at Oujda and Cadi Ayyad at Marrakesh with a total enrolment of 99,637 students and 3,146 teaching staff in 1984.

Health. In the public sector, 1984, there were 1,048 medical centres and dispensaries, 5,258 doctors, 63 chemists and 4,424 (1983) registered nurses. In the private sector, 1984, there were 1,971 doctors, 6,713 (1983) chemists and 709 registered nurses. There were 14,847 qualified nurses in 1983.

DIPLOMATIC REPRESENTATIVES

Of Morocco in Great Britain (49 Queen's Gate Gdns., London, SW7 5NE)
Ambassador: Abdeslam Zenined, GCVO.

Of Great Britain in Morocco (17 Blvd de la Tour Hassan, Rabat)
Ambassador: John Macrae, CMG.

Of Morocco in the USA (1601 21st St., NW, Washington, D.C., 20009)
Ambassador: Ali Bengelloun.

Of the USA in Morocco (2 Ave. de Marrakech, Rabat)
Ambassador: E. Michael Ussery.

Of Morocco to the United Nations
Ambassador: Aziz Hasbi.

Further Reading

Statistical Information: The Service Central des Statistiques (BP 178, Rabat) was established in 1942. Its publications include: *Annuaire de Statistique Générale.—La Conjoncture Économique Marocaine* (monthly; with annual synthesis).—*Bulletin économique et social du Maroc* (trimestral)

Bulletin Official (in Arabic and French). Rabat. Weekly

Findlay, A. M. and A. M. and Lawless, R. I., *Morocco.* [Bibliography] Oxford and Santa Barbara, 1984

Kinross, Lord and Hales-Gary, D., *Morocco.* London, 1971

National Library: Bibliothèque Générale et Archives, Rabat.

MOZAMBIQUE

Capital: Maputo
Population: 14·9m. (1988)
GNP per capita: US$100 (1988)

República de Moçambique

HISTORY. Trading settlements were established by Arab merchants at Sofala (Beira), Quelimane, Angoche and Mozambique Island in the fifteenth century. Mozambique Island was visited by Vasco da Gamba's fleet on 2 March 1498, and Sofala was occupied by Portuguese in 1506. At first ruled as part of Portuguese India, a separate administration was created in 1752, and on 11 June 1951 Mozambique became an Overseas Province of Portugal. Following a decade of guerrilla activity, Portugal and the nationalists jointly established a transitional government on 20 Sept. 1974. Independence was achieved on 25 June 1975. In March 1984 the Republic of South Africa and Mozambique signed a non-agression pact.

In Nov. 1990 the government and the RENAMO rebel movement began talks on ending the civil war.

AREA AND POPULATION. Mozambique is bounded east by the Indian ocean, south by South Africa, south-west by Swaziland, west by South Africa and Zimbabwe and north by Zambia, Malawi and Tanzania. It has an area of 799,380 sq. km (308,642 sq. miles) and a population, according to the census of 1980, of 11,673,725. Estimate (1988) 14,907,000 of whom (1986) 882,814 lived in the capital, Maputo. Other chief cities are Beira (1986 population, 269,700) and Nampula (182,553). The areas, populations and capitals of the provinces are:

Province	*Sq. km*	*Census 1980*	*Estimate 1987*	*Capital*
Cabo Delgado	82,625	940,000	1,109,921	Pemba
Niassa	129,056	514,100	607,670	Lichinga
Nampula	81,606	2,402,700	2,837,856	Nampula
Zambézia	105,008	2,500,200	2,952,251	Quelimane
Tete	100,724	831,000	981,319	Tete
Manica	61,661	641,200	756,886	Chimoio
Sofala	68,018	1,065,200	1,257,710	Beira
Inhambane	68,615	997,600	1,167,022	Inhambane
Gaza	75,709	990,900	1,138,724	Xaixai
Province of Maputo	25,756	491,800	544,692	Maputo
City of Maputo	602	755,300	1,006,765	

The main ethnolinguistic groups are the Makua/Lomwe (52% of the population), mainly in the 4 provinces in the north, the Malawi (12%), Shona (6%) and Yao (3%) in Tete, Manica and Sofala, and the Thonga (24%) in the 3 provinces in the south. Portuguese remains the official language, but vernaculars are widely spoken throughout the country.

CLIMATE. A humid tropical climate, with a dry season from June to Sept. In general, temperatures and rainfall decrease from north to south. Maputo. Jan. 78°F (25·6°C), July 65°F (18·3°C). Annual rainfall 30" (760 mm). Beira. Jan. 82°F (27·8°C), July 69°F (20·6°C). Annual rainfall 60" (1,522 mm).

CONSTITUTION AND GOVERNMENT. Under the Constitution adopted at independence on 25 June 1975, the directing power of the state was vested in the Mozambique Liberation Front (*Frente de Liberação de Moçambique*, FRELIMO), the liberation movement, which in Feb. 1977 was reconstituted as sole political Party.

On 2 Nov. 1990 the People's Assembly unanimously voted a new constitution, which came into force on 30 Nov. This changed the name of the state to 'Republic of Mozambique' and that of the parliament to 'Assembly of the Republic', legalized opposition parties, provided for universal secret elections and introduced a bill of rights including the right to strike, press freedoms and habeas corpus. The 250-member People's Assembly had been elected in Dec. 1986. The Speaker is Marcelino dos Santos.

The Council of Ministers in June 1989 consisted of:

President, and Commander-in-Chief of the Armed Forces: Joaquim Alberto Chissano.

Prime Minister: Mário da Graça Machungo.

Foreign Affairs: Pascoal Manuel Mocumbi. *Finance:* Abdul Magid Osman. *Defence:* Gen. Alberto Chipande.

National flag: Horizontally green, black, yellow with the black fimbriated in white; a red triangle based on the hoist, charged with a yellow star surmounted by an open white book and a crossed rifle and hoe in black.

Local Government. The capital of Maputo and 10 provinces, each under a Governor who is automatically a member of the Council of Ministers, are sub-divided into 112 districts.

DEFENCE. Selective conscription for 2 years is in force.

Army. The Army consists of 1 tank brigade and 7 infantry brigades, 7 anti-aircraft artillery battalions and many support units. Equipment includes T-34/-54/-55 main battle tanks. Strength (1991) 60,000. There are also 5,000 Border Guards and various militias.

Navy. The small flotilla based principally at Maputo, with subsidiary bases at Beira, Nacala, Pemba and Inhambane comprises 20 inshore patrol craft of mixed origins, 3 ex-Soviet inshore minesweepers and 2 landing craft. 4 of the patrol craft are based at Metangula on Lake Nyasa. Naval personnel in 1990 totalled 1,000.

Air Force. The Air Force is reported to have about 20 MiG-17 and 30 MiG-21 fighters, probably flown by Cuban pilots, An-26 turboprop transports, and a few C-47 piston-engined transports. About 6 Mi-24 armed helicopters and 10 Mi-8 transport helicopters, a small number of L-39 jet trainers, Zlin 326 primary trainers and a few ex-Portuguese Air Force Alouette liaison helicopters. Personnel (1991) 6,000, with 43 combatant aircraft and 12 armed helicopters.

INTERNATIONAL RELATIONS

Membership. Mozambique is a member of UN, OAU, SADCC and is an ACP state of EEC.

ECONOMY

Policy. In 1990 the government abandoned economic planning in favour of a market economy.

Budget. In 1987 the revenue was US$277·87m.; expenditure, US$427·91m. Foreign debt (1986) US$3,200m.

Currency. The unit of currency is the *metical* (MZM) of 100 *centavos*. The *metical* was established at par with the former *escudo* in 1980. In March 1991, £1 = 1,970 *meticais*; US$1 = 1,038 *meticais*.

Banking. Most banks had been nationalized by 1979. The *Banco de Moçambique* (bank of issue) and the *Banco Popular de Desenvolvimento* (state investment bank) each have a capital of 1,000m. meticais.

Weights and Measures. The metric system is in force.

ENERGY AND NATURAL RESOURCES

Electricity. Production (1986) 1,640m. kwh. Capacity (1986) 2,225,000 kw. Supply 220 volts; 50 Hz. The hydro-electric dam at Cabora Bassa on the Zambezi is the largest producer in Africa.

Minerals. Coal is the main mineral being exploited. Output was 380,000 tonnes in 1983. Coal reserves (estimate) 400m. tonnes. Small quantities of bauxite, gold, titanium, fluorite and colombo-tantalite are produced. Iron ore deposits and natural gas are known to exist.

Agriculture. Production in tonnes (1988): Cereals, 530,000; tea, 5,000; maize, 334,000; bananas, 82,000; sisal, 3,000; rice, 55,000; groundnuts, 65,000; copra, 69,000; vegetables, 198,000; citrus, 42,000; potatoes, 65,000; cashews, 30,000; sunflower seed, 20,000; cotton (lint), 32,000; sugar, 50,000.

Livestock 1988: 1·36m. cattle, 375,000 goats, 119,000 sheep, 160,000 pigs, 20,000 asses.

Forestry. Forests covered (1988) 19% of land area. Production (1985) 35,000 cu. metres of cut timber.

Fisheries. In 1984 the prawn catch was 5,800 tonnes; other fish (1986) 31,900 tonnes.

INDUSTRY. Although the country is overwhelmingly rural, there is some substantial industry in and around Maputo (steel, engineering, textiles, processing, docks and railways).

FOREIGN ECONOMIC RELATIONS

Commerce. Imports in 1987 totalled US$645m. and exports US$96m. In 1986 12% of imports came from the USSR, 12% from the Republic of South Africa and 12% from the USA. 21% of exports were to Spain, 22% to the USA and 23% to Japan. Shrimps made up 48% of exports; cashews, 12%; sugar, 10%; copra, 3% and petroleum products, 5%.

Total trade between Mozambique and UK (British Department of Trade returns, in £1,000 sterling):

	1986	*1987*	*1988*	*1989*	*1990*
Imports to UK	1,335	6,580	5,574	14,582	10,709
Exports and re-exports from UK	13,175	21,168	24,218	20,268	28,992

COMMUNICATIONS

Roads. There were, in 1984, 20,000 km of roads, of which 5,000 km were tarred. Motor vehicles, in 1980, included 99,400 passenger cars and 24,700 lorries and buses. The Government is devoting effort to constructing a new North/South road link, and to improving provincial rural feeder road systems.

Railways. The Mozambique State Railways consist of 5 independent networks known as the Maputo, Mozambique, Sofala (Beira), Inhambane and Gaza, and Quelimane systems. The Maputo system has a link at Komatipoort with the Republic of South Africa, Swaziland and Zimbabwe railways; the Sofala system links with Zimbabwe at Machipanda (near Umtali); and the Mozambique system links with Malaŵi at Entre Lagos. Total route-km (1986), 2,988 km (1,067 mm gauge), and 143 km (762 mm gauge). In 1989, 6·8m. passengers and 400m. tonne-km of goods were carried.

Aviation. There are international airports at Maputo, Beira and Nampula with regular services to European and Southern African destination by several foreign airlines and by *Linhas Aéreas de Moçambique*, who also serve 13 domestic airports.

Shipping. The total tonnage handled by Mozambique ports (1987) was 2·7m. The principal ports are Maputo, Beira, Nacala and Quelimane.

Telecommunications. Maputo is connected by telegraph with the Transvaal system. Quelimane has telegraphic communication with Chiromo. Number of telephones (1983), 59,000.

Radio Moçambique broadcasts 5 programmes in Portuguese, English and Tsonga as well as 4 regional programmes in 8 languages. Number of receivers (1986): Radio, 500,000; TV 02, 20,000.

Cinemas. There were 60 in 1987.

Newspapers. There are 2 daily newspapers: *Noticias*, published in Maputo, and *Diario de Mozambique* in Beira.

JUSTICE, RELIGION, EDUCATION AND WELFARE

Justice. The 1990 constitution provides for an independent judiciary, habeas corpus, and an entitlement to legal advice on arrest. The death penalty was abolished in Nov. 1990.

Religion. About 60% of the population follow traditional animist religions, while some 18% are Christian (mainly Roman Catholic) and 16% Moslem.

Education. In 1987 there were 1,370,528 pupils in 4,105 primary schools and (1986) 144,015 in 171 secondary schools. Private schools were permitted to function in 1990. The *Universidade Eduardo Mondlane* had 2,500 students in 1985. Literacy rate (1986) 30%.

Health. There were (1987) 1,156 hospitals and medical centres with 11,671 beds; there were 327 doctors, 1,112 midwives and 2,871 nursing personnel. In 1987 there were 138 dentists and 301 pharmacists.

DIPLOMATIC REPRESENTATIVES

Of Mozambique in Great Britain (21 Fitzroy Sq., London W1P 5HJ)
Ambassador: Armado Alexandre Panguene.

Of Great Britain in Mozambique (Ave. Vladimir I. Lenine 310, Maputo)
Ambassador: Maeve G. Fort, CMG.

Of Mozambique in the USA (1990 M. St., NW, Washington, D.C., 20036)
Ambassador: Valeriano Ferrao.

Of the USA in Mozambique (Ave Kaunda 193, Maputo)
Ambassador: Melissa F. Wells.

Of Mozambique to the United Nations
Ambassador: Pedro Comissario Afonso.

Further Reading

Darch, C., *Mozambique*. [Bibliography] Oxford and Santa Barbara, 1987
Hanlon, J., *Mozambique: The Revolution under Fire*. London, 1984
Henriksen, T. H., *Mozambique: A History*. London and Cape Town, 1978
Houser, G. and Shore, H., *Mozambique: Dream the Size of Freedom*. New York, 1975
Isaacman, A., *A Luta Continua: Building a New Society in Mozambique*. New York, 1978.
—*Mozambique: From Colonization to Revolution, 1900–1982*. Aldershot and Boulder, 1984
Mondlane, E., *The Struggle for Mozambique*. London, 1983
Munslow, B., *Mozambique: The Revolution and its Origins*. London and New York, 1983

NAMIBIA

Capital: Windhoek
Population: 1·29m. (1988)
GNP per capita: US$1,020 (1986)

Republic of Namibia

HISTORY. Britain annexed Walvis Bay in 1878, and incorporated it in the Cape of Good Hope in 1884. In 1884 South West Africa was declared a German protectorate. In 1915 the Union of South Africa occupied German South West Africa at the request of the Allied powers. On 17 Dec. 1920 the League of Nations entrusted South West Africa as a Mandate to the Union of South Africa, to be administered under the laws of the mandatory power. After World War II South Africa refused to place the territory under the UN Trusteeship system, and formally applied for its annexation to the Union. On 18 July 1966 the International Court of Justice decided that Ethiopia and Liberia had no legal right in applying for a decision on the international status of South West Africa, but in Oct. 1966 the General Assembly of the UN terminated South Africa's mandate, and established a UN Council for South West Africa in May 1967. However, South Africa continued to administer the territory, in defiance of various UN resolutions. It speeded up the implementation of the Odendaal Plan (1964), which required massive development aid and the formation of enlarged homelands for the various ethnic groups. In June 1968 the UN changed the name of the territory to Namibia. In 1971 the International Court of Justice ruled in an advisory opinion that South Africa's presence in Namibia was illegal. In Dec. 1973 the UN appointed a UN Commissioner for Namibia.

After negotiations between South Africa and the UN, a multi-racial Advisory Council was appointed in 1973. Representatives of all the population groups assembled in the Turnhalle in Windhoek for the Constitutional Conference, which on 17 Aug. 1976 decided that a multi-racial interim government was to be formed by early 1977, and that the country should become independent by 31 Dec. 1978. This interim government was rejected by the Western Five, (USA, Britain, Federal Republic of Germany, France and Canada), after which South Africa agreed to universal suffrage elections. An Administrator-General was appointed in Sept. 1977 to govern the territory until independence, and he moved to abolish all laws based on racial discrimination – a precondition for elections. In April 1978 South Africa accepted a plan for UN-supervised elections leading to independence, which was endorsed in UN Security Council Resolution 435 of 27 July 1978. After the final plans for the UN-supervised elections were published, South Africa announced on 20 Sept. 1978 that it was going ahead with internally sponsored elections for a Constitutent Assembly. In the elections held on 4-8 Dec. 1978 the Democratic Turnhalle Alliance (DTA) gained 41 of the 50 seats in a percentage poll of 82%, in spite of the fact that the South West Africa People's Organisation (SWAPO) instructed its members not to take part in the elections.

A 12-member Ministers' Council was instituted, and in Sept. 1981 it was enlarged to 15 members and given executive authority on all matters except constitutional issues, security and foreign affairs. On 11-13 Nov. 1980 elections were held for the second-tier Representative Authorities, which each control certain administrative functions for a specific ethnic group, but no specific geographical area. In Jan. 1983 the Ministers' Council and the National Assembly were dissolved and executive and legislative powers reverted to the Administrator-General.

On 13 Sept. 1983 the Multi-Party Conference (MPC) was formed. In May 1984 talks were held in Lusaka between the MPC and SWAPO, which were followed in July 1984 by talks between the Administrator-General and SWAPO. SWAPO was again invited to take part in constitutional talks with the MPC, but again refused. The MPC then petitioned the Republic of South Africa for a form of self-government for Namibia, and on 17 June 1985 the Transitional Government of National Unity was installed. Negotiations began again in May and July 1988 between Angola, Cuba and the Republic of South Africa. A peaceful settlement was agreed and the Geneva Protocol was signed on 5 Aug. 1988. In Dec. it was agreed that Cuban troops should withdraw from Angola and South African troops from Namibia by 1 April 1989. The Transitional Government of National Unity resigned on 28 Feb. 1988 to make provision for the implementation of UN Security Council Resolution 435. The UN Transition Assistance Group (UNTAG) supervised elections for the constituent assembly in Nov. 1989. Independence was achieved on 21 March 1990.

AREA AND POPULATION. The area, including the Caprivi-Strip, is 823,145 sq. km. Namibia lays claim to the enclave of Walvis Bay, administered by the Republic of South Africa (1,124 sq. km.).

The country is bounded in the north by Angola and Zambia, west by the Atlantic ocean, south and south-east by South Africa and east by Botswana. The Caprivi Strip, about 300 km long, extends eastwards up to the Zambezi river, projecting into Zambia and Botswana and touching Zimbabwe. The rainfall increases steadily from less than 50 mm. in the west and south-west up to 600 mm. in the Caprivi Strip.

The population at the censuses in 1970 and 1981 and estimates 1988, were:

	1970	*1981*	*1988*
Ovambos	342,455	506,114	641,000
Whites	90,658	76,430	82,000
Damaras	64,973	76,179	97,000
Hereros	55,670	76,296	97,000
Namas	32,853	48,541	62,000
Kavangos	49,577	95,055	120,000
Caprivians	25,009	38,594	48,000
Coloureds	28,275	42,254	52,000
Basters	16,474	25,181	32,000
Bushmen	21,909	29,443	37,000
Tswanas	4,407	6,706	8,000
Other	...	12,403	12,000
	732,260	1,033,196	1,288,000

Namibia is divided into 26 districts of which one is the capital, Windhoek (population 114,500, estimate 1988). Towns with populations over 5,000: Swakopmund, 15,500; Rehoboth, 15,000; Rundu, 15,000; Keetmanshoop, 14,000; Tsumeb, 13,500; Otjiwarongo, 11,000; Grootfontein, 9,000; Okahandja, 8,000; Mariental, 6,500; Gobabis, 6,500; Khorixas, 6,500; Lüderitz, 6,000.

The other districts are (with chief town where name differs): Bethanian, Bushmanland (Tsumkwe), Caprivi East (Katima Mulilo), Damaraland (Khorixas), Gobabis, Grootfontein, Hereroland East (Otjinene), Hereroland West (Okakarara), Kaokoland (Opuwo), Karasburg, Karibib, Kavango (Rundu), Keetmanshoop, Lüderitz, Maltahöhe, Mariental, Namaland (Gibeon), Okahandja, Omaruru, Otjiwarongo, Outjo, Owambo (Ondangwa), Rehoboth, Swakopmund, Tsemeb.

English and Afrikaans are the official languages. German is also spoken.

CONSTITUTION AND GOVERNMENT. For history of the administration from 1949–1985 *see* THE STATESMAN'S YEAR-BOOK 1986–87 p. 1087.

At the elections 7–11 Nov. 1989 voting was for the 72 seats in the Constituent Assembly. South West Africa People's Organization (SWAPO) won 41 seats; Democratic Turnhalle Alliance (DTA) 21; United Democratic Front, 4; Action Christian Nation (ACN) 3; Namibia Patriotic Front (NPF) 1; Federal Convention of Namibia (FCN) 1; Namibia National Front (NNF) 1. Swapo-Democrats (SWAPO-D), Christian Democratic Action (CDA) and Namibia National Democratic Party (NNDP) won no seats.

On 9 Feb 1990 with a unanimous vote the Constituent Assembly approved the Constitution which stipulated a multi-party republic, an independent judiciary and an executive *President* who may serve a maximum of two 5-year terms. The bicameral legislature consists of a 78-member *National Assembly*, elected for 5-year terms by proportional representation, and a *National Council* consisting of 2 members from each geographical region elected for 6-year terms from members of regional councils.

President: Sam Nujoma.

In Feb. 1991 the Government consisted of:

Prime Minister: Hage Geingob.

Minister of Home Affairs: Hifikepunye Pohamba. *Foreign Affairs*: Theo-Ben Gurirab. *Defence*: Peter Mueshihange. *Finance*: Otto Herrigel. *Education, Culture Youth and Sport*: Nahas Angula. *Information and Broadcasting*: Hidipo Hamutenya. *Health and Social Services*: Nicky Iyambo. *Labour, Public Service and Manpower Development*: Hendrik Witbooi. *Mines and Energy*: Andimba Toivo ya Toivo. *Justice*: Ngarikutuke Tjiriange. *Local Government and Housing*: Libertine Amathila. *Wildlife, Conservation and Tourism:* Nico Bessinger. *Trade and Industry:* Ben Amathila. *Agriculture, Fisheries, Water and Rural Development*: Gerhard Hanekom. *Works, Transport and Communications*: Richard Kapelwa Kabajani. *Lands, Resettlement and Rehabilitation*: Marco Hausiku. *Attorney-General*: Hartmut Ruppel.

National Flag: Divided diagonally blue over green by a red white-edged stripe; in the canton a yellow sun of 12 rays.

Local government is carried out by elected regional and local authority councils. A *Council of Traditional Chiefs* advises the President on the utilization and control of communal land.

DEFENCE. The UK is training a Namibian Defence Force, which is composed of former members of the South West African Territorial Force and the People's Liberation Army of Namibia. Initial strength was about 9,000.

INTERNATIONAL RELATIONS

Membership. Namibia is a member of the Commonwealth.

ECONOMY

Budget. In 1989-90 revenue was R2,116·6m. and expenditure, R1,959·3m. Tax revenue totalled R1,312·6m. and included taxes on income and profits, R805·2m.

Currency. The monetary unit is the South African *Rand*.

Banking and Finance. The South African Reserve Bank branch in Windhoek performs the functions of a central bank. Commercial banks include First National Bank, Boland Bank, Nedbank, Standard Bank, Bank of South West Africa/Namibia and Bank of Windhoek Ltd (the only locally-owned bank). There is a Land and Agricultural Bank in Windhoek. Total assets of commercial and general banks were R1,960·7m. at 31 Dec. 1989.

A Post Office Savings Bank was established in 1916. The number of accounts opened in 1985–86 was 3,398. The balance due to holders as at 31 March 1986 amounted to R2,983,790.

ENERGY AND NATURAL RESOURCES

Electricity. Production (1986) 692m. kwh.

Water. The 12 most important dams have a total capacity of 589·2m. cu. metres. Rainfall increases steadily from less than 50 mm. in the west and south-west up to 600 mm. in the Caprivi Strip.

The Kunene River and the Okavango, which form portions of the northern border of the country, the Zambezi, which forms the eastern boundary of the Caprivi-Strip, the Kwando or Mashi, which flows through the Caprivi-Strip from the north between the Okavango and the Zambezi, and the Orange River in the south, are the only permanently running streams. But there is a system of great, sandy, dry riverbeds throughout the country, in which water can generally be obtained by sinking shallow wells. In the Grootfontein area there are large supplies of underground water, but except for a few springs, mostly hot, there is no surface water in the country.

Minerals. Diamonds of 1,009,520 carats were recovered in 1986 from open cast mines north of the Orange river. A new open-cast diamond mining area will start production here in 1990, with another to be developed near Elizabeth Bay, south of Lüderitz. The largest open groove uranium mine in the world started operations near Swakopmund in 1976. The mine has a production capacity of 5,000 short tons of uranium oxide concentrate per year and an estimated average of 60m. tons of ore has been processed annually since 1979. Total value of mineral exports, 1988, R1,542·6m.; diamonds, R653·5m.

Agriculture. Namibia is essentially a stock-raising country, the scarcity of water and poor rainfall rendering crop-farming, except in the northern and north-eastern parts, almost impossible. Generally speaking, the southern half is suited for the raising of small stock, while the central and northern parts are more suited for cattle. In 1986 there were 314 registered hunting farms, 25 guest farms and 20 safari farms. Guano is harvested from the coast, converted into fertilizer in the Republic of South Africa and most of it exported to Europe. In 1986, 16% of the active labour force worked in the agricultural sector, while 70% of the population was directly or indirectly dependent on agriculture for their living.

Livestock (1988): 2·05m. cattle, 6·4m. sheep, 2·5m. goats. In 1987, 246,163 head of cattle, 102,037 beef carcasses and 786,611 head of small stock were exported, and 770,627 karakul pelts were produced.

In 1988, 70,000 tonnes of cows' milk and 70,000 tonnes of cheese were produced. Principal crops (1988 in tonnes): Wheat, 1,000; maize, 48,000; sunflower seed (1987), 525, sorghum; 7,000; vegetables, 28,000.

Forestry. Forests cover 18m. ha (22% of the land area).

Fisheries. Value of catches, 1988-89: Pelagic fish, R182·7m.; crayfish, R53,298,968. After independence a 200-mile exclusive economic zone was declared.

INDUSTRY. Of the estimated total of 350 undertakings (66% of which are in Windhoek), the most important are meat processing, the supply of specialized equipment to the mining industry, the assembly of goods from predominantly imported materials and the manufacture of metal products and construction material. Small industries, including home industries, textile mills, leather and steel goods, have expanded. Products manufactured locally include chocolates, beer, leather shoes and delicatessen meats and game meat products.

Labour. In 1988 there were 184,983 economically active persons, 67·2% male. The estimated unemployment rate was 20%. The main employers were government services, agriculture and mining.

FOREIGN ECONOMIC RELATIONS

Commerce. Total imports (in R1,000), 1987, 1,712.9. Total exports, 1989: 2,671·6 including agricultural exports, 293·7; fish, 64·9; diamonds, 814; other minerals, 1212·8.

Total trade between Namibia and UK (British Department of Trade returns, in £1,000 sterling):

	1986	*1987*	*1988*	*1989*	*1990*
Imports to UK	6,826	7,681	10,729	4,568	349
Exports and re-exports from UK	2,915	3,909	3,259	4,264	4,246

COMMUNICATIONS

Roads. In 1988 the total national road network was 41,762 km, including 4,500 km of tarred roads. In 1986 there were 103,715 registered motor vehicles.

Railways. The Namibia system connects with the main system of the South African railways at Aramsvlei. The total length of the line inside Namibia was 2,349 km of 1,065 mm gauge in 1990. In 1989 railways carried 232,000 passengers and 19·4m. tonnes of freight.

Aviation. In 1987–88 the Territory's 2 major airports handled about 190,217 passengers and 2·2m. kg of freight on international flights and 10,000 passengers and 88,000 kg of freight on internal flights.

Shipping. The bulk of the direct imports into the country is landed at Walvis Bay which handles 750,000 tons of cargo a year.

In 1985 Walvis Bay harbour handled 764 vessels and Lüderitz, 152 vessels.

Telecommunications. In 1987 there were 71 post offices and 16 postal agencies, and 1,070 private bag services distributed by rail or road transport.

There were (1987) 69,273 telephones. There were 1,012 telex users.

In 1987, 57,683 radio licences and 28,500 television licences were issued.

Newspapers (1989). There are 5 daily and 6 weekly newspapers.

JUSTICE, RELIGION, EDUCATION AND WELFARE

Justice. There is a Supreme Court, a High Court and a number of magistrates' and lower courts. An Ombudsman is appointed. Judges' appointments are approved by the National Assembly.

Religion. About 90% of the population is Christian.

Education (1988). In 1989–90, R143·6m. was spent on education. There were 1,153 schools for all races, 374,269 pupils and 12,525 teachers. This included 1,118 primary and senior secondary schools, 3 centres for the handicapped, 1 technical school and 2 agricultural schools, 3 technical institutes and 3 agricultural colleges. There were 4 teachers' training colleges and an academy.

Health (1988). There were 68 hospitals and 171 clinics. The ratio of beds per population was 5·5 per 1,000. There were 270 general practitioners, 30 specialists and 40 dentists. Nursing staff numbered 4,350.

DIPLOMATIC REPRESENTATIVES

Of Namibia in Great Britain (34 South Molton St., London W1P 5HJ)
Acting High Commissioner: Niilo Taapopi.

Of Great Britain in Namibia (116A Leutwein St., Windhoek)
High Commissioner: Francis Richards.

Of Namibia in the USA
Ambassador: (Vacant).

Of the USA in Namibia (14 Lossen St., Windhoek)
Chargé d'affaires: Roger A. McGuire.

Of Namibia to the United Nations
Ambassador: (Vacant).

Further Reading

Namibia Information Services, *Namibia: The Economy*. Windhoek, 1987
Human Rights and Namibia. London, 1986
Herbstein, D. and Evenston, J., *The Devils are Among Us: The War for Namibia*. London, 1989
Katjavivi, P.H., *A History of Resistance in Namibia*. London, 1988
Rotberg, R. I., *Namibia: Political and Economic Prospects*. Lexington, 1983
Schoeman, E. R. and H. S., *Namibia*. [Bibliography] Oxford and Santa Barbara, 1984
Soggot, D., *Namibia: The Violent Heritage*. New York, 1986
Thomas, W. H., *Economic Development in Namibia*. Munich, 1978
van der Merwe, J. H., *National Atlas of South West Africa*. Windhoek, 1983

NAURU

Population: 8,100 (1983)
GNP per capita: US$9,091 (1985)

Republic of Nauru

HISTORY. The island was discovered by Capt. Fearn in 1798, annexed by Germany in Oct. 1888, and surrendered to Australian forces in 1914. It was administered under a mandate, effective from 17 Dec. 1920, conferred on the British Empire and approved by the League of Nations until 1 Nov. 1947, when the UN General Assembly approved a trusteeship agreement with the governments of Australia, New Zealand and the UK as joint administering authority. Independence was gained in 1968.

AREA AND POPULATION. The island is situated 0° 32' S. lat. and 166° 56' E. long. Area, 5,263 acres (2,130 hectares). It is an oval-shaped upheaval coral island of approximately 12 miles in circumference, surrounded by a reef which is exposed at low tide. There is no deep water harbour but offshore moorings, reputedly the deepest in the world, are capable of holding medium-sized vessels, including 30,000 tonne capacity bulk carriers. On the seaward side the reef dips abruptly into the deep waters of the Pacific at an angle of 45°. On the landward side of the reef there is a sandy beach interspersed with coral pinnacles. From the sandy beach the ground rises gradually, forming a fertile section ranging in width from 150 to 300 yd and completely encircling the island. There is an extensive plateau bearing phosphate of a high grade, the mining rights of which were vested in the British Phosphate Commissioners until 1 July 1970, subject to the rights of the Nauruan landowners. In July 1970 the Nauru Phosphate Corporation assumed control and management of the enterprise. It is chiefly on the fertile section of land between the sandy beach and the plateau that the Nauruans have established themselves, as the plateau has been mined out, and the near absence of top soil prevents regeneration of fruit-bearing trees or crops.

At the census held on 13 May 1983 the population totalled 8,100, of whom 5,285 were Nauruans.

Vital statistics, 1982: Births, 286 (224 Nauruan); deaths, 77 (42 Nauruan).

CLIMATE. A tropical climate, tempered by sea breezes, but with a high and irregular rainfall, averaging 82" (2,060 mm). Jan. 81°F (27·2°C), July 82°F (27·8°C). Annual rainfall 75" (1,862 mm).

CONSTITUTION AND GOVERNMENT. A Legislative Council was established by the Nauru Act, passed by the Australian Parliament in Dec. 1965 and was inaugurated on 31 Jan. 1966. The trusteeship agreement terminated on 31 Jan. 1968, on which day Nauru became an independent republic but having special relationship with the Commonwealth. An 18-member Parliament is elected on a 3-yearly basis.

President and Minister for Foreign Affairs: Kenas Aroi.

National flag: Blue with a narrow horizontal gold stripe across the centre, beneath this near the hoist a white star of 12 points.

INTERNATIONAL RELATIONS

Membership. Nauru is a member of the South Pacific Forum.

ECONOMY

Currency. The Australian dollar is in use.

Budget. For year ending 30 June 1989 (estimate): revenue, $A57·35m.; expenditure, $A59·23m., including on health, $A3·12m.; education, $A3·5m.

INDUSTRY. The interests in the phosphate deposits were purchased in 1919 from the Pacific Phosphate Company by the governments of the UK, Australia and New Zealand at a cost of £3·5m., and a Board of Commissioners representing the three governments was appointed to manage and control the working of the deposits. In 1967 the British Phosphate Corporation agreed to hand over the phosphate industry to Nauru for approximately $A20m. over 3 years. Nauru took over the industry in July 1969. It is estimated that the deposits will be exhausted by 1995–97. Phosphate sales amounted to $A1·4m. in 1988-89. In May 1989 Nauru filed a claim against Australia for environmental damage caused by the mining.

FOREIGN ECONOMIC RELATIONS

Commerce. The export trade consists almost entirely of phosphate shipped to Australia, New Zealand, the Philippines and Japan. The imports: food, building construction materials, machinery for the phosphate industry and medical supplies.

Total trade between Nauru and UK (British Department of Trade returns, in £1,000 sterling):

	1986	*1987*	*1988*	*1989*	*1990*
Imports to UK	148	674	642	662	54
Exports from UK	1,239	394	759	549	1,145

COMMUNICATIONS

Aviation. There is an airfield on the island capable of accepting medium size jet aircraft. Air Nauru, a wholly owned government subsidiary, operates services with Boeing 737 aircraft to Melbourne, Sydney, Honiara, Guam, Tarawa, Port Vila, Suva, Nadi, Manila, Truk, Palau and Auckland.

Shipping. The Nauru Local Government Council, through its agency the Nauru Pacific Shipping Line, owns 3 ships and 1 fishing boat. These ships ply between Australia, the Pacific Islands, the USA, New Zealand, Japan and Singapore. Other shipping coming to the island consists of vessels under charter to the phosphate industry.

Telecommunications. There were 2,000 telephones in 1989 and 5,500 radio receivers in 1984. International telephone, telex and fax communications are maintained by Intelsat satellite. a satellite earth station was commissioned in 1990.

Cinemas. In 1989 there were 3 cinemas with seating capacity of 500.

JUSTICE, RELIGION AND EDUCATION

Justice. The highest Court is the Supreme Court of Nauru. It is the Superior Court of record and has the jurisdiction to deal with constitutional matters in addition to its other jurisdiction. There is also a District Court which is presided over by the Resident Magistrate who is also the Chairman of the Family Court and the Registrar of Supreme Court. The laws applicable in Nauru are its own Acts of Parliament. A large number of British statutes and much common law has been adopted insofar as is compatible with Nauruan custom.

Religion. The population is mainly Roman Catholic or Protestant.

Education. Attendance at school is compulsory for all children between the ages of 6 and 17. In June 1989 there were 10 infant and primary schools and 2 secondary schools. There were 165 teachers and 2,707 pupils in infant, primary and secondary schools. In addition, there is a trade school with 4 instructors and an enrolment of 88 trainees. Scholarships are available for Nauruan children to receive secondary and higher education and vocational training in Australia and New Zealand. In 1989, 99 Nauruans were receiving secondary and tertiary education abroad.

DIPLOMATIC REPRESENTATIVES

Of Great Britain in Nauru
High Commisioner: A. B. P. Smart (resides in Suva).

Of Nauru in the USA
Ambassador: T. W. Star (resides in Melbourne).

Further Reading

Macdonald, B., *Trusteeship and Independence in Nauru.* Wellington, 1988
Packett, C. N., *Guide to the Republic of Nauru.* Bradford, 1970
Viviani, N., *Phosphate and Political Progress.* Canberra, 1970
Williams, M. and Macdonald, B., *the Phosphateers.* Melbourne Univ. Press, 1985

NEPAL

Capital: Kathmandu
Population: 18m. (1990)
GNP per capita: US$170 (1988)

Nepal Adhirajya

(Kingdom of Nepal)

HISTORY. From 1846 to 1951 Nepal was virtually ruled by the Rana family, a member of which always held the office of prime minister, the succession being determined by special rules. The last Rana prime minister (and, until 18 Feb. 1951, Supreme C.-in-C.) was HH Maharaja Mohan Shumsher Jung Bahadur Rana, who resigned in Nov. 1951. The 15 feudal chieftanships were integrated into the kingdom on 10 April 1961.

Following two months of popular pro-democracy demonstrations, on 16 April 1990 King Birendra dismissed the government and proclaimed the abolition of the *panchayat* system of nominated councils. On 9 Nov. 1990 the King proclaimed a constitution which relinquished his absolute powers.

AREA AND POPULATION. Nepal, is bounded on the north by Tibet, on the east by Sikkim and West Bengal, on the south and west by Bihar and Uttar Pradesh. There are 3 geographical regions: The fertile Tarai plain in the south; a central belt containing the Mahabharat Lekh and Churia Hills and the basins of the Inner Tarai; and the Himalayas in the north. Area 56,827 sq. miles (147,181 sq. km); population (estimate, 1990), 18m.; (census, 1981) 15,022,839 of whom 52·4% were Nepali-speaking and 18·5% Bihari-speaking.

Capital, Kathmandu, 75 miles from the Indian frontier; population (census 1981) 235,160. Other towns include Patan (also called Lalitpur), 79,875; Morang (Biratnagar), 93,544; Bhadgaon (Bhaktapur), 48,472.

The aboriginal stock is Tibetan with a considerable admixture of Hindu blood from India. They were originally divided into numerous hill clans and petty principalities, one of which, Gurkha, became predominant in 1559 and has since given its name to men from all parts of Nepal.

CLIMATE. The rainfall is high, with maximum amounts from May to Sept., but conditions are very dry from Nov. to Jan. The range of temperature is moderate. Káthmándu. Jan. 50°F (10°C), July 76°F (24·4°C). Annual rainfall 57" (1,428 mm).

RULING KING. The sovereign is HM Maharajadhiraja **Birendra Bir Bikram Shah Dev** (b. 1946), who succeeded his father Mahendra Bir Bikram Shah Dev on 31 Jan. 1972.

CONSTITUTION AND GOVERNMENT. On 18 Feb. 1951 the King proclaimed a constitutional monarchy, and on 16 Dec. 1962 a new Constitution of the 'Constitutional Monarchical Hindu State'. The village and town *panchayat*, recognized as the basic units of democracy, elect the district *panchayat*, these elect the zonal *panchayat*, and these finally the 112 members of the national *panchayat*.

In 1990 the *panchayat* system of nominated national and local councils was abolished and a 30-year ban on opposition parties was lifted.

Under the constitution of 9 Nov. Nepal became a constitutional monarchy based on multi-party democracy. *Parliament* has 2 chambers: a 205-member House of Representatives (*Pratinidhi Sabha*) elected for 5-year terms, and a 60-member House of Estates (*Rashtriya Sabha*), of which 10 members are nominated by the king.

Elections were scheduled for May 1991. Until then a provisional government of Social Democrats and Communists was in place.

Prime Minister: Krishna Prasad Bhattarai.

National flag: Two triangular parts of red, with a blue border all round, bearing symbols of the moon and the sun in white.

National anthem: 'May glory crown our illustrious sovereign' (1952).

Local Government: The country is administratively divided into 14 zones (Bagmati, Bheri, Dhaulagiri, Gandaki, Janakpur, Karnali, Kosi, Lumbini, Mahakali, Mechi, Narayani, Rapti, Sagarmatha and Seti) and thence into 75 districts and over 3,500 villages.

DEFENCE. The King is commander-in-chief of the armed forces, but shares supreme military authority with the National Defence Council, of which the Prime Minister is chairman.

Army. The Army consists of 1 Royal Guard, 7 infantry brigades, 1 artillery regiment, engineer, parachute and garrison battalions, 1 cavalry and 1 reconnaissance squadron. Equipment includes 25 Ferrets. Strength of all services (1991) about 35,000, and there is also a 28,000-strong paramilitary police force.

Air Force. Independent of the army since 1979, the Air Force has 3 Skyvan transport aircraft, 1 Puma helicopter and 2 Chetak helicopters. An H.S. 748 turboprop transport and 1 Super Puma and 1 Puma helicopter are operated by the Royal Flight. There are no combatant aircraft.

INTERNATIONAL RELATIONS

Membership. Nepal is a member of the UN and the Colombo Plan.

ECONOMY

Budget. The general budget for the fiscal year 1987–88 envisaged current expenditure of NRs 4,307m. Domestic revenue were estimated at NRs 5,875m.

Currency. The unit of currency is the *Nepalese rupee* (NPR) of 100 *pais*. 50 *pais* = 1 *mohur*. The rupee is 171 grains in weight, as compared with the Indian rupee, which weighs 180 grains. Coins of all denominations are minted. The Rastra Bank also issues notes of 1, 5, 10, 100 and 1,000 rupees. In March 1991, US$1 = 30·41 *rupees*; £1 = 57·69 *rupees*.

ENERGY AND NATURAL RESOURCES

Electricity. Production (1986) 395m. kwh. A hydro-electric power scheme on the Karnali river costing US$4,500m. was being planned in 1986.

Agriculture. Nepal has valuable forests in the southern part of the country. In the northern part, on the slopes of the Himálayas, there grow large quantities of medicinal herbs which find a world-wide market. Forests covered (1988) 2·3m. ha, 17% of the land area; 5·4m. acres is covered by perpetual snow; 9·6m. acres is under paddy, 2·9m. maize and millet, 800,000 wheat. Production (1988 in 1,000 tonnes): Rice, 2,787; maize, 890; wheat, 745; sugar-cane, 816; potatoes, 566; millet, 160.

Livestock (1988); Cattle, 6,374,000, including about 675,000 cows; 2·9m. buffaloes; sheep, 833,000; goats, 5,125,000; pigs, 479,000; poultry, 10m.

Fisheries. Catch (1986) 9,400 tonnes.

INDUSTRY. Industries, such as jute- and sugar-mills, match, leather, cigarette, and shoe factories, and chemical works have been established, including two industrial estates at Pátan and Balaju. Production (1986 in 1,000 tonnes): Jute goods, 20·5; sugar, 18·5; cement, 10·4.

FOREIGN ECONOMIC RELATIONS

Commerce. The principal articles of export are food grains, jute, timber, oilseeds, ghee (clarified butter), potatoes, medicinal herbs, hides and skins, cattle. The chief imports are textiles, cigarettes, salt, petrol and kerosene, sugar, machinery, medicines, boots and shoes, paper, cement, iron and steel, tea.

Imports and exports in NRs 1,000:

	1985	*1986*	*1987*	*1988*
Imports	7,742,000	9,341,200	11,020,300	13,940,000
Exports	2,741,000	3,079,000	3,059,700	4,080,000

Total trade between Nepal and UK (British Department of Trade returns, in £1,000 sterling):

	1986	*1987*	*1988*	*1989*	*1990*
Imports to UK	5,966	8,331	9,384	8,306	7,039
Exports and re-exports from UK	4,672	8,707	4,968	7,802	4,099

Tourism. There were 248,000 tourists in 1987.

COMMUNICATIONS

Roads. With the co-operation of India and the USA 900 miles of motorable roads are being constructed, including the East-West Highway through southern Nepal. A road from the Tibetan border to Káthmándu was recently completed with Chinese aid. There are about 1,300 miles motorable roads. A ropeway for the carriage of goods covers the 14 miles from Dhursing above Bhimphedi into the Káthmándu valley. A road connects Káthmándu with Birgung.

Railways. Railways (762 mm gauge) connect Jayanagar on the North Eastern Indian Railway with Janakpur and thence with Bizalpura (54 km).

Aviation. The Royal Nepal Airline Corporation has linked Kathmandu, the capital, with 11 districts of Nepal; and in 1984, 30 airfields were in regular use. The airline carried 424,000 passengers and 2,900 tonnes of freight in 1983–84. The Royal Nepalese Airline Corporation has services between Kathmandu and Calcutta, Patna, New Delhi, Bangkok, Rangoon and Dacca, employing Boeing 727 jet aircraft.

Telecommunications. Kathmandu is connected by telephone with Birganj and Raxaul (North Eastern Indian Railway) on the southern frontier with Bihar; and with the eastern part of the Terai foothills; an extension to the western districts is being completed. Number of telephones (1980) 11,800. Under an agreement with India and the USA, a network of 91 wireless stations exists in Nepal, with further stations in Calcutta and New Delhi. Radio Nepal at Kathmandu broadcasts in Nepali and English. In 1986 there were 2m. radio receivers and 27,000 television receivers.

Newspapers. In 1987 there were 58 daily newspapers.

JUSTICE, RELIGION, EDUCATION AND WELFARE

Justice. The Supreme Court Act, established a uniform judicial system, culminating in a supreme court of a Chief Justice and no more than 6 judges. Special courts to deal with minor offences may be established at the discretion of the Government.

Religion. Hinduism is the religion of 90% of the people. Buddhists comprise 5% and Moslems 3%. Christian missions are permitted, but conversion is forbidden.

Education. In 1985 there were 1,818,668 primary school pupils, 501,063 secondary school pupils and in 1984, 55,555 students at the Tribhuvan University (founded 1960.

In 1981, 23% of the population were literate.

Health. There were about 420 doctors and 2,586 hospital beds in 1979.

DIPLOMATIC REPRESENTATIVES

Of Nepal in Great Britain (12a Kensington Palace Gdns., London, W8 4QU)
Ambassador: Maj.-Gen. Bharat Kesher Simha (accredited 14 July 1988).

Of Great Britain in Nepal (Lainchaur, Kathmandu)
Ambassador: T. J. B. George.

Of Nepal in the USA (2131 Leroy Pl., NW, Washington, D.C., 20008)
Ambassador: Mohan Man Sainju.

Of the USA in Nepal (Pani Pokhari, Kathmandu)
Ambassador: Julia Chang Bloch.

Of Nepal to the United Nations
Ambassador: Jai Pratap Rana.

Further Reading

Statistical Information: A Department of Statistics was set up in Kathmandu in 1950.

Baral, L. S., *Political Development in Nepal.* London, 1980
Bezruchka, S., *A Guide to Trekking in Nepal.* Leicester, 1981
Whelpton, J., *Nepal.* [Bibliography] Oxford and Santa Barbara, 1990

THE NETHERLANDS

Capital: Amsterdam
Seat of Government: The Hague
Population: 14·89m. (1990)
GNP per capita: US$14,530 (1988)

Koninkrijk der Nederlanden

(Kingdom of the Netherlands)

HISTORY. William of Orange (1533–84), as the German count of Nassau, inherited vast possessions in the Netherlands and the Princedom of Orange in France. He was the initiator of the struggle for independence from Spain (1568–1648); in the Republic of the United Netherlands he and his successors became the 'first servants of the Republic' with the title of 'Stadhouder' (governor). In 1689 William III acceded to the throne of England, becoming joint sovereign with Mary II, his wife. William III died in 1702 without issue, and after a stadhouderless period a member of the Frisian branch of Orange–Nassau was nominated hereditary stadhouder in 1747; but his successor, Willem V, had to take refuge in England, in 1795, at the invasion of the French Army. In Nov. 1813 the United Provinces were freed from French domination.

The Congress of Vienna joined the Belgian provinces, the 'Austrian Netherlands' before the French Revolution, to the Northern Netherlands. The son of the former stadhouder Willem V was proclaimed King of the Netherlands at The Hague on 16 March 1815 as Willem I. The union was dissolved by the Belgian revolution of 1830, and the treaty of London, 19 April 1839, constituted Belgium an independent kingdom.

Netherlands Sovereigns

Willem I	1815–1840 (died 1843)	Wilhelmina	1890–1948 (died 1962)
Willem II	1840–1849	Juliana	1948–1980
Willem III	1849–1890	Beatrix	1980–

AREA AND POPULATION. The Netherlands is bounded north and west by the North Sea, south by Belgium and east by the Federal Republic of Germany.

The total area of the Netherlands is 41,864 sq. km (16,163 sq. miles), of which 33,934 sq. km (13,102 sq. miles) is land area.

On 14 June 1918 a law was passed concerning the reclamation of the Zuiderzee. The work was begun in 1920; the following sections have been completed: 1. The Noordholland–Wieringen Barrage (2·5 km), 1924; 2. The Wieringermeer Polder (210 sq. km), 1930 (inundated by the Germans in 1945, but drained again in the same year); 3. The Wieringen–Friesland Barrage (30 km), 1932; 4. The Noordoost Polder (501 sq. km), 1942; 5. Oost Flevoland (604 sq. km), 1957; 6. Zuidelijk Flevoland (499 sq. km), 1967.

The reclamation of the Markerwaard is still a subject of political discussion. A portion of what used to be the Zuiderzee behind the barrage will remain a freshwater lake: Ijsselmeer (1,400 sq. km). The 'Delta-project', completed in 1986, comprises (semi) enclosure dams in the estuaries between the islands in the southwestern part of the country, excluding the sea-entrances to the ports of Rotterdam and Antwerp. *See* map in THE STATESMAN'S YEAR-BOOK, 1959.

Growth of census population:

1829	2,613,298	1909	5,858,175	1960	11,461,964
1849	3,056,879	1920	6,865,314	1971	13,060,115
1869	3,579,529	1930	7,935,565		
1889	4,511,415	1947	9,625,499		

Area, density and estimated population on 1 Jan. 1990:

Province	Land area (in sq. km) 1990	Population 1990	Population 1989	Density per sq. km 1990
Groningen	2,345·79	553,862	555,200	236
Friesland	3,359·00	599,151	599,190	179
Drenthe	2,655·46	441,028	439,066	166
Overijssel	3,339·65	1,020,424	1,014,949	306
Flevoland [1]	1,411·50	211,507	202,678	150
Gelderland	5,014·76	1,804,209	1,794,678	360
Utrecht	1,363·37	1,015,515	1,004,632	747
Noord-Holland	2,662·79	2,376,015	2,365,160	891
Zuid-Holland	2,876·62	3,219,839	3,200,408	1,122
Zeeland	1,792·57	355,947	355,585	198
Noord-Brabant	4,942·55	2,189,481	2,172,604	442
Limburg	2,169·16	1,103,960	1,099,622	509
Central Population Register [2]	—	1,636	1,468	—
Total	33,933·22	14,892,574	14,805,240	435

[1] The new province Flevoland, former Ijsselmeerpolders, established on 1 Jan. 1986. The Noordoostpolder (drained in 1942) and the Zuidelijke Ijsselmeerpolders (drained in 1957) are parts of the former Zuiderzee, now called Ijsselmeer.

[2] The Central Population Register includes persons who are residents of the Netherlands but who have no fixed residence in any particular municipality (living in caravans and houseboats, population on inland vessels, etc.).

Of the total population on 1 Jan. 1990, 7,358,482 were males, 7,534,092 females.

Vital statistics for calendar years:

	Live births Total	Live births Illegitimate	Still births	Marriages	Divorces	Deaths	Net migration
1985	178,136	14,766	1,054	82,747	34,044	122,704	+ 24,147
1986	184,513	16,220	1,060	87,337	29,836	125,307	+ 32,669
1987	186,667	17,385	1,036	87,400	27,788	122,199	+ 43,924
1988	186,647	18,951	1,038	87,843	27,870	124,163	+ 35,447
1989	188,979	20,177	1,100	90,248	28,250	128,905	+ 39,207

Population of municipalities with over 20,000 inhabitants on 1 Jan. 1990:

Aalsmeer	22,167
Achtkarspelen	27,542
Alkmaar	89,649
Almelo	62,190
Almere	71,086
Alphen a/d Rijn	61,132
Amersfoort	99,403
Amstelveen	69,982
Amsterdam	695,162
Apeldoorn	147,586
Arnhem	130,220
Assen	49,650
Baarn	24,773
Barneveld	42,335
Bergen op Zoom	46,870
Best	22,125
Beuningen	22,237
Beverwijk	35,151
De Bilt	32,174
Borne	21,434
Borsele	20,242
Boxtel	25,144
Breda	123,025
Brummen	20,782
Brunssum	29,804
Bussum	31,740
Capelle a/d Ijssel	57,574
Castricum	22,378
Culemborg	21,532
Delft	88,739
Delfzijl	31,962
Deurne	29,518
Deventer	66,888
Doetinchem	41,647
Dongen	21,244
Dongeradeel	24,430
Dordrecht	109,285
Dronten	24,733
Edam-Volendam	24,766
Ede	93,377
Eindhoven	191,467
Elburg	20,657
Emmen	92,807
Enschede	146,010
Epe	34,004
Ermelo	25,827
Etten-Leur	32,304
Franekeradeel	20,837
Geldermalsen	22,143
Geldrop	25,719
Geleen	33,666
Gendringen	20,271
Gilze en Rijen	22,872
Goes	32,034
Gorinchem	28,700
Gouda	64,611
's-Gravenhage	441,506
Groningen	167,872
Haaksbergen	22,854
Haarlem	149,269
Haarlemmermeer	95,782
Hardenberg	32,161
Harderwijk	35,389
Heemskerk	33,362
Heemstede	26,334
Heerenveen	37,930
Heerhugowaard	35,799
Heerlen	94,046
Heiloo	20,386
Den Helder	61,647
Hellendoorn	34,526
Hellevoetsluis	34,728
Helmond	68,159
Hengelo	75,993
's-Hertogenbosch	91,113
Hilversum	84,608
Hoogeveen	45,764
Hoogezand-Sappemeer	34,463
Hoorn	57,384
Houten	25,502
Huizen	41,966
Ijsselstein	20,225
Kampen	32,704
Katwijk	39,857
Kerkrade	53,127
Krimpen a/d Ijssel	27,477
Landgraaf	40,187
Langedijk	20,968

Leeuwarden	85,570	Putten	20,940	Utrecht	230,358
Leiden	110,423	Raalte	27,102	Valkenswaard	29,991
Leiderdorp	22,577	Renkum	33,578	Veendam	28,271
Leidschendam	32,992	Rheden	45,691	Veenendaal	48,343
Lelystad	57,638	Ridderkerk	45,999	Veghel	25,904
Leusden	27,272	Rijssen	24,143	Veldhoven	39,035
Lisse	21,124	Rijswijk	48,010	Velsen	58,520
Loon op Zand	21,727	Roermond	38,721	Venlo	63,918
Losser	22,562	De Ronde Venen	31,223	Venray	34,292
Maarssen	38,701	Roosendaal en		Vlaardingen	73,852
Maassluis	33,249	Nispen	60,206	Vlissingen [1]	43,949
Maastricht	117,008	Rosmalen	27,256	Voorburg	40,116
Meerssen	20,541	Rotterdam	579,179	Voorschoten	22,325
Meppel	23,755	Rucphen	21,378	Voorst	23,633
Middelburg	39,343	Schiedam	69,417	Vught	23,882
Naaldwijk	27,898	Schijndel	21,509	Waalwijk	28,708
Nieuwegein	58,774	Sittard	45,401	Waddinxveen	25,088
Nijkerk	25,619	Skarsterlân	24,017	Wageningen	32,492
Nijmegen	144,748	Sliedrecht	23,039	Wassenaar	26,159
Noordoostpolder	38,074	Smallingerland	50,229	Weert	40,262
Noordwijk	25,210	Sneek	29,299	Weststellingwerf	24,398
Nuenen c.a.	21,055	Soest	41,469	Wierden	22,343
Nunspeet	24,853	Spijkenisse	67,229	Wijchen	34,206
Oldebroek	21,487	Stadskanaal	32,979	Winterswijk	27,919
Oldenzaal	29,803	Steenwijk	20,979	Woerden	34,713
Oosterhout	48,395	Stein	26,583	Zaanstad	130,007
Ooststellingwerf	24,799	Terneuzen	34,983	Zeist	59,469
Opsterland	26,511	Tiel	32,016	Zevenaar	26,955
Oss	51,218	Tilburg	156,421	Zoetermeer	96,292
Oud-Beijerland	20,526	Tytsjerksteradiel	30,220	Zutphen	30,996
Papendrecht	27,347	Uden	35,512	Zwijndrecht	41,884
Purmerend	58,718	Uithoorn	22,563	Zwolle	94,131

[1] Also known as Flushing

Urban agglomerations as at 1 Jan. 1989: Rotterdam, 1,039,566; Amsterdam, 1,038,382; The Hague, 683,631; Utrecht, 525,989; Eindhoven, 381,788; Arnhem, 299,310; Heerlen-Kerkrade, 267,156; Enschede-Hengelo, 250,189; Nijmegen, 241,981; Tilburg, 227,050; Haarlem, 213,963; Groningen, 206,415; Dordrecht-Zwijndrecht, 204,429; 's-Hertogenbosch, 194,759; Leiden, 185,478; Geleen-Sittard, 178,842; Maastricht, 161,281; Breda, 157,331; Zaanstreek, 141,834; Velsen-Beverwijk, 125,644; Hilversum, 102,603.

CLIMATE. A cool temperate maritime climate, marked by mild winters and cool summers, but with occasional continental influences. Coastal temperatures vary from 37°F (3°C) in winter to 61°F (16°C) in summer, but inland the winters are slightly colder and the summers slightly warmer. Rainfall is least in the months Feb. to May, but inland there is a well-defined summer maximum in July and Aug.

The Hague. Jan. 37°F (2·7°C), July 61°F (16·3°C). Annual rainfall 32·8" (820 mm). Amsterdam. Jan. 36°F (2·3°C), July 62°F (16·5°C). Annual rainfall 34" (850 mm). Rotterdam. Jan. 36·5°F (2·6°C), July 62°F (16·6°C). Annual rainfall 32" (800 mm).

REIGNING QUEEN. Beatrix Wilhelmina Armgard, born 31 Jan. 1938 daughter of Queen Juliana and Prince Bernhard; married to Claus von Amsberg on 10 March 1966; succeeded to the crown on 1 May 1980, on the abdication of her mother. *Offspring:* Prince Willem-Alexander, born 27 April 1967; Prince Johan Friso, born 25 Sept. 1968; Prince Constantijn, born 11 Oct. 1969.

Mother of the Queen: Queen Juliana Louise Emma Marie Wilhelmina, born 30 April 1909, daughter of Queen Wilhelmina (born 31 Aug. 1880, died 28 Nov. 1962) and Prince Henry of Mecklenburg-Schwerin (born 19 April 1876, died 3 July 1934); married to Prince Bernhard Leopold Frederick Everhard Julius Coert Karel Godfried Pieter of Lippe-Biesterfeld (born 29 June 1911) on 7 Jan. 1937. Abdicated in favour of her daughter, the Reigning Queen, on 30 April 1980.

Sisters of the Queen: Princess Irene Emma Elisabeth, born 5 Aug. 1939, married to Prince Charles Hugues de Bourbon-Parma on 29 April 1964, divorced 1981 (*sons:* Prince Carlos Javier Bernardo, born 27 Jan. 1970; Prince Jaime Bernardo, born 13 Oct. 1972; *daughters:* Princess Margarita Maria Beatriz, born 13 Oct. 1972; Princess Maria Carolina Christina, born 23 June 1974); Princess Margriet Francisca, born in Ottawa, 19 Jan. 1943, married to Pieter van Vollenhoven on 10 Jan. 1967 (*sons:* Prince Maurits, born 17 April 1968; Prince Bernhard, born 25 Dec. 1969; Prince Pieter-Christiaan, born 22 March 1972; Prince Floris, born 10 April 1975); Princess Maria Christina, born 18 Feb. 1947, married to Jorge Guillermo on 28 June 1975 (*sons:* Bernardo, born 17 June 1977; Nicolas Daniel Mauricio, born 6 July 1979; *daughter:* Juliana, born 8 Oct. 1981).

CONSTITUTION AND GOVERNMENT. According to the Constitution of the Kingdom of the Netherlands, the Kingdom consists of the Netherlands, Aruba and the Netherlands Antilles. Their relations are regulated by the 'Statute' for the Kingdom, which came into force on 29 Dec. 1954. Each part enjoys full autonomy; they are united, on a footing of equality, for mutual assistance and the protection of their common interests.

The first Constitution of the Netherlands after its restoration as a Sovereign State was promulgated in 1814. It was revised in 1815 (after the addition of the Belgian provinces, and the assumption by the Sovereign of the title of King), 1840 (after the secession of the Belgian provinces), 1848, 1884, 1887, 1917, 1922, 1938, 1946, 1948, 1953, 1956, 1963, 1972 and 1983.

The Netherlands is a constitutional and hereditary monarchy. The royal succession is in the direct male or female line in the order of primogeniture. The Sovereign comes of age on reaching his/her 18th year. During his/her minority the royal power is vested in a Regent—designated by law—and in some cases in the Council of State.

The central executive power of the State rests with the Crown, while the central legislative power is vested in the Crown and Parliament (the *Staten-Generaal*), consisting of 2 Chambers. After the 1956 revision of the Constitution the Upper or First Chamber is composed of 75 members, elected by the members of the Provincial States, and the Second Chamber consists of 150 deputies, who are elected directly from all Netherlands nationals who are aged 18 or over on polling day. Members of the States-General must be Netherlanders or recognized as Netherlands subjects and 21 years of age or over; they may be men or women. They receive an allowance.

First Chamber (as constituted in 1987): Labour Party, 26; Christian Democratic Appeal, 26; People's Party for Freedom and Democracy, 12; Democrats '66, 5; Party of Political Radicals, 1; Communist Party, 1; Pacifist Socialist Party, 1; Calvinist Party, 1; Reformed Political Federation, 1; Calvinist Political Union, 1.

Second Chamber (elected on 6 Sept. 1989): Christian Democratic Appeal, 54; Labour Party, 49; People's Party for Freedom and Democracy, 22; Democrats, 66, 12; Green Left, 6; Calvinist Party, 3; Reformed Political Federation, 1; Calvinist Political Union, 2; Centre Democrats, 1.

The revised Constitution of 1917 has introduced an electoral system based on universal suffrage and proportional representation. Under its provisions, members of the Second Chamber are directly elected by citizens of both sexes who are Netherlands subjects not under 18 years (since 1972).

The members of the First Chamber and of the Second Chamber are elected for 4 years, and retire in a body. The Sovereign has the power to dissolve both Chambers of Parliament, or one of them, subject to the condition that new elections take place within 40 days, and the new House or Houses be convoked within 3 months.

Both the Government and the Second Chamber may propose Bills; the First Chamber can only approve or reject them without inserting amendments. The meetings of both Chambers are public, though each of them may by a majority vote decide on a secret session. It is a fixed custom, that Ministers and Secretaries of State, on their own initiative or upon invitation of the Parliament, attend the sessions to defend their policy, their budget, their proposals of Bills, etc., when these are in discussion. A Minister or Secretary of State, however, cannot be a member of Parliament at the same time.

The Constitution can be revised only by a Bill declaring that there is reason for introducing such revision and containing the proposed alterations. The passing of this Bill is followed by a dissolution of both Chambers and a second confirmation by the new States-General by two-thirds of the votes. Unless it is expressly stated, all laws concern only the realm in Europe, and not the oversea part of the kingdom, the Netherlands Antilles.

Every act of the Sovereign has to be covered by a responsible Minister.

The Ministry, a coalition of Christian Democrats and Liberals, was composed as follows in Jan. 1991:

Prime Minister: Ruud Lubbers (CDA).

Deputy Prime Minister and Finance: Wim Kok (PVDA). *Foreign Affairs:* Hans van den Broek (CDA). *Economic Affairs:* J. Andriessen (CDA). *Defence:* Relus ter Beek (PVDA). *Development Aid Co-operation:* Jan Pronk (PVDA). *Home Affairs:* Ien Dales (PVDA). *Justice:* E. Hirsch-Ballin (CDA). *Agriculture and Fisheries:* vacant. *Welfare, Public Health and Culture:* Hedy d'Ancona (PVDA). *Education and Science:* Jo Ritzen (PVDA). *Transport and Public Works:* Hanja Maij-Weggen (CDA). *Housing, Physical Planning and Environment:* Hans Alders (PVDA). *Social Affairs and Employment:* Bert de Vries (CDA).

There are also 11 state secretaries.

The Council of State *(Raad van Staat)*, appointed by the Crown, is composed of a vice-president and not more than 28 members. The Queen is president, but the day-to-day running of the council is in the hands of the vice-president. The Council can be consulted on all legislative matters. Decisions of the Crown in administrative disputes are prepared by a special section of the Council.

The Hague is the seat of the Court, Government and Parliament; Amsterdam is the capital.

National flag: Three horizontal stripes of red, white, blue.

National anthem: Wilhelmus van Nassoue (words by Philip Marnix van St Aldegonde, *c.* 1570).

Local Government. The kingdom is divided into 12 provinces and 672 municipalities. Each province has its own representative body, the Provincial States. The members must be 21 years of age or over; they are directly elected for 4 years. The electoral register is the same as for the Second Chamber. The members retire in a body and are subject to re-election. The total number of members is 748; provincial membership varies according to the population of the province, from 83 for Zuid-Holland to 39 for Flevoland. The Provincial States are entitled to issue ordinances concerning the welfare of the province, and to raise taxes pursuant to legal provisions. The provincial budgets and the provincial ordinances and resolutions relating to provincial property, loans, taxes, etc., must be approved by the Crown. The members of the Provincial States elect the First Chamber of the States-General. They meet twice a year, as a rule in public. A permanent commission composed of 6 of their members, called the 'Deputy States', is charged with the executive power and, if required, with the enforcement of the law in the province. Deputy as well as Provincial States are presided over by a Commissioner of the Queen, appointed by the Crown, who in the former assembly has a deciding vote, but attends the latter in only a deliberative capacity. He is the chief magistrate in the province. The Commissioner and the members of the Deputy States receive an allowance.

Elections to the Provincial States were held in March 1991; turn-out was 58.1%.

Each municipality forms a Corporation with its own interests and rights, subject to the general law, and is governed by a Municipal Council, directly elected from the Netherlands inhabitants, and, under certain circumstances, non-Netherlands inhabitants of the municipality who are 18 years of age or over, for 4 years. All Netherlands inhabitants and non-Netherlands inhabitants who meet certain requirements aged 21 or over are eligible, the number of members varying from 7 to 45, according to the population. The Municipal Council has the right to issue bye-laws concerning the communal welfare. The Council may levy taxes pursuant to legal provisions; these ordinances must be approved by the Crown. All bye-laws may be vetoed by the Crown. The Municipal Budget and resolutions to alienate municipal property require the approbation of the Deputy States of the province. The Council meets in public as often as may be necessary, and is presided over by a Burgomaster, appointed by the Crown. The day-to-day administration is carried out by the Burgomaster and 2–7 Aldermen *(wethouders)*, elected by and from the Council; this body is also charged with the enforcement of the law. The Burgomaster may suspend the execution of a resolution of the council for 30 days, but is bound to notify the Deputy States of the province. In maintaining public order, the Burgomaster acts as the chief of police. The Burgomaster and Aldermen receive allowances.

DEFENCE

Army. Service is partly voluntary and partly compulsory; the voluntary enlistments are of small proportion to the compulsory. The total peacetime strength amounts to 65,204, including Military Police. The number of regulars is 23,124. The Army also employs 11,775 civilians. The legal period of active service for national servicemen is 20-22 months; the actual service period is 14 months for reserve-officers and n.c.o.s and 12 months for other ranks. The balance is spent as 'short leave'. After their period of actual service or short leave, conscript personnel are granted long leave. However, they will be liable to being called up for refresher training or in case of mobilization until they have reached the age of 35 (n.c.o.s 40, reserve officers 45).

The 1st Netherlands Army Corps is assigned to NATO. It consists of 10 brigades and Corps troops. The active part of the Corps comprises 2 armoured brigades and 4 armoured infantry brigades, grouped in two divisions and 40% of the Corps troops. Part of this force is stationed in Germany. The peacetime strength of the active brigades is 80% of the war-authorized strength.

The mobilizable part of the Corps comprises 1 armoured brigade, 2 armoured infantry brigades, 1 infantry brigade and the remaining Corps troops.

The mechanized brigades comprise tank battalions (Leopard I improved and Leopard 2), armoured infantry battalions (YPR-765), medium artillery battalions (155 mm self-propelled), armoured engineer units and armoured anti armour units. The Corps troops comprise headquarters units, combat-support units, including Engineer and Corps artillery (203 mm, 155 mm and Lance and MLRS) and service-support units. Helicopter squadrons are also available.

The National Territorial Command forces consist of territorial brigades, security forces, some logistical units and staffs. The major part of these units is mobilizable. Some units in the Netherlands may be assigned to the UN as peace-keeping forces. The army is responsible for the training of these units. In time of war, the civil defence operations will be closely co-ordinated with the local civilian authorities.

Navy. The principal headquarters and main base of the Royal Netherlands Navy is at Den Helder, with minor bases at Vlissingen (Flushing), Curaçao (Netherlands Antilles) and Oranjestad (Aruba).

The modern and effective combatant fleet, all built in home shipyards, and largely equipped with indigenous sensors and imported weapons, comprises 5 diesel submarines including the first of the new Zeeleeuw class, 4 guided-missile destroyers armed with US Standard SM1-MR surface-to-air missiles, 10 frigates each with 1 or 2 Lynx anti-submarine helicopters, 15 coastal minehunters and 11 coastal minesweepers. There are 2 multi-purpose support ships (each carrying up to 3 helicopters), 3 survey ships, 2 training ships and a torpedo tender, plus numerous service vessels.

The first ship of 8 new *Karel Doorman* class frigates commenced sea trials in 1990.

The Marine corps has 12 small amphibious craft, but is integrated operationally with the UK Marines for its NATO tasks.

The Naval air service operates 13 Orion P-3C, 17 Westland Lynx SH-14B/C for embarked service and 5 Lynx UH-14A for search and rescue, utility and transport.

In 1990 personnel totalled 16,500 officers and other ranks, including 1,400 in the Naval Air Service, 560 women (who serve in all classes of ships except submarines) and 2,800 in the Royal Netherlands Marine Corps.

Air Force. The Royal Netherlands Air Force (RNLAF) was established 1 July 1913. Its strength (1991) was 19,553 personnel and it has a first-line combat force of 9 squadrons of aircraft and 2 groups of surface-to-air missiles in Germany. All squadrons are operated by Tactical Air Command. Aircraft operated are F-16A/B (7 squadrons for air defence and ground attack, 1 for tactical reconnaissance), and NF-5A/B fighter-bombers (1 squadron, to be re-equipped with F-16s by 1991). Also under control of Tactical Air Command is 1 squadron of the USAF, flying F-15C/D Eagles in the air defence role. 3 squadrons of Alouette III and Bölkow Bö 105C helicopters are under control of the Royal Netherlands Army, but flown and maintained by the RNLAF for use in the communications and observation roles. Also operated is 1 squadron of F.27 Friendship/Troopship transport aircraft, and another (based in Curaçao) with F.27 maritime patrol aircraft.

Training of RNLAF pilots is undertaken in the USA and the Netherlands. The surface-to-air missile force consists of 4 squadrons of Patriot with 160 missiles and 11 squadrons with Hawks, of which 7 are for airfield defence.

INTERNATIONAL RELATIONS

Membership. The Netherlands is a member of the UN, EC, OECD, Council of Europe, WEU and NATO. The Schengen Accord of June 1990 abolished border controls between the Netherlands and Belgium, France, Germany and Luxembourg. Italy acceded in Nov. 1990.

ECONOMY

Budget. The revenue and expenditure of the central government (ordinary and extraordinary) were, in 1m. guilders, for calendar years:

	1983	*1984*	*1985*	*1986*	*1987*	*1988*	*1989*
Revenue [1]	115,002	127,918	138,605	159,689	156,111	151,904	148,699
Expenditure[2]	146,622	157,709	162,085	167,321	170,275	173,097	172,456

[1] Without the revenue of loans. [2] Without redemption of loans.

The revenue and expenditure of the Agriculture Equalization Fund, the Fund for Central Government roads, the Property Acquisition Fund and of the Investment Account Fund (established in 1978) have been incorporated in the general budget.

The national debt, in 1m. guilders, was on 31 Dec.:

	1985	*1986*	*1987*	*1988*	*1989*
Internal funded debt	208,484	219,466	234,474	263,949	287,155
„ floating „	19,799	19,969	16,683	10,524	6,544
Total	228,283	239,435	251,157	274,473	293,699

Currency. The monetary unit is the *gulden* (NLG; written as fl[orin]; in English, 'guilder') of 100 *cents*. It is tied to the German Deutschmark. In March 1991 the rate of exchange was US$1 = 1·73 guilders; £1 = 3·29 guilders.

Legal tender are bank-notes, silver 10-guilder pieces, 5-guilder pieces, nickel 2½- and 1-guilder pieces, 25-cent, 10-cent pieces and bronze 5-cent pieces.

Banking and Finance. The central bank and bank of issue is the Netherlands Bank (*Governor* Willem Duisenberg), which was nationalized on 1 Aug. 1948. The capital amounts to 75m. guilders.

There is a stock exchange in Amsterdam.

Weights and Measures. The metric system of weights and measures was adopted in the Netherlands in 1820.

ENERGY AND NATURAL RESOURCES

Electricity. Production of electrical energy (in 1m. kwh.) in 1985, 62,936; 1986, 67,148; 1987, 68,437; 1988, 69,016; 1989, 73,151. Supply 220 volts; 50 Hz.

Gas. Production of manufactured gas (milliard k joule): 1978, 181,033; 1979, 233,553; 1980, 210,011; 1981, 197,586; 1982, 244,438; 1983, 258,515; 1984,

267,643. Production of natural gas in 1950, 8m. cu. metres; 1955, 139; 1960, 384; 1970, 31,688; 1980, 91,153; 1985, 80,721; 1986, 74,037; 1987, 74,247; 1988, 65,610; 1989, 71,715.

Minerals. On 1 Jan. 1975 all coalmines were closed.

The production of crude petroleum (in 1,000 tonnes) amounted in 1943 (first year) to 0·2; 1953, 820; 1970, 1,919; 1978, 1,402; 1979, 1,316; 1980, 1,280; 1981, 1,348; 1982, 1,637; 1983, 2,589; 1984, 3,102; 1985, 3,729; 1986, 4,628; 1987, 4,291; 1988, 4,272; 1989, 3,814; 1990, 4,142.

There are saltmines at Hengelo and Delfzijl; production (in 1,000 tonnes), 1950, 412·6; 1960, 1,096; 1970, 2,871; 1978, 2,939; 1979, 3,951; 1980, 3,464; 1981, 3,578; 1982, 3,191; 1983, 3,124; 1984, 3,674; 1985, 4,154; 1986, 3,763; 1987, 3,979; 1988, 3,693; 1989, 3,756.

Agriculture. The net area of all holdings was divided as follows (in ha):

	1986	*1987*	*1988*	*1989*	*1990*
Field crops	763,068	787,078	789,798	795,822	799,434
Grass	1,141,978	1,124,472	1,114,009	1,098,823	1,096,496
Market gardening	72,352	66,971	70,415	71,281	71,294
Land for flower bulbs	15,564	16,432	16,420	16,698	16,319
Flower cultivation	6,216	6,377	6,623	7,054	7,243
Nurseries	7,037	7,523	7,911	8,478	8,883
Fallow land	6,367	5,410	6,493	5,722	5,939
Total	2,012,589	2,014,263	2,011,669	2,003,878	2,005,608

The net areas under special crops were as follows (in ha):

Products	*1989*	*1990*	*Products*	*1989*	*1990*
Autumn wheat	130,738	135,104	Colza	6,275	8,415
Spring wheat	8,894	5,499	Flax	5,258	5,535
Rye	6,826	8,604	Agricultural seeds	25,696	26,314
Autumn barley	7,806	9,941	Potatoes, edible [1]	104,919	112,481
Spring barley	42,393	30,447	Potatoes, industrial [2]	60,204	62,838
Oats	7,787	3,401	Sugar-beet	123,757	124,995
Peas	15,913	11,703	Fodder-beet	2,532	3,023

[1] Including early and seed pototoes. [2] Including seed potatoes.

The yield of the more important products, in tonnes, was as follows:

Crop	*Average 1960–69*	*Average 1970–79*	*1988*	*1989*	*1990* [1]
Wheat	630,054	701,934	827,139	1,046,770	1,075,853
Rye	289,503	103,442	28,271	33,424	36,219
Barley	388,444	327,345	302,290	250,712	218,834
Oats	385,164	144,855	59,541	32,055	16,104
Field beans	1,847	...	56,791	29,823	15,067
Peas	61,808	19,972	107,518	72,095	57,287
Colza	11,763	32,797	24,153	22,953	25,508
Flax, unrippled	159,257	43,620	31,967	31,341	39,590
Potatoes, edible	2,508,369	3,084,356	4,413,192	4,376,244	4,658,423
Potatoes, industrial	1,469,799	2,554,555	2,329,304	2,479,372	2,377,816
Sugar-beet	4,045,153	5,546,689	6,737,330	7,678,508	8,623,400
Fodder-beet	1,678,285	348,117	165,649	232,519	292,086

[1] Provisional figures.

Livestock, May 1990: 4,926,023 cattle, 13,915,048 pigs; 69,592 horses and ponies; 1,702,406 sheep, 95,451,720 poultry.

In 1989 the production of butter, under state control, increased to 180,154 tonnes; in 1988, that of cheese, under state control, increased to 581,757 tonnes. Export value (processed and unprocessed) of arable crops: 17,501m. guilders; animal produce, 19,100m. guilders and horticultural produce, 12,487m. guilders.

Fisheries. The total produce of fish landed from the sea and inshore fisheries in 1981 was valued at 595m. guilders; the total weight amounted to 399,438 tonnes. In 1981 the herring fishery had a value of 26m. guilders and a weight of 16,710 tonnes. The quantity of oysters produced in 1981 amounted to 573 tonnes (10m. guilders).

INDUSTRY. Numbers employed (in 1,000) and turnover (in 1m. guilders) in manufacturing enterprises with 10 employees and more, excluding building:

Class in industry	*Numbers employed* 1987	1988 [1]	*Turnover* 1987	1988 [1]
Mining and quarrying	17·8	14·7	9·3	9·5
Manufacturing industry	238·2	253·8	811·2	814·2
Foodstuffs and tobacco products	67·3	69·7	132·6	133·3
Textile industry	5·0	5·1	23·0	22·2
Clothing	1·4	1·4	9·7	9·9
Leather and footwear	0·9	0·9	5·8	5·4
Wood and furniture industry	4·5	4·9	25·3	26·7
Paper industry	7·1	7·7	24·7	24·9
Graphic industry, publishers	13·3	14·2	64·0	65·2
Petroleum industry	16·7	14·7	9·3	8·9
Chemical industry, artificial yarns and fibre industry	36·7	41·4	87·6	87·9
Rubber and synthetic materials processing industry	6·9	7·3	28·1	28·8
Building industry, earthenware and glass	6·4	7·4	29·2	29·9
Basic metal industry	7·8	9·8	30·0	29·7
Metal products (excl. machinery and means of transport)	12·6	14·2	72·4	75·9
Machinery	14·3	14·7	78·7	80·4
Electrical industry	23·5	24·4	121·5	117·2
Means of transport	12·2	14·1	57·8	55·9
Instrument making and optical industry	1.0	1·1	7·2	7·4
Other industries	0·7	0·8	4·4	4·9
Public utilities	18·5	16·3	...	...

[1] Provisional.

Labour. In Jan. 1991 job exchanges were moved from government control to joint control by employers, trade unions and local authorities.

Unemployment was 343,000 at the end of 1990, with 125,000 job vacancies.

FOREIGN ECONOMIC RELATIONS. On 5 Sept. 1944 and 14 March 1947 the Netherlands signed agreements with Belgium and Luxembourg for the establishment of a customs union. On 1 Jan. 1948 this union came into force and the existing customs tariffs of the Belgium–Luxembourg Economic Union and of the Netherlands were superseded by the joint Benelux Customs Union Tariff. It applies to imports into the 3 countries from outside sources, and exempts from customs duties all imports into each of the 3 countries from the other two. The Benelux tariff has 991 items and 2,400 separate specifications.

Commerce. Returns of special imports and special exports for calendar years (in 1,000 guilders):

	Imports	*Exports*		*Imports*	*Exports*
1959	14,968,454	13,702,927	1986	185,052,790	197,286,108
1969	39,955,406	36,205,110	1987	184,843,632	188,017,411
1979	134,885,386	127,689,416	1988	195,801,221	203,777,722
1985	216,008,008	226,017,400	1989	220,985,736	228,544,316

Value of the trade with leading countries (in 1,000 guilders):

Country	*Imports* 1988	1989	*Exports* 1988	1989
Belgium–Luxembourg	28,756,911	31,245,287	30,010,794	33,401,293
France	14,415,093	16,792,158	21,939,850	24,811,452
Germany (Fed. Rep.)	51,675,196	56,782,526	53,179,932	59,118,154
Indonesia	814,132	933,307	822,805	403,209
Italy	7,366,879	8,072,051	13,067,921	14,883,468
Kuwait	1,943,455	2,416,177	201,786	264,250
Sweden	4,393,096	4,859,371	3,827,246	4,515,046
UK	15,125,293	17,445,287	21,981,940	25,269,472
USA	15,002,474	18,592,563	8,768,109	10,393,687
Venezuela	128,588	171,241	307,933	178,004

Total trade between the Netherlands and UK (British Department of Trade returns, in £1,000 sterling):

	1986	1987	1988	1989	1990
Imports to UK	6,615,851	7,148,036	8,279,747	9,585,699	10,483,576
Exports and re-exports from UK	5,442,503	5,856,164	5,583,280	6,515,325	7,516,576

Tourism. There were 3·54m. foreign visitors in 1989 to hotels: 0·68m. from the Federal Republic of Germany, 0·66m. from the UK and 0·42m. from the USA. Total income from tourism (1988) US$2,858m.

COMMUNICATIONS

Roads. In 1988 the length of the Netherlands network of surfaced inter-urban roads was 55,100 km, of which 2,060 km were motor highways. Number of private cars (1989), 5·4m.

Railways. All railways are run by the mixed company 'N.V. Nederlandse Spoorwegen'. Route length in 1989 was 2,828 km, of which 1,957 km were electrified. Passengers carried (1989), 239m.; goods transported, 19·4m. tonnes.

Aviation. The Royal Dutch Airlines (KLM) was founded on 7 Oct. 1919. Revenue traffic, 1989–90: Passengers, 7·2m.; freight, 338m. kg; mail, 18m. kg.

Sea-going Shipping. Survey of the Netherlands mercantile marine as at 1 Jan. (capacity in 1,000 GRT):

	1989		*1990*	
Ships under Netherlands flag	*Number*	*Capacity*	*Number*	*Capacity*
Passenger ships [1]	4	77	4	77
Freighters (100 GRT and over)	367	2,060	359	2,047
Tankers	57	668	55	646
	428	2,804	718	2,771

[1] With accommodation for 13 or more cabin passengers.

In 1989, 46,349 sea-going ships of 406m. gross tons entered Netherlands ports.

Total goods traffic by sea-going ships in 1988 (with 1989 figures in brackets), in 1m. tonnes, amounted to 267 (280) unloaded, of which 121 (128) tankshipping, and 88 (93) loaded, of which 31 (33) tankshipping. The total seaborne freight traffic at Rotterdam was 274m. (290m.) and at Amsterdam 28m. (29m.) tonnes.

The number of containers (including flats) at Rotterdam in 1988 (with 1989 figures in brackets) was: Unloaded from ships, 1,062,661 (1,183,961) and 1,122,541 (1,222,728) loaded into ships.

Inland Shipping. The total length of navigable rivers and canals is 5,016 km, of which 2,391 km is for ships with a capacity of 1,000 and more tonnes. On 1 Jan. 1990 the inland fleet used for transport (with carrying capacity in 1,000 tonnes) was composed as follows:

	Number	*Capacity*
Self-propelled barges	5,255	4,277
Dumb barges	305	288
Pushed barges	722	1,547
	6,282	6,113

In 1989, 293m. (1988: 285m.) tonnes of goods were transported on rivers and canals, of which 203m. (194m.) was international traffic. Goods transport on the Rhine across the Dutch–German frontier near Lobith amounted to 130m. (126m.) tonnes.

Telecommunications. On 1 Jan. 1990 there were 6·7m. telephone connexions (45 per 100 inhabitants). Number of telex lines, 26,000. *Nederlandse Omroep Stichting* (NOS) provides 5 programmes on medium-waves and FM in co-operation with broadcasting organizations. Regional programmes are also broadcast.

Advertisements are transmitted. NOS broadcasts 3 TV programmes. Advertisements, 1986–87 were restricted to 5·5% of the transmission time in the evening. Television sets (1 Jan. 1988) totalled 4·7m.; holders of television licences may, in addition, have wireless receiving sets.

Cinemas (end 1988). There were 443 cinemas with a seating capacity of 104,000.

Newspapers (Sept. 1986). There were 85 daily newspapers with a total circulation of nearly 4·6m.

JUSTICE, RELIGION, EDUCATION AND WELFARE

Justice. Justice is administered by the High Court of the Netherlands (Court of Cassation), by 5 courts of justice (Courts of Appeal), by 19 district courts and by 63 cantonal courts; trial by jury is unknown. The Cantonal Court, which deals with minor offences, is formed by a single judge; the more serious cases are tried by the district courts, formed as a rule by 3 judges (in some cases one judge is sufficient); the courts of appeal are constituted of 3 and the High Court of 5 judges. All judges are appointed for life by the Sovereign (the judges of the High Court from a list prepared by the Second Chamber of the States-General). They can be removed only by a decision of the High Court.

At the district court the juvenile judge is specially appointed to try children's civil cases and at the same time charged with administration of justice for criminal actions committed by young persons between 12 and 18 years old, unless imprisonment of more than 6 months ought to be inflicted; such cases are tried by 3 judges.

Number of sentences, and cases in which prosecution was evaded by paying a fine to the public prosecutor (excluding violation of economic and tax laws):

Major offences		*Minor offences*	
1987	97,361	1987	915,329
1988	102,348	1988	825,190
1989	107,059	1989[1]	751,401

In addition, prosecution was evaded by paying a fine to the police in about 1·95m. cases in 1988.

[1] Provisional.

Police. There are both State and Municipal Police. In 1989 the State Police, about 7,500 strong, served 554, and the Municipal Police, about 20,400 strong, served 148 municipalities. The State Police includes ordinary as well as water, mounted and motor police. The State Police Corps is under the jurisdiction of the Police Department of the Ministry of Justice, which also includes the Central Criminal Investigation Office, which deals with serious crimes throughout the country, and the International Criminal Investigation Office, which informs foreign countries of international crimes.

Religion. Entire liberty of conscience is granted to the members of all denominations. The royal family belong to the Dutch Reformed Church.

The number of adherents of the Churches according to survey estimates of 1988 was: Roman Catholics, 5,297,000; Dutch Reformed Church, 2,751,000; Reformed Churches, 1,177,000; other creeds, 824,000; no religion, 4,723,000.

The government of the Reformed Church is Presbyterian. On 1 July 1972 the Dutch Reformed Church had 1 synod, 11 provincial districts, 54 classes, 147 districts and 1,905 parishes.

Their clergy numbered 2,000. The Roman Catholic Church had, Jan. 1973, 1 archbishop (of Utrecht), 6 bishops and 1,815 parishes and rectorships. The Old Catholics had (1 July 1972) 1 archbishop (Utrecht), 2 bishops and 29 parishes. The Jews had, in 1970, 46 communities.

Education. Statistics for the scholastic year 1988–89:

	Full-time Pupils/Students			*Part-time[1] Pupils/Students*		
	Schools	*Total*	*Female*	*Schools*	*Total*	*Female*
Basic schools	8,426	1,428,577	705,924	—	—	—
Special schools	1,001	105,090	33,616	—	—	—
Secondary general schools	1,305	718,341	376,997	80	90,775	64,683
Secondary vocational schools:						
Junior—						
Technical, nautical	576	112,801	5,811	5	877	73
Agricultural	196	24,373	7,438	93	8,021	1,784
Domestic science	707	59,851	55,847	—	—	—
Other	242	75,452	37,860	—	—	—

[1] Including apprenticeship schemes, young workers' educational institutes.

	Full-time Pupils/Students			Part-time[1] Pupils/Students		
	Schools	Total	Female	Schools	Total	Female
Senior—						
Technical, nautical	128	83,280	9,081	43	8,027	418
Agricultural	65	18,700	3,736	48	6,163	1,302
Service trade and health care training	132	72,593	64,980	26	9,711	6,695
Other	206	123,977	59,321	343	177,345	62,401
Third level non-university training:						
Technical, nautical	62	42,651	5,240	16	4,311	471
Agricultural	18	8,256	1,929	1	253	25
Arts	47	16,615	9,374	32	4,554	2,323
Teachers' training	73	27,275	18,317	49	22,000	11,062
Other	133	74,333	43,072	66	24,176	12,867

[1] Including apprenticeship schemes, young workers' educational institutes.

Academic Year 1988–89

	Schools	Full-time Students Total	Full-time Students Female	Part-time Students Total	Part-time Students Female
University education:					
Humanities	21	25,804	16,295	1,391	767
Social sciences		70,636	29,434	10,936	4,513
Natural sciences		13,088	3,575	246	52
Technical sciences		24,040	2,716	...	...
Medical sciences		16,864	8,607	271	177
Agricultural sciences		5,667	2,262	73	31

Health. On 1 Jan. 1989 there were 35,853 doctors and about 66,647 licensed hospital beds.

DIPLOMATIC REPRESENTATIVES

Of the Netherlands in Great Britain (38 Hyde Park Gate, London, SW7 5DP)
Ambassador: Joop Hoekman.

Of Great Britain in the Netherlands (Lange Voorhout, 10, The Hague)
Ambassador: Sir Michael Jenkins, KCMG.

Of the Netherlands in the USA (4200 Linnean Ave., NW, Washington, D.C., 20008)
Ambassador: Johan H. Meesman.

Of the USA in the Netherlands (Lange Voorhout, 102, The Hague)
Ambassador: C. Howard Wilkins Jr.

Of the Netherlands to the United Nations
Ambassador: Robert J. Van Schaik.

Further Reading

Statistical Information: The 'Centraal Bureau voor de Statistiek' at Voorburg and Heerlen, is the official Netherlands statistical service. *Director-General of Statistics:* Prof. Dr W. Begeer.

The Bureau was founded in 1899. Prior to that year, statistical publications were compiled by the 'Centrale commissie voor de statistiek', the 'Vereniging voor staathuishoudkunde en statistiek' and various government departments. These activities have gradually been taken over and co-ordinated by the Central Bureau, which now compiles practically all government statistics.

Its current publications include:

Statistical Yearbook of the Netherlands. From 1923/24 (preceded by *Jaarcijfers voor het Koninkrijk der Nederlanden, 1898–1922);* latest issue, 1990 (in English)
Statistisch jaarboek (Statistical Year Book). From 1899/1924 (1 vol.); latest issue, 1991
CBS Select (Statistical Essays). From 1980; latest issue, 1990
Statistisch Bulletin (From 1945; weekly statistical bulletin)
Maandschrift (From 1944; monthly bulletin)

90 Jaren Statistiek In Tijdreeksen (historical series of the Netherlands 1899–1989)
Nationale Rekeningen (National Accounts). From 1948–50; latest issue, 1990
Statistisch Magazine. From 1981
Statistische onderzoekingen. From 1977
Regionaal Statistisch Zakboek (Regional Pocket Yearbook). From 1972, latest issue 1989
Environmental Statistics of the Netherlands, 1987 (in English)

Other Official Publications

Central Economic Plan. Centraal Plan bureau, The Hague (Dutch text), annually, from 1946
Netherlands. Organization for Economic Co-operation and Development. Paris, annual from 1964
Staatsalmanak voor het Koninkrijk der Nederlanden. Annual. The Hague, from 1814
Staatsblad van het Koninkrijk der Nederlanden. The Hague, from 1814
Staatscourant (State Gazette). The Hague, from 1813
Atlas van Nederland. Government Printing Office, The Hague, 1970 and supplements up to and including 1973
Basic Guide to the Establishing of Industrial Operations in the Netherlands 1976. Ministry of Economic Affairs, The Hague, 1976

Non-Official Publications

Jansonius, H., *Nieuw Groot Nederlands—Engels Woordenboek Voor Studie en Praktijk.* 3 vols. Leiden, 1973 (Vols. 1–3)
King, P. K. and Wintle, M., *The Netherlands.* [Bibliography] Oxford and Santa Barbara, 1988
Pyttersen's Nederlandse Almanak. Zaltbommel, annual, from 1899
A Compact Geography of the Netherlands. Utrecht, 1980
National Library: De Koninklijke Bibliotheek, Prinz Willem Alexanderhof 5, The Hague. *Director:* Dr C. Reedijk.

ARUBA

HISTORY. Discovered by Alonzo de Ojeda in 1499, the island of Aruba was claimed for Spain but not settled. It was acquired by the Dutch in 1634, but apart from garrisons was left to the indigenous Caiquetios (Arawak) Indians until the 19th century. From 1828 it formed part of the Dutch West Indies and, from 1845, part of the Netherlands Antilles, with which on 29 Dec. 1954 it achieved internal self-government.

Following a referendum in March 1977, the Dutch government announced on 28 Oct. 1981 that Aruba would proceed to independence separately from the other islands. Aruba was constitutionally separated from the Netherlands Antilles from 1 Jan. 1986, and full independence has been promised by the Netherlands after a 10-year period.

AREA AND POPULATION. The island, which lies in the southern Caribbean 24 km north of the Venezuelan coast and 68 km west of Curaçao, has an area of 193 sq. km (75 sq. miles) and a population at the 1981 census of 60,312; estimate (1988) 62,500. The chief towns are Oranjestad, the capital (20,000) and Sint Nicolaas, site of the former oil refinery (17,000). Dutch is the official language, but the language usually spoken is Papiamento, a creole language. Unlike other Caribbean islands, over half the population is of Indian stock, with the balance chiefly of Dutch, Spanish and mestizo origin.

CLIMATE. Aruba has a tropical marine climate, with a brief rainy season from Oct. to Dec. Oranjestad. Jan. 79°F (26·0°C), July 84°F (29·0°C). Annual rainfall 17" (432 mm).

CONSTITUTION AND GOVERNMENT. Under the separate constitution inaugurated on 1 Jan. 1986, Aruba is an autonomous part of the Kingdom of the Netherlands with its own legislature, government, judiciary, civil service and police force. The Netherlands is represented by a Governor appointed by the monarch. The unicameral legislature *(Staten)* consists of 21 members; at the general elections held on 6 Jan. 1989, 10 seats were won by the *(Movimento Electoral di Pueblo*, 8 by the *Arubaanse Volks Partij*, and 1 each by 3 smaller parties with whom the AVP formed a coalition government.

Governor: Felipe B. Tromp.
Prime Minister, Minister of General Affairs: Nelson O. Oduber.
Deputy Prime Minister, Public Works and Health: Pedro P. Kelly.
Economic Affairs and Tourism: Daniel I. Leo. *Justice:* Hendrik S. Croes. *Social Affairs and Education:* Fredis J. Refunjol. *Transport and Communications:* Euladio D. Nicolaas. *Finance:* Guillermo P. Trinidad.

Flag: Blue, with 2 narrow horizontal yellow stripes, and in the canton a red 4-pointed star fimbriated in white.

ECONOMY

Budget. The 1984 budget totalled 207m. guilders revenue and 278m. guilders expenditure.

Currency. From 1 Jan. 1986 the currency has been the Aruban florin, at par with the Netherlands Antilles guilder. In March 1991, £1 = 3·40 *Aruban florins*; US$1 = 1·79 *Aruban florins*.

Banking. As well as the Aruba Bank, there are local branches of the Algemene Bank Nederland, Barclays Bank International, Caribbean Mercantile Bank and Citibank.

ENERGY AND NATURAL RESOURCES

Electricity. Generating capacity totals 310,000 kw. Production (1986) 945m. kwh.

Oil. The Exxon refinery dominated the economy from 1929–85, when it was closed, resulting in unemployment reaching 40% by the end of 1985.

Minerals. Gold, first discovered in 1825, is still found but in uneconomic quantities.

EXTERNAL ECONOMIC RELATIONS

Commerce. Total trade between Aruba and UK (British Department of Trade returns, in £1,000 sterling):

	1988	*1989*	*1990*
Imports to UK	133	653	50
Exports and re-exports from UK	7,315	12,751	11,386

Tourism. Tourism is now the main economic sector. In 1986 there were 181,000 tourists.

COMMUNICATIONS

Roads. In 1984 there were 380 km of surfaced highways. In 1984 there were 23,409 passenger cars and 582 commercial vehicles.

Aviation. There is an international airport (Prinses Beatrix) served by numerous airlines.

Telecommunications. In 1983 there were 5 radio stations and 1 television station. In 1983 there were 17,000 telephones.

JUSTICE RELIGION, EDUCATION AND WELFARE

Justice. The Aruban judiciary is now separated from that of the Netherlands Antilles. There is a Court of First Instance and a Court of Appeal situated in Oranjestad.

Religion. In 1981, 89% of the population were Roman Catholic and 7% Protestant.

Education. In 1983 there were 33 elementary schools with 6,763 pupils, 10 junior high schools with 3,082 pupils and 4 senior schools and colleges with 881 students.

Health. In 1985 there were 59 doctors, 16 dentists, 9 pharmacists, 189 nursing personnel and one hospital with 279 beds.

THE NETHERLANDS ANTILLES

De Nederlandse Antillen

HISTORY. Bonaire and Curaçao islands, originally populated by Arowak Indians, were discovered in 1499 by Alonso de Ojeda, and claimed for Spain. They were settled in 1527, and the indigenous population exterminated and replaced by a slave-worked plantation economy. The 3 Windward Islands, inhabited by Caribs, were discovered by Columbus in 1493. They were taken by the Dutch in 1632 (Saba and Sint Eustatius), 1634 (Curaçao and Bonaire) and 1648 (the southern part of Sint Maarten, with France acquiring the northern part). With Aruba, the islands formed part of the Dutch West Indies from 1828, and the Netherlands Antilles from 1845, with internal self-government being granted on 29 Dec. 1954. Aruba was separated from 1 Jan. 1986.

AREA AND POPULATION. The Netherlands Antilles comprise two groups of islands, the Leeward group (Curaçao and Bonaire) being situated 100 km north of the Venezuelan coast and the Windward Islands situated 800 km away to the north-east, at the northern end of the Lesser Antilles. The total area is 800 sq. km (308 sq. miles) and the Census population in 1981 was 235,707. Estimate (1988) 192,866 (excluding Aruba). Willemstad is the capital.

The areas, populations and chief towns of the islands are:

Island	*Sq. km*	*1989 Estimate*	*Chief town*	*1981 Census*
Bonaire	288	10,797	Kralendijk	1,200
Curaçao	444	146,096	Willemstad	50,000
Saba	13	1,112	The Bottom	–
Sint Eustatius	21	1,861	Oranjestad	–
Sint Maarten [1]	34	29,821	Philipsburg	6,000

[1] The southern part belongs to the Netherlands Antilles, the northern to France.

Dutch is the official language, but the languages usually spoken are Papiamento (a creole language) on Curaçao and Bonaire, and English in the Windward Islands.

Vital statistics (1989), Live births, 3,504; marriages, 1,226; deaths, 1,204.

CLIMATE. All the islands have a tropical marine climate, with very little difference in temperatures over the year. There is a short rainy season from Oct. to Jan. Willemstad. Jan. 79°F (26·1°C), July 82°F (27·8°C). Annual rainfall 23" (582 mm).

CONSTITUTION AND GOVERNMENT. On 29 Dec. 1954, the Netherlands Antilles became an integral part of the Kingdom of the Netherlands but are fully autonomous in internal affairs, and constitutionally equal with the Netherlands and Aruba. The Sovereign of the Kingdom of the Netherlands is Head of State and Government, and is represented by a Governor.

The executive power in internal affairs rests with the Governor and the Council of Ministers, who together form the Government. The Ministers are responsible to a unicameral legislature *(Staten)* consisting of 22 members (since 1986, 14 from Curaçao, 3 from Bonaire, 3 from Sint Maarten, and 1 each from Saba and Sint Eustatius) elected by universal suffrage. In general elections held on 16 March 1990, 1 seat was won by the *Democratische Partij* (DP), 7 by the *Nationale Volks Partij* (NVP), 2 by the *Movimento Antijas Nobo* (MAN), 3 by the combination *Sosial Independiente/Frerhe Obrero y Liberashon* (SI/FOL), 3 by the *Union Patriotico Bonairiano* (UPB), 2 by the *Democratic Party of St. Maarten Patriotic Alliance* (DPSXM), 1 for *Nos Patria*, 1 for *St. Maarten Patriotic Alliance* (SPA), 1 for the *Windward Island People's Movement* (WIPM), and 1 for the *Democratic Party of St. Eustatius* (DP St. Eustatius).

The executive power in external affairs is vested in the Council of Ministers of the Kingdom, in which the Antilles is represented by a Minister Plenipotentiary with full voting powers. On each of the insular communities, local autonomous power is divided between an Island Council (elected by universal suffrage), the Executive Council and the Lieut.-Governor, responsible for law and order.

Governor: Dr Jaime M. Saleh.

The Cabinet in Nov. 1990 was composed as follows:
Prime Minister: Maria-Liberia Peters (NVP).
Deputy Prime Minister, Transport and Communications: Louis Gumbs (DPSXM). *Justice:* Ivo Knoppel. *Finance:* Gilbert de Paula. *Economic Affairs and Education:* Chuchu Smits (NVP). *Social and Labour Affairs:* Eithel Pietersz (SI/FOL). *Developmental Affairs:* Jopie Giskus (UPB). *Public Health and Environmental Affairs:* Stanley Inderson (SI/FOL).

Flag: White, with a red vertical strip crossed by a blue horizontal strip bearing 5 white stars.

ECONOMY

Budget. The central budget for 1989 envisaged 298·7m. NA guilders revenue and 327·7m. NA guilders expenditure.

Currency. The unit of currency is the *Netherlands Antilles guilder* (ANG) of 100 *cents.* There are notes of 250, 100, 50, 25, 10, 5, $2^1/_2$ and 1 *guilder*, and coins of $2^1/_2$ and 1 *guilder* and 25, 10, 5, $2^1/_2$ and 1 *cent*. The official rate of exchange was £1 = 3·40 *NA guilder*; US$1 = 1·80 *NA guilder* in March 1991.

Banking. At 31 Dec. 1989 the Bank of the Netherlands Antilles had total assets and liabilities of 542·5m. NA guilders; commercial banks, 3,272·9m. NA guilders.
Post office savings banks had deposits of 6,837m. NA guilders in 1987.

ENERGY AND NATURAL RESOURCES

Electricity. Production (1989) totalled 738m. kwh.

Oil. The economy was formerly based largely on oil refining at the Shell refinery on Curaçao, but following an announcement by Shell that closure was imminent, this was sold to the Netherlands Antilles government in Sept. 1985, and leased to Petróleos de Venezuela to operate on a reduced scale.

Minerals. About 100,000 tons of calcium phosphate are mined annually. Calcium carbonate (limestone) has been mined since 1980, when mining of calcium phosphate ceased. Production, 1988, 375,000 tons.

Agriculture. Livestock (1988): Cattle, 8,000; goats, 23,000. Figures include Aruba. (Curaçao, 1990: cows, 350; goats, 48,000; pigs, 5,700; sheep, 9,000).

Fisheries. Catch (1982) 11,000 tonnes.

INDUSTRY AND TRADE

Industry. Curaçao has one of the largest ship-repair dry docks in the western hemisphere. Curaçao has a paint factory, 2 cigarette factories, a textile factory, a brewery and some smaller industries. Bonaire has a textile factory and a modern equipped salt plant. Sint Maarten has a rum factory and fishing is important. Sint Eustatius and Saba are of less economic importance.

Labour. In 1988 the economically active population numbered 73,101 (Curaçao, 1989: 58,938), the working population 58,165, (Curaçao, 1989: 43,770).

Commerce. There is a Free Zone on Curaçao, Total imports (1987) amounted to 2,703m. (crude and petroleum products, 1,889m.) NA guilders, total exports to 2,354m. (crude and petroleum products, 2,241m.) NA guilders.
Total trade between the Netherlands Antilles and UK (British Department of Trade returns, in £1,000 sterling):

	1986 [1]	*1987* [1]	*1988*	*1989*	*1990*
Imports to UK	78,509	5,133	7,823 [1]	5,115	43,552
Exports and re-exports from UK	17,260	19,635	20,089	19,396	23,800

[1] Excluding Aruba.

Tourism. In 1989, 718,935 tourists visited the islands (Sint Maarten, 488,720; Curaçao, 193,032; Bonaire, 37,183) excluding 596,522 cruise passengers (Curaçao, 117,391; Sint Maarten, 472,022; Bonair, 7,109).

COMMUNICATIONS

Roads. In 1984, the Netherlands Antilles had 820 km of surfaced highway distributed as follows: Curaçao, 550; Bonaire, 210; Sint Maarten, 3. Number of motor vehicles (31 Dec. 1986): 51,462.

Aviation. There are international airports on Curaçao (Hato Airport), Bonaire (Flamingo Field) and Sint Maarten (Princess Juliana Airport). In 1988 Curaçao handled 769,000 passengers, Bonaire 200,000, Sint Maarten 951,000, Sint Eustatius 28,772 and Saba 15,392.

Shipping (1989). 4,555 ships (totalling 29,286,000 GRT) entered the port of Curaçao; 809 ships (5,461,000 GRT) entered the port of Bonaire: 2,742 ships (15,062,000 GRT) entered the port of St. Maarten. In 1986 Curaçao handled 172,904 passengers, Bonaire 3,898 and Sint Maarten 1,021,896.

Telecommunications. Number of telephones, 1989, 49,560. At 31 Dec. 1986 there were 17 radio transmitters (6 on Bonaire, 8 on Curaçao and 1 each on Saba, Sint Eustatius and Sint Maarten) and 6 TV channels (5 on Curaçao, 1 on Sint Maarten). These stations broadcast in *Papiamento*, Dutch, English and Spanish and are mainly financed by income from advertisements. In addition, Radio Nederland and Trans World Radio have powerful relay stations operating on medium- and short-waves from Bonaire. There were (1984, including Aruba) 160,000 radio and 57,000 TV receivers.

Newspapers. In 1989 there were 10 daily newspapers. Total circulation 94,000 (1988).

JUSTICE, RELIGION, EDUCATION AND WELFARE

Justice. There is a Court of First Instance, which sits in each island, and a Court of Appeal in Willemstad.

Religion. In 1981, 85% of the population were Roman Catholics, 9·7% were Protestants (Sint Maarten and Sint Eustatius being chiefly Protestant).

Education. In 1987 there were 22,073 pupils in primary schools, 9,396 pupils in general secondary schools, 4,962 pupils in junior and senior secondary vocational schools, and 803 students in vocational colleges and universities.

Health. In 1988 there were 227 doctors, 47 dentists and 1,596 hospital beds; (1987) 1,465 nursing personnel.

DIPLOMATIC REPRESENTATIVE

USA Consul-General: Sharon Wilkinson.

Further Reading

Statistical Information: Statistical publications (on population, trade, cost of living, etc., are obtainable on request from the Statistical Office, Willemstad, Curaçao. *Statistical Jaarboek 1970* (text in Dutch, English and Spanish).

De West Indische Gids. The Hague. Monthly from 1919

NEW ZEALAND

Capital: Wellington
Population: 3·39m. (1990)
GNP per capita: US$11,126 (1988)

HISTORY. The first European to discover New Zealand was Tasman in 1642. The coast was explored by Capt. Cook in 1769. From about 1800 onwards, New Zealand became a resort for whalers and traders, chiefly from Australia. By the Treaty of Waitangi, in 1840, between Governor William Hobson and the representatives of the Maori race, the Maori chiefs ceded the sovereignty to the British Crown and the islands became a British colony. Then followed a steady stream of British settlers.

The Maoris are a branch of the Polynesian race, having emigrated from the eastern Pacific before and during the 14th century. Between 1845 and 1848, and between 1860 and 1870, misunderstandings over land led to war, but peace was permanently established in 1871.

AREA AND POPULATION. New Zealand lies south-east of Australia in the south Pacific, Wellington being 1,983 km from Sydney by sea. There are two principal islands, the North and South Islands, besides Stewart Island, Chatham Islands and small outlying islands, as well as the territories overseas (*see* pp. 000–00).

New Zealand (*i.e.*, North, South and Stewart Islands) extends over 1,750 km from north to south. Area, excluding territories overseas, 267,844 sq. km comprising North Island, 114,821 sq. km; South Island, 149,463 sq. km; Stewart Island, 1,746 sq. km; Chatham Islands, 963 sq. km; minor islands, 833 sq. km. Growth in census population, exclusive of territories overseas:

	Total population	*Average annual increase %*		*Total population*	*Average annual increase %*
1858	115,462	—	1926	1,408,139	2·06
1874	344,984	—	1936	1,573,810	1·13
1878	458,007	7·33	1945[1]	1,702,298	0·83
1881	534,030	5·10	1951[1]	1,939,472	2·37
1886	620,451	3·05	1956[1]	2,174,062	2·31
1891	668,632	1·50	1961[1]	2,414,984	2·12
1896	743,207	2·13	1966[1]	2,676,919	2·10
1901[1]	815,853	1·89	1971[1]	2,862,631	1·34
1906	936,304	2·75	1976[1]	3,129,383	1·71
1911	1,058,308	2·52	1981[1]	3,175,737	0·20
1916[1]	1,149,225	1·50	1986[1]	3,307,084	0·82
1921	1,271,644	2·27			

The census of New Zealand is quinquennial, but the census falling in 1931 was abandoned as an act of national economy, and owing to war conditions the census due in 1941 was not taken until 25 Sept. 1945.

[1] Excluding members of the Armed Forces overseas.

The areas and populations of local government regions (with principal centres) at 4 March 1986 were as follows [1]:

Local Government Region (and principal centre)	*Area [2] (sq. km)*	*Total Population 1981 census*	*1986 census*	*Intercensal change (%)*
Northland (Whangarei)	12,604	113,994	126,999	11·4
Auckland (Auckland) [1]	5,201	827,408	887,448	7·3
Thames Valley (Thames–Coromandel)	4,666	54,343	58,665	8·0
Bay of Plenty (Tauranga)	9,126	172,480	187,462	8·7
Waikato (Hamilton)	13,241	221,850	228,303	2·9
Tongariro (Taupo)	12,085	40,089	40,793	1·8
East Cape (Gisborne)	11,461	53,295	53,968	1·3
Hawke's Bay (Napier, Hastings)	12,396	137,840	140,709	2·1
Taranaki (New Plymouth)	7,876	103,798	107,600	3·7
Wanganui (Wanganui)	9,171	68,702	69,439	1·1

Local Government Region (and principal centre)	*Area* [2] *(sq. km)*	*Total Population 1981 census*	*1986 census*	*Intercensal change (%)*
Manawatu (Palmerston North)	6,669	113,238	115,500	2·0
Horowhenua (Levin)	1,614	49,296	53,592	8·7
Wellington (Wellington)	1,379	323,162	328,163	1·5
Wairarapa (Masterton)	6,894	39,689	39,608	−0·2
Total, North Island [2]	*114,383*	*2,319,184*	*2,438,249*	*5·1*
Nelson Bays (Nelson)	10,197	65,934	69,648	5·6
Marlborough (Blenheim)	12,882	37,557	38,225	1·8
West Coast (Greymouth)	22,893	34,178	34,942	2·2
Canterbury (Christchurch)	17,465	336,846	348,712	3·5
Aorangi (Timaru)	19,910	84,772	81,294	−4·1
Clutha–Central Otago	28,982	45,402	48,771	7·4
Coastal–North Otago (Dunedin)	10,590	138,164	137,393	−0·6
Southland (Invercargill)	27,716	107,905	104,618	−3·0
Total, South Island [2]	*150,635*	*850,758*	*863,603*	*1·3*
Total, New Zealand [2]	265,018	3,169,942	3,301,852	4·2

[1] Excludes Great Barrier Island and Chatham Island Counties.
[2] Excludes Extra County Islands.

New Zealand-born residents made up 84·5% of the population at the 1986 census. Foreign-born (provisional): UK, 196,872; Australia, 46,839; Netherlands, 24,159; Samoa, 33,864; Cook Islands, 15,540; others (including USA and Ireland), 187,644.

Estimated population on 31 Dec. 1989, 3,384,600 (1,711,000 females).

Maori population: 1896, 42,113; 1936, 82,326; 1945, 98,744; 1951, 115,676; 1961, 171,553; 1971, 227,414; 1976, 270,035; 1981, 279,255; 1986, 294,201. Estimate, 1989: 306,200 (152,300 females). Population increase, 1989, 0·9%.

Populations of main urban areas as at 31 March 1990 were as follows:

Auckland	864,700	Invercargill	51,700
Christchurch	303,400	Nelson	45,800
Dunedin	106,400	New Plymouth	48,300
Hamilton	105,000	Rotorua	54,200
Hastings	55,800	Tauranga	64,000
Napier	52,300	Timaru	28,200
Palmerston North	69,300	Wanganui	41,100
Wellington	325,700	Whangarei	44,100
Gisborne	31,900		

Vital statistics for calendar years:

	Total live births	*Ex-nuptial births*	*Deaths*	*Marriages*	*Divorces (decrees absolute)*
1987	55,254	15,798	27,419	24,443	8,709
1988	57,546	17,623	27,408	23,485	8,674
1989	58,091	19,230	27,042	22,733	. . .

Birth rate, 1988, 17·34 per 1,000; death rate, 8·09 per 1,000; marriage rate, 22·08 per 1,000; infant mortality, 10·19 per 1,000 live births. Population increase 1989, 0·8%. Expectation of life, 1990: Males 71 years; females, 77.

In 1990 there were 52,001 immigrants (46,233 in 1989) and 56,019 emigrants (70,941 in 1989).

CLIMATE. Lying in the cool temperate zone, New Zealand enjoys very mild winters for its latitude owing to its oceanic situation, and only the extreme south has cold winters. The situation of the mountain chain produces much sharper climatic contrasts between east and west than in a north-south direction. Observations for 1983: Auckland. Jan. 65·5°F (18·6°C), July 50°F (10·2°C). Annual rainfall 41·5" (1,053 mm). Christchurch. Jan. 61·3°F (16·3°C), July 42·4°F (5·8°C). Annual rainfall 29" (737 mm). Dunedin. Jan. 57·4°F (14·1°C), July 43·2°F (6·2°C). Annual rainfall 38·1" (968 mm). Hokitika. Jan. 56·1°F (13·4°C), July 43·5°F (6·4°C). Annual rainfall 132·2" (3,357 mm). Rotorua. Jan. 61·2°F (16·2°C), July 43·7°F (6·5°C). Annual rainfall 49·9" (1,268 mm). Wellington. Jan. 59·9°F (15·5°C), July 46·4°F (8·0°C). Annual rainfall 51·2" (1,300 mm).

CONSTITUTION AND GOVERNMENT. Definition was given to the status of New Zealand by the (Imperial) Statute of Westminster of Dec. 1931, which had received the antecedent approval of the New Zealand Parliament in July 1931. The Governor-General's assent was given to the Statute of Westminster Adoption Bill on 25 Nov. 1947.

The powers, duties and responsibilities of the Governor-General and the Executive Council under the present system of responsible government are set out in Royal Letters Patent and Instructions thereunder of 11 May 1917, published in the *New Zealand Gazette* of 24 April 1919. In the execution of the powers vested in him the Governor-General must be guided by the advice of the Executive Council.

The following is a list of Governors-General, the title prior to June 1917 being Governor:

Earl of Liverpool	1917–20	Viscount Cobham	1957–62
Viscount Jellicoe	1920–24	Sir Bernard Fergusson	1962–67
Sir Charles Fergusson, Bt	1924–30	Sir Arthur Porrit, Bt	1967–72
Lord Bledisloe	1930–35	Sir Denis Blundell	1972–77
Viscount Galway	1935–41	Sir Keith Holyoake	1977–80
Sir Cyril Newall	1941–46	Sir David Beattie	1980–85
Lord Freyberg, VC	1946–52	Sir Paul Reeves	1985–90
Lord Norrie	1952–57		

National flag: The British Blue Ensign with 4 stars of the Southern Cross in red, edged in white, in the fly.

National anthems: God Save the Queen; God Defend New Zealand (words by Thomas Bracken, music by John J. Woods).

Since Nov. 1977 both 'God Save the Queen' and 'God Defend New Zealand' have equal status as national anthems.

Parliament consists of the House of Representatives, the former Legislative Council having been abolished since 1 Jan. 1951.

The statute law on elections and the life of Parliament is contained in the Electoral Act, 1956. In 1974 the voting age was reduced from 20 to 18 years.

The House of Representatives from Aug. 1987 consists of 97 members, including 4 members representing Maori electorates, elected by universal adult suffrage for 3-year terms. (At a referendum of 27 Oct. 1990 continuation of the 3-year term was favoured by a large majority). The 4 Maori electoral districts cover the whole country and adult Maoris of half or more Maori descent are the electors. From 1976 a descendant of a Maori is entitled to register either for a general or a Maori electoral district.

At the elections of 27 Oct. 1990, 677 candidates stood. The National Party won 68 seats with 48·7% of the votes cast; the Labour Party, 28, with 34·5%; the New Labour Party, 1, with 5·2%.

Governor-General: Dame Catherine Tizard, DBE.

The National Party government formed in Dec. 1990 consisted of:

Prime Minister: Jim Bolger (b.1935).

Deputy Prime Minister, Minister for External Relations and Trade, Foreign Affairs: Don McKinnon. *Labour, Immigration, State Services, Pacific Island Affairs:* Bill Birch. *Finance:* Ruth Richardson. *Attorney-General, Leader of the House:* Paul East. *Agriculture, Forestry, Racing:* John Falloon. *State-owned Enterprises:* Doug Kidd. *Commerce and Industry:* Philip Burdon. *Health, Environment, Research, Science and Technology:* Simon Upton. *Police, Tourism, Recreation and Sport:* John Banks. *Social Welfare and Womens Affairs:* Jenny Shipley. *Defence, Local Government, Television and Radio:* Warren Cooper. *Justice, Disarmament and Arms Control, Arts and Culture:* Doug Graham. *Education:* Lockwood Smith. *Employment:* Maurice McTigue. *Transport, Statistics and Lands:* Rob Storey. *Maori Affairs:* Winston Peters. *Conservation:* Denis Marshall. *Housing and Energy:* John Luxton. *Revenue, Customs and Government Superannuation Fund:* Wyatt Creech.

There are also 5 Ministers outside the Cabinet.

The Prime Minister (provided with residence) had in 1989 a salary of

NZ$147,000 plus a tax-free expense allowance of $26,000 per annum; Ministers with portfolio, $103,000 plus a tax-free expense allowance of $10,750 per annum; Minister without portfolio, $83,000 plus a tax-free expense allowance of $8,500 per annum; Parliamentary Under-Secretaries, $80,000 plus an expense allowance of $8,500 per annum. In addition, Ministers and Parliamentary Under-Secretaries not provided with residence at the seat of Government receive $2,000 per annum house allowance. An allowance of up to $220 per day while travelling within New Zealand on public service is payable to Ministers.

The Speaker of the House of Representatives receives $97,000 plus an expense allowance of $14,250 per annum in addition to his electorate allowance, and residential quarters in Parliament House, and the Leader of the Opposition $103,000 plus expense allowance of $10,750 per annum, and allowances for travelling and housing.

Members were paid $57,000 per annum, plus an expense allowance of $5,500 plus an electoral allowance varying from $7,600 to $18,600 according to the area of electorate represented.

There is a compulsory contributory superannuation scheme for members; retiring allowances are payable to a member after 9 years' service and the attainment of 45 years of age.

Dollimore, H. N., *The Parliament of New Zealand and Parliament House.* 3rd ed. Wellington, 1973

Scott, K. J., *The New Zealand Constitution.* OUP, 1962

Local Government. Since the local government reform of Nov. 1989, territorial local authorities consist of 20 cities and 59 districts. There are also 14 regional authorities. Chatham Islands remains outside this system. Territorial and regional councils are directly elected. A city must have a minimum of 50,000 persons, be predominantly urban in character, be a distinct entity and a major centre of activity within the region. A district, on the other hand, serves a combination of rural and urban communities. There is no distinction in structural status or responsibility between a city council and a district council. There are a few other local authorities created for specific functions.

DEFENCE. The control and co-ordination of defence activities is obtained through the Ministry of Defence. This is a unitary department combining not only all joint-Service functions but also the former Departments of Army, Navy and Air.

Defence spending was reduced by 4% at the budget of July 1990, and by a further NZ$20m. in Dec. 1990.

Army. The Chief of the General Staff commands the Army, assisted by the General Staff and the staffs of Defence Headquarters. A regular force battalion is stationed in Singapore.

There are 2 infantry battalions, 1 artillery battery, 1 light armoured squadron. Equipment includes 26 Scorpion light tanks.

Regular personnel, in 1991, totalled 5,200, territorial personnel totalled 6,300.

Navy. The Royal New Zealand Navy is 2,400 strong (with 500 Reserve personnel) and includes 4 frigates of British Leander type, 1 12,400-tonne fleet replenishment ship with helicopter facilities, 4 inshore patrol craft, 2 survey vessels, and 1 diver support ship. The 7 Wasp helicopters for embarked service are Air Force owned and operated. The main base and Fleet headquarters is at Auckland.

Air Force. The Chief of Air Staff and Air Officer Commanding commands the Royal New Zealand Air Force (RNZAF). Maritime (P-3B Orion), long and medium-range transport (Boeing 727, C-130H Hercules, Andover, F.27 Friendship) and helicopter (Iroquois, Wasp) squadrons are based at RNZAF Base Auckland, and Hobsonville; and offensive support (A-4 Skyhawk) at RNZAF Base Ohakea. Flying training units (Airtrainer, Strikemaster, TA-4 Skyhawks, Sioux) are located at RNZAF Bases Wigram and Ohakea; ground training is carried out at RNZAF Bases Auckland, Woodbourne and Wigram.

The strength in 1991 was 4,000 regular personnel with 36 combatant aircraft.

INTERNATIONAL RELATIONS

Membership. New Zealand is a member of the UN, the Commonwealth, OECD, South Pacific Forum and the Colombo Plan.

ECONOMY

Budget. The following tables of revenue and expenditure relate to the Consolidated Account, which covers the ordinary revenue and expenditure of the government—*i.e.*, apart from capital items, commercial and special undertakings, advances, etc. Total revenue and expenditure of the Consolidated Account, which covers ordinary revenue and expenditure of the New Zealand government (*i.e.* apart from capital items, commercial and special undertakings, advances, etc.), in NZ$1m., year ended 31 March:

	1988	*1989*
Revenue	29,871·7	32,150·6
Expenditure	30,476·8	32,151·2

Taxation receipts in 1988–89 for all purposes amounted to $22,864m., giving an average of $6,807 per head of mean population. Included in the total taxation is $561m. National Roads Fund taxation.

The gross public debt at 31 March 1989 was $39,601m., of which $23,008m. was held in New Zealand, $3,569m. in Europe, $7,323m. in USA and $5,701m. in Canada, Australia and other sources. The gross annual interest charge on the public debt at 31 March 1989 was $4,487m.

New Zealand System of National Accounts. This replaces the National Income and Expenditure Accounts which have been produced since 1948.

National Accounts aggregates for 4 years are given in the following table (in NZ$1m.):

Year ended 31 March	*Gross domestic product*	*Gross national product*	*National income*
1986	44,861	42,817	39,180
1987	53,079	50,865	46,768
1988	59,257	56,506	51,944
1989	63,805	61,075	55,960

Currency. The monetary unit is *the New Zealand dollar* (NZD), of 100 *cents*. There are notes of NZ$5, 10, 20, 50 and 100; and coins of 5c, 10c, 20c, 50c, NZ$1 and NZ$2. Inflation was 5% at the end of 1990. In March 1991, £1 = 3·17NZ$; US$1 = 1·67NZ$.

Banking and Finance. The central bank and bank of issue is the Reserve Bank (*Governor*, Don Brash).

The financial system comprises a central bank (the Reserve Bank of New Zealand), registered banks, and other financial institutions. Registered banks including banks from abroad, which have to satisfy capital adequacy and managerial quality requirements. Other financial institutions include the regional trustee banks, now grouped under Trust Bank, building societies, finance companies, merchant banks and stock and station agents. The number of registered banks (1990, 22) grows as other financial institutions apply for, and satisfy the requirements for registration as a bank.

The primary functions of the Reserve Bank are the formulation and implementation of monetary policy to achieve the economic objectives set by the Government, and the promotion of the efficiency and soundness of the financial system, through the registration of banks, and supervision of financial institutions. The state owns 52% of the Bank of New Zealand, whose assets were NZ$17,900m. in 1989-90; deposits amounted to NZ$16,210m.

On 31 March 1989 the funding (financial liabilities including deposits) and claims (financial assets including loans) for each institutional group were in NZ$ millions:

Institutional Group	*Funding* NZ$	*Funding* Foreign Currency	*Claims* NZ$	*Claims* Foreign Currency
Registered banks	30,808	5,374	29,249	3,740
Other financial institutions	*20,924*	*3,857*	*23,370*	*1,627*
Total (net of inter-institutional claims and funds)	*45,777*	*9,231*	*45,253*	*5,367*

There is a stock exchange in Wellington.

Weights and Measures. The metric system of weights and measures operates.

ENERGY AND NATURAL RESOURCES

Electricity. On 1 April 1987 the former Electricity Division of the Ministry of Energy became a state-owned enterprise, the Electricity Corporation of N.Z. Ltd., which has 39 power stations (30 hydro-electric and 9 thermal, with a total nominal capacity of 7,247 mw) producing 96% of the country's electricity. The other 4% comes from supply authorities' own generation schemes. Supply 230 volts; 50 Hz.

Statistics for 4 years ended 31 March are:

	1986	*1987*	*1988*	*1989*
Total sales revenue ($1m.)	1,022	1,196	1,317	1,434
Total sales volume (gwh)	24,241	25,187	25,772	26,436
Generation (gwh) (nett)	25,957	26,948	27,498	28,189
Number of employees	5,107	5,079	4,403	4,106
Production/total staff employed (gwh/person)	5·15	5·30	5·80	6·63

Natural Gas. In 1989 there were 4 gasfields in production: Kapuni (on stream 1970), Maui (1979), McKee (mainly crude oil) (1984), Kaimiro (1984).

Minerals. Production of minerals in 1988 included 2,404 kg of gold, 1,255 tonnes of bentonite, 87,892 tonnes of clay for bricks, tiles, etc., 29,649 tonnes of potters' clays, 2,351,000 tonnes of iron sand concentrate, 708,404 tonnes of limestone for agriculture and 310,577 tonnes of limestone for industry, 1,255,720 tonnes of limestone, marl, etc., for cement, 25,000 tonnes of pumice, 16,000 tonnes of serpentine, 55,000 tonnes of silica sand and 2,401,000 tonnes of coal. Macraes hard rock gold mine started production in Nov. 1990. Deposits are some 1,235m. troy oz.; annual initial output 55,000 troy oz.

Agriculture. Two-thirds of the surface of New Zealand is suitable for agriculture and grazing. The total area under cultivation at 30 June 1988 was 17,746,065 ha. (including residential area and domestic orchards). There were 13,770,601 ha. of grassland, lucerne and tussock, 88,961 ha. of land for horticulture, 330,676 ha. of grain or fodder crops and 1,265,104 ha. of plantations.

The largest freehold estates are held in the South Island. The extent of occupied holdings as at 30 June 1988 (exclusive of holdings within borough boundaries) was as follows:

Size of holdings (ha.)	*Number of farms*	*Area (ha.)*	*Size of holdings (ha.)*	*Number of farms*	*Aggregate area (ha.)*
Under 5	10,851	31,182	400–799	4,395	2,389,912
5–19	16,477	157,622	800–1,199	1,211	1,160,296
20–39	8,596	235,550	1,200–1,999	921	1,398,745
40–59	7,487	359,649	2,000–3,999	564	1,544,234
60–99	10,073	777,712	4,000 and over	484	5,415,761
100–199	11,447	1,639,339			
200–399	9,557	2,685,111	Total	82,063	17,795,113

The area and yield for each of the principal crops are given as follows (area and yield for threshing only, not including that grown for chaff, hay, silage, etc.):

Crop years	Wheat Area (1,000 ha.)	Wheat Yield (1,000 tonnes)	Maize Area (1,000 ha.)	Maize Yield (1,000 tonnes)	Barley Area (1,000 ha.)	Barley Yield (1,000 tonnes)
1986	91·4	379·7	19·5	187·7	138·6	556·2
1987 [1]	83·0	336·8	19·0	176·1	102·5	400·6
1988 [1]	50·6	206·0	16·0	136·9	83·0	356·1
1989 [1]	37·8	135	14·9	138·7	86·5	326·8

[1] Area sown.

Private air companies are carrying out such aerial work as top-dressing, spraying and crop-dusting, seed-sowing, rabbit poisoning, aerial photography and surveying, and dropping supplies to deer cullers and dropping fencing materials in remote areas. In 1988, 1,723,485 tonnes of fertilizer was spread.

Livestock 1990 (in 1,000): Dairy cattle, 3,422; beef cattle, 4,651; sheep, 58,334; deer, 951; goats, 1,108; pigs (1989), 411. Total meat produced in the year ended 30 Sept. 1988 was estimated at 1·21m. tonnes (including 554,000 tonnes of beef and 417,700 tonnes of lamb). Total liquid milk produced in the year ended 31 May 1988 was 6,921m. litres.

Production of wool for 1987–88, 346,400 tonnes.

Agricultural Statistics. Dept. of Statistics, Wellington. Annual.

Forestry. Of the 6·2m. ha. of indigenous forest, most is protected in National Parks or State Forests. Declining quantities of indigenous timber are being produced from restricted areas of State Forest and from privately owned forest. There are just over 1m. ha. of productive exotic forest, and this produces far more timber than the indigenous forests. Introduced pines form the bulk of the large exotic forest estate and among these radiata pine is the best multi-purpose tree, reaching log size in 25–30 years. Other species planted are Douglas fir and Eucalyptus species. The table below shows production of rough sawn timber in 1,000 cu. metres for years ending 31 March:

	Indigenous Rimu and Miro	Indigenous Beech	Indigenous Total	Exotic Exotic Pines	Exotic Douglas Fir	Exotic Total	All Species Total
1985–86	96	13	133	2,044	183	2,265	2,398
1986–87	85	8	112	1,764	174	1,966	2,079
1987–88	62	9	85	1,557	163	1,737	1,822

Forest industries consist of 300 saw-mills, 6 plywood and veneer plants, 3 particle board mills, 8 pulp and paper mills and 4 fibreboard mills.

The basic products of the pulp and paper mills are mechanical and chemical pulp which are converted into newsprint, kraft and other papers, paperboard and fibreboard. Production of woodpulp, 31 March 1988, amounted to 1·21m. tonnes and of paper (including newsprint paper and paperboard) to 699,000 tonnes.

Fisheries. The total value of New Zealand Fisheries exports during the year ended 30 June 1989 was $789·9m., an increase of $178·9m. over the previous year.

	Exports, 1988 Quantity tonnes	Exports, 1988 Value $ (1m.)	Exports, 1989 Quantity tonnes	Exports, 1989 Value $ (1m.)
Fish	109,054	406·2	150,025	537·1
Squid	32,038	54·2	79,083	124·2
Crayfish	2,424	88·5	2,446	73·3
Mussels	5,496	21·7	6,119	26·6
Other fish	...	40·4	...	28·7
Total	149,012	611·0	237,673	789·9

INDUSTRY. Major industrial developments in recent years have included the establishment of an oil refinery, an iron and steel industry using New Zealand iron sands, a petro-chemical industry and an aluminium smelter using hydro-electric power.

Statistics of manufacturing industries:

Production year	*Persons engaged*	*Salaries and wages paid (NZ$1,000)*	*Cost of materials (NZ$1,000)*	*Sales and other income (NZ$1,000)*	*Value added (NZ$1,000)*
1986–87	300,063	6,091,996	17,068,922	33,331,340	10,571,806

The following is a statement of the provisional value of the products (including repairs) of the principal industries for the year 1986–87 (in NZ$1,000):

Industry group	*Purchases & operating expenses*	*Sales and other income*	*Value added*	*Additions to fixed tangible assets*
		(NZ$1,000)		
Food, beverage and tobacco manufacturing	8,819,221	9,203,149	2,558,848	558,534
Textile, wearing apparel, leather industries	2,895,136	3,050,800	1,022,716	90,679
Wood and wood products (including furniture)	2,049,450	2,164,985	742,505	86,216
Paper and paper products, printing and publishing	3,373,133	3,632,622	1,305,913	286,007
Chemicals and chemical, petroleum, coal, rubber and plastic products	3,749,973	4,196,454	1,511,459	1,590,900
Non-metallic mineral products	1,137,708	1,260,637	429,018	63,904
Basic metal industries	1,321,356	1,305,817	338,752	343,073
Fabricated metal products, machinery and equipment	7,622,760	8,154,538	2,545,426	396,190
Other manufacturing industries	3,333,346	362,338	117,169	19,914
Total	31,302,084	33,331,340	10,571,806	3,435,417

Labour. There were 965,300 full-time jobs in Nov. 1990. Unemployment was 7·5% of the workforce. The weekly average wage in Nov. 1989 was NZ$547·63 for men, NZ$426·51 for women.

Trade Unions. In March 1989 there were 168 industrial unions of workers with a total of 649,857 members. Compulsory trade union membership was made illegal in 1991, and the national wage award system was replaced by local wage agreements.

FOREIGN ECONOMIC RELATIONS

Foreign debt was NZ$47,600m. at the end of 1989. In 1990 New Zealand and Australia completed the Closer Economic Relations Agreement (initiated in 1983), which provides for mutual free trade in goods.

Commerce. Trade (excluding specie and bullion) in NZ$1m. for 12 months ended 30 June:

	Total merchandise imported (v.f.d.) [1]	*Exports of domestic produce*	*Re-exports*	*Total merchandise exported (f.o.b.)*
1985–86	10,468·3	10,139·0	432·7	10,571·7
1986–87	10,803·4	11,723·9	383·3	12,107·2
1987–88	10,625·1	12,104·1	347·4	12,451·5
1988-89	11,402·4	14,484·7	422·5	14,907·2

[1] Value for duty.

The principal imports for the 12 months ended 30 June 1989:

Commodity	*Value (NZ$1m. v.f.d.)*
Fruit	92·4
Sugar and sugar confectionery	77·0
Beer, wine and spirits	83·9
Crude petroleum oil	432·8
Inorganic chemicals (excluding aluminium oxide)	122·4
Aluminium oxide	191·5
Knitted or crocheted fabrics and articles	94·8

Commodity	*Value (NZ$1m. v.f.d.)*
Glass and glassware	91·5
Iron and steel	243·9
Articles of iron and steel	162·9
Copper and articles of copper	111·3
Aluminium and articles of aluminium	126·2
Tools, implements and articles of base metals	146·3
Machinery and mechanical appliances	1,769·2
Organic chemicals	195·4
Pharmaceutical products	286·3
Plastics and articles of plastic	547·9
Rubber and articles of rubber	149·6
Paper, paperboard and articles thereof	263·8
Printed books, newspapers etc.	215·1
Cotton yarn and fabrics	104·5
Man-made filaments and fibres	197·4
Electrical machinery and equipment	1,252·6
Motor cars, station wagons, utilities	844·5
Trucks, buses and vans	192·6
Aircraft	224·5
Ships and boats	77·3
Optical, photographic, technical and surgical equipment	420·9

The principal exports of New Zealand produce for the 12 months ended 30 June 1989 were:

Commodity	*Value (NZ$1m.f.o.b.)*	*Commodity*	*Value (NZ$1m.f.o.b.)*
Live animals	212·1	Fresh apples	154·9
Meat, fresh, chilled or frozen		Forest products	
Beef and veal	1,279·6	Sawn timber and logs	316·8
Lamb and mutton	1,007·9	Paper and paper products	265·9
Dairy products		Wood pulp	398·8
Milk, cream and yoghurt	934·3	Aluminium and articles thereof	339·2
Butter	609·2	Casein and caseinates	878·4
Cheese	319·8	Plastic materials and articles thereof	135·3
Raw hides, skins and leather	725·2	Iron and steel and articles thereof	316·9
Wool	1,795·3	Machinery and mechanical appliances	329·8
Sausage casings	122·5	Electrical machinery and equipment	183·3
Fish, fresh, chilled or frozen	537·2		
Vegetables	166·1		
Fresh kiwifruit	455·1		

The following table shows the trade with different countries for the year ended 30 June (in NZ$1m.):

Countries	*Imports v.f.d. from* 1988	1989	*Exports and re-exports f.o.b. to* 1988	1989
Australia	2,266·6	2,459·9	2,073·8	2,609·6
Bahrain	9·2	3·3	8·4	–
Belgium	83·2	75·3	257·6	272·1
Canada	181·2	227·7	216·9	261·2
China	112·2	125·2	435·3	539·1
Fiji	16·1	–	88·5	141·6
France	177·6	165·8	188·7	204·8
Germany, Fed. Rep. of	597·9	497·0	294·3	307·6
Greece	6·8	–	60·7	–
Hong Kong	178·6	202·6	177·6	247·8
India	38·1	–	51·4	–
Iran	34·3	–	207·0	130·6
Italy	209·4	196·0	250·7	316·8
Japan	1,864·9	2,109·6	2,078·2	2,661·2
Korea, Republic of	199·0	280·0	287·5	468·8
Kuwait	20·0	–	15·3	–
Malaysia	57·6	72·2	163·6	247·5
Netherlands	158·2	124·7	170·7	171·1
Peru	–	–	–	22·9
Philippines	19·4		90·8	159·7

Countries	*Imports v.f.d. from* 1988	1989	*Exports and re-exports f.o.b. to* 1988	1989
Saudi Arabia	247·6	343·9	99·7	–
Singapore	128·4	138·2	160·8	174·9
Sweden	121·8	169·7	26·6	–
Switzerland	–	106·5	–	–
Taiwan	–	372·8	–	281·4
UK	1,014·6	882·6	1,062·2	1,036·4
USSR	11·0	–	146·6	351·4
USA	1,683·0	1,906·0	1,803·0	2,008·2
Venezuela	–	–	–	114·4

Total trade between New Zealand and UK was as follows (British Department of Trade returns, in £1,000 sterling):

	1986	*1987*	*1988*	*1989*	*1990*
Imports to UK	455,694	487,332	443,081	436,772	438,615
Exports and re-exports from UK	343,145	378,368	300,016	399,295	439,608

Tourism. There were 961,470 touristsin the year to 31 July 1990 (including 337,981 from Australia. 137,071 from the USA, 104,102 from Japan and 84,926 from the UK). Tourist earnings for the year ended 31 March 1990 were NZ$2,551m. (NZ$2,277m. in 1988-89).

COMMUNICATIONS

Roads. Total length of formed roads and streets at 31 March 1989 was 92,974 km. There were 14,057 bridges of over 3 metres in length with a total length of 314,000 metres. The network of state highways comprised 11,523 km, including the principal arterial traffic routes.

Total expenditure on roads, streets and bridges by the central government and local authorities combined for the financial year 1988–89 amounted to $849m.

At 31 March 1989 motor vehicles licensed numbered 2,217,259, of which 1,438,704 were cars and 10,633 omnibuses, public taxis and service vehicles. Included in the remaining numbers were 89,459 motor cycles, 1,211 power cycles, 289,225 trucks, 341,280 trailers and caravans and 7,904 farm tractors and other farm equipment.

In 1989 there were 18,052 traffic casualties, of which 728 were fatal.

Railways. On 31 March 1988 there were 4,202 km of 1,067 mm gauge railway open for traffic (525 km electrified). In 1988 89, railways carried 8·8m. tonnes and 26·9m. passengers. Operating revenue during 1987–88, $646,821,000 and operating expenses $684,117,000. Three rail/road ferries maintain a regular service between the North and South Islands.

Aviation. International services are operated to and from New Zealand by a previously state-owned company, Air New Zealand Ltd, and by a number of overseas companies. There are various flights from Auckland to Los Angeles taking in Fiji, Hawaii, Rarotonga and Tahiti, and flights to Japan, Thailand and South Korea. In Nov. 1990 Air New Zealand's fleet included 8 Boeing 767s and 5 Boeing 747s. Air New Zealand Ltd, Mt Cook Airlines and Ansett are the major domestic carriers.

Domestic scheduled services during the 12 months ended Dec. 1987: Passengers carried, 3,782,000. International services: Passengers carried, 3,001,000; mail, 4,385 tonnes; freight, 117,769 tonnes.

Shipping. Container ships operate from all major ports, serving all the major trading areas.

Entrances and clearances of vessels from overseas:

	Entrances		*Clearances*	
	No.	*Tons*	*No.*	*Tons*
1985	2,932	14,607,000	2,935	14,613,000
1986	2,519	13,388,000	2,527	13,365,000
1987	3,060	14,113,000	3,050	14,107,000
1988	3,298	27,844,000	3,334	27,247,000

Telecommunications. The provision of postal and telecommunication services is the responsibility of two state-owned enterprises: New Zealand Post, which began operations on 1 April 1987, and the Telecom Corporation of New Zealand, formed in 1987. New Zealand Post restarted a telegram service in 1990. There are also 2 independent telegraph companies. In 1989 there were 470 post offices, and 336 post shops with 8,700 staff.

The New Zealand Broadcasting Corporation has been superseded. Radio New Zealand operates sound services. Television New Zealand operates 2 channels. A third, TV3, is commercial. Radio New Zealand International broadcasts in 14 languages. There are (1990) 59 medium-wave broadcasting stations, 28 FM broadcasting transmitters and 1 100 kw short-wave transmitter. Some commercial material is broadcast by both sound and TV services. Number of TV receiving licences at 31 March 1988 was 949,810.

Cinemas. There were in 1987, 121 cinemas.

Newspapers. There were (1987), 34 daily newspapers (10 morning and 24 evening) with a combined circulation of 1,134,835. Seven of these newspapers (2 each in Auckland, Wellington and Christchurch and 1 in Dunedin) had a circulation of 711,538.

JUSTICE, RELIGION, EDUCATION AND WELFARE

Justice. The judiciary consists of the Court of Appeal, the High Court and District Courts. All exercise both civil and criminal jurisdiction. Other special courts include the Maori Land Court, Family Courts and Children's and Young Persons' Courts. In Aug. 1990 prisons and corrective training institutions contained 4,062 prisoners. The death penalty for murder was replaced by life imprisonment in 1961.

The Criminal Injuries Compensation Act, 1963, which came into force on 1 Jan. 1964, provided for compensation of persons injured by certain criminal acts and the dependants of persons killed by such acts. However, this has now been phased out in favour of the Accident Compensation Act, 1972, except in the residual area of property damage caused by escapers. The Offenders Legal Aid Act 1954 provides that any person charged or convicted of any offence may apply for legal aid which may be granted depending on the person's means and the gravity of the offence etc. Since 1970 legal aid in civil proceedings (except divorce) has been available for persons of small or moderate means.

Police. The police in New Zealand are a national body maintained wholly by the central government. The total authorized establishment at 31 March 1989 was 5,328, the proportion of police to population being 1 to 625. The total cost of police services for the year 1988–89 was NZ$479m., equivalent to $144 per head of population. In New Zealand the police do not control traffic.

Ombudsmen. The office of Ombudsman was created in 1962. From 1975 additional Ombudsmen have been authorized. There are currently two. Ombudsmen's functions are to investigate complaints under the Ombudsman Act, the Official Information Act and the Local Government Official Information and Meetings Act from members of the public relating to administrative decisions of central, regional and local government.

During the year ended 31 March 1989, a total of 3,511 complaints were received, 593 of which were sustained.

Religion. No direct state aid is given to any form of religion. For the Church of England the country is divided into 7 dioceses, with a separate bishopric (Aotearoa) for the Maoris. The Presbyterian Church is divided into 23 presbyteries and the Maori Synod. The Moderator is elected annually. The Methodist Church is divided into 10 districts; the President is elected annually. The Roman Catholic Church is divided into 4 dioceses, with the Archbishop of Wellington as Metropolitan Archbishop.

Religious denomination	*Number of clergy (April 1977)*	*Number of adherents 1981 census*	*Number of adherents 1986 census* [1]
Church of England	780	814,740	784,059
Presbyterian	686	523,221	586,530
Roman Catholic (including 'Catholic' undefined)	931	456,858	495,300
Methodist	349	148,512	152,955
Baptist	254	50,043	67,716
Brethren	187	24,324	
Ratana	142	35,781	
Protestant (undefined)	—	16,986	
Salvation Army	241	20,490	
Latter-day Saints (Mormon)	162	37,686	
Congregationalist	10	3,825	
Seventh-day Adventist	55	11,523	871,689
Ringatu	88	6,114	
Christian (undefined)	—	101,901	
Jehovah's Witnesses	125	13,737	
Hebrew	7	3,360	
All other religious professions	—	279,768	
Agnostic	—	24,201	
Atheist	—	21,528	
Not specified	—	108,015	59,385
Object to state	—	473,115	244,152
Total	4,712	3,175,737	3,261,786

[1] Provisional.

Education. New Zealand has 7 universities, the University of Auckland, University of Waikato (at Hamilton), Victoria University of Wellington, Massey University (at Palmerston North), the University of Canterbury (at Christchurch), the University of Otago (at Dunedin) and Lincoln University (near Christchurch). The number of students in 1988 was 72,313. There were 6 teachers' training colleges with 4,502 students in 1988.

At 1 July 1988 there were 315 state secondary schools with 14,506 full-time teachers and 217,272 pupils. There were also 35 area high schools with 3,208 scholars in the secondary division. At 1 July 1988, 70,045 part-time pupils attended technical classes, and 33,601 received part-time instruction from the technical correspondence institute. At 1 July 1988, 1,171 pupils received tuition from the secondary department of the correspondence school. There were 18 registered private secondary schools with 451 teachers and 12,132 pupils.

At 1 July 1988, there were 2,316 state primary schools (including intermediate schools and departments), with 398,189 pupils; the number of teachers was 18,214. A correspondence school for children in remote areas and those otherwise unable to attend school had 1,683 primary pupils. There were 78 registered private primary schools with 356 teachers and 12,053 pupils.

Education is compulsory between the ages of 6 and 15. Children aged 3 and 4 years may enrol at the 568 free kindergartens maintained by Free Kindergarten Associations, which receive government assistance. There are also 644 play centres which also receive government subsidy. In July 1988 there were 42,537 and 14,628 children on the rolls respectively. There are also 618 childcare centres with 15,701 children, 534 *kohanga reo* (providing early childhood education in the Maori language) with 11,125 children, and a number of other smaller providers of early childhood care and education.

Total budgeted expenditure in 1988–89 on education was NZ$3,568m.

The universities are autonomous bodies. All state-funded primary and secondary schools are controlled by boards of trustees. Education in state schools is free for children under 19 years of age. All educational institutions are reviewed every 3 years by teams of educational reviewers.

Report of the Minister of Education ('E.1. Report'). Annually. Wellington, Government Printer

NZ Committee on Secondary Education. *Towards Partnership.* Dept. of Education, 1976

Health. At 30 June 1988 there were 8,980 doctors on the medical register. At 31 March 1988 there were 23,744 public hospital beds, of which 2,052 were for maternity cases.

Social Welfare. New Zealand's record for progressive legislation reached back to 1898, when it was second to Denmark in introducing non-contributory old-age pensions. Large reductions in welfare expenditure were introduced by the government in Dec. 1990. (For previous provisions *see* THE STATESMAN'S YEAR-BOOK, 1990–91, pp. 928–30).

The July 1990 budget announced that in April 1991 a new Universal Benefit would replace the former Unemployment, Widows' and Domestic Purposes Benefits. A Family Benefit for families on the lowest incomes was to be NZ$49·36 for the first child and NZ$28·31 for subsequent children. Child allowance for single persons with one child was to be NZ$213·14 per week; with two or more children, NZ$228·87 per week.

Under the Guaranteed Retirement Income scheme (GRI) introduced in April 1990, a married couple receive NZ$288·10 per week; a single person, NZ$172·86. Persons living alone received an additional NZ$14·40 per week from Oct. 1990. GRI increases annually in line with the Consumer Price Index, or the average ordinary-time wage, whichever is the lower. Eligibility is at 60 years.

Benefit reductions in Dec. 1990 included the abolition of the universal NZ$6 per week child allowance, and a cut in unemployment benefit for a single man from NZ$135 to NZ$108 per week (NZ$100 to persons under 25 years). Persons made redundant become eligible for benefit only after 26 weeks.

Social Welfare Benefits and War Pensions:

Benefits	*Number in force at 31 March 1990*	*Total payments 1989–90 (NZ$1,000)*
SOCIAL WELFARE:		
Monetary—		
Retirement pension	493,715	4,539,578
Widows	12,847	132,111
Invalids	27,550	287,762
Miners and orphans	5,189	21,652
Domestic purposes	94,381	1,326,604
Unemployment	134,328	1,411,390
Sickness	18,944	258,445
War pensions	25,412	111,927
Total	812,366	8,089,469

Family benefits in 1990: 440,168 were in force; expenditure was NZ$446,487,000.

Health benefits in 1990: Payments for private hospitals, NZ$55,023,000; health benefits, NZ$321,235,000; pharmaceutical, NZ$516,822.

Reciprocity with Other Countries. There are reciprocal arrangements between New Zealand and Australia in respect of age, invalids', widows', family, unemployment and sickness benefits, and between New Zealand and the UK in respect of family, age, superannuation, widows', orphans', invalids', sickness and unemployment benefits.

MINOR ISLANDS

The minor islands (total area, 320 sq. miles, 829 sq. km) included within the geographical boundaries of New Zealand (but not within any local government area) are the following: Kermadec Islands (34 sq. km), Three Kings Islands (8 sq. km), Auckland Islands (62 sq. km), Campbell Island (114 sq. km), Antipodes Islands (606 sq. km), Bounty Islands (1 sq. km), Snares Islands (3 sq. km), Solander Island (1 sq. km). With the exception of meteorological station staff on Raoul Island in the

Kermadec Group (5 in 1986) and Campbell Island (10 in 1986) there are no inhabitants.

The **Kermadec Islands** were annexed to New Zealand in 1887, have no separate administration and all New Zealand laws apply to them. Situation, 29° 10' to 31° 30' S. lat., 177° 45' to 179° W. long., 1,000 miles NNE of New Zealand. The largest of the group is Raoul or Sunday Island, 29 sq. km, smaller islands being Macaulay and Curtis, while Macaulay Island is 3 miles in circuit.

TERRITORIES OVERSEAS

Territories Overseas coming within the jurisdiction of New Zealand consist of Tokelau and the Ross Dependency.

Tokelau. Situated some 480 km to the north of Western Samoa between 8° and 10° S. lat., and between 171° and 173° W. long., are the 3 atoll islands of Atafu, Nukunonu and Fakaofo of the Tokelau (Union) group. Formerly part of the Gilbert and Ellice Islands Colony, the group was transferred to the jurisdiction of New Zealand on 11 Feb. 1926. By legislation enacted in 1948, the Tokelau Islands were declared part of New Zealand as from 1 Jan. 1949. The area of the group is 1,011 ha; the population at 10 Oct. 1986 was 1,690.

By the Tokelau Islands Act 1948 the Tokelau Group was included within the territorial boundaries of New Zealand; legislative powers are now invested in the Governor-General in Council. The inhabitants are British subjects and New Zealand citizens. In Dec. 1976 the territory was officially renamed 'Tokelau', the name by which it has customarily been known to its inhabitants.

From 8 Nov. 1974 the office of Administrator was invested in the Secretary of Foreign Affairs. Certain powers are delegated to the district officer in Apia, Western Samoa.

Because of the very restricted economic and social future in the atolls, the islanders agreed to a proposal put to them by the Minister of Island Territories in 1965 that over a period of years most of the population be resettled in New Zealand. Up to March 1975, 528 migrants entered New Zealand as permanent residents under Government sponsorship. At the request of the people the scheme has now been suspended.

New Zealand Government aid to Tokelau totalled \$3·3m. for the year ended 31 March 1987.

Ross Dependency. By Imperial Order in Council, dated 30 July 1923, the territories between 160° E. long. and 150° W. long. and south of 60° S. lat. were brought within the jurisdiction of the New Zealand Government. The region was named the Ross Dependency. From time to time laws for the Dependency have been made by regulations promulgated by the Governor-General of New Zealand.

The mainland area is estimated at 400,000–450,000 sq. km and is mostly ice-covered. In Jan. 1957 a New Zealand expedition under Sir Edmund Hillary established a base in the Dependency. In Jan. 1958 Sir Edmund Hillary and 4 other New Zealanders reached the South Pole.

The main base—Scott Base—at Pram Point, Ross Island—is manned throughout the year, about 12 people being present during winter. Vanda Station in the dry ice-free Wright Valley is manned every summer.

Quartermain, L. B., *New Zealand and the Antarctic*. Wellington, 1971

SELF-GOVERNING TERRITORIES OVERSEAS

THE COOK ISLANDS

HISTORY. The Cook Islands, which lie between 8° and 23° S. lat., and 156° and 167° W. long., were proclaimed a British protectorate in 1888, and on 11 June 1901 were annexed and proclaimed part of New Zealand. In 1965 the Cook Islands became a self-governing territory in 'free association' with New Zealand.

AREA AND POPULATION. The islands within the territory fall roughly into two groups—the scattered islands towards the north (Northern group) and the islands towards the south known as the Lower group. The names of the islands with their populations as at the census of 1986 were as follows:

Lower Group—	*Area sq. km*	*Population*	*Northern Group—*	*Area sq. km*	*Population*
Rarotonga	67·2	9,678	Nassau	1·2	118
Mangaia	51·8	1,235	Palmerston (Avarau)	2·0	66
Atiu	26·9	955	Penrhyn (Tongareva)	9·8	496
Aitutaki	18·0	2,391	Manihiki (Humphrey)	5·4	508
Mauke (Parry Is.)	18·4	637	Rakahanga (Reirson)	4·1	283
Mitiaro	22·3	272	Pukapuka (Danger)	5·1	760
Manuae and Te au-o-tu	6·2	–	Suwarrow (Anchorage)	0·4	6
Takutea	1·3	–			
			Total	293	17,463

The population in 1988 was 17,700. Birth rate (per 1,000), 24·3; death rate, 5·3.

CONSTITUTION AND GOVERNMENT. The Cook Islands Constitution Act 1964, which provides for the establishment of internal self-government in the Cook Islands, came into force on 4 Aug. 1965.

The Act establishes the Cook Islands as fully self-governing but linked to New Zealand by a common Head of State, the Queen, and a common citizenship, that of New Zealand. It provides for a ministerial system of government with a Cabinet consisting of a Premier and 6 other Ministers. The New Zealand Government is represented by a New Zealand Representative and the position of a Queen's Representative has recently been created by changes in the Constitution. New Zealand continues to be responsible for the external affairs and defence of the Cook Islands, subject to consultation between the New Zealand Prime Minister and the Prime Minister. The changed status of the Islands does not affect the consideration of subsidies or the right of free entry into New Zealand for exports from the group. The capital is Rarotonga, which was devastated by a hurricane in Jan. 1987.

The unicameral Parliament comprises 24 members elected for a term of 5 years; at general elections held in Jan. 1989, the Cook Islands Party won 12 seats, the Democratic Coalition Party 10, and the Democratic Tumu Party, 2 seats. There is also an advisory council composed of hereditary chiefs, the 15-member House of Ariki, without legislative powers.

Prime Minister: Hon. Geoffrey A. Henry.

ECONOMY AND TRADE

Budget. Revenue, 1988–89, NZ$55·08m. (NZ$28·23m. from taxation); expenditure, NZ$55·83m. Revenue is derived chiefly from customs duties which follow the New Zealand customs tariff, income tax and stamp sales.

Grants from New Zealand, mainly for medical, educational and general administrative purposes totalled NZ$7m. in 1982–83.

Currency. The Cook Island *dollar* is at par with the New Zealand *dollar*.

Electricity. 14·31m. KWH were generated in 1988.

Agriculture. Livestock (1988): Pigs, 18,000; goats, 3,000.

Fisheries. Catch (1984) 800 tonnes.

Commerce. Exports, mainly to New Zealand, were valued at NZ$6·6m. in 1988. Main items exported were fresh fruit and vegetables, clothing and footwear. Imports totalled NZ$64·5m. in 1988. Main items imported were foodstuffs, manufactured goods (including transport equipment), petrol and petroleum products.

COMMUNICATIONS

Roads. In 1984 there were 280 km of roads and 1,417 vehicles.

Aviation. New Zealand has financed the construction of an international airport at Rarotonga which became operational for jet services in Sept. 1973.

Shipping. A fortnightly cargo shipping service is provided between New Zealand, Niue and Rarotonga.

Telecommunications. Wireless stations are maintained at all the permanently inhabited islands. In 1983 there were 2,052 telephones. There are 2 radio stations on Rarotonga with (1983) 10,000 receivers.

Newspapers. The *Cook Islands News* (circulation 2,000) is the sole daily newspaper.

JUSTICE, RELIGION, EDUCATION AND HEALTH

Justice. There is a High Court and a Court of Appeal, from which further appeal is to the Privy Council in the UK.

Religion. Some 60% of the population belong to the Cook Islands Congregational Church, about 20% are Roman Catholics, and the rest chiefly Mormons and Seventh-Day Adventists.

Education. In 1986 there were 30 primary schools with 165 teachers and 3,183 pupils, and 8 secondary schools with 146 teachers and 2,156 pupils on Rarotonga, Aitutaki, Mangaia, Atiu, Mauke and Pukapuka.

Health. All Cook Islanders receive free medical and surgical treatment in their villages, the hospital and the tuberculosis sanatorium. Cook Islands Maori patients in the hospital and the sanatorium and all schoolchildren receive free dental treatment. In 1982 there were 18 doctors, 8 dentists and 65 nursing personnel. In 1981 there were 8 hospitals and clinics with 154 beds.

NIUE

History. Captain James Cook sighted Niue in 1774 all called it Savage Island. Christian missionaries arrived in 1846. Niue became a British Protectorate in 1900 and was annexed to New Zealand in 1901. Internal self-government was achieved in free association with New Zealand on 19 Oct. 1974, New Zealand taking responsibility for external affairs and defence. Niue is a member of the South Pacific Forum.

Area and Population. Niue is the largest uplifted coral island in the world. Distance from Auckland, New Zealand, 1,343 miles; from Rarotonga, 580 miles. Area, 258 sq. km; height above sea-level, 220 ft. Population (census, 1986) 2,531; estimate 31 Dec. 1988 was 2,190. During 1988 births registered numbered 55, deaths 14. Migration to New Zealand is the main factor in population change. The capital is Alofi (811 inhabitants in census, 1986).

Constitution and Government. There is a Legislative Assembly of 20 members, 14 elected from 14 constituencies and 6 elected by all constituencies.

Premier: Sir Robert R. Rex, CMG, OBE.

Budget. Financial aid from New Zealand, 1987–88, totalled $8,500,000.

Agriculture. The most important products of the island are coconuts, honey, limes and root crops.

Trade. Exports, 1985, $175,924 (main export, coconut cream); imports, $3,753,384.

Communications. There is a wireless station at Alofi, the port of the island. A weekly commercial air service links Niue with New Zealand. Telephones (1986) 460.

Justice. There is a High Court under a Chief Justice, with a right of appeal to the New Zealand Supreme Court.

Religion. 75% of the population belong to the Congregational (Ekalesia Niue); 10% are Mormons and 5% Roman Catholics.

Education. There were 7 government schools with 702 pupils in 1987.

Health. In 1986 there were 3 doctors, 3 dentists, 7 midwives and 27 nursing personnel. There is a 25-bed hospital at Alofi.

DIPLOMATIC REPRESENTATIVES

Of New Zealand in Great Britain (New Zealand Hse, Haymarket, London, SW1Y 4TQ)
High Commissioner: vacant.

Of Great Britain in New Zealand (Reserve Bank of New Zealand Bldg., 2 The Terrace, Wellington, 1)
High Commissioner: D. J. Moss, CMG.

Of New Zealand in the USA (37 Observatory Cir., NW, Washington, D.C., 20008)
Ambassador: H. H. (Tim) Francis.

Of the USA in New Zealand (29 Fitzherbert Terrace, Wellington)
Ambassador: Della M. Newman.

Of New Zealand to the United Nations
Ambassador: Terence O'Brien.

Further Reading

Statistical Information: The central statistical office for New Zealand is the Department of Statistics (Wellington, 1).

The beginning of a statistical service may be seen in the early 'Blue books' prepared annually from 1840 onwards under the direction of the Colonial Secretary, and designed primarily for the information of the Colonial Office in England. A permanent statistical authority was created in 1858. The Department of Statistics functions under the Statistics Act 1975 and reports to Parliament through the Minister of Statistics. A comprehensive statistical service has been developed to meet national requirements, and close contact is maintained with the United Nations Statistical Office and other international statistical organizations; through the Conference of Asian Statisticians assistance is being given with the development of statistics in the region. The oldest publications consist of *(a)* census results from 1858 onwards and *(b)* annual volumes of statistics (first published 1858 but covering years back to 1853). Main current publications:

New Zealand Official Yearbook. Annual, from 1893
Catalogue of New Zealand Statistics. 1972
Statistical Reports of New Zealand. Annual
Monthly Abstract of Statistics. From 1914
Pocket Digest of Statistics. Annual, 1927–31, 1938 ff.

Parliamentary Reports of Government Departments. Annual
Dictionary of New Zealand Biography. vol 1 (to 1868). Wellington, 1990
Encyclopaedia of New Zealand. 3 vols. Wellington, 1966
National Bibliography. Wellington
Alley, R., *New Zealand and the Pacific.* Boulder, 1984
Bedggood, D., *Rich and Poor in New Zealand.* Sydney, 1980
Bush, G., *Local Government and Politics in New Zealand.* Sydney, 1980
Easton, B., *Social Policy and the Welfare State in New Zealand.* Auckland, 1980
Grover, R. R., *New Zealand.* [Bibliography] Oxford and Santa Barbara, 1981
Hawke, G. R., *The Making of New Zealand: An Economic History.* CUP, 1985
Morrell, W. P. and Hall, D. O. W., *A History of New Zealand Life.* Christchurch and London, 1957
Oliver, W. H. (ed.) *The Oxford History of New Zealand.* OUP, 1981
Robson, J. L. (ed.) *New Zealand: The Development of its Laws and Constitution.* 2nd ed. London, 1967
Sinclair, K., *A History of New Zealand.* Rev. ed. London, 1980 –. (ed.) *The Oxford Illustrated History of New Zealand.* OUP, 1990
Thakur, R., *In Defence of New Zealand.* Wellington, 1984
Wards, I., *A Descriptive Atlas of New Zealand.* Wellington, Government Printer, 1976

NICARAGUA

Capital: Managua
Population: 3·75m. (1990)
GNP per capita: US$830 (1987)

República de Nicaragua

HISTORY. Active colonization of the Pacific coast was undertaken by Spaniards from Panama, beginning in 1523. After links with other Central American territories, and Mexico, Nicaragua became completely independent in 1838, but subject to a prolonged feud between the 'Liberals' of León and the 'Conservatives' of Granada. Mosquitia remained an autonomous kingdom on the Atlantic coast, under British protection until 1860.

On 5 Aug. 1914 the Bryan–Chamarro treaty between Nicaragua and the US was signed, under which the US in return for US$3m. acquired a permanent option for a canal route through Nicaragua and a 99-year option for a naval base in the Bay of Fonseca on the Pacific coast and Corn Islands on the Atlantic coast. It was ratified by Nicaragua on 7 April 1916 and by the US on 22 June 1916. US Marines finally left in 1933. The Bryan–Chamarro treaty was abrogated on 14 July 1970 and the Corn Islands handed back in 1971.

The 46-year political domination of Nicaragua by the Somoza family ended on 17 July 1979, after the 17 years long struggle by the Sandinista National Liberation Front flared into civil war. A Government Junta of National Reconstruction was established by the revolutionary government on 20 July 1979 and a 51-member Council of State later created; both were dissolved on 10 Jan. 1985 following new Presidential and legislative elections.

On 9 Jan. 1987 the President signed the new Constitution, but immediately reimposed a state of emergency, suspending many of the liberties granted under the Constitution.

In Nov. 1989, following infiltration into Nicaragua by some 2,000 Contras, the ceasefire was ended. On 7 Nov. 1989 the Security Council of the UN voted to establish a UN Observer Group in Central America.

AREA AND POPULATION. Nicaragua is bounded north by Honduras, east by the Caribbean, south by Costa Rica and west by the Pacific. Area 127,849 sq. km (49,363 sq. miles) or 118,558 sq. km (45,775 sq. miles) if the lakes are excluded. The coastline runs 540 km on the Atlantic and 350 km on the Pacific. Population at the census of April 1971 was 1,877,972. Estimate (1990) 3·75m. Population density was 28·8 per sq. km in 1990.

In 1984, births, 139,800; marriages, 13,600; deaths, 30,700.

The population is of Spanish and Amerindian origins with an admixture of Afro-Americans on the Caribbean coast. The main ethnic groups in 1980 were: Mestizo, 69%; white, 14%; black, 8%; Amerindian, 4%.

Area, 1985 populations and chief towns of the former 6 regions and 3 special zones:

Region	*Capital*	*Sq. km*	*1985*	*Special Zone*	*Capital*	*Sq. km*	*1985*
1	Estelí	7,598	334,717	Zelaya Norte	Rosita	59,094	325,454
2	León	9,896	545,321	Zelaya Sur	Bluefields	[1]	[1]
3	Managua	3,597	903,998	Rio San Juan	San Carlos	7,448	34,330
4	Jinotepe	4,726	514,113				
5	Juigalpa	9,929	209,218				
6	Matagalpa	16,370	406,913				

[1] Included in Zelaya Norte.

The capital is Managua, situated on the lake of the same name, 180 ft above sea level, with (1985) 682,111 inhabitants. Other cities: León, 100,982; Granada, 88,636; Masaya, 74,946; Chinandega, 67,792; Matagalpa, 36,983; Estelí, 30,635; Tipitapa, 30,078; Chichigalpa, 28,889; Juigalpa, 25,625; Corinto, 24,250; Jinotepe, 23,538.

CLIMATE. The climate is tropical, with a wet season from May to Jan. Temperatures vary with altitude. Managua. Jan. 79°F (26°C), July 86°F (30°C). Annual rainfall 45" (1,140 mm).

CONSTITUTION AND GOVERNMENT. The National Assembly drafted and approved on 19 Nov. 1986 the new Constitution which was promulgated on 9 Jan. 1987. It provided for a unicameral *National Assembly* comprising 90 members directly elected by proportional representation, together with unsuccessful presidential election candidates obtaining a minimum level of votes.

The *President* and Vice-President are directly elected for a 6-year term commencing on the 10 Jan. following their date of election.

Under Article 185 of the Constitution, the President is empowered to declare a state of emergency and suspend certain of the civil rights provisions enshrined therein; this was done by the President immediately upon the promulgation of the Constitution.

Elections were held on 25 Feb 1990 and Violeta Barrios de Chamorro of the National Opposition Union (UNO) defeated Daniel Ortega Saavedra of the Sandinista National Liberation Front (FSLN).

President and Minister of Defence: Violeta Barrios de Chamorro (elected 25 Feb. 1990, took office 25 April 1990).

Minister of the Interior: Carlos Hurtado Cabrera. *Foreign Affairs:* Enrique Dreyfus Morales. *Finance:* Emilio Pereira Alegria. *Education:* Sofonias Cisneiros Leiva. *Agriculture:* Roberto Rondón Sacasa. *Economy and Development:* Silvio de Franco Montalván. *Construction and Transport:* Jaime Icabalceta Mayorga. *Health:* Ernesto Salmarón Bermudez. *Labour:* Francisco Rosales Arguello. *Presidency Minister:* Antonio Lacayo Oyanguren. *Agrarian Reform:* Boanerges Matus. *Director of the Nicaraguan Repatriation Institute:* Jaime Cuadra.

National flag: Three horizontal stripes of blue, white, blue, with the national arms in the centre.

National anthem: Salve a ti Nicaragua (words by S. Ibarra Mayorga, 1937).

Local government. There are 16 departments (chief town in brackets if name differs): Boaco; Carazo (Jinotepe); Chinandega; Chontales (Juigalpa); Esteli; Granada; Jinotega; León; Madriz (Samoto); Managua; Masaya; Matagalpa; Nueva Segovia (Ocotal); Río San Juan (San Carlos); Rivas; Zelaya (Bluefields).

DEFENCE. Conscription was ended in 1990, and the armed forces cut from 70,000 to 28,000. The 1991 budget cut defence spending by 10%.

Army. The Army is organized into 2 armoured, 2 motorized infantry, 2 frontier and 1 artillery brigades, 20 infantry and 4 engineer battalions. Equipment includes 130 T-54/-55 main battle tanks. Strength (1991) 57,000; 22,000 reservists and militia.

Navy. The Marina de Guerra Sandinista was (1990) some 600 strong and operates 18 inshore patrol craft of mixed Soviet and North Korean origins, 8 small inshore minesweepers and 3 minor landing craft.

Air Force. Formed in June 1938 as the Nicaraguan Army Air Force, the Air Force has been semi-independent since 1947. Its combat units are reported to have 4 L-39 Albatros light jet attack/trainers, 4 T-33 armed jet trainers, and 3 T-28 armed piston-engined trainers but confirmation is not available. Other equipment includes 2 C-47s, 2 Spanish-built Aviocar transports and smaller communications aircraft and helicopters, including 20 Mi-8/17s, 2 Mi-2s and 5 Mi-24 gunships and 6 SF.260s for counter-insurgency duties. Personnel (1991) 3,000, with 16 combatant aircraft and 7 armed helicopters.

INTERNATIONAL RELATIONS

Membership. Nicaragua is a member of the UN, OAS and the CACM.

ECONOMY

Budget. Estimates for 1991: Revenue, US$349m.; expenditure, US$499m. US$91m. of the deficit was to be covered by foreign loans.

Currency. The monetary unit is the *córdoba* (NIC), of 100 *centavos*. There are notes in denominations from 1,000 córdobas to 1 córdoba. Coins are 5 and 1 *córdobas* and 50, 25, 10 and 5 *centavos*. A 'gold córdoba', with parity with the US dollar, was introduced in 1990, and devalued to 5 = US$1 in March 1991. In a series of devaluations in 1990 the value of the ordinary currency was reduced by 98·4%. In March 1991, US$1 = 5·2m. *córdobas*; £1 = 9·87m. new *córdobas*.

Banking and Finance. The Central Bank of Nicaragua came into operation on 1 Jan. 1961 as an autonomous bank of issue, absorbing the issue department of the National Bank. Its *Governor* is Raul Lacayo. In July 1979 private financial banking was nationalized and branches of foreign banks were prohibited from receiving deposits.

Weights and Measures. Since 1893 the metric system of weights and measures has been recommended.

ENERGY AND NATURAL RESOURCES

Electricity. Installed capacity for electric energy was 398,000 kw. in 1986 and 1,200 kwh. was produced. Supply 120 volts; 60 Hz.

Minerals. Production of gold in 1980 was 67,000 troy oz.; of silver, 167,000 troy oz.; of copper, 3,000 tonnes. Large deposits of tungsten in Nueva Segovia were reported in 1961.

Agriculture. Agriculture is the principal source of national wealth, finding work for 65% of the labour force.

Of the total land area (about 36·5m. acres), about 17·5m. acres are under timber 900,000 acres are used for grazing and 2·1m. acres are arable. The unit of area used locally is the *manzana* (= 1·73 acres). Of the arable only 1·2m. acres are actively cultivated, 780,000 in annual crops such as cotton and rice and the remainder in perennial crops such as coffee and sugar-cane, or in two harvests a year in the cases of maize, sorghum and beans.

The products of the western half are varied, the most important being cotton, coffee, now under the aegis of the new *Instituto del Café*, sugar-cane, cocoa, maize, sesame and beans. Production (1988): Coffee, 43,000 tonnes; sugar-cane, 1,932,000 tonnes; seed cotton, 130,000 tonnes.

There were about 1·7m. head of cattle in 1988 and 745,000 pigs.

Forestry. Timber production has been declining, though the forests, which cover 10m. acres, contain mahogany and cedar, which were formerly largely exported, three varieties of rosewoods, guayacán (*lignum vitae*) and dye-woods. Production of sawn wood in 1983, 222,000 tonnes.

Fisheries. On the Atlantic coast fisheries are an important subsistence activity. Catch (1984) 4,300 tonnes.

INDUSTRY. Chief local industries are cane sugar, cooking oil, cigarettes, beer, leather products, plastics, textiles, chemical products, metal products, cement (100,000 tonnes in 1982), strong and soft drinks, soluble coffee, dairy products, meat, plywood. Production of oil products (1983) 489,000 tonnes.

Labour. In 1980 there were some 813,000 persons gainfully employed.

FOREIGN ECONOMIC RELATIONS

Commerce. The foreign trade of Nicaragua, in US$1m. (1984): Exports, 390m. consisting of cotton, coffee, chemical products, meat, sugar; imports, 750m.

Total trade between Nicaragua and UK (British Department of Trade returns, in £1,000 sterling):

	1986	*1987*	*1988*	*1989*	*1990*
Imports to UK	1,307	717	725	918	1,899
Exports and re-exports from UK	7,349	7,883	6,856	6,985	6,515

Tourism. In 1985 there were about 100,000 visitors, mainly from the USA.

COMMUNICATIONS

Roads. In 1984, 4,000 km were paved, out of a total of 25,000 km. The whole 368·5 km of the Nicaraguan section of the Pan-American Highway is now paved. The all-weather Roosevelt Highway linking Managua with the river port Rama was completed in 1968, to provide the first overland link with the Atlantic coast. There are paved roads to San Juan del Sur, Puerto Sandino and Corinto. In 1986 there were 78,000 vehicles in use including 46,000 cars.

Railways. The Pacific Railroad of Nicaragua, owned and operated by the Government, has a total length of 334 km, all single-track, and connects Corinto, Chinandega, León, Managua, Masaya and Granada. Passengers carried (1986) 3·5m. and 2·5m. tonnes of freight.

Aviation. LANICA, the Nicaraguan airline has daily flights to Miami and 6 flights a week to Guatemala and to the inner cities of Blue fields, Puerto Cabezas and the mining towns of Siuna and Bonanza. PANAM and TACA (Transportes Aéreos Centroamericanos), COPA (Compañía Panameña de Aviacíon), have daily services to Panama, Mexico, the other Central American countries and USA. SAM (Servicio Aéreo de Medellín) has 3 flights a week to Nicaragua and Colombia.

Shipping. The Pacific ports are Corinto (the largest), San Juan del Sur and Puerto Sandino through which pass most of the external trade. The chief eastern ports are El Bluff (for Bluefields) and Puerto Cabezas. The merchant marine consists solely of the Mamenic Line with 8 vessels. In 1980, 471,000 tonnes of goods were loaded and 1·14m. tonnes unloaded at Nicaraguan ports.

Telecommunications. In 1984 there were 51,237 telephones.

The Tropical Radio Telegraph Company maintains a powerful station at Managua, and branch stations at Bluefields and Puerto Cabezas. The Government operates the National Radio with 47 broadcasting stations: There are 31 commercial stations and some 70 others. Number of radio sets in 1986 was 870,000 and television sets 200,000. There are 2 television stations at Managua.

Newspapers. In 1984 there were 3 daily newspapers (2 in Managua and 1 in León), with a total circulation of about 105,000.

JUSTICE, RELIGION, EDUCATION AND WELFARE

Justice. The judicial power is vested in a Supreme Court of Justice at Managua, 5 chambers of second instance (León, Masaya, Granada, Matagalpa and Bluefields) and 153 judges of inferior tribunals.

Religion. The prevailing form of religion is Roman Catholic, but religious liberty is guaranteed by the Constitution. The republic constitutes 1 archbishopric (seat at Managua) and 7 bishoprics (León, Granada, Estelí, Matagalpa, Juigalpa, Masaya and Puerto Cabezas). Protestants, established principally on the Atlantic coast, numbered 54,100 in 1966.

Education. There were, in 1986, 4,526 primary schools, with a total of 556,684 pupils and 17,199 teachers; and 119,000 pupils in secondary schools. The illiteracy rate was 12% in 1983. In 1987 there were 26,878 students in higher education. Universities were restructured in 1990 to form 2 state universities and 2 religious universities (the Jesuit UCA and the Protestant UPOLI).

Health. In 1984 there were 2,172 doctors, 222 dentists, 5,649 nursing personnel and 49 hospitals with 5,045 beds.

DIPLOMATIC REPRESENTATIVES

Of Nicaragua in Great Britain (8 Gloucester Rd., London, SW7 4PP)
Ambassador: Roberto Parrales.

Of Great Britain in Nicaragua
Ambassador and Consul-General: W. Marsden (resides in San José).

Of Nicaragua in the USA (1627 New Hampshire Ave., NW, Washington, D.C., 20009)
Chargé d'Affaires: Leonor de Huper.

Of the USA in Nicaragua (Km. 4½ Carretera Sur., Managua)
Ambassador: (Vacant).

Of Nicaragua to the United Nations
Ambassador: Dr Roberto Mayorga-Cortes.

Further Reading

Dirección General Estadística y Censos, *Boletín de Estadística* (irregular intervals); and *Indicadores Economicos.*
Boletín de la Superintendencia de Bancos. Banco Central, Managua
Booth, J. A., *The End of the Beginning: The Nicaraguan Revolution.* Boulder, 1982
Christian, S., *Nicaragua: Revolution in the Family.* New York, 1985
Gilbert, D., *Sandinistas: The Party and the Revolution.* Oxford, 1988
McGinnis, J., *Solidarity with the People of Nicaragua.* New York, 1985
Rosset, P. and Vandermeer, J., (eds.) *The Nicaragua Reader: Documents of a Revolution under Fire.* New York, 1984
Spalding, R. J., *The Political Economics of Revolutionary Nicaragua.* London, 1987
Walker, T. W., *Nicaragua: The Land of Sandino.* Boulder, 1982.—*Nicaragua: The First Five Years.* New York, 1985
Woodward, R. L., *Nicaragua.* [Bibliography] Oxford and Santa Barbara, 1983

National Library: Biblioteca Nacional, Managua, D.N.

NIGER

Capital: Niamey
Population: 7·45m. (1990)
GNP per capita: US$310 (1988)

République du Niger

HISTORY. Niger was occupied by France between 1883 and 1899, and constituted a military territory in 1901, which became a part of French West Africa in 1904. It became an autonomous republic within the French Community on 18 Dec. 1958 and achieved full independence on 3 Aug. 1960.

On 15 April 1974 the first President, Hamani Diori, was overthrown in a military coup led by Lieut.-Col. Seyni Kountché, who suspended the constitution, dissolved the National Assembly and banned political groups.

AREA AND POPULATION. Niger is bounded north by Algeria and Libya, east by Chad, south by Nigeria, south-west by Benin and Burkina Faso, and west by Mali. Area, 1,267,000 sq. km, with a population at the 1977 census of 5,098,657. Estimate (1990) 7,445,000. of which 18.8% live in urban areas. Population density 5.4 per sq. km. The major towns (populations 1983) are: Niamey, the capital (399,100 inhabitants), Zinder (82,800), Maradi (65,100), Tahoua (41,900), Agadez (27,000). Arlit (28,000), Akouta (26,000). The population is composed chiefly of Hausa (54%), Songhai and Djerma (23%), Fulani (10%), Beriberi-Manga (9%) and Tuareg (3%).

The official language is French. Hausa is understood by 85% of the population. Growth rate, 1985-90, 3%; infant mortality, 135 per 1,000; expectation of life, 44.5 years.

Vital statistics (1985): Births, 330,000; deaths, 150,000.

CLIMATE. Precipitation determines the geographical division into a southern zone of agriculture, a central zone of pasturage and a desert-like northern zone. The country lacks water, with the exception of the south-western districts, which are watered by the Niger and its tributaries, and the southern zone, where there are a number of wells. Niamey, 95°F (35°C). Annual rainfall varies from 22" (560 mm) in the south to 7" (180 mm) in the Sahara zone.

CONSTITUTION AND GOVERNMENT. The country is administered by a Supreme Military Council (SMC) of 12 officers led by the President, who appoints a Council of Ministers to assist him. A system of elected Development Councils at all levels has been created, culminating in a 150-member National Development Council with limited legislative powers charged with drafting a new constitution.

The Council of Ministers, in Feb. 1991, included:

Head of State, President of SMC, Defence and Interior: Col. Ali Seybou (took office 14 Nov. 1987).

Prime Minister: Alio Mahamidou.

Foreign Affairs and Co-operation: Mahamat Sani Bako.

National flag: Three horizontal strips of orange, white and green, with an orange disc in the middle of the white strip.

Local government: Niger is divided into 7 *départements* (Agadez, Diffa, Dosso, Maradi, Niamey, Tahoua and Zinder), each under a prefect, sub-divided into 32 *arrondissements*, each under a sub-prefect, and some 150 communes.

DEFENCE. Selective military service for 2 years operates.

Army. The Army consists of 2 armoured reconnaissance squadrons, 6 infantry, 1 engineer and 1 parachute company. Equipment includes 10 M-8, 18 AML-90 and

18 AML-60-7 armoured cars. Strength (1991) 3,200. There are additional paramilitary forces of some 4,500 men.

Air Force. The Air Force had (1991) over 100 officers and men, 2 C-130H and 3 Noratlas transports, 1 Boeing 737 VIP transport, 2 Cessna Skymasters and 3 Do 28D Skyservants and 1 Do 228 for communications duties. There are no combatant aircraft.

INTERNATIONAL RELATIONS

Membership. Niger is a member of the UN, OAU and is an ACP state of the EEC.

ECONOMY

Policy. The 10-year plan (1981–90) provided for an investment of 520,000m. francs CFA in the first phase (1981–85) with a prime aim of obtaining selfsufficiency in food and developing the mining sector.

Budget. The 1988 budget balanced at 114,310 francs CFA.

Currency. The unit of currency is the *franc CFA* (XAF), with a parity rate of 50 francs CFA to 1 French franc.

Banking. The *Banque Centrale des États de l'Afrique de l'Ouest* is the bank of issue, and there are 9 commercial banks in Niamey.

ENERGY AND NATURAL RESOURCES

Electricity. Production (1986) amounted to 265m. kwh. Supply 220 volts; 50 Hz.

Minerals. Large uranium deposits are mined at Arlit and Akouta. Concentrate production (1986) 3,108 tonnes. Phosphates are mined in the Niger valley, and coal reserves are being exploited by open-cast mining (production, 1985, 61,000 tonnes). Salt and natron are produced at Manga and Agadez, tin ore in Aïr, iron ore at Say.

Agriculture. The chief foodcrops in 1988 (in 1,000 tonnes) were: Millet, 1,783; rice, 50; sorghum, 603; cassava, 212; sugar-cane, 112; onions, 126. The main cash crops are ground-nuts (41), cotton and gum arabic.

Livestock (1988): Cattle, 3·5m.; horses, 296,000; asses, 512,000; sheep, 3·5m.; goats, 7·55m.; camels, 417,000; chickens, 17m.

Forestry. There were (1988) 2·5m. ha of forest. Production (1986) 4·01m. cu. metres.

Fisheries. Catch (1986) 2,400 tonnes.

INDUSTRY. Some small manufacturing industries, mainly in Niamey, produce textiles, food products, furniture and chemicals.

Trade Unions. The sole national body is the *Union Nationale des Travailleurs du Niger*, which has 15,000 members in 31 unions.

FOREIGN ECONOMIC RELATIONS

Commerce. Imports in 1983 were valued at 123,288m. francs CFA and exports at 113,896m. francs CFA of which uranium formed 83%. France provided 33% of imports and Nigeria 32%, while 48% of exports went to France, 23% to Japan and 11% to Nigeria.

Total trade between Niger and UK (British Department of Trade returns, in £1,000 sterling):

	1986	*1987*	*1988*	*1989*	*1990*
Imports to UK	848	10,556	1,359	1,472	1,161
Exports and re-exports from UK	10,367	7,026	7,552	6,862	10,780

Tourism. There were 27,000 tourists in 1986.

COMMUNICATIONS

Roads. In 1987 there were 19,000 km of roads. Niamey and Zinder are the termini of two trans-Sahara motor routes; the Hoggar–Aïr–Zinder road extends to Kano and the Tanezrouft-Gao-Niamey road to Benin. A 648-km 'uranium road' runs from Arlit to Tahoua. There were (1987), 9,000 private cars and 21,000 goods vehicles and vans.

Aviation. There are international airports at Niamey, Zinder and Maradi. Air Niger operates domestic services to over 20 other public airports.

Shipping. Sea-going vessels can reach Niamey (300 km. inside the country) between Sept. and March.

Telecommunications. There were (1983) 159 post offices and (1985) 11,824 telephones. In 1986 there were 300,000 radio and 25,000 television receivers.

Newspapers. In 1986 there was 1 daily newspaper, *Le Sahel*, with a circulation of 3,000.

JUSTICE, RELIGION, EDUCATION AND WELFARE

Justice. There are Magistrates' and Assize Courts at Niamey, Zinder and Maradi, and justices of the peace in smaller centres. The Court of Appeal is at Niamey.

Religion. In 1983, 97% of the population was Sunni Moslem and the remainder mainly followed animist beliefs. There were about 30,000 Christians.

Education. There were, in 1986, 294,000 pupils and 7,600 teachers in 2,000 primary schools, 51,000 and 1,900 teachers in secondary schools, and 2,400 students and 120 teachers in the technical and teacher-training colleges. In 1984 there were 2,863 students and 314 teaching staff at the University of Niamey.

Health. In 1982 there were 2 hospitals, 36 medical centres and 116 dispensaries. In 1980 there were 136 doctors, and (in 1978) 10 dentists, 12 pharmacists, 88 midwives and 1,080 nursing personnel.

DIPLOMATIC REPRESENTATIVES

Of Niger in Great Britain
Ambassador: Sandi Yacouba (resides in Paris).

Of Great Britain in Niger
Ambassador: (Vacant).

Of Niger in the USA (2204 R. St., NW, Washington, D.C., 20008)
Ambassador: Col. Moumouni Adamou Djermakoye.

Of the USA in Niger (PO Box 11201, Niamey)
Ambassador: Carl C. Cundiff.

Of Niger to the United Nations
Ambassador: Col. Moumouni Adamo Djermakoye.

Further Reading

Bonardi, P., *La République du Niger*. Paris, 1960
Fugelstad, F., *A History of Niger, 1850–1960*. OUP, 1984
Séré de Rivières, E., *Histoire du Niger*. Paris, 1965

NIGERIA

Capital: Lagos
Population: 118·7m. (1988)
GNP per capita: US$290 (1988)

Federal Republic of Nigeria

HISTORY. The Federal Republic comprises a number of areas formerly under separate administrations. Lagos, ceded in Aug. 1861 by King Dosunmu, was placed under the Governor of Sierra Leone in 1866. In 1874 it was detached, together with Gold Coast Colony, and formed part of the latter until Jan. 1886, when a separate 'colony and protectorate of Lagos' was constituted. Meanwhile the United African Company had established British interests in the Niger valley, and in July 1886 the company obtained a charter under the name of the Royal Niger Company. This company surrendered its charter to the Crown on 31 Dec. 1899, and on 1 Jan. 1900 the greater part of its territories was formed into the protectorate of Northern Nigeria. Along the coast the Oil Rivers protectorate had been declared in June 1885. This was enlarged and renamed the Niger Coast protectorate in 1893; and on 1 Jan. 1900, on its absorbing the remainder of the territories of the Royal Niger Company, it became the protectorate of Southern Nigeria. In Feb. 1906 Lagos and Southern Nigeria were united into the 'colony and protectorate of Southern Nigeria', and on 1 Jan. 1914 the latter was amalgamated with the protectorate of Northern Nigeria to form the 'colony and protectorate of Nigeria', under a Governor. On 1 Oct. 1954 Nigeria became a federation under a Governor-General. In 1967, 12 states were created and in 1976 this was increased to 19 and to 21 in 1987. On 1 Oct. 1960 Nigeria became sovereign and independent and a member of the Commonwealth and on 1 Oct. 1963 Nigeria became a republic.

President Shagari was elected in Aug. 1983. Military coups took place in Dec. 1983 and Aug. 1985.

AREA AND POPULATION. Nigeria is bounded north by Niger, east by Chad and Cameroon, south by the Gulf of Guinea and west by Benin. It has an area of 356,669 sq. miles (923,773 sq. km). Census population, Nov. 1963, 55,670,052. The results of the 1973 census have been officially repudiated. There is considerable uncertainty over the total population, but one estimate based on electoral registration in 1978 is 95m. Estimate (1988) 118·7m.

There were (1988) 21 states and a Federal Capital Territory (Abuja):

States	*Area (in sq. km)*	*Population 1988*	*States*	*Area (in sq. km)*	*Population 1988*
Akwa Ibom	7,081	5,077,540	Katsima	24,192	5,389,950
Anambra	17,675	7,879,900	Kwara	66,869	3,685,100
Bauchl	64,605	5,326,800	Lagos	3,345	4,569,400
Bendel	35,500	5,391,700	Niger	65,037	2,214,700
Benue	45,174	5,317,500	Ogun	16,762	3,397,900
Borno	116,400	6,567,200	Ondo	20,959	5,980,700
Cross River	20,156	2,505,766	Oyo	37,705	11,412,300
Gongola	91,390	5,708,200	Plateau	58,030	4,385,100
Imo	11,850	8,046,500	Rivers	21,850	3,768,100
Kaduna	46,053	3,689,850	Sokoto	102,535	9,944,100
Kano	43,285	12,351,100	Abuja (FCT)	7,315	523,900

The populations (1983) of the largest towns were as follows:

Lagos	1,097,000	Abeokuta	308,800	Kaduna	247,100
Ibadan	1,060,000	Port Harcourt	296,200	Mushin	240,700
Uyo	1,000,000 [1]	Zaria	274,000	Maiduguri	230,900
Ogbomosho	527,400	Ilesha	273,400	Enugu	228,400
Kano	487,100	Onitsha	268,700	Ede	221,900
Oshogbo	344,500	Ado-Ekiti	265,800	Aba	216,000
Ilorin	343,900	Iwo	261,600	Ife	214,500

[1] 1988.

Ila	189,700	Offa	142,300	Effon-Alaiye	110,600
Oyo	185,300	Owo	132,600	Kumo	107,000
Ikerre-Ekiti	176,800	Calabar	126,000	Shomolu	106,800
Benin City	165,900	Shaki	125,800	Oka-Akoko	103,500
Iseyin	157,000	Ondo	122,600	Ikare	101,700
Katsina	149,300	Akure	117,300	Sapele	100,600
Jos	149,000	Gusau	114,100	Minna	98,900
Sokoto	148,000	Ijebu-Ode	113,100	Warri	91,100
Ilobu	143,800				

A new federal capital is being constructed at Abuja at a central site some 500 km from Lagos. Several ministries are already in operation there.

CLIMATE. Lying wholly within the tropics, temperatures everywhere are high. Rainfall varies very much, but decreases from the coast to the interior. The main rains occur from April to Oct. Lagos. Jan. 81°F (27·2°C), July 78°F (25·6°C). Annual rainfall 72" (1,836 mm). Ibadan. Jan. 80°F (26·7°C), July 76°F (24·4°C). Annual rainfall 45" (1,120 mm). Kano. Jan. 70°F (21·1°C), July 79°F (26·1°C). Annual rainfall 35" (869 mm). Port Harcourt. Jan. 79°F (26·1°C), July 77°F (25°C). Annual rainfall 100" (2,497 mm).

CONSTITUTION AND GOVERNMENT. Under the Constitution drafted and ratified in 1977–78, Nigeria is a sovereign, federal republic comprising 22 states and a federal capital district. Following the coup of Aug. 1985 a 29-member Armed Forces Ruling Council (AFRC) was sworn in on 30 Aug. 1985. As part of the process of demilitarization and democratization the government has created 2 parties, the Social Democratic Party (SDP) and the National Republican Convention (NRC). Presidential elections have been announced for Oct. 1991.

President, Defence, Chairman of AFRC and C.-in-C. of the Armed Forces: Gen. Ibrahim Badamisi Babangida; *Vice-President*: Vice-Adm. Augustus Aikhomu.

On 12 Sept. 1985 the AFRC appointed a National Council of Ministers comprising the following in Jan. 1991:

Agriculture and Natural Resources: Shettima Mastapha. *Aviation:* Tonye Graham-Douglas. *Budget and Planning:* Chu Okongwu. *Communications:* A. O. Ige. *Culture and Social Welfare:* Maj.-Gen. Y. Y. Kure. *Defence:* Lieut.-Gen. Sani Abacha. *Education:* Babs Fafunwa. *Employment, Labour and Productivity:* Bunu Sherif Musa. *External Affairs:* Maj.-Gen. Ike Nwachukwu. *Federal Capital Territory:* Maj.-Gen. Gado Nasko. *Finance and Economic Development:* Alhaji Abubakar Alhaji. *Health:* Olikoye Ransome-Kuti. *Industries:* Air Vice-Marshal M. Yahaya. *Information:* Alex Akinyele. *Internal Affairs:* Maj.-Gen. A. B. Mamman. *Justice:* Prince Bola Ajibola. *Mines, Power and Steel:* Air Vice-Marshal Nura M. Imam. *Petroleum Resources:* Jubril Aminu. *Science and Technology:* Gordian Ezekwe. *Youth and Sports:* Air-Cmdre. A. Ikazobor. *Water Resources:* Alhaji Abubakar Hashidu. *Trade and Tourism:* S. J. Ukpanah. *Transport:* Cmdre. L. Gworm. *Works and Housing:* Brig. Mamman Kontagora.

National flag: Three vertical strips of green, white, green.

Local Government: Each of the 22 states is administered by a military governor, who appoints and presides over a State Executive Council. Local elections took place in Dec. 1990. The SDP won control of 232 authorities, the NRC of 206.

DEFENCE. Restructuring of the armed forces began in Sept. 1990 with the retirement of 22 senior officers.

Army. The Army consists of 1 armoured division, 2 mechanized divisions and 1 airborne and amphibious forces division, each with supporting artillery and engineer and reconnaissance units. Equipment includes 60 T-55 and 72 Vickers Mk 3 main battle tanks. Strength (1991) 80,000 men.

Navy. The Nigerian Navy comprises 1 German-built MEKO-type frigate with a helicopter and one frigate-type training ship, 3 British-built corvettes, 6 fast missile craft, 2 minehunters, and some 420 inshore patrol craft. There are also 2 German-built tank landing ships, 1 survey ship and some 15 service craft. The Navy has a small aviation element equipped with 2 Lynx anti-submarine helicopters. Naval personnel in 1989 totalled 5,000.

The Nigerian police also operate about 80 small patrol launches.

Air Force. The Nigerian Air Force was established in Jan. 1964. Pilots were trained initially in Canada, India and Ethiopia. The Air Force was built up subsequently with the aid of a Federal Republic of Germany mission; much first-line equipment has since been received from the Soviet Union.

It has 14 MiG-21 supersonic jetfighters, 15 Jaguar attack aircraft and MiG-21U fighter-trainers, and 22 Alpha Jet light attack/trainers. About 20 BO 105 twin-turbine helicopters have been acquired from the Federal Republic of Germany for search and rescue, while 2 F.27MPAs are used for maritime patrol. Transport units operate 9 C-130H-30 and C-130H Hercules 4-turboprop heavy transports, 5 twin-turboprop Aeritalia G222s, 2 Puma and 2 Super Puma helicopters, 3 DO 228s, a Boeing 727 and a Gulfstream II for VIP use, 18 Dornier 128-6 twin-turboprop and 18 DO 28D twin-piston utility aircraft, 2 Navajos and a Navajo Chieftain. Training types include 25 Bulldog primary trainers, 12 MB 339 jets for instrument training, and 22 L-39 Albatros advanced trainers. Personnel (1991) total about 9,500, with 95 combatant aircraft and 16 armed helicopters.

INTERNATIONAL RELATIONS

Membership. Nigeria is a member of the UN, the Commonwealth, ECOWAS, OAU, OPEC and is an ACP state of the EEC.

ECONOMY

Budget. The 1991 budget provided for capital expenditure of ₦9,700, recurrent expenditure of ₦12,300m. and revenue of ₦38,800m.

Currency. The unit of currency is the *naira* (NGN) of 100 *kobo*. Notes in circulation ₦20, ₦10, ₦5, ₦1, 50k. Coins, 25k, 10k, 5k, 1k, ½k.

The currency is non-convertible and subject to exchange controls. Inflation was 15% at the end of 1990. In March 1991, £1 = ₦18·50; US$1 = ₦9·75.

Banking. The Central Bank is the bank of issue. There were 130 banks in 1990 (81 in 1989), in 20 of which central or state governments held a controlling interest.

Weights and Measures. The metric system is in force.

ENERGY AND NATURAL RESOURCES

Electricity. The National Electric Power Authority generated 10,730m. kwh. in 1986. Supply 230 volts; 50 Hz.

Oil. There are refineries at Port Harcourt, Warri and at Kaduna. Oil represents 95% of exports. Production, 1990, 90·81m. tonnes.

Gas. Natural gas is being used at electric power stations at Afam, Ughelli and Utorogu. Reserves: 2,600,000m. cu. metres.

Water. Eleven River Basin Development Authorities have been established for water resources development.

Minerals. Production: Tin, 1980, 2,527 tonnes; columbite, 1977 (the world's largest producer), 800 tonnes; coal (1981) 114,875 tonnes. There are large deposits of iron ore, coal (reserves estimate 245m. tonnes), lead and zinc. There are small quantities of gold and uranium.

Agriculture. Of the total land mass, 75% is suitable for agriculture, including arable farming, forestry, livestock husbandry and fisheries. Main food crops are millet and sorghum in the north, plantains and oil palms in the south, and maize, yams, cassava and rice in much of the country, the north being, however, the main food producing area. Production, 1988 (in 1,000 tonnes): Millet, 4,000; sorghum,

4,940; plantains, 1,800; maize, 1,500; yams, 16,000; cassava, 14,000; rice, 1,400; groundnuts, 720; cotton lint, 57; palm kernal, 370; palm oil, 750.

Cocoa production was an estimated 160,000 tonnes in 1990; cocoa processing capacity is 90,000 tonnes a year.

Livestock (1988). There were 12·2m. cattle, 13·2m. sheep, 26m. goats, 1·3m. pigs and 190m. poultry.

Forestry. In 1988 there were 14m. ha of woodland, 16% of the total land area. There are plywood factories at Epe, Sapele and Calabar, and numerous saw-mills. The most important timber species include mahogany, iroko, obeche, abwa, ebony and camwood.

Fisheries. The total catch (1984) was 373,800 tonnes.

INDUSTRY. Timber and hides and skins are major export commodities. Industrial products include soap, cigarettes, beer, margarine, groundnut oil, meat and cake, concentrated fruit juices, soft drinks, canned food, metal containers, plywood, textiles, ceramic products and cement (3m. tonnes, 1985). Of growing importance is the local assembly of motor vehicles, bicycles, radio equipment, electrical goods and sewing machines. In 1982, the Delta Steel Plant opened at Ovwian—Aladja.

Two petrochemical plants (one at Ekpan near Warri in Bendel State producing about 35,000 tonnes of polypropylene and 18,000 tonnes of carbon black annually, and one at Kaduna producing 30,000 tonnes of linear-alkyl benzene annually) were commissioned in 1988.

Labour. The government doubled the minimum wage to ₦230 per month in 1991.

Trade Unions. There is a central labour Trade Union, the Nigerian Labour Congress.

FOREIGN ECONOMIC RELATIONS. Foreign exchange reserves were US$3,000m. in 1990. Foreign debt was US$34,000m.

Commerce. Total trade in ₦m. for 4 years; oil 97% of exports in 1988.

	1984	*1985*	*1986*	*1987*
Imports (c.i.f.)	7,200	8,300	6,700	15,694
Exports and re-exports (f.o.b.)	8,700	12,600	6,800	29,578

Total trade between Nigeria and UK (according to British Department of Trade returns, in £1,000 sterling):

	1986	*1987*	*1988*	*1989*	*1990*
Imports to UK	329,036	159,386	128,123	129,406	297,436
Exports and re-exports from UK	566,176	481,568	330,476	388,777	499,838

Tourism. There were 340,000 foreign visitors in 1985.

COMMUNICATIONS

Roads (1980). There were 108,000 km of maintained roads and 633,268 vehicles were registered.

Railways. There are 3,505 route-km of line 1,067 mm gauge, which in 1989 carried 1.5m. tonnes of freight and carried 9·9m. passengers.

Aviation. There is an extensive system of internal and international air routes, serving Europe, USA, Middle East and South and West Africa. Regular services are operated by Nigerian Airways (WAAC), British Caledonian, UTA, KLM, SABENA, Swissair, PANAM and other lines. In 1981, 2·3m. passengers were carried on domestic and international routes.

Shipping. The principal ports are Lagos, Port Harcourt, Warri and Calabar. There is an extensive network of inland waterways.

Telecommunications. Postal facilities are provided at 1,667 offices and agencies; telegraph, money order and savings bank services are provided at 280 of these.

Most internal letter mail is carried by air at normal postage rates. External telegraph services are owned and operated by Nigerian External Telecommunications (NITEL), at Lagos, from which telegraphic communication is maintained with all parts of the world. There were 708,390 telephones in use in 1982, of which 249,150 were in Lagos and 33,138 in Ibadan. There is also a telex service.

Federal and some state governments have established commercial corporations for sound and television broadcasting, which are widely used in schools. In 1985 there were 15·7m. radio and 500,000 television receivers.

Cinemas (1974). There were 120 cinemas, with a seating capacity of 60,000. Mobile cinemas are used by the Federal and States Information Services.

Newspapers. In 1989 there were 18 daily and 30 weekly newspapers. The aggregate circulation is about 1m., of which the *Daily Times* (Lagos) has about 400,000. (Another 4 dailies were published in Lagos, 4 in Ikeja, 3 in Enugu, and 4 in Ibadan.)

JUSTICE, RELIGION, EDUCATION AND WELFARE

Justice. The highest court is the Federal Supreme Court, which consists of the Chief Justice of the Republic, and up to 15 Justices appointed by AFRC. It has original jurisdiction in any dispute between the Federal Republic and any State or between States; and to hear and determine appeals from the Federal Court of Appeal, which acts as an intermediate appellate Court to consider appeals from the High Court.

High Courts, presided over by a Chief Justice, are established in each state. All judges are appointed by the AFRC. Magistrates' courts are established throughout the Republic, and customary law courts in southern Nigeria. In each of the northern States of Nigeria there are the Sharia Court of Appeal and the Court of Resolution. Moslem Law has been codified in a Penal Code and is applied through Alkali courts.

Religion. Moslems, 48%; Christians, 34% (17% Protestants and 17% Roman Catholic); others, 18%. Northern Nigeria is mainly Moslem; Southern Nigeria is predominantly Christian and Western Nigeria is evenly divided between Christians, Moslems and animists.

Education. In 1982–83 there were 15,021,100 primary school pupils, and 2,421,625 secondary grammar/commercial school pupils.

In 1989 there were 9 teacher training colleges, 41 government 'Unity' colleges and 10 polytechnics.

In 1989 there were 16 federal and 8 state universities.

Health. Most tropical diseases are endemic to Nigeria. Blindness, yaws, leprosy, sleeping sickness, worm infections, malaria are major health problems which, however, are yielding to remedial and preventative measures. In co-operation with the World Health Organization river blindness and malaria are being tackled on a large scale, while annual campaigns are undertaken against the danger of smallpox epidemics. Dispensaries and travelling dispensaries are found in most parts of the country.

In 1980 there were 8,000 doctors and 75,000 hospital beds.

DIPLOMATIC REPRESENTATIVES

Of Nigeria in Great Britain (9 Northumberland Ave., London, WC2 5BX)
High Commissioner: Christopher Macrae.

Of Great Britain in Nigeria (11 Eleke Cres., Victoria Island, Lagos)
High Commissioner: (Vacant).

Of Nigeria in the USA (2201 M. St., NW, Washington, D.C., 20037)
Ambassador: Hamzat Ahmadu.

Of the USA in Nigeria (2 Eleke Cres., Lagos)
Ambassador: Lannon Walker.

Of Nigeria to the United Nations
Ambassador: Prof. Ibrahim A. Gambari.

Further Reading

Nigeria Digest of Statistics. Lagos, 1951 ff. (quarterly)
Annual Abstract of Statistics. Federal Office of Statistics. Lagos, 1960 ff.
Nigeria Trade Journal. Federal Ministry of Commerce and Industries (quarterly)
Achebe, C., *The Trouble with Nigeria*. London, 1984
Adamolekun, L., *Politics and Administration in Nigeria*. Ibadan, 1986
Barbour, K. M. (ed.) *Nigeria in Maps*. London, 1982
Burns, A., *History of Nigeria*. 8th ed. London, 1978
Crowder, M. and Abdullahi, G., *Nigeria, an Introduction to its History*. London, 1979
Ikoku, S. G., *Nigeria's Fourth Coup: Options for Modern Statehood*. Enugu, 1984
Kirk-Greene, A. and Rimmer, D., *Nigeria since 1970*. London, 1981
Myers, R. A., *Nigeria*. [Bibliography] Oxford and Santa Barbara, 1989
Nwabueze, B. O., *The Presidential Constitution of Nigeria*. Lagos and London, 1982
Oyediran, O., *Nigerian Government and Politics under Military Rule, 1966–1979*. New York, 1980
Oyovbaine, S.E., *Federalism in Nigeria: A Study in the Development of the Nigerian State*. London, 1985
Shaw, T. M. and Aluko, O., *Nigerian Foreign Policy: Alternative Perceptions and Projections*. London, 1984
Simmons, M. and Obe, O. A., *Nigerian Handbook 1982–83*. London, 1982
Tijjani, A. and Williams, D. (eds.) *Shehu Shagari: My Vision of Nigeria*. London, 1981
Van Apeldoorn, G. J., *Perspectives on Drought and Famine in Nigeria*. London, 1981
Williams, D., *President and Power in Nigeria*. London, 1982
Zartman, I. W., *The Political Economy of Nigeria*. New York, 1983

NORWAY

Capital: Oslo
Population: 4·2m. (1989)
GNP per capita: US$20,020 (1988)

Kongeriket Norge

(Kingdom of Norway)

HISTORY. By the Treaty of 14 Jan. 1814 Norway was ceded to the King of Sweden by the King of Denmark, but the Norwegian people declared themselves independent and elected Prince Christian Frederik of Denmark as their king. The foreign Powers refused to recognize this election, and on 14 Aug. a convention proclaimed the independence of Norway in a personal union with Sweden. This was followed on 4 Nov. by the election of Karl XIII (II) as King of Norway. Norway declared this union dissolved, 7 June 1905, and Sweden agreed to the repeal of the union on 26 Oct. 1905. The throne was offered to a prince of the reigning house of Sweden, who declined. After a plebiscite, Prince Carl of Denmark was formally elected King on 18 Nov. 1905, and took the name of Haakon VII.

Norwegian Sovereigns

Inge Baardssøn	1204	Erik of Pomerania	1389
Haakon Haakonssøn	1217	Kristofer af Bavaria	1442
Magnus Lagabøter	1263	Karl Knutssøn	1449
Eirik Magnussøn	1280	Same Sovereigns as in Denmark	1450–1814
Haakon V Magnussøn	1299	Christian Frederik	1814
Magnus Erikssøn	1319	Same Sovereigns as in Sweden	1814–1905
Haakon VI Magnussøn	1343	Haakon VII	1905
Olav Haakonssøn	1381	Olav V	1957
Margrete	1388		

AREA AND POPULATION. Norway is bounded north by the Arctic ocean, east by the USSR, Finland and Sweden, south by the Skagerrak Straits and west by the North Sea.

Fylker (counties)	*Area (sq. km)*	*Census population 1 Nov. 1980*	*Population 1 Jan. 1990*	*Pop. per sq. km (total area) 1990*
Oslo (City)	454·0	452,023	458,364	1,009·6
Akershus	4,916·5	369,193	414,503	84·3
Østfold	4,183·4	233,301	237,981	56·9
Hedmark	27,388·4	187,223	186,884	6·8
Oppland	25,259·7	180,765	182,350	7·2
Buskerud	14,927·3	214,571	224,701	15·1
Vestfold	2,215·9	186,691	197,207	89·0
Telemark	15,315·1	162,050	162,981	10·6
Aust-Agder	9,211·7	90,629	96,880	10·5
Vest-Agder	7,280·3	136,718	144,026	19·8
Rogaland	9,140·7	305,490	335,753	36·7
Hordaland	15,633·8	391,463	409,124	26·2
Sogn og Fjordane	18,633·5	105,924	106,540	5·7
Møre og Romsdal	15,104·2	236,062	238,346	15·8
Sør-Trøndelag	18,831·4	244,760	250,344	13·3
Nord-Trøndelag	22,463·4	125,835	126,858	5·6
Nordland	38,327·1	244,493	239,532	6·2
Troms	25,953·8	146,818	146,594	5·6
Finnmark	48,637·3	78,331	74,148	1·5
Mainland total	323,877·5 [1]	4,092,340	4,233,116	13·1

Svalbard and Jan Mayen have an area of 63,080 sq. km. Persons staying on Svalbard and Jan Mayen are registered as residents of their home Norwegian municipality.

[1] 125,049 sq. miles.

On 1 Nov. 1980, 2,874,990 persons lived in densely populated areas and 1,197,939 in sparsely populated areas.

Population of the principal towns at 1 Jan. 1990:

Oslo	458,364	Sandnes	43,340	Gjøvik	27,275
Bergen	211,826	Sandefjord	38,019	Halden	26,527
Trondheim	137,346	Bodø	36,536	Moss	26,083
Stavanger	97,570	Ålesund	35,888	Lillehammer	25,816
Kristiansand	64,888	Porsgrunn	35,751	Harstad	24,657
Drammen	51,978	Haugesund	31,275	Molde	22,782
Tromsø	50,548	Ringerike	31,209	Kongsberg	22,507
Skien	47,679	Fredrikstad	27,600	Steinkjer	22,384

Vital statistics for calendar years:

	Marriages	*Divorces*	*Births*	*Still-born*	*Outside marriage* [1]	*Deaths*
1986	20,513	7,891	52,514	268	14,673	43,560
1987	21,081	8,417	54,027	237	16,705	44,959
1988	21,744	8,772	57,526	270	19,407	45,354
1990	...	9,238	59,303	292	21,588	45,173

[1] Excluding still-born.

CLIMATE. There is considerable variation in the climate because of the extent of latitude, the topography and the varying effectiveness of prevailing westerly winds and the Gulf Stream. Winters along the whole west coast are exceptionally mild but precipitation is considerable. Oslo. Jan. 24°F (–4·7°C), July 63°F (17·3°C). Annual rainfall 29·1" (740 mm). Bergen. Jan. 35°F (1·4°C), July 60°F (15·3°C). Annual rainfall 83" (2,108 mm). Trondheim. Jan. 26°F (–3·5°C), July 57°F (14°C). Annual rainfall 32·1" (870 mm).

REIGNING KING. Harald V, born 21 Feb. 1937, married on 29 Aug. 1968 to Sonja Haraldsen. He succeeded on the death of his father, King Olav V, on 21 Jan. 1991. *Offspring:* Princess Märtha Louise, born 22 Sept. 1971; Crown Prince Haakon Magnus, born 20 July 1973.

Women have been eligible to succeed to the throne since 1990. There is no coronation ceremony.

CONSTITUTION AND GOVERNMENT. Norway is a constitutional and hereditary monarchy. The royal succession is in direct male line in the order of primogeniture. In default of male heirs the King may propose a successor to the Storting, but this assembly has the right to nominate another, if it does not agree with the proposal.

The Constitution, voted by the constituent assembly at Eidsvoll on 17 May 1814 and modified at various times, vests the legislative power of the realm in the *Storting* (Parliament). The royal veto may be exercised; but if the same Bill passes two Stortings formed by separate and subsequent elections it becomes the law of the land without the assent of the sovereign. The King has the command of the land, sea and air forces, and makes all appointments.

National flag: Red with a blue white-bordered Scandinavian cross.

National anthem: Ja, vi elsker dette landet (Yes, we love this land; words by B. Bjørnson, 1865; tune by R. Nordraak, 1865).

The 165-member Storting assembles every year. The meetings take place *suo jure*, and not by any writ from the King or the executive. They begin on the first weekday in Oct. each year, until June the following year. Every Norwegian subject of 18 years of age is entitled to vote, unless he is disqualified for a special cause. The mode of election is direct and the method of election is proportional. The country is divided into 19 districts, each electing from 4 to 15 representatives.

At the elections for the Storting held in 1989 the following parties were elected: Labour, 63; Conservative, 37; Centre Party, 11; Christian Democratic Party, 14; Socialist Left Party, 17; Party of Progress, 22; Future for Finmark, 1.

The Storting, when assembled, divides itself by election into the *Lagting* and the *Odelsting*. The former is composed of one-fourth of the members of the Storting, and the other of the remaining three-fourths. Each Ting (the Storting, the Odelsting and the Lagting) nominates its own president. Most questions are decided by the Storting, but questions relating to legislation must be considered and decided by the

Odelsting and the Lagting separately. Only when the Odelsting and the Lagting disagree, the Bill has to be considered by the Storting in plenary sitting, and a new law can then only be decided by a majority of two-thirds of the voters. The same majority is required for alterations of the Constitution, which can only be decided by the Storting in plenary sitting. The Storting elects 5 delegates, whose duty it is to revise the public accounts. The Lagting and the ordinary members of the Supreme Court of Justice (the *Høyesterett*) form a High Court of the Realm (the *Riksrett*) for the trial of ministers, members of the *Høyesterett* and members of the Storting. The impeachment before the *Riksrett* can only be decided by the Odelsting.

The executive is represented by the King, who exercises his authority through the Cabinet or Council of State *(Statsråd)*, composed of a Prime Minister (*Statsminster*) and (at present) 17 ministers *(Statsråder)*. The ministers are entitled to be present in the Storting and to take part in the discussions, but without a vote.

A Coalition Government was formed and took office on 16 Oct. 1989. This government resigned on 29 Oct. 1990 over the question of joining the EEC, and Gro Harlem Brundtland (b. 1949) formed a minority Labour government of 19 ministers:

Prime Minister: Gro Harlem Brundtland.

Foreign Affairs: Thorvald Stoltenberg. *Education, Research and Church Affairs:* Gudmund Hernes. *Environment:* Torbjørn Berntsen. *Industry:* Ole Knapp. *Petroleum and Energy:* Finn Kristensen. *Local Government and Labour:* Kjell Borgen. *Development Cooperation:* Grete Faremo. *Trade and Shipping:* Eldrid Nordbøe. *Fisheries:* Oddrun Pettersen. *Defence:* Johan Jørgen Holst. *Transport and Communications:* Kjell Opseth. *Justice and the Police:* Kari Gjesteby. *Finance:* Sigbjørn Johnsen. *Child and Family Affairs:* Matz Sandmann. *Health and Social Affairs:* Tove Veierød. *Agriculture:* Gunhild Øyangen. *Cultural Affairs:* Åse Kleveland. *Government Administration:* Tove Strand Gerhardsen.

The official language is Norwegian, which has 2 versions: Bokmål (or Riksmål) and Nynorsk (or Landsmål).

Local Government. For the purposes of administration the country is divided into 19 counties *(fylker)*, in each of which the central government is represented by a county governor *(fylkesmannen)*. The counties are divided into 448 municipalities, each of which usually corresponds in size to a parish *(prestegjeld)*. The municipalities are administered by municipal councils *(kommunestyrer)*, whose membership may vary between 13 and 85 councillors, and by a committee *(formannskap)* which is elected by and from the members of the council. The council is four times the size of the committee. The council elects a chairman and a vice-chairman from among the committee members.

Each of the 18 counties forms a county district *(fylkeskommune)*, while the remaining one, Oslo, comprises an urban district. The supreme authority in a county district is the county council *(fylkesting)*. The members of the county council are elected directly by the electors of the county and the number of representatives varies between 25 and 85. In a county district the county committee *(fylkesutvalg)* occupies a position corresponding to that of the committee *(formannskap)* in the primary districts. The county committee is elected by and from among the members of the county council. The number of county committee members is one-fourth of the membership of the county council, but must be not more than 15. The county council elects from among the members of the county committee a county sheriff *(fylkesordfører)* and a deputy sheriff.

DEFENCE. Service is universal and compulsory, liability in peace-time commencing at the age of 19 and continuing till the age of 44. The service period in the Army, Coastal Artillery and the Air Force is 12 months, and periodic refresher training, in the Navy, 15 months and limited refresher training. The Norwegian Defence forces are organized into 2 integrated regional commands, Northern and Southern.

Army. Under the 2 principal subordinate commands (Commander Land Forces North Norway COMLANDNON, and Commander Allied Land Forces South Norway COMLANDSONOR), the Army is organized in 5 regional commands and 16 territorial commands.

In Defence Command North Norway the largest standing element is Brigade North. There are also 2 infantry battalions and 1 tank platoon, 1 self-propelled field artillery battery and 1 AD battery in the north. Defence Command South Norway comprises 1 infantry battalion, 1 tank company and 1 self-propelled field artillery battery. Equipment includes 78 Leopard I/A5 and 55 M-48A5 main battle tanks. Strength (1990) 22,000 (including 15,000 conscripts). The fast mobilization force numbers 165,000, organized under the 2 principal subordinate commands, (North and South Norway).

In the war time command structure there are 5 regional commands, 16 territorial commands, 13 brigades, 28 independent infantry battalions, 7 independent artillery battalions and 50–60 independent units as tank squadrons, infantry companies, engineer companies and signal units.

There is also a Land Home Guard of 75,000.

Navy. The Royal Norwegian Navy has 3 components: The Navy, Coast Guard and Coastal Artillery. Main Naval combatants include 12 coastal submarines (including the first 2, of a new German-built ULA class), 5 frigates, 2 corvettes, 36 missile torpedo-boats, 5 coastal minesweepers, 1 minehunter and 2 minelayers. Auxiliaries comprise 1 submarine missile craft support ship, 1 Royal Yacht and some 10 small general-purpose tenders. The Coastal Artillery man 32 fortresses and other static defence systems.

The personnel of the navy totalled 5,300 in 1990, of whom 3,500 were conscripts, and 2,000 served in coast artillery. The main naval base is at Bergen (Håkonsvern), with subsidiary bases at Horten, Ramsund and Tromsø.

The naval elements of the Home Guard on mobilization can muster some 7,000 personnel, and man 2 tank landing craft and about 400 requisitioned fishing vessels.

The 13 Coast Guard offshore patrol vessels (of which 3 are armed, and of frigate capability) are Navy-subordinated, and assist other government agencies in rescue service, environmental patrols, surveillance and police duties. The coast guard numbered 675 in 1990.

Air Force. The Royal Norwegian Air Force comprises the Air Force and the Anti-air Artillery. The Air Force consists of 4 squadrons of F-16 Fighting Falcons, 1 squadron of F-5 fighter-bombers, 1 maritime patrol squadron of P-3N and P-3C Orions, 1 squadron of C-130 Hercules transports and DA-20 Jet Falcons equipped for EW duties, 1 squadron with DHC-6 Twin Otter light transports and 2 squadrons of Bell 412SP helicopters. The Anti-air Artillery deploy 4 Nike surface-to-air missile batteries and several light anti-aircraft artillery units. 6 NOAH (Norwegian adapted Hawk missiles) batteries provide area and airfield defence co-ordinated with 10 SAM batteries with the mobile missile system RBS-70. Finally 27 batteries with 40 mm Bofors AA-guns and 12·7 mm machine guns. 9 Westland Sea King helicopters are used for search and rescue duties; 6 Lynx helicopters are operated for the Coast Guard; 17 O-1 Bird Dogs provide artillery spotting for the Army.

Total strength (1990) is about 9,500 personnel, including 4,800 conscripts.

Home Guard. The Home Guard is organized in small units equipped and trained for special tasks. Service after basic training is 1 week a year. The total strength is approximately 80,000.

The Home Guard consists of the Land Home Guard (LHG), Sea Home Guard (SHG) and Anti-Air Home Guard (AAHG) organized in 18 Home Guard Districts. The LHG is divided into 83 LHG sub-districts and 470 local units. The SHG is divided into 5 SHG sub-districts and 33 local units. The AAHG is divided into 2 AAHG sub-districts organized in 8 AAHG batteries and 1 reinforced battery.

In case of preparedness, mobilization or war, the Land HG is subordinate to The Land Defence District or The Land Defence, Sea HG is subordinate to The Naval District and the Anti-Air HG is subordinate to the Air Station.

INTERNATIONAL RELATIONS

Membership. Norway is a member of UN, NATO, EFTA, OECD, the Council of Europe and the Nordic Council.

ECONOMY

Budget. Current revenue and expenditure for years ending 31 Dec. (in 1,000 kroner):

	1985 [1]	*1986* [1]	*1987* [1]	*1988* [1]	*1989* [1]	*1990* [1 2]
Revenue	222,994,000	246,466,000	256,991,000	268,317,000	288,193,000	297,137,000
Expenditure	198,332,000	225,143,000	248,689,000	263,745,000	283,333,000	305,685,000

[1] Including National Insurance. [2] Voted budget.

National debt [1] for years ending 31 Dec. (in 1,000 kroner):

1981	107,662,000	1984	115,805,000	1987	165,248,000
1982	103,799,400	1985	142,392,600	1988	166,471,000
1983	92,406,100	1986	194,287,500	1989	176,546,000

[1] At the rate of par on foreign loans: including treasury bills (in 1m. kroner) which amounted to 35,111 in 1985, 48,975 in 1986, 24,644 in 1987, 22,980 in 1988, and 28,174,000 in 1989.

Currency. The unit of currency is the *Norwegian krone* (NOK) of 100 *øre*. National bank-notes of 50, 100, 500 and 1,000 *kroner* are legal means of payment. In March 1991, US$1 = 6 *kroner*; £1 = 11·38 *kroner*.

On 30 June 1990 the nominal value of the coin in circulation was 1,956m. kroner; notes in circulation, 27,690m. kroner.

Since Oct. 1990 the krone has been fixed to the ecu in the European Monetary System of the EEC in the narrow band of 2·25%.

Banking. Norges Bank is the central bank. Supreme authority is vested in the Executive Board consisting of 7 members appointed by the King and the Supervisory Council consisting of 15 members elected by the Storting. The *Governor* is Hermod Skanland. It is the only bank of issue.

At the end of 1989 there were 28 private joint-stock banks. Their total amount of capital and funds was 14,923m. kroner (capital 9,230m., funds 5,693m.). Deposits amounted to 245,824m. kroner, of which 184,118m. kroner were on ordinary notice, and 161,706m. kroner on special terms.

The number of savings banks at the end of 1989 was 151. The total amount of capital and funds of the savings banks amounted to 10,840m. kroner, of which 638m. kroner were capital certificate funds. Total deposits amounted to 183,716m. kroner, of which 143,193m. kroner were on ordinary terms and 40,523m. kroner on special terms.

There is a stock exchange in Oslo.

Weights and Measures. The metric system of weights and measures has been obligatory since 1875.

ENERGY AND NATURAL RESOURCES

Electricity. Norway is a large producer of hydro-electric energy. The potential total hydro-electric power at regulated mean water flow is estimated at 170,000m. kwh. annually.

By the end of 1988 the capacity of the installations for production of thermo-electric energy was 251 mw. and the capacity for production of hydro-electric energy was 25,841 mw. In 1989 the total production of electricity amounted to 119,099m. kwh. of which 99·6% was produced by hydro-electric plants.

Most of the electricity is used for industrial purposes, especially by the chemical and basic metal industries for production of nitrate of calcium and other nitrogen products, carbide, ferrosilicon and other ferro-alloys, aluminium and zinc. The paper and pulp industries are also big consumers of electricity. Supply 130, 150, 220 and 230 volts; 50 Hz.

Oil. In 1963 sovereignty was proclaimed over the Norwegian continental shelf and in 1966 the first exploration well was drilled. By 1989 production was almost 7 times the domestic consumption of petroleum and is valued at about 12% of the GNP. Production (1990) 81m. tonnes.

Gas. Production (1989) 1,128,330m. cu. ft.

Minerals. Production and value of the chief concentrates, metals and alloys were:

	1987		*1988*	
Concentrates and minerals	*Tonnes*	*1,000 kroner*	*Tonnes*	*1,000 kroner*
Copper concentrates	102,471	303,282	82,830	287,173
Pyrites	355,686	77,819	306,842	62,704
Titanium ore	852,323	...	898,035	...
Zinc and lead concentrates	47,471	69,369	38,195	84,465
Metals and alloys				
Copper	30,101	...	31,730	...
Nickel	44,564	...	52,545	...
Aluminium	853,213	8,880,670	838,224	11,331,473
Ferro-alloys	776,945	2,705,960	863,682	3,973,330
Pig-iron	377,671	...	390,751	...
Zinc	116,593	...	122,203	...
Lead and tin	17	...	9	...

Agriculture. Norway is a barren and mountainous country. The arable soil is found in comparatively narrow strips, gathered in deep and narrow valleys and around fiords and lakes. Large, continuous tracts fit for cultivation do not exist. Of the total area, 75% is unproductive, 22% productive forest and 3% under cultivation.

	Area [1] *(ha)*			*Produce* [1] *(tonnes)*		
Principal crops	*1987*	*1988*	*1989*	*1987*	*1988*	*1989*
Wheat	57,980	43,610	37,320	249,000	148,300	139,600
Rye	960	720	786	3,600	2,100	...
Barley	162,740	172,960	174,920	566,500	542,000	613,800
Oats	122,310	126,950	133,720	465,900	373,700	423,400
Potatoes	17,610	18,540	18,770	370,300	482,600	455,100
Hay	422,560	426,050	430,290	2,889,400	3,010,200	2,859,800

Livestock, 1989 [1]: 18,000 horses, 951,200 cattle (339,700 milch cows), 2,209,700 sheep (1988), 91,400 goats, 712,000 pigs, 3,848,100 hens.

Fur production in 1988–89 was as follows (1987–88 in brackets): Silver fox, 320,400 (223,300); silver-blue fox, 59,300 (170,300); blue fox, 359,200 (295,700); mink, 566,800 (509,000).

[1] Holdings with at least 5 decares agricultural area in use.

Forestry. About 80% of the productive forest area consists of conifers and 20% of broadleaves. The annual increment (estimate, 1987) is about 19m. cu. metres with bark. The area of productive forests is 66,600 sq. km. Forests in public ownership cover 8,470 sq. km of this area. Between 1979–80 and 1988–89 an annual average of 9·2m. cu. metres was cut for sale: 8·9m. for industrial use, 0·4m. for fuel. Of industrial use, 3·6m. cu. metres in the lumber industry, 3·6m. as pulp, 0·2m. as particle board, about 0·5m. in other industries or exported. About 0·7m. cu. metres are consumed annually on farms.

Fisheries. The total number of registered fishermen in 1989 was 28,655, of whom 7,207 had another chief occupation. In 1989, the number of fishing vessels (all with motor) was 18,515, and of these, 10,043 were open boats.

The value of sea fisheries in 1m. kroner in 1989 was: Cod, 1,264; capelin, 86; mackerel, 284; coal-fish (saithe), 430; deep-water prawn, 780; haddock, 212; herring, 388; dogfish, 22. The catch totalled in 1989, 1·8m. tons, valued at 7,332m. kroner.

Fish farming is a growth industry, exports (1989) 3,486m. kroner.

INDUSTRY. Industry is chiefly based on raw materials produced within the country (wood, fish, etc.) and on water power, of which the country possesses a large amount. Crude petroleum and natural gas production, the manufacture of paper and paper products, industrial chemicals and basic metals are the most important export manufactures. In the following table are given figures for industrial establishments in 1988, excluding one-man units. Electrical plants, construction and building industry are not included. The values are given in 1m. kroner.

Industries	*Establish-ments*	*Number of Employees*	*Gross value of produc-tion*	*Value added*
Coalmining	1	557	134·2	–8·4
Crude petroleum and natural gas	15	14,138	65,489·9	45,769·0
Metal-mining	9	2,278	1,309·0	397·4
Other-mining	449	3,256	2,629·5	1,140·0
Food manufacturing	2,159	48,758	59,971·3	7,992·3
Beverages	56	4,669	5,628·4	3,677·2
Tobacco	3	936	3,197·3	2,635·7
Textiles	417	7,476	3,395·6	1,278·8
Clothing, etc.	258	3,191	1,185·4	502·9
Footwear	27	542	192·6	84·7
Leather	45	608	285·8	89·7
Wood	1,412	19,470	13,637·3	4,219·6
Furniture and fixtures	511	8,501	4,468·5	1,579·1
Pulp and paper	128	12,369	16,602·9	4,592·5
Printing and publishing	1,918	35,673	20,602·7	8,762·1
Chemical, industrial	56	8,040	14,216·1	4,906·0
Chemical, other	149	5,954	6,004·4	2,256·7
Petroleum, refined	3	1,189	8,022·0	819·6
Petroleum and coal	74	1,466	1,995·1	435·5
Rubber	73	1,582	981·7	398·0
Plastics	325	6,534	4,934·7	1,638·6
Ceramics	39	1,034	341·4	193·6
Glass	67	1,996	1,265·2	493·4
Other mineral products	501	8,083	7,442·3	2,643·0
Iron, steel and ferro-alloys	45	9,253	10,615·3	3,209·4
Non-ferrous metals	57	12,364	23,852·3	7,930·3
Metal products, except machinery	1,782	26,785	13,541·6	5,650·2
Machinery and equipment	1,245	37,725	42,656·5	10,126·1
Electrical apparatus and supplies	500	19,596	13,985·7	5,162·0
Transport equipment	861	23,810	16,755·2	5,302·5
Professional and scientific instruments, photographic and optical goods	75	1,720	1,170·9	490·3
Other manufacturing industries	294	2,883	1,241·0	545·3
Total (all included)	13,554	332,436	367,751·8	134,913·0

Income at factor cost (in 1m. kroner):

	1986	*1987*	*1988*
Net domestic product	441,157	480,497	501,942
Less Indirect taxes	99,922	107,059	107,042
Add Subsidies	29,569	31,515	33,638
	370,804	404,953	428,538
Industries			
Agriculture	10,198	11,684	11,175
Forestry	2,788	3,182	3,675
Fishing and fish breeding	3,519	3,187	3,707
Crude petroleum and natural gas production	27,066	24,755	15,529
Manufacturing, mining and quarrying	71,366	78,011	87,361
Electricity supply	11,429	12,385	14,659
Construction	25,374	32,534	33,593
Wholesale and retail trade	41,649	43,919	44,275
Hotels and restaurants	7,709	8,730	9,413
Financial services	24,287	29,691	29,875
Business services	22,292	25,008	27,450

Labour. The labour force (i.e. employed persons plus non-employed persons seeking work aged 16–74) averaged 2,155,000 (69·8%) persons in 1989, of whom 2,049,000 (66·4%) were in employment.

Distribution of employed persons by occupation in 1989 showed 459,000 (22%) in technical, physical science, humanistic and artistic work; 131,000 (6%) administrative executive work; 228,000 (11%) clerical; 215,000 (10%) sales; 131,000 (6%) agriculture, forestry, fishing etc.; 9,000 (0·4%) mining and quarrying;

134,000 (7%) transport and communication; 423,000 (21%) manufacturing; 273,000 (13%) service, and 46,000 (2%) military and occupation not specified.

Non-employed persons seeking work averaged 106,000 (4·9%) in 1989.

Source: Labour Force Sample Surveys.

FOREIGN ECONOMIC RELATIONS

Commerce. Total imports and exports in calendar years (in 1,000 kroner):

	1985	*1986*	*1987*	*1988*	*1989*
Imports	132,563,356	150,052,325	152,041,081	151,100,812	163,380,270
Exports	170,732,779	133,847,404	144,543,413	146,165,546	187,146,395

Trading according to countries was as follows (in 1,000 kroner):

	1988		*1989*	
Countries	*Imports*	*Exports*	*Imports*	*Exports*
Argentina	230,356	116,193	192,251	35,340
Australia and New Zealand	737,023	883,943	597,610	926,489
Belgium and Luxembourg	3,805,489	3,672,093	4,261,916	4,699,200
Brazil	877,436	421,891	999,513	580,049
Canada	2,546,566	2,114,310	3,513,550	4,129,914
China	712,908	438,419	1,140,629	717,180
Czechoslovakia	264,969	220,631	285,918	191,407
Denmark	11,430,379	7,777,145	10,858,697	8,754,191
Fed. Republic of Germany	20,517,675	18,105,178	20,560,346	20,970,435
Finland	5,259,429	3,321,102	4,909,094	3,997,781
France	5,012,644	10,525,918	5,335,596	16,591,540
Hong Kong	1,666,557	434,156	1,761,424	435,498
India	219,566	354,319	237,452	298,956
Italy	5,044,164	3,926,226	4,719,492	4,457,723
Japan	6,904,203	2,780,334	6,056,124	3,133,239
Korea	1,402,501	574,750	1,245,660	477,643
Netherlands	5,912,971	9,884,347	5,422,182	12,418,117
Panama	2,776,003	464,413	5,503,599	442,015
Poland	384,114	517,154	537,859	482,201
Portugal	1,454,868	949,742	1,922,318	1,038,481
Spain	1,829,012	1,265,969	1,775,175	1,937,814
Sweden	26,539,775	17,250,450	24,804,672	23,152,820
Switzerland	2,456,967	1,505,305	2,373,391	1,645,274
UK	11,721,879	38,130,979	12,124,448	50,098,570
USA	10,002,548	8,854,188	12,121,541	12,364,456
USSR	1,114,382	895,783	1,932,436	1,182,714

Principal items of import in 1989 (in 1,000 kroner): Machinery, transport equipment, etc., 69,800,259; fuel oil, etc., 6,368,863; base metals and manufactures thereof, 14,453,753; chemicals and related products, 13,233,744; textiles, 3,276,198.

Principal items of export in 1989 (in 1,000 kroner): Machinery and transport equipment, 25,042,018; base metals and manufactures thereof, 32,173,342; crude oil and natural gas, 73,540,191; edible animal products, 11,116,329; pulp and paper, 9,594,313.

Total trade between Norway and UK (British Department of Trade returns, in £1,000 sterling):

	1986	*1987*	*1988*	*1989*	*1990*
Imports to UK	3,265,157	3,290,339	3,074,000	3,637,119	4,235,348
Exports and re-exports from UK	1,147,790	1,220,844	1,053,613	1,056,506	1,289,789

COMMUNICATIONS

Roads. On 31 Dec. 1989 the length of the public roads (including roads in towns) was 88,174 km. Of these, 52,996 km were main roads; 61,026 km had some kind of paving, mostly bituminous and oil-gravel treatment, the rest being gravel-surfaced.

Number of registered motor vehicles (31 Dec. 1989) was 2,343,204, including 1,612,674 passenger cars (including taxis), 300,212 lorries and vans, 20,199 buses, 202,187 motor cycles and mopeds. The scheduled bus and lorry services in 1987 drove 4,199m. passenger-km.

Railways. The length of state railways on 31 Dec. 1989 was 4,044 km; of private companies, 16 km. On 2,426 km of state and 16 km of private railways electric traction is installed. Total receipts of the state railways and road traffic in 1989 were 3,072m. kroner; total expenses, 4,346m. kroner. The state railways carried 23·7m. tonnes of freight and 33·8m. passengers.

Aviation. Det Norske Luftfartselskap (DNL) started its post-war activities on 1 April 1946. On 1 Aug. 1946 DNL, together with DDL (Danish Airlines) and ABA/SILA (Swedish Airlines), formed the 'Scandinavian Airlines System'—SAS. The 3 companies remained independent units, but all services were co-ordinated. In 1951 a new agreement was signed (retroactive from 1 Oct. 1950) according to which the 3 national companies became holding partners in a new organization which took over the entire operational system. Denmark and Norway hold each two-sevenths and Sweden three-sevenths of the capital, but they have joint responsibility towards third parties.

On 31 Dec. 1989 there were 848 registered engine-driven aircraft. Scheduled air services are run by SAS, Braathens South-American and Far East Air transport service (SAFE) and Wideroes Flyveselskap service. The Norwegian share of the scheduled air service run by SAS is two-sevenths of the SAS service on international routes and the total SAS service in Norway.

Air transport on domestic routes only:

	1,000 km flown	*Passengers carried*	*1,000 passenger-km*	*Post, luggage, freight and passengers (1,000 ton-km) Total*	*Of which post*
1986	44,171	5,764,926	2,271	210,000	8,000
1987	45,882	6,360,417	2,495	231,000	8,000
1988	47,436	6,421,708	2,553	239,000	8,000
1989	44,050	6,003,917	2,442	229,000	7,000

Shipping. The Norwegian International Shipping Registry was set up in 1987. In 1989 495 ships were registered (439 Norwegian); in 1990 841 ships were on the Register, totalling 37·4m. DWT. The total registered mercantile marine on 1 Jan. 1989 was 1,532 vessels, 13m. gross tons (steam and motor vessels above 100 gross tons). These figures do not include fishing and catching boats, tugs, salvage vessels, icebreakers and similar special types of vessels, totalling 787 vessels of 370,000 gross tons.

Vessels entering Norway from foreign countries 1985	*Total No.*	*Net tons*
Norwegian	6,970	17,470
Foreign	10,013	31,264
Total entered	16,983	48,734

Goods (in 1,000 tonnes) in 1989 discharged, 18,369; loaded, 82,886, of which 13,447 was Swedish iron ore shipped from Narvik.

Telecommunications. Number of telephone connexions on 31 Dec. 1989 was 2,070,249 (48·9 per 100 of population). Receipts, 14,553·1m. kroner; expenses, 12,491·1m. kroner (interest on capital included) for State Telecommunications. *Norsk Rikskringkasting* is a non-commercial enterprise operated by an independent state organization and broadcasts 1 programme (P1) on long-, medium-, and short-waves and on FM and 1 programme (P2) on FM. Local programmes are also broadcast. It broadcasts 1 TV programme from 2,259 transmitters. Colour programmes are broadcast by PAL system. Number of television licences, 1,467,331.

Cinemas. There were 426 cinemas with a seating capacity of 110,913 in 1987.

Newspapers. There were 61 daily newspapers with a combined circulation of 2,087,737 in 1988.

JUSTICE, RELIGION, EDUCATION AND WELFARE

Justice. The judicature is common to civil and criminal cases. The same professional judges, who are legally educated, preside over both kinds of cases. These judges are as such state officials. The participation of lay judges and jurors, both summoned for the individual case, varies according to the kind of court and kind of case.

The 96 city or district courts of first instance are in criminal cases composed of one professional judge and 2 lay judges, chosen by ballot from a panel elected by the local authority. In civil cases 2 lay judges may participate. These courts are competent in all cases except criminal cases where the maximum penalty exceeds 6 years imprisonment.

In every community there is a Conciliation Board *(Forliksråd)* composed of 3 lay persons elected by the district council. A civil lawsuit usually begins with mediation by the Board which can pronounce judgement in certain cases.

The 5 high courts, or courts of second instance are composed of 3 professional judges. Additionally, in civil cases 2 or 4 lay judges may be summoned. In serious criminal cases, which are brought before high courts in the first instance a jury of 10 lay persons is summoned to determine whether the defendant is guilty according to the charge. In less serious criminal cases the court is composed of 2 professional and 3 lay judges. In civil cases, the court of second instance is an ordinary court of appeal. In criminal cases in which the lower court does not have judicial authority, it is itself the court of first instance. In other criminal cases it is an appeal court as far as the appeal is based on an attack against the lower court's assessment of the facts when determining the guilt of the defendant. An appeal based on any other alleged mistakes is brought directly before the Supreme Court.

The Supreme Court *(Høyesterett)* is the court of last resort. There are 18 Supreme Court judges. Each individual case is heard by 5 judges. Some major cases are determined in plenary session. The Supreme Court may in general examine every aspect of the case and the handling of it by the lower courts. However, in criminal cases the Court may not overrule the lower court's assessment of the facts as far as the guilt of the defendant is concerned.

The Court of Impeachment *(Riksretten)* is composed of 5 judges of the Supreme Court and 10 members of Parliament.

All serious offences are prosecuted by the State. The Public Prosecution Authority *(Påtalemyndigheten)* consists of the Attorney General *(Riksadvokaten)*, 18 district attorneys *(statsadvokater)* and legally qualified officers of the ordinary police force. Counsel for the defence is in general provided for by the State.

Religion. There is complete freedom of religion, the Evangelical Lutheran Church, however, being the national church, endowed by the State. Its clergy are nominated by the King. Ecclesiastically Norway is divided into 11 *Bispedømmer* (bishoprics), 96 *Prostier* (provostships or archdeaconries) and 624 *Prestegjeld* (clerical districts). There were 197,645 members of registered and unregistered religious communities outside the Evangelical Lutheran Church, subsidized by central government and local authorities in 1990. The Roman Catholics are under a Bishop at Oslo, a Vicar Apostolic at Trondheim and a Vicar Apostolic at Tromsø.

Education. In Norway the children normally start their school attendance the year they are 7 years of age and finish compulsory school the year they complete 16 years of age.

On 1 Sept. 1989 the number of primary schools and pupils were as follows: 3,442 primary schools, 482,964 pupils; 84 special schools for the handicapped, 2,427 pupils.

On 1 Oct. 1988 the number of pupils in upper secondary schools, *i.e.*, folk high schools, secondary general schools and vocational schools, was 209,065.

There are in Norway 4 universities and 19 institutions equivalent to universities. In autumn 1989 the total number of students was 57,329. The University of Oslo, founded in 1811, had 25,816 students. The University of Bergen, founded in 1948, had 11,940 students. The University of Trondheim consists of the Norwegian Institute of Technology, founded in 1910, and the College of Arts and Science, founded in 1925. At each of them the number of students was in autumn 1989, 6,605 and 4,907 respectively. The University of Tromsø was established in 1968; 3,017 students were registered in autumn 1989. The other university institutions had 5,044 students.

On 1 Oct. 1988 there were at other schools of higher education, 63,721 students. These included 12,877 at colleges for teachers, 7,936 at colleges for engineers and 10,461 at district colleges.

In 1985–86 there were 6,67.23 Norwegian students and pupils attending foreign universities and schools.

Health. In 1986 there were 9,443 doctors and (1987.2) 66,37.23 hospital beds.

Social Security. In 1989, about 120,800m. kroner were paid under different social insurance schemes, amounting to approximately 23% of the net national income.

The National Insurance Act of 17.2 June 1966, which came into force on 1 Jan. 1967.2, replaced the schemes relating to old age pensions, disability benefits, widows' and mothers' pensions, benefits to unmarried women, 'survivors' benefit for children and rehabilitation aid. Schemes relating to health insurance, unemployment insurance and occupational injury insurance were revised and incorporated in National Insurance Scheme on 1 Jan. 197.21. As from 1 Jan. 1981, benefits to divorced and separated supporters also are covered by the National Insurance Scheme.

The following conspectus gives a survey of schemes established by law. Some municipalities grant additional benefits to old-age, disablement and survivor's pensions.

Type of scheme	*Introduced* [1]	*Scope*	*Principal benefits as from 1 Oct. 1990*
National insurance	1967.2 (1990)		
Medical care and sickness cash benefits [2]	1911	All residents	Medical benefits: all hospital expenses; cost share of expense of medical consultation, important medicines, travel expenses, etc. (such costs exceeding 880kr. a calendar year are paid in full by the National Insurance).
		Nearly all wage-earners	Daily sickness allowances: kr. 65 to 7.285 per day cash (5 days a week). The present sickness allowance scheme (established 197.28) entitles employees to a daily allowance equal to 100% of their gross earned income (within certain limits) from and including the first day of absence; self-employed persons, ordinarily 65% of gross earned income as from the 15th day. Supplementary insurance available
		All female residents giving birth	Maternity allowances: same as sickness allowances for 140 days (or 80% of allowance for 17.25 days) (time sharing with the father is possible) or a lump sum of kr. 8,7.250 per child
Unemployment benefits [2]	1939	Nearly all wage-earners	Daily allowance during unemployment kr. 52 to 408 per day, excluding supplement for supported child(ren) (six days a week). Contributions to training and retraining, removal expenses, wage subsidies
Rehabilitation benefits [3]	1961	Persons unfit for work because of disablement and persons who have a substantially limited general functional capacity	Training; treatment; rehabilitation allowance grants and loans Full rehabilitation allowance equals old age pension (however, no special supplement is granted, see below.)
Disability benefits [3]	1961	All residents	*A basic grant* and *an assistance grant* to persons with special needs. Basic grant: kr. 4,800 to kr. 15,960 per annum. Assistance grant: kr. 7.2,980, may be increased for children below 18 years of age to a maximum of kr. 44,688 per annum

For notes *see* p. 000.

Type of scheme	Introduced [1]	Scope	Principal benefits as from 1 Oct. 1990
		All residents between 16 and 67 years of age	*Disability pension* to persons between 16 and 67 years of age, occupationally disabled by at least 50%, unfit for rehabilitation. Full disability pension equals old age pension
Occupational injury benefits [1] (industrial workers 1895; fishermen 1909; seamen 1913; military personnel 1953, combined in the act of occupational injury insurance 1960)	1895	All employed persons, drafted military personnel, school children and students; self-employed on a voluntary basis	The ordinary benefits of the National Insurance, alternative calculation of pensions etc. which in many cases are more favourable for the insured person—or his survivors than the ordinary rules *An occupational injury compensation,* alone or in addition to a disability pension
Old age pensions [3]	1937	All persons above 67 years of age	Basic pensions: Single, kr. 34,000; couples, kr. 51,000 per annum; supplementary pensions based on previous pensionable income; supplement for supported spouse kr. 17,000 per annum; supplement for supported child(ren) kr. 8,500 to kr. 4,250 per child per annum; *see below* under 'Special supplement' and 'Compensation supplement'
Death grants	1967	All residents	A certain amount fixed by the Storting, for the time being kr. 4,000
Survivors' benefits [3]	1965	All residents	Full pension = kr. 34,000 per annum + 55% of the supplementary pension due to the deceased, *transitional benefits,* child care allowance and educational allowances (*see below* under 'Special supplement' and 'Compensation supplement')
Children's pension [3]	1958	Under 18 (20) years of age, after loss of one or both parents	40% of basic amount (kr. 13,600) for first child, 25% (kr. 8,500) for each additional child. If both parents are dead, full survivors' pension for first, 40% of basic amount for second, 25% third, etc., child
Benefits to unmarried supporters [3]	1965	Unmarried mothers or fathers	An additional maternity benefit of kr. 9,680, transitional benefit, full amount kr. 34,000 per annum, child care allowance and educational allowances (*see below* under 'Special supplement' and 'Family allowances')
Benefits to divorced and separated supporters [4]	1972	Divorced and separated supporters	Same kind of benefits as unmarried supporters above
Benefits to unmarried persons forced to live at home [3]	1965	Unmarried persons under 67 years of age having stayed at home for at least 5 years to give necessary care and attention to parents or other near relatives	Transitional benefit or a pension kr. 34,000 per annum, educational allowances (*see below* under 'Special supplement' and 'Compensation supplement')

For notes *see* p. 961.

Type of scheme	Introduced [1]	Scope	Principal benefits as from 1 Oct. 1990
Special supplement to National Insurance pensions or transitional benefits	1969 (1989)	Pensioners and persons with transitional allowance on basic rates	Full special supplement, 58% of basic amount, *i.e.* kr. 19,720. For a married pensioner the rate may be different. If the pensioner supports a spouse who is 60 years or older, the rate is 106·5%, *i.e.*kr. 36,210. If the spouse has a pension of his/her own, the rate is 53·25%, *i.e.*kr. 18,105
Compensation supplement to National Insurance pensions or transitional benefits	1970 (1989)	Pensioners, persons with transitional benefits (except unmarried, divorced and separated supporters) or rehabilitation allowances	Full compensation supplement kr. 500 for single persons and kr. 750 for married couples per annum
Family allowances	1946 (1989)	All families with children under 16 years of age	Kr. 8,748 per annum for the first child, kr. 9,240 for the second, kr. 10,656 for the third, kr. 11,280 for the fourth and kr. 11,664 for the fifth and each additional child. Single supporters receive benefits for one child more than the actual number. Families resident in certain districts north of the Arctic Circle receive an additional amount of kr. 3,600 per child
War pensions	1946 (1989)	War victims, 1939–45	Pensions up to kr. 150,720 per annum for single pensioners/ couples (excluding supplement for supported child(ren); widows' and children's pensions)
Special pension schemes:		Persons with at least: [5]	Maximum old-age pension:
Forestry workers	1952 (1989)	750 premium weeks (1,500 „ „)	Kr. 34,000 per annum (for supported spouse an additional 33⅓%, 10% supplement per child, maximum 5 children)
Fishermen	1958 (1989)	750 premium weeks (1,500 „ „)	Kr. 34,000 per annum (for supported spouse an additional 50%, 30% supplement per child)
Seamen	1948 (1989)	150 months service (360 „ „)	Kr. 111,409 [6] per annum (officers) Kr. 79,578 [6] „ „ (others) (no spouse supplement, an additional 10% per child)

[1] Date of latest revision of law in brackets.
[2] Transferred to national insurance scheme and revised in 1971.
[3] Transferred to national insurance scheme and revised in 1967.
[4] Transferred to national insurance scheme and revised in 1981.
[5] Requirements for maximum pensions in brackets.
[6] Supplements for service during war not included.

Provisions have been laid down for the integration of more than one benefit, pension, etc., so as to limit the total amount.

As a main rule all running benefits are taxable, while lump sums are not taxed. Certain tax modifications apply to all pensioners and pensioners with no other income than minimum benefits are not charged for tax.

SVALBARD

An archipelago situated between 10° and 35° E. long. and between 74° and 81° N. lat. Total area, 62,000 sq. km (24,000 sq. miles).

The main islands of the archipelago are Spitsbergen (formerly called Vest-spitsbergen), Nordaustlandet, Edgeøya, Barentsøya, Prins Karls Forland, Bjørnøya, Hopen, Kong Karls Land, Kvitøya, and many small islands. The arctic climate is tempered by mild winds from the Atlantic.

The archipelago was probably discovered by Norsemen in 1194 and rediscovered by the Dutch navigator Barents in 1596. In the 17th century the very lucrative whale-hunting caused rival Dutch, British and Danish–Norwegian claims to sovereignty and quarrels about the hunting-places. But when in the 18th century the whale-hunting ended, the question of the sovereignty of Svalbard lost its significance; it was again raised in the 20th century, owing to the discovery and exploitation of coalfields. By a treaty, signed on 9 Feb. 1920 in Paris, Norway's sovereignty over the archipelago was recognized. On 14 Aug. 1925 the archipelago was officially incorporated in Norway.

Coal is the principal product. Of the 3 Norwegian and 3 Soviet mining camps, 2 Norwegian and 2 Soviet camps are operating. Total population on 31 Dec. 1988 was 3,646, of which 1,055 were Norwegians, 2,579 Soviet citizens, and 12 Poles. In 1987, 473,279 tonnes of coal were exported from the Norwegian and 462,942 tonnes from the Soviet mines.

Norwegian and foreign companies have been prospecting for oil. So far 5 deep drillings have been made, but oil and gas finds have not been reported.

There are Norwegian meteorological and/or radio stations at the following places: Bjørnøya (since 1920), Hopen (1945), Isfjord Radio (1933), Longyearbyen (1930), Svalbard Lufthavn (1975) and Ny-Ålesund (1961). A research station, administered by Norsk Polarinstitutt, was erected at Ny-Ålesund in 1968 for various observations and investigations. An airport near Longyearbyen (Svalbard Lufthavn) opened in 1975.

Norsk Polarinstitutt, Skrifter, Oslo, from 1948 (under different titles from 1922)
Greve, T., *Svalbard: Norway in the Arctic.* Oslo, 1975
Hisdal, V., *Geography of Svalbard.* Norsk Polarinstitutt, Oslo, rev. ed., 1984
Orvin, A. K., 'Twenty-five Years of Norwegian Sovereignty in Svalbard 1925–1950' (in *The Polar Record,* 1951)

JAN MAYEN

This bleak, desolate and mountainous island of volcanic origin and partly covered by glaciers, is situated 71° N. lat. and 8° 30' W. long., 300 miles NNE of Iceland. The total area is 380 sq. km (147 sq. miles). Beerenberg, its highest peak, reaches a height of 2,277 metres. Volcanic activity, which had been dormant, was reactivated in Sept. 1970.

The island was possibly discovered by Henry Hudson in 1608, and it was first named Hudson's Tutches (Touches). It was again and again rediscovered and renamed. Its present name derives from the Dutch whaling captain Jan Jacobsz May, who indisputably discovered the island in 1614. It was uninhabited, but occasionally visited by seal hunters and trappers, until 1921 when Norway established a radio and meteorological station. On 8 May 1929 Jan Mayen was officially proclaimed as incorporated in the Kingdom of Norway. Its relation to Norway was finally settled by law of 27 Feb. 1930. A LORAN station (1959) and a CONSOL station (1968) have been established.

BOUVET ISLAND

Bouvetøya

This uninhabited volcanic island, mostly covered by glaciers and situated 54° 25' S. lat. and 3° 21' E. long., was discovered in 1739 by a French naval officer, Jean Baptiste Loziert Bouvet, but no flag was hoisted till, in 1825, Capt. Norris raised the Union Jack. In 1928 Great Britain waived its claim to the island in favour of Norway, which in Dec. 1927 had occupied it. A law of 27 Feb. 1930 declared Bouvetøya a Norwegian dependency. The area is 50 sq. km (19 sq. miles). From 1977 Norway has had an automatic meteorological station on the island, and 5 men operated a meteorological station there during the 1978–79 season.

PETER I ISLAND
Peter I Øy

This uninhabited island, situated 68° 48' S. lat. and 90° 35' W. long., was sighted in 1821 by the Russian explorer, Admiral von Bellingshausen. The first landing was made in 1929 by a Norwegian expedition which hoisted the Norwegian flag. On 1 May 1931 Peter I Island was placed under Norwegian sovereignty, and on 24 March 1933 it was incorporated in Norway as a dependency. The area is 180 sq. km (69 sq. miles).

QUEEN MAUD LAND
Dronning Maud Land

On 14 Jan. 1939 the Norwegian Cabinet placed that part of the Antarctic Continent from the border of Falkland Islands dependencies in the west to the border of the Australian Antarctic Dependency in the east (between 20° W. and 45° E.) under Norwegian sovereignty. The territory had been explored only by Norwegians and hitherto been ownerless. Since 1949 expeditions from various countries have explored the area. In 1957 Dronning Maud Land was given the status of a Norwegian dependency.

DIPLOMATIC REPRESENTATIVES

Of Norway in Great Britain (25 Belgrave Sq., London, SW1X 8QD)
Ambassador: Kjell Eliassen, GCMG (accredited 15 Feb. 1989).

Of Great Britain in Norway (Thomas Heftyesgate 8, 0244 Oslo, 2)
Ambassador: David Ratford, CMG, CVO.

Of Norway in the USA (2720 34th St., NW, Washington, D.C., 20008)
Ambassador: Kjeld Vibe.

Of the USA in Norway (Drammensveien 18, 0244 Oslo, 2)
Ambassador: Loret Miller Ruppe.

Of Norway to the United Nations
Ambassador: Martin Huslid.

Further Reading

Statistical Information: The Central Bureau of Statistics, Statistisk Sentralbyrå (Skippergaten 15, P.B.8131 Dep.N-0033, Oslo 1), was founded in 1876 as an independent state institution. *Acting director general:* Arne Øien. The earliest census of population was taken in 1769. The Sentralbyrå publishes the series *Norges Offisielle Statistikk,* Norway's official statistics (from 1828), and *Social Economic Studies* (from 1954). The main publications are:

- *Statistisk Årbok for Norge* (annual, from 1880; from 1952 bilingual Norwegian–English)
- *Economic survey* annual, from 1935; with English summary from 1952, now published in *Økonomiske Analyser* (annual)
- *Historisk Statistikk 1978* (historical statistics; bilingual Norwegian–English)
- *Statistisk Månedshefte* (monthly, from 1880; with English index)
- *Sosialt Utsyn 1989* (social survey). Irregular
- *Miljóstatistikk 1988* (environmental statistics). Irregular

Norges Statskalender. From 1816; annual from 1877

Facts about Norway. Ed. by Aftenposten. 20th ed. Oslo, 1986–87
Arntzen, J. G. and Knudsen, B. B., *Political Life and Institutions in Norway*. Oslo, 1981
Derry, T. K., *A History of Modern Norway, 1814–1972*. OUP, 1973.—*A History of Scandinavia*. London, 1979
Glässer, E., *Norwegen* [Bibliography] Darmstadt, 1978
Gleditsch, Th., *Engelsk–norsk ordbok*, 2nd ed. Oslo, 1948
Greve, T., *Haakon VI of Norway, Founder of a New Monarchy*. London, 1983
Grønland, E., *Norway in English, Books on Norway . . . 1742–1959*. Oslo, 1961
Haugen, E., *Norwegian–English Dictionary*, Oslo, 1965
Helvig, M., *Norway: Land, People, Industries, a Brief Geography*. 3rd ed. Oslo, 1970
Holtedahl, O. (ed.) *Geology of Norway*. Oslo, 1960
Hornby, A. S. and Svenkerud, H., *Oxford engelsk-norsk ordbok*. Oslo, 1983
Hove, O., *The System of Education*. Oslo, 1968
Imber, W., *Norway*. Oslo, 1980
Knudsen, O., *Norway at Work*. Oslo, 1972
Larsen, K., *A History of Norway*. New York, 1948
Midgaard, J., *A Brief History of Norway*. Oslo, 1969
Nielsen, K. and Nesheim, A., *Lapp Dictionary: Lapp–English–Norwegian*. 5 vols., Oslo 1963
Orvik, N. (ed.) *Fears and Expectations: Norwegian Attitudes Toward European Integration*. Oslo, 1972
Paine, R., *Coast Lapp Society*. 2 vols. Tromsø, 1957–65
Popperwell, R. G., *Norway*. London, 1972
Sather, L. B., *Norway*. [Bibliography] Oxford and Santa Barbara, 1986
Selbyg, A., *Norway Today: An Introduction to Modern Norwegian Society*. Oslo, 1986

National Library: The University Library, Drammensvein 42b, 0255 Oslo. *Director:* Ben Rugaas.

OMAN

Capital: Muscat
Population: 2m. (1990)
GNP per capita: US$4,200 (1989)

Sultanate of Oman

HISTORY. Oman was dominated by Portugal from 1507–1649. The Al-Busaid family assumed power in 1744 and have ruled to the present day. The Sultanate of Oman was known as the Sultanate of Muscat and Oman until 1970.

AREA AND POPULATION. Oman is bounded in the north-east by the Gulf of Oman and south-east by the Arabian Sea (a coastline of some 1,700 km), south-west by Yemen and north-west by Saudi Arabia and the United Arab Emirates. There is an enclave at the northern tip of the Musandam Peninsula between the United Arab Emirates of Ras al-Khaimah in the west and Fujairah in the south-east.

The port of Gwadur and a small tract of country on the Baluchistan coast of the Gulf of Oman were handed over to Pakistan on 8 Sept. 1958.

The **Kuria Muria** islands were ceded to the UK in 1854 by the Sultan of Muscat and Oman. On 30 Nov. 1967 the islands were retroceded to the Sultan of Muscat and Oman, in accordance with the wishes of the population.

The Sultanate extends inland to the borders of the Rub' al Khali ('Empty Quarter') across three geographical divisions—a coastal plain, a range of hills and a plateau. The coastal plain varies in width from 10 miles near Suwaiq to practically nothing in the vicinity of Mutrah and Muscat, where the hills descend abruptly into the sea. These hills are for the most part barren. The plateau has an average height of 1,000 ft.; with the exception of oases there is little or no cultivation. North-west of Muscat the coastal plain, known as the Batinah, is fertile and prosperous. Whereas the coastline between Muscat and the southern province of Dhofar is barren, Dhofar itself is highly fertile. Its principal town is Salalah on the coast which is served by the port of Raysut.

The area has been estimated at about 105,000 sq. miles (300,000 sq. km) and the population (1990) 2m., chiefly Arabs. The capital is Muscat. Estimated population of the Capital area (comprising Muscat, Mutrah, Ruwi and Seeb), 1987, 400,000. Other principal towns are Nizwa, 10,000 and Salalah, 10,000.

The country is divided into 7 planning regions:

Region	*Population 1990*	*Regional centres*	*Population 1990*
Muscat	444,472	Muscat	...
Southern (Janubiah)	216,546	Salalah	...
Interior (Dakhiliah)	253,684	Nizwa,	62,880
		Sumail	44,721
Sharqiyah	290,784	Ibra,	21,967
		Sur	59,963
Batinah	581,968	Sohar,	91,521
		Rustaq	66,205
Dhahirah	180,781	Al-Buraimi	40,160
Musandam	31,766	Khasab	19,702

CLIMATE. Oman has a desert climate, with exceptionally hot and humid months from April to Oct., when temperatures may reach 117°F (47°C). From Dec. to the end of March, the climate is more pleasant. Light monsoon rains fall in the south from June to Sept., with highest amounts in the western highland region. Muscat. Jan. 72°F (22·2°C), July 91°F (33·3°C). Annual rainfall 4·0" (99·1 mm). Salalah. Jan. 72°F (22·2°C), July 78°F (25·6°C). Annual rainfall 3·3" (81·3 mm).

RULER. The present Sultan is Qaboos bin Said (born Nov. 1940). He took over from his father Said bin Taimur, on 23 July 1970 in a Palace coup.

CONSTITUTION AND GOVERNMENT. Oman is an absolute monarchy and there is no formal constitution. The Sultan legislates by decree and appoints a Cabinet to assist him; and he is nominally Prime Minister and Minister of Foreign Affairs, Defence and Finance. The other Ministers were in Feb. 1991:

Deputy Prime Ministers: Sayyid Fahr bin Taimur bin Faisal Al Said (*Security and Defence*), Sayyid Fahd bin Mahmud bin Muhammad Al Said (*Legal Affairs*), Qais bin Abdul Mun'im al Zawawi (*Financial and Economic Affairs*). *Agriculture and Fisheries:* Muhammed bin Abdullah bin Zaher al Hinai. *Civil Service:* Ahmad bin Abdul Nabi Macki. *Commerce and Industry:* Salim bin Abdullah al Ghazali. *Communications:* Hamud bin Abdullah al Harthy. *Education and Youth:* Yahya bin Mahfudh al Manthari. *Electricity and Water:* Mohamed bin Ali al Qatabi. *Environment:* Sayyid Shabib bin Taimur Al Said. *Health:* Ali bin Muhammed bin Musa al Raisi. *Housing:* Malik bin Sulaiman al Ma'mari. *Information:* Abdul Aziz bin Muhammed al Rowas. *Interior:* Sayyid Badr bin Saud bin Harib Al Bu Saidi. *Justice, Awqaf and Islamic Affairs:* Sayyid Hilal bin Saud bin Harib Al Bu Saidi. *National Heritage and Culture:* Sayyid Faisal bin Ali Al Said. *Petroleum and Minerals:* Said bin Ahmad al Shanfari. *Posts, Telegraphs and Telephones:* Ahmad bin Suweidan al Baluchi. *Regional Municipalities:* Amour bin Shuwin al Hosni. *Social Affairs:* Mustahail bin Ahmed al Ma'ashani. *Labour and Vocational Training:* Sayid Mutasim bin Hamood al Busaidy. *President, Diwan of the Royal Court:* Sayyid Saif bin Hamad bin Saud. *President of the Palace Office:* Maj.-Gen. Ali bin Majid al Mamari.

In 1981 the Sultan established a 45-member State Consultative Council composed of government officials and private citizens appointed by the Sultan. The number of Council members was increased to 55 in 1983. It meets 4 times a year.

National flag: Red, with a white panel in the upper fly and a green one in the lower fly, and in the canton the national emblem in white.

Local government: Oman is divided into 7 regions *(see above)* and sub-divided into 51 governorates *(wilayats)*, each under a governor *(wali)*.

DEFENCE

Army. The Army consists of 2 headquarter brigades; 1 armoured, 1 reconnaissance and 2 artillery regiments; 8 infantry regiments; 1 special force, 1 engineer regiment and 1 parachute regiment. Equipment includes 6 M-60A1 and 33 Chieftain main battle tanks. Strength (1991) about 20,000. (Regiments are of battalion size.)

Navy. The Navy, which is based principally at Seeb (HQ) and Wudam comprises 4 fast missile craft, 4 coastal and 4 inshore patrol craft. Auxiliaries include 1 training ship, 1 logistic support ship, 1 troop transport and 1 survey craft. There are also 2 specially adapted amphibious ships and 3 craft. Naval personnel in 1990 totalled 2,500.

The marine police coastguard, 400 strong in 1990, operate 11 coastal patrol boats, 2 logistics support craft, 3 inshore patrol boats and 8 launches.

The wholly separate Royal Yacht Squadron consists of a 3,800-tonne yacht and an 11,000-tonne support ship.

Air Force. The Air Force, formed in 1959, had in 1987 two strike/interceptor squadrons of Jaguars, a ground attack/interceptor squadron of Hunters, a squadron of Strikemaster light jet training/attack aircraft, 1 DC-8, 3 BAC One-Eleven and 2 Gulfstream VIP transports, 3 C-130H Hercules, 6 Defender and 15 Skyvan light transports, 35 Agusta-Bell 205, 212, 214B and JetRanger, and Bell 214 ST helicopters for security duties, 2 Super Puma VIP helicopters and 2 Bravo piston-engined trainers. Air defence force has batteries of Rapier low-level surface-to-air missiles. Personnel (1991) about 3,000, with 57 combatant aircraft.

INTERNATIONAL RELATIONS

Membership. Oman is a member of the UN, the Arab League, the Islamic Conference Organisation and the Gulf Co-operation Council.

Treaties. The Treaty of Friendship, Commerce and Navigation between Britain and the Sultan signed on 20 Dec. 1951, reaffirmed the close ties which have existed between the British Government and the Sultanate of Oman for over a century and a half. A Memorandum of Understanding signed in June 1982 provided for regular consultations on international and bilateral issues.

ECONOMY

Policy. The fourth 5-year plan is running from 1991 to 1995.

Budget. Revenue (1989) R.O. 1,482m. (82% from oil); expenditure, 1,644m.

Currency. The *Rial Omani* (OMR) was introduced in Nov. 1972 replacing the *Rial Saidi*. It is divided into 1,000 *baiza*. There are notes of 100, 200 and 500 *baiza* and 1, 5, 10, 20 and 50 *Rial Omani* and coins of 2, 5, 10, 25, 50, 100, 250 and 500 *baiza*. The exchange rate in March 1991 was £1 = 728 *baiza*; US$1 = 384 *baiza*.

Banking. In 1990 there were 24 commercial banks operating, of which 13 were foreign institutions. There are 3 specialized banks: The Oman Development Bank, the Oman Housing Bank and the Oman Bank for Agriculture and Fisheries. The Central Bank of Oman commenced operations in 1975.

Weights and Measures. The metric system is in operation. Transactions in the former measurements are now illegal.

ENERGY AND NATURAL RESOURCES

Electricity. Production (1989) 3,927m. kwh. Supply 240 volts; 50 Hz.

Oil. The economy of Oman is dominated by the oil industry, which provides nearly all Government revenue. In 1937 Petroleum Concessions (Oman) Ltd, a subsidiary of the Iraq Petroleum Co., was granted a 75-year oil concession extending over the whole of Oman, although it relinquished Dhofar in 1950. In 1951 the company's name was changed to Petroleum Development (Oman) Ltd. The company (PDO) regained the Dhofar concession area in 1969. When some of the IPC partners withdrew from Oman in 1960, Shell took over the management of PDO with an 85% interest (minority interests were held by Compagnie Française des Pétroles, 10% and Gulbenkian, 5%). At the beginning of 1974 the Oman Government bought a 25% share in PDO, increasing this retroactively to 60% in July. A Joint Management Committee was established. Other companies active in exploration activities in Oman, with mixed success, include Amoco, Elf-Acquitaine and a consortium of Deminex, Agip and Hispanoil with BP as operator.

Oil in commercial quantities was discovered in 1964 and production began in 1967. Production in 1990 was 33·06m. tonnes. Total proven reserves were estimated in 1988 to be 4,071m. bbls, or sufficient for 19 years at the current rate of production. Since the first oil refinery became operational in 1982, Oman has been self-sufficient in most oil-derived products.

Oman is not a member of OPEC or OAPEC.

Gas. Production (1988) 7m. cu. metres per day. In 1989 reserves were estimated at 283,000m. cu. metres.

Water Resources. Oman relies on a combination of water and desalination plants for its water. Two desalination plants at Ghubriah, built in 1972 and 1982, provide most of the water needs of the capital area.

Minerals. Production of refined copper at the smelter at Sohar was 14,963 tonnes in 1989.

Agriculture. About 41,000 hectares are under cultivation. In the valleys of the interior, as well as on the Batinah coastal plain, date cultivation has reached a high level, and there are possibilities of agricultural development subject to present water resources and soil surveys. The crop of dates was 97,000 tonnes in 1988, most of which is exported to India. Other main crops are limes, bananas, coconuts, mangoes and alfalfa. Camels (82,000 in 1988) are bred in large numbers by the inland tribes.

Fisheries. Catch (1989) 110,285 tonnes.

INDUSTRY. In 1989 manufacturing accounted for only 4·2% of GDP. Apart from oil production, copper mining and smelting and cement production there are light industries, mainly food processing and chemical products. The government gives priority to import substitute industries.

FOREIGN ECONOMIC RELATIONS

Commerce. Main imports include machinery and transport equipment, manufactured goods, food and live animals, petroleum products and chemicals.

Total imports, 1989: R.O. 868m.; exports, R.O. 1,512m. (of which oil: R.O. 1,344m.).

Total trade between Oman and UK (British Department of Trade returns, in £1,000 sterling):

	1986	*1987*	*1988*	*1989*	*1990*
Imports to UK	87,235	49,487	146,751	84,009	89,445
Exports and re-exports from UK	399,647	249,916	344,875	298,974	272,072

COMMUNICATIONS

Roads. A network of adequate graded roads links all the main sectors of population, and only a few mountain villages are not accessible by motor vehicles. In 1990 there were 4,553 km of asphalt roads and 20,147 km of graded roads. In 1989 there were 94,830 registered motor vehicles.

Aviation. Gulf Air run regional services in and out of Seeb international airport (20 miles from Muscat) to Bahrain, Doha, Abu Dhabi, Dubai, Karachi, Bombay and operate daily flights to and from London. Other airlines serving Muscat are British Airways, KLM, Thai International, British Caledonian, Air Tanzania, MEA, Kuwait Airlines, PIA, Air India, Iran Air, TMA (cargo) and Trade Winds (cargo). Domestic flights are provided by Oman Aviation Services.

Shipping. In Mutrah a deep-water port (named Mina Qaboos) was completed in 1974 at a cost of R.O. 18·2m. It provides 12 berths, 9 of which are deep-water berths, warehousing facilities and a harbour for dhows and coastal vessels. The annual handling capacity has been raised to 1·5m. tons. Mina Raysut, the port of Salalah, has a capacity of 1m. tons per year.

Telecommunications. In 1989 there were 71 post offices and sub-post offices. Omantel maintain a telegraph office at Muscat and an automatic telephone exchange (23,000 lines, 1984) which includes Mutrah, Bait-al-Falaj and Mina al-Fahal, the oil company terminal. A high-frequency radio link with Bahrain was opened in Aug. 1972 providing communications with other parts of the world. Internally, there are radio telephone, telex and telegraph services direct between Salalah and Muscat, and a VHF radio link between Seeb international airport and Muscat. The airport is also served by a SITA telex system. Radio Oman broadcasts daily for 17 hours in Arabic and 2 hours in English.

A colour television service covering Muscat and the surrounding area started transmission in Nov. 1974. A television service for Dhofar opened in 1975. Total number of televisions, 23,500 and radios, 800,000 in 1985.

Newspapers. There were (1989) 2 Arabic and 1 English daily newspapers and 1 English weekly newspaper.

EDUCATION AND WELFARE

Education. In 1989–90, there were 741 schools with 323,468 pupils and 13,695 teachers. Plans have been implemented for the development of technical and agricultural training and craft training at intermediate and secondary level. Oman's first university, the Sultan Qaboos University, opened in Sept. 1986 and in 1990 there were 2,550 students and 337 teachers. There are programmes to combat adult illiteracy.

Health. In 1989 there were 47 hospitals with 3,360 beds, 88 health centres, 1,392 doctors, 96 dentists, 235 pharmacists and 3,866 nursing staff.

DIPLOMATIC REPRESENTATIVES

Of Oman in Great Britain (44A Montpelier Sq., London, SW7 1JJ)
Ambassador: Abdalla Bin Mohamed Al-Dhahab.

Of Great Britain in Oman (PO Box 300, Muscat)
Ambassador: Sir Terence Clark, KBE, CMG, CVO.

Of Oman in the USA (2342 Massachusetts Ave., NW, Washington, D.C., 20008)
Ambassador: Awadh Bader Al-Shanfari.

Of the USA in Oman (PO Box 50202 Madinat Qabos, Muscat)
Ambassador: Richard Boehm.

Of Oman to the United Nations
Ambassador: Salim Bin Mohammed Al-Khussaiby.

Further Reading

Oman in 10 years. Ministry of Information. Oman, 1980
Oman: A MEED Practical Guide. London, 1984
Carter, J. R. L., *Tribes of Oman*. London, 1981
Clements, F. A., *Oman: The Reborn Land*. London and New York, 1980.—*Oman*. [Bibliography] Oxford and Santa Barbara, 1981
Graz, L., *The Omani's: Sentinels of the Gulf*. London, 1982
Hawley, D., *Oman and its Rennaissance*. London, 1977
Peterson, J. E., *Oman in the Twentieth Century*. London and New York, 1978
Peyton, W. D., *Oman before 1970: The End of an Era*. London, 1985
Pridham, B. R., (ed.) *Oman: Economic, Social and Strategic Developments*. London, 1987
Shannon, M. O., *Oman and South-Eastern Arabia: A Bibliographic Survey*. Boston, 1978
Skeet, I., *Muscat and Oman: The End of an Era*. London, 1974
Thesiger, W., *Arabian Sands*. London, 1959
Townsend, J., *Oman*. London, 1977
Ward, P., *Travels in Oman*. Cambridge, 1987
Wikan, U., *Behind the Veil in Arabia: Women in Oman*. Johns Hopkins Univ. Press, 1982
Wilkinson, J. C., *The Imanate Tradition of Oman*. CUP, 1987

PAKISTAN

Capital: Islamabad
Population: 105·4m. (1989)
GNP per capita: US$350 (1988)

Islamic Republic of Pakistan

HISTORY. Pakistan was constituted as a Dominion on 14 Aug. 1947, under the provisions of the Indian Independence Act, 1947. The Dominion consisted of the following former territories of British India: Baluchistan, East Bengal (including almost the whole of Sylhet, a former district of Assam), North-West Frontier, West Punjab and Sind; and those States which had acceded to Pakistan.

On 23 March 1956 an Islamic republic was proclaimed after the Constituent Assembly had adopted the draft constitution on 29 Feb.

On 7 Oct. 1958 President Mirza declared martial law in Pakistan, dismissed the central and provincial Governments, abolished all political parties and abrogated the constitution of 23 March 1956. Field Marshal Mohammad Ayub Khan, the Army Commander-in-Chief, was appointed as chief martial law administrator and assumed office on 28 Oct. 1958, after Maj.-Gen. Iskander Mirza had handed all powers to him. His authority was confirmed by a ballot in Feb. 1960. He proclaimed a new constitution on 1 March 1962.

On 25 March 1969 President Ayub Khan resigned and handed over power to the army under the leadership of Maj.-Gen. Agha Muhammad Yahya Khan who immediately proclaimed martial law throughout the country, appointing himself chief martial law administrator on the same day. On 29 March 1970 the Legal Framework Order was published, defining a new constitution: Pakistan to be a federal republic with a Moslem Head of State; the National Assembly and Provincial Assemblies to be elected in free and periodical elections, the first of which was held on 7 Dec. 1970.

At the general election the Awami League based in East Pakistan and led by Sheikh Mujibur Rahman gained 167 seats and the Peoples' Party 90. Martial law continued pending the settlement of differences between East and West, which developed into civil war in March 1971. The war ended in Dec. 1971 and the Eastern province declared itself an independent state, Bangladesh. On 20 Dec. 1971 President Yahya Khan resigned and Z. A. Bhutto became President and chief martial law administrator. On 30 Jan. 1972, Pakistan withdrew from the Commonwealth, rejoining on 1 Oct. 1989.

A new Constitution was adopted by the National Assembly on 10 April 1973 and enforced on 14 Aug. 1973. It provided for a federal parliamentary system with the President as constitutional head and the Prime Minister as chief executive. President Bhutto stepped down to become Prime Minister and Fazal Elahi Chaudhry was elected President.

The Chief of the Army Staff, Gen. M. Zia-ul-Haq, proclaimed martial law on 5 July 1977 and the armed forces took control of the administration; scheduled elections were postponed. Mr Bhutto was hanged (for conspiracy to murder) on 4 April 1979. Gen. M. Zia-ul-Haq succeeded Fazal Elahi Chaudhry as President in Sept. 1978.

With the proclamation of martial law the Constitution was kept in abeyance, but not abrogated.

National elections were held in Feb. 1985 on the basis of the 1973 Constitution, amended to provide wider presidential powers. On 19 Dec. 1984 a referendum had been held to determine whether the President should continue in office for a 5-year term, following the elections; results were announced as 98% in favour.

The Pakistan People's Party won 47 seats in the new Assembly, the Muslim League 17 and the Jamaat Islami Party, 9. In March 1985 the President set up a new

National Security Council, led by himself; he assumed power to appoint and dismiss ministers and retained the final decision on legislation.

In April 1985 the Council was replaced by a Federal Cabinet. On 30 Dec. 1985 martial law ended. On 6 Aug. 1990 the President, accusing the government of corruption and undermining the constitution, dismissed the Prime Minister, Benazir Bhutto, and all her cabinet, dissolved the National Assembly and declared a state of emergency. New governors were appointed for all four provinces. In Sept. Benazir Bhutto was brought to trial on charges of misconduct and abuse of power.

Governors-General of Pakistan: Quaid-I-Azam Mohammed Ali Jinnah (14 Aug. 1947–11 Sept. 1948); Khawaja Nazimuddin (14 Sept. 1948–18 Oct. 1951; took over the premiership after the assassination of Liaquat Ali Khan); Ghulam Mohammad (19 Oct. 1951–6 Aug. 1955); Maj.-Gen. Iskander Mirza (assumed office of President on 6 Oct. 1955, elected President on 5 March 1956).

Presidents of Pakistan: Maj.-Gen. Iskander Mirza (23 March 1956–28 Oct. 1958); Field Marshal Mohammad Ayub Khan (28 Oct. 1958–25 March 1969); Maj.-Gen. Agha Muhammad Yahya Khan (31 March 1969–20 Dec. 1971); Zulfiqar Ali Bhutto (20 Dec.1971–14 Aug. 1973); Fazal Elahi Chaudhry (14 Aug. 1973–16 Sept. 1978); Gen. Mohammad Zia ul-Haq (16 Sept. 1978–17 Aug. 1988); Ghulam Ishaq Khan (acting 17 Aug. 1988, confirmed 12 Dec. 1988).

AREA AND POPULATION. Pakistan is bounded north-west by Afghanistan, north by the USSR and China, east by India and south by the Arabian Sea. The total area of Pakistan is 307,293 sq. miles (796,095 sq. km); population (1981 census), 84·25m.; males, 44,232,000; females, 40,021,000. Density, 105·8 per sq. km. Estimate (1989) 105·4m. Urban population (1987), 28·3%.

The population of the principal cities is:

Census of 1981

Islamabad	201,000	Multan	730,000	Jhang	195,000
Karachi	5,103,000	Gujranwala	597,000	Sukkur	191,000
Lahore	2,922,000	Peshawar	555,000	Bahawalpur	178,000
Faisalabad	1,092,000	Sialkot	296,000	Kasur	155,000
Rawalpindi	928,000	Sargodha	294,000	Gujrat	154,000
Hyderabad	795,000	Quetta	285,000	Okara	154,000

Population of the provinces (census of 1981) was (1,000):

	Area (sq. km)	*1981 census population Total*	*Male*	*Female*	*Urban*	*1981 density per sq. km (number)*	*Estimated total 1985*
North-west Frontier Province	74,521	11,061	5,761	5,300	1,665	148	12,287
Federally admin. Tribal Areas	27,219	2,199	1,143	1,056	–	81	2,467
Fed. Cap. Territory Islamabad	907	340	185	155	204	376	379
Punjab	205,344	47,292	24,860	22,432	13,051	230	53,840
Sind	140,914	19,029	9,999	9,030	8,243	135	21,682
Baluchistan	347,190	4,332	2,284	2,048	677	12	4,908

By Jan. 1987 there were 3m. Afghan refugees in Pakistan, of whom most were in the North-west Frontier Province, and small numbers in Baluchistan and the Punjab.

Language. The commonest languages are Urdu and Punjabi. Urdu is the national language while English is used in business and in central government. Provincial languages are Punjabi, Sindhi, Pushtu (North-West Frontier Province), Baluchi and Brahvi.

CLIMATE. A weak form of tropical monsoon climate occurs over much of the country, with arid conditions in the north and west, where the wet season is only from Dec. to March. Elsewhere, rain comes mainly in the summer. Summer temperatures are high everywhere, but winters can be cold in the mountainous north. Islamabad. Jan. 50°F (10°C), July 90°F (32·2°C). Annual rainfall 36" (900 mm). Karachi. Jan. 61°F (16·1°C), July 86°F (30°C). Annual rainfall 8" (196 mm). Lahore. Jan. 53°F (11·7°C), July 89°F (31·7°C). Annual rainfall 18" (452 mm).

Multan. Jan. 51°F (10·6°C), July 93°F (33·9°C). Annual rainfall 7" (170 mm). Quetta. Jan. 38°F (3·3°C), July 80°F (26·7°C). Annual rainfall 10" (239 mm).

CONSTITUTION AND GOVERNMENT. Under the Constitution of 1973 Parliament is bi-cameral, comprising a Senate of 63 members (14 from each province elected by the members of the Provincial Assemblies 2 from the federal capital area elected by the National Assembly and 5 from tribal areas), and a National Assembly of 207 directly elected Moslem males, 20 women elected by the National Assembly and 10 religious minority representatives.

The Constitution obliges the Government to enable the people to order their lives in accordance with Islam. The Constitution (Ninth Amendment) Bill, 1986, consolidated Islam as the basis of law. An Ombudsman was appointed in Jan. 1983.

Following the President's dismissal of Benazir Bhutto's government in Aug. 1990, elections were held in Oct. 1990 for the 217 contestable seats in the National Assembly. The 8-party coalition of the Islamic Democratic Alliance (IDA) won 105 seats, and the Pakistan Democratic Alliance, headed by Benazir Bhutto's Pakistan People's Party (PPP), won 45. The electorate was 49m.; turn-out was low. There were 1,331 candidates.

Elections to 42 seats of the Senate were held in March 1991. The IDA won 30 seats, the PPP, 5.

President, Head of State: Ghulam Ishaq Khan.

On 6 Nov. 1990 Nawaz Sharif (b.1949) was elected *Prime Minister* by 153 votes to 39. His cabinet of 18 ministers includes: *Finance*: Sartaj Aziz. *Industry*: Shujaat Hussain.

National flag: Green, charged at the centre, with a white crescent and white 5-pointed star, a white vertical stripe at the mast to one-quarter of the flag.

Provincial and local government. Pakistan comprises the Federal Capital Territory (Islamabad), the provinces of the Punjab, the North-West Frontier (NWFP), Sind and Baluchistan, and the tribal areas of the north-west. The provincial capitals are Peshawar (NWFP), Lahore (Punjab), Karachi (Sind) and Quetta (Baluchistan). Provincial governors are appointed by the President and are assisted by elected provincial assemblies. Elections for all 4 assemblies were held in Oct. 1990.

Within the provinces there are divisions administered by Commissioners appointed by the President; the divisions are divided into districts and agencies administered by Deputy Commissioners or Political Agents who are responsible to the Provincial Governments.

The tribal areas (Khyber, Kurram, Malakand, Mohmand, North Waziristan, South Waziristan) are administered by political agents responsible to the federal government.

Kashmir. Pakistan controls the northern and western portions of Kashmir, an area of about 84,160 sq. km with a population of about 2·8m. in 1985. Under a United Nations resolution of 1949 its future was to be decided by plebiscite; it is still a disputed territory.

The people of Azad Kashmir (the west) have their own Assembly (42 members including 2 women), their own Council (of 14 members), High Court and Supreme Court. There is a Parliamentary form of Government with a Prime Minister as the executive head and the President as the Constitutional head. Elections to the Legislative's 40 general seats are to be held within 10 days of the general elections in Pakistan, according to a presidential proclamation of 8 Oct. 1977. The seat of government is Muzaffarabad.

The Pakistan Government is directly responsible for Gilgit, Diamir and Baltistan (the north).

DEFENCE

Army. The Army consists of 2 armoured and 19 infantry divisions; 7 independent armoured, 4 independent infantry, 7 artillery and 4 anti-aircraft brigades; 3 armoured reconnaissance regiments and 1 Special Services Group. Equipment includes 500 M-47/-48, 50 T-54/-55 and 1,300 Chinese Type-59 and -69 main battle tanks. The Army has an air component with about 150 fixed-wing aircraft for transport, reconnaissance and observation duties and 120 helicopters for anti-armour operations, transport, liaison and training. Strength (1991) 500,000, with a further 500,000 reservists. There are also 164,000 men in paramilitary units: National Guard, Frontier Corps, Pakistan Rangers, Coast Guard and Frontier Constabulary.

Navy. 10 ex-US frigates form the core of the surface fleet. The smaller craft are mostly of Chinese origin.

The combatant fleet comprises 6 French-built diesel submarines, about 6 midget submarines for swimmer delivery, 1 UK-built 'County' class destroyer, *Babur*, converted to carry up to to 4 Sea King anti-submarine helicopters, 2 ex-US Second World War vintage destroyers, 4 ex-US Brooke class guided missile frigates armed with Standard SM-1 surface-to-air missiles, 6 other frigates, 8 fast missile craft, 4 hydrofoil torpedo craft, 4 coastal and 9 inshore patrol craft, and 3 coastal minesweepers. Auxiliaries include 2 fleet replenishment tankers, 1 survey ship and 1 salvage tug, as well as a static ex-US repair ship. There are about a dozen minor auxiliaries.

The Air force operates 5 Atlantic and 1 Fokker F-27 Friendship for maritime patrol and transport duties, whilst the Navy operates 6 Sea King helicopters and 4 Alouette III anti-submarine and liaison helicopters. All destroyers and frigates have helicopter decks capable of operating an Alouette.

The principal naval base and dockyard are at Karachi. Naval personnel in 1990 totalled 20,000.

A navy-subordinated Maritime Safety Agency 2,000 strong (1990) operates 2 ex-naval destroyers and 4 fast inshore patrol craft on economic exclusion zone protection duties.

Air Force. The Pakistan Air Force came into being on 14 Aug. 1947. It has its headquarters at Peshawar and is organized within 3 air defence sectors, in the northern, central and southern areas of the country. Air defence units include 2 squadrons of F-16 Fighting Falcons, 2 squadrons of F-7P Skybolts and at least 6 squadrons of Chinese-built F-6s (MiG-19). Tactical units include 5 squadrons of Mirage III-EP/5 supersonic fighters and 6 with A-5 fighter-bombers, 1 squadron equipped with Mirage III-RP reconnalssance aircraft, and 1 with C-130 Hercules turboprop transports. Flying training schools are equipped with Masshaq (Saab Supporter) armed piston-engined primary trainers, T-37B/C jet trainers supplied by the USA, Mirage III-DPs and Chinese-built FT-5s (two-seat MiG-17s) and FT-6s (two-seat MiG-19s). A VIP transport squadron operates the Presidential F27 turboprop aircraft, 3 four-jet Boing 707s, 3 twin-jet Falcon 20s and a Puma helicopter. There is a flying college at Risalpur and an aeronautical engineering college at Korangi Creek. Total strength in 1991 was 470 combat aircraft and 30,000 all ranks.

INTERNATIONAL RELATIONS

Membership. Pakistan is a member of the UN, the Commonwealth, the Colombo Plan, and Regional Co-operation for Development.

External Debt (30 June 1989), US$19,983·17m.

ECONOMY

Policy. Since 1991 investors have no longer been required to seek government permission to set up industrial units, except in arms and alcohol production.

Budget. The following table shows the budget for the years 1987–88 and 1988–89 in Rs 1m.:

		1988–89
	Revised	*Budget*
Revenue receipts	121,239·8	134,993·9
of which taxes	89,018·6	98,611·9
Capital receipts	71,704·4	66,414·3
of which External	27,515·6	32,040·4
Revenue expenditure	146,233·4	158,606·9
Capital expenditure	39,068·7	43,884·3

Main items of expenditure on revenue account (Rs 1m.):

	1988–89	
	Revised	*Budget*
Defence	45,295·1	48,321·5
Debt servicing	29,343·5	34,201·2
Development	25,628·4	26,776·0
Administration	5,210·6	5,925·9
Social, including health and education	4,538·2	5,853·5

Currency. The monetary unit is the *Pakistan rupee* (PKR) of 100 *paisas*. There are notes of R1, 5, 10, 50 and 100; and coins of 1, 5, 10, 25 and 50 paisas.

Total monetary assets on 30 June 1988 amounted to Rs 269,437m. Currency in circulation, Rs 87,782m. In March 1991 Rs 42·50 = £1; Rs 22·40 = US$1.

Banking and Finance. As from 1 Jan. 1985, banks and other financial institutions abandoned, in conformity with Islamic doctrine, the payment of interest on new transactions. This does not apply to international business, but does apply to the domestic business of foreign banks operating in Pakistan. Investment partnerships, between bank and customer, replaced straight loans at interest.

The State Bank of Pakistan is the central bank; it came into operation as the Central Bank on 1 July 1948 with an authorized capital of Rs 30m. and was nationalized in Jan. 1974. At end June 1988 total assets or liabilities of the issue department amounted to Rs 91,206m. and those of the banking department Rs 82,253m.; total deposits, Rs 68,163m. It is the sole bank of issue for Pakistan, custodian of foreign exchange reserves and banker for the federal and provincial governments and for scheduled banks. It also manages the rupee public debt of federal and provincial governments. It provides short-term loans to the Government and commercial banks and short and medium-term loans to specialized banks. The Bank's subsidiary Federal Bank for Co-operatives makes loans to provincial co-operative banks.

In 1991 there were 10 Pakistani and 20 foreign banks, the former nationalized since 1974. It was announced in Nov. 1990 that 51% of the equity of state-owned banks was to be privatized in 2 phases. Total liabilities or assets of all scheduled banks stood at Rs 481,456·7m., of which time liabilities, Rs 115,184·8m., on the last working day of June, 1988. The National Bank of Pakistan acts as an agent of the State Bank for transacting Government business and managing currency chests at places where the State Bank has no offices of its own.

Weights and Measures. The metric system is in general use.

ENERGY AND NATURAL RESOURCES

Electricity. Installed capacity of the state power system (1986–87) by type of generation: Thermal 3,263 mw., hydro-electric, 2,898 mw.; the Karachi Electric Supply Corporation had 17·9%. Total generated electrical energy in 1986–87, 28,236m. kwh; 15,241m. kwh of this was hydro-electricity, the main source being the Tarbela Dam. By June 1986 21,846 villages (of a total 43,244) had access to electric power. Supply 230 volts; 50 Hz.

Oil. Oil comes mainly from the Potowar Plain, from fields at Meyal, Tut, Balkassar, Joya Mair and Dhullian. Production in 1990 was 3·1m. tonnes. Oil reserves were also found at Dhodak in Dec. 1976. Exploitation is mainly through government incentives and concessions to foreign private sector companies. The Pak-Arab refinery pipeline runs 865 km. from Karachi to Multan; capacity, 4·5m. tonnes of oil annually.

Gas. Gas pipelines from Sui to Karachi (345 miles) and Multan (200) supply natural gas to industry and domestic consumers. A pipeline between Quetta and Shikarpur was constructed in 1982. There are 4 other productive fields. Reserves (1983), 500,000m. cu. metres; production in 1987–88 was 12,383m. cu. metres.

Water. The Indus water treaty of 1960, concluded between India and Pakistan, has created the basis for a large-scale development programme. The Indus Basin Development Fund Agreement has been subscribed by Australia, Canada, Federal Republic of Germany, New Zealand, UK and USA and is administered by the International Bank; the works to be constructed call for expenditure of US$1,000m. The main purpose of the treaty is the division of the water power of the Indus and its 5 tributaries between India and Pakistan. After the construction of some 460 miles of canals, the Indus and the 2 western tributaries will serve Pakistan and the entire flow of the 3 eastern tributaries will be released for use in India.

The largest project is the construction of the Tarbela Dam, an earth-and-rock filled dam on the river Indus, 485 ft high, which has a gross storage capacity of 11·1m. acre feet of water for irrigation.

The Lloyd Barrage and Canal Construction Scheme, consists of a barrage across the river Indus at Sukkur and 7 canals—4 on the left and 3 on the right bank. Another barrage across the Indus, $4^1/_2$ miles north of Kotri, called the Ghulam Muhammad Barrage, was completed in 1955. The Taunsa barrage on the Indus, 80 miles downstream of Kalabagh, was completed in 1958. The Gudu barrage, 10 miles from Kashmore, was completed in 1962.

The province of the Punjab set up in 1949 the Thal Development Authority to colonize the Thal desert between the Indus and Jhelum rivers.

The Chashma canal will carry water 172 miles across Dera Ismail Khan from the Chashma barrage on the Indus. The Mangla Dam on the Jhelum was inaugurated in Nov. 1967.

Minerals. The main agencies are the Pakistan Mineral Development Corporation, the Resource Development Corporation and the Gemstone Corporation of Pakistan. Coal is mined at Sharigh and Harnai on the Sind–Pishin railway and in the Bolan pass, also in Sor Range and Degari in the Quetta–Pishin district and in the Punjab; total recoverable reserves, about 480m. tonnes, mainly low-grade. A further 55m. tonnes was found at Lakhra in 1980 and reserves of over 500m. tonnes were found in the 300 sq. mile Thatta Sadha field in 1981. Copper ore reserves at Saindak, in Balúchistán, 412m. tons, containing (1984 estimate) 1·69m. tons of copper; 2·24m. oz. of gold; 2·2m. oz. of silver. Chromite is extracted in and near Muslimbagh. Limestone is quarried generally. Gypsum is mined in the Sibi district and elsewhere; reserves (1983), about 370m. tonnes. Iron ore is being worked in Kalabagh and elsewhere; reserves, about 400m. tonnes, low-grade. A further 18m. tonnes, high-grade, has been found in Baluchistan. Uranium has been found in Dera Ghazi Khan.

Production (tonnes, 1987–88): Coal, 2·73m.; chromite, 8,628; limestone, 7·61m.; gypsum, 404,042; rock salt, 502,281; fire clay, 133,869. Other minerals of which useful deposits have been found are magnesite, sulphur, barites, marble, bauxite, antimony ore, bentonite, celestite, dolomite, fireclay, fluorite, fuller's earth, phosphate rock, silica sand and soapstone.

Agriculture. The entire area in the north and west is covered by great mountain ranges. The rest of the country consists of a fertile plain watered by 5 big rivers and their tributaries. Agriculture is dependent almost entirely on the irrigation system based on these rivers. Areas irrigated, 1987: Punjab, 11·8m. ha; Sind, 3·3m.; NWFP, 840,000; Baluchistan, 520,000. It employs (1987) about 50% of labour and provides about 22% of GNP. The main crops are wheat, cotton, maize, sugar-cane and rice, while the Quetta and Kalat divisions (Baluchistan) are known for their fruits and dates.

Pakistan is self-sufficient in wheat, rice and sugar. Areas harvested, 1987–88: Wheat, 7·3m. ha; rice, 1·96m. ha; sugar, 841,600 ha.

Production, 1987–88, in 1,000 tonnes: Rice (cleaned), 3,240·9; wheat, 12,675·1; sugar-cane, 33,013·4; cotton, 1,468·5; cottonseed, 2,937; maize, 1,126·9; potatoes, 563·2.

An ordinance of Jan. 1977 reduced the upper limit of land holding to 100 irrigated or 200 non-irrigated acres; it also replaced the former land revenue system with a new agricultural income tax, from which holders of up to 25 irrigated or 50 unirrigated acres are exempt. Of about 4m. farms, 89% are of less than 25 acres. Of the surveyed area of 156m. acres, cultivated land accounts for 63m. acres, of which 11m. acres consist of fallow land, so that the net area sown is 52m. acres.

Livestock (estimate, 1988): Cattle, 17,156,000; buffaloes, 14·02m.; sheep, 27,479,000; goats, 33,018,000; poultry, 151m.

Forestry. In 1986–87 the forest area was 2·9m. ha, some 4% of the total land area. The government considers a 20-25% coverage desirable for economic growth and environmental stability. 14·4m. cu. ft of timber and 19·2m. cu. ft of firewood were produced. Forest lands are also used as national parks, wildlife and game reserves.

Fisheries. In 1987 landings were 336,100 tonnes of marine and 96,100 of inland water fish.

INDUSTRY. Manufacturing (1987–88) contributed about 17% to GNP. In 1972 public sector companies were re-organized under a Board of Industrial Management. Government policy since 1977 has been to encourage private industry, particularly small industry. The public sector, however, is still dominant in large industries. Steel, cement, fertilizer and vegetable ghee are the most valuable public sector industries.

A public sector steel-mill (Pakistan Steel) has been built at Port Qasim near Karachi, capacity 1·1m. tonnes; production of coke and pig-iron began in autumn 1981 and of steel in 1983.

Production 1987–88 (tonnes): Refined sugar, 1·77m.; vegetable products, 685,549; jute textiles, 113,602; soda ash, 134,106; sulphuric acid, 78,723; caustic soda, 61,344; chip board and paper board, 70,027; bicycles, 661,183 units; cotton cloth, 280·9m. sq. metres; cotton yarn, 685·5m. kg.; cement, 7·04m.; steel billets 271,367; hot-rolled steel sheets and coils, 475,621; cold-rolled, 154,550; mild steel products, 867,565.

Labour. The 1981 census gave the total work force as 22·62m. Estimates (1985–86) give 28·9m., employed workforce 27·86m. In 1988 51·15% were engaged in agriculture, forestry and fishing, 12·69% in manufacturing; the textile industry was the largest single manufacturing employer. Services employed 11·39%; commerce, 11·92%; construction, 6·38%; transport, storage and communication, 4·89%.

FOREIGN ECONOMIC RELATIONS. Foreign exchange reserves were US$500m. in Sept. 1990. Most foreign exchange controls were removed in Feb. 1991. Foreign investors may repatriate both capital and profits.

Commerce. Total value of exports, 1987–88: Rs 78,444·6m.; imports: Rs 111,381·9m. (In 1986–87, exports were Rs 63,267·9m., imports, Rs 92,430·8m.). The value of the chief articles imported and exported (in Rs 1m.):

Imports	*1986–87*	*1987–88*	*Exports*	*1986–87*	*1987–88*
Minerals, fuels, lubricants	14,806·2	18,057·5	Cotton cloth	5,931·1	8,539·5
Machinery and transport equipment	27,543·5	32,869·0	Cotton yarns	8,765·6	9,597·4
Edible oils	5,003·4	8,977·0	Rice	5,052·6	6,404·4
Chemicals	15,773·1	17,612·5	Leather	...	5,041·5
Raw cotton	7,675·8	10,758·6	Carpets, tapestries	3,419·5	4,418·2

Of exports (1987–88), Rs 24,530·4m. went to the European Community; Rs 9,582·3m. to the middle east, of which Rs 3,892·1m. was to Saudi Arabia; Rs 8,603·4m. went to USA. Of imports, Rs 29,379·8m. came from the European Community; Rs 12,471·3m. from USA; Rs 20,898·5m. from the middle east, of which Rs 5,621·8m. was from Saudi Arabia.

Total trade between Pakistan and UK (British Department of Trade returns, in £1,000 sterling):

	1986	1987	1988	1989	1990
Imports to UK	131,296	167,315	175,337	216,110	236,448
Exports and re-exports from UK	227,064	252,978	263,300	233,532	251,841

Tourism. In 1987 there were 424,900 tourist arrivals spending US$172·8m.; 189,300 came from India; 110,200 from Europe, including 73,000 from UK.

COMMUNICATIONS

Roads. In 1987–88 Pakistan had 108,530 km of roads, of which 46,143 km were all-weather roads. The Karakoram highway to the Chinese border, through Kohistan and the Hunza valley, was opened in 1978. An all-weather road linking Skardu and the remote NE Indus valley to the highway was built in 1980.

In 1987 there were 2·22m. vehicles registered, including 1·06m. motor-cycles and 514,837 cars, jeeps and station wagons.

Railways. Pakistan Railways had (1988) a route length of 8,775 km (of which 290 km electrified) mainly on 1,676 mm. gauge, with some metre gauge and narrow gauge line. In 1987–88 there were 81·2m. passengers and 11·6m. tonnes of freight.

Aviation. Karachi is served by British Airways, KLM, PANAM, Lufthansa, Swissair, SAS, Iran National Airlines, Air France, Garuda, Gulf Air and by Philippine, Japanese, Chinese, East African, Syrian, Iraqi, Kuwait, Jordanian, Saudi Arabian, Romanian, Egyptian and Soviet airlines.

Pakistan International Airlines (founded 1955; 62% of shares are held by the Government) had 8 Boeing 747s, 8 Airbus A300-B4s, 6 Boeing 707s, 6 Boeing 737-300s, 9 Fokker F-27s, 2 Twin Otters and 5 Cessna Trainers in 1987. Services operate to 30 home and 38 international airports, including London, New York, Frankfurt, Paris, Amsterdam, Copenhagen, İstanbul, Athens, Rome, Cairo, Tripoli, Nairobi, Dhahran, Damascus, Amman, Baghdad, Riyadh, Tokyo, Peking (Beijing), Zahedan, Singapore, Manila, Kuala Lumpur, Bangkok, Colombo, Bombay, Delhi, Dacca, Tehrán, Káthmándu, the Maldive Islands and Jiddah.

At Pakistan airports, 1987–88, there were 10m. passengers (including 6·3m. on domestic flights) and 180,577 tonnes of cargo (61,294).

Shipping. There is a seaport at Karachi, dry-cargo-handling capacity 6m. tonnes a year, oil-handling, 10m. The second port, 26 miles east of Karachi, is Port Muhammad Bin Qasim; it has iron and coal berths for Pakistan Steel Mills, multi-purpose berths, bulk-cargo handling, oil and container-traffic terminals. International shipping entered and cleared (1987–88): Karachi 1,901 and 1,888 vessels; Port Qasim 152 and 154. Cargo handled: Karachi 17·7m. tonnes, Port Qasim 3·72m. Coastal shipping (Pakistani and Arabian craft), total 823 vessels entered (239·1m. NRT), 793 cleared (298·4m.). The Pakistan National Shipping Corporation had 26 vessels in 1988, of 410,234 DWT. National flag carriers now operate between Pakistan and UK; USA and Canada; the Far East; the (Persian) Gulf, Arabian Gulf, Red Sea, Black Sea and Mekran Coast; Continental Europe and the Middle East. The Karachi Shipyard and Engineering Works Ltd construct all types of vessels up to 27,000 DWT and repairs all types; dry-dock and under-water repairs can be done on vessels up to 29,000 DWT, above-water repairs on vessels and drilling rigs of all sizes.

Telecommunications. The telegraph and telephone system is government-owned. Telephones, 1988, numbered 740,000; a nationwide dialling system is in operation between 46 cities. In 1988 there were 12,226 post offices. Pakistan has international telephone connections by 102 satellite, 7 HF, 4 microwave and 10 carrier circuits, and an international direct-dialling exchange. The Pakistan Broadcasting Corporation had 18 radio stations in 1988 and 5 TV stations (Lahore, Karachi, Peshawar, Quetta and Rawalpindi–Islamabad). In 1988 there were 1·51m. radio licences and 1·51m. TV sets, and 235,100 video recorders were in use.

Cinemas (1986). There were about 850 cinemas.

Newspapers. Newspapers and periodicals numbered 1,826 in 1988; 177 were dailies, 368 weeklies, 126 twice-weeklies, 776 monthlies and 374 quarterlies. Titles by language (and average circulation) in 1988: Urdu, 1,343 (263m.); English, 379 (387,741); Sindhi, 72 (64,823). Titles are also published in Pushtu, Punjabi, Baluchi and Brahvi.

JUSTICE, RELIGION, EDUCATION AND WELFARE

Justice. The Central Judiciary consists of the Supreme Court of Pakistan, which is a court of record and has three-fold jurisdiction, namely, original, appellate and advisory. There are 4 High Courts in Lahore, Peshawar, Quetta and Karachi. Under the Constitution, each has power to issue directions of writs of *Habeas Corpus, Mandamus, Certiorari* and others. Under them are district and sessions courts of first instance in each division; they have also some appellate jurisdiction. Criminal cases not being sessions cases are tried by district magistrates and subordinate magistrates. There are subordinate civil courts also.

The Constitution provides for an independent judiciary, as the greatest safeguard of citizens' rights. The Laws (Continuance in Force) (Eleventh Amendment) Order, 1980, prescribed the date of 14 Aug. 1981 by which the judiciary shall be separated from the executive. There is an Attorney-General, appointed by the President, who has right of audience in all courts.

A Federal Shariat Court at the Supreme Court level has been established to decide whether any law is wholly or partially un-Islamic. After the dismissal of Benazir Bhutto's government in Aug. 1990 a presidential ordinanace decreed that the criminal code must conform to Islamic law.

Religion. Religious groups (1981 census): Moslems, 96·68%; Christians, 1·55%; Hindus, 1·51%; Parsees, Buddhists, and others. There is a Minorities Wing at the Religious Affairs Ministry to safeguard the constitutional rights of religious minorities.

Education. At the census of 1981, 23·3% of the population were able to read and write. Estimate (1985), 26%. Adult literacy programmes have been established.

The principle of free and compulsory primary education has been accepted as the responsibility of the state; duration has been fixed provisionally at 5 years. About 49% of children aged 5-9 are enrolled at school. Present policy stresses vocational and technical education, disseminating a common culture based on Islamic ideology. Figures for 1987–88 in 1,000:

	Total pupils	*Female pupils*	*Total teachers*	*Women teachers*	*Institutions*
Primary	7,606	2,498	186·3	59·4	83,872
Middle	2,133	594	61·2	18·5	6,458
High	695	190	82·2	25·7	5,008
Colleges	502	153	35·2	14·4	680
Universities	65	10	4·0	0·6	22

Health. In 1988 there were 710 hospitals and 3,616 dispensaries (52,866 beds) and 55,346 doctors. There were 998 maternity and child welfare centres.

Distribution by province:

	Hospitals	*Dispensaries*	*Mother and child centres*
Punjab	258	1,154	448
Sind	251	1,557	154
NWFP	152	590	325
Baluchistan	45	267	68

DIPLOMATIC REPRESENTATIVES

Of Pakistan in Great Britain (35 Lowndes Sq., London, SW1X 9JN)
High Commissioner: Humayun Khan.

Of Great Britain in Pakistan (Diplomatic Enclave, Ramna 5, Islamabad)
High Commissioner: N. J. Barrington, CMG, CVO.

Of Pakistan in the USA (2315 Massachusetts Ave., NW, Washington, D.C., 20008)
Ambassador: Zulfiqar Ali Khan.

Of the USA in Pakistan (Diplomatic Enclave, Ramna, 5, Islamabad)
Ambassador: Robert B. Oakley.

Of Pakistan to the United Nations
Ambassador: Jamsheed K. A. Marker.

Further Reading

Pakistan Statistical Yearbook. Karachi
Pakistan Yearbook., Karachi
Ahmed, A. S., *Religion and Politics in Muslim Society: Order and Conflict in Pakistan*. CUP, 1973
Ali, T., *Can Pakistan Survive? The Death of the State*. Harmondsworth, 1983
Bhutto, B., *Daughter of the East*. London, 1988
Burki, S. J., *Pakistan Under Bhutto*. London, 1980
Choudbury, G. W., *Pakistan: Transition from Military to Civilian Rule*. London, 1988
Gilmartin, D., *Empire and Islam: Punjab and the making of Pakistan*. London, 1988
Hyman, A. *et al Pakistan: Zia and After*. London, 1989
Jennings, Sir Ivor, *Constitutional Problems in Pakistan*. CUP, 1957
Noman, O., *The Political Economy of Pakistan, 1947-85*. London and New York, 1988
Taylor, D., *Pakistan*. [Bibliography] Oxford and Santa Barbara, 1989
Waseem, N., *Pakistan under Martial Law, 1977-85*. Lahore, 1987

PANAMA

Capital: Panama City
Population: 2·32m. (1990)
GNP per capita: US$2,240 (1987)

República de Panamá

HISTORY. A revolution, supported by the USA, led to the separation of Panama from the United States of Colombia and the declaration of its independence on 3 Nov. 1903. The *de facto* Government was on 5 Nov. recognized by the USA, and soon afterwards by the other Powers. In 1924 Colombia agreed to recognize the independence of Panama. On 8 May 1924 diplomatic relations between Colombia and Panama were established. On 1 Oct. 1979 Panama assumed sovereignty over what was previously known as the Panama Canal Zone and now called the Canal Area. For the treaties regulating the relations between Panama and the USA *see* pp. 983–84.

Elections, the first to be held in Panama for 16 years, were held in May 1984. Nicholas Barletta was elected president and took office in Nov. 1984, but he resigned in Sept. 1985 and was succeeded by one of his vice-presidents.

On 26 Feb. 1988 the Legislative Assembly deposed Eric Arturo Delvalle and appointed Manuel Solis Palma as acting President in his place. Elections on 9 May 1989 were annulled by the Electoral Court. The Council of State elected Francisco Rodríguez and Dr Carlos Ozores as Provisional President and Vice-President. They were sworn in on 1 Sept. 1989 but Gen. Manuel Noriega remained *de facto* leader.

In May 1989 a further 2,000 US troops were sent to Panama and a US-backed coup attempt in Oct. failed. On 15 Dec. Gen. Noriega declared a 'state of war' with the US. On 20 Dec. the US invaded Panama to remove Gen. Noriega from power and he surrendered on 3 Jan. 1990. US troops started to withdraw on 2 Jan.

President Endara Gallimany was elected on 9 May 1989.

AREA AND POPULATION. Panama is bounded north by the Caribbean, east by Colombia, south by the Pacific and west by Costa Rica. Extreme length is about 480 miles (772 km); breadth between 37 (60) and 110 miles (177 km); coastline, 726 miles (1,160 km) on the Atlantic and 1,060 (1,697 km) on the Pacific; total area is 29,761 sq. miles (77,082 sq. km); population according to the census of 13 May 1990 was 2,315,047. Over 75% are of mixed blood and the remainder Indians, negroid, white and Asiatic. In 1988, 52% were urban. Over 93% speak Spanish, the official language, 3% speak Guaymí and 2% Kuna (both Amerindian languages).

The largest towns (census, 1990) are Panama City, the capital on the Pacific coast (578,461); its suburb San Miguelito (242,529); Colón, the port on the Atlantic coast (140,732); and David (102,517).

The areas and populations of the 9 provinces and the Special Territory were:

Province	*Sq. km*	*Census 1980*	*Census 1990*	*Capital*
Bocas del Toro	9,506	53,579	92,731	Bocas del Toro
Chiriquí	8,924	287,801	368,023	David
Veraguas	11,226	173,195	202,904	Santiago
Herrera	2,185	81,866	93,360	Chitré
Los Santos	4,587	70,200	76,604	Las Tablas
Coclé	4,981	140,320	172,165	Penonomé
Colón	7,205	166,439	202,007	Colón
San Blas (Special Territory)	3,206			El Porvenir
Panama	11,400	830,278	1,064,221	Panama City
Darién	15,458	26,497	43,032	La Palma

Vital statistics (1988): Births, 58,093; marriages, 10,112; deaths, 10,416. Crude birth rate (per 1,000): 25·0.

CLIMATE. A tropical climate, unvaryingly with high temperatures and only a short dry season from Jan. to April. Rainfall amounts are much higher on the north side of the isthmus. Panama City. Jan. 79°F (26·1°C), July 81°F (27·2°C). Annual rainfall 70" (1,770 mm). Colón. Jan. 80°F (26·7°C), July 80°F (26·7°C). Annual rainfall 127" (3,175 mm). Balboa Heights. Jan. 80°F (26·7°C), July 81°F (27·2°C). Annual rainfall 70" (1,759 mm). Cristóbal. Jan. 80°F (26·7°C), July 81°F (27·2°C). Annual rainfall 130" (3,255 mm).

CONSTITUTION AND GOVERNMENT. The 1972 Constitution, as amended in 1978 and 1983, provides for a president and two vice-presidents to be elected by direct popular vote and a 67-seat Legislative Assembly to be elected on a party basis; in 28 of the 40 constituencies the party winning the vote obtaining one seat; in the other 12, the 39 remaining seats being allocated on a system of proportional party representation. There are also 510 Representatives elected, one member for each electoral district.

The President elected on 9 May was sworn in by an electoral tribunal on 27 Dec. 1989. By-elections were held in Jan. 1991 for the 9 seats vacant because the 1989 were invalidated.

President: Guillermo Endara Gallimany.

Vice Presidents: Ricardo Arias Calderón (also *Minister of the Interior*); Guillermo Ford (also *Minister of Planning*).

National flag: Quarterly: first a white panel with a blue star, second red, third blue, fourth white with a red star.

National anthem: Alcanzamos por fin la victoria (words by J. de la Ossa; tune by Santos Jorge, 1903).

Local government: The 9 provinces and a Special Territory (another is envisaged) are sub-divided into 67 municipal districts and are further sub-divided into 510 *corregimientos* (electoral districts).

DEFENCE. All armed forces were disbanded in 1990. Previous strengths were:

Army. The Army (National Guard) numbered (1990) 3,500 men organized in 8 light infantry companies, equipped with 16 V-150 and 13 V-300 armoured cars. There is one air-borne group. There was (1990) a para-military force of 11,000.

Navy. Divided between both coasts, the National Maritime Service, a coast guard rather than a navy comprised 2 patrol craft, 1 smaller craft, 4 utility landing craft, and 1 logistic support vessel. In 1990 personnel totalled 380.

Air Force. Prior to the US intervention in late 1989 the service had 5 CASA 212, 2 Islander, 1 CN-235 and 2 Twin Otter transports, 4 Cessna and 2 DHC-3 Otter liaison aircraft, a Falcon 20 and 2 Boeing 727s for VIP transport, 25 UH-1B/H Iroquois and twin-engined UH-1N helicopters plus a Super Puma for official use. Four Chilean-built Pillan trainers were used for training. Personnel (1990) 500.

INTERNATIONAL RELATIONS

Membership. Panama is a member of the UN, OAS and Non-aligned Countries.

ECONOMY

Budget. The 1988 budget provided for expenditure of 847m. balboas and revenue of 605m. balboas. Public sector debt was US$3,771m. in 1989.

Currency. The monetary unit is the *balboa* (PAB). Other coins are the half-balboa (equal to 50 cents US); the quarter and tenth of a balboa piece; a cupro-nickel coin of 5 cents, and a copper coin of 1 cent. US coinage is also legal tender. The only paper currency used is that of the USA. In March 1991, US$1 = 1 *balboa*; £1 = 1·90 *balboas*.

Banking and Finance. There is no statutory central bank. The Government accounts are handled through the *Banco Nacional de Panama*. The number of commercial banks was 132 in June 1986. Leading banks are the Citibank, Lloyds Bank International (Bahamas) Ltd., and the Chase Manhattan Bank of New York. Other foreign-owned banks include the Bank of America, as well as Canadian.

Weights and Measures. English weights and measures are in general use; the metric system is the official system.

ENERGY AND NATURAL RESOURCES

Electricity. Production (1988) 2,558m. kwh. Supply 110 and 120 volts; 60 Hz.

Minerals. There are known to be copper deposits in the provinces of Chiriquí, Colón and Darién. The most important, containing possibly the largest undeveloped reserves in the world, is Cerro Colorado (Chiriquí) on which a feasibility study was undertaken by the Rio Tinto Zinc Corporation Ltd. The deposit has estimated reserves of 1,300m. tonnes, with an average grade of 0·76% copper.

Agriculture. Of the whole area (1981) 15·6% is cultivated, 57·6% is natural or artificial pasture land and 8·6% is fallow. Of the remainder only a small part is cultivated, though the land is rich in resources. About 60% of the country's food requirements are imported. Production in 1988 totalled 900,000 tonnes of bananas and 107,000 tonnes of raw sugar. Oranges (36,000 tonnes) and mangoes (28,000 tonnes) are also produced. Most important food crop, for home consumption, is rice, grown on 80% of the farms; Panama's *per capita* consumption is very high. Production of rice was 166,000 tonnes in 1988. Other products are maize (97,000 tonnes in 1988), cocoa (1,000 tonnes), coffee (13,000 tonnes) and coconuts (22,000 tonnes). Beer, whisky, rum, 'seco', anise and gin are produced. Coffee is mainly grown in the province of Chiriquí, near the Costa Rican frontier. The country has great timber resources, notably mahogany. Livestock (1988): 1,502,000 cattle, 240,000 pigs and 7m. poultry.

Forestry. Production (1986) 2·05m. cu. metres.

Fisheries. The catch in 1988 was 92,951 tonnes.

INDUSTRY. Local industries include cigarettes, clothing, food processing, shoes, soap, cement factories; foreign firms are being encouraged to establish industries, and a petrol refinery is operating at Colón.

FOREIGN ECONOMIC RELATIONS. Foreign debt was some US$6,000m. in May 1990.

Commerce. Imports and exports for 4 calendar years (in 1,000 balboas):

	Imports	*Exports*		*Imports*	*Exports*
1986	1,275,245	326,864	1988	795,454	291,786
1987	1,307,755	336,158	1989	985,100	349,800

Total trade between Panama and UK (British Department of Trade returns, in £1,000 sterling):

	1986	*1987*	*1988*	*1989*	*1990*
Imports to UK	4,950	4,919	12,230	6,818	4,056
Exports and re-exports from UK [1]	44,975	40,020	32,497	32,875	35,552

[1] Including new ships built for foreign owners and registered in Panama.

Tourism. In 1989, 211,000 people visited Panama.

COMMUNICATIONS

Roads. Panama had in 1988, 9,651 km of roads. The road from Panama City westward to the cities of David and Concepción and to the Costa Rican frontier, with several branches, is part of the Pan-American Highway. A concrete highway connects Panama City and Colón.

In 1988 there were 176,400 registered motor vehicles.

Railways. The *Ferrocarril de Panama* (Panama Railroad) (1,524 mm gauge) (through the Canal area), which connects Ancón on the Pacific with Cristóbal on the Atlantic, is the principal railway. It is 190 km long and runs along the banks of the Canal. As most vessels unload their cargo at Cristóbal (Colón), on the Atlantic side, the greater portion of the merchandise destined for Panama City is brought overland by the *Ferrocarril de Panama*. The United Brands Company runs 376 km of railway, and the Chiriquí National Railroad 171 km.

Aviation. Eastern Airlines, Swissair, Varig, JAL, Alitalia, KLM, Iberia Airlines, Aeromexico, VIASA, Air France and other international companies operate at Tocumén Airport, 12 miles from Panama City. Air Panama provides services between Panama City and New York, Los Angeles, Miami, Central America and some countries in South America. The *Compañía Panameña de Aviación* (COPA) and *Aerolineas Las Perlas* provide a local service between Panama City and the provincial towns. COPA also provides an international service to Central America and some countries in Latin America.

Shipping. Ships under Panamanian registry in 1990 numbered 11,500 of 58m. gross tons; most of these ships elect Panamanian registry because fees are low and labour laws lenient. All the international maritime traffic for Colón and Panama runs through the Canal ports of Cristóbal, Balboa and Bahia Las Minas (Colón); Almirante is used for both the provincial and international trade. There is an oil transfer terminal at Puerto Armuelles on the Pacific coast.

Panama Canal. On 18 Nov. 1903 a treaty between the USA and the Republic of Panama was signed making it possible for the US to build and operate a canal connecting the Atlantic and Pacific oceans through the Isthmus of Panama. The treaty granted the US in perpetuity the use, occupation and control of a Canal Zone, approximately 10 miles wide, in which the US would possess full sovereign rights 'to the entire exclusion of the exercise by the Republic of Panama of any such sovereign rights, power or authority'. In return the US guaranteed the independence of the republic and agreed to pay the republic $10m. and an annuity of $250,000. The US purchased the French rights and properties—the French had been labouring from 1879 to 1899 in an effort to build the Canal—for $40m. and in addition, paid private landholders within what would be the Canal Zone a mutually agreeable price for their properties.

Two new treaties between Panama and USA were agreed on 10 Aug. and signed on 7 Sept. 1977. One deals with the operation and defence of the canal until the end of 1999 and the other guarantees permanent neutrality.

The USA maintains operational control over all lands, waters and installations, including military bases, necessary to manage, operate and defend the canal until 31 Dec. 1999. A new agency of the US Government, the Panama Canal Commission, operates the canal, replacing the Panama Canal Co. A policy-making board of 5 US citizens and 4 Panamanians serves on the Commission's board of directors. Until 31 Dec. 1989 the canal administrator was a US citizen and the deputy was Panamanian. After that date the position was reversed.

Six months after the exchange of instruments of ratification Panama assumed general territorial jurisdiction over the former Canal Zone and became able to use portions of the area not needed for the operation and defence of the canal. Panamanian penal and civil codes became applicable. At the same time Panama assumed responsibility for commercial ship repairs and supplies, railway and pier operations, passengers, police and courts, all of which were among other areas formerly administered by the Panama Canal Company and the Canal Zone Government.

66% of the electorate of Panama agreed to the ratification of the treaties when a referendum was held on 23 Oct. 1977 and on 18 April 1978 the treaty was ratified by the US Congress. The treaty went into effect on 1 Oct. 1979.

At the end of 1962 the US completed the construction of a high-level bridge over the Pacific entrance to the Canal, and the flags of Panama and the US were flown jointly over areas of the Canal Zone under civilian authority. Following the devaluation of the dollar in 1972 and 1973, the annuity was adjusted proportionally to US$2·1m. and US$2·33m. respectively.

In 1986 a tripartite commission, formed by Japan, Panama and the USA, began studies on alternatives to the Panama Canal. Options are: To build a sea-level canal, to enlarge the existing canal with more locks, to improve the canal alongside upgraded rail and road facilities, to continue with the existing facilities.

The Panama Canal Commission, a US Government Agency, is concerned primarily with the actual operation of the Canal. On 8 July 1974, 18 Nov. 1976, 10 Oct. 1979 and 12 March 1983 tolls were increased. These were the first increases of toll rates in the history of the Canal. Tolls were raised again on 1 Oct. 1989. The new rates are US$2.01 a Panama Canal ton for vessels carrying passengers or cargo and US$1·60 per ton for vessels in transit in ballast. A Panama Canal ton is equivalent to 100 cu. ft of actual earning capacity. The new toll rate for warships, hospital ships and supply ships, which pay on a displacement basis, is US$1·12 a ton.

The changes were designed to continue the approximately break-even financial operating results after paying its own expenses and paying interest on the net direct investment of the US in the Canal.

Administrator of the Panama Canal Commission: Gilberto Guardia Fábrega.

US military personnel assigned permanently in Panama in Sept. 1989 were approximately 10,000. The total permanent workforce employed by the Panama Canal Commission in Sept. 1990 was 7,232, comprising 921 US citizens, 6,231 Panamanians and 74 others.

The Canal was opened to commerce on 15 Aug. 1914. It is 85 ft above sea-level. It is 51·2 statute miles in length from deep water in the Caribbean Sea to deep water in the Pacific Ocean, and 36 statute miles from shore to shore. The channel ranges in bottom-width from 500 to 1,000 ft; the widening of Gaillard Cut to a minimum width of 500 ft was completed in 1969. Normally, the average time of a vessel in Canal waters is about 24 hours, 8–12 of which are in transit through the Canal proper. A map showing the Panama, Suez and Kiel canals on the same scale will be found in THE STATESMAN'S YEAR-BOOK, 1959 and a further map in the 1978–79 edition.

Particulars of the ocean-going commercial traffic through the canal are given as follows (vessels of 300 tons Panama Canal net and 500 displacement tons and over; cargo in long tons):

Fiscal year ending 30 Sept.	*North-bound (Pacific to Atlantic)*		*South-bound (Atlantic to Pacific)*		*Total*		*Tolls levied*[1] *(in US$)*
	Vessels	*Cargo*	*Vessels*	*Cargo*	*Vessels*	*Cargo*	
1987	5,766	61,683,921	6,464	87,006,459	12,230	148,690,380	329,858,775
1988	5,807	65,504,306	6,427	90,978,335	12,234	156,482,641	339,319,326
1989	5,678	63,360,524	6,311	88,275,589	11,989	151,636,113	329,696,838
1990	5,667	66,107,105	6,274	90,965,873	11,941	157,072,978	355,557,957

[1] All annual tolls figures have been revised to show total tolls collected instead of oceangoing commercial tolls.

In the fiscal year ending 30 Sept. 1990, 13,325 ships passed through the Canal. Transits by flag included 1,866 Panamanian; 1,479 Liberian; 660 Norwegian; 611 US; 585 Greek; 542 Cypriot; 501 Japanese; 500 Soviet; 404 UK; 372 Bahamian; 364 Filipino; 337 Ecuadorian.

Statistical Information: The Panama Canal Commission Office of Public Affairs.

Annual Reports on the Panama Canal, by the Administrator of the Panama Canal Commission.
Rules and Regulations Governing Navigation of the Panama Canal. The Panama Canal Commission, Miami, Florida *or* Washington, DC
Cameron, I., *The Impossible Dream*. London, 1972
Le Feber, W., *The Panama Canal: The Crisis in Historical Perspective*. OUP, 1978
McCullough, D., *The Path Between the Seas*. New York and London, 1978

Telecommunications. There are telegraph cables from Panama to North America and Central and South American ports, and from Colón to the USA and Europe. There is also inter-continental communication by satellite. There were (1985) 97 licensed commercial broadcasting stations, nearly all operated by private companies, one of which functions in the canal. There are 6 television stations, one of them run by the US Army at Fort Clayton. In 1985 there were 295,000 radio and 400,000 television sets. In 1988 there were 241,900 telephones.

Newspapers. There were (1989) 1 English language and 5 Spanish language daily morning newspapers and 1 English/Spanish evening newspaper.

JUSTICE, RELIGION, EDUCATION AND WELFARE

Justice. The Supreme Court consists of 9 justices appointed by the executive. There is no death penalty. The police force numbered 12,000 in 1991.

Religion. 85% of the population is Roman Catholic, 5% Protestant, 4·5% Moslem. There is freedom of religious worship and separation of Church and State. Clergymen may teach in the schools but may not hold public office.

Education. Elementary education is compulsory for all children from 7 to 15 years of age, with an estimated 543,453 students in schools in 1988. The University of Panama at Panama City, inaugurated on 7 Oct. 1935, and the Catholic university Sta. Maria La Antigua, inaugurated on 27 May 1965, had a combined enrolment of 51,058 students in 1988.

Health. In 1988 there were 2,761 doctors, 527 dentists and 2,514 nursing personnel. There were 58 hospitals, 178 health centres and 435 health sub-centres with a total of 7,776 beds.

DIPLOMATIC REPRESENTATIVES

Of Panama in Great Britain (119 Crawford St., London, W1H 1AF)
Ambassador: Teodoro F. Franco (accredited 3 April 1990).

Of Great Britain in Panama (Apartado 889, Panama City 1)
Ambassador: John Grant MacDonald, CBE.

Of Panama in the USA (2862 McGill Terr., NW, Washington, D.C., 20008)
Ambassador: Eduardo Vallarino.

Of the USA in Panama (Apartado 6959, Panama City 5)
Ambassador: Dean R. Hinton.

Of Panama to the United Nations
Ambassador: César Pereira Burgos.

Further Reading

Statistical Information: The Comptroller-General of the Republic (Contraloria General de la República, Calle 35 y Avenida 6, Panama City) publishes an annual report and other statistical publications.

Jorden, W. J., *Panama Odyssey*. Univ. of Texas Press, 1984
Langstaff, E. DeS., *Panama*. [Bibliography] Oxford and Santa Barbara 1982
Ropp, S. C., *Panamanian Politics*. New York, 1982
Sahota, G. S., *Poverty Theory and Policy: a Study of Panama*. Johns Hopkins Univ. Press, 1990

National Library: Biblioteca Nacional, Departamento de Información. Calle 22, Panama.

PAPUA NEW GUINEA

Capital: Port Moresby
Population: 3·8m. (1990)
GNP per capita: US$770 (1988)

HISTORY. To prevent that portion of the island of New Guinea not claimed by the Netherlands or Germany from passing into the hands of a foreign power, the Government of Queensland annexed Papua in 1883. This step was not sanctioned by the Imperial Government, but on 6 Nov. 1884 a British Protectorate was proclaimed over the southern portion of the eastern half of New Guinea, and in 1887 Queensland, New South Wales and Victoria undertook to defray the cost of administration, and the territory was annexed to the Crown the following year. The federal government took over the control in 1901; the political transfer was completed by the Papua Act of the federal parliament in Nov. 1905, and on 1 Sept. 1906 a proclamation was issued by the Governor-General of Australia declaring that British New Guinea was to be known henceforth as the Territory of Papua. The northern portion of New Guinea was a German colony until the First World War. It became a League of Nations mandated territory in 1921, administered by Australia, and later a UN Trust Territory (of New Guinea).

The Papua New Guinea Act 1949–1972 provides for the administration of the UN Australian Trust Territory of New Guinea in an administrative union with the Territory of Papua, in accordance with Art. 5 of the New Guinea Trusteeship Agreement, under the title of Papua New Guinea.

Australia granted Papua New Guinea self-government on 1 Dec. 1973 and, on 16 Sept. 1975, Papua New Guinea became a fully independent state.

In Jan. 1991 peace talks between the government and the secessionist Bougaineville Revolutionary Army (BRA) ended 2 years of fighting. Weapons were to be surrendered to an international peace-keeping force.

AREA AND POPULATION. Papua New Guinea extends from the equator to Cape Baganowa in the Louisiade Archipelago to 11° 40' S. lat. and from the border of West Irian to 160° E. long. with a total area of 462,840 sq. km. According to the census the 1980 population was 3,010,727. Estimate (1990) 3·8m. Port Moresby, 152,100; Lae, 79,600; Rabaul (1980), 14,954; Madang, 24,700; Wewak, 23,200; Goroka, 21,800; Mount Hagen (1980), 13,441. Area and population of the provinces:

Provinces	*Sq.km*	*Census 1980*	*Estimate 1987*	*Capital*
Milne Bay	14,000	127,975	153,800	Alotau
Northern	22,800	77,442	92,200	Popondetta
Central	29,500	116,964	135,000	Port Moresby
National Capital District	240	123,624	145,300	—
Gulf	34,500	64,120	72,600	Kerema
Western	99,300	78,575	93,600	Daru
Southern Highlands	23,800	236,052	262,400	Mendi
Enga	12,800	164,534	180,100	Wabag
Western Highlands	8,500	265,656	304,800	Mount Hagen
Chimbu	6,100	178,290	186,800	Kundiawa
Eastern Highlands	11,200	276,726	310,300	Goroka
Morobe	34,500	310,622	364,400	Lae
Madang	29,000	211,069	251,100	Madang
East Sepik	42,800	221,890	260,000	Wewak
West Sepik	36,300	114,192	130,100	Vanimo
Manus	2,100	26,036	30,500	Lorengau
West New Britain	21,000	88,941	110,600	Kimbe
East New Britain	15,500	133,197	157,800	Rabaul
New Ireland	9,600	66,028	78,900	Kavieng
North Solomons	9,300	128,794	159,100	Arawa

Vital statistics (1987, estimate): Crude birth rate, 35 per 1,000; crude death rate, 13.

CLIMATE. There is a monsoon climate, with high temperatures and humidity the year round. Port Moresby is in a rain shadow and is not typical of the rest of Papua New Guinea. Jan. 82°F (27·8°C), July 78°F (25·6°C). Annual rainfall 40" (1,011 mm).

CONSTITUTION AND GOVERNMENT. Papua New Guinea has a Westminster type of government. A single legislative house, known as the National Parliament, is made up of 109 members from all parts of the country. The members are elected under universal suffrage and general elections are held every 5 years. All persons over the age of 18 who are Papua New Guinea citizens are eligible to vote and stand for election. Voting is by secret ballot and follows the preferential system.

The first Legislative Council was established in 1951. It was abolished in 1964 and replaced with the House of Assembly.

In the general elections held in June-July 1987, 26 seats were won by the Pangu Party, 18 by the People's Democratic Movement, 12 by the National Party, 32 by other parties and 21 by independents. A PDM-led government held office until 4 July 1988, when it was defeated in Parliament and replaced by one led by the Pangu Party.

Governor-General: Sir Serei Eri.

The Cabinet in Feb. 1991 was as follows:

Prime Minister: Rt. Hon. Rabbie Namaliu.

Deputy Prime Minister, Public Service: Ted Diro. *Agriculture and Livestock:* Tom Pais. *Finance and Planning:* Paul Pora. *Tourism and Culture:* Aruru Matiabe. *Minerals and Energy:* Patterson Lowa. *Forests:* Karl Stack. *Provincial Affairs:* John Momis. *Transport:* Anthony Temo. *Justice:* Bernard Narakobi. *Education:* Utula Samana. *Defence:* Benias Sabumei. *Communications:* Brown Sinamoi. *Works and Supply:* Paul Wanjik. *Fisheries and Marine Resources and Minister of State, Assisting the Prime Minister:* Akoka Doi. *Environment and Conservation:* Jim Waim. *Foreign Affairs:* Michael Somare. *Lands and Physical Planning:* Karl Swokin. *Health:* Beona Motawiya. *Labour and Employment:* Toni Ila. *Police:* Mathias Ijape. *Home Affairs and Youth:* Matthew Bendumb. *Trade and Industry:* John Giheno. *Correctional Services:* Melchior Pep. *Housing:* Michael Singan. *Administrative Services:* Theodore Tuyo. *Civil Aviation:* Bernard Vogae.

The seat of the Government is at Port Moresby.

National flag: Diagonally ochre-red over black, on the red a bird of paradise in gold, and on the black 5 stars of the Southern Cross in white.

Local government: In 1950 the first village council was formed which established the basis of an extensive local government system. A system of provincial government was introduced in 1976 and, since then, the importance of lower-level local government has diminished.

DEFENCE. The Papua New Guinea Defence Force has a total strength of 3,500 (1991) consisting of land, maritime and air elements. The Army is organized in 2 infantry and 1 engineer battalions. The Navy, based at Port Moresby and Manus, is all of Australian build and comprises 5 inshore patrol craft and 2 tank landing craft. Personnel numbered 300 in 1990. The Defence Force has an Air Transport Squadron with (1990) about 100 personnel. Current equipment comprises 5 C-47 transports, and 4 Australian-built N22B Nomads and 3 Israeli-built Aravas for both transport and border patrol duties. The Aravas were being offered for sale late in 1989.

INTERNATIONAL RELATIONS

Membership. Papua New Guinea is a member of the UN, the Commonwealth, the Colombo Plan, the South Pacific Commission and the South Pacific Forum and is an ACP state of the EEC.

ECONOMY

Budget. Revenue (in K1,000) for calendar years was:

Source	*1988*	*1989*	*1990*
Customs, excise and export tax	246,000	301,000	369,100
Other taxes	263,000	266,160	319,900
Foreign government grants [1]	189,865	190,550	182,715
Loans	180,667	198,809	144,450
Other revenue	107,341	122,000	135,000
Total	986,873	1,078,519	1,151,165

[1] Mainly from Australia.

Expenditure (in K1,000) for the same periods:

Source	*1986*	*1987*	*1988*
Consumption	513,350	538,250	530,590
Capital	138,830	71,438	81,042
Other expenditure [1]	178,930	254,317	298,501
Total	831,100	864,005	910,133

[1] Includes transfers to provincial governments.

Currency. The unit of currency is the *kina* (PGK) of 100 *toea*. In March 1991, £1 = K1·79; US$1 = K0·95.

Banking and Finance. The Bank of Papua New Guinea assumed the central banking functions formerly undertaken by the Reserve Bank of Australia on 1 Nov. 1973.

A national banking institution which has been named the Papua New Guinea Banking Corporation has been established. This bank has assumed the Papua New Guinea business of the Commonwealth Trading Bank of Australia except where certain accounts give rise to special financial or contractual problems.

The subsidiaries of 3 Australian commercial banks also operate in Papua New Guinea. These are the Australia and New Zealand Banking Group (PNG) Ltd, the Bank of New South Wales (PNG) Ltd, and the Bank of South Pacific Ltd, all of which offer trading and savings facilities. As from 1 Nov. 1973 these banks operated under Papua New Guinea banking legislation.

In 1983, two additional commercial banks Indosuez Niugini Bank Ltd and Niugini Lloyds International Bank Ltd began operating, each with 51% national ownership, and the remaining 49% held by the affiliate of a major international bank.

In addition to these five commercial banks, the Agriculture Bank of Papua New Guinea (formerly the Development Bank) has provided long-term development finance with a particular attention to the needs of small-scale enterprises since 1967. The country's first merchant bank, Resources and Investment Finance Ltd (RIFL), specializing in large-scale financial services began business in late 1979. Its shares are owned by the Hong Kong and Shanghai Banking Corporation, the Commonwealth Trading Bank of Australia and the Papua New Guinea Banking Corporation.

On 30 June 1987 commercial banks deposits totalled K762·2m.

Weights and Measures. The metric system is in force.

ENERGY AND NATURAL RESOURCES

Electricity. In 1986 installed capacity was 494,300 mw, production 1,602·4m. kwh.

Oil. The Iagifu field in the Southern Highlands had (1988) potential recoverable reserves of 500m. bbls.

Minerals. Copper is the main mineral product. Gold, copper and silver are the only minerals produced in quantity. The Misima open-pit gold mine, first mined in 1888, was opened in 1989. Production is forecast at 210,000 oz a year with a life of 10 years. The Porgera gold mine opened in 1990 with an expected life of 20 years. Major copper deposits in Bougainville have proven reserves of about 800m. tonnes;

mining was halted by secessionist rebel activity. Copper and gold deposits in the Star Mountains of the Western Province are being developed by Ok Tedi Mining Ltd at the Mt. Fubilan mine. Production of gold commenced in 1984 and of copper concentrates in 1987. In 1986, B.C.L. produced 586,552 tonnes of copper concentrate containing approximately 178,593 tonnes of copper, 16,367 kg of gold and 50,385 kg of silver; Ok Tedi Mining Ltd produced 18,277 kg of gold and 5,677 kg of silver.

Agriculture. At 31 Dec. 1983, the total area of larger holdings was 397,081 hectares, of which 180,000 hectares were for agricultural purposes, the principal crops being coffee, copra, cocoa and palm oil. Minor commercial crops include pyrethrum, tea, peanuts and spices. Locally consumed food crops include sweet potatoes, maize, taro, bananas, rice and sago. Tropical fruits grow abundantly. There is extensive grassland. A newly-established sugar industry has made the country self-sufficient in this commodity while a beef-cattle industry is being developed.

Production (1988, in 1,000 tonnes): Coffee, 72; copra, 155; cocoa beans, 36; palm oil, 156.

Livestock (1988): Cattle, 101,000; pigs, 1·7m.; goats, 12,000; poultry, 3m.

Forestry. Timber production is of growing importance for both local consumption and export. In 1986, 1·7m. cu. metres of logs were harvested; logs exported, 1·3m. cu. metres.

Production of sawn timber, 1986, 84,000 cu. metres, exports, 7,438 cu. metres; exports of woodchips, 81,037 tonnes.

Fisheries. Tuna, both skipjack and yellowfin species, is the major fisheries resource; in 1980 the catch was 33,000 tonnes but has diminished sharply since then due to oversupply conditions on world markets. Exports of various crustacea, 1986, 1,575 tonnes, value K10·47m.

INDUSTRY. Secondary and service industries are expanding for the local market. The main industries were (1988) food processing, beverages, tobacco, timber products, wood, and fabricated metal products. In 1985 there were 707 factories employing 27,195 persons. Value of output K695m.

Labour. In 1980 about 733,000 were gainfully employed.

FOREIGN ECONOMIC RELATIONS. Australian aid amounts to an annual $A300m.

Commerce. Imports (in K1,000) for calendar years:

	1986	*1987*	*1988*
Food and live animals	162,809	171,524	181,777
Beverages and tobacco	8,481	11,888	15,456
Crude materials, inedible, except fuels	6,945	7,824	8,577
Mineral fuels, lubricants and related materials	93,444	112,047	98,183
Oils and fats (animal and vegetable)	3,453	3,608	3,346
Chemicals	81,568	84,595	84,404
Manufactured goods, chiefly by material	149,046	181,570	205,720
Machinery and transport equipment	307,997	339,631	424,738
Miscellaneous manufactured articles	75,973	87,636	99,137
Commodities and transactions of merchandise trade, not elsewhere specified	12,353	12,550	12,352
Total imports	902,069	1,012,874	1,133,691

Exports (in K1,000) for calendar years:

	1987	*1988*	*1989*
Coconut and copra products—			
Copra	15,113	19,486	15,484
Copra (coconut) oil	14,486	17,456	15,179
Copra cake and pellets	1,034	1,262	1,597
Total	30,633	38,204	32,260

	1987	*1988*	*1989*
Coffee beans	134,643	113,512	138,070
Cocoa beans	56,359	46,017	45,048
Crude rubber	3,078	4,401	3,177
Tea	5,571	6,439	6,037
Pyrethrum extract	249	148	–
Forest and timber products			
Logs	103,028	91,013	91,602
Sawn timber	1,259	1,039	1,386
Other	6,780	6,238	5,566
Total	111,067	98,290	95,554
Crocodile skins	1,879	877	928
Crayfish and prawns	10,509	7,321	7,320
Gold	140,573	112,096	61,158
Copper concentrate	538,315	702,756	691,004
Other domestic produce	35,726	37,640	14,551
Total domestic produce	1,069,262	1,169,253	1,205,935
Re-exports	17,665	34,484	59,667
Total exports	1,086,927	1,203,737	1,265,602

Of exports in 1988, Japan took 41%, Federal Republic of Germany, 22% and Australia, 6%; of imports (1987), Australia furnished about 43%, Singapore, 7% and Japan, 19%.

Total trade between Papua New Guinea and UK (British Department of Trade returns, in £1,000 sterling):

	1986	*1987*	*1988*	*1989*	*1990*
Imports to UK	38,474	46,045	44,291	47,839	34,849
Exports and re-exports from UK	12,084	16,693	20,521	15,822	8,793

Tourism. In 1988, there were 40,529 visitors of which 10,648 were tourists.

COMMUNICATIONS

Roads. In 1985 there were approximately 19,736 km of roads including approximately 1,200 km paved. Motor vehicles numbered (1986) 45,713 including 16,499 cars and station wagons.

Aviation. Frequent air services operate to and from Australia (Sydney, Brisbane and Cairns), and there are regular flights to Djayapura (Indonesia), Manila and Singapore. A service is also maintained to Honiara in the Solomon Islands. In addition to Air Niugini, the national flag carrier, Qantas operates in and out of Papua New Guinea. There are a total of 177 airports and airstrips with scheduled services.

Shipping. There are regular shipping services between Australia and Papua New Guinea ports, and also services to New Zealand, Japan, Hong Kong, US west coast, Singapore, Solomon Islands, Vanuatu, Taiwan, Philippines and Europe. Small coastal vessels run between the various ports. In 1985 cargo discharged from overseas was 1·5m. tonnes; cargo loaded for overseas was 2·1m. tonnes.

Telecommunications. Telephones numbered 63,212 on 31 Dec. 1986. The National Broadcasting Commission operates three networks. A national service is relayed throughout the country by a series of transmitters on medium- and short-wave bands. Local services operate in each of the 19 provinces, mainly on short-wave, while the larger urban centres are also covered by a commercial FM network relayed from Port Moresby. Two commercial television stations broadcast to Port Moresby which had plans (1987) to extend their services to other areas. In 1985 there were 230,000 television and (1986) 225,000 radio receivers.

Newspapers. In 1986 there was one daily newspaper with a circulation of 28,000.

JUSTICE, RELIGION, EDUCATION AND WELFARE

Justice. In 1983, over 1,500 criminal and civil cases were heard in the National Court and an estimated 120,000 cases in district and local courts.

Police. Total uniformed strength at 31 Dec. 1986, 4,756.

Religion. At the 1980 Census, Protestants formed 64% of the population and Roman Catholics 33%.

Education. At 30 June 1986 about 374,950 children attended 2,461 primary schools and 60,052 enrolled in 234 secondary, technical and vocational schools. The University of Papua New Guinea and the Papua New Guinea University of Technology had 3,029 students enrolled in full-time courses in 1986.

Health. In 1986, there were 19 hospitals, 459 health centres, 2,231 aid posts and 283 doctors.

DIPLOMATIC REPRESENTATIVES

Of Papua New Guinea in Great Britain (14 Waterloo Pl., London, SW1R 4AR)
High Commissioner: Philip Bouraga, CBE.

Of Great Britain in Papua New Guinea (Kiroki St., Port Moresby)
High Commissioner: E. J. Sharland.

Of Papua New Guinea in the USA (1330 Connecticut Ave., NW, Washington D.C., 20036)
Ambassador: Margaret Taylor.

Of the USA in Papua New Guinea (Armit St., Port Moresby)
Ambassador: Robert W. Farrand.

Of Papua New Guinea to the United Nations
Ambassador: Renagi Lohia.

Further Reading

The Territory of Papua. Annual Report. Commonwealth of Australia. 1906–1940–41 and from 1945–46
The Territory of New Guinea. Annual Report. Commonwealth of Australia. 1914–1940–41 and from 1946–47
Papua New Guinea, Annual Report. From 1970–71
Hasluck, P., *A Time for Building.* Melbourne Univ. Press, 1976
McConnell, F., *Papua New Guinea.* [Bibliography] Oxford and Santa Barbara, 1988
Ross, A. C. and Langmore, J., *Alternative Strategies for Papua New Guinea.* OUP, 1974
Ryan, P. (ed.) *Encyclopaedia of Papua and New Guinea.* Melbourne Univ. Press, 1972
Skeldon, R. (ed.) *The Demography of Papua New Guinea.* Institute of Applied Social and Economic Research, 1979

PARAGUAY

Capital: Asunción
Population: 4·16m. (1990)
GNP per capita: US$1,180 (1988)

República del Paraguay

HISTORY. The Republic of Paraguay gained its independence from Spain on 14 May 1811. In 1814 Dr José Gaspar Rodríguez de Francia was elected dictator, and in 1816 perpetual dictator by the National Assembly. He died 20 Sept. 1840. In 1844 a new constitution was adopted, under which Carlos Antonio López (first elected in 1842, died 10 Sept. 1862) and his son, Francisco Solano López, ruled until 1870. During the devastating war against Brazil, Argentina and Uruguay (1865–70) Paraguay's population was reduced from about 600,000 to 232,000. Argentina, in Aug. 1942, and Brazil, in May 1943, voided the reparations which Paraguay had never paid. Further severe losses were incurred during the war with Bolivia (1932–35) over territorial claims in the Chaco. A peace treaty by which Paraguay obtained most of the area her troops had conquered was signed in July 1938.

AREA AND POPULATION. Paraguay is bounded north-west by Bolivia, north-east and east by Brazil, south-east, south and south-west by Argentina. The area of the Oriental province is officially estimated at 159,827 sq. km (61,705 sq. miles) and the Occidental province at 246,925 sq. km (95,337 sq. miles), making the total area of the republic 406,752 sq. km (157,042 sq. miles).

The population (Census 1982) was 3,035,360; estimate (1990) 4,157,287. In 1984 the capital, Asunción (and metropolitan area), had 729,307 inhabitants; other principal cities: Presidente Stroessner (110,000), Pedro Juan Caballero (80,000), Encarnación (31,445), Pilar (26,352), Concepción (25,607).

The capital district and 19 departments had the following populations in 1982:

Asunción (city) / Central	729,307	Misiones	79,278
		Neembucu	70,689
Caaguazú	299,227	Amambay	68,422
Itapua	263,021	Canendiyú	65,807
Paraguari	202,152	*Oriente*	*2,959,568*
Cordillera	194,826	Presidente Hayes	43,787
San Pedro	189,751	Boquerón	14,685
Alto Paraná	188,351	Alto Paraguay	4,535
Guairá	143,374	Chaco	286
Concepción	135,068	Nueva Asunción	231
Caazapá	109,510	*Occidente*	*63,524*

Number of births, 1986, was 109,626; deaths, 11,519.

The population is overwhelmingly *mestizo* (mixed Spanish and Guaraní Indian) forming a homogeneous stock. There are some 46,700 unassimilated Indians of other tribal origin, in the Chaco and the forests of eastern Paraguay. There are some small traces of Negro descent. 40·1% of the population speak only Guaraní; 48·2% are bilingual (Spanish/Guaraní); and 6·4% speak only Spanish.

Mennonites who arrived in 3 groups (1927, 1930 and 1947) are settled in the Chaco and Oriental Paraguay and were estimated in 1969 to number 13,000, of whom 2,000 came from Canada and 11,000 from Germany. The Japanese colonists in the Oriental section, who first came in 1935, were reckoned to number 7,000 in 1983. An agreement with Korea was signed in 1966 and there were (1988) about 7,575 Korean families living in Paraguay.

CLIMATE. A tropical climate, with abundant rainfall and only a short dry season from July to Sept., when temperatures are lowest. Asunción. Jan. 81°F (30°C), July 64°F (17·8°C). Annual rainfall 53" (1,316 mm).

CONSTITUTION AND GOVERNMENT. A new constitution replacing that of 1940 was drawn up by a Constituent Convention in which all legally recognized political parties were represented and was signed into law on 25 Aug. 1967. It provides for a two-chamber parliament consisting of a 36-seat Senate and a 72-seat House of Deputies, each elected for a 5-year term. Two-thirds of the seats in each House are allocated to the majority party (since 1954 the *Partido Colorado)* and the remaining one-third shared among the minority parties in proportion to the votes cast. Voting is compulsory for all citizens over 18. The President is directly elected for a 5-year (renewable) term; he appoints the Cabinet and during parliamentary recess can govern by decree through the Council of State, the members of which are representatives of the Government, the armed forces and other bodies. Gen. Stroessner was deposed in a *coup* on 3 Feb. 1989. At the presidential elections held on 1 May 1989 Gen. Rodríguez received 74·18% of the vote.

President: Gen. Andrés Rodríguez, assumed office 3 Feb. 1989; inaugurated after election on 15 May 1989.

The following is a list of past presidents since 1948, with the date on which each took office:

Dr J. Natalicio González, 15 Aug. 1948 (deposed).
Gen. Raimundo Rolón, 30 Jan. 1949.
Dr Felipe Molas López, 26 Feb. 1949[1] (resigned).
Dr Federico Chávez, 16 July 1950 (resigned).
Tomás Romero Pereira, 4 May 1954.
Gen. Alfredo Stroessner, 11 July 1954 (deposed).

[1] Provisional, *i.e.*, following a coup d'état.

The Cabinet in Jan. 1991 was composed as follows:

Foreign Affairs: Dr Alexis Frutos Vaesken. *Interior:* Gen. Orlando Machuca Vargas. *Finance:* Enzo Debernardi. *Public Health and Social Welfare:* Cynthia Prieto. *Justice and Labour:* Dr Hugo Estigarribia. *Public Works and Communications:* Gen. Porfirio Pereira Ruiz Díaz. *Industry and Commerce:* Pedro Antonio Zuccolillo. *Education and Worship:* Dr Angel R. Seifart. *Without Portfolio:* Dr Juan Ramón Chaves. *Defence:* Brig.-Gen. Angel Juan Souto Hernández. *Agriculture and Livestock:* Dr Raúl Torres. *Secretary-General of the Presidency:* Conrado Pappalardo.

National flag: Red, white, blue (horizontal); the white stripe charged with the arms of the republic on the obverse, and, on the reverse, with a lion and the inscription *Paz y Justicia*—the only flag in the world with different obverse and reverse.

National anthem: ¡Paraguayos, república o muerte! ('Paraguayans, republic or death!' words by F. Acuña de Figueroa; tune by F. Dupey).

The country is divided into 2 provinces: the 'Oriental', east of Paraguay River, and the 'Occidental', west of the same river. The Oriental section is divided into 14 departments and the capital. The more important departments are supervised by a *Delegado* appointed by and directly responsible to the central government. The Occidental province, or Chaco, is divided into 5 departments.

DEFENCE. The army, navy and air forces are separate services under a single command. The President of the Republic is the active Commander-in-Chief. The armed forces totalled (1991) about 16,000 (9,800 conscripts). Conscription is for 18 months (2 years in the navy). There are some 45,000 reserves.

Army. The Army consists of 1 cavalry division, 8 infantry divisions and supporting artillery, engineer and signals units. Equipment includes 3 M-4A3 main battle and 18 M-3A1 light tanks. Strength (1991) 12,500 (including 8,600 conscripts).

Navy. The flotilla comprises 6 armoured river defence gunboats (the average age of which exceeds 40 years), 1 converted landing ship with helicopter deck, 7 river patrol boats, 1 ocean-going transport and training ship, and about 12 service craft. There are 2 AT-6G naval counter-insurgency aircraft, 1 Dakota transport and 3 helicopters. Personnel in 1990 totalled 2,500 including 500 marines, of whom 1,000 were conscripts.

Air Force. The Air Force came into being in the early thirties. After operating only transport and training aircraft for a number of years, it received 9 Xavante light jet strike/training aircraft from Brazil in 1980. Other types in service include about 6 C-47 and 4 Aviocar twin-engined transports, 1 Convair C-131A, a Twin Otter, an Otter, 8 Brazilian-built Uirapuru primary trainers, 12 T-6 Texan, 5 Brazilian-supplied Universal armed basic trainers, 5 Tucano advanced trainers and a number of light aircraft and helicopters. HQ and flying school are at Campo Grande, Asunción. Personnel (1991) 1,000 (700 conscripts), with 20 combat aircraft.

INTERNATIONAL RELATIONS

Membership. Paraguay is a member of the UN, OAS and LAIA.

ECONOMY

Budget. In 1989 the central budget balanced at Gs. 815,796,996.

Currency. The *guaraní* was established on 5 Oct. 1943 equal to 100 old paper pesos. Total monetary circulation was Gs.81,531m. in Dec. 1983. There were (1988) two official rates of exchange; a rate Gs.400 for the import of oil and by-products and Gs.550 for other goods. Inflation was an annualized 36% in 1990. Rate of exchange, March 1991: 1,321 *guaranís* = US$1; 2,507 *guaranís* = £1.

Banking and Finance. The Banco Central del Paraguay opened 1 July 1952 to take over the central banking functions previously assigned to the National Bank of Paraguay, which had opened in March 1943 and been reorganized as the Banco del Paraguay in Sept. 1944 with a monetary, a banking and a mortgage department. The Banco del Paraguay closed in Nov. 1961 and has been replaced, with the aid of a US loan of US$3m., by the Banco Nacional de Fomento.

The Banco Nacional de Fomento, Lloyds Bank, Banco Exterior do Brasil, Citibank, Banco de Asunción, Banco Exterior SA, Banco Unión SA, Banco Paraguayo de Comercio, Banco Real del Paraguay SA, Banco Aleman Transatlantico, Banco Holandés Unido, Banco Nacional del Estado de São Paulo, Yegros y Azara, Interbanco, Banco Paraná and Banco de Inversiones all have agencies in Asunción and branches in some main towns.

Weights and Measures. The metric system was officially adopted on 1 Jan. 1901.

ENERGY AND NATURAL RESOURCES

Electricity. Electricity requirements are supplied by Acaray hydro-electric power plant. Production in 1988 was 13,535m. kwh. Supply 220 volts; 50 Hz.

Itaipú, the largest hydro-electric dam in the world, a joint effort of the governments of Brazil and Paraguay, was inaugurated in 1982 and it is estimated that the whole project will be completed in 1990. Eventually it will have 18 turbogenerators, each with a capacity of 700,000 kw. In 1984 the first turbine started generating power.

The Yacyretá project is being carried out by the Binational Commission Yacyretá which was created by a treaty between the governments of Argentina and Paraguay. Work is being carried out on this project and it is hoped that the plant will be in full operation by the end of this decade. Initially 20 turbines each of 135,000 kw generating capacity will be installed giving the plant an initial output of 2·7m. kw.

Oil. The oil refinery at Villa Elisa, which has been in operation since 1966, has a production of about 3,500 bbls a day. Exploration for petroleum in the Chaco yielded negative results but prospecting was continuing in 1988.

Minerals. Iron, manganese and other minerals have been reported but have not been shown to be commercially exploitable. There are large deposits of limestone, and also salt, kaolin and apatite. National and international firms have acquired licences to prospect for oil and natural gas in the Chaco.

Agriculture. In 1981 it was estimated that agriculture absorbs some 51·4m. ha. In 1989, the main agricultural products (in 1,000 tonnes) were: Mandioca (cassava),

3,978; soybeans, 1,614; maize, 1,211; cotton, 630; wheat, 432; rice, 93; tobacco, 2; sugar-cane, 2,909; poroto (green beans), 46.

Wheat, soybeans, cotton, sugar, tobacco, coffee are increasing in importance, as are also essential oils and oilseeds. *Yerba maté*, or strongly flavoured Paraguayan tea, continues to be produced but is declining in importance.

Livestock (1988). Paraguay had about 7,780,000 cattle, 328,000 horses, 2,108,000 pigs, 430,000 sheep.

Forestry. In 1988, 39% of the land area was forested (15·6m. hectares). In the Oriental section there are reserves of hardwoods and cedars that have scarcely been exploited. Palms, tung and other trees are exploited for their oils. The Japanese are experimenting with mulberries for silk growing. Pines and firs have been introduced under a UN project. In 1986, 181,355 tons of timber were exported.

INDUSTRY. Production, 1988 (1,000 tons): Frozen meat, 15·5; cotton fibre, 187·4; sugar, 98·1; rice, 34·8; wheat flour, 104·5; edible oil, 39·7; industrial oil, 12·9; tung oil, 6·9; sawn timber, 629·7; cement, 255·6; soybean, peanut and coconut flour, 405; cigarettes (1m. packets), 46,598; matches (1,000 boxes), 8,979. There are 3 meat-packing plants and other factories producing vegetable oils. A textile industry in Pilar and Asunción meets a large part of local needs.

Trade Unions. Trade unionists number about 30,000 (*Confederación Paraguaya de Trabajadores* and *Confederación Cristiana de Trabajadores*).

FOREIGN ECONOMIC RELATIONS

Commerce. Imports and exports (in US$1m.):

	1985	*1986*	*1987*	*1988*	*1989*
Imports	442·3	509·4	517·5	494·7	1,009·4
Exports	303·9	232·5	353·4	509·8	660·8

Chief exports in 1989 included (in US$1,000): Soybeans, 382,967; cotton fibres, 306,920; meat, 96,116; coffee, 40,340; vegetable oil, 16,537; sawn wood, 31,611; cake and expellers, 10,460; tobacco, 2,147; hides, 24,026; tung oil, 6,662; essential oils, 24,686.

Chief imports 1989 (in US$1,000): Fuels and lubricants, 115,004; machinery, 211,647; chemical and pharmaceutical products, 42,543; transport and accessories, 61,718; drinks and tobacco, 45,516; foodstuffs, 19,790; iron and manufactures, 19,650; agricultural implements and accessories, 12,010; paper, cardboard and paper products, 17,751; metal products, 7,550.

Imports and exports (in US$), by country, 1989:

Country	*Imports*	*Exports*
Algeria	49,475	...
Argentina	67,752	48,976
Belgium	6,138	35,693
Brazil	177,150	328,473
Federal Republic of Germany	29,117	23,280
France	9,842	7,600
Italy	5,729	24,146
Japan	82,102	...
Netherlands	...	186,892
Spain	4,285	21,093
Sweden	1,459	...
Switzerland	6,133	73,779
UK	26,902	5,341
Uruguay	6,487	10,582
USA	93,838	89,659

Total trade between Paraguay and UK (British Department of Trade returns, in £1,000 sterling):

	1986	*1987*	*1988*	*1989*	*1990*
Imports to UK	1,455	1,409	1,950	8,898	10,077
Exports and re-exports from UK	31,010	25,409	22,024	19,282	32,035

Tourism. Visitors numbered 300,000 in 1989.

COMMUNICATIONS

Roads. In 1986 there were 23,606 km of roads, of which 2,159 were paved. The principal paved roads are Route No. 2/7 running from Asunción to the bridge over the Paraná at Puerto Presidente Stroessner, and thence down to the ocean at Paranaguá; and Route No. 1 to Encarnación in the south. The other main arteries are Coronel Oviedo-Pedro Juan Caballero road (unpaved from Coronel Oviedo) in the north and the Trans-Chaco road which starts from the bridge across the river Paraguay north of Asunción and ends at Nueva Asunción on the Bolivian border. Unpaved roads are closed when it rains. In the Argentine, a paved road starts from Pilcomayo, opposite Asunción, and provides good communication with Buenos Aires. In 1987 there were 90,000 vehicles (36,900 cars, 24,300 lorries, 2,700 buses and 26,100 jeeps and taxis).

Railways. The President Carlos Antonio López (formerly Paraguay Central) Railway runs from Asunción to Encarnación, on the Río Alto Paraná, with a length of 441 km (1,435 mm gauge), and connects with Argentine Railways over the Encarnación-Posadas bridge opened in 1989. In 1986, traffic amounted to 156,231 tonnes and 348,535 passengers.

Aviation. International services are operated by 8 airlines (1 domestic and 7 foreign) and internal routes by military airlines and some small private lines.

Shipping. In flood the Paraguay River, which divides the country into two distinct parts, is navigable for 12ft-draught vessels as far as Concepción, 180 miles north of Asunción, and for smaller vessels for a further distance of 600 miles northward. Drought conditions often restrict navigation to lighter traffic. The Paraná River is navigable by large boats from Corrientes up to Puerto Aguirre, at the mouth of the Yguazú River. Boats of a few hundred tons capacity navigate the tributary rivers.

Asunción, the chief port, is 950 miles from the sea. The cargo fleet includes 25 vessels of 300–1,000 tons, 3 tankers of 1,100–1,700 tons, 2 passenger river boats and 1 ocean-going freighter of 713 tons.

Telecommunications. In 1985 there were 382 postal offices and 88,730 telephones. In Dec. 1984 there were 266,200 television and 624,000 radio receivers. There are 4 television stations.

Cinemas (1986). Cinemas numbered 6 in Asunción. The larger country towns usually have an outdoor cinema.

Newspapers (1988). There were 5 daily newspapers in Asunción.

JUSTICE, RELIGION, EDUCATION AND WELFARE

Justice. The highest court is the Supreme Court with 5 members. There are special Chambers of Appeal for civil and commercial cases, and criminal cases. Judges of first instance deal with civil, commercial and criminal cases in 6 departments. Minor cases are dealt with by Justices of the Peace.

The Attorney-General represents the State in all jurisdictions, with representatives in each judicial department and in every jurisdiction. In matters of revenue, taxes, etc., the State is represented by the *Abogado del Tesoro*.

Religion. Religious liberty is guaranteed by the 1967 constitution. Article 6 thereof recognizes Roman Catholicism as the official religion of the country. The same article states that relations between Paraguay and the Holy See shall be regulated by concordats or other bilateral agreements, but no such agreements have yet been negotiated.

The Roman Catholic Church is organized into the Archdiocese of Asunción, 3 other dioceses (San Juan Bautista de las Misiones, Concepción and Villarrica); 4 Prelatures (Coronel Oviedo, Encarnación, Alto Paraná and Caacupé); and 2 Vicariates Apostolic (Chaco and Pilcomayo). The bishops meet in a Conference of Paraguayan Bishops. Only civil marriages are legally valid. There are numerous non-catholic communities, the largest of whom are the Mennonites. There is a small Anglican church in Asunción, with missions in the Chaco, which comes under the jurisdiction of an Anglican Bishop resident in Asunción.

Education. Education is free and nominally compulsory. In 1987 there were 4,101 primary schools (public and private) with 579,687 pupils and 28,136 teachers. In 1985 there were 740 secondary schools with (1987) 148,516 students and (1982) 2,448 teachers. The National University in Asunción had, in 1987, 18,711 students and (1985) 2,694 professors; the Catholic University had 10,409 students and (1984) 900 professors.

Health. In 1982 there were 2,201 doctors. In 1979 there were 855 dentists, 860 pharmacists, 783 midwives and 2,636 nursing personnel. In 1985 there were 3,380 hospital beds.

DIPLOMATIC REPRESENTATIVES

Of Paraguay in Great Britain (51 Cornwall Gdns, London, SW7 4AQ)
Ambassador: Anthony Espinoza.

Of Great Britain in Paraguay (Calle Presidente Franco, 706, Asunción)
Ambassador and Consul-General: T. H. Steggle, CMG.

Of Paraguay in the USA (2400 Massachusetts Ave., NW, Washington, D.C., 20008)
Ambassador: Dr Marcos Martínez Mendieta.

Of the USA in Paraguay (1776 Mariscal López Ave., Asunción)
Ambassador: Timothy Towell.

Of Paraguay to the United Nations
Ambassador: Alfredo Cañete.

Further Reading

Gaceta Official, published by Imprenta Nacional, Estrella y Estero Bellaco, Asunción
Anuario Daumas. Asunción
Anuario Estadístico de la República del Paraguay. Asunción. Annual
Lewis, P. H., *Paraguay under Stroessner.* Univ. of North Carolina Press, 1980
Maybury-Lewis, D. and Howe, J., *The Indian Peoples of Paraguay: Their Plight and Their Prospects.* Cambridge, Mass., 1980
Nickson, R. A., *Paraguay.* [Bibliography] Oxford and Santa Barbara, 1987

National Library: Biblioteca Nacional, De la Rosidenta, Asunción.

PERU

República del Perú

Capital: Lima
Population: 22·33m. (1990)
GNP per capita: US$1,470 (1987)

HISTORY. The Republic of Peru, formerly the most important of the Spanish vice-royalties in South America, declared its independence on 28 July 1821; but it was not till after a war, protracted till 1824, that the country gained its actual freedom.

On 3 Oct. 1968 a military junta overthrew the government of President Fernando Belaúnde Terry and installed Gen. Juan Velasco Alvarado as President of a 'Revolutionary Government' with a cabinet composed entirely of officers of the armed services. Gen. Velasco was ousted in bloodless coup in Aug. 1975 and was replaced by Gen. Francisco Morales Bermudez.

Civilian government was restored in July 1980.

AREA AND POPULATION. Peru is bounded north by Ecuador and Colombia, east by Brazil and Bolivia, south by Chile and west by the Pacific Ocean. Area 1,285,216 sq. km (496,093 sq. miles).

The long-standing dispute with Chile over the provinces of Tacna and Arica (*see* THE STATESMAN'S YEAR-BOOK, 1928, p. 1198) reached an amicable settlement on 3 June 1929 at Lima, Tacna going to Peru and Arica to Chile. In response to demands by Bolivia for permanent access to the Pacific Coast, proposals for a Bolivian corridor to the sea and a new Bolivian port to be built in the disputed area have been put forward by Chile and Peru. To date, little progress has been made. One result has been increased tension along the Chilean–Peruvian border, there is no sign of a settlement of the border dispute, and the armed forces of both countries remain on the alert in the disputed border area. Fighting broke out between Peruvian and Ecuadorean Forces, in early 1981, along part of the disputed border (the Cordillera del Condor) which has to date not been adequately mapped. A number of proposals for settling the issue permanently have been put forward but a final settlement is unlikely to be reached in the near future. For an account of the settlement of other boundary disputes, *see* THE STATESMAN'S YEAR-BOOK, 1948, p. 1173.

Census population, 1981, 17,005,210. Estimate (1990), 22,332,100 (11,249,300 male). Vital statistics 1989: Births, 730,000; deaths, 190,000; infant deaths (under 1 year), 60,800. Birth rate per 1,000 in 1989, 33.5; death rate, 8.7; infant mortality rate per 1,000 live births, 83·3. Expectation of life in 1989: males, 60.8 years; females, 64.7.

Area and population of the 24 departments and the constitutional province of Callao, together with their capitals:

Department	*Sq. km*	*Estimate 1990*	*Capital*	*Estimate 1990*
Amazonas	39,249	335,300	Chachapoyas	14,000
Ancash	35,041	983,200	Huaraz	65,600
Apurímac	20,895	371,700	Abancay	29,200
Arequipa	63,345	965,000	Arequipa	634,500
Ayacucho	43,814	566,400	Ayacucho	101,600
Cajamarca	34,023	1,270,600	Cajamarca	92,600
Callao [1]	147	588,600	Callao [2]	...
Cuzco	71,892	1,041,800	Cuzco	275,000
Huancavelica	22,131	375,700	Huancavelica	27,400
Huánuco	37,722	609,200	Huánuco	86,300
Ica	21,328	542,900	Ica	152,300
Junín	44,410	1,113,600	Huancayo	207,600
La Libertad	24,795	1,243,500	Trujillo	532,000
Lambayeque	14,231	935,300	Chiclayo	426,300
Lima	34,802	6,707,300	Lima [2]	...
Loreto	368,852	654,100	Iquitos	269,500

[1] Constitutional province.
[2] Lima/Callao metropolitan area 6,404,500.

Department	*Sq. km*	*Estimate 1990*	*Capital*	*Estimate 1990*
Madre de Dios	85,183	49,000	Puerto Maldonado	21,200
Moquegua	15,734	134,100	Moquegua	31,500
Pasco	25,320	282,900	Pasco	77,000
Piura	35,892	1,494,300	Piura	324,500
Puno	72,012	1,023,500	Puno	99,600
San Martín	51,253	460,000	Moyobamba	26,000
Tacna	16,063	209,800	Tacna	150,200
Tumbes	4,669	144,200	Tumbes	64,800
Ucayali	102,411	230,100	Pucallpa	153,000

[1] Constitutional province.
[2] Lima/Callao metropolitan area 6,404,500.

The official languages are Spanish (spoken by 68% of the population) and Quechua (spoken by 27%); 3% speak Aymara.

In 1991 there were some 100,000 Peruvians of Japanese origin.

CLIMATE. There is a very wide variety of climate, ranging from equatorial to desert, (or perpetual snow on the high mountains). In coastal areas, temperatures vary very little, either daily or annually, though humidity and cloudiness show considerable variation, with highest humidity from May to Sept. Little rain is experienced in that period. In the Sierra, temperatures remain fairly constant over the year, but the daily range is considerable. There the dry season is from April to Nov. Desert conditions occur in the extreme south, where the climate is uniformly dry, with a few heavy showers falling between Jan. and March. Lima. Jan. 74°F (23·3°C), July 62°F (16·7°C). Annual rainfall 2" (48 mm). Cuzco. Jan. 56°F (13·3°C), July 50°F (10°C). Annual rainfall 32" (804 mm).

CONSTITUTION AND GOVERNMENT. The new Constitution, which became effective when a civilian government was installed in July 1980, provides for a Legislature consisting of a *Senate* (60 members) and a *Chamber of Deputies* (180 members) and an Executive formed of the President of the Republic and a Council of Ministers appointed by him. Elections are held every 5 years with the President and Congress elected, at the same time, by separate ballots. All citizens over the age of 18 are eligible to vote. Voting is compulsory.

In June 1990 Alberto Fujimori (b.1938; change 90 Movement) was elected president with 56% of votes cast.

Presidents since 1963:

Gen. Nicolás Lindley López, 3 March–28 July 1963.
Fernando Belaúnde Terry, 28 July 1963–3 Oct. 1968.[1]
Gen. Juan Velasco Alvarado, 3 Oct. 1968–29 Aug. 1975.[1]
Gen. Francisco Morales Bermudez, 29 Aug. 1975–28 July 1980.
Fernando Belaúnde Terry, 28 July 1980–28 July 1985.
Alan García Pérez, 28 July 1985–27 July 1990

[1] Deposed.

President: Alberto Fujimori (sworn in 28 July 1990).

The 11-member Cabinet in Feb. 1991 included:

Prime Minister and Economy: Carlos Coloña Bher.

Defence: Gen. Jorge Torres Aciego. *Education:* Gloria Helfer Palacios. *Foreign Affairs*: Adm. Raúl Sanchez Sotomayor. *Interior*: Gen. Adolfo Alvarado Fournier. *Energy and Mines*: Fernando Sanchez Albaverg. *Industry*: Guido Pennano. *Justice*: Augusto Antonioli Vasquez. *Labour*: Carlos Torres y Torres Lara.

There are 24 departments divided into 179 provinces (plus the constitutional province of Callao) and 1,764 districts; the province of Callao has some of the functions of a department.

National flag: Three vertical strips of red, white, red, with the national arms in the centre.

National anthem: Somos libres, seámoslo siempre ('We are free, let us always be so'; words by J. de la Torre Ugarte; tune by J. B. Alcedo, 1821).

DEFENCE

Army. There is selective conscription for 2 years. The country is divided into 5 military regions.

The Army comprises (1991) approximately 80,000 men (60,000 conscripts) and 188,000 reserves. There are 2 armoured, 1 cavalry, 8 infantry, 1 airborne and 1 jungle divisions with supporting artillery, engineer and helicopter battalions. There is an air element of 35 Mil Mi-8 and Mi-17, 2 Mi-6 and 1 Alouette III helicopter, plus about a dozen fixed-wing transport and liaison aircraft. Equipment includes 350 T-54/-55 main battle and 110 AMX-13 light tanks, over 300 light armoured fighting vehicles and 105-mm./130-mm./155-mm. field artillery.

There is a para-military national police force of 70,000 personnel.

Navy. The principal ships of the Navy are the former Netherlands cruisers *Almirante Grau* and *Aguirre* built in 1953. *Almirante Grau*'s main armament is 8 152 mm guns and 8 Otomat surface-to-surface missiles. *Aguirre* has been converted to a helicopter cruiser and mounts only 4 152 mm guns, the after two turrets having been removed in favour of a hangar and flight deck capable of supporting 3 SH-3D Sea King helicopters.

There are 11 diesel submarines, 6 built in West Germany (1974-82), and 5 ex-US over 30 years old. Other combatants include 2 modernized former British Daring class and 6 ex-Netherlands Friesland class destroyers of 1950s vintage, 4 Italian Lupo class frigates, 6 French-built fast missile craft and 4 tank landing ships. Major auxiliaries include 5 tankers, 2 transports, 1 survey ship and 1 ocean tug, and 30 minor auxiliaries and service craft. A river flotilla of 10 patrol craft police the Upper Amazon, based at Puerto Maldonado and Iquitos.

The Naval Aviation branch comprises 8 S-2 Trackers and 3 Super-King Air anti-submarine aircraft based ashore, 6 Sea King and 6 AB-212 anti-submarine helicopters for service afloat plus 15 miscellaneous transport and utility aircraft.

Callao is the main base, where the dockyard is located and most training takes place. Smaller ocean bases exist at Paita and Talara.

Naval personnel in 1990 totalled 25,000 (12,000 conscripts) including the Naval Air Arm and 2,500 Marines.

The Coast Guard, 600 strong in 1990, includes 6 coastal patrol craft, 5 inshore and 10 river patrol craft.

Air Force. The operational force consists of 5 combat groups. No. 6 Group has 2 squadrons of Mirage 5 jet fighters; No. 9 Group has 2 squadrons of Canberra light jet bombers; No. 7 Group has 2 squadrons of A-37B light attack aircraft; No. 12 Group has Soviet-built Su-22 variable-geometry fighter bombers in 2 operational squadrons; No. 11 Group has one squadron of Su-22s and one with Mirage 2000s. Other aircraft in service include medium transports (1 F.28 Fellowship, 15 An-32, 14 C-130/L-100 Hercules), light transports (16 Twin Otter, 1 twin-jet Falcon and 12 Turbo-Porter), helicopters (2 Mi-6 and 6 Mi-8, 24 Mi-24 gunships, Bell 47G, 206, 212, 214ST, 412 and UH-1, BO 105 and Alouette III), 70 training aircraft (including Aermacchi MB 339, T-37 and T-41D) and a small number of miscellaneous types for photographic and communications duties. There are military airfields at Talara, Chiclayo, Piura, Pisco, Lima (2), Iquitos and La Joya, and a seaplane base at Iquitos. All officers and pilots are trained at the Air Academy at Lima (Las Palmas). In 1991 there were some 15,000 personnel (7,000 conscripts) and 116 combat aircraft.

INTERNATIONAL RELATIONS

Membership. Peru is a member of the UN, OAS, the Andean Group and LAIA.

ECONOMY

Budget. The budget for 1987 envisaged expenditure of 92,539m. intis and revenue of 66,424m. intis.

Currency. The monetary unit is the new *sol*, which replaced the inti in 1990. In March 1991, £1 = 1·06 *soles*; US$1 = 0·56 *soles*.

Banking and Finance. The bank of issue is the Banco Central de Reserva, which was established in 1922. The government's fiscal agent is the Banco de la Nación.

There were, in 1991, 12 commercial banks (of which 7 were state-owned), 2 foreign commercial banks, 5 development banks, 6 regional commercial banks and a savings bank.

Weights and Measures. The metric system is in use.

ENERGY AND NATURAL RESOURCES

Electricity. In 1989 the production of electric energy was 13,736m. kwh (10,518m. kwh hydro-electric). Supply 220 volts; 60 Hz.

Oil. Proven oil reserves in 1989 amounted to 406m. bbls. Output amounted to 5·9m. tonnes in 1989.

Minerals. Lead, copper, iron, silver, zinc and petroleum are the chief minerals exploited. Mineral production (in 1,000 tonnes, 1989) of iron, 2,908; zinc, 598; copper, 364; lead, 192; silver, 1,840,000 kg; gold, 3,790,000 kg.

Agriculture. There are 4 natural zones: The coast strip, with an average width of 80 km; the Sierra or Uplands, formed by the coast range of mountains and the Andes proper; the Montaña or high wooded region which lies on the eastern slopes of the Andes, and the jungle in the Amazon Basin, known as the Selva. In 1984 irrigation was increasing the amount of cultivable acreage in the arid coastal sections of the country, using the abundance of water flowing from the Andes mountains.

Production in 1989 (in 1,000 tonnes): Sugar-cane, 6,333; potatoes, 1,691; seed cotton, 322; coffee, 106; rice, 1,092; maize, 1,010.

Livestock (in 1,000), 1989: Alpacas, 2,700; cattle, 4,100; pigs, 2,400; sheep, 13,100; poultry, 55,000.

Forestry. There were 84·5m. ha of forest area in 1989, made up of 74m. ha of natural forest, 253,646 ha of planted forest and 10·25m. ha of land suitable for reforestation. The forests contain valuable hardwoods; oak and cedar account for about 40%. In 1989 roundwood removals totalled 8·5m. cu metres.

Fisheries. Production (1989 in tonnes) 6,639,000, including anchoveta, 3,712,000; sardine, 2,400,000.

INDUSTRY. About 70% of Peru's manufacturing industries are located in or around the Lima/Callao metropolitan area. Products include pig-iron, blooms, billets, largets, round and round-deformed bars, wire rod, black and galvanized sheets and galvanized roofing sheets. Refractories are manufactured at Lima.

The Government has a monopoly of the import and/or local manufacture and sale of guano, salt, alcohol and explosives.

Labour. In 1990 the workforce numbered 7,661,800, of whom 2,605,000 worked in agriculture, 183,900 in mining, 804,500 in manufacturing, 23,000 in electricity production, 283,000 in building, 1,195,200 in commerce, 337,100 in transport, 183,900 in finance and 2,045,700 in services. In Aug. 1990 private-sector salaries were increased 333%, and the minimum monthly wage became 16m. intis.

Trade Unions. Trade unions have about 2m. members (approximately 1·5m. in peasant organizations and 500,000 in industrial). The major trade union organization is the *Confederación de Trabajadores del Perú*, which was reconstituted in 1959 after being in abeyance for some years. The other labour organizations recognized by the Government are the *Confederación General de Trabajadores del Perú*, the *Confederación Nacional de Trabajadores* and the *Central de Trabajadores de la Revolución Peruana.*

FOREIGN ECONOMIC RELATIONS

Commerce. The value of trade has been as follows (in US$1m.):

	1983	*1984*	*1985*	*1986*	*1987*	*1988*	*1989*
Imports	2,722	2,140	1,806	2,596	3,068	2,790	2,140
Exports	3,015	3,147	2,978	2,531	2,605	2,691	3,542

In 1989, imports (in US$1,000) were mainly from the USA (407,938), Argentina (105,444) and the Federal Republic of Germany (96,258); exports were mainly to the USA (447,189) and Japan (94,251). 15·2m. bbls of oil were exported in 1989.

Total trade between Peru and UK (British Department of Trade returns, in £1,000 sterling):

	1987	*1988*	*1989*	*1990*
Imports to UK	91,689	90,844	125,538	96,654
Exports and re-exports from UK	49,324	31,384	29,707	29,233

Tourism. There were 333,594 visitors in 1989.

COMMUNICATIONS

Roads. In 1986 there were 69,942 km of roads, of which 7,459 km were paved and 13,538 km gravel. In 1989 there were 612,249 registered motor vehicles, including 328,638 cars, 44,152 station wagons, 140,080 vans, 20,612 buses and 67,566 lorries.

Railways. Total length (1986), 1,672 km on 1,435- and 914-mm gauges. In 1986 railways carried 2·3m. tonnes of freight and 3·3m. passengers.

Aviation. In 1991 there were 30 airports. 182 civil aircraft were registered in 1989, of which 103 were in commercial use.

Shipping. In 1989 there were 51 sea-going vessels and 579 lake and river craft.

Telecommunications. In 1988 there were 2,305 post offices and 2,123 telegraph offices. An earth satellite ground communication station at Lurin connects Peru through Intelsat. III to the USA and Europe. In 1988 there were 702,037 telephones and 3,791 teleprinters. Radio receivers (1987) 5·2m. and television receivers 1·6m.

Newspapers. The main Lima newspapers are *El Comercio, Expreso, República, Hoy, El Nacional, La Crónica, La Tercera, Extra, El Universal, Página Libre, Onda, Novedades* and *Gestión.*

JUSTICE, RELIGION, EDUCATION AND WELFARE

Justice. The Peruvian judicial system is a pyramid at the base of which are the justices of the peace who decide minor criminal cases and civil cases involving small sums of money. The apex is the Supreme Court with a President and 12 members; in between are the judges of first instance, who usually sit in the provincial capitals, and the superior courts.

Religion. Religious liberty exists, but the Roman Catholic religion is protected by the State, and since 1929 only Roman Catholic religious instruction is permitted in schools, state or private. In 1972 there were 1 Roman Catholic cardinal, 7 archbishops, 14 bishops, 3 vicars-general, 8 vicars apostolic, 2,672 priests, 506 cloistered monks and 4,558 members of religious orders.

Education. Elementary education is compulsory and free for both sexes between the ages of 7 and 16; secondary education is also free.

In 1987 there were 3,763,730 pupils in primary schools and 1,732,466 pupils in secondary schools.

In 1989 the number of students at the 27 state and 19 private universities was 445,758.

Health. There were in 1989, 368 hospitals and 1,019 health centres.

DIPLOMATIC REPRESENTATIVES

Of Peru in Great Britain (52 Sloane St., London, SW1X 9SP)
Ambassador: Felipe Valdivieso - Belaúnde (accredited 20 July 1989).

Of Great Britain in Peru (Edificio El Pacifico Washington, Ave. Arequipa, Lima)
Ambassador: D. Keith Haskell, CVO.

Of Peru in the USA (1700 Massachusetts Ave., NW, Washington, D.C., 20036)
Ambassador: Cesar G. Atala.

Of the USA in Peru (PO Box 1995, Lima)
Ambassador: Anthony C. E. Quainton.

Of Peru to the United Nations
Ambassador: Dr Ricardo V. Luna.

Further Reading

The official gazette is *El Peruano*, Lima.

Anario Estadistico del Perú. Annual.—*Perú: Compendio Estadístico*. Annual.—*Boletin de Estadistica Peruana*. Quarterly.—*Demarcación Política del Perú*. (Dirección Nacional de Estadística), Lima

Estadística del Comercio Exterior (*Superintendencia de Aduanas*). Lima

Banco Central de Reserva. Monthly Bulletin.—*Renta Nacional del Perú*. Annual, Lima

Figueroa, A., *Capitalist Development and the Peasant Economy of Peru*. CUP, 1984

Fisher, J., *Peru*: [Bibliography]. Oxford and Santa Barbara, 1989

Hemming, J., *The Conquest of the Incas*. London, 1970

McClintock, C. and Lowental, A. F., (eds.) *The Peruvian Experiment Reconsidered*. Princeton Univ. Press, 1983

Mejía Baca, J. and Tauro, A., *Diccionário Enciclopédico del Perú*. 3 vols. 1966

Thorpe, R. and Bertram, G., *Peru 1890–1977: Growth and Policy in an Open Economy*. London, 1978

National Library: Avenida Abancay, Lima.

PHILIPPINES

Capital: Manila
Population: 60·5m. (1990)
GNP per capita: US$734 (1989)

Republika ng Pilipinas

HISTORY. Before the Spanish discovery of the Philippines, the native Filipinos came in contact with India, China and Arabia. According to the early records of China, 'some Filipinos from the country of Ma-i arrived in Canton and sold their merchandise' as early as 982. The Philippine islands were discovered by Magellan in 1521 and conquered by Spain in 1565. Following the Spanish–American war, the islands were ceded to the USA on 10 Dec. 1898, after the Filipinos had tried in vain to establish an independent republic in 1896.

The Philippines acquired self-government as a Commonwealth of the USA by Act of Congress signed by President Roosevelt on 24 March 1934 and ratified by plebiscite on 14 May 1935. This provided for independence after a 10-year transitional period, at the end of which the Philippines became completely independent on 4 July 1946.

AREA AND POPULATION. The Philippines is situated between 21° 25' and 4° 23' N. lat. and between 116° and 127° E. long. It is composed of 7,100 islands and islets, 2,773 of which are named. Approximate land area, 115,830 sq. miles (300,000 sq. km). The largest islands (in sq. km) are Luzon (104,684), Mindanao (94,627), Samar (13,079), Negros (12,706), Palawan (11,784), Panay (11,515), Mindoro (9,735), Leyte (7,215), Cebu (4,421), Bohol (3,864), Masbate (3,268).

Census population 1990 was 60,477,000 (preliminary). Estimate (1991) 62,868,000 (based on 1980 census).

The area and population (in 1,000)of the 14 regions are as follows (from north to south):

Region	*Sq. km*	*Estimate 1990*	*Region*	*Sq. km*	*Estimate 1990*
Ilocos	12,840	3,548	Central Visayas	14,951	4,593
Cagayan Valley	26,838	2,342	Eastern Visayas	21,432	3,048
Central Luzon	18,231	6,191	Northern Mindanao	28,328	3,503
National Capital	636	7,832	Southern Mindanao	31,693	4,453
Southern Tagalog	46,924	8,261	Central Mindanao	23,293	3,121
Bicol	17,633	3,911	Western Mindanao	18,685	3,145
Western Visayas	20,223	3,379	Cordillero Administrative	18,294	1,149

City populations (1990 census, in 1,000) are as follows; all on Luzon unless indicated in parenthesis.

Manila	1,587 [1]	Cadiz (Negros)	120
Quezon City	1,632 [1]	Lipa	160
Davao (Mindanao)	850	Baguio	183
Cebu (Cebu)	610	Silay (Negros)	92
Caloocan	746 [1]	Mandaue (Cebu)	180
Zamboanga (Mindanao)	449	Lucena	151
Bacolod (Negros)	364	Calbayog (Samar)	113
Iloilo (Panay)	311	Ormoc (Leyte)	129
Cagayan de Oro (Mindanao)	340	Tacloban (Leyte)	138
Angeles	236	San Carlos	124
Butuan (Mindanao)	228	Legaspi	121
Iligan (Mindanao)	227	Dagupan	122
Olongapo	192	San Carlos (Negros)	106
General Santos (Mindanao)	250	Naga	115
Batangas	184		
Cabanatuan	173		
San Pablo	161		

[1] City within Metropolitan Manila.

In 1980 the national language, Pilipino (based on Tagalog, a Malayan dialect) was spoken by 55% of the population, but as a mother tongue by only 23·8%; among the 76 other indigenous languages spoken, all of the Malayo-Polynesian family,

Cebuano was spoken as a mother tongue by 24·4%, Ilocano by 11·1%, Hiligaynon by 8% and Bikol by 5%.

CLIMATE. Some areas have an equatorial climate while others experience tropical monsoon conditions, with a wet season extending from May to Nov. Mean temperatures are high all year, with very little variation. Manila. Jan. 77°F (25°C), July 82°F (27·8°C). Annual rainfall 82" (2,083 mm).

CONSTITUTION AND GOVERNMENT. Presidential elections were held on 7 Feb. 1986. Ferdinand E. Marcos was opposed by Corazón Aquino. The elections proved to be fraudulent and although Marcos was proclaimed President, by the National Assembly, on 15 Feb., on 25 Feb. he fled the country. President Corazón Aquino was sworn in on 25 Feb.

On 25 March 1986 the President abolished the Parliament and declared a provisional government. A new Constitution was ratified by referendum in 1987 with 78·5% of the voters endorsing it. It aims 'to secure to ourselves and our posterity the blessings of independence and democracy under the rule of law and a regime of truth, justice, freedom, love, equality and peace'.

At congressional elections held on 11 May 1987, 24 senators were elected in the Upper House and 200 congressmen in the House of Representatives.

In Feb. 1991 the government included:

President: Corazón Aquino.

Vice President: Salvador Laurel.

Executive Secretary, Presidential Co-ordinator for Political and Security Affairs: Oscar Orbos. *Defence:* Fidel Ramos. *Local Government:* Luis Santos. *Foreign Affairs:* Raul Manglapus. *Justice:* Franklin Drilon. *Finance:* Jesus Estanislao. *Trade and Industry:* Peter Garrucho. *Public Works and Highways:* José de Jesus. *Agrarian Reform:* Benjamin Leong. *Agriculture:* Senen Bacani. *Social Welfare:* Mita Pardo de Tavera. *Education:* Isidro Carino. *Science:* Ceferino Follosco. *Budget:* Guillermo Carague. *Press:* Tomas Gomez. *Economic Planning:* Cayetano Pedranga. *Labour:* Ruben Torres. *Presidential Spokesman:* Adolfo Azcuna. *Speaker:* Ramon Mitra.

National flag: Horizontally blue over red, with a white triangle based on the hoist bearing a gold sun of 8 rays and 3 gold stars.

National hymn: 'Land of the Morning', lyric in English by M. A. Sane and C. Osias, tune by Julian Felipe (1898); 'Pambansang Awit ng Pilipinas', Tagalog lyric by the Institute of National Language, music by Julian Felipe.

Local Government. The country is administratively divided into 14 regions, 73 provinces, 60 cities, 1,532 municipalities, 21 municipal districts and 41,322 *barangays* (1990). On 14 Nov. 1975 the name of provincial boards and city or municipal boards or councils was changed into *Sangguniang Bayan*.

DEFENCE. In Nov. 1990 the USA announced it would withdraw its air forces after the expiry of the US-Philippine military-base agreement of March 1947 due to end on 16 Sept. 1991. An extension of the agreement granting the USA the use of several army, navy and air force bases was under discussion in Feb. 1991. In 1990 there were some 16,000 US soldiers stationed in the Philippines. The Philippines is a signatory of the S.E. Asia Collective Defence Treaty.

The Chief of Staff of the Armed Forces has overall command over the Army, Air Force, Navy and Constabulary.

Army. The Army comprises 8 infantry divisions, 3 engineer brigades, 1 special services brigade, 1 light armoured regiment and 8 artillery battalions. Equipment includes 41 Scorpion light tanks. Strength (1991) 68,000, with reserves totalling 100,000.

Navy. The Philippine navy consists principally of ex-US ships completed in 1944 and 1945, and serviceability and spares are a problem. A modernization programme, based on acquisition of a substantial number of much smaller patrol craft of US design is planned, of which the first is on trials.

The present fleet includes 2 US frigates, 8 offshore patrol vesels (ex-US minesweepers and escorts), 4 ex-US coastal patrol craft, and about 40 inshore patrol craft. There are 5 tank landing ships and 2 medium landing ships, and some 30 landing craft. Auxiliaries include 3 repair ships, 2 oilers, 2 yachts/search-and-rescue craft and 1 transport, as well as some 20 minor auxiliaries. There are 65 patrol craft and search-and-rescue craft in the coastguard.

Navy personnel in 1990 totalled 25,000 including 10,000 marines and 2,000 in the coastguard.

Air Force. The Air Force had (1991) a strength of 15,500, with 26 combat aircraft and 71 armed helicopters, and was built up with US assistance. Its fighter-bomber wing is equipped with 1 squadron of F-5As. A strike wing is equipped with armed trainers, 2 squadrons having T-28s and 1 squadron SF.260WPs. Other units include a maritime patrol squadron with F27 Maritimes and HU-16 Albatross amphibians and 7 transport squadrons (1 with C-130/L-100 Hercules, 1 with F27s, 1 with Nomads, 1 with C-47s, 2 with UH-1 Iroquois helicopters and 1 with S-76 helicopters). Training aircraft include T-41s, T-34s and T-33 jets, plus S. 211s from Italy being delivered 1989-90. Two S-70 helicopters are used as VIP transports.

Constabulary. Public order is maintained partly through the Philippine constabulary and partly through the local police forces. The constabulary is part of the Armed Forces and has some 45,000 personnel.

INTERNATIONAL RELATIONS

Membership. The Philippines is a member of the UN and the Colombo Plan.

ECONOMY

Policy. A development plan, 1987–92, aimed at an average growth rate of 6·8%.

Budget. The revenues and expenditures of the central government for calendar years were, in 1m. Philippine pesos, as follows:

	1986	*1987*	*1988*	*1989*	*1990*
Revenue	79,245	103,214	128,253	149,865	179,539
Expenditure	114,505	155,503	190,689	227,421	233,500

Expenditure (1990) included (in 1m. pesos): National defence, 22,580; education, health and social services, 52,591; economic development, 49,933; debt service, 36,819.

At Oct. 1989 the total internal public debt outstanding of the national and local governments and monetary institutions, including those of the government corporations, stood at P.137,249·6m.

Currency. The unit of currency is the *Philippine peso* (PHP) of 100 *centavos*. There are notes of 2, 5, 10, 20, 50, 100 and 500 pesos and coins of 1, 5, 10, 25 and 50 centavos and 1 and 5 pesos. Total money supply, June 1990, was P.69,788m. Inflation was an annualized 13.1% in Nov. 1990.

In March 1991, £1 = 51 *pesos*; US$1 = 26·88 *pesos*.

Banking and Finance. In 1990 there were 962 head offices and 2,603 branches of commercial banks, with 23 overseas. Total deposits of the commercial banks at 31 Dec. 1989 were P.252,391·0m. Total number of Philippine banking institutions, 31 Dec. 1989, 3,588 with total assets P.637,978·2m. and total deposits of P.286,652·2m.

Under the law passed 15 June 1948 the Central Bank of the Philippines was created to have sole control of the credit and monetary supply, independent of the Treasury. It has a capital of P.10m. furnished solely by the Government. Its total assets, at 31 Dec. 1987 were P.325,185·1m. Central Bank's total assets at 31 Dec. 1989 were P.385,889·7m. The Governor is José Cuisia.

Weights and Measures. The metric system of weights and measures was established by law in 1869, and since 1916 has come into general use but there are local units including the picul (63·25 kg) for sugar and fibres, and the cavan (16·5 gallons) for cereals.

ENERGY AND NATURAL RESOURCES

Electricity. Government and private electric systems furnish the Philippines with electric power, with total installed capacity of 6,865m. mw (1989); production 25,931m. kwh. Supply 110 and 220 volts; 60 Hz.

Minerals. Mineral production in 1989, provisional (in tonnes): Nickel metal, 18,049; zinc metal, 1,345; copper metal, 196,422; cobalt metal (1986), 90; coal, 1,344,676; salt, 488,676; gold, 29,992 kg; silver, 50,630 kg; silica sand, 184,890. Other minerals include chromite, cement, rock asphalt, sand and gravel.

Agriculture. In 1980 the total area was 30m. ha, of which 9·7 (30·11%) was farm area. The rest was comprised of commercial and non-commercial forests, open grassland, mangrove and marshes, and cultivated land.

The average size of the farm was 2·63 ha in 1980. The principal products are coconuts, unhusked rice (palay), sugar-cane, maize and root crops, bananas and pineapples. As of Oct. 1989 9,720,000 persons were employed in agriculture (44% of the working population).

The products (in 1,000 tonnes) are (1989, provisional): Rough rice, 9,459; coconuts, 11,810; sugar-cane, 17,950; shelled corn, 4,522; bananas, 3,190; tobacco, 80; abaca fibre, 88.

Minor crops are fruits, nuts, vegetables, onions, beans, coffee, cacao, peanuts, ramie, rubber, maguey, kapok, abaca and tobacco.

Livestock, estimated in 1989 (in 1,000): 2,826 carabaos (water buffaloes), 1,666 cattle, 7,775 pigs, 2,201 goats and 72,437 poultry.

Forestry. The forests covered about 15·88m. ha, or 53% of the total land area. Out of these forest lands, 15·0m. ha. or 94·4% have been classified into: Forest Reserve, 3,271,504 ha; timber land, 10,015,427 ha; National Parks, 1,342,416 ha; civil reservation, 165,935 ha; Military and Naval reservation, 130,330; fish ponds, 75,478 ha; and unclassified forest lands, 881,157 ha.in 1988. Log production, 1988, 3,809,200 cu. metres.

Fisheries. Fish production from all sources was 2,101,000 tonnes in 1989.

INDUSTRY. Manufacturing is a major source of economic development contributing 25·1% to GNP in 1989. Leading growth sectors were food manufacturing, textile, footwear and wearing apparel, machinery except electrical, fabricated metal products, wood and cork products, industrial chemicals and other chemical products, furniture and fixtures and publishing and allied industries. In 1987 (annual survey), there were 5,000 large manufacturing establishments, of which 1,165 were engaged in food; 414 wearing apparel; 111 footwear; 297 textile; 366 publishing and allied industries; 300 machinery except electrical; 258 fabricated metal products; 295 industrial chemicals and other chemical products; 254 wood and cork products; 162 plastic products and 145 transport equipment.

Labour. The non-agricultural labour force as of Oct. 1989 was 12,141,000 out of a total of 22,154,000 employed.

FOREIGN ECONOMIC RELATIONS. Foreign debt was US$27,616m. at the end of 1989.

Commerce. The values of imports and exports (f.o.b.) for calendar years are stated as follows in US$1m.:

	1986	*1987*	*1988*	*1989*
Imports	5,044	6,737	8,159	10,419
Exports	4,842	5,720	7,074	7,821

The principal exports in 1988 were (in US$1m.): Garments, 1,575; electronics, 1,388; coconut oil (crude), 377; bars, rods and slabs of copper, 330; shrimps and prawns, 231; lumber, 136; bananas, 146; copper concentrates, 237.

Main imports in 1989 (in US$1m.): Petroleum products and related materials, 1,315; textile yarns, fabrics, made-up articles and related products, 452; machinery, apparatus and appliances, 570; cereals and cereal preparations, 339; iron and steel,

743; general industrial machinery and equipment, 310; artificial resins, plastic materials, cellulose esters and ethers, 289; motor vehicles, 475; special transactions and commodities not classified according to kind, 1,683.

For over a half-century the foreign trade has been chiefly with the USA.

Total trade between the Philippines and UK (British Department of Trade returns, in £1,000 sterling):

	1986	*1987*	*1988*	*1989*	*1990*
Imports to UK	182,852	202,707	223,571	233,128	220,706
Exports and re-exports from UK	79,809	113,784	123,974	137,367	158,030

Tourism. In 1988, 1,189,719 tourists visited the Philippines spending US$1,469m.

COMMUNICATIONS

Roads. In 1989 highways totalled 159,069 km; of this, 10,146 km were concrete; 12,602, asphalt; 8,631, earth; 127,689, gravel. In 1989 there were registered 1,415,723 motor vehicles of all types.

Railways. The National Railway totals 805 km of 1,067 mm gauge on Luzon. In 1989, 1,004,711 passengers and 53,182 tonnes of freight. The light railway in Manila carried 101m. passengers in 1987.

Aviation. The Philippine Air Lines, Inc., in 1989 carried 5,911,595 international and domestic passengers. In 1990 there were 86 national and 125 private airports.

Shipping. In 1989 there were 164 public and 234 private ports. In 1988, 80,512 vessels of 69,562,000 net tons entered and 80,610 vessels of 69,064,000 net tons cleared all ports.

Telecommunications. In 1989 there were in operation 2,116 post offices. The Philippine Long Distance Telephone Co. had 931,742 telephone connections. Other major operators had 56,148 connexions.

Radio stations in 1989 numbered 40,435, television stations, 69.

Newspapers (1989). There were 234 registered publications (186 published in Manila); 32, daily newspapers; 1, weekly tabloid; 58, magazines; 7, foreign publications; and 48, provincial publications.

JUSTICE, RELIGION, EDUCATION AND WELFARE

Justice. There is a Supreme Court which is composed of a chief justice and 14 associate justices; it can declare a law or treaty unconstitutional by the concurrent votes of the majority sitting. There is an intermediate appellate court, which consists of a presiding appellate justice and 49 associate appellate justices. There are 13 regional trial courts, one for each judicial region, with a presiding regional trial judge in its 720 branches. There is a metropolitan trial court in each metropolitan area established by law, a municipal trial court in each of the other cities or municipalities and a municipal circuit trial court in each area defined as a municipal circuit comprising one or more cities and/or one or more municipalities.

The Supreme Court may designate certain branches of the regional trial courts to handle exclusively criminal cases, juvenile and domestic relations cases, agrarian cases, urban land reform cases which do not fall under the jurisdiction of quasijudicial bodies and agencies and/or such other special cases as the Supreme Court may determine.

Local police forces are supplemented by the Philippine Constabulary, which is part of the armed forces (*see* p. 1006).

Religion. In 1970 there were 31,169,488 Roman Catholics, 1,433,688 Aglipayans, 1,584,963 Moslems, 1,122,999 Protestants, 475,407 members of the Iglesia ni Kristo, 33,639 Buddhists and 863,302 others.

The Roman Catholics are organized in 12 archbishoprics, 30 bishoprics, 12 prelatures nullius, 4 apostolic vicariates, 4 apostolic prefectures and some 1,633 parishes. The Philippine Independent Church, founded in 1902, and comprising about 3·9% of the population, denies the spiritual authority of the Roman Pontiff. It is divided into two groups, one of which has accepted ordinations by the Episcopalian Church.

Education. Formal education consists of 3 levels: Elementary, secondary and further education. Public elementary education is free and public elementary schools are established in almost every *barangay* or *barrio*. The majority of the secondary and post-secondary schools are private, sectarian or non-sectarian. The number of years required to complete the elementary and secondary levels are 6 and 4 years respectively, while the tertiary level requires at least 4 years for an academic degree. Pre-school education is also offered mostly in private schools to children from ages 3–6.

Non-formal education consists of adult literacy classes, agricultural and farming training programmes, occupation skills training, youth clubs, and community programmes of instructions in health, nutrition, family planning and co-operatives.

Public and private schools in 1988–89 enrolled 9,972,571 pupils in primary schools, 3,737,104 in secondary schools and 1,308,000 students in further education. The University of the Philippines (founded in 1908) had 15,316 students in 1984.

Health. In 1985 there were 51,461 registered physicians and (1987) 87,697 hospital beds.

DIPLOMATIC REPRESENTATIVES

Of the Philippines in Great Britain (9A Palace Green, London, W8 4QE)
Ambassador: Tomas T. Syquia.

Of Great Britain in the Philippines (115 Esteban St., Manila)
Ambassador: Keith MacInnes, CMG.

Of the Philippines in the USA (1617 Massachusetts Ave., NW, Washington, D.C., 20036)
Ambassador: Emmanuel N. Pelaez.

Of the USA in the Philippines (1201 Roxas Blvd., Manila)
Ambassador: Nicholas Platt.

Of the Philippines to the United Nations
Ambassador: Sedfrey Ordoñez.

Further Reading

Philippine Yearbook 1987. National Statistics Office, Manila, 1987
Bresnan, J. (ed.) *Crisis in the Philippines: The Marcos Era and Beyond.* Princeton Univ. Press, 1986
Karnow, S., *In Our Image: America's Empire in the Philippines.* New York, 1989
May, R. J. and Nemenzo, F. (eds.), *The Philippines after Marcos.* London and Sydney, 1985
Poole, F. and Vanzl, M., *Revolution in the Philippines.* New York, 1984
Richardson, J. A., *Philippines.* [Bibliography] Oxford and Santa Barbara, 1989
Seagrove, S., *The Marcos Dynasty.* London, 1989

PITCAIRN ISLAND

Only settlement: Adamstown
Population: 59 (1990)

HISTORY. It was discovered by Carteret in 1767, but remained uninhabited until 1790, when it was occupied by 9 mutineers of HMS *Bounty*, with 12 women and 6 men from Tahiti. Nothing was known of their existence until the island was visited in 1808. In 1856 the population having become too large for the island's resources, the inhabitants (194 in number) were, at their own request, removed to Norfolk Island; but 43 of them returned in 1859–64.

AREA AND POPULATION. Pitcairn Island (1·75 sq. miles; 4·6 sq. km) is situated in the Pacific Ocean, nearly equidistant from New Zealand and Panama (25° 04' S. lat., 130° 06' W. long.). Adamstown is the only settlement. The population on 31 Dec. 1990 was 59. The uninhabited islands of Henderson (12 sq. miles), Ducie (1½ sq. miles) and Oeno (2 sq. miles) were annexed in 1902 and are included in the Pitcairn group.

CLIMATE. An equable climate, with average annual rainfall of 80" (2,000 mm), spread evenly throughout the year. Mean monthly temperatures range from 75°F (24°C) in Jan. to 66°F (19°C) in July.

CONSTITUTION. Pitcairn was brought within the jurisdiction of the High Commissioner for the Western Pacific in 1898 and transferred to the Governor of Fiji in 1952. When Fiji became independent in Oct. 1970, the British High Commissioner in New Zealand was appointed Governor.

The Local Government Ordinance of 1964 constitutes a Council of 10 members, of whom 6 are elected, 3 are nominated (1 by the 6 elected members and 2 by the Governor) and the Island Secretary is an *ex-officio* member. The Island Magistrate, who is elected triennially, presides over the Council; other members hold office for only 1 year. Liaison between Governor and Council is through a Commissioner in the Auckland, New Zealand, office of the British Consulate-General.

Governor: D. J. Moss, CMG (resides in Wellington).
Island Magistrate: Brian Young (elected Dec. 1987).

Flag: British Blue Ensign with the whole arms of Pitcairn in the fly.

BUDGET. In 1989 the island earned $958,733 and spent $923,355.

CURRENCY. The Pitcairn *dollar* has the same value as the New Zealand dollar.

TRADE. Fruit, vegetables and curios are sold to passing ships; fuel oil, machinery, building materials, flour, sugar and other foodstuffs are imported.

ROADS. There were (1989) 6 km of roads. In Aug. 1989 motor cycles provided the sole means of personal automotive transport; there were 4 2-wheelers, 16 3-wheelers and four 4-wheeled motor cycles.

JUSTICE. The Island Court consists of the Island Magistrate and 2 assessors.

EDUCATION. In 1990 there was 1 teacher and 12 pupils.

Further Reading

A Guide to Pitcairn. Pitcairn Island Administration, Auckland, revised ed. 1990
Ball, I., *Pitcairn: Children of the Bounty.* London, 1973
Ross, A. S. C. and Moverly, A. W., *The Pitcairnese Language.* London, 1964

POLAND

Capital: Warsaw
Population: 37·93m. (1990)
GNP per capita: US$1,850 (1988)

Rzeczpospolita Polska

(Polish Republic)

HISTORY. In 1966 Poland celebrated its millennium, but modern Polish history begins with the partitions of the once-powerful kingdom between Russia, Austria and Prussia in 1772, 1793 and 1795. For 19th century events *see* THE STATESMAN'S YEAR-BOOK 1980–81.

On 10 Nov. 1918 independence was proclaimed by Józef Piłsudski, the founder of the Polish Legions during the war. On 28 June 1919 the Treaty of Versailles recognized the independence of Poland.

On 1 Sept. 1939 Germany invaded Poland, on 17 Sept. 1939 Soviet troops entered eastern Poland, and on 29 Sept. 1939 the fourth partition of Poland took place. After the German attack on the USSR, Germany occupied the whole of Poland. By March 1945 the country had been liberated by the USSR. For the establishment of the Communist regime *see* THE STATESMAN'S YEAR-BOOK, 1990–91.

In 1970 the Federal Republic of Germany recognized Poland's western boundary as laid down by the Potsdam Conference of 1945 (the 'Oder–Neisse line'), and reaffirmed this recognition in March 1990.

After riots in Poznań in June 1956 nationalist anti-Stalinist elements gained control of the Communist Party, under the leadership of Władysław Gomułka. In Dec. 1970 strikes and riots in Gdańsk, Szczecin and Gdynia led to the replacement of Gomułka by Edward Gierek. The raising of meat prices on 1 July 1980 resulted in a wave of strikes which broadened into generalized wage demands and eventually acquired a political character. Workers in Gdańsk, Gdynia and Sopot elected a joint strike committee, led by Lech Wałęsa. On 31 Aug. the Government and Wałęsa signed the 'Gdańsk Agreements' permitting the formation of independent trade unions.

On 5 Sept. Gierek was replaced by Stanisław Kania. On 17 Sept. various trade unions decided to form a national confederation ('Solidarity') and applied for legal status, which was granted on 24 Oct.

On 9 Feb. 1981 the Defence Minister, Gen. Wojciech Jaruzelski, became Prime Minister. At Solidarity's first national congress (4–10 Sept. and 2–8 Oct. 1981) Wałęsa was re-elected chairman and a radical programme of action was adopted. On 18 Oct. Kania was replaced as Party leader by Jaruzelski. On 13 Dec. 1981 the Government imposed martial law (*stan wojenny*) and set up a 20-member Military Council of National Salvation (WRON). Solidarity was proscribed and its leaders detained. Martial law was approved by the Sejm on 26 Jan. 1982. Wałęsa was released in Nov. 1982. On 8 Oct. the Sejm voted a law dissolving all registered trade unions including Solidarity. These were replaced by workplace unions.

Martial law was lifted in July 1983. In Nov. 1985 Jaruzelski resigned the Prime Ministership in favour of Zbigniew Messner, and was elected Chairman of the Council of State. Following strikes and demands for the reinstatement of Solidarity, Messner and his government resigned in Sept. 1988. Mieczysław Rakowski was appointed Prime Minister on 27 Sept.

After the parliamentary elections of June 1989 Czesław Kiszczak was elected Prime Minister on 2 Aug. 1989, but was unable to form a government against the opposition of Solidarity, and resigned on 14 Aug. Tadeusz Mazowiecki, a Solidarity member, was elected Prime Minister by the Sejm on 24 Aug. by 378 votes to 4, with 41 abstentions.

AREA AND POPULATION. Poland is bounded in the north by the Baltic Sea and Russia, east by Lithuania, Belorussia and the Ukraine, south by Czechoslovakia and west by Germany. On 14 Nov. 1990 Germany signed a treaty with Poland confirming Poland's existing western frontier and renouncing German claims to territory lost as a result of the Second World War. Poland comprises an area of 312,683 sq. km (120,628 sq. miles). The country is divided into 49 voivodships (*wojewodztwo*) and these in turn are divided into 822 towns and 2,121 wards (*gmina*). The capital is Warsaw (Warszawa).

Area (in sq. km) and population (in 1,000) in 1989 (1984 % urban in brackets).

Voivodship	*Area*	*Population*	*Voivodship*	*Area*	*Population*
Biała Podlaska	5,348	304 (32·5)	Opole	8,535	1,010 (50·9)
Białystok	10,055	688 (57·7)	Ostrołęka	6,498	393 (30·9)
Bielsko–Biała	3,704	895 (48·9)	Piła	8,205	476 (53·9)
Bydgoszcz	10,349	1,104 (62·8)	Piotrków	6,266	639 (45·3)
Chełm	3,866	246 (39·9)	Płock	5,117	513 (45·7)
Ciechanów	6,362	426 (33·0)	Poznan	8,151	1,323 (69·7)
Częstochowa	6,182	773 (51·2)	Przemyśl	4,437	404 (35·7)
Elbląg	6,103	476 (58·6)	Radom	7,294	745 (44·5)
Gdańsk	7,394	1,418 (76·2)	Rzeszów	4,397	716 (37·7)
Gorzów	8,484	497 (60·4)	Siedlce	8,499	648 (28·7)
Jelenia Góra	4,378	515 (65·3)	Sieradz	4,869	408 (33·1)
Kalisz	6,512	707 (44·5)	Skierniewice	3,960	417 (42·2)
Katowice	6,650	3,954 (87·7)	Słupsk	7,453	410 (53·8)
Kielce	9,211	1,124 (44·4)	Suwałki	10,490	467 (49·9)
Konin	5,139	466 (38·6)	Szczecin	9,981	964 (73·9)
Koszalin	8,470	503 (61·0)	Tarnobrzeg	6,283	594 (34·6)
Kraków (Cracow)	3,254	1,223 (69·1)	Tarnów	4,151	665 (34·2)
Krosno	5,702	496 (32·8)	Toruń	5,348	656 (60·8)
Legnica	4,037	510 (66·6)	Wałbrzych	4,168	738 (88·5)
Leszno	4,154	383 (46·1)	Warsaw	3,788	2,416 (73·0)
Łódź	1,523	1,139 (91·4)	Włocławek	4,402	427 (44·9)
Łomża	6,684	345 (35·7)	Wrocław	6,287	1,123 (72·4)
Lublin	6,792	1,011 (55·5)	Zamośc	6,980	488 (24·9)
Nowy Sącz	5,576	691 (35·5)	Zielona Góra	8,868	655 (59·0)
Olsztyn	12,327	746 (56·4)			

Population (in 1,000) of the largest towns (1985):

Warsaw	1,649	Bydgoszcz	361	Gliwice	213
Łódź	849	Lublin	324	Kielce	201
Kraków (Cracow)	716	Sosnowiec	255	Zabrze	198
Wrocław (Breslau)	636	Częstochowa	247	Toruń	186
Poznań	553	Białystok	245	Tychy	182
Gdańsk (Danzig)	467	Gdynia	243	Bielsko-Biala	174
Szczecin (Stettin)	391	Bytom	239	Ruda Słąska	165
Katowice	363	Radom	214	Olsztyn	147

At the census of 6 Dec. 1984 the population was 37,026,000 (18m. males; 60% urban). Population on 31 Dec. 1989, 37,932,000 (19·43m. females; 23·36m. urban), density, 121 per sq. km. Vital statistics, 1989 (per 1,000): Marriages, 6·8; divorces, 1·2; live births, 14·9; deaths, 10·1; infant mortality (per 1,000 live births), 15·9.

The rate of natural growth, 1989, 4·8 per 1,000. Expectation of life in 1984 was 66·8 years. In 1984, 55% of the population was under 30.

Ethnic minorities are not identified. There were estimated to be 1·2m. Germans in 1984. In 1989 there were 2,200 immigrants and 26,600 emigrants. There is a large Polish diaspora, some 65% in USA. About 250,000 Poles settled abroad between 1981 and 1988, 153,000 illegally.

CLIMATE. Climate is continental, marked by long and severe winters. Rainfall amounts are moderate, with a marked summer maximum. Warsaw. Jan. 25°F (–3·9°C), July 66°F (18·9°C). Annual rainfall 22·1" (550 mm). Gdańsk. Jan. 29°F (–1·7°C), July 63°F (17·2°C). Annual rainfall 22" (559 mm). Kraków. Jan. 27°F (–2·8°C), July 67°F (19·4°C). Annual rainfall 29" (729 mm). Poznań. Jan. 30°F (–1·1°C), July 67°F (19·4°C). Annual rainfall 21" (523 mm). Szezecin. Jan. 30°F

(–1·1°C), July 65°F (18·3°C). Annual rainfall 22" (550 mm). Wrocław. Jan. 30°F (–1·1°C), July 66°F (18·9°C). Annual rainfall 23" (574 mm).

CONSTITUTION AND GOVERNMENT. The present Constitution was adopted on 22 July 1952. Amendments were adopted in 1976 and 1983.

The authority of the republic is vested in the *Sejm* (Parliament of 460 members), elected for 4 years by all citizens over 18. The Sejm elects a *Council of State* and a *Council of Ministers*.

The titular head of state is the *President,* Lech Wałęsa sworn in 22 Dec. 1990.

Talks between the Communist Party (PUWP), Solidarity and others in Feb.–March 1989 resulted in the establishment of a 100-member upper house (Senate), the legalization of Solidarity and Rural Solidarity, and the holding of parliamentary elections at which Solidarity and other opposition groups were free to contest all seats in the Senate and 35% of seats in the Sejm. The Senate has power of veto which only a two-thirds majority of the Sejm can overrule.

At the elections of 4 and 18 June 1989 Solidarity (S) won 99 seats in the Senate and 161 in the Sejm. Only 2 of a government-sponsored 'National List' of 35 candidates qualified for election by gaining more than 50% of votes. The PUWP were allotted 173 seats, and their coalition partners the United Peasant's Party (UPP) 76; the Democratic Party (DP), 27; the Christian Democrats, 23.

Elections were scheduled for 31 Oct. 1991.

A Political Council consultative to the presidency consisting of representatives of all the major political tendencies was set up in Jan. 1991.

At the first round of the presidential elections on 26 Nov. 1990 Lech Wałęsa polled 39.96% of the vote (failing to reach the 50% plus 1 vote necessary to win outright); Stanisław Tymiński, 23.1%, and the Prime Minister, Tadeusz Mazowiecki, 18.08%; the latter announced that on this showing he and his government would resign. At the second round turn-out was 53.4%; 75% of votes were cast for Wałęsa. A new government was formed in Jan. 1991 consisting of:

Prime Minister: Jan Krzystof Bielecki.

Deputy Prime Minister and Minister of Finance: Leszek Balcerowicz. *Labour and Social Policy*: Michał Boni. *Justice*: Wiesław Chrzanowski. *Chairman of the Central Planning Office*: Jerzy Eysymontt. *Construction and Regional Development*: Adam Glapiński. *Education*: Robert Głębocki. *Defence*: Vice-Adm. Piotr Kołodziejczyk. *Foreign Economic Relations*: Dariusz Ledworowski. *Privatization*: Janusz Lewandowski. *Interior*: Henryk Majewski. *Environment*: Maciej Nowicki. *Culture*: Marek Roztworowski. *Foreign Affairs*: Krzysztof Skubiszewski. *Health*: Władysław Sidorowicz. *Communications*: Jerzy Ślezak. *Agriculture and Food*: Adam Tański. *Transport*: Ewaryst Waligórski. *Industry*: Andrzej Zawiślak. *Chief of the Office of the Council of Ministers*: Krzysztof Żabiński.

In Jan. 1990 the PUWP dissolved itself and formed a new party, the Social Democracy of the Polish Republic. *Chairman:* Aleksander Kwaśniewski (b. 1964); *Secretary:* Leszek Miller.

Local government is carried out by councils elected every 4 years at voivodship and community level. Communities of fewer than 40,000 inhabitants elect councils on a first-past-the-post system; larger communities have a proportional party-list system. It was admitted in 1990 that the elections of June 1988 were undemocratic, and new elections were held on 27 May for 2,348 councils; turn-out was 42%.

National flag: Horizontally white over red, with the arms of Poland on the white strip.

National anthem: Jeszcze Polska nie zginęla ('Poland has not yet perished'; words by J. Wybicki, 1797; tune by M. Ogiński, 1796).

DEFENCE. A National Defence Committee was set up in Nov. 1983 with Gen. Jaruzelski at its head. Poland is divided into 3 military districts: Warsaw (the eastern part of Poland); Pomerania (Baltic coast, part of central Poland; headquarters at Bydgoszcz); Silesia (Silesia and southern Poland; headquarters at Wrocław).

Armed forces are divided into army and air force (18 months conscription), navy (2 years), anti-aircraft, rocket and radio-technological units (3 years) and internal security forces (2 years). The military age extends from the 19th to the 50th year. The strength of the armed forces was (1990) 312,800 (204,000 conscripts), plus 43,500 security and frontier forces.

3-year civilian duty as a conscientious alternative to conscription was introduced in 1988. Reductions in defence spending and personnel were announced in 1989.

Army. The Army includes 9 mechanized divisions, 1 airborne, 1 coastal defence and 6 artillery brigades; 4 anti-tank regiments; 4 surface-to-surface missile brigades; 1 air defence brigade. Equipment includes 2,150 T-54/-55 and 750 T-72 main battle tanks and 60 PT-76 light tanks. Strength (1991) 206,600 (including 168,000 conscripts).

Navy. The fleet comprises 3 ex-Soviet diesel submarines, 1 ex-Soviet guided missile destroyer armed with SA-N-1 Goa surface-to-air and SS-N-2C Styx anti-ship missiles, 1 small frigate, 4 missile corvettes, 11 smaller fast missile craft, 8 inshore patrol craft, 19 coastal and 13 inshore minesweepers, 25 medium landing ships and 16 landing craft. Auxiliaries include 3 support tankers, 2 intelligence vessels, 3 survey vessels, and 2 training ships together with about 60 minor auxiliaries.

The Fleet Air Arm operates 11 shore-based Mi-14 Haze helicopters and a further 10 transport and utility helicopters. Naval-manned coast defences provide 6 artillery battalions and 3 missile batteries.

Personnel in 1990 totalled 20,000 including 6,000 conscripts. 2,300 of these serve in naval aviation and 4,000 in coast defence. Bases are at Gdynia, Gdańsk and Świnoujscie.

A para-military border guard service operates 18 inshore patrol craft and some 30 boats.

Air Force. The Air Force had a strength (1991) of some 86,200 (30,000 conscripts) with 516 combat aircraft and 100 armed helicopters. There are 11 air defence regiments (33 squadrons) with about 400 MiG-21, MiG-23 and MiG-29 supersonic interceptors, and 6 regiments (18 squadrons) operating variable-geometry MiG-23BM and Su-20 close-support fighters. There are also reconnaissance, ECM, transport, helicopter (including Mi-2s for observation and Mi-24 gunships) and training units. Soviet 'Guideline' 'Goa', 'Ganef', 'Gainful' and 'Gaskin' surface-to-air missiles are operational.

In 1990 there were some 40,000 Soviet troops stationed in Poland.

INTERNATIONAL RELATIONS

Membership. Poland is a member of the UN, IMF, OIEC and the Warsaw Pact.

ECONOMY

Policy. For planning history until 1989 *see* THE STATESMAN'S YEAR-BOOK 1989–90, p.1012-13. Wide-ranging measures to convert the economy into a market-oriented system were passed by Parliament in Dec. 1989, including the commercialization of interest and exchange rates, the abolition of price subsidies, the termination of wages indexation and the encouragement of foreign investment. Legislation of July 1990 envisages the transfer of state enterprises into private ownership through the issue of 'privatization bonds'.

Budget. Budget in 1m. złotys, for calendar years:

	1984	*1985*	*1986*	*1987*	*1988*	*1989*
Revenue	3,299,700	3,854,200	4,902,700	5,850,400	10,080,800	30,090,100
Expenditure	3,367,800	3,979,200	4,193,200	5,029,800	8,423,000	29,619,200

Main items of 1989 revenue (in 1m. złotys): State enterprises, 23,962,300; finance and insurance, 2,856,900; private sector and personal taxes, 2,462,400. Expenditure: The economy, 11,919,000; welfare, 4,017,700; education, 3,506,100; defence, 2,118,000. 1990 budget estimates halve subsidies but increase allocations to health, education and the environment.

Currency. The currency unit is the *złoty* (PLZ), divided into 100 *groszy*. The currency consists of notes of 10, 20, 50, 100, 500, 1,000, 2,000 and 5,000 złotys; and of coins of 10, 20 and 50 groszy and 1, 2, 5, 10, 20 and 50 złotys. The złoty was substantially devalued in 1989. Inflation was 250% at the end of 1990 (640% in 1989). In Dec. 1989 a US$1,000m. Currency Stabilization Fund was established with the agreement of the IMF. The złoty became convertible on 1 Jan. 1990. In March 1991, £1 sterling = 18,044 złotys, US$1 = 9,512 złotys.

Banking and Finance. The National Bank of Poland (established 1945) is the central bank and bank of issue. The banking system is being commercialized with IMF advice. The General Savings Bank (Powszechna Kasa Oszczędności) exercises central control over savings activities.

Other foreign-exchange banks are the Polish Welfare Bank (Bank Polska Kasa Opieki SA) and the Commercial Bank of Warsaw (Bank Handlowy w Warszawie SA). An Export Development Bank was established in 1986. A stock exchange is due to open in 1991.

Deposits in savings institutions amounted to 7,917·3m. złotys in 1989.

A stock exchange was due to open in 1991.

Weights and Measures. The metric system is in general use.

ENERGY AND NATURAL RESOURCES

Electricity. Electricity production (1989) 145,000m. kwh. In 1989, 70% of electricity was produced by coal-powered thermal plants. Supply 127 and 220 volts; 50 Hz. A nuclear power station is being built at Zarnowiec.

Minerals. Poland is a major producer of coal (reserves of some 120,000m. tonnes), copper (56m. tonnes) and sulphur. Production in 1989 (in tonnes): Coal, 178m.; brown coal, 71·8m.; copper ore (1988) 401,000; silver, 1,003. Oil was discovered 80 km off the port of Leba in 1985. Total oil reserves amount to some 100m. tonnes. Crude oil production was 130,000 tonnes in 1989, natural gas 5,377m. cu. metres.

Agriculture. In 1989 there were 18·73m. ha of agricultural land, of which 14·27m. ha were in private hands, 3·5m. in state farms, 705,000 in co-operatives and 57,000 in agricultural associations. 14·41m. ha were arable, 265,000 orchards, 2·5m. meadows, 1·6m. pasture lands.

Although collectivization had been largely abandoned by the Communist government, procurement remained a state monopoly, and prices were centrally-fixed. There were 2,004 co-operatives in 1989, 1,231 state farms and 173 agricultural associations. In Dec. 1987 a private, Catholic, Foundation for the Development of Polish Agriculture was set up to aid farmers with Western finance. Rural Solidarity (*Chairman:* Josef Slisz) was re-legalized in 1989. A compulsory contributory pension scheme was introduced in 1978 for farmers who turned over their farms to their successors or the State. There were 2·73m. private holdings in 1989, of which 809,000 were less than 2 ha.

	Area (1,000 ha)		*Total Yield (1,000 tonnes)*		
Crops	*1988*	*1989*	*1988*	*1989*	*(from private sector)*
Wheat	2,179	2,195	7,528	8,462	(5,702)
Rye	2,325	2,275	5,501	6,216	(5,167)
Barley	1,250	1,175	3,804	3,909	(2,721)
Oats	850	803	2,222	2,185	(1,692)
Potatoes	1,866	1,077	34,707	34,390	(31,345)
Sugar-beet	412	423	14,069	14,374	(12,025)

Livestock (1989, in thousands): 10,733 cattle (4,994 cows), 18,835 pigs, 4,409 sheep, 973 horses. Milk production was 15,925m. litres; meat, 3,139,000 tonnes.

Tractors in use in 1989: 1,153,000 (in 15-h.p. units).

Forestry. In 1989, 8·68m. ha were forests (predominantly coniferous). 75,000 ha were afforested, and 22·67m. cu. metres of timber gained.

Fisheries. In 1985 the fishing fleet had 93 deep-sea vessels totalling 314,000 GRT. The catch was 650,600 tonnes.

INDUSTRY

Production. Output declined by 14% in 1990. Production in 1989 (in 1,000 tonnes): Coke, 16,500; rolled steel, 11,276; cement, 17,100; sulphuric acid (100%), 4,865; fertilizers, 2,727; electrolytic copper, 390; zinc, 164; sugar, 1,712; plastics, 723. In 1989, 283 ships over 100 DWT were built (224 in 1988), 286,000 cars, 43,900 lorries and 9,100 buses.

Output of light industry in 1989: Cotton fabrics, 756m. metres; woollen fabrics, 96·7m. metres; synthetic fibres, 238,000 tonnes; shoes (1988), 168m. pairs; household glass, 68,700 tonnes; paper, 1,406,000 tonnes; washing machines 811,000, refrigerators 516,000, and TV sets 763,000.

Labour. In 1989 the total number in employment was 17·1m., of whom 5·08m. worked in the private sector (3·56m. of these in agriculture), and including in industry 4·86m., agriculture, 4·53m.; trade, 1·43m., building 1·32m. and transport and communications, 1·1m. Average wage in the state sector in 1990, 893,070 złotys per month. Unemployment benefit of an initial 70% of previous wages was introduced in Dec. 1989. There were 1,124,753 unemployed (8.3% of the workforce) in Dec. 1990. Workers made redundant are entitled to one month's wages. There is a statutory 42-hour working week which may be compulsorily extended in certain workplaces, with 38 free Saturdays a year.

Trade Unions. Founded in Aug. 1980 the 'independent self-governing union' organization Solidarity (Chairman, Lech Wałęsa) was dissolved in Oct. 1982 along with all other trade unions. New official unions (OPZZ) established in 1983 took over Solidarity's funds in 1985. OPZZ (Chairman, Alfred Miodowicz) had 5m. members in 1990. There are also some 4,000 small unions not affiliated to OPZZ. Solidarity was re-legalized in May 1989 and successfully contested the parliamentary elections in June. It had 2·3m. members in 1991; its chairman is Marian Krzaklewski.

FOREIGN ECONOMIC RELATIONS. Foreign trade deals should be made directly with the appropriate foreign trade enterprise. Information may be obtained from the Polish Chamber of Foreign Trade, Trebacka 4, 00–950 Warsaw. Joint ventures with Western firms are encouraged both at home and abroad. Since Jan. 1989 Western investors may own 100% of companies on Polish soil.

In Feb. 1990 the IMF granted a loan of US$725m., and Western creditor nations agreed to a rescheduling of debts. Foreign debt was US$45,200m. in Nov. 1990. Offers of aid to the Solidarity government in 1989 included DM3,000m. from Federal Germany, US$200m. from USA and US$150m. from UK. Poland does not accept liability for the £495,000 debts of pre-war Danzig (Gdańsk).

Commerce. Trade statistics for calendar years (in 1m. złotys; trade with convertible currency areas in brackets):

	1986	*1987*	*1988*		*1989*	
Imports	1,964,000	2,875,600	5,272,300	(3,145,700)	14,864,200	(8,908,500)
Exports	2,115,600	3,236,500	6,011,700	(3,611,800)	19,476,200	(11,561,700)

Main imports in 1989 (in tonnes): Crude oil, 15m.; iron ore, 13·44m.; fertilizers, 5·36m.; wheat, 1·8m.; passenger cars, 33,200 units; machinery and electronic equipment.

Main exports in 1989 (in tonnes): Coal, 28·9m.; coke, 3·16m.; copper, 157,000; sulphur, 3·64m.; ships, 186,000 DWT.

41% of Poland's trade was with Comecon countries in 1988. A trade agreement with the USSR for 1986–90 gave the USSR a wide role in the Polish economy, particularly in the supply of oil, and rescheduled Poland's 5,000m. rouble debt beyond 1990. Soviet exports include plant and equipment and raw materials; Polish exports, machinery, ships, coal, chemicals and consumer goods. Since Jan. 1991 trade with the USSR has been conducted in convertible currency. Germany and the UK are Poland's major Western trading partners.

Total trade between Poland and UK (British Department of Trade returns £1,000 sterling):

	1986	*1987*	*1988*	*1989*	*1990*
Imports to UK	309,746	303,418	328,013	330,163	357,164
Exports and re-exports from UK	182,841	181,451	175,685	196,446	221,536

In Feb. 1987 the US restored Poland's most-favoured-nation status. A trade agreement was signed with the European Community in Sept. 1989.

Tourism. In 1988, 4,196,000 tourists visited Poland (1,104,000 from the West) and 6,924,000 Polish citizens made visits abroad (1,665,000 to the West). More liberal passport regulations were introduced for Polish citizens in 1987.

COMMUNICATIONS

Roads. In 1989 Poland had 159,000 km of hard-surfaced roads. There were 4·85m. passenger cars (4·77m. private), 977,000 lorries (452,000 private) 91,000 buses and 1·41m. motor cycles. Public road transport carried 2,504m. passengers and 105m. tonnes of freight in 1988. There were 37,538 road accidents in 1989 (4,851 fatal).

Railways. Length of standard gauge routes was 24,287 km (11,015 km electrified) in 1990. In 1989 55,800m. passenger-km and 110,990m. tonne-km of freight were carried.

Aviation. In 1990 the state airline 'Lot' had 29 aircraft including 2 Western-built, and operated 9 internal and 34 international routes. 2·02m. passengers were flown in 1988. There are British Airways, SABENA, KLM, PANAM, Alitalia, Swissair, Air France, Austrian Airlines and Lufthansa services to Okęcie (Warsaw) airport.

Shipping. The principal ports are Gdynia, Gdańsk (Danzig) and Szczecin (Stettin). Ocean-going services are grouped into Polish Ocean Lines based on Gdynia and operating regular liner services, and the Polish Shipping Company based on Szczecin and operating cargo services. Poland also has a share in the Gdynia America Line. 30·8m. tonnes of freight and 453,000 passengers were carried in 1988.

In 1989 the merchant marine had 249 vessels totalling 4·1m. GRT (including 45 container ships, 9 ferries and 8 tankers and 16 vessels over 30,000 tons). There are regular lines to London, Hull, China, Indonesia, Australia, Vietnam and some African and Latin-American countries.

There are 3,997 km of navigable inland waterways. In 1989 there were 69 passenger vessels, 413 tugs and 1,380 barges. 15·5m. tonnes of freight and 6·5m. passengers were carried in 1988.

Pipeline. In 1989 there were 2,021 km of oil pipeline; 43m. tonnes were transported in 1988.

Telecommunications. In 1989 there were 8,273 post offices. There were 2·63m. telephones of which 1·98m. were private and 32,000 telex subscribers in 1987.

Polskie Radio i Telewizja broadcasts 3 radio programmes and 2 TV programmes. Colour programmes are transmitted by the SECAM system. Links with the West are provided through the Eutelstat satellite. There were 84 transmitting stations in 1989. Radio licences in 1989, 11·12m.; TV licences, 10·05m.

Cinemas and Theatres. In 1989 there were 1,792 cinemas, 92 theatres and 50 concert halls. Cinema attendance was 69·9m.; theatre, 7·1m. 25 full-length films were made.

Newspapers and Books. In 1989 there were 99 newspapers with an overall circulation of 9·63m. and 2,811 other periodicals. 10,391 book titles were published in 1989 in 217·2m copies. In 1990 there were 32,400 public libraries.

JUSTICE, RELIGION, EDUCATION AND WELFARE

Justice. The penal code was adopted in 1969. Espionage and treason carry the severest penalties. For minor crimes there is provision for probation sentences and fines.

There exist the following courts: The Supreme Court; 29 voivodship courts, district and special courts. Judges and lay assessors are elected. The State Council elects the judges of the Supreme Court for a term of 5 years, and appoints the Prosecutor-General. The office of the Prosecutor-General is separate from the judiciary. An ombudsman's office was established in 1987.

Family courts were established (1977) for cases involving divorce and domestic relations but divorce suits were transferred to the voivodship courts in 1990. Crimes reported in 1983 (and 1984) 466,205 (538,930) including 478 (593) homicides and 1,875 (2,184) rapes.

Religion. In 1978, 93% of the population was baptized into the Catholic Church, and 78% of the population attended church regularly. According to a survey published in the Communist Party journal *Nowe drogi* in 1985, 90% of the population held religious beliefs. Church–State relations are regulated by three laws of May 1989 which guarantee religious freedom, grant the Church radio and TV programmes and permit it to run schools, hospitals and old age homes. The Church has a university (Lublin), an Academy of Catholic Theology and in 1983 46 seminaries.

The archbishop of Warsaw and Gniezno is the primate of Poland (since 1981, Cardinal Józef Glemp). The Vatican considers the archbishoprics of Lwów and Vilnius (incorporated in the USSR in 1940) as still being under Polish jurisdiction. In 1983 there were 5 archbishoprics, 27 dioceses and 7,496 parishes, 84 bishops, 37,132 monks and nuns and 14,498 churches and 4,201 chapels. In 1986 there were 3 cardinals and 22,381 priests. In Oct. 1978 Cardinal Karol Wojtyla, archbishop of Cracow, was elected Pope as John Paul II.

On 28 June 1972 the Vatican adjusted the Church boundaries, to coincide with the State's western frontier ('Oder–Neisse line') and the 4 apostolic administrators in the former German territories became bishops.

Figures for other churches in 1983: Polish Autocephalous Orthodox, 5 dioceses, 218 parishes, 301 churches, 226 priests, 1 monastery, 1 nunnery, 600,000 adherents. Lutheran, 6 dioceses, 121 parishes, 173 churches, 153 chapels, 100 parsons (100,000 adherents in 1975). Uniate, 3 dioceses, 85 parishes, 98 churches, 90 priests (200,000 adherents in 1975). Old-Catholic Mariavite, 3 dioceses, 42 parishes, 55 churches, 29 priests (30,000 adherents in 1975). Methodist, 5 districts, 60 parishes, 57 chapels, 36 parsons (4,133 adherents in 1975). United Evangelical, 200 congregations, 56 chapels, 180 parsons. Seventh-day Adventist, 123 communities, 123 churches, 61 parsons. Baptist, 128 congregations, 58 chapels, 58 parsons (2,300 adherents in 1975). Jews, 16 congregations, 10 synagogues (12,000 adherents in 1978). Epiphany World Mission, 9 chapels and 426 priests. In 1985 there were 2,500 Moslems with 3 mosques and 5 priests.

Education. Basic education from 7 to 15 is free and compulsory. Free secondary education is then optional in general or vocational schools. Primary schools are organized in complexes based on wards under one director ('gmina collective schools'). In 1989–90 there were: Nursery schools, 26,358 with 1·32m. pupils and 91,000 teachers; primary schools, 18,283 with 5,229,000 pupils and 293,000 teachers; secondary schools, 1,177 with 463,000 pupils and 23,000 teachers; vocational schools, 9,366 with 1,755,000 pupils and 85,000 teachers, and 98 institutions of higher education (including 11 universities, 18 polytechnics, 9 agricultural schools, 6 schools of economics, 10 teachers' training colleges and 11 medical schools) with 378,400 students and 61,475 teaching staff.

Religious (Catholic) instruction was introduced in all schools in 1990; for children of dissenting parents there are classes in ethics.

Health. In 1989 there were 716 hospitals (including 43 mental hospitals) with 254,000 beds, 6,687 dispensaries and 3,321 health centres. There were 79,200 doctors, 18,000 dentists, 16,300 pharmacists and 197,800 nurses.

Social Security. In 1984, 76,955m. złotys were paid in family allowances and 77,830m. złotys in sick pay. In 1989 2·26m. retirement pensions were paid (monthly average 110,100 złotys), 2·15m. disability pensions (91,500 złotys), 1m. dependants' pensions (90,500 złotys) and 1·36m. farmers' retirement pensions (72,700 złotys).

DIPLOMATIC REPRESENTATIVES

Of Poland in Great Britain (47 Portland Pl., London, W1N 3AG)
Ambassador: Tadeusz de Virion

Of Great Britain in Poland (Aleje Roz No. 1, Warsaw)
Ambassador: S. J. Barrett, CMG.

Of Poland in the USA (2640 16th St., NW, Washington, D.C., 20009)
Ambassador: Jan Kinast.

Of the USA in Poland (Aleje Ujazdowskie 29/31, Warsaw)
Ambassador: John R. Davis, Jr.

Of Poland to the United Nations
Ambassador: Stanisław Pawlak.

Further Reading

Statistical Information: The Central Statistical Office, Warsaw (Wawelska 1–3), publishes *Rocznik statystyczny* (annual, 1930–39; 1947–); *Poland: Statistical Data.* (annual, 1977–); *Wiadomości statystycznie* (quarterly, 1957–).

Constitution of the Polish People's Republic. Warsaw, 1964
Ascherson, N., *The Struggles for Poland.* London, 1987
Ash, T. G., *The Polish Revolution: Solidarity 1980–82.* London, 1983
Beneš, V. L. and Pounds, N. G. J., *Poland.* London, 1970
Bielasiak, J. and Simon, M. D. (eds.) *Polish Politics: Edge of the Abyss.* New York, 1984
Brandys, K., *Warsaw Diary 1978–1981.* New York, 1984
Bromke, A., *Poland: the Protracted Crisis.* Oakville (Ontario), 1983.—*The Meaning and Uses of Polish History.* New York, 1987
Brumberg, A., *Poland: Genesis of a Revolution.* New York, 1983
Bulas, K. and others, *English–Polish and Polish–English Dictionary.* 2 vols. The Hague, 1959
Burda, A., *Parliament of the Polish People's Republic.* Wrocław, 1978
Davies, N., *Poland, Past and Present: A Select Bibliography of Works in English.* Newtonville, 1977.—*God's Playground: A History of Poland.* 2 vols. OUP, 1981.—*Heart of Europe: a Short History of Poland.* OUP, 1984
De Weydenthal, J. B., et al. *The Polish Drama, 1980–1982.* Lexington, 1983
Dziewanowski, M. K., *Poland in the Twentieth Century.* Columbia Univ. Press, 1977
Eringer, R., *Strike for Freedom: The Story of Lech Wałesa and Polish Solidarity.* New York, 1982
Gieysztor, A., and others, *History of Poland. 2nd ed. Warsaw, 1979*
Halecki, O., *A History of Poland.* 4th ed. London, 1983
Jaruzelski, W., *Jaruzelski, Prime Minister of Poland: Selected Speeches.* Oxford, 1985
Kanka, A. G., *Poland: An Annotated Bibliography of Books in English.* New York, 1988
Karpiński, J., *Countdown: the Polish Upheavals of 1956, 1968, 1970, 1976, 1980.* New York, 1982
Kieniewicz, S. (ed.) *History of Poland.* 2nd ed. Warsaw, 1979
Landau, Z., *The Polish Economy in the Twentieth Century.* London, 1985
Leslie, R. F., (ed.) *The History of Poland since 1863.* CUP, 1980
Lewański, R. C., *Poland.* [Bibliography] Oxford and Santa Barbara, 1984
Lipski, J. J., *KOR: A History of the Workers' Defense Committee in Poland, 1976–1981.* Univ. of California Press, 1985
Michnik, A., *Letters from Prison and Other Essays.* London, 1985
Misztal, B., (ed.) *Poland after Solidarity.* New Brunswick, 1985
Potel, J.-I., *The Summer Before the Frost: Solidarity in Poland.* London, 1982
Preibisz, J. M., (ed.) *Polish Dissident Publications: An Annotated Bibliography.* New York, 1982
Raina P., *Independent Social Movements in Poland.* London, 1981.—*Poland 1981: Towards Social Renewal.* London, 1985
Ruane, K., *The Polish Challenge.* London, 1982
Singer, D., *The Road to Gdansk: Poland and the USSR.* New York and London, 1981
Staniszkis, J., *Poland's Self-Limiting Revolution.* Princeton, 1984
Steven, S., *The Poles.* London, 1982
Szczypiorski, A., *The Polish Ordeal: The View from Within.* London, 1982
Taras, R., *Poland: Socialist State, Rebellious Nation.* Boulder, 1986
Wałęsa, L., *A Path of Hope.* London, 1989
Wedel, J., *The Private Poland.* New York, 1986
Weschler, L., *Solidarity: Poland in the Season of its Passion.* New York, 1982
Who's Who in Poland. New York, 1983
Wielka Encyklopedia Powszechna. 13 vols. Warsaw, 1962–70
Woodall, J., (ed.) *Policy and Politics in Contemporary Poland: Reform, Failure and Crisis.* London, 1982

National Library: Biblioteka Narodowa, Rakowiecka 6, Warsaw.

PORTUGAL

Capital: Lisbon
Population: 10·30m. (1988)
GNP per capita: US$4,260 (1990)

República Portuguesa

HISTORY. Portugal has been an independent state since the 12th century, apart from one period of Spanish rule (1580–1640). The monarchy was deposed on 5 Oct. 1910 and a republic established.

A *coup* on 28 May 1926 established a military provisional government from 1 June. A corporatist constitution was adopted on 19 March 1933 under which a civil dictatorship governed until a fresh *coup* on 25 April 1974 established a Junta of National Salvation.

Following an attempted revolt on 11 March 1975, the Junta was dissolved and a Supreme Revolutionary Council formed which ruled until 25 April 1976 when constitutional government was resumed; the SRC was renamed the Council of the Revolution, becoming a consultative body until its abolition in 1982.

AREA AND POPULATION. Mainland Portugal is bounded north and east by Spain and south and west by the Atlantic ocean. The Atlantic archipelagoes of the Azores and of Madeira form autonomous but integral parts of the republic, which has a total area of 91,985 sq. km (35,516 sq. miles) and census populations:

1940	7,755,423	1960	8,889,392	1981	9,833,014
1950	8,510,240	1970	8,648,369		

The areas and populations of the districts and Autonomous Regions are:

Districts:	*sq. km*	*Census 1981*	*Estimate 31 Dec. 1988*
Aveiro	2,808	622,988	670,100
Beja	10,225	188,420	175,400
Braga	2,673	708,924	778,200
Bragança	6,608	184,252	183,900
Castelo Branco	6,675	234,230	221,200
Coimbra	3,947	436,324	446,600
Evora	7,393	180,277	172,800
Faro	4,960	323,534	342,900
Guarda	5,518	205,631	194,100
Leiria	3,515	420,229	436,200
Lisboa	2,761	2,069,467	2,128,700
Portalegre	6,065	142,905	136,200
Porto	2,395	1,562,287	1,683,200
Santarém	6,747	454,123	459,900
Setúbal	5,064	658,326	798,900
Viana de Castelo	2,225	256,814	266,700
Vila Real	4,328	264,381	261,500
Viseu	5,007	423,648	421,400
Total mainland	88,944	9,336,760	9,777,900
Autonomous Regions:			
Azores	2,247	243,410	253,600
Madeira	794	252,844	273,200

At the 1981 census, 29·7% of the population was urban (living in towns of 10,000 and more) and 48·2% were male. The chief cities at 31 Dec. 1987 (and census, 1981) are Lisbon, the capital 830,500 (817,627) and Porto 350,000 (330,199); other population aggregates are Amadora 95,518 (93,663), Setúbal 77,885 (76,812), Coimbra 74,616 (71,782), Braga 63,033 (63,771), Vila Nova de Gaia 62,469 (60,962), Barreiro 50,863 (50,745), Funchal 44,111 (48,638), Almada 42,607 (41,468), Queluz 42,241 (41,112), Odivelas 38,322 (38,546), Evora 34,851 (34,072), Agualva-Cacem 34,341 (34,041) and Oeiras 32,529 (32,046).

The Azores islands lie in the mid-Atlantic ocean, between 1,200 and 1,600 km west of Lisbon. They are divided into 3 widely separated groups with clear channels between, São Miguel (759 sq. km) together with Santa Maria (97 sq. km) being the most easterly; about 100 miles north-west of them lies the central cluster of Terceira (382 sq. km), Graciosa (62 sq. km), São Jorge (246 sq. km), Pico (446 sq. km) and Faial (173 sq. km); still another 150 miles to the north-west are Flores (143 sq. km) and Corvo (17 sq. km), the latter being the most isolated and primitive of the islands. São Miguel contains over half the total population of the archipelago.

Madeira comprises the island of Madeira (745 sq. km), containing the capital, Funchal; the smaller island of Porto Santo (40 sq. km), lying 46 km. to the northeast of Madeira; and two groups of uninhabited islets, Ilhas Desertas (15 sq. km), being 20 km. south-east of Funchal and Ilhas Selvagens (4 sq. m), near the Canaries.

Vital statistics for calendar years:

	Live-births	*Still-births*	*Marriages*	*Divorces*	*Deaths*	*Emigrants*
1984	142,805	1,664	69,875	7,034	97,227	6,556
1985	130,492	1,510	68,461	8,988	97,339	7,149
1986	126,748	1,390	69,271	8,411	95,828	6,253
1987	123,218	1,230	71,656	8,948	95,423	8,108
1988	122,121	1,152	71,098	...	98,236	9,540

In 1988 the births included 63,020 boys and 59,101 girls; deaths, 51,527 males and 46,709 females. In 1988, 4,886 emigrants went to France, 2,112 to USA and 889 to Oceania.

CLIMATE. Because of westerly winds and the effect of the Gulf Stream, the climate ranges from the cool, damp Atlantic type in the north to a warmer and drier Mediterranean type in the south. July and Aug. are virtually rainless everywhere. Inland areas in the north have greater temperature variation, with continental winds blowing from the interior. Lisbon. Jan. 52°F (11°C), July 72°F (22°C). Annual rainfall 27·4" (686 mm). Porto. Jan. 48°F (8·9°C), July 67°F (19·4°C). Annual rainfall 46" (1,151 mm).

CONSTITUTION AND GOVERNMENT. A new Constitution, replacing that of 1976, was approved by the Assembly of the Republic (by 197 votes to 40) on 12 Aug. 1982 and promulgated in Sept. It abolished the (military) Council of the Revolution and reduced the role of the President of the Republic.

Portugal is a sovereign, unitary republic. Executive power is vested in the *President* of the Republic, directly elected for a 5-year term (for a maximum of 2 consecutive terms). At the presidential elections of Jan. 1991 Mario Soares was elected against 3 opponents by 70.4% of the votes cast. Presidents since 1926:

Marshal António Oscar de Fragoso Carmona, 29 Nov. 1926–18 April 1951 (died).

Dr Antonio de Oliveira Salazar (acting), 18 April 1951–22 July 1951.

Marshal Francisco Higino Craveiro Lopez, 22 July 1951–9 Aug. 1958.

Rear-Adm. Américo Deus Rodrigues Tomaz, 9 Aug. 1958–25 April 1974. (deposed).

Gen. Antonio Sebastião Ribeiro de Spinola, 25 April 1974–30 Sept. 1974 (resigned).

Gen. Francisco da Costa Gomes, 30 Sept. 1974–14 July 1976.

Gen. Antonio Ramalho Eanes, 14 July 1976–9 March 1986.

President of the Republic: Mario Soares, elected 16 Feb. 1986 (took office 9 March 1986); elected for a 2nd term Jan. 1991.

The President appoints a Prime Minister and, upon the latter's nomination, other members of the Council of Ministers, as well as Secretaries and Under-Secretaries of State, who are outside the Council.

The Social Democrat government was composed in Jan. 1991 of:

Prime Minister: Anibal Cavaço Silva.

Deputy Prime Minister, Defence: Carlos Brito. *Minister of State and Justice:* Fernando Nogueira. *Parliamentary Affairs:* Antonio Capucho. *Finance:* Miguel Beleza. *Planning and Territorial Administration:* Luis Valente de Oliveira. *Interior:* Manuel Pereira Godinho. *Foreign Affairs:* João de Deus Pinheiro. *Agriculture, Fisheries and Alimentation:* Arlindo Cunha. *Industry and Energy:* Luis Mira Amaral. *Education:* Roberto Carneiro. *Public Works, Transport and Communication:* João Oliveira Martins. *Health:* Arlindo Carvalho. *Labour and Social Security:* José Silva Peneda. *Trade and Tourism:* Joaquim Ferreira do Amaral. *Youth:* Antonio Couto dos Santos. *Environment:* Ferrando Ferreira Real.

There is a unicameral legislature, the Assembly of the Republic, comprising 250 deputies elected for 4 years by universal adult suffrage under a system of proportional representation. At the General Election of 19 July 1987, there were 148 seats won by the *Partido Social Democrata* (PSD), 60 by the *Partido Socialista* (PS), 7 by the Democratic Renewal Party, 31 by the Communist Party and 4 by the Christian Democrats.

National flag: Vertical green and red, with the red of double width, and over all on the dividing line the national arms.

National anthem: A Portuguesa (words by Lopes de Mendonça, 1890; tune by Alfredo Keil).

Local government: Since 1976, the archipelagoes of the Azores and of Madeira are Autonomous Regions with their own legislatures and governments. Pending the formation of other regional governments, Continental Portugal is divided into 18 districts. Regions and districts are divided into 305 municipal authorities *(concelhos)* and sub-divided into 4,050 parishes. Each level is governed by an assembly elected by direct universal suffrage under a system of proportional representation, with an executive body responsible to the assembly.

DEFENCE. Military service is compulsory for 12–15 months in the Army and Navy and 18–20 months in the Air Force. Reserves for all services number about 190,000.

Army. The Army consists of 1 brigade, 2 cavalry regiments, 1 armoured regiment, 14 infantry regiments, 1 commando regiment and 3 independent battalions, 1 special forces brigade, 1 field, 1 air-defence and 1 coast artillery regiments, 2 engineer and 1 signals regiments and 1 regiment of military police. Equipment includes 86 M-48A5 main battle tanks and 132 M113 armed personnel carriers. Strength (1991) 44,000 (35,000 conscripts). Paramilitary forces are the National Republican Guard (19,000), Public Security Police (17,000), and the Border Guard (8,500).

Navy. The Navy is organized into 3 commands: Continental, based at Lisbon and Portimão; Azores; and Madeira. The combatant fleet comprises 3 French-built Daphne class diesel submarines, 8 small frigates, 6 offshore and 14 coastal patrol vessels. Auxiliaries include 1 tanker, 1 transport, 1 survey ship, 1 sail training ship and 1 ocean tug. There are 6 small amphibious craft and some 20 service vessels. The first of 3 frigates of West German MEKO design the *Vasco da Gama*, has commenced trails. Naval personnel in 1990 totalled 13,000 (4,500 conscripts) including 2,700 marines.

Air Force. Formed in 1912, the Air Force has been independent since 1952, when it was combined with the naval air service and given equal status with the Army and Navy. In 1991, it had a strength of about 11,000 (3,600 conscripts).

Equipment comprises 2 strike squadrons with 40 A-7P Corsair IIs; 2 squadrons of G.91Rs for ground attack; 1 squadron of P-3P Orion maritime patrol aircraft now forming; 1 squadron of 5 C-130H Hercules and 4 squadrons of CASA 212 Aviocars for transport and search and rescue operations; 32 Cessna 337 Skymasters and a force of Puma and Alouette III helicopters. Other aircraft in service include Chipmunk piston-engined trainers, T-37C jet basic trainers, T-33, T-38A Talon and G.91T jet advanced trainers. Delivery of 18 Epsilon trainers (to replace the Chipmunks) began early in 1989.

INTERNATIONAL RELATIONS

Membership. Portugal is a member of the UN, EC, OECD, NATO, WEU and the Council of Europe.

ECONOMY

Policy. Large-scale privatization is in train. The main objective of the 1989-92 medium-term plan is the modernization of the economy and society.

Budget. The 1989 budget balanced at 2,656,560m. escudos. 1991 budget estimates: Revenue 3,273,300m. excudos; expenditure, 3,911,000m. escudos. Expenditure on welfare, 35.2%; education, 15.2%..

Currency. The unit of currency is the *escudo* (PTE) of 100 *centavos*, which contains 0·06651 gramme of fine gold. It was stabilized on 9 June 1931, and the paper currency re-linked to gold when the notes of the Bank of Portugal became payable in gold or its equivalent in foreign currency. 1,000 *escudos* is called a *conto*.

There are notes of 5,000, 1,000, 500 and 100 *escudos*; cupronickel coins of 50, 25, 20, 5 and 2½ *escudos*; nickel-brass coins of 1 *escudo*; bronze coins of ½ *escudo*. Inflation was an annualized 13% in Oct. 1990. In March 1991, £1 = 254·40 *escudos*; US$1 = 134·10 *escudos*.

Banking and Finance. Since 1931 the central bank and bank of issue has been the Banco de Portugal, founded 19 Nov. 1846 and nationalized on 13 Sept. 1974. Its capital is fixed at 200m. escudos. Its *Governor* is Jose Alberto Tavares Moreira. Banks and insurance companies were nationalized in 1975 but are now being privatized. From Feb. 1984 new private banks were allowed to operate. The National Development Bank began operations on 4 Jan. 1960.

In Dec. 1988 there were 27 banks (6 foreign) operating in Portugal: 22 commercial banks, 2 investment banks and 3 savings banks. In March 1988 commercial banks' total credits were 1,777,184m. escudos and deposits 3,730,027m. escudos; investment banks' total credits 266,675m. escudos and deposits 163,822m. escudos; savings banks' total credits 1,335,841m. escudos and deposits 1,886,075m. escudos.

Ceilings on bank lending were removed in Jan. 1991.

There are stock exchanges in Lisbon and Oporto.

Weights and Measures. The metric system is the legal standard. The arroba (of 14·69 kg) is sometimes used locally.

ENERGY AND NATURAL RESOURCES

Electricity. Total production of electrical power in 1986 was 20,355m. kwh.; the installed capacity totalled 7,730,645 kva. of which 3,350,106 was hydro-electric. Supply 110 and 220 volts; 50 Hz.

Minerals. Portugal possesses considerable mineral wealth. Production in tonnes:

	1985	*1986*	*1987*		*1985*	*1986*	*1987*
Coal	238,414	209,501	228,648	Gold (refined)	0·229	0·303	0·320
Cupriferous pyrites	355,519	321,514	279,061	Uranium	139	131	167
Tin ores	379	300	90	Wolframite	2,977	2,764	2,011
Kaolin	104,055	70,567	66,736				

Uranium mining commenced in Aug. 1979. Annual production, 115 tonnes; reserves, 7,000 tonnes.

Agriculture. About 30% of the workforce is engaged in agriculture. The following figures show the area (in 1,000 ha) and production (in 1,000 tonnes) of the chief crops:

	1986		*1987*		*1988*	
Crop	*Area*	*Quantity*	*Area*	*Quantity*	*Area*	*Quantity*
Wheat	315·0	499·7	323·0	532·5	275	401
Maize	252·7	611·4	256·9	640·4	230	663
Oats	194·1	152·7	196·9	155·2	168	76
Barley	87·1	89·6	83·7	79·4	73	48
Rye	124·4	99·9	128·4	108·2	124	73
Rice	32·3	149·4	32·2	144·4	33	151
Dried beans	198·4	44·4	195·5	44·1	162	47
Potatoes	118·8	1,067·2	123·0	1,112·4	124	795

Wine production (in tonnes), 1988, 368,000; olive oil (tonnes), 22,000. In 1987, 76,839 tonnes of port wine were exported.

Livestock (1988). 29,000 horses, 90,000 mules, 175,000 asses, 1,387,000 cattle, 745,000 goats, 5·22m. sheep and 2·8m. pigs.

Forestry. Forest area covers 3m. ha, of which 1·38m. are pine, 680,390 cork oak, 534,370 other oak, 243,180 eucalyptus, 30,230 chestnut and 160,890 other species.

Portugal is a major producer of cork; 79,357 tonnes in 1987. Most of it is exported crude. Production of resin was 108,439 tonnes in 1986.

Fisheries. The fishing industry for the continent and adjacent isles is of importance. At 31 Dec. 1987 there were 41,844 men and boys employed, with 17,980 registered boats. The sardine catch, 1987, was 90,416 tonnes valued at 2,881,221 contos. The most important centres of the sardine industry are at Matosinhos, Figueira di Foz, Peniche, Setúbal, Portimão and Olhão.

INDUSTRY. The main groups are textiles, shoes, leather goods, wood and cork products and ceramics; these are produced mainly by small companies.

Labour. The maximum working week was 44 hours in 1991; the minimum monthly wage for industrial and farm workers was 40,100 escudos. Unemployment was 5% in 1990.

Trade Unions. An agreement between trade unions, employers and the government for 1991 involved a voluntary wage ceiling, a commitment to labour peace, improvements in working conditions and a 15% increase in pension and social security payments.

FOREIGN ECONOMIC RELATIONS

Commerce. Imports for consumption and exports (exclusive of coin and bullion and re-exports) for calendar years, in 1m. escudos:

	1984	*1985*	*1986*	*1987*	*1988*
Imports	1,160,633	1,326,528	1,442,493	1,965,315	2,555,163
Exports	760,580	971,747	1,082,261	1,311,003	1,581,231

Principal exports in 1988 (in 1m. escudos): Textiles, 480,985; pulp and paper, 125,254; wood and cork, 110,425; foodstuffs and wine, 91,242; chemicals, 69,143; minerals, 57,676.

The distribution of the imports and exports (in 1m. escudos):

	Imports (c.i.f.)			*Exports (f.o.b.)*		
From or to	*1986*	*1987*	*1988*	*1986*	*1987*	*1988*
Angola	11,196	5,614	4,499	13,785	14,612	29,337
Belgium-Lux.	41,682	63,628	104,906	37,037	39,106	104,906
France	145,157	220,721	293,986	164,235	207,268	239,724
Germany, Fed. Rep. of	205,420	294,270	372,329	158,627	200,948	231,583
Italy	114,487	171,591	236,038	42,915	51,727	65,734
Mozambique	389	1,361	1,029	3,073	4,486	4,649
Netherlands	57,053	79,636	122,902	72,232	84,983	92,672
Spain	157,060	230,601	335,752	71,681	118,438	176,697
UK	108,281	158,468	210,831	154,010	184,451	228,314
USA	100,592	94,777	110,412	75,557	84,325	93,743

Total trade between Portugal (excluding the Azores and Madeira) and UK (British Department of Trade returns, in £1,000 sterling):

	1986	*1987*	*1988*	*1989*	*1990*
Imports to UK	768,470	847,980	928,015	1,040,706	1,176,161
Exports and re-exports from UK	472,078	699,915	810,537	915,682	1,033,268

Tourism. Tourism is of increasing importance for the invisible balance of payments. In 1988 there were 16,076,681 visitors.

COMMUNICATIONS

Roads (1987). There were 22,375 km of road. There were 2,838,732 motor cars registered in 1988 and 120,819 motor cycles. In 1988 there were 93,408 road accidents, with 2,566 fatalities.

Railways. In 1989 total railway length was 3,588 km (1,668 mm and metre gauges), of which 461 km of broad-gauge was electrified. In 1989, 232m. passengers were carried and 7.9m. tonnes of freight.

Aviation. There are international airports at Portela (Lisbon), Pedras Rubras (Porto), Faro (Algarve), Santa Maria and Lages (Azores) and Funchal (Madeira). Services connect Lisbon with most major centres in North and South America, Western Europe and Africa. Airlines in 1988 carried 2·8m. passengers and 50,214 tonnes of freight. The national airline changed its name to Air Portugal in 1979.

Shipping. In 1988, 13,601 vessels of 77·1m. tonnes entered the ports (continental and islands). In 1987, 4,637 were Portuguese, 338 British and 601 Spanish. In 1986 the merchant marine consisted of 65 transport vessels of 1,469,051 gross tons.

Telecommunications (1987). The number of post offices was 17,835. The State owned 7,693,529 km of telephone line through the *Telefones de Lisboa e Porto* (nationalized in 1977). Number of telephones was 2,071,544 (1987).

Radio Difusão Portuguesa broadcasts 3 programmes on medium-waves and on FM as well as 3 regional services. *Radiotelevisão Portuguesa* broadcasts 2 commercial TV programmes. *Radio Renancença* is a commercial, nationwide network. In addition there are 6 local, commercial stations, operating on medium-waves. Radio Trans Europe is a high-powered short-wave station, retransmitting programmes of different broadcasting organizations, *e.g.*, IBRA, Radio Canada and Deutsche Welle. Radio Free Europe also has relay facilities on short-waves in Portugal. Number of receivers: Radio (1984), 2,155,000; TV (1987), 1,618,313.

Cinemas (1987). There were 358 cinemas with a seating capacity of 163,112.

Newspapers (1987). There were 31 daily newspapers with a combined circulation of 162,649m.; 14 of these, with a combined circulation of 103,458m., appeared in Lisbon.

JUSTICE, RELIGION, EDUCATION AND WELFARE

Justice. Portuguese law distinguishes civil (including commercial) and penal, labour, military, administrative and fiscal branches, having low courts and high courts.

The republic is divided for civil and penal cases into 217 *comarcas*; in every comarca there is at least one court or tribunal. In the comarca of Lisbon there are 39 lower sub divisional courts *(juizos)* (22 for criminal procedure and 17 for civil or commercial cases); in the comarca of Porto there are 20 such courts (11 for criminal and 9 for civil or commercial cases); at Braga, Coimbra, Loures, Setúbal, Sintra and Vila Nova de Gaia there are 4 functioning courts; at Almada, Cascais, Funchal, Guimarães, Leiria, Matosinhos, Oeiras, Santarém, Torres Vedras, Viana do Castelo, Vila do Conde, Vila da Feira and Viseu there are 3 courts; 22 comarcas have 2 courts each. There are 4 courts of appeal *(Tribunal de Relação)* at Lisbon, Coimbra, Evora and Porto, and a Supreme Court in Lisbon *(Supremo Tribunal de Justiça)*.

Capital punishment was abolished completely in the Constitution of 1976.

The prison population as at 1 Jan. 1988 was 8,275.

Religion. In 1981, 94·5% of the population were Roman Catholic, but there is freedom of worship, both in public and private, with the exception of creeds incompatible with morals and the life and physical integrity of the people.

Education. Compulsory education has been in force since 1911. Adult illiteracy was 20% in 1990 according to official figures. In 1986–87 there were 10,165 public primary schools with 787,759 pupils and 41,518 teachers. In 1986–87 private elementary schools numbered 662 with 50,216 pupils and 2,506 teachers. Basic preparatory schools numbered 1,865 with 395,064 pupils and 28,699 teachers. In 1985–86 there were 499 secondary schools, with 647,391 pupils and 53,881 teachers. There were also 27 schools which taught art activities (cinema, music and theatre) with 15,165 students. There are 18 universities, of which 8 are in Lisbon: The University of Lisbon (1930), the private Portuguese Catholic University, also with faculties and sections at Braga, Porto and Viseu (1968), the New University of Lisbon (1973), the private International University (1984), the private Autonomous University of Lisbon 'Luis de Camoes' (1986), the private Lusiada University (1986) and the Open University (1988); the other 10 are Coimbra (founded 1290), Porto (1911), Aveiro (1973), Minho, at Braga and Guimaraes (1973), Evora (1979), Azores, at Agra do Heróismo, Horto and Ponta Delgado (1980) and Algarve, at Faro (1983) Beira Interior, at Covilha (1986), Tras-os-Montes e Alto Douro, at Vila Real (1986) and the private Portucaleuse University, at Porto (1986). Including other colleges, there were 107,485 students in higher education in 1985–86 with 12,749 teaching staff.

Health. In 1987 there were 229 hospitals, 366 health centres, 26,381 doctors, 392 dentists, 607 stomatologists, 4,728 pharmacists and 25,777 nursing personnel.

DIPLOMATIC REPRESENTATIVES

Of Portugal in Great Britain (11 Belgrave Sq., London, SW1X 8PP)
Ambassador: António Vaz-Pereira LVO (accredited 12 July 1989).

Of Great Britain in Portugal (35-37 Rua de S. Domingos à Lapa, Lisbon)
Ambassador: H. J. Arbuthnott, CMG.

Of Portugal in the USA (2125 Kalorama Rd., NW, Washington, D.C., 20008)
Ambassador: João Eduardo M. Pereira Bastos.

Of the USA in Portugal (Ave. das Forcas Armadas, 1600 Lisbon)
Ambassador: Everett E. Briggs.

Of Portugal to the United Nations
Ambassador: Fernando José Reino.

Further Reading

Statistical Information: The Instituto Nacional de Estatistica (Avenida António José de Almeida, Lisbon) was set up in 1935 in succession to the Direcção-Geral de Estatistica. The Centro de Estudos Económicos and the Centro de Estudos Demográficos were affiliated to the Instituto in 1944. The main publications are:

Anuário Estatistíco. Annuaire statistique. Annual, from 1875
Estatísticas do Comércio Externo. 2 vols. Annual from 1967 (replacing *Comércio Externo,* 1936–66, and *Estatística Comercial*, 1865–1935)
Censo da População de Portugal. 1864 ff. Decennial (latest ed. 1972)
Estatística da Organização Corporativa. 1938–49. Estatísticas da Organização Corporativa e Previdência Social. 1950 ff.
Estatísticas das Finanças, Publicas and *Estatísticas Nometárias.* 1969 ff. (replacing *Estatísticas Financeiras.* 1947–68 and *Situação Bancária*, 1919–46)
Estatísticas Agrícolas. Statistique Agricole. 1943–64; replaced by *Estatísticas Agri colas e Alimentares.* From 1965. Annual
Estatísticas Industrials. 1967 ff. (replacing *Estatística Industrial. Statistique Industrielle.* 1943–66)
Estatísticas Demográficas. From 1967 (replacing *Anuário Demográfico*, 1929–66)
Boletim Mensal do Instituto Nacional de Estatística. Monthly since 1929
Centro de Estudos Económicos. Revista. 1945 ff.
Centro de Estudos Demográficos. Revista. 1945 ff.
Estatísticas das Contribuiçôes e Impostos. Annual from 1967 (replacing *Anuário Estatístico das Contribuiçôes e Impostos*, 1936–66)
Estatisticas da Cultura, Reveio e Resporto, 1979 ff.
Estatísticas da Educação. 1940 ff.
Estatísticas da Justica. 1968 ff. (replacing *Estatísticas Judiciária.* 1936–66)
Estatísticas das Sociedades. 1939 ff.
Estatísticas da Saúde, 1969 ff.
Estatísticas do Turismo. 1969 ff.
Estatísticas do Energia. 1969 ff.

Azevedo, Gonzaga de, *Historia de Portugal.* 6 vols. Lisbon, 1935–44
Ferreira, H. G. and Marshall, M. W., *Portugal's Revolution: Ten Years On.* CUP, 1986
Ferreira, J. A., *Dictionario inglês-portugês.* 2 vols. Porto, 1948
Gallagher, T., *Portugal: A Twentieth Century Interpretation.* Manchester Univ. Press, 1983
Graham, L. S. and Wheeler, D. L., (eds.) *In Search of Modern Portugal: The Revolution and its Consequences.* Univ. of Wisconsin Press, 1983
Harvey R., *Portugal: Birth of a Democracy.* London, 1978
Robertson, I., *Blue Guide: Portugal.* London, 1982
Rogers, F. M., *Atlantic Islanders of the Azores and Madeiras.* North Quincy, 1979
Taylor, J. L., *Portuguese-English Dictionary.* London, 1959
Unwin, P. T. H., *Portugal.* [Bibliography] Oxford and Santa Barbara, 1987

National Library: Biblioteca Nacional de Lisboa, Campo Grande, Lisbon. *Director:* A. H. C. Marques.

MACAO

HISTORY. Macao was visited by Portuguese traders from 1513 and became a Portuguese colony in 1557; it remains a Portuguese-administered territory by virtue of a Sino-Portuguese treaty of 1 Dec. 1887. It was an Overseas Province of Portugal, 1961–74. Discussions on the future of Macao were taking place with the People's Republic of China in 1986–87 and in 1999 Macao will be handed to China.

AREA AND POPULATION. The territory, which lies at the mouth of the Canton (Pearl) River, comprises a peninsula (6·05 sq. km) connected by a narrow isthmus to the People's Republic of China, on which is built the city of Santa Nome de Deus de Macao, and the islands of Taipa (3·78 sq. km), linked to Macao by a 2-km bridge, and Colôane (7·09 sq. km) linked to Taipa by a 2-km causeway (total area, 16·92 sq. km (6 sq. miles). The population (Census, 1981) was 261,680, Estimate (1990) 440,000. The official language is Portuguese, but Cantonese is used by virtually the entire population.

Vital statistics (1987): Births, 7,565; marriages, 2,472; deaths, 1,321.

CONSTITUTION AND GOVERNMENT. By agreement with Beijing in 1974, Macao is a Chinese territory under Portuguese administration. An 'organic statute' was published on 17 Feb. 1976. It defined the territory as a collective entity, *pessoa colectiva,* with internal legislative authority which, while remaining subject to Portuguese constitutional laws, would otherwise enjoy administrative, economic and financial autonomy. The Governor is appointed by the Portuguese President, who also appoints up to 5 Secretaries-Adjunct on the Governor's nomination. The Legislative Assembly of 17 deputies, chosen for a 3-year term, comprises 6 members directly elected by universal suffrage, 6 indirectly elected by economic, cultural and social bodies and 5 appointed by the Governor. In April 1990 the Portuguese parliament unanimously approved laws passed by the Legislative Assembly to widen its powers and those of the governor.

Governor: Vacant.

ECONOMY

Budget. In 1987, revenue was 2,488,700,000 *patacas* and expenditure 2,390,800,000 *patacas.*

Currency. The unit of currency is the *pataca* (MOP) of 100 *avos* which is tied to the *Hong Kong dollar* at the rate of 103 *patacas* = HK$100. In March 1991, £1 = 15·28 *patacas*; US$1 = 8·05 *patacas.*

Banking. The bank of issue is the Instituto Emissor de Macau. Commercial business is handled (1987) by 22 banks with 94 branches in Macao, 8 of which are local (with 81·5% of total resident deposits and 67·4% of total domestic credit at 31 Dec. 1984) and 14 foreign (including 4 offshore banking units). Total banks' deposits, 1987, 14,111·5m. patacas.

INDUSTRY AND TRADE

Industry. In 1985 the number of establishments for food products was 74 and output in 1,000 patavos was 108,853; textiles (130) 1,330,626; clothing (444) 2,836,832; plastics (67) 523,128.

Labour. The estimated total labour force in 1984 was 178,000, 44% of whom were employed in manufacturing, 33% in commerce and services and 8% in construction.

Commerce. The trade, mostly transit, is handled by Chinese merchants. Imports, in 1987, were 9,107·1m. patacas and exports, 11,233·5m. patacas.

In 1987, 43% of imports came from Hong Kong and 21% from China. 33% of exports went to USA, 36% to EEC (mainly Federal Republic of Germany, France and UK); clothing and textiles accounted for 73·5% of exports, toys 9·9%.

Total trade between Macao and UK (British Department of Trade returns, in £1,000 sterling):

	1986	*1987*	*1988*	*1989*	*1990*
Imports to UK	45,286	45,896	41,116	45,299	44,809
Exports and re-exports from UK	6,522	5,617	4,348	7,498	11,398

Tourism. There were 5,100,500 visitors in 1987. 82·2% were from Hong Kong and 5·1% from Japan.

COMMUNICATIONS

Roads. In 1984 there were 90 km of roads. In 1987 there were 35,925 vehicles, of which 20,391 were passenger cars and 4,099 commercial vehicles.

Shipping. Macao is served by Portuguese, British and Dutch steamship lines. In 1987, 39,239 vessels of 11·5m. gross tons entered the port. In 1987, 4·84m passengers embarked and 4·7m disembarked. Regular services connect Macao with Hong Kong, 65 km to the north-east.

Post and Broadcasting. The territory has 1,577 km of telephone line (55,643 instruments in 1987). One government and 1 private commercial radio station are in operation on medium-waves broadcasting in Portuguese and Chinese. Number of receivers (1977), 70,000. Macao receives television broadcasts from Hong Kong and in 1984 a public bilingual TV station began operating. There were (1979) 50,000 receivers.

Newspapers. In 1987, there were 8 newspapers (2 in Portugese and 6 in Chinese).

JUSTICE, RELIGION, EDUCATION AND WELFARE

Justice. There is a court of First Instance, from which there is appeal to the Court of Appeal and then the Supreme Court, both in Lisbon.

In 1987 there were 4,717 cases of crimes known to the police, of which 3,454 were against property. There were 29,558 cases in courts pending on 1 Jan. and presented during 1987, of which 4,840 were in district court, 10,195 in criminal court and 3,467 in administrative court. At 31 Dec. 1987 there were 326 prisoners, and 37 addicts in the centre for rehabilitation of drugs-abusers.

Religion. The majority of the Chinese population are Buddhists. About 6% are Roman Catholic.

Education. In 1986–87 education was provided at 60 kindergartens (16,516 pupils; 458 teachers), 74 primary schools (31,914; 1,118), 30 secondary schools (14,913; 851), 5 special schools (88; 31), 5 teacher-training schools (61; 26), 5 higher schools (6,891; 70) and 88 adult schools (23,088; 629). The University of East Asia, established in 1981 on Taipa, had 1,165 students in 1983.

Health. In 1987 there were 2 hospitals with 1,242 beds; there were 179 doctors and (1982) 26 pharmacists, 10 midwives and 315 nursing personnel.

Further Reading

Anuário Estatístico de Macau. Macao, Annual
Macau in Figures. Macao, Annual.
Education Survey, 1984–85, Macao, 1986
Brazáo, E., *Macau*. Lisbon, 1957
Edmonds, R.L., *Macau*. [Bibliography] Oxford and Santa Barbara, 1989

QATAR

Capital: Doha
Population: 371,863 (1987)
GNP per capita: US$11,610 (1988)

Dawlat Qatar

(State of Qatar)

HISTORY. The State of Qatar declared its independence from Britain on 3 Sept. 1971, ending the Treaty of 3 Nov. 1916 which was replaced by a Treaty of friendship between the 2 countries.

AREA AND POPULATION. The State of Qatar, which includes the whole of the Qatar peninsula, extends on the landward side from Khor al Odeid to the boundaries of the Saudi Arabian province of Hasa. The territory includes a number of islands in the coastal waters of the peninsula, the most important of which is Halul, the storage and export terminal for the offshore oilfields. Area, 11,437 sq. km; population census (1981) 244,534; estimate in 1987 371,863. In 1987 only 25% were Qatari, with a large majority coming from Pakistan and India.

The capital is Doha (population 1986, 217,294), which is the main port. Other towns are Dukhan, the centre of oil production, Umm Said, oil-terminal of Qatar, and Ruwais, Wakra, Al-Khour, Umm Salal Mohammad and Umm-Bab.

Vital statistics (1988): Live births, 10,842; deaths, 861; marriages, 1,333; divorces, 385.

The official language is Arabic.

CLIMATE. The climate is hot and humid. Doha. Jan. 62°F (16·7°C), July 98°F (36·7°C). Annual rainfall 2·5" (62 mm).

RULER. *The Amir:* HH Shaikh Khalifa bin Hamad Al-Thani, assumed power on 22 Feb. 1972. On 31 May 1977, HH Shaikh Hamad bin Khalifa Al-Thani was appointed Heir Apparent of the State of Qatar, and the portfolio of Minister of Defence was added to his existing responsibility of Commander-in-Chief of the Armed Forces.

Minister of Foreign Affairs: Abdullah bin Khalifa al-Attiyah.

There is no Parliament, but the Council of Ministers is assisted by a 30-member nominated Advisory Council.

Local government: Qatar is divided into 9 municipalities.

Flag: Maroon, with white serrated border on hoist.

DEFENCE

Army. The Army consists of 1 Royal Guard regiment, 1 tank and 3 mechanized infantry battalions, 1 artillery regiment and 1 surface-to-air missile battery. Equipment includes 24 AMX-30 tanks. Personnel (1991) 6,000.

Navy. The navy has 3 French-built fast missile craft and 6 British-built inshore patrol craft, 1 tank landing craft and some 30 boats. There are also 3 quadruple shore-based Exocet missile batteries. Personnel in 1990 totalled 700.

Air Force. The Air Force has 1 squadron of Mirage F1 fighters and 12 Commando, 16 Gazelle and 6 Super Puma helicopters and 6 Alpha Jet armed trainers and Tigercat surface-to-air missile systems. Personnel (1990) 300.

INTERNATIONAL RELATIONS

Membership. Qatar is a member of the UN, the Arab League and the Gulf Co-operation Council.

ECONOMY

Budget. Revenue (1987–88) 6,745m. riyals; expenditure 12,217m. riyals.

Currency. The unit of currency is the *Qatari riyal* (QAR) of 100 *dirhams*, introduced in 1973. There are coins of 1, 5, 10, 25 and 50 *dirhams*, and banknotes of 1, 5, 10, 50, 100 and 500 *riyals*. In March 1991, £1 = 6·89 *riyals*, US$1 = 3·63 *riyals*.

Banking and Finance. The 13 banks operating in Qatar in 1989, included 5 national banks: Qatar National Bank, The Commercial Bank of Qatar, Doha Bank, the Islamic Bank of Qatar and Al Ahli Bank. There are 2 Arab banks: Arab Bank Limited and Bank of Oman. The other 6 foreign banks were: Banque Paribas, the British Bank of the Middle East, Chartered Bank, Bank Saderat Iran, Grindlays Bank and the United Bank. The Qatar National Bank was established in 1965 with capital of 56m. riyals, 50% of which was contributed by the Government and 50% by the private sector. Deposits in commercial banks were 1,241·8m. riyals by Dec. 1987. Government deposits 331m. riyals and private sector's savings deposits 1,240·1m. riyals in 1987.

Weights and Measures. The metric system is in general use.

ENERGY AND NATURAL RESOURCES

Electricity. Production (1988) 4,592·3m. kwh (generation of Abu Samra not included). Supply 240 volts; 50 Hz.

Oil. On 9 Feb. 1977 Qatar gained national control over its 2 natural resources, oil and gas, with the signing of an agreement with Shell Qatar over the procedure for the transfer to the State of the company's remaining 40% share. A similar agreement had been reached with the Qatar Petroleum Co. on 16 Sept. 1976.

The Qatar General Petroleum Corporation (QGPC) had been established by decree in July 1974 to assume overall responsibility for the State's domestic and foreign oil interests and operations. On 16 Oct. 1976 the Qatar Petroleum Producing Authority (QPPA) was established to serve as the executive arm of the QGPC—but in 1980 it was merged into the QGPC, which now directly oversees oil production through two operational divisions, Onshore and Offshore. The National Oil Distribution Company (NODCO) had a daily throughput capacity of 62,000 bbls a day in 1984 following the opening of a 50,000 bbls a day refinery at Umm Said to supplement the existing refinery.

Production, 1990, 19·4m. tonnes. Proven reserves (1986) 3,300m. bbls.

Gas. The North West Dome oilfield is being developed which contains 12% of the known world gas reserves. Production (1986) 229,100m. cu. ft.

Water Resources. Two main desalination stations, at Ras Abu Aboud and Ras Abu Fontas, together have a daily capacity of 167·6m. gallons of potable water. A third station is planned at Al Wasil, with a capacity of 40m. gallons a day. Total water production 1988 (well field and distillate) 17,542·5m. gallons.

Agriculture. 10% of the working population is engaged in agriculture. The Ministry of Agriculture is implementing a long-term policy aimed at ensuring self-sufficiency in agricultural products. The number of farms rose from 120 in 1960 to 841 in 1985. Production (1988) in tonnes: Cereals, 3,224; fruits and dates, 8,409; vegetables, 20,927; green fodder, 72,612; meat, 1,734 milk, 18,501; eggs, 1,522.

Livestock (1988): Cattle, 9,516; camels, 22,706; sheep, 122,259; goats, 87,396; chickens, 1,786,467; horses, 1,041; deer (1987), 3,463.

Fisheries. The produce of local fisheries in 1984 met 77·2% of Qatar's requirements. The state-owned Qatar National Fishing Company has 3 trawlers and its refrigeration unit processes 10 tonnes of shrimps a day. Catch (1988) 2,880 tonnes; value (1987) 19·55m riyals.

INDUSTRY. The Qatar Fertiliser Co. plant was opened in 1974 (production, 1988, 724,900 tonnes of ammonia and 779,600 tonnes of urea), the Qatar Steel Co. factory in 1978 (output, 1987, 483,833 tonnes of steel, 482,270 tonnes of sponge iron and (1988) 533,000 tonnes of reinforcing steel bars) and the Qatar Petrochemicals Co. plant in 1981 (production, 1988, 256,500 tonnes of ethylene, 171,400 tonnes of polyethylene and 37,000 tonnes of sulphur), all in the Umm Said industrial zone. Other production (1987, in tonnes): Cement, 791,200; unslaked lime, 13,500; flour, 26,200; bran, 6,600; organic fertilizer, 27,700. Two natural gas liquids plants produced 315,724 tonnes of propane, 223,384 tonnes of butane and 182,592 tonnes of gasoline in 1987.

Labour. The economically active population (15 years and above) in March 1986 totalled 200,238, of whom 6,283 were engaged in agriculture and fishing, 4,807 in mining and quarrying, 13,914 in manufacturing, 5,266 in electricity, gas and water, 40,523 in building and construction, 21,964 in trade, restaurants and hotels, 7,357 in transport and communications, 3,157 in finance, insurance and real estate and 96,466 in social and community services.

FOREIGN ECONOMIC RELATIONS

Commerce. In 1987 exports totalled 7,224m. riyals, and imports, 4,000m. riyals, (1988, 4,613m. riyals). Main imports in 1987 (in 1,000 riyals) were machinery and transport equipment (1,666,892), manufactured goods (1,218,517) and food and live animals (706,201). In 1987 Japan provided 16·3% of imports, the UK 16%, the USA 11·9% and the Federal Republic of Germany 7·2%.

Total trade between Qatar and UK (British Department of Trade returns, in £1,000 sterling):

	1986	*1987*	*1988*	*1989*	*1990*
Imports to UK	29,587	13,765	3,888	4,342	5,004
Exports and re-exports from UK	112,143	105,087	88,920	89,256	98,504

Tourism. In 1988 tourists stayed 226,134 nights in hotels.

COMMUNICATIONS

Roads. In 1981 there were about 800 miles of road. In 1988 there were 154,963 registered vehicles including 2,502 motorcycles.

Aviation. Gulf Air (owned equally by Qatar, Bahrain, Oman and the UAE), operates daily services from Bahrain; British Airways, Middle East and about 15 other airlines operate regular international flights from Doha airport. In 1988, 520,478 passengers arrived, 508,843 departed and 453,126 were in transit; 9,996 aircraft arrived and 9,996 departed.

Shipping. In 1987, 395 vessels, 1,101,925 tonnes of cargo and 1,854 containers were handled.

Telecommunications. There were 26 post offices in Doha and other towns in 1988. Qatar Broadcasting Service, using 12 transmission stations, broadcasts for 41 hours a day in Arabic, English, French and Urdu. Telephone and radiotelephone services connect Qatar with Europe and America; there were 129,291 telephones in 1988. In 1987 there were 75,000 radios and 111,000 television receivers.

Cinemas. In 1987 there were 4 cinemas.

Newspapers. In 1987 there were 4 daily and 2 weekly newspapers and 6 magazines.

JUSTICE, RELIGION, EDUCATION AND WELFARE

Justice. The Judiciary System is administered by the Ministry of Justice which comprises three main departments: Legal affairs, courts of justice and land and real estate register. There are 5 Courts of Justice proclaiming sentences in the name of H. H. the Amir: The Court of Appeal, the Labour Court, the Higher Criminal Court, the Civil Court and the Lower Criminal Court.

All issues related to personal affairs of Moslems under Islamic Law embodied in the Holy Quran and Sunna are decided by Sharia Courts.

Religion. The population is almost entirely Moslem.

Education. There were, in 1988, 35,133 pupils at 97 primary schools, 12,817 pupils at 43 preparatory schools, 8,064 pupils at 29 secondary schools and 894 male students at 3 specialist schools. There were 48 Arab and foreign private schools with 18,346 pupils in 1987–88. The University of Qatar had 5,621 students in 1989.

Students abroad (1988) numbered 881. In 1986–87, 3,435 men and 2,507 women attended evening classes.

Health. There were 3 hospitals (including 1 for women and 1 for gynaecology and obstetrics) with a total of 937 beds in 1987. There were 21 health centres in 1988. In 1987 there were 560 doctors, 62 dentists, 140 pharmacists and 1,418 qualified nurses.

DIPLOMATIC REPRESENTATIVES

Of Qatar in Great Britain (27 Chesham Pl., London, SWIX 8HG)
Ambassador: Abdulrahman Abdulla Al-Wohaibi (accredited 20 Dec. 1989).

Of Great Britain in Qatar (Doha, Qatar)
Ambassador and Consul-General: G. H. Boyce.

Of Qatar in the USA (600 New Hampshire Ave., NW, Washington, D.C., 20037)
Ambassador: Dr Hamad Abdelaziz Al-Kawari.

Of the USA in Qatar (Fariq Bin Omran, Doha)
Ambassador: Marc Hambley.

Of Qatar to the United Nations
Ambassador: Dr Hassan Ali Hussain Alni'ma.

Further Reading

Annual Statistical Abstract. 8th ed. Doha, 1988
El Mallakh, R., *Qatar: The Development of an Oil Economy*. New York, 1979
Unwin, P. T. H., *Qatar*. [Bibliography] Oxford and Santa Barbara, 1982

ROMANIA

Capital: Bucharest
Population: 23m. (1990)
GNP per capita: US$2,540 (1981)

HISTORY. 1918 is celebrated as the year of foundation of the 'unitary national Romanian state'. For the history and constitution of Romania from 1859 to 1947, *see* THE STATESMAN'S YEAR-BOOK, 1947, pp. 1187–89. On 30 Dec. 1947 King Michael abdicated under Communist pressure and parliament proclaimed the 'People's Republic'. The former king now lives in exile.

Since the accession to power in 1965 of Nicolae Ceauşescu Romania had been taking a relatively independent stand in foreign affairs while becoming increasingly repressive and impoverished domestically.

An attempt by the authorities on 16 Dec. 1989 to evict a protestant pastor, László Tőkés, from his home in Timişoara provoked a popular protest which escalated into a mass demonstration against the government. Despite the use of armed force against the demonstrators, the uprising spread to other areas. On 21 Dec. the government called for an official rally in Bucharest, but this turned against the régime. A state of emergency was declared, but the Army went over to the uprising, and Nicolae and Elena Ceauşescu fled the capital. A dissident group which had been active before the uprising, the National Salvation Front (NSF), proclaimed itself the provisional government. Suggestions of Soviet involvement have been denied.

The Ceauşescus were captured, and after a secret two-hour trial by military tribunal, summarily executed on 25 Dec. on four charges of genocide, undermining the power of the state, undermining the economy and embezzlement. Fighting by pro-Ceauşescu 'Securitate' forces continued until 27 Dec. It is estimated that 7,689 people were killed in the uprising.

On 26 Dec. Ion Iliescu, leader of the NSF, and Petre Român, were sworn in as President and Prime Minister respectively. The Provisional Government was at once recognized by many countries throughout the world, including the UK, USA and USSR.

AREA AND POPULATION. Romania is bounded north and north-east by the USSR, east by the Black Sea, south by Bulgaria, south-west by Yugoslavia and north-west by Hungary. The area of Romania is 237,500 sq. km (91,699 sq. miles). Pre-war Romania had an area of 113,918 sq. miles. Population at censuses: 1930, 18,057,208 (14,280,729 within present-day Romania); 1948, 15,872,624 (48·3% male); 1966, 19,103,163 (49% male, 38·2% urban); 1977, 21,559,910 (49·3% male, 47·5% urban).

In 1987 the population was 22,940,430 (49·3% male; 51·3% urban), density per sq. km, 96. Population estimate, 1990: 23m. Vital statistics, 1985 (per 1,000 population): Live births, 15·8; deaths, 10·9; marriages, 7·1; divorces, 1·43; stillborn (per 1,000 live births), 7·8; infant mortality (per 1,000 live births), 25·6. Expectation of life in 1984, 66·9 years. Measures designed to raise the birthrate were immediately abolished by the post-Ceauşescu government, and abortion and contraception legalized. Population growth rate per 1,000 was 4·9 in 1985 and 5·2 in 1984.

Administratively, Romania is divided into 41 counties (*judeţ*), 237 towns (*oraş*) (of which 55 are municipalities) and 2,705 local authorities (*comune*). The capital is Bucharest (Bucureşti), a municipality with county status.

District	*Area in sq. km*	*Population 1987*	*Capital*	*Population 1985*
Alba	6,231	425,903	Alba Iulia	64,369
Arad	7,652	504,556	Arad	185,892
Argeş	6,801	671,954	Piteşti	154,112
Bacău	6,606	717,946	Bacău	175,299
Bihor	7,535	657,707	Oradea	208,507
Bistriţa-Năsăud	5,305	322,501	Bistriţa	73,429
Botoşani	4,965	460,211	Botoşani	104,836

District	Area in sq. km	Population 1987	Capital	Population 1985
Braşov	5,351	695,160	Braşov	346,640
Brăila	4,724	400,832	Brăila	234,600
Buzău	6,072	522,685	Buzău	132,311
Caraş-Severin	8,503	407,402	Reşiţa	104,362
Călăraşi	5,075	347,312	Călăraşi	68,226
Cluj	6,650	740,929	Cluj-Napoca	309,843
Constanţa	7,055	726,059	Constanţa	323,236
Covasna	3,705	233,049	Sf. Gheorghe	65,868
Dîmboviţa	4,035	563,621	Tîrgovişte	88,663
Dolj	7,413	771,971	Craiova	275,098
Galaţi	4,425	635,425	Galaţi	292,805
Giurgiu	3,810	325,150	Giurgiu	65,792
Gorj	5,641	380,582	Tîrgu Jiu	85,058
Harghita	6,610	359,205	Miercurea-Ciuc	45,651
Hunedoara	7,016	559,619	Deva	76,934
Ialomiţa	4,449	304,809	Slobozia	44,797
Iaşi	5,469	793,369	Iaşi	314,156
Maramureş	6,215	546,035	Baia Mare	135,536
Mehedinţi	4,900	327,309	Drobeta-Turnu Severin	97,862
Mureş	6,696	616,401	Tîrgu Mureş	157,411
Neamţ	5,890	570,204	Piatra-Neamţ	107,581
Olt	5,507	531,323	Slatina	73,982
Prahova	4,694	868,779	Ploieşti	234,021
Satu Mare	4,405	412,227	Satu Mare	128,115
Sălaj	3,850	267,517	Zalău	54,676
Sibiu	5,422	507,850	Sibiu	176,928
Suceava	8,555	685,661	Suceava	92,690
Teleorman	5,760	504,623	Alexandria	51,267
Timiş	8,692	731,667	Timişoara	318,955
Tulcea	8,430	269,808	Tulcea	84,353
Vaslui	5,297	457,699	Vaslui	62,372
Vîlcea	5,705	427,059	Rîmnicu Vîlcea	93,271
Vrancea	4,863	390,055	Focşani	83,562
Bucharest [1]	1,521	2,298,256	Bucharest [2]	1,975,808

[1] Total conurbation. [2] Central area.

The last official figures on the size of the ethnic minorities were published in 1977. Estimates for 1990: Hungarians, 2·5m. (mainly in Transylvania); Germans, 200,000; Gypsies, 2·3m.; Jews, 30,000. The agricultural 'systematisation' (*see* Agriculture, p. 1036) bore particularly hardly upon ethnic Hungarians, who had not been allowed to emigrate. Some 120,000 Germans had emigrated by 1988. The official language is Romanian.

CLIMATE. A continental climate with a large annual range of temperature and rainfall showing a slight summer maximum.

Bucharest. Jan. 27°F (–2·7°C), July 74°F (23·5°C). Annual rainfall 23·1" (579 mm). Constanţa. Jan. 31°F (–0·6°C), July 71°F (21·7°C). Annual rainfall 15" (371 mm).

CONSTITUTION AND GOVERNMENT. For the Communist Constitution and government *see* THE STATESMAN'S YEAR-BOOK, 1989-90, pp. 1033-34.

The head of state is the *President*, elected by direct vote. The bicameral parliament consists of a 396-member *National Assembly* and a 119-member *Senate*; both are elected from 41 constituencies by modified proportional representation, the number of seats won in each constituency being determined by the proportion of the total vote.

Presidential and parliamentary elections were held on 20 May 1990. A 60-member team of observers from 19 countries concluded that there had been many irregularities but not enough to invalidate the results.

Ion Iliescu was elected President with 85% of the vote. The National Salvation Front (NSF) gained 66% of the vote and 233 seats in the National Assembly; the

Democratic Union of Hungarians gained 7% and 29 seats; Liberals, 6% and 29; Greens, 3% and 12; National Peasants, 3% and 12; others, 15% and 81.

The new government will hold office for 2 years and draw up a new constitution. In Feb. 1991 it consisted of:

Prime Minister, Petre Român (b. 1947).

Adrian Severin (b. 1954), *Deputy Prime Minister and Minister for Reform and Relations with Parliament*; Teodor Stolojan (b. 1943), *Finance*; Adrian Năstase (b. 1950), *Foreign Affairs*; Victor Stănculescu (b. 1928), *Defence*; Dorel Viorel Ursu, *Interior*; Bogdan Mărinescu, *Health*; Ioan Ţîpu, *Agriculture and Food*; Andrei Chirică, *Communications*; Victor Babiuc, *Justice*; Vacant, *Resources and Industry*; Constantin Fota, *Trade and Tourism*; Doru Pană, *Public Works and Transport*; Valeriu Eugen Pop, *Environment*; Ştefan Gheorghe, *Education*; Cătălin Zamfir, *Labour and Social Security*; Bogdan Niculescu Duvăz, *Youth and Sport*; Andrei Pleşu (ind.), *Culture*. The *Speaker* is Dan Marţian.

More than 30 parties compaigned for the May 1990 elections, including the NSF (reconstituted as a party), the National Peasant Party (*Chairman:* Corneliu Coposu) and the National Liberal Party (*Chairman:* Radu Campeanu).

Local government is carried out by People's Councils at the administrative levels mentioned on p. 1033. 57,584 councillors were elected from among 117,349 candidates on 15 Nov. 1987.

National flag: Three vertical strips of blue, yellow and red.

National anthem: Trei culori ('Three colours'). A new anthem is under consideration.

DEFENCE. Military service is compulsory for 12 months in the Army and Air Force and 24 months in the Navy.

Army. The 4 Army Areas consist of 2 tank and 8 motor rifle divisions; 4 mountain, 2 artillery, 4 anti-aircraft and 2 surface-to-surface missile brigades; and 4 artillery, 5 anti-tank and 4 airborne regiments. Equipment includes 1,060 T-34, 757 T-55, 30 T-72, 556 TR-80 and 414 TR-580 main battle tanks. Strength (1991) 126,000 (95,000 conscripts), and 178,000 reservists. There are a further 45,000 men in paramilitary border guard and internal security forces.

Navy. The fleet comprises 1 ex-Soviet diesel submarine, 1 Romanian-built missile-armed destroyer with hangar for 2 helicopters, 4 frigates, 3 corvettes, 6 fast missile craft, 42 fast torpedo craft, 4 offshore, 2 coastal and 6 inshore patrol vessels, 2 minelayer/mine countermeasure support ships and 40 small minesweepers. The Danube flotilla counts 3 river monitors (100 mm guns) and some 40 river patrol craft. Auxiliaries include 2 logistic ships, 1 oceanographic ship, 1 training ship and 2 tugs.

There is a substantial coastal defence force organized into 10 batteries of artillery with about 100 guns (130 mm, 150 mm and 152 mm).

Headquarters of the Navy is at Mangalia, and of the Danube flotilla at Brăila. Personnel in 1990 totalled 9,000 (2,500 conscripts) including 2,000 in Coastal Defence.

Air Force. The Air Force numbered some 28,000 (10,000 conscripts), with 370 combat aircraft in 3 air divisions (7 regiments) in 1991. These were organized into 12 interceptor squadrons with MiG-21 and MiG-23 fighters, 6 ground-attack and close-support squadrons with MiG-17 fighters, and 1 reconnaissance squadron of Il-28s. There were also more than 150 training aircraft, 20 An-24/26/30 transports and more than 150 helicopters (Mi-2, Mi-4, Mi-8, Mi-14, Alouette and Puma). Under delivery were 185 IAR-93 close-support/interceptors to replace the MiG-17s and Skyfox anti-armour helicopters. 'Guideline' and 'Gainful' surface-to-air missiles were operational, and short-range surface-to-surface missiles have been displayed.

INTERNATIONAL RELATIONS

Membership. Romania is a member of the UN, IMF, OIEC and Warsaw Pact.

ECONOMY

Policy. For planning under Ceauşescu *see* THE STATESMAN'S YEAR-BOOK, 1989–90, p. 1035). Romania was committed to intensive industrialization and agriculture had been neglected. Severe shortages resulted from the diversion of resources to pay off foreign debt.

A law of Aug. 1990 establishes procedures for transforming state-owned enterprises (including farms) into shareholding companies with government-appointed directors. 30% of these companies' shares are to be distributed for a nominal price to the public; the remainder are to be sold at market prices to domestic and foreign investors under the supervision of the recently-established National Privatization Agency.

In Nov. 1990 a policy of removing subsidies and matching consumer to producer prices caused prices to double on most items: bread, meat, heat and light continued to be subsidized. On 12 Nov. the Prime Minister was given special powers for a 6-month period to run the economy by decree, including the power to change taxation and negotiate foreign loans.

Budget. Revenue and expenditure (in 1m. lei) for calendar years:

	1982	*1983*	*1984*	*1985*	*1986*	*1988* [1]
Revenue	288,511	301,908	308,917	363,180	340,914	433,094
Expenditure	288,511	301,908	308,917	342,545	340,914	433,094

[1] Estimates.

In 1985 sources of revenue (in 1m. lei) included: Profit payments of state enterprises 29,527; turnover tax, 93,666; personal taxes, 4,251; insurance contributions, 40,009; taxes on enterprise wage funds, 47,125. Expenditure: National economy, 172,559; social and cultural, 90,412; defence, 12,113.

Revenue and expenditure of local councils (included above) was 63,054m. lei and 60,560m. lei in 1985.

Romania has settled UK claims arising out of the peace treaty and on defaulted bonds.

Currency. The monetary unit is the *leu*, pl.*lei* (ROL) of 100 *bani*. On 1 Feb. 1954 the gold content of the leu was to 0·148112 gramme of fine gold. Exchange rates (March 1991): £1 = 67·55 lei; US$1 = 35·61 lei.

Bank-notes of 1, 5, 10, 25, 50 and 100 *lei* are issued by the National Bank, and there are coins of 5, 10, 15 and 25 *bani* and 1, 3 and 5 *lei*.

Banking and Finance. The National Bank of Romania (founded 1880, nationalized 1946) is the State Bank under the Minister of Finance. Its *Governor* is Mugul Isarescu. Half its profits are allotted to the State budget. There are also a Bank of Investments, a Foreign Trade Bank, an Agriculture and Food Industry Bank and a Savings Bank. In 1974 the American bank Manufactures Hanover Trust Co. opened a branch in Bucharest, the first Western bank to do so in a Communist country.

Weights and measures. The Gregorian calendar was adopted in 1919. The metric system is in use. Tubes and pipes are measured in *tol* (= 1 inch).

ENERGY AND NATURAL RESOURCES

Electricity. Installed electric power 1984: 18,829,000 kw.; output, 1987, 74,079m. kwh (11,209m. kwh hydroelectric). Supply 220 volts; 50 Hz. There are two joint Romanian–Yugoslav hydro-electric power plants on the Danube at the 'Iron Gates' with a combined yearly output of 22,250m. kwh. A nuclear power programme has been subject to cut-backs and delays. A nuclear powere plant is under construction at Cernăvoda. In Oct. 1985 a state of emergency was declared in the energy sector and its administration handed over to the military. This was still in force in 1989.

Oil. The oilfields are in the Prahova, Băcau, Gorj, Crişana and Argeş districts. Oil production in 1990 was 8·23m. tonnes. Oil reserves are expected to be exhausted by the mid-1990s. Refining capacity was enlarged from 16m. tonnes per annum in 1970 to 30m. tonnes in 1985. Crude oil has to be imported.

Minerals. The principal minerals are oil and natural gas, salt, brown coal, lignite, iron and copper ores, bauxite, chromium, manganese and uranium. Salt is mined in the lower Carpathians and in Transylvania; production in 1987 was 5·4m. tonnes.

Output, 1987 (and 1986) (in 1,000 tonnes): Iron ore, 2,281 (2,431); coal, 51,524 including lignite, 41,579 (47,518, including lignite 38,012); methane gas (cu. metres), 25,301m. (26,763m.).

Agriculture. There were 15·09m. ha of agricultural land in 1987, including (in 1,000 ha): Arable, 10,080; meadows and pasture, 4,407; vineyards and fruit trees, 606. In 1985 there were 2·7m. ha of irrigated land.

Production in 1988 (in 1,000 tonnes): Wheat, 9,000; rye, 60; barley, 2,200; maize, 19,500; potatoes, 8,000; sunflower seeds, 1,190; sugar-beet, 6,500.

Livestock (1988, in 1,000's): 7,182 cattle, 15,224 pigs, 18,793 sheep, 135,956 poultry, 693 horses. Romania is a major sheep-rearing country.

In 1985 there were 4,363 collective farms, with 9·1m. ha of land (7·2m. arable; 1·4m. private plots). State farms numbered 419, with 2m. ha of land, of which 1·65m. ha were arable. A further 2·4m. ha of land were in the hands of other state agricultural organizations.

A law of Feb. 1991 provides for the restitution of collectivized land to its former owners or their heirs up to a limit of 10 ha. Land may be resold, but there is a limit of 100 ha on total holdings. Landless peasants are to receive a distribution from the residue. State farms are to remain nationalized; peasants will receive shares in their equity worth up to 10 ha. Local authorities are to manage the redistribution of land. Collective farms may if they wish become private co-operative associations.

Forestry. Total forest area was 6·34m. ha in 1988, representing 28% of the land area.

INDUSTRY. Output of main products in 1987 (and 1986) (in tonnes): Pig-iron, 8,673 (9,329); steel, 13,885 (14,276); steel tubes, 1,394 (1,565); coke, 5,826 (5,182); rolled steel, 9,675 (10,207); chemical fertilizers, 2,897 (3,278); washing soda, 894 (895); caustic soda, 817 (846); paper, 712 (768); cement, 13,583 (14,216); sugar, 646 (489); edible oils, 392 (339). Fabrics (in 1m. sq. metres): Cotton, 710 (731); woollens, 139 (140); man-made fibres, 286,818 (302,681). In 1,000 units: Radio sets, 618 (580); TV sets, 484 (530); washing machines, 242 (263); motor cars, 129,330 (124,372). It was estimated that there was a fall in production of 60% in 1990.

Labour. The employed population in 1986 was 10·7m., of whom 3m. worked in agriculture and 4·8m. industry and building. In 1985 39·4% of the total workforce, and 42·6% of the industrial workforce, were women. Wages were increased by 10% in 1988. A 5-day working week was introduced in Dec. 1989. Men retire at 62, women at 57. A minimum monthly wage of 2,300 lei was set in Nov. 1990.

Trade Unions. In Dec. 1990 the principal trade union federations were the Inter-Union Alliance (1·8m. members), Cartel Alfa (1·6m.), the Convention of Non-Affiliated Trade Unions (1m.), Fraţia (0·7m.), and the former official union (UGSR), renamed National Confederation of Free Trade Unions (CNSLR), with 3m. members.

FOREIGN ECONOMIC RELATIONS. In June 1990 a 10-year treaty of commercial and economic co-operation was signed with the EEC. In July 1990 the USA extended its trade agreement with Romania for 3 years, but did not grant most-favoured-nation status.

Foreign investors may establish joint ventures or 100%-owned domestic companies in all but a few strategic industries. After an initial 2-year exemption, profits are taxed at 30%, dividends at 10%.

Commerce. In 1985 exports totalled 192,295m. lei and imports 148,362m. lei.

Principal exports in 1985 were (in 1,000 tonnes): Petroleum products, 9,691; cement, 2,477; cereals, 842; oilfield equipment, 6,110m. lei; equipment for cement mills, 274m. lei; equipment for chemical factories, 904m. lei; shipbuilding, 966m. lei. Principal imports (in 1,000 tonnes): Iron ore, 15,207; industrial coke, 1,898; rolled ferrous metals, 696; electrical equipment, 4,809m. lei; motor cars, 1,303 units, and industrial and agricultural equipment.

In 1985 Romania's main trading partners (trade in 1m. lei) were: USSR, 74,333; Egypt, 22,304; Federal Republic of Germany, 19,486; Italy, 16,866; Iran, 16,758; German Democratic Republic, 16,737; USA, 15,645.

Total trade between Romania and UK (British Department of Trade returns, in £1,000 sterling):

	1986	*1987*	*1988*	*1989*	*1990*
Imports to UK	86,730	92,526	100,906	117,685	61,215
Exports and re-exports from UK	82,011	55,688	50,111	38,141	85,879

Tourism. In Jan. 1990 citizens were granted the right to travel freely.

COMMUNICATIONS

Roads. There were in 1985, 14,666 km of national roads of which 12,239 km were modernized. Freight carried, 362m. tonnes; passengers, 837m.

Railways. Length of standard-gauge route in 1987 was 11,275 km, of which 3,411 km were electrified. In 1985 there were 472 km of narrow-gauge lines. Freight carried in 1985, 283m. tonnes; passengers, 460m.

Aviation. TAROM (*Transporturi Aeriene Române*), the state airline, operates all internal services, and also services to Amsterdam, Athens, Beijing, Beirut, Belgrade, Berlin, Brussels, Budapest, Cairo, Cologne, Copenhagen, Düsseldorf, Frankfurt, Istanbul, London, Moscow, Paris, Prague, Rome, Sofia, Tel-Aviv, Vienna, Warsaw and Zürich. Bucharest is also served by British Airways, PANAM, SABENA, Aeroflot, Air France, Interflug, ČSA, MALEV, Austrian Air Lines, SAS, Lot, TABSO, El Al, Alitalia, Lufthansa and Swissair.

Bucharest's airports are at Băneasa (internal flights) and Otopeni (international flights). Air transport in 1985 carried 2·5m. passengers and 29,000 tonnes of freight. TAROM had 32 aircraft in 1990.

Shipping. The main ports are Constanța on the Black Sea and Galați and Brăila on the Danube. A new port has been constructed at Agigea on the Black Sea and the 64 km canal between the Danube and the Black Sea was opened in 1984. The largest shipyard is at Galați.

In 1985 the mercantile marine (NAVROM) owned some 200 sea-going ships. In 1985 sea-going transport carried 25·72m. tonnes of freight; river transport, 18·4m. tonnes and 1·84m. passengers.

Telecommunications. There were 4,979 post offices in 1985. Number of telephone subscribers, 1·96m. *Radio-televiziunea Românа* broadcasts 3 programmes on medium-waves and FM. There are also 6 regional programmes, and radio and TV transmission in Hungarian and German (restored since Dec. 1989). As a result of the energy crisis in 1984 TV broadcasting was reduced to 22 hours a week, but had been increased to 80 hours a week by Feb. 1990. Links with the West are provided by Eutelsat satellite. Radio receiving sets in 1986 3·19m.; TV sets, 3·86m.

Cinemas and Theatres. There were, in 1987, 5,454 cinemas and 150 theatres and concert halls. 27 full-length feature films were made in 1985.

Newspapers and Books. There were, in 1987, 36 daily and 24 weekly newspapers and 435 periodicals, including 11 dailies and 3 weeklies in minority languages. There were 7,181 public libraries in 1987. 3,063 book titles were published in 1985 in 66·3m. copies. (376 titles in minority languages).

JUSTICE, RELIGION, EDUCATION AND WELFARE

Justice. Justice is administered by the Supreme Court, the 41 county courts, and lower courts. Lay assessors (elected for 4 years) participate in most court trials, collaborating with the judges. The *Procurator-General* exercises 'supreme supervisory power to ensure the observance of the law' by all authorities, central and local, and all citizens. The Procurator-General in 1990 was Gheorghe Robu. The Procurator's Office and its organs are independent of any organs of justice or administration, and only responsible to the Grand National Assembly (which appoints the Procurator-General for 4 years) and between its sessions, to the State Council. The Ministry of the Interior is responsible for ordinary police work. State security is the responsibility of the State Security Council. A new penal code came into force on 1 Jan. 1969. An amnesty of Jan. 1988 abolished or reduced the sentences of all convicts. All political prisoners were released on 23 Dec. 1989. The death penalty was abolished in Dec. 1989.

Religion. Churches functioned in accordance with art. 30 of the Communist Constitution. Churches administer their own affairs and run seminaries for the training of priests. Expenses and salaries are paid by the State. There are 14 Churches, the largest being the Romanian Orthodox Church, which claimed some 16m. members in 1985. It is autocephalous, but retains dogmatic unity with the Eastern Orthodox Church. It is administered by the consultative Holy Synod and National Ecclesiastical Assembly and the executive National Ecclesiastical Council and Patriarchal Administration. It is organized into 12 dioceses grouped into 5 metropolitan bishoprics (Hungaro-Wallachia; Moldavia-Suceava; Transylvania; Olt; Banat) and headed by Patriarch Teoctist Arapaşu. There are some 11,800 churches, 2 theological colleges and 6 'schools of cantors', as well as seminaries.

The Uniate (Greek Catholic) Church (which severed its connexion with the Vatican in 1698) was suppressed in 1948. It had 1·6m. adherents and 1,818 priests. Estimates for 1973: 700,000 adherents and 600 priests.

Other churches: Serbs have a Serbian Orthodox Vicariate at Timişoara. In 1986 there were 1·2m. Roman Catholics, mainly among the Hungarian and German minorities. There are 8 dioceses. In 1985 6 were vacant. There is a bishop of Alba Iulia and an Apostolic Administrator was appointed to Bucharest in Oct. 1984. There were 734 priests in 1982. The Church has not secured approval for a Statute and has no hierarchical ties with the Vatican.

Calvinists (600,000; mainly Hungarian) have bishoprics at Cluj and Oradea; Lutherans (150,000, mainly Germans) a bishopric at Sibiu and Unitarians (60,000, Hungarians) a bishopric at Cluj. These sects share a seminary at Cluj. In 1987 there were about 200,000 Baptists and 300,000 other neo-Protestants.

In 1989 there were 20,000 Jews under a Chief Rabbi. There were 120 synagogues in 1987.

There were 40,000 Moslems in 1983 and they have a Muftiate at Constanţa.

Education. Education is free and compulsory from 6 to 16, consisting of 8 years of primary school and 2 years of secondary (gymnasium). Further secondary education is available at *lycées*, professional schools or advanced technical schools.

In 1987–88 there were 12,291 kindergartens with 31,300 teachers and 828,079 children; 13,895 primary and secondary schools with 141,609 teachers and 3,027,196 pupils; 981 *lycées* with 43,805 teachers and 1,228,490 pupils; 764 professional schools with 2,419 teachers and 278,003 pupils; and 322 advanced technical schools with 1,146 teachers and 22,879 pupils. In 1983–84 there were 3,130 schools for 340,773 pupils of ethnic minorities with 15,922 teachers.

There are universities at Iaşi (founded 1860), Bucharest (1864), Cluj (1919), Timişoara (1962), Craiova (1965) and Braşov (1971). In 1987–88 there were in all 44 institutes of higher education, with 157,041 (7,062 foreign) students and 12,036 teachers. In 1983–84 there were 11,568 students at institutes of higher education for ethnic minorities with some 1,000 teachers.

The Academy, with seat at Bucharest, has 2 branches at Iaşi and Cluj.

Health. In 1987 there were 214,253 hospital beds and 48,271 doctors (including 7,212 dentists). Under the Ceauşescu régime health standards severely declined and medical services were neglected.

Social Security. In 1987 3·26m. pensioners drew an average monthly pension of 2,106 lei.

DIPLOMATIC REPRESENTATIVES

Of Romania in Great Britain (4 Palace Green, London, W8 4QD)
Ambassador: Sergiu Celac.

Of Great Britain in Romania (24 Strada Jules Michelet, Bucharest)
Ambassador: M. W. Atkinson, CMG, MBE.

Of Romania in the USA (1607 23rd St., NW, Washington, D.C., 20008)
Ambassador: Virgil Constantinescu.

Of the USA in Romania (7–9 Strada Tudor Arghezi, Bucharest)
Ambassador: Alan Green, Jr.

Of Romania to the United Nations
Ambassador: Aurel D. Munteanu.

Further Reading

Anuarul Statistic al R.S.R. Bucharest, annual
Atlas Geografic Republica Socialistă Romania. Bucharest, 1965
Dicționar Enciclopedic Român. Bucharest, 1962–66
Economic and Commercial Guide to Romania. Bucharest, annual since 1969
Mic Dicționar Enciclopedic. Bucharest, 1973
Revista de Statistică. Bucharest, monthly
Romania: An Encyclopaedic Survey. Bucharest, 1980
Romania, the Industrialization of an Agrarian Economy under Socialist Planning: Report of a Mission sent to Romania by the World Bank. Washington, 1979
Deletant, A. and D., *Romania* [Bibliography]. Oxford and Santa Barbara, 1985
Fischer-Galati, S. A., *Rumania: A Bibliographical Guide.* Library of Congress, 1963.—*The New Rumania.* Mass. Inst. of Technology, 1968.—*The Socialist Republic of Rumania.* Baltimore, 1969.—*Twentieth Century Rumania.* New York, 1970
Gilberg, T., *Nationalism and Communism in Romania: the Rise and Fall of Ceaușescu's Personal Dictatorship.* Oxford, 1990
Giurescu, C. C. (ed.) *Chronological History of Romania.* 2nd ed. Bucharest, 1974
King, R. R., *History of the Romanian Communist Party.* Stanford, 1980
Morariu, T., *et al, The Geography of Rumania.* 2nd ed. Bucharest, 1969
Pacepa, I., *Red Horizons.* London, 1988
Shafir, M., *Romania: Politics, Economics and Society.* London, 1985
Stanciu, I. G. and Cernovodeanu, P., *Distant Lands: The Genesis and Evolution of Romanian–American Relations.* Boulder, 1985
Turnock, D., *An Economic Geography of Romania.* London, 1974.—*The Romanian Economy in the Twentieth Century.* London 1986

RWANDA

Capital: Kigali
Population: 6·71m. (1988)
GNP per capita: US$310 (1988)

Republika y'u Rwanda

HISTORY. From the 16th century to 1959 the Tutsi kingdom of Rwanda shared the history of Burundi (*see* p. 258). In 1959 an uprising of the Hutu destroyed the Tutsi feudal hierarchy and led to the departure of the Mwami Kigeri V. Elections and a referendum under the auspices of the UN in Sept. 1961 resulted in an overwhelming majority for the republican party, the Parmehutu (*Parti du Mouvement de l'Emancipation du Bahutu*), and the rejection of the institution of the Mwami. The republic proclaimed by the Parmehutu on 28 Jan. 1961 was recognized by the Belgian administration (but not by the UN) in Oct. 1961. Internal self-government was granted on 1 Jan. 1962, and by decision of the General Assembly of the UN the Republic of Rwanda became independent on 1 July 1962.

In Oct. 1990 rebel Tutsi forces of the Patriotic Rwandan Front (FPR) invaded from Uganda. A ceasefire was signed in March 1991.

AREA AND POPULATION. Rwanda is bounded south by Burundi, west by Zaïre, north by Uganda and east by Tanzania. A mountainous state of 26,338 sq. km (10,169 sq. miles), its western third drains to Lake Kivu on the border with Zaïre and thence to the Congo river, while the rest is drained by the Kagera river into the Nile system.

The population was 4,819,317 at the 1978 Census, of whom over 90% were Hutu, 9% Tutsi and 1% Twa (pygmy); latest estimate (1988) 6,710,000. In 1988 there were about 20,000 refugees in Rwanda, all from Burundi.

The areas and populations (1978 Census) of the 10 prefectures are:

Prefecture	*Sq. km*	*Census 1978*	*Prefecture*	*Sq. km*	*Census 1978*
Cyangugu	2,226	331,380	Kigali	3,251	698,063
Kibuye	1,320	337,729	Kibungo	4,134	360,934
Gisenyi	2,395	468,786	Gitarama	2,241	602,752
Ruhengeri	1,762	528,649	Gikongoro	2,192	369,891
Byumba	4,987	519,968	Butare	1,830	601,165

Kigali, the capital, had 156,650 inhabitants in 1981; other towns (1978) being Butare (21,691), Ruhengeri (16,025) and Gisenyi (12,436). Kinyarwanda, the language of the entire population, and French are official languages, and Kiswahili is spoken in the commercial centres, where most of the 1,200 Europeans and 750 Asians reside.

Vital statistics (1975): Live births, 113,154; deaths, 41,385; marriages, 13,899.

CLIMATE. Despite the equatorial situation, there is a highland tropical climate. The wet seasons are from Oct. to Dec. and March to May. Highest rainfall occurs in the west, at around 70" (1,770 mm), decreasing to 40–55" (1,020–1,400 mm) in the central uplands and to 30" (760 mm) in the north and east. Kigali. Jan. 67°F (19·4°C), July 70°F (21·1°C). Annual rainfall 40" (1,000 mm).

CONSTITUTION AND GOVERNMENT. A new Constitution was approved by referendum on 17 Dec. 1978; under it, the *Mouvement revolutionnaire national pour le développement* (MRND) founded 5 July 1975 becomes the sole political organization. Executive power is vested in a President, elected by universal suffrage for a (renewable) 5-year term. He presides over a Council of Ministers, whom he appoints and dismisses.

Legislative power rests with a National Development Council of 70 deputies, elected for a 5-year term; elections were held on 26 Dec. 1983.

President: Maj.-Gen. Junéval Habyarimana (took office July 1975; elected Dec. 1978 and re-elected Dec. 1983).

Foreign Affairs and Co-operation: Casimir Bizimungu.

National flag: Three equal vertical panels of red, yellow and green (left to right), the letter 'R' in black superimposed on the centre panel.

Local government: The 10 prefectures, each under an appointed Prefect, are divided into 143 communes, each with an appointed Burgomaster and an elected Council.

DEFENCE

Army. The Army consists of 1 commando battalion, 1 reconnaissance, 8 infantry and 1 engineer companies. Equipment includes 12 AML-60 armoured cars. Strength (1991) about 5,000. There is a paramilitary gendarmerie of some 1,200.

Air Force. The Air Force currently operates 2 Guerrier armed light aircraft, 2 Noratlas, 2 Islander light transports, 6 Gazelle and 4 Alouette III helicopters. A Caravelle is operated on VIP duties. Personnel (1991) 200.

INTERNATIONAL RELATIONS

Membership. Rwanda is a member of the UN, OAU and is an ACP state of the EEC. With Burundi and Zaïre it forms part of the Economic Community of Countries of the Great Lakes.

ECONOMY

Budget. The budget for 1989 balanced at 27,500m. Rwanda francs.

Currency. The unit of currency is the *Rwanda franc* (RWF) of 100 *centimes*. In March 1991 £1 = 231.98 Rwanda francs; US$1 = 122.29 Rwanda francs.

Banking. The Development Bank of Rwanda *(Banque Rwandaise de Développement—BRD)* had a capital (1983) of 1,000m. Rwanda francs. Other banks are the Central Bank *(Banque Nationale du Rwanda)*; 2 commercial banks which are majority foreign owned—the *Banque Commerciale du Rwanda* and the *Banque de Kigali*; the People's Bank, the Savings Association and the *Caisse Hypothécaire*.

ENERGY AND NATURAL RESOURCES

Electricity. 4 hydro-electric installations and 1 thermal plant produced 110m. kwh in 1986, but over half of the country's needs come from Zaïre. Supply 220 volts; 50 Hz.

Minerals. Cassiterite and wolframite are mined east of Lake Kivu. Production (1983): Cassiterite, 1,526 tonnes; wolfram, 429 tonnes. About 1m. cu. metres of natural gas are obtained from under the lake each year.

Agriculture. Subsistence agriculture accounts for most of the gross national product. Staple food crops (production 1988, in 1,000 tonnes) are sweet potatoes (800), cassava (390), dry beans (143), sorghum (177), potatoes (183), maize (88), peas and groundnuts. The main cash crops are *aravica* coffee (42), tea (8) and pyrethrum. There is a pilot rice-growing project.

Long-horned Ankole cattle, 639,000 head in 1980, play an important traditional role. Efforts are being made to improve their present negligible economic value. There were (1988) 660,000 cattle, 1·2m. goats, 360,000 sheep and 92,000 pigs.

INDUSTRY. There are about 100 small-sized modern manufacturing enterprises in the country. Food manufacturing is the dominant industrial activity (64%) followed by construction (15·3%) and mining (9%). There is a large modern brewery.

FOREIGN ECONOMIC RELATIONS. With Burundi and Zaire Rwanda forms part of the Economic Community of the Great Lakes.

Commerce. In 1984 imports amounted to 27,122m. Rwanda francs and exports to 15,543m. of which coffee comprised 83%, tea 4% and tin 6%; Belgium provided 14% of imports, Kenya 13% and Japan 10%.

Total trade between Rwanda and UK (British Department of Trade returns, in £1,000 sterling):

	1986	*1987*	*1988*	*1989*	*1990*
Imports to UK	7,487	4,291	8,434	2,991	2,128
Exports and re-exports from UK	1,681	2,526	1,636	1,790	1,915

Tourism. In 1984 there were 20,000 visitors to national parks.

COMMUNICATIONS

Roads. There were (1982) 6,760 km of roads. There are road links with Burundi, Uganda, Tanzania and Zaïre. There were in 1982 6,188 cars and 7,168 commercial vehicles.

Aviation. There are international airports at Kanombe, for Kigali, and at Kamembe, with services to Bujumbura, Bukavu, Entebbe, Goma, Lubumbashi, Athens and Brussels.

Telecommunications. Telephones (1983) 6,598. In 1983 there were 2 radio stations and 155,000 receivers.

JUSTICE, RELIGION, EDUCATION AND WELFARE

Justice. A system of Courts of First Instance and provincial courts refer appeals to Courts of Appeal and a Court of Cassation situated in Kigali.

Religion. The population was (1983) predominantly Roman Catholic (56%); there is an archbishop (Kigali) and 3 bishops. 23% of the population follow traditional religions, 12% are Protestants and 9% Moslems.

Education. In 1985 there were 790,198 pupils attending primary schools with 14,005 teachers. There were secondary, technical and teacher-training schools with 45,000 students and 1,082 teachers. The National University, opened at Butare, with sites at Butare and Ruhengeri, in 1963, had 1,577 students in 1984.

Health. In 1983 there were 170 hospitals and health centres with (1980) 9,015 beds; there were also 164 doctors, 1 dentist, 10 pharmacists, 464 midwives and 525 nursing personnel.

DIPLOMATIC REPRESENTATIVES

Of Rwanda in Great Britain
Ambassador: (Vacant).

Of Great Britain in Rwanda
Ambassador: R. L. B. Cormack, CMG (resides in Kinshasa).

Of Rwanda in the USA (1714 New Hampshire Ave, NW, Washington, D.C., 20009)
Ambassador: Aloys Uwimana.

Of the USA in Rwanda (Blvd. de la Revolution, Kigali)
Ambassador: Leonard H. O. Spearman, Sr.

Of Rwanda to the United Nations
Ambassador: Oswald Rukashaza.

ST CHRISTOPHER (ST KITTS)—NEVIS

Capital: Basseterre
Population: 43,410 (1987)
GNP capita: US$2,770 (1988)

Federation of St Christopher and Nevis

HISTORY. St Christopher (known to its Carib inhabitants as *Liamuiga*) and Nevis were discovered and named by Columbus in 1493. They were settled by Britain in 1623 and 1628 respectively, but ownership was disputed with France until 1713. They formed part of the Leeward Islands Federation from 1871 to 1956, and part of the Federation of the West Indies from 1958 to 1962. In Feb. 1967 the colonial status was replaced by an 'association' with Britain, giving the islands full internal self-government, while Britain remained responsible for defence and foreign affairs. St Christopher–Nevis became fully independent on 19 Sept. 1983.

AREA AND POPULATION. The islands form part of the Lesser Antilles in Eastern Caribbean. Population, estimate (1986) 43,700.

	sq. km	*Census 1980*	*Chief town*	*Census 1980*
St Christopher	174	33,881	Basseterre	14,283
Nevis	93	9,428	Charlestown	1,243
	267	43,309		

In 1980, 94% of the population were black and 36% were urban. English is the official and spoken language.

CLIMATE. A pleasantly healthy climate, with a cool breeze throughout the year, low humidity and no recognized rainy season. Average annual rainfall is about 55" (1,375 mm).

CONSTITUTION AND GOVERNMENT. The 1983 Constitution described the country as 'a sovereign democratic federal state'. It allowed for a unicameral Parliament consisting of 11 elected Members (8 from St Kitts and 3 from Nevis) and 3 appointed Senators. Nevis was given its own Island Assembly and the right to secession from St Kitts. At the General Elections held on 21 March 1989, 6 seats in St Kitts were won by the People's Action Movement and 2 by the Labour Party, and in Nevis 2 seats were won by the Nevis Reformation Party and 1 by the Concerned Citizens Movement.

Governor-General: Sir Clement Athelston Arrindell, GCMG, GCVO.

Prime Minister and Minister of Finance, Home and Foreign Affairs: Rt. Hon. Dr Kennedy Alphonse Simmonds.

Deputy Prime Minister and Minister of Tourism and Labour: Michael O'Powell. *Education, Youth, Community Affairs, Communications, Works, Public Utilities and Sports:* Sidney E. Morris. *Agriculture, Lands, Housing and Development:* Hugh C. Heyliger. *Trade and Industry:* Fitzroy P. Jones. *Health and Women's Affairs:* Constance Mitcham. *Minister in the Office of the Prime Minister:* Joseph Parry. *Minister in the Ministry of Finance:* Richard Caines. *Attorney-General:* Tapley Seaton. *Natural Resources and the Environment:* Simeon Daniel. The Prime Minister of *Nevis* is Simeon Daniel.

Flag: Diagonally green, black, red, with the black fimbriated in yellow and charged with two white stars.

INTERNATIONAL RELATIONS

Membership. St Christopher–Nevis is a member of the UN, the OAS, the Commonwealth and is an ACP state of EEC.

ECONOMY

Budget. The 1990 budget envisaged expenditure at EC$93,235,249 and revenue at EC$98,969,309.

Currency. The East Caribbean *dollar* (XCD) (of 100 *cents*) is in use. In March 1991, £1 = EC$5·12; US$1 = EC$2·70.

Banking. The National Bank operates 4 branches in St. Kitts and Nevis. The main office is located in Basseterre. Other banks include Barclay's Bank International, with a sub-branch in Nevis, Royal Bank of Canada, and the Nevis Co-operative Banking Co. Ltd and the Bank of Nevis in Charlestown. Branches of the Bank of Nova Scotia are located in Basseterre and Charlestown. Commercial banks' assets (1988) EC$418·6m.; deposits EC$289·8m.

ENERGY AND NATURAL RESOURCES

Electricity. Production (1989) 42m. kwh.

Agriculture. The main crops are sugar and cotton. There are 30 sugar estates and 124 acres of cotton. Most of the farms are small-holdings and there are a number of coconut estates amounting to some 1,000 acres under public and private ownership. Sugar production (1989) 24,777 long tonnes. 35,185 lbs of cotton and 287,020 lbs of copra were produced in 1987, and 6,587 lbs of cotton lint in 1988-89.

Livestock (1988): Cattle, 7,000; pigs, 10,000; sheep, 15,000; goats, 10,000; donkeys, (1987) 1,116; poultry, (1987) 50,116.

Fisheries. Catch (1988) 2·5m. lbs.

INDUSTRY. The main employer of labour is the sugar industry. In 1989 construction was a major industry. Other industries are clothing and assembly of electronic equipment.

FOREIGN ECONOMIC RELATIONS

Commerce. Imports, (1988) EC$255·7m. mainly from the USA and UK; exports, EC$76·6m. Chief export was sugar, with 14,873 long tons (EC$20,717,387) to the UK and 6,895 long tons (EC$9,005,747). to the USA.

Total trade between St Christopher (St Kitts)–Nevis and UK (British Department of Trade returns, in £1,000 sterling):

	1987	*1988*	*1989*	*1990*
Imports to UK	4,677	4,271	4,866	4,513
Exports and re-exports from UK	7,041	8,025	5,887	6,477

Tourism. In 1988, there were 123,200 tourists, 53,600 arriving by sea. In 1989 there were 22 hotels with 1,353 beds.

COMMUNICATIONS

Roads. There were (1983) about 305 km of roads, and (1988) 4,903 licensed vehicles.

Railways. There are 36 km of railway operated by the sugar industry.

Aviation. There is an airport at Golden Rock (St Kitts). 98,263 passengers arrived by air in 1987. There is an airfield on Nevis (Newcastle).

Shipping. A deep water port was opened in 1981 at Bird Rock with accommodation for cargo, tourist, roll-on-roll-off ships and bulk sugar and molasses loading. 1,428 tourists arrived by sea in 1985.

Post and Telecommunications. There is a general post office in Basseterre. Five branches are on the island. Charlestown has a general post office, and there are two branches in Nevis. There were 9,367 telephones in 1990. In 1985 there were 5,000 television and 21,000 radio receivers.

JUSTICE, RELIGION, EDUCATION AND WELFARE

Justice. Justice is administered by the Supreme Court and by Magistrates' Courts.They have both civil and criminal jurisdiction.

Religion. In 1985, 36·2% were Anglican, 32·3% Methodist, 7·9% other Protestant, and 10·7% Roman Catholic.

Education. Primary education is compulsory for all children between the ages of 5 and 14, but no pupil is required to leave school before the age of 16 years. There is an Extra-Mural Department of the University of the West Indies, a Technical College and a Teachers' Training College.

In 1988 there were 1,357 pupils in nurseries and pre-schools, 7,473 pupils in primary schools, 4,273 in secondary schools, and (1989) 211 students in the Technical and Teacher's Training Colleges.

Health. In 1990 there were 27 doctors, 4 hospitals with 258 beds and 17 health clinics.

DIPLOMATIC REPRESENTATIVES

Of St Christopher and Nevis in Great Britain (10 Kensington Ct., London W8)
High Commissioner: Richard Gunn.

Of Great Britain in St Christopher and Nevis
High Commissioner: E. T. Davies, CMG (resides in Bridgetown).

Of St Christopher and Nevis in the USA (2501 M. St., NW, Washington, D.C., 20037)
Chargé d'Affaires: Erstein M. Edwards.

Of St Christopher and Nevis to the United Nations
Ambassador: Dr William Herbert.

Further Reading

National Accounts. Statistics Division, Ministry of Development (annual)
St Kitts and Nevis Quarterly. Statistics Division, Ministry of Development

Gordon, J., *Nevis: Queen of the Caribees*. London, 1985

Library: Public Library, Basseterre. *Librarian:* Miss V. Archibald.

ST HELENA

Capital: Jamestown
Population: 5,564 (1988)

HISTORY. The island was administered by the East India Company from 1659 and became a British colony in 1834.

AREA AND POPULATION. St Helena, of volcanic origin, is 1,200 miles from the west coast of Africa. Area, 47 sq. miles (121·7 sq. km), with a cultivable area of about 600 acres (243 ha). Population (1988) 5,564. The port of the island is Jamestown, population (1976) 1,516.

In 1982 there were: Births, 123; deaths, 52; marriages, 26.

CLIMATE. A mild climate, with little variation. Temperatures range from 75–85°F (24–29°C) in summer to 65–75°F (18–24°C) in winter. Rainfall varies between 13" (325 mm) and 37" (925 mm) according to altitude and situation.

GOVERNMENT. The Government of St Helena is administered by a Governor, with the aid of a Legislative Council consisting of the Governor, 2 *ex-officio* members (the Government Secretary and the Treasurer) and 12 elected members. Committees of the Legislative Council are responsible for the general oversight of the activities of government departments and have, in addition, statutory and administrative functions.

The Governor is also assisted by an Executive Council consisting of the 2 *ex-officio* members and the chairmen of the 6 Council committees.

Governor and C.-in-C.: R. F. Stimson.
Government Secretary: E. C. Brooks, OBE.

Flag: The British Blue Ensign with the shield of the colony in the fly.

FINANCE AND TRADE

Budget. In 1984 revenue was £4·34m. and expediture £3·91m.

Commerce. Total trade between Ascension and St Helena and UK (British Department of Trade returns, in £1,000 sterling):

	1986	*1987*	*1988*	*1989*	*1990*
Imports to UK	380	189	205	504	555
Exports and re-exports from UK	8,196	8,065	6,103	7,208	7,429

Banking. Savings-bank deposits on 31 Dec. 1982, £1,467,079, belonging to 3,800 depositors.

COMMUNICATIONS

Roads. There were (1988) 94 km of all-weather motor roads. There were 1,301 vehicles in 1987.

Shipping. There is a service from Cardiff (UK) 6 times a year, and links with South Africa and neighbouring islands.

Telecommunications. The Cable & Wireless Ltd cable connects St Helena with Cape Town and Ascension Island. There is a telephone service with 85 miles of wire and (1982), 310 telephones.

St Helena Government Broadcasting Station broadcasts in English on medium-waves. Number of radio receivers (1988), 2,400.

JUSTICE, RELIGION, EDUCATION AND WELFARE

Justice. Police force, 32; cases dealt with by police magistrate, 205 in 1981.

Religion. There are 10 Anglican churches, 4 Baptist chapels, 3 Salvation Army halls, 1 Seventh Day Adventist church and 1 Roman Catholic church.

Education. Three pre-school playgroups, 7 primary, 3 senior and 1 secondary schools controlled by the Government had 1,188 pupils in 1987.

Health. There were 3 doctors, 1 dentist and 54 hospital beds in 1982.

Ascension is a small island of volcanic origin, of 34 sq. miles (88 sq. km), 700 miles north-west of St Helena. In Nov. 1922 the administration was transferred from the Admiralty to the Colonial Office and annexed to the colony of St Helena. There are 120 hectares providing fresh meat, vegetables and fruit. Population, 31 March 1988, was 1,007 (excluding military personnel).

The island is the resort of sea turtles, which come to lay their eggs in the sand annually between Jan. and May. Rabbits are more or less numerous on the island, which is, besides, the breeding ground of the sooty tern or 'wideawake', these birds coming in vast numbers to lay their eggs every eighth month. There is also a small herd of feral donkeys.

Cable & Wireless Ltd own and operate a cable station, connecting the island with St Helena, Sierra Leone, St Vincent, Rio de Janeiro and Buenos Aires. There is an airstrip (Miracle Mile) near the settlement of Georgetown which was being extended in 1985.

Administrator: M. T. S. Blick.

Tristan da Cunha, is the largest of a small group of islands in the South Atlantic lying 1,320 miles (2,124 sq. km) south-west of St Helena, of which they became dependencies on 12 Jan. 1938. Tristan da Cunha has an area of 98 sq. km and a population (1988) of 313, all living in the settlement of Edinburgh. Inaccessible Island (10 sq. km) lies 20 miles west and the 3 Nightingale Islands (2 sq. km) lie 20 miles south of Tristan da Cunha; they are uninhabited. Gough Island (90 sq. km) is 220 miles south of Tristan and has a meteorological station.

Tristan consists of a volcano rising to a height of 6,760 ft, with a circumference at its base of 21 miles. The volcano, believed to be extinct, erupted unexpectedly early in Oct. 1961. The whole population was evacuated without loss and settled temporarily in the UK. In 1963 they returned to Tristan where they all dwell in the settlement of Edinburgh. Before the disaster occurred the habitable area was a small plateau on the north west side of about 12 sq. miles, 100 ft above sea-level. Only about 30 acres was under cultivation, three-quarters of it for potatoes. There were apple and peach trees. Potatoes remain the chief crop, cattle, sheep and pigs are now reared, and fish are plentiful.

Population in 1880, 109; in 1988, 306. The original inhabitants were shipwrecked sailors and soldiers who remained behind when the garrison from St Helena was withdrawn in 1817.

At the end of April 1942 Tristan da Cunha was commissioned as HMS *Atlantic Isle*, and became an important meteorological and radio station. In Jan. 1949 a South African company commenced crawfishing operations. An Administrator was appointed at the end of 1948 and a body of basic law brought into operation. The Island Council, which was set up in 1932, in 1982 consisted of a Chief Islander, 3 nominated and 7 elected members under the chairmanship of the Administrator.

Administrator: R. Perry.

Further Reading

Crawford, A., *Tristan da Cunha and the Roaring Forties*. Edinburgh, 1982
Cross, A., *Saint Helena*. Newton Abbot, 1980
Munch, P. A., *Sociology of Tristan da Cunha*. Oslo, 1945.—*Crisis in Utopia*. New York, 1971

ST LUCIA

Capital: Castries
Population: 146,600 (1988)
GNP per capita: US$1,540 (1988)

HISTORY. St Lucia was discovered about 1500 A.D. Attempts to colonize the island by the English took place in 1605 and 1638. The French settled in 1650 and St Lucia was ceded to Britain in 1814. Self-government was achieved in 1967 and independence on 22 Feb. 1979.

AREA AND POPULATION. St Lucia is a small island of the Lesser Antilles situated in the Eastern Caribbean between Martinique and St Vincent, with an area of 238 sq. miles (617 sq. km); population (census, 1980) 120,300. Estimate (1988) 146,600. The capital is Castries (population, 1988, 52,868), and Vieux Fort, the second town and port 12,951 in 1984. Life expectancy (1985) was 68·6 (men) and 75·5 (women).

CLIMATE. The climate is tropical, with a dry season lasting from Jan. to April, a wet season from May to Aug., followed by an Indian summer for two months, but most rain falls in Nov. and Dec. Amounts vary over the year, according to altitude, from 60" (1,500 mm) to 138" (3,450 mm). Temperatures are uniform at about 80°F (26·7°C).

CONSTITUTION AND GOVERNMENT. There is a 17-seat House of Assembly elected for 5 years; an 11-seat Senate appointed by the Governor-General, 6 on the advice of the Prime Minister, 3 on the advice of the Leader of the Opposition, and 2 'after consultation with appropriate religious, economic or social bodies or associations'.

At the elections in April 1987, the United Workers' Party gained 9 seats, and the St Lucia Labour Party, 8.

Acting Governor-General: Stanislaus James OBE.

Prime Minister, Minister of Finance, Planning, and Home Affairs: Rt Hon. John George Melvin Compton.

Deputy Prime Minister and Minister of Trade, Industry and Tourism: George Mallet. *Foreign Affairs:* Neville Cenac. *Health, Labour, Information and Broadcasting:* Romanus Lansiquot. *Education and Culture:* Louis George. *Community Development, Social Affairs, Youth and Sport:* Stephenson King. *Agriculture, Lands, Fisheries and Co-operatives:* Ferdinand Henry. *Communications, Works and Transport:* Gregory Avril. *Attorney-General and Minister of Legal Affairs:* Parry Husbands. *Minister of State in the Prime Minister's Office:* Desmond Brathwate.

Flag: Blue with a design of a black triangle edged in white, bearing a smaller yellow triangle, in the centre.

Local government: In 1986 the 10 *quartiers* were replaced by 8 administrative regions.

INTERNATIONAL RELATIONS

Membership. St Lucia is a member of the UN, OAS, Caricom, the Commonwealth and is an ACP state of the EEC.

ECONOMY

Planning. The aim of the Development Plan, 1977–90, was to develop agriculture to diversify production and to contain rural-urban drift.

Budget. The budget in 1989–90 amounted to EC$370·3m. expenditure; revenue, EC$358·7m.

Banking. There are Barclays Bank International with 4 branches and 2 agencies, the Royal Bank of Canada with 1 branch, the Bank of Nova Scotia with 3 branches, the Canadian Imperial Bank of Commerce and the St Lucia Co-operative bank with 2 branches each, the National Development Bank with 1 branch and the National Commercial Bank with 3 branches.

INDUSTRY. In 1990, laundry soap, coconut meal, rum, beverages, electronic assembly and clothing were the chief products.

Agriculture. Bananas, cocoa, coconuts, mace, nutmeg and citrus fruit are the chief products. Livestock (1988): Cattle, 13,000; pigs, 12,000; sheep, 15,000; goats, 12,000.

FOREIGN ECONOMIC RELATIONS

Commerce. Value of imports (1986), EC$419·3m.; of exports, EC$213·2m., including coconut oil, cocoa beans, copra and bananas. Main items of imports were artificial silk and cotton piece-goods, cement, plastic goods, iron and steel products, hardware, motor vehicles, agricultural machinery, fertilizers, wheat flour, codfish and rice, meat and meat preparations.

Total trade between St Lucia and UK (British Department of Trade returns, in £1,000 sterling):

	1987	*1988*	*1989*	*1990*
Imports to UK	40,908	58,385	48,746	55,737
Exports and re-exports from UK	13,196	19,750	19,601	17,573

Tourism. The total number of visitors during 1987 was 202,336.

COMMUNICATIONS

Roads. The island has 500 miles of main and secondary roads, and 2,084 commercial vehicles and 8,629 cars in 1986.

Aviation. The island is served on a scheduled basis by Leeward Islands Air Transport, British West Indian Airways, Eastern Airline, British Airways, Pan Am, Caribbean Airways and Air Canada. There are 2 airfields—Hewanorra International Airport, with 9,000 ft runway, and Vigie.

Shipping. There are 2 ports, Castries and Vieux Fort.

Post and Broadcasting. There were (1986) 13,654 telephone instruments coupled to 7,960 exchange lines; 157 telex machines, and telegram service. There were 5,000 TV and 99,000 radio receivers in 1988.

Cinemas. There were 8 cinemas in 1986.

JUSTICE, RELIGION, EDUCATION AND WELFARE

Justice. The island is divided into 2 judicial districts, and there are 9 magistrates' courts. Appeals lie with the Eastern Caribbean Supreme Court of Appeal.

Religion. In 1989 over 82% of the population was Roman Catholic.

Education (1985–86). 79 primary schools, with 32,273 pupils on roll. Primary education is free and compulsory by law, but the legislation is not enforced. There are 12 secondary schools with 5,665 pupils. There is 1 technical college with (1985–86) 223 students and 1 teachers' college with (1985–86) 123 students.

Health. Victoria Hospital (in Castries) has 213 beds; there is also a 162-bed mental hospital, 3 other hospitals (150 beds) and 29 health centres. In 1984 there were 58 doctors, 5 dentists and 236 nursing personnel.

DIPLOMATIC REPRESENTATIVES

Of St Lucia in Great Britain (10 Kensington Ct., London, W8)
High Commissioner: Richard Gunn.

Of Great Britain in St Lucia
High Commissioner: E. T. Davies, CMG (resides in Bridgetown).

Of St Lucia in the USA (2100 M St., NW, Washington, D.C., 20037)
Ambassador: Dr Joseph E. Edmunds.

Of St Lucia to the United Nations
Ambassador: Dr Charles S. Flemming.

Further Reading

Ellis, G., *St Lucia: Helen of the West Indies.* London, 1985

Library: The Central Library, Castries. *Acting Librarian:* Frances Niles.

ST VINCENT AND THE GRENADINES

Capital: Kingstown
Population: 113,950 (1989)
GNP per capita: US$1,100 (1988)

HISTORY. The date of discovery of St Vincent was 22 Jan. 1498. In 1969 St Vincent became a self-governing Associated State of UK and acquired full independence on 27 Oct. 1979.

AREA AND POPULATION. St Vincent is an island of the Lesser Antilles, situated in the Eastern Caribbean between St Lucia and Grenada, from which latter it is separated by a chain of small islands known as the Grenadines. The total area of 388 sq. km (150 sq. miles) comprises the island of St Vincent itself (345 sq. km) and the Northern Grenadines (43 sq. km) of which the largest are Bequia, Mustique, Canouan, Mayreau and Union.

The population at the 1980 Census was 97,845; latest estimate (1989) was 113,950 of whom 5,503 lived in the Northern, and 2,963 in the Southern Grenadines. The capital, Kingstown, had 29,372 inhabitants in 1989 (including suburbs). The population is mainly of black (82%) and mixed (13·9%) origin, with small white, Asian and Amerindian minorities.

Vital statistics (1989): Live births, 2,537; deaths, 712; marriages (1987), 416.

CLIMATE. The climate is tropical marine, with north-east Trades predominating and rainfall ranging from 150" (3,750 mm) a year in the mountains to 60" (1,500 mm) on the south-east coast. The rainy season is from June to Dec., and temperatures are equable throughout the year.

CONSTITUTION AND GOVERNMENT. The House of Assembly consists of 15 elected members, directly elected for a 5-year term from single-member constituencies, and 6 Senators appointed by the Governor-General (4 on the advice of the Prime Minister and 2 on the advice of the Leader of the Opposition). At the General Elections held 16 May 1989, the New Democratic Party won all 15 contested seats.

Governor-General: Sir David Jack.

Prime Minister and Minister of Finance and Foreign Affairs: Rt. Hon. James Fitz-Allen Mitchell.

Agriculture, Industry and Labour: Allan Cruickshank. *Education, Youth and Women's Affairs:* John Horne. *Housing, Community Development and Local Government:* Louis Jones. *Health and Environment:* Burton Williams. *Attorney General, Minister of Justice, Information and Culture:* Parnell Campbell. *Communications and Works:* Jeremiah Scott. *Trade and Tourism:* Herbert Young.

There are 2 Ministers of State.

National Flag: Three vertical stripes of blue, yellow, green, with the yellow of double width and charged with three green diamonds.

INTERNATIONAL RELATIONS

Membership. St Vincent and the Grenadines is a member of UN, OAS, Caricom, the Commonwealth and is an ACP state of the EEC.

ECONOMY

Budget. Revenue (estimate), 1989–90, EC$128·38m.; expenditure, EC$123·56m. Public debt at the end of the financial year 1988–89 was EC$122·57m.

Currency. The currency in use is the *East Caribbean dollar* (XCD). In March 1991, £1 = EC$5·12; US$1 = EC$2·70.

Banking and Finance. There are branches of Barclays Bank PLC, the Caribbean Banking Corporation, the Canadian Imperial Bank of Commerce, the Bank of Nova Scotia. Locally-owned banks: the National Commercial Bank, St Vincent Co-operative Bank and the St Vincent Agricultural Credit and Loan Bank.

ENERGY AND NATURAL RESOURCES

Electricity. Production (1987) was 48,116,190 kwh. Supply 230 volts; 50 Hz.

Agriculture. Agriculture accounted for 20·8% of GDP in 1987. According to the 1985–86 census of agriculture, 29,649 acres of the total acreage of 85,120 were classified as agricultural lands; 5,500 acres were under forest and woodland and all other lands accounted for 1,030 acres. The total arable land was about 8,932 acres, of which 4,016 acres were under temporary crops, 2,256 acres under temporary pasture, 2,289 acres under temporary fallow and other arable land covering 371 acres. 16,062 acres were under permanent crops, of which approximately 5,500 acres were under coconuts and 7,224 acres under bananas; the remainder produce cocoa, citrus, mangoes, avocado pears, guavas and miscellaneous crops. The sugar industry was closed down in 1985 although some sugar-cane will be grown for rum production. Production (1988, in tonnes): Coconuts, 25,000; bananas, 40,000.

Livestock (1988): Cattle, 7,000; pigs, 9,000; sheep, 15,000; goats, 5,000.

INDUSTRY. Industries include assembly of electronic equipment, manufacture of garments, electrical products, animal feeds and flour, corrugated galvanized sheets, exhaust systems, industrial gases, concrete blocks, plastics, soft drinks, beer and rum, wood products and furniture, and processing of milk, fruit juices and food items.

Labour. The Department of Labour is charged with looking after the interest and welfare of all categories of workers, including providing advice and guidance to employers and employees and their organizations and enforcing the labour laws.

FOREIGN ECONOMIC RELATIONS

Commerce (1989). Imports, EC$344·18m.; exports, EC$201·34m.

Principal exports, 1989 (in EC$1,000): Eddoes and dasheen, 8,576; sweet potatoes, 5,113; tannias, 1,922; bananas, 89,933; tobacco, 540; coconut, 741; plantain, 1,830; ginger, 1,063; flour, 18,773.

Total trade between St Vincent and the Grenadines and UK (British Department of Trade returns, in £1,000 sterling):

	1987	*1988*	*1989*	*1990*
Imports to UK	20,208	29,709	31,570	37,906
Exports and re-exports from UK	8,529	8,011	11,075	9,514

Tourism. There were 128,615 visitors in 1989.

COMMUNICATIONS

Roads. There were (1989) 53 miles of highway, 19 miles of concrete road, 245 miles of oiled asphalt road and 217 miles of earth track. Vehicles registered (1987) 8,500.

Aviation. Scheduled services are operated daily by LIAT and Air Martinique. Non-scheduled services are operated by Mustique Airways, Tropical Air Services, Aero-Services and St Lucia Airways. Passengers are able to travel daily through the chain of islands stretching as far north as San Juan, Puerto Rico and south to Trinidad. Connexions to the USA, Canada, South America and Europe are possible *via* Barbados, Antigua, Trinidad and St Lucia.

Shipping (1987): 36 auxiliary sailing vessels of 1,510 NRT entered and cleared. 659 motor vessels of 805,261 NRT entered and cleared. 47 tankers of 41,798 NRT bringing 18,925·13 tons of fuel entered.

Telecommunications. There is a General Post Office at Kingstown and 49 district post offices. There is an automatic telephone system with (1989) 12,000 subscribers; 7,950 stations and a digital radio link to Bequia, Mustique and Union Island; VHF links Petit St Vincent and Palm Island. In 1987 there were 12,000 TV and 60,000 radio receivers.

Cinemas. There were 2 cinemas in 1987 with a seating capacity of 1,825.

JUSTICE, RELIGION, EDUCATION AND WELFARE

Justice (1986). There were 3,699 criminal matters disposed of in the 3 magisterial districts which comprise 11 courts. 192 cases were dealt with in the 1987 Criminal Assizes in the High Court. Strength of police force (1982), 525 (including 12 officers).

Religion. At the 1980 Census, 42% of the population was Anglican, 21% Methodist and 12% Roman Catholic.

Education. In 1989 there were 64 primary schools (52 rural) with 25,152 pupils, 21 secondary schools (13 rural) and 1 school for special needs.

Health. In 1989 there was a general hospital in Kingstown with 204 beds, 4 rural hospitals, 2 private hospitals and 35 clinics. There were 40 doctors, 2 dentists, 208 registered nurses, 46 auxiliary nurses and 35 community health aides.

Library: St Vincent Public Library, Kingstown. *Librarian:* Mrs Lorna Small.

DIPLOMATIC REPRESENTATIVES

Of St Vincent and the Grenadines in Great Britain (10 Kensington Ct, London, W8)
High Commissioner: Richard Gunn.

Of Great Britain in St Vincent and the Grenadines
High Commissioner: E. T. Davies, CMG (resides in Bridgetown).

Of St Vincent and the Grenadines to the USA and the UN
Ambassador: Kingsley C. A. Layne.

Further Reading

Price, N., *Behind the Planter's Back*. London, 1988

SAN MARINO

Capital: San Marino
Population: 22,746 (1988)

Repubblica di San Marino

HISTORY. On 22 March 1862 San Marino concluded a treaty of friendship and co-operation, including a *de facto* customs union with the kingdom of Italy, preserving the independence of the ancient republic, although completely surrounded by Italian territory. The treaty was renewed on 27 March 1872, 28 June 1897 and 31 March 1939, with several amendments 1942–85.

The republic has extradition treaties with Belgium, France, the Netherlands, UK and USA.

AREA AND POPULATION. San Marino is a land-locked state in central Italy, 20 km from the Adriatic. The frontier line is 38·6 km in length, area is 61·19 sq. km (24·1 sq. miles) and the population (31 Dec. 1988), 22,746; some 11,000 citizens live abroad. The capital, San Marino, had 4,363 inhabitants (1986); the largest town is Serravalle (7,109), an industrial centre in the north.

CONSTITUTION AND GOVERNMENT. The legislative power is vested in the Great and General Council of 60 members elected every 5 years by popular vote, 2 of whom are appointed every 6 months to act as regents *(Capitani reggenti)*.

The elections held on 29 May 1988 gave 27 seats to the Christian Democrats, 18 to the Communists, 15 to Socialist parties.

The regents (who are Heads of State) exercise executive power together with the Congress of State *(Congresso di Stato)*, which comprises the regents, 3 secretaries of state and 7 ministers, and through Commissions on social welfare, public works, etc.

National flag: Horizontally white over light blue, with the national arms over all in the centre.

DEFENCE. Military service is not obligatory, but all citizens between the ages of 16 and 55 can be called upon to defend the State. They may also serve as volunteers in the Military Corps.

ECONOMY. The budget (ordinary and extraordinary) for the financial year ending 31 Dec. 1989 balanced at 259,275,271,797 lire.

Wheat, barley, maize and vines are grown. The chief exports are wood machinery, chemicals, wine, textiles, tiles, varnishes and ceramics.

Italian currency is in general use, but the republic issues its own postage stamps and coins.

In 1987, 3m. tourists visited San Marino.

COMMUNICATIONS

Roads. A bus service connects San Marino with Rimini. There are 237 km of roads and (1987) 16,540 passenger cars and 3,225 commercial vehicles.

Telecommunications. In 1986 there were 11,707 telephones. In 1983 there were 8 post offices. In 1987 there were 10,600 radio and 6,608 television receivers.

Cinemas. In 1987 there were 7 cinemas with a seating capacity of 1,000.

JUSTICE, RELIGION, EDUCATION AND WELFARE

Justice. Law is administered by a Commissioner for civil cases and a Commissioner for criminal cases (acting with a penal judge), from whom appeals can be made to a civil appeals judge and a criminal appeals judge respectively. The highest legal authority is, in certain cases, the *Consiglio dei XII*. Civil marriage was instituted in Sept. 1953 and divorce allowed in April 1986.

Religion. 95% of the population are Roman Catholic.

Education. In 1985 there were 13 elementary schools with 1,411 pupils and 158 teachers, 4 secondary schools with 1,248 pupils and 183 teachers. There is also a foreign languages school, a technical school and a trade and handicraft school.

Health. In 1987 there were 149 hospital beds and 60 doctors.

DIPLOMATIC REPRESENTATIVES

British Consul-General (resides at Florence): M. L. Croll.
Consul-General in London: Lord Forte.

Further Reading

Information: Office of Cultural Affairs and Information of the Department of Foreign Affairs.

Garbelotto, A., *Evoluzione storica della costituzione di S. Marino.* Milan, 1956
Matteini, N., *The Republic of San Marino.* San Marino, 1981
Packett, C. N., *Guide to the Republic of San Marino.* Bradford, 1970
Rossi, G., *San Marino.* San Marino, 1954

SÃO TOMÉ E PRÍNCIPE

Capital: São Tomé
Population: 115,600 (1988)
GNP per capita: US$280 (1987)

República Democrática de São Tomé e Príncipe

HISTORY. The islands of São Tomé and Príncipe, were discovered in 1471 by Pedro Escobar and João Gomes, and from 1522 constituted a Portugese colony. On 11 June 1951 it became an overseas province of Portugal.

On 26 Nov. 1974 the Government of Portugal and the liberation movement of São Tomé e Príncipe signed an agreement granting independence to the archipelago on 12 July 1975.

AREA AND POPULATION. The republic, which lies about 200 km off the west coast of Gabon, in the Gulf of Guinea, comprises the main islands of São Tomé (845 sq. km) and Príncipe and several smaller islets including Pedras Tinhosas and Rolas. It has a total area of 1,001 sq. km (387 sq. miles). Total population (census, 1981) 96,611. Estimate (1988) 115,600.

The areas and populations of the 2 provinces were as follows:

Province	*Sq. km*	*Census 1981*	*Estimate 1987*	*Chief town*	*Estimate 1984*
São Tomé	859	91,356	106,900	São Tomé	34,997
Príncipe	142	5,255	6,100	São António	1,000

The official language is Portuguese, but 90% speak Fang, a Bantu language.

Vital statistics (1985): Births, 3,700; deaths, 900.

CLIMATE. The tropical climate is modified by altitude and the effect of the cool Benguela current. The wet season is generally from Oct. to May, but rainfall varies very much, from 40" (1,000 mm) in the hot and humid north-east to 150–200" (3,800–5,000 mm) on the plateau. São Tomé Jan. 79°F (26·1°C), July 75°F (23·9°C). Annual rainfall 38" (951 mm).

CONSTITUTION AND GOVERNMENT. A new constitution was approved by 72% of the votes cast at a referendum in Aug. 1990. It abolishes the monopoly status of the *Movimento de Libertação de São Tomé e Príncipe*. The *President* is elected by the People's Assembly for a 4-year term; he is also head of government and appoints a Cabinet of Ministers to assist him. The 55-member *People's Assembly* is also elected for 4 years.

At the elections of Jan. 1991 the Democratic Convergence Party won.

At the presidential elections of Feb. 1991 the sole candidate, Miguel Trovoada (b.1946; ind) was elected by 80% of votes cast.

President, Commander-in-Chief: Miguel Trovoada.

Flag: Three horizontal stripes of green, yellow, green, with the yellow of double width and bearing 2 black stars; in the hoist a red triangle over all.

Local government: São Tomé province comprises 6 districts, while Príncipe province forms a seventh district.

INTERNATIONAL RELATIONS

Membership. São Tomé e Príncipe is a member of the UN, OAU and is an ACP state of the EEC.

ECONOMY

Budget. In 1986 the budget balanced at 1,092m. dobra.

Currency. The unit of currency is the *dobra* (STD), introduced in 1977, divided into 100 *centavos.* In March 1991, £1 = 285·98 *dobra*; US$1 = 150·75 *dobra.*

Banking. *Banco Nacional de São Tomé e Príncipe* (established, 1975) is the central bank.

ENERGY AND NATURAL RESOURCES

Electricity. Production (1986) 3m. kwh.

Agriculture. About 38% of the area is under cultivation. Production (1988 in tonnes): Coconuts, 37,000; copra, 4,000; bananas, 3,000; palm oil, 250. Food crops include cassava, sweet potatoes and yams. In 1988 there were 4,000 goats, 2,000 sheep, 3,000 pigs and 3,000 cattle.

Fisheries. The fishing industry is being developed, to exploit the rich tuna shoals. Catch (1986) 2,800 tonnes.

FOREIGN ECONOMIC RELATIONS

Commerce. Imports in 1984 amounted to 485·9m. dobras and exports to 539·6m. dobras the main exports being cocoa (80%), copra (15%), coffee, bananas and palm-oil. Portugal provided 30% of imports while the German Democratic Republic took 35% of exports, the Netherlands 18% and Portugal 15%.

Total trade between São Tomé e Príncipe and UK (British Department of Trade returns, in £1,000 sterling):

	1986	*1987*	*1988*	*1989*	*1990*
Imports to UK	327	205	20	4	114
Exports and re-exports from UK	455	329	416	819	879

COMMUNICATIONS

Roads. There were 288 km of roads (198 paved) in 1975.

Aviation. São Tomé airport is linked by regular services to Douala, Lisbon, Luanda, Cabinda, Libreville, Malabo and Brazil, as well as to Príncipe.

Telecommunications. There were (1986) 28,000 radio receivers and 2,200 telephones.

Newspapers. In 1986 there were 2 weekly newspapers.

JUSTICE, RELIGION, EDUCATION AND WELFARE.

Justice. Members of the Supreme Court are appointed by the People's Assembly.

Religion. About 80% of the population are Roman Catholic.

Education. In 1984 there were 19,086 pupils and 517 teachers in 63 primary schools, 6,186 pupils and 300 teachers in 11 secondary schools, and 370 students and 35 teachers in 2 technical schools.

Health. In 1981 there were 38 doctors and 118 nursing personnel.

DIPLOMATIC REPRESENTATIVES

Of São Tomé and Príncipe to Great Britain
Ambassador: (Vacant) (resides in Brussels).

Of Great Britain in São Tomé and Príncipe
Ambassador: J. G. Flynn (resides in Luanda).

Of São Tomé and Príncipe in the USA and to the United Nations
Ambassador: Joaquim Rafael Branco.

SAUDI ARABIA

Capital: Riyadh
Population: 12m. (1988)
GNP per capita: US$6,170 (1988)

Al-Mamlaka al-'Arabiya as-Sa'udiya

(Kingdom of Saudi Arabia)

HISTORY. Saudi Arabia was founded by Abdul Aziz ibn Abdur-Rahman al-Faisal Al Sa'ud, GCB, GCIE (born about 1880; died 9 Nov. 1953), who had been proclaimed King of the Hejaz on 8 Jan. 1926 and had in 1927 changed his title of Sultan of Nejd and its Dependencies to that of King of the Hejaz and of Nejd and its Dependencies. By a treaty of 20 May 1927 the UK recognized the independence of Hejaz, Nejd, Asir and Al-Hasa, which became the State of the Kingdom of Saudi Arabia by decree of 23 Sept. 1932.

Following the Iraqi invasion of Kuwait in Aug. 1990 Saudi Arabia invited the the UN-supported coalition forces to base themselves on its territory. There were Iraqi missile attacks on Saudi Arabian targets.

AREA AND POPULATION. Saudi Arabia, which occupies over 70% of the Arabian peninsula, is bounded in the west by the Red Sea, east by the Persian Gulf and the United Arab Emirates, north by Jordan, Iraq and Kuwait and south by Yemen and Oman. The total area is estimated to be 849,400 sq. miles (2·2m. sq. km). Riyadh is the political, and Mecca the religious, capital.

The principal cities of the Western Province (formerly *Hejaz*) are Jiddah (561,104 inhabitants at the 1974 Census; estimate (1986) 1·4m.), Mecca (618,006), Taif (204,857) and Medina (500,000); of the Central Province (formerly *Nejd*) are Riyadh, the national capital (666,840; estimate, 1988, 2m.), Buraidah (184,000), Ha'il (92,000), Uneiza and Al-Kharj; of the Northern Province are Tabouk (99,000), Al-Jawf and Sakaka; of the Eastern Province (formerly *Al-Hasa*) are Dammam (127,844), Hofuf (101,271), Haradh (100,000), Al-Mobarraz (54,325), Al-Khobar (48,817) and Qatif; and of the Southern Province (formerly *Asir*) are Khamis-Mushait (49,581), Najran (47,501), Jisan (32,814) and Abha (155,406). New industrial cities are being built at Jubail and Yanbu on the Gulf. Taif, about 3,800ft above sea-level and some 50 miles from Mecca, is a summer resort.

The total population was (1974 census) 7,012,642, of which 5,128,655 were categorized as settled and 1,883,987 as nomadic. Estimate (1988) 12m.

The Neutral Zone (3,560 sq. miles, 5,700 sq. km.), jointly owned and administered by Kuwait and Saudi Arabia from 1922 to 1966, was partitioned between the two countries in May 1966, but the exploitation of the oil and other natural resources will continue to be shared.

CLIMATE. A desert climate, with very little rain and none at all from June to Dec. The months May to Sept. are very hot and humid, but winter temperatures are quite pleasant. Riyadh. Jan. 58°F (14·4°C), July 108°F (42°C). Annual rainfall 4" (100 mm). Jiddah. Jan. 73°F (22·8°C), July 87°F (30·6°C). Annual rainfall 3" (81 mm).

KING. Fahd ibn Abdul Aziz, Custodian of the two Holy Mosques, succeeded in May 1982, after King Khalid's death. *Crown Prince:* Prince Abdullah ibn Abdul Aziz, half-brother of the King.

National flag: Green, with the text 'There is no God but Allah and Mohammed is his prophet' in white Arabic script, and beneath this a white sabre.

CONSTITUTION AND GOVERNMENT. Constitutional practice derives from Koranic Shariah law. There is no formal Constitution.

The King has the post of Prime Minister.

Deputy Prime Minister and Commander of the National Guard: Prince Abdullah ibn Abdul Aziz.

Second Deputy Prime Minister and Minister of Defence and Aviation, and Inspector General: Prince Sultan ibn Abdul Aziz.

Public Works and Housing: Prince Miteb ibn Abdul Aziz. *Interior:* Prince Naif ibn Abdul Aziz. *Foreign Affairs:* Prince Saud al Faisal. *Labour and Social Affairs:* Muhammad al-Ali al-Fayiz. *Communications:* Hussein Ibrahim al Mansouri. *Finance and National Economy:* Muhammad Ali Aba'l Khail. *Information:* Ali ibn Hasan al-Shaer. *Industry and Electricity:* Dr Abdul Aziz al Zamil. *Commerce:* Dr Sulaiman Abdul Aziz al Sulaim. *Justice:* Muhammad ibn Jubair. *Education and Acting Higher Education:* Dr Abdul Aziz al Abdullah al Khuwaiter. *Petroleum and Mineral Resources and Planning:* Hisham Nazer. *Haj Affairs, Waqfs:* Abdul Wahhab Ahmad Abdul Wasi. *Municipal and Rural Affairs:* Khalid ibn Mohammed al Anqari. *Agriculture and Water:* Dr Abdul Rahman ibn Abdul Aziz ibn Hasan al Shaikh. *Health:* Faisal ibn Abdul Aziz al Hejailan. *Posts and Telecommunications:* Dr Alawi Darwish Kayyal. There are 8 Ministers of State.

There are provisions for the setting up of certain advisory councils, comprising a consultative Legislative Assembly in Mecca, municipal councils in each of the towns of Mecca, Medina and Jiddah, and village and tribal councils throughout the provinces. The country is divided for administrative purposes into 14 Regions (Emirates).

DEFENCE. The US maintains a Military Mission (with an Air Force element) as do France and Pakistan. Personnel are trained in Saudi Arabia, France, Pakistan, UK and the USA. The UK has training missions with the National Guard and the Navy.

Army. The Army comprises 2 armoured brigades, 4 mechanized brigades, 1 airborne brigade, 1 Royal Guard regiment, 5 artillery battalions and 1 infantry brigade. Equipment includes 300 AMX-30, 50 M-60A1 and 200 M-60A3 main battle tanks. There are surface-to-air units with Stinger and Hawk. 18 helicopters are in service. Strength (1990) was approximately 40,000. There is a para-military Frontier Force (approximately 10,500).

Navy. The Royal Saudi Naval Forces, comprise 4 French-built 2,900-tonnes frigates armed with Otomat anti-ship missiles, 4 smaller US-built missile frigates, 9 fast missile craft, 3 German-built torpedo craft and 4 US-built coastal minesweepers. Auxiliaries include 2 French-built replenishment tankers each embarking 2 helicopters, 3 ocean tugs and a Royal Yacht. There are numerous minor auxiliaries and boats.

Naval Aviation forces operate 24 Dauphin helicopters, both ship and shore based, and there is a regiment of some 1,500 marines.

The main naval bases are at Jiddah (Red Sea) and Jubail (The Gulf). Naval personnel in 1990 totalled 9,500 including 1,500 marines.

The Coast Guard operates some 40 inshore patrol craft, 24 hovercraft and over 300 boats of various types.

Air Force. Formed as a small army support unit in 1932, the Air Force has been built up considerably with British and US assistance since 1946. Complete re-equipment began in 1966 and delivery of 58 F-15 Eagles to equip 3 air superiority squadrons was made in 1982–84; they operate in conjunction with 5 E-3A Sentry AWACS aircraft and 8 KC-707 flight refuelling tankers. Current combat units include 3 squadrons of F-5E Tiger II supersonic fighter-bombers and RF-5E Tigereye reconnaissance aircraft, supported by a conversion unit with F-5B/F combat trainers. One squadron has formed with 24 Tornado strike aircraft with 23 on order, plus an air defence unit with 24 Tornado interceptors. Two squadrons of Strikemaster light jet attack/trainers are based at the King Faisal Air Academy, Riyadh, together with 12 Reims/Cessna FR172 piston-engined primary trainers, PC-9 basic trainers, Hawk advanced trainers and Jetstream navigation trainers. Other types in current service include 50 C-130E/H and KC-130H Hercules transports and tankers, 1 Boeing 747 SP, 1 Boeing 747-200, 1 Boeing 737, 3 Boeing 707, 4 CN-235s and 2 JetStar VIP jet transports, more than 60 Agusta-Bell 205, 212 and JetRanger helicopters, 2 Agusta AS-61A-4 VIP transport helicopters and communications aircraft. Personnel (1991), about 18,000 with 189 combat aircraft.

Air Defence Force. This separate Command was formerly part of the Army, which retains a point air defence capability. In 1989 there were French and Pakistani training missions. Equipment comprises approximately 18 Crotale missile systems, 15 batteries of Improved Hawk surface-to-air missiles, 30 mm Oerlikon and 20 mm Vulcan guns.

National Guard. The National Guard comprises 2 mechanized brigades (trained by the US), 1 ceremonial cavalry squadron. Additionally there are a number of regular and irregular units, the total strength of the National Guard amounting to approximately 56,000 (10,000 active). The National Guard's primary role is the protection of the Royal Family and vital points in the Kingdom. It does not come under command of the Ministry of Defence and Aviation. UK provides small advisory teams to the National Guard in the fields of general training and communications.

INTERNATIONAL RELATIONS

Membership. Saudi Arabia is a member of UN, the Arab League, the Gulf Co-operation Council and OPEC.

ECONOMY

Policy. The fifth 5-year development plan (1990–95) aims to increase manpower by an overall 3·5% and emphasizes industrial growth and economic development.

Budget. In 1986 the financial year became the calendar year. The 1990 budget provided for expenditure of 143,000m. rials and revenue of 118,000m. rials. The 1991 budget was postponed following Iraq's invasion of Kuwait.

There is no public debt.

Currency. The unit of currency is the *rial* (SAR) of 100 *halalas*. In March 1991, £1 = 7·10 *rials*; US$1 = 3·74 *rials*.

Banking and Finance. The Saudi Arabian Monetary Agency, established in 1953, is the central bank and the government's fiscal agent. There were 12 commercial banks with 958 branches, 5 special credit institutions and a variety of other financial institutions in 1990. The Saudi Arabian Agricultural Bank with 70 branches and offices extended 755m. rials in credit services to farmers during 1989. In 1989 total deposits in commercial banks were US$146,300m. and total assets were 233,600m. rials.

ENERGY AND NATURAL RESOURCES

Electricity. 57,108m. kwh. was generated by the main electricity companies in 1989. A programme of research and development of solar energy has produced a photovoltaic power system with a capacity in 1988 of 50 kw to provide electricity for 2 villages. Supply 127 and 220 volts; 50 and 60 Hz.

Oil. The first general geologic–geographical survey of Saudi Arabia was completed in 1961 under the joint sponsorship of the Saudi Arabian and US governments but surveying continues. Proven reserves (1989) 255,000m. bbls.

Oil production began in 1938 by Aramco, which is now 100% state-owned and accounts for about 97% of total crude oil production, with Getty and the Arabian Oil Co. accounting for the remainder.

Crude oil production in 1990 was 320·72m. tonnes. Crude oil exports in 1989 were 176m tonnes. 1989 oil exports earned US$26,000m.

Production comes from 14 major oilfields, mostly in the Eastern Region, the most important of which are Ghawar (the world's largest oilfield in operation), Abqaiq, Safaniyah (the largest offshore field) and Berri.

New fields have been discovered onshore at Farhah and Assahba and deeper pools offshore at Marjan, Safaniya and Zuluf, and during 1989 48 new wells were drilled and 5 seismic explorations conducted.

There is a pipeline from the eastern oilfields to the Red Sea oil terminal at Yanbu with a link to the Iraqi oilfields (cut after the Iraqi invasion of Kuwait in Aug. 1990).

In 1990 there were 5 domestic refineries: Ras Tanura, refining capacity 530,000 bbls per day (Aramco); Riyadh, 134,000 bbls per day, Jiddah, 91,000 bbls per day and Yanbu, 170,000 bbls per day (Petromin); Rasal-Khafji, 30,000 bbls per day (Arabian Oil Co.); as well as 3 joint venture export refineries: Yanbu, 250,000 bbls per day (Petromin/Mobil Oil); Jubail, 250,000 bbls per day (Petromin/Shell Saudi Arabia); Rabigh, 325,000 bbls per day (Petromin/Petrola International). Aramco has added a 300 tonne a day sulphur plant to Ras Tanura and operates a 400 tonnes a day desulphurization plant at Jubail.

Gas. In 1989 production of liquefied natural gas from oilfield—associated and dissolved gas was 420,946 bbls per day.

Water Resources. Intensive efforts are under-way to provide adequate supplies of water for urban, industrial, rural and agricultural use. Most investment however has gone into seawater desalination. In 1991 28 plants had the capacity to produce 1·9m. cu. metres a day.

Minerals. Production began in 1988 at Mahd Al-Dahab gold mine. Deposits of iron, phosphate, bauxite, uranium and copper have been found.

Agriculture. Since 1970 the Government has spent substantially on desert reclamation, irrigation schemes, drainage and control of surface water and control of moving sands. Undeveloped land has been distributed to farmers and there are research and extension programmes. Large scale private investment has concentrated on wheat, poultry and dairy production.

Production, 1988 (in 1,000 tonnes): Dates, 517; tomatoes, 465; water melons, 745; wheat, 3,000; barley, 186; grapes, 112; milk, 508; poultry meat, 248; eggs, 455.

Livestock estimates for 1988 include 630,000 cattle, 200,000 camels, 4m. sheep and 2·6m. goats.

Fisheries. Saudi Fisheries, established in 1981, has introduced a wide variety of fish to the domestic market and opened up a thriving export business in shrimps. Annual catch about 10,000 tonnes.

INDUSTRY. The Government encourages the establishment of manufacturing industries. Its policy includes the provision of industrial estates and loans covering 50% of capital investment. The Government has also established two industrial poles at Jubail and Yanbu, linked by gas and oil pipelines, to be the focus of heavy industrial development. Both have petrochemical complexes producing ethylene and methanol. In 1988 there were 12 major industries (petrochemical, urea and ammonia fertilizer, steel, gas and plastics) and over 65 support and light manufacturing businesses in operation in Jubail, and 8 heavy industries (natural gas liquids fractionation, refining, petrochemical, lube additives, crude oil and chemical terminals) and 21 light and support industries in operation in Yanbu.

Labour. The expatriate labour force grew by an average of 11·7% a year between 1980 and 1985. The proportion of non-Saudis in the total labour force rose from 28·2% in 1975 to 60% by 1985. In 1988, 95% of the total labour force was employed in the non-oil sector.

FOREIGN ECONOMIC RELATIONS

Commerce. Exports in 1988 (in 1m. rials) 88,896 of which crude oil, 62%; refined oil, 23%; petro-chemicals, 11%. Total imports (1988) 81,582m. rials. Major export destinations in 1988 included: Japan, USA, Singapore. Major import sources in 1984 included: USA, Japan, UK, Federal Republic of Germany, Italy and France.

Total trade between Saudi Arabia and UK (British Department of Trade returns, in £1,000 sterling):

	1986	*1987*	*1988*	*1989*	*1990*
Imports to UK	435,930	383,143	614,144	502,416	794,633
Exports and re-exports from UK	1,507,062	1,978,440	1,713,423	2,432,941	2,012,585

Tourism. In 1989 there were nearly 774,560 pilgrims to Mecca from abroad.

COMMUNICATIONS

Roads. The main regions and population centres are linked by asphalted roads, of which there were 33,576 km in 1987 and 59,226 km of graded, unpaved agricultural roads. An additional 2,021 km of roads were under construction including the Trans-Peninsula Expressway. There are road links with Yemen, Jordan, Kuwait and Qatar, and a causeway link to Bahrain. In 1986 there were 2·25m. passenger cars, 2·25m. commercial vehicles and about 41,000 buses. Women may not drive.

Railways. There is a railway from Riyadh to Dammam on the Gulf (571 km, 1,435 mm gauge) via Dhahran and the oilfields Abqaiq, Ithmaniya and Haradh. A 'dry port' at Riyadh station opened in 1981, and a new 465 km Dammam-Riyadh direct line was opened throughout in 1985. There are plans to extend the line via Medina to Jiddah. That section of the Hejaz Railway which is in Saudi Arabian territory is not now in working order, but studies have been initiated to restore the whole line from Damascus to Medina. In 1989 railways carried some 0·3m. passengers and 1·6m. tonnes of freight.

Aviation. Saudi Arabian Air Lines, a government-owned company operates regular internal air services, and international routes to Africa, the Middle East, Europe and the Far East, as well as special flights for pilgrims. There are 3 major international airports at Jiddah, Dhahran and Riyadh and 20 domestic airports. King Fahd International Airport in Eastern Province is due to be completed in 1990. In 1987, 21m. passengers and 332,000 tonnes of cargo were carried.

Shipping. The ports of Dammam and Jubail on the Gulf and Jiddah, Yanbu and Jizan on the Red Sea had 143 deep-water piers by 1985 and discharged 35·9m. freight tonnes. Aramco operates a deepwater oil terminal at Ras Tanura.

Telecommunications. Number of telephones (1988), 1,099,000. Number of post offices (1988) 603. In 1988 there were (estimate) 3·2m. radio receivers and 3·6m. television receivers.

Newspapers. In 1988 there were 8 daily newspapers in Arabic and 3 in English and 15 weekly or monthly magazines.

JUSTICE, RELIGION, EDUCATION AND WELFARE

Justice. The religious law of Islam is the common law of the land, and is administered by religious courts, at the head of which is a chief judge, who is responsible for the Department of Sharia (legal) Affairs. Sharia courts are concerned primarily with family inheritance and property matters. The Committee for the Settlement of Commercial Disputes is the commercial court. Other specialized courts or committees include one dealing exclusively with labour and employment matters; the Negotiable Instruments Committee, which deals with cases relating to cheques, bills of exchange and promissory notes, and the Board of Grievances, whose preserve is disputes with the government or its agencies and which also has jurisdiction in trademark-infringement cases and is the authority for enforcing foreign court judgements.

Religion. About 92% are Sunni Moslems and 8% Shiites.

Education. Schooling is in three stages, primary, intermediate and secondary which is to prepare older pupils for university; pre-primary schools are being introduced. Education is free in all these stages; monthly scholarships are paid to students in higher education and certain allowances are paid at general education level. Girls' education is administered separately. In 1987 there were 512 pre-primary schools with 60,590 pupils, 4,662 primary schools with 1,460,283 pupils and 90,535 teachers, and 3,526 intermediate/secondary schools with 635,606 students and 43,361 teachers. In 1988 there were 3,526 pupils in 30 special education institutes for mentally retarded and physically handicapped children. In 1986–87 there were 64,888 students in 1,305 schools in the programme to combat illiteracy.

In 1987 there were 27 vocational centres, where 2,820 primary school graduates were instructed in basic trades. There were also 8 technical and 22 commercial secondary schools, taking 11,310 intermediate school graduates, and 2 technical and 3 commercial higher institutes (649 students), 21 more advanced industrial, commercial and agricultural education institutes.

University courses concentrating on science, engineering, agriculture and medicine, but also covering education, commerce and arts, are available at the King Abdul Aziz University, Jiddah, King Saud University, Riyadh and King Faisal University, Dammam and Hofuf. There are two branches of King Saud University at Abha and Qaseem. King Abdul Aziz University had a branch campus at Taif. Specialized engineering studies are available at the King Fahd University of Petroleum and Minerals, Dhahran, and Arabic and Sharia law studies at the Islamic University, Medina, Imam Mohammad bin Saud University, Riyadh and the Um-AlQura University, Makkah. There were 113,939 university students (46,355 women) and 5,500 post-graduate students in 1986–87.

Welfare. The Ministry of Health is responsible for medical services, serving both Saudi citizens, foreign residents and pilgrims. In 1988 there were 224 hospitals with 35,797 beds, 2,258 primary health care centres and in 1988, 18,048 doctors, 38,434 nurses and midwives, 8,858 technical assistants. There were also 73 private hospitals (10,244 beds) employing 6,096 doctors. The Jiddah Quarantine Centre, designed by WHO and primarily for pilgrims, can take 2,400 patients.

DIPLOMATIC REPRESENTATIVES

Of Saudi Arabia in Great Britain (30 Belgrave Sq., London, SW1X 8QB)
Ambassador; Sheikh Nasser H. Almanqour, GCVO.

Of Great Britain in Saudi Arabia (PO Box 94351, Riyadh)
Ambassador: Sir Alan Munro, KCMG.

Of Saudi Arabia in the USA (601 New Hampshire Ave., NW, Washington, D.C., 20037)
Ambassador: HRH Prince Bandar bin Sultan.

Of the USA in Saudi Arabia (PO Box 9041, Riyadh)
Ambassador: Charles W. Freeman, Jr.

Of Saudi Arabia to the United Nations
Ambassador: Samir Shihabi.

Further Reading

Anderson, N., *The Kingdom of Saudi Arabia.* (Rev. ed.). London, 1982
Clements, F. A., *Saudi Arabia.* [Bibliography] Oxford and Santa Barbara, 1988
Hajrah, H. H., *Land Distribution in Saudi Arabia.* London, 1982
Holden, D. and Johns, R., *The House of Saud.* London and New York, 1981
Looney, R. E., *Saudi Arabia's Development Potential.* Lexington, 1982
McMaster, B., *The Definitive Guide to Living in Saudi Arabia.* London, 1980
Niblock, T., *State, Society and Economy in Saudi Arabia.* New York, 1981
Presley, J. R., *A Guide to the Saudi Arabian Economy.* London, 1984
Quandt, W. B., *Saudi Arabia in the 1980's: Foreign Policy, Security and Oil.* Washington, 1981
Safran, N., *Saudi Arabia: The Ceaseless Quest for Security.* Harvard Univ. Press, 1985

SENEGAL

Capital: Dakar
Population: 7·17m. (1990)
GNP per capita: US$630 (1988)

République du Sénégal

HISTORY. France established a fort at Saint-Louis in 1659 and later acquired other coastal settlements from the Dutch; the interior was occupied in 1854–65. Senegal became a territory of French West Africa in 1902 and an autonomous state within the French Community on 25 Nov. 1958. On 4 April 1959 Senegal joined with French Sudan to form the Federation of Mali, which achieved independence on 20 June 1960, but on 22 Aug. Senegal withdrew from the Federation and became a separate independent republic. Senegal was a one-Party state from 1966 until 1974, when a pluralist system was re-established. Léopold Sédar Senghor, President since independence, resigned on 31 Dec. 1980 and was succeeded by his Prime Minister, Abdou Diouf. From 1 Feb. 1982 Senegal joined with Gambia to form a Confederation of Senegambia.

AREA AND POPULATION. Senegal is bounded by Mauritania to the north and north-east, Mali to the east, Guinea and Guinea-Bissau to the south and the Atlantic to the west with The Gambia forming an enclave along that shore. Area, 196,192 sq. km; population (census, 1976), 4,907,507; (estimate, 1990) 7·17m. (38% urban).

The areas (in sq. km), populations and capitals of the 10 regions:

Region	*sq. km*	*1984 Estimate*	*Capital*	*1985 Estimate*
Dakar	550	1,380,700	Dakar	1,382,000
Diourbel	4,359	501,000	Diourbel	55,307 [1]
Fatick	7,935	506,500	Fatick	...
Kaolack	16,010	741,600	Kaolack	132,400
Kolda	21,011	517,600	Kolda	...
Louga	29,188	493,900	Louga	37,665 [2]
Saint-Louis	44,127	612,100	Saint-Louis	91,500
Tambacounda	57,602	355,000	Tambacounda	29,054 [1]
Thiès	6,601	837,900	Thiès	156,200
Ziguinchor	7,339	361,000	Ziguinchor	79,464 [1]

[1] 1976 [2] 1979.

Ethnic groups are the Wolof (36% of the population), Serer (19%), Fulani (13%), Tukulor (9%), Diola (8%), Malinké (6%), Bambara (6%) and Sarakole (2%).

Growth rate (1985–90), 2·7%; infant mortality, 128 per 1,000 live births; expectation of life, 45·8 years.

CLIMATE. A tropical climate with wet and dry seasons. The rains fall almost exclusively in the hot season, from June to Oct., with high humidity. Dakar. Jan. 72°F (22·2°C), July 82°F (27·8°C). Annual rainfall 22" (541 mm).

CONSTITUTION AND GOVERNMENT. Under the Constitution promulgated on 7 Mar. 1963 (as subsequently amended) there are simultaneous elections by universal adult suffrage for 5-year terms for both the Presidency and for the unicameral 120-member National Assembly; for the latter 60 members are elected in single-member constituencies and 60 by a form of proportional representation.

On 14 Nov. 1981, President Diouf of Senegal and President Jawara of The Gambia issued a joint communiqué proposing the establishment of a confederation, to be known as *Senegambia.* Both parliaments ratified the agreement and the Confederation formally came into existence on 1 Feb. 1982.

The agreement stated that each confederal state shall maintain its independence and sovereignty and calls for the integration of the armed security forces, economic and monetary union, co-operation in the fields of communications and external relations, and the establishment of joint institutions (*i.e.* President, Vice President,

Council of Ministers, Confederal Parliament). The President of the Confederation would be President Diouf, and the Vice President President Jawara, The Confederal Parliament would have one third Gambian representation and two thirds Senegalese.

President Jawara said in Nov. 1981 that 'the Confederation would not compromise any of the agreements which link The Gambia direct to Britain and the rest of the Commonwealth'.

President of the Republic: Abdou Diouf (took office in Jan. 1981, re-elected 1983 and 1988).

The Council of Ministers was composed as follows in Dec. 1990:

Foreign Affairs: Ibrahima Fall. *Defence:* Medoune Fall. *Interior:* André Sonko. *Economy and Finance:* Serigne Lamine Diop. *Culture:* Moustapha Kâ. *National Education:* Ibrahima Niang. *Higher Education:* Hakhir Thiam. *Rural Development:* Cheikh Abdoul Khadre Cissokho. *Industrial Development and Handicrafts:* Famara Ibrahima Sagna. *Housing and Urban Affairs:* Momodou Abbas Bâ. *Commerce:* Seydina Oumar Sy. *Planning and Co-operation:* Djibo Kâ. *Communications:* Robert Sagna. *Justice, Keeper of the Seals:* Seydou Madani Sy. *Civil Service and Labour:* Moussa N'Doye. *Public Health:* Mme. Therese King. *Social Development:* Ndioro Ndiaye. *Water Resources:* Samba Yella Diop. *Youth and Sports:* Abdoulaye Makhtar Diop. *Equipment:* Alassane Dialy Ndiaye. *Tourism:* Malik Sy.

Ministers-Delegate: Farba Lo *(Relations with National Assembly)*, Fatou Ndongo Dieng *(Emigration)*, Moussa Toure *(Finance and Economy)*, Mbaye Diouf *(Rural Development, Animal Resources)*, Moctar Kebe *(Rural Development, Protection of the Environment)*.

National flag: Three vertical strips of green, yellow, red, with a green star in the centre.

The official language is French.

Local Government. Senegal is divided into 10 *régions,* each with an appointed governor and an elected regional assembly. They are divided into 30 *départements,* each under an appointed *Préfet,* and thence into 99 *arrondissements.*

DEFENCE. There is selective conscription for 2 years.

Army. The Army had a strength of 8,500 (1991), organized in 6 infantry battalions, 1 engineer, 1 armoured, 1 airborne, 1 commando and 1 artillery battalions, and minor units. Equipment includes 67 armoured cars. There is also a paramilitary force of gendarmarie and customs.

Navy. The flotilla includes 2 coastal patrol craft, 8 inshore patrol craft, 2 tank landing craft, 2 smaller amphibious craft, and about 6 service craft. Personnel (1990) totalled 700, and bases are at Dakar and Casamance.

Air Force. The Air Force, formed with French assistance, has 4 Rallye Guerrier and 5 Magister armed trainers and 1 Twin Otter for maritime patrol, 1 Boeing 727 transport, 6 F.27 twin-turboprop transports, 2 Broussard and 1 Cessna 337 liaison aircraft, 2 Puma, 1 Gazelle and 2 Alouette II helicopters, plus 4 Rallye trainers. Personnel (1991) 500, with 9 combat aircraft.

INTERNATIONAL RELATIONS

Membership. Senegal is a member of the UN, OAU and is an ACP state of the EEC.

ECONOMY

Policy. The Seventh 4-year Development Plan (1985–89) provided 645,000m. francs CFA for investment in the productive sector, improved infrastructure and for reducing foreign debt.

Budget. The budget for 1987–88 balanced at 337,660m. francs CFA.

Currency. The currency is the *franc CFA* (XOF), a parity value of 50 *francs CFA* to 1 French *franc.*

Banking. The bank of issue is the *Banque Centrale des États de l'Afrique de l'Ouest.* The principal commercial bank is the *Union Sénégalaise de la Banque pour le Commerce et l'Industrie* (established 1961 with assistance from Crédit Lyonnais) in which the Senegalese government has the majority share-holding; also state controlled is the *Banque Nationale de Développement du Sénégal.* There are 3 private banks.

ENERGY AND NATURAL RESOURCES

Electricity. Production (1986) was 737m. kwh. Supply 110 volts; 50 Hz.

Minerals. Production of phosphates (1987) 2,022,300 tonnes. Titanium ores and zirconium are extracted from coastal (sand) deposits. Iron ore deposits amounting to an estimated 980m. tonnes have been located at La Faleme.

Agriculture. Of the total area (19·7m. ha), 5·35m. were under cultivation, 5·84m. were pasture, 5·45m. were forested and 3·03m. were uncultivated land in 1981. Production, 1989 (in tonnes): Groundnuts for oil, 703,362; groundnuts for consumption, 19,536; cotton, 45,000; sorghum, 594,200; rice paddy, 146,405; maize, 123,327; manioc, 54,885.

Livestock (1988): 3,792,000 sheep, 1·15m. goats, 2,608,000 cattle, 470,000 pigs, 210,000 asses, 8,000 camels and 208,000 horses.

Forestry. There were (1988) 5·9m. ha of forest representing 31% of the land area. Production (1986) amounted to 4·1m. cu. metres.

Fisheries. The 1986 catch totalled 255,400 tonnes.

INDUSTRY. Dakar has numerous industrial works. A major ship-repairing complex has been constructed there for vessels of up to 28,000 tonnes. Cement production (1983) 395,300 tonnes; petroleum products, 336,000; groundnut oil, 217,000.

Trade Unions. There are two major unions, the *Union Nationale des Travailleurs Sénégalais* (government-controlled) and the *Conféderation Nationale des Travailleurs Sénégalais* (independent) which broke away from the former in 1969.

FOREIGN ECONOMIC RELATIONS

Commerce. In 1986 imports totalled 332,929m. francs CFA and exports 214,793m. francs CFA; 30% of imports came from France and 30% of exports went to France. In 1985 petroleum products provided 22% of exports, fisheries 22%, phosphates 10% and cotton fabrics 4%.

Total trade between Senegal and UK (British Department of Trade returns, in £1,000 sterling):

	1986	*1987*	*1988*	*1989*	*1990*
Imports to UK	13,881	11,307	11,284	6,820	5,002
Exports and re-exports from UK	12,328	11,878	14,840	13,448	14,884

Tourism. In 1987, 235,466 tourists visited Senegal.

COMMUNICATIONS

Roads. The length of roads (1989) was 9,971 km of which 3,476 km was bitumenized. In 1984 there were 73,665 passenger cars and 36,144 commercial vehicles.

Railways. There are 4 railway lines: Dakar-Kidira (continuing in Mali), Thiès-Saint-Louis (193 km), Guinguinéo-Kaolack (22 km), and Diourbel-Touba (46 km). Total length (1986), 905 km (metre gauge). In 1986–87 railways carried 800,000 passengers and 1·4m. tonnes of freight.

Aviation. In 1984 230m. passenger-km and 17·4m. tonne-km of freight were flown. There are major airports at Yoff, Saint-Louis, Tambacounda and Ziguinchor.

Shipping. In 1986 the merchant marine numbered 148 vessels of 41,651 DWT. There is a river service on the Senegal from Saint-Louis to Podor (363 km) open throughout the year, and to Kayes (924 km) open from July to Oct. The Senegal

River is closed to foreign flags. The Saloum River is navigable as far as Kaolack, the Casamance River as far as Ziguinchor.

Telecommunications. There were, in 1983, 530 post offices. Telephones in 1986 numbered 54,000. In 1985 there were 11 radio stations with 450,000 radio receivers and 2 television stations with 55,000 receivers.

Newspapers. The main daily is *Le Soleil,* circulation (1989) 30,000.

JUSTICE, RELIGION, EDUCATION AND WELFARE

Justice. There are *juges de paix* in each *département* and a court of first instance in each region. Assize courts are situated in Dakar, Kaolack, Saint-Louis and Ziguinchor, while the Court of Appeal resides in Dakar.

Religion. The population (1980) was 91% Moslem, 6% Christian (mainly Roman Catholic) and 3% animist.

Education. In 1986-87 there were 610,946 pupils in elementary schools, 102,771 pupils in middle schools (general and technical) and 34,098 pupils in secondary schools (general, 30,005; technical, 4,093). In 1986-87 there were 12,028 teachers in private and public schools. The University in Dakar, established on 24 Feb. 1957, had 15,324 students in 1987. A second university was being built (1985) at St Louis. In 1987 32% adult literacy was claimed.

Health. In 1978 there were 44 hospitals with 7,092 beds; and in 1981, 449 doctors, 70 dentists, 139 pharmacists, 326 midwives and 1,766 state nursing personnel.

DIPLOMATIC REPRESENTATIVES

Of Senegal in Great Britain (11 Phillimore Gdns., London, W8 7QG)
Ambassador: Seydou Masani Sy.

Of Great Britain in Senegal (20 Rue du Docteur Guillet, Dakar)
Ambassador: R. C. Beetham, LVO.

Of Senegal in the USA (2112 Wyoming Ave., NW, Washington, D.C., 20008)
Ambassador: Ibra Deguene Ka.

Of the USA in Senegal (Ave. Jean XXIII, Dakar)
Ambassador: George E. Moose.

Of Senegal to the United Nations
Ambassador: Absa Claude Diallo.

Further Reading

Crowder, M., *Senegal: A Study in French Assimilation.* OUP, 1962
Gellar, S., *Senegal.* Boulder, 1982.—*Senegal: An African Nation between Islam and the West.* Aldershot, 1983
Samb, M. (ed.) *Spotlight on Senegal.* Dakar, 1972

SEYCHELLES

Capital: Victoria
Population: 67,378 (1990)
GNP per capita: US$3,590 (1988)

Republic of Seychelles

HISTORY. The islands were first colonized by the French in 1756, in order to establish plantations of spices to compete with the Dutch monopoly. They were captured by the English in 1794 and incorporated as a dependency of Mauritius in 1814. In Nov. 1903 the Seychelles archipelago became a separate colony. Internal self-government was achieved on 1 Oct. 1975 and independence as a republic within the Commonwealth on 29 June 1976. The first President, James Mancham, was deposed in a *coup* on 5 June 1977 and replaced by his Prime Minister.

AREA AND POPULATION. The Seychelles consists of 115 islands in the Indian ocean, north of Madagascar, with a combined area of 175 sq. miles (455 sq. km) in two distinct groups. The Granitic group of 32 islands cover 92 sq. miles (239 sq. km); the principal island is Mahé, with 59 sq. miles (153 sq. km) and 59,500 inhabitants at the 1987 census, the other inhabited islands of the group being Praslin, La Digue, Silhouette, Fregate and North, which together have 7,100 inhabitants.

The Outer or Coralline group comprises 83 islands spread over a wide area of ocean between the Mahé group and Madagascar, with a total land area of 83 sq. miles (214 sq. km) and a population of about 400. The main islands are the Amirante Isles (including Desroches, Poivre, Daros and Alphonse), Coetivy Island and Platte Island, all lying south of the Mahé group; the Farquhar, St Pierre and Providence Islands, north of Madagascar; and Aldabra, Astove, Assumption and the Cosmoledo Islands, about 1,000 km south-west of the Mahé group. Aldabra (whose lagoon covers 55 sq. miles), Farquhar and Desroches were transferred to the new British Indian Ocean Territory in 1965, but were returned by Britain to the Seychelles on the latter's independence in 1976. Population (1990, estimate) 67,378. Vital statistics (1989): Births, 1,581; deaths, 588. Life expectancy was 69 years in 1990; infant mortality, 17 per 1,000 live births.

The official languages are Creole, English and French but 95% of the population speak Creole.

CLIMATE. Though close to the equator, the climate is tropical. The hot, wet season is from Dec. to May, when conditions are humid, but south-east trades bring cooler conditions from June to Nov. Temperatures are high throughout the year, but the islands lie outside the cyclone belt. Victoria. Jan. 80°F (26·7°C), July 78°F (25·6°C). Annual rainfall 95" (2,375 mm).

CONSTITUTION AND GOVERNMENT. A new Constitution came into force on 5 June 1979, under which the Seychelles People's Progressive Front is the sole legal Party and nominates all candidates for election. There is a unicameral *People's Assembly* comprising 23 members elected for 5 years with 2 further nominated members. There is an *Executive President* directly elected for a 5-year term, who nominates and leads a Council of Ministers.

President: France Albert René (re-elected for a 3rd, 5-year term June 1989).

Education: Simone Testa. *Information, Culture and Sports:* Sylvette Frichot. *Tourism and Transport:* Jacques Hodoul. *Finance:* James Michel. *Health:* Ralph Adam. *Employment and Social Affairs:* William Herminie. *Agriculture and Fisheries:* Jeremy Bonnelame. *Planning and External Relations:* Danielle De St Jorre. *Administration and Manpower:* Joseph Belmont. *Community Development:* Esme Jumeau.

National flag: Divided horizontally red over green by a wavy white stripe, with red of double width.

DEFENCE. The Defence Force comprises all services. Personnel (1989) 1,300 organized in 1 infantry battalion, 2 artillery troops and a marine group, 200 strong, based at Port Victoria, which operates 5 fast inshore patrol craft and a tank landing craft. The Air Wing with 2 Islanders, 1 Defender and 1 Merlin IIB for transport and 2 Chetak helicopters. There is also a People's Militia (5,000).

INTERNATIONAL RELATIONS

Membership. Seychelles is a member of the UN, Commonwealth, OAU, Non-Aligned Movement and is an ACP state of the EEC.

ECONOMY

Policy. There is a 1990–94 development plan.

Budget, in 1m. rupees, for calendar years:

	1986	*1987*	*1988*	*1989*
Recurrent revenue	515·6	639·2	763·8	896·8
Recurrent expenditure	591·1	641·8	744·0	904·1

Currency. The unit of currency is the *Seychelles rupee* (SCR) divided into 100 *cents.* In March 1991, £1 = 10 *rupees;* US$1 = 5·27 *rupees.*

Banking and Finance. Central Bank of Seychelles, Development Bank of Seychelles and Seychelles Savings Bank have head offices and Barclays Bank, Standard Bank, Bank of Credit and Commerce International, Banque Francaise Commerçiale, Habib Bank and Bank of Baroda, have branches in Victoria and Mahé.

ENERGY AND NATURAL RESOURCES

Electricity. Production (1989) 94·3m. kwh.

Agriculture. Coconuts are the main cash crop (production, 1988, 19,000 tonnes). Other main crops produced for export are cinnamon bark (1989, 249 tonnes) and copra (1989, 1,337 tonnes). Tea production, 1989, 150 tonnes. Crops grown for local consumption include cassava, sweet potatoes, yams, sugar-cane, bananas and vegetables. The staple food crop, rice, is imported.

Livestock (1988): Cattle, 2,000; pigs, 15,000; goats, 4,000.

Fisheries. Seychelles is located in abundant tuna fishing grounds, and fishing is a major industry. Catch (1989) 4,392 tonnes.

INDUSTRY. Local industry is expanding, the largest development in recent years being the brewery (output, 1989, 5,243,000 litres). Other main activities include production of soft drinks (4,378,000 litres in 1989), cigarettes (58m. in 1989), tuna canning and paints, dairy, processing of cinnamon and coconuts.

FOREIGN ECONOMIC RELATIONS

Commerce. Total trade, in 1m. rupees, for calendar years:

	1985	*1986*	*1987*	*1988*	*1989*
Imports (less re-exports)	704·7	652·0	633·9	823·0	925·8
Domestic exports	21·9	13·9	35·8	73·9	67·8

Principal imports (1989): Manufactured goods, Rs 255·1m.; food, beverages and tobacco, Rs 170·6m.; petroleum products, Rs 169·1m., machinery and transport equipment, Rs 242·6m. mainly (1989) from UK (14·8%), Republic of South Africa (13·1%), France (9·5%) and Italy (4·4%). Principal exports (1989): Copra, Rs 2·5m.; fresh and frozen fish, Rs 13·1m.; cinnamon bark, Rs 1·4m.; canned tuna, Rs 43·8m. mainly (1989) to France (63%), Réunion (16·2%) and Pakistan (6·3%).

Total trade between Seychelles and UK (British Department of Trade returns, in £1,000 sterling):

	1987	*1988*	*1989*	*1990*
Imports to UK	884	1,297	993	8,353
Exports and re-exports from UK	10,770	10,478	10,741	14,955

Tourism. Tourism is the main foreign exchange earner. Visitor numbers were nearly 100,000 in 1990, (86,000 in 1989).

COMMUNICATIONS

Roads. In 1990 there were 196 km of tarmac roads and 89 km of earth roads on Mahé.

Aviation. Air Seychelles operates 3 services a week between Europe and Seychelles, regular services from Mahé to Praslin and Fregate Islands and a weekly service to Singapore. British Airways operates 2 services a week between London, Bahrain, Mauritius and Seychelles. Air France operates 3 services a week. Kenya Airways operates a service twice a week. Aeroflot has 2 flights a month. South African Airways operate a service to Johannesburg. In 1989 aircraft movements were 2,117; passenger movements, 371,000 (including domestic flights); freight loaded, 430 tonnes, unloaded, 1,653 tonnes.

Shipping. The main port is Victoria, which is also a tuna-fishing and fuel and services supply centre. Shipping (1989), goods unloaded, 364,500 tonnes, goods loaded, 8,900 tonnes. There are regular cargo vessels from Australia and the Far East, South Africa and Europe. The vessel *Cinq Juin* travels to and from Mauritius and visits the outlying islands.

Telecommunications. Services operated by Cable & Wireless Ltd provide telegraphic communications with all parts of the world by satellite. Telephones in Jan. 1983 numbered 4,512. There are 2 radio stations and (1983) 18,000 receivers. There were 3,500 television sets in 1987 and Radio Television Seychelles runs radio and television services in Creole, English and French.

Cinema. In 1989 there was 1 cinema with seating capacity of 200.

Newspaper. In 1990 there was 1 daily newspaper.

JUSTICE, RELIGION, EDUCATION AND WELFARE

Justice. The police force numbered 492 all ranks and 69 special constabulary.

Religion. 90% of the inhabitants are Roman Catholic and 8% Anglican.

Education. Education is free from 6 to 15 years. In 1990 there were 14,440 pupils and 767 teachers in primary schools, 2,787 pupils and 157 teachers in secondary schools and 1,609 students and 171 teachers in the Polytechnic. In 1983, a total of 239 students were undergoing training overseas, mainly in the UK; 153 were in university, 39 teacher-training and 6 nursing. 85% adult literacy was claimed in 1991.

Health. In 1990 there were 49 doctors, 12 dentists, 299 nurses and 436 hospital beds. The health service is free.

DIPLOMATIC REPRESENTATIVES

Of Seychelles in Great Britain (111 Baker St., London, W1M 1FE)
Acting High Commissioner: Sylvestre Radegonde.

Of Great Britain in Seychelles (Victoria Hse., Victoria, Mahé)
High Commissioner: G. W. P. Hart, OBE.

Of Seychelles in the USA and to the United Nations
Chargé d'affaires: Marc C. Marengo.

Of the USA in Seychelles (Victoria Hse., Victoria, Mahé)
Ambassador: James B. Moran.

Further Reading

Statistical Information: Information Office, 52 Kingsgate House, Victoria, Mahé.
Agricultural Survey 1980. Government Printer
Seychelles in Figures. Statistics Division, Mahé, 1989
Benedict, M. and Benedict, B., *Men, Women and Money in Seychelles*. Univ. of California Press, 1983
Franda, M., *The Seychelles: Unquiet Islands*. Boulder, 1982
Lionnet, G., *The Seychelles*. Newton Abbot, 1972
Mancham, J. R., *Paradise Raped: Life, Love and Power in the Seychelles*. London, 1983

SIERRA LEONE

Capital: Freetown
Population: 4·14m. (1990)
GNP per capita: US$240 (1988)

Republic of Sierra Leone

HISTORY. The Colony of Sierra Leone originated in the sale and cession, in 1787, by native chiefs to English settlers, of a piece of land intended as a home for natives of Africa who were waifs in London, and later it was used as a settlement for Africans rescued from slave-ships. The hinterland was declared a British protectorate on 21 Aug. 1896. Sierra Leone became independent as a member state of the Commonwealth on 27 April 1961, and a republic on 19 April 1971.

AREA AND POPULATION. Sierra Leone is bounded on the north-west, north and north-east by the Republic of Guinea, on the south-east by Liberia and on the south-west by the Atlantic ocean. The coastline extends from the boundary of the Republic of Guinea to the north of the mouth of the Great Scarcies River to the boundary of Liberia at the mouth of the Mano River, a distance of about 212 miles (341 km). The area of Sierra Leone is 27,925 sq. miles (73,326 sq. km). Population (census 1985), 3,517,530, of whom about 2,000 were Europeans, 3,500 Asiatics and 30,000 non-native Africans. Estimate (1990), 4,140,000. The capital is Freetown, with 469,776 inhabitants in 1985.

Vital statistics (1986); Live births, 75,862; deaths, 6,272.

Sierra Leone is divided into 3 provinces and the Western Area:

	Sq. km	*Census 1985*	*Capital*	*Estimate 1988*
Western Area	557	554,243	Freetown	469,776
Southern province	19,694	740,510	Bo	26,000
Eastern province	15,553	960,551	Kenema	13,000
Northern province	35,936	1,262,226	Makeni	12,000

The principal peoples are the Mendes (34% of the total) in the south, the Temnes (31%) in the north and centre, the Konos, Fulanis, Bulloms, Korankos, Limbas and Kissis.

CLIMATE. A tropical climate, with marked wet and dry seasons and high temperatures throughout the year. The rainy season lasts from about April to Nov., when humidity can be very high. Thunderstorms are common from April to June and in Sept. and Oct. Rainfall is particularly heavy at Freetown because of the effect of neighbouring relief. Freetown. Jan. 80°F (26·7°C), July 78°F (25·6°C). Annual rainfall 135" (3,434 mm).

CONSTITUTION AND GOVERNMENT. For earlier Constitutional history *see* THE STATESMAN'S YEAR-BOOK 1978–79, p. 1046. Following a referendum in June 1978, a new Constitution was instituted under which the ruling All People's Congress (APC) became the sole legal Party. The 124-member Parliament comprises 105 members directly elected for a 5-year term (latest elections, 31 May 1986), together with 12 Paramount Chiefs representing the 12 districts and 7 members appointed by the President. The President is elected for a 7-year term by the National Delegates' Conference of the APC; he appoints and leads a Council of Ministers.

In Feb. 1991 the Cabinet consisted of:

President, Minister of Defence and Responsibility for the Public Services: Maj.-Gen. Dr Joseph Saidu Momoh.

First Vice-President: Abu Bakarr Kamara. *Second Vice-President:* Salia Jusu Sherriff.

Minister of Finance: T. Taylor-Morgan. *Attorney-General and Minister of Justice:* Dr Abdulai Conteh. *Foreign Affairs:* Dr Alhaji Abdul Karim Koroma. *Education,*

Cultural Affairs and Sports: Dr Moses Dumbuya. *Trade:* Joseph Bandabla Dauda. *Transport and Communications:* Philipson Kamara. *Industries and State Enterprises:* Ben Kanu. *Health:* Dr Wiltshire Johnson. *Information and Broadcasting:* V.I.V. Mambu. *Agriculture:* M. O. Bash Taqi. *Mines:* Birch Momodu Conteh. *Internal Affairs:* Ahmed Sesay. *Works:* J. E. Laverse. *Labour:* M. L. Sidique. *Economic Planning and National Development:* Dr Sheka Kanu. *Energy and Power:* Dr Sheku Sesay. *Tourism:* A. M. Iscandri. *Social Welfare and Rural Development:* Alhaji Musa Kabia. *Lands, Housing and Environment:* Dominic Musa. *Minister of State and Leader of the House:* E. R. Ndomohina. *Minister of State and Inspector-General of Police:* Bambay Kamara. *Minister of State Party Affairs:* E. T. Kamara.

National flag: Three horizontal stripes of green, white, blue.

Local Government. The provinces are administered through the Ministry of Internal Affairs and divided into 148 Chiefdoms, each under the control of a Paramount Chief and Council of Elders known as the Tribal Authorities, who are responsible for the maintenance of law and order and for the administration of justice (except for serious crimes). All of these Chiefdoms have been organized into local government units, empowered to raise and disburse funds for the development of the Chiefdom concerned.

DEFENCE

Army. The Army consists of 2 infantry battalions, 2 artillery batteries and 1 engineer squadron. Equipment includes 10 armoured personnel carriers and 3 helicopters. Strength (1991), 3,000 officers and men.

Navy. The small flotilla comprises 2 ex-Chinese fast inshore patrol craft, 3 very small inshore craft and 3 utility landing craft. Personnel in 1990 totalled 150.

INTERNATIONAL RELATIONS

Membership. Sierra Leone is a member of the UN, OAU, ECOWAS, the Commonwealth, the Mano River Union and is an ACP state of the EEC.

ECONOMY

Budget. Revenue and expenditure (in 1,000 leone) for years ending 30 June:

	1985–86	*1986–87*	*1987–88*	*1988–89*
Revenue	375,500	1,254,500	1,990,400	3,500,000
Expenditure	566,400	1,828,300	3,960,800	6,630,000

Currency. The unit of currency is the *leone* (SLL) of 100 *cents*. There are notes of 50 cents and 1, 2, 5, 10 and 20 *leone*, and coins of 1, 5, 10, 20 and 50 *cents*.

In March 1991, £1 = 348·80 *leone*; US$1 = 83·87 *leone*.

Banking. The bank of issue is the Bank of Sierra Leone (established 1964). The Standard Chartered Bank Sierra Leone, the National Commercial Bank, International Bank of Credit and Commerce, International Bank of Trade and Industry and Barclays Bank Sierra Leone have their headquarters at Freetown; the Standard Chartered Bank has 14, Barclays Bank 12 and the National Commercial Bank, 8 branches and agencies.

The Post Office Savings Bank had 94,910 depositors with total credit balance of nearly Le. 3,455,469 in 1983.

ENERGY AND NATURAL RESOURCES

Electricity. Production (1986) 85m. kwh. Supply 230 volts; 50 Hz.

Minerals. The chief minerals mined are diamonds (314,000 carats, 1987), bauxite (1·3m. tonnes), and rutile (113,900 tonnes). Molybdenite is being prospected.

Agriculture. In the western area farming is largely confined to the production of cassava and garden crops, such as maize, vegetables and mangoes, for local consumption. In the regions the principal products include rice, which is the staple food of the country, cassava, groundnuts and export crops such as palm-kernels, cocoa beans, coffee, ginger and piassava. Cattle production is important in the northern part of the country, and most of the poultry, eggs and pork are produced in the Western Area. Production (1988, in 1,000 tonnes): Rice, 430; cassava, 116; palm oil, 44; palm kernels, 30; coffee, 9; cocoa, 11.

Livestock (1988): Cattle, 330,000; goats, 180,000; sheep, 330,000; chickens, 6m.

Fisheries. The estimated tonnage of catch of all species of fish during 1986 was 53,000 tonnes.

INDUSTRY. Four pioneer oil-mills for the expressing of palm-oil are operated by the Sierra Leone Produce Marketing Board. Government also operates 4 rice-mills, and there are a number of privately owned mills. At Kenema the Government Forest Industries Corporation produces sawn timber, joinery products (including prefabricated buildings) and high-class furniture. In addition, there is a smaller privately owned saw-mill at Panguma, Kenema and Hangha, and several small furniture workshops are used internally. Village industries include fishing, fish curing and smoking, weaving and hand methods of expressing palm-oil and cracking palm kernels.

Labour. A large proportion of the population is engaged in agriculture and about 125,000 workers are in wage-earning employment. The number of workers in establishments employing 6 or more persons was 64,092 in 1982, distributed as follows: Services, 24,142; mining and quarrying, 6,170; transport, storage and communications, 4,814; construction, 9,721; commerce, 6,870; manufacturing, 9,407; agriculture, forestry and fishing, 5,834; electricity and water services, 24,142.

FOREIGN ECONOMIC RELATIONS

Commerce. Total trade (in 1,000 leone) for 1988: Imports, 5,215; exports, 3,317.

Total trade between Sierra Leone and UK (British Department of Trade returns, in £1,000 sterling):

	1986	*1987*	*1988*	*1989*	*1990*
Imports to UK	11,599	12,679	14,462	15,899	7,011
Exports and re-exports from UK	17,403	16,221	14,256	20,402	21,365

Tourism. Tourism is being developed and is a major growth industry. In 1986 there were 194,000 tourists.

COMMUNICATIONS

Roads. There were (1978) about 7,500 miles of main roads, of which 1,000 miles are surfaced with bitumen. A programme to improve the road system was initiated in 1988.

Motor vehicles licensed in 1987, passenger cars, 25,000; commercial vehicles, 18,200.

Railways. The government railway closed in 1974. An 84-km mineral line of 1,067-mm gauge connecting Marampa with the port of Pepel has been rehabilitated. It carries about 2·7m. tonnes annually.

Aviation. Freetown Airport (Lungi), situated north of Freetown in the Port Loko District, is the only international airport in Sierra Leone.

The airport is served by Sierra Leone Airlines, Ghana/Nigeria Airways, Union de Transport Aériens, KLM, Air Afrique and Aeroflot.

Sierra Leone Airlines provide domestic flights daily (except Sundays) from Hastings (14 miles from Freetown) to Gbangbatoke, Bo, Kenema, Yengema; twice weekly to Bonthe, and occasional charter flights to Marampa and Port Loko. Domestic air taxi services also operate.

Shipping. During 1986 the total imports handled by the port of Freetown amounted to 1,990 tonnes and exports 990 tonnes.

Bonthe-Sherbro, 80 miles south of Freetown, is used for the shipment of rutile and bauxite. Pepel lies some 12 miles from Freetown and exports iron ore.

Telecommunications. Number of telephones (1981) 220,000. Telegraphic facilities are provided at 58 offices.

There were (1983) 37 post offices and 76 postal agencies.

The number of private wireless-licence holders (1986, estimate) was 820,000 and 31,000 television sets.

Newspapers. In 1987 there was one daily newspaper with a circulation of 12,000.

JUSTICE, RELIGION, EDUCATION AND WELFARE

Justice. The High Court has jurisdiction in civil and criminal matters. Subordinate courts are held by magistrates in the various districts. Native Courts, headed by court Chairmen, apply native law and custom under a criminal and civil jurisdiction. Appeals from the decisions of magistrates' courts are heard by the High Court. Appeals from the decisions of the High Court are heard by the Sierra Leone Court of Appeal. Appeal lies from the Sierra Leone Court of Appeal to the Supreme Court which is the highest court.

Religion. The Moslem community was estimated to comprise 39% of the population in 1980, while 52% followed traditional tribal religions; Protestants were 6% and Roman Catholics 2% of the total. The Temne people are mainly Moslem and the Mende chiefly animists. Spiritualist churches were growing in 1985.

Education (1984). There were over 1,267 registered primary schools; total enrolment (1982) 276,911. Primary education is partially free but not compulsory though parents and guardians are urged to send their children and wards to school. School attendance varies considerably in different parts of the country. There were (1984) 184 secondary schools with (1982) 66,464 pupils; 71 of these schools are fully assisted by the Government. Technical education was provided in 4 technical institutes, 2 trade centres and in the technical training establishments of the mining companies. There is also a rural institute.

Fourah Bay College (1,400 students) and Njala University College are the 2 constituent colleges of the University of Sierra Leone. The Institute of Education, which is part of the University, is now responsible for teacher education, educational research and curriculum development in the country.

There is a paramedical school at Bo in the Southern region.

Health (1984). In the Western Area there are 13 government hospitals (1,108 beds and 217 cots), including a maternity hospital, a children's hospital and an infectious diseases hospital near Freetown. There are 6 government health centres in the Western Area. Three private hospitals are located in Freetown with 108 beds. A mental hospital at Kissy has accommodation for 224 patients. In the provinces there are 14 government hospitals, 6 hospitals associated with mining companies and 7 mission hospitals. There is a school of nursing in Freetown. There are 156 government dispensaries and health treatment centres and two military hospitals with 124 beds.

DIPLOMATIC REPRESENTATIVES

Of Sierra Leone in Great Britain (33 Portland Pl., London, W1N 3AG)
High Commissioner: Caleb Aubee.

Of Great Britain in Sierra Leone (Standard Chartered Bank of Sierra Leone Ltd Bldg., Lightfoot Boston St., Freetown)
High Commissioner: D. W. Partridge, CMG.

Of Sierra Leone in the USA (1701 19th St., NW, Washington, D.C., 20009)
Ambassador: Dr George Carew.

Of the USA in Sierra Leone (Corner Walpole and Siaka Stevens St., Freetown)
Ambassador: Johnny Young.

Of Sierra Leone to the United Nations
Ambassador: Dr Thomas Kargbo.

Further Reading

Atlas of Sierra Leone. Ed. Survey and Lands Dept. Freetown, 1953
Background to Sierra Leone. Freetown, 1980

Cole, B. P., *Sierra Leone Directory of Commerce, Industry and Tourism.* 1985
Fyfe, C., *A History of Sierra Leone.* OUP, 1962.—Fyfe, C. and Jones, E. (ed.) *Freetown.* Sierra Leone Univ. Press and OUP, 1968
Fyfe, C. N. and Jones, E. D., *A Krio–English Dictionary.* OUP and Sierra Leone Univ. Press, 1980
Kup, A. P., *Sierra Leone.* Newton Abbot, 1975
Porter, A. T., *Creoledom: A Study in the Development of Freetown Society.* OUP, 1963
Riley, S. P., *Sierra Leone.* [Bibliography] Oxford and Santa Barbara, 1989

SINGAPORE

Population: 2·69m. (1989)
GNP per capita: US$9,955 (1989)

Republic of Singapore

HISTORY. For the early history of the settlement (1819) and colony (1867) *see* THE STATESMAN'S YEAR-BOOK, 1959, pp. 246 f.

By an agreement entered into between the Governments of Malaysia and of the State of Singapore on 7 Aug. 1965, effective on 9 Aug. 1965, Singapore ceased to be one of the 14 states of the Federation of Malaysia and became an independent sovereign state. On 22 Dec. 1965 it became a republic. The separation was ratified by the Constitution and Malaysia (Singapore Amendment) Act of the Malaysian Parliament on 9 Aug. The 2 governments agreed to enter into a treaty on external defence and mutual assistance. The Singapore Government retains its executive authority and legislative powers under its State Constitution and took over the powers of the Malaysian Government under the Malaysian Constitution in Singapore. The sovereignty and jurisdiction of the head of the Malaysian State was transferred to the Singapore Government. Civil servants working in Singapore for the Federal Departments became Singapore civil servants. Singapore citizens ceased to be Malaysian citizens.

Singapore accepted responsibility for international agreements entered into by the Malaysian Government on its behalf.

AREA AND POPULATION. The Republic of Singapore consists of Singapore Island itself, and some 58 islets.

Singapore Island is situated off the southern extremity of the Malay peninsula, to which it is joined by a 1,056-metre causeway carrying a road, railway and water pipeline. The Straits of Johore between the island and the mainland are about three-quarters of a mile wide. The island is some 26·1 miles (42 km) in length and 14·3 miles (23 km) in breadth, and about 240·4 sq. miles (625·6 sq. km) in area, including some 58 adjacent islets, 20 of which are inhabited.

Census of population (1980): 1,856,237 Chinese, 351,508 Malays, 154,632 Indians and 51,568 others; total 2,413,945. Estimate (June 1989), 2,038,000 Chinese, 408,800 Malays, 174,300 Indians and 64,300 others; total 2,685,400. Density, 4,293 per sq. km; growth rate, 1988, 1·5%; infant mortality, 1988, 7 per 1,000 live births; life expectancy, 1990, 71·2 years.

CLIMATE. The climate is equatorial, with uniformly high temperatures and no defined wet or dry season, rain being plentiful throughout the year, especially from Nov. to Jan., generally the cooler months. Jan. 78·1°F (25·6°C), July 80·8°F (27·1°C). Annual rainfall 93·2" (2,369 mm).

CONSTITUTION AND GOVERNMENT. By a constitutional amendment the name of the state was changed to 'Republic of Singapore', the head of state was named 'President of Singapore' and the legislative assembly was renamed 'Parliament'.

Parliament is unicameral consisting of 81 members, elected by secret ballot from single-member and group representation constituencies and 1 non-constituency member of Parliament, and is presided over by a Speaker, chosen by Parliament from its own members who are neither ministers nor parliamentary secretaries or from among persons who are not members of Parliament but who are qualified for election as members of Parliament. In the latter case, the Speaker has no vote. The present Speaker is an elected Member of Parliament. With the customary exception of those serving criminal sentences, all citizens over 21 are eligible to vote irrespective of sex, race, education or property qualification. Voting in an election is compulsory. For the general election held on 3 Sept. 1988, Singapore was divided into 55 electoral divisions, of which 42 were single-member constituencies and 13 were group representation constituencies (GRC). Each GRC returned 3 Members of Parliament, one of whom must be from the Malay community, the Indian and other minority communities. There is a common roll without communal electorates. Citizenship is acquired by birth and descent; it can also be acquired by registration or by naturalization.

A Presidential Council for minority rights was established under Part IVA of the Constitution enacted on 9 Jan. 1970. The general function of the Council is to consider and report on matters affecting persons of any racial or religious community in Singapore as referred to it by Parliament or the Government. The Council will draw attention to any bill or subsidiary legislation which in its opinion is a differentiating measure.

Parliament is composed of 80 People's Action Party members, 1 Singapore Social Democratic Party member and 1 non-constituency member of Parliament from the Workers' Party.

President of Singapore: Wee Kim Wee (re-elected for a second term, Sept. 1989).

The People's Action Party Cabinet at Feb. 1991 was composed as follows:
Prime Minister and Minister for Defence: Goh Chok Tong.

First Deputy Prime Minister and Minister for Trade and Industry: Brig.-Gen. Lee Hsien Loong. *Second Deputy Prime Minister:* Ong Teng Cheong. *National Development:* S. Dhanabalan. *Education:* Dr Tony Tan Keng Yam. *Environment:* Dr Ahmad Mattar. *Communications and Second Minister for Defence (Policy):* Dr Yeo Ning Hong. *Law and Home Affairs:* S. Jayakumar. *Finance:* Dr Richard Hu Tsu Tau. *Labour:* Lee Yock Suan. *Foreign Affairs and Community Development:* Wong Kan Seng. *Information and the Arts:* George Yeo. *Acting Minister for Health:* Dr Yeo Cheow Tong.

There are 7 Ministers of State.

National flag: Horizontally red over white, charged in the upper left canton with a crescent and a circle of 5 stars, all in white.

Malay, Chinese (Mandarin), Tamil and English are the official languages; Malay is the national language and English is the language of administration.

DEFENCE. The Ministry of Defence comprises 5 major divisions: general staff, manpower, logistics, security and intelligence and finance. Compulsory military service in peace-time for all male citizens and permanent residents was introduced in 1967. Periods of service are officers/n.c.o.s. 30 months, other ranks 24 months. Reserve liability is to 40 for men, 50 for officers.

An agreement with the USA in Nov. 1990 provided for an increase in US use of naval and air force facilities.

Army. The Army consists of the 1st and 2nd People's Defence Force (PDF) Commando and 3 divisions: The 3rd (Tiger) division, the 6th (Cobra) division and the 9th (Panther) division, the latter 2 being reservist formations. Standard infantry weapons are the SAR-80 assault rifle, AR-15 (M-16) rifle, Ultimax 100 light machine gun, 60 mm and 81 mm mortars, 84 mm Carl Gustav anti-tank guns and the Jeep-mounted 106 mm recoilless guns. Most of these weapons and the ammunition are manufactured locally. Strength (1991) 45,000 (including 30,000 conscripts) and 170,000 reserves. Paramilitary forces number 11,600.

Navy. The small, relatively modern Navy operates 6 German-designed fast missile corvettes, 6 German-designed fast missile craft, 20 inshore patrol craft, 2 old ex-US coastal minesweepers, 5 ex-US tank landing ships and 8 small landing craft. Naval personnel in 1990 numbered 5,000 (1,800 conscripts) and the naval base is on Pulau Brani.

The Marine Police operates some 60 patrol boats, some armed.

Air Defence Command. The formation of an Air Defence Command began in 1968. The Republic of Singapore Air Force now has 2 squadrons of F-5E supersonic fighters supported by 2-seat F-5Fs; 4 fighter-bomber squadrons equipped with A-4S Skyhawks, supported by TA-4S two-seat trainers; 1 squadron of Hawker

Hunter jet fighters and reconnaissance-fighters, supported by Hunter 2-seat trainers; a squadron of Strikemaster armed trainers; a radar unit, anti-aircraft guns and Bloodhound, Rapier and Hawk surface-to-air missile squadrons; a transport squadron of C-130 Hercules (including 4 equipped as flight refuelling tankers); a squadron of Skyvans equipped for search and rescue; a squadron of Bell UH-1s and AS 332M Super Pumas helicopters; and training units equipped with SF.260MS piston-engined basic trainers, a fleet of new-generation trainers, the SIAI-Marchetti S.211 jets, AS 350 Ecureuil helicopters, plus four E-2C Hawkeye AWACS aircraft. Eight F-16 Fighting Falcons entered service in mid-1989. Personnel strength (1989) about 6,000 (3,000 conscripts), with 193 combat aircraft and 6 armed helicopters.

INTERNATIONAL RELATIONS

Membership. Singapore is a member of UN, the Commonwealth, the Colombo Plan and ASEAN.

Treaties. Singapore has a Five-Power Defence Agreement with Australia, Malaysia, New Zealand and the UK.

ECONOMY

Policy. The GNP in 1989, at current cost was S$56,347·4m., an increase of 11·9% over 1988.

Budget. Public revenue and expenditure for financial years (in S$1m.):

	1986	*1987*	*1988*	*1989*
Revenue	10,970·4	10,470·9	13,632·0	15,328·5
Expenditure [1]	6,281·9	8,465·9	10,817·5	12,959·1

[1] Payments from Consolidated Revenue Account.

Currency. The unit of currency is the *Singapore dollar* (SGD) divided into 100 *cents*. Gross circulation in Dec. 1989 was S$6,735·55m. In March 1991, £1 = 3·29 *dollars*; US$1 = 1·73 dollars.

Banking and Finance. The Monetary Authority of Singapore performs the functions of a central bank, except the issuing of currency which is the responsibility of the Board of the Commissioner of Currency.

The Development Bank of Singapore was established as a fully licensed bank in 1968, and is the largest local bank in terms of assets. Primarily it provides long-term financing of manufacturing and other industries. At 31 Dec. 1989 it had a paid up capital of S$431·1m. and shareholders' funds amounting to S$2,746·3m.

There were 139 commercial banks with 415 banking offices operating in Singapore in 1989. The total assets/liabilities amounted to S$96,400m. as at Dec. 1988. Total deposits of non-bank customers amounted to S$42,500m. while loans and advances including bills financing, totalled S$41,800m.

There were 67 merchant banks operating in Singapore at 31 Dec. 1989. Of these, 66 had an Asian Currency Unit each and were engaged actively in Asian dollars transactions. Their main functions included underwriting, portfolio fund management, financial advisory services and loan syndication.

In Dec. 1989, the Singapore Post Office Savings Bank had 3,643,523 savings accounts and a total deposit balance of all accounts of S$13,049m.

There is a stock exchange.

Weights and Measures. The metric system or the International System of Units (SI) was introduced in 1971.

ENERGY AND NATURAL RESOURCES

Electricity. The Public Utilities Board is responsible for the provision of electricity, piped gas and water. Electrical power is generated by 4 oil-fired power stations, with a total generating capacity of 3,371 mw at the end of 1988. Production (1989) 14,039m. kwh. Supply 230 volts; 50 Hz.

Oil. Singapore is the largest oil refining centre in Asia.

Agriculture. Only 3% of Singapore's total area is used for farming. Agriculture employed only 1% of the labour force in 1989. Most food is imported but Singapore is self-sufficient in eggs, and 10,000 tonnes (5·6%) of vegetables were produced for domestic consumption in 1988.

Fisheries. As the prospect of increasing fish production from inshore waters is poor, in 1967 various projects were introduced with the aim of making Singapore self-sufficient in fish as well as a major fishing base in the region.

The Jurong fishing port and fish market began operating 26 Feb. 1969. A Fishery Training Institute was established at Changi with the assistance of the United Nations Development Programme (Special Fund) to train youths and fishermen in modern fishing techniques. At Changi, too, a Marine Fisheries Research Department was set up under the sponsorship of the South-East Asian Fisheries Development Centre. Research on fish culture and ornamental fish was carried out at the Freshwater Fisheries Section at Sembawang. The total local supply of fresh fish in 1989 was 13,110 tonnes.

INDUSTRY. The largest industrial area is the Jurong Industrial Estate with 1,934 factories employing 107,837 workers in March 1989.

Production, 1989 (in S$1m.), totalled 6,321·5m., including machinery and appliances, 29,649·3; petroleum, 9,243·2; food and beverages, 2,804·6; chemical products, 3,183·6; transport equipment, 3,128; fabricated metal products, 3,404·9; paper products and printing, 2,807; wearing apparel, 1,759·1; rubber processing, 128·2.

Labour. In 1989, 1,277,254 persons were employed, of whom 1,093,650 were employees, 70,041 were employers, 95,992 were self-employed and 17,571 were unpaid family workers. The majority were working in manufacturing, 369,857; trade, 291,490.

The Employment Act and the Industrial Relations Act provide principal terms and conditions of employment such as hours of work, sick leave and other fringe benefits. A new labour legislation was introduced allowing youths of 14-16 years to work in industrial establishments, and also children from 12-14 years to be employed in approved apprenticeship schemes. A trade dispute may be referred to the Industrial Arbitration Court which was established in 1960.

The Ministry of Labour operates an employment service to assist job seekers to obtain employment and employers to recruit workers. In addition it provides the handicapped with specialized on-the-job training. The Central Provident Fund was established in 1955 to make provision for employees in their old age. On 31 Dec. 1989 there were 2·1m. members with S$32,500m. standing to their credit in the fund. The total number of contributors to the fund in 1988 was 963,786.

Trade Unions. There were 92 registered trade unions comprising 86 employee unions, 5 employer unions and 1 federation of employee unions at 31 Dec. 1989. The total membership of employee unions numbered 212,874, of whom 208,625 belonged to 70 employee unions and 4 co-operatives affiliated to the National Trades Union Congress. Members of employer unions numbered 1,207.

FOREIGN ECONOMIC RELATIONS

Commerce. Imports and exports (in S$1m.), by country, 1989:

	Imports (c.i.f.)	*Exports (f.o.b.)*
Australia	1,637·5	2,550·3
China	3,310·8	2,334·5
France	2,167·4	1,369·4
Germany, Federal Republic of	3,505·2	3,199·0
Hong Kong	2,738·8	5,505·4
Italy	1,574·4	1,173·4
Japan	20,669·4	7,447·7
Malaysia	12,784·0	11,914·8

	Imports (c.i.f.)	*Exports (f.o.b.)*
Saudi Arabia	4,657·5	476·1
Taiwan	4,372·8	2,262·0
Thailand	2,443·3	4,805·7
UK	2,715·5	2,927·0
USA	16,605·3	20,290·8

The major trading countries for 1989 were US (20·1%), the EEC (15·6%), Japan (15·3%), and Malaysia (13·4%). In 1989, imports (S$96,864m.) increased by 10%. Exports increased by 10% from S$79,051·3m. in 1988 to S$87,116m. in 1989.

Exports (1989, in S$1m.): Machinery and transport equipment, 43,142·2 (of which electrical machinery, 20,471·9; transport equipment, 2,731·2; non-electric machinery, 19,939·1); mineral fuels, 13,443; crude materials, 3,721·4 (including rubber); chemicals (1988), 5,198·9; food, beverages and tobacco (1988), 3,837·9; clothing (1988), 2,495·4; animal and vegetable oils, 1,016·1; textiles, 1,544·8; scientific and optical instruments (1988), 1,558·3; metal goods, 1,025·9; iron and steel, 861·5.

Exports of orchids were valued at S$16m., and of aquarium fish at S$57·9m., in 1989.

Imports (1989, in S$1m.): Machinery and transport equipment, 42,837.6 (of which electrical machinery, 19,809·6; transport equipment, 6,228·9; non-electric machinery, 16,799·1); mineral fuels, 13,407·5; food, beverages and tobacco, 5,476·7; chemicals, 7,411·9; crude materials, 2,662·6 (of which rubber, 1,266·7); textiles, 3,123·3; iron and steel, 3,034·7; animal and vegetable oils, 924·1; metal goods, 1,873; scientific and optical instruments, 2,571·3; non-metal mineral goods, 1,276·5; paper and paperboard and related articles, 1,151·9.

In the following table (British Department of Trade returns, in £1,000 sterling) the imports include produce from Sabah, Sarawak and other eastern places, transhipped at Singapore, which is thus entered as the place of export:

	1986	*1987*	*1988*	*1989*	*1990*
Imports to UK	462,878	473,814	579,368	903,248	1,021,148
Exports and re-exports from UK	547,419	602,627	632,452	773,866	1,040,188

Tourism. There were 4·83m. visitors in 1989, spending nearly S$5,000m. The average length of stay was 3·3 days. At 31 Dec. 1989 there were 64 gazetted hotels with a total of 22,607 rooms.

COMMUNICATIONS

Roads. There were (1990) 2,836 km of public roads, of which 2,752 km are asphalt-paved. In Dec. 1989 motor vehicles numbered 520,537, of which 257,371 were private cars, 9,126 buses, 120,996 motor cycles and scooters, 13,787 public cars including taxis, school taxis and private hire cars.

Railways. A 16-mile (25·8-km) main line runs through Singapore, connecting with the States of Malaysia and as far as Bangkok. Branch lines serve the port of Singapore and the industrial estate at Jurong. A metro opened in 1987 and was fully operational by 1990.

Aviation. In 1990 Singapore Airlines (SIA) flew to 57 destinations in 37 countries. 49 international airlines operated 1,500 scheduled flights a week, totalling 79,037 commercial aircraft movements at Singapore International Airport in Changi ('Airtropolis') in 1988. Changi Airport has routes to 110 destinations in 53 countries. Freight handled (1988) 511,541 tonnes and there were 12,569,788 passengers.

Shipping. The economy is dependent on shipping and entrepôt trade. A total of 38,942 vessels of 430·7m. GRT entered Singapore during 1989. Singapore is one of the world's largest container ports.

Telecommunications. In 1990, 91 post offices and 44 postal agencies were in operation. Telephones numbered 1·27m. and fax machines 18,500 in 1988. In 1988 there were 647,717 radio and 554,133 TV licences.

Cinemas (1990). There were 52 cinemas with a total seating capacity of 46,959.

Newspapers (1989). There were 7 daily newspapers, in 4 languages, with a total daily circulation of 777,052.

JUSTICE, RELIGION, EDUCATION AND WELFARE

Justice. There is a Supreme Court in Singapore which consists of the High Court, the Court of Appeal and the Court of Criminal Appeal. The Supreme Court is composed of a Chief Justice and 7 Judges. An appeal from the High Court lies to the Court of Appeal in civil matters and to the Court of Criminal Appeal in criminal matters. The High Court has original civil and criminal jurisdiction as well as appellate civil and criminal jurisdiction in respect of appeals from the Subordinate Courts. There are 17 district courts, 13 magistrates' courts, 1 juvenile and 1 coroner's court and a small claims tribunal.

Penalties for drug trafficking and abuse are severe. The death penalty is mandatory for possession of morphine in excess of 30 grammes or diamorphine in excess of 15 grammes.

Religion. In Aug. 1988, 41·7% of the population aged 15 years and above were Buddhists and Taoists, 18·7% Christians, 16% Moslems and 4·9% Hindus.

Education. Statistics of schools in 1989:

	Schools	*Pupils*	*Teachers*
Primary			
Government schools	158	196,186	7,954
Government-aided schools	53	61,504	2,276
Private schools	1	143	...
Secondary			
Government schools	116	145,587	6,834
Government-aided schools	44	51,971	2,338
Private schools	4	1,518	64

The National University of Singapore was established on 8 Aug. 1980 following the merger of the University of Singapore and the Nanyang University. The National University of Singapore has 8 faculties: Arts and social sciences, law, science, medicine, dentistry, engineering, architecture and building, and business administration. Post-graduate studies are offered in all the faculties and there are 3 post-graduate schools for medical, dental and management studies. Total enrolment for 1989–90 was 16,626 students.

The Nanyang Technological Institute, situated in the former Nanyang University, was established on 8 Aug. 1981. It had an enrolment of 5,482 students in 1989–90, and is scheduled for development into the Nanyang Technological University by 1991. The Singapore Polytechnic had 14,735 students and the Ngee Ann Polytechnic 12,371 students in 1989–90. The Institute of Education, established on 1 April 1973, is the only institution responsible for teacher education and for promoting research in education. There were 1,413 students in 1989.

The Vocational and Industrial Training Board is responsible for vocational training and continuing education. It runs 15 training institutes and centres offering full-time and part-time courses. The total student enrolment for 1989 was 29,066.

Literacy in the population over 10 years was 87·2% in 1988.

Health. There were 7 government hospitals with 5,765 beds and 2 government restricted hospitals with 2,159 beds in 1989. There were 3,397 doctors, 593 dentists and 9,237 nurses registered. There are 10 private hospitals with 1,792 beds.

DIPLOMATIC REPRESENTATIVES

Of Singapore in Great Britain (2 Wilton Cres., London, SW1X 8RW)
High Commissioner: Abdul Aziz Mahmood.

Of Great Britain in Singapore (Tanglin Rd, Singapore, 1024)
High Commissioner: Gordon Duggan.

Of Singapore in the USA (1824 R. St., NW, Washington, D.C., 20009)
Ambassador: S. R. Nathan.

Of the USA in Singapore (30 Hill St., Singapore, 0617)
Ambassador: Robert D. Orr.

Of Singapore to the United Nations
Ambassador: Chan Heng Chee.

Further Reading

Statistical Information: The Department of Statistics (PO Box 3010, Maxwell Road, Singapore 9050) was established 1 Jan. 1922. Its publications include: *Singapore Trade Statistics: Imports and Exports* (monthly), *Monthly Digest of Statistics, Yearbook of Statistics, Singapore Demographic Bulletin* (monthly), *Census of Population 1980. Singapore Yearbook of Labour Statistics. Chief Statistician:* Khoo Chian Kim.

National Library. *Books About Singapore*. Singapore. Biennial
Singapore. Constitution. The Constitution of Singapore. Singapore, 1966
The Budget for the Financial Year 1989–90. Singapore, 1989
Singapore. Economic Committee, The Singapore Economy: new directions: report of the Economic Committee, Ministry of Trade and Industry, Singapore, 1986
Singapore Yearbook. Singapore, Information Division, Ministry of Communications and Information
Singapore. Government Gazette (published weekly with supplement)
Economic Survey of Singapore. Ministry of Trade and Industry, Singapore (Quarterly and Annual)
Singapore Facts and Pictures. Singapore, Information Division, Ministry of Communications and Information, 1989
Singapore Government Directory. Singapore, Information Division, Ministry of Communications and Information, 1989
Singapore: An Illustrated history, 1941–48. Ministry of Culture, Singapore, 1984
The Statutes of the Republic of Singapore. Rev. 12 vols., 1985 (with annual supplements). Singapore, Law Revision Commission, 1986—.
Clammer, J. R., *Singapore: Ideology, Society, Culture.* Singapore, 1985
Drysdale, J., *Singapore: Struggle for Success.* Singapore, 1984
Krause, L. B., *The Singapore Economy Reconsidered.* Singapore, 1988
Lim, L., *Trade, Employment and Industrialisation in Singapore.* Singapore, 1989
Myint, S., *The Principles of Singapore Law.* Singapore, 1987
Quah, J. S. T., *Government and Politics of Singapore.* OUP, 1985
Quah, S. R. and Quah, J. S. T., *Singapore* [Bibliography] Oxford and Santa Barbara, 1988
Saw, S. H., *New Population and Labour Force Projections and Policy Implications for Singapore.* Singapore, 1987
Soon, T. W., *Singapore's New Education System; Education Reform for National Development.* Singapore, 1988
Tan, C. H., *Financial Markets and Institutions in Singapore.* 5th ed. Singapore, 1987
Turnbull, C. M., *A History of Singapore, 1819–1975.* OUP, 1982
You, P. S. and Lim, C. Y. (eds.) *Singapore: Twenty-five years of Development.* Singapore, 1984

National Library: National Library, Stamford Rd, Singapore, 0617. *Director:* Mrs Yoke-Lan Wicks.

SOLOMON ISLANDS

Capital: Honiara
Population: 308,796 (1989)
GNP per capita: US$430 (1988)

HISTORY. The Solomon Islands were discovered in 1568 by Alvaro de Mendana, on a voyage of discovery from Peru; 200 years passed before European contact was again made with the Solomons. The southern Solomon Islands were placed under British protection in 1893; the eastern and southern outliers were added in 1898 and 1899. Santa Isabel and the other islands to the north were ceded by Germany in 1900. Full internal self-government was achieved on 2 Jan. 1976 and independence on 7 July 1978.

AREA AND POPULATION. The Solomon Islands lie within the area 5° to 12° 30' S. lat. and 155° 30' to 169° 45' E. long. The group includes the main islands of Guadalcanal, Malaita, New Georgia, San Cristobal (now Makira), Santa Isabel and Choiseul; the smaller Florida and Russell groups; the Shortland, Mono (or Treasury), Vella La Vella, Kolombangara, Ranongga, Gizo and Rendova Islands; to the east, Santa Cruz, Tikopia, the Reef and Duff groups; Rennell and Bellona in the south; Ontong Java or Lord Howe to the north; and innumerable smaller islands. The land area of the Solomons is estimated at 10,640 sq. miles (27,556 sq. km). The larger islands are mountainous and forest clad, with flood-prone rivers of considerable energy potential. Guadalcanal has the largest land area and the greatest amount of flat coastal plain.

Population of the Solomon Islands was (census, 1986) 285,796. Growth rate (1989) 3·5%.

The islands are administratively divided into 7 provinces. These provinces are (with 1987 estimated population): Western Province (62,300), Guadalcanal, including Honiara (71,300), Central (20,600), Malaita (80,700), Makira and Ulawa (20,800), Temotu (15,300), Isabel (15,500).

The capital, Honiara, on Guadalcanal, is the largest urban area, with an estimated population in 1989 of 33,749.

English is the official language but there are at least 87 vernacular languages.

CLIMATE. An equatorial climate with only small seasonal variations. South-east winds cause cooler conditions from April to Nov., but north-west winds for the rest of the year bring higher temperatures and greater rainfall, with annual totals ranging between 80" (2,000 mm) and 120" (3,000 mm).

CONSTITUTION AND GOVERNMENT. The Solomon Islands is a constitutional monarchy with the British Sovereign (represented locally by a Governor-General, who must be a Solomon Island citizen) as Head of State. Legislative power is vested in the single-chamber National Parliament composed of 36 members, elected by universal adult suffrage for four years. Executive authority is effectively held by the Cabinet, led by the Prime Minister.

At the elections of 22 Feb. 1989, the People's Alliance Party gained 21 seats, the United Party 3, the National Front for Progress 3 and the Liberation Party 3; 6 seats went to independents.

The Governor-General is appointed for up to five years, on the advice of Parliament, and acts in almost all matters on the advice of the Cabinet. The Prime Minister is elected by and from members of Parliament. Other Ministers are appointed by the Governor-General on the Prime Minister's recommendation, from members of Parliament. The Cabinet is responsible to Parliament. Emphasis is laid on the devolution of power to provincial governments, and traditional chiefs and leaders have a special role within the arrangement.

Governor General: Sir George Lepping, GCMG, MBE.
Prime Minister: Solomon Mamaloni.

Deputy Prime Minister and Minister for Home Affairs: Danny Philip. *Foreign Affairs and Trade Relations:* Sir Baddeley Devesi GCMG, GCVO. *Finance and Economic Affairs:* Christopher Abe. *Commerce and Industries:* Edmund Andersen. *Provincial Government:* Nathaniel Waena. *Police and Justice:* Allen Kamakeza. *Transport, Works and Utilities:* Michael Maina. *Education and Human Resource Development:* Albert Laore. *Posts and Communications:* Ben Gale. *Health:* Nathaniel Supa. *Natural Resources:* Allen Paul. *Agriculture and Lands:* Abraham Kapei. *Tourism and Aviation:* Victor Ngele. *Housing and Government Services:* Allen Qurusu.

National flag: Divided blue over green by a diagonal yellow band, and in the canton 5 white stars.

DEFENCE. The marine wing of the police operates 3 inshore patrol craft and 3 small landing craft with about 50 personnel in 1990.

INTERNATIONAL RELATIONS

Membership. The Solomon Islands is a member of the UN, the Commonwealth, South Pacific Forum and is an ACP state of the EEC.

ECONOMY

Policy. The Government's Programme of Action for 1990–94 aims for economic and constitutional reforms, emphasizing the needs of national resource management, health and education.

Budget. The budget for 1989 envisaged expenditure of SI$115m. and revenue of SI$110·5m.

Currency. The *Solomon Island dollar* (SBD) was introduced in 1977. In March 1991, US$1 = 2·58 *dollars*; £1 = 4·90 *dollars*.

Banking. In 1988 there were 3 commercial banks: Australia and New Zealand Banking Group, National Bank of Solomon Islands and Westpac Banking Corporation.

Weights and Measures. The metric system is in force.

ENERGY AND NATURAL RESOURCES

Electricity. Production (1987) 24,205,117 kwh. Supply 240 volts; 50 Hz.

Minerals. There are reserves of bauxite and phosphate, and there is a small industry extracting gold (36,241 grams refined, in 1989) and silver (7,414) by panning.

Agriculture. Land is held either as customary land (88% of holdings) or registered land. Customary land rights depend on clan membership or kinship. Only Solomon Islanders own customary land; only Islanders or government members may hold perpetual estates of registered land. Coconuts, cocoa, rice and other minor crops are grown. Main food crops: coconut, cassava, sweet potato, yam, taro and banana. Solomon Islands Plantations Ltd has a plantation of 5,519 ha of oil-palm. Production of copra (1989), 27,228 tonnes; palm oil, 13,591; cocoa, 2,640; palm kernels, 3,310.

Rice production (1988): 6,000 tonnes.

Livestock (1988): Cattle, 13,000; pigs, 52,000.

Forestry. Forests cover about 2·4m. ha, with (1987) an estimated 10·4m. cu. metres of commercial timber. Production (1989) of logs, 286,760 cu. metres; sawn timber, 4,660 cu. metres.

Fisheries. Catch of tuna (1987) 32,210 tonnes.

INDUSTRY. Industries include palm oil milling, rice milling, fish canning, fish freezing, saw milling, food, tobacco and soft drinks. Other products include wood and rattan furniture, fibreglass articles, boats, clothing and spices.

FOREIGN ECONOMIC RELATIONS. The Government's Programme of Action for 1990–94 aims to encourage foreign investment, particularly in manufacturing and tourism.

Commerce. Total exports (1988) SI$170·6m. The main imports (1988, in SI$1m.) were machinery and transport equipment, 62; minerals, fuels and lubricants, 24·7; manufactured goods, 40·2; food, 34·8. Total imports SI$203·3m. Main exports included fish products, 78·4; wood products, 39·8; cocoa beans, 7·4; copra, 15·4; palm oil products, 14. In 1988 imports were mainly from Australia (45·5%), Japan (16·2%), New Zealand (8·2%), Singapore (5·4%), the UK (5·3%) and the USA (5%). Value of exports (in SI$m.) to main destinations in 1988: Japan (58·8%), Thailand (24·8%), UK (24·7%), USA (12·7%), Australia (8%) and South Korea (5·4%). Imports and exports by region, 1988: South Asia, 31·3% and 56·6%; Oceania, 56·9% and 17·4%; EEC, 7·7% and 21·1%.

Total trade between Solomon Islands and UK (British Department of Trade returns, in £1,000 sterling):

	1987	*1988*	*1989*	*1990*
Imports to UK	4,461	5,153	6,404	6,903
Exports and re-exports from UK	1,566	2,576	1,088	523

Tourism. In 1988, there were 10,679 visitors of whom 50·3% were tourists.

COMMUNICATIONS

Roads. In 1987 there were 1,300 km of motorable roads of which 100 km of bitumen-topped roads; the rest were coral or gravel. In 1986 there were 3,629 vehicles, of which about 1,827 were commercial vehicles.

Aviation. (1988) An international airport 13 km from Honiara is served by Air Nauru, Air Niugini, Air Pacific and Solomon Islands Airline. There are 27 airfields. Solomon Islands Airline also provides inter-island transport and scheduled flights to Kieta in Papua New Guinea.

Shipping. There are international ports at Honiara, and Yandina in the Russell group. Shipping services are maintained with Australia, New Zealand, UK and Asia. Honiara port handled about 261 overseas vessels in 1989. In 1989 the merchant marine comprised 234 vessels of 1,579 GRT.

Post and Broadcasting. In addition to the general post office, there are 9 post offices, 4 sub post offices and 95 Postal Agencies. Number of telephones (1988), 2,500. Solomon Islands Broadcasting Corp. transmits 118 hours a week from Honiara, Gizo and Lata. In 1987 there were about 35,000 radio receivers.

Newspapers. In 1988 there were 3 weekly newspapers.

JUSTICE, RELIGION, EDUCATION AND WELFARE

Justice. Civil and criminal jurisdiction is exercised by the High Court of Solomon Islands, constituted 1975. A Solomon Islands Court of Appeal was established in 1982. Jurisdiction is based on the principles of English law (as applying on 1 Jan. 1981). Magistrates' courts can try civil cases on claims not exceeding $2,000, and criminal cases with penalties not exceeding 14 years' imprisonment. Certain crimes, such as burglary and arson, where the maximum sentence is for life, may also be tried by magistrates. There are also local courts, which decide matters concerning customary titles to land; decisions may be put to the Customary Land Appeal Court. There is no capital punishment.

Religion. At the 1986 census, 33·9% of the population were Anglican, 19·2% Roman Catholic, 17·6% South Sea Evangelical and 23·5% other Protestant.

Education. In 1989 there were 51,436 pupils and 2,248 teachers in 468 primary schools, and 5,556 pupils and 307 teachers in 12 provincial and 8 national secondary schools.

Training of teachers and trade and vocational training is carried out at the college of Higher Education. There were 459 students on overseas scholarships in 1989.

Health. In 1988 there were 8 hospitals, 31 doctors, 464 registered nurses and 283 nursing aides.

DIPLOMATIC REPRESENTATIVES

Of the Solomon Islands in Great Britain (resides in Honiara).
High Commissioner: Wilson Ifunaoa (accredited 12 Feb. 1987).

Of Great Britain in the Solomon Islands (Soltel House, Mendana Ave., Honiara)
High Commissioner: (Vacant).

Of the USA in the Solomon Islands
Ambassador: Robert W. Farrand (resides in Port Moresby).

Of the Solomon Islands to the United Nations
Ambassador: Francis Bugotu.

Further Reading

Solomon Islands Hand Book 1983. Government Information Service, Honiara, 1983
Bennett, J. A., *Wealth of the Solomons: A History of a Pacific Archipelago, 1800–1978*. Univ. of Hawaii Press, 1987
Kent, J., *The Solomon Islands*. Newton Abbot, 1972

SOMALIA

Capital: Mogadishu
Population: 6·26m. (1988)
GNP per capita: US$170 (1988)

Jamhuriyadda Dimugradiga Somaliya

(Somali Democratic Republic)

HISTORY. The Somali Republic came into being on 1 July 1960 as a result of the merger of the British Somaliland Protectorate, which became independent on 26 June 1960, and the Italian Trusteeship Territory of Somalia.

On 21 Oct. 1969 Maj.-Gen. Mohammed Siyad Barre took power in a coup, suspended the Constitution and formed a Supreme Revolutionary Council to administer the country, which was renamed the Somali Democratic Republic. After 12 years of civil war involving 5 factions, prominent amongst them the United Somali Congress (USC), the Somali National Movement (SNM) and the Somali Patriotic Movement (SPM), rebel forces had fought their way into Mogadishu by the end of 1990. Mohamed Siyad Barre fled on 27 Jan. 1991.

AREA AND POPULATION. Somalia is bounded north by the Gulf of Aden, east and south by the Indian ocean, and west by Kenya, Ethiopia and Djibouti. Total area 637,657 sq. km (246,201 sq. miles). Census population (1975) 3,253,024 of whom 15% urban. Estimate (1988) 6·22m. In Aug. 1987 there were 700,000 refugees from Ethiopia.

The capital is Mogadishu (1m. including a floating population of about 250,000), other large towns being Hargeisa (400,000), Baidoa (300,000), Burao (300,000), Kismaayo (200,000), Merca (100,000), Kisimayu (70,000) and Berbera (65,000).

CLIMATE. Much of the country is arid, though rainfall is more adequate towards the south. Temperatures are very high on the northern coasts. Mogadishu. Jan. 79°F (26·1°C), July 78°F (25·6°C). Annual rainfall 17" (429 mm). Berbera. Jan. 76°F (24·4°C), July 97°F (36·1°C). Annual rainfall 2" (51 mm).

CONSTITUTION AND GOVERNMENT. The Constitution came into force in 1984. The sole legal Party was the Somali Revolutionary Socialist Party (SRSP). The Executive President was elected for a 7-year term by direct popular vote. The People's Assembly consisted of 171 members elected for a 5-year term from a single list of 171 SRSP candidates.

Following the deposition of President Barre, Umar Arteh Ghaleb (USC) declared himself provisional prime minister.

National flag: Light blue with a white star in the centre.

The national language is Somali. Arabic is also an official language and English and Italian are extensively spoken.

Local Government. There are 18 regions, sub-divided into 84 districts.

DEFENCE

Army. The Army consists of 4 tank, 45 mechanized and infantry, 4 commando and 1 surface-to-air missile, 3 field artillery brigades. Equipment includes 140 T-34/-54/-55, 123 M-47 and 30 Centurion main battle tanks. Strength (1990) 61,300. There are additional paramilitary forces: Police (8,000), Border Guards (1,500) and People's Militia (20,000).

Navy. The flotilla includes 2 fast missile craft, 4 fast torpedo boats, 2 inshore patrol craft, 1 medium landing ship and 4 minor landing craft. All are former Soviet naval units. Personnel totalled 2,000 in 1990. Bases are at Mogadishu, Berbera and Kisimayu.

Air Force. Formed with a nucleus of aircraft taken over from the former Italian Air Corps of Somalia, in 1960, the Air Corps was built up with Soviet aid. Current equipment includes 6 MiG-21 and 20 F-6 (Chinese-built MiG-19) supersonic fighters, 8 Hunter fighter-bombers (including 1 trainer), about 8 MiG-17 jetfighters and 2 MiG-15UTI two-seat advanced trainers, and small transport, helicopter and training units. Support equipment includes 2 Aeritalia G222, 6 Aviocar and 2 An-26 twin-turboprop transports, 5 SIAI-Marchetti SF.260W armed trainers and 4 Agusta-Bell 212 helicopters from Italy, plus 3 Islander and 2 P-166 light transports. Serviceability of most aircraft is reported to be low. Personnel (1990) 2,500.

INTERNATIONAL RELATIONS

Membership. Somalia is a member of the UN, OAU, the Arab League, the Islamic League and is an ACP state of the EEC.

ECONOMY

Budget. The budget for 1989 balanced at Som.Sh.18,055m.

Currency. The unit of currency is the *Somali shilling* (SOS) of 100 *cents*. There are notes of 5, 10, 20 and 100 shillings and coins of 1, 5, 10, 50 cents and 1 shilling. In March 1991 £1 = 4,971·97 Som.Sh.; US$1 = 2,620·96 Som.Sh.

Banking. The bank of issue is the Central Bank of Somalia (founded in 1960 as the Somali National Bank). All foreign banks were nationalized in May 1970, and the Commercial and Savings Bank of Somalia and the Somali Development Bank, both state-owned, are the only other banks.

Weights and Measures. The metric system is in use.

ENERGY AND NATURAL RESOURCES

Electricity. Electricity production (1986) was 137m. kwh. Supply 220 volts; 50 Hz.

Minerals. Deposits of iron ore in the south and gypsum in the north are known to exist. Beryl and columbite are also found in the north. None are commercially exploited. Several firms hold exploration and drilling licences for oil. Uranium is found in the Juba area.

Agriculture. Somalia is essentially a pastoral country, and about 80% of the inhabitants depend on livestock-rearing (cattle, sheep, goats and camels). In Southern Somalia, especially along the Shebeli and Juba rivers, there are banana and sugar-cane plantations with a cultivated area of some 90,000 ha. Estimated production, 1988 (in 1,000 tonnes): Sugar-cane, 450; bananas, 120; maize, 260; sorghum, 220; grapefruit, 28; seed cotton, 6. Fresh fruit and oil seeds are grown in increasing quantities.

Livestock (1988): 20m. goats; 13·5m. sheep; 6·68m. camels; 5m. cattle; 1,000 horses, 25,000 asses and 23,000 mules.

Forestry. Production (1986) 4·5m. cu. metres.

Fisheries. 21 co-operatives, including 4,000 full-time and 10,000 part-time fishermen, caught some 16,500 tonnes in 1986.

INDUSTRY. A few small industries existed in 1986 including sugar refining, food processing, textile and petroleum refining. Production (1985): Textiles, 3·4m. yards; sugar, 39,400 tonnes; flour and pasta, 11,700 tonnes.

FOREIGN ECONOMIC RELATIONS. Foreign debt was US$1,750m. in 1988.

Commerce. In 1983 imports were Som.Sh.2,844m. and exports Som.Sh.1,423m. The chief exports are fresh fruit, livestock, hides and skins.

In 1984, 20% of imports came from Italy, 20% from USA and 13% from Saudi Arabia, while 59% of exports went to Saudi Arabia.

Total trade between the Somali Republic and UK (British Department of Trade returns, in £1,000 sterling):

	1986	*1987*	*1988*	*1989*	*1990*
Imports to UK	740	825	1,151	508	510
Exports and re-exports from UK	9,139	11,417	10,379	10,508	11,865

COMMUNICATIONS

Roads. Somalia has no developed transport system. Internal freight and passenger transport is almost entirely by means of road haulage. In 1985 there were 17,215 km of roads (2,500 km were paved), 17,754 passenger cars and 9,533 commercial vehicles.

Aviation. There is a commercial national airline, Somali Airlines. Mogadishu airport is used by Alitalia, Alyemda, Air Tanzania, PIA, Saudi Airways and Kenya Airways.

Shipping. There are 4 deep-water harbours at Kisimayu, Berbera, Marka and Mogadishu. The merchant fleet (1985) amounted to 26 vessels of 28,053 gross tons.

Telecommunications. Number of telephones (1985), about 6,000. The state radio stations transmit in Somali, Arabic, English and Italian from Mogadishu, and Hargeisa. There were 250,000 radios in 1986.

JUSTICE, RELIGION, EDUCATION AND WELFARE

Justice. There are 84 district courts, each with a civil and a criminal section. There are 8 regional courts and 2 Courts of Appeal (at Mogadishu and Hargeisa), each with a general section and an assize section. The Supreme Court is in Mogadishu.

Religion. The population is almost entirely Sunni Moslems.

Education. The nomadic life of a large percentage of the population inhibits education progress. In 1985 there were 194,335 pupils and 9,676 teachers in primary schools, there were 37,181 pupils and 2,320 teachers in secondary schools, and in 1984 613 students with 30 teachers at teacher-training establishments. The National University of Somalia in Mogadishu (founded 1959) had 15,562 students in 1986.

Health. In 1986 there were 450 doctors, 180 pharmacists, 2 dentists, 556 midwives and 1,834 nursing personnel.

DIPLOMATIC REPRESENTATIVES

Of Somalia in Great Britain (60 Portland Pl., London, W1N 3DG)
Ambassador: (Vacant).

Of Great Britain in Somalia (Waddada Xasan Geedd Abtoow 7/8, Mogadishu)
Ambassador: Ian McCluney, CMG.

Of Somalia in the USA (600 New Hampshire Ave., NW, Washington, D.C., 20037)
Ambassador: Abdikarim Ali Omar.

Of USA in Somalia (Corso Primo Luglio, Mogadishu)
Ambassador: James K. Bishop.

Of Somalia to the United Nations
Ambassador: Abdillahi Said Osman.

Further Reading

Background to the Liberation Struggle of the Western Somalis. Ministry of Foreign Affairs, Mogadishu, 1978
DeLancey, M. W., *et al. Somalia.* [Bibliography] Oxford and Santa Barbara, 1988
Legum, C. and Lee, B., *Conflict in the Horn of Africa.* London, 1977

SOUTH AFRICA

Republiek van Suid-Afrika—Republic of South Africa

Capital: Pretoria
Population: 30·19m. (1989)
GNP per capita: US$2,290 (1988)

HISTORY. The Union of South Africa was formed in 1910 and comprised the former self-governing British colonies of the Cape of Good Hope, Natal, the Transvaal and the Orange Free State.

The Union remained a member of the British Commonwealth until it became a republic on 31 May 1961.

By 1989 the restrictions of apartheid were being gradually removed, and the government announced its willingness to consider the extension of Black South Africans' political rights. In Feb. 1990 a 30-year ban on the African National Congress (ANC) was lifted and its deputy president and *de facto* leader, Nelson Mandela, released from prison.

Since 1990 there has been violent unrest in some homelands associated with demands for re-integration into South Africa.

In Aug. 1990 the ANC suspended, and in Feb. 1991 renounced, the use of armed action in the interests of a negotiated peaceful settlement.

The State of Emergency imposed in June 1986 was lifted in June 1990 (Oct. in Natal). The Separate Amenities Act racially segregating public facilities was repealed as of 15 Oct. 1990 by 105 votes to 38 with 1 abstention in the white House of Assembly, and unanimously in the Indian and Coloured assemblies. Relevant municipal by-laws are to be rescinded automatically.

Factional violence continued throughout 1990 between supporters of the ANC and the Zulu Inkatha Party, but after talks in Jan. 1991 between Nelson Mandela and the Inkatha leader Chief Mangosuthu Buthelezi, a joint plea to end the conflict was issued.

On 1 Feb. 1991 President de Klerk announced before parliament that the last instruments of apartheid, the Land Act, the Group Areas Act and the Population Registration Act, would be abolished within months.

AREA AND POPULATION. South Africa is bounded north by Namibia, Botswana and Zimbabwe, north-east by Mozambique and Swaziland, east by the Indian ocean, south and west by the South Atlantic. Lesotho forms an enclave between the Orange Free State and Natal. Area without the 'independent' homelands (Transkei, Bophuthatswana, Venda and Ciskei) was (1989) 347,860 sq. miles (1,127,200 sq. km), divided between the provinces as follows: Cape Province, 198,760 (644,060); Natal, 28,310 (91,740); Transvaal, 81,930 (265,470); Orange Free State, 38,860 (125,930).

On 25 Dec. 1947 the Union formally took possession of Prince Edward Island and, on 30 Dec., of Marion Island, about 1,200 miles south-east of Cape Town.

The census taken in 1904 in each of the 4 colonies was the first simultaneous census taken in South Africa. In 1911 the first Union census was taken.

	All races			*Whites*		*Non-whites*	
	Total	*Whites*	*Non-Whites*	*Males*	*Females*	*Males*	*Females*
1904	5,174,827	1,117,234	4,057,593	635,317	481,917	2,046,370	2,011,223
1911	5,972,757	1,276,319	4,696,438	685,206	591,113	2,383,879	2,312,559
1921	6,927,403	1,521,343	5,406,060	783,006	738,337	2,753,188	2,652,872
1936	9,587,863	2,003,334	7,584,529	1,017,557	985,777	3,818,211	3,766,318
1946	11,415,925	2,372,044	9,043,881	1,194,201	1,177,843	4,610,862	4,433,019
1951	12,671,452	2,641,689	10,029,763	1,322,754	1,318,935	5,109,331	4,920,432
1960	15,994,181	3,080,159	12,914,022	1,534,923	1,545,236	6,504,317	6,409,705
1970	21,402,470	3,726,540	17,675,930	1,856,180	1,870,360	8,689,920	8,986,010
1980[1]	24,885,960	4,528,100	20,357,860	2,265,400	2,262,700	10,393,780	9,964,080
1985[2]	23,391,245	4,574,339	18,816,906	2,254,801	2,319,538	9,293,081	9,523,825
1986[2]	27,607,000	4,832,000	...	...	...	...	...

[1] Excludes the 'independent' homelands except Ciskei (677,820).
[2] Excludes the 'independent' homelands.

Official population estimates (without the 'independent' homelands), 30 June 1990, (in 1,000; females in brackets): Whites, 5,018 (2,528); Coloureds, 3,214 (1,634): Asians, 956 (481); Blacks, 21,609 (10,373). The numerically leading Black nations (1980) are the Zulu (5,682,520), Xhosa (2,987,340), Sepedi (North Sotho) (2,347,600), Seshoeshoe (South Sotho) (1,742,060), Tswana (1,357,360). Population, (1985) of the Black national areas: Kwa Zulu, 3,738,334; Gazankulu, 496,200; Lebowa, 1,833,144; Qwaqwa, 180,924; Ka Ngwane, 391,205; Kwa Ndebele, 235,511. These places are included in the land area figures for the provinces where they lie, but their inhabitants are not included in the provincial population figures. Annual growth rate 1980–90, 2·07% (Black, 2·39%; Coloured, 1·78%; Asian, 1·72%; White, 1·05%). Urban population was 56% in 1985.

Vital statistics for calendar years:

	Whites					*Asians and Coloureds*		
	Births	*Deaths*	*Marriages*	*Immi-grants*	*Emigrants*	*Births*	*Deaths*	*Marriages*
1987	70,431	40,194	41,033	7,953	11,174	103,642	33,867	24,433
1988	69,189	40,194	41,219	10,400	7,767	97,277	32,353	21,879
1989	70,964	35,060	44,124	11,270	4,911	103,128	29,651	24,648

Marriages and divorces in 1989: Whites, 44,124 and 18,637; Coloureds, 18,111 and 4,729; Asians, 6,537 and 1,282; Mixed, 2,144 and 187.

Births in 1989: Whites, 70,964 (females, 34,744); Coloureds, 82,484 (41,233); Asians, 20,644 (10,086).

Deaths in 1989: Whites, 35,060 (females, 16,091); Coloureds, 24,333 (10,386); Asians, 5,318 (2,165). Infant deaths: Whites, 611; Coloureds, 2,899; Asians, 252.

Of the 11,270 immigrants in 1989, 6,322 were from Europe (of whom 3,371, UK); 2,917 from Africa (of whom 1,448, Zimbabwe); 520 from the Americas and 1,356 from Asia: Of the 4,911 emigrants 1,920 went to Europe (of whom 1,420 to UK); 1,275 to Australia; 256 to Africa.

The registration of Black essential data was introduced on a compulsory basis many years ago. However, despite serious efforts on the part of the registering authorities, the Blacks are still largely reluctant to have their essential data registered. Consequently no complete vital statistics are available for this population group.

Urban areas, according to the 1985 census:

Urban Area	*Total*	*White*	*Coloured*	*Asian*	*Black*
Johannesburg/Randburg	1,609,408	515,670	121,860	57,775	914,103
Cape Peninsula	1,911,521	542,705	1,068,921	18,389	281,506
Durban/Pinetown/Inanda	982,075	307,930	59,925	490,857	123,363
East Rand	1,038,108	399,445	33,390	17,472	587,801
Pretoria/Wonderboom/ Soshanguve	822,925	432,267	21,215	18,017	351,426
Port Elizabeth/Uitenhage	651,993	173,273	172,186	7,346	299,188
West Rand	647,334	233,460	19,206	7,631	387,037
Vanderbijlpark/Vereeniging/ Sasolburg	540,142	167,905	15,321	4,529	352,387
Bloemfontein	232,984	95,271	20,152	35	117,526
Pietermaritzburg	192,417	60,161	13,771	57,006	61,479
Free State Goldfields	320,319	69,387	6,246	2	244,184
Kimberley	149,667	33,782	50,214	1,202	64,469
East London/King William's Town	193,819	77,827	29,008	2,921	84,063

In 1986 (estimate), of the 4·8m. Whites Afrikaans was spoken by 2·7m., English by 1·75m. The remainder included Portuguese, 70,000; German, 43,000; Greek, 20,000; Italian, 15,000; Dutch, 14,000. Nguni languages (mainly Zulu, Xhosa, Swazi and South Ndebele) are spoken by about 13·6m.; Sotho languages (Southern, Northern or Sepedi and Western or Tswana) by about 8m.; Tsongo languages by about 1·2m. and Venda by 550,000. Fanakilo is a pidgin language developed mainly on the mines.

Afrikaans and English are the official languages.

CLIMATE. The climate is healthy and invigorating, with abundant sunshine and relatively low rainfall. The factors controlling this include the latitudinal position, the oceanic location of much of the country, and the existence of high plateaus. The south-west has a Mediterranean climate, with rain mainly in winter, but most of the country has a summer maximum, though quantities show a clear decrease from east to west. Temperatures are remarkably uniform over the whole country. Pretoria. Jan. 70°F (21·1°C), July 52°F (11·1°C). Annual rainfall 31" (785 mm). Bloemfontein. Jan. 73°F (22·8°C), July 47°F (8·3°C). Annual rainfall 23" (564 mm). Cape Town. Jan. 69°F (20·6°C), July 54°F (12·2°C). Annual rainfall 20" (508 mm). Durban. Jan. 75°F (23·9°C), July 62°F (16·7°C). Annual rainfall 40" (1,008 mm). Johannesburg. Jan. 68°F (20°C), July 51°F (10·6°C). Annual rainfall 28" (709 mm).

CONSTITUTION AND GOVERNMENT. On 2 Nov. 1983 a referendum among white voters approved the South Africa Constitution Bill which had previously been passed in the House of Assembly by 119 votes to 35. Turnout for the referendum was 2,062,469 (76·02%), of whom 1,360,223 voted in favour.

The new constitution became effective on 4 Sept. 1984. It provides for a tricameral parliament: The House of Assembly with 178 members of whom 166 are directly elected and 8 indirectly elected by White voters; the House of Representatives with 85 members of whom 80 are directly elected by Coloured voters; the House of Delegates with 45 members of whom 40 are directly elected by Indian voters. The term for all members is 5 years.

These houses choose (from their majority parties) respectively 50 White, 25 Coloured and 13 Indian members of an electoral college which elects an executive President. The President initiates legislation and resolves disputes between houses. He is helped by a 60-member President's Council: 20 members are elected by the House of Assembly, 10 by the House of Representatives and 5 by the House of Delegates; 15 are MPs nominated by himself and 10 are MPs nominated by Opposition parties.

The President appoints a Ministers' Council for each house, choosing 5 members from the majority party; a member chosen from outside the house must become a member of it within one year, and enjoy majority-party support. The Councils handle the affairs of their own population group and administer the departments established for that group. The President also appoints a Cabinet; any member appointed from outside Parliament must become a member of one of the three houses within one year. Any Ministers' Council member may be appointed a Cabinet member for a specific purpose or for an indefinite period. Any Ministers' Council may co-opt a Cabinet member in the same way, providing that member qualifies as a member of the Council in question.

Each house legislates on its own community affairs; the three houses have co-responsibility for national affairs. The State President, on the Cabinet's advice, decides whether a certain matter is a community or a national affair.

To hold an office of profit under the State (with certain exceptions) is a disqualification for membership of either House, as are also insolvency, crime and insanity. Pretoria ls the seat of government, and Cape Town is the seat of legislature.

The state of the parties on 4 Sept. 1984: in the House of Assembly, National Party, 114; Progressive Federal Party, 26; Conservative Party, 17; New Republic Party, 8; South African Party, 3. In the House of Representatives, Labour Party, 76; others, 4. In the House of Delegates, National People's Party 18; Solidarity, 17; others, 5.

Indians voting in the elections to the new House of Delegates in Aug. 1984, 20·3% of registered voters; Coloured voters to the new House of Representatives, 30·9%.

At the House of Assembly elections of 6 Sept. 1989, the Nationalist Party won 93 seats; the Conservative Party, 39; and the Democratic Party (formed from a merger of the Progressive Federal Party, the New Republic Party and Independents), 33.

President: Frederik Willem de Klerk (sworn in, 20 Sept. 1989).

The Cabinet in March 1991 was in order of seniority as follows:

Foreign Affairs: R. F. 'Pik' Botha. *Constitutional Development and Planning and National Education:* Gerrit Viljoen. *Defence:* Gen. Magnus Malan. *Mineral and*

Energy Affairs and Public Enterprises: Dawie de Villiers. *Justice:* Kobie Coetsee. *Finance:* Barend du Plessis. *Manpower:* Eli Louw. *Law and Order:* Adriaan Vlok. *Environment and Water:* Gert Kotze. *Education and Development Aid:* Stoffel van der Merwe. *Home Affairs:* Gene Louw. *Trade and Industry and Tourism:* Kent Durr. *Transport and Public Works and Land Affairs:* George Bartlett. *Planning and Provincial Affairs:* Hernus Kriel. *National Health and Population Development:* Rina Venter. *Agriculture:* Jacob de Villers. *Administration and Privatization:* Vacant.

The Chairman of the President's Council is Willie van Niekerk.

The Prime Minister receives an annual salary of R43,000 and a reimbursive allowance of R20,000; a member of the Cabinet an annual salary of R23,500 and a reimbursive allowance of R6,500; and a Deputy Minister an annual salary of R19,000 and a reimbursive allowance of R6,500.

The English and Afrikaans languages are both official, subject to amendments carried by a two-thirds majority in joint session of both Houses of Parliament.

National flag: Three horizontal stripes of orange, white, blue, with the flags of the Orange Free State and the Transvaal, and the Union Jack side by side in the centre.

National anthem: The Call of South Africa/Die Stem van Suid-Afrika (words by C. J. Langenhoven, 1918; tune by M. L. de Villiers, 1921).

Provincial Administration. In each of the 4 provinces there is an Administrator appointed by the State President-in-Council for 5 years. Until 1986 there were provincial councils, each council electing an executive committee of 4 (either members or not of the council), the Administrator acting as chairman. Provincial councils were abolished in 1986; local governments remain, comprising municipal councils, management boards and other local committees, all of which have authority to deal with local matters, of which provincial finance, education (primary and secondary, other than higher education and technical education), hospitals, roads and bridges, townships, horse and other racing, and game and fish preservation are the most important. All ordinances passed by the local councils are subject to the veto of the State President-in-Council.

Black Administration. In 1959 the main ethnic groups received legislative recognition by the passing of the Promotion of Bantu Self-Government Act, which provided *inter alia* for the various ethnic groups to develop into self-governing national units.

As the Act envisaged eventual political autonomy for each of the various national units and representation in the highest White governing bodies was regarded as a retarding factor, the representation of Blacks by Whites in Parliament and the Cape Provincial Administration was abolished with effect from 30 June 1960.

Territorial Authorities were established between 1968 and 1970, and were converted to Legislative Assemblies in 1971.

Each national unit also has an Executive Council. These Councils, each headed by a Chief Councillor, consist of 6 members, except in the case of the South Sotho, where there are only 4. Each of these Councillors is responsible for the administration of a Department. A civil service has been established in each instance, staffed by citizens of the respective homelands. White officials will serve the homeland governments on secondment, until trained Black citizens are able to take over all duties.

There are (1991) 10 homelands of which 4 are recognised by the South African government as Independent:

The Transkei, territory of the Xhosa nation, became independent on 26 Oct. 1976 (*see* p. 1110), Bophuthatswana on 6 Dec. 1977 (*see* p. 1108), Venda on 13 Sept. 1979 (*see* p. 1111) and Ciskei on 4 Dec. 1981 (*see* p. 1114).

There are (1991) 6 territories with a degree of self-government but still forming part of the Republic: Kwa Zulu, Gazankulu (Machangana-Tsonga people), Lebowa (North Sotho), Qwaqwa (South Sotho), Ka Ngwane (Swazi) and Kwa Ndebele (Southern Ndebele).

DEFENCE. The South African Defence Force comprises a Permanent Force, a

Citizen Force and a Commando organization. The Permanent Force consists of professional soldiers, airmen and seamen who are responsible for the administration and training of the whole Defence Force in peace-time, but who are gradually absorbed into the Citizen Force in time of war. The Permanent Force and the Citizen Force consist of Army, Air Force and Naval components; the Commando organization is an army and air organization.

Every white male citizen between 18 and 65 is liable to undergo training and to render personal service in time of war. Those between the ages of 16 and 25 are liable to undergo a compulsory course of peace training.

The S.A. Defence Force is administered by the Chief of the Defence Force, his advisers being the Chief of the Army, Chief of the Air Force and Chief of the Navy, Chief of Staff Operations, Chief of Staff Personnel, the Chief of Staff Management Services and the Surgeon-General.

Army. South Africa is divided into 11 territorial Commands. Within the various Commands are training units, of which members of the Permanent Force form the permanent staff. Courses of various types are held also at the S.A. Military College. The Army includes 1 armoured, 1 mechanized, 4 motorized and 1 parachute brigade; 1 special reconnaissance regiment and supporting artillery, engineer and signals units. Equipment includes some 250 Centurion/Olifant main battle tanks. Strength in 1991 was estimated at 19,900 regular personnel (12,000 white, 2,500 women) and 41,000 conscripts with an Active Reserve of 150,000. Paramilitary forces are Commandos (130,000) and 60,000 men and women of the South African Police with 37,000 reserves.

Navy. The Navy has its headquarters at Pretoria where operational control is now centralized. The navy includes 3 French-built diesel submarines, 9 fast missile armed patrol craft, 9 coastal minesweepers, 1 British-built survey ship, 2 fleet replenishment ships and a naval-manned Antarctic supply ship, the latter three all with helicopter facilities. There are additionally some 6 service craft. The Marine force of 900 (in 1989) is being disbanded.

Navy personnel in 1990 totalled 5,500 (1,500 conscripts) including marines.

Air Force. There is 1 bomber squadron with 5 Canberra B.12 and 2 Canberra T.4; 1 bomber squadron with 6 Buccaneer Mk.50; 1 coastal patrol squadron with 18 Piaggio P.166S; 1 coastal patrol squadron with C-47s; 1 fighter-bomber squadron with 30 Mirage F1-AZ ground attack aircraft; 2 fighter-bomber squadrons with Atlas Cheetahs (locally modified Mirage IIIs) including some equipped for reconnaissance; and 1 squadron with Mirage F1-CZ interceptors. Transport squadrons have 9 Transall C-160s, 7 C-130B Hercules, more than 40 C-47s, 7 C-54s, 4 Boeing 707s, 1 Viscount, 4 twin-jet HS.125s and 4 twin-turboprop Merlin IVA light transports. Four helicopter squadrons and No. 22 Flight have more than 80 Alouette IIIs, 60 Pumas, 8 Wasps, and 14 Super Frelons. T-6Gs are used for primary training, followed by advanced training on Impalas, Atlas Cheetahs and Mirage IIIEZ/DZ, weapons training on Impalas, and multi-engine/crew training on C-47s. Built under licence in the Republic of South Africa, about 150 two-seat Impala Mk. 1s have been followed by 75 single-seat Impala Mk. 2s, based on the Aermacchi MB.326M and 326K respectively. Three squadrons operate C4M Kudu and AM.3C Bosbok liaison aircraft. South African industry is currently modernizing the Mirage combat aircraft (under the name 'Cheetah') and developing an armed helicopter derived from the Puma.

The Citizen Force has 3 squadrons of Impalas for counter-insurgency duties and C4M Kudu and AM.3C Bosbok liaison aircraft. CF personnel have additional functions in regular SAAF squadrons, notably those equipped with C-47 transports and P.166 light transport/coastal patrol aircraft. Total strength (1991) was about 11,000 (4,000 conscripts).

INTERNATIONAL RELATIONS

Membership. South Africa is a member of the UN.

ECONOMY

Budget. Total revenue and expenditure of the central government's State Revenue Account in R1m.:

	1987–88	*1988–89*	*1989-90*	*1990-91*
Revenue	38,794	48,071	61,385	69,468
Expenditure	46,319	55,926	65,180	71,546

The main sources of State Revenue 1990–91 were income tax, R38,660m.; general sales tax, R18,500m.; excise duties, R2,750m.; customs duties, R2,100m. Main expenditure: Education, R13,346m.; defence, R10,292m.; economic services, R8,566m.; interest on public debt, R11,123m.; health, R7,024m.; other social, R7,483m.

Public debt on 31 March 1989, R81,124m., of which R2,033m. was foreign debt; internal debt, R79,091m.

Currency. The unit of currency is the *rand* (ZAR) of 100 *cents*, introduced in 1959. The coins are: *Gold coins*. 2 rand; 1 rand. *Silver coins*. 50 cents; 20 cents; 10 cents; 5 cents. *Bronze coins*. 2 cents; 1 cent. In March 1991, £1 = R4·92; US$1 = R2·59.

Banking and Finance. In Dec. 1920 a Central Reserve Bank was established at Pretoria. It commenced operations in June 1921, and began to issue notes in April 1922. The bank has branches in Pretoria (Head Office), Johannesburg, Cape Town, Durban, Port Elizabeth, East London, Bloemfontein, Pietermaritzburg and Windhoek (Namibia). Total deposits, 31 March 1987, R3,957m.; assets, R12,158m. Its *Governor* is Chris Stals.

At 31 Dec. 1987 there were 15 commercial banks with total liabilities, R51,764m.; 24 general banks (formerly hire-purchase and savings banks), R397m.; 8 merchant banks, R6,038m.; 4 discount houses, R862m. The Land and Agricultural Bank had (March 1987) R8,342m. total liabilities; Post Office Savings Bank deposits, R3,356m.

The Deposit-Taking Institutions Act of Feb. 1991 standardized the requirements of banks and building societies and brought capital adequacy requirements into line with the Basle Concordat.

Weights and Measures. The metric system is in force.

ENERGY AND NATURAL RESOURCES

Electricity. The total capacity of the power plants controlled by supply agency Eskom was 28,086,000 kw at the end of 1986. There were 21 coal-fired stations, 3 hydro-electric stations and 3 gas-turbine stations. Production (1986) 145,394m. kwh of which Eskom generated 133,644m. kwh. Net production (sent out from plants for consumption), 133,293, of which Eskom, 123,643. Supply 220 and 240 volts; 50 Hz.

Oil. In 1987 reserves were found to be sufficient to yield 25,000 bbls of diesel and petrol a day for 30 years from gas produced at sea and converted on land.

Water. Government activities are governed by the Water Act, 1956 (as amended), which is administered by the Directorate of Water Affairs. A Water Research Commission was established in 1971 to co-ordinate and promote research; it is responsible for hydrological research, major water resource development, water pollution control. The combined average flow of South Africa's rivers is about 53,500m. cu. metres annually, most of it lost by evaporation and spillage.

In 1989, 2 major storage dams controlled 7,300m. cu. metres of the annual flow of 7,500m. cu. metres. An 82·5 km long tunnel to transfer water from the Orange River to the Great Fish River valley had been completed.

In Oct. 1986 South Africa signed a treaty with Lesotho to allow damming the Orange River head waters within Lesotho and diverting the collected water through tunnels into the Vaal River system of the OFS. Lesotho is to receive royalties and hydro-electric power in exchange.

Minerals. Value of the main mineral production sales (in R1,000):

	1986	*1987*	*1988*	*1989*
Asbestos	99,064	88,410	108,281	158,087
Chrome ore	212,794	242,413	312,495	432,220
Coal	5,245,943	4,788,544	5,916,659	7,032,146
Copper	550,178	618,711	937,582	1,333,538
Fluorspar	62,104	63,438	83,737	112,227
Gold	17,287,356	17,492,636	19,686,986	20,096,273
Iron ore	473,510	472,559	564,583	826,278
Lime and limestone	237,311	272,538	320,419	369,960
Manganese	271,024	176,947	353,841	721,012
Silver	72,087	74,188	79,469	71,037

Total value of all minerals sold (1989), R37,506·4m.

Mineral production (tonnes) 1986: Coal, 170m.; iron ore, 24·5m.; phosphates, 2·9m.; manganese ore, 3·7m.; chromite, 3m.; asbestos, 138,000; copper, 196,000; lime and limestone, 14·3m.; fluorspar, 334,000; gold, 635,233 kg; silver, 216,599 kg; diamonds, 10·1m. carats.

South Africa is a major producer of gold. Reserves were estimated at US$1,275m. in 1989. Production was estimated at 605 tonnes in 1990.

At 31 Dec. 1986 the number of persons engaged in mining was 752,264. Of these, 553,668 were engaged in goldmining.

Minerals. A Quarterly Report of Production and Sales. Department of Mineral and Energy Affairs. Pretoria, from 1936

Mining Statistics. Department of Mineral and Energy Affairs, Pretoria, from 1966

Agriculture. Much of the land suitable for mechanical farming has unreliable rainfall. Good rainfall in 1989 followed 7 years of drought and crop failure. Of the total area natural pasture occupies 58% (71·3m. ha); about 14m. ha are suitable for dry-land farming, of which 10·6m. are actually cultivated. There are some 65,000 farms.

In 1990, agriculture, forestry and fisheries contributed 5·1% to GDP.

Production (1989, in 1,000 tonnes): Maize, 12,061; sorghum, 466; wheat, 2,720; groundnuts, 146; sunflower seed, 431; sugar-cane, 18,200; oranges, 477; potatoes, 1,245; vegetables, 3,153; grapes, 1,456; apples, 503.

Livestock, in 1,000 (1989): 8,500 cattle, 28,616 sheep, 2,870 goats, 1,161 pigs.

The 1989 production of red meat was 889,000 tonnes, poultry meat 546,000 tonnes, wool, 94,000 tonnes, eggs, 200,000 tonnes, milk, 1·2m. tonnes.

Cotton-growing is now undertaken by many farmers, the plant being found a better drought resistant than either tobacco or maize. Viticulture and fruit-growing are important. Gross value of production (1988–89), R1,831m.

In 1988–89 the gross value of agricultural production (excluding homelands) was R17,944m. (field crops, R6,749m.; livestock products, R8,116m.; horticultural products, R3,129m.).

Forestry. The commercial forests occupy about 1·62m. ha, of which 148,000 ha are indigenous trees and the rest exotic trees (pine, gum, wattle). On 31 March 1986 there were 613,747 ha of pines and other softwoods, 387,236 ha of eucalypts, 124,228 ha of wattle and 8,013 ha of other hardwoods.

Production, 1985-86, of sawn timber, 1·66m. cu. metres (value R313m.); pulp, paper and paperboard, 1·39m. tonnes (R1,227m.).

Local production meets South Africa's needs of mining timber, firewood, round poles, wooden boxes, crates, particle boards, fibre board and sawn softwood, 30% of its requirements for sawn hardwood and more than 80% of its paper requirements. Rayon pulp, newsprint, other pulp and paper products, pulpwood chips and wattle tanning extract are the main exports.

The Republic is self-sufficient in newsprint and exports pulp and paper.

Fisheries. In 1986 sea fisheries landed 573,000 tons, of which 390,000 tons were pelagic shoal fish, 78% anchovy; trawl fisheries caught 191,000 tons, 72% hake. Total output, wholesale value, R585m. The fishing fleet consists of about 4,420 vessels. About 22,000 people are employed in the fishing industry and its ancillary activities. 10,100 seal pups and 321 bulls were culled in 1986.

INDUSTRY. Net value of sales of the principal groups of industries (in R1m.) in 1989: Processed food, 20,070; beverages and tobacco, 7,873; vehicles, 11,138; basic metals, 18,152; chemicals and products, 26,462; non-electrical machinery, 6,687; electrical machinery, 7,233; fabricated metal products except machinery, 8,933; printing and publishing, 3,084; wood and cork products except furniture, 2,459; clothing, 3,403; paper and products, 7,638; textiles, 5,956; total net value including other groups, 151,317. Manufacturing industry contributed R52,289m. to GDP of R206,804m. in 1989. (25·6% of GDP at current prices in 1990).

Labour. In 1990 the workforce (excluding the 'independent' homelands of Transkei, Bophuthatswana, Venda and Ciskei) numbered (in 1,000; females in brackets): Whites, 2,049 (660); Coloureds, 1,241 (517); Asians, 350 (90); Blacks, 7,433 (2,411).

Industrial employment (except mining) at March 1990: Manufacturing employed 1,457,200 workers; construction, 412,900; trade and accommodation services, 810,167.

Average monthly earnings of white employee, 1984, R1,402; of black, R364.

Trade Unions. In 1988 there were 209 registered trade unions in 10 federations with an estimated total membership of 2,084,323. There were 40 White unions, 26 Coloured and Asian and 28 Black. Ninety-three unions were mixed and 22 did not specify their composition.

The Industrial Conciliation Amendment Act (1979) provides for freedom of association to all workers irrespective of race. Unions were barred from political activity in Feb. 1988. Secondary and repeat strikes are banned, and unions are financially liable for illegal strike action. Work-days lost through strikes: 1987, 5·82m.; 1988, 914,000.

FOREIGN ECONOMIC RELATIONS

Commerce. South Africa, Botswana, Lesotho, Swaziland and Transkei are members of a customs union and the foreign trade statistics shown below represent the combined imports and exports of these countries. The total value of the imports and exports was as follows (in R1m.):

	Imports		*Exports*
1988	39,483·9	1988	49,724·0
1989	44,741·3	1989	58,198·8
1990	44,206·6	1990	...

The principal commodity groups of imports and exports (in R1m.) in 1989 were:

Imports		*Exports*	
Machinery	12,767·4	Minerals and products	...
Vehicles and aircraft	4,827·2	Base metals	6,428·7
Chemical products	5,124·7	Precious stones, metals and coins	3,641·7
Base metals	1,873·4	Textiles	229·1
Scientific and special equipment	...	Chemical products	1,731·9
Resins and plastics	...	Food, beverages and tobacco	2,465·8
Textiles	1,144·5	Vegetable products	1,048·7

Gold exports totalled R19,228·5m. in 1989, some 33% of all exports.

In 1987 Japan was South Africa's main export market, with 11·6% of all exports, and Federal Germany the major source of imports (18·3%). In 1986 the geographical origin of South Africa's imports and the Direction of its export trade were mainly as follows:

	Imports %	*Exports %*
Africa	2	4
Europe	42	23
USA	13	9
Japan	10	8

Total trade between South Africa and UK (British Department of Trade returns, in £1,000 sterling):

	1986	*1987*	*1988*	*1989*	*1990*
Imports to UK	829,305	658,162	807,669	884,607	1,078,546
Exports and re-exports from UK	849,557	948,584	1,074,826	1,038,342	1,113,397

Tourism. In 1989, 930,393 tourists visited South Africa, of whom 460,634 were from African countries and 332,279 from Europe (129,982 from the UK and 79,435 from the Federal Republic of Germany).

COMMUNICATIONS. In 1990 South African Transport Services became Transnet, a public company comprising railways, harbours, pipelines and road transport, set up, with the government as sole shareholder, as a first step to possible privatization.

Roads. The railway administration operates the long-distance road motor services, together with private operators.

There were at 31 March 1987, 228,268 km of roads, of which 182,968 km were national and provincial roads (52,438 km surfaced) and 45,300 km municipal roads and streets (36,200 surfaced).

South African Transport Services carried 11·7m. passengers and 4·12m. tonnes of goods by road in 1986-87.

Motor vehicles in operation on 30 June 1989 included 3,316,706 passenger cars, 1,252,104 commercial vehicles, 181,466 minibuses, 28,000 buses and 303,251 motorcycles.

Railways. Railway history in South Africa begins in 1860 with the line Durban–Point. With the formation of the Union in 1910, the state-owned lines in the 4 provinces (12,194 km) were amalgamated into one state undertaking. In 1990 South African Railways, renamed Spoornet, became part of Transnet.

In 1988-89 there were 23,259 km of 1,065 mm gauge (8,440 km electrified) and 360 km of 762 mm gauge. Railways caried 568m. passengers and 165m. tonnes of freight.

Aviation. Civil aviation in South Africa is controlled by the Department of Transport, which administers the following state-owned airports: Jan Smuts Airport, Johannesburg; D. F. Malan Airport, Cape Town; Louis Botha Airport, Durban; J. B. M. Hertzog Airport, Bloemfontein; Ben Schoeman Airport, East London; H. F. Verwoerd Airport, Port Elizabeth; B. J. Vorster Airport, Kimberley; P. W. Botha Airport, George; Pierre van Ryneveld Airport, Upington. At other airports the Department provides air navigation services.

South African Airways, as the national air carrier, operate scheduled international air services within Africa and to Europe, Latin America, Israel and the Far East. 13 independent operators provide internal flights which link up with SAA's internal network.

During 1986-87 South African Airways carried 4,220,317 passengers (3,741,963 on internal flights) and 75,269 tonnes of freight and mail (25,596).

In March 1990 there were 215 licensed aerodromes, of which 155 were public and 105 private, and 55 approved helistops.

Shipping. The main ports are Durban, Cape Town, Saldanha, Richards Bay, Port Elizabeth and East London. Smaller ports are Mossel Bay, Port Nolloth, Walvis Bay and Lüderitz. During 1988 the main ports handled 97m. tonnes of cargo.

Telecommunications. On 31 March 1989 there were 2,180 money-order post offices and postal agencies.

In March 1988 the international telex switchboard served 31,604 telex subscribers. Line capacity of automatic telephone exchanges (1989), 2·4m.; there were (1989) 4,744,000 telephones.

The South African Broadcasting Corporation broadcasts (1990) 23 radio services in 16 languages and 4 TV services in 7 languages. An external radio service broadcasts in 7 languages. There were (1988) about 2m. television viewers. An independent TV company, N-Met, was permitted to broadcast news from 1 Jan. 1991.

Cinemas (1990). There were approximately 1,200.

Newspapers (1987). There are 39 main newspapers, of which 10 were Afrikaans, 27 English, 1 Zulu and English and 1 Xhosa and English. There were 6 Afrikaans and 14 English daily newspapers.

JUSTICE, RELIGION, EDUCATION AND WELFARE

Justice. The common law of the republic is the Roman–Dutch law—that is, the uncodified law of Holland as it was at the date of the cession of the Cape in 1806. The law of England as such is not recognized as authoritative, though by statute the principles of English law relating to evidence and to mercantile matters, *e.g.*, companies, patents, trademarks, insolvency and the like, have been introduced. In shipping and insurance, English law is followed in the Cape Province, and it has also largely influenced civil and criminal procedure throughout the republic. In all other matters, family relations, property, succession, contract, etc., Roman–Dutch law rules, English decisions being valued only so far as they agree therewith.

The Supreme Court of South Africa is constituted as follows: (i) The Appellate Division, consisting of the Chief Justice and as many Judges of Appeal as the State President may stipulate, is the highest court and its decisions are binding on all courts. It has no original jurisdiction, but is purely a Court of Appeal. (ii) The Provincial Divisions: In each province there is a provincial division of the Supreme Court, while in the Cape there are three such divisions possessing both original and appellate jurisdiction. (iii) The Local Divisions: There is a local division each in the Transvaal and Natal exercising the same original jurisdiction within limited areas as the provincial divisions. The judges hold office till they attain the age of 70 years. No judge can be removed from office except by the State President upon an address from all Houses of Parliament on the ground of misbehaviour or incapacity. The circuit system is fully developed.

The Black appeal courts have been abolished. Black divorce courts have jurisdiction to some extent concurrent with that of the Supreme Court in cases in which the parties are Black.

Each province is further divided into districts with a magistrate's court having a prescribed civil and criminal jurisdiction. From this court there is an appeal to the provincial divisions of the Supreme Court, and thence to the appellate division. Magistrates' convictions carrying sentences above a prescribed limit are subject to automatic review by a judge. In addition, several regional divisions consisting of a number of districts have been constituted. Convictions of such courts are not subject to automatic review by a judge.

Courts of Black affairs commissioners were abolished in 1984. All criminal and civil cases are dealt with by judges (in the Supreme Courts) and magistrates (in the lower courts). Judges and magistrates are entitled to take judicial cognizance of customary (indigenous) laws and must, where relevant, apply them. A limited civil and criminal jurisdiction is conferred upon the Black chief or headman over his own tribe.

It was announced in Dec. 1990 that political exiles who fled South Africa before 8 Oct. 1990 were free to return and immune from prosecution.

Religion. The latest figures are still those of the 1980 population census results as regards religious denominations: *Whites:* Nederduits Gereformeerde Kerk, 1,695,875; Anglicans, 461,543; Methodists, 420,957; Roman Catholics, 388,336; Nederduits Hervormde Kerk, 258,769; Presbyterians, 129,771; Gereformeerde Kerk, 127,235; Apostolics, 125,501; other Christians, 608,139; Jews, 117,963. *Blacks:* Methodists, 11,657,787; Black independent churches, 5,124,566; Nederduits Gereformeerde Kerk, 1,120,461; Roman Catholics, 1,731,623; Anglican, 815,346; Lutheran, 742,421; other Christian churches, 915,312; non-Christian churches, 37,557. *Coloureds and Asians:* Nederduits Gereformeerde Kerk, 678,573; Hindus, 524,913; Anglican, 369,728; Roman Catholic, 286,740; Islam 342,248.

Membership of the white branch of the Nederduits Gereformeerde Kerk was opened to all races in 1986.

Education. Primary and secondary public education, other than that specifically provided elsewhere, falls under the Provincial Administration. In terms of the National Education Policy Act, 1967, the Minister of Education, Arts and Science may, after consultation with the Provincial Administrators and the National Advisory Education Council, determine general educational policy within the framework of the Act. Black education is the responsibility of the Department of Black Education and Training, while education for Coloureds and Indians is controlled by the Department of Internal Affairs.

Public primary and secondary schools in 1988: Schools for Whites had 902,314 pupils and 53,534 teachers. For Coloureds, 837,350 pupils and 35,649 teachers. For Indians, 233,910 pupils and 11,405 teachers. For Blacks, 4,965,428 pupils and 132,743 teachers. A non-racial school (100 pupils) opened near Durban in 1987. Special schools (1988) for 4,847 Black pupils had 720 teachers; for 13,414 White pupils, 2,504 teachers; for 5,967 Coloured pupils, 798 teachers; for 5,847 Indian pupils, 456 teachers.

Private Schools. To a certain extent the activities of private schools are controlled by government regulations. Their pupils generally sit for the state schools' examinations. These schools make provision for kindergarten, elementary and preparatory, general primary, secondary and commercial education.

Higher Education. In March 1988 tertiary-level students included 196,787 whites, 20,039 coloureds, 10,057 Indians and 53,715 Blacks.

There were 158,143 whites, 16,856 coloureds, 10,507 Indians and 50,957 Blacks were at university and Colleges of Education. There are 17 universities in the republic: (1) The University of Cape Town. (2) The University of Natal in Durban and Pietermaritzburg. (3) The University of the Orange Free State at Bloemfontein (teaching in Afrikaans). (4) Potchefstroom University for Christian Higher Education, Potchefstroom (Afrikaans). (5) The University of Pretoria (Afrikaans). (6) Rhodes University, Grahamstown, C.P. (7) The University of Stellenbosch (Afrikaans). (8) The University of the Witwatersrand, Johannesburg. (9) The University of South Africa, with its seat in Pretoria, which conducts a Division of External Studies by means of correspondence and vacation courses (English and Afrikaans); it is also an examining body. (10) The University of Port Elizabeth (English and Afrikaans). (11) Rand Afrikaans University, Johannesburg (All may enrol, white, black, coloured or Asian students).

The University of Fort Hare (12), the University of the North (13) near Pietersburg and the University of Zululand (14) near Empangeni, Natal, are operated by the Department of Education and Training and provide education at university level for Blacks, the University of the Western Capo (15), Bellville (Cape), offers university facilities to the Coloured population and is administered by the Department of Internal Affairs as is the University for Indians (16), the University of Durban-Westville, at Durban. The Medical University of South Africa (17) is for Black students.

Technical and Vocational Education. Technical, vocational and special education for persons other than those for whom specific provision is made: The Department of National Education is responsible for the maintenance, management and control of or the payment of subsidies to colleges for advanced technical education, technical colleges, technical institutes, special schools, schools of industries and reform schools. Colleges for advanced technical education provide education on an advanced level for a variety of technical, commercial and general courses of study as well as secondary education on a part-time basis. Technical colleges and technical institutes are mainly responsible for the training of apprentices and the education, on a part-time basis, of persons not subject to compulsory school attendance. Special schools for handicapped children cater for the educational needs of those who are blind, partially sighted, deaf, hard of hearing, epileptic, cerebral palsied and physically handicapped. Children found to be in need of care by a children's court, are admitted to schools of industries and reform schools.

The Department of Internal Affairs has taken over all schools of this nature for Coloureds.

In 1988, technical and training colleges (except Colleges of Education) had 62,510 white students; 6,022 coloured; 5,529 Indian; 10,367 black.

Health. In 1988 there were 20,947 medical practitioners of whom 5,960 were specialists, 3,581 dental specialists and dentists, 141,459 nurses. In 1987 there were 737 hospitals. In 1987 there were 24,178 beds in psychiatric hospitals; 95,839 mentally ill were treated as in-patients, 290,550 consultations were performed for out-patients.

All public health services rendered by government bodies are free, or charged according to the patient's means.

Social Welfare. Under the Social Pensions Act, 1973, pensions and allowances are made to aged, blind, disabled and war veterans, subject to a means test. Family allowances are paid to families with 3 or more children and inadequate income, and to mothers alone with one or more children and inadequate income.

Welfare Services. South Africa is not a welfare state, yet provides many services for the community. Welfare work on behalf of the Government is done by the Departments of Health and Welfare, Co-operation and Development, and Internal Affairs.

In 1989 there were over 1,600 voluntary organizations. The work of all these bodies is co-ordinated by the South African Welfare Council and regional welfare boards set up under the National Welfare Act, 1978.

The Child Care Act, 1983 which superseded the Children's Act, 1960 is designed to protect children against neglect, abuse, ill-treatment and exploitation. The Act provides for preventive child care services, foster care, adoption and residential care, and also for various children's allowances and financial assistance to children's homes and creches.

Welfare services for the aged are mainly provided by voluntary bodies with government subsidies; the same principle applies to the care of the handicapped, but there are State settlements for the permanently handicapped, and State sheltered-employment programmes for handicapped adults.

The National Advisory Board on Rehabilitation Matters advises and brings together the voluntary and government agencies working on drug abuse and alcoholism.

In all fields of welfare, State subsidies enable voluntary bodies to employ professional social workers.

DIPLOMATIC REPRESENTATIVES

Of South Africa in Great Britain (South Africa Hse., Trafalgar Sq., London, WC2N 5DP)
Ambassador: (Vacant).

Of Great Britain in South Africa (255 Hill St., Arcadia, Pretoria, 0002)
Ambassador: Sir Robin Renwick, KCMG.

Of South Africa in the USA (3051 Massachusetts Ave., NW, Washington, D.C., 20008)
Ambassador: Piet G. Koornhof.

Of the USA in South Africa (225 Pretorius St., Pretoria)
Ambassador: William L. Swing.

Of South Africa to the United Nations
Ambassador: Jeremy B. Shearar.

Further Reading

Statistical Information: The Central Statistical Service (Private Bag X44, Pretoria 0001)

The Customs and Excise Office, Pretoria, publishes *Monthly Abstract of Trade Statistics* (from 1946) and *Trade and Shipping of the Union of South Africa* (annually, 1910–55); *Foreign Trade Statistics* (annually, from 1956)

Benson, M. *Nelson Mandela: The Man and the Movement*. New York, 1986
Bindman, G., (ed.) *South Africa: Human Rights and the Rule of Law*. London, 1988
Bissell, R. E. and Crocker, C. A., *South Africa in the 1980s*. Boulder, 1979
Böhning, W. R., *Black Migration to South Africa*. Geneva, 1981
Branford, J., *A Dictionary of South African English*. Rev. ed. OUP, 1980
Davenport, T. R. H., *South Africa: A Modern History*. 3rd ed. CUP, 1986
Goldenhuys, D., *The Diplomacy of Isolation: South African Foreign Policy Making*. Johannesburg, 1984

Hill, C. R., *Change in South Africa: Blind Alleys and New Directions*. London, 1983
Lewis, S. R., *The Economics of Apartheid*. New York, 1989
Meli, F., *South Africa belongs to us*. Indiana Univ. Press, 1989
Musiker, R., *South Africa*, [Bibliography] Oxford and Santa Barbara, 1980
Nattrass, N. and Ardington, E. (eds.), *The Political Economy of South Africa*. Cape Town and OUP, 1990
Oxford History of South Africa. OUP, Vol. 1, 1969; Vol. 2 1971
Sparks, A., *The Mind of South Africa*. London, 1990
Thompson, L., *The Political Mythology of Apartheid*. Yale Univ. Press, 1985.—*A History of South Africa*. Yale Univ. Press, 1990
Venter, D. J., *South Africa, Sanctions and Multinationals*. London, 1989

PROVINCE OF THE CAPE OF GOOD HOPE

Kaapprovinsie

HISTORY. The colony of the Cape of Good Hope was founded by the Dutch in the year 1652. Britain took possession of it from 1795 to 1803 and again in 1806, and it was formally ceded to Great Britain by the Convention of London, 13 Aug. 1814. Letters patent issued in 1850 declared that in the colony there should be a Parliament which should consist of the Governor, a Legislative Council and a House of Assembly. On 31 May 1910 the colony was merged in the Union of South Africa, thereafter forming an original province of the Union.

AREA AND POPULATION. The following table gives the population of the Cape of Good Hope [1] (area (1980) 646,332 sq. km) at the last census:

	All races			Whites		Non-Whites	
	Total	*Males*	*Females*	*Males*	*Females*	*Males*	*Females*
1936	3,527,865	1,663,169	1,864,796	396,058	394,993	1,267,011	1,469,803
1946	4,051,424	1,924,334	2,127,090	433,849	436,300	1,490,485	1,690,790
1951	4,426,726	2,110,674	2,316,052	463,917	471,168	1,646,757	1,844,884
1960	5,360,234	2,553,245	2,806,989	493,370	507,398	2,059,875	2,299,591
1970 [2]	4,293,726	2,151,629	2,142,097	546,761	567,448	1,604,868	1,579,649
1980 [3]	5,091,360	2,575,460	2,515,900	624,360	639,360	1,950,780	1,876,540
1986 [1]	4,901,261	2,371,906	2,529,355	...	...	...	...

[1] Including Walvis Bay. [2] Excluding Transkei.
[3] Excluding Transkei, Ciskei and Bophuthatswana.

Present area, 641,379 sq. km (247,637 sq. miles), including the enclave of Walvis Bay 1,124 sq. km (434 sq. miles) on the coast of Namibia which forms an administrative part of the Cape Province.

Of the non-White population in 1985, 31,989 were Asians, 1,402,307 were Blacks and 2,397,424 Coloureds.

Vital statistics for calendar years:

	Births	*Deaths*	*Marriages*
1985	90,484	44,283	27,375
1986	87,121	37,445	27,897
1987	88,164	51,088	25,225
1988	81,855	53,759	23,383

ADMINISTRATION. In June 1986 the provincial councils were abolished. Cape Town is the seat of the provincial administration.

Administrator: J. W. H. Meiring.

The province is divided into 111 magisterial districts and 35 divisions. Each division has a council of at least 6 members (15 in the Cape Division) elected quinquennially by the owners or occupiers of immovable property. The duties devolving upon divisional councils include the construction and maintenance of roads and bridges, local rating, vehicle taxation (except motor vehicle taxation) and preservation of public health. There are 216 municipalities, each governed by a mayor and councillors. Municipal elections are held biennially.

FINANCE. In 1989–90 revenue amounted to R2,935,566,000 and expenditure to R2,935,566,000.

MINING. For mineral production, *see* pp. 1096-97.

AGRICULTURE. Viticulture in the republic is almost exclusively confined to the Cape Province, but practically all other forms of agricultural and pastoral activity are pursued.

INDUSTRY. The province has brick, tile and pottery works, saw-mills, engineering works, foundries, grain-mills, distilleries and wineries, clothing factories, furniture, boot and shoe factories, etc.

RELIGION. From the 1980 population census, Nederduits Gereformeerde Kerk, 1,336,637; Gereformeerde Kerk, 12,576; Nederduits Hervormde Kerk, 110,560; Anglican, 567,715; Presbyterian, 109,521; Methodist, 529,853; Roman Catholic, 390,969; Apostolic Faith Mission, 62,113; Lutheran, 113,879; Islam, 170,000; Hindu, 6,629; Independent Churches, 458,524; other Christian Churches, 869,703; Jews, 32,349.

EDUCATION. On 1 April 1986 the Education Department came within the jurisdiction of the Central Government. Education is compulsory for all White children. Primary and secondary education is free to the end of the calendar year in which the age of 19 years is attained.

Whites (1985). There were 828 government and aided schools with 14,205 teachers and 238,853 pupils; 8 teacher-training colleges with 291 lecturers and 1,841 students; 53 private schools with 13,859 pupils.

Coloureds (1985). There were 1,776 government and aided schools with 26,583 teachers and 657,391 pupils; 13 teacher-training colleges with 6,709 students; 18 private schools with 2,652 pupils.

Black (1985). There were 1,137 government schools with 7,105 teachers and 318,541 pupils and 17 private schools with 118 teachers and 6,120 pupils.

Asians (1985). There were 8 government schools with 201 teachers and 5,400 pupils.

PROVINCE OF NATAL

HISTORY. Natal was annexed to Cape Colony in 1844, placed under separate government in 1845, and on 15 July 1856 established as a separate colony. By this charter partially representative institutions were established, and in 1893 the colony attained responsible government. The province of Zululand was annexed to Natal on 30 Dec. 1897. The districts of Vryheid, Utrecht and part of Wakkerstroom, formerly belonging to the Transvaal, were annexed in Jan. 1903. On 31 May 1910 the colony was merged in the Union of South Africa as an original province of the Union.

AREA AND POPULATION. The province (including Kwa Zulu, 36,073 sq. km) has an area of 91,785 sq. km, with a seaboard of about 576 km. The climate is sub-tropical on the coast and somewhat colder inland. The province is divided into 45 magisterial districts.

The census returns of population (excluding Kwa Zulu) were:

		All races		*Whites*		*Non-Whites*	
	Total	*Males*	*Females*	*Males*	*Females*	*Males*	*Females*
1960	2,979,034	1,443,561	1,535,473	166,404	222,750	1,227,157	1,362,468
1970	4,236,770	2,009,410	2,227,360	171,005	214,960	1,794,430	2,004,610
1980	2,676,340	1,360,600	1,315,740	276,240	285,620	1,084,360	1,030,120
1985	2,145,018	1,072,426	1,072,592	274,987	285,234	797,629	787,358

Of the non-White population in 1985, 659,703 were Asians, 95,743 Coloureds and 829,541 Blacks. Population of Kwa Zulu, *see* p. 1092.

ADMINISTRATION. State of parties Oct. 1990: National Party, 10; Democratic Party, 10.

The seat of provincial government in Natal is Pietermaritzburg. In April 1978 the area of East Griqualand was transferred to Natal from Cape Province.

Administrator: Cornelius Johannes van Rooyen Botha.

FINANCE. In 1988–89 revenue amounted to R1,478,605,796 and expenditure to R1,434,163,171. Tax incentives encourage industrial development.

MINING. The province is rich in mineral wealth, particularly coal. For figures of mineral production, *see* p. 1096-97.

AGRICULTURE. Sugar, timber (wattle, pine and gum) and livestock production (beef and dairy cattle, pigs, sheep and poultry) are the mainstays of agriculture. Cultivated pastures are increasingly important.

INDUSTRY. There are 4 highly industrialized development zones: Durban-Pinetown, Pietermaritzburg, Newcastle and Richards Bay. The road and rail networks are good and electricity is supplied from a grid. There are deep-water natural harbours at Durban and Richards Bay. Durban is an international port. Richards Bay is a terminal for ore, coal and wood-chip export. Important industries include metallurgical plants, cereal mills, sugar refineries, tannin extraction plants, pulp-mills, explosives and fertilizer plants, milk-processing plants, meat-processing factories, foundries, paper and fibre-processing plants and clothing factories.

EDUCATION. The Department of Education and Culture controls primary and secondary education for Whites. Control was transferred from the province to central government on 1 April 1986, and the classification of government-aided schools changed to private although they continue to receive a subsidy.

Whites (1989). There were 261 government schools with 98,966 pupils; 2 residential teacher-training colleges with 893 students; 1 correspondence teacher-training college with 458 pupils; 52 private schools with 11,290 pupils; 11 special schools and training centres with 1,426 pupils and 9 technical colleges with 3,668 pupils.

Coloureds (1989). There were 65 state and state-aided schools with 1,386 teachers and 30,565 pupils; 18 state subsidized pre-primary schools with 15 teachers and 1,000 pupils; 4 special schools with 155 pupils and 22 teachers; 1 teacher-training college with 301 students and 32 lecturers; 1 technical college with 42 full-time lecturers and 14 part-time lecturers.

Blacks (1990). There were 1,147 schools with 5,952 teachers and 236,182 pupils. These schools are situated in Natal and KwaZulu.

Asians (1990). There were 447 state and state-aided primary and secondary schools with 11,959 teachers and 249,713 pupils; 35 private pre-primary schools with 2,462 children; 1 school of industry with 149 pupils; 16 special schools and training centres with 1,635 pupils; 3 technical colleges with 2,416 full-time and 7,487 part-time students; 2 Colleges of Education with 833 students and 1 pre-vocational school with 262 pupils.

PROVINCE OF THE TRANSVAAL

HISTORY. The Transvaal was one of the territories colonized by the Boers who left the Cape Colony during the Great Trek in 1834 and following years. In 1852, by the Sand River Treaty, Great Britain recognized the independence of the Transvaal, which, in 1853, took the name of the South African Republic. In 1877 the republic was annexed by Great Britain, but the Boers took up arms towards the end of 1880. In 1881 peace was made and self-government, subject to British suzerainty and certain stipulated restrictions, was restored to the Boers. The London Convention of 1884 removed the suzerainty and a number of these restrictions but reserved to Great Britain the right of approval of the Transvaal's foreign relations, excepting with regard to the Orange Free State. In 1886 gold was discovered on the Witwatersrand, and this discovery, together with the great influx of foreigners which it occasioned, gave rise to many grave problems. Eventually, in 1899, war broke out between Great Britain and the Transvaal. Peace was concluded on 31 May 1902, the Transvaal and the Orange Free State both losing their independence. The Transvaal was governed as a crown colony until 12 Jan. 1907, when responsible government came into force. On 31 May 1910 the Transvaal became one of the four provinces of the Union.

AREA AND POPULATION. The area of the province is 262,499 sq. km or 101,351 sq. miles, including Gazankulu, Lebowa, Ka Ngwane and Kwa Ndebele. The province is divided into 53 districts. The following table shows the population, excluding Gazankulu, Lebowa, Ka Ngwane and Kwa Ndebele in 1985, at each of the last censuses:

		All races		*Whites*		*Non-Whites*	
	Total	*Males*	*Females*	*Males*	*Females*	*Males*	*Females*
1936	3,341,470	1,846,576	1,494,894	424,470	396,286	1,422,108	1,098,608
1946	4,283,038	2,374,323	1,908,715	541,053	522,068	1,833,270	1,386,647
1951	4,812,838	2,619,314	2,193,524	737,194	731,111	2,575,119	2,230,053
1960	6,270,711	3,310,948	2,959,763	735,845	729,730	2,575,103	2,230,034
1970	6,478,904	3,507,753	2,971,151	957,291	946,802	2,550,462	2,024,349
1980	8,376,042	4,581,054	3,794,988	1,192,484	1,176,055	3,388,570	2,618,933
1985	7,532,179	4,008,070	3,524,109	1,224,064	1,237,300	2,784,006	2,286,809

Of the non-White population in 1985, 4,674,290 were Black, 126,201 Asians and 270,324 Coloureds. Population of Gazankulu, Lebowa, Ka Ngwane and Kwa Ndebele, *see* p. 1092.

Important towns of the province are listed on p. 1092.

ADMINISTRATION. The seat of provincial government is at Pretoria, which is also the administrative capital of the Republic of South Africa.

Administrator: D. J. Hough.

FINANCE. In 1989–90 revenue amounted to R3,377,227,103 and expenditure to R3,292,499,420.

MINING. For mineral production, *see* p. 1096-97. Gold output in 1983 was 15,807,760 oz. worth R7,483,932,210.

AGRICULTURE. The province is in the main a stock-raising country, though there are considerable areas well adapted for agriculture, including the growing of tropical crops.

INDUSTRY. The province has iron and brass foundries and engineering works, grain-mills, breweries, brick, tile and pottery works, tobacco, soap, and candle factories, coach and wagon works, clothing factories, etc.

RELIGION. From the 1980 population census. Nederduits Gereformeerde Kerk, 1,239,484; Gereformeerde Kerk, 95,021; Nederduits Hervormde Kerk, 225,850; Anglican, 509,400; Presbyterian, 135,701; Methodist, 684,284; Roman Catholic, 753,982; Apostolic Faith Mission, 139,393; Lutheran, 312,484; Islam, 74,504; Hindu, 37,249; independent churches, 1,972,759; other Christian churches, 20,257; Jews, 77,759.

EDUCATION. All education for Whites except that of universities is under the provincial authority. The province has been divided for the purposes of local control and management into 21 school districts. Instruction in government schools, both primary and secondary, is free. The medium of instruction is the home language of the pupil. The teaching of the other language begins at the earliest stage at which it is appropriate on educational grounds. Both languages are taught as examination subjects to every pupil.

Whites (1988). There were 984 public schools with 27,400 teachers and 504,032 pupils; 6 teacher-training colleges with 7,560 students; 115 private schools with 2,187 teachers and 33,831 pupils.

Coloureds (1988). There were 103 state and state-aided schools with 2,956 teachers and 74,607 pupils; 1 teacher-training college with 562 students.

Asians (1988). There were 81 public schools with 1,409 teachers and 32,412 pupils; 1 teacher-training college with 31 teachers and 126 students.

Blacks (1988). There were 4,295 public and private school sections with 25,779 teachers and 957,322 pupils (homelands excluded).

PROVINCE OF THE ORANGE FREE STATE

Oranje-Vrystaat

HISTORY. The Orange River was first crossed by Europeans in the middle of the 18th century. Between 1810 and 1820, settlements were made in the southern parts of the Orange Free State, and the Great Trek greatly increased the number of settlers during and after 1836. In 1848, Sir Harry Smith proclaimed the whole territory between the Orange and Vaal rivers as a British possession called the 'Orange River Sovereignty'. However, in 1854, by the Convention of Bloemfontein, British sovereignty was withdrawn and the independence of the country was recognized.

During the first 5 years of its existence the Orange Free State was much harassed by incessant raids by the Basutos. These were at length conquered, but, owing to the intervention of the British Government, the treaty of Aliwal North incorporated only part of the territory of the Basutos in the Orange Free State.

On account of the treaty with the South African Republic, the Orange Free State took a prominent part in the South African War (1899–1902) and was annexed on 28 May 1900 as the Orange River Colony. Crown colony government continued until 1907, when responsible government was introduced. On 31 May 1910 the Orange River Colony was merged in the Union of South Africa as the province of the Orange Free State, and on 31 May 1961 became a province of the Republic of South Africa.

AREA AND POPULATION. The area of the province is 127,993 sq. km or 49,418 sq. miles, including Qwaqwa. The province is divided into 43 administrative and 49 magisterial districts. The population has varied as follows:

	All races			*Whites*		*Non-Whites*	
	Total	*Males*	*Females*	*Males*	*Females*	*Males*	*Females*
1936	772,060	381,903	390,157	101,872	99,106	280,031	291,051
1946	879,071	432,896	446,175	101,874	100,203	331,022	345,972
1951	1,016,570	519,166	497,404	115,637	112,015	403,529	385,389
1960	1,386,202	731,486	654,716	139,304	137,103	601,182	553,613
1970	1,716,350	899,140	817,210	148,110	148,030	751,030	669,180
1980	1,931,860	1,039,220	892,640	166,380	159,840	872,840	732,800
1989	2,349,556	1,246,523	1,103,033	183,679	188,219	1,062,844	914,814

Of the non-White population in 1989, 1,908,414 were Black, 69,184 Coloureds and 60 Indians.

ADMINISTRATION. Provincial councils were abolished on 30 June 1986.

For the Whites there are 71 municipal councils and 6 village management boards. For the coloured 9 management committees and for the Blacks, 4 city councils, 8 town councils, 56 village committees and 2 local authority committees.

Administrator: L. J. Botha.

FINANCE. In 1988–89 revenue was R957m. and expenditure R871m.

MINING. For mineral statistics, *see* p. 1096. The output of gold in 1988 was 171,512 kg valued at R5,462·7m.

AGRICULTURE. The province consists of undulating plains, affording excellent grazing and wide tracts for agricultural purposes. The rainfall is moderate. The Orange Free State is the largest grain-producing province in the Republic and is also an important sheep- and cattle-farming region.

INDUSTRY. The more important manufacturing industries in the province are the oil-from-coal factory at Sasolburg (as well as industries based on its by-products); grain mills and brick, tile and pottery works. Fertilizers, agricultural implements, blankets, woollen products, clothing, hosiery, cement and pharmaceutical products are also manufactured.

EDUCATION. Primary, secondary and vocational education and the training of teachers are controlled and financed by the Department of Education and Culture Administration: House of Assembly for Whites and Administration; House of Representatives for Coloureds; Department of Education and Training for Blacks.

Education is free in all public schools up to the university matriculation standard. Attendance is compulsory for White and Coloured between the ages of 7 and 16, but exemption may be granted in special cases. Attendance is not compulsory for Black children, except in areas/communities/towns where a request for compulsory education had been made. In these cases education is compulsory up to Standard 5 or the age of 16. The home language of the pupil is the medium of instruction up to Standard 2; thereafter he has an option of Afrikaans, English or his home language in Black schools.

Further education and training are given at 2 universities (UOFS and Vista), 3 teachers' training colleges, 1 technikon, 1 agricultural college, 2 nursing colleges, 5 technical colleges and numerous training centres.

Whites (1989). There were 211 government and aided schools with 4,460 teachers and 75,711 pupils.

Coloureds (1989). There were 47 government and aided schools with 750 teachers and 17,381 pupils.

Blacks (1989). There were 2,687 government schools with 10,574 teachers and 414,329 pupils.

BOPHUTHATSWANA

HISTORY. Bophuthatswana was first to obtain self-government under the Bantu Homeland Constitution Act of 1971 and was the second black homeland to ask the Republic of South Africa for full independence, which was granted on 6 Dec. 1977.

AREA AND POPULATION. The total area is 44,000 sq. km.

In 1985 there was a *de jure* population of 3·2m., of which 47% lived in the White areas. The remaining 53% (1,740,600) lived in the homeland. Estimate (1989) 3·2m. The capital is Mmabatho.

CONSTITUTION AND GOVERNMENT. The Bophuthatswana Government is a compromise between the traditional chief-in-council system and a democratic electoral system. There are 72 elected and 24 nominated members in the Legislative Assembly. Self-government was granted in 1972. Each regional authority (coinciding with the 12 districts of the country) nominates 2 members, and each district elects 6 members to the National Assembly and 12 designated by the President on account of their special knowledge, qualifications or experience.

Executive power vests in the President, who is directly elected by general suffrage of persons who are registered as voters, and he appoints his Cabinet.

The first general election was held in Oct. 1972, 2 political parties taking part. Kgosi Lucas Mangope's Bophuthatswana National Party (BNP) won 20 of the 24 contested seats, but in 1974 he formed the Bophuthatswana Democratic Party which in the 1987 elections won 66 seats; the People's Progressive Party, 6 seats.

Members of regional authorities are elected from among the tribal and community authorities in their areas.

The Cabinet in Nov. 1990 consisted of:

President, Minister of Law and Order, Audit and Public Service: Dr Kgosi Lucas Manyane Mangope (took office 6 Dec. 1977; re-elected for another 7 years as from 11 Nov. 1984).

Population Development: T. M. Molatlhwa. *Internal Affairs:* Kgosi S. V. Suping. *Finance:* L. G. Young. *Posts and Telecommunications and Broadcasting:* M. Z. Masilo. *Manpower and Coordination:* S. M. Seodi. *State Affairs and Civil Aviation:* R. Cronje. *Foreign Affairs:* G. S. M. Nkau. *Health and Social Welfare:* Dr N. C. O. B. Khaole. *Water Affairs:* T. M. Tlhabane. *Economic Planning, Energy Affairs and Mines:* E. B. Keikelame. *Agriculture and Natural Resources:* P. H. Moeketsi. *Parliamentary Affairs, Local Government and Housing:* H. F. Tlou. *Education:* K. C. V. A. Sehume. *Justice and Transport:* S. G. Mothibe. *Public Works:* S. C. Kgobokoe.

There were 6 Deputy Ministers.

Flag: Blue, crossed by a diagonal orange stripe, and in the canton a white disc charged with a leopard's face in black and white.

DEFENCE. The Air Wing of the Defence Force has 2 Partenavia P-68 patrol aircraft, 2 Aviocar transports, and 1 Alouette III, 2 BK-117 and 1 Ecureuil helicopters. There is an Army Force of 3,100 with 2 infantry battalions.

INTERNATIONAL RELATIONS

Aid. The Republic of South Africa granted aid of R607m. in 1990–91.

ECONOMY

Budget. The 1989–90 budget balanced at R2,300m.

Currency. South African Rand.

Banking and Finance. The financial system is controlled by legislation inherited from South Africa on independence, and commercial banks have strong direct links with South African banks which in certain instances are controlled by overseas banking companies.

In 1990 there were 3 commercial banks with branches in all major commercial and agricultural centres offering a full range of banking services. The Agricultural Bank of Bophuthatswana provides finance to farmers. The government-funded Agricultural Development Fund provides loan finance and subsidy support to agricultural co-operative societies. The Bophuthatswana Building Society grants loans for house building.

NATURAL RESOURCES

Water. The Department of Water Affairs controls and maintains 2,833 reservoirs, 6,845 boreholes and 648 earth dams.

Minerals. The territory is particularly rich in minerals. In 1990 there were 46 mines. Minerals include platinum, asbestos, gold, calcite, granite, chrome, vanadium, limestone and diamonds.

Exploration for more platinum, chrome and coal is currently being carried out both by the private sector and by the Mining and Geological Survey Division of the Department of Economic Planning. The platinum mines around Rustenburg produce about 66% of the free world's total production. The major chrome mines are near Rustenburg and Marico, while vanadium is mined in the Odi district near Brits. The Rustenburg, Western and Impala Platinum mines which are shared with the Republic of South Africa produce about 1·9m. oz. a year.

AGRICULTURE. Bophuthatswana is a semi-arid area of bushveld and grass veld suitable for stock farming. The annual rainfall is 300 mm in the west and 700 mm in the east and there are 4 river catchment areas—those of the Molopo, Ngotwane, Sehujwane and Madikwe rivers.

Although the land tenure system militates against establishing large farms, some land which is suitable for farming is leased by the Government to successful farmers.

Livestock (1988): Cattle, 467,355; sheep, 268,351; goats, 530,430; pigs, 8,039; poultry, 196,396.

Only 6·6% of the territory is suited to dryland farming, but crop yields have shown a steady improvement in recent years. In Ditsobotla district, 36,926 ha of fertile land has been developed by 3 primary co-operatives comprising 190 Batswana farmers. Silkworm farming was being tried in 1983. By 1981 the country was self sufficient in maize and exported the surplus. Three rice projects are successfully expanding and vegetable production was flourishing in 1987. The budget for 1990–91 is R182m.

INDUSTRY. The first industries were started on an agency basis at Babelegi; the fastest growing industrial area in the homeland, in 1977 it covered 183 hectares and by March 1985 more than R234m. had been invested in the project. Other industries are situated at Mmabatho, Garankuwa, Selosesha, Mafikeng and Mogwase. South African border industries are also promoted by the government, notably at Rosslyn where 128 industries had been established by Dec. 1975.

Labour. 56,000 persons were employed in mining in 1988.

COMMUNICATIONS

Roads. Total length (1988) 6,300 km, of which 1,300 km are tarred.

Aviation. Mmabatho International Airport was opened in 1984.

Telecommunications. There were 29,636 telephones and 253 telex lines at 30 Sept. 1990, and 44 post offices.In 1989 there was 1 television station and 2 radio stations (Radio-Bop broadcasts in English and Radio Mmabatho in Setswana), and (1990) 63,001 television licences.

EDUCATION AND WELFARE

Education. Education is not compulsory but is free apart from nominal contributions to school funds and hostel fees at post-primary schools. Medium of instruction from Grade I to Standard 2 is in Setswana; from Standard 3 to senior standards is in English. Afrikaans is taught as a subject. The education is controlled by the Department of Education with a budget of R506m. in 1990-91.

In 1989 there were 28,439 children in kindergartens, 328,698 in primary schools, 125,542 in middle schools, 76,747 in high schools, 1,094 in schools for the mentally handicapped, 1,092 for the physically handicapped, 3,751 in colleges of education (2 new colleges of education opened in 1990), 1,638 in adult education and 2,330 in university. The number of teachers was 16,058 excluding lecturers.

Health. In 1989 there were 12 hospitals, 204 static clinics, 197 mobile clinics, 6,303 hospital and clinic beds, 178 doctors and 6,039 nurses. The health budget in 1990–91 was R184m.

Further Reading

Five Years of Independence: Republic of Bophuthatswana. Mafikeng, 1983
A Nation on the March
Bophuthatswana at a Glance

TRANSKEI

HISTORY. Transkei is the homeland of the Xhosa nation and was granted self-government by the Republic of South Africa in 1963. Over 1·5m. Transkeians live permanently in the Republic of South Africa but were deprived of their South African citizenship on independence.

AREA AND POPULATION. The total area is 16,910 sq. miles (43,798 sq. km). Population (1985 estimate) 2,876,122. The capital is Umtata (population (1976) 24,805; 20,196 Blacks, 1,067 Coloured and 3,542 Whites). Other towns include Gcuwa, Kwabhaca, Umzimvubu and Lusikisiki.

CONSTITUTION AND GOVERNMENT. The Status of Transkei Bill of 1976 gave Transkei a unicameral National Assembly instead of the then existing Legislative Assembly. Independence was achieved 26 Oct. 1976.

General elections were held on 29 Sept. 1976 and the Transkei National Independence Party gained 69 of the 75 elective seats in the National Assembly. Members were elected for a 5-year period. In addition there are 75 traditional (co-opted) members (70 chiefs and 5 paramount chiefs).

President: Paramount Chief T. N. Ndamase.

In Sept. 1987 Chief George Mantanzima the Prime Minister, resigned and was succeeded by Stella Sigcau who in turn was ousted in a bloodless military coup, led by Major-Gen. Bantu Holomisa in Jan. 1988.

Flag: Three horizontal stripes of ochre, white, green.

FINANCE. In 1985 government income was R872m. and expenditure R984m.

MINERALS. Coal, titanium and black granite are mined.

AGRICULTURE. Notable examples of successful commercial enterprises in agriculture are the Magwa and Majola tea estates, with approximately 1,700 hectares planted, and various fibre plantations. 70,000 hectares of land are under indigenous forests and 61,000 hectares have been put under exotic plantations. There are 28 sawmills in the country.

Livestock (1976): Cattle, 1·3m.; sheep, 2·5m.; goats, 1·25m.

COMMUNICATIONS

Roads. There are above 8,800 km of roads.

Railways. There is a 209 km railway line linking Umtata with the port of East London in the Republic of South Africa.

Aviation. An international airport exists at Umtata.

Shipping. A start was made in 1978 on a 'free port' at Mnganzana but has since been abandoned.

Telecommunications. There were 11,498 telephones in 1978.

EDUCATION AND WELFARE

Education. In 1985 there were 690,000 pupils in primary schools and 193,000 pupils in secondary schools. The national university was inaugurated in Umtata in 1977 and has a brance in Butterworth.

Health. There were (1987) 31 hospitals with a total of 7,561 beds.

DIPLOMATIC REPRESENTATIVES

No country, other than the Republic of South Africa, has recognized Transkei as an independent state.

VENDA

HISTORY. Traditionally the territory of the Vhavenda, the country was granted self-government in 1973, and became the third Black homeland to be granted independence by the Republic of South Africa on 13 Sept. 1979.

Brig. Gabriel Ramushwana seized power in a bloodless coup in April 1990.

AREA AND POPULATION. The total area is 7,460 sq. km. In 1985, census, the *de jure* population of Venda was estimated at 651,393, the *de facto* population at 459,986. The capital is Thohoyandou. The other main towns are Sibasa, Makwarela, Makhado, Vuwani, Mutale and Masisi.

Vital statistics, 1987: Birth rate was 39·1 per 1,000 population; crude death rate, 10·3; infant mortality rate 56·9 per 1,000 live births.

CONSTITUTION AND GOVERNMENT. Executive power is vested in the President, who is elected for the duration of each Parliament, which consists of the President and the National Assembly; legislative power is vested in Parliament. In addition to the National Assembly there is an Executive Council, or Cabinet, and a judiciary independent of the Executive. The National Assembly consists of 45 members elected by popular vote, 15 members designated by 5 district councils, 6 members nominated by the President and 27 chiefs as *ex officio* members, and a representative of the Paramount Chief. A new Assembly must be elected after every 5 years, but it may be dissolved at any time by the President. All existing tribal, community and regional councils were retained with their status and powers unchanged, like those of the tribal leaders.

The *President* is Brig. Gabriel Ramushwana, who seized power in April 1990.

Flag: Three horizontal stripes of green, yellow, and brown, with a brown V on the yellow stripe, and a blue vertical strip in the hoist.

DEFENCE. The Venda Defence Force was formed in 1983. It includes a small aviation component operating 1 Alouette III and 1 BK-117 helicopters.

INTERNATIONAL RELATIONS

Aid. The Republic of South Africa granted aid of R45m. in 1981–82.

ECONOMY

Budget. The 1989–90 budget envisaged expenditure of R776m.

Currency. South African Rand.

NATURAL RESOURCES

Water. In 1989 there were 4 major dams with a total capacity of 26·1m. cu. metres, and a purification plant.

Minerals. Venda is relatively poor in mineral resources, although there are large supplies of stone for construction. Coal is the most important mineral; there are large deposits in the west near Makhado. In 1988 further development was planned of the trial coal mine in the east at Tshikondeni to increase production from 208,000 to 750,000 tons a year.

Agriculture. About 85% of Venda is suitable only for the raising of livestock because of insufficient rainfall and poor soils, while some 10% is suited to dry-land crop production. Over 10,965 hectares have been given over to forest, mainly pine and eucalyptus. Eighteen irrigation schemes are being developed and there is extensive reclamation and conservation of eroded or overgrazed land. Only maize is grown on a comparatively large scale, but tea, sisal, groundnuts, coffee and subtropical fruits are increasing in importance. Over 80% of the working population are engaged in agriculture.

INDUSTRY AND TRADE

Industry. Industrial development is still in its early stages, and since Venda's location is unfavourable, the Government is concentrating on the promotion of agro-industries utilizing local produce, and small-scale industries. A chutney factory has recently been established, in addition to a tea processing plant, a furniture factory and several saw-mills. A copper-chrome arsenate preservation plant has been established at Phiphidi. At Shayandima a 20-hectare industrial area has been prepared. In 1989 the 460-ha Shayandima industrial area at Thohoyandou had over 70 developed sites with 43 industries, and 21 new factories under construction. There was a second major industrial area at Muraleni, and commercial complexes at Makhado. In 1986 there were 159 manufacturing establishments, mainly small labour-intensive firms with a total employment of 3,016 and 906 commercial establishments with employment of 3,803.

Labour. In 1986, 45,000 migrant workers earned R180m. in the Republic of South Africa. In 1985 an estimated 6,500 border commuters worked in the Republic of South Africa, income R26m.

Commerce. Venda is a member of the South African Customs Union and trade is mainly with the Republic of South Africa. Exports include sub-tropical fruit, tea, coffee, timber, clothing, furniture and pottery. Petroleum products, machinery, motor vehicles, food, clothing and furniture are imported.

Tourism. In 1989 there were 3 National Parks, 2 caravan parks and 2 holiday resorts.

COMMUNICATIONS

Roads. There were (1989) 2,100 km of roads, of which 300 km had a permanent surface.

Aviation. An airline, inaugurated in 1981, operates between Nwangundu in Thohoyandu and Johannesburg *via* Pietersburg and Pretoria.

Telecommunications. In 1989 there were 17 post offices, 21 postal agencies and 14 money order offices, and telex and fax facilities in all urban areas. There were 3 automatic and 13 manual telephone exchanges, and 15 telephone agencies. In 1989 the government-owned Radio Thohoyandou broadcast 24 hours daily in Venda and English on MW and FM, and South African television programmes were received through its transposers.

Newspapers. In 1989 there was 1 newspaper published weekly in Venda and English, with a circulation of 33,000.

JUSTICE, EDUCATION AND WELFARE

Justice. The Supreme Court acts as the Court of Appeal for the 5 magistrates' courts and 2 sub-offices, 2 periodical courts and the one Regional Court. Appeals from the Supreme Court are heard in the Republic of South Africa Appeal Court.

Education. The Department of Education assumed responsibility for education on independence. Education is free up to Standard 2, and pupils are taught in the native tongue, Luvenda, for the first 4 years (up to Standard 2), after which English is gradually introduced. Secondary education comprises Standards 6 to 10.

In 1989 there were 661 schools with 227,569 pupils and (1988) 7,200 teachers, 4 teacher training colleges, 3 trade schools, 1 technical high school and 1 special school. The University of Venda was established in 1981; 4,500 students (1988).

Health. In 1989 there were 3 general hospitals (1,433 beds), 2 maternity hospitals (38 beds), 2 health centres (80 beds), 51 clinics, 1 chronic ill-health institution (412 beds) and 508 rural care groups. There were about 35 doctors in the general hospitals and 15 private doctors in different areas, and 1,411 nurses.

Welfare. In 1986-87 the Government spent R20·6m. on social pension payments to 34,388 pensioners; civil pensions' payments were R1,982,127 to 301 beneficiaries.

Further Reading

Venda 1983. Dept. of Information and Broadcasting. Sibasa, 1984

CISKEI

HISTORY. On 4 Dec. 1981 the Republic of South Africa gave independence to Ciskei, the fourth of the tribal homelands.

Brig. Oupo Gqozo seized power in a bloodless coup in March 1990.

AREA AND POPULATION. Ciskei lies between latitudes 32° and 33°35' and longitudes 26°20' and 27°48', and has a coastal boundary between East London and Port Alfred. The total area is about 9,000 sq. km. The population was (1987) 2m. but only 1m. live in Ciskei. The remainder are resident and workers in the Republic of South Africa.

Populations of towns (1987): Mdantsane, 350,000; Zwelitsha, 55,000; Sada, 38,000; Dimbaza, 25,000 and Litha, 9,500. The capital, Bisho, houses 8,000 people, although the development is still going on.

CONSTITUTION AND GOVERNMENT. In 1981 Ciskei became an independent democratic republic. The Government had consisted of a President, an Executive Council and a National Assembly of Hereditary Chiefs, elected and nominated members and the Paramount Chief's representatives. On 4 March 1990, in a bloodless coup, the President-for-life, Dr Lennox Sebe was deposed. The Constitution was suspended. The coup was led by Brig. Oupo Gqozo. A constitutional amendment of Feb. 1991 relinquished sovereignty, and made over constitutional, financial and judicial control to the Republic of South Africa.

Flag: Blue, a broad diagonal band from lower hoist to upper fly, charged with a black crane.

National Anthem: Nkosi Sikelel' i Afrika, composed by Enoch Sontonga.

DEFENCE. There is a Ciskei Defence Force. Its aviation element is equipped with 2 Skyvan and 3 Islander transports, and 3 BK-117 and 1 BO 105 helicopters, plus 2 Cessna 152 trainers.

ECONOMY

Budget. The 1987–88 budget balanced at R859m.

Currency. South African Rand.

ENERGY AND NATURAL RESOURCES

Electricity. Ciskei is totally dependent on power supply lines maintained by the Republic of South Africa.

Minerals. Mineral resources are mainly undeveloped and in 1988 only two mines existed in Ciskei, one producing dolorite, the other rutile ilmenite, leucoxene and zircon.

Agriculture. In 1977–78, total agricultural production was valued at R8·26m.

In 1986, the dryland products included (in tons): Maize, 3,125; wheat, 131; sorghum, 325; sunflower, 8·7. Horticultural crops included (1986, in tons): Potatoes, 979·9; cabbage, 5,135·8; carrots, 981·1; brussel sprouts, 356; onions, 4·8; pumpkins, 102·4; cauliflower, 11·6; peas, 28; dry beans, 83·3; spinach, 1·9; beetroot, 8·5.

Livestock (1986): 11,442 cattle, 76,294 sheep, 77,568 goats, 3,743 pigs, 14,742,814 poultry.

Forestry. In 1983–84, 5,500 ha were planted mainly with conifers. The indigenous forest covered some 18,000 ha. In 1984–85 (estimate), production of timber was valued at R600,000.

INDUSTRY AND TRADE

Industry. In 1988 total investment was R467m. The chief manufactures include textiles, timber products, electronic components, steel products, food and leather goods.

Commerce. International trade is mainly with the Republic of South Africa and no separate figures are available. The main exports are pineapples, timber and manufactured goods.

Tourism. Tourism is an important and developing industry.

COMMUNICATIONS

Roads. In 1988 there were 448 km of tarred roads and 2,556 km of gravel roads.

Railways. There are two main railway lines serving the southern part of Ciskei.

Aviation. Ciskei uses East London's airport and there is a new international airport at Bulembu, near Bisho.

Shipping. Ciskei has no harbour of its own but has full access to the facilities of East London in the Republic of South Africa.

Telecommunications. All major centres have post offices and manual and automatic telephone exchanges; telex facilities are available. There were (1987–88) 21,095 telephones. Radio Ciskei broadcasts from Bisho daily.

Newspapers (1988). There were three Ciskeian newspapers: *Umthombo*; *Imvo*, first published in 1884; *Umtha*, an agricultural newspaper.

JUSTICE, RELIGION, EDUCATION AND WELFARE

Justice. The Supreme Court acts as Court of Appeal for the eight Magistrates' Courts, which in turn act as Courts of Appeal for the Chiefs' Courts. Appeals from the Supreme Court are heard by the Appellate Division of Ciskei in Bisho.

Religion. In 1988 (estimate) the population was 27% Methodists, 20% Independent, 16% Presbyterian, 12% Anglicans, 7% Roman Catholics and 5% Dutch Reformed Church.

Education. In 1986–87 there were 545 primary schools with 200,752 pupils and 4,369 teachers; 158 post primary schools with 59,414 students and 1,809 teachers; 3 training colleges with 1,677 students and 97 teachers and 1 vocational school with 174 students and 20 teachers. The University of Fort Hare had a total of 2,304 students in 1981.

Health. In 1987–88, there were 8 hospitals with 2,910 beds, and a total of 2,952 nursing staff.

Social Welfare. Pensions paid in 1984–85:

	Beneficiaries	*Amount (R1,000)*
Old age	42,573	20,435
Blind	564	270
Disability	5,421	2,602
War veterans	72	38
Leprosy	11	5

Further Reading

Charlton, N., *Ciskei: Economics and Politics of Dependence in a South African Homeland.* London, 1980
Pauw, B. A., *Christianity and the Xhosa Tradition.* OUP, 1975
Van der Kooy, R. (ed.) *The Republic of Ciskei: A Nation in Transition.* Pretoria, 1981

SOUTH GEORGIA AND SOUTH SANDWICH ISLANDS

HISTORY. South Georgia was probably first sighted by a London merchant, Antonio de la Roche, and then in 1756 by a Spanish Captain, Gregorie Jerez. The first landing and exploration was undertaken by Captain James Cook, who formally took possession in the name of George III on 17 Jan. 1775. British sealers arrived in 1788 and American sealers in 1791. Sealing reached its peak in 1800. A German team was the first to carry out scientific studies there in 1882–83. Whaling began in 1904 when the Compania Argentina de Pesca formed by C. A. Larsen, a Norwegian, established a station at Grytviken. Six other stations were established up to 1912. Whaling ceased in 1966 and the civil administration was withdrawn. Argentine forces invaded South Georgia on 3 April 1982. A British naval task force recovered the Island on 25 April 1982.

AREA AND POPULATION. South Georgia lies 800 miles south-east of the Falkland Islands and has an area of 1,450 sq. miles. The South Sandwich Islands are 470 miles south-east of South Georgia and have an area of 130 sq. miles. There has been no permanent population in South Georgia since the whaling station at Leith was abandoned in 1966. There is a small military garrison. The British Antarctic Survey have a biological station on Bird Island. The South Sandwich Islands are uninhabited.

CLIMATE. The climate is wet and cold with strong winds and little seasonal variation. 15°C is occasionally reached on a windless day. Temperatures below –15°C at sea level are unusual.

CONSTITUTION AND GOVERNMENT. Under the new Constitution which came into force on 3 Oct. 1985 the Territories ceased to be dependencies of the Falkland Islands. Executive power is vested in a Commissioner who is the officer for the time being administering the Government of the Falkland Islands. The Commissioner is obliged to consult the officer for the time being commanding Her Majesty's British Forces in the South Atlantic on matters relating to defence and internal security (except police). The Commissioner whenever practicable consults the Executive Council of the Falkland Islands on the exercise of functions that in his opinion might affect the Falkland Islands. There is no Legislative Council. Laws are made by the Commissioner.

Commissioner: W. H. Fullerton, CMG.

Economy. The total revenue of the Territories (estimate, 1988–89) £268,240, mainly from philatelic sales and investment income. Expenditure estimate £194,260.

Communications. There is occasional direct sea communication between the Falkland Islands and South Georgia and the South Sandwich Islands by means of the Royal Research Ships *John Biscoe* and *Bransfield* and the ice patrol vessel *HMS Endurance*. Royal Fleet Auxiliary ships, which serve the garrison, run regularly to South Georgia. Mail is dropped from military aircraft.

Justice. There is a Supreme Court for the Territories and a Court of Appeal in the United Kingdom. Appeals may go from that court to the Judicial Committee of the Privy Council. There is no magistrate permanently in residence. The Officer Commanding the garrison is usually appointed a magistrate.

Further Reading

Headland, R. K., *The Island of South Georgia*. CUP, 1985

SPAIN

Capital: Madrid
Population: 39·54m. (1990)
GNP per capita: US$8,620 (1989)

Reino de España

(Kingdom of Spain)

HISTORY. Although Spain has traditionally been a monarchy there have been two Republics, the first in 1873, which lasted for 11 months, and the second 1931–39; both were democratically and peacefully proclaimed. Part of the army rebelled against the republican government on 18 July 1936, thus beginning the Spanish Civil War, *see* THE STATESMAN'S YEAR-BOOK, 1939, pp. 1325–26. The new regime was led by Gen. Franco, who had been proclaimed Head of State and Government in 1936, and its institutions were based on single party rule, with the *Falange* as the only legal political organization.

In July 1969, Prince Don Juan Carlos de Borbón y Borbón, grandson of Alfonso XIII, was sworn in as successor to the Head of State and he had the title of HRH Prince of Spain until he became King.

Gen. Francisco Franco y Bahamonde died on 20 Nov. 1975 and on 22 Nov. Prince Juan Carlos de Borbón y Borbón took the oath as Juan Carlos I, King of Spain.

AREA AND POPULATION. Spain is bounded north by the Bay of Biscay and the Pyrenees (which form the frontier with France and Andorra), east and south by the Mediterranean and the Straits of Gibraltar, south-west by the Atlantic and west by Portugal and the Atlantic. Continental Spain has an area of 492,592 sq. km, and including the Balearic and Canary Islands and the towns of Ceuta and Melilla 504,750 sq. km (194,884 sq. miles). Population (mid-decennial census, 1986), 38,891,313. Estimate (1990) 39,541,782 (20,124,818 female).

The growth of the population has been as follows:

Census year	*Population*	*Rate of annual increase*	*Census year*	*Population*	*Rate of annual increase*
1860	15,655,467	0·34	1950	27,976,755	0·81
1910	19,927,150	0·72	1960	30,903,137	0·88
1920	21,303,162	0·69	1970	33,823,918	0·94
1930	23,563,867	1·06	1981	37,746,260	1·15
1940	25,877,971	0·98			

Area and population of the autonomous communities and provinces, mid-decennial census of 1 April 1986:

Autonomous community Province	*Area (sq. km)*	*Population*	*Per sq. km*	*Autonomous community Province*	*Area (sq. km)*	*Population*	*Per sq. km*
Andalusia	*87,268*	*6,875,628*	*78*	Zaragoza	17,194	845,832	49
Almería	8,774	448,592	51	*Asturias*	*10,565*	*1,114,115*	*106*
Cádiz	7,385	1,054,503	142	*Baleares*	*5,014*	*754,777*	*151*
Córdoba	13,718	745,175	54	*Basque Country, The*	*7,261*	*2,133,002*	*296*
Granada	12,531	796,857	63	Álava	3,047	275,703	92
Huelva	10,085	430,918	43	Guipúzcoa	1,997	688,894	344
Jaén	13,498	633,612	47	Vizcaya	2,217	1,168,405	531
Málaga	7,276	1,215,479	168	*Canary Islands*	*7,273*	*1,614,882*	*221*
Sevilla	14,001	1,550,492	110	Palmas, Las	4,065	855,494	213
Aragón	*47,669*	*1,214,729*	*25*	Santa Cruz de Tenerife	3,208	759,388	237
Huesca	15,671	220,824	14				
Teruel	14,804	148,073	10				

Autonomous community / *Province*	*Area (sq. km)*	*Population*	*Per sq. km*	*Autonomous community* / *Province*	*Area (sq. km)*	*Population*	*Per sq. km*
Cantabria	*5,289*	*524,670*	*99*	Tarragona	6,283	531,281	84
Castilla-La Mancha	*79,226*	*1,665,029*	*21*	*Extremadura*	*41,602*	*1,088,543*	*26*
Albacete	14,858	342,278	23	Badajoz	21,657	664,516	30
Ciudad Real	19,749	477,967	24	Cáceres	19,945	424,027	21
Cuenca	17,061	210,932	12	*Galicia*	*29,434*	*2,785,394*	*94*
Guadalajara	12,190	146,008	12	Coruña, La	7,876	1,102,376	141
Toledo	15,368	487,844	31	Lugo	9,803	399,232	40
Castilla-León	*94,147*	*2,600,330*	*27*	Orense	7,278	399,378	55
Ávila	8,048	179,207	22	Pontevedra	4,477	884,408	197
Burgos	14,269	363,530	25	*Madrid*	*7,995*	*4,854,616*	*607*
León	15,468	528,502	34	*Murcia*	*11,317*	*1,014,285*	*89*
Palencia	8,029	188,472	23	*Navarra*	*10,421*	*512,676*	*49*
Salamanca	12,336	366,668	29	*Rioja, La*	*5,034*	*262,611*	*52*
Segovia	6,949	151,520	21	*Valencian Community*	*23,305*	*3,772,002*	*161*
Soria	10,287	97,565	9	Alicante	5,863	1,254,920	216
Valladolid	8,202	503,306	61	Castellón	6,679	437,320	66
Zamora	10,559	221,560	21	Valencia	10,763	2,079,762	194
Catalonia	*31,930*	*5,977,008*	*187*	*Ceuta* [1]	*18*	*71,403*	*3,996*
Barcelona	7,773	4,598,249	591	*Melilla* [1]	*14*	*55,613*	*3,972*
Gerona	5,886	490,667	83				
Lérida	12,028	356,811	29	*Total*	*504,750*	*38,891,313*	*77*

[1] Ceuta and Melilla are municipalities on the northern coast of Morocco. They are to gain full provincial status in 1991.

The capitals of the autonomous communities are as follows: Andalusia, cap. Sevilla (Seville); Aragón, cap. Zaragoza (Saragossa); Asturias, cap. Oviedo; Baleares (Balearic Islands), cap. Palma de Mallorca; The Basque Country, cap. Vitoria; Canary Islands, dual and alternative capital, Las Palmas and Santa Cruz de Tenerife; Cantabria, cap. Santander; ; Castilla-La Mancha, cap. Toledo; Castilla-León, cap. Valladolid; Catalonia, cap. Barcelona; Extremadura, cap. Mérida; Galicia, cap. Santiago de Compostela; Madrid, cap. Madrid; Murcia, cap. Murcia (but regional parliament in Cartagena); Navarra, cap. Pamplona; La Rioja, cap. Logroño; Valencian Community, cap. Valencia.

The capitals of the provinces are in the towns from which they take the name, except in Álava (capital Vitoria), Asturias (Oviedo), Baleares (Palma de Mallorca), Cantabria (Santander), Guipúzcoa (San Sebastián), La Rioja (Logroño), Navarra (Pamplona) and Vizcaya (Bilbao).

On 1 April 1986 there were 19,771,007 females and 19,120,306 males.

By decree of 21 Sept. 1927 the islands which form the Canary Archipelago were divided into 2 provinces, under the name of their respective capitals: Santa Cruz de Tenerife and Las Palmas de Gran Canaria. The province of Santa Cruz de Tenerife is constituted by the islands of Tenerife, La Palma, Gomera and Hierro, and that of Las Palmas by Gran Canaria, Lanzarote and Fuerteventura, with the small barren islands of Alegranza, Roque del Este, Roque del Oeste, Graciosa, Montaña Clara and Lobos. The area of the islands is 7,273 sq. km; population (mid-decennial census 1986), 1,614,882. Places under Spanish sovereignty in Morocco are: Alhucemas, Ceuta, Chafarinas, Melilla and Peñón de Vélez.

The following were the registered populations of principal towns at mid-decennial census 1986:

Town	*Population*	*Town*	*Population*	*Town*	*Population*
Albacete	127,169	Baracaldo	112,854	Cornellá	86,467
Alcalá de Henares	150,221	Barcelona	1,694,064	Coruña, La	241,808
Alcorcón	137,225	Bilbao	378,221	Elche	173,392
Algeciras	97,213	Burgos	163,910	Ferrol, El	88,101
Alicante	265,543	Cáceres	79,342	Fuenlabrada	119,463
Almería	156,838	Cádiz	154,051	Gerona	67,578
Avila	44,618	Cartagena	168,809	Getafe	130,971
Badajoz	126,340	Castellón	129,813	Gijón	259,226
Badalona	223,444	Córdoba	304,826	Granada	280,592

Town	Population	Town	Population	Town	Population
Hospitalet	276,865	Orense	102,455	Santa Cruz de Tenerife	211,389
Huelva	135,427	Oviedo	190,651	Santander	188,539
Jerez de la Frontera	180,444	Palencia	76,707	Santiago de Compostela	104,045
Jaén	102,826	Palma de Mallorca	321,112	Sevilla	668,356
Laguna, La	114,223	Palmas, Las	372,270	Tarragona	109,557
Leganés	167,088	Pamplona	183,703	Tarrasa	159,530
León	137,414	Reus	83,251	Torrejón de Ardoz	79,877
Lérida	111,507	Sabadell	185,960	Valencia	738,575
Logroño	118,770	Salamanca	166,615	Valladolid	341,194
Lugo	77,728	San Baudilio del Llobregat	75,388	Vigo	263,998
Madrid	3,123,713	San Fernando	84,940	Vitoria	207,501
Málaga	595,264	San Sebastián	180,043	Zaragoza	596,080
Mataró	99,642	Santa Coloma de Gramanet	133,515		
Móstoles	175,802				
Murcia	309,504				

Vital statistics for calendar years:

	Marriages	*Births*	*Deaths*
1984	192,406	465,709	295,425
1985	193,128	451,373	308,430
1986	203,394	434,490	306,613
1987	210,098	421,799	309,364
1988	214,898	415,844	318,848

On 31 Dec. 1988 the number of foreigners legally registered was 360,032 (largest foreign community, British, 64,081).

Languages. The Constitution states that 'Castilian is the Spanish official language of the State', but also that 'All other Spanish languages will also be official in the corresponding Autonomous Communities'.

Catalan is spoken by a majority of people in Catalonia (64%, 1986) and Baleares (70·8%), and by one half in Valencian Community (49%, where it is frequently called Valencian); in Aragón, a narrow strip close to Catalonia and Valencian Community boundaries, speaks Catalan.

Galician, a language very close to Portuguese, is spoken by a majority of people in Galicia (90%, 1986); Basque, by a significant minority in the Basque Country (24·5%). Basque is also spoken by a small minority in north-west Navarra (12%).

In bilingual communities, both Spanish and the regional language are taught in the schools and universities.

CLIMATE. Most of Spain has a form of Mediterranean climate with mild, moist winters and hot, dry summers, but the northern coastal region has a moist, equable climate, with rainfall well-distributed throughout the year, mild winters and warm summers, though having less sunshine than the rest of Spain.

Madrid. Jan. 41°F (5°C), July 77°F (25°C). Annual rainfall 16·8" (419 mm). Barcelona. Jan. 46°F (8°C), July 74°F (23·5°C). Annual rainfall 21" (525 mm). Cartagena. Jan. 51°F (10·5°C), July 75°F (24°C). Annual rainfall 14·9" (373 mm). La Coruña. Jan. 51°F (10·5°C), July 66°F (19°C). Annual rainfall 32" (800 mm). Sevilla. Jan. 51°F (10·5°C), July 85°F (29·5°C). Annual rainfall 19·5" (486 mm). Palma de Mallorca (Balearic Islands). Jan. 51°F (11°C), July 77°F (25°C). Annual rainfall 13·6" (347 mm). Santa Cruz de Tenerife (Canary Islands). Jan. 64°F (17·9°C), July 76°F (24·4°C). Annual rainfall 7·72" (196 mm).

KING. Juan Carlos I, born 5 Jan. 1938. The eldest son of Don Juan, Conde de Barcelona. Juan Carlos was given precedence over his father as pretender to the Spanish throne in an agreement in 1954 between Don Juan and Gen. Franco. Don Juan resigned his claims to the throne in May 1977. King (then Prince) Juan Carlos married, in 1962, Princess Sophia of Greece, daughter of the late King Paul of the Hellenes and Queen Frederika. *Offspring:* Elena, born 20 Dec. 1963; Cristina, 13 June 1965; Felipe, Prince of Asturias, Heir to the throne, 30 Jan. 1968.

CONSTITUTION AND GOVERNMENT. The *Cortes* (Parliament) was freely elected on 15 June 1977. The text of the new Constitution was approved by referendum on 6 Dec. 1978, and came into force 29 Dec. 1978. It established a parliamentary monarchy, with King Juan Carlos I as head of state. Legislative power is vested in the Cortes, a bicameral parliament composed of the *Congress of Deputies* (lower house) and the *Senate* (upper house). The Congress of Deputies has not less than 300 nor more than 400 members (350 in the general elections of 1977, 1979, 1982, 1986 and 1989), all elected in a proportional system reflecting the population of every province. The members of the Senate are elected in a majority system: The 47 mainland provinces elect 4 senators each, regardless of population; the island provinces electing 5 (Baleares, Las Palmas) or 6 (Santa Cruz de Tenerife); and Ceuta and Melilla, 2 senators each. There are 208 senators, to whom are added some other members of the upper house elected by the parliaments of the autonomous communities. Deputies and senators are elected in universal (but not compulsory), direct, free, equal and secret suffrage, for a term of 4 years, liable to dissolution. Executive power is vested in the President of the Government (*Prime Minister*) and a Cabinet; the Prime Minister is elected by the Congress of Deputies.

A general election took place on 29 Oct. 1989.

In Feb. 1991 the composition of the 350-member Congress of Deputies was: Spanish Workers Socialist Party (PSOE), 175; Popular Party (PP, conservative), 107; United Left (IU, communist dominated coalition), 17; Convergence and Union (CiU, Catalan nationalists), 18; Social and Democratic Centre (CDS, centrist), 14; Basque Nationalist Party (PNV), 5; Herri Batasuna (HB, Basque separatists), 4; Andalusian Party (PA, Andalusian regionalists), 2; Eusko Alkartasuna (EA) and Euskadiko Eskerra (EE), both non-radical Basque separatists, 2 each; Valencian Union (UV, Valencian regionalists), 2; two conservative regional parties from Aragón and the Canaries, 1 each. The Speaker (*Presidente*) is Félix Pons Irazazábal (PSOE).

Senate: 208 members, excluding those elected by regional parliaments (250 including them): PSOE, 106; PP, 78; CiU, 10; PNV, 4; HB, 3; CDS, 2; IU, 1; four different groups from the Canaries, 4 in all. Speaker (*Presidente*) of the Senate, Juan José Laborda (PSOE).

The Council of Ministers was composed as follows in Feb. 1991:

President of the Government (Prime Minister): Felipe González Márquez (Secretary-General of PSOE).

Vice-President of the Government: Narcís Serra i Serra. *Foreign Affairs:* Francisco Fernández Ordóñez. *Economy and Finance:* Carlos Solchaga Catalán. *Industry, Commerce and Tourism:* Claudio Aranzadi Martínez. *Interior:* José Luis Corcuera. *Defence:* Julián García Vargas. *Public Administration:* Juan Manuel Eguiagaray. *Education and Science:* Javier Solana Madariaga. *Public Works and Transport:* José Borrell. *Justice:* Tomas de la Quadra Salcedo. *Culture:* Jordi Solé Tura. *Agriculture, Fisheries and Food:* Pedro Solbes. *Health and Consumers Affairs:* Julián García Valverde. *Labour and Social Security:* Luis Maritínez Noval. *Social Affairs:* Matilde Fernández. *Minister, Government Spokeswoman:* Rosa Conde. *Relations with the Cortes and Secretary of the Cabinet:* Virgilio Zapatero.

National flag: Three horizontal stripes of red, yellow, red, with the yellow of double width, and charged near the hoist with the national arms.

National anthem: Marcha real.

Regional and local government. The Constitution of 1978 establishes a semi-federal system of regional administration, with the *autonomous community (comunidad autónoma)* as its basic element. There are 17 autonomous communities, each of them having a Parliament, elected by universal vote, and a regional government; all possess exclusive legislative and executive power in many matters, as listed in the national Constitution and in their own fundamental law *(estatuto de autonomía)*. The Basque Country and Catalonia elected their first parliaments in March 1980, Galicia in Oct. 1981 and Andalusia in May 1982. All others in May 1983. Further elections were held in the autonomous communities 1984–90. In elections to the regional parliament in *Andalusia* in June 1990, the PSOE won 61 out of 109 seats; the PP, 27; the United Left, 11; the Andalusian Party, 10. Turn-out was 55%.

In elections to the regional parliament in the *Basque Country* in Oct. 1990, the Basque Nationalist Party (PNV) won 22 of the 75 seats; PSOE, 16; Herri Batasuna,

13; Eusko Alkartasuna (EA), 9; Euskadiko Ezquerra (EE), 6; the Popular Party, 6; Alaversa Union, 3. A PNV-EA-EE coalition government was formed in Jan. 1991.

There are 7 autonomous communities composed of only one province: Asturias, Cantabria, La Rioja, Navarra, Baleares, Murcia and Madrid. The other 10 are formed by 2 or more provinces. In all, there are in Spain 50 provinces, since the administrative division established in 1833; Ceuta and Melilla, municipalities in the northern coast of Morocco, are scheduled to achieve full provincial status in 1991. The *Provincial Council (Diputación Provincial)* is the administrative organ of the province, except in the 7 autonomous communities composed of one only province, where there are only the regional legislative and executive powers. The provincial council is indirectly elected. Each of the 7 main islands of the Canaries (provinces of Las Palmas and Santa Cruz de Tenerife) has a directly elected corporation, the *Cabildo Insular,* to rule its special interests; in the main islands of the Balearics there is also an elected *Consell Insular*.

The provinces are constituted by the association of municipalities (8,063 on 10 June 1987). Municipalities are autonomous in their own sphere. At their head stands the municipal council *(Ayuntamiento),* members of which are elected in a universal ballot every 4 years, and they, in turn, elect one of them as Mayor *(Alcalde).*

DEFENCE. On 26 Sept. 1953 the US and Spain signed three agreements covering the construction and use of military facilities in Spain by the US, economic assistance, and military end-item assistance. These agreements were renewed several times, the last in July 1982. The American naval and air base at Rota (near Cádiz) is connected by pipelines with the American bomber bases at Morón de la Frontera (near Seville), Torrejón (near Madrid) and Zaragoza. The US will withdraw from Torrejón in 1991 (withdrawal began in Aug. 1988).

Length of service is 12 months which may be extended to from 16 to 36 months for volunteers. Since early 1989 women are accepted in all sections of the armed forces.

In March 1986 a referendum was conducted to establish whether Spain should remain in NATO. 52·5% of the voters were for the resolution.

Army. The Army is divided into 2 principal parts: 8 Regional Operation Commands (including 2 overseas) and the General Reserve Force. The former consist of 1 armoured, 1 mechanized, 2 mountain and 1 motorized divisions; 2 armoured cavalry, 1 parachute and 1 air-portable brigades; 1 infantry regiment and supporting artillery, engineer and signals units. The General Reserve Force comprises an airborne brigade with air defence, artillery and engineer units. There are also the Royal Guard unit, and the Army Aviation forces. Equipment includes 299 AMX-30, 329 M-47E, 46 M-47E2 and 164 M-48 tanks. The aviation element of the Army consists of 183 helicopters (60 armed). Strength (1991) 274,500 (including 200,900 conscripts). Of these 5,600 are stationed on the Balearic Islands, 10,000 on the Canary Islands and 15,800 in Ceuta and Melilla. The paramilitary Civil Guard number 63,000 men. Immediate army reserves number 142,700.

Navy. The accession of Spain to NATO, even though not fully integrated into the military structure, has provided the Navy with a key operational role in support of NATO sea lines of communication on the Canaries-Gibraltar-Balearics axis. The main task force, 'Grupo Alfa', is centred on the flagship, *Príncipe de Asturias*, escorted by new and modernized frigates.

The 17,000-tonne *Príncipe de Asturias*, a light vertical/short take-off and landing aircraft carrier built to a US design was commissioned in 1989. The *Príncipe de Asturias* air group comprises 8 AV-8B Matador, 8 Sea King anti-submarine helicopters, 2 Sea King early warning helicopters and about 4 AB-212 light helicopters.

There are also 8 French-designed submarines (4 Daphne class, 4 Agosta class), 4 old ex-US destroyers, 4 US-design Santa María guided missile frigates with Standard SM-1 surface-to-air missiles, 5 other guided missile frigates with Standard, and 6 smaller frigates, 4 offshore patrol vessels, 19 coastal and 37 inshore patrol craft, 4 ocean minesweepers, 8 coastal minesweepers, 2 amphibious troop transports, 3 tank landing ships and 11 landing craft. Major auxiliaries include 1 transport, 6 ocean tugs, 1 training ship, 4 water carriers and 6 survey ships. There are about 80 minor auxiliaries and service craft.

The Navy is being renewed and modernized; 2 frigates have been ordered. A fleet replenishment ship is being designed in co-operation with the Netherlands, and mine countermeasures vessels will start building shortly to the British Sandown class design.

The Naval Air Service operates 22 EAV-8 and EAV-8B Harrier-II attack aircraft, 39 Sea King, AB-212 and Hughes 500 anti-submarine helicopters, 3 radar early warning Sea Kings and a few additional training and utility aircraft. The Air force operates 6 Orion maritime patrol aircraft on anti-submarine tasks.

There are 7,500 marines, who provide 1 amphibious regiment and garrison regiments at the main bases. Main naval bases are at Ferrol, Rota, Cádiz, Cartagena, Palma de Mallorca, Mahón and Las Palmas (Canary Islands).

In 1990 personnel totalled 34,400 (23,800 conscripts) including marines.

Air Force. The Air Force is organized as an independent service, dating from 1939. It is administered through 4 operational commands. These comprise Air Combat Command which controls interceptor squadrons (including USAF elements) and the control and warning radar network, Tactical and Transport Commands, and Air Command of the Canaries. Strength (1991) 33,700 (18,600 conscripts), with 59,200 immediate reserves and 221 combat aircraft.

The Tactical Air Command has 2 fighter-bomber squadrons of Spanish-built Northrop SF-5s, 1 aero-naval co-operation squadron with P-3 Orion anti-submarine aircraft, and a liaison flight at Tablada with CASA 127s. Air Combat Command has 2 squadrons of Mirage III-Es, 1 squadron of RF-4C Phantom IIs, 3 squadrons of F-18 Hornets and 2 squadrons of Mirage F1-Cs, plus a flight of CASA/Dornier Do27/127 liaison aircraft. Five KC-130H tankers support the fighter squadrons. Three wings of Air Transport Command operate C-130 Hercules, Caribou and Spanish-built CASA Aviocars. Air Command of the Canaries has 3 squadrons, equipped with Aviocar transports; Mirage F1 fighter-bombers; F27 Maritime aircraft and Super Puma helicopters for search and rescue. Other equipment includes 2 Boeing 707s, 2 CN-235s, 5 Falcons and helicopters for VIP transport; and aircraft for photographic, firefighting, target towing and research duties. Air-sea rescue units have Aviocars and Super Puma helicopters.

American-built F33 Bonanza and Chilean-built Pillan piston-engined aircraft are used for basic training, after which pupil pilots progress to CASA C-101 jet aircraft. Two-seat versions of operational types are used as advanced trainers. Other training types include Beechcraft Barons for instrument flying and liaison duties.

INTERNATIONAL RELATIONS

Membership. Spain is a member of the UN, the Council of Europe, NATO, WEU, the EC and OECD.

ECONOMY

Budget. Revenue and expenditure in 1m. pesetas:

	1986	*1987*	*1988*	*1989*	*1990*
Revenue	7,164,232	8,113,442	8,939,237	10,644,507	12,629,510
Expenditure	7,164,232	8,113,442	8,939,237	10,644,507	12,629,510

The budget is made up as follows (in 1m. pesetas):

Revenue (1990)		*Revenue (1990) continued*	
Direct taxes	4,880,000	Real estate income	724,631
Indirect taxes	4,413,000	Deficit (financed with public	
Levies and various revenues	531,000	debt, treasury loans, etc)	1,672,183
Current transactions	408,696		

Expenditure (1990)		*Expenditure (1990) continued*	
H.M. House	795	Constitutional Court	1,121
Cortes (Parliament)	12,818	Council of State	565
Court of Accounts	2,721	Public Debt	2,364,682

Expenditure (1990) continued	
Civil Service Pensions	543,261
General Council of the Judicial Power	1,533
Relations with the Cortes and Secretariat of the Cabinet	21,901
Ministry of Foreign Affairs	67,120
„ Justice	188,049
„ Defence	870,434
„ Finance	404,162
„ Interior	431,090
„ Public Works and Housing	597,141
„ Education and Science	975,263
„ Labour and Social Security	1,011,439

Expenditure (1990) continued	
Ministry of Industry and Energy	202,241
„ Agriculture and Food	198,215
„ Transport, Tourism and Communications	584,201
„ Culture	49,123
„ Public Administration	35,750
„ Health and Consumer Affairs	1,310,415
„ Social Affairs	35,014
„ the Government Spokeswoman	1,824
Regional governments	1,800,864
Regional Compensation Fund	239,802
Expenses in several ministries	294,308
Financial relations with EEC	383,653

Currency. The unit of currency is the *peseta* (ESP), notionally divided into 100 *céntimos* (not in use since 1984).

Bank-notes of 10,000, 5,000, 2,000, 1,000, 500, 200 and 100 *pesetas* and coins of 1 *peseta* (copper and aluminium), 2, 5, 10, 25, 50, 100, 200 and 500 *pesetas* (nickel and copper) are in circulation. In Dec. 1988 the circulation of bank-notes was 3,413,500m. *pesetas* and of coins, 214,000m. *pesetas*.

In March 1991, £1 = 181·35 *pesetas*; US$1 = 95·60.

Inflation rate in Dec. 1987, 4·6%; 1988, 5·8%; 1989, 6·9%; 1990, 6·7%.

Banking and Finance. On 1 Jan. 1922 the Bank of Spain (Governor, Mariano Rubio) came under the Bank Ordinance Law, according to which the Government participate in its net profits.

The 9 largest banks are: Banco Bilbao Vizcaya; Banco Central; Banco Español de Crédito; Banco Hispano Americano; Banco de Santander; Banco Popular Español; Banco Exterior de España; Banco Pastor; Banco de Sabadell. All are privately owned except the Banco Exterior de España.

Spanish banks deposits, 30 June 1988, amounted to 19,053,135m pesetas; foreign banks, 402,405m.; savings banks, 14,152,285m.; rural (farmers) savings banks, 698,896m.

There are stock exchanges in Madrid, Barcelona, Bilbao and Valencia.

Weights and Measures. On 1 Jan. 1859 the metric system of weights and measures was introduced.

ENERGY AND NATURAL RESOURCES

Electricity. Electric power-stations in 1989 had a total installed capacity of 45·5m. kw. The total output 1989, amounted to 147,500m. kwh of which 19,600m. hydro-electric and 56,100m. nuclear. There were 10 nuclear power stations, with a net capacity of 7·5m. kw (Jan. 1989), which produced 36% of electricity in 1990. Supply 110 and 220 volts; 50 Hz.

Oil. Crude oil production (1990) 0·83m. tonnes.

Gas. Production of natural gas in 1989 was 1,512m. cu. metres.

Minerals. Spain has a relatively wide range of minerals but most of them are found in small or moderate quantities. Production of the principal minerals (in 1,000 tonnes; net metal content):

	1988	*1989*		*1988*	*1989*
Anthracite	5,271	5,573	Lead	71	62
Coal	9,211	8,951	Zinc	247	266
Lignite	17,288	21,927	Tin [1]	59	64
Uranium [1]	306	255	Wolfram [1]	101	73
Iron	1,940	2,127	Fluorspar	151	156
Pyrites	1,060	894	Potassium salts	1,360	1,582
Copper	9	25			

[1] Tonnes.

Agriculture. In 1988 the total value of agricultural produce was 1,852·3m. pesetas; of livestock, 1,141·3m. Land under cultivation in 1989 (in 1,000 ha) included: Cereals, 7,715; vegetables, 433; potatoes, 233. In 1989, 690,000 tractors and 54,600 harvesters were in use.

Principal crops	*Area (in 1,000 ha)* 1986	1987	1988	1989	*Yield (in 1,000 tonnes)* 1986	1987	1988	1989
Wheat	2,096	2,174	2,332	2,295	4,292	5,774	6,514	5,456
Barley	4,334	4,377	4,175	4,257	7,331	9,533	12,070	9,308
Oats	384	378	335	345	422	502	537	494
Rye	223	222	222	227	220	321	357	337
Rice	79	78	80	59	494	482	499	341
Maize	525	526	535	516	3,405	3,338	3,577	3,224
Potatoes	289	303	280	274	4,857	5,550	4,578	5,230
Sugar-beet	195	184	194	171	7,629	7,638	9,056	7,434
Sunflower	936	978	894	950	844	926	1,123	869

In 1986, 1,574,000 ha were under vines; production of wine was (1989) 30·3m. hectolitres. The area under onions was 27,000 ha, yielding 1,011,000 tonnes. Production of oranges and mandarines was 4,105,000 tonnes, lemons, 605,000. Other products are esparto, flax, hemp and pulse. Spain has important industries connected with the preparation of wine and fruits.

Industrial crops (1989 in 1,000 tonnes): Cotton, 194; olive oil, 466; tobacco, 41.

Livestock products (1989 in 1,000 tonnes): Pork, 1,743; beef, 453; mutton, 204; poultry meat, 839; goat meat, 18; rabbit meat, 70; cows' milk, 5,637m. litres; sheep's milk, 263m. litres; goats' milk, 401m. litres; eggs, 846m. dozen.

Livestock (1988): Horses, 250,000; asses, 131,000; mules, 110,000; cattle, 4·98m.; sheep, 17,894,000; goats, 2·9m.; pigs, 16,941,000; poultry, 55m.

Forestry. Total forests (1989) 15·7m. ha; production, 1988, 8,736,000 cu. metres of wood. Other forest products (1988 in tonnes): Resins, 16,972; cork, 82,680; esparto, (1987) 6,425. Value of forest products, 1987: 116·4m. pesetas.

Fisheries. The total catch amounted in 1989 to 983,779 tonnes, including 115,761 tonnes of molluscs, 30,080 of crustaceans and 97,454 from nurseries; total value, 235,445m. pesetas. The main fishing region is the North-West (Galicia), with 59·7% of the catch. The Spanish fishing fleet in 1986 consisted of 17,464 vessels of 649,457 tonnes, with a total crew of 94,246.

INDUSTRY. The industrial sector represented 72·3% of export value, 38·6% of GNP and 24·2% of employment in 1987. In 1986, the principal textile productions were (in 1,000 tonnes): Wool yarn, 26; cotton yarn, 105; fabrics yarn, 191; wool cloth, 11; cotton cloth, 81; fabrics cloth, 74. In 1986, 2·7m. tonnes of writing, printing, packing and other paper were produced. The production of cement reached 27,375,000 tonnes in 1989. Steel production (1989) 12,770,000 tonnes; the three great blast-furnaces concentrations are in Bilbao area, Avilés (Asturias) and Sagunto (Valencia). The chemical industry is located in the areas of Madrid, Barcelona and Bilbao; sulphuric acid production (1986), 3·4m. tonnes; nitrogenous fertilizers, 829,000 tonnes; plastics (1989), 1,934,000 tonnes. The 9 oil refineries refined (1989) 49·8m. tonnes of crude oil. In 1986 1·23m. TV sets were manufactured. 953,067 refrigerators and 1,354,000 washing machines were manufactured in 1988. Spain has important toy and shoe industries, toys especially in Alicante and Barcelona provinces and shoes in Alicante province and the Balearic islands.

Spanish shipyards launched 325,083 BRT in 1989. In 1989, 1,639,000 cars and 407,000 industrial and commercial vehicles were built.

Labour. The monthly minimum wage for workers was 53,250 pesetas (Jan. 1991). The average monthly wage for workers in industry and services was 118,106 pesetas in 1989.

The economically active population numbered 14,841,600 in Dec. 1989. Of these, 12,258,300 were employed: 1,597,200 in agriculture and fishing, 2,898,000 in manufactures, 1,155,300 in construction industry and 6,607,800 in trade, transport and other public and personal services. 17·3% of the active population was unemployed at the end of 1989 (2,560,800 persons).

Trade Unions. The Constitution guarantees the establishment and activities of trade unions provided they have a democratic structure. The two most important trade unions are *Unión General de Trabajadores* (UGT), founded in 1888 by Pablo Iglesias (who had founded in 1879 the Spanish Workers Socialist Party, PSOE), and *Comisiones Obreras*, which was gradually established 1958–63, then as a clandestine labour organization.

FOREIGN ECONOMIC RELATIONS

Commerce. Foreign trade of Spain (Peninsula, Baleares, Canaries, Ceuta, Melilla) (in 1m. pesetas):

	1985	*1986*	*1987*	*1988*	*1989*
Imports	5,073,239	4,890,768	6,029,838	7,039,516	8,458,361
Exports	4,104,143	3,800,225	4,195,623	4,686,376	5,257,628

In 1989 the most important imports were (in 1m. pesetas): Nuclear reactors, boilers and mechanical engineering, 1,370,800 (16·21% of total); crude petroleum and other fuels, 1,001,609 (11·84%); vehicles and tractors, 964,719 (11·41%); electric engines and tools, 733,929 (8·68%); steel and iron foundry, 308,614 (3·65%); organic chemicals, 279,835 (3·31%); optical instruments and tools, 257,919 (3·05%); plastics, 208,668 (2·47%); fish, shellfish and molluscs, 199,675 (2·36%); aircraft, 189,967 (2·25%).

The most important exports in 1989 (in 1m. pesetas) were: Vehicles, 947,111 (18·01%); nuclear reactors, boilers and mechanical engineering, 545,613 (10·38%); refined petroleum and other fuels, 257,652 (4·90%); steel and iron foundries, 241,180 (4·59%; electric engines and tools, 230,282 (4·38%); fresh fruits, 227,146 (4.32%); organic chemicals, 139,618 (2·66%); shoes, 135,304 (2·57%); plastics, 132,452 (2·52%); steel, iron and foundry manufactures, 124,406 (2·37%).

Distribution of Spanish foreign trade (in 1m. pesetas) according to main origin and destination, for calendar years:

	Imports		*Exports*	
	1988	*1989*	*1988*	*1989*
EEC	3,998,825	4,828,375	3,074,843	3,509,760
Germany, Federal Republic	1,138,357	1,358,988	561,996	623,640
France	947,517	1,155,451	865,142	1,024,586
Italy	675,484	881,712	453,721	508,062
UK	499,423	549,364	458,931	524,229
Netherlands	243,869	276,760	229,762	238,710
Belgium–Luxembourg	230,178	267,431	158,899	170,130
Portugal	146,224	196,668	262,128	327,592
USA	626,439	765,280	368,871	387,356
Japan	361,057	404,826	55,565	71,905
Latin America	375,305	389,180	142,188	188,061
Mexico	128,642	134,556	27,429	48,229
EFTA	376,828	475,246	195,758	207,776
Sweden	131,912	166,850	45,645	48,525
Switzerland	105,876	131,636	30,775	80,657
COMECON	180,892	212,993	61,844	80,874
USSR	129,494	153,006	31,104	47,180
Nigeria	109,334	153,245	13,122	9,815
Libya	77,075	91,879	14,347	9,762
Saudi Arabia	53,060	69,158	51,869	42,494
Iraq	48,060	77,954	18,010	20,747
Iran	56,643	98,204	8,895	17,622

Total trade between Spain and UK (British Department of Trade returns, in £1,000 sterling):

	1987	*1988*	*1989*	*1990*
Imports to UK	2,099,139	2,482,360	2,772,011	2,884,691
Exports and re-exports from UK	2,164,221	2,691,662	3,137,941	3,750,143

Total trade of the Spanish territories and UK (British Department of Trade returns, in £1,000 sterling):

	Imports to UK			*Exports from UK*		
	1988	*1989*	*1990*	*1988*	*1989*	*1990*
Canary Islands	77,491	74,532	86,023	90,834	89,852	92,886
North Africa	34	57	56	3,599	4,640	5,933

Tourism. In 1989, 54,057,355 tourists visited Spain (from France, 22·2%; Portugal,

18·6%; UK, 13·6%; Federal Republic of Germany, 12·5%; Morocco, 4·8%). Receipts of foreign currency (1989) US$16·17m. Hotel and similar beds, 1,733,105 (Jan. 1990). There were about 52m. tourists in 1990.

COMMUNICATIONS

Roads. In 1986 the total length of highways and roads of all classes was 318,225 km. The main network in 1988 comprised 2,344 km of motorways (1,806 km toll motorways), 510 km of other four-lane highways and 17,621 km of first class roads. Number of cars (1988) was 10,788,975, lorries and vans, 2,034,728, buses, 44,178 and motorcycles (1987), 845,612. There were in Dec. 1986 12,345,589 driving licences (3,370,450 drivers were women).

Railways. The total length of the state railways in 1989 was 12,710 km, mostly broad (1,676-mm) gauge (6,226 km electrified). In 1941 the broad gauge railways, passed into state ownership; they are under a board known as the *Red Nacional de Ferrocarriles Españoles* (RENFE). The differential gauge of Spanish railways had strategic origins; passengers therefore must change at the frontier stations unless aboard variable-gauge trains. A high-speed standard-gauge railway from Madrid to Seville started construction in 1989. In 1988 freight carried was 36·6m. tonnes and 194·5m. passengers. There are several regional railways including Basque, Catalan and FEVE (narrow gauge) railways.

Aviation. The most important Spanish airline is 'Iberia': it maintains a regular service with Europe, America, Africa and the Middle and Far East. Its fleet included 6 B-747s (for 430 passengers each), 8 DC-10s (for 266), 6 Airbus-300Bs (for 253), 35 B-727s (for 161) and 30 DC-9s (for 110) in 1985. 'Aviaco' operates mainly internal flights. There are 43 airports open to civil traffic; those of Madrid, Palma de Mallorca and Barcelona are the most active. A small airport in Seo de Urgel, in the Pyrenees, used especially for the air service of Andorra was opened in 1982.

Aircraft movements in 1987, 309,385 internal and 293,177 international. In 1989 70·8m passengers and 408,600 tonnes of freight were carried.

Shipping. The merchant navy in 1989 had 430 vessels of a gross tonnage of 3·2m.

In 1987, 82,174 ships entered Spanish ports, carrying 14·1m. passengers and discharging and loading 215·7m. tonnes of cargo.

Telecommunications. The receipts of the post office in 1988 were 100,930m. pesetas; expenses, 119,370m. pesetas. There were in 1988, 12,597 post offices and (Nov. 1987) 15,350,464 telephones, these all privately operated.

Radio Nacional de España broadcasts 5 programmes on medium-waves and FM, as well as many regional programmes; it has one commercial programme. The greatest radio audience is that of an independent network, *Sociedad Española de Radiodifusión* (SER); *Cadena de Ondas Populares Españolas* (COPE) belongs to the Roman Catholic church. Two independent radio networks were established in 1982 covering the whole of Spain, *Antena 3* and *Radio 80*. *Televisión Española* broadcasts 2 programmes. There were in 1990 the following regional TV networks: *TV3* (1983) and *Canal 33* (1989), both broadcasting in Catalan; *ETB1* (1983) and *ETB2* (1987), both Basque, the first one broadcasting in Basque; *Televisión de Galicia* (1985), in Galician; *TM3* (1989), for the area of Madrid; *Canal 9* (1989), mostly in Valencian (Catalan); and *Tele-Sur* (1989), for Andalusia. *Radio Exterior* broadcasts abroad, and *Televisión Española* has an international channel. In 1990 3 nationwide commercial TV networks: Antena 3, Tele 5 and Canal Plus. Colour transmissions are carried by PAL system. Number of receivers (1986): Radio, 11·5m.; television, 12·5m. (about 90% colour sets).

Cinemas (1986). There were 2,640 cinemas with an audience of 87·3m.

Newspapers (1988). There were about 76 daily newspapers with a total daily circulation of about 5m. copies. In 1988 the following dailies had a daily circulation of more than 100,000 copies: *El País* (Madrid, 376,230), *La Vanguardia* (Barcelona, 202,741), *ABC* (Madrid, 267,772), *Marca* (Madrid, [sports], 159,915), *El Periódico* (Barcelona, 157,192), *Diario 16* (Madrid, 139,956) and *El Correo Español-El Pueblo Vasco* (Bilbao, 125,555).

JUSTICE, RELIGION, EDUCATION AND WELFARE

Justice. Justice is administered by *Tribunales* and *Juzgados* (Tribunals and Courts), which conjointly form the *Poder Judicial* (Judicial Power). Judges and magistrates cannot be removed, suspended or transferred except as set forth by law. The Constitution of 1978 has established a new organ, the *Consejo General del Poder Judicial* (CGPJ, General Council of the Judicial Power), formed by 1 President and 20 magistrates, judges, attorneys and lawyers, governing the Judicial Power in full independence from the other two powers of the State, the Legislative (Cortes) and the Executive (President of the Government and his Cabinet); all members of the CGPJ, magistrates, etc., have been appointed by the Cortes since 1985. Its President is that of the *Tribunal Supremo*.

The Judicature is composed of the *Tribunal Supremo* (Supreme High Court); 17 *Tribunales Superiores de Justicia* (Upper Courts of Justice, 1 for each autonomous community); 52 *Audiencias Provinciales* (Provincial High Courts); *Juzgados de Primera Instancia* (Courts of First Instance), *Juzgados de Instrucción* (Courts of Judicial Proceedings, not passing sentences) and *Juzgados de lo Penal* (Penal Courts, passing sentences).

The *Tribunal Supremo* consists of a President (appointed by the King, on proposal from the *Consejo General del Poder Judicial*) and various judges distributed among 7 chambers: 1 for trying civil matters, 3 for administrative purposes, 1 for criminal trials, 1 for social matters and 1 for military cases. The *Tribunal Supremo* has disciplinary faculties; is court of cassation in all criminal trials; for administrative purposes decides in first and second instance disputes arising between private individuals and the State, and in social matters resolves in the last instance.

The jury system, re-established by the art. 125 of the Constitution, had not been applied by Jan. 1991, pending its parliamentary regulation.

The *Tribunal Constitucional* (Constitutional Court) has power to solve conflicts between the State and the Autonomous Communities, to determine if legislation passed by the Cortes is contrary to the Constitution and to protect constitutional rights of the individuals violated by any authority. Its 12 members are appointed by the King in the following way: 4, on proposal of the Congress of Deputies; 4, on proposal of the Senate; 2 on proposal of the *Consejo General del Poder Judicial;* and 2 on proposal of the Cabinet. It has a 9 year term, a third of the membership renewed every 3 years.

The death penalty was abolished in 1978 by the Constitution (art. 15). Divorce is again legal since July 1981 and abortion since Aug. 1985.

The prison population was, on 7 Nov. 1989, 31,918.

Religion. Roman Catholicism is the religion of the majority. There are 11 metropolitan sees and 52 suffragan sees, the chief being Toledo, where the Primate resides.

The archdioceses of Madrid-Alcalá and Barcelona depend directly from the Vatican.

The Constitution guarantees full religious freedom and states that no religion has an established legal condition (art. 16); so, since 29 Dec. 1978 there has been no official religion in Spain. A report issued in 1982 by the Episcopal Conference of the Roman Catholic Church claims that 82·76% of all children born in 1981 were baptized in that church.

There are about 250,000 other Christians, including several Protestant denominations, Jehovah Witnesses (about 60,000) and Mormons. The British and Foreign Bible Society was, on 10 March 1963, allowed to resume its activities.

The first synagogue since the expulsion of the Jews in 1492 was opened in Madrid on 2 Oct. 1959. The number of Jews is estimated at about 15,000.

There is a growing Moslem community, with about 450,000 members. Most of them are foreign citizens, but there are also Spanish Moslems, mainly in Ceuta and Melilla.

Education. Primary education is compulsory and free between 6 and 14 years of age, but school-leaving age is being extended to 16.

In 1987–88 pre-primary education (under 6 years) was undertaken by 37,961 schools, with 39,513 teachers and 1,331,431 pupils. Primary or basic education (6 to 14 years): 182,499 schools, 191,036 teachers and 6,695,326 pupils. Secondary education (14-17 years) is conducted on two branches: Middle schools *(Institutos)*, and vocational and technical centres *(Formación Profesional)*, with 2,752 and 2,230 school units, 80,937 and 51,927 teachers and 1,049,450 and 772,325 pupils. For adult education there were (in 1986–87) 602 school units, with 543 teachers and (1985–86) 145,062 students. For the physically or mentally disabled there were (1987–88) 4,923 school units, with 5,514 teachers and 41,231 pupils.

In 1990 there were in all 36 universities: 25 State Universities, in Madrid, Barcelona, Valencia, Granada, Sevilla, Santiago de Compostela, Zaragoza, Bilbao (University of the Basque Country), Oviedo, Valladolid, Salamanca (founded in 1215), La Laguna (Canaries), Murcia, Málaga, Córdoba, Badajoz-Cáceres (University of Extremadura), Cádiz, León, Santander, Alicante, Palma de Mallorca, Albacete–Ciudad Real (University of Castilla–La Mancha), Alcalá de Henares, Pamplona, and in the southern area of Madrid (Carlos III University, 1989); 4 Polytechnic Universities, in Madrid, Barcelona, Valencia and Las Palmas (Canaries); 2 Autonomous Universities, in Madrid and Barcelona; 4 private (Catholic) universities, in Deusto (Bilbao), Pamplona, Salamanca and Madrid (University of Comillas); and the *Universidad Nacional de Educación a Distancia* (Open University), which teaches by mail, radio and TV, with its central seat at Madrid (74,388 students, 1988–89). There were 1,028,336 university students (1988–89) including 33,500 students at private universities.

Health. In 1987 there were 131,080 doctors, 5,722 dentists, 31,118 pharmacists, 147,462 nurses, 6,103 midwives. In 1988 there were 861 hospitals with 180,688 beds.

Social Security. The social services budget was 5,467,797m. pesetas in 1989, and covered retirement pensions (59·3% of that budget), health and hospital services (29·7%) and other allowances and aids. There is a minimum pension for every retired citizen with yearly earnings under 520,000 pesetas.

In 1990 the system of contributions to the social security and employment scheme was: For pensions, sickness, invalidity, maternity and children, a contribution of 28·8% of the basic wage (24% paid by the employer, 4·8% by the employee); for unemployment benefit, a contribution of 6·3% (5·2% paid by the employer, 1·1% by the employee). There are also minor contributions for a Fund of Guaranteed Salaries, working accidents and professional sicknesses, and vocational training.

DIPLOMATIC REPRESENTATIVES

Of Spain in Great Britain (24 Belgrave Sq., London SW1X 8QA)
Ambassador: Felipe de la Morena.

Of Great Britain in Spain (Calle de Fernando el Santo, 16, Madrid, 4)
Ambassador: Sir Patrick Fearn, KCMG.

Of Spain in the USA (2700 15th St., NW, Washington, D.C., 20009)
Ambassador: Jaime de Ojeda y Eiseley.

Of the USA in Spain (Serrano 75, Madrid)
Ambassador: Joseph Zappala.

Of Spain to the United Nations
Ambassador: Francisco Villar Ortiz de Urbina.

Further Reading

Statistical Information: The Instituto Nacional de Estadística (Paseo de la Castellana, 183, Madrid) combines the administrative work of a government department attached to the Presidency of the Government with a centre of statistical studies.

Bell, D. (ed.) *Democratic Politics in Spain: Spanish Politics after Franco.* London, 1983
Carr, R., *Modern Spain, 1875–1980.* OUP, 1980
Collins, R., *The Basques.* Oxford, 1986
Donaghy, P. J. and Newton, M. T., *Spain: A Guide to Political and Economic Institutions.* CUP, 1987

Enciclopedia Universal Ilustrada. 70 vols., 10 appendices, 10 supplements. Madrid
Gunther, R. (et al) *Spain after Franco: The Making of a Competitive Party System*. Univ. of California Press, 1986
Harrison, J., *The Spanish Economy in the Twentieth Century*. London, 1985
Hooper, J., *The Spaniards: A Portrait of The New Spain*. London, 1986
Maravall, J., *The Transition to Democracy in Spain*. London, 1982
Morris, J., *Spain*. London, 1979
Preston, P., *The Triumph of Democracy in Spain*. London and New York, 1986
Shields, G. J., *Spain*. [Bibliography] Oxford and Santa Barbara, 1985
Shubert, A., *A Social History of Modern Spain*. London, 1990

National Library: Biblioteca Nacional, Madrid.

FORMER PROVINCE IN AFRICA (WESTERN SAHARA)

The colony of Spanish Sahara became a Spanish province in July 1958. On 14 Nov. 1975 Spain, Morocco and Mauritania had reached agreement on the transfer of power over Western Sahara to Morocco and Mauritania on 28 Feb. 1976. Morocco occupied al-Aaiún in late Nov. and on 12 Jan. 1976 the Spanish army withdrew from Western Sahara which had ceased to be a Spanish province on 31 Dec. 1975. The country was partitioned by Morocco and Mauritania on 28 Feb. 1976; Morocco reorganized its sector into 3 provinces. In Aug. 1979 Mauritania withdrew from the territory it took over in 1976. The area was taken over by Morocco and reorganized into a fourth province.

A liberation movement, *Frente Polisario*, launched an armed struggle against Spanish rule on 20 May 1973 and, in spite of occupation of all western centres by Moroccan troops, Saharawi guerrillas based in Algeria continue to attempt to liberate their country. They have renamed it the Saharawi Arab Democratic Republic and hold most of the desert beyond a defensive line built by Moroccan troops encompassing Smara, Bu Craa and Laâyoune. A ceasefire was agreed in Aug. 1988. In Sept. 1989 Polisario's guerrillas ended the lull in fighting with battles on 7 and 11 Oct. – Morocco and Polisario failed to agree on how the referendum (part of UN plan) should be held.

In 1982 the Saharawi Arab Democratic Republic became a member of the Organization of African Unity (OAU).

President: Mohammed Abdelaziz.

Area 266,769 sq. km (102,680 sq. miles). The population at the census held by Morocco in Sept. 1982 was 163,868; estimate (1986) 180,000. Another estimated 165,000 Saharawis live in refugee camps around Tindouf in south-west Algeria. The main towns (1982 census) are Laâyoune (al-Aaiún), the capital (96,784), Dakhla (17,822) and as-Smara (17,753). The population is Arabic-speaking, and virtually entirely Sunni Moslem.

Rich phosphate deposits were discovered in 1963 at Bu Craa. Morocco holds 65% of the shares of the former Spanish state-controlled company. While production reached 5·6m. tonnes in 1975, exploitation has been severely reduced by guerrilla activity but in 1984 produced 1m. tonnes. After a nearly complete collapse, production and transportation of phosphate resumed in 1978, ceased again, and then resumed in 1982. There are about 6,100 km of motorable tracks, but only about 500 km of paved roads. There are airports at Laâyoune and Dakhla. As most of the land is desert, less than 19% is in agricultural use, with about 2,000 tonnes of grain produced annually. There are (1983) about 22,000 sheep, as well as goats and camels raised. Electricity produced (1983) 78m. kwh.

Further Reading

Damis, J., *Conflict in Northwest Africa: The Western Sahara Dispute*. Stanford, 1983
Hodges, T., *Western Sahara: The Roots of a Desert War*. London and Westport, 1984
Sipe, L. F., *Western Sahara: A Comprehensive Bibliography*. New York, 1984
Thompson, V. and Adloff, R., *The Western Saharans: Background to Conflict*. London, 1980

SRI LANKA

Capital: Colombo
Population: 16·81m. (1989)
GNP per capita: US$367 (1989)

Democratic Socialist Republic of Sri Lanka

HISTORY. A monarchical form of government continued until the beginning of the 19th century when the British subjugated the Kandyan Kingdom in the central highlands.

In 1505 the Portuguese had formed settlements in the west and south, which were taken from them about the middle of the next century by the Dutch. In 1796 the British Government annexed the foreign settlements to the presidency of Madras. In 1802 Ceylon was constituted a separate colony.

Ceylon became an independent Commonwealth state on 4 Feb. 1948 and became a republic in 1972 as Sri Lanka.

War between northern Tamil separatists and government forces began in 1983. A state of emergency ended on 11 Jan. 1989, but violence continued.

AREA AND POPULATION. Sri Lanka is an island in the Indian Ocean, south of the Indian peninsula from which it is separated by the Palk Strait. On 28 June 1974 the frontier between India and Sri Lanka in the Palk Strait was redefined, giving to Sri Lanka the island of Kachchativu. Area (in sq. km.) and census population on 17 March 1981.

Provinces	*Area*	*Population*	*Provinces*	*Area*	*Population*
Western	3,708·61	3,919,807	North-Central	10,723·59	849,492
Central	5,583·50	2,009,248	Uva	8,487·91	914,522
Southern	5,559·15	1,882,661	Sabaragamuwa	4,901·55	1,482,031
Northern	8,882·11	1,109,404			
Eastern	9,951·26	975,251	Total	65,609·86	14,846,750
North-Western	7,812·18	1,704,334			

Population (1981 census), 14,846,750, an increase of 17% since 1971. Population (in 1,000) according to ethnic group and nationality at the 1981 census: 10,980 Sinhalese, 1,887 Sri Lanka Tamils, 1,047 Sri Lanka Moors, 39 Burghers, 47 Malays, 819 Indian Tamils, 28 others. Non-nationals of Sri Lanka totalled 635,150.

Vital statistics, 1989 (provisional): Birth-rate (per 1,000 population), 21·3; death-rate, 6·2; infant mortality (per 1,000 live births) (1988, provisional), 19·4.

The urban population was 21·5% of the total in 1981. The principal towns and their population according to the census of 1981 are: Colombo (the capital), 587,647; Dehiwela-Mt. Lavinia, 173,529; Moratuwa, 134,826; Jaffna, 118,224; Kotte, 101,039; Kandy, 97,872; Galle, 76,863; Negombo, 60,762; Trincomalee, 44,313; Batticaloa, 42,963; Matara, 38,843; Ratnapura, 37,497; Anuradhapura, 35,981; Badulla, 33,068; Kalutara, 31,503. Population of the Greater Colombo area, 1980, about 1m.

Sinhala and Tamil are the official languages; English is in use.

CLIMATE. Sri Lanka has an equatorial climate with low annual temperature variations, but it is affected by the north-east Monsoon (Dec. to Feb.) and the south-west Monsoon (May to Sept.). Rainfall is generally heavy but never lasts long; it is heaviest in the south-west and central highlands while the north and east are relatively dry. Thirty-year averages, 1951–80: Colombo. Jan. 79·7°F (26·5°C), July 81·1°F (27·3°C). Annual rainfall 99·5" (2,527 mm). Trincomalee. Jan. 78·6°F (25·9°C), July 86·2°F (30·1°C). Annual rainfall 63·60" (1,615 mm). Kandy. Jan. 73·9°F (23·3°C), July 75·9°F (24·4°C). Annual rainfall 76·6" (1,947 mm). Nuwara Eliya. Jan. 58·5°F (14·7°C), July 60·3°F (15·7°C). Annual rainfall 80·04" (2,044 mm).

CONSTITUTION AND GOVERNMENT. A new constitution for the Democratic Socialist Republic of Sri Lanka was promulgated in Sept. 1978.

The Executive *President* is directly elected by the people and has to receive more than one-half of the valid votes cast. His term of office is six years and he shall not hold the office for more than two consecutive terms. He is the Head of the State, the Head of the Executive and of the Government and the Commander-in-chief of the Armed Forces. He does not have any veto power over legislation; even in a time of public emergency, he must act with Parliamentary control and approval.

Parliament consists of one chamber, composed of 225 members (196 elected and 29 from the National List). Election is by proportional representation by universal suffrage at 18 years. The term of Parliament is 6 years. The Prime Minister and other Ministers, who must be members of Parliament, are appointed by the President.

Elections were held on 15 Feb. 1989.

The Cabinet was as follows in Feb. 1991:

President, Buddha Sasana, Defence, Policy Planning and Implementation: Ranasinghe Premadasa (assumed office 2 Jan. 1989).

Prime Minister, Finance: D. B. Wijetunga.

Reconstruction, Rehabilitation and Social Welfare: A. M. S. Adikari. *Posts and Telecommunications:* Alick Aluvihare. *Education and Higher Education:* Lalith Athulath Mudali. *Power and Energy:* K. D. M. C. Bandara. *Housing and Construction:* B. Sirisena Cooray. *Lands, Irrigation and Mahaweli Development:* P. Dayaratne. *Agricultural Development and Research:* R. M. Dharmadasa Banda. *Justice:* A. C. S. Hameed. *Foreign Affairs:* Harold Herat. *Health and Women's Affairs:* Mrs. Renuka Herath. *Ports and Shipping:* Rupasena Karunatilleke. *Cultural Affairs and Information:* W. J. M. Lokubandara. *Food and Co-operatives:* Weerasinghe Mallimarachchi. *Youth Affairs and Sports:* C. Nanda Mathew. *Transport and Highways:* Wijayapala Mendis. *Trade and Commerce:* Abdul Razak Munsoor. *Public Administration, Provincial Councils and Home Affairs:* Festus Perera. *Fisheries and Aquatic Resources:* M. Joseph Michael Perera. *Environment and Parliamentary Affairs and Chief Government Whip:* M. Vincent Perera. *Labour and Vocational Training:* G. M. Premachandra. *Tourism and Rural Industrial Development:* S. Thondaman. *Industries, Science and Technology and Leader of the House of Parliament:* Ranil Wickremasinghe. *Handlooms and Textile Industries:* U. B. Wijekoon. *Plantation Industries:* Ranjan Wijeratne.

National flag: A yellow field bearing 2 panels; in the hoist 2 vertical strips of green and orange; in the fly, dark red with a gold lion holding a sword and in each corner a gold 'bo' leaf.

National anthem: 'Sri Lanka Matha...Apa Sri Lanka'.

Local government: For purposes of general administration, the island is divided into 25 districts, administered by government agents. There are 12 Municipal Councils and 24 District Councils. There are 9 Provincial Councils, consisting of a governor, appointed by the President, a Chief Minister, a Board of Ministers and members elected for 5-year terms. There were 455 elected members in 1991.

DEFENCE

Army. The Army was constituted on 16 Oct. 1949. It consists of 3 infantry divisions, 10 infantry brigades, 3 armoured reconnaissance regiments, 3 field artillery regiments, 3 engineer regiments, 3 signal regiments and service units. Equipment includes 18 Saladin armoured cars and 15 Ferret scout cars. Strength (1991) 67,000 including active reservists and a Volunteer Force of 1 artillery regiment, 12 infantry battalions and service units.

Navy. The naval force comprises 3 Surveillance Command Ships (ex-mercantile), 2 locally-built coastal patrol craft, 36 inshore patrol craft of varying types plus about 30 small fast patrol boats and service craft. There are 2 mechanized landing craft of 270 tonnes full load. The main naval base is at Trincomalee. Personnel in 1990 numbered 8,000, with a reserve of about 1,000.

Air Force. The Air Force was formed on 10 Oct. 1950. Its flying bases are at Katunayake and China Bay, Trincomalee. Equipment of 4 squadrons comprises 9 SF.260 and 4 Cessna 150/152 trainers, 3 HS748, 6 Chinese-built Y-12s, 2 Chinese-built Y-8s (An-12s), 1 Super King Air, 3 Cessna Skymasters, 1 Cessna 421 and a Cessna Cardinal for general transport and utility purposes; and 2 Dauphin, 10 Bell 212, 4 Bell 412 and 8 JetRanger helicopters for internal security operations. Total strength (1991) about 6,000 with 9 combat aircraft and 14 armed helicopters. There is also an Air Force Reserve numbering about 1,000.

INTERNATIONAL RELATIONS

Membership. Sri Lanka is a member of the UN, the Commonwealth, the Non-Aligned Movement, the South Asian Association for Regional Co-operation and the Colombo Plan.

ECONOMY

Policy. The 1990–94 plan aims at a 5·3% annual growth rate. Investment allocated is mainly for completion of projects in priority areas such as power, irrigation, road rehabilitation, water supply and telecommunications. Total public investment is about Rs200,900m.

Budget. Revenue and expenditure of central government in Rs 1m. for financial years ending 31 Dec.:

		Expenditure		
Year	*Revenue*	*Recurrent*	*Capital*	*Total*
1987	44,900	38,816	29,013	67,829
1988	45,675	49,093	41,794	90,887
1989 [1]	56,750	56,658	34,730	91,388

[1] Estimate.

The principal sources of revenue in 1989 were (in Rs 1m.): General sales and tax, 14,658; import levies, 15,708; export duties, 1,217; selective sales taxes, 6,283.

The principal items of recurrent expenditure in 1989 (in Rs 1m.): Finance, 21,963; defence, 6,673; public administration, 5,783; education, 5,423; agriculture, 3,509; health, 3,479; labour and social services, 2,777. Capital expenditure on finance, 4,782; Mahaweli development, 3,730; power and energy, 3,195; transport and highways, 2,601; defence, 2,119.

Currency. The unit of currency is the *Sri Lankan rupee* (LKR) of 100 *cents*.

Notes and coins issued by the Central Bank are legal tender except notes of Rs 50 and Rs 100 dated before 25 Oct. 1970. Currency notes are issued in the denominations of Rs 2, 5, 10, 20, 50, 100, 500 and 1,000. Coins are issued in the denominations of 1, 2, 5, 10, 25 and 50 cents; Rs 1, 2, 5 and 10. The total circulation was Rs 21,126m. on 31 Dec. 1989. In March 1991, £1 = Rs 77·00; US$1 = Rs 40·59.

Banking and Finance. The narrow money supply (M1) at 31 Dec. 1989 stood at Rs 35,337·9m.

The Central Bank of Sri Lanka is the bank of issue. The main commercial banks are: The Bank of Ceylon and the People's Bank (state-managed), the State Bank of India, Grindlays Bank, the Hongkong and Shanghai Banking Corporation, the Standard Chartered Bank, the Commercial Bank of Ceylon Ltd., the Hatton National Bank Ltd., the Habib Bank (Overseas) Ltd., Indo-Suez Bank, Bank of Credit and Commerce International Ltd., American Express Bank Ltd., the Indian Overseas Bank Ltd., Citibank NA, Sampath Bank Ltd., Seylan Trust Bank Ltd., Algemene Bank Nederlands NV, Amsterdam-Rotterdam Bank NV, Bank of Oman Ltd., Deutsche Bank AG, Habib Bank AG, Zurich, Indian Bank, Overseas Trust Bank Ltd and Emirates Bank International Ltd. Total assets of 24 commercial banks at 31 Dec. 1989, Rs 106,351·9m.

The monopoly in all insurance business enjoyed by the state-owned Ceylon Insurance Corporation and the National Insurance Corporation is broad based with the participation of a large number of assurance companies.

Sri Lanka National Savings Bank at 31 Dec. 1989 had a balance to depositors' credit of Rs 19,902·3m. Sri Lanka State Mortgage and Investment Bank, National Development Bank, Development Finance Corporation, the National Housing Authority and the Housing Development Finance Corporation of Sri Lanka Ltd. are the main long-term credit institutions.

Weights and Measures. The metric system has been established.

ENERGY AND NATURAL RESOURCES

Electricity. Installed capacity of electric energy (1989), 1,240,650 kw. Energy produced, 2,858m. kwh; the main source was thermal power as the water levels of the reservoirs were not sufficient to operate the hydro power plants at full capacity. Supply 230 volts; 50 Hz.

Water. The Mahaweli Ganga irrigation scheme is (1989) irrigating 41,000 ha of new land and 45,576 ha of land already cultivated. The supply of water to the city of Colombo and the Greater Colombo Area is carried out by the National Water Supplies and Drainage Board, set up in 1974. Consumption within Colombo city limits is estimated at 10,000m. gallons a year.

Minerals. Gems are among the chief minerals mined and exported. Precious and semi-precious stones are found mainly in the Ratnapura district in the south-east. The most important are sapphire, ruby, chrysoberyl, beryl, topaz, spinel, garnet, zircon and tourmaline. Value of gemstones exported in 1989, Rs 2,204m.

Graphite is also important; production in 1989 was 3,987 tonnes. Production of ilmenite, 1989, 321,798 tonnes. Some rutile is also produced (5,589 tonnes in 1989).

Salt extraction is the oldest industry and is controlled by the National Salt Corporation. The method is solar evaporation of sea-water. Production, 1989, 148,589 tonnes.

Agriculture. About 2m. ha are under cultivation. Agriculture engages 47·5% of the labour force. Main crops in 1989: Paddy (2,063,000 tonnes from 726,958 ha), rubber (111,000 tonnes), tea (207,000 tonnes) and coconuts (2,483m. nuts).

Livestock in 1989 (estimate): 1,819,900 cattle, 967,000 buffaloes, 94,400 swine, 518,300 goats, 29,800 sheep, 8,833,400 poultry.

Fisheries. Production in 1989 was 205,286 tonnes including 157,411 tonnes of coastal water fish, 39,720 tonnes of fresh water fish and 8,155 tonnes from deep-sea fisheries. In 1989 there were 27,167 fishing craft, of which 15,136 were not motorized.

INDUSTRY. The main industries are food, beverages and tobacco; textiles, clothing and leather goods; chemicals, petroleum, rubber and plastics.

The Greater Colombo Economic Commission has two Investment Promotion Zones: Katunayake and Biyagama.

Trade Unions. The registration and control of trade unions are regulated by the Trade Unions Ordinance (Ch. 138 of the Legislative Enactments). In 1989 there were 949 registered trade unions with a membership of 1,496,001.

FOREIGN ECONOMIC RELATIONS. Foreign debt in Dec. 1989 was Rs 125,656·9m.

Commerce. The values of total imports and exports (imports excluding bullion, specie and postal articles; exports, including re-exports and ship's stores) for calendar years (in Rs 1,000):

	1985	*1986*	*1987*	*1988*	*1989*
Imports	49,068,542	51,281,508	59,749,717	70,320,427	75,352,750
Exports	35,034,947	34,092,261	39,860,638	47,092,044	55,511,162

Principal exports in 1989 (in Rs 1m.): Tea, 13,664; rubber, 3,112; copra, coconut oil and desiccated coconut, 1,920; other crops, 2,408; textiles and garments, 17,631; precious and semi-precious stones, 5,430.

Principal imports (Rs 1m.) in 1989 were petroleum, 8,376m.; machinery and equipment, 6,278m.; vehicles and transport equipment, 1,833; food and beverages, 13,136.

In 1989 the principal sources of imports were (in Rs 1m.): Japan, 9,350; USA, 4,939; UK, 4,512; Iran, 3,479; South Korea, 3,410; Singapore, 3,402; Federal Germany, 2,564; India, 2,313; Saudi Arabia, 1,645.

Principal export destinations 1989 were (in Rs 1m.): USA, 14,417; Federal Germany, 2,564; Japan, 3,208; UK, 3,186; Pakistan, 1,619; Saudi Arabia, 1,200.

Total trade between Sri Lanka and UK (British Department of Trade returns, in £1,000 sterling):

	1986	*1987*	*1988*	*1989*	*1990*
Imports to UK	51,860	53,817	56,661	63,527	63,362
Exports and re-exports from UK	83,315	84,680	92,528	92,465	88,496

Tourism. 184,732 tourists visited the country in 1989.

COMMUNICATIONS

Roads. There are 25,749 km. of motorable roads, of which 82% are blacktopped, including 6,493 km of first-class nationally-maintained roads. Number of motor vehicles, 31 Dec. 1989, 714,058, comprising 163,779 private cars and cabs, 103,426 lorries, 86,425 tractors, 307,392 motor cycles and 38,603 buses.

Railways. In 1989 there were 1,453 km of railway, of which 1,394 km were 1,676 mm gauge and 59 km 762 mm gauge. In 1989 railways ran 7,337m. passenger-km and 170·6m. tonne-km.

Aviation. Air Lanka operates international services. Foreign airlines which operate scheduled services to Sri Lanka are Indian Airlines, Aeroflot, KLM, Singapore Airlines, Thai Airways International, Pakistan International Airlines, Gulf Air, Kuwait Airways, Saudi Air, Emirates, UTA French Airlines, Royal Jordanian Airlines and Balkan Bulgarian Airlines; various others operate charter services.

Internal services are operated by Upali, Air Taxis and Consolidated Engineering.

Shipping. In 1989, merchant vessels totalling 33·9m. GRT entered the ports. The Sri Lanka Shipping Corporation began functioning as ship-owners, charterers, brokers and shipping agents in 1971. The Sri Lanka Port Authority was established in 1979.

Telecommunications. In 1989 there were 511 post offices and 3,330 sub-post offices. In 1982 there were 1,900 telegraph offices and 109,900 telephones. Throughout the Greater Colombo Area inter-dialling facilities are now available between 52 stations.

The Overseas Telecommunication Service operates telegraph and telephone services to most parts of the world. Broadcasting is provided by the Sri Lanka Broadcasting Corporation, which assumed the functions of Radio Ceylon on 5 Jan. 1967.

Cinemas. In 1989 there were 365 cinemas. The National Film Corporation established in 1971 has exclusive rights to import films and arrange distribution of foreign and local films. Films released, 1989, 119.

Newspapers. There are 5 main newspaper groups: Associated Newspapers of Ceylon Ltd (5 daily and 3 weekly papers and other periodicals); Express Newspapers (Ceylon) Ltd (2 daily and 2 weekly papers); Independent Newspapers Ltd. (3 daily and 3 weekly papers and other periodicals); Upali Newspapers Ltd. (2 daily, 2 weekly papers and other periodicals); Wijeya Publications (2 weekly papers and other periodicals).

There are 6 daily and 5 weekly papers in Sinhala; 5 daily and 4 weekly in Tamil; 4 daily and 4 weekly in English.

JUSTICE, RELIGION, EDUCATION AND WELFARE

Justice. The systems of law which obtain in Sri Lanka are the Roman-Dutch law, the English law, the Tesawalamai, the Moslem law and the Kandyan law.

The Kandyan law applies to the Kandyan Sinhalese in respect of all matters relating to inheritance, matrimonial rights and donations. The law of Tesawalamai is applied to all inhabitants of Jaffna, in all matters relating to inheritance, marriages, gifts, donations, purchases and sales of land. The Moslem law is applied to all Moslems in respect of succession, donations, marriage, divorce and maintenance. These customary and religious laws have been modified in many respects by local enactments.

The courts of original jurisdiction are the High Court, District Courts, Magistrates' Courts and Primary Courts. The High Court tries major crimes and also exercises admiralty jurisdiction. The 13th Amendment to the Constitution established Provincial High Courts which exercise original criminal jurisdiction of the High Court in respect of offences committed within the province and appellate and revisionary jurisdiction in respect of appeals from the Magistrates' Courts and the Primary Courts within the province. The Provincial High Courts also have the power to issue orders in the nature of Habeas Corpus, in respect of persons illegally detained within the province and issue Writs of Certiorari, Prohibition, Procedendo, Mandamus and Quo Warranto pertaining to matters within the province. The District Court has unlimited civil jurisdiction in civil, revenue, trust, insolvency and testamentary matters, over persons and estates of persons of unsound mind, and wards. The Magistrates' Courts exercise criminal jurisdiction carrying the power to impose terms of imprisonment not exceeding 2 years and fines not exceeding Rs 1,500. The Primary Courts which were established in 1978 exercise civil jurisdiction where the value of the subject matter does not exceed Rs 1,500 and also have jurisdiction in respect of by-laws of local authorities and matters relating to the recovery of revenue of such local authorities. Primary Courts exercise exclusive criminal jurisdiction in respect of offences which may be prescribed by regulation by the Minister. The Primary Courts have the power to impose sentences of imprisonment not exceeding three months and fines not exceeding Rs 250.

The Constitution of 1978 provided for the establishment of two superior courts, the Supreme Court and the Court of Appeal.

The Supreme Court is the highest and final superior court of record and exercises jurisdiction in respect of constitutional matters, jurisdiction for the protection of fundamental rights, final appellate jurisdiction in election petitions and jurisdiction in respect of any breach of the privileges of Parliament. Parliament may provide by law that the Supreme Court exercises the power to grant and issue any of the orders in the nature of Writs of Certiorari, Prohibition, Procedendo, Mandamus or Quo Warranto. The Court of Appeal has appellate jurisdiction to correct all errors in fact or law committed by any court, tribunal or institution; it can grant and issue orders in the nature of the above Writs, and of Writs of Habeas Corpus and Injunctions; it can also try election petitions in respect of election of members of Parliament.

Police. The strength of the police service in 1989 was 25,886.

Religion. Buddhism was introduced from India in the 3rd century B.C. and is the religion of 69·3% of the inhabitants. There were (1981) 10,288,325 Buddhists, 2,297,806 Hindus, 1,130,568 Christians, 1,121,717 Moslems and 8,334 others.

Education. Education is free from school year 1 to university and is imparted in the medium of the mother tongue. In 1981 about 87% of the population (10 years old and older) was literate.

In 1989 there were 10,272 schools including 9,805 government schools, 430 Pirivenas and 37 private schools. The government schools had 146,997 teachers and 4·06m. students from year 1 to 13. Ministry of Education expenditure (1989), Rs 5,618·7m. Education is administered by 8 provisional education directors.

The overall control of the education regions is vested in the Ministry of Education and Higher Education.

There are 9 universities: Peradeniya, Colombo, Jaffna, Sri Jayawardenepura, Moratuwa, Kelaniya, Eastern, Ruhuna and an Open University. Dumbara Campus comes under Peradeniya University. There are 9 institutes (5 for postgraduate and 4 for undergraduate studies).

In 1988 there were 29,781 students and 1,932 teachers in the 8 universities excluding the Open University, which had 13,231 students. Postgraduate institutes had 832 students, the others, 2,102. There were 29 institutions for technical education, 13 of which had grade I status; total enrolment (1988), 19,094.

Health. In 1989 there were 507 hospitals, including 83 maternity homes, and 361 central dispensaries. Hospitals had 46,620 beds and there were 2,456 Department of Health doctors. Total state budget expenditure on health, 1989, Rs 5,038m.

Social Security. The activities of the Department of Social Services include:
(1) Payment of Public Assistance, monthly allowance, tuberculosis assistance and leprosy allowance to all needy persons.
(2) Relief for those affected by widespread distress, such as floods, drought, cyclone.
(3) Custodial care and welfare services to the elderly and infirm.
(4) Vocational training, rehabilitation, aids and appliances for the physically handicapped.
(5) Custodial care, vocational training and rehabilitation for socially handicapped persons.
(6) Distribution of Food Stamps.
(7) Financial assistance to voluntary institutions that provide welfare services.

DIPLOMATIC REPRESENTATIVES

Of Sri Lanka in Great Britain (13 Hyde Park Gdns., London, W2 2LU)
High Commissioner: Gen. D. S. Attygalle.

Of Great Britain in Sri Lanka (190 Galle Rd., Kollupitiya, Colombo 3)
High Commissioner: D. A. S. Gladstone, CMG.

Of Sri Lanka in the USA (2148 Wyoming Ave., NW, Washington, D.C., 20008)
Ambassador: W. S. L. De Alwis.

Of the USA in Sri Lanka (210 Galle Rd., Kollupitiya, Colombo 3)
Ambassador: Marion V. Creekmore, Jr.

Of Sri Lanka to the United Nations
Ambassador: Daya Perera.

Further Reading

The Sri Lanka Year Book. Department of Census and Statistics. Colombo, Annual
Census Publications from 1871
Economic Atlas. Department of Census and Statistics. Colombo, 1980
Performance 1985. Ministry of Plan Implementation, Colombo. 1985
Review of the Economy. Central Bank of Ceylon. Annual
Statistical Pocket-Book. Department of Census and Statistics. Colombo, 1984
Statistical Abstract. Department of Census and Statistics, Colombo, 1982

Coomaraswamy, R., *Sri Lanka: The Crisis of the Anglo-American Constitutional Traditions in a Developing Society.* Colombo, 1984
de Silva, K. M. (ed.) *Sri Lanka: A Survey.* London, 1977.—*A History of Sri Lanka.* London, repr. 1982.—*Managing Ethnic Tensions in Multi-Ethnic Societies: Sri Lanka 1880–1985.* New York, 1986
Ferguson's *Ceylon Directory.* Annual (from 1858)
International Commission of Jurists, ed., *Sri Lanka: A Mounting Tragedy of Errors.* London, 1984
Johnson, B. L. C. and Scrivenor, M. le M., *Sri Lanka: Land, People and Economy.* London, 1981
Manogaran, C., *Ethnic Conflict and Reconciliation in Sri Lanka.* Univ. Hawaii Press, 1987
Manor, J., *Sri Lanka: In Change and Crisis.* London, 1984
Moore, M., *The State and Peasant Politics in Sri Lanka.* CUP, 1985
Piyadasa, L., *Sri Lanka: The Holocaust and After.* London, 1984
Poonambalam, S., *Dependent Capitalism in Crisis: The Sri Lankan Economy 1948–80.* London, 1981

Ratnasuriya, M. D. and Wijeratne, P. B. F., *Shorter Sinhalese-English Dictionary*. Colombo, 1949
Richards, P. and Gooneratne, W., *Basic Needs, Poverty and Government Policies in Sri Lanka*. Geneva, 1981
Samaraweera, V., *Sri Lanka*. [Bibliography] Oxford and Santa Barbara, 1987
Schwarz, W., *The Tamils of Sri Lanka*. London, 1983
Tambiah, S. J., *Sri Lanka: Ethnic Fratricide and the Dismantling of Democracy*. London, 1986
Wilson, A. J., *Politics in Sri Lanka 1947-73*. London, 1974.—*The Gaullist System in Asia: the Constitution of Sri Lanka*. London, 1980.—*The Break-Up of Sri Lanka: The Sinhalese-Tamil Conflict*. London, 1988

SUDAN

Capital: Khartoum
Population: 25·56m. (1987)
GNP per capita: US$340 (1988)

Jamhuryat es-Sudan

(Republic of Sudan)

HISTORY. Sudan was proclaimed a sovereign independent republic on 1 Jan. 1956. On 19 Dec. 1955 the Sudanese parliament passed unanimously a declaration that a fully independent state should be set up forthwith, and that a Council of State of 5 should temporarily assume the duties of Head of State. The Codomini, the UK and Egypt, gave their assent on 31 Dec. 1955.

For the history of the Condominium and the steps leading to independence, *see* THE STATESMAN'S YEAR-BOOK, 1955, pp. 340–341; for subsequent political history *see* THE STATESMAN'S YEAR-BOOK, 1990–91, pp. 1135–36.

On 30 June 1989 Brig.-Gen. (later Lieut.-Gen.) Omar Hassan Ahmad al-Bashir overthrew the civilian government in a military coup, and pledged himself to ending the 6-year old civil war.

AREA AND POPULATION. Sudan is bounded north by Egypt, north-east by the Red Sea, east by Eritrea and Ethiopia, south by Kenya, Uganda and Zaïre, west by the Central African Republic and Chad, north-west by Libya. Sudan covers an area of 967,500 sq. miles (2,505,813 sq. km) and the population at the census of 14 Feb. 1983 was 20,564,364; latest estimate (1987) 25·56m. The chief cities (census, 1983) are the capital, Khartoum (476,218), its suburbs Omdurman (526,287) and Khartoum North (341,146), Port Sudan (206,727), Wadi Medani (141,065), al-Obeid (140,024), Kassala (98,751 in 1973), Atbara (73,009), al-Qadarif (66,465 in 1973), Kosti (65,257 in 1973) and Juba (56,737 in 1973).

The northern and central thirds of the country are populated by Arab and Nubian peoples, while the southern third is inhabited by Nilotic and Negro peoples; Arabic, the official language, is spoken by 51%, Darfurian by 6% and other northern languages by 12%, while Nilotic languages (chiefly Dinka and Nuer) are spoken by 18%, Nilo-Hamitic by 5%, Sudanic by 5% and others by 3%. In 1987 there were 975,000 refugees in Sudan (337,544 from Ethiopia).

The area and population (census, 1983) of the regions are as follows:

Region	*Sq. km*	*1983*	*Region*	*Sq. km*	*1983*
Northern	183,941	1,083,024	Dafur	196,555	3,093,699
Eastern	129,086	2,208,209	Equatoria [1]	76,495	1,406,181
Central	53,716	4,012,543	Bahr al-Ghazal [1]	77,625	2,265,510
Kurdufan	146,932	3,093,294	Upper Nile [1]	92,269	1,599,605
Khartoum (province)	10,883	1,802,299			

[1] Re-united in 1985 as Southern Region.

CLIMATE. Lying wholly within the tropics, the country has a continental climate and only the Red Sea coast experiences maritime influences. Temperatures are generally high throughout the year, with May and June the hottest months. Winters are virtually cloudless and night temperatures are consequently cool. Summer is the rainy season inland, with amounts increasing from north to south, but the northern areas are virtually a desert region. On the Red Sea coast, most rain falls in winter. Khartoum. Jan. 74°F (23·3°C), July 89°F (31·7°C). Annual rainfall 6" (157 mm). Juba. Jan. 83°F (28·3°C), July 78°F (25·6°C). Annual rainfall 39" (968 mm). Port Sudan. Jan. 74°F (23·3°C), July 94°F (34·4°C). Annual rainfall 4" (94 mm). Wadi Halfa. Jan. 60°F (15·6°C), July 90°F (32·2°C). Annual rainfall 0·1" (2·5 mm).

CONSTITUTION AND GOVERNMENT. The constitution was suspended after the 1989 coup. In Feb. 1991 the government included:

Prime Minister, Defence: Lieut.-Gen. Omar Hassan Ahmad al-Bashir.

Deputy Prime Minister: Brig.-Gen. Zubir Mohammed Saleh. *Foreign Affairs:* Ali Sahlul. *Finance and Economic Planning:* Abdul-Rahim Hamdi. *Relief and Displaced Persons:* Peter Orat.

National flag: Three horizontal stripes of red, white, black, with a green triangle based on the hoist.

Regional and local government: In Feb. 1991 a federal system of 9 states (Khartoum, Central, Kordofan, Darfur, Northern, Eastern, Bahr al-Ghazal, Upper Nile and Equatoria) was set up, each under a governor, a deputy governor and a cabinet of ministers. The states are subdivided into 66 provinces and 218 districts.

DEFENCE

Army. The Army is organized in 1 Republican Guard brigade, 2 armoured, 1 parachute, 20 infantry brigades and 1 airborne division, with 3 artillery and 1 engineer regiments, and 2 Air Defence brigades (including 1 surface-to-air missile). Equipment includes 155 T-54 and T-55, 40 T-62 and 20 M-60A3 main battle tanks. Strength (1991) 68,000. Paramilitary forces are National Guard (500) and Border Guard (2,500).

Navy. The Navy operates in the Red Sea and also on the River Nile. It comprises 2 inshore patrol craft transferred in the 1970s from the Iranian coastguard, 4 riverine patrol craft, 2 ex-Yugoslav landing craft and some boats. The flotilla suffers from lack of maintenance and spares. Personnel in 1990 totalled 500.

Air Force. The Air Force was built up with Soviet and Chinese assistance, and is now receiving equipment from the USA. Two combat squadrons are equipped with about 10 MiG-21 fighters, 6 Northrop F-5E, 2 MiG-23, 10 F-6 (Chinese-built MiG-19) and 12 F-5 (Chinese-built MiG-17) fighter-bombers. There is 1 transport squadron, with 5 C-130H Hercules, 6 Aviocars and 3 DHC-5D Buffalo turboprop transports; 2 hellcopter squadrons have 12 AB.212s, 12 Romanian-built Pumas, 6 Mi-8s; there are 3 Jet Provost, 3 Strikemaster and 1 F-5F jet armed trainers, and some Chinese-built FT-2 (MiG/ISUII) advanced trainers. Personnel totalled (1991) about 6,000, with 53 combat aircraft.

INTERNATIONAL RELATIONS

Membership. Sudan is a member of the UN, OAU, the Arab League and is an ACP state of the EEC.

ECONOMY

Budget. The 1989–90 budget envisaged revenue of £S8,600m. and expenditure of £S21,600m.

Currency. The monetary unit is the *Sudanese pound* (SDP) of 100 *piastres* and 1,000 *milliemes*. There are notes of £S10, £S5, £S1, 50 and 25 *piastres* and coins of P. 10, 5, 2; m/ms 10, 5, 2, 1. In March 1991, £1 = £S21·73; US$1 = £S11·45.

Banking. The Bank of Sudan opened in Feb. 1960 with an authorized capital of £S1·5m. as the central bank and bank of issue. All foreign banks were nationalized in 1970. The application of Islamic law from 1 Jan. 1991 put an end to the charging of interest in official banking transactions.

Weights and Measures. The metric system is in use.

ENERGY AND NATURAL RESOURCES

Electricity. Production (1986) 1,210m. kwh. Supply 240 volts; 50 Hz.

Oil. Two oil wells in the south-west produce 15,000 bbls per day of high quality oil. Production of petrol products (1985) 1,019 tonnes.

Minerals. Minerals known to exist include: Gold, graphite, sulphur, chromium-ore (estimate, 9,900m. tonnes in 1982), iron-ore, manganese-ore, copper-ore, zinc-ore, fluorspar, natron, gypsum and anhydrite, magnesite, asbestos, talc, halite, kaolin, white mica, coal, diatomite (kieselguhr), limestone and dolomite, pumice, lead-ore, wollastonite, black sands, vermiculite pyrites.

Gold is being exploited on a small scale at Gabeit and at Abirkateib (in Kassala Province); alluvial gold is occasionally exploited in Southern Fung and Equatoria.

Processed and scrap white mica have been mined since the late fifties; it went out of production for almost a decade, but started again in 1970 when 170 tonnes were produced; 1982, 200 tonnes. A big deposit of vermiculite and a medium-sized deposit of pyrophyllite are known to occur in the Sinkat District. Reserves of metallurgical grade chromite occur in the Ingessana Hills, Blue Nile Province. Huge reserves of chrysotile asbestos are proved in this vicinity and also in Qala El Nahal area, Kassala Province. Deposits of magnesite, with or without talc, are known to occur in the Ingessana Hills and Qala El Nahal areas in addition to other occurrences in the Halaib area, Red Sea Province.

Agriculture. The Sudan is a predominantly agricultural country. Cotton is by far the most important cash crop on which the Sudan depends for earning foreign currency. The two types of cotton grown in the Sudan are: (*a*) long staple sakellaridis and sakel types (derivatives of sakellaridis), grown in Gezira, White Nile, Abdel Magid and private pump schemes; (*b*) short staple, mainly American types, in Equatoria and Nuba Mountains, generally by rain cultivation.

Production (1988) in 1,000 tonnes: Sorghum, 4,640; sugar-cane, 4,500; groundnuts, 527; seed cotton, 394; millet, 550; wheat, 181; sesame, 278; cotton seed, 290.

One of the largest sugar complexes in the world was opened at Kenana in March 1981. It is capable of processing 330,000 tonnes a year.

Livestock (1988): Cattle, 22·5m.; sheep, 18·5m.; goats, 13·5m.; poultry, 29m.

The government's policy of self-sufficiency and disengagement from the west, coupled with drought, resulted in a food shortage of between 0·5m. and 1m. tonnes of grain, which was officially acknowledged in Jan. 1991.

Forestry. Gum arabic, mainly hashab gum from *Acacia senegal*, is the sole forest produce exported on a major scale. Production (1983) 38·16m. cu. metres.

FOREIGN ECONOMIC RELATIONS

Commerce. Total trade for calendar years, in US$1,000:

	1984	*1985*	*1986*
Imports	556,000	1,237,000	1,055,000
Exports	519,000	544,000	497,000

In 1983, Saudi Arabia provided 14·3% of imports and the UK 10%, while 17·1% of exports went to Saudi Arabia and 10% to Italy; cotton formed 49% by value of exports and groundnuts 2%, sesame 9% and gum arabic 9%.

Total trade between Sudan and UK (British Department of Trade returns, in £1,000 sterling):

	1986	*1987*	*1988*	*1989*	*1990*
Imports to UK	12,826	18,850	9,910	9,532	9,016
Exports and re-exports from UK	83,335	75,322	86,480	60,602	63,670

Tourism. There were 42,000 visitors in 1986.

COMMUNICATIONS

Roads. In 1982 there were about 3,000 km of tarmac roads, including the new 1,190 km road from Khartoum to Port Sudan, and 45,000 km of tracks. There were 99,400 passenger cars and 17,500 commercial vehicles in 1985.

Railways. The main railway lines run from Khartoum to El Obeid *via* Wadi Medani, Sennar Junction, Kosti and El Rahad (701 km); El Rahad to Nyala *via* Abu Zabad, Babanousa and Ed-Daein (698 km); Sennar Junction to Kassala *via* Gedaref (455 km) and to Roseires *via* Singa (220 km); Kassala to Port Sudan *via* Haiya Junction and Sinkat (550 km); Khartoum to Wadi Halfa *via* Shendi, El Dammer,

Atbara, Berber and Abu Hamad Junction (924 km); Abu Hamad to Karima (248 km); Atbara to Haiya Junction (271 km); Babanousa to Wau (444 km). The main flow of exports and imports is to and from Port Sudan *via* Atbara and Kassala. The total length of line open for traffic (1982) was 4,786 km. The gauge is 1,067 mm. In 1987, the railways carried 357m. passenger-km and 699m. tonne-km of freight.

Aviation. Sudan Airways is a government-owned airline, with its headquarters in Khartoum, operating domestic and international services. In 1980 Sudan Airways carried 519,000 passengers and 6·8m. ton-kg of mail and freight.

Shipping. Supplementing the railways are regular river steamer services of the Sudan Railways, between Karima and Dongola, 319 km; from Khartoum to Kosti, 319 km; from Kosti to Juba, 1,436 km, and from Kosti to Gambeila, 1,069 km. Port Sudan is the country's only seaport; it is equipped with 13 berths.

Telecommunications. Number of telephones in 1983 was 68,838 (44,756 in Greater Khartoum). Radio receivers (1982) 5m. The television service broadcasts for 35 hours per week. There were (1982) 1m. TV receivers.

Cinemas. In 1975 there were 58, seating capacity 112,000 and also 43 mobile units.

Newspapers. In 1985 there were 2 daily newspapers with a circulation of 120,000.

JUSTICE, RELIGION, EDUCATION AND WELFARE

Justice. The judiciary is a separate and independent department of state directly and solely responsible to the President of the Republic. The general administrative supervision and control of the judiciary is vested in the High Judicial Council.

Civil Justice is administered by the courts constituted under the Civil Justice Ordinance, namely the High Court of Justice—consisting of the Court of Appeal and Judges of the High Court, sitting as courts of original jurisdiction—and Province Courts—consisting of the Courts of Province and District Judges. The law administered is 'justice, equity and good conscience' in all cases where there is no special enactment. Procedure is governed by the Civil Justice Ordinance.

Justice in personal matters for the Moslem population is administered by the Mohammedan law courts, which form the Sharia Divisions of the Court of Appeal, High Courts and Kadis Courts; President of the Sharia Division is the Grand Kadi. The religious law of Islam is administered by these courts in the matters of inheritance, marriage, divorce, family relationship and charitable trusts. In Dec. 1990 the government announced that Sharia would be applied in the northern parts of the country.

Criminal Justice is administered by the courts constituted under the Code of Criminal Procedure, namely major courts, minor courts and magistrates' courts. Serious crimes are tried by major courts, which are composed of a President and 2 members and have the power to pass the death sentence. Major Courts are, as a rule, presided over by a Judge of the High Court appointed to a Provincial Circuit or a Province Judge. There is a right of appeal to the Chief Justice against any decision or order of a Major Court, and all its findings and sentences are subject to confirmation by him.

Lesser crimes are tried by Minor Courts consisting of 3 Magistrates and presided over by a Second Class Magistrate, and by Magistrates' Courts.

Religion. In 1980 about 73% of the population was Moslem. The population of the 12 northern provinces is almost entirely Moslem (Sunni), while the majority of the 6 southern provinces are animist (18%) or Christian (9%).

Education (1985). 6,707 primary schools had 1·7m. pupils; there were 490,583 pupils in 2,167 secondary schools and 28,985 in tertiary education. In 1979 Khartoum University with 10 faculties had 8,777 students. The Khartoum branch of Cairo University with 4 faculties had about 5,000 students and the Islamic University of Omdurman with 3 faculties had 1,472 students. Juba University, founded in 1975 with 5 faculties had 425 students.

Health. In 1981 the Ministry of Health maintained 158 hospitals (with 17,205 beds), 887 dispensaries, 1,619 dressing stations and 220 health centres. There were 2,122 doctors and 12,871 nurses.

DIPLOMATIC REPRESENTATIVES

Of Sudan in Great Britain (3 Cleveland Row, London, SW1A 1DD)
Ambassador: Sayed El Rashid Abushama (accredited 6 Dec. 1989).

Of Great Britain in Sudan (PO Box No. 801, Khartoum)
Ambassador: Allan Ramsay, CMG.

Of Sudan in the USA (2210 Massachusetts Ave., NW, Washington, D.C., 20008)
Ambassador: Abdalla Ahmed Abdalla.

Of the USA in Sudan (Sharia Ali Abdul Latif, Khartoum)
Ambassador: James R. Cheek.

Of Sudan to the United Nations
Ambassador: Lieut.-Gen. Joseph Lagu.

Further Reading

Sudan Almanac. Khartoum (annual)
Daly, M. W., *Sudan*. [Bibliography] Oxford and Santa Barbara, 1983
Gurdon, C., *Sudan in Transition: A Political Risk Analysis*. London, 1986
Halasa, A. *et al The Return to Democracy in Sudan*. Geneva, 1986
Holt, P. M., *A Modern History of the Sudan*. New York, 3rd ed. 1979
Khalid, M., *The Government They Deserve: the Role of the Elite in Sudan's Political Evolution*. London, 1990
Woodward, P., *Sudan, 1898-1989: the Unstable State*. London, 1991

SURINAME

Capital: Paramaribo
Population: 416,839 (1990)
GNP per capita: US$2,450 (1988)

Republic of Suriname

HISTORY. At the peace of Breda (1667) between Great Britain and the United Netherlands, Suriname was assigned to the Netherlands in exchange for the colony of New Netherland in North America, and this was confirmed by the treaty of Westminster of Feb. 1674. Since then Suriname has been twice in British possession, 1799–1802 (when it was restored to the Batavian Republic at the peace of Amiens) and 1804–16, when it was returned to the Kingdom of the Netherlands according to the convention of London of 13 Aug. 1814, confirmed at the peace of Paris of 20 Nov. 1815. On 25 Nov. 1975, Suriname gained full independence and was admitted to the UN on 4 Dec. 1975. On 25 Feb. 1980 the Government was ousted in a coup, and a National Military Council (NMC) established. A further coup on 13 Aug. replaced several members of the NMC, and the State President.

Suriname returned to democracy in Jan. 1988 following elections held in Nov. 1987. On 24 Dec. 1990 a military coup removed President Ramsewak Shankar and his cabinet from office.

AREA AND POPULATION. Suriname is situated on the north coast of South America and bounded on the north by the Atlantic ocean, on the east by the Marowijne River, which separates it from French Guiana, on the west by the Corantijn River, which separates it from Guyana, and on the south by forests and savannas, which separate it from Brazil.

Area, 163,820 sq. km. Census population (1980), 354,860. Estimate (1987) 415,000. The capital, Paramaribo, had (1988 estimate) 192,109 inhabitants.

Suriname is divided into 10 districts (with chief town): Brokopondo (Brokopondo), Commewijne (Nieuw Amdterdam), Coronie (Totness), Marowijne (Albina), Nickerie (Nieuw Nickerie), Para (Onverwacht), Paramaribo (Paramaribo), Saramacca (Groningen), Sipalwini (local authority in Paramaribo), Wanica (Lelydorp).

The official languages are Dutch and English. English is widely spoken next to Hindi, Javanese and Chinese as inter-group communication. A vernacular, called 'Sranan Tongo' or 'Surinamese', is used as a lingua franca. In 1976 it was announced that Spanish would become the nation's principal working language.

CLIMATE. The climate is equatorial, with uniformly high temperatures and rainfall. There is no recognized dry season. Paramaribo. Jan. 80°F (26·7°C), July 81°F (27·2°C). Annual rainfall 89" (2,225 mm).

CONSTITUTION AND GOVERNMENT. A new Constitution was approved by referendum in Sept. 1980. Elections took place 25 Nov. 1987. The Front for Democracy and Development won 40 of the 51 seats in the National Assembly.

After the coup of Dec. 1990 Johan Kraag (National Party) was named provisional president by the National Assembly. Elections for president, vice-president and National Assembly were scheduled for 25 May 1991.

Flag: Horizontally green, red, green with the red of double width with yellow 5-pointed star in centre of red bar.

DEFENCE

Army. Armed forces of the Republic of Suriname consist of 1 infantry and 1 military police battalions with a strength of about 2,700 in 1990. Equipment includes 2 PC-7 armed trainers, 3 Defender twin-engined light transports operated alongside 1 Bell 205, 2 Alouette III and 1 Cessna 206 liaison aircraft. Officers' ranks were abolished in Feb. 1986.

Navy. The flotilla comprises 3 32m and 3 22m inshore patrol craft, as well as 3 river patrol boats, all built in the Netherlands. In 1990 personnel totalled 250.

INTERNATIONAL RELATIONS

Membership. Suriname is a member of the UN, OAS and is an ACP state of the EEC.

ECONOMY

Policy. For 15 years from independence (i.e. to 1990) approximately 3,500m. guilders was available from the Netherlands to carry out an extensive social and economic development programme.

Budget. 1989 revenue was (in 1m. Sf) 836·6, made up of direct taxes, 316·9; indirect taxes, 230; bauxite levy and other revenues, 191·8; grants, 50·4; aid, 47·5. Total expenditure was 1,206·5, made up of wages, 562·8; materials, 278·1; transfers, 149·8; interest, 134·6; development expenditure, 62·5; loans, 18·7.

Currency. The unit of currency is the *Suriname guilder* (SRG) of 100 *cents*. Notes ranging from 5 to 1,000 *Suriname guilders* are legal tender. Currency notes of 1·00 and 2·50 guilders are issued by the Government. In March 1991, US$1 = 1·79 Sf; £1 sterling = 3·39 Sf.

Banking and Finance. The Central Bank of Suriname is a bankers' bank and also a bank of issue; the Surinaamsche Bank, the Algemene Bank Nederland and the Handels-, Kredieten Industriebank, are commercial banks; the Suriname People's Credit Bank operates under the auspices of the Government; Surinaamse Postspaarbank (postal savings bank); Surinaamse Hypotheekbank NV (mortgage bank); Surinaamse Investerings Mij. NV (investment bank); Agentschap van de Maatschappij tot financiering van het Nationaal Herstel NV (long-term investments); National Development Bank; The Agrarian Bank.

Weights and Measures. The metric system is in force.

ENERGY AND NATURAL RESOURCES

Electricity. Production (1986) 1,610m. kwh.

Minerals. Bauxite is the most important mineral; it is being mined in the Suriname and Marowijne districts but in 1987 several mines were closed by attacks by anti-government rebels. Fresh deposits have been found in the western areas. The ore is exported mainly to USA and the Dominican Republic, but partly processed locally into alumina and aluminium. Production (1987 in 1,000 tonnes): Bauxite, 2,522.

Agriculture. Agriculture is restricted to the alluvial coastal zone; cultivated area in 1982, 87,442 ha. The staple food crop is rice; 72,571 ha of paddy were planted in 1982, chiefly in the Nickerie, Commewijne, Saramacca and Coronie districts.

Production (1988, in 1,000 tonnes): Sugar-cane, 45; rice, 300; oranges, 9; grapefruit, 2; coconuts, 11; palm oil, 6·8; cassava, 3.

Livestock (1988): 74,000 head of cattle, 4,000 sheep, 6,000 goats, 20,000 pigs, 6m. poultry.

Forestry. Forests cover 14·9 ha, 42% of the land area. Production in 1986 was 196,000 cu. metres.

Fisheries. The fish catch in 1987 amounted to 2,321 tonnes.

INDUSTRY. In 1981, there were 3 large bauxite plants, 1 alumina and 1 aluminium smelting plants, sugar- and rice-mills, 3 paint factories, 2 fruit-juice plants, 3 shrimp freezing plants, a plywood factory, timber-mills, a milk pasteurization plant, a butter and margarine factory and a number of various medium and small industries. Shortage of skilled personnel inhibits expansion.

FOREIGN ECONOMIC RELATIONS

Commerce. In 1988 imports totalled 249·9m. Suriname guilders and exports, 535m.

Principal imports in 1988 (in 1m. Suriname guilders): Raw materials, 249·9; investment goods, 115·4; fules and lubricants, 90·3; foodstuffs, 41·5; cars and motorcycles, 32·3; textiles, 10·6.

Principal exports in 1988 (in 1m. Suriname guilders): Alumina, 535; rice, 71·7; shrimps, 55·8; bananas, 36·2; aluminium, 26·5; wood and wood products, 5·6.

Total trade between Suriname and UK (British Department of Trade returns, in £1,000 sterling):

	1986	*1987*	*1988*	*1989*	*1990*
Imports to UK	15,554	12,488	11,256	16,366	10,094
Exports and re-exports from UK	9,743	7,974	6,107	6,777	10,564

Tourism. Visitors totalled 8,440 in 1987.

COMMUNICATIONS

Roads. There are 1,335 km of main roads. Two of them lead from Paramaribo to the bauxite centres of Smalkalden (29 km) and Paranam (30 km) and to the airport of Zanderij (49 km). Another main road runs across the districts of Saramacca (71 km) and Coronie (68 km), a fourth across the Commewijne district (41 km) and a fifth in the Marowijne district, from the bauxite centre Moengo to Albina (45 km). The 'East–West connexion' is almost completed, linking the Corantijn and the Marowijne rivers (375 km).

In 1987 there were 32,000 passenger cars, 11,000 trucks, 2,000 buses and 1,100 motor cycles.

Railways. There is a single-track railway, running from Onverwacht to Bronsweg (86 km); part of the track, from Paramaribo to Onverwacht (34 km) has been removed. Another single-track railway runs from Apoera to the Bakhuis Mountains.

Aviation. Regular air services are maintained by KLM, SLM, Aero Cubano and Cruzeiro do Sul. The international airfield at Zanderij is capable of handling all types of planes.

Suriname Airways Ltd provides daily services between all major districts and maintains also a charter service.

Shipping. The Royal Netherlands Steamship Co. plies between Amsterdam, Rotterdam, Antwerp, Hamburg and Paramaribo, and New York, Baltimore, New Orleans and Paramaribo. Regular sailings are made to Georgetown, Ciudad Bolivar and most Caribbean ports. The Suriname Navigation Co. maintains services from Paramaribo to Georgetown and Cayenne, and once a month to the Caribbean area. A French and an Italian company maintain passenger services to Europe. The Alcoa Steamship Co. has a fortnightly service to New York, Baltimore, Mobile and New Orleans; a Japanese line sails once a month from Hong Kong and Yokohama to Paramaribo; the Boomerang Line maintains a monthly freight and passenger service between Suriname and Australia.

Telecommunciations. In 1985 there were 36,000 telephones. Wireless telephone connects Suriname with the Netherlands, USA, Curaçao, Guyana, French Guiana and Trinidad. There are 6 broadcasting and 1 television stations. In 1986 there were 246,000 radios and 48,000 TV sets.

Cinemas. In 1981 there were 18 cinemas and 1 drive-in cinema.

Newspapers (1987). There are 2 daily newspapers.

JUSTICE, RELIGION, EDUCATION AND WELFARE

Justice. There is a court of justice, whose members are nominated by the President. There are 3 cantonal courts.

Religion. There is entire religious liberty. At the end of 1983 the main religious bodies were: Hindus, 97,170; Roman Catholics, 80,922; Moslems, 69,638;

Moravian Brethren, 55,625; Reformed, 6,265; Lutheran, 2,695; Jehovah's Witnesses, 1,626; Seventh Day Adventists, 1,061; others, 24,627.

Education. In 1986–87 there were 301 primary schools with 3,954 teachers and 59,633 pupils, and there were 1,588 teachers and 23,217 pupils at 89 secondary schools. There was also a University with (1986) 1,070 students and a teacher training college with 1,500 students.

Health. There were (1985) 1,964 hospital beds and 219 physicians.

DIPLOMATIC REPRESENTATIVES

Of Suriname in Great Britain
Ambassador: Cyrill Bisoendat Ramkisor.

Of Great Britain in Suriname
Ambassador: R. D. Gordon (resides in Georgetown).

Of Suriname in the USA (4301 Connecticut Ave., NW, Washington, D.C., 20008)
Ambassador: Willem A. Udenhout.

Of the USA in Suriname (Dr Sophie Redmondstraat 129, Paramaribo)
Ambassador: (Vacant).

Of Suriname to the United Nations
Ambassador: Kriesnadath Nandoe.

Further Reading

Statistical Information: The General Bureau of Statistics in Paramaribo was established on 1 Jan. 1947. Its publications comprise trade statistics, *Suriname in Figures* (including, from 1953, the former *Handelsstatistiek*) and *Statistische Berichten.*

Economische Voorlichting Suriname. Ministry of Economic Affairs, Paramaribo
Annual Report of the Central Bank of Suriname
Hoefte, R. A. L., *Suriname*: [Bibliography]. Oxford and Santa Barbara, 1990

SWAZILAND

Capital: Mbabane
Population: 681,059 (1986)
GNP per capita: US$790 (1988)

Kingdom of Swaziland

HISTORY. The Swazi migrated into the country to which they have given their name, in the last half of the 18th century. They settled first in what is now southern Swaziland, but moved northwards under their chief, Sobhuza, known also to the Swazi as Somhlolo. Sobhuza died in 1838 and was succeeded by Mswati. The further order of succession has been Mbandzeni and Bhunu, whose son, Sobhuza II, was installed as King of the Swazi nation in 1921 after a long minority.

The independence of the Swazis was guaranteed in the conventions of 1881 and 1884 between the British Government and the Government of the South African Republic. In 1890, soon after the death of Mbandzeni, a provisional government was established representative of the Swazis, the British and the South African Republic Governments. In 1894 the South African Republic was given powers of protection and administration. In 1902, after the conclusion of the Boer War, a special commissioner took charge, and under an order-in-council in 1903 the Governor of the Transvaal administered the territory, through the Special Commissioner. Swaziland became independent on 6 Sept. 1968.

On 25 April 1967 the British Government gave the country internal self-government. It changed the country's status to that of a protected state with the Ngwenyama, Sobhuza II, recognized as King of Swaziland and head of state. King Sobhuza died on 21 Aug. 1982. On 25 April 1986, King Mswati III was installed as King of Swaziland.

AREA AND POPULATION. Swaziland is bounded on the north, west and south by the Transvaal Province, and on the east by Mozambique and Zululand. The area is 6,705 sq. miles (17,400 sq. km).

The country is divided geographically into 4 longitudinal regions running from north to south; 3 of roughly equal width—Highveld (westernmost), Middleveld, Lowveld—and the Lubombo plateau in the east. The mountainous region on the west rises to an altitude of over 6,000 ft (1,800 metres). The Middleveld is mostly between 1,700 and 3,000 ft, while the Lowveld has an average height of not more than 1,000 ft (300 metres).

Population (census 1986), 681,059. Mbabane, the administrative capital (1986, 38,290). The main urban areas with 1986 census populations are: Manzini (18,084); Big Bend (9,676); Mhlume (6,509); Havelock Mine (4,850); Nhlangano (4,107); Pigg's Peak (3,223) and Siteki (2,271). 31,072 citizens abroad. In early 1988 there were 14,550 refugees living in the country.

CLIMATE. A temperate climate with two seasons. Nov. to March is the wet season, when temperatures range from mild to hot, with frequent thunderstorms. The cool, dry season from May to Sept. is characterised by clear, bright sunny days. Mbabane. Jan. 68°F (20°C), July 54°F (12·2°C). Annual rainfall 56" (1,402 mm).

CONSTITUTION AND GOVERNMENT. Britain's protection ended at independence, when a Constitution similar to the 1967 Constitution was brought into force. The general elections (by universal adult franchise) in April 1967 gave the royalist and traditional Imbokodvo National Movement all 24 seats. The Parliament consists of a House of Assembly, with 24 elected and 6 nominated members and the Attorney-General, who has no vote, and a Senate comprising 12 members, 6 of whom are elected by the House of Assembly and 6 appointed by the King. The executive authority is vested in the King and exercised through a Cabinet presided over by the Prime Minister, and consisting of the Prime Minister, the Deputy Prime Minister and up to 8 other ministers. In April 1973 the King assumed supreme power and the Constitution was suspended and in 1976 it was abolished. On 28 Oct. 1983 a general election took place to elect an electoral college of 80 members.

His Majesty the King: Mswati III (crowned 25 April 1986).

In Feb. 1991, the Cabinet was composed as follows:

Prime Minister: Obed M. Dlamini.

Foreign Affairs: George M. Mamba. *Labour and Public Service:* B. M. Nsibandze. *Agriculture and Co-operatives:* H. S. Mamba. *Commerce, Industry and Tourism:* N. D. Ntiwane. *Works and Communications:* Wilson C. Mkhonta. *Education:* Chief Sipho Shongwe. *Finance:* B.S. Dlamini. *Health:* Dr F. Friedman. *Justice:* Reginald Dladla. *Interior and Immigration:* E. S. Shabalala. *Natural Resources, Land Utilization and Energy:* Prince Nqaba Dlamini.

National flag. Horizontally 5 unequal stripes of blue, yellow, crimson, yellow, blue; in the centre of the crimson strip an African shield of black and white, behind which are 2 assegais and a staff, all laid horizontally.

Local Government. The country is divided into the 4 regions of Shiselweni, Lubombo, Manzini and Hhohho. They are administered by Regional Administrators.

DEFENCE

Army Air Wing. First military aircraft acquired by Swaziland, in mid-1979, were 2 Israeli-built Arava light twin-turboprop transports with underwing weapon attachments for light attack duties.

INTERNATIONAL RELATIONS

Membership. Swaziland is a member of UN, OAU, the Commonwealth and is an ACP state of EEC.

ECONOMY

Budget. Revenue and expenditure (in 1,000 emalangeni) for financial years ending 31 March:

	1987–88	*1988–89* [1]	*1989–90* [1]
Revenue	337,310	361,052	449,211
Expenditure	315,726	370,568	450,234

[1]Estimate.

Currency. The unit of currency is the *lilangeni* (plural *emalangeni*) (SZL) but Swaziland remains in the rand monetary area. In March 1991, £1 = 4·92 *emalangeni;* US$1 = 2·59 *emalangeni*.

Banking. Barclays Bank International and the Standard Bank Ltd maintain branches at Mbabane and Manzini; sub-branches and agencies are operated in 17 other places. Bank rates are those in force throughout South Africa and are prescribed by the main South African offices of the 2 banks. The Swazi Bank, a statutory body, was opened in 1965. It specializes in credit for agriculture and low-cost housing. Its head office is in Mbabane and it has branches or agencies at 3 other places. The Bank of Credit and Commerce International opened in 1978; its head office is in Manzini and it has a branch in Mbabane. The Union Bank opened in 1988. Its head office is in Mbabane.

ENERGY AND NATURAL RESOURCES

Electricity. Production (1986) 120m. kwh. Supply 230 volts; 50 Hz.

Minerals. Swaziland produces asbestos from the Havelock Mine (22,804 tonnes in 1988). Coal is mined at Mpaka (165,122 tonnes in 1989). Quarry stone is also mined (107,205 cu. metres in 1988).

A railway has been built from the Ngwenya haematite deposits to Goba, in Mozambique, chiefly for the transportation of iron ore. The extensive deposits of low-volatile bituminous coal in the Lowveld are being worked to provide coal for the railway, sugar-mills and export.

Agriculture. In 1987–88 the cultivated area was 165,464 hectares, the grazing area 1,105,274 hectares and the commercial forest area 102,625 hectares. Production (1987–88, in 1,000 tonnes): Sugar-cane, 3,870; citrus, 68; rice, 4; seed cotton, 26; maize, 113; sorghum, 1; pineapples, 35; tomatoes, 4; potatoes, 6. Tobacco is also grown. It is usually necessary to import maize from South Africa. Sugar, first produced in 1958, and woodpulp and other forest products are the two main agricultural exports.

Livestock (1988): Cattle, 640,000; goats, 284,000; sheep, 26,000; poultry, 1m.

FOREIGN ECONOMIC RELATIONS.

Swaziland has a customs union with South Africa and receives a *pro rata* share of the dues collected.

Commerce. In 1988 exports (in E1,000) were 1,024,896, including sugar, 295,337; unbleached wood pulp, 163,544; canned fruits, 43,688; asbestos, 22,110. Imports: 1,398,972, including machinery and transport euqipment, 469,805; minerals, fuels and lubricants, 165,644; manufactured items, 214,783; food (1987), 119,727.

Total trade between Swaziland and UK (British Department of Trade returns, in £1,000 sterling):

	1986	*1987*	*1988*	*1989*	*1990*
Imports to UK	48,194	36,901	27,973	31,368	34,473
Exports and re-exports from UK	3,922	2,257	1,564	1,358	2,719

Tourism. There were 201,438 visitors in 1989.

COMMUNICATIONS

Roads. There is daily communication by railway motor-buses and interstate transport between Swaziland and South Africa. There are also Swazi owned taxis and buses which operate between the two countries. Total length of roads (1988) 2,779 km of which 719 km were tarred.

Railways. In 1989 the system comprised 301 km of route, and carried 5·5m. tonnes of freight.

Aviation. The country's chief airport is at Matsapa, near Manzini. It is served by Royal Swazi National Airways connecting with Johannesburg, Durban, Lusaka, Nairobi, Harare and Gaborone. Lesotho National Airways flies to Harare and Maputo through Matsapa. In 1986 Zambian Airways inaugurated their weekly flight to Matsapa *via* Gaborone.

Post and Broadcasting. There were (1987) 71 post offices, 2 telegraph stations and 29 postal agencies. In 1988 there 22,414 telephones, 10,529 exchange connexions and 357 telex exchange connexions. In 1986 there were over 96,000 radio sets and over 12,000 television receivers.

Cinemas. There were 5 cinemas in 1980 with a total seating capacity of 1,625.

Newspapers. There were in 1987 two daily newspapers.

JUSTICE, RELIGION, EDUCATION AND WELFARE

Justice. The judiciary is headed by the Chief Justice. A High Court having full jurisdiction and subordinate courts presided over by Magistrates and District Officers are in existence.

There is a Court of Appeal with a President and 3 Judges. It deals with appeals from the High Court. There are 16 Swazi courts of first instance, 2 Swazi courts of appeal and a Higher Swazi Court of Appeal. The channel of appeal lies from Swazi Court of first instance to Swazi Court of Appeal, to Higher Swazi Court of Appeal, to the Judicial Commissioner and thence to the High Court of Swaziland.

Religion. In 1984 there were about 120,000 Christians and about 30,000 adults holding traditional beliefs. A large number of churches and missionary societies are established throughout the country and, in addition to evangelism, are doing important work in the fields of education and medicine. In the larger centres there are churches of several denominations—Protestant, Roman Catholics and others.

Education. In 1988 there were 606 schools with 152,895 pupils in primary classes and 35,278 in secondary and high school classes. The then Swaziland Agricultural College and University Centre at Luyengo was opened in Oct. 1966. The College is now the Faculty of Agriculture at the University of Swaziland, which is situated in Matsapa. Technical and vocational training classes are run at the Government Swaziland College of Technology (SCOT), the Swaziland Institute of Management and Public Administration (SIMPA), the Gwamile Vocational Commercial Training Institute (VOCTIM), Mpaka Vocational Centre and the Manzini Industrial Training Centre. The Government also operates a Police College, Institute of Health Sciences, the Nazarene Prison College and the Nursing College which trains para-medical staff for the hospitals and clinics. There were 3 teacher training colleges with 501 students in 1987–88. There were 1,313 students enrolled in all the vocational centres except SIMPA, and 1,427 at the University of Swaziland, in 1987–88.

Health. In 1984 there were 80 doctors, 13 dentists and 1,608 hospital beds.

DIPLOMATIC REPRESENTATIVES

Of Swaziland in Great Britain (58 Pont St., London SW1X 0AE)
High Commissioner: Mboni N. Dlamini.

Of Great Britain in Swaziland (Allister Miller St., Mbabane)
High Commissioner: Brian Watkins.

Of Swaziland in the USA (3400 International Dr., NW, Washington, D.C., 20008)
Ambassador: Absalom V. Mamba.

Of the USA in Swaziland (PO Box 199, Mbabane)
Ambassador: (Vacant).

Of Swaziland to the United Nations
Ambassador: Dr Timothy L. L. Dlamini.

Further Reading

Booth, A., *Swaziland: Tradition and Change in a Southern African Kingdom.* Aldershot and Boulder, 1984
Grotpeter, J. J., *Historical Dictionary of Swaziland.* Metuchen, 1975
Jones, D., *Aid and Development in Southern Africa.* London, 1977
Matsebula, J. S. M., *A History of Swaziland.* London, 1972
Nyeko, B., *Swaziland.* [Bibliography] Oxford and Santa Barbara, 1982

SWEDEN

Capital: Stockholm
Population: 8·5m. (1989)
GNP per capita: US$21,761 (1989)

Konungariket Sverige

(Kingdom of Sweden)

HISTORY. Organized as an independent unified state in the 10th century, Sweden became a constitutional monarchy in 1809. In 1809 she also ceded Finland to Russia. In 1815 German possessions were ceded to Prussia and Sweden was united with Norway, which union lasted until 1905.

AREA AND POPULATION. Sweden is bounded west and north-west by Norway, east by Finland and the Gulf of Bothnia, south-east by the Baltic Sea and south-west by the Kattegat. The first census took place in 1749, and it was repeated at first every third year, and, after 1775, every fifth year. Since 1860 a general census has been taken every 10 years and, in addition, in 1935, 1945, 1965, 1975 and 1985.

Latest census figures: 1940, 6,371,432 (annual increase since 1935: 0·38%); 1950, 7,041,829 (1·1% since 1945); 1960, 7,495,316 (0·64% since 1950); 1965, 7,766,424 (1·04% since 1960); 1970, 8,076,903 (1·04% since 1965); 1975, 8,208,544 (1·02% since 1970); 1980, 8,320,438 (1·01% since 1975); 1985, 8,360,178.

Counties (Län)	*Land area: sq. km*	*Census population 1 Nov. 1985*	*Estimated population 31 Dec. 1989*	*Pop. per sq. km 31 Dec. 1989*
Stockholm	6,488	1,577,596	1,629,631	251
Uppsala	6,989	251,754	264,738	37
Södermanland	6,060	249,885	253,363	41
Östergötland	10,562	393,668	399,506	37
Jönköping	9,944	300,892	306,590	30
Kronoberg	8,458	174,025	176,589	20
Kalmar	11,170	238,406	239,564	21
Gotland	3,140	56,180	56,840	18
Blekinge	2,941	151,055	149,960	50
Kristianstad	6,089	280,516	286,654	47
Malmöhus	4,938	750,294	771,361	156
Halland	5,454	240,090	250,959	46
Göteborg and Bohus	5,141	715,831	735,672	143
Älvsborg	11,395	426,769	437,516	38
Skaraborg	7,938	270,530	274,546	34
Värmland	17,583	279,503	282,375	16
Örebro	8,519	270,384	271,523	31
Västmanland	6,302	254,858	256,510	40
Kopparberg	28,194	284,029	286,667	10
Gävleborg	18,191	289,452	288,223	15
Västernorrland	21,678	262,555	260,488	12
Jämtland	49,443	134,161	134,789	2
Västerbotten	55,401	245,302	250,134	4
Norrbotten	98,911	262,443	262,838	2
Total	410,928[1]	8,360,178	8,527,036	20

[1] Total area of Sweden, 449,964 sq. km.

On 31 Dec. 1989 there were 4,212,080 males and 4,314,956 females.

On 31 Dec. 1989 aliens in Sweden numbered 456,049. Of these, 123,867 were Finns, 39,591 Yugoslavs, 35,144 Iranians, 35,046 Norwegians, 28,081 Danes, 24,152 Turks, 19,129 Chileans, 14,736 Poles, 12,020 West Germans, 9,167 Britons, 7,501 Americans, 6,722 Greeks, 6,101 Ethiopians, 6,007 Iraqis and 4,781 Lebanese.

Vital statistics for calendar years:

	Total living births	To mothers single, divorced or widowed	Stillborn	Marriages	Divorces	Deaths exclusive of still-born
1987	104,699	52,218	412	41,223	18,426	93,307
1988	112,080	57,090	422	44,229	17,746	96,743
1989	116,023	60,077	423	108,919	18,862	92,110

Expectation of life in 1990: males, 74; females, 80.

Immigration: 1983, 27,495; 1984, 31,486; 1985, 33,134; 1986, 39,487; 1987, 42,688; 1988, 51,092; 1989, 65,811. Emigration: 1983, 25,269; 1984, 22,825; 1985, 22,041; 1986, 24,495; 1987, 20,679; 1988, 21,461; 1989, 21,479.

In 1860 the urban population numbered 435,000 (11% of the total population) and on 31 Dec. 1965, 4,177,212 (54%); including other densely populated areas, the urbanized population in 1965 was 77·4%.

On 15 Sept. 1980, population in densely populated areas was 6,910,431 (83·1%).

Population of largest communities, 31 Dec. 1989:

Stockholm	672,187	Halmstad	79,362	Kalmar	55,801
Göteborg	431,840	Karlstad	76,120	Kungsbacka	53,124
Malmö	232,908	Skellefteå	74,720	Falun	53,110
Uppsala	164,754	Huddinge	73,107	Mölndal	51,767
Linköping	120,562	Kristianstad	71,123	Solna	51,427
Örebro	120,353	Växjö	68,849	Sollentuna	50,606
Norrköping	119,921	Botkyrka	68,255	Trollhättan	50,602
Västerås	118,386	Luleå	67,903	Hässleholm	48,794
Jönköping	110,860	Nyköping	65,135	Varberg	48,193
Helsingborg	108,359	Nacka	63,114	Skövde	47,181
Borås	101,231	Haninge	62,178	Uddevalla	46,988
Sundsvall	93,404	Örnsköldsvik	59,255	Borlänge	46,424
Umeå	90,004	Karlskrona	58,768	Norrtälje	44,811
Eskilstuna	89,460	Östersund	57,733	Motala	41,710
Gävle	88,081	Gotland	56,840	Sandviken	40,015
Lund	86,412	Täby	56,553	Västervik	39,602
Södertälje	81,460	Järfälla	56,386		

Befolkningsförändringar (Population Changes). Annual. 3 vols. Statistics Sweden, Stockholm
Folkmängd 31 Dec. (Population). Annual. 2 vols. Statistics Sweden, Stockholm

CLIMATE. North Sweden suffers from severe winters, with snow lying for 4–7 months. Summers are fine but cool, with long daylight hours. Further south, winters are less cold, summers are warm and rainfall generally well-distributed over the year, though with a slight summer maximum. Stockholm. Jan. 24·4°F (–4·1°C), July 59·9°F (17·3°C). Annual rainfall 25" (622 mm).

REIGNING KING. Carl XVI Gustaf, born 30 April 1946, succeeded on the death of his grandfather Gustaf VI Adolf, 15 Sept. 1973, married 19 June 1976 to *Silvia* Renate Sommerlath, born 23 Dec. 1943 (Queen of Sweden). *Daughter* and *Heir Apparent:* Crown Princess Victoria Ingrid Alice Désirée, Duchess of Västergötland, born 14 July 1977; *son:* Prince Carl Philip Edmund Bertil, Duke of Värmland, born 13 May 1979; *daughter:* Princess Madeleine Thérèse Amelie Josephine, Duchess of Hälsingland and Gästrikland, born 10 June 1982.

Sisters of the King. Princess Margaretha, born 31 Oct. 1934, married 30 June 1964 to Mr John Ambler; Princess Birgitta (Princess of Sweden), born 19 Jan. 1937, married 25 May 1961 (civil marriage) and 30 May 1961 (religious ceremony) to Johann Georg, Prince of Hohenzollern; Princess Désirée, born 2 June 1938, married 5 June 1964 to Baron Niclas Silfverschiöld; Princess Christina, born 3 Aug. 1943, married 15 June 1974 to Tord Magnuson.

Uncles of the King. Sigvard, Count of Wisborg, born on 7 June 1907; Prince Bertil, Duke of Halland, born on 28 Feb. 1912, married 7 Dec. 1976 to Lilian May Davies, born 30 Aug. 1915 (Princess of Sweden, Duchess of Halland); Carl Johan, Count of Wisborg, born on 31 Oct. 1916.

Aunt of the King. Princess Ingrid (Princess of Sweden), born 28 March 1910, married 24 May 1935 to Frederik, Crown Prince of Denmark (King Frederik IX), died 14 Jan. 1972.

The following is a list of the kings and queens of Sweden, with the dates of their accession from the accession of the House of Vasa:

House of Vasa		*House of Pfalz-Zweibrücken* (contd.)		*House of Bernadotte*	
Gustaf I	1521	Carl XII	1697	Carl XIV Johan	1818
Eric XIV	1560	Ulrica Eleonora	1719	Oscar I	1844
Johan III	1568			Carl XV	1859
Sigismund	1592	*House of Hesse*		Oscar II	1872
Carl IX	1599	Fredrik I	1720	Gustaf V	1907
Gustaf II Adolf	1611			Gustaf VI Adolf	1950
Christina	1632	*House of Holstein-Gottorp*		Carl XVI Gustaf	1973
House of Pfalz-Zweibrücken		Adolf Fredrik	1751		
		Gustaf III	1771		
Carl X Gustaf	1654	Gustaf IV Adolf	1792		
Carl XI	1660	Carl XIII	1809		

The royal family of Sweden have a civil list of 18·47m. kronor; this does not include the maintenance of the royal palaces.

CONSTITUTION AND GOVERNMENT. Sweden's present Constitution came into force in 1975 and replaced the 1809 Constitution. Under the present Constitution Sweden is a representative and parliamentary democracy. Parliament (*Riksdag*) is declared to be the central organ of government. The executive power of the country is vested in the Government, which is responsible to Parliament. The King is Head of State, but he does not participate in the government of the country. Since 1971 Parliament has consisted of one chamber. It has 349 members, who are elected for a period of 3 years in direct, general elections.

Every man and woman who has reached the age of 18 years on election-day itself, and who is not under wardship has the right to vote and to stand for election.

The manner of election to the *Riksdag* is proportional. The country is divided into 28 constituencies. In these constituencies 310 members are elected. The remaining 39 seats constitute a nation-wide pool intended to give absolute proportionality to parties that receive at least 4% of the votes. A party receiving less than 4% of the votes in the country is, however, entitled to participate in the distribution of seats in a constituency, if it has obtained at least 12% of the votes cast there.

The *Riksdag*, elected 1988, has 156 Social Democrats, 66 Conservatives, 42 Centre Party, 44 Liberals, 21 Communists and 20 Green Party.

The Social Democratic Cabinet was composed as follows in Oct. 1990:

Prime Minister: Ingvar Carlsson.

Deputy Prime Minister: Odd Engstrom. *Finance:* Allan Larsson. *Health and Social Affairs:* Ingela Thalen. *Special responsibility for international development co-operation, Ministry of Foreign Affairs:* Lena Hjelm-Wallén. *Foreign Affairs:* Sten Andersson. *Higher Education, with special responsibility for cultural affairs and the mass media:* Bengt Göransson. *Foreign Trade:* Anita Gradin. *Environment:* Birgitta Dahl. *Defence:* Roine Carlsson. *Agriculture:* Mats Hellström. *Public Administration:* Bengt Johansson. *Transport and Communications:* Georg Andersson. *Special responsibility for family policy, the disabled and elderly, Ministry of Health and Social Affairs:* Bengt Lindqvist. *Labour, with special responsibility for immigrant affairs:* Maj-Lis Lööw. *Housing:* Ulf Lönnqvist. *Labour:* Mona Sahlin. *Industry and Energy:* Rune Molin. *Assistant Minister of Finance:* Erik Åsbrink. *Justice:* Laila Freivalds. *Special responsibility for church, equality and consumer affairs, Ministry of Public Administration:* Margot Wallström. *Special responsibility for comprehensive schools, adult education, Ministry of Education:* Göran Persson.

Ministerial decisions are formally made by the Cabinet collectively and not (with some exceptions) by individual ministers.

Public administration in Sweden is characterized by a unique degree of functional decentralization. The Ministries are not really administrative agencies. Their main function is to prepare the decisions of the Cabinet; such decisions may concern bills for the *Riksdag*, general government directives and higher appointments. Only to a small extent does the Cabinet make individual administrative decisions. The routine administrative work is attended to by the central boards (*centrala ämbetsverk*). Each board is in principle subordinate to the government; its sphere of activity depends on the appropriations granted by the *Riksdag*. The Government often asks the boards' opinion on proposed measures.

National flag: Blue with a yellow Scandinavian cross.

National anthem: Du gamla, du fria, du fjällhöga nord ('Thou ancient, thou free, thou mountainous north'; words by R. Dybeck, 1844; folk-tune).

The official language is Swedish. The capital is Stockholm.

Regional and Local Government. For national administrative purposes Sweden is divided into 24 counties (*län*), in each of which the central government is represented by a state county administrative board (*länsstyrelse*). The governor (*landshövding*), appointed by the government, is chairman of the board, which in addition to the governor has 14 members elected by the county council.

Local government and the levying of local taxes are based on the Instrument of Government (the Swedish Constitution) and are regulated by the local government act and special acts. According to the local government act Sweden is divided into municipalities in which all men and women who have reached the age of 18 on election-day itself, and not under wardship, are entitled to elect the municipal council. These councils are named *kommunfullmäktige*. The number of municipalities has, since 1951, been reduced from about 2,500 to 284. The municipalities deal with a great variety of different tasks such as social welfare, education and culture, public health, town planning, housing etc. Each county, except Gotland, which consists of only one municipality, has a county council (*landsting*) elected by men and women who enjoy local suffrage. The county councils chiefly administer the health services and medical care. The municipalities of Gothenburg and Malmö do not belong to county councils. The parishes, 2,563 in 1990, are the local units of the Church of Sweden and have the same status in public law as the municipalities. The parochial church council (*kyrkofullmäktige*) is the supreme decision-making body in most parishes, whose members are publicly elected. Small parishes have instead the parish meeting, a form of direct democracy.

Boalt, G., *The Political Process.* Stockholm, 1984
Gustafsson, A., *Local Government in Sweden.* Stockholm, 1988
Hadenius, S., *Swedish Politics During the 20th Century.* Stockholm, 1988
Lindström, E., *The Swedish Parliamentary System.* Stockholm, 1983
Peterson, C.-G., *Local Self-Government and Democracy in Transition.* Stockholm, 1989
Strömberg, L. and Westerstahl, J., *The New Swedish Communes.* Gothenburg, 1984
Vinde, P., *Swedish Government Administration.* 2nd rev. ed. Stockholm, 1978

DEFENCE. A Supreme Commander is, under the Government, in command of the three services. He is assisted by the Defence Staff under a chief of staff.

The military forces are recruited on the principle of national service, supplemented by voluntarily enlisted personnel who form the permanent cadres for training purposes, staff duties, etc.

Liability to service commences at the age of 18, and lasts till the end of the 47th year. The period of training for the Army and Navy is $7^1/_2$-12 months and for the Airforce 8-12 months.

The territorial organization consists of 6 military commands each one under a general officer commanding.

Army. The C.-in-C. of the Swedish Army has at his disposal the Army Staff under a chief of staff. The peace-time Army consists for training purposes of 16 infantry, 2 cavalry, 6 armour, 4 artillery, 5 AA, 3 engineer, 2 signal and 3 Army Service Corps units, most of which are called 'regiments' (*regementen*). The Army Aviation Corps comprises 2 Battalions operating 6 Bulldog aircraft and 18 JetRanger helicopters for observation, 20 armed BO 105 helicopters, 12 AB.204B transport helicopters, plus 26 Hughes 300C helicopters and 2 DO 27 aircraft for training and observation duties.

The Army is organized and equipped with regard to the varying geographical and climatic conditions of the country. The voluntary Home Guard (*Hemvärnet*) with a total strength of more than 125,000 men ready for action within 2 hours, raised during the War continues to be in force.

Sweden's ground forces, total 850,000 men (including the voluntary Home Guard), can be said to consist of an Army which for the most part is on indefinite leave, but which on short notice can be ready for action. One of the basic principles of the Swedish system of mobilization is the local recruitment of as many units as possible. The storage of equipment and supplies is decentralized on more than 3,000 places.

The active personnel of the Army comprises (1991) about 44,500 (37,700 conscripts).

Navy. The C.-in-C. of the Navy is assisted by the Chief of Naval Staff and the Chief of Naval Material. THe main operational commander is the Commander-in-Chief, Coastal Fleet. Naval forces are divided between 2 branches: Navy and Coastal Defence Artillery. There are 4 Naval Command Areas, covering southern, eastern, western and northern coasts. The coastal defence areas are the Stockholm archipelago, Blekinge, Göteborg, Gotland and Norrland, covered by a coastal artillery brigade each.

The Navy operates 12 small diesel submarines, 1 57m Göteborg and 2 50m Stockholm class missile craft, (which act as leaders for smaller craft), 28 other missile craft, 11 inshore patrol craft, 3 minelayers, 6 minehunters, 4 coastal minesweepers and 18 inshore minesweepers. Auxiliaries include 1 mine countermeasures support ship, 1 electronic intelligence gatherer, 1 surveying vessel, 6 icebreakers, 2 tugs and 1 salvage vessel, as well as numerous service craft and boats.

As well as an extensive inventory of artillery up to 120mm calibre, and coast defence missiles, the coastal defence artillery also operate 9 coastal and 16 inshore minelayers, 18 small patrol craft and some 140 small amphibious craft.

The Naval Air Arm comprises 14 Boeing Vertol 107 helicopters and 9 AB-206 Jet-Ranger helicopters, plus 1 Aviocar fixed-wing aircraft for anti-submarine warfare and electronic surveillance.

The personnel of the navy in 1990 totalled 12,000 (6,300 conscripts) of whom 2,600 serve in coastal artillery.

A separate civil Coast Guard, 550 strong, operate some 70 inshore cutters, patrol boats and service craft and 4 aircraft.

Air Force. The C-in-C. of the Swedish Air Force has at his disposal the Air Staff under a chief of staff.

The combat force consists of 3 fighter-interceptor, 3 ground-attack and 3 mixed interceptor/reconnaissance wings (*flottiljer*), each with 2-3 squadrons of 12-15 aircraft, including 6 reconnaissance squadrons (*divisioner*). Total peace-time strength of the combat units is 20 squadrons with nearly 400 first-line aircraft.

Night and all-weather fighters are the Swedish-built Saab J35 Draken, equipping 3 squadrons, and JA37 Viggen, equipping 8 squadrons. The ground-attack wings have 6 squadrons of Saab AJ37 Viggens, and there is provision for 4 light ground-attack squadrons of twin-jet Saab-105s (Sk60s), which could be drawn in wartime from training units. The 3 reconnaissance squadrons have SF37 (photo) and SH37 (maritime, radar) Viggen reconnaissance aircraft; and there are transport, helicopter and other support units. The Sk60 is the Air Force's standard advanced trainer, to which pupils progress after initial training on piston-engined Bulldogs. Other trainers in service include the Sk61 Bulldog, Sk35C Draken and Sk37 Viggen.

Active strength (1991) 8,000 (5,000 conscripts), with 415 combat aircraft.

INTERNATIONAL RELATIONS

Membership. Sweden is a member of the UN and EFTA. On 12 Dec. 1990 Parliament approved application for membership of the EC.

ECONOMY

Budget. Revenue and expenditure of the total budget (Current and Capital) for financial years ending 30 June (in 1m. kr.):

	Revenue	Expenditure		Revenue	Expenditure
1984–85	260,596	329,136	1987–88	332,552	336,669
1985–86	275,099	321,901	1988–89	367,707	349,600
1986–87	320,105	335,267	1989–90	401,563	396,600

The preliminary revenue and expenditure for the financial year 1 July 1989 to 30 June 1990 was as follows (in 1m. kr.):

Revenue		*Expenditure*	
Taxes:		Royal Household and residences	52
Taxes on income, capital gains and profits	107,423	Justice	6,352
		Foreign Affairs	14,035
		Defence	32,591
Statutory social security fees	55,023	Health and Social Affairs	106,211
		Transport and Communications	18,103
Taxes on property	23,159	Ministry of Finance	27,468
Value-added tax	100,214	Education and Cultural Affairs	50,949
Other taxes on goods and services	68,297	Agriculture	5,558
		Labour	28,283
Total revenue from taxes	354,117	Housing and Physical Planning	23,874
		Industry	3,038
Non-tax revenue	37,465	Civil Service Affairs	13,515
Capital revenue	1,199	Ministry of Environment and Energy	2,020
Loan repayment	5,405		
Computed revenue	3,377	Parliament and agencies	586
Total revenue	401,563	Interest on National Debt, etc.	63,696
		Unforeseen expenditure	12
		Changed appropriation of short-term credits	248
		Total expenditure	396,600

On 31 Dec. 1989 the national debt amounted to 600,047m. kr.

A reform of Jan. 1990 moved the burden of taxation from income to services and goods by reducing tax to 31% of annual incomes below 180,000 kr.

Riksgäldskontoret (National Debt Office), *årsbok*. Annual. Stockholm, from 1920
Riksskatteverket (National Tax Board), *årsbok*. Annual. Stockholm, from 1971
The Swedish Budget. Ministry of Economic Affairs and Ministry of the Budget, from 1962/63

Currency. The unit of currency is the Swedish *krona* (SEK), of 100 *öre*. There are notes for 5, 10, 50, 100, 500, 1,000 and 10,000 krona. Inflation was an annualized 11·5% in Nov. 1990. In March 1991, £1 = 10·81 *krona*; US$1 = 5·70 *krona*.

Banking and Finance. The central bank and bank of issue is the *Riksbank*. The *Governor* of the *Riksbank* is appointed for 5 years by 8 trustees, 7 of whom are appointed by Parliament. The *Governor* is Bengt Dennis. The bank's capital and reserve fund are provided by its constitution. On 31 Dec. 1989 its note circulation amounted to 66,079m. kr.; its gold and foreign-exchange reserves totalled 60,704m. kr. There are 24 commercial banks. On 31 Dec. 1989 their total deposits amounted to 363,239m. kr.; advances to the public amounted to 582,347m. kr.

On 31 Dec. 1989 there were 109 savings banks; their total deposits amounted to 155,426m. kr.; advances to the public were 168,649m. kr. Co-operative banks had total deposits of 45,692m. kr.; advances to the public were 40,055m. kr.

Sveriges Riksbank. Annual report. Stockholm, 1989
Skandinaviska Enskilda Banken, Kvartalskrift. Quarterly Review (in English). Stockholm, from 1920
Bosworth, B. and Rivlin, A. M., (eds.) *The Swedish Economy*. Washington, D.C., 1987

Weights and Measures. The metric system is obligatory.

ENERGY AND NATURAL RESOURCES

Electricity. Sweden is rich in hydro-power resources. The total electric energy net production in 1988 was 141,110m. kwh. About 49% of this energy was produced in hydro-electric plants and 47% in 12 nuclear power plants. A referendum of 1980 called for the phasing out of nuclear power by 2010. The remaining 4% was produced in conventional thermal power plants. Supply 220 volts; 50 Hz.

Minerals. Sweden is one of the leading exporters of iron ore. The largest deposits are found north of the polar circle in the area of Kiruna and Gällivare-Malmberget. The ore is exported via the Norwegian port of Narvik and the Swedish port of Luleå. There are also important resources of iron ore in southern Sweden (Bergslagen). The most important fields are Grängesberg and Stråssa and the ores are shipped via the port of Oxelösund. Some of the southern deposits have, in contrast to the fields in North Sweden, a low phosphorus content.

There are also some deposits of copper, lead and zinc ores especially in the Boliden area in the north of Sweden. These ores are often found together with pyrites. Non-ferrous ores, except zinc ores, are used in the Swedish metal industry and barely satisfy domestic needs.

The total production of iron ores amounted to 26·2m. tons in 1988; the production of copper ore was 306,228 tons, of lead ore 229,229 tons, of zinc ore 451,197 tons.

There are also deposits of raw materials for aluminium not worked at present. In southern Sweden there are big resources of alum shale, containing oil and uranium.

Agriculture. According to the farm register which is revised annually the following data was provided for 1989. The number of farms in cultivation of more than 2 ha of arable land, was 98,553; of these there were 56,304 of 2-20 ha; 38,388 of 20-100 ha; 3,861 of above 100 ha. Of the total land area of Sweden (41,161,500 ha), 2,853,116 [1] ha were arable land, 331,426[1] ha cultivated pastures and (1988) 22,535,284 ha forests.

	Area (1,000 ha) [1]			Production (1,000 tonnes)		
Chief crops	*1987*	*1988*	*1989*	*1987*	*1988*	*1989*
Wheat	335·6	258·9	291·8	1,558	1,296	1,751
Rye	42·2	35·3	70·7	137	128	319
Barley	580·5	566·7	500·9	1,907	1,879	1,870
Oats	424·6	446·6	432·7	1,440	1,330	1,455
Mixed grain	45·8	38·3	36·0	...	...	...
Peas and vetches	59·0	45·4	37·2	...	...	...
Potatoes	37·9	38·8	36·0	958	1,283	1,179
Sugarbeet	51·3	51·3	50·6	1,699	2,439	2,654
Tame hay	676·6	699·0	709·7	4,488	4,435	4,624
Oil seed	169·7	149·8	169·4	296	293	417

Area of rotation meadows for pasture was (in 1,000 ha[1]): 1984, 182; 1985, 181; 1986, 180; 1987, 175; 1988, 182; 1989, 185.

Tota8l production of milk (in 1,000 tonnes): 1984, 3,821; 1985, 3,724; 1986, 3,566; 1987, 3,513; 1988, 3,498; 1989, 3,563. Butter production in the same years was (in 1,000 tonnes): 78, 75, 68, 66, 62, 69; and cheese 116, 115, 113, 114, 123, 117.

Livestock (1989): Cattle, 1·7m.; sheep, 401,000; pigs, 2·3m.; poultry, 11m.

Number of farm tractors in 1986, 183,828; combines in 1986, 47,089.

The number of pelts produced in 1988–89 was: Fox, 43,245; mink, 1·57m.; others, 6,013.

[1] Figures refer to holdings of more than 2 ha of arable land.

Forestry. In 1985–89 the forests covered an area of 23·4m. ha, i.e. roughly 57% of the country's land area. Municipal and State ownership accounts for one-fourth of the forests, companies own another fourth, and the remaining half is in private hands. In the felling seasons, 1987–88 and 1988–89 respectively, 53m. and 55·4m. cu. metres (solid volume excluding bark) of wood were removed from the forests in Sweden. The sawmill, wood pulp and paper and paperboard industries are all of great importance. The number of sawmills in 1984 was about 2,500, producing 12·1m. cu. metres of sawn wood. In 1989 the production of sawn soft-wood was about 11·3m. cu. metres. The production of woodpulp in 1989 was 10·3m. tons (dry weight).

Fisheries. In 1988 the total catch of the sea fisheries was 231,826 tonnes.

INDUSTRY. The most important sector of Swedish manufacturing is the production of metals, metal products, machinery and transport equipment, covering almost half of the total value added by manufacturing. Production of high-quality steel is an old Swedish speciality. A large part of this production is exported. The production of ordinary steel is slightly decreasing and is still short of domestic demand. The total production of steel amounted to 4·7m. tons in 1986. There is also a large production of other metals (aluminium, lead, copper) and rolled semi-manufactured goods of these metals.

These basic metal industries are an important basis for the production of more developed metal products, machinery and equipment, which are to a large extent sold on the world market, *i.e.*, hand tools, mining drills, ball-bearings, turbines, pneumatic machinery, refrigerating equipment, machinery for pulp and paper industries, etc., sewing machines, machine tools, office machinery, high-voltage electric machinery, telephone equipment, cars and trucks, ships and aeroplanes.

Another important manufacturing sector is based on Sweden's forest resources. This sector includes saw-mills, plywood factories, joinery industries, pulp- and paper-mills, wallboard and particle board factories, accounting for about 20% of the total value of manufacturing. A fast increasing sector is the chemical industry, especially the petro-chemical branch. Minerals industries include production of building materials, decorative arts products of glass and china.

	No. of establishments		*Average no. of wage-earners*		*Sales value of production (gross) in 1m. kr.*	
Industry groups	*1987*	*1988*	*1987*	*1988*	*1987*	*1988*
Mining and quarrying	*100*	*95*	*7,249*	*6,786*	*5,601*	*6,275*
Metal-ore mining	34	32	6,198	5,743	4,867	5,468
Other mining	66	63	1,051	1,043	735	808
Manufacturing	*9,012*	*9,005*	*531,100*	*529,058*	*560,874*	*607,209*
Manufacture of food, beverages and tobacco	817	809	50,638	51,431	76,453	82,033
Textile, wearing apparel and leather industries	592	567	22,414	20,686	11,463	11,387
Manufacture of wood products including furniture	1,335	1,303	45,268	45,743	38,224	42,418
Manufacture of paper and paper products, printing and publishing	1,077	1,074	65,383	65,578	85,781	93,972
Manufacture of chemicals and chemical, petroleum, coal, rubber and plastic products	719	730	43,100	42,347	73,669	75,654
Manufacture of non-metallic mineral products, except products of petroleum and coal	368	370	15,898	16,089	12,752	13,730
Basic metal industries	161	179	34,267	34,064	40,040	48,582
Manufacture of fabricated metal products, machinery and equipment	3,847	3,788	251,495	250,434	220,953	237,667
Other manufacturing industries	96	95	2,637	2,686	1,538	1,765
Electricity and gas	*691*	*703*	*10,165*	*10,175*	*79,442*	*83,029*
Electricity, gas and steam	691	703	10,165	10,175	79,442	83,029

Arbetsmarknadsstatistik (Labour Market Statistics). Monthly. National Labour Market Board, Stockholm, from 1963

Arbetsmarknadsstatistisk Årsbok (Year Book of Labour Statistics). Statistics Sweden, Stockholm, from 1973

Johansson, Ö., *The Gross Domestic Product of Sweden and its Composition 1861–1955.* Stockholm, 1967

Thalberg, B. and Marno, N., eds., *Economic Growth, Welfare and Industrial Relations: A Comparative Study of Japan and Sweden.* Tokyo, 1984

Jordbruksekonomiska meddelanden (Journal of Agricultural Economics, published monthly by the National Agricultural Market Board). Stockholm, from 1939

Jordbruksstatistisk årsbok (Yearbook of Agricultural Statistics). Statistics Sweden, Stockholm, from 1965

The Swedish Economy. Ministry of Economic Affairs and National Institute of Economic Research. Stockholm, from 1960

Trade Unions. The Swedish Federation of Trade Unions (LO) had 24 member unions with a total membership of 2,275,720 in 1988; the Swedish Central Organization of Salaried Employees (TCO) had 21, with 1,259,681; the Swedish Confederation of Professional Associations (SACO-SR) had 25, with 309,299.

FOREIGN ECONOMIC RELATIONS

Commerce. The imports and exports of Sweden, unwrought gold and coin not included, have been as follows (in 1m. kr.):

	1983	*1984*	*1985*	*1986*	*1987*	*1988*	*1989*
Imports	200,368	218,569	244,654	232,614	257,870	280,650	315,061
Exports	210,516	242,811	260,481	265,103	281,433	305,056	332,145

Imports and exports by products (in 1m. kr.):

	Imports		*Exports*	
	1988	*1989*	*1988*	*1989*
Food and live animals chiefly for food	15,563	15,786	4,822	5,382
Cereals and cereal preparations	927	964	1,168	1,288
Vegetables and fruit	5,379	5,487	459	405
Coffee, tea, cocoa, spices and manufactures thereof	2,744	2,616	687	797
Feeding stuff for animals (not including unmilled cereals)	1,203	1,243	128	129
Beverages and tobacco	2,154	2,353	372	450
Crude materials, inedible, except fuels	12,793	13,565	28,181	31,382
Hides, skins and furskins, raw	615	601	1,107	1,152
Crude rubber (including synthetic and reclaimed)	508	461	199	174
Cork and wood	3,468	3,395	9,950	10,878
Pulp and waste paper	673	839	12,129	13,357
Textile fibres (other than wool tops and other combed wool) and their wastes (not manufactured into yarn or fabric)	376	362	216	209
Crude fertilizers and crude minerals (excluding coal, petroleum and precious stones)	1,551	1,616	465	506
Metalliferous ores and metal scrap	3,733	4,396	3,761	4,739
Mineral fuels, lubricants and related materials	19,176	24,231	6,641	9,209
Coal, coke and briquettes	1,388	1,667	114	86
Petroleum, petroleum products and related materials	16,837	21,191	5,763	7,922
Chemicals and related products, n.e.s.	28,162	30,176	21,822	24,119
Artificial resins and plastic materials, and cellulose esters and ethers	8,875	9,218	6,460	6,687
Manufactured goods classified chiefly by material	47,226	52,998	81,263	87,314
Paper, paperboard, and articles of paper pulp, of paper or of paperboard	3,772	4,177	33,832	35,768
Textile yarn, fabrics, made-up articles, n.e.s., and related products	7,174	7,338	3,444	3,575
Non-metallic mineral manufactures, n.e.s.	4,479	5,266	3,099	3,065
Iron and steel	10,219	11,867	19,311	21,968
Non-ferrous metals	7,008	8,307	6,158	6,518
Machinery and transport equipment	111,143	126,409	130,761	141,052
Power generating machinery and equipment	6,441	7,267	9,164	9,564
Machinery specialized for particular industries	9,982	11,633	15,241	17,009
Metal working machinery	3,288	3,597	3,221	3,493
General industrial machinery and equipment, n.e.s. and machine parts, n.e.s.	15,501	17,455	21,132	24,006
Office machines and automatic data processing machines	14,017	15,805	8,388	9,126
Telecommunications and sound recording and reproducing apparatus and equipment	8,210	9,488	12,343	14,227

	Imports 1988	Imports 1989	Exports 1988	Exports 1989
Electrical machinery apparatus and appliances, n.e.s., and electrical parts thereof (including non-electrical counterparts, n.e.s., of electrical household type equipment)	17,895	19,349	12,925	13,373
Road vehicles (including air cushion vehicles)	30,875	32,839	43,800	44,840
Other transport equipment	4,934	8,618	4,550	5,415
Miscellaneous manufactured articles	42,558	47,006	28,787	30,257

Principal import and export countries (in 1m. kr.):

	Imports from 1988	Imports from 1989	Exports to 1988	Exports to 1989
Belgium-Luxembourg	9,071	9,824	12,677	12,565
Denmark	18,676	21,708	21,074	22,090
Federal Republic of Germany	59,714	63,244	37,005	42,280
Finland	19,582	21,189	20,040	23,233
France	14,104	16,745	16,093	17,712
Italy	11,313	12,976	12,100	14,752
Netherlands	11,371	13,165	14,623	16,625
Norway	17,013	22,101	28,531	27,301
Switzerland	5,542	5,824	7,203	7,557
USSR	4,533	5,149	1,771	2,458
UK	24,122	25,486	34,230	37,238
USA	21,074	25,774	30,092	30,921

Total trade between Sweden and UK (British Department of Trade returns, in £1,000 sterling):

	1986	1987	1988	1989	1990
Imports to UK	2,756,536	2,952,453	3,366,524	3,747,600	3,594,547
Exports and re-exports from UK	2,307,900	2,322,235	2,195,032	2,350,122	2,712,775

Historisk Statistik för Sverige, 3: Utrikeshandel [Foreign Trade], *1732–1970*. Statistics Sweden, Stockholm, 1972

Under the title *Utrikeshandel* (Foreign trade), Statistics Sweden issue a series of annual (*årsstatistik*), quarterly (*kvartalsstatistik*) and monthly (*månadsstatistik*) statistical reports.

Tourism. In 1989 foreign visitors spent 16,358m. kr., and stayed 3,366,899 nights in hotels, 961,113 in holiday villages and youth hostels and 3,256,009 camping. Earnings from tourism (1987) 12·88m. kr.

COMMUNICATIONS

Roads. On 1 Jan. 1989 there were 205,000 km of public roads comprising State-administered roads, 98,548 km, municipal, 32,000 km, private roads with subsidies, 77,106 km, of which 69,819 km were surfaced. Motor vehicles on 31 Dec. 1988 included 3,482,656 passenger cars, 281,387 buses and lorries and 32,536 motor cycles (all in use).

Railways. At the end of 1989 the total length of railways was 11,501 km; 7,464 km were electrified which carried 87m. passengers and 56m. tonnes of freight.

Aviation. Commercial air traffic is maintained in (1) Sweden and other parts of the world by Scandinavian Airlines System (SAS), of which AB Aerotransport (ABA = Swedish Air Lines) is the Swedish partner (DDL = Danish Air Lines and DNL = Norwegian Air Lines being the other two); (2) only within Sweden by Linjeflyg AB. Scandinavian Airlines System have a joint paid-up capital of about 12,177m. Sw. kr. Capitalization of ABA, 3,761m. Sw. kr., of which 50% is owned by the Government and 50% by private enterprises. Capitalization of Linjeflyg, 880m. Sw. kr., of which 50% is owned by SAS and 50% by ABA.

In scheduled air traffic during 1989 the total number of km flown was 113m.; passenger-km, 8,496·7m.; goods, 182m. tonne-km; mail, 21·8m. tonne-km. These figures represent the Swedish share of the SAS traffic (Swedish domestic and three-sevenths of international traffic) and the Linjeflyg traffic.

Shipping. The Swedish mercantile marine consisted on 30 June 1990 of 443 vessels of 2m. gross tons (only vessels of at least 100 gross tons, and excluding fishing vessels and tugs). Stockholm and Göteborg, with together 179 vessels of 1·4m. gross tons in Dec. 1989, are the two major home ports for the Swedish mercantile marine.

Vessels entered from and cleared for foreign countries, exclusive of passenger liners and ferries, with cargoes and in ballast, in 1989, are as follows (only vessels of at least a gross tonnage of 75): With cargoes, 27,285 with a gross tonnage of 123·9m.; in ballast, 13,424 with a gross tonnage of 52·8m.

Telecommunications. On 1 Jan. 1989 there were 5,601,000 main telephone lines.

Number of combined radio and television reception fees paid at the end of 1988 was 3,314,000, of which 3m. included extra fees for colour television. As from 1 April 1978, special sound broadcasting licences were discontinued.

Sveriges Radio AB is a non-commercial semi-governmental corporation, transmitting 3 programmes on long-, medium-, and short-waves and on FM. There are also regional programmes. It also broadcasts 2 TV programmes. Colour programmes are broadcast by PAL system.

The overseas radio-telegraph and radio-telephone services are conducted by the Swedish Telecommunications Administration.

The number of post offices at the end of 1987 was 2,128. For receipts of the post and telecommunication services *see* the section on Economy.

Cinemas (1988). There were 1,100 cinemas.

Newspapers (1988). There were 175 daily newspapers with a total circulation of 4·8m.

JUSTICE, RELIGION, EDUCATION AND WELFARE

Justice. The administration of justice is entirely independent. The *Justitiekansler*, or Attorney-General (a government appointment) and the *Justitieombudsmän* (4 judicial Commissioners appointed by Parliament), exercise a check on the administration. In 1968 a reform was carried through which meant that the offices of the former *Justitieombudsman* (Ombudsman for civil affairs) and the *Militieombudsman* (Ombudsman for military affairs) were turned into one sole institution with 3 Ombudsmen, each styled *Justitieombudsman*. They exert a general supervision over all courts of law, the civil service, military laws and the military services. In 1989–90 they received altogether 3,668 cases; of these, 176 were instituted on their own initiative and 3,477 on complaints.

The *Riksåklagaren* (a government appointment) is the chief public prosecutor.

There is a 3-tier hierarchy of courts: the Supreme Court (*högsta domstolen*); 6 intermediate courts of appeal (*hovrätter*) and 100 district courts (*tingsrätter*). There is also a Housing Appeal Court and 12 rent and tenancy tribunals. Of the district courts 27 also serve as real estate courts and 6 as water rights courts.

District courts are courts of first instance and deal with both civil and criminal cases. Each member of the court has an individual vote and is legally responsible for the decision. In the voting, the majority rules. When the votes are evenly divided in a criminal case, the opinion implying the least severe sentence applies, and in cases where there is no opinion that could be considered the mildest, the Chair has the casting vote, as is also the case in family civil cases and matters; petty cases are tried by the judge alone. Civil cases are tried as a rule by 3 to 4 judges or in minor cases by 1 judge. Disputes of greater consequence relating to the Marriage Code or the Code relating to Parenthood and Guardianship are tried by a judge and a jury (*nämnd*) of 3-4 lay assessors. When cases concerning real estate are being tried the court consists of 2 qualified lawyers, 1 specialist on technical matters and 2 lay assessors.

More serious criminal cases are tried by a judge and a jury of 5 members (lay assessors) in felony cases, and of 3 members in misdemeanour cases. The cases in courts of appeal are generally tried by 4 or 5 judges, but the same cases, which are tried with a judge and a jury in the first instance, are tried by 3 or 4 judges and a jury of 2-3 members. In cases concerning real estate the court consists of a specialist on technical matters in place of one of the judges and in water-right cases of 3 or 4 judges and 1 or 2 specialists on technical water matters.

Those with low incomes can receive free legal aid out of public funds. In criminal cases a suspected person has the right to a defence counsel, paid out of public funds.

The Attorney-General and the Judicial Commissioner for the Judiciary and Civil Administration supervise the application in the public sector of acts of Parliament and regulations. The Attorney-General is the government's legal adviser and also the Public Prosecutor.

There were 80 penal and correctional institutions for offenders in 1989 with an average population of 4,364 male and 252 female inmates (including offenders in remand prison). Besides, there were 456 children or young people registered for care in treatment and/or residential homes on 31 Dec. 1988, admitted under the 'Care of Young Persons' Act.

Anderman, S., (ed.) *Law and the Weaker Party: An Anglo-Swedish Comparative Study*. Abingdon, 1981–83

Bruzelius, A. and Ginsburg, R. B., *The Swedish Code of Judicial Procedure*. South Hackensack, Rev. ed., 1979

Strömholm, S., *An Introduction to Swedish Law*. Stockholm, 1981

al-Wahab, I., *The Swedish Institution of Ombudsmen*. Stockholm, 1979

Justitieombudsmännens ämbetsberättelse avgiven till Riksdagen. Annual. Stockholm

The Penal Code of Sweden: As Amended 1 Jan. 1972. South Hackensack, 1972

Rättsstatistisk årsbok (Year Book of Legal Statistics). Statistics Sweden, Stockholm, from 1975

Religion. The overwhelming majority of the population belong to the Evangelical Lutheran Church, which is the established national church. In 1989 there were 13 bishoprics (Uppsala being the metropolitan see) and 2,563 parishes. The clergy are chiefly supported from the parishes and the proceeds of the church lands. The nonconformists mostly still adhere to the national church. The largest denominations, on 1 Jan. 1988, were: Pentecost Movement, 98,134; The Mission Covenant Church of Sweden, 79,136; Salvation Army, 29,159; Swedish Evangelical Mission, 23,222; Swedish Baptist Church, 20,720; Orebro Missionary Society, 22,176; Swedish Alliance Missionary Society, 13,382; Holiness Mission, 6,031.

There were also 135,470 Roman Catholics (under a Bishop resident at Stockholm).

Parliament and Convocation (*Kyrkomötet*) decided in 1958 to admit women to ordination as priests.

Education. By the Swedish Higher Educational Act of 1977 a unified educational system was created by integrating institutions which had previously been administered separately. This new *högskola* includes not only traditional university studies but also those of various former professional colleges as well as a number of study programmes earlier offered by the secondary school system. One of the goals of the 1977 university reform was to introduce an increased element of vocational training into part of Swedish higher education and to widen admission. A Certificate of Education (B.Sc., M.Sc., U.C. etc.) is awarded on completion of a general study programme. This certificate states the number of courses taken as well as the points and grades obtained on each course in the study programme.

In autumn 1989 there were, in these new integrated institutions for higher education, *högskola*, about 164,900 enrolled for undergraduate studies of whom 116,200 were distributed by sector as follows: Education for technical professions, 35,700; education for social work, economic and administrative professions, 33,800; education for medical and paramedical professions, 22,200; education for the teaching professions, 18,500; and education for information, communication and cultural professions, 6,000. The number of students enrolled for post-graduate studies was 13,000.

In autumn term in the school year 1989–90 there were 578,500 pupils in primary education (grades 1–6 in compulsory comprehensive schools). Secondary education at the lower stage (grades 7–9 in compulsory comprehensive schools) comprised 316,000 pupils. In secondary education at the higher stage (the integrated upper secondary school), there were 246,000 pupils (excluding about 7,600 pupils in the fourth year of the technical line regarded as third-level education). The folk high schools, 'people's colleges', had 15,500 pupils in courses of more than 15 weeks.

In municipal adult education there were 125,300 pupils (corresponding to a gross number of 269,300 participants). Basic education for adults had 25,300 pupils.

There are also special schools for pupils with visual and hearing handicaps (about 660 in 1989–90) and for those who are mentally retarded (about 10,500 pupils).

Education Policy for Planning: Goals for Educational Policy in Sweden. OECD, Paris, 1980
Science and Technology Policies in Sweden. Ministry of Education and Cultural Affairs, Stockholm, 1986
The Swedish Folk High School. Swedish National Board of Education, Stockholm, 1986
Yearbook of Educational Statistics 1986, Statistics Sweden, Stockholm, 1986
Boucher, L., *Tradition and Change in Swedish education.* OUP, 1982
Düring, A., *Swedish Research.* Stockholm, 1985
Götberg, B. and Svärd, S., *The Swedish 'Folk High School': Its Background and its Present Situation.*
Kim, L., *Widened Admission to Higher Education in Sweden.* Stockholm, 1982
Marklund, S., *Educational Administration and Educational Development.* Univ. of Stockholm, 1979.—*The Democratization of Education in Sweden.* Univ. of Stockholm, 1980
Paulston, C. B., *Swedish Research and Debate about Bilingualism.* Stockholm, 1983
Stenholm, B., *The Swedish School System.* Stockholm, 1984
Sundgvist, A., *New Rules for Swedish Study Circles.* Stockholm, 1983
Ueberschlag, G., *La Folkhögskola.* Paris, 1981

Social Welfare. The social security schemes are greatly expanding. Supported by a referendum, the Diet in 1958 and 1959 decided that the national pensions should be increased successively until 1968 and supplementary pensions paid from 1963. These pensions are of invariable value. In 1969 the Diet decided that as from 1 July 1969 an increment to the basic pension was to be paid to persons without supplementary pensions, and this amount is to be successively increased in a 10-year period. The basic and supplementary pensions consist of old-age and family pensions, as well as pensions paid to the disabled. The financing of the supplementary system is based on the current-cost method.

The most important social welfare schemes are described in the conspectus below.

Type of scheme	*Introduced*	*Scope*	*Principal benefits*
Sickness insurance (compulsory–current law, 1962)	1955	All residents	Hospital fees, most private doctors charge the insured person normally 70 kr., district physicians and doctors in hospitals charge the insured person only 60 kr. for full medical treatment, some reimbursement of cost of transportation as well as costs of physiotherapy, convalescent care, etc., medicines at reduced prices or free of charge. During sickness daily allowance 90% of the yearly income in between 6,000 and 222,700 kr. There is generally no maximum benefit period. Dental care is available to all residents from 20 years of age, the maximum payable by the patient being 60% up to 3,000 kr. and 25% thereafter. Before 20 years of age dental care is given free through the national dental service.
Employment injury insurance (compulsory–current law, 1976)	*1901*	All employed persons	Medical treatment, medicine and medical appliances, hospital care, sickness benefit 100% of the yearly income in between 6,000 and 222,700 kr. (first 90 days covered by sickness insurance), disability annuities, funeral benefit and survivor's pensions.

Type of scheme	*Introduced*	*Scope*	*Principal benefits*
Unemployment insurance (current law, 1973)	1935	Members of recognized unemployment insurance societies (about 70% of all employees)	174-495 kr. per day subject to tax.
Basic pensions (current law, 1962)			
Old-age	1914	All citizens	Payable from the age of 65 or, at a reduced rate, from the age of 60. 76,330 kr. per annum for married couples, 43,362 kr. for others (including the special increment of 29,700 kr. and 14,850 kr. respectively for those without supplementary pension); about half of them receive municipal housing supplement.
Disability	1914	All citizens	Payable before the age of 65. Full pension 58,212 kr. per annum (including the special increment of 29,700 kr.).
Survivors	1948	All citizens	New rules came into force on 1 Jan. 1990. Since then both men and women are entitled to 'readjustment grants' for one year of 43,362 kr. (including the special increment of 14,850 kr.). If the survivor after one year is unable to support him/herself, a special survivor's pension can be granted of the same amount. There is a means test every 3 years. Child pension is payable before the age of 18, sometimes until the age of 20 for studies. The pension amounts to 7,425 kr. (fatherless or motherless) and 14,850 kr. (orphans).
Supplementary pensions (current law, 1962)			
Old-age	1960	All gainfully occupied persons	Payable from the same age as the basic pension (*see above*). The pension is in principle 60% of the insured person's average annual earnings during the best 15 years except an amount corresponding to the basic pension and subject to a ceiling.
Disability	1960	All gainfully occupied persons	Payable before the age of 65. Full pension corresponds in principle to supplementary old-age pension.
Survivors	1960	All gainfully occupied persons	Payable to widow and children, before the age of 18, of a deceased person as a certain percentage of the deceased's supplementary pension.

Type of scheme	*Introduced*	*Scope*	*Principal benefits*
Partial pensions (current law, 1979)	1976	All employees between 60–65 years of age	The pension is payable between 60-65 years of age. The insured must have reduced his working time by 5 hours on an average a week and the part-time work must thereafter comprise at least 17 hours per week. Furthermore the insured must have worked during at least 75 days in the last 12 months and gained a right to supplementary pension for 10 years after the age of 45. The partial pension is paid out by 65% of the loss of income in connection with the change-over to part-time work.
Parents benefit	1974	All resident parents in connection with confinement	Parents cash benefit of 60 kr. a day during 450 days until the child reaches 8 years of age. Employed parents entitled to daily parents cash benefit of 90% of the daily income (in between 6,000–222,700 kr. yearly) for 360 days. Maximum daily parents cash benefit 549 kr. and for the last 90 days 60 kr. a day will be paid.
Temporary parents benefit	1974	All resident parents	Temporary parents cash benefit with the same amount as for parents cash benefit for care of each child which is ill during 60 days for the parents together until the child reaches 12 years of age or if ill 16 years of age.
Children's allowances	1948	All children below 16	From 1 Jan. 1990 6,720 kr. per annum. An additional allowance is paid out for the third child with one-half of an allowance and 190% of a full allowance for the fourth child, 240% for the fifth child and 160% for each additional child.
		Children at school 16–18	560 kr. per month during school-courses.

Total social expenditure, including also hygiene, care of the sick and social assistance, amounted to 345,737m. kr. in 1987, representing 34% of the GDP.

The Cost and Financing of the Social Services in Sweden, 1981. Stockholm, 1983

Ministry of Health and Social Affairs, *The Evolution of the Swedish Health Insurance*. Stockholm, 1978

Socialnytt (Official Journal of the National Board of Health and Welfare). Stockholm, from 1968

Social Insurance Statistics. Facts 1986. National Social Insurance Board, Stockholm, 1986

The Swedish Health Services in the 1990s. The National Board of Health and Welfare, Stockholm, 1985

Forsberg, M., *The Evolution of Social Welfare Policy in Sweden*. Stockholm, 1984

Heclo, H., *Modern Social Politics in Britain and Sweden: From Relief to Income Maintenance*. New Haven, 1974

Lagerström, L., *Pension Systems in Sweden*. Stockholm, 1976.—*Social Security in Sweden*. Stockholm, 1976

DIPLOMATIC REPRESENTATIVES

Of Sweden in Great Britain (11 Montagu Pl., London, W1H 2AL)
Ambassador: Lennart Eckerberg.

Of Great Britain in Sweden (Skarpögatan 6-8, 115 27 Stockholm)
Ambassador: Sir John Ure, KCMG, LVO.

Of Sweden in the USA (600 New Hampshire Ave., NW, Washington, D.C., 20037)
Ambassador: Anders Thunborg.

Of the USA in Sweden (Strandvägen 101, 115 27 Stockholm)
Ambassador: Charles E. Redman.

Of Sweden to the United Nations
Ambassador: Jan Eliasson.

Further Reading

Statistical Information: Statistics Sweden, (Statistiska, Centralbyrån, S-11581 Stockholm) was founded in 1858, in succession to the Kungl. Tabellkommissionen, which had been set up in 1756. *Director-General:* Sten Johansson. Its Publications include:

Levnadsförhållanden, årsbok (Living Conditions). Annual. From 1975.—*Rapport.* From 1976
Statistisk årsbok för Sverige (Statistical Abstract of Sweden). From 1914
Siffror om Sverige (Sweden). From 1971. Also in English as *Sweden*
Historisk statistik för Sverige (Historical Statistics of Sweden). 1955 ff. (4 vols. to date)
Allmän månadsstatistik (Monthly Digest of Swedish Statistics). From 1963
Statistiska meddelanden (Statistical Reports). From 1963

Andersson, L., *A History of Sweden.* Stockholm, 1962
Atlas över Sverige. Stockholm, 1953–71. [Publ. in separate parts dealing with population, economics, etc.]
Publications on Sweden. Stockholm, 1988
Documents on Swedish Foreign Policy. Stockholm, Annual.
Grosskopf, G., *The Swedish Tax System.* Stockholm, 1986
Gullberg, I. E., *Swedish–English Dictionary of Technical Terms.—Svensk-Engelsk Fackordbok.* Stockholm, 2nd ed. 1977
Hadenius, S., *Swedish Politics during the Twentieth Century.* Stockholm, 1985
Hansson, I., Jonung, L., Myhrman, J. and Söderström, H. T., *Sweden – the Road to Stability.* Stockholm, 1985
Heelo, H. and Madsen, H., *Policy and Politics in Sweden: Principled Pragmatism.* Philadelphia, 1987
Hellberg, T. and Jansson, L. M., *Alfred Nobel.* Stockholm, 1984
Linton, M., *The Swedish Road to Socialism.* London, 1985
Meyerson, P-M., *Eurosclerosis, The Case of Sweden.* Stockholm, 1985
Nordic Council, *Yearbook of Nordic Statistics.* From 1962 (in English and one Nordic Language)
Olivecrona, G., (ed.) *Sweden In Fact.* Stockholm, 1986
Sather, L. B. and Swanson, A., *Sweden.* [Bibliography] Oxford and Santa Barbara, 1987
Scott, F. D., *Sweden: The Nation's History.* Univ. of Minnesota Press, 1983
Söderström, H. T., *Getting Sweden Back to Work.* Stockholm, 1986
Turner, B., *Sweden.* London, 1976
Sveriges statskalender. Published by Vetenskapsakademien. Annual, from 1813

National Library: Kungliga Biblioteket, Stockholm. *Director:* Lars Tynell.

SWITZERLAND

Capital: Bern
Population: 6·7m. (1989)
GNP per capita: US$27,260 (1988)

Schweizerische Eidtgenossenschaft— Confédération Suisse— Confederazione Svizzera

HISTORY. On 1 Aug. 1291 the men of Uri, Schwyz and Unterwalden entered into a defensive league. In 1353 the league included 8 members and in 1513, 13. Various territories were acquired either by single cantons or by several in common, and in 1648 the league became formally independent of the Holy Roman Empire, but no addition was made to the number of cantons till 1798. In that year, under the influence of France, the unified Helvetic Republic was formed. This failed to satisfy the Swiss, and in 1803 Napoleon Bonaparte, in the Act of Mediation, gave a new Constitution, and out of the lands formerly allied or subject increased the number of cantons to 19. In 1815 the perpetual neutrality of Switzerland and the inviolability of her territory were guaranteed by Austria, France, Great Britain, Portugal, Prussia, Russia, Spain and Sweden, and the Federal Pact, which included 3 new cantons, was accepted by the Congress of Vienna. In 1848 a new Constitution was passed. The 22 cantons set up a Federal Government (consisting of a Federal Parliament and a Federal Council) and a Federal Tribunal. This Constitution, in turn, was on 29 May 1874 superseded by the present Constitution. In a national referendum held in Sept. 1978, 69·9% voted in favour of the establishment of a new canton, Jura, which was established on 1 Jan. 1979.

AREA AND POPULATION. Switzerland is bounded in the west and north-west by France, north by Germany, east by Austria and south by Italy. Area and population, according to the census held on 1 Dec. 1980 and estimate 31 Dec. 1989.

Canton	*Area (sq. km)*	*Census 1 Dec. 1980*	*Estimate 31 Dec. 1989*
Zürich (Zurich) (1351)	1,729	1,122,839	1,144,900
Bern (Berne) (1553)	6,049	912,022	937,400
Luzern (Lucerne) (1332)	1,492	296,159	314,800
Uri (1291)	1,076	33,883	33,500
Schwyz (1291)	908	97,354	108,100
Obwalden (Obwald) (1291)	491	25,865	28,300
Nidwalden (Nidwald) (1291)	276	28,617	32,000
Glarus (Glaris) (1352)	685	36,718	37,300
Zug (Zoug) (1352)	239	75,930	84,000
Fribourg (Freiburg) (1481)	1,670	185,246	204,300
Solothurn (Soleure) (1481)	791	218,102	223,500
Basel-Stadt (Bâle-V.) (1501)	37	203,915	400
Basel-Landschaft (Bâle-C.) (1501)	428	219,822	229,000
Schaffhausen (Schaffhouse) (1501)	298	69,413	71,000
Appenzell A.-Rh. (Rh.-Ext.) (1513)	243	47,611	900
Appenzell I.-Rh. (Rh.-Int.) (1513)	172	12,844	500
St Gallen (St Gall) (1803)	2,014	391,995	414,700
Graubünden (Grisons) (1803)	7,106	164,641	169,000
Aargau (Argovie) (1803)	1,405	453,442	490,400
Thurgau (Thurgovie) (1803)	1,013	183,795	201,600
Ticino (Tessin) (1803)	2,811	265,899	283,000
Vaud (Waadt) (1803)	3,218	528,747	572,000
Valais (Wallis) (1815)	5,226	218,707	243,700
Neuchâtel (Neuenburg) (1815)	797	158,368	158,600
Genève (Genf) (1815)	282	349,040	373,000
Jura (1979)	837	64,986	65,000
Total	41,293[1]	6,365,960	6,673,900

[1] 15,943 sq. miles.

German, French and Italian are the official languages; Romansch (spoken mostly in Graubünden) is a national language. German is spoken by the majority of inhabitants in 19 of the 26 cantons above (French names given in brackets), French in 6 (Fribourg, Vaud, Valais, Neuchâtel, Jura and Genève, for which the German names are given in brackets), and Italian in 1 (Ticino). In 1980, 65% spoke German, 18·4% French, 9·8% Italian, 0·8% Romansch and 6% other languages; counting only Swiss nationals, the percentages were 73·5, 20·1, 4·5, 0·9 and 1.

At the end of 1989 the 5 largest cities were Zürich (342,900); Basel (165,600); Geneva (169,600); Berne (134,400); Lausanne (122,600). At the end of 1988 the population figures of conurbations were: Zürich, 838,700; Basel, 358,500; Geneva, 389,000; Bern, 298,700; Lausanne, 262,900; other towns 1985, (and their conurbations, 1986), were Winterthur, 84,400 (107,812); St Gallen, 73,200 (125,879); Luzern, 60,600 (160,594); Biel, 52,000 (82,544).

The number of foreigners resident in Switzerland in Dec. 1989 was 1,066,139.

Vital statistics for calendar years:

	Live births					
	Total	*Illegitimate*	*Marriages*	*Divorces*	*Still births*	*Deaths*
1986	76,300	4,300	40,200	11,400	330	60,100
1987	76,500	4,500	43,000	11,600	340	59,500
1988	80,300	. . .	45,700	12,700	. . .	60,600
1989	81,180	. . .	45,066	12,720	. . .	60,882

In 1983 there were 91,300 emigrants and 88,000 immigrants; in 1984, 85,000 and 97,000; in 1985, 85,000 and 99,000; in 1986, 85,000 and 107,000; in 1987, 86,300 and 112,700; in 1988, 91,500 and 125,000.

CLIMATE. The climate is largely dictated by relief and altitude and includes continental and mountain types. Summers are generally warm, with quite considerable rainfall; winters are fine, with clear, cold air. Bern. Jan. 32°F (0°C), July, 65°F (18·5°C). Annual rainfall 39·4" (986 mm).

CONSTITUTION AND GOVERNMENT. Switzerland is a republic. The highest authority is vested in the electorate, *i.e.*, all Swiss citizens over 18 (20 until a referendum of March 1991). This electorate—besides electing its representatives to the Parliament—has the voting power on amendments to, or on the revision of, the Constitution. It also takes decisions on laws and international treaties if requested by 50,000 voters or 8 cantons (facultative referendum), and it has the right of initiating constitutional amendments, the support required for such demands being 100,000 voters (popular initiative).

The Federal Government is supreme in matters of peace, war and treaties; it regulates the army, the railway, telecommunication systems, the coining of money, the issue and repayment of bank-notes and the weights and measures of the republic. It also legislates on matters of copyright, bankruptcy, patents, sanitary policy in dangerous epidemics, and it may create and subsidize, besides the Polytechnic School at Zürich and at Lausanne, 2 federal universities and other educational institutions. There has also been entrusted to it the authority to decide concerning public works for the whole or great part of Switzerland, such as those relating to rivers, forests and the construction of national highways and railways. By referendum of 13 Nov. 1898 it is also the authority in the entire spheres of common law. In 1957 the Federation was empowered to legislate on atomic energy matters and in 1961 on the construction of pipelines of petroleum and gas.

National flag: Red with a white couped cross.

National anthem: Trittst im Morgenrot daher (words by Leonard Widmer, 1808–68; tune by Alberik Zwyssig, 1808–54); adopted by the Federal Council in 1962. A new anthem was being sought to celebrate Switzerland's 700th anniversary in 1991.

The legislative authority is vested in a parliament of 2 chambers, a *Ständerat*, or Council of States, and a *Nationalrat*, or National Council.

The *Ständerat* is composed of 46 members, chosen and paid by the 23 cantons of the Confederation, 2 for each canton. The mode of their election and the term of membership depend entirely on the canton. Three of the cantons are politically divided—Basel into Stadt and Land, Appenzell into Ausser-Rhoden and Inner-Rhoden, and Unterwalden into Obwalden and Nidwalden. Each of these 'half-cantons' sends 1 member to the State Council.

The *Nationalrat*—after the referendum taken on 4 Nov. 1962—consists of 200 National Councillors, directly elected for 4 years, in proportion to the population of the cantons, with the proviso that each canton or half-canton is represented by at least 1 member. The members are paid from federal funds at the rate of 150 francs for each day during the session and a nominal sum of 10,000 francs per annum.

In 1987 the 200 members were distributed among the cantons [1] as follows:

Zürich (Zurich)	35	Appenzell—Outer- and Inner-Rhoden	3
Bern (Berne)	29	St Gallen (St Gall)	12
Luzern (Lucerne)	9	Graubünden (Grisons)	5
Uri	1	Aargau (Argovie)	14
Schwyz	3	Thurgau (Thurgovie)	6
Unterwalden–Upper and Lower	2	Ticino (Tessin)	8
Glarus (Glaris)	1	Vaud (Waadt)	17
Zug (Zoug)	2	Valais (Wallis)	7
Fribourg (Freiburg)	6	Neuchâtel (Neuenburg)	5
Solothurn (Soleure)	7	Genève (Genf)	11
Basel (Bâle)—town and country	13	Jura	2
Schaffhausen (Schaffhouse)	2		

[1] The name of the canton is given in German, French or Italian, according to the language most spoken in it, and alternative names are given in brackets.

Composition of the National Council in 1987: Social Democrats, 42; Radicals, 51; Christian-Democratic People's Party, 42; Swiss People's Party, 25; Liberals, 9; Independents, 8; National Campaign/Vigilance, 3; Evangelical Party, 3; Progressive Organizations, 4; Environmentalists, 9; Others, 4.

Council of States (1987): Christian Democrats, 19; Radicals, 14; Social Democrats, 5; Swiss People's Party, 4; Liberals, 3; Independents, 1.

A general election takes place by ballot every 4 years. Every citizen of the republic who has entered on his 20th year is entitled to a vote, and any voter, not a clergyman, may be elected a deputy. Laws passed by both chambers may be submitted to direct popular vote, when 50,000 citizens or 8 cantons demand it; the vote can be only 'Yes' or 'No'. This principle, called the *referendum*, is frequently acted on.

Women's suffrage, although advocated by the Federal Council and the Federal Assembly, was on 1 Feb. 1959 rejected, but in a subsequent referendum, held on 7 Feb. 1971, women's suffrage was carried.

The chief executive authority is deputed to the *Bundesrat*, or Federal Council, consisting of 7 members, elected from 7 different cantons for 4 years by the *Vereinigte Bundesversammlung*, *i.e.*, joint sessions of both chambers. The members of this council must not hold any other office in the Confederation or cantons, nor engage in any calling or business. In the Federal Parliament legislation may be introduced either by a member, or by either House, or by the Federal Council (but not by the people). Every citizen who has a vote for the National Council is eligible for becoming a member of the executive.

The *President* of the Federal Council (called President of the Confederation) and the Vice-President are the first magistrates of the Confederation. Both are elected by the Federal Assembly for 1 calendar year from among the Federal Councillors. and are not immediately re-eligible to the same offices. The Vice-President, however, may be, and usually is, elected to succeed the outgoing President.

President of the Confederation. (1991): Flavio Cotti.

The 7 members of the Federal Council—each of whom has a salary of 203,000 francs per annum, while the President has 215,000 francs—act as ministers, or chiefs of the 7 administrative departments of the republic. The city of Berne is the seat of the Federal Council and the central administrative authorities.

The Federal Council was composed as follows in 1990:

Foreign Affairs: René Felber.

Interior: Flavio Cotti.
Justice and Police: Arnold Koller.
Military: Kaspar Villiger.
Finance: Otto Stich.
Public Economy: Jean-Pascal Delamuraz.
Transport, Communications and Energy: Adolf Ogi.

Local Government. Each of the 26 cantons and demi-cantons is sovereign, so far as its independence and legislative powers are not restricted by the federal constitution; all cantonal governments, though different in organization (membership varies from 5 to 11, and terms of office from 1 to 5 years), are based on the principle of sovereignty of the people.

In 21 cantons a body chosen by universal suffrage, usually called *der Grosse Rat*, or *Kantonsrat*, exercises the functions of a parliament. In all the cantonal constitutions except those of the 5 cantons which have a *Landsgemeinde*, the referendum has a place. By this principle, where it is most fully developed, as in Zürich, all laws and concordats, or agreements with other cantons, and the chief matters of finance, as well as all revisions of the Constitution, must be submitted to the popular vote. In the 5 cantons of Appenzell, Glarus and Unterwalden the people exercise their powers direct in the *Landsgemeinde*, *i.e.*, the assembly in the open air of all citizens of full age. In all the cantons the *popular initiative* for constitutional affairs, as well as for legislation, has been introduced, except in Lucerne, where the *initiative* exists only for constitutional affairs. In most cantons there are districts (*Amtsbezirke*) consisting of a number of communes grouped together, each district having a Prefect (*Regierungsstatthalter*) representing the cantonal government. In the larger communes, for local affairs, there is an Assembly (legislative) and a Council (executive) with a president, mayor or syndic, and not less than 4 other members. In the smaller communes there is a council only, with its officials.

DEFENCE. There are fortifications in all entrances to the Alps and on the important passes crossing the Alps and the Jura. Large-scale destructions of bridges, tunnels and defiles are prepared for an emergency.

Army. Switzerland depends for defence upon a *national militia*. Service in this force is compulsory and universal, with few exemptions except for physical disability. Those excused or rejected pay certain taxes in lieu. Liability extends from the 20th to the end of the 50th year for soldiers and of the 55th year for officers. The first 12 years are spent in the first line, called the *Auszug*, or *Élite*, the next 10 in the *Landwehr* and 8 in the *Landsturm*. The unarmed *Hilfsdienst* comprises all other males between 20 and 50 whose services can be made available for non-combatant duties of any description.

The initial training of the Swiss militia soldier is carried out in recruits' schools, and the periods are 118 days for infantry, engineers, artillery, etc. The subsequent trainings, called 'repetition courses', are 20 days annually; but after going through 8 courses further attendance is excused for all under the rank of sergeant. The *Landwehr* men are called up for training courses of 13 days every 2 years, and the *Landsturm* men have to undergo a refresher course of 13 days.

The Army is divided into 3 field corps each of 1 armoured and 2 infantry divisions and support groups, a corps with 3 mountain divisions, and independent redoubt-, fortress- and territorial-brigades. Strength on mobilization (1991): 565,000, and 400,000 reserves.

The administration of the Swiss Army is partly in the hands of the Cantonal authorities, who can promote officers up to the rank of captain. But the Federal Government is concerned with all general questions and makes all the higher appointments.

In peace-time the Swiss Army has no general; only in time of war the Federal Assembly in joint session of both Houses appoints a general.

The Swiss infantry are armed with the Swiss automatic rifle and with machine-guns, bazookas and mortars. The field artillery is armed with a Q.F. shielded 10·5 Bofors and field howitzers of 10·5 cm calibre. The heavy artillery is armed with guns of 10·5 cm and howitzers of 15 cm calibre. Equipment includes 130 Leopard,

150 Centurion and P3-61/-68 tanks and 1,350 M-63/-73/-64 armoured personnel carriers.

Air Corps. The Air Corps is part of the Army. It has 3 flying regiments. The fighter squadrons are equipped with Swiss-built F-5E Tiger IIs (7 squadrons), Mirage IIIS supersonic interceptor/ground-attack (2 squadrons), Mirage IIIRS fighter/reconnaissance (1 squadron), and Hunter interceptor/ground-attack (9 squadrons) aircraft. Bloodhound surface-to-air missile batteries are operational.

Training aircraft are Pilatus P-3 and PC-7 Turbo-Trainer and Vampire; there are also communications and transport aircraft and helicopters. The Vampires were being replaced, in 1989, by Hawk trainers. Personnel (1991), 60,000 on mobilization, with 271 combat aircraft.

INTERNATIONAL RELATIONS

Membership. Switzerland is a member of OECD, EFTA and the Council of Europe. In a referendum in 1986 the electorate voted against joining the UN.

ECONOMY

Budget. Revenue and expenditure of the Confederation, in 1m. francs, for calendar years:

	1985	*1986*	*1987*	*1988*	*1989*	*1990*
Revenue	22,200	25,200	24,902	27,881	28,031	30,264
Expenditure	22,900	23,200	23,861	26,633	27,555	29,607

The public debt, including internal debt, of the Confederation in 1980 amounted to 24,409m. francs; 1981, 24,677m.; 1982, 24,968m.; 1983, 25,249m.; 1984, 27,700m.; 1985, 29,300m.; 1986, 28,200m.; 1987, 27,200m.

Schweizerisches Finanz-Jahrbuch. Bern. Annual. From 1899

Currency. The unit of currency is the *Swiss franc* (CHF) of 100 *Rappen* or *centimes*. On 10 May 1971 there was a revaluation to 0·21759 gramme of fine gold.

The legal gold coins are 20- and 10-franc pieces; cupro-nickel coins are 5, 2, 1 and ½ franc, 20, 10 and 5 centimes; bronze, 2 and 1 centime. Notes are of 1,000, 500, 100, 50, 20, 10 and 5 francs.

On 10 July 1981 the notes in circulation (of francs of nominal value) was as follows: In 1,000 franc notes, 8,685·1m. francs; in 500, 4,201·9m. francs; in 100, 6,687·3m. francs; in 50, 1,058·3m. francs, and in lower denominations 1,195·8m.

Inflation was 6·1% in Sept. 1990.

In March 1991, £1 = 2·54 *francs*; US$1 = 1·34 *francs*.

Banking and Finance. The National Bank, with headquarters divided between Bern and Zürich, opened on 20 June 1907. It has the exclusive right to issue banknotes. In 1984 the condition of the bank was as follows (in 1m. francs): Gold, 11,904, foreign exchange (currency), 38,800; currency in circulation, 26,500. The *Governor* is Marcus Lusser.

On 31 Dec. 1988 there were 1,675 banking institutions with total assets of 915,800m. Swiss francs. They included 29 cantonal banks (179,700m. francs), 5 big banks (483,500m.), 213 regional and saving banks (82,400m.), 1,243 loan and *Raiffeisen* banks (28,100m.), 205 other banks (142,100m.). In 1991 the 10 largest banks in order of capitalization were: Union Bank of Switzerland, Swiss Bank Corporation, Crédit Suisse, Swiss Volksbank, Zürcher Kantonalbank, Bank Leu, Banca della Svizzera Italiana, Banque Cantonale Vaudoise, Bank Julius Baer.

Money laundering was made a criminal offence in Aug. 1990. Complete secrecy about clients' accounts remains intact.

On 31 Dec. 1988 the total amount of savings deposits, deposit and investment accounts in Swiss banks was 197,600m. francs.

The stock exchange system is being reformed under federal legislation of 1990 on securities trading and capital market services. The 4 smaller exchanges are being abandoned and activity concentrated on the major exchanges of Zurich, Basel and Geneva, which are increasingly harmonizing their operations.

Weights and Measures. The metric system is legal.

ENERGY AND NATURAL RESOURCES

Electricity. The total production of energy amounted to 51,656m kwh. in 1989 of which 30,485m. kwh. were generated by hydro-electric plants. In 1990 37% was nuclear-produced, but in Sept. 1990 54% of citizens voted for a 10-year moratorium on the construction of new nuclear plants. Supply 220 volts; 50 Hz.

Gas. The production of gas in 1986 was 54·52m. cu. metres.

Minerals. There are 2 salt-mining districts; that in Bex (Vaud) belongs to the canton, but is worked by a private company, and those at Schweizerhalle, Rheinfelden and Ryburg are worked by a joint-stock company formed by the cantons interested. The output of salt of all kinds in 1982 was 361,964 tonnes.

Agriculture. Of the total area of the country of 4,129,315 ha, about 1,057,794 ha (25·6%) are unproductive. Of the productive area of 3,071,521 ha, 1,051,991 ha are wooded. The agricultural area, in 1985, totalled 1,076,339 ha, of which 287,049 ha arable land, 13,450 ha vineyards, 7,229 ha intensive fruit growing and 642,194 ha permanent meadow and pasture land. In 1985 there were 119,731 farms. The gross value of agricultural products was estimated at 7,243·1m. francs in 1980 and 8,775m. francs in 1986.

Area harvested, 1988 (in 1,000 ha): Cereals, 186; coarse grains, 92; potatoes, 19; sugar-beet, 15. Production, 1988 (in 1,000 tonnes): Potatoes, 748; sugar-beet, 923; wheat, 553; barley, 299; maize, 237; tobacco, 1.

The fruit production (in 1,000 tonnes) in 1988 was: Apples, 540; pears, 229; plums, 33; cherries, 35; nuts, 6.

Wine is produced in 18 of the cantons. In 1988 Swiss vineyards yielded 117 tonnes of wine.

Livestock (1988): 49,000 horses, 367,000 sheep, 1,837,000 cattle (including about 798,000 milch cows), 1,940,000 pigs, (1985) 6m. poultry.

Forestry. Of the forest area of 999,795 ha, 56,876 were owned by the Federation or the cantons, 636,069 by communes and 306,850 by private persons or companies in 1982. Production (1987) 4,570 cu. metres of softwood and 1,158 cu. metres of hardwood.

INDUSTRY. The chief food producing industries, based on Swiss agriculture, are the manufacture of cheese, butter, sugar and meat. The production in 1986 was (in tonnes): Cheese, 130,900; butter, 37,300; sugar, 9,800; meat, 37,600. There are 46 breweries, producing in 1978, 4·05m. hectolitres of beer. Tobacco products in 1986: Cigars, 278m.; cigarettes (1982), 26,497m.

Among the other industries, the manufacture of textiles, wearing apparel and footwear, chemicals and pharmaceutical products, bricks, glass and cement, the manufacture of basic iron and steel and of other metal products, the production of machinery (including electrical machinery and scientific and optical instruments) and watch and clock making are the most important. In 1981 there were 8,738 factories with 693,243 workers. In 1982, 41,200 were working in textile industries, 45,000 in the manufacture of clothing and footwear, 70,200 in chemical works, 194,700 in the construction industry, 168,600 in manufacture of metal products, 252,000 in the manufacture of machinery and 55,300 in watch and clock making and in the manufacture of jewellery.

Production in 1982 was: Woollen and blended yarn, 15,467 tonnes; woollen and blended cloth, 7,534 metres; footwear (1981), 5·87m. pairs; cement, 4,099,874 tonnes; raw aluminium, 75,256 tonnes; chocolate, 76,605 tonnes, 25·38m. watches and clocks were exported (1981).

Labour. In 1988, the total working population was 3,572,300, of which 208,600 were active in agriculture and forestry, 1,230,200 in manufacture and construction and 2,133,600 in services. 15,136 persons (6,737 females) were unemployed in 1989.

The foreign labour force with permit of temporary residence was 954,940 in Aug. 1990 (301,881 women). Of these 289,401 were Italian, 122,954 Yugoslav, 119,122 French, 92,558 German, 91,613 Portuguese and 89,515 Spanish.

Trade Unions. The Swiss Federal Union of Administrative and Public Service Workers had, in 1985, a membership of 123,300. The Federation of Trade Unions had about 443,000 members.

FOREIGN ECONOMIC RELATIONS

Commerce. The special commerce, excluding gold (bullion and coins) and silver (coins), was (in 1m. Swiss francs) as follows:

	1982	*1983*	*1984*	*1985*	*1986*	*1987*	*1988*	*1989*
Imports	58,060	61,064	69,024	74,750	73,513	75,171	82,399	95,209
Exports	52,659	53,724	60,654	66,624	67,004	67,477	74,064	84,268

The following table, in 1m. francs, shows the distribution of the special trade of Switzerland among the principal countries:

	Imports from				*Exports to*			
Countries	*1985*	*1986*	*1987*	*1988*	*1985*	*1986*	*1987*	*1988*
Federal Rep. of Germany	22,912·7	24,267·1	25,806·0	28,056·0	13,103·2	14,146·2	14,367·8	15,481·3
France	8,344·2	8,423·6	8,109·1	8,745·7	5,552·5	6,065·0	6,166·1	6,935·8
Italy	7,243·0	7,487·4	7,641·9	8,356·5	4,956·4	5,161·3	5,568·0	6,159·7
Netherlands	3,412·6	3,069·9	3,015·9	3,465·3	1,767·4	1,829·8	1,880·0	2,059·0
Belgium–Luxembourg	3,009·4	2,593·1	2,570·4	2,779·8	1,344·5	1,450·8	1,629·4	1,639·5
UK	5,425·2	5,375·0	4,577·8	4,691·4	5,298·9	5,182·1	5,038·5	5,820·0
Denmark	677·6	713·0	787·8	834·2	889·8	904·3	817·7	893·5
Portugal	244·1	271·6	276·0	298·1	377·8	413·2	462·6	535·4
Ireland	354·2	402·9	409·0	361·5	153·1	150·2	118·2	162·0
Spain	1,089·8	944·5	925·6	1,014·8	1,186·4	1,098·7	1,200·2	1,390·2
Greece	135·1	127·4	113·6	114·8	406·0	348·4	347·8	375·2
EEC Total	51,514·0	53,675·5	54,233·0	58,718·1	33,471·7	36,750·0	37,596·2	41,451·7
Austria	2,666·1	2,896·9	2,903·3	3,181·8	2,582·6	2,605·2	2,558·1	2,693·1
Norway	302·5	285·0	360·3	383·9	560·0	586·0	493·4	491·8
Sweden	1,377·2	1,330·6	1,483·4	1,699·0	1,317·3	1,300·2	1,327·8	1,363·4
Finland	418·5	454·0	484·9	536·4	530·0	562·9	573·9	607·9
Iceland	66·9	64·5	81·0	106·0	20·3	19·6	20·3	24·2
EFTA	5,075·4	5,031·0	5,312·7	5,907·2	5,388·0	5,073·8	4,973·5	5,180·4
Gibraltar, Malta	4·1	5·4	10·8	4·6	25·0	24·5	20·8	24·1
German Dem. Republic	133·3	129·4	115·1	131·8	189·8	243·0	352·4	492·0
Poland	134·2	101·3	104·9	104·3	300·2	264·3	261·1	291·5
Czechoslovakia	194·6	163·4	152·1	166·1	310·2	324·4	310·2	355·2
Hungary	351·2	271·1	237·8	234·2	335·1	321·7	318·3	325·2
Yugoslavia	197·7	167·9	163·1	157·3	462·3	512·4	424·2	456·2
Bulgaria	33·4	23·2	18·3	21·1	233·3	279·2	229·5	181·4
Romania	48·9	38·9	29·8	26·0	84·8	52·3	29·0	17·7
USSR	1,196·4	722·0	409·5	300·0	636·5	535·2	710·3	810·8
Turkey	200·1	228·6	201·7	198·3	590·1	667·9	677·6	666·0
Other European countries	23·2	14·4	12·4	11·0	45·1	38·6	44·2	49·7
Europe Total	60,196·3	60,572·1	61,001·3	65,980·2	43,258·5	45,087·3	45,947·4	50,301·9
Egypt	58·2	27·0	21·4	21·1	395·9	291·3	278·6	282·4
Sudan	2·9	1·7	...	6·4	44·9	36·5	...	51·9
Libya	949·1	410·7	409·0	292·5	170·4	117·4	113·8	87·5
Tunisia	21·6	33·5	...	43·9	52·0	50·2	...	38·8
Algeria	417·6	166·3	154·0	92·1	242·3	200·7	125·6	139·4
Morocco	23·6	25·2	...	30·8	90·2	81·1	...	118·7
Côte d'Ivoire	67·3	56·5	...	32·5	46·2	55·3	...	37·6
Guinea	1·8	0·2	...	1·1	11·4	8·2	...	4·6

Countries	*Imports from* 1985	1986	1987	1988	*Exports to* 1985	1986	1987	1988
Ghana	30·3	30·1	...	28·0	21·5	32·8	...	19·9
Nigeria	439·0	147·8	112·7	40·8	344·6	279·7	153·5	248·2
Zaïre	6·2	10·0	...	7·0	38·0	41·2	...	26·5
Angola	6·4	5·6	...	4·0	37·3	23·0	...	14·6
S Africa, Rep. of	171·4	154·3	395·4	800·3	482·9	430·9	404·7	470·6
Zambia	5·7	10·6	...	20·2	19·2	8·0	...	12·2
Zimbabwe	34·3	19·4	...	12·9	32·8	37·1	...	21·1
Tanzania	3·9	1·7	...	4·3	26·6	22·9	...	18·8
Kenya	35·0	40·7	...	23·2	35·6	43·7	...	45·9
Other African countries	117·5	101·2	...	97·3	216·4	223·4	...	199·1
Africa Total	2,391·8	1,242·5	1,393·2	1,558·5	2,308·2	1,983·4	1,679·5	1,837·7
Syria	3·1	6·5	...	1·9	95·3	59·1	...	40·5
Lebanon	55·4	93·2	...	105·3	81·4	75·5	...	135·1
Israel	260·3	233·6	235·7	262·7	843·0	749·3	797·7	1,028·0
Iraq	1·2	1·1	...	0·5	256·5	169·0	...	265·9
Kuwait	2·4	1·2	...	1·6	189·1	111·3	...	103·6
Iran	66·7	87·4	77·1	75·4	475·6	420·0	327·5	290·3
Saudi Arabia	307·7	188·7	192·1	288·2	1,410·7	981·6	1,073·5	919·9
UAE	96·3	7·1	40·6	14·0	342·0	224·3	205·2	243·0
Pakistan	46·9	54·0	...	60·1	197·8	259·2	...	234·1
India	173·8	173·3	185·4	197·8	381·4	549·9	354·5	355·2
Thailand	155·7	200·7	...	208·4	248·5	201·8	...	401·5
Malaysia	72·2	54·9	...	64·1	142·2	144·0	...	119·2
Singapore	93·8	87·1	116·0	137·4	457·7	415·6	482·6	582·7
China	218·0	185·3	238·7	297·6	589·1	738·3	613·6	596·7
Hong Kong	802·7	722·1	772·2	873·5	1,086·4	1,305·7	1,392·3	1,730·0
Taiwan	233·7	277·1	...	534·4	265·6	260·7	...	501·6
Korea, Rep. of	227·9	244·7	...	415·4	252·8	280·5	...	410·2
Korea, Dem. People's Rep.	...	...	...	2·1	...	...	...	7·2
Japan	2,960·2	3,418·6	3,448·4	4,117·0	1,122·2	2,171·5	2,573·8	3,184·3
Philippines	41·0	31·7	...	31·2	101·2	104·6	...	115·0
Indonesia	70·2	64·4	...	50·1	155·9	193·6	...	223·3
Other Asian countries	73·6	97·4	...	200·2	543·4	464·6	...	456·3
Asia Total	5,962·8	6,230·1	6,664·4	7,939·0	10,237·8	9,880·1	10,448·4	11,943·5
Canada	274·7	240·9	293·5	305·6	759·8	719·5	633·8	757·4
USA	4,390·9	3,970·1	3,993·6	4,560·7	6,870·8	6,343·0	5,917·5	6,294·4
Mexico	43·6	40·4	38·8	56·1	358·5	341·3	242·8	327·1
Guatemala	47·3	55·3	...	28·8	28·1	17·2	...	21·0
Honduras	50·5	43·6	...	32·1	20·2	15·5	...	25·1
Costa Rica	68·4	63·3	...	46·5	15·2	17·6	...	14·0
Panama	217·8	161·6	258·0	144·5	233·6	176·9	185·8	150·2
Cuba	14·5	14·4	...	13·6	65·8	40·7	...	44·0
Colombia	140·6	145·2	...	87·2	160·9	127·1	...	134·4
Venezuela	17·3	9·2	9·2	13·6	190·0	215·2	181·7	276·2
Brazil	421·9	304·6	291·4	363·5	473·5	557·1	489·3	544·8
Uruguay	24·0	29·3	...	25·9	29·3	27·3	...	24·9
Argentina	132·0	83·5	74·3	102·3	293·1	223·7	242·3	184·9
Chile	18·1	21·2	...	11·2	83·0	95·0	...	100·7
Bolivia	2·5	0·7	...	1·0	9·4	11·9	...	6·0
Peru	35·7	34·8	...	25·6	86·0	126·4	...	75·7
Ecuador	23·5	20·0	...	13·9	68·4	67·4	...	60·7
Other American countries	126·7	89·1	...	958·0	338·5	230·9	...	262·3
Australia and Oceania	149·5	140·6	133·6	130·9	735·1	699·5	689·3	676·9

Custom receipts (in 1,000 francs): 1980, 3,170,700; 1981, 3,243,631; 1982, 3,243,000; 1983, 3,382,000; 1984, 3,393,000; 1985, 3,449,000.

Total trade between Switzerland (including Liechtenstein) and UK for calendar years (British Department of Trade, in £1,000 sterling):

	1986	*1987*	*1988*	*1989*	*1990*
Imports to UK	2,989,112	3,298,009	3,840,643	4,125,731	4,252,783
Exports and re-exports from UK	1,575,247	1,835,851	1,854,918	2,245,354	2,358,528

Tourism. Tourism is an important industry. In 1989, overnight stays in hotels and sanatoria were 35,246,000 and in other accommodation (1988) 39,266,000 (34,496,000 by foreign visitors).

COMMUNICATIONS

Roads. There were (1984) 70,926 km of main roads, including 1,300 km of 'national roads' for motor cars only. Motor vehicles, as at 30 Sept. 1989, numbered 3,642,000, including 2,900,000 private cars, 248,000 trucks, 262,000 motor cycles, 29,000 buses and 203,000 commercial and agricultural vehicles.

Railways. Railway history in Switzerland begins in 1847. In 1987 the length of the general traffic railways was 5,020 km, and of special lines (funiculars etc.), 814 km. The operating receipts of general traffic lines amounted to (1986) 4,504,500,000 francs; operating expenses, 5,074,800,000 francs. Traffic (1987) was 12,494m. passenger-km and 7,184 tonnes-km of goods were carried.

There are many privately-owned lines, the most important of which are the Bern–Lotschberg–Simplon (115 km) and Rhaetian (363 km) networks.

Aviation. In 1985 Swiss aviation on domestic and international routes carried 7,498,000 passengers. Routes covered 327,022 km in 1987.

The air transport organization Swissair (founded in 1931) in 1982 carried 189,139 tonnes of freight and 7,168,567 passengers. Its fleet consisted of 53 aircraft in Jan. 1983.

Shipping. In 1987 there were 1,208 km of navigable waterway. A merchant marine was created in 1941, the place of registry of its vessels being Basel. In 1985 it consisted of 39 vessels with a total of 225,434 GRT.

Pipeline. In 1987 there were 244 km of oil pipeline.

Telecommunications. In 1988 there were 3,847 post offices and 5,879,200 telephones. In 1988 there were 35,300 telex, 13,304 fax and 14,474 videotext subscribers.

Radio communication is furnished by 3 main medium-wave stations and 1 short-wave station. There are 3 television studios and more than 100 transmitters. TV programmes are financed by licence fees and advertisements. Advertisements are limited to 15 minutes each day. All stations are operated by the Federal Post, Telephone and Telegraph (PTT) services. Radio-telegraph circuits are operated by Radio Suisse SA, radio-telephone circuits by the PTT. Radio licences, 1988, 2,590,200; television licences, 2,338,300.

In 1988 PTT revenue was 106% of expenses.

Cinemas (1986). There were 428 cinemas with a seating capacity of 122,000.

Newspapers (1988). There were 112 daily newspapers (85 German language, 19 French, 7 Italian and 1 multi-lingual).

JUSTICE, RELIGION, EDUCATION AND WELFARE

Justice. The Federal Tribunal (*Bundesgericht*), which sits at Lausanne, consists of 26-28 members, with 11-13 supplementary judges, appointed by the Federal Assembly for 6 years and eligible for re-election; the President and Vice-President serve for 2 years and cannot be re-elected. The President has a salary of 170,000 francs a year, and the other members 158,000 francs. The Tribunal has original and final jurisdiction in suits between the Confederation and cantons; between cantons and cantons; between the Confederation or cantons and corporations or individuals, the value in dispute being not less than 8,000 francs; between parties who refer their case to it, the value in dispute being at least 20,000 francs; in such suits as the constitution or legislation of cantons places within its authority; and in many classes of railway suits. It is a court of appeal against decisions of other federal authorities, and of cantonal authorities applying federal laws. The Tribunal also tries persons accused of treason or other offences against the Confederation. For this purpose it is divided into 4 chambers: Chamber of Accusation, Criminal Chamber (*Cour d'Assises*), Federal Penal Court and Court of Cassation. The jurors who serve in the Assize Courts are elected by the people, and are paid 100 francs a day when serving.

On 3 July 1938 the Swiss electorate accepted a new federal penal code, to take the place of the separate cantonal penal codes. The new code, which abolished capital punishment, came into force on 1 Jan. 1942.

Religion. There is complete and absolute liberty of conscience and of creed. No one is bound to pay taxes specially appropriated to defraying the expenses of a creed to which he does not belong. No bishoprics can be created on Swiss territory without the approbation of the Confederation.

According to the census of 1 Dec. 1980 Roman Catholics numbered 3,030,069 (47·6%) of the population; Protestants, 2,822,266 (44·3%) and others, 513,625 (8·1%). In 1960 Protestants were in a majority in 10 of the cantons and Catholics in 12. Of the more populous cantons, Zürich, Bern, Vaud, Neuchâtel and Basel (town and land) were mainly Protestant, while Luzern, Fribourg, Ticino, Valais and the Forest Cantons are mainly Catholic. The Roman Catholics are under 6 Bishops, viz., of Basel (resident at Solothurn), Chur, St Gallen, Lugano, Lausanne–Geneva–Fribourg (resident at Fribourg) and Sitten (Sion), all of them immediately subject to the Holy See. The Old Catholics have a theological faculty at the university of Bern.

Education. Education is administered by the cantons and is compulsory. Before the year 1848 most of the cantons had organized a system of primary schools, and since that year elementary education has steadily advanced. In 1874 it was made obligatory for the whole country (the school age varying in the different cantons) and placed under the civil authority. In some cantons the cost falls almost entirely on the communes, in others it is divided between the canton and communes. In all the cantons primary instruction is free. In 1988–89 there were 134,804 pupils in nursery schools and 696,516 in primary schools.

In most cantons there are also secondary schools for youths of from 12 to 15, gymnasia, higher schools for girls, teachers' seminaries, commercial and administrative schools, trade schools, art schools, technical schools, schools for the instruction of girls in domestic economy and other subjects, agricultural schools, schools for horticulture, for viticulture, for arboriculture and for dairy management. There are also institutions for the blind, the deaf and dumb and feeble-minded. In 1988–89 there were 308,189 pupils in secondary schools.

There are 7 universities in Switzerland. These universities are organized on the model of those of Germany, governed by a rector and a senate, and divided into faculties (theology, jurisprudence, philosophy, medicine, etc.). In 1988–89 the Federal Institute of Technology at Zürich (founded in 1855) had 11,004 matriculated students; the Federal Institute of Technology at Lausanne, independent of the university since 1946, had 3,431 students; the St Gall School of Economics and Social Sciences, founded in 1899, had 3,845 matriculated students.

University statistics in the winter of 1986–87:

	Theology	*Humanities etc*	*Law*	*Economics*	*Medicine*	*Science*	*Teaching staff (1985–86)*
Basel (1460)	223	1,687	881	848	1,761	1,275	625
Zürich (1523 & 1833)	358	7,463	3,138	2,239	3,354	2,101	1,661
Bern (1528 & 1834)	374	2,696	1,657	848	1,798	1,628	723
Genève (1559[1] & 1873[1])	130	4,578	995	2,411	1,506	1,645	913
Lausanne (1537[1] & 1890[2])	85	1,678	889	1,405	1,503	875	476
Fribourg (1889)	504	1,999	995	1,129	225	506	548
Neuchâtel (1866 & 1909)	52	870	310	444	57	524	240

[1] Founded as an academy. [2] Reorganized as a university.

These numbers are exclusive of 'visitors', but inclusive of women students. In 1988–89 there were 80,629 students attending universities.

Health. In 1988 there were 18,667 doctors, 37,360 (1980) nurses, 4,750 dentists and 12,300 physiotherapists. There were (1988) 435 hospitals and 1,417 pharmacies.

Social Security. The Federal Insurance Law against illness and accident, of 13 June 1911, entitles all Swiss citizens to insurance against illness; foreigners may be admitted to the benefits. Compulsory insurance against illness does not exist as yet, but cantons and communities are entitled to declare insurance obligatory for certain classes or to establish public benefit (sick fund) associations, and to make employers responsible for the payment of the premiums of their employees.

Unemployment insurance is based since 13 June 1976 upon a Constitution amendment which stipulates unemployment insurance as compulsory for all wage-earners.

Insurance against accident is compulsory for all officials, employees and workmen of all the factories, trades, etc., which are under the federal liability law.

On 6 July 1947 a federal law was accepted by a referendum, providing compulsory old age and widows and widowers insurance for the whole population, as from 1 Jan. 1948. In March 1985 the number of normal pensioners was 1,033,000.

DIPLOMATIC REPRESENTATIVES

Of Switzerland in Great Britain (16–18 Montagu Pl., London, W1H 2BQ)
Ambassador: Franz E. Muheim (accredited 14 June 1989).

Of Great Britain in Switzerland (Thunstrasse 50, 3005 Bern)
Ambassador: Christopher Long, CMG.

Of Switzerland in the USA (2900 Cathedral Ave., NW, Washington, D.C., 20008)
Ambassador: Edouard Brunner.

Of the USA in Switzerland (Jubilaeumstrasse 93, 3005, Bern)
Ambassador: Joseph Gildenhorn.

Further Reading

Statistical Information: Bureau fédéral de statistique (Hallwylstr. 15, 3003 Bern) was established in 1860. *Director:* Carlo Malaguerra. Its principal publications are:

Annuaire statistique de la Suisse. From 1891
Bibliographie Suisse de statistique et d'économie politique. Annual, from 1937

Swiss Confederation
Annuaire; Budget; Message du Budget; Compte d'Etat (annual) *Feuille Fédérale; Recueil des Lois fédérales* (weekly)
Recueil systématique des lois et ordonnances, 1848–1947 (in German, French and Italian). Bern, 1951
Sammlung der Bundes- und Kantonsverfassungen (in German, French and Italian). Bern, 1937

Federal Department of Economics
La vie économique (and supplements). Monthly. From 1928
Legislation sociale de la Suisse. Annual, from 1928

Meier, H. K. and Meier, R. A., *Switzerland.* [bibliography] London and Santa Barbara, 1990
Schwarz, U., *The Eye of the Hurricane: Switzerland in World War Two*. Boulder, 1980
Wildblood, R., *What makes Switzerland tick?* London, 1988

National Library: Bibliothèque Nationale Suisse, Hallwylstr.15, 3003, Bern. *Director:* Dr Jean Frédéric Janslin.

SYRIA

Capital: Damascus
Population: 11·3m. (1988)
GNP per capita: US$1,670 (1988)

Jumhuriya al-Arabya as-Suriya

(Syrian Arab Republic)

HISTORY. For the history of Syria from 1920 to 1946 *see* THE STATESMAN'S YEAR-BOOK , 1957, pp. 1408–9. Complete independence was achieved on 12 Apr. 1946. Syria merged with Egypt to form the United Arab Republic from 2 Feb. 1958 until 29 Sept. 1961, when independence was resumed following a coup the previous day. Lieut.-Gen. Hafez al-Assad became Prime Minister following the fifth coup of that decade on 13 Nov. 1970, and assumed the Presidency on 22 Feb. 1971.

AREA AND POPULATION. Syria is bounded by the Mediterranean and Lebanon on the west, by Israel and Jordan on the south, by Iraq on the east and by Turkey on the north. The frontier between Syria and Turkey (Nisibim-Jeziret ibn Omar) was settled by the Franco-Turkish agreement of 22 June 1929.

The area of Syria is 185,180 sq. km (71,498 sq. miles), of which 35,000 sq. km have been surveyed. The census of 1981 gave a total population of 9,046,144 (47% urban). Estimate (1988) 11,338,000. of whom 50% were urban. There were 282,673 registered Palestinian refugees in 1987

Area and population (1981 Census) of the 14 districts *(mohafaza)* are:

	Sq. km	*1981 Census*		*Sq. km*	*1981 Census*
Damascus (City)	105	1,112,214	Idlib	6,097	579,581
Damascus (District)	18,032	917,364	Hasakah	23,334	669,887
Aleppo	18,500	1,878,701	Raqqah	19,616	348,383
Homs	42,223	812,517	Suwaydá	5,550	199,114
Hama	8,883	736,412	Dará	3,730	362,969
Lattakia	2,297	554,384	Tartous	1,892	443,290
Dayr az-Zawr	33,060	409,130	Qunaytirah	1,861	26,258

Principal towns (census 1981), Damascus (the capital), 1,112,214; Aleppo, 985,413; Homs, 346,871; Lattakia, 196,791; Hama, 177,208.

Vital statistics, 1987: Births, 421,328; deaths, 43,571; marriages, 102,626; divorces, 7,249.

Arabic is the official language, spoken by 89% of the population, while 6% speak Kurdish (chiefly Hasakah governorate), 3% Armenian and 2% other languages.

CLIMATE. The climate is Mediterranean in type, with mild wet winters and dry, hot summers, though there are variations in temperatures and rainfall between the coastal regions and the interior, which even includes desert conditions. The more mountainous parts are subject to snowfall. Damascus. Jan. 45°F (7°C), July 81°F (27°C). Annual rainfall 9" (225 mm). Aleppo. Jan. 43°F (6·1°C), July 83°F (28·3°C). Annual rainfall 16" (401 mm). Homs. Jan. 45°F (7·2°C), July 83°F (28·3°C). Annual rainfall 12" (300 mm).

CONSTITUTION AND GOVERNMENT. A new Constitution was approved by plebiscite on 12 March 1973 and promulgated on 14 March. It confirmed the Arab Socialist Renaissance *(Ba'ath)* Party, in power since 1963, as the 'leading party in the State and society'. Legislative power is held by a 250-member People's Council, elected for a 4-year term. At the elections on 22 May 1990, 150 seats went to the National Progressive Front, a coalition of the Ba'ath Party and four smaller ones and the remainder to independents. 9,765 candidates stood.

President: Lieut.-Gen. Hafez al-Assad (re-elected for further 7-year terms in 1978 and 1985).

First Vice-President: Abdul Halim Khaddam *(Political and Foreign Affairs). Second Vice-President:* Rifaat al-Assad *(Defence and Security). Third Vice-President:* Mohammed Zuhair Mashrqa *(Party Affairs).*

Prime Minister: Mahmoud Zubi.

Deputy Prime Ministers: Gen. Mustafa Tlass *(Defence)*; Salim Yassin *(Economic Affairs)*; Mahmud Qaddur *(Public Affairs). Education:* Ghassan Halabi. *Higher Education:* Kamal Sharaf. *Interior:* Mohammad Harbah. *Transport:* Yusuf al-Ahmed. *Information:* Mohammad Salman. *Local Administration:* Ahmed Diab. *Supply and Internal Trade:* Hassan Saqqa. *Economy and Foreign Trade:* Mohammad al-Imadi. *Culture:* Najah al-Attar. *Foreign Affairs:* Farooq ash-Shar'. *Tourism:* Adnan Quli. *Health:* Iyad al-Shatti. *Waqfs (Religious Endowments):* Abdel-Majid Tarabulsi. *Irrigation:* Abd ar-Rahman Madani. *Electricity:* Kamil al-Baba. *Oil and Mineral Resources:* Antonios Habib. *Construction:* Marwan Farra. *Housing and Utilities:* Mohammad Nur Antabi. *Agriculture and Agrarian Reform:* Mohammad Ghabbash. *Finance:* Khaled al-Mahayni. *Industry:* Antoine Jubran. *Communications:* Murad Quwatli. *Justice:* Khalid Ansari. *Presidential Affairs:* Wahib Fadil. *Labour and Social Affairs:* Haydar Buzu.

There are 7 Ministers of State.

National flag: Three horizontal stripes of red, white, black, with 2 green stars on the white stripe.

Local Government: Syria is administratively divided into 14 districts *(mohafaza)* (*see* area and population above). These are divided into 59 *mantika*, which are sub-divided into 179 smaller administrative units *(nahia)*, each covering a number of villages.

DEFENCE. Military service is compulsory for a period of 30 months.

Army. The Army is organized into 5 armoured and 3 mechanized divisions, 1 special forces division, 7 independent special forces regiments, 2 artillery, 3 surface-to-surface missile brigades and 3 coastal defence brigades. Equipment includes 2,050 T-54/-55, 1,000 T-62 and 950 T-72/-72M main battle tanks. Strength (1991) about 300,000 (including 130,000 conscripts) and reserves 50,000. There are a further 25,000 men in paramilitary forces.

Navy. The Navy includes 3 ex-Soviet 'Romeo'-class diesel submarines, 2 small frigates, 12 fast missile craft, 8 inshore patrol craft, 2 minesweepers, 6 inshore minesweepers, and 3 medium landing ships (all ex-Soviet). A small naval aviation branch operates 17 Soviet-type anti-submarine helicopters. Personnel in 1990 totalled 6,000. The main base is at Tartus, which also provides facilities for the Soviet Mediterranean Squadron.

Air Force. The Air Force, including Air Defence Command, was believed (1991) to have about 40,000 personnel and 558 combat aircraft, including over 500 first-line jet combat aircraft, made up of about 200 MiG-21, 80 MiG-23 and 30 MiG-25 supersonic interceptors, 60 MiG-23, 40 Su-7, 60 Su-22 and 50 MiG-17 fighter-bombers, plus some MiG-25 reconnaissance aircraft. Sixty MiG-29 interceptors are being delivered by the USSR. Training units have Spanish-built Flamingo piston-engined primary trainers and Czechoslovakian L-29 Delfin and L-39 jet basic trainers. There are also transport units with Il-76, An-12, An-24/26, Il-14 and other types, and helicopter units with Soviet-built Mi-6s, Mi-8s, Mi-14s and Mi-24 gunships, and French-built Gazelles. 'Guideline', 'Goa', 'Gainful' and 'Gaskin' surface-to-air missiles are widely deployed in Syria by Air Defence Command, and 'Gammon' long-range surface-to-air missiles in Lebanon.

INTERNATIONAL RELATIONS

Membership. Syria is a member of the UN and Arab League.

ECONOMY

Budget. The consolidated budget for the calendar year 1988 balanced at £Syr.61,875m.

Currency. The monetary unit is the *Syrian pound* (SYP) of 100 *piastres*. In March 1991, £1 = £Syr.39·85; US$1 = £Syr.21·01.

Banking and Finance. The Central Bank has the sole right to issue currency. Other banks were nationalized in March 1963. Number of branches, 1 Jan. 1987: Central Bank of Syria, 10; Commercial Bank of Syria, 35; Industrial Bank, 11; Agricultural Co-operative Bank, 64; Real Estate Bank, 13; Popular Credit Bank, 44. Total deposits at specialized banks, 1987 (in £Syr.1m.): Commercial Bank of Syria, 23,403·3; Industrial Bank, 1,369; Agricultural Co-operative Bank, 1,882; Real Estate Bank, 5,810·1; Popular Credit Bank, 4,298·7.

Weights and Measures. The metric system is legal, though former weights and measures may still be in use: 1 *okiya* = 0·47 lb.; 6 *okiyas* = 1 *oke* = 2·82 lb.; 2 *okes* = 1 *rottol* = 5·64 lb.; 200 *okes* = 1 *kantar*.

ENERGY AND NATURAL RESOURCES

Electricity. Production (1988), 8,161m. kwh.

Oil. A branch of the Iraq Petroleum Co.'s oil pipeline from Kirkuk crosses Syria between Makaleb in the east and Nahr el Kebir valley in the west. The Iraq Petroleum Co. has constructed a new pipeline from Kirkuk to the small fishing port of Banias (south of Lattakia), which came into use in April 1952; the Trans-Arabian Pipeline Co.'s line to Sidon crosses southern Syria. Crude oil production (1990), 20·29m. tonnes. Reserves (1983) 1,521m. bbls.

Gas. Gas reserves (1982), 700,000m. cubic ft. Production (1983), 75·86m. cu. metres.

Water. In 1987 there were 3 main dams, at Al-Rastan (storage capacity 250m. cu. metres), Mouhardeh (50m. cu. metres) and Taldo (15m. cu. metres), and 29 surface dams. Production of drinking water, 1988, 501·37m. cu. metres.

Minerals. Phosphate deposits have been discovered at two places near al-Shargiya and at Khneifis. Production, 1988, 2,186,000 tonnes; other minerals were salt, 127,000 tonnes and gypsum 179,000 tonnes. There are indications of lead, copper, antimony, nickel, chrome and other minerals widely distributed. Sodium chloride and bitumen deposits are being worked.

Agriculture. In 1987, 129,000 ha were under cotton, 1,183,000 ha under wheat and 1,570,000 ha under barley. The cultivable area in 1987 was 6,133,000 ha, and there were 8,277,000 ha of steppe and pasture. In 1987 there were 52,400 tractors.

Production of principal crops, 1988 (in 1,000 tonnes): Wheat, 2,067; barley, 2,836; maize, 105; seed cotton, 446; olives, 439; lentils, 171; millet, 6; sugar-beet, 368; potatoes, 353; tomatoes, 517; grapes, 515.

Production, of animal products 1987 (in tonnes): Milk, 1,108,000; butter, 2,924; cheese, 62,181; chicken meat, 64,250; wool, 13,284; hair, 688; honey, 590; silk cocoons, 84; 1,283m. eggs.

Livestock (1988): Cattle, 723,000; horses, 43,000; mules, 30,000; asses, 200,000; sheep, 13,304,000; goats, 1,078,000; poultry, 12m.

Forestry. In 1987 there were 534,000 ha of forest. The artificial forestry area was 25,586 ha, producing 30,406,000 woody plants, 1,509 tonnes of charcoal, 57,660 tonnes of firewood and 26,900 tonnes of industrial wood.

Fisheries. The total catch in 1986 was 4,800 tonnes.

INDUSTRY. Public sector industrial production in 1988 included (in tonnes): Cotton yarn, 36,744; cotton and mixed textiles, 21,018; mixed woollen yarn, 1,817; manufactured tobacco, 17,056; cement, 3,481; iron bars, 15,455; asbestos (1987),

21,684; vegetable oil, 22,838; electrical engines, 16,590; refrigerators, 9,158; water meters, 30,780; tractors, 1,198 (1987, units); woollen carpets, 520,000 sq. metres.

Trade Unions. In 1987 there were 198 trade unions with 312,003 members.

Labour. In 1984 the labour force was 2,356,000 (out of a total population of 9,616,000), of whom 2,246,000 were employed (1,329,000 urban). In 1987, 137,941 people were employed in the industrial public sector.

FOREIGN ECONOMIC RELATIONS

Commerce. Trade in calendar years in £Syr.1m. was as follows:

	1984	*1985*	*1986*	*1987*
Imports	16,154	15,570	10,709	27,915
Exports	7,275	6,427	5,199	15,192

Main imports, 1987 (in £Syr.1,000) included: Petroleum and products, 5,343,278; wheat, 730,764; iron tubes and pipes (not cast iron), 706,174; refined sugar, 637,898; yarn of continuous synthetic fibres, 549,272; direct current generators, 531,584; special purpose motor lorries, trucks and vans, 511,372. Main exports included: Petroleum and products, 7,871,220; raw cotton, 877,224; printed woven cotton fabrics, 577,433.

In 1987, imports (in £Syr.1,000) came mainly from France, 2,737,676; USSR, 2,317,606, Iran, 2,294,879; Federal Republic of Germany, 2,284,403; Italy, 1,883,869; Libya, 1,575,212; USA, 1,470,980. Exports went mainly to Italy, 4,718,628; USSR, 3,165,821; France, 1,507,082; Romania, 1,311,369.

Total trade between Syria and UK (British Department of Trade returns, in £1,000 sterling):

	1986	*1987*	*1988*	*1989*	*1990*
Imports to UK	31,298	24,937	36,100	55,258	85,874
Exports and re-exports from UK	55,511	34,053	24,647	38,537	38,245

Tourism. In 1987, there were 1,217,564 visitors.

COMMUNICATIONS

Roads. In 1988 there were 22,738 km of asphalted roads, 6,155 km of paved non-asphalted road and 1,559 km of earth roads. The first-class roads are capable of carrying all types of modern motor transport and are usable all the year round, while the second-class roads are usable during the dry season only, *i.e.*, for about 9 months. In 1988 there were 331,439 motor vehicles, including 112,337 cars and taxis, 4,197 buses, 7,808 mini-buses, 36,002 goods vehicles and 75,464 motorcycles.

Railways. In 1988 the network totalled 1,751 km of 1,435 mm gauge (Syrian Railways) and 127 km of 1,050 mm gauge (Hedjaz-Syrian Railway). In 1988 Syrian Railways carried 4,349,000 passengers and 5,992,000 tonnes of freight.

Aviation. In 1988, 11,204 aircraft arrived at Damascus, Aleppo, Al-Kamishli, Lattakia and Deir Ez-Zor airports; 659,790 passengers arrived, 726,441 departed and 127,520 were in transit; 2,915,966 kg of freight was unloaded and 3,412,936 kg loaded.

Shipping. The amount of cargo discharged in 1980 was 2·6m. tons and the amount loaded 430,000 tons.

Post and Broadcasting. Number of telephones (1988), 507,989; of these, 184,555 were in Damascus and 81,602 in Aleppo. There were 2m. radio sets in 1985 and 400,000 television receivers.

Cinemas. In 1985 there were 85 cinemas with 47,840 seats.

Newspapers. There were (1984) 3 national daily newspapers in Damascus; other dailies and periodicals appear in Hama, Homs, Aleppo and Lattakia.

JUSTICE, RELIGION, EDUCATION AND WELFARE

Justice. Syrian law is based on both Islamic and French jurisprudence. There are 2 courts of first instance in each district, one for civil and 1 for criminal cases. There is also a Summary Court in each sub-district, under Justices of the Peace. There is a Court of Appeal in the capital of each governorate, with a Court of Cassation in Damascus.

Religion. The population is composed 90% of Sunni Moslems and there are also Shi'ites and Ismailis. There are also Druzes and Alawites. Christians include Greek Orthodox, Greek Catholics, Armenian Orthodox, Syrian Orthodox, Armenian Catholics, Protestants, Maronites, Syrian Catholics, Latins, Nestorians and Assyrians. There are also Jews and Yezides.

Education. The Syrian University was founded in 1924, although the faculties of law and of medicine had existed previously. In 1986-87 there were 4 universities with 138,743 students.

In 1986-87 there were 766 kindergartens with 70,859 children; 9,315 primary schools with 85,583 teachers and 2,158,594 pupils; 1,922 intermediate and secondary schools with 37,541 teachers and 855,453 pupils. In 1987, 21 teachers' colleges had 1,167 teachers and 10,076 students; 143 schools for professional education had 7,245 teachers and 56,664 students.

Health. In 1987 there were 12,606 hospital beds (1 per 870 persons) in 206 hospitals, and 566 health centres; there were also 8,146 doctors, 2,456 dentists, 2,960 pharmacists, 3,049 midwives and 9,786 nursing personnel.

DIPLOMATIC REPRESENTATIVES

Of Great Britain in Syria (11 Mohammad Kurd Ali St., Damascus)
Chargé d'Affaires: M. E. Cribbs.

Of Syria in the USA (2215 Wyoming Ave., NW, Washington, D.C., 20008)
Chargé d'Affaires: Bushra Kanafani.

Of the USA in Syria (Abu Rumaneh, Al Mansur St., Damascus)
Ambassador: Edward P. Djerejian.

Of Syria to the United Nations
Ambassador: Dia-Allah Al-Fattal.

Diplomatic relations between Syria and the UK, broken off in Oct. 1986, were restored in Nov. 1990.

Further Reading

Statistical Information: There is a Central Statistics Bureau affiliated to the Council of Ministers, Damascus. It publishes a monthly summary and an annual Statistical Abstract (in Arabic and English).

Abd-Allah, U. F., *The Islamic Struggle in Syria*. Berkeley, 1983
Barthélemy, A., *Dictionnaire arabe-français. Dialectes de Syrie*. 4 vols. Paris, 1935–50
Devlin, J. F., *Syria: Modern State in an Ancient Land*. Boulder, 1983
Maoz, M. and Yaniv, A., *Syria under Assad*. New York, 1986
Seale, P., *The Struggle for Syria*. London, 1986.—*Asad of Syria: The Struggle for the Middle East*. London, 1989
Seccombe, I. J., *Syria*. [Bibliography] Oxford and Santa Barbara, 1987

TANZANIA

Capital: Dodoma
Population: 24·8m. (1989)
GNP per capita: US$160 (1988)

Jamhuri ya Muungano wa Tanzania

(United Republic of Tanzania)

HISTORY. German East Africa was occupied by German colonialists from 1884 and placed under the protection of the German Empire in 1891. It was conquered in the First World War and subsequently divided between the British and Belgians. The latter received the territories of Ruanda and Urundi and the British the remainder, except for the Kionga triangle, which went to Portugal. The country was administered as a League of Nations mandate until 1946 and then as a UN trusteeship territory until 9 Dec. 1961.

Tanganyika achieved responsible government in Sept. 1960 and full self-government on 1 May 1961. On 9 Dec. 1961 Tanganyika became a sovereign independent member state of the Commonwealth of Nations. It adopted a republican form of government on 9 Dec. 1962. For history from the end of the 17th century until 1884 *see* THE STATESMAN'S YEAR-BOOK 1982–83, p. 1170.

On 24 June 1963 Zanzibar became an internal self-governing state and on 9 Dec. 1963 she became independent. On 24 June 1963 the Legislative Council was replaced by a National Assembly.

On 12 Jan. 1964 the sultanate was overthrown and the sultan sent into exile by a revolt of the Afro-Shirazi Party leaders who established the People's Republic of Zanzibar.

On 26 April 1964 Tanganyika, Zanzibar and Pemba combined to form the United Republic of Tanganyika and Zanzibar (named Tanzania on 29 Oct.).

AREA AND POPULATION. Tanzania is bounded north-east by Kenya, north by Lake Victoria and Uganda, north-west by Rwanda and Burundi, west by Lake Tanganyika, south-west by Zambia and Malaŵi and south by Mozambique. Total area 945,037 sq. km (364,881 sq. miles including the offshore islands of Zanzibar (1,660 sq. km) and Pemba (984 sq. km) and inland water surfaces (59,050 sq. km)). The census of Aug. 1978 gave 17,551,925 for the United Republic, of which 17,076,270 were counted in mainland Tanzania and 475,655 in Zanzibar and Pemba. Estimate (1989) 24·8m.

The chief towns (1978 census populations) are Dar es Salaam, the chief port and former capital (757,346), Zanzibar Town (110,669), Mwanza (110,611), Dodoma, the capital (45,703), Tanga (103,409), Arusha (55,281), Mbeya (76,606), Morogoro (61,890), Mtwara (48,510), Tabora (67,392), Iringa (57,182), and Kigoma (50,044).

The United Republic is divided into 25 administrative regions of which 20 are in mainland Tanzania, 3 in Zanzibar (Zanzibar North, Zanzibar West, Zanzibar South) and 2 in Pemba (Pemba North, Pemba South). The 1985 estimated population of the islands was 571,000, of which 45% (256,950) were in Pemba and 55% (314,050) in Zanzibar.

The estimated populations of the 20 mainland regions were as follows in 1985:

Arusha	1,183,000	Lindi	604,000	Rukwa	603,000
Dar es Salaam	1,394,000	Mara	862,000	Ruvuma	691,000
Dodoma	1,171,000	Mbeya	1,335,000	Shinyanga	1,662,000
Iringa	1,100,000	Morogoro	1,134,000	Singida	730,000
Kagera	1,298,000	Mtwara	878,000	Tabora	1,089,000
Kigoma	782,000	Mwanza	1,736,000	Tanga	1,236,000
Kilimanjaro	1,093,000	Pwani	578,000		

Kiswahili is the national language and English is the official language.

CLIMATE. The climate is very varied and is controlled very largely by altitude and distance from the sea. There are three climatic zones: the hot and humid coast, the drier central plateau with seasonal variations of temperature, and the semi-temperate mountains. Dodoma. Jan. 75°F (23·9°C), July 67°F (19·4°C). Annual rainfall 23" (572 mm). Dar es Salaam. Jan. 82°F (27·8°C), July 74°F (23·3°C). Annual rainfall 43" (1,064 mm).

CONSTITUTION AND GOVERNMENT. A permanent Constitution was approved in April 1977. The country is a one-party state. The Tanganyika African National Union and the Afro-Shirazi Party in Zanzibar merged into one revolutionary party, *Chama cha Mapinduzi,* in Feb. 1977.

The *President* is head of state, chairman of the party and commander-in-chief of the armed forces. The second vice-president is head of the executive in Zanzibar. The Prime Minister and first vice-president is also the leader of government business in the National Assembly.

According to the Constitution of 1977, as amended in Oct. 1984, the *National Assembly* is composed of a total of 244 members: 169 Members of Parliament elected from the Constituencies (119 from the mainland and 50 from Zanzibar); 15 National Members elected by the National Assembly; 15 women members elected by the National Assembly, 5 from Zanzibar; 5 members elected by the House of Representatives in Zanzibar; 25 ex-officio Members (20 Regional Commissioners from the mainland and 5 from Zanzibar) and 15 Nominated Members (by the President), 5 from Zanzibar.

In Dec. 1979 a separate Constitution for Zanzibar was approved. Although at present under the same Constitution as Tanzania, Zanzibar has, in fact, been ruled by decree since 1964.

At the presidential elections of Oct. 1990 Ali Hassan Mwinyi, the sole candidate, gained 95·5% of votes cast.

The Government in Feb. 1991 consisted of:

President: Ali Hassan Mwinyi (b. 1925; elected Oct. 1990 for a second 5-year term).

Prime Minister and First Vice President: Joseph S. Warioba.

President of Zanzibar and Second Vice President: Salmin Amur. *Without Portfolio:* Rashid Kawawa, Gertrude Mongella. *Deputy Prime Minister, Defence and National Service:* Salim Ahmed Salim. *Finance, Economic Affairs and Planning:* Cleopa D. Msuya *Foreign Affairs:* Benjamin Mkapa. *Agriculture and Livestock Development:* Jackson Makweta. *Local Government, Community Development, Co-operatives and Marketing:* Paul Bomani. *Communications and Works:* Steven A. Kibona. *Labour, Culture and Social Services:* Christian Kisanji. *Home Affairs:* Maj.-Gen. Muhiddin Kimario. *Education:* Amrani H. Mayagila. *Minerals and Energy:* Al Noor Kassum. *Lands, Natural Resources and Tourism:* Arcado Ntagazwa. *Industries and Trade:* Joseph Rwegasira. *Health:* Dr Aaron Chiduo. *Attorney-General and Justice:* Damian Lubuva. *Water:* Dr Pius Ng'wandu. There are 9 Ministers of State.

National flag: Divided diagonally green, black, blue, with the black strip edged in yellow.

DEFENCE

Army. The Army consists of 8 infantry, 1 tank brigade; 2 artillery, 2 anti-aircraft, 2 mortar, 1 surface-to-air missile, 2 anti-tank and 2 signals battalions. Equipment includes 30 Chinese Type-59 and 30 T-62 main battle tanks. Strength (1991), 45,000 (25,000 conscripts). There is also a Citizen's Militia of 100,000.

Navy. There are 4 ex-Chinese torpedo-armed hydrofoils and 10 inshore patrol craft of mixed Chinese and North Korean origins. 4 British-built inshore patrol craft are based permanently in Zanzibar and 4 armed patrol boats on Lake Victoria Nyanza. Personnel in 1990 totalled some 800.

Air Force. The Tanzanian People's Defence Force Air Wing was built up initially with the help of Canada, but combat equipment has been acquired from China. Personnel totalled about 1,000 in 1991, with about 10 F-7 (MiG-21), 10 F-6 (MiG-19) and 8 F-4 (MiG-17) jet fighters; 1 F28 Fellowship VIP transport; 5 Buffalo twin-engined STOL transports; 4 HS 748 turboprop transports; 2 Cessna 404 and 6 Cessna 310 liaison aircraft; 4 Agusta-Bell AB.205 transport helicopters, and 2 JetRanger and 2 Bell 47G light helicopters; and Piper Cherokee and FT-2 (Chinese-built MiG-15 UTI) trainers.

INTERNATIONAL RELATIONS

Membership. Tanzania is a member of the UN, OAU, the Commonwealth, Non-Aligned Movement and is an ACP state of the EEC.

ECONOMY

Budget. In 1988–89 revenue US$627m., capital expenditure US$284m. and recurrent expenditure US$903m.

Currency. The monetary unit is the *Tanzanian shilling* (TZS) of 100 *cents*. There are coins of 5, 10, 20, 50 cents, 1 Sh., 5 Sh., 20 Sh. and 1,500 Sh.; and notes of 10 Sh., 20 Sh., 50 Sh., 100 Sh. and 200 Sh. In March 1991, £1 = Sh. 376·69; US$ = Sh. 198·57.

Banking and Finance. On 14 June 1966 the central bank, the Bank of Tanzania, with a government-owned capital of Sh. 20m., began operations.

On 6 Feb. 1967 all commercial banks with the exception of National Co-operative Banks were nationalized and their interests vested in the National Bank of Commerce on the mainland and the Peoples' Bank in Zanzibar.

Weights. The metric system is in force.

ENERGY AND NATURAL RESOURCES

Electricity. Production (1986) 830m. kwh. Supply 230 volts; 50 Hz.

Minerals. Production (1986): Diamonds, 38,000 grammes; gold, 46,900 grammes; salt, 15,300 tonnes. Large deposits of coal and tin exist but mining is on a small scale. Exploration is going on to establish economic deposits of copper, cobalt and nickel, and feasibility studies to exploit iron ore deposits in south-western Tanzania.

Agriculture. Production of main agricultural crops in 1988 (in 1,000 tonnes) was: Sisal, 28; seed cotton, 245; sugar-cane, 1,190; coffee, 51; tobacco, 13; maize, 2,339; wheat, 79; cashew nuts, 25; citrus, 33. Production of sisal has been declining since 1967. The Tanganyika Sisal Corporation has embarked on a diversification programme by introducing various new crops. Crops already planned are cardamom, beans, cashew nuts, citrus, cocoa, coconuts, cotton, maize and timber. Cattle ranching, dairying and twine spinning have also been introduced.

Zanzibar used to provide the greater part of the world's supply of cloves, but in 1989 only contributed 10% of world production.

A 10-year programme to rehabilitate the coconut industry started in 1980. By 1985 over 23m. trees were under plantation on the mainland and Zanzibar. Chillies, cocoa, limes, other tropical fruits and coil tobacco are also cultivated. The chief food crops are rice, bananas, cassava, pulses, maize and sorghum.

Livestock (1988, including Zanzibar): 13·5m. cattle, 4·7m. sheep, 6·6m. goats, 30m. poultry.

Forestry. Total forested land 43m. ha (48% of the land area). Total production (1983) 114,900 cu. metres.

Fisheries. A Fisheries Development Co. is catching sardines and tuna for export. Catch (1986) 309,900 tonnes of which, inland waters, 265,800 tonnes.

INDUSTRY. Industry is limited and is mainly textiles, petroleum and chemical products, food processing, tobacco, brewing and paper manufacturing.

FOREIGN ECONOMIC RELATIONS

Commerce. Total trade (in Sh. 1m.):

	1982	*1983*	*1984*	*1985*	*1986*	*1987*
Imports	7,781	8,877	11,953	17,962	30,270	57,971
Exports	4,117	4,138	5,661	5,937	10,963	18,512

Imports and exports (in Tanzanian Sh. 1m.), by country, 1987:

Country	*Imports*	*Exports*	*Country*	*Imports*	*Exports*
Bahrain	1,279·6	23·0	India	1,181·3	1,119·7
Belgium	1,056·0	359·6	Italy	5,195·9	609·8
China	557·4	18·8	Japan	6,533·9	726·1
Denmark	2,813·6	15·5	Netherlands	2,842·2	1,426·5
Federal Republic of Germany	7,217·9	2,267·1	Singapore	444·3	590·5
			Thailand	3·8	119·3

Major export items 1987 (in Sh. 1m.): Coffee, 5,792·6; cotton, 2,831·8; sisal, 321·7; cloves, 264·7; tea, 825·4; tobacco, 864·2; cashew nuts, 439; diamonds, 576·9.

Total trade between Tanzania and UK (British Department of Trade returns, in £1,000 sterling):

	1987	*1988*	*1989*	*1990*
Imports to UK	26,400	26,386	22,641	25,575
Exports and re-exports from UK	91,874	88,686	93,036	84,694

Tourism. In 1987 there were about 103,000 visitors.

COMMUNICATIONS

Roads. In 1988 there were 82,000 km of roads and (1983) 43,248 cars and 12,579 licensed commercial vehicles of which 11,290 were trucks and 1,289 buses.

Railways. On 23 Sept. 1977 the independent Tanzanian Railway Corporation was formed following the break-up of the East African Railways administration. The network totals 2,600 km (metre-gauge), excluding the Tan-Zam Railway 969 km in Tanzania (1,067 mm gauge) operated by a separate administration. In 1989, the state railway carried some 2m. passengers and 0·9m. tonnes of freight and the Tan-Zam Railway carried 1·5m. passengers and 1·2m. tonnes of freight.

Aviation. There are 53 aerodromes and landing strips maintained or licensed by Government; of these, 2 are of international standards category (Dar es Salaam and Kilimanjaro) and 18 are suitable for Dakotas. Air Tanzania Corporation provide regular and frequent services to all the more important towns within the territory and to Mozambique, Zambia, Seychelles, Comoro, Rwanda, Burundi and Madagascar.

There is an all-weather landing-ground in Zanzibar and a smaller all-weather landing-ground in Pemba.

Shipping. In 1985, 635,000 tonnes of freight were loaded and 2·6m. unloaded.

Telecommunications. In 1988 there were 63,000 direct telephone lines and 1,400 telex lines. There are 2 broadcasting stations (1 for mainland Tanzania and 1 for Zanzibar) and colour television operates in Zanzibar. In 1986 there were 13,000 television receivers (on Zanzibar only) and 2m. radio receivers.

Newspapers (1985). There were 3 dailies, 2 weeklies and several monthly magazines.

JUSTICE, RELIGION, EDUCATION AND WELFARE

Justice. The Judiciary is independent in both judicial and administrative matters and is composed of a 4-tier system of Courts: Primary Courts; District and Resident Magistrates' Courts; the High Court and the Court of Appeal. The Chief Justice is head of the Court of Appeal and the Judiciary Department. The Court's main registry is at Dar es Salaam; its jurisdiction includes Zanzibar. The Principal Judge is head of the High Court, also headquartered at Dar es Salaam, which has resident judges at 7 regional centres.

Religion. In 1984 some 40% were Christian, including Roman Catholics under the Archbishops of Dar es Salaam and Tabora, Anglicans under the Archbishop of Tanzania, and Lutherans. Moslems amount to 33%, but reach 66% in the coastal towns; Zanzibar is 96% Moslem and 4% Hindu. Some 23% follow traditional religions.

Education. In 1987 there were 10,302 primary schools with 3,169,202 pupils, and 288 (1988) secondary schools (175 private) with 127,703 students.

Technical and vocational education is provided at several secondary and technical schools and at the Dar es Salaam Technical College.

There were, in 1987, 63 teachers' colleges, including the college at Chang'ombe for secondary-school teachers, with 11,667 students.

The University of Dar es Salaam, independent since 1970, has faculties of law, arts, social sciences, medicine, engineering, commerce and management. Sokoine University of Agriculture, established in 1984, has faculties of agriculture, forestry and veterinary medicine. The total number of students in both universities was 3,395 in 1987.

Health. In 1984 there were 1,065 doctors and 152 hospitals with 22,800 beds.

DIPLOMATIC REPRESENTATIVES

Of Tanzania in Great Britain (43 Hertford St., London, W1)
High Commissioner: Vacant.

Of Great Britain in Tanzania (Hifadhi Hse., Samora Ave., Dar es Salaam)
High Commissioner: J. T. Masefield, CMG.

Of Tanzania in the USA (2139 R. St., NW, Washington, D.C., 20008)
Ambassador: Ali A. Karume.

Of the USA in Tanzania (36 Laibon Rd., Dar es Salaam)
Ambassador: Edward DeJarnette, Jr.

Of Tanzania to the United Nations
Ambassador: Anthony B. Nyakyi.

Further Reading

Atlas of Tanganyika. 3rd ed. Dar es Salaam, 1956
Tanganyika Notes and Records. Tanganyika Society, Dar es Salaam. (Twice yearly, from 1936) *The Economic Development of Tanganyika. Report... by the International Bank.* Johns Hopkins Univ. Press and OUP, 1961
Ayany, S. G., *A History of Zanzibar.* Nairobi, 1970
Coulson, A., *Tanzania: A Political Economy.* OUP, 1982
Darch, C., *Tanzania.* [Bibliography] Oxford and Santa Barbara, 1985
Hood, M., (ed.) *Tanzania and Nyerere.* London, 1988
Nyerere, J., *Freedom and Development.* New York, 1976
Resnick, I. N., *The Long Transition: Building Socialism in Tanzania.* New York and London, 1981
Yeager, R., *Tanzania: An African Experiment.* Aldershot, 1982

THAILAND

Capital: Bangkok
Population: 55·9m. (1989)
GNP per capita: US$1,000 (1988)

Prathes Thai, or Muang-Thai

(Kingdom of Thailand)

HISTORY. Until 24 June 1932 Siam was an absolute monarchy. A coup of that date resulted in the constitution of 1932. Numerous coups have followed.

On 23 Feb. 1991 a military junta seized power, deposing the prime minister.

AREA AND POPULATION. Thailand is bounded west by Burma, north and east by Laos and south-east by Cambodia. In the south it becomes a peninsula bounded west by the Indian Ocean, south by Malaysia and east by the Gulf of Thailand. Area is 513,115 sq. km (198,456 sq. miles).

At the census taken in 1980 the registration gave a population of 46,961,338, of whom 30·4% lived in the Central region, 35·2% in the North-East region, 12·5% in the South region, 21·9% in the North region. Estimate (1989) 55,888,393 (27,837,050 females).

Vital statistics, 1989: Births, 1,017,218 (495,543 females); deaths, 242,881 (102,491 females).

Thailand is divided into 73 provinces and Bangkok, the capital. Provinces with over 1m. population 1989 were Nakhon Ratchasima (2,360,797), Ubol Ratchathani (1,902,177), Udon Thani (1,799,261), Khon Kaen (1,666,671), Buriram (1,422,177), Nakhon Sithamnaraj (1,411,966), Chiangmai (1,361,320), Sri Saket (1,313,192), Surin (1,272,597), Roi Et (1,214,641), Nakhon Sawan (1,081,502), Songkhla (1,073,586), Chaiyaphum (1,042,763) and Chiangpai (1,027,647).

Population of Bangkok in 1989, 5,832,843. Other towns (1980 census): Chiangmai (101,595), Hat Yai (93,519), Khon Kaen, (85,863), Phitsanulok (79,942), Nakhon Ratchasima (78,246), Udon Thani (71,142), Songkhla (67,945), Nakhon Sawan (63,935), Nakhon Sithamnaraj (63,162), Ubol Ratchathani (50,788), Ayutthaya (47,189), Nakhon Pathom (45,242), Lampang (42,301) and Ratchaburi (40,404).

Thai is the national language. Chinese dialects are also spoken in Bangkok and the north and north-east and some Malay in the south.

CLIMATE. The climate is tropical, with high temperatures and humidity. Over most of the country, 3 seasons may be recognized. The rainy season is June to Oct., the cool season from Nov. to Feb. and the hot season is March to May. Rainfall is generally heaviest in the south and lightest in the north east.

Bangkok. Jan. 78°F (25·6°C), July 83°F (28·3°C). Annual rainfall 56" (1,400 mm).

REIGNING KING. Bhumibol Adulyadej, born 5 Dec. 1927, younger brother of King Ananda Mahidol, who died on 9 June 1946. King Bhumibol married on 28 April 1950 Princess Sirikit, and was crowned 5 May 1950. Children: Princess Ubol Ratana (born 5 April 1951, married Aug. 1972 Peter Ladd Jensen), Crown-Prince Vajiralongkorn (born 28 July 1952, married 3 Jan. 1977 Soamsawali Kitiyakra), Princess Maha Chakri Sirindhorn (born 2 April 1955), Princess Chulabhorn (born 4 July 1957, married 7 Jan. 1982 Virayudth Didyasarin).

CONSTITUTION AND GOVERNMENT. Following the deposition of Chatichai Choonhavan's government (*see* THE STATESMAN'S YEAR-BOOK, 1990–91, pp. 1185–86) in Feb. 1991, martial law was declared. The King appointed Gen. Sunthorn Kongsompong president of a 6-member National Council for the Maintenance of Order, and approved a provisional constitution granting it extensive powers. A legislative assembly of 294 members, of whom 148 were allotted to the military, was installed in March to prepare for elections and approve a constitution being drawn up by a constitutional commission.

Prime Minister: Anand Panyarachun.

Deputy Prime Ministers: Sanoh Unakul; Meechai Ruechupan; Pao Sarasin. *Defence:* Adm. Prapat Krisanachan. *Foreign:* Arsa Sarasin. *Interior:* Gen. Isaraponse Noonpakdi. *Finance:* Suthee Singsaneh. *Industry:* Sippanond Ketthat. *Trade:* Amaret Sila-on. *Agriculture:* Anat Arpapirom. *Justice:* Prapas Uaychai. *Education:* Kor Sawadpanit.

National flag: Five horizontal stripes of red, white, blue, white, red, with the blue of double width.

Local Government. Thailand is divided into 73 provinces *(changwads)*, each under the control of a *changwad* governor. The *changwads* are subdivided into 655 districts *(amphurs)* and 88 sub-districts *(king amphurs)*, 6,633 communes *(tambons)* and 59,458 villages *(moobans)*.

DEFENCE. Under the Military Service Act of 1954 every able-bodied man between the ages of 21 and 30 is liable to serve 2 years with the colours; 7 years in the first reserve; 10 years in the second reserve; 6 years in the third reserve.

Army. The Army is organized in 4 Regions and includes 1 cavalry, 1 mechanized infantry, 7 infantry, 2 special forces, 1 artillery and 1 anti-aircraft divisions; 19 engineer and 8 independent infantry battalions; and 4 reconnaissance companies. Equipment includes 100 M-48A5 and about 60 Chinese Type-69 main battle tanks. There is also an Army Aviation force including about 100 transport helicopters, and over 62 O-1 Bird Dog observation aircraft and 4 C-47 and 1 Short 330 twin-turboprop transport. Strength (1991) 190,000 (80,000 conscripts, with 500,000 reserves for all the armed forces).

Navy. The Royal Thai Navy is, next to the Chinese, the most significant naval force in the South China Sea. The combatant fleet includes 5 small frigates, 2 modern missile-armed 950-tonne corvettes, 6 German and Italian-built fast missile craft, 14 coastal and 30 inshore patrol craft, and about 40 riverine patrol boats. There is 1 mine countermeasures support vessel, 2 coastal minehunters and 4 coastal minesweepers. Amphibious capability is provided by 7 tank landing ships and 3 medium landing ships as well as 39 landing craft. Major auxiliaries are 1 small tanker, 2 surveying ships, and 2 training ships. Minor auxiliaries and service craft number about 12.

The Naval air element, all shore based includes 3 F-27 Friendship, 5 N24A Nomad and 2 CL-215s for maritime patrol, 10 Cessna T-337 armed light transports and 14 Bell utility and search-and-rescue helicopters.

Naval personnel in 1990 totalled 50,000 including 20,000 marines and 900 Naval Air Arm. The main bases are at Bangkok, Sattahip, Songkla and Phan Nga, with the riverine forces based at Nakhon Pathom.

A separate coast guard force, the Royal Thai Marine Police, numbers 1,700 and operates 3 coastal patrol craft, 32 riverine and inshore craft and numerous boats.

Air Force. The Royal Thai Air Force was reorganized with the assistance of a US Military Air Advisory Group. It had a strength (1991) of 43,000 personnel and 158 combat aircraft, and is made up of a headquarters and Combat, Logistics Support, Training and Special Services Groups. Combat units comprise 1 squadron of F-16 and 2 squadrons of F-5E/F interceptors, 1 squadron of F-5A/B fighter-bombers and RF-5A reconnaissance aircraft, 1 squadron with A-37B light jet attack aircraft, 2 with OV-10 Bronco light reconnaissance/attack aircraft, and 1 with AU-23A Peacemakers and 1 squadron with C-47s for security duties. Three Aravas are used for electronic intelligence gathering and 3 Learjets for combat support. There are transport units equipped with a total of about 70 C-130H/H-30 Hercules, HS 748, C-123B Provider, C-47 and smaller aircraft, including 20 Australian-built Missionmasters; there are 25 UH-1H and 17 S-58T helicopters; 20 O-1 Bird Dog observation aircraft; training units with Airtrainer CT/4 primary trainers built in New Zealand, Italian-built SF.260MTs, T-37 and Fantrainer intermediate and T-33A advanced trainers.

INTERNATIONAL RELATIONS

Membership. Thailand is a member of UN, ASEAN and the Colombo Plan.

ECONOMY

Policy. The Sixth 5-year Development Plan (1987–91) envisages emphasis on development of the production system, with specific attention being paid to providing employment and expanding the industrial base.

Budget. Expenditure, 1989: 248,200m. baht; revenue: 309,200m. baht. Government expenditure in 1988: economic services, 30,924; social services, 65,647; defence, 44,149; general administration and services, 28,059; unallocatable items, 54,310.

Currency. The unit of currency is the *baht* (THB) of 100 *satang*. Coins are in denominations of 1, 2, 5 *baht* and 25 and 50 *satang*. Currency notes are for 5, 10, 20, 50, 100, and 500 *baht*.

On 28 Feb. 1990 the total amount of notes in circulation was 136,584·8m. baht. In March 1991, £1 = 47·50 *baht*; US$1 = 25·04 *baht*.

Banking and Finance. In 1942 the Bank of Thailand was established under the Bank of Thailand Act, B.E. 2485 (1942) and began operations on 10 Dec. 1942, with the functions of a central bank; total assets and liabilities of the Bank of Thailand at 28 Feb. 1990, 403,011m. baht. The Bank has its banking activities entirely separate from the management of the note issue. Its *Governor* is Vijit Supinit.

The Bank also took over the note issue previously performed by the Treasury Department of the Ministry of Finance. Although the entire capital is owned by the Government, the Bank is an independent body.

Banks incorporated under Thai law include the Bangkok Bank Ltd, the Bangkok Bank of Commerce Ltd, the Bank of Asia, the Bank of Ayudhya Ltd, Bangkok Metropolitan Bank Ltd, the Laem Thong Bank Ltd, the Siam City Bank Ltd, the Siam Commercial Bank Ltd, First Bangkok City Bank Ltd, Union Bank of Bangkok Ltd and the Government Housing Bank. Foreign banks include the Chartered Bank, the Hongkong and Shanghai Banking Corporation, Indosuez, Bank of Canton Ltd, Bank of America, N.T. & S.A., the Mitsui Bank Ltd, Bharat Overseas Bank Ltd, The Chase Manhattan Bank, United Malayan Banking Corporation and the Bank of Tokyo Ltd, Nakornthon Bank, Thai Farmers' Bank, Thai Military Bank Ltd, Thai Danu Bank Ltd.

Total assets and liabilities of commercial banks at 28 Feb. 1990, 1,485,216·7m. baht. Deposits, 1989: 1,117,900m. baht.

There is a Government Savings Bank.

Weights and Measures. The metric system was made compulsory by a law promulgated on 17 Dec. 1923. The actual weights and measures prescribed by law are: Units of weight: 1 *standard picul* = 60 kg; 1 *standard catty* (1/100 picul) = 600 grammes; 1 *standard carat* = 20 centigrammes. Units of length: 1 *sen* = 40 metres; 1 *wah* (1/20 sen) = 2 metres; 1 *sauk* (1/2 wah) = 0·50 metre; 1 *keup* (1/2 sauk) = 0·25 metre. Units of square measure: 1 *rai* (1 sq. sen) = 1,600 sq. metres: 1 *ngan* (1/4 rai) = 400 sq. metres; 1 *sq. wah* (1/100 ngan) = 4 sq. metres. Units of capacity: 1 *standard kwien* = 2,000 litres; 1 *standard ban* (1/2 kwien) = 1,000 litres; 1 *standard sat* (1/50 ban) = 20 litres; 1 *standard tannan* (1/20 sat) = 1 litre.

Legislation passed in 1940 provided that the calendar year shall coincide with the Christian Year, and that the year of the Buddhist era (B.E.) 2484 shall begin on 1 Jan. 1941. (The New Year's Day was previously 1 April) (B.E.).

ENERGY AND NATURAL RESOURCES

Electricity. In 1987 the principal sources of energy generation were natural gas (50%), lignite (24%), hydro (17%) and heavy oil (7%). Installed capacity was 55%

thermal, 30% hydro, 11% combined cycle and 4% gas turbine. Annual hydro capacity, 26,204 mw. Supply 220 volts; 50 Hz.

Oil. There is extensive oil and gas exploration in the Gulf of Thailand. In 1987 the Sirikit oil field, which came on stream in 1983, remained Thailand's only significant find. Proven oil reserves in 1987 were less than 160m. bbls. Production of crude oil (1990) 1·82m. tonnes providing 15% of needs.

Gas. Production of natural gas (1989) 211,398m. cu. ft. Estimated reserves, 1986, 12,922,000m. cu. ft.

Minerals. The mineral resources include cassiterite (tin ore), wolfram, scheelite, antimony, coal, copper, gold, iron, lead, manganese, molybdenum, rubies, sapphires, silver, zinc and zircons. Production, 1989 (in 1,000 tonnes): Iron ore, 177·4; manganese ore, 10; tin concentrates, 20·4; lead ore, 58; antimony ore, 1·2; zinc ore, 412·6; lignite, 8,995; gypsum, 5,477·2; wolfram ore (tungsten), 1; fluorite ore, 97·9; marl, 564.

Agriculture. The chief produce is rice, a staple of the national diet. The area under paddy is about 18m. acres. In 1987 40% of the total land area was cultivated.

Output of the major crops in 1989 was (in 1,000 tonnes): Paddy, 21,400; maize, 4,100; sugar-cane, 33,560; jute and kenaf, 164·7; tobacco, 28·5; tapioca-root, 22,312; soybeans, 610; coconut, 1,140; mung beans, 355; cotton, 103; groundnuts, 177; sesame, 28·7; castor seeds, 34; kapok and bambax fibre, 42.

Livestock, 1988 (in 1,000): Horses, 19; buffaloes, 6,000; cattle, 5,000; pigs, 4,260; sheep, 95; goats, 80; poultry, 101,000.

Forestry. About 28% of the land area (14·4m. ha) was under forest in 1988. In the north, mixed deciduous forests with teak growing in mixture with several other species predominate. In the north-east hardwood is found in most parts. In all other regions of the country tropical evergreen forests are found, with the timber yang the main crop (a source of yang oil). Most of the teak timber exploited in northern Thailand is floated down to Bangkok.

Output of main forestry products in 1989: Teak, 26,200 cu. metres; yang and other woods, 892,600 cu. metres. By-products in 1989: Firewood, 426,000 cu. metres; charcoal, 325,500 cu. metres.

Rubber production in 1989: 1,131,000 tonnes.

Fisheries. In 1989 the catch of sea fish was 2·6m. tonnes including marine prawns and shrimps, 0·23m. tonnes; of freshwater fish, 165,000 tonnes.

INDUSTRY. Production of manufactured goods in 1989 included 15,024,622 tonnes of cement, 180,085,000 litres of beer, 2,299,798 bottles of soft drinks, 37,365 tonnes of cigarettes, 200,616 tonnes of galvanized iron sheets, 149,478 tonnes of tin plate, 213,536 automobiles, 587,216 motorcycles, 59,427 tonnes of tyres, 202,347 tonnes of synthetic fibre, 191,633 tonnes of jute products, 140,370 tonnes of paper, 143,644 tonnes of detergent, 13,188m. litres of petroleum products, 3,836,766 tonnes of sugar and 938m. integrated circuits.

Labour. In 1988, 28·2m. persons out of a labour force of 29·9m. were employed: 17·9m. in agriculture and 2·8m. in manufacturing.

FOREIGN ECONOMIC RELATIONS

Commerce. The foreign trade (in 1m. baht) was as follows:

	1985	*1986*	*1987*	*1988*	*1989*
Imports (c.i.f.)	251,169	241,358	334,209	513,114	662,679
Exports (f.o.b.)	193,366	233,383	299,853	403,570	515,745

Main exports by category in 1989, in 1m. baht: Manufactures, 195,973; food, 173,352; machinery, 91,710; raw materials, 35,330. Imports: Machinery, 251,001; manufactures, 181,156; chemicals, 74,204; mineral fuel and lubricant, 59,819.

In 1987 exports (in 1m. baht) included: Garments, 35,900; rice, 22,668; tapioca, 20,719; rubber, 20,392; jewellery, 19,722; integrated circuits, 15,173; canned seafood, 13,220; fabrics, 8,683; sugar, 8,583; footwear, 5,918.

1987 imports (in 1m. baht) included: Chemicals, 36,045; iron and steel, 23,693; non-electrical machinery and parts, 49,485; electrical machinery and parts, 31,988; vehicles and parts, 15,240; fuel and lubricants, 44,457.

In 1989 exports (in 1m. baht) were mainly to USA (111,788), Japan (87,993) and Singapore (36,840); imports were mainly from Japan (200,937), USA (74,673) and Singapore (50,867).

Total trade between Thailand and UK (British Department of Trade returns, in £1,000 sterling):

	1986	*1987*	*1988*	*1989*	*1990*
Imports to UK	182,756	239,430	321,241	443,144	484,276
Exports and re-exports from UK	158,195	206,571	279,717	427,484	416,648

Tourism. In 1990 5·37m. foreigners visited Thailand. Tourist revenue was 110,000m. baht.

COMMUNICATIONS

Roads. In 1988 there were 15,899 km of state highways and 25,895 km of provincial highways.

Railways. In 1988 the State Railway totalled 3,924 km (metre gauge). In 1989 it carried 84m. passengers and 7m. tonnes of freight.

Aviation. There are international airports at Bangkok, Chiangmai in the north and Phuket and Hat Yai in the south. Thai Airways Co. Ltd (TAC), is the sole Thai air transport enterprise. In 1959 Thai Airways and SAS set up Thai Airways International, to operate international air services. In 1990, 8·3m. passengers were carried. Thai Airways International had 58 aircraft in 1990. There are plans to privatize it.

Shipping. In 1987, 4,296 vessels of 21,706,798 NRT entered and 4,072 of 20,929,467 NRT cleared the port of Bangkok.

The port of Bangkok, about 30 km from the mouth of the Chao Phya River, is capable of berthing ocean-going vessels of 10,000 gross tons and 28 ft draught. Bangkok is now a port of entry for Laos, and goods arriving in transit are sent up by rail to Nong Khai and ferried across the river Mekhong to Vientiane.

Telecommunications. In 1985 there were 576,082 telephones, of which 389,096 were in Bangkok.

In 1985, there were 275 radio stations and 11 television stations,7,629,998 radios and 4,122,000 televisions.

Cinemas (1988). There were 584 cinemas with a seating capacity of 401,584.

Newspapers (1989). There are 23 daily newspapers in Bangkok, including 2 in English and 7 in Chinese, with a combined circulation of about 2m.

JUSTICE, RELIGION, EDUCATION AND WELFARE

Justice. The judicial power is exercised in the name of the King, by *(a)* courts of first instance, *(b)* the court of appeal *(Uthorn)* and *(c)* the Supreme Court *(Dika)*. The King appoints, transfers and dismisses judges, who are independent in conducting trials and giving judgment in accordance with the law.

Courts of first instance are subdivided into 20 magistrates' courts *(Kwaeng)* with limited civil and minor criminal jurisdiction; 85 provincial courts *(Changwad)* with unlimited civil and criminal jurisdiction; the criminal and civil courts with exclusive jurisdiction in Bangkok; the central juvenile courts for persons under 18 years of age in Bangkok.

The court of appeal exercises appellate jurisdiction in civil and criminal cases from all courts of first instance. From it appeals lie to Dika Court on any point of law and, in certain cases, on questions of fact.

The Supreme Court is the supreme tribunal of the land. Besides its normal appellate jurisdiction in civil and criminal matters, it has semi-original jurisdiction over general election petitions. The decisions of Dika Court are final. Every person has the right to present a petition to the Government who will deal with all matters of grievance.

Religion. In 1983 there were 47,049,223 Buddhists, 1,869,427 Moslems, 267,381 Christians and 64,369 Hindus, Sikhs and others.

Education. Primary education is compulsory for children between the ages of 7–14 and free in local municipal schools. In 1984 there were 532,097 students enrolled at pre-primary level, 7,229,064 at primary level, 1,304,520 at lower secondary level, 945,260 at upper secondary level and 361,819 in higher education. In 1980 there were 36 teachers' training colleges with 5,317 teachers and 63,983 students and about 180 government vocational schools and colleges with 11,240 teachers and 208,088 students. There are 8 schools for deaf children, 2 for the blind, 1 for multiple-handicapped and 2 for the mentally retarded. In 1984 the 36 teacher training colleges were regionally consolidated into 8 United Colleges also offering 4-year programmes in science and technology, management, social development, agriculture, arts and journalism. In 1986 there were 14 universities 3 of which were private: Chulalongkorn University (1916), Thammasat University (1934), Universities of Medical Science, Agriculture and Fine Arts; Ramkamhaeng University (1971)—all in Bangkok; Chiengmai University (1964), the Khon Kaen University (1966) in the north-east and Prince of Songkhla University (1968) in the south.

Health. The Primary Health Care Programme had provided health services in 95% of villages in 1986. In 1982 there were 434 hospitals and 6,496 health centres. In 1982 there were 6,550 physicians, 1,122 dentists and (1981) 2,680 pharmacists.

DIPLOMATIC REPRESENTATIVES

Of Thailand in Great Britain (30 Queen's Gate, London, SW7 5JB)
Ambassador: Sudhee Prasasvinitchai (accredited 4 Nov. 1986).

Of Great Britain in Thailand (Wireless Rd., Bangkok)
Ambassador: M. R. Melhuish, CMG.

Of Thailand in the USA (2300 Kalorama Rd., NW, Washington, D.C., 20008)
Ambassador: Vitthya Vejjajiva.

Of the USA in Thailand (95 Wireless Rd., Bangkok)
Ambassador: Daniel A. O'Donohue.

Of Thailand to the United Nations
Ambassador: Nitya Pibulsonggram.

Further Reading

Thailand Statistical Yearbook. National Statistical Office, Bangkok
Thailand in Brief. 7th ed. Bangkok, 1985
Girling, J. I. S., *Thailand: Society and Politics.* Cornell Univ. Press, 1981
Morrell, D. and Samudavanija, C., *Political Conflict in Thailand.* Cambridge, Mass., 1981
Watts, M., *Thailand.* [Bibliography] Oxford and Santa Barbara, 1986

TOGO

Capital: Lomé
Population: 3·4m. (1990)
GNP per capita: US$370 (1988)

République Togolaise

HISTORY. A German protectorate from July 1884, Togo was occupied by British and French forces in Aug. 1914 and subsequently partitioned between the two countries on 20 July 1922 under a League of Nations mandate. British Togo subsequently joined Ghana. The French mandate was renewed by the UN as a trusteeship on 14 Dec. 1946. On 28 Oct. 1956 a plebiscite was held to determine the status of the territory. Out of 438,175 registered voters, 313,458 voted for an autonomous republic within the French Union and the end of the trusteeship system. The trusteeship was abolished on the achievement of independence on 27 April 1960.

On 13 Jan. 1963 the first President Sylvanus Olympio was murdered by n.c.o.s. of the army. Nicolas Grunitzky, a former prime minister and Olympio's brother-in-law, was appointed President. On 13 Jan. 1967 in a bloodless coup the army under Lieut.-Col. Étienne Eyadéma made President Grunitzky 'voluntarily withdraw'. On 14 April 1967 Col. Eyadéma assumed the Presidency. There was a return to constitutional government on 13 Jan. 1980.

AREA AND POPULATION. Togo is bounded west by Ghana, north by Burkina Faso, east by Benin and south by the Gulf of Guinea. The area is 56,785 sq. km. The population of Togo in 1981 (census) was 2,700,982; 1990 (estimate) 3·4m. (24·9% urban). The capital is Lomé (population, 1983, 366,476), other towns (1981, population) being Sokodé (48,098), Kpalimé (31,800), Atakpamé (27,100), Bassar (21,800), Tsévié (17,000) and Aného (14,000).

The areas, populations and chief towns of the 5 regions are:

Region	*Sq. km*	*Census 1981*	*Chief town*
Des Savanes	8,602	326,826	Dapaong
De La Kara	11,630	432,626	Kara
Centrale	13,182	269,174	Sokodé
Des Plateaux	16,975	561,656	Atakpamé
Maritime	6,396	1,039,700	Lomé

The south is largely populated by Ewe-speaking peoples (forming 47% of the population) and related groups, while the north is mainly inhabited by Hamitic groups speaking Voltaic (Gur) languages such as Kabre (22%), Gurma (14%) and Tem (4%). The official language is French but Ewe and Kabre are also taught in schools.

Population growth in 1990 was 3% per annum; infant mortality was 10%.

CLIMATE. The tropical climate produces wet seasons from March to July and from Oct. to Nov. in the south. The north has one wet season, from April to July. The heaviest rainfall occurs in the mountains of the west, south-west and centre. Lomé. Jan. 81°F (27·2°C), July 76°F (24·4°C). Annual rainfall 35" (875 mm).

CONSTITUTION AND GOVERNMENT. Following approval in a referendum on 30 Dec. 1979, a new Constitution came into force on 13 Jan. 1980, when the Third Togolese Republic was proclaimed. There is an Executive President, directly elected for a 7-year term, and a National Assembly of 79 deputies, elected on a regional list system for a 5-year term. Elections to the Assembly were held in March 1990. There were 230 candidates. All candidates must belong to the *Rassemblement du peuple togolais*, the sole legal Party since 1969.

The government in Nov. 1990 included:

President, Minister of Defence: Gen. Gnassingbé Eyadéma (re-elected for a further 7-year term in Dec. 1986).

Foreign Affairs and Co-operation: Yaovi Adodo. *Rural Development:* Koffi Walla. *Economy and Finance:* Komlan Alipui. *Planning and Mines:* Barry Moussa Barque. *Posts and Telecommunications:* Ayeva Nassirou. *Public Works, Labour and Civil Service:* Bitokotipou Yagninim.

National flag: Five horizontal stripes of green and yellow, a red quarter with a white star.

Local Government: There are 5 regions, each under an inspector appointed by the President; they are divided into 21 *prefectures,* each administered by a district chief assisted by an elected district council.

DEFENCE. Armed forces numbered (1991) about 5,900, all forming part of the Army. There is selective conscription for 2 years.

Army. The Army consists of 2 infantry, 1 Presidential Guard and 1 parachute commando regiments, with artillery and logistic support units. Equipment includes 9 Scorpion light tanks and 2 T-54/-55 main battle tanks. Strength (1991) 4,000, with a further 750 in a paramilitary gendarmerie.

Navy. In 1990 the Naval wing of the Army operated 2 inshore patrol craft from the naval base at Lomé. Naval personnel number 100.

Air Force. An Air Force, established with French assistance, has 6 Brazilian-built EMB-326 Xavante (Aermacchi MB.326) armed jet trainers; 5 Alpha Jet advanced trainers, with strike capability, 1 Boeing 707, 1 DC-8 and 1 twin-turbofan F28 Fellowship for VIP use, 2 turboprop Buffalo transports; 2 Beech Barons and 2 Cessna 337s for liaison; 3 Epsilon basic trainers; 1 Puma and 2 Lama helicopters. Personnel (1991), 250, with 16 combat aircraft.

INTERNATIONAL RELATIONS

Membership. Togo is a member of the UN, OAU and ECOWAS, and is an ACP state of the EEC.

ECONOMY

Budget. The ordinary budget for 1988 balanced at 89,692m. francs CFA.

Currency. The unit of currency is the *franc* CFA with a parity rate of 50 *francs* CFA to 1 French *franc*. The rate of exchange (March 1991) was 496·12 francs CFA to £1; US$1 = 261·53.

Banking and Finance. The bank of issue is the *Banque Centrale des Etats de l'Afrique de l'Ouest*. Seven commercial and 3 development banks are based in Lomé.

ENERGY AND NATURAL RESOURCES

Electricity. Production (1986) 203m. kwh. There is a hydro-electric plant at Kpalime. Supply 127 and 220 volts; 50 Hz.

Minerals. A Mines Department was set up in 1953 after the discovery of very rich deposits of phosphate and bauxite; mining began in 1961. Output of phosphate rock (1985) 2·5m. tonnes. Other mineral deposits are limestone, estimated at 200m. tons; iron ore, estimated at 550m. tons with iron content varying between 40% and 55%, and marble estimated at 20m. tonnes. Salt production (1982) 600,000 tonnes.

Agriculture. Inland the country is hilly, rising to 3,600 ft, with streams and waterfalls. There are long stretches of forest and brushwood, while dry plains alternate with arable land. Maize, yams, cassava, plantains, groundnuts, etc., are cultivated; oil palms and dye-woods grow in the forests; but the main commerce is based on coffee, cocoa, palm-oil, palm-kernels, copra, groundnuts, cotton, manioc. There are considerable plantations of oil and cocoa palms, coffee, cacao, kola, cassava and cotton. Production, 1988 (in 1,000 tonnes): Cassava, 410; tomatoes, 7; yams 378; maize, 296; sorghum, 120; millet, 50; seed cotton, 67; rice, 27; groundnuts, 17; coffee, 11.

Livestock (1988): Cattle, 290,000; sheep, 1m.; swine, 300,000; horses, 1,000; asses, 3,000; goats, 900,000.

Forestry. In 1988 forests covered 25% of the land surface (1·4m. ha). Roundwood production (1987) 813,000 cu. metres.

Fisheries. Catch (1986) 14,800 tonnes.

INDUSTRY. There is a cement works (production, 1983; 232,000 tonnes); a second is being built in co-operation with Ghana and Côte d'Ivoire with a capacity of 1·2m. tonnes per annum. An oil refinery of 1m. tonne capacity opened in Lomé in 1978 and a steel mill (20,000 tonne capacity) in 1979. Industry, though small, is developing and there are about 40 medium sized enterprises in the public and private sectors, including textile and food processing plants.

FOREIGN ECONOMIC RELATIONS. A free trade zone was established in 1990.

Commerce (in 1m. francs CFA):

	1981	*1982*	*1983*	*1984*	*1985*
Imports	117,769	128,354	108,141	118,460	129,406
Exports	56,241	58,173	61,921	83,588	85,380

In 1985, of the exports, phosphates amounted to 38%, cotton 11%, coffee 11% and cocoa beans 6% by value; 22% of exports went to France and 18% to the Netherlands. Of the imports, France supplied 27%, the Netherlands, 11% and UK, 10%.

Total trade between Togo and UK (British Department of Trade returns, in £1,000 sterling):

	1986	*1987*	*1988*	*1989*	*1990*
Imports to UK	5,008	2,579	690	2,022	3,454
Exports and re-exports from UK	17,488	15,431	22,231	15,009	13,038

Tourism. There were about 121,000 tourists in 1988.

COMMUNICATIONS

Roads. There were, in 1986, 7,850 km of roads, of which 1,500 km were paved. In Dec. 1987 there were 44,120 passenger cars and 22,000 commercial vehicles.

Railways. There are 4 metre-gauge railways connecting Lomé, with Aného (continuing to Cotonou in Benin), Kpalime, Tabligbo and (*via* Atakpamé) Blitta; total length 525 km. In 1986 the railways carried 6·3m. tonne-km and 60m. passenger-km.

Aviation: Air services connect Tokoin airport, near Lomé, with Paris, Dakar, Abidjan, Douala, Accra, Lagos, Cotonou and Niamey and by internal services with Sokodé, Mango, Dapaong, Atakpamé and Niamtougou.

Shipping. In 1983, vessels landed 654,000 tonnes and cleared 683,000 tonnes at Lomé; 31,058 containers passed through the port in 1981. The merchant marine comprised (1985) 11 vessels of 77,989 DWT. In 1981 some 2·2m. tonnes of phosphate were loaded at the port of Kpéme.

Telecommunications. There were (1983) 388 post offices and 11,105 telephones. Togo is connected by telegraph and telephone with Ghana, Benin, Côte d'Ivoire and Senegal, and by wireless telegraphy with Europe and America. There were 16,000 television receivers and 680,000 radio receivers in 1986.

Newspapers. There was (1989) 1 daily newspaper (circulation 10,000).

JUSTICE, RELIGION, EDUCATION AND WELFARE

Justice. The Supreme Court and two Appeal Courts are in Lomé, one for criminal cases and one for civil and commercial cases. Each receives appeal from a series of local tribunals.

Religion. In 1980, 28% of the population were Catholics, 17% Moslem (chiefly in the north) and 9% Protestant; while 46% follow animist religions.

Education. In 1986 there were 474,998 pupils and 10,209 teachers in 2,345 primary schools, 86,327 pupils in secondary schools, and 5,050 students and 198 teachers in technical schools and 374 students and 22 teachers at the teacher-training college. In 1990 about 50% of children of school age were attending school. The University of Benin at Lomé (founded in 1970) had 4,500 students and 308 teaching staff in 1986.

Health. In 1981 there were 61 hospitals with 4,500 beds; and in 1985, 168 doctors, 7 dentists, 51 pharmacists, 559 midwives (1980) and 1,116 nursing staff.

DIPLOMATIC REPRESENTATIVES

Of Togo in Great Britain (30 Sloane St., London, SW1)
Chargé d'Affaires: Djibril Akanga.

Of Great Britain in Togo
Ambassador and Consul-General: A. M. Goodenough, CMG (resides in Accra).

Of Togo in the USA (2208 Massachusetts Ave., NW, Washington, D.C., 20008)
Ambassador: Ellom-Kodjo Schuppius.

Of the USA in Togo (Rue Pelletier Caventou, Lomé)
Ambassador: Rush W. Taylor, Jr.

Of Togo to the United Nations
Ambassador: Soumi-Biova Pennaneach.

Further Reading

Cornevin, R., *Histoire du Togo*. 3rd ed., Paris, 1969
Feuillet, C., *Le Togo en general*. Paris, 1976
Piraux, M., *Le Togo aujourd' hui*. Paris, 1977

TONGA

Capital: Nuku'alofa
Population: 95,200 (1988)
GNP per capita: US$800 (1988)

Kingdom of Tonga

HISTORY. The Kingdom of Tonga attained unity under Taufa'ahau Tupou (George I) who became ruler of his native Ha'apai in 1820, of Vava'u in 1833 and of Tongatapu in 1845. By 1860 the Kingdom had become converted to Christianity (George himself having been baptized in 1831). In 1862 the King granted freedom to the people from arbitrary rule of minor chiefs and gave them the right to the allocation of land for their own needs. These institutional changes, together with the establishment of a parliament of chiefs, paved the way towards the democratic constitution under which the Kingdom is now governed, and provided a background of stability against which Tonga was able to develop her agricultural economy.

The Kingdom continued up to 1899 to be a neutral region in accordance with the Declaration of Berlin, 6 April 1886. By the Anglo-German Agreement of 14 Nov. 1899 subsequently accepted by the USA, the Tonga Islands were left under the Protectorate of Great Britain. A protectorate was proclaimed on 18 May 1900, and a British Agent and Consul appointed. On 4 June 1970 the UK Government ceased to have any responsibility for the external relations of Tonga.

The Tongatapu group was discovered by Tasman in 1643.

AREA AND POPULATION. The Kingdom consists of some 169 islands and islets with a total area of 289 sq. miles (748 sq. km; including inland waters), and lies between 15° and 23° 30' S. lat and 173° and 177° W. long., its western boundary being the eastern boundary of Fiji. The islands are split up into the following groups reading from north to south: The Niuas, Vava'u, Ha'apai, Tongatapu and 'Eua. The 3 main groups, both from historical and administrative significance, are Tongatapu in the south, Ha'apai in the centre and Vava'u in the north.

The capital is Nuku'alofa on Tongatapu, population (1986) 29,018.

There are 5 divisions comprising 23 districts:

Division	*Sq. km*	*Census 1986*	*Capital*
Niuas	72	2,368	Hihifo
Vava'u	119	15,175	Neiafu
Ha'apai	110	8,919	Pangai
Tongatapu	261	63,794	Nuku'alofa
'Eua	87	4,393	Ohonua

Census population (1986) 94,649 (males, 47,611); estimate (1988) 95,200.

CLIMATE. Generally a healthy climate, though Jan. to March is hot and humid, with temperatures of 90°F (32·2°C). Rainfall amounts are comparatively high, being greatest from Dec. to March. Nuku'alofa. Jan. 78°F (25·6°C), July 70°F (21·1°C). Annual rainfall 63" (1,576 mm). Vava'u. Jan. 80°F (26·7°C), July 73°F (22·8°C). Annual rainfall 110" (2,750 mm).

CONSTITUTION AND GOVERNMENT. The present Constitution is almost identical with that granted in 1875 by King George Tupou I. There is a Privy Council, Cabinet, Legislative Assembly and Judiciary. The legislative assembly, which meets annually, is composed of 9 nobles elected by their peers, 9 elected representatives of the people and the Privy Councillors (numbering 11); the King appoints one of the 9 nobles to be the Speaker. The elections are held triennially. In 1960, women voted for the first time.

King: HM King Taufa'ahau Tupou IV, GCVO, GCMG, KBE, born 4 July 1918, succeeded on 16 Dec. 1965 on the death of his mother, Queen Salote Tupou III; his coronation took place on 4 July 1967.

In Feb. 1991 the government included:

Prime Minister and Minister of Agriculture: HRH Prince Fatafehi Tu'ipelehake, KCMG, KBE, younger brother of the King.

Acting Deputy Prime Minister and Minister of Lands: Dr S. L. Kavaliku. *Foreign Affairs and Defence:* HRH Crown Prince Tupouto'a. *Works and Civil Aviation:* Dr Slangi Kavaliku. *Health:* Dr Sione Tapa. *Labour, Commerce and Industry:* Baron Vaea. *Finance:* James Cocker: *Attorney-General and Minister of Justice:* Tevita Tupou.

National flag: Red with a white quarter bearing a red couped cross.

INTERNATIONAL RELATIONS

Membership. Tonga is a member of the Commonwealth and the South Pacific Forum, and is an ACP state of the EEC.

ECONOMY

Budget. Recurrent revenue and expenditure in T$1,000:

	1987–88 [1]	*1988–89* [1]	*1989–90* [1]
Revenue	29,846	35,860	43,720
Expenditure	29,846	35,957	43,720

[1] Estimate.

The principal sources of revenue are import dues, income tax, sales tax, port and service tax, wharfage and philatelic revenue.

Public debt at 30 June 1987, T$44·5m. of which T$40·9m. was external debt.

Currency. The unit of currency is the *pa'anga* (TOP) of 100 *seniti*. There are notes of T$50, 20, 10, 5, 2 and 1 and coins of T$2, T$1 and *seniti* 50, 20, 10, 5, 2 and 1. In March 1991, £1 = 2·44 *pa'anga*; US$1 = 1·29 *pa'anga*.

Banking and Finance. The Bank of Tonga and the Tonga Development Bank are both situated in Nuku'alofa (Tongatapu) with branches in the main islands 'Eua, Ha'apai, Vava'u and the Niuas.

ENERGY AND NATURAL RESOURCES

Electricity. Production (1986) 8m. kwh. Supply 230 volts; 50 Hz.

Agriculture. Production (1988, in 1,000 tonnes) consisted of coconuts (53), fruit and vegetables (21), copra (6) and cassava (17).

Livestock (1988): Cattle, 8,000; horses, 9,000; pigs, 65,000; goats, 11,000; poultry (1982), 175,000.

Fisheries. Catch (1982) 2,500 tonnes.

FOREIGN ECONOMIC RELATIONS

Commerce. In 1988, imports were valued at T$70,688,883 while exports and re-exports were T$9,502,664 and T$1,052,628.

Main imports (1988, in T$): Food 17,740,693, beverages and tobacco 3,302,660, crude materials 2,635,054, fuel and lubricants 6,853,259, oils and fats 178,927, chemicals 4,603,950, manufactured goods 13,453,825, machinery and transport equipment 15,472,034, miscellaneous manufactured articles 6,028,649.

Main exports (1988, in T$): Coconut oil 1,101,656, vanilla beans 1,384,837, bananas 658,362, dessicated coconut 403,250, water melons 19,169, knitted clothes 733,219, tarotaruas 99,286; fish 2,295,046, cassava 157,584, yams, 253,379, footwear 105,806, tapa cloth 102,345.

Principal destinations for Tongan exports/re-exports in 1988 were: New Zealand (T$3,313,202), Australia (T$1,738,191), USA (T$1,729,788), UK (T$28,170). Of 1988 imports (in T$), New Zealand furnished 21,313,446; Australia, 20,184,246; Japan, 5,401,330; Singapore, 3,451,779; USA, 5,338,115; Fiji, 7,190,968; China (Mainland), 2,068,269; UK, 766,370.

Total trade between Tonga and UK (British Department of Trade returns, in £1,000 sterling):

	1987	*1988*	*1989*	*1990*
Imports to UK	100	145	28	239
Exports and re-exports from UK	2,013	856	831	1,296

Tourism. There were 39,550 visitors in 1987.

COMMUNICATIONS

Roads. In 1987–88 there were over 5,000 registered motor vehicles and (1988) 1,242 km of roads (291 km paved).

Aviation. International air service connexions to Tongatapúare now provided by Air New Zealand, Polynesian Airlines, Air Pacific and Hawaiian Air with 4 flights per week to Auckland, 3 to Apia, 4 to Suva and 2 to Nadi. Hawaiian Air provides a twice weekly service to Hawaii via Pagopago. Internal air service flights are operated during the week to 'Eua, Ha'apai, Vava'u and Niuatoputapu by Friendly Island Airways.

Shipping. Pacific Forum Line maintains a four weekly service New Zealand–Fiji–Samoas–Tonga from Sydney, Australia–Noumea–Fiji–Samoas–Tonga. Warner Pacific Line maintains a monthly service New Zealand–Tonga–Samoas–Tonga–New Zealand and a monthly service Tonga–New Zealand–Australia–Funufuti–Tarawa–Samoas–Tonga.

Telecommunications. Telephones numbered 3,500 in 1986 and there were 65,000 radio receivers. The operation of the International Telecommunication Services is undertaken by Cable and Wireless, under an agreement between the Company and the Government. The operation and development of the National Telecommunication Network and Services and the responsibilities of the Tonga Telecommunication Commission.

JUSTICE, RELIGION, EDUCATION AND WELFARE

Justice. Since the lapse of British extra-territorial jurisdiction British and foreign nationals charged with an offence against the laws of Tonga (the enforcement of which is a responsibility of the Minister of Police) are fully subject to the jurisdiction of the Tongan courts to which they are already subject in all civil matters.

Religion. The Tongans are Christian, 40,516 (1986) being adherents of the Free Wesleyan Church.

Education. In 1987 there were 102 government and 11 denominational primary schools, with a total of 16,715 pupils. There were 8 government and 48 mission schools and 1 private school offering secondary education, with a total roll of 14,137. There was one government teacher-training college; 5 government technical and vocational schools and 3 non-government technical and vocational schools. 201 students were undertaking tertiary training overseas under an official scholarship in 1985.

Health. In 1988–89 there were 45 doctors, 11 dentists, 2 pharmacists, 37 midwives, 266 nursing personnel and 4 hospitals with 307 beds.

DIPLOMATIC REPRESENTATIVES

Of Tonga in Great Britain (New Zealand Hse., Haymarket, London, SW1Y 4TE)
High Commissioner: S. M. Tuita (accredited 6 June 1989).

Of Great Britain in Tonga (Nuku'alofa)
High Commissioner: W. L. Cordiner.

Further Reading

Luke, Sir Harry, *Queen Salote and Her Kingdom.* London, 1954
Packett, C. N., *Travel and Holiday Guide to Tongatapu Island.* Bradford, 1984

TRINIDAD AND TOBAGO

Capital: Port-of-Spain
Population: 1·24m. (1988)
GNP per capita: US$3,350 (1988)

Republic of Trinidad and Tobago

HISTORY. Trinidad was discovered by Columbus in 1498 and colonized by the Spaniards in the 16th century. During the French Revolution a large number of French families settled in the island. In 1797, Great Britain being at war with Spain, Trinidad was occupied by the British and ceded to Great Britain by the Treaty of Amiens in 1802. Trinidad and Tobago were joined in 1889.

Under the Bases Agreement concluded between the governments of the UK and the USA on 27 March 1941, and the concomitant Trinidad–US Bases Lease of 22 April 1941, defence bases were leased to the US Government for 99 years. On 8 Dec. 1960 the US agreed to abandon 21,000 acres of leased land and the US has since given up the remaining territory, except for a small tracking station.

On 31 Aug. 1962 Trinidad and Tobago became an independent member state of the Commonwealth. A Republican Constitution was adopted on 1 Aug. 1976.

During an attempted coup in July 1990 by a Moslem sect the prime minister was taken hostage and wounded.

AREA AND POPULATION. The island of Trinidad is situated in the Caribbean Sea, about 12 km off the north-east coast of Venezuela; several islets, the largest being Chacachacare, Huevos, Monos and Gaspar Grande, lie in the Gulf of Paria which separates Trinidad from Venezuela. The smaller island of Tobago lies about 31 km further to the north-east. Altogether, the islands cover 5,124 sq. km (1,978 sq. miles) of which Trinidad (including the islets) has 4,821 sq. km (1,861 sq. miles) and Tobago 303 sq. km (117 sq. miles). Population (census 1980): 1,079,800. (Trinidad, 1,039,100; Tobago, 40,700); estimate (1988) 1,243,000 (Trinidad, 1,198,000, Tobago, 45,000). Capital, Port-of-Spain, 58,400; other important towns, San Fernando (34,200) and Arima (24,600). Those of African descent are 40·8% of the population, Indians, 40·7%, mixed races, 16·3%, European, Chinese and others, 2·2%. English is spoken generally. Estimated population in 1988, 1·24m.

Vital statistics (rate per 1,000), 1983: Births, 29·2; deaths, 6·6; infant deaths, 12·6. Proportion of population under 15 years (1984) 39·2%.

Tobago is situated about 30·7 km north-east of Trinidad. Main town is Scarborough.

Principal goods shipped from Tobago to Trinidad are copra, cocoa, livestock and poultry, fresh vegetables, coconut oil and coconut fibre.

CLIMATE. A tropical climate whose dry season runs from Jan. to June, with a wet season for the rest of the year. Temperatures are uniformly high the year round. Port-of-Spain. Jan. 78°F (25·6°C), July 79°F (26·1°C). Annual rainfall 65" (1,631 mm).

CONSTITUTION AND GOVERNMENT. The 1976 Constitution provides for a bicameral legislature of a *Senate* and a *House of Representatives.* The Senate consists of 31 members, 16 being appointed by the President on the advice of the Prime Minister, 6 on the advice of the Leader of the Opposition and 9 at the discretion of the President.

The House of Representatives consists of 36 (34 for Trinidad and 2 for Tobago) elected members and a Speaker elected from within or outside the House.

The Prime Minister is appointed by the President, and there is a Cabinet.

At the general elections in 1986 the National Alliance for Reconstruction (NAR) won 33 seats; the People's National Movement won 3 seats. In 1990 the United National Congress (founded in 1989 and joined by 6 former NAR members) became the official Opposition.

President: Noor Mohammed Hassanali.

In Feb. 1991 the Cabinet included:
Prime Minister and Minister of Finance and Economy: Arthur N. R. Robinson. *Justice and National Security:* Joseph Toney. *Planning and Mobilization:* Winston Dookeran. *Health:* Selwyn Richardson. *Industry, Enterprise and Tourism:* Dr Bhoendradatt Tewarie. *Food Production, Marine Exploitation, Forestry and the Environment:* Lincoln Myers. *Works and Infrastructure:* Dr Carson Charles. *Community Development, Welfare and the Status of Women:* Gloria Henry. *Sport, Youth, Culture and the Creative Arts:* Jennifer Johnson. *Energy, Labour, Employment and Manpower Resources:* Dr Albert Richards. *Public Utilities and Settlements:* Pamela Nicholson.

Local Government: Trinidad is divided into 3 municipalities, 8 counties and Tobago, which has a 15-member elected House of Assembly with limited powers of self-government. Elections due in Sept. 1990 were postponed for a year.

National flag: Red with a diagonal black strip edged in white.

DEFENCE. The Defence Force has a regular and a reserve infantry battalion and a support battalion equipped with 81mm mortars, and there is also a small air element, equipped with 1 Cessna 402 light transport. Personnel in 1991 totalled 2,650.

The Coast Guard operates 9 inshore patrol craft, the Police, 5. Of total defence personnel (1990), 600 were coastguard.

INTERNATIONAL RELATIONS

Membership. Trinidad and Tobago is a member of the UN, the Commonwealth, OAS, CARICOM and is an ACP state of the EEC.

ECONOMY

Budget. The 1989 budget envisaged current expenditure (in TT$) as 4,627·9m. and capital expenditure at 1,324·6m.

Currency. The currency is the *Trinidad and Tobago dollar* (TTD) of 100 *cents*. There are coins of 1, 5, 10, 25 and 50 cents and TT$1, and banknotes of TT$1, 5, 10, 20 and 100. Foreign exchange reserves were TT$480·4m, in Dec. 1989. Inflation was 11·4% at the end of 1989. £1 = TT$8·07; US$1 = TT$4·25 (March 1991).

Banking and Finance. Banks operating: Republic Bank of Trinidad and Tobago Ltd; Royal Bank of Trinidad and Tobago Ltd; Bank of Commerce, Trinidad and Tobago Ltd; Bank of Nova Scotia; United Bank of Trinidad and Tobago Ltd; National Commercial Bank of Trinidad and Tobago; Workers' Bank of Trinidad and Tobago; Trinidad Co-operative Bank Ltd. A Central Bank began operations in Dec. 1964.

Government savings banks are established in 69 offices, with a head office in Port-of-Spain. There is a stock exchange.

ENERGY AND NATURAL RESOURCES

Electricity. In 1986, 3,182m. kwh was generated. Supply 115 and 230 volts; 60 Hz.

Oil. Oil production is one of Trinidad's leading industries and represented (1986) 71·6% of exports. Commercial production began in 1909; production of crude oil in 1990 was 7·3m. tonnes. Trinidad also possesses 2 refineries, with rated distillation capacity of 305,000 bbls annually; crude oil is imported from Venezuela, Indonesia, Ecuador, Nigeria, Brazil, and Saudi Arabia and refined in Trinidad. The 'Pitch Lake' is an important source of asphalt; production, 1986, 5,360,700 cu. metres.

Gas. In 1985 production was 7,413m. cu. ft., of which 1,601m. cu. ft. was flared and lost.

Agriculture. Hectares under cultivation and care include (1984): Cocoa, 21,000; sugar, 18,000. Sugar production in 1988 was 91,000 (1987: 85,000) tonnes. The territory is still largely dependent on imported food supplies, especially flour, dairy products, meat and rice. Areas have been irrigated for rice, and soil and forest conservation is practised.

Livestock (1988): Cattle, 78,000; sheep, 12,000; goats, 50,000; pigs, 84,000; poultry, 8m.

Fisheries. The catch in 1986, 14,800 tonnes.

INDUSTRY. In 1985, 474,300 tonnes of iron and steel were produced. Other manufacturing includes ammonia (production, 1985, 1,323,500 tonnes), fertilizers (1986 production, 1,888,000 tonnes), cement (338,000 tonnes, 1986), rum (2,307,000 proof gallons, 1986), beer (20,716 litres, 1986), cigarettes (920,000 kg, 1986).

Labour. The working population in 1986 was 471,300. Unemployment in 1989 was 22%.

Trade Unions. About 30% of the labour force belong to unions.

FOREIGN ECONOMIC RELATIONS. The Foreign Investment Act of 1990 permits foreign investors to acquire land and shares in local companies, and to form companies.

Commerce. Exports in 1986 were TT$4,962·2m. of which TT$3,504·4m. was mineral fuels and products and chemicals, TT$766·8m. USA took 61·5% of exports. Imports totalled TT$4,902·8m. of which TT$1,792·9m. was for machinery and transport of which the USA supplied 41·8%.

Total trade of Trinidad and Tobago with UK (British Department of Trade returns, in £1,000 sterling):

	1986	*1987*	*1988*	*1989*	*1990*
Imports to UK	41,662	38,600	35,728	37,426	45,058
Exports and re-exports from UK	79,029	57,016	39,868	45,881	49,894

Tourism. In 1986, 182,640 foreigners visited Trinidad and Tobago spending (estimate) TT$293·9m.

COMMUNICATIONS

Roads. There were (1985) about 6,435 km of main and local roads. Motor vehicles registered in 1985 totalled 336,769, including 127,716 private cars, 26,392 hired and rented cars, and 33,846 goods vehicles.

Aviation. There is an international airport at Piarco. The following airlines operate scheduled passenger, mail and freight services. British West Indian Airways (BWIA), Air Canada, PANAM, KLM, Linea Aeropostal Venezolana, Leeward Islands Air Transport, Caribair, British Airways, American Airlines, Guyana Airways, ALM Antillean Airline, Cruzeiro (Brazil), Caribbean Airways and Viasa. A scheduled air services agreement was signed with the USA in 1990. BWIA fly to Cologne, Frankfurt, London, Stockholm and Zurich.

Shipping. In 1985 12·6m. tons of cargo were handled. A deep-water harbour at Scarborough (Tobago) was opened in 1991.

Telecommunications. International communications to all parts of the world are provided by Trinidad and Tobago External Telecommunications Co. Ltd (TEXTEL) by means of a satellite earth station and various high quality radio circuits. The marine radio service is also maintained by TEXTEL. Number of post offices (1984), 69; postal agencies, 166; number of telephones (1986), 182,325. Broadcasting is overseen by the Telecomunications Authority. As well as the National Broadcasting Service Radio 610, Radio Trinidad and Trinidad and Tobago Television, there are 4 independent TV channels and 7 radio, as well as community and cable services. There were 500,000 radio and 300,000 television receivers in 1985.

Cinemas (1986). There are 57 cinemas and 3 drive-in cinemas.

Newspapers (1986). There are 4 daily newspapers with a total daily circulation (1984) of 166,380, 2 Sunday newspapers with a total circulation (1984) of 161,832, and 3 weekly newspapers.

JUSTICE, RELIGION, EDUCATION AND WELFARE

Justice. The High Court consists of the Chief Justice and 11 puisne judges. In criminal cases a judge of the High Court sits with a jury of 12 in cases of treason and murder, and with 9 jurors in other cases. The Court of Appeal consists of the Chief Justice and 3 Justices of Appeal; there is a limited right of appeal from it to the Privy Council. There are 3 High Courts and 12 magistrates' courts. There is an *Ombudsman* (George Edoo).

Religion. In 1980, 15% of the population were Anglicans (under the Bishop of Trinidad and Tobago), 33·6% Roman Catholics (under the Archbishop of Port-of-Spain), 25% Hindus and 5·9% Moslems.

Education. In 1985–86 there were 172,424 pupils enrolled in primary schools, 12,622 in government secondary schools, 17,576 in assisted secondary schools, 39,188 in junior secondary schools, 21,614 in senior comprehensive schools, 3,564 in composite schools and 4,419 in technical and vocational schools. The University of the West Indies campus in St Augustine had 2,684 full- and part-time students in 1984–85.

Health. In 1985 there were 1,103 physicians, 129 dentists, 496 pharmacists and 31 hospitals and nursing homes with 4,087 beds. There were 3,344 nurses and midwives and 980 nursing assistants in government institutions.

DIPLOMATIC REPRESENTATIVES

Of Trinidad and Tobago in Great Britain (42 Belgrave Sq., London, SW1X 8NT)
High Commissioner: P. L. U. Cross.

Of Great Britain in Trinidad and Tobago (Furness Hse., 90 Independence Sq., Port-of-Spain)
High Commissioner: Sir Martin Berthoud, KCVO, CMG.

Of Trinidad and Tobago in the USA (1708 Massachusetts Ave., NW, Washington, D.C., 20036)
Ambassador: Angus Albert Khan.

Of the USA in Trinidad and Tobago (15 Queen's Park West, Port-of-Spain)
Ambassador: Charles A. Gargano.

Of Trinidad and Tobago to the United Nations
Ambassador: Dr Marjorie R. Thorpe.

Further Reading

Statistical Information: The Central Statistical Office, Government of Trinidad and Tobago, 2 Edward St., Port-of-Spain. *Director:* J. Harewood. Publications include *Annual Statistical Digest, Quarterly Economic Report, Annual Overseas Trade Report, Population and Vital Statistics Annual Report, Report on Education Statistics.*

Facts on Trinidad and Tobago. Ministry of Information, Port-of-Spain, 1983
Immigration Guidelines. Government Printer, Port-of-Spain, 1980
Oil and Energy, Trinidad and Tobago. Government Printer, Port-of-Spain, 1980
Trinidad and Tobago Year Book. Port-of-Spain. Annual (from 1865)
Chambers, F., *Trinidad and Tobago.* [Bibliography] Oxford and Santa Barbara, 1986
Cooper, St G. C. and Bacon, P. R. (eds.) *The Natural Resources of Trinidad and Tobago.* London, 1981

Central Library: The Central Library of Trinidad and Tobago, Queen's Park East, Port-of-Spain. *Acting Librarian:* Mrs L. Hutchinson.

TUNISIA

Capital: Tunis
Population: 7·75m. (1988)
GNP per capita: US$1,230 (1988)

Al-Jumhuriya at-Tunisiya

(Republic of Tunisia)

HISTORY. Tunisia was a French protectorate from 1883 and achieved independence on 20 March 1956. The Constituent Assembly, elected on 25 March 1956, abolished the monarchy (of the Bey of Tunis) on 25 July 1957 and proclaimed a republic.

AREA AND POPULATION. The boundaries are on the north and east the Mediterranean Sea, on the west Algeria and on the south Libya. The area is about 164,150 sq. km (63,378 sq. miles), including that portion of the Sahara which is to the east of the Djerid (salt marsh), extending towards Ghadamès.

At the census of 30 March 1984 there were 6,966,173 inhabitants (3,547,487 males and 3,419,026 females) of whom 52·8% were urban. Estimate (1988) 7,745,500.

The census populations of the 23 *gouvernorats* were as follows as at 30 March 1984:

	Sq. km	*1984*		*Sq. km*	*1984*
Aryanah	1,558	374,192	Qasrayn (Kassérine)	8,066	297,959
Bajah (Béja)	3,558	274,706	Qayrawan (Kairouan)	6,712	421,607
Banzart (Bizerta)	3,685	394,670	Qibili (Kebili)	22,084	95,371
Bin Arus	761	246,193	Safaqis (Sfax)	7,545	577,992
Jundubah (Jendouba)	3,102	359,429	Sidi Bu Zayd (Sidi Bouzid)	6,994	288,528
Kaf (Le Kef)	4,965	247,672	Silyanah (Siliana)	4,631	222,038
Madaniyin (Médénine)	8,588	295,889	Susah (Sousse)	2,621	322,491
Mahdiyah (Mahdia)	2,966	270,435	Tatawin (Tataouine)	38,889	100,329
Munastir (Monastir)	1,019	278,478	Tawzar (Tozeur)	4,719	67,943
Nabul (Nabeul)	2,788	461,405	Tunis	346	774,364
Qabis (Gabès)	7,175	240,016	Zaghwan (Zaghouan)	2,768	118,743
Qafsah (Gafsa)	8,990	235,723			

Tunis, the capital, had (census, 1984) 596,654 inhabitants: Sfax, 231,911; Aryanah, 98,655; Bizerta, 94,509; Djerba, 92,269; Gabès, 92,258; Sousse, 83,509; Kairouan, a holy city of the Moslems, 72,254; Bardo, 65,669; La Goulette, 61,609; Gafsa, 60,970; Béja, 46,708; Kasserine, 47,606; Nabeul, 39,531; Mahdia, 36,828; Monastir, 35,546; Le Kef, 34,509; Tataouine, 30,371; Medenine, 26,602; Jendouba, 23,249; Tozeur, 21,604; Sidi Bouzid, 19,218; Siliana, 12,433; Kébili, 11,780; Zaghouan, 10,149.

Vital statistics (1986). Birth rate, 31·7 per 1,000 population; death rate, 6·7 per 1,000.

The official language is Arabic but the use of French is widespread.

CLIMATE. The climate ranges from warm temperate in the north, where winters are mild and wet and the summers hot and dry, to desert in the south. Tunis. Jan. 48°F (8·9°C), July 78°F (25·6°C). Annual rainfall 16" (400 mm). Bizerta. Jan. 52°F (11·1°C), July 77°F (25°C). Annual rainfall 25" (622 mm). Sfax. Jan. 52°F (11·1°C), July 78°F (25·6°C). Annual rainfall 8" (196 mm).

CONSTITUTION AND GOVERNMENT. The Constitution was promulgated on 1 June 1959. The *President* and the *National Assembly* are elected simultaneously by direct universal suffrage for a period of 5 years. The President cannot be re-elected more than 3 times consecutively.

Elections were held on 2 Nov. 1986, when all 125 seats in the Chamber of Deputies were won by the National Front, an alliance of the Constitutional Democratic Assembly (CDA) and the *Union générale des travailleurs tunisiens*. The elections were boycotted by opposition parties.

President of the Republic: Zine El Abidine Ben Ali (appointed 2 April 1989).

The Cabinet in March 1991 included:

Prime Minister: Hamed Karoui.

Justice: Mustapha Bouaziz. *Foreign Affairs:* Habib Ben Yahia. *Secretary General of the Presidency:* Mohamed El Jeri. *Defence and Interior:* Abdallah Kallal. *Planning and Finance:* Mohamed Ghannouchi. *Agriculture:* Nouri Zorgati. *Equipment and Housing:* Ahmed Friaa. *Tourism and Handicrafts:* Mohamed Jegham. *Economy:* Sadok Rabah. *Education, Higher Education and Scientific Research:* Mohamed Charfi. *Public Health:* Daly Jazi. *Social Affairs:* Ahmed Smaoui. *Youth and Infancy:* Hamouda Ben Slama. *Secretary General of the Government:* Taoufik Cheikhrouhou.

There were 12 Secretaries of State.

Local Government. The country is divided into 23 governorates, sub-divided into 199 districts and then into communes and imadas. At the elections of June 1990 there were 3,774 CDA candidates and 328 independents. Independents won seats on 12 out of 245 councils and gained control of 1. Turn-out was 79·37%. The 6 legal opposition parties boycotted the elections.

Flag: Red with a white circle in the middle, on which is a 5-pointed red star encircled by a red crescent.

DEFENCE. Selective conscription is 1 year.

Army. The Army consists of 2 mechanized, 1 Sahara and 1 parachute commando brigades; 1 armoured reconnaissance, 3 field, 2 anti-aircraft, 1 anti-tank and 1 engineer regiments. Equipment includes 14 M-48, 30 M-60A1 and 54 M-60A3 main battle, and 40 AMX-13, 42 Kuerassier and 10 M-41 light tanks. Strength (1991) 30,000 (25,000 conscripts). There are also the paramilitary Public Order Brigade (3,500) and National Guard (10,000).

Navy. The Navy consists of 1 frigate (ex-US, vintage 1943), 3 1985-built fast missile craft and 3 older craft with short range missiles, 2 ex-US-coastal minesweepers used as patrol ships, 14 inshore patrol craft and 1 large tug. In 1990 naval personnel totalled 4,500 (700 conscripts). Forces are based at Bizerta, Sfax and Kelibia.

Air Force. Equipment of the Air Force, acquired from various Western sources, includes 1 squadron of Aermacchi M.B.326K/L jet light attack aircraft; 1 squadron of F-5E/F Tiger II fighters; 12 SF.260W piston-engined light trainer/attack aircraft; 2 C-130H Hercules transports, 2 S.208 liaison aircraft, 6 SF.260M trainers, 7 M.B.326B jet trainers, 6 UH-1H, 18 AB.205, 6 Ecureuil and about 12 Alouette II and III helicopters. Personnel (1991) about 3,500 (700 conscripts), with 50 combat aircraft.

INTERNATIONAL RELATIONS

Membership. Tunisia is a member of the UN, OAU, the Islamic Conference and the Arab League.

ECONOMY

Policy. A seventh development plan (1987–91) envisaged investment of 8,000m. dinars.

Budget (in dinars). Budget estimates, 1988, revenue, 3,287m.; expenditure, 3,148m.

Currency. The unit of currency is the *Tunisian dinar* (TND) of 1,000 *millimes*.

There are coins of 1, 2, 5, 10, 20, 50, 100 and 500 *millimes*, and notes of 500 *millimes*, 1 *dinar*, 5 and 10 *dinars*. £1 = 1·64 *dinar*; US$1 = 0·87 *dinar* (March 1991).

Banking and Finance. The Central Bank of Tunisia is the bank of issue. In 1988 there were 9 development banks, 10 deposit banks and 9 off-shore banks.

Weights and Measures. The metric system of weights and measures has almost entirely taken the place of those of Tunisia, but corn is still sold in *kaffis* and *wibas*. The *kfiz* (of 16 *wiba*, each of 12 *sa'*) = 16 bushels. The *ounce* = 31·487 grammes.

ENERGY AND NATURAL RESOURCES

Electricity. Electrical energy generated was 3,820m. kwh. in 1986. Supply 127 and 220 volts; 50 Hz.

Oil. Crude oil production (1990) 4·42m. tonnes.

Gas. Natural gas production (1984) 430m. cu. metres.

Water. In 1989 there were 15 dams (total capacity 945m. cu. metres) and 3 were being built (259m. cu. metres). In 1986, 257,000 ha were irrigated.

Minerals. Mineral production (in 1,000 tonnes) in 1987: Calcium phosphate, 6,200; iron ore, 291; lead ore (concentrated), 3·4; zinc ore (concentrated), 10·7; salt, 422; barytine, 18; spath fluor, 43.

Agriculture. There are 5 agricultural regions: The *north*, mountainous with large fertile valleys; the *north-east*, with the peninsula of Cap Bon, suited for the cultivation of oranges, lemons and tangerines; the *Sahel*, where olive trees abound; the *centre*, a region of high table lands and pastures, and the *desert* of the south, where dates are grown.

Some 40% of the population are employed in agriculture, which contributed 12·2% of GDP in 1989. Large estates predominate; smallholdings are tending to fragment, partly owing to inheritance laws. There were some 0·4m. farms in 1990 (0·32m. in 1960). Of the total area of 15,583,000 ha, about 9m. ha are productive, including 2m. under cereals, 3·6m. used as pasturage, 900,000 forests and 1·3m. uncultivated. The main crops are cereals and olive oil. Production, 1988 (in 1,000 tonnes): Wheat, 225; barley, 63; olive oil, 71; olives, 320; citrus fruits, 214; dates, 40; almonds, 35; potatoes, 180; tomatoes, 370; pimentoes, 160; melons, 354; chick-peas, 21; sugar-beet, 267; tobacco, 5. Wine (1988) 49,000 tonnes.

Other products are apricots, pears, apples, peaches, plums, figs, pomegranates, almonds, shaddocks, pistachios, esparto grass, henna and cork.

Livestock (1988): Horses, 56,000; asses, 220,000; mules, 76,000; cattle, 612,000; sheep, 5·9m.; goats, 1,115,000; camels, 184,000; pigs, 4,000.

Fisheries. In 1980, 6,209 boats with 22,555 men were engaged in fishing. In 1987 the catch amounted to 99,180 tonnes.

INDUSTRY. Production, 1987 (in 1,000 tonnes): Superphosphate, 1,030; phosphoric acid, 593; cement, 3,215; lime, 527. 2,010 cars, 450 lorries, 1,240 vans, 220 buses and coaches, 330 tractors, 23,320 radio and 58,460 television sets were produced in 1987.

Trade Unions. The Union Générale des Travailleurs Tunisiens won 27 seats in the parliamentary elections (1 Nov. 1981). There are also the Union Tunisienne de l'Industrie, du Commerce et de l'Artisanat (UTICA, the employers' union) and the Union National des Agriculteurs (UNA, farmers' union).

FOREIGN ECONOMIC RELATIONS. In Feb. 1989 Tunisia signed a treaty of economic co-operation with the other countries of Maghreb: Algeria, Libya, Mauritania and Morocco.

Commerce. The imports and exports for calendar years (in 1,000 dinars) were as follows:

	1982	*1983*	*1984*	*1985*	*1986*	*1987*
Imports	2,008,000	2,116,100	2,472,500	2,287,000	2,308,300	2,509,000
Exports	1,188,000	1,263,900	1,396,800	1,443,000	1,387,600	1,770,600

Exports to France in 1987 totalled 384·1m. dinars, and imports from France,

687·2m. dinars and exports to USA were valued at 32·1m. dinars and imports from USA were valued at 149·1m. dinars.

In 1987 the main exports (in 1m. dinars) were: Clothing, 354·5; hosiery, 90·3; phosphoric acid, 69·8; electric machines, 66·8; fish and molluscs, 66·7; olive oil, 65·6.

Total trade between Tunisia and UK (British Department of Trade returns, in £1,000 sterling):

	1986	*1987*	*1988*	*1989*	*1990*
Imports to UK	17,292	14,714	36,062	43,266	40,959
Exports and re-exports from UK	39,824	24,943	30,780	31,148	40,800

Tourism. Tourism is important. In 1989 there were 3·2m. visitors spending TD855m..

COMMUNICATIONS

Roads. In 1987 there were 18,952 km of roads. Number of motor vehicles, 1987, 506,000.

Railways. In 1989 there were 2,241 km of railways (492 km of 1,435 mm gauge and 1,739 km of metre-gauge), of which 21 km were electrified. 29m. passengers and 10·9m. tonnes of freight were carried in 1989. A suburban railway links Tunis and La Marsa, and a light rail network opened in Tunis in 1985.

Aviation. The national airline is Tunis-Air. In 1990 the 5 countries of the Maghreb decided to merge their airlines into Air Maghreb. There are 5 international airports, the main one at Tunis-Carthage. In 1987, 4,429,000 passengers and 21,688 tonnes of freight were carried.

Shipping. The main port is Tunis, and its outer port is Tunis-Goulette. These two ports and Sfax, Sousse and Bizerta are directly accessible to ocean going vessels. The ports of La Skhirra and Gabès are used for the shipping of Algerian and Tunisian oil.

In 1983, 5,370 ships of 19,224,000 tons entered Tunisian ports.

Telecommunications. There were, in 1983, 218,808 telephones. There were, in 1978, 403 post offices, and 6 wireless transmitting stations. Wireless sets in use in 1985 were 1·15m. Television began in 1966 and in 1985 there were 400,000 sets.

Cinemas (1987). There were 80 cinemas.

Newspapers. There were (1987) 2 Arabic and 4 French daily newspapers.

JUSTICE, RELIGION, EDUCATION AND WELFARE

Justice. There are 51 magistrates' courts, 13 courts of first instance, 3 courts of appeal (in Tunis, Sfax and Sousse) and the High Court in Tunis.

A Personal Status Code was promulgated on 13 Aug. 1956 and applied to Tunisians from 1 Jan. 1957. This raised the status of women, made divorce subject to a court decision, abolished polygamy and decreed a minimum marriage age.

Religion. The constitution recognizes Islam as the state religion. There are about 20,000 Roman Catholics, under the Prelate of Tunis. The Greek Church, the French Protestants and the English Church are also represented.

Education. All education was in 1956 made dependent on the Ministry of National Education. The 208 independent koranic schools have been nationalized and the distinction between religious and public schools has been abolished. All education is free from primary schools to university. A teachers' training college (*école normale supérieure*) was established in 1955. There are also a high school of law, 2 centres of economic studies, 2 schools of engineering, 2 medical schools, a faculty of agriculture, 2 institutes of business administration and one school of dentistry.

In 1987–88 there were 3,605 primary schools with 43,189 teachers and 1,338,905 pupils; 436 secondary schools with 22,373 teachers and 437,604 pupils. In 1980–81 there were 60,137 students at technical and vocational schools and 4,101 students in teacher-training. In 1988 there were 3 universities: The University of Tunis (38,829 students and 5,019 teaching staff in 1984–85), the University of Sousse and the University of Sfax.

Health. In 1987 there were 36 general hospitals (22 university and 14 regional), 20 specialized institutions, centres and university hospitals, and (1988) 92 district hospitals. In 1986 there were 15,814 beds.

Social Security. A system of social security was set up in 1950 (amended 1963, 1964 and 1970).

DIPLOMATIC REPRESENTATIVES

Of Tunisia in Great Britain (29 Prince's Gate, London, SW7 1QG)
Ambassador: Dr Abdelaziz Hamzaoui.

Of Great Britain in Tunisia (5 Place de la Victoire, Tunis)
Ambassador and Consul-General: S. P. Day, CMG.

Of Tunisia in the USA (1515 Massachusetts Ave., NW, Washington, D.C., 20005)
Ambassador: (Vacant).

Of the USA in Tunisia (144 Ave. de la Liberté, Tunis)
Ambassador: Robert H. Pelletreau, Jr.

Of Tunisia to the United Nations
Ambassador: Ahmed Ghezal.

Further Reading

Statistical Information: Institut National de la Statistique (27 Rue de Liban, Tunis) was set up in 1947. Its main publications are: *Annuaire statistique de la Tunisie* (latest issue, 1975).
Lawless R. I. *et al.*, *Tunisia.* [Bibliography] Oxford and Santa Barbara, 1982
Ling, D. L., *Tunisia: From Protectorate to Republic.* Indiana Univ. Press, 1967
Rudebeck, L., *The Tunisian Experience: Party and People.* London, 1970
Salem, N., *Habib Bourguiba, Islam and the Creation of Tunisia.* London, 1984

TURKEY

Capital: Ankara
Population: 50·67m. (1985)
GNP per capita: US$1,434 (1989)

Türkiye Çumhuriyeti

(Republic of Turkey)

HISTORY. The Turkish War of Independence (1919–22), following the disintegration of the Ottoman Empire, was led and won by Mustafa Kemal (Atatürk) on behalf of the Grand National Assembly which first met in Ankara on 23 April 1920. On 20 Jan. 1921 the Grand National Assembly voted a constitution which declared that all sovereignty belonged to the people and vested all power, both executive and legislative, in the Grand National Assembly. The name 'Ottoman Empire' was later replaced by 'Turkey'. On 1 Nov. 1922 the Grand National Assembly abolished the office of Sultan and Turkey became a republic on 29 Oct. 1923.

Religious courts were abolished in 1924, Islam ceased to be the official state religion in 1928, women were given the franchise and western-style surnames were adopted in 1934.

On 27 May 1960 the Turkish Army, directed by a National Unity Committee under the leadership of Gen. Cemal Gürsel, overthrew the government of the Democratic Party. The Grand National Assembly was dissolved and party activities were suspended. Party activities were legally resumed on 12 Jan. 1961. A new constitution was approved in a referendum held on 9 July 1961 and general elections were held the same year.

On 12 Sept. 1980, the Turkish armed forces overthrew the Demirel Government (Justice Party). Parliament was dissolved and all activities of political parties were suspended. The Constituent Assembly was convened in Oct. 1981, and prepared a new Constitution which was enforced after a national referendum on 7 Nov. 1982.

AREA AND POPULATION. Turkey is bounded west by the Aegean Sea and by Greece, north by Bulgaria and the Black Sea, east by the USSR and Iran, and south by Iraq, Syria and the Mediterranean.

The area (including lakes) is 779,452 sq. km (300,947 sq. miles). Area in Europe (Trakya), 23,764 sq. km. Area in Asia (Anadolu), 755,688 sq. km; population (census 1985), 50,664,458.

Some 12m. Kurds live in Turkey. Limited use of the Kurdish language (not in schools or publications) was sanctioned in Feb. 1991.

The census population is given as follows:

	Total		*Total*		*Total*
1927	13,648,270	1950	20,947,188	1970	35,605,176
1935	16,158,018	1955	24,064,763	1975	40,347,719
1940	17,820,950	1960	27,754,820	1980	44,736,957
1945	18,790,174	1965	31,391,421	1985	50,664,458

Vital statistics, 1988: Marriages, 448,144; divorces, 22,513; deaths, 152,236.

The population of the provinces, at the census in 1985, was as follows:

Adana	1,725,940	Bolu	504,778	Gaziantep	966,490
Adıyaman	430,728	Burdur	248,002	Gireşun	502,151
Afyonkarahisar	666,978	Bursa	1,324,015	Gümüşhane	283,753
Ağri	421,131	Çanakkale	417,121	Hakkari	182,645
Amasya	358,289	Çankırı	263,964	Hatay	1,002,252
Ankara	3,306,327	Çorum	599,204	Isparta	382,844
Antalya	891,149	Denizli	667,478	Içel	1,034,085
Artvin	226,338	Diyarbakir	934,505	Istanbul	5,842,985
Aydin	743,419	Edirne	389,638	Izmir	2,317,829
Balıkesir	910,282	Elâziğ	483,715	Kahramanmaraş	840,472
Bilecik	160,909	Erzincan	299,985	Kars	722,431
Bingöl	241,548	Erzurum	856,175	Kastamonu	450,353
Bitlis	300,843	Eskişehir	597,397	Kayseri	864,060

Kırklareli	297,098	Nevşehir	278,129	Sivas	772,209
Kirşehir	260,156	Niğde	560,386	Tekirdağ	402,721
Kocaeli	742,245	Ordu	763,857	Tokat	679,071
Konya	1,769,050	Rize	374,206	Trabzon	786,194
Kütahya	543,384	Sakarya	610,500	Tunceli	151,906
Malatya	665,809	Samsun	1,108,710	Uşak	271,261
Manisa	1,050,130	Şanliurfa	795,034	Van	547,216
Mardin	652,069	Siirt	524,741	Yozgat	545,301
Muğla	486,290	Sinop	280,140	Zonguldak	1,044,945
Muş	339,492				

65% of the population was urban in 1990. (Istanbul, 8m.).

The population of towns of over 100,000 inhabitants, at the census of Oct. 1985, was as follows:

Istanbul	5,494,916	Diyarbakir	305,259	Denizli	171,360
Ankara	2,251,533	Samsun	280,068	Trabzon	155,960
Izmir	1,489,817	Antalya	258,139	Sakarya	155,041
Adana	776,000	Erzurum	252,648	Balikesir	152,402
Bursa	614,133	Malatya	251,257	Manisa	126,319
Gaziantep	466,302	Kocaeli	236,144	Van	121,306
Konya	438,859	K. Maraş	212,206	Kütahya	120,354
Kayseri	378,458	Şanliurfa	206,385	Zonguldak	119,125
Eskişehir	367,328	Sivas	197,266	Hatay	109,233
Içel	314,105	Elaziğ	181,253	Isparta	101,784

CLIMATE. Coastal regions have a Mediterranean climate, with mild, moist winters and hot, dry summers. The interior plateau has more extreme conditions, with low and irregular rainfall, cold and snowy winters and hot, almost rainless summers. Ankara. Jan. 32·5°F (0·3°C), July 73°F (23°C). Annual rainfall 14·7" (367 mm). Istanbul. Jan. 41°F (5°C), July 73°F (23°C). Annual rainfall 28·9" (723 mm). Izmir. Jan. 46°F (8°C), July 81°F (27°C). Annual rainfall 28" (700 mm).

CONSTITUTION AND GOVERNMENT. The Turkish Grand National Assembly was dissolved on 12 Sept. 1980. The National Security Council took over its functions and powers. On 23 Oct. 1981 a Consultative Assembly was inaugurated, to prepare a new Constitution to replace that of 1961. The Assembly began its work in Oct. 1981 under the presidency of Sadi Irmak and on 7 Nov. 1982 a national referendum established that 98% of the electorate were in favour of the new Constitution. The Presidency is not an executive position, and the President may not be linked to a political party.

Turkish men and women are entitled to vote at the age of 21 to elect members of a single-chamber parliament.

Elections were held on 29 Nov. 1987. Of the 450 seats in the Grand National Assembly the Motherland Party won 292; The Social Democratic Populist Party, 99; The True Path Party, 59.

President: Turgut Özal.

The Cabinet in Feb. 1991 was composed as follows:

Prime Minister: Yildirim Akbulut.

Justice: Oltan Sungurlu. *Defence:* Mehmet Yazar. *Interior:* Abdulkadir Aksu. *Foreign Affairs:* Ahmet Kurtcebe Alptemocin. *Customs and Finance:* Adnan Kahveci. *Education:* Avni Akyol. *Public Works and Housing:* Cengiz Altinkaya. *Health:* Halil Sivgin. *Labour:* Imren Aykut. *Transportation and Communications:* Cengiz Tuncer. *Agriculture, Forestry and Rural Affairs:* Lutfullah Kayalar. *Industry and Commerce:* Sükrü Yürür. *Energy and Natural Resources:* Fahrettin Kurt. *Tourism:* Ilhan Akuzum. *Culture:* Namik Kemal Zeybek.

There are 14 Ministers of State.

National flag: A white crescent and star on red.

National anthem: Korkma! Sönmez bu şafaklarda yüzen al sancak (words by Mehmed Akif Ersoy; tune by Zeki Güngör; adopted 12 March 1921).

Local Government. The Constitution of 1921 provided for the administrative division of the country into *İl*, (province, now 67 in number), divided into *İlçe* (district), subdivided in their turn into *Bucak* (township or commune). At the head of each *Il* is a *Vali* representing the Government. Each *Il* has its own elective council.

The district is regarded as a mere grouping of townships or communes for certain purposes of general administration. The township or commune is an autonomous entity and possesses an elective council charged with the administration of such matters as are not reserved to the State.

At local elections in June 1990 the Motherland Party won 31 of the 51 districts contested, the Social Democratic Populist Party, 11, and the True Path Party, 5.

DEFENCE. There is a Supreme Council of National Security, under the chairmanship of the Prime Minister, which co-ordinates the resources in case of war. Besides the Minister of National Defence and the Chief of the General Staff, the heads of economic Ministries are members of this council.

Conscription in the Army, Air Force and Navy is 18 months at the age of 20.

Army. The Army consists of 13 infantry, and 1 mechanized divisions, 10 infantry, 7 armoured, 6 mechanized, 1 parachute and 2 commando brigades; 5 coastal defence battalions. Equipment includes 1,130 M-48A5, 523 M-47, 1,980 M48A5 T1/T2 and 81 Leopard main battle tanks. Army Aviation has 163 aircraft and 273 helicopters. Strength (1991) 525,000 (475,000 conscripts), and reserves number 950,000. There is also a paramilitary gendarmerie cum national guard of 70,000.

Navy. Current strength includes 15 diesel submarines (6 of German design built 1975-89 and 9 ex-US built 1944-45, 12 ex-US destroyers (1943-46), 10 frigates of which 4 are modern German MEKO-type, 4 ex-German Type 120 Köln class, and 2 locally built in the 1970s. Light forces comprise 16 fast missile craft, 2 fast torpedo craft, 7 coastal and 21 inshore patrol craft. Mine warfare forces include 6 minelayers and 22 coastal and 11 inshore minesweepers. Amphibious lift is provided by 7 tank landing ships and over 70 smaller craft. Major auxiliaries in service are 1 replenishment and 6 support tankers, 5 depot ships, 3 salvage/rescue ships, 1 survey ship and 1 training ship. Minor auxiliaries, coastal freighters and service craft number about 120.

The main naval bases are at Gölcük in the Gulf of İzmit, at İskenderun, at Taskizak (İstanbul) and at İzmir.

The naval air component operates 22 S-2 mixed Air Force and Naval-manned Tracker anti-submarine aircraft and 15 helicopters for anti-submarine and patrol duties. There is a Marine Brigade some 4,000 strong.

Personnel in 1990 totalled 55,000 (42,000 conscripts) including marines.

The separate Coast Guard numbers about 1,000 and performs coastal police duties with a force of 28 inshore patrol vessels, 4 transports and numerous boats.

Air Force. The Air Force is under the control of the General Staff and, operationally, under 6 ATAF. It is organized as 2 tactical air forces, with headquarters at Eskisehir and Diyarbakir, each having a flight of C-47s, UH-1H helicopters, T-33s. Combat aircraft comprise F-104G and F-104S Starfighters in 7 squadrons; F-5As in 3 squadrons; F-16A/Bs in 2 squadrons; RF-5As in 1 squadron; F-4E and RF-4E Phantoms in 6 squadrons; plus Nike-Hercules surface-to-air missile batteries. The 4 transport squadrons are equipped with Transall C-160, C-130 Hercules, Citation, Viscount and C-47 aircraft, and UH-IH helicopters. Training types include T-33A, T-37 and T-38 advanced trainers, T-34 basic and T-41 primary trainers. Delivery of 160 F-16 Fighting Falcons began late in 1987. Personnel strength (1991), 67,400, with 455 combat aircraft.

INTERNATIONAL RELATIONS

Membership. Turkey is a member of the UN, OECD, NATO and Council of Europe and an Associate of the EEC.

ECONOMY

Policy. The development plan for 1985–90 envisaged an investment of TL14,412,900m. Privatization of state enterprises is in train and 13 co-ordinated by the Public Participation Fund.

Budget. The budget for 1988–89 envisaged expenditure of TL20,800,000m. and revenue of TL18,400,000m.

Currency. The unit of currency is the *Turkish lira* (TRL) of 100 *kuruş*. There are coins of TL5, 10, 25, 50, 100 and 500 and notes of TL1,000, 5,000, 10,000, 20,000 and 50,000. In March 1991, US$1 = TL3,369; £1 = TL6,391. The lira is fully convertible. Annualized inflation was 55% in Dec. 1990.

Banking and Finance. The Turkish banking system is composed of the Central Bank (Merkez Bankası; *Governor*, Rüsdu Saracoğlu) and 64 other banks. The Central Bank's assets were TL28,327,000m. at the end of 1989. The assets and liabilities of deposit money banks in 1988 were TL61,401,000m.

There is a stock exchange in Istanbul.

Weights and Measures. The metric system is in use. The Gregorian calendar has been in exclusive use since 26 Dec. 1925.

ENERGY AND NATURAL RESOURCES

Electricity. The potential hydro-electric power in Turkey is estimated at 56,000m. kwh. In 1986 the electrical power plants (hydro-electric or thermal) produced 38,490m. kwh. Supply 220 volts; 50 Hz.

Oil. Oil is being produced in Garzan and Raman by the Turkish Petroleum Co. Under the oil law of 14 Oct. 1954 private companies can explore and produce oil. Crude oil production (1990) was 3·4m. tonnes. The 3 refineries refined 12m. tons of crude oil in 1975. With a fourth refinery, introduced in 1973, total refining capacity now reaches 24m. tons a year. The oil pipeline Batman–Iskenderun (494 km) was opened on 4 Jan. 1967. Imports (refined locally) in 1983 were 14·3m. tonnes.

Minerals. Turkey is rich in minerals, and is a major producer of chrome.

Production of principal minerals (in 1,000 tonnes) was:

	1985	*1986*	*1987*	*1988*
Coal	7,260	7,015	7,084	6,688
Lignite	39,437	45,470	46,481	39,025
Chrome	877	1,040	1,049	1,225
Copper concentrate	161	119	137	168
Refined sulphur	43	40	39	30
Iron	3,995	5,249	5,366	5,481
Boron	1,543	1,636	1,629	2,044

Of the Government organizations producing these ores, Zonguldak coal mines operate under the Turkish State Coal Exploitation; while the copper mines at Murgul and Ergani, the Eastern chromite mines, Keçiborlu sulphur, Emet colemanite, Küre pyrite and cupriferous pyrite, Keban argentiferous lead mines operate under the Etibank.

Agriculture. The number of people aged 12 and over engaged in agriculture and animal husbandry (including hunting) in 1985 was 12,037,883.

In 1990 there were some 28m. ha of agricultural land and 3m. smallholdings. In 1987, 24,318,000 ha were crop land, 18,744,000 ha of it sown and 5,574,000 ha fallow; vineyards, fruit orchards and olive groves occupied 2,963,000 ha; forest occupied 20,199,000 ha.

The soil for the most part is very fertile; the principal products are cotton, tobacco, cereals (especially wheat), figs, silk, dried fruits, liquorice root, nuts, almonds, mohair, skins and hides, furs, wool, gums, canary seed, linseed and sesame. The South-Eastern Anatolian Irrigation Project (CAP) is expected to produce 1·6m. ha of fertile land. The production of olives for olive oil was estimated at 0·6m. tonnes in 1990 (1·1m. tonnes in 1988). Sugar production (refined) in 1985 was 1,429,586 tonnes. Agricultural production (in tonnes) in 1988 included 3·35m. grapes, 740,000 oranges and 360,000 lemons, 353,000 hazelnuts, 1·95m. apples, 5·25m. tomatoes, tea (fresh leaves, 1988) 752,662.

Turkey produced 600 tonnes of flax fibre, 4,950 tonnes of hemp fibre and 536,786 tonnes of cotton lint in 1988. Agricultural tractors numbered 654,636 in 1988.

Production (in 1,000 tonnes) of principal crops:

	1985	1986	1987	1988	1989
Wheat	17,000	19,000	18,900	20,500	11,500
Barley	6,500	7,000	6,900	7,500	4,900
Maize	1,900	2,300	2,400	2,000	...
Rye	360	350	380	280	...
Tobacco	170	158	185	212	252
Oats	314	300	325	276	...
Rice	162	165	165	158	...

Estimated production in 1990 (in tonnes): Sultanas, 0·13m.; sunflower seeds, 0·85m.; soya beans, 0·2m.; pistachios, 8,000; hazelnut, 0·34m.; cotton, 0·62m.; wheat, 14m.; barley, 6m.; tobacco, 0·21m.

Livestock (1988): 40m. sheep, 13·1m. goats, 12m. cattle, 1·2m. asses, 620,000 horses, 540,000 buffaloes.

In 1988 Turkey produced 62,000 tonnes of wool, 245,000 tonnes of cattle meat and 305,000 tonnes of sheep meat and 290,000 tonnes of poultry.

Forestry. The most wooded Ils are Kastamonu, Aydın, Bursa, Bolu, Trabzon, Konya and Balikesir. In 1987 total forest land was 20,199,000 ha, 26% of the land area. Produce (1,000 cu. metres) in 1988: Logs, 3,571; pit props, 529; industrial wood, 373; poles, 123. Also 5,176,699 tonnes of firewood.

Fisheries. Catch (1987): Sea fish, 562,697 tonnes; crustaceans and molluscs, 20,156 tonnes; fresh water fish, 41,760 tonnes. Aquaculture production, 1987, 3,300 tonnes (mainly carp and trout). There were (1987) 8,594 fishing boats.

INDUSTRY.

In 1990 55 state enterprises accounted for about 30% of production. Production in 1988 (in tonnes): 8,993,023 of fuel oil; 6,558,826 of motor oil; 4,461,959 of crude iron; 453,596 of pig iron; 8,009,073 of crude steel; 3,822,497 of super phosphate; 3,143,902 of coke; 22,674,724 of cement and 367,201 of paper. In 1988, 120,796 passenger cars were produced and 31,327 tractors. There are steel works at Karabük, Ereğli and Iskenderun.

Labour. Economically active population aged 12 and over, 1985, 20,556,786, of whom 12,118,533 were engaged in agriculture, forestry, hunting and fishing, 2,185,369 in manufacturing, 1,382,636 in trade, restaurants and hotels and 2,847,289 in services.

Trade Unions. The trade-union movement began in 1947. There are 4 national confederations (including Türk-Is and Disk) and 6 federations. There are 35 unions affiliated to Türk-Iş and 17 employers' federations affiliated to Disk, whose activities were banned on 12 Sept. 1980. In 1988, labour unions totalled 80 and employers' unions, 49. Some 2·2m. workers belonged to unions in 1990. Membership is forbidden to civil servants (including schoolteachers).

FOREIGN ECONOMIC RELATIONS.

Foreign debt in 1990 was US$41,000m. Direct foreign investment in 1989 was US$663m.

Commerce. Imports and exports (in US$1m.) for calendar years:

	1985	1986	1987	1988	1989
Imports	11,343	11,105	14,158	14,335	15,762
Exports	7,958	7,457	10,190	11,662	11,627

Exports (1989) in US$1m.: Textiles, 3,605; iron and steel products, 1,349; chemical products, 779; leather clothing, 604; plastic material and rubber, 351; hazelnuts, 266; machinery, 191; petroleum products, 243; processed agricultural products, 1,349; mining and quarrying products, 413; tobacco (1988), 266.

Imports (1989) in US$1m.: Machinery, 2,188; chemical products, 2,101; iron and steel products, 2,217; electrical equipment, 1,028; transport equipment, 796; plastic material and rubber, 484; mining and quarrying products, 2,902; processed agricultural products, 707; crude oil (1988), 2,434.

In 1988 imports (in US$1m.) were: From Federal Republic of Germany, 2,054·4;

USA, 1,519·7; Iraq, 1,436·5; Italy, 1,005·7; France, 828·8; UK, 739·1; Iran, 659·8; Japan, 554·8; Belgium, 477·8; USSR, 442·6. Exports: Federal Republic of Germany, 2,149; Iraq, 986·1; Italy, 954·7; USA, 760·6; UK, 576·1; Iran, 545·7; France, 498·5; Saudi Arabia, 355·2; Netherlands, 351·1; USSR, 291·4.

Total trade between Turkey and UK (British Department of Trade returns, in £1,000 sterling):

	1986	*1987*	*1988*	*1989*	*1990*
Imports to UK	406,605	579,366	509,636	533,769	550,803
Exports and re-exports from UK	433,753	513,479	477,539	434,562	606,829

Tourism. The number of foreign visitors was 4,511,193m. in 1989, including 2·3m. on organized tours; earnings from tourism in 1988, US$1,997m. There were 150,159 tourist beds in 1990.

COMMUNICATIONS

Roads. In 1988 there were 30,999 km of state highways (including 125 km of motorway in 1989) and 27,852 km of provincial roads; 55,887 km were surfaced. In 1988 there were 1,309,557 cars, 474,886 trucks and pick-ups, 169,055 buses and minibuses and 420,891 motorcycles.

Railways. Total length of railway lines in 1989 was 8,430 km (1,435 mm gauge) of which 567 km were electrified; 146m. passengers and 13·6m. tonnes of freight were carried.

Aviation. In 1988 the Turkish Airlines fleet of 31 planes flew 3,806,196 passengers (1,663,777 on international flights) and carried 341,791 tonnes (152,187) of freight.

Shipping. In 1985 the gross tonnage of cargo ships totalled 690,784; passenger ships 131,325 and tankers 186,267. The main ports are: Istanbul, Izmir, Samsun, Mersin, Iskenderun and Trabzon.

Coastal shipping, 1988: 24,996 vessels handled; 934,432 passengers entered, 933,044 cleared; 25·6m. tons of goods entered, 20·2m. cleared. International shipping: 14,058 vessels handled; 640,078 passengers entered, 618,988 cleared; 43·5m. tons of goods entered, 87·1m. cleared.

Post and Broadcasting. Number of telephones in 1986 was 2·28m.; Istanbul, 566,745; Ankara, 248,824.

In 1984 there were 6,023,000 licensed radio sets. There were 6,933,285 television receivers.

Newspapers. In 1988, 13 dailies were published in Ankara, 29 dailies in Istanbul, 5 dailies in Izmir, 4 dailies in Bursa and 3 dailies in Konya.

JUSTICE, RELIGION, EDUCATION AND WELFARE

Justice. The unified legal system consists of: (1) justices of the peace (single judges with limited but summary penal and civil jurisdiction); (2) courts of first instance (single judges, dealing with cases outside the jurisdiction of (3) and (4)); (3) central criminal courts (a president and 2 judges, dealing with cases where the crime is punishable by imprisonment over 5 years); (4) commercial courts (3 judges); (5) state security courts, to prosecute offences against the integrity of the state (a president and 4 judges, 2 of the latter being military).

The civil and military Courts of Cassation sit at Ankara.

The Council of State is the highest administration tribunal; it consists of 5 chambers. Its 31 judges are nominated from among high-ranking personalities in politics, economy, law, the army, etc.

The Military Court of Cassation in Ankara is the highest military tribunal. The Military Administrative Court deals with the judicial control of administrative acts and deeds concerning military personnel.

The Constitutional Court, set up under the Constitution, can review and annul legislation and try the President of the Republic, Ministers and senior judges. It consists of 15 regular and 5 alternate members.

The Civil Code and the Code of Obligations have been adapted from the corresponding Swiss codes. The Penal Code is largely based upon the Italian Penal Code, and the Code of Civil Procedure closely resembles that of the Canton of Neuchâtel. The Commercial Code is based on the German.

Religion. Freedom of religion is guaranteed by the Constitution. Although Islam is not the official state religion, Moslems (mainly Sunni) form 98·2% of the population. There are some 17m. Shi'ites (Alevis). The administration of the Moslem religious organizations is in charge of the Presidency of Religious Affairs, attached to the Prime Minister's office. The Turkish Republic is a secular state.

Istanbul is the seat of the (Ecumenical Patriarch, who is the head of the Orthodox Church in Turkey. The Armenian Church (Gregorian) is ruled by a Patriarch in Istanbul who is subordinate to the Katholikos of Etchmiadzin, the spiritual head of all Armenians. The Armenian Apostolic Church is ruled by the Patriarch of Cilicia. The Chaldeans (Nestorian Uniats) have a Bishop at Mardin. The Syrian Uniats have a See of Mardin and Amida, but it is united with their Patriarchate of Antioch (residence, Damascus). Greek Uniats (Byzantine Rite) have as their Ordinary in Istanbul, the Titular Bishop of Gratianopolis. The Latins have an Apostolic Delegate in Istanbul and an Archbishop in Izmir, but their Patriarch of Istanbul is titular and non-resident. There is a Grand Rabbi (Hahambaşi) in Istanbul for the Jews, who are nearly all Sephardim.

A law passed in Dec. 1934 forbids the wearing of clerical garb for those other than religious leaders except in places of worship and during divine service. The constitution forbids the political exploitation of religion or any impairment of the secular character of the republic.

Education. Elementary education is compulsory and co-educational and, in state schools, free. All children from 7 to 12 are to receive primary instruction, which may be given in state schools, schools maintained by communities, or private schools, or, subject to certain tests, at home. The state schools are under the direct control of the Ministry of Education. They include primary schools, secondary or middle schools, and *lycées* or secondary schools of a superior kind. There are also training schools for male and female teachers, and technical schools. The important non-Moslem communities in Istanbul maintain their own schools, which, like all 'private' schools, are subject to the supervision of the Ministry of Education.

Literacy of the population of 6 years and over was 77·3% in 1985.

Religious instruction in schools, hitherto prohibited, was made optional in elementary and middle schools in May 1948. There are many training schools for Moslem clergy as well as a Faculty of Theology in Ankara.

Statistics for 1987–88	*Number*	*Teachers*	*Students*
Primary schools (state and private)	50,455	220,943	6,880,304
Secondary schools (state and private)	5,001	42,551	1,870,515
High schools (state and private)	1,436	57,834	697,227
Vocational and technical schools	2,236	47,157	720,567
Faculties (university and higher education)	343	27,196	503,623

In 1989 there were 29 universities with 5,600 teaching staff and 550,000 students. In 1987–88 there were 152 other institutes of higher education.

Health. Public health is the responsibility of the Ministry of Health and Social Welfare, established in 1920; social insurance for workers comes under the Workers' Insurance Institution attached to the Ministry of Labour. A law promulgated in 1961 and implemented from 1963 provided for the nationalization of the health services within 15 years. In 1986, 2·8m. workers and employees were covered by social insurance, including free medical care.

In 1989 there were 42,502 doctors, 9,639 dentists and 37,694 nurses, and 113,010 beds in 777 hospitals and 111 health centres.

DIPLOMATIC REPRESENTATIVES

Of Turkey in Great Britain (43 Belgrave Sq., London, SW1X 8PA)
Ambassador: Nurver Nureş (accredited 16 Feb. 1989).

Of Great Britain in Turkey (Sehit Ersan Caddesi 46/A, Cankaya, Ankara)
Ambassador: Sir Timothy Daunt, KCMG.

Of Turkey in the USA (1606 23rd St., NW, Washington, D.C., 20008)
Ambassador: Nüzhet Kandemir.

Of the USA in Turkey (110 Ataturk Blvd., Ankara)
Ambassador: Morton Abramowitz.

Of Turkey to the United Nations
Ambassador: Mustafa Akşin.

Further Reading

Statistical Information: The State Institute of Statistics in Ankara consists of a research bureau and 10 sections dealing with agriculture, education, foreign trade, etc. It published an *Annuaire Statistique/Istatistik Yiliği* (1928–53) and *Aylık Istatistik Bülteni*, Monthly Bulletin of Statistics.

The Turkish Constitution, 1971. Ankara, 1972
Resmî Gazete, Official Gazette. Ankara
Konjonktür. Ministry of Commerce (three times a year, from 1940)
Turkish Daily News. Ankara
Banque Centrale de la République de Turquie. *Bulletin Mensuel* (from Jan. 1953)
Barchard, D., *Turkey and the West*. London, 1985
Dodd, C. H., *The Crisis of Turkish Democracy*. Beverley, 1983
Goodwin, G., *A History of Ottoman Architecture*. London, 1971
Güclü, M., *Turkey*. [Bibliography] Oxford and Santa Barbara, 1981
Hale, W., *The Political and Economic Development of Modern Turkey*. London, 1981
Hesper, M., *The State Tradition in Turkey*. Beverley, 1985
Kazancigil, A. and Ozbudun, E., (eds.) *Atatürk: Founder of a Modern State*. London, 1981
Kinross, Lord, *Atatürk*. London, 1964
Lewis, B., *The Emergence of Modern Turkey*. OUP, 1968
Mackenzie, K., *Turkey in Transition: The West's Neglected Ally*. London, 1984
Rustow, D. A., *Turkey: America's Forgotten Ally*. New York, 1987
Sezer, D. B., *Turkey's Security Policies*. London, 1981
Tachau, F., *Turkey: The Politics of Authority, Democracy and Development*. New York, 1984
Weiker W., *The Modernization of Turkey*. New York, 1981

State Library: MilliKütüphane Müdürlüğü, Ankara.

THE TURKS AND CAICOS ISLANDS

Capital: Grand Turk
Population: 11,696 (1990)

HISTORY. After a long period of rival French and Spanish claims the islands were eventually secured to the British Crown by the appointment in 1766 of a Resident British Agent, and became a separate colony in 1973 after association at various times with the colonies of the Bahamas and Jamaica.

AREA AND POPULATION. The Turks and Caicos Islands are geographically part of the Bahamas extremity, of which they form the south-eastern archipelago. There are upwards of 30 small cays; area 192 sq. miles (430 sq. km). Only 6 are inhabited; the largest, Grand Caicos, is 30 miles long by 2 to 3 miles broad. The seat of government is at Grand Turk, 7 miles long by 1·25 broad. Population, 1990 census (provisional), 11,696: Grand Turk, 3,720; South Caicos, 1,220; Middle Caicos, 275; North Caicos, 1,305; Providenciales, 4,963; Salt Cay, 213.

Vital statistics (1989): Births, 192; deaths, 58: There were 49 marriages in 1985.

CLIMATE. An equable and healthy climate as a result of regular trade winds, though hurricanes are sometimes experienced. Grand Turk. Jan. 76°F (24·4°C), July 83°F (28·3°C). Annual rainfall 29" (725 mm).

CONSTITUTION AND GOVERNMENT. A new Constitution was introduced in Aug. 1976, providing for an Executive Council and a Legislative Council. The Governor retains responsibility for external affairs, internal security, defence and certain other matters. The Executive Council comprises 3 official members: The Chief Secretary, the Financial Secretary and the Attorney-General; a Chief Minister and 3 other ministers from among the elected members of the Legislative Council; and is presided over by the Governor. The Legislative Council consists of a Speaker, the 3 official members of the Executive Council, 13 elected members and 2 appointed members. At general elections held on 3 March 1988 for the 13 elective seats on the Legislative Council, 11 seats were won by the People's Democratic Movement.

Governor: M. J. Bradley, QC.
Chief Minister: Oswald Skipping

Flag: British Blue Ensign with the shield of the Colony in the fly.

ECONOMY

Budget. 1990–91 total revenue US$46,281,000 and expenditure, US$46,224,000.

Currency. The currency in circulation is US dollars.

Banking. In 1990 there were 3 commercial banks: Barclays Bank PLC, Bank of Nova Scotia and Turks and Caicos Banking Company have offices on Grand Turk and Providenciales.

Total assets of all 5 banks at 31 Dec. 1989: US$128,641,000; deposits, US$105,683,000.

LABOUR. In 1989, out of a total population of 4,885 aged 14 or over, 4,043 were working, 573 unemployed and 269 economically inactive.

COMMERCE (1987–88). Exports, US$4,133,900, and imports, US$33,212,700. Principal imports 1987–1988 (in US$1,000): Food, drink and tobacco, 6,883·2;

manufactured goods, 20,109·3; raw materials, 1,342·2; fuel, 2,911·1. Origin of imports (1985–86 in US$): USA, 26,149,337; UK, 558,378. The main exports are lobster products (US$1,380,200 in 1987–88), dried and fresh frozen conch (US$2,278,000 in 1987–88). All lobster, conch and other fish exports go to the USA after processing in plants in South Caicos and Providenciales.

Total trade between Turks and Caicos Islands and UK (British Department of Trade returns, in £1,000 sterling):

	1986	*1987*	*1988*	*1989*	*1990*
Imports to UK	86	31	66	74	8
Exports and re-exports from UK	1,025	496	710	731	1,719

The Islands joined CARICOM in 1990.

Tourism. Number of visitors, 1989, 48,535, of whom 32,898 were from the USA.

COMMUNICATIONS

Aviation. There is a 6,335 ft paved airfield on Grand Turk. On South Caicos there is a 6,000 ft paved airfield and on Providenciales a 7,000 ft paved airstrip. There are small paved and unpaved airstrips on the other 3 inhabited islands. Pan American World Airways operate passenger services to Miami. Turks and Caicos National Airlines operates daily service to the islands and a number of flights a week to Cap Haitien (Haiti), the Dominican Republic and the Bahamas. Turks Air Ltd and Caicos Caribbean operate regular weekly cargo services from Miami. There are 5 local charter operators, operating charters to the Bahamas and the Caribbean.

Shipping. Registered shipping (1985), 168 sailing vessels of 2,445 tons and 49 motor vessels of 5,517 tons.

Telecommunications. Air-mail is received 4 times weekly from Miami and dispatched twice weekly to Miami. Surface mail from all parts of the world is routed *via* the US arriving weekly from Miami, Florida. There is no regular outgoing surface mail and this is sent as accumulated. Cable & Wireless (West Indies) provide internal and international cable, telephone, telex, telegraph and facsimile services. There were (1988) 1,359 telephones. North Caicos and Salt Cay are linked with the Providenciales and Grand Turk exchanges respectively. The Government operates a radio broadcasting service from Grand Turk to the Islands, call sign Radio Turks and Caicos (RTC), for a total of 98 hours a week on 1,460 KHZ medium wave. Number of receivers, approximately 12,000.

Newspapers. The *Turks and Caicos News* is published weekly.

JUSTICE, RELIGION, EDUCATION AND WELFARE

Justice. Laws are a mixture of Statute and Common Law. There is a Magistrates Court and a Supreme Court. Appeals lie from the Supreme Court to the Court of Appeal which sits in Nassau, Bahamas. There is a further appeal in certain cases to the Privy Council in London. In 1989 the prison population was 159.

Religion. The Christian faith predominates with Anglican, Methodist, Baptist. Church of God of Prophecy and New Testament Church of God being the largest group.

Education. Education is free and compulsory up to 15 years of age in the 14 government primary and 4 government secondary schools. In 1989–90 there were 1,401 pupils and 73 teachers in the primary schools and 903 pupils and 81 teachers in the secondary schools. There were also 2 private primary schools. Expenditure on education 1988–89 was US$1,878,003.

Health. In 1989 there were 6 doctors, 1 dentist, 43 nurses and midwives, 24 hospital beds and 10 district clinics.

TUVALU

Capital: Fongafale
Population: 8,229 (1985)
GNP per capita: US$500 (1984)

HISTORY. Formerly the Ellice Islands, a British Protectorate since 1892. On the recommendation of a Commissioner, appointed by the British Government, to consider requests that the island group be separated from the Gilbert Islands, a referendum was held in 1974. There was a large majority in favour of separation and this took place in Oct. 1975. Independence was achieved on 1 Oct. 1978.

AREA AND POPULATION. Tuvalu (formerly the Ellice Islands) lies between 5° 30' and 11° S. lat. and 176° and 180° E. long. and comprises Nanumea, Nanumanga, Niutao, Nui, Vaitupu, Nukufetau, Funafuti (administrative centre), Nukulaelae and Niulakita. Population (census 1985) 8,229 and 1,500 work abroad, mainly in Nauru. Area approximately $9^1/_2$ sq. miles (24 sq. km). The population is of a Polynesian race.

CLIMATE. A pleasant but monotonous climate with temperatures averaging 86°F (30°C), though trade winds from the east moderate conditions for much of the year. Rainfall ranges from 120" (3,000 mm) to over 160" (4,000 mm). Funafuti. Jan. 84°F (28·9°C), July 81°F (27·2°C). Annual rainfall 160" (4,003 mm).

CONSTITUTION AND GOVERNMENT. The Constitution provides for a Prime Minister and 4 other Ministers to be elected from among the 12 elected members of the House of Parliament, for which general elections took place in Sept. 1985. The Cabinet, chaired by the Prime Minister, consists of the 4 ministers and 2 *ex-officio* members, the Attorney-General and the Secretary to Government, who are also *ex-officio* members of the House of Assembly.

Governor-General: Sir Tupua Leupena, GCMG, MBE.
Prime Minister, Minister of Foreign Affairs, Local Government and Social Services: Bikenibeu Paeniu.
Deputy Prime Minister, Finance: Kitiseni Lopati. *Commerce and Natural Resources:* Lale Seluka. *Works and Communications:* Solomona M. Tealofi.

National flag: Light blue with the Union Jack in the canton, and 9 gold stars in the fly arranged in the same pattern as the 9 islands.

Local Government. There is a town council on Funafuti and island councils on the 7 other atolls, each consisting of 6 elected members including a president. Since 1966 Members of Parliament have been *ex-officio* members of Island Councils. The island of Niulakita is administered as part of Niutao.

INTERNATIONAL RELATIONS

Membership. Tuvalu is a member of the Commonwealth and the South Pacific Forum and is an ACP state of the EEC.

ECONOMY

Budget. In 1988 the budget envisaged revenue of $A4,701,594.

Currency. The unit of currency is the Australian *dollar* although Tuvaluan coins up to $A1 are in local circulation.

Banking. The Tuvalu National Bank was established at Funafuti in 1980 and is a joint venture between the Tuvalu Government and Wespac International.

ENERGY AND NATURAL RESOURCES

Electricity. Production (1986) 3m. kwh.

Agriculture. Coconut palms are the main crop. Production of coconuts (1988), 3,000 tonnes. Fruit and vegetables are grown for local consumption.

Fisheries. Sea fishing is excellent but is largely unexploited although (1988) Japanese, Taiwanese and South Korean vessels have been granted licences to fish. The USSR was refused a licence.

INDUSTRY AND TRADE

Industry. The main sources of income are from overseas remittances from Tuvaluans working abroad, philatelic and copra sales, and handicrafts.

Employment. A significant number of the population are employed in the phosphate industry on Nauru. The remainder are engaged in harvesting coconuts and fishing.

Commerce. Commerce is dominated by co-operative societies, the Tuvalu Co-operative Wholesale Society being the main importer. Imports (1984) $A3·96m.

Total trade between Tuvalu and UK (British Department of Trade returns, in £1,000 sterling):

	1986	*1987*	*1988*	*1989*	*1990*
Imports to UK	88	2	1	—	—
Exports and re-exports from UK	78	106	105	162	506

Tourism. In 1979 there were 474 visitors.

COMMUNICATIONS

Aviation. Tuvalu is linked to the outside world by Fiji Air which operates three times a week, on Monday, Wednesday and Friday, and Air Marshal once a week on Saturdays from Kiribati and Sundays from Fiji.

Shipping. Funafuti is the only port and a deep-water wharf was opened in 1980. Inter-island communication is by ship.

Post and Broadcasting. The Tuvalu Broadcasting Service transmits daily in Tuvaluan and English and all islands have daily radio communication with Funafuti. There were 120 telephones and 2,500 radio receivers in 1985.

JUSTICE, RELIGION, EDUCATION AND WELFARE

Justice. There is a High Court presided over by the Chief Justice of Fiji. Appeals lie to the Fiji Court of Appeal.

Religion. The majority of the population are Christians mainly Protestant but with small groups of Roman Catholics, Seventh Day Adventists, Jehovah's Witnesses, Mormons and Bahai's. There are some Moslems.

Education. In 1985 there was 1 secondary school jointly administered by the Government and the Church with 250 pupils. In addition there were 9 primary schools with (1985, inclusive of 326 pupils in community training centres) 924 pupils run by Island Councils and subsidized by the central government. In 1979, a maritime school was opened on Amatuku islet. Tuvaluans requiring further education must seek it abroad.

Health. In 1984 there was 1 central hospital with 36 beds situated at Funafuti. There were 4 doctors.

DIPLOMATIC REPRESENTATIVES

Of Great Britain in Tuvalu
High Commissioner: A. B. P. Smart (resides in Suva).

Of Tuvalu in the USA
Ambassador: Gregory Polson (resides in Tuvalu).

UGANDA

Capital: Kampala
Population: 17m. (1989)
GNP per capita: US$280 (1988)

Republic of Uganda

HISTORY. Uganda became a British Protectorate in 1894, the province of Buganda being recognized as a native kingdom under its Kabaka. In 1961 Uganda was granted internal self-government with federal status for Buganda.

Uganda became a fully independent member of the Commonwealth on 9 Oct. 1962. Full sovereign status was granted by the Uganda Independence Act, 1962. Uganda became a republic on 8 Sept. 1967.

In 1971, President Milton Obote was overthrown by troops led by Gen. Idi Amin.

In April 1979 a force of the Tanzanian Army and Ugandan exiles advanced into Uganda taking Kampala on 11 April. On 14 April Dr Yusuf Lule was sworn in as President and the country was administered, initially, by the Uganda National Liberation Front. Godfrey Lukongwa Binaisa, was appointed President by the National Consultative Council on 20 June 1979. He was deposed in May 1980 by the Military Commission, the military arm of Uganda National Liberation Front.

Milton Obote again became President when the Uganda People's Congress won the elections of Dec. 1980; he was deposed on 27 July 1985.

Lieut.-Gen. Tito Okello became head of State on 29 July 1985 but the National Resistance Army of Yoweri K. Museveni, the armed wing of the National Resistance Movement, was not prepared to co-operate with the new regime. A ceasefire between the National Resistance Army of Yoweri K. Museveni, the armed wing of the National Resistance Movement, and government forces was agreed on 17 Dec. 1985 and Yoweri Museveni was installed as President on 27 Jan. 1986.

AREA AND POPULATION. Uganda is bounded on the north by Sudan, on the east by Kenya, on the south by Tanzania and Rwanda, and the west by Zaïre. Total area 91,343 sq. miles (236,860 sq. km), including 15,217 sq. miles (39,459 sq. km) of swamp and water.

At the 1980 census the population was 12,630,076; 12% lived in urban areas, the largest towns being Kampala, the capital (458,423), Jinja (45,060), Masaka (29,123), Mbale (28,039), Mbarara (23,155), Entebbe (20,472) and Gulu (14,958).

The country is administratively divided into 33 districts, which are grouped in 4 geographical regions (which do not have administrative status): Central Region (Kampala, Luwero, Masaka, Mpigi, Mubende, Mukono, Rakai); Eastern Region (Iganga, Jinja, Kamuli, Kapchorwa, Kumi, Mbale, Soroti, Tororo); Northern Region (Apac, Arua, Gulu, Kitgum, Kotido, Lira, Moroto, Moyo, Nebbi); and Western Region (Bundibugyo, Bushenyi, Hoima, Kabale, Kabarole, Kasese, Masindi, Mbarara, Rukungiri).

Population estimate, 1989: 17m.

About 70% of the population speak Bantu languages, the major groups being the Baganda (18%), Banyoro (14%), Banyankole (8%), Bagisu (10%), Basoga (8%) and Bachiga (7%). About 16% were Nilotic groups in the north, chiefly the Lango (6·5%) and Acholi (4%), and the rest mainly Nilo-Hamitic, predominantly Teso (8%) and Karamojong (3%) in the northeast. The official language is English, but Kiswahili is also widely used as a lingua franca.

CLIMATE. Although in equatorial latitudes, the climate is more tropical, because of its elevation, and is characterized the year round by hot sunshine, cool breezes and showers of rain. The wettest months are March to June and there is no dry season. Temperatures vary little over the year. Kampala. Jan. 74°F (23·3°C), July 70°F (21·1°C). Annual rainfall 46" (1,150 mm). Entebbe. Jan. 72°F (22·2°C), July 69°F (20·6°C). Annual rainfall 60" (1,506 mm).

CONSTITUTION AND GOVERNMENT. In Oct. 1963 the post of Governor-General was replaced by that of President as head of state, elected for a 5-year term by the National Assembly. The President's salary in 1990 was 20,000 Uganda shillings per month. The national legislature is the 278-member National Resistance Council. Elections were held in Feb.-March 1989. In Oct. 1989 the Council extended its period of office for five years from 26 Jan. 1990. In Feb. 1991 the government was composed as follows:

President, Minister of Defence: Yoweri Museveni (sworn in 27 Jan. 1986).
Prime Minister: George Adyebo (b. 1947).
First Deputy Prime Minister: E. Kategaya. *Second Deputy Prime Minister, Minister of Foreign Affairs and Regional Co-operation:* Dr P. K. Semwogerere. *Third Deputy Prime Minister:* Abubaker Mayanja Kakyama. *Finance:* Dr C. Kiyonga. *Co-operatives and Marketing:* J. F. Wapakabhulo. *Animal Industry and Fisheries:* Dr M. Kagonyera. *Health:* Z. Kaheru. *Public Service and Cabinet Affairs:* Tom Rubale. *Industry and Technology:* Dr E. T. Adriko. *Works:* Dan Kigozi. *Internal Affairs:* Ibrahim Mukiibi. *Information and Broadcasting:* Kintu Musoke. *Planning and Economic Development:* Joshua Mayanja Nkangi. *Commerce:* Paul Etyang. *Rehabilitation:* Adoko Nekyon. *Lands and Surveys:* Ben Okello Luwum. *Water and Mineral Development:* Henry Kajura. *Justice and Attorney-General:* Dr G. Kanyeihamba. *Tourism and Wildlife:* Sebagereka Sam. *Education:* Amanya Mushega. *Agriculture:* Victoria Sekitoleko. *Transport and Communications:* Dr Ruhakana Rugunda. *Energy:* Richard Kaijuka. *Labour:* Stanley Okurut. *Environment Protection:* Moses Kintu. *Constitutional Affairs:* Samuel K. Njuba. *Housing and Urban Development:* Ssebaana Kizito. *Local Government:* Jaberi Bidandi Ssali.

National flag: Six horizontal stripes of black, yellow, red, black, yellow, red, in the centre a small white disc bearing a representation of a Balearic Crested Crane.

Local government: The 33 districts are divided into 152 counties, which are in turn divided into sub-counties which form the basic administrative units.

DEFENCE

Army. The National Resistance Army had a strength of about 70,000 in 1991 and is loosely organized in 6 brigades and some battalions. Equipment includes some BTR-60 armoured personnel carriers and 7 helicopters.

Navy. A small lake patrol was initiated in 1977.

Air Force. Since 1979, the service has been in a period of decline. As far as was known in early 1989, the equipment received from the East Bloc (MiG-17 and MiG-21 combat aircraft and L-29 jet trainers) was in storage. It is understood that some aircraft of Western European origin are still serviceable, including a small number of AS.202 Bravo and SF.260 trainers and about 6 Agusta-Bell helicopters, plus 3 Mi-8 transport helicopters, donated by Libya. The Police Air Wing still operates 2 fixed-wing aircraft and 7 Bell helicopters.

INTERNATIONAL RELATIONS

Membership. Uganda is a member of UN, OAU, Islamic Conference Organization, the Non-Aligned Movement, the Commonwealth and is an ACP state of EEC.

ECONOMY

Budget. In 1988–89 revenue was 56,690m. Uganda Sh. and expenditure, 88,240m. Uganda Sh.

Currency. The monetary unit is the *Uganda shilling* (UGS) divided into 100 *cents*. In May 1987 a new 'heavy' shilling was introduced worth 100 old shillings. In March 1991, £1 = 1,145·36 Uganda shillings; US$1 = 603·77 Uganda shillings.

Banking. The Bank of Uganda was established on 16 May 1966. The Uganda Credit and Savings Bank, established in 1950, was on 9 Oct. 1965 reconstituted as the Uganda Commercial Bank, with its capital fully owned by the Government.

Barclays Bank of Uganda Ltd. has 4 branches, Standard Bank Uganda Ltd. has 1 branch, Bank of Baroda Uganda Ltd. has 3 branches and the Libyan Arab Uganda Bank for Foreign Trade and Development has 3 branches, the Uganda Commercial Bank has 184 branches. The Co-operative Bank is owned by the Co-operative Movement. There are 2 Development Banks; the East African Development Bank and the Uganda Development Bank.

ENERGY AND NATURAL RESOURCES

Electricity. Industrial expansion is based on hydro-electric power provided by the Owen Falls scheme, which has a capacity of 150,000 kwh. Production (1986) 287m. kwh.

Minerals. Production, 1988: Gold, 26·3 grammes; tin, 63·8 tonnes.

Agriculture. In 1989, agriculture was one of the priority areas for increased production, with many projects funded both locally and externally. Coffee, cotton, tea and tobacco are the principal exports. Production (1988) in 1,000 tonnes: Tobacco, 4; coffee, 184; cotton seed, 18; tea, 2; sugar-cane, 900.

Livestock (1988): Cattle, 3·91m.; sheep, 1·74m.; goats, 2·8m.; pigs, 440,000; poultry, 15m.

Forestry. Woodland covers 29% of the land area (5·7m. hectares) and exploitable forests consist almost entirely of hardwoods. 40% of the hardwood timber is used locally and 30% is exported to Kenya, Rwanda and the UK. There is also a small percentage of mature softwood plantation out of which 10% of softwood timber is exported to Rwanda and 20% used locally.

Fisheries. With its 13,600 sq. miles of lakes and many rivers, Uganda possesses one of the largest fresh-water fisheries in the world. In 1988 fish production was 214,700 tonnes of which 50% came from Lake Victoria. Fish farming (especially carp and tilapia) is a growing industry.

FOREIGN ECONOMIC RELATIONS

Commerce. In 1987 imports were US$605·5m. and exports, US$319·4m.

Total trade between Uganda and UK (British Department of Trade returns, in £1,000 sterling):

	1986	*1987*	*1988*	*1989*	*1990*
Imports to UK	50,870	37,076	30,487	20,985	12,124
Exports and re-exports from UK	26,046	38,545	35,340	39,218	39,506

Tourism. There were 35,000 tourists in 1986.

COMMUNICATIONS

Roads. There were (1985) 7,582 km of all-weather roads maintained by the Ministry of Works, of which 1,934 km are two-lane bitumenized highways, and some 19,640 km of other roads, maintained by district governments.

Railways. In Aug. 1977 Uganda Railways was formed following the break-up of the East African Railways administration. The network totals 1,286 km (metre gauge). In 1989 railways carried 1·5m. passengers and 453,000 tonnes of freight.

Aviation. The International Airport, at Entebbe, has direct flights to Europe, Zimbabwe, Sudan, Kenya, Burundi, Ghana, Ethiopia, Zaïre, Nigeria, USSR, and Rwanda by Sudan Airways, Air Congo, SABENA, Air France, Ethiopian Airlines, Air Zaïre and Aeroflot. Eleven other government airfields are used for internal communications.

Posts and Broadcasting. There were 54,400 telephones in use in 1983. There were 600,000 radio receivers and about 90,000 television sets in 1986.

Newspapers. There were 5 daily newspapers in 1989 with a circulation of 35,000.

JUSTICE, RELIGION, EDUCATION AND WELFARE

Justice. The High Court of Uganda, presided over by the Chief Justice and 15 puisne judges, exercises original and appellate jurisdiction throughout Uganda.

Subordinate courts, presided over by Chief Magistrates and Magistrates of the first, second and third grade, are established in all areas: Jurisdiction varies with the grade of Magistrate. Chief and first-grade Magistrates are professionally qualified; second- and third-grade Magistrates are trained to diploma level at the Law School, Entebbe. Chief Magistrates exercise supervision over and hear appeals from second- and third-grade courts.

The Supreme Court of Uganda hears appeals from the High Court.

Religion. About 62% of the population are Christian and 6% Moslem.

Education. In 1989 there were 2,633,764 pupils in 7,905 primary schools (of which 7,420 were Government-aided schools and 485 private schools); 240,334 students in 774 secondary schools; 13,174 students in 94 primary teacher training colleges; 3,208 students in 24 technical institutes; 1,819 students in 10 national teachers colleges; 1,009 students in technical colleges; 1,628 students in 5 colleges of commerce; 1,037 students in the Institute of Teacher Education, Kyambogo; 504 students in the Uganda Polytechnic, Kyambogo; 800 students in the National College of Business Studies, Nakawa; 5,565 students in Makerere University, Kampala; 163 in the Islamic University, Mbale; 50 students in the University of Science and Technology, Mbarara. There are also 3 agricultural colleges, 1 forestry college, 1 fisheries institute, 1 land survey school and training institutes under different ministries which offer pre-service courses in different fields.

Health. In 1989 there were 81 hospitals and 20,136 hospital beds. The Ministry of Health has 16 schools for training nurses, midwives, medical assistants, environmental and laboratory personnel, and other health staff, 105 health centres, 89 dispensaries with maternity units, 87 dispensaries, 35 maternity units, 371 subdispensaries, 14 leprosy centres and 169 aid posts.

DIPLOMATIC REPRESENTATIVES

Of Uganda in Great Britain (Uganda Hse., Trafalgar Sq., London, WC2N 5DX)
High Commissioner: Prof. George Kirya.

Of Great Britain in Uganda (10/12 Parliament Ave., Kampala)
High Commissioner: Charles A. K. Cullimore.

Of Uganda in the USA (5909 16th St., NW, Washington, D.C., 20011)
Ambassador: Stephen K. Katenta Apuuli.

Of the USA in Uganda (Parliament Ave., Kampala)
Ambassador: John A. Burroughs Jr.

Of Uganda to the United Nations
Ambassador: Perezi Karukubiro Kamunanwire.

Further Reading

Collison, R. L., *Uganda.* [Bibliography] Oxford and Santa Barbara, 1981
Jørgensen, J. J., *Uganda: A Modern History.* London, 1981

UNION OF SOVIET SOCIALIST REPUBLICS

Capital: Moscow
Population: 290·1m. (1991)

Soyuz Sovetskikh Sotsialisticheskikh Respublik

HISTORY. For the 1917 revolution *see* THE STATESMAN'S YEAR-BOOK, 1990–91, p. 1223.

On 25 Jan. 1918 the third All-Russian Congress of Soviets proclaimed Russia a Republic of Soviets (i.e. councils) of Workers', Soldiers' and Peasants' Deputies; and on 10 July 1918 the fifth Congress adopted a Constitution for the Russian Soviet Federal Socialist Republic (RSFSR). In the course of the ensuing civil war Soviet Republics were set up in the Ukraine, Belorussia and Transcaucasia. These first entered into treaty relations with the RSFSR and then, on 30 Dec. 1922, joined with it to form the Union of Soviet Socialist Republics (USSR).

AREA AND POPULATION. The area of the USSR in April 1990 was 22·4m. sq. km (8·65m. sq. miles). The census population on 15 Jan. 1970 was 241·7m. (111·4m. males, 130·3m. females; 136m. urban, 105·7m. rural). The census population on 12 Jan. 1989 was 286·7m. (135·5m. males, 151·2m. females, 188·8m. urban, 97·9m. rural). The increase of 25·2m. in urban population between 1979 and 1989 was due to natural increase (14·6m.) and migration from rural areas and the urbanization of large rural centres (10·6m.). Consequently, despite a natural increase in rural areas, there was a net decrease of 0·9m. over this period.

In 1989 workers (in industry and state-owned agriculture) accounted for 58·8% of total population, collective farmers for 11·7%, office workers for 29·3% and others (including the self-employed and clerics) for 20·2%.

The areas (in 1,000 sq. km) and population (in 1m., in Jan. 1990) of the constituent republics are as follows (capitals in brackets):

Constituent Republics	*Area*	*Population*	*Constituent Republics*	*Area*	*Population*
RSFSR (Moscow)	17,075	148·0	Tadzhikistan (Dushanbe)	143	5·3
Ukraine (Kiev)	604	51·8	Kirgizia (Frunze)	199	4·4
Uzbekistan (Tashkent)	447	20·3	Lithuania (Vilnius)	65	3·7
Kazakhstan (Alma-Ata)	2,717	16·7	Armenia (Yerevan)	30	3·3
Belorussia (Minsk)	208	10·3	Turkmenistan (Ashkhabad)	488	3·6
Azerbaijan (Baku)	87	7·1	Latvia (Riga)	64	2·7
Georgia (Tbilisi)	70	5·5	Estonia (Tallinn)	45	1·6
Moldavia (Kishinev)	34	4·4			

Nationalities. The most numerous nationalities at the 1989 census were: 145·2m. Russians, 44·2m. Ukrainians, 16·7m. Uzbeks, 10m. Belorussians, 8·1m. Kazakhs, 6·8m. Azerbaijanians, 6·6m. Tatars, 4·6m. Armenians, 4m. Georgians, 3·4m. Moldavians, 4·2m. Tajiks, 3m. Lithuanians, 2·7m. Turkmenians, 2·5m. Kirghiz, 2m. Germans, 1·8m. Chuvashes, 1·5m. Latvians, 1·5m. Bashkirs, 1·4m. Jews, 1·2m. Mordovians, 1·1m. Poles, 1m. Estonians. The great majority (in each case 71-99%) indicated the language of their nationality as their native tongue; exceptions were the Mordovians (67%), Germans (49%), Poles (31%) and Jews (11%).

The following tables show the growth of the population:

1897 (Russian Empire)	126,900,000	1959 (census)	208,826,650
1913 (Russian Empire)	170,900,000	1970 (census)	241,720,134
1913 (present frontiers)	159,153,000	1979 (census)	262,436,227
1939 (census)	170,557,093	1989 (census)	286,717,000

The following was the population on 1 Jan. 1989 of the larger towns (in 1,000):

Astrakhan	509	Krasnodar	620	Rostov-on-Don	1,020
Baku	1,757	Krasnoyarsk	912	Ryazan	515
Barnaul	602	Krivoi Rog	713	Samara	1,257
Bishbek	616	Leningrad	5,020	Saratov	905
Chelyabinsk	1,143	Lvov	790	Sverdlovsk	1,367
Dnepropetrovsk	1,179	Minsk	1,589	Tashkent	2,073
Donetsk	1,110	Moscow	8,967	Togliatti	630
Dushanbe	595	Naberezhnye Chelny	501	Tomsk	502
Gomel	500	Nikolaev	503	Tula	540
Irkutsk	626	Nizhni Novgorod	1,438	Ufa	1,083
Izhevsk	635	Novokuznetsk	600	Ulyanovsk	625
Karaganda	614	Novosibirsk	1,436	Vilnius	582
Kazan	1,094	Odessa	1,115	Vladivostok	648
Kemerovo	520	Omsk	1,148	Volgograd	999
Khabarovsk	601	Orenburg	547	Voronezh	887
Kharkov	1,611	Penza	543	Yaroslavl	633
Kiev	2,587	Perm	1,091	Yerevan	1,199
Kishinev	565	Riga	915	Zaporozhye	884

Narodnoe khozyaistvo SSSR. Moscow, annual
Naselenie SSSR. Moscow, annual
Sovetskii Soyuz. Geograficheskoe opisanie, 22 vols. Moscow, 1966–72
Cole, J. P., *Geography of the Soviet Union*. London, 1984
Howe, G. Melvyn, *The Soviet Union: a Geographical Survey* (2nd ed.). London, 1983
Symons, L., (ed.) *The Soviet Union: a Systematic Geography*. London, 1983
Wixman, R., *The Peoples of Russia and the USSR*. London, 1984

CLIMATE. The USSR comprises several different climatic regions, ranging from polar conditions in the north, through sub-arctic and humid continental, to sub-tropical and semi-arid conditions in the south. Rainfall amounts are greatest in areas bordering the Baltic, Black Sea, Caspian Sea and eastern coasts of Asiatic Russia. In most cases, there is a summer maximum.

Moscow. Jan. 15°F (–9·4°C), July 65°F (18·3°C). Annual rainfall 25·2" (630 mm). Arkhangelsk. Jan. 5°F (–15°C), July 57°F (13·9°C). Annual rainfall 20·1" (503 mm). Kiev. Jan. 21°F (–6·1°C), July 68°F (20°C). Annual rainfall 22" (554 mm). Leningrad. Jan. 17°F (–8·3°C), July 64°F (17·8°C). Annual rainfall 19·5" (488 mm). Vladivostok. Jan. 6°F (–14·4°C), July 65°F (18·3°C). Annual rainfall 24" (599 mm).

CONSTITUTION AND GOVERNMENT. The Union of Soviet Socialist Republics (USSR) was formed by the union of the Russian Soviet Federal Socialist Republic (RSFSR), the Ukrainian Soviet Socialist Republic (Ukrainian SSR), the Belorussian SSR and the Transcaucasian SSR; the Treaty of Union was adopted by the first Soviet Congress of the USSR on 30 Dec. 1922. In Oct. 1924 the Uzbek and Turkmen Autonomous SSRs and in Dec. 1929 the Tajik Autonomous SSR were declared constituent republics of the USSR.

On 5 Dec. 1936 a new constitution was adopted. The Transcaucasian Republic was split into the Armenian SSR, the Azerbaijan SSR and the Georgian SSR, each of which became constituent republics of the USSR. The Kazakh SSR and the Kirghiz SSR, previously autonomous republics within the RSFSR, also became constituent republics.

In Sept. 1939 Soviet troops occupied Poland to the 'Curzon line', which in 1919 had been drawn on ethnographical grounds as the eastern frontier of Poland, and incorporated it into the Ukrainian and Belorussian SSRs. In Feb. 1951 some districts of the Drogobych Region of the Ukraine and the Lublin Voivodship of Poland were exchanged.

On 31 March 1940 territory ceded by Finland was joined to that of the Autonomous SSR of Karelia to form the Karelo-Finnish SSR, which was admitted into the Union as the 12th Union Republic, but downgraded to the status of an Autonomous Republic within the the RSFSR in 1956.

On 2 Aug. 1940 the Moldavian SSR was constituted as the 13th Union Republic. It comprised the former Moldavian Autonomous SSR and Bessarabia (44,290 sq. km, ceded by Romania on 28 June 1940), except for the districts of Khotin,

Akerman and Ismail, which, together with Northern Bukovina (10,440 sq. km), were incorporated in the Ukrainian SSR. The Soviet-Romanian frontier thus constituted was confirmed by the peace treaty with Romania, signed on 10 Feb. 1947. On 29 June 1945 Ruthenia (Sub-Carpathian Russia, 12,742 sq. km) was by treaty with Czechoslovakia incorporated into the Ukrainian SSR.

On 3, 5 and 6 Aug. 1940 Lithuania, Latvia and Estonia were incorporated in the USSR as the 14th, 15th and 16th Union Republics respectively.

After the defeat of Germany in 1945 it was agreed by the UK, the USA and the USSR (by the Potsdam declaration) that part of East Prussia should be embodied in the USSR. The area (11,655 sq. km), which includes the town of Königsberg (renamed Kaliningrad) was joined to the RSFSR in April 1946.

By the peace treaty with Finland, signed on 10 Feb. 1947, the province of Petsamo (Pechenga), ceded to Finland on 14 Oct. 1920 and 12 March 1946, was returned to the USSR. On 19 Sept. 1955 the USSR renounced its treaty rights to the naval base of Porkkala-Udd.

In 1945, after the defeat of Japan, the southern half of Sakhalin (36,000 sq. km) and the Kurile Islands (10,200 sq. km) were, by agreement with the Allies, incorporated in the USSR. This is still a matter of contention with Japan.

According to the 1977 Constitution the USSR is a socialist state of the whole people, the political units of which are the Soviets (Councils) of People's Deputies. All central and local authority is vested in these Soviets. The economic foundation of the USSR is the socialist system of economy and the socialist ownership of the means of production. There are two forms of socialist property: (1) state property (property of the whole people); (2) co-operative and collective farm (*kolkhoz*) property (property of individual collective farms and property of co-operative associations). The land, mineral deposits, waters, forests, mills, factories, mines, railways, water and air transport, banks, means of communication, state farms (*sovkhozy*), as well as municipal enterprises and the principal dwelling-house properties in the cities and industrial localities, are state property, but the land occupied by collective farmers is secured to them in perpetuity so long as they use it in accordance with the laws of the country. The members of the *kolkhozy* may have small plots of land attached to their dwellings for their own use. Peasants unwilling to enter a kolkhoz may retain their individual farms, but they are not allowed to employ hired labour. The right of personal property of citizens in their income from work and in their savings, in their dwellings and domestic and personal effects, as well as the right of inheritance of such property, are protected by law. The constitution recognizes the right of all citizens to work, rest, leisure, education, health protection, housing, maintenance in old age, sickness or incapacity, without distinction of sex, race or nationality, and lays down that any direct or indirect restriction of the rights of, or conversely, the establishment of direct or indirect privileges for, citizens on account of their race, or nationality, as well as the advocacy of racial or national exclusiveness, or hatred or contempt, is punishable by law. The franchise is enjoyed by all citizens of the USSR who have reached the age of 18, irrespective of sex, with the exception of the legally certified insane or incompetent or those serving terms of imprisonment. Candidates for election as a People's Deputy of the USSR must be 21 years of age; for sub-national levels of government the minimum age for candidates is 18. A member of any Soviet may be recalled by a majority of electors.

The USSR consists of 15 Union Republics, each inhabited by a major nationality which gives its name to the republic. These are divided into 120 territories and regions, and these again into 3,217 districts, 2,200 towns, 603 urban districts and 4,042 urban settlements (1 Jan. 1990). Within the districts there are 43,095 rural Soviets (usually each including a number of villages). The territories and regions also include a number of smaller nationalities, forming their own self-governing units– 20 Autonomous Soviet Socialist Republics, 8 Autonomous Regions and 10 Autonomous Areas.

In 1990 the Fourth Congress of People's Deputies approved the outlines of a new 'union treaty' whose more detailed provisions remained to be negotiated.

A referendum was scheduled for 17 March 1991 on the desirability of maintaining the USSR as a reformed federation of equal sovereign republics.

Under amended constitutional provisions which came into effect in Dec. 1988 the highest body of state authority of the USSR is the *Congress of People's Deputies* of the USSR (for earlier arrangements see THE STATESMAN'S YEAR-BOOK, 1989-90, pp. 1226–27). The Congress is exclusively empowered to adopt and amend the Constitution and to determine the national and state structure of the USSR; it also establishes the 'guidelines of the domestic and foreign policies of the USSR', including long-term state plans and programmes (Art. 108). The Congress consists of 2,250 deputies, 750 of whom are elected by territorial electoral districts with equal numbers of voters, and 750 of whom are elected by national-territorial electoral districts (32 from each union republic, 11 from each autonomous republic, 5 from each autonomous region and 1 from each autonomous area). A further 750 deputies are elected by public organizations including the Communist Party and the trade unions on the basis of the Law on Elections of the People's Deputies of the USSR, which was also approved in Dec. 1988. Regular sessions of the Congress of People's Deputies are convened at least once a year; the first, following elections in March 1989, met from 25 May to 9 June 1989. At those elections 89·8% of the registered electorate were reported to have voted and 1,958 deputies were returned, 87·6% of whom were members or candidate members of the CPSU; 18·6% were industrial workers, 11·2% were collective farmers, and 17·1% were women. The vacancies that remained were subsequently filled at repeat votes (*povtornoe golosovanie*) or repeat elections (*povtornye vybory*), which under the electoral law must be held within 2 months of the original elections.

The powers of the Congress of People's Deputies also include the election of the Chairman of the USSR Supreme Soviet and the endorsement of the chairman of the Cabinet of Ministers, the chairman of the Supreme Court, the Procurator-General and the chairman of the Supreme Court of Arbitration. The Congress, by secret ballot from among its members, elects a 542-member *Supreme Soviet* of the USSR, which is described in the Constitution as the 'permanent legislative, and control body of state authority of the USSR' (Art. 111). The USSR Supreme Soviet consists of 2 chambers, the Soviet of the Union and the Soviet of Nationalities, each of which has equal numbers of deputies and equal powers. The Soviet of the Union (chairman, I. D. Laptev) is elected from among deputies representing territorial districts and public organizations, taking into account the size of the electorate in the republic or region in question. The Soviet of Nationalities (chairman, R. N. Nishanov) is elected by deputies representing national-territorial districts and public organizations, on the basis of 11 from each union republic, 4 from each autonomous republic, 2 from each autonomous region and 1 from each autonomous area. One-fifth of the members of the Soviet of the Union and the Soviet of Nationalities are re-elected annually by the Congress of People's Deputies.

The Supreme Soviet is convened by its Presidium for spring and autumn sessions which last, 'as a rule', 3 or 4 months each. Special sessions may also be convened. The Supreme Soviet, under the Constitution (Art. 113), approves the appointment of the Prime Minister and other members of the Cabinet of Ministers on the nomination of the President. It approves nominations to the Security Council of the USSR and the Soviet high command, deals with national-level policy on economic, financial, social and cultural questions, approves the state plan and budget, ratifies and denounces international treaties and authorizes the deployment of Soviet armed forces further to those obligations. In addition to commissions attached to each chamber, the USSR Supreme Soviet establishes the following committees: International affairs; defence and state security; legislation and legality; the Soviets and self-management; economic reform; agrarian questions and food; construction and architecture; science, education, culture and upbringing; public health; women, the family, motherhood and childhood; veterans and invalids; youth; ecology and the rational use of natural resources; and *glasnost'* (openness) and communications from citizens.

The *Presidium* of the USSR Supreme Soviet is headed by the chairman of the USSR Supreme Soviet, who is elected from among the deputies by secret ballot for a maximum of 2 5-year terms. It includes the chairmen of the Soviet of the Union and the Soviet of Nationalities and their deputies, the chairmen of the standing commissions and committees, 1 further deputy from each union republic, 2 representatives of the autonomous republics, and 1 representative of the autonomous regions and areas. The Presidium, under the Constitution (Art. 118), is responsible for preparing for sessions of the Congress and of the Supreme Soviet; it co-ordinates the work of the commissions and committees, and organizes nationwide discussion of draft laws and 'other vital state issues'. The Presidium, additionally, is responsible for the publication of the laws and other acts of the Congress, Supreme Soviet and President.

The office of *President* was established for the first time by the Third Congress of People's Deputies in March 1990. The President, under the Constitution (Art. 127), is the 'head of the Soviet state'. Any Soviet citizen between the ages of 35 and 65 may be elected to the post for a maximum of 2 terms. The President is elected for 5 years by universal, direct and secret ballot; the election is valid if at least half of those entitled to vote exercise their rights. To secure election a candidate must obtain more than 50% of the votes cast, 'in the USSR overall and in a majority of the union republics'. The President represents the USSR nationally and internationally; he nominates the prime minister and members of the Cabinet of Ministers, chairs the Security Council of the USSR, and heads a Council of the Federation which is responsible for the co-ordination of state institutions and nationality matters. On 16 March 1990 Mikhail Gorbachev was elected President (exceptionally, by the Congress of People's Deputies rather than a nationwide ballot).

The *USSR Cabinet of Ministers* was formed in Dec. 1990, replacing the former Council of Ministers. According to the Constitution (Art. 128), it is an 'executive and administrative organ' subordinate to the President of the USSR. The Cabinet consists of a Prime Minister, his deputies and ministers. Its composition is approved by the Supreme Soviet on the proposal of the President. The heads of government of the union republics are also full members. The Cabinet of Ministers is responsible both to the President and to the USSR Supreme Soviet. A newly formed Cabinet presents a programme of the action it proposes to the Supreme Soviet, and accounts for its work at least once a year. The Cabinet must resign if the Supreme Soviet adopts a vote of no confidence in its activity by a two-thirds majority. The Cabinet of Ministers is empowered to deal with all matters of state administration that do not fall within the competence of other bodies. In practice this includes the conduct of a wide variety of government business, including economic management, foreign relations, defence and social welfare.

Soon after the adoption of the 1936 Constitution the constituent republics adopted their own constitutions based in all essentials upon the Constitution of the Union but adapted where necessary to local requirements. In April 1978 the Supreme Soviets of the Union Republics similarly adopted new republican constitutions based upon the new Constitution of the USSR approved by the Supreme Soviet in Oct. 1977. Article 73 of the 1977 Constitution of the USSR reserves to the central government the spheres of war and peace, diplomatic relations, defence, foreign trade, state security, economic planning, education, the basic principles of legislation, and other matters of 'all-Union significance'. The right of the constituent republics to withdraw from the Union is, however, formally recognized in Article 72, and (after a referendum and other formalities) by a law on secession of 1990. Union Republics have their own Congresses of People's Deputies, Supreme Soviets, Presidiums and Councils of Ministers, and exercise a wide range of devolved powers in local matters.

There are 20 Autonomous Republics in the USSR, which are similarly governed by their own Congresses of People's Deputies, Supreme Soviets, Presidiums and Councils of Ministers exercising devolved powers over local matters. Most (16) are in the RSFSR; 2 are in Georgia and 1 each in Azerbaijan and Uzbekistan. Five Autonomous Regions are in the RSFSR, 1 each in Azerbaijan, Georgia, and Tajikistan. All 10 Autonomous Areas are in the RSFSR. Elections are held every five years to the Supreme Soviets of Union and Autonomous Republics. At elections in Feb. 1985, 10,190 deputies were elected; 3,830 (37·6%) were women, 3,495 (34·3%) were non-Party, 3,605 (35·4%) were industrial workers and 1,557 (15·3%) were collective farmers. Further elections were held in 1989–90.

Regions and territories, districts, towns and rural areas are similarly governed by their own Soviets, elected for a term of 2½ years. At the June 1987 elections, 2,321,766 deputies were elected to these Soviets; 1,146,329 (49·4%) were women, 1,317,009 (56·7%) were non-Party, 976,552 (42·1%) were industrial workers and 562,052 (24·2%) were collective farmers. In 162 districts elections were conducted, as an experiment, with more candidates nominated than seats available. On 1 Jan. 1988 there were 52,602 rural and urban Soviets in the USSR with 2·3m. deputies and over 30m. voluntary co-opted members participating in the work of their standing committees.

On 24 Sept. 1990 the Supreme Soviet granted President Gorbachev, by 305 votes to 36, authority to rule by decree until 31 March 1992 in matters affecting the economy and public order.

State flag: Red, with sickle and hammer in gold in the upper corner near the staff, and above them a 5-pointed star bordered in gold.

National anthem: Soyuz nerushimy respublik svobodnykh ('Indestructible union of free republics'; words by S. Mikhalkov and G. El-Registan; music by A. V. Aleksandrov; 1944, revised 1977).

President of the USSR: M. S. Gorbachev.

Vice-President: Gennadi Yanaev.

Chairman of the USSR Supreme Soviet: A. I. Lukyanov.

Secretary of the Presidium: Tengiz Menteshashvili.

Chairman of the Cabinet of Ministers of the USSR (Prime Minister): Valentin Pavlov (b. 1947).

First Vice-Chairman: V. S. Murakhovsky.

Minister of Defence: Marshal D. T. Yazov. *Minister of Foreign Economic Relations:* K. F. Katushev. *Minister for Foreign Affairs:* Aleksandr Bessmertnykh. *Minister of Internal Affairs:* B. K. Pugo. *Minister of Justice:* S. G. Lushchikov. *Chairman, State Security Committee (KGB):* V. A. Kryuchkov. *Chairman, State Planning Committee (Gosplan):* Yu. D. Maslyukov.

Communist Party of the Soviet Union (CPSU). According to the Rules adopted at the 28th Party Congress in 1990, the CPSU is a 'political organization uniting citizens of the USSR on a voluntary basis for the realization of its programmatic aims, based on all-human values and a communist perspective'. Following amendments to Article 6 of the Constitution of the USSR in March 1990 the CPSU no longer enjoys a guaranteed monopoly of power, but takes part with other parties in the formation of state policy and the administration of public and social affairs. The Party Programme adopted at the 27th Congress in 1986 is no longer operative; until a new Programme is approved by a future conference or congress the CPSU is guided by a programmatic declaration, 'Towards a humane, democratic socialism', which was adopted by the 28th Congress in 1990. This defines the CPSU as a party of the 'socialist option and communist perspective' and incorporates both a commitment to a 'humane, democratic socialism' and a series of more specific 'urgent anti-crisis measures'.

The Party is organized on the territorial-industrial principle. The supreme organ is the Party Congress. Ordinary congresses are convened not less than once every 5 years. The Congress elects a Central Committee which meets at least every 6 months to carry on the work of the Party between congresses. The Central Committee forms standing commissions to conduct its work on a more regular basis. In 1988 six such commissions were formed, dealing with ideology, party matters, socio-economic affairs, agriculture, international affairs and legal affairs. In 1990 further commissions were formed on women and the family, sociopolitical questions, the renewal of primary party organizations, science education and culture, and military policy. In the intervals between congresses the Central Committee may convene party conferences for the discussion of 'urgent questions of policy and practical activity'. The 19th Party Conference, the first since 1941, met in Moscow in June-July 1988.

The Central Committee forms a Political Bureau *(Politburo)*, which is responsible for 'political and organizational questions' during the intervals between its meetings. The Politburo includes the General Secretary, the Deputy General Secretary, the first secretaries of the 15 republican party organizations and such additional members as the Central Committee may approve. The Politburo, which is directed by the General Secretary, is required to account for its actions once a year to the Central Committee. The Central Committee also elects a Secretariat, directed by the Deputy General Secretary, and responsible for the implementation of party decisions, and a Central Control Commission, which is responsible for party discipline. Similar rules hold for the republican, regional and district levels of the party organization. Party branches, called Primary Party Organizations, exist in factories, state and collective farms, units of the Soviet armed forces, in villages, offices, educational establishments etc. where there are at least 3 Party members. There were 443,192 Primary Party Organizations in Jan. 1990.

The Central Committee elected by the 28th Congress in July 1990 consisted of 412 full members; candidate membership has been discontinued. The General Secretary, who is elected by the Congress, is an *ex officio* member of the Central Committee, and so too is the Deputy General Secretary. At the 28th Congress M. S. Gorbachev and V. A. Ivashko respectively were elected General Secretary and Deputy General Secretary.

The Politburo in March 1991 consisted of: M. S. Gorbachev *(General Secretary)*, V. A. Ivashko *(Deputy General Secretary)*, L. E. Annus, M. M. Burokjavičius, A. S. Dzasokhov, I. T. Frolov, S. I. Gurenko, I. A. Karimov, P. K. Luchinsky, K. Makhkamov, A. A. Malofeev, A. M. Masaliev, A. N. Mutalibov, N. A. Nazarbaev, S. A. Niyazov, S. K. Pogosyan, I. K. Polozkov, Yu. A. Prokofyev, A. P. Rubiks, G. V. Semenova, O. S. Shenin, E.-A. A. Sillari and E. S. Stroev.

The Secretariat consisted of: M. S. Gorbachev *(General Secretary);* V. A. Ivashko *(Deputy General Secretary);* the following Secretaries: O. D. Baklanov, A. S. Dzasokhov, V. M. Falin, B. V. Gidaspov, A. N. Girenko, A. Kuptsov, P. K. Luchinsky, Yu. A. Manaenkov, G. V. Semenova, O. S. Shenin, E. S. Stroev; and the following members of the Secretariat: V. V. Aniskin, V. A. Gaivoronsky, I. I. Mel'nikov, A. I. Teplenichev and G. Turgunova.

Chairman of the Central Control Commission: Vacant.

Chairman of the Central Auditing Commission: G. F. Sizov.

In Jan. 1990 the Communist Party had 19,228,217 members (about 9% of the adult population). Of these, 28·2% were classified as workers, 7·8% as collective farmers and 44·3% as office workers; the remainder were students, pensioners, housewives, etc. Women accounted for 30·2% of the membership, and Russians for 59·3%. The party's youth wing, the Komsomol (All-Union Leninist Communist Union of Youth), had 36m. members in 1989. V. Zyukin was re-elected First Secretary of its Central Committee at its 21st Congress in 1990.

Istoriya Kommunisticheskoi partii Sovetskogo Soyuza, 7th ed. Moscow, 1985
KPSS v rezolyutsiyakh i resheniyakh s''ezdov, konferentsii i plenumov TsK, 9th ed., vol. 1ff. Moscow, 1983ff.
Resolutions and Decisions of the Communist Party of the Soviet Union, ed. R. H. McNeal, 5 vols. Toronto, 1974–82
Spravochnik partiinogo rabotnika. Moscow, annual
Izvestiya Tsk KPSS. Moscow, monthly
Hill, R. and Frank, P., *The Soviet Communist Party.* 3rd ed., London, 1987
Schapiro, L. B., *The Communist Party of the Soviet Union.* 2nd ed., London, 1970
White, S. (ed.) *Soviet Communism: Programme and Rules.* London, 1989

DEFENCE. Overall supervision of defence and security matters is exercised by the Defence Council of the USSR, headed by the General Secretary of the CPSU.

About 90% of the officers of the armed forces are members of the Communist Party or Young Communist League, and 50% have had an engineering and technical education.

Since 1989 it has been declared Soviet policy to reduce the size of the armed forces, to take part in international arms control negotiations and to adopt a more defensive operational stance. The Warsaw Pact has ceased to function as a military alliance, and Soviet troops have been withdrawn from some countries abroad. Conscription is for 2 years (3 years for sea-going naval personnel).

Total strength of the armed forces was 3,988,000 in 1991, with a probable 55m. reserves and a further 230,000 Committee of State Security (KGB) troops (167,000 conscripts).

Declared budgetary expenditure on defence (in 1m. rubles) for 1987, 26,600. Estimate for 1991: 96,562.

Army. The Army is thought to consist of 53 tank, 153 motor rifle, 7 airborne and 18 artillery divisions; 10 air assault brigades; and various independent tank, artillery, missile and engineer units. Equipment includes some 19,000 T-54/-55, 9,700 T-64, 10,000 T-720/L/-M and 4,000 T-80 main battle tanks, and 1,000 PT-76 light tanks. Strength (1991), 1,473,000 (1·1m. conscripts).

There are 5 operational rocket armies deploying 1,398 intercontinental ballistic missiles (SS-11,-13,-17,-18,-19-24,-25). Intermediate range ballistic missiles (SS-20) number 174, but are due to be eliminated in accordance with the Intermediate-Range Nuclear Forces Treaty. There are a further 112 medium range ballistic missiles, but these are being phased out. Personnel number 260,000, with reserves of 537,000.

Navy. There are signs that Soviet defence budget cuts are having an impact on Naval new construction, but the Fleet is still steadily and progressively modernizing and its overall combat capability has been maintained. The scrapping of older ships, particularly submarines, is now in full swing, and may be expected to continue for several years.

The wartime tasks of the Soviet Navy are largely defensive in strategic terms. The safe deployment and protection of the large force of strategic missile-firing submarines is the first priority; the defence of the Soviet homeland, in particular against the threat of sudden attack, the second; whilst interdiction of enemy shipping and protection of own shipping take lower priority.

Peacetime command of the Soviet Navy (with the exception of the missile submarines which form part of the Strategic Nuclear Force) is exercised by the Main Naval Staff in Moscow, through the Commanders of the 4 fleets into which the Navy is divided. The 4 fleets comprise the Northern Fleet (HQ Severomorsk), Baltic Fleet (HQ Kaliningrad), Black Sea Fleet (HQ Sevastopol) and the Pacific Fleet (HQ Vladivostok). The Northern and Pacific fleets are markedly stronger than the others, partly because strategic submarines are only deployed in their areas. All the operational aircraft carriers, and the 3 large cruisers of the Kirov class are deployed with these major fleets. Detached squadrons, found from the regional fleets, are deployed on a rotational basis into the Mediterranean Sea and Indian Ocean. A small flotilla of frigates and amphibious ships is also maintained in the Caspian Sea.

The overall strength of the Soviet Navy at the end of the indicated year was as follows:-

Category	*1985*	*1986*	*1987*	*1988*	*1989*	*1990*
Strategic Submarines	77	77	76	75	64	61
Nuclear Attack Submarines	121	118	127	127	130	104
Diesel Submarines	148	145	140	136	133	86
Aircraft Carriers	3	4	4	4	5	5
Cruisers	44	42	43	44	44	40
Destroyers	66	57	59	54	45	32
Frigates	175	167	168	166	171	148

In the tables and listings which follow, it should be noted that, in the west, Soviet ship classes and weapons are generally known by their official NATO nicknames. These may be recognized as follows: Surface ships are given names with an initial letter 'K' *e.g. Kynda*, *Kresta*, and submarines by letters from the phonetic alphabet, *e.g. Alfa*, *Kilo*. Surface-to-air missiles are numbered in the SA-N- series, and given nicknames beginning with an initial 'G', *e.g. Goa*, surface-to-surface missiles are numbered SS-N-3 etc., and have nicknames commencing with 'S', fighter aircraft 'F', bombers 'B', and all helicopters 'H'. This practice is slowly being discarded as more information on Soviet ship classes and weapon names becomes known in the west.

The Soviet force of Strategic Submarines is constituted as follows:-

Class	*No.*	*Tonnage (in 1,000)*	*Speed*	*Missiles*	*Other Weapons*
Typhoon	6	27·00	27	20 SS-N-20	Torpedoes
Delta-IV	6	12·35	24	16 SS-N-23	Torpedoes
Delta-III	14	11·90	24	16 SS-N-18	Torpedoes
Delta-II	4	11·50	24	16 SS-N-8	Torpedoes
Delta-I	18	11·00	25	12 SS-N-8	Torpedoes
Yankee-II	1	9·75	26	12 SS-N-17	Torpedoes
Yankee-I	12	9·75	26	16 SS-N-6	Torpedoes

This wide range of submarine demonstrates the Soviet preference for making small, incremental changes in operational capability. Only with the Typhoon class, completed between 1982 and 1989, and the largest submarine ever built, was this approach dropped. The SS-N-20 'Sturgeon' missile carried by the Typhoon carries 6 warheads to a maximum range of 4,500 nautical miles, while the SS-N-23 'Skiff' in the other currently-building class, the 'Delta-IV', carries 10 warheads over the same range. The other older missiles carry one to 3 warheads over ranges varying between 1,300 and 4,000 nautical miles. The USSR has announced that all 'Golf-IIs' were withdrawn before the end of 1990. Of the 6 in service in mid-1989, 3 were disposed of by Jan. 1990 and the remainder have been de-activated subsequently.

The Soviet fleet of about 200 attack submarines again comprises a wide range of classes. From the enormous 16,250-tonne 'Oscar' nuclear-powered missile submarine to the small diesel 'Whiskey' of 1,370 tonnes, there are over 20 classes of submarine in service with the navy. The difficulties in training personnel to operate, and the technical and logistic complications supporting such a diverse mix are self-evident. The inventory of anti-ship missile-firing submarines comprises 6 'Oscar', built 1982-89, 24 SS-N-19 'Shipwreck' missiles; 6 'Charlie-II', built 1973-80, 8 SS-N-9; 9 'Charlie-I', 1967-72, 8 SS-N-7 'Starbright'; and 22 'Echo-II', 1961-67, 8 SS-N-3 'Shaddock' or SS-N-12 'Sandbox'. The former are all nuclear-propelled, and there are additionally 14 diesel-powered 'Juliet' class built between 1961 and 1968 carrying 4 SS-N-3. Finally, there are 2 former strategic 'Yankee'-class submarines converted to fire the SS-N-21 'Sampson' land-attack cruise missile, which has a range of 1,600 nautical miles. The list of torpedo-firing boats is equally impressive. The types currently building are the Akula, nuclear-powered and of 8,100 tonnes, of which there are 5, the 'Sierra', nuclear-powered, 7,700 tonnes now numbering 2, and the 'Victor-III', nuclear-powered, 6,400 tonnes, the total of which is now 24. The diesel-powered 'Kilo' class, of which the Soviet Navy operates 15, is also building at 3 to 4 per year, but the majority have been exported. In addition to these classes there are a further 73 nuclear-powered and 71 diesel submarines on the active list. The disposal of a number of old diesel and the first generation of nuclear-powered boats proceeded apace through 1990.

Modern Soviet surface warships are assigned categories rather different from western ships. Ships which, in the west, would be called 'Aircraft Carriers' are termed 'Large Aircraft-Carrying Cruisers' by the Soviet Navy partly because they usually carry significant ship weaponry as well as aircraft, but also to exempt them from the prohibition on the movement of Aircraft Carriers through the Turkish Straits imposed by the Montreux Convention. Ships of cruiser size (7,500-8,000 tonnes full load and upwards) are divided into two categories; those optimized for anti-submarine warfare (ASW) and those for anti-surface ship operations. Ships of cruiser size in the former category are classified as 'Large Anti-Submarine Ships' while the missile-armed anti-surface warfare ships are classified 'Rocket Cruisers'. The tables following listing the principal surface ships of the Soviet Navy use the most appropriate western classifications:-

Aircraft Carriers

Completed	*Name*	*Tonnage (in 1,000)*	*Speed*	*Aircraft*	*Other Armament*
1989	Adm. Kuznetsov (formerly Tbilisi)	65·0	30	See below	Anti-Ship Missiles Anti-Air missiles.

Completed	*Name*	*Tonnage (in 1,000)*	*Speed*	*Aircraft*	*Other Armament*
1987	Adm. Gorshkov (formerly Baku)	37·7	32	13 Yak-38 V/STOL 16 Ka-25/27 hel	12 anti-ship missiles 4 SA-N-6 SAM launchers
Kiev Class					
1982	Novorossiisk	37·7	32	13 Yak-38 V/STOL	8 anti-ship missiles.
1978	Minsk	37·7	32	16 Ka-25/27 hel	4 SA-N-3 SAM launchers
1976	Kiev	37·7	32		1 twin ASW missile.

Cruisers

Completed	*Name*	*Tonnage (in 1,000)*	*Speed*	*Main Armament*	*Aircraft*
Kirov Class					
1988 1984 1980	Kalinin Frunze Kirov	28·4	33	20 SS-N-19 anti-ship missiles, 12 X 8 SA-N-6 SAM, 2 SS-N-14 ASW missiles (*Kirov*) 2 100-mm guns (*Kirov*), 1 X 2 130-mm gun (*Frunze, Kalinin*)	2 Ka-27 Helix, 1 Ka-25 Hormone helicopters.
Moskva Class (Helicopter Cruisers).					
1968 1967	Leningrad Moskva	16·50	31	1 X 2 ASW missile launcher. 2 X 2 SA-N-3 SAM launchers.	14 Ka-25 ASW helos.
Slava Class.					
1988 1986 1983	Chervona Ukraina Marshal Ustinov Slava	12·70	34	16 SS-N-12 anti-ship missiles 8 X 8 SA-N-6 Grumble SAM. 8 533mm Torpedo tubes	1 Ka-27 Helix helicopter
Nikolayev (or 'Kara') Class.					
1979 1978 1977 1976 1975 1974 1973	Tallin Tashkent Petropavlovsk Azov Kerch Ochakov Nikolayev	9·85	34	8 SS-N-14 Silex ASW missiles 2 X 2 SA-N-3 Goblet SAM 10 X 533mm Torpedo tubes	1 Ka-25 Hormone ASW helicopter
Kronshtadt ('Kresta II') Class.					
1977 1976 1975 1974 1973 1973 1972 1971 1970 1969	Adm. Yumashev Vasily Chapayev Mar. Timoshenko Adm. Isachenkov Adm. Oktyabrsky Mar. Voroshilov Adm. Makarov Adm. Nakhimov Adm. Isakov Khronshtadt	7·83	35	8 SS-N-14 ASW missiles 2 X 2 SA-N-3 Goblet SAM 10 533mm Torpedo tubes	1 Ka-25 Hormone ASW helicopter
Admiral Zozulya ('Kresta I') Class.					
1969 1968 1968 1967	Sevastopol V-Adm. Drozd Vladivostok Adm. Zozulya	7·70	34	4 SS-N-3 Shaddock anti-ship missiles 2 X 2 SA-N-1 Goa SAM 10 533mm Torpedo tubes	1 Ka-25 Hormone ASW helicopter
Udaloy Class					
1990 1988 1988 1986 1985 1985 1984 1983	Adm. Kharlamov Adm. Vinograd Adm. Levchenko Simferopol Mar. Shaposhnikov Adm. Tributs Adm. Spiridonov Adm. Zakorov	8·60	30	8 SS-N-14 Silex ASW missiles, 2 X 100mm guns, 8 X 533mm Torpedo tubes	2 X Ka-27 Helix ASW helicopters.

Completed	*Name*	*Tonnage (in 1,000)*	*Speed*	*Main Armament*	*Aircraft*
Udaloy Class (continued)					
1983	Mar. Vasilevsky				
1981	V-Adm. Kulakov				
1980	Udaloy				

Trials of the new aircraft carrier *Adm. Kuznetsov* (formerly the *Tbilisi*) commenced in late 1989. This ship appears to be a unique hybrid between the conventional aircraft carrier equipped with catapults and arrester gear and vertical/short take-off and landing carriers without flight deck machinery. Initial flight trials show she launches aircraft over a ski-jump bow, and recovers them into arrester wires. It remains to be seen how effective this method is in terms of aircraft weapon and fuel loads at launch, and it will be some time before the ship can be considered fully operational. Aircraft used for the initial trials in Nov. 1989 were the Su-27 'Flanker', the MiG-29 'Fulcrum' and the Su-25 'Frogfoot'. These aircraft are potentially much more effective than the Yak-38 'Forger' deployed in the earlier carriers.

The 'Kara', 'Kresta II' and Udaloy classes tabled above are classified as 'Large anti-submarine warfare ships'. The Kirov, Slava and 'Kresta I' cruiser classes above, and the 'Kynda' guided missile destroyers below are classified as 'Rocket Cruisers'. The Kirov class, of which a fourth unit is fitting out, are the largest combatant warships, apart from aircraft carriers, to be built for any navy since the Second World War. The ships have an unusual and ingenious machinery arrangement. The main propulsion outfit comprises 2 nuclear reactors for long-range cruising, boosted by oil-fired superheat boilers for high-speed work. *Azov*, nominally of the 'Kara' class, has a different guided missile outfit to serve as trials ship for the armament of subsequent classes. Among the older ships, of the 24 Sverdlov class cruisers planned, 14 were completed in the 1950s, but they no longer remain in operational service and the scrapping programme is gaining momentum.

Among the smaller ships the most impressive are the 12 Sovremenny class guided missile destroyers, of 7,900 tonnes, armed with 8 SS-N-22 'Sunburn' anti-ship missiles, 1 twin SA-N-7 'Gadfly' surface-to-air missile launcher, 4 130mm guns and a helicopter. Also in the anti-surface category are the 4 Grozny (or 'Kynda') class of 5,650 tonnes, with 8 SS-N-3 'Shaddock' anti-ship missiles, and the 4 remaining 'modified Kashin' class. There are a further 10 'Kashin', and 1 other destroyer, 32 large frigates and 116 smaller frigates. An additional 50 or so frigates and above are maintained in inactive reserve. A formidable defence force is headed by 70 missile corvettes, 86 fast missile craft, 30 hydrofoil and 3 conventional fast torpedo craft and numerous patrol classes totalling 205 hulls. Mine warfare constitutes an important element of Soviet naval strategy; large stocks (some hundreds of thousands) of modern mines are held, and all submarines and many surface ship classes are provided with mine-laying equipment. There are additionally 3 specific minelayers, 65 offshore, 120 coastal and 140 inshore mine countermeasure vessels.

Amphibious capability is provided by 3 large dock landing ships of the Ivan Rogov class, 24 Ropucha and 14 Alligator class tank landing ships, 36 medium landing ships, as well as some 140 minor craft including about 85 special purpose amphibious surface-effect vessels. Total amphibious lift available to the Soviet authorities is some 17,000 men. 750 main battle tank equivalents but operating facilities for only 10 helicopters.

Amphibious landing forces are found from the Soviet Naval Infantry, 17,000 strong, units of which are assigned to all fleets. Organized into a single division, 7,000 strong, plus 3 independent brigades, the force is equipped to relatively light scales. Principal equipment includes 230 main battle tanks, 150 amphibious light tanks, 90 artillery pieces and over 1,000 armoured personnel carriers. A separate force of 7,500 Coastal Defence troops man artillery and missile batteries positioned to defend the main naval bases and ports. Controversy was caused in 1991 by the nominal transfer of over 20,000 men and some 800 tanks from the Army to the Coastal Defence commands, thus evading controls imposed by the Conventional Armed Forces in Europe treaty.

The operational reach of the Soviet Navy is however limited by its poor capability for afloat support. A first class multi-purpose underway replenishment ship, the *Berezina*, was completed in 1977, but remains the sole example of her class. There are an additional 6 dual-purpose stores and fuel replenishment ships, 4 purpose-built tankers, and 10 tankers converted from a commercial design with limited underway replenishment capability. Second line support is provided by 14 tankers, and about 260 maintenance and logistic ships, 67 electronic intelligence gatherers, 76 other special-purpose auxiliaries, and 250 survey, research and space support ships.

There are 5 warship building yards in and near Leningrad, yards on the Black Sea at Nikolayev, Kerch and Sevastopol, at Severodvinsk in the North Sea Fleet region and at Komsomolsk-on-Amur in the Far East. The shipbuilding programme is believed to include further 'Delta-IV' strategic submarines, and attack submarines of the Akula, 'Sierra', 'Victor-III' and 'Kilo' classes. There is a further aircraft carrier similar to the *Admiral Kuznetsov* fitting out, and a third, rather larger unit on the building ways. A fourth heavy cruiser of the Kirov class is nearing completion, as is the last of 4 Slava class. Further Udaloys are expected, and the first of a new class of large frigates is starting trials. The replacement of coastal force units built in the 1950s and early 1960s continues at a steady pace.

Shore-based naval aviation forms a major element of all Soviet Fleets. In addition to the aircraft held on inventory for seaborne service, there are some 270 bombers, 330 maritime patrol, 180 fighter/ground attack aircraft plus helicopters. Main bomber types held are 130 Tu-26 'Backfire', 125 Tu-16 'Badger' and 15 Tu-22 'Blinder', all of which are armed principally with stand-off anti-ship missiles. Maritime reconnaissance and anti-submarine tasks fall predominantly to the force of 80 Tu-95 and Tu-142 'Bear' with 200 miscellaneous shorter range aircraft tasked to anti-submarine operations, electronic countermeasures, intelligence gathering and tankers. The helicopter inventory amounts to some 320, principally anti-submarine, 25 combat assault, and 25 mine countermeasures. There are over 400 training and transport aircraft.

The total personnel in 1990 numbered 410,000, of whom 245,000 were conscripts who serve 3 years if in seagoing categories, and 2 years if shore-based. Of the total, some 16,000 serve in the strategic submarine force, 68,000 in naval aviation, 15,000 marines or naval infantry, and 7,500 in coastal defence.

Coastguard, customs and border patrol duties are performed by the substantial maritime element of the KGB. Some 23,000 strong, this force operates some 5 large helicopter-carrying frigates of a modified naval Krivak class, 12 small frigates, 7 offshore, 50 coastal and 165 inshore patrol craft divided among all the Soviet coastal areas.

Air Force. The Soviet Air Force (excluding the strategic bomber force and Voyska PVO air defence force) was believed to have a personnel strength, in 1990, of over 448,000 officers and men. To supplement long-range rocket missiles (estimated at 1,398 emplaced ICBM, 600 MRBM/IRBM), the strategic bomber force has still about 125 Tupolev Tu-95 ('Bear')[1] 4-turboprop bombers, 50 Myasishchev M-4 4-jet bombers and flight-refuelling tankers ('Bison'), 300 twin-jet Tupolev Tu-16 ('Badger'), and 135 supersonic Tupolev Tu-22 ('Blinder') bombers, ECM and reconnaissance aircraft, and at least 200 Tupolev ('Backfire') swing-wing bombers. All types are used also by the Naval Air Force for long-range maritime reconnaissance; the Tu-16, Tu-95, Tu-22 and 'Backfire' can carry air-to-surface guided self-propelled cruise missiles and all 5 types have provision for flight refuelling. A new swing-wing strategic Tupolev bomber ('Blackjack'), larger and faster than the American B-1, is entering service.

The tactical air forces, under local army command in the field, have an estimated total of 6,000 ground attack, air combat, ECM and reconnaissance aircraft, including 2,600 MiG-23/27 ('Flogger') and 800 two-seat Sukhoi Su-24 ('Fencer') supersonic swing-wing aircraft, 300 twin-jet Yakovlev Yak-28 ('Brewer') reconnaissance aircraft, 1,000 swing-wing Su-17 and Su-22 ('Fitter-C/D/G/H/J'), and 600 MiG-21 ('Fishbed') fighter-bombers, 340 Su-15 ('Flagon'), 200 MiG-25 ('Foxbat') and MiG-31 ('Foxhound') interceptors, and an increasing number of new

Su-25 ('Frogfoot') twin-engined ground attack aircraft supported by 60 MiG-21 and 170 MiG-25 ('Foxbat') reconnaissance aircraft, and over 3,500 helicopters, including very large Mi-26 ('Halo') transports and over 1,000 heavily-armed Mi-24 ('Hind') assault helicopters, in gunship/transport versions. Electronic warfare duties are performed by a variety of aircraft, including Yak-28s and Mi-8 and Mi-17 helicopters. The Voyska PVO defence forces, organized as a separate service, have a total of 1,300 jet interceptors. A high proportion of the squadrons are equipped with MiG-23 ('Flogger'), Su-15 ('Flagon'), MiG-25 ('Foxbat') and improved MiG-31 ('Foxhound') all-weather interceptors, armed with air-to-air missiles plus the MiG-29 ('Fulcrum') and Su-27 ('Flanker') new-generation aircraft now entering service. The twin-jet Yak-28P ('Firebar') and Tu-28P ('Fiddler') make up the balance of the force. Early warning and fighter-control duties are performed by about 10 radar-carrying adaptations of the Tu-114 turboprop transport, redesignated Tu-126 ('Moss'), which are being replaced by a more effective radar-equipped AWACS version ('Mainstay') of the Il-76 transport. Very large numbers of surface-to-air guided missiles are operational, on some 10,000 launchers, including the new high-performance SA-10 (low-altitude) and SA-12 (high-altitude) with capability against cruise and submarine-launched missiles respectively, the older 'Guild', 'Guideline', 'Goa', 'Gainful' and 'Ganef', the long-range 'Gammon' and the 'Galosh' which is deployed around Moscow on 32 launchers and has anti-missile capability.

Soviet Air Force transport squadrons have 150 An-12 ('Cub') 4-turboprop transports and 100 An-24s ('Coke') and An-26s ('Curl'), with 50 An-22s ('Cock'), and 400 Il-76 ('Candid') heavy four-jet freighters. The very large four-jet An-124 ('Condor') is entering service to replace the An-22. Training aircraft include the piston-engined Yak-18 primary trainer and its Yak-52 successor, the Czech-built L-29 Delfin and L-39 jet basic trainers and versions of operational types such as MiG-21, MiG-23, MiG-25, MiG-15, Su-7, Su-15, Su-17, Yak-28 and Tu-22.

[1] Soviet aircraft and missiles are usually referred to by invented English names; *see* p. 1233.

Naval Air Force. With 1,100 fixed-wing aircraft and helicopters, the Soviet Navy has the world's second largest naval air arm. Under the control of the various naval commands, *i.e.*, Baltic, Black Sea and Pacific, the Naval Air Arm has an estimated 220 Tu-16 ('Badger') twin-jet bombers, and 160 'Backfire' swing-wing bombers, able to carry air-to-surface missiles, 40 supersonic twin-jet Tu-22 ('Blinder') maritime reconnaissance aircraft, about 70 Su-17 ('Fitter') shore-based fighters, and 90 Beriev M-12 ('Mail') maritime patrol amphibians. For reconnaissance, anti-subarine and electronic warfare there are about 100 Tu-95 and Tu-142 ('Bear') 4-engined bombers, 90 Tu-16s, and a few Tu-22s, plus a small number of Il-20s ('Coot-A') and 60 Il-38s ('May'). The Tu-142 also has an important targeting rôle for ships fitted with anti-shipping missile launchers. Over 250 anti-submarine and missile targeting/guidance helicopters, notably the Ka-27 ('Helix') and Ka-25 ('Hormone'), are carried in naval vessels, including 4 aircraft carriers (which also operate Yak-36 ('Forger') vertical take-off attack/reconnaissance aircraft) and 2 helicopter carriers. Several hundred transport, flight refuelling tanker ('Badger'), utility and training fixed-wing aircraft and 100 Mi-14 ('Haze') shore-based ASW helicopters are also under Navy control.

Berman, H. J. and Kerner, M. (ed.) *Soviet Military Law and Administration.* 2 vols. Harvard Univ. Press, 1955

Moynahan, B., *The Claws of the Bear: A History of the Soviet Armed Forces from 1917 to the Present.* London, 1989

Scott, H. F. and Scott, W. F., *The Armed Forces of the USSR.* 2nd ed. Boulder, 1981

Smith, M. J., *The Soviet Navy, 1941–1978: A Guide to Sources in English.* Oxford and Santa Barbara, 1981

Suvorov, V., *The Liberators: The Soviet Army.* London, 1981

Watson, B. W., *Red Navy at Sea.* Boulder, 1982

INTERNATIONAL RELATIONS

Membership. The USSR is a member of the UN, OIEC and the Warsaw Pact, and an observer at GATT.

ECONOMY

Policy. Planning is based on public ownership in industry and trade, and on mixed public and collective (co-operative) ownership in agriculture. For planning history, 1920–85, *see* THE STATESMAN'S YEAR-BOOK, 1990–91, pp. 1237–38.

The 12th Five-Year Plan, adopted in 1986, placed its main emphasis upon raising living and cultural standards. The plan covers the period 1986–90 and up to the year 2000, by which time real living standards are planned to increase by 1·6 to 1·8 times; manual labour should account for no more than 15–20% of all productive work; state and co-operative retail trade should increase by 1·8 times; and health, educational and other social expenditure should double. Over the same period the national income should approximately double and industrial production more than double, entirely as a result of increased productivity, which is planned to increase by 2·3 to 2·5 times. Greater economy was to be achieved in the use of energy and natural resources; investment was to be concentrated in priority areas; and scientific-technical progress was to be accelerated and related more closely to production. Continued emphasis was placed upon the Energy Programme, the Food Programme and the Complex Programme for the Development of Consumer Goods and Services, which were adopted between 1982 and 1985. In the 5-year period 1986–90 national income was to increase by 22%, industrial production by 25%, labour productivity by 12–25%, and real incomes by 14%.

In 1990 national income produced decreased by 4% (1981–85 average increase, 3·2%), gross industrial production fell by 1·2% (1981–85 average increase, 3·6%) and agricultural production fell by 2·3% (1981–85 average increase, 2·7%).

Private small businesses were made legal in Aug. 1990, and a State Property Fund was set up to oversee the transformation of large state enterprises into joint-stock companies.

In Oct. 1990 the Supreme Soviet voted by 333 to 12 with 34 abstentions for a programme to reduce state control over the economy and cut government expenditure.

State prices for consumer goods and services were raised by an average of 60% in April 1991. Blanket compensation payments were introduced for wage-earners and pensioners.

Narodnoe khozyaistvo SSSR. Moscow, annual
Resheniya partii i pravitel'stva po khozyaistvennym voprosam. Vol. 1ff. Moscow, 1967ff
Istoriya sotsialisticheskoi ekonomiki SSSR. 7 vols. Moscow, 1976–80
Nove, A., *An Economic History of the USSR*. 2nd ed., Harmondsworth, 1989.—*The Soviet Economic System*. 3rd ed., London, 1986
US Congress, Joint Economic Committee, *Gorbachev's Economic Plans*. 2 vols. Washington D.C., 1987

Budget. Revenue and expenditure in 1m. rubles for calendar years:

	1985	*1988*	*1989*	*1990*
Revenue	390,603	378,900	401,900	452,000
Expenditure	386,469	459,500	482,600	510,100

Budgetary spending in 1989 on the economy was 201,500m. rubles, on sociocultural purposes and science 149,300m., on defence 75,200m. and on administration 2·9m.; the budgetary deficit was 80,700m. rubles (in 1985, 13·9m.).

Social insurance expenditure from the state budget accounted for 61,109m. rubles in 1989 (35,296m. in 1980). Of this 45,487m. rubles were allocated to pensions and 13,023m. to other forms of income support.

National income produced was assessed at 656,800m. rubles in 1989 (462,200m. in 1980); GNP in current prices was 924,000m. rubles in 1989 (619,000m. in 1980).

Capital investment (1989) was 228,500m. rubles, including 200,800m. by state and co-operative enterprises, 18,100m. by collective farms and 4,300m. by individuals (on housing). A 5% sales tax was introduced by presidential decree to take effect from 1 Jan. 1990; 70% of the revenue goes to the constituent republics.

Currency. The unit of currency is the *ruble* (SUR) of 100 *kopeks*. The official exchange rates (March 1991) 1·08 *rubles* = £1; 0·57 *rubles* = US$1.

The gold holdings of the USSR were, in Dec. 1955, estimated at about 200m. fine oz. (US$7,000m.), or about 20% of the world total of monetary gold.

The currency in circulation is: (1) State Bank notes in denominations of 10, 25, 50 and 100 *rubles;* (2) Treasury notes in denominations of 1, 3 and 5 *rubles;* (3) cupro-nickel coins in denominations of 10, 15, 20 and 50 *kopeks* and 1 *ruble*; (4) cupro-zinc coins in denominations of 1, 2, 3 and 5 *kopeks.*

50- and 100-ruble notes were withdrawn from circulation in Jan. 1991 to reduce speculation and curb inflation.

In Aug. 1990 it became legal for Soviet citizens to hold hard currency. In Jan. 1991 foreign currency exchanges were set up in major cities under the aegis of the State Bank.

Banking and Finance. The State Bank *(Gosbank)* began operations on 16 Nov. 1921. The State Bank (*Chairman:* Viktor Gerashchenko), in addition to short-term credits, effects long-term investments in agriculture and in individual rural house building. In 1988 it was reorganized into 5 departments: Savings; foreign economic relations; industry and construction; agricultural industry; housing. The Bank for Financing Capital Investments (*Stroibank*) covers industry, transport, urban housing schemes and public utilities and individual housebuilding in towns.

Deposits in 75,300 savings banks were over 337,800m. rubles to the credit of 208m. depositors at 1 Jan. 1990.

Weights and Measures. The metric system is in use. The Gregorian Calendar was adopted as from 14 Feb. 1918.

ENERGY AND NATURAL RESOURCES

Electricity. There were (1983) 57 fuel-burning power stations of over 1m. kw. capacity, and these account for over 80% of the country's electricity.

Hydro-electric stations have been constructed on major rivers. Among them are the Bratsk (4·5m. kw.), Ust-Ilimsk, Central Siberia (3·6m. kw.), Krasnoyarsk (6m. kw.) and a 1·26m. kw. station on the River Pechora (Far North).

Total installed capacity of power stations in 1938 was 8·7m. kw. and 341m. kw. in 1989. Industry consumes about 70% of the total electricity. Over 35,000 small rural power stations have been closed in recent years owing to supply from State stations becoming available, but there are still many operating in the countryside. 800 towns and urban settlements were heated by central thermal plants.

The world's first commercial nuclear power station in Obninsk, built in 1954, was followed by the Beloyarsk, Novo-Voronezh, Leningrad, Kursk, Chernobyl, Armenian and Shevchenko nuclear stations. Soviet nuclear power plants so far have standard slow 1m. kw. reactors, but a 1·5m. kw. reactor has now been designed. A fast reactor is functioning at Shevchenko.

The general design for a nuclear thermal station has been developed, and practical experience in this field has been obtained at the Bilibino nuclear power station in the Arctic, which supplies electricity and heat to the inhabitants on the Chukchi Peninsula.

Soviet nuclear power stations had a capacity of 37·4m. kw. in 1989 (12·5m. in 1980) and produced 213,000m. kwh. of electricity (72·9m. in 1980).

Total electricity output in 1989 was 1,722,000m. kwh.

The country's integrated power grid is now in operation, covering over 900 power stations, which are handled by a central control panel in Moscow through (in 1989) 1,024,800 km. of cable of 35 kw. or greater capacity. A unified power grid with all the Communist countries of eastern Europe was built up between 1962 and 1967. Supply 127 and 220 volts; 50 Hz.

Oil. In the 1930s practically all Soviet oil came from the Caucasian fields, of which the Baku fields yielded 75-80% and the Grozny and Maikop fields between them 15%. Since then, the distribution has considerably changed. The Ural-Volga area, the 'Second Baku', has 4 large centres in operation, at Samarska Luka (Kuibyshev), Tuimazy (Bashkiria), Ishimbaev (Bashkiria) and Perm, producing nearly 100m. tonnes annually.

A large new oilfield has been developed in the Trans-Volga area of the Saratov region. The Tyumen (West Siberian) complex now accounts for over 50% of the USSR's oil output. In 1990 the USSR extracted 569·3m. tonnes of oil.

At the end of 1981 there were 70,800 km of pipeline, through which (in 1981) were conveyed 637·7m. tonnes of oil.

The 'Friendship' pipeline of 5,327 km from the oilfields near Kuibyshev to Poland and Germany (northern branch) and to Czechoslovakia and Hungary (southern branch) has an annual throughput of 50m. tonnes.

In 1989 the USSR exported 184·4m. tonnes of crude oil and oil products.

Meyerhoff, A. A., *The Oil and Gas Potential of the Soviet Far East.* Beaconsfield, 1981

Gas. A natural-gas pipeline from Gazli, near Khiva, to Voskresensk, near Moscow (2,750 km), with a planned capacity of 100m. cu. metres per day, began operating in Oct. 1967. Since then it has been extended to Czechoslovakia, where a 1,000 km extension, for transmission of Soviet gas to Austria, Italy and Germany, is under construction and another to Bulgaria. Another natural-gas pipeline, over 3,000 km from Medvezhye (Tyumen Region) to Moscow, began operating in Oct. 1974. A second pipeline from this region, linking the Urengoi deposit with Petrovsky in the Central European area of the USSR, became operational in 1980, and is to be continued to the southern Ukraine, to a total length of 3,000 km. A gas pipeline starting from Orenburg (Urals) across the Ukraine via Kremenchug and Vinnitsa to Czechoslovakia (2,750 km), supplies Czechoslovakia, Poland, Bulgaria and Hungary with 14,000m. cu. metres annually and Romania with 1,500m. A unified gas-grid exceeding 124,000 km now exists.

By Dec. 1981 construction work had begun on the 5,000 km Urengoi (West Siberia)-Uzhgorod-West Europe gas pipeline.

In 1988, 796,000m. cu. metres of gas were produced (in 1970, 197,900m.). Proven reserves are some 40,000,000m. cu. metres.

Minerals. Mining experts are trained in 6 mining, 3 oil and 1 peat institutes, the mining faculties of 17 higher educational establishments, oil faculties of 2 industrial institutes and a peat faculty at the Belorussian Polytechnical Institute.

The Soviet Union is rich in minerals. Soviet scientists claim that it contains 58% of the world's coal deposits, 58·7% of its oil, 41% of its iron ore, 76·7% of its apatite, 25% of all timber land, 88% of its manganese, 54% of its potassium salts and nearly one-third of its phosphates.

Estimated output (in tonnes) in 1962: Copper, 634,900; zinc, 399,000; lead, 363,000; tungsten, 10,500; antimony, 5,980; silver, 27m. fine oz. Output in 1963: Baryte, 199,500; magnesium, 31,745; aluminium, 961,400; manganese ore (1977), 8·6m.; graphite, 54,000; bauxite, 4·3m.; asbestos, 1·3m.; phosphate rock, 3·7m. (plus 7·4m. apatite); chromite, 1·23m.; gold, 12·5m. fine oz.; molybdenum, 12·5m. lb.; cadmium (1956), 160.

Output of iron and steel in the USSR (in 1m. tonnes):

	Pig-iron	*Ingot steel*	*Rolled steel*		*Pig-iron*	*Ingot steel*	*Rolled steel*
1913	4·2	4·2	3·5	1960	46·8	65·3	50·9
1928–29	4·0	4·8	3·9	1965	66·2	91·0	61·7
1932	6·2	5·9	4·4	1970	85·9	115·9	80·6
1940	14·9	18·3	13·1	1980	107·3	147·9	118·3
1946	10·0	13·4	9·6	1985	110·0	154·7	128·4
1950	19·2	27·3	20·9	1989	114·0	160·0	133·4

Coal production (in 1m. tonnes) was 29·1 in 1913, 165·9 in 1940, 261·1 in 1950, 509·6 in 1960, 624·1 in 1970, 716·4 in 1980, 740 in 1989.

The main centre of the atomic ore industry is at Ust-Kamenogorsk in the Altai Mountains. Uranium deposits are being worked near Taboshar (south-east of Tashkent), Andizhan (in the Tynya-Muyan Mountains), Slyudianka (near Lake Baikal), on the Kolyma River and in Southern Armenia.

Agriculture. The Soviet Union, up to about 1928 predominantly agricultural in character, has become an industrial-agricultural country. Of gross national product in 1988, industry accounted for 34%, services 20%, agriculture 18%, trade 12%, construction for 10% and transport and communications 6%. Of the total state land fund of 2,227·6m. ha, agricultural land in use in 1990 amounted to 1,055m., state forests and state reserves to 1,098m. ha. 19% of all gainfully employed in 1989 were engaged in agriculture and forestry (1913, 75%; 1940, 54%).

The total area under cultivation (including single-owner peasant farms, state farms and collective farms) was (in the same territory) 118·2m. ha in 1913, 150·6m. in 1940, 146·3m. in 1950, 203m. in 1960, 206·7m. in 1970, 217·3 in 1980, and 209·8m. in 1990.

Collective farms in 1990 possessed 101·2m. ha of cultivated land, of which 60·9m. were under crops of various kinds; state farms and other state agricultural undertakings possessed 120·7m. ha, of which 65·5m. were under crops; personal subsidiary holdings (private plots and allotments) accounted for 4·5m. ha.

State procurements (after consumption by farms) were, in 1m. tonnes, for the present area of the USSR:

	1950	*1960*	*1970*	*1989*		*1950*	*1960*	*1970*	*1989*
Grain	32·3	46·7	73·3	59·0	Meat[2] and fats	1·3	4·8	8·1	23·3
Raw Cotton[1]	3·5	4·3	6·9	8·6	Milk and milk products	11·4	29·1	48·0	78·1
Sugar-beet	19·7	52·2	71·4	91·9	Sunflower seed	1·1	2·3	4·6	5·6
Potatoes	14·0	13·7	18·1	14·6	Eggs (1,000m.)	3·5	10·5	22·1	55·8
Other vegetables	4·3	8·0	13·8	19·0					

[1] Seed-cotton unginned. [2] Slaughter weight.

Since 1954 grain crops have been measured in 'barn crop' (*i.e.*, net quantities delivered to barns) and not in 'gross harvest' or 'biological yield' (*i.e.*, calculated as growing crops) as previously. Average annual crops (in 1m. tonnes): 1909–13, 72·5; 1946–50, 64·8; 1951–55, 88·5; 1956–60, 121·5; 1961–65, 130·3; 1966–70, 167·5; 1971–75, 181·6; 1976–80, 205; 1981–85, 180·3; 1989, 211.

Other produce (in 1m. tonnes) in 1989: Milk, 108·5; sugar-beet, 97·4; potatoes, 72·2; vegetables, 28·7; meat (slaughter weight), 20·1; raw cotton, 8·6; sunflower seed, 7·1; wool, 0·5; eggs, 84,854m.

In 1990 there were 27,900 collective farms employing 11·8m. collective farmers. Total value of output, 82,100m. rubles. In 1985 they produced 89% of all sugar-beet, cotton 66%, milk 37%, meat 30%, potatoes 21%, other vegetables 24%, eggs 7%, sunflower seeds 74%, wool 30%. In Nov. 1969 the Third Congress of collective farmers adopted a new model constitution, considerably enlarging the planning powers of collective farms and making payments to their members a priority.

In 1990 there were 23,303 state farms employing 11·2m. workers (9·2m. engaged in agriculture) and producing an output valued at 80,900m. rubles.

Investments in agriculture in 1989 were 38,400m. rubles (including 25,300m. by the state and 13,100m. by collective farms). Total agricultural output in 1989 was valued at 225,100m. rubles (in 1983 prices).

In 1986 the total of irrigated land was 20·2m. ha. The total of land drained was 14·9m. ha in 1986. In 1986, 2,615m. rubles were spent on conservation measures (1,798m. on water resources and 263m. on the atmosphere).

In 1981, 84m. tonnes of mineral fertilizers were used. On 1 Jan. 1990 there were 2·7m. tractors, 689,000 grain combine harvesters and 1·1m. motorized ploughs.

An All-Union Academy of Agricultural Sciences, founded in 1929, has regional branches in Siberia and Central Asia and 310 research institutes.

Livestock (1 Jan. 1991), in 1m. head: Cattle, 116·2 (including 41·4 milch cows); pigs, 76·8; sheep and goats, 141·7. Since 1957 the enumeration of livestock has been made on 1 Jan. instead of 1 Oct., *i.e.*, after the winter sales and slaughter for the market. Percentage of farm production in 1985:

	Grain	*Cotton*	*Sugar-beet*	*Pota-toes*	*Other vegetables*	*Meat*	*Milk*	*Eggs*	*Wool*
State	48	35	12	18	46	42	32	66	44
Collective	51	65	88	22	25	30	39	6	30
Private[1]	1	0	0	60	29	28	29	28	26

[1] *i.e.*, household plots of collective farmers.

Forestry. Of the 814·3m. ha of forest land of the USSR in 1988, 795·3m. ha is administered and worked by the State; the remainder, 19m. ha in extent, is granted for use to the peasantry free of charge.

The largest forest areas are 515m. ha in the Asiatic part of USSR, 51·4m. along the northern seaboard, 25·4m. in the Urals and 17·95m. in the north-west.

On 24 Oct. 1948 a plan was published for planting crop-protecting forest belts, introducing crop rotation with grasses and building of ponds and water reservoirs in the steppe and forest-steppe areas of the European part of the USSR. By the middle of 1952 some 2·6m. ha had been planted with shelter-belt trees and 13,500 ponds and reservoirs had been built. The planting of the shelter belts in the Kamyshin-Volgograd and Belgorod-Don areas has in the main been completed. A Volga forest belt has been planted along 1,200 km of railway. Re-afforestation was carried out on 2·2m. ha of state land in 1989.

Fisheries. The fishing catch including whaling (in 1,000 tonnes): 1985, 12,400. There were 422 fishing co-operatives in 1985 with a total output valued at 772m. rubles.

Blandon, P., *Soviet Forest Industries*. Boulder, 1983
Shaffer, H. G., *Soviet Agriculture*. New York, 1977
Symons, L., *Russian Agriculture: A Geographic Survey*. London, 1972

INDUSTRY. The organization of industry is based on state ownership and control, administered by a separate ministry for each large industry.

Under the successive 5-year plans, large-scale modern industrial works have been constructed, namely: 1st, over 1,500; 2nd, 4,500; 3rd (up to June 1941), 3,000; wartime, 3,500 (apart from reconstruction of destroyed plants); 4th, 6,200; 5th, 3,200; 6th, 2,700; 7th (1959–65), 5,470; 8th (1966–70), 1,870; 9th (1971–75), 2,000; 10th (1976–80), 1,200.

Output of some heavy industries was as follows:

Industry	*1950*	*1960*	*1970*	*1980*	*1990*
Iron ore (1m. tonnes)	39·7	106·2	197·3	244·7	236·0
Oil (1m. tonnes)	37·9	148·0	353·0	603·2	570·0
Electric power (1,000m. kwh.)	91·2	292·0	740·9	1,295·0	1,728·0
Coal (1m. tonnes)	261·1	509·6	624·1	716·4	703·0
Steel (1m. tonnes)	27·3	65·3	115·9	147·9	154·0
Rolled steel (finished, 1m. tonnes)	18·0	43·7	80·6	102·9	112·0
Steam and gas turbines (1,000 kw.)	2,381·0	9,200·0	16,191·0	20,300·0	21,100·0[2]
Steel pipe (1m. tonnes)	2·0	5·8	12·4	18·2	19·5
Chemical fibres (1m. tonnes)	0·0	0·2	0·6	1·2	1·5
Mineral fertilizer (1m. tonnes)	1·3	3·3	13·1	24·8	31·7
Automobiles (1,000)	64·6	138·8	344·2	1,327·0	2,119·0
Tractors (1m. h.p.)	5·5	11·4	29·4	47·0	51·6[2]
Sulphuric acid (1m. tonnes)	2·1	5·4	12·1	23·0	27·3
Excavators (no.)	3,540·0	12,290·0	30,800·0	42,000·0	37,700·0
Timber (commercial, 1m.cu. metres)[1]	161·0	261·5	298·5	277·7	305·3[2]
Cement (1m. tonnes)	10·2	45·5	95·2	125·0	137·0

[1] Excluding collective farm production. [2] Production in 1988.

The process of industrial mechanization and the installation of automatic remote control is being pushed ahead. About 93% of Soviet pig-iron and 87% of the steel is produced in fully automatic furnaces. All hydro-electric plants (in terms of capacity) are fully automatic. Coal production in open-cast mines has been completely mechanized; hydraulic mining is coming into general use.

Output in some consumer industries was as follows:

Industry	*1950*	*1960*	*1970*	*1980*	*1990*
Cotton fabrics (1m. linear metres)	3,899	6,387	7,482	8,063	
Woollen fabrics (1m. linear metres)	156	342	496	564	12,700
Silk fabrics (1m. linear metres)	130	810	1,241	1,632	
Leather footwear (1m. pairs)	203	419	679	744	820
Clocks and watches (1m.)	8	26	40	67	...
Radio receivers (1m.)	1	4	8	9	9
Television sets (1m.)	–	2	7	8	11
Refrigerators (1,000)	1	530	4,140	5,925	6,500
Paper (1,000 tonnes)	1,193	2,334	4,185	5,288	6,200
Meat (slaughter weight, 1m. tonnes)	5	9	12	15	20

Industry–Cont.	*1950*	*1960*	*1970*	*1980*	*1990*
Butter (1,000 tonnes)	336	737	963	1,278	1,700
Granulated sugar (1,000 tonnes)	2,523	6,360	10,221	10,127	12,200
Canned foods (1m. tins)	1,113	4,864	10,678	15,268	20,400

Since 1945 the cotton industry has expanded, especially in the Urals, Central Asia and Siberia. Large mills have been built at Kamyshin, Kherson, Barnaul, Engels, Alma-Ata, Chernigov and Frunze.

Labour. Industrial and clerical workers engaged (1989) in the whole national economy were 115·4m., 51% of them women; a further 11·6m. were engaged in collective-farm agriculture. The 7-hour day (6 hours for miners underground and other heavy trades) was generally in operation by the end of 1960. The average working week since 1970 has been 39 hours and in industry 39·6 hours. The 5-day week (without reduction of total working hours) was introduced in 1967.

New 'Fundamentals of Labour Legislation', intended to codify and extend labour laws adopted in the last 40 years, were adopted by the Supreme Soviet in July 1970. They lay down, *inter alia,* the right to receive wages irrespective of the income of the enterprise concerned, the right to free vocational and advanced technical training; the right of trade unions to participate in and supervise management and planning, labour legislation, safety regulation and housing, fixing of working conditions and wages, etc. Pensioners in Jan. 1990 numbered 59·7m., including 44·3m. old age. Average monthly wages in the state sector were 240·4 rubles in 1989.

Trade Unions. Trade unions are organized on an industrial basis, all workers, whether white- or blue-collar, in every branch of a given industry being eligible for membership of the same union. Collective farmers may join trade unions.

Since 1933 the trade unions have carried out the functions of the former Labour Commissariat; they control and supervise the application of labour laws, introduce new labour laws for approval by the Government and administer social insurance and factory inspection. Social insurance is non-contributory. The All-Union Congress has met at irregular intervals; the 17th Congress met in 1982 and the 18th in 1987. The 19th Congress, in 1990, reorganized the Congress on a federal basis as a General Confederation of Trade Unions of the USSR.

In 1987 there were 31 unions. Contributions range from 0·5 to 6% of wages. There are 173 regional and Republican Trades Councils. Membership (1990) 142m. The right to strike is now legal, and unions are permitted to work outside the structure of the All-Union Central Council of Trade Unions. Since the late 1980s a widely supported independent union and workers' movement has developed. An independent coal-miners' union was formed in Oct. 1990.

Chairman, General Confederation of Trade Unions: V. Shcherbakov.

FOREIGN ECONOMIC RELATIONS. The legal basis for joint ventures with foreign partners is a Council of Ministers Decree of 13 Jan. 1987 with some subsequent additional regulations. Joint ventures benefit from an initial 2-year tax exemption after the first profits are made; thereafter tax is 30%. Either partner may own up to 99% of the equity. On 1 Jan. 1990, 1,274 joint enterprises had been registered, of which 307 had begun operations.

100% foreign investment ownership with repatriation of profits became legal in Oct. 1990.

A Union-Republican Foreign Currency Committee, comprising representatives of the External Economic Commission and the heads of government of the constituent republics was established in Nov. 1990 to centralize the management of foreign currency earnings, and enforce a monopoly of goods of state importance, including oil and gas, gold, precious stones and high technology items.

Commerce. Foreign trade is organized as a state monopoly. Importation and exportation of goods are effected under licences issued by the Ministry for Foreign Economic Relations and its respective departments in pursuance of a plan annually sanctioned by the Government. The right of purchasing goods for importation, and that of selling Soviet exports abroad, is vested in trade delegations and representatives of the appropriate state corporations in foreign countries.

There are 29 state import and export organizations, including chartering and tourist corporations (one, Vostokintorg, dealing with Mongolia, Sinkiang and Afghanistan). The Central Union of Consumers' Societies (Tsentrosoyuz) is also authorized to conduct foreign trade operations.

Foreign trade in 1990 was conducted with 145 foreign countries (in 1950, 45), and had by 1986 increased 45 times by value since 1950. Exports in 1989 were valued at 68,742m. rubles (37,958m. to the communist countries), and imports at 72,137m. rubles (40,588m. from the communist countries).

Soviet imports of machinery and equipment, between 1940 and 1987, rose from 32·4 to 40·9%, ores and concentrates fell from 26·6 to 8%, foodstuffs rose from 14·9 to 15·8% and manufactured consumer goods rose from 1·4 to 12·8% by value; exports of fuel and electricity increased from 13·2 to 42·1% and of machinery and equipment from 2 to 16·2% by value over the same period.

Main items of exports in 1989:

Crude oil (1m. tonnes)	127·0	Gas (1m. cu. metres)	101,000·0
Iron ore (1m. tonnes)	29·3	Tractors (1,000)	51·3
Rolled metal (1m. tonnes)	9·3	Motor cars (1,000)	365·0
Paper (1,000 tonnes)	668·0	Clocks and watches (1m.)	15·7
Cotton cloth (1,000 tonnes)	791·0	Grain (1m. tonnes)	1·3

Total trade between the USSR and UK (British Department of Trade returns, in £1,000 sterling):

	1987	*1988*	*1989*	*1990*
Imports to UK	875,431	732,115	833,369	917,619
Exports and re-exports from UK	491,615	511,653	681,599	606,013

Tourism. Tourist facilities for Soviet and foreign citizens are presently made available under state, trade union and other auspices, all of which come ultimately under the supervision of the State Committee on Tourism which is attached to the USSR Council of Ministers. The number of hotels available to such tourists was 948 in 1989, with a total accommodation of 453,000; the number of tourist bases, for the hire of equipment and shorter stays, was 8,052, with a total accommodation of 806,000. In 1988 these facilities were used by 32·7m. and 4·2m. tourists respectively. A total of 54m. citizens in 1988 made use of all forms of tourist accommodation, including sanatoria and boarding houses. In 1988 a further 218m. citizens took part in tourist excursions.

Visitors to the USSR from foreign countries are catered for by 'Intourist' and its offices abroad. In 1989 the USSR had 7·8m. foreign visitors, of whom 2·7m. were on tourist visits. In the same year 8m. Soviet citizens made tourist, business or other visits abroad.

COMMUNICATIONS

Roads. The total length of motor roads in 1990 was 868,300 km. Road freights by lorry amounted to 27,873m. tonnes in 1988. Passengers carried were 50,496m. in 1989. In 1987, 24,100 inter-urban bus routes had a total length of 3,642,000 km.

Railways. The length of railways in Jan. 1990 was 147,400 km, of which 51,700 km was electrified. In 1986, 47% of all domestic tonne-km of freight and 37% of all passenger-km of traffic went by rail. In 1989 railways carried 4,017m. tonnes of freight (representing 3,851,700 tonne-km) and carried 4,323m. passengers (representing 410,700m. passenger-km).

Operations are centred on 32 regions with headquarters at: Baku, Alma-Ata, Tyndin, Minsk, Irkutsk, Nizhni Novgorod, Khabarovsk, Donetsk, Chita, Tbilisi, Aktyubinsk, Novosibirsk, Kemerovo, Krasnoyarsk, Kuibyshev, Lvov, Kishinev, Moscow, Odessa, Leningrad, Riga, Saratov, Dnepropetrovsk, Sverdlovsk, Yaroslavl, Rostov-on-Don, Tashkent, Tselinograd, Voronezh, Kharkov and Chelyabinsk.

The Baikal-Amur Magistral (BAM) project was completed in 1985. This is a new main line to the east, sited well to the north of the existing Trans-Siberian route to the Pacific ports of Nakhodka and Vladivostok. It runs from Lena, on the Lena river, to Komsomolsk-on-Amur, 3,145 km distant. BAM is intended to become the principal route for export traffic to the eastern ports, easing the very heavy pressure on the Trans-Siberian line, which is only partially electrified and not double-track throughout.

Underground railways have been built in Moscow, Leningrad, Kiev, Tbilisi, Kharkov, Tashkent, Baku, Nizhni Novgorod, Minsk, Yerevan, Novosibirsk and Kuibyshev. Others are under construction at Omsk, Dnepropetrovsk and Sverdlovsk.

Aviation. In 1990 length of internal airlines was approximately 915,100 km; 3·2m. tonnes of freight were carried. Some 132m. passengers were carried in 1989. The Central Asian Airways in some instances provide the only means of communication across the desert and mountainous regions of the local republics. An 8,500-km air service was opened in Feb. 1941 between Moscow and Anadyr (Eastern Siberia), through Archangel, Igarka, Khatanga, Tiksi Bay and Cape Schmidt, *i.e.*, along the entire course of the Northern Sea Route. There are also other Arctic airlines, *e.g.*, Igarka-Gulf of Kozhevnikov; Igarka-Dickson Island; Yakutsk-Tiksi Bay; Yakutsk-Viluisk; Yakutsk-Verkhoiansk.

Direct air services are maintained throughout the year between Moscow and the capitals of all the constituent republics as well as London, New York, Montreal, Tokyo, Delhi, Rangoon, Belgrade, Peking, Pyongyang, Ulan Bator, Kabul, Tirana, Paris, Warsaw, Prague, Budapest, Bucharest, Sofia, Vienna, Berlin, Helsinki, Stockholm, Copenhagen, Jakarta, Dakar and Gander. Soviet air services reached 87 countries in 1981, and 20 foreign lines have regular services to the USSR, including British Airways, KLM, SAS, Air France, SABENA, Air India, PANAM. In 1990 the number of aircraft possessed by Aeroflot was still a state secret, but there were estimated to be 1,900 passenger jets. The first Soviet airbus, the 350-seater IL-86, began flights on civil aviation routes in 1981. The 120-seater YAK-42 will gradually replace the TU-134 and AN-24 on major shorter routes.

MacDonald, H., *Aeroflot: Soviet Air Transport Since 1923*. London, 1975

Shipping. In 1977 the Soviet mercantile marine comprised 7,000 self-propelled vessels, of which 80% were built between 1957 and 1966. By May 1977 the gross cargo capacity was (including fishing vessels) 20·8m. registered tonnes (16m. tonnes dead-weight).

Freights carried on domestic waterways were in 1989, 694m. tonnes; 127m. passengers were carried. The Soviet share in world marine tonnage was 2% in 1960 and 6% in 1977. Deep-sea ports are under construction at Vostochny (Far East) and Grigorevsky (Black Sea) with new deep-sea wharves at Ventspils (Latvia), Murmansk and Archangel (for Arctic traffic). Archangel is kept open by icebreakers all the year round from 1979. Foreign freights in 1977 totalled 14% of all Soviet seaborne trade.

The North Sea route affords convenient communication between the European USSR and the Far East along the Soviet coast, for the produce of the basins of the Ob, Yenissei, Lena and Kolyma rivers.

The length of navigable rivers and canals in exploitation was (1989) 122,500 km, of which the length of floatable rivers is 81,000 km. There are several thousand miles of canals and other artificial waterways; among them the Baltic and White Sea Canal (235 km), the Moscow-Volga Canal (130 km). Goods turnover on inland waterways was 239,591m. in 1989.

The Volga-Don Shipping Canal was opened for traffic in 1952. The Volga-Don waterway from Volgograd to Rostov is 540 km long, of which the Volga-Don canal comprises 101 km. The canal has transformed the section of the river from Kalach, where the Don is joined by the Volga-Don canal, to Rostov into a deep-water highway suitable for big Volga shipping. The canal links the White, Baltic, Caspian, Azov and Black Seas into a single water transport system. In Oct. 1964 the 2,430-km Baltic-Volga waterway, linking Klaipeda on the Baltic to Kakhovka at the mouth of the Dnieper and suitable for 5,000-tonne vessels, was begun. Reconstruction of the 18th-century Mariinsky canal system in north-west Russia was completed, providing a through waterway from Leningrad to Rybinsk (on the Upper Volga).

There is a train ferry between Ilichovsk and Varna in Bulgaria.

The first section of Vostochny port, in Wrangel Bay on the Pacific coast, is completed. It will be the country's largest deep-sea port.

In 1962 a canal was completed across the Kara-Kum desert in southern Turkmenistan. The canal, from Bussag on the river Amu-Darya to Archnan, northwest of Ashkhabad, through the Murgab oasis, 900 km long, supplies water to an area exceeding 200,000 ha, suitable for cotton, fruit, vineyards and livestock. An extension to the Caspian (500 km) is under construction: The complete system will irrigate 1m. ha.

An irrigation canal system (250 miles), bringing water from Kakhovka on the Dnieper to the North Crimea, is nearing completion. Work to divert water from the Pechora and Vychegda rivers (flowing into the White Sea) south to the Volga is in progress. Work has begun on a 300-mile canal which will supply water from the Irtysh to Karaganda in Central Kazakhstan, irrigating over 150,000 acres; the first 37 miles were opened in 1965 and another 45 miles in Dec. 1967. Most of the 11 reservoirs required had been completed by 1 Jan. 1972. Other irrigation canals under construction are Kuibyshev (279 km long, to supply over 100,000 ha) and Stavropol (481 km, irrigating 200,000 ha); the second section of the latter went into commission in Nov. 1974, 14 months ahead of schedule. In Sept. 1972 the Saratov Canal (irrigating 1m. ha) went into commission.

Telecommunications. In Jan. 1990 the number of post, telegraph and telephone offices was 91,000 and of general telephones 40·1m.

The international radio-telecommunications services are operated by the Ministry of Communications of the USSR. The Great Northern Telegraph Co., Ltd, of Denmark, operates cables connecting Denmark with Leningrad, whence connexion is made by means of a trans-Siberian landline with Vladivostok. From the latter place the Great Northern Telegraph Co. owns cables connecting with Japan, China and Hong Kong. Direct radio and telephone communication with India is provided for in an agreement concluded in 1955.

The Television and Radio Broadcasting Corporation produces 3 programmes in Moscow, broadcasting throughout the Union. In addition the regional radio stations produce 1, 2 or 3 programmes for the republics as well as local programmes for a town or region. The foreign service from Moscow is beamed to all parts of the world, in 64 languages. Several republics have their own foreign services. English is broadcast from Moscow, Kiev, Tashkent, Vilnius and Yerevan. There are 120 TV centres, several of them producing more than 1 programme. In Moscow there are 4 programmes. Colour programmes are broadcast by the SECAM system. A nationwide system of space telecommunications, consisting of satellites and ground stations, takes TV broadcasts to distant parts of the country.

Number of receivers, Jan. 1990: Radio, 84·8m. (1960, 28m); television, 92·4m. (1960, 5m.).

Cinemas and Theatres (Jan. 1990). There were 147,800 cinemas to which 3,205m. visits were made annually. In Jan. 1990 there were 713 theatres, to which 104·4m. visits were made.

Newspapers. In 1989, 8,811 newspapers with a total daily circulation of 230·5m. copies were published in 57 languages of the USSR. Day to day press censorship was abolished on 1 Aug. 1990.

JUSTICE, RELIGION, EDUCATION AND WELFARE

Justice. The basis of the judicial system is the same throughout the Soviet Union, but the constituent republics have the right to introduce modifications and to make their own rules for the application of the codes of laws. The *Supreme Court* of the USSR is the chief court and supervising organ for all constituent republics and is elected by the Congress of People's Deputies of the USSR for 5 years. *Chairman* (elected 1989) E. A. Smolentsev. Supreme Courts of the Union and Autonomous Republics and of the Autonomous Regions and Areas are elected by the Supreme Soviets of these republics, and Territorial, Regional and City Courts by the respective immediately superior Soviets, each for a term of 10 years. At the lowest level are the People's Courts, which are elected directly by immediately superior soviets of people's deputies and by the population.

Court proceedings are conducted in the local language with full interpreting facilities as required. All cases are heard in public, unless otherwise provided for by law, and the accused is guaranteed the right of defence.

Laws establishing common principles of legislation in various fields are adopted by the Supreme Soviet and are then enacted in more specific form and implemented by subordinate levels of state and judicial authority.

The Law Courts are divided into People's Courts and higher courts. The People's Courts consist of the People's Judge and 2 Assessors, and their function is to examine, as the first instance, most of the civil and criminal cases, except the more important ones, some of which are tried at the Regional Court, and those of the highest importance at the Supreme Court. The Regional Courts supervise the activities of the People's Courts and also act as Courts of Appeal from the decisions of the People's Court. Special chambers of the higher courts deal with offences committed in the Army and the public transport services.

Judges are elected for 10-year terms by panels of their colleagues. They are assisted by assessors, who serve on a rota basis and are elected directly by the citizens of each constituency for a 5-year term. In 1990 a contempt of court law was passed, and the option of trial by jury for serious offences introduced.

The People's Assessors are called upon for duty for 2 weeks in a year. The People's Assessors for the Regional Court must have had at least 2 years' experience in public or trade-union work. The list of Assessors for the Supreme Court is drawn up by the Supreme Soviet of the republic.

The Labour Session of the People's Court supervises the regulations relating to the working conditions and the protection of labour and gives decisions on conflicts arising between managements and employees, or the violation of regulations.

Disputes between State institutions must be referred to an arbitration commission. Disputes between Soviet State institutions and foreign business firms may be referred by agreement to a Foreign Trade Arbitration Commission of the All-Union Chamber of Commerce.

The *Procurator-General* of the USSR (N. S. Trubin, elected 1990) is appointed for 5 years by the USSR Congress of People's Deputies. All procurators of the republics, autonomous republics and autonomous regions are appointed by the Procurator-General of the USSR for a term of 5 years. The procurators supervise the correct application of the law by all state organs, and have special responsibility for the observance of the law in places of detention. The procurators of the Union republics are subordinate to the Procurator-General of the USSR, whose duty it is to see that acts of all institutions of the USSR are legal, that the law is correctly interpreted and uniformly applied; he has to participate in important cases in the capacity of State Prosecutor.

Capital punishment was abolished on 26 May 1947, but was restored on 12 Jan. 1950 for treason, espionage and sabotage, on 7 May 1954 for certain categories of murder, in Dec. 1958 for terrorism and banditry, on 7 May 1961 for embezzlement of public property, counterfeiting and attack on prison warders and, in particular circumstances, for attacks on the police and public order volunteers and for rape (15 Feb. 1962) and for accepting bribes (20 Feb. 1962). The sentence is carried out by a single shot to the head. There were 770 executions in 1985; 526 in 1986; 344 in 1987; 271 in 1988; 276 in 1989.

In view of criminal abuses, extending over many years, discovered in the security system, the powers of administrative trial and exile previously vested in the Ministry of the Interior security authorities (MVD) were abolished in 1953; accelerated procedures for trial on charges of high treason, espionage, wrecking, etc., by the Supreme Court were abolished in 1955; and extensive powers of protection of persons under arrest or serving prison terms were vested in the Procurator-General's Office (1955).

On 25 Dec. 1958 the age of criminal responsibility was raised from 14 to 16 years; deportation and banishment were abolished; and the burden of proof of guilt was placed upon the prosecutor. Secret trials and the charge of 'enemy of the people' were abolished. Articles 70 and 190 of the Criminal Code, which deal with 'anti-Soviet agitation and propaganda' and 'crimes against the system of administration' respectively, were however widely used against political dissidents in subsequent years.

Butler, W. E., *The Soviet Legal System. Selected Contemporary Legislation and Documents.* New York, 1978.—*Soviet Law*. 2nd ed. London, 1988
Feldbrugge, F. J. M. (ed.) *Encyclopedia of Soviet Law*. 2nd ed. Dordrecht, 1985
Hazard, J., Butler, W. E. and Maggs, P., *The Soviet Legal System*. 3rd ed. New York, 1977
Simons, W. B. (ed.) *The Soviet Codes of Law*. Alphen aan den Rijn, 1980

Religion. With the Revolution the Orthodox Church lost its position as the dominant religion and all religions were placed on an equal footing. Article 52 of the 1977 Soviet Constitution reads as follows: 'Citizens of the USSR are guaranteed freedom of conscience, that is, the right to profess or not to profess any religion, and to conduct religious worship or atheistic propaganda. Incitement of hostility or hatred on religious grounds is prohibited. In the USSR the church is separated from the state, and school from the church.'

By decree of 2 Feb. 1918 the Orthodox Church was disestablished; its property, together with that of all other denominations, was nationalized. The congregations themselves have to maintain their churches and clergy, regardless of confession or denomination. A minimum of 20 persons may request and receive the use of a church building, free of charge, except for maintenance, insurance, land taxes, etc. About two-thirds of all the churches have been closed since 1917, but about 20,000 churches and 18 religious seminaries were reported to be in operation in 1986. Religious instruction may be given in private, but otherwise only in church classes. The income of religious communities is not subject to taxation. Religious instruction in classes for persons under 18 is forbidden. The state supplies paper and printing facilities to all denominations for producing the Bible, the Koran, prayer books, missals, etc, although in very limited quantities. A freedom of conscience law, adopted in 1990, considerably extended these rights.

Relations between the religious communities of all creeds and the Government are maintained through a Council for Religious Affairs which is attached to the Council of Ministers of the USSR. (*Chairman*, Yuri Khristoradnov).

The Russian Orthodox Church, represented by the Patriarchate of Moscow, had, in 1990, an estimated 35-40m. adherents, 6,000 clergy and 6,500 churches. There are still many Old Believers, whose schism from the Orthodox Church dates from the 17th century. The Russian Church is headed by the Patriarch of Moscow and All Russia (Metropolitan Aleksei II (b. 1929) of Leningrad and Novgorod, elected June 1990), assisted by the Holy Synod, which has 7 members–the Patriarch himself and the Metropolitans of Krutitsy and Kolomna (Moscow), Leningrad and Kiev *ex officio*, and 3 bishops alternating for 6 months in order of seniority from the 3 regions forming the Moscow Patriarchate. The Patriarchate of Moscow maintains jurisdiction over a few parishes of Russian Orthodox abroad, in Tehran, Jerusalem, Germany, France (1 archbishop), the UK and in North and South America (2 bishops). There are 16 monasteries and nunneries, and 5 Orthodox academies and seminaries with 4 official publications.

The Armenian church has a patriarch (Catholicos), whose seat is at Etchmiadzin, and who is head of all the Armenian (Gregorian) communities throughout the world. There is an Armenian Orthodox academy and a seminary.

The Georgian Orthodox Church has its own organization under a Catholicos (Patriarch) who is resident in Tbilisi and who directs the church's seminary in Mtskheta.

Protestantism is represented chiefly by the Evangelical Christian Baptists, with over 512,000 baptized adult members and some 5,000 churches; the Lutherans are concentrated mainly in the Baltic States (350,000 in Estonia, 600,000 in Latvia), the Reformed in the Transcarpathian Region of the Ukraine (70,000). Both Baptists and Lutherans conduct theological courses. The Methodist Church functions in Estonia.

The Roman Catholics are most numerous in Lithuania, Belorussia and the western Ukraine, with an estimated 5m. adherents in total. There are 2 Roman Catholic arch-episcopates and 4 episcopates in Lithuania with 630 churches and a seminary at Kaunas providing a 5-year course. In 1946 the Uniate Church, which practises the Orthodox rite but acknowledges the Pope of Rome, was banned; it had some 3·5m. adherents. In 1990 the Soviet government indicated the ban was no longer in effect. The head of the Uniate Church is Cardinal Myroslav Lubachivsky. In Latvia there are an archepiscopate and 1 episcopate (Riga and Liepaja) of the Roman Catholic Church.

The Moslems (estimate 40-45m. members, mainly Sunnis), are divided into 4 administrative regions, 3 of them (Central Asia and Kazakhstan, European Russia and Siberia, Northern Caucasus) headed by a Mufti; the largest (Transcaucasia, with its centre at Baku) by a Sheikh-ul-Islam.

There is a Moslem academy and a madrasah in Central Asia. Several editions of the Koran have appeared in recent years.

There are various Jewish communities, the chief being in Moscow, Leningrad and Kiev. There were, in 1984, an estimated 69 synagogues, 35-40 rabbis, and one Yeshiva in Moscow. There are no official religious publications and the teaching of Hebrew is severely restricted. The Central Buddhist Council of the USSR is headed by a Lama with communities in Buryatia, Tuva, Kalmykia and in the national (minority) areas of the Chita and Irkutsk regions.

O religii i tserkvi: sbornik vazhneishikh vyskazivanii klassikov Marksizma-Leninizma, dokumentov KPSS i sovetskogo gosudarstva. 2nd ed., Moscow, 1981
Bordeaux, M., *Opium of the People. The Christian Religion in the USSR*. London, 1965.—*Religious Ferment in Russia*. London, 1968
Curtiss, J. S., *The Russian Church and the Soviet State, 1917–50*. New York, 1953
Ellis, J., *The Russian Orthodox Church: A Contempory History*. London, 1986
Kochan, L., (ed.) *Jews in Soviet Russia since 1917*. 3rd ed., Oxford, 1977
Lane, C., *Christian Religion in the Soviet Union*. London, 1978

Education. Education is free and compulsory from 7 to 16/17. There are 2 types of general schools, with an 8-year or a 10-year curriculum; the minimum school-leaving age is now 17. Pupils who leave an 8-year school continue their education at either a 10-year school or a vocational training school. A 10-year school pupil may also transfer to vocational school after the 8th year. Under directives adopted in 1984, there will be a gradual transition towards an 11-year school system, starting at 6, from 1986 onwards; efforts are also being made to improve pupils' preparation for employment and the status and working conditions of teachers.

In 1989–90 there were 135,000 primary and secondary schools. Pupils in general educational schools numbered 44·6m. (4·9m. of them in the tenth and eleventh forms) and the teachers 3m. Those at vocational and specialized technical secondary schools numbered 9·8m.

At the end of 1940 labour reserve schools (both vocational and industrial) were organized, admitting applicants from 14 to 17 years of age. From 1959 onwards these and other technical schools were reorganized as town and rural vocational and technical schools, at which pupils stay for a year longer than at general schools, combining completion of general secondary education with vocational training. From 1940 to 1977 inclusive they trained 35m. skilled workers. In 1978, 2·3m. graduated from such schools, including 628,000 for agriculture; 600,000 agricultural mechanics were trained in state and collective farms. Over 4,300 vocational training schools existed in 1981, training 2·17m. boys and girls, all of whom receive a full secondary education. In 1990, 17·2m. children of from 3 to 7 years of age attended kindergartens; this represented 57% of all children of the corresponding age.

In 1989–90 there were 4,539 technical colleges with 4·2m. students, and 904 universities, institutes and other places of higher education, with 5·2m. students (including 1·7m. taking correspondence or evening courses). Among the 65 university towns are: Moscow, Leningrad, Kharkov, Odessa, Tartu, Kazan, Saratov, Tomsk, Kiev, Sverdlovsk, Tbilisi, Alma-Ata, Tashkent, Minsk, Nizhni Novgorod and Vladivostok.

On 1 Jan. 1989 there were 1·5m. scientific workers in 5,111 places of higher education, research institutes and Academies of Sciences. There are 33,000 foreign students from 130 countries.

The Academy of Sciences of the USSR had 909 members and corresponding members. Total learned institutions under the USSR Academy of Sciences number 244, with 62,363 scientific staff. Each Union Republic (other than the RSFSR) has its own Academy of Sciences, with scientific staff numbering 49,988. There are also Siberian, Far Eastern and other branches of the USSR Academy. On 1 Jan. 1989 there were 97,569 post-graduate students in Academy and other higher educational institutions, 52% studying on a part-time basis.

The Academy of Pedagogical Sciences had 14 research institutes with 1,664 staff.

In 1989-90 over 101m. people were studying at schools, colleges and training or correspondence courses. 143 per 1,000 of the employed population had a higher education (1939, 13; 1970, 65).

Grant, N., *Soviet Education*. 4th ed., Harmondsworth, 1979
Matthews, M., *Education in the Soviet Union*. London, 1982

Health and Social Security. All health services are free of charge although payment is required for medicines; but private practice exists. The health service is administered by the Ministry of Health of the USSR, which supervises the work of the Health Ministries of the Union Republics and the Autonomous Republics.

In 1944 an Academy of Medical Sciences was formed; in 1989 it had 328 members and corresponding members working in 64 research institutes in which 7,835 staff were employed.

In Jan. 1990 there were 23,700 civil hospitals with 3·8m. beds. There were 3·4m. medical staff and 1,278,000 doctors (including dentists) in the health service. All confinements in towns and 75% in the country were in hospital.

There were 42,810 outpatients' clinics, apart from the 29,200 women's consultation centres and children's clinics.

The death-rate in the USSR in 1989 was 10 per 1,000, and the birth rate 17·6 per 1,000. Infant death rate was 22·7 (per 1,000 live births) in 1989, compared with 273 in 1913, 184 in 1940 and 81 in 1950. Average expectation of life, 69·5 (men 64·6, women, 74).

Social insurance is administered by the trade unions, through social insurance councils elected in places of work and social insurance sub-committees of factory committees: About 5m. volunteers are engaged in this work. 52·5m. people went to holiday sanatoria or rest homes in 1987.

Total number of holiday sanatoria providing toning-up treatment at resorts in 1989 was 2,323, with accommodation for 609,000; in addition, there were 3,517 overnight sanatoria at large plants for treatment of mild disorders without absence from work, accommodating 306,000. There were also 1,186 trade union-managed holiday hotels with a capacity of 372,000, holidays being partly or wholly at trade unions' expense. In 1987, 52m. citizens were systematically engaged in physical culture and sport; there were 3,799 stadiums seating 1,500 or more, 2,295 swimming pools and 80,000 sports halls.

State expenditure (in 1m. rubles) on health services and physical education: 1940, 0·9; 1970, 9,300; 1980, 14,800; 1989, 24,600.

Between 1950 and 1980 62,766,000 apartments (in towns) and houses (in rural areas) were built. In 1989, 2·1m. apartments and houses were built. Rents in the USSR have not been increased since 1928 and in 1988 accounted for about 3% of the expenditure of an average worker's family. By the end of 1989, 77% of all urban housing had a gas supply installed, 93% had running water, 90% had central heating and 86% had bathrooms. 60% of total housing space is publicly and 40% is privately owned.

DIPLOMATIC REPRESENTATIVES

Of the USSR in Great Britain (13 Kensington Palace Gdns., London, W8 4QX)
Ambassador: Leonid M. Zamyatin.

Of Great Britain in the USSR (Naberezhnaya Morisa Toreza 14, Moscow 72)
Ambassador: Sir Rodric Braithwaite, KCMG.

Of the USSR in the USA (1125 16th St., NW, Washington, D.C., 20036)
Ambassador: Viktor Komplektov.

Of the USA in the USSR (Ulitsa Chaikovskogo 19, Moscow)
Ambassador: Jack F. Matlock, Jr.

Of the USSR to the United Nations
Ambassador: Yuli M. Vorontsov.

The Ukraine and Belorussia also have ambassadors at the United Nations (*see* pp. 1265, 1267).

Further Reading

Narodnoe Khozvaistvo SSSR (National Economy of the USSR). Statistical Yearbook. Moscow
Pravda (Truth). Daily organ of the Central Committee of the Communist Party
Izvestiya (News). Daily organ of the Presidium of the Supreme Soviet of the USSR
Vedomosti Verkhovnovo Soveta. Bulletin of the Supreme Soviet of the USSR in the languages of the 15 republics; published weekly
Pravitelstvennyi Vestnik. Weekly publication of the Soviet government
Sovetskaya Torgovlya. Monthly publication of the Ministry of Trade of the USSR
Planovoye Khozyaistvo. Monthly. Moscow
Vestnik Statistiki. Monthly publication of the USSR Statistical Committee
Vneshnyaya Torgovlya. Published by the Ministry for Foreign Trade. Monthly. Moscow
Trud. The daily organ of the General Confederation of Trade Unions
Professionalnye Soyuzy. A trade union fortnightly. Moscow
Kommunist. A fortnightly organ of the Communist Party of the Soviet Union
Finansy SSSR. A monthly publication of the Ministry for Finance
Bolshaya Sovetskaya Entsiklopedia. 65 vols. Moscow, 1926–47; 2nd ed., 51 vols. Moscow, 1949–58; 3rd ed., Moscow, 1959–78; annual supplement (*Ezhegodnik*)
Soviet Union. A monthly pictorial. Moscow. (In English)
Soviet Studies; A Quarterly Review. Glasgow, quarterly.
The Current Digest of the Soviet Press. Published by Joint Committee on Slavic Studies. Columbus, Ohio, weekly.
Beloff, M., *The Foreign Policy of Soviet Russia, 1929–41*. 2 vols. 1947–49.—*Soviet Policy in the Far East*. Oxford, 1953.—*Soviet Policy in Asia, 1944–52*. Oxford, 1953
Bialer, S., *The Soviet Paradox: External Expansion, Internal Decline*. London, 1987
Brown, A. (ed.) *The Soviet Union: a Biographical Dictionary*. London, 1990
Byrnes, J. F. (ed.) *After Brezhnev. Sources of Soviet Conduct in the 1980s*. London, 1983
Cambridge Encyclopedia of Russia and the Soviet Union. CUP, 1982
Carr, E. H., *A History of Soviet Russia*. 14 vols. London, 1951–78
Clarke, R. A. and Matko, D. J. I., (eds.) *Soviet Economic Facts 1917–80*. London, 1983
Cracraft, J., *The Soviet Union Today*. Chicago, 2nd ed. 1988
Degras, J. (compiler), *Soviet Documents on Foreign Policy, 1917–41*. 3 vols. London, 1948–52
Edmonds, R., *Soviet Foreign Policy: the Brezhnev Years*. Oxford, 1983
Gorbachev, M., *Perestroika*. English ed. London, 1987
Hammond, T. T. (ed.) *Soviet Foreign Relations and World Communism: A Selected Bibliography*. Princeton, 1965
Heisbourg, F. (ed.) *The Strategic Implications of Change in the Soviet Union*. London, 1990
Hill, R. J., *The Soviet Union. Politics, Economics and Society*. London, 2nd ed., 1989
Hosking, G., *A History of the Soviet Union*. London, 1985
Hough, J. F. and Fainsod, M., *How the Soviet Union is Governed*. Rev. ed. Harvard Univ. Press, 1979
Hutchings, R., *The Soviet Budget*. London, 1983
Jensen, R. G. et al (eds.) *Soviet Natural Resources in the World Economy*. Univ. of Chicago Press, 1983
Jones, D. L., *Books in English in the Soviet Union 1917–73: A Bibliography*. London and New York, 1975
Kelley, D. R., (ed.) *Soviet Politics in the Brezhnev Era*. London, 1980
McCauley, M., *The Soviet Union since 1917*. London, 1981.—(ed.) *Gorbachev and Perestroika*. London, 1990
Nahaylo, B. and Swoboda, V., *Soviet Disunion: a History of the Nationalities Problem in the USSR*. London, 1990
Pares, Sir B., *A History of Russia*. London, 1962
Paxton, J., *Companion to Russian History*. London and New York, 1984
Pethybridge, R., *One Step Backwards, Two Steps Forwards: Soviet Society and Politics under the New Economic Policy*. OUP, 1990
Ra'anan, U. and Lukes, I. (eds.) *Gorbachev's USSR: a System in Crisis*. London, 1990
Riasanovsky, N. V., *A History of Russia*. 4th ed. OUP, 1984

Schapiro, L. and Godson, J., *The Soviet Worker*. London, 1981
Schmidt-Häuer, C., *Gorbachov: The Path to Power*. London, 1986
Slusser, R. M. and Triska, J. F., *A Calendar of Soviet Treaties, 1917–57*. Stanford Univ. Press, 1959—and Ginsburgs, G., *A Calendar of Soviet Treaties, 1958–1973*, Alphen aan den Rijn, 1981
Smith, H., *The New Russians*. London, 1990
Tauris Soviet Directory, The. London, 1989
Thompson, A., *Russia/USSR*. [Bibliography] Oxford and Santa Barbara, 1979
Treadgold, D. W., *Twentieth Century Russia*. 6th ed. Boston, 1987
Urban, M. E., *More Power to the Soviets: the Democratic Revolution in the USSR*. Aldershot, 1990.
Vernadsky, G., *A History of Russia*. 5th ed. Yale Univ. Press, 1961
Walker, M., *The Waking Giant: Gorbachev's Russia*. New York, 1987
White, S., *Gorbachev in Power*. CUP, 1990.—*et al* (eds.) *Developments in Soviet Politics*. London, 1990

RUSSIAN SOVIET FEDERAL SOCIALIST REPUBLIC (RSFSR)

Rossiiskaya Sovetskaya Federativnaya Sotsialisticheskaya Respublika

AREA AND POPULATION. The RSFSR occupies 17,075,000 sq. km (over 76% of the total area of the USSR) stretching from the Far North to the Black Sea in the south and from the Far East to Kaliningrad in the west. 82·6% of its population in Jan. 1979 were Russians, the rest being 38 national minorities such as the Tatars, Ukrainians, Jews, Mordovians, Chuvashis, Bashkirs, Poles, Germans, Udmurts, Buryats, Mari, Yakuts and Ossetians. The 2 principal cities are Moscow, the capital, with a population (Jan. 1989) of 8·9m. (without suburbs, 8,769,000) and Leningrad, the former capital, 5,020,000 (without suburbs, 4,456,000). Among other important cities are Nizhni Novgorod (formerly Gorky), Rostov-on-Don, Volgograd, Sverdlovsk, Novosibirsk, Chelyabinsk, Kazan, Omsk and Kuibyshev. Census population, Jan. 1989, 147,386,000.

The RSFSR contains great mineral resources: Iron ore in the Urals, the Kerch Peninsula and Siberia; coal in the Kuznets Basin, Eastern Siberia, Urals and the sub-Moscow Basin; oil in the Urals, Azov-Black Sea area, Bashkiria, and West Siberia. It also has abundant deposits of gold, platinum, copper, zinc, lead, tin and rare metals.

The RSFSR produces about 70% of the total industrial and agricultural output of the Soviet Union. Industrial and agricultural workers averaged 71·3m. in 1989.

CONSTITUTION AND GOVERNMENT. The RSFSR adopted its present constitution at a meeting of the Supreme Soviet in April 1978. In June 1990, pending the adoption of a new constitution, it adopted a declaration of republican sovereignty by 544 votes to 271.

Chairman, Supreme Soviet (i.e. *President of the Republic*)*:* B. N. Yeltsin.
Chairman, Council of Ministers (i.e. *Prime Minister*)*:* I. S. Silaev.

Boris Yeltsin was elected President by the Supreme Soviet by 535 votes to 478 in May 1990. The President's salary is 900 rubles per month.

The RSFSR consists of:

(1) *Territories (krai):* Altai, Khabarovsk, Krasnodar, Krasnoyarsk, Primorye, Stavropol.

(2) *Regions (oblast):* Amur, Archangel, Astrakhan, Belgorod, Briansk, Chelyabinsk, Chita, Irkutsk, Ivanovo, Kaluga, Kaliningrad, Kamchatka, Kemerovo, Kirov, Kostroma, Kuibyshev, Kurgan, Kursk, Leningrad, Lipetsk, Magadan, Moscow, Murmansk, Nizhni Novgorod, Novgorod, Novosibirsk, Omsk, Orel, Orenburg, Penza, Perm, Pskov, Rostov, Ryazan, Sakhalin, Saratov, Smolensk,

Sverdlovsk, Tambov, Tomsk, Tula, Tver, Tyumen, Ulyanovsk, Vladimir, Volgograd, Vologda, Voronezh, Yaroslavl.

(3) *Autonomous Soviet Republics:* Bashkir, Buryat, Chechen-Ingush, Chuvash, Daghestan, Kabardin-Balkar, Kalmyk, Karelian, Komi, Mari, Mordovian, North Ossetia, Tatar, Tuva, Udmurt, Yakut.

Subordinate to and within Territories and Regions are the following:

(4) *Autonomous Regions (avtonomnaya oblast):* Adygei, Gorno-Altai, Jewish, Karachayevo-Cherkess, Khakass.

(5) *Autonomous Areas (avtonomny okrug):* Agin-Buryat, Chukot, Evenki, Khanty-Mansi, KomiPermyak, Koryak, Nenets, Taimyr (Dolgano-Nenets), Ust-Ordyn-Buryat, Yamalo-Nenets.

On 4 March elections were held for a 1,068-seat Congress of People's Deputies, which elected a two-chamber parliament, the Supreme Soviet, from amongst its members.

A Russian Communist Party (dissolved in 1925) was reconstituted in 1990. It elected a First Secretary (I. K. Polozkov, b. 1935) and a Central Committee of 272 members.

Elections to local authorities were also held on 4 March 1990.

FINANCE. Revenue and expenditure balanced as follows (in 1m. rubles): 1988, 110,102; 1989 (plan), 126,471. These figures, and those for the other 14 Union Republics, include grants from the Union Budget. Since June 1990 the Government has been able to raise money from enterprises only by taxing profits. Prices are fixed only for monopolies; other firms may sell for whatever price they can obtain.

ECONOMY. A law of 31 Oct. 1990 places Russian economic resources under Russian control.

AGRICULTURE. In Dec. 1990 the Supreme Soviet voted to allow plots for the growing of agricultural products to be privately owned. They may only be resold back to the state, and only after 10 years.

INDUSTRY. Legislation of June 1990 renders the previously mandatory election of managers optional, and creates councils of employees empowered to reject or approve state plans.

EXTERNAL RELATIONS. In Nov. 1990 Russia concluded an agreement with the Ukraine to co-operate on defence and external policy, to co-ordinate pricing and exchange representatives.

Foreign investments and export contracts require approval by the Council of Ministers.

COMMUNICATIONS. Length of railways on 1 Jan. 1989 was 86,300 km, hard-surface motor roads, 620,000 km. In 1988 233,000m. tonne-km of freight was carried on inland waterways.

Newspapers. In 1988 there were 4,696 newspapers, 4,388 of them in Russian. Daily circulation of Russian-language newspapers, 150·1m., other languages, 2·8m.

EDUCATION. In 1988–89 there were 20·1m. pupils in 69,200 primary and secondary schools; 2,795,000 students in 507 higher educational establishments (including correspondence students) and 2,408,000 students in 2,583 technical colleges of all kinds (including correspondence students). 29·9m. children were attending preschool institutions. There were, on 1 Jan. 1989, 1,032,100 scientific staff in 3,036 learned and scientific institutions.

In 1957 a Siberian branch of the Academy of Sciences was organized, in charge of all scientific research institutions from the Urals to the Pacific. There are also Far Eastern and Urals divisions.

There is an Academy of Municipal Economy (with 5 research institutions and a staff of 485).

HEALTH. Doctors in 1988 numbered 688,300, and hospital beds 2m. There were 12,622 medical institutions.

BASHKIR AUTONOMOUS SOVIET SOCIALIST REPUBLIC

Area 143,600 sq. km (55,430 sq. miles), population (Jan. 1989) 3,952,000. Capital, Ufa. Bashkiria was annexed to Russia in 1557. It was constituted as an Autonomous Soviet Republic on 23 March 1919. A declaration of republican sovereignty was adopted in 1990. Population, census 1979, included 24·3% Bashkirians, 40·3% Russians, 24·5% Tatars, and 3·2% Chuvashes.

280 deputies were elected to the republican Supreme Soviet on 24 Feb. 1985, 108 of them women.

In 1988–89 there were 552,000 pupils in 3,164 schools. There is a state university and a branch of the USSR Academy of Sciences with 8 learned institutions (511 research workers). There were 67,200 students in 71 technical colleges and 51,600 in 9 higher educational establishments.

In Jan. 1989 there were 13,992 doctors and 53,500 hospital beds.

There are chemical, coal, steel, electrical engineering, timber and paper industries. There were 629 collective farms and 159 state farms in 1980. Crop area was 4,587,000 ha. Bashkiria is a major oil producer.

BURYAT AUTONOMOUS SOVIET SOCIALIST REPUBLIC

Area is 351,300 sq. km (135,650 sq. miles). The Buryat Republic, situated to the south of the Yakut Republic, adopted the Soviet system 1 March 1920. This area was penetrated by the Russians in the 17th century and finally annexed from China by the treaties of Nerchinsk (1689) and Kyakhta (1727). The population (Jan. 1989) was 1,042,000. Capital, Ulan-Ude (1989 census population, 353,000). The name of the republic was changed from 'Buryat-Mongol' on 7 July 1958. The population (1979 census) includes 23% Buryats and 72% Russians.

170 deputies were elected to the republican Supreme Soviet on 24 Feb. 1985, 60 of them women.

The main industries are coal, timber, building materials, fisheries, sheep and cattle farming. In 1980 there were 105 state and 61 collective farms. Crop area was 827,100 ha. Gold, molybdenum and wolfram are mined.

In 1988–89 there were 574 schools with 179,000 pupils, 21 technical colleges with 17,000 students and 4 higher educational institutions with 20,700 students. A branch of the Siberian Department of the Academy of Sciences had 4 learned institutions with 281 research workers.

In 1989 there were 4,017 doctors and 14,400 hospital beds.

CHECHENO-INGUSH AUTONOMOUS SOVIET SOCIALIST REPUBLIC

Area, 19,300 sq. km (7,350 sq. miles); population (Jan. 1989), 1,277,000. Capital, Grozny (1989 census population, 401,000). After 70 years of almost continuous fighting, the Chechens and Ingushes were conquered by Russia in the late 1850s. In 1918 each nationality separately established its 'National Soviet' within the Terek Autonomous Republic, and in 1920 (after the Civil War) were constituted areas within the Mountain Republic. The Chechens separated out as an Autonomous Region on 30 Nov. 1922 and the Ingushes on 7 July 1924. In Jan. 1934 the two regions were united, and on 5 Dec. 1936 constituted as an Autonomous Republic. This was dissolved in 1944, but reconstituted on 9 Jan. 1957: 232,000 Chechens and Ingushes returned to their homes in the next 2 years. The population (1979 census) includes 52·9% Chechens, 11·7% Ingushes, and 29·1% Russians.

175 deputies were elected to the republican Supreme Soviet on 24 Feb. 1985, 78 of them women.

The republic has one of the major Soviet oilfields, and a number of engineering works, chemical factories, building materials works and food canneries. There is timber, woodworking and furniture industry. In 1984 there were 122 state and 39 collective farms. Crop area was 453,900 ha.

There were, in 1988–89, 535 schools with 252,000 pupils, 12 technical colleges with 13,000 students and 3 places of higher education with 14,800 students.

In 1989 there were 3,676 doctors and 13,500 hospital beds.

CHUVASH AUTONOMOUS SOVIET SOCIALIST REPUBLIC

Area, 18,300 sq. km (7,064 sq. miles); population (Jan. 1989), 1,336,000. Capital, Cheboksary (1989 census population, 420,000). The territory was annexed by Russia in the middle of the 16th century. On 24 June 1920 it was constituted as an Autonomous Region, and on 21 April 1925 as an Autonomous Republic. The population (1979 census) includes Chuvashes (68·4%), Russians (26%), Tatars (2·9%) and Mordovians (1·6%).

200 deputies were elected to the republican Supreme Soviet on 24 Feb. 1985, 79 of them women.

The timber industry antedates the Soviet period. Other industries today include railway repair works, electrical and other engineering industries, building materials, chemicals, textiles and food industries; timber felling and haulage are largely mechanized. In 1985 there were 179 collective farms and 104 state farms. Grain crops account for nearly two-thirds of all sowings and fodder crops for nearly a quarter. Fruit and wine-growing are a developing branch of agriculture. Crop area was 732,400 ha.

In 1988–89 there were 208,000 pupils at 687 schools, 23,200 students at 24 technical colleges and 18,200 students at 3 higher educational establishments.

In 1988 there were 4,672 doctors and 18,500 hospital beds.

DAGESTAN AUTONOMOUS SOVIET SOCIALIST REPUBLIC

Area, 50,300 sq. km (19,416 sq. miles); population (Jan. 1989), 1,792,000. Capital, Makhachkala (1989 census population, 315,000). Over 30 nationalities inhabit this republic apart from Russians (11·6% at 1979 census); the most numerous are the Avartsy (25·7%), Dargintsy (15·2%), Lezginy (11·6%), Kumyki (12·4%), Laki (5·1%), Tabasarany (4·4%) and Azerbaijanis (4%). Annexed from Persia in 1723, Dagestan was constituted an Autonomous Republic on 20 Jan. 1921.

210 deputies were elected to the republican Supreme Soviet on 24 Feb. 1985, 84 of them women.

There are engineering, oil, chemical, woodworking, textile, food and other light industries. Agriculture is varied, ranging from wheat to grapes, with sheep farming and cattle breeding; in 1983 there were 249 collective farms and 262 state farms. Crop area was 427,800 ha. A chain of power stations is under construction in the Sulak River (total capacity 2·5m. kw.).

In 1988–89 there were 1,510 schools with 391,000 pupils, 23,000 students at 28 technical colleges and 5 higher education establishments with 26,000 students; and a branch of the USSR Academy of Sciences with 4 learned institutions (373 research workers). In 1989 there were 7,539 doctors and 22,700 hospital beds.

KABARDINO-BALKAR AUTONOMOUS SOVIET SOCIALIST REPUBLIC

Area, 12,500 sq. km (4,825 sq. miles); population (Jan. 1989) 760,000. Capital, Nalchik (1989 census population, 235,000). Kabarda was annexed to Russia in 1557. The republic was constituted on 5 Dec. 1936. Population (1979 census) includes Kabardinians (45·6%), Balkars (9%), Russians (35·1%).

160 deputies were elected to the republican Supreme Soviet on 24 Feb. 1985, 69 of them women.

Main industries are ore-mining, timber, engineering, coal, food processing, timber and light industries, building materials. Grain, livestock breeding, dairy farming and wine-growing are the principal branches of agriculture. There were, in 1983, 59 state and 66 collective farms.

In 1988–89 there were 239 schools with 123,000 pupils, 8,900 students in 10 technical colleges and 10,700 students at 2 higher educational establishments. In 1989 there were 3,573 doctors and 9,300 hospital beds.

KALMYK SOVIET SOCIALIST REPUBLIC

Area, 75,900 sq. km (29,300 sq. miles); population (Jan. 1989), 322,000. Capital, Elista (85,000). The population (1979 census) includes 41·5% Kalmyks, 42·6% Russians, 6·6% Kazakhs, Chechens and Dagestanis.

The Kalmyks migrated from western China to Russia (Nogai Steppe) in the early 17th century. The territory was constituted an Autonomous Region on 4 Nov. 1920, and an Autonomous Republic on 22 Oct. 1935; this was dissolved in 1943. On 9 Jan. 1957 it was reconstituted as an Autonomous Region and on 29 July 1958 as an Autonomous Republic once more. In Oct. 1990 the republic was renamed the Kalmyk Soviet Socialist Republic.

130 deputies were elected to the republican Supreme Soviet on 24 Feb. 1985, 54 of them women.

Main industries are fishing, canning and building materials. Cattle breeding and irrigated farming (mainly fodder crops) are the principal branches of agriculture. In 1983 there were 79 state and 23 collective farms. Crop area was 859,000 ha.

In 1988–89 there were 53,000 pupils in 245 schools, 6,000 students in 7 technical colleges and 5,000 in higher education. There were 1,372 doctors and 5,000 hospital beds in 1989.

KARELIAN AUTONOMOUS SOVIET SOCIALIST REPUBLIC

HISTORY. Karelia (formerly Olonets Province) became part of the RSFSR after 1917. In June 1920 a Karelian Labour Commune was formed and in July 1923 this was transformed into the Karelian Autonomous Soviet Socialist Republic (one of the autonomous republics of the RSFSR). On 31 March 1940, after the Soviet–Finnish war, practically all the territory (with the exception of a small section in the neighbourhood of the Leningrad area) which had been ceded by Finland to the USSR was added to Karelia and the Karelian Autonomous Republic was transformed into the Karelo-Finnish Soviet Socialist Republic as the 12th republic of the USSR. In 1946, however, the southern part of the republic, including its whole seaboard and the towns of Viipuri (Vyborg) and Keksholm, was attached to the RSFSR, reverting in 1956 to autonomous republican status within the RSFSR.

AREA AND POPULATION. The Karelian Autonomous Republic, capital Petrozavodsk (1989 census population, 270,000), covers an area of 172,400 sq. km, with a population of 792,000 (Jan. 1989). Karelians represent 11·1% of the population, Russians, 71·3%, Belorussians 8·1%, Ukrainians 3·2%, Finns 2·7% (1979 census).

150 deputies were elected to the republican Supreme Soviet on 24 Feb. 1985, 57 of them women.

NATURAL RESOURCES. Karelia is chiefly noted for its wealth of timber, some 70% of its territory being forest land. It is also rich in other natural resources, having large deposits of diabase, spar, quartz, marble, granite, zinc, lead, silver, copper, molybdenum, tin, baryta, iron ore, etc. Karelia takes first place in the USSR for the production of mica. It has 43,643 lakes, which, as well as its rivers, are rich in fish.

Agriculture. There were 9 collective farms and 59 state farms in 1983. The crop area was 78,900 ha (over 85% under fodder crops).

INDUSTRY. The republic has timber mills, paper-cellulose works, mica, chemical plants, power stations and furniture factories. Output, 1986: Timber, 11·1m. cu. metres; paper, 1·3m. tonnes; cellulose, 826,000 tonnes; electricity, 3,634m. kwh.; iron ore, 9·5m. tonnes.

The opening of the White Sea–Baltic Canal influenced economic development. New refrigerating plants, cellulose factories and timber mills began working in 1970.

COMMUNICATIONS. A railway between Petrozavodsk and Suoyarvi connects the capital and the Murmansk Railway with the main railway line Sortavala–Vyborg. A railway line was also laid between Kandalaksha and Kuolayarvi. Length of track, 1,600 km.

EDUCATION. In 1988–89 there were 112,000 pupils in 319 schools. There were 9,800 students in 2 places of higher education and 14,300 in 16 technical colleges.

HEALTH. In 1989 there were 4,020 doctors, and 12,200 hospital beds.

KOMI SOVIET SOCIALIST REPUBLIC

Area, 415,900 sq. km (160,540 sq. miles); population (Jan. 1989), 1,263,000. Capital, Syktyvkar (1989 census population, 233,000). Annexed by the princes of Moscow in the 14th century, the territory was constituted as an Autonomous Region on 22 Aug. 1921 and as an Autonomous Republic on 5 Dec. 1936. The population (1979 census) included Komi (25·3%), Russians (56·7%), Ukrainians and Belorussians (10·7%).

180 deputies were elected to the republican Supreme Soviet on 24 Feb. 1985, 59 of them women.

A declaration of sovereignty was adopted by the republican parliament in Sept. 1990, and the designation 'Autonomous' dropped from the republic's official name.

There are coal, oil, timber, gas, asphalt and building materials industries, and light industry is expanding. Livestock breeding (including dairy farming) is the main branch of agriculture. There were 56 state farms in 1983. Crop area, 92,000 ha.

In 1988–89 there were 192,000 pupils in 564 schools, 11,400 students in 3 higher educational establishments, 16,800 students in 19 technical colleges; and a branch of the Academy of Sciences with 4 learned institutions (297 research workers).

In 1989 there were 5,048 doctors and 17,700 hospital beds.

MARI SOVIET SOCIALIST REPUBLIC

Area, 23,200 sq. km (8,955 sq. miles); population (Jan. 1989), 750,000. Capital, Yoshkar-Ola (1989 census population, 242,000). The Mari people were annexed to

Russia, with other peoples of the Kazan Tatar Khanate, when the latter was overthrown in 1552. On 4 Nov. 1920 the territory was constituted as an Autonomous Region, and on 5 Dec. 1936 as an Autonomous Republic. The republic renamed itself the Mari Soviet Socialist Republic in Oct. 1990. The population (1979 census) included Mari (43·5%), Tatars (5·8%), Chuvashes (1·1%), Russians (47·5%).

150 deputies were elected to the republican Supreme Soviet on 24 Feb. 1985, 60 of them women.

There are over 300 factories. The main industries are metalworking, timber, paper, woodworking and food processing. In 1983 there were 89 collective farms and 82 state farms. Over 69% of cultivated land is grain, but flax, potatoes, fruit and vegetables are also expanding branches of agriculture, as is also livestock farming. 638,000 ha were under crops.

Estimated reserves of the Pechora coalfield are 260,000m. tonnes.

In 1988–89 there were 431 schools with 109,000 pupils; 13 technical colleges and 3 higher education establishments had 10,300 and 15,300 students respectively.

In 1989 there were 2,552 doctors and 10,400 hospital beds.

MORDOVIAN AUTONOMOUS SOVIET SOCIALIST REPUBLIC

Area, 26,200 sq. km (10,110 sq. miles); population (Jan. 1989), 964,000. Capital, Saransk (1989 census population, 312,000). By the 13th century the Mordovian tribes had been subjugated by the Russian princes of Ryazan and Nizhni-Novgorod. In 1928 the territory was constituted as a Mordovian Area within the Middle-Volga Territory, on 10 Jan. 1930 as an Autonomous Region and on 20 Dec. 1934 as an Autonomous Republic. The population (1979 census) included Mordovians (34·2%), Russians (59·7%), Tatars (4·6%)

175 deputies were elected to the republican Supreme Soviet on 24 Feb. 1985, 74 of them women.

The republic has a wide range of industries: Electrical, timber, cable, building materials, furniture, textile, leather and other light industries. Agriculture is devoted chiefly to grain, sugar-beet, sheep and dairy farming. In 1983 there were 78 state and 273 collective farms.

In 1988–89 there were 129,000 pupils in 839 schools, 15,600 students in 21 technical colleges and 20,500 attending 2 higher educational institutions. In 1989 there were 3,788 doctors and 14,500 hospital beds.

NORTH OSSETIAN AUTONOMOUS SOVIET SOCIALIST REPUBLIC

Area, 8,000 sq. km (3,088 sq. miles); population (Jan. 1989), 634,000. Capital, Ordzhonikidze (formerly Vladikavkaz; 1989 census population, 300,000). The Ossetians were annexed to Russia after the latter's treaty of Kuchuk-Kainardji with Turkey, and in 1784 the key fortress of Vladikavkaz was founded on their territory (given the name of Terek region in 1861). On 4 March 1918 the latter was proclaimed an Autonomous Soviet Republic, and on 20 Jan. 1921 this territory with others was set up as the Mountain Autonomous Republic, with North Ossetia as the Ossetian (Vladikavkaz) Area within it. On 7 July 1924 the latter was constituted as an Autonomous Region and on 5 Dec. 1936 as an Autonomous Republic. The population (1979 census) comprised Ossetians (50·5%), Russians (33·9%), Ingushi and other Caucasian nationalities (8·1%).

150 deputies were elected to the republican Supreme Soviet on 24 Feb. 1985, 68 of them women.

The main industries are non-ferrous metals (mining and metallurgy), maize-processing, timber and woodworking, textiles, building materials, distilleries and food processing. There is also a varied agriculture. In 1983 there were 38 state and 45 collective farms.

There were in 1988–89, 98,000 children in 209 schools, 12,800 students in 13 technical colleges and 17,900 students in 4 higher educational establishments (pedagogical, agriculture, medical and mining-metallurgical institutes). In 1989 there were 4,292 doctors and 8,100 hospital beds.

TATAR SOVIET SOCIALIST REPUBLIC (REPUBLIC OF TATARSTAN)

Area, 68,000 sq. km (26,250 sq. miles); population (Jan. 1989), 3,640,000. Capital, Kazan. From the 10th to the 13th centuries this was the territory of the Volga-Kama Bulgar State; conquered by the Mongols, it became the seat of the Kazan (Tatar) Khans when the Mongol Empire broke up in the 15th century, and in 1552 was conquered again by Russia. On 27 May 1920 it was constituted as an Autonomous Republic. The population (1979 census) included Tatars (47·7%), Chuvashes, Mordovians and Udmurts (5·9%), Russians (44%).

250 deputies were elected to the republican Supreme Soviet on 24 Feb. 1985, 97 of them women.

In Aug. 1990 the Supreme Soviet adopted a declaration of sovereignty and renamed the republic the Tatar Soviet Socialist Republic, or the Republic of Tatarstan.

The republic has engineering, oil and chemical, timber, building materials, textiles, clothing and food industries. In 1983, 557 collective and 250 state farms served a total area under crops of 3·4m. ha.

In 1988–89 there were 2,300 schools with 500,000 pupils, 61 technical colleges with 58,900 students and 13 higher educational establishments with 67,500 students (including a state university). There is a branch of the USSR Academy of Sciences with 5 learned institutions (512 research workers).

Doctors in 1989 numbered 13,979 and hospital beds 47,200.

TUVA AUTONOMOUS SOVIET SOCIALIST REPUBLIC

Area, 170,500 sq. km (65,810 sq. miles); population (Jan. 1989), 309,000. Capital, Kyzyl (80,000). Tuva was incorporated in the USSR as an autonomous region on 13 Oct. 1944 and elevated to an Autonomous Republic on 10 Oct. 1961. It is situated to the north-west of Mongolia, between 50° and 53°N. lat. and between 90° and 100°E. long. It is bounded to the east, west and north by Siberia, and to the south by Mongolia. The Tuvans are a Turkic people, formerly ruled by hereditary or elective tribal chiefs. (For the earlier history of the former TannuTuva Republic, *see* THE STATESMAN'S YEAR-BOOK, 1946, p. 798.) The population (1979 census) included Tuvans (60·5%) and Russians (36·2%).

130 deputies were elected to the republican Supreme Soviet on 24 Feb. 1985, 53 of them women.

Tuva is well-watered and hydro-electric resources are important. The Tuvans are mainly herdsmen and cattle farmers and there is much good pastoral land, but, in 1983, 371,000 ha were under crops. There are deposits of gold, cobalt and asbestos. The main exports are hair, hides and wool. There are 60 state farms. There are mining, woodworking, garment, leather, food and other industries.

In 1988–89 there were 155 schools with 66,000 pupils; 6 technical colleges with 3,900 students, and 1 higher education institution with 2,800 students.

In 1989 there were 1,125 doctors and 5,500 hospital beds.

UDMURT AUTONOMOUS SOVIET SOCIALIST REPUBLIC

Area, 42,100 sq. km (16,250 sq. miles); population (Jan. 1989), 1,609,000. Capital, Izhevsk. The Udmurts (formerly known as 'Votyaks') were annexed by the Russians in the 15th and 16th centuries. On 4 Nov. 1920 the Votyak Autonomous Region was constituted (the name was changed to Udmurt in 1932), and on 28 Dec. 1934 was raised to the status of an Autonomous Republic. The population (1979 census) included Udmurts (32·2%), Tatars (6·6%), Russians (58·3%).

200 deputies were elected to the republican Supreme Soviet on 24 Feb. 1985, 79 of them women.

Heavy industry includes the manufacture of locomotives, machine tools and other engineering products, timber and building materials. There are also light industries: Clothing, leather, furniture and food.

There were 96 state and 244 collective farms in 1983; crop area 1·4m. ha.

In 1988–89 there were 855 schools with 237,000 pupils; there were 22,600 students at 29 technical colleges and 23,700 at 5 higher educational institutions.

In 1989 there were 6,994 doctors and 21,100 hospital beds.

YAKUT AUTONOMOUS SOVIET SOCIALIST REPUBLIC

The area is 3,103,200 sq. km (1,197,760 sq. miles); population (Jan. 1989), 1,081,000. Capital, Yakutsk (187,000). The Yakuts were subjugated by the Russians in the 17th century. The territory was constituted an Autonomous Republic on 27 April 1922. The population (1979 census) included Yakuts (36·9%), other northern peoples (2·2%), Russians (50·4%).

205 deputies were elected to the republican Supreme Soviet on 24 Feb. 1985, 92 of them women.

The principal industries are mining (gold, tin, mica, coal) and livestock-breeding. The Soviet Soyuz-Zoloto Trust and a number of individual prospectors are working the fields. Silver- and lead-bearing ores and coal are worked; large diamond fields have been opened up. Timber and food industries are developing. There was 1 collective farm in 1985 and 88 state farms, with an area under crops of 107,100 ha. Trapping and breeding of fur-bearing animals (sable, squirrel, silver fox, etc.) are an important source of income. A severe climate and lack of railways are serious obstacles to the economic development of the republic. There are, however, 10,000 km of roads and internal air lines totalling 10,000 km including an air service between Irkutsk and Yakutsk.

In 1988–89 there were 194,000 pupils in 653 secondary schools, 10,300 students at 18 technical colleges and 7,900 attending 2 higher education institutions.

In 1989 there were 4,814 doctors and 16,400 hospital beds.

ADYGEI AUTONOMOUS REGION

Part of Krasnodar Territory. Area, 7,600 sq. km (2,934 sq. miles); population (Jan. 1989), 432,000. Capital, Maikop (149,000). Established 27 July 1922.

Chief industries are timber, woodworking, food processing and there is some engineering. Cattle breeding predominates in agriculture. There were 38 collective and 33 state farms in 1983.

In 1988–89 there were 164 schools with 59,000 pupils, 6 technical colleges with 7,000 students and a pedagogical institute with 5,200 students. In 1989 there were 1,422 doctors and 5,900 hospital beds.

GORNO-ALTAI AUTONOMOUS REGION

Part of Altai Territory. Area, 92,600 sq. km (35,740 sq. miles); population (Jan. 1989), 192,000. Capital, Gorno-Altaisk (39,000). Established 1 June 1922 as Oirot Autonomous Region; renamed 7 Jan. 1948.

Chief industries are gold, mercury and brown-coal mining, timber, chemicals and dairying. Cattle breeding predominates; pasturages and hay meadows cover over 1m. ha, but 142,000 ha are under crops. There were 20 collective and 37 state farms in 1983.

In 1988–89 there were 34,000 school pupils in 193 schools; 5 technical colleges had 4,300 students and 2,600 students were attending a pedagogical institute. There were 2,800 hospital beds and 735 doctors.

JEWISH AUTONOMOUS REGION

Part of Khabarovsk Territory. Area, 36,000 sq. km (13,895 sq. miles); population (Jan. 1989), 216,000 (1979 census, Russians, 84·1%; Ukrainians, 6·3%; Jews, 5·4%). Capital, Birobijan (82,000). Established as Jewish National District in 1928, became an Autonomous Region 7 May 1934.

Chief industries are non-ferrous metallurgy, building materials, timber, engineering, textiles, paper and food processing. There were 161,000 ha under cultivation in 1983; main crops are wheat, soya, oats, barley. There were 36 state farms and 2 collective farms in 1983.

In 1988–89 there were 35,000 pupils in 110 schools; students in 6 technical colleges numbered 5,400. There is a Yiddish national theatre, a Yiddish newspaper and a Yiddish broadcasting service. Doctors numbered 820 and hospital beds 3,100 in 1989.

KARACHAEVO-CHERKESS SOVIET SOCIALIST REPUBLIC

Part of Stavropol Territory. Area, 14,100 sq. km (5,442 sq. miles); population (Jan. 1989), 418,000. Capital, Cherkessk (113,000). A Karachai Autonomous Region was established on 26 April 1926 (out of a previously united Karachaevo-Cherkess Autonomous Region created in 1922), and dissolved in 1943. A Cherkess Autonomous Region was established on 30 April 1928. The present Autonomous Region was re-established on 9 Jan. 1957. The Region declared itself a Soviet Socialist Republic in Dec. 1990.

There are ore-mining, engineering, chemical and woodworking industries. The Kuban-Kalaussi irrigation scheme irrigates 200,000 ha. Livestock breeding and grain growing predominate in agriculture; crop area in 1983 was 196,000 ha. There were 15 collective farms and 37 state farms in 1983.

In 1988–89 there were 67,000 pupils in 178 secondary schools, 6 technical colleges with 5,400 students and 1 institute with 4,100 students. In 1989 there were 1,381 doctors and 4,700 hospital beds.

KHAKASS AUTONOMOUS REGION

Part of Krasnoyarsk Territory. Area, 61,900 sq. km (23,855 sq. miles); population (Jan. 1989), 569,000. Capital, Abakan (154,000). Established 20 Oct. 1930.

There are coal- and ore-mining, timber and woodworking industries. The region is linked by rail with the Trans-Siberian line.

In 1985, 1·8m. ha were under crops. Livestock breeding, dairy and vegetable farming are developed. There are 56 state farms.

In 1988–89 there were 89,000 pupils in 266 secondary schools, 7,900 students in 7 technical colleges and 6,100 students at a higher educational institution. In 1989 there were 1,913 doctors and 8,300 hospital beds.

AUTONOMOUS AREAS

Agin-Buryat Situated in Chita region (Eastern Siberia); area, 19,000 sq. km, population (1989), 77,000. Capital, Aginskoe. Formed 1937, its economy is basically pastoral.

Chukot Situated in Magadan region (Far East), its area of 737,700 sq. km in the far northeast. Population (1989), 158,000. Capital, Anadyr. Formed 1930. Population chiefly Russian, also Chukchi, Koryak, Yakut, Even. Minerals are extracted in the north, including gold, tin, mercury and tungsten.

Evenki Situated in Krasnoyarsk territory (Eastern Siberia); area, 767,600 sq. km, population (1989) 24,000, chiefly Evenks. Capital, Tura.

Khanty-Mansi Situated in Tyumen region (Western Siberia); area, 523,100 sq. km, population (1989) 1,269,000, chiefly Russians but also Khants and Mansi. Capital, Khanti-Mansiisk. Formed 1930.

Komi-Permyak Situated in Perm region (Northern Russia); area, 32,900 sq. km, population (1989) 159,000, chiefly Komi-Permyaks. Formed 1925. Capital, Kudymkar. Forestry is the main occupation.

Koryak Situated in Kamchatka region (Far East); area, 301,500 sq. km, population (1989) 39,000. Capital, Palana. Formed 1930.

Nenets Situated in Archangel region (Northern Russia); area, 176,700 sq. km, population (1989) 55,000. Capital, Naryan-Mar.

Taimyr Situated in Krasnoyarsk territory, this most northerly part of Siberia comprises the Taimyr peninsula and the Arctic islands of Severnaya Zemlya. Area, 862,100 sq. km, population (1989) 55,000, excluding the mining city of Norilsk which is separately administered. Capital, Dudinka.

Ust-Ordyn-Buryat Situated in Irkutsk region (Eastern Siberia); area, 22,400 sq. km, population (1989) 136,000. Capital, Ust-Ordynsk. Formed 1937.

Yamalo-Nenets Situated in Tyumen region (Western Siberia); area, 750,300 sq. km, population (1989) 487,000. Capital, Salekhard. Formed 1930.

Further Reading

Armstrong, T., *Russian Settlement in the North*. CUP, 1965
Dallin, D. J., *The Rise of Russia in Asia*. New York, 1949.—*Soviet Russia and the Far East*. London, 1949
Dukes, P., *A History of Russia: Medieval, Modern, Contemporary*. London, 1990
Kolarz, W., *The Peoples of the Soviet Far East*. London, 1954
Istoriya Sibiri s drevneishikh vremen do nashikh dnei. 5 vols., Leningrad, 1968–69

UKRAINE

Ukrainska Radyanska Sotsialistichna Respublika

HISTORY. The Ukrainian Soviet Socialist Republic was proclaimed on 25 Dec. 1917 and was finally established in Dec. 1919. In Dec. 1920 it concluded a military and economic alliance with the RSFSR and on 30 Dec. 1922 formed, together with the other Soviet Socialist Republics, the Union of Soviet Socialist Republics. On 1 Nov. 1939 Western Ukraine (about 88,000 sq. km) was incorporated in the Ukrainian SSR. On 2 Aug. 1940 Northern Bukovina (about 6,000 sq. km) ceded to the USSR by Romania 28 June 1940, and the Khotin, Akkerman and Izmail provinces of Bessarabia were included in the Ukrainian SSR, and on 29 June 1945 Ruthenia

(Sub-Carpathian Russia), about 7,000 sq. km, was also incorporated. From the new territories 2 new regions were formed, Chernovits and Izmail.

AREA AND POPULATION. The Ukraine is in south-west USSR; it has a Black Sea coast and western frontiers with Romania, Hungary, Poland and Czechoslovakia. It is bounded north by Belorussia and otherwise by the RSFSR. In 1938 the Ukrainian SSR covered an area of 445,000 sq. km (171,770 sq. miles); it now covers 603,700 sq. km (231,990 sq. miles).

Population, Jan. 1989, 51,704,000 (in 1979 census, 73·6% Ukrainians, 21·1% Russians, 1·3% Jews, 0·8% Belorussians).

The principal towns are the capital Kiev, Kharkov, Donetsk, Odessa, Dnepropetrovsk, Lvov, Zaporozhye and Krivoi Rog.

The Ukrainian SSR consists of the following regions: Cherkassy, Chernigov, Chernovtsy, Crimea (transferred from the RSFSR on 19 Feb. 1954, and elevated to the status of Autonomous Republic in 1991), Dnepropetrovsk, Donetsk, Ivan Franko, Khmelnitsky (formerly Kamenets-Podolsk), Kharkov, Kherson, Kiev, Kirovograd, Lvov, Nikolayev, Odessa, Poltava, Rovno, Sumy, Ternopol, Vinnitsa, Volhynia, Voroshilovgrad, Zakarpatskaya (Transcarpathia), Zaporozhye, Zhitomir.

CONSTITUTION AND GOVERNMENT. A new Constitution, based on that of the USSR, was adopted in April 1978. The 450-member Supreme Soviet was elected on 4 March 1990, Communists gaining 239 seats. In July 1990 it adopted a declaration of republican sovereignty by 355 votes to 4.

At local elections (21 June 1987), out of 527,799 deputies returned, 259,795 (49·2%) were women, 297,136 (56·3%) non-Party and 378,000 (72·1%) industrial workers and collective farmers. New elections were held on 4 March 1990.

Chairman, Supreme Soviet: Leonid Kravchuk (b. 1934; elected Aug. 1990 by 244 votes).

Chairman, Council of Ministers (Prime Minister): Vitold Fokin (Communist).

Foreign Minister: V. A. Kravtsev.

First Secretary, Communist Party: S. I. Gurenko.

FINANCE. Budget estimates (in 1m. rubles), 1988, 33,164; 1989 (plan), 36,885.

AGRICULTURE. The Ukraine contains some of the richest land in the USSR. It raises wheat, buckwheat, beet, sunflower, cotton, flax, tobacco, soya, hops, the rubber plant kok-sagyz, fruit and vegetables, and in 1985 produced 46% by value of the USSR's total agricultural output. The area under cultivation was 27m. ha in 1939 before the new territories were added, and 48·6m. ha in 1986.

Output (in 1m. tonnes) in 1988: Grain, 47·4; sugar-beet, 48·1; vegetables, 7·3; sunflower seed, 2·8; potatoes, 13·5; meat and fats, 4·3; milk, 24·3; 17,600m. eggs.

On 1 Jan. 1989 there were 25·6m. cattle, 19·5m. pigs, 9·2m. sheep and goats. In 1949 silver-fox breeding farms were started.

On 1 Jan. 1987 there were 2,466 state farms and 7,452 collective farms.

Irrigation networks supplied 1·82m. ha of land; 2·2m. ha were drained.

Tractors numbered 431,300 at 1 Jan. 1989 and combine harvesters, 115,300.

INDUSTRY. Coal in the Donets field (25,900 sq. km stretching from Donetsk to Rostov), estimated to contain 60% of the bituminous and anthracite coal reserves of the USSR, yielded, in 1988, 192m. tonnes—about 25% of the USSR production. Large seams have been found near Novo-Moskovsk (Dnepropetrovsk region), Kharkov, Lugansk (beyond the Don) and on the left bank of the Dnieper.

Combining coal from the Donets field with the iron-ore from the mines in Krivoi Rog has made possible the development of a large ferrous metallurgical industry. Output of steel was 56·5m. tonnes in 1988. Manganese is obtained at Nikopol; output in 1987, 7·2m. tons. Output of finished rolled metal products, 40m. tonnes in 1988; of steel pipe, 7·11m.

The Ukraine also contains oil, rich deposits of salt and various important chemicals. Oil output was 5·4m. tonnes in 1988, including natural gas.

There are chemical and machine-construction industries producing one-fifth of the total output of machinery and chemicals in the USSR. Output in 1988: Paper, 343,000 tonnes; synthetic fibre, 192,000 tonnes; sulphuric acid (1987), 4·2m. tonnes; caustic soda (1987), 489,000 tonnes; TV sets, 3·1m.; refrigerators, 753,000; washing machines, 533,000; vacuum cleaners, 904,000.

In Northern Bukovina there are deposits of gypsum, oil, alabaster, brown coal and timber. Output in 1988 of cardboard, 567,000 tonnes; of mineral fertilizers (re-calculated base), 5·6m. tonnes.

Consumer goods and food industries are important. Output in 1988 of knitwear, 346m. items; of motorcycles, 112,000; of granulated sugar, 6·1m. tonnes; of leather footwear, 191m. pairs; of preserves, 4,600m. standard jars.

There were 20·7m. industrial and office workers in 1987. There were 3·9m. collective farmers in 1985.

During the first 5-year plan (1929–32) the Dnieper power-station was built; destroyed during the War, it was restored during the fourth plan (1946–50). Another large hydro-electric station at Kakhovka began operations during the fifth plan (1951–55). Power output was 297,000m. kwh. in 1989.

EXTERNAL RELATIONS. In Nov. 1990 the Ukraine concluded an agreement with Russia to co-operate on defence, external policy and price co-ordination, and to exchange representatives.

COMMUNICATIONS. The total length of railways of the Ukrainian SSR in Jan. 1989 was 22,760 km, of hard-surface motor roads 219,900 km. In 1988, 11,040 tonne-km of freight was carried on inland waterways.

Airlines connect Kiev, Lvov, Chernovtsy and Odessa with Crimean and Caucasian spas, Kiev with Tbilisi, Odessa with Riga and Donetsk.

Newspapers (1988). Out of 1,794 newspapers, 1,261 were in Ukrainian. Daily circulation of Ukrainian-language newspapers, 15·9m., other languages, 8·2m.

RELIGION. The main churches are the Orthodox and Roman Catholic. The Uniate Church, which practises the Orthodox rite but acknowledges the Pope of Rome, was banned in 1946. There is also an Autocephalous Orthodox Church of Ukraine. (*Patriarch*, Mstislav; b.1898). There are also some Protestants as well as Jews and others.

EDUCATION. In 1988–89 the number of pupils in 21,500 primary and secondary schools was 7·1m.; 146 higher educational establishments had 854,000 students, and 737 technical colleges 792,400 students; 61% of children were attending pre-school institutions.

The Ukrainian Academy of Sciences was established in 1919; in 1989 it had 78 institutions with 17,256 scientific staff. There is an academy of building and architecture. Total scientific staff in all institutions was 219,300 in 1989.

HEALTH. Doctors numbered 221,700 in 1988, and hospital beds, 687,500.

DIPLOMATIC REPRESENTATIVE

Of the Ukraine to the United Nations
Ambassador: Gennadi I. Udovenko.

Further Reading

Allen, W. E. D., *The Ukraine: A History*. 2nd ed. Cambridge, 1963
Kubiojovyc, V. (ed.) *Encyclopedia of Ukraine*, 4 vols. Toronto, 1984ff
Magoci, P. R. and Matthews, G. J., *Ukraine: A Historical Atlas*. Univ. of Toronto Press, 1985

BELORUSSIA (WHITE RUSSIA)

Belaruskaya Sovietskaya Sotsialistychnaya Respublika

HISTORY. The Belorussian Soviet Socialist Republic was set up on 1 Jan. 1919.

AREA AND POPULATION. Belorussia is situated along the Western Dvina and Dnieper. It is bounded in the west by Poland, north by Latvia and Lithuania, east by the RSFSR and south by the Ukraine. The area is 207,600 sq. km (80,134 sq. miles). The capital is Minsk. Other important towns are Gomel, Vitebsk, Mogilev, Bobruisk, Grodno and Brest. On 2 Nov. 1939 western Belorussia was incorporated with an area of over 108,000 sq. km and a population of 4·8m. The population (Jan. 1989) was 10,200,000; 79·4% of this population in 1979 (census) were Belorussians, 4·2% Poles, 11·9% Russians, 2·4% Ukrainians and 1·4% Jews.

Belorussia comprises the following regions: Brest, Gomel, Grodno, Mogilev, Minsk, Vitebsk.

CONSTITUTION AND GOVERNMENT. A new Constitution was adopted in April 1978. The Supreme Soviet elected on 4 March 1990 consists of 360 seats, 50 of which are filled by public organizations. In July 1990 it adopted a declaration of republican sovereignty by 230 votes to nil with 120 abstentions.

At elections to regional, district, urban and rural Soviets (21 June 1987), of 85,375 deputies returned, 41,518 (48·6%) were women. New elections were held on 4 March 1990.

Chairman, Supreme Soviet: N. I. Dementei.
Chairman, Council of Ministers: M. V. Kovalev.
Foreign Minister: A. E. Gurinovich
First Secretary, Communist Party: A. A. Malofeev.

FINANCE. Budget estimates (in 1m. rubles), 1988, 8,893; 1989 (plan), 11,022.

NATURAL RESOURCES. Belorussia is hilly, with a general slope towards the south. It contains large tracts of marsh land, particularly to the south-west, and valuable forest land wooded with oak, elm, maple and white beech: There are over 6,500 peat deposits.

AGRICULTURE. Agriculturally, Belorussia may be divided into three main sections—Northern: Growing flax, fodder, grasses and breeding cattle for meat and dairy produce; Central: Potato growing and pig breeding; Southern: Good natural pasture land, hemp cultivation and cattle breeding for meat and dairy produce. The area under cultivation was 12·3m. ha in 1986. There were 7·3m. cattle, 5·1m. pigs and 570,400 sheep and goats on 1 Jan. 1989.

Output of main agricultural products (in 1,000 tonnes) in 1988: Grain, 6,922; meat, 1,169; milk, 7,501; eggs, 3,498m.; potatoes, 7,708; vegetables, 881; sugar-beet, 1,585.

On 1 Jan. 1987 there were 1,675 collective farms and 913 state farms. About 2·5m. ha of marsh land have been drained for agricultural use, 828,200 of these for crops. This reclaimed land is rich and yields good harvests of grain, fodder, potatoes, kok-sagyz and other crops. In Jan. 1989 there were 127,300 tractors and 34,300 grain combine harvesters.

INDUSTRY. There are food-processing, chemical, textile, artificial silk, flax-spinning, motor vehicle, leather, machine-tool and agricultural machinery industries.

In 1988 output was as follows: Chemical fibre, 437,000 tonnes; steel, 1·1m. tonnes; paper, 203,000 tonnes; bricks, 2,279m.; radio receivers, 798,000; televisions, 1,040,000; watches, 10·9m.; bicycles, 845,000; granulated sugar, 355,000 tonnes; preserves, 731m. jars; footwear, 46·9m. pairs.

Particular attention has been paid to the development of the peat industry with a view to making Belorussia as far as possible self-supporting in fuel. In 1988 2·3m. tonnes of peat briquettes were produced. There are rich deposits of rock salt.

Output of electricity in 1988, 38,100m. kwh.

The number of employees in 1988 was 4,328,000.

COMMUNICATIONS. In Jan. 1989 there were 5,580 km of railways, 90,300 km of motor roads (56,600 km hard-surface) and 1,815m. tonne-km of freight was carried on inland waterways.

Newspapers (1988). Of 216 newspapers published 130 were in Belorussian. Daily circulation of Belorussian-language newspapers, 1·7m., other languages, 3·6m.

EDUCATION. In 1988–89 there were 178,600 students in 33 places of higher education and 149,300 students in 138 technical colleges. There were (Jan. 1989) 44,100 scientific personnel in 178 institutions, and 562,300 specialists with a higher education employed in the national economy. The Belorussian Academy of Sciences controlled 32 learned institutions with 5,923 scientific staff. The number of children in 5,700 primary and secondary schools was 1·5m. in 1988–89. 71% of children attended pre-school institutions in Jan. 1989.

HEALTH. In 1988 there were 40,500 doctors and 137,400 hospital beds.

DIPLOMATIC REPRESENTATIVE

Of Belorussia to the United Nations
Ambassador: Gennadi N. Buravkin.

Further Reading

Belaruskaya Sovietskaya Entsyklapediya. Minsk, 1960–76
Lubachko, I. S., *Belorussia under Soviet Rule, 1917–57*. Lexington, 1972
Vakar, N. P., *Belorussia*. Harvard Univ. Press, 1956.—*A Bibliographical Guide to Belorussia*. Harvard Univ. Press, 1956

AZERBAIJAN

Azarbaijchan Soviet Sotsialistik Respublikasy

HISTORY. The 'Mussavat' (Nationalist) party, which dominated the National Council or Constituent Assembly of the Tatars, declared the independence of Azerbaijan on 28 May 1918, with a capital, first at Ganja (Elizavetpol) and later at Baku. On 28 April 1920 Azerbaijan was proclaimed a Soviet Socialist Republic. From 1922, with Georgia and Armenia it formed the Transcaucasian Soviet Federal Socialist Republic. In 1936 it assumed the status of one of the Union Republics of the USSR. In Jan. 1990 there were violent disturbances in Baku and on the Armenian border over the enclave of Nagorno-Karabakh.

AREA AND POPULATION. Azerbaijan covers an area of 86,600 sq. km (33,430 sq. miles) and has a population (Jan. 1989) of 7,029,000. Its capital is Baku. Other important towns are Kirovabad and Sumgait. Nakhichevan is the capital of the Autonomous Republic of the same name.

Azerbaijan includes the Nakhichevan Autonomous Republic and the Nagorno-Karabakh Autonomous Region. Situated in the eastern area of Transcaucasia, it is protected by mountains in the west and north, washed by the Caspian Sea in the east and bounded by Iran in the south. Its climate is inclined to drought.

In 1979 (census) 78·1% of the population were Azerbaijanis, who are mainly Shi'a Moslems. Other nationalities were Russians (7·9%), Armenians (7·9%) and Daghestanis (3·4%).

CONSTITUTION AND GOVERNMENT. Elections were held to the 350 seats in the Supreme Soviet in Sept. 1990. A new Constitution was adopted in April 1978.

At elections to the Nagorno-Karabakh regional Soviet and the district, urban and rural Soviets (21 June 1987), of 51,681 deputies returned, 24,859 (48·1%) were women, 28,484 (55·1%) non-Party and 35,047 (67·8%) industrial workers and collective farmers.

President: Ayaz Mutalibov (*First Secretary, Communist Party*).
Chairman, Council of Ministers (Prime Minister): Hasan Hasanov.

FINANCE. (in 1m. rubles). Budget estimates, 1988, 3,361; 1989 (plan), 3,808.

AGRICULTURE. The chief agricultural products are grain, cotton, rice, grapes, fruit, vegetables, tobacco and silk. The Mexican rubber plant *grayule* has been acclimatized. A new kind of high-yielding winter wheat has been produced for use in mountainous parts of the republic. Area under cultivation, 6·7m. ha.

Livestock on 1 Jan. 1989: Cattle, 2m.; pigs, 215,700; sheep and goats, 5·7m.

Output of main agricultural products (in 1,000 tonnes) in 1988: Grain, 1,417; cotton, 616; grapes, 1,247; vegetables, 880; tobacco, 60 (in 1987); potatoes, 165; tea, 22·4; meat, 190; milk, 1,067; eggs, 1,067m.; wool, 11·9.

Azerbaijan has become an important cotton-growing and sub-tropical base. About 70% of cultivated land is irrigated. On the irrigated land crops of Egyptian and Sea-Island cotton are obtained. Here, too, rice and lucerne are cultivated, and in the mountain valleys there are also orchards, vineyards and silk cultures.

In the south along the coast of the Caspian, where the climate is more moist, there are tea plantations, and citrus fruits and other sub-tropical plants are grown.

There were on 1 Jan. 1989, 608 collective farms, 808 state farms, 39,300 tractors and 4,600 grain combine harvesters.

INDUSTRY. The republic is rich in natural resources: Oil, iron, aluminium, copper, lead, zinc, precious metals, sulphur pyrites, limestone and salt. Iron and steel and aluminium works have been built at Sumgait.

The most important industry is the oil industry, especially in the Baku region. The largest producing area lies along the western shore of the Caspian Sea, north and south of Baku, where the largest refineries are located. Other wells lie west of Baku, and some have been drilled in the Caspian itself, off the Apsheron Peninsula. Baku is connected by a double pipeline with Batum on the Black Sea. All the oilfields have been electrified and are connected with Baku.

Azerbaijan has also copper, chemical, cement and building material, food, timber, salt, textiles and fishing industries. In 1988, 840,100 tonnes of steel were produced, 726,300 tonnes of iron ore, 1·2m. tonnes of cement, 5m. square metres of linoleum, 42·6m. items of knitwear, 236,200 tonnes of caustic soda, 20m. pairs of leather footwear, 106,000 tonnes of confectionery and 805·7m. standard jars of conserves.

Kirovabad, Nukha, Stepanakert, Nakhichevan and Lenkoran are also important industrial centres.

In 1988 electric power output was 23,500m. kwh. Output of gas was 10,989m. cubic metres in 1976. Pipelines from Karadag to Baku and Sumgait supply gas fuel for all oil-cracking factories and most engineering works.

Synthetic rubber works (Sumgait), tyre works and a worsted combine (Baku) and a large textile combine (Mingechaur) have been built.

The number of employees in 1988 was 2,115,000.

COMMUNICATIONS. Total length of railways in 1989, 2,070 km, of motor roads 30,000 km (28,200 km hard surface).

Newspapers (1988). There were 150 newspapers, 128 in the Azerbaijani language (circulation 2·4m.), other languages, (circulation 479,000).

EDUCATION. In 1988–89 there were 1·4m. pupils in 4,400 primary and secondary schools and 20% of children attended pre-school institutions. There were 77 technical colleges with 67,600 students, 16 higher educational institutions, including a state university at Baku, with 98,800 students (including correspondence students). The Azerbaijan Academy of Sciences, founded in 1945, has 30 research institutions with 4,296 research workers. There were 22,700 research workers in the republic as a whole in Jan. 1989.

HEALTH. In 1988 there were 27,600 doctors and 69,400 hospital beds.

NAKHICHEVAN AUTONOMOUS SOVIET SOCIALIST REPUBLIC

Area, 5,500 sq. km (2,120 sq. miles), population (Jan. 1989), 295,000. Capital, Nakhichevan (37,000). This territory, on the borders of Turkey and Iran, forms part of the Azerbaijan SSR although separated from it by the territory of Soviet Armenia. Its population, mainly Azerbaijanis, had a chequered history for 1,500 years under the ancient Persians, Arabs, Seljuk Turks, Mongols, Ottoman Turks and modern Persians before being annexed by Russia in 1828. On 9 Feb. 1924 it was constituted as an Autonomous Republic within Azerbaijan. Its Supreme Soviet, elected 24 Feb. 1985, has 110 members including 52 women.

The republic has silk, clothing, cotton, canning, meat-packing and other factories. Nearly 70% of the people are engaged in agriculture, of which the main branches are cotton and tobacco growing. Fruit and grapes are also produced in increasing quantity. There are 35 collective and 37 state farms. Crop area 37,400 ha.

In 1984–85 there were 219 primary and secondary schools with 66,000 pupils, and 2,100 were studying in higher educational institutions.

In Jan. 1983 there were 599 doctors and 2,500 hospital beds.

NAGORNO-KARABAKH AUTONOMOUS REGION

Area, 4,400 sq. km (1,700 sq. miles); population (Jan. 1989), 188,000. Capital, Stepanakert (33,000). Populated by Armenians (75·9%) and Azerbaijanis (23%), a separate khanate in the 18th century, it was established on 7 July 1923 as an Autonomous Region within Azerbaijan.

Main industries are silk, wine, dairying and building materials. Crop area is 67,200 ha; cotton, grapes and winter wheat are grown. There are 33 collective and 38 state farms.

In 1984–85 34,000 pupils were studying in primary and secondary schools, 2,400 in colleges and 2,100 in higher educational institutions. In Jan. 1983 there were 523 doctors and 1,800 hospital beds.

Following extensive public demonstrations in Armenia and Azerbaijan as well as Nagorno-Karabakh itself, the area was placed under a 'special form of administration' subordinate to the USSR government in 1989.

Further Reading

Baddeley, J. F., *The Rugged Flanks of Caucasus*. 2 vols. Oxford, 1941
Guseinov, I. A. et al, *Istoriya Azerbaidzhana*. 8 vols. Baku, 1958–63

GEORGIA

Sakartvelos Respublika (Republic of Georgia)

HISTORY. The independence of the Georgian Social Democratic Republic was declared at Tiflis on 26 May 1918 by the National Council, elected by the National Assembly of Georgia on 22 Nov. 1917. The independence of Georgia was recognized by the USSR on 7 May 1920. On 12 Feb. 1921 a rising broke out in Mingrelia, Abkhazia and Adjaria, and Soviet troops invaded the country, which, on 25 Feb. 1921, was proclaimed the Georgian Soviet Socialist Republic. On 15 Dec. 1922 Georgia was merged with Armenia and Azerbaijan to form the Trancaucasian Soviet Federal Socialist Republic. In 1936 the Georgian Soviet Socialist Republic became one of the constituent republics of the USSR. Following nationalist successes at elections in Oct. 1990, the Supreme Soviet resolved in Nov. 1990 to begin a transition to full independence and renamed the republic the 'Republic of Georgia'.

AREA AND POPULATION. Georgia is bounded west by the Black Sea and south by Turkey, Armenia and Azerbaijan. It occupies the whole of the western part of Transcaucasia and covers an area of 69,700 sq. km (26,900 sq. miles). Its population on 1 Jan. 1989 was 5,449,000. The capital is Tbilisi (Tiflis). Other important towns are Kutaisi (235,000), Rustavi (159,000), Batumi (136,000), Sukhumi (121,000), Poti (54,000), Gori (59,000).

Protected from the north by the Caucasian mountains and receiving in the west the warm, moist winds from the Black Sea into which most of its rivers flow, Georgia is outstanding for its fine, warm climate and its natural wealth, variety and beauty. It has the highest snow-capped peaks of the Caucasian mountains. Georgia contains valuable sulphur and other medicinal springs. Georgians, an ancient people, were (1979 census) 68·8% of the population; Armenians 9%; Russians, 7·4%; Azerbaijanis, 5·1%; Ossetians, 3·2%; Abkhazians, 1·7%.

CONSTITUTION AND GOVERNMENT. The Georgian Republic includes the Abkhazian ASSR, the Adjarian ASSR and the South Ossetian Autonomous Region.

The Supreme Soviet consists of 250 deputies. At the elections of Nov. 1990 the 7-party coalition Round Table-Free Georgia won 155 seats with 62% of the votes cast.

At elections to the district, rural and urban Soviets, and that of the South Ossetian region (21 June 1987), of 50,982 deputies returned 25,826 (50·7%) were women, 28,974 (56·8%) non-Party and 34,930 (68·5%) industrial workers and collective farmers.

Chairman, Presidium of the Supreme Soviet: Zviad Gamsakhurdia (b.1939; Round Table).

Chairman, Council of Ministers: T. Sigua.

First Secretary, Communist Party: Avtandil Margiari.

FINANCE (in 1m. rubles). Budget estimates, 1988, 3,360; 1989 (plan), 4,067.

AGRICULTURE. There are 3 main agricultural areas: (1) The moist subtropical area along the Black Sea Coast, where are cultivated tea, citrus fruits (lemons, oranges, mandarins, etc.), the tung tree (which yields special industrial oils), eucalyptus, bamboo, high-quality tobacco; (2) Imeretia (the Kutais region) where the chief cultures are grapes and silk, and (3) Kakhetia, along the Alazani (a tributary of the Kura river), famed for its orchards and wines. Land under cultivation was 4·6m. ha in 1986.

Output of main agricultural products (in 1,000 tonnes) in 1988: Grain, 714; tea leaf, 458; citrus fruit, 439; sugar-beet, 51; potatoes, 326; vegetables, 641; grapes, 621; meat, 182; milk, 743; eggs, 871m.; wool, 6.

On 1 Jan. 1986 there were 719 collective farms working over 66% of all agricultural land, 594 state farms working nearly 34% of such land. In the Colchis area 115,000 ha of extremely rich land have been reclaimed. There are 389,000 ha of irrigated land. 151,400 ha of marsh land have been drained. Tractors numbered 25,900 on 1 Jan. 1989; grain combines, 1,600.

Livestock on 1 Jan. 1989: Cattle, 1·5m.; pigs, 1·1m.; sheep and goats, 1·9m.

Georgia is rich in forest lands where fine varieties of timber are grown. Area covered by forests, 2·4m. ha.

INDUSTRY. The most important mining industry is the exploitation of the manganese deposits, the richest of which lie in the Chiatura region. Manganese deposits are calculated at 250m. tonnes, distributed over an area of 140 sq. km. The most important coal seams are at Tkvarcheli (deposits estimated at 250m. tonnes) and Tkibuli (deposits of 80m. tonnes). Other important minerals are baryta, the best in the USSR, fire-resisting and other clays, diatomite shale, oil, agate, marble, cement, alabaster, iron and other ores, building stone, arsenic, molybdenum, tungsten and mercury. In 1941 a goldfield was discovered. Output of coal in 1988 was 1·4m. tonnes.

The Transcaucasian Metallurgical Plant is at Rustavi (near Tbilisi) and there is a motor works at Kutaisi. There are factories for processing tea, creameries and breweries. There are also textile and silk industries.

In 1988, 1·8m. tonnes of manganese ore were produced, 1·4m. tonnes of steel, 186,000 tonnes of oil, 517,000 tonnes of steel pipe, 39,700 tonnes of chemical fibres, 28,500 tonnes of paper, 17·8m. pairs of footwear, 60·1m. knitwear garments, 55,700 colour televisions, 68,600 tonnes of confectionery, 458,200 tonnes of tea and 938m. jars of preserves.

Georgia's fast flowing rivers form an abundant source of energy. The hydro-electric station at Tblisi has an installed capacity of 1m. kw. Power output in 1987 was 14,500m. kwh.

There were 2,228,000 employees in 1988.

COMMUNICATIONS. Length of railways in 1989, 1,580 km; of motor roads 42,800 (with hard surface 37,600).

Newspapers (1988). Out of 148 newspapers, 139 were in Georgian. Daily circulation of Georgian-language newspapers, 3·1m., other languages, 568,000.

EDUCATION. In 1988–89 there were 900,000 pupils in 3,700 primary and secondary schools, 47,900 in 89 technical colleges and 85,600 students in 19 higher educational institutions. Tbilisi University has 16,300 students. In towns, 11 years' education is usual. In Abastuman there is an astro-physical observatory. In 1936 a branch of the Academy of Sciences of the USSR was formed in Tbilisi, and in Feb. 1941 a Georgian Academy of Sciences was opened, which in Jan. 1988 had 42 institutions with scientific staff totalling 6,107. There were in all 194 research institutions with 29,000 scientific staff.

In Jan. 1989, 44% of children were attending pre-school institutions.

HEALTH. There were 30,700 doctors and 58,700 hospital beds in 1988.

ABKHAZIAN AUTONOMOUS SOVIET SOCIALIST REPUBLIC

Area, 8,600 sq. km (3,320 sq. miles); population (Jan. 1989), 537,000. Capital Sukhumi (1989 census population, 121,000). This area, the ancient Colchis, included Greek colonies from the 6th century B.C. onwards. From the 2nd century B.C. onwards, it was a prey to many invaders—Romans, Byzantines, Arabs, Ottoman Turks—before accepting a Russian protectorate in 1810. However, from the 4th century A.D. a West Georgian kingdom was established by the Lazi princes in the territory (known to the Romans as 'Lazica') and by the 8th century the prevailing language was Georgian and the name Abkhazia. In March 1921 a congress of local Soviets proclaimed it a Soviet Republic, and its status as an Autonomous Republic, within Georgia, was confirmed on 17 April 1930.

Population (1979 census) Abkhazians, 17·1%, Georgians, 43·9% and Russians, 16·4%.

140 deputies were elected to the republican Supreme Soviet on 24 Feb. 1985, 57 of them women.

The Abkhazian coast (along the Black Sea) possesses a famous chain of health resorts—Gagra, Sukhumi, Akhali-Antoni, Gulripsha and Gudauta—sheltered by thickly forested mountains.

The republic has coal, electric power, building materials and light industries. In 1985 there were 89 collective farms and 56 state farms; main crops are tobacco, tea, grapes, oranges, tangerines and lemons. Crop area 43,900 ha.

Livestock, 1 Jan. 1987: 147,300 cattle, 127,900 pigs, 28,800 sheep and goats.

In 1986–87 about 100,000 pupils were engaged in study at all levels. A university has been opened in Sukhumi.

In Jan. 1985 there were 2,300 doctors and 6,000 hospital beds.

ADJARIAN AUTONOMOUS SOVIET SOCIALIST REPUBLIC

Area, 3,000 sq. km (1,160 sq. miles); population (Jan. 1989), 393,000. Capital, Batumi (1989 census population, 136,000). After a history similar to that of Abkhazia, it fell under Turkish rule in the 17th century, and was annexed to Russia (rejoining Georgia) after the Berlin Treaty of 1878. On 16 July 1921 the territory was constituted as an Autonomous Republic within the Georgian SSR.

Population (1979 census) Georgians, 80·1%, Russians, 9·8% and Armenians 4·6%.

110 deputies were elected to the republican Supreme Soviet on 24 Feb. 1985, 45 of them women.

The republic specializes in sub-tropical agricultural products. These include tea, mandarines and lemons, grapes, bamboo, eucalyptus, etc. Livestock (Jan. 1987): 133,400 cattle, 6,300 pigs, 11,600 sheep and goats. In 1980 there were 69 collective farms and 21 state farms.

There are shipyards at Batumi, modern oil-refining plant (the pipeline from the Baku oilfields ends at Batumi), food-processing and canning factories, clothing, building materials, drug factories, etc.

Health resorts are Kobuleti, Tsikhisdziri, Batumi on the coast and Beshumi in the hills. The sub-tropical climate and flora, and the combination of mountains and sea, make this republic (like Abkhazia) a favourite holiday area.

In 1986–87 79,800 pupils were engaged in study at all levels and 1,000 graduated from colleges.

In Jan. 1985 there were 1,430 doctors and 3,900 hospital beds.

SOUTH OSSETIAN AUTONOMOUS REGION

This area was populated by Ossetians from across the Caucasus (North Ossetia), driven out by the Mongols in the 13th century. The region was set up within the Georgian SSR on 20 April 1922. Area, 3,900 sq. km (1,505 sq. miles); population (Jan. 1989), 99,000 (1979 census, Ossetians, 66·4% and Georgians, 28·8%). Capital, Tskhinvali (34,000).

Main industries are mining, timber, electrical engineering and building materials. Crop area, chiefly grains, was 21,600 ha in 1985; other pursuits are sheepfarming (128,500 sheep and goats on 1 Jan. 1987) and vine-growing. There were 14 collective farms and 18 state farms.

In 1986–87 there were 18,543 pupils in elementary and secondary schools; there were 1,967 graduates from higher educational institutions and 837 from colleges.

In Jan. 1987 there were 511 doctors and 1,400 hospital beds.

Further Reading

Lang, D. M., *A Modern History of Georgia*. London, 1962. — *The Georgians*. London, 1966

Gvarjaladze, T. and I. (eds.) *English-Georgian and Georgian-English Dictionary*. Tbilisi, 1974

Suny, R. G., *The Making of the Georgian Nation*. London, 1989

Istoriya Gruzii. 3 vols. Tbilisi, 1962–73

ARMENIA

Haikakan Hanrapetoutioun (Republic of Armenia)

HISTORY. On 29 Nov. 1920 Armenia was proclaimed a Soviet Socialist Republic. The Armenian Soviet Government, with the Russian Soviet Government, was a party to the Treaty of Kars (March 1921), which confirmed the Turkish possession of the former Government of Kars and of the Surmali District of the Government of Yerevan. From 1922 to 1936 it formed part of the Transcaucasian Soviet Federal Socialist Republic. In 1936 Armenia was proclaimed a constituent republic of the USSR.

AREA AND POPULATION. Armenia covers an area of 29,800 sq. km (11,490 sq. miles). It is bounded in the north by Georgia, in the east by Azerbaijan and in the south and west by Turkey and Iran. It is a very mountainous country with but little forest land, has many turbulent rivers and a highly fertile soil, but is subject to drought. In Jan. 1989 the population was 3,283,000. Census (1979) 89·7% of the population were Armenians, the rest are Russians (2·3%), Kurds (1·7%), Azerbaijanians (5·3%). The capital is Yerevan. Other large towns are Leninakan (120,000) and Kirovakan (159,000).

CONSTITUTION AND GOVERNMENT. A new Constitution was adopted in April 1978. The Supreme Soviet has 259 seats. Elections took place on 20 May 1990. The Supreme Soviet adopted a declaration of sovereignty in Aug. 1990, voted to unite Armenia with Nagorny Karabakh and renamed Armenia the 'Republic of Armenia'.

At elections to the district, urban and rural Soviets (21 June 1987), of 27,776 deputies returned 13,758 (49·5%) were women, 15,681 (56·5%) non-Party and 19,149 (68·9%) industrial workers and collective farmers.

In Aug. 1990 the Supreme Soviet elected Levon Ter Petrosyan (b. 1945; leader, Armenian National Movement) its Chairman (i.e. *President of the Republic*) by 140 votes to 80. Vazgen Manukyan (Armenian National Movement) was elected Chairman of the Council of Ministers (i.e. *Prime Minister*) by 170 votes to 35. The *First Secretary of the Communist Party* is S. K. Pogosyan (Dec. 1990).

FINANCE. Budget estimates (in 1m. rubles), 1988, 2,243; 1989 (plan), 2,460.

AGRICULTURE. The chief agricultural area is the valley of the Arax and the area round Yerevan. Here there are considerable cotton plantations as well as orchards and vineyards. Sub-tropical plants, such as almonds and figs, are also grown. Olive groves and pomegranate plantations occupy large areas; experiments are being made to naturalize cork oak. In the mountainous areas the chief pursuit is livestock raising. Land under cultivation in Nov. 1986, 2·3m. ha.

Output of main agricultural products (in 1,000 tonnes) in 1988: Grain, 374; potatoes, 207; vegetables, 567; sugar-beet, 117; fruit, 241; grapes, 205; meat, 120; milk, 570; eggs, 621m.; wool, 4·1.

Area of irrigated land in 1982 was 284,000 ha.

There were, on 1 Jan. 1987, 280 collective farms, and these together with the 513 state farms tilled 99·9% of the total cultivated area. Livestock in Jan. 1989 included 317,000 pigs, 743,600 cattle and 1·5m. sheep and goats. There were 13,400 tractors and 1,900 grain and cotton combines in Jan. 1989.

INDUSTRY. Armenia contains large deposits of copper, zinc, aluminium, molybdenum and other metals. It is also rich in marble, granite, cement and other building materials. The mining of these minerals is becoming more and more important. Among other industries are the chemical, producing chiefly synthetic rubber and fertilizers, and the extraction and processing of building materials such as cement, pumice-stone, tuffs, marble, volcanic basalt and fire-proof clay, ginning- and textile-mills, carpet weaving, food, including wine-making, fruit, meat-canning and creameries. Machine-tool and electrical engineering works have also been established. Among the industrial centres are Yerevan, Leninakan, Alaverdi, Kafan, Kirovakan, Daval, Megri and Oktemberyan. Output of electricity in 1988 was 15,300m. kwh. A chain ('cascade') of 8 hydro-electric stations on the river Razdan, as it falls about 3,300 ft from the mountain lake Sevan to its junction with the Arax, has been completed.

In 1988 output included 76,200 centrifugal pumps, 146m. light bulbs, 138,700 km of light cable, 1·4m. cubic metres of ferroconcrete, 15,000 tonnes of synthetic fabric, 4·5m. clocks, 89,000 washing machines, 47,300 tonnes of confectionery and 490·3m. jars of preserves.

There were 1,363,000 employees in the state sector in 1988.

COMMUNICATIONS. Length of railways in Jan. 1989, 830 km; motor roads, 12,100 km (hard surface, 9,400).

Newspapers (1988). Out of 90 newspapers 79 appeared in Armenian. Daily circulation of Armenian-language newspapers, 1·5m.; other languages, 135,000.

EDUCATION. In 1988–89 there were 600,000 pupils in 1,400 primary and secondary schools; 65 technical colleges with 47,100 students; 13 higher educational institutions with 57,900 students (including correspondence students). Yerevan houses the Armenian Academy of Sciences, 43 scientific institutes, a medical institute and other technical colleges, and a state university. In Jan. 1989, 33 learned institutions with 3,330 scientific staff were under the Academy of Sciences; scientific workers in 101 institutions totalled 21,800.

In Jan. 1989 39% of children attended pre-school institutions.

HEALTH. In 1988 there were 13,800 doctors and 30,400 hospital beds.

Further Reading

Kurkjian, V., *A History of Armenia*. New York, 1958

Lang, D.M., *Armenia: Cradle of Civilization*. London, 1978.—*The Armenians. A People in Exile*. London, 1981

Walker, C. J., *Armenia*. 2nd ed. London, 1990

MOLDAVIA

Republica Sovietică Socialistă Moldovenească

HISTORY. The Moldavian Soviet Socialist Republic (in 1990 renamed Moldova), capital Kishinev, was formed by the union of part of the former Moldavian Autonomous Soviet Socialist Republic (organized 12 Oct. 1924), formerly included in the Ukrainian Soviet Socialist Republic, and the areas of Bessarabia (ceded by Romania to the USSR, 28 June 1940) with a mainly Moldavian population. As from 2 Aug. 1940 the MSSR includes the following regions of the former Moldavian Autonomous Soviet Socialist Republic: Grigoriopol, Dubossarsk, Kamensk, Rybnits, Slobodzeisk and Tiraspol, and the following districts of Bessarabia: Beltsk, Bendery, Kagulsk, Kishinev, Orgeev and Sorok. The republic, however, is divided not into regions but into 36 rural districts, 21 towns and 45 urban settlements.

AREA AND POPULATION. Moldavia is bounded in the east and south by the Ukraine and on the west by Romania. The area is 33,700 sq. km (13,000 sq. miles). In Jan. 1989 the population was 4,341,000, of whom (1979 census) 63·9% are Moldavians. Others include Ukrainians (14·2%), Russians (12·8%), Gagauzi (3·5%), Jews (2%). Apart from Kishinev, larger towns are Tiraspol (182,000), Beltsy (159,000) and Bendery (130,000). The Moldavian language (i.e., Romanian) was written in Cyrillic prior to the restoration of the Roman alphabet in 1989.

CONSTITUTION AND GOVERNMENT. A new Constitution was adopted in April 1978. Elections to the 380 seats in the Supreme Soviet were held on 25 Feb. 1990. A declaration of republican sovereignty was adopted in June 1990.

Elections to the district, urban and rural Soviets were also held on 25 Feb. 1990.

President of the Republic: M. I. Snegur.
Chairman of the Supreme Soviet: A. Moseanu

Chairman, Council of Ministers: M. Druk.
First Secretary, Communist Party: G. I. Eremei.

FINANCE. Budget estimates (in 1m. rubles), 1988, 3,000; 1989 (plan), 3,396.

AGRICULTURE. On 1 Jan. 1989 there were 368 collective farms and 473 state farms. All ploughing and sowing is mechanized. Livestock included (1 Jan. 1989) 1·1m. cattle, 1·9m. pigs and 1·3m. sheep and goats. There were 50,300 tractors and 4,700 combine harvesters in Jan. 1989. Land under cultivation (Nov. 1986) 2·9m. ha.

Output of main agricultural products (in 1,000 tonnes) in 1988: Grain, 3,052; sugar-beet, 2,272; vegetables, 1,281; fruit, 856; grapes, 1,120; meat, 334; milk, 1,491; eggs, 1,176m.

Moldavia has an equable climate and very fertile soil. It contains nearly one quarter of the vineyards of the USSR, and is also rich in fish in the south: Sturgeon, mackerel, brill.

INDUSTRY. There are canning plants, wine-making plants, woodworking and metallurgical factories, a factory of ferro-concrete building materials, and footwear and textile plants. Production in 1988 included 103,000 centrifugal pumps, 713,000 tonnes of steel, 22m. pairs footwear, 6·6m. items knitwear, 82,500 colour televisions, 155,900 refrigerators, 310,000 washing machines, 1,843m. jars of preserves. Food industries include processing of dairy produce. Electricity generated (1986) 17,700m. kwh.

There are lignite, phosphorites, gypsum and valuable building materials.

In 1988 there were 1,566,000 employees in the state sector.

COMMUNICATIONS. Length of railways in Jan. 1989, 1,150 km. There are 19,600 km of motor roads (13,700 hard surface). 263m. tonne-km of freight was carried on inland waterways.

Newspapers (1988). There were 195 newspapers, 81 in Moldavian. Daily circulation of Moldavian-language newspapers, 1,118,000; other languages, 1,223,000.

EDUCATION. In 1988–89 there were 700,000 pupils in 1,600 primary, secondary and special schools, 55,200 students in 51 technical colleges and 53,100 students in 9 higher educational institutions including the state university. A Moldavian Academy of Sciences was established in 1961; it had 17 research institutions and a scientific staff of 1,264 in Jan. 1989. In all, there are 68 learned institutions with 10,200 scientific staff. In Jan. 1989, 70% of children attended pre-school institutions.

HEALTH. In 1988 there were 17,100 doctors and 55,100 hospital beds.

Further Reading

Zlatova, Y. and Kotelnikov, V., *Across Moldavia* (English ed.). Moscow, 1959
Istoriya Moldavskoi SSR. 2nd ed. 2 vols. Kishinev, 1965–68

ESTONIA

Eesti Vabariik (Republic of Estonia)

HISTORY. The workers' and soldiers' Soviets in Estonia took over power on 8 Nov. 1917, were overthrown by the German occupying forces in March 1918, and were restored to power as the Germans withdrew in Nov. 1918, establishing the 'Estland Labour Commune'. It was overthrown with the assistance of British naval forces in May 1919, and a democratic republic proclaimed. In March 1934 this regime was, in turn, overthrown by a coup.

The secret protocol of the Soviet-German agreement of 23 Aug. 1939 assigned Estonia to the Soviet sphere of interest. An ultimatum (16 June 1940) led to the formation of a government acceptable to the USSR. On 21 July the Estonian parliament proclaimed the establishment of an Estonian Soviet Socialist Republic and applied to join the USSR; on 6 Aug. the Supreme Soviet of the USSR accepted the application. The incorporation has been accorded *de facto* recognition by the UK, but not by the USA, which continues to recognize an Estonian consul-general in New York.

On 30 March 1990 the Estonian Supreme Soviet proclaimed that the Soviet occupation of Estonia on 17 June 1940 has not disrupted the continuity of the former republic, and adopted, by 73 votes to 0 with 3 abstentions, a declaration calling for the eventual re-establishment of full sovereignty.

AREA AND POPULATION. Estonia is bounded west and north by the Baltic, east by the RSFSR and south by Latvia. Area, 45,100 sq. km (17,413 sq. miles); population, 1,573,000 (Jan. 1989). Census (1979) 64·7% were Estonians, 27·9% Russians, 2·5% Ukrainians and 1·6% Belorussians. In June 1990 the Supreme Soviet established entry quotas for 'foreign citizens'. The capital is Tallinn (1989 census population, 482,000). Other large towns are Tartu, Narva, Kohtla-Järve and Pärnu. There are 15 districts, 33 towns and 26 urban settlements.

CONSTITUTION AND GOVERNMENT. The Supreme Soviet, elected on 18 March 1990, consists of 105 deputies. In May 1990 it renamed the republic the 'Republic of Estonia', and restored the pre-1940 flag and national anthem. Alongside the Supreme Soviet, a Congress of Estonia elected by ethnic Estonians has been set up. In a ballot in March 1991 77·8% voted for an independent democratic republic.

The *Chairman of the Supreme Soviet* (i.e. President of the Republic) is Arnold Rüütel.

In Feb. 1991 the Government comprised the following ministers: *Prime Minister*, Edgar Savisaar; *Health*, Andres Ellamaa; *Construction*, Gennadii Golubkov; *Social Affairs*, Arvo Kuddo; *Ethnic Relations*, Artur Kuznetsov; *Interior*, Olev Laanjärv; *Trade*, Ants Laos; *Economic Affairs*, Jaak Leimann; *Agriculture*, Vello Lind; Endel Lippmaa (*without portfolio*); *Education*, Rein Loik; *Foreign Affairs*, Lenart Meri; *Finance*, Rein Miller; *Social Welfare*, Siiri Oviir; *Justice*, Jüri Raidla; *Material Resources*, Aleksander Sikkal; *Culture*, Lepo Sumera; *Communications*, Toomas Sõmera; *Industry and Energy*, Jaak Tamm; *Chancellor of State*, Raivo Vare; *Transport*, Tiit Vähi.

First Secretary, Communist Party: Enn-Arno Sillari.

BANKING AND FINANCE. Budget estimates (in 1m. rubles), 1988, 1,797; 1989 (plan), 2,035. A central bank, the Bank of Estonia (*governor*, Rein Otsason), was re-established in 1990. There are 10 commercial banks.

AGRICULTURE. Agriculture and dairy farming are the chief occupations. Area under cultivation was 2·6m. ha in Nov. 1986. There were 142 agricultural and 8 fishery collectives and 152 state farms in 1989 using 20,500 tractors and 3,300 grain combines.

On 1 Jan. 1989 there were 823,000 head of cattle, 138,100 sheep and goats, and 1·1m. pigs.

Output of main agricultural products (in 1,000 tonnes) in 1988: Grain, 591; potatoes, 716; vegetables, 129; meat, 225; milk, 1,290; eggs, 567m.

Some 22% of the land is covered by forests which provide material for sawmills, furniture, match and pulp industries, as well as wood fuel. Since 1945, 80,000 ha have been afforested. 966,700 ha of marsh had been reclaimed by 1977.

INDUSTRY. Estonia has rich high-quality shale deposits (particularly in the north-east) which are estimated at 3,700m. tonnes. Shale output was 23·3m. in

1988. A factory for the production of gas from shale and a pipeline (208 km long) from Kohtla-Järve supplies shale gas to Leningrad and Tallinn. Estonian factories are now turning out agricultural and peat-digging machines, complex control and measuring instruments.

In the neighbourhood of Tallinn, phosphorites have been found, and in 1947 a plant for refining and for the production of super-phosphates was started. Estonia also contains valuable peat deposits, and some of her electrical stations work on peat. There are 350 rural electric stations. Electricity generated (1988) 17,500m. kwh. Output of paper in 1988 was 94,000 tonnes; leather footwear, 7m. pairs; knitwear, 22·8m. garments; preserves, 323m. jars.

In 1988 there were 695,000 employees in the state sector.

In 1990 there were some 5,600 enterprises of which 51% were state-owned, 32% co-operatives, 5% joint stock companies and 1·4% joint ventures.

EXTERNAL ECONOMIC RELATIONS. On 12 April 1990 Estonia, Latvia and Lithuania concluded a Baltic Economic Co-operation Agreement.

Joint ventures are permitted, but non-Estonians may not own more than 50% of the equity without government permission. New ventures enjoy a 2-year tax exemption. In Feb. 1991 there were 246 joint ventures from 27 countries.

COMMUNICATIONS. Length of railways in 1989, 1,030 km. Estonia has 20 ports, but Tallinn handles four-fifths of the total sea-going transport. Length of motor roads, 30,100 km (hard surface, 28,900 km). Airlines link Tallinn with Moscow, Leningrad, Riga and the Estonian islands.

Newspapers (1988). There were 52 newspapers, 36 of them in Estonian. Daily circulation of Estonian-language newspapers, 1,420,000; other languages, 261,000.

EDUCATION. Estonia has retained an 11-year school curriculum, when it was reduced to 10 years elsewhere in the USSR. In 1988–89 pupils in 600 primary, secondary and special schools numbered 200,000. There were 24,300 students in 6 higher educational establishments, including Tartu (Dorpat) University, founded in 1632, and 20,600 students in 36 technical colleges.

The Estonian Academy of Sciences, founded in 1946, had 24 institutions with 1,312 scientific staff in Jan. 1989; in all, 7,100 scientific staff were working in 72 institutions.

In Jan. 1989 68% of children attended pre-school institutions.

HEALTH. In 1988 there were 7,600 doctors and 19,200 hospital beds.

Further Reading

Istoriya Estonskoi SSR. 3 vols. Tallin, 1961–74

Küng, A., *A Dream of Freedom*. Cardiff, 1980

Misiuras, R.-J. and Taagepera, R., *The Baltic States: Years of Dependence 1940–1980*. Farnborough, 1983

Parming, T. and Jarvesro, E., (eds.) *A Case Study of a Soviet Republic*. Boulder, 1978

Raun, T. U., *Estonia and the Estonians*. Stanford, 1987

LATVIA

Latvijas Republika (Republic of Latvia)

HISTORY. In the part of Latvia unoccupied by the Germans, the Bolsheviks won 72% of the votes in the Constituent Assembly elections (Nov. 1917). Soviet power was proclaimed in Dec. 1917, but was overthrown when the Germans occupied all Latvia (Feb. 1918). Restored when they withdrew (Dec. 1918), it was overthrown once more by combined British naval and German military forces (May–Dec. 1919), and a democratic government set up. This régime was in turn replaced when a coup took place in May 1934.

The secret protocol of the Soviet–German agreement of 23 Aug. 1939 assigned Latvia to the Soviet sphere of interest. An ultimatum (16 June 1940) led to the formation of a government acceptable to the USSR. On 21 July a People's Diet proclaimed the establishment of the Latvian Soviet Socialist Republic and applied to join the USSR, whose Supreme Soviet accepted the application on 5 Aug. The incorporation has been accorded *de facto* recognition by the UK, but not by the USA, which continues to recognize the Chargé d'Affaires in Washington, D.C.

On 4 May 1990 the Latvian Supreme Soviet declared, by 138 votes to nil with 58 abstentions, that the Soviet occupation of Latvia on 17 June 1940 was illegal, and resolved to re-establish the authority of the Constitution of 1922. A transition period was set for the restoration of independence.

AREA AND POPULATION. Latvia is bounded north by Estonia and the Baltic Sea, west by the Baltic, south by Lithuania and Belorussia and east by the RSFSR. Latvia has a total area of 63,700 sq. km (24,595 sq. miles). Population, Jan. 1989, 2,681,000, of whom (1979 census) 53·7% are Latvians and 32·8% Russians. There are 26 districts, 56 towns and 37 urban settlements.

The capital is Riga; other principal towns are Daugavpils (Dvinsk), Liepāja, Jurmala, Jelgava (Mitau) and Ventspils (Windau).

CONSTITUTION AND GOVERNMENT. A new Constitution was adopted in April 1978. On 18 March 1990 elections were held to the 201-member Supreme Soviet. The Popular Front won a majority. A Congress of Latvia, elected by ethnic Latvians, has been set up alongside the Supreme Soviet. In a ballot in March 1991, 73·6% voted for an independent democratic republic.

In Dec. 1989 elections were held to district, urban and rural Soviets.

Chairman, Presidium of the Supreme Soviet (i.e. *President of the Republic*): A. V. Gorbunov (b. 1942); *Vice-President:* Dainis Ivans.

Chairman, Council of Ministers (i.e. *Prime Minister*): Ivars Godmanis.

First Secretary, Communist Party: A. P. Rubiks.

An independent section renamed itself the Democratic Labour Party of Latvia in Sept. 1990; Chairman, I. I. Kezbers.

FINANCE. Budget estimates (in 1m. rubles), 1988, 2,733; 1989 (plan), 3,133.

AGRICULTURE. Latvia is now no longer mainly an agricultural country. The urban population, 35% of the total in 1939, was 71% in Jan. 1986.

Forest lands (2·4m. ha) produced in 1983 4·2m. cubic metres of timber. Area under cultivation was 3·9m. ha in 1986. 1·8m. ha of marsh land had been drained (1983). Cattle and dairy farming are the chief agricultural occupations. Oats, barley, rye, potatoes and flax are the main crops.

After the establishment of the Soviet regime about 960,000 ha were distributed among the landless peasants or those with very small holdings. On 1 Jan. 1989 there were 248 state farms and 331 (including 11 fishery) collective farms. There were 38,100 tractors and 7,400 grain combine harvesters.

Livestock (Jan. 1989): Cattle, 1·5m; sheep and goats, 167,000; pigs, 1·8m.

Output of main agricultural products (in 1,000 tonnes) in 1988: Grain, 1,413; sugar-beet, 459; potatoes, 1,110; vegetables, 214; meat, 340; milk, 1,984; eggs, 920m.

INDUSTRY. Latvia is a major producer of electric railway passenger cars and long-distance telephone exchanges, paper and woollen goods, sawn timber, and mineral fertilizers.

Industrial output in 1988 (in 1,000 tonnes) included: Steel, 559,000; paper, 153; hosiery, 78·3m. pairs; knitwear, 42·4m. garments; leather footwear, 10·3m. pairs; radio receivers, 1·8m.; washing machines, 657,000; railway carriages, 633; buses, 17,600; synthetic fibre, 51·9; jars of preserves, 431m. Electricity generated (1988) 5,100m. kwh.

Peat deposits extend over 645,000 ha or about 10% of the total area, and it is estimated that total deposits are 3,000–4,000m. tons; output of briquettes in 1988, 55,200 tonnes. There are also gypsum deposits; amber is frequently found in the coastal districts.

In 1988 employees in the state sector numbered 1,239,000.

EXTERNAL ECONOMIC RELATIONS. On 20 April 1990 Latvia, Estonia and Lithuania concluded a Baltic Economic Co-operation Agreement.

COMMUNICATIONS. In Jan. 1989 the length of railways was 2,380 km, and motor roads, 58,300 km (hard surface, 31,800 km). Riga is the largest port in the Baltic after Leningrad. In 1986, 211m. tonne-km of freight was carried on inland waterways.

Newspapers (1988). There were 121 newspapers (72 in Latvian). Daily circulation of Latvian-language newspapers, 1·7m., other languages 645,000.

RELIGION. The Latvian Lutheran Church numbered 600,000 members in 1956.

EDUCATION. In 1988–89 there were 900 primary and secondary schools, with a total of 400,000 pupils: 63% of children attended pre-school institutions. 10 places of higher education had 44,200 students, 57 technical colleges had 40,000 students; there were also 21 music and art schools, 3 teachers' training colleges and an agricultural academy. In 1946 an Academy of Sciences was opened which in Jan. 1989 had 15 research institutes with a staff of 1,812 scientific workers; there were over 14,000 scientific workers in 101 research institutions.

HEALTH. There were 13,400 doctors and 37,400 hospital beds in 1988.

Further Reading

Latvian Academy of Sciences, *Istoriya Latviiskoi SSR*. Riga. 3 vols. 1952–58
Bilmanis, A., *A History of Latvia*. Princeton Univ. Press, 1951
Roze, B. and K., *Latviska–Angliska Vārdnicā*. Göppingen, 1948
Spekke, A., *History of Latvia*. Stockholm, 1951
Turkina, E., *Angliski–Latviska Vārdnicā*. Riga, 1948.—*Latviešu-Anglu Vārdnicā*. Riga, 1962

LITHUANIA

Lietuvos Respublika (Republic of Lithuania)

HISTORY. In 1914–15 the German army occupied the whole of Lithuania. On its withdrawal (Dec. 1918) Soviets were elected in all towns and a Soviet republic was proclaimed. In the summer of 1919 it was overthrown by Polish, German and nationalist Lithuanian forces, and a democratic republic established. In Dec. 1926 this regime was in turn overthrown by a coup.

The secret protocol of the Soviet–German frontier treaty of 28 Sept. 1939 assigned the greater part of Lithuania to the Soviet sphere of influence. In Oct. 1939 the province and city of Vilnius (in Polish occupation 1920–39) were ceded by the USSR. An ultimatum (16 June 1940) led to the formation of a government acceptable to the USSR. A people's Diet, elected on 14–15 July, proclaimed the establishment of the Lithuanian Soviet Socialist Republic on 21 July and applied for admission to the USSR, which was effected by decree of the USSR Supreme Soviet on 3 Aug. and included also those parts of Lithuania which had been reserved for inclusion in Germany. This incorporation has been accorded *de facto* recognition by the UK, but not by the USA, which continues to recognize a Lithuanian Chargé d'Affaires in Washington, D.C. In March 1990 the newly-elected Lithuanian Supreme Soviet, by 120 votes to nil, proclaimed independence based on the continuing validity of the act of independence of 16 Feb. 1918. This decision was not accepted by the USSR government.

Massive price rises in Jan. 1991 triggered demonstrations from ethnic Russians and led the Prime Minister, Kazimiera Prunskiene, to resign, a decision approved by parliament by 72 votes to 8 with 22 abstentions. Initially dispatched to Vilnius to enforce conscription, Soviet army units occupied key buildings in the face of mounting popular unrest. On 13 Jan. the army fired on demonstrators and there were fatal casualties.

AREA AND POPULATION. Lithuania is bounded north by Latvia, east and south by Belorussia, west by Poland, the Kaliningrad area of the RSFSR and the Baltic Sea. The total area of Lithuania is 65,200 sq. km (25,170 sq. miles) and the population (Jan. 1989) 3,690,000, of whom 80% were Lithuanians, 8·6% Russians and 7·7% Poles (1979 census).

The capital is Vilnius (Vilna). Other large towns are Kaunas (Kovno), Klaipeda (Memel), Siauliai (145,000) and Panėvežys (126,000). There are 44 rural districts, 92 towns and 22 urban settlements.

CONSTITUTION AND GOVERNMENT. At the elections to the 141-member Supreme Soviet of 24 Feb. 1990, the nationalist movement Sajudis won a large majority. In Dec. 1989, by an 85% vote, the Lithuanian Communist Party asserted its independence from the Soviet Party (CPSU). A minority organization retained its association. At a ballot in March 1991 90·5% voted for an independent democratic republic.

At elections to district, urban and rural Soviets (21 June 1987), of 28,354 deputies returned, 13,680 (48·2%) were women, 15,321 (54%) non-Party and 18,197 (64·1%) industrial workers and collective farmers.

Chairman, Presidium of the Supreme Soviet (i.e. *President of the Republic):* Vytautas Landsbergis.

*Chairman, Council of Ministers (*i.e., *Prime Minister):* Gediminas Valaorius.

First Secretary, (CPSU): Communist Party: Mikolas Burokjavičius.

Chairman, Democratic Labour Party of Lithuania: A. K. Brazauskas.

FINANCE. Budget estimates (in 1m. rubles), 1988, 3,962; 1989 (plan), 4,581.

AGRICULTURE. Lithuania before 1940 was a mainly agricultural country, but has since been considerably industrialized. The population was 66% urban in Jan. 1986. Resources consist of timber and agricultural produce. Of the total area, 49·1% is arable, 22·2% meadow and pasture, 16·3% forests and 12·4% unproductive.

Area under cultivation in Nov. 1986, 4·6m. ha. By 1981 over 2·7m. ha of swamps had been drained. Output of main agricultural products (in 1,000 tonnes) in 1988: Grain, 3,046; potatoes, 1,850; sugar-beet, 1,213; vegetables, 370; meat, 526; milk, 3,166; eggs, 1,356m. On 1 Jan. 1989 there were 2·4m. cattle, 2·7m. pigs, 78,000 sheep and goats.

Forests cover 1·55m. ha; 70% of the forests consist of conifers, mostly pines. Peat reserves total 4,000m. cubic metres.

Between 1940 and 1947 about 575,500 ha were distributed among the landless and poor peasant farmers. In 1988 there were 49,100 tractors and 11,500 grain combines serving 737 collective farms and 311 state farms.

INDUSTRY. There are heavy engineering, shipbuilding and building material industries. Industrial output included, in 1988: Synthetic fibres, 14,400 tonnes; fuel pumps, 339,000; ferroconcrete, 2·6m. cubic metres; cement, 3·4m. tonnes; sulphuric acid, 430,000 tonnes; paper, 123,000 tonnes; carpet, 6·9m. square metres; tape recorders, 176,000; televisions, 655,000; leather footwear, 11·4m. pairs; granulated sugar, 239,000 tonnes; felled timber, 1·4m. cubic metres; knitwear, 61·7m. garments; hosiery, 103m. pairs; electric power, 26,000m. kwh. In 1988 there were 1,590,000 employees in the state sector. In 1990 oil production started from a small field at Kretinga.

EXTERNAL ECONOMIC RELATIONS. On 20 April 1990 Lithuania, Estonia and Latvia concluded a Baltic Economic Co-operation Agreement.

COMMUNICATIONS. Length of railways in Jan. 1989, 1,990 km. Vilnius has one of the largest airports of the USSR. There are 42,500 km of motor roads (33,100 km hard surface) and 161m. tonne-km of freight was carried on inland waterways in 1987. Klaipeda has an ice-free harbour and fishery base.

Newspapers (1988). Of 147 newspapers, 114 were in Lithuanian. Daily circulation of Lithuanian-language newspapers, 2·6m.; other languages, 312,000.

RELIGION. The predominant religion is Roman Catholic. In 1956, the Lithuanian Lutheran Church had 215,000 members.

EDUCATION. In 1988–89 there were 500,000 pupils in 2,200 primary and secondary schools. The University of Vytautas the Great, at Kaunas, was opened on 16 Feb. 1922. On 15 Jan. 1940 certain faculties were transferred to Vilnius to join the ancient University of Vilnius (founded 1570). In 1988–89 there were 12 higher educational institutions with 66,300 students: in 66 technical colleges of all kinds there were 55,800 students. The Lithuanian Academy of Sciences, founded in 1941, had 12 institutions with a total scientific staff of 1,966 in Jan. 1989; there were 88 scientific institutions with 15,400 research personnel. 61% of children in Jan. 1989 were attending pre-school institutions.

JUSTICE. Trial by jury has been introduced for capital offences.

HEALTH. In 1988 there were 16,600 doctors and 46,800 hospital beds.

Further Reading

Jurgėla, C. R., *History of the Lithuanian Nation*. New York, 1948
Kantantas, A. and F., *A Lithuanian Bibliography*. Univ. of Alberta Press, 1975
Peteraitis, V., *Lithuanian–English Dictionary*. 2 vols. Chicago, 1960
Suziedlis, S., (ed.) *Encyclopedia Lituanica*. 6 vols. Boston, 1970–78
Vardys, S., (ed.) *Lithuania under the Soviets: Portrait of a Nation, 1940–45*. New York, 1965

SOVIET CENTRAL ASIA

Soviet Central Asia (a geographical term) embraces Kazakhstan, Uzbekistan, Turkmenistan, Tajikistan and Kirghizia.

Turkestan (by which name part of this territory was then known) was conquered by the Russians in the 1860s. In 1866 Tashkent was occupied and in 1868 Samarkand, and subsequently further territory was conquered and united with Russian Turkestan. In the 1870s Bokhara was subjugated, the emir, by the agreement of 1873, recognizing the suzerainty of Russia. In the same year Khiva became a vassal state to Russia. Until 1917 Russian Central Asia was divided politically into the Khanate of Khiva, the Emirate of Bokhara and the Governor-Generalship of Turkestan.

In the summer of 1919 the authority of the Soviet Government became definitely established in these regions. The Khan of Khiva was deposed in Feb. 1920, and a People's Soviet Republic was set up, the medieval name of Khorezm being revived. In Aug. 1920 the Emir of Bokhara was deposed, and a similar regime was set up in Bokhara. The former Governor-Generalship of Turkestan was constituted an Autonomous Soviet Socialist Republic within the RSFSR on 11 April 1921.

In the autumn of 1924 the Soviets of the Turkestan, Bokhara and Khiva Republics decided to redistribute the territories of these republics on a nationality basis; at the same time Bokhara and Khiva became Socialist Republics. The redistribution was completed in May 1925, when the new states of Uzbekistan, Turkmenistan and Tajikistan were accepted into the USSR as Union Republics. The remaining districts of Turkestan populated by Kazakhs were united with Kazakhstan which was established as an ASSR in 1925 and became a Union Republic in 1936. Kirghizia, until then part of the RSFSR, was established as a Union Republic in 1936.

Further Reading

Akiner, S., *The Islamic Peoples of the Soviet Union.* Rev. ed. London, 1986
Bennigsen, A. and Broxup, M., *The Islamic Threat to the Soviet State.* London, 1983
Nove, A. and Newth, J. A., *The Soviet Middle East.* London, 1967
Rwykin, M., *Moscow's Muslim Challenge.* New York, 1982
Wheeler, G., *The Modern History of Soviet Central Asia.* London, 1964.—*The Peoples of Soviet Central Asia.* London, 1966

KAZAKHSTAN

Kazak Soviettik Sotzialistik Respublikasy

HISTORY. On 26 Aug. 1920 Uralsk, Turgai, Akmolinsk and Semipalatinsk provinces formed the Kirgiz (in 1925 renamed Kazakh) Autonomous Soviet Socialist Republic within the RSFSR. It was made a constituent republic of the USSR on 5 Dec. 1936. To this republic were added the parts of the former Governorship of Turkestan inhabited by a majority of Kazakhs. It consists of the following regions: Aktyubinsk, Alma-Ata, Chimkent, Dzhambul, Dzhezkazgan, East Kazakhstan, Guryev, Karaganda, Kokchetav, Kustanai, Kzyl-Orda, Mangyshlak, North Kazakhstan, Pavlodar, Semipalatinsk, Taldy-Kurgan, Tselinograd, Turgai, Uralsk.

AREA AND POPULATION. Kazakhstan is bounded on the west by the Caspian Sea and the RSFSR, on the east by China, on the north by the RSFSR and on the south by Uzbekistan and Kirghizia. The area of the republic is 2,717,300 sq. km (1,049,155 sq. miles). It is the next in size to the RSFSR, is far larger than all the other Central Asian Soviet Republics combined and stretches nearly 3,000 km from west to east and over 1,500 km from north to south. Population (Jan. 1989) 16,538,000, of whom 57% live in urban areas. The Kazakhs form 36%, Russians 40·8% and Ukrainians 6·1% of the population (1979 census), as a result of the industrialization of the country since 1941 and the opening of virgin lands since 1945. The population includes over 100 nationalities.

The capital is Alma-Ata, formerly Verny; other large towns are Karaganda, Semipalatinsk, Chimkent and Petropavlovsk. In all there are 82 towns, 197 urban settlements and 221 rural districts.

CONSTITUTION AND GOVERNMENT. The Supreme Soviet elected in 1985 consisted of 510 deputies. New elections were held on 25 March 1990. A declaration of state sovereignty was adopted in Oct. 1990.

At elections to the regional, district, urban and rural Soviets (21 June 1987), out of 131,074 deputies returned, 64,717 (49·4%) were women. New elections were held in Dec. 1989.

President: N. A. Nazarbaev.
Chairman, Council of Ministers (i.e. *Prime Minister):* U. Karamanov.
First Secretary, Communist Party: N. A. Nazarbaev.

FINANCE. The budget (in 1m. rubles) balanced as follows: 1988, 12,697; 1989 (plan), 14,254.

AGRICULTURE. Kazakh agriculture has changed from primarily nomad cattle breeding to production of grain, cotton and other industrial crops. In Nov. 1986 218·3m. ha were under cultivation—over 20% of the total cultivated area of the USSR. 2,047,000 ha of land have an irrigation network.

The 'Ukrainka' winter wheat has been transformed into a spring wheat suitable for cultivation in Kazakhstan. Tobacco, rubber plants and mustard are also cultivated. Kazakhstan has rich orchards and vineyards, which accounted for 95,000 ha of cultivated land in 1985. Between 1954 and 1959, over 23m. ha of virgin and long fallow land were opened up, 544 new state grain farms being organized for the purpose. State purchases of grain were 14·6m. in 1987.

Kazakhstan is noted for its livestock, particularly its sheep, from which excellent quality wool is obtained. Livestock on 1 Jan. 1989 included 9·7m. cattle, 36·5m. sheep and goats and 3·2m. pigs.

There were, on 1 Jan. 1988, 388 collective farms and 2,140 state farms with 222,300 tractors and 100,900 grain combine harvesters. There were 5,293 rural power stations of 307,800 kwh. capacity.

Output of main agricultural products (in 1m. tonnes) in 1988: Grain, 22·6; sugar-beet, 1·3; potatoes, 2·3; vegetables, 1·4; fruit, 0·3; grapes, 0·1; meat, 1·5; milk, 5·3; eggs, 4,204m.; wool, 0·1.

INDUSTRY. Kazakhstan is extremely rich in mineral resources. Coal and tungsten in Karaganda (in the centre), oil along the river Emba (in the west), copper, lead and zinc—Kazakhstan contains about one-half of the total deposits of these three metals contained in the USSR—Iceland spar (in the south), nickel and chromium in the Kustanai and Semipalatinsk regions, molybdenum and other minerals.

In 1943 big deposits of manganese were found in Eastern Kazakhstan; coal seams were also discovered there. In South Kazakhstan copper and bauxite deposits have been found.

Coal, oil, non-ferrous metallurgy, heavy engineering and chemical industries have brought Kazakhstan to the third place among the industrial republics of the USSR. Production (1m. tonnes) in 1988 included oil, 25·5; steel, 6·8; cement, 8·4; synthetic fibres, 21·8; gas, 7,100m. cubic metres, footwear, 38·7m. pairs; jars of preserves, 468·5m.; knitwear, 108·4m. items. The Leninogorsk and Chimkent lead plants, the Balkhash, Irtysh and Karaskpai copper-smelting works and others supply the country with non-ferrous metals. A meat-packing plant has been built in Semipalatinsk, a fish cannery in Guryev, a chemical plant in Aktyubinsk, a tractor works at Pavlodar, and a superphosphate plant in Dzhambul. The oil industry in Emba and Aktyubinsk yields high-quality aviation oil.

Aviation plays an important part in agriculture. About 14m. ha were in 1984 treated from the air (destruction of pests, surface feeding of sugar-beet plantations, pollination of orchards, etc.).

Among recent enterprises are a large textile combine at Kustanai, hosiery factories at Djezkazgan, Leninogorsk and Aktyubinsk, a sugar factory at Aksu, meat canneries at Djetygar and Kzyl-Orda.

Electric power output in 1988 was 88,000m. kwh.

There were, in 1988, 6,586,000 employees in the state sector.

COMMUNICATIONS

Roads. In 1989 there were 152,700 km of motor roads (103,300 km hard surface).

Railways. In 1989 the total length of railways in operation was 14,550 km. Over 600 km of narrow-gauge line and 700 km of broad-gauge line were built in the virgin lands area in 1951-57.

Inland waterways. In 1987 3,761m. tonne-km of freight was carried on inland waterways.

Newspapers (1988). Of 453 newspapers, 170 were in the Kazakh language. Daily circulation of Kazakh-language newspapers, 2m.; other languages, 4·7m.

EDUCATION. In 1988–89 there were 3·2m. pupils at 8,600 elementary and secondary schools; 247 technical colleges with 269,200 students, 55 higher educational institutions with 276,900 students, and 207 research institutes with 41,300 scientific personnel. The Kazakh Academy of Sciences, founded in 1945, had, in 1989, 31 institutions, the scientific staff of which numbered 4,465. There were 41,400 scientific workers in 1989. 53% of children were attending pre-school institutions in Jan. 1989.

HEALTH. In 1988 there were 65,800 doctors and 221,600 hospital beds.

Further Reading

Istoriya Kazakhskoi SSR. 2 vols. Alma-Ata, 1957–59
Olcott, M. B., *The Kazakhs*. Stanford, 1987

TURKMENISTAN

Tiurkmenostan Soviet Sotsialistik Respublikasy

HISTORY. The Turkmen Soviet Socialist Republic was formed on 27 Oct. 1924 and covers the territory of the former Trans-Caspian Region of Turkestan, the Charjiui vilayet of Bokhara and a part of Khiva situated on the right bank of the Oxus. In May 1925 the Turkmen Republic entered the Soviet Union as one of its constituent republics. In Aug. 1990 the Turkmen Supreme Soviet unanimously adopted a declaration of sovereignty.

AREA AND POPULATION. Turkmenistan is bounded on the north by the Autonomous Kara-Kalpak Republic, a constituent of Uzbekistan, by Iran and Afghánistán on the south, by the Uzbek Republic on the east and the Caspian Sea on the west. The principal Turkmen tribes are the Tekkés of Merv and the Tekkés of the Attok, the Ersaris, Yomuds and Goklans. All speak closely related varieties of a Turkic language (of the south-western group); many are Sunni Moslems.

The country passed under Russian control in 1881, after the fall of the Turkoman stronghold of Gök Tépé. Census (1979) 68·4% of the population were Turkmenians, most of whom were nomads before the First World War. 12·6% are Russians living mostly in urban areas, and 8·5% Uzbeks. There are also Kazakhs (2·9%), Tatars, Ukrainians, Armenians and others.

The area of Turkmenistan is 488,100 sq. km (186,400 sq. miles), and its population in Jan. 1989 was 3,534,000.

There are 5 regions: Chardzhou, Mary, Ashkhabad, Tashauz and Krasnovodsk, comprising 42 rural districts, 15 towns and 74 urban settlements.

The capital is Ashkhabad (Poltoratsk; 1989 census population, 398,000); other large towns are Chardzhou, Mary (Merv), Nebit-Dag and Krasnovodsk.

CONSTITUTION AND GOVERNMENT. A new Constitution was adopted in April 1978. Elections to the Supreme Soviet were held on 7 Jan. 1990.

Elections to regional, district, urban and rural Soviets were held on 7 Jan. 1990.

President of the Republic: S. A. Niyazov (elected Oct. 1990).
Chairman, Council of Ministers: Kh. Akhmedov.
First Secretary, Communist Party: S. A. Niyazov.

FINANCE. Budget estimates (in 1m. rubles), 1988, 1,683; 1989 (plan), 1,934.

AGRICULTURE. The main occupation of the people is agriculture, based on irrigation. Turkmenistan produces cotton, wool, Astrakhan fur, etc. It is also famous for its carpets, and produces a special breed of Turkoman horses and the famous Karakul sheep.

There were 350 collective farms and 134 state farms in 1989, with 43,800 tractors and 1,600 grain combines. There were 608 rural power stations.

A considerable area is under Egyptian cotton, and from it has been evolved an original Soviet long-fibred cotton.

The main grain grown is maize. Sericulture, fruit and vegetable growing are also important; dates, olives, figs, sesame and other southern plants are grown. There is fishing in the Caspian. 34·7m. ha were under cultivation in Nov. 1986.

Between 1958 and 1970 the Kara-Kum Canal was extended to 860 km. In 1971 the fourth section, to reach the Caspian, was begun to reach 1,000 km. By 1982 over 1,011,000 ha had been irrigated.

Livestock on 1 Jan. 1989: Cattle, 774,300; pigs, 243,300; sheep and goats, 4·9m.

Output of main agricultural products (in 1,000 tonnes) in 1988: Grain, 435; cotton, 1,341; vegetables, 373; fruit, 50; grapes, 164; meat, 106; milk, 395; eggs, 323m.; wool, 16.

INDUSTRY. Turkmenistan is rich in minerals, such as ozocerite, oil, coal, sulphur and salt. Industry is being developed, and there are now chemical, tailoring, textile, light, food, agricultural implements, cement and other factories, oil refineries, as well as ore-mining.

In the Kara-Kum Desert deposits of magnesium, minerals and coal have been discovered, as well as some 50 new saltmines. Here a new oil town, Nebit-Dag, has sprung up. On the Kara-Bogaz bay a sulphate industry has been developed. Industrial output in 1988 included oil, 5·7m. tonnes; ferroconcrete, 0·8m. cubic metres; 10·9m. items knitwear, 5·6m. pairs of footwear, 64·3m. jars of preserves. Electric power output was 12,847m. kwh. in 1988.

In 1988 there were 855,000 employees in the state sector.

COMMUNICATIONS. Length of motor roads in 1989, 21,400 km (17,100 km hard surface). Motor communication exists between Ashkhabad and Meshed (Iran).

Length of railways, 2,120 km. The line Chardzhou–Kungrad crosses the Chardzhou and Tashauz regions of Turkmenia and runs across Uzbekistan. Another line connects Chardzhou and Urgench. Inland waterways, 1,300 km.

Airlines connect Leninsk and Tashauz, and Ashkhabad and remote areas in the west, north and east.

Newspapers (1988). Of 72 newspapers, 56 were in the Turkmen language. Daily circulation of Turkmen-language newspapers, 874,000; in all languages, 1,142,000.

EDUCATION. In 1988–89 there were 1,700 primary and secondary schools with 800,000 pupils, 9 higher educational institutions with 39,600 students, 37 technical colleges with 35,800 students, and 11 music and art schools. The Turkmen Academy of Sciences, founded in 1951, directs the work of 15 learned institutions with a staff of 1,114 scientific staff; there were 58 research institutions in all, with 5,700 research workers, in Jan. 1989.

In Jan. 1989, 31% of children were attending pre-school institutions.

HEALTH. In 1988 there were 12,400 doctors and 38,700 hospital beds.

Further Reading

Istoriya Turkmenskoi SSR. 2 vols. Ashkhabad, 1957

UZBEKISTAN

Ozbekiston Soviet Sotsialistik Respublikasy

HISTORY. In Oct. 1917 the Tashkent Soviet assumed authority, and in the following years established its power throughout Turkestan. The semi-independent Khanates of Khiva and Bokhara were first (1920) transformed into People's Republics, then (1923–24) into Soviet Socialist Republics and finally merged in the Uzbek SSR and other republics.

The Uzbek Soviet Socialist Republic was formed on 27 Oct. 1924 from lands formerly included in Turkestan. It includes a large part of the Samarkand region, the southern part of the Syr Darya, Western Ferghana, the western plains of Bukhara, the Kara-Kalpak ASSR and the Uzbek regions of Khorezm. In May 1925 Uzbekistan, by the decision of the Congress of Soviets of the USSR, was accepted as one of the constituent republics of the Soviet Union.

On 20 June 1990 the Uzbek Supreme Soviet adopted a declaration of sovereignty.

AREA AND POPULATION. Uzbekistan is bordered on the north by the Kazakh Soviet Socialist Republic, on the east by the Kirghiz Soviet Socialist Republic and the Tadzhik Soviet Socialist Republic, on the south by Afghánistán and on the west by the Turkmen Soviet Socialist Republic. The Uzbeks, who form 68·7% (1979 census) of the population, were the ruling race in Central Asia until the arrival of the Russians during the third quarter of the 19th century. The several native states over which Uzbek dynasties formerly ruled were founded in the 15th century upon the ruins of Tamerlane's empire. The Uzbek speak Jagatai Turkish, which is related to Osmanli and Azerbaijan Turkish; many are Sunni Moslems. Russians numbered (census 1979) 10·8%, Tadzhiks, 3·9%, Tatars 4·2%.

The area of Uzbekistan is 447,400 sq. km (172,741 sq. miles). The population in Jan. 1989 was 19,906,000 (41% urban). The country comprises the following regions: Andizhan, Bukhara, Dzhizak, Ferghana, Kashkadar, Khorezm, Namangan, Navoi, Samarkand, Surkhan-Darya, Syr-Darya, Tashkent and the Autonomous Soviet Socialist Republic of Kara Kalpakia. The capital of the Republic is Tashkent; other large towns are Samarkand, Andizhan, Namangan. There are 124 towns, 97 urban settlements and 155 rural districts.

On 19 Sept. 1963 the Supreme Soviet of the USSR confirmed decisions of the Supreme Soviets of Kazakhstan and Uzbekistan, transferring over 40,000 sq. km from the former to the latter to ensure more efficient use of the 'Hungry Steppe'.

CONSTITUTION AND GOVERNMENT. A new Constitution was adopted in April 1978. Elections tq the 500-member Supreme Soviet were held on 18 Feb. 1990.

Elections to the regional, district, urban and rural Soviets were also held on 18 Feb. 1990.

President of the Republic: I. A. Karimov.
Vice-President: S. R. Mirsaidov.
First Secretary, Communist Party: I. A. Karimov.

FINANCE. Budget estimates (in 1m. rubles), 1988, 9,012; 1989 (plan), 10,029.

AGRICULTURE. Uzbekistan is a land of intensive farming, based on artificial irrigation. It is the chief cotton-growing area in the USSR. About 3·7m. ha of collective and state farmland have irrigation networks, totalling over 150,000 km in length, and all are in full use.

In 1939 the Ferghana Canal (270 km) was built. During 1940, among the irrigation canals completed were: The North Ferghana Canal (165 km), and Andreyev South Ferghana Canal (108 km) and the first section of the Tashkent Canal (63 km). A canal from the Amu-Darya to Bokhara across the Kzyl-Kum and Ust-Urt deserts (180 km) was completed in 1965. A 200-km canal joining the river Zeravshan with the Kashka Darya at the village of Paruz was completed in Aug. 1955; it is part of the Iski–Angara Canal. The first section (93 km) of a canal irrigating the southern 'Hungry Steppe' was opened in 1960; 500,000 ha of this desert were under cultivation in 1967.

Agriculture flourishes, particularly in the well-watered, warm, rich oases areas, such as the Ferghana valley, Zeravshan, Tashkent and Khorezm, where cotton, fruit, silk and rice are cultivated. In the higher-lying plains grain is grown; the wide desert and semi-desert area of Western Uzbekistan is mainly given to pasture land and the breeding of the Karakul sheep; there is a Karakul institute at Samarkand.

Orchards occupied 206,000 ha and the vineyards 133,000 ha in 1985. The Central Asian Branch of the Scientific Research Institute of Viticulture in Tashkent has produced new frost resistant grapes by crossing the wild Amur grape with Central Asian and European types. In 1989 there were 856 collective farms and 1,085 state farms, with 179,500 tractors and 19,200 cotton picking and grain combines. Ploughing, cotton-sowing and cultivation are completely mechanized; cotton picking over 46%.

Uzbekistan provides 65% of the total cotton, 50% of the total rice and 60% of the total lucerne grown in the USSR. The area under cultivation was 33·1m. ha in 1986.

Livestock on 1 Jan. 1988: 4·1m. cattle, 8·7m. sheep and goats and 708,300 pigs.

Output of main agricultural products (in 1,000 tonnes) in 1988: Grain, 2,199; cotton, 5,365; potatoes, 308; vegetables, 2,760; fruit, 617; grapes, 640; meat, 428; milk, 2,760; eggs, 2,329m.; wool, 25.

Afforestation over an area of 50,000 ha has been carried out to protect the Bokhara and Karakul oases from the advancing Kzyl-Kum sands and to stop the sand-drifts in a number of districts of Central Ferghana.

INDUSTRY. Of its mineral resources, in addition to oil and coal, copper and building materials and ozocerite deposits are now also exploited.

There are over 1,600 factories and mills. Output in 1988 included 5·5m. tonnes of coal, 1m. tonnes of steel, 22,400 tractors, 25,600 tonnes of paper, 5·6m. tonnes of cement, 1·4m. Karakul skins, 106m. items of knitwear, 42m. pairs of footwear, 1,198m. jars of preserves. Gold is being worked at Muruntau, Chadak and Kochbulak.

The Tashkent power station (2m. kw.) was completed in 1971. Power output in 1988 was 50,600m. kwh. Two natural-gas pipelines (Djaikak–Tashkent, Ferghana–Kokand) and a third from Bokhara to the Urals are operating. Natural gas output (1988) was 39,900m. cubic metres.

In 1988 there were 5,038,000 employees in the state sector.

COMMUNICATIONS. The total length of railway in 1989 was 3,500 km. Branches lead to Karshe-Kitab, Kerki-Termez, Jalal-Abad, Namangan, Andijan and other centres. In 1947–55 a new line was built from Chardzhou to Kungrad.

The Great Uzbek Highway was completed in April 1941. Total length of motor roads in 1989 was 70,800 km (hard surface, 59,700 km). Inland waterways, 1,100 km.

Newspapers (1988). There were 196 newspapers in the Uzbek language out of a total of 290. Daily circulation of Uzbek-language newspapers, 4·8m.; in all languages, 6·4m.

EDUCATION. In 1988–89 there were 8,200 elementary and secondary schools with 4·6m. pupils, 43 higher educational establishments with 308,900 students and 246 technical colleges with 291,300 students. Uzbekistan has an Academy of Sciences, founded in 1943, with 37 institutions and 4,297 academic staff; there were 188 research institutes with a scientific staff of 40,200 in Jan. 1989. There are universities and medical schools in Tashkent and Samarkand. In Jan. 1989, 36% of children were attending pre-school institutions.

The Uzbek Arabic script was in 1929 replaced by the Latin alphabet which in 1940 was superseded by one based on the Cyrillic alphabet.

HEALTH. In 1988 there were 70,300 doctors and 242,400 hospital beds.

Further Reading

Istoriya Uzbekskoi SSR. 4 vols. Tashkent, 1967–68
Waterson, N., (ed.) *Uzbek-English Dictionary*. London, 1980

KARAKALPAK AUTONOMOUS SOVIET SOCIALIST REPUBLIC

Area, 164,900 sq. km (63,920 sq. miles); population (Jan. 1989), 1,214,000. Capital, Nukus (1989 census population, 169,000). The Karakalpaks are first mentioned in written records in the 16th century as tributary to Bokhara, and later to the Kazakh Khanate. In the second half of the 19th century, as a result of the Russian conquest of Central Asia, they came under Russian rule. On 11 May 1925 the territory was constituted within the then Kazakh Autonomous Republic (of the Russian Federation) as an Autonomous Region. On 20 March 1932 it became an Autonomous Republic within the Russian Federation, and on 5 Dec. 1936 it became part of the Uzbek SSR. Census (1979) Karakalpaks were 31·1% of population, Uzbeks, 31·5% and Kazakhs, 26·9%.

185 deputies were elected to its Supreme Soviet on 24 Feb. 1985, of whom 69 were women and 118 Communists.

Its manufactures are in the field of light industry—bricks, leather goods, furniture, canning, wine. In Jan. 1987 cattle numbered 348,600 and sheep and goats, 523,900. There were 38 collective and 124 state farms. The total cultivated area in 1985 was 350,400 ha.

In 1986–87 there were 286,800 pupils at schools, 21,400 at technical colleges, and 6,200 at Nukus University. There is a branch of the Uzbek Academy of Sciences with 190 scientific staff.

There were 2,600 doctors and 12,800 hospital beds.

TAJIKISTAN

Respublikai Sovieth Sotsialistii Tojikiston

HISTORY. The Tajik Soviet Socialist Republic was formed from those regions of Bokhara and Turkestan where the population consisted mainly of Tajiks. It was admitted as a constituent republic of the Soviet Union on 5 Dec. 1929. In Aug. 1990 the Tajik Supreme Soviet adopted a declaration of republican sovereignty.

AREA AND POPULATION. Tajikistan is situated between 39° 40' and 36° 40' N. lat. and 67° 20' and 75° E. long., north of the Oxus (Amu-Darya). On the west and north it is bordered by Uzbekistan and by the Kirghiz Soviet Socialist Republic; on the east by Chinese Turkestan and on the south by Afghanistan. It includes three regions (Khudzand [1], Kurgan-Tyube and Kulyab) and 43 rural districts, 18 towns and 49 urban settlements, together with the Gorno-Badakhshan Autonomous Region. Its highest mountains are Communism Peak (7,495 metres) and Lenin Peak (7,127 metres). Even the lowest valleys in the Pamirs are not below 3,500 metres above sea-level. The huge mountain glaciers are the source of many rapid rivers—the tributaries of the Amu-Darya, which flows from east to west along the southern border of Tajikistan. About 58·8% of the population are Tajiks. They speak an Iranian language, akin to Persian, and they are considered to be the descendants of the original Aryan population of Turkestan. Unlike the Persians, the Tajiks are mostly Sunni Moslems. Of the rest, 22·9% are Uzbeks living in the north-west of the republic. Russians and Ukrainians number 10·4% (1979 census).

The area of the territory is 143,100 sq. km (55,240 sq. miles). Population (Jan. 1989), 5,112,000. The capital is Dushanbe. Other large towns are Khudzand [1] (153,000), Kurgan-Tyube, Kulyab.

[1] Formerly Leninabad.

CONSTITUTION AND GOVERNMENT. A new Constitution was adopted in April 1978. Elections to the 230-member Supreme Soviet were held on 25 Feb. 1990.

Elections to the district, urban and rural Soviets and the regional Soviet of Gorno-Badakhshan were held in Dec. 1989.

Chairman of the Supreme Soviet: K. M. Makhkamov.
Chairman, Council of Ministers: I. Kh. Khaeev.
First Secretary, Communist Party: K. M. Makhkamov.

FINANCE. Budget estimates (in 1m. rubles), 1988, 2,109; 1989 (plan), 2,375.

AGRICULTURE. The occupations of the population are mainly farming, horticulture and cattle breeding. Area under cultivation in Nov. 1986 was 9·6m. ha. There are 43,000 km of irrigation canals: The irrigation networks cover about 634,000 ha of land.

Tajikistan grows many varieties of fruit, including apricots, figs, olives, pomegranates, a local variety of lemons and oranges, and in the south sugar-cane has been grown. Even on the highest mountain plateaux of the Pamirs, 'the roof of the world', the biological station of Tajikistan (3,860 metres above sea-level) has succeeded in raising crops of 60 varieties of barley, 10 varieties of oats, 4 of wheat, as well as vegetables. Eucalyptus and geranium are grown for the perfumery industry. Jute, rice and millet are also grown.

Tajikistan contains rich pasture lands, and cattle breeding is a very important branch of its agriculture. Livestock on 1 Jan. 1989: 1·3m. cattle, 3·3m. sheep and goats and 212,200 pigs.

The Gissar sheep is famous in the south for its meat and fat; the Karakul sheep is widely bred for its wool.

There were 157 collective farms and 299 state farms in 1989, with 34,100 tractors and 1,600 cotton and grain combine harvesters.

Output of main agricultural products (in 1,000 tonnes) in 1988: Grain, 381; cotton, 963; potatoes, 183; vegetables, 556; fruit, 208; grapes, 178; meat, 116; milk, 598; eggs, 602m.; wool, 5·4.

INDUSTRY. The original small-scale handicraft industries have been replaced by big industrial enterprises, including mining, engineering, food, textile, clothing and silk factories.

There are rich deposits of brown coal, lead, zinc and oil (in the north of the republic), rare elements, such as uranium, radium, arsenic and bismuth. Asbestos, mica, corundum and emery, lapis lazuli, potassium salts, sulphur and other minerals have been found in other parts of the republic.

Industrial output in 1988 included 271,000 tonnes of oil, 235m. cubic metres of gas, 673,000 tonnes of coal, 1·1m. tonnes of cement, 15·3m. items knitwear, 10·3m. pairs footwear, 349m. jars of preserves.

There are 80 big electrical stations. The hydro-electric Varzob station began to operate in 1954, that at Kairak-Kum on the Syr Darya River was completed in 1957 and 2 more at Murgab in 1964. Output in 1988 was 18,844m. kwh.

In 1988 there were 1,162,000 employees in the state sector.

COMMUNICATIONS

Roads. In Jan. 1989 there were 29,600 km of motor roads. Of these, 18,300 km are hard surface, including the Osh–Khorog (700 km), Yasui–Bazar–Charm (107 km) and Dushanbe–Khorog in the Pamirs (557 km) roads.

Railways. A railway line between Termez and Dushanbe (258 km) connects the republic with the railway system of the USSR. The mountainous nature of the republic makes ordinary railway construction difficult; accordingly 345 km of narrow gauge railways have been constructed (Kurgan–Tyube–Piandzh and Dushanbe–Kurgan–Tyube, connecting Dushanbe with the cotton-growing Vakhsh valley are particularly important). Length of railways, 1989, 480 km.

Aviation. Dushanbe is connected by air with Moscow, Tashkent, Baku and the regional and district centres of the republic.

Shipping. A steamship line on the Amu-Darya runs between Termez, Sarava and Jilikulam on the river Vakhsh (200 km).

Newspapers (1988). There were 74 newspapers, 62 in Tajik. Daily circulation of Tajik-language newspapers, 1,175,000; in all languages, 1,585,000.

EDUCATION. In 1988–89 there were 3,000 primary and secondary schools with 1·2m. pupils, 10 higher educational institutions with 58,600 students and 41 technical colleges with 42,100 students; the Tajik State University had 12,467 students. In Jan. 1989, 16% of children were attending pre-school institutions. In 1951 an Academy of Sciences was established; it has 16 institutions, the scientific staff of which numbers 1,499; there are 61 research institutions in all, with 9,100 scientific personnel in Jan. 1989. The Pamir research station is the highest altitude meteorological observatory in the world.

In 1940 a new alphabet based on Cyrillic was introduced.

HEALTH. There are 325 hospitals as well as maternity homes, clinics and special institutes to combat tropical diseases. There were 14,500 doctors in 1988 and 53,500 hospital beds.

GORNO-BADAKHSHAN AUTONOMOUS REGION

Comprising the Pamir massif along the borders of Afghánistán and China, the region was set up on 2 Jan. 1925. Area, 63,700 sq. km (24,590 sq. miles); population (Jan. 1989), 161,000 (83% Tadjiks, 11% Kirghiz). Capital, Khorog (14,800). The inhabitants are predominantly Ismaili Moslems.

Mining industries are developed (gold, rock-crystal, mica, coal, salt). Wheat, fruit and fodder crops are grown and cattle and sheep are bred in the western parts. In 1987 there were 74,700 cattle, 343,300 sheep and goats. Total area under cultivation, 18,400 ha.

In 1986 3,494 pupils completed secondary education.

Further Reading

Academy of Science of Tajikistan, *Istoriya Tajikskogo Naroda*. 3 vols. Moscow, 1963–65
Luknitsky, P., *Soviet Tajikistan* [In English]. Moscow, 1954

KIRGHIZIA

Kyrgyz Sovietik Respublikasy

HISTORY. After the establishment of the Soviet regime in Russia, Kirghizia became part of Soviet Turkestan, which itself became an Autonomous Soviet Socialist Republic within the RSFSR in April 1921. In 1924, when Central Asia was reorganized territorially on a national basis, Kirghizia was separated from Turkestan and formed into an autonomous region within the RSFSR. On 1 Feb. 1926 the Government of the RSFSR transformed Kirghizia into an Autonomous Soviet Socialist Republic within the RSFSR, and finally in Dec. 1936 Kirghizia was proclaimed one of the constituent Soviet Socialist Republics of the USSR.

AREA AND POPULATION. The territory of Kirghizia covers 198,500 sq. km (76,640 sq. miles), and its population in Jan. 1989 was 4,291,000. The republic comprises 6 regions: Djalal-Abad, Issyk-Kul, Naryn, Osh, Talas and Chu. There are 18 towns, 31 urban settlements and 40 rural districts. Its capital is Bishbek (formerly Frunze). Other large towns are Osh (213,000), Przhevalsk (56,000), Kyzyl-Kiya, Tokmak.

Kirghizia is situated on the Tien-Shan mountains and bordered on the east by China, on the west by Kazakhstan and Uzbekistan, on the north by Kazakhstan and in the south by Tajikistan. The Kirghizians are of Turkic origin and form 47·9% (1979 census) of the population; the rest are Russians (25·9%), Ukrainians (3·1%), Uzbeks (12·1%) and Tatars (2%).

CONSTITUTION AND GOVERNMENT. The Supreme Soviet elected in 1985 consisted of 350 deputies. New elections were held on 25 Feb. 1990. A new Constitution was adopted in April 1978.

Kirghizia declared itself independent in Dec. 1990.

At elections to the regional, district, urban and rural Soviets (21 June 1987), of the 28,063 deputies returned, 13,652 (48·6%) were women. New elections were held on 25 Feb. 1990.

President of the Republic: A. Akaev.
Chairman, Council of Ministers: A. D. Dzhumagulov.
First Secretary, Communist Party: A. M. Masaliev.

FINANCE. Budget estimates (in 1m. rubles), 1988, 2,388; 1989 (plan), 2,692.

AGRICULTURE. Kirghizia is famed for its livestock breeding. On 1 Jan. 1989 there were 1·2m. cattle, 411,000 pigs, 10·4m. sheep and goats. Yaks are bred as meat and dairy cattle, and graze on high altitudes unsuitable for other cattle.

Crossed with domestic cattle, hybrids are produced much heavier than ordinary Kirghiz cattle and giving twice the yield of milk. The Kirghizian horse is famed for its endurance, but it is of small stature; it has in recent years been crossed with Don, Arab and other breeds.

On 1 Jan. 1986 there were 176 collective and 290 state farms. Area under cultivation (Nov. 1986), 16·1m. ha. There were 28,000 tractors and 4,200 grain combine harvesters in 1989.

Kirghizia raises wheat sufficient for its own use and other grains and fodder, particularly lucerne; also sugar-beet, hemp, kenaf, kendyr, tobacco, medicinal plants and rice. Sericulture, fruit, grapes and vegetables and bee-keeping are major branches of Kirghiz agriculture. Agriculture is highly mechanized; nearly all the area under crops is worked by tractors. In 1983 irrigation networks in collective and state farms covered 974,000 ha; practically all were in use. A canal in the western Tien-Shan ranges and a reservoir in the Urto-Tokoi mountains are being constructed.

Output of main agricultural products (in 1,000 tonnes) in 1988: Grain, 1,758; cotton, 79; potatoes, 332; vegetables, 548; fruit, 139; grapes, 28; meat, 220; milk, 1,063; eggs, 663m.; wool, 38·2.

INDUSTRY. Kirghizia contains over 500 large modern industrial enterprises including sugar refineries, tanneries, cotton and wool-cleansing works, flour-mills, a tobacco factory, food, timber, textile, engineering, metallurgical, oil and mining enterprises.

Production in 1988 included 331m. light bulbs, 49,500 centrifugal pumps, 28·8m. pairs hosiery, 233,700 washing machines, 1·2m. cubic metres of ferroconcrete, 11·6m. pairs of footwear, 175m. jars of preserves and 377,600 tonnes of granulated sugar.

Hydro-electric power stations are being built in the Central Tien-Shans and the cotton-growing districts in the Osh Region, the Chui valley and on the shore of Lake Issyk-Kul. Power output (1988) was 14,000m. kwh.

There were, in 1988, 1,248,000 employees in the state sector.

COMMUNICATIONS. In the north a railway runs from Lugovaya through Frunze to Rybachi on Lake Issyk-Kul. Towns in the southern valleys are linked by short lines with the Ursatyevskaya–Andizhan railway in Uzbekistan. Total length of railway (Jan. 1989) is 370 km. Most of the traffic is by road; there were 28,700 km of motor roads (25,900 hard surface) in 1989. A road tunnel through the Tien-Shan mountains at an altitude of 9,600 ft, connecting Frunze and Osh, is being constructed. Inland waterways, 600 km. Airlines link Frunze with Moscow and Tashkent.

Newspapers (1988). Of 119 newspapers with a daily 1·6m. circulation, 65 with 939,000 circulation are in the Kirghiz language.

EDUCATION. Kirghizia had 1,700 primary and secondary schools with 900,000 pupils in 1988–89; 30% of children were attending pre-school institutions. There were also 10 higher educational institutions with 57,100 students, 47 technical and teachers' training colleges with 49,200 students, as well as music and art schools. The Kirghiz Academy of Sciences was established in 1954. In 1989 there were 18 research institutes, with 1,560 scientific staff, operating under its auspices; altogether there were 10,100 scientific staff in 1989. A university was opened in 1951. In 1940 a new alphabet, based on Cyrillic, was introduced.

HEALTH. In 1987 there were 14,900 doctors and 50,200 hospital beds.

Further Reading

Istoriya Kirgizskoi SSR. 5 vols. Frunze, 1984 ff.
Ryazantsev, S. N., *Kirghizia*. Moscow, 1951

UNITED ARAB EMIRATES

Federal Capital: Abu Dhabi
Population: 1·6m. (1988)
GNP per capita: US$15,720 (1988)

HISTORY. From Sha'am, 35 miles south-west of Ras Musam dam, for nearly 400 miles to Khor al Odeid at the south-eastern end of the peninsula of Qatar, the coast, formerly known as the Trucial Coast, of the Gulf (together with 50 miles of the coast of the Gulf of Oman) belongs to the rulers of the 7 Trucial States. In 1820 these rulers signed a treaty prescribing peace with the British Government. This treaty was followed by further agreements providing for the suppression of the slave trade and by a series of other engagements, of which the most important are the Perpetual Maritime Truce (May 1853) and the Exclusive Agreement (March 1892). Under the latter, the sheikhs, on behalf of themselves, their heirs and successors, undertook that they would on no account enter into any agreement or correspondence with any power other than the British Government, receive foreign agents, cede, sell or give for occupation any part of their territory save to the British Government.

British forces withdrew from the Gulf at the end of 1971 and the treaties whereby Britain had been responsible for the defence and foreign relations of the Trucial States were terminated, being replaced on 2 Dec. 1971 by a treaty of friendship between Britain and the United Arab Emirates. The United Arab Emirates (formed 2 Dec. 1971) consists of the former Trucial States: Abu Dhabi, Dubai, Sharjah, Ajman, Umm al Qaiwain, Ras al Khaimah (joined in Feb. 1972) and Fujairah. The small state of Kalba was merged with Sharjah in 1952.

AREA AND POPULATION. The Emirates are bounded north by the Gulf and Oman, east by the Gulf of Oman and Oman, south and west by Saudi Arabia, north-west by Qatar. The area of these states is approximately 32,300 sq. miles (83,657 sq. km). The total population at census (1985), 1,622,393. Estimate (1988) 1·6m. In 1980, 69% were male and 72% lived in urban areas. About one-tenth are nomads.

Population of the 7 Emirates, 1985 census: Abu Dhabi, 670,125; Ajman, 64,318; Dubai, 419,104; Fujairah, 54,425; Ras al-Khaimah, 116,470; Sharjah, 268,722; Umm al Qaiwain, 29,229.

The chief cities (1980 census) are Dubai (265,702), Abu Dhabi, the provisional federal capital (242,975), Sharjah (125,149) and Ras al-Khaimah (42,000).

CLIMATE. The country experiences desert conditions, with rainfall both limited and erratic. The period May to Nov. is generally rainless, while the wettest months are Feb. and March. Temperatures are very high in the summer months. Dubai. Jan. 74°F (23·4°C), July 108°F (42·3°C). Annual rainfall 2·4" (60 mm). Sharjah. Jan. 64°F (17·8°C), July 91°F (32°C). Annual rainfall 4·2" (105 mm).

GOVERNMENT. The Emirates is a federation, headed by a Supreme Council which is composed of the 7 rulers and which in turn appoints a Council of Ministers. The Council of Ministers drafts legislation and a federal budget; its proposals are submitted to a federal National Council of 40 elected members which may propose amendments but has no executive power.

President: HH Sheikh Zayed bin Sultan al Nahyan, Ruler of Abu Dhabi.

Members of the Supreme Council of Rulers:

HH Sheikh Maktoum bin Rashid al-Maktoum, *Vice President* and Ruler of Dubai.
HH Sheikh Sultan bin Mohammed al-Qasimi, Ruler of Sharjah.
HH Sheikh Saqr bin Mohammed al-Qasimi, Ruler of Ras al-Khaimah.
HH Sheikh Rashid bin Ahmed al-Mualla, Ruler of Umm al Qaiwain.
HH Sheikh Hamad bin Mohammed al Sharqi, Ruler of Fujairah.
HH Sheikh Humaid bin Rashid al-Nuaimi, Ruler of Ajman.

The Council of Ministers in Feb. 1991 was:

Prime Minister: HH Sheikh Maktoum bim Rashid al-Maktoum.
Deputy Prime Minister: HH Sheikh Sultan bin Zayed al-Nahyan.
Interior: HE Major General Hamouda bin Ali. *Finance and Industry:* Sheikh Hamdan bin Rashid al-Maktoum. *Defence:* Sheikh Mohammed bin Rashid al-Maktoum. *Economy and Commerce:* HE Saeed Ghobash. *Information and Culture:* HE Khalfan bin Mohammed Al-Roumi. *Communications:* Mohammed Saeed al-Mualla. *Public Works and Housing:* HE Rakad bin Salem bin Rakad. *Education:* HE Hamad Abdul Rahman al-Madfa. *Petroleum and Mineral Resources:* HE Yousuf bin Omeir bin Yousuf. *Electricity and Water:* Humaid bin Nasser al-Oweis. *Health:* HE Ahmed bin Saeed al-Badi. *Labour and Social Affairs:* HE Saif al-Jarwan. *Planning:* HE Sheikh Humaid al-Mualla. *Agriculture and Fisheries:* HE Saeed al-Raghbani. *Islamic Affairs and Endowments:* HE Sheikh Mohammed bin Ahmed al-Khazraji. *Foreign Affairs:* HE Rashid Abdullah al-Noami. *Justice:* HE Dr Abdullah bin Omran Taryam. *Higher Education:* HE Sheikh Nahyan bin Mubarak al-Nahyan. *Youth and Sports:* HE Sheikh Faisal bin Khaled bin Mohammed al-Qassimi.

National flag: Three horizontal stripes of green, white, black, with a vertical red strip in the hoist.

DEFENCE

Army. The Army consists of 1 Royal Guard, 1 armoured, 1 mechanized infantry, 2 infantry, 1 artillery and 1 air defence brigades. Equipment includes 95 AMX-30 and 36 Lion OF-40 Mk 2 main battle tanks. The strength was (1990) 40,000.

Navy. The combined naval flotilla of the Emirates includes 2 German-built missile corvettes, 6 German-built fast missile craft, 9 British-built inshore patrol craft, 2 tank landing craft, 2 transports, 1 maintenance ship and 3 service craft. Personnel in 1990 numbered 1,500 officers and ratings. A new base is being constructed at Taweela.

The Coast Guard flotilla comprises 28 inshore patrol craft and some 30 boats.

Air Force. Formation of an air wing in Abu Dhabi, to support land forces, began in 1968 with the purchase of some light STOL transports and helicopters. Expansion has been rapid. Current equipment includes 23 Mirage 5 supersonic fighter-bombers, 3 Mirage 5R tactical reconnaissance aircraft and 3 Mirage 5D 2-seat trainers (to be replaced by Mirage 2000s, which are now entering service); 4 C-130 Hercules and 5 Buffalo turboprop transports; 4 CASA C-212 Aviocar ECM/elint aircraft; about 40 Gazelle, Alouette III, Puma, Super Puma and Ecureuil helicopters; 23 PC-7 Turbo-Trainers and 15 Hawk light attack/trainers. Initial personnel were mostly British but considerable assistance is now being received from Arab countries and from Pakistan. The air wing became the Air Force of Abu Dhabi in 1972, in which year 3 JetRanger helicopters were transferred to the air wing of the Union Defence Force, since combined with the Dubai Police Air Wing to form a single component of the United Emirates Air Force. Current equipment of the Dubai Air Wing of the UEAF, bought mainly in Italy, comprises 3 Aermacchi MB 326K jet light attack aircraft, 1 piston-engined SF.260W armed basic trainer, 5 SF.260TP turboprop trainers, and 2 MB 326L, 5 MB 339 and 8 Hawk jet trainers, 6 Bell 205A-1, 3 Bell 212, 4 Bell 214 and 6 JetRanger helicopters and 1 Cessna 182 liaison aircraft, plus 2 L-100-30 Hercules transports and a variety of other types for VIP use. Sharjah formed a small aviation force, the Amiri Guard Air Wing, at the end of 1984. The service is essentially an internal security and transport force operating 1 Short 330 and 1 Skyvan for transport duties and 3 JetRanger helicopters. Personnel (1991) 2,500, with 91 combat aircraft and 19 armed helicopters.

INTERNATIONAL RELATIONS

Membership. The UAE is a member of the UN, Gulf Co-operation Council and of the Arab League.

ECONOMY

Budget. Revenue is principally derived from oil-concession payments. Federal expenditure (1989) was DH 14,645·1m. and public revenue (1988) 21,600m.

Currency. The unit of currency is the *dirham* (AED) of 100 *fils*. There are notes of 5, 10, 50, 100 and 500 *dirham* and coins of 1 and 5 *dirham* and 1, 5, 10, 25 and 50 *fils*. Rate of exchange, March 1991: £1 = 6·95 *dirham*; US$1 = 3·67 *dirham*.

Banking and Finance. The UAE Central Bank was established in 1980. In 1989 there were 47 local and foreign banks. Foreign banks are restricted to 8 branches each.

ENERGY AND NATURAL RESOURCES

Electricity. Production (1986) 16,440m. kwh. Supply in Abu Dhabi 230 volts; Dubai 220 volts and in the remaining Emirates 240 volts; all 50 Hz.

Oil. Total production of crude oil (1985) 442·3m. bbls. Reserves (1988) 200,000m. bbls.

Abu Dhabi. Ownership in 1976 was as follows: *ADPC*, 60% Government; 9·5% BP; 9·5% Shell; 9·5% CFP; 4·75% Mobil; 2% Partex. *ADMA*, 60% Government; 26·7% BP/Japan Oil Development Co.; 13·3% CFP. A Japanese company, Abu Dhabi Oil Co. (ADOCO) began production from its Mubarraz field in 1973. There are other companies which have concessions in the State: Japan's Middle East Oil; a US consortium led by Pan Ocean Oil and Sunningdale Oils of Canada. A State Petroleum Co., the Abu Dhabi National Oil Co. (ADNOC), was formed in 1971 and began to set up its own tanker fleet known as the Abu Dhabi National Tankers Co. (ADNATCO). Proven reserves (1988) 31,000m. bbls. Oil production, 1990, 78·96m. tonnes.

Dubai. In July 1975 Dubai decided to take full control of all foreign oil and gas operations in the State. The companies were to remain however. A Dubai producing group was set up to comprise the foreign interests–US and continental companies. Dubai Petroleum Co. (DPC–a subsidiary of Continental Oil) has a 30% interest in this group; the other members are Dubai Marine Areas (*Compagnie Française des Pétroles*) with 50%; Deutsche Texaco with 10%; Dubai Sun Oil 5%; and Delfzee Dubai Petroleum (Wintershall) 5%. Oil production (1990) 20·9m. tonnes.

Sharjah. In Sharjah the concession is given to Crescent Oil, its shareholders are: Ashland Oil, Skelly Oil, Kerr-McGee, Cities Services and Juniper. Other oil concessions have recently been given to the Crystal Oil Co. of USA and the Reserves Oil and Gas Co. Oil production, 1990, 1·8m. tonnes.

Ajman. An oil concession was awarded to United Refining in 1974.

Umm al Qawain. The concession here was given to US Occidental Petroleum; another was awarded to a consortium led by the US company United Refinery.

Ras al-Khaimah. The Dutch oil firm Vitol took over Union's concession in 1973. Shell began prospecting in 1969 but pulled out in 1971. A concession in the same area was awarded to Peninsula Petroleum, a subsidiary of the US California Time Group, in 1973. Oil production (1990) 400,000 tonnes.

Gas. Abu Dhabi has reserves of natural gas, nationalized in 1976. The Abu Dhabi Gas Liquefaction Plant at Das Island (51% ADNOC) has a capacity of 2m. tons LNG, 1m. tons LPG, 220,000 tons of light distillate and 230,000 tons of pelletized sulphur. Gas exports (1986) DH4,500m.

Water. Production of drinking water by desalination of sea water (1986) 11,600m. gallons. In 1986 the solarpowered Umm al Nar station produced 15,000 gallons a day. The first phase of the biggest solar-operated water production plant in the Gulf region (with an estimated daily capacity of 21m. gallons and 265 mw of electricity) was completed at Al Taweela in 1987, the second phase (40m. gallons and 400 mw) in 1990.

Agriculture. The fertile Buraimi Oasis, known as Al Ain, is largely in Abu Dhabi territory. By 1988, 2,620 farms had been set up on 12,565 ha of land reclaimed from sand dunes. Owing to lack of water and good soil there is little agriculture in the rest of UAE. Cultivated area (1985) 320,000 ha. Production (1988): Red meat, 18,000 tonnes; poultry, 7,000 tonnes; dates, 68,000 tonnes; vegetables, 285; wheat, 2.

Livestock (1988): Cattle, 50,000; camels, 120,000; sheep, 430,000; goats, 850,000.

Fisheries. Sharjah exports shrimps and prawns; a fishmeal plant is operating in Ras al-Khaimah and plants are planned for Ajman and Sharjah. Catch (1986) 72,400 tonnes.

INDUSTRY. A fertilizer plant at Ruwais in Abu Dhabi, opened in 1984, produced 343,000 tonnes of ammonia and 353,000 tonnes of urea in 1985. Umm al-Nar has a plant producing salt, hydrochloric acid, chlorine, caustic soda and distilled water.

There were about 190 industrial and commercial companies in the Jebel Ali industrial zone in Dubai by 1988, including an aluminium smelter and power and desalination plant, opened in 1979, and a lubricants plant with an annual capacity of 30,000 tonnes, opened in 1988. Production of aluminium in 1986, 155,605 tonnes, nearly all of which was exported.

There were 8 cement plants in 1987 (3 of them in Ras al-Khaimah), with a total annual capacity of 8m. tonnes. The home market for cement amounted to 25% of the total installed capacity of 6m. tonnes in 1986.

The 2 main steel rolling mills are in Dubai and Sharjah. Plastics are produced at factories in Dubai and Sharjah and mechanical dies and tools, sportswear and equipment, clothing and knitwear in Dubai. Fujairah has rockwool and ceramics factories. Ship repairs and steel fabrication are carried on in Ajman. There is a petrochemical complex on Das Island in Abu Dhabi.

FOREIGN ECONOMIC RELATIONS. There is a free zone at the port of Jebel Ali.

Commerce. Imports in 1988 for UAE were DH31,000m. Exports and re-exports (non-oil) totalled DH13,500m. Oil exports accounted for DH28,000m.

Total trade between the UAE (excluding Abu Dhabi) and UK (British Department of Trade returns, in £1,000 sterling):

	1986	*1987*	*1988*	*1989*	*1990*
Imports to UK	59,428	81,218	58,651	77,755	105,072
Exports and re-exports from UK	413,651	329,008	334,506	415,982	494,559

Total trade between Abu Dhabi and UK (British Department of Trade returns, in £1,000 sterling):

	1986	*1987*	*1988*	*1989*	*1990*
Imports to UK	14,584	13,771	25,566	87,248	76,414
Exports and re-exports from UK	168,111	149,989	128,838	155,439	170,165

Tourism. In 1987 there were 85 hotels and 18,000 visitors.

COMMUNICATIONS

Roads. In 1984 there were 2,200 km of roads and 230,000 vehicles.

Aviation. In 1991 there were 6 international airports. Gulf Air is run by a consortium of Abu Dhabi, Bahrain, Doha and Muscat. A number of cargo airlines also fly regularly to the country's major airports. An air-taxi service, Emirates Air Services, operates between Abu Dhabi and Dubai. Dubai set up its own, Emirates, airline in 1985. It flies to Saudi Arabia, Europe, India, Singapore and Manila.

Shipping. In 1987 there were 7 commercial sea ports. Jebel Ali is the largest. Abu Dhabi has dry docks and there are smaller ports at Sharjah, Ras al-Khaimah and Fujairah. Jebel Ali is a port and industrial estate 35 km south-west of Dubai city and had (1982) 66 berths.

Telecommunications. In 1990 there were 367,333 telephones. The Cable and Wireless Station at Jebel Ali in the State of Dubai links the system with the international communication network.

Television stations are at Abu Dhabi and Dubai, with extension of the service well advanced to the rest of the Emirates. Stations for The Voice of the Gulf Cooperation Council, a 6-state radio station, began broadcasting from Abu Dhabi in Aug. 1985. Estimated radios (1984) 190,000 and television sets over 110,000.

Newspapers (1990). There are a number of daily and weekly publications mostly in Arabic, but some in English, notably the dailies *Emirates News* of Abu Dhabi, *The Gulf News*, and the *Khaleej Times* both of Dubai.

JUSTICE, RELIGION, EDUCATION AND WELFARE

Justice. UAE subjects and citizens of all Arab and Moslem states are subject to the jurisdiction of the local courts. In the local courts the rules of Islamic law prevail. A new code of law is being produced for Abu Dhabi. In Dubai there is a court run by a *qadi*, while in some of the other States all legal cases are referred immediately to the Ruler or a member of his family, who will refer to a *qadi* only if he cannot settle the matter himself. In Abu Dhabi a professional Jordanian judge presides over the Ruler's Court.

Religion. Nearly all the inhabitants are Moslem of the Sunni, and a small minority of the Shi'ite sects.

Education In 1986–87 there were 122,543 pupils in primary schools, 36,810 in preparatory schools and 20,753 in secondary schools. There were 1,712 students in religious schools, 597 in technical schools and (1987–88) 2,075 at university. In 1990 there were 380,000 pupils altogether.

Health. In 1984 there were 28 hospitals (4,853 beds) and 119 clinics. There were 1,840 physicians.

DIPLOMATIC REPRESENTATIVES

Of the UAE in Great Britain (30 Prince's Gate, London, SW7 1PT)
Ambassador: Dr Khalifa Mohamed Sulaiman, GCVO (accredited 18 Nov. 1988).

Of Great Britain in the UAE
Ambassador: Graham Burton, CMG (British Embassy, Abu Dhabi).

Of the UAE in the USA (600 New Hampshire Ave., NW, Washington, D.C., 20037)
Ambassador: Abdulla bin Zayed Al-Nahayyan.

Of the USA in the UAE (Al-Sudan St., Abu Dhabi)
Ambassador: Edward S. Walker, Jr.

Of the UAE to the United Nations
Ambassador: Mohammed Hussain Al-Shaali.

Further Reading

Alkim, H. al-, *The Foreign Policy of the UAE*. Saqi, 1989
Clements, F. A., *United Arab Emirates*. [Bibliography] Oxford and Santa Barbara, 1983
Heard-Bey, F., *From Trucial States to United Arab Emirates*. London, 1982
Mallakh, R.S., *The Economic Development of the United Arab Emirates*, London, 1981
Soffan, L. U., *Women of the United Arab Emirates*. London, 1980
Taryam, A. O., *The Establishment of the United Arab Emirates*. London, 1987
Whelan, J., *UAE: a MEED Practical Guide*. 3rd ed. London, 1990

UNITED KINGDOM OF GREAT BRITAIN AND NORTHERN IRELAND

Capital: London
Population: 57·24m. (1989)
GNP per capita: US$12,800 (1988)

'Great Britain' is the geographical name of that island of the British Isles which comprises England, Scotland and Wales (so called to distinguish it from 'Little Britain' or Brittany). By the Act of Union, 1801, Great Britain and Ireland formed a legislative union as the United Kingdom of Great Britain and Ireland. Since the separation of Great Britain and Ireland in 1921 Northern Ireland remained within the Union which is now the United Kingdom of Great Britain and Northern Ireland. The United Kingdom (UK) does not include the Channel Islands or the Isle of Man which are direct dependencies of the Crown with their own legislative and taxation systems. England and Wales form an administrative entity, with some special arrangements for Wales (*see* pp. 1310–11).

GREAT BRITAIN

AREA AND POPULATION. Area (in sq. km) and population (present on census night) at the census taken 5 April 1981:

Divisions	*Area*	*Total*
England	130,357	46,362,836
Wales	20,761	2,791,851
Scotland	78,762	5,130,735
	229,880	54,285,422

Population at the 4 previous decennial censuses:

Divisions	*1931*	*1951*	*1961*	*1971*
England [1]	37,359,045	41,159,213	43,460,525	46,019,000
Wales	2,158,374	2,598,675	2,644,023	2,731,000
Scotland	4,842,980	5,096,415	5,178,490	5,228,963
Army, Navy and Merchant Seamen abroad	434,532	—	—	—
Total	44,794,931	48,854,303	51,283,038	53,978,963

[1] Areas now recognised as part of Gwent, Wales, formed the English county of Monmouthshire until 1974.

Population (usually resident) at the census of 1981:

Divisions	*Males*	*Females*	*Total*
England	22,288,395	23,483,561	45,771,956
Wales	1,336,323	1,413,317	2,749,640
Scotland	2,428,472	2,606,843	5,035,315
Great Britain	26,053,190	27,503,721	53,556,911

In 1981 in Wales 21,283 persons 3 years of age and upwards were able to speak Welsh only, and 482,266 able to speak Welsh and English: These totals represent 19% of the total population. In Scotland in 1981, 79,307 of the usually resident population could speak Gaelic (1·7%); 3,313 could read or write Gaelic, but could not speak it.

At the census of 1981, in England and Wales, there were 17,706,492 private households; in Great Britain, 19,500,113.

The age distribution in 1981 of the 'usually resident' population of England and Wales and Scotland was as follows (in 1,000):

Age-group	*England and Wales*	*Scotland*	*Great Britain*
Under 5	2,910	308	3,219
5 and under 10	3,207	344	3,551
10 ,, 15	3,846	425	4,271
15 ,, 20	4,020	447	4,467
20 ,, 25	3,564	394	3,959
25 ,, 35	6,931	701	7,632
35 ,, 45	5,885	588	6,473
45 ,, 55	5,474	575	6,049
55 ,, 65	5,410	541	5,951
65 ,, 70	2,426	241	2,667
70 ,, 75	2,062	204	2,265
75 ,, 85	2,280	221	2,501
85 and upwards	507	46	552
Total	48,522	5,035	53,557

At 30 June 1989 the estimated population of the UK was 57,236,000 (29,330,000 females), and of Great Britain, 55,653,000 (28,524,000 females). Age and sex distribution (UK, in 1,000 persons/females): Under 5, 3,808/1,857; 5-14, 7,017/3,416; 15-59, 34,549/18,808; 60-64, 2,914/1,511; over 65, 8,954/5,383.

Population densities (persons per sq. km), 1989: UK, 236; England, 366; Wales, 138.

England and Wales: The census population, (present on census night) of England and Wales 1801 to 1981:

Date of enumeration	*Population*	*Pop. per sq. mile*	*Date of enumeration*	*Population*	*Pop. per sq. mile* [1]
1801	8,892,536	152	1891	29,002,525	497
1811	10,164,256	174	1901	32,527,843	558
1821	12,000,236	206	1911	36,070,492	618
1831	13,896,797	238	1921	37,886,699	649
1841	15,914,148	273	1931	39,952,377	685
1851	17,927,609	307	1951	43,757,888	750
1861	20,066,224	344	1961	46,104,548	791
1871	22,712,266	389	1971	48,749,575	323
1881	25,974,439	445	1981	49,154,687	325

[1] Per sq. km from 1971

The birth places of the 1981 'usually resident' population were: England, 41,552,500; Wales, 2,758,026; Scotland, 752,188; Northern Ireland, 209,042; Ireland, 579,833; Commonwealth, 1,429,407; foreign countries, 1,209,091.

At June 1989 the estimated population of England and Wales was 50,562,500 (25,893,400 females); England, 47,689,400 (24,413,800). Age and sex distribution (in 1,000 persons/females): Under 5, 3,156/1,540; 5-14, 5,774/2,810; 15-59, 28,813/14,303; 60-64, 2,423/1,252; over 65, 7,523/4,509.

Eight 'standard regions' are identified in England for statistical purposes. They have no administrative significance. Population (in 1,000) in 1989: East Anglia, 2,045; East Midlands, 3,999; West Midlands, 5,216; North, 3,073; North West, 6,380; South East, 17,384 (including Greater London, 6,756); South West, 4,652; Yorkshire and Humberside, 4,940.

England and Wales are divided (apart from Greater London) into 53 counties (6 of them 'metropolitan') subdivided into 369 districts. Greater London comprises 32 boroughs and the City of London.

Area in sq. km of counties and population estimate 30 June 1989:

ENGLAND *Metropolitan counties*	*Area sq. km*	*Population*	*Metropolitan counties*—contd.	*Area sq. km*	*Population*
Greater Manchester	1,286	2,582,400	Tyne and Wear	540	1,128,100
Merseyside	652	1,448,000	West Midlands	899	2,615,400
South Yorkshire	1,560	1,295,200	West Yorkshire	2,039	2,066,600

Non-metropolitan counties	Area sq. km	Population (in 1,000)
ENGLAND		
Avon	1,338	952·8
Bedfordshire (Beds)	1,235	513·1
Berkshire (Berks)	1,256	748·4
Buckinghamshire (Bucks)	1,883	634·4
Cambridgeshire (Camb)	3,409	665·0
Cheshire	2,322	958·6
Cleveland	583	552·9
Cornwall and Isles of Scilly	3,546	464·1
Cumbria	6,809	491·6
Derbyshire	2,631	929·4
Devon	6,715	1,029·9
Dorset	2,654	656·8
Durham	2,436	596·9
East Sussex	1,795	711·8
Essex	3,674	1,532·0
Gloucestershire (Gloucs)	2,638	529·5
Hampshire (Hants)	3,772	1,546·0
Hereford and Worcester	3,927	675·3
Hertfordshire (Herts)	1,634	987·4
Humberside (Humb)	3,512	856·3
Isle of Wight (IOW)	381	130·5
Kent	3,732	1,523·6
Lancashire (Lancs)	3,043	1,390·8
Leicestershire (Leics)	2,553	891·9
Lincolnshire (Lincs)	5,885	586·9

Non-metropolitan counties—contd.	Area sq. km	Population (in 1,000)
Norfolk	5,355	748·5
Northamptonshire (Northants)	2,367	576·1
Northumberland	5,033	303·6
North Yorkshire (N. Yorks)	8,317	722·3
Nottinghamshire (Notts)	2,164	1,014·8
Oxfordshire (Oxon)	2,611	577·6
Shropshire (Salop)	3,490	403·2
Somerset (Som)	3,458	460·9
Staffordshire (Staffs)	2,716	1,039·9
Suffolk	3,800	641·1
Surrey	1,655	1,000·0
Warwickshire	1,981	483·1
West Sussex	2,016	704·9
Wiltshire (Wilts)	3,481	558·4
WALES		
Clwyd	2,425	411·1
Dyfed	5,765	352·6
Gwent	1,376	446·9
Gwynedd	3,868	240·8
Mid Glamorgan (M. Glam)	1,019	538·1
Powys	5,077	116·8
South Glamorgan (S. Glam)	416	404·1
West Glamorgan (W. Glam)	815	362·8

County districts with populations of over 90,000 (estimate, 30 June 1989):

ENGLAND	
Allerdale (Cumbria)	96·8
Amber Valley (Derbyshire)	113·3
Arun (W. Sussex)	130·7
Ashfield (Notts)	109·4
Ashford (Kent)	95·6
Aylesbury Vale (Bucks)	147·3
Barnsley (S. Yorks)	221·7
Basildon (Essex)	157·0
Basingstoke and Deane (Hants)	141·4
Bassetlaw (Notts)	105·5
Beverley (Humberside)	115·2
Birmingham (W. Midlands)	992·5
Blackburn (Lancs)	135·7
Blackpool (Lancs)	143·1
Bolton (Greater Manchester)	265·0
Bournemouth (Dorset)	154·3
Bracknell Forest (Berks)	104·6
Bradford (W. Yorks)	467·7
Braintree (Essex)	118·0
Breckland (Norfolk)	104·1
Brighton (E. Sussex)	143·1
Bristol (Avon)	372·6
Broadland (Norfolk)	105·3
Broxtowe (Notts)	110·0
Burnley (Lancs)	90·9
Bury (Greater Manchester)	176·4
Calderdale (W. Yorks)	197·4
Cambridge	99·0
Canterbury (Kent)	131·8
Carlisle (Cumbria)	103·1
Charnwood (Leics)	149·3
Chelmsford (Essex)	151·4
Cherwell (Oxon)	123·3
Chester (Cheshire)	114·2
Chesterfield (Derbyshire)	100·2
Chichester (W. Sussex)	105·9
Chorley (Lancs)	96·7
Colchester (Essex)	151·9
Coventry (W. Midlands)	304·1
Crewe and Nantwich (Cheshire)	100·1
Dacorum (Herts)	133·0
Darlington (Durham)	100·0
Derby	216·6
Doncaster (S. Yorks)	293·3
Dover (Kent)	107·1
Dudley (W. Midlands)	305·4
Easington (Durham)	95·2
East Devon	118·6
East Hampshire	102·3
East Hertfordshire	119·2
Eastleigh (Hants)	102·2
East Lindsey (Lincs)	119·2
East Staffordshire	96·9
Elmbridge (Surrey)	107·3
Epping Forest (Essex)	111·6
Erewash (Derbyshire)	108·2
Exeter (Devon)	102·3
Fareham (Hants)	101·4
Gateshead (Tyne and Wear)	205·8
Gedling (Notts)	111·0
Gillingham (Kent)	94·6
Gloucester	90·5
Great Grimsby (Humberside)	90·2
Great Yarmouth (Norfolk)	90·1
Guildford (Surrey)	122·9

ENGLAND—*contd.*

Halton (Cheshire)	124·8
Harrogate (N. Yorks)	147·9
Havant (Hants)	116·3
Hinckley and Bosworth (Leics)	97·6
Horsham (W. Sussex)	108·6
Hove (E. Sussex)	91·1
Huntingdonshire (Cambs)	149·1
Ipswich (Suffolk)	113·7
King's Lynn and West Norfolk	134·2
Kingston upon Hull (Humberside)	245·1
Kirklees (W. Yorks)	375·5
Knowsley (Merseyside)	157·5
Lancaster	130·8
Langbaurgh on Tees (Cleveland)	144·6
Leeds (W. Yorks)	711·7
Leicester	279·7
Lewes (E. Sussex)	91·3
Lichfield (Staffs)	93·0
Liverpool (Merseyside)	265·9
Luton (Beds)	169·9
Macclesfield (Cheshire)	151·7
Maidstone (Kent)	137·4
Manchester	443·6
Mansfield (Notts)	100·8
Mendip (Som)	94·0
Mid-Bedfordshire	114·4
Middlesbrough (Cleveland)	142·7
Mid-Sussex (W. Sussex)	119·7
Milton Keynes (Bucks)	182·3
Newark and Sherwood (Notts)	103·6
Newbury (Berks)	139·0
Newcastle under Lyme (Staffs)	118·1
Newcastle upon Tyne (Tyne and Wear)	277·6
New Forest (Hants)	163·3
Northampton	184·0
Northavon (Avon)	133·7
North Bedfordshire	137·3
North-East Derbyshire	96·8
North Hertfordshire	113·5
North Norfolk	95·8
North Tyneside (Tyne and Wear)	192·7
North Wiltshire	113·7
Norwich (Norfolk)	117·5
Nottingham	273·5
Nuneaton and Bedworth (Warwickshire)	116·7
Oldham (Greater Manchester)	220·8
Oxford	116·5
Peterborough (Cambs)	153·8
Plymouth (Devon)	255·0
Poole (Dorset)	131·5
Portsmouth (Hants)	183·9
Preston (Lancs)	128·4
Reading (Berks)	130·0
Reigate and Banstead (Surrey)	115·0
Rochdale (Greater Manchester)	207·7
Rochester upon Medway (Kent)	147·7
Rotherham (S. Yorks)	253·7
Rushcliffe (Notts)	101·1
Ryedale (N. Yorks)	91·6
St Albans (Herts)	128·4
St Edmundsbury (Suffolk)	91·9
St Helens (Merseyside)	188·8
Salford (Greater Manchester)	234·6
Salisbury (Wilts)	100·7

ENGLAND—*contd.*

Sandwell (W. Midlands)	295·6
Scarborough (N. Yorks)	106·2
Sedgemoor (Som)	97·3
Sefton (Merseyside)	299·6
Selby (N. Yorks)	93·6
Sevenoaks (Kent)	105·9
Sheffield (S. Yorks)	526·5
Shrewsbury and Atcham (Salop)	90·8
Slough (Berks)	101·0
Solihull (W. Midlands)	204·4
Southampton (Hants)	197·5
South Bedfordshire	109·5
South Cambridgeshire	118·9
Southend on Sea (Essex)	166·0
South Kesteven (Lincs)	105·8
South Lakeland (Cumbria)	101·2
South Norfolk	101·7
South Oxfordshire	130·1
South Ribble (Lancs)	101·6
South Somerset	142·7
South Staffordshire	109·1
South Tyneside (Tyne and Wear)	155·8
Stafford	119·1
Staffordshire Moorlands	97·8
Stockport (Greater Manchester)	291·3
Stockton on Tees (Cleveland)	176·9
Stoke on Trent (Staffs)	137·2
Stratford on Avon (Warwickshire)	105·8
Stroud (Gloucs)	110·5
Suffolk Coastal	112·8
Sunderland (Tyne and Wear)	167·2
Swale (Kent)	116·8
Tameside (Greater Manchester)	218·2
Taunton Deane (Som)	94·8
Teignbridge (Devon)	110·5
Tendring (Essex)	132·1
Test Valley (Hants)	102·6
Thamesdown (Wilts)	170·2
Thanet (Kent)	131·3
Thurrock (Essex)	125·6
Tonbridge and Malling (Kent)	100·4
Torbay (Devon)	120·0
Trafford (Greater Manchester)	215·3
Tunbridge Wells (Kent)	99·2
Vale of White Horse (Oxon)	112·0
Vale Royal (Cheshire)	114·0
Wakefield (W. Yorks)	314·2
Walsall (W. Midlands)	263·5
Warrington (Cheshire)	187·9
Warwick	115·2
Waveney (Suffolk)	107·1
Waverley (Surrey)	109·4
Wealden (E. Sussex)	135·7
Welwyn Hatfield (Herts)	92·1
West Lancashire	104·6
West Oxfordshire	95·7
West Wiltshire	106·1
Wigan (Greater Manchester)	309·6
Winchester (Hants)	95·8
Windsor and Maidenhead (Berks)	125·3
Wirral (Merseyside)	336·2
Wokingham (Berks)	148·5
Wolverhampton (W. Midlands)	249·9
Woodspring (Avon)	189·8
Worthing (W. Sussex)	98·7
Wrekin (Salop)	136·1

ENGLAND—*contd.*		WALES—*contd.*	
Wychavon (Hereford and Worcestor)	101·4	Newport (Gwent)	128·4
Wycombe (Bucks)	157·6	Ogwr (Mid-Glam)	137·6
Wyre (Lancs)	103·7	Rhymney Valley (Mid-Glam)	104·2
Wyre Forest (Hereford & Worcestor)	95·6	Swansea (W. Glam)	186·4
York (N. Yorks)	101·1	Taff Ely (Mid-Glam)	96·3
		Torfaen (Gwent)	92·6
WALES		Vale of Glamorgan	119·1
Cardiff (S. Glam)	284·9	Wrexham Maelor (Clwyd)	116·8

The following table shows the distribution of the urban and rural population of England and Wales in 1951, 1961, 1971, and 1981.

		Population		*Percentage*	
	England and Wales	*Urban districts* [1]	*Rural districts* [1]	*Urban*	*Rural*
1951	43,757,888	35,335,721	8,422,167	80·8	19·2
1961	46,071,604	36,838,442	9,233,162	80·0	20·0
1971	48,755,000	38,151,000	10,598,000	78·2	21·5
1981	49,011,417	37,686,863	11,324,554	76·9	23·1

[1] As existing at each census.

Conurbations. These are aggregates of local-authority areas with high population densities. In April 1981 there were 6 in England and Wales, with a population of 14·7m. (30% of total population): Greater London, 6·7m.; Tyneside, 0·7m.; W. Yorks., 1·67m.; S.E. Lancs., 2·24m.; Merseyside, 1·13m.; W. Midlands, 2·24m.

Greater London Boroughs. Total area 1,580 sq.km. Estimated population on 30 June 1989, 6,756,400. By borough:

Barking and Dagenham	147,400	Hammersmith and Fulham	148,500	Lewisham	226,700
Barnet	310,400	Haringey	189,900	Merton	164,000
Bexley	220,000	Harrow	193,800	Newham	207,100
Brent	254,700	Havering	232,600	Redbridge	232,200
Bromley	299,400	Hillingdon	235,300	Richmond upon Thames	163,700
Camden	183,700	Hounslow	195,900	Southwark	219,800
Croydon	317,300	Islington	169,500	Sutton	168,900
Ealing	293,800	Kensington and Chelsea	130,600	Tower Hamlets	163,900
Enfield	262,100	Kingston upon Thames	136,100	Waltham Forest	211,800
Greenwich	213,500	Lambeth	238,300	Wandsworth	256,200
Hackney	191,800			Westminster, City of	173,400

The City of London (677 acres) is administered by its Corporation which retains some independent powers. Resident population (1989 estimate) 4,300.

Scotland: Area 78,762 sq. km, including its islands, 186 in number, and inland water 1,580 sq. km.

Population (including military in the barracks and seamen on board vessels in the harbours) at the dates of each census:

Date of enumeration	*Population*	*Pop. per sq. mile*	*Date of enumeration*	*Population*	*Pop. per sq. mile* [1]
1811	1,805,864	60	1901	4,472,103	150
1821	2,091,521	70	1911	4,760,904	160
1831	2,364,386	79	1921	4,882,497	164
1841	2,620,184	88	1931	4,842,980	163
1851	2,888,742	97	1951	5,096,415	171
1861	3,062,294	100	1961	5,179,344	174
1871	3,360,018	113	1971	5,229,963	68
1881	3,735,573	125	1981	5,130,735	66
1891	4,025,647	135			

[1] per sq. km from 1971.

The 1981 population present on census night included 2,466,000 males, 2,664,000 females.

At 30 June 1989 the estimated population of Scotland was 5,090,700 (2,630,327 females). Age and sex distribution (in 1,000, persons/females): Under 5, 325/159; 5-14, 630/307; 15-59, 3,111/1,556; 60-64, 264/141; over 65, 761/468.

Population density 1989: 66 persons per sq.km.

Scotland is divided into 9 regions (subdivided into 53 districts) and 3 island authority areas. Area of regions and population estimate of regions and districts in June 1989:

Regions (area sq. km) and Districts	*Population (in 1,000) 1989*
Borders (4,662)	102·7
Berwickshire	18·9
Ettrick and Lauderdale	33·9
Roxburgh	34·9
Tweeddale	15·0
Central (2,590)	271·4
Clackmannan	47·2
Falkirk	143·1
Stirling	81·2
Dumfries and Galloway (6,475)	147·6
Annandale and Eskdale	36·3
Nithsdale	57·6
Stewartry	23·3
Wigtown	30·4
Fife (1,308)	344·8
Dunfermline	129·8
Kirkcaldy	146·7
North East Fife	68·3
Grampian (8,550)	503·5
Aberdeen City	210·7
Banff and Buchan	84·4
Gordon	74·1
Kincardine and Deeside	49·8
Moray	84·5
Highland (26,136)	201·9
Badenoch and Strathspey	10·9
Caithness	26·6
Inverness	62·3
Lochaber	19·1
Nairn	10·2
Ross and Cromarty	48·3
Skye and Lochalsh	11·6
Sutherland	13·0
Lothian (1,756)	742·9
East Lothian	84·1
Edinburgh City	433·2
Midlothian	80·8
West Lothian	144·8
Strathclyde (13,856)	2,311·2
Argyll and Bute	66·4
Bearsden and Milngavie	40·7
Clydebank	47·2
Clydesdale	58·4
Cumbernauld and Kilsyth	62·8
Cumnock and Doon Valley	43·0
Cunninghame	137·2
Dumbarton	79·9
East Kilbride	82·3
Eastwood	60·3
Glasgow City	695·6
Hamilton	107·3
Inverclyde	94·4
Kilmarnock and Loudoun	81·0
Kyle and Carrick	113·3
Monklands	104·7
Motherwell	146·7
Renfrew	200·6
Strathkelvin	89·4
Tayside (7,668)	392·5
Angus	95·1
Dundee City	172·5
Perth and Kinross	124·9
Island Authority Areas	
Orkney Islands (974)	19·4
Shetland Islands (1,427)	22·2
Western Isles (2,901)	30·6

The birthplaces of the 1981 usually resident population were: Scotland, 4,548,708; England, 297,784; Wales, 12,733; Northern Ireland, 33,927; Ireland 27,018; Commonwealth, 48,515; foreign countries, 65,384.

The population of the Central Clydeside conurbation in 1989 was 1,637,630.

Isle of Man and Channel Islands:

Islands	*Area in sq. km*	*Population 1961*	*1971*	*1986*
Isle of Man	572	48,151	56,289	55,482
Jersey	116	57,200	69,329	80,212 [1]
Guernsey, Herm and Jethou	64	47,178	53,734	64,282
Alderney	8			
Sark, Brechou and Lihou	6			

[1] 1985.

Vital statistics for England and Wales:

	Total live births	*Live births outside marriage*	*Total*	*Deaths under 1 year*	*Marriages*	*Divorces, annulments and dissolutions*
1984	636,818	110,465	566,881	6,037	349,186	144,501
1985	656,417	126,250	590,734	6,141	346,389	160,300
1986	661,018	141,345	581,203	6,313	347,924	153,903
1987	681,511	158,431	566,994	6,308	351,761	151,007
1988	693,577	177,352	571,408	6,270	348,492	152,633
1989	687,725	185,804	576,872	5,808	...	150,872

Expectation of life, 1988: UK, males, 72·2 years, females, 77·9; England and Wales, males, 72·4, females, 78·1.

Birth rate, 1989, per 1,000 population, 13·6; death rate, 11·4; marriage (1988), 13·9; divorce rate per 1,000 married couples, 12·7; infant mortality per 1,000 live births, 8·4; sex ratio, 1,051 male births to 1,000 female. Average age of first marriage, 1988: Males, 26, females, 24.

In the UK in 1988 some 21% of unmarried females between the ages of 18 and 49 were cohabiting.

Vital statistics for Scotland:

	Estimated resident population at 30 June[1]	*Total births*	*Live births outside marriage*	*Deaths*	*Marriages*	*Divorces, annulments and dissolutions*
1982	5,166,557	66,196	9,395	65,022	34,942	11,288
1983	5,150,405	65,078	9,581	63,454	34,962	13,238
1984	5,145,722	65,106	10,640	62,345	36,253	11,915
1985	5,136,509	66,676	12,362	63,967	36,385	13,373
1986	5,121,013	65,812	13,547	63,467	35,790	12,800
1987	5,112,129	66,241	15,125	62,014	35,813	12,133
1988	5,094,001	66,212	16,224	61,957	35,599	11,472
1989	5,090,700	63,480	16,476	65,017	35,326	11,659

[1] Includes merchant navy at home and forces stationed in Scotland.

Birth rate, 1989, per 1,000 population, 12·5; death rate, 12·8; marriage, 14; divorce rate per 1,000 married couples, 10; infant mortality per 1,000 live births, 8·7; sex ratio, 1,049 male births to 1,000 female. Average age of first marriage in 1988: Males, 30, females 27·7. Expectation of life, 1988: Males, 70·3 years, females, 76·5.

Emigration and Immigration. During the last hundred years the UK has most often been a net exporter of population. Throughout the period 1881–1931 there was a consistent net loss from migration, though the fifteen years 1931–46 brought a reversal of the trend as a result of immigration from Europe. Since the Second World War the loss has largely continued. However, during the five years 1956–1961, increased immigration particularly from the new Commonwealth and Pakistan, resulted in a net gain.

Since 1964 migration figures have been available from the International Passenger Survey. This is a sample survey conducted by the Office of Population Censuses and Surveys, covering all the principal air and sea routes between the UK and overseas, except those to and from the Republic of Ireland. For the years 1970–79 the survey shows an average annual net loss for the UK of 36,000; and for 1980–89, 2,000.

The table below, derived from the International Passenger survey, summarizes migration statistics for 1989 (in 1,000):

By country of last or future intended residence		*Into UK*	*Out from UK*	*Balance*
All Countries		250	205	+44
Australia, Canada, New Zealand		48	55	−6
India, Bangladesh, Sri Lanka		16	5	+11
Other Commonwealth		43	29	+14
EC		55	45	+10
USA		31	30	+1
Republic of South Africa		12	6	+5
Rest of World		45	35	+10
By sex/age in 1989				
Males	0–14	21	16	+5
	15–24	29	23	+6
	25–44	47	56	−9
	45 and over	12	13	−1
	All ages	110	108	+1

By country of last or future intended residence		Into UK	Out from UK	Balance
Females	0–14	26	18	+9
	15–24	46	26	+19
	25–44	56	45	+11
	45 and over	12	9	+4
	All ages	140	97	+43

CLIMATE. The climate is cool temperate oceanic, with mild conditions and rainfall evenly distributed over the year, though the weather is very changeable because of cyclonic influences. In general, temperatures are higher in the west and lower in the east in winter and rather the reverse in summer. Rainfall amounts are greatest in the west, where most of the high ground occurs.

London. Jan. 40°F (4·5°C), July 64°F (18°C). Annual rainfall 24" (600 mm). Aberdeen. Jan. 39°F (4°C), July 57°F (14°C). Annual rainfall 33" (823 mm). Belfast. Jan. 40°F (4·5°C), July 61°F (16·1°C). Annual rainfall 34·6" (865 mm). Birmingham. Jan. 38°F (3·3°C), July 61°F (16·1°C). Annual rainfall 30" (749 mm). Cardiff. Jan. 40°F (4·4°C), July 61°F (16·1°C). Annual rainfall 42·6" (1,065 mm). Edinburgh. Jan. 38°F (3·5°C), July 58°F (14·5°C). Annual rainfall 28" (708 mm). Glasgow. Jan. 39°F (4°C), July 60°F (15·5°C). Annual rainfall 37·2" (930 mm). Manchester. Jan. 41°F (5°C), July 62°F (16·5°C). Annual rainfall 34·1" (853 mm).

QUEEN, HEAD OF THE COMMONWEALTH. Elizabeth II Alexandra Mary, born 21 April 1926 daughter of King George VI and Queen Elizabeth; married on 20 Nov. 1947 Lieut. Philip Mountbatten (formerly Prince Philip of Greece), created Duke of Edinburgh, Earl of Merioneth and Baron Greenwich on the same day and created Prince Philip, Duke of Edinburgh, 22 Feb. 1957; succeeded to the crown on the death of her father, on 6 Feb. 1952. Offspring: *Charles* Philip Arthur George, Prince of Wales (Heir Apparent), born 14 Nov. 1948, married Lady Diana Spencer on 29 July 1981. Offspring: *William* Arthur Philip Louis, born 21 June 1982; *Henry* Charles Albert David, born 15 Sept. 1984. Princess *Anne* Elizabeth Alice Louise, the Princess Royal, born 15 Aug. 1950, married Mark Anthony Peter Phillips on 14 Nov. 1973. Offspring: *Peter* Mark Andrew, born 15 Nov. 1977; *Zara* Anne Elizabeth, born 15 May 1981. Prince *Andrew*, Albert Christian Edward, created Duke of York, 23 July 1986, born 19 Feb. 1960, married Sarah Margaret Ferguson on 23 July 1986. Offspring: Princess *Beatrice* Mary, born 8 Aug. 1988; Princess *Eugenie* Victoria Helena, born 23 March 1990. Prince *Edward* Antony Richard Louis, born 10 March 1964.

The Queen Mother: Queen Elizabeth, born 4 Aug. 1900, daughter of the 14th Earl of Strathmore and Kinghorne; married the Duke of York, afterwards King George VI, on 26 April 1923.

Sister of the Queen: Princess Margaret Rose, born 12 Aug. 1930; married Antony Armstrong-Jones (created Earl of Snowdon, 3 Oct. 1961) on 6 May 1960; divorced, 1978. Offspring: *David* Albert Charles (Viscount Linley), born 3 Nov. 1961; Lady *Sarah* Frances Elizabeth Armstrong-Jones, born 1964.

Children of the late Duke of Gloucester (died 10 June 1974): William Henry Andrew Frederick, born 18 Dec. 1941, died 28 Aug. 1972; Richard Alexander Walter George, Duke of Gloucester, born 26 Aug. 1944, married Birgitte van Deurs on 8 July 1972 (offspring: Alexander Patrick Gregers Richard Windsor, Earl of Ulster, born 24 Oct. 1974; Davina Elizabeth Alice Benedikte Windsor, born 19 Nov. 1977; Rose Victoria Birgitte Louise Windsor, born 1 March 1980).

Children of the late Duke of Kent (died 25 Aug. 1942): Edward George Nicholas Patrick, Duke of Kent, born 9 Oct. 1935; married Katharine Worsley on 8 June 1961 (offspring: George Philip Nicholas, Earl of St Andrews, born 26 June 1962, married Sylvania Tomaselli on 9 Jan. 1988 (offspring: Lord Downpatrick, born 2 Dec. 1988); Lady Helen Windsor, born 28 April 1964; Lord Nicholas Charles Edward Jonathan Windsor, born 25 July 1970). Alexandra Helen Elizabeth Olga Christabel, born 25 Dec. 1936; married 24 April 1963, Angus Ogilvy (offspring: James Robert Bruce, born 29 Feb. 1964; Marina Victoria Alexandra, born 31 July 1966). Michael George Charles Franklin, born 4 July 1942; married Marie-Christine von Reibnitz on 30 June 1978 (offspring: Lord *Frederick* Michael George David Louis Windsor, born 6 April 1979; Lady *Gabriela* Marina Alexander Ophelia Windsor, born 23 April 1981).

The Queen's legal title rests on the statute of 12 and 13 Will. III, ch. 3, by which the succession to the Crown of Great Britain and Ireland was settled on the Princess Sophia of Hanover and the 'heirs of her body being Protestants'. By proclamation of 17 July 1917 the royal family became known as the House and Family of Windsor. On 8 Feb. 1960 the Queen issued a declaration varying her confirmatory declaration of 9 April 1952 to the effect that while the Queen and her children should continue to be known as the House of Windsor, her descendants, other than descendants entitled to the style of Royal Highness and the title of Prince or Princess, and female descendants who marry and their descendants should bear the name of Mountbatten-Windsor. For the Royal Style and Titles of Queen Elizabeth *see* Commonwealth section.

By letters patent of 30 Nov. 1917 the titles of Royal Highness and Prince or Princess are restricted to the Sovereign's children, the children of the Sovereign's sons and the eldest living son of the eldest son of the Prince of Wales.

Provision is made for the support of the royal household, after the surrender of hereditary revenues, by the settlement of the Civil List soon after the beginning of each reign. (For historical details, *see* THE STATESMAN'S YEAR-BOOK, 1908, p. 5, and 1935 p. 4). The Civil List Act of 1 Jan. 1972 provided for a decennial, and the Civil List (Increase of Financial Provision) Order 1975 for an annual review of the List, but in July 1990 it was again fixed for one decade.

The Civil List of 1991-2000 provides for an annuity of £7,900,000 to the Queen; £230,500 to the Princess Royal; £360,000 to Prince Philip; £640,500 to Queen Elizabeth (the Queen Mother); £220,000 to the Princess Margaret; £250,000 to the Duke of York; £100,000 to Prince Edward. The income of the Prince of Wales derives from the Duchy of Cornwall.

Sovereigns of Great Britain, from the Restoration (with dates of accession):

House of Stewart

Charles II 29 May 1660
James II 6 Feb. 1685

House of Stewart-Orange

William and Mary 13 Feb. 1689
William III 28 Dec. 1694

House of Stewart

Anne 19 March 1702

House of Hanover

George I 1 Aug. 1714
George II 11 June 1727
George III 25 Oct. 1760
George IV 29 Jan. 1820
William IV 26 June 1830
Victoria 20 June 1837

House of Saxe-Coburg and Gotha

Edward VII 22 Jan. 1901

House of Windsor

George V 6 May 1910
Edward VIII 20 Jan. 1936
George VI 11 Dec. 1936
Elizabeth II 6 Feb. 1952

CONSTITUTION AND GOVERNMENT. The supreme legislative power is vested in Parliament, which consists of the Crown, the House of Lords and the House of Commons and dates in its present form from the middle of the 14th century. A Bill which is passed by both Houses and receives Royal Assent becomes an Act of Parliament and part of statute law.

Parliament is summoned, and a General Election is called, by the sovereign on the advice of the Prime Minister. A Parliament may last up to 5 years, normally divided into annual sessions. A session is ended by prorogation, and all Bills which have not been passed by both Houses then lapse. A Parliament ends by dissolution, either by will of the sovereign or by lapse of the 5-year period.

Under the Parliament Acts 1911 and 1949, all Money Bills (so certified by the Speaker of the House of Commons), if not passed by the Lords without amendment, may become law without their concurrence within 1 month of introduction in the Lords. Public Bills, other than Money Bills or a Bill extending the maximum duration of Parliament, if passed by the Commons in 2 successive sessions and rejected each time by the Lords, may become law without their concurrence provided that 1 year has elapsed between Commons second reading in the first session and third reading in the second session, and that the Bill reaches the Lords at least 1 month before the end of the second session. No Act has been passed in this way since 1949, because the Lords today respect the privileges of the elected House, especially as regards taxes and public spending, and act mainly as a revising chamber.

Peerages are created by the sovereign, without limit of number. They are held for life, and may or may not be hereditary. The House of Lords consisted (on 31 Dec. 1990) of: (1) 763 hereditary peers (including 20 women) sitting by virtue of creation or descent, other than those who have disclaimed their titles for life under the provisions of the Peerage Act, 1963; (2) life peers (non-hereditary being *(a)* 18 Lords of Appeal (active and retired), under the Appellate Jurisdiction Act, 1876, as amended; *(b)* 357 peers (including 53 women) under the Life Peerages Act, 1958; (3) 2 archbishops and 24 diocesan bishops of the Church of England, who leave the House on retirement. The full House thus consists of 1,184, though the average daily attendance is only 321.

The House of Commons consists of members (of both sexes) representing constituencies determined by the Boundary Commissions. Persons under 21 years of age, Clergy of the Church of England and of the Scottish Episcopal Church, Ministers of the Church of Scotland, Roman Catholic clergymen, civil servants, members of the regular armed forces, policemen, most judicial officers and other office-holders named in the House of Commons (Disqualification) Act are disqualified from sitting in the House of Commons. No peer eligible to sit in the House of Lords can be elected to the House of Commons unless he has disclaimed his title, but Irish peers and holders of courtesy titles, who are not members of the House of Lords, are eligible.

The Representation of the People Act 1948, abolished the business premises and University franchises, and the only persons entitled to vote at Parliamentary elections are those registered as residents or as service voters. No person may vote in more than one constituency at a general election. Persons may apply on certain grounds to vote by post or by proxy.

All persons over 18 years old and not subject to any legal incapacity to vote and who are either British subjects or citizens of Ireland are entitled to be included in the register of electors for the constituency containing the address at which they were residing on the qualifying date for the register and are entitled to vote at elections held during the period for which the register remains in force.

Members of the armed forces, Crown servants employed abroad, and the wives accompanying their husbands, are entitled, if otherwise qualified, to be registered as 'service voters' provided they make a 'service declaration'. To be effective for a particular register, the declaration must be made on or before the qualifying date for that register. In certain circumstances, British subjects living abroad may also vote.

The House of Commons (Redistribution of Seats) Acts 1944, 1949 and 1958, provided for the setting up of Boundary Commissions for England, Wales, Scotland and Northern Ireland. The Commissions are required to make general reports at intervals of not less than 10 and not more than 15 years and to submit reports from time to time with respect to the area comprised in any particular constituency or constituencies where some change appears necessary. Any changes giving effect to reports of the Commissions are to be made by Orders in Council laid before Parliament for approval by resolution of each House. The Parliamentary electorate of the United Kingdom and Northern Ireland in the register in 1990 numbered 43,663,423, of whom 36,388,575 were in England, 2,207,542 in Wales, 3,936,704 in Scotland and 1,130,602 in Northern Ireland.

At the general election held in 1987, 650 members were returned, 523 from England, 72 from Scotland, 38 from Wales and 17 from Northern Ireland. Every constituency returns a single member.

In Aug. 1911 provision was first made for the payment of a salary of £400 per annum to members of the Commons, other than those already in receipt of salaries as officers of the House, as Ministers or as officers of Her Majesty's household. As from 1 Jan. 1991 the salaries of members are £28,970 per annum. There is an office costs allowance of up to £27,166 per annum and a living allowance, for an additional home, of up to £10,570 per annum. Members of the House of Lords are unsalaried but may recover expenses incurred in attending sittings of the House within maxima for each day's attendance of £26 for day subsistence, £68 for night subsistence and £27 for secretarial and research assistance and office expenses. Additionally, Members of the House who are disabled may recover the extra cost of attending the House incurred by reason of their disablement. In connection with attendance at the House and parliamentary duties within the UK Lords may also recover the cost of travelling to and from home.

The following is a table of the duration of Parliaments called since Nov. 1935.

Reign	*When met*	*When dissolved*	*Duration (years and days)*	
George V, Edward VIII and George VI	26 Nov. 1935	15 June 1945	9	205
George VI	1 Aug. 1945	3 Feb. 1950	4	188
,,	1 Mar. 1950	5 Oct. 1951	1	219
George VI and Elizabeth II	31 Oct. 1951	6 May 1955	3	188
Elizabeth II	7 June 1955	18 Sept. 1959	4	105
,,	20 Oct. 1959	25 Sept. 1964	4	341
,,	27 Oct. 1964	10 Mar. 1966	1	134
,,	18 Apr. 1966	29 May 1970	4	81
,,	29 June 1970	8 Feb. 1974	3	225
,,	12 Mar. 1974	20 Sept. 1974	0	224
,,	22 Oct. 1974	7 April 1979	4	167
,,	9 May 1979	13 May 1983	4	4
,,	15 June 1983	18 May 1987	3	338
,,	25 June 1987	—	—	—

The executive government is vested nominally in the Crown, but practically in a committee of Ministers, called the Cabinet, which is dependent on the support of a majority in the House of Commons.

The head of the Ministry is the Prime Minister, a position first constitutionally recognized, and special precedence accorded to the holder, in 1905. His colleagues in the Ministry are appointed on his recommendation, and he dispenses the greater portion of the patronage of the Crown.

Heads of the Administrations since 1937 (C. = Conservative, L. = Liberal, Lab. = Labour, Nat. = National, Coal. = Coalition, Care. = Caretaker):

N. Chamberlain (Nat.)	28 May 1937	Sir Alec Douglas-Home (C.)	18 Oct. 1963
W. S. Churchill (Coal.)	10 May 1940	H. Wilson (Lab.)	16 Oct. 1964
W. S. Churchill (Care.)	23 May 1945	E. Heath (C.)	19 June 1970
C. R. Attlee (Lab.)	26 July 1945	H. Wilson (Lab.)	12 Mar. 1974
W. S. Churchill (C.)	26 Oct. 1951	J. Callaghan (Lab.)	5 Apr. 1976
Sir Anthony Eden (C.)	6 Apr. 1955	M. Thatcher (C.)	4 May 1979
H. Macmillan (C.)	10 Jan. 1957	J. Major (C.)	22 Nov. 1990

In March 1991 the Government consisted of the following members:

(*a*) Members of the Cabinet

1. *Prime Minister, First Lord of the Treasury and Minister for the Civil Service:* Rt Hon. John Major, MP, born 1943. (Salary £50,724 per annum.)

2. *Lord President of the Council, Leader of the House of Commons and Deputy Prime Minister:* Rt Hon. John MacGregor, OBE MP, born 1937. (£38,105.)

3. *Lord Chancellor:* Rt Hon. The Lord Mackay of Clashfern, QC, born 1927. (£91,500.)

4. *Secretary of State for Foreign and Commonwealth Affairs:* Rt Hon. Douglas Hurd, CBE, MP, born 1930. (£38,105.)

5. *Chancellor of the Exchequer:* Rt Hon. Norman Lamont, MP, born 1942. (£38,105.)

6. *Secretary of State for the Home Department:* Rt Hon. Kenneth Baker, QC, MP, born 1934. (£38,105.)

7. *Secretary of State for Wales:* Rt Hon. David Hunt, MBE, MP, born 1942. (£38,105.)

8. *Secretary of State for Defence:* Rt Hon. Tom King, MP, born 1933. (£38,105.)

9. *Secretary of State for Trade and Industry:* Rt Hon. Peter Lilley, MP, born 1943. (£38,105.)

10. *Chancellor of the Duchy of Lancaster:* Rt Hon. Chris Patten, MP, born 1944. (£28,970.)

11. *Secretary of State for Health:* Rt Hon. William Waldegrave, QC, MP, born 1946. (£38,105.)

12. *Secretary of State for Education and Science:* Rt Hon. Kenneth Clark, QC, MP, born 1940. (£38,105.)

13. *Secretary of State for Scotland:* Rt Hon. Ian Lang, QC, MP, born 1940. (£38,105.)

14. *Secretary of State for Transport:* Rt Hon. Malcolm Rifkind, QC, MP, born 1946. (£38,105.)

15. *Secretary of State for Energy:* Rt Hon. John Wakeham, MP, born 1932. (£38,105.)

16. *Lord Privy Seal and Leader of the House of Lords:* Rt Hon. The Lord Waddington, QC, born 1929. (£48,381.)

17. *Secretary of State for Social Security:* Rt Hon. Antony Newton, OBE, MP, born 1937. (£38,105.)

18. *Secretary of State for the Environment:* Rt Hon. Michael Heseltine, MP, born 1933. (£38,105.)

19. *Secretary of State for Northern Ireland:* Rt Hon. Peter Brooke, MP, born 1934. (£38,105.)

20. *Minister of Agriculture, Fisheries and Food:* Rt Hon. John Gummer, MP, born 1939. (£38,105.)

21. *Chief Secretary to the Treasury:* Rt Hon. David Mellor, QC, MP, born 1937. (£38,105.)

22. *Secretary of State for Employment:* Rt Hon. Michael Howard, QC, MP, born 1941. (£38,105.)

(*b*) Law Officers

23. *Attorney-General:* Rt Hon. Sir Patrick Mayhew, QC, MP, born 1929. (£40,492.)

24. *Lord Advocate:* Rt Hon. The Lord Fraser of Carmyllie, QC, born 1945. (£48,457.)

25. *Solicitor-General:* Rt Hon. Sir Nicholas Lyell, QC, MP, born 1938. (£33,201.)

26. *Solicitor-General for Scotland:* Alan Rodger, QC, born 1944. (£42,433.)

(*c*) Ministers not in the Cabinet

27. *Parliamentary Secretary, Treasury (Chief Whip):* Rt Hon. Richard Ryder, OBE, MP, born 1949. (£31,517.)

28. *Minister of State, Privy Council Office, Minister for the Arts:* Rt Hon. Tim Renton, MP, born 1932. (£37,715.)

29. *Minister of State, Foreign and Commonwealth Office, Minister for Overseas Development:* Rt Hon. Lynda Chalker, MP, born 1942. (£31,715.)

30. *Minister of State, Foreign and Commonwealth Office:* Rt Hon. The Earl of Caithness, born 1948. (£43,010.)

31. *Minister of State, Foreign and Commonwealth Office:* Hon. Douglas Hogg, MP, born 1945. (£26,962.)

32. *Minister of State, Foreign and Commonwealth Office:* Hon. Tristan Garel-Jones, MP, born 1941. (£26,962.)

33. *Financial Secretary, Treasury:* Hon Francis Maude, MP, born 1953. (£26,962.)

34. *Paymaster General (Northern Ireland Office):* The Rt Hon. Lord Belstead, JP, born 1932. (£39,641.)

35. *Minister of State, Home Office:* Rt Hon. John Patten, MP, born 1945. (£29,962.)

36. *Minister of State, Home Office:* Angela Rumbold, CBE, MP, born 1932. (£29,962.)

37. *Minister of State, Home Office:* Rt Hon. The Earl Ferrers, DL, born 1929. (£43,010.)

38. *Minister of State, Welsh Office:* Sir Wyn Roberts, MP, born 1930. (£26,962.)

39. *Minister of State, Ministry of Defence, Armed Forces:* Hon. Archie Hamilton, MP, born 1941. (£26,962.)

40. *Minister of State, Ministry of Defence, Defence Procurement:* Rt Hon. Alan Clark, MP, born 1928. (£26,962.)

41. *Minister of State, Department of Trade and Industry, Minister for Industry and Enterprise:* The Lord Hesketh, born 1950. (£43,010.)

42. *Minister of State, Department of Trade and Industry, Minister for Industry and Enterprise:* Rt Hon. Tim Sainsbury, born 1932. (£26,962.)

43. *Minister of State, Department of Trade and Industry, Corporate Affairs:* John Redwood, MP, born 1951. (£26,962.)

44. *Minister of State, Department of Health, Minister for Health:* Virginia Bottomley, MP, born 1948. (£26,962.)

45. *Minister of State, Department of Education and Science:* Tim Eggar, MP, born 1951. (£26,962.)

46. *Minister of State, Scottish Office:* Michael Forsyth, MP, born 1954. (£26,962.)

47. *Minister of State, Department of Transport, Minister for Public Transport:* Roger Freeman, FCA, MP, born 1942. (£26,962.)

48. *Minister of State, Department of Transport, Minlster for Aviation and Shipping:* The Lord Brabazon of Tara, born 1946. (£43,010.)

49. *Minister of State, Department of Social Security, Minister for Social Security and Disabled People:* Rt Hon. Nicholas Scott, MBE, MP, born 1933. (£26,962.)

50. *Minister of State, Department of the Environment, Minister for the Environment and Countryside:* David Trippier, RD, MP, born 1946. (£26.962.)

51. *Minister of State, Department of the Environment, Minister for Local Government and Inner Cities:* Michael Portillo, MP, born 1953. (£26,962.)

52. *Minister of State, Department of the Environment, Minister for Housing and Planning:* Sir George Young, MP, born 1941. (£26,962.)

53. *Minister of State, Northern Ireland Office:* Dr Brian Mawhinney, MP, born 1940. (£26,962.)

54. *Minister of State, Ministry of Agriculture, Fisheries and Food:* The Baroness Trumpington, born 1922. (£43,010.)

55. *Minister of State, Treasury:* Gillian Shephard, MP, born 1940. (£26,962.)

Leader of the Opposition in the House of Commons: Rt Hon. Neil Kinnock, MP, born 1942. (£34,937.)

Leader of the Opposition in the House of Lords: Rt Hon. The Lord Cledwyn of Penrhos, born 1916. (£36,066.)

Cabinet Ministers, Ministers of State, Parliamentary Secretaries and the Leader of the Opposition who are also Members of Parliament, receive additionally a reduced Parliamentary salary of £21,809.

The Constitution of the House of Commons after the 1987 general election was as follows: Conservative, 375; Labour, 229; Liberals, 17, SDP, 5; Others, 24.

Ball, A., *British Political Parties: The Emergence of a Modern Party System*. 1981
Butler, D. and Butler, G., *British Political Facts, 1900–85*. London, 1986
Butler, D. and Kavanagh, D., *The British General Election of 1987*. 1988
Drewry, G. (ed.), *The New Select Committees*. OUP, 1985
King, A. (ed.), *The British Prime Minister*. Rev. ed. London, 1985.—*British Members of Parliament*. London, 1974
Mackintosh, J. P., *The British Cabinet*. 3rd ed. London, 1977.—*The Government and Politics of Britain*. 4th ed. London, 1977
May, Sir T. E., *Treatise on the Law, Privileges, Proceedings and Usage of Parliament*. 20th ed., London, 1983
Norton, P., *Parliament in the 1980s*. Oxford, 1985
Parker, F. K., *Conduct of Parliamentary Elections*. London, 1983
Pelling, H., *A Short History of the Labour Party*. London, 1976
Shell, D., *The House of Lords*. Oxford, 1988
Silk, E. P., *How Parliament Works*. London, 1987
The Times Guide to the House of Commons, June 1987. London, 1987

National flag: The combined crosses of St George (red), St Andrew (white) and St Patrick (red), the red fimbriated in white, all on a blue ground.

European Parliament: On 15 June 1989 Great Britain elected 81 representatives to the European Parliament, of which 66 came from England, 8 from Scotland and 4 from Wales, each constituency returning a single member by a first past the post system. Northern Ireland returned 3 members by single transferable vote. The seats were won as follows: Labour 45, Conservative 32, Scottish Nationalists 1, Ulster Unionists 1, Democratic Unionists 1, Social, Democratic and Labour Party 1.

Local Government. Local Administration is carried out by four different types of bodies, namely: (i) local branches of some central ministries, such as the Department of Health and Social Security (now two separate departments); (ii) local sub-managements of nationalized industries; (iii) specialist authorities such as electricity boards; and (iv) the system of local government described below. The phrase 'local government' has come to mean that part of the local administration conducted by elected councils.

There are two separate systems, one for England and Wales and one for Scotland, but both systems are financed by a charge on individuals known as the Community Charge paid at a flat rate by each adult, varying from one area to another, levied locally, supplemented by a new streamlined government grant system and a nationwide uniform tax on business property - the Uniform Business Rate.

Local Government: England and Wales—*Outside London*. England and Wales have slightly differing systems. Each country has three types of councils namely, county, district and English parish or Welsh Community Councils. In addition, England has some metropolitan district councils.

Councillors are elected by their local electors for 4 years. The chairman of the council is one of the councillors elected by the rest. In a district with the status of borough his title is mayor, or in a city, Lord Mayor. Any parish or community council can by simple resolution adopt the style 'town council' and the status of town for the parish or community. The chairman of the council will be known as the town mayor.

Counties and Districts: There are 47 non-metropolitan counties (of which 8 are in Wales). The 6 metropolitan counties (Greater Manchester, Merseyside, South Yorkshire, Tyne and Wear, West Yorkshire and West Midlands) have no councils, the metropolitan districts having most of the county functions. Within the counties there are 369 districts (36 metropolitan and 333 non-metropolitan, of which 37 are in Wales).

Parishes and Communities: There are some 10,000 parishes within the English districts, of which 8,000 or so have councils. About 300 are former small boroughs or urban districts which became successor parishes.

In Wales, parishes are known as communities. Unlike England, where some urban areas are not in any parish, communities have been established for the whole of Wales. There is one for each former parish, county borough, borough or urban district (or part thereof where the former area is divided by a new boundary). There are about 1,000 communities altogether, of which 800 or so have councils.

The Local Government Act 1972 laid down the boundaries for all the counties and districts in England and Wales except the English non-metropolitan districts.

Permanent Local Government Boundary Commissions for England and for Wales advise the Secretaries of State on boundaries and electoral arrangements.

Local government functions may be classified into county, district and parish or community functions, but whereas county and district functions are distinct, the parish and community functions are mostly concurrent with those of the districts. Arrangements may, however, be made so that any council may discharge functions of any other as its agent.

The following is the classification of powers given above: *Parish and Community Functions.* Allotments, burial and cremation, halls, meeting places and entertainments, facilities for exercise and recreation, public lavatories, street lighting, offstreet vehicle parking, footpaths, the support of local arts and crafts, the encouragement of tourism and the right to be consulted by the district council on planning applications and certain byelaws. *District Functions.* In addition to the Parish and Community functions, aerodromes, civic restaurants, housing, markets, refuse collection, the administration of planning control, the formulation of local plans, sewerage on behalf of the water authority, museums, the licensing of places of entertainment and refreshment, and the constitutional oversight of parishes and communities. *County Functions.* The formulation of structure plans, traffic, transportation and roads, education, public libraries and museums, youth employment and social services.

There are, in addition, a number of special arrangements. Four district councils in Wales are designated as library authorities and Welsh district councils have powers in relation to allotments currently with community councils. The county councils in England and Wales separately or jointly appoint the fire and police authorities, and the bodies responsible for national parks. In Metropolitan counties, there are no county councils and all functions are performed by the districts (in some cases jointly). The total number of local government electors in England and Wales was 38,539,032 in 1990.

Greater London. From 1965–86 London was governed by the Greater London Council, covering the whole metropolitan area, and by 32 London boroughs and the Corporation of the City of London, each with responsibilities in its own area. The GLC was abolished on 1 April 1986. The individual borough councils are the education authorities. Fire services in Greater London are the responsibility of the London Fire and Civil Defence Authority, whose members are appointed by the boroughs and the City. Flood prevention is the responsibility of the Thames Water Authority. Waste regulation for the whole of Greater London is the function of the London Waste Regulation Authority. Waste collection is the responsibility of the boroughs. Waste disposal is the responsibility of the boroughs acting individually or in groups. Except in the City, the police authority is the Metropolitan Police, which is responsible to central government. London Regional Transport is likewise responsible to central government for passenger transport. Other local government functions are the responsibility of the boroughs, acting either individually or jointly, and the City.

Net current expenditure for all London authorities in 1988–89 was estimated at £4,832m. (including £978m. for ILEA but excluding Metropolitan Police). Gross capital expenditure (excluding leasing) for all London authorities and the London Residuary Body was estimated at £1,300m. in 1987–88.

Saint, A., (ed.) *Politics and the People of London.* London, 1989

Scotland. For local government purposes, mainland Scotland is divided on a two-tier basis into 9 regions and 53 districts. Functions are allocated between regional and district councils in the same way (with minor exceptions) as they are allocated between county and district councils in England. The 3 islands areas of Orkney,

Shetland and the Western Isles have single-tier councils responsible for virtually all functions. The members of each council are elected for a 4-year term, elections for regional and islands councils alternating with elections for district councils at 2-year intervals. Each council elects a chairman for the 4-year term. In some cases the chairman is called 'Convener' or 'Provost', and the chairman of Edinburgh, Glasgow, Aberdeen and Dundee District Councils are titled 'Lord Provost'.

Over 1,000 community councils have been established under schemes drawn up by district and island councils. These community councils cannot claim public funds as of right nor do they have specific powers conferred by statute: Consequently they are not local authorities in the sense that English parish councils or Welsh community councils are.

As in England and Wales, a permanent Local Government Boundary Commission advises the Secretary of State on local authority boundaries and electoral constituencies.

The total number of local government electors in Scotland was 3,936,737 in 1990.

DEFENCE. The Defence Council was established on 1 April 1964 under the chairmanship of the Secretary of State for Defence, who is responsible to the Sovereign and Parliament for the defence of the realm. Vested in the Defence Council are the functions of commanding and administering the Armed Forces. The Secretary of State heads the Ministry of Defence as a Department of State. There are 4 subordinate Ministers; 2 Ministers of State and 2 Parliamentary Under-Secretaries of State.

Defence Council membership comprises the Secretary of State, the 4 Ministers mentioned above, the Chief of the Defence Staff, the 3 single Service Chiefs of Staff, the Vice-Chief of Defence Staff, the Chief of Defence Procurement, the Chief Scientific Adviser, the Permanent Under-Secretary of State and the Second Permanent Under Secretary of State.

There are 3 Service Boards, each of which enjoys delegated powers for the administration of matters relating to the naval, military and air forces respectively.

Defence policy decision making is a collective Governmental responsibility. Important matters of policy are considered by the full Cabinet or, more frequently, by the Defence and Oversea Policy Committee under the chairmanship of the Prime Minister. Other members of this Committee include the Secretary of State for Defence, the Foreign and Commonwealth Secretary and the Home Secretary.

The Procurement Executive. An important development in 1971 was the creation of a Procurement Executive to combine the Defence Procurement responsibilities of the Ministry of Defence and the former Ministry of Aviation Supply.

Service Strengths at 1 Jan. 1990, all ranks, males and females, UK personnel only: Royal Navy and Royal Marines, 83,500; Army, 152,900; Royal Air Force, 89,600; total, 306,000. In Jan. 90 the Ministry of Defence employed 171,800 civilians (140,600 in the UK).

Defence Budget (Plans): 1990–91, £21,223m; 1991–92, £22,360m 1992–93 £22,430.

Army. Control of the British Army is vested in the Defence Council and is exercised through the Army Board. The Secretary of State for Defence is Chairman of the Army Board. The other civilian members are the 4 subordinate Ministers; the Controller Establishments, Research and Nuclear Programmes and the Second Permanent Under Secretary of State.

The Military members of the Army Board are the Chief of the General Staff, the Adjutant General, the Quartermaster General and the Master General of the Ordnance. The Chief of the General Staff is the professional head of his Service and the professional adviser to Ministers on the Army aspects of military matters. He is responsible for the fighting efficiency of his Service; for Army advice on the conduct of operations; and for the issuing of such single Service operational orders as may be appropriate resulting from defence policy decisions. He is also responsible for the Territorial Army. The Chief of the General Staff is a member of the Chiefs of Staff Committee which is chaired by the Chief of the Defence Staff, who is responsible to HM Government for professional advice on strategy and military operations and on the military implication of defence policy. The Adjutant-General is responsible for recruiting and selection of army manpower; for the administration and individual training of military personnel; for the discipline of the Army; for pay and allowances and pensions; for legal services; for the veterinary and remount services; for the Army Cadet Forces; for questions of Army welfare and education including school children overseas; and for resettlement and sports. The Quartermaster-General is responsible for logistic planning for the Army; for the storage, distribution, maintenance, repair and inspection of equipment, stores and ammunition; for development of stores; for supply, transport and accommodation; for the development, production and inspection of clothing; for military movements and transportation; for the Army postal, catering, salvage and fire services; and for questions connected with canteens, institutes and military labour. The Master General of the Ordnance is a member of both the Army Board and of the Procurement Executive Management Board. He is responsible to the Chief of Defence Procurement for the financial and technical management of the approved programme for the procurement of land service equipment for the Armed Services, and to the Army Board for the co-ordination of the Army's total equipment programme.

Headquarters United Kingdom Land Forces at Wilton commands all Army units in UK except Ministry of Defence controlled units. The Ministry of Defence retains direct operational control of units in Northern Ireland. Command by HQ United Kingdom Land Forces is exercised through 9 district headquarters. There are 3 major overseas Commands: Land Forces British Army of the Rhine, Hong Kong and Cyprus. There are also garrisons in Berlin, Gibraltar, Falkland Islands, Brunei and Belize. The Army Air Corps has some 300 helicopters and 25 fixed-wing aircraft.

The strength of the Regular Army (less the Brigade of Gurkhas and locally enlisted personnel) on 1 Jan. 1989 was 155,500 men and 6,500 women. Strength of reserve forces were: Regular reserves, 173,100; territorial army, 72,800; Home Service Force, 3,000.

The Territorial Army role is to provide a national reserve for employment on specific tasks at home and overseas and to meet the unexpected when required; and, in particular, to complete the Army Order of Battle of NATO committed forces and to provide certain units for the support of NATO Headquarters, to assist in maintaining a secure UK base in support of forces deployed on the Continent of Europe and to provide a framework for any future expansion of the Reserves. In addition, men who have completed service in the Regular Army normally have some liability to serve in the Regular Reserve. All members of the TA and Regular Reserve may be called out by a Queen's Order in time of emergency of imminent national danger and most of the TA and a large proportion of the Regular Reserve may be called out by a Queen's Order when warlike operations are in preparation or in progress. There is a special reserve force in Northern Ireland, the Ulster Defence Regiment, 6,300 strong, which gives support to the regular army.

Men, women and juniors enlist in the Army for 22 years' active and reserve service. However, under a scheme introduced in May 1981 they are entitled to give 12 months' notice (18 months' for women) to leave active service provided they serve for a minimum of 3 years. Alternatively, they can agree to serve for 6 or 9 years to receive the benefit of higher rates of pay. Those enlisting in certain technical trades must agree to serve for a minimum of 6 years. Recruits under the age of $17^1/_2$ on reaching the age of 18 are entitled either to confirm their original engagement or to reduce their period of service to 3 years.

Women serve in both the Regular Army and the TA in the Queen Alexandra's Royal Army Nursing Corps, the Ulster Defence Regiment and the Women's Royal Army Corps, employments including communications, motor transport, clerical and catering duties. Some officers of the Women's Royal Army Corps are employed on the staffs of military headquarters.

Blaxford, G., *The Regiments Depart: A History of the British Army 1945–70*. London, 1971
Brereton, J. M., *The British Soldier*. London, 1985
Johnson, F. A., *Defence by Ministry: The British Ministry of Defence 1944–1974*. London, 1980
Strawson, J., *Gentlemen in Khaki: The British Army 1890-1990*. London, 1989

Navy. Control of the Royal Navy is vested in the Defence Council and is exercised through the Admiralty Board, chaired by the Secretary of State for Defence. The other civilian members are the Ministers and Under Secretaries of State for the Armed Forces and Defence Procurement; the Second Permanent Under Secretary of State; and the Controller, Research and Development Establishments, Research and Nuclear. The naval members are the Chief of Naval Staff and First Sea Lord responsible for management, fighting efficiency, planning and operational advice; the Chief of Naval Personnel and Second Sea Lord, responsible for the manning of the Fleet and all personnel aspects; the Controller of the Navy, responsible for procurement of ships, their weapons and equipment; and the Chief of Fleet Support, responsible for all aspects of logistic support, stores, fuels and transport, naval dockyards, the Royal Fleet Auxiliary and Royal Maritime Auxiliary services.

The Commander-in-Chief Fleet, headquartered at Northwood, commands the fleet. Naval Air Stations are commanded by the Flag Officer Naval Aviation. The command of all other naval establishments in the UK, except those under the Commandant General Royal Marines, is exercised by the Commander-in-Chief. Naval Home Command from Portsmouth, through Area Flag Officers. Main naval bases are at Devonport, Rosyth, Portsmouth, and Faslane, with a training base at Portland, and minor bases overseas at Hong Kong and Gibraltar.

The Royal Naval Reserve (RNR) and the Royal Marines Reserve (RMR) in 1990 numbered 5,770 and 1,100 respectively. The RNR provides trained personnel in war to undertake Naval Control of Shipping, to man mine counter-measures vessels, HQ Command and Communications, and Rotary Wing Aircrew. The main roles of the RMR are reinforcement and other specialist tasks with the UK-Netherlands Amphibious Force. In addition, men who have completed service in the Royal Navy and the Royal Marines have a commitment to serve in the Royal Fleet Reserve, currently 25,600 strong. The Royal Naval Auxiliary Service (RNXS) is a civilian auxiliary some 3,200 strong who man Port Headquarters and provide crews for patrol and administrative craft in wartime.

Royal Navy ratings enlist to complete 22 years active service (at the end of which there is selective re-engagement open to senior, chief and charge specialists for a further 5 or 10 years) with the option to leave at 18 months notice on completion of a minimum of 2 and a half years productive service. Those who leave before completing 22 years have a liability for up to 3 years service in the Royal Fleet Reserve. Royal Marine ranks, Women's Royal Naval Service (WRNS) and Queen Alexandra's Royal Naval Nursing Service (QARNNS) ratings enlist to complete an initial 9 year engagement but they may apply to re-engage to complete 14 years and 22 years. As from 6 Feb. 1990, all new entrants to the WRNS are liable for sea service except in submarines; the first sea-going WRNS joined the frigate *Brilliant* in Oct. 1990, and there are now WRNS in 4 operational ships. No peacetime role exists for QARNNS at sea except for the Medical Assistant branch; in war they put to sea in hospital ships.

The roles of the Royal Navy are first, to deploy the national strategic nuclear deterrent, second to contribute to the NATO maritime strategy of forward defence, third to provide maritime defence of the UK and fourth to meet national maritime objectives outside the NATO area. A review of future fleet strength is under way in response to the changed international situation, and is already leading to a reduction in numbers and altered balance.

The strategic deterrent is provided by the 4 nuclear-powered strategic missile submarines of the Resolution class (Resolution, Repulse, Renown and *Revenge*) each of 8,600 tonnes submerged displacement, completed between 1967 and 1969 and deploying 16 Polaris A3TK missiles each. These ships are to be replaced, commencing in 1994, by 4 substantially larger units of the Vanguard class (*Vanguard, Vengeance, Victorious* and *Venerable*), 15,250 tonnes, of which the first 3 have been ordered and which will deploy 16 US-built Trident-2 D5 UGM-133A missiles with British warheads.

The strength of the fleet's major non-strategic units at the end of each of the last 8 years was as follows:

	1983	*1984*	*1985*	*1986*	*1987*	*1988*	*1989*	*1990*
Nuclear Submarines	12	13	14	14	15	15	16	14
Other Submarines	16	15	15	14	12	11	11	9
Aircraft Carriers	3	3	3	2[1]	2[1]	2[1]	2[1]	2[1]
Destroyers	13	13	15	14	13	13	13	13
Frigates	46	48	42	39	36	35	36	35

[1] Following Government policy, of the 3 Carriers held, only 2 are kept in operational status.

The nuclear-powered submarine force, saw an unexpected decline in numbers in 1990, partly in response to the defence review but also through nuclear reactor defects. It now numbers 14 of three main classes. All are armed with torpedoes and Harpoon anti-ship missiles. There are 6 Trafalgar class, (5,300 tonnes) completed 1983-1990 (with 1 further ship fitting-out), 6 Swiftsure (4,800 tonnes) completed 1973-79, and 2 Valiant/Churchill of 4,900 tonnes completed 1966-71. 3 ships of this class were stricken in 1990. Other submarines are of diesel-electric propulsion and comprise the first of 4 Upholder class (2,400 tonnes) completed in 1989 and 8 Oberon class (completed 1960-67).

The principal surface ships are the Light vertical/short take-off and landing Aircraft Carriers of the Invincible class, (*Invincible, Illustrious* and *Ark Royal*), 20,900 tonnes, completed 1980-85, embarking an air group of 8 Sea Harrier vertical/short take-off and landing fighters, 9 anti-submarine Sea King and 3 radar early warning Sea King helicopters, and armed with 1 twin Sea Dart surface-to-air missile system. 2 of these ships are maintained in the operational fleet, with the third either in refit or reserve. (As from May, 1989, *Illustrious* was in reserve in Portsmouth).

The 13 destroyers comprise 12 Type 42 (completed 1976-85), and *HMS Bristol*, the sole Type 82 (completed 1973), now employed as the Dartmouth Training Ship. All are armed with 1 twin Sea Dart surface-to-air missile system. Frigates comprise 14 Type 22 (1979-89), the first Norfolk class (Type 23) accepted in late 1989, 6 Amazon (Type 21), completed 1974-78, and the last 14 of the 26 Leander class built between 1963 and 1970.

The lightly-armed patrol force comprises 1 ice patrol ship, 13 other offshore patrol vessels (including 3 in the Hong Kong squadron), and 28 inshore patrol craft mostly employed on training duties. Mine countermeasures capability is provided by 13 offshore hunter/sweepers, 12 offshore minesweepers, 9 coastal minehunters and 2 coastal minesweepers. Amphibious lift for the Royal Marines is provided by 1 dock landing ship (with a second in reserve) and 5 tank landing ships (civil manned, and in peacetime employed on army freighting), supported by about 32 small amphibious craft.

Comprehensive support to the fleet is provided by 34 major auxiliaries including 4 replenishment and 4 support tankers, 2 ammunition ships, 1 repair ship, 1 transport, 3 ocean tugs, 6 survey ships, 4 trials ships, 1 aviation training ship, 1 chartered training ship, and the Royal Yacht. Second-line support is provided by about 200 harbour and coastal service craft and minor auxiliaries.

Ships under construction or on order include the final nuclear powered Trafalgar class submarines, 3 further Upholder class submarines, 9 Norfolk class frigates, 5 coastal minehunters and 2 large general purpose replenishment ships.

The Fleet Air Arm has 350 aircraft of which 280 are active, in 14 operational squadrons. The operational inventory comprises 41 Sea Harrier vertical/short take-off and landing fighter aircraft, 76 Sea King and 83 Lynx anti-submarine helicopters, 10 Sea King airborne early warning helicopters and 35 Sea King (commando transport version). There are 7 training and second-line squadrons, equipped with about 50 fixed wing aircraft of various types and 25 training helicopters.

The total number of male and female personnel (including Royal Marines) was (in 1,000) on 31 March: 1988, 65·7; 1989, 65·5; 1990, 63.2; 1991 (estimated), 62.7. The estimated total of 62,700 includes 7,600 marines and 3,400 women.

Sharpe, R. G. (ed.) *Jane's Fighting Ships*. London, annual

Air Force. In May 1912 the Royal Flying Corps first came into existence with military and naval wings, of which the latter became the independent Royal Naval Air Service in July 1914. On 2 Jan. 1918 an Air Ministry was formed, and on 1 April

1918 the Royal Flying Corps and the Royal Naval Air Service were amalgamated, under the Air Ministry, as the Royal Air Force.

In 1937 the units based on aircraft carriers and naval shore stations again passed to the operational and administrative control of the Admiralty, as the Fleet Air Arm. In 1964 control of the RAF became a responsibility of the Ministry of Defence.

The Royal Air Force is administered by the Air Force Board, of which the Secretary of State for Defence is Chairman. The Minister of State for the Armed Forces is Vice-Chairman, and normally acts as Chairman on behalf of the Secretary of State. Other members of the Board are the Minister of State for Defence Procurement, the Under-Secretary of State for the Armed Forces, the Under-Secretary of State for Defence Procurement, the Chief of the Air Staff, Air Member for Personnel, Air Member for Supply and Organization, Controller of Aircraft, Second Permanent Under-Secretary of State and Controller R & D Establishments, Research and Nuclear. The RAF is organized into commands:

Home Commands. Strike and Support Commands. The Air Training Corps and the Air Sections of the Combined Cadet Force are under the administrative control of Support Command and functionally controlled by the Ministry of Defence.

The RAF College, which trains all candidates for commissions, is at Cranwell. The RAF Staff College is at Bracknell. The Department of Air Warfare is at Cranwell. The RAF Central Flying School is at Scampton. The trained personnel strength in Sept. 1990, including WRAF, was 83,173.

Strike Command itself is responsible for transport and air-to-air refuelling. VC10, Tristar and Hercules aircraft are used for air refuelling as well as strategic and tactical transport; the Victor solely for air refuelling. However, day-to-day functioning and organization of most operations is delegated to 3 Groups. Nos 1 and 38 Groups merged in late 1983 to form a new No 1 Group, responsible for the strike/attack, reconnaissance, tanker and battlefield support. The Tornado GR1 and Jaguar are used in the strike, attack and reconnaissance roles. Battlefield support forces comprise Harrier GR5s, Chinook, Puma and Wessex support helicopters. No 11 Group controls the air defence forces: Tornado F3 and Phantom supersonic all-weather interceptors, Bloodhound surface-to-air missiles, and ground environment radars, the associated communication systems, and the Ballistic Missile Early Warning System at Fylingdales. No 11 Group also controls the Hawks of the Tactical Weapons Units which, in war, would supplement air defence fighters at bases throughout the UK. UK air defence is undergoing major improvements. The Boeing E-3 will enter service in 1991, replacing the Shackleton, and in the ground environment, there are new radars and communications systems entering service. No 18 Group is responsible for maritime air operations. ASW is the duty of the Nimrod Mk 2, which also has a capability against surface ships, although Buccaneers provide the main offensive force against a maritime surface threat. No 18 Group also operates Canberras in a multitude of roles, including photo-reconnaissance, target towing and ECM training, as well as Nimrod special-purpose aircraft. Search and rescue units are equipped with Sea King and Wessex helicopters. RAF Regiment short-range air defence squadrons, armed with Rapier, and the field squadrons form part of 1 Group, as does The Queen's Flight, which has 3 BAe 146s and 2 Wessex helicopters. The Military Air Traffic Operations organization also has the status of a Group. Strike Command has NATO commitments, but is available for overseas reinforcement. The training element of RAF Support Command utilizes Bulldog and Chipmunk primary trainers, Jet Provost basic trainers (now being replaced by turboprop Tucanos), Hawk advanced trainers, Jetstreams for multi-engine pilot training, twin-jet Dominies for training navigators and other non-pilot aircrew, and Gazelle and Wessex helicopters.

Overseas Commands. Royal Air Force Germany. Small units in Gibraltar, the Falkland Islands, Belize, Cyprus and Hong Kong.

Squadrons of RAF Germany, which form part of NATO's 2nd Allied Tactical Air Force under SACEUR, have Tornado GR1, Harrier GR5, Phantom fighters, Chinook and Puma Helicopters, Andover communications aircraft, and Rapier surface-to-air missile squadrons of the RAF Regiment.

A flight of Phantom aircraft, a squadron of Chinook and Sea King helicopters for transport and search and rescue, and a flight of Hercules tankers are based in the Falkland Islands; a squadron of Wessex helicopters is based in Hong Kong and Cyprus.

The Royal Air Force, 1939–45. Vols. I, II, III. HMSO, 1953–54
Taylor J. W. R. (ed.) *Jane's All the World's Aircraft*. London. Annual from 1909

INTERNATIONAL RELATIONS

Membership. The UK is a member of the UN, Commonwealth, the EC, OECD, the Council of Europe, WEU, NATO and the Colombo Plan.

ECONOMY

Budget. Revenue and expenditure for years ending 31 March, in £1m. sterling:

Revenue	*Estimated in the Budgets*	*Actual receipts into the Exchequer*	*More than estimates*
1988	168,800	173,700	4,900
1989	184,900	190,900	6,000
1990	206,400	203,400	– 3,000
1991	218,600	216,600	– 2,000

The Budget estimate of ordinary revenue for 1991–92 is £226,500m.

Expenditure	*Budget and supplementary estimates*	*Actual payments out of the Exchequer*	*More than estimates*
1988	173,500	171,800	–1,700
1989	182,900	179,100	–3,800
1990	194,300	197,700	3,400
1991	212,700	216,000	3,300

The Budget estimate of ordinary expenditure for 1991–92 is £234,800m.

Revenue in detail for 1990–91 and the expenditure, are given below, as is the budget estimate for 1991–92 (in £1m.):

Sources of revenue	*Net receipts 1990–91*	*Budget estimate 1991–92*
Inland Revenue:		
Income tax	55,500	59,600
Corporation tax	21,600	19,500
Petroleum revenue tax	900	—
Capital Gains tax	1,900	1,400
Inheritance tax	1,300	1,300
Stamp duties	1,700	2,100
Total Inland Revenue	82,900	83,900
Customs and Excise:		
Value Added Tax	30,800	35,700
Petrol, etc. duties	9,600	10,900
Tobacco duties	5,600	6,100
Alcohol duties	4,900	5,200
Betting and gaming duties	1,000	1,000
Car tax	1,400	1,300
Customs duties	1,700	1,700
Agricultural levies	100	200
Total Customs and Excise	55,300	62,200
Vehicle Excise duties	3,000	3,000
Miscellaneous receipts:		
Interest and dividends	6,400	6,100
Oil royalties	600	500
Total Government Receipts	216,600	226,500

The following are the branches of expenditure for year ended 31 March 1991 and the estimates for the year 1991–92 (in £1m.):

	Estimates 1990–91	Estimates 1991–92
Social Security	51,800	58,200
Defence	22,100	22,800
Health and Personal Social Services	22,500	24,900
Northern Ireland	5,900	6,400
Privatization proceeds	–5,300	–5,500
Planning total	180,400	205,000
Interest Payments	17,600	16,700
Other Adjustments	3,400	3,900
Total	216,000	234,800

A single graduated income tax came into operation on 6 April 1973, replacing the existing income tax and surtax.

Rates of Personal Tax from 6 April 1991	%
Income between	
£0–£23,700	25
Over £23,700	40

Under the tax system, the amounts of the personal allowances are adjusted so that they retain their equivalent in relation to earned income. Independent taxation of husband and wife was introduced on 6 April 1990.

Personal Allowances	*1991–92* £
Single person / Wife's earned income	3,295
Married couple's allowance	1,720
Age allowance (age 65 to 74):	
Single	4,020
Married couple's allowance	2,355
Age allowance (age 75 or over):	
Single	4,180
Married couple's allowance	2,395

Deductions of tax under PAYE ('pay as you earn') extend over the full range of unified tax rates and not merely the basic rate. Similarly, assessment on business profits and on other income which was directly assessed to tax, such as rents and interest on bank deposits, are made by reference to the full scale of rates, including where appropriate the investment income surcharge.

The standard rate of 25% is the rate at which tax is deducted from payments of interest, etc., and corresponds under the corporation tax system, to the tax credit on dividends. Where an individual's total income is such that he is liable on this taxed investment income at rates exceeding 25%, or if his investment income is high enough to make him liable to the surcharge, the higher rate or surcharge liability on this taxed investment income will in general be assessed separately after the end of the tax year.

Corporation Tax. Corporation Tax applies, with certain exceptions, to trades or businesses carried on by bodies corporate or by unincorporated societies or other bodies. Corporation Tax for companies was 34% for 1990–91 and 33% for 1991–92. Small companies (i.e. with profits under £0·25m.), 1991–92, 25%.

Capital Gains Tax. Gains resulting from the disposal of capital assets (other than British Government and Government guaranteed securities and certain exempted forms of property such as a private car and personal residences) are taxed under the Finance Act 1965. In 1991–92 exemption was granted for all gains made in a financial year which in total did not exceed £5,500 and most trusts on the first £2,750. In 1988 the base was brought forward from 1965 to 1982.

Inheritance Tax. Formerly Capital Transfer Tax. From 18 March 1986 there is no lifetime charge on gifts between individuals. From 1989 a flat rate of 40% was introduced with a threshold in 1991–92 of £140,000.

Value Added Tax. Value Added Tax (VAT) was introduced from 1 April 1973 at the rate of 10% on the supply of goods (with certain exceptions) and services. From 18 June 1979 the rate of tax was fixed at 15%. It was raised to 17·5% from 1 April 1991. From 20 March 1991 the registration limits became £35,000 per annum.

Kay, J. A. and King, M. A., *The British Tax System*. OUP, 1980

Local Taxation. The Community Charge was introduced in Scotland in 1989 and in England and Wales in 1990 (*see* p. 1310).

The introduction of the Community Charge ('poll tax') changed the basis of levying local revenue from the ownership of residential or business property at a national variable rate ('rateable value'), to personal residence at a flat rate (with reliefs rebating liability by up to 80%). The amount of the charge is set by the local authorities, subject to central government ceilings ('rate-capping'), and varies considerably from authority to authority. A uniform business rate applies nationally to business premises and second residences. The average charge paid in 1991 was £385.

A Government review of local government in 1991 concluded that the level of the Community Charge was unsustainably high, and the Budget of March 1991 provided for its reduction by £140.

Local authority estimated receipts (in £1m.) for 1990–91 (and forecasts for 1991–92) were £58,500 (£66,500), made up of: Community Charge and domestic rates, £11,500 (£7,300); non-domestic rates, £12,500 (£14,100); current grants from central government, £27,400 (£35,400); capital grants from central government, £2,200 (£2,900); other, £4,900 (£6,900). Expenditure was £61,500 (£66,300), made up of: Current expenditure on goods and services, £43,500 (£47,300); current grants and subsidies, £6,800 (£8,000); interest, £5,100 (£5,500); capital expenditure and net lending, £6,100 (£5,500).

Central government support for local authorities (in £1m.), 1990–91 estimates (and 1991–92 plans) was £42,600 (£52,500), including: Revenue/rate support grant, £13,100 (£13,600); non-domestic rate payments, £12,100 (£14,300); current specific grants, £12,200 (£18,900); capital grants, £1,100 (£1,500); credit approvals, £4,000 (£4,300).

The 1991 Budget provided for additional central government support to local authorities in order to reduce the Community Charge, to be financed mainly from an increase in value-added tax from 15% to 17·5%. The Government is to pay a new grant ('Community Charge Grant') which wlll reimburse local authorities for the gross cost of reducing charges in 1991–92 by £140, estimated at £5,600m. 90% of this grant is to be paid in 1991–92, and the remainder in 1992–93.

In Scotland, revenue support grant replaced rate support grants when the community charge was introduced on 1 April 1989. It was paid under the Abolition of Domestic Rates Etc (Scotland) Act 1987, as amended by the Local Government and Housing Act 1989.

Gross National Product:

	1946	*1960*	*1970*	*1980*	*1989*
Expenditure (£1m.)					
Consumers' expenditure	7,273	16,939	31,773	135,738	328,453
Central and local government final consumption	2,282	4,206	8,961	48,424	99,426
Gross domestic fixed capital formation	925	4,190	9,462	39,411	100,472
Value of physical increase in stocks and work in progress	–126	562	425	–2,706	3,102
Total domestic expenditure at market prices	10,354	25,897	50,581	220,867	531,453
Exports of goods and services	1,775	5,153	11,533	63,158	123,396
Less Imports of goods and services	–2,083	–5,549	–11,122	–57,913	–142,527
Less Taxes on expenditure	–1,573	–3,378	–8,416	–36,882	–80,136
Subsidies	384	493	884	5,308	5,668
Gross domestic product at factor cost	8,855	22,616	43,460	194,538	438,774

Factor incomes (£1m.)	*1946*	*1960*	*1970*	*1980*	*1989*
Income from employment	5,758	15,174	30,404	136,050	284,399
Income from self-employment [1]	1,126	2,008	3,735	17,581	53,126
Gross trading profits of companies [1]	1,476	3,730	5,935	27,708	65,639
Gross trading surplus of public corporations [1]	20	534	1,447	6,222	6,576
Gross trading surplus of other public enterprises [1]	86	189	151	242	192
Rent [2]	429	1,086	2,833	13,390	31,568
Total domestic income before providing for depreciation and stock appreciation	8,895	22,863	44,837	203,304	445,340
Less Stock appreciation	–125	–122	–1,090	–6,456	–7,598
Residual error	...	–125	–287	–2,310	1,032
Gross domestic product at factor cost	8,770	22,616	43,460	194,538	438,774
Net property income from abroad	85	233	559	–273	4,582
Gross national product	8,855	22,849	44,019	194,265	443,356
Less Capital consumption	...	–2,047	–4,420	–27,223	–56,186
National income	...	20,802	39,599	167,042	387,170

[1] Before providing for depreciation and stock appreciation.
[2] Before providing for depreciation.

National Economic Development Council. The NEDC, which first met in 1962, is the national forum for economic consultation between government, management and unions. It includes leading representatives of the Government, CBI and TUC, chairmen of nationalized industries and independent members. It meets under the chairmanship of the Chancellor of the Exchequer, other Secretaries of State and occasionally, the Prime Minister. The Sector Groups and Working Parties, like the NEDC, bring together representatives of management unions, Government and experts in the field to study the efficiency and prospects of individual industries and sectors and to suggest ways in which these could be improved and advantage taken of new opportunities. The National Economic Development Office (NEDO) provides the professional staff for the NEDC and the Sector Groups and Working Parties and undertakes its own self-initiated research.

Currency. The unit of currency is the *pound sterling* (GBP) of 100 *pence*. A gold standard was adopted in 1816, the sovereign or twenty-shilling piece weighing 7·98805 grammes 0·916⅔ fine. Currency notes for £1 and 10*s.* were first issued by the Treasury in 1914, replacing the circulation of sovereigns. The issue of £1 and 10*s.* notes was taken over by the Bank of England in 1928. The issue of 10*s.* notes ceased on the issue of the 50p coin in 1969.

In March 1991, £1 = US$ 1·90; US$ = £0·53.

Coinage. The sovereign (£1) weighs 123·27447 grains, or 7·98805 grammes, 0·916⅔ (or eleven-twelfths) fine, and consequently it contains 113·00159 grains or 7·32238 grammes of fine gold. On 15 Feb. 1971 (Decimalization Day) a decimal currency system was introduced retaining the *pound sterling* as the major unit but now divided into 100 *new pence* instead of 240 old pence. The decimal coins are the £1 (22·5 mm diameter, 9·5 grammes weight); 50p (equilateral curved heptagon, 30 mm diameter, 13·5 grammes); 20p (equilateral curved heptagon 21·4 mm diameter, 5 grammes); 10p (28·5 mm, 11·31 grammes); 5p (18·0 mm, 3·25 grammes); 2p (25·9 mm, 7·12 grammes) and 1p (20·3 mm, 3·56 grammes). The Decimal Currency Act, 1967 and the Proclamation of 27 Dec. 1968 required that the 50p, 10p and 5p be made of cupro-nickel and the 2p, 1p and ½p of mixed metal; copper, tin and zinc (bronze). The Decimal Currency Act, 1969, provided that the coins of the Queen's Maundy Money should continue to be made in silver to a millesimal fineness of 925.

By Proclamation dated 28 July 1971, which came into force on 30 Aug. 1971, the crown, double-florin, the florin, the shilling and the sixpence were treated as coins of the new currency and as being of the denominations respectively of 25, 20, 10, 5 and 2½ new pence. The sixpence was demonetised on 30 June 1980, the ½p on 31 Dec. 1984 and the 5p/shilling on 31 Dec. 1990. A smaller 5p coin was issued on 27 June 1991.

The Coinage Act, 1971, specified that the legal tender limits for coins were: Gold coins, for payment of any amount; coins of cupro-nickel and silver of denominations of more than 10p, for payment of any amount not exceeding £10; coins of cupro-nickel and silver of not more than 10p, for payment of any amount not exceeding £5; coins of bronze, for payment of any amount not exceeding 20p. The £1 coin is legal tender to any amount.

UK coins issued in the 12 months up to March 1990 totalled £126m.

Coins in circulation at 31 March 1990: £1 911m.; 50p 676m.; 20p 1,295m.; 10p 1,510m.; 5p 2,320m.; 2p 3,500m.; 1p 5,600m.

Bank-notes. The Bank of England issues notes in denominations of £5, £10, £20 and £50 for the amount of the fiduciary note issue. Under the provisions of the Currency and Bank Notes Act, 1954, which came into force on 22 Feb. 1954, the amount of the fiduciary note issue was fixed at £1,575m., but this figure might be altered by direction of HM Treasury after representations made by the Bank of England.

All Bank of England notes are legal tender in England and Wales. The banks in Scotland and Northern Ireland have certain note-issuing powers.

The total amount of Bank of England notes issued at 24 Dec. 1990 was £17,530m., of which £17,523,758,790 were in the hands of other banks and the public and £6,241,210 in the Banking Department of the Bank of England.

Banking and Finance. The Bank of England, Threadneedle Street, London, is the Government's banker and the 'banker's bank'. It has the sole right of note issue in England and Wales and manages the National Debt. The Bank operates under royal charters of 1694 and 1946 and the Bank of England Act, 1946. The capital stock has, since 1 March 1946, been held by the Treasury. The *Governor* is Robin Leigh-Pemberton.

The statutory return is published weekly. End-Dec. figures for the past 4 years are as follows (in £1m.):

	Notes in circulation	*Notes and coin in Banking Department*	*Public deposits (government)*	*Other deposits* [1]
1987	14,542	8	100	3,144
1988	15,949	1	91	3,106
1989	17,071	9	62	4,444
1990	17,524	6	42	8,169

[1] Including Special Deposits.

The fiduciary note issue was £17,530,000,000 at 24 Dec. 1990. All the profits of the note issue are passed on to the National Loans Fund.

Official reserves of gold and convertible currencies, SDR and reserve position in the IMF at the end of Dec. 1989 were US$38,645m.

The value of paper debit bank clearings for 1987, £8,324,927m. Paper credit clearings for 1987, £91,980m. Automatic direct debits, 1987, £126,835m.; automatic credit transfers, 1987, £229,509m.

The following statistics relate to the London and Scottish banks' groups at 31 Dec. 1990. Total deposits (sterling and currency), £349,845m.; sterling market loans £63,673m.; advances (sterling and currency), £243,907m.; sterling investments £12,806m.

Total net profits from the operations of the main London clearing bank groups in 1990 amounted to £842m., of which £879m. was paid in gross dividends and £309m. transferred to reserves.

The clearing banks cover all aspects of banking business in UK including corporate business, and are also actively involved in international banking.

National Savings Bank. Statistics for 1987 and 1988:

	Ordinary accounts		*Investment accounts*	
	1988	*1989*	*1988*	*1989*
Accounts open at 31 Dec.	15,741,178 [1]	15,762,005 [1]	4,300,148	4,521,105
Amounts—	*£1,000*	*£1,000*	*£1,000*	*£1,000*
Received	651,528	596,433	1,856,470	1,382,085
Interest credited	65,976 [2]	64,467 [2]	686,615	792,423
Paid	727,899	728,104	1,800,697	2,068,926
Due to depositors at 31 Dec.	1,646,556	1,579,352	7,733,400	7,838,982
Average amount due to each depositor in active accounts	£104·60	£100·20	£1,798·40	£1,733·87

[1] Excluding non-computerized accounts, amounting to £98m. in 1988 and £97·8m. in 1989.
[2] The interest credited to depositors for the Ordinary account for 1989 has been calculated on the same basis as 1988. Interest of 5% a year payable on accounts with a minimum balance of £500 and 2½% on accounts with a minimum balance of less than £500. Interest is earned on each whole pound on depost for complete calendar months.

The amount due to depositors in Ordinary Accounts on 1 Jan. 1991 was approximately £1,495,258,252 and in Investment Accounts £8,535,906,300.

The banking arm of the Post Office, Girobank (founded 1968) was sold to a building society in 1990.

Bank of England Quarterly Bulletin. Bank of England
Bank of England Annual Report. Bank of England
British Banking and other Financial Institutions. HMSO, 1977
Central Statistical Office, Financial Statistics. HMSO (monthly)
The Royal Mint. 6th ed. HMSO, 1977
Sayers, R. H., *The Bank of England 1891–1944*. CUP, 1976

Weights and Measures. Conversion to the metric system, which will replace the imperial system, is in progress.

ENERGY AND NATURAL RESOURCES

Electricity. The electricity industry was vested in the British Electricity Authority on 1 April 1948. Following the re-organization of the electricity supply industry after the passing of the Electricity Act, 1957, the statutory bodies comprising the electricity service in England and Wales were the Electricity Council, the Central Electricity Generating Board and the 12 Area Electricity Boards. The Electricity Council functioned from Jan. 1958 as the central council for the supply industry in England and Wales for consultation on, and formulation of, general policy.

The Electricity Bill of Nov. 1988 proposed the restructuring and transfer to the private sector of the electricity supply industry – it was enacted in July 1989.

The Office of Electricity Regulation (Offer) was set up under the Act to protect consumer interests following privatization.

Generators. The Central Electricity Generating Board, which was responsible for the generation and bulk supply of electricity to the 12 Area Boards in England and Wales was replaced by 4 companies under the provisions of the 1989 Electricity Act: National Power, PowerGen, Nuclear Electric and the National Grid Company. National Power and PowerGen were privatized in Feb. 1991. Nuclear Electric, responsible for nuclear power generation, is to remain in state ownership. The wholesale market created by the generators is termed 'the pool'.

Suppliers. The 12 Area Electricity Boards have been replaced under the 1989 Electricity Act by 12 successor companies which were privatized in Nov.–Dec. 1990. These are Eastern Electricity; East Midlands Electricity; London Electricity; Manweb; Midlands Electricity; Northern Electricity; Norweb; Seeboard; Southern Electric; South Wales Electricity; South Western Electricity; Yorkshire Electricity.

The number of power stations owned by the Generating Board in England and Wales on 31 March 1987 was 78 with a total output capacity, of 52,363 mw. Total number of customers in England and Wales on 31 March 1987 was 21,715,000 (on 31 March 1986, 21,487,941).

Electricity sold in England and Wales in 1986–87 amounted to 219,551m. units. Operating profit before MWCA in 1986–87 was £1,150m. Coal used for electricity generation in 1986–87 amounted to 77m. tonnes (79m. tonnes in 1985–86). Total fuel (coal equivalent) used in 1985–86 amounted to 100·8m. tonnes and in 1986–87 to 100m. tonnes. Ten nuclear stations of total output capacity 5,029 mw provided 16·4% of total units supplied in 1986–87. Eight of these are gas cooled graphite-moderated stations using natural uranium fuel canned in magnesium alloy (Magnox) and 2 are advanced gas-cooled stations (AGR).

The number of persons employed by the Generating Board, the Electricity Council and Area Boards at the end of March 1987 was 131,067.

Scottish Hydro-Electric plc, with head office in Perth, the nationalized authority responsible for the generation, transmission, distribution and sale of electricity to its (1988) 596,960 customers was to be privatized alongside Scottish Power plc in May 1991. It supplies the district north and west of a line joining the firths of Clyde and Tay as well as all the island groups extending to the Outer Hebrides, Orkney and Shetland. On the mainland it operates generating stations with a total installed generating capacity of 3,216 mw consisting of 1,762 mw of hydro power and pumped storage, together with 1,320 mw of steam. Diesel stations with a total installed capacity of 102 mw supply the principal island groups together with 32 mw gas turbine. A 1,320 mw of oil/gas fired thermal plant is now operating at Peterhead. The main transmission system consists of 5,097 circuit km of 275 kv and 132 kv lines linking the power stations and the bulk supply points serving the distribution networks. The system control centre at Pitlochry co-ordinates the operation of the transmission system and power stations. The number of staff at 31 March 1989 was 3,917.

Scottish Power plc, with head office in Glasgow, was formally vested in 1990 to take over the non-nuclear operations of the former South of Scotland Electricity Board. The area served stretches north of a line from Holy Island in Northumberland to the Solway Firth to a northern boundary running from the Firth of Clyde to the Firth of Tay. Within this area of approximately 21,000 sq. km (8,000 sq. miles) is located the main industry and population concentrations of Scotland, with 4m. of the total population of 5·1m. Scottish Power provides a full electricity service to its area. It operates 4 coal-fired, 8 hydro, 1 pumped storage station and one gas-fired power station with a maximum sent-out capacity of 4,467 mw. A further 2,000 mw oil-fired station is on care and maintenance. The company transmits and distributes electricity throughout its area to 1·7m. domestic, commercial, industrial and agricultural customers. It operates 75 retail shops, which also provide full customer services. During 1989-90 Scottish Power had a turnover of £1,132m. and produced a total of 19,740m. units of electricity, which included the production of the nuclear power stations now operated by Scottish Nuclear Ltd. Scottish Power has approximately 9,500 employees.

Scottish Nuclear Ltd was formally vested in 1990 to take over and operate the nuclear assets of the former South of Scotland Electricity Board. Initially envisaged as part of the privatization of electricity supply, it is now to remain under government control. With 2,300 employees, it generates electricity at the 2 nuclear power stations at Hunterston, Ayrshire, and Torness, East Lothian. Both plants have two 650 mw Advanced Gas-Cooled Reactors. Scottish Nuclear is also undertaking the decommissioning of the Magnox power station located at Hunterston. During 1988-89, these 3 nuclear power stations generated over 14·5m. units of electricity and for much of the year supplied over 60% of the electricity consumed in the whole of Scotland.

Oil. Production 1989, in 1,000 tonnes (1988 in brackets): Throughput of crude and process oils, 87,699 (85,662); refinery use, 5,816 (5,484). Refinery output: Gases, 1,658 (1,649); naphtha, 2,073 (1,856); motor spirit, 27,237 (26,409); kerosene, 9,436 (9,014); diesel oil, 23,294 (23,925); fuel oil, 13,020 (12,495); lubricating oils,

1,050 (970); bitumen, 2,393 (2,295). Total output of refined products, 81,392 (79,837). Estimated crude oil, 1990, 93·47m. tonnes.

Gas. Following the Gas Act of 1986, British Gas plc became the successor company to the British Gas Corporation. Its primary activities are the purchase, distribution and sale of gas, supported by a broad range of services to customers. It also explores for and produces hydrocarbons. It is organized into a headquarters and twelve Regions.

British Gas explores for gas through 3 wholly owned subsidiary companies: Gas Council (Exploration) Limited (UK onshore and Denmark offshore); Hydrocarbons Great Britain Limited (Irish Sea and Cardigan Bay); Hydrocarbons Ireland Limited, (offshore Eire). British Gas owns and operates two gas fields, Morecambe and Rough field. The latter is used as a gas store and both have been developed to help meet peak winter demand.

In 1986–87, British Gas sold 18,894m. therms of gas to over 17m. customers. Just over 50% of the gas went to domestic customers, the rest to industrial and commercial enterprizes. The industry won 269,000 new customers in the period and made a before-tax profit of £1,062m. with a turnover of £7,610m.

In March 1986, there were 89,000 people employed directly by the industry. British Gas spends £74m. each year on its research and development programme and its international consultancy service works in about 20 countries.

Gas reserves are some 590,000m. cu. metres.

Minerals. Coal. The number of British Coal Corporation producing collieries at 25 March 1989 was 86. Statistics of the coalmining industry for recent years are as follows:

	1985–86	1986–87	1987–88	1988-89
Output, 1m. tonnes:				
BCC mines (inc. tip and capital coal)	88·4	88·0	82·4	85·0
Opencast	14·1	13·3	15·1	16·8
Licensed	2·0	2·0	2·1	1·7
Total	104·5	103·3	99·6	103·5
Employees, 1,000:				
Colliery industrial manpower	138·5	107·7	89·0	80·1
Other industrial manpower	19·3	14·6	11·9	10·8
Non-industrial staff	21·8	19·2	16·4	14·1
Total	179·6	141·5	117·3	105·0
Productivity, tonnes:				
Output per man-year	571	700	789	978
Overall output per manshift	2·72	3·29	3·62	4·14
Consumption, 1m. tonnes:				
Power stations	86·0	82·4	86·2	80·7
Coke ovens	11·5	10·9	10·8	10·9
Domestic	8·9	8·1	7·0	6·3
Other inland	12·0	11·0	11·5	11·3
Total inland	118·4	112·4	115·5	109·2
Imports	12·1	9·9	9·8	12·0
Exports	3·3	2·2	2·2	1·8

Total stocks of coal at 31 March 1989 amounted to 37m. tonnes (28m. tonnes consumer stocks, 9m. tonnes BCC stocks). Operating profit made by British Coal for the year ended March 1989 amounted to £498m. Interest payable was £432m. The overall deficit for 1988–89 was £203m. Deficit grants ceased in 1987-88.

Production of coke (including coke breeze), 1988–89, 1·4m. tonnes.

The UK is among the 10 largest steel producing countries in the world. Output in recent years was as follows (in 1m. tonnes):

	Pig-iron	Crude steel	Finished steel products	Home consumption Crude steel equivalent
1987	12·1	17·4	12·4	15·0
1988	13·2	19·0	14·7	17·5
1989	12·8	18·7	14·9	17·4
1990	12·5	17·8	14·2	...

Exports of finished steel products were 6·8m. tonnes in 1990 and imports 5·2m. tonnes.

With turnover for the year to March 1990 of £5,113m., British Steel plc is the largest steel producer in the UK, the second largest in Europe and the fourth largest in the non-Communist world in terms of crude steel production. The number of UK employees at 31 Dec. 1990 was some 52,000. UK steel producers, other than British Steel plc, are represented by BISPA (British Independent Steel Producers Association). There are approximately 50 companies in membership of BISPA, who account for almost one quarter of UK liquid steel production, and approximately one third of the UK output of finished steel products. For some products such as wire rod, reinforcement steel, bright bars, wire and high speed tool and engineering steels, these companies account for nearly all UK production.

Production of non-ferrous metals (in 1,000 tonnes) in 1988 (and 1989): Refined copper, 124 (119); refined lead, 373·8 (347·2); tin metal, 13·8 (11·2); primary aluminium, 300·2 (297·3); slab zinc, 92·8 (79·8).

Agriculture. In 1988 (and 1989) agricultural land in the UK totalled (in 1,000 ha) 18,575 (18,553), comprising common grazing, 1,216 (1,236), and agricultural holdings, 17,359 (17,317). Land use of the latter: All grasses 6,774 (6,785); crops, 5,253 (5,202); rough grazing, 4,712 (4,710); bare fallow, 58 (65); other, 562 (620). Area sown to crops: Cereals, 3,896 (3,866); fodder crops, 393 (337); horticultural crops, 209 (208); others, 576 (612).

The number of workers employed in agriculture, forestry and fishing in the UK was, in June 1989, 300,000. Of these, 276,000 (77,200 female) were solely engaged in agriculture, including 88,300 (34,300 female) seasonal and casual workers. These figures do not include farmers, partners and directors. There were some 257,000 farm holdings in 1989, some 75% owner-occupied. Average size of holdings, 107·3 ha.

Principal crops in the UK as at June in each year:

	Wheat	Barley	Oats	Horticultural crops	Potatoes	Fodder crops	Sugar-beet	Rape for oilseed
				Area (1,000 ha)				
1985	1,902	1,965	133	213	191	229	269	296
1986	1,997	1,916	97	212	178	239	205	299
1987	1,994	1,830	99	199	177	356	202	388
1988	1,886	1,878	120	209	180	293	201	347
1989	2,083	1,652	119	192	175	337	197	321
				Total product (1,000 tonnes)				
1984	14,970	11,070	515	3,777	7,395	7,085	9,015	925
1985	12,050	9,740	615	3,763	6,895	6,655	7,715	895
1986	13,910	10,010	505	3,869	6,446	7,325	8,120	965
1987	11,940	9,230	450	3,788	6,713	6,939	7,990	1,326
1988	11,600	8,800	600	3,882	6,899	5,673	8,152	...

Livestock in the UK as at June in each year (in 1,000):

	1985	1986	1987	1988	1989
Cattle	12,865	12,533	12,158	11,872	11,977
Sheep	35,628	37,016	38,701	40,942	42,967
Pigs	7,865	7,937	7,942	7,980	7,509
Poultry	128,968	120,740	128,628	130,809	120,198

Forestry. On 31 March 1990 the area of productive woodland in Britain was 2,130,000 ha of which the Forestry Commission managed 864,000 ha and the private sector 1,266,000 ha.

The Forestry Commission employed 7,525 staff in 1990. In addition a further

14,930 were employed in private forestry with an estimated 10,040 engaged in the wood processing industry.

In 1989–90 a total of 6·6m. cu. metres of timber was thinned and felled.

New Planting (1989–90) 19,700 ha (4,100, Forestry Commission; 15,600, private woodlands).

James, N. D. G., *A History of English Forestry*. London, 1981

Fisheries. Quantity (in 1,000 tonnes) and value (in £1,000) of fish of British taking landed in Great Britain (excluding salmon and sea-trout):

Quantity	*1985*	*1986*	*1987*	*1988*	*1989*
Wet fish	687·2	629·3	677·3	645·5	580·4
Shell fish	74·8	87·6	111·0	96·5	91·3
	762·1	716·9	788·3	742·0	671·8
Value					
Wet fish	258,904	284,161	338,965	310,412	299,354
Shell fish	64,920	77,519	95,941	92,481	94,992
	323,825	361,680	434,906	402,893	394,346

In 1990 the fishing fleet of England and Wales comprised 5,417 vessels including 1,664 trawlers and that of Scotland, 2,424 vessels including 394 trawlers. Major fishing ports: (England) Fleetwood, Grimsby, Hull, Lowestoft, North Shields; (Wales) Milford Haven; (Scotland) Aberdeen, Mallarg, Lerwick, Peterhead.

INDUSTRY. Statistics (UK, unless otherwise stated) of a cross-section of industrial production (in 1,000 tonnes):

	1987	*1988*	*1989*
Sulphuric acid	2,158	2,270	2,148
Synthetic resins	1,629	1,590	...
Cotton single yarn	42	35	28
Wool tops	83	80	69
Woollen yarn	77	78	75
Man-made fibres (rayon, nylon, etc.)	277	280	273
Newsprint	497	541	569
Other paper and board	3,682	3,802	3,880
Cement	14,311	16,506	...
Fertilizers	5,153	5,227	4,980

Engineering. Manufacturers' sales (in £1m.) for 1989 (and 1988): Motor vehicles and engines, 12,204 (10,928); railway and tramway vehicles, 391 (462); boilers and process plant, 1,986 (1,654); mechanical lifting and handling equipment, 2,626 (2,236); refrigerating, space-heating, ventilating and air conditioning equipment, 1,842 (1,599); construction and earth-moving equipment, 1,426 (1,265), wheeled tractors, 1,236 (1,231); industrial (including marine) engines, 988 (880).

Electrical Goods. Manufacturers' sales (in £1m.) for 1989 (and 1988): Radio and electronic capital goods, (3,358 in 1988); basic electrical equipment, 3,036 (2,919); electronic data processing equipment, 5,740 (5,186); telephone and telegraph apparatus and equipment, 2,192 (1,978); domestic electrical appliances, 1,553 (1,816).

Textile Manufacturers. Production of woven cloth for 1989 (and 1988): Cotton (1m. metres), 206 (219); man-made fibres (1m. metres), 217 (213); woven woollen and worsted fabrics (1m. sq. metres), deliveries, 85 (89).

Construction. Total value (in £1m.) of constructional work in Great Britain in 1989 (and 1988) was 46,174 (40,546), including new work, 27,315 (23,420), of which housing, 8,067 (8,469). Housing for public authorities, 979 (922); for private developers, 7,088 (7,547).

Annual Abstract of Statistics. HMSO
Statistical Summary of the Mineral Industry. HMSO, annual

Labour. In June 1990 the UK workforce (*i.e.* all persons in employment plus the claimant unemployed) totalled (in 1,000) 28,508, of whom 26,765 were in employment, 22,756 (10,776 females) were employees, 3,240 were self-employed and 308 were in HM Forces. UK employees by form of employment in June 1989 (in

1,000): Agriculture and fishing, 300; energy and water supply, 471; manufacturing industry, 5,235; construction, 1,062; distributive and catering trades, 4,609; transport and communications, 1,362; business and finance, 2,675; public administration, 1,650; education, 1,797; health, 1,485; recreation and culture, 527; others, 1,584. Registered unemployed in UK (in 1,000; figures adjusted for seasonality and discontinuities): 1985, 3,036 (females, 921); 1986, 3,107 (959); 1987, 2,822 (851); 1988, 2,295 (687); 1989, 1,784 (507); 1990, 1,639. In Oct. 1990 507,800 persons (103,500 females) had been unemployed for more than a year. In Nov. 1990 there were 145,400 job vacancies.

Workers (in 1,000) involved in industrial stoppages (and working days lost): 1985, 791 (6·4m.); 1987, 887 (3·5m.); 1988, 790 (3·7m.); 1989, 727 (4·1m.).

Trade Unions. In Sept. 1990 there were 76 unions affiliated to the Trades Union Congress (TUC) with a total membership of 8,416,832 (8,652,318 in 1989) (3m. of them women). The unions affiliated to the TUC in 1990 ranged in size from the Transport and General Workers' Union, with 1,270,776 members, to the Sheffield Wool Shear Workers' Society with 15 members. The 6 largest unions, however, account for more than half the total membership.

The TUC's executive body, the General Council, is elected at the annual Congress. It is composed of 55 members made up of 33 members nominated by unions with a membership of over 200,000, entitled to automatic representation in proportion to their size, and 9 members elected from unions with a numerical membership of 100,000 up to 199,999. Eight members are elected from unions with a numerical membership of less than 100,000 and 4 women members are elected to represent women workers in smaller unions. Unions with a total membership of over 200,000 of which 100,000 or over are women must nominate at least one woman to represent women workers.

The General Secretary is elected by the Congress but is not subject to annual re-election. The TUC General Council appoints committees, which draw upon the services of specialist departments in preparing policies on economic, education, international, employment, industrial organization, equal rights, and social questions.

The TUC is affiliated to the International Confederation of Free Trade Unions, the Trade Union Advisory Committee of OECD, the Commonwealth Trade Union Council and the European Trade Union Confederation. The TUC provides a service of trade union education. It provides members to serve, with representatives of employers, on joint committees advising the Government on issues of national importance (e.g., National Economic Development Council) and on the managing boards of such bodies as the Health and Safety Commission; and Advisory, Conciliation and Arbitration Service.

FOREIGN ECONOMIC RELATIONS.

On 8 Oct. 1990 the UK entered the Exchange-Rate Mechanism (ERM) of the EC's European Monetary System (*see* p. 46), initially with the pound sterling having a fluctuation margin of 6%.

Commerce. Value of the imports and exports of merchandise (excluding bullion and specie and foreign merchandise transhipped under bond) of the UK for 6 recent years (in £1,000):

	Total imports	*Total exports*		*Total imports*	*Total exports*
1985	78,705,170	70,511,345	1988	106,412,879	81,476,249
1986	86,066,650	73,009,049	1989	120,787,729	93,249,123
1987	94,015,696	79,851,395	1990	126,165,755	103,910,969

The value of goods imported is generally taken to be that at the port and time of entry, including all incidental expenses (cost, insurance and freight) up to the landing on the quay. For goods consigned for sale, the market value in this country is required and recorded in the returns. For exports, the value at the port of shipment (including the charges of delivering the goods on board) is taken. Imports are entered as from the country whence the goods were consigned to the UK, which may, or may not, be the country whence they were last shipped. Exports are credited to the country of ultimate destination as declared by the exporters.

Trade according to countries for 1989 and 1990 (in £1,000):

	Imports from		*Exports to*	
	1989 [1]	*1990* [1]	*1989* [1]	*1990* [1]
Foreign countries				
Europe and Overseas Possessions—				
Albania	605	413	1,957	4,512
Austria	933,971	957,789	598,099	705,850
Belgium and Luxembourg	5,700,534	5,732,427	4,872,641	5,648,625
Bulgaria	34,272	32,787	86,209	45,022
Czechoslovakia	156,649	135,988	131,418	133,158
Denmark and Faroe Islands	2,260,382	2,310,965	1,215,573	1,421,595
Finland	1,893,163	1,175,766	925,784	1,041,739
France	10,785,429	11,758,481	9,461,648	10,885,803
German Dem. Rep.	168,742	128,498	106,455	57,013
Germany (Fed. Rep. of)	20,005,276	19,907,062	11,110,623	13,169,405
Greece	395,086	400,476	571,409	682,887
Hungary	105,221	102,741	117,947	121,837
Iceland	196,678	259,430	69,497	88,537
Italy	6,701,683	6,735,496	4,630,896	5,612,751
Netherlands	9,585,699	10,483,576	6,515,325	7,561,576
Netherlands Antilles	5,768	43,552	32,147	35,186
Norway	3,637,119	4,235,348	1,056,506	1,289,789
Poland	330,163	357,164	196,446	221,536
Portugal, Azores and Madeira	1,040,706	1,176,161	915,682	1,033,268
Romania	117,685	61,215	38,141	85,879
Spain	2,772,011	2,884,691	3,137,941	3,750,143
Canary Islands	74,532	86,023	89,852	92,886
Sweden	3,747,600	3,594,547	2,350,122	2,712,775
Switzerland and Liechtenstein	4,125,731	4,252,783	2,245,354	2,358,528
Turkey	533,769	550,803	434,562	606,829
USSR	833,369	917,691	681,599	606,013
Yugoslavia	202,405	189,421	219,866	260,972
European Communities	53,494,966	65,855,511	47,140,164	55,024,710
EFTA	14,534,262	15,075,672	7,246,363	8,179,218
Africa—				
Algeria	177,456	259,959	74,368	73,831
Angola	1,286	5,142	24,785	29,284
Burundi	1,974	541	2,738	2,804
Cameroon	11,362	8,241	24,836	20,652
Côte d'Ivoire	65,943	69,849	29,434	26,941
Egypt	212,727	145,323	296,272	298,262
Ethiopia	12,772	19,465	44,148	41,403
Liberia	12,776	13,240	15,148	8,639
Libya	104,546	151,605	239,191	244,850
Mali	2,305	1,835	7,102	8,819
Mauritania	15,387	14,525	4,005	2,997
Morocco	96,138	106,425	84,475	118,599
Mozambique	14,582	10,709	20,268	28,992
Rwanda	2,991	2,128	1,790	1,195
South Africa	6,820	1,078,546	13,448	1,113,397
Senegal	884,607	5,002	1,038,342	14,884
Sudan	9,532	9,016	60,602	63,670
Tunisia	43,266	40,959	31,148	40,800
Zaïre	9,069	7,337	28,419	23,801
Asia and Oceania—				
Afghanistan	4,813	9,194	5,376	7,816
Bahrain	61,018	48,459	138,529	127,309
Burma	3,484	4,582	12,217	15,951
China	530,720	583,425	417,911	465,585
Fiji	69,558	61,863	10,221	8,168
Indonesia	273,102	327,877	184,032	194,274
Iran	250,548	279,135	257,149	384,713
Iraq	55,175	101,557	450,495	293,393
Israel	479,840	506,106	502,411	567,712
Japan	7,108,441	6,761,592	2,259,823	2,631,326
Jordan	16,462	14,788	110,684	109,483
Korea (South)	1,164,723	963,829	493,945	620,690
Kuwait	150,364	108,970	228,711	181,480

[1] Provisional figures.

Foreign countries	Imports from 1989 [1]	Imports from 1990 [1]	Exports to 1989 [1]	Exports to 1990 [1]
Asia and Oceania—(contd.)				
Lebanon	11,054	6,249	48,474	53,266
Pakistan	216,110	236,448	233,532	251,841
Philippines	233,128	220,706	137,367	158,030
Qatar	4,342	5,004	89,256	98,504
Saudi Arabia	502,416	794,633	432,941	2,012,585
Syria	65,256	88,874	38,537	38,245
Thailand	443,144	484,276	427,484	416,648
America—				
Argentina	98,490	144,205	13,585	35,953
Bolivia	17,666	12,387	6,148	6,234
Brazil	817,545	719,849	338,634	328,234
Chile	193,280	222,469	96,003	128,056
Colombia	70,715	82,507	61,733	60,469
Costa Rica	24,113	17,468	12,780	14,556
Cuba	34,388	30,924	53,255	37,568
Dominican Republic	11,223	17,440	25,519	19,668
Ecuador	19,319	19,527	29,410	30,155
El Salvador	2,133	1,261	9,594	10,415
Guatemala	6,950	42,034	52,324	17,551
Haiti	803	1,271	6,566	6,807
Honduras	12,121	11,661	5,518	7,345
Mexico	165,295	172,144	205,130	262,952
Nicaragua	918	1,899	6,985	6,515
Panama	6,818	4,056	32,875	35,552
Paraguay	8,898	10,077	19,282	32,035
Peru	125,538	96,654	29,707	29,233
Puerto Rico	117,628	123,087	79,851	69,593
Uruguay	52,185	51,859	26,119	31,192
USA	12,888,890	14,354,516	12,098,549	12,998,506
Venezuela	111,072	101,717	124,672	204,921
Total (including some not specified above)	106,859,689	110,987,934	78,101,944	87,695,185
Commonwealth countries				
In Europe—				
Cyprus	145,047	154,065	173,092	204,857
Gibraltar	4,560	5,048	69,350	69,073
Malta	42,194	50,541	132,287	141,298
In Africa				
West Africa:				
Gambia	2,340	3,158	16,563	17,815
Ghana	92,208	105,118	121,076	162,057
Nigeria	129,406	297,436	388,777	499,838
Sierra Leone	15,899	7,011	20,402	21,365
Southern Africa:				
Botswana	13,135	18,854	34,582	24,777
Lesotho	734	1,288	795	642
Malawi	27,890	24,666	30,604	33,575
Namibia	4,568	349	4,264	0,000
Swaziland	31,368	34,473	1,358	2,719
Zambia	21,565	19,308	119,057	92,832
Zimbabwe	85,792	86,280	87,013	83,718
East Africa:				
Kenya	154,313	149,474	208,464	223,080
Mauritius	216,190	233,936	43,528	50,746
Tanzania	22,641	25,575	93,036	84,694
Uganda	20,985	12,124	39,218	39,506
Seychelles	993	8,353	10,741	14,955
St Helena	504	555	7,208	7,429
In Asia—				
Bangladesh	52,527	72,515	78,270	70,584
Hong Kong	2,036,976	1,972,154	1,111,517	1,238,023
India	701,985	799,438	1,382,436	1,264,189
Malaysia	676,258	775,667	441,762	601,909
Singapore	903,248	1,021,148	773,866	1,040,188
Sri Lanka	63,527	63,362	92,465	88,496

[1] Provisional figures.

Commonwealth countries	Imports from 1989 [1]	Imports from 1990 [1]	Exports to 1989 [1]	Exports to 1990 [1]
In Oceania—				
Australia	864,965	1,039,080	1,711,241	1,645,620
Nauru	662	54	549	1,145
New Zealand	436,772	483,615	399,295	439,608
Papua New Guinea	47,839	34,849	15,822	8,793
Western Samoa	1,376	295	296	427
In America—				
Bahamas	17,681	15,053	22,543	22,917
Barbados	22,308	24,294	38,136	35,811
Belize	24,272	22,734	11,842	12,439
Bermuda	4,517	12,849	77,122	28,114
Canada	2,174,339	2,259,099	2,165,731	1,901,939
Falkland Islands	5,375	4,817	10,200	11,309
Guyana	54,523	53,892	13,216	15,294
Jamaica	95,516	136,535	61,355	58,702
Leeward Islands (Anguilla; St. Kitts-Nevis; Antigua and Barbuda; Montserrat)	10,209	7,991	34,895	29,735
Trinidad and Tobago	37,426	45,058	45,881	49,894
Windward Islands (Dominica; St. Lucia; St. Vincent and the Grenadines)	104,025	117,126	39,403	36,794
Total, Commonwealth countries (including some not specified above)	9,648,838	10,679,250	10,432,399	10,904,245
Ireland	4,279,202	4,498,571	4,714,780	5,311,539
Grand Total	120,787,729	126,165,755	93,249,123	103,910,969

[1] Provisional figures.

Imports and exports for 1988 and 1989 (Great Britain and Northern Ireland) (in £1,000):

Import values c.i.f. *Export values f.o.b.*	Total imports 1989 [1]	Total imports 1990 [1]	Domestic exports 1989 [1]	Domestic exports 1990 [1]
0. *Food and Live Animals*				
Live animals (excluding zoo animals, dogs and cats)	286,533	290,674	265,738	257,975
Meat and meat preparations	1,826,899	1,887,821	699,590	609,155
Dairy products and eggs	786,423	913,676	501,896	458,148
Fish and fish preparations	885,003	968,965	449,958	505,315
Cereals and cereal preparations	722,189	785,063	951,332	1,045,466
Fruit and vegetables	2,727,077	2,964,873	281,250	263,747
Sugar, sugar preparations, honey	603,642	639,242	228,238	240,291
Coffee, tea, cocoa, spices	941,570	904,423	387,715	438,653
Feeding stuff for animals	582,258	624,598	228,742	238,917
Miscellaneous food preparations	400,802	429,901	233,962	266,890
Total of Section 0	9,762,395	10,409,237	4,228,421	4,324,557
1. *Beverages and Tobacco*				
Beverages	1,322,059	1,529,780	1,802,190	2,112,771
Tobacco and tobacco manufactures	345,445	377,246	524,153	657,472
Total of Section 1	1,667,504	1,907,026	2,326,343	2,770,244
2. *Crude Materials, Inedible, except Fuels*				
Hides, skins and furskins, undressed	149,241	100,499	253,922	188,815
Oil seeds, oil nuts and oil kernels	238,949	273,042	37,194	67,266
Crude rubber (including synthetic and reclaimed)	250,167	244,899	211,610	221,863
Wood and cork	1,429,033	1,409,978	27,762	27,717
Pulp and waste paper	896,286	777,341	51,745	53,079

[1] Provisional figures.

Import values c.i.f. *Export values f.o.b.*	*Total imports* 1989 [1]	1990 [1]	*Domestic exports* 1989 [1]	1990 [1]
2. *Crude Materials, Inedible, except Fuels*—Contd.				
Textile fibres and their waste	681,179	548,875	498,141	494,510
Crude fertilizers and crude minerals (excluding fuels)	360,836	344,709	368,927	369,947
Metalliferous ores and metal scrap	1,573,765	1,479,233	711,652	633,515
Crude animal and vegetable materials, not elsewhere specified	518,125	542,667	103,101	105,876
Total of Section 2	6,097,580	5,721,243	2,264,073	2,162,586
3. *Mineral Fuels, Lubricants and Related Materials*				
Coal, coke and briquettes	537,842	654,771	111,892	122,014
Petroleum and petroleum products	4,674,403	6,254,923	5,511,771	7,477,620
Gas, natural and manufactured	717,888	824,546	144,431	176,518
Total [2] of Section 3	6,235,124	7,839,960	5,768,094	7,801,368
4. *Animal and Vegetable Oils and Fats*	384,948	377,370	83,644	87,743
5. *Chemicals*				
Chemical elements and compounds	3,637,917	3,593,336	4,394,766	4,303,304
Dyeing, tanning and colouring materials	612,639	651,629	1,063,251	1,193,499
Medicinal and pharmaceutical products	1,061,634	1,157,805	2,016,300	2,258,096
Essential oils and perfume; toilet and cleansing preparations	681,827	756,071	1,003,434	1,161,840
Fertilizers, manufactured	217,187	286,227	105,185	110,197
Plastic materials	2,059,770	3,227,404	1,244,955	2,124,162
Total [2] of Section 5	10,440,540	10,834,619	12,349,574	13,182,512
6. *Manufactured Goods Classified Chiefly by Material*				
Leather and dressed furs	242,672	240,736	326,498	311,784
Rubber	827,073	880,447	801,636	872,787
Wood and cork (excluding furniture)	967,028	949,087	91,038	114,228
Paper, paperboard	4,015,994	4,016,552	1,239,817	1,539,386
Textile yarn, fabrics	3,769,721	3,936,197	2,205,028	2,446,974
Non-metallic mineral manufactures	3,567,041	3,602,140	3,198,613	3,191,300
Iron and steel	2,787,870	2,676,693	2,893,572	3,035,980
Non-ferrous metals	3,069,877	3,003,621	1,967,544	2,193,182
Manufactures of metal, not elsewhere specified	2,483,082	2,593,488	1,786,499	2,115,354
Total of Section 6	21,730,357	21,898,961	14,510,245	15,820,974
7. *Machinery and Transport Equipment*				
Boilers, engines, motors and power-units	3,487,336	3,518,388	4,738,901	5,251,433
Agricultural and Industrial machinery	8,972,689	8,874,665	8,559,173	9,690,584
Office machinery	7,552,324	7,714,644	6,115,925	6,341,244
Electrical machinery, apparatus, not elsewhere specified	10,374,203	10,410,547	7,273,050	8,335,937
Transport equipment	15,513,094	16,771,327	11,002,980	12,536,256
Total of Section 7	45,899,646	47,289,572	37,690,028	42,155,433

[1] Provisional figures.
[2] Includes items not specified here.

Import values c.i.f. *Export values f.o.b.*	*Total imports* *1989* [1]	*1990* [1]	*Domestic exports* *1989* [1]	*1990* [1]
8. *Miscellaneous Manufactured Articles*				
Prefabricated buildings, sanitary, plumbing, heating and lighting fixtures	371,728	394,498	222,255	260,363
Furniture	1,099,567	1,111,997	460,832	533,186
Travel goods, handbags and similar articles	292,973	309,127	56,304	69,887
Clothing	3,542,262	3,905,902	1,444,837	1,699,392
Footwear	973,211	1,169,085	227,579	274,439
Scientific instruments; cameras, watches and clocks	3,994,402	4,071,459	3,927,625	4,108,709
Miscellaneous manufactured articles, not elsewhere specified	6,783,537	7,920,066	5,433,210	6,401,044
Total of Section 8	17,057,680	18,252,133	11,772,643	13,347,020
9. *Commodities and Transactions not Classified According to Kind*				
Total of Section 9	1,511,954	1,635,634	2,256,059	2,258,531
Total [2] of all classes	120,787,729	126,165,755	93,249,123	103,910,969

[1] Provisional figures. [2] Includes items not specified here.

Tourism. There were 17·3m. overseas visitors in 1989 spending £6,945m. in the UK and an estimated £1,600m. in fares to British carriers. Provisional figures for 1990: 17·7m. visitors spent £7,475m.

COMMUNICATIONS

Roads. Central government responsibility for highways in England rests with the Secretary of State for Transport. His responsibilities are administered by the Department of Transport through a number of Directorates at Headquarters together with 9 Regional Offices. For Welsh and Scottish roads, central government responsibility rests with the Secretaries of State for Wales and Scotland respectively.

The Secretary of State is the highway authority responsible for all trunk roads. The Shire County Councils, the Metropolitan District Councils, the London Borough Councils and the Common Council of the City of London are the highway authorities responsible for local roads in their own areas.

The Secretary of State has powers to provide roads designed for limited classes of motor traffic, and to confirm schemes for the provision of such special roads by local authorities. The former have the status of trunk roads; the latter principal roads. 2,995 km of motorway were open to traffic in Great Britain in 1989 (2,550 km of trunk motorway in England, 233 km in Scotland, 120 km in Wales and 92 km of principal motorway). Public highways in Great Britain in 1989, excluding lengths of unsurfaced roads (green lanes), totalled 356,517 km (England, 271,837 km; Wales, 33,213 km; Scotland, 51,465 km). There were 12,715 km of all-purpose trunk roads, 2,992 km of trunk and principal motorways, 35,034 km of principal roads (excluding motorways) and 305,744 km of other roads.

Motor vehicles for which licences were current under the Vehicles (Excise) Act, 1971, at 31 Dec. 1989, numbered 24,196,000, including 19,248,000 private cars, 875,000 mopeds, scooters and motor cycles, 122,000 public transport vehicles and 2,704,000 goods vehicles. New vehicle registrations in 1989, 2,828,900.

Road casualties in Great Britain numbered in 1989, 341,592 including 5,373 killed; in 1987, 311,473 including 5,125 killed.

Railways. The British Railways Board as a public authority owns and manages British Rail: The national rail network, British Rail Maintenance Ltd, British Rail Property Board, European Passenger Services Ltd. and Transportation Systems and Market Research Ltd. (Transmark). The role of the Board is to determine policies, establish the organization to carry them out, monitor performance and take major decisions to meet objectives set by the Secretary of State for Transport.

The Group turnover 1990–91 was £3,485m. and 134,361 staff were employed, of whom 128,476 were involved in the railway business.

The management of the railways is the responsibility of the Chief Executive. He establishes plans and budgets for the achievement of objectives set by the Board, monitors and achieves results against the plans and budgets, and directs the organization and deployment of manpower resources. He is assisted by Managing Directors and other Board members with responsibility for functions such as Engineering, Research, Finance and Planning, Marketing, Operating, Productivity and Personnel.

In the year ending 31 March 1990, British Rail carried 143·1m. tonnes of freight and parcels and 746·4m. passenger journeys were made.

The rail business is split into 5 sectors: InterCity, Network Southeast, Regional Railways, Freight and Parcels. A director is responsible for efficient operation and budgeting within his sector, each of which bears its fair share of the fixed costs of operation, such as signalling and track maintenance. The day-to-day running of the rail network has been the responsibility of 6 regional general managers, but is scheduled to pass to the business sectors.

		1988–89	*1989–90*
Passenger Receipts and Traffic			
Receipts	£m.	1,780·8	1,882·7
Passenger journeys	m.	763·7	746·4
Passenger miles (estimated)	m.	21,327·0	20,706·0
Freight Train Traffic			
Receipts	£m.	655·0	671·9
Traffic	m. tonnes	149·5	143·1
Net tonne miles (trainload and wagonload)	m.	11,249·0	10,403·0
Locomotives			
Diesel		1,920	1,835
Electric		260	260
High Speed Trains			
Power cars		197	197
Passenger carriages		722	718
Coaching vehicles		14,258	13,115
Freight vehicles (excluding brake vans)		24,922	21,970
Stations		2,561	2,610
Route open for traffic	miles	10,314	10,307
Electrified	miles	. . .	2,834

The London Regional Transport (formerly London Transport Executive) is the authority responsible for the operation of the capital's Underground and bus services. Overall policy and financial control is exercised by the Secretary of State for Transport. In April 1989, London Underground had 245 route miles of railway open for traffic and also operated over 10 route miles owned by British Rail. Rolling stock owned: Underground, 3,950; buses, 4,825. In the financial year 1988–89, the number of train miles run in passenger service was 32·1m.; number of bus miles run in passenger service was 170m. The number of passenger journeys was: Underground 815m.; buses 1,244m.

Aviation. British Airways is engaged in the provision of air transport services for passengers, cargo and mail worldwide, both on scheduled and charter services. It operates long and short haul international services, as well as an extensive domestic network. In 1988–89, it carried 24·6m. passengers and 459,000 tonnes of freight, and at 31 March 1989 it had a fleet of 211 aircraft and employed 48,760 staff.

In addition to British Airways, there were in 1987 about 55 other UK air transport operators.

Following the Civil Aviation Act 1971, the Civil Aviation Authority (CAA) was established as an independent public body responsible for the economic and safety regulation of British civil aviation. It also runs the National Air Traffic Services in conjunction with the Ministry of Defence. CAA established a wholly-owned subsidiary, Highlands and Islands Airports Ltd, on 1 April 1986 to own and operate eight airports in the Scottish Highlands and Islands.

In addition to the public transport operators there are a number of companies engaged in miscellaneous aviation activities such as crop-spraying, aerial survey and photography, and flying instruction.

Operating and traffic statistics of UK airlines on scheduled services during the calendar year 1989 (and 1988): Aircraft km flown, 486m. (443m.); revenue passengers carried, 35m. (31m.); cargo (freight and mail) carried 453,430 (435,071) tonnes.

Traffic between UK airports and places abroad in 1989 (and 1988) on all services included 933,902 (695,781) air transport aircraft movements.

There were 13,972 and 14,353 civil aircraft registered in the UK at 31 Dec. 1989 and 1990 respectively.

Shipping. The UK-owned merchant fleet (trading vessels over 500 GRT) in Dec. 1990 totalled 581 ships of 15·3m. DWT and 9·8m. GRT. The UK-registered fleet totalled 337 ships of 4·2m. DWT and 3·7m. GRT.

The average age of the UK-owned fleet was 13 years. Total gross earnings in 1989 were £4,076m. The net contribution to the UK balance of payments was £1,143m.; there were gross import savings of £1,070m.

Inland Waterways. There are approximately 3,500 miles of navigable canals and river navigations in Great Britain. Of these, British Waterways is responsible for some 380 miles of commercial waterways (maintained for freight traffic) and some 1,160 miles of cruising waterways (maintained for pleasure cruising, fishing and amenity). British Waterways is also responsible for a further 600 miles of canals, of which in 1968 some 350 miles were no longer navigable and whose future has been considered in conjunction with local authorities. As a result, some 215 miles have been restored for cruising or as local amenities. The Board's external turnover for the 12 months to 31 March 1990 was £24·1m. Freight traffic was 4·16m. tonnes.

The most important of the river navigations and canals managed by other authorities include the rivers Thames, Great Ouse and Nene, the Norfolk Broads and the Manchester Ship Canal.

Hadfield, C., *British Canals*. 6th ed. Newton Abbot, 1979

Post and Telecommunications. The Post Office operates as a group of 3 distinct businesses: Royal Mail (letter delivery), Royal Mail Parcelforce (parcel delivery), and Post Office Counters (retailing and agency services). Every area of the country is served by regional offices for each of the businesses. Royal Mail collects and delivers 58m. letters a day to the 24m. UK addresses. Other services include electronic mail, guaranteed parcel deliveries (same-day and overnight to UK addresses) and swift deliveries to 100 other countries. The British Postal Consultancy Service provides advice to administrations abroad.

In 1989–90 there were 20,871 post offices and some 100,000 posting boxes. Staff numbered 211,670. 14,718m. letters and 191·5m. parcels were posted. Group turnover was £4459·4m., pre-tax profit, £116·4m., and profit retained, £2·9m.

	1985–86 (1m.)	*1986–87 (1m.)*	*1987–88 (1m.)*	*1988–89 (1m.)*
Correspondence (incl. registered items) posted	11,700	12,500	13,500	13,700
Parcels handled	194	192	197	191

Income (1988–89) £3,914·8m. Profit retained, £100m. British Telecom (BT) was established in 1981 to take over the management of telecommunications from the Post Office. At 30 Sept. 1989 there were 7,062 local exchanges, 345 trunk exchanges and 5 international exchanges operated by British Telecom. At 30 Sept. 1989 there were 5,473,000 business and 19,018,000 residential telephone connexions and 105,000 telex connexions. In 1990 British Telecom's modernization programme will continue. By the end of Sept. 1989 there were more than 2,546 digital exchanges in operation and more than 730,000 km of optical fibre had been installed in the network.

At 31 Dec. 1989 about 330,000 customers were connected to Cellnet, the cellular mobile radio network launched in 1985 and run jointly by BT and Securicor. In 1989 BT owned and operated 6 cable and satellite TV systems at The Barbican (London), Bracknell, Berks, Irvine (Scotland), Milton Keynes, Swindon and Washington (Tyne and Wear). At 31 May 1989 BT employed a total staff of 235,400.

Daunton, M. J., *Royal Mail: The Post Office since 1840*. London, 1985

Broadcasting. Radio and television services are provided by the BBC and by the Independent Broadcasting Authority (IBA) and its programme contractors. The BBC, constituted by Royal Charter until 31 Dec. 1996, has responsibility for providing domestic and external broadcast services, the former financed from the television licence revenue, the latter by Government grant. The domestic services include 2 national television services, 4 national radio network services and an expanding local radio service.

The IBA provides an independent television service on a regional basis, with programmes provided by its programme contractors. The 1981 Act provided for the establishment of the fourth television channel (Channel 4) and of the Welsh Fourth Channel Authority (S4C) which provides a Welsh service on that channel in Wales; they started broadcasting in Nov. 1982. The IBA also provides independent local radio services. All these services are financed by the sale of broadcast advertising time.

The BBC's domestic radio services are available on LF, MF and VHF; those of the IBA on MF and VHF. The television services of the 2 authorities BBC1, BBC2, ITV, and Channel 4 are broadcast at UHF in 625-line definition and in colour.

The broadcasting authorities, whose governing bodies are appointed (by HM the Queen in the case of the BBC and by the Home Secretary in the case of the IBA and S4C) as trustees for the public interest in broadcasting, are independent of government in matters of programme content and are publicly accountable to Parliament for the discharge of their responsibilities.

Cable services are regulated by the Cable Authority which was established by Parliament in 1984 to oversee the development of cable in the UK. Five direct broadcasting by satellite (DBS) channels began broadcasting in 1989. They were authorized under the Cable and Broadcasting Act 1984; they are uplinked from this country and will be subject to IBA regulation. Satellite services are also receivable direct from other countries. Most existing satellite services received from abroad are used to feed cable systems and are therefore subject to Cable Authority regulation

In 1981 the Broadcasting Complaints Commission was set up to consider and adjudicate upon complaints of unfair or unjust treatment in broadcast programmes or of unwarranted infringement of privacy in or in the making of programmes. The number of broadcast receiving licences in force on 31 March 1988 was 19·3m., including 17·1m. for colour.

Cinemas. In 1990 cinemas had a total seating capacity of 0·46m. (0·44m. in 1989). Admissions were 91m. (88m. in 1989, from a low point of 54m. in 1984).

Newspapers. In 1987 there were 14 national dailies.

In Jan. 1991 the Press Complaints Commission replaced the former Press Council. It has 15 members (*Chairperson* Lord McGregor of Durris) including 7 editors. It is funded (£1·5m. in 1991) by the newspaper industry.

Benn's Media Directory. Tunbridge Wells, Annual

JUSTICE, RELIGION, EDUCATION AND WELFARE

Justice. *England and Wales*. The legal system of England and Wales, divided into civil and criminal courts has at the head of the superior courts, as the ultimate court of appeal, the House of Lords, which hears each year a number of appeals in civil matters, including a certain number from Scotland and Northern Ireland, as well as some appeals in criminal cases. In order that civil cases may go from the Court of Appeal to the House of Lords, it is necessary to obtain the leave of either the Court of Appeal or the House itself, although in certain cases an appeal may lie direct to the House of Lords from the decision of the High Court. An appeal can be brought from a decision of the Court of Appeal or the Divisional Court of the Queen's Bench Division of the High Court in a criminal case provided that the Court is satisfied that a point of law 'of general public importance' is involved, and either the Court or the House of Lords is of the opinion that it is desirable in the public interest that a further appeal should be brought. As a judicial body, the House of Lords consists of the Lord Chancellor, the Lords of Appeal in Ordinary, commonly called Law Lords, and such other members of the House as hold or have held high judicial office. The final court of appeal for certain of the Commonwealth countries is the Judicial Committee of the Privy Council which, in addition to Privy Counsellors who are or have held high judicial office in the UK, includes others who are or have been Chief Justices or Judges of the Superior Courts of Commonwealth countries.

Civil Law. The main courts of original civil jurisdiction are the county courts for less important cases, and the High Court for the more important ones.

There are some 270 county courts located throughout the country, each in its own district, and presided over by a circuit judge. In 1991 they had a general jurisdiction to determine all actions founded on contract or tort involving sums of not more than £5,000 and can also deal with other classes of case, such as landlord and tenant, probate, equity and admiralty, up to certain limits. Certain matters, such as actions of libel and slander, are entirely reserved for the High Court. In addition, certain designated county courts have jurisdiction in matrimonial, bankruptcy and patents proceedings. Divorce proceedings must now commence in these courts and, subject to limited exceptions, are determined in the county court.

The High Court has both appellate and original jurisdiction, covering virtually all civil causes not determined in the county court. The judges of the High Court are attached to one of its 3 divisions: Chancery; Queen's Bench; and Family; each with its separate field of jurisdiction. The Heads of the 3 divisions are the Lord Chief Justice (Queen's Bench), the Vice Chancellor (Chancery), and the President of the Family Division. In addition there are over 80 High Court judges, called puisne judges. For the hearing of cases at first instance, the High Court judges sit singly. Appellate jurisdiction is usually exercised by Divisional Courts consisting of 2 (sometimes 3) judges, though in certain circumstances a judge sitting alone may hear the appeal.

The Restrictive Practices Court was set up in 1956 under the Restrictive Trade Practices Act, and is responsible for deciding whether a restrictive trade agreement is in the public interest. It is presided over by a High Court judge, but laymen sit on the bench also. Another specialist court is the Employment Appeal Tribunal, with similar composition, which hears appeals in employment cases from lower tribunals.

The Court of Appeal (Civil Division) hears appeals in civil actions from the High Court and county courts and certain special courts such as the Restrictive Practices Court and the Employment Appeal Tribunal. Its President is the Master of the Rolls, aided by up to 28 Lords Justices of Appeal sitting in 6 or 7 divisions of 2 or 3 judges each.

Civil proceedings are instituted by the aggrieved person, but, as they are a private matter, they are frequently settled by the parties to a dispute through their lawyers before the matter actually comes to court. In some cases, at the instance of either party, a jury may sit to decide questions of fact and award of damages.

Criminal Law. At the base of the system of criminal courts in England and Wales are the magistrates' courts which try over 97% of criminal cases. In general, in exercising their summary jurisdiction, they have power to pass a sentence of up to six months imprisonment and to impose a fine of up to £2,000 on any one offence. They also deal with the preliminary hearing of cases triable only at the Crown Court. In addition to dealing summarily with over 2m. cases, which include thefts, assaults, road traffic infringements, drug abuse, etc, they also have a limited civil jurisdiction.

Magistrates' courts normally comprise three lay justices. Although unpaid they are entitled to loss of earnings and travel and subsistence allowance. They undergo training after appointment and they are advised by a professional justices' clerk. In central London and in some provincial areas full-time stipendiary magistrates have been appointed. Generally they possess the same powers as the lay bench, but they sit alone. On 1 Jan. 1991 the total strength of the lay magistracy was 29,062 including 12,964 women. Justices are appointed on behalf of the Queen by the Lord Chancellor, except in Greater Manchester, Merseyside and Lancashire where they are appointed by the Chancellor of the Duchy of Lancaster.

Justices are selected and trained specially to sit in Juvenile and domestic courts. Juvenile courts deal with cases involving persons under 17 years of age charged with criminal offences (other than homicide and other grave offences) or brought before the court as being in need of care or control. These courts normally sit with three justices, including at least one man or one woman, and are accommodated separately from other courts.

Domestic Proceedings courts deal with matrimonial applications, custody, guardianship and maintenance of children, and adoption. These courts normally sit with three justices including at least one man or one woman.

Above the magistrates' courts is the Crown Court. This was set up by the Courts Act 1971 to replace quarter sessions and assizes. Unlike quarter sessions and assizes, which were individual courts, the Crown Court is a single court which is capable of sitting anywhere in England and Wales. It has power to deal with all trials on indictment and has inherited the jurisdiction of quarter sessions to hear appeals, proceedings on committal of persons from the magistrates' courts for sentence, and certain original proceedings on civil matters under individual statutes.

The jurisdiction of the Crown Court is exercisable by a High Court judge, a Circuit judge or a Recorder or Assistant Recorder (part-time judges) sitting alone, or, in specified circumstances, with justices of the peace. The Lord Chief Justice has given directions as to the types of case to be allocated to High Court judges (the more serious cases) and to Circuit judges or Recorders respectively.

Appeals from magistrates' courts go either to a Divisional Court of the High Court (when a point of law alone is involved) or to the Crown Court where there is a complete re-hearing on appeals against conviction. Appeals from the Crown Court in cases tried on indictment lie to the Court of Appeal (Criminal Division). Appeals on questions of law go by right, and appeals on other matters by leave. The Lord Chief Justice or a Lord Justice sits with judges of the High Court to constitute this court.

There remains as a last resort the invocation of the royal prerogative exercised on the advice of the Home Secretary. In 1965 the death penalty was abolished for murder.

All contested criminal trials, except those which come before the magistrates' courts, are tried by a judge and a jury consisting of 12 members. The defence may challenge any potential juror for cause. The prosecution may ask that any number may 'stand by' until the jury panel is exhausted, and only then need to show cause. The jury decides whether the accused is guilty or not. The judge is responsible for summing up on the facts and explaining the law; he sentences convicted offenders. If, after at least 2 hours of deliberation, a jury is unable to reach a unanimous verdict it may, on the judge's direction, provided that in a full jury of 12 at least 10 of its members are agreed, bring in a majority verdict. The failure of a jury to agree on a unanimous verdict or to bring in a majority verdict may involve the retrial of the case before a new jury.

The Employment Appeal Tribunal. The Employment Appeal Tribunal which is a superior Court of Record with the like powers, rights, privileges and authority of the High Court, was set up in 1976 to hear appeals on questions of fact and law against decisions of industrial tribunals and of the Certification Officer. The appeals are heard by a High Court Judge sitting with 2 members (in exceptional cases 4) appointed for their special knowledge or experience of industrial relations either on the employer or the trade union side, with always an equal number on each side. The great bulk of their work is concerned with the problems which can arise between employees and their employers.

Military Courts. Offences by persons subject to service law against the system of military law created under the powers of the Army Act, Air Force Act or Naval Discipline Act are dealt with either summarily or by courts-martial.

The Personnel of the Law. All judicial officers except the Lord Chancellor (who is a member of the Cabinet) are independent of Parliament and the Executive. They are all appointed by the Crown on the advice of the Prime Minister or the Lord Chancellor and hold office until retiring age. The legal profession is divided; barristers, who advise on legal problems and can conduct cases before all courts, usually act for the public only through solicitors, who deal directly with the legal business brought to them by the public and have rights to present cases before certain courts. Long-standing members of both professions are eligible for appointment to most judicial offices. Only barristers, however, are eligible for appointment direct to the High Court and above.

Legal Aid. Broadly there are 3 kinds of legal aid. Firstly there is legal advice and assistance, otherwise known as the 'Green Form' scheme. This includes advice and help on any question of English law, both civil and criminal, but does not normally cover any form of representation before a court or tribunal. As an extension of the scheme, however, assistance by way of representation has been available for certain proceedings, chiefly civil, in magistrates' courts. Legal advice and assistance also provides for duty solicitor schemes at magistrates' courts and police stations. Under the magistrates' courts schemes, initial advice, and representation where necessary, is available to unrepresented defendants at court, from duty solicitors either in attendance at courts or on call. The scheme covers advice to a defendant in custody, making a bail application, representing a defendant in custody on a guilty plea, and certain other cases. The advice and assistance at police stations scheme enables any person who has been arrested and taken to a police station, or who is assisting the police with their enquiries, to receive advice and assistance, from either a duty solicitor or the person's own solicitor. The cost of these schemes, which are not subject to means test or contribution, is met from the Legal Aid fund and in 1989–90 amounted to £37·5m. Secondly, under Part IV of the Legal Aid Act 1988, there is legal aid for civil court proceedings. Under regulations, aid is available to those of low or moderate means either free or subject to a contribution, depending on means. In 1989–90 there were over 1·5m. payments for advice and assistance under the Legal Advice and Assistance Scheme and around 300,000 civil legal aid certificates were issued. The cost of legal aid in civil cases is met from (*a*) contributions from assisted persons; (*b*) the operation of the statutory charge which gives the Law Society a first charge on money or property recovered or preserved for an assisted person; (*c*) costs recovered from opposing parties and (*d*) a grant from the Exchequer. The net cost of civil legal aid to the state (excluding administration costs of the scheme) in the year 1989–90 amounted to £165·1m. and the cost of the legal advice and assistance scheme was £78·6m. of which £16·2m. was accounted for by assistance by way of representation. Thirdly under Part V of the Legal Aid Act 1988 a court dealing with criminal proceedings may order legal aid to be given if it considers it is desirable in the interests of justice and if it also considers that the defendant (or appellant) requires financial assistance in meeting the costs he may incur. The interests of justice are statutorily defined to include, for example, situations where the defendant is in real danger of going to prison or losing his job, where substantial questions of law are to be argued or where the defendant is unable to follow the proceedings and explain his case due to inadequate knowledge of English, mental illness or other mental or physical disability. Legal aid must be granted, subject to means, in the following circumstances: where a person is committed for trial on a charge of murder, where the prosecutor appeals or applies for leave to appeal from the criminal division of the Court of Appeal or the Courts-Martial Appeal Court to the House of Lords, and in certain circumstances where the court is considering depriving a defendant of his liberty.

The costs of legal aid in criminal proceedings are paid by the central government, but courts have power to require legally aided persons to contribute towards the cost of legal aid given to them. The net cost of legal aid in criminal proceedings in the year 1989–90 was £319·93m., £133·63m. of this was for legal aid in the higher courts which is paid for out of the Lord Chancellor's vote and £148·8m. for legal aid in the magistrates' courts which is paid from the legal aid fund.

Police. The authorized establishment of the police force in England and Wales in Dec. 1990 was 127,588: the actual strength was 112,577 men and 14,513 women. In addition there were 15,902 special constables (including 5,419 women). The estimated total expenditure on the police service in England and Wales for 1988–89 was £4,347m.

SCOTLAND. The High Court of Justiciary is the supreme criminal court in Scotland and has jurisdiction in all cases of crime committed in any part of Scotland, unless expressly excluded by statute. It consists of the Lord Justice-General, the Lord Justice-Clerk and 22 other judges, who are the same judges as of the Court of Session, the Scottish supreme civil court. One judge is seconded to the Scottish Law Commission. The Court, which is presided over by the Lord Justice-General, whom failing, the Lord Justice-Clerk, exercises an appellate jurisdiction as well as one of first instance, sits as business requires in Edinburgh both as a Court of Appeal (the *quorum* being 3 judges) and as a court of first instance and on circuit as a court of first instance. The decisions of the Court in either case are not subject to review by the House of Lords. One judge sitting with a jury of 15 persons can, and usually does, try cases, but 2 or more (with a jury) may do so in important or complex cases. It has a privative jurisdiction over cases of treason, murder, rape, deforcement of messengers and breach of duty by magistrates. It also, in practice, is the only court which tries serious crimes against person or property and generally those cases in which a sentence greater than imprisonment for 3 years is likely to be imposed. Moreover, the Court has inherent power to try and to punish all acts which are plainly criminal though previously unknown and not dealt with by any statute.

The appellate jurisdiction of the High Court of Justiciary extends to all cases tried on indictment, whether in the High Court or the Sheriff Court, and persons so convicted may appeal to the Court against conviction or sentence or both except that there is no appeal against any sentence fixed by law. By such an appeal, a person may bring under review of the High Court of Justiciary any alleged miscarriage of justice including any alleged miscarriage of justice on the basis of the existence and significance of additional evidence which was not heard at the trial and which was not available and could not reasonably have been made available at the trial. It is also a court of review from courts of summary criminal jurisdiction, and on the final determination of any summary prosecution a convicted person may appeal to the Court by way of stated case on questions of law, etc., but not on questions of fact, except in relation to a miscarriage of justice alleged by the person accused on the basis of the existence and significance of additional evidence which was not heard at the trial and which was not available and could not reasonably have been made available at the trial. The Lord Advocate may refer a point of law which has arisen during a trial on indictment in which accused has been acquitted for the opinion of the Court. A prosecutor may appeal only on a point of law. A further or complementary form of process of review which can be resorted to by convicted persons in these courts is by Bill of Suspension (and Liberation), but it is of strictly limited application. A prosecutor in cases tried on indictment or under summary criminal procedure may also bring under review a decision in law, prior to final judgment of the case, by way of Bill of Advocation. The Court also hears appeals under the Courts-Martial (Appeals) Act 1951.

The Sheriff Court has an inherent universal criminal jurisdiction (as well as an extensive civil one) limited in general to crimes and offences committed within a sheriffdom (a specifically defined region), which has, however, been curtailed by statute or practice under which the High Court of Justiciary has exclusive jurisdiction in relation to the crimes above-mentioned. This Court is presided over by a Sheriff-Principal or Sheriff, and when trying cases on indictment sits with a jury of

15 persons. His power of awarding punishment involving imprisonment is restricted to 3 years in the maximum, but he may under certain statutory powers remit the prisoner to the High Court for sentence. The Sheriff also exercises a wide summary criminal jurisdiction and when doing so sits without a jury; and he has concurrent jurisdiction with every other court within his Sheriff Court District in regard to all offences competent for trial in summary courts. The great majority of offences which come before the courts are of a minor nature and, as such, are disposed of in the Sheriff Summary Courts or in the District Courts (*see* below). In cases to be tried on indictment either in the High Court of Justiciary or in the Sheriff Court, the judge may, and in some cases must, before the trial, hold a Preliminary Diet to decide questions of a preliminary nature, whether to the competency or relevancy or otherwise. Any decision at a preliminary diet can be the subject of an appeal to the High Court of Justiciary prior to the trial.

District Courts in each local authority district have jurisdiction in minor offences occurring within the district. These courts are presided over by lay magistrates, known as justices, and have limited powers of fine and imprisonment. In Glasgow District there are also 4 Stipendiary Magistrates who have the same sentencing powers as Sheriffs.

The Court of Session, presided over by the Lord President (the Lord Justice-General in criminal cases), is divided into an Inner House comprising 2 divisions of 4 judges each with mainly appellate function, and an Outer House comprising 15 single judges, sitting individually at first instance; it exercises the highest civil jurisdiction in Scotland, with the House of Lords as a court of appeal.

Police. The police forces in Scotland at the end of 1989 had an authorized establishment of 13,877; the strength was 12,656 men and 1,158 women. There were 5,025 part-time special constables. The total police net expenditure in Scotland was £358,565,000 for 1988–89.

Civil Judicial Statistics

England and Wales	1987	1988
Appellate Courts		
Judicial Committee of the Privy Council	56	61
House of Lords	125	90
Court of Appeal	1,614	1,645
High Court of Justice (appeals and special cases from inferior courts)	2,436	2,151
Courts of First Instance (excluding Magistrates' Courts and Tribunals)		
High Court of Justice:		
Chancery Division [1]	22,868	27,054
Queen's Bench Division [2]	229,399	235,721
Family Division: Principal Registry matters [3]	1,471	1,435
District Registry wardships	2,500	2,636
Official Referee's	1,187	1,363
County courts: Matrimonial suits [4]	186,675	186,333
Other [5]	2,437,178	2,348,220
Restrictive Practices Court	5	4

Scotland	1987	1988	1989
House of Lords (Appeals from Court of Session)	12	4	–
Court of Session—			
General Department	8,938	8,977	10,806
Sheriff's Ordinary Cause	79,875	84,254	81,548
Sheriff's Summary Cause	146,158	133,157	70,725

[1] Including Companies Court, Bankruptcy petitions and Patents Court.
[2] Including Admiralty Court.
[3] Adoption, guardianship and wardship.
[4] Including petitions filed at Principal Registry.
[5] Plaint, Admiralty, Bankruptcy and Companies, Adoption, Guardianship and miscellaneous.

CRIMINAL STATISTICS

ENGLAND AND WALES

	Total number of offenders		Indictable offences [1]	
	1988	1989	1988	1989
Aged 10 and over [2]				
Proceeded against in magistrates' courts [3]	1,863,181	1,864,143	494,479	449,056
Found guilty at magistrates' courts	1,464,287	1,448,913	295,183	256,451
Found guilty at the Crown Court	91,053	85,666	91,053	83,096
Cautioned [4]	235,401	238,078	140,703	136,001
Aged 10 and under 17				
Proceeded against in magistrates' courts [3]	61,513	55,444	47,629	36,750
Found guilty at magistrates' courts	45,204	38,973	34,801	25,105
Found guilty at the Crown Court	1,646	1,400	1,646	1,355
Cautioned [4]	101,375	96,627	82,818	72,832

[1] Includes offences which can be tried either at the Crown Court or at magistrates' courts.
[2] Includes other offenders, e.g. companies, public bodies.
[3] Almost all defendants are initially proceeded against at magistrates' courts.
[4] Offenders who, on admission of guilt, are given an oral caution by or on the instruction of a senior police officer as an alternative to court proceedings. Such cautions are not given for motoring offences.

CRIMINAL STATISTICS

SCOTLAND

	All Crimes and Offences		Crimes[1]	
	1988	1989 [2]	1988	1989 [2]
All persons and companies				
Proceeded against in all courts	196,554	192,469	64,417	62,700
Charge proved	177,024	171,809	56,032	53,115
Children (aged 8–15)				
Proceeded against in all courts	429	366	283	240
Given formal police warning/ referred to reporter	23,816	22,882	16,564	16,369

[1] Crimes are generally the more serious criminal acts and offences the less serious. 'Crimes' are not equivalent in coverage to 'indictable/triable either way offences'. [2] Provisional.

Average population in prisons, youth custody centres and detention centres (1989) in England and Wales was 48,610 (convicted 39,814; untried 8,576, and 220 non-criminal prisoners); in Scotland (1989), 4,986 (sentenced, 4,216; remanded, 770).

Criminal statistics, England and Wales, 1989. HMSO, Cm1322
Prison statistics, England and Wales, 1989. HMSO, Cm1221
Paterson, A., *The Law Lords*. London, 1982

Religion. The Anglican Communion has originated from the Church of England and parallels in its fellowship of autonomous churches the evolution of British influence beyond the seas from colonies to dominions and independent nations. There is no terrestrial head of the Anglican Communion; the Archbishop of Canterbury presides as *primus inter pares* at the decennial meetings of the bishops of the Anglican Communion at the Lambeth Conference. The last Conference was held in Canterbury in 1988 and was attended by 518 bishops.

The Anglican Communion consists of 28 member Churches or Provinces. These are Australia, Brazil, Burma, Burundi, Rwanda and Zaïre, Canada, Central Africa, Council of Churches of East Asia, England, Indian Ocean, Ireland, Japan, Jerusalem and the Middle East, Kenya, Melanesia, New Zealand, Nigeria, Papua New Guinea, Scotland, Southern Africa, Southern Cone of America, Sudan, Tanzania, Uganda, USA, Wales, West Africa, West Indies. There are also areas which come under the metropolitical jurisdiction of the Archbishop of Canterbury. These are Bermuda, Ceylon, the Diocese of Europe, Falkland Islands, The Council of the Churches of

East Asia (which includes the Church in Korea), The Diocese of Hong Kong and Macao, Sabah, Kuching, Singapore, West Malaysia, The Lusitanian Church (Portugal) and The Spanish Reformed Episcopal Church.

England and Wales. The established Church of England, which baptizes about 30% of the children born in England (*i.e.* excluding Wales but including the Isle of Man and the Channel Islands), is Protestant Episcopal. Civil disabilities on account of religion do not attach to any class of British subject. Under the Welsh Church Acts, 1914 and 1919, the Church in Wales and Monmouthshire was disestablished as from 1 April 1920, and Wales was formed into a separate Province.

The Queen is, under God, the supreme governor of the Church of England, with the right, regulated by statute, to nominate to the vacant archbishoprics and bishoprics. The Queen, on the advice of the First Lord of the Treasury, also appoints to such deaneries, prebendaries and canonries as are in the gift of the Crown, while a large number of livings and also some canonries are in the gift of the Lord Chancellor.

There are 2 archbishops (at the head of the 2 Provinces of Canterbury and York), and 42 diocesan bishops including the bishop of the diocese of Europe, which is part of the Province of Canterbury. Each archbishop has also his own particular diocese, wherein he exercises episcopal, as in his Province he exercises metropolitan, jurisdiction. In Dec. 1990 there were 68 suffragan and assistant bishops, 40 deans and provosts of cathedrals and 108 archdeacons. The *General Synod*, which replaced the Church Assembly in 1970 in England, consists of a House of Bishops, a House of Clergy and a House of Laity, and has power to frame legislation regarding Church matters. Each House has a veto over the others. The first two Houses consist of the members of the Convocations of Canterbury and York, each of which consists of the diocesan bishops and elected representatives of the suffragan bishops, 6 for Canterbury province and 3 for York (forming an Upper House), deans, provosts, and archdeacons, and a certain number of proctors elected as the representatives of the inferior clergy, together with, in the case of Canterbury Convocation, 4 representatives of the Universities of Oxford, Cambridge, London and the Southern Universities and in the case of York 2 representatives for the Universities of Durham and Newcastle and the other Northern Universities; the chaplains in the Forces and 2 representatives of the Religious Communities (forming the Lower House). The House of Laity is elected by the lay members of the Deanery Synods but also includes 3 representatives of the Religious Communities and *ex-officio* Church Commissioners and Ecclesiastical Judges. Every Measure passed by the General Synod must be submitted to the Ecclesiastical Committee, consisting of 15 members of the House of Lords nominated by the Lord Chancellor and 15 members of the House of Commons nominated by the Speaker. This committee reports on each Measure to Parliament, and the Measure receives the Royal Assent and becomes law if each House of Parliament resolves that the Measure be presented to the Queen.

Parochial affairs are managed by annual parochial church meetings and parochial church councils. At 31 Dec. 1989 there were 13,155 ecclesiastical parishes, inclusive of the Isle of Man and the Channel Islands. These parishes do not, in many cases, coincide with civil parishes. Although most parishes have their own churches, not every parish nowadays can have its own incumbent or minister. In Dec. 1990 there were 6,734 beneficed clergymen excluding dignitaries, 1,331 other clergymen of incumbent status and 1,703 assistant curates working in the parishes.

Women were admitted to Holy Orders for the first time in the Church of England in 1987. At 31 Dec. 1990 there were 596 full-time stipendiary women deacons, 532 of whom were in the parochial ministry.

Private persons possess the right of presentation to over 2,000 benefices; the patronage of the others belongs mainly to the Queen, the bishops and cathedrals, the Lord Chancellor, and the universities of Oxford and Cambridge. In addition to the 9,768 parochial incumbents and (male) assistant curates, there were (1990) 387 dignitaries and cathedral clergymen, 329 non-parochial clergymen working within the diocesan framework and approximately 2,000 non-parochial clergymen outside the framework.

In 1988 there were estimated to be 1·6m. Easter and 1·7m. Christmas Communicants. Reversing a decline that began in 1968, Sunday attendances increased by 1·5% in 1988 to 1,165,000.

Of the 40,393 buildings registered for the solemnization of marriages at 30 June 1990, 16,563 belonged to the Established Church and the Church in Wales and 23,830 to other religious denominations. Of the 348,492 marriages celebrated in 1988 (351,761 in 1987), 34% were in the Established Church and the Church in Wales, 17·6% in buildings of other denominations and 48·5% were civil marriages in Register Offices.

Roman Catholics in England and Wales were estimated at 4,305,608 in 1990. There were 5 archdioceses and 18 dioceses, 6,261 clergy and 2,842 parish churches and 1,174 other churches open to the public. Convents, 1,263.

The Unitarians have about 230 places of worship and 8,000 members. The Salvation Army, had, in British Territory, 1988, over 1,800 officers. They operate eventide homes, centres for the homeless, homes for children and adolescents and alcoholic rehabilitation centres.

The following is a summary of recent statistics of certain churches:

Denomination	*Full members*	*Ministers in charge*	*Local and lay preachers*
Methodist	450,406	3,399	13,378
Independent Methodist	3,870	131	—
Wesleyan Reform Union	3,026	23	145
United Reform	126,000	1,000	—
Baptist	167,466	2,111	—
Calvinistic Methodist Church of Wales	65,237	146	—
Society of Friends	18,010	—	—

There were (1989) about 410,000 Jews in the UK with about 295 synagogues; Moslems (900,000); Sikhs (175,000); Hindus (140,000).

Scotland. The Church of Scotland, which was reformed in 1560, subsequently developed a presbyterian system of church government which was established in 1690 and has continued to the present day.

The supreme court is the General Assembly, which now consists of some 1,250 members, ministers and elders in equal numbers, commissioned by presbyteries. It meets annually in May, under the presidency of a Moderator appointed by the Assembly. The Queen is normally represented by a Lord High Commissioner, but has occasionally attended in person. The royal presence in a special throne gallery in the hall but outside the Assembly symbolises the independence from state control of what is nevertheless recognised as the national Church in Scotland.

There are also 12 synods, roughly co-terminous with Regional Councils, and 46 presbyteries in Scotland, roughly co-terminous with District Councils, together with 1 presbytery of England, 1 presbytery of Europe, and 1 presbytery of Jerusalem. At the base of this conciliar structure of Church courts are the kirk sessions, of which there were 1,700 on 1 Dec. 1989, with a total of 804,468 members.

The Episcopal Church of Scotland is a province of the Anglican Church and is one of the historic Scottish churches. It consists of 7 dioceses. As at 31 Dec. 1990 it had 258 churches and missions, 287 clergy and 57,934 members, of whom 35,281 were communicants.

There are in Scotland some small outstanding Presbyterian bodies and also Baptists, Congregationalists, Methodists and Unitarians.

The Roman Catholic Church which celebrated the centenary of the restoration of the Hierarchy in 1978, had in Scotland (1987) 1 cardinal, 2 archbishops and 9 bishops, 1,066 clergy, 472 parishes, and 798,150 adherents.

The proportion of marriages in Scotland according to the rites of the various Churches in 1989 was: Church of Scotland, 40%; Roman Catholic, 12·4%; Episcopal, 1·5%; United Free, 0·3%; others, 4·5%; civil, 41·4%.

Education (England and Wales). *The Publicly Maintained System of Education:* Compulsory schooling begins at the age of 5 and the minimum leaving age for all pupils is 16[1]. No tuition fees are payable in any publicly maintained school (but it is open to parents, if they choose, to pay for their children to attend other schools). The post-school stage, which is voluntary, includes universities, polytechnics and other further and higher education establishments (including those which provide courses for the training of teachers), as well as adult education and the youth service. Financial assistance is generally available to students on higher education courses in the university and non-university sectors and to some students on other courses in further education.

Nursery Education. Provision for children under 5 is made in either nursery schools or in nursery or infant classes in primary schools. In the public sector no fees are payable. In Jan. 1990 there were 564 maintained nursery schools and 4,688 primary schools with nursery classes. There were 51,582 pupils under 5 attending nursery schools and 525,696 pupils under 5 in nursery and infant classes. About 51% of all these children were attending part-time.

Primary Schools. These provide for pupils from the age of 5 up to the age of 11. In Jan. 1990 there were 18,952 primary schools in England of which 2,738 were infant schools providing for pupils up to the age of about 7, the remainder mainly taking pupils from age 5 through to 11. Nearly all primary schools take both boys and girls. 20% of primary schools had 100 full time pupils or less.

There are 1,718 primary schools in Wales. In those primary schools (and some secondary schools) which are in the predominantly Welsh-speaking areas, the main language of instruction is Welsh. There are also 'Welsh', or, more accurately, bilingual schools in mainly English-speaking parts of Wales. Generally children transfer from primary to secondary schools at 11.

[1] As a result of the Education (School Leaving Dates) Act 1976, one of the two former leaving dates was amended. This means that pupils whose dates of birth fall between 1 Feb. and 31 Aug. (inclusive) cease to be of compulsory school age on the Friday before the last Monday in May. Some of these pupils will leave school before their 16th birthdays. Pupils whose dates of birth fall between 1 Sept. and 31 Jan. (inclusive) remain of compulsory school age until the end of the Easter term following their 16th birthdays.

Middle Schools. A number of local education authorities operate a middle school system. These provide for pupils from the age of 8, 9 or 10 up to the age of 12, 13 or 14. In Jan. 1990 there were 1,093 middle schools in England deemed either primary or secondary according principally to the age range of the school concerned. This number is 20 fewer than in 1989.

Secondary Schools. These usually provide for pupils from the age of 11 upwards. In Jan. 1990 there were 3,453 secondary schools in England and 230 in Wales. In England some local education authorities have retained selection at age 11 for entry to grammar schools of which there were 150 such schools in 1990. There were a small number of technical schools in 1987 which specialise to a greater or lesser extent in technical studies. There were 214 secondary modern schools in 1989 providing a general education up to the minimum school leaving age of 16, although exceptionally some pupils may be allowed to stay on beyond that age in these schools.

Almost all local education authorities operate a system of comprehensive schools to which pupils are admitted without reference to ability or aptitude. In Jan. 1990 there were 3,082 such schools in England with just over 2·5m. pupils. With the development of comprehensive education various patterns of secondary schools have come into operation. Principally these are: 1. all through schools with pupils aged 11 to 18 or 11 to 16; pupils over 16 being able to transfer to an 11 to 18 school or a sixth form college providing for pupils aged 16 to 19. (There were 113 sixth form colleges in England in 1990). 2. local education authorities operating a three-tier system involving middle schools where transfer to secondary school is at ages 12, 13 or 14. These correspond to 12 to 18, 13 to 18 and 14 to 18 comprehensive schools respectively; or 3. in areas where there are no middle schools a two-tier system of junior and senior comprehensive schools for pupils aged 11 to 18 with optional transfer to these schools at age 13 or 14.

There were a number of other secondary schools of various combinations of grammar, technical or modern in Wales in 1988. There were 41 secondary using Welsh as a teaching medium, of these 16 are designated bilingual schools.

Grant Maintained Schools. Since 1988 all local education authority maintained secondary, middle and primary schools with 300 or more registered pupils can apply for Grant Maintained status and receive direct grants from the Department of Education and Science. The governing body of such a school is responsible for all aspects of school management, including the deployment of funds, employment of staff and provision of most of the educational support services for staff and pupils. In Jan. 1991 there were 50 Grant Maintained schools in England and Wales.

City Technology Colleges. New legislation in 1988 enabled the Secretary of State for Education and Science, in partnership with sponsors from business and industry, to fund the establishment of City Technology Colleges. These are secondary schools for 11-18 year olds, having a broad curriculum with an emphasis on science and technology. The schools are independent of local education authorities. Their capital costs are shared between central Government and sponsors with Government meeting all recurrent costs. They do not charge fees.

Assisted Places Scheme. In order to give able children a wider range of educational opportunity the Government set up, in 1981, the Assisted Places Scheme to give help with tuition fees at certain independent schools to parents who could not otherwise afford them. In the school year 1989–90, the 278 participating schools offered a total of 5,706 assisted places, 4,520 for entry at age 11, 12, and 13, and 984 for entry at sixth form level. A further 17 schools joined the Scheme in Sept. 1990, providing an extra 69 places for entry at age 11, 12 or 13.

Special Education. The majority of children with special educational needs attend special schools, including hospital and non-maintained special schools and independent schools under arrangements made by local education authorities. The total number of children with statements under the 1981 Education Act is around 138,800.

Of maintained special schools, 1,110 are day schools, 156 are mainly boarding schools and there are 50 hospital special schools. Attendance is compulsory from 5–16. In addition, the Act's definition of special educational needs applies to children under 5 who are likely to have a learning difficulty when over this age, or whose learning difficulty would be likely to persist if special educational provision were not made for them. Authorities also have a duty to make special educational provision either in a school or in a college of further education for children aged 16–18 who have been assessed as being in need of, and who want, such provision. In addition to the provision in ordinary and special schools, authorities can make special arrangements for educating children at home, in small groups or in hospitals. There are also some establishments which provide further education, P.E. vocational training and for assessment for employment purely for disabled school leavers.

Ancillary Services. Local education authorities may provide registered pupils at any school maintained by them with milk, meals and refreshment and they may make such charges as they think fit for anything they provide. For pupils whose parents are in receipt of supplementary benefit or family income supplement, however, authorities are required to ensure that such provision is made for the pupil at midday as appears to them to be requisite and anything which is provided must be free of charge. Facilities must also be provided, free of charge, for consuming any meals or other refreshments which pupils bring to school themselves.

Further and Higher Education (Non-University). In Nov. 1987 there were about 475 institutions in England providing courses of further education, ranging from shorthand instruction to degree-level, postgraduate work and courses of teacher-training. Course enrolments numbered 609,308 full-time (including 76,907 sandwich students) and 1·6m. part-time and evening (including 498,629 students released by their employers). There were in addition 2,412 Adult Education Centres (formerly known as Evening Institutes), which provided mainly part-time courses of non-advanced general education and were attended by 1,371,037 students. In April 1989, 29 polytechnics and 55 colleges of higher education were brought together under the Polytechnics and Colleges Funding Council to create a new sector of higher education in England. The institutions offer both further and higher education courses, many leading to degrees of a standard comparable to those in universities or to professional qualifications. They cater for a mixture of full-time, part-time and sandwich students. Enrolments to the sector in 1988 totalled 293,000. In Wales the polytechnic and 4 other higher education institutions are scheduled to become independent of the local authorities in April 1992 and be funded by the Welsh Office.

Courses were also provided by the Workers' Educational Association, the University extramural departments and the Welsh National Council of YMCAs.

Education at institutions of further education is not free, but fees are generally low, and are remitted for most students under the age of 18 by the local authority.

The Youth Service. The Youth Service forms part of the education system and is concerned with promoting the personal development and social education of young people through a wide range of leisure-time activities. A duty is laid upon local education authorities by the provisions of the 1944 Education Act to secure the adequacy of such facilities for young people in their area. The Education Reform Act 1988 retained the force of these provisions. To this end they either provide, maintain and staff youth clubs, centres and other facilities themselves or assist voluntary agencies to do so.

Grants to voluntary agencies to help meet the cost of regional and national capital projects and to national voluntary bodies in support of a range of programmes of work and training expenses are made by the Government. Grants are also made to support the work of the 4 National Youth Service Bodies on the basis of annual work programmes.

Awards to Students. Local education authorities in England and Wales are responsible for making mandatory awards to suitably qualified students taking first-degree and comparable courses, courses of initial teacher-training and certain other advanced level courses. These awards cover fees and maintenance but the maintenance grants are subject to the income of the student and his parents or spouse. In addition scholarships may be available both from universities and other sources. The authorities may also give discretionary awards to students who do not qualify for mandatory awards including those taking non-degree level courses.

In 1986–87 there were 441,997 full value awards current, 44% at universities and 34,551 mandatory awards for initial teacher-training courses. Lesser value awards, which are paid below the full rate of the student's fees and maintenance, were also made by the authorities. There were 115,694 such awards taken up in the academic year 1986–87.

The Research Council gave over 6,600 new awards in 1987–88 and there were more than 13,000 current awards in that academic year. In 1988–89 the British Academy gave 924 new awards and the Department 594 state bursaries and 70 state scholarships.

Teachers. To attain qualified teacher status, for work in maintained schools in England and Wales, teachers must have successfully completed a course of professional training. This can be either by completion of a recognized course of initial teacher training at an higher education institution or, in the case of mature entrants and overseas trained teachers, a period of 'on the job' training as a licensed teacher. EC nationals who are recognized as qualified teachers in other member states will usually be entitled, on application, to automatic qualified teacher status.

In Nov. 1990 there were about 41,000 students on initial teacher-training courses.

On 1 Jan. 1990, 424,000 teachers were employed by local education authorities in maintained nursery, primary and secondary schools in England and Wales.

Finance. Total current and capital expenditure on education in England (including Universities GB, and Mandatory Awards England and Wales) from public funds is estimated at £21,667m. for 1990–91 as compared with £19,677m. for 1989–90.

Scotland. The statistics on schools relate to education authority and grant-aided schools. All teachers employed in these schools require to be qualified; figures given are full-time equivalents.

Nursery Education. In Sept. 1989 there were 633 nursery schools and departments, with a total enrolment of 42,269 pupils.

Primary Education. In Sept. 1989 there were 2,378 primary schools and departments and the number on the registers was 437,072. In Sept. 1989, 22,186 teachers were employed in primary schools and departments.

Secondary Education. In Sept. 1989 there were 429 secondary schools with 298,587 pupils. Of these schools, 423 were all-comprehensive and 6 part-selective. All but 40 schools provided a full range of Scottish Certificate of Education courses and non-certificate courses. Pupils who start their secondary education in schools which do not cater for a full range of courses may be transferred at the end of their second or fourth year to schools where a full range of courses is provided. There were 24,143 teachers in secondary schools at Sept. 1989.

Special Schools. In Sept. 1989 there were 338 special schools and departments. 8,386 children were under instruction.

Further Education. In 1988–89 there were 181 colleges and centres of further education. with 267,571 students, of whom 65,406 attended full-time (advanced courses, 32,641; non-advanced, 32,735) and 202,165 part-time (advanced courses, 22,527; non-advanced, 179,000).

Teacher Training. In Sept. 1989 there were 3,845 students in 5 colleges of education on pre-service courses of teacher-training.

Finance. Total expenditure on education met from revenue in 1988–89 was £2,012m. (excluding university education and loan charges).

Independent Schools. Outside the state system of education there were in England 2,283 independent schools in Jan. 1990, ranging from large 'public' schools to small local ones. There were (Jan. 1990) 539,512 full-time and 19,233 part-time pupils in these schools. In Wales (1990) 12,075 full-time pupils attended 67 independent schools. Fees are charged by all these schools, which receive no grant from central government sources. All independent schools in England (and Wales) are required to be registered by the Department of Education and Science (and the Welsh Office) and are liable to the inspection by HM Inspectors. The term 'public schools' refers to independent schools in membership of the Headmasters' Conference, Governing Bodies Association or the Governing Bodies of Girls' Schools Association. Qualifications under which a school may be represented at the Headmasters' Conference include the measure of independence enjoyed by the governing body and the amount of advanced courses undertaken. Some of these schools are for boarders only, but the majority include non-resident 'day-pupils'. In Scotland there were 121 independent schools, with a total of 33,071 pupils in Sept. 1989. A small number of the Scottish independent schools are of the 'public school' type but they are not known as 'public schools' since in Scotland this term is used to denote education authority (*i.e.*, state) schools.

The earliest of the schools were founded by, and attached to, medieval churches. Many were founded as 'grammar' (classical) schools in the 16th century, receiving charters from the reigning sovereign. Reformed mainly in the middle of the 19th century, among the best-known are Eton College, founded in 1440 by Henry VI; Winchester College (1394) founded by William of Wykeham, Bishop of Winchester; Harrow School, founded in 1560 as a grammar school by John Lyon, a yeoman; and Charterhouse (1611). Among the earliest foundations are King's School, Canterbury, founded 600; King's School, Rochester (604) and St Peter's, York, (627).

Universities. In *England* there are 34 traditional degree-giving universities. In addition there are the London and Manchester Business Schools and the Open University.

In *Wales* there is 1 university, the University of Wales, with constituent colleges at Aberystwyth, Bangor, Cardiff, Lampeter and Swansea. The University of Wales College of Medicine is a college of the University. The University of Wales College of Cardiff was formed in 1988 by the merger of University College Cardiff and the University of Wales Institute of Science and Technology.

In *Scotland* there are 8 universities, St Andrews, Glasgow, Aberdeen and Edinburgh Universities date from the 15th and 16th centuries while the others, Strathclyde, Heriot-Watt, Stirling and Dundee have been formally established since the early 1960s.

All these universities and colleges are independent, self-governing institutions, although they receive substantial aid from the State (in the case of the Open University by direct grant from the Department of Education and Science, and the traditional universities through the Universities Funding Council). The Universities Funding Council, is a non-departmental public body with full executive responsibility for distributing to universities funds provided for that purpose by the Secretary of State for Education and Science and voted by Parliament. It has 15 members, from higher education and elsewhere. The Council also advises the Secretary of State on matters relating to universities. The Government receives advice on the universities' requirements for central computing facilities from the Computer Board for the Universities and Research Councils whose members are also drawn from the universities and industry.

The Royal College of Art and the Cranfield Institute of Technology are primarily postgraduate institutions which award higher degrees under charters granted in 1967 and 1969 respectively.

The Open University received its Royal Charter on 1 June 1969 and is an independent, self-governing institution, awarding its own degrees at undergraduate and postgraduate level. It is financed by the Government through the Department of Education and Science and by the receipt of students' fees.

Tuition is by means of correspondence textbooks, audio and video cassettes, radio and television broadcasts and residential schools. Students can also attend one of over 250 local study centres for weekly, etc, classes. No formal qualifications are required for entry to undergraduate or associate student courses. Anyone resident in the EC aged 18 or over may apply, though some courses are not available outside the UK. There are about 140 undergraduate courses; many are available on a one-off basis to associate students.

In 1990 there were over 72,000 undergraduates, over 4,700 postgraduates and over 20,000 short course and associate students 65,000 packs of learning materials were sold. The university has some 3,000 full-time staff working at its Milton Keynes headquarters and in 13 regional centres throughout the country. There are 5,800 part-time tutors and counsellors.

The University of Buckingham opened in in 1976 and received a Royal charter in 1983. It is self-governing and independent of the state system. It offers 2-year courses towards its own honours degrees, the academic year commencing in Jan. and consisting of four 10-week terms. There are 4 Schools of Studies with 11 academic departments: Accounting, Business, and Economics; Humanities; Law; and Sciences. Postgraduate opportunities are offered in all the schools of studies. In 1991, there were 850 full-time students.

All universities charge fees, but financial help is available to students from several sources. The universities themselves provide scholarships of various kinds and local education authorities and the Scottish Office Education Department make loans to help suitable students to attend university. The amount of aid given generally depends upon the parents' means. The majority of university students receive some form of financial assistance. Awards known as state studentships are offered on a competitive basis by the Department of Education and Science to candidates considered by the universities and other higher education institutions to be qualified for postgraduate studies in the humanities; similar awards, tenable at universities or other higher education institutions, are offered by the Research Councils to students studying topics within the broad spectrum of agriculture and food; the biological sciences; man's natural environment; science and engineering and the social sciences at postgraduate level.

Academic staff and students (full-time and sandwich) in 1989–90:

University	*Students*	*Staff*	*University*	*Students*	*Staff*
Aston	3,733	298	Oxford	13,079	2,058
Bath	4,077	527	Reading	7,205	911
Birmingham	10,021	1,486	Salford	4,372	412
Bradford	4,760	501	Sheffield	9,073	1,161
Bristol	7,777	1,247	Southampton	6,975	1,204
Brunel	3,050	379	Surrey	3,870	561
Cambridge	13,219	2,075	Sussex	5,057	600
City	3,323	390	Warwick	6,906	894
Durham	5,338	631	York	4,078	574
East Anglia	4,518	522			
Essex	3,546	377	*Wales—*		
Exeter	5,752	598	Aberystwyth	3,617	388
Hull	5,818	522	Bangor	3,328	414
Keele	3,288	345	Cardiff	8,279	900
Kent	4,622	504	St David's, Lampeter	854	76
Lancaster	5,139	606	Swansea	5,272	496
Leeds	11,407	1,452	Univ. of Wales		
Leicester	5,657	811	College of Medicine	950	360
Liverpool	8,688	1,327			
London Business School	308	82	*Scotland—*		
London	46,014	9,293	Aberdeen	6,087	724
Loughborough	5,614	752	Dundee	3,762	523
Manchester Business School	273	48	Edinburgh	10,862	1,812
Manchester	12,249	1,845	Glasgow	11,523	1,643
Univ. of Manchester Inst. of			Heriot-Watt	4,396	440
Science and Technology	4,652	645	St Andrews	3,939	423
Newcastle	8,364	1,223	Stirling	3,416	372
Nottingham	8,004	1,146	Strathclyde	8,368	1,008

Number of women students: 143,096 (England, 109,892; Wales, 10,246; Scotland, 22,958. There are colleges exclusively for women at Oxford and Cambridge. Total number of full-time or sandwich students, 334,479 (England, 259,826; Wales, 22,300; Scotland, 52,353).

The British Council. The British Council promotes Britain abroad. Established in 1934 and incorporated by Royal Charter in 1940, it is Britain's principal agency for cultural relations overseas. An independent, non-political organization managed by a Director General and governed by a Board, it is represented in 90 countries, where it has 154 offices, 118 libraries and 56 English teaching centres. Its headquarters are in London and there are offices in Edinburgh, Cardiff, Belfast and 21 other university centres in Britain.

The Council's estimated expenditure for 1991–92 is £395m. This is made up of government grants (£120m.), revenue from English teaching and client-funded services (£91m.) and programmes, principally in education and training, which are managed on behalf of the British government and other clients (£184m.).

Each year the Council brings to Britain some 38,000 professional visitors, students and trainees from overseas and sends abroad 4,000 British specialists on advisory visits or teaching appointments. It is involved with about 1,000 arts events from Britain, and runs a programme of short courses, seminars and summer schools for 2,000 specialists from 100 countries, notably in medicine, science, literature and the arts, education and English language teaching.

Chairman: Sir David Orr, MC.
Director-General: Sir Richard Francis, KCMG.
Headquarters: 10 Spring Gdns., London, SW1A 2BN.

British Council. *Annual Report and Accounts.*
Donaldson, F., *The British Council: the First Fifty Years.* London, 1984.

National Insurance. The National Insurance Act, 1946, came into operation on 5 July 1948, repealing the existing schemes of health, pensions and unemployment insurance. This Act, along with later legislation, was consolidated as the National Insurance Act, 1965.

The Social Security Act 1975 introduced, from 6 April 1975, a new system of national insurance contributions to replace the previous system of flat-rate and graduated contributions. Since 6 April 1975, Class 1 contributions have been related to the employee's earnings and are collected with PAYE income tax, instead of by affixing stamps to a card. Class 2 and Class 3 contributions remain flat-rate, but, in addition to Class 2 contributions, those who are self-employed may be liable to pay Class 4 contributions, which for the year 1990–91 will be at the rate of 6·3% on profits or gains between £5,450 and £18,200, which are assessable for income tax under Schedule D. The non-employed and others whose contribution record is not sufficient to give entitlement to benefits are able to pay a Class 3 contribution voluntarily to qualify for a limited range of benefits. Class 2 weekly contributions for 1990–91 for men and women are £4·55. Class 3 contributions are £4·45 a week.

From 6 April 1978 the Social Security Pensions Act 1975 introduced earnings-related retirement, invalidity and widows' pensions. Employee's national insurance contribution liability depends on whether he is in contracted-out or not contracted-out employment.

Full rate contributions (contribution table leters A or D or Mariner's equivalents) for non contracted-out employment in 1990–91: On earnings between £46 and £79.99 a week the employee pays 2% on the first £46 and 9% on the remainder, the employers pay 5% on all earnings; on earnings between £80 and £124.99 a week the employee pays 2% on the first £46 and 9% on the remainder, the employer pays 7% on all earnings; on earnings between £125 and £174.99 a week the employee pays 2% on the first £46 and 9% on the remainder, the employer pays 9% on all earnings; on earnings between £175 and £350 a week the employee pays 2% on the first £46 and 9% on the remainder, the employer pays 10·45% on all earnings; on earnings of over £350 a week the employee pays 2% on the first £46 and 9% on earnings between £46 and £350 but the employer pays 10·45% of all earnings. For contracted-out employment in 1990–91: On earnings between £46 and £79.99 a week the employee pays 2% on the first £46 and 7% on the remainder and the employer pays 5% on the first £46 and 1·2% on the remainder; on earnings between £80 and £124.99 a week the employee pays 2% on the first £46 and 7% on the remainder and the employer pays 7% on the first £46 and 3·2% on the remainder; on earnings between £125 and £174.99 a week the employee pays 2% on the first £46 and 7% on the remainder and the employer pays 9% on the first £46 and 5·2% on the remainder; on earnings between £175 and £350 a week the employee pays 2% on the first £46 and 7% on the remainder and the employer pays 10·45% on the first £46 and 6·65% on the remainder; on earnings of over £350 a week the employee pays 2% on the first £46 and 7% on earnings between £46 and £350 and the employer pays 10·45% on the first £46, 6·65% on earnings between £46 and £350 and 10·45% on the remainder.

Reduced rate contributions (contribution table letters B or E) for non contracted-out and contracted-out employment in 1990-91: On earnings between £46 and £350 a week the employee pays 3·85% of the full amount, including that part which is below £46; on earnings over £350 a week the employee pays 3·85% of £350. The employer pays contributions as shown in the preceding paragraph - there is no equivalent reduced rate for employers.

The State supplements the contributions paid by contributors and employers, from general taxation. Contributions and supplement together with interest on investments form the income of the National Insurance Fund from which benefits are paid.

Statutory Sick Pay (SSP). Employers are now responsible for paying statutory sick pay (SSP) to their employees for up to 28 weeks in any period of incapacity for work. Basically, all employees aged 16 years and over are covered by the scheme whenever they are sick for 4 or more days consecutively. For most employees SSP completely replaces their entitlement to State sickness benefit which is not payable as long as any employer's responsibility for SSP remains.

Benefits. Qualification for any benefit depends upon fulfilment of the appropriate contribution conditions. Persons who are incapable of work as the result of an industrial accident may get sickness benefit followed by invalidity benefit without having to satisfy the contributions conditions. Employed persons may qualify for all the benefits; self-employed may not qualify for unemployment benefit.

Sickness Benefit. From 11 April 1991 the rate is £39·60 a week plus £24·50 a week for an adult dependant.

Unemployment Benefit is paid through the local unemployment benefit offices of the Department of Employment. The rate is £41·40 a week plus £25·55 a week for an adult dependant.

Invalidity Benefit replaces sickness benefit after 168 days of entitlement. It comprises a basic invalidity pension of £52·00 weekly and an invalidity allowance of £11·10 if incapacity began before age 40: £6·90 if incapacity began between 40 and 49 or £3·45 if it began between 50 and 59 (54 for women). Increases are: £31·25 for an adult dependant plus £9·70 for a child for whom the higher rate of child benefit is payable and £10·70 for each other child for whom child benefit is payable. Invalidity allowance is reduced or extinguished by the amount of any additional invalidity pension and/or guaranteed minimum pension to which there is title.

Maternity Benefit. Statutory maternity pay may be payable to a woman from her employer if she has been employed by him for 6 months into the 15th week before the baby is expected and her earnings were above the lower earnings limit. If she has been employed by the same employer for at least 2 years, payment for the first 6 weeks of maternity absence may be at 90% of her average earnings. Payment for the remainder of the period is at a standard rate of £44·50. Women who do not qualify for statutory maternity pay may be entitled to maternity allowance from DSS if they satisfy a test of recent work and contributions paid. From April 1991, the weekly rate is £40·60. Both statutory maternity pay and maternity allowance can be paid for up to 18 weeks. Payment can start at the earliest 11 weeks before the expected week of confinement but the woman has some choice in deciding when to give up work and still retain title to the full 18 weeks.

Widow's Benefits. From 11 April 1988 the three main widow's benefits, will be: Widow's payment, widowed mother's allowance, widow's pension.

A widow cannot get any widow's benefits based on her husband's NI if: She had been divorced from the man who has died; or she was living with the man as if she were married to him, but without being legally married to him; or she is living with another man as if she is married to him. A widow can only get widow's benefits if her husband has paid enough NI contributions.

Widow's Payment is a single tax-free payment of £1,000. A widow may be able to get this benefit if her husband has paid enough NI contributions and: She was under 60 when her husband died; or her husband was not getting a State Retirement Pension when he died.

Widowed Mother's Allowance: A widow may be able to get a widowed mother's allowance if her husband has paid enough NI contributions and: She is receiving child benefit for one of her children; or her husband was receiving child benefit, or she is expecting her husband's baby, or if she was widowed before 11 April 1988 she has a young person under 19 living with her for whom she was receiving Child Benefit.

A widow entitled to a widowed mother's allowance will get an amount based on her husband's NI contributions. The maximum will be £52·00 a week. She will also get £9·70 a week for her eldest dependent child and £10·70 for each subsequent child and she may also get an additional pension based on her husband's earnings since 1978. Widowed mother's allowance is usually paid as long as the widow is getting child benefit. It is taxable.

Widow's Pension: A widow may be able to get a widow's pension if her husband has paid enough NI contributions. She must be 45 or over (40 or over if widowed before 11 April 1988) when her husband died or when her widowed mother's allowance ends. A widow cannot get a widow's pension at the same time as a widowed mother's allowance. A widow who is entitled to a widow's pension will get an amount that depends on her age when her husband died or when her widowed mother's allowance ends. If she was 55 or over (50 or over if widowed before 11 April 1988) she will get the full rate of widow's pension. The maximum amount of widow's pension will be £52·00 a week. She may also get an additional pension based on her husband's earnings since 1978. Widow's pension is usually paid until the widow is entitled to state retirement pension, when she is 60 or older. Widow's pension is taxable.

Guardian's Allowance. A person responsible for an orphan child may be entitled to a guardian's allowance of £10·70 a week in addition to child benefit. Normally both the child's parents must be dead but when they never married or were divorced, or one is missing, or serving a long sentence of imprisonment, the allowance may be paid on the death of one parent only.

Retirement Pension. In order to receive a retirement pension, subject to satisfying the contributions before 1 Oct. 1989, men over 65, and women over 60, whether retired from regular employment or not, must make a claim. From 6 April 1979 a woman divorced over the age of 60 must satisfy the retirement conditions before a pension is payable. The standard rates of basic pensions are £52·00 a week for a man or woman on his or her own contributions and £31·25 for a married woman through her husband's contributions. Proportionately reduced pensions are payable where contribution records are deficient. For a person who reaches pension age on or after 6 April 1979, additional pension may also be payable. This is based on the earnings on which he or she has paid Class I or Class II contributions in each complete tax year between April 1978 and pension age. If the person has been a member of a contracted-out occupational pension scheme, that scheme will be responsible for paying the whole or part of the additional pension. An increase of £31·25 a week may be payable for a dependent wife. A tapered earnings rule (£45·09) applies to claims made before 16 Sept. 1985. From that date the earnings rule will apply in these circumstances. When the spouse/ woman looking after the claimant's child is living with the claimant an adult dependant's allowance will only be payable if the dependant's earnings do not exceed the standard rate of unemployment benefit for a person under pensionable age (currently £41·40). If she does not reside with the beneficiary an increase is not payable if she earns more than £31·25 a week. In addition £9·70 a week may be payable for the eldest child for whom child benefit is payable and £10·70 for each subsequent child. In certain circumstances an increase of £31·25 a week may be payable for a woman having care of the pensioner's children. In addition, a man who had paid graduated contributions receives 6·81p per week for every £7·50 of graduated contributions paid, and a woman 6·81p per week for every £9 paid. Although no further graduated contributions have been paid after April 1975, pension already earned will be paid along with the basic pension in the normal way.

Before 1 Oct. 1989 if, after being awarded a retirement pension, a man under 70 or a woman under 65 earned more than £75 in a calendar week the pension for the next pension week, including any increase for dependants, was reduced by 5p for every 10p earned between £75 and £79 and by 5p for every 5p earned over £79. If retirement was postponed after minimum pension age increments of all components of the pension could be earned for periods of deferred retirement. From 6 April 1979 increments were earned at the rate of one-seventh penny per £1 of basic pension for every 6 days (excluding Sundays) for which pension had been foregone. Any days for which another benefit was paid did not count. These increments had to be at least 1% of the pension rate unless the minimum was earned under the arrangements which applied before 6 April 1979. On 1 Oct 1989 this 'earnings rule' was abolished, and the pension for which a person has qualified may be paid in full whether a person continues in work or not irrespective of the amount of earnings.

At the age of 80 an age addition of £0·25 a week is payable. In addition non-contributory pensions are now payable, subject to residence conditions, to persons aged 80 and over who do not qualify for a retirement pension or qualify for one at a low rate. The rates of these pensions, which are financed by Exchequer funds, are £31·25 a week for a single person and £18·70 for a married woman. These amounts do not include the £0·25 age addition. From 22 Dec. 1984 the lower rate of category D retirement pension payable to married women was abolished.

The Industrial Injuries Provisions of the Social Security Act, 1975. The Industrial Injuries Act, which also came into operation on 5 July 1948, with its later amending Acts, was consolidated as the National Insurance (Industrial Injuries) Act, 1965. This legislation was incorporated in the Social Security Act, 1975. The scheme provides a system of insurance against 'personal injury by accident arising out of and in the course of employment' and against certain prescribed diseases and injuries due to the nature of the employment. It takes the place of the Workmen's Compensation Acts and covers persons who are employed earners under the Social Security Act. There are no contribution conditions for the payment of benefit. Three types of benefit are provided:

(1) Disablement benefit. This is payable where, as the result of an industrial accident or prescribed disease, there is a loss of physical or mental faculty. The loss of faculty will be assessed as a percentage by comparison with a person of the same age and sex whose condition is normal. If the assessment is between 14-100% benefit will be paid as weekly pension; 14-19% are payable at the 20% rate. The rates vary from £16·98 (20% disabled) to £84·90 (100% disablement). Assessments of less than 14% do not normally attract basic benefit except for certain progressive chest diseases. Pensions for persons under 18 are at a reduced rate. When injury benefit was abolished for industrial accidents occurring and prescribed diseases commencing on or after 6 April 1983, a common start date was introduced for the payment of disablement benefit 90 days (excluding Sundays) after the date of the relevant accident or onset of the disease. The following increases can be paid with disablement benefit: Constant attendance allowance – where the disability for which the claimant is receiving disablement benefit is assessed at 100% and is so severe that they need constant care and attention. There are 4 rates depending on the amount of attendance needed. Exceptionally severe disablement allowance – where the claimant is in receipt of constant attendance allowance at one of the two higher rates and the need for attendance is likely to be permanent.

Reduced earnings allowance is now a separate benefit. Entitlement exists if the claimant has not retired and cannot go back to their normal job or do another job for the same pay because of the effects of the disability caused by an accident or disease which occurred on or before 30 Sept. 1990. It can be paid whether or not disablement benefit is paid, providing the disablement benefit assessment is 1% or more (*e.g.* where disablement is assessed at less than 14%) and on top of 100% disablement benefit. From 1 Oct. 1989, if a claimant is of pensionable age (60 for a woman, 65 for a man) they can continue to receive REA if they are in regular employment, or in some cases if they are receiving Sickness Benefit, Invalidity Benefit or Unemployment Benefit. It will not matter whether or not they receive State Retirement Pension. If they are not in regular employment then entitlement to REA will cease. In most cases it will be replaced by Retirement Allowance.

(2) *Death Benefit.* This is payable to the widow of a person who died before 11 April 1988 as the result of an industrial accident or a prescribed disease. Benefit is a weekly pension of either £52·00 or £15·60 depending on such factors as age and entitlement to a child's allowance. A child allowance of £10·70 per child may be payable to the widow if she is entitled to child benefit for children of the deceased. Deaths which occurred on or after 11 April 1988 – a widow is entitled to full widow's benefits even if her late husband did not satisfy the contribution condition, if he died as a result of an industrial accident or prescribed disease.

Allowances may be paid to people who are suffering from pneumoconiosis or byssinosis or certain other slowly developing diseases due to employment before 5 July 1948. They must at any time have been entitled to benefit for the disabled under the Industrial Injuries provision of the Social Security Act or compensation under Workmen's Compensation Acts or received damages through the courts.

In certain cases supplementation allowances are payable to people who are getting or are entitled to compensation under the Workmen's Compensation Acts.

War Pensions. The number of beneficiaries in receipt of war (1914–18) pensions or allowances as at 31 Dec. 1989 was 6,163. The number of beneficiaries in receipt of war (1939–45 and later) pensions or allowances in payment as at 31 Dec. 1989 was 245,814. The expenditure for both wars for 1988–89 was £610·34m.

National Insurance Fund. At 1 April 1988 the balance of the National Insurance Fund amounted to £7,287,620,000. Income during the period 1 April 1988 to 31 March 1989, consisting of contributions from insured persons and employers, payments from the Exchequer and interest on investments, etc., was £29,825,327,000. Payments of benefit in respect of unemployment were £1,106,745,000; injury and sickness, £191,960,000; invalidity, £3,359,358,000; maternity, £26,870,000; widows, £850,164,000; guardian's allowance and child's special allowance, £1,352,000; retirement pension, £19,237,593,000; disablement benefits, £454,973,000; death benefits, £58,610,000. Included in these figures are the following estimated amounts of additional component, £777,104,000; earnings related supplement having ceased. Administrative and other payments cost approximately £1,168,039,000. The balance at 31 March 1989 was £10,368,808,000.

From 1 April 1975 the National Insurance Reserve Fund and the Industrial Injuries Fund were merged with the National Insurance Fund. All basic scheme contributions payable under the 1975 Social Security Act are paid into the single fund out of which the existing range of benefits is financed. The National Insurance Fund receives a Treasury Supplement; for 1988–89 this was set at a level of 5% of total contribution income. Payment of Disablement Benefit has come out of the General Consolidated Fund since April 1990.

Child Benefit. Child benefit is a tax-free cash allowance for children. The weekly rate for the eldest qualifying child was £8·25 from 6 April 1991, rising to £9·25 from Oct. 1991. Benefit for subsequent children from Oct. 1991 is £7·50. From April 1992 child benefit is to be indexed. Child benefit is payable for children under 16, for 16 and 17 year olds registered for work or training and for those under 19 receiving full-time non-advanced education. *One Parent Benefit* is a tax-free cash allowance for certain people bringing up children alone. It is payable for the first or only child in the family in addition to child benefit. The weekly rate from 9 April 1990 is £5·60.

Family Credit. Family Credit is a tax-free benefit for working families with children. To be able to get Family Credit there must be at least one child under 16 in the family (or under 19 if in full-time education up to, and including, A level or equivalent standard). The claimant or partner (if there is one) must be working at least 24 hours a week to qualify. They may be employed or self-employed, a lone parent or a couple. The claim should be made by the woman in two parent families. The amount of family credit payable depends on the income of the claimant and partner, how many children there are in the family and their ages. The same rates of benefit are paid for one-parent families as for two-parent families. Family Credit is not payable if the claimant (or claimant and partner together) have savings or capital of over £8,000. Benefit is reduced if savings or capital of more than £3,000 is held.

Family Credit is paid at the same rate for 26 weeks. The amount of the award will usually stay the same even if earnings, or other circumstances, change during that period.

Attendance allowance. This is a tax-free non-contributory allowance for severely disabled people who require a lot of help from another person. There are 2 rates, the higher rate of £41·65 a week for those who require attention or supervision by day and night, and the lower rate of £27·80 a week for those who need the attendance either by day or night. In addition to the medical requirements a simple test of residence and presence in Great Britain must also be satisfied.

Invalid Care Allowance. This is a non-contributory taxable benefit which may be paid to those who stay at home to care for a person who is receiving attendance allowance or constant attendance allowance. Current rate £31·25 a week, with increases for dependants.

Income Support. Under the Social Security Act, 1986, benefit is payable to any persons in Great Britain aged 18 years or over (excluding persons at school or college or anyone directly involved in a trade dispute) who are not in full-time work or who work for less than 24 hours per week and who are without resources, or whose resources (including national insurance benefits) need to be supplemented in order to meet their requirements. Income Support is not payable if the claimant (or claimant and partner together) have savings or capital over £8,000. Benefit is reduced if savings or capital of more than £3,000 is held. A person who is excluded from benefit under the normal rules may, nevertheless, receive payments to meet urgent need. The general standards by reference to which income support is granted are determined by statutory regulations approved by Parliament. Persons dissatisfied with the benefit granted may appeal to an independent Appeal Tribunal.

National Health. The National Health Service (NHS) in England and Wales started on 5 July 1948 under the National Health Service Act, 1946. There are separate Acts for Scotland and for Northern Ireland, where the Health Services are run on similar lines to those in England and Wales.

The NHS is a charge on the national income in the same way e.g. as the armed forces. Every person normally resident in this country is entitled to use any complete part of the services, and no insurance qualification is necessary. Most of the cost of running the service is met from the national exchequer, *i.e.*, from taxes.

Since Sept. 1957 a small weekly National Health Service contribution has been payable by contributors and where applicable by their employers. For convenience this contribution is collected with the National Insurance contribution and for 1991–92 is estimated to be £4,098m. for Great Britain.

Organization. Under the provisions of the NHS Act, 1977 and the Health Service Act, 1980, the administration of the NHS in England and Wales is organized under a system of regional and district health authorities accountable to the Secretary of State for the Social Services and the Secretary of State for Wales. In Scotland the National Health Service is administered under the National Health Service (Scotland) Act, 1978, by 15 Health Boards and a Common Services Agency, all accountable to the Secretary of State for Scotland.

There are 190 district health authorities in England responsible for the administration and development of health services in their district. 14 regional health authorities, each consisting of a number of health districts, are responsible for allocating resources between the district health authorities in their regions and for monitoring their performance. The regional authorities are responsible for developing strategic plans and priorities and for carrying out certain executive functions.

The National Health Service and Community Care Act, 1990, provided for a major restructuring of the existing organization of the NHS. From 1 April 1991, health authorities became the purchasers of health care, concentrating on their responsibilities to plan and obtain services for their local residents by the placement of health service contracts with the appropriate units. Day-to-day management tasks became the responsibility of hospitals and other units, with whom the contracts are placed, in their capacity as providers of care. Provider units will be able to choose to become NHS Trusts, with greater control over their own affairs. Some general medical practitioners (GPs) will be able to join the GP fund holding scheme, purchasing a range of care directly for their patients.

Services. The NHS broadly consists of hospital and specialist services, general medical, dental and ophthalmic services, pharmaceutical services, community health services and school health services. All these services are free of charge except for such things as prescriptions, spectacles, dental and optical examination, dentures and dental treatment, amenity beds in hospitals and for some of the community services, for which charges are made with certain exemptions.

The total cost of the Health and Personal Social Services (England) is estimated at £23,665m. for 1989–90 (Local Authority Personal Social Service being £3,750m.).

The number of abortions performed in England and Wales 1989 under the provisions of the Abortion Act, 1967, was 183,974 (183,798 in 1988). Of these, 170,463 abortions were to England and Wales residents, of which 113,001 were to single women, 38,138 to married women, and 19,324 were to widowed, divorced or separated women and to women who did not state their marital status.

The number of abortion notifications received in Scotland in 1989 under the provisions of the Abortion Act, 1967, was 10,159, of which 10,143 related to Scottish residents. Of these 10,143 notifications, 6,643 (5·5%) were to single women, 2,242 (22·1%) were to married women, and 1,158 (11·4%) were to widowed, divorced or separated women and to women who did not state their marital status.

In Great Britain in 1989 there were 33,291 general medical practitioners (GPs) and 17,830 general dental practitioners and (1986) 287,700 qualified nurses and mid wives. There were (1989) 356,400 average daily available hospital beds in the UK.

Personal Social Services. Under the Local Authority Social Services Act, 1970, and in Scotland the Social Work (Scotland) Act, 1968, the welfare and social work services provided by local authorities were made the responsibility of a new local authority department—the Social Services Department in England and Wales, and Social Work Departments in Scotland headed by a Director of Social Work. The social services thus administered include: the fostering, care and adoption of children, welfare services and social workers for the mentally disordered, the disabled and the aged, and accommodation for those needing residential care services. In Scotland the social work departments' functions also include the supervision of persons on probation, of adult offenders and of persons released from penal institutions or subject to fine supervision orders.

The number of supported residents in residential accommodation for the elderly and younger disabled was as follows:

England (31 March)	*Residential accommodation Adults and Children*	*Scotland (31 March)*	*Residential accommodation Adults and Children*
1988	107,130	1987	14,348
1989	103,539	1988	14,381

England and Wales. Expenditure and income relating to the personal social services administered by local authorities (in £1,000 sterling):

Year ended 31 March	*Gross current expenditure*	*Income from sales, fees and charges*	*Net current expenditure*
1988	3,610,297	460,087	3,150,210
1989	3,984,012	470,463	3,513,549

Capital Spending

Year ended 31 March	*Gross expenditure*	*Income from sales of fixed assets*	*Net expenditure*
1984	95,903	17,940	77,963
1985	106,708	23,041	83,667
1986	107,913	27,366	80,547
1987 [1]	103,871	23,662	80,209

[1] Provisional.

Scotland. The total local authority expenditure for 1987–88 in respect of residential accommodation and welfare services under the Social Work (Scotland) Act, 1968, was £409·5m. Central Government expenditure on social work totalled £8·1m.

Klein, R., *The Politics of the National Health Service.* London, 1983
Watkin, B., *The National Health Service.* London, 1978

DIPLOMATIC REPRESENTATIVES

Of the USA in Great Britain (Grosvenor Sq., London, W1A 1AE)
Ambassador: Raymond Seitz

Of Great Britain in the USA (3100 Massachusetts Ave., NW, Washington, D.C., 20008)
Ambassador: Sir Robin Renwick, KCMG.

Of Great Britain to the United Nations
Ambassador: Sir David Hannay.

Great Britain's permanent representative to the European Communities: Sir John Kerr, KCMG.

Further Reading

Publications of Public Departments and Reports, etc. of Royal Commissions and Parliamentary Committees. HM Stationery Office (HMSO).
Central Statistical Office. *Annual Abstract of Statistics*. HMSO.—*Monthly Digest of Statistics*. HMSO
Central Office of Information. *Britain: An Official Handbook*. HMSO, annual.
Directory of British Associations. Beckenham, annual
Government Statistical Service. *Social Trends*. HMSO.—*Regional Statistics*. HMSO
Government Statistics: A Brief Guide to Sources. HMSO, 1984
Barr, N., *et al. The State of Welfare: the Welfare State in Britain since 1974*. Oxford, 1990
Catterall, P., *British History, 1945–1987: an Annotated Bibliography*. Oxford, 1991
Gamble, A., *Britain in Decline: Economic Policy, Political Strategy and the British State*. 3rd ed. London, 1990
Griffith, J.A.G. and Ryle, M., *Parliament: Functions, Practices and Procedures*. London, 1990
Hanson, A.H. and Walles, M., *Governing Britain: a Guidebook to Political Institutions*. 5th ed. London, 1990
Hennessy, P., *Whitehall*. London, 1989
Institute of Contemporary British History. *Contemporary Britain: an Annual Review*. Oxford, from 1990
Kendall, M. G. (ed.), *The Source and Nature of the Statistics of the United Kingdom*. 2 vols. London, 1952–1957
Lever, W. F., *Industrial Change in the United Kingdom*. Harlow, 1987
McIntosh, M., *Managing British Defence*. London, 1990
Mitchell, B. R., *Abstract of British Historical Statistics*. OUP, 1962
Morgan, K.O., *The People's Peace: British History, 1945-89*. OUP, 1990
Oxford History of England. 15 vols. OUP, 1936–75
Thompson, F.M.L. (ed.) *The Cambridge Social History of Britain, 1750-1950*. 3 vols. CUP, 1990
Waller, R. (ed.), *The Almanack of British Politics*. London, 1987

Scotland

Scottish Council (Development and Industry). *Inquiry into the Scottish Economy, 1900–61*. Edinburgh, 1961
Scottish Office. *Scottish Economic Bulletin*. HMSO (quarterly).—*Scottish Abstract of Statistics*. HMSO (annual)
The New Scottish Local Authorities: Organisation and Management Structures. HMSO, 1973
Brand, J., *The National Movement in Scotland*. London, 1978
Campbell, R. H., *The Rise and Fall of Scottish Industry, 1707–1939*. Edinburgh, 1981
Donaldson, G. (ed.) *The Edinburgh History of Scotland*. 4 vols. Edinburgh, 1965–75
Grant, E., *Scotland*. [Bibliography] Oxford and Santa Barbara, 1982
Hogg, A. and Hutcheson, A. MacG., *Scotland and Oil*. 2nd ed. Edinburgh, 1975
Johnston, T. L., *Structure and Growth in the Scottish Economy*. London, 1971
Kellas, J. G., *The Scottish Political System*. 3rd ed. CUP, 1984
Monies, G., *Local Government in Scotland*. Edinburgh, 1985

Wales

Wales: The Way Ahead (Cmnd 3334.) HMSO, 1971
Wales: Employment and the Economy. Cardiff, 1972
Digest of Welsh Statistics. HMSO (annual)
Huws, G. and Roberts, H., *Wales* [Bibliography]. Oxford and Santa Barbara, 1990
Jenkins, G. H., *The Foundations of Modern Wales 1642–1780*. Oxford, 1988
Williams, D., *A History of Modern Wales*. New ed. London, 1977
Williams, G., (ed.) *Social and Cultural Change in Contemporary Wales*. London, 1978

NORTHERN IRELAND

AREA AND POPULATION. Area (revised by the Ordnance Survey Department) and population were as follows:

District	*Population (usually resident) 1981 Census* [1]	*Population estimate 30 June 1989*	*Land area (ha)*
Antrim	45,016	48,100	41,510
Ards	57,792	64,500	36,789
Armagh	49,223	49,000	66,733
Ballymena	54,813	57,200	63,384
Ballymoney	22,946	23,900	41,687
Banbridge	30,110	31,900	44,174
Belfast	314,270	296,900	11,140
Carrickfergus	28,625	30,400	8,484
Castlereagh	60,785	58,000	8,426
Coleraine	46,739	48,500	47,763
Cookstown	28,257	27,600	51,207
Craigavon	73,260	77,700	27,945
Derry (Londonderry)	89,101	99,500	37,258
Down	53,193	57,200	63,835
Dungannon	43,883	43,700	76,266
Fermanagh	51,594	50,400	169,952
Larne	29,076	29,100	33,744
Limavady	26,964	29,800	58,523
Lisburn	83,998	97,400	43,595
Magherafelt	32,494	32,900	56,186
Moyle	14,396	15,100	49,378
Newry and Mourne	76,574	88,900	88,589
Newtownabbey	72,246	72,900	15,956
North Down	66,264	71,900	7,329
Omagh	44,288	44,900	112,354
Strabane	36,279	35,600	86,090
Northern Ireland	1,532,186	1,583,000	1,348,297

[1] Arising from difficulties during the Census taking, a number of households were not enumerated. The population effect of this non-enumeration is estimated at about 50,000 and is included in this column.

Chief town (population, estimate 1989): Belfast, 296,900.
Vital statistics for calendar years:

	Marriages	*Divorces*	*Births*	*Deaths*
1985	10,343	1,669	27,635	15,955
1986	10,225	1,539	28,152	16,065
1987	10,363	1,514	27,865	15,334
1988	9,958	1,550	27,767	15,813
1989 [1]	10,619	1,818	26,080	15,844

[1] Provisional.

CONSTITUTION AND GOVERNMENT. Northern Ireland is part of the United Kingdom. As such it shares in the written and unwritten constitution of the United Kingdom and is subjected to the fundamental constitutional provisions which apply to the rest of the United Kingdom. However, in the Northern Ireland Constitution Act 1973 and the Northern Ireland Act 1982, Parliament provides for a measure of devolved government in Northern Ireland. This can only be introduced if both Houses of Parliament agree that the arrangements for devolution are likely to command widespread acceptance throughout the community in Northern Ireland.

Such matters as the Crown, Parliament, international relations, the armed forces and the raising of taxes cannot be devolved in any circumstances and remain the responsibility of the UK Parliament and Government. In the event of agreement on widely-acceptable arrangements for devolution, powers over a range of social and economic matters would be devolved first. The Northern Ireland Assembly would have power to make laws on these subjects and Members of the Assembly would be appointed as heads of the relevant Northern Ireland government departments. Such powers were devolved on 1 Jan. 1974, following an agreement among the Northern Ireland political parties to form a power-sharing Executive. This collapsed on 28 May 1974.

In the interim and in the absence of devolved arrangements which command widespread acceptance, Northern Ireland is governed by 'direct rule' under the provisions of the Northern Ireland Act 1974. This provides for Parliament to approve all laws for Northern Ireland and places the Northern Ireland departments under the direction and control of a UK Cabinet Minister, the Secretary of State for Northern Ireland.

A 78-member Assembly was elected by proportional representation in 1982. In May 1984 the Assembly set up a Committee on Devolution to consider and report on how the Assembly might be strengthened and progress made towards legislative and executive devolution. The Assembly was dissolved on 23 June 1986, having failed in its statutory duty to make proposals for devolution likely to command widespread acceptance throughout the community.

Since the last Assembly was dissolved in 1986 the Government has continued to express the hope that a new Assembly would be established which would contribute to the better government and administration of Northern Ireland. To this end dialogue has been continuing since late 1989 between the Government and the local constitutional political parties as a means of exploring the extent of the common ground which now appears to exist between them. This approach is viewed by the Government as a necessary prelude to discussions about arrangements for the transfer of powers and responsibilities to locally elected representatives in Northern Ireland.

In Nov. 1985 the governments of the UK and the Republic of Ireland entered into a formal Agreement which is designed to promote peace and stability in Northern Ireland, help to reconcile the two major traditions in Ireland, create a new climate of friendship and co-operation between the people of the two countries and improve co-operation in combating terrorism. Under the Agreement an Intergovernmental Conference was established in which the Irish Government will put forward views and proposals concerning stated aspects of Northern Ireland affairs; in which the promotion of cross-border co-operation will be discussed; and in which determined efforts will be made to resolve any differences between the two governments. A Secretariat was also established by the two governments to service the Conference.

What began ostensibly as a Civil Rights campaign in 1968 escalated into a full-scale offensive designed to overthrow the State. This offensive was originally mounted by an illegal organization, the Irish Republican Army (not to be confused with the legitimate Army of the Republic of Ireland). At times counter-measures have required the services of over 20,000 regular troops, in addition to the Royal Ulster Constabulary, the RUC Reserve and the part-time Ulster Defence Regiment.

Secretary of State for Northern Ireland: Rt Hon. Peter Brooke, MP.

Local Government. Northern Ireland has a single-tier system of 26 district councils based on main centres of population.

The district councils are responsible for the provision of a wide range of local services including refuse collection and disposal, street cleansing, litter prevention, consumer protection, environmental health, miscellaneous licensing including dog control, the provision and management of recreational and cultural facilities, the promotion of tourist development schemes and the enforcement of building regulations. They have in addition both a representative role in which they send forward representatives to sit as members of statutory bodies including the Northern Ireland Housing Council, the Fire Authority and the Area Boards for health and personal social services and education and libraries; and a consultative role under which the Department of Environment (NI) and the Northern Ireland Housing Executive, among others, have an obligation to consult them regarding the provision of the regional services for which these bodies are responsible.

The Government's policy for the future development of the Province is contained in the *Regional Physical Development Strategy 1975–95* which was published in May 1977. Basically the policy advocates that the main town in each District Council area should be developed to fulfil its function as the prime centre in the district and for any other specialized rôles it may have such as an industrial centre, port or tourist resort. The Strategy also recognizes that the smaller towns and villages have an important rôle to play, depending on the availability of services, as locations for smaller scale industries service centres and as dormitory centres for people not wishing to live in the towns where they find employment.

The Regional Strategy provides a framework within which development plans can be prepared for all the districts. Since its adoption of the Strategy the Department has been engaged in formulating the detailed policies and proposals for future communications, the location of industry, housing and major services in the light of anticipated population growth and distribution.

A development plan sets down the broad policies and proposals for the development or other use of land in the area covered by the plan over a period of up to 15 years ahead. Development plans covering almost all of Northern Ireland have been published and work is progressing on the remaining areas, together with review of some earlier plans.

FINANCE. There exists a separate Northern Ireland Consolidated Fund from which is met the expenditure of Northern Ireland Departments. Its main sources of revenue are: *(i)* The Northern Ireland attributed share of UK taxes; *(ii)* A non-specific grant in aid of Northern Ireland's revenue, payable by the Secretary of State for Northern Ireland; *(iii)* Rates and other receipts of Northern Ireland Departments.

The general principle underlying the financial arrangements is that Northern Ireland should have parity of taxation and services with Great Britain.

Since the financial year 1987–88 the income of the Northern Ireland Consolidated Fund has been as follows (in £ sterling):

	1988–89	*1989–90* [1]	*1990–91* [1] *(in 1,000)*
Attributed share of UK taxes	2,383,344,413	2,698,742,228	2,766
Payments by UK Government:			
Grant in Aid	1,300,000,000	1,150,000,000	1,000
Refund of value added tax	28,914,872	29,000,000	33
Regional and district rates	276,500,000	309,000,000	320
Other receipts	339,206,178	292,000,000	295
Total	4,327,965,463	4,478,742,228	4,414

[1] Provisional.

The public debt at 31 March 1990 was as follows: Ulster Savings Certificates, £137,622,102; Ulster Development Bonds, £26,581; borrowing from UK Government, £1,357,605,846; borrowing from Northern Ireland Government Funds, £53,223,451; European Investment Bank Loan, £12,707,614; total, £1,561,186,094.

The above amount of public debt is offset by equal assets in the form of loans from Government to public and local bodies and of cash balances.

ENERGY AND NATURAL RESOURCES

Electricity. The planning, generation and distribution of electricity supplies are the responsibility of Northern Ireland Electricity. The installed capacity of the system is 2,400 mw largely provided from 4 thermal power-stations.

Sales of electricity in the year ended 31 March 1990 amounted to 5,667m. units supplied to a total of 598,651 consumers.

Water Supplies and Sewerage. The Department of the Environment Water Service is responsible for water supply and sewerage. Some 670 megalitres of water are supplied per day to approximately 97% of the population. Approximately 92% of the population live in property which is connected to sewers or modern septic tanks.

The Department is also responsible for the conservation and planned development of water resources.

Minerals. The output of minerals (in 1,000 tonnes) during 1988 was approximately: Basalt and igneous rock (other than granite), 7,324; grit and conglomerate, 2,870; limestone, 2,409; sand and gravel, 3,871; and other minerals (rocksalt, fireclay, diatomite, granite, chalk, clay and shale), 870. There are lignite deposits of 1,200m. tonnes near Crumlin in County Antrim.

Agriculture. Estimated gross output in 1989:

		Quantity (1,000)	Value (£m.)			Quantity (1,000)	Value (£m.)
Fat cattle and calves	head	436	296·2	Other crops	tonnes	19	1·6
Fat sheep and lambs	head	1,280	63·0	Fruit	tonnes	31	5·9
Fat pigs	head	1,107	78·0	Vegetables	tonnes	29	7·5
Poultry (tonnes)		63	45·6	Mushrooms	tonnes	8	9·5
Eggs: for human consumption (dozen)		63,000	26·2	Flowers		—	6·5
Wool (tonnes)		3,000	2·9	Other items		—	33·6
Milk (litres)		1,295	237·0	Total receipts			853·2
Other livestock products		...	9.9	Value of changes in stocks due to volume			–3·9
Potatoes		229	20·7				
Barley		69	7·4	Gross output			849·3
Wheat		14	1·5				

Area (in 1,000 ha) of crops at June census (1989 and 1990):

	1989	1990		1989	1990
Oats	2·8	2·9	Crop silage	3·3	3·3
Wheat	4·7	5·5	Other crops	1·3	0·3
Barley	40·2	37·3	Fruit	1·9	1·9
Other cereals and pulses	0·3	0·1	Grass for mowing or grazing	764·8	770·3
Potatoes	10·3	10·5	Rough grazing (excluding common land)	189·3	190·1
Turnips, swedes, kale and cabbage[1]	0·7	0·8			
Vegetables	1·4	1·4			

[1] Stock feeding only.

Livestock (1,000) at June census (1989 and 1990):

	1989	1990		1989	1990
Dairy cows	277	279	Total sheep	2,317	2,432
Beef cows	244	238	Breeding sows	58	61
Total cattle	1,467	1,511	Total pigs	589	614
Breeding ewes	1,085	1,152	Total poultry	9,824	10,362

INDUSTRY

Labour. The main sources of employment statistics are the Census of Employment, which was last conducted in Sept. 1989, and the Quarterly Employment Enquiry. In June 1990 there were 525,590 employees in employment, of whom 271,430 were males. The average level of seasonally-adjusted unemployment between Jan. and Sept. 1990 was 14% of the workforce, 97,400.

In June 1990 employment in manufacturing and construction amounted to 129,520, just under 25% of the total employees in employment. Of this number, 19,260 were engaged in the food, drink and tobacco industries, 17,230 in clothing and footwear, 10,430 in aircraft, shipbuilding and other transport equipment (except motor vehicles), 9,490 in textiles, 25,660 in construction and 47,540 in other branches of manufacturing.

Training and Placement. The Training and Employment Agency, launched on 2 April 1990, has responsibility for all training and employment activities previously carried out by the Department of Economic Development and for the functions of the Northern Ireland Training Authority and a number of Industrial Training Boards. The Agency is the first 'Next Steps' Agency to be set up in Northern Ireland. The Agency has some 1,700 staff and a budget of approximately £170m. It also has a 12-member Advisory Board which advises Ministers and the Agency on the formulation of training and employment policy and aims to develop collaboration between employers and the Agency.

The Agency's overall aim is, within available resources, to assist economic growth by ensuring that its training and employment functions help firms become more competitive; by increasing the skills of the workforce to enable individuals to acquire the competencies required for increased competitiveness; and by providing other like services which Ministers deem desirable for Northern Ireland's economic development. The Agency's main programmes and services are as follows:

Action for Community Employment (ACE): Jobs are provided for the long-term unemployed and offer one year's work in employment of community benefit such as environmental improvement, help to the aged and disadvantaged, and energy conservation. In 1990-91 the Agency is providing 10,000 ACE places through community organizations known as ACE Sponsors.

Job Training Programme (JTP) is an employer-based training programme which parallels Employment training in Great Britain. It aims to address the needs of the long-term unemployed by offering opportunities to them to refresh, enhance and update existing skills or to acquire skills in a new field thus enabling participants to compete more effectively for available jobs or to progress to self-employment. In 1990–91 the Agency is aiming to provide 3,300 JTP places which are delivered by Managing Agents drawn mainly from the private sector.

Youth Training Programme (YTP) is an integrated two-year programme aimed at all 16- and 17-year olds. Its purpose is to strengthen the economy by offering training and relevant work experience to young people; and, assist personal effectiveness by helping young people to make the transition from school to adult life. The Programme is delivered by Training Organizations including Community Workshops, Employers, Further Education Colleges and the Agency's Training Centres. In 1990–91 the Agency is aiming to provide 15,500 YTP places.

The Employment Service provides a comprehensive all-age guidance and placement service for the adult unemployed, young people, disabled persons and employers delivered through the Agency's 29 Offices located across Northern Ireland. In 1989–90 the Employment Service placed 46,322 people in employment and 18,836 in training.

The Agency provides a range of schemes designed to improve and develop management skills both for existing managers and graduates seeking to follow managerial careers in industry. It also delivers the Enterprise Allowance Scheme which provides financial assistance to certain categories of unemployed people who wish to start up their own business.

The Training Advisory Service promotes the benefits of training in industry and offers advice tailored to the needs of individual companies and industrial sectors. The Manpower Training Scheme offers financial support to companies seeking to introduce comprehensive training programmes. The Scheme aims to improve the overall competitiveness of Northern Ireland industry.

The Agency's network of 12 Training Centres located across Northern Ireland provide high quality off-the-job industrial skills training for young persons and adults. The Centres also provide Sponsored Training for Industry. Where an individual company identifies a particular training need or problem, a package tailored to the company's specific needs can be designed. Subject to the expertise available, this training can be provided in the Training Centre or in-company.

To supplement the Training Centres facilities, arrangements have been made for the use of spare training capacity in industry and commerce to attach people to firms for training courses. By this means a wide variety of training is made available and this has been further supplemented by use of spare capacity in other training agencies and in Colleges of Further Education.

The Department of Economic Development administers an Entry to Management Programme for unemployed trainees and a Management Development Programme for private sector firms. The former Programme contains training opportunities schemes for those wishing to enter or re-enter management or to set up new businesses – at the peak time of the training year up to 250 people can be in training. The latter Programme is designed to encourage companies to develop management structures and to train individual managers to a high level of competence. Each year about 2,000 grants are awarded to support training courses or training places in companies. Also, up to 2,100 places were available in the financial year 1988–89 under the Enterprise Allowance Scheme, to encourage unemployed people to set up in business, by paying them £40 a week for up to 52 weeks as a business receipt to compensate for loss of unemployment or income support.

TOURISM. Tourism earns a substantial amount of revenue for Northern Ireland

and total spending by some 824,000 visitors in 1986 was £82m. Altogether tourism provides over 9,000 full-time jobs. The Northern Ireland Tourist Board has the main responsibility for promoting tourist traffic to and within Northern Ireland.

Scenic beauty, scientific and nature interest, and wildlife are protected by the Department of the Environment under the Access to the Countryside (NI) Order 1983, the Nature Conservation and Amenity Lands (NI) Order 1985 and the Wildlife (NI) Order 1985. The Department is advised by the Council for Nature Conservation and the Countryside. Nine Areas of Outstanding Natural Beauty have been designated, where special attention is given to the amenity aspects of planning applications. Country Parks have been established at Crawfordsburn, Redburn and Scrabo, Co. Down, at the Roe Valley and Ness Wood, Co. Derry, and at Castle Archdale, Co. Fermanagh. At The Birches in N. Armagh there is a Peatlands Park. The Lagan Valley between Belfast and Lisburn is Northern Ireland's first Regional Park. Countryside Information Centres are located at Portrush, Co. Antrim and Newcastle, Co. Down and a visitor centre at the Quoile Pondage National Nature Reserve, near Downpatrick, Co. Down. Forty-five National Nature Reserves have been declared, and more are being acquired.

The Department is advised by the Historic Monuments Council on the exercise of its powers under the Historic Monuments Act (NI) 1971 in respect of the conservation of historic monuments and the preservation of objects of archaeological or historic interest. At present there are some 167 monuments in State care and approximately 1,000 are scheduled. The Department, advised by the Historic Buildings Council, under the Planning (NI) Order 1972 is also responsible for listing buildings of special architectural or historic interest and for designating areas of similar interest the character or appearance of which it is desirable to preserve or enhance. To date some 7,725 buildings have been listed and 28 conservation areas have been designated. Grants may be payable by the Department to assist in the repair or maintenance of listed buildings and for schemes of enhancement in conservation areas.

COMMUNICATIONS

Roads. Most bus services are operated by two other subsidiaries, Ulsterbus Ltd and Citybus Ltd. Ulsterbus runs services outside the Belfast area while all the services within the Belfast area are run by Citybus.

The Department of the Environment (NI) administers a licensing system for professional hauliers with the objective of maintaining standards and conditions necessary for the safe operation of vehicles and fair competition between hauliers. The level of services provided and the rates charged by the industry are determined by the normal economic forces of supply and demand. At 31 March 1990 there were 1,494 professional hauliers and 3,009 vehicles licensed to engage in road haulage.

The number of motor vehicles licensed at 31 Dec. 1990 was 500,490, comprising private cars, 456,611; motor cycles, 9,460; hackney vehicles, 2,962; goods vehicles, 23,492; special machines, 7,965. In addition, there were 17,166 vehicles which were not subject to licence duty.

At 1 April 1988 the total mileage of roads was 14,812, graded for administrative purposes as follows: Motorway 69 miles; Class I dual carriageway, 81 miles; Class I single carriageway, 1,283 miles; Class II, 1,774 miles; Class III, 2,936 miles; unclassified, 8,669 miles.

Railways. All train services are operated by the Northern Ireland Railways Co. Ltd which is a subsidiary of the Northern Ireland Transport Holding Co. The number of track km operated is 357; passenger route miles, 210. In 1989–90 railways carried 5·2m. passengers.

Aviation. Northern Ireland Airports Ltd operate the region's principal facility at Belfast International Airport. In 1989 it handled 2·2m. passengers and 33,000 tonnes of freight and mail. A major development programme is in progress. A three-phase project to improve and expand the existing passenger terminal is nearing completion and a new £7m. cargo development was due to open in 1991.

Belfast City Airport offers scheduled air services to 15 other regional centres in the UK and to Dublin. In 1989 it handled 0·5m. passengers. A programme of improvements to the terminal and other facilities has begun.

There are 3 other licensed airfields in Northern Ireland and of these Eglinton has some scheduled services; otherwise these airfields are used principally by flying clubs, by private owners and by expanding air taxi businesses flying to destinations in Ireland, the UK and continental Europe.

Shipping. Passenger services operate between Larne and (i) Cairnryan and (ii) Stranraer. Conventional cargo services have given way in many cases to container, unit load and drive on/drive off services. The latter type of service now operates from Belfast, Larne and Warrenpoint to various ports in the UK.

JUSTICE, RELIGION, EDUCATION AND WELFARE

Justice. The Lord Chancellor has responsibility for the administration of all courts in Northern Ireland through the Northern Ireland Court Service, and is responsible for the appointment of judges and resident magistrates.

The court structure in Northern Ireland has 3 tiers–the Supreme Court of Judicature of Northern Ireland (comprising the Court of Appeal, the High Court and the Crown Court), the County Courts and the Magistrates' Courts. There are 22 Petty Sessions districts which when grouped together for administration purposes form 7 County Court Divisions and 4 Circuits.

The County Court has general civil jurisdiction subject to an upper monetary limit of £5,000. Appeals from the Magistrates' Courts lie to the County Court, while appeals from the County Court lie to the High Court or, on a point of law, to the Court of Appeal by way of case stated. Circuit Registrars have jurisdiction to deal with most defended actions up to £1,000 and most undefended actions up to £5,000. They also deal, by an informal arbitration procedure, with small claims whose value does not exceed £500. An appeal from the decision of a Circuit Registrar lies to the High Court other than in small claims cases.

Police. The police force consists of the Royal Ulster Constabulary, supported by the Royal Ulster Constabulary Reserve, a mainly part-time force.

Religion. According to the census of 1981 of the total enumerated population of 1,481,959 there were: Roman Catholics, 414,532; Presbyterians, 339,818; Church of Ireland, 281,472; Methodists, 58,731. Those belonging to other Churches and of no stated denomination numbered 387,406. 18·5% of the enumerated population failed to answer the voluntary question on religion.

Education. Public education, other than university education, is administered centrally by the *Department of Education for Northern Ireland* and locally by 5 Education and Library boards. The Department is concerned with the whole range of education from nursery education through to higher education and continuing education; for sport and recreation; for youth services; for the arts and culture (including libraries) and for the development of community relations with and between schools. District councils are the main providers of sport, recreation and community facilities and are supported in this provision by grant from the Department.

Each *Education and Library Board* is the local education authority for its area. Boards were first appointed in 1973, the year of local government reorganization, and are reappointed every 4 years following the District Council elections. Boards were last reconstituted on 1 July 1989. The membership of each Board consists of District councillors, representatives of transferors of schools, representatives of trustees of maintained schools and other persons who are interested in the service for which the Board is responsible. Boards have a duty, amongst other things, to ensure that there are sufficient schools of all kinds to meet the needs of their areas. They are wholly responsible for the schools under their management and equip, maintain and meet other running costs of the maintained schools. The Boards are responsible for costs associated with capital works at controlled schools whereas voluntary schools, including maintained and voluntary schools, can receive grant-aid from the Department of Education of up to 85% of approved expenditure. Most voluntary grammar schools can receive the same rate of grant on the purchase of equipment. The Boards award university and other scholarships; they provide school milk and meals; free books and transport for pupils; they enforce school attendance; provide a curriculum advisory and support service to all schools in their area; regulate the employment of children and young people; and secure the provision of youth and recreational facilities. They are also required to develop a comprehensive and efficient library service for their area. Board expenditure is funded at 100% by the Department of Education.

The Education Reform (NI) Order 1989 made provision for the setting up of a *Council for Catholic Maintained Schools* with effect from April 1990. The Council has responsibility for all maintained schools under Roman Catholic Management which are under the auspices of the diocesan authorities and of religious orders. The main objective of the Council is to promote high standards of education in the schools for which it is responsible. Its functions include providing advice on matters relating to its schools, the employment of teaching staff and administration of appointment procedures, the promotion of effective management and the promotion and co-ordination of effective planning and rationalization of school provision in the Catholic Maintained sector. The membership of the Council consists of trustee representatives appointed by the Northern Bishops, parents, teachers, and persons appointed by the Head of the Department of Education in consultation with the Bishops.

Universities. There are 2 universities: The Queen's University of Belfast and the University of Ulster. The Queen's University of Belfast (founded in 1849 as a college of the Queen's University of Ireland and reconstituted as a separate university in 1908) had 109 professors, 246 readers and senior lecturers, 558 lecturers and tutors and 7,682 full-time students in 1988–89. The University of Ulster, formed on 1 Oct. 1984, has campuses in Belfast, Coleraine, Jordanstown and Londonderry. In 1988–89 the University had 53 professors, 221 readers and senior lecturers, 558 lecturers and demonstrators and 8,293 full-time students.

Nursery Education is provided in nursery schools or nursery classes in primary schools. There were 85 nursery schools in 1988–89, with 4,868 pupils and 153 teachers.

Primary Education is from 4 to 11 years. In 1988–89 there were 978 primary schools with 184,241 pupils and 7,920 teachers.

Secondary Education is from 11 to 18 years. In 1988–89 there were 71 grammar schools with 53,131 pupils and 3,507 teachers and 174 secondary schools with 89,968 pupils and 6,337 teachers.

Further Education. There were 26 institutions of further education in 1988–89 with 2,448 full-time and 2,073 part-time teachers and an enrolment of 15,619 full-time, 23,935 part-time day and 17,154 evening students on vocational courses; and 46,023 students on non-vocational (mostly evening) courses.

Special Education. The Education and Library Boards provide for children with special educational needs up to the age of 19. This provision may be in primary or secondary schools or in special units attached to schools. In 1988–89 there were 54 special schools with 4,018 pupils.

Teacher training takes place at both universities and at 2 colleges of education: Stranmillis, and St. Mary's, the latter mainly for the primary school sector, in respect of which 4-year (Hons) BEd courses and one-year Postgraduate Certificate in Education (PGCE) courses are available. The training of teachers for secondary schools is provided, in the main, in the education departments of the 2 universities, but 4-year (Hons) BEd courses are also available in the colleges for intending secondary teachers of religious education, business studies and craft, design and technology. There were a total of 1,816 students (314 men and 1,502 women) in training at the 2 colleges and the 2 universities during 1988–89. There were 21,781 full-time teachers (8,478 men and 13,303 women) in grant-aided schools and institutions of further education. The principal initial teacher-training courses are the Bachelor of Education (3 year and 4 year honours), general or honours BA and

BSc. degrees with education (3, 4 and 5 year) and the one year Certificate of Education for graduates. There were 1,816 students (314 men and 1,502 women) in training at the 2 Colleges of Education and the 2 Universities during 1988–89.

Expenditure by the Department of Education (1988–89) £812m.

Health and Personal Social Services. Under the provisions of the Health and Personal Social Services (NI) Order 1972, the Department of Health and Social Services is responsible for the provision of integrated health and personal social services in Northern Ireland, designed to promote the physical and mental health of the people of Northern Ireland through the prevention, diagnosis and treatment of illness, and also to promote their social welfare. Four Health and Social Services Boards, Eastern, Northern, Southern and Western, established under the above Order, administer health and personal social services, as the Department directs, within their designated areas.

Social Security. The social security schemes in Northern Ireland are similar to those in force in Great Britain.

National Insurance. During the year ended 31 March 1990, £10·5m. sickness benefit was paid to an average of 9,617 persons and £31·2m. unemployment benefit was paid to an average of 17,090 persons. Widows' benefits amounting to £31·5m. were paid to an average of 12,188 persons and retirement pensions totalling £453·2m. were paid to an average of 214,768 persons. Invalidity pensions and allowances totalling £157·3m. were paid to an average of 49,098 persons. Industrial disablement benefit amounting to £13·2m. was paid to an average of 5,540 persons. Maternity allowance totalling £0·8m. was paid to an average of 564 persons. Receipts of the Northern Ireland Insurance Fund in the year ended 31 March 1990 were £745·3m. and payments were £733·6m.

Child Benefit. During the year ended 31 March 1990, £174m. was paid to an average of 216,819 families.

Income Support. In 1989–90 £378m. was paid to an average of 198,505 persons.

Family Credit. In 1989–90, £29m. was paid to an average of 14,131 persons.

Further Reading

Northern Ireland Social Security Statistics
Census of Population Reports, Northern Ireland. Belfast, HMSO, 1981
Northern Ireland: A Trade Directory. Belfast, HMSO, 1st ed. 1985
Reports on the Census of Production of Northern Ireland. Belfast, HMSO
The Statutes Revised: Northern Ireland. HMSO, 1982
Arthur, P. and Jeffery, K., *Northern Ireland since 1968.* Oxford, 1988
Bell, G., *The Protestants of Ulster.* London, 1976
Flackes, W. D., *Northern Ireland: Political Directory 1968–88.* London, 1989
Kelly, K., *The Longest War: Northern Ireland and the IRA.* Dingle, Westport and London, 1982
Kenny, A., *The Road to Hillsborough.* London, 1986
McGarry, J. and O'Leary, B., (eds.) *The Future of Northern Ireland.* Oxford, 1991
Shannon, M. O., *Northern Ireland.* [Bibliography] Oxford and Santa Barbara, 1991
Wallace, M., *British Government in Northern Ireland: From Devolution to Direct Rule.* Newton Abbot, 1982
Watt, D. (ed.) *The Constitution of Northern Ireland.* London, 1981
Whyte, J., *Interpreting Northern Ireland.* Oxford Univ. Press, 1990

ISLE OF MAN

AREA AND POPULATION. Area, 221 sq. miles (572 sq. km); resident population census April 1986, 64,282. The principal towns are Douglas (population, 20,368), Ramsey (5,778), Peel (3,660), Castletown (3,019). Vital statistics, 1989: Births, 817; deaths, 988; marriages, 420.

CONSTITUTION AND GOVERNMENT. The Isle of Man is a Crown dependency administered in accordance with its own laws by the High Court of *Tyn-*

wald, consisting of the President of Tynwald, elected by the Court and the *Legislative Council*, composed of the Lord Bishop of Sodor and Man, the Attorney-General (who does not vote) and 8 members selected by the *House of Keys*; and the House of Keys, a representative assembly of 24 members chosen by adult suffrage. The Isle of Man is not bound by Acts of the UK Parliament unless specially mentioned in them or applied by Order in Council although the UK is responsible for conducting its foreign affairs. The office of elected president replaced that of lieutenant governor in 1990.

A Council of Ministers was instituted in 1990. This replaced the former Executive Council and consists of the Chief Minister and the ministers of the 9 major departments of Government. Elections for the House of Keys were due in Nov. 1991.

President: Sir Charles Kerruish (elected July 1990).
Chief Secretary: J. F. Kissack.

In March 1991 the *Chief Minister* was Miles Walker. *Treasury Minister:* Don Gelling. *Health:* Jim Cain.

Flag: Red, with 3 steel-coloured legs armoured and spurred (knees and spurs, yellow) in the centre.

ECONOMY

Budget. The Isle of Man levies its own taxes. Revenue is derived from customs duties, value added tax and from income tax. In 1990–91 the budget allowed for expenditure of £263m. Income tax was 15% of the first £8,000 of taxable income and 20% on the balance. There are no inheritance or capital gains taxes. A non-resident company duty of £450 was introduced on 6 April 1987 on every company incorporated in the Isle of Man which trades and is controlled outside the island.

The Island currently makes an annual contribution to the UK Government towards the cost of defence and other common services provided by the UK Government. That contribution currently amounts to about £1·5m.

Currency. The Isle of Man Government issues its own notes and coin on a par with £ sterling. £50, £20, £10, £5, £1, and £5, £2, £1, 50p, 20p, 10p, 5p, 2p and 1p coins are issued. Various commemorative coins have been minted together with legal tender gold coins and a platinum bullion coin.

Banking and Finance. Government regulation of the banking sector is exercised through the Financial Supervision Commission. The Commission was established in 1983 and is responsible for the licensing and supervision of banks, deposit-takers and certain financial intermediaries giving financial advice and receiving client monies for investment and management. As at 30 Sept. 1990 there were 60 licensed banking institutions, 53 investment businesses and 5 UK Building Societies with Isle of Man licences. As at 30 Sept. 1989 the deposit base was £5,284m.

Agriculture. The area farmed is about 117,000 acres out of a total land area of around 140,000 acres. About 66,000 acres is devoted to grass whilst a further 38,000 acres are accounted for by rough grazing. Barley accounts for most of the remaining land under cultivation and some barley is exported. There are approximately 152,000 sheep, 33,000 cattle, 61,000 poultry and 6,000 pigs on farms in the Island. Agriculture contributes less than 3% of the Island's GNP.

External Economic Relations. A special relationship exists with the EEC providing for free trade and the adoption of external trade policies with third countries.

Tourism. In 1988–89 tourism contributed around 9% of national income; there were 325,574 visitors during the 1990 summer season.

COMMUNICATIONS

Roads. There are 500 miles of good roads. The International TT Motor Cycle Races and cycle races take place annually. Omnibus services operate to all parts of the island.

In 1989–90 there were 48,659 licensed vehicles on the roads, including 2,494 motorcycles.

Railways. Several novel transport systems operate on the Island during the summer season, including 100-year-old horse-drawn trams, and the Manx Electric Railway, linking Douglas, Ramsey and Snaefell Mountain (2,036 ft). The Isle of Man Steam Railway also operates between Douglas and Port Erin.

Aviation. Ronaldsway Airport handles scheduled services operated by Manx Airlines and Jersey European to and from London, Manchester, Belfast, Dublin, Glasgow, Liverpool, Blackpool, Birmingham, etc. Air taxi services also operate.

Shipping. Car ferries of the Isle of Man Steam Packet Co. link the Island with Heysham throughout the year and similar services operate to Liverpool, Fleetwood, Stranraer, Dublin and Belfast during the summer season.

Telecommunications. The first constitutionally licensed commercial radio station in the British Isles, Manx Radio, is operated by Government on medium and VHF wavelengths from Douglas.

Newspapers. In 1990 there were 3 weekly newspapers and 1 twice weekly newspaper.

JUSTICE AND EDUCATION

Police. The police force numbered 209 all ranks in 1990.

Education. Education is compulsory between the ages of 5 and 16. In 1989 there were 32 primary schools with 5,458 pupils in attendance. The net expenditure on education for 1989–90 amounted to £28·5m. There are 7 secondary schools, 5 provided by the Board of Education (4,327 registered pupils), 1 direct grant school for girls (61 senior and 168 junior registered pupils), 1 independent co–educational public school (218 senior and 134 junior registered pupils), 1 college of further education (425 full-time pupils in 1990–91), and 1 special school (31 pupils).

Further Reading

Additional information is available from: Economic Affairs Division, 14 Hill St, Douglas, Isle of Man.

Publications: *Isle of Man Key Facts 1990, Isle of Man Digest of Economic and Social Statistics 1988, Isle of Man Census Reports 1981*. 3 vols, *Isle of Man Interim Census Report 1986, Isle of Man Family Expenditure Survey 1981–82, Isle of Man Passenger Survey Reports 1985–1989, Isle of Man National Income Estimates 1988–89, Isle of Man General Index of Retail Prices* (Monthly), *Isle of Man Earnings Survey 1988*.
Tynwald Companion 1985. Isle of Man Government, 1985
Kinvig, R. H., *History of the Isle of Man*. Oxford, 1945.—*The Isle of Man: A Social, Cultural and Political History*. Liverpool Univ. Press, 1975
Robinson, V. and McCarroll, D., (eds.) *The Isle of Man: Celebrating a Sense of Place*. Liverpool Univ. Press, 1990
Solly, M., *The Isle of Man: A Low Tax Area*. London, 1984
Stenning, E. H., *Portrait of the Isle of Man*. London, 1984

CHANNEL ISLANDS

AREA. The Channel Islands are situated off the north-west coast of France and are the only portions of the 'Duchy of Normandy' now belonging to the Crown of England, to which they have been attached since the Conquest. They consist of Jersey (28,717 acres), Guernsey (15,654 acres) and the following dependencies of Guernsey–Alderney (1,962), Brechou (74), Great Sark (1,035), Little Sark (239), Herm (320), Jethou (44) and Lihou (38), a total of 48,083 acres, or 75 sq. miles (194 sq. km).

CLIMATE. The climate is mild, with an average temperature for the year of 11·5°C. Average yearly rainfall totals: Jersey, 862·9mm; Guernsey, 858·9mm. The wettest months are in the winter. Highest temperatures recorded: Jersey, 34·8°C.; Guernsey, 31·7°C. Maximum temperatures usually occur in July and Aug. (daily maximum 20·8°C. in Jersey, slightly lower in Guernsey). Lowest temperatures recorded: Jersey, 10·3°C.; Guernsey, –7·4°C. Jan. and Feb. are the coldest months (mean temperature approximately 6°C.).

CONSTITUTION. The Lieut.-Governors and Cs.-in-C. of Jersey and Guernsey are the personal representatives of the Sovereign, the Commanders of the Armed Forces of the Crown and the channel of communication between the Crown and the insular governments. They are appointed by the Crown and have a voice but no vote in the Assemblies of the States (the insular legislatures). The Secretaries to the Lieut.-Governors are their staff officers.

The Bailiffs are appointed by the Crown and are Presidents both of the Assembly of the States and of the Royal Courts of Jersey and Guernsey. They have in the States a casting vote. The official languages are French and English, but English is the main language. In the country districts of Jersey and Guernsey and throughout Sark some people also speak a Norman-French dialect; that of Alderney has died out.

EXTERNAL ECONOMIC RELATIONS. The Channel Islands are not members of the EC, but participate in ERM through their monetary union with the UK. From 1958 the trade of the Channel Islands with the UK has been regarded as internal trade.

COMMUNICATIONS

Road. Omnibus services operate in all parts of Jersey and Guernsey.

Aviation. Scheduled air services are maintained by British Airways, Aer Lingus, Air UK, Jersey European, British Midland, Aurigny Air Services, Dan-Air, Brymon Airways, NLM City Hopper and other companies between the islands and airports in the UK, Ireland, the Netherlands, France, Germany, Norway, Portugal, Switzerland, Gibraltar, Spain, Finland and Belgium.

Shipping. Passenger and cargo services between Jersey, Guernsey and England are maintained by British Channel Island Ferries; between Guernsey, Jersey and England and St Malo by the Commodore Shipping Co., Emeraude Ferries connect Jersey with St Malo; between Guernsey, Jersey, Alderney, England and France by Condor Ltd (hydrofoil), and between Guernsey and Alderney and England and Guernsey and Sark by local companies.

Telecommunications. Postal and overseas telephone and telegraph services are maintained by the respective Postal Administrations of each bailiwick. The local telephone services are maintained by the insular authorities. There were, in 1989, 47,647 telephone lines in Jersey and 54,529 rented telephones in Guernsey.

There is an independent television station in Jersey and local radio stations, BBC Radio Jersey and Guernsey, opened in 1982.

JUSTICE AND RELIGION

Justice. Justice is administered by the Royal Courts of Jersey and Guernsey, each of which consists of the Bailiff and 12 Jurats, the latter being elected by an electoral college. There is an appeal from the Royal Courts to the Courts of Appeal of Jersey and of Guernsey. A final appeal lies to the Privy Council in certain cases. A stipendiary magistrate in each, Jersey and Guernsey, deals with minor civil and criminal cases.

Church. Jersey and Guernsey each constitutes a deanery under the jurisdiction of the Bishop of Winchester. The rectories (12 in Jersey; 10 in Guernsey) are in the gift of the Crown. The Roman Catholic and various Nonconformist Churches are represented.

Further Reading

Ambrière, F., *Les Iles Anglo-Normandes*. Paris, 1971
Coysh, V., *The Channel Islands: A New Study*. Newton Abbot, 1977
Cruickshank, C., *The German Occupation of the Channel Islands*. London, 1975
Jee, N., *The Landscape of the Channel Islands*. Chichester, 1982

Lemprière, R., *Portrait of the Channel Islands.* London, 1970.—*History of the Channel Islands.* Rev. ed. London, 1980
Uttley, J., *The Story of the Channel Islands.* London, 1966

JERSEY

POPULATION (1989), 82,809. In the year ended 31 Dec. 1989 there were 1,158 births and 896 deaths. The town is St Helier on the south coast.

CONSTITUTION. The States consist of 12 Senators (elected for 6 years, 6 retiring every third year), 12 Constables (triennial) and 29 Deputies (triennial), all elected on universal suffrage by the people.

The island legislature is 'The States of Jersey'. The States comprises the Bailiff, the Lieut.-Governor, 12 Senators, the Constables of the 12 parishes of the island, 29 Deputies, the Dean of Jersey, the Attorney-General and the Solicitor-General. They all have the right to speak in the Assembly, but only the 53 elected members (the Senators, Constables and Deputies) have the right to vote; the Bailiff has a casting vote. General elections for Senators and Deputies are held every third year. Except in specific instances, enactments passed by the States require the sanction of The Queen-in-Council. The Lieut.-Governor has the power of veto on certain forms of legislation.

Flag: White with a red diagonal cross. In the top centre of the flag a shield of the arms of Jersey ensigned with the Plantagenet Crown.

Lieut.-Governor and C.-in-C. of Jersey: Air Marshal Sir John Sutton, KCB.
Secretary and ADC to the Lieut.-Governor: Cdr D. M. L. Braybrooke, LVO, RN (Retd).

Bailiff of Jersey and President of the States: Sir Peter Crill, CBE.
Deputy Bailiff: V. A. Tomes.

ECONOMY

Budget (year ending 31 Dec. 1989). Revenue, £297,865,800; expenditure, £223,625,000. The standard rate of income tax is 20p in the pound. No super-tax or death duties are levied. Parochial rates of moderate amount are payable by owners and occupiers.

Banking and Finance. Bank deposits totalled £42,100m. in Sept. 1990.

Currency. The States issue bank-notes in denominations of £50, £20, £10, £5 and £1.

INDUSTRY AND TRADE

Industry. Principal activities: Tourism; total number of hotel and guesthouse bedrooms (1990), 23,069; expenditure of tourists (1990), £270m. Agriculture, total output (1988), £36·4m. and total exports, £30·7m. Light industry, mainly electrical goods, textiles and clothing. Total exports (1980), £29m. Banking and finance, total bank deposits and balances due to parent companies by deposit-taking institutions (1990), £40,400m.

Commerce. Since 1980 the Customs have ceased recording imports and exports. Principal imports: Machinery and transport equipment, manufactured goods, food, mineral fuels, and chemicals. Principal exports: Machinery and transport equipment, food, and manufactured goods.

Tourism. 0·88m. tourists spent £270m. in 1989. There were 23,625 tourist beds.

COMMUNICATIONS

Aviation. The Jersey airport is situated at St Peter. It covers approximately 375 acres. Number of aircraft movements excluding local flying (1990) 60,107; number of passengers: 1,890,714; cargo and mail, 8792 tonnes.

Shipping (1990). All vessels arriving in Jersey from outside Jersey waters report at St Helier or Gorey on first arrival. There is a harbour of minor importance at St Aubin. Number of commercial vessels entering St Helier, 26,472 number of visiting yachts (1990), 12,097. Passengers arrived in 1990, 491,145.

Post and Broadcasting. In 1988 there were 47,647 telephones and 24 post offices.

EDUCATION (1990). There were 5 States secondary schools and 1 high school, and 24 States primary schools; 4,506 pupils attended the primary schools, 3,557 the secondary schools. There were 8 private primary schools with 1,288 pupils and 8 private secondary schools with 848 pupils. Highlands College offers full- and part-time courses to Ordinary and National Certificate and Diploma levels or similar standards and, together with Les Quennevais Adult Community Centre, evening classes in technical and recreational subjects.

Further Reading

Balleine, G. R., *Biographical Dictionary of Jersey*. London, 1948.—*A History of the Island of Jersey*. Rev. ed. Chichester, 1981.—*The Bailiwick of Jersey*. 3rd ed. London, 1970
Bois, F. de L., *The Constitutional History of Jersey*. Jersey, 1970
Carre, A. L., *English–Jersey Language Vocabulary*. Jersey, 1972
Le Maistre, F., *Dictionnaire Jersiais-Français*. Jersey, 1966

States of Jersey Library: Halkett Place, St Helier. *Librarian:* J. K. Antill, FLA.

GUERNSEY

POPULATION. Census population (1986) 55,482. Births during 1989 were 729; deaths, 595. The town is St Peter Port.

CONSTITUTION. The government of the island is conducted by committees appointed by the States.

The States of Deliberation, the Parliament of Guernsey, is composed of the following members: The Bailiff, who is President *ex officio;* 12 Conseillers; H.M. Procureur and H.M. Comptroller (Law Officers of the Crown), who have a voice but no vote; 33 People's Deputies elected by popular franchise; 10 Douzaine Representatives elected by their Parochial Douzaines; 2 representatives of the States of Alderney.

The States of Election, an electoral college, elects the Jurats and Conseillers. It is composed of the following members; The Bailiff (President *ex officio*); the 12 Jurats or 'Jurés-Justiciers'; the 12 Conseillers; H.M. Procureur and H.M. Comptroller; the 33 People's Deputies; 34 Douzaine Representatives; and (for the election of Conseillers) 4 representatives of the States of Alderney.

Since Jan. 1949 all legislative powers and functions (with minor exceptions) formerly exercised by the Royal Court have been vested in the States of Deliberation. Projets de Loi (Bills) require the sanction of The Queen-in-Council.

Flag: White bearing a red cross of St George, with an argent with a cross gules superimposed on the cross.

Lieut.-Governor and C.-in-C. of Guernsey and its Dependencies: Lieut.-Gen. Sir Michael Wilkins, KCB, OBE.
Secretary and ADC to the Lieut.-Governor: Capt. D. P. L. Hodgetts.

Bailiff of Guernsey and President of the States: Sir Charles Frossard.
Deputy Bailiff of Guernsey: G. M. Dorey.

BANKING AND FINANCE (year ending 31 Dec. 1989). Revenue, including

Alderney, £129,639,543; expenditure, including Alderney, £112,025,191. The standard rate of income tax is 20p in the pound. States and parochial rates are very moderate. No super-tax or death duties are levied.

There were 72 banks in Sept. 1990.

COMMERCE (1989). Principal imports: Petrol and oils, 146,174,198 litres. Principal exports: Tomatoes, £6,510,319; flowers and fern, £25,305,647; sweet peppers, £112,980; other vegetables, £1,337,436; plants, £1·8m.

Tourism. 0·25m. tourists spent £92m. in 1989.

COMMUNICATIONS

Aviation. The airport in Guernsey, situated at La Villiaze, has a landing area of approximately 124 acres and a tarmac runway of 4,800 ft. In 1989, passenger arrivals totalled 857,425.

Shipping. The principal harbour is that of St Peter Port, and there is a harbour at St Sampson's (used mainly for commercial shipping). In 1989 passenger arrivals totalled 386,980. Ships registered in Guernsey at 31 Dec. 1989 numbered 1,333 and 316 fishing vessels. In 1989, 13,362 yachts visited Guernsey.

EDUCATION. There are 2 public schools in the island: Elizabeth College, founded by Queen Elizabeth in 1563, for boys, and the Ladies' College, for girls. The States grammar school provides for education up to University entrance requirements, and there are numerous modern secondary and primary schools and a College of Further Education. The total number of school children was (1989) 8,133. Facilities are available for the study of art, domestic science and many other subjects of a technical nature. There is also a convent school with boarding facilities for girls.

ALDERNEY. Population (1986 census, 2,130). The island has an airport. The Constitution of the island (reformed 1987) provides for its own popularly elected President and States (12 members), and its own Court. The town is St Anne's.

Flag: White with a red cross with the island badge in the centre.

President of the States: J. Kay-Mouat.
Clerk of the States: D. V. Jenkins.
Clerk of the Court: A. Johnson.

SARK. Population (1986 estimate, 550). The Constitution is a mixture of feudal and popular government with its Chief Pleas (parliament), consisting of 40 tenants and 12 popularly elected deputies, presided over by the Seneschal. The head of the island is the Seigneur. Sark has no income tax. Motor vehicles, except tractors, are not allowed.

Flag: White with a red cross and a red first quarter bearing two gold lions.

The Seigneur: J. M. Beaumont.
Seneschal: L. P. de Carteret.

Further Reading

Carteret, A. R. de, *The Story of Sark.* London, 1956
Coysh, V., *Alderney.* Newton Abbot, 1974
Durand, R., *Guernsey, Present and Past.* Guernsey, 1933.—*Guernsey under German Rule.* London, 1946
Hathaway, S., *Dame of Sark: An Autobiography.* London, 1961
Le Huray, C. P., *The Bailiwick of Guernsey.* London, 1952
Marr, L. J., *A History of Guernsey.* Chichester, 1982
Wood, A. and M. S., *Islands in Danger.* 2nd ed. London, 1957
Wood, J., *Herm, Our Island Home.* London, 1973

UNITED STATES OF AMERICA

Capital: Washington, D.C.
Population: 249·63m. (1990)
GNP per capita: US$19,780 (1988)

HISTORY. The Declaration of Independence of the 13 states of which the American Union then consisted was adopted by Congress on 4 July 1776. On 30 Nov. 1782 Great Britain acknowledged the independence of the USA, and on 3 Sept. 1783 the treaty of peace was concluded and was ratified by the USA on 14 Jan. 1784.

AREA AND POPULATION. Estimated population on 1 July 1989 was (in 1,000) 248,762, including males, 121,445; females, 127,317; White, 209,326 (106,774 females); Black, 30,788 (16,136 females); other races, 8,647 (4,407 females); persons of Hispanic origin, 20,528 (10,190 females). At the census of 1 April 1990 the population was 249,632,692. Population of USA at each census from 1790 to 1980, and for USA including Alaska and Hawaii, from 1960. Residents of Puerto Rico, Guam, American Samoa, the Virgin Islands of the USA, Northern Mariana Islands, the remainder of the Trust Territory of the Pacific Islands, Midway, Wake, Johnston and US population abroad are excluded from the figures of this table. Residents of Indian reservations are excluded prior to 1890.

	White	Black [1]	Other races [2]	Total	Decennial increase %
1790	3,172,464 [3]	757,208	—	3,929,672	—
1800	4,306,446	1,002,037	—	5,308,483	35·1
1810	5,862,073	1,377,808	—	7,239,881	36·4
1820	7,866,797	1,771,562	—	9,638,359	33·1
1830	10,537,378	2,328,642	—	12,866,020	33·5
1840	14,195,805	2,873,648	—	17,069,453	32·7
1850	19,553,068	3,638,808	—	23,191,876	35·9
1860	26,922,537	4,441,830	78,954 [4]	31,443,321	35·6
1870 [5]	33,589,377	4,880,009	88,985	38,558,371	22·6
1870 [5]	*34,337,292*	*5,392,172*	*88,985*	*39,818,449*	*26.6*
1880	43,402,970	6,580,793	172,020	50,155,783	30·1
1890	55,101,258	7,488,676	357,780	62,947,714	25·5
1900	66,868,508	8,834,395	509,265	76,212,168	21·0
1910	81,812,405	9,828,667	587,459	92,228,531	21·0
1920	94,903,540	10,463,607	654,421	106,021,568	14·9 [6]
1930	110,395,753 [7]	11,891,842	915,065	123,202,660	16·1 [6]
1940	118,357,831	12,865,914	941,384	132,165,129	7·3
1950	135,149,629	15,044,937	1,131,232	151,325,798	14·5
1960 [8]	158,831,732	18,871,831	1,619,612	179,323,175	18·5
1970	177,748,975	22,580,289	2,882,662	203,211,926	13·3
1980	188,371,622	26,495,025	11,679,158	226,545,805	11·4

[1] Seventeen southern states (including D.C.) in 1900 had 7,922,969 Blacks (89·7% of the total Black population); in 1920, 8,912,231 (85·2%); in 1940, 9,904,619 (77%); in 1950, 10,225,407 (68%); in 1960, 11,311,607 (59·9%); in 1970, 11,969,961 (53%); in 1980, 14,048,000 (53%).

[2] 1870: 63,199 Chinese, 55 Japanese and 25,731 Indians; 1880, 105,465 Chinese, 148 Japanese and 66,407 Indians; 1890, 107,488 Chinese, 2,039 Japanese and 248,253 Indians; 1900, 118,746 Chinese, 85,716 Japanese, 237,196 Indians, 67,607 other races; 1910, 94,414 Chinese, 152,745 Japanese, 276,927 Indians, 2,767 Filipino, 60,606 other races; 1920, 85,202 Chinese, 220,596 Japanese, 244,437 Indians, 26,634 Filipino, 77,552 other races; 1930, 343,352 Indians, 102,159 Chinese, 278,743 Japanese, 108,424 Filipino, 82,387 other races; 1940, 345,252 Indians, 106,334 Chinese, 285,115 Japanese, 98,535 Filipino, 106,148 other races; 1950, 357,499 Indians, 326,379 Japanese, 150,005 Chinese, 122,707 Filipino, 174,642 other races; 1960, 523,591 Indians, 464,332 Japanese, 237,292 Chinese, 176,310 Filipino, 218,087 other races;

[*Footnotes continued on p. 1374.*]

Population at the 1980 census comprised 110,053,161 males and 116,492,644 females; 167,054,638 were urban and 59,491,167 were rural. Black, 12,519,189 males and 13,975,836 females.

Age distribution by sex of the population (excluding armed forces overseas, US population abroad and outlying areas) at the 1980 census:

Age-group	*Male*	*Female*	*Total*
Under 5	8,362,009	7,986,245	16,348,254
5–9	8,539,080	8,160,876	16,699,956
10–14	9,316,221	8,925,908	18,242,129
15–19	10,755,409	10,412,715	21,168,124
20–24	10,663,231	10,655,473	21,318,704
25–34	18,381,903	18,699,936	37,081,839
35–44	12,569,719	13,064,991	25,634,710
45–54	11,008,919	11,790,868	22,799,787
55–59	5,481,863	6,133,391	11,615,254
60–64	4,669,892	5,417,729	10,087,621
65–74	6,756,502	8,824,103	15,580,605
75 and over	3,548,413	6,420,409	9,968,822
Total	110,053,161	116,492,644	226,545,805

The following table includes population statistics, the year in which each of the original 13 states ratified the constitution, and the year when each of the other states was admitted into the Union. Postal abbreviations for the names of the states are shown in brackets. Land area includes land temporarily or partially covered by water, and lakes, etc., of less than 40 acres.

Geographic divisions and states		*Land area: sq. miles 1980*	*Estimated population 1 July 1989 (in 1,000)*	*Census population 1 April 1980*	*Pop. per sq. mile, 1980*
United States		3,539,289	248,239	226,545,805	64·0
New England		63,012	13,047	12,348,493	196·0
Maine (1820)	*(Me.)*	30,995	1,222	1,124,660	36·3
New Hampshire (1788)	*(N.H.)*	8,993	1,107	920,610	102·4
Vermont (1791)	*(Vt.)*	9,273	567	511,456	55·2
Massachusetts (1788)	*(Mass.)*	7,824	5,913	5,737,037	733·3
Rhode Island (1790)	*(R.I.)*	1,055	998	947,154	897·8
Connecticut (1788)	*(Conn.)*	4,872	3,239	3,107,576	637·8
Middle Atlantic		99,733	37,726	36,786,790	368·9
New York (1788)	*(N.Y.)*	47,377	17,950	17,558,072	370·6
New Jersey (1787)	*(N.J.)*	7,468	7,736	7,364,823	986·2
Pennsylvania (1787)	*(Pa.)*	44,888	12,040	11,863,895	264·3

1970, 792,730 Indians, 591,290 Japanese, 435,062 Chinese, 343,060 Filipino, 720,520 other races; 1980, 1,364,033 Indians, 700,974 Japanese, 806,040 Chinese, 774,652 Filipino, 8,033,459 other races.

[3] Made up of Anglo-Scottish, 89·1%; German, 5·6%; Dutch, 2·5%; Irish, 1·9%; French, 0·6%.

[4] 34,933 Chinese and 44,021 Indians.

[5] Enumeration in 1870 incomplete. Figures in italics represent estimated corrected population.

[6] Between the 1910 census (15 April 1910) and the 1920 census (1 Jan. 1920), the period covered was 116 months (less than a full decade). Adjusting for this, the exact rate of increase for the decade was 15·4%. Similarly correcting for the 123 months between the 1920 and 1930 censuses, the true rate of increase was 15·7%.

[7] Figures for 1930 have been revised to include Mexicans (1,422,533), who were classified with 'Other Races' in the 1930 census reports.

[8] Figures for 1960 strictly comparable with those given for other years (*i.e.*, excluding Alaska and Hawaii) are: White, 158,454,956; Black, 18,860,117; other races, 1,149,163; total, 178,464,236; decennial increase, 18·4%.

Geographic divisions and states		Land area: sq. miles 1980	Estimated population 1 July 1989 (in 1,000)	Census population 1 April 1980	Pop. per sq. mile, 1980
East North Central		243,961	42,298	41,682,217	170·9
Ohio (1803)	*(Oh.)*	41,004	10,907	10,797,630	263·3
Indiana (1816)	*(Ind.)*	35,932	5,593	5,490,224	152·8
Illinois (1818)	*(Ill.)*	55,645	11,658	11,426,518	205·3
Michigan (1837)	*(Mich.)*	56,954	9,273	9,262,078	162·6
Wisconsin (1848)	*(Wis.)*	54,426	4,867	4,705,767	86·5
West North Central		508,132	17,851,389	17,183,453	33·8
Minnesota (1858)	*(Minn.)*	79,548	4,353	4,075,970	51·2
Iowa (1846)	*(Ia.)*	55,965	2,840	2,913,808	52·1
Missouri (1821)	*(Mo.)*	68,945	5,159	4,916,686	71·3
North Dakota (1889)	*(N.D.)*	69,300	660	652,717	9·4
South Dakota (1889)	*(S.D.)*	75,952	715	690,768	9·1
Nebraska (1867)	*(Nebr.)*	76,644	1,611	1,569,825	20·5
Kansas (1861)	*(Kans.)*	81,778	2,513	2,363,679	28·9
South Atlantic		266,910	43,115	36,959,123	138·5
Delaware (1787)	*(Del.)*	1,932	673	594,338	307·6
Maryland (1788)	*(Md.)*	9,837	4,694	4,216,975	428·7
Dist. of Columbia (1791)	*(D.C.)*	63	604	638,333	10,132·3
Virginia (1788)	*(Va.)*	39,704	6,098	5,346,818	134·7
West Virginia (1863)	*(W. Va.)*	24,119	1,857	1,949,644	80·8
North Carolina (1789)	*(N.C.)*	48,843	6,571	5,881,766	120·4
South Carolina (1788)	*(S.C.)*	30,203	3,512	3,121,820	103·4
Georgia (1788)	*(Ga.)*	58,056	6,486	5,463,105	94·1
Florida (1845)	*(Fla.)*	54,153	12,671	9,746,324	180·0
East South Central		178,824	15,406	14,666,423	82·0
Kentucky (1792)	*(Ky.)*	39,669	3,727	3,660,777	92·3
Tennessee (1796)	*(Tenn.)*	41,155	4,940	4,591,120	111·6
Alabama (1819)	*(Al.)*	50,767	4,118	3,893,888	76·7
Mississippi (1817)	*(Miss.)*	47,233	2,621	2,520,638	53·4
West South Central		427,271	27,002	23,746,816	55·6
Arkansas (1836)	*(Ark.)*	52,078	2,406	2,286,435	43·9
Louisiana (1812)	*(La.)*	44,521	4,382	4,205,900	94·5
Oklahoma (1907)	*(Okla.)*	68,655	3,224	3,025,290	44·1
Texas (1845)	*(Tex.)*	262,017	16,991	14,229,191	54·3
Mountain		855,193	13,513	11,372,785	13·3
Montana (1889)	*(Mont.)*	145,388	806	786,690	5·4
Idaho (1890)	*(Id.)*	82,412	1,014	943,935	11·5
Wyoming (1890)	*(Wyo.)*	96,989	475	469,557	4·8
Colorado (1876)	*(Colo.)*	103,595	3,317	2,889,964	27·9
New Mexico (1912)	*(N. Mex.)*	121,335	1,528	1,302,894	10·7
Arizona (1912)	*(Ariz.)*	113,508	3,556	2,718,215	23·9
Utah (1896)	*(Ut.)*	82,073	1,707	1,461,037	17·8
Nevada (1864)	*(Nev.)*	109,894	1,111	800,493	7·3
Pacific		896,253	38,283	31,799,705	35·5
Washington (1889)	*(Wash.)*	66,511	4,761	4,132,156	62·1
Oregon (1859)	*(Oreg.)*	96,184	2,820	2,633,105	27·4
California (1850)	*(Calif.)*	156,299	29,063	23,667,902	151·4
Alaska (1959)	*(Ak.)*	570,833	527	401,851	0·7
Hawaii (1960)	*(Hi.)*	6,425	1,112	964,691	150·1

Geographic divisions and states	*Land area: sq. miles 1980*	*Estimated population 1 July 1988 (in 1,000)*	*Census population 1 April 1980*	*Pop. per sq. mile, 1980*
Outlying Territories, total	4,691	...	3,565,376	760
Puerto Rico (1898)	3,515	3,291	3,196,520	909
Virgin Islands (1917)	132	103·2	96,569	731
American Samoa (1900)	77	39·5	32,297	419
Guam (1898)	209	133	105,979	507
Northern Marianas (1947)	184	21·2	16,780	91
Marshall Islands (1947)	70	...	30,873	441
Micronesia, Fed. States (1947)	271	...	73,160	270
Palau (1947)	192	...	12,116	63
Midway Islands (1867)	2	...	453	226
Wake Island (1898)	3	...	302	100
Johnston and Sand Islands (1858)	...	...	...	...

The 1980 census showed 9,323,946 foreign-born Whites. The 9 countries contributing the largest numbers who were foreign-born were Mexico, 2,199,221; Germany, 849,384; Canada, 842,859; Italy, 831,922; UK, 669,149; Cuba, 607,814; Philippines, 501,440; Poland, 418,128; USSR, 406,022.

Increase or decrease of native White, and foreign-born White, population from 1860 to 1980, by decades:

	Native White			*Foreign-born White*		
	Total	*Increase*	*Per cent increase*	*Total*	*Increase or decrease (–)*	*Per cent. change*
1860	22,825,784	5,513,251	31·8	4,096,753	1,856,218	82·8
1870	28,095,665	5,269,881	23·1	5,493,712	1,396,959	34·1
1880	36,843,291	8,747,626	31·1	6,559,679	1,065,967	19·4
1890	45,979,391	9,018,732 [1]	24·5	9,121,867	2,562,188	39·1
1900	56,595,379	10,615,988	23·1	10,213,817	1,091,950	12·0
1910	68,386,412	11,791,033	20·8	13,345,545	3,131,728	30·7
1920	81,108,161	12,721,749	18·6	13,712,754	367,209	2·8
1930	96,303,335	15,195,174	18·7	13,983,405	270,651	2·0
1940	106,795,732	10,492,397	10·9	11,419,138	–2,564,267	–18·3
1950	124,780,860	17,985,128	16·8	10,161,168	–1,257,970	–11·0
1960	149,543,638	24,762,778	19·8	9,293,992	– 867,176	– 8·5
1970	169,385,451	19,841,813	13·3	8,733,770	– 560,222	– 6·0
1980	179,711,066	10,325,615	6·0	9,323,946	590,176	6·7

[1] Exclusive of population specially enumerated in 1890 in Indian Territory and on Indian reservations.

Population of cities with over 100,000 inhabitants at the census of 1980, and estimate at 1 July 1988:

Cities	*Census 1980*	*Estimate 1988*	*Cities*	*Census 1980*	*Estimate 1988*
New York, N.Y.	7,071,639	7,352,700	Boston, Mass.	562,994	577,830
Los Angeles, Calif.	2,968,528	3,352,710	Columbus, Ohio	565,032	569,570
Chicago, Ill.	3,005,072	2,977,520	New Orleans, La.	557,927	531,700
Houston, Tex.	1,611,382	1,698,090	Cleveland, Ohio	573,822	521,370
Philadelphia, Pa.	1,688,210	1,647,000	El Paso, Tex.	425,259	510,970
San Diego, Calif.	875,538	1,070,310	Seattle, Wash.	493,846	502,200
Detroit, Mich.	1,203,369	1,035,920	Denver, Colo.	492,694	492,200
Dallas, Tex.	904,599	987,360	Nashville-Davidson Tenn.	455,651	481,400
San Antonio, Tex.	810,353	941,150			
Phoenix, Ariz.	790,183	923,750	Austin, Tex.	372,564	464,690
Baltimore, Md.	786,741	751,400	Kansas City, Mo.	448,028	438,950
San José, Calif.	629,402	738,420	Oklahoma City, Okla.	404,014	434,380
San Francisco, Calif.	678,974	731,600	Fort Worth, Tex.	385,164	426,610
Indianapolis, Ind.	700,807	727,130	Atlanta, Ga.	425,022	420,220
Memphis, Tenn.	646,170	645,190	Portland, Ore.	396,666	418,470
Jacksonville, Fla.	540,920	635,430	Long Beach, Calif.	361,496	415,040
Washington, D.C.	638,332	617,000	St. Louis, Mo.	452,804	403,700
Milwaukee, Wis.	636,292	599,380	Tucson, Ariz.	338,636	385,720

Cities	Census 1980	Estimate 1988	Cities	Census 1980	Estimate 1988
Albuquerque, N.M.	332,336	378,480	Fremont, Calif.	131,945	166,590
Honolulu, Hawaii	367,878	376,110	Amarillo, Tex.	149,230	166,010
Pittsburgh, Pa.	423,960	375,230	Tacoma, Wash.	158,501	163,960
Miami, Fla.	346,681	371,100	Chattanooga, Tenn.	169,520	162,670
Cincinnati, Ohio	385,410	370,480	Hialeah, Fla.	145,254	162,080
Tulsa, Okla.	360,919	368,330	Glendale, Calif.	139,060	161,210
Charlotte, N.C.	315,474	367,860	Kansas City, Kan.	161,148	160,630
Virginia Beach, Va.	262,199	365,300	Newport News, Va.	144,903	160,100
Oakland, Calif.	339,337	356,860	Huntsville, Ala.	142,513	159,450
Omaha, Nebr.	314,255	353,170	Bakersfield, Calif.	105,611	157,650
Minneapolis, Minn.	370,951	344,670	Worcester, Mass.	161,799	156,190
Toledo, Ohio	354,635	340,760	Providence, R.I.	156,804	156,160
Sacramento, Calif.	275,741	338,220	Orlando, Fla.	128,291	155,950
Newark, N.J.	329,248	313,800	Syracuse, N.Y.	170,105	153,610
Buffalo, N.Y.	357,870	313,570	Salt Lake City, Utah	163,034	152,740
Fresno, Calif.	217,491	307,090	Springfield, Mass.	152,319	150,320
Wichita, Kan.	279,838	295,320	Winston-Salem, N.C.	131,885	148,690
Norfolk, Va.	266,979	286,500	Modesto, Calif.	106,963	148,670
Colorado Springs Colo.	215,105	283,110	San Bernardino, Calif.	118,794	148,420
			Chesapeake, Va.	114,486	147,800
Louisville, Ky.	298,694	281,880	Savannah, Ga.	141,658	145,980
Tampa, Fla.	271,578	281,790	Fort Lauderdale, Fla.	153,279	145,610
Mesa, Ariz.	152,404	280,360	Warren, Mich.	161,134	145,410
Birmingham, Ala.	284,413	277,280	Springfield, Mo.	133,116	142,690
Corpus Christi, Tex.	232,134	260,930	Flint, Mich.	159,611	141,620
St. Paul, Minn.	270,230	259,110	Tempe, Ariz.	106,919	140,440
Arlington, Tex.	160,113	257,460	Glendale, Ariz.	97,172	140,170
Anaheim, Calif.	219,494	244,670	Bridgeport, Conn.	142,546	139,770
Santa Ana, Calif.	204,014	239,540	Paterson, N.J.	137,970	138,620
St. Petersburg. Fla.	238,647	235,450	Torrance, Calif.	129,881	137,940
Baton Rouge, La. 2/	220,394	235,270	Garden Grove, Calif.	123,307	135,310
Rochester, N.Y.	241,741	229,780	Rockford, Ill.	139,712	134,500
Lexington-Fayette, Ky.	204,165	225,700	Irving, Tex.	109,943	133,000
			Gary, Ind.	151,968	132,460
Akron, Ohio	237,177	221,510	Pasadena, Calif.	118,072	132,010
Aurora, Colo.	158,588	218,720	Hartford, Conn.	136,392	131,300
Anchorage, Alaska	174,431	218,500	Hampton, Va.	122,617	130,800
Shreveport, La.	206,989	218,010	Oxnard, Calif.	108,195	130,080
Jersey City, N.J.	223,532	217,630	Evansville, Ind.	130,496	128,210
Richmond, Va.	219,214	213,300	Chula Vista, Calif.	83,927	126,240
Riverside, Calif.	170,591	210,630	Tallahassee. Fla.	81,548	125,640
Las Vegas, Nev.	164,674	210,620	Lansing, Mich.	130,414	124,960
Mobile, Ala.	200,452	208,820	Laredo, Tex.	91,449	124,730
Jackson, Miss.	202,895	201,250	New Haven, Conn.	126,089	123,840
Montgomery, Ala.	177,857	193,510	Ontario, Calif.	88,820	123,380
Des Moines, Iowa	191,003	192,910	Topeka, Kan.	118,690	122,360
Stockton, Calif.	148,283	190,680	Scottsdale, Ariz.	88,622	121,740
Lubbock, Tex.	173,873	188,090	Pomona, Calif.	92,742	120,470
Lincoln, Nebr.	171,932	187,890	Hollywood, Fla.	121,323	120,140
Huntington Beach, Calif.	170,505	186,880	Lakewood, Colo.	113,808	119,340
			Plano, Tex.	72,331	118,790
Raleigh, N.C.	150,255	186,720	Macon, Ga.	116,896	117,940
Grand Rapids, Mich.	181,843	185,370	Pasadena, Tex.	112,560	116,880
Yonkers, N.Y.	195,351	183,000	Sunnyvale, Calif.	106,618	116,180
Greensboro, N.C.	155,642	181,970	Durham, N.C.	101,149	115,430
Garland, Tex.	138,857	180,450	Reno, Nev.	100,756	115,130
Little Rock, Ark.	159,159	180,090	Independence, Mo.	111,797	115,090
Fort Wayne, Ind.	172,391	179,810	Sterling Heights, Mich.	108,999	114,720
Madison, Wis.	170,616	178,180	Beaumont, Tex.	118,102	114,210
Dayton, Ohio	193,549	178,000	Erie, Pa.	119,123	112,800
Columbus, Ga.	169,441	177,680	Oceanside, Calif.	76,698	112,630
Knoxville, Tenn.	175,045	172,080	Boise City, Idaho	102,249	111,030
Spokane, Wash.	171,300	170,900	Cedar Rapids, Iowa	110,243	110,300

Cities	Census 1980	Estimate 1988	Cities	Census 1980	Estimate 1988
Fullerton, Calif.	102,246	109,740	Waterbury, Conn.	103,266	104,520
Peoria, Ill.	124,160	109,560	Brownsville, Tex.	84,997	104,510
Abilene, Tex.	98,315	109,110	Inglewood, Calif.	94,162	103,920
Ann Arbor, Mich.	107,969	108,440	Berkeley, Calif.	103,328	103,660
Alexandria, Va.	103,217	108,400	Hayward, Calif.	93,582	103,600
Santa Rosa, Calif.	83,320	108,220	Waco, Tex.	101,261	103,420
Concord, Calif.	103,763	108,040	Thousand Oaks, Calif.	77,072	101,530
Eugene, Ore.	105,662	108,030	Youngstown, Ohio	115,510	101,150
Portsmouth, Va.	104,577	107,500	Livoria, Mich.	104,814	101,100
Overland Park, Kan.	81,784	106,860	Salinas, Calif.	80,479	101,090
South Bend, Ind.	109,727	106,190	Pueblo, Colo.	101,686	101,070
Orange, Calif.	91,450	105,710	Vallejo, Calif.	80,303	100,730
Allentown, Pa.	103,758	105,200	Stamford, Conn.	102,466	100,260
Elizabeth, N.J.	106,201	105,150	Irvine, Calif.	62,134	100,130

Vital Statistics: Vital statistics are based on records of births, deaths, fœtal deaths, marriages and divorces filed with registration officials of states and cities. Figures for the US include Alaska beginning with 1959 and Hawaii beginning with 1960.

Annual collection of mortality records from a national death-registration area was inaugurated in 1900. A national birth-registration area was established in 1915. These areas, which at their inception comprised 10 states and the District of Columbia, expanded gradually until 1933, when both the birth- and death-registration areas covered the entire continental US. Marriage and divorce statistics are compiled from reports furnished by state and local officials. Data on annulments are included in the divorce statistics. The marriage-registration area was established in 1957 with 30 states and 3 other areas. The divorce-registration area was established in 1958 with 14 states and 2 other areas. In Jan. 1980 the marriage-registration area included 42 states and D.C., and the divorce-registration area included 30 states.

	Live births [1]	Deaths [2]	Marriages [3]	Divorces [4]	Maternal deaths	Deaths under 1 year [5]
1900	—	343,217	709,000	56,000	—	—
1910	2,777,000	696,856	948,000	83,000	—	—
1920	2,950,000	1,118,070	1,274,476	170,505	16,320	170,911
1930	2,618,000	1,327,240	1,126,856	195,961	14,915	143,201
1940	2,559,000	1,417,269	1,595,879	264,000	8,876	110,984
1950	3,632,000	1,452,454	1,667,231	385,144	2,960	103,825
1960	4,257,850 [7]	1,711,982	1,523,000	393,000	1,579	110,873
1970	3,731,386 [7]	1,921,031	2,158,802	708,000	803	74,667
1980	3,612,258	1,989,841	2,390,252	1,189,000	334	45,526
1985	3,760,561	2,086,440	2,412,625	1,190,000	295	40,030
1986	3,756,547	2,105,361	2,407,099	1,178,000	272	38,891
1987	3,809,394	2,123,323	2,421,000 [8]	1,157,000 [8]	251	38,408
1988 [8]	3,913,000	2,171,000	2,389,000	1,183,000	300	38,700

[1] Figures through 1959 include adjustment for under-registration (the 1959 registered count was 4,244,796); beginning 1960 figures represent number registered.
[2] Excluding fœtal deaths and deaths among the armed forces overseas.
[3] Estimates for all years except 1970.
[4] Includes reported annulments. Estimated for all years.
[5] Deaths for 1979–81 (Ninth Revision, International Classification of Diseases, 1975). Deaths from complications of pregnancy, childbirth and the puerperium. Deaths for 1968–78 were classified according to the Eighth Revision, International Classification of Diseases, adopted, 1965. Deaths for 1958–67 were classified according to the Seventh Revision of the International Lists of Diseases and Causes of Death, those for 1949–57 according to the Sixth Revision and those for 1939–48, according to the Fifth Revision.
[6] Excluding fœtal deaths. [7] Based on a 50% sample. [8] Provisional.

The crude birth rate, based on total live-birth estimates per 1,000 total population, fell from 29·5 in 1915 to 18·4 in 1933; it rose to a peak of 26·6 in 1947—its highest for 25 years. This peak reflects demobilization (1945–46), the record marriage rate that followed, and the high levels of employment and income. The decrease in the following 3 years was moderate. In 1951 the rate moved upward and levelled off in

1957 at about 25 per 1,000 population. Since 1957 the crude birth rate declined every year to 18·4 live births per 1,000 population in 1966. The crude birth rate for 1988 was 15·9. Estimated number of illegitimate births in 1986 was 878,477, a ratio of 233·9 illegitimate births per 1,000 registered live births.

Deaths, excluding fœtal deaths (per 1,000 population), declined from 17·2 in 1900 to 10 in 1946. The death rate has been below 10 per 1,000 since 1947, fluctuating slightly from year to year, mainly under the impact of occurrences of outbreaks of severe respiratory diseases. The rate for 1970, 9·5; 1980, 8·8; 1981, 8·6; 1982, 8·6; 1983, 8·6; 1984, 8·7; 1985, 8·7; 1986, 8·7; 1987, 8·7; 1988, 8·8.

Leading causes of death, 1988, per 100,000 population: Diseases of heart, 312·2; malignant neoplasms, 198·6; cerebrovascular diseases, 61·1; accidents, 39·7; suicides, 12·3; homicides, 9.

Deaths from AIDS (HIV infection) in 1988 (provisional) 16,210.

The marriage rates per 1,000 population for selected years are: 1920, 12; 1932, 7·9; 1946, 16·4; 1951, 10·4; 1961, 8·5; 1970, 10·6; 1975, 10; 1980, 10·6; 1981, 10·6; 1982, 10·8; 1983, 10·5; 1984, 10·5; 1985, 10·1; 1986, 10; 1987, 9·9; 1988, 9·7. The divorce rates per 1,000 population for selected years are: 1920, 1·6; 1946, 4·3; 1951, 2·5; 1961, 2·3; 1971, 3·7; 1979, 5·3; 1980, 5·2; 1981, 5·3; 1982, 5; 1983, 4·9; 1984, 5; 1985, 5; 1986, 4·8; 1987, 4·8; 1988, 4·8.

Maternal mortality rates (deaths of mothers from conditions associated with deliveries and complications of pregnancy, childbirth and the puerperium) per 100,000 live births, were 1915–19, 727·9 and thereafter declined: 493·9 for 1935–39; 376 for 1940; 207·2 for 1945; 83·3 for 1950; 47 for 1955; 37·1 for 1960; 31·6 for 1965; 21·5 for 1970; 12·8 for 1975; 9·2 for 1980; 8·5 for 1981; 8·9 for 1982; 8 for 1983; 7·2 for 1986. The 1986 rate for white women was 4·9 and for all other women 16.

The infant mortality rates, per 1,000 live births were: 1915–19, 95·7; 1920–24, 76·7; 1925–29, 69; 1930–34, 60·4; 38·3 in 1945; 29·2 in 1950; 26·4 in 1955; 26 in 1960; 20 in 1970; 16·1 in 1975; 12·6 in 1980; 10·6 in 1985; 10·4 in 1986; 10 in 1987; 9·9 in 1988. In 1984 the rate for whites was 9·4; for all other, 16·1.

Immigration: The Immigration and Nationality Act, as amended, provides for the numerical limitation of most immigration. Public Law 96–212, the Refugee Act of 1980, reduced the worldwide numerical limitation to 280,000 for 1980 and 270,000 thereafter, with a maximum of 20,000 visas available for one country. The colonies and dependencies of a foreign state are limited to 5,000 per year, chargeable to the country limitation of the mother country. Visas are allocated under a system of 6 preference categories, 4 of which are designed to reunite close relatives of US citizens and resident aliens of the US, and 2 for skilled and professional workers. Visa numbers not used in the preference categories are made available to qualified non-preference immigrants. The non-preference category has not been available since 1978 due to high demand in other categories. Immigrants not subject to any numerical limitation are spouses, children, and parents of US citizens, who are 21 years of age or older; certain former US citizens; ministers of religion; certain long-term US government employees; and refugees adjusting to immigrant status.

Immigrant data for 1989 include 478,814 aliens who were admitted as permanent residents under the legalization programme created by the Immigrant Reform and Control Act of 1986. These aliens have resided in the U.S. since before 1982 and have qualified as temporary residents under the first phase of the legalization programme; in the fiscal year 1989, they began qualifying for permanent status.

Immigrant aliens admitted to US for permanent residence, by country or region of birth.

Country or region of birth	*Immigrants admitted* 1986	1987	1988	1989
All countries	601,708	601,516	643,025	1,090,924
Europe	62,512	61,174	64,797	82,891
Germany, Fed. Rep.	6,991	7,210	6,645	6,708
Greece	2,512	2,653	2,458	2,491
Italy	3,089	2,784	2,949	2,910
Poland	8,481	7,519	9,507	15,101

Country or region of birth	Immigrants admitted 1986	1987	1988	1989
Portugal	3,766	3,912	3,199	3,958
Spain	1,591	1,578	1,483	1,550
UK	13,657	13,497	13,228	14,090
Yugoslavia	2,011	1,827	1,941	2,496
Other Europe	20,414	20,194	23,387	33,787
Asia	268,248	257,684	264,465	312,149
China and Taiwan	38,530	37,772	38,387	46,246
Hong Kong	5,021	4,706	8,546	9,740
India	26,227	27,803	26,268	31,175
Japan	3,959	4,174	4,512	4,849
Korea (North and South)	35,776	35,849	34,703	34,222
Philippines	52,558	50,060	50,697	57,034
Thailand	6,204	6,733	6,888	9,332
Other Asia	99,973	90,587	94,464	119,551
North America	207,714	216,550	250,009	607,398
Canada	11,039	11,876	11,783	12,151
Mexico	66,533	72,351	95,039	405,172
Cuba	33,114	28,916	17,558	10,046
Dominican Republic	26,175	24,858	27,189	26,723
Haiti	12,666	14,819	34,806	13,658
Jamaica	19,595	23,148	20,966	24,523
Trinidad and Tobago	2,891	3,543	3,947	*,***
Other Caribbean	7,191	7,615	7,891	8,588
Central America	28,380	29,296	30,715	101,034
Other North America	130	128	115	109
South America	41,874	44,385	41,007	58,926
Colombia	11,408	11,700	10,322	15,204
Ecuador	4,516	4,641	4,716	7,532
Other South America	25,950	28,044	25,969	36,180
Africa	17,463	17,724	18,882	25,166
Australia and New Zealand	1,964	1,844	2,024	2,335
Other countries	1,933	2,155	1,841	2,059

The total number of immigrants admitted from 1820 up to 30 Sept. 1989 was 54,366,607; this included 7,060,894 from the Federal Republic of Germany, and from Italy 5,345,773.

Aliens coming to the US for temporary periods of time are classified as non-immigrants. During fiscal year 1989, a total of 16,144,577 non-immigrants were admitted. This total includes multiple entry documents but excludes border crossers, crewmen and insular travellers. Tourists numbered 12,114,584, with 7,034,219 coming from Mexico, Japan, the UK, the Caribbean, Germany and Canada. There were 859,521 aliens expelled during fiscal year 1989. Of this number, 28,965 were deported and 830,556 were required to depart without formal orders of deportation.

During fiscal year 1989, 233,727 persons became US citizens through naturalization, including 210,673 naturalized under the general provisions of 5-year residence in the US, 20,443 spouses and children of US citizens, 1,954 members of US Armed Forces and 92 under other provisions. The new citizens included 9,514 from Cuba, 24,802 from the Philippines, 17,443 from China and Taiwan, 11,301 from Korea, 7,865 from the UK, 2,492 from Italy, 18,520 from Mexico, 6,455 from Jamaica, and 19,357 from Vietnam.

CLIMATE. For temperature and rainfall figures, see entries on individual states as indicated by regions, below, of mainland USA.

Pacific Coast. The climate varies with latitude, distance from the sea and the effect of relief, ranging from polar conditions in North Alaska through cool to warm temperate climates further south. The extreme south is temperate desert. Rainfall everywhere is moderate. *See* Alaska, California, Oregon, Washington.

Mountain States. Very varied, with relief exerting the main control; very cold in the north in winter, with considerable snowfall. In the south, much higher temperatures and aridity produce desert conditions. Rainfall everywhere is very variable as a result of rain-shadow influences. *See* Arizona, Colorado, Idaho, Montana, Nevada, New Mexico, Utah, Wyoming.

High Plains. A continental climate with a large annual range of temperature and moderate rainfall, mainly in summer, although unreliable. Dust storms are common in summer and blizzards in winter. *See* Nebraska, North Dakota, South Dakota.

Central Plains. A temperate continental climate, with hot summers and cold winters, except in the extreme south. Rainfall is plentiful and comes at all seasons, but there is a summer maximum in western parts. *See* Mississippi, Missouri, Oklahoma, Texas.

Mid-West. Continental, with hot summers and cold winters. Rainfall is moderate, with a summer maximum in most parts. *See* Indiana, Iowa, Kansas.

Great Lakes. Continental, resembling that of the Central Plains, with hot summers but very cold winters because of the freezing of the lakes. Rainfall is moderate with a slight summer maximum. *See* Illinois, Michigan, Minnesota, Ohio, Wisconsin.

Appalachian Mountains. The north is cool temperate with cold winters, the south warm temperate with milder winters. Precipitation is heavy, increasing to the south but evenly distributed over the year. *See* Kentucky, Pennsylvania, Tennessee, West Virginia.

Gulf Coast. Conditions vary from warm temperate to sub-tropical, with plentiful rainfall, decreasing towards the west but evenly distributed over the year. *See* Alabama, Arkansas, Florida, Louisiana.

Atlantic Coast. Temperate maritime climate but with great differences in temperature according to latitude. Rainfall is ample at all seasons; snowfall in the north can be heavy. *See* Delaware, District of Columbia, Georgia, Maryland, New Jersey, New York, North Carolina, South Carolina, Virginia.

New England. Cool temperate, with severe winters and warm summers. Precipitation is well distributed with a slight winter maximum. Snowfall is heavy in winter. *See* Connecticut, Maine, Massachusetts, New Hampshire, Rhode Island, Vermont. *See* also Hawaii and Outlying Territories.

CONSTITUTION AND GOVERNMENT. The form of government of the USA is based on the constitution of 17 Sept. 1787.

By the constitution the government of the nation is composed of three co-ordinate branches, the executive, the legislative and the judicial.

The National Government has authority in matters of general taxation, treaties and other dealings with foreign Powers, foreign and inter-state commerce, bankruptcy, postal service, coinage, weights and measures, patents and copyright, the armed forces (including, to a certain extent, the militia), and crimes against the USA; it has sole legislative authority over the District of Columbia and the possessions of the US.

The 5th article of the constitution provides that Congress may, on a two-thirds vote of both houses, propose amendments to the constitution, or, on the application of the legislatures of two-thirds of all the states, call a convention for proposing amendments, which in either case shall be valid as part of the constitution when ratified by the legislatures of three-fourths of the several states, or by conventions in three-fourths thereof, whichever mode of ratification may be proposed by Congress. Ten amendments (called collectively 'the Bill of Rights') to the constitution were added 15 Dec. 1791; two in 1795 and 1804; a 13th amendment, 6 Dec. 1865, abolishing slavery; a 14th in 1868, including the important 'due process' clause; a 15th, 3 Feb. 1870, establishing equal voting rights for white and coloured; a 16th, 3 Feb. 1913, authorizing the income tax; a 17th, 8 April 1913, providing for popular election of senators; an 18th, 16 Jan. 1919, prohibiting alcoholic liquors; a 19th, 18 Aug. 1920, establishing woman suffrage; a 20th, 23 Jan. 1933, advancing the date of the President's and Vice-President's inauguration and abolishing the 'lameduck' sessions of Congress; a 21st, 5 Dec. 1933, repealing the 18th amendment; a 22nd, 26 Feb. 1951, limiting a President's tenure of office to 2 terms, or to 2 terms plus 2 years in the case of a Vice-President who has succeeded to the office of a President;

a 23rd, 30 March 1961, granting citizens of the District of Columbia the right to vote in national elections; a 24th, 4 Feb. 1964, banning the use of the poll-tax in federal elections; a 25th, 10 Feb. 1967, dealing with Presidential disability and succession; a 26th, 22 June 1970, establishing the right of citizens who are 18 years of age and older to vote.

National flag: Seven red and 6 white alternating stripes, horizontal; with a blue canton, extending down to the lower edge of the 4th red stripe from the top, and displaying 50 white 5-pointed stars, one for each state. The stars have one point directed vertically upward, and they are arranged in 6 rows of 5 each, alternating with 5 rows of 4 each. On the admission of additional states, stars are added, effective on 4 July following the date of admission. Congress, by law of 22 Dec. 1942, has codified 'existing rules and customs' pertaining to the display of the flag, for civilians.

National anthem: The Star-spangled Banner, 'Oh say, can you see by the dawn's early light' (words by F. S. Key, 1814; tune by J. S. Smith; formally adopted by Congress 3 March 1931).

National motto: 'In God we trust'; formally adopted by Congress 30 July 1956.

Presidency. The executive power is vested in a president, who holds office for 4 years, and is elected, together with a vice-president chosen for the same term, by electors from each state, equal to the whole number of senators and representatives to which the state may be entitled in the Congress. The President must be a natural-born citizen, resident in the country for 14 years, and at least 35 years old.

The presidential election is held every fourth (leap) year on the Tuesday after the first Monday in November. Technically, this is an election of presidential electors, not of a president directly; the electors thus chosen meet and give their votes (for the candidate to whom they are pledged, in some states by law, but in most states by custom and prudent politics) at their respective state capitals on the first Monday after the second Wednesday in December next following their election; and the votes of the electors of all the states are opened and counted in the presence of both Houses of Congress on the sixth day of January. The total electorate vote is one for each senator and representative.

If the successful candidate for President dies before taking office the Vice-President-elect becomes President; if no candidate has a majority or if the successful candidate fails to qualify, then, by the 20th amendment, the Vice-President acts as President until a president qualifies. The duties of the Presidency, in absence of the President and Vice-President by reason of death, resignation, removal, inability or failure to qualify, devolve upon the Speaker of the House under legislation enacted 18 July 1947. And in case of absence of a Speaker for like reason, the presidential duties devolve upon the President *pro tem.* of the Senate and successively upon those members of the Cabinet in order of precedence, who have the constitutional qualifications for President.

The presidential term, by the 20th amendment to the constitution, begins at noon on 20 Jan. of the inaugural year. This amendment also installs the newly elected Congress in office on 3 Jan. instead of—as formerly—in the following December. The President's salary is $200,000 per year, plus $50,000 to assist in defraying expenses resulting from official duties. Also he may spend up to $100,000 non-taxable for travel and $20,000 for official entertainment. The office of Vice-President carries a salary of $115,000, plus $10,000 allowance for travel, all taxable.

The President is C.-in-C. of the Army, Navy and Air Force, and of the militia when in the service of the Union. The Vice-President is *ex-officio* President of the Senate, and in the case of 'the removal of the President, or of his death, resignation, or inability to discharge the powers and duties of his office', he becomes the President for the remainder of the term.

President of the United States: George Bush, of Texas, born at Milton, Massachusetts, in 1924; Vice-President, 1981–89.

Vice President: Dan Quayle, of Indiana; born 1947.

At the Presidential election on 8 Nov. 1988 total vote cast, including men and women in the armed services, was 91,585,872, of which George Bush (R.) received

48,881,011 (53·4%), Michael Dukakis (D.) 41,828,350 (45·67%), Ron Paul (Libertarian) 431,499 (0·47%), Lenora Fulani (New Alliance) 218,159 (0·24%). Electoral college votes: Bush 426; Dukakis 112.

Presidents of the USA

Name	*From state*	*Term of service*	*Born*	*Died*
George Washington	Virginia	1789–97	1732	1799
John Adams	Massachusetts	1797–1801	1735	1826
Thomas Jefferson	Virginia	1801–09	1743	1826
James Madison	Virginia	1809–17	1751	1836
James Monroe	Virginia	1817–25	1759	1831
John Quincy Adams	Massachusetts	1825–29	1767	1848
Andrew Jackson	Tennessee	1829–37	1767	1845
Martin Van Buren	New York	1837–41	1782	1862
William H. Harrison	Ohio	Mar.–Apr. 1841	1773	1841
John Tyler	Virginia	1841–45	1790	1862
James K. Polk	Tennessee	1845–49	1795	1849
Zachary Taylor	Louisiana	1849–July 1850	1784	1850
Millard Fillmore	New York	1850–53	1800	1874
Franklin Pierce	New Hampshire	1853–57	1804	1869
James Buchanan	Pennsylvania	1857–61	1791	1868
Abraham Lincoln	Illinois	1861–Apr. 1865	1809	1865
Andrew Johnson	Tennessee	1865–69	1808	1875
Ulysses S. Grant	Illinois	1869–77	1822	1885
Rutherford B. Hayes	Ohio	1877–81	1822	1893
James A. Garfield	Ohio	Mar.–Sept. 1881	1831	1881
Chester A. Arthur	New York	1881–85	1830	1886
Grover Cleveland	New York	1885–89	1837	1908
Benjamin Harrison	Indiana	1889–93	1833	1901
Grover Cleveland	New York	1893–97	1837	1908
William McKinley	Ohio	1897–Sept. 1901	1843	1901
Theodore Roosevelt	New York	1901–09	1858	1919
William H. Taft	Ohio	1909–13	1857	1930
Woodrow Wilson	New Jersey	1913–21	1856	1924
Warren Gamaliel Harding	Ohio	1921–Aug. 1923	1865	1923
Calvin Coolidge	Massachusetts	1923–29	1872	1933
Herbert C. Hoover	California	1929–33	1874	1964
Franklin D. Roosevelt	New York	1933–Apr. 1945	1882	1945
Harry S. Truman	Missouri	1945–53	1884	1972
Dwight D. Eisenhower	New York	1953–61	1890	1969
John F. Kennedy	Massachusetts	1961–Nov. 1963	1917	1963
Lyndon B. Johnson	Texas	1963–69	1908	1973
Richard M. Nixon	California	1969–74	1913	—
Gerald R. Ford	Michigan	1974–77	1913	—
James Earl Carter	Georgia	1977–81	1924	—
Ronald Reagan	California	1981–89	1911	—
George Bush	Texas	1989–	1924	—

Vice-Presidents of the USA

Name	From state	Term of service	Born	Died
John Adams	Massachusetts	1789–97	1735	1826
Thomas Jefferson	Virginia	1797–1801	1743	1826
Aaron Burr	New York	1801–05	1756	1836
George Clinton	New York	1805–12 [1]	1739	1812
Elbridge Gerry	Massachusetts	1813–14 [1]	1744	1814
Daniel D. Tompkins	New York	1817–25	1774	1825
John C. Calhoun	South Carolina	1825–32 [1]	1782	1850
Martin Van Buren	New York	1833–37	1782	1862
Richard M. Johnson	Kentucky	1837–41	1780	1850
John Tyler	Virginia	Mar.–Apr. 1841 [1]	1790	1862

[1] Position vacant thereafter until commencement of the next presidential term.

Name	*From state*	*Term of service*	*Born*	*Died*
George M. Dallas	Pennsylvania	1845–49	1792	1864
Millard Fillmore	New York	1849–50 [1]	1800	1874
William R. King	Alabama	Mar.–Apr. 1853 [1]	1786	1853
John C. Breckinridge	Kentucky	1857–61	1821	1875
Hannibal Hamlin	Maine	1861–65	1809	1891
Andrew Johnson	Tennessee	Mar.–Apr. 1865 [1]	1808	1875
Schuyler Colfax	Indiana	1869–73	1823	1885
Henry Wilson	Massachusetts	1873–75 [1]	1812	1875
William A. Wheeler	New York	1877–81	1819	1887
Chester A. Arthur	New York	Mar.–Sept. 1881 [1]	1830	1886
Thomas A. Hendricks	Indiana	Mar.–Nov. 1885 [1]	1819	1885
Levi P. Morton	New York	1889–93	1824	1920
Adlai Stevenson	Illinois	1893–97	1835	1914
Garret A. Hobart	New Jersey	1897–99 [1]	1844	1899
Theodore Roosevelt	New York	Mar.–Sept. 1901 [1]	1858	1919
Charles W. Fairbanks	Indiana	1905–09	1855	1920
James S. Sherman	New York	1909–12 [1]	1855	1912
Thomas R. Marshall	Indiana	1913–21	1854	1925
Calvin Coolidge	Massachusetts	1921–Aug. 1923 [1]	1872	1933
Charles G. Dawes	Illinois	1925–29	1865	1951
Charles Curtis	Kansas	1929–33	1860	1935
John N. Garner	Texas	1933–41	1868	1967
Henry A. Wallace	Iowa	1941–45	1888	1965
Harry S. Truman	Missouri	1945–Apr. 1945 [1]	1884	1972
Alben W. Barkley	Kentucky	1949–53	1877	1956
Richard M. Nixon	California	1953–61	1913	—
Lyndon B. Johnson	Texas	1961–Nov. 1963 [1]	1908	1973
Hubert H. Humphrey	Minnesota	1965–69	1911	1978
Spiro T. Agnew	Maryland	1969–73	1918	—
Gerald R. Ford	Michigan	1973–74	1913	—
Nelson Rockefeller	New York	1974–77	1908	1979
Walter Mondale	Minnesota	1977–81	1928	—
George Bush	Texas	1981–89	1924	—
Danforth Quayle	Indiana	1989–	1947	—

[1] Position vacant thereafter until commencement of the next presidential term.

Cabinet. The administrative business of the nation has been traditionally vested in several executive departments, the heads of which, unofficially and *ex officio*, formed the President's Cabinet. Beginning with the Interstate Commerce Commission in 1887, however, an increasing amount of executive business has been entrusted to some 60 so-called independent agencies, such as the Veterans Administration, Housing and Home Finance Agency, Tariff Commission, etc.

All heads of departments and of the 60 or more administrative agencies are appointed by the President, but must be confirmed by the Senate.

The Cabinet consisted of the following (March 1991):

1. *Secretary of State* (created 1789). James Addison Baker III, of Texas, lawyer; Presidential Chief of Staff 1981–85; Secretary of the Treasury 1985–88; born 1930.

2. *Secretary of the Treasury* (1789). Nicholas F. Brady, investment banker; born 1930.

3. *Secretary of Defense* (1947). Richard Cheney, of Wyoming; congressman; White House Chief of Staff 1975–76; born 1940.

4. *Attorney-General* (Department of Justice, 1870). Richard Thornburgh, of Pennsylvania; lawyer, academic administrator; governor of Pennsylvania 1979–87; born 1932.

5. *Secretary of the Interior* (1849). Manuel Lujan, Jr., of New Mexico; congressman; born 1928.

6. *Secretary of Agriculture* (1889). Edward R. Madigan, of Illinois; congressman; member of the House of Energy and Commerce Committee; Republican chief deputy whip; born 1936.

7. *Secretary of Commerce* (1903). Robert A. Mosbacher, Sr., of Texas; oil and gas producer; former co-chairman, Republican National Finance Committee; born 1927.

8. *Secretary of Labor* (1913). Lynn Morley Martin, of Illinois; congresswoman; teacher; born 1939.

9. *Secretary of Health and Human Services* (1953). Louis W. Sullivan, of Georgia; medical school president; born 1933.

10. *Secretary of Housing and Urban Development* (1966). Jack F. Kemp, of New York; congressman; born 1935.

11. *Secretary of Transportation* (1967). Samuel K. Skinner, of Chicago; regional transport authority chairman; lawyer; born 1938.

12. *Secretary of Energy* (1977). James D. Watkins, naval officer; Chief of Naval Operations 1982–86; born 1927.

13. *Secretary of Education* (1979). Andrew Lamar Alexander, of Tennessee; lawyer; academic administrator; governor of Tennessee, 1979-87; chairman, National Governors' Association; born 1940.

14. *Veterans' Affairs* (1989). Edward J. Derwinski, of Chicago; government official; born 1926.

Each of the above Cabinet officers receives an annual salary of $138,900 and holds office during the pleasure of the President.

Congress: The legislative power is vested by the Constitution in a Congress, consisting of a Senate and House of Representatives.

Electorate: By amendments of the constitution, disqualification of voters on the ground of race, colour or sex is forbidden. The electorate consists of all citizens over 18 years of age. Literacy tests have been banned since 1970. In 1972 durational residency requirements were held to violate the constitution. In 1973 US citizens abroad were enfranchised.

With limitations imposed by the constitution, it is the states which determine voter eligibility. In general states exclude from voting: Persons who have not established residency in the jurisdiction in which they wish to vote; persons who have been convicted of felonies whose civil rights have not been restored; persons declared mentally incompetent by a court.

Illiterate voters are entitled to receive assistance in marking their ballots. Minority-language voters in jurisdictions with statutorily prescribed minority concentrations are entitled to have elections conducted in the minority language as well as English. Disabled voters are entitled to accessible polling places. Voters absent on election days or unable to go to the polls are generally entitled under state law to vote by absentee ballot.

The constitution guarantees citizens that their votes will be of equal value under the 'one person, one vote' rule.

Senate: The Senate consists of 2 member from each state, chosen by popular vote for 6 years, one-third retiring or seeking re-election every 2 years. Senators must be no less than 30 years of age; must have been citizens of the USA for 9 years, and be residents in the states for which they are chosen. The Senate has complete freedom to initiate legislation, except revenue bills (which must originate in the House of Representatives); it may, however, amend or reject any legislation originating in the lower house. The Senate is also entrusted with the power of giving or withholding its 'advice and consent' to the ratification of all treaties initiated by the President with foreign Powers, a two-thirds majority of senators present being required for approval. (However, it has no control over 'international executive agreements' made by the President with foreign governments; such 'agreements', representing an important but very recent development, cover a wide range and are actually more numerous than formal treaties.) It also has the power of confirming or rejecting major appointments to office made by the President, but it has no direct control over the appointment by the President of 'personal representatives' or 'personal envoys' on missions abroad. Members of the Senate constitute a High Court of Impeachment, with power, by a two-thirds vote, to remove from office and disqualify any civil officer of the USA impeached by the House of Representatives, which has the sole power of impeachment.

The Senate has 16 Standing Committees to which all bills are referred for study, revision or rejection. The House of Representatives has 22 such committees. In both Houses each Standing Committee has a chairman and a majority representing the majority party of the whole House; each has numerous sub-committees. The jurisdictions of these Committees correspond largely to those of the appropriate executive departments and agencies. Both Houses also have a few special Committees with limited duration; there were (1991) 4 Joint Committees.

House of Representatives: The House of Representatives consists of 435 members elected every second year. The number of each state's representatives is determined by the decennial census, in the absence of specific Congressional legislation affecting the basis. The states, in 1991, had the following representatives:

Alabama	7	Indiana	10	Nebraska	3	South Carolina	6
Alaska	1	Iowa	6	Nevada	2	South Dakota	1
Arizona	5	Kansas	5	New Hampshire	2	Tennessee	9
Arkansas	4	Kentucky	7	New Jersey	14	Texas	27
California	45	Louisiana	8	New Mexico	3	Utah	3
Colorado	6	Maine	2	New York	34	Vermont	1
Connecticut	6	Maryland	8	North Carolina	11	Virginia	10
Delaware	1	Massachusetts	11	North Dakota	1	Washington	8
Florida	19	Michigan	18	Ohio	21	West Virginia	4
Georgia	10	Minnesota	8	Oklahoma	6	Wisconsin	9
Hawaii	2	Mississippi	5	Oregon	5	Wyoming	1
Idaho	2	Missouri	9	Pennsylvania	23		
Illinois	22	Montana	2	Rhode Island	2		

The constitution requires congressional districts within each state to be substantially equal in population. Final decisions on congressional district boundaries are taken by the state legislatures and governors. By custom the representative lives in the district from which he is elected.

Representatives must be not less than 25 years of age, citizens of the USA for 7 years and residents in the state from which they are chosen. The District of Columbia, Guam, American Samoa and the Virgin Islands have one non-voting delegate each. The House also admits a 'resident commissioner' from Puerto Rico, who has the right to speak on any subject and to make motions, but not to vote; he is elected in the same manner as the representatives but for a 4-year term. Each of the two Houses of Congress is sole 'judge of the elections, returns and qualifications of its own members'; and each of the Houses may, with the concurrence of two-thirds, expel a member. The period usually termed 'a Congress' in legislative language continues for 2 years, terminating at noon on 3 Jan.

The salary of a senator is $102,000 per annum, with tax-free expense allowance and allowances for travelling expenses and for clerical hire. The salary of the Speaker of the House of Representatives is $155,000 per annum, with a taxable allowance. The salary of a Member of the House is $125,100. Salaries are under review.

No senator or representative can, during the time for which he is elected, be appointed to any *civil* office under authority of the USA which shall have been created or the emoluments of which shall have been increased during such time; and no person holding *any* office under the USA can be a member of either House during his continuance in office. No religious text may be required as a qualification to any office or public trust under the USA or in any state.

The 102nd Congress (1991–93) was constituted (Feb. 1991) as follows: Senate, 56 Democrats, 44 Republicans; House of Representatives, 267 Democrats, 167 Republicans, 1 independent.

Indians: By an Act passed on 2 June 1924 full citizenship was granted to all Indians born in the USA, though those remaining in tribal units were still under special federal jurisdiction. Those remaining in tribal units constitute from one-half to three-fourths of the Indian population. The Indian Reorganization Act of 1934 gave the tribal Indians, at their own option, substantial opportunities to self-government and of self-controlled corporate enterprises empowered to borrow money, buy land, machinery and equipment; these corporations are controlled by democratically elected tribal councils; by 1945 roughly a third of the Indians had taken advantage of this Act. Recently a trend towards releasing Indians from federal supervision has resulted in legislation terminating supervision over specific tribes. Indian lands (1981) amounted to 52,473,000 acres, of which 41,062,000 was tribally owned and 10·96m. in trust allotments. Indian lands are held free of taxes. Total Indian population at the 1980 census was 1,418,195, of which Oklahoma, Arizona, California and New Mexico accounted for 628,400.

State and Local Government: The Union comprises 13 original states, 7 states which were admitted without having been previously organized as territories, and 30 states which had been territories—50 states in all. Each state has its own constitution (which the USA guarantees shall be republican in form), deriving its authority, not from Congress, but from the people of the state. Admission of states into the Union has been granted by special Acts of Congress, either (1) in the form of 'enabling Acts' providing for the drafting and ratification of a state constitution by the people, in which case the territory becomes a state as soon as the conditions are fulfilled, or (2) accepting a constitution already framed, and at once granting admission.

Each state is provided with a legislature of two Houses (except Nebraska, which since 1937 has had a single-chamber legislature), a governor and other executive officials, and a judicial system. Both Houses of the legislature are elective, but the senators (having larger electoral districts usually covering 2 or 3 counties compared with the single county or, in some states, the town, which sends 1 representative to the Lower House) are less numerous than the representatives, while in 38 states their terms are 4 years; in 12 states the term is 2 years. Of the 4-year senates, Illinois, Montana and New Jersey provide for two 4-year terms and one 2-year term in each decade. Terms of the lower houses are usually shorter; in 45 states, 2 years.

Members of both Houses are paid at the same rate, which varies from $100 a year in New Hampshire to $57,500 a year in New York. The trend is towards annual sessions of state legislatures; in 1991, 43 met annually (in 1939, only 4), and 7 (Arkansas, Kentucky, Montana, Nevada, North Dakota, Oregon and Texas) biennially.

The Governor has power to summon an extraordinary session, but not to dissolve or adjourn. The duties of the two Houses are similar, but in many states money bills must be introduced first in the Lower House. The Senate sits as a court for the trial of officials impeached by the other House, and often has power to confirm or reject appointments made by the Governor.

State legislatures are competent to deal with all matters not reserved for the federal government by the federal constitution nor specifically prohibited by the federal or state constitutions. Among their powers are the determination of the qualifications for the right of suffrage, and the control of all elections to public office, including elections of members of Congress and electors of President and Vice-President; the criminal law, both in its enactment and in its execution, with unimportant exceptions, and the administration of prisons; the civil law, including all matters pertaining to the possession and transfer of, and succession to, property; marriage and divorce, and all other civil relations; the chartering and control of all manufacturing, trading, transportation and other corporations, subject only to the right of Congress to regulate commerce passing from one state to another; labour; education; charities; licensing; fisheries within state waters, and game laws (apart from the hunting of migratory birds, which is a federal concern under treaties with Canada and Mexico). Taxes on income were left to the states until 1913, when the 16th amendment authorized the imposition of federal taxes on income without regard to apportionment.

The Governor is elected by direct vote of the people over the whole state. His term of office varies in the several states from 2 to 4 years, and his salary from $35,000 (Arkansas, Maine) to $100,000 (New York). His duty is to see to the faithful administration of the law, and he has command of the military forces of the state. He may recommend measures but does not present bills to the legislature. In some states he presents estimates. In all but one of the states (North Carolina) the Governor has a veto upon legislation, which may, however, be overridden by the two Houses, in some states by a simple majority, in others by a three-fifths or two-thirds majority. In some states the Governor, on his death or resignation, is succeeded by a Lieut.-Governor who was elected at the same time and has been presiding over the state Senate. In several states the Speaker of the Lower House succeeds the Governor.

The chief officials by whom the administration of state affairs is carried on (secretaries, treasurers, members of boards of commissioners, etc.) are usually chosen by the people at the general state elections for terms similar to those for which governors hold office.

Local Government. The chief unit of local government is the county, of which there were (1991) 3,042 with definite functions; in addition, Rhode Island has 5 'counties' which have no functions; Alaska does not have 'counties' as such and, since Oct. 1960, there has been no active county government in Connecticut. Louisiana has 61 'parishes'. The counties maintain public order through the sheriff and his deputies, who may, in a crisis, be drawn temporarily from willing citizens; in many states the counties maintain the smaller local highways; other functions are the granting of licences and the apportionment and collection of taxes. In a few states they also manage the schools.

The unit of local government in New England is the rural township, governed directly by the voters, who assemble annually or oftener if necessary, and legislate in local affairs, levy taxes, make appropriations and appoint and instruct the local officials (selectmen, clerk, school-committee, etc.). Townships are grouped to form counties. Where cities exist, the township government is superseded by the city government.

The **District of Columbia,** ceded by the State of Maryland for the purposes of government in 1791, is the seat of the US Government. It includes the city of Washington, and embraces a land area of 61 sq. miles. The Reorganization Plan No. 3 of 1967 instituted a Mayor Council form of government with appointed officers. In 1973 an elected Mayor and elected councillors were introduced; in 1974 they received power to legislate in local matters. Congress retains power to enact legislation and to veto or supersede the Council's acts. Since 1961 citizens have had the right to vote in national elections. On 23 Aug. 1978 the Senate approved a constitutional amendment giving the District full voting representation in Congress. This has still to be ratified.

The **Commonwealth of Puerto Rico, American Samoa, Guam and the Virgin Islands** each have a local legislature, whose acts may be modified or annulled by Congress, though in practice this has seldom been done. Puerto Rico since its attainment of commonwealth status on 25 July 1952, enjoys practically complete self-government, including the election of its governor and other officials. The conduct of foreign relations, however, is still a federal function and federal bureaux and agencies still operate in the island.

General supervision of territorial administration is exercised by the Office of Territories in the Department of Interior.

Congress and the Nation, 4 vols., Congressional Quarterly, Washington, from 1965.—*Congressional Ethics,* Rev. ed., 1980.—*Congressional Quarterly Almanac,* annual
Constitution of the US, National and State. 2 vols. [with subsequent amendments]. Dobbs Ferry, 1962
Political profiles. 5 vols. New York, from 1978
Adrian, C. R., *State and Local Government*. 4th ed. New York, 1977
Barone, M. (ed.) *The Almanac of American Politics*. New York and London, Annual
Brenner, P., *The Limits and Possibilities of Congress*. New York, 1983
Seymour – Ure, C., *The American President: Power and Communication*. London, 1982

DEFENCE. The President is C.-in-C. of the Army, Navy and Air Force.

The National Security Act of 1947 provides for the unification of the Army, Navy and Air Forces under a single Secretary of Defense with cabinet rank. The President is also advised by a National Security Council and the Office of Civil and Defense Mobilization.

The major components of the Department of Defense are the Office of the Secretary of Defense and the Joint Chiefs of Staff, who provide immediate staff assistance and advice to the Secretary; the departments of the Army, Navy and Air Force, each separately organized under a civilian head (not of cabinet rank); and the unified and specified commands.

Army. *Secretary of the Army:* Michael P. W. Stone.

Central Administration. The Secretary of the Army is the head of the Department of the Army. Subject to the authority of the President as C.-in-C. and of the Secretary of Defense, he is responsible for all affairs of the Department.

The Secretary of the Army is assisted by the Under Secretary of the Army, 5 Assistant Secretaries of the Army (Civil Works, Financial Management, Installations, Logistics and Environment, Manpower and Reserve Affairs, Research, Development and Acquisition), General Counsel, Administrative Assistant, Director for Information Systems for Command, Control, Communications and Computers, Inspector General, Auditor General, Chief of Legislative Liaison, Chief of Public Affairs, Director for Small and Disadvantaged Business Utilization, Chairman of the Army Reserve Forces Policy Committee and the Army Staff headed by the Chief of Staff, US Army. The Office of the Under Secretary of the Army includes a Deputy Under Secretary (Operations Research).

The Chief of Staff, Army, in his role as a member of the Joint Chiefs of Staff, takes part in the planning and supervision of the operational forces under the command of the Commanders-in-Chief. The Vice Chief of Staff assists and advises the Chief of Staff.

The Army General Staff is the principal element of the Army Staff and includes the Offices of the Chief of Staff, Deputy Chief of Staff for Operations and Plans, Deputy Chief of Staff for Personnel, Deputy Chief of Staff for Logistics, and Deputy Chief of Staff for Intelligence. Other elements of the Army Staff are the offices of the Judge Advocate General, Surgeon General, Chief of Chaplains, Chief, Army Reserve, Chief, National Guard Bureau, and Chief of Engineers.

The Army consists of the Active Army, the Army National Guard of the US, the Army Reserve and civilian workforce; and all persons appointed to or enlisted into the Army without component; and all persons serving under call or conscription, including members of the National Guard of the States, etc., when in the service of the US. The strength of the Active Army was (1990) 732,403 (including 83,153 women).

The US Army Forces Command, with headquarters at Fort McPherson, Georgia, commands the Third US Army; five continental US Armies, and all assigned Active Army and US Army Reserve troop units in the continental US, Alaska, Panama, the Commonwealth of Puerto Rico, and the Virgin Islands of the USA. The headquarters of the continental US Armies are: First US Army, Fort George G. Meade, Maryland; Second US Army, Fort Gillem, Georgia; Fourth US Army, Fort Sheridan, Illinois; Fifth US Army, Fort Sam Houston, Texas; Sixth US Army, Presidio of San Francisco, California. The US Army Training and Doctrine Command, with headquarters at Fort Monroe, Virginia, co-ordinates and integrates the total combat development effort of the Army as well as developing, managing, establishing and verifying the training of individuals of the US Army and authorized foreign nationals. The US Army Health Services Command, with headquarters at Fort Sam Houston, Texas, provides health services in the continental US for the US Army and provides professional education and training for medical personnel of the US Army and authorized foreign national personnel. The US Army Materiel Command, with headquarters in Alexandria, Virginia, is responsible for US Army activities dealing with equipment development, procurement, delivery, supply and maintenance. The US Army Information Systems Communications Command, with headquarters at Fort Huachuca, Arizona, provides worldwide communication automation support to the Department of the Army and supports the Defense Communications Systems. The US Army Military District of Washington, with headquarters at Fort McNair, Washington, D.C., provides support to the Department of the Army and the Department of Defense at the seat of Government. The US Army Space Command, with headquarters in Colorado Springs, Colorado, is the Army component to the US Space Command.

Nearly 40% of the Active Army is deployed outside the continental US. Several divisions, most of which are located in the USA, keep equipment in the Federal Republic of Germany and can be flown there in 48–72 hours. Headquarters of US Seventh and Eighth Armies are in Europe and Korea respectively.

Operational Commands and Weapons. The larger commands are the theater army and corps. The typical theater army may consist of a variable number of corps composed of combat forces of armour, infantry, air defense artillery, aviation and field artillery units; combat support forces of aviation, engineer, intelligence and signal elements; and combat service support forces. A typical corps consists of a variable number and mixture of infantry, mechanized infantry, armoured, air assault, or airborne divisions; one or more separate infantry, mechanized infantry or armoured brigades; one or more armoured cavalry regiments; corps artillery (155-mm howitzer, 203-mm howitzer, multiple launch rocket system (MLRS), *Lance* missile battalions); corps air defense brigade (*Hawk, Chaparral, Patriot* and *Avenger* battalions), corps aviation brigade and combat support and combat service support forces.

US Army Divisions have a common base (containing command, divisional artillery, air defense artillery, combat support and combat service support units) aviation brigade, and a varying mixture of combat manoeuvre battalions (usually 9 or 10 in number in 3 brigades) to make up airborne, infantry, armoured, mechanized infantry and air assault divisions. Divisions can in this way be 'tailored' to fit a variety of strategic or tactical situations. An infantry division, with about 16,500 soldiers, may have 8 infantry battalions, an armoured battalion and a mechanized infantry battalion; a mechanized infantry division, with about 17,300 soldiers, may have 5 mechanized infantry battalions and 5 armoured battalions; an armoured division, with about 17,300 soldiers, may have 4 mechanized infantry battalions and 6 armoured battalions; an airborne division, with 13,100 soldiers, may have 9 infantry (airborne) battalions. The air assault division is a highly specialized force capable of battlefield helicopter operations for infantry, field artillery, air defense artillery and necessary support forces.

The 10,800-man light infantry divisions consist of 9 infantry battalions and offer rapid strategic force projection. Light divisions can operate in all environments and are general purpose forces. Special operations forces consist of special forces, rangers, special operations aviation psychological operations, and civil affairs units. The units are designed, equipped, and trained for special missions.

Small arms include the M-9 (9mm pistol), the M-16 series rifle and the M-249 Squad Automatic Weapon both of which fire a 5·56-mm cartridge. The standard generalpurpose machine-gun is the M-60 (23 lb.; 550 rounds of 7·62-mm per minute). Infantry weapons also include M-203 grenade launcher attachment for the M-16A1 rifle, which fire a 40-mm grenade up to 400 metres, the *TOW* and *Dragon* anti-tank missile systems, and the M-72 rocket, a light anti-tank weapon.

Combat vehicles of the US Army are the tank, armoured personnel carrier, infantry fighting vehicle, and the armoured command vehicle. The first-line tanks are the M1A1 Abrams tank with a 120mm main gun, and both the M1 Abrams and the M60A3 tanks with 105-mm main armament. The standard armoured infantry personnel carrier is the M2 Bradley Fighting Vehicle (BFV), which is replacing the older M113. Both carry a mechanized infantry squad, but the BFV mounts a 25-mm Bushmaster gun and *TOW* missile launchers. The M3 version of the BFV is being used as the ground scout vehicle in armoured cavalry regiments, armoured and mechanized infantry divisional cavalry squadrons and in scout platoons of armoured and mechanized infantry battalions.

The approved calibres of artillery are: Light, 105-mm howitzer, medium 155-mm howitzer; the heavy, 203-mm howitzer. The Multiple Launch Rocket System

(MLRS) is a 227-mm rapid fire rocket system used in a non-nuclear counterfire role. The 107-mm mortar, the 81-mm mortar and the 60-mm mortar are used by the combat manoeuvre elements. The 120mm mortar will replace the 107mm mortar. The *TOW* is the primary anti-tank weapon. Forward-area air-defence weapons, including the *Chaparral, Stinger* and *Avenger* 20-mm gun, provide the capability of low-altitude defence against high-performance aircraft.

The Army has three categories of missiles—surface-to-surface (field artillery) and surface-to-air (air defence artillery) and anti-tank. Surface-to-surface missiles are: *Pershing II*, terminally-guided, nuclear warhead, range about 1,000 miles (1,800 km) operational (being phased out under the terms of the Intermediate Nuclear Forces Treaty between the US and USSR); *Lance*, guided, nuclear warhead, storable, liquid propellant, operational. Surface-to-air missiles, for air defence, are: *Patriot*, guided, conventional warhead, operational; *Hawk*, homing type, low-to-mid-altitude, field operational (product improvements continue to improve the effectiveness of the system); *Chaparral*, infra-red homing, low-altitude, forward area, operational (improvements to the basic system are under development); *Stinger*, hand-held or mobile-launched, infra-red homing, low-altitude, forward area, operational. Anti-tank missiles are: *TOW*, tube launched, optically tracked, wire guided, anti-armour, forward area, operational; *Hellfire*, laser-guided, anti-armour, operational and *Dragon*, wire-guided, medium anti-armour, forward area, operational.

The Army employs rotary- and fixed-wing aircraft as organic elements of its ground formations where their use is required on a full-time basis and their immediate and constant availability is essential. The front line commander exploits the benefits of aviation technology to perform traditional land battle tasks in the third dimension. This concept of airmobility for ground formation utilizes aerial vehicles as a highly integrated team to perform all five functions of land combat: reconnaissance, command and control, logistics and that inseparable combination, firepower and manoeuvre.

The Army has over 8,000 aircraft, all but about 500 of them helicopters. The principal types are 3,100 UH-1 Iroquois Huey and 1,100 UH-60 Black Hawk utility helicopters, 1,600 OH-58 Kiowa observation helicopters, 1,000 AH-1 Cobra and 800 AH-64 Apache attack helicopters, and 450 CH-47 Chinook cargo helicopters.

Enlistment, Terms of Service. Since 1974 the Army has operated an 'all volunteer' system making it, in effect, an all-regular force both regular and reserve components. Terms of service may be 2, 3, 4, 5 or 6 years. Men and women who enlist incur an 8-year obligation and must serve in the reserve components any part of the period not served on active duty. Over 95% of recruits enlisting in the Army have a high school education, over 50% of the Army is married, and 11·4% of the active force is filled by women. Women serve in both combat support and combat service support units.

The National Guard is the only reserve military component with a dual mission: A state and federal rôle. Enlistment is voluntary. The members are recruited by each state, but are equipped and paid by the federal government (except when performing state missions). Training is supervised by the active Army (FORSCOM), and unit organization parallels that for the active army; training facilities are made available by the USA and each state. As the organized militia of the several states, the District of Columbia, Puerto Rico and the Territories of the Virgin Islands and Guam, the Guard may be called into service for local emergencies by the chief executives in those jurisdictions; and may be called into federal service by the President to thwart invasion or rebellion or to enforce federal law. In its role as a reserve component of the Army, the Guard is subject to the order of the President in the event of national emergency.

The Army Reserve is designed to supply qualified and experienced units and individuals in an emergency. US Army Forces Command is charged with the command, support and training supervision of US Army Reserve units. Members of units are assigned to the Ready Reserve, which is subject to call by the President in case of national emergency without declaration of war by Congress. The Standby Reserve and the Retired Reserve may be called only after declaration of war or national emergency by Congress.

Defense 88. Dept. of Defense, Washington, D.C.
Coker, C., *US Military Power in the 1980s*. London, 1984
Kinnell, S., *Military History of the United States: An Annotated Bibliography*. Oxford and Santa Barbara, 1986

Navy. *Secretary of the Navy:* H. Lawrence Garrett, III.

The Department of the Navy is administered under the Secretary of Defense by the Secretary of the Navy, assisted by the Under Secretary; 4 Assistant Secretaries, for Financial Management; for Shipbuilding and Logistics; for Manpower and Reserve Affairs; and for Research, Engineering and Systems, as well as by the Chief of Naval Operations and the Commandant of the Marine Corps. The 3 divisions of the Department of the Navy are:

Navy Department, comprised of staff offices of the Secretary for Legislative Affairs, Information, the Judge Advocate General, Auditor General, Program Appraisal, General Counsel, Naval Research and Comptroller; offices of the Chief of Naval Operations which include the Vice Chief, the Assistant Vice Chief/ Director of Naval Administration, 3 Assistant Chiefs, 5 Deputy Chiefs and 6 Directors; Naval Inspector General; the Surgeon General; Bureau of Naval Personnel; and Headquarters U.S. Marine Corps.

The Shore Establishment comprises commands dealing with air, naval acquisition support, space and warfare systems, facilities engineering, sea (including ordnance) and supply systems and other commands: Space, Medical, Education and Training, Data Automation, Telecommunications, Intelligence, Oceanography, Legal Service, Security Group, and Investigative Service; as well as supporting establishment of the Marine Corps and Marine Corps Reserve.

The Operating Forces are the Military Sealift Command, U.S. Naval Forces Europe, the Atlantic and Pacific Fleets including Fleet Marine Forces; operating forces of the Marine Corps, the Mine Warfare Command, Operational Test and Evaluation Force, Naval Forces Southern and Central Commands, and the Naval Reserve Forces.

Major shore activities include 8 shipyards, 27 air stations and facilities, 2 amphibious bases, 5 submarine bases and 13 naval stations and bases.

The authorized budget for the Department of the Navy (which includes funding both for the Navy and Marine Corps) for current and recent fiscal years: 1984, \$82,088m.; 1985, \$99,015m.; 1986, \$99,113m.; 1987, \$93,500m.; 1988, \$100,281m.; 1989, \$97,407m.; 1990, \$101,670m. and 1991, \$105,051m.

The Navy personnel total in 1990 was 590,500, including 50,000 women who are eligible to serve at sea in support ships. The U.S. Marine Corps totalled 195,300 (10,500 women).

The operational strength of the United States Navy at the end of the year indicated was as follows:

Category	*1983*	*1984*	*1985*	*1986*	*1987*	*1988*	*1989*	*1990*
Strategic Submarines	34	35	37	36	36	36	36	34
Nuclear Attack Submarines	90	94	98	97	96	95	97	93
Diesel Submarines	5	4	4	4	4	4	3	nil
Aircraft Carriers [1]	13	13	13	14	14	14	14	14
Amphibious Carriers	12	12	12	12	12	12	13	13
Battleships	1	2	2	3	3	4	4	2
Cruisers	28	29	29	31	36	38	41	44
Destroyers	68	68	68	68	68	68	68	58
Frigates	90	94	101	109	116	112	100	98

[1] Omits one Aircraft Carrier in 'Service Life Extension Program' (SLEP), a three-year refit, not counted to operational total.

Ships in inactive reserve are not included; but those serving as Naval Reserve Force training ships are. Amphibious Carriers are those ships of the Wasp, Tarawa, and Iwo Jima classes capable of operating AV-8 Harrier-type aircraft as well as helicopters.

A principal part of the US naval task is to deploy the seaborne leg of the United States' strategic deterrent 'triad': This task is performed by the squadrons deploying nuclear-powered strategic ballistic missile-carrying submarines (SSBN), the strength and armament of which is as follows:

Strategic Submarines

Class	No.	Tonnage (in 1,000)	Speed	Missiles	Other Weapons
Tennessee	4	19·00	24	24 Trident D-5	Torpedoes
Ohio	8	19·00	24	24 Trident C-4	Torpedoes
Benjamin Franklin	12	8·12	25	6 with 16 Trident C-4 6 with 16 Poseidon C-3	Torpedoes
James Madison	8	8·12	25	6 with 16 Trident C-4 2 with 16 Poseidon C-3	Torpedoes
Lafayette	6	8·12	25	16 Poseidon C-3	Torpedoes

The Lafayette, Madison and Franklin classes comprise the first generation of SSBN, most of which were initially equipped with Polaris missiles, with maximum range between 1,500 and 2,500 nautical miles. These missiles were replaced between 1970 and 1977 with Poseidon C-3 missiles of similar maximum range, but deploying greatly increased numbers of warheads (10 per missile). 12 of these submarines were modernized between 1978 and 1982 to carry the Trident-1 C-4 missile, which is of similar size to the Poseidon, but with a range of 4,000 nautical miles, and delivering 8 warheads per missile. The second generation Ohio and Tennessee class submarines, with a much larger hull, are designed to deploy the Trident-2 D-5 missile, with a maximum range of 6,500 nautical miles, carrying a similar number of warheads but with substantially improved targetting accuracy. Sea trials of this weapon began in March 1989 but a technical fault, now corrected, delayed operational deployment until March 1990. The Ohio class will be retrofitted with the Trident-2 in due course, and a total of 20 of this larger class, completing at one per year, is anticipated.

The listed total of 93 nuclear-powered attack submarines (SSN) comprises 45 of the Los Angeles class (7,040 tonnes) in three major batches: A basic design (31 ships) completed 1976-85, a small group of 8 ships additionally equipped with vertical-launch missile tubes for Tomahawk cruise missiles completed 1985-89, and the current building programme of which 6 ships have been completed, known as 'Improved' Los Angeles incorporating cruise missile tubes, a new command system, and several important additional technical modifications. There are also 37 Sturgeon class (5,040 tonnes) completed 1967-75, 8 Permit class (4,370 tonnes) completed 1963-67, and 3 others. The last remaining diesel submarines, built in the late 1950s, have been decommissioned.

The table below lists the principal operational surface ships:

Aircraft Carriers

Completed	Name	Tonnage (in 1,000)	Speed	Aircraft
Nimitz Class				
1989	George Washington	97·8	33[1]	All carriers, except *Roosevelt* and *Midway* carry a standard Air Wing of 86 aircraft:-
1986	Theodore Roosevelt	97·8	33[1]	24 F/A-18 Hornet fighter/bombers.
1982	Carl Vinson	92·9	33[1]	10 A-6E Intruder bombers.
1977	Eisenhower	92·9	33[1]	24 F-14 Tomcat fighters.
1975	Nimitz	92·9	33[1]	4 EA-6B Prowler electronic warfare aircraft.
Kitty Hawk Kennedy Class				4 E-2C Hawkeye airborne early warning.
1968	John F Kennedy	82·5	32	10 S-3A Viking anti-submarine aircraft.
1965	America	81·0	33	4 KA-6D Tankers.
1962	Constellation	83·1	34	6 SH-3A Sea King anti-submarine helicopters.
1961	Kitty Hawk	82·4	34	*Roosevelt* carries an experimental air wing. *Midway*, much smaller, carries no F-14, 36 F/A-18 and 14 A-6E.
1962	Enterprise	91·5	33[1]	
Forrestal Class				
1959	Independence	81·9	33	
1957	Ranger	82·5	33	
1956	Saratoga	81·7	33	
1955	Forrestal	80·5	33	
1945	Midway	65·0	32	

[1] Indicates nuclear propulsion

Amphibious Carriers

Completed	Name	Tonnage (in 1,000)	Speed	Aircraft
Wasp Class (LHD)				
1989	Wasp	41·2	23	6-8 AV-8 Harriers and up to 42 helicopters.
Tarawa Class (LHA)				
1981	Pelileu			
1980	Nassau			Normal Air group is 30 aircraft, e.g.
1978	Belleau Wood	40·0	24	6 AV-8 Harriers, and 24 mixed helicopters,
1977	Saipan			principally CH-53E, CH-46 and gunships.
1976	Tarawa			
Iwo Jima Class (LPH)				
1970	Inchon			
1968	New Orleans			
1965	Tripoli			
1965	Guam	18·8	21	4 AV-8 plus maximum of 16 mixed helicopters, or 20 helicopters only.
1963	Guadalcanal			
1962	Okinawa			
1961	Iwo Jima			

Battleships

Completed	Name	Tonnage (in 1,000)	Speed	Main Armament	Aircraft
Iowa Class					
1944	Missouri	58·25	33	9 x 406 mm, 12 x 127 mm guns. 32 Tomahawk cruise missiles. 16 Harpoon anti-ship missiles.	None.
1944	Wisconsin				

Cruisers

Completed	Name	Tonnage (in 1,000)	Speed	Main Armament	Aircraft
Ticonderoga (Aegis) Class					
1990	Chosin				
1990	Gettysburg				
1990	Cowpens				
1989	Chancellorsville				
1989	Normandy				
1989	Princeton				
1989	Philippine Sea			Standard SM-2 ER SAM,	
1988	Lake Champlain			2 x 2 launchers in first	
1988	San Jacinto	9·6	32	5 ships; 2 x 61-cell vertical launcher systems	2 SH-60B Sea-hawk LAMPS-III helicopters.
1987	Leyte Gulf			for Standard, Tomahawk	
1987	Antietam			and Harpoon in remainder.	
1987	Mobile Bay			2 x 127 mm guns in all.	
1986	Bunker Hill				
1986	Thomas S. Gates				
1986	Valley Forge				
1985	Vincennes				
1984	Yorktown				
1983	Ticonderoga				
Virginia Class [1]					
1980	Arkansas			2 x 2 Standard SM-2 SAM.	
1978	Mississippi			8 Tomahawk cruise missiles.	
1977	Texas	11·45	31	8 Harpoon anti-ship and ASROC anti-submarine	None
1976	Virginia			missiles. 2 x 127 mm guns.	
California Class [1]					
1974	South Carolina	10·7	31	As for *Virginia*, without Tomahawk.	None
1973	California				

Com-pleted	*Name*	*Tonnage (in 1,000)*	*Speed*	*Main Armament*	*Aircraft*
Miscellaneous [1]					
1961	Long Beach	17·4	30	1 or 2 x 2 SM-2 ER SAMs. ASROC anti-submarine missiles. 8 x Tomahawk (Long Beach only).	None
1967	Truxtun	8·9	30		
1962	Bainbridge	9·25	30		
Belknap Class					
1967	Biddle				
1967	Sterett				
1967	Horne				
1966	Fox				
1966	Wm. H. Standley	8·2	33	Standard SM-2 ER SAMs ASROC anti-submarine missiles 8 Harpoon missiles 1 x 127 mm Gun.	1 SH-2F Sea-sprite LAMPS-I helicopter.
1966	Jouett				
1966	Wainwright				
1965	Jos. L. Daniels				
1964	Belknap				
Leahy Class					
1964	Reeves				
1964	Rich. K. Turner				
1963	Dale				
1963	Halsey				
1963	England	8·3	32	2 x 2 SM-2 ER SAMs ASROC anti-submarine missiles 8 Harpoon missiles	None
1963	Gridley				
1963	Worden				
1963	Harry E. Yarnell				
1962	Leahy				

[1] Indicates nuclear-powered.

The target of '15 deployable carriers' set in 1986 was officially amended to 14 as a result of budgetary pressure in 1989. Of the 15 listed in the table, *Kitty Hawk* is undergoing a three-year 'service life extension' refit and so does not count to the authorized deployable total. However, before the *George Washington* commissioned in Nov. 1989, the *Coral Sea* was withdrawn from the fleet, and de-activated in April 1990. *Midway*, scheduled to decommission in early 1991, will probably only be retained until no longer needed for Middle East operations. In addition the training carrier *Lexington* is maintained in service, but is classified as an auxiliary.

The Wasp (LHD-1), and the 5 ships of the Tarawa (LHA-1) class are in many aircraft carriers in other principal navies and are capable of sea control tasks. The 7 ships of the Iwo Jima class are also capable of operating vertical/short take-off and landing aircraft but do not normally do so. All are, however, configured, trained and equipped primarily for amphibious operations.

In addition to the previously listed principal surface ships, there are 27 guided-missile destroyers, 31 anti-submarine destroyers of the Spruance class, 51 guided-missile frigates of the Oliver Hazard Perry class, 47 other frigates, 6 hydrofoil missile patrol craft and 24 inshore patrol craft. Mine warfare has been somewhat neglected over the past decades, but two new classes are now building. There are now 7 new mine countermeasure vessels of the Avenger class in service, and the first of a new Osprey class coastal minehunter building, together with 18 old ocean minesweepers (completed between 1954 and 1958, mostly employed on reserve training).

Amphibious capability comprises some 66 ships. In addition to the 13 amphibious aircraft carriers listed above, there are 2 amphibious command ships, 27 dock landing ships, 20 tank landing ships and 5 amphibious transports. There are 80 amphibious craft including 16 air-cushion landing craft (hovercraft) and 55 utility landing craft, and several hundred minor personnel and vehicle transports. The total oceanic lift capability of the amphibious forces amounts to over 50,000 men, 1,300 main battle tank equivalents, and operating facilities for about 180 helicopters.

Specially trained and equipped amphibious expeditionary forces are provided by the US Marine Corps, some 195,000 strong, which although administratively part of the Department of the Navy, ranks as a separate armed service, with the Commandant of the Corps serving in his own right as a member of the Joint Chiefs of Staff. The Marine Corps is organized into 3 divisions each some 55,000 strong, which are subdivided into Marine Expeditionary Brigades, (18,000) and Marine Expeditionary Units (some 6,000 strong). In peace time Marine Expeditionary Units are permanently deployed afloat in the Eastern Atlantic/Mediterranean and the West Pacific/Indian Ocean. The principal equipment of the US Marine Corps consists of 700 M-60A1 tanks, 420 LAV-25 armoured infantry fighting vehicles, 800 armoured personnel carriers, and over 1,000 artillery pieces of calibres between 105 mm and 203 mm. Additional heavy equipment for US-based Marine forces units, beyond that which can be embarked in the amphibious shipping, is provided in 2 squadrons each of 13 large cargo ships prepositioned at Diego Garcia (Indian Ocean) and in the Mediterranean. In addition the Corps includes an autonomous aviation element numbering some 500 combat aircraft and 540 helicopters. There are 200 F/A 18 Hornet, 175 AV-8 and AV-8B Harriers, 60 A-4 Skyhawks, 60 A-6 attack and electronic warfare, 40 KC-130 tankers, and a miscellany of other support and training aircraft. Helicopters include 200 CH-46E and 160 CH-53 transport, as well as 100 AH-1 Cobra attack helicopters of various types. Harriers and helicopters are normally employed afloat in the amphibious aircraft carriers and other suitable ships. The Hornets and other fixed wing aircraft are normally based ashore, but may be embarked in other aircraft carriers, given the operational need.

The Navy is provided with global, long-term sustainability through a force of some 56 underway replenishment ships, including 28 tankers, 4 multi-purpose fast replenishment ships, 11 stores ships and 13 ammunition ships. Second-line support is provided by 2 repair ships, 21 depot ships, 4 support tankers, 9 tugs, 2 hospital ships and 3 fast cargo vessels. Special purpose auxiliaries include 2 command ships, 17 ocean surveillance ships, 5 missile and space support ships, and 20 survey and oceanographic vessels. Of these 150 major auxiliaries, about half are operated by the civilian-manned Military Sealift Command. In addition there are some hundreds of minor auxiliaries, and several thousand service craft.

Major warship building yards involved in the current building programme are located at Groton, Conn. (submarines), Newport News, Va., (submarines and aircraft carriers), Pascagoula, Miss. (cruisers and amphibious ships), Bath, Me. (cruisers and destroyers) and New Orleans, La., (amphibious and auxiliary ships). No major ships are currently being built in west coast shipyards. The future construction programme is in some doubt due to budgetary restrictions.

Naval Aviation. The principal function of the naval aviation organization is to provide and train the 13 Air Wings maintained for service in the Aircraft Carriers. As shown in the ship tables, these usually consist of 80 fixed wing and 6 rotary wing aircraft. In addition, 2 carrier air wings are provided from the reserves, in some cases with slightly older aircraft. The main carrier-borne combat aircraft on inventory are 370 F-14 fighters, 240 A-6E Intruder attack aircraft, 210 F/A-18 Hornet dual-purpose fighter/attack aircraft and 130 S-3A Viking anti-submarine aircraft. Supporting roles are performed by 80 EA-6B electronic warfare aircraft, 90 E-2C Hawkeye airborne early warning aircraft, 60 KA-6D tankers, and 100 SH-3A Sea King helicopters for inner-zone anti-submarine defence. The reserve air wings have some A-7 Corsair attack aircraft on strength, of which holdings are still over 200. Helicopters held for embarkation in cruisers and below are of two types, the older SH-2F Seasprite LAMPS-I aircraft of which there are some 100 and the SH-60B Seahawk LAMPS-III of which there are 120. A different version of this latter aircraft, the SH-60F Oceanhawk is now in production as a replacement for the elderly Sea Kings in the Aircraft Carriers. The principal tasks of the shore-based elements of US naval aviation are maritime reconnaissance and anti-submarine warfare, for which there are holdings of about 370 P-3C Orion aircraft. Additional tasks include electronic warfare (12 EP-3), electronic intelligence (14 EA-3) and mine countermeasures for which 40 MH- and RH-53 helicopters are held. Finally there are some 650 training aircraft of types not previously mentioned, and 110 aircraft and 90 helicopters for transport and other miscellaneous duties.

The US Coast Guard operates under the Department of Transportation in time of peace and as a part of the Navy in time of war or when directed by the President. The act of establishment stated the Coast Guard 'shall be a military service and branch of the armed forces of the United States at all times'. The Coast Guard did operate as part of the Navy during the First and Second World Wars. It also had some units serving in Vietnam. It comprises 250 ships including cutters of destroyer, frigate, corvette and patrol vessel types, 2 powerful icebreakers, and para-military auxiliaries and tenders, plus over 2,000 rescue and utility craft. It also maintains 70 fixed-wing aircraft and 130 helicopters. The Coast Guard missions include maintenance of aids to navigation, enforcement of maritime laws, enforcement of international treaties, environmental protection (especially waterway pollution), commercial vessel safety programmes, recreational boating safety, search and rescue efforts and military readiness. In the new construction programme are 34 patrol boats. The strength of personnel in 1989 was 5,077 officers, 1,342 warrant officers and 30,255 enlisted personnel and 817 cadets.

Air Force. *Secretary of the Air Force:* Donald B. Rice.

The Department of the Air Force was activated within the Department of Defense on 18 Sept. 1947, under the terms of the National Security Act of 1947. It is administered by a Secretary of the Air Force, assisted by an Under Secretary and 3 Assistant Secretaries (Space; Acquisition; and Manpower, Reserve Affairs and Logistics). The USAF, under the administration of the Department of the Air Force, is supervised by a Chief of Staff, who is a member of the Joint Chiefs of Staff. He is assisted by a Vice Chief of Staff, Assistant Vice Chief of Staff, and 4 Deputy Chiefs of Staff (Personnel; Programs and Resources; Plans and Operations; and Logistics and Engineering).

The USAF consists of active duty Air Force officers and enlisted personnel, civilian employees, the Air National Guard and the Air Force Reserve. For operational purposes the service is organized into 13 major commands, 16 separate operating agencies and 7 direct reporting units. The Strategic Air Command, equipped with long-range bombers and with intercontinental ballistic missiles, is maintained primarily for strategic air operations anywhere on the globe. Tactical Air Command is the Air Force's mobile strike force, able to deploy US general-purpose air forces anywhere in the world for tactical air combat operations. The Military Airlift Command provides air transportation of personnel and cargo for all military services on a worldwide basis; and is also responsible for Air Force audio-visual products, weather service, Air Force special operations forces, and aerospace rescue and recovery operations.

The other major commands are the Air Force Systems Command, Air Force Logistics Command, Air Force Communications Command, Electronic Security Command, Air Training Command, Alaskan Air Command, Pacific Air Forces, Air Force Space Command, United States Air Forces in Europe, and Air University. The Alaskan, Pacific and European commands conduct, control and co-ordinate offensive and defensive air operations according to tasks assigned by their respective theatre commanders.

The separate operating agencies are the Air Force Accounting and Finance Center, Air Force Audit Agency, Air Force Commissary Service, Air Force Engineering and Services Center, Air Force Inspection and Safety Center, Air Force Intelligence Service, Air Force Office of Security Police, Air Force Military and Personnel Agency, Air Force Office of Medical Support, Air Force Management Engineering Agency, Air Force Service Information and News Center, Air Force Legal Services Center, Air Force Office of Special Investigations, Air Force Operational Test and Evaluation Center, Air Force Reserve, and Air Reserve Personnel Center. Air Force direct reporting units are the Air Force Academy, Air National Guard, Air Force Technical Applications Center, Air Force District of Washington, D.C., Air Force Civilian Personnel Management Center and USAF Historical Research Center.

Of the fighter and interceptor aircraft in service, the F-15 Eagle, F-16 Fighting Falcon, F-111 and F-4 Phantom II fly faster than the speed of sound in level flight and can carry a variety of armament. The E-3 Sentry (AWACS) is a large long-range airborne warning and control aircraft; the EF-111A Raven is a radar jamming aircraft produced by conversion of the F-111A fighter. The subsonic A-7 Corsair II, the A-10 Thunderbolt and the AC-130H are close air support aircraft. The OA-37 and the OV-10 are observation aircraft. Strategic bombers are the B-52 Stratofortress and the B-1B heavy bombers. The Strategic Air Command also operates the KC-10A Extender and the KC-135 Stratotanker for aerial refuelling and the U-2 and TR-1 for reconnaissance. Primary transports include the C-141 Starlifter the C-5 Galaxy, KC-10A Extender and the turboprop-powered C-130 Hercules. Intercontinental ballistic missiles in USAF service are the Minuteman II and III and Peacekeeper.

In 1989, the Air Force had about 579,000 military personnel. The service operates approximately 9,400 aircraft in the active Air Force, the Air National Guard and the Air Force Reserve.

INTERNATIONAL RELATIONS

Membership. The USA is a member of the UN, OAS, NATO, OECD and the Colombo Plan.

ECONOMY

Budget. The budget covers virtually all the programmes of federal government, including those financed through trust funds, such as for social security, Medicare and highway construction. Receipts of the Government include all income from its sovereign or compulsory powers; income from business-type or market-orientated activities of the Government is offset against outlays. Budget receipts and outlays (in $1m.):

Year ending 30 June	*Receipts* [2]	*Outlays* [2]	*Surplus (+) or deficit (–)*
1950	39,443	42,562	– 3,119
1955	65,451	68,444	– 2,993
1960	92,492	92,191	+ 301
1970	192,807	195,649	– 2,842
1985 [1]	734,057	946,316	–212,260
1988	908,954	1,064,044	–155,090
1989	990,691	1,142,643	–151,952
1990	1,073,451	1,197,236	–123,785
1991 [3]	1,170,232	1,233,331	–63,099

[1] From 1977 the fiscal year changed from a 1 July–30 June basis to a 1 Oct.–30 Sept. basis.
[2] From 1970, revised to include Medicare premiums and collections.
[3] July 1990 estimates.

Budget receipts, by source, for fiscal years (in $1m.):

Source	*1989* [1]	*1990* [1]	*1991* [2]
Individual income taxes	445,690	489,444	528,489
Corporation income taxes	103,583	112,030	129,665
Social insurance taxes and contributions	359,416	385,362	421,449
Excise taxes	34,084	36,154	37,634
Estate and gift taxes	8,745	9,279	9,809
Customs	16,334	18,615	18,615
Miscellaneous	22,839	24,397	24,572
Total	990,691	1,073,451	1,170,232

[1] Includes off-budget receipts. [2] July 1990 estimates.

Budget outlays, by function, for fiscal years (in $1m.):

Source	*1989* [1]	*1990* [1]	*1991* [2]
National defence	303,559	296,342	303,251
International affairs	9,574	14,554	18,172
General science, space, and technology	12,838	14,145	16,609
Energy	3,702	3,194	3,029
Natural resources and environment	16,182	17,499	18,168
Agriculture	16,948	14,571	14,938
Commerce and housing credit	27,719	22,688	17,184
Transportation	27,608	29,250	29,758
Community and regional development	5,361	8,776	7,825
Education, training, employment and social services	36,648	37,652	41,005
Health	48,390	57,819	63,698
Medicare	84,964	96,616	98,615
Income security	136,031	146,601	153,738
Social Security	232,542	248,462	264,811
Veterans' benefits and services	30,066	28,888	30,308
Administration of justice	9,422	10,489	12,608
General government	9,124	10,560	11,282
Net interest	169,137	175,591	172,979
Allowances	...	...	–1,070
Undistributed offsetting receipts	–37,212	–36,462	–43,578
Total budget outlays	1,142,643	1,179,375	1,233,331

[1] Includes outlays of off-budget Federal entities and programmes.
[2] July 1990 estimates.

Budget outlays, by agency, for fiscal years (in $1m.):

Agency	*1988* [1]	*1989* [1]	*1990* [2]
Legislative branch	1,852	2,094	2,490
The Judiciary	1,337	1,493	1,754
Executive Office of the President	121	124	145
Funds appropriated to the President	7,253	4,302	11,075
Agriculture	44,003	48,414	45,897
Commerce	2,279	2,571	3,455
Defence—Military	281,935	294,876	286,899
Defence—Civil	22,029	23,427	24,727
Education	18,246	21,608	22,360
Energy	11,166	11,387	12,670
Health and Human Services, except Social Security	159,071	172,301	190,173
Health and Human Services, Social Security	214,489	227,473	242,947
Housing and Urban Development	18,938	19,772	20,122
Interior	5,147	5,308	5,035
Justice	5,246	6,232	7,114
Labor	21,870	22,657	24,458
State	3,421	3,722	3,930
Transportation	26,404	26,689	27,208
Treasury	202,386	230,573	249,480
Environmental Protection Agency	4,871	4,906	5,492
General Services Administration	–281	–462	196
National Aeronautics and Space Administration	9,092	11,036	12,587
Office of Personnel Management	29,191	29,073	33,775
Small Business Administration	–54	83	–1,077
Veterans Affairs	29,271	30,041	27,956
Other Independent Agencies	23,444	32,323	14,584
Allowances	...	...	1,889
Undistributed offsetting receipts	–78,863	–89,155	–97,967
Total budget outlays	1,064,044	1,142,869	1,179,375

[1] Includes outlays of off-budget Federal entities and programmes.
[2] July 1989 estimates.

National Debt: Federal debt held by the public (in $1m.), and *per capita* debt (in $1) on 30 June to 1970 and then on 30 Sept.:

	Public debt	Per capita [2]		Public debt	Per capita [2]
1919 [1]	25,485	243	1970	283,198	1,381
1920	24,299	228	1980	709,291	3,114
1930 [1]	16,185	132	1985	1,499,362	6,266
1940	42,772	324	1986	1,736,163	7,183
1950	219,023	1,444	1987	1,888,134	7,738
1960 [3]	236,840	1,310	1988 [4]	2,050,196	8,321

[1] On 31 Aug. 1919 gross debt reached its First World War (1914–18) peak of $26,596,702,000, which was the highest ever reached up to 1934; on 31 Dec. 1930 it had declined to $16,026m., the lowest it has been since the First World War. On the 30 Nov. 1941, just preceding Pearl Harbor, debt stood at $61,363,867,932. The highest Second World War debt was $279,764,369,348 on 28 Feb. 1946.

[2] *Per capita* figures, beginning with 1960, have been revised; they are based on the Census Bureau's estimates of the total population of the US, including Alaska and Hawaii.

[3] Debt figures since 1956 exclude the unamortized discount or premium on all Treasury debt securities held by the public.

[4] July 1988 estimate.

State and Local Finance: Revenue of the 50 states and all local governments (82,237 in 1987) from their own sources amounted to $827,622m. in 1988–89; in addition they received $125,839m. in revenue from fiscal aid, shared revenues and reimbursements from the federal government, bringing total revenue from all sources to $953,461m. Of the revenue from state and local sources, taxes provided $468,586m., of which property taxes (mainly imposed by local governments) yielded $142,526m. or 30% of all tax revenue; and sales taxes, both general sales taxes and selective excises, provided $166,079m. (35%).

State tax revenue totalled $284,042m. in 1989. Largest sources of state tax revenue are general sales taxes (imposed during 1989 by 45 states), motor fuel sales taxes (all states), individual income (44 states), motor vehicle and operators' licences (46 states), corporation income (46 states), tobacco products (all states) and alcoholic beverage sales taxes (all states).

General revenue of local units from own sources in 1988–89 totalled $293,363m. In addition they received $175,246m. from state and federal aids. Property taxes provided 26% of total revenue.

Total expenditures of state and local governments were $890,668m. in 1988–89, of which approximately 72% was for current operation. Education took $263,881m. in current and capital expenditure; highways, $58,074m.; welfare (chiefly public assistance), $94,989m., and health and hospitals, $67,734m. Capital outlays (construction, equipment and land purchases) totalled $111,765m.

Gross debt of state and local governments totalled $798,281m. or $3,216 *per capita* at the close of their 1988–89 fiscal year. Total cash and investment assets of state and local governments were $1,362,001m. 46% of all assets are employee retirement funds.

US Bureau of the Census, *Governmental Finances in 1986–87*. Washington, D.C., 1988
American Economic Association, *Readings in Fiscal Policy*. Homewood, Ill., 1985

National Income. The Bureau of Economic Analysis of the Department of Commerce prepares detailed estimates on the national income and product of the United States. The principal tables are published monthly in *Survey of Current Business;* the complete set of national income and product tables are published in the *Survey* regularly each July, showing data for recent years. *The National Income and Product Accounts of the United States, 1929–1982: Statistical Tables* (1986) and the July 1987, July 1988, July 1989 and July 1990 *Survey* contain complete sets of tables from 1929 through 1989. The conceptual framework and statistical methods underlying the US accounts were described in *National Income, 1954*. The July 1987 *Survey* provides a current overview of concepts and estimating procedures as well as a comprehensive directory to information on the US national accounts. Subsequent limited changes were described in the July 1988 *Survey*.

These latest figures [1] in $1,000m. for various years are as follows:

[1] The inclusion of statistics for Alaska and Hawaii beginning in 1960 does not significantly affect the comparability of the data.

	1929 [2]	*1933* [3]	*1960*	*1970*	*1980*	*1988*	*1989*
I. Gross National Product	103·9	56·9	515·3	1,015·5	2,732·0	4,873·6	5,220·8
(a) Personal consumption expenditures	77·3	45·8	330·7	640·0	1,732·6	3,238·2	3,450·1
(b) Gross private domestic investment	16·7	1·6	78·2	148·8	437·0	747·1	771·2
(c) Net exports of goods and services	1·1	0·4	5·9	8·5	32·1	–74·1	–46·1
(d) Government purchases of goods and services	8·9	8·3	100·6	218·2	530·3	962·5	1,025·6
1. GNP *less* capital consumption allowances with capital consumption adjustment, indirect business tax and non-tax liability, business transfer payments, statistical discrepancy, *plus* subsidies less current surplus of government enterprises, equals:							
2. National Income	84·7	39·4	424·9	832·6	2·203·5	3,984·9	4,222·3
which, *less* corporate profits with inventory valuation and capital consumption adjustments, contributions for social insurance, wage accruals less disbursements, *plus* government transfer payments to persons, interest paid by government to persons and business less interest received by government, interest paid by consumers, personal dividend income, business transfer payments, equals:							
3. Personal income whereof	84·3	46·3	409·4	831·8	2,258·5	4,070·8	4,384·8
4. Personal tax and non-tax payments take	2·6	1·4	50·5	116·2	340·5	591·6	658·8
leaving							
5. Disposable personal income divided into	81·7	44·9	207·5	715·6	1,918·0	3,479·2	3,725·5
(e) Personal outlays [4]	79·2	46·5	338·1	657·9	1,781·1	3,333·6	3,553·7
(f) Personal saving	2·6	–1·6	20·8	57·7	136·9	145·6	171·8
IA. GNP in constant (1982) $s	709·6	498·5	1,665·3	2,416·2	3,187·1	4,016·9	4,117·7
(a) Personal consumption expenditures	471·4	378·7	1,005·1	1,492·0	2,000·4	2,606·5	2,656·8
(b) Gross private domestic investment	139·2	22·7	260·5	381·5	509·3	...	...
(c) Net exports of goods and services	4·7	–1·4	–4·0	–30·0	57·0	...	...
(d) Government purchases of goods and services	94·2	98·5	403·7	572·6	620·5	780·5	798·1
II. National Income composed of	84·7	39·4	424·9	832·6	2,203·5	3,984·9	4,223·3
Compensation of employees	*51·1*	*29·6*	*296·7*	*618·3*	*1,638·2*	*2,905·1*	*3,079·9*
(g) Salaries and wages	50·5	29·0	272·8	551·5	1,372·0	2,432·1	2,573·2
(h) Supplements to wages and salaries	0·7	0·6	23·8	66·8	266·3	474·0	505·8
Proprietors' income [5]	*14·4*	*5·4*	*52·1*	*80·2*	*180·7*	*354·2*	*379·3*
(i) Farm [5]	6·1	2·5	11·6	14·7	20·5	43·7	48·6
(j) Business and professional [5]	8·3	2·9	40·5	65·4	160·1	310·5	330·7
Personal income from rents [6]	*4·9*	*2·0*	*15·3*	*18·2*	*6·6*	*16·3*	*8·2*
Net interest	*4·7*	*4·1*	*11·3*	*41·2*	*200·9*	*371·8*	*445·1*
Corporate profits with inventory valuation and capital consumption adjustments	*9·6*	*–1·5*	*49·5*	*74·7*	*177·2*	*337·6*	*311·6*
(k) Tax liabilities	1·4	0·5	22·7	34·4	84·8	136·2	135·1
(l) Inventory valuation adjustment	0·5	–2·1	–0·2	–6·6	–43·1	–27·0	–21·7
(m) Capital consumption adjustment	–0·9	–0·3	–0·3	5·2	–16·8	47·8	25·2
(n) Dividends	5·8	2·0	12·9	22·5	54·7	110·0	123·5
(o) Undistributed profits	2·8	–1·6	14·3	19·2	97·6	70·5	49·1

[2] Peak year between First and Second World Wars. [3] Low point of the depression.

[4] Includes personal consumption expenditures, interest paid by consumers and personal transfer payments to foreigners (net).

[5] With inventory valuation and capital consumption adjustments.

[6] With capital consumption adjustment.

Currency. Prior to the banking crisis that occurred early in 1933, the monetary system had been on the gold standard for more than 50 years. An Act of 14 March 1900 required the Secretary of the Treasury to maintain at a parity with gold all forms of money issued by the USA. For a description of these, *see* THE STATESMAN'S YEAR-BOOK, 1934. For information 1934–74 *see* THE STATESMAN'S YEAR-BOOK, 1988–89.

Under the Coinage Act of 1965, all coins and currencies of the USA, regardless of when coined or issued, are legal tender for all debts, public and private.

Only one of the eight kinds of notes outstanding is now significant: Federal Reserve notes in denominations of $1, $2, $5, $10, $20, $50 and $100. The issue of *(a)* $500, $1,000, $5,000 and $10,000 Federal Reserve notes; of *(b)* silver certificates, and of *(c)* $100, $5 and $2 US notes have been discontinued, although they are still outstanding. The following issues were stopped many years ago and have been in process of retirement: (1) Federal Reserve Bank notes; (2) National Bank notes; (3) Treasury notes of 1890; (4) fractional currency.

Federal Reserve notes are obligations of the USA and a first lien on the assets of the Federal Reserve Banks, through which they are issued. Each of the 12 banks issues them against the security of an equal volume of collateral.

Inflation was 6·1% in 1990 (4·6% in 1989, 4·4% in 1988).

In March 1991 $1 = £0·53 sterling; £1 sterling = $1·90.

Banking and Finance. The Federal Reserve System, established under The Federal Reserve Act of 1913, comprises the Board of 7 Governors, the 12 regional Federal Reserve Banks with their 25 branches, and the Federal Open Market Committee. The 7 members of the Board of Governors are appointed by the President with the consent of the Senate. Each Governor is appointed to a full term of 14 years or an unexpired portion of a term, one term expiring every 2 years. The Board exercises broad supervisory authority over the operations of the 12 Federal Reserve Banks, including approval of their budgets and of the appointments of their presidents and first vice presidents; it designates 3 of the 9 directors of each Reserve Bank including the Chairman and Deputy Chairman. The Board has supervisory and regulatory responsibilities over banks that are members of the Federal Reserve System, bank holding companies, bank mergers, Edge Act and agreement corporations, foreign activities of member banks, international banking facilities in the U.S., and activities of the U.S. branches and agencies of foreign banks. The Board also assures the smooth functioning and continued development of the nation's vast payments system. Another area of the Boards responsibilities involves the implementation by regulation of major federal laws governing consumer credit. The 12 members of the Federal Open Market Committee include the 7 members of the Board of Governors and 5 of the 12 Federal Reserve Bank presidents. The latter serve 1-year terms on the Committee in rotation except for the President of the Federal Reserve Bank of New York, who is a permanent member. The Federal Open Market Committee influences credit market conditions, money and bank credit, by buying or selling US Government securities; and it also supervises System operations in foreign currencies for the purpose of helping to safeguard the value of the dollar in international exchange markets and facilitating co-operation and efficiency in the international monetary system. The Board also influences credit conditions through powers to set reserve requirements, to approve discount rates at Federal Reserve Banks, and to fix margin requirements on stock-market credit.

The Reserve Banks advance funds to depository institutions, issue Federal Reserve notes, which are the principal form of currency in the US, act as fiscal agent for the Government, and afford nationwide cheque-clearing and fund transfer arrangements. They may increase or reduce the country's supply of reserve funds by buying or selling Government securities and other obligations at the direction of the Federal Open Market Committee. The purchase and sale of securities in the open market is conducted by the Federal Reserve Bank of New York. Their capital stock is held by the member banks, but it carries no voting rights except in the election of directors.

From 1968, the Congress passed a number of consumer financial protection acts, the first of which was the Truth in Lending Act, for which it has directed the Board to write implementing regulations and assume partial enforcement responsibility. Others include the Equal Credit Opportunity Act, Home Mortgage Disclosure Act, Consumer Leasing Act, Fair Credit Billing Act, and Electronic Fund Transfer Act. To manage these responsibilities the Board has established a Division of Consumer and Community Affairs. To assist it, the Board consults with a Consumer Advisory Council, established by the Congress as a statutory part of the Federal Reserve System.

The Consumer Advisory Council was established by Congress in 1976 at the suggestion of the Board of Governors. Representing both consumer/community and financial industry interests, the Council meets several times a year to advise the Board on its implementation of consumer regulations and other consumer related matters.

Another statutory body, the Federal Advisory Council, consists of 12 members (one from each district); it meets in Washington four times a year to advise the Board of Governors on general business and financial conditions.

Following the passage of the Monetary Control Act of 1980, the Board of Governors established the Thrift Institutions Advisory Council to provide information and views on the special needs and problems of thrift institutions. The group is comprised of representatives of mutual savings banks, savings and loan associations, and credit unions.

Banks which participate in the federal deposit insurance fund have their deposits insured against loss up to $100,000 for each account. The fund is administered by the Federal Deposit Insurance Corporation established in 1933; it obtains resources through annual assessments on participating banks. All members of the Federal Reserve System are required to insure their deposits through the Corporation, and non-member banks may apply and qualify for insurance.

Board of Governors of the Federal Reserve System. *The Federal Reserve System: Purposes and Functions.* 7th ed., 1984.—*Federal Reserve Bulletin.* Monthly.—*Annual Report.*—*Annual Statistical Digest.*—*The Federal Reserve Act, As Amended Through 1984*

Meek, P., *U.S. Monetary Policy and Financial Markets.* New York, 1982

Timberlake, R. H., *The Origins of Central Banking in the United States.* Cambridge, Massachusetts, 1978

Weights and Measures. The metric system is to be introduced in the early 1990s. British weights and measures are usually employed, but the old Winchester bushel and wine gallon are used instead of the new or Imperial standards: *Wine gallon* = 0·83268 Imperial gallon; *Bushel* = 0·9690 Imperial bushel. Instead of the British cwt of 112 lb., one of 100 lb. is used; the *short* or *net ton* contains 2,000 lb.; the *long* or *gross ton*, 2,240 lb.

ENERGY AND NATURAL RESOURCES

Electricity. In 1990 19% of electricity was produced by 112 nuclear reactors. Production (public utilities only, 1985) 2,679,857,000m. kwh.

Minerals. Total value of non-fuel minerals produced in 1988 was estimated at $30,022m. ($26,317m. in 1987). Details are given in the following tables. Oil production was 409·63m. tonnes in 1990.

Production of metallic minerals (long tons, 2,240 lb.; short tons, 2,000 lb.):

Metallic minerals	*1987* *Quantity*	*Value ($1,000)*	*1988* *Quantity*	*Value ($1,000)*
Bauxite (dried equiv.) tonnes	575,574	10,916	587,889	10,566
Copper (recoverable content), tonnes	1,243,638	2,261,833	1,419,645	3,771,570
Gold (recoverable content), troy oz.	4,947,040	2,216,027	6,459,539	2,831,281
Lead (recoverable content), tonnes	311,381	246,720	384,983	315,222
Molybdenum (content of concentrate), 1,000 lb.	69,868	179,286	99,738	266,899
Silver (recoverable content), 1,000 troy oz.	39,896,541	279,675	53,415,677	349,339
Zinc (recoverable content), tonnes	216,320	199,924	244,314	324,249
Total metals	—	*7,423,000*	—	*10,219,000*

The US is wholly or almost wholly dependent upon imports for industrial diamonds, bauxite, tin, chromite, nickel, strategic-grade mica and long-fibre asbestos; it imports the bulk of its tantalum, platinum, manganese, mercury, tungsten, cobalt and flake graphite, and substantial quantities of antimony, cadmium, arsenic, fluorspar, zinc and bismuth.

Precious metals are mined mainly in Nevada, Idaho, Montana, Utah and Arizona (in order of combined output of gold and silver).

Statistics of important non-metallic minerals and mineral fuels are:

Non-metallic minerals	*1987* Quantity	Value ($1,000)	*1988* Quantity	Value ($1,000)
Boron minerals, short tons	1,385,000	475,092	1,267,000	429,667
Cement:				
Portland, 1,000 short tons	74,868	3,646,561	74,074	3,575,906
Masonry, 1,000 short tons	3,680	259,926	3,574	243,941
Clays, 1,000 short tons	47,657	1,202,284	49,069	1,400,820
Gypsum, 1,000 short tons	15,612	106,977	16,390	109,205
Lime, 1,000 short tons	15,733	786,125	17,293	828,007
Phosphate rock, 1,000 tonnes	40,954	793,280	48,389	887,809
Potassium salts, 1,000 tonnes (K_2O equivalent)	1,485	195,700	1,427	240,300
Salt (common), 1,000 short tons	36,493	684,170	37,997	680,174
Sand and gravel, 1,000 short tons	923,210	3,366,600	951,880	3,514,000
Stone, 1,000 short tons	1,201,284	5,438,753	1,248,989	5,754,289
Sulphur (Frasch-process), 1,000 tonnes	3,610	386,834	4,341	430,814
Total non-metallic minerals	—	*18,894,000*	—	*19,803,000*

Mineral fuels	*1987*		*1988*	
Coal: Bitum. and lignite, 1,000 short tons	915,200	21,050,000	946,700	20,827,400
Pennsylv. anthracite,[1] 1,000 short tons	3,000	160,000	3,600	158,976
Gas: Natural gas,[2] 1m. cu. ft	16,540,000	28,970,000	16,990,000	28,713,100
Petroleum (crude), 1,000 bbls of 42 gallons	3,047,378	46,930,000	2,971,100	37,376,438

[1] Includes a small quantity of anthracite mined in states other than Pennsylvania.
[2] Value at wells.

Minerals Yearbook. Bureau of Mines. Washington, D.C. Annual from 1932–33; continuing the *Mineral Resources of the United States* series (1866–1931); from 1977 in 3 vols. *(Metals and Minerals; Area Reports, Domestic; and Area Reports, International)*

Agriculture. Agriculture in the USA is characterized by its ability to adapt to widely varying conditions, and still produce an abundance and variety of agricultural products. From colonial times to about 1920 the major increases in farm production were brought about by adding to the number of farms and the amount of land under cultivation. During this period nearly 320m. acres of virgin forest were converted to crop land or pasture, and extensive areas of grass lands were ploughed. Improvident use of soil and water resources was evident in many areas.

During the next 20 years the number of farms reached a plateau of about 6·5m., and the acreage planted to crops held relatively stable around 330m. acres. The major source of increase in farm output arose from the substitution of power-driven machines for horses and mules. Greater emphasis was placed on development and improvement of land, and the need for conservation of basic agricultural resources was recognized. A successful conservation programme, highly co-ordinated and on a national scale—to prevent further erosion, to restore the native fertility of damaged land and to adjust land uses to production capabilities and needs—has been in operation since early in the 1930s.

Following the Second World War the uptrend in farm output has been greatly accelerated by increased production per acre and per farm animal. These increases are associated with a higher degree of mechanization; greater use of lime and fertilizer; improved varieties, including hybrid maize and grain sorghums; more effective control of insects and disease; improved strains of livestock and poultry; and wider use of good husbandry practices, such as nutritionally balanced feeds, use of superior sites and better housing. During this period land included in farms decreased slowly, crop land harvested declined somewhat more rapidly, but the number of farms declined sharply.

Some significant changes during these transitions are:

All land in farms totalled less than 500m. acres in 1870, rose to a peak of over 1,200m. acres in the 1950s and declined to 991m. acres in 1989, even with the addition of the new States of Alaska and Hawaii in 1960. The number of farms declined from 6·35m. in 1940 to 2,173m. in 1989, as the average size of farms doubled. The average size of farms in 1989 was 456 acres, but ranged from a few acres to many thousand acres. In 1987, 595,000 farms (690,329 in 1978) were less than 50 acres; 645,000 (814,689), 50–179 acres; 678,000 (811,468), 180–999 acres; and 162,000 (162,156) 1,000 acres or more.

Farms operated by owners in 1987 were 1,239,000; by part-owners, 609,000; by tenants, 240,000. The average size of farms in 1982 was 227 acres for full-owners, 794 acres for part-owners and 428 acres for tenants.

In 1988 (with 1970 figures in parentheses) large-scale, highly mechanized farms with sales of agricultural products totalling $20,000 and over per farm made up 40·7% (17·6%) of all farms and accounted for 79·9% of all farmland. Farms selling between $19,999 and $5,000 worth of products per farm were 25·2% (24·9%) of all farms and accounted for 15·7% of farmland. Operators in every sales category received off-farm income, but operators selling less than $20,000 per year received more of their average income from non-farm sources than from farming in 1986. In 1988 the average net farm income for farms with sales of $500,000 and over was $714,414; for farms with sales between $100,000–$499,999, $70,825; for farms with sales between $40,000–$99,999, $17,420; and for farms with sales of less than $40,000, $1,290. The average net farm income in 1987 for all farms was $26,067. In 1988, farms with sales of less than $40,000 accounted for 42·3% of total farm cash income in the US. Farms with sales of $40,000–$99,999 contributed 12·2% of total cash income; farms with sales of $100,000–$499,999, 29·3%; farms with sales of $500,000 and over, 21·5%.

A century ago three-quarters of the total US population was rural, and practically all rural people lived on farms. In April 1988 27% of the population was rural. Farm residents accounted for 2% of the total population.

During the week of July 10–16, 1988, there were 3·52m. people working on farms and ranches. The workforce comprised 1·43m. self-employed farm operators, 591,000 unpaid workers, 1·20m. workers hired directly by farm operators and 303,000 Agricultural Service employees.

Cash receipts from farm marketings and government payments (in $1m.):

	Crops	*Livestock and livestock products*	*Government payments*	*Total*
1932	1,996	2,752	—	4,748
1945	9,655	12,008	742	22,405
1950	12,356	16,105	283	28,744
1960	15,259	18,989	702	34,950
1970	20,976	29,563	3,717	54,256
1980	71,746	67,991	1,286	141,022
1987	63,751	75,717	16,747	156,215
1988	72,569	78,862	14,480	165,911

Realized gross farm income (including government payments), in $1m., was 174,891 in 1984, 166,364 in 1985, 160,422 in 1986, 171,625 in 1987 and 177,626 in 1988; net farm income amounted to 45,664 in 1988. Farm real estate debt, excluding debt in operator dwellings, was $103,585m. in 1984, $97,591m. in 1985, $88,561m. in 1986, $81,063m. in 1987 and $76,697m. in 1988.

US agricultural exports, fiscal year, totalled: 1982–83, $34,769m.; 1983–84, $38,027m.; 1984–85, $31,201m.; 1985–86, $26,324m.; 1986–87, $28,700m. (12% of all exports); 1987–88, $37,100m. (12% of all exports).

Total area of farm land under irrigation in 1987 was 46,386,000 acres.

According to census returns and estimates of the Economic Research Service, the acreage and specified values of farms has been as follows (area in 1,000 acres; value in $1,000; cash receipts in $1m.):

	Farm area	*Crop land available for crops*	*Value, land, bldgs,[2] machinery, livestock*	*Cash receipts*
1910	878,798	432,000	41,089,000	…
1930	990,112 [1]	480,000	57,815,000	…
1940	1,065,114 [1]	467,000	41,829,000	…

[1] Includes Alaska and Hawaii.

[2] Real estate, livestock and machinery, excluding crops.

	Farm area	Crop land available for crops	Value, land, bldgs,[2] machinery, livestock	Cash receipts
1950	1,161,420[1]	478,000	104,800,000	28,461
1959	1,123,508[1]	458,100	155,700,000	33,647
1969	1,062,893[1]	472,100	241,200,000	48,179
1978	1,014,777[1]	471,000	728,700,000	112,360
1982	986,797[1]	489,000	903,800,000	142,595
1988	995,000	...	686,400,000	150,431

[1] Includes Alaska and Hawaii.
[2] Real estate, livestock and machinery, excluding crops.

The areas and production of the principal crops for 3 years were:

	1986			1987			1988		
	Harvested 1,000 acres	Production 1,000	Yield per acre	Harvested 1,000 acres	Production 1,000	Yield per acre	Harvested 1,000 acres	Production 1,000	Yield per acre
Corn for grain (bu.)	69,159	8,249,864	119·3	59,208	7,072,073	119·4	58,164	4,921,000	84·6
Oats (bu.)	6,860	386,356	56·3	6,925	374,000	54·0	...	...	...
Barley (bu.)	12,007	610,522	50·8	10,057	529,530	52·7	7,500	291,000	38·6
All wheat (bu.)	60,723	2,081,635	34·4	55,960	2,107,480	37·7	53,174	1,811,000	34·1
Rice (cwt.)[1]	2,360	133,356	5,651	2,333	129,603	5,555	2,900	160,000	2,900
Soybeans for beans (bu.)	58,292	1,940,101	33·3	56,977	1,922,762	33·7	57,383	1,539,000	26·8
Flaxseed (bu.)	683	11,538	16·9	463	7,444	16·1	...	...	...
All Cotton[1] (bales)	8,468	9,731·1	552	10,035	14,759·9	706	11,891	15,466,000	623
Potatoes (cwt.)	1,220	361,511	296	1,279	385,462	301	...	...	...
Tobacco (lb.)	582	1,163,940	2,001	587	1,190,674	2,028	632	1,348,000	2,134

[1] Yield in lb.

Corn (Maize). The chief corn-growing states (1988) were (estimated production, corn for grain in 1,000 bu.): Iowa, 899,000; Nebraska, 818,000; Illinois, 701,000; Indiana, 415,000; Minnesota, 348,000; Ohio, 255,000; Montana, 154,000; Kansas, 144,000; South Dakota, 132,000; Wisconsin, 131,000; Texas, 130,000.

Wheat. The chief wheat-growing states (1988) were (estimated production in 1,000 bu.): Kansas, 323,000; Oklahoma, 173,000; Washington, 125,000; North Dakota, 103,000; Texas, 90,000; Colorado, 80,000; Missouri, 78,000; Idaho, 76,000; Nebraska, 72,000.

Cotton. Leading production, 1988, by state (in 1,000 bales, 480 lb. net weight) was: Texas, 5,260; California, 2,853; Mississippi, 1,830; Arizona, 1,120; Arkansas, 1,050; Louisiana, 950; Tennessee, 590; Alabama, 380; Oklahoma, 290.

Tobacco. Production (1,000 lb.) of the chief tobacco-growing states was, in 1988: N. Carolina, 553,000; Kentucky, 337,000; S. Carolina, 100,000; Virginia, 91,000; Tennessee, 91,000; Georgia, 86,000.

Fruit. Production, in 1,000 tonnes:

	1985	1986	1987	1988
Apples	3,918	3,954	5,226	4,554
Citrus Fruit	10,525	11,051	11,968	12,641
Grapes	5,607	5,225	5,250	5,984

Dairy produce. In 1988, production of milk was 145,527m. lb.; cheese solid, 5,572m. lb.; butter, 1,208m. lb.; ice-cream, 882m. gallons; non-fat dry milk, 978m. lb.; cottage cheese, 1,204m. lb.

Livestock (31 Dec. 1988): Cattle and calves, 99,484,000; sheep and lambs, 10,745,000; hogs and pigs (1 Dec. 1988), 55·3m.

On 31 Dec. 1988 there were 355,489,000 chickens, excluding broilers. In 1987 240·3m. turkeys were raised; 5,002·9m. broilers were produced, 1 Dec. 1986–30 Nov. 1987. Eggs produced, same period, 69,492m. (value $3,177m.).

Value of production (in $1m.) was:

	1986	*1987*	*1988*
Cattle and calves	20,935·3	24,629·3	27,426
Sheep	443·9	498·9	...
Hogs and pigs	9,555·8	10,426·8	9,128

Total value of livestock, excluding poultry and goats and, from 1961, horses and mules (in $1m.) on farms in the USA on 1 Jan. was: 1930, 6,061; 1933 (low point of the agricultural depression), 2,733; 1970, 22,886; 1980, 60,598; 1985, 45,594; 1988, 64,945; 1989, 60,400.

In 1987 the production of shorn wool was 85·8m. lb. from 11m. sheep (average 1970–74, 320m. lb. from 18·2m. sheep); of pulled wool, 1·15m. lb. (1970–74, 10·1m. lb.).

Forestry. In 1977 the US forest lands, including Alaska and Hawaii, capable of producing timber for commercial use, covered 482,485,900 acres (more than one-fifth of the land area), classified as follows: Saw-timber stands, 215,435,700 acres; pole timber stands, 135,609,900 acres, seedling and sapling stands, 115,032,100 acres; non-stocked and other areas, 16,408,200 acres. Ownership of commercial forest land is distributed as follows: Federal government, 99,410,400 acres; state, county, municipal and Indian, 36,311,200 acres; privately owned, 346,764,300 acres, including 115,777,100 acres on farms. Of the saw-timber stand (2,578,940m. bd ft) Douglas fir constitutes 514,317; Southern pine, 321,563; Western yellow (ponderosa and jeffrey) pine, 192,070; other softwoods, 957,458; hardwoods, 255,189. In 1976 growing stock timber removals amounted to 14,229,023,000 cu. ft compared to net annual growth of about 21,664,316,000 cu. ft. Saw-timber removals amounted to 65,176,618,000 bd ft against an annual growth of 74,620,832,000 bd ft. The net area of the 156 national forests and other areas in USA and Puerto Rico administered by the US Department of Agriculture's Forest Service, including commercial and non-commercial forest land, was in Oct. 1986, 191m. acres.

Fire takes a heavy annual toll in the forest; total area burned over in 1986 was 3,191,125 acres; 1,500m. acres of land are now under organized fire-protection service. Federal land that was planted or seeded in forest and wind barrier nursery stock in the year ending 30 Sept. 1986 was 300,640 acres.

Land Areas of National Forest System. Forest Service, US Dept. of Agriculture, 1985
Report of the Forest Service, 1985

Fisheries. Total US catch (edible and industrial), 1988, 3·3m. tonnes valued at $3,520m.; harvest outside the US and joint venture operations (mostly Alaskan pollock, and tuna), 1·7m. tonnes valued at $490m.; foreign catch in the 200 mile wide US fishery zone (mostly Alaskan pollock, 73%; Pacific flounders, 13% and Pacific cod, 6%), 1·2m. tonnes.

Major species caught, 1988: Menhaden, 2,086m. lb, value $105·7m. (29% of total US catch); Alaskan pollock, 1,257m. lb, $95·3m.; salmon, 606·1m. lb, $910·7m.; crabs, 4,566m. lb, $383·6m.; shrimp, 330·9m. lb, $506m.; cod, 343·2m. lb, $81·4m. Major landing areas, 1988: By value (in $1m.): Alaska, 1,339; Louisiana, 317·3; Massachusetts, 274; California, 199·3; Texas, 175·7.

Exports, 1988, totalled $2,275m.; imports, $8,872m. *Per capita* consumption, 1988, 15 lb edible meat; estimated live weight equivalent about 45 lb *per capita*.

Tennessee Valley Authority. Established by Act of Congress, 1933, the TVA is a multiple-purpose federal agency which carries out its duties in an area embracing some 41,000 sq. miles, in 201 counties (aggregate population, about 4·7m.) in the 7 Tennessee River Valley states: Tennessee, Kentucky, Mississippi, Alabama, North Carolina, Georgia and Virginia. In addition, 76 counties outside the Valley are served by TVA power distributors. Its 3 directors are appointed by the President, with the consent of the Senate; headquarters are in Knoxville, Tenn. There were 25,844 employees in Aug. 1989.

In the 1930s and 1940s, the Tennessee Valley offered the world a model of the first effort to develop all resources of a major river valley under one comprehensive programme, the Tennessee Valley Authority. The multipurpose development of the Tennessee River for flood control, navigation, and electric power production was the first big task for TVA. But there were other needs; controlling erosion on the land, introducing better fertilizers and new farming practices, eradicating malaria, demonstrating ways electricity could lighten the burdens in the home and increase production on the farm, and a multitude of potential job-producing enterprises.

In the depression year, 1933, the *per capita* income in the Valley was $168, compared with the national average of $375. Through the years, TVA has placed a strong emphasis on the economic development of the Valley. In recent years average income levels in the region have been nearly 80% of the national level.

TVA supplies electric power to 160 local distribution systems serving 3m. customers. The power system originated with the water-power development of the Tennessee River, but has become predominantly a coal-fired system as power requirements have outgrown the region's hydro-electric potential. In fiscal year 1988, the TVA system generated 95,000m. kwh. Installed capacity in 1988 was 32·1m. kw, with another 5·2m. kw under construction at TVA's nuclear plants.

Power operations are financially self-supporting from revenues. In fiscal year 1986 power revenues were $4,639m. Power facilities are financed from revenues and the sale of revenue bonds and notes, and TVA is repaying appropriations previously invested in power facilities. Other TVA resource development programmes continue to be financed from congressional appropriations.

Annual Report of the TVA. Knoxville, 1934 to date

Clapp, G.R., *The TVA; An Approach to the Development of a Region*. Univ. of Chicago Press, 1955

Lilienthal, D. E., *TVA; Democracy on the March*. 20th Anniversary ed. New York and London, 1953

Tennessee Valley Authority. *A History of the Tennessee Valley Authority*. Knoxville, Tennessee, 1982

INDUSTRY. The following table presents industry statistics of manufactures as reported at various censuses from 1909 to 1982 and from the Annual Survey of Manufactures for years in which no census was taken. The figures for 1958 to 1982 include data for some establishments previously classified as non-manufacturing. The figures for 1939, but not for earlier years, have been revised to exclude data for establishments classified as non-manufacturing in 1954. The figures for 1909–33 were previously revised by the deduction of data for industries excluded from manufacturing during that period.

The statistics for 1958, 1963, 1967, 1972, 1977 and 1982 relate to all establishments employing 1 or more persons anytime during the year; for 1950, 1956–57, 1959–62, 1966 and 1968–74 on a representative sample of manufacturing establishments of 1 or more employees; for 1929 through 1939, those reporting products valued at $5,000 or more; and for 1909 and 1919, those reporting products valued at $500 or more. These differences in the minimum size of establishments included in the census affect only very slightly the year-to-year comparability of the figures.

The annual Surveys of Manufactures carry forward the key measures of manufacturing activity which are covered in detail by the Census of Manufactures. The estimate for 1950 is based on reports for approximately 45,000 plants out of a total of more than 260,000 operating manufacturing establishments; those for 1956–57 on about 50,000, and those for 1959–62, 1966 and 1968–74 on about 60,000 out of about 300,000. Included are all large plants and representative samples of the much more numerous small plants. The large plants in the surveys account for approximately two-thirds of the total employment in operating manufacturing establishments in the US.

	Number of establishments	*Production workers (average for year)*	*Production workers' wages total ($1,000)*	*Value added by manufacture ($1,000)*
1909	264,810	6,261,736	3,205,213	8,160,075
1919	270,231	8,464,916	9,664,009	23,841,624
1929	206,663	8,369,705	10,884,919	30,591,435

	Number of establish-ments	*Production workers (average for year)*	*Production workers' wages total ($1,000)*	*Value added by manufacture ($1,000)*
1933	139,325	5,787,611	4,940,146	14,007,540
1939	173,802	7,808,205	8,997,515	24,487,304
1950	260,000	11,778,803	34,600,025	89,749,765
1960	...	12,209,514	55,555,452	163,998,531
1963	306,317	12,232,041	62,093,601	192,082,900
1967	305,680	13,955,300	81,393,600	261,983,800
1970	...	13,528,000	91,609,000	300,227,600
1972	312,662	13,526,500	105,494,700	353,974,200
1973	...	14,233,100	118,332,300	405,623,500
1974	...	13,970,900	124,983,200	452,468,400
1975	...	12,567,900	121,427,200	442,485,800
1977	350,757	13,691,000	157,163,700	585,165,600
1978	...	14,228,700	176,416,800	657,412,000
1979	...	14,537,800	192,881,500	747,480,500
1980	...	13,900,100	198,164,000	773,831,300
1982	348,385	12,400,600	204,787,200	824,117,700
1984	...	12,572,800	231,783,900	983,227,700
1985	...	12,171,100	235,731,700	999,065,800
1986	...	11,800,000	237,000,000	1,035,000,000
1987	358,061	12,259,500	251,533,000	1,166,554,900

For comparison of broad types of manufacturing, the industries covered by the Census of Manufactures have been divided into 20 general groups according to the *Standard Industrial Classification*.

Code No.	*Industry group*	*Year*	*Production workers (average for year)*	*Production workers' wages, total ($1,000)*	*Value added by manu-facture* [1] *($1,000)*
20.	Food and kindred products	1985	993,600	17,427,700	104,140,000
		1986	990,000	17,789,000	112,191,000
		1987	1,029,500	18,894,800	122,072,600
21.	Tobacco products	1985	36,900	440,900	11,893,700
		1986	34,000	912,000	12,725,000
		1987	32,700	992,500	14,260,500
22.	Textile mill products	1985	565,300	7,609,200	20,193,300
		1986	555,000	7,898,000	22,232,000
		1987	580,200	8,766,800	26,013,900
23.	Apparel and other textile products	1985	904,000	9,003,000	27,728,400
		1986	863,000	8,949,000	28,451,000
		1987	913,300	9,910,200	33,310,800
24.	Lumber and wood products	1985	514,200	7,835,800	21,065,500
		1986	512,000	8,135,000	23,239,000
		1987	581,100	9,516,500	28,590,900
25.	Furniture and fixtures	1985	380,000	5,345,500	16,478,800
		1986	376,000	5,556,000	17,659,000
		1987	408,000	6,230,100	20,239,100
26.	Paper and allied products	1985	462,100	10,783,400	40,387,200
		1986	458,000	11,297,000	43,925,000
		1987	465,700	11,758,700	49,725,800
27.	Printing and publishing	1985	742,100	13,554,400	73,054,300
		1986	738,000	14,099,000	78,150,000
		1987	796,900	15,669,900	89,207,900
28.	Chemical and allied products	1985	476,000	11,602,000	95,257,500
		1986	458,000	11,756,000	100,013,000
		1987	464,300	12,327,100	121,241,800
29.	Petroleum and coal products	1985	83,500	2,533,900	17,111,600
		1986	82,000	2,598,000	17,496,000
		1987	76,500	2,462,800	18,398,900

[1] Figures represent adjusted value added.

Code No. Industry group	Year	Production workers (average for year)	Production workers' wages, total ($1,000)	Value added by manufacture [1] ($1,000)
30. Rubber and miscellaneous plastics products	1985	578,400	9,799,200	35,708,300
	1986	572,000	10,124,000	37,236,000
	1987	640,900	11,644,700	44,293,100
31. Leather and leather products	1985	124,800	1,342,200	4,107,500
	1986	110,000	1,213,000	3,611,000
	1987	107,400	1,281,700	4,274,900
32. Stone, clay and glass products	1985	403,800	8,196,200	28,841,800
	1986	399,000	8,352,000	30,677,000
	1987	402,700	8,742,500	33,076,400
33. Primary metal industries	1985	571,000	14,277,900	38,081,900
	1986	529,000	13,472,000	38,092,000
	1987	541,000	14,162,700	46,471,200
34. Fabricated metal products	1985	1,103,500	21,976,800	69,161,500
	1986	1,050,000	21,817,000	68,621,000
	1987	1,083,700	22,914,800	75,502,900
35. Machinery (except electrical)	1985	1,236,600	26,510,500	110,234,100
	1986	1,141,000	25,422,000	108,365,000
	1987	1,145,900	26,077,700	119,214,400
36. Electric and electronic equipment	1985	1,233,100	23,658,800	109,861,500
	1986	1,160,000	23,361,000	112,422,000
	1987	1,003,800	19,757,800	95,958,100
37. Transportation equipment	1985	1,179,600	33,171,400	120,953,100
	1986	1,169,000	33,626,000	125,706,000
	1987	1,206,300	34,755,100	135,782,700
38. Instruments and related products	1985	348,000	6,192,600	40,278,300
	1986	335,000	6,704,000	40,005,000
	1987	509,300	11,655,000	71,847,200
39. Miscellaneous manufacturing	1985	234,600	3,415,300	14,031,600
	1986	236,000	3,520,000	14,622,000
	1987	270,100	4,011,900	17,431,600

[1] Figures represent adjusted value added.

Iron and Steel: Output of the iron and steel industries (in net tons of 2,000 lb.), according to figures supplied by the American Iron and Steel Institute, was:

	Furnaces in blast 31 Dec.	Pig-iron (including ferro-alloys)	Raw steel	Steel by method of production[1]			
				Open hearth	Bessemer	Electric [2]	Basic Oxygen
1932 [3]	44	9,835,227	15,322,901	13,336,210	1,715,925	270,044	...
1939	195	35,677,097	52,798,714	48,409,800	3,358,916	1,029,067	...
1944 [4]	218	62,866,198	89,641,600	80,363,953	5,039,923	4,237,699	...
1950	234	66,400,311	96,336,075	86,262,509	4,534,558	6,039,008	...
1960	114	68,566,384	99,281,601	86,367,506	1,189,196	8,378,743	3,346,156
1970	152	87,933,000	131,514,000	48,022,000	—	20,162,000	63,330,000
1980	...	70,329,000	111,835,000	13,054,000	—	31,166,000	67,617,000
1988	...	55,745,000	99,924,000	5,118,000	—	36,846,000	57,960,000
1989	...	55,873,000	97,943,000	4,442,000	—	35,154,000	58,348,000

[1] The sum of these 4 items should equal the total in the preceding column; any difference appearing is due to the very small production of crucible steel, omitted prior to 1950.
[2] Includes crucible production beginning 1950. [3] Low point of the depression.
[4] Peak year of war production.

The iron and steel industry in 1989 employed 124,215 wage-earners (compared with 449,888 in 1960), who worked an average of 41 hours per week and earned an average of $17.69 per hour: total employment costs were $5,544m. and total employment costs for 44,635 salaried employees were $2,592m.

Annual Statistics Report. American Iron and Steel Institute

Labour. The Bureau of Labor Statistics estimated that in 1989 the labour force was 125,557,000 (66·8% of those 16 years and over); the resident armed forces accounted for 1,688,000 and the civilian labour force for 123,869,000, of whom 117,342,000 were employed and 6,528,000—or 5·3%—were unemployed. The following table shows civilian employment by industry and sex and percentage distribution of the total:

Industry Group	*Male*	*Female*	*Total*	*Percentage distribution*
Employed (1,000 persons):	64,315	53,027	117,342	100·0
Agriculture, forestry and fisheries	2,654	725	3,378	2·9
Mining	602	117	719	0·6
Construction	6,992	687	7,680	6·5
Manufacturing:				
Durable goods	9,384	3,420	12,805	10·9
Non-durable (including not specified)	5,181	3,666	8,847	7·5
Transportation, communication and other public utilities	5,800	2,294	8,094	6·9
Wholesale and retail trade	12,795	11,435	24,230	20·6
Finance, insurance and real estate	3,247	4,742	7,989	6·8
Services	14,486	23,561	38,048	32·4
Private households	160	949	1,108	0·9
Other services	14,327	22,613	36,939	31·5
Professional services	7,886	16,724	24,609	20·6
Public administration	3,173	2,381	5,553	4·7

Source: U.S. Department of Labour, Bureau of Labor Statistics

A total of 51 strikes and lockouts of 1,000 workers or more occurred in 1989, involving 452,000 workers and 17m. idle days; the number of idle days was 0·07% of the year's total working time of all workers.

There are 3 federal agencies which provide formal machinery for the adjustment of labour disputes: (1) The Federal Mediation and Conciliation Service, now an independent agency, whose mediation services are available 'in any labor dispute in any industry affecting commerce'; under Executive Order 11491, as amended, to federal agencies and organizations of federal employees involved in negotiation disputes; and in state and local government collective bargaining disputes when adequate dispute resolution machinery is not available to the parties. Its aim is to prevent and minimize work stoppages. (2) The National Mediation Board (1934) provides much the same facilities for the railroad and air-transport industries pursuant to the Railway Labor Act. (3) The National Railroad Adjustment Board (1934) acts as a board of final appeal for grievances arising over the interpretation of existing collective agreements under the Railway Labor Act; its decisions are binding upon both sides and enforceable by the courts.

Trade Unions. The American labour movement comprises about 90 national and international labour organizations plus a large number of small independent local or single-firm labour organizations. In 1989 total membership was approximately 17m. The American Federation of Labor (founded 1881 and taking its name in 1886) and the Congress of Industrial Organizations merged into one organization, named the AFL–CIO, in Dec. 1955, representing 14·1m. workers in 1990.

Unaffiliated or independent labour organizations, inter-state in scope, had an estimated total membership excluding all foreign members (1990) of about 3m.

Labour organizations represented 18·6% (19·2m.) of employed persons in 1989; 16·4% (17) were actual members of unions.

The National Labor Relations Act, as amended by the Labor–Management Relations (Taft–Hartley) Act, 1947 (*see* THE STATESMAN'S YEAR-BOOK, 1955, p. 617), was amended by the Labor–Management Reporting and Disclosure Act, 1959, and again amended in 1974. The 1959 Act requires extensive reporting and disclosure of certain financial and administrative practices of labour organizations, employers and labour relations consultants. In addition, certain powers are vested in the Secretary of Labor to prevent abuses in the administration of trusteeships by labour organizations, to provide minimum standards and procedures for the election of union officers and to establish rules prescribing minimum standards for determining the adequacy of union procedures for the removal of officers. Other provisions impose a fiduciary responsibility upon union officers and provide for the exclusion of those convicted of certain named felonies from office for specified periods; more stringently regulate secondary boycotts and banning of 'hot' cargo agreements; put limitations upon organizational and recognition picketing and permit States to assert jurisdiction over labour disputes where the National Labor Relations Board declines to act. The Act also contains a 'Bill of Rights' for union members (enforceable directly by them) dealing with such things as equal rights in the nomination and election of union officers, freedom of speech and assembly subject to reasonable union rules, and safeguards against improper disciplinary action.

FOREIGN ECONOMIC RELATIONS. On 1 Jan. 1989 the Canada-USA Free Trade Agreement came into effect, providing for the phased removal of tariff and other barriers.

Commerce. Total value of imports and exports of merchandise by yearly average or by year (in $1m.):

	Exports *Total* [1]	*Exports* *US mdse.*	*General imports*		*Exports* [2] *Total* [1]	*Exports* [2] *US mdse.*	*General imports* [2]
1951–55	15,333	15,196	10,832	1985	213,146	206,925	345,276
1956–60	19,204	19,029	13,650	1986	227,159	206,376	365,438
1961–65	24,006	24,707	17,659	1987	254,122	243,859	406,241
1970	43,224	42,590	39,952	1988	322,426	310,049	440,952
1984	217,888	212,057	325,726	1989	363,983	349,650	472,977

[1] Excludes re-exports. [2] Includes US Virgin Islands trade with foreign countries.

For a description of how imports and exports are valued, see *Explanation of Statistics of Report FT990, Highlights of US Export and Import Trade,* Bureau of the Census, US Department of Commerce, Washington, D.C., 1946.

The 'most favoured nation' treatment in commerce between Great Britain and US was agreed to for 4 years by the treaty of 1815, was extended for 10 years by the treaty of 1818, and indefinitely (subject to 12 months' notice) by that of 1827.

Imports and exports of gold and silver bullion and specie in calendar years (in $1,000):

	Gold *Exports*	*Gold* *Imports*	*Silver* *Exports*	*Silver* *Imports*
1932	809,528	363,315	13,850	19,650
1940	4,995	4,749,467	3,674	58,434
1944	959,228	113,836	126,915	23,373
1955	7,257	104,592	8,331	72,932
1960	1,647	335,032	25,789	57,438
1965	1,285,097	101,669	54,061	64,769
1970	36,887	227,472	53,003	58,838
1975	429,278	406,583	104,086	274,106
1980	2,787,431	2,508,520	1,326,878	1,336,009
1985	919,400	2,109,500	81,746	855,528
1987	1,034,186	1,052,941	79,123	460,235

The domestic exports of US produce, including military, and the imports for consumption by economic classes for 3 calendar years were (in $m.):

	Exports (US merchandise)			*Imports for consumption*		
	1987	*1988*	*1989*	*1987*	*1988*	*1989*
Food and live animals	19,179	26,182	29,724	20,267	20,110	20,685
Crude materials	20,416	25,151	26,947	11,295	13,624	15,370
Machinery and transport equipment	108,596	135,082	148,800	176,893	196,017	205,761
Chemicals	26,381	32,281	36,485	16,046	19,580	20,752
Total of the above main groups	174,572	218,696	241,956	224,501	249,311	262,568

Leading exports of US merchandise are listed below for the calendar year 1988: Special category merchandise is included. Data for major subdivisions of certain classes are also given:

Commodity	*$1m.*	*Commodity*	*$1m.*
Machinery, total	88,432	Chemicals	32,300
Power generating machinery	12,818	Chemical elements and compounds	12,950
Metalworking machinery	1,925	Plastic materials and resins	7,277
Agricultural machines and tractors	1,956	Soybeans	4,816
Office machinery and computers	23,128	Cotton	1,975
Telecommunications apparatus	6,544	Textiles and apparel	3,650
Electrical machinery and apparatus	21,602	Tobacco and cigarettes	3,897
Electrical power apparatus and switchgear	4,206	Iron and steel-mill products	2,017
Road motor vehicles (and parts)	25,178	Non-ferrous base metals and alloys	3,041
Aircraft and spacecraft (and parts)	20,004	Pulp, paper and products	7,894
Grains and preparations	12,281	Coal	3,960
Wheat (and flour)	5,080	Fruits and vegetables	3,488
		Petroleum and products	3,679
		Firearms of war and ammunition	2,609

Chief imports for 27 commodity classes for consumption for the calendar year 1988:

Commodity	*$1m.*	*Commodity*	*$1m.*
Petroleum products, crude and refined	37,469	Wool and other hair	328
Petroleum	25,654	Metal manufactures n.e.s.	8,979
Petroleum products	11,815	Diamonds (excl. industrial)	4,306
Non-ferrous metals	10,066	Rubber	1,023
Copper	1,860	Textile yarn, fabrics and products	6,302
Aluminium	3,442	Clothing	21,418
Nickel	1,220	Cotton fabrics, woven	979
Lead	859	Machinery, total	113,595
Tin	315	Agricultural machinery and tractors	2,124
Paper, paperboard and products	8,333	Office machinery	22,586
Newsprint	4,462	Coffee	2,287
Wood pulp	2,506	Chemicals and related products	19,475
Fertilizers	1,021	Chemicals	10,336
Sugar	438	Oils and fats	763
Iron and steel-mill products	10,299	Cocoa beans	405
Cattle, meat and preparations	3,327	Glass, pottery and china	2,934
Automobiles and parts	74,082	Footwear	8,022
Fish (and shellfish)	861	Toys and sports goods	6,714
Fruit and vegetables	4,439	Furs, undressed	154
Alcoholic beverages	3,148	Telecommunications apparatus	21,087
		Artworks and antiques	2,044
		Natural and manufactured gas	2,578

Total trade beween the USA and the UK (British Department of Trade returns, in £1,000 sterling):

	1987	*1988*	*1989*	*1990*
Imports to UK	9,136,015	10,767,750	12,888,890	14,357,516
Exports and re-exports from UK	11,014,242	10,544,077	12,098,549	12,998,506

Imports and exports by selected countries for the calendar years 1988 and 1989 (in $1m.):

Country	*General imports* 1988	1989	*Exports incl. re-exports* [1] 1988	1989
UK	17,976	18,242	18,364	20,866
France	12,509	13,029	9,970	11,585
Federal Republic of Germany	26,362	24,834	14,348	16,883
Italy	11,576	11,946	6,775	7,232
Netherlands	4,559	4,796	10,117	11,393
EEC	84,939	85,129	75,755	86,592
USSR	586	703	2,769	4,271
Canada	81,398	88,210	71,622	78,639
Mexico	23,260	27,186	20,628	24,969
China	8,511	11,989	5,021	5,807
Japan	89,519	93,586	37,725	44,584
South Korea	20,105	19,742	11,232	13,478
Taiwan	24,714	24,327	12,129	11,323
Australia	3,541	3,898	6,973	8,347
Hong Kong	10,238	9,739	5,687	6,304

[1] 'Special category' exports are included in these totals.

Imports and exports by continents, groupings and selected countries for the calendar years 1987 and 1988 (in $1m.):

Area and country	General imports 1987	General imports 1988	Exports incl. re-exports[1] 1987	Exports incl. re-exports[1] 1988
Colombia	2,232	2,167	1,412	1,758
Ecuador	1,266	1,231	621	684
Mexico	20,271	23,277	14,582	20,643
Paraguay	22	37	183	194
Peru	769	656	814	798
Uruguay	344	275	92	100
Venezuela	5,579	5,228	3,586	4,611
Dominican Republic	1,163	1,417	1,142	1,362
Haiti	395	384	459	479
Bahamas	416	411	782	741
Netherlands Antilles	521	411	507	432
Jamaica	395	444	601	758
Trinidad and Tobago	815	719	361	328
Europe				
Western Europe	95,496	100,515	69,718	87,995
OECD Countries	94,636	99,558	69,091	87,236
Denmark	1,779	1,666	893	970
Greece	480	529	402	649
Ireland	1,112	1,373	1,810	2,182
Portugal	664	691	581	752
Spain	2,839	3,205	3,148	4,217
Turkey	821	983	1,483	1,843
EFTA countries				
Austria	929	1,085	549	748
Norway	1,404	1,452	842	932
Sweden	4,758	4,995	1,894	2,705
Switzerland	4,249	4,638	3,151	4,207
Finland	999	1,206	515	763
Iceland	286	190	84	98
Yugoslavia	797	847	461	534
Poland	296	378	239	304
Asia	174,452	190,729	73,268	99,705
Near East	10,811	11,511	9,502	10,857
Bahrain	63	99	205	281
Iran	1,668	9	54	73
Iraq	495	1,488	683	1,156
Israel	2,639	2,978	3,130	3,248
Kuwait	522	464	505	690
Lebanon	33	40	97	123
Saudi Arabia	4,433	5,594	3,373	3,799
Other Asia	83,582	92,414	41,497	56,918
Bangladesh	370	369	193	258
India	2,529	2,952	1,463	2,498
Indonesia	3,394	3,188	767	1,056
Malaysia	2,921	3,711	1,897	2,139
Pakistan	405	461	733	1,093
Philippines	2,264	2,682	1,599	1,880
Singapore	6,201	7,996	4,053	5,770
Sri Lanka	417	424	77	124
Thailand	2,220	3,218	1,544	1,964
Vietnam	...	...	23	16
Oceania	4,136	4,824	6,526	8,242
New Zealand and W. Samoa	1,053	1,168	821	946

[1] 'Special category' exports are included in these totals.

Area and country	General imports 1987	General imports 1988	Exports incl. re-exports [1] 1987	Exports incl. re-exports [1] 1988
Africa	11,939	10,863	6,283	7,431
Algeria	1,999	1,813	426	733
Egypt	465	221	2,210	2,340
Ethiopia	74	54	136	181
Morocco	50	92	383	428
Ghana	249	202	115	117
Liberia	88	108	70	68
Nigeria	3,573	3,298	295	356
Kenya	79	64	95	92
Zaïre	308	365	104	125
South Africa, Republic of	1,346	1,530	1,281	1,690

[1] 'Special category' exports are included in these totals.

US Department of Commerce. Report FT 990, *Highlights of US Export and Import Trade* (ceased publication 1989). FT 925, *US Merchandise Trade*. Monthly from 1990.

Tourism. In 1988, 33,859,000 visitors travelled to the USA and spent over US$29,202,000 (excluding transportation paid to US international carriers). They came mainly from Canada (13,843,000), Mexico (7,505,000), Europe (5,772,000) and Asia/Japan (3,719,000). Expenditure by US travellers in foreign countries for 1988 was over US$32,112,000. (excluding transportation paid to foreign flag international carriers).

COMMUNICATIONS

Roads. On 31 Dec. 1989 the total US public road [1] mileage, including rural and urban roads, amounted to 3,876,501 miles, of which 3,507,002 miles were surfaced roads. The total mileage cited includes 706,404 miles of rural roads under control of the states, 2,238,108 miles of local rural roads, 179,240 miles of federal park and forest roads, and 752,749 miles of urban roads and streets. Expenditures for construction and maintenance amounted to $68,590m. in 1988.

By the end of 1988, toll roads administered by state and local toll authorities, totalled 5,020 miles (including some under construction).

Motor vehicles registered in the calendar year 1989 were (Federal Highways Administration) 191,694,462, including 143,081,443 automobiles, 625,040 buses, 43,554,064 trucks and 4,433,915 motorcycles.

Inter-city trucks (private and for hire) averaged 704,000m. revenue net ton-miles in 1989. Of the 615,669 buses in service in 1987, 486,753 were school buses. Inter-city service operated a total of 19,887 buses and carried a total of 334m. revenue passengers in 1988.

There were 45,555 deaths in 40,718 road accidents in 1989.

[1] Public road mileage excludes that mileage not open to public travel, not maintained by public authority, or not passable by standard four-wheel vehicles. This excluded mileage was reported to the US Federal Highway Administration prior to 1981.

Railways. Railway history in the USA commences in 1828, but the first railway to convey both freight and passengers in regular service (between Baltimore and Ellicott's Mills, Md., 13 miles) dates from 24 May 1830. Mileage rose to a peak of 266,381 miles in 1916, falling thereafter to 222,164 in 1969 (these include some duplication under trackage rights and some mileage operated in Canada by US companies). The ordinary gauge is 4 ft 8½ in. (about 99·6% of total mileage).

In addition to the independent railroad companies, railway service is provided by the National Railroad Passenger Corporation (Amtrak), which is federally assisted. Amtrak was set up on 1 May 1971 to maintain a basic network of inter-city passenger trains, and is responsible for almost all non-commuter services with 40,000 miles of route including 1,256 km owned (555 electrified). Amtrak carried 21·4m. passengers in 1989.

The Consolidated Rail Corporation (Conrail) was established on 1 April 1976 with federal assistance to run freight services in the industrial north-east. It was returned to the private sector in 1985. There are in addition some 400 minor railways (short lines) which provide local freight connections. Outside the major conurbations there are almost no regular passenger services other than those provided by Amtrak.

The following table, based on the figures of the Interstate Commerce Commission, shows some railway statistics for 4 calendar years:

Classes I and II Railroads	*1960*	*1970*	*1980* [2]	*1986* [1]
Mileage owned (first main tracks)	223,779	204,621	157,078	135,782
Revenue freight originated (1m. short tons)	1,421	1,572	1,537	1,306
Freight ton-mileage (1m. ton-miles)	591,550	771,012	932,748	867,722
Passengers carried (1,000)	488,019	289,469	281,503	[3]
Passenger-miles (1m.)	31,790	10,786	6,557	[3]
Operating revenues ($1m.)	9,587	12,209	28,708	26,204
Operating expenses ($1m.)	7,135	9,806	26,761	24,896
Net railway operating income ($1m.)	1,055	506	1,364	507
Net income after fixed charges ($1m.)	855	126	2,029	1,579
Class I Railroads:				
Locomotives in service	40,949	27,086	28,240	21,045
Steam locomotives	25,640	—	—	—
Freight-train cars (excluding caboose cars)	1,721,269	1,423,921	1,101,343	713,954
Passenger-train cars	57,146	11,177	2,219	672
Average number of employees	1,220,784	566,282	458,996	275,817
Average wage per week ($1)	72.59	188.71	474.21	690.27

[1] Class I railroads only. From 1981, Class II railroads were no longer required to file annual reports.
[2] Data for National Railroad Passenger Corporation excluded.
[3] This data has been discontinued.

Aviation. In civil aviation there were, on 31 Dec. 1989, 700,010 certificated pilots (including 142,544 student pilots), 274,834 registered civil aircraft and 455,263,066 passengers.

Airports (Landing Facilities 17,446) on 31 Dec. 1989: Air carrier, 632; general aviation, 16,814. Of these airports, 12,946 were conventional land-based, while 414 were seaplane bases, 4,014 were heliports and 70 stolports (STOL—Short Take-Off and Landing).

Statistics from the Department of Transportation indicate that for 1988 US flag carriers in scheduled international service had 35·4m. enplanements with 493·7m. aircraft miles (excluding all-cargo) for a total of 93,992m. revenue passenger-miles. The non-scheduled airlines had a total of 14,191m. revenue passenger-miles internationally and domestically. Domestically US scheduled airlines in 1988 had 419·2m. enplanements with a total of 3,571·3m. aircraft miles for 329,309m. revenue passenger-miles. (A revenue passenger-mile is one paying passenger carried per mile.)

Shipping. On 1 June 1989 the US merchant marine included 669 sea-going vessels of 1,000 gross tons or over, with aggregate dead-weight tonnage of 25m. This included 241 tankers of 15·8m. DWT.

On 1 June 1989 US merchant ocean-going vessels were employed as follows: Active, 378 of 17·5m. DWT, of which 151 of 6·5m. tons were foreign trade, 165 of 9·5m. tons in domestic trade and 62 of 1·5m. tons in other US agency operations. Inactive vessels totalled 7·2m. DWT; 51 of 3·5m. DWT privately owned were laid up and 240 of 3·7m. tons were Government-owned National Defense reserve fleet. Of the total vessels in the US fleet, 421 of 21m. DWT were privately owned.

US exports and imports carried on dry cargo and tanker vessels in the year 1988 totalled 718·8m. long tons, of which 30·8m. long tons or 3·9% were carried in US flag vessels.

Telecommunications. Until the beginning of 1984 the telephone business was largely in the hands of the American Telephone and Telegraph Company (AT & T) and its telephone operating subsidiaries, which together were known as the Bell System. Pursuant to a government anti-trust suit, the Bell System was broken up, with the telephone operating companies being divested from AT & T to create seven regional companies for providing local service. There are also many hundreds of smaller telephone companies having no common ownership affiliation with the Bell companies, but which connect with them for universal service, countrywide and worldwide. In addition, several new entrants have begun to compete with AT & T in the long-distance telephone market. The message telegraph and telex services are in the hands of The Western Union Telegraph Company, and the international record carriers, which compete with the telephone industry in providing leased private lines. Western Union also provides an inter-city telephone service. Total exchange access lines in 1987, 126,725,000.

The US Postal Service superseded the Post Office Department on 1 July 1971. Postal business for the years ended 30 Sept. included the following items:

	1986	*1987*	*1988*	*1989*
Number of post offices	39,270	40,030	40,117	40,031
Operating revenue ($1,000)	30,102,691	31,528,112	35,035,753	38,415,092
Operating expenses ($1,000)	30,716,595	32,519,689	36,119,186	38,370,758

In 1987 there were 91m. households with television and (1988) 520m. radio receivers in use. In 1986 there were over 10,000 authorized radio stations and (1988) 1,342 television stations with 46 national cable networks.

Cinemas. Cinemas increased from 17,003 in 1940 to 20,239 in 1950 and decreased to 20,200 in 1984, of which 2,832 were drive-ins.

Newspapers. Of the daily newspapers being published in the USA in 1971, 339 were morning papers with a circulation of 26,116,000, and 1,425 were evening papers with a circulation of 36,115,000. The 590 Sunday papers had a total circulation of 49·7m.

JUSTICE, RELIGION, EDUCATION AND WELFARE

Justice. Legal controversies may be decided in two systems of courts: The federal courts, with jurisdiction confined to certain matters enumerated in Article III of the Constitution, and the state courts, with jurisdiction in all other proceedings. The federal courts have jurisdiction exclusive of the state courts in criminal prosecutions for the violation of federal statutes, in civil cases involving the government, in bankruptcy cases and in admiralty proceedings, and have jurisdiction concurrent with the state courts over suits between parties from different states, and certain suits involving questions of federal law.

The highest court is the Supreme Court of the US, which reviews cases from the lower federal courts and certain cases originating in state courts involving questions of federal law. It is the final arbiter of all questions involving federal statutes and the Constitution; and it has the power to invalidate any federal or state law or executive action which it finds repugnant to the Constitution. This court, consisting of 9 justices who receive salaries of $118,600 a year (the Chief Justice, $124,000), meets from Oct. until June every year. For the term ended June, 1989 it disposed of 4,932 cases, deciding 276 on their merits. In the remainder of cases it either summarily affirms lower court decisions or declines to review. A few suits, usually brought by state governments, originate in the Supreme Court, but issues of fact are mostly referred to a master.

The US courts of appeals number 13 (in 11 circuits composed of 3 or more states and 1 circuit for the District of Columbia and 1 Court of Appeals for the Federal Circuit); the 168 circuit judges receive salaries of $102,500 a year. Any party to a suit in a lower federal court usually has a right of appeal to one of these courts. In addition, there are direct appeals to these courts from many federal administrative agencies. In the year ending 30 June 1990, 43,364 appeals were filed in the courts of appeals, including 1,466 in the Federal Circuit.

The trial courts in the federal system are the US district courts, of which there are 89 in the 50 states, 1 in the District of Columbia and 1 each in the Commonwealth of Puerto Rico and the Territories of the Virgin Islands, Guam and the Northern Marianas. Each state has at least 1 US district court, and 3 states have 4 apiece.

Each district court has from 1 to 27 judgeships. There are 575 US district judges ($96,600 a year), who received 217,879 civil cases and 66,340 criminal defendants from 1 July 1989 to 30 June 1990.

In addition to these courts of general jurisdiction, there are special federal courts of limited jurisdiction. The US Claims Court (16 judges at $96,600 a year) decides claims for money damages against the federal government in a wide variety of matters; the Court of International Trade (9 judges at $96,600) determines controversies concerning the classification and valuation of imported merchandise.

The judges of all these courts are appointed by the President with the approval of the Senate; to assure their independence, they hold office during good behaviour and cannot have their salaries reduced. This does not apply to judges in the Territories, who hold their offices for a term of 10 years or to judges of the US Claims Court. The judges may retire with full pay at the age of 70 years if they have served a period of 10 years, or at 65 if they have 15 years of service, but they are subject to call for such judicial duties as they are willing to undertake. 11 US judges up to 1990 have been involved in impeachment proceedings, of whom 6 district judges and 1 commerce judge were convicted and removed from office.

Of the 217,879 civil cases filed in the district courts in the year ending 30 June 1990, about 118,576 arose under various federal statutes (such as labour, social security, tax, patent, securities, antitrust and civil rights laws); 43,759 involved personal injury or property damage claims; 46,039 dealt with contracts; and 9,505 were actions concerning real property.

Of the 47,962 criminal cases filed in the district courts in the year ending 30 June 1990, 2.390 were charged with alleged infractions of the immigration laws; 243, the transport of stolen motor vehicles; 3,391 larceny and theft; 9,579, embezzlement and fraud; and 2,592 narcotics laws.

Persons convicted of federal crimes are either fined, released on probation under the supervision of the probation officers of the federal courts, confined in prison for a period of up to 6 months and then put on probation (known as split sentencing) or confined in one of the following institutions: 3 for juvenile and youths; 7 for young adults; 7 for intermediate term adults; 7 for short-term adults; 2 for females; 1 hospital and 15 community service centres. In addition, prisoners are confined in centres operated by the National Institutes of Mental Health. In addition, prisoner drug addicts may be committed to US Public Health Service hospitals for treatment. Prisoners confined in Federal and State Prisons at 30 June 1990, numbered 755,425.

The state courts have jurisdiction over all civil and criminal cases arising under state laws, but decisions of the state courts of last resort as to the validity of treaties or of laws of the US, or on other questions arising under the Constitution, are subject to review by the Supreme Court of the US. The state court systems are generally similar to the federal system, to the extent that they generally have a number of trial courts and intermediate appellate courts, and a single court of last resort. The highest court in each state is usually called the Supreme Court or Court of Appeals with a Chief Justice and Associate Justices, usually elected but sometimes appointed by the Governor with the advice and consent of the State Senate or other advisory body; they usually hold office for a term of years, but in some instances for life or during good behaviour. Their salaries range from $55,425 to $115,161 a year. The lowest tribunals are usually those of Justices of the Peace; many towns and cities have municipal and police courts, with power to commit for trial in criminal matters and to determine misdemeanours for violation of the municipal ordinances; they frequently try civil cases involving limited amounts.

The death penalty is illegal in Alaska, Hawaii, Iowa, Kansas, Maine, Massachusetts, Michigan, Minnesota, New York, North Dakota, Rhode Island, Vermont, West Virginia and Wisconsin. The death penalty is legal in 36 states. Until 1982 it had fallen into disuse and had been abolished *de facto* in many states. The US Supreme Court had held the death penalty, as applied in general criminal statutes, to contravene the eighth and fourteenth amendments of the US constitution, as a cruel and unusual punishment when used so irregularly and rarely as to destroy its deterrent value.

There were no executions 1968–76. In 1977 a convicted murderer requested that he should be executed and after a lengthy legal dispute the sentence was carried out at Utah state prison. 120 persons were executed between 1977 and 1989. On 31 Dec. 1989, 2,250 prisoners were reported under sentence of death.

The total number of civilian executions carried out in the US from 1930 to 1989 was 3,979.

A Guide to Court Systems. Institute of Judicial Administration. New York, 1960
The United States Courts. Administrative Office of the US Courts, Washington, D.C., 20544
Blumberg, A. S., *Criminal Justice: Issues and Ironies.* 2nd ed. New York, 1973
Huston, L. A. and others, *Roles of the Attorney General of the United States.* New York, 1968
McCloskey, R. G., *The Modern Supreme Court.* Harvard Univ. Press, 1972
McLauchlan, W. P., *American Legal Processes.* New York, 1977
Walker, S. E., *Popular Justice.* New York, 1980

Religion. *The Yearbook of American and Canadian Churches for 1990,* published by the National Council of the Churches of Christ in the USA, New York, presents the latest figures available from official statisticians of church bodies. The large majority of reports are for the calendar year 1988, or a fiscal year ending 1988. The 1988 reports indicated that there were 145,383,738 (143,830,806 in 1987) members with 350,481 local churches. There were 335,389 clergymen serving in local congregations in 1988. The principal religious bodies (numerically or historically) or groups of religious bodies are shown below:

Denominations	*Local churches*	*Total membership* [3]
Summary:		
Protestant bodies	320,264	79,328,686
Roman Catholic Church	23,091	54,918,949
Jews [1]	3,416	5,935,000
Eastern Churches	1,689	4,077,011
Old Catholic, Polish National Catholic and Armenian	431	826,889
Buddhists	100	100,000
Miscellaneous [2]	1,130	197,203
1987 totals	350,481	145,383,738

[1] Includes Orthodox, Conservative and Reformed bodies.
[2] Includes non-Christian bodies such as Spiritualists, Ethical Culture, Unitarian-Universalists.
[3] Membership figures are not strictly comparable, as definitions of membership vary from body to body.

Protestant Church Membership	*Total membership*
Baptist bodies	
Southern Baptist Convention	14,812,844
National Baptist Convention, USA	5,500,000
National Baptist Convention of America, Inc.	2,668,799
National Primitive Baptist Convention	250,000
American Baptist Churches in the USA	1,549,563
American Baptist Association	250,000
Conservative Baptist Association of America	204,496
Regular Baptist Churches	260,000
Free Will Baptists	204,382
Baptist Missionary Association of America	227,897
Christian Church (Disciples of Christ)	1,073,119
Christian Churches and Churches of Christ	1,070,616
Church of the Nazarene	552,264
Churches of Christ	1,626,000
The Episcopal Church	2,455,422
Latter-Day Saints:	
Church of Jesus Christ of Latter-Day Saints	4,000,000
Reorganized Church of Jesus Christ of Latter-Day Saints	190,950
Lutheran Bodies :	
Evangelical Lutheran Church in America	5,251,534
The Lutheran Church-Missouri Synod	2,604,278
Wisconsin Evangelical Lutheran Synod	418,691
Methodist Bodies:	
United Methodist Church	9,055,575
African Methodist Episcopal Church	2,210,000
Protestant Church Membership	*Total membership*

Lutheran Bodies—contd.	
African Methodist Episcopal Zion Church	1,220,260
Christian Methodist Episcopal Church	718,922
Pentecostal Bodies:	
The Church of God in Christ	3,709,661
Assemblies of God	2,147,041
Church of God (Cleveland, Tenn.)	582,203
United Pentecostal Church, International, Inc.	500,000
Presbyterian Bodies:	
Presbyterian Church (USA)	2,929,608
Presbyterian Church in America	208,349
Reformed Churches:	
Reformed Church in America	333,798
Christian Reformed Church	224,408
The Salvation Army	433,448
Seventh-day Adventist Church	687,200
United Church of Christ	1,644,787

Yearbook of American and Canadian Churches. Annual, from 1951. New York
Greeley, A., *Religious Change in America*. Harvard Univ. Press, 1989

Education. Under the system of government in the USA, elementary and secondary education is committed in the main to the several states. Each of the 50 states and the District of Columbia has a system of free public schools, established by law, with courses covering 12 years plus kindergarten. There are 3 structural patterns in common use; the K8-4 plan, meaning kindergarten plus 8 elementary grades followed by 4 high school grades; the K6–3–3 plan, or kindergarten plus 6 elementary grades followed by a 3-year junior high school and a 3-year senior high school; and the K6–6 plan, kindergarten plus 6 elementary grades followed by a 6-year high school. All plans lead to high-school graduation, usually at age 17 or 18. Vocational education is an integral part of secondary education. In addition, some states have, as part of the free public school system, 2-year colleges in which education is provided at a nominal cost. Each state has delegated a large degree of control of the educational programme to local school districts (numbering 15,376 in school year 1988–89), each with a board of education (usually 3 to 9 members) selected locally and serving mostly without pay. The school policies of the local school districts must be in accord with the laws and the regulations of their state Departments of Education. While regulations differ from one jurisdiction to another, in general it may be said that school attendance is compulsory from age 7 to 16.

The Census Bureau estimates that in Nov. 1979 only 1m. or 0·6% of the 170m. persons who were 14 years of age or older were unable to read and write; in 1930 the percentage was 4·8. In 1940 a new category was established—the 'functionally illiterate', meaning those who had completed fewer than 5 years of elementary schooling; for persons 25 years of age or over this percentage was 2·4 in March 1988 (for the non-white population alone it was 5·1%); it was 1% for white and 1·2% for non-whites in the 25–29-year-old group. The Bureau reported that in March 1988 the median years of school completed by all persons 25 years old and over was 12·7, and that 20·3% had completed 4 or more years of college. For the 25–29-year-old group, the median school years completed was 12·8 and 22·7% had completed 4 or more years of college.

In the autumn of 1988, 13,043,000 students (5,999,000 men and 7,045,000 women) were enrolled in 3,565 colleges and universities; 2,376,000 were first-time students. About 30% of the population between the ages of 18 and 24 were enrolled in colleges and universities.

Public elementary and secondary school revenue is supplied from the county and other local sources (44·1% in 1987–88), state sources (49·5%) and federal sources (6·3%). In 1987–88 expenditure for public elementary and secondary education totalled about $172,800m., including $159,200m. for current operating expenses, $10,700m. for capital outlay and $2,900m. for interest on school debt. The current expenditure per pupil in average daily attendance was $4,243. The total cost per pupil, also including capital outlay and interest, amounted to $4,610. Estimated total expenditures, for private elementary and secondary schools in 1987–88 were about

$15,100m. In 1987–88 college and university spending totalled $126,100m., of which about $80,900m. was spent by institutions under public control. The federal government contributed about 13% of total current-fund revenue; state governments, 29%; student tuition and fees, 24%; and all other sources, 34%.

Vocational education below college grade, including the training of teachers to conduct such education, has been federally aided since 1918. Federal support for vocational education in 1987–88 amounted to about $864m. Many public high schools offer vocational courses in addition to their usual academic programmes.

Summary of statistics of regular schools (public and private), teachers and pupils in autumn 1988 (compiled by the US National Center for Education Statistics):

Schools by level	*Number of schools 1988–89*	*Teachers autumn 1988*	*Enrolment autumn 1988*
Elementary schools:			
Public	61,531	1,324,000	24,417,000
Private	20,252 [1]	251,000 [2]	4,036,000 [2]
Secondary schools:			
Public	22,785	993,000	15,775,000
Private	7,387 [1]	94,000 [2]	1,206,000 [2]
Higher education:			
Public	1,582	524,000 [2]	10,156,000
Private	1,983	217,000 [2]	2,887,000
Total	115,520	3,403,000	58,477,000

[1] Data for 1985–86. [2] Estimated.

Most of the private elementary and secondary schools are affiliated with religious denominations. Of the children attending private elementary and secondary schools in 1985, nearly 3·1m. or 55·4% were enrolled in Roman Catholic schools. About 1·6m. or 28·7% were in schools affiliated with other religious groups.

During the school year 1987–88 high-school graduates numbered about 2,797,000 (about 49·3% boys and 50·7% girls). Institutions of higher education conferred 993,362 bachelor's degrees during the year 1987–88, 476,842 to men and 516,520 to women; 298,733 master's degrees, 144,923 to men and 153,810 to women; 34,839 doctorates, 22,592 to men and 12,247 to women; and 70,415 first professional degrees, 45,289 to men and 25,129 to women.

During the academic year, 1988–89, 366,650 foreign students were enrolled in American colleges and universities. The percentages of students coming from various areas in 1988–89 were: South and East Asia, 52·2; Middle East, 11; Latin America, 12·3; Africa, 7·3; Europe, 11·7; North America, 4·6; Oceania, 1.

School enrolment, Oct. 1988, embraced 96% of the children who were 5 and 6 years old; more than 99% of the children aged 7–13 years; 95% of those aged 14–17 and 56% of those aged 18 and 19.

The US National Center for Education Statistics estimates the total enrolment in the autumn of 1990 at all of the country's elementary, secondary and higher educational institutions (public and private) at 59·8m. (59·4m. in the autumn of 1989); this was 23·8% of the total population of the USA as of 1 Sept. 1990.

The number of teachers in regular public and private elementary and secondary schools in the autumn of 1990 was expected to increase slightly to 2,785,000. The average annual salary of the public school teachers was about $31,200 in 1989–90.

Digest of Education Statistics. Annual. Dept. of Education, Washington 20208, D.C. (from 1962)

American Community, Technical and Junior Colleges. 9th ed. American Council on Education. Washington, 1984

American Universities and Colleges. 12th ed. American Council on Education. Washington, 1983

Health and Welfare. Admission to the practice of medicine (for both doctors of medicine and doctors of osteopathic medicine) is controlled in each state by examining boards directly representing the profession and acting with authority conferred by state law. Although there are a number of variations, the usual time now required to complete training is 8 years beyond the secondary school with up to 3 or more years of additional graduate training. Certification as a specialist may require between 3 and 5 more years of graduate training plus experience in practice. In academic year 1987–88 the 142 US schools (15 osteopathic and 127 allopathic) graduated 17,451 physicians. About 36% of first-year students were women. In Dec. 1988 the estimated number of active physicians (MD and DO—in all forms of practice) in the US, Puerto Rico and outlying US areas was 573,583 (1 active physician to 434 population). The distribution of physicians throughout the country is uneven, both by state and by urban–rural areas.

In 1987–88 the 58 dental schools graduated 4,581 dentists. Active dentists in Dec. 1988 numbered 146,800 (1 active dentist to 1,678 population).

In academic year 1987–88, there were 1,443 registered nursing programmes in the US and 64,915 graduates. In Dec. 1988 registered nurses employed full- or part-time were 1 to 144 population.

Number of hospitals listed by the American Hospital Association in 1984 was 6,872, with 1,339,000 beds and 37,938,000 admissions during the year; average daily census was 970,000. Of the total, 341 hospitals with 112,000 beds were operated by the federal government; 1,662 with 203,000 beds by state and local government; 3,366 with 717,000 beds by non-profit organizations (including church groups); 786 with 100,000 beds are proprietary. The categories of non-federal hospitals are 5,814 short-term general and special hospitals with 1,020,000 beds; 131 non-federal long-term general and special hospitals with 30,000 beds; 579 psychiatric hospitals with 175,000 beds; 7 tuberculosis hospitals with 1,000 beds.

Social welfare legislation was chiefly the province of the various states until the adoption of the Social Security Act of 14 Aug. 1935. This as amended provides for a federal system of old-age, survivors and disability insurance; health insurance for the aged and disabled; supplemental security income for the aged, blind and disabled; federal state unemployment insurance; and federal grants to states for public assistance (medical assistance for the aged and aid to families with dependent children generally) and for maternal and child-health and child-welfare services. The Social Security Administration of the Department of Health and Human Services has responsibility for the programmes—old-age, survivors and disability insurance and supplemental security income. The Family Support Administration has federal responsibility for the programmes—aid to families with dependent children, low income energy assistance, child support enforcement, refugee and entry assistance and community services block grant. The Health Care Financing Administration, an agency of the same Department, has federal responsibility for health insurance for the aged and disabled. The Office of Human Development Services has federal responsibility for social service programmes for such groups as the elderly, children, youth, native Americans and persons with developmental disabilities, and its Public Health Service supports maternal and child-health services. Unemployment insurance is the responsibility of the Department of Labor.

The Social Security Act provides for protection against the cost of medical care through the two-part programme of health insurance for people 65 and over and for certain disabled people under 65, who receive disability insurance payments or who have permanent kidney failure (Medicare). During fiscal year 1987, payments totalling $49,967m. were made under the hospital part of Medicare on behalf of 31,852,860 people. During the same period, $29,937m. was paid under the voluntary medical insurance part of Medicare on behalf of 31,169,960 people.

In 1989 about 130m. persons worked in employment covered by old-age, survivors and disability insurance.

In June 1989 over 38·9m. beneficiaries were on the rolls, and the average benefit paid to a retired worker (not counting any paid to his dependants) was about $539 per month.

In 1987 an average of 11m. persons (adults and children) were receiving payments under aid to families with dependent children (average monthly payment, $374 per family). Total payments under aid to families with dependent children were $16,827m. for the calendar year 1988. The role of Child Support Enforcement is to ensure that children are supported by their parents. Money collected is for children who live with only one parent because of divorce, separation or out-of-wedlock birth. In 1988, nearly $4,613m. was collected on behalf of these children.

In June 1989, about 4·5m. persons were receiving supplementary security income payments, including 1·4m. persons aged 65 or over; 83,000 blind persons, and over 3m. disabled persons. Payments, including supplemental amounts from various states, totalled $13,800m. in 1988.

In 1986, federal appropriations for the social services block grant amounted to $2,700m. In addition, 1989 federal appropriations for human development and family social services to selected target groups totalled $4,117m. Included in this amount were $3,333m. for children and youth; $748m. for the elderly; $95m. for persons with developmental disabilities; and $30m. for native Americans. During 1989, the Public Health Services awarded a total of $554·3m. for maternal and child health services, $465·3m. as block grants to the States, $82·1m. for special projects of regional and national significance, and $6·9m. for genetic screening. Other block grants awarded by the Public Health Service in 1988 included $88m. for preventive health; $487m. for alcohol, drug abuse and mental health; $155m. for alcohol and drug abuse treatment and rehabilitation. In 1989, $414·8m. was awarded for community health centres; $45·6m. for migrant health centres; $20·6m. for efforts to reduce infant mortality; $3·2m. for black lung clinics; and $135·1m. for family planning. Other block grants awarded by the Family Support Administration included $316·9m. for community services block grant programmes for fiscal year 1989, and $1,380m. for the low income home energy assistance programme (LIHEAP).

DIPLOMATIC REPRESENTATIVES

Of the USA in Great Britain (Grosvenor Sq., London, W1A 1AE)
Ambassador: Raymond Seitz.

Of Great Britain in the USA (3100 Massachusetts Ave., Washington, D.C., 20008)
Ambassador: Sir Robin Renwick, KCMG.

Of the United States to the United Nations
Ambassador: Thomas Pickering.

Further Reading

I. Statistical Information

The Office of Management and Budget, Washington, D.C. 20503 is part of the Executive Office of the President; it is responsible for co-ordinating all the statistical work of the different Federal Government agencies. The Office does not collect or publish data itself. The main statistical agencies are as follows:

(1) Data User Services Division, Bureau of the Census, Department of Commerce, Washington, D.C. 20233. Responsible for decennial censuses of population and housing, quinquennial census of agriculture, manufactures and business; current statistics on population and the labour force, manufacturing activity and commodity production, trade and services, foreign trade, state and local government finances and operations. (*Statistical Abstract of the United States*, annual, and others).

(2) Bureau of Labor Statistics, Department of Labor, 441 G Street NW, Washington, D.C. 20212. (*Monthly Labor Review* and others).

(3) Information Division, Economic Research Service, Department of Agriculture, Washington, D.C. 20250. (*Agricultural Statistics*, annual, and others).

(4) National Center for Health Statistics, Department of Health and Human Services, 3700 East-West Highway, Hyattsville Md. 20782. (*Vital Statistics of the United States*, monthly and annual, and others).

(5) Bureau of Mines Office of Technical Information, Department of the Interior, Washington, D.C. 20241. (*Minerals Yearbook*, annual, and others).

(6) Office of Energy Information Services, Energy Information Administration, Department of Energy, Washington, D.C. 20461.

(7) Statistical Publications, Department of Commerce, Room 5062 Main Commerce, 14th St and Constitution Avenue NW, Washington, D.C. 20230; the Department's Bureau of Eco-

nomic Analysis and its Office of Industry and Trade Information are the main collectors of data.

(8) Center for Education Statistics, Department of Education, 555 New Jersey Avenue NW, Washington, D.C. 20208.

(9) Public Correspondence Division, Office of the Assistant Secretary of Defense (Public Affairs P.C.), The Pentagon, Washington, D.C. 20301-1400.

(10) Bureau of Justice Statistics, Department of Justice, 633 Indiana Avenue NW, Washington, D.C. 20531.

(11) Public Inquiry, APA 200, Federal Aviation Administration, Department of Transportation, 800 Independence Avenue SW, Washington, D.C. 20591.

(12) Office of Public Affairs, Federal Highway Administration, Department of Transportation, 400 7th St. SW, Washington, D.C. 20590.

(13) Statistics Division, Internal Revenue Service, Department of the Treasury, 1201 E St. NW, Washington, D.C. 20224.

Statistics on the economy are also published by the Division of Research and Statistics, Federal Reserve Board, Washington, D.C. 20551; the Congressional Joint Committee on the Economy, Capitol; the Office of the Secretary, Department of the Treasury, 1500 Pennsylvania Avenue NW, Washington, D.C. 20220.

II. Other Official Publications

Guide to the Study of the United States of America. General Reference and Bibliography Division, Library of Congress. 1960.

Historical Statistics of the United States, Colonial Times to 1957: A Statistical Abstract Supplement. Washington, 1960.—*Continuation to 1962 and Revisions,* 1965.

United States Government Manual. Washington. Annual.

The official publications of the USA are issued by the US Government Printing Office and are distributed by the Superintendent of Documents, who issued in 1940 a cumulative *Catalog of the Public Documents of the... Congress and of All the Departments of the Government of the United States.* This *Catalog* is kept up to date by *United States Government Publications, Monthly Catalog* with annual index and supplemented by *Price Lists.* Each *Price List* is devoted to a special subject or type of material, *e.g., American History* or *Census.* Useful guides are Schmeckebier, L. F. and Eastin, R. B. (eds.) *Government Publications and Their Use.* 2nd ed., Washington, D.C., 1961; Boyd, A. M., *United States Government Publications.* 3rd ed. New York, 1949, and Leidy, W. P., *Popular Guide to Government Publications.* 2nd ed. New York and London, 1963.

Treaties and other International Acts of the United States of America (Edited by Hunter Miller), 8 vols. Washington, 1929–48. This edition stops in 1863. It may be supplemented by *Treaties, Conventions... Between the US and Other Powers, 1776–1937* (Edited by William M. Malloy and others). 4 vols. 1909–38. A new Treaty Series, *US Treaties and Other International Agreements* was started in 1950.

Writings on American History. Washington, annual from 1902 (except 1904–5 and 1941–47).

III. Non-Official Publications

A. Handbooks

National Historical Publications Commission. *Guide to Archives and Manuscripts in the United States,* ed. P. M. Hamer. Yale Univ. Press, 1961

Adams, J. T. (ed.) *Dictionary of American History.* 2nd ed. 7 vols. New York, 1942

Dictionary of American Biography, ed. A. Johnson and D. Malone. 23 vols. New York, 1929–64.—*Concise Dictionary of American Biography.* New York, 1964

Current Biography. New York, annual from 1940; monthly supplements

Handlin, O. and others. *Harvard Guide to American History.* Cambridge, Mass., 1954

Herstein, S. R. and Robbins, N., *United States of America.* [Bibliography] Oxford and Santa Barbara, 1982

Lord, C. L. and E. H., *Historical Atlas of the US.* Rev. ed. New York, 1969

Who's Who in America. Chicago, 1899–1900 to date; monthly Supplement. 1940 to date

B. General History

Barck, Jr, O. T. and Blake, N. M., *Since 1900: A History of the United States.* 5th ed. New York, 1974

Brogan, H., *The Longman History of the United States of America.* London, 1985

Carman, H. J. and others, *A History of the American People.* 3rd ed. 2 vols. New York, 1967

King, A. (ed.) *The New American Political System.* 2nd ed. Washington, DC, 1990

Morison, S. E. with Commager, H. S., *The Growth of the American Republic*. 2 vols. 5th ed. OUP, 1962–63
Nicholas, H. G., *The Nature of American Politics*. OUP, 1980
Scammon, R. N. (ed.) *American Votes: A Handbook of Contemporary American Election Statistics*. Washington, D.C., 1956 to date (biennial)
Schlesinger, J., *America at Century's End*. Columbia Univ. Press, 1989
Snowman, D., *America Since 1920*. London, 1978
Watson, R. A., *The Promise and Performance of American Democracy*. 2nd ed. New York, 1975

C. Minorities
Burma, J. J., *Spanish-speaking Groups in the US*. Duke University Press, 1954, repr. 1974
McNickle, D., *The Indian Tribes of the United States*. OUP, 1962.—*Native American Tribalism*. OUP, 1973
Sklare, M., *The Jew in American Society*. New York, 1974

D. Economic History
The Economic History of the United States. 9 vols. New York, 1946 ff.
Bining, A. C. and Cochran, T. C., *The Rise of American Economic Life*. 4th ed. New York, 1963
Dorfman, J., *The Economic Mind in American Civilization*. 5 vols. New York, 1946–59
Friedman, M. and Schwartz, A. J., *A Monetary History of the United States, 1867–1960*. New York, 1963
Marmor, T. R. *et al.*, *America's Misunderstood Welfare State*. New York, 1990

E. Foreign Relations
Documents on American Foreign Relations. Princeton, from 1948. Annual
The United States in World Affairs. 1931 ff. Council on Foreign Relations. New York, from 1932. Annual
Agnew, J., *The United States in the World Economy*. CUP, 1987
Bartlett, R. (ed.) *The Record of American Diplomacy; Documents and Readings in the History of American Foreign Relations*. 4th ed. New York, 1964
Beloff, M., *The United States and the Unity of Europe*. London, 1963, repr. 1976
Connell-Smith, G., *The United States and Latin America*. London, 1975
Schwab, G., (ed.) *United States Foreign Policy at the Crossroads*. Westport, 1982
Vance, C., *Hard Choices: Critical Years in America's Foreign Policy*. New York, 1983

F. National Character
Degler, C. N., *Out of Our Past: The Forces That Shaped Modern America*. Rev. ed. New York, 1970
Duigan, P. and Rabushka, A., (eds.) *The United States in the 1980s*. Stanford, 1980
Fawcett, E. and Thomas, T., *America and the Americans*. London, 1983

National Library: The Library of Congress. Washington 25, D.C. *Librarian:* Lawrence Quincy Mumford, AB, MA, BS.

STATES AND TERRITORIES

For information as to State and Local Government, see under UNITED STATES, *pp.* 1386–88.

Against the names of the Governors and the Secretaries of State, (D.) stands for Democrat and (R.) for Republican.

Figures for the revenues and expenditures of the various states are those of the Federal Bureau of the Census unless otherwise stated, which takes the original state figures and arranges them on a common pattern so that those of one state can be compared with those of any other.

Official publications of the various states and insular possessions are listed in the *Monthly Check-List of State Publications*, issued by the Library of Congress since 1910. Their character and contents are discussed in J. K. Wilcox's *Manual on the Use of State Publications* (1940). Of great importance bibliographically are the publications of the Historical Records Survey and the American Imprints Inventory, which record local archives, official publications and state imprints. These publications supplement those of state historical societies which usually publish journals and monographs on state and local history. An outstanding source of statistical data is the material issued by the various state planning boards and commissions, to which should be added the annual *Governmental Finances* issued by the US Bureau of the Census.

The Book of the States. Biennial. Council of State Governments, Lexington, 1953 ff.
State Government Finances. Annual. Dept. of Commerce, 1966 ff.

ALABAMA

HISTORY. Alabama, settled in 1702 as part of the French Province of Louisiana, and ceded to the British in 1763, was organized as a Territory, 1817, and admitted into the Union on 14 Dec. 1819.

AREA AND POPULATION. Alabama is bounded north by Tennessee, east by Georgia, south by Florida and the Gulf of Mexico and west by Mississippi. Area, 51,998 sq. miles, including 1,562 sq. miles of inland water. Census population, 1 April 1990, 4,040,587, an increase of 146,699 over that of 1980. Estimate (1989) 4,241,653. Births, 1989, 62,530 (14·7 per 1,000 population); deaths, 38,924 (9·2); infant deaths (under 1 year), 756 (12·1 per 1,000 live births); marriages, 43,158 (10·2); divorces, 24,985 (5·9).

Population in 5 census years was:

	White	*Black*	*Indian*	*Asiatic*	*Total*	*Per sq. mile*
1910	1,228,832	908,282	909	70	2,138,093	41·4
1930	1,700,844	944,834	465	105	2,646,248	51·3
1960	2,283,609	980,271	1,726	915	3,266,521	64·0
			All others			
1970	2,533,831	903,467	6,867		3,444,165	66·7
1980	2,872,621	996,335	24,932		3,893,888	74·9

Of the total population in 1980, 49% were male, 61% were urban and 65% were 21 years or older.

The large cities (1990 census) were: Birmingham, 265,968 (metropolitan area, 907,810); Mobile, 196,278 (476,923); Montgomery (the capital), 187,106 (292,517); Huntsville, 159,789 (238,912); Tuscaloosa, 777,759 (150,522).

CLIMATE. Birmingham. Jan. 46°F (7·8°C), July 80°F (26·7°C). Annual rainfall 54" (1,346 mm). Mobile. Jan. 52°F (11·1°C), July 82°F (27·8°C). Annual rainfall 63" (1,577 mm). Montgomery. Jan. 49°F (9·4°C), July 81°F (27·2°C). Annual rainfall 53" (1,321 mm). *See* Gulf Coast, p. 1382. The growing season ranges from 190 days (north) to 270 days (south).

CONSTITUTION AND GOVERNMENT. The present constitution dates from 1901; it has had 524 amendments (at 29 Nov. 1990). The legislature consists of a Senate of 35 members and a House of Representatives of 105 members, all elected for 4 years. The Governor and Lieut.-Governor are elected for 4 years.

The state is represented in Congress by 2 senators and 7 representatives. Applicants for registration must take an oath of allegiance to the United States and fill out a questionnaire to the satisfaction of the registrars. In the 1988 presidential election Bush polled 809,663 votes, Dukakis, 547,347.

Montgomery is the capital.

Governor: Guy Hunt (R.), 1991–95 ($70,223).
Lieut.-Governor: Jim Folsom, Jr. (D.) ($2,100 a month plus allowances).
Secretary of State: Billy Joe Camp (D.) ($50,634).

BUDGET. The total net revenue for the fiscal year ending 30 Sept. 1988 was $15,601m. ($3,548m. from tax, $1,411m. from federal payments); total net expenditure was $15,595m. ($2,495m. on education, $545m. on highways, $528m. on public welfare, $612m. on health).

The outstanding debt on 30 Sept. 1988 amounted to $2,513m.

Per capita income (1988) was $12,604.

ENERGY AND NATURAL RESOURCES

Minerals. Principal minerals (1986): Coal, limestone, sand and gravel, petroleum (21·1m. bbl.) and natural gas (146,606m. cu. ft.). Total mineral output (1986) was valued at $2,001m. of which fuels, $1,440m.

Agriculture. The number of farms in 1989 was 47,000, covering 10·6m. acres; average farm had 219 acres and was valued at about $193,000.

Cash receipts from farm marketings, 1989: Crops, $790,872,000m.; livestock and poultry products, $1,932,392,000m.; and total, $2,723,264,000m. Principal sources: greenhouses and nurseries, peanuts, cotton, pototoes and other vegetables, soybeans; corn, wheat, pecans, hay, peaches and other fruit are also important. In 1989, poultry accounted for the largest percentage of cash receipts from farm marketings; cattle and calves were second, horticulture third, peanuts fourth.

Forestry. Area of national forest lands, Oct. 1990, 651,200 acres; state-owned forest, 211,600; industrial forest, 5,499,400; private non-industrial forest, 15,270,600; other government-owned forest, 344,900.

INDUSTRY. Alabama is predominantly industrial. In 1989 manufacturing establishments employed 383,800 workers; government, 314,700; trade, 349,100; services, 302,400; transport and public utilities, 80,100 (total non-agricultural workforce 1·6m.).

TOURISM. In 1986 about 28·6m. travelled to or through Alabama from other states. In 1989 total estimated tourist revenues amounted to $2,800m.

COMMUNICATIONS

Roads. Paved roads of all classes at July 1990 totalled 64,938 miles; total highways, 90,535 miles. Registered motor vehicles, 1990, 3,623,204.

Railways. At Dec. 1989 the railways had a length of 5,554 miles including side and yard tracks.

Aviation. In 1988 the state had 103 public-use airports. Nine airports are for commercial service, two are relief airports for Birmingham and the rest, general aviation.

Shipping. There are 1,200 miles of navigable inland water and 50 miles of Gulf Coast. The only deep-water port is Mobile, with a large ocean-going trade; total tonnage (1989), 37·2m. tons. The docks can handle 34 ocean-going vessels at once. The 9-ft channel of the Tennessee River traverses North Alabama for 200 miles; the Tennessee-Tombigbee waterway (232 miles), connects the Tennessee River with the Tombigbee River for access to the Gulf of Mexico. The Warrier– Tombigbee system (476 miles) connects the Birmingham industrial area to the Gulf.
The Coosa-Alabama River system reaches central Alabama as far north as Montgomery from Mobile and the Gulf Intracoastal Waterway. The Chattahoochee River runs for 261 miles. The Alabama State Docks also operates a system of 10 inland docks; there are several privately-run inland docks.

JUSTICE, RELIGION, EDUCATION AND WELFARE

Justice. The prison population on 30 Sept. 1990 was 15,074.

From 1 Jan. 1927 to 13 July 1990 there were 161 executions (electrocution): 129 for murder, 25 for rape, 5 for armed robbery, 1 for burglary and 1 for carnal knowledge. Before 1 Jan. 1927, persons executed in Alabama were hanged locally by the sheriffs in the counties of their conviction.

In 41 counties the sale of alcoholic beverage is permitted, and in 26 counties it is prohibited; but it is permitted in 7 cities within those 26 counties.

Religion. Chief religious bodies (in 1980) are: Southern Baptist Convention (about 1,182,018), Churches of Christ (113,919), United Methodist (about 344,790), Roman Catholic (106,123), African Methodist Episcopal Zion (139,714), Christian Methodist Episcopal (about 53,493) and Assemblies of God (48,610).

Education. In the school year 1989–90 the 1,294 public elementary and high schools required 39,416 teachers to teach 714,691 students enrolled in grades K-12. In 1989-90 there were 16 public senior institutions with 120,822 students and 4,596 faculty members. In 1989-90 the 12 community colleges had 40,814 students and

1,011 faculty members; 10 junior colleges had 16,270 students and 320 faculty members; 17 technical colleges had 11,766 students and 487 faculty members.

Health. In 1987 there were 137 hospitals (21,404 beds) licensed by the State Board of Health. In 1990 there were 2,493 patients in hospitals for mental diseases and 1,318 residents in facilities for the mentally retarded.

Welfare. In July 1990 Alabama paid supplements (to federal welfare payments) to 6,097 recipients of old-age assistance, receiving an average of $54.01 each; 4,312 permanently and totally disabled, $58.16; 104 blind, $57.06. Combined state–federal aid to dependent children was paid to 44,907 families, average $113.92 per family.

Further Reading

Alabama Official and Statistical Register. Montgomery. Quadrennial
Alabama County Data Book. Alabama Dept. of Economic and Community Affairs. Annual
Directory of Health Care Facilities. Alabama State Board of Health
Economic Abstract of Alabama. Center for Business and Economic Research, Univ. of Alabama, 1987
McCurley, R. L., Jr., ed., *The Legislative Process*. Alabama Law Institute, 3rd ed., 1984
Thigpen, R. A., *Alabama Government Manual*. Alabama Law Institute, 7th ed., 1986
Wiggins, S. W., (ed.) *From Civil War to Civil Rights, 1860–1960*. Univ. of Alabama Press, 1987

ALASKA

HISTORY. Discovered in 1741 by Vitus Bering, its first settlement, on Kodiak Island, was in 1784. The area known as Russian America with its capital (1806) at Sitka was ruled by a Russo-American fur company and vaguely claimed as a Russian colony. Alaska was purchased by the United States from Russia under the treaty of 30 March 1867 for $7·2m. It was not organized until 1884, when it became a 'district' governed by the code of the state of Oregon. By Act of Congress approved 24 Aug. 1912 Alaska became an incorporated Territory; its first legislature in 1913 granted votes to women, 7 years in advance of the Constitutional Amendment.

Alaska officially became the 49th state of the Union on 3 Jan. 1959.

AREA AND POPULATION. Alaska is bounded north by the Beaufort Sea, west and south by the Pacific and east by Canada. It has the largest area of any state, being more than twice the size of Texas. The gross area (land and water) is 591,004 sq. miles; the land area is 586,412 sq. miles of which 85% was in federal ownership in 1984. Census population, 1 April 1980, was 401,851, including military personnel, an increase of 33·5% over 1970. Estimate (1987), 537,800. Births, 1984, were 12,247 (24·5 per 1,000 population); deaths, 1,993 (4); infant deaths, 147 (12 per 1,000 live births); marriages, 6,519 (13); divorces, 3,904 (7·8).

Population in 5 census years was:

	White	*Black*	*All Others*	*Total*	*Per sq. mile*
1940	39,170	...	33,354	72,524	0·13
1950	92,808	...	35,835	128,643	0·23
1960	174,649	...	51,518	226,167	0·40
1970	236,767	8,911	54,704	300,382	0·53
1980	309,728	13,643	78,480	401,851	0·70

Of the total population in 1980, 53·01% were male, 64·34% were urban and 68·57% were aged 21 years or over.

The largest city is Anchorage, which had a 1980 census area population of 174,430 (1987 estimate, 231,422). Other census area populations, 1980 (and 1987 estimate), Fairbanks North Star, 53,983 (73,164); Juneau, 19,528 (25,369); Kenai Peninsula, 25,282 (39,170); Ketchikan Gateway, 11,316 (12,432); Kodiak Island, 9,939 (13,658); Matanuska-Susitna 17,816 (37,027). There are 14 boroughs and 148 incorporated cities.

CLIMATE. Anchorage. Jan. 12°F (–11·1°C), July 57°F (13·9°C). Annual rainfall 15" (371 mm). Fairbanks. Jan. –11°F (–23·9°C), July 60°F (15·6°C). Annual rainfall 12" (300 mm). Sitka. Jan. 33°F (0·6°C), July 55°F (12·8°C). Annual rainfall 87" (2,175 mm). *See* Pacific Coast, p. 1381.

CONSTITUTION AND GOVERNMENT. An important provision of the Enabling Act is that the state has the right to select 103·55m. acres of vacant and unappropriated public lands in order to establish 'a tax basis'; it can open these lands to prospectors for minerals, and the state is to derive the principal advantage in all gains resulting from the discovery of minerals. In addition, certain federally administered lands reserved for conservation of fisheries and wild life have been transferred to the state. Special provision is made for federal control of land for defence in areas of high strategic importance.

The constitution of Alaska was adopted by public vote, 24 April 1956. The state legislature consists of a Senate of 20 members (elected for 4 years) and a House of Representatives of 40 members (elected for 2 years). The state sends 2 senators and 1 representative to Congress. The franchise may be exercised by all citizens over 18.

The capital is Juneau.

In the 1988 presidential election Bush polled 102,381 votes, Dukakis, 62,205.

Governor: Walter J. Hickel (ind.), 1991–95 ($81,648).

ECONOMY

Budget. Total state government revenue for the year ended 30 June 1989 (Annual Financial Report figures) was $3,168·5m. Total expenditure was $3,185·5m.

In 1976 a Permanent Fund was set up for the deposit of at least 25% of all mineral-related revenue; total assets at 30 June 1989, $9,200m.

General obligation bonds at 30 June 1989, $386·1m.

Per capita income (1988) was $19,514.

ENERGY AND NATURAL RESOURCES

Oil and Gas. Commercial production of crude petroleum began in 1959 and by 1961 had become the most important mineral by value. Production: 1961, 6·3m. bbls (of 42 gallons); 1977, 171m. bbls; 1981, 587m. bbls; 1985, 666m. bbls; 1988, 738m. bbls, value $122·29m. Oil comes mainly from Prudhoe Bay, the Kuparuk River field and several Cook Inlet fields. Natural gas (liquid) production, 1988, 20·3m. bbls. Alaska receives approximately 85% of its general revenue from petroleum taxes and royalties. Revenue to the state from oil production in 1984 was $2,861·7m. (78% of general fund revenues) from corporate petroleum tax $265·1m. and from royalties $1,047·5m., severance tax, $1,393·1m., property tax, $131m., bonus sale, $10·1m., rents, $3·8m., intergovernmental receipts, $11·1m.

Oil from the Prudhoe Bay arctic field is now carried by the Trans-Alaska pipeline to Prince William Sound on the south coast, where a tanker terminal has been built at Valdez.

Minerals. Value of production, 1989 estimates: Gold (8,852 kg) $108,723,694; silver (162,102 kg) $27,360,852; lead (8,698 tonnes) $7,672,009; zinc (18,007 tonnes) $29,383,386; tin (87,988 kg) $672,000; jade and soapstone (51·7 tonnes) $1·14m.; sand and gravel (13·1m. tonnes) $39,875,000; building stone (2·6m. tonnes) $20·34m.; coal (1,317,574 tonnes) $41,464,800. Total value, $276,983,741.

Agriculture. In some parts of the state the climate during the brief spring and summer (about 100 days in major areas and 152 days in the south-eastern coastal area) is suitable for agricultural operations, thanks to the long hours of sunlight, but Alaska is a food-importing area. In 1987 about 1·4m. acres was farmland; Crops covered 29,134 acres and the balance was idle in pasture or uncleared land. In 1990 (preliminary) there were 8,200 cattle and calves, 700 hogs and pigs, 2,500 sheep and lambs and (1989) 5,000 poultry.

Total value of agricultural products in 1988: $30m. of which $19·5m. was from crops (mainly hay and potatoes) and $10·5m. from livestock and poultry.

There were about 34,000 reindeer in western Alaska in 1990. Sales of reindeer meat and by-products in 1990 (preliminary) were valued at $1,706,000.

Forestry. Of the 129m. forested acres of Alaska, 21m. acres are classified as timberland or commercial forest. The interior forest covers 115m. acres; more than 13m. acres are considered commercial forest, of which 3·4m. acres are in designated parks or wilderness and unavailable for harvest. The coastal rain forests provide the bulk of commercial timber volume; of their 13·6m. acres, 7·6m. acres support commercial stands, of which 1·9m. acres are in parks or wilderness and unavailable for harvest. In 1988, more than 390m. bd ft of timber were harvested from publicly owned or managed lands; lumber was the second most valuable product exported, with a value of $527m. (over 24% of all exports).

Fisheries. The catch for 1988 was 2,639m. lb. of fish and shellfish having a value to fishermen of $1,339m. The most important species are salmon, crab, herring, halibut and pollock.

INDUSTRY. Main industries with employment, 1988: Government, 66,600; trade, 41,900; services, 42,900; contract construction, 8,700; manufacturing, 14,800; mining including oil and gas, 9,500; transport, communication and utilities, 17,200; finance, insurance and property, 10,700.

The major manufacturing industry was food processing, followed by timber industries. Total non-agricultural employment, 1988, 212,300. Total wages and salaries, 1987, $5,759·86m.

TOURISM. About 742,800 tourists visited the state in 1988.

COMMUNICATIONS

Roads. Alaska's highway and road system, 1990, totalled 12,272 miles, including 10,462 miles rural. Registered motor vehicles, 1990, 363,743.

The Alaska Highway extends 1,523 miles from Dawson Creek, British Columbia, to Fairbanks, Alaska. It was built by the US Army in 1942, at a cost of $138m. The greater portion of it, because it lies in Canada, is maintained by Canada.

Railways. There is a railway of 111 miles from Skagway to the town of Whitehorse, the White Pass and Yukon route, in the Canadian Yukon region (this service operates seasonally). The government-owned Alaska Railroad runs from Seward to Fairbanks, a distance of 471 miles. This is a freight service with only occasional passenger use. A passenger service operates from Anchorage to Fairbanks via Denali National Park in the tourist season.

Aviation. In 1986 the state had 988 airports, of which 294 were state owned. Commercial passengers by air from Alaska's largest international airports Anchorage and Fairbanks in 1988 numbered 1,375,500 at Anchorage and 251,495 at Fairbanks. General aviation aircraft in the state per 1,000 population was about ten times the US average.

Shipping. Regular shipping services to and from the US are furnished by 2 steamship and several barge lines operating out of Seattle and other Pacific coast ports. A Canadian company also furnishes a regular service from Vancouver, B.C. Anchorage is the main port.

A 1,435 nautical-mile ferry system for motor cars and passengers (the 'Alaska Marine Highway') operates from Bellingham, Washington and Prince Rupert (British Columbia) to Juneau, Haines (for access to the Alaska Highway) and Skagway. A second system extends throughout the south-central region of Alaska linking the Cook Inlet area with Kodiak Island and Prince William Sound.

JUSTICE, RELIGION, EDUCATION AND WELFARE

Justice. There is no death penalty in Alaska. In 1988 there were 2,588 prisoners in state and federal institutions.

Religion. Many religions are represented, including the Russian Orthodox, Roman Catholic, Episcopalian, Presbyterian, Methodist and other denominations.

Education. Total expenditure on public schools in 1987 was $693,643,154. In 1988 there were about 3,100 elementary and 2,800 secondary school teachers, average salary, $41,000. During 1988 there were 104,956 pupils at public schools, 5,440 at private schools. The Bureau of Indian Affairs schools had 691 pupils in 1985. The University of Alaska (founded in 1922) had (Autumn 1988) 29,102 students: Fairbanks, 8,079; Anchorage, 17,062; Southeast, 3,961. Other colleges had 2,361 students in Autumn 1988.

Health. In 1983 there were 26 acute care hospitals with 1,800 beds, of which 7 were federal public health hospitals; 1 mental hospital; 24 mental health clinics.

Welfare. Old-age assistance was established under the Federal Social Security Act; in 1985 aid to dependent children covered a monthly average of 6,400 households; payments, an average of $501 per month; aid to the disabled was given to a monthly average of 2,300 persons receiving on average $251 per month. An average of 1,100 aged per month received $166.

Further Reading

Statistical Information: Department of Commerce and Economic Development, Economic Analysis Section, Juneau; Department of Labor, Research and Analysis, Juneau.

Alaska Blue Book, Department of Education, Juneau. Biennial
Alaska Industry–Occupation Outlook to 1992, Department of Labor, Juneau.
Alaska Economy, The. Division of Economic Enterprise, Juneau. Annual
Alaska Statistical Review. Office of the Governor, Juneau. Biennial
Annual Financial Report, Department of Administration, Juneau.
Gardey, J., *Alaska: The Sophisticated Wilderness.* London, 1976
Hulley, Clarence C., *Alaska Past and Present.* Portland, Oregon, 1970
Hunt, W. R., *Alaska, a Bicentennial History.* New York, 1976
Pearson, R. W. and Lynch, D. F., *Alaska, a Geography.* Boulder, 1984
Thomas, L., Jr., *Alaska and the Yukon.* New York, 1983
Tourville, M., *Alaska, a Bibliography, 1570–1970.* 1971

State Library: P.O. Box G, Juneau, Alaska 99811. *Director:* Karen R. Crane.—Alaska Historical Library P.O. Box G, Juneau. *Librarian:* Kay Shelton.

ARIZONA

HISTORY. Arizona was settled in 1752, organized as a Territory in 1863 and became a state on 14 Feb. 1912.

AREA AND POPULATION. Arizona is bounded north by Utah, east by New Mexico, south by Mexico, west by California and Nevada. Area, 113,508 sq. miles, including 492 sq. miles of inland water. Of the total area in 1985, 28% was Indian Reservation, 17% was in individual or corporate ownership, 16% was held by the US Bureau of Land Management, 15% by the US Forest Service, 13% by the State and 10% by others. Census population on 1 April 1980 was 2,718,425, an increase of 53·4% over 1970. Estimate (1987) 3,469,000. Births, 1986, 60,575; deaths, 25,035; infant deaths (1983), 509; marriages, 36,025; divorces, 23,062.

Population in 5 census years:

	White	*Black*	*Indian*	*Chinese*	*Japanese*	*Total*	*Per sq. mile*
1910	171,468	2,009	29,201	1,305	371	204,354	1·8
1930	378,551	10,749	43,726	1,110	879	435,573	3·8
1960	1,169,517	43,403	83,387	2,937	1,501	1,302,161	11·3
				All others			
1970	1,604,498	53,344		117,557		1,775,399	15·6
1980	2,260,288	74,159		383,768		2,718,215 [1]	23·9

[1] Preliminary.

Of the population in 1980, 1,375,214 were male, 2,278,728 were urban and 1,872,447 were aged 20 and over.

The 1980 census population of Phoenix was 789,704 (1986 estimate, 881,640); Tucson, 330,537 (384,385); Scottsdale, 88,412 (108,447); Tempe, 106,743 (132,942); Mesa, 152,453 (239,587); Glendale, 97,172 (122,392).

CLIMATE. Phoenix. Jan. 52°F (11·1°C), July 90°F (32·2°C). Annual rainfall 8" (191 mm). Yuma. Jan. 55°F (12·8°C), July 91°F (32·8°C). Annual rainfall 3" (75 mm). *See* Mountain States, p. 1381.

CONSTITUTION AND GOVERNMENT. The state constitution (1910, with 103 amendments) placed the government under direct control of the people through the Initiative, Referendum and the Recall. The state Senate consists of 30 members, and the House of Representatives of 60, all elected for 2 years. Arizona sends to Congress 2 senators and 5 representatives. In the 1988 presidential election Bush polled 694,379 votes, Dukakis, 447,272.

The state capital is Phoenix. The state is divided into 15 counties.

Governor: J. Fife Symington (R.), 1991–95 ($75,000).

BUDGET. General revenues, year ending 30 June 1987 (US Census Bureau figures), were $2,422m. (taxation, $2,431m.); general expenditures, $2,384m. (education, $1,484m.; transport $15·8m., and public health and welfare, $458·6m.).

Per capita income (1986) was $13,090.

NATURAL RESOURCES

Minerals. The mining industries of the state are important, but less so than agriculture and manufacturing. By value the most important mineral produced is copper. Production (1986) 874,715 short tons; gold and silver are both largely recovered from copper ore. Other minerals include sand and gravel and lead. Total value of minerals mined in 1986 was $1,566·3m.

Agriculture. Arizona, despite its dry climate, is well suited for agriculture along the water-courses and where irrigation is practised on a large scale from great reservoirs constructed by the US as well as by the state government and private interests. Irrigated area, 1984, 1·07m. acres. The wide pasture lands are favourable for the rearing of cattle and sheep, but numbers are either stationary or declining compared with 1920.

In 1987 Arizona contained 8,400 farms and ranches with 852,866 acres of crop land, out of a total farm and pastoral area of 38m. acres. The average farm was estimated at 4,405 acres. Farming is highly commercialized and mechanized and concentrated largely on cotton picked by machines and by Indian, Mexican and migratory workers.

Area under cotton (1986), 322,800 acres; 823,000m. bales (of 480 lb.) of cotton were harvested.

Cash income, 1986, from crops, $838m.; from livestock, $714m. Most important cereals are wheat, corn and barley; other crops include oranges, grapefruit and lettuce. On 1 Jan. 1985 there were 1,050,000 all cattle, 82,000 milch cows, 306,000 sheep.

Forestry. The national forests in the state had an area (1983) of 11·22m. acres.

INDUSTRY. In 1986 there were 3,747 manufacturing establishments with 172,047 production workers, earning $1,947m.

TOURISM. In 1982 15·7m. tourists visited Arizona; direct employment, 71,700; indirect, 114,600; state tax revenue, $204m.

COMMUNICATIONS

Roads. In 1990 there were 57,389 miles of public roads and streets and 2,775,270 motor vehicles were registered.

Aviation. Airports, 1984, numbered 251, of which 82 were for public use; 6,079 aircraft were registered.

JUSTICE, RELIGION, EDUCATION AND WELFARE

Justice. A 'right-to-work' amendment to the constitution, adopted 5 Nov. 1946, makes illegal any concessions to trade-union demands for a 'closed shop'.

The Arizona state and federal prisons 31 Dec. 1985 held 8,518. There have been no executions since 1963; from 1930 to 1963 there were 38 executions (lethal gas) all for murder, and all men (28 whites, 10 Negro).

Religion. The leading religious bodies are Roman Catholics and Mormons (Latter Day Saints); others include Methodists, Presbyterians, Baptists and Episcopalians.

Education. School attendance is compulsory to grade 9 (from 1985–86) and to grade 10 (from 1986–87). In autumn 1986 there were 532,694 pupils enrolled in grades K-12. In 1986 spending on public schools was $1,589m. or $499 per capita. The state maintains 3 universities: the University of Arizona (Tucson) with an enrolment of 30,437 in autumn 1986; Arizona State University (Tempe) with 40,735; Northern Arizona University (Flagstaff) with 13,354.

Health. In 1985 there were 88 hospitals reported by the State Department of Health; capacity 13,890 beds; the hospitals had 1,522 physicians and dentists, 8,437 registered nurses and 1,503 licensed practical nurses.

Social Security. Old-age assistance (maximum depending on the programme) is given, with federal aid, to needy citizens 65 years of age or older. In June 1985, federal Social Security Insurance payments went to 10,500 aged ($158 each), and 22,000 disabled ($251); 71,900 people in 25,200 families received aid for families with dependent children.

Further Reading

Arizona Statistical Review. 42nd ed. Valley National Bank, Phoenix, 1986
Comeaux, M. L., *Arizona: a Geography*. Boulder, 1981
Faulk, O. B., *Arizona: A Short History*. Univ. Oklahoma Press, 1970
Goff, J. S., *Arizona Civilization*. 2nd ed. Cave Creek, 1970
Mason, B. B. and Hink, H., *Constitutional Government of Arizona*. 7th ed.Tempe, 1982

State Library: Department of Library, Archives and Public Records, Capitol, Phoenix 85007. *Director:* Sharon G. Turgeon.

ARKANSAS

HISTORY. Arkansas was settled in 1686, made a territory in 1819 and admitted into the Union on 15 June 1836. The name originated with the Quapaw Indian tribe. The constitution, which dates from 1874, has been amended 59 times.

AREA AND POPULATION. Arkansas is bounded north by Missouri, east by Tennessee and Mississippi, south by Louisiana, south-west by Texas and west by Oklahoma. Area, 53,187 sq. miles (1,109 sq. miles being inland water). Census population on 1 April 1980 was 2,286,435, an increase of 18·9% from that of 1970. Estimate (1988) 2,395,000. Births, 1988, were 35,017 (14·6 per 1,000 population); deaths, 24,883 (10·4); infant deaths, 375 (10·7 per 1,000 live births); marriages, 34,935 (14·6); divorces 16,747 (7).

Population in 5 census years was:

	White	*Black*	*Indian*	*Asiatic*	*Total*	*Per sq. mile*
1910	1,131,026	442,891	460	72	1,574,449	30·0
1930	1,375,315	478,463	408	296	1,854,482	35·2
1960	1,395,703	388,787	580	1,202	1,786,272	34·0
			All others			
1970	1,565,915	352,445	4,935		1,923,295	37·0
1980	1,890,332	373,768	22,335		2,286,435	43·9

Of the total population in 1980, 48·3% were male, 51·6% were urban, 60·2% were 21 years of age or older.

Little Rock (capital) had a population of 158,461 in 1980; Fort Smith, 71,626; North Little Rock, 64,288; Pine Bluff, 56,636; Fayetteville, 36,608; Hot Springs, 35,781; Jonesboro, 31,530; West Memphis, 28,138. The population of the largest standard metropolitan statistical areas: Little Rock–North Little Rock, 393,774; Fayetteville–Springdale, 178,609; Fort Smith (Arkansas portion), 132,064; Pine Bluff, 90,718; Memphis (Arkansas portion), 49,499; Texarkana (Arkansas portion), 37,766.

CLIMATE. Little Rock. Jan. 42°F (5·6°C), July 81°F (27·2°C). Annual rainfall 49" (1,222 mm). *See* Gulf Coast, p. 1382.

GOVERNMENT. The General Assembly consists of a Senate of 35 members elected for 4 years, partially renewed every 2 years, and a House of Representatives of 100 members elected for 2 years. The sessions are biennial and usually limited to 60 days. The Governor and Lieut.-Governor are elected for 4 years. The state is represented in Congress by 2 senators and 4 representatives.

In the 1988 presidential election Bush polled 463,754 votes, Dukakis, 344,991.

The state is divided into 75 counties; the capital is Little Rock.

Governor: Bill Clinton (D.), 1991–95 ($35,000).

FINANCE

Budget. The state and local government revenue for the fiscal year 1988 was $5,585m., of which taxation furnished $2,665m. and federal aid, $1,028m. General expenditure was $5,236m., of which education took $1,959m.; highways, $484m., and public welfare, $559m.

Long-term debt (state and local governments) for the financial year 1988 was $4,327m.

Per capita income (1989) was $12,901.

Banking. In 1989 total bank deposits were $16,434·7m.

ENERGY AND NATURAL RESOURCES

Minerals. In 1988 crude petroleum amounted to 13,455,729 bbls; natural gas, 146,894,144m. cu. ft; the state is an important source of bauxite, bromine, clays, construction, sand, gravel and crushed stone. It is one of four states producing tripoli and vanadium and one of two shipping gallium. In 1980 non-fuel mineral production was $307m.

Agriculture. In 1989 47,000 farms had a total area of 15m. acres; average farm was 319 acres; 7·6m. acres were harvested cropland; 2,406,338 acres were irrigated.

In 1989, Arkansas ranked first in the production of broilers (920·5m. birds, value $1·500m.) and rice (41·3% of US total production, with a yield of 5,600 lb per acre), fourth in turkeys (19·8m. birds) and sixth in eggs (3,400m. eggs, value $237·4m.). 851,000 bales of cotton were harvested and soybean production yielded 76·8m. bu. in 1989. Dairy farmers received $112·3m. for the sale of milk in 1989.

Livestock in Jan. 1989 included 1·75m. all cattle and calves, total value was $437·6m.

INDUSTRY. In Aug. 1990 total employment averaged 1,060,500 (51,700 agricultural, 234,700 manufacturing, 215,200 wholesale and retail trade, 147,800 government). The Arkansas Department of Labor estimated that 192,000 factory production workers earned an average $353.08 per week (41·2 hours). In the manufacturing group, food and kindred products employed 49,000, electric and electronic equipment, 21,700 and lumber and wood products, 21,100.

COMMUNICATIONS

Roads. Total road mileage, 82,789 miles. State-maintained highways (1989) total 16,179 miles; local county highways, 49,548 miles; city streets, 9,744 miles; federal roads, 1,654 miles; roads not publicly maintained, 5,664 miles. In 1989 there were 1,653,032 registered motor vehicles.

Railways. In 1989 there were in the state 3,169 miles of commercial railway.

Aviation. Six air carrier and 2 commuter airlines serve the state; there were, in 1990, 167 airports (92 public-use and 75 private).

Waterways. There are about 1,000 miles of navigable streams, including the Mississippi, Arkansas, Red, White and Ouachita Rivers. The Arkansas River/Kerr-McClellan Channel flows diagonally eastward across the state and gives access to the sea *via* the Mississippi River.

RELIGION, EDUCATION AND WELFARE

Religion. Main protestant churches in 1980: Baptist (603,844), Methodist (214,925), Church of Christ (90,671), Assembly of God (53,555). Roman Catholics (1980), 56,911.

Education. In the school year 1988–89 public elementary and secondary schools had 458,538 enrolled pupils and about 22,365 classroom teachers. Average salaries of teachers in elementary schools was $20,719, secondary $22,152. In 1987–88 expenditure on elementary and secondary education was $1,335m.

An educational TV network provides a full 12-hour-day telecasting; it has 5 stations (1990).

Higher education is provided at 33 institutions: 10 state universities, 1 medical college, 12 private or church colleges, 11 community or junior colleges. Total enrolment in institutions of higher education in 1989, was 82,823.

There were (1988–89) 24 vocational-technical schools with 48,085 students, including extension class students. Total expenditure (1987–88), $32·5m.

Health. There were 102 licensed hospitals (12,732 beds) in 1990, and 255 licensed nursing homes (23,894 beds).

Social Welfare. In 1988 457,320 persons drew social security payments; 258,700 were retired workers; 43,620 were disabled workers; 67,470 were widows and widowers; 43,620 were wives and husbands. In Dec. 1988 monthly payments were $193m., $134m. to retired workers and their dependants, $36m. to survivors, and $34m. to disabled workers and their dependants.

State prisons in June 1990 had 6,455 inmates.

Further Reading

Current Employment Developments. Arkansas Department of Labor, Little Rock, 1990
Arkansas State and County Economic Data. Regional Economic Analysis, Univ. Arkansas, Little Rock, 1989
Arkansas Vital Statistics. Arkansas Department of Health, Little Rock, 1990
Governmental Finances. U.S. Dept. of Commerce, Bureau of the Census, 1987–88
Agricultural Statistics for Arkansas. U.S. Dept. of Agriculture, Crop Reporting Service, Little Rock, 1988
Statistical Summary for the Public Schools of Arkansas. Dept. of Education, Little Rock, 1987-89
Ferguson and Atkinson, *Historic Arkansas*. Little Rock, 1966

CALIFORNIA

HISTORY. California, first settled in July 1769, was from its discovery until 1846 politically associated with Mexico. On 7 July 1846 the American flag was hoisted at Monterey, and a proclamation was issued declaring California to be a portion of the US. On 2 Feb. 1848, by the treaty of Guadalupe–Hidalgo, the territory was formally ceded by Mexico to the US, and was admitted to the Union 9 Sept. 1850 as the thirty-first state, with boundaries as at present.

AREA AND POPULATION. Area, 158,693 sq. miles (2,120 sq. miles being inland water). In 1985 the federal government owned 48m. acres (48% of the land area); in 1984, 570,000 acres were under jurisdiction of the Bureau of Indian Affairs, of which 501,000 acres were tribal. Public lands, vacant in 1975, totalled 15,607,125 acres, practically all either mountains or deserts.

Census population, 1 April 1980, 23,667,902, an increase of 18·5% over 1970, making California the most populous state of the USA (New York: 17,557,288). Estimate (1989) 29,063,200. Births in 1988, 532,708 (18·8 per 1,000 population); deaths, 215,185 (7·6); infant deaths, 4,559 (8·6 per 1,000 live births); marriages (1989), 234,120 (8·1); divorces, 124,889 in 1989 (4·3).

Population in 5 census years was:

	White	*Black*	*Japanese*	*Chinese*	*Total (incl. all others)*	*Per sq. mile*
1910	2,259,672	21,645	41,356	36,248	2,377,549	15·0
1930	5,408,260	81,048	97,456	37,361	5,677,251	35·8
1960	14,455,230	883,861	157,317	95,600	15,717,204	99·0
1970	17,761,032	1,400,143	213,280	170,131	19,953,134	125·7
			All others			
1980	18,030,893	1,819,281	3,817,728		23,667,902	149·1

Of the 1980 population 49·3% were male, 91·3% were urban and 67·2% were 21 years old or older.

The largest cities with 1980 census population are:

Los Angeles	2,966,850	Anaheim	219,494	Fremont	131,945
San Diego	875,538	Fresno	217,289	Torrance	129,881
San Francisco	678,974	Santa Ana	204,023	Garden Grove	123,307
San José	629,546	Riverside	170,591	San Bernardino	118,794
Long Beach	361,334	Huntington Beach	170,505	Pasadena	118,550
Oakland	339,337	Stockton	149,779	Oxnard	108,195
Sacramento	275,741	Glendale	139,060		

Urbanized areas (1980 census): Los Angeles–Long Beach, 9,477,926; San Francisco–Oakland, 3,191,913; San Diego, 1,704,352; San José, 1,243,900; Sacramento, 796,266; San Bernardino–Riverside, 703,316; Oxnard–Ventura–Thousand Oaks, 378,420; Fresno, 331,551.

CLIMATE. Los Angeles. Jan. 55°F (12·8°C), July 70°F (21·1°C). Annual rainfall 15" (381 mm). Sacramento. Jan. 45°F (7·2°C), July 74°F (23·3°C). Annual rainfall 19" (472 mm). San Diego. Jan. 55°F (12·8°C), July 69°F (20·6°C). Annual rainfall 10" (259 mm). San Francisco. Jan. 50°F (10°C), July 59°F (15°C). Annual rainfall 22" (561 mm). Death Valley. Jan. 52°F (11°C), July 100°F (38°C). Annual rainfall 1·6" (40 mm). *See* Pacific Coast, p. 1381.

CONSTITUTION AND GOVERNMENT. The present constitution became effective from 4 July 1879; it has had numerous amendments since 1962. The Senate is composed of 40 members elected for 4 years—half being elected each 2 years—and the Assembly, of 80 members, elected for 2 years. Two-year regular sessions convene in Dec. of each even-numbered year. The Governor and Lieut.-Governor are elected for 4 years.

California is represented in Congress by 2 senators and 45 representatives.

In the 1988 presidential election Bush polled 5,054,917 votes, Dukakis, 4,702,233.

The capital is Sacramento. The state is divided into 58 counties.

Governor: Pete Wilson (R.), 1991–95 ($85,000).

ECONOMY

Budget. For the year ending 30 June 1989 total General Fund revenues were $36,782m.; total General Fund expenditures were $35,897m. ($19,260m. for education, $11,312m. for health and welfare).

The long-term state debt (general obligation bonds outstanding) was $10,232m. on 30 June 1990.

Per capita personal income (1989) was $19,929.

Banking. In 1988 there were more than 440 banks, of which 18 were foreign-owned, 11 out-of-state and 400 independent. Total loans, 1989 (preliminary), $223,812m., of which real estate loans were almost $105,000m. In Dec. 1989 (preliminary) all insured commercial banks had demand deposits of $62,446m. and time and savings deposits of $168,821m. Savings and loan associations had savings capital of $255,000m. at 31 Dec. 1989 (preliminary).

ENERGY AND NATURAL RESOURCES

Electricity. In 1987 hydro-power produced 21%, gas 33% coal and nuclear power 18% each, and oil, geothermal, biomass, wind, solar and other sources 8% of electricity needs.

Minerals. Crude oil output was estimated at 331m. bbls in 1989. Proved reserves were an estimated 4,900m. bbls in 1989. Output of natural gas was 336,015·1m. cu. ft; of natural gas liquids from wells, 102,883 bbls in 1989. Gold output was 27,705 K (1989 preliminary); asbestos, boron minerals, diatomite, tungsten, sand and gravel, salt, magnesium compounds, clays, cement, copper, silver, gypsum, calcium chloride, wollastonite and iron ore are also produced. The value of all the minerals produced was $2,839m. in 1989 (preliminary). Mining employed 40,300 in 1989.

Agriculture. Extending 700 miles from north to south, and intersected by several ranges of mountains, California has almost every variety of climate, from the very wet to the very dry, and from the temperate to the semi-tropical.

In 1987 there were 83,217 farms, comprising 31m. acres; average farm, 368 acres. Cotton, fruit, livestock and vegetables are important. Cash receipts, 1988, from crops, $11,894m.; from livestock and poultry, $4,704m. Dairy produce, cattle, horticultural products, grapes, and cotton lint (in that order) are the main sources of farm income.

Production of cotton lint, 1989, was 645,100 short tons; other field crops included (in 1m. short tons): Sugar-beet, 5·0; hay and alfalfa, 8·5; rice, 1·6; wheat, 1·6. Principal crops 1989 (in 1,000 short tons): Wine, table and raisin grapes, 5,400; lettuces, 2,900; tomatoes, 9,100; almonds, 245: in 1987, peaches, 734; pears, 337; apricots, 110; prunes, 228; plums, nectarines, avocados, olives and almonds. Citrus fruit crops 1989, were (in 1,000 short tons): Oranges, 2,200; lemons, 615·6; grapefruit, 279·5.

On 1 Jan. 1988 the farm animals were: 1·1m. milch cows, 4·9m. all cattle, 775,000 sheep and 140,000 swine.

Forestry. There were (1989) 16·3m. acres of productive forest land, from which about 4,000m. bd ft are harvested annually. Lumber production, 1989, 5,300m. bd ft.

Fisheries. The catch in 1989 was 484·6m. lb.; leading species were mackerel, tuna and sea urchin.

INDUSTRY. In 1989, manufacturing employed 2,162,400. The fastest-growing industries were petroleum products, clothing, stone, clay and glass products. The aerospace industry is important, as is food-processing. In 1989 the civilian labour force was 14,518,000, of whom 13,780,000 were employed.

Tourism. In 1988 there were 116m. tourists, 32% from other states and 6% from abroad.

COMMUNICATIONS

Roads. In 1989 California had 60,688 miles of roads inside cities and 103,610 miles outside. In 1989 there were about 16·6m. registered cars and about 5·2m. commercial vehicles.

Railways. Total mileage of railways in 1986, was 8,044 miles. There are 2 systems: Amtrak and Southern Pacific Railroad commuter trains. Amtrak carries about 1·7m. passengers per year on the intra-state routes. Southern Pacific carries about 5·4m. on a commuter route. Amtrak services run from San Francisco and Los Angeles. Southern Pacific runs the Caltrains commuter route from San Francisco to San José. There is a metro (BART) and light rail (Muni) system in San Francisco. There is a light rail line in San Diego and Sacramento and another under construction in San José.

Aviation. In 1986 there were 283 public airports and 739 private airstrips.

Shipping. The chief ports are San Francisco and Los Angeles.

JUSTICE, RELIGION, EDUCATION AND WELFARE

Justice. State prisons, 1 Jan. 1990, had 81,297 male and 6,000 female inmates. From 1893 to 1942, 307 inmates were executed by hanging. From 1938 to 1976, 194 inmates were executed by lethal gas. No further death sentences were passed until 1980.

Religion. The Roman Catholic Church is much stronger than any other single church; next are the Jewish congregations, then Methodists, Presbyterians, Baptists and Episcopalians.

Education. Full-time attendance at school is compulsory for children from 6 to 16 years of age for a minimum of 175 days per annum, and part-time attendance is required from 16 to 18 years. In autumn 1989 there were 5·3m. pupils enrolled in both public and private elementary and secondary schools. Total state expenditure on public education, 1988–89, was $19,323m.

Community Colleges had 1,382,944 students in autumn 1989.

California has two publicly supported higher education systems: The University of California (1868) and the California State University and Colleges. In autumn 1989, the University of California with campuses for resident instruction and research at Berkeley, Los Angeles, San Francisco and 6 other centres, had 164,605 students. California State University and Colleges with campuses at Sacramento, Long Beach, Los Angeles, San Francisco and 15 other cities had 360,838 students. In addition to the 28 publicly supported institutions for higher education there are 117 private colleges and universities which had a total estimated enrolment of 151,844 in the autumn of 1987.

Health. In 1990 there were 502 general hospitals; capacity, 105,938 beds. On 30 June 1990 state hospitals for the mentally disabled had 4,913 patients.

Social Security. On 1 Jan. 1974 the federal government (Social Security Administration) assumed responsibility for the Supplemental Security Income/State Supplemental Program which replaced the State Old-Age Security. The SSI/SSP provides financial assistance for needy aged (65 years or older), blind or disabled persons. An individual recipient may own assets up to $2,000; a couple up to $3,000, subject to specific exclusions. There are federal, state and county programmes assisting the aged, the blind, the disabled and needy children. In 1989 5,634 families per month were receiving an average of $400 per family in General Relief.

Further Reading

California Almanac, 1984–85. Fay, J. S., (ed.) Oxford, 1984
California Government and Politics. Hoeber, T. R., et al, (eds.) Sacramento, Annual
California Handbook. California Institute, 1981
California Statistical Abstract. 31st ed. Dept. of Finance, Sacramento, 1990
Economic Report of the Governor. Dept. of Finance, Sacramento, Annual
Lavender, D. S., *California.* New York, 1976

State Library: The California State Library, Library-Courts Bldg, Sacramento 95814.

COLORADO

HISTORY. Colorado was first settled in 1858, made a Territory in 1861 and admitted into the Union on 1 Aug. 1876.

AREA AND POPULATION. Colorado is bounded north by Wyoming, north-east by Nebraska, east by Kansas, south-east by Oklahoma, south by New Mexico and west by Utah. Area, 104,090 sq. miles (496 sq. miles being inland water). Federal lands, 1974, 23,974,000 acres (36% of the land area).

Census population, 1 April 1980, was 2,889,964, an increase of 680,368 or 30·8% since 1970. Estimated (1989), 3,317,000. Births, 1989, were 52,874 (15·9 per 1,000 population); deaths, 21,481 (6·5); infant deaths (1988), 505 (9·5 per 1,000 live births); marriages (1988), 31,350 (9·3); dissolutions (1988), 18,660 (5·6).

Population in 5 census years was:

	White	*Black*	*Indian*	*Asiatic*	*Total*	*Per sq. mile*
1910	783,415	11,453	1,482	2,674	799,024	7·7
1930	1,018,793	11,828	1,395	3,775	1,035,791	10·0
1950	1,296,653	20,177	1,567	5,870	1,325,089	12·7
1970	2,112,352	66,411	8,836	10,388	2,207,259	21·3
			All others			
1980	2,571,498	101,703	216,763		2,889,964	27·7

Of the total population in 1980, 49·6% were male, 80·6% were urban; 68% were aged 20 years or older. Large cities with 1980 census population (and 1989 estimate): Denver, 492,365 (498,234); Colorado Springs, 215,150 (282,528); Aurora, 158,588 (216,353); Lakewood, 112,860 (120,479); Pueblo, 101,686 (105,501); Arvada, 84,576 (91,511); Boulder, 76,685 (82,981); Fort Collins, 65,092 (83,555); Wheat Ridge, 30,293 (28,821); Greeley, 53,006 (62,288); Westminster, 50,211 (67,620).

Main metropolitan areas (1989): Denver–Boulder, 1,850,813; Fort Collins, 182,979; Colorado Springs, 397,250; Greeley, 143,436; Pueblo, 132,947; Front Range Urban Area, 2,707,425.

CLIMATE. Denver. Jan. 31°F (–0·6°C), July 73°F (22·8°C). Annual rainfall 14" (358 mm). Pueblo. Jan. 30°F (–1·1°C), July 83°F (28·3°C). Annual rainfall 12" (312 mm). *See* Mountain States, p. 1381.

CONSTITUTION AND GOVERNMENT. The constitution adopted in 1876 is still in effect with (1989) 115 amendments. The General Assembly consists of a Senate of 35 members elected for 4 years, one-half retiring every 2 years, and of a House of Representatives of 65 members elected for 2 years. Sessions are annual, beginning 1951. The Governor, Lieut.-Governor, Attorney-General, Secretary of State and Treasurer are elected for 4 years. Qualified as electors are all citizens, male and female (except convicted, incarcerated criminals), 18 years of age, who have resided in the state and the precinct for 32 days immediately preceding the election. The state is divided into 63 counties. The state sends to Congress 2 senators and 6 representatives.

In the 1988 presidential election Bush polled 727,633 votes, Dukakis, 621,093.

The capital is Denver.

Governor: Roy Romer (D.), 1991–95 ($60,000).

BUDGET. The state's total budget, 1990–91, is $5,237m., of which taxation furnishes $2,675m. and federal grants $1,180m. Education takes $2,265m.; health, welfare and rehabilitation, $1,538m., and highways, $438m. Total state and local taxes *per capita* (1985) were $2,167.

The state has no general obligation debt. The net long-term debt (in revenue bond) on 30 June 1985 was $139m.

Per capita personal income (1989) was $17,494.

ENERGY AND NATURAL RESOURCES

Minerals. Colorado has a variety of mineral resources. Among the most important are crude oil, metals and coal. Total value of mineral production in 1989, $1,859m. In 1989, 19,800 people were employed in mining: 12,400 in extracting oil and natural gas; 3,400 in metals; 3,000 in coal and 1,000 other.

Agriculture. In 1989 farms numbered 27,000, with a total area of 33·5m. acres. 5·7m. acres were harvested crop land; average farm (1989), 1,241 acres. Cash income, 1988, from crops $1,037m.; from livestock, $2,655m. In 1989 there were 1·5m. acres under irrigation.

Production of principal crops in 1989: Corn for grain, 134·8m. bu. (from 0·93m. acres); wheat for grain, 62·1m. bu. (2·27m.); barley for grain, 12·2m. bu. (0·16m.); hay, 3·45m. tons (1·5m.); dry beans, 3·11m. cwt (0·18m.); oats and sorghum, 14·4m. bushels (0·38m.); vegetables, 375,000 tons (0·02m.).

In 1987 the number of farm animals was: 76,285 milch cows, 2,946,334 all cattle, 708,070 sheep, 258,725 swine. The wool clip in 1987 yielded 3·9m. lb. of wool.

INDUSTRY. In 1989 1,502,100 were employed in non-agricultural sectors, of which 371,700 were in trade; 401,000 in services; 259,900 in government; 195,900 in manufacturing; 62,800 in construction; 93,800 in transport and public utilities; 19,800 in mining; 97,200 in finance, insurance and property. In manufacturing the biggest employers were non-electrical machinery, foods and kindred products, and printing.

TOURISM. In 1985 about 20m. people spent holidays in Colorado, of whom about 3% were Colorado residents. Overall expenditure, $4,500m.

COMMUNICATIONS

Roads. In 1990 there were 77,361 miles of road and 3,153,838 registered motor vehicles.

Railways. In 1982 there were in the state 4,500 miles of main-track and branch railway.

Aviation. There were (1984) 233 airports in the state. Of these, 68 are publicly owned and open to the public; 16 are privately owned and open to the public; 149 are private and not open to the public.

JUSTICE, RELIGION, EDUCATION AND WELFARE

Justice. At 30 Sept. 1989 there were 7,570 people committed to the State Department of Corrections, inmates of the State Penitentiary, the State Reformatory and other institutions. In 1967 there was 1 execution; since 1930 executions (by lethal gas) numbered 47, including 41 whites, 5 Negroes and 1 other; all were for murder.

Colorado has a Civil Rights Act (1935) forbidding places of public accommodation to discriminate against any persons on the grounds of race, religion, sex, colour or nationality. No religious test may be applied to teachers or students in the public schools, 'nor shall any distinction or classification of pupils be made on account of race or colour'. In 1957 the General Assembly prohibited discrimination in employment of persons in private industry and in 1959 adopted the Fair Housing Act to discourage discrimination in housing. A 1957 Act permits marriages between white persons and Negroes or mulattoes.

Religion. In 1984 the Roman Catholic Church had 550,300 members; the ten main Protestant denominations had 350,900 members; the Jewish community had 45,000 members. Buddhism is among other religions represented.

Education. In autumn 1989 the public elementary and secondary schools had 562,755 pupils and 31,954 teachers; teachers' salaries averaged $30,758. Enrolments in state universities, Sept. 1988, were: University of Colorado (Boulder), 24,057 students; University of Colorado (Denver), 10,048; University of Colorado

(Colorado Springs), 5,583; Colorado State University (Fort Collins), 19,386; Colorado School of Mines (Golden), 2,319; University of Northern Colorado (Greeley), 9,167; University of Southern Colorado (Pueblo), 3,971; Western State College (Gunnison), 2,434; Adams State College (Alamosa), 2,487; Metropolitan State College (Denver), 15,638; Fort Lewis College (Durango), 3,843; Mesa College (Grand Junction), 4,006.

Health. Approved hospitals, 1983, numbered 98. In 1983, there were 25 public mental health centres and clinics.

Social Security. A constitutional amendment, adopted 1956, provides for minimum old age pensions of $100 per month, which may be raised on a cost-of-living basis; for a $5m. stabilization fund and for a $10m. medical and health fund for pensioners. In 1984 the maximum monthly retirement pension (for citizens of 65 and older) was $703; maximum monthly benefit for a disabled worker, $854.

Further Reading

Directory of Colorado Manufacturers, 1986. Business Research Division, School of Business, Univ. of Colorado, Boulder, 1987

State of Colorado Business Development Manual. Office of Business Development, Denver, 1986

Economic Outlook Forum, 1986. Colorado Division of Commerce and Development, and the College of Business, Univ. of Colorado, Denver, 1987

Griffiths, M. and Rubright, L., *Colorado: a Geography.* Boulder, 1983

Sprague, M., *Colorado: A History.* New York, 1976

State Library: Colorado State Library, State Capitol, Denver, 80203.

CONNECTICUT

HISTORY. Connecticut was first settled in 1634 and has been an organized commonwealth since 1637. In 1629 a written constitution was adopted which, it is claimed, was the first in the history of the world formed under the concept of a social compact. This constitution was confirmed by a charter from Charles II in 1662, and replaced in 1818 by a state constitution, framed that year by a constitutional convention.

AREA AND POPULATION. Connecticut is bounded north by Massachusetts, east by Rhode Island, south by the Atlantic and west by New York. Area, 5,018 sq. miles (147 sq. miles being inland water).

Census population, 1 April 1980, 3,107,576, an increase of 2·5% since 1970. Estimate (1987) 3,277,980. Births (1987) were 46,941 (14·3 per 1,000 population); deaths, 28,249 (8·6); infant deaths, 410 (8·7 per 1,000 live births); marriages, 27,106 (16·5); divorces, 12,052 (7·4).

Population in 5 census years was:

	White	*Black*	*Indian*	*Asiatic*	*Total*	*Per sq. mile*
1910	1,098,897	15,174	152	533	1,114,756	231·3
1930	1,576,700	29,354	162	687	1,606,903	328·0
1960	2,423,816	107,449	923	3,046	2,535,234	517·5
			All others			
1970	2,835,458	181,177	15,074		3,031,709	629·0
1980	2,799,420	217,433	4,533	18,970	3,107,576	634·3

Of the total population in 1980, 1,498,005 persons were male, 2,449,774 persons were urban. Those 19 years old or older numbered 2,228,805.

The chief cities and towns are (1989 government figures):

Bridgeport	141,986	New Britain	75,740
Hartford	133,060	West Hartford	61,700
New Haven	128,360	Danbury	70,690
Waterbury	111,630	Greenwich	60,750
Stamford	109,910	Bristol	63,600
Norwalk	81,770	Meriden	61,520

Larger urbanized areas, 1980 census: Hartford, 726,114; Bridgeport, 395,455; New Haven, 417,592; Waterbury, 228,178; Stamford, 198,854.

CLIMATE. New Haven: Jan. 28°F (–2·2°C), July 72°F (22·2°C). Annual rainfall 46" (1,151 mm). *See* New England, p. 1382.

CONSTITUTION AND GOVERNMENT. The 1818 Constitution was revised in June 1953 effective 1 Jan. 1955. On 30 Dec. 1965 a new constitution went into effect, having been framed by a constitutional convention in the summer of 1965 and approved by the voters in Dec. 1965.

The 1965 Constitution provides for 30 to 50 members of the Senate (instead of 24 to 36) and for 125 to 225 members of the House of Representatives, to be elected from assembly districts, rather than 2 or 1 from each town, as in the former constitution. The convention has added a new provision for a 3-day session following each regular or special session, solely to reconsider bills vetoed by the Governor.

The General Assembly consists of a Senate of 36 members and a House of Representatives of 151 members. Members of each House are elected for the term of 2 years (annual salary $16,760, plus mileage and expenses; $4,500 if State Senator, and $3,500 if State Representative). Legislative sessions are annual. The Governor and Lieut.Governor are elected for 4 years. All citizens (with necessary exceptions and the usual residential requirements) have the right of suffrage.

Connecticut is one of the original 13 states of the Union. The state is represented in Congress by 2 senators and 6 representatives.

In the 1988 presidential election Bush polled 747,082 votes, Dukakis, 674,873. The state capital is Hartford.

Governor: Lowell P. Weicker (ind.), 1991–95 ($78,000).

BUDGET. For the year ending 30 June 1989 (state government figures) general revenues were $5,511m. (taxation, $4,327m., and federal aid, $686m.); general expenditures were $6,372m. (education, $1,655m., transportation, $573m., and public welfare, $1,403m.).

The total operating deficit on 30 June 1989 was $259m.

Per capita income, 1989, was $23,866.

NATURAL RESOURCES

Minerals. The state has some mineral resources: crushed stone, sand, gravel, clay, dimension stone, feldspar and quartz; total production in 1988 was valued at $118m.

Agriculture. In 1988 the state had 4,000 farms with a total area of about 440,000 acres; average farm was of 110 acres, valued at $3,208 per acre. Total cash receipts, 1988, were $382m., including $202m. from crops and $180m. from livestock and products (mainly from dairy products and eggs). Principal crops are hay, greenhouse and nursery products, tobacco, potatoes, sweet corn, apples, peaches, berries, vegetables and small fruit.

Livestock (1989): 77,000 all cattle (value $48·1m.), 8,000 sheep ($792,000), 7,000 swine ($540,000) and 6·5m. poultry ($16·9m.).

Forestry. The state had (1989) 139,377 acres of state forest land, which is about 4·3% of the total land area (3.205,760 acres).

INDUSTRY. Total non-agricultural labour force in 1989 was 1,683,400. The main employers are manufacturers (370,830 workers mainly in transport equipment, non-electrical machinery and fabricated metals); trade (385,360 workers); services (413,070) and government (209,110).

COMMUNICATIONS

Roads. The state (1 Jan. 1989) maintains 4,044 miles of highways, all surfaced. Motor vehicles registered at 1 Oct. 1990 numbered 2·6m.

Railways. In 1981 there were 950 miles of railway track.

Aviation. In 1988 there were 61 airports (26 commercial including 6 state-owned, and 67 heliports and 9 seaplane bases).

JUSTICE, RELIGION, EDUCATION AND WELFARE

Justice. In 1990 there were no executions; since 1930 there have been 22 executions (19 by electrocution, 3 by hanging), all for murder. In 1989 there were 8,899 inmates in 19 prison facilities. The total supervised population was 13,236.

The Civil Rights Act makes it a punishable offence to discriminate against any person or persons 'on account of alienage, colour or race' and to hold up to ridicule any persons 'on account of creed, religion, colour, denomination, nationality or race'. Places of public resort are forbidden to discriminate. Insurance companies are forbidden to charge higher premiums to persons 'wholly or partially of African descent'. Schools must be open to all 'without discrimination on account of race or colour'.

Religion. The leading religious denominations (1989) in the state are the Roman Catholic (1,375,557 members), United Churches of Christ (135,000), Protestant Episcopal (79,969), Jewish (108,000), Methodist (37,178), Baptist (38,000), Presbyterian and Greek Orthodox.

Education. Elementary instruction is free for all children between the ages of 4 and 16 years, and compulsory for all children between the ages of 7 and 16 years. In 1989 there were 574 public elementary schools, 304 secondary schools and 54 combined. In 1989 there were 486,326 pupils and 33,994 elementary and secondary teachers. Expenditure of the state on public schools, 1989, $1,308m. Mean salary of teachers in public schools, 1989, $38,131.

Connecticut has 47 colleges, of which one state university, 4 state colleges, 5 technical colleges and 12 regional community colleges are state funded. The University of Connecticut at Storrs, founded 1881, had 1,210 faculty and 25,882 students in 1988. Yale University, New Haven, founded in 1701, had 2,106 faculty and 10,983 students. Wesleyan University, Middletown, founded 1831, had 285 faculty and 3,428 students. Trinity College, Hartford, founded 1823, had 148 faculty and 2,043 students. Connecticut College, New London, founded 1915, had 153 faculty and 1,969 students. The University of Hartford, founded 1877, had 273 faculty and 7,703 students. The regional community colleges (2-year course) had 36,511 students.

Health. Hospitals listed by the American Hospital Association, 1990, numbered 63, with 16,134 beds. The state operated one general hospital, one veterans' hospital (614 patients in Jan. 1989), 7 hospitals for the mentally ill (1,882 patients in Oct. 1988), 2 training schools for the mentally retarded (and 6 regional centres) and a state-aided institution for the blind.

Social Security. Disbursements during the year ending 30 June 1989 amounted to $74·6m. in aid to the aged and disabled, (21,334 persons per month receiving an average of $307·76). In other areas of welfare, there was an average of 37,883 cases for aid to families with dependent children comprising 105,642 recipients.

Further Reading

The Register and Manual of Connecticut. Secretary of State. Hartford. Annual

The Structure of Connecticut's State Government. Connecticut Public Expenditure Council. Hartford, 1973

Adams, V. Q., *Connecticut: The Story of Your State Government.* Chester, 1973

Halliburton, W. J., *The People of Connecticut.* Norwalk, 1985

Roth, David M. (ed.) *Series in Connecticut History.* 5 vols., Chester, 1975

Smith, Allen R., *Connecticut, a Thematic Atlas.* Newington, 1974

Van Dusen, Albert E., *Connecticut.* New York, 1961

State Library: Connecticut State Library, 231 Capitol Avenue, Hartford, 06015. *State Librarian:* Richard G. Akeroyd.

DELAWARE

HISTORY. Delaware, permanently settled in 1638, is one of the original 13 states of the Union, and the first one to ratify the Federal Constitution.

AREA AND POPULATION. Delaware is bounded north by Pennsylvania, north-east by New Jersey, east by Delaware Bay, south and west by Maryland. Area 2,044 sq. miles (112 sq. miles being inland water). Census population, 1 April 1980 was 594,338, an increase of 46,234 or 8·4% since 1970. Estimate (1989), 673,000. Births in 1989, 11,492; deaths, 5,968; infant deaths, 109; marriages, 5,940; divorces, 2,987.

Population in 5 census years was:

	White	*Black*	*Indian*	*Asiatic*	*Total*	*Per sq. mile*
1910	171,102	31,181	5	34	202,322	103·0
1930	205,718	32,602	5	55	238,380	120·5
1960	384,327	60,688	597	410	446,292	224·0
			All others			
1970	466,459	78,276	3,369		548,104	276·5
1980	488,002	96,157	10,179		594,338	290·8

Of the total population in 1980, 48·4% were male, 70·7% were urban and 65·7% were 21 years old or older.

The 1980 census figures show Wilmington with population of 70,195; Newark, 25,247; Dover, 23,507; Elsmere Town, 6,493; Milford City, 5,366; Seaford City, 5,256.

CLIMATE. Wilmington. Jan. 32°F (0°C), July 75°F (23·9°C). Annual rainfall 43" (1,076 mm). *See* Atlantic Coast, p. 1382.

CONSTITUTION AND GOVERNMENT. The present constitution (the fourth) dates from 1897, and has had 51 amendments; it was not ratified by the electorate but promulgated by the Constitutional Convention. The General Assembly consists of a Senate of 21 members elected for 4 years and a House of Representatives of 41 members elected for 2 years. The Governor and Lieut.Governor are elected for 4 years.

With necessary exceptions, all adult citizens, registered as voters, who are *bona fide* residents, and have complied with local residential requirements, have the right to vote.

Delaware is represented in Congress by 2 senators and 1 representative, elected by the voters of the whole state.

In the 1988 presidential election Bush polled 130,581 votes, Dukakis, 99,479.

The state capital is Dover. Delaware is divided into 3 counties.

Governor: Michael N. Castle (R.), 1989–92 ($80,000).
Lieut.-Governor: Dale E. Wolf (R.), ($35,100).
Secretary of State: Michael Harkins (R.) ($73,700) (appointed by the Governor).

FINANCE. For the year ending 30 June 1990 total revenue was $1,438·6m., of which federal grants were $282m. Total expenditure was $1,170·2m.

On 30 June 1990 the total debt was $456·3m.

Per capita income (1989) was $19,116.

ENERGY AND NATURAL RESOURCES

Minerals. The mineral resources of Delaware are not extensive, consisting chiefly of clay products, stone, sand and gravel and magnesium compounds.

Agriculture. Delaware is mainly an industrial state, but 590,000 acres is in farms; 475,000 acres of this is harvested annually. There were 3,000 farms in 1989. The average farm was valued (land and buildings) at $436,000 in 1988. The main product is broilers, accounting for $458·49m. receipts, out of total farm receipts of $705·4m. in 1989.

The chief field crops are corn and soybeans.

INDUSTRY. In 1989 manufacturing establishments employed 72,600 people; main manufactures were chemicals, transport equipment and food.

COMMUNICATIONS

Roads. The state in 1989 maintained 4,796 miles of roads and streets and 1,388 miles of federally-aided highways. There were also 622 miles of municipal maintained streets. Vehicles registered in year ended 30 June 1990, 565,000.

Railways. In 1989 the state had 285 miles of railway.

Aviation. Delaware had 11 airports, all of which were for general use in 1989.

JUSTICE, RELIGION, EDUCATION AND WELFARE

Justice. State prisons, 30 Sept. 1989–30 Sept. 1990, had daily average of 3,546 inmates. The death penalty was illegal from 2 April 1958 to 18 Dec. 1961. Executions since 1930 (by hanging) have totalled 12 (none since 1946).

Religion. Membership, 1979–80: Methodists, 60,489; Roman Catholics, 103,060; Episcopalians, 18,696; Lutherans, 10,000.

Education. The state has free public schools and compulsory school attendance. In Sept. 1989 the elementary and secondary public schools had 97,808 enrolled pupils and 5,982 classroom teachers. Another 22,016 children were enrolled in private and parochial schools. Appropriation for public schools (financial year 1988–89) was about $379·7m. Average salary of classroom teachers (financial year 1988–89), $33,377. The state supports the University of Delaware at Newark (1834) which had 904 full-time faculty members and 20,477 students in Sept. 1989, Delaware State College, Dover (1892), with 147 full-time faculty members and 2,603 students, and the 4 campuses of Delaware Technical and Community College (Wilmington, Stanton, Dover and Georgetown) with 224 full-time faculty members and 9,309 students.

Health. In 1989 there were 7 short-term general hospitals. During financial year 1990 the average daily census in state mental hospitals was 407.

Social Security. In 1974 the federal Supplemental Security Income (SSI) programme lessened state responsibility for the aged, blind and disabled. SSI payments in Delaware (1989), $19·68m. Provisions are also made for the care of dependent children; in 1989 there were 19,114 recipients in 7,434 families (average monthly payment per family, $278). The total state programme for the year ending 30 June 1989 was $24,826,000 for the care of dependent children.

Further Reading

Information: Division of Historical and Cultural Affairs, Hall of Records, Dover.
Delaware Data Book. Delaware Development Office. Dover, 1990
State Manual, Containing Official List of Officers, Commissions and County Officers. Secretary of State, Dover. Annual
Hoffecker, C. E., *Delaware: a Bicentennial History.* New York, 1977
Smeal, L., *Delaware Historical and Biographical Index.* New York, 1984
Weslager, C. A., *Delaware Indians, a History.* Rutgers Univ. Press, 1972
Topical History of Delaware. Division of Historical and Cultural Affairs. Dover, 1977

DISTRICT OF COLUMBIA

HISTORY. The District of Columbia, organized in 1790, is the seat of the Government of the US, for which the land was ceded by the states of Maryland and Virginia to the US as a site for the national capital. It was established under Acts of Congress in 1790 and 1791. Congress first met in it in 1800 and federal authority over it became vested in 1801. In 1846 the land ceded by Virginia (about 33 sq. miles) was given back.

AREA AND POPULATION. The District forms an enclave on the Potomac River, where the river forms the south-west boundary of Maryland. The area of the District of Columbia is 68·68 sq. miles, 6 sq. miles being inland water.

Census population, 1 April 1980, was 638,333, a decrease of 16% from that of 1970. Estimate (1983) 623,000. Metropolitan statistical area of Washington, D.C.–Md–Va. (1980), 3m. Density of population in the District, 1980, 10,453 per sq. mile. Births, 1984, in the District were 19,123 (30·7 per 1,000 population); resident deaths, 8,302 (13·3); infant deaths, 393 (20·6 per 1,000 live births); marriages, 5,488 (8·8); divorces, 2,874 (4·6).

Population in 5 census years was:

	White	*Black*	*Indian*	*Chinese and Japanese*	*Total*	*Per sq. mile*
1910	236,128	94,446	68	427	331,069	5,517·8
1930	353,981	132,068	40	780	486,869	7,981·5
1960	345,263	411,737	587	3,532	763,956	12,523·9
			All others			
1970	209,272	537,712	9,526		756,510	12,321·0
1980	171,768	448,906	17,659		638,333	10,184·0

CLIMATE. Washington. Jan. 34°F (1·1°C), July 77°F (25°C). Annual rainfall 43" (1,064 mm). *See* Atlantic Coast, p. 1382.

GOVERNMENT. Local government, from 1 July 1878 until Aug. 1967, was that of a municipal corporation administered by a board of 3 commissioners, of whom 2 were appointed from civil life by the President, and confirmed by the Senate, for a term of 3 years each. The other commissioner was detailed by the President from the Engineer Corps of the Army. Reorganization Plan No. 3 of 1967 submitted by the President to Congress on 1 June 1967 abolished the Commission form of government and instituted a new Mayor Council form of government with officers appointed by the President with the advice and consent of the Senate. On 24 Dec. 1973 the appointed officers were replaced by an elected Mayor and councillors, with full legislative powers in local matters as from 1974. Congress retains the right to legislate, to veto or supersede the Council's acts. The 23rd amendment to the federal constitution (1961) conferred the right to vote in national elections; in the 1984 presidential election Mondale polled 172,459 votes, Reagan, 26,805. Since 1971 the District has had a delegate (two, by 1987) in Congress who may vote in Committees but not on the House floor.

BUDGET. The District's revenues are derived from a tax on real and personal property, sales taxes, taxes on corporations and companies, licences for conducting various businesses and from federal payments.

The District of Columbia has no bonded debt not covered by its accumulated sinking fund. *Per capita* personal income, 1985, $18,186.

INDUSTRY. The District's main industries (1985) are government service (263,000 workers); services (214,000); wholesale and retail trade (64,000); finance, real estate, insurance (35,000), communications, transport and utilities (26,000); total workforce, 1985, 629,000.

TOURISM. About 17m. visitors stay in the District every year and spend about $1,000m.

COMMUNICATIONS

Roads. Within the District are 340 miles of bus routes. There are 1,102 miles of streets maintained by the District; of these, 673 miles are local streets, 262 miles are major arterial roads. In 1990, 258,934 motor vehicles were registered.

Railways. There is a rapid rail transit system including a town subway system. This coordinates with the bus system and connects with Union railway station and the National Airport. Nine rail lines serve the District.

Aviation. The District is served by 3 general airports; across the Potomac River in Arlington, Va., is National Airport, in Chantilly, Va., is Dulles International Airport and in Maryland is Baltimore—Washington International Airport.

JUSTICE, RELIGION, EDUCATION AND WELFARE

Justice. Since 1958 there have been no executions; from 1930 to 1957 there were 40 executions (electrocution) including 3 whites for murder and 35 Negroes for murder and 2 for rape. The death penalty was declared unconstitutional in the District of Columbia on 14 Nov. 1973. At 31 Dec. 1985 there were 6,404 prisoners in state and federal institutions.

The District's Court system is the Judicial Branch of the District of Columbia. It is the only completely unified court system in the United States, possibly because of the District's unique city-state jurisdiction. Until the District of Columbia Court Reform and Criminal Procedure Act of 1970, the judicial system was almost entirely in the hands of Federal Government. Since that time, the system has been similar in most respects to the autonomous systems of the states.

Religion. The largest churches are the Protestant and Roman Catholic Christian churches; there are also Jewish, Eastern Orthodox and Islamic congregations.

Education. In 1983–84 there were about 89,000 pupils in secondary and elementary schools. Expenditure on public schools, 1986, $404m. or $645 per capita; public school teachers' average salary was $34,000. Higher education is given through the Consortium of Universities of the Metropolitan Washington Area, which consists of six universities and three colleges: Georgetown University, founded in 1795 by the Jesuit Order (11,688 students in 1985–86); George Washington University, non-sectarian founded in 1821 (17,948); Howard University, founded in 1867 (11,184); Catholic University of America, founded in 1887 (6,805); American University (Methodist) founded in 1893 (8,032); University of D.C., founded 1976 (12,080); Gallaudet College, founded 1864 (2,128); Trinity College, founded 1897 (926). There are altogether 18 institutes of higher education.

All benefit from such facilities as the 12 museums of the Smithsonian Institution, the Library of Congress, National Archives, and the Legal Libraries of the US Supreme Court and Department of Justice.

Social Security. The District government provides primary health care for residents, mainly through its Department of Human Services. In 1983 there were 17 hospitals with 8,700 beds. The welfare programme of aid to families with dependent children gave money to 55,900 recipients in 21,600 families in 1985; 4,100 aged and 11,600 disabled also received aid, total payments $43·8m.

Further Reading

Statistical Information: The Metropolitan Washington Board of Trade publications.
Reports of the Commissioners of the District of Columbia. Annual. Washington

FLORIDA

HISTORY. European men, probably Spaniards but possibly English, saw Florida for the first time in the period 1497–1512. John Cabot first charted the cape now called Florida in 1498. Juan Ponce de Leon sighted Florida on 27 March 1513. Going ashore between 2 and 8 April in the vicinity of what is now St Augustine, he named the land 'Pasqua de Flores' because his landing was 'in the time of the Feast of Flowers'. The first permanent settlement was Spanish and was made at St

Augustine, 8 Sept. 1565; it is the oldest permanent settlement in the US. In 1763 Florida was ceded to England; back to Spain in 1783, and to the US in 1821. Florida became a Territory in 1821 and was admitted into the Union on 3 March 1845.

AREA AND POPULATION. Florida is a peninsula bounded west by the Gulf of Mexico, south by the Straits of Florida, east by the Atlantic, north by Georgia and north-west by Alabama. Area, 58,664 sq. miles, including 4,510 sq. miles of inland water. Census population, 1 April 1980, was 9,746,324, an increase of 43·4% since 1970. Estimate (1 July 1989) 12,671,000. Births in 1989 were 189,375; deaths, 132,249; infant deaths, 1,915; marriages, 138,325; divorces and other dissolutions, 79,882.

Population in 5 federal census years was:

	White	*Black*	*All Others*	*Total*	*Per Sq. Mile*
1940	1,381,986	514,198	1,230	1,897,414	35·0
1950	2,166,051	603,101	2,153	2,771,305	51·1
1960	4,063,881	880,168	7,493	4,952,788	91·5
1970	5,719,343	1,041,651	28,449	6,789,443	125·6
1980	8,319,448	1,342,478	84,398	9,746,324	180·1

Of the population in 1980, 48% of the total were male; 84·3% were urban and 72·4% were 20 years of age or over.

The largest cities in the state, 1980 census (and 1989 estimates) are: Jacksonville, 540,898 (647,440); Miami, 346,931 (371,444); Tampa, 271,523 (287,917); St Petersburg, 236,893 (246,769); Fort Lauderdale, 153,256 (150,631); Hialeah, 145,254 (172,964); Orlando, 128,394 (166,181); Hollywood, 117,188 (126,380); Miami Beach, 96,298 (98,047); Clearwater, 85,450 (101,082); Tallahassee, 81,548 (130,284); Gainesville, 81,371 (85,663); West Palm Beach, 62,530 (74,284); Pompano Beach, 52,618 (71,181); Coral Springs, 37,349 (73,814); Lakeland, 47,406 (72,787).

CLIMATE. Jacksonville. Jan. 55°F (12·8°C), July 81°F (27·2°C). Annual rainfall 54" (1,353 mm). Key West. Jan. 70°F (21·1°C), July 83°F (28·3°C). Annual rainfall 39" (968 mm). Miami. Jan. 67°F (19·4°C), July 82°F (27·8°C). Annual rainfall 60" (1,516 mm). Tampa. Jan. 61°F (16·1°C), July 81°F (27·2°C). Annual rainfall 51" (1,285 mm). *See* Gulf Coast, p. 1382.

CONSTITUTION AND GOVERNMENT. The 1968 Legislature revised the constitution of 1885. The state legislature consists of a Senate of 40 members, elected for 4 years, and House of Representatives with 120 members elected for 2 years. Sessions are held annually, and are limited to 60 days. The Governor is elected for 4 years, and can hold two terms in office. Two senators and 19 representatives are elected to Congress.

In the 1988 presidential election Bush polled 2,535,503 votes and Dukakis, 1,630,647.

The state capital is Tallahassee. The state is divided into 67 counties.

Governor: Lawton Chiles (D.), 1991–95 ($103,909).
Lieut.-Governor: Kenneth 'Buddy' MacKay (D.), 1991–95 ($94,040).
Secretary of State: Jim Smith (R.), 1991–95 ($94,040).

FINANCE. There is no state income tax on individuals. For the year ending 30 June 1989 the state had a total revenue of $33,742m. and total expenditure of $32,279m. General revenue fund expenditure was $8,429m.

Net long-term debt, 30 June 1989, amounted to $4,456m.

Per capita personal income (1989) was $17,647.

NATURAL RESOURCES

Minerals. Chief mineral is phosphate rock, of which marketable production in 1989 was 38·2m. tonnes. This was approximately 80% of US and 30% of the world supply of phosphate in 1989.

Agriculture. In 1990, there were 41,000 farms; net income per farm was $71,695 in 1989. Total value of all farm land and buildings (1990), $23,801m. There were 732,767 acres in citrus groves in 1990 and 10·2m. acres of other farms and ranches. Total cash receipts from crops and livestock (1989), $6,203m., of which crops provided $4,982m. Oranges, grapefruit, melons and vegetables are important. Other crops are indoor and landscaping plants, soybeans, sugar-cane, tobacco and peanuts. On 1 Jan. 1990 the state had 1·9m. cattle, including 0·18m. milch cows, and 0·14m. swine.

The national forests area in Sept. 1989 was 1,122,372 acres. There were 14,982,607 acres of commercial forest.

Fisheries. Florida has extensive fisheries for oysters, shrimp, red snapper, crabs, mackerel and mullet. Catch (1989, preliminary), 175m. lb. valued at $180m.

INDUSTRY. In 1989 there were 15,500 manufacturers. They employed 536,439 persons. The metal-working, lumber, chemical, woodpulp, food-processing and instruments industries are important.

TOURISM. During 1989, 38·7m. tourists visited Florida. They spent $25,690m. making tourism one of the biggest industries in the state. There were (1989) 146 state parks, 15 state forests, 2 national parks, 8 national memorials, monuments, seashores and preserves and 4 national forests. The state parks were visited by 15·2m. people in 1988–89, 1·3m. of them campers.

COMMUNICATIONS

Roads. The state (1990) had 107,962·3 miles of highways, roads, and streets all of which were in the state and local system (67,574·1 miles being county roads), and 19,849·7 miles were federally-aided roads (1,429·6 miles interstate).

In 1989–90, 14,179,240m. vehicle licence plates were issued.

Railways. In 1990 there were 3,197 miles of railway.

Aviation. In 1990 Florida had 129 public use airports (15 international) of which 23 have scheduled commercial service.

JUSTICE, RELIGION, EDUCATION AND WELFARE

Justice. From 1968–90 there have been 25 executions, by electrocution, for murder; from 1930-68 there were 168 executions (electrocution), including 130 for murder, 37 for rape and 1 for kidnapping. State prisons, 1990, had 43,818 inmates.

Religion. The main Christian churches are Roman Catholic, Baptist, Methodist, Presbyterian and Episcopalian.

Education. Attendance at school is compulsory between 7 and 16.

In 1989 the public elementary and secondary schools had 1,775,529 enrolled pupils. Total expenditure on public schools (1988–89) was $11,580·6m. The state maintains 28 community colleges, with a full-time equivalent enrolment of 177,672 in 1989-90.

There are 9 universities in the state system, namely the University of Florida at Gainesville (founded 1853) with 36,242 students in 1989; the Florida State University (founded at Tallahassee in 1857) with 28,439; the University of South Florida at Tampa (founded 1960) with 32,348; Florida A. & M. University at Tallahassee (founded 1887) with 7,504; Florida Atlantic University (founded 1964) at Boca Raton with 11,828; the University of West Florida at Pensacola with 7,840; the University of Central Florida at Orlando with 20,443; the University of North Florida at Jacksonville with 7,806; Florida International University at Miami with 20,203.

Health. State-licensed general hospitals, 1990, numbered 222 with 51,993 beds.

Social Security. From 1974 aid to the aged, blind and disabled became a federal responsibility. The state continued to give aid to families with dependent children and general assistance. Monthly payments 1989–90: Aid to 4,208 blind averaged

$258.99; aid to 129,411 dependent children averaged $90.98; aid to 128,017 disabled averaged $257.05; aid to 85,694 aged averaged $203.11.

Further Reading

Florida Population: Summary of the 1980 Census. Univ. of Florida Press, 1981
Report. Florida Secretary of State. Tallahassee. Biennial
Report of the Comptroller. Tallahassee. Biennial
Morris, A., *The Florida Handbook*. Tallahassee. Biennial
Fernald, E. A. (ed.) *Atlas of Florida*. Florida State Univ., 1981
Tebeau, C. W., *A History of Florida*. Univ. Miami Press, rev. ed., 1980

State Library: Gray Building, Tallahassee. *Librarian:* Barratt Wilkins.

GEORGIA

HISTORY. Georgia (so named from George II) was founded in 1733 as the 13th original colony; she became the 4th original state.

AREA AND POPULATION. Georgia is bounded north by Tennessee and North Carolina, north-east by South Carolina, east by the Atlantic, south by Florida and west by Alabama. Area, 58,910 sq. miles, of which 854 sq. miles are inland water. Census population, 1 April 1980, was 5,464,265. Estimate (1987), 6,222,000. Births, 1986, were 98,175 (16 per 1,000 population); deaths, 49,336 (8·1); infant deaths, 1,225 (12·5 per 1,000 live births); marriages, 70,866 (11·6); divorces and annulments, 33,957 (5·5).

Population in 5 census years was:

	White	*Black*	*Indian*	*Asiatic*	*Total*	*Per sq. mile*
1910	1,431,802	1,176,987	95	237	2,609,121	44·4
1930	1,837,021	1,071,125	43	317	2,908,506	49·7
1960	2,817,223	1,122,596	749	2,004	3,943,116	67·7
			All others			
1970	3,391,242	1,187,149	11,184		4,589,575	79·0
1980	3,948,007	1,465,457	50,801		5,464,265	92·7

Of the 1980 population, 2,641,030 were male, 3,406,171 were urban and those 20 years of age and over numbered 3,601,895.

The largest cities are: Atlanta (capital), with population, 1980 census, of 422,293 (urbanized area, 2,010,368); Columbus, 168,598 (238,593); Savannah, 133,672 (225,581); Macon, 116,044 (251,736); Albany, 74,471 (112,257).

CLIMATE. Atlanta. Jan. 43°F (6·1°C), July 78°F (25·6°C). Annual rainfall 49" (1,234 mm). *See* Atlantic Coast, p. 1382.

CONSTITUTION AND GOVERNMENT. A new constitution was ratified in the general election of 2 Nov. 1976, proclaimed on 22 Dec. 1976 and became effective 1 Jan. 1977. The General Assembly consists of a Senate of 56 members and a House of Representatives of 180 members, both elected for 2 years. The Governor and Lieut.-Governor are elected for 4 years. Legislative sessions are annual, beginning the 2nd Monday in Jan. and lasting for 40 days.

Georgia was the first state to extend the franchise to all citizens 18 years old and above. The state is represented in Congress by 2 senators and 10 representatives.

Registered voters, 1986, numbered 2,575,815. At the 1988 presidential election Bush polled 1,081,331 votes, Dukakis, 714,792.

The state capital is Atlanta. Georgia is divided into 159 counties.

Governor: Zell Miller (D.), 1991–95 ($82,530).

BUDGET. For the fiscal year ending 30 June 1987 general revenue was $8,368m.

(taxes, $5,290m.; federal aid, $2,027m.); general expenditure was $8,079m. (education, $3,148m.; medical care and public assistance, $1,285m.).

On 30 June 1987 total liability was $4,390m.

Estimated *per capita* personal income (1987), was $14,098.

NATURAL RESOURCES

Minerals. Georgia is the leading producer of kaolin. The state ranks first in production of crushed and dimensional granite, second in production of fuller's earth and marble (crushed and dimensional).

Agriculture. In 1987, 49,000 farms covered 13m. acres; average farm was of 265 acres; total value, land and buildings, 1986, $11,094m. For 1986 cotton output was 185,000 bales (of 480 lb.). Other crops include tobacco, corn, wheat, soybeans, peanuts and pecans. Cash income, 1987, $3,500m: from crops, $1,300m.; from livestock, $1,800m.

On 1 Jan. 1986 farm animals included 1·65m. all cattle, including 119,000 milch cows, and 1·1m. swine.

Forestry. The forested area in 1987 was 24m. acres.

INDUSTRY. In 1987 the state's manufacturing establishments had 569,400 workers; the main groups were textiles, apparel, food and transport equipment. Trade employed 692,200, services 536,100, government, 476,000.

TOURISM. In 1987 tourists spent $8,670m.

COMMUNICATIONS

Roads. In 1990 there were 108,010 miles of road and 5,270,487 motor vehicles registered.

Railways. In 1976 there were 5,417 miles of railways. A metro opened in Atlanta in 1979.

Aviation. In 1988 there were 118 public and 168 private airports.

Shipping. The principal port is Savannah.

JUSTICE, RELIGION, EDUCATION AND WELFARE

Justice. State and federal prisons, 31 Dec. 1985, had 16,118 inmates. Since 1964 there have been two executions (for murder). From 1924 to 1964 there were 415 executions (electrocution), including 75 whites and 268 Negroes for murder, 3 whites and 63 Negroes for rape and 6 Negroes for armed robbery.

Under a Local Option Act, the sale of alcoholic beverages (not including malt beverages and light wines) is prohibited in more than half the counties.

Religion. An estimated 78% of the population are church members. Of the total population, 74·3% are Protestant, 3·2% are Roman Catholic and 1·5% Jewish.

Education. Since 1945 education has been compulsory; tuition is free for pupils between the ages of 6 and 18 years. In 1987 there were 1,289 public elementary schools and 361 public secondary schools; in autumn 1987 they had 1·1m. pupils and 60,509 teachers. Teachers' salaries averaged $27,606 in 1987–88. Expenditure on public schools (1987), $2,394m. or $438 per capita and $2,939 per pupil.

The University of Georgia (Athens) was founded in 1785 and was the first chartered State University in the US (26,547 students in 1987–88). Other institutions of higher learning include Georgia Institute of Technology, Atlanta (11,771), Emory University, Atlanta (8,884), Georgia State University, Atlanta (22,116) and Mercer University, Macon (3,416). The Atlanta University Center, devoted primarily to Negro education, includes Clark College (1,860) and Morris Brown College (1,257, co-educational, Morehouse (2,160), a liberal arts college for men, Interdenominational Theological Center, a co-educational theological school, and Spelman College, the first liberal arts college for Negro women in the US. Atlanta University serves as the graduate school centre for the complex. Wesleyan College near Macon is the oldest chartered women's college in the US.

Health. Hospitals licensed by the Department of Human Resources, 1985, numbered 173 with 26,051 beds.

Social Security. In Dec. 1985, 60,300 persons were receiving SSI old-age assistance of an average $128 per month; 82,500 families were receiving as aid to dependent children an average of $186 per family; aid to 89,500 disabled persons was $217 monthly.

Further Reading

Georgia History in Outline. Univ. of Georgia Press, Athens, 1978

Bonner, J. C. and Roberts, L. E. (eds.) *Studies in Georgia History and Government*. Reprint Company, Spartanburg, 1940 Repr.

Pound, M. B. and Saye, A. B., *Handbook on the Constitution of the U.S. and Georgia*. Univ. of Georgia Press, Athens, 1978

Rowland, A. R., *A Bibliography of the Writings on Georgia History*. Hamden, Conn., 1978

Saye, A. B., *A Constitutional History of Georgia, 1732–1968*. Univ. of Georgia, Athens, Rev. ed., 1970

State Library: Judicial Building, Capital Sq., Atlanta. *State Librarian:* John D. M. Folger.

HAWAII

HISTORY. The Hawaiian Islands, formerly known as the Sandwich Islands, were discovered by Capt. James Cook in Jan. 1778. During the greater part of the 19th century the islands formed an independent kingdom, but in 1893 the reigning Queen, Liliuokalani (died 11 Nov. 1917), was deposed and a provisional government formed; in 1894 a Republic was proclaimed, and in accordance with the request of the Legislature of the Republic, and a resolution of the US Congress of 6 July 1898 (signed 7 July by President McKinley), the islands were on 12 Aug. 1898 formally annexed to the US. On 14 June 1900 the islands were constituted as a Territory of Hawaii.

Statehood was granted to Hawaii on 18 March 1959, effective 21 Aug. 1959.

AREA AND POPULATION. The Hawaiian Islands lie in the North Pacific Ocean, between 18° 56' and 28° 25' N. lat. and 154° 49' and 178° 22' W. long., about 2,090 nautical miles south-west of San Francisco. There are 136 named islands and islets in the group, of which 7 major and 8 minor islands are inhabited. The land and inland water area of the state is 6,471 sq. miles, with census population, 1 April 1980, of 964,691, an increase of 194,778 or 25·4% since 1970; density was 150·1 per sq. mile.

The principal islands are Hawaii, 4,035 sq. miles and population, 1980, 92,053 (estimate, 1988, 117,500); Maui, 735 and 62,823 (84,100); Oahu, 618 and 762,534 (838,500); Kauai, 558 and 38,856 (49,100); Molokai, 264 and 6,049 (6,700); Lanai, 141 and 2,119 (2,200); Niihau, 71 and 226 (207); Kahoolawe, 46 (uninhabited). The capital Honolulu, on the island of Oahu, had a population in 1980 of 365,048 and Hilo on the island of Hawaii, 35,269. Estimated state population, 1989, 112,100.

Figures for racial groups, 1980, are: 331,925 White, 239,734 Japanese, 132,075 Filipinos, 118,251 Hawaiian, 55,916 Chinese, 17,453 Korean, 17,687 Black, 51,650 all others. In 1986, 31·2% of the population (outside barracks and other institutions) was of mixed race. Of the total, 92·3% were citizens of the US.

Inter-marriage between the races is common. Of the 9,709 resident marriages in 1988, 42·9% were between partners of different race. Births, 1987, were 18,555; deaths, 6,149; infant deaths, 168; marriages, 16,567; divorces and annulments, 4,419.

CLIMATE. All the islands have a tropical climate, with an abrupt change in conditions between windward and leeward sides, most marked in rainfall. Temperatures vary little. Honolulu. Jan. 71°F (21·7°C), July 78°F (25·6°C). Annual rainfall 31" (775 mm).

CONSTITUTION AND GOVERNMENT. The constitution took effect on 21 Aug. 1959. Amended 1968 and 1978.

The Legislature consists of a Senate of 25 members elected for 4 years, and a House of Representatives of 51 members elected for 2 years. The constitution provides for annual meetings of the legislature with 60-day regular sessions. The Governor and Lieut.-Governor are elected for 4 years. The registered voters, 1988, numbered 443,742.

The state sends to Congress 2 senators and 2 representatives.

In the 1988 presidential election Dukakis polled 192,364 votes, Bush, 158,625.

Governor: John Waihee (D.), 1991–95 ($94,780).

BUDGET. Revenue is derived mainly from taxation of sales and gross receipts, real property, corporate and personal income, and inheritance taxes, licences, public land sales and leases. For the year ending 30 June 1988 state general fund receipts amounted to $2,036·2m.; special fund receipts, $1,107·7m., and federal grants, $438·3m. (included as $8·7m. of general funds and $429·6m. of special funds). State expenditures were $2,980·7m. (education, $886·2m.; highways, $78·6m.; public welfare, $380·8m.; figures include both special and general funds).

Net long-term debt, 31 Dec. 1988, amounted to $3,382·3m.

Estimated *per capita* personal income (1988) was $16,753.

NATURAL RESOURCES

Minerals. Total value of mineral production, 1988, amounted to $78,225,000. Cement shipped from plants amounted to 410,000 short tons; stone, 6,300,000 short tons.

Agriculture. Farming is highly commercialized, aiming at export to the American market, and highly mechanized. In 1987 there were 4,870 farms with an acreage of 1·72m.

Sugar and pineapples are the staple crops. Income from crop sales, 1988, was $485m., and from livestock, $88·6m. The sugar crop was valued at $209·9m.; pineapples, $107·4m.; other crops, $168·2m.

Forestry. In 1988 there were 840,540 acres of forest reserve land, including 327,845 in private ownership.

INDUSTRY. In 1987 manufacturing establishments employed 15,300 production workers who earned an estimated $254·6m. Defence is the second-largest industry; US armed forces spent $1,892m. in Hawaii in 1988.

COMMERCE. In 1988 imports were $1,118m.; exports, $131m.

TOURISM. Tourism is outstanding in Hawaii's economy. Tourist arrivals numbered 1·1m. in 1967, and reached 6·1m. in 1988. Tourist expenditures, $380m. in 1967, contributed $9,200m. to the state's economy in 1988.

COMMUNICATIONS

Roads. In 1990 there were 4,082 miles of roads (2,663 miles rural) and 736,393 registered motor vehicles.

Aviation. There were 7 commercial airports in 1989; passengers arriving from overseas in 1988 numbered 6·65m., and there were 9m. passengers between the islands.

Shipping. Several lines of steamers connect the islands with the mainland USA, Canada, Australia, the Philippines, China and Japan. In 1989, 2,024 overseas and 3,101 inter-island vessels entered the port of Honolulu.

Post. There were 530,022 telephone access lines at 31 Dec. 1988.

Broadcasting. In 1989, Hawaii had 47 commercial and 2 other radio stations, 17 commercial and 2 other TV stations.

JUSTICE, RELIGION, EDUCATION AND WELFARE

Justice. There is no capital punishment in Hawaii.

Religion. The residents of Hawaii are mainly Christians, though there are many Buddhists. A sample survey in 1979 showed that 31% were Roman Catholic, 34% Protestant, 12% Buddhist, 2·5% Latter Day Saints.

Education. Education is free, and compulsory for children between the ages of 6 and 18. The language in the schools is English. In 1988–89 there were 235 public schools (167,899 pupils with 8,973 teachers) and 141 private schools (35,459 pupils and 2,512 teachers) ranging from kindergarten through the 12th grade. The University of Hawaii-Manoa, founded in 1907, had 18,477 day students in 1988; total attendance at all campuses of the University of Hawaii system, 42,767; 9,612 at private colleges.

Social Security. During 1988 5,123 people were receiving old-age assistance of an average $217 per month; 13,396 families, $453 in aid to dependent children; 7,008 disabled people, $288. Social Security beneficiaries, 141,730, receiving aggregate monthly payments of $67·5m.

Further Reading

Government in Hawaii. Tax Foundation of Hawaii. Honolulu, 1988
Guide to Government in Hawaii. 8th ed. Legislative Reference Bureau. State of Hawaii, Honolulu, 1989
Atlas of Hawaii. Hawaii Univ., rev. ed. Honolulu, 1983
State of Hawaii Data Book. Hawaii Dept. of Business and Economic Development, 1989
Allen, G. E., *Hawaii's War Years*. 2 vols. Hawaii Univ. Press, 1950–52
Bell, R. J., *Last Among Equals: Hawaiian Statehood and American Politics*. Honolulu, 1984
Kuykendall, R. S. and Day, A. G., *Hawaii, A History*. Rev. ed. New Jersey, 1961
Morgan, J. R., *Hawaii*. Boulder, 1982
Pukui, M. K. and Elbert, S. H., *Hawaiian–English Dictionary*. Rev. ed. Honolulu, 1986

IDAHO

HISTORY. Idaho was first permanently settled in 1860, although there was a mission for Indians in 1836 and a Mormon settlement in 1855. It was organized as a Territory in 1863 and admitted into the Union as a state on 3 July 1890.

AREA AND POPULATION. Idaho is bounded north by Canada, east by the Rocky Mountains of Montana and Wyoming, south by Nevada and Utah, west by Oregon and Washington. Area, 83,564 sq. miles, of which 1,153 sq. miles are inland water. In 1983 the federal government owned 34,282,000 acres (65% of the state area). Census population, 1 April 1980, 943,935, an increase of 32·4% since 1970. Estimate (1984) 1,001,000.

Births, 1984, 17,996 (18 per 1,000 population); deaths, 7,229 (7·2); infant deaths, 174 (9·7 per 1,000 live births); marriages, 13,264 (13·3); divorces, 6,210 (6·2).

Population in 5 census years was:

	White	*Black*	*Indian*	*Asiatic*	*Total*	*Per sq. mile*
1910	319,221	651	3,488	2,234	325,594	3·9
1930	438,840	668	3,638	1,886	445,032	5·4
1960	657,383	1,502	5,231	2,958	667,191	8·1
1970	693,375	3,655	5,413	2,526	713,008	8·5
			All others			
1980	901,641	2,716	39,578		943,935	11·3

Of the total 1980 population, 471,155 were male, 509,702 were urban and those 20 years of age or older 600,242.

The largest cities are Boise (capital) with 1980 census population of 102,160 (1984 estimate, 107,188); Pocatello, 46,340 (45,334); Idaho Falls, 39,734 (41,774); Lewiston, 27,986 (28,050); Twin Falls, 26,209 (28,168); Nampa, 25,112 (27,347).

CLIMATE. Boise. Jan. 29°F (–1·7°C), July 74°F (23·3°C). Annual rainfall 12" (303 mm). *See* Mountain States, p. 1381.

CONSTITUTION AND GOVERNMENT. The constitution adopted in 1890 is still in force; it has had 104 amendments. The Legislature consists of a Senate of 42 members and a House of Representatives of 84 members, all the legislators being elected for 2 years. The Governor, Lieut.-Governor and Secretary of State are elected for 4 years. Voters are citizens, over the age of 18 years. The state is represented in Congress by 2 senators and 2 representatives.

In the 1988 presidential election Bush polled 253,467 votes, Dukakis, 147,420.

The state is divided into 44 counties. The capital is Boise.

Governor: Cecil D. Andrus (D.), 1991–95 ($50,000).

BUDGET. For the year ending 30 June 1985 (State Auditor's Office) general revenues were $551·1m. and general expenditures, $555·5m. (which includes $3·4m. outstanding obligations).

Per capita personal income (1985) was $11,120.

NATURAL RESOURCES

Minerals. Production of the most important minerals (1984): Silver, 18·87m. troy oz.; copper, 3,701 tonnes; antimony, 557 short tons. There is some gold, lead, zinc and vanadium. Non-metallic minerals include phosphate rock (4·7m. tonnes), lime (87,000 short tons), garnet, gypsum, perlite, pumice, tungsten, molybdenum, crushed stone (1·8m. short tons), sand and gravel and dimension stone. Value of total mineral output was $412m. in 1984.

Agriculture. Agriculture is the leading industry, although a great part of the state is naturally arid. Extensive irrigation works have been carried out, bringing an estimated 4m. acres under irrigation; 83 reservoirs have a total capacity of 10·4m. acre-ft, 7·3m. acre-ft of which is primarily used for irrigation.

In 1985 there were 24,600 farms with a total area of 14·7m. acres (27% of the land area); average farm had 598 acres with land and buildings valued at approximately $749 per acre.

In 1984 there were 51 soil conservation districts, managed by local farmers and ranchers, covering most of the state.

Cash receipts from marketings, 1985, was $2,063m. ($1,200m. from crops and $862m. from livestock). The most important crops are potatoes and wheat—potatoes leading all states; in 1985 the production amounted to 103m. cwt, cash receipts $323m.; wheat, 72m. bu., $235m. Other crops are sugar-beet, alfalfa, barley, field peas and beans, onions and apples. On 1 Jan. 1985 the number of sheep was 313,000; milch cows, 165,000; all cattle, 1·78m.; swine, 112,000.

Forestry. In 1983 a total of 20,635,700 acres (37·6% of the state's area) was in forests; 13,540,600 acres of this was commercial (non-reserved) forest. The volume of sawtimber in commercial forests was 139,600m. bd ft. The stumpage value of forest products was about $124m., and about $531m. was added by processing. Ownership of commercial forests is 70% federal, 6·5% state and local government, 0·5% Indian, 22·3% private. Some 16,100 workers are involved in forestry.

INDUSTRY. In 1985 85,000 were employed in trade, 70,000 in government, 66,000 in services, 55,000 in manufacturing.

TOURISM. Money spent by travellers in 1984 was about $1,200m. Estimated state and local tax receipts from tourism, $48m. Jobs generated, 25,000 (pay-roll over $300m.).

COMMUNICATIONS

Roads. In 1990 there were 61,317 miles of roads (58,911 miles rural) and 1,039,045 registered motor vehicles.

Railways. The state had (1985) 1,910 miles of railways (including 2 Amtrak routes).

Aviation. There were 68 municipally owned airports in 1985.

Shipping. Water transport is provided from the Pacific to the Port of Lewiston, by way of the Columbia and Snake rivers, a distance of 464 miles.

JUSTICE, RELIGION, EDUCATION AND WELFARE

Justice. The death penalty may be imposed for first degree murder, but the judge must consider mitigating circumstances before imposing a sentence of death. Since 1926 only 4 men (white) have been executed, by hanging (1 in 1926, 2 in 1951 and 1 in 1957). At 1 Oct. 1985 14 prison inmates (13 men and 1 woman) were under sentence of death. Execution is now by lethal injection. The state prison system, 1 Oct. 1985, had 1,260 inmates.

Religion. The leading religious denominations are the Church of Jesus Christ of Latter Day Saints (Mormon Church), Roman Catholics, Methodists, Presbyterians, Episcopalians and Lutherans.

Education. In 1984–85 public elementary schools (grades K to 6) had 118,647 pupils and 5,481 classroom teachers; secondary schools had 92,053 pupils and 4,980 classroom teachers.

Average salary, 1984–85, of elementary and secondary classroom teachers, $20,032. The University of Idaho, founded at Moscow in 1889, had 459 professors and 8,970 students in 1984–85. There are 9 other institutions of higher education; 5 of them are public institutions with a total enrolment (1984–85) of 21,914 (excluding vocational-technical colleges).

Social Welfare. Old-age assistance is granted to persons 65 years of age and older. In Aug. 1985, 1,014 persons were drawing an average of $105.86 per month; 6,023 families with 10,858 children were drawing an average of $243.85 per case (or $90.10 per eligible person); 28 blind persons, $73.21; 569 children were receiving $248.88 per child for foster care; 1,827 permanently and totally disabled persons, $133.69.

Health. In Sept. 1985 skilled nursing covered 4,761 beds; intermediate care, 107; intermediate care for the mentally retarded 528. Hospitals had 3,547 beds and home health agencies totalled 36.

Further Reading

Idaho Blue Book. Secretary of State. Boise, 1983–84
Idaho. Idaho First National Bank
Idaho Almanac. Division of Economic and Community Affairs, 1977
Idaho's Yesterdays. State Historical Society. Quarterly

ILLINOIS

HISTORY. Illinois was first discovered by Joliet and Marquette, two French explorers, in 1673. In 1763 the country was ceded by the French to the British. In 1783 Great Britain recognized the United States' title to the land that became Illinois; it was organized as a Territory in 1809 and admitted into the Union on 3 Dec. 1818.

AREA AND POPULATION. Illinois is bounded north by Wisconsin, north-east by Lake Michigan, east by Indiana, south-east by the Ohio River (forming the boundary with Kentucky), west by the Mississippi River (forming the boundary with Missouri and Iowa). Area, 56,400 sq. miles, of which 652 sq. miles are inland water. Census population, 1980, 11,426,518, an increase of 2·71% since 1970. Estimate (1988), 11,544,000. Births in 1988 were 184,708; deaths, 105,038); infant deaths, 2,077; marriages 78,302; divorces, 45,736; annulments, 175.

Population in 5 census years was:

	White	*Black*	*Indian*	*All others*	*Total*	*Per sq. mile*
1910	5,526,962	109,049	188	2,392	5,638,591	100·6
1930	7,295,267	328,972	469	5,946	7,630,654	136·4
1960	9,010,252	1,037,470	4,704	28,732	10,081,158	180·3
			All others			
1970	9,600,381	1,425,674	87,921		11,113,976	199·4
1980	9,233,327	1,675,398	517,793		11,426,518	203·0

Of the total population in 1980, 5,537,737 were male, 9,518,039 persons were urban and 5,597,360 were 18 years of age or older.

The most populous cities with population (1980 census), are:

Chicago	3,005,072
Rockford	139,712
Peoria	124,160
Springfield (cap.)	99,637
Decatur	94,081
Joliet	77,956
Aurora	81,293
Evanston	73,706
Waukegan	67,653
Arlington Heights	66,116

Standard Metropolitan Statistical Area population, 1980 census (and 1988 estimate): Chicago, 7,102,378 (6,216,300); East St Louis, 565,874 (1987, 570,400); Peoria, 365,864 (340,400); Rockford, 279,514 (282,200); Springfield, 176,089 (191,700); Decatur, 131,375 (123,700).

CLIMATE. Chicago. Jan. 25°F (–3·9°C), July 73°F (22·8°C). Annual rainfall 33" (836 mm). *See* Great Lakes, p. 1382.

CONSTITUTION AND GOVERNMENT. The present constitution became effective 1 July 1971. The General Assembly consists of a House of Representatives of 118 members, elected for 2 years and a Senate of 59 members who are divided into three groups; in one, they are elected for terms of four years, four years, and two years; in the next, for terms of four years, two years, and four years; and in the last, for terms of two years, four years, and four years. Sessions are annual. The Governor and Lieut.-Governor are elected as a team for 4 years; the Comptroller and Secretary of State are elected for 4 years. Electors are citizens 18 years of age, having the usual residential qualifications.

The state is divided into legislative districts, in each of which 1 senator is chosen; each district is divided into 2 representative districts, in each of which 1 representative is chosen.

Illinois is represented in Congress by 2 senators and 22 representatives.

In the 1988 presidential election Bush polled 2,298,648 votes, Dukakis, 2,180,657.

The capital is Springfield. The state has 102 counties.

Governor: Jim Edgar (R.), 1991–95 ($88,825).

BUDGET. For the year ending 30 June 1990 general revenues were $12,841m. and general expenditures were $12,987m.

Total net long-term debt, 30 June 1989, was $14,992m.

Per capita personal income (1989) was $18,824.

ENERGY AND NATURAL RESOURCES

Minerals. Chief mineral product is coal; 42 operative mines had an output (1989) of 60,131,053 tons. Mineral production also included: Crude petroleum, fluorspar, tripoli, lime, sand, gravel and stone. Total value of mineral products, 1988, was $2,807·9m.

Agriculture. In 1990, 83,000 farms had an area of 28·5m. acres; the average farm was 343 acres.

Cash receipts, 1989, from crops, $4,459,087,000; from livestock and livestock products, $2,248,498,000. Illinois is a large producer of maize and soybeans, the state's leading cash commodities. Output, 1989: Soybeans, 354m. bu; wheat, 105·02m. bu; maize, 1,322·25m. bu. In Jan. 1990 there were 195,000 milch cows, 1·95m. cattle and calves; 159,000 sheep and lambs and 5·7m. swine. The wool clip was 1,038,000 lb. in 1988.

Forestry. National forest area under the US Forest Service administration, Sept. 1985, was 262,291 acres. Total forest land, 5·2m. acres.

INDUSTRY. In 1987, 18,440 manufacturing establishments employed 986,879 workers; annual payroll, $26,593,839,000. Largest industry was non-electrical machinery. Gross state product, 1989, $257,599m.

LABOUR. In 1989 there were 5,197,000 employees, of whom 982,000 were in manufacturing, 1,275,000 in trade, 1,279,000 in services, 738,000 in government.

COMMUNICATIONS

Roads. In 1989 there were 6,293,250 passenger cars, 1,412,142 trucks and buses, 11,300 taxis, liveries and ambulances, 566,445 trailers and semi-trailers, 223,032 motor cycles and 1,131,059 other vehicles registered in the state. At 31 Dec. 1989 there were 13,218·48 miles of state primary roads of which 1,676·53 miles were interstate; 3,673·33 miles of state supplementary roads and 284·81 miles of toll roads and toll bridges.

Railways. There were, on 1 Dec. 1989, 7,621 miles of Class I railway. Chicago is served by Amtrak long-distance trains on several routes, and by a metro (CTA) system, and by 7 groups of commuter railways controlled by the Northeast Illinois Railroad Corporation (now called METRA).

Shipping. In 1988 the seaport of Chicago handled 22,893,740 short tons of cargo.

Aviation. There were (1989) 131 public airports and 714 restricted landing areas.

JUSTICE, RELIGION, EDUCATION AND WELFARE

Justice. In June 1989 the total average daily prison population was 21,271. There was 1 execution in 1990 (98 in 1928–62),

A Civil Rights Act (1941), as amended, bans all forms of discrimination by places of public accommodation, including inns, restaurants, retail stores, railroads, aeroplanes, buses, etc., against persons on account of 'race, religion, colour, national ancestry or physical or mental handicap'; another section similarly mentions 'race or colour.'

The Fair Employment Practices Act of 1961, as amended, prohibits discrimination in employment based on race, colour, sex, religion, national origin or ancestry, by employers, employment agencies, labour organizations and others. These principles are embodied in the 1971 constitution.

The Illinois Human Rights Act (1979), prevents unlawful discrimination in employment, real property transactions, access to financial credit, and public accommodations, by authorizing the creation of a Department of Human Rights to enforce, and a Human Rights Commission to adjudicate, allegations of unlawful discrimination.

Religion. Among the larger religious denominations are: Roman Catholic (3·6m.), Jewish (50,000), Presbyterian Church, USA (200,000), Lutheran Church in America (200,000), Lutheran Church Missouri Synod (325,000), American Baptist (105,000), Disciples of Christ (75,000), and United Methodist (505,000), Southern

Baptist (265,000), United Church of Christ (192,000), Church of Nazarene (50,000), Assembly of God (63,000).

Education. Education is free and compulsory for children between 7 and 16 years of age. In autumn 1989 public school elementary enrolments were 1,278,557 pupils and 60,439 teachers; secondary enrolments, 518,798 pupils and 28,973 teachers. Enrolment (1989–90) in non-public schools was 249,922 elementary and 68,737 secondary. Teachers' salaries, 1989–90, averaged $32,815. Total enrolment in 189 institutions of higher education (autumn 1989) was 714,392.

Colleges and universities with over 3,000 students:

Founded	*Name*	*Place*	*Control*	*Autumn 1989 Enrolment*
1851	Northwestern University	Evanston	Methodist	16,807
1857	Illinois State University	Normal	Public	23,107
1867	University of Illinois	Urbana	Public	61,531
1867	Chicago State University [1]	Chicago	Public	6,032
1869	Southern Illinois University	Carbondale	Public	35,916
1870	Loyola University	Chicago	Roman Catholic	14,292
1890	University of Chicago	Chicago	Non-Sect.	10,680
1895	Eastern Illinois University	Charleston	Public	11,068
1895	Northern Illinois University	DeKalb	Public	24,443
1897	Bradley University	Peoria	Non-Sect.	5,658
1899	Western Illinois University	Macomb	Public	13,238
1940	Illinois Institute of Technology [2]	Chicago	Non-Sect.	6,300
1945	Roosevelt University	Chicago	Non-Sect.	6,437
1961	Northeastern Illinois University [3]	Chicago	Public	10,293

[1] Formerly Illinois Teachers College (South).
[2] Illinois Institute of Technology formed in 1940 by merger of two older technical schools.
[3] Formerly Illinois Teachers' College (North).

Health. In 1988 hospitals listed by the American Hospital Association numbered 258, with 61,750 beds. At June 1990 state institutions had 4,496 developmentally disabled and 3,385 mentally ill residents.

Social Security. State-administered Supplemental Security Income (SSI) was paid to 53,148 recipients in financial year 1990; gross income-maintenance payments (no adjustments) totalled $60·7m.; medical payments, $166·6m. Aid to families with dependent children was paid to 209,822 families, average monthly payment per family, $324; total payments, $815·6m.; medical payments, $484·4m.

Further Reading

Blue Book of the State of Illinois. Edited by Secretary of State. Springfield. Biennial

Angle, P. M. and Beyer, R. L., *A Handbook of Illinois History*. Illinois State Historical Society, Springfield, 1943

Clayton, J., *The Illinois Fact Book and Historical Almanac 1673–1968*. Southern Illinois Univ., 1970

Howard, R. P., *Illinois: A History of the Prairie State*. Grand Rapids, 1972.—*Mostly Good and Competent Men: Illinois Governors, 1818–1988*. Springfield, 1989

Pease, T. C., *The Story of Illinois*. 3rd ed. Chicago, 1965

The Illinois State Library: Springfield, Il.62756. *State Librarian:* Jim Edgar.

INDIANA

HISTORY. Indiana, first settled in 1732–33, was made a Territory in 1800 and admitted into the Union on 11 Dec. 1816.

AREA AND POPULATION. Indiana is bounded west by Illinois, north by Michigan and Lake Michigan, east by Ohio and south by Kentucky across the Ohio River. Area, 36,185 sq. miles, of which 253 sq. miles are inland water. Census population, 1 April 1980, was 5,490,224, an increase of 294,832 or 5·7% since 1970. Estimate (1989) 5,593,000. In 1988 live births were 81,000 (14·7 per 1,000 population); deaths 50,000 (9·1); infant deaths, 895 (11 per 1,000 live births); (1986) marriages 49,900 (9·1).

Population in 5 census years was:

	White	*Black*	*Indian*	*Asiatic*	*Total*	*Per sq. mile*
1910	2,639,961	60,320	279	316	2,700,876	74·9
1930	3,125,778	111,982	285	458	3,238,503	89·4
1960	4,388,554	269,275	948	2,447	4,662,498	128·9
			All others			
1970	4,820,324	357,464	15,881		5,193,669	143·9
1980	5,004,394	414,785	71,045		5,490,224	152·8

Of the total in 1980, 2,665,805 were male, 3,525,298 were urban and 3,545,431 were 21 years of age or older.

The largest cities with census population, 1980 (and 1988 estimates), are: Indianapolis (capital), 711,539 (727,130); Fort Wayne, 172,196 (179,810); Gary, 151,953 (132,460); Evansville, 130,496 (128,210); South Bend, 109,727 (106,190); Hammond, 93,714 (84,630); Muncie, 77,216 (73,320); Anderson, 64,695 (60,720); Terre Haute, 61,125 (56,330); Bloomington (54,850).

CLIMATE. Indianapolis. Jan. 29°F (–1·7°C), July 76°F (24·4°C). Annual rainfall 41" (1,034 mm). *See* The Mid-West, p. 1382.

CONSTITUTION AND GOVERNMENT. The present constitution (the second) dates from 1851; it has had (as of Nov. 1983) 34 amendments. The General Assembly consists of a Senate of 50 members elected for 4 years, and a House of Representatives of 100 members elected for 2 years.

A constitutional amendment of 1970 allows the legislators to set the length and frequency of sessions, which are currently held annually. The Governor and Lieut.-Governor are elected for 4 years. The state is represented in Congress by 2 senators and 10 representatives.

In the 1988 presidential election Bush polled 1,280,292 votes, Dukakis, 850,851.

The state capital is Indianapolis. The state is divided into 92 counties and 1,008 townships.

Governor: Evan Bayh (D.), 1989–92 ($66,000 plus expenses).
Lieut.-Governor: Frank O'Bannon (D.), 1988–92 ($51,000 plus expenses).
Secretary of State: Joseph Hogsett (D.), 1988–92 ($46,000).

BUDGET. In the fiscal year 1987–88 (US Census Bureau figures) total revenues were $9,744,252,000 ($1,907,967,000 from federal government, $5,311,824,000 from taxes), total expenditures were $8,847·76m. ($3,660,862,000 for education, $1,446·67m. for public welfare and $903,246,000 for highways).

Total long-term debt, on 30 June 1988, was $3,085,427,000.

Per capita personal income (1988) was $14,924.

ENERGY AND NATURAL RESOURCES

Minerals. The state produced 36,188,000 short tons of crushed stone and 27,212,000 short tons of dimension stone in 1989; the output of coal was 33·6m. short tons in 1988; petroleum, 5m. bbls (of 42 gallons) in 1984.

Agriculture. Indiana is largely agricultural, about 75% of its total area being in farms. In 1987, 70,506 farms had 16,170,895 acres (average, 229 acres). Cash income, 1987, from crops, including nursery and greenhouse crops, $2,127,135; from livestock, poultry and their products, $1,940,549.

The chief crops (1987) were corn for grain or seed (619,049,978 bu.), corn for silage or green chop (1,961,381 tons), wheat for grain (30,789,151 bu.), oats for grain, (4,317,321 bu.), soybeans for beans (169,749,051 bu.), hay (alfalfa, other tame small grain, wild, grass silage, etc.) (1,892,466 tons).

The livestock on 1 Jan. 1987 included 2,031,915 all cattle, 163,867 milch cows,

82,757 sheep and lambs, 4,372,294 hogs and pigs, 26,787,315 chickens. In 1987 the wool clip yielded 537,966 lb. of wool from 76,056 sheep and lambs.

Forestry. In 1988 there were 4·3m. acres of forest and (1987) 12 state forests and Hoosier National Forest (187,812 acres).

INDUSTRY. Manufacturing establishments employed, in 1988, 648,012 workers, earning $20,282,963,000. The steel industry is the largest in the country.

COMMUNICATIONS

Roads. In 1990 there were 91,744 miles of road (73,941 miles rural) and 4,322,302 registered motor vehicles.

Railways. In 1989 there were 3,796 miles of mainline railway and 861·5 miles of secondary track.

Aviation. Of airports, 1990, 115 were for public use and 486 were for private use.

JUSTICE, RELIGION, EDUCATION AND WELFARE

Justice. In 1963–80 there were no executions; there have since been 4, for murder. State correctional institutions, financial year 1987–88, had an average daily population of 11,889.

The Civil Rights Act of 1885 forbids places of public accommodation to bar any persons on grounds not applicable to all citizens alike; no citizen may be disqualified for jury service 'on account of race or colour'. An Act of 1947 makes it an offence to spread religious or racial hatred.

A 1961 Act provided 'all ... citizens equal opportunity for education, employment and access to public conveniences and accommodations' and created a Civil Rights Commission.

Religion. Religious denominations include Methodists, Roman Catholic, Disciples of Christ, Baptists, Lutheran, Presbyterian churches, Society of Friends.

Education. School attendance is compulsory from 7 to 16 years. In 1989–90 public and parochial schools and nursery schools had 921,433 pupils and 54,196 teachers. Teachers' salaries averaged $29,161 (1989–90). Total expenditure for public schools, 1988, $2,784,938,952.

The principal institutions for higher education are (1987–88):

Founded	*Institution*	*Control*	*Students (full-time)*
1801	Vincennes University	State	8,228
1824	Indiana University, Bloomington	State	33,421
1837	De Pauw University, Greencastle	Methodist	2,404
1842	University of Notre Dame	R.C.	9,811
1850	Butler University, Indianapolis	Independent	3,723
1859	Valparaiso University, Valparaiso	Evangelical Lutheran Church	3,690
1870	Indiana State University, Terre Haute	State	11,161
1874	Purdue University, Lafayette	State	33,303
1898	Ball State University, Muncie	State	19,110
1902	University of Indianapolis, Indianapolis	Methodist	1,471
1963	Indiana Vocational Technical College, Indianapolis	State	4,760
1985	University of Southern Indiana	State	4,624

Health. Hospitals listed by the Indiana State Board of Health (1988) numbered 124 (23,929 beds in 1981). In 1989 there were 3,612 patients in state mental hospitals.

Social Security. Old-age assistance, assistance to the blind and to the disabled were transferred from state to federal programmes in June 1974. In July–Dec. 1989, state supplemental assistance and/or Federal Supplemental Security assistance was paid to an average of 11,165 aged persons per month (total $8,817,094,000), 1,163 blind ($1,717,006) and 42,814 disabled ($61,940,133).

Further Reading

Indiana State Chamber of Commerce. *Here is Your Indiana Government.* 22nd ed. Indianapolis, 1985

State Library: Indiana State Library, 140 North Senate, Indianapolis 46204. *Director:* C. Ray Ewick.

IOWA

HISTORY. Iowa, first settled in 1788, was made a Territory in 1838 and admitted into the Union on 28 Dec. 1846.

AREA AND POPULATION. Iowa is bounded east by the Mississippi River (forming the boundary with Wisconsin and Illinois), south by Missouri, west by the Missouri River (forming the boundary with Nebraska), north-west by the Big Sioux River (forming the boundary with South Dakota) and north by Minnesota. Area, 56,375 sq. miles, including 310 sq. miles of inland water. Census population, 1 April 1980, 2,913,808, an increase of 3·17% since 1970. Estimate, 1989, 2,840,000. Births, 1989, were 38,361; deaths, 27,583; infant deaths, 319; marriages (1988), 25,090; dissolutions of marriages, 10,808.

Population in 5 census years was:

	White	*Black*	*Indian*	*Asiatic*	*Total*	*Per sq. mile*
1870	1,188,207	5,762	48	3	1,194,020	21·5
1930	2,452,677	17,380	660	222	2,470,939	44·1
1960	2,728,709	25,354	1,708	1,022	2,757,537	49·2
			All others			
1970	2,782,762	32,596	10,010		2,825,368	50·5
1980	2,839,225	41,700	32,882		2,913,808	51·7

At the census of 1980, 1,415,705 were male, 1,708,232 were urban and 1,971,502 were 20 years of age or older.

The largest cities in the state, with their census population in 1980 are: Des Moines (capital), 191,003; Cedar Rapids, 110,243; Davenport, 103,264; Sioux City, 82,003; Waterloo, 75,985; Dubuque, 62,321; Council Bluffs, 56,449; Iowa City, 50,508; Ames, 45,775; Cedar Falls, 36,322; Clinton, 32,828; Mason City, 30,144; Burlington, 29,529; Fort Dodge, 29,423; Ottumwa, 27,381.

CLIMATE. Cedar Rapids. Jan. 18·5°F (–7·5°C), July 74·3°F (23·5°C). Annual rainfall 36" (903 mm). Des Moines. Jan. 18·6°F (–7·5°C), July 76·3°F (29·6°C). Annual rainfall 31" (773 mm). *See* The Mid-West, p. 1382.

CONSTITUTION AND GOVERNMENT. The constitution of 1857 still exists; it has had 45 amendments. The General Assembly comprises a Senate of 50 and a House of Representatives of 100 members, meeting annually for an unlimited session. Senators are elected for 4 years, half retiring every second year: Representatives for 2 years. The Governor and Lieut.-Governor are elected for 4 years. The state is represented in Congress by 2 senators and 6 representatives. Iowa is divided into 99 counties; the capital is Des Moines.

In the 1988 presidential election Dukakis polled 670,557 votes, Bush, 545,355.

Governor: Terry Branstad (R.), 1991–95 ($72,500).
Lieut.-Governor: Joy Corning (R.), 1991–95 ($25,100).
Secretary of State: Elaine Baxter (D.) ($55,700).

BUDGET. For fiscal year 1988-89 state tax revenue was $2,849·2m. General expenditures were $2,222·2m. for education, $825·8m. for public welfare, and $702·98m. for transport.

On 30 June 1988 the net long-term debt was $399·49m.

Per capita personal income (1989) was $15,447.

ENERGY AND NATURAL RESOURCES

Minerals. Production in 1988: Crushed stone 29·2m. tons; sand and gravel, 11·88m. tons; gypsum, 2·05m. tons; cement 2·03m. short tons; coal, 429,871 short tons. The value of mineral products in 1988, was $290·3m.

Agriculture. Iowa is the wealthiest of the agricultural states, partly because nearly the whole area (93·5%) is arable and included in farms. Large-scale commercial farming has not developed; the average farm in 1989 was 319 acres.

Cash farm income (1988 estimate) was $9,074m.; from livestock, $5,045·1m., and from crops, $4,028·9m. Production of corn was 1,445·5m. bu., value $3,107·8m. and soybeans, 322·9m. bu., value $1,759·5m. On 1 Dec. 1989 livestock included swine, 13·5m. (leading all states); milch cows, 308,000; all cattle, 4·7m., and sheep and lambs, 490,000. The wool clip (1989) yielded 3·4m. lb. of wool.

INDUSTRY. In 1989 manufacturing establishments employed 234,600 people: Trade, 306,200; services, 271,200.

COMMUNICATIONS

Roads. On 1 Jan. 1989 number of miles of streets and highways was 112,712. In 1990 there were 1·9m. licensed drivers and 3·02m. registered vehicles.

Railways. The state, 1989, had 4,414 miles of track, and 6 Class I railways.

Aviation. Airports (1989), numbered 350, including 107 lighted airports and 95 all-weather runways. There were approximately 2,500 private aircraft.

JUSTICE, RELIGION, EDUCATION AND WELFARE

Justice. There is now no capital punishment in Iowa. State prisons, 12 Nov. 1990, had 3,941 inmates.

Religion. Chief religious bodies in 1989 were: Roman Catholic (539,482 members); United Methodists, 261,613; American Lutheran, 153,539 baptised members; United Presbyterians, 86,763; United Church of Christ, 50,840.

Education. School attendance is compulsory for 24 consecutive weeks annually during school age (7–16). In 1989–90 521,114 were attending primary and secondary schools; 46,043 pupils attending non-public schools. Classroom teachers numbered 30,000 in 1988 with average salary of $25,900 (1989); in 1987–88 the state spent an average $3,846 on each elementary and secondary school student. Leading institutions for higher education (1990–91) were:

Founded	*Institution*	*Control*	*Full-time Professors*	*Students*
1843	Clarke College, Dubuque	Independent	7	876
1846	Grinnell College, Grinnell	Independent	39	1,281
1847	University of Iowa, Iowa City	State	477	28,045
1851	Coe College, Cedar Rapids	Independent	23	1,250
1852	Wartburg College, Waverly	Evangelical Lutheran	25	1,440
1853	Cornell College, Mount Vernon	Independent	31	1,140
1858	Iowa State University, Ames	State	511	25,339
1876	Univ. of Northern Iowa, Cedar Falls	State	143	12,638
1881	Drake University, Des Moines	Independent	106	8,029
1894	Morningside College, Sioux City	Methodist	19	1,366

Health. In 1988, the state had 137 hospitals (17,757 beds). In 1989-90 the state-run hospitals served 4,628 patients and had an average daily census of 692.

Social Security. Iowa has a Civil Rights Act (1939) which makes it a misdemeanour for any place of public accommodation to deprive any person of 'full and equal enjoyment' of the facilities it offers the public.

Supplemental Security Income (SSI) assistance is available for the aged (65 or older), the blind and the disabled. As of June 1990, 7,658 elderly persons were drawing an average of $125 per month, 1,066 blind persons $255 per month, and 23,532 disabled persons $267 per month. Aid to dependent children was received by 34,316 cases representing 96,406 recipients.

Further Reading

Statistical Information: State Departments of Health, Public Instruction and Social Services; State Aeronautics and Commerce Commissions; Iowa Department of Economic Development; Crop and Livestock Reporting Services, Des Moines; Iowa Dept. of Transportation, Ames; Geological Survey, Iowa City; Iowa College Aid Commission.

Annual Survey of Manufactures. US Department of Commerce
Government Finance. US Department of Commerce
Official Register. Secretary of State. Des Moines. Biennial
Petersen, W. J., *Iowa History Reference Guide.* Iowa City, 1952
Smeal, L., *Iowa Historical and Biographical Index.* New York, 1984
Vexler, R. I., *Iowa Chronology and Factbook.* Oceana, 1978

State Library of Iowa: Des Moines 50319.

KANSAS

HISTORY. Kansas, settled in 1727, was made a Territory (along with part of Colorado) in 1854, and was admitted into the Union with its present area on 29 Jan. 1861.

AREA AND POPULATION. Kansas is bounded north by Nebraska, east by Missouri, with the Missouri River as boundary in the north-east, south by Oklahoma and west by Colorado. Area, 82,277 sq. miles, including 499 sq. miles of inland water. Census population, 1 April 1980, 2,364,236, an increase of 5·1% since 1970. Estimate (1985) 2,450,000. Vital statistics, 1984: Births, 38,570 (15·8 per 1,000 population); deaths, 21,742 (8·9); infant deaths, 336 (8·7 per 1,000 live births); marriages, 24,795 (10·2); divorces 12,915 (5·3).

Population in 5 federal census years was:

	White	*Black*	*Indian*	*Asiatic*	*Total*	*Per sq. mile*
1870	346,377	17,108	914	—	364,399	4·5
1930	1,811,997	66,344	2,454	204	1,880,999	22·9
1960	2,078,666	91,445	5,069	2,271	2,178,611	26·3
			All others			
1970	2,122,068	106,977	17,533		2,249,071	27·5
1980	2,168,221	126,127	69,888		2,364,236	28·8

Of the total population in 1980, 1,156,941 were male, 1,575,899 were urban and those 20 years of age or older numbered 1,620,368.

Cities, with 1980 census population, are Wichita, 279,835; Kansas City, 161,148; Topeka (capital), 115,266; Overland Park, 81,784; Lawrence, 52,738.

CLIMATE. Dodge City. Jan. 29°F (–1·7°C), July 78°F (25·6°C). Annual rainfall 21" (518 mm). Kansas City. Jan. 30°F (–1·1°C), July 79°F (26·1°C). Annual rainfall 38" (947 mm). Topeka. Jan. 28°F (–2·2°C), July 78°F (25·6°C). Annual rainfall 35" (875 mm). Wichita. Jan. 31°F (–0·6°C), July 81°F (27·2°C). Annual rainfall 31" (777 mm). *See* Mid-West, p. 1382.

CONSTITUTION AND GOVERNMENT. The year 1861 saw the adoption of the present constitution; it has had 78 amendments. The Legislature includes a Senate of 40 members, elected for 4 years, and a House of Representatives of 125 members, elected for 2 years. Sessions are annual. The Governor and Lieut.-Governor are elected for 4 years. The right to vote (with the usual exceptions) is possessed by all citizens. The state is represented in Congress by 2 senators and 5 representatives.

The state was the first (of 42 states) to establish in 1933 a Legislative Council; this is now called the Legislative Coordinating Council and has 7 members.

In the 1988 presidential election Bush polled 552,659 votes, Dukakis, 422,056.

The capital is Topeka. The state is divided into 105 counties.

Governor: Joan Finney (D.), 1991–95 ($65,000).

BUDGET. For the year ending 30 June 1986 (Governor's Budget Report) general revenue fund was $1,863m. General expenditures were $1,738m.

Bonded debt outstanding for 1982 amounted to $316·9m.

Per capita personal income (1985) was $13,775.

ENERGY AND NATURAL RESOURCES

Minerals. Important minerals are coal, petroleum (75m. bbl. in 1985), natural gas (513,000m. cu. ft.), lead and zinc.

Agriculture. Kansas is pre-eminently agricultural, but sometimes suffers from lack of rainfall in the west. In 1985, 72,000 farms covered 48m. acres; average farm, 667 acres.

Cash income, 1985, from crops was $2,478m.; from livestock and products, $3,264m.

Kansas is a great wheat-producing state. Its output in 1985 was 433·2m. bu. valued at $1,321m. Other crops in 1985 (in bushels) were maize, 140m. ($351m.); sorghum, 207m.; soybeans, 44m.; oats and barley. The state has an extensive livestock industry, comprising, on 1 Jan. 1986, 115,000 milch cows, 5·8m. all cattle, 210,000 sheep and lambs 1·5m. swine.

INDUSTRY. Employment distribution (1985): Total workforce 975,000, of which 245,000 were in trade; 191,000 in government; 187,000 in services; 174,000 in manufacturing; 65,000 in transport and utilities; 53,000 in finance, insurance and real estate; 44,000 in construction. The slaughtering industry, other food processing, aircraft, the manufacture of transport equipment and petroleum refining are important.

COMMUNICATIONS

Roads. In 1990 there were 133,156 miles of roads (124,169 miles rural) and 1,986,647 registered motor vehicles.

Railways. There were 7,273 miles of railway in Jan. 1982.

Aviation. There were 384 airports and landing strips in 1983, of which 168 were public.

JUSTICE, RELIGION, EDUCATION AND WELFARE

Justice. There were 4,748 prisoners in state institutions, 31 Dec. 1985. The death penalty (by hanging) for murder was abolished in 1907 and restored in 1935; there have been no executions since 1968; executions 1934 to 1968 have been 15 (all for murder).

For the various Civil Rights Acts forbidding racial or political discrimination, *see* THE STATESMAN'S YEAR-BOOK, 1955, p. 666. The 1965 Kansas Act against Discrimination declared that it is the policy of the state to eliminate and prevent discrimination in all employment relations, and to eliminate and prevent discrimination, segregation or separation in all places of public accommodations covered by the Act.

Religion. The most numerous religious bodies are Roman Catholic, Methodists and Disciples of Christ.

Education. In 1982–83 organized school districts had 1,519 elementary and secondary schools which had 407,074 pupils and 26,053 teachers. Average salary of public school teachers, 1986, $22,800 (elementary and secondary). There were 20 independent colleges, 20 community colleges, 2 Bible colleges, 1 municipal university.

Kansas has 6 state-supported institutions of higher education: Kansas State University, Manhattan (1863), had 17,570 students in 1985–86; The University of Kansas, Lawrence, founded in 1865, had 24,774; Emporia State University, Emporia, had 5,344; Pittsburg State University, Pittsburg, had 5,096; Fort Hays State University, Hays, had 5,657 and Wichita State University, Wichita, had 16,902. The state also supports a two-year technical school, Kansas Technical Institute, at Salina.

Health. In 1983 the state had 165 hospitals (18,300 beds) listed by the American Hospital Association; hospitals had an average daily occupancy rate of 70·3%.

Social Security. In Dec. 1985, 20,900 persons received state and federal aid under programmes of aid to the aged or disabled, and 66,800 in 22,700 families received aid to dependent children. Average monthly payment to the aged, $121; the disabled, $206, per family with dependent children, $303 (1984).

Further Reading

Annual Economic Report of the Governor. Topeka
Directory of State Officers, Boards and Commissioners and Interesting Facts Concerning Kansas. Topeka, Biennial
Drury, J. W., *The Government of Kansas.* Lawrence, Univ. of Kansas, 1970
Zornow, W. F., *Kansas: A History of the Jayhawk State.* Norman, Okla., 1957

State Library: Kansas State Library, Topeka.

KENTUCKY

HISTORY. Kentucky, first settled in 1765, was originally part of Virginia; it was admitted into the Union on 1 June 1792 and its first legislature met on 4 June.

AREA AND POPULATION. Kentucky is bounded north by the Ohio River (forming the boundary with Illinois, Indiana and Ohio), north-east by the Big Sandy River (forming the boundary with West Virginia), east by Virginia, south by Tennessee and west by the Mississippi River (forming the boundary with Missouri). Area, 40,409 sq. miles, of which 740 sq. miles are water. Census population, 1980 3,660,777, an increase of 13·6% since 1970. Estimate (1988) 3,727,000. Births in 1987, 51,358 (13·8 per 1,000 population); deaths, 34,579 (9·3); infant deaths, 497 (9·7 per 1,000 live births); marriages, 46,917 (12·6); divorces, 19,797 (5·3).

Population in 5 census years was:

	White	*Black*	*All others*	*Total*	*Per sq.mile*
1930	2,388,364	226,040	185	2,614,589	65·1
1950	2,742,090	201,921	795	2,944,806	73·9
1960	2,820,083	215,949	2,124	3,038,156	76·2
1970	2,981,766	230,793	6,147	3,218,706	81·2
1980	3,379,006	259,477	22,294	3,660,777	92·3

Of the total population in 1980, 1,789,039 were male, 1,862,183 were urban and 2,359,614 were 21 years old or older.

The principal cities with census population in 1980 are: Louisville, 298,694 (urbanized area, 654,938); Lexington-Fayette, 204,165; Owensboro, 54,450; Covington, 49,585; Bowling Green, 40,450; Paducah, 29,315; Hopkinsville, 27,318; Ashland, 27,064; Frankfort (capital), 25,973.

CLIMATE. Kentucky has a temperate climate. Temperatures are moderate during both winter and summer, precipitation is ample without a pronounced dry season, and there is little snow during the winter. Lexington. Jan. 33°F (0·6°C), July 76°F (24·4°C). Annual rainfall 43" (1,077 mm). Louisville. Jan. 34°F (1·1°C), July 78°F (25·6°C). Annual rainfall 43" (1,077 mm). *See* Appalachian Mountains, p. 1382.

CONSTITUTION AND GOVERNMENT. The constitution dates from 1891; there had been 3 preceding it. The 1891 constitution was promulgated by convention and provides that amendments be submitted to the electorate for ratification. The General Assembly consists of a Senate of 38 members elected for 4 years, one half retiring every 2 years, and a House of Representatives of 100 members elected for 2 years. A constitutional amendment approved by the voters in Nov. 1979, changes the year in which legislators are elected from odd to even numbered years and establishes an organizational session of the legislature, limited to ten legislative days, in odd-numbered years. The amendment provides for regular sessions limited to 60 legislative days between the first Tuesday after the first Monday of Jan. and 15 April of even numbered years. The Governor and Lieut.-Governor are elected for 4 years. All citizens are (with necessary exceptions) qualified as electors; the voting age was reduced from 21 to 18 years in 1955. Registered voters, Aug. 1990: 1,829,474. In the 1988 presidential election Bush polled 734,281 votes, Dukakis, 580,368.

The state is represented in Congress by 2 senators and 7 representatives.

The capital is Frankfort. The state is divided into 120 counties.

Governor: Wallace G. Wilkinson (D.), 1987–91 ($74,649). [1]
Lieut.-Governor: Brereton Jones (D.) ($63,462). [1]
Secretary of State: Brerner Ehrler (D.) ($63,462). [1]

[1] 1990. Salaries are revised annually by the percentage change in the Consumer Price Index.

BUDGET. For the fiscal year ending 30 June 1990 revenues received within the five major operating funds amounted to $6,860m. Included in this figure are $3,561m. General Fund revenues and $1,689·6m. Federal Fund revenues. Total expenditures amounted to $6,352·8m. including education and humanities, $1,742·3m.; human resources benefits payments, $1,156·7m.; and transport, $630·9m.

The general obligation bonded indebtedness on 30 June 1990 was $70·7m.

Per capita personal income (1989) was $13,777.

ENERGY AND NATURAL RESOURCES

Minerals. The principal mineral product of Kentucky is coal, 157·9m. short tons mined in 1988, value $4,136m. Output of petroleum, 5·5m. bbls (of 42 gallons); natural gas, 73,629m. cu. ft; stone, 50·7m. short tons, value $207·9m.; clay, 840,317 short tons, value $3·2m.; sand and gravel, 6·3m. short tons, value $15m. Total value of non-fuel mineral products in 1988 was $344,979,000. Other minerals include fluorspar, ball clay, lead, zinc, silver, cement, lime, industrial sand and gravel, oil shale and tar sands.

Agriculture. In 1989, 96,000 farms had an area of 14·2m. acres. The average farm was 148 acres.

Cash income, 1989, from crops, $1,257·7m., and from livestock, $1,670m. The chief crop is tobacco: Production, in 1989, 355m. lb., ranking second to N. Carolina in US. Other principal crops include hay, corn, soybeans, wheat, fruit and vegetables, barley, sorghum grain, oats and rye.

Stock-raising is important in Kentucky, which has long been famous for its horses. The livestock in 1989 included 211,000 milch cows, 2·4m. cattle and calves, 35,000 sheep, 975,000 swine.

Forestry. Total forests area, 1978, 12,160,800 acres. Total commercial forest land, 1978, 11,901,900 acres; 92% is privately owned.

INDUSTRY. In 1989 the state's 3,661 manufacturing plants had 211,400 production workers; value added by manufacture in 1986 was $15,909·1m. The leading manufacturing industries (by employment) are non-electrical machinery, electrical machinery, apparel and transportation equipment.

TOURISM. In 1989 tourist expenditure was $4,308m., producing over $321m. in tax revenues and generating 118,444 jobs. The state had (1989) 863 hotels and motels, 232 campgrounds and 45 state parks.

COMMUNICATIONS

Roads. In 1990 the state had over 69,711 miles of federal, state and local roads. There were over 2·8m. motor vehicle registrations in 1990.

Railways. In 1988 there were 3,521 miles of railway.

Aviation. There are (1990) 69 publicly-used airports and 2,279 registered aircraft in Kentucky.

Shipping. There is an increasing amount of barge traffic on 1,090 miles of navigable rivers. There are 6 river ports and 3 planned.

JUSTICE, RELIGION, EDUCATION AND WELFARE

Justice. There are 11 prisons within the Department of Adult Institutions and one privately-run adult institution; average daily population (1989–90), 8,957, including 6,287 in prison, 448 in a private prison, 1,356 in jails awaiting incarceration, 523 in local community centres.

There has been no execution since 1962. A session of Congress in 1976 limited the death penalty to cases of kidnap and murder.

Total executions, 1911–62, were 162; 144 were for murder, 7 for rape, 6 for criminal offences, 5 for armed robbery. There were (1990) 29 people under death sentences.

Religion. The chief religious denominations in 1980 were: Southern Baptists, with 883,096 members, Roman Catholic (365,277), United Methodists (234,536), Christian Churches and Church of Christ (81,222) and Christian (Disciples of Christ) (78,275).

Education. Attendance at school between the ages of 5 and 15 years (inclusive) is compulsory, the normal term being 175 days. In 1989–90, 24,280 teachers were employed in public elementary and 11,563 in secondary schools, in which 433,557 and 197,131 pupils enrolled respectively. Expenditure on elementary and secondary day schools in 1989–90 was $2,344m.; public school classroom teachers' salaries (1989–90) averaged $26,275.

There were also 4,004 teachers working in private elementary and secondary schools with 64,433 students.

The state has 25 universities and senior colleges, 3 junior colleges and 14 community colleges, with a total (autumn 1989) of 162,216 students. Of these universities and colleges, 23 are state-supported, and the remainder are supported privately. The largest of the institutions of higher learning are (autumn 1989): University of Louisville, with 23,182 students; University of Kentucky, 22,957; Western Kentucky University, 14,821; Eastern Kentucky University, 14,268; Northern Kentucky University, 10,332; Murray State University, 8,013; Morehead State University, 7,962; Kentucky State, 2,190. Five of the several privately endowed colleges of standing are Berea College, Berea; Centre College, Danville; Transylvania University, Lexington; Georgetown College, Georgetown; and Bellarmine College, Louisville.

Health. In 1990 the state had 129 licensed hospitals (19,265 beds). There were 360 licensed long-term care facilities (30,185) and 475 licensed family care homes (1,345).

Welfare. In July 1990 there were 268,884 persons receiving financial assistance; 107,832 of these persons received the Federal Supplemental Security Income (SSI); 28,353 of them were aged, 1,906 blind, 77,573 disabled. Also, in the all state funded Supplementation programme, payments were made in July 1990 to 6,459 persons, of which 3,137 were aged, 85 blind and 3,237 disabled. The average State Supplementation payment was $133.66 to aged, $76.32 to blind and $139.63 to disabled.

In the Aid to Families with Dependent Children Programme as of July 1990, aid was given to 154,593 persons in 58,319 families. The average payment per person was $87.04, per family $230.73.

In addition to money payments, medical assistance, food stamps and social services are available.

Further Reading

Kentucky Economic Statistics. Cabinet for Economic Development, Frankfort
Kentucky Statistical Abstract. Univ. of Kentucky, Center for Business and Economic Research
Lee, L. G., *A Brief History of Kentucky and its Counties*. Berea, 1981

LOUISIANA

HISTORY. Louisiana was first settled in 1699. That part lying east of the Mississippi River was organized in 1804 as the Territory of New Orleans, and admitted into the Union on 30 April 1812. The section west of the river was added very shortly thereafter.

AREA AND POPULATION. Louisiana is bounded north by Arkansas, east by Mississippi, with the Mississippi River forming the boundary in the north-east, south by the Gulf of Mexico and west by Texas, with the Sabine River forming most of the boundary. Area, 52,453 sq. miles, including lakes, rivers and coastal waters inside 3-mile limit; land area, 44,873 sq. miles. Census population, 1 April 1980, 4,205,900, an increase of 15·5% since 1970. Estimate (1987) 4,460,578. Births, 1986, 77,944 (17·3 per 1,000 population); deaths, 36,287 (8·1); infant deaths, 925 (11·9 per 1,000 live births); marriages, 37,459 (8·4); divorces, 15,164.

Population in 5 census years was:

	White	*Black*	*Indian*	*Asiatic*	*Total*	*Per sq. mile*
1910	941,086	713,874	780	648	1,656,388	36·5
1930	1,322,712	776,326	1,536	1,019	2,101,593	46·5
1960	2,211,715	1,039,207	3,587	2,004	3,257,022	72·2
			All others			
1970	2,541,498	1,086,832	12,976		3,641,306	81·1
1980	2,911,243	1,237,263	55,466		4,203,972[1]	93·5

[1] Preliminary.

Of the 1980 total, 2,039,894 were male, 2,885,535 were urban; those 20 years of age or older numbered 2,699,100.

The largest cities with their 1980 census population (and 1987 estimate) are: New Orleans, 557,482 (555,641); Baton Rouge (capital), 219,486 (242,184); Shreveport, 205,815 (217,718); Lafayette, 81,961 (91,084); Lake Charles, 75,051 (76,599); Kenner, 66,382 (74,851).

CLIMATE. New Orleans. Jan. 54°F (12·2°C), July 83°F (28·3°C). Annual rainfall 58" (1,458 mm). *See* Gulf Coast, p. 1382.

CONSTITUTION AND GOVERNMENT. The present constitution dates from 1974.

The Legislature consists of a Senate of 39 members and a House of Representatives of 105 members, both chosen for 4 years. Sessions are annual; a fiscal session is held in odd years. The Governor and Lieut.-Governor are elected for 4 years.

A Governor may serve a second consecutive term. Qualified electors are all registered citizens with the usual residential qualifications.

In the 1988 presidential election Bush polled 880,660 votes, Dukakis, 715,475.

The state sends to Congress 2 senators and 8 representatives. Louisiana is divided into 64 parishes (corresponding with the counties of other states).

Governor: Charles E. 'Buddy' Roemer, Jr. (R.), 1988–92 ($73,440).

Lieut.-Governor: Paul Hardy (R.), 1988–92 ($63,367).
Secretary of State: W. Fox McKeithen (D.), 1988–92 ($60,169).

BUDGET. For the fiscal year ending 30 June 1987 (Louisiana State Budget Office figures) general revenues were $7,381,332,298, of which $1,885,922,784 were federal funds; total expenditures were $7,582,740,576 (education, $2,435,062,145; transport and development, $230,935,484; health, hospitals and public welfare, $2,092,812,284).

Per capita personal income (1986) was $11,191.

ENERGY AND NATURAL RESOURCES

Minerals. The yield in 1987 of crude petroleum was 144m. bbls; marketed production of natural gas, 1,572,835,903m. cu. ft. Rich sulphur mines are found in the state, and wells for the extraction of sulphur by means of hot water and compressed air are in operation; output, 1986, 524,000 tonnes.

Louisiana is the USA's main salt producer. Output of salt (1986) was 11·6m. short tons.

Agriculture. The state is divided into two parts, the uplands and the alluvial and swamp regions of the coast. A delta occupies about one-third of the total area. Manufacturing is the leading industry, but agriculture is important. In 1986 there were about 36,000 farms with annual average sales of at least $1,000; average farm, 278 acres; average value per acre $1,256.

Cash income, 1986, from crops $1,371·69m.; from livestock, $502·7m. Crops by value: Soybeans, $189·9m.; rice, $110·9m.; cotton lint, $179·7m.; sugar-cane, $115·2m..

In 1985 the state contained 89,910 milch cows, 1·2m. all cattle, 25,114 sheep and 133,349 swine.

Fisheries. The catch in 1986 was 1,700m. lb., value $321·5m.

Forestry. Forests, 13·9m. acres, represent 49% of the state's area. Income from manufactured products exceeds $2,500m. annually. In 1986 pulpwood cut, 5·1m. cords; sawtimber cut, 1,500m. bd ft.

INDUSTRY. The manufacturing industries are chiefly those associated with petroleum, chemicals, lumber, food, paper. In 1987 167,600 were employed in manufacturing, 368,500 in trade and 327,200 in service industries.

TOURISM. Travellers spent an estimated $4,000m. in 1987. Tourism is the second most important industry for state income.

COMMUNICATIONS

Roads. In 1990 there were 58,521 miles of roads (46,277 miles rural) and 2,967,097 registered motor vehicles.

Railways. In 1986 there were 3,347 miles of track in the state.

Aviation. In 1988 there were 386 commercial and private airports.

Shipping. In 1984 New Orleans handled 43·9m. short tons of cargo. The Mississippi and other waterways provide 7,500 miles of navigable water.

JUSTICE, RELIGION, EDUCATION AND WELFARE

Justice. State and federal prisons, Nov. 1988, had 16,121 inmates. Execution is by electrocution; there were 135 between 1930 and 1961, 15 between 1977 and 1987.

Religion. The Roman Catholic Church is the largest denomination in Louisiana. The leading Protestant Churches are Southern Baptist and Methodist.

Education. School attendance is compulsory between the ages of 7 and 15, both inclusive. In 1986–87 there were 804,645 pupils in public elementary and secondary schools. In 1987 the 42,019 instructional staff had an average salary of $20,235. There are 17 four-year public colleges and universities and 11 non-public four-year institutions of higher learning. There are 47 state trade and vocational-technical schools. Superior instruction is given in the Louisiana State University with 54,912 students (1987). Tulane University in New Orleans had 10,302; The Roman Catholic Loyola University in New Orleans had 5,210; Dillard University in New Orleans had 1,218; and the Southern University System, 5,210.

Health. In 1988 the state had 186 licensed hospitals and 3 state mental hospitals.

Social Security. In Dec. 1985, assistance was being given to 49,400 elderly persons; 78,800 families with dependent children; 74,700 disabled people. Aid was from state and federal sources.

Further Reading

Davis, E. A., *Louisiana, the Pelican State.* Louisiana State Univ. Press, Baton Rouge, 1975
Kniffen, F. B., *Louisiana, its Land and People.* Louisiana State Univ. Press, Baton Rouge, 1968

State Library: The Louisiana State Library, Baton Rouge, Louisiana. *State Librarian:* Thomas F. Jaques.

MAINE

HISTORY. After a first attempt in 1607, Maine was settled in 1623. From 1652 to 1820 it was part of Massachusetts and was admitted into the Union on 15 March 1820.

AREA AND POPULATION. Maine is bounded west, north and east by Canada, south-east by the Atlantic, south and south-west by New Hampshire. Area, 33,265 sq. miles, of which 2,269 are inland water. Of the state's total area, about 17·2m. acres (87%) are in timber and wood lots. Census population, 1 April 1980 1,125,027, an increase of 13·29% since 1970. Estimate (1986) 1,174,000. In 1986 live births numbered 16,717 (14·3 per 1,000 population); deaths, 10,796 (9·2); infant deaths, 146 (8·9 per 1,000 live births); marriages, 10,887 (9·2); divorces 5,621 (4·8).

Population for 5 census years was:

	White	*Black*	*Indian*	*Asiatic*	*Total*	*Per sq. mile*
1910	739,995	1,363	892	121	742,371	24·8
1930	795,185	1,096	1,012	130	797,423	25·7
1950	910,846	1,221	1,522	185	913,774	29·4
			All others			
1970	985,276	2,800	3,972		992,048	31·0
1980	1,109,850	3,128	12,049		1,125,027	36·3

Of the total population in 1980, 48·5% were male, 40·7% were urban and 60·5% were 21 years or older.

The largest city in the state is Portland with a census population of 61,572 in 1980. Other cities (with population in 1980) are: Lewiston, 40,481; Bangor, 31,643; Auburn, 23,128; South Portland, 22,712; Augusta (capital), 21,819; Biddeford, 19,638; Waterville, 17,779.

CLIMATE. Average maximum temperatures range from 56·3°F in Waterville to 48·3°F in Caribou, but record high (since *c.* 1950) is 103°F. Average minimum ranges from 36·9°F in Rockland to 28·3°F in Greenville, but record low (also in Greenville) is –42°F. Average annual rainfall ranges from 48·85" in Machias to 36·09" in Houlton. Average annual snowfall ranges from 118·7" in Greenville to 59·7" in Rockland. *See* New England, p. 1382.

CONSTITUTION AND GOVERNMENT. The constitution of 1820 is still in force, but it has been amended 153 times. In 1951, 1965 and 1973 the Legislature approved recodifications of the constitution as arranged by the Chief Justice under special authority.

The Legislature consists of the Senate with 35 members and the House of Representatives with 151 members, both Houses being elected simultaneously for 2 years. Apart from these legislators and the Governor (elected for 4 years), no other state officers are elected. The Justices of the Supreme Judicial Court give their opinion upon important questions of law and upon solemn occasions when required by the Governor, Senate or House of Representatives. The suffrage is possessed by all citizens, 18 years of age; persons under guardianship for reasons of mental illness have no vote. Indians residing on tribal reservations and otherwise qualified have the vote in all county, state and national elections but retain the right to elect their own tribal representative to the legislature.

In the 1988 presidential election Bush polled 304,087 votes, Dukakis, 240,508.

The state sends to Congress 2 senators and 2 representatives.

The capital is Augusta. The state is divided into 16 counties.

Governor: John R. McKernan (R.), 1991–95 ($35,000).

BUDGET. For the financial year ending 30 June 1986 general revenue was $932m. and expenditure was $927m.

Total net long-term debt on 30 June 1984 was $294·5m.

Per capita personal income (1987) was $13,720.

NATURAL RESOURCES

Minerals. Minerals include sand and gravel, stone, lead, clay, copper, peat, silver and zinc. Mineral output, 1986, was valued at $46m.

Agriculture. In 1986, 7,800 farms occupied 2m. acres; the average farm was 194 acres.

Cash receipts, 1985, $378m., of which $80m. came from potatoes; Maine is the third largest producer of potatoes (about 7% of the country's total of 325·7m. cwt). Other important items include eggs ($94m.), dairy products ($107·5m.) and poultry ($29·7m.); these with potatoes provide 78% of receipts. Sweet corn, peas and beans, oats, hay, apples and blueberries are also grown. On 1 Jan. 1983 the farm animals included 57,000 milch cows, 146,000 all other cattle, and 14,000 sheep.

Forestry. Lumber, wood turnings and pulp are important. In 1982 the cut of softwood was 769,195m. bd ft; hardwood, 150,878m. bd ft, and pulpwood, 3,417,586 cords. Spruce and fir, white pine, hemlock, white and yellow birch, sugar maple, northern white cedar, beech and red oak are the most important species cut. There were (1982) 17,600,000 acres of commercial forest (98% in private ownership). National forests comprise 37,500 acres; other federal, 35,800; state forests, 163,000 acres; municipal, 75,200 acres. Wood products industries are of great economic importance; in 1982 the lumber, wood and paper industries' production was valued at $3,355,731. There were (1982) 342 primary manufacturers and over 1,400 secondary.

Fisheries. In 1983, 202,657,000 lb. of fish and shellfish (valued at $107,889,000 were landed; the catch included 21,976,000 lb. of lobsters (valued at $51,234,000). 1·97m. lb. of scallops ($10·8m.); 4·14m. lb. of soft clams ($7·24m.); 12·31m. lb of dabs ($6·0m.); 42·4m. lb. of menhaden ($846,000); 40m. lb. of herring ($2·14m.).

INDUSTRY. Total non-agricultural workforce, 1985, 459,000. Manufacturing employed 106,000; trade, 108,000; services, 95,000; government, 86,000; the main manufacture is paper at 47 plants, producing about 34% of manufacturing value added.

LABOUR. The four largest employers are government, education, health and tourism.

TOURISM. In 1987 there were about 4·8m. tourists (including state residents on holiday), generating nearly $1,000m. in business. Eating, drinking and accommodation produce 12·4% of sales tax.

COMMUNICATIONS

Roads. In 1990 there were 22,240 miles of roads (19,781 miles rural) and 939,301 registered motor vehicles.

Railways. In 1984 there were 1,516 miles of mainline railway tracks.

Aviation. Licensed airports, 1984, numbered 76, including 37 commercial public airports, 12 non-commercial and 4 commuter airports, 15 commercial and 4 non-commercial seaplane bases, and 4 air-carrier airports. There were also 2 military airports and 23 private landing strips.

JUSTICE, RELIGION, EDUCATION AND WELFARE

Justice. The state's penal system in Sept. 1984 held 435 adults in the State Prison, 237 in the Correctional Center and 332 juveniles in the Youth Center. There is no capital punishment. Inmates serving life sentences are eligible for parole consideration after 15 years, less remission for good conduct, provided they were imprisoned before the passage of a new Criminal Code by the 107th Maine Legislature, which abolished the parole system.

Religion. The largest religious bodies are: Roman Catholic (270,283 members), Baptists (36,808 members) and Congregationalists (40,750 members), and other Christian Churches (34,066 members).

Education. Education is free for pupils from 5 to 21 years of age, and compulsory from 7 to 17. In 1983–84 the 756 public schools (610 elementary, 105 secondary and 41 combined elementary and secondary) had 12,283 staff and 209,753 enrolled pupils. In 1983–84 there were 126 private schools with 1,035 teachers and 15,461 pupils. Public school teachers' salaries, 1983–84, averaged $17,328. Total public expenditure on public elementary and secondary education in 1982–83, $461,252,847.

The state University of Maine, founded in 1865, had (1983–84) 1,003 teaching staff and 28,591 students at 7 locations; Bowdoin College, founded in 1794 at Brunswick, (107 and 1,371); Bates College at Lewiston, (104 and 1,424); Colby College at Waterville, (125 and 1,733); Husson College, Bangor, (31 and 1,465); Westbrook College at Westbrook, (56 and 1,120); Unity College at Unity, (23 and 325), and the University of New England (formerly St Francis College) at Biddeford, (55 and 848).

Health. In 1984 the state had 42 general hospitals (4,571 beds for acute care); 3 hospitals for mental diseases, acute and psychiatric care (541 beds); 144 nursing homes (10,220 beds).

Social Security. Supplemental Security Income (SSI) (maximum payment for single person, $324·30 per month) is administered by the Social Security Administration. It became effective on 1 Jan. 1974 and replaces former aid to the aged, blind and disabled, administered by the state with state and federal funds. SSI is supplemented by Medicaid for nursing home patients or hospital patients. State payments for SSI recipients for 1985 totalled $42·3m., covering 22,000 cases. Aid to families with dependent children is granted where one or both parents are disabled or absent and income is insufficient; aid was being granted in Aug. 1985 to 20,100 families (58,300 children) with an average payment per family of $321 per month. Payments under Maine Medicaid Assistance programme totalled $217m. for the financial year 1983–84. There is a programme of assistance for catastrophic illness. Child welfare services include basic child protective services, enforcing child support, establishing paternity and finding missing parents, foster home placements, adoptions; services in divorce cases and licensing of foster homes, day care and residential treatment services, and public guardianship. There are also protective services for adults.

Further Reading

Maine Register, State Year-Book and Legislative Manual. Tower Publishing, Portland. Annual
Banks, R., *Maine Becomes A State.* Wesleyan U.P., 1970
Caldwell, B., *Rivers of Fortune.* Gannett, 1983
Calvert, M. R., *Dawn over the Kennebec.* Private Pr., 1983
Clark, C., *Maine.* New York, 1977

MARYLAND

HISTORY. Maryland, first settled in 1634, was one of the 13 original states.

AREA AND POPULATION. Maryland is bounded north by Pennsylvania, east by Delaware and the Atlantic, south by Virginia and West Virginia, with the Potomac River forming most of the boundary, and west by West Virginia. Chesapeake Bay almost cuts off the eastern end of the state from the rest. Area, 10,460 sq. miles, of which 623 sq. miles are inland water; in addition, water area under Maryland jurisdiction in Chesapeake Bay amounts to 1,726 sq. miles. Census population, 1 April 1980, 4,216,975, an increase since 1970 of 293,078 or 7·5%. Estimate (1986) 4,463,000. In 1985 births were 67,985 (15·5 per 1,000 population); deaths, 36,607 (8·3); infant deaths, 811 (11·9 per 1,000 live births); marriages, 46,063 (10·5); divorces, 16,187 (3·7).

Population for 5 federal censuses was:

	White	*Black*	*Indian*	*Asiatic*	*Total*	*Per sq. mile*
1920	1,204,737	244,479	32	413	1,449,661	145·8
1930	1,354,226	276,379	50	871	1,631,526	165·0
1960	2,573,919	518,410	1,538	5,700	3,100,689	314·0
			All others			
1970	3,194,888	499,479	28,032		3,922,399	396·6
1980	3,158,838	958,150	99,987		4,216,975	428·7

Of the total population in 1980, 2,042,810 were male, 3,386,555 persons were urban and those 20 years old or older numbered 2,890,196.

The largest city in the state (containing 16·9% of the population) is Baltimore, with 786,741 in 1980 (and 751,400 in 1988); Baltimore metropolitan area, 2·3m. Maryland residents in the Washington, D.C., metropolitan area total more than 1·7m. Other cities (1980) are Dundalk (71,293); Towson (51,083); Silver Spring (72,893); Bethesda (62,736). Incorporated places, estimate 1986: Rockville, 46,900; Bowie, 35,740; Hagerstown, 33,670; Frederick, 33,800; Annapolis, 33,360; Gaithersburg, 32,350; Cumberland, 23,230; Cambridge, 11,070.

CLIMATE. Baltimore. Jan. 36°F (2·2°C), July 79°F (26·1°C). Annual rainfall 41" (1,026 mm). *See* Atlantic Coast, p. 1382.

CONSTITUTION AND GOVERNMENT. The present constitution dates from 1867; it has had 125 amendments. The General Assembly consists of a Senate of 47, and a House of Delegates of 141 members, both elected for 4 years, as are the Governor and Lieut.-Governor. Voters are citizens who have the usual residential qualifications. At the 1988 presidential election Bush polled 834,202 votes, Dukakis, 793,939.

Maryland sends to Congress 2 senators and 8 representatives.

The state capital is Annapolis. The state is divided into 23 counties and Baltimore City.

Governor: William D. Schaefer (D.), 1991–95 ($75,000).

BUDGET. For the fiscal year ending 30 June 1989 general revenues were $8,820,102,000 ($6,369,830,000 from taxation). General expenditures,

$8,567,633,000, including $1,902,965,000 for education and $2,480,021,000 for public welfare and health; $1,475,634,000 for transport.

Total authorized long-term state debt, 30 June 1989 was $3,007·36m. (Issued and outstanding, $2,005·36m.; authorized but not issued, $1,002m.)

Per capita personal income (1989) was $21,013.

ENERGY AND NATURAL RESOURCES

Minerals. Value of non-fuel mineral production, 1989, was $367m. Sand and gravel (18·5m. short tons) and stone (33·4m. short tons) account for 73% of the total value. Coal is the leading mineral commodity by value followed by, stone, sand and gravel and Portland cement. Output of coal was 3.3m. short tons, valued at about $83m. Natural gas is produced from 1 field in Garrett County; 34m. cu. ft in 1989. A second gas field in the same county is used for natural gas storage.

Agriculture. Agriculture is an important industry in the state. In 1988 there were approximately 16,000 farms with an area of 2·4m. acres (37% of the land area).

Farm animals, 1 Jan. 1989, were: Milch cows, 109,000; all cattle, 328,000; swine, 170,000; sheep, 35,000; chickens (not broilers), 4·8m. The most important crops, 1988, were: Corn for grain, 27·3m. bu.; soybeans, 14·1m. bu.; tobacco, 12m. lb., and hay, 619,000 bu.

Cash receipts from farm marketings, 1988, were $1,221m.; from livestock and livestock products, $767m., and crops, $454m. Dairy products and broilers are important.

INDUSTRY. In 1987 manufactories had 139,600 production workers earning $2,994·3m.; value added by manufacture, $14,020m. Chief industries are printing and publishing, food and kindred products, instruments and related products, chemicals and products.

TOURISM. Tourism is one of the state's leading industries. In 1988 tourists spent over $5,875m.

COMMUNICATIONS

Roads. The state highway department maintained, 1 Jan. 1990, 5,205 miles of highways, of which 83 miles were toll roads. The 23 counties maintained 18,578 miles of highways, and the 159 municipalities (including the city of Baltimore) maintained 4,102 miles of streets and alleys. Total mileage, 1 Jan. 1990, of public highways, streets and alleys, 27,885 miles. In 1989, an estimated 3·5m. automobiles were registered.

Railways. Railways, in 1990, had 1,068 miles of line.

Aviation. There were, 1990, 46 commercially licensed aiports.

Shipping. In 1989 Baltimore was the seventh largest US seaport in value of trade, eighth in tonnage handled.

JUSTICE, RELIGION, EDUCATION AND WELFARE

Justice. Prisons on 10 Oct. 1990 had about 16,277 men and 775 women; the total equalled 360 per 100,000 population, a high rate, which may be explained by the fact that Maryland incarcerates domestic relations law violators in state prisons; state prisons also receive a considerable number of persons committed for misdemeanours by magistrates' courts of the counties as well as from Baltimore's court system.

Since 1930 there have been 68 executions (by lethal gas since 1957; earlier by hanging)—7 whites and 37 Negroes for murder, and 6 whites and 18 Negroes for rape. Last execution was June 1961.

Maryland's prison system has conducted a work-release programme for selected prisoners since 1963. All institutions have academic and vocational training programmes.

In accordance with the 1950 Supreme Court decisions declaring segregation unconstitutional, the University of Maryland and other public and private colleges began admitting Black students in Sept. 1956; elementary and secondary schools followed.

Religion. Maryland was the first US state to give religious freedom to all who came within its borders. Present religious affiliations of the population are approximately: Protestant, 32%; Roman Catholic, 24%; Jewish, 10%; remaining 34% is nonrelated and other faiths.

Education. Education is compulsory from 6 to 16 years of age. In Sept. 1989 the public elementary schools (including kindergartens and secondary schools) had 698,806 pupils. Teachers and principals in the elementary and secondary schools numbered 44,029. Teachers' average salary in 1988–89 was $34,159. Current expenditure by local school boards on education, 1988–89, was $3,480·8m., of which the state's contribution was $1,387·9m.

In 1990 there were 33 degree-granting 4-year institutions and 23 2-year colleges. The largest was the University of Maryland system, with 104,584 students (Sept. 1990), consisting of 11 campuses with the highest enrolment at College Park (34,837) and Towson State University (15,034).

Health. In Sept. 1990, 86 hospitals (19,503 beds) were licensed by the State Department of Health and Mental Hygiene.

The Maryland State Department of Health, organized in 1874, was in 1969 made part of the Department of Health and Mental Hygiene which performs its functions through its central office, 23 county health departments and the Baltimore City Health Department. For the financial year 1989 the department's budget was $1,774·7m., of which $1,212·7m. were general funds and $45.5m. special funds appropriated by the General Assembly. The balance of the budget, $516·5m., derives from federal funds.

During financial year 1990 Maryland's programme of medical care for indigent and medically indigent patients covered about 437,000 persons. The programme, which covers in-patient and out-patient hospital services, laboratory services, skilled nursing home care, physician services, pharmacy services, dental services and home health services, cost approximately $1,138m.

Social Security. Under the supervision of the Department of Human Resources, local social service departments administer public assistance for needy persons. In March 1990 families with dependent children received $24,968,328 (186,313 recipients, average actual monthly payment $134.01); general public assistance payments were $3,836,260 (19,039 recipients, average actual monthly payments $201.49).

Further Reading

Statistical Information: Maryland Department of Economic and Employment Development, Baltimore City, 21202.

Maryland Manual: A Compendium of Legal, Historical and Statistical Information Relating to the State of Maryland. Annapolis. Biennial

DiLisio, J. E., *Maryland.* Boulder, 1982

Papenfuse, E. C., et al., *Maryland, a New Guide to the Old Line State.* Johns Hopkins Univ. Press, 1976

Rollo, V. F., *Maryland's Constitution and Government.* Maryland Hist. Press, Rev. ed., 1982

State Library: Maryland State Library, Annapolis. *Director:* Michael S. Miller.

MASSACHUSETTS

HISTORY. The first permanent settlement within the borders of the present state was made at Plymouth in Dec. 1620, by the Pilgrims from Holland, who were separatists from the English Church, and formed the nucleus of the Plymouth Colony. In 1628 another company of Puritans settled at Salem, forming eventually the Massachusetts Bay Colony. In 1630 Boston was settled. In the struggle which ended in the separation of the American colonies from the mother country, Massachusetts took the foremost part, and on 6 Feb. 1788 became the sixth state to ratify the US constitution.

AREA AND POPULATION. Massachusetts is bounded north by Vermont and New Hampshire, east by the Atlantic, south by Connecticut and Rhode Island and west by New York. Area, 8,284 sq. miles, 460 sq. miles being inland water.The census population 1 April 1980, was 5,737,037, an increase of 47,867 or 0·8% since 1970. Estimate (1985) 5,819,087. Births, 1985 were 82,872 (14·2 per 1,000 population); deaths, 54,935 (9·4 per 1,000); infant deaths (1984), 739 (9·3 per 1,000 live births); marriages, 51,648 (8·9); divorces, 19,794 (3·4).

Population at 4 federal census years was:

	White	*Black*	*Other*	*Total*	*Per sq. mile*
1950	4,611,503	73,171	5,840	4,690,514	598·4
1960	5,023,144	111,842	13,592	5,148,578	656·8
1970	5,477,624	175,817	35,729	5,689,170	725·8
1980	5,362,836	221,279	152,922	5,737,037	732·0

Of the total population in 1980, 47·6% were male, 83·8% were urban and 32% were 21 years old or older.

In 1985 the population of the principal towns and cities was:

Boston	571,980	Lowell	93,343	Framingham	64,999
Worcester	160,489	Fall River	92,560	Lawrence	64,970
Springfield	151,015	Quincy	83,845	Leominster	64,768
New Bedford	98,900	Newton	82,384	Waltham	57,609
Brockton	98,040	Lynn	79,207	Medford	57,191
Cambridge	93,405	Somerville	75,802	Chicopee	55,936

The largest of 10 standard metropolitan statistical areas, 1980 census were: Boston, 2,763,357; Springfield–Chicopee–Holyoke, 530,668; Worcester, 372,940.

CLIMATE. Boston. Jan. 28°F (–2·2°C), July 71°F (21·7°C). Annual rainfall 41" (1,036 mm). *See* New England, p. 1382.

CONSTITUTION AND GOVERNMENT. The constitution dates from 1780 and has had 116 amendments. The legislative body, styled the General Court of the Commonwealth of Massachusetts, meets annually, and consists of the Senate with 40 members, elected biennially, and the House of Representatives of 160 members, elected for 2 years. The Governor and Lieut.-Governor are elected for 4 years. The state sends 2 senators and 11 representatives to Congress.

At the 1988 presidential election Dukakis polled 1,387,398 votes, Bush, 1,184,323.

Electors are all citizens 18 years of age or older.

The capital is Boston. The state has 14 counties, 39 cities and 312 towns.

Governor: William F. Weld (R.), 1991–95 ($75,000).

BUDGET. For the fiscal year ending 30 June 1986 the total revenue of the state was $9,569·6m. ($7,488·3m. from taxes, $1,201·7m. from federal aid, $879·6m. from other sources); total expenditures, $9,692·7m. ($1,389·3m. for education, $418·7m. for highway transport and highway construction and $3,659·6m. for human services).

The net long-term debt on 30 June 1986 amounted to $3,645m.

Per capita personal income (1986) was $17,516.

NATURAL RESOURCES

Minerals. There is little mining within the state. Total mineral output in 1985 was valued at $114·5m., of which most came from sand, gravel, crushed stone and lime.

Agriculture. On 1 Jan. 1986 there were approximately 6,000 farms (11,179 in 1959) with an area of 598,900 acres.

Cash income, 1986, totalled \$425·2m.; dairy, \$76·3m.; greenhouse and nursery, \$118m.; poultry, \$30·8m.; vegetables, \$38·8m.; tobacco, \$7m.; cranberries, \$98·6m.; other fruit, \$23·2m.; potatoes, \$2·6m. Total from crops, \$295·2m., from livestock, \$130m.

Principal 1986 crops include cranberries, 1·69m. bbls; apples, 2·1m. bu. in 1985; potatoes, 825,000 cwt in 1985. On 1 Jan. 1982 farms in the state had 48,000 milch cows, 98,000 all cattle, 49,000 swine. In 1982 farms produced 145,000 turkeys and 0·8m. chickens.

Forestry. About 68% of the state is forest. State forests cover about 256,000 acres. Total forest land covers about 3m. acres. Commercially important hardwoods are sugar maple, northern red oak and white ash; softwoods are white pine and hemlock. About 240m. bd ft of timber are cut annually.

Fisheries. The 1985 catch amounted to 296m. lb. of fish and shellfish valued at \$232m.

INDUSTRY. In 1986, manufacturing establishments employed an average of 637,740 workers. The 3 most important manufacturing groups, based on employment, were electric and electronic equipment, machinery (except electrical), printing and publishing. Service industries employed 875,736 and trade, 697,257. Total non-agricultural employment, 2,685,611.

COMMUNICATIONS

Roads. In 1990 there were 33,807 miles of public roads (13,201 miles rural) and 3,804,458 registered motor vehicles.

Railways. In 1984 there were 1,310 miles of mainline railway.

Aviation. There were, in 1983, 52 aircraft landing areas for commercial operation, of which 27 were publicly owned.

Shipping. The state has 3 deep-water harbours, the largest of which is Boston (port trade (1983), 16,767,585 short tons). Other ports are Fall River and New Bedford.

JUSTICE, RELIGION, EDUCATION AND WELFARE

Justice. On 31 Dec. 1985 state penal institutions held 5,447 inmates. There have been no executions since 1947.

Religion. The principal religious bodies are the Roman Catholics, Jewish Congregations, Methodists, Episcopalians and Unitarians.

Education. A regulation effective from 1 Sept. 1972 makes school attendance compulsory for ages 6–16. In 1985–86 expenditure by cities and towns on public schools was \$3,521m. or \$605 per capita, including debt retirement and service payments. In 1985–86 there were 56,400 classroom teachers and approximately 900,000 pupils.

Within the state there were (1982) 126 degree-granting institutions of higher learning (including 89 colleges and universities). Some leading institutions are:

Year opened	*Name and location of universities and colleges*	*Students 1988*
1636	Harvard University, Cambridge [1]	16,871
1839	Framingham State College	4,303
1839	Westfield State College	6,053
1840	Bridgewater State College	6,539
1852	Tufts University, Medford [1], [3]	6,297
1854	Salem State College	6,364
1861	Mass. Institute of Technology, Cambridge [1]	9,158
1863	University of Massachusetts, Amherst [1]	26,233

[1] Co-educational. [3] Includes Jackson College for women.
[2] For women only. [4] Includes Forsyth Dental Center School.

Year opened	Name and location of universities and colleges	Students 1988
1863	Boston College (RC), Chestnut Hill [1]	12,858
1865	Worcester Polytechnic Institute, Worcester [1]	4,022
1869	Boston University, Boston [1]	22,373
1874	Worcester College	4,899
1894	Fitchburg State College	5,212
1894	University of Lowell [1]	10,445
1895	Southeastern Massachusetts University	5,031
1898	Northeastern University, Boston [1, 4]	20,618
1899	Simmons College, Boston [2]	2,594
1905	Wentworth Institute of Technology	3,350
1906	Suffolk University	5,978
1917	Bentley College	5,611
1919	Western New England College	3,686
1919	Babson College	3,163
1947	Merrimack College	2,300
1948	Brandeis University, Waltham [1]	3,484
1964	University of Massachusetts, Boston	8,027

[1] Co-educational. [3] Includes Jackson College for women.
[2] For women only. [4] Includes Forsyth Dental Center School.

Health. In 1984 the state had 177 hospitals (with 41,200 beds); average daily census, 1982, 32,736, including patients in public and private mental hospitals and institutions for the mentally retarded.

Social Security. The Department of Public Welfare had an appropriation of $1,828m. in financial year 1984 and paid $388m. in aid to families with dependent children (average 95,798 families per month); other main items were general relief (average 27,242 cases), Supplemental Security Income (average 105,402 cases) and Medical Assistance only (average 65,841 cases).

Further Reading

Annual Reports. Massachusetts and US Boards, Commissions, Departments and Divisions, Boston, annual
Manual for the General Court. By Clerk of the Senate and Clerk of the House of Representatives, Boston, Mass. Biennial
Hart, Albert B., (ed.) *Commonwealth History of Massachusetts, Colony, Province and State*. 5 vols., New York, 1966
Levitan, D. with Mariner, E. C., *Your Massachusetts Government*. Newton, Mass., 1984
Higher Education Publications, Washington, D.C., 1983

MICHIGAN

HISTORY. Michigan, first settled by Marquette at Sault Ste Marie in 1668, became the Territory of Michigan in 1805, with its boundaries greatly enlarged in 1818 and 1834; it was admitted into the Union with its present boundaries on 26 Jan. 1837.

AREA AND POPULATION. Michigan is divided into two by Lake Michigan. The northern part is bounded south by the lake and by Wisconsin, west and north by Lake Superior, east by the North Channel of Lake Huron; between the two latter lakes the Canadian border runs through straits at Sault Ste Marie. The southern part is bounded west and north by Lake Michigan, east by Lake Huron, Ontario and Lake Erie, south by Ohio and Indiana. Area, 58,527 sq. miles, of which 56,954 sq. miles are land area, 1,573 sq. miles are inland water. Census population, 1 April 1980, 9,262,078, an increase of 380,252 or 4·3% since 1970. Estimate (1986) 9,145,000. In 1985 births were 138,902 (15·2 per 1,000 population); deaths, 78,515 (8·7); infant deaths, 1,575 (11·4 per 1,000 live births); marriages, 79,022 (17·4); divorces, 38,775 (8·5).

Population of 5 federal census years was:

	White	*Black*	*Indian*	*Asiatic*	*Total*	*Per sq. mile*
1910	2,785,247	17,115	7,519	292	2,810,173	48·9
1930	4,663,507	169,453	7,080	2,285	4,842,325	84·9
1960	7,085,865	717,581	9,701	10,047	7,823,194	137·2
			All others			
1970	7,833,474	991,066	50,543		8,875,083	156·2
1980	7,872,241	1,199,023	190,814		9,262,078	162·6

Of the total population in 1980, 4,516,189 were male, 6,551,551 persons were urban and those 20 years old or older numbered 6,146,694. 162,440 were of Spanish origin.

Population of the chief cities (census of 1 April 1980) was:

Detroit	1,203,339	Dearborn	90,660	Royal Oak	70,893
Grand Rapids	181,843	Westland	84,603	Dearborn Heights	67,706
Warren	161,134	Kalamazoo	79,722	Troy	67,102
Flint	159,611	Taylor	77,568	Wyoming	59,616
Lansing (capital)	130,414	Saginaw	77,508	Farmington Hills	58,056
Sterling Heights	108,999	Pontiac	76,715	Roseville	54,311
Ann Arbor	107,316	St Clair Shores	76,210		
Livonia	104,814	Southfield	75,568		

Larger standard metropolitan areas, 1980 census: Detroit, 4,353,413; Grand Rapids, 601,680; Flint, 521,589; Lansing, 471,565.

CLIMATE. Detroit. Jan. 22·1°F (–5·5°C), July 72°F (22·2°C). Annual rainfall 32" (813 mm). Grand Rapids. Jan. 23·8°F (–4·6°C), July 72·6°F (22·5°C). Annual rainfall 33·6" (833 mm). Lansing. Jan. 21·7°F (–5·7°C), July 71°F (21·7°C). Annual rainfall 30·8" (782 mm). *See* Great Lakes, p. 1382.

CONSTITUTION AND GOVERNMENT. The present constitution was adopted in April 1963 and became effective on 1 Jan. 1964. The Senate consists of 38 members, elected for 4 years, and the House of Representatives of 110 members, elected for 2 years. The Governor and Lieut.-Governor are elected for 4 years. Electors are all citizens over 18 years of age meeting the usual residential requirements. The state sends to Congress 2 senators and 18 representatives.

At the 1988 presidential election Bush polled 1,969,435 votes, Dukakis, 1,673,496.

The capital is Lansing. The state is organized in 83 counties.

Governor: John Engler (R.), 1991–95 ($100,077).

BUDGET. For the financial year ending 30 Sept. 1986, the general fund revenue was $12,769,500,000 (taxation, $9,270,600,000, and federal aid, $3,298,600,000); total revenue, $13,607,400,000; special revenue funds, $837,900,000; general expenditures, $12,235,600,000.

Per capita personal income (1985 estimate) was $13,608.

ENERGY AND NATURAL RESOURCES

Minerals. Most important minerals by value of production are iron ore, petroleum and cement. Output (1985): Iron ore, 12·69m. long tons; Portland cement, 4·75m. short tons; petroleum, 31·5m. bbls; sand and gravel, 41·35m. short tons; lime, 534,000 short tons; natural gas, 153,484,651m. cu. ft; Salt, 991,000 short tons. Mineral output in 1984 was valued at $2,695·2m.

Agriculture. The state, formerly agricultural, is now chiefly industrial. In 1985 it contained 63,000 farms with a total area of 11m. acres; the average farm was 175 acres. Cash income, 1985, from crops, $1,729·6m.; from livestock and products, $1,237m. Principal crops are maize (production, 1985, 287·6m. bu. of grain), oats (26·1m. bu.), wheat (45m. bu.), sugar-beet (2·33m. tons); soybeans (34·6m. bu.), hay (5·7m. tons). On 1 Jan. 1986 there were in the state 108,000 sheep, 397,000 milch cows, 1·41m. all cattle and 1·19m. swine; 8·9m. chickens and 38,000 (1985) turkey breeder hens. In 1985 the wool clip yielded 902,000 lb. of wool.

Forestry. The forests of Michigan consist of 18·4m. acres, about 51% of total state land area. About 17·5m. acres of this total is commercial forest, 64% of which is privately owned, 20% state forest, 14% federal forest and 1·5% in various public ownerships. Three-fourths of the timber volume is hardwoods, principally hard and soft maples, aspen, oak and birch. Christmas trees are another important forest crop.

Michigan leads in the number of state parks and public campsites. There are 83 state parks and recreation areas, 6 state forests, 3 national forests and 3 national parks. There are 169 state forest campgrounds and 64 state game areas.

INDUSTRY. Transport equipment and non-electrical machinery are the most important manufactures. The state ranks first in 19 manufacturing categories; among principal products are motor vehicles and trucks, cement, chemicals, furniture, paper, cereal, baby food and pharmaceuticals. Total non-agricultural labour force, 1986, 4,386,000, of which 975,000 are in manufacturing.

COMMUNICATIONS

Roads. In 1990 there were 117,996 miles of roads (90,968 miles rural) and 7,138,583 registered motor vehicles.

Railways. On 1 Jan. 1986 there were 4,770 miles of railway and 67 miles of active car-ferry routes.

Aviation. Airports (1986) numbered 245 licensed airports and 22 air carrier airports.

JUSTICE, RELIGION, EDUCATION AND WELFARE

Justice. The 1963 Constitution provides that no person shall be denied the equal protection of the law; nor shall any person be denied the enjoyment of his civil or political rights or be discriminated against in the exercise thereof because of religion, colour or national origin. A Civil Rights Commission was established, and its powers and duties were implemented by legislation in the extra session of 1963. Earlier statutory enactments guaranteeing civil rights in specific areas are as follows. An Act of 1885, last amended in 1956, orders all places of public accommodation and resort, etc., to furnish equal accommodations without discrimination. An Act of 1941, as last amended, forbids the Civil Service in counties with population exceeding 1m. to discriminate against employees or applicants on the ground of political, racial or religious opinions or affiliations. An Act of 1881 incorporated into the school code of 1955 forbids any discrimination in school facilities. An Act of 1893 incorporated in the Insurance code of 1956 prohibits insurance companies from discriminating between white and coloured persons.

In 1951 the legislature restored the unique one-man grand jury system abandoned in 1949.

Religion. Roman Catholics make up the largest body; largest Protestant denominations, Lutherans, United Methodists, United Presbyterians, Episcopalians.

Education. Education is compulsory for children from 6 to 16 years of age. The operating expenditure for graded and ungraded public schools for the fiscal year 1985, was $5,704m. In 1984–85 there were 567 school districts (elementary and secondary schools) with 1,678,458 pupils and 75,193 teachers. Teachers' salaries in 1985 averaged $28,440.

In 1985 there were 98 institutes of higher education with 508,000 students.

Universities and students (autumn 1986):

Founded	*Name*	*Students*
1817	University of Michigan	34,947
1849	Eastern Michigan University	21,349
1855	Michigan State University	44,088
1884	Ferris State College	11,274

Founded	*Name*	*Students*
1885	Michigan Technological University	6,326
1868	Wayne State University	34,764
1892	Central Michigan University	17,993
1889	Northern Michigan University	7,852
1903	Western Michigan University	21,747
1946	Lake Superior State College	2,660
1959	Oakland University	12,707
1960	Grand Valley State College	8,321
1965	Saginaw Valley College	5,377

Social Welfare. Old-age assistance is provided for persons 65 years of age or older who have resided in Michigan for one year before application; assets must not exceed various limits. In 1974 federal Supplementary Security Income (SSI) replaced the adults' programme. In Jan. 1987 aid was supplied to a monthly average of 418,572 dependent children in 188,972 families at $463.86 per family.

Health. In 1983 the state had 231 hospitals (47,812 beds) licensed by the state and 12 psychiatric hospitals, 7 centres for developmental disabilities, 5 centres for emotionally disturbed children.

In 1986 the Medicaid programme disbursed (with federal support) $1,642·9m. to 469,226 persons.

Further Reading

Michigan Manual. Dept of *Management and Budget.* Lansing. Biennial

Bureau of Business Research, Wayne State University. *Michigan Statistical Abstract.* Detroit, 1983

Bald, F. C., *Michigan in Four Centuries.* 2nd ed. New York, 1961

Blanchard, J. J., *Economic Report of the Governor 1985.* Lansing, 1985

Catton. B., *Michigan—a Bicentennial History.* Norton, New York, 1976

Lewis, F. E., *State and Local Government in Michigan.* Lansing, 1979

Dunbar, W. F. and May, G. S., *Michigan: A History of the Wolverine State.* Grand Rapids, 1980

Sommers, L. (ed.), *Atlas of Michigan.* East Lansing, 1977

State Library Services: Library of Michigan, Lansing 48909. *State Librarian:* James W. Fry.

MINNESOTA

HISTORY. Minnesota, first explored in the 17th century and first settled in the 20 years following the establishment of Fort Snelling (1819), was made a Territory in 1849 (with parts of North and South Dakota), and was admitted into the Union, with its present boundaries, on 11 May 1858.

AREA AND POPULATION. Minnesota is bounded north by Canada, east by Lake Superior and Wisconsin, with the Mississippi River forming the boundary in the south-east, south by Iowa, west by South and North Dakota, with the Red River forming the boundary in the north-west. Area, 84,402 sq. miles, of which 4,854 sq. miles are inland water. Census population, 1 April 1980, 4,075,970, an increase of 7·1% since 1970. Estimate (1988), 4,306,550. Births in 1988, 66,745 (15·5 per 1,000 population); deaths, 35,436 (8·2); infant deaths, 521 (7·8 per 1,000 live births); marriages, 33,654 (7·8); divorces (1987), 14,931 (3·5).

Population in 5 census years was:

	White	*Black*	*Indian*	*Asiatic*	*Total*	*Per sq. mile*
1910	2,059,227	7,084	9,053	344	2,075,708	25·7
1930	2,542,599	9,445	11,077	832	2,563,953	32·0
1960	3,371,603	22,263	15,496	3,642	3,413,864	42·7
			All others			
1970	3,736,038	34,868	34,163		3,805,069	47·6
1980	3,935,770	53,344	86,856		4,075,970	51·4

Of the 1980 population, 1,997,826 were male; 2,725,270 were urban; those 21 years of age or older numbered 2,656,947.

The largest cities are Minneapolis, 370,951; St Paul (capital), 270,230 (Minneapolis–St Paul standard metropolitan statistical area, 2,113,533 in 1980); Duluth, 92,811; Bloomington, 81,831; Rochester, 57,890.

CLIMATE. Duluth. Jan. 8°F (–13·3°C), July 63°F (17·2°C). Annual rainfall 29" (719 mm). Minneapolis-St. Paul. Jan. 12°F (–11·1°C), July 71°F (21·7°C). Annual rainfall 26" (656 mm). *See* Great Lakes, p. 1382.

CONSTITUTION AND GOVERNMENT. The present constitution dates from 1858; it has had 109 amendments. The Legislature consists of a Senate of 67 members, elected for 4 years, and a House of Representatives of 134 members, elected for 2 years. The Governor and Lieut.-Governor are elected for 4 years. The state sends to Congress 2 senators and 8 representatives.

In the 1988 presidential election Dukakis polled 1,109,471 votes, Bush 962,337.

The capital is St Paul. There are 87 counties, four containing less than 400 sq. miles, the largest being 6,092 sq. miles.

Governor: Arne Carlson (R.), 1991–95 ($98,914).

BUDGET. The general fund budget for the 1989–91 2-year period was $13,686m.; tax relief $1,966m., education $7,121m., public welfare $1,940m., transport $207m.

Net long-term debt, 30 June 1989, was $1,416m.

Per capita personal income (1988) was $16,787.

NATURAL RESOURCES

Minerals. The iron ore and taconite industry is the most important in the USA. Production of usable iron ore in 1988 was 42m. tons, value $1,278m. Other important minerals are sand and gravel, crushed and dimension stone, lime and manganiferous ore. Total value of mineral production, 1988, $1,391m.

Agriculture. In 1989 there were 90,000 farms with a total area of 30m. acres (60% of the land area); the average farm was of 333 acres. Average value of land and buildings (1989) $192,245. Commercial farms in 1987 numbered 85,079; 12% of the farms were operated by tenant-farmers. Cash receipts, 1988, from crops, $2,743m.; from livestock, $3,364m. In 1988 Minnesota ranked second in sugar-beets, spring wheat, processing sweet corn, oats, dry milk, cheese, mink and turkeys. Other important products are wild rice, butter, eggs, flaxseed, milch cows, milk, corn, barley, swine, cattle for market, soybeans, honey, potatoes, rye, chickens, sunflower seed and dry edible beans. Of livestock, cattle represents 16% of total farm income, swine 12% and milk 20%. Of crops, corn represents 15% and soybeans 19%. On 1 Jan. 1989 the farm animals included 3·15m. all cattle, 855,000 milch cows, 237,000 sheep and lambs, 4·26m. swine and 12·8m. chickens. Turkey production, 1988, 38·5m. In 1988 the wool clip amounted to 1·89m. lb. of wool from 255,000 sheep.

Forestry. Forests of commercial timber cover 14m. acres, of which 53% is government-owned. The value of forest products in 1987 was $4,400m.: $1,300m. from primary processing, of which $901m. was from pulp and paper; and $3,100m. from secondary manufacturing. Logging, pulping, saw-mills and associated industries employed 53,700 in 1987.

INDUSTRY. In 1986 manufacturing establishments employed 369,000 workers; value added by manufacture was $19,800m. Largest manufacturing industry is computers and non-electric machinery (81,000 employees); then food products and kindred products (45,000), printing and publishing (43,000).

TOURISM. In 1987, travellers spent about $5,500m. The industry employed about 108,000.

COMMUNICATIONS

Roads. In 1990 there were 129,553 miles of roads (115,458 miles rural) and 3,283,292 registered motor vehicles.

Railways. There are 3 Class I and 16 Class II and smaller railroads operating, with total mileage of 5,044.

Aviation. In 1989 there were 141 airports for public use and 12 public seaplane bases.

JUSTICE, RELIGION, EDUCATION AND WELFARE

Justice. A Civil Rights Act (1927) forbids places of public resort to exclude persons 'on account of race or colour' and another section forbids insurance companies to discriminate 'between persons of the same class on account of race'. Contractors on public works may have their contracts cancelled if 'in the hiring of common or skilled labour' they are found to have discriminated on the grounds of 'race, creed or colour'. The state's penal reformatory system on 1 Oct. 1989 held 3,005 adult men and women. There is no death penalty in Minnesota.

Religion. The chief religious bodies are: Lutheran with 1,088,304 members in 1980; Roman Catholic, 1,041,781; Methodist, 146,422. Total membership of all denominations, 2,653,161.

Education. In 1988, there were 61,442 kindergarten students, 340,967 elementary students, and 318,714 secondary students enrolled in 1,511 public schools. There were 82,165 kindergarten, elementary, and secondary students enrolled in 572 private schools. The University of Minnesota, chartered in 1851 and opened in 1869, had a total enrolment in 1988 of 54,515 students on all campuses. The 18 public community colleges (2-year) had a total enrolment of 49,589. There are seven state universities (4-year) at Bemidji, Mankato, Marshall, Moorhead, St Cloud, Winona, Minneapolis and St Paul. Enrolment in all institutions of higher education, 1988, 251,304.

Health. In 1989 the state had 163 general acute hospitals with 19,229 beds. Patients resident in institutions under the Department of Human Services in Aug. 1989 included 1,343 people with mental illness, 1,405 people with mental retardation, 265 with chemical dependency and 486 in state nursing homes.

Social Security. Programmes of old age assistance, aid to the disabled, and aid to the blind are administered under the federal Supplemental Security Income (SSI) Programme. Minnesota has a supplementary programme, Minnesota Supplemental Aid (MSA) to cover individuals not eligible for SSI, to supplement SSI benefits for others whose income is below state standards, and to provide one-time payments for emergency needs such as major home repair, essential furniture or appliances, moving expenses, fuel, food and shelter.

Further Reading

Statistical Information: Current information is obtainable from the State Planning Agency (300 Centennial Office Building, 658 Cedar Street, St Paul 55155); non-current material from the Reference Library, Minnesota Historical Society, St Paul 55101.

Legislative Manual. Secretary of State. St Paul. Biennial
Manufacturers' Directory. Nelson Name Service, Minneapolis, Biennial
Minnesota Agriculture Statistics. Dept. of Agric., St Paul. Annual
Minnesota Pocket Data Book 1985–86, St Paul, 1985

MISSISSIPPI

HISTORY. Mississippi, settled in 1716, was organized as a Territory in 1798 and admitted into the Union on 10 Dec. 1817. In 1804 and in 1812 its boundaries were extended, but in March 1817 a part was taken to form the new Territory of Alabama, leaving the boundaries substantially as at present.

AREA AND POPULATION. Mississippi is bounded north by Tennessee, east by Alabama, south by the Gulf of Mexico and Louisiana, west by the Mississippi River forming the boundary with Louisiana and Arkansas. Area, 47,689 sq. miles, 457 sq. miles being inland water. Census population, 1 July 1980, 2,520,638, an increase of 13·6% since 1970. Births, occurring in the state, 1989, were 42,309; deaths, 24,475; infant deaths, 458; marriages, 24,240; divorces, 12,945.

Population of 6 federal census years was:

	White	*Black*	*Indian*	*Asiatic*	*Total*	*Per sq. mile*
1910	786,111	1,009,487	1,253	263	1,797,114	38·8
1930	998,077	1,009,718	1,458	568	2,009,821	42·4
1950	1,188,632	986,494	2,502	1,286	2,178,914	46·1
1960	1,257,546	915,743	3,119	1,481	2,178,141	46·1
			All others			
1970	1,393,283	815,770	7,859		2,216,912	46·9
1980	1,615,190	887,206	18,242		2,520,638	53·0

Of the population in 1980, 1,213,878 were male, 1,192,805 were urban and 1,601,157 were 20 years old or older.

The largest city (1980) is Jackson, 202,895. Others are: Biloxi, 49,311; Meridian, 46,577; Hattiesburg, 40,829; Greenville, 40,613; Gulfport, 39,676; Pascagoula, 29,318; Columbus, 27,383; Vicksburg, 25,434; Tupelo, 23,905.

CLIMATE. Jackson. Jan. 47°F (8·3°C), July 82°F (27·8°C). Annual rainfall 49" (1,221 mm). Vicksburg. Jan. 48°F (8·9°C), July 81°F (27·2°C). Annual rainfall 52" (1,311 mm). *See* Central Plains, p. 1381.

CONSTITUTION AND GOVERNMENT. The present constitution was adopted in 1890 without ratification by the electorate; 94 amendments by 1988.

The Legislature consists of a Senate (52 members) and a House of Representatives (122 members), both elected for 4 years, as are also the Governor and Lieut.-Governor. Electors are all citizens who have resided in the state 1 year, in the county 1 year, in the election district 6 months before the next election who have been registered according to law. In the 1988 presidential election Bush polled 551,745 votes, Dukakis, 360,892.

The state is represented in Congress by 2 senators and 5 representatives.

The capital is Jackson; there are 82 counties.

Governor: Ray Mabus (D.), 1988–92 ($75,600).
Lieut.-Governor: Bradford Johnson Dye (D.) ($40,800).
Secretary of State: Dick Molpus (D.) ($54,000).

BUDGET. For the fiscal year ending 30 June 1989 the general revenues were $5,391,165,868 (taxation, $2,373,140,438; federal aid, $1,177,055,491; other state resources, $1,840,969,938), and general expenditures were $5,415,338,112 ($1,434,363,972 for education, $373,451,710 for highways and $1,031,233,151 for public welfare).

On 30 June 1989 the total net long-term debt was $532,617,308.

Per capita personal income (1988) was $11,090 (lowest in US).

ENERGY AND NATURAL RESOURCES

Minerals. Petroleum and natural gas account for about 90% (by value) of mineral production. Output of petroleum, 1989, was 28,462,215 bbls and of natural gas 202,178,969m. cu. ft. There are 6 oil refineries. Value of oil and gas products sold 1990 was $693,009,759.

Agriculture. Agriculture is the leading industry of the state because of the semi-tropical climate and a rich productive soil. In 1990 there were 82 soil conservation districts covering 30m. acres. In 1990 farms numbered 40,000 with an area of 13·3m. acres. Average size of farm was 325 acres. This compares with an average farm size of 138 acres in 1960.

Cash income from all crops and livestock during 1988, including government payments, was $2,640,777,000. Cash income from crops was $1,209,405,000 and from livestock and products, $1,176,272,000. The chief product is cotton, cash income (1989) $457,865,000 from 1m. acres producing 1,566,000 bales of 732 lb. Soybeans, rice, corn, hay, wheat, oats, sorghum, peanuts, pecans, sweet potatoes, peaches, other vegetables, nursery and forest products continue to contribute.

On 1 Jan. 1989 there were 1,390,000 head of cattle and calves on Mississippi farms. Milch cows totalled 63,000, beef cows, 717,000; hogs and pigs (1989), 180,000. Of cash income from livestock and products, 1989, $258,548,000 was credited to cattle and calves. Cash income from poultry and eggs, 1989, totalled $691,364,000; dairy products, $109,291,000; swine, $33,012,000.

Forestry. In 1989 income from forestry amounted to $716,675,686; output of logs, lumber, etc., was 1,859,970 bd ft; pulpwood, 7,249,518 cords; distillate wood, 333 tons. There are about 16,990,100 acres of forest (56% of the state's area). National forests area, 1987, 1,212,100 acres.

INDUSTRY. In 1989 the 3,462 manufacturing establishments employed 243,715 workers, earning $4,542,036,498. The average annual wage was $18,637.

TOURISM. Total receipts, 1989, $1,500m. from about 2·4m. tourists.

COMMUNICATIONS

Roads. The state in July 1990 maintained 10,359 miles of highways, of which 10,350 miles were paved; 1,779,403 cars were registered.

Railways. The state in 1990 had 2,948 miles of railway.

Aviation. There were 80 public airports in 1990, 73 of them general. There were also 5 privately owned airports.

JUSTICE, RELIGION, EDUCATION AND WELFARE

Justice. In 1989 there were no executions; from 1955 to 1989 executions (by gas-chamber) totalled 35 (25 for murder, 9 for rape and 1 for armed robbery). As of 30 Sept. 1990, the state prisons had 8,011 inmates.

Religion. Southern Baptists in Mississippi (1989), 672,832 members; Negro Baptists (1987), about 477,000; United Methodists (1989) 186,554; Roman Catholics (1990), 99,857 in Biloxi and Jackson dioceses.

Education. Attendance at school is compulsory as laid down in the Education Reform Act of 1982. The public elementary and secondary schools in 1989–90 had 502,020 pupils and 27,506 classroom teachers.

In 1989, teachers' average salary was $24,364. The expenditure per pupil in average daily attendance, 1989–90, was $2,960.

There are 15 universities and senior colleges, of which 8 are state-supported. The University of Mississippi, at Oxford (1844), had, 1989–90, 828 instructors and 12,423 students; Mississippi State University, Starkville, 904 instructors and 13,994 students; Mississippi University for Women, Columbus, 158 instructors and 2,109 students; University of Southern Mississippi, Hattiesburg, 689 instructors and 12,999 students; Jackson State University, Jackson, 340 instructors and 7,152 students; Delta State University, Cleveland, 241 instructors and 3,848 students; Alcorn State University, Lorman, 161 instructors and 2,847 students; Mississippi Valley State University, Itta Bena, 142 instructors and 1,691 students. State support for the 8 universities (1989–90) was $314,901,119.

Junior colleges had (1989–90) 62,844 students and 2,446 instructors. The state appropriation for junior colleges, 1989–90, was $72,695,877.

Health. In 1989 the state had 110 acute general hospitals (12,530 beds) listed by the State Department of Health; 10 hospitals with facilities for care of the mentally ill had 2,867 beds.

Social Security. The state Medicaid commission paid (1990) $591,943,397 for medical services, including $70,158,321 for drugs, $62,282,045 for skilled nursing home care, $197,163,856 for hospital services. There were 76,447 persons eligible for Aged Medicaid benefits and 80,561 persons eligible for Disabled Medicaid benefits at 30 June 1990. In June 1990, 60,766 families with 129,979 dependent children received $7,225,005 in the Aid to Dependent Children programme. The average monthly payment was $120·44 per family or $56·26 per child.

Further Reading

1980 Census of Population and Housing: Mississippi.
Mississippi Official and Statistical Register. Secretary of State. Jackson. Biennial
Bettersworth, J. K., *Mississippi: A History*. Rev. ed. Austin, Tex., 1964

Mississippi Library Commission: PO Box 10700 Jackson, MS. 39289–0700. *Director:* David M. Woodburn.

MISSOURI

HISTORY. Missouri, first settled in 1735 at Ste Genevieve, was made a Territory on 1 Oct. 1812, and admitted to the Union on 10 Aug. 1821. In 1837 its boundaries were extended to their present limits.

AREA AND POPULATION. Missouri is bounded north by Iowa, east by the Mississippi River forming the boundary with Illinois and Kentucky, south by Arkansas, south-east by Tennessee, south-west by Oklahoma, west by Kansas and Nebraska, with the Missouri River forming the boundary in the north-west. Area, 69,697 sq. miles, 752 sq. miles being water.

Census population, 1 April 1980, 4,916,766, an increase since 1970 of 5·1%. Estimate (1988), 5,139,000. Births, 1989, were 75,712 (14·7 per 1,000 population); deaths, 49,684 (9·7); infant deaths, 769 (10·2 per 1,000 live births); marriages, 51,508 (10); divorces, 24,681 (4·8).

Population of 5 federal census years was:

	White	*Black*	*Indian*	*Asiatic*	*Total*	*Per sq. mile*
1910	3,134,932	157,452	313	638	3,293,335	47·9
1930	3,403,876	223,840	578	1,073	3,629,367	52·4
1960	3,922,967	390,853	1,723	3,146	4,319,813	62·5
			All others			
1970	4,177,495	480,172	19,732		4,677,399	67·0
1980	4,345,521	514,276	56,889		4,916,686	71·3

Of the total population in 1980, 2,365,487 were male, 3,350,746 persons were urban and those 18 years of age or older numbered 3,554,203.

The principal cities at the 1980 census (and estimates, 1988) are:

St Louis	453,085 (403,700)	Columbia	62,061 (64,330)
Kansas City	448,159 (438,953)	Florissant	55,372 (60,560)
Springfield	133,116 (142,690)	University City	42,738 (41,600)
Independence	111,806 (115,090)	Joplin	38,893 (41,630)
St Joseph	76,691 (73,490)	St Charles	37,379 (42,260)

Metropolitan areas, 1980: St Louis, 2,356,000; Kansas City, 1,327,000.

CLIMATE. Kansas City. Jan. 30°F (–1·1°C), July 79°F (26·1°C). Annual rainfall 38" (947 mm). St Louis. Jan. 32°F (0°C), July 79°F (26·1°C). Annual rainfall 40" (1,004 mm). *See* Central Plains, p. 1381.

CONSTITUTION AND GOVERNMENT. A new constitution, the fourth, was adopted on 27 Feb. 1945; it has been amended 27 times. The General Assembly consists of a Senate of 34 members elected for 4 years (half for re-election every 2 years), and a House of Representatives of 163 members elected for 2 years. The Governor and Lieut.-Governor are elected for 4 years. Missouri sends to Congress 2 senators and 9 representatives.

Voters (with the usual exceptions) are all citizens and those adult aliens who, within a prescribed period, have applied for citizenship. In the 1988 presidential election Bush polled 1,081,163 votes, Dukakis, 1,004,040.

Jefferson City is the state capital. The state is divided into 114 counties and the city of St Louis.

Governor: John D. Ashcroft (R.), 1989–93 ($81,000).
Lieut.-Governor: Mel Carnahan (D.), 1989–93 ($48,600).
Secretary of State: Roy D. Blunt (R.), 1989–93 ($64,800).

BUDGET. For the year 1988 the total revenues from all funds were $8,150m. (federal revenue, $1,567m., general revenue, $7,016m.).

Total outstanding debt, 1988, was $4,569m.

Per capita personal income (1989) was $16,431.

NATURAL RESOURCES

Minerals. Principal minerals are lead (ranks first in USA), zinc (ranks second), clays, coal, iron ore, and stone for cement and lime manufacture. Value of production (1986) $748·6m.

Agriculture. In 1989 there were 108,000 farms in Missouri producing crops and livestock on 30·4m. acres. Production of principal crops, 1989: Corn, 219·8m. bu.; soybeans, 123·9m. bu.; wheat, 86·95m. bu.; sorghum grain, 45·3m. bu.; oats, 3·6m. bu.; rice, 4·1m. cwt; cotton, 269,000 bales (of 480 lb.). Cash receipts from farming, 1989, $3,940m. to which livestock sales contributed $2,170m. and soybeans $755m.

Forestry. Forest land area, 1990, 12·9m. acres.

INDUSTRY. The largest employer in 1988 was manufacturing, in which the transport equipment industry employed 68,557 workers. Other large industries are food and kindred products, electrical equipment and supplies, apparel and related products and non-electrical machinery, leather products, chemicals, paper, metal industries, stone, clay, glass, rubber and plastic products. Wholesale and retail trade employed 559,900 as of May 1989.

LABOUR. The State Board of Mediation has jurisdiction in labour disputes involving only public utilities. The Prevailing Wage Law (1959) provides that no less than the local hourly rate of wages for work of a similar character shall be paid to any workmen engaged in public works. The Industrial Commission has authority to inspect records and to institute actions for penalties described in the Act. There is a state programme for industrial safety in hand, under the Federal Occupational and Health Act. In May 1990 (preliminary) the annual average number of employed was 2,668,100, and 121,000 were unemployed; the unemployment rate was 4·5%.

COMMUNICATIONS

Roads. In 1990 there were 120,077 miles of roads (104,230 miles rural) and 3,843,982 registered motor vehicles.

Railways. The state has 9 Class I railways; approximate total mileage, 6,646. There are 10 other railways (switching, terminal or short-line), total mileage 435, in 1989.

Aviation. In 1990 there were 140 public airports and 225 private airports.

Shipping. Ten major barge lines (1990) operated on about 1,000 miles of navigable waterways including the Missouri and Mississippi Rivers. Boat shipping seasons: Missouri River, April–end Nov.; Mississippi River, all seasons.

Post and Broadcasting. There were 146 commercial radio stations and 30 TV stations in 1990.

Newspapers. There were (1990) 50 daily and 276 weekly newspapers.

JUSTICE, RELIGION, EDUCATION AND WELFARE

Justice. State prisons in 1990 had an average of 11,593 inmates including 462 females. The median age was 28 in 1988, 56% between age 15 and 29. The death penalty was reinstated in 1978. The first execution since 1965 was on 1 Jan. 1989 (by lethal injection). Since 1930 executions (by lethal gas) have totalled 42, including 32 for murder, 7 for rape and 3 for kidnapping. The Missouri Law Enforcement Assistance Council was created in 1969 for law reform. With reorganization of state government in 1974 the duties of the Council were delegated to the Department of Public Safety.

Religion. Chief religious bodies (1980) are Catholic, with 800,228 members, Southern Baptists (700,053), United Methodists (270,469), Christian Churches (175,101), Lutheran (157,928), Presbyterian (38,254). Total membership, all denominations, about 2·6m. in 1980.

Education. School attendance is compulsory for children from 7 to 16 years for the full term. In the 1989–90 school year, public schools (kindergarten through grade 12) had 807,934 pupils. Total expenditure for public schools in 1988–89, $2,842,233,745. Salaries for teachers (kindergarten through grade 12), 1988–89, averaged $27,271. Institutions for higher education include the University of Missouri, founded in 1839 with campuses at Columbia, Rolla, St Louis and Kansas City, with 3,614 accredited teachers and 45,660 students in 1989–90. Washington University at St Louis, founded in 1857, is an independent co-ed university with 6,637 students in 1989–90. St Louis University (1818), is an independent Roman Catholic co-ed university with 3,657 students in 1989–90. Sixteen state colleges had 102,666 students in 1989–90. Private colleges had (1989–90) 29,131 students. Church-affiliated colleges (1989–90) had 29,948 students. Public junior colleges had 50,520 students. There are about 90 secondary and post-secondary institutions offering vocational courses, and about 294 private career schools. There were 220,500 students in higher education in autumn 1989.

Health. There were 10 state mental health hospitals and centres and 3 children's hospitals in 1990, admitting 21,583 patients.

Social Security. In 1988 the number of recipients of medicaid was 379,000. The number of recipients of Aid to families with Dependent Children was 202,000 with an average monthly payment per family of $263.

Further Reading

Missouri Area Labor Trends, Department of Labour and Industrial Relations, monthly
Missouri Farm Facts, Department of Agriculture, annual
Report of the Public Schools of Missouri. State Board of Education, annual
Statistical Abstract for Missouri. College of Business and Public Administration, Columbia, 1985

MONTANA

HISTORY. Montana, first settled in 1809, was made a Territory (out of portions of Idaho and Dakota Territories) in 1864 and was admitted into the Union on 8 Nov. 1889.

AREA AND POPULATION. Montana is bounded north by Canada, east by North and South Dakota, south by Wyoming and west by Idaho and the Bitterroot Range of the Rocky Mountains. Area, 147,138 sq. miles, including 1,551 sq. miles of water, of which the federal government, 1986, owned 28,236,000 acres or

30·3%. US Bureau of Indian Affairs (1982) administered 5·03m. acres, of which 2,820,000 were allotted to tribes. Census population, 1 April 1980, 786,690, an increase of 13·3% since 1970. Estimate (1986), 819,000. Births, 1986, were 12,728 (15·5 per 1,000 population); deaths, 6,738 (8·2); infant deaths, 122 (9·8 per 1,000 live births); marriages, 6,739 (8·2); divorces 4,307 (5·3).

Population in 5 census years was:

	White	*Black*	*Indian*	*Asiatic*	*Total*	*Per sq. mile*
1910	360,580	1,834	10,745	2,870	376,053	2·6
1930	519,898	1,256	14,798	1,239	537,606	3·7
1950	572,038	1,232	16,606	—	591,024	4·1
1970	663,043	1,995	27,130	1,099	694,409	4·7
1980	740,148	1,786	37,270	2,503	786,690	5·3

Of the total population in 1980, 392,625 were male, 416,402 persons (52·9%) were urban. Persons 20 years of age or older numbered 524,836. Median age, 29 years. Households, 283,742.

The largest cities, 1980 (and 1986 estimate) are Billings, 66,798 (80,310); Great Falls, 56,725 (57,310). Others: Butte-Silver Bow, 37,205 (33,380); Missoula, 33,388 (33,960); Helena (capital), 23,938 (24,670); Bozeman, 21,645 (23,490); Anaconda-Deer Lodge County, 12,518 (10,700); Havre, 10,891 (10,840); Kalispell, 10,648 (11,890).

CLIMATE. Helena. Jan. 18°F (–7·8°C), July 69°F (20·6°C). Annual rainfall 13" (325 mm). *See* Mountain States, p. 1381.

CONSTITUTION AND GOVERNMENT. A new constitution was ratified by the voters on 6 June 1972, and fully implemented on 1 July 1973; the Senate to consist of 50 senators, elected for 4 years, one half at each biennial election. The 100 members of the House of Representatives are elected for 2 years.

The Governor and Lieut.-Governor are elected for 4 years. Montana sends to Congress 2 senators and 2 representatives.

In the 1988 presidential election Bush polled 189,598 votes, Dukakis, 168,120.

The capital is Helena. The state is divided into 56 counties.

Governor: Stan Stephens (R.), 1989–93 ($50,452).

Lieut.-Governor: Allen Kolstad (R.), 1989–93 ($36,141).

Secretary of State: Mike Cooney (D.), 1989–93 ($33,342).

BUDGET. Total state revenues for the year ending 30 June 1985 were $1,738,000,000; total expenditures were $1,557,000,000 ($436m. for education, $239m. for highways and $184m. for public welfare).

Total net long-term debt on 30 June 1985 was $157,225,000.

Per capita personal income (1986) was $11,904.

ENERGY AND NATURAL RESOURCES

Electricity. Electric power generated in April 1986 was 1,112 gwh., of which 796 gwh. was hydro-electric and 310 gwh. from coal-fired plants; 1 from oil-fired, and 4 gwh. from other sources.

Minerals (1985). Output of crude petroleum, 30·2m. bbls; copper, 15,092 tonnes; sand and gravel, 9,000 short tons; phosphate rock, undisclosed; silver, 4m. troy oz.; gold, 160,262 troy oz.; zinc, undisclosed; natural gas, 46,592m. cu. ft; coal, 33·3m. short tons. Value of total mineral production, $1,198·8m., with petroleum ($761·9m.) the first, coal ($417·4m.) the second, natural gas ($95·5m.) the third and gold ($50·9m.) the fourth most important commodity.

Agriculture. In 1986 there were 23,300 farms and ranches (50,564 in 1935) with an area of 60·8m. acres (47,511,868 acres in 1935). Large-scale farming predominates; in 1986 the average size per farm was 2,609 acres. Income from all farm marketings was $1,145m. in 1986 (crops, $493m.; livestock, $652m.). Irrigated area harvested in 1986 was 1·6m. acres; non-irrigated, 7·8m. acres.

The chief crops are wheat, amounting in 1986 to 138·5m. bu.; barley, 85m. bu.; oats, 4·1m. bu.; sugar-beet, hay, potatoes, alfalfa, dry beans, flax and cherries. In 1986 there were 24,000 milch cows, 2·4m. all cattle; 190,000 swine and 423,000 sheep.

Forestry. Total forest area (1986), 22·6m. acres. In 1986 there were 16·8m. acres within 11 national forests.

INDUSTRY. In 1987 manufacturing establishments numbering 1,223 had 20,900 production workers; value added by manufacture was (1986) $907·4m.

LABOUR (March 1988). Work force, 402,900; total employed, 366,000; total non-agricultural workers, 336,000; agricultural workers, 29,000. Workers employed by major industry group: Mining, 5,900 (average net weekly earnings, $533.32); contract construction, 6,900 ($499.22); manufacturing, 20,100 ($404.80); transport and public utilities, 18,900 ($433.81; wholesale/retail trade, 70,900 ($197.78); finance/insurance/real estate, 12,500 ($264.54); services, 64,700 ($230.08); government, 70,200 (no income figures available). Average weekly earnings for all workers in private non-agricultural industries $270.19. Total unemployed 36,000 (9·2% of the work force in March 1988 as compared to 5·5% nationally for that month).

There were 13 work stoppages in 1987 involving 9,920 workers, with a total of 68,164 man days idle during the year.

COMMUNICATIONS

Roads. In 1990 there were 71,360 miles of roads (69,092 miles rural) and 741,197 registered motor vehicles.

Railways. In Oct. 1988 there were 3,400 route miles of railway in the state.

Aviation. There were 129 airports open for public use in Jan. 1988, of which 122 were publicly owned.

JUSTICE, RELIGION, EDUCATION AND WELFARE

Justice. At 31 Dec. 1987 the Montana State Prison at Deer Lodge held 961 inmates and the Women's Correctional Facility at Warm Springs, 36. Since 1943 there have been no executions; total since 1930 (all by hanging) was 6; 4 whites and 2 Negroes, for murder.

Religion. The leading religious bodies are (1987): Roman Catholic with 162,000 members; Lutheran, 68,654; Methodist (Yellowstone Conference, including N. Wyoming, Montana, and Salmon, Idaho), 21,609 (church estimates).

Education. In Oct. 1987 public elementary and secondary schools had 152,207 pupils. Public elementary and secondary school teachers (9,659 in 1987) had an average salary of $23,774. Expenditure on public school education (1986–87) was $475·9m. This included $26·33m. for Special Education.

The Montana University system consists of the Montana State University, at Bozeman (autumn 1987 enrolment: 9,878 students), the University of Montana, at Missoula, founded in 1895 (8,472), the Montana College of Mineral Science and Technology, at Butte (1,746), Northern Montana College, at Havre (1,658), Eastern Montana College, at Billings (3,926) and Western Montana College, at Dillon (992).

Social Security. In Aug. 1988, 4,892 persons over age 65 were receiving in medical assistance an average of $940 per year per person; 55 blind persons, $558, 6,035 totally disabled, $767; 9,290 families received in aid-to-dependent children assistance an average of $313. Aid was from state and federal sources.

Health. In Aug. 1988 the state had 60 hospitals (3,354 beds) listed by the Montana Board of Health. Four centres for mental illness and developmental disabilities had 703 patients.

Further Reading

Montana Agricultural Statistics. U.S. Dept. of Agriculture, Montana Crop and Livestock Reporting Service. Biennial from 1946
Montana Employment and Labor Force. Montana Dept. of Labor and Industry. Monthly from 1971
Montana Federal-Aid Road Log. Montana Dept. of Highways and US Dept. of Transportation, Federal Highway Administration. Annual from 1938
Montana Vital Statistics. Montana Dept. of Health and Environmental Sciences. Annually from 1954
Statistical Report. Montana Dept. of Social and Rehabilitation Services. Monthly from 1947
Lang, W, L. and Myers, R. C., *Montana, Our Land and People*. Pruett, 1979
Malone, M. P. and Roeder, R. B., *Montana, A History of Two Centuries*. Univ. of Washington Press, 1976
Spence, C. C., *Montana, a History*. New York, 1978

NEBRASKA

HISTORY. The Nebraska region was first reached by white men from Mexico under the Spanish general Coronado in 1541. It was ceded by France to Spain in 1763, retroceded to France in 1801, and sold by Napoleon to the US as part of the Louisiana Purchase in 1803. Its first settlement was in 1847, and on 30 May 1854 it became a Territory and on 1 March 1867 a state. In 1882 it annexed a small part of Dakota Territory, and in 1908 it received another small tract from South Dakota.

AREA AND POPULATION. Nebraska is bounded north by South Dakota, with the Missouri River forming the boundary in the north-east and the boundary with Iowa and Missouri to the east; south by Kansas, south-west by Colorado and west by Wyoming. Area, 77,355 sq. miles, of which 711 sq. miles are water. Census population, 1980: 1,569,825, an increase of 5·7% since 1970. Estimate (1987), 1,594,000. Births, 1987, were 23,813 (14·9 per 1,000 population); deaths, 14,820 (9·3); infant deaths, 204 (8·6 per 1,000 live births); marriages, 11,808 (7·4): divorces, 6,189 (3·9).

Population in 5 census years was:

	White	*Black*	*Indian*	*Asiatic*	*Total*	*Per sq. mile*
1910	1,180,293	7,689	3,502	730	1,192,214	15·5
1920	1,279,219	13,242	2,888	1,023	1,296,372	16·9
1960	1,374,764	29,262	5,545	1,195	1,411,330	18·3
			All others			
1970	1,432,867	39,911	10,715		1,483,791	19·4
1980	1,490,381	48,390	31,054		1,569,825	20·5

Of the total population in 1980, 48·8% were male,62·9% were urban 65·6% were 21 years of age or older. The largest cities in the state are: Omaha, with a census population, 1980, of 313,911 (estimate, 1986, 349,270); Lincoln (capital), 171,932 (183,050); Grand Island, 33,180 (39,100); North Platte, 24,509 (22,490); Fremont, 23,979 (23,780); Hastings, 23,045 (22,990); Bellevue, 21,813 (32,200); Kearney, 21,158 (22,770); Norfolk, 19,449 (20,260).

The Bureau of Indian Affairs, in June 1987, administered 65,000 acres, of which 23,000 acres were allotted to tribal control.

CLIMATE. Omaha. Jan. 22°F (–5·6°C), July 77°F (25°C). Annual rainfall 29" (721 mm). *See* High Plains, p. 1381.

CONSTITUTION AND GOVERNMENT. The present constitution was adopted in 1875; it has been amended 184 times. By an amendment adopted in Nov. 1934 Nebraska has a single-chambered legislature (elected for 4 years) of 49 members—the only state in the Union to have one. The Governor and Lieut.-Governor are elected for 4 years. Amendments adopted in 1912 and 1920 provide for legislation through the initiative and referendum and permit cities of more than 5,000 inhabitants to frame their own charters. A 'right-to-work' amendment adopted 5 Nov. 1946 makes illegal the 'closed shop' demands of trade unions. Nebraska is represented in Congress by 2 senators and 3 representatives.

In the 1988 presidential election Bush polled 389,394 votes, Dukakis, 254,426.

The capital is Lincoln. The state has 93 counties.

Governor: Ben Nelson (R.), 1991–95 ($58,000).

BUDGET. For the fiscal year ending 30 June 1986 (US Census Bureau figures) the state's revenues were $2,334m. (taxation, $1,119m. and federal aid, $561m.); general expenditures were $2,205m. ($690m. for education, $353m. for highways and $361m. for public welfare).

The state has a bonded indebtedness limit of $100,000.

Per capita personal income (1987) was $14,328.

ENERGY AND NATURAL RESOURCES

Minerals. The total output of minerals, 1987, was valued at $191·5m., petroleum (6·1m. bbls) and sand and gravel (10·4m. tons) being the most important.

Agriculture. Nebraska is one of the most important agricultural states. In 1986 it contained approximately 55,000 farms, with a total area of 47·1m. acres. The average farm was 856 acres.

In 1986, 7·9m. acres were irrigated and 71,587 irrigation wells were registered.

Cash income from crops (1987), $1,975m., and from livestock, $4,848m. Principal crops, with estimated 1987 yield: Maize, 812·2m. bu. (ranking third in US); wheat, 85·8m. bu.; sorghums for grain, 109·2m. bu.; oats, 17·3m. bu.; soybeans, 81·9m. bu. About 750 farms grow sugar-beet for 3 factories; output, 1987, 1·1m. short tons. On 1 Jan. 1988 the state contained 5·5m. all cattle (ranking third in US), 100,000 milch cows, 180,000 sheep and 4m. swine.

Forestry. The area of national forest, 1986, was 352,000 acres.

INDUSTRY. In 1986 there were 1,800 manufacturing establishments; 62,600 production workers earned $1,141·2m. and value added by manufacturing was $5,362·6m. The chief industry is meat-packing.

COMMUNICATIONS

Roads. In 1990 there were 92,459 miles of roads (87,509 miles rural) and 1,361,724 registered motor vehicles.

Railways. In 1988 there were 4,013 miles of railway.

Aviation. Airports (1988) numbered 354, of which 101 were publicly owned.

JUSTICE, RELIGION, EDUCATION AND WELFARE

Justice. A 'Civil Rights Act' revised in 1969 provides that all people are entitled to a 'full and equal enjoyment of the accommodations, advantages, facilities and privileges' of hotels, restaurants, public conveyances, amusement places and other places. The state university is forbidden to discriminate between students 'because of age, sex, color or nationality'. An Act of 1941 declares it to be 'the policy of this state' that no trade union should discriminate, in collective bargaining, 'against any person because of his race or color'.

The state's prisons had, 10 Oct. 1988, 2,132 inmates (134 per 100,000 population). From 1930 to 1962 there were 4 executions (electrocution), 3 white men and 1 American Indian, all for murder, and none since.

Religion. The Roman Catholics had 337,855 members in 1985; Protestant Churches, 737,361; Jews, 7,865 members. Total, all denominations, 1,083,081.

Education. School attendance is compulsory for children from 7 to 16 years of age. Public elementary schools, autumn 1986, had 147,149 enrolled pupils. Teachers' salaries, 1987–88, averaged $23,246. Estimated public school expenditure for year ending 30 Aug. 1987 was $936m. Total enrolment in 27 institutions of higher education, autumn 1987, was 100,454 students. The largest institutions were (1987):

Opened	*Institution*	*Students*
1867	Peru State College, Peru (State)	1,396
1869	Univ. of Nebraska, Lincoln (State)	25,722
1872	Doane College, Crete (UCC)	796
1878	Creighton Univ., Omaha (RC)	5,827
1882	Hastings College (Presbyterian)	894
1883	Midland Lutheran College, Fremont (Lutheran)	836
1887	Nebraska Wesleyan Univ. (Methodist)	1,359
1891	Union College, Lincoln (Seventh Day Adventist)	578
1894	Concordia Teachers' College, Seward (Lutheran)	816
1905	Kearney State College, Kearney (State)	9,075
1908	Univ. of Nebraska, Omaha (State)	14,210
1910	Wayne State College, Wayne (State)	2,899
1911	Chadron State College, Chadron (State)	2,250
1923	College of St. Mary	1,256
1966	Bellevue College, Bellevue (Private)	1,922

The state holds 1·52m. acres of land as a permanent endowment of her schools; permanent public school endowment fund in Aug. 1988 was $94·9m.

Health. In 1988 the state had 114 hospitals and 565 patients in mental hospitals.

Social Security. The administration of public welfare is the responsibility of the County Divisions of Welfare with policy-forming, regulatory, advisory and supervisory functions performed by the State Department of Public Welfare. In 1987 public welfare provided financial aid and/or services as follows: for 7,680 individuals who were aged, blind or disabled, with an average state supplement of $58.65; for 16,315 families with dependent children, with an average payment of $318.31 per family; for 88,390 individuals who had medical needs, $1,937.02, per individual; for 3,280 children in need of child welfare services; $1·8m. was spent on medically-handicapped children. The amount of aid is based on need in accordance with State assistance standards; the programme of aid to families with dependent children is limited to a maximum maintenance payment of $300 for 1 child plus $75 for each additional child.

Further Reading

Agricultural Atlas of Nebraska. Univ. of Nebraska Press, 1977
Climatic Atlas of Nebraska. Univ. of Nebraska Press, 1977
Economic Atlas of Nebraska. Univ. of Nebraska Press, 1977
Nebraska. A Guide to the Cornhusker State. Univ. of Nebraska Press, 1979
Nebraska Statistical Handbook, 1988–89. Nebraska Dept. of Econ. Development, Lincoln
Nebraska Blue-Book. Legislative Council. Lincoln. Biennial
Olson, J. C., *History of Nebraska*. Univ. of Nebraska Press, 1955

State Library: State Law Library, State House, Lincoln. *Librarian:* Reta Johnson.

NEVADA

HISTORY. Nevada, first settled in 1851, when it was a part of the Territory of Utah (created 1850), was made a Territory in 1861, enlarged in 1862 by an addition from Utah Territory and admitted into the Union on 31 Oct. 1864 as the 36th state. In 1866 and 1867 the area of the state was significantly enlarged at the expense of the Territories of Utah and Arizona.

AREA AND POPULATION. Nevada is bounded north by Oregon and Idaho, east by Utah, south-east by Arizona, with the Colorado River forming most of the boundary, south and west by California. Area 110,561 sq. miles, 667 sq. miles being water. The federal government in 1987 owned 59,891,667 acres, or 85·1% of the land area. Vacant public lands, 47,738,597 acres. The Bureau of Indian Affairs controlled 1·15m. acres.

Census population on 1 April 1980, 800,508, an increase of 311,770 since 1970. Estimate (1989) 1,111,000. Births, 1989, were 19,993 (17·9 per 1,000 population); deaths, 8,537 (7·7); marriages, 114,334 (102·9); divorces, 13,303 (11·9); infant deaths, 163 (8·2 per 1,000 live births).

Population in 5 census years was:

	White	*Black*	*Indian*	*All others*	*Total*	*Per sq. mile*
1910	74,276	513	5,240	1,846	81,875	0·7
1930	84,515	516	4,871	1,156	91,058	0·8
1960	263,443	13,484	6,681	1,670	285,278	2·6
1970	449,850	27,579	7,329	3,980	488,738	4·4
1980	700,360	50,999	13,308	35,841	800,508	7·2

Of the total population in 1980, 405,060 were male, 683,062 were urban and 556,776 were 20 years of age or older.

The largest cities are Las Vegas, with population at the 1980 census of 164,674 (1989 estimate, 262,600); Reno, 100,756 (127,190); North Las Vegas, 42,739 (52,420); Sparks, 40,780 (55,460); Carson City, 32,022 (39,420); and Henderson, 24,363 (67,150). Clark County (Las Vegas, North Las Vegas and Henderson) and Washoe County (Reno and Sparks) together had 82% of the total state population in 1980 (88·6% in 1989).

CLIMATE. Las Vegas. Jan. 44°F (6·7°C), July 85°F (29·4°C). Annual rainfall 4" (112 mm). Reno. Jan. 32°F (0°C), July 69°F (20·6°C). Annual rainfall 7" (178 mm). *See* Mountain States, p. 1381.

CONSTITUTION AND GOVERNMENT. The constitution adopted in 1864 is still in force, with 112 amendments by 1990. The Legislature meets biennially (and in special sessions) and consists of a Senate of 21 members elected for 4 years, half their number retiring every 2 years, and an Assembly of 42 members elected for 2 years. The Governor, Lieut.-Governor, Attorney-General, Secretary of State, Treasurer and Controller are elected for 4 years, the Governor being limited to 2 consecutive terms. Qualified electors are all citizens with the usual residential qualification. Nevada is represented in Congress by 2 senators and 2 representatives. A Supreme Court of 5 members is elected for 6 years on a non-partisan ballot. The state is represented in Congress by 2 senators and 2 representatives.

In the 1988 presidential election Bush polled 306,040 votes, Dukakis, 132,738.

The state capital is Carson City. There are 16 counties, 18 incorporated cities and 44 unincorporated communities and 1 city-county (the Capitol District of Carson City).

Governor: Bob Miller (D.), 1991–94 ($90,000).
Lieut.-Governor: Sue Wagner, 1991-94 ($20,000).
Secretary of State: Cheryl Lau, 1991-94 ($62,500).

BUDGET. For the fiscal year ending 30 June 1990, state general fund revenues were $799·3m.; budget expenditures were $761·5m. from the general fund ($1,750m. including federal funds and all other categories). Education (57·5% of the total), followed by human resources (21·2%) and public safety (9·6%), received the largest appropriations.

State bonded indebtedness on 30 June 1989, was $100·8m. The state has no franchise tax, capital stock tax, special intangibles tax, stock transfer tax, admissions tax, gift tax, or income tax. Taxes on gambling and the state's 2% share of the sales tax support nearly 80% of the general fund.

Per capita personal income (1989) was $18,827.

ENERGY AND NATURAL RESOURCES

Electricity. In Aug. 1988 electricity power stations served 433,313 residential customers, 64,314 commercial, and 623 industrial customers.

Minerals. Production, 1989 was $1,944·57m. In order of value: Gold ($1,611·02m.), silver ($127·76m.), sand and gravel ($50·93m.), barite ($5·05m.), gypsum ($1·5m.). Petroleum produced, 3·2m. bbls. Other minerals are iron ore, mercury, lime, lithium, gemstones, lead, molybdenum, fluorspar, perlite, pumice, clays, talc, salt, tungsten, magnesite, diatomite and zinc.

Agriculture. In 1988, an estimated 2,500 farms had a farm area of 8·9m. acres under cultivation (9·2m. in 1960). Farms averaged 3,560 acres. Area under irrigation (1989) was 569,800 acres compared with 542,976 acres in 1959.

Gross income, 1989, from crops, livestock and government payments, $281·3m. Cattle, hay, dairy products, potatoes and sheep are the principal commodities in order of cash receipts. Total value of crops produced, $79·6m. In Jan. 1989 there were 19,000 milch cows, 490,000 beef cattle, 87,000 sheep and lambs.

Forestry. The area of national forests (1988) under US Forest Service administration was 5,150,090 acres. National forests: Toiyabe (3,243,260 acres); Humboldt (2,468,812).

INDUSTRY. The main industry is the service industry (43·1% of employment), especially tourism and legalized gambling; others include mining and smelting, livestock and irrigated agriculture and construction. In 1989 there were 988 manufacturing establishments with 26,243 employees, and 2,664 construction firms with 38,133 employees.

Gaming industry gross revenue for financial year 1989, $4,589,005,000 from 2,400 licensed operators, manufacturers and gaming service companies.

LABOUR. The annual average unemployment for 1989 was 5% of the work force. All industries employed 582,300 workers. Main industries and employees, 1989: Service industries, 251,100; retail trade, 97,000; government, 70,800; insurance and real estate, 25,500; transport, 18,200; public works and utilities, 12,400; mining, 13,600; manufacturing, 25,400.

COMMUNICATIONS

Roads. Highway mileage (federal, state and local) totalled 51,888 in 1989, of which 13,341 miles were surfaced; motor vehicle registrations in 1989 numbered 886,594.

Railways. In 1989 there were 1,275 miles of main-line railway. Nevada is served by Southern Pacific, Union Pacific and Western Pacific railways, and Amtrak passenger service for Las Vegas, Elko, Reno and Sparks.

Aviation. There were 77 civil airports and heliports in 1989. During 1989 McCarran International Airport (Las Vegas) handled 16m. passengers and Reno-Cannon International Airport handled 3·3m. passengers.

Post. In Dec. 1989 there were 82 telephone exchanges, and 689,785 telephones in service.

JUSTICE, RELIGION, EDUCATION AND WELFARE

Justice. Prohibition of marriage between persons of different race was repealed by statute in 1959. It is illegal for persons operating public accommodation or selling houses, employers of 15 or more employees, labour unions, and employment agencies to discriminate on the basis of race, colour, religion or national origin. A Commission on Equal Rights of Citizens is charged with enforcing these laws.

Between 1924 and 1961 executions (by lethal gas—the first state to adopt this method, in 1921), numbered 31. Capital punishment was abolished in 1972 and re-introduced in 1978; there have since been 5 executions, 2 by lethal gas (in 1979 and 1985) and 3 by lethal injection (2 in 1989 and 1 in 1990).

Religion. Roman Catholics are the most numerous religious group, followed by members of the Church of Jesus Christ of Latter-day Saints (Mormons) and various Protestant churches.

Education. School attendance is compulsory for children from 7 to 17 years of age. In 1989 the 213 public elementary schools had 109,468 pupils; there were 98 secondary public schools with 76,533 pupils. There were 4,331 elementary teachers (average salary $29,920), 3,139 secondary teachers ($31,943). There were 80 private schools (8,973 pupils). The University of Nevada, Reno, had, in 1989–90, 407 full-time instructors and 11,317 students (regular, non-degree and correspondent), and University of Nevada, Las Vegas, 537 instructors and 16,009 students. Two-year community colleges operate as part of the University of Nevada system in Reno, Carson City, Elko, Fallon and Las Vegas. There were (1989–90) 492 instructors and 32,649 students.

Health. At 30 June 1990 the state had 30 hospitals (3,725 beds) and 29 nursing units (3,141 beds).

Social Security. In 1988 benefits were paid to 146,360 persons: 98,500 retired (aged 62 and over) workers (average payment $537 per month); 13,970 widows and widowers ($500); 11,420 disabled workers ($551), 10,380 wives and husbands ($266), 10,670 children ($270). Social Security beneficiaries represented 13·8% of the population.

Further Reading

Information: Bureau of Business and Economic Research (Univ. of Nevada-Reno).

Bushnell, E. and Driggs, D. W., *The Nevada Constitution: Origin and Growth*. Univ. of Nevada Press, 5th ed., 1980
Hulse, J. W., *The Nevada Adventure, A History*. Univ. of Nevada Press, 2nd ed., 1969
Laxalt, R., *Nevada: A History*. New York, 1977
Mack, E. M. and Sawyer, B. W., *Here is Nevada: A History of the State*. Sparks, Nevada, 1965
Paher, S. W., *Nevada, an Annotated Bibliography*. Nevada, 1980

State Library: Nevada State Library, Carson City. *State Librarian:* Mildred J. Heyer.

NEW HAMPSHIRE

HISTORY. New Hampshire, first settled in 1623, is one of the 13 original states of the Union.

AREA AND POPULATION. New Hampshire is bounded in the north by Canada, east by Maine and the Atlantic, south by Massachusetts and west by Vermont. Area, 9,279 sq. miles, of which 286 sq. miles are inland water. Census population, 1 April 1980, 920,610, an increase of 24·8% since 1970. Estimate (1989), 1,107,000 (544,000 male; 374,000 over 20 years), an increase of 20·3% since 1980. Births, 1988, were 17,363 (16 per 1,000 population); deaths, 8,770 (8·1); infant deaths, 147 (8·5 per 1,000 live births); marriages, 11,116 (10·2); divorces, 4,899 (4·5).

Population at 5 federal censuses was:

	White	*Black*	*Indian*	*Asiatic*	*Total*	*Per sq. mile*
1910	429,906	564	34	68	430,572	47·7
1930	464,351	790	64	88	465,293	51·6
1960	604,334	1,903	135	549	606,921	65·2
			All others			
1970	733,106	2,505	2,070		737,681	81·7
1980	910,099	3,990	6,521		920,610	101·9

The largest city in the state is Manchester, with a 1989 population of 101,960. The capital is Concord, with 37,342. Other cities are: Nashua, 81,536; Dover, 26,476; Rochester, 25,735; Portsmouth, 25,063; Keene, 22,724; Laconia, 16,926; Claremont, 14,111; Lebanon, 12,523; Berlin, 11,962; Somersworth, 10,916; Franklin, 8,383.

CLIMATE. Manchester. Jan. 22°F (–5·6°C), July 70°F (21·1°C). Annual rainfall 40" (1,003 mm). *See* New England, p. 1382.

CONSTITUTION AND GOVERNMENT. While the present constitution dates from 1784, it was extensively revised in 1792 when the state joined the Union. Since 1775 there have been 16 state conventions with 49 amendments adopted to amend the constitution.

The Legislature consists of a Senate of 30 members, elected for 2 years, and a House of Representatives, restricted to between 375 and 400 members, elected for 2 years. The Governor and 5 administrative officers called 'Councillors' are also elected for 2 years.

Electors must be adult citizens, able to read and write, duly registered and not paupers or under sentence for crime. New Hampshire sends to the Federal Congress 2 senators and 2 representatives.

In the 1988 presidential election Bush polled 280,533 votes, Dukakis, 163,205.

The capital is Concord. The state is divided into 10 counties.

Governor: Judd Gregg (R.), 1991–93 ($72,146).

Secretary of State: William M. Gardner (D.) ($50,675).

BUDGET. The state government's general revenue for the fiscal year ending 30 June 1987 (US Census Bureau figures) was $1,382m. ($563m. from taxes, $327m. from federal aid); general expenditures, $1,295m. ($292m. on education, $244m. on public welfare, $183m. on highways).

Per capita personal income (1989) was $20,251.

NATURAL RESOURCES

Minerals. Minerals are little worked; they consist mainly of sand and gravel, stone, and clay for building and highway construction. Value of mineral production, 1988, $47m.

Agriculture. In 1988, there were 2,515 farms occupying 426,237 acres; average farm was 169 acres. Average value per acre, $2,112. The US Soil Survey estimates that the state has 164,167 acres of excellent soil, 486,615 acres of fair soil, 530,630 of poor soil and 3,843,798 of non-arable soil. Only 636,195 acres (11% of the total area) show moderate erosion.

Cash income, 1987, from crops, $38m., and livestock and products, $72m. The chief field crops are hay and vegetables; the chief fruit crop is apples. Livestock on farms, 1987: 55,000 all cattle; 25,000 milch cows; 9,182 sheep; 6,610 swine; 460,000 poultry; 26,000 turkeys; about 30,000 horses.

Forestry. In 1988 forest land totalled 5m. acres; national forest, 735,000 acres.

Fisheries. The 1988 catch was 8·4m. lb., worth $5·6m.

INDUSTRY. Principal manufactures: Machinery, metal products, textiles and shoes.

Labour. In 1988 657,653 persons were in employment (excluding agriculture), of whom 169,148 worked in services, 127,895 in trade and 124,928 in manufacturing.

COMMUNICATIONS

Roads. In 1990 there were 14,803 miles of roads (12,387 miles rural) and 953,642 registered motor vehicles.

Railways. In 1988 the length of railway in the state was 608 miles.

Aviation. In 1988 there were 15 public and 19 private airports.

JUSTICE, RELIGION, EDUCATION AND WELFARE

Justice. The state prison held 940 persons on 1 June 1988. Since 1930 there has been only one execution (by hanging)—a white man, for murder, in 1939.

Religion. The Roman Catholic Church is the largest single body. The largest Protestant churches are Congregational, Episcopal, Methodist and United Baptist Convention of N.H.

Education. School attendance is compulsory for children from 6 to 14 years of age during the whole school term, or to 16 if their district provides a high school. Employed illiterate minors between 16 and 21 years of age must attend evening or special classes, if provided by the district.

In 1990 the public elementary and secondary schools had 171,696 pupils and 10,572 teachers. Public school salaries, 1990, averaged $28,986. Total expenditure on public schools in 1989–90 was estimated at $934m.

Of the 4-year colleges, the University of New Hampshire (founded in 1866) had 12,196 students in 1989–90; New Hampshire College (1932), 6,472; Keene State College (1909), 4,290; Rivier College (1933), 2,603; Dartmouth College (1769), 4,601. Total enrolment, 1989-90, in the 29 institutions of higher education, was 64,045.

Health. In 1987 the state had 37 hospitals.

Social Security. The Division of Human Services handles public assistance for (1) aged citizens 65 years or over, (2) needy aged aliens, (3) needy blind persons, (4) needy citizens between 18 and 64 years inclusive, who are permanently and totally disabled, (5) needy children under 18 years, (6) Medicaid and the medically needy not eligible for a monthly grant.

In May 1988, 1,298 persons were receiving old-age assistance of an average $87 per month; 2,761 permanently and totally disabled, $133 per month; 4,003 families with dependent children, $439 per month.

Further Reading

Delorme, D. (ed.) *New Hampshire Atlas and Gazetteer*. Freeport, 1983
Morison, E. E. and E. F., *New Hampshire*. New York, 1976
Squires, J. D., *The Granite State of the United States: A History of New Hampshire from 1623 to the present*. 4 vols., New York, 1956

NEW JERSEY

HISTORY. New Jersey, first settled in the early 1600s, is one of the 13 original states in the Union.

AREA AND POPULATION. New Jersey is bounded north by New York, east by the Atlantic with Long Island and New York City to the north-east, south by Delaware Bay and west by Pennsylvania. Area (US Bureau of Census), 7,787 sq. miles (319 sq. miles being inland water). Census population, 1 April 1990, 7,730,188, an increase of 365,365 since 1980. Population density, 1990, 1,037·6 per sq mile. Vital statistics, 1988 (per 1,000): Births, 17,481 (15·2); deaths, 72,668 (9·4); marriages, 61,063 (7·9); divorces, 28,919 (3·5).

Population at 5 federal censuses was:

	White	*Black*	*Indian*	*Hispanics*	*Asiatic*	*Others*	*Total*
1910	2,445,894	89,760	168	—	1,345	—	2,537,167
1930	3,829,663	208,828	213	—	2,630	122	4,041,334
1960	5,539,003	514,875	1,699	—	8,778	2,427	6,066,782
1980	6,127,467	925,066	8,394	—	103,847	200,048	7,364,823
1990	6,130,465	1,036,825	14,970	739,861	272,521	275,407	7,730,188

Of the population in 1980, 3,533,012 were male, 6,557,377 persons were urban, 5,116,581 were 20 years of age or older.

Census population of the larger cities and towns in 1990 was:

Newark	275,221	Irvington	61,018	Parsippany-Troy Hills	48,478
Jersey City	228,537	Union City	58,012	Middletown	68,183
Paterson	140,891	Vineland	54,780	Union Township	50,024
Elizabeth	110,002	Passaic	58,041	Bloomfield	45,066
Trenton (capital)	88,675	Woodbridge	93,086	Atlantic City	37,986
Camden	87,992	Hamilton	86,553	Plainfield	46,567
Clifton	71,742	Edison	88,680	Hoboken	33,397
East Orange	73,552	Cherry Hill	69,348	Montclair	37,729
Bayonne	61,444				

Largest urbanized areas (1980) were: Newark, 1,963,000; Jersey City, 555,483; Paterson-Clifton-Passaic, 447,785; Trenton (NJ–Pa.), 305,678.

CLIMATE. Jersey City. Jan. 31°F (–0·6°C), July 75°F (23·9°C). Annual rainfall 41" (1,025 mm). Trenton. Jan. 32°F (0°C), July 76°F (24·4°C). Annual rainfall 40" (1,003 mm). *See* Atlantic Coast, p. 1382.

CONSTITUTION AND GOVERNMENT. The legislative power is vested in a Senate and a General Assembly, the members of which are chosen by the people, all citizens (with necessary exceptions) 18 years of age, with the usual residential qualifications, having the right of suffrage. The present constitution, ratified by the registered voters on 4 Nov. 1947, has been amended 38 times. In 1966 the Constitutional Convention proposed, and the people adopted, a new plan providing for a 40-member Senate and an 80-member General Assembly. This plan, as certified by the Apportionment Commission and modified by the courts, provides for 40 legislative districts, with 1 senator and 2 assemblymen elected for each. Assemblymen serve 2 years, senators 4 years, except those elected at the election following each census, who serve for 2 years. The Governor is elected for 4 years.

The state sends to Congress 2 senators and 14 representatives.

In the 1988 presidential election Bush polled 1,743,192 votes, Dukakis, 1,320,352.

The capital is Trenton. The state is divided into 21 counties, which are subdivided into 567 municipalities—cities, towns, boroughs, villages and townships.

Governor: James J. Florio (D.), 1990–94 ($85,000).
Secretary of State: Joan M. Harberle ($95,000).

BUDGET. For the year ending 30 June 1990 (budget figures) general revenues were $16,789·4m. general expenditures were $17,103m.

Total net long-term debt, 27 Nov. 1990, was approximately $2,500m.

Per capita personal income (1989) was $23,764.

NATURAL RESOURCES

Minerals. In 1988 the chief minerals were stone (19,300,000 short tons, value $123,500,000) and sand and gravel (18,318,000, $74,183,000); others are clays (16,484, $368,482), peat (43,000, $797,000) and gemstones. New Jersey is a leading producer of greensand marl, magnesium compounds and peat. Total value of mineral products, 1988, was $241,832,000.

Agriculture. Livestock raising, market-gardening, fruit-growing, horticulture and forestry are pursued. In 1987, 9,032 farms had a total area of 894,426 acres; and the average farm had 99 acres valued at $3,969 per acre.

Market value of agricultural products sold, 1987: Crops, including nursery and greenhouse, $370·58m.; livestock, poultry and their products, $125,423,000.

Leading crops are tomatoes (value, $15·8m., 1986), corn for grain ($18·4m.), peaches ($23·6m.), all hay ($30·3m.), blueberries ($23·2m.), soybeans ($16·1m.), white potatoes ($11·9m.), sweet corn ($14·1m.), peppers ($12·4m.), cranberries ($17·2m.).

Farm animals on 1 Jan. 1987 included 35,000 milch cows, 90,000 all cattle, 14,000 sheep and lambs and (1 Dec. 1986) 40,000 swine.

INDUSTRY. In 1990 the top 100 corporate employers employed 80,994 workers. The unemployment rate in Nov. 1989 was 4·7%.

In July 1989 there were 3,721,100 employees on non-agricultural payrolls; 2,500 in mining, 184,800 in construction, 658,800 in manufacturing, 242,700 in transportation and public utilities, 889,800 in wholesale and retail trade, 246,900 in finance, insurance and real estate, 945,500 in services, 550,100 in government.

COMMUNICATIONS

Roads. In 1989 there were about 2,254 miles of state and interstate highways. At 1 Jan. 1989 there were 6,712 miles of county highways, 24,302 miles of municipal roads and 929 miles of other road.

Railways. In Sept. 1985, the state had 1,882·05 route miles of railway.

Aviation. There were (1985) 119 airports, 162 heliports and 13 seaplane bases (total 294, of which 67 were publicly owned).

JUSTICE, RELIGION, EDUCATION AND WELFARE

Justice. State prisons in Aug. 1988 had 15,199 inmates. The last execution (by electrocution) was in 1963; it was the 160th, all for murder. Future executions would be by lethal injection.

The constitution of New Jersey forbids discrimination against any person on account of 'religious principles, race, color, ancestry or national origin'. The state has had, since 1945, a 'fair employment act', *i.e.*, a Civil Rights statute forbidding any employer, public or private (with 6 or more employees), to discriminate against any applicant for work (or to discharge any employee) on the grounds of 'race, creed, color, national origin or ancestry'. Trade unions may not bar Blacks from membership.

Religion. The Roman Catholic population of New Jersey in 1990 was 3·1m. In 1984 the five largest Protestant sects were United Methodists, 150,000; United Presbyterians, 174,000; Episcopalians, 147,000; Lutherans, 89,000; American Baptists, 74,000. There were 40,000 African Methodists and 4,000 Christian Methodist Episcopalians. In 1989 there were 411,000 Jews.

Education. Elementary instruction is compulsory for all from 6 to 16 years of age and free to all from 5 to 20 years of age. In 1988 public elementary schools had 733,179 and secondary schools had 347,692 enrolled pupils; public colleges in 1986 had 253,354 students, including 107,250 in community colleges, and independent colleges had 41,736. Average salary of 78,335 elementary and secondary classroom teachers in public schools 1987–88 was $30,778.

In 1988: Rutgers, the State University (founded as Queen's College in 1766) had, 47,719 students; Princeton (founded in 1746) had 6,264; Fairleigh Dickinson (1941), had 5,308; Montclair State College, 12,673; Glassboro State College, 8,500; Trenton State College, 7,779.

Health. In 1989 the state had 123 hospitals (36,617 beds), listed by the American Hospital Association.

Social Security. In the financial year 1987 gross expenditure for all social welfare was $834,446,000. Average monthly social security payment was $559·40.

Further Reading

Legislative District Data Book. Bureau of Government Research. Annual
Manual of the Legislature of New Jersey. Trenton. Annual
Boyd, J. P. (ed.) *Fundamentals and Constitutions of New Jersey, 1664–1954.* Princeton, 1964
Cunningham, J. T., *New Jersey: America's Main Road.* Rev. ed. New York, 1976
Kull, I. Stoddard (ed.) *New Jersey, a History.* New York, 1930

State Library: 185 W. State Street, Trenton, CN 520. N.J. 08625. *State Librarian:* Barbara F. Weaver.

NEW MEXICO

HISTORY. The first European settlement was established in 1598. Until 1771 New Mexico was the Spanish kings' 'Kingdom of New Mexico'. In 1771 it was annexed to the northern province of New Spain. When New Spain won its independence in 1821, it took the name of Republic of Mexico and established New Mexico as its northernmost department. When the war between the US and Mexico was concluded on 2 Feb. 1848 New Mexico was recognized as belonging to the US, and on 9 Sept. 1850 it was made a Territory. Part of the Territory was assigned to Texas; later Utah was formed into a separate Territory; in 1861 another part was transferred to Colorado, and in 1863 Arizona was disjoined, leaving to New Mexico its present area. New Mexico became a state in Jan. 1912.

AREA AND POPULATION. New Mexico is bounded north by Colorado, north-east by Oklahoma, east by Texas, south by Texas and Mexico and west by Arizona. Land area 121,335 sq. miles (258 sq. miles water). Public lands, administered by federal agencies (1975) amounted to 26·7m. acres or 34% of the total area. The Bureau of Indian Affairs held 7·3m. acres; the State of New Mexico held 9·4m. acres; 34·4m. acres were privately owned.

Census population, 1 April 1980, 1,303,303, an increase of 286,248 or 28% since 1970. Estimate (1989) 1,528,000. Vital statistics, 1988: Births, 26,935 (17·9 per 1,000 population); deaths, 10,381; infant deaths, 268 (9·9 per 1,000 live births); marriages, 13,039; divorces in 1987, 7,943 (5·3).

The population in 5 census years was:

	White	*Black*	*Indian*	*Asian and Pacific Island*	*Other*	*Total*	*Per sq. mile*
1910	304,594	1,628	20,573	506		327,301	2·7
1940	492,312	4,672	34,510	324		531,818	4·4
1960	875,763	17,063	56,255	1,942		951,023	7·8
1970	915,815	19,555	72,788	7,842 [1]		1,016,000	8·4
1980	1,164,053	24,406	106,119	6,825	1,491	1,302,894	10·7

[1] Includes unspecified races, 1970.

Of the 1980 total, 642,157 were male, 939,963 persons were urban; 884,987 were 18 years of age or older.

Before 1930 New Mexico was largely a Spanish-speaking state, but since 1945 an influx of population from other states has reduced the percentage of persons of Spanish origin or descent to 36·6% (1980).

The largest cities are Albuquerque, with census population, 1980, 332,336 (and 1988 estimate, 378,480); Santa Fé (capital), 49,299 (59,300); Las Cruces, 45,086 (56,000); Roswell, 39,676 (43,230); Farmington, 32,677 (38,470).

CLIMATE. Santa Fé. Jan. 29°F (–1·7°C), July 68°F (20°C). Annual rainfall 15" (366 mm). *See* Mountain States, p. 1381.

CONSTITUTION AND GOVERNMENT. The constitution of 1912 is still in force with 105 amendments. The state Legislature, which meets annually, consists of 42 members of the Senate, elected for 4 years, and 70 members of the House of Representatives, elected for 2 years. The Governor and Lieut.-Governor are elected for 4 years. The state sends to Congress 2 senators and 3 representatives.

In the 1988 presidential election Bush polled 270,341 votes, Dukakis 244,497.

The state capital is Santa Fé. For local government the state is divided into 33 counties.

Governor: Bruce King (D.), 1991–95 ($63,000).

BUDGET. For the year ending 30 June 1987 (US Census Bureau figures) the states general revenues were $3,268m. ($1,573m. from taxation and $566m. from federal government); general expenditures, $3,074m. (education, $1,298m.; highways, $382m., and public welfare, $317m.).

Per capita personal income (1989) was $13,140.

ENERGY AND NATURAL RESOURCES

Minerals. New Mexico is the country's largest domestic source of uranium, perlite and potassium salts. Production of recoverable U_3O_8 was 2·3m. lb. in 1988; perlite,

706,000 short tons; potassium salts, 1·35m. short tons; petroleum, 71·2m. bbls (of 42 gallons); natural gas, 781,000 cu. ft; copper, 321,650 short tons; coal, 21·7m. short tons marketed. The value of the total mineral output (1988) was $3,680m. An average of 15,400 persons were employed monthly in the mining industry in 1988.

Agriculture. New Mexico produces cereals, vegetables, fruit, livestock and cotton. Dry farming and irrigation have proved profitable in periods of high prices. There were 14,000 farms and ranches covering 44·5m. acres in 1988; in the 1987 US Census of Agriculture average farm (or ranch) was valued (land and buildings) at $582,012; 3,767 farms and ranches were of 1,000 acres and over.

Cash income, 1988 (preliminary), from crops, $370·8m., and from livestock products, $910·3m. Principal crops are wheat (7m. bu. from 290,000 acres), hay (1·2m. tons from 275,000 acres) and sorghum/grains (8·7m. bu. from 145,000 acres). Farm animals on 1 Jan. 1989 included 63,000 milch cows, 1·35m. all cattle, 516,000 sheep and 26,000 swine (1988). National forest area (1986) covered 9·3m. acres.

INDUSTRY. Average monthly non-agricultural employment during 1989 was 560,400: 42,100 were employed in manufacturing, 144,600 in government. Value of manufactures shipments, 1986, $3,776·4m.; leading industries, food and kindred products, transport and equipment, lumber and wood.

COMMUNICATIONS

Roads. In 1990 there were 54,807 miles of roads (49,367 miles rural) and 1,294,521 registered motor vehicles.

Railways. On 31 Dec. 1987 there were 2,062 miles of railway.

Aviation. There were 71 public-use airports in Dec. 1988.

JUSTICE, RELIGION, EDUCATION AND WELFARE

Justice. The number of state prison inmates in Oct. 1989 was 2,924, and there were 380 in juvenile centres in 1988; there were also 78 New Mexico prisoners held outside the state in 1989. The death penalty (by electrocution formerly, and now by lethal injection) has been imposed on 8 persons since 1933, 6 whites and 2 Negroes, all for murder. The last execution was in 1961.

Since 1949 the denial of employment by reason of race, colour, religion, national origin or ancestry has been forbidden. A law of 1955 prohibits discrimination in public places because of race or colour. An 'equal rights' amendment was added to the constitution in 1972.

Religion. There were (1975) approximately 356,530 Protestant Church members and 315,470 Roman Catholics.

Education. Elementary education is free, and compulsory between 6 and 17 years or high-school graduation age. In 1988–89 the 88 school districts had an estimated enrolment of 316,332 students in elementary and secondary schools of which private and parochial schools had 24,134. There were 15,759 FTE teachers receiving an average salary of $24,620. Public expenditure for elementary and secondary schools was $1,103m. (1987-88).

The state-supported 4-year institutes of higher education are (1988–89 [1]):

	Full-time Faculty	*Students*
University of New Mexico, Albuquerque	1,936	28,258
New Mexico State University, Las Cruces	838	20,027
Eastern New Mexico University, Portales	267	8,260
New Mexico Highlands University, Las Vegas	110	2,234
Western New Mexico University, Silver City	71	1,800
New Mexico Institute of Mining and Technology, Socorro	83	1,129

[1] Figures include branches outside main campus in cities listed.

Health. In 1988 the state had 49 short-term hospitals (4,637 beds).

Social Security. In Dec. 1986, 17,622 persons were receiving federal supplemental security income for the disabled (average $257.29 per month); 9,322 persons were receiving old-age assistance (average $140.43 per month); 511 persons were receiving aid to the blind (average $239.21 per month). A monthly average of 50,831 people received aid to families with dependent children (average $83.64 per month).

Further Reading

New Mexico Business (monthly; annual review in Jan.–Feb. issue). Bureau of Business and Economic Research, Univ. of N.M., Albuquerque
New Mexico Progress Economic Review (annual). Sunwest, Albuquerque
New Mexico Statistical Abstract: 1989. Bureau of Business and Economic Research, Univ. of N.M., Albuquerque, 1989
Beck, W., *New Mexico: a History of Four Centuries*. Univ. of Oklahoma, 1979
Garcia, C., Haine, P. and Rhodes, H., *State and Local Government in New Mexico*. Albuquerque, 1979
Jenkins, M. and Schroeder, A., *A Brief History of New Mexico*. Univ. of New Mexico, 1974
Muench, D. and Hillerman, T., *New Mexico*. Belding, Portland, Oregon, 1974
Williams, J. L., *New Mexico in Maps*. Univ. of New Mexico, 1986

NEW YORK STATE

HISTORY. From 1609 to 1664 the region now called New York was claimed by the Dutch; then it came under the rule of the English, who governed the country until the outbreak of the War of Independence. On 20 April 1777 New York adopted a constitution which transformed the colony into an independent state; on 26 July 1788 it ratified the constitution of the US, becoming one of the 13 original states. New York dropped its claim to Vermont after the latter was admitted to the Union in 1791. With the annexation of a small area from Massachusetts in 1853, New York assumed its present boundaries.

AREA AND POPULATION. New York is bounded west and north by Canada with Lake Erie, Lake Ontario and the St Lawrence River forming the boundary; east by Vermont, Massachusetts and Connecticut, south-east by the Atlantic, south by New Jersey and Pennsylvania. Area, 49,108 sq. miles (1,731 sq. miles being water). Census population, 1 April 1980, 17,557,288, a decrease of 3·7% since 1970. Estimate (1985) 17,783,000. Births in 1984 were 251,062 (14·2 per 1,000 population); deaths, 168,852 (9·5); infant deaths, 2,789 (11·1 per 1,000 live births); marriages, 168,860 (9·5); divorces, 61,075 (3·4, includes all dissolutions).

Population in 5 census years was:

	White	*Black*	*Indian*	*Asiatic*	*Total*	*Per sq. mile*
1910	8,966,845	134,191	6,046	6,532	9,113,614	191·2
1930	12,143,191	412,814	6,973	15,088	12,588,066	262·6
1960	15,287,071	1,417,511	16,491	51,678	16,782,304	350·2
			All others			
1970	15,834,090	2,168,949	233,828		18,236,967	380·3
1980	13,961,106	2,401,842	1,194,340		17,557,288	367·0

Of the 1980 population, 8,338,961 were male, 14,857,202 were urban; those 20 years of age or older numbered 12,232,284. Aliens registered in Jan. 1980 numbered 801,411.

The population of New York City, by boroughs, census of 1 April 1980 was: Manhattan, 1,427,533; Bronx, 1,169,115; Brooklyn, 2,230,936; Queens, 1,891,325; Staten Island, 352,121; total, 7,071,030. The New York metropolitan statistical area had, in 1980, 9,080,777.

Population of other large cities and incorporated places census, April 1980, was:

Buffalo	357,002	Albany (capital)	101,767	Schenectady	67,877
Rochester	241,509	Utica	75,435	Mount Vernon	66,023
Yonkers	194,557	Niagara Falls	71,344	Troy	56,614
Syracuse	170,292	New Rochelle	70,345	Binghamton	55,745
White Plains	46,999	N. Tonawanda	35,760	Lindenhurst	26,919
Rome	43,826	Elmira	35,327	Rockville Center	25,405
Hempstead	40,404	Auburn	32,548	Newburgh	23,438
Freeport	38,272	Poughkeepsie	29,757	Garden City	22,927
Jamestown	35,775	Watertown	27,861	Massapequa Park	19,779
Valley Stream	35,769				

Other large urbanized areas, census 1980; Buffalo, 1·2m.; Rochester, 970,313; Albany–Schenectady–Troy, 794,298.

CLIMATE. Albany. Jan. 24°F (–4·4°C), July 73°F (22·8°C). Annual rainfall 34" (855 mm). Buffalo. Jan. 24°F (–4·4°C), July 70°F (21·1°C). Annual rainfall 36" (905 mm). New York. Jan. 30°F (–1·1°C), July 74°F (23·3°C). Annual rainfall 43" (1,087 mm). *See* Atlantic Coast, p. 1382.

CONSTITUTION AND GOVERNMENT. The present constitution dates from 1894; a later constitutional convention, 1938, is now legally considered merely to have amended the 1894 constitution, which has now had 93 amendments. The Constitutional Convention of 1967 (4 April through 26 Sept.) was composed of 186 delegates who proposed a new state constitution; however this was rejected by the registered voters on 7 Nov. 1967. The Senate consists of 60 members, and the Assembly of 150 members, both elected every 2 years. The Governor and Lieut.-Governor are elected for 4 years. The right of suffrage resides in every adult who has been a citizen for 90 days, and has the residential qualifications; new voters must establish, by certificates or test, that they have had at least an elementary education. The state is represented in Congress by 2 senators and 34 representatives. In the 1988 presidential election Dukakis polled 3,228,304 votes, Bush, 2,975,276. The state capital is Albany. For local government the state is divided into 62 counties, 5 of which constitute the city of New York. New York leads in state parks and recreation areas, covering 252,984 acres in 1979.

Cities are in 3 classes, the first class having each 175,000 or more inhabitants and the third under 50,000. Each is incorporated by charter, under special legislation. The government of New York City is vested in the mayor (Edward Koch), elected for 4 years, and a city council, whose president and members are elected for 4 years. The council has a President and 37 members, each elected from a state senatorial district wholly within the city. The mayor appoints all the heads of departments, except the comptroller, who is elected. Each of the 5 city boroughs (Manhattan, Bronx, Brooklyn, Queens and Richmond) has a president, elected for 4 years. Each borough is also a county bearing the same name except Manhattan borough, which, as a county, is called New York, and Brooklyn, which is Kings County.

Governor: Mario Cuomo (D.), 1991-95 ($130,000).

BUDGET. The state's general revenues for the financial year ending 31 March 1982 were $16,142m. ($14,959m. from taxes); general expenditures were $16,126m. ($5,298m. for education, $8,049m. for social services, $1,893m. for transport).

Per capita personal income was $14,121 in 1984.

The assessed valuation in 1980 of taxable real property in New York City was $38,056m. The assessed valuation of the state was $86,741m.

ENERGY AND NATURAL RESOURCES

Minerals. Production of principal minerals in 1980: Sand and gravel (22,000 short tons), salt (5,500 short tons), zinc (33,629 tonnes), petroleum (824,296 bbls), natural gas (15,680m. cu. ft). The state is a leading producer of titanium concentrate, talc, abrasive garnet, wollastonite and emery. Quarry products include trap rock, slate, marble, limestone and sandstone. Value of mineral output in 1980 $497·9m.

Agriculture. New York has large agricultural interests. In 1985 it had 45,000 farms, with a total area of 9m. acres; average farm was 200 acres; average value per acre, $808.

Cash income, 1985, from crops $719m. and livestock, $1,845m. Dairying, with 18,500 farms, 1981, is an important type of farming with produce at a market value of $1,383m. Field crops comprise maize, winter wheat, oats and hay. New York ranks second in US in the production of apples, and maple syrup. Other products are grapes, tart cherries, peaches, pears, plums, strawberries, raspberries, cabbages, onions, potatoes, maple sugar. Estimated farm animals, 1986, included 2m. all cattle, 968,000 milch cows, 55,000 sheep, 130,000 swine and 8m. chickens.

INDUSTRY. The main employers (1982 census) are service industries (997,800), trade (1,381,000) and manufacture (1,418,800). Leading industries were clothing, non-electrical machinery, printing and publishing, electrical equipment, instruments, food and allied products and fabricated metals.

COMMUNICATIONS

Roads. In 1990 there were 110,964 miles of roads (73,263 miles rural). The New York State Thruway extends 559 miles from New York City to Buffalo. The Northway, a 176-mile toll-free highway, is a connecting road from the Thruway at Albany to the Canadian border at Champlain, Quebec.

Motor vehicle registrations in 1990 were 10,020,539.

Railways. There were in 1981, 3,891 miles of Class I railways. New York City has NYCTA and PATH metro systems, and commuter railways run by Metro-North, New Jersey Rail and Long Island Rail Road.

Aviation. There were 472 airports and landing areas in 1986.

Shipping. The canals of the state, combined in 1918 in what is called the Improved Canal System, have a length of 524 miles, of which the Erie or Barge canal has 340 miles. In 1981 the canals carried 807,925 tons of freight.

JUSTICE, RELIGION, EDUCATION AND WELFARE

Justice. The State Human Rights Law was approved 12 March 1945, effective 1 July, 1945. The State Division of Human Rights is charged with the responsibility of enforcing this law. The division may request and utilize the services of all governmental departments and agencies; adopt and promulgate suitable rules and regulations; test, investigate and pass judgment upon complaints alleging discrimination in employment, in places of public accommodation, resort or amusement, education, and in housing, land and commercial space; hold hearings, sub-poena witnesses and require the production for examination of papers relating to matters under investigation; grant compensatory damages and require repayment of profits in certain housing cases among other provisions; apply for court injunctions to prevent frustration of orders of the Commissioner.

On 30 Dec. 1984, 33,155 persons were in state prisons.

In 1963–81 there were no executions. Total executions (by electrocution) from 1930 to 1962 were 329 (234 whites, 90 Negroes, 5 other races; all for murder except 2 for kidnapping).

In 1985 murders reported in New York were 1,688; total violent crimes, 165,145. Police strength (sworn officers) in 1985 was 61,009 (39,193 New York City).

Religion. The churches are Roman Catholic, with 6,367,576 members in 1981, Jewish congregations (about 2m. in 1981) and Protestant Episcopal (299,929 in 1980).

Education. Education is compulsory between the ages of 7 and 16. In 1985 the public elementary and secondary schools had 2,605,363 pupils; classroom teachers numbered 175,256 in public schools. Total expenditure on public schools in 1985 was $13,244m. Teachers' salaries, 1985, averaged $29,200.

The state's educational system, including public and private schools and secondary institutions, universities, colleges, libraries, museums, etc., constitutes (by legislative act) the 'University of the State of New York', which is governed by a Board of Regents consisting of 15 members appointed by the Legislature. Within the framework of this 'University' was established in 1948 a 'State University' which controls 64 colleges and educational centres, 30 of which are locally operated community colleges. The 'State University' is governed by a board of 16 Trustees, appointed by the Governor with the consent and advice of the Senate.

Higher education in the state is conducted in 296 institutions (642,000 full-time and 371,000 part-time students in autumn 1982); 573,000 students are in public-control colleges and 439,000 in private.

In autumn 1980 the institutions of higher education in the state included:

Founded	*Name and place*	*Teachers*	*Students*
1754	Columbia University, New York	3,965	17,410
1795	Union University, Schenectady and Albany	178	2,071
1824	Rensselaer Polytechnic Institute, Troy	442	6,145
1831	New York University, New York	2,615	45,000
1846	Colgate University, New York	205	2,550
1846	Fordham University, New York	958	14,653
1847	University of the City of New York, New York	12,426	172,683
1848	University of Rochester, Rochester	1,549	11,159
1854	Polytechnic Institute of New York	242	4,583
1856	St Lawrence University, Canton	173	2,375
1857	Cooper Union Institute of Technology, New York	161	872
1861	Vassar College, Poughkeepsie	230	2,364
1863	Manhattan College, New York	291	3,498
1865	Cornell University, Ithaca	1,863	17,866
1870	Syracuse University, Syracuse	1,100	11,819
1948	State University of New York	13,228	372,415

The Saratoga Performing Arts Centre (5,100 seats), a non-profit, tax-exempt organization, which opened in 1966, is the summer residence of the New York City Ballet and the Philadelphia Orchestra—two groups which present special educational programmes for students and teachers.

Health. In 1981 the state had 278 hospitals (67,798 beds), 585 skilled nursing homes (62,435 beds) and 241 other institutions (24,302 beds). In 1986 mental health facilities had 21,836 patients and institutions for the mentally retarded had 10,581 patients.

Social Security. The federal Supplemental Security Income programme covered aid to the needy aged, blind and disabled from 1 Jan. 1975. In the state programme for 1980, $4,543m. was paid in Medicaid to 2,288,000 people; aid to dependent children in 1985 went to 1,109,610 recipients, average benefits $371 per family per month.

Further Reading

New York Red Book. Albany, 1979–80
Legislative Manual. Department of State, 1980–81
Managing Modern New York: the Carey Era. Rockefeller Institute, Albany, 1985
New York State Statistical Yearbook, 1986–87. Rockefeller Institute, Albany
Connery, R. and G. B., *Governing New York State: The Rockefeller Years.* Academy of Political Science, New York, 1974
Ellis, D. M., *History of New York State.* Cornell Univ. Press, 1967
Flick, A. (ed.) *History of the State of New York.* Columbia Univ. Press, 1933–37

State Library: The New York State Library, Albany 12230. *State Librarian and Assistant Commissioner for Libraries:* Joseph Shubert.

NORTH CAROLINA

HISTORY. North Carolina, first settled in 1585 by Sir Walter Raleigh and permanently settled in 1663, was one of the 13 original states of the Union.

AREA AND POPULATION. North Carolina is bounded north by Virginia, east by the Atlantic, south by South Carolina, south-west by Georgia and west by Tennessee. Area, 52,669 sq. miles, of which 3,826 sq. miles are inland water. Census population, 1 April 1980, 5,874,429, an increase of 15·5% since 1970. Estimated population (1986), 6,331,000.

Births, 1984, were 86,705 (14·1 per 1,000 population); marriages, 52,123 (8·5); deaths, 51,496 (8·4); infant deaths, 1,099 (12·7 per 1,000 live births); divorces and annulments, 29,125 (4·7).

Population in 6 census years was:

	White	*Black*	*Indian*	*Asiatic*	*Total*	*Per sq. mile*
1910	1,500,511	697,843	7,851	82	2,206,287	45·3
1930	2,234,958	918,647	16,579	92	3,170,276	64·5
1950	2,983,121	1,047,353	3,742	—	4,061,929	82·7
1960	3,399,285	1,116,021	38,129	2,012	4,556,155	92·2
			All others			
1970	3,901,767	1,126,478	53,814		5,082,059	104·1
1980	4,453,010	1,316,050	105,369		5,874,429	111·5

Of the total population in 1980, 2,852,012 were male, 2,818,794 were urban and 3,976,359 were 20 years old or older; 14·8% were non-white.

Cities (with census population in 1980) are: Charlotte, 314,447; Greensboro, 155,642; Winston-Salem, 131,885; Raleigh (capital), 149,771; Durham, 100,831; High Point, 64,107; Asheville, 53,281; Fayetteville, 59,507.

CLIMATE. Climate varies sharply with altitude; the warmest area is in the south east near Southport and Wilmington; the coldest is Mount Mitchell (6,684 ft). Raleigh. Jan. 42°F (5·6°C), July 79°F (26·1°C). Annual rainfall 46" (1,158 mm). *See* Atlantic Coast, p. 1382.

CONSTITUTION AND GOVERNMENT. The present constitution dates from 1971 (previous constitution, 1776 and 1868/76); it has had 19 amendments. The General Assembly consists of a Senate of 50 members and a House of Representatives of 120 members; all are elected by districts for 2 years.

The Governor and Lieut.-Governor are elected for 4 years. The Governor may succeed himself but has no veto. There are 19 other executive heads of department, 8 elected by the people and 9 appointed by the Governor. All registered citizens with the usual residential qualifications have a vote.

The state is represented in Congress by 2 senators and 11 representatives.

In the presidential election of 1988 Bush polled 1,232,132 votes, Dukakis, 890,034.

The capital is Raleigh, established in 1792.

Governor: James G. Martin (R.), 1989–93 ($100,000, plus $11,500 annual expenses).

Lieut.-Governor: Jim Gardner (R.) ($61,044, plus $11,500 annual expenses).

Secretary of State: Rufus Edmiston (D.) ($61,044).

BUDGET. General revenue for the year ending 30 June 1986 was $4,910·9m. General expenditure was $4,971·9m.

On 30 June 1986 the net total long-term debt amounted to $757m.

Per capita personal income (1985–86) was $11,903.

NATURAL RESOURCES

Minerals. Mining production in 1985 was valued at $474·7m. Principal minerals were stone, sand and gravel, phosphate rock, feldspar, lithium minerals, olivine, kaolin and talc.

North Carolina ranked first in the production of scrap mica, feldspar, lithium minerals, olivine and phrophyllite. It is also the leading producer of bricks, making more than 1,000m. bricks a year.

Agriculture. In 1985 there were 76,000 farms in North Carolina covering 10·8m. acres; average size of farms was 142 acres and total estimated value $18,500m.

Cash receipts from farming (1984), $4,125m., of which $2,198m. was from crops and $1,927m. from livestock, dairy and poultry products. Main crop production: flue-cured tobacco, maize, soybeans, peanuts, wheat, sweet potatoes and apples.

On 1 Jan. 1985 farms had 1·17m. all cattle, 2·3m. swine and 20·2m. chickens.

Forestry. Commercial forest covered 18·5m. acres (60% of land area), in 1984. Main products are hardwood veneer and hardwood plywood, furniture woods, pulp, paper and lumber.

Fisheries. Commercial fish catch, 1985, amounted to 215m. lb.; value approximately $65m. The catch is mainly of menhaden, crabmeat, bay scallops, flounder, croaker, shrimps, sea trout, spots and clams.

INDUSTRY. North Carolina's manufacturing establishments in 1985 had 827,400 workers. The leading industries by employment are textiles, clothing, furniture, electrical machinery and equipment, non-electrical machinery, and food processing.

In 1985 investment in new and expanded industry was $2,758m. About 576,200 are employed in trade, 422,800 in government and 427,600 in services.

TOURISM. Total receipts of the travel industry, $4,500m. in 1985.

COMMUNICATIONS

Roads. In 1990 there were 94,228 miles of roads (75,165 miles rural) and 5,113,224 registered motor vehicles.

Railways. The state in 1986 contained 3,682 miles of railway operating in 91 of the 100 counties. There are 22 Class I, II and III rail companies.

Aviation. In 1986 there were 82 public airports of which 14 are served by major airlines.

Shipping. There are 2 ocean ports, Wilmington and Morehead City.

JUSTICE, RELIGION, EDUCATION AND WELFARE

Justice. Total executions 1910–86, 365. There was one execution (by lethal injection) in 1986. Prison population at 31 Oct. 1986, 17,700.

Religion. Leading denominations are the Baptists (48·9% of church membership), Methodists (20·7%), Presbyterians (7·7%), Lutherans (3%) and Roman Catholics (2·7%). Total estimate of all denominations in 1983 was 2·6m.

Education. School attendance is compulsory between 6 and 16.

Public school enrolment, 1985–86, was 1,080,887; elementary and secondary schools numbered 1,968. Instructional staff (1986) consisted of 57,630 classroom teachers; average salary $22,476. Expenditure for public schools was $2,770m., 65·5% from state, 25·2% from local and 9·3% from federal sources.

In autumn 1985–86 state-supported colleges and universities included 58 community and technical colleges with 654,000 full and part time students. The 16 senior universities are all part of the University of North Carolina system, the largest campus being North Carolina State University and Raleigh, with 23,400 students. The university system was founded in 1789 at Chapel Hill and first opened in 1792. Its 1986 autumn enrolment was 130,000 students.

In addition to the state-supported institutions there were 7 private junior colleges with an enrolment of 2,585 and 31 private senior institutions with a total enrolment of 19,009. The total undergraduate enrolment in private institutions for 1985 was 21,594.

Health. In Oct. 1986 the state had 160 hospitals (34,438 beds).

Social Security. In June 1982 there were 900,070 persons receiving $300·4m. in social security benefits. Of that number 496,020 were retired, receiving $186·67m.; 85,640 were disabled ($34·7m.); 318,410 others received $79m.

Further Reading

North Carolina Manual. Secretary of State. Raleigh. Biennial
Clay, J. W. *et al* (eds.), *North Carolina Atlas: Portrait of a Changing Southern State*. Univ. of North Carolina Press, 1975
Corbitt, D. L., *The Formation of the North Carolina Counties*. Raleigh, 1969
Lefler, H. T. and Newsome, A. R., *North Carolina: The History of a Southern State*. Univ. of N.C., Chapel Hill, 1973

NORTH DAKOTA

HISTORY. North Dakota was admitted into the Union, with boundaries as at present, on 2 Nov. 1889; previously it had formed part of the Dakota Territory, established 2 March 1861.

AREA AND POPULATION. North Dakota is bounded north by Canada, east by the Red River (forming a boundary with Minnesota), south by South Dakota and west by Montana. Land area, 69,262 sq. miles, and 1,403 sq. miles of water. The Federal Bureau of Indian Affairs administered (1971) 850,000 acres, of which 153,000 acres were assigned to tribes. Census population, 1 April 1990 (preliminary), 634,223, a decrease of 18,494 or 2·8% since 1980. Births in 1988 were 10,111 (15·2 per 1,000 population); deaths, 5,664 (8·5); infant deaths, 107; marriages, 4,996; divorces, 2,365.

Population at 5 census years was:

	White	*Black*	*Indian*	*Asiatic*	*Total*	*Per sq. mile*
1910	569,855	617	6,486	98	577,056	8·2
1930	671,851	377	8,617	194	680,845	9·7
1960	619,538	777	11,736	274	632,446	9·1
			All others			
1970	599,485	2,494	15,782		617,761	8·9
1980	625,557	2,568	24,692		652,717	9·4

Of the total population in 1980, 328,126 were male, 317,821 were urban and 419,234 were 21 years old or older. Estimated outward migration, 1970–80, 16,983.

The largest cities are Fargo with population (census), 1980, of 61,383; Grand Forks, 43,765; Bismarck (capital), 44,485, and Minot, 32,843.

CLIMATE. Bismarck. Jan. 8°F (–13·3°C), July 71°F (21·1°C). Annual rainfall 16" (402 mm). Fargo. Jan. 6°F (–14·4°C), July 71°F (21·1°C). Annual rainfall 20" (503 mm). *See* High Plains and Mid-West (SW North Dakota is in the Plains, the rest in the mid-west lowlands), p. 1381-82.

CONSTITUTION AND GOVERNMENT. The present constitution dates from 1889; it has had 95 amendments. The Legislative Assembly consists of a Senate of 53 members elected for 4 years, and a House of Representatives of 106 members elected for 2 years. The Governor and Lieut.-Governor are elected for 4 years. Qualified electors are (with necessary exceptions) all citizens and civilized Indians. The state sends to Congress 2 senators elected by the voters of the entire state and 1 representative.

In the 1988 presidential election Bush polled 165,517 votes, Dukakis, 127,081.

The capital is Bismarck. The state has 53 organized counties.

Governor: George A. Sinner (D.), 1989–93 ($60,862 plus expenses).

FINANCE. General revenue of state and local government year ending 30 June 1989, was $1,052m.; general expenditures, $1,055m., taxation provided $598m. and federal grants, $431m.; education took $621m.; highways, $157m., and public welfare, $232m.

Total net long-term debt (local government) on 30 June 1982, $325m.

Per capita personal income (1985) was $13,004.

ENERGY AND NATURAL RESOURCES

Minerals. The mineral resources of North Dakota consist chiefly of oil which was discovered in 1951. Production of crude petroleum in 1987 was 41·4m. bbls; of natural gas, 71,612m. cu. ft. Output of lignite coal was 25·2m. short tons. Total value of mineral output, 1984, $1,724m.

Agriculture. Agriculture is the chief pursuit of the North Dakota population. In 1985 there were 33,000 farms (61,963 in 1954) with an area of 41m. acres (41,876,924 in 1954); the average farm was of 1,242 acres. The greater number of farms are cash-grain or livestock farms with annual sales of $20,000–$39,999.

Cash income, 1986, from crops, $1,423m., and from livestock, $676m. North Dakota leads in the production of barley, sunflowers, flaxseed, wheat, pinto beans, rye and durum. Other important products are sugar-beet, potatoes, hay, oats and maize.

The state has also an active livestock industry, chiefly cattle raising. On 1 Jan. 1985 the farm animals were: 97,000 milch cows, 2m. all cattle, 215,000 sheep and 250,000 swine. The wool clip yielded (1984), 1·6m. lb. of wool from 180,000 sheep.

Forestry. National forest area, 1977, 422,000 acres, of which 115,000 acres are federally owned or managed.

INDUSTRY. From 1970 to 1985 agricultural employment fell from 46,554 to 51,480; non-agricultural jobs rose from 175,700 to 314,900. In 1988, 68,200 were employed in trade, 64,700 in government, 63,600 in services, 16,400 in transport and utilities, 16,400 in manufacturing.

COMMUNICATIONS

Roads. The state highway department maintained, in 1989, 8,290 miles of highway; local authorities, 75,000 miles, and municipal, 3,250 miles. Car and truck registrations in 1989 numbered 716,967.

Railways. In 1989 there were 4,800 miles of railway.

Aviation. Airports in 1990, there were 100 public use airports and 475 private use airstrips.

JUSTICE, RELIGION, EDUCATION AND WELFARE

Justice. The state penitentiary, on 31 Dec. 1987, held 410 inmates. The State Farm, a minimum custody institution, held 40 inmates. There is no death penalty.

Religion. The leading religious denominations are the Roman Catholics, with 230,600 members in 1980; Combined Lutherans, 288,500; Methodists, 36,500; Presbyterians, 19,500, and the United Church of Christ, 15,000.

Education. School attendance is compulsory between the ages of 7 and 16, or until the 17th birthday if the eighth grade has not been completed. In Oct. 1988 the public elementary schools had 84,238 pupils; secondary schools, 32,896 pupils. State expenditure on public schools, 1988, $424m. or $663 per capita. Teachers (4,441 in elementary and 2,376 in secondary schools) earned an average $22,249 in 1988.

The university of North Dakota in Grand Forks, founded in 1883, had 12,280 students in 1989; North Dakota State University in Fargo, 9,432 students. Total enrolment in the 8 public institutions of higher education, 1989, 35,311.

Health. In 1987 the state had 52 hospitals (4,047 beds), and 95 nursing homes (6,728).

Social Security. In 1989 7,237 received SSI payments, including 2,294 aged (average $122 per month). 4,861 disabled ($209); total paid, $15·8m.; 15,049 recipients in 5,408 families received Aid to Families with Dependent Children.

Further Reading

North Dakota Growth Indicators, 1984. 20th ed. Economic Development Commission, Bismarck, 1985
North Dakota Blue Book. Secretary of State, Bismarck, 1981
Statistical Abstract of North Dakota, 1983. Bureau of Business and Economic Research, Univ. of North Dakota, 1983
Glaab, C. L. et al, *The North Dakota Political Tradition*. Iowa State Univ. Press, 1981
Jelliff, T. B., *North Dakota: A Living Legacy*. Fargo, 1983
Robinson, E. B., *History of North Dakota*. Univ. of Nebraska Press, 1966

OHIO

HISTORY. The first organized white settlement was in 1788; Ohio unofficially entered the Union on 19 Feb. 1803; entrance was made official, retroactive to 1 March 1803, on 8 Aug. 1953.

AREA AND POPULATION. Ohio is bounded north by Michigan and Lake Erie, east by Pennsylvania, south-east and south by the Ohio River (forming a boundary with West Virginia and Kentucky) and west by Indiana. Area, 41,330 sq. miles, of which 325 sq. miles are inland water. Census population, 1 April 1980 10,797,630, an increase of 145,402 or 1·4% since 1970. Estimate (1986) 10,752,000. In 1987 births numbered 157,820 (14·6 per 1,000 population); deaths, 99,177 (9·2); infant deaths, 1,469 (9·3 per 1,000 live births); marriages, 95,882 (8·9); divorces, 49,294 (4·6).

Population at 5 census years was:

	White	*Black*	*Indian*	*Asiatic*	*Total*	*Per sq. mile*
1910	4,654,897	111,452	127	645	4,767,121	117·0
1930	6,335,173	309,304	435	1,785	6,646,697	161·6
1960	8,909,698	786,097	1,910	8,692	9,706,397	236·9
			All others			
1970	9,646,997	970,477	34,543		10,652,017	260·0
1980	9,597,458	1,076,748	123,424		10,797,630	263·2

Of the total population in 1980, 5,217,027 were male, 7,918,259 persons were urban. Those 20 years old or older numbered 7,294,471.

Census population of chief cities on 1 April 1980 was:

Cleveland	573,822	Hamilton	63,189	Cuyahoga Falls	43,890
Columbus	565,032	Lakewood	61,963	Mentor	42,065
Cincinnati	385,457	Kettering	61,186	Newark	41,200
Toledo	354,635	Euclid	59,999	Marion	37,040
Akron	237,177	Elyria	57,538	East Cleveland	36,957
Dayton	193,444	Cleveland Heights	56,438	North Olmsted	36,486
Youngstown	115,436	Warren	47,381	Upper Arlington	35,648
Canton	93,077	Mansfield	53,927	Lancaster	34,953
Parma	92,548	Lima	47,381	Garfield Heights	34,938
Lorain	75,416	Middletown	43,719	Zanesville	28,655
Springfield	72,563				

Urbanized areas, 1980 census: Cleveland, 1,898,825; Cincinnati, 1,401,491; Columbus (the capital), 1,093,316; Dayton, 830,070; Akron, 660,328; Toledo, 791,599; Youngstown-Warren, 531,350; Canton, 404,421.

CLIMATE. Cincinnati. Jan. 33°F (0·6°C), July 78°F (25·6°C). Annual rainfall 39" (978 mm). Cleveland. Jan. 27°F (–2·8°C), July 71°F (21·1°C). Annual rainfall 35" (879 mm). Columbus. Jan. 29°F (–1·7°C), July 75°F (23·9°C). Annual rainfall 34" (850 mm). *See* Great Lakes, p. 1382.

CONSTITUTION AND GOVERNMENT. The question of a general revision of the constitution drafted by an elected convention is submitted to the people every 20 years. The constitution of 1851 had 141 amendments by 1983.

In the 118th General Assembly the Senate consisted of 33 members and the House of Representatives of 99 members. The Senate is elected for 4 years, half each 2 years; the House is elected for 2 years; the Governor, Lieut.-Governor and Secretary of State for 4 years. Qualified as electors are (with necessary exceptions) all citizens 18 years of age who have the usual residential qualifications. Ohio sends 2 senators and 21 representatives to Congress.

In the 1988 presidential election Bush polled 2,411,719 votes, Dukakis, 1,934,922.

The capital (since 1816) is Columbus. Ohio is divided into 88 counties.

Governor: George V. Voinovich (R.), 1991–95 ($65,000).

BUDGET. For the year ending 30 June 1987 general revenue fund income was 11,183·9m. and expenditure, $10,550·7m.

The bonded debt on 30 June 1986 was $3,378m.

Per capita personal income (1986) was $13,933 (current dollars).

ENERGY AND NATURAL RESOURCES

Minerals. Ohio has extensive mineral resources, of which coal is the most important by value: Output (1987) 35·4m. short tons. Production of crude petroleum, 1987, 12m. bbls; natural gas, 167,000m. cu. ft. Other minerals include stone, clay, sand and gravel. Value of minerals, 1986, $329·57m.

Agriculture. Ohio is extensively devoted to agriculture. In 1987, 89,000 farms covered 15·8m. acres; average farm value per acre, $942.

Cash income 1987, from crop and livestock and products, $3,422m. The most important crops in 1983 were: Maize (232m. bu.), wheat (58·6m. bu.), oats (15·4m. bu.), soybeans (101·7m. bu.). In 1987 there were 2·15m. swine, 1·8m. all cattle and 300,000 sheep.

Forestry. State forest area, 1982, 195,000 acres; total forest, 6,147,000 acres.

INDUSTRY. In May 1987, manufacturing employed 1,091,000 workers; non-manufacturing, 3,315,000. The largest industry was manufacturing of non-electrical machinery, then transport equipment and fabricated metals.

COMMUNICATIONS

Roads. In 1990 there were 113,439 miles of roads (82,126 miles rural) and 9,513,918 registered motor vehicles.

Railways. Class I railroads operated 6,102 miles in 1986.

Aviation. Ohio had (1985) 194 commercial airports including one seaplane base; 597 non-commercial airports; 31 commercial heliports and 222 non-commercial. There were 5,825 licensed aeroplanes at 31 Dec. 1984.

JUSTICE, RELIGION, EDUCATION AND WELFARE

Justice. A Civil Rights Act (1933) forbids inns, restaurants, theatres, retail stores and all other places of public resort to discriminate against citizens on grounds of 'colour or race'; none may be denied the right to serve on juries on the grounds of 'colour or race'; insurance companies are forbidden to discriminate between 'white persons and coloured, wholly or partially of African descent'.

A state Civil Rights Commission (created 1959) has general administrative powers to prevent discrimination because of race, colour, religion, national origin or ancestry in employment, labour organization membership, use of public accommodations and in obtaining 'commercial housing' or 'personal residence'. Ohio has no *de jure* segregation in the public schools.

On 31 Dec. 1987 the Department of Rehabilitation and Correction was operating 17 adult correction facilities with average inmate population of 23,949. Total executions (by electrocution) since 1930 were 170, all for murder. There have been no executions since 1963. The Department of Rehabilitation and Correction was created in July 1972, and has established probation services in counties where services would otherwise be inadequate or non-existent.

Religion. Many religious faiths are represented, including (but not limited to) the Baptist, Jewish, Lutheran, Methodist, Presbyterian and Roman Catholic.

Education. School attendance during full term is compulsory for children from 6 to 18 years of age. In autumn 1987 public schools had 1·8m. enrolled pupils and 99,642 full-time equivalent classroom teachers. Teachers' salaries (1987–88) averaged (estimate) $28,191. Operating expenditure on elementary and secondary schools for 1987 was $6,100m.: state average per pupil, $3,769. Universities and colleges had a total enrolment (autumn 1985) of 514,745 students of whom 135,481 were in private colleges. State appropriation to state universities 1984–85, $1,100m. Average annual charge (undergraduate) at 4-year institutions: $4,081 (state); $7,432 (private).

Main bodies, 1988: (figures are for main campus in named city):

Founded	*Institutions*	*Enrolments*
1804	Ohio University, Athens (State)	16,182
1809	Miami University, Oxford (State)	16,012
1819	University of Cincinnati (State)	22,509
1826	Case Western Reserve University, Cleveland (Indep.)	8,352
1850	University of Dayton (R.C.)	10,693
1870	University of Akron (State)	18,321
1870	Ohio State University, Columbus (State)	47,887
1872	University of Toledo (State)	15,753
1887	Sinclair Community College, Dayton	16,247
1908	Youngstown University (State)	15,252
1910	Bowling Green State University (State)	16,206
1910	Kent State University (State)	16,468
1962	Cuyahoga Community College District (State/local)	11,928
1964	Cleveland State University (State)	12,067
1964	Wright State University (State)	14,580

Health. In 1987 the state had 228 hospitals listed by the American Hospital Association. State facilities for the severely mentally retarded had 2,862 resident in 1984.

Mentally retarded who do not need constant supervision occupy 1,024 group homes (7,993 beds) in residential areas (1983). In 1988 17 psychiatric hospitals had a daily average of 3,823 residents. In 1984, general hospitals had 74 units (3,080 beds) for the mentally ill and 56 beds for mentally retarded. There were 399 community mental health agencies in 1988.

Social Security. Public assistance is administered through 6 basic programmes: Aid to dependent children, emergency assistance, Medicaid, general relief, food stamps and social services; 49% of the costs (except general relief and adult emergency assistance) are met by the federal government.

In 1987 (preliminary) Medicaid cost $2,377m. and served an average 1·32m. people. Aid to dependent children cost $832m., to 668,000 people. Food stamps cost $691m. General relief cost $211·8m., receipts varying from county to county. Optional State Supplement is paid to aged, blind or disabled adults. Free social services are available to those eligible by income or circumstances.

Further Reading

Official Roster: Federal State, County Officers and Department Information. Secretary of State, Columbus. Biennial

Rosebloom, E. H. and Weisenburger, F. P., *A History of Ohio.* State Arch. and Hist. Soc., Columbus, 1953

Shkurti, W. J. and Bartle, J. (eds.) Benchmark Ohio. Ohio State Univ. Press, 1989

OKLAHOMA

HISTORY. An unorganized area in the centre of the present state was thrown open to white settlers on 22 April 1889. The Territory of Oklahoma, organized in 1890 to include this area and other sections, was opened to white settlements by runs or lotteries during the next decade. In 1893 the Territory was enlarged by the addition of the Cherokee Outlet, which fixed part of the present northern boundary. On 16 Nov. 1907 Oklahoma was combined with the remaining part of the Indian Territory and admitted as a state with boundaries substantially as now.

AREA AND POPULATION. Oklahoma is bounded north by Kansas, northeast by Missouri, east by Arkansas, south by Texas (the Red River forming part of the boundary) and, at the western extremity of the 'panhandle', by New Mexico and Colorado. Area 69,957 sq. miles, of which 1,301 sq. miles are water. Census population, 16 Aug. 1990 (preliminary), 3,123,799, an increase of 98,313 or 3% since 1980. Births, 1988, 47,279; deaths, 29,766; infant deaths (1987) 726; marriages, 32,923; divorces and annulments, 23,048.

The population at 5 federal censuses was:

	White	*Black*	*Indian*	*Other*	*Total*	*Per sq. mile*
1930	2,130,778	172,198	92,725	339	2,396,040	34·6
1960	2,107,900	153,084	68,689	1,414	2,328,284	33·8
1970	2,280,362	171,892	97,179	10,030	2,559,253	37·2
1980	2,597,783	204,658	169,292	53,557	3,025,486	43·2
1990 [1]	...	...	...	...	3,123,799	44·6

[1] Preliminary.

In 1980, 1,476,719 were male, 2,035,082 were urban and those 20 years of age or older numbered 2,052,729. The US Bureau of Indian Affairs is responsible for 37 Indian tribes, 201,456 Indians on 1,229,341 acres (1984).

The most important cities with population, 1990 (preliminary) are Oklahoma City (capital), 441,154; Tulsa, 364,572; Norman, 79,579; Lawton, 79,544; Broken Arrow, 57,281; Midwest City, 52,037; Edmond, 51,930; Enid, 45,175; Moore, 40,037; Muskogee, 37,440; Stillwater, 36,543; Bartlesville, 34,195.

CLIMATE. 1988: Oklahoma City. Jan. 34·2°F (1·2°C), July 81·6°F (27·5°C). Annual rainfall 31·94" (8,113 mm). Tulsa. Jan. 34·8°F (1·5°C), July 82·6°F (27·5°C). Annual rainfall 33·22" (8,438 mm). *See* Central Plains, p. 1381.

CONSTITUTION AND GOVERNMENT. The present constitution, dating from 1907, provides for amendment by initiative petition and legislative referendum; it has had 139 amendments (as of Oct. 1990).

The Legislature consists of a Senate of 48 members, who are elected for 4 years, and a House of Representatives elected for 2 years and consisting of 101 members. The Governor and Lieut.-Governor are elected for 4-year terms; the Governor can only be elected for two terms in succession. Electors are (with necessary exceptions) all citizens 18 years or older, with the usual qualifications.

The state is represented in Congress by 2 senators and 6 representatives.

In the 1988 presidential election Bush polled 678,244 votes, Dukakis, 483,373.

The capital is Oklahoma City. The state has 77 counties.

Governor: David Walters (D.), 1991–95 ($70,000).

BUDGET. Total revenue for the year ending 30 June 1989 was $6,072,418,369. Total expenditure, $5,614,402,347.

Bonded indebtedness for the year ending 30 June 1989, $70·75m.

Per capita personal income (1989) was $15,483.

ENERGY AND NATURAL RESOURCES

Minerals. Production of mineral fuels, 1989: Petroleum, 117·97m. bbls; natural gas, 2,197,137m. cu. ft.; coal, 1,768,292 tons. In 1989 there were 96,344 oilwells and 27,443 natural gaswells in production. Non-fuel mineral production (short tons),

1988: Cement, (1987) 1,456,000; gypsum, 2,173,000; sand and gravel, 10,541,000; stone, 26,307,746; clays, 754,054; iodine, 2,238,152 lb.; solar salt, 75,000. Other minerals are tripoli, feldspar, refined germanium, helium, lime and pumice. Value of non-fuel mineral production, 1988, $220,137,000.

Agriculture. In 1987 the state had 70,228 farms with a total area of 31,541,977 acres; average farm was 499 acres. Harvested crop land was 24,443,459 acres; irrigated land, 478,437 acres. Operators by principal occupation: Farming, 33,052; other, 37,176. Livestock, 1 Jan. 1990: Cattle, 5·3m.; sheep, 142,000; pigs, 230,000.

Total market value of agricultural products sold, 1989, $3,023m. The major cash grain is winter wheat (value, 1989, $585m.). Other crops include barley, oats, rye, grain, corn, soybeans, grain sorghum, cotton, peanuts and peaches. Value of cattle and calves produced, 1989, $1,379m.; catfish, $1m.; racehorses, $63m. Other livestock included hogs, sheep and goats. Livestock, 1 Jan. 1990: cattle, 5·3m.; sheep, 142,000; pigs, 230,000.

The Oklahoma Conservation Commission works with 91 conservation districts, universities, state and federal government agencies. The early work of the conservation districts, beginning in 1937, was limited to flood and erosion control: since 1970, they include urban areas also.

Irrigated production has increased in the Oklahoma 'panhandle'. The Ogalala aquifer is the primary source of irrigation water there and in western Oklahoma, a finite source because of its isolation from major sources of recharge. Declining groundwater levels necessitate the most effective irrigation practices.

Forestry. There are 8·5m. acres of forest, one half considered commercial. The forest products industry is concentrated in the 18 eastern counties. There are 3 forest regions: Ozark (oak, hickory); Ouachita highlands (pine, oak); Cross-Timbers (post oak, black jack oak). Southern pine is the chief commercial species, at almost 80% of saw-timber harvested annually. Replanting is essential.

INDUSTRY. Nominal output grew by an estimated 6·3% to $57,400m. in 1989. Manufacturing is the most important sector, representing about 14·7% of total output in 1988; mining, primarily oil and gas related, 8·6% in 1989.

Labour. Total labour force, May 1989, 1,513,600. Establishment employment, 1989, 1,139,000: Manufacturing, 164,000; construction (1988), 32,000; mining, 44,000. Average unemployment rate, 1989, 5·9%.

TOURISM. In 1989, 16,816,546 tourists visted the 72 state parks and 10 museums and monuments. Travellers spent almost $3,000m.

COMMUNICATIONS

Roads. In 1990 there were 111,669 miles of roads (99,578 miles rural) and 2,568,454 registered motor vehicles.

Railways. In 1989 Oklahoma had 4,278 miles of railway operated by 17 companies.

Aviation. Airports, 1989, numbered 423, of which 131 were publicly owned. Four cities were served by commercial airlines.

Shipping. The McClellan-Kerr Arkansas Navigation System provides access from east central Oklahoma to New Orleans through the Verdigris, Arkansas and Mississippi rivers. In 1989, 51,052,303 tons were shipped inbound and outbound on 1,249 barges; 157,400 tons shipped internal. Total tonnage (1989) of traffic on the System, 8,357,435 tons; the Oklahoma segment of the System handled 4,032,732 tons. Commodities shipped, 1989 were mainly chemical fertilizer, farm produce, petroleum products, iron and steel, coal, sand and gravel.

Broadcasting. In 1990 there were 117 radio and 18 television broadcasting stations, and 16 cable-TV companies.

Newspapers. In 1990 there were 47 daily and 190 weekly newspapers.

JUSTICE, RELIGION, EDUCATION AND WELFARE

Justice. Penal institutions, 27 Sept. 1990, held 10,185 inmates (8,944 of them male). There were 15 penal institutions, 8 community treatment centres and 7 probation and parole centres.

The death penalty was suspended in 1966 and re-imposed in 1976. Since 1915 there have been 84 (53 whites, 27 Negroes, 4 other races) executions. Electrocution was replaced (1977) by lethal injection.

Religion. The chief religious bodies in 1980 were Baptists, 674,766; United Methodists, 248,635; Roman Catholics, 122,820; Churches of Christ, about 80,000; Assembly of God, 63,992; Disciples of Christ, 45,070; Presbyterian, 38,605; Lutheran, 33,664; Nazarene, 22,090; Episcopal, 21,500.

Education. In 1988–89 there were 605,771 pupils enrolled in grades Kindergarten–12. There were 40,052 teachers at elementary and secondary schools on average salaries of $23,521. Total expenditure on the 609 school districts, $1,661,743,679. In 1988–89 total expenditure for vocational-technical education was $107,459,457; there were 32,945 students enrolled.

Institutions of higher education with over 4,000 students:

Founded	*Name*	*Place*	*1988–89 Enrolment*
1891	Oklahoma State University	Stillwater, Okla. City, Okmulgee	34,588
1891	Central State University	Edmond	19,901
1892	University of Oklahoma	Norman, Okla. City, Tulsa	29,897
1894	University of Tulsa	Tulsa	5,128
1903	Southwestern Oklahoma State University	Weatherford	7,165
1909	East Central Oklahoma State University	Ada	5,808
1909	Northeastern Oklahoma State University	Tahlequah	11,335
1909	Southeastern Oklahoma State University	Durant	4,985
1909	Cameron University	Lawton	8,038
1909	Rogers State College	Claremore	5,379
1950	Oklahoma Christian University of Science and Arts	Oklahoma City	4,681
1968	Rose State College	Midwest City	15,196
1969	Tulsa Junior College	Tulsa	28,065
1970	Oklahoma City Community College	Oklahoma City	16,500

Total enrolment in Oklahoma State System of higher education, 1988–89, 112,680; total expenditure, $409,524,000.

Health. In 1989 there were 148 hospitals; 59 alcoholism treatment centres, 25 end state renal disease facilities, 80 home health agencies, 8 hospices, 58 independent laboratories, 19 ambulatory surgical centres, 10 HIV laboratories, 25 outpatient physical therapy/speech pathology facilities, 40 physical therapists in independent practice and 4 portable X–ray units.

Welfare. In 1988–89 the Oklahoma Department of Human Services provided for medical services, $690,516,055; assistance payments and services, $264,238,290; field services, $18,485,527; Oklahoma Medical Center, $164,172,790; children and youth services, $83,906,918; mentally retarded and developmental disability, $94,102,868; rehabilitation, $43,335,543; the ageing, $25,761,599; administration, $29,837,178; management information, $13,847,381; construction and special projects, $8,199,418.

In 1988–89, payments and benefits were: Grants and energy, $184,399,170; medical payments, $685,839,185; food stamps and commodities, $181,185,160; payroll and rent, $353,472,861; day care, $18,918,539. In 1990 there were 401,000 military veterans.

Further Reading

Directory of Oklahoma. Dept. of Libraries, Oklahoma City (irregular), 1989–90
Chronicles of Oklahoma. Oklahoma Historical Society, Oklahoma City (from 1921, quarterly)

Oklahoma Business Directory. Omaha, 1989
Gibson, A. M., *The History of Oklahoma*. Rev. ed., Oklahoma Univ. Press, 1984
Morris, J. W. *et al.*, *Historical Atlas of Oklahoma*. 3rd ed. Oklahoma Univ. Press, 1986
Strain, J. W., *Outline of Oklahoma Government*. Rev. ed., Central State Univ., Edmond, 1983

State Library: Oklahoma Dept. of Libraries, 200 N.E. 18th Street, Oklahoma City 73105. *State Librarian and State Archivist:* Robert L. Clark, Jr.

OREGON

HISTORY. Oregon was first settled in 1811 by the Pacific Fur Co. at Astoria, a provisional government was formed on 5 July 1834; a Territorial government was organized, 14 Aug. 1848, and on 14 Feb. 1859 Oregon was admitted to the Union.

AREA AND POPULATION. Oregon is bounded north by Washington, with the Columbia River forming most of the boundary, east by Idaho, with the Snake River forming most of the boundary, south by Nevada and California and west by the Pacific. Area, 97,073 sq. miles, 889 sq. miles being inland water. The federal government owned (1985) 30,110,212 acres (48·88% of the state area). Census population, 1 April 1980, 2,633,105, an increase of 541,720 or 26% since 1970. Estimated population (1990), 2,828,214. In 1986 births numbered 38,850 (14·6 per 1,000 population); deaths, 23,328 (8·8); infant deaths 368 (9·5 per 1,000 live births); marriages, 22,015 (8·3), and divorces, 15,774 (5·9).

Population at 5 federal censuses was:

	White	*Black*	*Indian*	*Asiatic*	*Total*	*Per sq. mile*
1910	655,090	1,492	5,090	11,093	672,765	7·0
1930	938,598	2,234	4,776	8,179	953,786	9·9
1960	1,732,037	18,133	8,026	9,120	1,768,687	18·4
1970	2,032,079	26,308	13,510	13,290	2,091,385	21·7
1980	2,490,610	37,060	27,314	34,775	2,633,105	27·3

Of the total population in 1980, 1,296,566 were male, 1,788,354 persons were urban. Those 18 years and older numbered 1,910,048.

The US Bureau of Indian Affairs (area headquarters in Portland) administers (1988) 768,665·2 acres, of which 633,613·36 acres are held by the US in trust for Indian tribes, and 135,052·36 acres for individual Indians.

The largest towns, according to 1980 census figures (and 1989 estimates), are: Portland, 366,383 (432,175); Eugene, 105,664 (109,785); Salem (the capital), 89,233 (99,860); Corvallis, 40,960 (43,715); Medford, 39,603 (45,290); Springfield, 41,621 (41,460); Beaverton, 31,926 (44,265); Albany, 26,678 (28,030). Metropolitan areas (1989): Portland, 1,202,200; Eugene-Springfield, 280,000; Salem, 271,800.

CLIMATE. Portland. Jan. 39°F (3·9°C), July 67°F (19·4°C). Annual rainfall 44" (1,100 mm). *See* Pacific Coast, p. 1381.

CONSTITUTION AND GOVERNMENT. The present constitution dates from 1859; some 250 items in it have been amended. The Legislative Assembly consists of a Senate of 30 members, elected for 4 years (half their number retiring every 2 years), and a House of 60 representatives, elected for 2 years. The Governor is elected for 4 years. The constitution reserves to the voters the rights of initiative and referendum and recall. In Nov. 1912 suffrage was extended to women.

The state sends to Congress 2 senators and 5 representatives.

In the 1988 presidential election Bush polled 517,920 votes, Dukakis, 575,151.

The capital is Salem. There are 36 counties in the state.

Governor: Barbara Roberts (D.), 1991–95 ($75,000).

BUDGET. Oregon has 2-year financial periods. Total resources for the biennium

1989-91 were $25,424,202,000 (federal funds, 1,980m.; taxes, $2,066m.); total expenditures, $14,360m. (education, $3,868m.; economic development and consumer services, $3,199·5m.; human resources, $3,563m.).

In 1989 the outstanding debt was $5,773m.

Per capita personal income (1989) was $15,785.

ENERGY AND NATURAL RESOURCES

Electricity. On 1 Jan. 1984 four privately owned utilities, 11 municipally owned utilities, 18 co-operatives and 6 utility districts provided electricity in the state. The privately owned companies provided 77% of the electricity. Hydroelectricity plants (130 in 1988) have an installed capacity of 5·1m. kw., of which multipurpose federal projects like the Bonneville Power Administration accounted for 3,011 mw. and the Trojan Nuclear plant 1,104mw. Boardman coal-fired plant produced no energy in 1987.

Minerals. Oregon's mineral resources include gold, silver, nickel copper, lead, mercury, chromite, sand and gravel, stone, clays, lime, silica, diatomite, expansible shale, scoria, pumice and uranium. There is geothermal potential. Metallurgical plant produces $1,000m. worth (approximately) per annum.

Agriculture. Oregon, which has an area of 61,557,184 acres, is divided by the Cascade Range into two distinct zones as to climate. West of the Cascade Range there is a good rainfall and almost every variety of crop common to the temperate zone is grown; east of the Range stock-raising and wheat-growing are the principal industries and irrigation is needed for row crops and fruits. In 1987 38,490 were employed in farming.

There were, in 1989, 37,000 farms with an acreage of 17·8m.; average farm size was 481 acres; most are family-owned corporate farms. Average value per acre (1989), $466.

Cash receipts from crops in 1988 amounted to $2,100m., and from livestock and livestock products, $682m., of which cattle made most. Principal crops are hay (2·8m. tons), wheat (46·9m. bu.), potatoes, grass, seed, pears, onions, greenhouse and farmforest products.

Livestock, 1 Jan. 1987: Milch cows, 92,000; cattle and calves, 1·36m.; sheep and lambs, 490,000; swine, 100,000.

Forestry. About 28·2m. acres is forested, almost half of the state. Of this amount, 22·4m. is commercial forest land suitable for timber production; ownership is as follows (acres): US Forestry Service, 10·9m.; US Bureau of Land Management, 1·8m.; other federal, 175,000; State of Oregon, 774,000; other public (city, county), 110,000; private owners, 8·3m., of which the forest industry owns 5·6m., non-industrial private owners, 2·7m., Indians, 335,000. Oregon's commercial forest lands provided a 1987 harvest of 8,200m. bd ft of logs, as well as the benefits of recreation, water, grazing, wildlife and fish. Trees vary from the coastal forest of hemlock and spruce to the state's primary species, Douglas-fir, throughout much of western Oregon. In eastern Oregon, ponderosa pine, lodgepole pine and true firs are found. Here, forestry is often combined with livestock grazing to provide an economic operation. Along the Cascade summit and in the mountains of northeast Oregon, alpine species are found.

Forest production in 1988 was worth $11,313,810.

Fisheries. All food and shellfish landings in the calendar year 1988 amounted to a value of $98m. The most important are: shrimp, salmon, ground fish, crab, tuna.

INDUSTRY. Forest products manufacturing is Oregon's leading industry, and in 1987 employed 80,000. The second most important industry is high technology. Gross State product, 1987, $41,300m. Manufacturing employed 204,900; trade, 276,300; services, 242,200; government, 204,500.

TOURISM. In 1989, the total income from tourism was estimated to be $2,054m.

COMMUNICATIONS

Roads. The state maintains (1988) 7,520 miles of primary and secondary highways, almost all surfaced; counties maintain 27,734 miles, and cities 7,316 miles; there were 52,450 miles in national parks and federal reservations. Registered motor vehicles, 31 Dec. 1988, totalled 2·6m.

Railways. The state had (1986) 5 common carrier railways with a total mileage of 2,700.

Aviation. In 1988 there were 3 public-use and 85 personal-use heliports; 225 personal-use airports; 107 public-use airports including 35 state-owned airports.

Shipping. Portland is a major seaport for large ocean-going vessels and is 101 miles inland from the mouth of the Columbia River. In 1988 the port handled 8·7m. short tons of cargo; main commodities for this and other Columbia River ports are grain and petroleum.

Post and Broadcasting. In Dec. 1988 there were 178 commercial radio stations and 23 educational radio stations. There were 17 commercial television stations and 6 educational television stations. There were also 5 campus limited radio stations and 1 subscription radio station.

Newspapers. In 1988 there were 22 daily newspapers with a circulation of more than 650,000 and 100 non-daily newspapers.

JUSTICE, RELIGION, EDUCATION AND WELFARE

Justice. There are 8 correctional institutions in Oregon. Total inmates, 1988, 4,197. The sterilization law, originally passed in 1917, was amended in 1967. The amendments changed the number of persons on the Board of Social Protection from 15 to 7 and provided that the Public Defender would automatically represent all persons examined. The basis on which a person would be subject to examination by the Board are: *(a)* if such person would be likely to procreate children having an inherited tendency to mental retardation or mental illness, or *(b)* if such person would be likely to procreate children who would become neglected or dependent because of the person's inability by reason of mental illness or mental retardation to provide adequate care.

Religion. The chief religious bodies are Catholic, Baptist, Lutheran, Methodists, Presbyterian and Mormon.

Education. School attendance is compulsory from 7 to 18 years of age if the twelfth year of school has not been completed; those between the ages of 16 and 18 years, if legally employed, may attend part-time or evening schools. Others may be excused under certain circumstances. In 1988–89 the public elementary and secondary schools had 483,960 students. Total expenditure on elementary and secondary education (1988-89) was $1,830,677,679; teachers' average salary (1989), $29,500.

Leading state-supported institutions of higher education (autumn 1989) included:

	Students
University of Oregon, Eugene	18,567
Oregon Health Sciences University:	1,317
Oregon State University, Corvallis	16,230
Portland State University, Portland	16,750
Western Oregon State College, Monmouth	3,856
Southern Oregon State College, Ashland	5,196
Eastern Oregon State College, La Grande	2,008
Oregon Institute of Technology, Klamath Falls	3,147

Total enrolment in state colleges and universities, 1989, 67,071. Largest of the privately endowed universities are Lewis and Clark College, Portland, with (1989) 3,418 students; University of Portland, 2,417 students; Willamette University,

Salem, 2,225 students; Reed College, Portland, 1,348 students, and Linfield College, McMinnville, 2,164 students. In 1989 there were 75,395 students (full-time equivalent) in community colleges.

Health. In 1988 there were 78 licensed hospitals; there were 2 state hospitals for mentally ill (937 patients), 1 for the mentally retarded (1,200) and 1 with both programmes (150).

Social Security. The State Adult and Family Services Division provides cash payments, medical care, food stamps, day care and help in finding jobs. In 1990 there were 85,947 people on low incomes, many of them children in single-parent families, benefiting from the Aid to Families with Dependent Children Programme; 213,733 people received food stamps.

There is also a Children's Services Division.

A system of unemployment benefit payments, financed by employers, with administrative allotments made through a federal agency, started 2 Jan. 1938.

Further Reading

Oregon Blue Book. Issued by the Secretary of State. Salem. Biennial
Federal Writers' Project. *Oregon: End of the Trail.* Rev. ed. Portland, 1972
Baldwin, E. M., *Geology of Oregon.* Rev. ed. Dubuque, Iowa, 1976
Carey, C. H., *General History of Oregon, prior to 1861.* 2 vol. (1 vol. reprint, 1971) Portland, 1935
Corning, H. M. (ed.), *Dictionary of Oregon History.* New York, 1956
Dicken, S. N., *Oregon Geography.* 5th ed. Eugene, 1973.—with Dicken, E. F., *Making of Oregon: a Study in Historical Geography.* Portland, 1979.—with Dicken, E. F., *Oregon Divided: A Regional Geography.* Portland, 1982
Dodds, G. B., *Oregon: A Bicentennial History.* New York, 1977
Friedman, R., *Oregon for the Curious.* 3rd ed. Portland, 1972
Highsmith, R. M. Jr. (ed.), *Atlas of the Pacific Northwest.* Corvallis, 1973
McArthur, L. A., *Oregon Geographic Names.* 4th ed., rev. and enlarged. Portland, 1974
Patton, Clyde P., *Atlas of Oregon.* Univ. Oregon Press, Eugene, 1976

State Library: The Oregon State Library, Salem. *Librarian:* Wesley Doak.

PENNSYLVANIA

HISTORY. Pennsylvania, first settled in 1682, is one of the 13 original states in the Union.

AREA AND POPULATION. Pennsylvania is bounded north by New York, east by New Jersey, south by Delaware and Maryland, south-west by West Virginia, west by Ohio and north-west by Lake Erie. Area, 45,308 sq. miles, of which 420 sq. miles are inland water. Census population, 1 April 1980, 11,863,895, an increase of 63,129 or 0·5% since 1970. Estimate (1988) 12,002,100. Births, 1988, 165,169; deaths, 125,337; infant deaths, 1,615; marriages, 87,963; reported divorces, 39,001.

Population at 5 census years was:

	White	*Black*	*Indian*	*All others*	*Total*	*Per sq. mile*
1910	7,467,713	193,919	1,503	1,976	7,665,111	171·0
1930	9,196,007	431,257	523	3,563	9,631,350	213·8
1960	10,454,004	852,750	2,122	10,490	11,319,366	251·5
			All others			
1970	10,745,219	1,015,884	39,663		11,800,766	262·9
1980	10,652,320	1,046,810	164,765		11,863,895	264·3

Of the total population in 1980, 47·9% were male, 69·3% were urban and 68·1% were 21 years of age or older.

The population of the larger cities and townships, 1980 census, was:

Philadelphia	1,688,210	Scranton	88,117	Lancaster	54,725
Pittsburgh	423,938	Reading	78,686	Harrisburg	53,264
Erie	119,123	Bethlehem	70,419	Wilkes-Barre	51,551
Allentown	103,758	Altoona	57,078	York	44,619

Larger urbanized areas, 1980 census: Philadelphia (in Pennsylvania), 3,682,709; Pittsburgh, 2,263,894; Northeast, 640,396, Allentown–Bethlehem–Easton (in Pennsylvania), 551,052; Harrisburg, 446,576.

CLIMATE. Philadelphia. Jan. 32°F (0°C), July 77°F (25°C). Annual rainfall 40" (1,006 mm). Pittsburgh. Jan. 31°F (–0·6°C), July 74°F (23·3°C). Annual rainfall 37" (914 mm). *See* Appalachian Mountains, p. 1382.

CONSTITUTION AND GOVERNMENT. The present constitution dates from 1968. The General Assembly consists of a Senate of 50 members chosen for 4 years, one-half being elected biennially, and a House of Representatives of 203 members chosen for 2 years. The Governor and Lieut.-Governor are elected for 4 years. Every citizen 18 years of age, with the usual residential qualifications, may vote. The state sends to Congress 2 senators and 23 representatives. Registered voters in May 1990, 5,705,079.

In the 1988 presidential election Bush polled 2,291,297 votes, Dukakis, 2,183,928.

The state capital is Harrisburg. The state is organized in counties (numbering 67), cities, boroughs, townships and school districts.

Governor: Robert P. Casey (D.), 1991–95 ($85,000).

BUDGET. Total revenues for 1990-91 were $11,961m.; general fund expenditure, $11,924·9; transport, $1,549·6m.; public welfare, $3,216·3m.).

In 1989-90 outstanding long-term debt (excluding highway bonds) amounted to $3,013m.

Per capita personal income (1989) was $16,233.

ENERGY AND NATURAL RESOURCES

Minerals. Pennsylvania is almost the sole producer of anthracite coal. Production (1989): Anthracite, 3,375,315 tons, with 2,443 employees; bituminous coal, 68,305,235 tons, with 13,644 employees; crude petroleum, 2,601,982 bbls; natural gas, 191,774m. cu. ft.

Agriculture. Agriculture, market-gardening, fruit-growing, horticulture and forestry are pursued within the state. In 1988 there were 55,000 farms with a total farm area of 8·3m. acres (4·5m. acres in crops). Cash income, 1989, from crops, $954·7m., and from livestock and products, $2,358m.

Pennsylvania ranks first in the production of mushrooms (284·8m. lb., value $205·1m. in 1987). Other crops are (1988) tobacco (18·2m. lb., $20·5m.), wheat (1988, 9m. bu.), oats (1988, 13m. bu.), maize, barley and potatoes. On 1 Jan. 1989 there were on farms: 1·92m. cattle and calves, including 717,000 milch cows, 134,000 sheep, 970,000 swine. Milk production, 1988, was 10,204m. lb., and eggs (1988) numbered 5,300m. valued at $185·69m. Pennsylvania is also a major fruit producing state; in 1988 apples totalled 520m. lb.; peaches, 80m. lb.; tart cherries, 9m. lb.; sweet cherries, 1,200 tons; and grapes, 58,000 tons. Other important items are soybeans (7·2m. bu.), vegetables for processing (50,000 tons), fresh vegetables (1·5m. cwt) and broiler-chickens (120·6m.).

Forestry. In 1990 state forest land and state park land totalled 1,976,435 acres as of 3 Jan.; state game lands, 1,333,580·6 acres as of 31 Aug.

INDUSTRY. Pennsylvania is third in national production of iron and steel. Output of steel, 1989, 11,869,968 net tons.

In 1989, manufacturing employed 1,050,286 workers; services, 1,277,983; trade, 1,188,857; government, 668,249.

COMMUNICATIONS

Roads. Highways and roads in the state (federal, local and state combined) totalled (1989) 116,277·62 miles. Registered motor vehicles for 1989 numbered 8,605,747.

Railways. In 1990, 57 railways operated within the state with a line mileage of about 5,500.

Aviation. There were (30 June 1990) 146 public airports, 291 private and 10 public heliports, 339 airports for personal use and 5 seaplane bases.

Shipping. Trade at the ports of Philadelphia (1989): Imports 60,651,352 short tons of bulk cargo and 5,581,840 of general cargo; exports, 3,182,266 of bulk cargo and 2,342,100 of general cargo.

Post and Broadcasting. Broadcasting stations comprised (1989) 50 television stations and 357 radio stations.

Newspapers. There were (1989) 97 daily and 303 weekly newspapers.

JUSTICE, RELIGION, EDUCATION AND WELFARE

Justice. No executions took place in 1963–89; since 1930 there have been 149 executions (electrocution), all for murder.

State prison population, on 30 July 1990, was 20,819.

Religion. The chief religious bodies in 1977 were the Roman Catholic, with 3,717,667 members; Protestant, 3,150,920 (1971); and Jewish, 469,078. The 5 largest Protestant denominations (by communicants) were: Lutheran Church in America, 766,276; United Methodist, 728,915 (1971), United Presbyterian Church in the USA, 573,905 (1971); United Church of Christ, 257,138; Episcopal, 193,399 (1971).

Education. School attendance is compulsory for children 8–17 years of age. In 1989–90 the public kindergartens and elementary schools had 911,302 pupils (Grades K-6); public secondary schools had 743,969 pupils. Non-public schools had 215,903 elementary pupils (Grades K-6) and 125,326 secondary pupils (Grades 7-12. Average salary, public school professional personnel, men $37,186; women $32,682; for classroom teachers, men $35,161, women $32,251.

Leading senior academic institutions included:

Founded	*Institutions*	*Faculty (Autumn 1989)*	*Students (Autumn 1989)*
1740	University of Pennsylvania (non-sect.)	1,007	22,016
1787	University of Pittsburgh	1,326	28,362
1832	Lafayette College, Easton (Presbyterian)	159	2,303
1833	Haverford College	83	1,159
1842	Villanova University (R.C.)	534	11,388
1846	Bucknell University (Baptist)	226	3,423
1851	St Joseph's University, Philadelphia (R.C.)	164	6,170
1852	California University of Pennsylvania	317	6,748
1855	Pennsylvania State University	1,704	37,718
1855	Millersville University of Pennsylvania	333	7,791
1863	LaSalle University, Philadelphia (R.C.)	208	6,478
1864	Swarthmore College	151	1,304
1866	Lehigh University, Bethlehem (non-sect.)	393	6,610
1871	West Chester University of Pennsylvania	465	11,815
1875	Indiana University of Pennsylvania	660	13,861
1878	Duquesne University, Pittsburgh (R.C.)	280	6,901
1884	Temple University, Philadelphia	1,194	32,713
1885	Bryn Mawr College	136	1,839
1888	University of Scranton (R.C.)	231	5,111
1891	Drexel University, Philadelphia	448	11,959
1900	Carnegie-Mellon University, Pittsburgh	489	7,090

Health. In 1989 the state had 300 hospitals (68,414 beds) listed by the State Health Department, excluding federal hospitals and mental institutions.

Social Security. During the year ending 30 June 1990 the monthly average number of cases receiving public assistance was: Aid to families with dependent children, 175,737; blind pension, 2,415; general assistance, 129,747.

Payments for medical assistance for 1989–90 totalled $2,579,729,762. Under the medical assistance programme payments are made for inpatient hospital care ($832,075,756); private nursing home care ($542,439,081); public long term care ($275,022,045); other medical care ($930,192,880).

Further Reading

Crop and Livestock Summary. Pennsylvania Dept. of Agriculture. Annual

Encyclopaedia of Pennsylvania, New York, 1984

Pennsylvania Manual. General Services, Bureau of Publications, Harrisburg. Biennial

Pennsylvania State Industrial Directory. Harris, Ohio. Annual

Cochran, T. C., *Pennsylvania*, New York, 1978

Klein, P. S. and Hoogenboom, A., *A History of Pennsylvania*. New York, 1973

League of Women Voters of Pennsylvania, *Key to the Keystone State*. Philadelphia, 1972

Majumdar, S. K. and Miller, E. W., *Pennsylvania Coal: Resources, Technology and Utilisation*. Pennsylvania Science, 1983

Pennsylvania Chamber of Commerce, *Pennsylvania Government Today*. State College, Pa., 1973

Weigley, R. F., (ed.) *Philadelphia: A 300-year History*. New York, 1984

Wilkinson, N. B., *Bibliography of Pennsylvania History*. Pa. Historical & Museum Commission. Harrisburg, 1957

RHODE ISLAND

HISTORY The earliest settlers in the region which now forms the state of Rhode Island were colonists from Massachusetts who had been driven forth on account of their non-acceptance of the prevailing religious beliefs. The first of the settlements was made in 1636, settlers of every creed being welcomed. In 1647 a patent was executed for the government of the settlements, and on 8 July 1663 a charter was executed recognizing the settlers as forming a body corporate and politic by the name of the 'English Colony of Rhode Island and Providence Plantations, in New England, in America'. On 29 May 1790 the state accepted the federal constitution and entered the Union as the last of the 13 original states.

AREA AND POPULATION. Rhode Island is bounded north and east by Massachusetts, south by the Atlantic and west by Connecticut. Area, 1,214 sq. miles, of which 165 sq. miles are inland water. Census population, 1 April 1980, 947,154 a decrease of 0·3% since 1970. Estimate (1987), 986,000.

Births, 1986, were 13,324; deaths (excluding foetal deaths), 9,587; infant deaths, 125; marriages, 8,103; divorces, 3,683.

Population of 5 census years was:

	White	*Black*	*Indian*	*Asiatic*	*Total*	*Per sq. mile*
1910	532,492	9,529	284	305	542,610	508·5
1930	677,026	9,913	318	240	687,497	649·3
1960	838,712	18,332	932	1,190	859,488	812·4
1970	914,757	25,338	1,390	5,240	949,723[1]	905·0
			All others			
1980	896,692	27,584	22,878		154	903·0

[1] Through tabulation errors there were 2,998 people unaccounted for, as to race and sex, in 1970.

Of the total population in 1980, 451,251 were male, 824,004 were urban and 665,054 were 20 years of age or older.

The chief cities and their population (census, 1980) are Providence, 156,804; Warwick, 87,123; Cranston, 71,992; Pawtucket, 71,204; East Providence, 50,980; Woonsocket, 45,914; Newport, 29,259; North Providence (town), 29,188; Cumberland (town), 27,069. The Providence–Pawtucket–Warwick Standard Metropolitan Statistical Area had a population of 919,216 in 1980.

CLIMATE. Providence. Jan. 28°F (–2·2°C), July 72°F (22·2°C). Annual rainfall 43" (1,079 mm). *See* New England, p. 1382.

CONSTITUTION AND GOVERNMENT. The present constitution dates from 1843; it has had 42 amendments. The General Assembly consists of a Senate of 50 members and a House of Representatives of 100 members, both elected for 2 years, as are also the Governor and Lieut.-Governor. Every citizen, 18 years of age, who has resided in the state for 30 days, and is duly registered, is qualified to vote.

Rhode Island sends to Congress 2 senators and 2 representatives.

At the 1988 presidential election Dukakis polled 216,668 votes, Bush, 169,730.

The capital is Providence. The state has 5 counties (unique in having no political functions) and 39 cities and towns.

Governor: Bruce Sundlun (D.), 1991–93 ($69,900).

BUDGET. For the fiscal year ending 30 June 1987 (Office of the State Controller) total revenues were $1,585·7m. (taxation, $1,032·8m., and federal aid, $361·1m.); general expenditures were $1,529·1m. (education, $442·6m.; and public welfare, $453·1m.)

Total net long-term debt on 30 June 1986 was $261·8m.

Per capita personal income (1987) was $15,555.

NATURAL RESOURCES

Minerals. The small mineral output, mostly stone, sand and gravel, was valued (1987) at an estimated $18m.

Agriculture. While Rhode Island is predominantly a manufacturing state, agriculture contributed $110m. to the general cash income in 1987; it had 697 farms with an area of 73,000 acres (11% of the total land area), of which 31,000 acres were crop land; the average farm was 86 acres.

Fisheries. In 1987 the catch was 90m. lb (live weight) valued at $76·5m.

INDUSTRY. Total non-agricultural employment in Oct. 1989 was 459,100, of which 112,300 were manufacturing, 346,800 non-manufacturing. Average weekly earnings for production workers in manufacturing, $359.99; value added by manufacture (1985), $4,289m. Principal industries are metals and machinery, jewellery–silverware and transport equipment.

COMMUNICATIONS

Roads. In 1990 there were 5,884 miles of roads (1,484 miles rural) and 670,576 registered motor vehicles.

Aviation. In 1988 there were 6 state-owned airports. Theodore Francis Green airport at Warwick, near Providence, is served by 8 airlines, and handled over 2m. passengers and 20m. lb. of freight in 1988.

Shipping. Waterborne freight through the port of Providence (1988) totalled 10·6m. tons.

Broadcasting. There are 24 radio stations and 5 television stations; there are 8 cable television companies.

JUSTICE, RELIGION, EDUCATION AND WELFARE

Justice. The state's penal institutions, Aug. 1988, had 1,290 inmates (131 per 100,000 population).

The death penalty is illegal, except that it is mandatory in the case of murder committed by a prisoner serving a life sentence.

Religion. Chief religious bodies are (estimated figures Sept. 1988): Roman Catholic with 550,000 members; Protestant Episcopal (baptized persons), 50,000; Baptist, 22,500; Congregational, 12,000; Methodist, 10,000; Jewish, 24,000.

Education. In 1987–88 the 240 public elementary schools had 3,702 teachers and total enrolment of 60,582 pupils; about 25,000 pupils were enrolled in private and parochial schools. The 58 senior and vocational high schools had 3,678 teachers and 59,011 pupils. Teachers' salaries (1987) averaged $23,400. Local expenditure, for schools (including evening schools) in 1987–88 totalled $580·6m.

There are 11 institutions of higher learning in the state, including 1 junior college. The state maintains Rhode Island College, at Providence, with 600 faculty members, and 5,600 full-time students (1987), and the University of Rhode Island, at South Kingstown, with over 900 faculty members and over 14,000 students (including graduate students). Brown University, at Providence, founded in 1764, is now non-sectarian; in 1987 it had over 600 full-time faculty members and 7,000 full-time students. Providence College, at Providence, founded in 1917 by the Order of Preachers (Dominican), had (1987) 210 professors and 5,400 students. The largest of the other colleges are Bryant College, at Smithfield, with 160 faculty and 5,000 students, and the Rhode Island School of Design, in Providence, with about 155 faculty and 1,800 students.

Health. In 1988 the state had 22 hospitals (over 7,000 beds), including 4 mental hospitals.

Social Security. In 1987 aid to dependent children was granted to 44,000 children in 15,000 families at an average payment per family of $380 per month, and the state also had a general assistance programme. (All other aid programmes were taken over by the federal government.)

Further Reading

Rhode Island Manual. Prepared by the Secretary of State. Providence
Providence Journal Almanac: A Reference Book for Rhode Islanders. Providence. Annual
Rhode Island Basic Economic Statistics. Rhode Island Dept. of Economic Development. Providence, 1987
McLoughlin, W. G., *Rhode Island: a History*. Norton, 1978
Wright, M. I. and Sullivan, R. J., *Rhode Island Atlas*. Rhode Island Pubs., 1983

State Library: Rhode Island State Library, State House, Providence 02908. State Librarian: Elliott E. Andrews.

SOUTH CAROLINA

HISTORY. South Carolina, first settled permanently in 1670, was one of the 13 original states of the Union.

AREA AND POPULATION. South Carolina is bounded in the north by North Carolina, east and south-east by the Atlantic, south-west and west by Georgia. Area, 31,113 sq. miles, of which 909 sq. miles are inland water. Census population, 1 April 1980, 3,121,833, an increase of 20·5% since 1970. Estimate July 1989 3,519,000. Births, 1989, were 51,239 (16·3 per 1,000 population); deaths, 29,563 (8·4); marriages, 54,693 (15·5); divorces and annulments, 15,115 (4·3); infant deaths, 731 (12·8 per 1,000 live births).

The population in 5 census years was:

	White	Black	Indian	Asiatic	Total	Per sq. mile
1910	679,161	835,843	331	65	1,515,400	49·7
1930	944,049	793,681	959	76	1,738,765	56·8
1960	1,551,022	829,291	1,098	946	2,382,594	78·7
			All others			
1970	1,794,432	789,040	3,588		2,587,060	83·2
1980	2,150,507	948,623	22,703		3,121,833	100·3

Of the total population in 1980, 49% were male, 54·1% were urban and 55% were 25 years old or older. Median age, 28.

Populations of large towns in 1988 (with those of associated metropolitan areas): Columbia (capital), 94,810 (465,500); Charleston, 81,030 (510,800); Greenville, 59,190; Spartanburg, 45,550 (Greenville–Spartanburg, 621,300).

CLIMATE. Columbia. Jan. 47°F (8·3°C), July 81°F (27·2°C). Annual rainfall 45" (1,125 mm). *See* Atlantic Coast, p. 1382.

CONSTITUTION AND GOVERNMENT. The present constitution dates from 1895, when it went into force without ratification by the electorate. The General Assembly consists of a Senate of 46 members, elected for 4 years, and a House of Representatives of 124 members, elected for 2 years. The Governor and Lieut.-Governor are elected for 4 years. Only registered citizens have the right to vote. South Carolina sends to Congress 2 senators and 6 representatives.

At the 1988 presidential election Bush polled 599,871 votes, Dukakis 367,511.

The capital is Columbia.

Governor: Carroll Campbell (R.), 1991–95 ($98,000).

BUDGET. For the fiscal year ending 30 June 1990 general revenues were $3,294m.; general expenditures were $0,000·8m.

Per capita personal income (1989) was $12,934.

NATURAL RESOURCES

Minerals. Non-metallic minerals are of chief importance: Value of mineral output in 1988 was $221·9m., chiefly from limestone for cement, clay, stone, sand and gravel. Production of kaolin, vermiculite, scrap mica and fuller's earth is also important.

Agriculture. In 1989 there were 25,500 farms covering a farm area of 5·3m. acres. The average farm was of 208 acres. Of the 20,517 farms of the 1987 Census of Agriculture, there were 936 of 1,000 acres or more, average farm 232 acres; owners operated 12,624 farms; tenants 1,460. There were 1,905 farms with $100,000 or more in value of sales.

Cash receipts from farm marketing in 1988 amounted to $620·7m. for crops and $488·1m. for livestock, including poultry. Chief crops are tobacco ($158·9m.), soybeans ($125·5m.), and corn ($42m.). Production, 1988: Cotton, 140,000 bales; peaches, 290m. lb.; soybeans, 18·2m. bu.; tobacco, 100m. lb.; eggs, 1,432,000m. Livestock on farms, 1989: 621,000 all cattle, 450,000 swine.

Forestry. The forest industry is important; total forest land (1987), 12·3m. acres. National forests amounted to 606,000 acres.

INDUSTRY. A monthly average of 386,694 workers were employed in manufacturing in 1988, earning $8,190m. Major sectors are textiles (27·6%), apparel (11·7%) and chemicals (9·2%).

Tourism is important; tourists spent an estimated $4,623m. in 1987, and tourism employed 97,223.

COMMUNICATIONS

Roads. Total highway mileage in the combined highway system in Aug. 1990 was 41,273 miles. Motor vehicle registrations numbered 2·5m. in 1989.

Railways. In 1989 the length of railway in the state was about 2,600 miles.

Aviation. In 1988 there were 152 aircraft facilities including 131 airports, 20 heliports and 1 seaplane base. Registered general aviation numbered 1,988 in 1988.

Shipping. The state has 3 deep-water ports.

JUSTICE, RELIGION, EDUCATION AND WELFARE

Justice. At 31 Dec. 1988 penal institutions held 13,745 prisoners under State and federal jurisdiction.

Education. In 1988–89 the total public-school enrolment (K-12) was 631,656; there were 364,675 white pupils and 266,981 non-white pupils. The total number of teachers was 35,063; average salary was $25,498.

For higher education the state operates the University of South Carolina, founded at Columbia in 1801, with (autumn 1989), 25,692 enrolled students; Clemson University, founded in 1889, with 16,072 students; The Citadel, at Charleston, with 3,669 students; Winthrop College, Rock Hill, with 5,388 students; Medical University of S. Carolina, at Charleston 2,672 students; S. Carolina State College, at Orangeburg, with 4,748 students, and Francis Marion College, at Florence, with 3,883 students; the College of Charleston has 6,778 students and Lander College, Greenwood, 2,307. There are 16 technical institutions (36,713).

There are also 479 private kindergartens, elementary and high schools with total enrolment (1988–89) of 44,705 pupils, and 31 private and denominational colleges and junior colleges with (autumn 1989) enrolment of 26,130 students.

Health. In 1989 the state had 370 non-federal health facilities with 33,139 beds licensed by the South Carolina Department of Health and Environmental Control.

Social Security. In 1989 there were 517,000 recipients of social security benefits. The average monthly expenditure in benefits was $222m.

Further Reading

South Carolina Legislative Manual. Columbia. Annual

South Carolina Statistical Abstract. South Carolina Budget and Control Board, Columbia. Annual

Jones, L., *South Carolina: A Synoptic History for Laymen*. Lexington, 1978

State Library: South Carolina State Library, Columbia.

SOUTH DAKOTA

HISTORY. South Dakota was first visited by Europeans in 1743 when Verendrye planted a lead plate (discovered in 1913) on the site of Fort Pierre, claiming the region for the French crown. Beginning with a trading post in 1794, it was settled from 1857 to 1861 when Dakota Territory was organized. It was admitted into the Union on 2 Nov. 1889.

AREA AND POPULATION. South Dakota is bounded north by North Dakota, east by Minnesota, south-east by the Big Sioux River (forming the boundary with Iowa), south by Nebraska (with the Missouri River forming part of the boundary) and west by Wyoming and Montana. Area, 77,116 sq. miles, of which 1,164 sq. miles are water. Area administered by the Bureau of Indian Affairs, 1985, covered 5m. acres (10% of the state), of which 2·6m. acres were held by tribes. The federal government, 1987, owned or managed 954,000 acres.

Census population, 1 April 1980, 690,178, an increase of 3·5% since 1970. Estimate (1990) 693,294. Births, 1988, were 11,185; deaths, 6,567; infant deaths, 112; marriages, 7,328; divorces, 2,649.

Population in 5 federal censuses was:

	White	*Black*	*Indian*	*Asiatic*	*Total*	*Per sq. mile*
1910	563,771	817	19,137	163	583,888	7·6
1930	669,453	646	21,833	101	692,849	9·0
1960	653,098	1,114	25,794	336	680,514	8·9
			All others			
1970	630,333	1,627	34,297		666,257	8·8
1980	638,955	2,144	49,079		690,178	9·0

Of the total population in 1980, 340,370 were male, 320,223 were urban and 441,851 were 21 years of age or older.

Population of the chief cities (census of 1980) was: Sioux Falls, 81,071; Rapid City, 46,340; Aberdeen, 25,973; Watertown, 15,632; Mitchell, 13,917; Brookings, 14,915; Huron, 13,000.

CLIMATE. Rapid City. Jan. 25°F (–3·9°C), July 73°F (22·8°C). Annual rainfall 19" (474 mm). Sioux Falls. Jan. 14°F (–10°C), July 73°F (22·8°C). Annual rainfall 25" (625 mm). *See* High Plains, p. 1381.

CONSTITUTION AND GOVERNMENT. Voters are all citizens 18 years of age or older who have complied with certain residential qualifications. The people reserve the right of the initiative and referendum. The Senate has 35 members, and the House of Representatives 70 members, all elected for 2 years; the Governor and Lieut.-Governor are elected for 4 years. The state sends 2 senators and 1 representative to Congress.

In the 1988 presidential election Bush polled 165,516 votes, Dukakis, 145,632.

The capital is Pierre (population, 1990, 12,836). The state is divided into 66 organized counties.

Governor: George S. Mickelson, (R.), 1991–95 ($60,816).

BUDGET. For the fiscal year ending 30 June 1991 the estimated general fund revenues were $453,813,852 ($241,137,581 from sales and use tax); expenditure was also $453,813,852 ($156,856,053 on state aid to education).

Per capita personal income (1989) was $12,755.

NATURAL RESOURCES

Minerals. The mineral products include gold (356,103 troy oz. in 1985, second largest yield of all states), silver (96,000 troy oz. in 1987). Mineral products, 1986, were valued at $232,866, including gold and silver.

Agriculture. In 1989 there were 35,000 farms, average size 1,266 acres. Farm units are large; in 1982 there were only 4,024 farms of 50 acres or less, compared with 10,165 exceeding 1,000 acres. 17,371 farms sold produce valued at $40,000 or over in 1985.

South Dakota ranks first in the US as producer of rye (3·2m. bu. in 1989), second in sunflower seed (275·8m. bu.) and flaxseed (3m. bu.), and fourth in oats (44m. bu.). The other important crops are all wheat (83·1m. bu.), sorghum for grain (11·6m. bu.) and corn for grain (190·8m. bu.). The farm livestock on 1 Jan. 1989 included 3·38m. cattle, 0·59m. sheep, 1·72m. hogs.

Forestry. National forest area, 1988, 1,997,000 acres.

INDUSTRY. In 1987, manufacturing establishments had 26,259 workers. Food processing was by far the largest industry with 96 plants employing 7,686 workers. Construction had 1,580 companies employing 7,336. There were 176 printing and publishing plants employing 2,597 workers. Also significant were mining (58 establishments employing 2,061), dairy, lumber and wood products, machinery, transport equipment, electronics, stone, glass and clay products.

COMMUNICATIONS

Roads. In 1990 there were 73,378 miles of roads (71,622 miles rural) and 705,386 registered motor vehicles.

Railways. In 1987 there were 2,005 miles of railway in operation. The state owns 969 miles of track.

Aviation. In 1989 there were 66 general aviation airports and 9 commercial airports.

JUSTICE, RELIGION, EDUCATION AND WELFARE

Justice. The State prisons had, in 1988, 1,020 inmates under state and federal correction. The death penalty was illegal from 1915 to 1938; since 1938, one person has been executed, in 1949 (by electrocution), for murder.

Religion. The chief religious bodies are: Lutherans, Roman Catholics, Methodist, Disciples of Christ, Presbyterian, Baptist and Episcopal.

Education. Elementary and secondary education are free from 6 to 21 years of age. Between the ages of 8 and 16, attendance is compulsory. In 1988–89 133,793 pupils were attending elementary and high (including parochial) schools (8,235 full-time equivalent classroom teachers).

Teachers' salaries (1988–89) averaged an estimated $20,522. Total expenditure on public schools, $494,563,007.

Higher education (spring 1990): The School of Mines at Rapid City, established 1885, had 2,012 students; the State University at Brookings, 6,909 students; the University of South Dakota, founded at Vermillion in 1882, 6,041; Northern State University, Aberdeen, had 2,648; Black Hills State University at Spearfish, 2,333; Dakota State University at Madison, 926. The 10 private colleges had 7,914 students. The federal Government maintains Indian schools on its reservations and 1 outside of a reservation at Flandreau.

Health. In 1988 there were 54 licensed hospitals (3,540 beds).

Social Security. In financial year 1988–89, 4,581 disabled persons received a total average monthly benefit of $195,104; 45 blind persons received $15,291. Aid to dependent children was $2,975,522, to 13,213 children.

Further Reading

Governor's Budget Report. South Dakota Bureau of Finance and Management. Annual
South Dakota Historical Collections. 1902–82
South Dakota Legislative Manual. Secretary of State, Pierre, S.D. Biennial
Berg, F. M., *South Dakota: Land of Shining Gold*. Hettinger, 1982
Karolevitz, R. F., *Challenge: the South Dakota Story*. Sioux Falls, 1975
Milton, John R., *South Dakota; a Bicentennial History*. New York, W. W. Norton, 1977
Schell, H. S., *History of South Dakota*. 3rd ed. Lincoln, Neb., 1975
Vexler, R. I., *South Dakota Chronology and Factbook*. New York, 1978

State Library: South Dakota State Library, 800 Governor's Drive, Pierre, S.D., 57501–2294. *State Librarian:* Dr Jane Kolbe.

TENNESSEE

HISTORY. Tennessee, first settled in 1757, was admitted into the Union on 1 June 1796.

AREA AND POPULATION. Tennessee is bounded north by Kentucky and Virginia, east by North Carolina, south by Georgia, Alabama and Mississippi and west by the Mississippi River (forming the boundary with Arkansas and Missouri). Area, 42,144 sq. miles (989 sq. miles water). Census population, 1 April 1980, 4,591,120, an increase of 665,102 or 16·9% since 1970. Estimate (1988), 4,895,000.

Vital statistics, 1988: Births, 70,685 (14·3 per 1,000 population); deaths, 45,728 (9·2); infant deaths 762 (10·8 per 1,000 live births); marriages, 65,329 (26·4); divorces, 31,287 (12·6).

Population in 6 census years was:

	White	*Black*	*Indian*	*Asiatic*	*Total*	*Per sq. mile*
1910	1,711,432	473,088	216	53	2,184,789	52·4
1930	2,138,644	477,646	161	105	2,616,556	62·4
1950	2,760,257	530,603	339	334	3,291,718	78·8
1960	2,977,753	586,876	638	1,243	3,567,089	85·4
			All others			
1970	3,293,930	621,261	8,496		3,923,687	95·3
1980	3,835,452	725,942	29,726		4,591,120	111·6

Of the population in 1980, 2,216,600 were male, 2,773,573 were urban and those 21 years of age or older numbered 3,026,398.

The cities, with population, 1980 (and estimates 1988), are Memphis, 646,356 (645,190); Nashville (capital), 455,651 (481,380); Knoxville, 175,030 (172,080); Chattanooga, 169,565 (162,670); Clarksville, 54,777 (72,620); Jackson, 49,131 (53,320); Johnson City, 39,753 (45,420); Murfreesboro, 32,845 (45,820); Kingsport, 32,027 (31,440); Oak Ridge, 27,662 (27,710). Standard metropolitan areas 1980 (1988): Memphis, 810,043 (971,930); Nashville, 850,505 (971,800); Knoxville, 476,517 (599,600); Chattanooga, 320,761 (438,100); Johnson City–Bristol–Kingsport, 343,041 (442,300); Clarksville, 83,342 (158,900); Jackson, 74,546 (78,200).

CLIMATE. Memphis. Jan. 41°F (5°C), July 82°F (27·8°C). Annual rainfall 49" (1,221 mm). Nashville. Jan. 39°F (3·9°C), July 79°F (26·1°C). Annual rainfall 48" (1,196 mm). *See* Appalachian Mountains, p. 1382.

CONSTITUTION AND GOVERNMENT. The state has operated under 3 constitutions, the last of which was adopted in 1870 and has been since amended 22 times (first in 1953). Voters at an election may authorize the calling of a convention limited to altering or abolishing one or more specified sections of the constitution. The General Assembly consists of a Senate of 33 members and a House of Representatives of 99 members, senators elected for 4 years and representatives for 2 years. Qualified as electors are all citizens (usual residential and age (18) qualifications). Tennessee sends to Congress 2 senators and 9 representatives.

In the 1988 presidential election Bush polled 939,434 votes, Dukakis, 677,715.

For the Tennessee Valley Authority *see* p. 1409.

The capital is Nashville. The state is divided into 95 counties.

Governor: Ned McWherter (D.), 1991–95 ($85,000).

BUDGET. For 1988–89 total revenue was $6,636m.; general expenditure, $5,987m.

Total net long-term debt on 30 June 1989 amounted to $651·9m.

Per capita personal income (1988) was $14,694.

ENERGY AND NATURAL RESOURCES

Minerals. Total value added by mining 1987: Metal mining, $50·1m.; coal mining, $145·7m.; oil and gas extraction, $59·5m.; non-metallic minerals (except fuels, $203·1m.

Agriculture. In 1989, 91,000 farms covered 12·6m. acres. The average farm was of 131 acres (only a few states had a smaller average) valued, land and buildings, at $1,126.

Cash income (1988) from crops was $965·3m.; from livestock, $1,080·4m. Main crops were cotton, tobacco and soybeans.

On 1 Jan. 1989 the domestic animals included 202,000 milch cows, 2·3m. all cattle, 10,000 sheep, 900,000 swine.

Forestry. Forests occupy 13,258,000 acres (50% of total land area). The forest industry and industries dependent on it employ about 40,000 workers, earning $150m. per year. Wood products are valued at over $500m. per year. National forest system land (1986) 626,000 acres.

INDUSTRY. The manufacturing industries include iron and steel working, but the most important products are chemicals, including synthetic fibres and allied products, electrical equipment and food. In 1987, manufacturing establishments employed 485,000 workers; value added by manufactures was $27,079m.

TOURISM. In 1988 43·1m. out-of-state tourists spent $4,883m.

COMMUNICATIONS

Roads. In 1990 there were 84,081 miles of roads (68,854 miles rural) and 4,315,702 registered motor vehicles.

Railways. The state had (1985) 2,857 miles of track.

Aviation. The state is served by 11 major airlines. In 1985 there were 74 public airports and 78 private; there were 71 heliports and 2 military air bases.

JUSTICE, RELIGION, EDUCATION AND WELFARE

Justice. There has been no execution since 1960; since 1930 there have been 66 ex-executions (by electrocution) for murder and 27 for rape. A US Supreme Court ruling prohibits the use of capital punishment under present Tennessee law, except for first degree murder.

Prison population, 30 June 1990, 8,424.

Religion. The leading religious bodies are the Southern Baptists, Methodists and Negro Baptists.

Education. School attendance has been compulsory since 1925 and the employment of children under 16 years of age in workshops, factories or mines is illegal.

In 1988–89 there were 1,672 public schools with a net enrolment of 860,004 pupils; 49,634 teachers earned an average salary of $25,619. Total expenditure for operating public schools (kindergarten to Grade 12) was $2,659m. Tennessee has 49 accredited colleges and universities, 18 2-year colleges and 28 vocational schools. The universities include the University of Tennessee, Knoxville (founded 1794), with 25,187 students in 1989–90; Vanderbilt University, Nashville (1873) with 9,059, Tennessee State University (1912) with 7,362, the University of Tennessee at Chattanooga (1886) with 7,362, Memphis State University (1912), 20,613 and Fisk University (1866) with 891.

Health. In 1986 the state had 146 hospitals with 27,274 beds. State facilities for the mentally retarded had 1,994 resident patients and mental hospitals had 1,742 in 1989.

Social Security. In 1988 Tennessee paid $4,102m. to retired workers and their survivors and to disabled workers. Total beneficiaries: 527,000 retired; 163,000 survivors and 107,000 disabled. 479,000 people received $890m. in Medicaid. Supplemental Security Income ($327m.) was paid to 133,600. 193,000 people (1988) received aid to dependent children ($130m.).

Further Reading

Tennessee Dept. of Finance and Administration, Annual Report, Annual
Dept. of Education Annual Report for Tennessee, Annual
Tennessee Blue Book. Secretary of State, Nashville
Tennessee Statistical Abstract, Center for Business and Economic Research, Univ. of Tennessee. Annual

Corlew, R. E., *Tennessee: A Short History*. Univ. Tennessee, 2nd ed., 1981
Davidson, D., *Tennessee: Vol. I, The Old River Frontier to Secession*, Univ. Tennessee, 1979
Dykeman, W., *Tennessee*, Rev. Ed., New York, 1984

State Library: State Library and Archives, Nashville. *Librarian:* Edwin Gleaves. *State Historian:* Wilma Dykeman.

TEXAS

HISTORY. In 1836 Texas declared its independence of Mexico, and after maintaining an independent existence, as the Republic of Texas, for 10 years, it was on 29 Dec. 1845 received as a state into the American Union. The state's first settlement dates from 1686.

AREA AND POPULATION. Texas is bounded north by Oklahoma, north-east by Arkansas, east by Louisiana, south-east by the Gulf of Mexico, south by Mexico and west by New Mexico. Area, 266,807 sq. miles (including 4,790 sq. miles of inland water). Census population, 1 April 1980 (provisional), 14,228,383, an increase of 27% since 1970. Estimate (1988), 16,841,000. Vital statistics for 1984: Births, 306,192 (19·2 per 1,000 population); deaths, 119,531 (7·5); infant deaths, 3,178 (10·4 per 1,000 live births); marriages, 207,631 (13); divorces, 98,074 (6·1).

Population for 5 census years was:

	White	*Black*	*Indian*	*Asiatic*	*Total*	*Per sq. mile*
1910	3,204,848	690,049	702	943	3,896,542	14·8
1930	4,967,172	854,964	1,001	1,578	5,824,715	22·1
1960	8,374,831	1,187,125	5,750	9,848	9,579,677	36·5
			All others			
1970	9,717,128	1,399,005	80,597		11,196,730	42·7
1980	11,197,663	1,710,250	1,320,470		14,228,383	54·2

Of the population in 1980, 6,998,301 were male, 11,327,159 persons were urban. Those 20 years old and older numbered 9,357,309. A census report, 1980, showed, 2,985,643 persons of Spanish origin.

The largest cities, with census population in 1980, are:

Houston	1,595,138	Amarillo	149,230	Odessa	90,027
Dallas	904,078	Beaumont	118,102	Garland	138,857
San Antonio	785,882	Wichita Falls	94,201	Laredo	91,449
Fort Worth	385,164	Irving	109,943	San Angelo	73,240
El Paso	425,259	Waco	101,261	Galveston	61,902
Austin (capital)	345,496	Arlington	160,113	Midland	70,525
Corpus Christi	231,999	Abilene	98,315	Tyler	70,508
Lubbock	173,979	Pasadena	112,560	Port Arthur	61,195

Larger urbanized areas, 1980: Houston, 2,891,146; Dallas-Fort Worth, 2,964,342; San Antonio, 1,070,245.

CLIMATE. Dallas. Jan. 45°F (7·2°C), July 84°F (28·9°C). Annual rainfall 38" (945 mm). El Paso. Jan. 44°F (6·7°C), July 81°F (27·2°C). Annual rainfall 9" (221 mm). Galveston. Jan. 54°F (12·2°C), July 84°F (28·9°C). Annual rainfall 46" (1,159 mm). Houston. Jan. 52°F (11·1°C), July 83°F (28·3°C). Annual rainfall 48" (1,200 mm). *See* Central Plains, p. 1381.

CONSTITUTION AND GOVERNMENT. The present constitution dates from 1876; it has been amended 326 times. The Legislature consists of a Senate of 31 members elected for 4 years (half their number retire every 2 years), and a House of Representatives of 150 members elected for 2 years.

The Governor and Lieut.-Governor are elected for 4 years. Qualified electors are all citizens with the usual residential qualifications. Texas sends to Congress 2 senators and 27 representatives.

In the 1988 presidential election Bush polled 3,014,007 votes, Dukakis, 2,331,286.

The capital is Austin. The state has 254 counties.

Governor: Ann W. Richards (D.), 1991–95 ($93,432).

BUDGET. In the fiscal year ending 31 Aug. 1987 general revenues were $23,617m. ($10,266·2m. from taxes, $4,078·1m. federal aid); general expenditures (1981-82), $21,334m. ($8,743m. on education, $2,506m. on highways, $2,067m. on hospitals, $1,741m. on public welfare).

Net long-term debt, 31 Aug. 1985, was $4,009m.

Per capita personal income (1985) was $13,483.

ENERGY AND NATURAL RESOURCES

Minerals. Production, 1988: Crude petroleum, 728m. bbls, natural gas 4,500m. cubic ft.; other minerals include natural gasoline, butane and propane gases, helium, crude gypsum, granite and sandstone, salt and cement. Total value of mineral products in 1982, $45,388m., of which $43,834 was for fuels.

Agriculture. Texas is one of the most important agricultural states of the Union. In 1988 it had 156,000 farms covering 136m. acres; average farm was of 846 acres valued, land and buildings, at $591 per acre. Large-scale commercial farms, highly mechanized, dominate in Texas; farms of 1,000 acres or more in number far exceed that of any other state. But small-scale farming persists.

Soil erosion is serious in some parts. For some 97,297,000 acres drastic curative treatment has been indicated and for 51,164,000 acres, preventive treatment.

Production, 1985: Cotton, 3,945,000 bales (of 480 lb., value $981m.); maize (157m. bu., value $422m.), wheat (187·2m. bu., value $580m.), oats, barley, soybeans, peanuts, oranges, grapefruit, peaches, potatoes, sweet potatoes.

Cash income, 1988, from crops was $3,027m.; from livestock, $6,059m.

The state has a very great livestock industry, leading in the number of all cattle, 13·7m. on 1 Jan. 1989, and sheep, 1·9m.; it also had 355,000 milch cows, and 560,000 swine.

Forestry. There were (1988) 22,032,000 acres of forested land.

INDUSTRY. In 1988 manufacturing establishments employed 970,267 workers; trade employed 1,667,000; government, 1·1m.; services, 1·4m.; construction, 337,379; finance, insurance and real estate, 427,656; transport and public utilities, 372,391. Chemical industries along the Gulf Coast, such as the production of synthetic rubber and of primary magnesium (from sea-water), are increasingly important.

COMMUNICATIONS

Roads. In 1990 there were 305,692 miles of roads (217,044 miles rural) and 12,564,555 registered motor vehicles.

Aviation. In 1988 there were 307 public and 1,308 private airports.

Shipping. The port of Houston, connected by the Houston Ship Channel (50 miles long) with the Gulf of Mexico, is the largest inland cotton market in the world. Cargo handled 1987, 112,546,187 tons.

JUSTICE, RELIGION, EDUCATION AND WELFARE

Justice. In Dec. 1988 the state prison held 39,221 men and women. Execution is by lethal injection; there were 300 between 1930 and 1968; between 1977 and 1986 there were 8.

Texas has adopted 11 laws governing the activities of trade unions. An Act of 1955 forbids the state's payment of unemployment compensation to workers engaged in certain types of strikes.

Religion. The largest religious bodies are Roman Catholics, Baptists, Methodists, Churches of Christ, Lutherans, Presbyterians and Episcopalians.

Education. School attendance is compulsory from 6 to 17 years of age.

In autumn 1988 public elementary and secondary schools had 3,057,147 enrolled pupils; in 1986 there were 175,500 classroom teachers whose salaries averaged $24,500. Total public school expenditure, 1987, $11,529m.

The largest institutions of higher education, with faculty numbers and student enrolment, 1988–89, were:

Founded	*Institutions*	*Control*	*Faculty*	*Students*
1845	Baylor University, Waco	Baptist	636	11,774
1852	St Mary's University, San Antonio	R.C.	209	3,932
1869	Trinity University, San Antonio	Presb.	255	2,573
1873	Texas Christian University, Fort Worth	Christian	519	6,725
1876	Texas A. and M. Univ., College Station	State	2,240	38,764
1876	Prairie View Agr. and Mech. Coll., Prairie View	State	297	5,812
1879	Sam Houston State University	State	365	12,359
1883	University of Texas System (every campus)	State	6,328	131,732
1890	University of North Texas, Denton	State	884	26,523
1891	Hardin-Simmons University, Abilene	Baptist	124	1,826
1889	East Texas State University, Commerce	State	363	7,811
1899	South West Texas State University, San Marcos	State	833	20,776
1903	Texas Woman's University, Denton	State	520	9,408
1906	Abilene Christian University, Abilene	Church of Christ	275	4,186
1911	Southern Methodist University, Dallas	Methodist	650	8,929
1923	Stephen F. Austin State University	State	517	12,783
1923	Texas Technical University, Lubbock	State	1,444	25,009
1925	Texas Arts and Industries University, Kingsville	State	234	5,872
1934	University of Houston, Houston	State	2,100	32,280
1947	Texas Southern University, Houston	State	544	9,214
1951	Lamar University, Beaumont	State	545	12,041

Health. In 1988, the state had 553 hospitals (80,914 beds) listed by the American Hospital Association; on 1 Jan. 1987 mental hospitals had 3,863 resident patients and state institutions for the mentally retarded, 8,134 resident patients.

Social Security. Aid is from state and federal sources. Old-age assistance (SSI) was being granted in Dec. 1985 to 123,400 persons, who received an average of $133 per month; aid was given to 127,100 disabled ($217) and 398,900 dependent children (average payment per family, $142 per month).

Further Reading

Texas Almanac. Dallas. Biennial

Texas Factbook. Univ. of Texas, 1983

Benton, W. E., *Texas, its Government and Politics*. 4th ed., Englewood Cliffs, 1977

Cruz, G. R. and Irby, J. A. (eds.) *Texas Bibliography*. Austin, 1982

Fehrenbach, T. R., *Lone Star: A History of Texas and the Texans*. London, 1986

Jordan, T. G. and Bean, J. L., Jr., *Texas*. Boulder, 1983

MacCorkle, S. A. and Smith, D., *Texas Government*. 7th ed. New York, 1974

Richardson, R. N., *Texas, the Lone Star State*. 3rd ed. New York, 1970

Legislative Reference Library: Box 12488, Capitol Station, Austin, Texas 78811. *Director:* Sally Reynolds.

UTAH

HISTORY. Utah, which had been acquired by the US during the Mexican war, was settled by Mormons in 1847, and organized as a Territory on 9 Sept. 1850. It was admitted as a state into the Union on 4 Jan. 1896 with boundaries as at present.

AREA AND POPULATION. Utah is bounded north by Idaho and Wyoming, east by Colorado, south by Arizona and west by Nevada. Area, 84,899 sq. miles, of which 2,826 sq. miles are water. The federal government (1967) owned 35,397,274 acres or 67·1% of the area of the state. The area of unappropriated and unreserved lands was 23,268,250 acres in 1974. The Bureau of Indian Affairs in 1974 administered 3,035,190 acres, all of which were allotted to Indian tribes.

Census population, 1 April 1980, 1,461,037, an increase of 38% since 1970. Estimate (1985), 1,645,000. Births in 1984 were 39,677 (24 per 1,000 population); deaths, 9,295 (5·6); infant deaths, 407 (10·3 per 1,000 live births); marriages, 17,579 (10·6); divorces, 8,134 (4·9).

Population at 5 federal censuses was:

	White	*Black*	*Indian*	*Asiatic*	*Total*	*Per sq. mile*
1910	366,583	1,144	3,123	2,501	373,851	4·5
1930	499,967	1,108	2,869	3,903	507,847	6·2
1960	873,828	4,148	6,961	5,207	890,627	10·8
1970	1,031,926	6,617	11,273	6,230	1,059,273	12·9
1980	1,382,550	9,225	19,256	15,076	1,461,037	17·7

Of the total in 1980, 724,501 were male, 1,232,908 persons were urban; 860,304 were 20 years of age or older.

The largest cities are Salt Lake City (capital), with a population (census, 1980) of 162,960; Provo, 74,007; Ogden, 64,444; Bountiful, 32,877; Orem, 52,399; Sandy City, 51,022 and Logan, 26,844.

CLIMATE. Salt Lake City. Jan. 29°F (–1·7°C), July 77°F (25°C). Annual rainfall 16" (401 mm). *See* Mountain States, p. 1381.

CONSTITUTION AND GOVERNMENT. Utah adopted its present constitution in 1896 (now with 61 amendments). It sends to Congress 2 senators and 3 representatives.

The Legislature consists of a Senate (in part renewed every 2 years) of 30 members, elected for 4 years, and of a House of Representatives of 75 members elected for 2 years. The Governor is elected for 4 years. The constitution provides for the initiative and referendum. Electors are all citizens, who, not being insane or criminal, have the usual residential qualifications.

The capital is Salt Lake City. There are 29 counties in the state.

In the 1988 presidential election Bush polled 426,858 votes, Dukakis, 206,853.

Governor: Norman Bangerter (R.), 1989–93 ($52,000).

Lieut.-Governor: W. Val Oveson (R.), 1989–93 ($35,500).

BUDGET. For the year ending 30 June 1982 general revenue was $2,490m. ($1,332m. from taxes, $612m. from federal aid) while general expenditures were $2,490m. ($1,104m. on education, $279m. on highways, $234m. on public welfare).

The net long-term debt on 30 June 1982 was about $2,171m.

Per capita personal income (1985) was $10,493.

ENERGY AND NATURAL RESOURCES

Minerals The principal minerals are: Copper, gold, petroleum, lead, silver and zinc. The state also has natural gas, clays, tungsten, molybdenum, uranium and phosphate rock.

Agriculture. In 1985 Utah had 14,000 farms covering 12m. acres, of which about 2m. acres were crop land and about 300,000 acres pasture. About 1m. acres had irrigation; the average farm was of 857 acres.

Of the total surface area, 9% is severely eroded and only 9·4% is free from erosion; the balance is moderately eroded.

Cash income, 1985, from crops, $138m. and from livestock, $409m. The principal crops are: Barley, wheat (spring and winter), oats, potatoes, hay (alfalfa, sweet clover and lespedeza), maize. In 1985 there were 515,000 sheep; 80,000 milch cows; 800,000 all cattle; 28,000 swine.

Forestry. Area of national forests, 1981, was 9,129,000 acres, of which 8·05m. acres were under forest service administration.

INDUSTRY. In 1985 manufacturing establishments had 94,000 workers. Leading manufactures by value added are primary metals, ordinances and transport, food, fabricated metals and machinery, petroleum products. Service industries employed 132,000; trade, 148,000; government, 138,000.

COMMUNICATIONS

Roads. In 1990 there were 42,971 miles of roads (37,430 miles rural) and 1,174,861 registered motor vehicles.

Railways. On 1 July 1974 the state had 1,734 miles of railways.

Aviation. In 1981 there were 57 public and 45 private airports.

JUSTICE, RELIGION, EDUCATION AND WELFARE

Justice. The number of inmates of the state prison in Dec. 1985 was 1,570. Since 1930 total executions have been 14 (13 by shooting, 1 by hanging—the condemned man has choice), all whites, and all for murder.

Religion. Latter-day Saints (Mormons) form about 73% of the church membership of the state; their church is a substantial property-owner. The Roman Catholic church and most Protestant denominations are represented.

Education. School attendance is compulsory for children from 6 to 18 years of age. There are 40 school districts. Teachers' salaries, 1985, averaged $21,500. There were (autumn 1983) 379,000 pupils in public elementary and secondary schools, and (1986) 16,700 classroom teachers, average salary, $22,550; estimated public school expenditure was $1,092m. or $664 per capita.

The University of Utah (1850) (24,770 students in 1985–86) is in Salt Lake City; the Utah State University (1890) (11,804) is in Logan. The Mormon Church maintains the Brigham Young University at Provo (1875) with 26,894 students. Other colleges include: Westminster College, Salt Lake City (1,302); Weber State College, Ogden (11,117); Southern Utah State College, Cedar City (2,587); College of Eastern Utah, Price (1,132); Snow College, Ephraim (1,328); Dixie College, St George (2,234).

Health. In 1983, the state had 44 hospitals (5,400 beds) listed by the Utah Department of Social Services. Mental hospitals had 317 resident patients on 1 Jan. 1980; state facilities for the mentally retarded had 763.

Social Security. In Dec. 1985 the state department of public welfare provided assistance to 37,800 persons receiving aid to dependent children at an average $322 per family per month; aid to the aged, the blind and disabled is provided from federal funds; there were 1,900 aged recipients in 1985 (average $150 per month), 6,600 disabled ($224).

Further Reading

Compiled Digest of Administrative Reports. Secretary of State, Salt Lake City. Annual
Statistical Abstract of Government in Utah. Utah Foundation, Salt Lake City. Annual
Utah Agricultural Statistics. Dept. of Agriculture, Salt Lake City. Annual
Utah: Facts. Bureau of Economic and Business Research, Univ. of Utah, 1975
Arrington, L., *Great Basin Kingdom: An Economic History of the Latter-Day Saints, 1830–1900.* Cambridge, Mass., 1958
Petersen, C. S., *Utah, a History.* New York, 1977

VERMONT

HISTORY. Vermont, first settled in 1724, was admitted into the Union as the fourteenth state on 4 March 1791. The first constitution was adopted by convention at Windsor, 2 July 1777, and established an independent state government.

AREA AND POPULATION. Vermont is bounded north by Canada, east by New Hampshire, south by Massachusetts and west by New York. Area, 9,614 sq. miles, of which 341 sq. miles are inland water. Census population, 1 April 1980, 511,456, an increase of 15% since 1970. Estimate (Jan. 1989) 567,000. Births, 1988, were 8,116 (14·6 per 1,000 population); deaths, 4,660 (8·4); infant deaths, 53 (6·5 per 1,000 live births); marriages, 6,125 (11); divorces, 2,588 (4·6).

Population at 5 census years was:

	White	*Black*	*Indian*	*Asiatic*	*Total*	*Per sq. mile*
1910	354,298	1,621	26	11	355,956	39·0
1930	358,966	568	36	41	359,611	38·8
1960	389,092	519	57	172	389,881	42·0
1970	442,553	761	229	787	444,732	48·0
1980	506,736	1,135	984	1,355	511,456	55·1

Of the population in 1980, 249,080 were male, 172,735 persons were urban; those 20 years of age or older numbered 343,666. The largest cities are Burlington, with a population (1988 estimate) of 37,725; Rutland, 18,378; Benrington, 16,593.

CLIMATE. Burlington. Jan. 17°F (–8·3°C), July 70°F (21·1°C). Annual rainfall 33" (820 mm). *See* New England, p. 1382.

CONSTITUTION AND GOVERNMENT. The constitution was adopted in 1793 and has since been amended. Amendments are proposed by two-thirds vote of the Senate every 4 years, and must be accepted by two sessions of the legislature; they are then submitted to popular vote. The state Legislature, consisting of a Senate of 30 members and a House of Representatives of 150 members (both elected for 2 years), meets in Jan. every year. The Governor and Lieut.-Governor are elected for 2 years. Electors are all citizens who possess certain residential qualifications and have taken the freeman's oath set forth in the constitution.

The state is divided into 14 counties; there are 251 towns and cities and other minor civil divisions. The state sends to Congress 2 senators and 1 representative, who are elected by the voters of the entire state.

In the 1988 presidential election Bush polled 123,166 votes, Dukakis, 116,419.

The capital is Montpelier (8,414, 1988 estimate).

Governor: Richard A. Snelling (R.), 1991–93 ($75,800).

BUDGET. The total revenue for the year ending 30 June 1988 was $1,096·1m.; total disbursements, $1,092·2m.

Total net long-term debt, 30 June 1986, was $254·7.

Per capita personal income (1988) was $15,302.

NATURAL RESOURCES

Minerals. Stone, chiefly granite, marble and slate, is the leading mineral produced in Vermont, contributing about 60% of the total value of mineral products. Other products include asbestos, talc, peat, sand and gravel. Total value of mineral products, 1984, $45m.

Agriculture. Agriculture is the most important industry. In 1988 the state had 7,100 farms covering 1·58m. acres; the average farm was of 223 acres. Cash income, 1988, from livestock and products, $376·9m.; from crops, $45m. The dairy farms produce about 2,387m. lb. of milk annually. The chief agricultural crops are hay, apples and silage. In 1989 Vermont had 297,000 cattle and calves, 17,000 sheep and lambs, 6,000 hogs and pigs, 300,000 poultry (1986).

Forestry. In 1989 the harvest was 84·2m. bd ft hardwood and 130·1m. bd ft softwood saw-logs, and 351,659 cords of pulpwood and boltwood. About 400,000 (1986) cords were cut for firewood.

The state is 76% forest, with 10% in public ownership. National forests area

(1986), 355,534 acres. State-owned forests, parks, fish and game areas, 250,000 acres; municipally-owned, 38,500 acres.

INDUSTRY. In 1986 service industries employed 65,000; manufacturing, 54,000; trade, 52,000; government, 35,000; construction, 20,000.

COMMUNICATIONS

Roads. The state had 14,089 miles of roads in 1989, including 7,475 miles of gravel, graded and drained, or unimproved roads. Motor vehicle registrations, 1988, 649,417, of which 315,275 were private.

Railways. There were, in 1988, 793 miles of railway, 291 of which was leased by the state to private operators.

Aviation. There were 18 airports in 1987, of which 11 were state operated, 1 municipally owned and 6 private. Some are only open in summer.

JUSTICE, RELIGION, EDUCATION AND WELFARE

Justice. In financial year 1989 prisons and centres had 761 (with another 110 on furlough) inmates; 700 of these were serving more than one year.

Religion. The principal denominations are Roman Catholic, United Church of Christ, United Methodist, Protestant Episcopal, Baptist and Unitarian–Universalist.

Education. School attendance during the full school term is compulsory for children from 7 to 16 years of age, unless they have completed the 10th grade or undergo approved home instruction. In 1989–90 the public schools had 94,779 pupils. Full-time teachers for public elementary schools (1986) numbered 2,900, secondary schools 3,500. Teachers' salaries, 1990–91, average base salary $19,629. Total expenditure on public schools, 1987–88, $334·7m.

In autumn 1985 there were 31,416 students in higher education. The University of Vermont (1791) had 11,096 students in 1986–87; Norwich University (1834, founded as the American Literary, Scientific and Military Academy in 1819), had 2,425; St Michael's College (1904), 2,130; there are 5 state colleges.

Health. In Sept. 1988 the state had 18 general hospitals (2,383 beds).

Social Security. Old-age assistance (SSI) was being granted in 1985 to 3,000 persons, drawing an average of $139 per month; aid to dependent children was being granted to 21,900 persons, drawing an average of $400 per family per month; and aid to the permanently and totally disabled was being granted to 6,200 persons, drawing an average of $260.

Further Reading

Legislative Directory. Secretary of State, Montpelier. Biennial
Vermont Annual Financial Report. Auditor of Accounts, Montpelier. Annual
Vermont Facts and Figures. Office of Statistical Co-ordination, Montpelier
Vermont Year-Book, formerly *Walton's Register.* Chester. Annual
Bassett T. (ed.) *Vermont: A Bibliography of its History,* Boston, 1981
Vermont Atlas and Gazetteer, Rev. ed., Freeport, 1983
Morrissey, C. T., *Vermont,* New York, 1981

State Library: Vermont Dept.of Libraries, Montpelier. *State Librarian:* Patricia Klinck.

VIRGINIA

HISTORY. The first English Charter for settlements in America was that granted by James I in 1606 for the planting of colonies in Virginia. The state was one of the 13 original states in the Union. Virginia lost just over one-third of its area when West Virginia was admitted into the Union (1863).

AREA AND POPULATION. Virginia is bounded north-west by West Virginia, north-east by Maryland, east by the Atlantic, south by North Carolina and Tennessee and west by Kentucky. Area, 40,767 sq. miles including 1,063 sq. miles of inland water. Census population, 1 April 1980, 5,346,818, an increase of 695,370 or 14·9% since 1970. Estimate 1988 5,996,000. In 1988 there were 87,002 births (15·1 per 1,000 population); 46,015 deaths (7·9); (1987) 850 infant deaths (11·5 per 1,000 live births); 67,073 marriages and 25,568 divorces.

Population for 5 federal census years was:

	White	*Black*	*Indian*	*Asiatic*	*Total*	*Per sq. mile*
1910	1,389,809	671,096	539	168	2,061,612	51·2
1930	1,770,441	650,165	779	466	2,421,851	60·7
1960	3,142,443	816,258	2,155	4,725	3,966,949	99·3
			All others			
1970	3,761,514	861,368	25,612		4,648,494	116·9
1980	4,230,000	1,008,311	108,517		5,346,818	134·7

Of the total population in 1980, 49% were male, 66% were urban and 59% were 21 years of age or older.

The population (census of 1980) of the principal cities was: Norfolk, 266,979; Virginia Beach, 262,199; Richmond, 219,214; Newport News, 144,903; Hampton, 122,617; Chesapeake, 114,226; Portsmouth, 104,577; Alexandria, 103,219; Roanoke, 100,427; Lynchburg, 66,743.

CLIMATE. Average temperatures in Jan. are 41°F in the Tidewater coastal area and 32°F in the Blue Ridge mountains; July averages, 78°F and 68°F respectively. Precipitation averages 36" in the Shenandoah valley and 44" in the south. Snowfall is 5-10" in the Tidewater and 25-30" in the western mountains. Norfolk. Jan. 41°F (5°C), July 79°F (26·1°C). Annual rainfall 46" (1,145 mm). *See* Atlantic Coast, p. 1382.

CONSTITUTION AND GOVERNMENT. The present constitution dates from 1971.

The General Assembly consists of a Senate of 40 members, elected for 4 years, and a House of Delegates of 100 members, elected for 2 years. The Governor and Lieut.-Governor are elected for 4 years. Qualified as electors are (with few exceptions) all citizens 18 years of age, fulfilling certain residential qualifications, who have registered. The state sends to Congress 2 senators and 10 representatives.

In the 1988 presidential election Bush polled 1,305,131 votes, Dukakis, 860,767.

The state capital is Richmond; the state contains 95 counties and 41 independent cities.

Governor: L. Douglas Wilder (D.), 1990–94 ($85,000).

BUDGET. General revenue for the year ending 30 June 1986 was $13,325m. (taxation, $8,125m., and federal aid, $2,275m.); general expenditures, $12,803m. ($5,102m. for education, $1,354m. for transport and $1,010m. for public welfare).

Total net long-term debt, 30 June 1986, amounted to $10,153m.

Per capita personal income (1987) was $16,517.

ENERGY AND NATURAL RESOURCES

Minerals. Coal is the most important mineral, with output (1984) of 35,500,000 short tons. Lead and zinc ores, stone, sand and gravel, lime and titanium ore are also produced. Total mineral output was $382m. in 1986.

Agriculture. In 1987 there were 50,000 farms with an area of 10m. acres; average farm had 192 acres and was valued at $10,667,000.

Income, 1986, from crops, $996m., and from livestock and livestock products, $1,127m. The chief crops are corn, hay, peanuts and tobacco.

Animals on farms on 1 Jan. 1987 included 150,000 milch cows, 1·86m. all cattle, 168,000 sheep and 360,000 swine (Dec. 1986).

Forestry. National forests, 1986, covered 1,637,000 acres.

INDUSTRY. The manufacture of cigars and cigarettes and of rayon and allied products and the building of ships lead in value of products.

TOURISM. Tourists spend about $4,100m. a year in Virginia, attracted mainly by the state's outstanding scenery, coastline and historical interest.

COMMUNICATIONS

Roads. In 1990 there were 67,282 miles of roads (52,228 miles rural) and 4,859,728 registered motor vehicles.

Railways. In 1985 there were 3,693 miles of railways.

Aviation. There were, in 1985, 81 airports, of which 58 were publicly owned.

JUSTICE, RELIGION, EDUCATION AND WELFARE

Justice. Executions (by electrocution) since 1940 totalled 70. Prison population, 31 Dec. 1987, 13,321 in federal and state prisons.

Religion. The principal churches are the Baptist, Methodist, Protestant-Episcopal, Roman Catholic and Presbyterian.

Education. Elementary and secondary instruction is free, and for ages 6–17 attendance is compulsory. No child under 12 may be employed in any mining or manufacturing work.

In 1985 the 135 school districts had, in primary schools, 665,000 pupils and 34,200 teachers and in public high schools, 303,000 pupils and 25,300 teachers. Teachers' salaries (1987) averaged $25,500. Total expenditure on education, 1987, was $3,667m. The more important institutions for higher education (1986) were:

Founded	*Name and place of college*	*Staff*	*Students*
1693	College of William and Mary, Williamsburg (State)	526	6,616
1749	Washington and Lee University, Lexington	194	1,804
1776	Hampden-Sydney College, Hampden-Sydney (Pres.)	74	825
1819	University of Virginia, Charlottesville (State)	1,772	17,149
1832	Randolph-Macon College, Ashland (Methodist)	102	1,013
1832	University of Richmond, Richmond (Baptist)	349	4,705
1838	Virginia Commonwealth University, Richmond	1,885	19,641
1839	Virginia Military Institute Lexington (State)	100	1,350
1865	Virginia Union University, Richmond	98	1,311
1868	Hampton University	297	4,483
1872	Virginia Polytechnic Institute and State University	2,209	22,345
1882	Virginia State University, Petersburg	263	3,583
1908	James Madison University, Harrisonburg	600	9,757
1910	Radford University (State)	365	7,500
1930	Old Dominion University, Norfolk	713	15,463
1956	George Mason University (State)	715	17,652

Health. In 1986 the state had 137 hospitals (31,005 beds) listed by the American Hospital Association.

Social Security. In 1938 Virginia established a system of old-age assistance under the Federal Security Act; in March 1986 persons in 778,000 cases were drawing an average grant of $246; aid to permanently and totally disabled, 92,000 cases, average grant $918.96; aid to dependent children, 154,000 persons, average grant $85.77; general relief, 6,642 persons, average grant $146.62.

Further Reading

Virginia Facts and Figures. Virginia Division of Industrial Development, Richmond. Annual
Dabney, V., *Virginia, the New Dominion.* 1971

Friddell, G., *The Virginia Way*. Burda, 1973
Gottmann, J., *Virginia in our Century*. Charlottesville, 1969
Morton, R. L., *Colonial Virginia*. 2 vols. Univ. Press of Virginia, 1960
Rouse, P. *Virginia: a Pictorial History*. Scribner, 1975
Rubin, L. D. Jr., *Virginia: a Bicentennial History*. Norris, 1977

State Library: Virginia State Library, Richmond 23219. *State Librarian:* Ella Gaines Yates.

WASHINGTON

HISTORY. Washington, formerly part of Oregon, was created a Territory in 1853, and was admitted into the Union as a state on 11 Nov. 1889. Its settlement dates from 1811.

AREA AND POPULATION. Washington is bounded north by Canada, east by Idaho, south by Oregon with the Columbia River forming most of the boundary, and west by the Pacific. Area, 68,192 sq. miles, of which 1,622 sq. miles are inland water. Lands owned by the federal government, 1977, were 12·4m. acres or 29·1% of the total area. Census population, 1 April 1980, 4,132,156, an increase of 718,906 or 21·1% since 1970. Estimated population (1987), 4,481,100. Births, 1986 were 69,431 (15·7 per 1,000 population); deaths, 34,166 (7·8); infant deaths (1985), 778 (10·2 per 1,000 live births); marriages, 43,255 (9·8); divorces and annulments, 26,405 (6·0).

Population in 5 federal census years was:

	White	*Black*	*Indian*	*Asiatic*	*Total*	*Per sq. mile*
1910	1,109,111	6,058	10,997	15,824	1,141,990	17·1
1930	1,521,661	6,840	11,253	23,642	1,563,396	23·3
1960	2,751,675	48,738	21,076	31,725	2,853,214	42·8
1970	2,351,055	71,308	33,386	53,420	3,409,169	51·2
1980	3,779,170	105,574	60,804	186,608	4,132,156	62·1

Of the total population in 1980, 2,052,307 were male, 3,037,014 persons were urban; 2,759,552 were 20 years of age or older.

There are 24 Indian reservations, the largest being held by the Yakima tribe. Indian reservations in Sept. 1979 covered 2,496,423 acres, of which 1,996,018 acres were tribal lands and 497,218 acres were held by individuals. Total Indian population, 1980, 60,804.

Leading cities are Seattle, with a population in 1980 (and 1987 estimate) of 491,897 (491,300); Spokane, 170,993 (172,100); Tacoma, 158,101 (158,900); Bellevue, 73,711 (82,070). Others : Yakima, 49,826; Everett, 54,413; Vancouver, 42,834; Bellingham, 45,794; Bremerton, 36,208; Richland, 33,578; Longview, 31,052; Renton, 30,612; Edmonds, 27,526; Walla Walla, 25,618. Urbanized areas (1980 census): Seattle–Everett, 1,600,944; Tacoma, 482,692; Spokane, 341,058.

CLIMATE. Seattle. Jan. 40°F (4·4°C), July 63°F (17·2°C). Annual rainfall 34" (848 mm). Spokane. Jan. 27°F (–2·8°C), July 70°F (21·1°C). Annual rainfall 14" (350 mm). *See* Pacific Coast, p. 1381.

CONSTITUTION AND GOVERNMENT. The constitution, adopted in 1889, has had 63 amendments. The Legislature consists of a Senate of 49 members elected for 4 years, half their number retiring every 2 years, and a House of Representatives of 98 members, elected for 2 years. The Governor and Lieut.-Governor are elected for 4 years. The state sends 2 senators and 7 representatives to Congress.

Qualified as voters are (with some exceptions) all citizens 18 years of age, having the usual residential qualifications.

In the 1988 presidential election Dukakis polled 844,544 votes, Bush, 800,182.

The capital is Olympia (population, 1980 census, 27,447). The state contains 39 counties.

Governor: Booth Gardner (D.), 1989–93 ($63,000).

Lieut.-Governor: Joel Pritchard (R.), 1989–93 ($28,600).
Secretary of State: Ralph Munro (R.), 1989–93 ($31,000).

BUDGET. For the 2-year budget period 1987–89 the state's total revenue is (projected) $19,923·6m.; general expenditure is (projected) $20,412·4m. (education, $8,497·5m.; transport, $2,072·8m., and human resources, $5,771·6m.).

Total outstanding debt in 1987 was $3,073m.

Per capita personal income (1986) was $14,625.

ENERGY AND NATURAL RESOURCES

Electricity. With about 20% of potential water-power resources of US, the state has ample developed and potential hydro-electricity.

Minerals. Mining and quarrying are not as important as forestry, agriculture or manufacturing. Uranium is mined but figures are not disclosed; other minerals include sand and gravel, stone, coal and clays.

Agriculture. Agriculture is constantly growing in value because of more intensive and diversified farming and because of the 1m.-acre Columbia Basin Irrigation Project.

In 1987 there were 37,000 farms with an acreage of 15·8m.; average farm was of 427 acres. Average value per acre (1985), $923.

Cash return from farm marketing, 1985, was $2,797m. (from crops, $1,865m.; from livestock and dairy products, $932m.). Wheat, cattle and calves, milk and apples are important.

On 1 Jan. 1985 animals on farms included 211,000 milch cows, 1·47m. all cattle, 53,000 sheep and 45,000 swine.

Forestry. Forests cover about 23m. acres, of which 9m. acres are national forest. In 1985, timber harvested from 486,506 acres cut, was 5,874·2m. bd ft. Acres planted or seeded, 1986, 171,641, not including natural re-seeding. Production of wood residues, 1986, included 695,927 tons of pulp and board.

Fisheries. Salmon and halibut are important; total fish catch, 1985, 210·3m. lb.; value, $108m.

INDUSTRY. In 1986 manufacturing employed 304,200 workers, of whom 85,000 were in aerospace and 58,700 in the forest products industry.

Abundance of electric power has made Washington the leading producer of primary aluminium; employment, 1986, 7,600; exported aluminium, $199·1m. worth. Aircraft exported, $5,641·9m.

In 1986 trade employed 434,700, service industries, 393,000; government, 349,300.

COMMUNICATIONS

Roads. In 1990 there were 81,439 miles of roads (65,011 miles rural) and 4,090,130 registered motor vehicles.

Railways. The railways had, in 1980, 6,057 miles.

Aviation. There were in 1979, 365 airports, 120 publicly owned. In 1986 Seattle–Tacoma Airport traffic was 13·6m. passengers, 65,975 tons of mail and 157,027 tons of freight and express.

JUSTICE, RELIGION, EDUCATION AND WELFARE

Justice. The adult population in state prisons in Dec. 1985 was 6,909. Since 1963 there have been no executions; total 1930–63 (by hanging) was 47, including 40 whites, 5 Blacks and 2 other races, all for murder, except 1 white for kidnapping.

Religion. Chief religious bodies are the Roman Catholic, United Methodist, Lutheran, Presbyterian, Latter-day Saints and Episcopalian.

Education. Education is given free to all children between the ages of 5 and 21 years, and is compulsory for children from 8 to 15 years of age. In autumn 1986 there were 761,760 pupils in public elementary and secondary schools. In 1986 there were 36,200 classroom teachers, average salary, $26,100. The total expenditure on public elementary and secondary schools for the school year 1986 was $3,124m. or $708 per capita.

The University of Washington, founded 1861, at Seattle, had, autumn, 1986, 33,226 students, and Washington State University at Pullman, founded 1890, for science and agriculture, had 15,888 students. Twenty-seven community colleges had (1986) a total enrolment of 134,522 state-funded students.

Health. In 1981 the 2 state hospitals for mental illness had a daily average of 1,204 patients; schools for handicapped children, 1,999 residents in Sept. 1981.

In 1983 the state had 122 general hospitals (16,200 beds); in 1981, 3 licensed psychiatric hospitals (181 beds) and 3 alcoholism hospitals (174 beds).

Social Security. Old-age assistance is provided for persons 65 years of age or older without adequate resources (and not in need of continuing home care) who are residents of the state. In Dec. 1985, 12,100 people were drawing an average of $157 per month; aid to 189,000 children in 67,900 families averaged $419 per family monthly; to 35,000 totally disabled, $266 monthly.

Further Reading

State of Washington Data Book. Office of Financial Management, Olympia, 1987
Swanson, T., *Political Life in Washington.* Pullman, 1985
Yates, R. and C., *Washington State Yearbook 1988.* Evgene, Oregon, 1988

State Library: Washington State Library, Olympia. *State Librarian:* Nancy Zussy.

WEST VIRGINIA

HISTORY. In 1862, after the state of Virginia had seceded from the Union, the electors of the western portion ratified an ordinance providing for the formation of a new state, which was admitted into the Union by presidential proclamation on 20 June 1863, under the name of West Virginia. Its constitution was adopted by the voters almost unanimously on 26 March 1863.

AREA AND POPULATION. West Virginia is bounded north by Pennsylvania and Maryland, east and south by Virginia, south-west by the Sandy River (forming the boundary with Kentucky) and west by the Ohio River (forming the boundary with Ohio). Area, 24,282 sq. miles, of which 102 sq. miles are water. Census population, 1 April 1980, 1,949,644, an increase of 11·8% since 1970. Estimate (1986), 1,919,000. Births, 1987, 22,280 (11·6 per 1,000 population); deaths, 19,669 (8·7); infant deaths, 217 (9·7 per 1,000 live births); marriages, 13,200 (6·8); divorces, 9,043 (4·8).

Population in 5 federal census years was:

	White	*Black*	*Indian*	*Asiatic*	*Total*	*Per sq. mile*
1910	1,156,817	64,173	36	93	1,221,119	50·8
1940	1,614,191	114,893	18	103	1,729,205	71·8
1960	1,770,133	89,378	181	419	1,860,421	77·3
1970	1,673,480	67,342	751	1,463	1,744,237	71·8
1980	1,874,751	65,051	1,610	5,194	1,949,644	80·3

Of the total population in 1980, 945,408 were male, 705,319 were urban; those 20 years of age or older numbered 1,319,566.

The 1980 census (and 1985 estimate) population of the principal cities was: Huntington, 63,684 (61,086); Charleston, 63,968 (59,371). Others: Wheeling, 43,070 (42,082); Parkersburg, 39,967 (39,399); Morgantown, 27,605 (27,786); Weirton, 24,736 (23,878); Fairmont, 23,863 (22,822); Clarksburg, 22,371 (21,379).

CLIMATE. Charleston. Jan. 34°F (1·1°C), July 76°F (24·4°C). Annual rainfall 40" (1,010 mm). *See* Appalachian Mountains, p. 1382.

CONSTITUTION AND GOVERNMENT. The present constitution was adopted in 1872; it has had 62 amendments.

The Legislature consists of the Senate of 34 members elected for a term of 4 years, one-half being elected biennially, and the House of Delegates of 100 members, elected biennially. The Governor is elected for 4 years and may succeed himself once. Voters are all citizens (with the usual exceptions) 18 years of age and meeting certain residential requirements. The state sends to Congress 2 senators and 4 representatives.

In the 1988 presidential election Dukakis polled 339,112 votes, Bush, 307,824.

The state capital is Charleston. There are 55 counties.

Governor: Gaston Caperton (D.), 1989–92 ($72,000).
Secretary of State: Ken Hechler (D.), ($43,200).

FINANCE. General revenues for the year ending 30 June 1987 were $3,225m. ($1,531m. from taxes, $877m. from federal funds); general expenditures were $3,355m. (education, $1,348m.; highways, $598m.; public welfare, $749m.).

Debts outstanding were $969·5m. on 30 June 1987.

Estimated *per capita* personal income (1988) was $10,959.

ENERGY AND NATURAL RESOURCES

Minerals. 38% of the state is underlain with mineable coal; 130·8m. short tons of coal were produced in 1986. Petroleum output, 3m. bbls; natural gas production was 135,431m. cu. ft. Salt, sand and gravel, sandstone and limestone are also produced. The total value of mineral output in 1986 was $4,837m.

Agriculture. In 1988 the state had 20,500 farms with an area of 3·6m. acres; average size of farm was 176 acres and valued at $542 per acre. Livestock farming predominates.

Cash income, 1987, from crops was $57·5m.; from government payments, $10·6m., and from livestock and products, $168·9m. Main crops harvested, 1987: Hay (1m. tons); all corn (3·6m. bu.); tobacco (2·5m. lb.). Area of main crops, 1987: hay, 630,000 acres; corn, 85,000 acres. Apples (185m. lb. in 1987) and peaches (17m. lb.) are important fruit crops. Livestock on farms, 1 Jan. 1988, included 490,000 cattle, of which 31,000 were milch cows; sheep, 91,000; hogs, 37,000; chickens, 721,000 excluding broilers. Production, 1987, included 32·8m. broilers, 108m. eggs; 2·4m. turkeys.

Forestry. State forests, 1987, covered 79,365 acres; national forests, 1,673,000 gross acres; 75% of the state is woodland.

INDUSTRY. In 1987, 1,645 manufactories had 86,088 production workers who earned $2,163m. Leading manufactures are primary and fabricated metals, glass, chemicals, wood products, textiles and apparel, and machinery.

In 1987 non-agricultural employment was 597,800 of whom 139,046 were in trade, 121,130 in government and 106,540 in service industries.

The first commercial coal liquefaction plant in the USA is being built near Morgantown with the co-operation of the governments of Federal Republic of Germany and Japan and the Gulf Oil Co.

COMMUNICATIONS

Roads. In 1990 there were 34,477 miles of roads (31,425 miles rural) and 1,213,950 registered motor vehicles.

Railways. In 1987 the state had 2,895 miles of railway, all operated by diesel or electric trains.

Aviation. There were 27 licensed airports in 1987.

Post and Broadcasting. There are 64 AM radio stations, 70 FM radio stations. Television stations number 9 VHF and 5 UHF.

Newspapers. Daily newspapers number 25; weekly newspapers 62.

JUSTICE, RELIGION, EDUCATION AND WELFARE

Justice. The state court system consists of a Supreme Court and 31 circuit courts. The Supreme Court of Appeals, exercising original and appellate jurisdiction, has 5 members elected by the people for 12-year terms. Each circuit court has from 1 to 7 judges (as determined by the Legislature on the basis of population and case-load) chosen by the voters within each circuit for 8-year terms.

Effective on 1 July 1967, the West Virginia Human Rights Act prohibits discrimination in employment and places of public accommodations based on race, religion, colour, national origin or ancestry.

There are 5 penal and correctional institutions which had, on 30 June 1987, 1,558 inmates. In 1965 the state legislature abolished capital punishment.

Religion. Chief denominations in 1987 were United Methodist (159,000 members, estimate), Baptists (116,000) and Roman Catholics (109,000).

Education. Public school education is free for all from 5 to 21 years of age, and school attendance is compulsory for all between the ages of 7 and 16 (school term, 200 days—180–185 days of actual teaching). The public schools are non-sectarian. In autumn 1987 public elementary and secondary schools had 344,604 pupils and 22,702 classroom teachers. Average salary of teachers in 1987, $21,736. Total 1986 expenditures for public schools, $1,196m.

Leading institutions of higher education in 1987:

Founded		*Full-time students*
1837	Marshall University, Huntington	12,033
1837	West Liberty State College, West Liberty	2,450
1867	Fairmont State College, Fairmont	5,432
1868	West Virginia University, Morgantown	17,270
1872	Concord College, Athens	2,380
1872	Glenville State College, Glenville	2,096
1872	Shepherd College, Shepherdstown	3,920
1891	West Virginia State College	4,503
1895	West Virginia Institute of Technology, Montgomery	2,814
1895	Bluefield State College, Bluefield	2,559
1901	Potomac State College of West Virginia Univ., Keyser	1,040
1972	West Virginia College of Graduate Studies	2,662
1976	School of Osteopathic Medicine, Lewisburg	233

In addition to the universities and state-supported schools, there are 3 community colleges (8,625 students in 1987), 10 denominational and private institutions of higher education (8,981 students in 1987) and 11 business colleges.

Health. In 1987 the state had 77 hospitals and 53 licensed personal care homes, 32 skilled-nursing homes and 3 mental hospitals.

Social Security. The Department of Human Services, originating in the 1930s as the Department of Public Assistance, is both state and federally financed. In the year ending 30 June 1988 day care for 4,735 children per month was provided; aid was given to 26,464 families with dependent children (average award, $231.64 per month); handicapped children's services conducted 8,389 examinations; 93,376 families per month received food stamps.

On 1 Jan. 1974 all blind, aged and disabled services were converted to the Federal Supplemental Security Income programme.

Further Reading

West Virginia Blue Book. Legislature, Charleston. Annual, since 1916

West Virginia Statistical Handbook, 1974. Bureau of Business Research, W. Va. Univ., Morgantown, 1974

Bibliography of West Virginia. 2 parts. Dept. of Archives and History, Charleston, 1939
West Virginia History. Dept. of Archives and History. Charleston. Quarterly, from 1939
Conley, P. and Doherty, W. T., *West Virginia History*. Charleston, 1974
Davis, C. J. and others, *West Virginia State and Local Government*. West Virginia Univ. Bureau for Government Research, 1963
Rice, O. K., *West Virginia: A History*. Univ. Press of Kentucky, Lexington, 1985
Williams, J. A., *West Virginia: A Bicentennial History*. New York, 1976

State Library: Division of Archives and History, Dept. of Culture and History, Charleston.

WISCONSIN

HISTORY. Wisconsin was settled in 1670 by French traders and missionaries. Originally a part of New France, it was surrendered to the British in 1763 and in 1783, when ceded to the US, became part of the North-west Territory. It was then contained successively in the Territories of Indiana, Illinois and Michigan. In 1836 it became part of the Territory of Wisconsin, which also included the present states of Iowa, Minnesota and parts of the Dakotas. It was admitted into the Union with its present boundaries on 29 May 1848.

AREA AND POPULATION. Wisconsin is bounded north by Lake Superior and the Upper Peninsula of Michigan, east by Lake Michigan, south by Illinois, west by Iowa and Minnesota, with the Mississippi River forming most of the boundary. Area, 56,154 sq. miles, including 1,439 sq. miles of inland water, but excluding any part of the Great Lakes. Census population, 1 April 1980 4,705,642, an increase of 6·5% since 1970. Estimated population (1990), 4,895,542. Births in 1988 were 70,711 (14·6 per 1,000 population); deaths, 42,979 (8·8); infant deaths, 598 (8·4 per 1,000 live births); marriages, 41,455 (8·5); divorces and annulments, 17,127 (3·5).

Population in 5 census years was:

	White	*Black*	*All others*	*Total*	*Per sq. mile*
1910	2,320,555	2,900	10,405	2,333,860	42·2
1930	2,916,255	10,739	12,012	2,939,006	53·7
1960	3,858,903	74,546	18,328	3,951,777	72·2
1970	4,258,959	128,224	30,750	4,417,933	80·8
1980	4,443,035	182,592	80,015	4,705,642	86·4

Of the total population in 1980, 49% were male, 64·2% were urban and 67% were 20 years old or older.

Population of the larger cities, 1980 census, was as follows:

Milwaukee	636,297	Appleton	58,913	Beloit	35,207
Madison	170,616	Oshkosh	49,620	Fond du Lac	35,863
Racine	85,725	La Crosse	48,347	Manitowoc	32,547
Green Bay	87,889	Sheboygan	48,085	Wausau	32,426
Kenosha	77,685	Janesville	51,071	Superior	29,571
West Allis	63,982	Eau Claire	51,509	Brookfield	34,035
Wauwatosa	51,308	Waukesha	50,365		

Population of larger urbanized areas, 1980 census: Milwaukee, 1,207,008; Madison, 213,678; Duluth–Superior (Minn.–Wis.), 132,585; Racine, 118,987; Green Bay, 142,747.

CLIMATE. Milwaukee. Jan. 19°F (–7·2°C), July 70°F (21·1°C). Annual rainfall 29" (727 mm). *See* Great Lakes, p. 1382.

CONSTITUTION AND GOVERNMENT. The constitution, which dates from 1848, has 125 amendments. The legislative power is vested in a Senate of 33 members (1991 term: 19 Democrats, 14 Republicans) elected for 4 years, one-half elected alternately, and an Assembly of 99 members (1991 term: 58 Democrats, 41 Republicans) all elected simultaneously for 2 years. The Governor and Lieut.-Governor are elected for 4 years. All 6 constitutional officers serve 4-year terms.

Wisconsin has universal suffrage for all citizens 18 years of age or over; but, as there is no official list of voters, the size of the electorate is unknown; 2,191,612 voted for President in 1988.

Wisconsin is represented in Congress by 2 senators and 9 representatives.

In the 1988 presidential election Dukakis polled 1,126,794 votes, Bush, 1,047,499.

The capital is Madison. The state has 72 counties.

Governor: Tommy G. Thompson (R.), 1991–95 ($86,149).
Lieut.-Governor: Scott McCallum (R.), 1991–95 ($46,360).
Secretary of State: Douglas La Follette (D.), 1991–95 ($42,089).

BUDGET. For the year ending 30 June 1990 (Wisconsin Bureau of Financial Operations figures) total revenue for all funds was $14,902,360,000 ($6,223,160,000 from taxation and $2,419,419,000 from federal aid). General expenditure from all funds was $12,752,292,000 ($4,044,485,000 for education, $3,676,043,000 for human resources).

Per capita personal income (1988) was $15,524.

ENERGY AND NATURAL RESOURCES

Electricity. There were, Dec. 1989, 87 hydro-electric power plants (16 of them municipal, 56 private in Wisconsin; 15 private outside the state) operated by public utilities with a total installed capacity of 504,072 kw.; output, 1989, was 1,492,535mwh. The 15 outside plants are in Michigan; installed capacity 99,990 kw., output 345,762mwh.

Fossil fuel and nuclear plants numbered 22 (3 municipal; 1 fossil fuel plant in Michigan); the former had a total installed capacity of 7,291,990 kw.; total output, (1989), 31,240,234mwh; the 2 nuclear plants had an installed capacity of 1,540,682 kw. and a total output (1989) of 10,832,221mwh.

There were also 27 internal combustion reciprocating plants (17 of them municipal), with a total installed capacity of 103,561 kw. and a total output of (1989) 5,833mwh., and 16 (1 municipal) internal combustion turbine plants with a total installed capacity of 1,257,450 kw.; total output was (1989) 55,865mwh.

There was a total of 152 plants, with a total installed capacity of 10,697,755 kw. and a total output of (1989) 43,626,688mwh.

Minerals. Construction sand and gravel, crushed stone and lime are the chief mineral products. Mineral production in 1988 was valued at $205m. This value included $60·1m. for sand and gravel, $98·3m. for crushed stone and about $24m. for lime. Value of all other minerals including industrial sand, dimension stone, crushed trap rock, peat and gemstones, $22·5m. There are plans to develop a 2m. ton copper (with small amounts of gold) deposit near Ladysmith.

Agriculture. The total number of farms has declined in the last 50 years, but farms have become larger and more productive. On 1 Jan. 1990 there were 81,000 farms with a total acreage of 17·6m. acres and an average size of 217·3 acres, compared with 142,000 farms with a total acreage of 22·4m. acres and an average of 158 acres in 1959.

Cash receipts from products sold by Wisconsin farms in 1989, $5,481m.; $4,752m. from livestock and livestock products and $909m. from crops.

Wisconsin ranked first among the states in 1989 in the number of milch cows, milk and butter production, output of all cheeses and of American, Brick, Muenster, Italian and Blue Mold Cheese. Production of cheese accounted for 32·9% of the nation's total. The state also ranked first in bulk whole and skim condensed sweetened milk, lactose, whey protein concentrate and dry whey. The state ranked first in 1988 in mink pelts. In crops the state ranked first in 1989 for snap beans, green beans, sweet corn for processing, and corn for silage. Production of the principal field crops in 1989 included: Corn for grain, 310·8m. bu.; corn for silage, 9·9m. tons; oats, 46·9m. bu.; all hay, 8·1m. tons. Other crops of importance 23·5m. cwt of potatoes, 11·4m. lb. of tobacco, 1·4m. bbls of cranberries, 1·6m. cwt of carrots and the processing crops of 810,200 tons of sweet corn, 130,100 tons of green peas and 281,300 tons of snap beans.

Forestry. Wisconsin has an estimated 15·3m. acres of forest land (about 42% of land area). Of 14·7m. acres of commercial forest (June 1988) national forests covered 1·2m. acres; state forests, 0·6m.; county and municipal forests, 2·3m.; forest industry, 1·2m.; private land, 9·1m.

Growing stock (1985), 15,500m. cu. ft, of which 11,900m. cu. ft is hardwood and 3,600m. cu. ft, softwood. Main hardwoods, aspen, maple, oak and birch; main softwoods, red pine, white pine, balsam fir, jack pine.

INDUSTRY. Wisconsin has much heavy industry, particularly in the Milwaukee area. Three fifths of manufacturing employees work on durable goods. Industrial machinery is the major industrial group (19% of all manufacturing employment) followed by food processing, fabricated metals, paper and paper products, printing and publishing, electrical machinery and rubber and miscellaneous plastics. Primary and secondary wood-product industries are high in value of product (over $91,000m. in 1986). Manufacturing establishments in 1990 provided 25% of non-farm wage and salary workers, 33% of all earnings. The total number of establishments was 9,333 in 1988; the biggest concentration (40% of employment) is in the south-east.

TOURISM. The tourist-vacation industry ranks among the first three in economic importance. The decline of lumbering and mining in the northern section of the state has increased dependency on the recreation industry. The Division of Tourism of the Department of Development spent $9,006,300 to promote tourism in financial year 1989–90.

COMMUNICATIONS

Roads. The state had on 1 Jan. 1990, 109,448 miles of highway. 76% of all roads in the state have a bituminous (or similar) surface. There are 11,882 miles of state trunk roads and 19,540 miles of county trunk roads.

On 1 July 1990 Wisconsin registered 3,871,406 motor vehicles.

Railways. On 1 Aug. 1987 the state had 4,224 road-miles of railway.

Aviation. There were, in 1990, 95 publicly operated airports. Eleven scheduled air carrier airports were served by 20 regional and national air carriers.

Shipping. Lake Superior and Lake Michigan ports handled 36·2m. tons of freight in 1986; 80% of it at Superior, one of the world's biggest grain ports, and much of the rest at Milwaukee and Green Bay.

JUSTICE, RELIGION, EDUCATION AND WELFARE

Justice. The state's penal, reformatory and correctional system on 31 July 1990 held 6,458 men and 304 women in 11 state-owned and other institutions for adult offenders; the probation and parole system was supervising 21,971 men and 5,835 women. Wisconsin does not impose the death penalty.

Religion. Wisconsin church affiliation, as a percentage of the 1980 population, was estimated at 32·2% Catholic, 20·06% Lutheran, 3·74% Methodist, 10·41% other churches and 32·6% un-affiliated.

Education. All children between the ages of 6 and 18 are required to attend school full-time to the end of the school term in which they become 18 years of age. In 1989–90 the public school grades kindergarten–8 had 521,691 pupils and 32,369 (full-time equivalent) teachers; school grades 9–12 had 250,672 pupils and 16,960 teachers. Private schools enrolled 142,729 students grades kindergarten–12. Public elementary teachers' salaries, 1988–89, averaged $29,856; junior high, $31,880; middle school, $31,744; high, $32,257.

In 1988–89 vocational, technical and adult schools had an enrolment of 436,746 and 3,434 (full-time equivalent) teachers. There is a school for the visually handicapped and a school for the deaf.

The University of Wisconsin, established in 1848, was joined by law in 1971 with the Wisconsin State Universities System to become the University of Wisconsin System with 13 degree granting campuses, 13 two-year campuses in the Center System, and the University Extension. The system had, in 1989–90, 7,258 full-time professors and instructors and 2,086 teaching assistants. In autumn 1989, 159,579 students enrolled (10,773 at Eau Claire, 4,776 at Green Bay, 8,984 at La Crosse, 43,695 at Madison, 24,857 at Milwaukee, 10,881 at Oshkosh, 5,265 at Parkside, 5,433 at Platteville, 5,236 at River Falls, 8,878 at Stevens Point, 7,322 at Stout, 2,533 at Superior, 10,270 at Whitewater and 11,006 in the Center System freshman-sophomore centres). There are also several independent institutions of higher education. These (with 1989–90 enrolment) include 2 universities (13,222), 18 liberal arts colleges (25,358), 4 technical and professional schools (4,622), and 4 theological seminaries (446).

The total expenditure, 1987–88, for all public education (except capital outlay and debt service) was $5,465m.

The state maintains an educational broadcasting and television service.

Health. In Oct. 1989 the state had 137 general and allied special hospitals (20,592 beds), 18 mental hospitals (2,161 beds), 9 treatment centres for alcoholism (342 beds). Patients in state mental hospitals and institutions for the mentally retarded in Dec. 1988 averaged 2,257. On 31 Dec. 1989 the state had 471 licensed nursing homes; the 1989 average daily census was 47,968 residents.

Social Security. On 1 Jan. 1974 the US Social Security administration assumed responsibility for financial aid (Supplemental Security Income) to persons 65 years old and over, blind persons and totally disabled persons, who satisfy requirements as to need. Recipients receive a federal payment plus a federally administered state supplementary payment, except for those who reside in a medical institution. In Aug. 1989, there were 80,900 SSI recipients in the state; payments were $489 for a single individual, $540 for an eligible individual with an ineligible spouse, and $745 for an eligible couple. A special payment level of $589 for an individual and $1,098 for a couple may be paid with special approval for SSI recipients who are developmentally disabled or chronically mentally ill, living in a non-medical living arrangement not his or her own home. All SSI recipients receive state medical assistance coverage.

Under the Aid to Families with Dependent Children programme, 78,944 families of 237,155 persons received an average of $464.15 per family in Sept. 1990. Medicaid cost $1,266·4m. in financial year 1988–89.

Further Reading

Dictionary of Wisconsin Biography. Wis. Historical Society, Madison, 1960
Wisconsin Blue Book. Wis. Legislative Reference Bureau, Madison. Biennial
Current, R. N., *Wisconsin, a History.* New York, 1977
Danziger, S. and Witte, J. F., *State Policy Choices: The Wisconsin Experience.* Univ. Wisconsin Press, 1988
Martin, L., *The Physical Geography of Wisconsin.* Univ. Wisconsin Press, 3rd ed., 1965
Nesbit, R. C., *Wisconsin, A History.* State Historical Society of Wisconsin, Madison, rev. ed., 1989
Robinson, A. H. and Culver, J. B., (eds.) *The Atlas of Wisconsin.* Univ. Wisconsin Press, 1974
Vogeler, I., *Wisconsin: A Geography.* Boulder, 1986

State Historical Society of Wisconsin: *The History of Wisconsin.* Vol. I [Alice E. Smith], Madison, 1973.—Vol. II [R. N. Current], Madison, 1976.—Vol. III [R. C. Nesbit], Madison, 1985.—Vol. VI [W. F. Thompson], Madison, 1988.—Vol. V (P. W. Glad), Madison, 1990
State Information Agency: Legislative Reference Bureau, State Capitol, Madison, Wis. 53702. *Chief:* Dr H. Rupert Theobald.

WYOMING

HISTORY. Wyoming, first settled in 1834, was admitted into the Union on 10 July 1890 as the 44th state. The name originated with the Delaware Indians.

AREA AND POPULATION. Wyoming is bounded north by Montana, east by South Dakota and Nebraska, south by Colorado, south-west by Utah and west by Idaho. Area 97,914 sq. miles, of which 868 sq. miles are water. The Yellowstone National Park occupies about 2·22m. acres; the Grand Teton National Park has 307,000 acres. The federal government in 1986 owned 49,838 sq. miles (50·9% of the total area of the state). The Federal Bureau of Land Management administers 17,546,188 acres.

Census population, 1 April 1980, 469,557, an increase of 41·25% since 1970. Estimate (1990) 483,000. Births in 1988 were 7,163 (15·9 per 1,000 population); deaths, 3,245 (6·4); marriages, 4,726 (9·9); divorces, 3,316 (6·7); infant deaths in 1987, 69 (9·2 per 1,000 live births).

Population in 5 census years was:

	White	*Black*	*Indian*	*Asiatic*	*Total*	*Per sq. mile*
1910	140,318	2,235	1,486	1,926	145,965	1·5
1930	221,241	1,250	1,845	1,229	225,565	2·3
1960	322,922	2,183	4,020	805	330,066	3·4
			All others			
1970	323,619	2,568	6,229		332,416	3·4
1980	446,488	3,364	19,705		469,557	4·8

Of the total population in 1980, 240,560 were male, 295,898 were urban and those over 21 years of age numbered 295,908.

The largest towns are Cheyenne (capital), with census population in 1980 of 58,429 (1990 estimate, 51,000); Casper, 59,287 (47,000); Laramie, 24,410 (27,000); Rock Springs, 19,458 (20,000); Gillette (17,500); Sheridan (15,000); Green River (13,000).

CLIMATE. Cheyenne. Jan. 25°F (–3·9°C), July 66°F (18·9°C). Annual rainfall 15" (376 mm). Yellowstone Park. Jan. 18°F (–7·8°C), July 61°F (16·1°C). Annual rainfall 18" (444 mm). *See* Mountain States, p. 1381.

CONSTITUTION AND GOVERNMENT. The constitution, drafted in 1890, has since had 43 amendments. The Legislature consists of a Senate of 30 members elected for 4 years, 15, retiring every 2 years, and a House of Representatives of 64 members elected for 2 years. The Governor is elected for 4 years.

The state sends to Congress 2 senators and 1 representative, elected by the voters of the entire state. The suffrage extends to all citizens, male and female, who have the usual residential qualifications.

In the 1988 presidential election Bush polled 106,814 votes, Dukakis, 67,077.

The capital is Cheyenne. The state contains 23 counties.

Governor: Mike Sullivan (D.), 1991–95 ($70,000).

ECONOMY

Budget. In the fiscal year ending 1 July 1989 (State Treasurer's figures) cash receipts were $1,656,132,900; general expenditures were $1,494,778,300.

Per capita personal income (1987) was $12,709.

Banking and Finance. In Sept. 1989 there were 55 state banks with a total of $1,846,407 deposits.

ENERGY AND NATURAL RESOURCES

Electricity. In 1988 there were 11 hydro-electric stations with a gross nameplate installed capacity of 281·0 mw, and 8 thermo-electric stations with a total installed capacity of 5668·7 mw.

Minerals. Wyoming is largely an oil-producing state. In 1989 the output of petroleum was valued at $1386·6m.; natural gas, $719·6m. Other mining: Coal,

$1,170·7m.; trona, uranium, iron ore, feldspar, gypsum, limestone, phosphate, sand, gravel and marble, taconite, bentonite and hematite.

Agriculture. Wyoming is semi-arid, and agriculture is carried on by irrigation (1·4 m. acres in 1989) and by dry farming (920,000 acres in 1989). In 1988 there were 8,700 farms and ranches; total land area in 1989 was 34·8m. acres. In 1987 13,162 people were employed on farms.

Total value, 1988, of crops produced, $283m.; of livestock produced, $407·5m. Principal commodities are wheat, cattle and calves, lambs and sheep, sugar-beet, barley, hay and wool. Animals on farms in 1989 included 10,000 milch cows, 1·3m. all cattle, 837,000 sheep and lambs and in 1988 21,000 hogs and pigs. Total egg production in 1988 was 3·6m.

Forestry. In 1989 there were 35,379 acres of timberland.

Fisheries. In 1989 the net production of fish hatch was 599,458.

INDUSTRY. In 1987 there were 531 manufacturing establishments. There were 964 mining companies or producers. A large portion of the manufacturing in the state is based on natural resources, mainly oil and farm products. Leading industries are food, wood products (except furniture) and machinery (except electrical). The Wyoming Industrial Development Corporation assists in the development of small industries by providing credit.

LABOUR. In 1987 the mining industry employed an average of 19,945 workers; construction, 17,318; manufacturing, 9,451; transportation and public utilities, 16,289. The total civilian labour force for 1987 was 254,630; non-agricultural, 241,468. The average unemployment rate was 6·3% in 1988 and average weekly earnings were $611 for mining (production workers) in 1987. In 1988 there were no work stoppages.

Trade Unions. There were 22,669 working members in trade unions (10·1% of total employment).

TOURISM. There are over 7m. tourists annually, mainly outdoor enthusiasts. The state has the largest elk and pronghorn antelope herds in the world, 10 fish hatcheries and numerous wild game. Receipts from hunters and fishermen in 1986, $14,628,081. In 1988, 5·2m. people visited the 6 national areas; 1·7m. people visited state parks and historic sites. In 1987 559,032 fishing, game and bird licences were sold. There were (1990) 12 operational ski areas.

COMMUNICATIONS

Roads. The roads in 1986 comprised 5,240 miles of federal highways, 349 miles of state highways and 914 miles of inter-state highway. There were (1988) 288,998 passenger vehicles, 179,669 lorries, and 20,050 motor cycles.

Railways. The railways, 1986, had a length of 2,615 mainline miles and 550 branch miles.

Aviation. There were 11 towns with commuter air services and 2 towns on jet routes in 1987.

Telecommunications. In 1989 there were 30 AM, 31 FM radio stations and 9 television stations.

Newspapers. (1989) there were 9 daily newspapers.

JUSTICE, RELIGION, EDUCATION AND WELFARE

Justice. The state penitentiary in July 1988 held 736 inmates, the Womens' Center, 49. There are 2 other state correctional institutions. There have been 14 executions in Wyoming, 8 by hanging and 6 by lethal gas.

Religion. Chief religious bodies are the Roman Catholic (with 45,917 members in

1974), Mormon (28,954 in 1971) and Protestant churches (83,327 in 1974). There were 5,000 members of the Eastern Orthodox Church in 1972.

Education. In 1988–89 public elementary and secondary schools had 97,793 pupils and 5,841 teachers. Enrolment in the parochial elementary and secondary schools was about 3,500. The average total expenditure per pupil for 1987–88 was $4,766.

The University of Wyoming, founded at Laramie in 1887, had in academic year 1989–90 12,289 students. There are 2-year colleges at Casper, Riverton, Torrington, Cheyenne, Powell, Rock Springs and Sheridan with credit course enrolment of 15,685 students in 1987–88.

Social Welfare. In Jan. 1974 the federal government assumed many of the previous state programmes including old age assistance, aid to the blind and disabled. In 1987 financial year, $16·2m. was distributed in food stamps; $17·6m. in aid to families with dependent children; $626,314 in general assistance; $1,189,902 in emergency assistance; $41m. in Medicaid. Total state expenditure on public assistance and social services programmes, financial year 1987, $123·5m.

Health. In 1989 the state had 30 hospitals with 2,133 beds, 30 registered nursing homes and 20 boarding homes with 3,280 beds.

Further Reading

Official Directory. Secretary of State. Cheyenne. Biennial
1987 Wyoming Data Handbook. Dept. of Administration and Fiscal Control. Division of Research and Statistics, Cheyenne, 1987
Brown, R. H., *Wyoming: A Geography*. Boulder, 1980
Larsen, T. A., *History of Wyoming*. Rev. ed. Univ. of Nebraska, 1979
Treadway, T., *Wyoming*. New York, 1982

OUTLYING TERRITORIES

Non-Self-Governing Territories: Summaries of Information Transmitted to the Secretary-General of the United Nations. Annual

GUAM

HISTORY. Magellan is said to have discovered the island in 1521; it was ceded by Spain to the US by the Treaty of Paris (10 Dec. 1898). The island was captured by the Japanese on 10 Dec. 1941, and retaken by American forces from 21 July 1944. Guam is of great strategic importance; substantial numbers of naval and air force personnel occupy about one-third of the usable land.

AREA AND POPULATION. Guam is the largest and most southern island of the Marianas Archipelago, in 13° 26' N. lat., 144° 43' E. long. The length is 30 miles, the breadth from 4 to 10 miles, and there are about 209 sq. miles (541 sq. km). Agaña, the seat of government is about 8 miles from the anchorage in Apra Harbour. The census on 1 April 1980 showed a population of 105,979, an increase of 20,983 or 24·7% since 1970; those of Guamanian ancestry numbered about 50,794; foreign-born, 28,572; density was 507 per sq. mile. Estimated population (1987), 130,400 (including 23,860 transient residents connected with the military). The Malay strain is predominant. The native language is Chamorro; English is the official language and is taught in all schools.

CLIMATE. Tropical maritime, with little difference in temperatures over the year. Rainfall is copious at all seasons, but is greatest from July to Oct. Agaña. Jan. 81°F (27·2°C), July 81°F (27·2°C). Annual rainfall 93" (2,325 mm).

CONSTITUTION AND GOVERNMENT. Guam's constitutional status is that of an 'unincorporated territory' of the US. Entry of US citizens is unrestricted; foreign nationals are subject to normal regulations. In 1949–50 the President transferred the administration of the island from the Navy Department (who held it from 1899) to the Interior Department. The transfer conferred full citizenship on the Guamanians, who had previously been 'nationals' of the US. There was a referendum on status, 30 Jan. 1982. 38% of eligible voters voted; 48·5% of those favoured Commonwealth status.

The Governor and his staff constitute the executive arm of the government. The Legislature is unicameral; its powers are similar to those of an American state legislature. At the general election of Nov. 1982, the Democratic Party won 14 seats and the Republicans 7. All adults 18 years of age or over are enfranchised. Guam returns one non-voting delegate to the House of Representatives.

Governor: Joseph F. Ada (R.), 1987–91.
Lieut.-Governor: Frank F. Blas.

ECONOMY

Budget. Total revenue (1989) $378m.; expenditure $369m.

Banking. Recent changes in banking law make it possible for foreign banks to operate in Guam.

NATURAL RESOURCES

Water. Supplies are from springs, reservoirs and groundwater; 65% comes from water-bearing limestone in the north. The Navy and Air Force conserve water in reservoirs. The Water Resources Research Centre is at Guam University.

Agriculture. The major products of the island are sweet potatoes, cucumbers, water melons and beans. In 1982 there were 140 full-time and 1,904 part-time farmers. Livestock (1988) included 2,000 cattle, 14,000 pigs, and (1984) 36,430 poultry. Commercial productions (1983) amounted to 6·6m. lb. of fruit and vegetables ($3·4m.), 567,000 doz. eggs ($811,093). There is an agricultural experimental station at Inarajan.

Fisheries. Fresh fish caught in 1982, 319,300 lb. Offshore fishing produced 100,687 lb., including 6,080 lb. of shrimps.

INDUSTRY AND TRADE

Industry. Guam Economic Development Authority controls three industrial estates: Cabras Island (32 acres); Calvo estate at Tamuning (26 acres); Harmon estate (16 acres). Industries include textile manufacture, cement and petroleum distribution, warehousing, printing, plastics and ship-repair. Other main sources of income are construction and tourism.

Labour. In 1983 51% of employment was in government, 18% in trade, 5% in construction, 13% in services, 4% in manufacturing, 5% in transport and 4% in finance.

Trade. Guam is the only American territory which has complete 'free trade'; excise duties are levied only upon imports of tobacco, liquid fuel and liquor. In the year ending 31 Dec. 1980 imports were valued at $544·1m. and accounted for 90% of trade.

Tourism. Tourism is developing; there were 1,900 visitors in 1964 and 407,100 in 1986.

COMMUNICATIONS

Roads. There are 419 miles of all-weather roads.

Aviation. Seven commercial airlines serve Guam.

Post and Broadcasting. Overseas telephone and radio dispatch facilities are available. In 1983 there were 23,442 telephones.

There are 4 commercial stations, a commercial television station, a public broadcasting station and a cable television station with 24 channels.

Newspapers. There is 1 daily newspaper, a twice-weekly paper, and 4 weekly publications (all of which are of military or religious interest only).

JUSTICE, RELIGION, EDUCATION AND WELFARE

Justice. The Organic Act established a District Court with jurisdiction in matters arising under both federal and territorial law; the judge is appointed by the President subject to Senate approval. There is also a Supreme Court and a Superior Court; all judges are locally appointed except the Federal District judge. Misdemeanours are under the jurisdiction of the police court. The Spanish law was superseded in 1933 by 5 civil codes based upon California law.

Religion. About 98% of the Guamanians are Roman Catholics; others are Baptists, Episcopalians, Bahais, Lutherans, Mormons, Presbyterians, Jehovah's Witnesses and members of the Church of Christ and Seventh Day Adventists.

Education. Elementary education is compulsory. There are Chamorro Studies courses and bi-lingual teaching programmes to integrate the Chamorro language and culture into elementary and secondary school courses. There were, Dec. 1983, 24 elementary schools, 6 junior high schools, 5 senior high schools, one vocational-technical school for high school students and adults and 1 school for handicapped children. There were 17,725 elementary school pupils, 7,418 junior high and 5,776 senior high school pupils. Department of Education staff included 1,258 teachers. The Catholic schools system also operates 3 senior high schools, 3 junior high and 5 elementary schools. The Seventh Day Adventist Guam Mission Academy operates a school from grades 1 through 12, serving over 100 students. St John's Episcopal Preparatory School provides education for 530 students between kindergarten and the 9th grade. The University of Guam (an accredited institution) had 2,774 students, 1983–84.

Health. There is a hospital, 8 nutrition centres, a school health programme and an extensive immunization programme. Emphasis is on disease prevention, health education and nutrition.

Further Reading

Report (Annual) of the Governor of Guam to the US Department of Interior
Guam Annual Economic Review. Economic Research Center, Agaña

Carano, P. and Sanchez, P. C., *Complete History of Guam*. Rutland, Vt., 1964

REPUBLIC OF PALAU

HISTORY. Under the Treaty of Versailles (1919) Japan was appointed mandatory to the former German possessions north of the Equator. In 1946 the USA agreed to administer the former Japanese-mandated islands of the Caroline, Marshall and Mariana groups (except Guam) as a Trusteeship for the UN; the trusteeship agreement came into effect on 18 July 1947. The Trust Territory was administered by the US Navy until 1951, when all the islands except Tinian and Saipan in the Marianas were transferred to the Secretary of the Interior. In 1962 the Interior Department assumed responsibility for them also. In April 1976 the US government separated the administration of the Northern Marianas (*see* below) from that of the rest of the Trust Territory. The rest was 3 entities, each with its own constitution: the Marshall Islands, the Federated States of Micronesia (Yap, Kosrae, Truk and Pohnpei) and the Republic of Palau. The US Congress agreed compacts of free association with all except Palau (*see* below) in 1985–86.

Palau is now the only remaining Trust Territory. The Republic lies west of the

Federated States of Micronesia, and has a land area of 192 sq. miles, divided between 26 larger islands and more than 300 islets. The largest island is Babelthuap (143 sq. miles). Population (1980 census) 12,116; 1988 estimate, 14,106. The language is Palauan.

The capital is Koror. The Republic has a bicameral parliament with an 18-member Senate, and 16-member House of Delegates, both elected for 4 years as are the president and vice-president. The Constitution, adopted in July 1980, provided for ultimate free-association status, but it also defines Palau as a nuclear-free zone; this is in conflict with the US intention of basing nuclear weapons on the islands, as part of the defence responsibility included in the Free Association Compact. To cancel the anti-nuclear clause and accept the Compact requires a 75% vote at referendum. This has not been achieved by successive referenda, gaining only 60% of votes cast at the 7th and latest, and Palau remains in Trust.

There is subsistence agriculture, craft-work and some commercial fishing.

REPUBLIC OF THE MARSHALL ISLANDS

On 21 Oct. 1986 the USA entered into a Compact of Free Association with this former Trust Territory. The Republic is a sovereign state responsible for its foreign policy; the USA controls defence policy (for a minimum of 15 years) and provides financial support. The constitution of 1 May 1979 is still in force; it provides for an elected assembly and an elected president, both serving four-year terms. There is also an advisory council of chiefs. The Republic is a member of the South Pacific Forum.

Population (July 1988), 40,609. The Marshallese are predominantly Micronesian and Christian. There are two indigenous languages; Japanese is also used, but the official language is English. The capital is Majuro. Kwajalein is a US missile-testing range and airfield.

The total area is 181·3 sq. km (land area).

FEDERATED STATES OF MICRONESIA

On 3 Nov. 1986 this island group, a former Trust Territory, entered into a Compact of Free Association with the USA. The Federation is a sovereign state; the USA controls defence (for a minimum period of 15 years) and provides financial support. The Federation is responsible for its own foreign policy. The capital is Kolonia.

Land area, 702 sq. km. Population (1990 estimate), 108,600. The Federation has 4 states: Kosrae, Pohnpei, Truk and Yap. There are 607 islands. The people are Micronesian and Polynesian; the main languages are Kosrean, Yapese, Pohnpeian and Trukese; the official language is English.

The federal congress is elected for four years, as are the president and vice-president. Each state has an elected governor and a unicameral assembly.

THE NORTHERN MARIANAS

The islands form a chain, extending 560 km north from Guam; there are 16 islands, all mountainous, with a combined land area of 477 sq. km (184 sq. miles). The islands were formerly part of the US-administered Trust Territory of the Pacific Islands. On 17 June 1975 the voters of the Northern Mariana Islands, in a plebiscite observed by the UN, adopted the covenant to establish a Commonwealth of the Northern Mariana Islands in Union with the USA. In April 1976 the US government approved the convenant and separated the administration of the Northern Marianas from that of the rest of the Trust Territory.

The Northern Marianas form a Commonwealth with an elected governor and lieutenant-governor, both serving 4-year terms; the bicameral parliament has a 9-member Senate, elected for four years, and a 15-member House of Representatives (elected for two). The people are US citizens; they elect a non-voting delegate to the US House of Representatives. The USA is responsible for defence.

The population, 1980 census, 16,780 (1988 estimate, 20,591). Saipan is the seat of government. The official language is English, 55% (1980) speak Chamorro.

AMERICAN SAMOA

HISTORY. The Samoan Islands were first visited by Europeans in the 18th century; the first recorded visit was in 1722. On 14 July 1889 a treaty between the USA, Germany and Great Britain proclaimed the Samoan islands neutral territory, under a 4-power government consisting of the 3 treaty powers and the local native government. By the Tripartite Treaty of 7 Nov. 1899, ratified 19 Feb. 1900, Great Britain and Germany renounced in favour of the US all rights over the islands of the Samoan group east of 171° long. west of Greenwich, the islands to the west of that meridian being assigned to Germany (now the Independent State of Western Samoa, *see* p. 1593). The islands of Tutuila and Aunu'u were ceded to the US by their High Chiefs on 17 April 1900, and the islands of the Manu'a group on 16 July 1904. Congress accepted the islands under a Joint Resolution approved 20 Feb. 1929. Swain's Island, 210 miles north of the Samoan Islands, was annexed in 1925 and is administered as an integral part of American Samoa.

AREA AND POPULATION. The islands (Tutuila, Aunu'u, Ta'u, Olosega, Ofu and Rose) are approximately 650 miles east-north-east of Fiji. The total area of American Samoa is 76·1 sq. miles (197 sq. km); population, 1980, 32,297, nearly all Polynesians or part-Polynesians. The island's 3 Districts are Eastern (population, 1980, 17,311), Western (13,227) and Manu'a (1,732). There is also Swain's Island, with an area of 1·9 sq. miles and 29 inhabitants (1980), which lies 210 miles to the north west. Rose Island (uninhabited) is 0·4 sq. mile in area. In 1981 there were 1,158 births and 153 deaths.

CLIMATE. A tropical maritime climate with a small annual range of temperature and plentiful rainfall. Pago-Pago. Jan. 83°F (28·3°C), July 80°F (26·7°C). Annual rainfall 194" (4,850 mm).

CONSTITUTION AND GOVERNMENT. American Samoa is constitutionally an unorganized unincorporated territory of the US administered under the Department of the Interior. Its indigenous inhabitants are US nationals and are classified locally as citizens of American Samoa with certain privileges under local laws not granted to non-indigenous persons. Polynesian customs (not inconsistent with US laws) are respected.

Fagatogo is the seat of the Government.

The islands are organized in 15 counties grouped in 3 districts; these counties and districts correspond to the traditional political units. On 25 Feb. 1948 a bicameral legislature was established, at the request of the Samoans, to have advisory legislative functions. With the adoption of the Constitution of 22 April 1960, and the revised Constitution of 1967, the legislature was vested with limited law-making authority. The lower house, or House of Representatives, is composed of 20 members elected by universal adult suffrage and 1 non-voting member for Swain's Island. The upper house, or Senate, is comprised of 18 members elected, in the traditional Samoan manner, in meetings of the chiefs.

Governor: Peter TaliColeman.
Lieut.-Governor: Galeá I. Poumele.

ECONOMY

Planning. The first formal Economic Development and Planning Office completed its first year in 1971. Much has been done to promote economic expansion within the Territory and a large amount of outside investment interest has been stimulated.

The Office initiated the first Territorial Comprehensive Plan. This plan when completed will, with periodic updating, provide a guideline to territorial development for the next 20 years. The planning programme was made possible under a Housing and Urban Development '701' grant programme, and Economic Development Administration '302' planning programmes.

The focus will be on physical development and the problems of a rapidly increasing population with severely limited labour resources.

Budget. The chief sources of revenue are annual federal grants from the US, and local revenues from taxes, and duties, and receipts from commercial operations (enterprise and special revenue funds), utilities, rents and leases and liquor sales. During the financial year 1983–84 the Government had a revenue of $76·6m. including local appropriations of $9·5m., federal appropriations of $39·6m. and enterprise funds of $17·5m.

Banking. The American Samoa branch of the Bank of Hawaii and the American Samoa Bank offer all commercial banking services. The Development Bank of American Samoa, government owned, is concerned primarily through loans and guarantees with the economic advancement of the Territory.

ENERGY AND NATURAL RESOURCES

Electricity. Net power generated (financial year 1981) was 72·2m. kwh., of which 23·1m. kwh. was supplied to large power users and 20·2m. kwh. to householders. All the Manu'a islands have electricity.

Agriculture. Of the 48,640 acres of land area, 11,000 acres are suitable for tropical crops; most commercial farms are in the Tafuna plains and west Tutuila. Principal crops are taro, bread-fruit, yams, bananas and coconuts. Production (1988 in 1,000 tonnes): Taro, 4; bananas, 1; fruit, 1; coconuts, 5.

Livestock (1988): Pigs, 11,000; (1984) goats, 8,000; poultry, 45,000.

INDUSTRY AND TRADE

Industry. Fish canning is important, employing the second largest number of people (after government). Attempts are being made to provide a variety of light industries. Tuna fishing and local inshore fishing are both expanding.

Commerce. In 1982 American Samoa exported goods valued at $186,782,060 and imported goods valued at $119,416,918. Chief exports are canned tuna, watches, pet foods and handicrafts. Chief imports are building materials, fuel oil, food, jewellery, machines and parts, alcoholic beverages and cigarettes.

COMMUNICATIONS

Roads. There are (1983) about 76 miles of paved roads and 16 miles of unpaved within the Federal Aid highway system. There are 21 miles of other unpaved roads. Motor vehicles registered, 1983, 3,657.

Aviation. South Pacific Island Airways and Polynesian Airlines operate daily services between American Samoa and Western Samoa. South Pacific Island Airways also operates between Pago Pago and Honolulu, and between Pago Pago and Tonga. The islands are also served by Air Nauru which operates between Pago Pago, Tahiti and Auckland, and Air Pacific (Fiji and westward). South Pacific and Manu'a Air Transport run local services.

Shipping. The harbour at Pago Pago, which nearly bisects the island of Tutuila, is the only good harbour for large vessels in Samoa. By sea, there is a twice-monthly service between Fiji, New Zealand and Australia and regular service between US, South Pacific ports, Honolulu and Japan.

Post and Broadcasting. A commercial radiogram service is available to all parts of the world through 2 principal trunks, United States and Western Samoa. Commercial phone and telex services are operated to all parts of the world on a 24-hour service. Number of telephones (Sept. 1983), 6,029; telex subscribers, 78.

JUSTICE, EDUCATION AND WELFARE

Justice. Judicial power is vested firstly in a High Court. The trial division has original jurisdiction of all criminal and civil cases. The probate division has jurisdiction of estates, guardianships, trusts and other matters. The land and title division decides cases relating to disputes involving communal land and Matai title court rules on questions and controversy over family titles. The appellate division hears appeals from trial, land and title and probate divisions as well as having original jurisdiction in selected matters. The appellate court is the court of last resort. Two American judges sit with 5 Samoan judges permanently. In addition there are temporary judges or assessors who sit occasionally on cases involving Samoan customs. There is also a District Court with limited jurisdiction and there are 69 village courts.

Education. Education is compulsory between the ages of 6 and 18. The Government (1983) maintains 24 consolidated elementary schools, 5 senior high schools with technical departments, 1 community college, special education classes for the handicapped and 92 Early Childhood Education Centres for pre-school children. Total elementary and secondary enrolment (1983), 8,300; in ECE schools, 1,611; classes for the handicapped, 68; total elementary and secondary classroom teachers, 480. Ten private schools had 2,108 students. Learning is by a variety of media including television.

Health. The Department of Health provides the only curative and preventive medical and dental care in American Samoa. It operates a general hospital (173 beds including 49 bassinets), 3 dispensaries on Tutuila, 4 dispensaries in the Manu'a group, 1 on Aunu'u and 1 on Swain's Island. A $3·5m. tropical medical centre was completed and placed in service in 1968. This now embraces the general hospital as well as preventive health services and out-patient clinics for surgery, obstetrics, gynaecology, emergencies, family practice, internal medicine, paediatrics; there are clinics for treatment of the eye, ear, nose and throat, dental and public health departments.

In 1983 there were 27 doctors, 7 dentists, 2 optometrists, 3 nurse anaesthetists, and 3 physician assistants. Total number of health service employees, 397.

OTHER PACIFIC TERRITORIES

Johnston Atoll. Two small islands 1,150 km south-west of Hawaii, administered by the US Air Force. Area, under 1 sq. mile; population (1980 census) 327, with Sand Island.

Midway Islands. Two small islands at the western end of the Hawaiian chain, administered by the US Navy. Area, 2 sq. miles; population (1980 census) 453.

Wake Island. Three small islands 3,700 km west of Hawaii, administered by the US Air Force. Area, 3 sq. miles; population (1980 census) 302.

COMMONWEALTH OF PUERTO RICO

HISTORY. Puerto Rico, by the treaty of 10 Dec. 1898 (ratified 11 April 1899), was ceded by Spain to the US. The name was changed from Porto Rico to Puerto Rico by an Act of Congress approved 17 May 1932. Its territorial constitution was determined by the 'Organic Act' of Congress (2 March 1917) known as the 'Jones Act', which ruled until 25 July 1952, when the present constitution of the Commonwealth of Puerto Rico was proclaimed.

AREA AND POPULATION. Puerto Rico is the most easterly of the Greater Antilles and lies between the Dominican Republic and the US Virgin Islands. The island has a land area of 3,459 sq. miles and a population, according to the census of 1980, of 3,196,520, an increase of 484,487 or 17·9% over 1970. Of the population in 1970 about 529,000 were bilingual, Spanish being the mother tongue and (with English) one of the two official languages. Urban population (1980) 2,134,365 (66·8%).

Vital statistics (1987): Births, 64,393 (19·5 per 1,000 population); deaths, 23,954 (7·3); deaths under 1 year, 916 (14·2 per 1,000 live births).

Chief towns, 1980 (and 1986 estimate) are: San Juan, 434,849 (431,227); Bayamón, 196,207 (211,616); Ponce, 189,046 (190,679); Carolina, 165,954 (162,888); Caguas, 117,959 (126,298); Mayaguez, 96,193 (98,861); Arecibo, 86,766 (90,960).

The Puerto Rican island of Vieques, 10 miles to the east, has an area of 51·7 sq. miles and 7,662 (8,084) inhabitants. The island of Culebra, with 1,265 (1,272) inhabitants, between Puerto Rico and St Thomas, has a good harbour.

CONSTITUTION AND GOVERNMENT. Puerto Rico has representative government, the franchise being restricted to citizens 18 years of age or over, residence (1 year) and such additional qualifications as may be prescribed by the Legislature of Puerto Rico, but no property qualification may be imposed. Women were enfranchised in 1932 (with a literacy test) and fully in 1936. Puerto Ricans do not vote in the US presidential elections, though individuals living on the mainland are free to do so subject to the local electoral laws. The executive power resides in a Governor, elected directly by the people every 4 years. Fourteen heads of departments form the Governor's advisory council, also designated as his Council of Secretaries. The legislative functions are vested in a Senate, composed of 27 members (2 from each of the 8 senatorial districts and 11 senators at large), and the House of Representatives, composed of 51 members (1 from each of the 40 representative districts and 11 elected at large). Puerto Rico sends to Congress a Resident Commissioner to the US, elected by the people for a term of 4 years, but he has no vote in Congress. Puerto Rican men are subject to conscription in US services.

On 27 Nov. 1953 President Eisenhower sent a message to the General Assembly of the UN stating 'if at any time the Legislative Assembly of Puerto Rico adopts a resolution in favour of more complete or even absolute independence' he 'will immediately thereafter recommend to Congress that such independence be granted'.

For an account of the constitutional developments prior to 1952, *see* THE STATESMAN'S YEAR-BOOK, 1952, p. 742. The new constitution was drafted by a Puerto Rican Constituent Assembly and approved by the electorate at a referendum on 3 March 1952. It was then submitted to Congress, which struck out Section 20 of Article 11 covering the 'right to work' and the 'right to an adequate standard of living'; the remainder was passed and proclaimed by the Governor on 25 July 1952.

At the election on 4 Nov. 1984 the Popular Democratic Party, headed by Rafael Hernández Colon, polled 822,783 votes (47·8% of the total); the New Progressive Party, headed by Carlos Romero Barceló, polled 768,742 votes (44·6% of the total); the Independence Party (full independence by constitutional means), 61,316 (3·6% of the total); Renewal Puerto Rican Party, 69,865 votes (3·6% of the total).

Governor: Rafael Hernández Colon (Popular Democratic Party).

ECONOMY

Budget. Central Government budget, year ending 30 June 1988: Balance at 1 July 1988, $31,441,000; receipts, $5,297,512,000; disbursements, $5,266,071,000.

Assessed value of property, 30 June 1989, was $6,670·2m., and bonded indebtedness, $3,497m.

The US administers and finances the postal service and maintains air and naval bases. US payments in Puerto Rico, including direct expenditures (mainly military), grants-in-aid and other payments to individuals and to business totalled: 1985–86, $3,961·8m.; 1986–87, $3,767·4m.; 1987-88, $3,976·1m.; 1988-89, £4,099·2m.

Banking. Banks on 30 June 1990 had total deposits of $23,505m. Bank loans were $12,645m. This includes 18 commercial banks, 2 government banks and 4 trust companies.

NATURAL RESOURCES

Minerals. There is stone, and some production of cement (1m. tons in 1989–90).

Agriculture. Farming is mainly of sugar-cane. Production of raw sugar, 96 degrees basis, 1990 crop year, was 68,086 tons.

Livestock (1989): Cattle, 585,501; pigs, 198,938; poultry, 10,352,936.

COMMERCE. In 1989–90 imports amounted to $15,721·6m., of which $10,801·2m. came from US; exports were valued at $19,305·4m., of which $16,780·5m. went to US.

In financial year 1990 the US took: Sugar, 11,567 short tons; cigarettes, cigars and cheroots, 987,410,870 units; other tobacco and products, 812,906 lb.; rum, 19,918,106 proof gallons.

Puerto Rico is not permitted to levy taxes on imports.

Total trade between Puerto Rico and UK (British Department of Trade returns, in £1,000 sterling):

	1986	*1987*	*1988*	*1989*	*1990*
Imports to UK	81,131	76,347	91,909	117,628	123,087
Exports and re-exports from UK	49,620	39,405	38,877	79,851	69,593

COMMUNICATIONS

Roads. The Department of Public Works had under maintenance at 31 Dec. 1988, 8,130 km of paved road. Motor vehicles registered 30 June 1989, 1,567,319.

Shipping. In financial year 1989–90, 10,118 American and foreign vessels of 76,257,363 gross tons entered and cleared Puerto Rico.

Telecommunications. In Jan. 1990 there were 104 broadcasting stations and 20 television companies. There were (1989) 945,051 telephones.

Newspapers. In 1990 there were 4 main newspapers, *El Nuevo Día* had a daily circulation of about 211,102 (Sept. 1990); *El Vocero,* 262,000 (Oct. 1990); *San Juan Star,* 47,000 (Oct. 1990); *El Mundo,* 85,000 (Oct. 1990).

JUSTICE AND EDUCATION

Justice. The Commonwealth Judiciary system is headed by a Supreme Court of 7 members, appointed by the Governor, and consists of a Superior Tribunal with 11 sections and 92 superior judges, a District Tribunal with 38 sections and 99 district judges, and 60 municipal judges all appointed by the Governor.

Education. Education was made compulsory in 1899, but in 1981, 3·6% of the children still had no access to schooling. The percentage of illiteracy in 1980 was 10·3% of those 10 years of age or older. Total enrolment in public day schools, 1989, was 661,576 (first school month). All private schools had a total enrolment of 129,220 pupils for 1988. All instruction below senior high school standard is given in Spanish only.

The University of Puerto Rico, in Río Piedras, 7 miles from San Juan, had 56,993 students in 1988–89 of which 4,243 were in 3 Regional Colleges and 52,750 in other colleges. Higher education is also available in the Inter-American University of Puerto Rico (38,379 students in 1988–89), the Catholic University of Puerto Rico (11,551), the Sacred Heart College (7,380) and the Fundacion Ana G. Méndez (17,854). These and other private colleges and universities had 24,746 students.

Further Reading

Statistical Information: The area of Economic Research and Social Analysis of the Puerto Rico Planning Board publishes: *(a)* annual *Economic Report to the Governor; (b) External Trade Statistics* (annual report); *(c) Reports on national income and balance of payments; (d) Socio-Economic Statistics* (since 1940); *(e) Puerto Rico Monthly Economic Indicators.* In addition there are annual reports by various Departments.
Annual Reports. Governor of Puerto Rico. Washington
Bloomfield, R. J., *Puerto Rico: The Search for a National Policy.* Boulder, 1985
Carr, R., *Puerto Rico: A Colonial Experiment.* New York Univ. Press, 1984

Cevallos, E., *Puerto Rico*. [Bibliography], Oxford and Santa Barbara, 1985
Crampsey, R. A., *Puerto Rico*. Newton Abbot, 1973
Dietz, J. L., *Economic History of Puerto Rico: Institutional Change and Capital Development*. Princeton Univ. Press, 1987
Falk, P. S., (ed.) *The Political Status of Puerto Rico*. Lexington, Mass., 1986

Commonwealth Library: Univ. of Puerto Rico Library, Rio Piedras. *Librarian:* José Lázaro.

VIRGIN ISLANDS OF THE UNITED STATES

HISTORY. The Virgin Islands of the United States, formerly known as the Danish West Indies, were named and claimed for Spain by Columbus in 1493. They were later settled by Dutch and English planters, invaded by France in the mid-17th century and abandoned by the French *c.* 1700, by which time Danish influence had been established. St Croix was held by the Knights of Malta between two periods of French rule.

They were purchased by the United States from Denmark for $25m. in a treaty ratified by both nations and proclaimed 31 March 1917. Their value was wholly strategic, inasmuch as they commanded the Anegada Passage from the Atlantic Ocean to the Caribbean Sea and the approach to the Panama Canal. Although the inhabitants were made US citizens in 1927, the islands are, constitutionally, an 'unincorporated territory'.

AREA AND POPULATION. The Virgin Islands group, lying about 40 miles due east of Puerto Rico, comprises the islands of St Thomas (28 sq. miles), St Croix (84 sq. miles), St John (20 sq. miles) and about 50 small islets or cays, mostly uninhabited. The total area of the 3 principal islands is 136 sq. miles, of which the US Government owns 9,599 acres as National Park.

The population, according to the census of 1 April 1985, was 110,800, an increase of 15,209 or 16% since 1980. Estimate (1987) 106,000. Population (1987) of St Croix, 52,740; St Thomas, 52,400; St John, 2,860. About 20–25% (1980) are native-born, 35–40% from other Caribbean islands, 10% from mainland USA and 5% from Europe. St Croix has over 40% of Puerto Rican origin or extraction, Spanish speaking. In 1987, live births were 2,375 and deaths, 558.

The capital and only city, Charlotte Amalie, on St Thomas, had a population (1985) of 52,660; there are two towns on St Croix. Christiansted with (1980) 2,856 and Frederiksted with 1,054.

CLIMATE. Average temperatures vary from 77°F to 82°F throughout the year; humidity is low. Average annual rainfall, about 45 inches. The islands lie in the hurricane belt; tropical storms with heavy rainfall can occur in late summer, but hurricanes rarely.

CONSTITUTION AND GOVERNMENT. The Organic Act of 22 July 1954 gives the US Department of the Interior full jurisdiction; some limited legislative powers are given to a single-chambered legislature, composed of 15 senators elected for 2 years representing the two legislative districts of St Croix and St Thomas-St John.

The Governor is elected by the residents. Since 1954 there have been four attempts to redraft the Constitution, to provide for greater autonomy. Each has been rejected by the electorate. The latest was defeated in a referendum in Nov. 1981, 50% of the electorate participating.

For administration, there are 15 executive departments, 14 of which are under commissioners and the other, the Department of Justice, under an Attorney-General. The US Department of the Interior appoints a Federal Comptroller of government revenue and expenditure.

The franchise is vested in residents who are citizens of the United States, 18 years of age or over. In 1986 there were 34,183 voters, of whom 26,377 participated in the local elections that year.

They do not participate in the US presidential election but they have a non-voting representative in Congress.

The capital is Charlotte Amalie, on St Thomas Island.

Governor: Alexander A. Farrelly ($62,400).
Lieut.-Governor: Derek M. Hodge ($57,000).
Administrator St Croix: Richard Roebuck, Jr.
Administrator St John: William Lomax.
Administrator St Thomas: Harold Robinson.

ECONOMY

Budget. Under the 1954 Organic Act finances are provided partly from local revenues—customs, federal income tax, real and personal property tax, trade tax, excise tax, pilotage fees, etc.—and partly from Federal Matching Funds, being the excise taxes collected by the federal government on such Virgin Islands products transported to the mainland as are liable.

Budget for financial year 1988, $303,575,186.

Currency and Banking. United States currency became legal tender on 1 July 1934. Banks are the Chase Manhattan Bank; the Bank of Nova Scotia; the First Federal Savings and Loan Association of Puerto Rico; Barclays Bank International; Citibank; First Pennsylvania Bank; Banco Popular de Puerto Rico, and the First Virgin Islands Federal Savings Bank.

ENERGY AND NATURAL RESOURCES

Electricity. The Virgin Islands Water and Power Authority provides electric power from generating plants on St Croix and St Thomas; St John is served by power cable and emergency generator.

Water. There are 6 de-salinization plants with maximum daily capacity of 8·7m. gallons of fresh water. Rain-water remains the most reliable source. Every building must have a cistern to provide rain-water for drinking, even in areas served by mains (10 gallons capacity per sq. ft of roof for a single-storey house).

Agriculture. Land for fruit, vegetables and animal feed is available on St Croix, and there are tax incentives for development. Sugar has been terminated as a commercial crop and over 4,000 acres of prime land could be utilized for food crops.

Livestock (1988): Cattle, 11,000; goats, 4,000; pigs, 3,000; sheep, 3,000, poultry (1986), 18,345.

Fisheries. There is a fishermen's co-operative with a market at Christiansted. There is a shellfish-farming project at Rust-op-Twist, St Croix.

INDUSTRY AND TRADE

Industry. The main occupations on St Thomas are tourism and government service; on St Croix manufacturing is more important. Manufactures include rum (the most valuable product), watches, pharmaceuticals and fragrances. Industries in order of revenue: Tourism, refining oil, watch assembly, rum distilling, construction.

Labour. In 1989 the total labour force was 43,340, of whom 13,200 were employed in government, 8,450 in retail trades, 4,430 in hotels and other lodgings, 3,550 self-employed and unpaid family workers, 2,570 in transportation and public utilities, 2,350 in manufacturing, 2,330 in construction, 1,940 in finance, insurance and real estate, 1,070 in wholesale trades, 1,050 in business services, 350 in legal services, 230 in personnel services and 150 in agriculture.

Commerce. Exports, calendar year 1987, totalled $2,057·7m. and imports $3,370·4m. The main import is crude petroleum, while the principal exports are petroleum products.

Total trade between the US Virgin Islands and UK (financial years, British Department of Trade returns, in £1,000 sterling):

	1987	*1988*	*1989*	*1990*
Imports to UK	2,674	75	150	317
Exports and re-exports from UK	6,503	5,281	4,664	26,725

Tourism. Tourism is the most important business. There were about 1·52m. visitors in 1986 spending $509·8m.; 728,700 came by air and 827,151 on cruise ships, mainly to St Thomas which has a good, natural deepwater harbour.

COMMUNICATIONS

Roads. The Virgin Islands have (1986) 660 miles of roads, and 48,800 motor vehicles registered.

Aviation. There is a daily cargo and passenger service between St Thomas and St Croix. Alexander Hamilton Airport on St Croix can take all aircraft except Concorde. Cyril E. King Airport on St Thomas takes 727-class aircraft. There are air connexions to mainland USA, other Caribbean islands, Latin America and Europe.

Shipping. The whole territory has free port status. There is an hourly boat service between St Thomas and St John.

Post and Broadcasting. All three Virgin Islands have a dial telephone system. In Dec. 1986 there were 39,232 telephones. Direct dialling to Puerto Rico and the mainland, and internationally, is now possible. Worldwide radio telegraph service is also available.

The islands are served by 10 radio stations and 4 television stations. In 1988 there were an estimated 103,500 radio receivers and 64,400 television receivers in use.

Newspapers. In 1989 there were 2 daily and 1 fortnightly papers and 1 magazine.

RELIGION AND EDUCATION

Religion. There are churches of the Protestant, Roman Catholic and Jewish faiths in St Thomas and St Croix and Protestant and Roman Catholic churches in St John.

Education. In 1988 there were 13,359 pupils and 873 teachers in elementary schools, and 10,661 pupils and 723 teachers in secondary schools; 33 non-public schools had 5,079 pupils. In autumn 1988 the University of the Virgin Islands had 2,196 full-time students, 4,654 part-time students and 575 graduate students. The College is part of the United States land-grant network of higher education.

Further Reading

Boyer, W. W., *America's Virgin Islands*. Durham, N.C., 1983

Dookhan, I., *A History of the Virgin Islands of the United States*. Caribbean Univ. Press, 1974

Lewis, G. K., *The Virgin Islands: A Caribbean Lilliput*. Northwestern University Press, Evanston, 1972

URUGUAY

Capital: Montevideo
Population: 3·11m. (1989)
GNP per capita: US$2,470 (1988)

República Oriental del Uruguay

HISTORY. The Republic of Uruguay, formerly a part of the Spanish Viceroyalty of Río de la Plata and subsequently a province of Brazil, declared its independence 25 Aug. 1825 which was recognized by the treaty between Argentina and Brazil signed at Rio de Janeiro 27 Aug. 1828. The first constitution was adopted 18 July 1830.

AREA AND POPULATION. Uruguay is bounded on the north-east by Brazil, on the south-east by the Atlantic, on the south by the Río de la Plata and on the west by Argentina. The area is 176,215 sq. km (68,037 sq. miles). The following table shows the area and the population of the 19 departments at census 1985:

Departments	*Sq. km*	*Census 1985*	*Capital*	*Census 1985*
Artigas	11,928	68,400	Artigas	34,551
Canelones	4,536	359,700	Canelones	17,316
Cerro-Largo	13,648	78,000	Melo	42,329
Colonia	6,106	112,100	Colonia	19,077
Durazno	11,643	54,700	Durazno	27,602
Flores	5,144	24,400	Trinidad	18,271
Florida	10,417	65,400	Florida	28,560
Lavalleja	10,016	61,700	Minas	34,634
Maldonado	4,793	93,000	Maldonado	33,498
Montevideo	530	1,309,100	Montevideo	1,247,920
Paysandú	13,922	104,500	Paysandú	75,081
Río Negro	9,282	47,500	Fray Bentos	20,431
Rivera	9,370	88,400	Rivera	56,335
Rocha	10,551	68,500	Rocha	23,910
Salto	14,163	107,300	Salto	80,787
San José	4,992	91,900	San José	31,732
Soriano	9,008	77,500	Mercedes	37,110
Tacuarembó	15,438	82,600	Tacuarembó	40,470
Treinta y Tres	9,529	45,500	Treinta y Tres	30,956

Total population, census (1985) 2,940,200 and estimate 1989 was 3,105,000. In 1985 Montevideo (the capital) had a census population of 1,246,500; Las Piedras, 58,221.

CLIMATE. A warm temperate climate, wlth mild winters and warm summers. The wettest months are March to June, but there is really no dry season. Montevideo. Jan. 72°F (22·2°C), July 50°F (10°C). Annual rainfall 38" (950 mm).

CONSTITUTION AND GOVERNMENT. There is a Senate of 31 members and a Chamber of Representatives of 99 members.

A National Constituent Assembly was installed on 1 July 1985 to consider reforms to the Constitution. On 26 Nov. 1989 the first free presidential and congressional elections for 18 years took place. Luis Ernesto Lacalle Herrara was elected President with 38% of votes cast, and the *Blanco* Party formed a minority government.

President: Luis Ernesto Lacalle Herrara (sworn in on 1 March 1990).

National flag: Nine horizontal stripes of white and blue, a white canton with the 'Sun of May' in gold.

National anthem: Orientales, la patria o la tumba ('Easterners, the fatherland or the tomb'; words by Francisco Acuña de Figueroa; music by Francisco José Deballi).

DEFENCE

Army. The Army consists of volunteers who enlist for 1-2 years service. There are 1 infantry and 1 engineer brigades, 15 infantry, 10 cavalry, 6 artillery and 6 engineer battalions. Equipment includes 17 M-24, 28 M-3A1 and 22 M-41 light tanks. Strength (1991) 17,200.

Navy. The navy has commenced replacing its major 1940-vintage ex-US ships with French frigates of the Commandant Rivière class as these are retired from the French navy. 2 has so far been transferred, and 1 more will be provided in 1991. The fleet presently consists of 2 frigates, 1 ex-French Rivière (built 1962–3) and 1 ex-US Dealey class (1954), 2 offshore patrol vessels, 3 fast inshore patrol craft (French-built, 1981), 2 other inshore patrol vessels and 1 coastal minesweeper. Auxiliaries comprise 1 freighting tanker, a sail training ship, a salvage ship and 2 service vessels. There are 5 small landing craft.

A naval aviation service 400 strong operates 6 S-2 Tracker anti-submarine aircraft, 1 maritime reconnaissance, 11 training aircraft and 4 general purpose helicopters. Personnel in 1990 totalled 4,500 including 500 naval infantry.

A separate coastguard, 1,900 strong, operates 3 inshore patrol craft.

Air Force. Organized with US aid, the Air Force had (1991) about 3,500 personnel and 21 combat aircraft, including 1 counter-insurgency squadron with 6 IA 58 Pucara, 4 AT-33 armed jet trainers and 8 A-37B light strike aircraft, a reconnaissance and training squadron with 10 T-6Gs, 3 transport squadrons with 2 turboprop F.27 Friendships, 5 Brazilian-built EMB-110 Bandeirantes (1 equipped for photographic duties), 5 CASA C-212 Aviocars and 6 Queen Airs, a search and rescue squadron with Cessna U-17A aircraft and Bell helicopters, and a number of Cessna 182 light aircraft for liaison duties. Basic training types are the T-41 and T-34.

INTERNATIONAL RELATIONS

Membership. Uruguay is a member of the UN, OAS and LAIA.

ECONOMY

Budget. The receipts and expenditure of the national accounts as approved by the National Council of Government (URN$1m.):

	1986	*1987*	*1988*
Revenue	150,000	270,939	456,675
Expenditure	161,000	292,988	510,651

External public debt US$5,888m. in Dec. 1987.

Currency. The unit of currency is the *Uruguayan nuevo peso* (UYP) of 100 *centésimos*. There are notes, of N$ 50, 100, 500, 1,000 and 5,000, and coins of N$ 1, 2, 5 and 10. In March 1991, US$1 = 1,722·40 *pesos*; £1 = 3,267·40 *pesos*.

Banking and Finance. The Bank of the Republic (founded 1896), whose president and directors are appointed by the Government, has a paid-up capital of N$1,852m. The Central Bank was inaugurated on 16 May 1967. In 1991 there were 21 banks, 3 state-supported and 18 foreign-owned.

The State Insurance Bank has a monopoly of new insurance business.

Weights and Measures. The metric system is in use.

ENERGY AND NATURAL RESOURCES

Electricity. Power output in 1986 was 3,730m kwh.

Oil. Petroleum production (1981) 185,000 tonnes.

Agriculture. Uruguay is primarily a pastoral country. Of the total land area of 46m.

acres some 41m. are devoted to farming, of which 90% to livestock and 10% to crops. Some large *estancias* have been divided up into family farms; the average farm is about 250 acres.

There were (1989) 10,548,000 cattle, 25,560,000m. sheep, 470,000 horses, 215,000 pigs, 14,000 goats and 9m. poultry.

1·83m. tonnes of beef and veal were produced in 1989, and 1·02m. tonnes of cow's milk; the wool clip in 1989 was 87,000 tonnes.

Agricultural products are raised chiefly in the departments of Paysandú, Río Negro, Colonia, San José, Soriano and Florida. The principal crops and their estimated yield (in tonnes) in 2 crop years were as follows:

	1988	*1989*		*1988*	*1989*
Wheat	414,000	473,000	Barley	204,000	195,000
Sugar beet	256,000	142,000	Maize	118,000	60,000
Oats	64,000	68,000	Rice	381,000	537,000

Uruguay is self-sufficient in rice, with a surplus for export.

Wine is produced chiefly in the departments of Montevideo, Canelones and Colonia, about enough for domestic consumption (74,000 tonnes in 1989). The country has some 6m. fruit trees, principally peaches, oranges, tangerines and pears.

Forestry. In 1986 roundwood removals were 2,663,000 cu. metres.

Fisheries. In 1987, the total catch was 134,900 tonnes.

INDUSTRY. Industries include meat packing, oil refining, cement manufacture, foodstuffs, beverages, leather and textile maufacture, chemicals, light engineering and transport equipment. Some 70,000 tonnes of sugar were refined in 1989. There are about 100 textile mills.

FOREIGN ECONOMIC RELATIONS

Commerce. The foreign trade (officially stated in US$, with the figure for imports based on the clearance permits granted and that for exports on export licences utilized) was as follows (in US$1,000):

	1985	*1986*	*1987*	*1988*
Imports	708·0	1,087·6	1,189·1	1,404·5
Exports	854·0	838·8	1,141·9	1,176·9

Of the imports in 1987 (in US$1m.) USA, 90; Brazil, 279; Argentina, 156; Federal Republic of Germany, 92; UK, 34. Of the exports in 1987 Brazil took 204; Argentina, 113; Federal Republic of Germany, 121; USA, 176; UK, 54.

Principal imports (1987) (in US$1,000): Mineral products, 189,000; chemical products, 176,000; machinery and appliances, 217,000. Exports: Textiles and textile products, 384,000; live animals and animal products, 257,000; skins and hides, 199,000; vegetable products, 99,000.

Total trade between Uruguay and UK (British Department of Trade returns, in £1,000 sterling):

	1986	*1987*	*1988*	*1989*	*1990*
Imports to UK	41,366	40,474	35,410	52,185	51,859
Exports and re-exports from UK	24,465	26,484	34,999	26,119	31,192

Tourism. There were 1,168,000 tourists in 1986.

COMMUNICATIONS

Roads. There were (1984) about 52,000 km of roads including 12,000 km of motorways.

Registered motor vehicles, 31 Dec. 1981, are estimated at 281,275 passenger cars and 47,102 trucks and buses.

Railways. The total railway system open for traffic was (1986) 2,991 km of 1,435 mm gauge. In 1988 it carried 1m. tonnes of freight.

Aviation. Carrasco, 22·5 km from Montevideo, is the most important airport. US, Argentine, Brazilian, Chilean, Dutch, French, Fed. German, Scandinavian and Paraguayan airlines fly to and from Uruguay. The state-operated civil airline PLUNA runs services in the interior of the country and to Brazil, Paraguay and Argentina, and Spain.

Shipping. In 1983 there were 13 merchant vessels and 3 tankers. River transport (1,270 km) is extensive, its main importance being to link Montevideo with Paysandú and Salto.

Telecommunications. The telephone system in Montevideo is controlled by the State; small companies operate in the interior. Telephone instruments, 1986, numbered 337,000. There are 1,277 post offices. Uruguay has 85 long-wave and 17 short-wave broadcasting stations. There were (1985) about 1·7m. wireless sets and 500,000 television receivers. There are 4 television stations in Montevideo and 11 in the interior.

Cinemas (1980). Cinemas numbered 85 with seating capacity of 47,000.

Newspapers (1984). There were 5 daily newspapers in Montevideo with aggregate daily circulation of about 210,000; most of the 25–30 provincial newspapers appear bi-weekly.

JUSTICE, RELIGION, EDUCATION AND WELFARE

Justice. The Ministry of Justice was created in 1977 to be responsible for relations between the Executive Power and the Judiciary and other jurisdictional entities. The Court of Justice is made up by 5 members appointed by the Council of the Nation at the suggestion of the Executive Power, for a period of 5 years. This court has original jurisdiction in constitutional, international and admiralty cases and hears appeals from the appellate courts, of which there are 4, each with 3 judges.

In Montevideo there are also 8 courts for ordinary civil cases, 3 for government *(Juzgado de Hacienda)*, as well as criminal and correctional courts. Each departmental capital has a departmental court; each of the 224 judicial divisions has a justice of peace court.

Religion. State and Church are separated, and there is complete religious liberty. The faith professed by 66% of the inhabitants is Roman Catholic although only 50% attend church.

Education. Primary education is obligatory; both primary and superior education are free.

In 1985–86 there were 356,002 primary school pupils, and 188,176 secondary school pupils.

The University of the Republic at Montevideo, inaugurated in 1849, has about 16,200 students; tuition is free to both native-born and foreign students; there are 10 faculties. There are 43 normal schools for males and females, and a college of arts and trades with about 33,000 students. There are also many religious seminaries throughout the Republic with a considerable number of pupils, a school for the blind, 2 for deaf and dumb and a school of domestic science.

Health. Hospital beds, 1983, numbered (estimate) 23,400; physicians numbered (1984) 5,736.

DIPLOMATIC REPRESENTATIVES

Of Uruguay in Great Britain (48 Lennox Gdns., London, SW1X 0DL)
Ambassador: Dr Luis Alberto Solé-Romeo.

Of Great Britain in Uruguay (Calle Marco Bruto 1073, Montevideo)
Ambassador: C. J. Sharkey, CMG, OBE.

Of Uruguay in the USA (1918 F. St., NW, Washington, D.C., 20006)
Ambassador: Juan Podesta Pinon.

Of the USA in Uruguay (Lauro Muller 1776, Montevideo)
Ambassador: Malcolm R. Wilkey.

Of Uruguay to the United Nations
Ambassador: Ramiro Piriz-Ballon.

Further Reading

The official gazette is the *Diario Oficial*
Statistical Reports of the Government. Montevideo. Annual and biennial
Anales de Instruccion Primaria. Montevideo. Quarterly

Finch, H., *Uruguay:* [Bibliography]. Oxford and Santa Barbara, 1989
Salgado, Jose, *Historia de la Republica O. del Uruguay.* 8 vols. Montevideo, 1943
Weinstein, M., *Uruguay: Democracy at the Crossroads.* Boulder, 1988

National Library: Biblioteca Nacional del Uruguay, Guayabo 1793, Montevideo. It publishes *Anuario Bibliografico Uruguayo.*

VANUATU

Capital: Vila
Population: 142,630 (1989)
GNP per capita: US$820 (1988)

Republic of Vanuatu

HISTORY. The group was administered for some purposes jointly, for others unilaterally, as provided for by Anglo-French Convention of 27 Feb. 1906, ratified 20 Oct. 1906, and a protocol signed at London on 6 Aug. 1911 and ratified on 18 March 1922. On 30 July 1980 the Condominium of the New Hebrides achieved independence and became the Republic of Vanuatu.

AREA AND POPULATION. The Vanuatu group, of 80 islands, lies roughly 500 miles west of Fiji and 250 miles north-east of New Caledonia. The estimated land area is 4,706 sq. miles (12,190 sq. km). The larger islands of the group are: (Espiritu) Santo, Malekula, Epi, Pentecost, Aoba, Maewo, Paama, Ambrym, Efate, Erromanga, Tanna and Aneityum. They also claim Matthew and Hunter islands, 67 islands were inhabited in 1990. Population at the census (1979) 112,596. Estimate (1989) 142,630. Vila (the capital) 19,400. There are 3 active volcanoes, on Tanna, Ambrym and Lopevi, respectively.

Language: The national language is Bislama (spoken by 82% of the population); English and French are also official languages.

CLIMATE. The climate is tropical, but moderated by oceanic influences and by trade winds from May to Oct. High humidity occasionally occurs and cyclones are possible. Rainfall ranges from 90" (2,250 mm) in the south to 155" (3,875 mm) in the north. Vila. Jan. 80°F (26·7°C), July 72°F (22·2°C). Annual rainfall 84" (2,103 mm). A cyclone hit Vila in Feb. 1987.

CONSTITUTION AND GOVERNMENT. Legislative power resides in a 46-member unicameral Parliament elected for a term of 4 years. In the latest elections on 30 Nov. 1987, 26 seats were won by the *Vanuaaku Pati* and 20 by the Union of Moderate Parties. There is also a Council of Chiefs, comprising traditional tribal leaders, to advise on matters of custom.

The President is elected for a 5-year term by an electoral college comprising Parliament and the presidents of the 11 regional councils. Executive power is vested in a Council of Ministers, responsible to Parliament, and appointed and led by a Prime Minister who is elected from and by Parliament.

President: Fred Timakata (elected Jan. 1989).

The cabinet in Feb. 1991 was composed as follows:

Prime Minister, Minister of Public Service, Planning and Information: Walter Hadye Lini, CBE.

Agriculture, Forestry and Livestock: Jack T. Hopa. *Education and Sport:* Sethy J. Regenvanu. *Finance and Housing:* Sela Molisa. *Foreign Affairs and Judicial Services:* Donald Kalpokas. *Health:* Jimmy Meto Chilia. *Home Affairs and Labour:* Iolu J. Abbil. *Lands, Geology, Minerals and Rural Water Supply:* William Mahit. *Trade, Commerce, Cooperatives, Industry and Energy:* Harold C. Qualao. *Public Works, Communications, Transport, Civil Aviation and Tourism:* Edward N. Natapei. *Attorney-General:* Silas Hakwa.

Flag: Red over green, with a black triangle in the hoist, the three parts being divided by fimbriations of black and yellow, and in the centre of the black triangle a boar's tusk overlaid by two crossed fern leaves.

DEFENCE. There is a paramilitary force with about 300 personnel. A naval service formed in 1987, and following training by the Royal Australian Navy operates 1 inshore patrol craft, and a former motor yacht, both lightly armed. Personnel numbered about 50 in 1990.

INTERNATIONAL RELATIONS

Membership. Vanuatu is a member of the UN, the Commonwealth and the South Pacific Forum and is an ACP state of the EEC.

ECONOMY

Budget. The budget for 1988 balanced at 3,938m. vatu.

Currency. The unit of currency is the *vatu* (VUV). March 1991: £1 = 203·00 *Vatu*; US$1 = 107·01.

Banking and Finance. The Finance Centre, established in 1970–71 and based primarily in Vila, consists of 4 international banks (including the Hongkong and Shanghai Banking Corporation) and 6 trust companies (including Melanesia International Trust Company Ltd, a Hongkong Bank group associate). In Aug. 1984 the Asian Development Bank opened a regional office in Vila. Commercial banks assets at 31 Dec. 1988, 20,900m. vatu.

Weights and Measures. The metric system is in force.

ENERGY AND NATURAL RESOURCES

Electricity. Production (1986) 20m. kwh.

Agriculture. The main commercial crops are copra, cocoa and coffee. Production, 1988: Copra, 29,552 tonnes; cocoa, 756 tonnes; coffee (1985), 65. In 1985 about 80% of the population were engaged in subsistence agriculture. Yams, taro, manioc, sweet potatoes and bananas are grown for local consumption. A large number of cattle are reared on plantations, and an upgrading programme using pure-bred Charolais, Limousins and Illawarras has begun. A beef industry is developing.

Livestock (1988): Cattle, 105,000; goats, 15,000; pigs, 79,000.

Forestry. In 1987 some 1,900 ha of plantation had been established. Production (1985) 37,900 cu. metres of logs and sawn timber.

Fisheries. The principal catch is tuna (1985, 3,962 tonnes) mainly exported to the USA. Small-scale commercial fishing (1985) over 200 tonnes.

INDUSTRY. Industries in 1987 included copra processing, meat canning and fish freezing, a saw-mill, soft drinks factories and a print works. Building materials, furniture and aluminium were also produced, and in 1984 a cement plant opened.

FOREIGN ECONOMIC RELATIONS

Commerce. Imports and exports were (in 1m. Vatu):

	1985	*1986*	*1987*	*1988*
Imports	7,378	6,105	7,638	7,361
Exports	3,262	1,841	1,942	2,066

In 1988 the main exports (in 1m. vatu) were: Copra, 953; beef and veal, 243; timber, 106; cocoa, 117. 52% of exports went to the Netherlands, 15% to Japan, 6% to France, 4% to Australia and 3% to New Caledonia. Australia (43%), Japan (9%), New Zealand (11%), France (5%), Fiji (7%), New Caledonia (4%), were the major sources of imports and principal imports (in 1m. vatu) were machinery and transport equipment (1,797), food and live animals (1,263), basic manufactures (1,430), manufactured articles (851), fuels and lubricants (584), chemicals (421) and beverages and tobacco (368).

Total trade between Vanuatu and UK (British Department of Trade returns, in £1,000 sterling):

	1987	*1988*	*1989*	*1990*
Imports to UK	15	5	52	47
Exports and re-exports from UK	1,058	856	363	1,796

Tourism. In 1988 there were 17,544 visitors to Vanuatu. In addition there were 50,932 tourists from cruise ships. Earnings from tourism 2,000m. vatu.

COMMUNICATIONS

Roads. In 1984 there were 1,062 km of roads in Vanuatu, of these about 250 km are paved, mostly on Efate Island and Espiritu Santo. There were 3,784 registered cars in Vanuatu (1988).

Aviation (1986). Air Vanuatu provides services to Australia; Air Nauru, Air Pacific, Air Caledonia, Solair and UTA serve Pacific routes; Air Melanisia provides regular services to 16 domestic airfields, and charter services. There are international airfields at Vila and Santo.

Shipping. Several international shipping lines serve Vanuatu, linking the country with Australia, New Zealand, other Pacific territories notably Hong Kong, Japan, North America and Europe. The chief ports are Vila and Santo. In 1977, 394 vessels arrived including 48 cruise ships carrying 40,412 visitors. 92,340 tons of cargo were exported and 102,867 tons discharged. Small vessels provide frequent inter-island services.

Telecommunications. Internal telephone and telegram services are provided by the Posts and Telecommunications and Radio Departments. There are automatic telephone exchanges at Vila and Santo; rural areas are served by a network of tele-radio stations. In 1983 there were 6 post offices and 3,000 telephones.

External telephone, telegram and telex services are provided by VANITEL, through their satellite earth station at Vila. There are direct circuits to Noumea, Sydney, Hong Kong and Paris and high quality communications are available on a 24-hour basis to most countries in the world. Air radio facilities are provided. Marine coast station facilities are available at Vila and Santo. Radio Vanuatu operates a service 7 days a week in, French, English and Bislama. In 1986 there were 4 radio stations and 18,000 receivers.

JUSTICE, RELIGION, EDUCATION AND WELFARE

Justice. A study was being made in 1980 which could lead to unification of the judicial system.

Religion. Over 80% of the population are Christians, but animist beliefs are still prevalent.

Education. There were (1988) 260 primary schools with 24,634 pupils, 11 government and denominational secondary schools with 2,000 pupils and Matevulu College. Tertiary education is provided at the Vanuatu Technical Institute and the Teachers College, while other technical and commercial training is through regional institutions in the Solomon Islands, Fiji and Papua New Guinea.

Health. In 1988 there were 12 hospitals (5 rural) with 419 beds, 37 health centres, 50 dispensaries, 23 doctors and 270 nurses.

DIPLOMATIC REPRESENTATIVES

Of Vanuatu in Great Britain
High Commissioner: (Vacant).

Of Great Britain in Vanuatu (Melitco Hse., Rue Pasteur, Vila)
High Commissioner: J. Thompson, MBE.

Of Vanuatu to the United Nations
Ambassador: Robert F. Van Lierop.

VATICAN CITY STATE

Stato della Città del Vaticano

HISTORY. For many centuries the Popes bore temporal sway over a territory stretching across mid-Italy from sea to sea and comprising some 17,000 sq. miles, with a population finally of over 3m. In 1859–60 and 1870 the Papal States were incorporated into the Italian Kingdom. The consequent dispute between Italy and successive Popes was only settled on 11 Feb. 1929 by three treaties between the Italian Government and the Vatican: (1) A Political Treaty, which recognized the full and independent sovereignty of the Holy See in the city of the Vatican; (2) a Concordat, to regulate the condition of religion and of the Church in Italy; and (3) a Financial Convention, in accordance with which the Holy See received 750m. lire in cash and 1,000m. lire in Italian 5% state bonds. This sum was to be a definitive settlement of all the financial claims of the Holy See against Italy in consequence of the loss of its temporal power in 1870. The treaty and concordat were ratified on 7 June 1929. The treaty has been embodied in the Constitution of the Italian Republic of 1947. A revised Concordat between the Italian Republic and the Holy See was subsequently negotiated and signed in 1984, and which came into force on 3 June 1985.

The Vatican City State is governed by a Commission appointed by the Pope. The reason for its existence is to provide an extra-territorial, independent base for the Holy See, the government of the Roman Catholic Church.

AREA AND POPULATION. The area of the Vatican City is 44 hectares (108·7 acres). It includes the Piazza di San Pietro (St Peter's Square), which is to remain normally open to the public and subject to the powers of the Italian police. It has its own railway station (for freight only), postal facilities, coins and radio. Twelve buildings in and outside Rome enjoy extra-territorial rights, including the Basilicas of St John Lateran, St Mary Major and St Paul without the Walls, the Pope's summer villa at Castel Gandolfo and a further Vatican radio station on Italian soil. *Radio Vaticana* broadcasts an extensive service in 34 languages from the transmitters in the Vatican City and in Italy.

The Vatican City has about 1,000 inhabitants.

CONSTITUTION. The Pope exercises sovereignty and has absolute legislative, executive and judicial powers. The judicial power is delegated to a tribunal in the first instance, to the Sacred Roman Rota in appeal and to the Supreme Tribunal of the Signature in final appeal.

The Pope is elected by the College of Cardinals, meeting in secret conclave. The election is by scrutiny and requires a two-thirds majority.

Name and family	*Election*	*Name and family*	*Election*
Benedict XIV *(Lambertini)*	1740	Leo XIII *(Pecci)*	1878
Clement XIII *(Rezzonico)*	1758	Pius X *(Sarto)*	1903
Clement XIV *(Ganganelli)*	1769	Benedict XV *(della Chiesa)*	1914
Pius VI *(Braschi)*	1775	Pius XI *(Ratti)*	1922
Pius VII *(Chiaramonti)*	1800	Pius XII *(Pacelli)*	1939
Leo XII *(della Genga)*	1823	John XXIII *(Roncalli)*	1958
Pius VIII *(Castiglioni)*	1829	Paul VI *(Montini)*	1963
Gregory XVI *(Cappellari)*	1831	John Paul I *(Luciani)*	1978
Pius IX *(Mastai-Ferretti)*	1846	John Paul II *(Wojtyla)*	1978

Supreme Pontiff: **John Paul II** (Karol Wojtyła), born at Wadowice near Kraków,

Poland, 18 May 1920. Archbishop of Kraków 1964–78, created Cardinal in 1967, elected Pope 16 Oct. 1978, inaugurated 22 Oct. 1978.

Pope John Paul II was the first non-Italian to be elected since Pope Adrian VI (a Dutchman) in 1522.

Secretary of State: Angelo Sodano.
Secretary for Relations with Other States: Jean-Louis Tauran.

Flag: Vertically yellow and white, with on the white the crossed keys and tiara of the Papacy.

ROMAN CATHOLIC CHURCH. The Roman Pontiff (in orders a Bishop, but in jurisdiction held to be by divine right the centre of all Catholic unity, and consequently Pastor and Teacher of all Christians) has for advisers and coadjutors the Sacred College of Cardinals, consisting in Jan. 1990 of 149 Cardinals appointed by him from senior ecclesiastics who are either the bishops of important Sees or the heads of departments at the Holy See. In addition to the College of Cardinals, the Pope has created a ' Synod of Bishops'. This consists of the Patriarchs and certain Metropolitans of the Catholic Church of Oriental Rite, of elected representatives of the national episcopal conferences and religious orders of the world, of the Cardinals in charge of the Roman Congregations and of other persons nominated by the Pope. The Synod meets as and when decided by the Pope. The next Synod (on the formation of priests) met in Oct. 1990.

The central administration of the Roman Catholic Church is carried on by a number of permanent committees called Sacred Congregations, each composed of a number of Cardinals and diocesan bishops (both appointed for 5-year periods), with Consultors and Officials. Besides the Secretariat of State and the Second Section of the Secretariat of State (Section for Relations with States) there are now 9 Sacred Congregations, viz.: Doctrine, Oriental Churches, Bishops, the Sacraments, Divine Worship, Clergy, Religious, Catholic Education, Evangelization of the Peoples and Causes of the Saints. Pontifical Councils have replaced some of the previously designated Secretariats and Prefectures and now represent the Laity, Christian Unity, the Family, Justice and Peace, Cor Unum, Migrants, Health Care Workers, Interpretation of Legislative Texts, Inter-Religious Dialogue, Non Believers, Culture, Preserving the Patrimony of Art and History, and, a new Commission, for Latin America. There are also Offices for the Apostolic Penitentiary, the Supreme Tribunal of the Apostolic Signature, the Roman Rota, the Apostolic Camera, the Patrimony of the Holy See, Economic Affairs, the Papal Household, Liturgical Celebrations, the Secret Archives, the Apostolic Library, the Academy of Sciences, the Polyglot Press, the Publishing House, Vatican Radio, the Vatican Television Centre, the Fabric of St Peter's, Papal Charities, Translation Centre, Central Labour Office, the Consistory, Council of Cardinals, Economic Questions and the Institute for Works of Religion (the IOR). The Pontifical Academy of Sciences was revived by Pius XI in 1936 with 70 members. The director of the Vatican Bank (Istituto per le Opere di Religione) is Giovanni Bodio.

DIPLOMATIC REPRESENTATIVES

In its diplomatic relations with foreign countries the Holy See is represented by the Secretariat of State and the Second Section (Relations with States) of the Council for Public Affairs of the Church. It maintains permanent observers to the UN in New York and Geneva and to UNESCO and FAO. The Holy See is a member of IAEA and the Vatican City State is a member of UPU and ITU. It therefore attends as a member those international conferences open to State members of the UN and specialized agencies.

Of the Holy See in Great Britain (54 Parkside, London, SW19 5NF)
Apostolic Pro-Nuncio: Archbishop Luigi Barbarito (accredited 7 April 1986).

Of Great Britain at the Holy See (91 Via Condotti, I–00187, Rome).
Ambassador: J. K. E. Broadley, CMG. *First Secretary:* P. J. McCormick.

Of the Holy See in the USA (3339 Massachusetts Ave., NW, Washington, D.C., 20008).
Apostolic Pro Nuncio: Agostino Cacciavillan.

Of the USA at the Holy See (Villino Pacelli, Via Aurelia 294, 00165, Rome).
Ambassador: Thomas Melady.

Further Reading

Acta Apostolicæ Sedis Romanæ. Rome
Annuario Pontificio. Rome. Annual
L'Attività della Santa Sede. Rome. Annual
The Catholic Almanac. Huntingdon. Annual
The Catholic Directory. London. Annual
The Catholic Directory for Scotland. Glasgow. Annual
Code of Canon Law. London, 1983
The New Catholic Encyclopædia. New York
Osservatore Romano. Vatican. Daily with weekly editions in English and other languages
Bull, G., *Inside the Vatican*. London, 1982
Cardinale, I., *The Holy See and the International Order*. Gerrards Cross, 1976
Hebblethwaite, P., *In the Vatican*. London, 1986
Mayer, F. *et al*, *The Vatican: Portrait of a State and a Community*. Dublin, 1980
Nichols, P., *The Pope's Divisions*. London, 1981
Walsh, M. J., *Vatican City State*. [Bibliography] Oxford and Santa Barbara, 1983

VENEZUELA

República de Venezuela

Capital: Caracas
Population: 9·25m. (1989)
GNP per capita: US$3,170 (1988)

HISTORY. Venezuela formed part of the Spanish colony of New Granada until 1821 when it became independent in union with Colombia. A separate, independent republic was formed in 1830.

AREA AND POPULATION. Venezuela is bounded north by the Caribbean, east by Guyana, south by Brazil, south-west and west by Colombia. The official estimate of the area is 912,050 sq. km (352,143 sq. miles); the frontiers with Colombia, Brazil and Guyana extend for 4,782 km and its Caribbean coastline stretches for some 3,200 km. Population (1981) census, 14,516,735. Estimate (1989) 19,246,000. The 1981 census excluded tribal Indians estimated at 53,350 (chiefly in Amazonas Territory) and illegal immigrants, estimated (1979) at about 3m. The official language is Spanish, spoken by all but 2·5% of the population.

The areas, populations and capitals of the 20 states and 4 federally-controlled areas are:

State	*Sq. km*	*Census 1981*	*Capital*	*Census 1981*
Anzoátegui	43,300	683,717	Barcelona	156,461
Apure	76,500	188,187	San Fernando	57,308
Aragua	7,014	891,623	Maracay	387,682
Barinas	35,200	326,166	Barinas	110,462
Bolívar	238,000	668,340	Ciudad Bolívar	182,941
Carabobo	4,650	1,062,268	Valencia	624,113
Cojedes	14,800	133,991	San Carlos	37,892
Falcón	24,800	503,896	Coro	96,339
Guárico	64,986	393,467	San Juan	57,219
Lara	19,800	945,064	Barquisimeto	523,101
Mérida	11,300	459,361	Mérida	143,805
Miranda	7,950	1,421,442	Los Teques	112,857
Monagas	28,900	388,536	Maturin	154,976
Nueva Esparta	1,150	197,198	La Asunción	10,375
Portuguesa	15,200	424,984	Guanare	64,025
Sucre	11,800	585,698	Cumaná	179,814
Táchira	11,100	660,234	San Cristóbal	198,793
Trujillo	7,400	433,735	Trujillo	31,774
Yaracuy	7,100	300,597	San Felipe	57,526
Zulia	63,100	1,674,252	Maracaibo	890,553
Ter. Amazonas	175,750	45,667	Puerto Ayacucho	28,248
Ter. Delta Amacuro	40,200	56,720	Tucupita	27,299
Federal District	1,930	2,070,742	Caracas	1,044,851
Federal Dependencies	120	850	—	—

Other large towns (1980) are Petare (334,800), Ciudad Guyana (314,041, census 1981), Baruta (180,100), Cabimas (138,529, census 1981), Acarigua (126,000), Maiquetiá (120,200), Valera (101,981, census 1981), Chacao (101,900), Puerto Cabello (94,000), Carúpano (82,000) and Puerto La Cruz (81,800).

Venezuela is the most urbanised Latin American nation; in 1985, 86% of the population lived in urban areas. Over half the population live in the valleys of Carabobo and Valencia (once the capital). At the 1981 census, 69% were of mixed ethnic origin (*mestizo*), 20% white, 9% black and 2% Amerindian.

Vital statistics (1986): 504,278 births, 100,002 marriages, 77,647 deaths. Life expectancy (1985) 65 males, 71 females, with 41% of population under 15 years.

CLIMATE. The climate ranges from warm temperate to tropical. Temperatures vary little throughout the year and rainfall is plentiful. The dry season is from Dec. to April. Caracas. Jan. 65°F (18·3°C), July 69°F (20·6°C). Annual rainfall 32" (833 mm). Ciudad Bolivar. Jan. 79°F (26·1°C), July 81°F (27·2°C). Annual rainfall 41" (1,016 mm). Maracaibo. Jan. 81°F (27·2°C), July 85°F (29·4°C). Annual rainfall 23" (577 mm).

CONSTITUTION AND GOVERNMENT. The constitution of 1961 provides for the election for a term of 5 years of a President, a National Congress, and state and municipal legislative assemblies by universal compulsory suffrage at 18 years. Voting is by proportional representation.

Congress consists of a Senate and a Chamber of Deputies. At least 2 Senators are elected for each State and for the Federal District. Senators must be Venezuelans by birth and over 30 years of age. Deputies must be native Venezuelans over 21 years of age; there is 1 for every 50,000 inhabitants. The territories, on reaching the population fixed by law, also elect deputies.

The President must be a Venezuelan by birth and over 30 years of age; he has a qualified power of veto.

The following is a list of presidents since 1945:

	Took Office		*Took Office*
Rómulo Betancourt	20 Oct. 1945	Rómulo Betancourt	13 Feb. 1959
Rómulo Gallegos	15 Feb. 1948	Raul Leoni	11 March 1964
Lieut.-Col. Carlos Delgado Chalbaud	24 Nov. 1948 [4]	Rafael Caldera	11 March 1969
Dr G. Suárez Flamerich	27 Nov. 1950 [2]	Carlos Andrés Pérez Rodríguez	12 March 1974
Col. Marcos Pérez Jiménez.	3 Dec. 1952 [1]	Dr Luis Herrera Campíns	12 March 1979
Rear-Adm. Wolfgang Larrazábal Ugueto	23 Jan. 1958 [2 3]	Dr Jaime Lusinchi	2 Feb. 1984
Dr Edgard Sanabria	14 Nov. 1958[3]	Carlos Andrés Perez Rodriguez	2 Feb. 1989

[1] Deposed. [2] Resigned. [3] Provisional. [4] Assassinated 13 Nov. 1950.

President: Carlos Andrés Perez Rodriguez, elected 4 Dec. 1988 with 54·56% of the votes, assumed office on 2 Feb. 1989.

The cabinet in March 1991 was composed as follows:

Interior: Alejandro Izaguirre. *Foreign Affairs:* Reinaldo Figueredo Planchart. *Finance:* Roberto Pocaterra. *Industrial Development:* Vacant. *Agriculture:* Eugenio de Armas. *Labour and Social Development:* German Lairet. *Justice:* Luis Beltran Guerra. *Transportation and Communications:* Edgar Elías Osuna. *Energy and Mines:* Celestino Armas. *Presidential Secretary:* Jesús Ramón Carmona Borjas. *Defence:* Gen. Filmo López Uzcategui.

At the Congressional elections held 4 Dec. 1983, 112 of the 200 seats in the Chamber of Deputies were won by Acción Democrática, 61 by COPEI (the Social Christians) and 27 by other parties.

The city of Caracas is the capital. The 20 states, autonomous and politically equal, have each a legislative assembly and a governor. The states are divided into 156 districts and 613 municipalities. There are also 2 federal territories with 7 departments, and a federal district with 2 departments and 2 parishes. Each district has a municipal council, and each municipio a communal junta. The federal district and the 2 territories are administered by the President of the Republic.

National flag: Three horizontal stripes of yellow, blue, red, with an arc of 7 white stars in the centre, and the national arms in the canton.

National anthem: Gloria al bravo pueblo (1811; words by Vicente Salias, tune by Juan Landaeta).

DEFENCE. There is selective conscription at age 18 for 24 months (30 months in the navy).

Army. The Army consists of 1 cavalry and 4 infantry divisions; 1 Ranger brigade, 1 airborne regiment with supporting regiments and groups. Equipment includes 81

AMX-30 main battle and 35 M-18 and 36 AMX-13 light tanks. Army aviation comprises 23 helicopters and aircraft. Strength (1991) 34,000.

Navy. The combatant fleet comprises 2 German-built submarines, 6 Italian-built Lupo class frigates, 6 fast missile craft, 7 riverine patrol craft, 5 tank landing ships and 2 craft. Auxiliaries comprise 1 logistic support, 2 transport, and a sail training ship, plus a few harbour service craft.

The Naval Air Arm, 2,000 strong, comprises 4 shore-based C-212 Aviocars for maritime reconnaissance, 8 AB-212 ship-borne anti-submarine helicopters, 2 Bell 47 helicopters for search-and-rescue and 11 miscellaneous transport and liaison aircraft.

Personnel in 1990 totalled 10,000 (4,000 conscripts) including the Marine Corps and the Coastguard. Main bases are at Caracas, Puerto Cabello and Punto Fijo.

The Coastguard, organizationally separate but under Naval operational control, is responsible for control of the economic exclusion zone and comprises 2 large frigate-type patrol craft, 2 ex-tugs and a number of boats.

The maritime elements of the National Guard, which is tasked with customs enforcement and internal security duties, operates some 70 patrol craft and boats of various sizes from 23m down.

Air Force. Formed in 1920, the Air Force of (1991) some 7,000 officers and men is a small, but well-equipped service with a total of about 200 aircraft. There are 8 combat squadrons. Two are equipped with 18 F-16A and 6 F-16B Fighting Falcons. Two have 14 Canadair CF-5A fighter-bombers and 6 two-seat CF-5Ds, and two share 9 Mirage III/5 single-seaters and 2 Mirage 5D trainers. Two bomber squadrons are equipped with 19 modernized Canberra jet-bombers and a single reconnaissance Canberra. Another operational squadron has 14 OV-10E Bronco twin-turboprop counter-insurgency aircraft. A helicopter force consists of more than 30 Bell 212s, 214STs and 412s, UH-1B/D/H Iroquois and Alouette IIIs. Transport units are equipped with 12 C-123 Providers, 6 C-130H Hercules, 5 C-47s and 8 Aeritalia G222s. Communications aircraft are Queen Airs and other types. Thirty Tucanos and 20 T-34A Mentors are used for training, together with 20 T-2D Buckeye advanced jet trainers, which have a secondary attack role. A battalion of paratroops comes within Air Force responsibility. There is a staff college and a cadet academy.

National Guard, a volunteer force of some 22,000 under the Ministry of Defence, is broadly responsible for internal security. It includes customs and forestry duties among its tasks.

INTERNATIONAL RELATIONS

Membership. Venezuela is a member of the UN, OAS, LAIA, OPEC and the Andean Group.

ECONOMY

Budget. The revenue and expenditure for calendar years were, in Bs.1m., as follows:

	1984	*1985*	*1986*	*1987*	*1988*
Revenue	102,808	118,039	109,000	165,000	180,000
Expenditure	103,539	113,307	105,000	165,000	180,000

Currency. The unit of currency is the *bolívar* (VEB) of 100 *céntimos*. There are notes of Bs 10, 20, 50, 100 and 500, and coins of 5, 12·5, 25, 50 céntimos and Bs 1, 2 and 5.

In March 1991, £1 = Bs.102·59; US$1 = 54·08.

Banking and Finance. The *Governor* of the Central Bank is Pedro Tinoco. The major banks include: Banco Provincial SAICA, Banco de Venezuela, Banco Consolidado, Banco Unión, Banco Mercantil, Banco Latino, Banco de Maracaibo, Banco Industrial de Venezuela, Bank of America.

There is a stock exchange in Caracas.

ENERGY AND NATURAL RESOURCES

Electricity. Production (1986) 50,240m. kwh. The Guri hydroelectric plant supplies 70% of the country's needs.

Oil. The oil-producing region around Maracaibo, covering some 30,000 sq. miles, produces about three-quarters of Venezuelan petroleum. Deposits in the Orinoco region are likely to prove one of the largest heavy oil reserves in the world. Nationalization of the privately owned oil sector in 1976 has proved successful. Crude oil production (1990) was 110·53m. tonnes.

Proven crude oil reserves in Jan. 1988 stood at 58,000m. bbls. However, these are considered conservative estimates and new fields off-shore have estimated reserves of 6,000–40,000m. bbls. In March 1988 a new field in the state of Monagas was confirmed estimated at 8,600m. bbls. The Orinoco tar sands belt has reserves variously estimated at between 700,000m. bbls. and 3,000,000m. bbls.

Gas. Production (1985) 33,059m. cu. metres.

Minerals. Bauxite is being exploited in the Guayana region by Bauxien, a state agency. There are important goldmines in the region south-east of Bolívar State, and new deposits have been discovered near El Callao (1959) and Sosa Méndez (1961) in the Guayana region. Output, 1982, amounted to 902 kg. Diamond output, from Amazonas territory, was 687,000 carats in 1977. Manganese deposits, estimated at several million tons, were discovered in 1954. Phosphate-rock deposits (yielding from 64 to 82% tricalcium phosphate) are found in the state of Falcón; reserves of 15m. tons of high-quality rock have been established. The state of Sucre has large sulphur deposits. Coal is worked in the states of Táchira, Aragua and Anzoátegui. Coal proven reserves in Zulia (160m. tons) are to be developed to service a new thermal power station in the Maracaibo area. An important nickel deposit (at Loma de Hierro near Tejerías) is estimated to equal 600,000 tons of pure nickel. Saltmines are now worked by the Government on the Araya peninsula. Asbestos and copper pyrite are being exploited. There were proven reserves (1984) of bauxite totalling 200m. tonnes and production of about 3m. per annum are scheduled from 1986.

Iron ore is exploited in Bolívar State by the Orinoco Mining Co. and Iron Mines of Venezuela, subsidiaries respectively of the US Steel Corp. and the Bethlehem Steel Co. Proven reserves at the end of 1980 were 1,800m. tonnes. National output of iron ore, 1985, 14·9m. tonnes of which 9m. was exported.

Agriculture. Venezuela is divided into 3 distinct zones—the agricultural, the pastoral and the forest zone. In the first are grown coffee, cocoa, sugar-cane, maize, rice, wheat (grown in the Andes), tobacco, cotton, beans, sisal, etc.; the second affords grazing for more than 6m. cattle and numerous horses; and in the third, which covers a very large portion of the country, tropical products, such as caoutchouc, balatá (a gum resembling rubber), tonka beans, dividivi, copaiba, vanilla, growing wild, are worked by the inhabitants. The 1988 livestock estimate showed cattle, 12,756,000; pigs, 2,707,000; goats, 1·4m.; sheep, 425,000; poultry, 57m. Area under cultivation is 5,530,898 acres. Over 50% of all farmers are engaged in subsistence agriculture and growth rates in agricultural production have not kept pace with the high population increase. Government has introduced a programme of price support, tax incentives and price increases.

Production (1988, in 1,000 tonnes): Rice, 385; maize, 1,400; cassava, 318; sugar-cane, 8,000; bananas, 1,050; oranges, 390; potatoes, 216; tomatoes, 145; coffee, 80; sesame seed, 67; tobacco, 16; cocoa, 15.

The coffee plantations number 62,673, covering 543,400 acres with 135m. bushes. The Venezuelan cocoa, from 13,000 plantations, is considered to be of high quality; it is grown chiefly in the states of Sucre and Miranda. The sugar industry has 6 government and 20 privately owned mills.

Forestry. Resources have been barely tapped; 600 species of wood have been identified.

Fisheries. Total catch (1986) was 283,600 tonnes.

INDUSTRY. Production (1985): Steel, 2·72m. tonnes; aluminium, 407,000; ammonia, 490,000; fertilizers, 650,000; cement, 5·12m.; paper, 550,000; vehicles (units) 116,000.

Labour. The labour force in 1990 was 6,655,000, of whom 758,000 worked in agriculture.

Trade Unions. The most powerful confederation of trade unions is the CTV (*Confederacion de Trabajadores de Venezuela*, formed 1947), which is dominated by the Accion Democratica party. Estimated membership, 1·1m. but claims 2m.

FOREIGN ECONOMIC RELATIONS

Commerce. Venezuela's exports and imports (in US$1m.):

	1984	*1985*	*1986*	*1987*
Exports	15,967	14,178	8,880	8,402
Imports	7,262	7,388	7,600	8,711

Main export markets in 1987 were the USA, Netherlands Antilles because of its oil refining and transhipment facilities, Japan and Colombia.

Principal imports are machinery and equipment, manufactured goods, chemical products, foodstuffs.

The USA supplied 47% of all imports in 1987, followed by Federal Republic of Germany, Japan, Italy and the UK.

Total trade between UK and Venezuela (British Department of Trade returns, in £1,000 sterling):

	1986	*1987*	*1988*	*1989*	*1990*
Imports to UK	96,339	91,749	76,563	111,072	101,717
Exports and re-exports from UK	170,101	157,760	177,787	124,672	204,921

Tourism. 692,400 tourists visited Venezuela in 1988.

COMMUNICATIONS

Roads. There were, 1985, 62,601 km of road fit for traffic the year round; of these 24,036 km are paved. There are 10,097 km of high-speed 4-lane motorway type. The motorway system runs from Caracas to Puerto Cabello via Valencia and will shortly be linked direct with one from La Guaira to Caracas.

Railways. Plans have existed since 1950 for large-scale railway construction but only the Puerto Cabello to Barquisimeto and Acarigua lines (336 km–1,435 mm gauge) has been completed. In 1989 it carried 37·6m. passenger-km and 38·6m. tonne-km. There is a metro in Caracas.

Aviation. In 1985 there were 7 international airports, 51 national and over 200 private airports. The chief Venezuelan airlines are LAV (Líneas Aéreas Venezolanas), a government-owned concern, and AVENSA (Aerovías Venezolanas). Both operate numerous internal services. VIASA operates international routes in conjunction with KLM. There are also 3 specialist air freight companies. In all there are over 100 commercial aircraft in operation. In addition to Venezuelan international services, a number of US and Latin American and European lines operate services to Venezuela. British Airways operates twice-weekly flights between London and Caracas.

Shipping. Foreign vessels are not permitted to engage in the coasting trade, except by special concessions or by contract with the Government. La Guaira, Maracaibo, Puerto Cabello, Puerto Ordaz and Guanta are the chief ports. In Dec. 1978 the merchant fleet had an aggregate gross tonnage of 824,000; this included tankers of 368,000 gross tons.

The principal navigable rivers are the Orinoco and its tributaries Apure and Arauca, from San Fernando to Tucupita through Ciudad Bolívar, Puerto Ordaz and San Félix; San Juan from Carípito to the Gulf of Paria; and Escalante in Lake Maracaibo.

Telecommunications. There were 1,165,699 telephones in 1985. An international telex service operates in the Caracas metropolitan zone. There is a submarine telephone link with USA.

In 1986 there were 6·7m. radio receivers and 77 radio stations. There were 3 television stations in Caracas (two privately owned), of which 2 cover, with relays, most of the country. In 1986 there were about 2·75m. homes with TV receivers.

Newspapers (1983). There were 25 leading daily newspapers with a circulation of over 1·7m.

JUSTICE, RELIGION, EDUCATION AND HEALTH

Justice. The Supreme Court, which operates in Divisions, each with 5 members, is elected by Congress for 5 years. The country is divided into 20 legal districts. They select their own President and Vice-President. The Federal Procurator-General is appointed for 5 years. There are lower federal courts.

Each state has a Supreme Court with 3 members, a superior court, or superior tribunal, courts of first instance, district courts and municipal courts. In the territories there are civil and military judges of first instance, and also judges in the municipios. Finally, there is an income-tax claims tribunal.

Religion. The Roman Catholic is the prevailing religion, but there is toleration of all others. There are 4 archbishops, 1 at Caracas, who is Primate of Venezuela, 2 at Mérida and 1 at Ciudad Bolívar. There are 19 bishops. In the state primary schools instruction is given only to those children whose parents expressly request it. Protestants number about 20,000.

Education. In 1987–88 there were 13,500 primary schools with 115,000 teachers and 2,900,000 pupils, 2,000 secondary schools with 63,000 teachers and 1,100,000 pupils. The number of students in higher education was 466,000 with 30,000 teaching staff in the 94 establishments.

Health. In 1983 there were 21,502 doctors and 43,650 beds in hospitals and dispensaries in 1979.

DIPLOMATIC REPRESENTATIVES

Of Venezuela in Great Britain (1 Cromwell Rd., London, SW7)
Ambassador: Dr Francisco Kerdel-Vegas, CBE (accredited 5 Nov. 1987).

Of Great Britain in Venezuela (Torre Las Mercedes, Avenida La Estancia, Chuao, Caracas 1060)
Ambassador: Giles Fitzherbert, CMG.

Of Venezuela in the USA (2445 Massachusetts Ave., NW, Washington, D.C., 20008)
Ambassador: Simon Alberto Consalvi.

Of the USA in Venezuela (Avenida Francisco de Miranda and Avenida Principal de la Floresta, Caracas)
Ambassador: (Vacant).

Of Venezuela to the United Nations
Ambassador: Dr Andrés Aguilar.

Further Reading

Statistical Information: The following are some of the principal publications:
Dirección General de Estadística, Ministerio de Fomento, *Boletín Mensual de Estadística.—Anuario Estadístico de Venezuela.* Caracas, Annual
Banco Central, *Memoria Annual* and *Boletin Mensual*
Ministerio de Sanidad y Asistencia Social, Dirección de Salud Pública, *Anuario de Epidemiología y Asistencia Social*

Bigler, G. E., *Politics and State Capitalism in Venezuela.* Madrid, 1981

Braveboy-Wagner, J. A., *The Venezuela-Guyana Border Dispute: Britain's Colonial Legacy in Latin America*. Boulder and Epping, 1984

Buitrón, A., *Causas y Efectos del Exodo Rural en Venezuela.—Efectos Económicos y Sociales de las Inmigraciones en Venezuela.—Las Inmigraciones en Venezuela*. Pan American Union, Washington, D.C., 1956

Ewell, J., *Venezuela: A Century of Change*. London, 1984

Lombard, J., *Venezuelan History: A Comprehensive Working Bibliography*. Boston, 1977.—*Venezuela: The Search for Order, the Dream of Progress*. OUP, 1982

Martz, J. D. and Myers, D. J., *Venezuela: The Democratic Experience*. New York, 1986

VIETNAM

Capital: Hanoi
Population: 65m. (1990)
GNP per capita: US$200 (1989)

Công Hòa Xã Hôi Chu Nghĩa Viêt Nam

(Socialist Republic of Vietnam)

HISTORY. Conquered by the Chinese in B.C. 111, Vietnam broke free from Chinese domination in 939, though at many subsequent periods it was a nominal Chinese vassal. (For subsequent history until the cessation of hostilities with the US in Jan. 1973 *see* THE STATESMAN'S YEAR-BOOK, 1989–90).

After the US withdrawal, hostilities continued between the North and the South until the latter's defeat in 1975.

(For details of the former Republic of Vietnam, *see* THE STATESMAN'S YEAR-BOOK, 1975–76). A Provisional Revolutionary Government established an administration in Saigon. A general election was held on 25 April 1976 for a National Assembly representing the whole country. Voting was by universal suffrage of all citizens of 18 or over, except former functionaries of South Vietnam undergoing 're-education', the last of whom (approximately 7,000) were released in Sept. 1987 and Feb. 1988. The unification of North and South Vietnam into the Socialist Republic of Vietnam took place formally on 2 July 1976. In 1978 Vietnam signed a 25-year treaty of friendship and co-operation with the USSR. Relations with China correspondingly deteriorated, an exacerbating factor being the Vietnamese military intervention in Cambodia in Dec. 1978. Occasional skirmishing along the China–Vietnam border continued into 1988. In 1988 Vietnam began the phased withdrawal of its 120,000 troops in Cambodia, claiming in Sept. 1989 that withdrawal was complete.

AREA AND POPULATION. The country has a total area of 329,566 sq. km and is divided administratively into 40 provinces. Areas and populations (in 1,000) at the census of Oct. 1979 were as follows:

Province	*Sq. km*	*1979*	*Province*	*Sq. km*	*1979*
Lai Chau	17,408	322,077	Thai Binh	1,344	1,506,235
Son La	14,656	487,793	Hai Phong (city) [1]	1,515	1,279,067
Hoang Lien Son	14,125	778,217	Ha Nam Ninh	3,522	2,781,409
Ha Tuyen	13,519	782,453	Thanh Hoa	11,138	2,532,261
Cao Bang	13,731	479,823	Nghe Tinh	22,380	3,111,989
Lang Son		484,657	Binh Tri Thien	19,048	1,901,713
Bac Thai	8,615	815,105	Quang Nam – Da Nang	11,376	1,529,520
Quang Ninh	7,076	750,055	Nghia Binh	14,700	2,095,354
Vinh Phu	5,187	1,488,348	Gia Lai – Kon Tum	18,480	595,906
Ha Bac	4,708	1,662,671	Dac Lac	18,300	490,198
Ha Son Binh	6,860	1,537,190	Phu Khanh	9,620	1,188,637
Hanoi (city) [1]	597	2,570,905	Lam Dong	10,000	396,657
Hai Hung	2,526	2,145,662	Thuan Hai	11,000	938,255
Dong Nai	12,130	1,304,799	Ben Tre	2,400	1,041,838
Song Be	9,500	659,093	Cuu Long	4,200	1,504,215
Tay Ninh	4,100	684,006	An Giang	4,140	1,532,362
Long An	5,100	957,264	Hau Giang	5,100	2,232,891
Dong Thap	3,120	1,182,787	Kien Giang	6,000	994,673
Thanh Pho – Ho Chi Minh [1]	1,845	3,419,978	Minh Hai	8,000	1,219,595
Tien Giang	2,350	1,264,498	Vung Tau – Con Dao [2]	—	91,160
				329,466	52,741,766

[1] Autonomous city. [2] Special area.

At the census of Oct. 1979 the population was 52,741,766 (25,580,582 male; 19·7% urban).

Population (1990), 65m. (Ho Chi Minh 4m.; Hanoi, 2m. (1979); growth rate (1988) 2·4% per annum. Density, 181 per sq. km. Sanctions are imposed on couples with more than two children.

84% of the population are Vietnamese (Kinh). There are also over 60 minority groups thinly spread in the extensive mountainous regions. The largest minorities are (1976 figures in 1,000): Tay (742); Khmer (651); Thai (631); Muong (618); Nung (472); Meo (349); Dao (294). In 1987 1m. Vietnamese were living abroad, mainly in the US. Following an agreement of July 1989 the US in Jan. 1990 began the phased immigration of some 94,000 families of former South Vietnamese soldiers and officials.

In 1990 some 70,000 persons emigrated (in 1989, 45,000; in 1988, 25,000). (For previous details *see* THE STATESMAN'S YEAR-BOOK, 1981–82). Between April 1975 and Aug. 1984 554,000 illegal emigrants ('boat people') succeeded in finding refuge abroad. In June 1988 the UK announced that Hong Kong would no longer accept 'boat people' who were not proven political refugees. In Feb. 1989, Vietnam agreed to accept their return but not their enforced repatriation, and a voluntary repatriation programme under the aegis of the UN High Commissioner of Refugees began. By Oct. 1989 there were 57,000 'boat people' in camps in Hong Kong, and the UK government announced it would embark on a programme of mandatory repatriation of up to 40,000 of them, giving each a resettlement allowance worth US$620. 51 persons were repatriated on 12 Dec. 1989, but the programme was then suspended. A meeting of the UN-sponsored Comprehensive Plan of Action for Indochinese Refugees in Jan. 1990 failed to agree a new repatriation programme, but in Sept. 1990 Vietnam, the UK and the UN High Commissioner for Refugees agreed on the repatriation of 'boat people' who had not volunteered, but were 'not opposed', to going home.

CLIMATE. The humid monsoon climate gives tropical conditions in the south and sub-tropical conditions in the north, though real winter conditions can affect the north when polar air blows south over Asia. In general, there is little variation in temperatures over the year. Hanoi. Jan. 62°F (16·7°C), July 84°F (28·9°C). Annual rainfall 72" (1,830 mm).

CONSTITUTION AND GOVERNMENT. A new Constitution was adopted in Dec. 1980. It states that Vietnam is a state of proletarian dictatorship and is developing according to Marxism–Leninism.

At the elections for the National Assembly held on 19 April 1987, 829 candidates stood and 496 were elected. Turn-out of voters was said to be 99·32%.

'The standing organ of the National Assembly and presidium of the Republic' is the State Council:

President (titular head of state): Vo Chi Cong. *Vice-Presidents:* Nguyen Huu Tho, Le Quang Do, Nguyen Quyet, Dam Quang Trung, Huynh Tan Phat, Mrs Nguyen Thi Dinh.

Chairman of the National Assembly: Le Quang Do.

All political power stems from the Communist Party of Vietnam (until Dec. 1976 known as the Workers' Party of Vietnam), founded in 1930; it had 2m. members in 1991. Its Politburo in Feb. 1991 consisted of Nguyen Van Linh *(First Secretary)*; Vo Chi Cong; Do Muoi *(Prime Minister)*; Vo Van Kiet; Le Duc Anh *(Minister of Defence)*; Nguyen Duc Tam; Nguyen Co Thach *(Deputy Prime Minister and Foreign Minister)*; Dong Si Nguyen *(Deputy Prime Minister)*; Nguyen Thanh Binh; Dao Duy Tung; Doan Khue; Mai Chi Tho *(Minister of the Interior)*. Ministers not in the Politburo include: Vo Nguyen Giap *(Deputy Prime Minister)*; Doan Duy Than *(Foreign Trade)*; Hoang Quy *(Finance)*; Tran Hoan *(Information)*, Pham Van Kai *(Chairman, State Planning Commission)*.

There were 2 puppet parties, the Democratic (founded 1944) and the Socialist (1946), which were unified with the trade and youth unions in the Fatherland Front. The Democratic Party was wound up in Oct. 1988.

National flag: Red, with a yellow 5-pointed star in the centre.

National anthem: 'Tien quan ca' ('The troops are advancing').

Local government is administered by people's councils, which appoint executive committees. Local elections were held with the National Assembly elections in April 1987.

DEFENCE. Men between 18 and 35 and women between 18 and 25 are liable for conscription of 3 years, specialists 4 years.

Army. The Army consists of 62 infantry, 3 mechanized, 8 engineer and 10 to 16 economic construction divisions, 10 armoured, 10 field artillery and 20 independent engineer brigades, and 15 independent infantry regiments. Equipment includes some 1,600 T-34/-54/-55 and Chinese Type-59 main battle and PT-76 and Chinese Type-62/63 light tanks. Strength was (1991) about 0·9m. Paramilitary forces are the Peoples' Defence Force (500,000), local forces of some 2·6m. and a tactical rear force of 500,000. In 1990 some 10-15,000 troops were still stationed in Laos but forces were withdrawn from Cambodia.

Navy. The equipment of the navy derives from two sources: ex-US equipment transferred to South Vietnam before or during the war, and ex-Soviet equipment transferred to North Vietnam during the war, or after unification in 1975. The latter is in general newer, and benefits from Soviet technical and logistic support in return for use of the main naval base at Cam Ranh Bay.

The fleet currently includes 5 ex-Soviet 'Petya' class frigates, 2 ex-US frigates (built 1943 and 1944), 8 Soviet-built fast missile craft, 16 fast torpedo craft, 5 patrol hydrofoils, 2 offshore and at least 30 inshore patrol craft, 3 coastal and 2 inshore minesweepers, 7 landing ships, and some 20 smaller amphibious craft. There may additionally still exist a proportion of the inshore fleet of 24 patrol craft, 25 coastguard cutters and over 350 riverine craft abandoned by the USA in 1975, but the continued operability of more than a few of these must be considered doubtful.

In 1990 personnel were estimated to number 13,000 plus an additional Naval Infantry force of 27,000.

Air Force. The Air Force, built up with Soviet and Chinese assistance, had (1991) about 12,000 personnel and 250 combat aircraft and 37 armed helicopters (plus many stored), including modern US types captured in war. There are reported to be 3 squadrons of variable-geometry MiG-23s, 6 squadrons of MiG-17s and Su-20s, over 150 MiG-21 interceptors; An-2, Li-2, C-47, An-24, An-26 and Il-14 transports; and a strong helicopter force with UH-1 Iroquois, Mi-6, Mi-8 and Mi-24 helicopters. 'Guideline', 'Goa' and 'Gainful' missiles are operational in large numbers.

INTERNATIONAL RELATIONS

Membership. Vietnam is a member of the UN, OIEC and IMF.

ECONOMY

Policy. Long-term forward planning gives priority to self-sufficiency in agriculture and stimulating regional industry. The fourth 5-year plan covered 1986–90. (For previous plans *see* THE STATESMAN'S YEAR-BOOK, 1985–86.).

Curtailment of Western aid, and resistance to Government measures have contributed to a shortage of consumer goods and widespread malnutrition. Small family businesses were legalized in 1986, and a law of April 1991 sanctions and protects all private business.

Reforms injecting free enterprise principles and reducing central control have been implemented.

The 'Draft Strategy for Socio-Economic Stabilization and Development to 2000' aims to double GDP through the 'socialist-oriented commodity economy, a market economy under state management' in which the state and collective sectors will play a 'predominant role'.

Currency. The unit of currency is the *dong* (VND). A currency reform of 14 Sept.

1985 substituted a new *dong* at a rate of 1 new *dong* = 10 (old) *dong*. Notes are issued for 1, 2, 5, 10, 20, 50, 100 and 500 *dong*. (For former currency *see* THE STATESMAN'S YEAR-BOOK, 1985–86). In a currency reform of March 1989 the *dong* was brought into line with free market rates. Inflation was 700% in 1988, but was significantly reduced in 1989. It was officially claimed to be 3·9% in Nov. 1990. In March 1991 £1 = 13,758 *dong*; US$1 = 7,253 *dong*.

Banking and Finance. The bank of issue is the National Bank of Vietnam (founded in 1951). There is also a Bank for Foreign Trade (Vietcombank). Some French banks are operating, and the Standard Chartered Bank has a representative office in Ho Chi Minh City. There were 7 foreign banks in 1991.

ENERGY AND NATURAL RESOURCES

Electricity. In 1988, 6,300m. kwh. of electricity were produced. A hydro-electric power station with a capacity of 2m. kw. was opened at Hoa-Binh in 1989.

Minerals. North Vietnam is rich in anthracite, lignite and hard coal: Total reserves are estimated at 20,000m. tonnes. Anthracite production in 1975 was 5m. tonnes. Coal production was 5·3m. tonnes in 1980. There are deposits of iron ore, manganese, titanium, chromite, bauxite and a little gold. Reserves of apatite are some of the biggest in the world. Offshore exploration for oil near Da Nang started in 1989. Crude oil production was 750,000 tonnes in 1988; 1990 estimate, 2.48m. tonnes.

Agriculture. In 1985, 62% of the population was engaged in agriculture. In 1984 there were some 23,000 production collectives and 268 agricultural co-operatives in the South accounting for 47% of the cultivated area. The intemperate collectivization of agriculture in the South after 1977 had disastrous effects which the Government tried to rectify by allowing peasants small private plots and the right to market some produce. These measures had only limited success, and in 1989 the Government abandoned virtually all its controls on the production and sale of agricultural produce, and switched to encouraging the household as the basic production unit. There were 105 state farms employing in all 70,000 workers and with 55,000 hectares arable and 50,000 hectares of pasture. The cultivated area in 1980 was 6·97m. ha (5·54m. ha for rice). Rice cultivation was deregulated in 1989. The 1990 harvest fell below 1989 through lack of fertilizer.

Production in 1,000 tonnes in 1988: Rice (15,200), soybeans (100), tea (35), rubber (61), maize (580), tobacco (40), potatoes (350), sweet potatoes (2,100) from 400,000 ha, sorghum (55) from 37,000 ha, dry beans (105) from 63,000 ha, coffee (14). Cereals production was 15,835,000m. tonnes in 1988. Other crops include sugar-cane and cotton.

Livestock (1988): Cattle 2,923,000; pigs, 12,051,000; goats, 414,000; poultry, 96m.

Animal products, 1988: Eggs, 171,000 tonnes, meat, 884,000 tonnes.

Forestry. There were (1988) 13m. ha of forest, representing 40% of the land area. 1,626,000 cu. metres of timber were produced in 1980.

Fisheries. Fishing is important, especially in Halong Bay. In 1976, 6m. tonnes of sea fish and 180,000 tonnes of freshwater fish were caught.

INDUSTRY. Next to mining, food processing and textiles are the most important industries; there is also some machine building. Older industries include cement, cotton and silk manufacture.

Private businesses were taken over in 1978. Foreign firms, principally French, are continuing to function, but all US property has been nationalized. There is little heavy industry. Most industry is concentrated in the Ho-Chi-Minh area.

Production (1980, in 1,000 tonnes) iron, 125; steel, 106; sulphuric acid, 6,700; caustic soda, 4,500; mineral fertilizer, 260; pesticides, 18,400; paper, 54,000; sugar, 94,000, cement, 705. 1,500 tractors were built in 1980, and 621 railway coaches. Footwear production, 200,000 pairs. Beer, 942,000 hectolitres.

Labour. Average wage (1984) 200 dong per month. Workforce (1985) 28·76m., of whom 17·91m. were in agriculture. There were some 3m. unemployed in 1990.

FOREIGN ECONOMIC RELATIONS. The EEC established relations in Oct. 1990. A US$1,000m. trade and co-operation agreement was signed with the USSR in Jan. 1991. The USSR supplies petroleum, steel, cotton and fertilizer in exchange for rubber, crude oil, rice, tea, coffee, meat, fruit and vegetables. In 1989 Vietnam's total indebtedness was estimated at US$9,000m (US$2,000m. to the West). In 1978 the IMF approved a virtually interest-free loan of US$90m. repayable over 50 years, but in April 1985 suspended all further credits to Vietnam. Sweden gives annual aid of US$47m. A law of Jan. 1988 regulates joint ventures with Western firms; full repatriation of profits and non-nationalization of investments are guaranteed. Offices may be opened in Vietnam.

Commerce. The USSR and Japan are Vietnam's main trading partners; others are Singapore and Hong Kong. Main exports are coal, farm produce, sea produce and livestock. Imports: Oil, steel, artificial fertilizers. Following the removal of rice cultivation from state control, Vietnam moved from being a net importer of rice to the world's third largest exporter in 1989. Rice exports in 1990 were some 1·7m. tonnes.

Trade between Vietnam and UK (British Department of Trade returns, in £1,000 sterling):

	1987	*1988*	*1989*	*1990*
Imports to UK	357	492	1,711	1,443
Exports and re-exports from UK	2,598	2,213	4,108	5,802

Tourism. Since 1988 Vietnamese have been permitted to travel abroad for up to 3 months for various specific reasons. Group travel to Communist countries has also been authorized.

COMMUNICATIONS

Roads. In 1986 there were about 65,000 km of roads described as 'main roads'.

Railways. Route length was 4,200 km in 1986. The Hanoi–Ho Chi Minh City line is being rebuilt in a programme of reconstruction and extension. About 50m. passengers and 10m. tonnes of freight are carried annually.

Aviation. Air Vietnam operates internal services from Hanoi to Ho Chi Minh City, Cao Bang, Na Son and Dien Bien, Vinh and Hue, and from Ho Chi Minh City to Ban Me Thuot and Da Nang, Can Tho, Con Son Island and Quan Long and from Hanoi to Bangkok in conjunction with Thai Airways. Aeroflot (USSR) operate regular services from Ho Chi Min City to Moscow and from Hanoi to Moscow, Rangoon and Vientiane, Interflug (German Dem. Rep.) to Berlin, Moscow and Dhaka, Philippine Airlines to Manila, and Air France to Paris.

Shipping. In 1986 there were 150 ships totalling 338,668 GRT. The major ports are Haiphong, which can handle ships of 10,000 tons, Ho Chi Minh City and Da Nang, and there are ports at Hong Gai and Haiphong Ben Thuy. There are regular services to Hong Kong, Singapore, Cambodia and Japan. In 1987 there were some 6,000 km of navigable waterways.

Cargo is handled by the Vietnam Ocean Shipping Agency; other matters by the Vietnam Foreign Trade Transport Corporation.

Telecommunications. In 1984 there were 6m. radios. There were 106,100 telephones in 1984. There were 2·25m. TV sets in 1984.

Cinemas and theatres. 116 films were produced in 1980 (including 10 full-length). There were 145 theatres.

Newspapers and books. The Party daily is *Nhan Dan* ('The People') circulation, 1985: 500,000. The official daily in the South is *Giai Phong*. Two unofficial dailies, *Cong Giao Va Dan Toc* (Catholic) and *Tin Sang* (independent) are also published. 2,564 books were published in 1980 totalling 90·9m. copies.

JUSTICE, RELIGION, EDUCATION AND WELFARE

Justice. A new penal code came into force 1 Jan. 1986 'to complete the work of the 1980 Constitution'. Penalties (including death) are prescribed for opposition to the people's power, and for economic crimes. There are the Supreme People's Court, local people's courts and military courts. The president of the Supreme Court is responsible to the National Assembly, as is the Procurator-General, who heads the Supreme People's Office of Supervision and Control.

Religion. Taoism is the traditional religion but Buddhism is widespread. At a Conference for Buddhist Reunification in Nov. 1981, 9 sects adopted a charter for a new Buddhist church under the Council of Sangha. The Hoa Hao sect, associated with Buddhism, claimed 1·5m. adherents in 1976. Caodaism, a synthesis of Christianity, Buddhism and Confucianism founded in 1926, has some 2m. followers. There are some 6m. Roman Catholics (mainly in the south). There is an Archbishopric of Hanoi and 13 bishops. There were 2 seminaries in 1989. In 1983 the Government set up a Solidarity Committee of Catholic Patriots. In Aug. 1988 the Government announced that all Catholic priests had been released from re-education camps, but were not yet permitted to resume their duties.

Education. Primary education consists of a 10-year course divided into 3 levels of 4, 3 and 3 years respectively. There were 500,000 teachers in 1988. Numbers of pupils and students in 1980–81: Nurseries, 2·66m.; primary schools, 12·1m.; complementary education, 2·19m.; vocational secondary education, 130,000. In 1980–81 there were 92,913 nurseries. There were 11,400 schools and 280 vocational secondary schools, with 357,000 and 13,000 teachers respectively.

In 1980–81 there were 83 institutions of higher education (including 3 universities: (Hanoi, Ho Chi Minh City, Central Highlands University at Ban Me Thuot), 13 industrial colleges, 7 agricultural colleges, 5 economics colleges, 9 teacher-training colleges, 7 medical schools and 3 art schools, in all with 16,000 teachers and 159,000 students. In 1981 there were 5,000 Vietnamese studying in the USSR.

Health. In 1975 there were 1,996 hospitals and dispensaries and 93 sanatoria. There were some 13,517 doctors and dentists in 1981 and 197,000 hospital beds.

DIPLOMATIC REPRESENTATIVES

Of Vietnam in Great Britain (12–14 Victoria Rd., London, W8)
Ambassador: Chau Phong (accredited 14 March 1990).

Of Great Britain in Vietnam (16 Pho Ly Thuong Kiet, Hanoi)
Ambassador: Peter Williams.

Of Vietnam to the United Nations
Ambassador: Trinh Xuan Lang.

Further Reading

Beresford, M., *National Unification and Economic Development in Vietnam*. London, 1989
Bui Phung, *Vietnamese-English Dictionary*. Hanoi, 1987
Chen, J. H.-M., *Vietnam: A Comprehensive Bibliography*. London, 1973
Dellinger, D., *Vietnam Revisited*. Boston (Mass.), 1986
Fforde, A., *The Limits of National Liberation: Problems of Economic Management in the Democratic Republic of Vietnam*. London, 1987
Harrison, J. P., *The Endless War: Fifty Years of Struggle in Vietnam*. New York, 1982
Higgins, H., *Vietnam*. 2nd ed. London, 1982
Ho Chi Minh, *Selected Writings, 1920–1969*. Hanoi, 1977
Hodgkin, T., *Vietnam: The Revolutionary Path:* London, 1981
Houtart, F., *Hai Van: Life in a Vietnamese Commune*. London, 1984
Karnow, S., *Vietnam: A History*. New York, 1983
Lawson, E. K., *The Sino-Vietnamese Conflict*. New York, 1984
Leitenberg, M. and Burns, R. D., *War in Vietnam*. 2nd ed. Oxford and Santa Barbara, 1982
Nguyen Tien Hung, C., *Economic Developments of Socialist Vietnam, 1955–80*. New York, 1977
Nguyen Van Canh, *Vietnam under Communism, 1975–1982*. Stanford Univ. Press, 1983
Post, K., *Revolution, Socialism and Nationalism in Vietnam*. vol. 1. Aldershot, 1989
Smith, R. B., *An International History of the Vietnam War*. London, 1983
Truong Nhu Tang, *Journal of a Vietcong*. London, 1986

BRITISH VIRGIN ISLANDS

Capital: Road Town
Population: 14,786 (1990)
GNP per capita: US$10,000 (1989)

HISTORY. The Virgin Islands were discovered by Columbus on his second voyage in 1493. The British Virgin Islands were first settled by the Dutch in 1648 and taken over in 1666 by a group of English planters. In 1774 constitutional government was granted. The Islands became a self-governing dependent territory of the UK in 1967.

AREA AND POPULATION. The British Virgin Islands form the eastern extremity of the Greater Antilles and, exclusive of small rocks and reefs, number 40, of which 15 are inhabited. The largest, with population (estimate, 1990), are Tortola, 12,533), Virgin Gorda, 1,283, Anegada, 192 and Jost Van Dyke, 157. Other islands in the group have a total population of 183; Marine population (estimate 1989), 124. Total area about 59 sq. miles (130 sq. km); population (1990, estimate), 14,786. Road Town, on the south-east of Tortola, is a port of entry; population (estimate 1990), 4,049.

CLIMATE. A pleasantly healthy sub-tropical climate with summer temperatures lowered by sea breezes. Nights are cool and rainfall averages 50" (1,250 mm).

CONSTITUTION AND GOVERNMENT. In 1950 representative government was introduced and in 1967 a new Constitution was granted (amended 1977). The Governor is responsible for defence and internal security, external affairs, the public service, and the courts. The Executive Council consists of the Governor, 1 *ex-officio* member who is the Attorney-General and 4 ministers in the Legislature. The Legislative Council consists of 1 *ex-officio* member who is the Attorney-General and 9 elected members, one of whom is the Chief Minister and Minister of Finance; the Speaker is elected from outside the Council.

Governor: J. Mark Herdman, LVO.
Chief Minister: H. Lavity Stoutt (Virgin Islands Party); elected in 1988.
Flag: The British Blue Ensign with the arms of the Territory in the fly.

INTERNATIONAL RELATIONS

Membership. The Islands are a member of CARICOM.

ECONOMY

Budget. In 1989 revenue (estimate) was US$41,400,000; expenditure, US$33,303,423.000.

Currency. The unit of currency is the US dollar.

Banking and Finance. Bank of Nova Scotia, Barclays Bank PLC, Chase Manhattan Bank NA, Royal Trust Company Ltd, First Pennsylvania Bank NA and Guyerzeller Bank (BVI) Ltd hold General Banking Licences and had total deposits of US$284·7m. at 31 Dec. 1989. 7 institutions hold restricted banking licences and there are a large number of trust companies providing financial services other than banking. Financial services are the most important industry after tourism.

ENERGY AND NATURAL RESOURCES

Electricity. Production, 1989, 46·5m. kwh.

Agriculture. Agricultural production is limited, with the chief products being livestock (including poultry), fish, fruit and vegetables. Production, 1989, in tonnes (value in US$1,000): Fruits, 623 (670·0); vegetables/root crop, 87 (174·9);

beef, 188 (676·8); mutton, 14 (112); pork, 8·5 (29·8); and 1,250 cases of eggs (93·8). In 1989 the Agriculture Department was extended to include an abattoir.

Livestock (1989): Cattle, 3,500; pigs, 3,000; sheep, 650 and goats, 12,000.

INDUSTRY. The construction industry is a significant employer.

FOREIGN ECONOMIC RELATIONS

Commerce. There is a very small export trade almost entirely with the Virgin Islands of the USA. In 1987 imports were US$77·3m. and exports US$3·1m.

Total trade between the British Virgin Islands and UK (British Department of Trade returns, in £1,000 sterling):

	1987	*1988*	*1989*	*1990*
Imports to UK	752	4,030	1,170	1,205
Exports and re-exports from UK	3,310	7,108	6,727	4,454

Tourism. Tourism is the most important industry and accounts for some 75% of GDP. There were 287,953 visitors in 1989, visitors spent US$124·7m.

COMMUNICATIONS

Roads. There were (1989) over 102 miles of roads and 5,489 licensed vehicles.

Aviation. Beef Island Airport, about 16 km from Road Town, is capable of receiving 80-seat short-take-off-and-landing jet aircraft. Air BVI operates internal flights and external flights to San Juan (main route), Puerto Rico; the USVI, Antiqua, Dominica, Dominion Republic and St Kitts. Other services to the BVI are Eastern Metro Express, LIAT and American Eagle.

Shipping. There are services to Europe, the USA and other Caribbean islands, and daily services by motor launches to the US Virgin Islands.

Telecommunications. There were (1990) nearly 6,291 telephones , 43 telex subscribers, 90 facsimile machine subscribers and an external telephone service links Tortola with Bermuda and the rest of the world. Radio ZBVI transmits 10,000 watts and British Virgin Islands Cable TV operates a cable system of 19 television channels.

RELIGION, EDUCATION AND WELFARE

Religion. There are Anglican, Methodist, Seventh-Day Adventist, Roman Catholic, Baptist Churches and other Christian churches in the Territory. The Jehovah's Witnesses are also represented.

Education. Primary education is provided in 16 government schools, three with secondary divisions, and 12 private schools. Total number of pupils (Dec. 1989) 1,912.

Secondary education to the GCE level and Caribbean Examination Council level is provided by the BVI High School and the secondary divisions of the schools on Virgin Gorda and Anegada. Total number of secondary level pupils (Dec. 1989) 1,147.

Government expenditure, 1989 (estimate), US$5m. In 1989 the total number of teachers in all Government schools was 113. In 1986 a branch of the Hull University (England) School of Education was established.

Health. In 1990 there were 14 doctors, 67 nurses, 50 public hospital beds and 1 private hospital with 10 beds. Expenditure, 1990 (estimate) was US$5·5m.

Further Reading

Economic Review 1987 – British Virgin Islands. Development Planning Unit, 1987
Dookham, I., *A History of the British Virgin Islands*. Epping, 1975
Harrigan, N. and Varlack, P., *British Virgin Islands: A Chronology*. London, 1971
Pickering, V. W., *Early History of the British Virgin Islands*. London, 1983

Library: Public Library, Road Town. *Librarian:* Bernadine Louis

WESTERN SAMOA

Capital: Apia
Population: 163,000 (1986)
GNP per capita: US$580 (1988)

Samoa i Sisifo—Independent State of Western Samoa

HISTORY. Western Samoa, a former German protectorate (1899–1914), was administered by New Zealand from 1920 to 1961, at first under a League of Nations Mandate and from 1946 under a UN Trusteeship Agreement. In May 1961 a plebiscite held under the supervision of the UN on the basis of universal adult suffrage voted overwhelmingly in favour of independence as from 1 Jan. 1962, on the basis of the Constitution, which a Constitutional Convention had adopted in Aug. 1960. In Oct. 1961 the UN General Assembly passed a resolution to terminate the trusteeship agreement as from 1 Jan. 1962, on which date Western Samoa became an independent sovereign state.

AREA AND POPULATION. Western Samoa lies between 13° and 15° S. lat. and 171° and 173° W. long. It comprises the two large islands of Savai'i and Upolu, the small islands of Manono and Apolima, and several uninhabited islets lying off the coast. The total land area is 1,093 sq. miles (2,830·8 sq. km), of which 659·4 sq. miles (1,707·8 sq. km) are in Savai'i, and 431·5 sq. miles (1,117·6 sq. km) in Upolu; other islands, 2·1 sq. miles (5·4 sq. km). The islands are of volcanic origin, and the coasts are surrounded by coral reefs. Rugged mountain ranges form the core of both main islands and rise to 3,608 ft in Upolu and 6,094 ft in Savai'i. The large area laid waste by lava-flows in Savai'i is a primary cause of that island supporting less than one-third of the population of the islands despite its greater size than Upolu.

The population at the 1981 census was 158,130, of whom 114,980 were in Upolu (including Manono and Apolima) and 43,150 in Savai'i. The capital and chief port is Apia in Upolu (population 33,170 in 1981). Estimate (1986) 163,000.

CLIMATE. A tropical marine climate, with cooler conditions from May to Nov. and a rainy season from Dec. to April. The rainfall is unevenly distributed, with south and east coasts having the greater quantities. Average annual rainfall is about 100" (2,500 mm) in the drier areas. Apia. Jan. 80°F (26·7°C), July 78°F (25·6°C). Annual rainfall 112" (2,800 mm).

CONSTITUTION AND GOVERNMENT. HH Malietoa Tanumafili II is the sole Head of State for life. Future Heads of State will be elected by the Legislative Assembly and hold office for 5-year terms.

The executive power is vested in the *Head of State*, who swears in the Prime Minister (who is appointed by members of the Legislative Assembly) and, on the Prime Minister's advice, the 8 Ministers to form the Cabinet.

The *Legislative Assembly* has 45 members elected from territorial constituencies on a franchise confined to matais or chiefs (of whom there were about 15,000 in 1988) and 2 members elected by universal adult suffrage from the individual voters roll. The Constitution also provides for a *Council of Deputies* of 3 members, of whom the chairman is the Deputy Head of State. In the elections held Feb. 1985, the Human Rights Protection Party won 31 seats.

The official languages are Samoan and English.

Head of State: HH Malietoa Tanumafili II, GCMG, CBE.
Deputy Head of State: Mataafa Faasuamaleaui Puela.

The cabinet in Feb. 1991 was composed as follows:

Prime Minister, Minister of Foreign Affairs, Internal Affairs, Broadcasting, Justice, Police and Prisons, Attorney General: Tofilau Eti Alesana. *Finance:* Tuilaepa Sailele. *Agriculture, Forests and Fisheries:* Pule Lameko. *Economic Affairs:* Tanuvasa Livigisitone. *Health:* Polataivao Fosi. *Education:* Patu Afaese. *Post Office and Telecommunications:* Jack Netzler. *Public Works:* Leia'taua Vaiao. *Lands and Survey:* Sifuiva Sione.

National flag: Red with a blue quarter bearing 5 white stars of the Southern Cross.

INTERNATIONAL RELATIONS. Under a treaty of friendship of 1962 New Zealand acts as the channel of communication between the Samoan Government and governments and international organizations outside the Pacific islands area. Liaison is maintained by the New Zealand High Commissioner in Apia.

Membership. Western Samoa is a member of the UN, the Commonwealth, the South Pacific Forum and is an ACP state of the EEC.

ECONOMY

Budget. In 1989 budgeted revenue was $WS101·7m.; expenditure, $WS81·6m.

Currency. The unit of currency is the *tala* (WST) of 100 *sene*. In March 1991, £1 = 4.33; US$1 = 2·28.

Banking and Finance. A Central Bank was established in 1984. In 1959 the Bank of Western Samoa was established with a capital of $WS500,000, of which $WS275,000 was subscribed by the Bank of New Zealand and $WS225,000 by the Government of Western Samoa. In 1977 the Pacific Commercial Bank was established jointly by Australia's Bank of New South Wales and the Bank of Hawaii.

ENERGY AND NATURAL RESOURCES

Electricity. Production (1986) 79m. kwh.

Agriculture. The main products (1988, in 1,000 tonnes) are coconuts (200), taro (40), copra (14), bananas (23), papayas (12), mangoes (6), pineapples (6) and cocoa beans (1).

Livestock (1988): Horses, 3,000; cattle, 27,000; pigs, 65,000; poultry 1m.

Fisheries. The total catch (1983) was 3,150 tonnes, valued at $WS5·1m.

INDUSTRY. Some industrial activity is being developed associated with agricultural products and forestry.

FOREIGN ECONOMIC RELATIONS

Commerce. In 1985, imports were valued at $WS115,074,000 and exports at $WS36,195,000. Principal exports were coconut oil (10,926 tonnes; $WS15,622,000), cocoa (581 tons; $WS2,356,000), taro (22,000 cases, $WS5,113,000), coconut cream ($WS2,833,000); fruit juice ($WS1,002,000); beer ($WS385,000) and cigarettes ($WS5,558,000). Chief imports in 1983 included food and live animals ($WS15,195,000), beverages and tobacco ($WS1,913,000), machinery and transport equipment ($WS14,968,000), mineral fuels, lubricants and other materials ($WS13,133,000), chemicals ($WS4,221,000) and miscellaneous manufactured articles ($WS5,279,000).

Total trade between Western Samoa and UK (British Department of Trade returns, in £1,000 sterling):

	1986	*1987*	*1988*	*1989*	*1990*
Imports to UK	622	531	1,323	1,376	295
Exports and re-exports from UK	433	1,650	757	296	427

Tourism. There were 49,710 visitors in 1986.

COMMUNICATIONS

Roads (1987). Western Samoa has 2,085 km of roads, 400 km of which are surfaced and 1,200 km plantation roads fit for light traffic. In 1984 there were 1,498 private cars, 1,909 pick-up trucks, 398 trucks, 187 buses, 297 taxis and 144 motor cycles.

Aviation. Western Samoa is linked by daily air service with American Samoa, which is on the route of the weekly New Zealand–Tahiti and New Zealand–Honolulu air services, with connexions to Fiji, Australia, USA and Europe. There are also services throughout the week to and from Tonga, Fiji, Nauru, the Cook Islands and New Zealand. Internal services link Upolu and Savai'i.

Shipping. Western Samoa is linked to Japan, USA, Europe, Fiji, Australia and New Zealand by regular shipping services.

Telecommunications. There is a radio communication station at Apia. Radio telephone service connects Western Samoa with American Samoa, Fiji, New Zealand, Australia, Canada, USA and UK. Telephone subscribers numbered 3,641 in 1984. In 1982 there were 70,000 radio receivers and about 2,500 television sets.

Cinemas. In 1989 there were 2 cinemas.

Newspapers. In 1985, there were 4 weeklies, circulation 12,000 and 2 monthlies (8,000); all were in Samoan and English.

RELIGION, EDUCATION AND WELFARE

Religion. In 1981, 47% of the population were Congregationalists, 22% Roman Catholic and 16% Methodist.

Education. In 1986 the total number of pupils in primary, junior and secondary schools was 51,940. The University of the South Pacific School of Agriculture is in Western Samoa. A National University was established in 1984.

Health. In 1988 there was 1 national hospital, 7 district hospitals, 9 health centres and 14 subcentres and 44 doctors.

DIPLOMATIC REPRESENTATIVES

Of Western Samoa in Great Britain
High Commissioner: Afamasaga Faamatala Toleafoa (resides in Brussels).

Of Great Britain in Western Samoa
High Commissioner: D. J. Moss, CMG (resides in Wellington)

Of the USA in Western Samoa
Ambassador: Della M. Newman (resides in Wellington).

Of Western Samoa in the USA and to the United Nations (1115 15th St., NW, Washington D.C. 20005)
Ambassador: Tuaopepe Fili Wendt.

Further Reading

Statistical Year-Book. Annual
Fox, J. W. (ed.) *Western Samoa.* Univ. of Auckland, 1963

YEMEN

Capital: Sana'a
Commercial capital: Aden
Population: 12m. (1990)
GNP per capita: US$540 (1988)

Jamhuriya al Yamaniya

(Republic of Yemen)

HISTORY. Following an agreement reached in Dec. 1989 on a constitution for a unified state, the (northern) Yemen Arab Republic and the (southern) People's Democratic Republic of Yemen were united as the Republic of Yemen on 22 May 1990. There were 25 opposition votes in the northern parliament, but none in the southern. For the pre-unification history of the two states, *see* THE STATEMAN'S YEAR-BOOK, 1990–91, p. 1596 and 1599.

AREA AND POPULATION. Yemen is bounded in the north by Saudi Arabia, east by Oman, south by the Gulf of Aden and west by the Red Sea. The territory includes the islands of Kamaran (181 sq. km) and Perim (300 sq. km) in the Red Sea and the island of Socotra (3,500 sq. km) in the Gulf of Aden. In the north the boundary between the Yemen and Saudi Arabia has been defined by the Treaty of Taif concluded in June 1934. This frontier starts from the sea at a point some 5 or 10 miles north of Maidi and runs due east inland until it reaches the hills some 30 miles from the coast, whence it runs northwards for approximately 50 miles so as to leave the Sa'da Basin within the Yemen. Thence it runs in an easterly and south-easterly direction until it reaches the desert area near Nejran. The area is about 531,000 sq. km with a population estimated at some 12m. in 1990. At the census of 1986 in the north the population was 8,105,974. There were 1,168,199 citizens working abroad mainly in Saudi Arabia and the United Arab Emirates not included in the census total. In 1990 Saudi Arabia began compulsory repatriation of Yemeni workers, then numbering some 1·5m. At the census of 1988 in the south the population was 2,345,266. The capital is Sana'a with a population of (1990) 0·5m. The commercial capital is the port of Aden, with a population of (1987) 417,366. Other important towns are the port of Hodeida (population, 155,110), Mukalla (154,360), Ta'iz (178,043), Ibb and Abyan.

CLIMATE. A desert climate, modified by relief. Sana'a. Jan. 57°F (13·9°C), July 71°F (21·7°C). Aden, Jan. 75°F (24°C), July 90°F (32°C). Annual rainfall 20" (508 mm) in the north, but very low in coastal areas: 1·8" (46 mm).

CONSTITUTION AND GOVERNMENT. The government is headed by a 5-member *Presidential Council*, of whom the chairman, Lieut.-Gen. Ali Abdullah Saleh (formerly President of the Arab Republic) was elected *President of the Republic* by a joint session of the Consultative Assembly of the Arab Republic and the Presidium of the Supreme People's Council of the People's Democratic Republic. The other members are Ali Salem Albidh (*Vice-President*), Abdulkarim Al-Arashy, Salem Saleh Muhammad and Abd Al-Aziz Abd Al-Ghani. The 301-member *General People's Congress* represents a merger of the former northern and southern assemblies. Multi-party elections by universal suffrage are due at the end of 1992. The new government (*Council of Ministers*) comprised 20 northerners and 19 southerners, and in Nov. 1990 included:.

Prime Minister: Haidar Abu-Bakr Al-Attas (formerly President of the People's Democratic Republic).

First Deputy Prime Minister: Hassan Mohd Maki. *Deputy Prime Ministers:* Brig.-Gen. Mugahed Yehya Abu-Shawarab *(reponsible for internal affairs)*, Brig.-Gen. Saleh Obeid (*security and defence*), Mohad Haiera Masdous (*development of the workforce and administrative reform*). *Minister of Construction and rehabilitation:*

Abdullah Hussein Al-Arashi. *Foreign Affairs:* Abdul Kareen Al-Iryani. *Emigrants' Affairs:* Brig.-Gen. Saleh Munsir Al-Saiyalli. *Industry:* Mohd Saeed Al-Attar. *Oil and Mineral Resources:* Saleh Abu-Bakr bin Husseinoon. *Supply and Trade:* Fadhle Mohsin Abdulla. *Local Government:* Mohd Saeed Abdulla. *Electricity and Water:* Abdul Wahab Mohmoud Abdul-Hameed. *Civil Service and Administrative reforms:* Mohd Khadam Al-Wajeah. *Planning and Development:* Farag bin Ghanem. *Communications:* Ahmed Mohd Al-Anasee. *Legal Affairs:* Ismaeal Ahemed Al-Wazeer. *Insurance and Social Affairs:* Ahmed Mohd Luqman. *Culture:* Hassan Ahmed Louzee. *Youth and Sport:* Mohd Ahmed Al-Kabab. *Education:* Mohd Abdulla Al-Gaifi. *Justice:* Abdul Wasa Sallam. *Information:* Mohd Ahmed Gurhoum. *Transport:* Saleh Abdulla Muthana. *Fish Resources:* Salem Mohd Gubran. *Housing and Planning:* Abdul Qawi Muthana Hadi. *Finance:* Arawee Assalami. *Health:* Mohd Ali Moqbil. *Agriculture and Water Resources:* Assadq Ameen Abu-Ras. *Tourism:* Mohmoud Abdulla Al-Arasee. *Interior and Security:* Col. Ghalib Muthar Al-Qamash. *Defence:* Brig. Hithem Qassam Tahar. *Labour:* Abdul Ruhman Dibyan. *Higher Education and Research:* Ahmed Salem Al-Qakhi.

National flag: Three horizontal stripes of red, white and black.

Local government: There are 11 provinces *(Liwa')* in the north: Sa'dah, Bayda, Sana'a, Hodeida, Hajjah, Jawf, Mahwit, Marib, Dhamar, Ibb and Ta'iz, and 6 governorates in the south: Aden, Lahej, Abyan, Shabwa, Hadhramaut and Mahra, divided into 30 provinces.

DEFENCE. Before the integration of the armies and air forces of the northern Arab Republic and the southern People's Democratic Republic, their strengths were:

Arab Republic:

Army. The Army consists of 3 armoured, 1 mechanized, 9 infantry, 2 para-commando, 1 Special Forces, 5 artillery brigades, 1 central guard force and 3 anti-aircraft artillery and 2 air defence battalions. Equipment includes 100 T-34, 480 T-54/-55, 20 T-62 and 64 M-60A1 main battle tanks. Strength (1989) 35,000.

Air Force. Built up with aid from both the USA and USSR, as well as Saudi Arabia, the Air Force is believed to be receiving many new Soviet aircraft. Current equipment includes 15 Su-22 fighter-bombers, 30 MiG-21 and 14 F-5 fighters, a total of 14 Il-14, An-12, An-24/26, C-130 Hercules and Skyvan transports, and over 30 Mi-8 and Agusta-Bell JetRanger and 212 helicopters. Personnel (1990) about 1,000.

People's Democratic Republic:

Army. The Army comprises 1 armoured, 3 mechanized, 9 infantry, 3 artillery, 2 rocket and 2 surface-to-surface missile brigades and 10 artillery battalions. Equipment includes 480 T-34/-54/-55/-62 main battle tanks. Strength (1990) about 24,000.

Air Force. Formed in 1967, the Air Force is now equipped mainly with aircraft of Soviet design. It has received about 40 MiG-21 fighters, 30 MiG-17 and 25 MiG-23 fighter-bombers, 30 Su-22 attack aircraft, 15 Mi-24 gunship helicopters, 4 An-24 and 2 An-26 twin-turboprop transports and about 30 Mi-8 and 5 Mi-4 helicopters. Personnel (1990) about 2,500.

Navy. No information is yet available on the outcome of the amalgamation of the navies of the two parts of the new republic. The North Yemen flotilla numbered about 500 at amalgamation and operated 3 US-built and 5 Soviet-built inshore patrol craft, 3 Soviet-built inshore minehunters and 4 small landing craft. The South Yemen navy, some 1,000 strong, comprised 6 fast missile craft, 2 fast torpedo craft, 1 tank landing ship, 4 medium landing ships and 5 small landing craft, all transferred from the Soviet Navy, and 5 boats. There is also a Soviet repair ship based in Aden, and a 4,500 tonne capacity floating dock, but they are the property of the Soviet Navy.

INTERNATIONAL RELATIONS

Membership. Yemen is a member of the UN and the Arab League.

ECONOMY

Policy. Development planning in the Arab Republic provided for investment of US$3,776m. (40% foreign aid), and concentrates principally on agricultural development; in the People's Democratic Republic expenditure of 998·2m. dinars was envisaged in the period 1986–91.

Budget. The Arab Republic's budget for 1989 provided for expenditure of 20,789m. riyals and revenue of 16,041m. riyals; that of the People's Democratic Republic, revenue of 354·3m. dinars and expenditure of 471·5m. dinars.

Currency. During the transitional period the northern *riyal* of 100 *fils* and the southern *dinar* of 1,000 *fils* coexist. In March 1991, 22·87 *riyal* = £1 and 12·05 *riyal* = US$1; 0·87 *dinars* = £1 and 0·46 *dinars* = US$1.

ENERGY AND NATURAL RESOURCES

Electricity. Production (1986) 556m. kwh.

Oil and Gas. The first large-scale oilfield and pipeline was inaugurated in 1987. There are reserves of 2,000m. bbls on the former north-south border. Production (1989) 10·85m. tonnes. Gas reserves are some 7,000m. cu. metres.

Minerals. The only commercial mineral being exploited is salt and (1985) production was 169,000 tons. Reserves (estimate) 25m. tonnes.

Agriculture. In the north, of a total area of 19·5m. ha, 1·3m. are arable or permanent crops. Cotton is grown in the Tihama, the coastal belt, round Bait al Faqih and Zabid. Fruit is plentiful, especially fine grapes from the Sana'a district. Production (1988, in 1,000 tonnes): Sorghum, 542; potatoes, 117; grapes, 133; dates, 15; wheat, 132; barley, 48; maize, 53.

In the south, agriculture is the main occupation of the people. This is largely of a subsistence nature, sorghum, sesame and millet being the chief crops, and wheat and barley widely grown at the higher elevations. Of increasing importance, however, are the cash crops which have been developed since the Second World War, by far the most important of which is the Abyan long-staple cotton.

Owing to the meagre rainfall, cultivation is largely confined to fertile valleys and flood plains on silt, built up and irrigated in the traditional manner. These traditional methods are being augmented and replaced by the use of modern earth moving machinery and pumps. Irrigation schemes with permanent installations are in progress. Production (1988, in tonnes): Wheat, 8,800; cotton, 2,200; sesame, 1,400; millet (1987), 17,683; maize, 3,439.

Livestock in 1988 (in 1,000): Cattle, 1,150; camels, 144; sheep, 3,612; goats, 3,136; poultry, 25,000.

Fisheries. Fishing is a major industry. Total catch (1986) 113,500 tonnes, catch in the south (1988), 80,600 tonnes.

INDUSTRY. There is very little industry. There are textile factories, and plastic, rubber and aluminium goods, and paint and matches are produced.

FOREIGN ECONOMIC RELATIONS

Commerce. Cotton and fish are major exports, the largest imports being food and live animals. A large transhipment and entrepôt trade is centred on Aden. Imports to the People's Democratic Republic were US$668m.; exports, US$2·2m.

Total trade between the former Arab Republic and the UK (British Department of Trade returns, in £1,000 sterling):

	1987	*1988*	*1989*	*1990*
Imports to UK	2,306	1,532	1,598	33,698
Exports and re-exports from UK	55,334	42,564	41,653	51,941

Total trade between the former People's Democratic Republic and the UK (British Department of Trade return, in £1,000 sterling):

	1987	*1988*	*1989*	*1990*
Imports to UK	1,056	1,827	5,029	2,540
Exports and re-exports from UK	28,271	20,862	17,246	18,889

Tourism. There were about 44,000 tourists in 1986.

COMMUNICATIONS

Roads. There were (1988) 39,200 km of roads, including 2,227 km of paved roads in the south, and 195,000 cars.

Aviation. There are 6 international airports: Seiyuun, Sana'a, Aden (Khormaksar), Mukalla (Riyan), Ta'iz and Hodeida. 6 airlines operate scheduled services: Air France, Middle East Airlines, Yemen Airlines, Aeroflot, Saudia and Air Djibouti.

Shipping. Because of its favourable geographical position and its efficient service to ships, Aden used to be one of the busiest oil-bunkering ports in the world, handling some 550 ships a month. There are 4 alongside berths and 1 ro-ro berth. In 1988 the port handled 1,900 ships. There are also ports at Hodeida, Mokha, Salif and Loheiya.

Telecommunications. There were about 70,000 telephones in 1988. In 1986 there were 94,000 television and 244,000 radio receivers.

JUSTICE, RELIGION, EDUCATION AND WELFARE

Justice. In the former People's Democratic Republic there was a Supreme Court and magistrate's courts. In some areas Islamic Law and common law are administered.

Religion. The population is predominantly Moslem of the Shi'ite Zaidi sect.

Education. In the Arab Republic there were (1985–86) 904,487 pupils at primary schools, 112,922 in secondary schools, and 11,616 at teacher-training establishments. In 1982 the University of Sana'a (founded in 1974) had 6,719 students. In the People's Democratic Republic there were (1987) 310,839 pupils attending 989 primary schools and 31,530 secondary school pupils attending 62 schools. A state university was founded in 1975 and the number of students is increasing. In 1985, 400,000 students were studying at schools at various levels.

Health. In 1986 there were 1,234 physicians and 60 hospitals and health centres with 5,986 beds in the north. In the south in 1988 there were 729 physicians and 32 hospitals with 3,372 beds.

DIPLOMATIC REPRESENTATIVES

Of Yemen in Great Britain (41 South St., London, W1Y 5PD)
Ambassador: Ahmed Abdo Rageh.

Of Great Britain in Yemen (129 Haddah Rd., Sana'a)
Ambassador: M. A. Marshall, CMG.

Of Yemen in the USA (600 New Hampshire Ave., NW, Washington, D.C., 20037)
Ambassador: (vacant).

Of the USA in Yemen (P.O. Box 1088, Sana'a)
Ambassador: Charles F. Dunbar.

Of Yemen to the United Nations
Ambassador: Abdalla Saleh Al-Ashtal.

Further Reading

Bidwell, R., *The Two Yemens*. Boulder and London, 1983
El Mallakh, R., *The Economic Development of the Yemen Arab Republic*. London, 1986
Ismael, T. Y. and Ismael, J. S., *The People's Democratic Republic of Yemen*. London, 1986
Peterson, J. E., *Yemen: The Search for a Modern State*. London, 1982
Smith, G. R., *The Yemens*. [Bibliography] Oxford and Santa Barbara, 1984
Thesiger, W., *Arabian Sands*. London, 1959

YUGOSLAVIA

Socijalistička Federativna Republika Jugoslavija

Capital: Belgrade
Population: 24·11m. (1990)
GNP per capita: US$2,680 (1988)

HISTORY. In 1917 the Yugoslav Committee in London drew up the Pact of Corfu, which proclaimed that all Yugoslavs would unite after the first world war to form a kingdom under the Serbian royal house. The Kingdom of Serbs, Croats and Slovenes was proclaimed on 1 Dec. 1918. In 1929 the name was changed to Yugoslavia. During the Second World War Tito's partisans set up a provisional government (AVNOJ) which was the basis of a Constituent Assembly after the war. On 29 Nov. 1945 Yugoslavia was proclaimed a republic.

The peace treaty with Italy, signed in Paris on 10 Feb. 1947, stipulated the cession to Yugoslavia of the greater part of the Italian province of Venezia Giulia, the commune of Zara and the island of Pelagosa and the adjacent islets.

By an agreement of 10 Nov. 1975 the city of Trieste ('Zone A') was recognized as Italian and the Adriatic coastal portion of the former Free Territory of Trieste ('Zone B') as Yugoslav. A free industrial zone was set up in the Fernetici–Sezana region on both sides of the frontier.

Dissensions in Kosovo between Albanians and Serbs, and in parts of Croatia between Serbs and Croats have brought inter-ethnic tensions into prominence since 1988. A government led by Ante Marković which took office in March 1989 has embarked on a radical programme of economic and political reform, but with the election of new national assemblies in all 6 republics during 1990, several of the latter came increasingly into conflict with the federal government. At the end of 1990 both Croatia and Slovenia proclaimed their right to secede from federal Yugoslavia. In Jan. 1991 the federal constitutional court ruled that Slovenia's declaration of independence, and Serbia's imposition of inter-republican tariffs, were illegal.

AREA AND POPULATION. Yugoslavia is bounded in the north by Austria and Hungary, north-east by Romania, east by Bulgaria, south by Greece and Albania, and west by the Adriatic Sea and Italy. There are 365 offshore islands in the Adriatic. The area is 255,804 sq. km. Population at the 1981 census: 22,424,711 (females, 11,340,933). Density, 87·7 per sq. km. Population estimate, 1990: 24,107,000.

Yugoslavia is a federation of 6 republics: Bosnia and Herzegovina (B), Croatia (C), Macedonia (Ma), Montenegro (Mo), Serbia (Se) and Slovenia (Sl); and 2 'autonomous provinces' within Serbia; Kosovo (K) and Vojvodina (V). For details *see* p. 1610. The federal capital is Belgrade (Beograd). Population (census, 1981) 1,470,073 and of other principal towns:

Banja Luka (B)	183,618	Priština (K)	210,040
Bitolj (Ma)	137,636	Prizren (K)	134,526
Čačak (Se)	110,676	Rijeka (C)	193,044
Čakovec (C)	116,825	Šabac (Se)	119,669
Gostivar (Ma)	101,028	Sarajevo (B)	448,519
Kragujevac (Se)	164,823	Skopje (Ma)	504,932
Kraljevo (Se)	121,622	Slavonski Brod (C)	106,400
Kruševac (Se)	132,972	Smederevo (Se)	107,366
Kumanovo (Ma)	126,188	Split (C)	180,571
Leskovac (Se)	159,001	Subotica (V)	154,611
Ljubljana (Sl)	305,211	Tetovo (Ma)	162,378
Maribor (Sl)	185,699	Titograd (Mo)	132,290
Mostar (B)	110,377	Titova Mitrovica (K)	105,322
Niš (Se)	230,711	Tuzla (B)	121,717
Novi Sad (V)	257,685	Uroševac (K)	113,680
Osijek (C)	158,790	Zadar (C)	116,174
Pančevo (V)	123,791	Zagreb (C)	1,174,512
Peć (K)	111,071	Zenica (B)	132,733
Prijedor (B)	108,868	Zrenjanin (V)	139,300

Population (1981 census) by ethnic group was *(i)* the 6 'leading nations': Serbs, 8,140,452; Croats, 4,428,005; Moslems, 1,999,957; Slovenes, 1,753,554; Macedonians, 1,339,729; Montenegrins, 579,023; *(ii)* of the 18 other 'nationalities': Albanians, 1,730,364; Hungarians, 426,866. 1,219,045 persons declared themselves 'Yugoslavs' (i.e. not professing any ethnic group). In 1986 about 460,000 nationals worked abroad. There were 181,000 Gypsies in 1986.

Vital statistics, 1987: Live births, 359,338; deaths, 214,666 (including 9,036 infantile); marriages, 163,469; divorces, 22,907.

Vital statistics, 1989 (per 1,000 population): Live births, 14·3; deaths, 9·1; marriages, 6·7; infant mortality, 24·3; natural increase, 5·2. Divorces per 1,000 marriages: 135·6. Expectation of life in 1982: Males, 68; females, 73.

The Yugoslav (*i.e.*, South Slav) languages proper are Slovene, Macedonian and Serbo-Croat, the latter having 2 variants (Serbian, or Eastern and Croatian, or Western) which are regarded as constituting one language. There are claims, largely politically-motivated, that Croatian is a separate language and Macedonian a dialect of Bulgarian. Macedonian is and Serbian may be written in the Cyrillic alphabet. There are also substantial Albanian and Hungarian-speaking minorities. Art. 246 of the Constitution lays down that 'The languages of the nations and nationalities and their alphabets shall be equal throughout the territory of Yugoslavia'. The sole use of Serbo-Croat is mandatory in the armed forces.

CLIMATE. Most parts have a central European type of climate, with cold winters and hot summers, but the whole coast experiences a Mediterranean climate with mild, moist winters and hot, brilliantly sunny summers with less than average rainfall. Belgrade. Jan. 32°F (0°C), July 72°F (22°C). Annual rainfall 24·4" (610 mm). Şarajevo. Jan. 31°F (–0·5°C), July 67°F (19·6°C). Annual rainfall 34" (856 mm). Šibenik. Jan. 45°F (7°C), July 78°F (25·5°C). Annual rainfall 32·5" (813 mm). Split. Jan. 47°F (8·5°C), July 78°F (25·6°C). Annual rainfall 35" (870 mm). Zagreb. Jan. 32°F (0°C), July 72°F (22°C). Annual rainfall 34·6" (865 mm).

CONSTITUTION AND GOVERNMENT. The Constitution passed on 31 Jan. 1946 declared the Federal Republic to be composed of 6 republics: Serbia, Croatia, Slovenia, Bosnia and Herzegovina, Macedonia and Montenegro.

On 13 Jan. 1953 a new Constitution affirmed the management of all public affairs by the workers and their representatives.

The Constitution promulgated 7 April 1963 set up the 2 socialist autonomous provinces of Kosovo and Vojvodina within the framework of Serbia.

Under this Constitution, social self-government was exercised by the representative bodies of communes, districts, autonomous provinces, republics and the Federation and the rights to self-government and distribution of income proclaimed in 1953 were extended to those employed in public services. The former Council of Producers was replaced by Councils of Working Communities representing employees in every field of social activity.

All the means of production and all natural resources were social property. Exceptions were peasants' holdings (up to 10 hectares of arable land) and handicrafts. Citizens could be owners of dwellings for personal and family needs.

A new Constitution was proclaimed on 21 Feb. 1974. This directly transfered economic and political decision making to the working people through the 'assembly system'. An assembly was defined as 'a body of social self-management and the supreme organ of power within the framework of the rights and duties of its socio-political community'. Assemblies were based upon the workplace or community.

In Jan. 1990 the Government announced an 8-point plan to rewrite the Constitution, abolish the Communist Party's monopoly of power, set up an independent judiciary, guarantee freedom of political association and institute economic reforms. Opposition parties were legalized in July 1990.

Speaker of the Federal Assembly: Slobodan Gligorijevič.

Every citizen over the age of 18 has the suffrage (16 if employed). The last elections were held from Jan. to April 1986.

The State Presidency is elected by the Federal Assembly every 5 years. It consists of: 8 representatives of the Republics and Autonomous Provinces. The one-year mandate as President (head of state) is rotated among the members of the Presidency from May of each year.

Membership of the state Presidency:

Bosnia and Herzegovina: Bogić Bogičević; *Croatia:* Štipe Mesić (Croat Democratic Union; President-elect from May 1991); *Macedonia:* Vasil Tupurkovski; *Montenegro:* Nenad Bućin; *Serbia:* Borisav Jović; *Slovenia:* Janez Drnovšek; *Kosovo:* vacant; *Vojvodina:* Dragutin Zelenović.

The Government is the Federal Executive Council of Chairman (i.e. Prime Minister), Vice-Chairmen, Ministers without Portfolio and Federal Secretaries, who are elected by the Federal Assembly every 4 years in conformity with equality of representation of the Republics and Autonomous Provinces. In March 1991 the Government comprised Ante Marković *(Prime Minister)* (b. 1925; Alliance of Reform Forces), Živko Pregl *(Deputy Prime Minister)*, Aleksandar Mitrović *(Deputy Prime Minister)*, Branko Zekan *(Finance)*, Budimir Lončar *(Foreign Affairs)*, Petar Gračanin *(Internal Affairs)*, Franc Horvat *(Foreign Economic Relations)*, Božo Marendić *(Development)*, Col.-Gen. Veljko Kadijević *(Defence)*, Radiša Gačić *(Labour)*, Stevan Santo *(Energy and Industry)*, Stevo Mirjanić *(Agriculture)*, Nazmi Mustafa *(Internal Trade)*, Vlado Kambovski *(Administration)*, Jože Slokar *(Transport and Communications)*, Nikola Gasoški, Sabrija Pojskić, Branimir Pajković, Veselin Vukotić *(without portfolio)*.

At an extraordinary congress in Jan. 1990 the League of Communists of Yugoslavia relinquished its monopoly of political activity by 1,573 votes to 27, but failed to abandon the principle of 'democratic centralism', whereupon the Slovene League severed its connection with it.

National flag: Three horizontal stripes of blue, white, red, with a large red, yellow-bordered star in the centre.

National anthem: Hej, Slaveni, jošte živi reč naših dedova—O Slavs, our ancestors' words still live.

Local Government. Within the federal framework of republics Yugoslavia is administratively divided into 533 communes (*opština*). 52,843 delegates were elected to commune assemblies in 1986 (9,260 women): 24,335 to Chambers of Associated Labour; 14,935 to Chambers of Local Communities; and 13,573 to Socio-Political Chambers.

DEFENCE. Military service for 12 months is compulsory. The General People's Defence Law of 1969 bases Yugoslavia's defence on the principle of a nation in arms ready to wage partisan war against any invader.

Army. The Army is divided into 4 Military Regions and comprises 2 infantry divisions; 1 airborne brigade and 29 brigades of armoured, mechanized, mountain and artillery forces. Equipment includes 850 T-54/-55, 300 M-84 and 45 M-47 main battle tanks. Strength (1991) 138,000 (including 93,000 conscripts), with a reserve of 440,000.

Navy. The Navy comprises 5 small diesel submarines, 6 midget submarines, 2 Soviet and 2 locally built frigates to similar designs armed with SS-N-2C Styx anti-ship missiles, 15 fast missile craft, 14 fast torpedo craft, 2 small corvette-style patrol vessels, 18 inshore patrol craft, 4 coastal minehunters, 10 inshore minesweepers, 6 river minesweepers, 10 tank landing craft with minelaying capability, and 25 minor landing craft. Auxiliaries include 3 transports, 1 survey ship, 1 salvage vessel, 1 headquarters ship, and 2 training ships (1 sail). Minor auxiliaries number about 25.

The Air Force operates 8 Ka-25 Hormone and 2 Ka-27 Helix anti-submarine helicopters plus 10 Mi-8 Hip and 15 Gazelle liaison helicopters, which are operationally assigned to the Navy. The Coast Defence Forces number 2,300 and man 25 coastal batteries and a few mobile missiles. A Marine force of 900 is divided into 2 'brigades'.

Personnel in 1990 totalled 10,000 (4,400 conscripts) including Coastal Defence and Marines. The main base is at Split.

Air Force. The Air Force is organized in 2 Air Corps, with HQ at Zagreb and Zemun. There are 2 fighter divisions equipped primarily with about 125 Russian-built MiG-21s, although now being joined by MiG-29s, 2 ground-attack divisions of locally-built Jastreb and Orao jet attack aircraft, and 2 squadrons of Jastreb jet reconnaissance aircraft. Transport units fly Il-14 and An-26 twin-engined aircraft, 4-turboprop An-12s, and a few other types in small numbers, notably CL-215 amphibians, C-47s, Turbo-Porters and Yak-40s, Mystère 50s and Learjets for VIP duties. Training types are the nationally-designed UTVA-75 primary trainer, Galeb jet basic trainer and the Super Galeb jet advanced trainer. A large number of Gazelle, Agusta-Bell 205, Mi-4 and Mi-8 helicopters are in service. 'Guideline' and 'Goa' surface-to-air missiles have been supplied by the USSR. Personnel (1991) 32,000 (4,000 conscripts), with 455 combat aircraft and 198 armed helicopters.

INTERNATIONAL RELATIONS

Membership. Yugoslavia is a member of UN and has special relationships with the OIEC and OECD. With Austria, Czechoslovakia, Hungary and Italy, Yugoslavia was an inaugural member of the 'Pentagonale' meeting on economic and political co-operation in June 1990.

ECONOMY

Policy. Reforms of the economic system which began in 1989 include curbs on the republics' powers by integrating taxation and raising policy-making to the federal level, the liberalization of imports and reduction of tariffs, the liberalization of prices except in the public infrastructure, the modification of the workers' councils system, the creation of limited companies and stock exchanges and equal treatment for foreign and domestic investors.

A second phase of economic reforms is aimed at completing a market-oriented fiscal system by 1995, including the establishment of a wage-bargaining structure and harmonization of taxation between republics. Gradual privatization ('democratization of capital') is expected to encourage private and foreign investment. Bonds will be made available to employees of self-managed enterprises.

Budget. Revenue and expenditure for 1987, 1,971,600m. old dinars. 459,609m. old dinars were allotted to defence in 1985.

Currency. The unit of currency is the *dinar* (YUD) of 100 *para*. The currency became convertible on 1 Jan. 1990 and a new 'heavy' dinar was introduced worth 10,000 old dinars. The new dinar was pegged at DM 7 throughout 1990, and at DM 9 from 1 Jan. 1991, a devaluation of 22·2%. For the dinar before 1990 *see* THE STATESMAN'S YEAR-BOOK, 1989-90 p. 1604. Inflation had reached 2,500% by the end of 1989. Currency in circulation in 1988 was 4,014,600m. old dinars. In March 1991, £1 = 26·27 *dinars*; US$1 = 13·85 *dinars*. International reserves, 1989: US$5,000m.

Banking and Finance. The National Bank is the bank of issue. There are also republican banks. In 1988 there were 243 'internal' banks, 155 'basic banks' and 10 'associated banks'. A reform programme which started in Feb. 1989 has transformed banks into shareholding companies, empowers the National Bank to impose solvency ratios on financial institutions and strengthens its control of the money supply. There are stock exchanges at Belgrade, Zagreb and Ljubljana. In 1988 credits amounted to 1,493,200m. old dinars. Savings deposits totalled 8,063,600m. old dinars in 1988, foreign exchange savings 39,243,100m.

Weights and Measures. The metric weights and measures have been in use since 1883. The *wagon* of 10 tonnes is used as a unit of measure for coal, roots and corn. The Gregorian calendar was adopted in 1919.

ENERGY AND NATURAL RESOURCES

Electricity. Output in 1989, 82,775m. kwh, of which 23,491m. were hydro-electric. There is a 664-mw nuclear power plant at Krško (opened 1981); output in 1989, 4,688 kwh. Construction of further nuclear plants was banned by law in June 1989.

Oil. Crude oil production (1989) 3·39m. tonnes; 1990 estimate, 3·25m. tonnes, about 20% of Yugoslavia's needs. Annual refining capacity is some 30m. tonnes.

Minerals. Yugoslavia has considerable mineral resources, including coal (chiefly brown coal), iron, copper ore, gold, lead, chrome, antimony and cement.

Mining output, in 1,000 tonnes, in 1989 (and 1988): Coal, 292 (362); brown coal, 12,063 (11,876); lignite, 62,276 (60,352); bauxite, 3,252 (3,034); salt, 368 (385); iron ore, 5,080 (5,545); copper ore, 30,078 (30,056); lead and zinc ore, 3,885 (3,847); antimony, 43 (38). In 1983, gold output was 4,238 kg; silver (1989), 133,000 kg.

Agriculture. The economically active agricultural population was 2,488,000 in 1981 (47·5% female). The total agricultural area was 14·18m. ha in 1989. The cultivated area was 9·81m. ha in 1989 of which 8·06m. were in private farms and 1·74m. in agricultural organizations, of which there were 3,203 in 1989. In 1984 only 6·5% of the 2·6m. private farms were more than 10 ha of land.

Area (in ha) and yield (in 1,000 tonnes) in 1989: Maize, 2·27m. (9,145); wheat, 1m. (5,599); sugar beet, 142,131 (6,797); rye, 37,000 (75); tobacco, 49,503 (57); sunflower, 204,396 (420); potatoes, 286,000 (2,359).

Livestock, 1989: Cattle, 4·76m.; pigs, 7·4m.; sheep, 7·56m.; poultry, 74·87m.

1989 yield of fruit (in 1,000 tonnes): Apples, 546; grapes, 1,022; plums (Yugoslavia is the world's largest producer), 819. 4·86m. hectolitres of wine were produced.

There were 1,065,000 tractors in 1989, of which 1,033,000 were in private hands.

Forestry. In 1988, 9·3m. ha were forested, 37% of the land area, and consisted largely of beech, oak and fir. 3·03m. ha were in private hands. Gross timber cut (1989): 21,542,000 cu. metres.

Fisheries. In 1988 the landings of fish were (in tonnes): Salt-water, 45,316; fresh-water, 26,449. The number of fishing craft was 387 motor vessels (13,401 GRT) and 1,458 sailing and rowing vessels.

INDUSTRY. The majority of industries are situated in the north-west. In 1988 there were 8,796 large industrial enterprises and 1,380 small businesses in the social sector, and 165,055 small businesses in the private sector.

Industrial output (in 1,000 tonnes) in 1989 (and 1988): Pig-iron, 2,899 (2,916); steel, 4,500 (4,485); cement, 8,560 (8,840); sulphuric acid, 1,634 (1,731); fertilizers, 2,508 (3,028); plastics, 742 (723). Fabrics (in 1m. sq. metres): Cotton, 339 (351); woollen, 100 (168). Sugar (1,000 tonnes), 960 (636). Motor cars (in 1,000s), 312 (305).

Labour. In 1989 (females in parentheses) there were 179,000 (69,000) employed in the private sector and 6·7m. (2·66m.) in the social sector. Of these 1·17m. worked in non-economic activities (e.g. education, social welfare). Amongst the economic activities 2·72m. worked in industry and mining, 675,000 in trade, 531,000 in building, 454,000 in transport and communications, 264,000 in financial services, 247,000 in tourism and 246,000 in agriculture. There were 1·2m. unemployed in 1989. Average monthly income per worker in 1989: 801·08 dinars. There were (1986) 6,086,600 trade union members.

Trade Unions. The Confederation of Trade Unions of Yugoslavia had 6,349,000 members in 1989.

FOREIGN ECONOMIC RELATIONS. Foreign indebtedness was US$17,600m. in 1989. In joint ventures the foreign partner may own up to 98% of the equity. International trade fairs are held in Zagreb in spring and autumn.

Commerce. Foreign trade, in 1m. dinars, for calendar years:

	1987	*1988*	*1989*
Imports	953	4,439	46,393
Exports	882	3,288	41,405

Structure of exports (and imports) in 1989 (%): Investment goods, 16 (15); intermediate goods, 52 (73·1); consumer goods, 31 (11·7). Largest suppliers in 1989 (goods in 1m. dinars): USSR, 6,734; Italy, 4,896; USA, 2,223; Austria, 1,994; Iraq, 1,790; Federal Republic of Germany, 1,307. Largest export markets: USSR, 8,983; Italy, 6,257; Federal Germany, 4,748; USA, 1,931.

Main exports as % share in 1989: Machinery and transport equipment, 27·6; other manufactures, 15; food and tobacco, 9·1; chemicals, 12; raw materials, 6·8; fuel, 1·9. Imports: Machinery and transport equipment, 27·3; chemicals, 17·9; raw materials, 10·8.

Total trade between Yugoslavia and UK (British Department of Trade returns, in £1,000 sterling):

	1986	*1987*	*1988*	*1989*	*1990*
Imports to UK	145,127	175,301	197,254	202,450	189,421
Exports and re-exports from UK	188,390	206,932	203,066	219,866	260,972

Tourism. In 1989, foreign tourists spent 49·18m. (1988: 52·35m.) nights in Yugoslavia.

COMMUNICATIONS

Roads. In 1988 there were 806 km of motorway, 73,527 km of asphalted roads and 33,663 km of macadamized roads. There were 3·09m. passenger motor cars, 88,228 motorcycles, 206,000 lorries and 28,000 buses. 804m. passengers and 125m. tonnes of freight were carried by public road transport in 1989. There were 65,392 road traffic casualties (4,555 deaths) in 1988.

Railways. In 1989 Yugoslavia had 9,567 km of railway, of which 3,782 km were electrified. 115·7m. passengers and 83·6m. tonnes of freight were carried in 1988.

Aviation. The national airline JAT (Jugoslovenski Aero Transport) operates 291 domestic and international routes totalling 455,122 km. in 1989. It had 48 aircraft in 1989. In 1989 5·6m. passengers and 48,897 tonnes of freight were carried. The chief airfields are Belgrade, Zagreb, Ljubljana, Sarajevo, Škopje, Dubrovnik, Split, Titograd, Tivat, Pula and Zadar.

Shipping. In 1989 Yugoslavia possessed 61 sea-going passenger vessels and 271 cargo vessels totalling 3·4m. tonnes. In 1989 8m. passengers were carried (7·9m. domestic) and 38·3m. tonnes of freight (35m. tonnes overseas).

International cargo handled at Yugoslav ports in 1987 totalled 30·85m. tonnes; domestic, 4·27m. tonnes.

Length of navigable waterways: Rivers, 1,673 km; canals, 664 km. There are 2 navigable lakes: Skadar (391 sq. km, of which 243 in Yugoslavia) and Ohrid (348 sq. km, of which 230 in Yugoslavia). In 1987 there were 1,156 river craft. 29,000 passengers and 19·27m. tonnes of cargo were carried in 1989.

Pipeline. An oil pipeline runs from Krk to Pančevo.

Telecommunications. There were 4,109 post offices and 4,550,000 telephone subscribers in 1989. *Jugoslovenska Radiotelevizija* consists of almost 250 main, relay and local stations operating on medium-waves and FM. In Aug. 1990 the central government launched the Yutel TV station with the aim of presenting a federal view of events. Number of receivers in 1989: Radio, 4·7m.; television, 4·07m.

Cinema and Theatre. In 1989 there were 1,165 cinemas with 482,000 seats and 65 theatres with 27,164 seats. 29 full-length films were made in 1989.

Newspapers and Books. In 1989 there were 28 dailies with a circulation of 2·1m., 2,481 other newspapers and 1,453 periodicals. 11,339 book titles (2,548 by foreign authors) were published in 1988.

JUSTICE, RELIGION, EDUCATION AND WELFARE

Justice. There are county tribunals, district courts, supreme courts of the constituent republics and a Supreme Court. There are also self-management courts, including courts of associated labour. In county tribunals and district courts the judicial functions are exercised by professional judges and by lay assessors constituted into collegia. There are no assessors at the supreme courts.

All judges are elected by the socio-political communities in their jurisdiction. The judges exercise their functions in accordance with the legal provisions enacted since the liberation of the country.

The constituent republics enact their own criminal legislation, but offences concerning state security and the administration are dealt with at federal level.

In 1987 258,000 crimes were reported, 163,000 charges made and 112,000 convictions obtained. 7,705 juveniles were sentenced.

Religion. Religious communities are separate from the State and are free to perform religious affairs. All religious communities recognized by law enjoy the same rights.

Serbia has been traditionally Orthodox and Croatia Roman Catholic. Moslems are found in the south as a result of the Turkish occupation. The 1953 percentage of the denominations was: Orthodox, 41·2%; Roman Catholic, 31·7%; Moslems, 12·3%; Protestants, 0·9%; without religion, 12·6%. 1984 estimates of believers: Orthodox, 9m.; Roman Catholic, 7m.; Moslems, 4m.

The Serbian Orthodox Church with its seat in Belgrade has 20 bishoprics within the country and 4 abroad, 3 in US and Canada and 1 in Hungary. The Serbian Orthodox Church numbers about 2,000 priests.

The Macedonian Orthodox Church with the Archbishop of Ohrid and Macedonia as its head in Skopje, has 4 bishoprics in the country and 1 abroad (American–Canadian–Australian). The Macedonian Orthodox Church numbers about 300 priests.

The Roman Catholic Church is divided into two provinces: Zagreb with 4 suffragan sees, and Sarajevo with 2 suffragan sees. In addition, the Roman Catholic Church has 4 archbishoprics, 10 independent bishoprics directly connected with the Vatican and 3 Apostolic Administrators. There is a National Conference of Bishops with the Archbishop of Zagreb, Cardinal Franjo Kuharič, at its head. The Roman Catholic Church has about 4,000 priests, 2 theological faculties and 15 seminaries. Relations with the Vatican are regulated by a 'Protocol' of 1966.

The Moslem Religious Union has 4 republic Superiorates in Sarajevo, Skopje, Titograd and Priština. The highest authority is the supreme synod of the Islamic Religious Community, which elects the Reis-ul-Ulema and the Supreme Islamic Superiorate. The Moslem religious community has about 2,000 priests.

The Protestant churches covering 4 independent Lutheran Churches, numbering about 150,000 believers, the Reformed Christian Church, numbering about 60,000 believers, include also several much smaller churches of Baptists, Methodists, Adventists, Nazarenes, etc., numbering together about 100,000 believers. The Protestant churches have about 450 priests.

Also there are independent Old Catholic Churches with Synodal Council at Zagreb.

The Jewish religion has about 35 communities making up a common league of Jewish Communities with its seat in Belgrade.

Education. Compulsory general education lasts 8 years, secondary 3–4 years. In 1988–89 there were 4,157 kindergartens with 46,413 teachers and 435,932 pupils, 11,910 primary schools with 141,584 teachers and 2,824,951 pupils; and 1,217 secondary schools with 59,128 teachers and 956,978 pupils.

Primary (and secondary) schools of ethnic minorities (1988–89): Albanian, 1,230 (87); Hungarian, 136 (26); Turkish, 65 (14); Bulgarian, 40 (nil); Romanian, 31 (2); Italian, 27 (7); Slovak, 21 (2).

In 1988–89 there were 314 institutes of higher education with 255,665 full-time students and 25,969 academic staff.

Health. In 1988 there were 55,140 doctors and dentists, and 142,957 hospital beds (11,031 psychiatric).

Social Security. There were 2·1m. pensioners in 1989. 100·4m. working days were lost through sickness in 1988. Health insurance benefits totalled 21,321·8m. dinars, old age pensions 8,076·1m. dinars and disability pensions, 5,219·4m. dinars in 1989. 2,628·5m. dinars were paid in child allowances in 1989. Consumption of food per capita in 1988: Meat, 597 kg.; cereals, 1,727 kg.; milk, 98·8 litres; vegetables and fruit, 171·7 kg. Daily consumption: 15,400 kilojoules.

DIPLOMATIC REPRESENTATIVES

Of Yugoslavia in Great Britain (5 Lexham Gdns., London, W8 5JJ)
Ambassador: Svetozar Rikanović.

Of Great Britain in Yugoslavia (46 Generala Ždanova, Belgrade)
Ambassador: P. E. Hall, CMG.

Of Yugoslavia in the USA (2410 California St., NW, Washington, D.C., 20008)
Ambassador: Dževad Mujezinović.

Of the USA in Yugoslavia (Belgrade)
Ambassador: Warren Zimmermann.

Of Yugoslavia to the United Nations
Ambassador: Darko Silović.

Further Reading

Statistical Information: The Federal Statistical Office (Savezni Zavod za Statistiku; Kneza Miloša 20, Belgrade) was founded in Dec. 1944. *Director:* Dr D. Grupković. Its publications include: *Statistički godišnjak Jugoslavije*, annual since 1954 with a separate volume of captions and editorial matter in English *Statistical Yearbook of Yugoslavia*; *Statistical Pocket-Book of Yugoslavia*, annual since 1955; *Statistics of Foreign Trade of the SFR of Yugoslavia*, annual since 1946.

The Assembly of the SFR of Yugoslavia. Belgrade, 1974
The Constitution of the Socialist Federal Republic of Yugoslavia. Belgrade, 1974
Alexander, S., *Church and State in Yugoslavia since 1945*. CUP, 1979
Artesien, P. F. R., *Joint Ventures in Yugoslav Industry*. Aldershot, 1985
Banac, I., *The National Question in Yugoslavia*. Cornell Univ. Press, 1985
Burg, S. L., *Conflict and Cohesion in Socialist Yugoslavia: Political Decision-Making since 1966*. Princeton Univ. Press, 1983
Čičin-Šain, A. and Ellis, M. (eds.), *Doing Business with Yugoslavia: Economic and Legal Aspects*. Belgrade, 1986
Cohen, L. J., *Political Cohesion in a Fragile Mosaic: The Yugoslav Experience*. Boulder, 1983
Dedijer, V., *et al., History of Yugoslavia*. New York, 1974
Djilas, M., *Memoir of a Revolutionary*. New York, 1973.—*Rise and Fall*. London, 1985
Drvodelić, M., *Croatian or Serbian-English Dictionary*. 4th ed. Zagreb, 1978
Filipović, R., *English-Croatian or Serbian Dictionary*. Zagreb, 1980.—*The New Foreign Exchange and Foreign Trade Regime of Yugoslavia*. Belgrade, 1986
Horton, J. J., *Yugoslavia*. [Bibliography] Oxford and Santa Barbara, 1978
Kotnik, J., *Slovensko–angleski slovar*. 4th ed. Ljubljana, 1959
Lydall, H., *Yugoslavia in Crisis*. OUP, 1989
McFarlane, B., *Yugoslavia: Politics, Economics and Society*. London, 1988
Milivojević, M. *et al.* (eds.) *Yugoslavia's Security Dilemmas: Armed Forces, National Defence and Foreign Policy*. Oxford, 1988
Milošević, D., *Investing in Yugoslavia and Other Forms of Long-Term Economic Co-operation with Yugoslav Enterprises*. 2nd ed. Belgrade, 1986
Pavlowitch, S. K., *The Albanian Problem in Yugoslavia*. London, 1982
Prout, C., *Market Socialism in Yugoslavia*. OUP, 1985
Ramet, P., *Nationalism and Federalism in Yugoslavia, 1963–1983*. Indiana Univ. Press, 1984.—*Yugoslavia in the 1980s*. Boulder, 1985
Seroka, J., *Political Organizations in Yugoslavia*. Durham, NC, 1986
Singleton, F., *Twentieth Century Yugoslavia*. London, 1976.—(with B. Carter) *The Economy of Yugoslavia*. London, 1982.—*A Short History of the Yugoslav Peoples*. CUP, 1985
Sirc, L., *The Yugoslav Economy under Self-Management*. London, 1979
Stojanović, R., (ed.) *The Functioning of the Yugoslav Economy*. New York, 1982
Tito, J. B., *The Essential Tito*. New York, 1970
Zimmerman, W., *Open Borders, Non-Alignment and the Political Evolution of Yugoslavia*. Princeton Univ. Press, 1987

REPUBLICS AND AUTONOMOUS PROVINCES

The Federal Republic of Yugoslavia comprises the 6 republics of Bosnia and Herzegovina, Croatia, Macedonia, Montenegro, Serbia and Slovenia, and the 2 autonomous provinces of Kosovo and Vojvodina within the Republic of Serbia.

Each republic has its own Constitution and Assembly.

Indicators (in %) for 1987:

	Population	*Workers*	*Social product*	*Investments*
Yugoslavia	*100*	*100*	*100*	*100*
Bosnia and Herzegovina	18·8	15·7	13·2	14·2
Croatia	19·9	23·6	25·6	21·9
Macedonia	8·8	7·7	5·4	4·2
Montenegro	2·7	2·5	1·9	2·0
Serbia	41·5	38·0	34·7	39·5
Slovenia	8·3	12·5	19·0	18·2

BOSNIA AND HERZEGOVINA

HISTORY. The country was settled by Slavs in the 7th century, the original clan system evolving between the 12th and 14th centuries into a principality under a *Ban,* during which time the Bogomil Christian heresy became entrenched. Bosnia was conquered by the Turks in 1463, and the majority of the Bogomils were converted to Islam. At the Congress of Berlin (1878) the territory was assigned to Austro-Hungarian administration under nominal Turkish suzerainty. Austria-Hungary's outright annexation in 1908 generated international tensions which contributed to the outbreak of the first world war.

AREA AND POPULATION. The republic is bounded in the north and west by Croatia, in the east by Serbia and in the south-east by Montenegro. It is virtually land-locked, having a coastline of only 20 km with no harbours. Its area is 51,129 sq. km. The capital is Sarajevo.

Population at the 1981 census: 4,124,256 (2,073,343 females), of whom the predominating ethnic groups were Moslems (1,630,033), Serbs (1,320,738) and Croats (758,140). Population density per sq. km, 1981: 80·7. Population, 1988, 4·44m.

Vital statistics:

	Live births	*Marriages*	*Deaths*	*Growth rate per 1,000*
1987	70,898	34,466	29,382	9·4
1988	70,711	34,700	29,555	9·3

CONSTITUTION AND GOVERNMENT. There is a 240-member bicameral National Assembly and 7-member collective presidency. Elections were held to both in Nov. and Dec. 1990. Moslem Democratic Action gained 86 National Assembly seats, the Serb Democratic Party, 70, and the Croat Democratic Union, 45. Alija Izetbegović (Moslem Democratic Action) was elected *President*; Jure Relivan (Croat Democratic Union) was appointed *Prime Minister*.

ECONOMY

Agriculture. In 1989 the cultivated area was 1·58m. ha. Yields (in 1,000 tonnes): Wheat, 424; maize, 798; potatoes, 343; plums, 166. Livestock in 1989 (1,000 head): Cattle, 884; sheep, 1,355; pigs, 608; poultry, 11,465. Timber cut in 1988: 7·05m. cu. metres.

Industry. Production (1989): Electricity, 14,372m. kwh; coal and lignite, 17·97m. tonnes; iron ore, 4·7m. tonnes; pig iron, 1·64m. tonnes; bauxite, 1·91m. tonnes; cement, 793,000 tonnes; cotton fabrics, 37m. sq. metres; cars, 34,000.

Employment. Population of working age, 1989, 3m. Non-agricultural workforce, 1·04m. (379,000 women), of whom 25,000 worked in private enterprise.

CROATIA

HISTORY. The Croats migrated to their present territory in the 6th century and were converted to Roman Catholicism. Croatia was united with Hungary by a personal union of thrones in 1091 and remained under Hungarian domination until after the first world war. For the duration of the second world war an independent fascist state was set up. In Feb. 1991 parliament ruled that henceforth Croatian law would take precedence over federal.

AREA AND POPULATION. Croatia is bounded in the north by Slovenia and Hungary and in the east by Serbia. It has an extensive Adriatic coastline well provided with ports, and includes the historical areas of Dalmatia, Istria and Slavonia, which no longer have administrative status. The capital is Zagreb. Its area is 56,538 sq. km. Population at the 1981 census was 4,601,469 (2,374,579 females), of whom the predominating ethnic groups were Croats (3,454,661) and Serbs (531,502). Population density per sq. km, 1981: 81·4. Population, 1988, 4·68m.

Vital statistics:

	Live births	*Marriages*	*Deaths*	*Growth rate per 1,000*
1987	59,209	31,395	53,080	1·3
1988	58,525	29,719	52,686	1·2

CONSTITUTION AND GOVERNMENT. There is a 3-chamber parliament (*Sabor*) of 365 members. Elections were held in April and May 1990. The electorate was 3·5m.; turn-out was 70%, The Croat Democratic Union gained 205 seats, the Party of Democratic Change (formerly Communists) 75. In May 1990 Franjo Tudjman (b. 1922; Croat Democratic Union) was elected *President* of Croatia by the Sabor. The *Prime Minister* was Josip Manolić in Feb. 1991.

A new constitution was adopted on 21 Dec. 1990 giving Croatia the right to secede from federal Yugoslavia.

ECONOMY

Agriculture. In 1989 the cultivated area was 2·02m. ha. Yields (in 1,000 tonnes): Wheat, 1,228; maize, 2,235; potatoes, 630; plums, 108. Livestock in 1989 (1,000 head): Cattle, 824; sheep, 743; pigs, 1,658; poultry, 16,458. Timber cut in 1989: 5·5m. cu. metres.

Industry. Production (1989): Electricity, 8,601m. kwh; coal and lignite, 197,000 tonnes; bauxite, 365; crude petroleum, 2·3m. tonnes; steel, 602,000 tonnes; plastics, 354,000 tonnes; cement, 2·9m. tonnes; cotton fabrics, 58m. sq. metres; sugar, 209,000 tonnes.

Employment. Population of working age, 1989: 3·05m. Non-agricultural workforce (1989), 1·51m. (653,000 women), of whom 51,000 worked in private enterprise.

MACEDONIA

HISTORY. The Slavs settled in Macedonia since the 6th century, who had been Christianized by Byzantium, were conquered by the non-Slav Bulgars in the 7th century and in the 9th century formed a Macedo-Bulgarian empire, the western part of which survived until Byzantine conquest in 1014. In the 14th century it fell to Serbia, and in 1355 to the Turks. After the Balkan Wars of 1912-13 Turkey was ousted, and Serbia received the greater part of the territory, the rest going to Bulgaria and Greece. In 1918 Yugoslav Macedonia was incorporated into Serbia as 'South Serbia'. Possession of this territory has long been a source of contention between Bulgaria and Yugoslavia.

AREA AND POPULATION. Macedonia is land-locked, and is bounded in the north by Serbia and Kosovo, in the east by Bulgaria, in the south by Greece and in the west by Albania. The capital is Skopje. Its area is 25,713 sq. km. Population at the 1981 census was 1,909,136 (940,993 females), of whom the predominating ethnic groups were Macedonians (1,279,323), Albanians (377,208) and Turks (86,591). Population density per sq. km, 1981, 74·2. Population, 1988, 2·09m.

Vital statistics:

	Live births	*Marriages*	*Deaths*	*Growth rate per 1,000*
1987	38,572	16,799	14,644	11·6
1988	37,379	46,580	14,565	11·2

CONSTITUTION AND GOVERNMENT. There is a 120-member single-chamber National Assembly. At the elections of Nov. and Dec. 1990 the Democratic Party for Macedonian National Unity gained 37 seats, the League of Communists–Party of Democratic Change, 31 and the Albanian-supported Party of Democratic Prosperity, 24. The *President* is Vladimir Mitkov.

ECONOMY

Agriculture. In 1989 the cultivated area was 668,000 ha. Yields (in 1,000 tonnes): Wheat, 314; maize, 137; cotton, 686; tobacco, 28. Livestock in 1989 (1,000 head): Cattle, 291; sheep, 2,378; pigs, 157; poultry, 4,406. Timber cut in 1989: 1·14m. cu. metres.

Industry. Production (1989): Electricity, 4,687m. kwh; lignite, 5·69m. tonnes; iron ore, 412,000 tonnes; pig-iron, 139,000 tonnes; steel, 224,000 tonnes; copper ore, 3·83m. tonnes; sulphuric acid, 92,000 tonnes; cement, 769,000 tonnes; cotton fabrics, 62m. sq. metres.

Employment. Population of working age, 1989: 1·35m. Non-agricultural workforce, 473,000 (180,000 women), of whom 14,000 worked in private enterprise.

MONTENEGRO

HISTORY. Montenegro emerged as a separate entity on the break-up of the Serbian Empire in 1355. It was never effectively subdued by Turkey. It was ruled by Bishop Princes until 1851, when a royal house was founded. The remains of King Nicholas I, (deposed 1918) were returned to Montenegro for reburial in Oct. 1989.

AREA AND POPULATION. Montenegro is a mountainous region which opens to the Adriatic in the south-west. It is bounded in the north-west by Bosnia and Herzegovina, in the north-east by Serbia and in the south-east by Albania. The capital is Titograd. Its area is 13,812, sq. km. Population at the 1981 census was 584,310 (294,571 females), of whom the predominating ethnic groups were Montenegrins (400,488), Moslems (78,080) and Albanians (37,735). Population density per sq. km, 1981: 42·3. Population, 1988, 632,000.

Vital statistics:

	Live births	*Marriages*	*Deaths*	*Growth rate per 1,000*
1987	10,567	4,358	3,990	10·4
1988	10,190	4,085	3,661	10·3

CONSTITUTION AND GOVERNMENT. There is a 125-member single-chamber National Assembly. At the elections of Dec. 1990 the electorate was 0·43m.; turn-out was 75%. The League of Communists gained 83 seats, the federal-oriented Alliance of Reform Forces, 17, the Albanian-supported Democratic Coalition, 13, and the National Party, 12. At the presidential elections turn-out was 65·8%. Momir Bulatović (Communist) was elected against one opponent with 76% of votes cast.

ECONOMY

Agriculture. In 1989 the cultivated area was 186,000 ha. Yields (in 1,000 tonnes): Wheat, 16; maize, 16; potatoes, 40. Livestock in 1989 (1,000 head): Cattle, 189; sheep, 488; pigs, 25. Timber cut in 1989: 882,000 cu. metres.

Industry. Production (1989): Electricity, 2,443m. kwh; lignite, 1·77m. tonnes; bauxite, 0·9m. tonnes; cement (1987), 155,000 tonnes.

Employment. Population of working age, 1989: 412,000. Non-agricultural work-force, 159,000 (62,000 women), of whom 5,000 worked in private enterprise.

SERBIA

HISTORY. The Serbs received Orthodox Christianity from the Byzantines. They threw off the latter's suzerainty to become a large prosperous medieval state, which was destroyed by the Turks at the Battle of Kosovo in 1389. After revolutions in 1804 and 1815 Serbia won increasing degrees of autonomy from Turkey; complete independence came with the Treaty of Berlin in 1878. Its prince took the title of king in 1881.

AREA AND POPULATION. Serbia is bounded in the north-west by Croatia, in the north by Hungary, in the north-east by Romania, in the east by Bulgaria, in the south by Macedonia and in the west by Albania, Montenegro and Bosnia and Herzegovina. It includes the Autonomous Provinces of Kosovo in the south and Vojvodina in the north. With these Serbia's area is 88,361 sq. km; without, 55,968 sq. km. The capital is Belgrade. Population at the 1981 census was (with Kosovo and Vojvodina) 9,313,676 (4,684,349 females), of whom the predominating ethnic group was Serbs (6,182,155). Population density per sq. km: 105·4 (without Kosovo and Vojvodina). 5,694,464 (2,876,909 females), of whom the predominating ethnic group was Serbs (4,865,283). Population density per sq. km, 101·7. Population, 1988: With Kosovo and Vojvodina, 9·76m.; without, 5·83m.

Vital statistics (without Kosovo and Vojvodina):

	Live births	*Marriages*	*Deaths*	*Growth rate per 1,000*
1987	73,076	38,331	58,651	2·5
1988	72,623	38,132	59,083	2·3

CONSTITUTION AND GOVERNMENT. At a referendum in July 1990 96·8% of the 5·33m. votes cast approved delaying parliamentary elections until a new constitution was adopted, and further reducing the autonomy of Kosovo and the Vojvodina. (Turn-out in the latter was 25% and 55% respectively). In Sept. a new constitution was adopted by the National Assembly by 64 votes to 6. It defines Serbia as a 'democratic' instead of a 'socialist' republic, lays down a framework for multi-party elections, and describes Serbia as 'united and sovereign on all its territory', thus stripping Kosovo and the Vojvodina of the attributes of autonomy granted by the 1974 federal constitution.

There is a 250-member single-chamber National Assembly. At the elections of Dec. 1990 the Socialist Party (reconstituted Communists) gained 194 seats, the Serbian Renewal Movement, 19, the Democratic Party, 7 and independents, 8. Allegations of irregularities at the polls were made by foreign observers. Slobodan Milošević was elected *President* of Serbia against 2 opponents with 65% of the votes cast.

In Feb. 1991 there was a government of 19 ministers including:

Prime Minister: Dragutin Zelenović.

Defence: Miodrag Jokić. *Interior:* Radmilo Bogdanović. *Serbs outside Serbia:* Stanko Cvijan.

ECONOMY [1]

Agriculture. In 1989 the cultivated area was 4·68m. ha. Yields (in 1,000 tonnes): Wheat, 3,390; maize, 5,905; potatoes, 882; sugar-beet, 4,946. Livestock in 1989: (in 1,000 head): Cattle, 2,026; sheep, 2,576; pigs, 4,574. Timber cut in 1989: 4·04m. cu. metres.

[1] Figures without Kosovo and Vojvodina.

Industry. (1989): Electricity, 40,103m. kwh.; coal and lignite, 42·69m. tonnes; pig-iron, 881,000 tonnes; steel, 886,000 tonnes; copper ore, 26·25m. tonnes; lorries (1988), 9,500; cars, 223,000; sulphuric acid, 1·08m. tonnes; plastics, 309,000 tonnes; cement, 2·93m. tonnes; sugar, 630,000 tonnes; cotton fabrics, 76,000 sq. metres; woollens, 42,000 sq. metres.

Employment. Population of working age, 1989: 6·31m. Non-agricultural work-force, 2·45m. (942,000 women), of whom 53,000 worked in private enterprise.

KOSOVO

HISTORY. Following Albanian-Serb conflicts the Kosovo and Serbian parliaments adopted constitutional amendments in March 1989 surrendering much of Kosovo's autonomy to Serbia. Renewed Albanian rioting broke out in 1990. The Prime Minister and 6 other ministers resigned in April 1990 over ethnic conflicts. In July 1990 114 of the 130 Albanian members of the National Assembly voted for full republican status for Kosovo, but the Serbian National Assembly declared this vote invalid and unanimously voted to dissolve the Kosovo Assembly. Direct Serbian rule was imposed. The *President* is Hisen Kajdomci.

AREA AND POPULATION. Area: 10,887 sq. km. The capital is Priština. Population at the 1981 census, 1,584,441 (766,048 females), of whom the predominating ethnic groups were Albanians (1,226,736), and Serbs (209,497). Population density per sq. km, 1981: 145·5. Population, 1987, 1·85m.

Vital statistics:

	Live births	*Marriages*	*Deaths*	*Growth rate per 1,000*
1987	56,221	13,644	10,307	24·8
1988	56,283	14,613	10,257	24·3

ECONOMY

Agriculture. The cultivated area in 1988 was 409,000 ha. Yields in 1989 (in 1,000 tonnes): Wheat, 320; maize, 374; potatoes, 83; plums, 14; grapes, 28. Livestock in 1989 (1,000 head): Cattle, 405; sheep, 407; pigs, 62; poultry, 4,537. Timber cut in 1989, 330,000 cu. metres.

Industry. Production (1989): Electricity, 5,531m. kwh; lignite, 10·67m. tonnes; sulphuric acid, 85,000 tonnes; cement, 316,000 tonnes.

Employment. Population of working age, 1989: 1·09m. Non-agricultural work-force, 226,000 (54,000 women), of whom 6,000 worked in private enterprise.

VOJVODINA

AREA AND POPULATION. Area: 21,506 sq. km. The capital is Novi Sad. Population at the 1981 census, 2,034,772 (1,041,392 females), of whom the predominating ethnic groups were Serbs (1,107,375) and Hungarians (385,356). Population density per sq. km, 1981: 94·6. Population, 1987, 2·05m.

Vital statistics:

	Live births	*Marriages*	*Deaths*	*Growth rate per 1,000*
1987	25,203	14,169	24,775	0·3
1988	24,848	13,577	24,533	0·2

ECONOMY

Agriculture. The cultivated area in 1989 was 1·63m. ha. Yields (in 1,000 tonnes): Wheat, 1,770; maize, 2,975; potatoes, 257; sugar-beet, 4,166. Livestock in 1989

(1,000 head): Cattle, 255; sheep, 329; pigs, 1,847; poultry, 9,609. Timber cut in 1989: 876,000 cu. metres.

Industry. Production (1989): Electricity, 1,510m. kwh.; crude petroleum, 1·09m. tonnes; sulphuric acid (1988), 55,000 tonnes; plastics (1988), 123,000 tonnes; cement, 1·3m. tonnes.

Employment. Population of working age, 1988: 1·35m. Non-agricultural workforce, 642,000 (257,000 women), of whom 18,000 worked in private enterprise.

SLOVENIA

HISTORY. The lands originally settled by Slovenes in the 6th century were steadily encroached upon by Germans. Slovenia developed as part of Austria-Hungary and gained independence only in 1918. A legal opposition group, the Slovene League of Social Democrats (leader, France Tomsič), was formed in Jan. 1989. In Oct. 1989 the Slovene Assembly voted a consitutional amendment giving it the right to secede from Yugoslavia. On 2 July 1990 the Assembly adopted a 'declaration of sovereignty' by 187 votes to 3, and in Sept. proclaimed its control over the territorial defence force on its soil. At a referendum on 23 Dec. 88·5% of participants voted for independence, which was formally declared on 26 Dec.

In Feb. 1991 parliament ruled that henceforth Slovenian law took precedence over federal.

AREA AND POPULATION. Slovenia is bounded in the north by Austria, in the north-east by Hungary, in the south-east by Croatia and in the west by Italy. There is a small strip of coast south of Trieste. Its area is 20,251 sq. km. The capital is Ljubljana. Population at the 1981 census: 1,891,864 (973,098 females), of whom the predominating ethnic group were Slovene (1,712,445). Population density per sq. km, 1981: 93·4. Population, 1988, 1·94m.

Vital statistics:

	Live births	*Marriages*	*Deaths*	*Growth rate per 1,000*
1987	25,592	10,307	19,837	3·0
1988	25,209	9,217	19,126	3·1

CONSTITUTION AND GOVERNMENT. There is a 240-member 3-chamber National Assembly. The *Speaker* is France Bučan. At the elections of April 1990 the 6-party Democratic United Opposition (Demos) won 55% of the vote and the Party of Democratic Renewal (formerly Communist), 18%. Milan Kučan (b. 1941) was elected *President* of Slovenia by 52% of the votes cast.

In Oct. 1990 the government included:

Prime Minister, Lojze Peterle; *Foreign*, Dimitri Rupel; *Interior*, Igor Bavčar; *Defence*, Janez Jansa. A new constitution is being drafted for promulgation in 1991. It will give Slovenia the powers of a sovereign state and its own economic system.

ECONOMY

Agriculture. In 1989 the cultivated area was 645,000 ha. Yields (in 1,000 tonnes): Wheat, 167; maize, 324; potatoes, 367. Livestock in 1989 (1,000 head): Cattle, 546; sheep, 24; pigs, 576; poultry, 13,269. Timber cut in 1989: 3·16m. cu. metres.

Industry. Production (1989): Electricity, 12,569m. kwh; lignite, 4·6m. tonnes; steel, 752,000 tonnes; lorries, 2,900; cars (1987), 66,000; sulphuric acid, 189,000 tonnes; sugar, 42,000 tonnes; cement, 1·18m. tonnes; cotton fabrics, 101m. sq. metres; woollens, 20m. sq. metres.

Employment. Population of working age, 1989: 1·26m. Non-agricultural workforce, 806,000 (376,000 women), of whom 31,000 worked in private enterprise.

ZAÏRE

Capital: Kinshasa
Population: 34·14m. (1990)
GNP per capita: US$170 (1988)

République du Zaïre

HISTORY. When the explorer Henry Stanley reached the mouth of the Congo in 1877, King Leopold II of the Belgians took the lead in exploring and exploiting the Congo Basin. The Berlin Conference of 1884–85 recognized King Leopold II as the sovereign head of the Congo Free State.

In 1908 the country was annexed to Belgium as the Belgian Congo, until the country became independent on 30 June 1960. The country's name was changed from Congo to Zaïre in Oct. 1971. For subsequent history to 1977 *see* THE STATESMAN'S YEAR-BOOK, 1980–81, p. 1613.

AREA AND POPULATION. Zaïre is bounded north by the Central African Republic, north-east by Sudan, east by Uganda, Rwanda, Burundi and Lake Tanganyika, south by Zambia, south-west by Angola, north-west by Congo. There is a 40-km Atlantic coastline separating Angola's province of Cabinda from the rest of that country.

The area is estimated at 2,344,885 sq. km (905,365 sq. miles). The population is composed almost entirely of Bantu groups, with minorities of Sudanese (in the north), Nilotes (northeast), Pygmies and Hamites (in the east). In the 1984 census the population was 29,671,407 (44% urban). Estimate (1990) 34,138,000. Population growth rate, 1989, 3%. In 1989 there were 340,689 refugees in Zaïre, mainly from Angola.

The area (in sq. km) and populations (census) 1984 of the regions were as follows, together with their chief towns:

Region	*Sq. km*	*Census 1984*	*Chief town*	*Census 1984*
Bandundu	295,658	3,682,845	Bandundu (Banningville)	96,841 [2]
Bas-Zaïre	53,920	1,971,520	Matadi	144,742
Equateur	403,293	3,405,512	Mbandaka (Coquilhatville)	125,263
Haut-Zaïre	503,239	4,206,069	Kisangani (Stanleyville)	282,650
Kasai Occidental	156,967	2,287,416	Kananga (Luluabourg)	290,898
Kasai Oriental	168,216	2,402,603	Mbuji-Mayi (Bakwanga)	423,363
Kinshasa City	9,965	2,653,558	Kinshasa (Leopoldville)	2,653,558
Kivu [1]	256,662	5,187,865	Bukavu (Costermansville)	171,064
Shaba	496,965	3,874,019	Lubumbashi (Elizabethville)	543,268

[1] Now divided into 3 regions.

Other large towns (1976): Likasi (194,465 in 1984); Kikwit (146,784 in 1984); Kalémié (172,297); Kamina (160,020); Ilebo (142,036); Boma (93,965) and Kolwezi (77,277).

French is the only official language, but of more than 200 languages spoken, 4 are recognized as national languages. Of these, Kiswahili is used in the east, Tshiluba in the south, Kikongo in the area between Kinshasa and the coast, while Lingala is spoken widely in and around Kinshasa and along the river; Lingala has become the *lingua franca* after French.

CLIMATE. Because of the size and the relief of the country, the climate is very varied, the central region having an equatorial climate, with year-long high temperatures and rain at all seasons. Elsewhere, depending on position north or south of the Equator, there are well-marked wet and dry seasons. The mountains of the east and south have a temperate mountain climate, with the highest summits having considerable snowfall. Kinshasa. Jan. 79°F (26·1°C), July 73°F (22·8°C). Annual rainfall 45" (1,125 mm). Kananga. Jan. 76°F (24·4°C), July 74°F (23·3°C). Annual rainfall 62" (1,584 mm). Kisangani. Jan. 78°F (25·6°C), July 75°F (23·9°C). Annual rainfall 68" (1,704 mm). Lubumbashi. Jan. 72°F (22·2°C), July 61°F (16·1°C). Annual rainfall 50" (1,237 mm).

CONSTITUTION AND GOVERNMENT. Under the Constitution of 1978 (as amended in 1980) the sole political party was the *Mouvement Populaire de la Révolution* (MPR), whose leader and President was automatically Head of State, of the National Executive Council and of the National Legislative Council. His nomination by the Political Bureau of the MPR (whose 38 members were all nominated by him) was confirmed for a 7-year term (renewable once) by election by universal adult suffrage (all Zaïreans acquiring automatic membership of the MPR at birth). In April 1990 President Mobutu announced the end of the Second Republic and the transition to a multi-party state. Presidential and legislative elections were scheduled for 1991 and also a referendum for a new constitution.

Former President: Joseph Kasavubu, 1 July 1960–25 Nov. 1965 (deposed).

President: Marshal Mobutu Sésé Séko Kuku Ngbendu wa Zabanga (took office 25 Nov. 1965, elected 1 Nov. 1970 and re-elected Dec. 1977 and July 1984).

The National Executive Council is composed of State Commissioners appointed by the President. In Feb. 1991 it was composed as follows:

Prime Minister: Lunda Bululu.

Deputy Prime Ministers: Nzanda Buana Kalemba *(responsible for Industry, Commerce and Trade),* Engulu Baanga Mpongo Bokolele Lokanga *(Territorial Administration and Decentralization). Defence, Territorial Security and Ex-Servicemen's Affairs:* Adm. Mavua Mudima. *Foreign Affairs:* Mushobekwa Kalimba wa Katana. *International Co-operation:* Buketi Bukayi. *Information and Press:* Ngongo Kamanda. *Planning:* Ilunga Ilukamba. *Finance:* Bombito Botombo. *Budget:* Mananga ma Pholo. *Agriculture, Rural and Community Development:* Onyembe Pene Mbutu. *Transport and Communications:* Kimosi Matuiku Basanla. *Land Affairs:* Okitakula Djambokota. *Higher Education, Universities and Scientific Research:* Kambayi Bwatshia. *Primary, Secondary and Professional Education:* Koli Elpmbe Motukoa. *Public Health, Telecommunications:* Lengelo Muyangandu. *Civil Liberties:* Sabi Ngampobu. *Youth, Sports and Leisure:* Nyamwisi Muvingi. *Environment, Nature Conservation and Tourism:* Diur Katonda. *Justice:* Muyabo Nkulu. *Culture and Arts:* Agbiano Gambe. *Parliamentary Relations:* Banza Mukalay Nsungu. *Public Works:* Bangala Baslla. *Employment and Social Services:* Mubuka Inyanza. *Women and Families:* Mitheo Lola Mara Tamba. *Civil Service:* Boshala Kantu wa Milandu. *Social Affairs:* Tshibangu Muyembe Kaza.

Parliament consists of a unicameral National Legislative Council comprising People's Commissioners (one per 150,000 inhabitants) elected by universal suffrage for a 5-year term. At the latest elections (Sept. 1987) 210 People's Commissioners were elected from a list of candidates presented by the MPR.

National flag: Green, with a yellow disc bearing an arm holding a flaming torch.

Local government: Zaïre is composed of the *ville neutre* of Kinshasa (administered by a Governor) and 10 regions, each under a Regional Commissioner and 6 Councillors; all are appointed by the President. The regions are divided into 41 sub-regions.

DEFENCE

Army. The Army is divided into 8 Military Regions and comprises 3 infantry brigades and 4 special brigades (1 parachute, 1 commando, 1 armoured and 1 Presidential Guard). Equipment includes 60 Chinese Type-62 tanks, and 95 AML-60 and 60 AML-90 armoured cars. Strength (1991) 22,000. There is a paramilitary gendarmerie which is responsible for security which numbered (1991) about 28,000, organized in 40 battalions.

Navy. The navy comprises 4 ex-Chinese inshore patrol craft and some 30 small boats divided among coastal, river and lake flotillas. Personnel in 1990 numbered 1,500 including 600 marines.

Air Force. The Air Force has been built up with training assistance from Italy. In

1990 it operated 3 Aermacchi MB.326GB and 3 MB.326K armed jet trainers, 1 C-130 Hercules and 1 DHC-5 Buffalo turboprop transport, 7 C-47, 4 C-54, 2 DC-6 piston-engined transports, 20 Bell 47, Alouette, Puma and Super Puma helicopters, 9 SIAI-Marchetti SF.260MC basic trainers and a variety of other transport and training aircraft. Personnel (1991) 2,400.

INTERNATIONAL RELATIONS

Membership. Zaïre is a member of the UN, OAU and is an ACP state of the EEC.

ECONOMY

Policy. The 5-year Development Plan, 1986–90, envisaged expenditure of US$5,000m. Emphasis is placed on food production and agricultural exports.

Budget. Revenue was budgeted at 607,000m. zaïres in 1990, and expenditure, 657,000m.

Currency. The unit of currency is the *zaïre* (ZRZ). There are coins of 1, 5 and 10 zaïres and notes of 10, 50, 100, 500, 1,000, 5,000 and 10,000 zaïres. In March 1991, £1 sterling = 6,006 *zaïre*; US$1 = 3,166 *zaïre*.

Banking and Finance. The central bank is Banque du Zaïre. A development bank with state backing is the Société Financière de Développement (SOFIDE). Commercial banks operating in Zaïre are Banque de Paris et des Pays-Bas, Banque de Kinshasa, National & Grindlays Bank, Barclays Bank SZPRL, First National City Bank, Union Zaïroise de Banques, Banque Commerciale Zaïroise, Banque du Peuple, Caisse Nationale d'Epargne et de Crédit Immobilier and Banque Internationale pour L'Afrique au Zaïre.

Weights and Measures. The metric system is in force.

ENERGY AND NATURAL RESOURCES

Electricity. Production (1989), 5,998m. kwh. A dam at Inga, on the Zaïre River near Matadi, has a potential capacity of 39,600 mw.

Oil. Offshore oil production began in Nov. 1975; crude production (1990) was 1·35m. tonnes.

Minerals. Production in 1989 (in 1,000 tonnes): Copper, 425·2; zinc, 54; cobalt, 9·5. Manganese, tin, gold and silver are also mined. The most important mining area is in the region of Shaba (formerly Katanga). The principal mining companies are the State-owned Gécamines and Sodimiza; the international Société Minière du Tenke-Fungurume which started production in 1976; and 2 diamond companies, MIBA and British Zaïre Diamond Distributors. Production (1989) 17,652 carats.

Agriculture. There were (1984) 5·65m. ha of arable land and 24·8m. ha of pastures and meadows. The main food crops (1988 production in 1,000 tonnes) are: Cassava, 16,254; plantains, 1,520; sugar-cane, 1,200; maize, 740; groundnuts, 400; bananas, 345; yams, 264; rice, 330. Cash crops (1988) include palm oil, 70; coffee, 95; palm kernels, 70; rubber, 17; seed cotton 77. There are also (1988) pineapples, 180; mangoes, 155; oranges, 150; papayas, 180.

Livestock (1988): Cattle, 1·4m.; sheep, 0·88m.; goats, 3·04m.; pigs, 0·8m.; poultry, 19m.

Forestry. Equatorial rain forests cover 55% of Zaïre's land surface, and 165,000 cu. metres of timber were produced in 1988.

Fisheries. The catch for 1986 was 150,000 tonnes, almost entirely from inland waters.

INDUSTRY. The main manufactures are foodstuffs, beverages, tobacco, textiles, rubber, leather, wood products, cement and building materials, metallurgy and metal extraction, metal items, transport vehicles, electrical equipment and bicycles.

FOREIGN ECONOMIC RELATIONS. With Burundi and Rwanda, Zaïre forms part of the Economic Community of the Great Lakes.

Commerce. Imports in 1989 totalled US$1,546·1m., exports US$2,101m. In 1989, 59% of the exports (by value) consisted of copper, 5·7% of coffee, 7·5% of crude petroleum, 11·9% of diamonds and 7·6% of cobalt. In 1987, 37% of all exports went to Belgium-Luxembourg, 18% to USA, 11% to Federal Republic of Germany and 11% to Italy, while 19·7% of imports came from Belgium, 9·3% from USA, 9% from France, 8·8% from Federal Republic of Germany and 8·7% from South Africa.

Total trade between Zaïre and UK (British Department of Trade returns, in £1,000 sterling):

	1986	*1987*	*1988*	*1989*	*1990*
Imports to UK	17,192	8,544	7,542	9,069	7,337
Exports and re-exports from UK	34,217	26,142	26,132	28,419	23,801

Tourism. There were 51,000 visitors in 1986 spending US$16·3m.

COMMUNICATIONS

Roads. In 1989 of 145,000 km of roads 2,370 km were asphalted and some 12,000 km motorable. In 1984 there were 25,000 passenger cars and 60,000 commercial vehicles.

Railways. There are two railway operators, the Zaïre National Railways (SNCZ) and the National Office of Transport and Communications (ONATRA), which leases two lines from SNCZ. Length in 1990 was 5,118 km on 3 gauges, of which 858 km is electrified. In 1988 SNCZ and ONATRA carried 4m. passengers and 5·8m. tonnes of freight.

Aviation. There are 4 international airports at Kinshasa (Ndjili), Lubumbashi (Luano), Goma and Bukavu. There are another 40 airports with regular scheduled internal services, and over 150 other landing strips.

10 international airlines operate in and out of Kinshasa from Europe and Africa. The national airline is Air Zaïre. It operates domestic routes and flights to Europe and Africa, including a weekly flight to Johannesburg via Lusaka (Zambia). South African Airways operate a weekly service from Johannesburg to Lubumbashi.

Shipping. The Zaïre River and its tributaries are navigable to 300-tonne vessels for about 14,500 km. Regular traffic has been established between Kinshasa and Kisangani as well as Ilebo, on the Lualaba (*i.e.*, the river above Kisangani), on some tributaries and on the lakes. Zaïre has only 40 km of sea coast. The merchant marine in 1988 comprised 4 vessels with a total tonnage of 60,562 GRT. Matadi and Boma are the main seaports; in 1989, Matadi handled 1·5m. tonnes of freight. Boma's traffic is negligible.

Telecommunications. In 1983 there were 362 post offices. Length of telegraph lines, 2,459 km. There were 15 broadcasting stations, 161 stations of wireless telegraphy and 206 telegraph offices; telephones numbered 31,855 in 1985. There is a ground satellite communications station outside Kinshasa. In 1987 there were 3·4m. radio and 16,000 television receivers.

Newspapers. There were (1989) 4 dailies: *Salongo* (mornings) and *Elima* (evenings) in Kinshasa; *Njumbe* in Lubumbashi and *Boyoma* in Kisangani.

JUSTICE, RELIGION, EDUCATION AND WELFARE

Justice. There is a Supreme Court at Kinshasa, 11 courts of appeal, 36 courts of first instance and 24 'peace tribunals'.

Religion. In 1988 there were about 15·7m. Roman Catholics, 9·4m. Protestants and 5·6m. Kimbanguistes, as well as some 450,000 Moslems and 2,000 Jews. The remaining inhabitants (about 1·1m.) chiefly adhere to animist beliefs.

Education. In 1987 there were 4,356,515 pupils in 10,819 primary schools and

1,066,351 pupils in 4,276 secondary schools. Secondary schools combine schools of general education, teacher training colleges and technical schools. In higher education there were in 1990 3 universities (Kinshasa, Kisangani and Lubumbashi), 14 teacher training colleges and 18 technical institutes in the public sector; and 13 university institutes, 4 teacher training colleges and 49 technical institutes in the private sector.

Health. In 1979 there were 1,900 doctors, 58 dentists, 414 pharmacists, 3,043 midwives, 14,661 nursing personnel and 942 hospitals and medical centres with 79,244 beds.

DIPLOMATIC REPRESENTATIVES

Of Zaïre in Great Britain (26 Chesham Pl., London, SW1X 8HH)
Ambassador: Nkema Liloo.

Of Great Britain in Zaïre (Ave. de l'Equateur, Kinshasa)
Ambassador: R. L. B. Cormack, CMG.

Of Zaïre in the USA (1800 New Hampshire Ave., NW, Washington, D.C., 20009)
Ambassador: Mukendi Tambo a Kabila.

Of the USA in Zaïre (310 Ave. des Aviateurs, Kinshasa)
Ambassador: William C. Harrop.

Of Zaïre to the United Nations
Ambassador: Bagbeni Adeito Nzengeya.

Further Reading

Atlas Général du Congo. Académie Royale, Brussels
Gran, G., *Zaïre: The Political Economy of Underdevelopment.* New York, 1979
MacGaffey, J., *Entrepreneurs and Parasites: The Struggle for Indigenous Capitalism in Zaïre.* CUP, 1988
Parfitt, T. W., *Zaïre:* [Bibliography]. Oxford and Santa Barbara, 1991
Young, C. and Turner, T., *The Rise and Decline of the Zaïrian State.* Univ. of Wisconsin Press, 1985

ZAMBIA

Capital: Lusaka
Population: 8·5m. (1990)
GNP per capita: US$290 (1988)

Republic of Zambia

HISTORY. The independent Republic of Zambia (formerly Northern Rhodesia) came into being on 24 Oct. 1964 after 9 months of internal self-government following the dissolution of the Federation of Rhodesia and Nyasaland on 31 Dec. 1963.

AREA AND POPULATION. Zambia is bounded by Tanzania in the north, Malaŵi in the east, Mozambique in the south-east and by Zimbabwe and South West Africa (Namibia) in the south. The area is 290,586 sq. miles (752,614 sq. km). Population (1980 census) 5,679,808 of which 43% urban; estimate (1990), 8·5m.

The republic is divided into 9 provinces. Their names, headquarters, area (in sq. km) and census population in 1980 were as follows:

Province	*Headquarters*	*Area*	*Population*	*Province*	*Headquarters*	*Area*	*Population*
Copperbelt	Ndola	31,328	1,248,888	Eastern	Chipata	69,106	656,381
Luapula	Mansa	50,567	412,798	Southern	Livingstone	85,283	686,469
Northern	Kasama	147,826	677,894	N.-Western	Solwezi	125,827	301,677
Central	Kabwe	94,395	513,835	Western	Mongu	126,386	487,988
Lusaka	Lusaka	21,898	693,878				

The seat of Government is at Lusaka (population, 1987, 818,994); other large towns are Kitwe (449,442), Ndola (418,142), Mufulira (192,323), Chingola (187,310), Luanshya (160,667), Kalulushi (89,065) and Chililabombwe (79,010) on the Copperbelt; Kabwe, the oldest mining township (190,752); Livingstone, the old capital (94,637); and other provincial capitals at Kasama, Mansa, Chipata, Mongu and Solwezi. In Jan. 1988 there were 146,000 refugees in Zambia including 97,000 Angolans.

The official language is English and the main ethnic groups are the Bemba (34%), Tonga (16%), Malawi (14%) and Lozi (9%).

CLIMATE. The climate is tropical, but has three seasons. The cool, dry one is from May to Aug., a hot dry one follows until Nov., when the wet season commences. Frosts may occur in some areas in the cool season. Lusaka. Jan. 70°F (21·1°C), July 61°F (16·1°C). Annual rainfall 33" (836 mm). Livingstone. Jan. 75°F (23·9°C), July 61°F (16·1°C). Annual rainfall 27" (673 mm). Ndola. Jan. 70°F (21·1°C), July 59°F (15°C). Annual rainfall 52" (1,293 mm).

CONSTITUTION AND GOVERNMENT. The Constitution provides for a President, elected in the first instance by the General Conference of the ruling party, the United National Independence Party, and thereafter by the electorate. On 13 Dec. 1972 President Kaunda signed a new Constitution based on one-party rule. In Dec. 1990 the National Assembly unanimously passed a constitutional amendment permitting opposition parties. Elections were scheduled for Oct. 1991.

In March 1991 the single political party was the United National Independence Party whose Central Committee took precedence over the legislative body, the National Assembly, which was led by the Prime Minister and consists of 125 elected members and up to 10 nominated members, including a cabinet of 18 ministers.

Presidential elections were held in Oct. 1988 and on 30 Oct. President Kaunda was sworn in for a sixth 5-year term.

The Cabinet in Feb. 1991 comprised:

President and Commander-in-Chief: Dr Kenneth David Kaunda.
Vice-President and Minister of Defence: Dodson Siatalimi.
Prime Minister: Gen. Malimba Masheke.
Foreign Affairs: L. Mwananshiku. *Finance and Planning:* vacant. *Attorney-General:* F. M. Chomba. *Higher Education, Science and Technology:* L. Goma.

Health: M. Muyunda. *Commerce and Industry:* R. Chongo. *Mines:* M. Muzungu. *Agriculture:* J. Mukando. *Home Affairs:* Gen. G. K. Chinkuli. *Labour and Social Services:* Lavu Mulimba. *Tourism:* P. Chitambala. *Information and Broadcasting:* A. Simuchimba. *Education, Sport and Youth:* E. Mwanangonze. *Water, Land and Natural Resources:* P. Malukutila. *Power, Transport and Communications:* E. Haimbe. *Works and Supply:* H. Y. Mwale.

National flag: Green, with in the fly a panel of 3 vertical strips of dark red, black and orange, and above these a soaring eagle in gold.
National anthem: Stand and Sing of Zambia, Proud and Free.

The 9 provinces (sub-divided into 53 districts) are administered by Central Committee Members for the provinces who are responsible for the overall government and Party administration of their respective areas.

DEFENCE

Army. The Army consists of 1 armoured regiment and 9 infantry battalions, with supporting artillery, engineer and signals units. Equipment includes some 30 main battle tanks and 88 armoured cars. Strength (1991) 15,000. There are also para-military police units numbering 1,200 men.

Air Force. Creation of the Zambian Air Force was assisted initially by an RAF mission. Training and expansion of the Air Force was next taken over by Italy, with the purchase of 23 Aermacchi M.B.326G armed jet basic trainers (of which 18 remain in service), 8 SIAI-Marchetti SF.260M piston-engined trainers and 15 Agusta-Bell 47G, 10 AB.205 and 2 AB.212 helicopters. Twelve F-6 (MiG-19) jet fighter-bombers and some BT-6 primary trainers have since been acquired from China, a squadron of 14 MiG-21 fighters, 3 Yak-40 light jet transports, 4 An-26 twin-turboprop transports and 6 Mi-8 helicopters from the Soviet Union, 5 DHC-5 Buffalo twin-turboprop transports from Canada, 6 C-47s built in the USA, 8 DO 28D Skyservant light transports from Germany, 15 Supporter armed light trainers from Sweden. Serviceability of most types is reported to be low. Personnel (1991) 1,200, with 81 combat aircraft.

INTERNATIONAL RELATIONS

Membership. Zambia is a member of the UN, the Commonwealth, SADCC, OAU and is an ACP state of the EEC.

ECONOMY

Budget. Revenue and expenditure for 1989 (in K1m.): Envisaged expenditure of 24,503 and revenue of 20,366.

Currency. The unit of currency is the *kwacha* (ZMK) of 100 *ngwee*. There are coins of 50, 20, 10, 5, 2 and 1 *ngwee* and banknotes of K20, K10, K5, K2 and K1. In March 1991, £1 = 95·83 *kwacha*; US$1 = 50·52 *kwacha*.

Banking and Finance. Barclays Bank has 25 branches, 6 sub-branches and 17 agencies; Standard Bank has 18 branches and 17 agencies; National & Grindlays, 10 branches and 1 sub-branch; Zambia National Commercial Bank, 10 branches and 1 in London; the post office saving bank has branches throughout the republic.

The Finance Development Corporation (FINDECO) controls the building societies, all insurance companies, one commercial bank and has shares in a second one. The Agricultural Finance Corporation provides loans to farmers, co-operatives, farmers' associations and agricultural societies.

ENERGY AND NATURAL RESOURCES

Electricity. The total installed capacity of hydro and thermal power stations, excluding Zambia's share of Kariba South, amounts to 1,924,700 kw and the energy production during 1986 amounted to some 11,100m. kwh. Zambia exports electricity to Zaïre, Zimbabwe and Angola.

Minerals. The total value of minerals produced (in 1,000 tonnes) in 1985 was: Copper, 543; zinc, 32; lead, 15; cobalt, 4·4; gold, 7,903 oz. Zambia is well-endowed with gemstones, especially emeralds, amethysts, aquamarine, tourmaline and garnets. In 1990 the government freed the gemstones trade from restrictions.

Agriculture. Although 70% of the population is dependent on agriculture only 10% of GDP is provided by the industry. Principal agricultural products (1988) were maize, 1,453,000 tonnes; sugar-cane, 1,318,000 tonnes; seed cotton, 44,000 tonnes; tobacco, 4,000 tonnes; groundnuts, 33,000 tonnes.

Livestock (1988): 2,684,000 cattle; 180,000 pigs; 80,000 sheep; 420,000 goats, and 15m. poultry.

Forestry. Forests covered (1988) 29·2m. ha, 39% of the total land area. Roundwood removals (1986) 9·9m. cu. metres.

Fisheries. Total catch (1986) 68,000 tonnes.

INDUSTRY. In Dec. 1984 there was a labour force of 2·27m. of which 63% were employed in agriculture, 2·6% in mining and quarrying and 2·1% in manufacturing.

FOREIGN ECONOMIC RELATIONS. In 1990 foreign debt was some US$7,000m.

Commerce. Trade in 1m. kwacha for 3 years:

	1985	*1986*	*1987*
Imports	2,089·5	4,447·7	6,227·5
Exports	1,486·1	3,074·4	8,058·6

In 1990, copper provided 90% of all exports (by value), cobalt 6%, zinc 2%. Official emerald exports in 1989 were valued at US$10m., but unofficial sales may have been a further US$200m.

Total trade between Zambia and UK (British Department of Trade returns, in £1,000 sterling):

	1987	*1988*	*1989*	*1990*
Imports to UK	30,310	24,822	21,565	19,308
Exports and re-exports from UK	75,178	85,746	119,057	92,832

Tourism. There were 121,000 visitors in 1987.

COMMUNICATIONS

Roads. There were (1984) 37,279 km of roads including over 5,592 km of tarred roads. In 1982 there were 33,000 commercial vehicles and 68,000 cars.

Railways. In 1985 the total route-km was 1,266 km (1,067 mm gauge). In 1988–89 the Zambian railways (excluding Tan-Zam) carried 2·1m. passengers and 4·4m. tonnes of freight. The Tan–Zam railway, giving Zambia access to Dar es Salaam, comprises 892 km of route in Zambia.

Aviation. There were (1982) 130 airports in Zambia (46 government owned). Lusaka is the principal international airport. Seven foreign airlines use Lusaka.

Telecommunications. There were (1982) 13 head post offices and 236 other post offices. In 1985 there were 74,500 telephones, and in 1986 528,000 radio and 66,000 television receivers.

Newspapers. There were (1989) 2 national daily papers: *The Times of Zambia* (circulation, 65,000) and *Zambia Daily Mail* (40,000), and *The Sunday Times* (74,000).

JUSTICE, RELIGION, EDUCATION AND WELFARE

Justice. The Judiciary consists of the Supreme Court, the High Court and 4 classes of magistrates' courts; all have civil and criminal jurisdiction.

The Supreme Court hears and determines appeals from the High Court. Its seat is at Lusaka.

The High Court exercises the powers vested in the High Court in England, subject to the High Court ordinance of Zambia. Its sessions are held where occasion requires, mostly at Lusaka and Ndola.

All criminal cases tried by subordinate courts are subject to revision by the High Court.

Religion. Freedom of worship is one of the constitutional rights of Zambian citizens. The Christian faith with 66% of the population has largely replaced traditional African religions. There are 20,000 Moslems.

Education. In 1986 there were 1·4m. pupils in 3,100 primary schools, secondary schools, 150,000 in 276 schools. In 1986 there were 5,400 students in technical colleges and 4,277 students were enrolled for teacher-training. In 1984 the University of Zambia had 3,621 full-time students.

Health. In 1981 there were 821 doctors, 52 dentists, 36 pharmacists, 866 midwives and 871 nursing personnel. There were also 636 hospitals and clinics with 20,638 beds.

DIPLOMATIC REPRESENTATIVES

Of Zambia in Great Britain (2 Palace Gate, London, W8 5LS)
High Commissioner: Edward M. Lubinda (accredited 23 Nov. 1989).

Of Great Britain in Zambia (Independence Ave., Lusaka)
High Commissioner: P. R. M. Hinchcliffe, CMG, CVO.

Of Zambia in the USA (2419 Massachusetts Ave., NW, Washington, D.C., 20008)
Ambassador: Dr Paul J. F. Lusaka.

Of the USA in Zambia (PO Box 31617, Lusaka)
Ambassador: Jeffrey Davidow.

Of Zambia to the United Nations
Ambassador: Peter Dingi Zuze.

Further Reading

General Information: The Director, Zambia Information Services, PO Box 50020, Lusaka.

Laws of Zambia. 13 vols. Govt. Printer, Lusaka
Beveridge, A. A. and Oberschall, A. R., *African Businessmen and Development in Zambia.* Princeton Univ. Press, 1980
Bliss, A. M. and Rigg, J. A., *Zambia.* [Bibliography] Oxford and Santa Barbara, 1984
Burdette, M. M., *Zambia: Between two Worlds.* Boulder, 1988
De Waal, V., *The Politics of Reconciliation: Zambia's First Decade.* London, 1990
Gertzel, C. (ed.) *The Dynamics of a One-Party State in Zambia.* Manchester Univ. Press, 1984
Kaunda, K. D., *Zambia Shall be Free.* London, 1962.—*Humanism in Zambia.* Lusaka. 2 vols. 1967 and 1974.—*Zambia's Economic Revolution.* Lusaka, 1968.—*Zambia's Guidelines for the Next Decade.* Lusaka, 1968.—*Letter to my Children.* Lusaka, 1973
Roberts, A., *A History of Zambia.* London, 1977

ZIMBABWE

Capital: Harare
Population: 9·37m. (1990)
GNP per capita: US$660 (1988)

Republic of Zimbabwe

HISTORY. Prior to Oct. 1923 Southern Rhodesia, like Northern Rhodesia, was under the administration of the British South Africa Co. In Oct. 1922 Southern Rhodesia voted in favour of responsible government. On 12 Sept. 1923 the country was formally annexed to His Majesty's Dominions, and on 1 Oct. 1923 government was established under a governor, assisted by an executive council, and a legislature, with the status of a self-governing colony. For the history of the period 1961–1979 including the period of unilateral declaration of independence *see* THE STATESMAN'S YEAR-BOOK, 1980–81, pp. 1623–25.

At the Commonwealth Conference held in Lusaka in Aug. 1979 agreement was reached for a new Constitutional Conference to be held in London and this took place between 10 Sept. and 15 Dec. 1979 at Lancaster House. It was attended by the various factions in Zimbabwe-Rhodesia, including Abel Muzorewa, Robert Mugabe and Joshua Nkomo, and was chaired by Lord Carrington. It achieved 3 objectives: (*i*) the terms of the Constitution for an independent Zimbabwe; (*ii*) terms for a return to legality: and (*iii*) a ceasefire. Lord Soames became Governor of Southern Rhodesia in Dec. 1979 and elections took place in March 1980, resulting in victory for the Zimbabwe African National Union (ZANU, PF). Rhodesia (Southern Rhodesia) became the Republic of Zimbabwe on 18 April 1980. The state of emergency in force since 1965 was lifted in July 1990.

AREA AND POPULATION. Zimbabwe is bounded north by Zambia, east by Mozambique, south by the Republic of South Africa and west by Botswana. The area is 150,872 sq. miles (390,759 sq. km). The capital is Harare (formerly Salisbury). The population was (1982 census) 7,539,300; 1990 estimate, 9,369,373.

There are 8 provinces:

Province	*Sq. km*	*Census 1982*	*Province*	*Sq. km*	*Census 1982*
Manicaland	35,219	1,099,202	Masvingo	55,777	1,031,697
Mashonaland Central	29,482	563,407	Matabeleland North	76,813	885,339
Mashonaland East	26,813	1,495,984	Matebeleland South	54,941	519,606
Mashonaland West	55,737	858,962	Midlands	55,977	1,091,844

Population of main urban areas (1982 census): Bindura, 18,243; Bulawayo, 414,800; Masvingo (Fort Victoria) 31,000; Kadoma (Gatooma) 45,000; Gweru (Gwelo) 79,000; Chegutu (Hartley) 26,617; Marondera (Marandellas) 37,092; Kwekwe (Que Que) 48,000; Redcliffe, 22,000; Harare (Salisbury) 656,100; Zvishavane (Shabani) 27,000; Chinhoyi (Sinoia) 24,322; Mutare (Umtali) 70,000; Hwange (Wankie) 39,000; Chitungwiza, 175,000.

In 1982 23% were urban and 51% under 15.

Vital statistics (1988): Birth rate, 39·5 per 1,000; death rate, 10·8 per 1,000; infant mortality, 23 per 1,000 live births; growth rate (1990), 3·5%. Life expectancy was 63 years in 1989.

The official language is English. Shona and Sindebele are the main spoken languages.

CLIMATE. Though situated in the tropics, conditions are remarkably temperate throughout the year because of altitude, and an inland position keeps humidity low. The warmest weather occurs in the three months before the main rainy season, which starts in Nov. and lasts till March. The cool season is from mid-May to mid-Aug. and, though days are mild and sunny, nights are chilly. Harare. Jan. 69°F (20·6°C), July 57°F (13·9°C). Annual rainfall 33" (828 mm). Bulawayo. Jan. 71°F (21·7°C), July 57°F (13·9°C). Annual rainfall 24" (594 mm). Victoria Falls. Jan. 78°F (25·6°C), July 61°F (16·1°C). Annual rainfall 28" (710 mm).

CONSTITUTION AND GOVERNMENT. The Constitution provides for a single chamber 150-member Parliament (*House of Assembly*), universal suffrage for citizens over the age of 18, an *Executive President* (elected for a 6-year term of office by Parliament), an independent judiciary enjoying security of tenure, a Declaration of Rights, derogation from certain of the provisions being permitted, within specified limits, during a state of emergency, and Independent Service Commissions exercising powers in respect of staffing and conditions of service in the Public Service, the uniformed forces and the judiciary.

Racial representation was abolished in 1987. No Parliament may continue in existence for more than 5 years. 120 members are elected by universal suffrage, 10 are chiefs elected by all the country's tribal chiefs, 12 are appointed by the President and 8 are provincial governors. The constitution can be amended by a two-thirds parliamentary majority.

At elections in April 1990, ZANU (PF) won 117 seats with 4·8m. votes (42%); Zimbabwe Unity, 2; ZANU (Ndonga), 1. At simultaneous presidential elections Robert Mugabe was elected by 2m. votes to 0·41m.

Executive President: Robert G. Mugabe (sworn in on 30 Dec. 1987, re-elected April 1990).

The Cabinet in Feb. 1991 comprised:

Vice-Presidents: Dr Joshua Nkomo, Simon Muzenda. *Senior Ministers:* Didymus Mutasa (*Political Affairs*), Dr Bernard Chidzero (*Finance, Economic Planning and Development*), Joseph Msika (*Local Government, Rural and Urban Development*). *Attorney-General:* Patrick Chinamasa. *Foreign Affairs:* Dr Nathan Shamuyarira. *Justice, Legal and Parliamentary Affairs:* Emmerson Mnangagwa. *Defence:* Richard Hove. *Home Affairs:* Moven Mahachi. *Lands, Agriculture and Rural Resettlement:* Dr Witness Mangwende. *Information, Posts and Telecommunications:* Victoria Chitepo. *Labour, Manpower Planning and Social Welfare:* John Nkomo. *Industry and Commerce:* Kumbairai Kangai. *Energy, Water Resources and Development:* Herbert Ushewokunze. *Mines:* Jonas Andersen. *Transport and National Supplies:* Dennis Norman. *Health:* Dr Timothy Stamps. *Community and Co-operative Development:* Joyce Mujuru. *Public Construction and National Housing:* Enos Chikowore. *Environment and Tourism:* Herbert Murerwa. *Higher Education:* David Karimanzira. *Education and Culture:* Fay Chung. *In President's Office for Sport Co-ordination:* David Kwidini. There are 8 Ministers of State.

National flag: Seven horizontal stripes of green, yellow, red, black, red, yellow and green; on a white black-edged triangle in the hoist a red star surmounted by the Zimbabwe Bird in yellow.

Local government: The first municipal elections were held in Nov. 1980.

DEFENCE

Army. The Army consists of 1 armoured, 1 engineer and 2 artillery regiments; 26 infantry with 1 commando and 2 parachute battalions. Equipment includes 8 T-54 and 35 Ch T-59 main battle tanks. Strength was (1991) 51,600, and there are a further 15,000 paramilitary police.

Air Force. The Air Force has a strength of (1991) about 3,000 personnel and 81 combat aircraft. Headquarters ZAF and the main ZAF stations are in Harare; the second main base is at Gweru, with many secondary airfields throughout the country. Equipment includes 1 squadron of F-7 (MiG-21) interceptors, 1 squadron of Hunter FGA.9 fighter-bombers, 1 squadron of Hawk training and light attack aircraft, a transport squadron with 11 turboprop CASA Aviocars, 6 twin-engined Islanders and 6 C-47s; a squadron with 15 Reims/Cessna 337 Lynx attack aircraft; a squadron with 14 SIAI-Marchetti SF.260W Genet and 15 SF.260C Genet trainers; a helicopter liaison/transport squadron with 40 Alouette II/IIIs, a helicopter casualty evacuation/transport squadron with 5 Agusta-Bell 205s and 12 Bell 412s. Nine Canberra bombers are in storage.

INTERNATIONAL RELATIONS

Membership. Zimbabwe is a member of UN, the Commonwealth, OAU, SADCC, the Non-Aligned Movement and is an ACP state of the EEC.

ECONOMY

Policy. The 5-year development plan (1986–90) emphasized greater public-sector involvement in all parts of the economy.

Budget. Revenue and expenditure (in Z$1,000):

	1985–86	*1986–87*	*1987–88*	*1988–89*
Revenue	2,616,185	2,997,000	3,784,856	4,211,000
Expenditure	3,136,738	3,828,528	4,295,736	5,015,801

Receipts during the year ended 30 June 1985 were (in Z$1,000): Income and profits tax, 1,066,584; taxes on goods and services, 1,137,808; miscellaneous taxes and other income, 311,757.

The gross amount of the public debt outstanding in June 1986 was Z$5,192,729,612.

Currency. The unit of currency is the *Zimbabwe dollar* (ZWD) divided into 100 *cents*. In March 1991, £1 = Z$5·27; US$1 = Z$2·78.

Banking and Finance. The Reserve Bank of Zimbabwe is the central bank; it became operative when the Bank of Rhodesia and Nyasaland ceased operations on 1 June 1965. It acts as banker to the Government and to the commercial banks and as agent of the Government for important financial operations. It is also the central note-issuing authority and co-ordinates the application of the Government's monetary policy. The Zimbabwe Development Bank, established in 1983 as a development finance institution, is 51% Government-owned.

The post office savings bank had Z$1,171·1m. deposits at 30 June 1988.

The 5 commercial banks are Barclays Bank of Zimbabwe Ltd, Grindlays Bank Ltd, Zimbabwe Banking Corporation Ltd, Standard Chartered Bank Zimbabwe Ltd, Bank of Credit and Commerce Zimbabwe (Pvt) Ltd. In 1986 they had 119 branches and 75 agencies. The 4 merchant banks are Standard Chartered Merchant Bank, Merchant Bank of Central Africa, RAL Merchant Bank and Syfrets Merchant Bank. There are 5 registered finance houses, 3 of which are subsidiaries of commercial banks. There is a stock exchange.

Weights and Measures. The metric system is in use but the US short ton is also used.

ENERGY AND NATURAL RESOURCES

Electricity. Production (1987) 7,606·3m. kwh.

Minerals. The total value of all minerals produced in 1987 was Z$896,691,000. Output (in 1,000 tonnes) and value (in Z$1,000):

	Output			*Value*		
	1986	*1987*	*1988*	*1986*	*1987*	*1988*
Asbestos	163·6	193·3	186·6	85,789	97,859	97,644
Gold (1,000 oz.)	478·0	472·0	481·0	292,770	349,931	379,631
Chrome ore	553·1	562·2	561·6	39,698	44,160	45,272
Coal	4,047·0	4,814·0	5,065·0	89,144	103,402	105,730
Copper	20·6	19·6	16·1	43,272	46,069	64,661
Nickel	9·7	10,912·0	11,489·0	60,672	73,153	198,029
Iron Ore	1,115·0	1,328·0	1,020·0	21,144	28,843	24,525
Silver (1,000 oz.)	840·0	813·0	704·0	10,612	15,790	13,253
Tin	1,019·0	1,037·0	855·5	10,568	11,547	11,162
Cobalt	76·0	107·0	122·0	2,379	1,370	2,766

Agriculture. Replacing a constitutional provision that permitted the government to acquire under-utilized land on a 'willing-seller willing-buyer' basis, legislation before parliament in Dec. 1990 provided for the compulsory purchase of land at a fixed price for peasant resettlement. 52,000 peasants have been resettled on 3m. ha of land purchased from white farmers. In 1990 some 4,000 farmers owned 12m. ha while 0·75m. peasants occupied 15m. ha of communal agricultural areas.

The most important food crop is maize, the staple food of a large proportion of the population; deliveries to the Grain Marketing Board in 1987 were 1·6m. tonnes. Milk production in 1988 was 244,009 tonnes.

Both citrus and deciduous fruit production are well established.

Tobacco is the most important single product, accounting for over 40% of the value of earnings from agricultural exports. In 1988 tobacco production was 112,000 tonnes.

Production, 1988 in 1,000 tonnes: Maize, 2,253; sorghum, 176; barley, 30; millet, 278; soyabeans, 102; groundnuts, 135; fruit, 135; vegetables, 148; seed cotton, 279; wheat, 229; tea, 17; coffee, 13; sugar-cane, 3.

Livestock (1988): Cattle, 5·7m.; pigs, 190,000; sheep, 580,000; goats, 1·65m.

Fisheries. Trout, prawns and bream are farmed to supplement supplies of fish caught in dams and lakes. In 1986 trout were caught at the rate of 200,000 a year, and the planned production of bream was 400–500 tonnes a year.

INDUSTRY. Metal products account for over 20% of industrial output. Important agro-industries include food processing, textiles, furniture and other wood products.

Labour. The labour force (1985) was 2·8m. In 1984, 1,036,400 were employed; of whom 271,200 were in agriculture, forestry and fishing and 166,300 in manufacturing. Unemployment was 1·2m. in 1990.

Trade Unions. There is a Zimbabwe Congress of Trade Unions (*Secretary General*, Morgan Tsvangirayi).

FOREIGN ECONOMIC RELATIONS. Import controls imposed in 1965 are being replaced from 1990 with an open general licence system,and tariffs are being restructured over five years. The Customs Agreement with the Republic of South Africa was extended in March, 1982 pending further discussion. Zimbabwe has also entered into Trade Agreements with Zambia, Mozambique, Tanzania, Angola and Swaziland and with countries outside Africa.

Commerce. Imports and exports (in Z$1,000):

	1984	*1985*	*1986*	*1987*	*1988*
Imports	1,200,700	1,447,000	1,686,000	1,741,763	2,155,000
Exports	1,453,000	1,545,343	2,206,000	1,892,240	2,863,000

Principal imports in 1984 (in Z$1,000): Machinery and transport equipment, 373,550; petroleum products, 256,924; chemicals, 178,111; manufactured goods, 177,851; miscellaneous manufactured goods, 78,615.

Principal exports in 1986 (in Z$1,000): Unmanufactured tobacco, 238,213; ferro-alloys, 210,079; asbestos, 82,741; cotton lint, 130,548.

In 1987, 13·3% of exports (excluding gold) went to the UK, 9·8% to the Federal Republic of Germany, 9·5% to the Republic of South Africa and 6·9% to the USA, while the Republic of South Africa provided 20·8% of imports, the UK 11·5%, the USA 9·4% and the Federal Republic of Germany 8·7%.

Total trade between Zimbabwe and UK (British Department of Trade returns, in £1,000 sterling):

	1986	*1987*	*1988*	*1989*	*1990*
Imports to UK	80,702	79,771	86,268	85,792	86,280
Exports and re-exports from UK	61,937	63,181	58,077	87,013	83,718

Tourism. In 1988, 451,000 tourists visited Zimbabwe. The main tourist areas are Victoria Falls, Kariba, Hwange, the Eastern Highlands and Great Zimbabwe. The Zimbabwe Tourist Development Corporation is in Harare and Victoria Falls.

COMMUNICATIONS

Roads. The Ministry of Transport is responsible for the construction and maintenance of all State roads and bridges, and all road bridges outside municipal areas.

The Ministry offers advice and help on roads and bridges, through Provincial Road Engineers, to district councils. State roads are those connecting all the main centres of population, international routes, major links in the system and main roads serving rural communities. The total length of roads is approximately 85,237 km including surfaced, 12,000; gravel, 46,187; earth, 27,000.

Number of motor vehicles, 1984: Passenger cars, 237,128; commercial vehicles, 17,058; motor cycles, 24,347; trailers, 33,227; tractors, 5,695.

Railways. Zimbabwe is served by the National Railways of Zimbabwe, which connect with the South African Railways to give access to the South African ports; with the Mozambique Railways to give access to the ports of Beira and Maputo; and with the Zambia railway system. In 1985 there were 3,394 km (1,067 mm gauge) of railways including 311 km electrified. In 1987-88 the railways carried 13·9m. tonnes of freight and 2·7m. passengers.

Aviation. Air Zimbabwe operates domestic services and also regular flights to Zambia, Kenya, Malawi, Botswana and South Africa, and to London, Frankfurt and Athens in Europe and also to Perth and Sydney in Australia in association with Qantas. The country is also served by British Airways, Kenya Airways, Ethiopian Airlines, Air Tanzania, Air Malawi, Zambian Airways, Balkan Bulgarian Airlines, Mozambique Airlines, South African Airways, Air Botswana, the Royal Swazi Airlines, TAP Air Portugal, Qantas, Lesotho Airways and Air India. Services by KLM, Swissair and UTA were temporarily suspended in 1986. In 1988, 760,420,000 passenger-km were flown by Air Zimbabwe.

Shipping. Zimbabwe outlets to the sea are Maputo and Beira in Mozambique, Dar-es-Salaam, Tanzania and the South African ports.

Telecommunications. At 31 Aug. 1986 there were 170 full post offices, 47 postal telegraph agencies and 86 postal agencies. At 30 June 1986 there were 251,344 telephones in Zimbabwe served by 96 exchanges; 2,102 telex connexions, served by 2 telex exchanges. Zimbabwe Broadcasting Corporation is an independent statutory body broadcasting a general service in English, Shona, N'debele, Nyanja, Tonga and Kalanga. There are 3 national semi-commercial services, Radio 1, 2 and 3, in English, Shona and N'debele. Radio 4 transmits formal and informal educational programmes. Zimbabwe Television broadcasts 2 channels 95 hours a week *via* 11 transmitters. In June 1986 there were 130,500 television and 450,000 radio licences.

JUSTICE, RELIGION, EDUCATION AND WELFARE

Justice. The general common law of Zimbabwe is the Roman Dutch law as it applied in the Colony of the Cape of Good Hope on 10 June, 1891, as subsequently modified by statute. Provision is made by statute for the application of African customary law by all courts in appropriate cases.

The Supreme Court consists of the Chief Justice and at least two (in 1985 there were three) permanent Supreme Court judges. It is Zimbabwe's final court of appeal. It exercises appellate jurisdiction in appeals from the High Court and other courts and tribunals; its only original jurisdiction is that conferred on it by the Constitution to enforce the protective provisions of the Declaration of Rights. The Court's permanent seat is in Harare but it sits regularly in Bulawayo also.

The High Court is also headed by the Chief Justice, supported by the Judge President and an appropriate number of High Court judges. It has full original jurisdiction, in both Civil and Criminal cases, over all persons and all matters in Zimbabwe. The Judge President is in charge of the Court, subject to the directions of the Chief Justice. The Court has permanent seats in both Harare and Bulawayo and sittings are held three times a year in three other principal towns.

Regional courts, established in Harare and Bulawayo but also holding sittings in other centres, exercise a solely criminal jurisdiction that is intermediate between that of the High Court and the Magistrates' courts.

Magistrates' courts, established in twenty centres throughout the country, and staffed by full-time professional magistrates, exercise both civil and criminal jurisdiction.

The tribal courts and district commissioners' courts of colonial days were abolished in 1981, to be replaced by a system of primary courts, consisting of village courts and community courts. By 1982 1,100 village and 50 community courts had been established. Village courts are presided over by officers selected for the purpose from the local population, sitting with two assessors. They deal with certain classes of civil cases only and have jurisdiction only where African customary law is applicable. Community courts are presided over by presiding officers in full-time public service who may be assisted by assessors. They have jurisdiction in all civil cases determinable by African customary law and also deal with appeals from village courts. They also have limited criminal jurisdiction in respect of petty offences against the general law.

Religion. The majority of the population adhere to traditional animist religion; but some 40% are Christian: Anglicans, Roman Catholics, Methodists and Presbyterians are represented.

Education. Education is compulsory. 'Manageable' school fees are due to be introduced in 1991; primary education had hitherto been free to all. All instruction is given in English. There are also over 3,800 private primary schools and over 950 private secondary schools, all of which must be registered by the Ministry of Education. In 1990 there were 2,273,890 pupils at primary schools and 951,259 pupils at secondary schools, together comprising 84·9% of the population between 5 and 19. In 1990 73·4% of the population was classed as literate.

There are 10 teachers' training colleges, 8 of which are in association with the University of Zimbabwe. In addition, there are 4 special training centres for teacher trainees in the Zimbabwe Integrated National Teacher Education Course. In 1990 there were 17,873 students enrolled at teachers' training colleges, 1,003 students at agricultural colleges and 20,943 students at technical colleges.

The University of Zimbabwe provides facilities for higher education. In 1990 the total enrolment of students in the 9 Faculties of Agriculture, Arts, Commerce and Law, Education, Engineering, Medicine, Science, Social Studies and Veterinary Science, was 9,255.

Health. In 1985 there were 162 hospitals, 1,062 static rural clinics and health centres and 32 mobile rural clinics operated by the Ministry of Health. All mission health institutions get 100% government grants-in-aid for recurrent expenditure. There is a medical school attached to the University of Zimbabwe in Harare, four government training schools attached to the 4 central hospitals for training state registered nurses, 14 training schools for medical assistants out of which 11 are administered by missions, and two for training maternity assistants, health assistants/health inspectors.

Social Services. It is a statutory responsibility of the government in many areas to provide: Processing and administration of war pensions and old age pensions; protection of children; administration of remand, probation and correctional institutions; registration and supervision of welfare organisations.

DIPLOMATIC REPRESENTATIVES

Of Zimbabwe in Great Britain (Zimbabwe Hse., 429 Strand, London, WC2R 0SA)
High Commissioner: Dr Stephen C. Chiketa.

Of Great Britain in Zimbabwe (Stanley Hse., Jason Mayo Ave., Harare)
High Commissioner: W. K. Prendergast, CMG.

Of Zimbabwe in the USA (2852 McGill Terr., NW, Washington, D.C., 20008)
Ambassador: Stanislaus Garikai Chigwedere.

Of the USA in Zimbabwe (172 Josiah Tongogara Ave., Harare)
Ambassador: J. Steven Rhodes.

Of Zimbabwe to the United Nations
Ambassador: S. Mumbengegwi.

Further Reading

Statistical Information: The Central Statistical Office, PO Box 8063, Causeway, Harare, Zimbabwe, originated in 1927 as the Southern Rhodesian Government Statistical Bureau. Ten years later its name was changed to Department of Statistics, and in 1948 it assumed its present title when it took over responsibility for certain Northern Rhodesian and Nyasaland statistics (which it relinquished in Dec. 1963 on the dissolution of the Federation). It publishes *Monthly Digest of Statistics*.

Akers, M., *Encyclopaedia Rhodesia*. Harare, 1973
Caute, D., *Under the Skin: The Death of White Rhodesia*. London, 1983
Davies, D. K., *Race Relations in Rhodesia*. London, 1975
Keppel-Jones, A., *Rhodes and Rhodesia: The White Conquest of Zimbabwe, 1884–1902*. Univ. of Natal Press, 1983
Linden, I., *The Catholic Church and the Struggle for Zimbabwe*. London, 1980
Martin, D. and Johnson, P., *The Struggle for Zimbabwe*. London, 1981.—*Destructive Engagement*. Harare, 1986
Meredith, M., *The Past is Another Century: Rhodesia 1890–1979*. London, 1979
Morris-Jones, W. H., (ed.) *From Rhodesia to Zimbabwe*. London, 1980
Nkomo, J., *Nkomo: The Story of My Life*. London, 1984
O'Meara, P., *Rhodesia: Racial Conflict or Co-Existence*. Cornell Univ. Press, 1975
Pollak, O. B. and Pollak, K., *Rhodesia/Zimbabwe* [Bibliography] Oxford and Santa Barbara, 1979
Schatzberg, M. G., *The Political Economy of Zimbabwe*. New York, 1984
Stoneham, C., *Zimbabwe's Inheritance*. London, 1982
Storeman, C., *Zimbabwe: Politics, Economics and Society*. London, 1988
Thornycroft, P., *A Field for Investment*. Harare, annual
Verrier, A., *The Road to Zimbabwe, 1890–1980*. London, 1986
Wiseman, H. and Taylor, A. M., *From Rhodesia to Zimbabwe: The Politics of Transition*. Elmsford, N.Y., 1981

Reference Library: National Archives of Zimbabwe, PO Box 8043, Causeway, Harare.

PLACE AND INTERNATIONAL ORGANIZATIONS INDEX

Italicised page numbers refer to extended entries

Salto, 1565, 1568
Salvador (Brazil), 229-30, 232, 235-6
Salvador, El, 52, 54, *453-7*
Salzburg, 167-8, 171-2
Salzgitter, 529, 534

PRODUCT INDEX

References are to production data

PERSON INDEX